CONN'S CURRENT THERAPY 2016

EDWARD T. BOPE, MD
Family Physician and Palliative Care Consultant
Columbus VAACC
Assistant Dean for VA Medical Students
and Clinical Professor, Family Medicine,
The Ohio State University
Columbus, Ohio

RICK D. KELLERMAN, MD
Professor and Chair
Department of Family and Community Medicine
University of Kansas School of Medicine–Wichita
Wichita, Kansas

Latest Approved Methods of Treatment for the Practicing Physician

ELSEVIER

ELSEVIER

1600 John F. Kennedy Blvd.
Ste 1800
Philadelphia, PA 19103-2899

Notices

Previous editions copyrighted 2015, 2014, 2013, 2012, 2011, 2010, 2009.

International Standard Book Number: 978-0-323-35535-3

Content Strategist: Suzanne Toppy
Content Development Strategist: Joan Ryan
Publishing Services Manager: Patricia Tannian
Project Manager: Ted Rodgers
Designer: Brian Salisbury

Printed in the United States of America

Last digit is the print number: 9 8 7 6 5 4 3 2 1

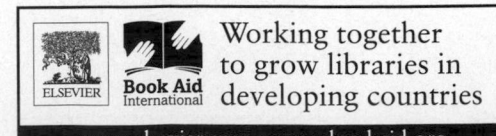

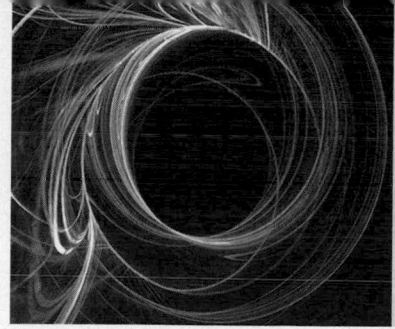

Contributors

Stoney Abercrombie, MD
AnMed Health Family Medicine Center, Anderson,
South Carolina
Antepartum Care

Jeremy S. Abramson, MD
Assistant Professor of Medicine, Harvard Medical School;
Director, Lymphoma Program, Massachusetts General
Hospital Cancer Center, Boston, Massachusetts
Hodgkin Lymphoma

Rodney D. Adam, MD
Department of Pathology, Aga Khan University Hospital,
Nairobi, Kenya; Professor Emeritus, University of Arizona
Health Sciences Center, Tucson, Arizona
Giardiasis

Paul C. Adams, MD
Professor of Medicine and Chief of Gastroenterology, University
of Western Ontario; Gastroenterologist, University Hospital,
London, Ontario, Canada
Hemochromatosis

Horacio E. Adrogué, MD
Associate Professor of Medicine, Division of Renal Disease and
Hypertension, The University of Texas Health Science Center at
Houston Medical School; Medical Director, Kidney and
Pancreas Transplant, Memorial Hermann Hospital, Texas
Medical Center, Houston, Texas
Hypertension

Lee Akst, MD
Assistant Professor, Department of Otolaryngology, The Johns
Hopkins University, Baltimore, Maryland
Hoarseness and Laryngitis

Brian K. Albertson, MD
University Physicians Group, Harrisburg, Pennsylvania
Osteomyelitis

Madson Q. Almeida, MD
Section on Endocrinology and Genetics, Program on
Developmental Endocrinology and Genetics, Eunice Kennedy
Shriver National Institute of Child Health and Human
Development, National Institutes of Health, Bethesda,
Maryland
Cushing's Syndrome

Kelley P. Anderson, MD
Clinical Adjunct Professor of Medicine, University of Wisconsin
School of Medicine and Public Health; Department of
Cardiology, Marshfield Clinic, Marshfield, Wisconsin
Heart Block

Emmanuel Andrés, MD, PhD
Service de Médecine Interne, Diabète et Maladies Métaboliques,
Clinique Médicale B, Hôpital Civil, Hôpitaux Universitaires de
Strasbourg, Strasbourg, France
Pernicious Anemia and Other Megaloblastic Anemias

Gregory M. Anstead, MD
Professor of Medicine, University of Texas Health Science Center
at San Antonio School of Medicine; Director,
Immunosuppression and Infectious Diseases Clinics, South
Texas Veterans Healthcare System, San Antonio, Texas
Coccidioidomycosis

Ann M. Aring, MD
Clinical Assistant Professor of Family Medicine, College of
Medicine and Public Health, The Ohio State University;
Associate Program Director, Family Medicine Residency,
Riverside Methodist Hospital, Columbus, Ohio
Rhinosinusitis

Juliet Aylward, MD
Clinical Associate Professor, University of Wisconsin School of
Medicine and Public Health; Staff Physician, University of
Wisconsin Hospitals and Clinics and Meriter Hospital,
Madison, Wisconsin
Premalignant Lesions

Cecilio Azar, MD
Associate in Medicine, Division of Gastroenterology, Department
of Internal Medicine, American University of Beirut Medical
Center, Beirut, Lebanon
Bleeding Esophageal Varices

Masoud Azodi, MD
Associate Professor, Division of Gynecology/Oncology, Yale
University School of Medicine, New Haven, Connecticut
Cancer of the Endometrium

Justin Bailey, MD
Clinical Instructor, Department of Family Medicine, University of
Washington, Seattle, Washington; Family Medicine Residency
of Idaho, Boise, Idaho
Gaseousness, Indigestion, Nausea, and Vomiting; Palpitations

Federico Balagué, MD
Professeur Titulaire, Rheumatology, Medical School, Geneva
University, Geneva, Switzerland; Adjunct Associate Professor,
Orthopedics, New York University, New York, New York;
Médecin Chef Adj Service de Rhumatologie, HFR-Hôpital,
Cantonal Fribourg, Switzerland
Spine Pain

Kurt T. Barnhart, MD
Professor of Obstetrics and Gynecology; Associate Chief, Penn Fertility Care; Director, Women's Health Clinical Research Center; and Assistant Dean, Clinical Research Operations, University of Pennsylvania School of Medicine, Philadelphia, Pennsylvania
Ectopic Pregnancy

Gina M. Basello, DO
Assistant Clinical Professor, Family and Social Medicine, Albert Einstein College of Medicine, Bronx, New York; Program Director, Family Medicine Residency Program and Associate Director, Palliative Care Fellowship Program, Jamaica Hospital Medical Center, Jamaica, New York
Fever

Julie M. Baughn, MD
Senior Associate Consultant, Pediatric Sleep Medicine, Mayo Clinic, Rochester, Minnesota
Pediatric Sleep Disorders

Sheryl Beard, MD
Clinical Assistant Professor, Department of Family and Community Medicine, University of Kansas School of Medicine–Wichita; Senior Associate Program Director, Via Christi Family Medicine Residency, Wichita, Kansas
Rhinitis

Ronen Ben-Ami, MD
Infectious Disease Unit, Tel Aviv Sourasky Medical Center, Tel Aviv, Israel
Cat Scratch Disease

Hassan Bencheqroun, MD
Interventional Pulmonary and Critical Care Medicine, Riverside, California
Pruritus

David I. Bernstein, MD
Professor of Medicine and Environmental Health, Division of Immunology, Allergy, and Rheumatology, University of Cincinnati College of Medicine, Cincinnati, Ohio
Hypersensitivity Pneumonitis

Kristin Schmid Biggerstaff, MD
Assistant Professor, Baylor College of Medicine; Glaucoma Staff, Michael E. DeBakey Veteran's Affairs Medical Center, Dallas, Texas
Glaucoma

John P. Bilezikian, MD
Professor, Department of Medicine, Columbia University College of Physicians and Surgeons; Attending Physician, New York–Presbyterian Hospital, New York, New York
Hyperparathyroidism and Hypoparathyroidism

B. Wayne Blount, MD, MPH
Market Medical Director for JenCare; adjunct faculty in Family and Preventive Medicine, Emory University School of Medicine, Atlanta, Georgia
Trigeminal Neuralgia

Stephen Boateng, DO
Rush University Medical Center, Division of Cardiovascular Medicine, Chicago, Illinois
Acute Myocardial Infarction; Tachycardias

Diana Bolotin, MD, PhD
Assistant Professor, Director of Dermatologic Surgery, The University of Chicago Department of Medicine, Section of Dermatology, Chicago, Illinois
Cancer of the Skin

Zuleika L. Bonilla-Martinez, MD
Wound Healing Fellow, Department of Dermatology and Cutaneous Surgery, University of Miami Miller School of Medicine, Miami, Florida
Venous Ulcers

Rachel A. Bonnema, MD, MS
Associate Professor of Medicine, Division of General Internal Medicine, University of Nebraska Medical Center, Omaha, Nebraska
Contraception

David Borenstein, MD
Clinical Professor of Medicine, The George Washington University Medical Center, Washington, District of Columbia
Spine Pain

Patrick Borgen, MD
Chief, Breast Service, Department of Surgery, Memorial Sloan Kettering Cancer Center, New York, New York
Breast Disease

Laurence A. Boxer, MD
Department of Pediatrics and Communicable Disease, University of Michigan C.S. Mott Children's Hospital, Ann Arbor, Michigan
Neutropenia

Krystene I. Boyle, MD
Clinical Instructor, Department of Obstetrics and Gynecology, University of Cincinnati College of Medicine; Clinical Fellow, Department of Obstetrics/Gynecology, Division of Reproductive Endocrinology, University of Cincinnati Medical Center, Cincinnati, Ohio
Menopause

Sylvia L. Brice, MD
Associate Professor of Dermatology, University of Colorado, Denver, Colorado
Viral Diseases of the Skin

Patricia D. Brown, MD
Professor of Medicine, Wayne State University School of Medicine; Associate Chief of Staff for Medicine, John D. Dingell VA Medical Center, Detroit, Michigan
Pyelonephritis

Patrick Brown, MD
Associate Professor of Oncology and Pediatrics, The Johns Hopkins University School of Medicine; Director, Pediatric Leukemia Program, Sidney Kimmel Comprehensive Cancer Center at Johns Hopkins, Baltimore, Maryland
Acute Leukemia in Children

Richard B. Brown, MD
Professor of Medicine, Tufts University School of Medicine, Boston, Massachusetts; Senior Clinician, Infectious Disease Division, Baystate Medical Center, Springfield, Massachusetts
Toxic Shock Syndrome

Susan C. Brunsell, MD
Executive Medicine Service, Walter Reed National Military
    Medical Center, Bethesda, Maryland
Uterine Leiomyomas

Peter Buckley, MD
Dean, Medical College of Georgia, Georgia Regents University,
    Augusta, Georgia
Schizophrenia

Irina Burd, MD, PhD
Instructor, Department of Obstetrics and Gynecology,
    University of Pennsylvania School of Medicine; Staff,
    Hospital of the University of Pennsylvania, Philadelphia,
    Pennsylvania
Menopause

Guenevere V. Burke, MD
Department of Emergency Medicine, The George Washington
    University School of Medicine and Health Sciences,
    Washington, District of Columbia
Amebiasis

Jennifer Burkmar, MD, MBA
Family Physician, Dekalb Medical Center, Resident
    Physician, Emory University School of Medicine,
    Atlanta, Georgia
Trigeminal Neuralgia

Samantha F. Butts, MD
Assistant Professor of Obstetrics and Gynecology, University
    of Pennsylvania School of Medicine, Philadelphia,
    Pennsylvania
Ectopic Pregnancy

Diego Cadavid, MD
Consultant in Immunology and Inflammatory Diseases,
    Massachusetts General Hospital, Boston,
    Massachusetts
Relapsing Fever

Thomas R. Caraccio, PharmD
Associate Professor of Emergency Medicine, Stony Brook
    University Medical Center School of Medicine, Stony Brook,
    New York; Assistant Professor of Pharmacology and
    Toxicology, New York College of Osteopathic Medicine,
    Old Westbury, New York
Medical Toxicology

Enrique V. Carbajal, MD
Associate Clinical Professor of Medicine, University of
    California–San Francisco School of Medicine, San Francisco,
    California; Department of Medicine, Veterans Affairs
    Central California Health Care System, Fresno,
    California
Premature Beats

Peter J. Carek, MD, MS
Professor and Chair, Department of Community Health and
    Family Medicine, University of Florida College, Gainesville,
    Florida
Osteoporosis

Petros E. Carvounis, MD
Director, Vitreoretinal Fellowship Program and Associate
    Professor, Cullen Eye Institute, Baylor College of Medicine,
    Houston, Texas
Uveitis

Donald O. Castell, MD
Professor of Medicine, Division of Gastroenterology and
    Hepatology, Medical University of South Carolina, Charleston,
    South Carolina
Gastroesophageal Reflux Disease (GERD)

William E. Cayley, Jr., MD, MDiv
Professor, University of Wisconsin Department of Family
    Medicine, Eau Claire Family Medicine Residency, Eau Claire,
    Wisconsin
Chest Pain

Sonia Cerquozzi, MD
Hematology Resident, University of Calgary, Calgary, Alberta,
    Canada
Polycythemia Vera

Alvaro Cervera, MD
University of Barcelona, Barcelona, Spain; National Stroke
    Research Institute, Heidelberg Heights, Victoria, Australia
Ischemic Cerebrovascular Disease

Toby C. Chai, MD
Professor of Surgery, Division of Urology, University of Maryland
    School of Medicine, Baltimore, Maryland
Urinary Incontinence

Lawrence Chan, MD
Professor of Medicine, Rutherford Chair, and Division Chief,
    Diabetes, Endocrinology, and Metabolism, Baylor College of
    Medicine; Chief, Diabetes, Endocrinology, and Metabolism,
    Baylor St. Luke's Medical Center, Houston, Texas
Hyperaldosteronism; Hyperlipidemia

Miriam Chan, BSc Pharm, PharmD
Clinical Assistant Professor of Family Medicine, College of
    Medicine and Public Health, The Ohio State University;
    Clinical Assistant Professor of Pharmacy, The Ohio State
    University College of Pharmacy; Program Director of
    Research and EBM Education, Medical Education, Riverside
    Methodist Hospital, Columbus, Ohio
*Popular Herbs and Nutritional Supplements; Drug Hypersensitivity
    Reactions*

Shingo Chihara, MD
Assistant Professor, Department of Internal Medicine, Division of
    Infectious Diseases, Southern Illinois University School of
    Medicine, Springfield, Illinois
Cough; Anthrax

Meera Chitlur, MD
Associate Professor of Pediatrics and Director, Hemophilia
    Treatment Center and Hemostasis Program, Division of
    Hematology/Oncology, Children's Hospital of Michigan,
    Detroit, Michigan
Hemophilia and Related Conditions

Saima Chohan, MD
Arizona Arthritis and Rheumatology Associates, Phoenix,
    Arizona
Gout and Hyperuricemia

Peter E. Clark, MD
Associate Professor of Urologic Surgery, Vanderbilt University
    School of Medicine, Nashville, Tennessee
Malignant Tumors of the Urogenital Tract

Matthew Cline, MD
AHEC Professor of Family Medicine, Medical University of South Carolina, Charleston, South Carolina
Antepartum Care

Keith K. Colburn, MD
Professor of Medicine and Chief of Rheumatology, Loma Linda University, Loma Linda, California
Bursitis, Tendinitis, Myofascial Pain, and Fibromyalgia

August Colenbrander, MD
Affiliate Senior Scientist, Smith-Kettlewell Rehabilitation Engineering Research Center (RERC), San Francisco, California
Vision Rehabilitation

John M. Conly, MD
Professor of Medicine, Microbiology, Immunology and Infectious Diseases, Pathology and Laboratory Medicine, University of Calgary, Calgary, Alberta, Canada
Methicillin-Resistant Staphylococcus aureus (MRSA)

Carlo Contini, MD
Full Professor of Infectious Diseases, Section of Infectious Diseases, Department of Medical Sciences, University of Ferrara, Ferrara, Italy
Toxoplasmosis

Patricia A. Cornett, MD
Associate Chair for Education, Medicine, University of California–San Francisco; Chief, Hematology/Oncology, San Francisco Veterans Affairs Medical Center, San Francisco, California
Hemolytic Anemia

Richard W. Crummer, MD
Clinical Assistant Professor and Director, Family Medicine Inpatient Service, State University of New York–Downstate, Brooklyn, New York
Tinnitus

Burke A. Cunha, MD
Professor of Medicine, Stony Brook University School of Medicine, Stony Brook, New York; Chief, Infectious Disease Division, Winthrop–University Hospital, Mineola, New York
Viral and Mycoplasmal Pneumonias

Cheston B. Cunha, MD
Assistant Professor of Medicine, Division of Infectious Diseases, Brown University Alpert School of Medicine; Medical Director, Antimicrobial Stewardship Program, Miriam Hospital and Rhode Island Hospital, Providence, Rhode Island.
Viral and Mycoplasmal Pneumonias

Gabriel P. Currie, MD
Resident Physician, Department of Dermatology, Medical College of Wisconsin, Milwaukee, Wisconsin
Erythema Multiforme; Stevens-Johnson Syndrome and Toxic Epidermal Necrolysis

Amy E. Curry, MD
Clinical Assistant Professor, Department of Family and Community Medicine, University of Kansas School of Medicine–Wichita; Associate Director, Via Christi Family Medicine Residency, Wichita, Kansas
Pelvic Inflammatory Disease

Beth A. Damitz, MD
Associate Professor, Department of Family and Community Medicine, Medical College of Wisconsin, Milwaukee, Wisconsin
Immunization Practices

Natalie C. Dattilo, PhD
Assistant Professor of Clinical Psychology in Clinical Psychiatry, Department of Psychiatry, Indiana University School of Medicine, Indianapolis, Indiana
Anxiety Disorders

Raul Davaro, MD
Associate Professor of Clinical Medicine, University of Massachusetts, Worcester, Massachusetts
Smallpox

Susan Davids, MD, MPH
Associate Professor of Medicine, Medical College of Wisconsin; Associate Program Director, Internal Medicine Residency, Clement J. Zablocki Veterans Affairs Medical Center, Milwaukee, Wisconsin
Acute Bronchitis

Susan A. Davidson, MD
Associate Professor, University of Colorado–Denver School of Medicine; Chief, Gynecologic Oncology, University of Colorado Hospital, Aurora, Colorado
Vulvar Neoplasia

Melinda V. Davis-Malesevich, MD
Resident, Bobby R. Alford Department of Otolaryngology–Head and Neck Surgery, Baylor College of Medicine, Houston, Texas
Obstructive Sleep Apnea

David de Berker, MRCP
Consultant Dermatologist and Honorary Clinical Senior Lecturer, Bristol Dermatology Centre, Bristol, United Kingdom
Diseases of the Nails

Alexei DeCastro, MD
Assistant Professor, Program Director, Trident/MUSC Family Medicine Residency; Department of Family Medicine, Medical University of South Carolina, Charleston, South Carolina
Osteoporosis

Prakash C. Deedwania, MD
Professor of Medicine, University of California–San Francisco School of Medicine, San Francisco, California; Chief, Cardiology Section, Veterans Affairs Central California Health Care System, Fresno, California
Premature Beats

Inna D'Empaire, MD
Associate Professor of Psychiatry, Kansas University School of Medicine–Wichita, Wichita, Kansas
Delirium

André de Leon, MD
Faculty, Eisenhower Family Medicine Residency, Physician, Eisenhower Medical Center, Rancho Mirage, California
Chronic Diarrhea

Tate de Leon, MD
Faculty, Eisenhower Family Medicine Residency, Physician, Eisenhower Medical Associates, La Quinta, California
Acute Diarrhea

Phyllis A. Dennery, MD
Professor of Pediatrics, University of Pennsylvania School of
Medicine; Werner and Gertrude Henle Chair and Chief,
Division of Neonatology, Children's Hospital of Philadelphia,
Philadelphia, Pennsylvania
Hemolytic Disease of the Fetus and Newborn

Clio Dessinioti, MD, MSc
Attending Dermatologist, Andreas Sygros Hospital, Athens,
Greece
Parasitic Diseases of the Skin

Edward Dick, MD, MPH
Medical Director, Family Physician in Private Practice, San
Antonio, Texas
Travel Medicine

Gretchen M. Dickson, MD, MBA
Assistant Professor, Department of Family and Community
Medicine, University of Kansas School of Medicine–Wichita;
Program Director, Wesley Family Medicine Residency, Wichita,
Kansas
Otitis Media

Sofia Dobrin, MD
Attending Physician, Department of Neurology, NorthShore
University HealthSystem; Clinician Educator, Pritzker School of
Medicine, University of Chicago, Chicago, Illinois
Seizures and Epilepsy in Adolescents and Adults

Geoffrey A. Donnan, MD
Department of Neurology, University of Melbourne Faculty of
Medicine, Dentistry, and Health Sciences; Florey Neuroscience
Institutes, Carlton South, Victoria, Australia
Ischemic Cerebrovascular Disease

Craig L. Donnelly, MD
Geisel School of Medicine at Dartmouth, Hanover,
New Hampshire; Chief, Child and Adolescent Psychiatry,
Dartmouth-Hitchcock Medical Center, Lebanon,
New Hampshire
Attention-Deficit/Hyperactivity Disorder

John N. Dorsch, MD
Associate Professor, Family and Community Medicine, University
of Kansas School of Medicine–Wichita, Wichita, Kansas
Red Eye; Dry Eye Syndrome

Douglas A. Drevets, MD
Professor and Chief, Section of Infectious Diseases, University of
Oklahoma Health Sciences Center; Staff Physician, Veterans
Affairs Medical Center, Oklahoma City, Oklahoma
Plague

Peter R. Duggan, MD
Associate Clinical Professor of Medicine, University of Calgary,
Calgary, Alberta, Canada
Polycythemia Vera

Maurice Duggins, MD
Clinical Associate Professor, Department of Family and
Community Medicine, University of Kansas School of
Medicine–Wichita; Associate Program Director, Via Christi
Family Medicine Residency, Wichita, Kansas
Erectile Dysfunction

Kim Eagle, MD
Albion Walter Hewlett Professor of Internal Medicine, Chief of
Clinical Cardiology, and Director, Cardiovascular Center,
University of Michigan Health System, Ann Arbor, Michigan
Angina Pectoris

Leigh M. Eck, MD
Associate Professor of Medicine, Department of Internal
Medicine, University of Kansas Medical Center, Kansas City,
Kansas
Thyroiditis

Genevieve L. Egnatios, MD
Affiliated Dermatology, Scottsdale, Arizona
Contact Dermatitis

Sean P. Elliott, MD, MS
Vice Chairman of Department of Urology, Associate Professor of
Urology, and Director of Urologic Reconstruction, University of
Minnesota School of Medicine, Minneapolis, Minnesota
Trauma to the Genitourinary Tract

Dirk M. Elston, MD
Director, Ackerman Academy of Dermatopathology, New York,
New York
Diseases of the Hair

E. Wesley Ely, MD, MPH
Professor of Medicine, Department of Allergy, Pulmonary and
Critical Care Medicine, Vanderbilt University Medical Center,
Nashville, Tennessee
Delirium

John M. Embil, MD
Professor of Internal Medicine (Section of Infectious Diseases) and
Medical Microbiology, University of Manitoba, Winnipeg,
Manitoba, Canada
Blastomycosis

Scott K. Epstein, MD
Dean for Educational Affairs and Professor of Medicine, Tufts
University School of Medicine, Boston, Massachusetts
Acute Respiratory Failure

Patricia Evans, MD
Residency Program Director, Department of Family Medicine,
Georgetown University, Washington, District of Columbia
Uterine Leiomyomas

Andrew M. Evens, DO, MSc
Professor of Medicine and Chief, Division of Hematology/
Oncology, Tufts University School of Medicine; Director,
Lymphoma Program, and Leader, Clinical Sciences Program,
Tufts Cancer Center, Boston, Massachusetts
Non-Hodgkin Lymphoma

Kinder Fayssoux, MD
Faculty, Eisenhower Family Medicine Residency, Physician,
Eisenhower Medical Associates, La Quinta, California
Bacterial Infections of the Urinary Tract in Women

Dorianne Feldman, MD
Assistant Professor of Physical Medicine and Rehabilitation,
The Johns Hopkins University School of Medicine, Baltimore,
Maryland
Rehabilitation of the Stroke Patient

Barri J. Fessler, MD, MSPH
Associate Professor of Medicine, Division of Clinical Immunology and Rheumatology, University of Alabama at Birmingham, Birmingham, Alabama
Polymyalgia Rheumatica and Giant Cell Arteritis

Terry D. Fife, MD
Associate Professor of Neurology, University of Arizona; Director, Balance Disorders and Otoneurology, Barrow Neurological Institute, Phoenix, Arizona
Ménière's Disease

David J. Finley, MD
Co-Director, Complex Airway Program, Surgeon, Thoracic Service, Memorial Sloan Kettering Cancer Center, New York, New York
Pleural Effusions and Empyema Thoracis

Robert S. Fisher, MD
Professor of Medicine, Gastroenterology Section and Digestive Disease Center, Temple University School of Medicine, Philadelphia, Pennsylvania
Irritable Bowel Syndrome

William E. Fisher, MD
Professor of Surgery, Baylor College of Medicine, Houston, Texas
Acute and Chronic Pancreatitis

Donald C. Fletcher, MD
Medical Director, Low Vision Rehabilitation, Envision, Wichita, Kansas
Vision Rehabilitation

Raja Flores, MD
Professor and Chairman, Department of Thoracic Surgery, Mount Sinai Medical Center, New York, New York
Pleural Effusions and Empyema Thoracis

Brian J. Flynn, MD
Associate Professor of Urology, University of Colorado–Denver School of Medicine, Aurora, Colorado
Urethral Strictures

Sarah Forsberg, PsyD
Postdoctoral Research Fellow, Child Psychiatry, Stanford University School of Medicine, Stanford, California
Eating Disorders

Jennifer Frank, MD
ThedaCare Physicians–Neenah West, Neenah, Wisconsin
Syphilis; Vaginal Bleeding Late in Pregnancy

Robert S. Freelove, MD
Clinical Associate Professor, Department of Family and Community Medicine, University of Kansas School of Medicine–Wichita, Wichita, Kansas; Program Director, Smoky Hill Family Medicine Residency, Salina, Kansas
Nongonococcal Urethritis

Ellen W. Freeman, PhD
Research Professor, Departments of Obstetrics/Gynecology and Psychiatry, University of Pennsylvania Perelman School of Medicine, Philadelphia, Pennsylvania
Premenstrual Syndrome

Theodore M. Freeman, MD
San Antonio Asthma and Allergy Clinic, San Antonio, Texas
Allergic Reactions to Insect Stings

Keith A. Frey, MD
Chief Physician Executive, Dignity Health Arizona, Phoenix, Arizona
Infertility

Aaron Friedman, MD
Ruben Bentson Professor and Chair, Pediatrics, University of Minnesota, Minneapolis, Minnesota
Parenteral Fluid Therapy for Infants and Children

Melissa Gaines, MD
Associate Professor of Internal Medicine, University of Kansas School of Medicine–Wichita, Wichita, Kansas
Constipation

R. Michael Gallagher, DO
Headache Consultant, Headache Center of Central Florida, Melbourne, Florida
Headache

John Garber, MD
Instructor in Medicine, Harvard Medical School; Fellow in Gastroenterology, Massachusetts General Hospital, Boston, Massachusetts
Acute and Chronic Viral Hepatitis

John D. Gazewood, MD, MSPH
Harrison Medical Teaching Associate Professor of Family Medicine, Residency Program Director, Medical Director, Family Medicine Practice at the Primary Care Center, University of Virginia Health System, Charlottesville, Virginia
Parkinson Disease

Khalil G. Ghanem, MD, PhD
Associate Professor of Medicine, The Johns Hopkins University School of Medicine, Baltimore, Maryland
Gonorrhea

Muhammad A. Ghazi, MD
Clinical Instructor, Department of Family Medicine, University at Buffalo, Buffalo, New York
Pruritus Ani and Vulvae

Donald L. Gilbert, MD, MS
Professor of Pediatrics and Neurology; Child Neurology Residency Program Director; Director, Movement Disorders and Tourette Syndrome Clinic; Co-Director, Transcranial Magnetic Stimulation Laboratory, Cincinnati Children's Hospital Medical Center, Cincinnati, Ohio
Gilles de la Tourette Syndrome

Robert Giusti, MD
Clinical Associate Professor of Pediatrics, Division of Pediatric Pulmonology, New York University School of Medicine; New York University Langone Medical Center, New York, New York
Cystic Fibrosis

Mark T. Gladwin, MD
Professor of Medicine, University of Pittsburgh School of Medicine; Chief, Division of Pulmonary, Allergy and Critical Care Medicine, University of Pittsburgh, Pittsburgh, Pennsylvania
Sickle Cell Disease

Stephen J. Gluckman, MD
Professor of Medicine, Perelman School of Medicine,
University of Pennsylvania, Philadelphia, Pennsylvania
Chronic Fatigue Syndrome

Andrew W. Goddard, MD
Professor of Psychiatry and Radiology, Indiana University School
of Medicine; Adjunct Professor, Purdue University Graduate
School; Director, Adult Psychiatry Clinic and Study Center;
Director, Adult Anxiety Program, IU Health Neuroscience
Center, Indianapolis, Indiana
Anxiety Disorders

Mark S. Gold, MD
Distinguished Professor and Chair, Psychiatry, Neuroscience,
Anesthesiology, and Community Health and Family Medicine,
University of Florida College of Medicine, Gainesville, Florida
Drug Abuse

Marlís González-Fernández, MD, PhD
Assistant Professor of Physical Medicine and Rehabilitation, The
Johns Hopkins University School of Medicine; Medical
Director, Outpatient Physical Medicine and Rehabilitation
Clinics, The Johns Hopkins Hospital, Baltimore, Maryland
Rehabilitation of the Stroke Patient

Aidar R. Gosmanov, MD, PhD, DMSc
Associate Professor of Medicine, Division of Endocrinology,
Diabetes, and Metabolism, The University of Tennessee Health
Science Center, Memphis, Tennessee
Diabetic Ketoacidosis

Luigi Gradoni, PhD
Research Director, Vector-Borne Diseases and International
Health, Istituto Superiore di Sanità, Rome, Italy
Leishmaniasis

Jane M. Grant-Kels, MD
Founding Chair, Department of Dermatology; Professor of
Dermatology, Pathology and Pediatrics; Dermatology
Residency Director and Assistant Dean of Clinical Affairs,
University of Connecticut School of Medicine; Director of
Dermatopathology and Director, Cutaneous Oncology and
Melanoma Center, University of Connecticut Health Center,
Farmington, Connecticut
Nevi

Leslie A. Greenberg, MD
Assistant Professor, Department of Family and Community
Medicine, University of Nevada School of Medicine in Reno,
Reno, Nevada
Keloids

William M. Greene, MD
Assistant Professor of Psychiatry, University of Florida,
Gainesville, Florida
Drug Abuse

Joseph Greensher, MD
Professor of Pediatrics, Stony Brook University Medical Center
School of Medicine, Stony Brook, New York; Medical Director
and Associate Chair, Department of Pediatrics, Long Island
Regional Poison and Drug Information Center, Winthrop-
University Hospital, Mineola, New York
Medical Toxicology

David Gregory, MD
Associate Clinical Professor of Family Medicine, University of
Virginia School of Medicine, Charlottesville, Virginia;

Assistant Clinical Professor of Family Medicine, Virginia
Commonwealth University School of Medicine, Richmond,
Virginia; Program Director, CENTRA-Lynchburg Family
Medicine Residency; Staff Physician in Family Medicine,
Lynchburg General Hospital and Virginia Baptist Hospital,
Lynchburg, Virginia
Resuscitation of the Newborn

Sriharsha Cherukumilli Grevich, MD
Pediatric Rheumatology Fellow, University of Washington,
Seattle, Washington
Rheumatoid Arthritis

Priya Grewal, MD
Assistant Professor, Division of Liver Diseases, Mount Sinai
School of Medicine, New York, New York
Cirrhosis

Robert Grossberg, MD
Associate Professor of Clinical Medicine, Infectious Diseases,
Albert Einstein College of Medicine and Montefiore Medical
Center, Bronx, New York
Fungal Diseases of the Skin

Eva C. Guinan, MD
Professor of Radiation Oncology and Director, Reactor Program,
Harvard Catalyst, Harvard Medical School, Boston,
Massachusetts
Aplastic Anemia

Tawanda Gumbo, MD
Associate Professor of Medicine, University of Texas
Southwestern Medical School; Attending Physician, Parkland
Memorial Hospital and University Hospital–St. Paul, Dallas,
Texas
Tuberculosis and Other Mycobacterial Diseases

Amita Gupta, MD, MHS
Associate Professor of Medicine (Division of Infectious Diseases)
and International Health, The Johns Hopkins University School
of Medicine, Baltimore, Maryland
HIV Disease

Rebat M. Halder, MD
Professor and Chair, Department of Dermatology, Howard
University College of Medicine, Washington, District of
Columbia
Pigmentary Disorders

Ronald Hall II, PharmD, MSCS
Associate Professor, Texas Tech University Health Sciences Center
School of Pharmacy, Dallas, Texas
Tuberculosis and Other Mycobacterial Diseases

Nicola A. Hanania, MD, MS
Associate Professor of Medicine, Section of Pulmonary, Critical
Care, and Sleep Medicine; Director, Asthma Clinical Research
Center, Baylor College of Medicine, Houston, Texas
Chronic Obstructive Pulmonary Disease

George D. Harris, MD, MS
Professor and Chair of Family Medicine, West Virginia University
Eastern Division, School of Medicine, Harper's Ferry,
West Virginia
Osteomyelitis

Kari R. Harris, MD
Assistant Professor of Pediatrics, University of Kansas School of
Medicine–Wichita, Wichita, Kansas
Adolescent Health

Adam L. Hartman, MD
Assistant Professor of Neurology, Pediatrics, and Molecular
   Microbiology and Immunology, The Johns Hopkins Hospital,
   Baltimore, Maryland
   Epilepsy in Infants and Children

Sean O. Henderson, MD
Professor and Chair, Emergency Medicine, Keck School of
   Medicine at the University of Southern California, Los Angeles,
   California
   Amebiasis

L. David Hillis, MD
Chair, Department of Medicine, University of Texas Health
   Science Center, San Antonio, Texas
   Congenital Heart Disease

Stacey A. Hinderliter, MD
Riverside Brentwood Pediatric Center, Newport News, Virginia
   Resuscitation of the Newborn

Molly Hinshaw, MD
Associate Professor of Dermatology, University of Wisconsin
   School of Medicine and Public Health, Madison, Wisconsin;
   Dermatopathologist, Dermpath Diagnostics, Brookfield,
   Wisconsin
   Cutaneous Vasculitis; Connective Tissue Disorders

Bryan Ho, MD
Assistant Professor of Neurology, Tufts Medical Center, Boston,
   Massachusetts
   Myasthenia Gravis

Vanessa Ho, MD
Faculty, Eisenhower Family Medicine Residency Program,
   Eisenhower Medical Center, La Quinta, California
   Hypopituitarism

Raymond J. Hohl, MD, PhD
Professor of Medicine and Pharmacology, Director, Penn State
   Hershey Cancer Institute, Hershey, Pennsylvania
   Thalassemia

Sarah A. Holstein, MD, PhD
Assistant Professor of Oncology, Roswell Park Cancer Institute,
   Buffalo, New York
   Thalassemia

Marisa Holubar, MD
Clinical Teaching Fellow, Warren Alpert Medical School of Brown
   University, Providence, Rhode Island
   Severe Sepsis

Laurie Hommema, MD
Program Director, Riverside Family Medicine, Columbus, Ohio
   Measles

Ahmad Reza Hossani-Madani, MD
Dermatologist, Kaiser Permanente, Upper Marlboro, Maryland
   Pigmentary Disorders

Steven A. House, MD
Associate Professor, Department of Family and Geriatric
   Medicine, University of Louisville; Program Director,
   University of Louisville/Glasgow Family Medicine Residency
   Program, Glasgow, Kentucky
   Pain

Sarah Houssayni, MD
Clinical Assistant Professor, Department of Family and
   Community Medicine, University of Kansas School of
   Medicine–Wichita; Pediatrics Faculty, Via Christi Family
   Medicine Residency, Wichita, Kansas
   Encopresis

Judith M. Hübschen, PhD
Scientist, Institute of Immunology, Centre de Recherche Public de
   la Santé/Laboratoire National de Santé, Luxembourg
   Rubella and Congenital Rubella

William J. Hueston, MD
Senior Associate Dean for Academic Affairs, Medical College of
   Wisconsin, Milwaukee, Wisconsin
   Hyperthyroidism; Hypothyroidism

Scott A. Hundahl, MD
Professor of Surgery, University of California–Davis School of
   Medicine, Sacramento, California; Chief of Surgery, Veterans
   Affairs Northern California Health Care System, Mather,
   California
   Tumors of the Stomach

Stephen P. Hunger, MD
Professor of Pediatrics, University of Colorado–Denver School of
   Medicine; Section Chief, Center for Cancer and Blood Disorders
   and Ergen Family Chair in Pediatric Cancer, The Children's
   Hospital, Aurora, Colorado
   Acute Leukemia in Children

Wendy S. Hupp, DMD
Interim Chair, Department of General Dentistry and Oral
   Medicine; Chair, Curriculum Committee; Associate Professor
   of Oral Medicine; University of Louisville School of Dentistry,
   Louisville, Kentucky
   Diseases of the Mouth

Gerald A. Isenberg, MD
Professor of Surgery and Director of Surgical Undergraduate
   Education, Jefferson Medical College of Thomas Jefferson
   University; Program Director, Colorectal Residency, Thomas
   Jefferson University Hospital, Philadelphia, Pennsylvania
   Tumors of the Colon and Rectum

Alan C. Jackson, MD
Professor of Medicine (Neurology) and Medical Microbiology,
   University of Manitoba Faculty of Health Sciences; Head,
   Section of Neurology, Winnipeg Regional Health Authority,
   Winnipeg, Manitoba, Canada
   Rabies

Kurt M. Jacobson, MD
Assistant Professor of Medicine, Cardiovascular Medicine
   Division, University of Wisconsin School of Medicine and
   Public Health, Madison, Wisconsin
   Mitral Valve Prolapse

James J. James, MD
Executive Director, Society for Disaster Medicine and Public
   Health, Washington, District of Columbia
   *Biologic Agents Reference Chart; Toxic Chemical Agents Reference Chart:
   Symptoms and Treatment*

Katarzyna Jamieson, MD
Associate Professor of Medicine, Division of Hematology and
Oncology, University of North Carolina, Chapel Hill,
North Carolina
Chronic Leukemias

James N. Jarvis, MD
Professor of Pediatrics and Section Chief, Pediatric Allergy/
Immunology/Rheumatology, University at Buffalo, Buffalo,
New York
Juvenile Idiopathic Arthritis

Roy M. John, MD, PhD
Clinical Associate Professor, Harvard Medical School; Associate
Director, Cardiac Electrophysiology Laboratory, Brigham and
Women's Hospital, Boston, Massachusetts
Cardiac Arrest: Sudden Cardiac Death

Lisa M. Johnson, MD
Assistant Professor, Department of Family Medicine and Rural
Health, Florida State University College of Medicine,
Tallahassee, Florida
Acne Vulgaris; Rosacea

Joshua S. Jolissaint, BA
University of Virginia School of Medicine, Charlottesville,
Virginia
Atelectasis

Gregory Juckett, MD, MPH
Professor of Family Medicine; Director, West Virginia University
International Travel Clinic, West Virginia University School of
Medicine, Morgantown, West Virginia
Campylobacter

Marc A. Judson, MD
Professor of Medicine and Chief, Division of Pulmonary and
Critical Care Medicine, Department of Medicine, Albany
Medical College, Albany, New York
Sarcoidosis

Tamilarasu Kadhiravan, MD
Associate Professor of Medicine, Department of Medicine,
Jawaharlal Institute of Postgraduate Medical Education and
Research–Puducherry, Puducherry, India
Typhoid Fever

Harmit Kalia, DO
Division of Gastroenterology and Hepatology, Albert Einstein
College of Medicine, Bronx, New York; University of Medicine
and Dentistry of New Jersey, Newark, New Jersey
Cirrhosis

Rick D. Kellerman, MD
Professor and Chair, Department of Family and Community
Medicine, University of Kansas School of Medicine–Wichita,
Wichita, Kansas
Chikungunya

Scott Kellermann, MD, MPH
Founder, Bwindi Community Hospital, Uganda
Chikungunya

Walter Kao, MD
Associate Professor of Medicine, University of Wisconsin School
of Medicine and Public Health; Attending Cardiologist, Heart

Failure and Transplant Program, University of Wisconsin
Hospitals and Clinics, Madison, Wisconsin
Congestive Heart Failure

Michael E. Karellas, MD
Department of Surgery/Urologic Oncology, Atlantic Health
Systems, Morristown Medical Center, Morristown, New Jersey
Renal Calculi

Dilip R. Karnad, MD
Consultant in Internal Medicine and Critical Care, Jupiter
Hospital, Thane, India
Tetanus

Andreas Katsambas, MD, PhD
Professor of Dermatology, Department of Dermatology,
University of Athens School of Medicine; Hygeia Hospital,
Athens, Greece
Parasitic Diseases of the Skin

Ben Z. Katz, MD
Professor of Pediatrics, Northwestern University Feinberg School
of Medicine; Division of Infectious Diseases, Ann and Robert H.
Lurie Children's Hospital of Chicago, Chicago, Illinois
Infectious Mononucleosis

Rebecca Katzman, MD
Resident, Family Medicine Residency of Idaho, Boise, Idaho
Palpitations

Daniel I. Kaufer, MD
Associate Professor, Department of Neurology, Division Chief,
Cognitive Neurology and Memory Disorders; Director, UNC
Memory Disorders Program; Co-Director, Carolina
Alzheimer's Network; University of North Carolina at Chapel
Hill, Chapel Hill, North Carolina
Alzheimer's Disease

Arthur Kavanaugh, MD
Professor of Medicine, University of California, San Diego, School
of Medicine, La Jolla, California
Rheumatoid Arthritis

Clive Kearon, PhD
Professor of Medicine, McMaster University Faculty of Health
Sciences; Attending Physician, Henderson General Hospital,
Hamilton, Ontario, Canada
Venous Thromboembolism

B. Mark Keegan, MD
Associate Professor and Section Chair, Multiple Sclerosis and
Autoimmune Neurology, Department of Neurology, Mayo
Clinic, Rochester, Minnesota
Multiple Sclerosis

Stephen F. Kemp, MD
Professor of Medicine and Pediatrics, Director, Allergy and
Immunology Fellowship Program, The University of Mississippi
Medical Center, Jackson, Mississippi
Anaphylaxis and Serum Sickness

Haejin Kim, MD
Division of Allergy and Clinical Immunology, Henry Ford Health
System, Detroit, Michigan
Hypersensitivity Pneumonitis

Jongoh Kim, MD
Assistant Professor of Medicine, Division of Diabetes, Endocrinology and Metabolism, Department of Medicine, Baylor College of Medicine, Houston, Texas
Hyperaldosteronism; Hyperlipidemia

Paul S. Kingma, MD, PhD
Associate Professor, The Perinatal Institute, Cincinnati Children's Hospital Medical Center, Cincinnati, Ohio
Care of the High-Risk Neonate

Robert S. Kirsner, MD, PhD
Professor, Vice Chairman, and Stiefel Laboratories Chair, Department of Dermatology and Cutaneous Surgery and Chief of Dermatology, University of Miami Miller School of Medicine, Miami, Florida
Venous Ulcers

Paul Knoll, MD
Surgery Resident, University of Colorado Denver, Aurora, Colorado
Urethral Strictures

Amanda Kolb, MD
Instructor, Department of Family Medicine, University of Virginia, Charlottesville, Virginia
Asthma in Children

Frederick K. Korley, MD
Robert E. Meyerhoff Assistant Professor of Emergency Medicine, The Johns Hopkins University School of Medicine; Staff, The Johns Hopkins Medical Institutions, Baltimore, Maryland
Disturbances Due to Cold

Adrienne N. Kovalsky, DO, MPH
Hospital Medicine, Colorado Springs, Colorado; Wailuku, Hawaii; Montana
High-Altitude Sickness

Robert A. Kratzke, MD
John Skoglund Chair of Lung Cancer Research, University of Minnesota Medical School; Associate Professor, University of Minnesota Medical Center, Minneapolis, Minnesota
Primary Lung Cancer

Eric H. Kraut, MD
Professor of Medicine and Director, Benign Hematology, Division of Hematology-Oncology, The Ohio State University, Columbus, Ohio
Platelet-Mediated Bleeding Disorders

Jeffrey A. Kraut, MD
Professor of Medicine, David Geffen School of Medicine at UCLA; Chief of Dialysis, Veterans Affairs Greater Los Angeles Healthcare System, Los Angeles, California
Chronic Kidney Disease

Marcus Kret, MD
Fellow, Division of Vascular and Endovascular Surgery, Stanford University School of Medicine, Stanford, California
Peripheral Arterial Disease

John N. Krieger, MD
Professor of Urology, University of Washington School of Medicine; Chief of Urology, Veterans Affairs Puget Sound Health Care System, Seattle, Washington
Bacterial Infections of the Male Urinary Tract

Lakshmanan Krishnamurti, MD
Professor of Pediatrics, Division of Hematology/Oncology, Children's Hospital of Pittsburgh of the University of Pittsburgh Medical Center, Pittsburgh, Pennsylvania
Sickle Cell Disease

Kumar Krishnan, MD
Assistant Professor of Medicine, Division of Gastroenterology, The Houston Methodist Hospital, Weill Cornell Medical College, Houston, Texas
Dysphagia and Esophageal Obstruction

Nathan Krug, MD
Lone Tree Medical Associates, Central City, Nebraska
Heat-Related Illness

Roshni Kulkarni, MD
Professor and Director, Pediatric Hematology/Oncology; Director (Pediatric), Michigan State University Center for Bleeding and Clotting Disorders, Department of Pediatrics and Human Development, Michigan State University College of Medicine, East Lansing, Michigan
Hemophilia and Related Conditions

Seema Kumar, MD
Associate Professor of Pediatrics, Mayo Clinic College of Medicine; Consultant, Division of Pediatrics, Endocrinology, and Metabolism, Department of Pediatrics, Mayo Clinic, Rochester, Minnesota
Obesity

Mary R. Kwaan, MD, MPH
Assistant Professor of Surgery, University of Minnesota Medical Center, Minneapolis, Minnesota
Hemorrhoids, Anal Fissure, and Anorectal Abscess and Fistula

Jennie H. Kwon, DO
Fellow in Infectious Diseases, Department of Medicine, Washington University School of Medicine, St. Louis, Missouri
Pseudomembranous Colitis

Robert A. Kyle, MD
Professor of Medicine, Laboratory Medicine, and Pathology, Mayo Clinic College of Medicine, Rochester, Minnesota
Multiple Myeloma

Lori M.B. Laffel, MD, MPH
Associate Professor of Pediatrics, Harvard Medical School; Chief, Pediatric, Adolescent, and Young Adult Section; Investigator, Section on Genetics and Epidemiology, Joslin Diabetes Center, Boston, Massachusetts
Diabetes Mellitus in Children

Richard A. Lange, MD
President and Dean, Paul L. Foster School of Medicine, Texas Tech University Health Sciences Center, El Paso, Texas
Congenital Heart Disease

Sarah Takach Lapner, MSc, MD
Clinical Lecturer, Department of Medicine, Division of Hematology, University of Alberta, Edmonton, Alberta, Canada
Venous Thromboembolism

Julius Larioza, MD
Assistant Professor of Medicine, Attending Physician, Bay State Medical Center, Springfield, Massachusetts
Toxic Shock Syndrome

Jerome Larkin, MD
Assistant Professor of Medicine, Warren Alpert Medical School at Brown University; Attending Physician, Rhode Island Hospital, Providence, Rhode Island
Severe Sepsis

David Larrabee, MD, MPH
Saint Vincent Medical Group, Shrewsbury, Massachusetts
Otitis Externa

Ryan Lasota, MD
Newman Family Medicine, Emporia, Kansas
Heat-Related Illness

Barbara A. Latenser, MD
Former Clara L. Smith Professor of Burn Surgery, University of Iowa Carver College of Medicine, Iowa City, Iowa
Burn Treatment Guidelines

Christine L. Lau, MD
Associate Professor, Division of Thoracic and Cardiovascular Surgery, University of Virginia Health System, Charlottesville, Virginia
Atelectasis

Susan Lawrence-Hylland, MD
Clinical Assistant Professor, Rheumatology Section, University of Wisconsin Hospital and Clinics, Madison, Wisconsin
Connective Tissue Disorders; Cutaneous Vasculitis

Miguel A. Leal, MD
Assistant Professor of Medicine, University of Wisconsin School of Medicine and Public Health, Madison, Wisconsin
Pericarditis

Jerrold B. Leikin, MD
Clinical Professor of Medicine, University of Chicago Pritzker School of Medicine; Professor of Medicine and Pharmacology, Rush Medical College, Chicago, Illinois; Director of Medical Toxicology, NorthShore University HealthSystem-OMEGA, Glenbrook Hospital, Glenview, Illinois
Disturbances Due to Cold

Scott M. Leikin, BA
Mount Sinai Medical Center, Chicago, Illinois
Disturbances Due to Cold

Alexander K.C. Leung, MBBS
Clinical Professor of Pediatrics, The University of Calgary; Pediatric Consultant, Alberta Children's Hospital, Calgary, Alberta, Canada
Nocturnal Enuresis

Jana Lewis, MD
Department of Surgery, Maimonides Medical Center, Brooklyn, New York
Breast Disease

Albert P. Lin, MD
Assistant Professor, Ophthalmology, Baylor College of Medicine; Staff Physician, Eye Care Line, Michael E. DeBakey VA Medical Center, Houston, Texas
Glaucoma

Janet C. Lindemann, MD, MBA
Professor of Family Medicine and Dean of Medical Student Education, Sanford School of Medicine, University of South Dakota, Sioux Falls, South Dakota
Fatigue

Jeffrey A. Linder, MD, MPH
Associate Professor of Medicine, Harvard Medical School; Associate Physician, Division of General Medicine and Primary Care, Brigham and Women's Hospital, Boston, Massachusetts
Influenza

James Lock, MD, PhD
Professor of Child Psychiatry and Pediatrics, Stanford University School of Medicine; Medical Director, Eating Disorder Program, Lucile Packard Children's Hospital, Stanford, California
Eating Disorders

Maya Lodish, MD
Deputy Director, Pediatric Endocrinology Fellowship; Staff Clinician, Eunice Kennedy Shriver National Institute of Child Health and Human Development, National Institutes of Health, Bethesda, Maryland
Cushing's Syndrome

M. Chantel Long, MD
Clinical Assistant Professor, Department of Family and Community Medicine, University of Kansas School of Medicine-Wichita, Wichita, Kansas; Associate Director, Smoky Hill Family Medicine Residency, Salina, Kansas
Condyloma Acuminata; Warts (Verrucae)

Michael F. Lynch, MD
Medical Epidemiologist, Division of Parasitic Diseases and Malaria, Malaria Branch, Center for Global Health, Centers for Disease Control and Prevention, Atlanta, Georgia
Malaria

James M. Lyznicki, MS, MPH
Senior Policy Analyst II, Science and Biotechnology, American Medical Association, Chicago, Illinois
Biologic Agents Reference Chart; Toxic Chemical Agents Reference Chart: Symptoms and Treatment

Kimberly E. Mace, PhD
Division of Parasitic Diseases and Malaria, Malaria Branch, Center for Global Health, Centers for Disease Control and Prevention, Atlanta, Georgia
Malaria

Bahaa S. Malaeb, MD
Assistant Professor, Genitourinary Trauma and Reconstructive Surgery, Department of Urology, University of Michigan, Ann Arbor, Michigan
Trauma to the Genitourinary Tract

Uma Malhotra, MD
Department of Infectious Diseases, Virginia Mason Medical Center, Seattle, Washington
Ebola Virus Disease

Michael A. Malone, MD
Co-Medical Director, Penn State Hershey Medical Group, Hershey, Pennsylvania
Vulvovaginitis

Paul Martin, MD
Chief, Division of Hepatology, University of Miami Miller School of Medicine, Miami, Florida
Cirrhosis

Vickie Martin, MD
Resident, Department of Obstetrics and Gynecology, Kingston
General Hospital, Kingston, Ontario, Canada
Amenorrhea

Jyoti S. Mathad, MD, MSc
Instructor, Division of Infectious Diseases and Center for Global
Health, Weill Cornell Medical College, New York, New York
HIV Disease

Pinckney J. Maxwell, IV, MD
Assistant Professor of Surgery, Colon and Rectal Surgery, Division
of Gastrointestinal & Laparoscopic Surgery, Medical
University of South Carolina, Charleston, South Carolina
Tumors of the Colon and Rectum

Laura Mayans, MD
Assistant Professor, Department of Family and Community
Medicine, University of Kansas School of Medicine–Wichita,
Wichita, Kansas
Varicella (ChickenPox)

Anthony L. McCall, MD, PhD
James M. Moss Professor of Diabetes, University of Virginia
School of Medicine; Endocrinologist, University of Virginia
Health Care System, Charlottesville, Virginia
Diabetes Mellitus in Adults

Laura J. McCloskey, PhD
Director of Laboratories; Associate Professor of Pathology,
Anatomy, and Cell Biology; and Director, Clinical
Immunology, Specimen Processing, and Referral Testing,
Jefferson Hospital for Neuroscience Laboratory, Jefferson
Infusion Center Laboratory, and Jefferson at the Navy Yard
Laboratory, Philadelphia, Pennsylvania
Reference Intervals for the Interpretation of Laboratory Tests

Christopher C. McGuigan, MBChB, MPH
Consultant in Health Protection, NHS Fife, Public Health
Department, Fife, United Kingdom
Psittacosis

Michael McGuigan, MD
Medical Director, Long Island Regional Poison and Drug
Information Center, Winthrop-University Hospital, Mineola,
New York
Medical Toxicology

Mick S. Meiselman, MD
Clinical Assistant Professor, University of Chicago Pritzker School
of Medicine; Section Chief, Advanced Therapeutic Endoscopy,
Department of Gastroenterology, NorthShore University
HealthSystem, Evanston, Illinois
Calculous Biliary Disease

Genevieve B. Melton-Meaux, MD
Associate Professor of Surgery, University of Minnesota Medical
School, Minneapolis, Minnesota
Hemorrhoids, Anal Fissure, and Anorectal Abscess and Fistula

Moises Mercado, MD
Professor of Medicine, Faculty of Medicine, Universidad Nacional
Autónoma de México; Head, Endocrine Service and
Experimental Endocrinology Unit, Hospital de Especialidades,
Centro Médico Nacional Siglo XXI, Institute Mexicano del
Seguro Social, Mexico City, Mexico
Acromegaly

Ryan Merrell, MD
Department of Neurology, NorthShore University HealthSystem,
Evanston, Illinois
Brain Tumors

Steven Meyers, MD
NorthShore Neurologic Institute, Department of Neurology,
NorthShore University HealthSystem, Evanston, Illinois
Acute Facial Paralysis

Brian Miller, MD, PhD, MPH
Associate Professor, Department of Psychiatry, Georgia Regents
University, Augusta, Georgia
Schizophrenia

Moben Mirza, MD
Assistant Professor, Division of Urologic Oncology, Department
of Urology, University of Kansas Medical Center, Kansas City,
Kansas
Hematuria

Howard C. Mofenson, MD
Professor of Pediatrics and Emergency Medicine, Stony
Brook University Medical Center School of Medicine, Stony
Brook, New York; Professor of Pharmacology and Toxicology,
New York College of Osteopathic Medicine, Old Westbury,
New York
Medical Toxicology

Kris M. Mogensen, MS, RD, LDN, CNSC
Team Leader Dietitian, Department of Nutrition, Brigham and
Women's Hospital; Instructor, Health Sciences (Nutrition),
Boston University College of Health and Rehabilitation
Sciences, Sargent College, Boston, Massachusetts
Parenteral Nutrition in Adults

Justin Moore, MD
Assistant Professor of Internal Medicine, University of Kansas
School of Medicine–Wichita, Wichita, Kansas
Adrenocortical Insufficiency

Enrique Morales, MD
Attending Nephrologist, Hospital 12 de Octubre, Madrid, Spain
Primary Glomerular Diseases

Jaime Morales-Arias, MD
Associate Professor of Pediatrics, Louisiana State University;
Director, Bleeding Disorders and Thrombosis Program,
Children's Hospital of New Orleans, New Orleans, Louisiana
Disseminated Intravascular Coagulation

Timothy I. Morgenthaler, MD
Associate Professor of Medicine, Pulmonary and Critical Care
Medicine, Center for Sleep Medicine, Mayo Clinic and
Foundation, Rochester, Minnesota
Sleep Disorders

Warwick L. Morison, MD
Professor of Dermatology, The Johns Hopkins University School
of Medicine, Baltimore, Maryland
Sunburn

Rami Mortada, MD
Assistant Professor, Division of Endocrinology, Kansas
University–Wichita, Wichita, Kansas
Diabetes Insipidus

Heather E. Moss, MD, PhD
Department of Ophthalmology and Visual Sciences, University of Illinois at Chicago, Chicago, Illinois
Optic Neuritis

Ladan Mostaghimi, MD
Clinical Associate Professor, University of Wisconsin School of Medicine and Public Health, Madison, Wisconsin
Psychocutaneous Medicine

Judd W. Moul, MD
James H. Semans Professor of Surgery, Department of Surgery, Division of Urologic Surgery; Director, Duke Prostate Center, Duke Cancer Institute, Duke University Medical Center, Durham, North Carolina.
Benign Prostatic Hyperplasia

Claude P. Muller, MD
Head of Department, Institute of Immunology, Centre de Recherche Public de la Santé/Laboratoire National de Santé, Luxembourg
Measles (Rubeola); Rubella and Congenital Rubella

Michael Murphy, MD
Professor of Dermatology, University of Connecticut School of Medicine; Attending Dermatopathologist, Department of Dermatology, University of Connecticut Health Center, Farmington, Connecticut
Nevi

Diya F. Mutasim, MD
Professor of Dermatology and Pathology, University of Cincinnati College of Medicine, Cincinnati, Ohio
Bullous Diseases

Alykhan S. Nagji, MD
Cardiothoracic Fellow, Department of Surgery, University of Virginia School of Medicine, Charlottesville, Virginia
Atelectasis

Tara J. Neil, MD
Assistant Professor, Department of Family and Community Medicine, University of Kansas School of Medicine–Wichita; Associate Program Director, Via Christi Family Medicine Residency, Wichita, Kansas
Postpartum Care

David G. Neschis, MD
Clinical Associate Professor of Surgery, University of Maryland School of Medicine, Baltimore, Maryland; Vascular Surgeon, The Maryland Vascular Center, Glen Burnie, Maryland
Aortic Disease: Aneurysm and Dissection

Theresa Nester, MD
Associate Professor of Laboratory Medicine, University of Washington Medical Center; Transfusion Service Medical Director, Puget Sound Blood Center, Seattle, Washington
Blood Component Therapy

David H. Neustadt, MD
Clinical Professor of Medicine, University of Louisville School of Medicine; Senior Attending, University Hospital, Jewish Hospital, Louisville, Kentucky
Osteoarthritis

Tam T. Nguyen, MD
Program Director, San Joaquin Hospital FM Residency Program, San Joaquin General Hospital, Chair, Family Medicine, San Joaquin General Hospital, French Camp, California
Papulosquamous Eruptions

Lucybeth Nieves-Arriba, MD
Case Western Reserve University School of Medicine; Gynecologic Oncology, Women's Health Institute, Cleveland Clinic, Cleveland, Ohio
Cancer of the Uterine Cervix

Andrei Novac, MD
Clinical Professor of Psychiatry and Founding Director, Traumatic Stress Program, University of California–Irvine, Irvine, California
Mood Disorders: Depression, Bipolar Disease, and Mood Dysregulation

Enrico M. Novelli, MD
Assistant Professor of Medicine, Department of Medicine, Division of Hematology/Oncology, Vascular Medicine Institute; Director, Adult Sickle Cell Anemia Program, University of Pittsburgh School of Medicine, Pittsburgh, Pennsylvania
Sickle Cell Disease

Jeffrey P. Okeson, DMD
Professor and Chair, Oral Health Science; Director, Orofacial Pain Program, College of Dentistry, University of Kentucky, Lexington, Kentucky
Temporomandibular Disorders

David L. Olive, MD
Professor of Obstetrics and Gynecology, University of Wisconsin School of Medicine and Public Health, Madison, Wisconsin
Endometriosis

Peck Y. Ong, MD
Associate Professor of Clinical Pediatrics, Department of Pediatrics, Keck School of Medicine of the University of Southern California; Attending Physician, Division of Clinical Immunology and Allergy, Children's Hospital Los Angeles, Los Angeles, California
Atopic Dermatitis

Bernhard Ortel, MD
Division Head, Dermatology, NorthShore University HealthSystem, Skokie, Illinois; Clinical Professor, University of Chicago Pritzker School of Medicine, Chicago, Illinois
Cancer of the Skin

Gary D. Overturf, MD
Professor Emeritus of Pediatrics and Pathology, University of New Mexico School of Medicine; Medical Director, Infectious Diseases, TriCore Reference Laboratories, Albuquerque, New Mexico
Bacterial Meningitis

Karel Pacak, MD, PhD, DSc
Professor of Medicine and Chief of the Section on Medical Neuroendocrinology, Eunice Kennedy Shriver National Institute of Child Health and Human Development, National Institutes of Health, Bethesda, Maryland
Pheochromocytoma

John E. Pandolfino, MD
Professor of Medicine, Gastroenterology, and Hepatology, Department of Medicine, Northwestern University Feinberg School of Medicine, Chicago, Illinois
Dysphagia and Esophageal Obstruction

Jotam Pasipanodya, MD
Research Scientist, University of Texas Southwestern Medical Center at Dallas, Dallas, Texas
Tuberculosis and Other Mycobacterial Diseases

Manish R. Patel, DO
Assistant Professor, University of Minnesota Medical Center, Minneapolis, Minnesota
Primary Lung Cancer

Peter D. Patrick, PhD
Department of Pediatrics, University of Virginia, Charlottesville, Virginia
Traumatic Brain Injury in Children

Paul Paulman, MD
Assistant Dean for Clinical Skills and Quality, Family Medicine, University of Nebraska College of Medicine, Omaha, Nebraska
Iron Deficiency Anemia

Gerson O. Penna, MD, PhD
Senior Researcher, Department of Tropical Medicine, University of Brasilia, Brasilia, Brazil
Leprosy

Maria Lucia Penna, MD, PhD
Professor, Department of Epidemiology and Biostatistics, Universidade Federal Fluminense, Rio de Janeiro, Brazil
Leprosy

Allen Perkins, MD, MPH
Professor and Chairman, Department of Family Medicine, University of South Alabama College of Medicine, Mobile, Alabama
Marine Poisonings, Envenomations, and Trauma

Georg A. Petroianu, MD, PhD
Professor and Chair, Department of Cellular Biology and Pharmacology, Herbert Wertheim College of Medicine, Florida International University, Miami, Florida
Hiccups

Vesna Petronic-Rosic, MD, MSc
Associate Professor and Dermatopathology Fellowship Program Director, The University of Chicago Section of Dermatology, Chicago, Illinois
Melanoma

Michael E. Pichichero, MD
Director of Research, Department of Immunology and Center for Infectious Disease, Rochester General Hospital Research Institute, Rochester, New York
Whooping Cough (Pertussis)

Claus A. Pierach, MD
Professor of Medicine, University of Minnesota Medical School, Abbott Northwestern Hospital, Minneapolis, Minnesota
Porphyrias

Mark Pietroni, MD
Medical Director, International Centre for Diarrhoeal Disease Research, Bangladesh, Dhaka, Bangladesh
Cholera

Jose A. Plaza, MD
Associate Professor, Department of Pathology, Medical College of Wisconsin; Director of Dermatopathology, Department of Pathology, Froedtert and The Medical College, Milwaukee, Wisconsin
Erythema Multiforme; Stevens-Johnson Syndrome and Toxic Epidermal Necrolysis

Daniel K. Podolsky, MD
Professor of Internal Medicine, University of Texas Southwestern Medical School; Philip O'Bryan Montgomery Jr., MD, Distinguished Presidential Chair in Academic Administration and Doris and Bryan Wildenthal Distinguished Chair in Medical Science, University of Texas Southwestern Medical Center, Dallas, Texas
Inflammatory Bowel Disease: Crohn's Disease and Ulcerative Colitis

Susan M. Pollart, MD, MS
Associate Professor of Family Medicine, University of Virginia School of Medicine, Charlottesville, Virginia
Asthma in Children

Andrew S.T. Porter, DO
Clinical Assistant Professor and Program Director, University of Kansas School of Medicine–Wichita Sports Medicine Fellowship at Via Christi; Associate Director, University of Kansas School of Medicine–Wichita Family Medicine Residency at Via Christi, Wichita, Kansas
Common Sports Injuries

Michael A. Posencheg, MD
Medical Director, Intensive Care Nursery and Newborn Nursery; Associate Professor of Clinical Pediatrics, Division of Neonatology and Newborn Services, Hospital of the University of Pennsylvania, Philadelphia, Pennsylvania
Hemolytic Disease of the Fetus and Newborn

Charles R. Powell, MD
Assistant Professor of Urology, Indiana University School of Medicine, Indianapolis, Indiana
Prostatitis

Manuel Praga, MD
Associate Professor of Medicine, Universidad Complutense; Head, Nephrology Department, Hospital 12 de Octubre, Madrid, Spain
Primary Glomerular Diseases

Daniel S. Pratt, MD
Assistant Professor of Medicine, Harvard Medical School; Director, Liver-Biliary-Pancreas Center, Massachusetts General Hospital, Boston, Massachusetts
Acute and Chronic Viral Hepatitis

Peter S. Rahko, MD
Professor of Medicine, University of Wisconsin School of Medicine and Public Health; Director of Echocardiography, University of Wisconsin Hospitals and Clinics, Madison, Wisconsin
Mitral Valve Prolapse

S. Vincent Rajkumar, MD
Professor of Medicine, Mayo Clinic College of Medicine, Rochester, Minnesota
Multiple Myeloma

Julio A. Ramirez, MD
Professor of Medicine, University of Louisville School of Medicine; Chief, Division of Infectious Diseases, Department of Veterans Affairs Medical Center, Louisville, Kentucky
Legionellosis (Legionnaires' Disease and Pontiac Fever)

Didier Raoult, MD, PhD
Aix Marseille Université, URMITE UMR 7278, Faculté de Médecine, Marseille, France
Q Fever

Anita Devi K. Ravindran, MD
Senior Lecturer in Medical Microbiology and Parasitology, Faculty of Medicine, SEGi University, Kota Damansara, Petaling Jaya, Selangor, Malaysia
Foodborne Illnesses

Elizabeth Reddy, MD
Infectious Disease faculty, Medical Director of DAC Clinic, Upstate Medical University, Syracuse, New York
Intestinal Parasites

Ian R. Reid, MD
Distinguished Professor of Medicine and Endocrinology, University of Auckland Faculty of Medical and Health Sciences School of Medicine, Auckland, New Zealand
Paget's Disease of Bone

Robert L. Reid, MD
Professor, Department of Obstetrics and Gynecology, Queen's University Faculty of Health Sciences; Chair, Division of Reproductive Endocrinology and Infertility, Kingston General Hospital, Kingston, Ontario, Canada
Amenorrhea

John D. Reveille, MD
Professor of Internal Medicine and Director, Rheumatology and Clinical Immunogenetics, The University of Texas Medical School, Houston, Texas
Ankylosing Spondylitis

Leslie Rickey, MD, MPH
Assistant Professor, Division of Urology, University of Maryland School of Medicine, Baltimore, Maryland
Urinary Incontinence

Jason R. Roberts, MD
Assistant Professor, Division of Gastroenterology, Hepatology, and Nutrition, University of Louisville School of Medicine, Louisville, Kentucky
Gastroesophageal Reflux Disease (GERD)

Malcolm K. Robinson, MD
Assistant Professor of Surgery, Harvard Medical School; Metabolic Support Service, Department of Surgery, Brigham and Women's Hospital, Boston, Massachusetts
Parenteral Nutrition in Adults

Michelle A. Roett, MD, MPH
Associate Professor and Program Director, Georgetown University–Providence Hospital Family Medicine Residency Program, Fort Lincoln Family Medical Center, Colmar Manor, Maryland
Ovarian Cancer

Jonathan Rosand, MD, MSc
Professor of Neurology, Harvard Medical School; Director, Division of Neurocritical Care and Emergency Neurology, Massachusetts General Hospital, Boston, Massachusetts
Intracerebral Hemorrhage

Peter G. Rose, MD
Case Western Reserve University School of Medicine; Section Head, Gynecologic Oncology, Women's Health Institute, Cleveland Clinic, Cleveland, Ohio
Cancer of the Uterine Cervix

Richard N. Rosenthal, MD
Professor of Psychiatry, Icahn School of Medicine at Mount Sinai, Medical Director of Addiction Psychiatry, Mount Sinai Behavioral Health System, New York, New York
Alcoholism

Alan R. Roth, DO
Assistant Clinical Professor, Family and Social Medicine, Albert Einstein College of Medicine, Bronx, New York; Chairman, Department of Family Medicine, Director, Palliative Medicine Fellowship Program, Jamaica Hospital Medical Center, Jamaica, New York
Fever

Anne-Michelle Ruha, MD
Clinical Associate Professor, Department of Emergency Medicine, University of Arizona College of Medicine, Tucson, Arizona; Director, Medical Toxicology Fellowship, Department of Medical Toxicology, Banner Good Samaritan Medical Center, Phoenix, Arizona
Spider Bites and Scorpion Stings

Kristen Rundell, MS, MD
Program Director, Family Medicine Residency Program, Riverside Methodist Hospital, Columbus, Ohio
Mumps; Drug Hypersensitivity Reactions

Richard Sadovsky, MD
Associate Professor of Family Medicine, Department of Family Medicine, State University of New York–Downstate, Brooklyn, New York
Tinnitus

Susan L. Samson, MD, PhD
Assistant Professor, Department of Medicine, Baylor College of Medicine; Attending Physician, Ben Taub General Hospital; Medical Director, The Pituitary Center at Baylor Clinic and St. Luke's Evangelical Hospital, Houston, Texas
Hyponatremia

Timothy Sanborn, MD
Clinical Professor of Cardiology, Department of Medicine, NorthShore University HealthSystem, Evanston, Illinois
Acute Myocardial Infarction

Sandeep Sangodkar, DO
Fellow, Cardiovascular Disease, University of New Mexico, Albuquerque, New Mexico
Hypertrophic Cardiomyopathy

Ravi Sarode, MD
Professor of Pathology, University of Texas Southwestern Medical School, Dallas, Texas
Thrombotic Thrombocytopenic Purpura

J. Terry Saunders, PhD
Assistant Professor of Medical Education in Internal Medicine, University of Virginia School of Medicine, Charlottesville, Virginia
Diabetes Mellitus in Adults

Ralph M. Schapira, MD
Professor and Vice Chair, Department of Medicine, Medical College of Wisconsin; Staff Physician, Milwaukee Veterans Affairs Medical Center, Milwaukee, Wisconsin
Acute Bronchitis

Michael Schatz, MD, MS
Clinical Professor, Department of Medicine, University of California–San Diego, School of Medicine, La Jolla, California; Departments of Allergy and Research and Evaluation, Kaiser Permanente, San Diego, California
Asthma in Adolescents and Adults

Rebecca B. Schechter, MD
Endocrinologist, Highland Park, Illinois
Thyroid Cancer

Stacey A. Scheib, MD
Resident Physician, Department of Obstetrics and Gynecology, Thomas Jefferson University Hospital, Philadelphia, Pennsylvania
Menopause

Lawrence R. Schiller, MD
Professor of Internal Medicine, Texas A&M University College of Medicine, Dallas Campus; Attending Physician, Digestive Health Associates of Texas; Program Director, Gastroenterology Fellowship, Baylor University Medical Center, Dallas, Texas
Malabsorption

Janet A. Schlechte, MD
Professor, Department of Internal Medicine, University of Iowa Hospital, Iowa City, Iowa
Hyperprolactinemia

Kim Schoessow, OTD, OTR/L
Assistant Professor of Occupational Therapy, MGH Institute of Health Professions, Boston, Massachusetts
Vision Rehabilitation

Kerrie Schoffer, MD
Assistant Professor in Neurology, Dalhousie University Faculty of Medicine; Neurologist, QEII Health Sciences Centre, Halifax, Nova Scotia, Canada
Peripheral Neuropathies

Jan Schovanek, MD
Program in Reproductive and Adult Endocrinology, Eunice Kennedy Shriver National Institute of Child Health and Human Development, National Institutes of Health, Bethesda, Maryland; Department of Internal Medicine III – Nephrology, Rheumatology and Endocrinology, Faculty of Medicine and Dentistry, Palacky University, Olomouc, Czech Republic
Pheochromocytoma

Sarina Schrager, MD, MS
Professor of Family Medicine, University of Wisconsin, Madison, Wisconsin
Abnormal Uterine Bleeding

Kevin Schroeder, MD
Program Director, Transitional Year; Medical Director of Acute Dialysis, Riverside Methodist Hospital, Columbus, Ohio
Acute Renal Failure

Dan Schuller, MD
Professor of Medicine, Texas A&M Health Science Center; Chief of Medical Critical Care, Director of Pulmonary and Critical Care Fellowship Program, Baylor University Medical Center, Dallas, Texas
Primary Lung Abscess

Amy Seery, MD
Assistant Professor, Department of Family and Community Medicine, University of Kansas School of Medicine–Wichita; Pediatrics Faculty, Via Christi Family Medicine Residency, Wichita, Kansas
Normal Infant Feeding

Steven A. Seifert, MD
Professor, University of New Mexico School of Medicine; Medical Director, New Mexico Poison Center, Albuquerque, New Mexico
Venomous Snakebite

Jeffery D. Semel, MD
Assistant Clinical Professor of Medicine, Pritzker School of Medicine, University of Chicago; Chief, Section of Infectious Diseases, NorthShore University HealthSystem, Chicago, Illinois
Pseudomembranous Colitis

Edward Septimus, MD
Medical Director, Infection Prevention and Epidemiology, Clinical Services Group, HCA, Nashville, Tennessee; Clinical Professor, Internal Medicine, Texas A&M Health Science Center College of Medicine, Bryan, Texas
Bacterial Pneumonia

Beejal Shah, MD
Endocrinology Fellowship Director, Department of Endocrinology, Banner Good Samaritan-Phoenix Veterans Administration Health Care System, Phoenix, Arizona
Hyponatremia

Samir S. Shah, MD
Director, Division of Hospital Medicine; Attending Physician, Hospital Medicine and Infectious Diseases, Cincinnati Children's Hospital Medical Center; Professor, Department of Pediatrics, University of Cincinnati College of Medicine, Cincinnati, Ohio
Viral Meningitis

Jamile M. Shammo, MD
Associate Professor of Medicine and Pathology, Division of Hematology/Oncology, Rush University Medical Center, Chicago, Illinois
Myelodysplastic Syndromes

Amir Sharafkhaneh, MD, PhD
Professor of Medicine, Section of Pulmonary, Critical Care, and Sleep Medicine; Director, Sleep Fellowship Program, Baylor College of Medicine, Houston, Texas
Chronic Obstructive Pulmonary Disease

Ala I. Sharara, MD
Professor of Medicine and Head, Division of Gastroenterology, American University of Beirut Medical Center, Beirut, Lebanon; Consulting Professor, Duke University Medical Center, Durham, North Carolina
Bleeding Esophageal Varices

Dan-Arin Silasi, MD
Associate Professor, Gynecologic Oncology, Yale University School of Medicine, New Haven, Connecticut
Cancer of the Endometrium

Lindsay R. Simon, MD
Doctor of Medicine, Office of the Chief Medical Examiner, New York, New York
Reference Intervals for the Interpretation of Laboratory Tests

Aaron Sinclair, MD
Assistant Professor, Department of Family and Community Medicine, University of Kansas School of Medicine–Wichita; Associate Director, Wesley Family Medicine Residency, Wichita, Kansas
Diverticula of the Alimentary Tract

Philip D. Sloane, MD, MPH
Elizabeth and Oscar Goodwin Distinguished Professor, Department of Family Medicine; Co-Director, Program on Aging, Disability, and Long-Term Care, Cecil G. Sheps Center for Health Services Research; University of North Carolina at Chapel Hill, Chapel Hill, North Carolina
Alzheimer's Disease

Zachary L. Smith, DO
Fellow, Division of Gastroenterology and Hepatology, Medical College of Wisconsin Milwaukee, Milwaukee, Wisconsin
Calculous Biliary Disease

Linda Speer, MD
Professor and Chair, Department of Family Medicine, University of Toledo College of Medicine, Toledo, Ohio
Dysmenorrhea

Abby L. Spencer, MD, MS
Vice Chairman of Education, Medicine Institute, Cleveland Clinic, Cleveland, Ohio
Contraception

Erik K. St. Louis, MD
Consultant and Head, Section of Sleep Neurology, Center for Sleep Medicine, Departments of Neurology and Medicine, Mayo Clinic and Foundation; Associate Professor of Neurology, Mayo Clinic College of Medicine; Associate Dean for Maintenance of Certification, Mayo School of Continuous Professional Development, Rochester, Minnesota
Sleep Disorders

Todd Stephens, MD
Clinical Assistant Professor, Department of Family and Community Medicine, University of Kansas School of Medicine–Wichita; Associate Program Director, Via Christi Family Medicine Residency, Wichita, Kansas
Genital Ulcer Disease: Chancroid, Granuloma Inguinale, and Lymphogranuloma

Dennis L. Stevens, MD, PhD
Professor of Medicine, University of Washington School of Medicine, Seattle, Washington; Chief, Infectious Diseases, Veterans Affairs Medical Center, Boise, Idaho
Bacterial Diseases of the Skin

Douglas F. Stickle, PhD
Professor, Department of Pathology, Jefferson Medical College; Director of Chemistry, Department of Pathology, Thomas Jefferson University Hospital, Philadelphia, Pennsylvania
Reference Intervals for the Interpretation of Laboratory Tests

Brenda Stokes, MD
Medical Staff, Central Health–Lynchburg General and Virginia Baptist Hospitals, Lynchburg, Virginia
Hypertensive Disorders of Pregnancy

Constantine A. Stratakis, MD, PhD
Program Head, Developmental Endocrinology and Genetics; Director, Pediatric Endocrinology Training Program, National Institutes of Health, Bethesda, Maryland
Cushing's Syndrome

Harris Strokoff, MD
Child and Adolescent Psychiatrist, Northwestern Counseling and Support Services, Saint Albans, Vermont
Attention-Deficit/Hyperactivity Disorder

Prabhakar P. Swaroop, MD
Assistant Professor of Internal Medicine, University of Texas Southwestern Medical Center at Dallas, Dallas, Texas
Inflammatory Bowel Disease: Crohn's Disease and Ulcerative Colitis

Masayoshi Takashima, MD
Director, The Sinus Center; Director, Sleep Medicine Fellowship–OTO Section; Associate Professor, Bobby R. Alford Department of Otolaryngology–Head and Neck Surgery, Baylor College of Medicine, Houston, Texas
Obstructive Sleep Apnea

Jie Tang, MD
Assistant Professor of Nephrology, University of Colorado School of Medicine, Denver, Colorado
Hypokalemia and Hyperkalemia

Janice C. Te, MD
Infectious Disease Fellow, The University of Oklahoma Health Sciences Center, Oklahoma City, Oklahoma
Plague

Joyce M.C. Teng, MD, PhD
Assistant Professor of Dermatology and Pediatrics, Stanford University School of Medicine, Lucile Packard Children's Hospital at Stanford, Stanford, California
Urticaria and Angioedema

Nathan Thielman, MD, MPH
Duke Global Health Institute, Duke University, Durham, North Carolina
Intestinal Parasites

David R. Thomas, MD
Professor Emeritus of Medicine, Division of Geriatric Medicine, Saint Louis University School of Medicine; Medical Director, Program for All-Inclusive Care of the Elderly, St. Louis, Missouri
Pressure Ulcers

Joanna Thomson, MD
Assistant Professor, Department of Pediatrics, University of Cincinnati College of Medicine; Attending Physician, Hospital Medicine, Cincinnati Children's Hospital Medical Center, Cincinnati, Ohio
Viral Meningitis

J. Brantley Thrasher, MD
Professor and the William L. Valk Chair, Department of Urology, Co-Director of Operative Services, University of Kansas Medical Center, Kansas City, Kansas
Hematuria

Kenneth Tobin, DO
Clinical Assistant Professor and Director, Chest Pain Center, University of Michigan Medical Center, Department of Internal Medicine, Division of Cardiovascular Disease
Angina Pectoris

Debra Tristram, MD
Professor, Department of Pediatrics, Albany Medical College, Albany, New York
Necrotizing Skin and Soft Tissue Infections

Arvid E. Underman, MD
Clinical Professor of Medicine and Microbiology, Keck School of Medicine of the University of Southern California, Los Angeles, California; Director of Graduate Medical Education, Huntington Hospital, Pasadena, California
Salmonellosis

George Van Buren, II, MD
Assistant Professor of Surgery, Division of Surgical Oncology, Michael E. DeBakey Department of Surgery, Baylor College of Medicine, Houston, Texas
Acute and Chronic Pancreatitis

David van Duin, MD, PhD
Associate Professor of Medicine, University of North Carolina, Chapel Hill, North Carolina
Histoplasmosis

Daniel J. Van Durme, MD, MPH
Professor and Chair, Department of Family Medicine and Rural Health; Director, Center on Global Health, Florida State University College of Medicine, Tallahassee, Florida
Acne Vulgaris; Rosacea

Brenda R. Velasco, MD
Allied GI Associates, Haddon Heights, New Jersey
Irritable Bowel Syndrome

Kyle Vincent, MD
Clinical Assistant Professor, Department of Surgery, University of Kansas School of Medicine–Wichita, Wichita, Kansas
Gastritis and Peptic Ulcer Disease

Donald C. Vinh, MD
Assistant Professor, Clinician-Scientist, Divisions of Infectious Disease and Allergy and Clinical Immunology, Departments of Medicine, Medical Microbiology, and Human Genetics, McGill University Health Centre–Montreal General Hospital, Montreal, Quebec, Canada
Blastomycosis

K.N. Viswanathan, MD
Senior Professor of Internal Medicine, Consultant in Internal and Tropical Medicine, Shri Sathya Sai Medical College and Research Institute (a unit of Sri Balaji Vidyapeeth University), Tamil Nadu, India
Foodborne Illnesses

Todd W. Vitaz, MD
Assistant Professor, Department of Neurological Surgery, University of Louisville School of Medicine; Director of Neurosurgical Oncology and Co-Director, Neurosciences ICU, Norton Hospital, Louisville, Kentucky
Head Injuries

Jatin M. Vyas, MD, PhD
Assistant Professor of Medicine, Harvard Medical School; Division of Infectious Diseases, Department of Medicine, Massachusetts General Hospital, Boston, Massachusetts
Rat-Bite Fever

Heather Wadams, MD, MHA
Department of Pediatrics, Mayo Clinic, Rochester, Minnesota
Obesity

Rahul Wadke, MD
Department of Internal Medicine, University of Chicago Northshore University HealthSystem, Evanston, Illinois
Atrial Fibrillation

Thomas W. Wakefield, MD
Stanley Professor of Surgery; Head, Section of Vascular Surgery, Department of Surgery; Director, Samuel and Jean Frankel Cardiovascular Center, University of Michigan, Ann Arbor, Michigan
Venous Thrombosis

Ellen R. Wald, MD
Professor and Chair, Department of Pediatrics, University of Wisconsin School of Medicine and Public Health; Pediatrician-in-Chief, American Family Children's Hospital, Madison, Wisconsin
Urinary Tract Infections in Infants and Children

Robin A. Walker, MD
Assistant Professor, Department of Family and Community Medicine, University of Kansas School of Medicine–Wichita; Associate Director, Wesley Family Medicine Residency Program, Wichita, Kansas
Epididymitis

Barry M. Wall, MD
Professor of Medicine, Division of Nephrology, Department of Medicine, University of Tennessee Health Science Center, Memphis, Tennessee
Diabetic Ketoacidosis

Stephen Waller, MD
Associate Professor of Infectious Diseases, University of Kansas Medical Center, Kansas City, Kansas
Rickettsial and Ehrlichial Infections (Rocky Mountain Spotted Fever and Typhus)

Anne Walling, MB, ChB
Professor, Department of Family and Community Medicine, University of Kansas School of Medicine–Wichita, Wichita, Kansas
Migraine Headache

Andrew Wang, MD
Professor of Medicine/Cardiology, Duke University Medical Center, Durham, North Carolina
Infective Endocarditis

Ernest Wang, MD
Associate Professor of Emergency Medicine, Evanston Hospital, NorthShore University HealthSystem, Evanston, Illinois
Disturbances Due to Cold

Ruth Weber, MD, MSEd
Clinical Associate Professor, Department of Family and Community Medicine, University of Kansas School of Medicine–Wichita; Associate Director, Wesley Family Medicine Residency, Wichita, Kansas
Pharyngitis

Cheryl Wehler, MD
Assistant Professor, Department of Psychiatry and Behavioral Sciences, University of Kansas School of Medicine–Wichita, Wichita, Kansas
Panic Disorder

David N. Weissman, MD
Adjunct Professor of Medicine and Microbiology (Immunology), West Virginia University School of Medicine; Director, Division of Respiratory Disease Studies, National Institute for Occupational Safety and Health, Morgantown, West Virginia
Pneumoconiosis: Asbestosis and Silicosis

Robert C. Welliver, Sr., MD
Professor of Pediatrics, CMRI Hobbs-Recknagel Endowed Chair in Pediatrics and Chief, Section on Infectious Diseases, Department of Pediatrics, University of Oklahoma Health Sciences Center, Oklahoma City, Oklahoma
Viral Respiratory Infections

Ryan Westergaard, MD, MPH
Assistant Professor of Medicine, University of Wisconsin-Madison, Madison, Wisconsin
HIV Disease

Meir Wetzler, MD
Professor of Medicine and Chief of Leukemia Section, Roswell Park Cancer Institute, Buffalo, New York
Acute Leukemia in Adults

Tracy L. Williams, MD
Assistant Professor, Department of Family and Community Medicine, University of Kansas School of Medicine–Wichita; Associate Program Director, Via Christi Family Medicine Residency, Wichita, Kansas
Chlamydia trachomatis

Nicholas Wilson, MD
Fellow in Gastroenterology, Temple University School of Medicine, Philadelphia, Pennsylvania
Irritable Bowel Syndrome

Elaine Winkel, MD
Associate Professor of Medicine, University of Wisconsin School of Medicine and Public Health; Attending Cardiologist, Heart Failure and Transplant Program, University of Wisconsin Hospital and Clinics, Madison, Wisconsin
Congestive Heart Failure

Jennifer Wipperman, MD, MPH
Assistant Professor, Department of Family and Community Medicine, University of Kansas School of Medicine-Wichita; Associate Program Director, Via Christi Family Medicine Residency, Wichita, Kansas
Dizziness and Vertigo

Gary S. Wood, MD
Professor and Chair, Department of Dermatology, University of Wisconsin School of Medicine and Public Health; Attending Physician, Veterans Affairs Medical Center, Madison, Wisconsin
Cutaneous T-Cell Lymphomas, Including Mycosis Fungoides and Sézary Syndrome

Jamie R.S. Wood, MD
Instructor in Pediatrics, Harvard Medical School; Research Associate, Sections on Genetics and Epidemiology and Vascular Cell Biology; Staff Physician, Pediatric, Adolescent, and Young Adult Section, Joslin Diabetes Center, Boston, Massachusetts
Diabetes Mellitus in Children

William F. Wright, DO
Assistant Professor, Medicine and Microbiology, Division of Infectious Diseases and Travel Medicine, Georgetown University School of Medicine, Washington, District of Columbia
Lyme Disease

Steve W. Wu, MD
Assistant Professor, University of Cincinnati College of Medicine; Assistant Professor, Cincinnati Children's Hospital Medical Center, Cincinnati, Ohio
Gilles de la Tourette Syndrome

Xinghong Yang, PhD
College of Veterinary Medicine, Infectious Diseases and Pathology, Gainesville, Florida
Brucellosis

Elizabeth Yeu, MD
Virginia Eye Consultants, Norfolk, Virginia
Vision Correction Procedures

James A. Yiannias, MD
Associate Professor, Department of Dermatology; Associate Medical Director, Center for Innovation; Medical Director, Connected Care, Mayo Clinic Scottsdale, Scottsdale, Arizona
Contact Dermatitis

Wei Zhou, MD
Professor of Surgery, Stanford University School of Medicine, Stanford, California
Peripheral Arterial Disease

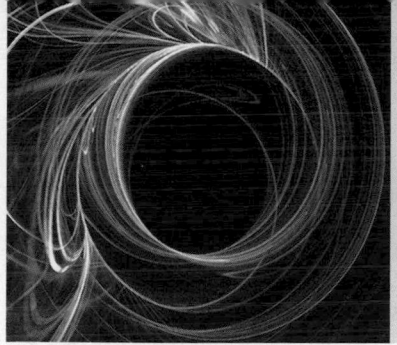

Preface

This is the sixty-eighth edition of *Conn's Current Therapy*. Much has changed in medicine and in the publishing industry since the first edition of Howard Conn's classic textbook. What has not changed is our dedication to providing current and easily accessible information to busy clinicians.

Conn's Current Therapy remains a bestselling source of pragmatic medical information available in print and electronic format. Each chapter is written by an expert who provides evidence-based content along with their own suggestions for moving evidence into practice.

We were pleased with the results of a recent survey of *Conn's Current Therapy* readers. A wide variety of health care professionals purchase *Conn's Current Therapy*. Half are practicing physicians and one fourth are academic physicians, residents and fellows. The remainder are from a wide variety of health professions, including physician assistants, nurse practitioners, allied health professionals, and laboratory directors. Many medical students have access to the book because their school library has purchased Clinical Key (www.clinicalkey.com), an online search engine that allows access to a wide variety of Elsevier medical publications, including *Conn's Current Therapy*.

About 60 percent of physicians who purchase *Conn's Current Therapy* are family physicians and internists. The remaining 40 percent are from the other specialties. In fact, the variety of physician specialists who use the book is remarkable. Subspecialists oftentimes use the book as a quick reference on topics outside their specialty area, a handy tool because so many patients have multiple co-morbid conditions. Some use the book to refresh their knowledge of both common and unusual conditions. Others use the book to review recent advances in clinical medicine and to review for maintenance of certification examinations.

We were pleased to learn that the Current Diagnosis and Current Therapy boxes were particularly popular. These boxes include clinical pearls of information on each topic. Readers can easily extract the most critical information for diagnosing and treating a particular condition. Similarly, information on differential diagnosis, medication dosages, laboratory evaluation, and ongoing monitoring was found to be useful and accessible.

Many of our readers are now accessing *Conn's Current Therapy* electronically. Those who purchase a hard copy of *Conn's Current Therapy* receive access to the enhanced Expert Consult eBook version of the book, which is downloadable to two devices of the reader's choice, such as a smart phone or tablet. Once downloaded, internet access is not necessary and you can take the book with you wherever you go. The eBook allows the reader to search all of the text, figures, and references from the book. We wonder what Howard Conn would have thought of the digital version of his book, which was first published in a loose-leaf format.

A rewarding aspect of editing *Conn's Current Therapy* is the opportunity to review information that is updated and topics that are added as medical knowledge evolves. This year is no different.

The 2016 edition has new chapters on Ebola, Chikungunya, dry eye, and adolescent health. Many chapters have had major revisions as new medical treatment guidelines have been released. We will continue to add other new pertinent topics in future editions.

We enjoy working with the talented authors of each edition. Each author works hard to write chapters that are accurate, up to date, and easily understood. Although we rotate authors on a regular basis to keep content fresh, some have been with us for several years as they do a particularly outstanding job on the chapters in their particular specialty area. Indeed, each chapter is an "expert consult." We also use international authors who add considerable expertise and bring important new perspectives to healthcare. We select new authors based on the recommendation of past authors, an individual's prominence in the medical literature, or their recognized clinical excellence. We also give designated up-and-coming clinical experts an opportunity to show us the way into the future of medical care.

Miriam Chan, PharmD, reviews each and every mention of a drug in the book. She checks drug indications, dosages, and formulations to be sure all are accurate and safe. The book uses both generic drug names and trade names that are familiar to the clinician. Footnotes are added when a drug has not been FDA approved for an indication or an author has suggested a drug dosage outside the usual FDA-approved range.

Senior Content Development Specialist Joan Ryan organizes and manages the manuscript submission process. She keeps us all on task. Joan helps us identify many of the new authors and communicates regularly with the existing authors about their chapters. We communicate almost daily with Joan, which is a pleasure due to her New Englander sense of humor. Her work to get the book ready for publication each year is critical.

The copy editors are outstanding and we appreciate their expertise. We sincerely thank them for their contribution to the process.

Ted Rodgers is the Project Manager and gets the book ready for final publication. This is Ted's second year with us and we appreciate his efforts to get everything in final order.

Suzanne Toppy is the Senior Content Strategist and we have appreciated her help as we try to keep *Conn's Current Therapy* accessible to both experienced and young clinician audiences. Suzanne has helped us envision how we can retain the historical value of *Conn's Current Therapy* and how health professionals will access information in the future.

Finally, we want to thank our practice partners, friends and family for their support and patience while we devote time to making *Conn's Current Therapy* a practical, useful, and clinically valuable "go-to" book.

Edward T. Bope, MD
Rick D. Kellerman, MD

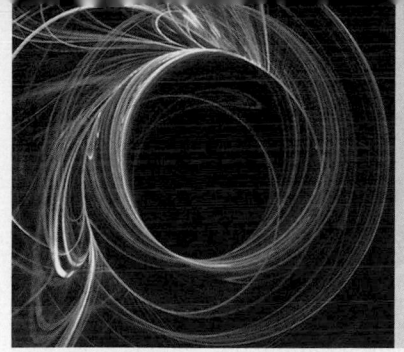

Contents

SECTION 4
Diseases of the Skin

SECTION 7
The Cardiovascular System

SECTION 8
The Digestive System

SECTION 9
Rheumatology and the Musculoskeletal System

Contents

SECTION 10
The Nervous System

SECTION 11
Endocrine and Metabolic Disorders

SECTION 16
Men's Health

SECTION 17
Women's Health

SECTION 18
Pregnancy and Antepartum Care

SECTION 19
Children's Health

Conn's Current Therapy 2016 uses a
standardized system of footnotes:

1. Not FDA approved for this indication.
2. Not available in the United States.
3. Exceeds dosage recommended by the manufacturer.
4. Not yet approved for use in the United States.
5. Investigational drug in the United States.
6. May be compounded by pharmacists.
7. Available as dietary supplement.
8. Orphan drug in the United States.
9. Available as homeopathic remedy.
10. Available in the United States from the Centers for Disease
Control and Prevention.

Contents

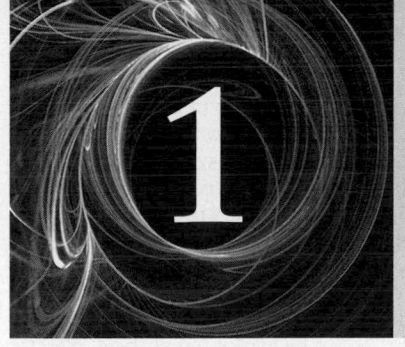

1

Symptomatic Care Pending Diagnosis

CHEST PAIN

Method of
William E. Cayley, Jr., MD, MDiv

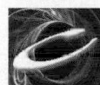

CURRENT DIAGNOSIS

- Initial evaluation of chest pain should include evaluation of clinical stability, a concise history and physical, and a chest x-ray and electrocardiogram (ECG) unless the cause is clearly not life-threatening.
- Chest pain described as exertional, radiating to one or both arms, similar to or worse than prior cardiac chest pain, or associated with nausea, vomiting, or diaphoresis indicates high risk for acute coronary syndrome. ECG identifies ST elevation myocardial infarction (STEMI), and cardiac biomarkers are essential for further evaluation of suspected chest pain in the absence of STEMI.
- The Wells, Geneva, and Pisa clinical prediction rules can help stratify a patient's risk of pulmonary embolism.
- Aortic dissection is an uncommon cause of chest pain, but patients with abrupt or instantaneous chest pain that is ripping, tearing, or stabbing should have evaluation for dissection with chest x-ray, computed tomography (CT), or magnetic resonance imaging.
- Esophageal rupture may be suspected in patients with pain, dyspnea, and shock following a forceful emesis, and prompt imaging with (CT) or esophagram is essential.
- Patients who have suspected tension pneumothorax and who are clinically stable should have a chest x-ray for confirmation before needle decompression is attempted.

CURRENT THERAPY

- Patients with STEMI require urgent reperfusion, and those with unstable angina or non–ST elevation myocardial infarction require admission for further monitoring and evaluation.
- Most patients with pulmonary embolism require admission for monitoring and anticoagulation, although outpatient treatment may be possible for low-risk patients after initial evaluation and anticoagulation.
- Prompt surgical consultation is required for patients with confirmed or suspected aortic dissection or esophageal rupture.
- Clinically unstable patients with suspected tension pneumothorax need immediate needle decompression.

Epidemiology

Chest pain is the chief complaint in 1% to 2% of all outpatient primary care visits. More than 50% of emergency department (ED) visits for chest pain are due to serious cardiovascular conditions such as acute coronary syndrome (ACS) or pulmonary embolism (PE), but these account for less than 15% of outpatient primary care encounters for chest pain, and up to 15% of chest pain episodes never reach a definitive diagnosis. Other potentially life-threatening etiologies for chest pain include PE, dissecting aortic aneurysm (AA), esophageal rupture, and tension pneumothorax. In outpatient primary care the most common causes of chest pain are musculoskeletal, gastrointestinal, angina due to stable coronary artery disease (CAD), anxiety or other psychiatric conditions, and pulmonary disease.

Initial Assessment

In initial evaluation of chest pain, it is important to obtain a clear history of the onset and evolution of chest pain, especially details such as location, quality, duration, and aggravating or alleviating factors. Initial physical examination should include vital signs, assessment of the patient's overall general condition, and examination of the heart and lungs. If there are any clinical signs of instability (altered mental status, hypotension, marked dyspnea, or other signs of shock) then initial stabilization and diagnosis must both be addressed simultaneously, consistent with current guidelines for emergency cardiovascular care. Unless the history and physical examination suggest an obviously nonthreatening cause of chest discomfort, most adults with chest pain should at least have basic diagnostic testing with an ECG and a chest x-ray. Several clinical prediction rules are available to help confirm or exclude some common causes of chest pain (Box 1).

Diagnosis and Treatment

Acute Coronary Syndrome

ACS includes acute myocardial infarction (MI) (ST-segment elevation and depression, Q wave and non–Q wave) or unstable angina. A review of prospective and retrospective studies correlating specific chest pain characteristics with the likelihood of ACS found that components of the patient history that increase the likelihood of ACS include radiation of pain to the right arm or shoulder, to both arms or shoulders, or to the left arm; or pain associated with exertion, diaphoresis, nausea, or vomiting; or pain described as pressure or as "worse than previous angina or similar to a previous MI." Similarly, components of the history that predicted decreased likelihood of ACS were pleuritic, positional, or sharp chest pain; pain in an inframammary location; or pain not associated with exertion. A physical examination finding of chest pain reproducibility with palpation also decreased the likelihood of ACS. Additional physical examination findings that may be helpful are the presence of hypotension or an S_3 on cardiac auscultation, both of which suggest increased likelihood of ACS. The Marburg Heart Score can help exclude CAD in primary care patients with chest pain - most patients with a score of 2 or less will not have CAD (Table 1). Recent studies have demonstrated that the presence or absence of typical cardiac risk factors (eg, diabetes, hypertension, smoking, high cholesterol, or family history) have little diagnostic value for determining the likelihood of ACS in patients over 40.

An ECG should be obtained promptly for any patient with suspected ACS. ST-segment elevation in two or more contiguous leads, or presumed new left bundle branch block, is diagnostic

TABLE 1 | Marburg Heart Score

FINDING	POINTS
Woman >64 years, man >54 years	1
Known CAD, cerebrovascular disease, or peripheral vascular disease	1
Pain worse with exercise	1
Pain not reproducible with palpation	1
Patient assumes pain is cardiac	1

Abbreviation: CAD = coronary artery disease.

Approximately 97% of patients with a MHS score of 2 or less will not have CAD. Approximately 23% of patients with a MHS score of 3 or more will have CAD.

Adapted from: Haasenritter J, Bösner S, Vaucher P, Herzig L, Heinzel-Gutenbrunner M, Baum E, Donner-Banzhoff N. Ruling out coronary heart disease in primary care: external validation of a clinical prediction rule. Br J Gen Pract. 2012 Jun;62(599):e415-21. doi: 10.3399/bjgp12X649106. http://www.ncbi.nlm.nih.gov/pmc/articles/PMC3361121/.

of ST-segment elevation MI (STEMI) and requires urgent revascularization with thrombolysis or angioplasty at an appropriate facility. Ischemic ST-segment depression more than 0.5 mm, dynamic T-wave inversion with chest discomfort, or transient ST-segment elevation of 0.5 mm or more are classified as unstable angina or non-ST-elevation MI (NSTEMI). However, none of these findings is sensitive enough that its absence can exclude MI, and patients whose chest pain is not low risk still require further assessment for ACS.

In patients with high-risk chest pain who do not have STEMI, elevated cardiac biomarkers distinguish NSTEMI from unstable angina. Cardiac troponins T and I are more sensitive for detecting NSTEMI than creatine kinase (CK) or the MB isoform (CK-MB).

Initial management of NSTEMI includes hospital admission for antiplatelet, antithrombin, and antianginal therapy. Patients with unstable angina should also be hospitalized for observation, and patients with either NSTEMI or unstable angina require risk stratification using the TIMI or GRACE risk scores (see Box 1). Patients with chest pain suspicious for CAD, but no definite initial diagnosis of STEMI or NSTEMI on initial presentation are often admitted to hospital for overnight observation and serial cardiac biomarker measurements at 6 and 12 hours after symptom onset to "rule out MI." However the ADAPT trial demonstrated a 2-hour accelerated protocol may allow for early discharge of low-risk patients. Specifically, for patients with a TIMI score of 0 and no new ischemic changes on ECG, normal values for all biomarkers at presentation and at 2 hours after arrival have a negative predictive value (NPV) 99.1% for major cardiac events.

Patients at low risk for ACS or MI can usually defer further testing unless there are other risk factors in their family or past medical history markedly increasing the likelihood of CAD. Current recommendations are that all other patients with chest pain suggesting CAD should have further non-invasive testing within 7 days, however a recent study of 4181 patients in an ED chest pain unit found that a reasonable alternative may be to test troponin levels twice over a 6 hour interval, with no stress testing done if both values are normal. Patients who can exercise and who have no left-bundle branch block, preexcitation, or significant resting ST depression on a resting ECG can be evaluated with an exercise stress ECG, and the Duke treadmill score can then be used to further quantify cardiac risk (see Box 1). Patients with baseline ECG abnormalities should have perfusion imaging performed along with a stress ECG, and patients who cannot exercise may be evaluated with a pharmacologic stress or vasodilator test (e.g., dobutamine [Dobutrex][1] or adenosine [Adenocard]). Patients at high risk for CAD or those with NSTEMI should generally proceed directly to angiography, which allows definitive assessment of coronary artery anatomy.

Pulmonary Embolism

There are no individual symptoms or physical examination findings that reliably diagnose or exclude pulmonary embolism (PE), but three clinical prediction rules have all been validated for use in determining likelihood of PE and therefore whether or not further testing is needed. The Wells prediction rule (Table 2) is based on the simplest combination of history and examination findings. The Geneva rule requires blood gas and chest x-ray findings. The Pisa rule is the most mathematically complicated and depends on clinical, ECG, and x-ray findings. The Wells rule has been the most widely studied, but a comparison of all three found the Pisa rule may be the most accurate for clinical diagnosis and for excluding PE. With the Wells and Geneva prediction rules, the likelihood of PE is approximately 10% in the low-probability category, 30% in the moderate-probability category, and 65% in the high-probability category. Routine tests done for patients with chest pain are not particularly helpful in diagnosing or excluding PE. The chest x-ray may be abnormal, but findings that typically occur with PE (atelectasis, effusion, or elevation of a hemidiaphragm) are nonspecific. ECG signs of right ventricular strain may be helpful if present, but their absence does not exclude PE. Hypoxia may be present, but up to 20% of patients with PE have a normal alveolar-arterial oxygen gradient.

Additional tests recommended for evaluating patients with suspected PE include D-dimer testing by enzyme-linked

---

[1]Not FDA approved for this indication.

TABLE 2 | Simplified Wells Scoring System for Pulmonary Embolism

CLINICAL FINDING	SCORE
Symptoms of deep vein thrombosis (DVT)	3.0
No alternative diagnosis more likely than PE	3.0
Heart rate >100 bpm	1.5
Immobilization greater than 3 days or surgery in past 4 weeks	1.5
Previous objectively diagnosed DVT or PE	1.5
Hemoptysis	1.0
Malignancy	1.0
Probability of PE: <2 points = low, 2–6 points = moderate, >6 points = high.	

Abbreviations: DVT = deep vein thrombosis; PE = pulmonary embolism.

Adapted from Miniati M, Bottai M, Monti S. Comparison of 3 clinical models for predicting the probability of pulmonary embolism. Medicine (Baltimore) 2005;84:107–114; Torbicki A, Perrier A, Konstantinides S, et al, ESC Committee for Practice Guidelines (CPG): Guidelines on the diagnosis and management of acute pulmonary embolism. Eur Heart J 2008;29:2276–315. http://eurheartj.oxfordjournals.org/content/29/18/2276.long.

immunosorbent assay (ELISA; sensitivity, >95%; specificity, approximately 40%) or latex agglutination (sensitivity, 85%–90%), compression ultrasonography, ventilation–perfusion scintigraphy, or computed tomography (CT) angiography. Patients with suspected high-risk PE (i.e., those with shock or hypotension) should have immediate CT angiography and treatment for PE if the CT is positive, though an echocardiographic finding of right ventricular overload may be used to justify treatment for PE in the unstable patient with high clinical suspicion for PE when CT angiography is not available. Patients who have suspected PE and who are not high risk (i.e., no shock or hypotension) and who have a high clinical probability (based on Wells, Geneva, or Pisa scoring) should also proceed directly to CT, with appropriate treatment if the scan is positive. Patients with low or intermediate clinical probability should initially have D-dimer testing; further testing or treatment for PE is unnecessary if the D-dimer is negative, and CT angiography should be performed if the D-dimer is positive.

Anticoagulation, with thrombolysis in high-risk patients, is the foundation of treatment for PE. Patients with shock or hypotension are high risk and require hemodynamic and respiratory support, thrombolysis or embolectomy, and then appropriate attention to anticoagulation. Normotensive patients with echocardiographic evidence of right ventricular dysfunction or serologic evidence of myocardial injury (elevated troponins or CK-MB) have intermediate risk and should be admitted for anticoagulation. Normotensive patients who have normal results on echocardiography and testing for myocardial injury are at low risk and often may be discharged early for management at home after initiation of anticoagulation. Anticoagulation for PE should be started at the time of diagnosis with unfractionated heparin, low-molecular-weight heparin, or fondaparinux (Arixtra) and continued for at least 5 days, with simultaneous initiation of oral anticoagulation with warfarin (Coumadin), titrated to maintain an international normalized ratio (INR) between 2.0 and 3.0. The newer anticoagulants dabigatran, rivaroxaban, or apixaban may be an option for patients who have difficulty maintaining steady anticoagulation with warfarin.

Aortic Dissection

Thoracic aortic dissection is a much less common cause of chest pain; prevalence estimates are 2 to 3.5 cases per 100,000 person-years. Up to 40% of patients die immediately, and 5% to 20% die during or shortly after surgery. Risk factors for acute thoracic aortic dissection include hypertension, presence of a pheochromocytoma, cocaine use, weight lifting, trauma or a rapid deceleration event, coarctation of the aorta, and certain genetic abnormalities. Pain due to acute aortic dissection is perceived as abrupt and severe in 84% to 90% of cases, and more than 50% of patients describe the pain as sharp or stabbing. No physical findings are sensitive or specific for detecting aortic dissection, because approximately equal percentages of patients are hypertensive, normotensive, or have hypotension or shock, and the most common physical findings (a murmur of aortic insufficiency or a pulse deficit) occur in less than half of patients.

In any patient with severe chest pain that is abrupt or instantaneous in onset or has a ripping, tearing, or stabbing quality, acute thoracic aortic dissection should be suspected. Physical examination should assess for a pulse deficit, a systolic pressure differential between limbs of greater than 20 mm Hg, a focal neurologic deficit, or a new aortic regurgitation murmur. It is also important to ask about a family history of connective tissue disease (including Marfan syndrome), about any family or personal history of aortic dissection or thoracic aneurysm, and about any known aortic valve disease or recent aortic interventions. D-dimer testing has been proposed as a way to screen for aortic dissection, but it is more important to obtain prompt imaging and surgical intervention for those in whom dissection is confirmed.

An ECG should be obtained in all patients with suspected aortic dissection in order to exclude STEMI (which can manifest with similar symptoms). In all low- and intermediate-risk patients, a prompt chest x-ray can help by either confirming an alternative diagnosis or confirming the presence of thoracic aortic disease.

High-risk patients should have prompt imaging with CT or magnetic resonance imaging (MRI), and those who are in shock or clinically unstable may be evaluated by bedside transesophageal echocardiography. If thoracic aortic dissection is confirmed on imaging, urgent surgical consultation is required. Medical therapy should be started with intravenous β-blockers. Patients with dissection of the ascending aorta require urgent surgery, while those with descending thoracic aortic dissection may be managed medically unless hypotension or other complications develop.

Esophageal Rupture

Esophageal rupture, or Boerhaave's syndrome, has a high mortality rate. Esophageal rupture is rare, and the most common cause is endoscopically induced injury, but it can happen in other settings as well. Common misdiagnoses include perforated ulcer, MI, PE, dissecting aneurysm, and pancreatitis. The "classic" presentation has been described as pain, dyspnea, and shock followed by forceful emesis, but history and physical are commonly nonspecific. Diagnosis most commonly is made by contrast esophagram or CT scan of the chest.

Patients whose rupture is diagnosed less than 48 hours after symptom onset should be treated surgically (especially if sepsis is present) or endoscopically. Those who present more than 48 hours after symptom onset may be considered for conservative treatment with hyperalimentation, antibiotics, and nasogastric suction.

Tension Pneumothorax

Tension pneumothorax is relatively rare among patients presenting with chest pain, but it is potentially life-threatening if not treated properly. Common symptoms and physical findings include chest pain, respiratory distress, decreased ipsilateral air entry, and tachycardia; hypoxia, tracheal deviation, and hypotension are less common.

Emergency needle decompression is usually recommended if tension pneumothorax is suspected, but this is ineffective in some cases and is associated with risks to the patient of pain, bleeding, infection, and cardiac tamponade. However, waiting for radiographic confirmation of the diagnosis is associated with up to a four-fold increase in mortality due to delay in decompression of the pneumothorax. Patients most likely to benefit from an immediate attempt at needle decompression are those with an oxygen saturation less than 92% while on oxygen, a decreased level of consciousness while on oxygen, a systolic blood pressure less than 90 mm Hg, or a respiratory rate less than 10. Patients without these signs of instability may be better managed by waiting for chest imaging to confirm or exclude the presence of a pneumothorax. While plain chest xrays have typically been used for diagnosing a pneumothorax, one study has found that pleural ultrasound may have higher sensitivity.

Other Causes of Chest Pain

A patient with chest pain and cough, fever, egophony, or dullness to percussion might have pneumonia, but none of these individual findings are specific enough to confirm the diagnosis. A large study in 1984 developed a decision rule (Table 3) using seven clinical findings to predict the likelihood of pneumonia. While there is ongoing debate over the reliability of pneumonia diagnosis based solely on history and physical examination and chest x-ray is usually considered the reference standard, a recent Cochrane review found two trials suggesting routine chest radiography does not affect the clinical outcomes in adults and children presenting suggestive of a lower respiratory tract infection. Thus, at least for clinically stable outpatients, treatment for pneumonia based on appropriate clinical findings alone may be reasonable.

Heart failure alone is an uncommon cause of chest pain, but it may accompany ACS or cardiac valve disease. A displaced apical impulse and a prior history of CAD support this diagnosis, and because virtually all patients with heart failure have exertional dyspnea, its absence is very helpful in excluding this diagnosis. An abnormal ECG and cardiomegaly on chest x-ray can increase the likelihood of heart failure among patients with chest pain, and B-natriuretic peptide (BNP) is now commonly used for detecting heart failure in patients presenting with acute dyspnea. One recent

TABLE 3 · Diehr Diagnostic Rule for Pneumonia in Adults with Acute Cough

SIGNS AND SYMPTOMS

FINDING	POINTS
Rhinorrhea	−2
Sore throat	−1
Night sweats	1
Myalgia	1
Sputum all day	1
Resp. rate >25	2
Temp. >100°F	2

Interpretation

SCORE	PROBABILITY OF PNEUMONIA
−3	5
−1	12
0	21
1	30
3	37

Adapted from Cayley Jr WE. Diagnosing the cause of chest pain. Am Fam Physician 2005;72:2012–21. http://www.aafp.org/afp/2005/1115/p2012.html.

study also found that bedside ultrasound may have high sensitivity and specificity for diagnosing acute cardiogenic pulmonary edema.

A 3-item questionnaire has been developed specifically to assess for panic disorder among patients with chest pain referred for cardiac evaluation (Table 4). However, even in patients with possible panic disorder, further cardiac testing should be done if there are significant cardiac risk factors.

Gastrointestinal disease can cause chest pain, but the history and physical examination are relatively inaccurate for diagnosing or excluding serious gastrointestinal pathology. However, if life-threatening cardiovascular or pulmonary causes of chest pain have been excluded, it is appropriate to try a course of high dose PPI (omeprazole 40 mg twice daily, lansoprazole 30 mg daily, or esomeprazole 40 mg twice daily) to evaluate for undiagnosed gastroesophageal reflux

TABLE 4

ITEM	0	1	2	3	4	5
When you are nervous, how often do you think "I am going to pass out?"		Never	Rarely	Half the time	Usually	Always
During the last 7 days, including today, how much have you been bothered by pains in the chest?	Not at all	A little bit	Moderately	Quite a bit	Extremely	
To what degree is your chest pain tiring or exhausting	None	Mild	Moderate	Severe		

Adapted from: Dammen T, Ekeberg O, Arnesen H, Friis S. The detection of panic disorder in chest pain patients. Gen Hosp Psychiatry. 1999 Sep-Oct;21 (5):323–32. PubMed PMID: 10572773. http://www.ncbi.nlm.nih.gov/pubmed/10572773.
Approximately 76% of patients with a score of 4 or less will not have panic disorder (PD).
Approximately 71% of patients with a score of 5 or more will have PD.

disease (GERD) as the cause of chest pain (even for patients without typical GERD symptoms.)

Chest wall pain can usually be diagnosed by history and examination if other etiologies have been excluded, and chest wall pain is more likely if the patient's pain is reproducible by palpation. Measurement of the sedimentation rate is not generally helpful in making the diagnosis, although in unusual situations radiography may be helpful.

References

Cao AM, Choy JP, Mohanakrishnan LN, Bain RF, van Driel ML. Chest radiographs for acute lower respiratory tract infections. Cochrane Database Syst Rev 2013 Dec 26;12:CD009119.

Cayley Jr WE. Chest pain–tools to improve your in-office evaluation. J Fam Pract 2014 May;63(5):246–51: 24795903.

Cayley Jr WE. Diagnosing the cause of chest pain. Am Fam Physician 2005;72:2012–21.

de Schipper JP, Pull ter Gunne AF, Oostvogel HJ, van Laarhoven CJ. Spontaneous rupture of the oesophagus: Boerhaave's syndrome in 2008. Literature review and treatment algorithm. Dig Surg 2009;26:1–6: 19145081.

Hiratzka LF, Bakris GL, Beckman JA, et al. American College of Cardiology Foundation/American Heart Association Task Force on Practice Guidelines. American Association for Thoracic Surgery. American College of Radiology. American Stroke Association. Society of Cardiovascular Anesthesiologists. Society for Cardiovascular Angiography and Interventions. Society of Interventional Radiology, Society of Thoracic Surgeons, Society for Vascular Medicine. 2010 ACCF/AHA/AATS/ACR/ASA/SCA/SCAI/SIR/STS/SVM guidelines for the diagnosis and management of patients with Thoracic Aortic Disease: a report of the American College of Cardiology Foundation/American Heart Association Task Force on Practice Guidelines. Circulation 2010;121:e266–e369. Erratum in Circulation 2010;122(4):e410.

Leigh-Smith S, Harris T. Tension pneumothorax–time for a re-think? Emerg Med J 2005;22:8–16.

Miniati M, Bottai M, Monti S. Comparison of 3 clinical models for predicting the probability of pulmonary embolism. Medicine (Baltimore) 2005;84:107–14.

O'Connor RE, Brady W, Brooks SC, et al. Part 10: acute coronary syndromes: 2010 American Heart Association guidelines for cardiopulmonary resuscitation and emergency cardiovascular care. Circulation 2010;122:S787–S817. Erratum in: Circulation 2011;123:e238.

Swap CJ, Nagurney JT. Value and limitations of chest pain history in the evaluation of patients with suspected acute coronary syndromes. JAMA 2005; 294:2623–9.

Torbicki A, Perrier A, Konstantinides S, et al. ESC Committee for Practice Guidelines (CPG). Guidelines on the diagnosis and management of acute pulmonary embolism. Eur Heart J 2008;29:2276–315.

Wong BC. Is proton pump inhibitor testing an effective approach to diagnose gastroesophageal reflux disease in patients with noncardiac chest pain?: a meta-analysis. Arch Intern Med. 2005 Jun 13;165(11):1222–8: 15956000.

Yelland M, Cayley Jr WE, Vach W. An algorithm for the diagnosis and management of chest pain in primary care. Med Clin North Am 2010;94:349–74.

CONSTIPATION

Method of
Melissa Gaines, MD

CURRENT DIAGNOSIS

- While constipation is a benign process, it is important to recognize signs of a serious condition.
- Classification of normal transit constipation, slow transit constipation, or pelvic floor dysfunction guides therapy.
- Clinical testing has low benefit, but colonoscopy or imaging can assess for organic causes.

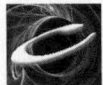

CURRENT THERAPY

- Initial therapy includes soluble dietary fiber to improve symptoms in chronic constipation.
- Osmotic laxatives are preferred while utilizing stimulant laxatives as rescue agents.
- Surgery is reserved for pelvic floor dysfunction after optimal therapies have failed.

Epidemiology

Constipation is common, with a prevalence of 1.9% to 27.2%, but the description of symptoms is variable. A thorough history and focused physical examination aids diagnosis. Treatment is directed toward relief of symptoms, alleviation of precipitating factors, and prevention of recurrence. While constipation is a benign process, it is important to recognize concerning signs for a more serious medical condition such as malignancy.

Risk Factors

Vulnerable populations include female, elderly, neurodegenerative disease, low-fiber diet, painful rectal disorders, hypothyroidism, and diabetes mellitus.

Pathophysiology

With aging, there is decreased rectal compliance, diminished rectal sensation, and decreased resting anal pressures, while colonic transit time is preserved. Normal transit constipation is a component of irritable bowel syndrome with normal transit time and stool frequency. Slow transit constipation is a condition with colonic dysmotility resulting from altered enteric nervous system. Defecatory disorders include structural disturbances of the pelvic floor. Pelvic floor dysfunction is the paradoxical contraction of the external anal sphincter and puborectalis muscles during defecation. Secondary causes of constipation are listed in Table 1.

Prevention

Provide an environment of privacy and comfort to allow for natural defecation. Prescribe an adequate fluid and fiber intake with specific amounts that vary depending on the patient's condition. Encourage physical activity, with a low to moderate level of exercise depending on the patient's functional status. Develop a routine for defecation with a prompt response to a call to defecate urgently. Recurrent fecal impaction can be prevented with polyethylene glycol (PEG, MiraLax).

Clinical Manifestations

Patients will complain using qualitative terms of hard stools, a feeling of incomplete voiding, straining, prolonged time for laxation, the need for additional maneuvers, abdominal bloating, and abdominal pain (Table 2). A change in bowel habit differentiates the current complaint from a serious medical condition. Red flags include acute onset, weight loss, abdominal pain or cramping,

rectal bleeding, nausea or vomiting, rectal pain, fever, or a change in stool caliber. Infants with abdominal distension and failure to pass meconium within 24 hours indicate Hirschsprung's disease. Patients should be asked if they have had loose stools or bowel incontinence to assess for fecal impaction. A medication review is required (see Table 1). Classification of patients with normal transit constipation, slow transit constipation, or pelvic floor dysfunction/defecatory disorders guides therapy.

Diagnosis

Diagnostic criteria have been established because the symptoms can vary (see Table 2). Conduct a physical examination that includes an assessment of vital signs, weight, volume status, auscultation of bowel sounds, abdominal percussion for tympani, and abdominal palpation for tenderness or mass. A rectal examination can detect resting rectal tone, fecal impaction, anorectal disorders, or rectal mass. Defecatory disorders show an increased resistance to the insertion of the examiner's finger with an impaired relaxation of the sphincter complex and reduced perineal descent during a Valsalva maneuver. Conduct laboratory testing on electrolytes, hemoglobin, thyroid-stimulating hormone, and fecal occult after initial measures fail. Red flag symptoms require imaging with CT of the abdomen and pelvis or an endoscopy to diagnose malignancy or fecal impaction. Anorectal testing with manometry and a rectal balloon expulsion test is appropriate for pelvic floor dysfunction or defecatory disorders. Hirschsprung's disease is diagnosed with barium enema, rectal manometry, or a rectal suction biopsy. Colonic transit rates with radiopaque markers (Sitz) on serial abdominal radiographs over 4 to 7 days diagnose slow transit constipation disorders.

Treatment

Nonpharmacologic therapies have limited benefit. Unless there are signs of dehydration, increasing fluid intake is not indicated. Moderate-intensity exercise improves symptoms of irritable bowel syndrome. Probiotics are not beneficial.

There is moderate evidence for pharmacologic agents (Table 3). Normal transit constipation responds to soluble dietary fiber supplements (e.g., psyllium [Metamucil]); however, these should not be used in the case of slow transit constipation or drug-induced constipation. Osmotic agents with PEG (Miralax) found to be superior to lactulose (Chronulac) are second line with titration for soft stools. Stimulant laxatives are used as rescue therapy if patients do not have a bowel movement for 2 days.

New classes of drugs to manage constipation include intestinal secretagogues, serotonin 5-HT$_4$ receptor antagonists, and opiate antagonists. Lubiprostone (Amitiza) requires a negative pregnancy test with contraception. Linaclotide (Linzess) is a 14-amino acid peptide similar to heat-stable enterotoxins that cause diarrhea. Lubiprostone and linaclotide are FDA-approved, but additional toxicology studies are required for the latter. None of the new highly selective serotonin 5-HT$_4$ receptor agonists are approved by the FDA. Methylnaltrexone (Relistor) is an opiate receptor antagonist administered subcutaneously that can cause laxation in patients on chronic opiate therapy.

Pelvic floor dysfunction or defecatory disorders respond to biofeedback therapy by utilizing manometry and visual or auditory feedback. Patients practice expelling a balloon and improve pelvic floor muscle coordination with Kegel exercises. Surgical intervention with subtotal colectomy with ileorectal anastomosis is indicated for slow transit constipation or defecatory disorders after failure of optimal medical management.

Complications

Fecal impaction a complication and a large bowel obstruction with colonic perforation has high mortality. Pediatric and geriatric patients are most susceptible with signs and symptoms of fecal incontinence, abdominal pain, abdominal distention, anorexia, weight loss, and delirium. Treatments for adults include a large-volume tap-water enema (500–1000 mL), local anesthetics administered topically with abdominal massage, a colonoscopy, or surgery. The prevention of recurrence requires maintenance bowel regimen with osmotic agents such as PEG (Miralax).

TABLE 1	Causes of Constipation
Dietary	Low-fiber diet, dementia, depression, anorexia, dehydration
Metabolic	Diabetes mellitus, hypercalcemia, hypokalemia, hypothyroidism, systemic sclerosis
Neurologic	Parkinson's disease, spinal cord disorder, multiple sclerosis, cerebrovascular disease (stroke)
Iatrogenic	Antacids, iron, anticholinergics, antidepressants, antipsychotics, opiates, antiepileptics
Painful anorectal condition	Anal fissure, hemorrhoids, abscess, fistula, pelvic floor dysfunction, malignancy

TABLE 2	Rome III Criteria

More than two present:
- Straining in more than 25% of defecations
- Hard or lumpy stool in more than 25% of defecations
- Sensation of incomplete evacuation
- Sensation of anorectal blockage
- Manual maneuvers
- Fewer than three defecations per week

Loose stools are rare without laxative use

Insufficient criteria for irritable bowel syndrome

Symptoms for 3 months with onset 6 months before diagnosis

TABLE 3 Drug Dosing and Adverse Effects

CLASS	DRUG NAME (BRAND)	ADULT DOSING	MECHANISM OF ACTION	TIME TO ONSET (h)	ADVERSE EFFECT
Fiber	Bran Psyllium (Metamucil) Methylcellulose (Citrucel) Calcium polycarbophil (FiberCon)	1 cup/day 1 tsp 1 tbsp or 1 tab twice daily 2–4 tabs/day	Increase water content and bulk of stool decreasing transit time	Unknown	Bloating excessive gas
Hyperosmolar agent	Sorbitol 70% Lactulose (Chronulac)	15–30 mL twice daily	Disaccharide metabolized by colonic bacteria into acetic acid and short-chain fatty acids	24–48	Sweet tasting, transient abdominal cramps, flatulence
Hyperosmolar agent	PEG-ES (GoLytely,* CoLyte*) PEG (Miralax)	8–32 oz daily 17 g (1 tbsp) qd	Osmotic effect increasing intraluminal fluids	0.5–1	Incontinence
Stimulant	Glycerin suppository Bisacodyl (Dulcolax) Senna (Senokot, Perdiem) Senna/docusate (Peri-Colace) Cascara†	1 daily 10 mg suppository or 5–10 mg PO 3 times a week 2–4 tabs twice daily 20–30 mg/day	Local rectal stimulation, secretory and prokinetic effect	8–12	Degeneration of Meissner's and Auerbach
Enemas	Mineral oil retention enema Tap water enema Sodium phosphate enema (Fleet)	199–250 mL daily PR 500–1000 mL PR 1 Unit PR	Evacuation induced by distended colon and mechanical lavage	6–8 for a mineral oil enema 5–15 min for all other enemas	Mechanical trauma, incontinence, rectal damage
Opioid antagonist	Methylnaltrexone (Relistor)	8–12 mg 1 dose SC every other day as needed	Opioid mu receptor antagonist in gut decreasing transit time	4	Diarrhea, intestinal perforation

*Not FDA approved for this indication.
†Available as dietary supplement.

References

Arshad A, Powell C. Easily missed? Hirschsprung's disease. Br Med J 2012;345:e5521.

Bharucha AE, Pemberton JH, Locke GR. American Gastroenterological Association technical review on constipation. Gastroenterology 2013;144:218–38.

Gallagher PF, O'Mahony D, Quigley EM. Management of chronic constipation in the elderly. Drugs Aging 2008;25:807–21.

Higgins PD, Johanson JF. Epidemiology of constipation in North America: A systematic review. Am J Gastroenterol 2004;99:750–9.

Larkin PJ, Sykes NP, Centeno C, et al. The management of constipation in palliative care: Clinical practice recommendations. Palliat Med 2008;22:796–807.

McCallum IJ, Ong S, Mercer-Jones M. Chronic constipation in adults. Br Med J 2009;338:b831.

Thomas J, Karver S, Cooney GA, et al. Methylnaltrexone for opioid-induced constipation in advanced illness. N Engl J Med 2008;358:2332–43.

Wald A. Management and prevention of fecal impaction. Curr Gastroenterol Rep 2008;10:299–501.

Gastroenterology. Rome criteria. Available at, http://www.romecriteria.org/; 2006.

Subacute Cough
- Postinfectious (e.g., viral upper respiratory infection, pertussis, exacerbation of underlying lung disorder)
- Noninfectious (same as chronic cough)

Chronic Cough
- Chronic upper airway cough syndrome secondary to rhinosinus disease
- Asthma
- Nonasthmatic eosinophilic bronchitis
- Gastroesophageal reflux disease
- Tuberculosis
- Others (e.g., ear wax or foreign body, lung cancer)

COUGH

Method of
Shingo Chihara, MD

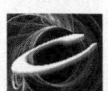

CURRENT DIAGNOSIS

Acute Cough
- Upper respiratory tract infection (e.g., common cold)
- Lower respiratory tract infection (e.g., pneumonia)
- Exacerbations of preexisting condition (e.g., asthma, bronchiectasis)
- Acute environmental exposure
- Pulmonary embolism
- Congestive heart failure

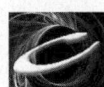

CURRENT THERAPY

Acute Cough (Symptomatic Treatment in Common Cold)
- Dexbrompheniramine 6 mg and pseudoephedrine 120 mg (Drixoral Cold and Sinus Tablets)[2] PO bid × 1 week
- Naproxen (Naprosyn, Aleve)[1] 500 mg × 1, then 500 mg PO tid × 5 days
- Ipratropium bromide nasal spray (Atrovent Nasal Spray 0.06%) 2 sprays in each nostril tid to qid × 4 days

Subacute Cough (Pertussis)
- Erythromycin (Ery-Tab) 500 mg PO qid × 14 days or trimethoprim-sulfamethoxazole (Bactrim DS)[1] 160 mg/800 mg PO bid × 14 days

Chronic Cough (Effective in Short-Term Symptomatic Relief in Chronic Bronchitis)

- Codeine 10–20 mg PO every 4–6 hours as needed
- Dextromethorphan (Robitussin Cough) 10–20 mg PO every 4 hours or 30 mg PO every 6–8 hours or 60 mg PO every 12 hours
- Empiric treatment of most likely etiology (e.g., asthma, gastroesophageal reflux disease)

[1]Not FDA approved for this indication.
[2]Not available in the United States.

Cough is a common reason patients seek care from their primary care physician. Lifestyle is often affected both physically and psychologically. Complications such as rib fractures, pneumothorax, vomiting, urinary incontinence, muscle pain, fatigue, depression, and syncope can result from excessive coughing.

Pathophysiology of Cough Reflex

Cough, which may be initiated voluntarily or reflexively, is a normal protective mechanism to clear the airway of secretions. Cough is mediated by the afferent vagus nerve, which innervates not only the airways but also other organs such as the ear canal and distal esophagus. (This is why ear wax and distal esophageal reflux can be etiologies for chronic cough.)

Cough has three phases. Initially, an inspiratory phase occurs. The compressive phase results when the glottis closes, the diaphragm relaxes, and the intrathoracic pressure rises. The expiratory phase occurs when muscles contract and air travels at high velocity through the airway, clearing any secretions or foreign material.

Patients in whom the cough reflex is compromised (e.g., the elderly, newborns, lung transplant recipients, or patients with paralysis or neuromuscular disorders) are at risk for aspiration pneumonia.

Although cough is a protective mechanism, when excessive, it can irritate the airways. A vicious cycle of coughing results when this mucosal damage precipitates the cough reflex.

Cough is classified according to its duration: acute if lasting less than 3 weeks, subacute if lasting 3 to 8 weeks, and chronic if lasting longer than 8 weeks. The etiology of cough is different depending on the duration of symptom.

Acute Cough

Self-limiting upper respiratory infection is the most common cause of acute cough, but it is necessary to rule out other serious etiologies such as congestive heart failure, pneumonia, and pulmonary embolism. The diagnosis for upper respiratory infection may be straightforward in a patient who is immunocompetent and has symptoms such as nasal congestion, runny nose, sore throat, lacrimation, and fever. If the chest examination is normal, chest x-ray is normal in 97% of such cases. The same cannot be said in immunocompromised patients, in whom the differential diagnosis broadens to include opportunistic infection such as Pneumocystis jirovecii or invasive aspergillosis.

Viral infection of the upper respiratory tract is the most common cause of acute cough, and antibiotics are not recommended. For reduction of cough, dexbrompheniramine plus pseudoephedrine (Drixoral Cold & Sinus)[2] and naproxen (Aleve, Naprosyn)[1] have been shown to be efficacious in randomized, double-blind studies. Relatively nonsedating histamine blockers have not been shown to reduce cough because they have minimal or no anticholinergic activity and the common cold is not mediated by histamine.

Subacute Cough

The etiologies of subacute cough are classified as postinfectious and noninfectious.

Postinfectious Cough

Postinfectious cough is a cough that follows a viral infection or infection with an atypical bacterium such as Mycoplasma pneumoniae. The cough lasts more than 3 weeks but less than 8 weeks, and the patient has a normal chest x-ray. Most cases are self-limiting. The pathogenesis is multifactorial, such as extensive mucosal damage in the airways, transient increase in cough receptor sensitivity, retained secretions, drainage of secretions to the larynx from the upper airways, and aggravation of reflux disease when intraabdominal pressure rises with coughing.

Bordetella pertussis is a pathogen that is a public health threat. It is highly contagious and can infect 70% to 100% of household members and 50% to 80% of school contacts. A classic presentation of pertussis consists of two phases: catarrhal phase (fever, conjunctivitis, rhinorrhea, malaise) and paroxysmal phase (worsening cough, shortness of breath, posttussive emesis). The diagnosis can be confirmed by polymerase chain reaction (PCR) test, culture, or serologies (acute and convalescent).

When B. pertussis infection is suspected, a macrolide (erythromycin [Ery-Tab] or azithromycin [Zithromax][1]) should be started. When drug treatment is started during the catarrhal phase, the bacteria are rapidly cleared from the nasal mucosa and there is a decrease in paroxysmal cough. There is less benefit when drug treatment is started later.

In recent years, pertussis has emerged as a cause of chronic cough in adults, who can transmit it to their infants. Since 2004, more than 3000 cases of infant pertussis and 19 deaths have been reported annually. Because infants younger than 2 months are too young to be vaccinated, the Advisory Committee on Immunization Practices (ACIP) recommends Tdap (tetanus toxoid, reduced diphtheria toxoid, and acellular pertussis vaccine [Adacel, Boostrix]) be given to unvaccinated pregnant women after 20 weeks' gestation, to postpartum mothers, and to family members who will come in contact with the infant. ACIP recommends Tdap instead of Td (tetanus and diphtheria toxoids vaccine, [Decavac] for any adult who is due for revaccination for Td, which is recommended to be given every 10 years.

Chronic Cough

The most common causes of chronic cough are chronic upper airway cough syndrome secondary to rhinosinus disease, asthma, gastroesophageal reflux disease (GERD), chronic bronchitis, eosinophilic bronchitis, and angiotensin-converting enzyme (ACE) inhibitors.

In some cases, multiple factors play a role, and therefore additive treatment is recommended. For example, a lack of response to a proton pump inhibitor does not rule out GERD as a component of chronic cough. Unfortunately, the character of the cough (productive, dry), the quality of the sound (barking, brassy), and the timing of cough (nighttime, with meals) are not useful in differentiating the cause of chronic cough.

The first step is to assess if the patient is taking an ACE inhibitor and if so, to stop the medication. The incidence of chronic cough in patients on ACE inhibitors is reported as 5% to 35%. The cough is typically dry and is more common in women, nonsmokers, and persons of Chinese origin. It can start within hours of the first dose of medication or can be delayed up to weeks or months after initiation. Most times the cough resolves within 1 to 4 weeks of cessation, but it can linger up to 3 months. The pathogenesis is thought to be protussive agents such as bradykinin and substance P, which are degraded by ACE and therefore accumulate in the airways in patients taking ACE inhibitors. An angiotensin-receptor blocker is an alternative to ACE inhibitors and does not have cough as a side effect.

Chronic Upper Airway Cough Syndrome Secondary to Rhinosinus Diseases

Previously known as postnasal drip syndrome, it is the most common cause of cough either by itself or in combination with another

[1]Not FDA approved for this indication.
[2]Not available in the United States.

[1]Not FDA approved for this indication.

diagnosis. Multiple mechanisms are postulated, such as mechanical stimulation of the afferent limb of the cough reflex by secretions and hypersensitivity of the cough reflex. A history of upper respiratory illness is often present with symptoms such as throat clearing, nasal discharge, and nasal congestion. A minority of patients have a silent chronic upper airway cough syndrome. It is recommended to give a trial of first-generation antihistamine before looking for other uncommon causes of cough.

Gastroesophageal Reflux Disease

Gastroesophageal reflux is the backflow of stomach contents into the esophagus. It can be physiologic and usually occurs during meals or postprandially in healthy persons. It is estimated that 7% to 10% of Americans have reflux symptoms every day; 20% have symptoms for more than a week and up to 36% for a month. The term *gastroesophageal reflux disease* (GERD) is used in those who have symptoms and/or evidence of tissue damage. GERD is one of the common causes of chronic cough. The prevalence ranges between 5% and 41%, but it is rising.

GERD can stimulate the afferent vagus nerve at multiple levels. Upper and lower upper respiratory tracts may be involved as well as the distal esophagus. The esophageal-bronchial cough reflex may be stimulated via the distal esophagus without airway involvement. There is increasing evidence that nonacid factors such as alkaline pH, pancreatic enzymes, bile, and esophageal dysmotility play a role in triggering cough. Cough itself worsens gastroesophageal reflux, and this can perpetuate the chronic cough.

When a patient has gastrointestinal symptoms such as heartburn and regurgitation, GERD should be considered as a cause of chronic cough, but in up to 75% of cases, the patient does not have gastrointestinal symptoms. Evidence of reflux may be seen with laryngoscopy (e.g., posterior laryngitis with red arytenoids and piled-up interarytenoid mucosa). Catheter-based 24-hour esophageal pH monitoring is considered the gold standard in diagnosing GERD. Antireflux medical therapy includes diet, lifestyle changes (no smoking, limiting vigorous exercise, no alcohol), acid suppression with proton pump inhibitors, and prokinetic agents. If rigorous medical therapy does not resolve symptoms after 3 months, then antireflux surgery must be considered.

Asthma

Asthma is a cause of chronic cough in about 25% of cases. Although wheezing and dyspnea are seen with asthma, cough is the predominant or sole symptom in a subgroup of patients, and this condition is called *cough-variant asthma*. As with other patients with asthma, thickening of the subepithelial layer is seen in patients with cough-variant asthma, but patients with cough-variant asthma are significantly more sensitive to the cough reflex. Spirometry and bronchoprovocation testing with inhaled methacholine (Provocholine) are helpful for diagnosis and resolution of symptoms, and response to specific therapy for asthma provides the definitive diagnosis.

Cough-variant asthma is treated as asthma with bronchodilators and inhaled corticosteroids first. Adding a leukotriene receptor antagonist is the next step. Systemic corticosteroids such as oral prednisone are reserved for difficult cases.

Nonasthmatic Eosinophilic Bronchitis

Nonasthmatic eosinophilic bronchitis accounts for about 10% of chronic cough. In these patients, there is no objective evidence of airflow obstruction, normal airway hyperresponsiveness, and sputum eosinophilia. This condition is rarely self-limiting and is treated with inhaled corticosteroids.

References

Bolser DC. Cough suppressant and pharmacologic protussive therapy: ACCP evidence-based clinical practice guidelines. Chest 2006;129(1 Suppl.): 238S–249S.

Centers for Disease Control and Prevention (CDC). Updated recommendations for use of tetanus toxoid, reduced diphtheria toxoid and acellular pertussis vaccine (Tdap) in pregnant women and persons who have or anticipate having close contact with an infant aged <12 months—Advisory Committee on Immunization Practices (ACIP), 2011. MMWR Morb Mortal Wkly Rep 2011 Oct 21;60:1424–6.

De Blasio F, Virchow JC, Polverino M, et al. Cough management: A practical approach. Cough 2011;7:7.

Dicpinigaitis PV. Chronic cough due to asthma: ACCP evidence-based clinical practice guidelines. Chest 2006;129(1 Suppl.):75S–79S.

Evans AT, Husain S, Durairaj L, et al. Azithromycin for acute bronchitis: A randomised, double-blind, controlled trial. Lancet 2002;359:1648–54.

Irwin RS. Chronic cough due to gastroesophageal reflux disease: ACCP evidence-based clinical practice guidelines. Chest 2006;129(1 Suppl.):80S–94S.

Irwin RS, Madison JM. The diagnosis and treatment of cough. N Engl J Med 2000;343:1715–21.

Jegoux F, Legent F, Beauvillain de Montreuil C. Chronic cough and ear wax. Lancet 2002;360:618.

Madison JM, Irwin RS. Cough: A worldwide problem. Otolaryngol Clin North Am 2010;43:1–13 vii.

Pavord ID, Chung KF. Management of chronic cough. Lancet 2008;371:1375–84.

Sperber SJ, Hendley JO, Hayden FG, et al. Effects of naproxen on experimental rhinovirus colds. A randomized, double-blind, controlled trial. Ann Intern Med 1992;117:37–41.

DIZZINESS AND VERTIGO

Method of
Jennifer Wipperman, MD

CURRENT DIAGNOSIS

- Benign paroxysmal positional vertigo
  - Repeated, brief episodes lasting less than 1 minute
  - Triggered by changes in head position
  - Positive Dix-Hallpike maneuver
- Vestibular neuritis
  - Single, severe, constant episode lasting days
  - Subacute onset
  - Positive head impulse test
  - Nystagmus is unilateral, horizontal, and spontaneous
- Ménière's disease
  - Recurrent episodes of vertigo lasting hours
  - May have unilateral hearing loss, tinnitus, or ear fullness
- Red flags for stroke include:
  - Sudden onset
  - Risk factors for stroke
  - Nystagmus with a central pattern
  - Negative head-thrust test
  - Additional neurologic signs
  - Inability to walk

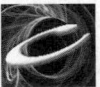

CURRENT THERAPY

- Benign paroxysmal positional vertigo
  - The canalith repositioning procedure (Epley maneuver) is the most effective treatment
  - Vestibular rehabilitation is effective
  - Consider observation with close follow-up if a patient will not tolerate the canalith repositioning procedure or if symptoms are mild
  - Avoid symptomatic medications
- Vestibular neuritis
  - Brief symptomatic care with benzodiazepines, antiemetics, and antihistamines
  - Early vestibular rehabilitation speeds recovery
  - Use of corticosteroids is controversial

The "dizzy" patient is often a frustrating phenomenon in clinical medicine. However, after a careful history and physical examination, most patients can be diagnosed and serious causes excluded. Peripheral causes of vertigo are usually benign, and include vestibular neuritis and benign paroxysmal positional vertigo (BPPV). Life-threatening central causes include stroke, vertebrobasilar insufficiency, demyelinating disease, and an intracranial mass. The first step in evaluating vertigo is differentiating among the four types of dizziness: near syncope or light-headedness, disequilibrium, psychogenic dizziness, and true vertigo. True vertigo is a false sense of motion, and patients typically report that "the room is spinning." This chapter will focus on the two most common causes of episodic vertigo: BPPV and vestibular neuritis.

Epidemiology

Vertigo is a common office complaint. In fact, 7.5 million Americans are evaluated for dizziness in ambulatory care settings each year, and approximately 50% of these cases are vertigo. In primary care office setting, BPPV and vestibular neuritis account for the majority of vertigo diagnoses, followed by vestibular migraine, Ménière's disease and vascular causes. BPPV is the most common vestibular disorder across the lifespan.

Risk Factors

BPPV is seven times more likely in individuals over age 60, and it is also more common in women. A history of prior head trauma and other vestibular disorders places patients at risk for BPPV. There are no identified risk factors for vestibular neuritis.

Pathophysiology

BPPV is thought to occur when calcium carbonate debris (otoconia) are dislodged and float freely in the semicircular canals of the inner ear. The posterior canal is most often involved. During head movement, loose otoconia move in the canal and cause a continued sense of motion for a few seconds until they settle. The pathophysiology of vestibular neuritis is uncertain. Evidence supports a viral infection, most likely HSV-1, which causes inflammation of the eighth cranial nerve. When hearing loss accompanies vertigo, the condition is called *acute labrynthitis*.

Clinical Manifestations

The history and physical examination are fundamental in the evaluation of vertigo. Key questions include the frequency and duration of attacks, triggers such as positional or pressure changes, prior head trauma, associated neurologic symptoms, hearing loss, and headache. A personal history of diabetes, hypertension, and hyperlipidemia are risk factors for stroke. BPPV, stroke, and

migraines can have a familial preponderance, and a family history of these disorders should be elicited. Many medications, including anticonvulsants and antihypertensives, cause dizziness.

BPPV causes brief, recurrent episodes that last less than 1 minute and are brought on by changes in head movement or position. Nausea and vomiting may be associated. Vestibular neuritis usually has a subacute onset over several hours, peaks in intensity for 1 to 2 days, and then gradually subsides over the next few weeks. Symptoms of vertigo are constant, and nausea and vomiting can be severe during the first few days. Patients with vestibular neuritis may have difficulty standing and veer toward the affected side. Although changes in position worsen the vertigo in vestibular neuritis, vertigo is always present at baseline. In BPPV, patients are normal between attacks.

General physical examination should include a thorough cardiovascular, ear, nose, throat, and neurologic examination. The neurologic examination can differentiate between benign (peripheral) and life-threatening (central) causes based on the ability to walk, type of nystagmus, results of the head-thrust test, and presence of associated neurologic signs (Table 1).

Patients with vestibular neuritis may have difficulty walking, but the inability to walk is a red flag for a central lesion. Nystagmus is unidirectional (always beats in the same direction) and horizontal in vestibular neuritis, and is suppressed by visual fixation. Having a patient focus on an object in the room will stop the nystagmus, which reappears if a blank sheet of paper is placed a few inches in front of the patient's face. Nystagmus in central causes is not suppressed by visual fixation, and may be direction-changing (nystagmus beats to the right when the patient looks right, and beats to the left when the patient looks left) or pure vertical. The head impulse test (Figure 1) is positive in peripheral causes like vestibular neuritis. The examiner holds the patient's head while the patient fixes her eyes on the examiner's nose, and then the examiner quickly moves the patient's head 10 degrees to the right and left. If a saccade (the eyes look away and then re-fixate on the examiner's nose) is found, this indicates a peripheral lesion on the side that the head is turned towards. Central lesions will not cause saccades and the head impulse test will be normal. HINTS (Head Impulse test, Nystagmus, Test of Skew) combines three physical examination findings which has been found to have a 97% sensitivity and 99% specificity for diagnosis a central cause of vertigo in the acute setting. If any of the tests indicate a central cause, including a positive head impulse test, nystagmus that is bidirectional, purely vertical or purely torsional, and vertical eye misalignment, then the HINTS test is considered positive.

The Dix-Hallpike maneuver is diagnostic of posterior canal BPPV (Figure 2). The patient should be warned that nausea and vomiting may occur. After the patient is placed in the head-hanging

TABLE 1	Differentiating Peripheral and Central Causes of Vertigo		
	PERIPHERAL CAUSES		**CENTRAL CAUSES**
	BPPV	*VESTIBULAR NEURITIS*	
History	Brief, recurrent attacks of vertigo lasting less than 1 minute Triggered by positional changes No vertigo between attacks	Subacute onset Constant and severe vertigo lasting days Nausea and vomiting may be severe	Sudden onset Risk factors for stroke May have severe headache
Nystagmus	Up-beating and torsional	Horizontal and unidirectional	Direction changing Pure vertical Pure torsional
Gait	Unaffected between episodes	May veer towards affected side	Unable to walk
Specialized physical examination tests	Positive Dix-Hallpike maneuver Positive supine roll test	Positive head thrust test Visual fixation stops nystagmus	Head-impulse test negative Visual fixation does not stop nystagmus
Additional neurologic signs	Rare	Rare	Common (e.g., dysarthria, aphasia, incoordination, weakness, or numbness)

Abbreviation: BPPV = benign paroxysmal positional vertigo.

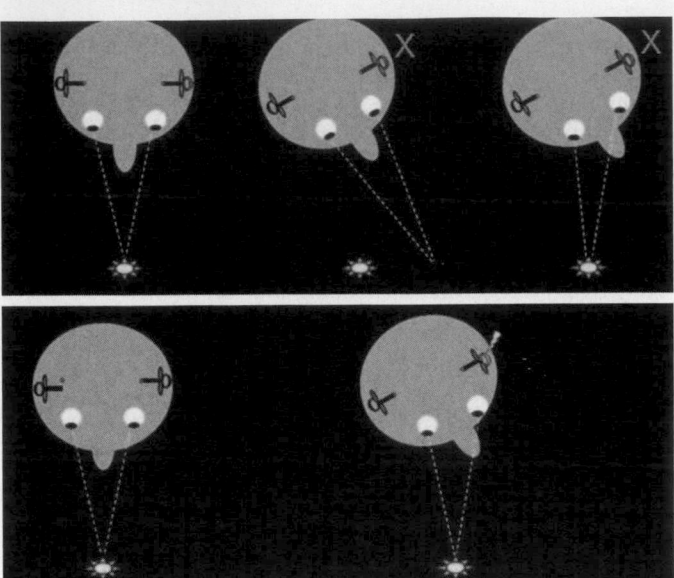

Figure 1. Head impulse test. Top panel shows a positive head-thrust test. The examiner moves the patient's head quickly 10 degrees to the side, in this case to the patient's left. A catch-up saccade is observed when the patient looks away and then refixes on the visual target, indicating a peripheral lesion on the left. Lower figure shows a normal head-thrust test. The patient maintains visual fixation during head movement. (Adapted from Seemungal BM, Bronstein AM. A practical approach to acute vertigo. Pract Neurol 2008; 8:211–21.)

position, there is a 5- to 20-second latency period before the nystagmus and symptoms appear. Both the nystagmus and vertigo will increase in severity and then resolve within 60 seconds. The nystagmus observed is up-beating and torsional. The maneuver should be repeated with the head held to the opposite side. The side that elicits the symptoms and nystagmus diagnoses BPPV in the ipsilateral ear. If both sides elicit symptoms, the patient may have bilateral BPPV. If the test is negative and BPPV is strongly suspected, the patient should lie supine and the examiner can turn the head to each side (supine roll test). This maneuver will cause symptoms and nystagmus in patients with horizontal canal BPPV.

Diagnosis

BPPV and vestibular neuritis are diagnosed clinically. Further diagnostic testing is indicated if the diagnosis is uncertain or a central cause is suspected. Audiometry may be abnormal in Ménière's disease. MRI is the best imaging test for central lesions because it includes the posterior fossa and is most sensitive for stroke. Vestibular function testing is useful if the diagnosis is unclear or in cases of refractory vertigo. Vestibular function testing includes several different specialized tests that evaluate the ocular and vestibular response to position changes and caloric stimulation. Video-oculographic recordings of nystagmus can magnify the eye and allow for repeated viewings for further study. Some patients with BPPV may have additional vestibular disorders causing vertigo that vestibular function testing can elucidate.

Differential Diagnosis

Ménière's disease migrainous vertigo is probably more common than once thought. is suspected in patients with the triad of tinnitus, fluctuating hearing loss, and vertigo. Episodes usually last hours, are disabling, and are recurrent over years. Migrainous vertigo features episodes lasting hours to days in patients with other migraine symptoms such as headache, photophobia, phonophobia, or aura. Central lesions such as stroke, vertebrobasilar insufficiency, or intracranial mass are most concerning. Red flags for stroke include sudden onset, risk factors for stroke, associated neurologic signs, inability to walk, negative head-thrust test, severe associated headache, and characteristic nystagmus. Posttraumatic vertigo may occur in patients after head trauma who present with vertigo,

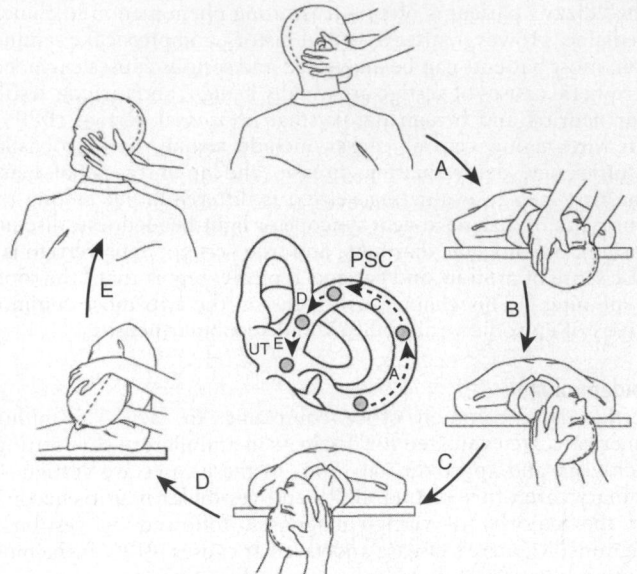

Figure 2. Treatment maneuver for posterior canal benign paroxysmal positional vertigo affecting the right ear. To treat the left ear, the procedure is reversed. The drawing of the labyrinth in the center shows the position of the particle as it moves around the posterior semicircular canal (PSC) and into the utricle (UT). The patient is seated upright, with head facing the examiner, who is standing on the right. **A,** The patient is rapidly moved to head-hanging right position (Dix-Hallpike test). This position is maintained until the nystagmus ceases. **B,** The examiner moves to the head of the table, repositioning hands as shown. **C,** The head is rotated quickly to the left with right ear upward. This position is maintained for 30 seconds. **D,** The patient rolls onto the left side while the examiner rapidly rotates the head leftward until the nose is directed toward the floor. This position is then held for 30 seconds. **E,** The patient is rapidly lifted into the sitting position, now facing left. The entire sequence should be repeated until no nystagmus can be elicited. After the maneuver, the patient is instructed to avoid head-hanging positions to prevent the particles from reentering the posterior canal. (Reprinted with permission from Rakel RE. Conn's Current Therapy 1995. Philadelphia, WB Saunders, 1995, p 839.)

tinnitus, and headache. A perilymphatic fistula is rare, but may be suspected in a patient with episodic vertigo after head trauma, heavy lifting, or barotrauma. Pressure changes with sneezing or coughing trigger vertigo attacks. Postural hypotension should be ruled out in all patients. An acoustic neuroma presents with slowly progressive, unilateral sensorineural hearing loss and tinnitus. Many patients may have an unsteady gait, but true vertigo is rare.

Treatment

Posterior canal BPPV is best treated with the *canalith repositioning procedure*, also known as the Epley maneuver (Figure 2). Studies have shown the procedure is safe and effective with an odds ratio of 4.2 (95% CI. 2.3-11.4) for symptom resolution. Patients should be warned that nausea or vomiting may occur during the procedure, and may be pre-treated with an antiemetic medication. The procedure can be repeated if unsuccessful. Posttreatment activity restrictions are unnecessary. Horizontal canal BPPV can be treated with the barbeque roll maneuver. Vestibular rehabilitation is another valuable treatment for BPPV, but it is less effective than the canalith repositioning procedure. It enhances central compensation for peripheral deficits and leads to faster symptom recovery than observation alone, though most patients will improve spontaneously after 4 to 6 weeks. Observation is an option if symptoms are mild or if a patient will not tolerate the canalith repositioning procedure or vestibular rehabilitation. However, observation is associated with higher recurrence rates than the canalith repositioning procedure. Vestibular-suppressant medications such as antihistamines and benzodiazepines are discouraged because they interfere with central compensation and increase the risk for falling. Surgery is rarely needed for BPPV, but may be helpful in refractory cases.

Vestibular neuritis is primarily treated with rest, vestibular suppressant medications, and vestibular rehabilitation. Patients may initially be admitted if symptoms, such as nausea and vomiting, are severe or if stroke is suspected. Treatment with antihistamines (dimenhydrinate [Dramamine][1] 50 mg every 6 hours), antiemetics (promethazine [Phenergan][1] 25 mg every 6 hours) or benzodiazepines (lorazepam [Ativan][1] 1 to 2 mg every 4 hours) may be used to treat severe symptoms. However, these should not be continued for more than 2 to 3 days because they inhibit central compensation. The use of corticosteroids is controversial. Although studies show that vestibular-function testing improves more quickly in patients treated with corticosteroids, there is conflicting evidence that corticosteroids hasten the recovery of clinical signs and symptoms of vestibular neuritis. A 2011 Cochrane review concluded that there is insufficient evidence to recommend corticosteroids for the treatment of vestibular neuritis. Finally, antiviral medications have not been proven effective for vestibular neuritis.

For patients with vestibular neuritis, vestibular rehabilitation should be started as soon as symptoms improve and a patient can tolerate the exercises. Exercises include balance and gait training as well as coordination of head and eye movements. Vestibular rehabilitation hastens recovery and improves balance, gait, and vision by increasing central compensation for vestibular dysfunction. Exercises may be home-based for compliant patients with mild symptoms, whereas formal referral may be more beneficial for patients with severe symptoms, or for the elderly.

Monitoring

Patients diagnosed with BPPV should be reassessed in 1 month regardless of treatment. Failure to improve warrants further evaluation for other etiologies, including central causes. Similarly, patients with vestibular neuritis should slowly improve over several weeks, and failure to do so suggests alternative diagnoses.

Complications

Patients with BPPV are at increased risk for falls. Thirty percent of elderly patients with BPPV have multiple falls in a year. Thus, patients should be assessed for fall risk, functional mobility, and balance. Home safety evaluation and home supervision should be considered. BPPV often recurs, with an estimated rate of 15% per year. Counseling patients about recurrence can lead to earlier recognition, earlier treatment and avoidance of falls. Patients with vestibular neuritis are at increased risk for BPPV and Ménière's disease. Vestibular neuritis rarely recurs.

---

[1]Not FDA approved for this indication.

References

Baloh RW. Vestibular neuritis. N Engl J Med 2003;348:1027–32.
Bhattacharyya N, Baugh RF, Orvidas L, et al. Clinical practice guideline: Benign paroxysmal positional vertigo. Otolaryngol Head Neck Surg 2008;139:S47–S81.
Chan Y. Differential diagnosis of dizziness. Otolaryngol Head Neck Surg 2009;17:200–3.
Epley JM. The canalith repositioning procedure: For treatment of benign paroxysmal positional vertigo. Otolaryngol Head Neck Surg 1992;107:399–404.
Fishman JM, Burgess C, Waddell A. Corticosteroids for the treatment of idiopathic acute vestibular dysfunction (vestibular neuritis). Cochran Database Syst Rev 2011;5: CD008607. Review.
Goudakos JK, Konstantinos DM, Franco-Vidal V, et al. Corticosteroids in the treatment of vestibular neuritis: A systematic review and meta-analysis. Otol Neurotol 2010;31:183–9.
Hamid M. Medical management of common peripheral vestibular diseases. Curr Opin Otolaryngol Head Neck Surg 2010;18:407–12.
Hillier SL, Holohan V. Vestibular rehabilitation for unilateral peripheral vestibular dysfunction. Cochrane Database Syst Rev 2007;4: CD005397.
Hilton M, Pinder D. The Epley (canalith repositioning) manoeuvre for benign paroxysmal positional vertigo. Cochrane Database Syst Rev 2004;2: CD003162.
Kerber KA. Vertigo and dizziness in the emergency department. Emerg Med Clin North Am 2009;27:39–50.
Leveque M, Labrousse M, Siedermann L, et al. Surgical therapy in intractable benign paroxysmal positional vertigo. Otolaryngol Head Neck Surg 2007;136:693–8.
Newman-Toker DE, Kerber KA, Hsieh YH, et al. HINTS outperforms ABCD2 to screen for stroke in acute continuous vertigo and dizziness. Acad Emerg Med 2013;20(10):986–96.
Seemungal BM, Bronstein AM. A practical approach to acute vertigo. Pract Neurol 2008;8:211–21.

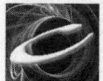

FATIGUE

Method of
Janet C. Lindemann, MD, MBA

CURRENT DIAGNOSIS

- The clinical evaluation of fatigue begins with a thorough medical and psychosocial history.
- Consider monitoring for a month before beginning a laboratory evaluation, because it usually does not yield a diagnosis. Initial evaluation should include a complete blood count (CBC), electrolytes, glucose, liver and kidney function tests, thyroid function tests, and urinalysis.
- Among the many possible causes of fatigue, the most common include depression, environmental stress, anemia, and diabetes. In many cases, a cause is not determined.

CURRENT THERAPY

- Any underlying cause discovered in the history, examination, or laboratory evaluation should be treated.
- If depression, anxiety, or environmental stress is suspected, early assessment and treatment is important.
- Symptom relief includes exercise, regular sleep habits, family discussion about the impact of fatigue, and a symptom and sleep diary.

Epidemiology

Fatigue or tiredness is a common complaint in the general population, representing the chief complaint in nearly 10% of patients presenting to a primary care physician and reported as a symptom in 21% of all patient encounters. While acute, prolonged, and chronic fatigue are relatively common, chronic fatigue syndrome is relatively rare.

Risk Factors

Risk factors for fatigue in adolescence include having depressive symptoms, being highly sedentary, and, conversely, being highly physically active. In adults, risk factors include age over 65 years, presence of one or more chronic medical conditions, and female gender. Precipitating factors include physical stresses such as infectious mononucleosis and psychological stresses such as job-related problems. Perpetuating factors include physical inactivity, emotional disorders, and disturbances of sleep.

Prevention

Because physical inactivity, psychological stress, and lack of sleep are predisposing and perpetuating factors for fatigue, it is helpful to advise patients about stress reduction, regular exercise, and proper sleep habits.

Clinical Manifestations

Fatigue is characterized by general malaise, vague physical discomfort, and an inability to perform routine activities. Acute fatigue is short-lived and generally attributable to physical exertion or an acute illness. Prolonged fatigue is defined as self-reported, persistent fatigue lasting 1 month or longer, whereas chronic fatigue is defined as similar symptoms lasting 6 months or more.

Diagnosis

The clinical evaluation begins with a thorough medical and psychosocial history. It is important to allow the patient to speak uninterrupted for the first minute or two of the interview, because this often provides pertinent clues. The history should include exploration of all medically unexplained symptoms, inquiry into work and life stressor issues, questions regarding alcohol and other substance use, and the current use of prescription, over-the-counter, and alternative therapies. A mental status examination and screening for depression and anxiety should follow. The Beck Depression Inventory or SIG-E-CAPS mnemonic (Sleep, Interest, Guilt, Energy, Concentration, Appetite, Psychomotor retardation, Suicidal) are useful screening tools. The challenge with the diagnostic workup for fatigue is that most laboratory tests do not yield a significant diagnosis. Repeated studies show that only about 15% of patients in primary care settings will have an organic cause for their fatigue (Harrison, Ponka), and laboratory results affect management in as little as 5% of patients (Rosenthal). The following recommendations for the laboratory investigation of fatigue are adapted from guidelines developed by Dutch, Canadian, and Australian general practice groups (Harrison):

- Consider monitoring for a month after initial presentation, while initiating conservative management.
- CBC, electrolytes, glucose, liver and kidney function tests, thyroid function tests, urinalysis.
- Clues from the history and examination may indicate the need for erythrocyte sedimentation rate, monospot, antinuclear antigen testing, or chest radiography.

Differential Diagnosis

The common causes of fatigue are represented in the mnemonic DEAD TIRED (Box 1). Depression, environmental factors such as lifestyle, anxiety, and anemia are among the most common causes of fatigue. Diabetes and other endocrine disorders, including thyroid disease, should be considered, as well as an undiscovered tumor. Many infections, especially those of viral origin, cause fatigue, as well as insomnia and sleep disorders such as obstructive sleep apnea. Rheumatologic disorders, such as rheumatoid arthritis, systemic lupus erythematosus, and fibromyalgia, are often accompanied by fatigue. Endocarditis, while rare, is a must-not-miss diagnosis, as are other cardiac conditions such as coronary artery disease. Finally, drugs, either prescription or of personal use or abuse, should be considered.

Chronic fatigue syndrome is a specific clinical diagnosis characterized by unexplained persistent or relapsing fatigue, not relieved by rest, that substantially limits daily activity. In addition, there must be at least four of the following: memory or concentration impairment, sore throat, tender cervical or axillary lymph nodes, muscle pain, multijoint pain without swelling or tenderness, new headaches, unrefreshing sleep, or postexertional malaise lasting more than 24 hours.

Treatment

The treatment of fatigue begins with acknowledging the patient's concern and providing reassurance and information about the natural course and most frequent causes of fatigue. Any underlying cause discovered in the history, examination, or laboratory evaluation should be treated. If depression, anxiety, or environmental stress is suspected, early assessment and treatment is important. In fatigue that remains unexplained, therapy should emphasize symptom relief and include exercise, regular sleep habits, family discussion about the impact of fatigue, and a symptom and sleep

diary. These same therapies, along with cognitive behavioral therapy, have been shown to have moderate benefit in chronic fatigue syndrome.

Monitoring

Ongoing fatigue can be monitored through a three question assessment:

- Are you experiencing fatigue?
- If so, how severe has it been, on average, during the past week? (0–3 is mild fatigue, 4–6 moderate, and 7–10 severe)
- How does fatigue interfere with your ability to function?

References

Beck A, Ward C, Mendelson M, et al. An inventory for measuring depression. Arch Gen Psychiatry 1961;4:561.

Gialamas A, Beilby JJ, Pratt NL, et al. Investigating tiredness in Australian general practice. Aust Fam Physician 2003;32:663.

Harrison M. Pathology testing in the tired patient: a rational approach. Aust Fam Physician 2008;37:908.

Poluri A, Mores J, Cook DB, et al. Fatigue in the elderly population. Phys Med Rehabil Clin N Am 2005;16:91.

Ponka D, Kirlew M. Top 10 differential diagnoses in family medicine: Fatigue. Can Fam Physician 2007;53:892.

Rosenthal TC, Majeroni BA, Pretorius R, Malik K. Fatigue: An overview. Am Fam Physician 2008;78:1173.

Sharpe M, Wilks D. Fatigue. BMJ 2002;325:480.

Viner RM, Clark C, Taylor SJ, et al. Longitudinal risk factors for persistent fatigue in adolescents. Arch Pediatr Adolesc Med 2008;162:469.

FEVER

Method of
Alan R. Roth, DO; and Gina M. Basello, DO

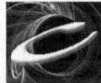

CURRENT DIAGNOSIS

- Fever is one of the most common clinical presentations encountered in primary care.
- Numerous endogenous and exogenous factors play a role in determining body temperature. Current standards define *fever* as an oral temperature of ≥ 100.4 °F (≥ 38 °C).
- Though temperature varies with measurement technique, in clinical practice, most recommendations refer to oral, rectal, and axillary temperature measurements, with rectal temperature being the standard of care in infants and young children.
- With improvement in modern techniques, tympanic thermometers are commonly used due to parental convenience and ease of use along with improved accuracy. They should not be used in young children.
- Fever is not an illness. It is the body's physiologic response to a disease process and has beneficial effects in fighting infection.
- All neonates with a fever should be admitted to the hospital for a full sepsis evaluation. For infants between 1 and 3 months of age, evidence-based guidelines, along with clinical evaluation, determine the diagnostic and therapeutic approach.
- *Fever of unknown origin* (FUO) is defined as a temperature greater than 100.9 °F (38.3 °C) for longer than 3 weeks with no identified cause after 3 days of hospitalization or three outpatient visits.
- FUO requires a systematic, thoughtful, and thorough evaluation based on the age of the patient and the existing clinical evidence, with repeated clinical assessments being essential.
- Hyperthermia is an unregulated, significant elevation of core body temperature above the normal diurnal range due to failure of thermoregulation from a hypothalamic insult, not a pyogenic source, and is considered a medical emergency. It is not synonymous with fever and often requires immediate intervention to avoid deleterious central nervous system (CNS) effects.

Box 1	Common Causes of Fatigue: DEAD TIRED		
D	Depression	T	Thyroid, Tumors
E	Environment/lifestyle	I	Infection, Insomnia
A	Anxiety, Anemia	R	Rheumatologic
D	Diabetes/endocrine	E	Endocarditis/cardiovascular
		D	Drugs (medications or substance abuse)

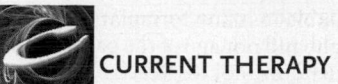

CURRENT THERAPY

- Treating a fever significantly increases the patient's level of comfort, activity, and oral feeding and fluid intake, in addition to decreasing the body temperature.
- Multiple randomized, controlled trials reveal that treating fever does not shorten or prolong the overall duration of illness or reduce the occurrence of febrile seizures.
- Many clinical recommendations state that a temperature less than 102.2 °F (39 °C) in healthy children does not require treatment. Antipyretics are known to provide comfort to children and their caregivers.
- Antipyretic treatment for children includes acetaminophen (Tylenol) 10 to 15 mg/kg every 4 to 6 hours or ibuprofen (Advil, Motrin) 10 mg/kg every 6 hours.
- Ibuprofen and acetaminophen have both been shown to reduce fever effectively and safely. Combination therapy has been shown in some studies to have an added benefit in both reduction of temperature and comfort without an increase in side effects, though caution should be taken to avoid dosing errors.
- Antipyretic therapy for adults and adolescents includes acetaminophen 650 to 1000 mg orally (PO) every 6 hours to a maximum of 3 g per day, ibuprofen 200 to 400 mg PO every 6 hours, or aspirin (ASA) 325 to 650 mg every 6 hours as needed (PRN) for fever.
- ASA should not be used in children due to the risk of Reye's syndrome.
- Sponge bathing should be done with tepid water and no alcohol. Recommendation: sponge bathing and other home remedies should not be used as sole treatment.

Fever is one of the most common clinical presentations encountered by primary care physicians and the most common complaint of acute visits for children in the ambulatory or emergency department setting. Fever is a symptom and one of the most reliable signs of illness rather than a disease process itself. Most causes of fever are secondary to acute viral illnesses such as upper respiratory infections (URIs), which account for 50 million visits to primary care providers annually. Less commonly, bacterial infections may cause pharyngitis, otitis, sinusitis, pneumonia, and urinary tract infections (UTIs). A cost-effective, evidence-based approach using clinical protocols, guidelines, and consensus recommendations to the diagnosis and management of febrile illness, including the appropriate use of antibiotic therapy, is the cornerstone of quality medical care for this presentation. Fever produces significant anxiety for patients, parents, and health care providers, which can lead to overtreatment. Typically, fever is transient and only requires treatment to provide patient comfort.

Definitions

The definition of fever is dependent on numerous endogenous and exogenous factors that play a role in determining body temperature, including age, time of day, site, and measuring device, as well as operator variables. Fever is an elevation of body temperature due to the adjustment of the hypothalamic-pituitary set point. This usually occurs in response to a pathologic stimulus. Fever is a beneficial physiologic mechanism that helps to promote an augmented immunologic response.

Despite individual variability, core body temperature is maintained at about 98.6 °F (37 °C). Diurnal variation results in lower body temperatures in the early morning and a temperature higher in the late afternoon or early evening, which is consistent with what is encountered in clinical practice.

In adults, a morning oral temperature of 98.9 °F (37.2 °C) or higher, or an evening temperature of 99.9 °F (37.7 °C) or higher defines a fever. Rectal temperatures are generally considered to be 0.7 °F (0.4 °C) higher than oral readings.

In infants and young children, rectal temperatures are still considered the standard of care and a rectal temperature greater than 100.4 °F (38 °C) is considered a fever.

Axillary temperatures of greater than 98.6 °F (37 °C) are regarded as a fever, though this measurement site is generally considered less accurate. An accurate measurement of body temperature is dependent on site, measuring device, and the clinical skills of the operator. Site selection should be determined by the age of the patient.

Young infants and older adults often have a diminished febrile response due to physiologic factors, thereby warranting the use of other clinical factors to guide diagnosis.

Recent technologic advances, including electronic devices, tympanic membrane scanning, and temporal artery scanning, have replaced the older mercury-in-glass thermometers. These devices offer faster results and minimal inconvenience to the patient and are becoming increasingly reliable. Chemical content or liquid crystal thermometers applied to the skin are neither accurate nor cost-effective.

Hyperthermia is an uncontrolled elevation of core body temperature that exceeds the body's ability to lose heat. In hyperthermia, the setting of the hypothalamic thermoregulatory center is unchanged, in contrast to fever. Hyperthermia requires urgent medical intervention because it could be rapidly fatal and does not respond to antipyretics. Common etiologies include heat stroke, neuromalignant syndrome, serotonin syndrome, malignant hyperthermia, endocrinopathy, and CNS damage.

Classic *fever of unknown origin* (FUO) is defined as a disorder with temperatures ≥ 100.9 °F (38.3 °C) that have persisted for at least 3 weeks, with no definitive cause elucidated after initial comprehensive inpatient or outpatient workup. The etiologies of FUO generally fall into four diagnostic categories: infectious, autoimmune or inflammatory, neoplastic, and miscellaneous.

Pathophysiology

Fever occurs as part of an inflammatory response to an inciting stimulus. The response includes the production of various cytokines that ultimately increase the production of prostaglandin E_2 (PGE_2), which resets the hypothalamic thermoregulatory set point at a higher level. Important pyogenic cytokines include interleukin-1 (IL-1), interleukin-6 (IL-6), tumor necrosis factor α (TNF-α), interferon-β (IFN-β), and interferon-γ (IFN-γ).

Risks and Benefits of Fever

Fever is known to enhance the immunologic response while suppressing the growth and replication of bacterial and viral infections. Though often uncomfortable for patients, caregivers, and health care providers, evidence supports the notion that fever is beneficial and ultimately protects against the development of asthma and other allergic disorders. In most instances, fever is not harmful. It does increase cardiac demand and metabolic needs, resulting in the common associated signs and symptoms of tachycardia, tachypnea, shivering, malaise, and diaphoresis.

The use of antipyretic agents has not been shown to either prolong or shorten the duration of illness. Febrile seizures cause significant anxiety for parents. They occur most commonly in children between the ages of 6 months and 6 years. Most febrile seizures are uncomplicated and have not been shown to be associated with significant bacteremia or to lead to the development of seizure disorder in older children. Antipyretic agents have not been shown to decrease the incidence of febrile seizures.

Diagnostic Evaluation of Fever

In most cases, the etiology of a febrile illness is a self-limiting viral infection. From 5% to 10% of fevers may be associated with a more serious bacterial infection such as pneumonia, UTI, bacteremia, meningitis, or bone and joint infections. At times, these conditions may be challenging to distinguish, and a thoughtful, systematic, evidence-based approach to the diagnostic evaluation will be most cost-effective while avoiding the inappropriate use of antibiotics.

All infants less than 28 days old with a fever should be admitted to the hospital for a full sepsis workup and empiric intravenous antibiotic therapy.

Young infants, 1 to 3 months of age, with a febrile illness can be especially challenging. Numerous studies addressing this challenging population have led to the development of multiple guidelines and clinical protocols that utilize risk stratification criteria. The use of these age-specific stratification criteria, along with clinical treatment guidelines, helps guide the clinician in the evaluation of febrile illness. Clinical judgment remains the cornerstone of good clinical care.

With the widespread use of *Haemophilus influenzae* type B (Hib) and pneumococcal vaccinations, the incidence of bacteremic illness has decreased significantly. Clinical judgment and a comprehensive assessment are required to guide appropriate diagnostic and therapeutic interventions. The increased use of rapid viral testing in the office and emergency department settings may alleviate the need for more invasive testing and antibiotic use because the risk of concurrent bacterial infection has been reported to be negligible.

In this age group, an initial workup that reveals a white blood cell (WBC) count of less than 5000 or greater than 15,000 indicates an increased likelihood of a significant bacterial illness (SBI). Blood cultures, urinalysis, urine culture, and cerebrospinal fluid (CSF) evaluation should then be obtained and accompanied by intravenous antibiotic therapy. Elevated C-reactive protein (CRP) or procalcitonin levels have also been associated with SBI in children with a febrile illness and have shown increased specificity and sensitivity when compared to the WBC count. Using a combination of these tests has not been proven to be beneficial.

Children age 3 to 36 months, who appear well and do not have any underlying medical history, require only a comprehensive clinical evaluation and do not warrant antibiotic therapy or diagnostic testing in most instances. Septic or ill-appearing children need a more aggressive evaluation, including complete blood count (CBC), inflammatory markers, urinalysis, urine culture, blood cultures, and a chest x-ray. High-risk children in this age group require empiric antibiotic therapy, and clinical judgment should guide the decision to hospitalize.

Classic FUO is defined as a disorder with temperatures greater than 100.9 °F (38.3 °C) that has persisted for at least 3 weeks with no clear etiology determined after 3 days of hospital evaluation or three outpatient visits. Common etiologic categories include infectious, neoplastic, inflammatory, and miscellaneous causes, of which drug fever has been shown to be the most prevalent.

The initial approach includes a thorough history, physical examination, and appropriate laboratory testing. The initial choice of imaging should be guided by clinical findings and most commonly includes a chest xray and a CAT scan of the abdomen and pelvis. If the etiology remains elusive, positron emission tomography (PET) scanning or invasive diagnostic testing should then be considered.

Differential Diagnosis

Hyperthermia is an unregulated, significant elevation of core body temperature above the normal diurnal range due to failure of thermoregulation from a hypothalamic insult, not a pyogenic source, and is considered a medical emergency. It is not synonymous with fever and often requires immediate intervention to avoid deleterious CNS effects. Since the hypothalamic set point remains unchanged, antipyretics are ineffective in hyperthermia. The most common etiology is the inability to regulate or dissipate excess body heat. Hyperthermia is a medical emergency that requires immediate treatment to prevent excessive morbidity and mortality.

Treatment

Though controversy exists regarding the necessity of lowering fever, antipyretics have been shown to effectively and safely reduce temperature and improve symptoms with minimal side effects.

Acetaminophen (Tylenol) is available in many formulations. Dosing should be based on body weight and not age of the patient. The dose is 10 to 15 mg/kg every 4 to 6 hours, not to exceed 3 g daily or 2 g in patients with renal or hepatic impairment. Ibuprofen (Advil, Motrin) is a nonsteroidal antiinflammatory drug (NSAID) that has both antiinflammatory and antipyretic effects. Dosing is 10 mg/kg every 6 to 8 hours in children and 200 to 400 mg every 6 hours in adolescents and adults. Ibuprofen is also available in multiple formulations, including a newer intravenous preparation (ibuprofen [Caldolor]) that may be beneficial in oral-intolerant hospitalized patients. Some studies suggest that ibuprofen may be a more effective antipyretic agent than acetaminophen.

In adults, aspirin (ASA) remains a therapeutic alternative for lowering fever at a dose of 325 to 650 mg every 4 to 6 hours. It should not be used in children with a febrile illness due to the risk of Reye's syndrome.

A combination of acetaminophen and ibuprofen in alternating doses has been shown in some studies to have an added benefit in both reduction of temperature and comfort without an increase in side effects, though caution should be taken to avoid dosing errors.

Nonpharmacologic therapies such as sponge bathing with tepid water and other environmental measures to control temperature, including adjusting room temperatures and sipping cool fluids to avoid dehydration, are used commonly and do provide symptom relief and comfort. These measures should never be used as the sole therapy for fever reduction.

References

Cunha BA. Fever of unknown origin: focused diagnostic approach based on clinical clues from the history, physical examination, and laboratory tests. Infect Dis Clin North Am 2007;21:1137–87.

Hernandez D, Nguyen V. Fever in infants <3 months old: what is the current standard? Pract J Pediatr Emerg Med 2011;16:1–15.

Herzog L, Phillips S. Addressing concerns about fever. Clin Pediatr 2011;50:383–90.

Huppler AR, Eickhoff JC, Wald ER. Performance of low-risk criteria in the evaluation of young infants with fever: review of the literature. Pediatrics 2010;125:228.

Jhavier R, Byington C, Klein J, Shapiro E. Management of the non-toxic appearing acutely febrile child: a 21st century approach. J Pediatr 2011;159:181–5.

Makoni M, Mukundan D. Fever. Curr Opin Pediatr 2010;22:100–6.

Roth AR, Basello GM. Fever. In Paulman PM, Harrison JD, Paulman MD, et al (eds): Signs and Symptoms in Family Medicine. Philadelphia: Mosby; 2012, pp 317–26.

Roth AR, Basello GM. Approach to the adult patient with fever of unknown origin. Am Fam Physician 2003;68:2223–8.

Sullivan J, Farrar HC. Clinical report: fever and antipyretic use in children. Pediatrics 2011;127:580–7.

Van den Bruel A, Thompson MJ, Haj-Hassan, et al. Diagnostic value of laboratory tests in identifying serious infections in febrile children; systematic review. BMJ 2011;342:3082.

GASEOUSNESS, INDIGESTION, NAUSEA, AND VOMITING

Method of
Justin Bailey, MD

Nausea is a vague, subjective feeling that vomiting (forceful expulsion of gastric contents) is imminent. Dyspepsia (based on ROME III criteria) can include postprandial fullness, early satiety, epigastric pain, burning, and reflux (return of gastric content to the lower esophagus or mouth, accompanied by a sour taste or "heartburn" sensation). Gaseousness can present with a variety of complaints including belching, bloating, abdominal pain, or flatulence.

Epidemiology

Nausea and vomiting (ICD-9 Code 787.01) is one of the top reasons patients see a primary care provider. Infectious diseases causing nausea and vomiting, gastroenteritis, diarrhea, and dehydration are leading causes of death in developing countries, and of sick days and reduction of employee productivity in the United States. Nausea and vomiting postoperatively and during cancer chemotherapy add significant costs, pain, and discomfort to hospital and ambulatory treatment. Dyspepsia occurs in an estimated 25% of the U.S. population every year, many of whom do not seek care. Gaseousness is ubiquitous in the population and is troubling to a small portion.

Risk Factors

Previous gastrointestinal surgery, certain medications, chemotherapeutic regimens, substance abuse, pregnancy, infectious diseases, medical conditions, and central nervous system disorders increase the risk for nausea and vomiting symptoms. Dyspepsia risk is increased significantly with ingestion of NSAIDs, tobacco use, *H. pylori* infection, obesity, anxiety, somatization, neuroticism, depression, and unemployment. Increased upper gastrointestinal gaseousness can be seen with air swallowing from gum chewing and eating quickly as well as consumption of foods that relax the lower esophageal sphincter (e.g., chocolate, fats, mints). Ingestion of lactose, fructose, sorbitol, undigested starches (e.g., bran) and carbonated beverages can all increase the risk of bloating and flatulence.

Pathophysiology

The pathophysiologic regulation of nausea and vomiting is complex and incompletely understood. Multiple neurotransmitters are involved, including acetylcholine, dopamine, histamine, and serotonin. The therapeutic action of antiemetics is often based on blocking the action of these neurotransmitters. Neurologic regulation of nausea and vomiting involves the chemoreceptor triggers in the fourth ventricle, the nucleus tractus solitarius in the medulla, motor nuclei that control the vomiting reflex, and vagal afferent nerves from the GI tract. The sympathetic and parasympathetic nervous systems are involved in conjunction with the smooth muscle cells and the enteric brain within the wall of the stomach and intestine.

The pathophysiology of dyspepsia is unclear, but probably has multiple causes. Delayed gastric motility can occur in up to 30% of patients with dyspepsia. Additionally, decreased gastric compliance can be seen in dyspeptic patients.

Sensations of lower tract gaseousness result from one of three different mechanisms: excess gas production, abnormal intestinal transit, and increased visceral sensitivity. Gas production caused by carbohydrate maldigestion, (e.g., lactose intolerance, poorly absorbed starches) results in bloating and a sensation of fullness. High-fiber diets, celiac disease, and small intestine bacterial overgrowth can increase gas production. Dysmotility associated with diabetes mellitus, scleroderma, amyloidosis, and endocrine disease may result in gastroparesis and chronic intestinal pseudo-obstruction. Additionally, previous Nissen fundoplication, fat intolerance, and various familial conditions may cause dysmotility. Increased visceral sensitivity is thought to be a main cause of pain and fullness in patients with functional bowel disorders such as irritable bowel syndrome (IBS) and functional dyspepsia.

Prevention

Once the diagnosis has been established, appropriate treatment of the underlying cause of the symptoms can be instituted. When the cause of nausea and vomiting is related to medication, the dose can be adjusted or the medication changed as appropriate.

Upper GI bloating and fullness is almost exclusively caused by excess air swallow and can be improved with altering behaviors such as gulping food and gum chewing. Lower GI symptoms can be prevented by avoiding problem foods such as milk products in patients with lactose intolerance.

Clinical Manifestations

Nausea and vomiting are extremely common and are associated with many conditions. Associated symptoms are helpful in sorting out causes. Many common historical associations are listed in Table 1.

The diagnosis of dyspepsia is based mainly on clinical symptoms. The Rome III criteria are listed in the opening paragraph.

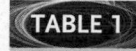

TABLE 1 Key Symptoms and Differential Vomiting, Dyspepsia, and Bloating

SYMPTOMS	DIFFERENTIAL
Abdominal Pain ± N/V • RUQ • Epigastric • RLQ • LLQ • Pelvic	Organic etiologies • Cholelithiasis, cholecystitis • Dyspepsia, pancreatitis, GERD, gastritis, MI • Appendicitis • Diverticulitis • PID, ovarian torsion, ectopic pregnancy
Abdominal pain + distention + N/V	Bowel obstruction
Abdominal distention associated with foods (lactose, wheat-based products, bran, legumes)	Lactose intolerance Celiac disease Carbohydrate malabsorption, Oligosaccharide fermentation (legumes)
Vomiting several hours after eating + succussion splash + N/V	Gastric obstruction Gastroparesis
Heartburn ± N/V	GERD, dyspepsia
Early morning + N/V	Pregnancy
Feculent vomiting + N/V	Intestinal obstruction Gastrocolic fistula
Vertigo + nystagmus + N/V	Vestibular neuritis
Dental erosions, parotid gland enlargement, lanugo like hair, callus on dorsal surface of hands	Bulimia
Positional N/V	Neurogenic

Abbreviations: GERD = gastroesophageal reflux disease; LLQ = left lower quadrant; MI = myocardial infarction; N/V = nausea and vomiting; PID = pelvic inflammatory disease; RLQ = right lower quadrant; RUQ = right upper quadrant.

Alarm symptoms that should raise suspicions for gastric cancer include unintended weight loss, persistent vomiting, progressive dysphasia, odynophagia, unexplained anemia, iron deficiency, hematemesis, palpable abdominal mass, lymphadenopathy, family history of gastric cancer, previous gastric surgery, or jaundice.

Gaseousness usually presents with abdominal fullness and bloating. Pain associated with the fullness is often relieved with eructation or flatulence (see Table 1).

Diagnosis

The first step in the assessment of patients with abdominal complaints is complete history of the duration of symptoms, the frequency of episodes, work environment, recent travel, household member illness, association of symptoms with certain foods or beverages (i.e., pain relief or worsening with food), and determination of the success or failure of what the patient has tried to alleviate the symptoms, all of which may offer diagnostic clues. Focused inquiries into surgeries, sexual activity, and other elements of a review of symptoms may be helpful. A complete review of medication usage, with particular attention to GI-irritating medications such as NSAIDs and over-the-counter medications, illicit drugs, and herbal products is important. Physical examination and diagnostic work-up can help isolate the cause (Table 2).

In patients with acute (<24 hours) nausea and vomiting, a laboratory workup is often unnecessary. Patients with the most commonly identified acute causes, such as acute gastroenteritis, vestibular neuritis, chemotherapy, medication, and alcohol ingestion, and those who are postoperative, can be started on symptomatic therapy. For persistent symptoms of nausea and vomiting, laboratory workup is guided by the history and physical examination and can include a complete blood count and differential, serum chemistries, renal function, liver function tests, serum

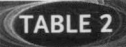

TABLE 2 Physical Examination: Nausea, Vomiting, Dyspepsia, and Gaseousness

FINDINGS	POSSIBLE ETIOLOGY
Fever	Infectious
Tachycardia, hypotension	Dehydration, volume depletion, sepsis (infectious), ectopic pregnancy, myocardial infarction, aortic aneurysm
Exophthalmos	Hyperthyroid
Papilledema	Increased intracranial pressure (tumors, subdural hemorrhage)
Bulging tympanic membrane	Otitis media, effusion
Thyromegaly	Hypothyroid
Lymphadenopathy	Infection, malignancy
Dry mucous membranes	Dehydration, volume depletion
Dental erosions	Bulimia
Abdominal distention	Obstruction, ileus, gastroparesis, irritable bowel, hepatic/spleenic flexure syndrome, postoperative gas-bloat syndrome
Absent bowel sounds	Ileus, perforation
Sense of abdominal distention without bloating	Irritable bowel syndrome
Abdominal bloating	Irritable bowel syndrome, obstruction
RUQ abdominal pain/guarding	Cholecysitis, cholelithiasis
RLQ/LLQ abdominal pain/ guarding	Appendicitis (RLQ), ovarian torsion, diverticulitis, ectopic pregnancy
Cervical motion tenderness	Pelvic inflammatory disease, endometriosis
Bladder tenderness	Urinary tract infection
Testicular pain	Torsion, epididymitis
Abnormal rectal examination	Fecal impaction, prostatitis, appendicitis, ovarian tumor, ectopic pregnancy, endometriosis
Delayed cap refill, poor skin turgor	Dehydration
Jaundice	Gallbladder disease, biliary obstruction

Abbreviations: LLQ = left lower quadrant; RLQ = right lower quadrant; RUQ = right upper quadrant.

protein and albumin, thyroid-stimulating hormone, amylase or lipase, drug screen, and a pregnancy test in women of childbearing age. Imaging should not be routine but should be directed by the history and physical findings as well as pertinent laboratory results. Useful studies may include acute abdominal series (chest x-ray, flat and upright views of the abdomen), abdominal computed tomography (CT), and abdominal ultrasound.

Similarly, in patients with dyspeptic symptoms, laboratory tests should be obtained based on the history and physical examination. Many therapies, such as discontinuing offending medications (e.g., NSAIDs) or acid suppression in patients without alarm symptoms, may be started without a laboratory work-up. Blood count chemistries and *H. pylori* testing can be considered if warranted. Alarm symptoms may warrant further imaging or direct visualization with esophagogastroduodenoscopy (EGD).

In gaseousness and bloating, the most sensitive work-up is the history and physical examination. Further work-up should be directed by initial findings. Patients with alarm symptoms such as weight loss, diarrhea, abdominal pain, distention, and anorexia may benefit from a malabsorption work-up including lactose tolerance test, stool fat, ova and parasites, stool culture, *C. difficile,* acute abdominal series, or EGD. A hydrogen breath test may be beneficial in selected patients to assess the relationship between specific foods and symptoms. Other blood work, tests, and imaging, such as CT, magnetic resonance imaging (MRI), and EGD are guided by availability of testing and the history, examination and laboratory findings.

Differential Diagnosis
Tables 3, 4, and 5 summarize the wide differential diagnosis of nausea and vomiting, dyspepsia, and gaseousness.

TABLE 3 Differential Diagnosis for Nausea and Vomiting

Central Nervous System
Multiple sclerosis, tumor, intracranial bleeding, infarction, abscess, meningitis, trauma, labyrinthitis, Ménière's disease, vestibular neuritis, motion sickness
Migraine headaches, seizure disorders

Gastrointestinal Disorders
Appendicitis, gastric bypass, gastroparesis, hepatobiliary disease cholecystitis, hepatitis, neoplasia
Ileus
Crohn's disease, ulcerative colitis
Irritable bowel syndrome
Ischemia: mesenteric, small bowel
Obstruction: scarring/adhesions from previous surgeries, small bowel obstruction, esophageal spasm
Pancreatitis
Peptic ulcer disease: esophagitis, gastritis, gastroesophageal reflux
Peritonitis

Endocrine
Addison's disease, diabetes (ketoacidosis, gastroparesis), hyperthyroidism, hypothyroidism, hyperparathyroidism, hypoparathyroidism, porphyria

Genitourinary
Nephritis, nephrolithiasis, torsion (ovary, testicle), uremia, kidney stone

Infectious Etiologies
Bacterial: *Campylobacter, Salmonella, Shigella,* Enterogenic *E. coli,*
Viral: rotavirus, Influenza
Otitis media: bacterial or viral
Sexually transmitted infection: cervicitis, epididymitis, pelvic inflammatory disease, prostatitis, urethritis; multiple organisms including gonorrhea and chlamydia
Urinary tract infection: lower (cystitis) or upper (pyelonephritis)

Pregnancy
Morning sickness, hyperemesis gravidarum, intrauterine and ectopic pregnancies

Psychiatric
Anorexia, anxiety, bulimia, depression

Medication Related
Acetaminophen (Tylenol)
Acyclovir (Zovirax)
Alcohol Abuse
Antibiotics: azithromycin (Zithromax), sulfasalazine (Azulfidine), erythromycin, metronidazole (Flagyl), sulfonamides (e.g., sulfamethoxazole-trimethoprim [Bactrim]), tetracycline
Antidepressants: Selective serotonin reuptake inhibitors (SSRIs)
Antihypertensives: β-blockers (atenolol [Tenormin], metoprolol [Lopressor]), calcium channel blockers, diuretics (hydrochlorothiazide)
Chemotherapeutic agents: cisplatinum (Cisplatin [Platinol]), cyclophosphamide (Cytoxan), nitrogen mustard (Mustargen), dacarbazine (DTIC-Dome), methotrexate (Trexall), vinblastine (Velban)
Diabetes treatment: metformin (Glucophage), sulfonylureas
Digoxin (Lanoxin)
Ergotamines: dihydroergotamine (Migranal), methysergide (Sansert)[2]
Ferrous gluconate, ferrous sulfate
Gout treatment: allopurinol (Zylprim)
Hormones: estrogen, progesterone and oral and injected contraceptives
Levodopa (L-dopa), carbidopa (Lodosyn)
Nicotine (patch, gum, smokeless tobacco, cigarette/pipe/cigar)
Nonsteroidal antiinflammatory: aspirin, ibuprofen (Motrin), naproxen (Naprosyn)
Opioids: codeine, heroin, hydrocodone, oxycodone, morphine, burprenorphine/naloxone (Suboxone)
Prednisone
Seizure medications: phenobarbital, phenytoin (Dilantin)
Theophylline (Uniphyl)

[2]Not available in the United States.

TABLE 4 Differential Diagnosis of Dyspepsia

Gastrointestinal Disorders	Medications
Functional or nonulcer (most common)	NSAIDs
Peptic ulcer disease	Antibiotics (macrolides and metronidazole)
Gastroesophogeal reflux	Corticosteroids
Gastritis	Digoxin
Pancreatitis	Narcotics
Gastroparesis	Theophylline
Gastric cancer	
Intestinal ischemia	**Respiratory**
Esophageal rupture	Pneumonia
Malabsorption	**Cardiac**
Lactase deficiency	Myocardial ischemia or pericarditis
Celiac	
Infectious	**Musculoskeletal**
Parasite infection	Abdominal hernia
H. pylori	**Psychiatric**
	Physical sexual abuse
Pregnancy	

Abbreviation: NSAIDs = nonsteroidal antiinflammatory drugs.

TABLE 5 Differential Diagnosis of Bloating and Gaseousness

Upper GI	**Gas-Producing Foods**
Air Swallowing	Beans, peas, lentils, broccoli, Brussels sprouts, cauliflower, cabbage, parsnips, leeks, onions, beer, coffee, pork
Small Bowel	
Pneumatosis cystoides intestinalis	
Carbohydrate Malabsorption	**Infectious**
Lactase deficiency	Parasites
Legumes (indigestible oligosaccharides)	Bacterial overgrowth
Fructose malabsorption	**Malabsorption**
Undigested starch (bran)	Celiac
	Crohn's disease
Irritable Bowel Syndrome	

Treatment

Antiemetics, hydration, and dietary changes are the first-line treatments for acute episodes of nausea and vomiting. Controlling the symptoms is often all that is necessary in acute, self-limited bouts of nausea and vomiting symptoms. If patients are dehydrated, oral rehydration can be accomplished by encouraging the patient to take small amounts (6 ounces or less) of cool water or electrolyte solutions on a frequent basis. If patients are unable to accomplish this, parenteral rehydration and antiemetics may be warranted.

Table 6 lists the common antiemetics agents, indications, dosages, side effects, and relative cost of medications.

Location of the cause with directed treatment is most effective for gaseousness. If no cause is found, it can be difficult to treat. Avoiding foods that are contributory, such as those containing lactose, fructose, sorbitol, high fiber, and starches, may be all that is necessary. Symptoms associated with increased sensitivity to normal levels of gas (i.e., IBS) can be difficult to treat. Therapeutic relationships, education, and dietary modification are the mainstays of IBS treatment. For moderate to severe symptoms, short-term treatment with antispasmotics, tricyclic antidepressants, and antidiarrheal agents may have some benefit. Medical treatments for bloating are listed in Table 7.

For most patients with dyspepsia, information can be powerful. Validation of symptoms and working toward a goal of management rather than cure are therapeutic. In patients with dyspepsia in which a concern for *H. pylori* exists, a test-and-treatment strategy can be effective. In other patients, proton pump inhibitors, H-2 receptor antagonists, prokinetic agents, and peppermint oil are all effective short-term therapies.

Monitoring

For patients who have complications related to nausea and vomiting, monitoring serum electrolytes, renal function, nutritional status, and other parameters may be necessary until hydration improves, electrolytes are replaced, and laboratory results and clinical status return to normal.

TABLE 6 Medications for Nausea and Vomiting

DRUG	USE	SIDE EFFECTS	DOSAGE	COST*
Anticholinergics Act as antimuscarinic agents		Sedation, dry mouth, dizziness, hallucinations, confusion, exacerbate narrow angle glaucoma, blurred vision.		
Scopalamine	Nausea associated with motion sickness		1–1.5 mg patch TD q3d	Patches: 4 ct = $60
Antihistamines		Sedation, dry mouth, confusion, urinary retention, blurred vision		
Diphenhydramine (Benadryl)	Nausea associated with motion sickness		50 mg PO q6h or 10–50 mg IV or IM	25-mg capsules: 50 ct = $6
Doxylamine (Aldex)	Nausea associated with pregnancy		5–10 mg PO qd	Capsules: 30 ct = $7
Hydroxyzine (Vistaril)	Nausea associated with motion sickness		25–100 mg q6h	100 mg: 30 ct = $20
Meclizine (Antivert)	Nausea associated with motion sickness		25–50 mg q6h	25 mg: 30 ct = $20
Promethazine (Phenergan)	Nausea associated with motion sickness		12.5–25 mg (PO, IM, IV, PR) q4–6h	50 mg: 30 ct = $22
Benzamides: Prokinetic agents; work on peripheral and central dopamine, weak 5-HT3		Sedation, hypotension, extrapyramidal effects, diarrhea, neuroleptic syndrome, supraventricular tachycardia, CNS depression		
Metoclopramide (Reglan)	2nd-line therapy for chemotherapy-induced nausea		10 mg (PO, IM, IV) q6h	10 mg: 30 ct = $6
Trimethobenzamide (Tigan)	Chemotherapy-induced nausea		250 mg PO q6h	30 ct = $65

Continued

TABLE 6 Medications for Nausea and Vomiting—cont'd

DRUG	USE	SIDE EFFECTS	DOSAGE	COST
Butyrophenones: Dopamine antagonists		Sedation, hypotension, extrapyramidal effects, tachycardia, dizziness, QT prolongation and torsades de pointes, neuroleptic malignant syndrome		
Droperidol (Inapsine)			0.625–1.25 mg (IM, IV) q4h	IV and IM only
Haloperidol (Haldol)			0.5–5 mg (PO, IM, IV) q8h	5 mg: 90 ct = $26
Phenothiazines: Dopamine antagonists		Sedation, hypotension, extrapyramidal effects, neuroleptic malignant syndrome, cholestatic jaundice		
Chlorpromazine (Thorazine)	Generalized nausea		10–25 mg (PO, IM, PR) q6h	10 mg: 30 ct = $12
Prochlorperazine (Compazine)	Generalized nausea		10 mg (PO, IM, IV) q6h; 25 mg q12h PR	10 mg: 30 ct = $30
5-Hydroxytryptamine type 3 (5-HT3): Serotonin Antagonists		Fever, constipation, diarrhea, dizziness, sedation, nervousness, altered liver function tests, headache, fatigue		
Dolasetron (Anzemet)	Chemotherapy-induced nausea		100 mg (PO, IV) q24h	100 mg: 5 ct = $360
Granisetron (Kytril)	Chemotherapy-induced nausea		2 mg (PO, IV) q24h	1 mg: 2 ct = $130
Ondansetron (Zofran)	Chemotherapy-induced nausea		4–8 mg (PO, IV) q8-12h	8 mg: 30 ct = $40
Palonosetron (Aloxi)	Prevention of chemotherapy-induced nausea		0.5 mg PO or 0.25 mg IV ×1	0.25 mg: $406
Neurokinin Receptor Antagonists Aprepitant capsule (Emend)	Prevention of postoperative nausea and vomiting (PO)	Headache, site reaction	40 mg PO × 1 prior to anesthesia	40 mg cap #1: $40
Fosaprepitant (Emend)	Prevention of chemotherapy-induced nausea		115 mg IV × 1, 125 mg PO ×1	115 mg: $223
Steroids		GI upset, anxiety, euphoria, flushing, insomnia		
Dexamethasone (Decadron)	Prophylaxis of chemotherapy-related nausea and vomiting		4 mg–10 mg (PO, IM, IV) q6–12h	4 mg: 90 ct = $20
Methylprednisolone (Medrol)			40–100 mg (PO, IM, IV) q24h	8 mg: 25 ct = $25
Cannabinoids		Vertigo, xerostomia, hypotension, dysphoria		
Dronabinol (Marinol)	Chronic or chemotherapy-induced nausea and vomiting		5 mg PO q2-4h; 4–6 per day	5 mg: 30 ct = $1200
Miscellaneous Erythromycin SE nausea, abdominal pain	Nausea associated with gastroparesis		250 mg PO q8h × 5–7 d	250 mg: 30 ct = $70
Ginger	Nausea associated with pregnancy		250 mg PO q6h or 1 g qd	250 mg: 60 ct = $8
Pyridoxine (vitamin B6)	Nausea associated with pregnancy (traditionally combined with doxylamine)		10 mg q6h	100 mg: 100 ct = $15

*Cost estimates from www.drugstore.com.

TABLE 7 Medications for Treatment of Gaseousness and Bloating

MEDICATION	INDICATION	DOSE	SIDE EFFECTS/COST
Rifaximin (Xifaxan)	Bloating (flatulence) from suspected bacterial overgrowth	200 mg PO tid × 7 d	Edema, nausea, dizziness, flatulence 200 mg: 30 ct = $355
Probiotics (multi component)	Bloating (flatulence)	Varies by preparation	Varies by preparation
Alpha-galactosidase (Bean-o)	Bloating associated with gas-producing foods	300–1200 mg with meals high in fermentable carbs	300 mg: 100 ct = $10
Simethicone	Bloating (flatulence) (indicated but not found to be effective)	80–120 mg qid prn	80 mg: 100 ct = $5
Bismuth subsalicylate	Odor from flatus	525 mg PO qid prn	525 mg: 15 ct = $5
Odor-neutralizing devices (briefs, pillows)	Odor from flatus	prn	Pillows: ~$25 Briefs: ~$20

Further testing is needed in patients with dyspepsia and alarm symptoms; however, in patients without alarm symptoms, no further testing is needed.

Complications

The complications of prolonged nausea and vomiting are dehydration, electrolyte disturbances (e.g., hypokalemia, hypophosphatemia and hypomagnesemia), depletion of vitamins and trace elements, metabolic alkalosis, and malnutrition. Usually these can be corrected with oral or intravenous hydration, correction of electrolyte deficiencies, and treatment of the underlying cause. In patients whose nausea and vomiting are accompanied by gastroenteritis, symptoms and clinical status may not return to baseline unless all electrolytes such as potassium, magnesium, phosphorus, and trace elements such as zinc are replaced.

Dyspeptic patients without alarm symptoms rarely have complications. In patients with chronic bloating, complications are uncommon.

References

Abraczinskas D. Intestinal gas and bloating, Available http://www.uptodate.com; November, 2013 [accessed 6.24.15].
ACOG Practice Bulletin No. 52: American College of Obstetrics and Gynecology. Nausea and vomiting in pregnancy. Obstet Gynecol 2004;103:803–14.
Bailey J. Effective Management of flatulence. Am Fam Phys 2009;79:1098–100.
Flake ZA, Scalley RD, Bailey AG. Practical selection of antiemetics. Am Fam Phys 2004;69:1169–74.
Hasler WL, Chey WD. Nausea and vomiting. Gastroenterology 2003;125:1860–7.
Kraft R. Nausea and vomiting. In Bope ET, Rakel RE, Kellerman R, (eds): Conn's Current Therapy 2010. Philadelphia, WB Saunders; 2010. pp 5–9.
Longstreth GF. Functional dyspepsia in adults, Available at http://www.uptodate.com; December 2014 [accessed 6.24.15].
Longstreth GF. Approach to the patient with dyspepsia, Available at http://www.uptodate.com; September 2014 [accessed 6.24.15].
Owings S. Gaseousness and Dyspepsia. In Bope ET, Rakel RE, Kellerman R, (eds): Conn's Current Therapy 2010. Philadelphia, WB Saunders; 2010. pp 9–11.
Talley NJ, Vakil NB, Moayyedi P. 2005 American Gastroenterological Association technical review on the evaluation of dyspepsia. Gastroenterology 2005;125:1756–80.

HEADACHE

Method of
R. Michael Gallagher, DO

Interest and understanding of the headache problem has increased during recent years, allowing physicians to help more sufferers. This interest was the result of Food and Drug Administration (FDA) approvals of medications for the treatment of headache and subsequent pharmaceutical company support of medical and community education. Although the more recently approved treatments are limited to migraine, the overall increase in headache awareness of medical professionals has resulted in help for patients afflicted with all types of headache.

- Headache is a disturbing and sometimes fearsome affliction that has plagued humankind throughout recorded history. It often is debilitating and particularly disturbing to the sufferer because the pain is located in the head, the very center of the body's cognitive and control functions. With its accompanying pain and debilitating symptoms, stress can mount and the headache can become all consuming.
- Headache is experienced by all age groups, from young children to the elderly. It is more common than asthma, diabetes, mental illness, and rheumatoid arthritis. In fact, the World Health Organization identifies severe migraine, along with psychosis and quadriplegia, as "one of the most debilitating chronic conditions."

Although the majority of Americans experience tension-type headaches (TTHAs) at some time in their lives, approximately 30 million experience migraine headache: 13% of women and 6% of men, predominantly in their most productive years between the ages of 13 and 55 years. *One out of every four households are affected by migraine headache.* Prepubescent boys and girls suffer equally; however, boys often outgrow their migraine attacks as they mature, and they are less subjected to hormonal influences. Smaller percentages of people, by comparison, suffer with other chronic headaches, such as cluster headache and chronic daily headache.

- No sure diagnostic tests are available to differentiate headache types. The headache condition can progress or change over time in frequency, severity, and debilitation. Each sufferer can be different and may require a detailed evaluation and individualized treatment plan; more frequent or prolonged attacks often necessitate a more comprehensive treatment plan. Thus, the headache problem can be a challenge for both the sufferer and the clinician.
- During the twentieth century, dramatic advancements were made in medicine. Longevity and quality of life improved for many individuals. Unfortunately, for headache sufferers, most of these advances were for maladies that killed or maimed rather than for nonlife-threatening conditions. It was not until the 1960s that even a reasonable preventive medication, propranolol (Inderal), was introduced, and by the 1980s only a handful of medications were available for wide use. Physicians had to improvise with medications and treatments that were originally designated for other medical conditions.

In the late 1980s and 1990s, epidemiologic, psychosocial, and pharmacologic research resulted in an increase in available headache information and treatment possibilities. The development of the triptans, serotonin agonists, brought a new awareness to both physicians and sufferers. Today, seven triptans and two relatively new preventive medications are available. In spite of this, a minority of migraine sufferers use these options, and more than 50% continue to self-treat without benefit of professional care.

In the past, surveys indicated that patients wanted their physician to believe their headache problem was real. They hoped that they would be taken seriously and that the physician would make a sincere attempt to help them. The headache patient has changed. The headache sufferer who seeks treatment today is more knowledgeable and interested in rapid relief and tolerability of medication.

Evaluation and Diagnosis

An accurate diagnosis is essential for effective management of patients with the more commonly encountered headaches. Because no biologic markers or diagnostic tests exist to determine headache type, the history is the single most important element in the evaluation of the headache patient. Various headache types sometimes have similar initial presentations, or patients may suffer with more than one type of headache (e.g., migraine and tension-type headache), which can be confusing at first, but the careful history usually differentiates the headache type. In general, little in the way of diagnostic testing is needed unless a physical cause is suspected. Some physicians prefer to perform simple laboratory tests to establish a baseline for medication toleration and monitoring as necessary (Table 1).

• The headache complaint on occasion can be a sign of a more serious medical condition, such as a tumor, infection, or aneurysm. For this reason, the clinician always must be cautious and diligent in establishing an accurate and timely diagnosis. Certain so-called red flags in the history require immediate attention. These include any complex of symptoms or history that does not fit a typical headache type; report of a significant neurologic deficit; significant or prolonged neurologic deficit with aura; late-onset migraine (in a patient older than 30 years); sudden onset of a new head pain without history of similar headaches; changes in headache character; headache associated with elevated temperature; or completely unresponsive attacks in the absence of analgesic or caffeine overuse. When any of these symptoms are present or physical examination reveals significant findings, further diagnostic evaluation with imaging studies and consultation is imperative.

The appropriate headache patient evaluation includes a thorough history; physical examination with special attention to the head and the neurologic, cardiovascular, and musculoskeletal systems; and diagnostic tests when appropriate. The history should include headache onset, location, pain character (e.g., pressure, throb), frequency, duration, associated symptoms, aura or prodrome, triggers, previous treatment, and family history. Certain clues in the history may lean toward the diagnosis of migraine, such as motion sickness; absence of headache during pregnancy; and headache relationship to menses, sun glare, oversleep, fatigue, fasting, foods, or alcohol.

Various diagnostic screening questionnaires and tools have been developed over the years to assist busy clinicians in establishing the diagnosis of migraine. Most are long and cumbersome and do not easily become a part of routine patient evaluation. A simple three-question screener for migraine is helpful for generalist clinicians. A "yes" answer to all three questions indicates a strong possibility of the migraine diagnosis:

1. Do you experience headaches severe enough to see a physician?
2. Are your headaches accompanied by other symptoms?
3. Are your headaches intermittent (i.e., nondaily)?

Note: This screener should not be substituted for a complete history; it should be used only for screening purposes.

Tension-Type Headache

Tension-type headache (TTHA) is the most common of headaches and first was believed to be caused by sustained muscle contraction of the neck, jaw, scalp, or facial muscles. However, consideration is being given to the possibility that sustained muscle contraction can, in fact, be an epiphenomenon to possible central disturbances rather than a primary process. Evidence suggests that altered levels of serotonin, substance P, and neuropeptide Y in the serum or platelets of patients with TTHA are responsible.

• TTHA is characterized by intermittent or persisting bilateral pain, usually described as a squeezing pressure or a band-like sensation around the head. Most patients experience their symptoms in the frontal, temporal, or occipital areas of the head. Location frequently varies with the attack, and tightness of the neck and shoulders is common. Intensity varies greatly. The attacks can last from hours to days, and in some extreme cases they may last for months. Aura, nausea, photophobia and phonophobia, and incapacitation are not typically associated with TTHA.

Many TTHA sufferers easily recognize the origin of their attacks. TTHA typically results from emotional upset, periods of stress, and major life changes. Anxiousness, poor adaptation skills, and anxiety and depression often are present. Physical causes, such as degenerative joint disease, trauma to the head or neck, awkward neck position, poor posture, temporomandibular joint dysfunction, bruxism, or heavy chewing also can precipitate attacks. Persons older than 50 years are prone to excessive muscle contraction because of arthritis of the neck and jaw, poor posture, or stress. TTHA that is consistently precipitated by tension or pathology of the neck frequently is referred to as a cervicogenic headache. In contrast to migraine headache, TTHA is more likely to begin in later life.

Migraine Headache

Migraine headache is a familial disease characterized by unilateral or bilateral paroxysmal headache lasting hours to days. Adult women experience attacks more than men by a ratio of 3:1. Children and the elderly experience migraine equally. Attacks occur from as infrequently as one or two per year to several times weekly. Associated symptoms usually occur and frequently include throbbing, nausea, vomiting, photophobia, phonophobia, fluid retention, and mood changes.

The two basic types of migraine headache are migraine with aura (previously called classic migraine) and migraine without aura (previously called common migraine). Migraine with aura is preceded by an aura, a transient neurologic symptom that usually is visual, such as scotoma, teichopsia, tunnel vision, or visual field deficit, lasting 5 to 30 minutes. However, aura can manifest as

TABLE 1	Current Diagnosis		
TYPE	**SYMPTOMS**	**FREQUENCY**	**DURATION**
Tension type	Bilateral variable pain Squeezing or band-like Tightness of neck and shoulders	Variable Recognizable cause	Hours to days
Migraine	Mostly unilateral Throbbing or constant pain Nausea, vomiting Photophobia/ phonophobia Fluid disturbances Mood changes Incapacitating Can be associated with aura	1–4/mo Can be cyclic	Hours to days
Cluster	Unilateral, severe boring or burning pain Ipsilateral lacrimation Scleral injection, eyelid droop Rhinorrhea Restlessness	Multiple daily or near daily	45–90 min Cycles of attacks
Chronic daily	Dull, whole headed Variable	Daily	Months

any neurologic deficit. Migraine without aura is more commonly experienced and comes on gradually or is present on awakening from sleep. In some patients, these headaches are associated with a nonspecific prolonged prodrome, such as mood changes, food cravings, or fluid retention hours before the pain.

The underlying cause of migraine headache is not clearly established, and various theories are proposed. Migraine appears to be of genetic origin and to be an inflammatory disease that causes disturbances in serotonin use and activity. Strong evidence indicates that the migrainous attack originates in the central nervous system by stimulation of the locus ceruleus and dorsal raphe nuclei. Resultant changes alter cerebral and extracranial blood flow; activate the trigeminovascular system; and cause vascular dilation, neurogenic inflammation, and pain. Various precipitants are known, and many sufferers report that migraine attacks frequently are associated with menstruation or are triggered by foods containing vasoactive amines, strong odors, too much or too little sleep, sun glare, stress, altitude, weather changes, exertion, or fasting (Boxes 1 and 2).

Some physicians classify migraine according to its precipitant or description (e.g., menstrual migraine, exertional migraine, coital migraine, cervicogenic migraine, cyclic migraine, "painless" or acephalic migraine). When a sufferer experiences headache for 50% of the month, it is referred to as chronic migraine. Regardless, the fundamentals of evaluation and treatment are similar.

Cluster Headache

The cause of cluster headache is unknown, and little credible research is available. Various possibilities or theories are suggested and include, but are not limited to, disturbances in histamine production or use; hypothalamic biorhythm dysfunction; or serotonin and neurotransmitter mechanisms similar to those of migraine.

Box 1	Common Migraine Dietary Triggers

- Dairy: ripened cheese (cheddar, brie, camembert), sour cream >½ cup
- Meats: processed lunch meats, hot dogs, sausage, bologna, salami, chicken liver
- Fish: pickled or dried herring
- Grains: sourdough bread
- Fruits: bananas, raisins, figs, avocado, citrus >½ cup
- Vegetables: broad and fava beans, onions, snow peas, garlic
- Other: chocolate, nuts, peanut butter, pickled foods, most Chinese food
- Beverages: most wines and alcohol, caffeine >200 mg
- Additives: MSG, soy sauce, meat tenderizers, aspartame, sulfites

---

Box 2	Migraine Triggers

- Altitude
- Alcohol
- Caffeine withdrawal
- Fluorescent or flickering lights
- Sun glare
- Weather changes
- Stress, stress letdown
- Foods
- Skipping meals
- Smoky environment
- Noisy environment
- Strong odors

Some authorities consider cluster headache one of the most severe pain conditions known to humankind.

- Cluster headache predominantly affects men, with a male-to-female ratio of 6:1. It occurs in well under 0.5% of the population. Onset later in life (after age 30 years) is common, and patients sometimes report head injury or a traumatic event occurring months before onset. Attacks occur on a daily or near-daily basis for weeks or months at a time and mysteriously disappear for months to years regardless of treatment, only to recur and cycle again. Although nonspecialist physicians only occasionally encounter the patient with cluster headaches, it is important to consider cluster headaches in the differential diagnosis.

The typical patient with a cluster headache experiences relatively brief attacks (45–90 minutes) of horrible unilateral head pain associated with ipsilateral lacrimation, scleral injection, rhinorrhea, or eyelid droop. The hallmark of the syndrome is its associated symptoms and its severe and intense pain. During attacks, most cluster patients move about, trying unsuccessfully to get more comfortable, similar to renal colic; this is in contrast to migraine sufferers, who prefer to lie quietly in a dark quiet room. Few triggers are identified, and alcohol almost always precipitates an attack during a cluster "on" cycle. A rare form of cluster headache, chronic cluster, does not cycle and continues on a daily or *near-daily* basis without cessation.

Chronic Daily Headache

A small percentage of headache sufferers present with chronic daily headache. The majority of these daily headaches are of the tension or migraine type. However, patients may present with daily nonincapacitating generalized headache. These headaches frequently are associated with major life changes (negative or positive), financial or relationship difficulties, and depression or emotional problems.

The assessment of the chronic daily headache patient is similar to other headache syndromes, but may require particular attention to mental health and medication rebounding issues.

Posttraumatic Headache

Posttraumatic headaches are headaches resulting from physical injury to the head. The trauma can be direct or the result of a contra-coux type injury encountered with whiplash or forced movement of the head or neck. The degree of injury and headache is not necessarily related to the degree of trauma. Seemingly minor injuries sometimes can result in significant and prolonged headache while apparent severe blows to the head sometimes do not result in significant headache.

Complicating the posttraumatic headache can be an associated spasm of shoulder, neck, and scalp muscles or reactive anxiety and depression. Patients with preexisting headaches may experience an increase in severity or frequency of headaches. It is not unusual for there to be a delay in the onset of headache.

It is imperative that the detailed evaluation of the posttraumatic headache patient include psychological and cognitive examination while keeping in mind that presumed trivial injuries can have significant sequela. The more frequent type of headache encountered is of the tension or chronic daily type. Migraine and cluster are reported.

Treatment

The doctor-patient relationship frequently is the key to successful treatment in the headache patient. Although to some this statement seems an obvious truism, its importance cannot be overemphasized.

Patients who experience frequent, near daily, or daily headaches invariably require a comprehensive treatment program that necessitates good communication. Anxious patients sometimes do not comprehend medical explanations or instructions; busy doctors sometimes do not have or take the time to ensure that the patient understands.

The two elements of headache treatment are abortive treatment, directed at attacks once they have begun, and prophylactic treatment, directed at preventing or reducing the frequency of attacks. In general, the abortive approach is used for patients who suffer infrequent attacks and for those who experience breakthrough attacks while undergoing prophylactic therapy.

Prophylactic therapy should be instituted when headaches are frequent, when headaches are unresponsive to abortive medication, or when there are contraindications to abortive medications.

- Headache treatment can include nonpharmacologic measures, such as physical exercise, stretching, stress avoidance, relaxation exercises, biofeedback, manipulation, massage, or cold/warm packs. Pharmacologic therapies can include a vast array of medicaments from over-the-counter (OTC) drugs to prescription drugs such as triptans, other vasoconstrictors, β-blockers, calcium channel blockers, antiepileptic agents, antidepressants, nonsteroidal anti-inflammatory drugs (NSAIDs), analgesics, muscle relaxants, anxiolytics, and others.

Treatment, whether prophylactic or abortive, should follow a definite plan incorporating the clinician and patient into a team focused on reducing the headache frequency, severity, and disability.

As mentioned earlier, impressions and physical findings should be explained to the patient in as much detail as necessary to ensure the patient's complete understanding. The complexity of the headache condition needs to be explained, emphasizing its chronicity, rather than its curability, and that the goal of treatment is disease control.

- The comprehensiveness of the treatment plan depends on the frequency of the patient's attacks. The more frequent and severe the attacks, the more detailed plan may be necessary. Patients experiencing infrequent attacks (e.g., once or twice monthly) may require only an abortive medication and little else. Patients with more frequent attacks may benefit from dietary restrictions, psychosocial intervention, biofeedback relaxation training, manipulation, and physical modality intervention, in addition to medication (Table 2).

TTHA Treatment

TTHA is often associated with emotional stress and muscle strain or tension of the shoulders and neck. Simple self-administered measures, such as stress avoidance, stretching, warm packs, or relaxation techniques, can be helpful in reducing or relieving attacks. More comprehensive professional intervention, such as manual manipulation, physical therapy, local injections, or biofeedback training, is a consideration for more frequent or severe cases. The ultimate goal is to restore normal function of involved muscles.

- Prophylactically, the use of OTC or prescription medications can be considered in addition to nonmedicinal measures for reducing the frequency and duration of attacks. NSAIDs, muscle relaxants, tricyclic antidepressants (TCA), selective serotonin reuptake inhibitors (SSRI), at the lowest effective doses, are more commonly used. Other categories of antidepressants are reported to be effective in some sufferers.
- Daily use of the longer-acting NSAIDs, such as naproxen[1] (Naprosyn) or celecoxib[1] (Celebrex), in the appropriately screened patient over a 2- to 3-week period, can be an effective preventative.

TCAs, such as nortriptyline[1] (Pamelor) or amitriptyline[1] (Elavil), in low doses at night over 1 to 3 months, are frequently effective, especially in patients with anxiety or mild depression. The SSRI drugs, such as fluoxetine[1] (Prozac) or sertraline[1] (Zoloft), similarly can be useful.

The muscle relaxant cyclobenzaprine[1] (Flexeril), at low doses, with a similar mechanism to the TCAs, can be administered at night for limited periods. Other muscle relaxants occasionally can be helpful. Potential side effects can limit the use of NSAIDs (gastrointestinal irritation) and the TCAs (fatigue and weight gain).

OnabotulinumtoxinA (Botox)[1] reportedly is helpful in the treatment of the tension-type headache, but controlled studies are limited. In this treatment, a diluted solution of botulinum toxin is injected into various muscles of the face, scalp, neck, or shoulders. It is imperative that these injections be administered by physicians skilled in the procedure to avoid complication and adverse events.

- Abortive or symptomatic treatment of TTHA can include simple OTC medications (e.g., aspirin or acetaminophen), NSAIDs (short acting), muscle relaxants, combination analgesics, and, in rare cases, opioid or opioid-like drugs. Limited studies have shown analgesic qualities of riboflavin (vitamin B_2)[2] 200 mg is recommended for patients who cannot tolerate NSAID type medications. Caution should be exercised in prescribing potentially habituating drugs. Daily or near-daily use of analgesics and especially those containing caffeine, can lead to analgesic rebound headache or medication overuse headache, which can compound the patient's headache problem.

Migraine Treatment

Migraineurs are unique individuals, and the effectiveness and tolerance of medications can vary from patient to patient. Medication changes, combinations of medications, and trial and error may be necessary in the early stages of treatment.

- Nonmedicinal measures for migraine sufferers include biofeedback stress reduction, caffeine and dietary restrictions, regimentation of meals and sleep, rest, exercise, stretching, and avoidance of work or activity overload. Strict limitation of caffeine to less than 200 mg/day is important to prevent caffeine headache (rebound headache) in most patients. Elimination of vasoactive foods, such as chocolate, aged cheese, and processed meats, and avoidance of fasting for more than 4 hours can be helpful for patients with more frequent attacks (see Box 1). Regular exercise and stretching, planned relaxation, regular sleep schedules, and following a healthy lifestyle are frequently included in a comprehensive treatment regimen. In some patients, especially children and adolescents, biofeedback stress reduction or psychotherapeutic intervention may be necessary.

TABLE 2	Current Therapy	
HEADACHE TYPE	**PRN**	**PROPHYLAXIS**
Tension type	OTC drugs NSAIDs Muscle relaxants Combination analgesics	Stress/trigger avoidance Stretching exercises Warm compresses Relaxation exercises Muscle relaxants Antidepressants
Migraine	NSAIDs* Triptans* Ergotamine* Dihydroergotamine (DHE-45)* Isometheptene* Combination analgesics	Biofeedback β-Blockers* Divalproex ER* Topiramate* TCA antidepressants Ca channel blockers
Cluster	Oxygen Triptans DHE-45 Ergotamine	No alcohol Ca channel blockers Divalproex NSAIDs Lithium Steroids

*FDA indication.
Abbreviations: NSAID = nonsteroidal anti-inflammatory drug; OTC = over-the-counter drug; TCA = tricyclic antidepressant.

[1]Not FDA approved for this indication.
[2]Not available in the United States.

- The more commonly used medications for prophylaxis are β-blockers, calcium channel blockers, antiepileptics (neurostabilizers), and the antidepressants. Treatment should be continued for a 6- to 8-week trial before discontinuation for ineffectiveness. The determination of which medication to use depends on comorbidities, interactions with concomitant medications, and tolerability.

β-Blockers such as propranolol and timolol (Blocadren) are nonselective and are approved by the FDA for migraine prevention. Other β-blockers, such as nadolol[1] (Corgard), metoprolol[1] (Lopressor), and atenolol[1] (Tenormin), also can be effective. The mechanism of action in migraine is not wholly understood, but it is thought to involve anxiolytic effects and vascular changes and stabilization. The usual dosage is recommended (e.g., timolol 10–30 mg/day, propranolol 120–160 mg/day), and many consider the nighttime dose the more significant.

Calcium channel antagonists are well tolerated in general and can be effective in many patients. They are believed to alter serotonin release and inhibit platelet serotonin uptake and release within the brain. Verapamil[1] (Calan) is considered the more effective and is commonly recommended to patients. Dosage can vary from 120 to 480 mg/day. Nimodipine[1] (Nimotop) is equally effective, but has been rarely used in the United States because of its high cost.

- Antiepileptic medications such as phenytoin[1] (Dilantin) and carbamazepine[1] (Tegretol) have been prescribed for migraine prevention over the years, with mixed results. Their use is now limited with the advent of newer, more easily tolerated agents, such as divalproex sodium (Depakote ER) and topiramate (Topamax).
- Divalproex sodium is effective in reducing migraine attacks and is particularly useful in patients with coexisting head injury, seizure disorders, and bipolar disorders. It is thought to improve inhibitory and excitatory amino acid imbalance in the brain. It is best to start with a lower dose and to gradually increase as needed and tolerated. The dosage of 500 to 1000 mg/day is more frequently prescribed. A commonly experienced side effect is sedation, which can sometimes be used to the patient's advantage when anxiolytic effects are needed.
- Topiramate is a preventive medication approved by the FDA for migraine prophylaxis. It has multiple mechanisms of action, but its exact mechanism in migraine headache is unknown.

Its effectiveness is believed to involve sodium ion channel stabilization, calcium ion channels, GABA (γ-aminobutyric acid) receptors, and neuronal membrane stabilization. The average daily dose is variable and ranges from 30 to 100 mg/day. A most unusual side effect of weight loss or appetite suppression can be used to the patient's advantage in preventing weight gain, which frequently accompanies migraine prophylactic medications.

The TCAs can be useful for patients who experience frequent attacks and for those who experience anxiety and depression. The TCAs inhibit synaptic reuptake of serotonin, thereby reducing neuron firing and release of neurotransmitters. Starting with a low dose in the evening and titrating up to efficacy and tolerability is recommended. Significant anticholinergic and sedation effects sometimes limit their use. The SSRIs are reported helpful in some patients, but their use in migraine prevention is limited.

Other medications have been utilized in migraine prophylaxis with varying success. These include NSAID's, cyproheptadine (Periactin),[1] clonidine (Catapres),[1] phenothiazines, anxiolytics, ergotamine (Ergomar), magnesium,[1] feverfew,[2] and others.

- In general, prophylactic medications should be taken for 6 to 8 weeks to determine efficacy. If effective, a course of 4 to 6 months is recommended before an attempt is made to discontinue medication.
- OnabotulinumtoxinA has been approved by the FDA for the treatment of chronic migraine. Multiple injections to the head and neck can be helpful for patients who experience symptoms for more than 14 days per month and it can be repeated after 3 months.

[1]Not FDA approved for this indication.
[2]Not available in the United States.

Because this treatment is administered by physicians in headache specialty and pain practices, simultaneous comprehensive treatment measures and medication can contribute to positive patient results. Side effects are relatively low when injected by experienced physicians; alteration of facial expressions is the most common. Proper administration of the toxin is imperative.

A large meta-analysis of 27 controlled clinical trials concluded that onabotulinumtoxinA injections showed a small to moderate benefit over placebo in patients experiencing chronic migraine and chronic daily headache. Patients with chronic tension type or episodic migraine showed no benefit.

- A trigeminal nerve stimulator, Cefaly device, was approved by the FDA in 2014. The Cefaly head-band apparatus can be self administered 20 minutes daily to reduce migraine frequency. Experience with this TENS device is limited.
- A variety of abortive treatment options are available for migraine sufferers. Although the triptans (Table 3) have generated much interest and are frequently prescribed, other medications continue to be used, including ergotamine and its derivatives, isometheptene, and NSAIDs. Many of the abortive medications carry significant prescribing limitations that must be taken into consideration. Vasoconstrictor medications are contraindicated in patients with cardiovascular or peripheral vascular disease. NSAIDs should not be used in those with gastrointestinal or bleeding disorders. As with all medications, the clinician must consider appropriate prescribing, contraindications, and side-effect information.
- The vasoconstrictor ergotamine is available in oral, rectal (with caffeine [Cafergot]), and sublingual forms (Ergomar). Ergotamine has a relatively long half-life and duration of action (up to 3 days) and should be used no more frequently than every 4 to 5 days to avoid ergotamine rebound headache. The ergot derivative dihydroergotamine (DHE-45, Migranal NS) is available for intramuscular, subcutaneous (SC), and intranasal use. Intravenous DHE-45 sometimes is used for intractable migraine (status migrainosus) in emergency departments and inpatient settings. The intranasal form (Migranal) is an effective treatment when administered correctly by the patient. Unfortunately, DHE-45 is not absorbed by the gastrointestinal tract, and unlike other abortive nasal sprays, any swallowed medication will be wasted. DHE-45 has a low headache recurrence rate of approximately 12%. All forms of ergotamine and DHE-45 are more effective when taken early in attacks.

Isometheptene is used in combination with dichloralphenazone and acetaminophen (Midrin). It is slow acting and more effective when taken early in attacks and when used for attacks preceded or

TABLE 3	Triptans		
MEDICATION	**BRAND NAME**	**HALF-LIFE (h)**	**FORM/ STRENGTH**
Sumatriptan	Imitrex	1.5	Oral: 25, 50, 100 mg NS: 5, 20 mg Injection: 6, 4 mg
	Treximet		Oral: Sumatriptan 85 mg + naproxen sodium 500 mg
	Zecuity		TD 6.5 mg
Naratriptan	Amerge	6	Oral: 1, 2.5 mg
Zolmitriptan	Zomig	3	Oral: 2.5, 5 mg MLT: 2.5, 5 mg NS: 2.5, 5 mg
Rizatriptan	Maxalt	2–3	Oral: 5, 10 mg MLT: 5, 10 mg
Almotriptan	Axert	3–4	Oral: 6.25, 12.5 mg
Frovatriptan	Frova	25	Oral: 5 mg
Eletriptan	Relpax	4	Oral: 20, 40 mg

MLT = oral disintegrating; NS = nasalspray; TD = transdermal.

accompanied by stress and muscle tension of the neck. Although isometheptene is considered less potent than ergotamine and triptans, it is preferred by many patients whose headaches have features of both migraine and tension type.

At the present time, seven serotonin agonists (triptans) are approved for abortive migraine treatment in the United States (see Table 3). As a category, the triptans are approximately 65% to 70% effective in published clinical trials. Their similarities are greater than their differences, but each triptan is not necessarily effective for all patients, and familiarity with their differences can be helpful to the treating physician. Half-life, onset and duration of action, adverse events, tolerability, recurrence of headache, and routes of administration may vary and allow the physician to match the medication to the individual patient. For example, a slower onset of action and longer-lasting triptan may be appropriate for slow-onset, longer-lasting migraine attacks.

- As with other headache treatments, oral triptan tablets are more effective in the early phases of migraines. It is thought that peripheral sensitization—allodynia—is a sign of later phase migraine, and treating the attack before this phenomenon occurs is important. When treatment is delayed or the patient awakens with severe migraine, the injection, nasal spray, or rapidly acting triptans may be more beneficial. Although triptans as a group are very effective, recurrence of headache, after initial relief, requiring retreatment is common and can be as high as 40%. The recurrence rate tends to be less with triptans having a longer half-life.

The ergotamines and triptans are contraindicated in patients with ischemic heart disease, uncontrolled hypertension, and cerebrovascular disease. Physicians initially were extremely cautious about recommending triptans to their patients when they were first introduced in the United States. However, significant human exposure to the triptans has shown that myocardial infarction or serious ischemia is rare. Chest pain following triptan use affects a small percentage of patients, and because its significance continues to be unclear, it is recommended that triptan use be held pending cardiac evaluation.

- Sumatriptan (Imitrex), the first triptan approved in the United States, is available in nasal spray (5, 20 mg), SC (6, 4 mg), oral formulations (25, 50, 100 mg), and transdermal (Zecuity; 6.5 mg). Its half-life is approximately 1.5 hours, and its duration of action is less than 4 hours. The injectable form produces rapid relief in 70% to 80% of patients, and it appears to be the most effective of all the available triptan forms. Conversely, it appears to cause the most side effects, and, for this reason, it should be used only for the more severe attacks. The oral forms are more favorable with regard to adverse effects, and their effectiveness is similar to that of other triptans (approximately 65%). Because of sumatriptan's short half-life and duration of action, recurrence of headache is common, necessitating repeat dosing.
- Zolmitriptan (Zomig) is available in 2.5 and 5 mg oral and oral disintegrating tablets (ZMT) and as 2.5 and 5 mg nasal sprays. The efficacy of oral zolmitriptan is approximately 65% and that of the nasal form is 70%. The half-life of oral zolmitriptan is 3 hours, and its duration of action is longer than the nasal form, which improves on the need to remedicate. The nasal spray has a biphasic absorption curve, which accounts for its favorable adverse effect profile over the 5 mg oral tablet.
- Naratriptan (Amerge) was the first to be approved of the gradual onset, longer-acting triptans. It is available as oral 1 and 2.5 mg tablets and has a half-life of 6 hours. Naratriptan is well tolerated by patients and often is used by patients with slow-onset migraine. Some specialists prescribe daily naratriptan[1] for limited periods for treatment of menstrual or intractable migraine attacks.
- Rizatriptan (Maxalt) is available as oral 5 and 10 mg tablets and as an oral disintegrating form (MLT). It's half-life is 2 to 3 hours and it has a favorable one-dose 2-hour response rate. Patients who are undergoing concomitant treatment with propranolol should take the lesser 5 mg rizatriptan dose because of higher resultant rizatriptan plasma levels.
- Almotriptan (Axert) is available in 6.25 and 12.5 mg tablets. It has a half-life of 3.5 hours and, because of a broad Tmax (time of maximal concentration) range of 1.4 to 3.8 hours, a relatively rapid onset of action. Almotriptan has favorable adverse effect and headache recurrence profile. Chest pain symptoms after almotriptan use were similar to placebo in clinical trials.
- Frovatriptan (Frova) is a long-acting triptan available in 2.5 mg oral tablets. It has the longest half-life of 25 hours and a favorable recurrence rate. Frovatriptan is frequently used for treatment of menstrual migraine and for attacks of longer duration. Some specialists prescribe daily frovatriptan[1] for a limited period for menstrual and prolonged migraine attacks.
- Eletriptan (Relpax) was the last triptan to be approved. It is available in 20 and 40 mg oral tablets and has a half-life of nearly 5 hours. Eletriptan has a relatively rapid onset but a longer duration of action and a favorable recurrence rate. In studies, some patients who were unresponsive to other triptans responded to eletriptan.

Various attempts have been made to compare triptans. Head-to-head trials mostly have compared one triptan to sumatriptan. A meta-analysis of 53 clinical trials published in 2001 compared the efficacy, recurrence, duration of action, and tolerability of all available triptans. Almotriptan and eletriptan were rated favorably across the major parameters of onset of action, efficacy, adverse events, and recurrence. In spite of efforts to adjust for variations in protocols and placebo response, specialists reached no clear consensus as to the validity or value of the meta-analysis or the preferability of one triptan over another.

- NSAIDs frequently are recommended for treatment of acute migraine and can be effective when taken early. Their effects on the physiology of pain, inflammation, and platelets are thought to be the mechanisms responsible. Some physicians recommend taking a NSAID with the first dose of a triptan for added efficacy. Various agents are used, but none of the rapid-acting NSAIDs appears to have significant efficacy superiority. Naproxen sodium 500 mg in combination with sumatriptan 85 mg (Treximet), OTC ibuprofen (Motrin, Advil), and aspirin combination with caffeine and acetaminophen (Excedrin Migraine) are approved by the FDA for treatment of acute migraine.
- Symptomatic treatment of pain may be necessary in patients who do not respond to recommended abortive treatment. Any effective analgesic can be appropriate, provided it is used infrequently and not on a daily or near-daily basis. In general, the more effective analgesics have antiinflammatory and sedative properties.

Cluster Headache Treatment
Cluster headache is one of the more unusual pain conditions occasionally encountered by physicians. Pain onset is rapid, and the duration of the attack is brief. For this reason, prophylactic treatment usually is the most practical. Abortive prescriptions frequently are given, but, for the most part, the cluster attack is resolving by the time medication is absorbed.

- Nonmedicinal prophylactic measures are extremely limited. The reduction of cigarette smoking and the addressing of individual stress and hostility during cluster periods should be part of any treatment program. There are no FDA-approved medications for the prophylactic treatment of cluster headache. Numerous medications can be helpful and include the calcium channel blockers verapamil (Calan, Isoptin, Verelan, Covera, Verap)[1] and nimodipine,[1] the neurostabilizers valproate

---

[1]Not FDA approved for this indication.

[1]Not FDA approved for this indication.

(Depakote)[1] and topiramate,[1] various NSAIDs, ergotamine,[1] lithium (Eskalith),[1] cyproheptadine,[1] combination H_1 and H_2 histamine antagonists, and, in extreme cases, short intervals of steroids. The addition of magnesium[1] 500 to 750 mg can be helpful in some sufferers. These medications are used in average therapeutic doses, and combinations of medications are commonly needed. The preventatives should be used during the cluster cycle and discontinued during off-cycle periods.

- Abortive treatment is less preferred for cluster headache, as noted previously. However, inhalation oxygen via facial mask at 6 L/min terminates cluster attacks in 75% to 80% of sufferers within 12 minutes. Other possibilities include sumatriptan[1] SC or nasal spray, zolmitriptan[1] nasal spray, ergotamine[1] sublingual, or DHE-45 injection[1] or nasal spray (Migranal).[1] The occasional patient reports relief with the oral triptans or potent analgesics. When triptans, ergotamine, or analgesics are used, appropriate prescribing and frequency guidelines should be followed. In general, with the exception of oxygen, daily as-needed medications should be avoided.

Chronic Daily and Posttraumatic Headache Treatment

The care of patients with chronic daily and posttraumatic headaches is determined by the type or types of headache being experienced. Treatment of each type follows what has been described above. In the patient experiencing posttraumatic headache, frequent follow-up visit monitoring is most appropriate. Extra care should be taken when prescribing medications, especially those that could affect cognitive function and recovery. Often, posttraumatic headache patients benefit with concomitant psychologic and cognitive professional support.

Conclusion

Headache continues to present a challenging problem for clinicians as well as for suffering patients. In spite of recent treatment advances and more public awareness, millions continue to needlessly endure pain and debilitation. Desperate sufferers in a quest for relief sometimes resort to unorthodox therapies or anxiolytics, habituative analgesics, or excessive caffeine that ultimately worsen their headache problems.

At first glance, the headache problem appears complex and difficult when, in actuality, most sufferers experience straightforward, easily diagnosed headaches. The interested generalist or specialist who takes the time to elicit a careful history can establish the headache diagnosis and direct a simple treatment plan that can make a tremendous difference in the headache sufferer's life.

---

[1]Not FDA approved for this indication.

References

Astin JA, Ernst E. The effectiveness of spinal manipulation for the treatment of headache disorders: A systematic review of randomized clinical trials. Cephalalgia 2002;22:617–23.

Diamond ML, Dalessio DJ, (eds): Diamond and Dalessio's The Practicing Physician's Approach to Headache. 5th ed. Philadelphia: WB Saunders; 1999.

Ferrari MD, Roon KI, Lipton RB, et al. Oral triptans (serotonin 5HT-IB/ID-agonists) in acute migraine treatment: A meta-analysis of 53 trials. Lancet 2001;358:1668–75.

Gallagher RM, Kunkel R. Migraine medication attributes important for patient compliance: Concerns about side effects may delay treatment. Headache 2003;43:36–43.

Goadsby PJ, Lipton RB, Ferreri MD. Migraine current understanding and treatment. N Engl J Med 2002;346:257–70.

Haberer LJ, Walls CM, Lener SE, et al. Distinct pharmacokinetic profile and safety of a fixed-dose tablet of sumatriptan and naproxen sodium for the acute treatment of migraine. Headache 2010;50:357–73.

Jackson JL, Kuriyama A, Hayashino Y, et al. Botulinum toxin A for prophylactic treatment of migraine and tension headaches in adults: A meta-analysis. JAMA 2012;307(16):1736–45.

Silberstein SD, Lipton EB, Dalessio DJ. Wolff's Headache and Other Head Pain. 7th ed. New York: Oxford University Press; 2001.

U.S. Food and Drug Administration. National Drug Code Directory.

Vernon H, McDermaid C, Hagino C. Systematic review of randomized clinical trials of complementary/alternative therapies in the treatment of tension-type and cervicogenic headache. Complement Ther Med 1999;7:142–55.

HEMATURIA

Method of
Moben Mirza, MD; and J. Brantley Thrasher, MD

CURRENT DIAGNOSIS

- Hematuria is defined as the presence of red blood cells in the urine. Hematuria can be gross (readily visible) or microscopic (detected by dipstick or microscopy). In the adult population, any unexplained hematuria should be presumed to be of malignant origin until proven otherwise. Urologic evaluation of the upper and lower urinary tract is compulsory for patients with gross hematuria. Patients with asymptomatic microscopic hematuria (>3 rbc/hpf) should undergo urologic evaluation once benign causes have been ruled out. The urologic evaluation includes urine analysis, serum creatinine, cystoscopy, and multiphasic computed tomography. Concurrent nephrologic evaluation should occur in select cases.

Epidemiology

Hematuria is a common clinical finding in adults. The prevalence of hematuria ranges from 0.2% to 16%. Prevalence varies based on age, gender, frequency of testing, threshold use to define hematuria, and study group characteristics (Davis et al., 2012). Transient microscopic hematuria may occur in up to 40% of patients; however, persistent microscopic hematuria in greater than three evaluated urine samples is limited to 2% of the population (Masahito, 2010). A wide range of causes can result in hematuria. Transient hematuria may be caused by vigorous exercise, sexual intercourse, mild trauma, menstrual contamination, and instrumentation. Patients with underlying urinary tract disease can have transient or persistent hematuria. The difference between gross and microscopic hematuria is that the chances of finding significant pathology are higher in patients with gross hematuria. For example, approximately 5% of patient with microscopic hematuria in contrast to 40% of patient with gross hematuria are found to have urologic malignancy on evaluation (Khadra et al., 2000). The most common cause of gross hematuria in adults older than age 50 is bladder cancer (Gerber & Brendler, 2011).

Risk Factors

Given the wide range of etiologies for hematuria, the risk factors are dependent on the etiology itself. The most concerning etiology of hematuria is urothelial malignancy. Smoking is the best-established and the most significant risk factor for the development of urothelial malignancies of the kidney, ureter, and bladder.

Pathophysiology

The presence of blood in the urine can be separated into glomerular and nonglomerular origin. Normal urine contains less than three red blood cells per high power field. The kidney does not excrete red blood cells under physiologic conditions. Therefore, presence of blood in the urine is due to pathology at the glomerulus (glomerular hematuria), allowing excretion of red blood cells into the urine or pathology in the urinary tract distal to the glomerulus (nonglomerular hematuria), which results in blood mixing into the already excreted urine. Nonglomerular hematuria can be further divided into medical and surgical disorders. Except for renal tumors, nonglomerular hematuria of medical/renal origin is due to tubulointerstitial, renovascular, or systemic disorders. Surgical nonglomerular hematuria or essential hematuria includes urologic tumors, stones, and urinary tract infections (Gerber & Brendler, 2011).

The urine dipstick commonly used for the detection of blood in the urine is dependent on the peroxidase-like activity of hemoglobin, which catalyzes the reaction and causes oxidation of the chromogen indicator. False positives can occur in states of hemoglobinuria and myoglobinuria, and microscopic examination of the urine for red blood cells can distinguish hematuria. Glomerular hematuria is suggested when dysmorphic erythrocytes, red blood cell casts, and proteinuria are present. Nonglomerular hematuria can be distinguished from glomerular hematuria in the presence of circular erythrocytes and the absence of erythrocyte casts. In the surgical and medical subcategories of nonglomerular hematuria, surgical hematuria is suggested by the absence of significant proteinuria.

Anticoagulation at normal therapeutic levels does not predispose patients to hematuria. Therefore, patients who have hematuria while receiving anticoagulation therapy should undergo evaluation similarly to patients who are not receiving anticoagulation therapy. In fact, super therapeutic anticoagulation may serve to unmask underlying pathology.

Prevention

Hematuria can be caused by a spectrum of causes. Prevention can be achieved by the prevention of what results in the pathologic state. For example, smoking is a modifiable risk factor in urothelial malignancy. Patients who have never smoked are at low risk for bladder cancer. Smoking cessation can also reduce the risk of developing bladder cancer. Liberal fluid intake and balanced sodium and protein intake can help prevent urolithiasis. Urinary tract infections can also be prevented by good voiding habits, facilitation of complete bladder emptying, and use of vaginal estrogen cream[1] in postmenopausal women.

---

[1]Not FDA approved for this indication.

Clinical Manifestations

The presentation of hematuria is often dependent on the cause. Certain characteristics of the presentation can help in the investigation. Is the hematuria gross or microscopic? Is the hematuria associated with pain? Are there any irritative voiding symptoms? Is there a presence of blood clots? Is it related to exercise? Is there any family history? Is there a presence of rash, arthritis, hemoptysis, upper respiratory infection, skin infection? Is there a history of radiation, diabetes, analgesic abuse? Is there a history of smoking or occupational exposures? Table 1 highlights findings in etiologies of hematuria. Patients with bladder cancer generally present with gross painless hematuria.

Diagnosis

The diagnosis and evaluation of hematuria starts with a careful history, physical examination, and microscopic urine analysis. The cause in an adult patient is urologic malignancy until proven otherwise. Some important questions are outlined in the clinical manifestation section. The physical examination should focus on blood pressure, a cardiovascular examination, an abdominal examination, a palpable mass, costovertebral angle tenderness, and a complete genitourinary examination inclusive of a prostate examination in the male and vaginal examination in the female patient. The assessment should help rule out causes such as infection, menstruation, vigorous exercise, medical renal disease, viral illness, trauma, or recent urologic procedures.

The urine should be collected as a midstream sample, and patients should be instructed to discard the initial 10 mL. The sample should be collected in a sterile cup after gently cleaning the urethral meatus with a sterilization towelette. Uncircumcised men should retract the foreskin before collection. Female patients should be asked to spread the labia adequately to allow cleansing

---

TABLE 1 Differential Diagnosis and Findings in Etiologies of Hematuria

DIAGNOSIS	FINDINGS	OTHER
Glomerular		
Familial Hematuria	Abnormal urine analysis	Family history
Systemic Lupus Erythematous	Elevated C3, C4, ANA	Rash, arthritis
Goodpasture Syndrome	Microcytic anemia	Hemoptysis, bleeding tendency
Poststreptococcal Glomerulonephritis	Elevated ASO titer, C3	Recent upper respiratory infection, rash
IgA Nephropathy	Normal ASO and C3, renal biopsy positive for IgA, IgG	Related to exercise
Nonglomerular Medical		
Exercise-Induced Hematuria	Abnormal urine analysis	After strenuous exercise
Papillary Necrosis	Gross hematuria, absence of urolithiasis on CT	Flank pain, African American, analgesic abuse, diabetes
Medullary Sponge Kidney, Polycystic Kidney Disease	Abnormal CT	Family history of renal cystic disease
Renovascular Disease	Renal artery embolus, vein thrombus, AV fistula	Atrial fibrillation, dehydration, bruit
Nonglomerular Surgical		
Urinary Tract Infection	Urine dip with LCE, Nit. Positive urine culture, elevated WBC	Dysuria, fever
Urolithiasis (renal, ureteral, or bladder stone)	Demonstrated on imaging such as CT, ultrasound, KUB	Flank pain, pelvic pain, vomiting, infection, renal obstruction
Urologic Tumor (kidney, ureter, bladder, urethra)	Demonstrated on CT, cystoscopy, ureteropyeloscopy	Constitutional, irritative symptoms, pain if obstruction, blood clots
Enlarged Prostate or Benign Prostatic hyperplasia	Enlarged prostate on examination or cystoscopy	Irritative and obstructive voiding symptoms
Radiation Cystitis	Generally gross hematuria, friable tissue on cystoscopy	Irritative voiding symptoms, history of pelvic radiation
Urothelial Strictures (ureter or urethra)	Demonstrated on ureteroscopy, pyelography, cystoscopy, or urethrography	Flank pain, renal insufficiency, bladder outlet obstruction

of the urethral meatus and avoid introital contamination. The following patients may require catheterization for collection: menstruating women, obese patients, patient with a nonintact urinary tract, and patients who do intermittent catheterization or have an indwelling urinary catheter (Davis et al., 2012). A urine dipstick can be performed in the office setting, but all samples should be sent for microscopic analysis. As mentioned previously, attention should be paid to dysmorphic erythrocytes, red blood cell casts, and the presence of protein. A urine culture should be performed based on the clinical presentation and findings of urine analysis. Urine cytology does need to be performed as part of the standard workup. The laboratory workup should include an evaluation of the serum creatinine (Davis et al., 2012). Additional helpful tests are serum electrolytes and a complete blood count.

Patients with a urinary tract infection should be treated appropriately and should have a urine analysis repeated in 2 to 6 weeks after treatment. Patients with an identified etiology such as urolithiasis should have a reevaluation of urine after the stone has been passed or treated.

A urologic evaluation of the upper and lower urinary tract is compulsory for patients with gross hematuria. Patients with asymptomatic microscopic hematuria (>3 rbc/hpf) should undergo urologic evaluation once benign causes have been ruled out. The urologic evaluation is especially important for patients with high risk factors for urothelial malignancy, such as age >35, irritative voiding symptoms, chemical exposures, smoking history, or history of urologic disorder or malignancy. Urologic evaluation should include a cystoscopy to evaluate the urethra and bladder. Multiphasic computed tomography with and without intravenous contrast should be performed to evaluate the upper tracts. Sufficient imaging phases should be performed. Ideally, a three-phase study including a noncontrast phase (e.g., stone disease), arterial phase (e.g., renal masses), and excretory phase (e.g., ureteral masses) should be performed (Sudakoff et al., 2008). The urologist can determine the appropriate study if contrasted CT cannot be performed because of allergy or renal insufficiency. Concurrent nephrologic evaluation should occur for patients who are suspected to have glomerular causes, and the evaluation may include further serum testing and renal biopsy (Davis et al., 2012).

Differential Diagnosis
The differential diagnosis of hematuria includes glomerular diseases, nonglomerular medical diseases, and nonglomerular surgical diseases. Table 1 shows a differential diagnosis for hematuria. Hematuria is considered to be from a malignant source until proven otherwise.

Therapy, Monitoring, and Complications
Therapy, monitoring, and complications for hematuria are dependent on the etiology. It is important that hematuria not be ignored even when treated empirically. For example, it is important to recheck a urine analysis after a course of antibiotics for a presumed urinary tract infection. Often, the transient nature of hematuria fools clinicians into thinking that an intervention or observation without the appropriate workup is adequate. Unfortunately, this can result in significant morbidity from the progression of disease, especially in the case of urothelial malignancies.

References
Davis R, Jones SJ, Barocas D, et al. Diagnosis, evaluation and follow-up of asymptomatic microscopic hematuria (AMH) in adults. AUA guideline. J Urol 2012;188(Suppl 6):2473.

Gerber GS, Brendler CB. Evaluation of the urologic patient: History, physical, and urinalysis. In Wein Campbell-Walsh Urology. 10th ed. Philadelphia: WB Saunders; 2011. pp 73–98.

Khadra MH, Pickard RS, Charlton M, et al. A prospective analysis of 1,930 patients with hematuria to evaluate current diagnostic practice. J Urol 2000;163:524.

Masahito J. Evaluation and management of hematuria. Prim Care 2010;37:461.

Sudakoff GS, Dunn DP, Guralnick ML, et al. Multidetector computerized tomography urography as the primary imaging modality for detecting urinary tract neoplasms in patients with asymptomatic hematuria. J Urol 2008;179:862.

HICCUPS
Method of
Georg A. Petroianu, MD, PhD

Mechanistic Description
Hiccup (Latin, *singultus*) is caused by an involuntary, usually repetitive and rhythmic, spasmodic contraction of the diaphragm (or hemidiaphragm) and accessory inspiratory muscles followed shortly (within 35 msec) by the sudden closure of the glottis. The forcefully inspired air meeting a closed glottis causes the typical hiccup sound. Occasional hiccups are generally perceived as being "funny"; however, hiccupping of extended duration can be incapacitating. Its most common direct consequence is esophagitis, due to concomitant relaxation of the lower esophageal sphincter favoring reflux, but extended hiccupping can also lead to wound dehiscence, depression, weight loss, malnutrition, insomnia, and exhaustion.

Classifications
Most classifications use arbitrary time limits to categorize hiccupping. Generally hiccups lasting less than 1 day are considered transient (acute), those lasting less than 1 week are labeled persistent, and hiccupping for more than 1 week is described as chronic. A simplified categorization draws the line at 48 hours: any hiccupping episode lasting longer is described as chronic. The practical value of these classifications is questionable; by the time the practitioner sees the patient, almost invariably the case involves persistent or chronic hiccup forms requiring drug therapy. The exceptions (in terms of time between appearance and presentation) are hiccup forms presenting immediately postoperatively or in critical care units. Brief episodes of hiccupping, as experienced by the vast majority of people at some point in time, are certainly physiologic. The point of transition to a pathologic form is not well defined. The rule of thumb of hiccup therapy, however, is that the longer the duration of the hiccupping, the less amenable it will be to nonpharmacologic interventions.

Etiologic classifications are also fraught with problems. Hiccup is not a disease, but a symptom. Literally, there is no known disease that has not been associated with hiccups. Although the categories psychogenic, organic, and idiopathic are most commonly used in practice, the situation most commonly encountered is that of hiccup of unknown (idiopathic) origin. In this context, "idiopathic" describes one's inability to demonstrate, rather than the absence of, an organic origin.

Epidemiology
During intrauterine life, hiccups are universally present, their incidence peaking in the third trimester. They can also be seen regularly in the newborn, the frequency of occurrence decreasing slowly over the first year of life. In adults, occasional transient hiccup is also so frequent that it can be viewed as physiologic. Persistent and chronic idiopathic singultus, the pathologic forms, are rare, their prevalence being estimated at 1 in 100,000. Males are almost exclusively affected (the male-to-female patient ratio is approximately 80:1), suggesting a hormone (estrogen) protective effect. The incidence increases with age. The psychogenic form, though less frequent overall by one order of magnitude, is believed to be more prevalent in females, with an even distribution among all age groups; however, data to support this view are almost nonexistent.

Pathophysiology
The universality of hiccups during fetal life begs the question of purposefulness. As early as 1887, it was suggested that hiccups might represent a necessary and vital primitive reflex that would permit intrauterine training of the diaphragm without aspiration of amniotic fluid. During intrapartum and postpartum maturation, higher centers would then suppress this primitive reflex. Immaturity or damage to the central nervous system would favor the persistence or reappearance of the reflex. The putative reflex

arch includes autonomic afferent fibers (the majority vagal fibers) from the digestive tract to a putative medullary hiccup center and motor efferent fibers via the phrenic nerve (diaphragm) and other branches of the vagus nerve to the intrinsic muscles of the larynx adducting the vocal cords. In an analogy with the vomiting center, the assumed role of the medullary hiccup center is to coordinate and fine-tune the sequence of events required for hiccupping; it is therefore a "pattern generator." The concept described, though useful for the purpose of designing a quasi-rational treatment protocol for hiccup, is neither proven nor generally accepted.

Another school of thought that questions the assumption that hiccupping is a reflex phenomenon suggests instead a similarity with cardiac arrhythmias: hiccups would therefore be due to arrhythmias of the breathing center. Still other researchers work on the assumption that hiccup is a myoclonic event, or that it represents brainstem seizures. These views are not necessarily mutually exclusive, because hiccup is not primarily a disease but a symptom, possibly representing different pathophysiologies.

Evaluation of the Hiccup Patient

Hiccup is a symptom associated with a multitude of pathologies. The practioner must take the hiccupping patient seriously, and for the purpose of finding and treating hidden pathology, persistent and chronic hiccups should be investigated. No consensus exists, however, concerning the extent of such investigations. Even the most enthusiastic users of modern imaging technologies will in most cases end up with a working diagnosis of chronic idiopathic singultus. Nonetheless, a detailed history, a thorough physical examination, and basic laboratory and diagnostic procedures are essential.

History

Ask about previous episodes, as well as precipitating and alleviating factors. The patient who describes vomiting as a "cure" for previous hiccup episodes gives a telltale sign that acidity is an etiologic factor, and omeprazole is a drug to consider. If the patient indicates that hyperventilation is a "sure bet" to worsen his or her hiccups, you can assume that drugs lowering the excitability of the nervous system are likely to help. Elucidating present drug consumption (medical and recreational) is essential: benzodiazepines, barbiturates, alcohol, and steroids are well-known hiccup inducers.

Physical Examination

Foreign bodies in the external auditory canal can induce hiccups, so look in the ears. Examine neck, chest, and abdomen, looking for possible sources of irritation (infection, neoplastic processes, or both) to the vagus and phrenic nerves and the diaphragm. Perform a neurologic examination, keeping in mind the association of hiccup with multiple sclerosis and intracranial processes.

Laboratory and Diagnostic Procedures

An upright chest x-ray, together with complete blood count (CBC) with differential, will help exclude neoplastic or infectious disease. An electrocardiogram (ECG) will help exclude pericarditis and malfunctioning pacemakers, and electrolyte and urea determinations will exclude known metabolic causes (hyponatremia and uremia).

To what extent magnetic resonance imaging (MRI), ultrasound scanning, or endoscopic examinations are necessary is a judgment call, and no generalizations are possible; they might occasionally be indicated.

Nonpharmacologic Interventions

A multitude of nonpharmacologic interventions to terminate hiccup belong to the public-domain hiccup "mythology" or have been described in the medical literature as case reports. Though usually effective in terminating bouts of acute hiccup, they are mostly ineffective in cases of hiccupping that has been present for an extended period. The common denominator of these maneuvers (also used to terminate paroxysmal supraventricular tachycardia) is their ability to directly or indirectly increase efferent vagal activity; the increased parasympathetic tone has a limiting effect on hiccupping. Interestingly, estrogens are also considered to be parasympathomimetic, which offers a plausible explanation of why the singultus prevalence in females is much lower than in males.

Pharmacologic Interventions

Probably only a few drugs in the *Physician's Desk Reference* have not been tried in the therapy of singultus, and anyone who looks hard enough at the literature will be able to find anecdotal support for the use of almost any drug. However, prospective controlled studies to support the use of a particular therapy are very few and rare.

Conceptually, all drugs potentially successful in the therapy of chronic hiccups work either by decreasing the input from the gastrointestinal tract to a (putative) hiccup center or by decreasing the excitability of the nervous system and therefore the output from the (putative) hiccup center.

Sedative-Hypnotics

Both benzodiazepine and barbiturate γ-aminobutyric acid receptor type A (GABA$_A$) agonists have been tried for treatment of hiccups. The consensus is that these substances not only are ineffective, but can actually worsen the clinical picture, producing a situation similar to the paradoxical excitation seen with the use of sedatives and explained by inhibitory effects on inhibitory centers.

Antiemetics

Following up on the analogy between the vomiting center and hiccup center as pattern generators, "setron" class antiemetics (5-HT$_3$ receptor antagonists) have been tried, with no success. Anecdotal evidence hints at possible worsening of the hiccup under the influence of ondansetron (Zofran).[1]

Analeptics

The use of analeptics derives from the concept that hiccup is a suppressed primitive reflex. Analeptics potentiate the central suppression. Although some success has been reported with methylphenidate (Ritalin),[1] caffeine produced failure.

Anticonvulsants

Anticonvulsants (phenytoin [Dilantin],[1] carbamazepine [Tegretol],[1] valproate [Depacon][1]) have been used to try to suppress hiccups. Considering the multitude of pharmacodynamic effects of anticonvulsants, it is not surprising that some success was achieved.

Antipsychotics

Historically, chlorpromazine (Thorazine) has been the most widely used drug for treatment of hiccup, and it is the only drug approved by the FDA for the disorder. Aliphatic phenothiazines such as chlorpromazine have strong sedative, hypotensive, and anticholinergic properties and mild to moderate extrapyramidal effects. For hiccup control, results are mixed at best, and in view of the side effects, routine use is not warranted. Haloperidol (Haldol),[1] a butyropherone derivative, has also been used for hiccup control; again, results are mixed at best, and the possibility of developing tardive dyskinesia weighs heavily against the routine use of this drug.

Antidepressants

The tertiary amine tricyclic antidepressant amitriptyline (Elavil)[1] is one of the oldest players in the therapy of hiccup; its use was being suggested in the mid-1960s. As with anticonvulsants, considering the multitude of pharmacodynamic effects of tricyclic antidepressants, it is not surprising that some success was achieved with these drugs. Their effectiveness is not related to their ability to inhibit monoamine uptake, but probably to their sodium channel blocking properties.

---

[1]Not FDA approved for this indication.

Calcium Channel Blockers

Nifedipine (Adalat)[1] is the dihydropyridine derivative most commonly used for hiccup control. Nimodipine (Nimotop)[1] has also been tried for the same purpose. Interestingly, anecdotal reports about the use of calcium for the same purpose also exist.

Sodium Channel Blockers

The local anesthetic class Ib antidysrhythmic lidocaine (Xylocaine)[1] and its oral analogue mexiletine (Mexitil)[1] have been used for hiccup control, with mixed results.

GABA$_B$ Agonists

Among the substances acting on the nervous system, baclofen (Lioresal)[1] has by far the best credentials in the treatment of chronic hiccup. It is one of the very few substances proven in clinical studies (albeit with small patient numbers) to be efficacious. This γ-aminobutyric acid receptor type B (GABA$_B$) agonist, normally used to lower an increased muscle tone (spasticity), has also been shown to suppress hiccups in an animal (cat) hiccup model. GABA$_B$ agonists, by reducing transmitter release, are generally able to depress complex reflexes.

Antacids

Lowering the acidity of the stomach using H$_2$-receptor blockers or proton pump inhibitors conceptually decreases the input from the gastrointestinal tract to the hiccup center. Omeprazole (Prilosec)[1] has been shown in a limited number of trials to be effective in hiccup treatment.

Gastrokinetic Drugs

One of the few reliable methods to induce a physiologic hiccup in humans is rapidly drinking an ice-cold can of beer on a hot summer day. Although it is highly debatable whether it has to be beer, stomach distention by carbon dioxide induces hiccups. Conversely, reducing stomach distention by using a gastrokinetic drug is helpful in alleviating hiccups. The strongest evidence available for the usefulness of a gastrokinetic drug was for cisapride (Propulsid); however, this selective serotonine 5-HT$_4$-receptor agonist was withdrawn from the market because of its propensity to prolong the QT interval and induce torsades de pointes. The available alternative is the related benzamide metoclopramide (Reglan),[1] a mixed dopamine receptor antagonist, 5-HT$_4$-receptor agonist, and cholinesterase inhibitor, with a long tradition in the treatment of hiccups, going back to the late 1960s.

Physical Interventions

Phrenic Nerve Destruction

Irreversible surgical destruction of the phrenic nerve cannot be recommended. Even if hiccup relief is achieved after unilateral local anesthetic blockade of the phrenic nerve without serious compromise in respiratory function, the long term effects of phrenic nerve destruction are unpredictable. Possible effects include both hiccup reappearance—even after bilateral phrenic nerve transection—and deterioration in respiratory function. More recently, diaphragmatic (phrenic) pacing has been described; however, experience is very limited.

Hypercapnia

Rebreathing in a paper bag is a well-known and reliable remedy for hyperventilation tetany. The increase in blood CO$_2$ levels (hypercapnia) thus induced leads to mild acidosis and thus to a liberation of calcium ions from the protein binding. The increase in plasma-free calcium decreases neuronal excitability, thus terminating not only the tetany, but possibly also hiccupping. A more high-tech version of this is the induction of normoxic hypercapnia in ventilated patients.

Positive End-Expiratory Pressure

Also practicable only in intubated patients is the application of high positive end-expiratory pressure (PEEP), a high-tech version of the Valsalva maneuver.

[1]Not FDA approved for this indication.

Nasogastric Tube

Gastric decompression via a nasogastric tube can terminate hiccups.

Treatment

The treatment algorithm described is based on the assumption that correctable organic causes have been excluded or treated.

We start therapy with omeprazole (Prilosec)[1] 20 to 40 mg orally (PO) daily. If after 7 days no satisfactory change has occurred, baclofen (Lioresal)[1] is introduced. With baclofen, a "start low, go very slow" approach is indicated in order to avoid excessive drowsiness, weakness, and fatigue. The maximum daily dose is 45 mg. Quite often, patients are already on a proton pump inhibitor (PPI) when presenting. In these cases, immediate introduction of baclofen and continuation of the PPI are recommended. In our experience, the time of response to the combination therapy omeprazole plus baclofen is unpredictable; however, all changes that we observed happened within the first 6 months, and the vast majority within the first 6 weeks. If the desired result is achieved, we continue therapy for another 6 months, after which a very cautious weaning from baclofen is attempted. In cases where the combination therapy omeprazole plus baclofen is not (or not entirely) satisfactory, the addition of gabapentin (Neurontin)[1] "on the top" can be attempted. As with baclofen, with gabapentin a "start low, go slow" approach is indicated, the maximum dose of 400 mg three times daily used in such cases being reached after 3 weeks. An inverse approach with PPI plus gabapentin as initial combination is also possible.

In addition to any pharmacologic therapy, the practitioner must convey to the patient the feeling that he or she understands and appreciates the seriousness of the condition. Compliance with the treatment is required from the patient, who must understand that success can take time. Lifestyle and habit changes are also required. The hiccup patient must limit the size of meals and avoid carbonated beverages and "gas-forming" foods.

The approach presented here represents our experience in the treatment of chronic singultus. The views expressed are neither guidelines nor regulations.

[1]Not FDA approved for this indication.

References

Jatzko A, Stegmeier-Petroianu A, Petroianu GA. Alpha-2-delta ligands for singultus (hiccup) treatment: three case reports. J Pain Symptom Manage 2007;33:756–60.

Petroianu G. Idiopathic chronic hiccup (ICH): phrenic nerve block is not the way to go. Anesthesiology 1998;89:1284–5.

Petroianu G, Hein G, Petroianu A, et al. Idiopathic chronic hiccup: combination therapy with cisapride, omeprazole, and Baclofen. Clin Ther 1997;19:1031–8.

Petroianu G, Hein G, Petroianu A, et al. ETICS study: empirical therapy of idiopathic chronic singultus. Z Gastroenterol 1998;36:559–66.

Petroianu G, Hein G, Stegmeier-Petroianu A, et al. Gabapentin "add-on therapy" for idiopathic chronic hiccup (ICH). J Clin Gastroenterol 2000;30:321–4.

HOARSENESS AND LARYNGITIS

Method of
Lee Akst, MD

CURRENT DIAGNOSIS

- The general term to describe vocal difficulty is dysphonia. Hoarseness is a specific term for rough voice quality, which is one type of dysphonia. Laryngitis signifies laryngeal inflammation, which is one possible cause of dysphonia.
- An accurate history and physical examination guide the diagnosis of voice complaints. Although many portions of the examination for dysphonia can be done in a general setting, videostroboscopy is often necessary for diagnosis and may be available only in specialized laryngology offices.

- The most common cause of acute hoarseness is viral laryngitis. Symptoms are self-limited and usually resolve within 2 weeks.
- Dysphonia persisting for longer than 2 weeks suggests the possibility of another diagnosis, such as vocal cord paralysis, neoplasm, phonotraumatic lesion, or chronic laryngitis.
- Indications for referral of a patient with voice complaints to an otolaryngologist include dysphonia that persists for longer than 2 weeks, that is of acute onset during voicing, or that is accompanied by other symptoms such as otalgia, dysphagia, or difficulty breathing.

CURRENT THERAPY

- Appropriate treatment of voice complaints depends on accurate diagnosis.
- Supportive therapy is all that is necessary for most cases of acute laryngitis associated with viral upper respiratory tract infections.
- Laryngopharyngeal reflux is a common cause of chronic laryngitis, and appropriate therapy often requires twice-daily administration of proton pump inhibitors for at least 2 months.
- Microlaryngeal phonosurgery may be indicated for some patients with benign phonotraumatic lesions.
- Vocal cord medialization can rehabilitate the voice in a patient with unilateral vocal cord paralysis.
- Many patients with dysphonia benefit from voice therapy, alone or in combination with other treatment strategies.

Voice is an essential component of communication. Vocal difficulty is very distressing to patients and can have a negative impact on physical, social, and emotional qualities of life. To understand the pathophysiology, evaluation, and treatment of voice complaints, it is important to understand the anatomy and physiology of normal voice production. Looking first at how good voice quality is achieved makes it readily apparent how alterations in vocal fold vibration, symmetry, or closure can lead to various vocal difficulties.

To aid discussion of voice complaints, clarification of terminology is necessary. Although "hoarseness" is a term that most patients use to describe any type of voice complaint and "laryngitis" is the presumptive explanation that many patients provide for their symptoms, each of these terms has a more precise meaning. Dysphonia is the general term for vocal difficulty. Hoarseness implies a rough or raspy change in voice quality and is one type of dysphonia. Other categories include limited vocal projection, strained vocal effort, and change in pitch—each of which may occur with or without vocal roughness. The term "laryngitis" specifically describes inflammation of the larynx. This inflammation may be acute or chronic, and again it describes some but certainly not all cases of dysphonia. This distinction will be made clear as the evaluation and management of dysphonia are described.

Normal Laryngeal Function

The larynx plays a central role in voice production by serving as a vibrating instrument that turns airflow from the lungs into sound. The sound is shaped into intelligible speech through the resonating and articulating functions of the pharynx and oral cavity. The ability of the larynx to create vibration and serve as a sound source is a function of its complex, layered microanatomy. The deeper layers of the vocal fold include the thyroarytenoid muscle and the vocal ligament, which position the more superficial layers of the superficial lamina propria and epithelium during phonation. Compared with the fibrous nature of the vocal ligament, the superficial lamina propria is a loose gelatinous layer whose pliability allows for voice production.

During inspiration (Figure 1A), the vocal folds are abducted so that air can move past the larynx without resistance. During phonation (Figure 1B), the vocal folds are held in an adducted position while the lungs drive air toward the larynx. Air pressure builds in the subglottis, beneath the vocal folds, until it overcomes the forces of vocal fold closure, pushes past the vocal folds, and generates negative pressure in its wake as it moves past the larynx. A combination of the vocal folds' intrinsic viscoelasticity and the negative pressure created through Bernoulli's effect draws the vocal fold edges back together, allowing subglottic pressure to rebuild and the cycle to repeat. Repeated cycles of opening and closing at the level of the vocal fold edges generate a so-called mucosal wave, which travels from the inferior edge of each vocal fold up across the medial and superior edges (Figure 1C). These waves may repeat hundreds of times each second, depending on pitch. This cycled opening and closing of the vocal folds during phonation imparts pressure waves to the air column that moves the vocal folds, generating sound. The ability of vocal folds to vibrate easily and symmetrically in this very rapid fashion allows for clear, smooth voicing.

Evaluation of Dysphonia

Central to the evaluation of dysphonia is the understanding that any disruption of vocal fold closure, symmetry, or vibration impairs the ability of the vocal folds to generate a clear sound source. Most voice complaints arise from anatomic or functional limitations in glottal closure or mucosal wave formation, although other parts of the respiratory tree are also responsible for components of the voice. General points concerning evaluation of dysphonia are discussed in this section, with specific causes discussed afterward.

History

A careful history can provide many clues that point toward the proper diagnosis in patients with dysphonia. Although many patients offer the complaint of "hoarseness" as a general term, a careful historian distinguishes between complaints related to voice

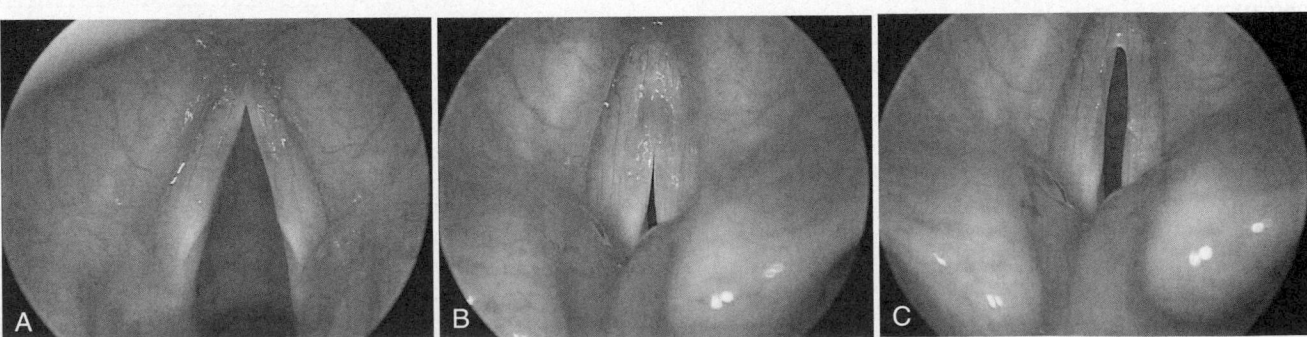

Figure 1. A, Normal vocal folds in abducted position for inspiration. B, Normal vocal folds in adducted position for phonation. C, Displacement of the vocal fold medial edges creates mucosal wave propagation during phonation and produces voice.

quality, vocal projection, vocal effort or strain, vocal fatigue, and so on. Two questions that can help a patient organize his or her own thoughts related to poor voice are "What abnormal things does your voice do now that it did not do before?" and "What normal things did your voice do before that it no longer can do?" The acuteness of onset, duration, severity, and progression of any complaint should be determined.

The history should also determine what other factors or events might have caused or exacerbated the dysphonia. Recent sources of laryngeal inflammation might include intubation, excessive voice use, or upper respiratory tract infection. Baseline conditions that foster chronic laryngeal inflammation include environmental allergies, rhinitis, and laryngopharyngeal reflux. Laryngopharyngeal reflux can exist in the absence of heartburn, with reflux-associated inflammation of the larynx and pharynx providing symptoms of globus pharyngeus, throat clearing, nonproductive cough, effortful swallowing, and even mild dysphagia in association with dysphonia.

Concerning the possibility of laryngeal malignancy, any patient with dysphonia should be asked about smoking and alcohol use, because these are risk factors for squamous cell carcinoma. Another important question in distinguishing inflammatory dysphonia from a mass lesion of the vocal fold concerns whether there are any periods of normal voice or the dysphonia is constant—inflammation may wax and wane, but dysphonia associated with mass lesions is usually progressive and unremitting. Finally, the history should elicit other possible head and neck complaints, including dyspnea, stridor, dysphagia, odynophagia, otalgia, sore throat, and pain with speaking (odynophonia). If hoarseness is associated with some of these symptoms for longer than 2 weeks, the suspicion of malignancy is increased.

Physical Examination

The physical examination for patients with dysphonia includes a complete head and neck evaluation with focus on the larynx and laryngeal function. Although much of the head and neck examination can be performed in a general setting, some portions of the laryngeal examination require specialized equipment found only in some otolaryngology offices that specialize in voice care. Routine head and neck evaluation should include systematic examination of the ears, nose, oral cavity, oropharynx, and neck.

Complaint of otalgia in the setting of an unremarkable ear examination suggests a possibility of referred pain from a lesion of the larynx or pharynx, and is concerning for possible malignancy. Edematous and erythematous nasal mucosa suggests rhinitis, with the possibility of postnasal drip contributing to laryngeal inflammation. Tremor of the tongue or palate might suggest neurologic disorder, whereas pharyngeal erythema and exudate suggest possible acute infection. Pachydermia (cobblestoning) of the posterior pharyngeal wall suggests the possibility of laryngopharyngeal reflux. Tenderness with manipulation of the hyoid bone suggests tension of the strap muscles and correlates closely with complaint of odynophonia and the possibility of muscle tension dysphonia. A neck mass might represent either metastatic lymphadenopathy from a laryngeal malignancy or a primary lesion which itself compresses the recurrent laryngeal nerve and causes paralytic dysphonia. Surgical scarring along the neck suggests the possibility that prior thyroid surgery, carotid endarterectomy, or anterior approach to the cervical spine might have led to vocal fold paralysis.

Laryngeal Examination

Beyond a general examination of the head and neck, there should be directed evaluation of the larynx and laryngeal function. The examiner should listen to the voice carefully, because vocal characteristics such as roughness, breathiness, strain, vocal breaks, and diplophonia (pitch instability, with two different pitches present simultaneously) can help guide the differential diagnosis of dysphonia. Visual examination of the larynx has many forms, ranging from mirror examination to flexible fiberoptic laryngoscopy to videostrobolaryngoscopy.

Mirror examination offers an adequate view of the vocal folds in many patients but may be limited by patient tolerance, physician inexperience, and the inherently limited ability of this technique to brightly illuminate the larynx or record the examination for later review. Flexible laryngoscopy is routinely available in almost all otolaryngology offices, is well tolerated by patients, and offers good views of the larynx that can be recorded with appropriate equipment. Mirror examination and flexible laryngoscopy are limited to observation of vocal fold motion and anatomy but cannot observe laryngeal function because they do not visualize vibration of the vocal folds. To examine vocal fold vibration, videostroboscopy uses a strobe light to create the impression of slow-motion analysis of mucosal waves. Stroboscopy is typically available only in selected otolaryngology practices in which laryngologists specialize in the treatment of voice disorders.

Other Testing

Videostroboscopic evaluation, combined with a thorough history and routine physical examination, can establish the diagnosis for almost all patients with voice complaints, but further testing is sometimes indicated. For instance, electromyography is used by some laryngologists for further evaluation of vocal fold paralysis or paresis. More commonly, radiographic studies are used for further evaluation of some voice complaints. Computed tomography (CT) scans are ordered most often in the evaluation of suspected laryngeal neoplasms and for patients with vocal fold paralysis.

In the case of neoplasm, CT scanning is useful to assess the extent of the primary lesion and to evaluate possible metastatic cervical lymphadenopathy. In patients with laryngeal malignancy, chest radiography is also important to assess for pulmonary metastases. For patients with vocal fold paralysis who do not have a clear history of surgical injury of the recurrent laryngeal nerve, a CT scan from skull base to thoracic inlet identifies possible lesions along the course of the recurrent laryngeal nerve. Central problems are less likely, but if they are suspected as a cause of vocal fold paralysis, then magnetic resonance imaging of the brain may be indicated as well.

Types of Dysphonia

Although not comprehensive, the conditions discussed here account for the vast majority of voice complaints. Some patients with voice complaints have more than one condition, and not every patient will fit neatly into a single category. Nevertheless, understanding how each of these conditions creates dysphonia, and knowing which particular history and physical examination findings might be associated with each cause, can help a physician to appropriately diagnose and manage voice complaints.

Acute Laryngitis

Acute laryngitis is the most common cause of hoarseness and dysphonia. It is most often viral in nature, and onset of laryngeal symptoms may be associated with other symptoms of upper respiratory tract infection, including fever, myalgia, sore throat, and rhinorrhea. Viral inflammation of the vocal folds leads to diminished and more effortful vocal fold vibration, yielding a voice characterized by increased effort and a harsh, strained quality with decreased projection. Characteristic findings on laryngoscopy include vocal fold edema and erythema with decreased amplitude of the mucosal wave. Treatment of acute viral laryngitis is supportive, with counseling for hydration, humidification, and mucolytics. Symptoms generally are self-limited and resolve within 2 weeks. During this time, patients should be instructed to use the voice in a comfortable fashion, rather than straining or pushing to get loudness, because pushing behaviors may lead to the development of persistent muscle tension dysphonia.

Bacterial or fungal infections also cause acute laryngitis in rare cases. With appropriate physical findings and in the right clinical setting, antibiotic or antifungal therapy may be used to treat these conditions. Amoxicillin-clavulanate (Augmentin) is often the antibiotic of choice, and fluconazole (Diflucan) is a commonly used antifungal agent.

Chronic Laryngitis

Chronic laryngitis is the nonspecific condition of prolonged laryngeal inflammation; the term itself does not indicate an etiology for the inflammation. Among the many possible sources for this inflammation are mechanical irritation from traumatic coughing or prolonged speaking, chemical irritation from environmental irritants (e.g., smoking, inhaled medications), and irritation from postnasal drip or laryngopharyngeal reflux. More than one cause may exist simultaneously. Issues related to cigarette use, excessive voice use, medication effect, and rhinitis can be identified with careful history taking. Laryngopharyngeal reflux is a very common source of chronic laryngitis. It may manifest with several nonspecific symptoms, such as throat irritation, globus pharyngeus, frequent throat clearing, and nonproductive cough, with or without accompanying heartburn. Because vocal fold inflammation increases with continued mechanical trauma, the hoarseness of chronic laryngitis typically gets worse with prolonged voice use and improves with voice rest. Examination findings in chronic laryngitis include generalized laryngeal edema and erythema, and careful inspection may also reveal interarytenoid hyperplasia, subglottic edema, laryngeal ventricular obliteration, and an increase in thick glottic secretions.

Treatment of chronic laryngitis is tailored to the cause of the inflammation. Vocal hygiene with moderate voice use and instructions to reduce throat clearing and coughing may diminish mechanical irritation, and smoking cessation is recommended to any smoker with laryngeal complaints. Several studies have suggested that an appropriate trial of proton pump inhibitors for treatment of laryngopharyngeal reflux includes twice-daily therapy for at least 2 months, in contrast to the once-daily dosing often used for typical heartburn complaints. Lifestyle counseling to limit consumption of caffeine, carbonation, alcohol, and acidic foods can improve reflux, and attention to hydration and humidification decreases the viscosity of glottic secretions. For patients who are troubled by vocal difficulties associated with chronic laryngitis, referral to a speech–language pathologist for voice therapy can improve compliance with suggested lifestyle changes and help foster vocal improvement.

Vocal Fold Paralysis

The dysphonia in cases of vocal fold paralysis usually relates to poor vocal fold closure (Figure 2). The result is a breathy voice with limited projection and increased vocal effort. The farther from midline the immobile vocal fold, the more air leaks through the incompetent glottal valve without being turned into sound. Patients whose immobile vocal fold sits in a lateral position may have severely weak and breathy voices, whereas patients whose immobile vocal fold sits near midline may have a perceptually near-normal conversational voice and complain only of mild increase in effort, vocal fatigue, or problems with loud projection. Because of their glottal insufficiency, patients may complain of "running out of air" with prolonged speech. Impaired glottal

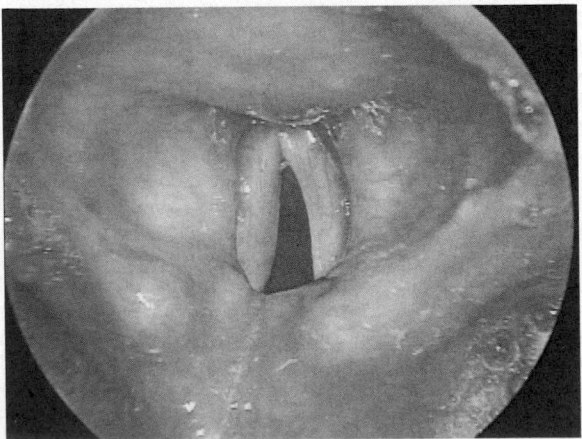

Figure 2. Vocal fold paralysis prevents the right vocal fold from closing to midline and creates dysphonia.

closure may also decrease airway protection during swallowing, so patients with vocal fold paralysis need to be questioned about aspiration as well. Whereas rehabilitation of poor voice may be elective, patients with increased aspiration risk need prompt therapy.

Evaluation of vocal fold paralysis includes identification of the cause of paralysis. Surgical injury to the recurrent laryngeal nerve accounts for almost half of all cases of unilateral vocal fold paralysis, and cervical or thoracic neoplasm and idiopathic paralysis account for most of the remaining cases. In a patient without a clear surgical history explaining the paralysis, CT scanning from skull base to mediastinum can identify any possible lesions along the course of the recurrent laryngeal nerve. In those patients whose histories suggest other possible causes (e.g., central neurologic injury, Lyme disease), further investigations, such as magnetic resonance imaging of the brain or blood work may be indicated as well. Some physicians perform laryngeal electromyography to help with the prognosis of paralysis or to differentiate neurologic injury from cricoarytenoid joint fixation; however, this study is neither standardized nor routine in many practices. Although flexible laryngoscopy alone may be satisfactory to document vocal fold immobility, stroboscopy can be added to investigate the impact of glottal insufficiency on vocal cord vibration and possible vocal fold flutter.

Treatment of vocal fold paralysis might include any combination of voice therapy, injection laryngoplasty, transcervical medialization laryngoplasty, and laryngeal reinnervation. Depending on the cause of the paralysis, some patients experience gradual recovery with synkinetic reinnervation or recovery of purposeful vocal fold motion over a period of several months. Based on the degree of voice and swallowing handicap, treatment of patients with vocal fold paralysis may be optional rather than necessary. Voice therapy can help teach patients to produce a stronger voice despite the paralysis, but by itself will not help a paralyzed vocal cord to recover motion. Various medialization techniques have been developed to help reposition an immobile vocal fold in the midline, where the contralateral mobile vocal fold can provide for complete glottal closure and lead to improved voice and swallowing. Injection medialization can be performed in the office or in the operating room, with temporary or permanent materials; if recovery of vocal fold motion is thought possible, then temporary injection is preferred. Transcervical medialization is a permanent but reversible surgical technique performed by otolaryngologists that repositions an immobile vocal fold in the midline. Laryngeal reinnervation offers the possibility of midline positioning of the immobile vocal fold with restored tone and bulk of the vocal fold musculature; however, because results may not mature for several months, this technique is less commonly performed than either injection or transcervical medialization.

Phonotraumatic Lesions: Nodules, Polyps, and Cysts

During vibration, vocal folds are subject to the shearing stresses of vibration. Although vocal fold structure is designed to accommodate these stresses in most circumstances, patients with vocal abuse or excessive voice use are at risk for development of lesions as the result of cumulative phonotrauma. Depending on the location and nature of these lesions, they are categorized as nodules, polyps, or cysts.

Vocal fold nodules are areas of fibrovascular scarring that are located just beneath the epithelium, at the level of the basement membrane and superficial lamina propria. They are typically bilateral and symmetrical, sitting at the junction of the anterior one third and the posterior two thirds of each vocal fold. Polyps are typically unilateral lesions that may be edematous or fibrous in nature and may contain hemorrhage (Figure 3). They usually are exophytic and extend outward from the vocal fold epithelium, although the fibrous base of a polyp may extend into the superficial lamina propria of a vocal fold. In contrast to an epithelial-based lesion such as a polyp, a vocal fold cyst is a subepithelial encapsulated lesion that sits entirely within the vocal fold; its size may exert a mass effect that deforms the medial edge of the

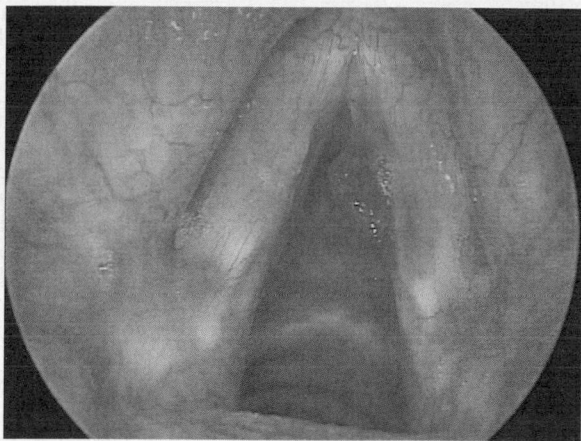

Figure 3. A large right hemorrhagic polyp, which can impair vocal fold vibration.

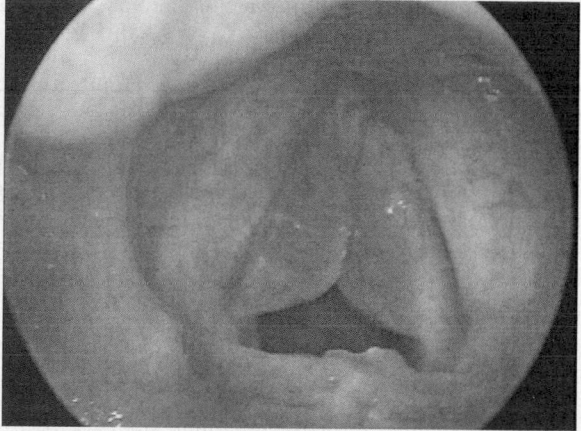

Figure 4. Symmetrical polypoid degeneration of the bilateral vocal folds, characteristic of Reinke's edema.

involved vocal fold. These cysts are occasionally noted as congenital lesions in children, but in adults they are more often caused by traumatic occlusion of the ducts of the seromucinous glands within the larynx.

Nodules, polyps, and cysts cause dysphonia by disturbing vocal fold vibration, leading to rough voice quality. These lesions get larger as traumatic voice use accumulates, and vocal roughness usually becomes more severe and more constant as the lesions progress. Because vibration is more easily disturbed at high pitch, performers with these lesions may notice that high pitch is affected first. Effort of phonation often increases, but projection remains intact. Lesions large enough to limit vocal fold closure may also cause a slightly breathy voice quality. Because patients with excessive voice use are at risk for these lesions, a history of social and occupational voice demands is valuable in cases of suspected phonotrauma.

Treatment for these lesions always begins with voice therapy designed to modify the patient's voice use so as to diminish trauma. Voice therapy may be all that is necessary to allow resolution of some early traumatic changes, particularly in the case of edematous nodules. If dysphonia persists despite voice therapy and other conservative measures, surgery may be considered. Surgery with the goal of voice preservation and restoration (phonosurgery) is typically performed by otolaryngologists who specialize in the care of persons with vocal difficulties. The goal of phonosurgery for these lesions is to remove the lesion that impairs vibration while preserving as much of the remaining, pliable superficial lamina propria as possible, so that vocal fold vibration can be restored.

Reinke's Edema

Reinke's edema, also known as polypoid corditis, is a benign swelling of the vocal folds that is most commonly seen in patients with a long-term smoking history. The edema, a reaction to long-term irritation, accumulates within the superficial lamina propria. The edema is most often bilateral and occurs diffusely along the entire length of the vocal fold, rather than being limited to a more discrete area, as is seen with phonotraumatic polyps (Figure 4). As vocal fold mass increases with disease progression, the pitch of the voice decreases, and this is the change in voice most associated with Reinke's edema. A classic presentation of this condition is a female in her fifth or sixth decade of life who provides a long history of smoking and progressive deepening of her voice. In rare circumstances, the vocal folds gradually accumulate enough edema to compromise the airway, so breathing complaints should be evaluated as well.

Because a significant smoking history is also a risk factor for vocal fold leukoplakia and malignancy, good visualization of the vocal folds is necessary to evaluate for other lesions in these patients. If benign edema of the vocal folds is truly the only lesion noted, management depends on the degree to which voice quality

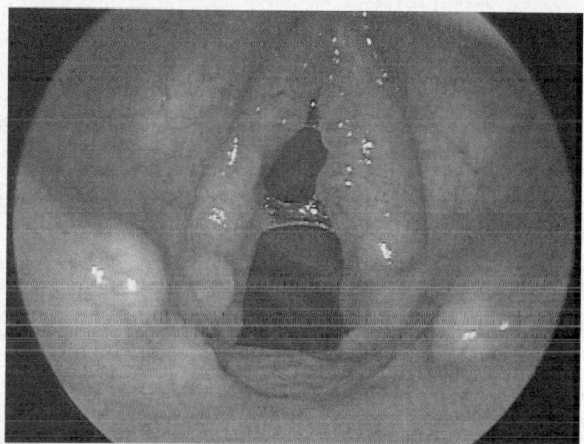

Figure 5. Recurrent respiratory papillomatosis, whose presence along each vocal fold medial edge disrupts sound production.

is disturbing to the patient or the degree to which the airway is narrowed. Smoking cessation can lead to stabilization of pitch at its current level, and phonosurgery to remove excess vocal fold mass can help lead to normalization of pitch and improve the airway. Phonosurgery may be performed with cold instruments or with the pulsed photoangiolytic lasers, an emerging therapy; in either case, there is a risk of creating a vocal fold scar that might limit vocal fold vibration even as vocal fold contours are improved.

Recurrent Respiratory Papillomatosis

Recurrent respiratory papillomatosis (Figure 5) is a benign laryngeal neoplasm that is caused by the human papilloma virus. It is the most common source of hoarseness in children, although adults also may be affected. As the lesions grow on the laryngeal epithelium, they create hoarseness and sometimes effortful voice by disrupting vocal fold vibration, particularly if the lesions are located along the medial edge of either vocal fold. Large and bulky lesions may lead to airway compromise, and advanced disease may spread throughout the mucosa of the upper aerodigestive tract rather than being limited to the larynx. Although accurate diagnosis depends on histopathologic analysis, a diagnosis of benign papilloma can be suspected from the characteristic appearance of the vascular fronds, which can be seen under magnified visualization in the office or in the operating room.

Treatment of recurrent respiratory papillomatosis is surgery, which is performed with a carbon dioxide laser, microdebrider, cold instruments, or the emerging technology of pulsed potassium titanyl phosphate (KTP) laser. As its name implies, the condition is recurrent: Even though surgery may reduce or remove the papilloma temporarily, the tissue continues to harbor the papilloma virus, and the disease usually grows back. Because repeated surgeries are expected, the goal of any single procedure is to remove as much disease as possible while limiting surgical scarring of the vocal folds. Scarring created as a result of surgery is cumulative, and over time patients develop persistent dysphonia caused as much by repeated surgeries as by recurrence of the disease. An ability to treat epithelial lesions while limiting scarring at the level of the superficial lamina propria is one main advantage of pulsed laser photoangiolysis; that these pulsed laser procedures can be performed in the office as well as the operating room is another. To help limit the need for repeated surgical procedures, adjunct medical therapies such as interferon and cidofovir are sometimes used for treatment of advanced disease.

Vocal Cord Cancer

In 2008, an estimated 12,250 new cases of laryngeal cancer and 3,670 deaths attributable to laryngeal cancer occurred in the United States. The annual incidence of laryngeal cancer is 6.4 cases per 100,000 for men and 1.3 cases per 100,000 for women. Smoking is the single largest risk factor for laryngeal cancer, and excessive alcohol use has a synergistic effect as a risk factor as well. Survival rates for laryngeal cancer depend on the stage of the tumor at the time of diagnosis, which is a function of tumor size and possible tumor spread to the cervical lymph nodes or distant metastatic sites. Cancers that occur on the medial edge of the vocal fold produce dysphonia while still small, and many laryngeal cancers are diagnosed early.

The dysphonia associated with laryngeal cancer is constant, progressive, and unremitting, without the intermittent vocal improvement that may occur in inflammatory conditions. The presence of dysphagia, odynophagia, otalgia, hemoptysis, or unexplained weight loss further increases the index of suspicion for malignancy. Cervical lymphadenopathy is associated with advanced tumors. Diagnosis may be suspected on the basis of laryngeal examination and is confirmed with biopsy. The presence or absence of mucosal waves on the involved vocal fold on videostroboscopic examination can help predict the depth of the lesion. Both a CT scan of the neck and chest radiographs are indicated to assess for tumor size and spread. Early cancers are treated with surgery or radiation therapy, with similar cure rates. Emerging technologies such as pulsed photoangiolytic lasers may allow for surgical treatment of early disease with better preservation of surrounding normal tissue. More advanced tumors are usually treated with a combination of radiation therapy and surgery or chemotherapy.

Leukoplakia, or a raised white plaque on the epithelial surface, is a visual marker for the likely presence of dysplasia or carcinoma in situ. As a very early lesion, vocal fold leukoplakia may manifest with mild dysphonia or may be found incidentally on head and neck examination performed for other reasons. This early disease may take many years before progressing to invasive carcinoma, and recognition of leukoplakia presents an opportunity for early treatment to prevent progression of disease. Pulsed laser photoangiolysis has emerged as a state-of-the-art therapy for treatment of this epithelial lesion with preservation of the underlying vocal fold pliability.

Neurologic Disorders and the Voice

Neurologic conditions that affect the voice usually do so by causing poor coordination of vocal fold motion. Spasmodic dysphonia, for instance, leads to involuntary spasms that bring the vocal folds either tightly together (adductor spasmodic dysphonia) or apart (abductor spasmodic dysphonia) during phonation. These spasms lead to vocal breaks that are strained or breathy, respectively. Although the cause of spasmodic dysphonia is thought to lie within the central nervous system, the gold standard treatment of botulinum toxin is targeted at the end organ. Injection of botulinum toxin (Botox)[1] into appropriate laryngeal muscles can weaken these muscles and diminish the spasm.

Vocal fold tremor is a neurologic disorder that is distinct from spasmodic dysphonia. Its hallmark is tremulous voice quality caused by tremor of the larynx, which may occur both during phonation and at rest. Vocal fold tremor may exist alone or as part of systemic tremor. Botulinum toxin[1] can decrease the amplitude of the tremor but may exacerbate the loss of projection that many tremor patients also have as a complaint. Medications such as anxiolytics or β-blockers that are used to treat systemic tremor may also improve the voice in patients with vocal fold tremor without worsening hypophonia.

Functional Voice Disorders

Functional dysphonia may exist by itself or in combination with an anatomic or neurologic source of dysphonia. The most common form of functional voice disorder is muscle tension dysphonia, which describes inappropriate hyperfunction of the supraglottic muscles. This hyperfunction often occurs in response to another source of hoarseness, as the patient tries to force out a strained voice with improved projection rather than accept the limited voice quality that may accompany the other disorder. The hyperfunction may then become an entrenched habit separate from the original pathology. In this sense, a classic scenario for muscle tension dysphonia is a patient who strains to speak more loudly during an acute laryngitis episode and whose strained, squeezed voice pattern persists even after the acute laryngitis has resolved. Patients with muscle tension dysphonia may complain of odynophonia as tension in the involved supraglottic muscles leads to muscular pain with prolonged speaking. Once other lesions have been evaluated, the treatment of muscle tension dysphonia is expert voice therapy with an emphasis on decreased hyperfunction.

Presbylaryngis

Presbylaryngis is the term that is used to describe the aging voice. It typically manifests in the seventh or eighth decade but can develop earlier. Acoustically, presbylaryngis results in a characteristic thinned voice, often with decreased projection and increased vocal strain. The condition occurs as cumulative voice use leads to traumatic thinning of the superficial lamina propria, particularly at the mid-cord level. This loss of superficial lamina propria leads to deficiency at the medial edge of each vocal fold, and a spindle-shaped defect in glottal closure may be noticed with close evaluation. Many patients with a complaint of presbylaryngis find that appropriate voice therapy to address breath support and vocal projection leads to satisfactory improvement in the voice without altering the vocal fold anatomy. For those patients who remain unsatisfied with their voice after therapy, vocal fold medialization procedures can restore straight vocal cord edges and may lead to improved projection; however, currently available injectables and implants that address contour defects cannot restore pliability.

Conclusion

Understanding the anatomy and physiology of normal voice production provides a framework through which dysphonia can be evaluated. Application of this knowledge during the history and physical examination guides the diagnosis of hoarseness and allows clinicians to distinguish among conditions as varied as acute laryngitis, benign phonotraumatic lesions, vocal fold paralysis, and laryngeal cancer as part of a differential diagnosis. Videostrobolaryngoscopy allows evaluation of vocal fold function

---

[1]Not FDA approved for this indication.

as well as structure and can confirm diagnosis. As with any condition, accurate diagnosis directs appropriate therapy. Because no further evaluation or management is necessary for acute viral laryngitis, many patients with hoarseness require no more than a careful history and physical examination. However, if dysphonia persists for longer than 2 weeks or is accompanied by other laryngopharyngeal symptoms that are not thought to be related to an upper respiratory tract infection, referral should be made to an otolaryngologist for further evaluation.

References

Koufman JA, Aviv JE, Casiano RR, et al. Laryngopharyngeal reflux: Position statement of the committee on speech, voice, and swallowing disorders of the American Academy of Otolaryngology-Head and Neck Surgery. Otolaryngol Head Neck Surg 2002;127:32–5.

Merati AL, Heman-Ackah YD, Abaza M, et al. Common movement disorders affecting the larynx: A report from the neurolaryngology committee of the AAO-HNS. Otolaryngol Head Neck Surg 2005;133:654–65.

Swibel Rosenthal LH, Benninger MS, Deeb RH. Vocal fold immobility: A longitudinal analysis of etiology over 20 years. Laryngoscope 2007;117:1864–70.

Wilson JA, Deary IJ, Millar A, et al. The quality of life impact of dysphonia. Clin Otolaryngol 2002;27:179–82.

Zeitels SM, Casiano RR, Gardner GM, et al. Management of common voice problems: Committee report. Otolaryngol Head Neck Surg 2002;126:333–48.

Zeitels SM, Healy GB. Laryngology and phonosurgery. N Engl J Med 2003;349:882–92.

PAIN

Method of
Steven A. House, MD

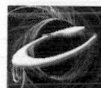

CURRENT DIAGNOSIS

- Always use history and physical examination and consider imaging or laboratory studies to rule out life- or function-threatening pathologies before merely providing symptomatic treatment.

Acute Pain

- Acute pain has a sudden onset, is usually nociceptive (somatic, visceral) in nature, and likely is due to apparent injury or medical condition.
- It can last up to 3 months and can demonstrate hypersympathetic signs of tachycardia, elevated blood pressure, dilated pupils, or diaphoresis.

Chronic Pain

- Chronic pain is usually gradual in onset, lasts more than 3 months, and rarely serves any purpose. It can manifest with hyperalgesia (hurts more than it should) or allodynia (hurts when it should not, e.g., light touch).
- Vegetative symptoms such as depression, fatigue, or anorexia may be present.
- A significant neuropathic component may be present.
- Psychiatric and social or socioeconomic issues may be exacerbating factors.
- Examples can include headaches, low back pain, osteoarthritis, and fibromyalgia.

Quality

- Quality of the pain (e.g., sharp, dull, radiating, deep, superficial, lancinating, tingling, burning) is an important factor in determining the best management modalities.
- Quality plays a role in ruling in or ruling out severe disease that can require urgent surgical or other interventions rather than analgesics or adjunctive medications or therapies.

Severity

- Severity of the pain can be rated on a variety of scales such as numerical (0–5, 0–10), analogue (marked on a line with a range from no pain to the worst possible pain), or facial expression (smiles to grimaces, available for children and the elderly or patients with dementia).
- Functional scales (fully satisfactory function to debilitated) may be more helpful in determining the impact of the pain on the person's life.

CURRENT THERAPY

Acute pain commonly responds to simple analgesics of the nonopioid, opioid, or combination varieties. Rest, ice, compression, and elevation (RICE) are helpful for acute inflammatory conditions and injuries.

Adjuvant medications are drugs that are used for pain but do not have pain treatment as their primary indication.

- Chronic pain, because of its complexity, often requires multiple modalities. Pharmacologic options include nonopioid, opioid, adjuvant, or homeopathic medications. Nonpharmacologic options include physical therapy, chiropractic care, transcutaneous electrical nerve stimulation (TENS) unit, acupuncture, or surgical or anesthesia interventions.
- Opioids are generally safer for long-term use, but the individual's risk for falls must be considered in the elderly from the GI and cardiac standpoint, as opioids can increase this risk, and the risk of overdose may rise with increasing age.
- Adjuvant medications are often the most effective agents in neuropathic pain.
- The patient *must* be involved in and cooperative with the treatment plan. Honesty and trust are necessary components of a therapeutic physician–patient relationship.
- Do not underestimate the placebo effect. If the patient feels that a harmless treatment is beneficial, take advantage of it.
- If the patient is not improving adequately, consult a surgeon if the source of pain is an operable condition, or consult a pain specialist if surgical intervention is not appropriate.
- Controlled substance agreements and ongoing drug testing as well as use of prescription-monitoring programs available in most states are important in appropriate monitoring of therapy.

Epidemiology

Approximately 50 million Americans experience chronic pain, with annual expenditures and overall economic impact estimated at $85 to $90 billion. Pain is the most common symptom that causes patients to pursue medical evaluation and management. The prevalence of several common pain syndromes including headaches, facial pain, abdominal pain, pelvic pain, and low back pain is slightly higher in women than in men because there are gender variations in the perception, coping, and reporting of pain. Pain tends to be undertreated in women, people of color, children, and the elderly, and it is underreported in nonverbal or cognitively impaired children and adults.

Risk Factors

Traumatic injury is a cause of acute pain and a risk factor for chronic pain. Patients who have mastectomy, laminectomy, thoracotomy, or amputations are at risk for pain syndromes. Chronic musculoskeletal conditions such as arthritis, spinal stenosis, degenerative disk disease, or fibromyalgia; infectious diseases including HIV or varicella zoster; neuropathies from diagnoses such as diabetes, B_{12} deficiency, or multiple sclerosis; treatment with certain chemotherapies or isoniazid (INH) without adequate vitamin B_6; psychiatric disorders such as depression, anxiety, or posttraumatic stress disorder (PTSD), especially as a consequence of domestic violence; or autoimmune disorders including lupus and rheumatoid arthritis can predispose the individual to chronic pain. Although the risk of pain increases with age, pain should not be considered a usual part of aging until it is appropriately evaluated. A motor vehicle accident or work-related injury or other condition where secondary gain is a possibility, especially if there is no apparent injury, raises the consideration of malingering.

Pathophysiology

Injury or potential injury is detected by nociceptors in the peripheral nervous system, and the signal is then transmitted through the dorsal horn of the spinal cord up to the brain for processing. The three primary classes of opioid receptors are the mu, kappa, and delta receptors, and they are located in areas throughout the central and peripheral nervous system. Upon binding these receptors, opioids block calcium channels and modulate the nociceptive pathways. The Hyperstimulation of chronic pain and the resultant increase in intracelluar calcium are neurotoxic due to lowering neuronal firing threshold and increasing firing frequency. This neurotoxicity can lead to ongoing pain in the absence of physical insult. Neuropathic pain can result from chronic pain or from physical or pathophysiologic injury or changes to the nerve, as in diabetic neuropathy or other neuropathies.

Prevention

The best prevention is a safe and healthy lifestyle. The combination of healthy diet and exercise has been demonstrated to improve pain in osteoarthritis better than either intervention alone, and maintaining a healthy weight can help to prevent the arthritis in the first place. Smoking and obesity have been associated with chronic pain. Regarding safety, wearing seat belts while driving or using appropriate safety equipment at work and during recreational activities can help to reduce the severity of injuries should they occur. Proper body mechanics are important as well.

Clinical Manifestations

Manifestations of pain depend upon the location and underlying cause. In the acute setting, the patient can have tachycardia, elevated blood pressure, or diaphoresis, whereas chronic pain can manifest with vegetative symptoms of depression, fatigue, anorexia, or insomnia.

Diagnosis

Pain is most commonly a symptom rather than a disease in and of itself, so it behooves the provider to pursue treatable causes, especially red flag conditions, in addition to providing symptomatic treatment. The history regarding onset (shorter or longer than 3 months), exacerbating or remitting factors, quality, radiation, severity, and timing of the pain (constant vs. intermittent), in addition to any associated signs or symptoms such as fever, nausea, vomiting, or diarrhea, can help the provider in that regard. The physical examination is a key component in ruling out life- or function-threatening disorders. Is there tenderness, swelling, bruising, erythema, or deformity? Are strength, reflexes, and sensation intact? Does the patient demonstrate a consistent demeanor (grimace or other signs of pain) and gait (antalgic vs. normal) when moving from the waiting area to the examination room and out to the parking lot? The choice to use laboratory studies or imaging is determined by the location of the pain and the structures or organs that might be in that area. When determining severity, "What does the pain keep you from doing?" (which uses function as the measure of impairment and treatment efficacy rather than a subjective pain score to guide therapy) may be a much more helpful question than "How bad is your pain?" If function is not improving, that could be considered a treatment failure, and medications and therapy should be adjusted rather than continuing the same regimen.

Differential Diagnosis

The differential diagnosis for all types of pain is far too extensive for the brevity of this chapter, but in addition to the plethora of physical diagnoses to be considered, the provider has to consider that chronic fatigue, depression, and domestic abuse can manifest as a chronic pain syndrome.

Treatment

Nonpharmacologic

Physical therapy, TENS units, chiropractic care, and regular exercise have shown benefit in certain conditions. Surgery may be required, and interventions such as vertebroplasty, nerve blocks, and epidural injections may also be of benefit. Aerobic exercise and water therapy are helpful for fibromyalgia, but the patient must not overexert because this can exacerbate the pain.

Pharmacologic

Nonopioid Analgesics

Acetaminophen (Tylenol) is generally a safe and effective medication as long as the total daily dose for adults remains less than 3 g/day.

Numerous NSAIDs are available, but none has been shown to be superior to another except for the convenience of dosing daily versus every 6 hours. All are generally safe in the acute setting but should be used with caution if needed long term, and they should be avoided altogether for long-term use in the elderly or patients with cardiovascular, renal, or peptic ulcer disease. This caution includes the cyclooxygenase (COX)-2–specific drugs. Naproxen seems to have the best cardiac profile while the COX-2 drugs tend to have the best GI profile. Misoprostol or proton pump inhibitors can be used for GI prophylaxis.

Topical agents such as diclofenac (Flector 1.3% Patch, Voltaren 1% Gel), menthol, camphor, lidocaine, and capsaicin (Zostrix, Qutenza) are effective in some patients.

Opioids (see Table 1)

For patients with inadequate response to the non-opioid analgesics, opioids are an option (Table 1). Opioids are generally a safer option in the elderly as compared to NSAIDs, but they should be avoided in patients with untreated sleep apnea because of increased risk for complications.

Tramadol (Ultram) is a weak mu agonist and an inhibitor of norepinephrine and serotonin uptake, a quality that gives it a niche in the treatment of neuropathic and radicular pain.[1] It is the only opioid studied for fibromyalgia[1] in a randomized trial. A recent study has demonstrated an increased risk for hypoglycemia, notably in the first 30 days of treatment with tramadol.

Codeine is a prodrug that has to be converted to morphine to be effective, and about 10% of the population lacks the cytochrome P450 2D6 enzyme that makes the conversion. Owing to the need for conversion, doses exceeding 60 mg do not increase benefit because the enzyme system is saturated. Use caution when prescribing codeine to children as deaths have been reported, even with the use of age- and weight-appropriate dosages, as a result of the hypermetabolism of codeine to morphine. The mu agonists do not technically have a ceiling dose; however, the dose should be limited to the lowest effective dose. (See the warning in the last paragraph in this section.) In the purely palliative or hospice patient, the dosage may be titrated to effect until the pain is relieved or side effects limit the dosage.

Morphine is the prototype for the opioids. It is extremely versatile, it can be given via almost any route, and it is available in multiple dosages and preparations ranging from liquid to daily sustained release. Hydromorphone (Dilaudid) shares similar qualities but is more potent. Hydrocodone is only available in the oral form and in combination with acetaminophen (Lortab, Norco). It was the number-one prescribed drug in the United States in 2011 at more than 136 million prescriptions, with generic levothyroxine (Synthroid, Levoxyl) as a distant second.

---

[1]Not FDA approved for this indication.

TABLE 1   Opioid Analgesics

OPIOID	ADMINISTRATION		PROPERTIES
	PARENTERAL	**ORAL**	
Buprenorphine			
Butrans transdermal patch: 5, 10, 20 µg/h weekly patches Subutex* SL tab and film: 2, 8 mg Buprenex injection: 0.3 mg/mL	0.3 mg (IV) Patch: MED <30 mg/day = 5 µg/h patch 30–80 mg/day = 10 µg/h patch; >80 mg/day: do not use	Oral buprenorphine, with or without naloxone (Suboxone, Subutex) is limited to treatment of opiate addiction Requires training, approval, and new DEA number	Partial agonist Can cause QT prolongation C-III
Codeine			
Tablet: 15, 30, 60 mg Oral solution: 15 mg/5 mL	130 mg	180 mg	Prodrug converted by liver to morphine About 10% of population cannot convert, and some are rapid metabolizers, resulting in increased levels of morphine Ceiling dose is 60 mg/dose
Fentanyl			
Duragesic 72 h patch: 12.5, 25, 50, 75, 100 µg/h	~100 µg/h	—	Patch for those who cannot swallow Patient *must* have subcutaneous fat because drug is lipophilic
Actiq or Oralet lozenge: 200, 400, 600, 800, 1200, 1600 µg Fentora buccal tab or Abstral SL tab: 100, 200, 300, 400, 600, 800 µg Subsys sublingual spray: 100, 200, 400, 600, 800 µg/spray.	No conversion for lozenges or buccal tabs; various formulations are not bioequivalent, so use caution when switching from one formulation to another; *must* start at lowest dose and titrate	~ ½ × daily morphine dose, disregarding units, e.g., 200 mg morphine PO/day = 100 µg/h patch	Lozenge or buccal tab for transmucosal use No cheap forms available Buccal formulations *only* indicated for breakthrough cancer pain in the opioid tolerant; Can be rapidly fatal in opioid naïve patients.
Hydrocodone			
Tab: 2.5, 5, 7.5, 10 mg with a max of 325 mg APAP per tablet (Norco, Lortab) as of 2014. (Lorcet no longer available) or with 200 mg ibuprofen (Vicoprofen 7.5/200; Ibudone 5/200, 10/200; Reprexain 2.5/200, 5/200, 10/200); Zohydro ER: 10, 15, 20, 30, 40, 50 mg/cap q 12 hours Solution: with APAP 7.5/325, 10/300, 10/325 per 15 mL	N/A	20 mg	CII as of 2014, so refills and phone orders are no longer allowed. Metabolized to hydromorphone and others
Hydromorphone (Dilaudid)			
Tab: 2, 4, 8 mg Liquid: 1 mg/mL Suppository: 3 mg SR† 24-h tab (Exalgo): 8, 12, 16 mg Injection (Dilaudid-HP): 1, 2, 4, 10 mg/mL	1.5 mg	7.5 mg	Good alternative to morphine, especially if using SC by continuous infusion (>20 mg/h) Active glucuronide metabolites
Meperidine (Demerol)			
Tab: 50, 100 mg Syrup: 50 mg/5 mL	100 mg	300 mg	Indicated for *acute* use *only* (i.e., <48 h) Contraindicated with MAOI and/or renal disease: Neurotoxic metabolite normeperidine can cause seizures and death

Continued

Pain

TABLE 1 Opioid Analgesics—cont'd

OPIOID	ADMINISTRATION		PROPERTIES
	PARENTERAL	ORAL	
Methadone (Dolophine)			
Tab: 5, 10, 40 mg Oral liquid: 1, 2, 10 mg/mL*40 mg dispersible tab (Methadose) – restricted use in US, mostly for detox or addiction maintenance dosing		Variable conversion ratios (see Table 2): converted by oral morphine equivalent dose	At least 3 mechanisms: mu agonist, NMDA receptor antagonist, norepinephrine–serotonin reuptake inhibition The longest-acting opioid Cheap: ~1¢ /mg Can cause QT prolongation Torsades de pointes is more likely with IV dosing STRONGLY consider risks before prescribing. Safety guidelines available from the American Pain Society.
Morphine			
Tab: 15, 30 mg Liquid: 10, 20, or 100 mg/5 mL (Roxanol) SR[†] 12-h tab (MS Contin): 15, 30, 60, 100, 200 mg SR[†] 12-h tab (Oramorph SR): 15, 30, 60, 100 mg SR[†] 24-h cap (Kadian): 10, 20, 30, 50, 60, 80, 100, 200 mg SR[†] 24-h cap (Avinza): 30, 45, 60, 75, 90, 120 mg SR[†] cap with naltrexone (Embeda): 20/0.8, 30/1.2, 50/2, 60/2.4, 80/3.2, 100/4 mg Suppository: 5, 10, 20, 30 mg	10 mg	30 mg	Numerous routes; very cheap, readily available; active metabolites, morphine-6-glucuronide 10 × more potent than morphine Avinza and Kadian capsules may be opened and beads sprinkled in applesauce, but the beads should not be crushed Avinza may be opened into apple juice and injected via gastric tube Kadian may be opened into water and given by gastric tube
Oxycodone			
Tab: 5, 10, 15, 20, 30 mg Liquid: 5 mg/5 mL or 20 mg/mL (OxyFast) SR[†] 12-h tab (generic, OxyContin): 10, 15, 20, 30, 40, 60, 80 mg SR[†] 12-h w/naltrexone (Targiniq ER 10/5, 20/10, 40/20) Multiple combinations w/APAP (Percocet, Endocet, Tylox) SR[†] 12-h w/APAP 7.5/325 (Xartemis XR)	N/A	20 mg	Equal potency but a little more bioavailable than morphine Caution in liver disease: T½ extends up to 4 × normal. Metabolized to oxymorphone: 40 × more potent than oxycodone ER/LA Opioids require REMS
Oxymorphone			
Tab: 5, 10 mg (Opana); in opioid-naïve patients, starting dose >20 mg/day is not recommended	1 mg	10 mg	Potentiated by cimetidine (Tagamet), MAOIs, and other CNS depressants
SR[†] tab (Opana ER): 5, 7.5, 10, 15, 20, 30, 40 mg, dosed q12h	1 mg	10 mg	10% bioavailability Caution with CrCl < 50 or with liver impairment Take 1 h before or 2 h after food (food increases absorption)

*Only approved in the United States for the treatment of opioid dependence.
[†]Sustained-release formulations should never be crushed.
Abbreviations: APAP = acetaminophen (*N*-acetyl-*p*-aminophenol); CNS = central nervous system; CrCl = creatinine clearance; MED = morphine equivalent dose; MAOI = monoamine oxidase inhibitor; NMDA = *N*-methyl-D-aspartate; TIRF-REMS = Transmucosal Immediate-Release Fentanyl Risk-Evaluation and Mitigation Strategy.

Methadone (Dolophine) is the longest acting of the opioids at a half-life of 23 hours, although the duration of action can be variable. It is active as an *N*-methyl-D-aspartate (NMDA) receptor antagonist, inhibits norepinephrine and serotonin uptake, and is an agonist at the mu receptor. Therefore, methadone can be effective when other opioids fail, especially in the case of chronic or neuropathic pain,[1] where the NMDA-receptor is more of a factor in pain control. It must be used with caution (Table 2) because it can prolong the QT interval and has an increased dose-dependent risk of respiratory depression as compared to other opioids. It is only approved in the United States for the treatment of opioid dependence.

Meperidine (Demerol) is relatively weak compared to morphine and others, and it is limited by poor oral bioavailability, a 48-hour acute pain indication, and the neurotoxicity of one of its metabolites, normeperidine (renally cleared, so it is contraindicated in renal patients). Other opioids are safer and more effective, so its use should be limited.

The mixed agonist-antagonists such as nalbuphine (Nubain), pentazocine (Talwin), and butorphanol (Stadol) tend to have a higher incidence of hallucination and confusion, and, because they are

[1]Not FDA approved for this indication.

TABLE 2	Morphine and Methadone Equivalents	
MORPHINE (DAILY REQUIREMENT)		**METHADONE EQUIVALENT**
<500 mg		5:1
500–1000 mg		10:1
>1000 mg		20:1

Acute pain: methadone = morphine (1:1). Chronic pain: The above conversion is for illustration of the complexity of methadone use. A more-detailed table should be referenced before prescribing, and methadone should be used with extreme caution because of the risk for cardiac complications and respiratory depression.

agonists at kappa and delta receptors and antagonists at the mu receptor, they can produce withdrawal symptoms in patients who are routinely taking mu agonists. The partial agonist buprenorphine (Butrans patch, Subutex,[1] Buprenex) is dose limited because it has a maximal effective dose as well as a potential to cause QT prolongation.

Patients who are taking opioids on a chronic basis should use a stimulant laxative such as senna with or without docusate because fiber and dietary modification are usually inadequate for opioid-induced constipation, and fiber can aggravate the problem. Bisacodyl should not be used chronically due to its potential to damage the myenteric plexus of the gut.

As a word of caution, recent research has demonstrated a twofold to threefold increase in all-cause mortality with chronic opioid use, especially if using more than 200 mg/day morphine equivalent and/or sustained-release or long-acting (methadone) preparations. Additionally, risk of overdose death is increased to 3.7 to 4.6-fold at doses of 50-100 mg/day MED as compared to MED of less than 20 mg/day. The risk of postoperative respiratory depression increases with age. The risks of using chronic opioids likely outweigh the benefits in the management of headache, fibromyalgia and chronic low back pain according to a 2014 position paper from the American Academy of Neurology.

Adjuvant Drugs

Adjuvant medications are drugs that are useful in the management of pain but do not have pain treatment as an indication. Some adjuvant medications such as duloxetine (Cymbalta) and pregabalin (Lyrica) have received an FDA indication for diabetic peripheral neuropathic pain. Tricyclic antidepressants are useful for chronic pain and they have the benefit, unlike duloxetine, of working at the lowest doses rather than having to titrate to the maximum dose to gain benefit.

Several anticonvulsants have demonstrated efficacy in the management of pain, most notably gabapentin (Neurontin),[1] pregabalin (Lyrica), and carbamazepine (Tegretol).[1] Others have been tested in trials, but these three have the most evidence to support their use. Gabapentin and pregabalin have the benefit of not requiring monitoring of blood levels or for marrow, liver, or renal toxicities.

Corticosteroids can be beneficial in inflammatory conditions, nerve or spinal cord compression, or increased intracranial pressure due to neoplasms. Any can help, but blood pressure elevations and fluid retention can be problematic in all but dexamethasone (Decadron),[1] which lacks mineralocorticoid activity. Steroids also have the downside of elevating blood glucose and, in long-term use, causing osteoporosis.

Muscle relaxants may be beneficial if muscle spasm is a source of pain, but there is insufficient evidence to determine relative efficacy or safety. Of these, two stand out: metaxalone (Skelaxin), which lacks the black-box warning for the operation of heavy equipment, and tizanidine (Zanaflex), which can antagonize α_1 receptors in the spinal cord to provide additional pain relief. In chronic use, the patient will need to be monitored for anemia and leukopenia with metaxalone and for liver abnormalities with tizanidine.

Calcitonin (Miacalcin)[1] has shown very modest benefit for pain due to osteoporotic vertebral compression fractures, but it shows no benefit for compression fractures due to bone metastasis.

---

[1]Not FDA approved for this indication.

Ziconotide (Prialt) has demonstrated benefit as well as safety for long-term pain management, but it is limited to only intrathecal use owing to gastrointestinal side effects.

Regarding alternative medications, riboflavin,[1,7] butterbur,[1,7] and coenzyme Q10 (CoQ10)[1,7] are effective for migraine prophylaxis. Glucosamine sulfate[7] (not HCl), S-adenosylmethionine (SAM-e),[1,7] methylsulfonylmethane (MSM),[1,7] and willow bark[1,7] are likely effective for arthritic and low-back pain.

Numerous medications in multiple drug classes have been studied for fibromyalgia, but many of the trials are small and/or of poor quality. Of these drugs, duloxetine (Cymbalta), pregabalin (Lyrica) and milnacipran (Savella) have received an FDA indication for fibromyalgia; and gabapentin (Neurontin),[1] ondansetron (Zofran),[1] and naltrexone (Depade, ReVia)[1] demonstrated modest benefit. Gabapentin (Neurontin)[1] has been beneficial using a single dose of 1200 mg preoperatively, notably in combination with celecoxib, in reducing postoperative opioid requirements in mastectomy, laminectomy, and thoracotomy patients.

Monitoring

Controlled-substance agreements are beneficial in setting the boundaries for the use of opioid pain relievers (Figure 1). Routine visits are necessary to document ongoing need for and adequate response to the prescribed regimen. Routine drug screening is beneficial for monitoring compliance with the opioid as well as nonopioid medications. However, the provider needs to be aware of the metabolites of the different drugs. Hydromorphone (Dilaudid) and oxymorphone (Opana) are metabolites of hydrocodone (Lortab, Norco) and oxycodone (Percocet, Endocet, OxyContin), respectively. Drug screening is not specifically recommended in the documentation guidelines released by the Federation of State Medical Boards, but other guidelines do recommend it. Most states have prescription-monitoring programs that allow providers to monitor for the use of multiple providers and pharmacies to obtain controlled medications. Rules governing the prescribing and use of controlled substances vary among states, so the provider should be knowledgeable of local regulations as well as Federal DEA requirements.

Complications

The Centers for Disease Control and Prevention (CDC) reported in 2011 that opioid pain relievers were involved in 73.8% of the 20,044 prescription drug overdose deaths, and this is believed to be an underestimate. Overdose death rates were three times greater in non-Hispanic whites and in American Indians and Alaska Natives than in blacks and Hispanic whites. The death rates were highest in the 35- to 54-years age range, producing a YPLL (years of potential life lost) comparable to that of motor vehicle accidents. Medicaid populations are at greater risk of opioid overdose than non-Medicaid populations, and prescription drug overdose death rates are higher in the more rural and impoverished counties.

In addition to the deaths, there is a significant cost burden of substance abuse treatment admissions, with the 2008 rates being six times the 1999 rate. Nonmedical use of opioids represents up to $72.5 billion in health care costs. By 2010, opioids were sold in such a volume that every American adult could be treated for a month with hydrocodone 5 mg every 4 hours. Incidentally, 1999 is the year that several organizations began promoting "pain as the fifth vital sign," with no secondary improvement in the quality of pain management. Drug addiction is very real, and about 15% of patients may be genetically predisposed to addiction; therefore, clinicians should strongly consider this in their risk/benefit analysis before exposing a patient to these powerful medications. Using a tool such as the Opioid Risk Tool may be helpful in determining the risk of addiction in a particular individual.

Long-term safety of opioids has not been demonstrated, and chronic use has been associated with sleep disorders, adrenal suppression, and hypogonadism (and secondary erectile dysfunction and depression).

---

[1]Not FDA approved for this indication.
[7]Available as dietary supplement.

Controlled Substances Agreement

1. **Purpose: This agreement is provided to prevent misunderstandings about policies regarding medications designated by the DEA as "controlled substances" that you will be taking for pain management or other medical conditions.** This protects both you and your provider(s) and helps to ensure compliance with federal and/or state laws regarding such substances.

2. **I understand that my provider is consenting to treat me based on this Agreement.**

3. **I understand that if I break this Agreement, my provider will stop prescribing these medications.** In the event of an Agreement violation, my provider may choose to taper me off of my medication, discontinue the medication and prescribe another medication to treat the withdrawal symptoms, or discontinue the medication and refer me to a detoxification program. This choice will be made by my provider.

4. If the medicine prescribed is a pain medication, I will communicate fully and honestly with my provider about the character and intensity of my pain, the effect that my pain has on my daily life, and how well the medication is helping to relieve my pain. I will take the medication ONLY as prescribed - any changes in dose or frequency need to be authorized by my provider BEFORE I make any changes. **I will only use the medication for the treatment of my physical pain and NOT for emotional or psychological distress (i.e., to get high).**

5. My physician may prescribe other medications (adjuvant medications) or non-pharmacological therapies (physical therapy, TENS unit, etc.) to help with certain aspects of pain such as muscle spasm, burning, tingling, or radiating pain. **I will comply with this treatment with the same diligence as is expected for my controlled medication.**

6. **I will not use ANY illegal controlled substances, including, but not limited to, marijuana, cocaine, methamphetamine, and/or heroin.** Any such use of any such illicit substances may result in **IMMEDIATE TERMINATION OF ANY AND ALL CONTROLLED SUBSTANCES** by the provider. Additionally, I understand that alcohol, although legal, should not be used in conjunction with my medication as the combination could be fatal.

7. **I will not share, sell, or trade my medications to anyone.** Altering a prescription in any manner, selling medications to others, or misrepresenting myself to a pharmacy is a serious offense. **Such infractions are felonies and will be reported to the police.** In addition, any such misuse will result in **IMMEDIATE TERMINATION OF ANY AND ALL CONTROLLED SUBSTANCES** by the provider.

8. **I will not attempt to obtain ANY controlled medications, including, but not limited to, narcotic pain medications, controlled stimulants, or antianxiety medications, from ANY other provider or physician, ER or urgent care center, or another individual. I will take my medications and ONLY my medications.** Any such attempt will result in **IMMEDIATE TERMINATION OF ANY AND ALL CONTROLLED SUBSTANCES** by the provider.

9. **I am responsible for my own medications. This responsibility begins as soon as I am given the written prescription. I will safeguard my written prescription and medications from loss or theft.** Lost or stolen medications will NOT be replaced under any circumstances. (Carry with you only the amount of medication you will need while away from home. Your medication should be secured at home in a lock box or safe. **These medications can be rapidly fatal to children, adolescents, or others who do not need the medication.)**

10. **I understand that refills of my prescriptions will be made at the time of an office visit or during regular office hours and never during evenings or weekends when the office is closed.** (If you fail to come to a scheduled appointment without notifying us PRIOR to that appointment, you will not be given a refill until you are seen.)

11. **I authorize my provider and my pharmacy to cooperate fully with any city, state and/or federal law enforcement agency** in the investigation of any possible misuse, sale, or other diversion of my medications.

12. **I agree to submit to a blood or urine test at my cost, if requested by my provider,** in order to determine my compliance with my medication program. Refusal to submit to this testing will result in the **IMMEDIATE TERMINATION OF ANY AND ALL CONTROLLED SUBSTANCES** by the provider.

13. I understand that the use of these medications may adversely affect my ability to drive, operate machinery, or perform certain tasks or occupations, and I agree, given that risk, not to use these medications under these circumstances.

14. I understand that a healthy lifestyle can be helpful in achieving control of pain, depression, and / or anxiety. **I will strive toward smoking cessation, a healthy diet, and exercise as my condition allows.**

15. **I agree to these guidelines, and they have been fully explained to me.** All of my questions and concerns regarding treatment have been adequately answered. A copy of this Agreement will be given to me, and a signed copy will be placed in my medical record.

NOTE: NO REFILLS WILL BE MADE UNDER ANY CIRCUMSTANCES WHATSOEVER DURING EVENINGS OR ON WEEKENDS.

I agree to use _____ pharmacy, *and only this pharmacy*, for my prescriptions for controlled substances.

This Agreement entered on this date: _____

Patient / Parent / Guardian signature: _____

Provider signature: _____

Witness: _____

Figure 1. Controlled substances agreement.

References

Argoff C. Tailoring chronic pain treatment to the patient: Long-acting, short-acting and rapid-onset opioids, Medscape Neurology & Neurosurgery March 26, 2007; Available at http://www.medscape.com/viewarticle/554015; [accessed 6.24.15].

Chou R, Peterson K, Helfand M. Comparative efficacy and safety of skeletal muscle relaxants for spasticity and musculoskeletal conditions. J Pain Sympt Manage 2004; 28:140–75.

Fournier JP, Azoulay L, Yin H, Montastruc JL, Suissa S. Tramadol Use and the Risk of Hospitalization in Patients with Noncancer Pain. JAMA Intern Med 2015;175 (2):186–93.

Franklin GM. Opioids for Chronic Noncancer Pain: A Position Paper of the American Academy of Neurology. Neurology 2014;83:1277–84.

Gomes T, Mandani MM, Dhalla IA, Paterson JM, Juurlink DN. Opioid dose and drug-related mortality in patients with nonmalignant pain. Arch Intern Med 2011;171(6):686–91.

Jellin JM, Gregory PJ, et al. Pharmacist's Letter/Prescriber's Letter Natural Medicines Comprehensive Database. 12th ed Stockton, CA: Therapeutic Research Faculty; 2009.

Mularski RA, White-Chu F, Overbay D, et al. Measuring pain as the 5th vital sign does not improve quality of pain management. J Gen Intern Med 2006; 21:607–12.

Partners Against Pain. Gender and pain management. Available at http://www.partnersagainstpain.com/hcp/pain-management-resources/gender-pain.aspx [accessed 6.22.15].

Paulozzi LJ, Jones CM. Vital signs: Overdoses of prescription opioid pain relievers—united states, 1999–2008. MMWR 2011;60:1487–92.

Pletcher MJ, Kertesz SG, Kohn MA, Gonzales R. Trends in opioid prescribing by race/ethnicity for patients seeking care in US emergency departments. JAMA 2008;299:70–8.

Traynor LM, Thiessen CN, Traynor AP. Pharmacotherapy of fibromyalgia. Am J Health Syst Pharm 2011;68:1307–19.

Webster LR, Webster RM. Predicting aberrant behaviors in opioid-treated patients: preliminary validation of the opioid risk tool. Pain Med 2005; 6:432–42.

PALPITATIONS

Method of
Rebecca Katzman, MD; and Justin Bailey, MD

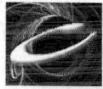

CURRENT DIAGNOSIS

- History and physical examination
- Electrocardiogram
- Complete blood count (CBC)
- Thyroid-stimulating hormone (TSH)
- Complete metabolic panel

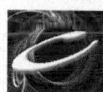

CURRENT THERAPY

- Dependent on underlying etiology. See Table 7.

Palpitations are the unpleasant sensation or awareness of one's own heartbeat. Patients may feel a racing heart, skipped heartbeats, or pounding in the chest or neck. Palpitations have been described as a "flip-flop" or "fluttering" in the chest. Palpitations may be due to cardiac arrhythmia, nonarrhythmic cardiac disease, drugs, other medical conditions, or psychiatric disease. Cardiac arrhythmias and anxiety account for a majority of cases. Palpitations may be completely benign or a manifestation of a potentially fatal arrhythmia.

Epidemiology

Palpitations (ICD-9-CM 785.1, ICD-10-CM R00.2) are a common presenting complaint in a primary care office or the emergency department. They affect all genders and ages. Up to 16% of patients in general medical settings report palpitations, and up to 18% of cardiology outpatient visits are for cardiac arrhythmias. The most common etiologies are cardiac arrhythmias (43%) and anxiety/psychiatric (31%). In outpatient clinics psychiatric etiologies are slightly more common; in emergency department settings cardiac causes are increasingly likely. The underlying cause of palpitations in 15% of patients cannot be identified.

Nearly 90% of patients who have palpitations have recurrent symptoms of palpitations. Overall, 1-year mortality does not appear to be significantly increased, but patients report a moderate impact on their quality of life.

Although arrhythmias are frequently found to be the underlying cause of palpitations, it is important to note that many patients with arrhythmias do not have any symptoms.

Differential Diagnosis

The differential for palpitations is broad, but can generally be broken down into cardiac versus noncardiac causes. Cardiac causes may be further divided into structural or arrhythmic causes. Noncardiac causes include medications and drugs, high output states, and certain medical conditions. Gastroesophageal reflux or esophageal spasm may present as a brief intermittent episode of tightness or pounding in the chest. See Table 1 for a full listing of causes.

Psychiatric causes may account for up to one third of presentations; however, it is important to note that psychiatric illness can coexist with cardiac or other medical causes, and palpitations can occur with panic attacks, generalized anxiety, depression, and somatization.

Cardiac arrhythmias often present as palpitations. Nearly any arrhythmia or change from a sinus rhythm can produce this sensation. A less common condition in otherwise healthy patients is inappropriate sinus tachycardia (IST), demonstrated by an elevated resting heart rate, an exaggerated heart rate response to exercise, or both. IST is thought to be due to abnormal autonomic control and response. Long QT syndrome, both congenital/familial and medication induced, may predispose to ventricular tachyarrhythmias, including the often-fatal Torsades de pointes.

Risk Factors

Structural cardiac disease, including valvular disease, may predispose patients to arrhythmias and palpitations. Table 2 lists symptoms and risk factors that indicate an increased likelihood that palpitations are due to an underlying arrhythmia.

Pathophysiology

An arrhythmia is caused by the disruption of the normal electrical impulse that originates at the sinoatrial node and is conducted to the atrioventricular node, then through the His-Purkinje system to depolarize the ventricles. Disruption may occur anywhere along this pathway. Underlying structural disease, prior ischemia, congenital abnormalities in myocytes, or electrical pathways affect a normal electrical conduction pathway. Palpitations that are due to supraventricular or ventricular tachyarrhythmias often result from sympathetic stimulation and catecholamine surges.

Palpitations involving skipped or premature beats are often a sensation that results from the following episode of systole, when stroke volume is increased secondary to the prolonged length of the preceding diastole and increased ventricular inotropy.

Clinical Assessment

The keys to evaluation are a history and physical, a 12-lead electrocardiogram (ECG), and a basic laboratory evaluation including an evaluation of the thyroid gland. Clinicians must identify which patients are more likely to have underlying arrhythmia and require further evaluation. A good clinical history includes age of onset, description of palpitations, frequency, duration, timing, position, and associated symptoms, including dizziness, presyncope, and syncope. The clinical history should include a thorough medication review, including over-the-counter medications, alcohol and tobacco use, and illicit substance use. An increasing number of medications are being found to cause QT prolongation, especially when

TABLE 1 Differential Diagnosis for Palpitations

NONCARDIAC			CARDIAC
Medications		*Arrhythmias*	Atrial fibrillation
Prescription	Digoxin (Lanoxin)		Atrial flutter
	Beta agonists (Albuterol [Proventil])		Benign ectopy (premature ventricular contractions, premature atrial contraction)
	Terbutaline		Nonsustained ventricular tachycardia
	Digitalis (digoxin)		
Over-the-counter	Caffeine		Supraventricular tachyarythmias (ex atrioventricular reentrant tachycardia)
	Antihistamines		Inappropriate sinus tachycardia
	Pseudoephedrine (Sudafed)		Long QT syndrome
	Ephedrine, Ephedra[a]		Torsades de pointes
	Atropine		
	Diphenoxylate/atropine [Lomotil]		
Drugs of abuse	Cocaine	*Structural abnormalities*	Mitral regurgitation
	Amphetamines		Aortic insufficiency
	Alcohol		Mitral valve prolapse
	Nicotine		Hypertrophic obstructive cardiomyopathy
Medical causes	Thyrotoxicosis	*Other*	Pericarditis
	Pheochromocytoma		Pacemaker-mediated tachycardia
	Anemia		Vasovagal syncope
	Hypoglycemia		
	Mastocytosis		
	Gastroesophogeal reflux		
	Esophogeal spasm		
High output states	Fever		
	Pregnancy		
	Paget's disease		
	Extra cardiac shunt		
	Exercise		
	Stress		
Psychiatric	Panic attack		
	Generalized anxiety		
	Depression		
	Somatization		

[a]Dietary supplement banned by the U.S. FDA.

TABLE 2 Risk Factors for Palpitations

Increased likelihood of underlying arrhythmia
Known structural or valvular cardiac disease
Visible neck pulsations
Palpitations that affect sleep
Palpitations that occur at work
Subjective feeling of irregular heart rate
Duration of palpitations more than 5 min
Male gender
Older age
Decreased likelihood of underlying arrhythmia
Family history of panic disorder
Duration of palpitations less than 5 min

used in combination, and may predispose the patient to ventricular arrhythmias (see Tables 3 and 4). A physical examination should be performed but may be limited, as clinicians rarely have the opportunity to examine a patient during an episode of palpitations.

Diagnostic Testing
A 12-lead ECG should be performed in all patients. It is appropriate to do limited laboratory evaluation with a complete blood count (CBC), thyroid-stimulating hormone (TSH), and complete metabolic panel (CMP or Chem-14) to identify anemia, thyroid

TABLE 3 History and Physical Examination Clues to the Etiology of Palpitations

CLUES FROM HISTORY OR EXAMINATION	SUGGESTED DIAGNOSIS
Onset in childhood or adolescence	Accessory pathway rhythms: AV nodal reentrant tachycardia Wolff Parkinson White Idiopathic ventricular tachyarrhythmia
Onset in older adult Description of irregular rate	Atrial fibrillation
Feeling of "fluttering"	Prolonged tachyarrhythmia
Pounding in the neck Exaggerated "a" wave in jugular venous pulse	Atrioventricular dissociations
Midsystolic click followed by late systolic murmur	Mitral valve prolapse
Holosystolic murmur along left sternal border that increases with valsalva	Hypertrophic obstructive cardiomyopathy Left ventricle outflow tract obstruction
Pale conjunctiva	Anemia
Exophthalmos Goiter	Thyrotoxicosis
Gravid abdomen	Pregnancy

TABLE 4	Medications That Cause QT Prolongation

Cardiac Antiarrhythmics Amiodarone (Cordarone)
   Disopyramide (Norpace)
   Procainamide
   Quinidine
   Sotalol (Betapace)
   Diuretics
   Sympathomimetics
   Vasodilators

Antibiotics Fluoroquinolones
   Macrolides

Psychiatric Phenothiazines Chlorpromazine (Thorazine)
   Promethazine (Phenergan)
   Prochlorperazine (Compazine)
   Fluphenazine (Prolixin)
   Trifluoperazine (Stelazine)
   Selective serotonin reuptake inhibitors
   Tricyclic antidepressants
   Haloperidol (Haldol)

Other Amphetamines
   Anticholinergics
   Antihistamines
   Protease inhibitors
   Methadone (Dolophine)

TABLE 6	Diagnostic Considerations in the Evaluation of Palpitations

FINDINGS	FURTHER EVALUATION
Arrhythmia or predisposition to arrhythmia seen on ECG	Echocardiogram to look for structural heart disease
Palpitations brought on by exertion	Exercise stress test (avoid dobutamine if suspect arrhythmia)
Suspected arrhythmia, but none identified on ECG	Ambulatory cardiac monitoring – Holter monitor (24–48 h) – Continuous loop event recorder – Implantable loop recorder
Associated dizziness, syncope, presyncope	Referral to cardiologist for electrophysiology study
Known cardiac dysfunction, structural or valvular abnormality	Referral to cardiologist for electrophysiology study
Family history of sudden cardiac death	Referral to cardiologist for electrophysiology study

TABLE 5	ECG Findings Suggestive of Diagnosis of Palpitations

ECG FINDINGS	SUGGESTED DIAGNOSIS
Irregularly irregular rhythm Absent P waves	Atrial fibrillation
Delta wave Short PR interval Widened QRS	Wolff Parkinson White
Short PR	AV nodal reentrant tachycardia
QT interval > 460 msec in women, > 440 msec in men	Predisposition to ventricular tachyarrhythmias, including Torsades de pointes
Left ventricular enlargement with left atrial abnormality	May be a focus for atrial fibrillation

disease, and electrolyte abnormalities that predispose to arrhythmias. Etiology can be determined in 40% of patients from this limited evaluation (see Tables 5 and 6).

Traditionally, ambulatory cardiac monitoring has been done via a Holter monitor. Patients keep a diary of the time and characteristics of their symptoms. This method is appropriate for patients who have daily palpitations. The monitor is worn for 24 to 48 hours. If symptoms are not present during the time the monitor is being worn, the test will be unrevealing. In addition, Holter monitoring may uncover arrhythmias (most commonly benign ectopy) that are unrelated to patient symptoms.

If arrhythmia is suspected in a patient but 24 to 48 hours is insufficient time to record an event, it is recommended that the patient be evaluated with a continuous loop event recorder for 2 weeks. These ambulatory monitors record continuously, but only save data from the specific interval when the patient activates the monitor (e.g., 2 min before and after an episode of palpitations). These monitors frequently send information transtelephonically rather than keeping data stored within the device itself. In patients with infrequent palpitations but known severe heart disease, an implantable loop recorder is an option. These monitors are implanted subcutaneously, typically in the left pectoral region, and usually left in place for 1 year. As with other loop event recorders, they save

data when activated by the patient and can send information transtelephonically.

Panic disorder or anxiety is a diagnosis of exclusion. A patient with anxiety or other psychiatric illness may have a significant underlying arrhythmia. The catecholamine increase in patients with psychiatric disorder in times of stress or intense emotional experience may be proarrhythmogenic. These patients should undergo evaluation for arrhythmia, especially in the presence of risk factors, before having all of their symptoms attributed to their psychiatric illness.

Patients who have palpitations associated with dizziness, presyncope, or syncope in whom the diagnosis is not apparent, should be referred for evaluation by a cardiologist. This sort of palpitation is the kind most likely to be associated with ventricular tachycardia or other serious arrhythmia.

Palpitations may occur more frequently during pregnancy, which is a high output state. Postpartum cardiomyopathy is a structural disease that is unique to this population. Because pregnant women also have an increased risk of new arrhythmias, including atrial fibrillation, persistent palpitations should be evaluated thoroughly.

Treatment

Treatment should be focused toward the underlying cause of the palpitation.

Discussion of the management of specific causes of palpitations, including anemia, thyrotoxicosis, and hypoglycemia, can be found elsewhere. Chronic management of atrial fibrillation is also beyond the scope of this article.

Table 7 outlines the treatment of specific causes of palpitations. Referral to a cardiologist is appropriate for patients with supraventricular tachyarrhythmias, long QT syndrome, or palpitations associated with syncope/presyncope, as these are more likely to be ventricular arrhythmias.

Patients with potentially malignant ventricular tachyarrhythmias (e.g., frequent premature ventricular depolarizations, up to 3–10 per hour with some repetitive forms) are at increased risk for sudden cardiac death, but there is little evidence that treating with antiarrhythmics decreases mortality; in fact, some evidence suggests that these drugs actually increase mortality via proarrhythmic mechanisms. In these patients, consider a referral to a cardiologist for evaluation for an implantable cardiac defibrillator.

TABLE 7	Treatment of Specific Causes of Palpitations
CAUSES OF PALPITATIONS	**TREATMENT**
Due to Medication or Drug	Stop Offending Agent
Premature atrial contractions	Decrease caffeine and alcohol Tobacco cessation
Ectopy (PACs)	Beta blockers for prevention of ectopy – *Metoprolol* [Toprol XL][a] 50 mg PO daily – *Atenolol* [Tenormin][a] 50 mg PO daily
Narrow complex SVT	Vagal maneuvers (carotid massage, valsalva, dive reflex) help during episode
Hospitalized patient with prolonged SVT	*Adenosine* [Adenoscan] 6 mg IV bolus over 1 to 2 s, increased up to 12 mg IV every 1 to 2 min as needed for 2 doses
Atrial fibrillation with rapid ventricular response	*Metoprolol* [Lopressor][a] 2.5 to 5 mg IV bolus over 2 min, repeated at 5 min intervals to a total of 15 mg *Esmolol* [Brevibloc] 0.5 mg/kg IV over 1 min, followed by 50 µg/kg/min continuous infusion with re-bolusing and increasing rate of infusion by 50 µg/kg/min every 4 min up to a maximum infusion rate of 200 µg/kg/min *Verapamil* [Isoptin] 5 to 10 mg IV over 2 to 3 min, repeated every 15 to 30 min as necessary *Diltiazem* [Cardizem], 0.25 mg/kg IV over 2 min with a second bolus of 0.35 mg/kg 15 min later if first dose is tolerated but does not produce desired reduction in heart rate. Diltiazem can then be run as a continuous infusion at a rate of 5 to 15 mg/h
Regular supraventricular tachyarrhythmias, such as WPW or AV nodal reentrant tachycardia	Radiofrequency ablation in electrophysiology laboratory

[a]Not FDA approved for this indication.

References

Abbott AV. Diagnostic approach to palpitations. Am Fam Physician 2005;71:743–50.

Chan T, Worster A. The clinical diagnosis of arrhythmias in patients presenting with palpitations. Ann Emerg Med 2011;57:303–4.

Crawford MH, Bernstein SJ, Deedwania PC, et al. ACC/AHA guidelines for ambulatory electrocardiography: Executive summary and recommendations. Circulation 1999;100:886–93.

Tayal U, Dancy M. Palpitations. Medicine 2013;41:118–24.

Weber BE, Kapoor WN. Evaluation and outcomes of patients with palpitations. Am J Med 1996;100:138–48.

Wexler AK, Pleister A, Raman S. Outpatient approach to palpitations. Am Fam Physician 2011;84:63–9.

PHARYNGITIS

Method of
Ruth Weber, MD, MSEd

CURRENT DIAGNOSIS

- Patients prioritize symptom relief over microbiologic cure.
- Most pharyngitis is viral; microbiologic confirmation is required for group A β-hemolytic streptococcus pharyngitis diagnosis.
- In adults, throat culture is not necessary if rapid antigen detection test is negative.
- Stop presumptive antibiotic therapy if throat culture results are negative for group A β-hemolytic streptococcus.

CURRENT THERAPY

- Penicillin is the drug of choice for group A β-hemolytic streptococcus pharyngitis. A first-generation cephalosporin or macrolide is indicated if the patient is allergic to penicillin.
- Treatment is necessary for 10 days to eradicate group A β-hemolytic streptococcus from the pharynx.
- Amoxicillin can be substituted for penicillin. Patients older than 12 years may be treated with once-daily amoxicillin (Moxatag).
- Patients are not infectious after 24 hours of appropriate antibiotic treatment.

Epidemiology

Pharyngitis is common and has substantial medical and societal costs. "Sore throat" accounts for over 7 million outpatient visits by children annually. The estimated total cost of pharyngitis in children is $540 million per year.

An estimated 30% of childhood pharyngitis is caused by group A β-hemolytic streptococcus (GABHS). In temperate climates, pharyngitis occurs in outbreaks during winter and early spring, predominantly involving children 5 to 15 years of age. GABHS is uncommon in preschool-aged children and in adults. Group C β-hemolytic streptococcus pharyngitis occurs mainly in college students and young adults.

Of other causes of pharyngitis (Table 1), gonococcal pharyngitis is most common in older adolescents and young adults. Transmission is by oral-genital contact. If gonococcal pharyngitis is diagnosed in a prepubertal child, sexual abuse must be considered.

Risk Factors

The major risk factors for GABHS pharyngitis are age and exposure such as in crowded schools or through household contacts.

TABLE 1	Pharyngitis: Distribution of Causative Organisms (All Age Groups)
PATHOGEN	**PERCENTAGE OF POPULATION**
Group A β-hemolytic streptococcus	15–30
Rhinovirus	20
Adenovirus	2–5
Coronavirus	2–5
Coxsackievirus	2–5
Group C β-hemolytic streptococcus	2–5
Herpes simplex virus	2–5
Influenza virus	2–5
Chlamydia trachomatis	<1
Corynebacterium diphtheriae	<1
Epstein-Barr virus	<1
Human immunodeficiency virus	<1
Arcanobacterium haemolyticum	<1
Mycoplasma spp.	<1
Neisseria gonorrhoeae	<1

Oral sexual activity is implicated in gonococcal pharyngitis. Swimming pools have been implicated in transmission of group C and D β streptococcal pharyngitis.

Pathophysiology

Pathogenic strains of *Streptococcus pyogenes* can be differentiated by Lancefield antigens and by hemolysis on blood agar. The strain containing group A antigen and displaying β hemolysis causes pharyngitis (GABHS). The M protein is responsible for virulence. The M protein cross-reacts with cardiac myosin and laminin, potentially causing rheumatic heart disease. More than 100 M-protein serotypes have been identified. Some streptococcus strains produce erythrogenic toxins, causing the rash of scarlet fever. Patients develop lifelong immunity to one serotype after infection, but reinfection with a different serotype is possible.

Prevention

GABHS is transmitted by droplet spread. No evidence supports other forms of transmission. Patients and household/close contacts should be educated on minimizing droplet spread to reduce the transmission of GABHS.

Phase I trials have been completed on a multivalent vaccine targeting streptococcus M proteins that cause pharyngitis, invasive disease, and rheumatic fever.

Clinical Manifestations

The type of pharyngitis cannot be identified by history and clinical findings. Microbiologic confirmation is necessary to diagnose GABHS pharyngitis.

Group A β-Hemolytic Streptococcal Pharyngitis

In patients age 3 years to adult, sudden onset of sore throat, pain on swallowing, and fever (101°F–104°F) suggest GABHS pharyngitis. Nausea and vomiting can also occur in school-aged children. Clinical signs can include tonsillar erythema with or without exudate, anterior cervical lymphadenitis, soft palate petechiae, red swollen uvula, and scarletiniform rash. Infants rarely present with exudative pharyngitis but have coryza with excoriation and crusting of the nares. Posttonsillectomy patients with GABHS can have milder symptoms and clinical signs.

Patients with suppurative complications of GABHS have unusually severe symptoms, with neck swelling, drooling, and "hot potato" voice. The clinician must look for peritonsillar abscess and infections in the parapharyngeal and submandibular spaces (Ludwig's angina).

Scarlet Fever

Some strains of GABHS produce a pyogenic exotoxin that causes scarlet fever in susceptible patients. The clinical signs and symptoms are identical to GABHS pharyngitis plus development of the characteristic rash within 24 to 48 hours of symptom onset. The fine, papular, bright red rash blanches with pressure, begins on the neck, and spreads to the extremities and trunk. It is more pronounced in creases and feels rough, with a goose-pimple appearance. The punctate rash spares the face, but patients have flushed cheeks and forehead with pallor around the mouth. The rash fades in 3 to 4 days and is followed by desquamation. After desquamation of an initial white coating, the tongue has a classical strawberry appearance caused by edematous papillae.

Poststreptococcal Glomerulonephritis

Renal symptoms of hypertension, edema, and hematuria can occur 1 to 3 weeks after GABHS pharyngitis. Glomerulonephritis is an autoimmune response to M proteins. It is not preventable by antibiotics.

Viral Pharyngitis

Coryza, hoarseness, cough, diarrhea, viral exanthem, anterior stomatitis, and conjunctivitis can indicate a viral etiology for pharyngitis. Adenovirus infections can cause fever for 7 days, and conjunctivitis can persist for 14 days. Adenoviral outbreaks are often associated with swimming pools.

Enterovirus pharyngitis (coxsackievirus, echovirus, enterovirus) occurs in summer and fall. Fever, cervical adenopathy, and erythema of the tonsils are common, but exudates are rare. Herpangina (Coxsackie virus A/B) manifests with fever and painful papulovesicular lesions in the posterior oropharynx that resolve in 7 days. Hand-foot-and-mouth disease (Coxsackie virus A-16) manifests with painful vesicles and ulcers in the mouth plus painful vesicles on the palms, soles, and occasionally trunk. Lesions resolve in 7 days.

Primary oral herpes simplex infection occurs in young children. It manifests as acute gingivostomatitis, with ulcerating vesicles on the anterior mouth and lips but not on the posterior pharynx. High fever with intense pain is common, and dehydration can occur. Symptoms last for 14 days.

Diagnosis

It is necessary to obtain microbiologic confirmation of infection before treating GABHS pharyngitis. If the clinical symptoms suggest GABHS pharyngitis, a throat culture or rapid antigen detection test (RADT) are indicated. If the clinical symptoms suggest viral pharyngitis, the pretest probability of GABHS infection is low, and a diagnostic test should not be performed.

Several methods for determining the probability of GABHS infection have been proposed. The Centor criteria (for adults) are widely accepted. A score of 1 is given for each of the following characteristics: tonsillar exudate, tender anterior cervical adenopathy, history of fever, and an absence of cough. A score of 3 or more indicates a positive predictive value for GABHS of 40% to 60%. A score of 0 to 1 indicates a positive predictive value for GABHS of 1% to 5%.

Throat culture is the gold standard for diagnosing GABHS infection. The tonsils and the posterior pharynx should be aggressively swabbed. Other areas of the mouth should not be touched when obtaining the culture. The culture should be obtained before beginning antibiotic therapy, because even a single dose of antibiotics can cause the culture to be negative. The swab is plated on a sheep's blood agar plate and incubated. The plate must be read at both 24 and 48 hours of incubation. When done correctly, the throat culture has 90% to 95% sensitivity. Although throat culture is considered the gold standard for diagnosing GABHS infection, it does not differentiate a carrier state from clinical infection.

RADT has high specificity but low sensitivity. The many tests available have different performance characteristics. In children aged 5 to 15, a throat culture should be performed if the RADT test is negative to identify patients who have a false-negative RADT result. In adults, throat culture is not necessary after a negative RADT because of the low incidence of GABHS and extremely low risk of acute rheumatic fever. The use of RADT has allowed clinicians to begin antibiotic therapy early in those with a positive test. This decreases the risk of spread of GABHS, allows earlier return to school or work, and modestly improves clinical signs and symptoms.

Streptococcal antibody testing has no value in the acute diagnosis of GABHS pharyngitis. Testing has some value in confirming prior GABHS infection in patients in whom acute rheumatic fever or acute poststreptococcal glomerulonephritis is suspected. The two antibodies that can be identified are antistreptolysin O (ASO) and antideoxyribonuclease B (ARB). Positive, elevated, or increasing titers are confirmation of recent GABHS infection. ASO titers rise within a week of infection and peak 3 to 6 weeks after infection. ARB titers rise within 1 to 2 weeks of infection and peak at 6 to 8 weeks. In some patients titers remain elevated for prolonged periods, therefore a doubling of the titer in 6 weeks in necessary for diagnosing prior GABHS infection.

Differential Diagnosis

Infectious Mononucleosis
Classically a triad of severe sore throat, lymphadenopathy, and fever (up to 104°F) in 15- to 25-year-olds, mononucleosis begins with a prodrome of chills, sweats, fever, and malaise. Clinical signs include enlarged tonsils; posterior and anterior cervical, axillary and inguinal adenopathy; and hepatosplenomegally. Approximately 15% of patients present with jaundice and 5% with rash. Patients with mononucleosis who are treated with amoxicillin (Amoxil)[1] often develop a pruritic maculopapular rash. Complete blood count (CBC) shows an absolute lymphocytosis with greater than 10% atypical lymphocytes. Within 2 to 3 weeks, the heterophile antibody test (Mono Spot) becomes positive. The antibody test has a higher false-negative rate in children than in adults. If a false-negative test is suspected, an IgM antibody to viral capsid antigen is indicated to confirm the diagnosis.

Acute Retroviral Syndrome
Primary infection with HIV can manifest as a syndrome of fever, nonexudative pharyngitis, arthralgia, myalgia, and lymphadenopathy. Some 40% to 80% of patients develop a rash. HIV antibodies are negative. Assay for HIV type 1 RNA or p24 antigen is positive.

Neisseria gonorrhea
N. gonorrhea pharyngitis is usually asymptomatic and associated with oral sexual practices. The diagnosis is confirmed by isolating the organism on Thayer-Martin medium. All patients should be screened and treated for coinfection with chlamydia.

Lemierre's Syndrome
Lemierre's syndrome is a rare etiology of severe pharyngitis caused by Fusobacterium necrophorum. Infection spreads from the pharynx to include the surrounding tissues, with subsequent thrombophlebitis of the internal jugular vein.

Treatment
A major therapeutic decision is to determine if the patient needs an antibiotic in addition to symptomatic treatment.

The goal of treatment of viral pharyngitis is control of symptoms, especially relief of pain. Nonsteroidal antiinflammatory drugs are slightly superior than acetaminophen (Tylenol) for pain relief. No evidence supports the use of Chinese herbs for symptom relief. Oral steroids can relieve pain, but the risks of use outweigh the benefit. Many patients mistakenly believe that antibiotic therapy relieves pain. Ancillary treatment options include rest, adequate fluid intake, and antipyretic medications.

The goals of antibiotic treatment of GABHS pharyngitis are to decrease infectivity and prevent suppurative and other complications, especially acute rheumatic fever. Symptoms generally improve within 3 to 4 days without treatment. Delay of treatment of GABHS pharyngitis for up to 9 days after symptoms begin does not appear to increase the risk of acute rheumatic fever, and a delay of 24 to 48 hours while awaiting culture results does not increase the risk of acute rheumatic fever. Early treatment of GABHS pharyngitis does reduce infectivity, lessens morbidity, and promotes early return to normal activities. Nevertheless, criteria for initiating antibiotics remain controversial.

The choice of antibiotic is determined by the bacteriology of GABHS, clinical efficacy, patient adherence to treatment regimen, adverse effects, and cost. It is not recommended to initiate antibiotics while awaiting throat culture result in children. However if an antibiotic is started it must be discontinued if the culture is negative.

Penicillin remains the antibiotic of choice for GABHS pharyngitis. GABHS has never shown resistance to penicillin or cephalosporins. Amoxicillin[1] can replace penicillin for treatment. (Liquid amoxicillin has a better taste than liquid penicillin.) In the penicillin-allergic patient, a first-generation cephalosporin or macrolide may be substituted. In some areas of the United States up to 8% of GABHS is resistant to macrolides and less than 1% is resistant to clindamycin (Cleocin).[1] Antibiotics should be given for 10 days to eradicate GABHS from the pharynx. At this time, short-course (≤5 days) treatment cannot be recommended, except with azithromycin (Zithromax).

No clear evidence supports antibiotic treatment for group C or group G streptococcal pharyngitis. Treatment might shorten the course of infection. Treatment options are identical to those for GABHS pharyngitis.

Treatment Regimens
- Oral penicillin: PenicillinVK (Veetids)[1]: 40 mg/kg/day (up to adult dose of 1000 mg/day) in divided doses two or three times daily for 10 days.
- Amoxicillin[1]: 50 mg/kg/day (up to adult dose of 1000 mg/day) twice daily for 10 days; FDA has approved amoxicillin ER tab (Moxatag) for patients older than 12 years at 775 mg once a day.
- Penicillin G benzathine (Bicillin-LA): Patients weighing less than 27 kg, 600,000 units IM; patients weighing 27 kg or more, 1.2 million units IM once. Penicillin G is used for patients who are unlikely to complete a full 10-day course of oral medication and for those with a personal or family history of rheumatic fever.
- First-generation oral cephalosporin: Cephalexin (Keflex) 25 to 50 mg/kg/day (up to adult dose of 1000 mg/day) twice daily for 10 days. This regimen should be used if the patient is allergic to penicillin; shorter courses are not FDA approved.
- Macrolides should be used if the patient is allergic to penicillin: Erythromycin 20 to 40 mg/kg/day (up to adult dose of 1000 mg/day) in three or four doses for 10 days. Azithromycin (patients older than 6 months): Day 1: 10 mg/kg once (up to adult dose of 500 mg); days 2 to 5: 5 mg/kg once daily (up to adult dose of 250 mg/day). The dose of azithromycin is not established in infants younger than 6 months.

Tetracycline, sulfonamides, and older fluroquinalones are not recommended because of high rates of resistance. All patients should be considered infectious until they have completed 24 hours of antibiotic therapy.

Monitoring
In general, follow-up throat cultures or RADT for patients successfully treated for GABHS pharyngitis (i.e., test for cure) are not necessary. An additional RADT or throat culture is required if symptoms do not abate, symptoms recur, or the patient had previous rheumatic fever.

Patients who have repeated symptomatic episodes of GABHS have either recurrent new infections or are carriers of GABHS, with repeated superimposed viral infections.

GABHS carriers have positive cultures for GABHS without clinical symptoms. Approximately 20% of school-aged children are carriers. GABHS carrier status is suspected if the clinical picture is of viral pharyngitis but the patient has positive RADT or cultures both when symptomatic and when asymptomatic. Carriers do not respond to antibiotics and have no serologic response to ASO and anti-DNA B. These patients do not need to be identified or treated. These patients do not develop rheumatic fever and are not important in the spread of GABHS to others.

Patients with repeated GABHS pharyngitis have a clinical picture of recurrent bacterial pharyngitis. They respond to antibiotics and have negative RADT and culture when they are asymptomatic. They have a serologic response to ASO and anti-DNA B. Prophylactic antibiotics are not recommended for these patients. Tonsillectomy may be considered when infection attack rates do not decrease over time and no other explanation

---

[1]Not FDA approved for this indication.

[1]Not FDA approved for this indication.

of recurrent infection can be found. Meta-analyses have found inconclusive evidence of benefit from tonsillectomy compared to nonsurgical treatment.

Patients with GABHS pharyngitis who remain symptomatic and continue to have positive cultures should receive a second course of antibiotics, with either the same antimicrobial agent or intramuscular penicillin. If a patient experiences repeated infections and there is concern that the GABHS infection is being spread among close contacts, all close and family contacts should be cultured and only those who are positive should be treated. Family pets are not reservoirs and do not spread disease.

Mass screening should be considered in outbreaks of GABHS in a closed or semiclosed community or in outbreaks of acute rheumatic fever or poststreptococcal glomerulonephritis.

Non-GABHS pharyngitis (i.e., group C or G β-hemolytic streptococcus) is not associated with rheumatic fever, and no evidence supports treatment or follow-up culture.

Complications

The complications of GABHS pharyngitis can be classified as suppurative and nonsuppurative.

Suppurative complications occur when the infection spreads to cause conditions such as lateral pharyngeal abscess, cervical lymphandenitis, sinusitis, otitis media, retropharyngeal abscess, Lemierre's syndrome, and mastoiditis. Appropriate treatment of GABHS with antibiotics decreases these complications.

Nonsuppurative complications include acute rheumatic fever, acute poststreptococcal glomerulonephritis, and poststreptococcal reactive arthritis. Acute rheumatic fever occurs 2 to 3 weeks after GABHS pharyngitis. It is not seen after GABHS skin infections. Starting antibiotics within 9 days of symptoms can prevent acute rheumatic fever. Acute poststreptococcal glomerulonephritis can occur 10 days after pharyngeal infection and 21 days after skin infection. Antibiotics do not alter the attack rate. Poststreptococcal reactive arthritis is similar to other reactive arthritis, and the attack rate is not altered by antibiotics.

Potential complications from treatment of GABHS pharyngitis include anaphylactic reaction to antibiotics and antibiotic resistance.

References

ESCMID Sore Throat Guideline Group, Pelucchi C, Grigoryan L, et al. Guideline for the management of acute sore throat, Clin Microbiol Infect 2012;18(Suppl 1):1–28.http://www.ncbi.nlm.nih.gov/puhmed/22432746.
Kociolek L, Shulman S. In the clinic pharyngitis, Ann Intern Med 2012;157. ITC3-1–ITC3-16, Downloaded from, http://annals.org.
Shulman ST, Bisno AL, Clegg HW, et al. Clinical practice guideline for the diagnosis and management of group A streptococcal pharyngitis: 2012 update by the Infectious Diseases Society of America. Clin Infect Dis 2012;55:e86–e102.

PRURITUS

Method of
Hassan Bencheqroun, MD

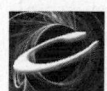

CURRENT DIAGNOSIS

- A careful history and physical examination will reveal a clear exposure, a sick contact, a recent travel, or clues to a systemic disease.
- Antihistamines are effective in treating histamine-mediated pruritus, but they are less effective in mechanisms involving serotonin, leukotrienes, etc.
- Initial testing in the absence of improvement with nonpharmacologic methods or antihistamine should include complete blood counts, thyroid-stimulating hormone, renal and liver panel, human immunodeficiency virus (HIV) test, and chest radiograph.

- Chronic pruritus may precede a systemic illness, especially in older adults. Hodgkin lymphoma is the malignant disease most strongly associated with pruritus and occurs in up to 30% of patients diagnosed with pruritus.

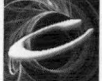

CURRENT THERAPY

- Acute and localized pruritus may resolve with nonpharmacologic methods, such as skin hydration with hypoallergenic, alcohol-free, and fragrance-free moisturizing creams; decreasing the length of showers and baths as well as the temperature of the water; identifying material that may irritate the skin either in jewelry or clothing items; and avoiding scratching.
- Wound care of scratch lesions includes any cellulitic portions.
- First-line pharmacologic treatments may include the use of antihistamine and antipruritic creams. Antipruritic agents may be used as second-line treatments.
- In the absence of improvement, the management of chronic pruritus should be directed at the underlying cause.

Pruritus is defined as an unpleasant sensory perception that causes the desire to scratch. While it shares similarities with pain, the neurophysiology of pruritus is distinct: pain causes withdrawal, whereas pruritus induces the reflex of reaching out and scratching.

Classification

Pruritus can be distinguished as acute or chronic, with the latter defined by the International Forum for the Study of Itch (IFSI) as lasting for 6 or more weeks.

Despite many classifications over the years, there is no uniform, clinically based classification of pruritic diseases to assist in the diagnosis and management of patients with pruritus. The classification chosen for this chapter focuses on clinical signs and distinguishes between the disease with and without primary or secondary skin lesions.

1. Group 1: Pruritus of primary diseased, inflamed skin
2. Group 2: Pruritus of primary nondiseased, noninflamed skin
3. Group 3: Pruritus with chronic secondary scratch lesions

Pathophysiology

The sensation of pruritus stems from a number of different causes. It is generally transmitted through slow-conducting unmyelinated C fibers and free nerve endings located superficially in the skin, which appear to be more sensitive to pruritogenic substances than pain receptors. Histamine, neuropeptide substance P, serotonin (a key component in several diseases), bradykinin, mast cell tryptase, and other unknown mediators (e.g., in uremic pruritus, cholestatic pruritus), may be involved in the genesis of pruritus. Impulses are transmitted from the dorsal root ganglion to the spinothalamic tract. Pruritus then generates a spinal reflex response, the scratch, which is as innate as a deep tendon reflex. Other pathogenic mechanisms include neuropathic (e.g., herpes zoster) and immune-mediated (atopic dermatitis). Lastly, opioids are known to modulate the sensation of pruritus, both peripherally and centrally.

Clinical Manifestations

Pruritus is among the most common symptoms in dermatology. Other associated symptoms depend on the etiology and may include urticarial skin lesions, dry skin, jaundice, and thyroid-related symptoms. Left untreated, itch and its associated scratching increase the risk of chronic skin changes and secondary infection.

Differential Diagnosis

The patient's work-up further places him or her in one of the following categories:

1. Primary diseased, inflamed skin
   - *Inflammatory:* Atopic and contact dermatitis, psoriasis, dry skin, drug reactions
   - *Infectious:* Mycotic, bacterial and viral infections, folliculitis, scabies, pediculosis, arthropod reactions, and insect bites
   - *Autoimmune:* Bullous dermatoses, especially dermatitis herpetiformis, bullous pemphigoid, and dermatomyositis
   - *Dermatoses of pregnancy*
   - *Neoplasms:* Cutaneous T-cell-lymphoma (especially erythrodermic variants), cutaneous B-cell lymphoma, leukemic infiltrates of the skin
2. Primary nondiseased, noninflamed skin
   - Endocrine and metabolic diseases: Chronic renal failure, liver diseases/cholestasis, hyperthyroidism, malabsorption, perimenopausal pruritus
   - Infectious diseases: HIV infection, helminthosis, parasitosis
   - Hematologic and lymphoproliferative diseases, iron deficiency, polycythaemia vera, Hodgkin and Non-Hodgkin lymphoma
   - Visceral neoplasms of the cervix, prostate, or colon, carcinoid syndrome
   - Pregnancy: Pruritus gravidarum with and without cholestasis
   - Drug-induced pruritus: Opioids, ACE-inhibitors, amiodarone, hydrochlorothiazide, estrogens, simvastatin, hydroxyethyl starch, allopurinol
3. Pruritus with chronic secondary scratch lesions (The underlying origin may be a systemic disease or a skin disease.)
   - Neurogenic origin (without neuronal damage), such as hepatic itch
   - Neuropathic diseases (neuronal damage causes itch)
   - Multiple sclerosis, neoplasms, abscesses, cerebral or spinal infarcts, brachioradial pruritus, postherpetic neuralgia, vulvodynia, small fiber neuropathy
   - Somatoform pruritus (e.g., obsessive-compulsive disorders)

Therapy

- Basic measures to lessen drying of skin: Limit bathing to short, cool showers with soap applied only to oily skin areas. A mild moisturizing cream is preferably applied immediately after bathing to lock in moisture. The patient's home should be humidified, especially during dry, cold winter months. Avoid contact irritants, such as wool, fiberglass, and detergents.
- Nonspecific therapy: A wheal and flare response is a marker of histamine-induced pruritus in patients with urticaria or an allergic dermatitis. These patients benefit from long-acting antihistamines. Concurrent H1 and H2 blockers increase therapeutic effectiveness.
- Treatment specific: Itching gradually recedes as the primary systemic condition improves.

Complications

Pruritus is accompanied by intense scratching. Skin may thicken, displaying lichen simplex chronicus: a localized skin thickening often appearing over the posterior neck, extremities, scrotum, vulva, anus, and buttocks. In prurigo nodularis, a variant of lichen simplex chronicus, some nodules develop over areas within easy scratching reach, such as the extensor arms and legs. Impetigo may result from superinfected excoriations in patients with atopic dermatitis.

References

Ikoma A, Rukwied R, Ständer S, et al. Neurophysiology of pruritus: Interaction of itch and pain. Arch Dermatol 2003;139:1475–8.

Ständer S, Weisshaar E, Mettang T, et al. Clinical classification of itch: A position paper of the International Forum for the Study of Itch. Acta Derm Venereol 2007;87:291–4.

Zirwas MJ, Seraly MP. Pruritus of unknown origin: A retrospective study. J Am Acad Dermatol 2001;45:892–6.

Cho YL, Liu HN, Huang TP, Tarng DC. Uremic pruritus: Roles of parathyroid hormone and substance P. J Am Acad Dermatol 1997;36:538–43.

Ganesh E, Maxwell LG. Pathophysiology and management of opioid-induced pruritus. Drugs 2007;67:2323–33.

Krajnik M, Zylicz Z. Understanding pruritus in systemic disease. J Pain Symptom Manage 2001;21:151–68.

Reamy B. A diagnostic approach to pruritus. Am Fam Physician 2011;84:195–202.

Moses S. Pruritus. Am Fam Physician 2003;68:1135–42.

RHINITIS

Method of
Sheryl Beard, MD

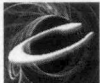

CURRENT DIAGNOSIS

- Rhinitis presents as nasal congestion, sneezing, itching, rhinorrhea, and postnasal drainage.
- Patients with palatal and nasal itching should be considered for allergic disease.
- Allergic rhinitis is confirmed by positive skin-prick testing and IgE reactivity.
- Nonallergic rhinitis patients lack allergic evidence for disease.
- Nonallergic rhinitis conditions have multiple presentations.

CURRENT THERAPY

- Avoidance therapy should be first-line treatment for all forms of rhinitis.
- Second generation oral antihistamines have good therapeutic efficacy for allergic rhinitis.
- Intranasal corticosteroids are the mainstay of treatment for nonallergic rhinitis and moderate-to-severe allergic rhinitis.
- Consultation with an allergy specialist should be considered in cases with multiple treatment failures.
- Patients whose allergic rhinitis is uncontrolled on multiple therapies should be considered for immunotherapy.

Introduction

Rhinitis is defined as inflammation of the nasal mucous membranes. Rhinitis presents as nasal congestion, sneezing, itching, rhinorrhea, and postnasal drainage; it can be divided into allergic and nonallergic rhinitis. Mixed rhinitis has components of both allergic and nonallergic disease. Allergic rhinitis is nasal inflammation that is mediated by IgE to environmental allergens. Nonallergic rhinitis is defined by non–IgE-mediated perennial symptoms. Nonallergic rhinitis shares symptoms with allergic rhinitis, but is only distinguishable by negative allergy tests. Nonallergic rhinitis is also known as perennial nonallergic rhinitis, idiopathic rhinitis, and vasomotor rhinitis.

Most research still classifies allergic rhinitis according to its seasonality or its perennial nature. Seasonal allergic rhinitis is commonly caused by pollen allergens; perennial allergic rhinitis is mainly caused by dust mites and animal dander. Allergic rhinitis can be further classified as mild, moderate, or severe. Mild rhinitis is rhinitis that does not impair work, school, daily functioning, or sleep. Moderate to severe rhinitis interferes with activities of daily living, quality of life, and/or sleep. Severe rhinitis is so marked that normal functioning cannot take place without treatment. Episodic allergic rhinitis occurs with sporadic inhalant aeroallergen exposure not typically encountered by the patient's usual indoor and outdoor environments. An example of episodic allergic rhinitis is a child who is allergic to cats but is not normally exposed, but then visits a household with cats and develops symptoms.

The Allergic Rhinitis and its Impact on Asthma Guidelines: Revised 2010 (ARIA) discouraged the use of the terms seasonal and perennial rhinitis in favor of intermittent and persistent rhinitis. Intermittent rhinitis can be defined as nasal symptoms lasting less than 4 weeks' duration and fewer than 4 days per week. Persistent rhinitis is rhinitis lasting more than 4 weeks' duration or more that 4 days per week.

No standard classification exists for nonallergic rhinitis. A variety of conditions present with similar symptoms and are called nonallergic rhinitis. Nonallergic rhinitis includes vasomotor rhinitis, gustatory rhinitis, nonallergic rhinitis with eosinophilia syndrome (NARES), occupational rhinitis, hormonal rhinitis, drug-induced rhinitis, and atrophic rhinitis. Another entity classified in or out of nonallergic rhinitis is infectious rhinitis.

Local allergic rhinitis is a newly defined entity found in nonatopic patients. Local allergic rhinitis is characterized by local inflammatory reactions including local eosinophils and localized IgE in response to aeroallergens. Local allergic rhinitis does not show significant skin-prick testing reactions, and patients have negative systemic IgE reactions to aeroallergens.

Rhinitis may be viewed by some as a trivial disease, but it places a significant financial burden on society. The estimated direct and indirect costs to society of rhinitis were around $11.58 billion in 2002.

Epidemiology/Risk Factors

The National Health and Nutrition Survey (NHANES II and III) suggests that the overall prevalence of IgE sensitivity might be increasing. Of the patients evaluated for rhinitis in the United States, 43% (58 million people) have allergic disease, 23% (19 million people) have nonallergic disease, and 34% (26 million people) have mixed rhinitis. Seventy percent of allergic patients develop the disease in childhood (20 years and younger) as opposed to nonallergic rhinitis patients, 70% of whom develop disease in adulthood. Approximately two thirds of nonallergic rhinitis patients have vasomotor rhinitis, and one-third have NARES. Nonallergic rhinitis has a female predominance.

The prevalence of local allergic rhinitis is largely unknown. In a small study of rhinitis patients, the prevalence of local allergic rhinitis was 25.7%, nonallergic rhinitis was 11.2%, and allergic rhinitis was 63.1%. Local allergic rhinitis is associated with asthma and conjunctivitis, and commonly begins in childhood.

Pathophysiology

Allergic

Allergic rhinitis is the result of an IgE mediated, type I hypersensitivity allergic reaction in response to an inhaled allergen. Allergens are proteins derived from airborne particulate matter, including dust-mite feces, pollens, animal dander, and cockroach particles. Antigen-presenting cells (APCs) engulf allergens in the nose and break them into antigenic peptides. APCs present these peptides to naïve T cells (T_H0). T_H0 cells differentiate once activated, into the T_H2 subtype. The T_H2 lymphocytes generate cytokines that regulate B-lymphocytes and sequester inflammatory cells (including eosinophils).

B-lymphocytes produce IgE. IgE attaches to mast cells and basophils and renders them sensitized. Once sensitized and cells are exposed to allergen, the mast cells and basophils degranulate. Degranulation of these cells releases a host of mediators including histamine and prostaglandin. Histamine stimulates histamine type I (H1) receptors on nerve endings that cause pruritus, sneezing and increased secretions. These symptoms constitute the early-phase response of allergic rhinitis. The early-phase response occurs within minutes of allergen exposure and dissipates within 1 hour.

Eosinophils produce IL-5, which acts to promote activation and survival of other eosinophils. Eosinophils also produce toxic products that damage local mucosal cells. The damage done by these cells is what constitutes the late-phase reaction. The late-phase reaction occurs several hours after allergen exposure and is characterized by nasal congestion.

Nonallergic Rhinitis

The nasal mucosa has two major functions; one is trapping inhaled particles through mucus production and the second is humidifying inhaled air through a complex vascular system. The mucus glands and the vascular system are regulated by the parasympathetic and the adrenergic nervous systems. Sensory nerves are stimulated by irritants in the nose through the use of a sensory receptor called a *nociceptor*. The nociceptive signal generates a neural reflex in the central nervous system (CNS) controlling sympathetic and parasympathetic tone in the nasal mucosa. Parasympathetic stimulation results in mucus production. Sympathetic stimulation causes vasoconstriction, which empties venous cavities. Lack of sympathetic tone causes venous engorgement and nasal congestion.

Symptomatic nonallergic rhinitis is an exaggeration of a normal defensive mechanism. Inflammation in the nose causes an upregulation of this neural activity, resulting in the exaggerated response (also known as neural hyperresponsiveness). Hyperresponsive parasympathetic efferent nerves trigger glandular activation in the nasal mucosa, leading to vasodilation and mucus production. Excessive mucus production anteriorly causes rhinorrhea and posteriorly causes postnasal drip. This hyperresponsiveness can be due to structural or functional components of the nasal mucosa altered through genetic or pathologic factors. The exact mechanisms of nonallergic rhinitis conditions are poorly understood because of their multiple presentations.

Infectious Rhinitis/Rhinosinusitis

Acute sinusitis (rhinosinusitis) most commonly occurs as a complication of viral upper-respiratory infections (URIs) Viral URIs cause nasal mucosal edema, which leads to obstruction of the sinus openings and ciliary impairment. Bacteria proliferate in the stagnant mucus as well as the low–oxygen-tension environment of the sinus cavities. Chronic rhinosinusitis is the result of long-term obstruction and/or dysfunction of the sinuses. Chronic inflammation leads to chronic low grade infections.

Prevention

Environmental control of allergens can improve the severity of allergic rhinitis and can reduce the need for medications. Environmental control should be thorough if treatment is sought, but the full beneficial effects of the change may take weeks to months. Mild disease can usually be managed with avoidance measures. Complete avoidance of allergen, particularly pollen, is usually not feasible.

Reduction of dust mite allergen exposure can be done in the following ways: remove carpets and soft toys, use covers impermeable to allergen for mattresses and pillows, vacuum beds weekly, and wash bedding at 60 degrees Celsius (140 degrees Fahrenheit). Pet dander avoidance can only be effectively managed by removing the pet and carefully cleaning all carpets, furniture and mattresses.

Clinical Manifestations

If the patient presents with symptoms of palatal itching, nasal itching, ocular symptoms, or sneezing, consideration should be given to an allergic cause.

The presentation of nonallergic rhinitis is dependent on the type of nonallergic rhinitis. Overall, patients with nonallergic rhinitis lack other allergic conditions.

The vasomotor rhinitis patient will present with predominantly nasal obstruction and rhinorrhea. Typically, symptoms are triggered by temperature, exercise, and environmental stimuli (odors, smoke, and dust).

NARES patients generally have more intense symptoms than vasomotor rhinitis or allergic disease patients. NARES patients present with paroxysms of flares to include sneezing, watery rhinorrhea, nasal itching, congestion, and some anosmia. NARES patients have eosinophils on a nasal smear, but lack other allergic evidence by skin-prick testing.

Gustatory rhinitis sufferers complain of nasal congestion and rhinorrhea associated with ingestion of foods and, sometimes, alcoholic beverages.

Nasal crusting, dryness, and fetor are the characteristics of atrophic rhinitis. These findings are due to glandular cell atrophy. Patients will have abnormally wide nasal cavities and may have squamous metaplasia.

Occupational rhinitis patients have components of allergic and nonallergic disease. Patients present with nasal congestion and rhinorrhea triggered by an occupational exposure. Symptoms are present during duty and generally improve away from the work environment. Substances leading to symptoms include irritating chemicals, grain dust, ozone, lab animal antigens, and wood. Often occupational rhinitis co-exists with occupational asthma.

Hormonal rhinitis manifests as nasal congestion during pregnancy or the menstrual cycle. Pregnant women are six times more likely to have rhinitis and sinusitis than nonpregnant women. Rhinitis usually resolves two weeks postdelivery.

Drug-induced rhinitis occurs with certain medications. ACE inhibitors, phosphodiesterase-5 selective inhibitors, alpha-receptor antagonists, and phentolamine are common triggers. Patients present with rhinorrhea and nasal congestion.

Rhinitis medicamentosa is a condition that presents with severe congestion. It is caused by prolonged and repetitive use of topical nasal decongestants. It can also be associated with cocaine use.

Anatomic rhinitis is more likely in patients who present with unilateral nasal symptoms.

Infectious rhinitis presents with sinus tenderness, erythema to the mucosa, postnasal drainage and sometimes periorbital edema.

Diagnosis

The diagnosis of allergic rhinitis, nonallergic rhinitis, and infectious rhinitis is based largely on history and physical examination. Other diagnostic testing can be performed to aid in providing a more definitive diagnosis or to rule out other causes.

Allergic rhinitis is confirmed by IgE reactivity to environmental allergen sensitivity through skin-prick testing. When skin-prick testing is difficult to interpret or if it is not feasible, serum–allergen-specific IgE testing can be used. Nasal smears looking for eosinophils are not recommended for routine use in the diagnosis of allergic rhinitis.

Other testing available for evaluation of rhinitis includes nasal endoscopy, rhinomanometry, and radiologic imaging. Fiberoptic nasal endoscopy is reserved for those with atypical symptoms or an inadequate response to treatment. Rhinomanometry measures airflow obstruction in the upper airway. Rhinomanometry provides an objective measurement of nasal congestion. Rhinomanometry is used to evaluate clinical response to interventions and assess anatomic severity, such as in patients with obstructive sleep apnea. Radiologic imaging, such as computerized tomography (CT) and magnetic resonance imaging (MRI), is used to evaluate anatomic structure. Imaging may not correlate well with nasal function and is expensive.

If a provider suspects a cerebrospinal fluid (CSF) leak, the rhinorrhea can be evaluated for beta transferrin protein, which is present only in CSF.

History

The best diagnostic tool in the evaluation of rhinitis is the history. Information regarding previous evaluation and treatment should be elicited. A positive family history of rhinitis points towards allergic disease. The history of symptoms should include questions regarding congestion; sneezing; rhinorrhea; sore throat; dry throat; cough; itchy, red, or tearing eyes; voice changes; sinus symptoms of drainage; pressure or pain; snoring; ear pain or loss of hearing; and smelling difficulty.

When gathering the details of each symptom, evaluate the onset (such as those in childhood), frequency (episodic versus continual), pattern (seasonality), characteristics of secretions, triggers, severity (to include quality of life evaluation), and associated geographic location or environment (home versus work). Once a trigger is identified, history needs to be gathered even further to evaluate the possibility of modifying the exposure.

Physical Examination

As with any disease process, the physical examination provides clues into the diagnosis. Although the physical examination in rhinitis patients should focus on the nasal mucosa, other body areas should be examined to rule out other processes. For example, the tympanic membranes should be examined for mobility, retraction, erythema, and Eustachian tube dysfunction.

Examination of the eyes in allergic rhinitis might show that the conjunctiva have edema, erythema, and/or cobblestoning. Excessive lacrimation could be another finding. Darkening of the skin of the lower eyelids is prevalent in allergic disease and is also called "allergic shiners."

Allergic and nonallergic nasal mucosa may have a similar appearance. The nasal mucosa may appear boggy with a bluish appearance or be erythematous. Excessive watery-clear mucus might be present. Turbinate hypertrophy is another physical examination finding in rhinitis. Other nasal mucosa findings to look for are nasal polyps, sinusitis, septal deviation, septal perforation, and crusting.

Looking for elongated facies, mouth breathing, and a high arch in the palate may provide a clue to the severity of the nasal obstruction. The tonsils and adenoids should be examined for enlargement. Posterior nasal drainage and cobblestoning in the oropharynx are common findings in rhinitis patients.

The skin examination provides useful information in the patient with rhinitis. Atopic dermatitis or urticaria may be findings associated with allergic disease. The skin should be evaluated for dermatographism. Patients with dermatographism cannot be evaluated for allergic disease using skin-prick testing.

Differential Diagnosis

Many different pathologic conditions can present similarly to rhinitis. Conditions to keep in mind while evaluating and treating a patient for rhinitis include: nasal polyps, ciliary dyskinesia syndrome, anatomic abnormalities such as deviated septum or tumors, nasal turbinate hypertrophy, cerebrospinal fluid rhinorrhea, pharyngonasal reflux, systemic disorders such as Wegener's disease, aspirin intolerance, and other medication side effects.

Treatment

Overall

Current guidelines in treatment of rhinitis do not take cost into consideration. However, the individual treatment goals should be based on factors such as age, route of administration preference (i.e., nasal versus oral), severity, seasonality, side effects, cost, benefit to comorbid conditions, and onset of action. For example, onset of action is an important consideration for an individual who has more episodic symptoms. Also, individual patients respond differently to treatment regimens within a given group.

Avoidance

Due to the lack of high-quality evidence, implementation of avoidance measures is largely based on panel recommendations. In addition, the ubiquitous nature of allergens may limit the effectiveness of the avoidance measures. For dust mites, encasing pillows and bedding in dust mite resistant materials may be beneficial. Pollen is seasonal and can be minimized by keeping the windows closed, using air conditioning, and limiting outdoor exposure. Using particulate filters in the home can also assist in reducing overall allergen load of pollens and dust. Avoiding basements and lowering household humidity may reduce the amount of mold exposure patients receive. Pet avoidance can only be reached by ridding the house of the pet altogether. Other, less-effective measures include limiting exposure of the pet to the house and/or bedroom.

Intranasal Corticosteroid (INS)

Intranasal corticosteroids are first-line treatment for moderate to severe allergic rhinitis and most nonallergic rhinitis conditions. All allergic rhinitis symptoms can be treated with INS. The intranasal corticosteroids bedesonide aerosol, fluticasone propionate aqueous, and beclomethasone aqueous preparations all have a Federal Drug Administration (FDA) treatment indication of nonallergic rhinitis. Intranasal corticosteroid side effects include irritation, bleeding, and perforation of the nasal septum; rarely, local candidiasis is seen with INS use. They are safe to use in pregnancy. No single INS preparation is more efficacious than, or has any relevant difference from, any other. INS has negligible hypothalamic-pituitary-adrenal axis suppression, and systemic burden is clinically insignificant.

Intranasal Anticholinergic (IP)

Ipratropium bromide, a specific intranasal anticholinergic, inhibits parasympathetic function in the nasal mucosa. The parasympathetic blockade reduces the output of secretions from seromucus glands in the nose. Ipratropium can be used in treatment of anterior watery rhinorrhea but has a very limited role in reducing postnasal drip, nasal congestion, or sneezing. Topical ipratropium prior to ingestion of food can be used as pretreatment of gustatory rhinitis and is effective in treatment of the common cold and skier's nose. Side effects of IP include nasal dryness, burning, irritation, stuffy nose, headache, and dry mouth.

Intranasal Antihistamine (INA)

Azelastine is a nasal spray approved by the FDA for allergic and vasomotor rhinitis, and is the only intranasal antihistamine available in the United States. INA has faster onset of action than intranasal corticosteroids. INA should be taken twice per day for maximum clinical benefit and may benefit those with nasal congestion. INA does not produce a significant amount of sedation, but side effects include headache, epistaxis, bitter taste, and nasal irritation.

Nasal Cromolyn

Cromolyn should be considered for early mild rhinitis, but should not be considered a first-line treatment in allergic rhinitis. Nasal cromolyn can be used prior to allergen exposure for prophylaxis of episodic allergic rhinitis. Cromolyn is mostly void of side effects. Cromolyn inhibits mast cell degranulation and is administered three to four times a day. Cromolyn has very limited usefulness for nonallergic rhinitis conditions.

Nasal Saline

Using nasal saline to irrigate the nasal cavities may remove mucus, enhance ciliary movement, improve sinus opening, and remove allergic and irritant particles. Several devices exist including: the neti pot, a nasally adapted plastic bottle, and a pulse irrigator. Evidence suggests that hypertonic saline provides modest benefit over isotonic saline, although it might be more irritating.

Topical Decongestants

Topical decongestants reduce congestion, but have no effect on itching, sneezing, or rhinorrhea. Oxymetazoline, a common topical decongestant, causes nasal vasoconstriction. Vasoconstriction can cause tissue hypoxemia and inflammation, leading to severe rebound nasal congestion. Topical decongestants are not recommended for continued use because they can cause rhinitis medicamentosa.

Oral Antihistamines

Oral antihistamines block H1 receptors, thereby reducing nasal and palatal itching, rhinorrhea, sneezing, conjunctivitis, and urticaria. Nasal congestion is not treated well with oral antihistamines. First-generation oral antihistamines are poorly selective for H1 receptors. The sedative effects of these antihistamines result from crossing the blood–brain barrier; they have been linked to industrial accidents and contribute to loss of function at work and school. For these reasons, first-generation antihistamines have limited usefulness. Second generation H1 antagonists have excellent evidence for therapeutic efficacy. These medications may have some role in the treatment of nonallergic rhinitis because of their anticholinergic properties, but consideration must be given to these systemic properties, including dry mucous membranes, blurry vision, constipation, tachycardia, and urinary retention. A combination of intranasal corticosteroid treatment with oral antihistamines may be effective for sneezing and rhinorrhea in NARES.

Leukotriene Receptor Antagonists (LTRA)

Leukotriene receptor antagonists were originally studied in the treatment of asthma. The only LTRA approved by the FDA for treatment of allergic rhinitis is montelukast. Montelukast is clinically efficacious in both perennial and seasonal allergic rhinitis. Montelukast is approved for children 6 months and older and has a pregnancy category B rating. The oral antihistamine loratadine and montelukast have similar efficacy, and can have additional benefit when used together. Although rare, montelukast has been associated with adverse psychiatric behavior, including suicidality. LTRA have no role in nonallergic rhinitis.

Oral Decongestants

Oral decongestants such as pseudoephedrine reduce nasal congestion. Oral decongestants have a sales restriction in many states. Side effects include insomnia, anorexia, irritability, and palpitations. Blood pressure elevation is rarely a concern in controlled hypertensive patients or in normotensive patients. Oral decongestants should be considered last-line treatment for nonallergic rhinitis conditions.

Systemic Corticosteroids

Few studies are available to support the use of systemic steroids in the treatment of rhinitis. Oral corticosteroids may have a role for severe resistive rhinitis, but not as first-line treatment. Short-term use of 5 to 7 days of oral corticosteroids is the standard, but they should not be used for longer than 3 weeks because of the risk for adverse effects. Oral steroids should be used as first-line treatment for severe nasal polyposis, a subset of anatomic rhinitis. Systemic steroids should not be used in children or pregnant women. Intraturbinate injections of corticosteroids have no role in the treatment of rhinitis. Parenteral corticosteroids are contraindicated because of long-term effects.

Surgery

Surgery can reduce nasal obstruction caused by septal deviation, turbinate hypertrophy, or adenoid hypertrophy. Procedures that can be performed include nasal polypectomy, septoplasty, reductive hypertrophic turbinate surgery, adenoidectomy, and endoscopic sinus surgery. Two nerves can be transected to decrease the parasympathetic nerve supply to the nasal mucosa: the vidian nerve, through endoscopic resection; and the anterior ethmoid nerve, through electrocoagulation, which leads to reduced nasal secretions.

Anti IgE

Omalizumab is a monoclonal antibody available for the treatment of poorly controlled asthma, but it might have a role in the treatment of allergic rhinitis. Omalizumab binds to IgE, hindering its relationship with inflammatory cells. Omalizumab only binds to circulating IgE and not bound IgE. Due to its high cost, reports of anaphylaxis, and its injectable only formulation, omalizumab has a limited role in allergic rhinitis treatment.

Immunotherapy

Allergen extract immunotherapy has been used in the treatment of respiratory allergic disease since 1911, and its efficacy has been documented since the 1970s. The amount of allergen in each immunotherapy dose is slowly increased with each dose until a maintenance phase is reached. Immunotherapy is an effective treatment for allergic rhinitis and is the only treatment proven to alter the course of allergic disease.

Subcutaneous immunotherapy uses the injectable form of allergen extract and is the only immunotherapy that is FDA approved. Adequate treatment usually consists of a 3- to 4-year course of immunotherapy. Subcutaneous immunotherapy is indicated in those patients for whom medications and avoidance measures are inadequate, as well as those with only a few relevant allergens. The inherent risk of subcutaneous immunotherapy is systemic anaphylaxis. The rate of significant systemic reactions in rhinitis patients is approximately 5%.

Studies for local-route immunotherapy (noninjected), many of which were carried out in Europe, have only been undertaken in adults. Local routes of immunotherapy include sublingual, local nasal, oral, and bronchial. Local-route immunotherapy has no known life-threatening reactions. Indications for local-route immunotherapy are the same as those for subcutaneous immunotherapy.

Sublingual immunotherapy is not FDA approved in the United States for the treatment of allergic rhinitis, although there is significant use in Europe. Sublingual immunotherapy formulations in the United States are low dose compared to those used in Europe. Nonmedical allergy providers, such as homeopaths, use the majority of sublingual formulations. Some medical allergy providers use subcutaneous extracts as sublingual therapy, but this is an off-label use.

Use of local nasal immunotherapy is used mostly in Europe. Oral and bronchial immunotherapy are not supported by evidence.

Monitoring

The provider should consider stepping down treatment when the patients' symptoms have been controlled. The Total Nasal Symptoms Score [TNSS] is a subjective assessment of the patient's specific symptoms, including rhinorrhea, nasal congestion, sneezing, and pruritus, and can be used to assess effectiveness of medications. The Rhinoconjunctivitis Quality of Life Questionnaire can also be used. Consideration for referral to an allergist might be extended to patients who have had a prolonged course, secondary infections, polyps, or other comorbid conditions including chronic sinusitis and asthma, or if immunotherapy is a consideration.

Complications

Rhinitis is associated with multiple complications including fatigue, decline in cognitive function, loss of productivity, headache, and disturbance of sleep. Patients with mild disease may experience these in mild form. Patients with moderate to severe disease may experience these complications in addition to impairment of activities, leisure, and work or school functioning.

References

Brozek J, Bousquet J, Baena-Cagnani C, et al. Allergic rhinitis and its impact on asthma (ARIA) guidelines: 2010 revision. J Allergy Clin Immunol 2010;126:466–76.

Chaaban M, Corey J. Pharmacotherapy of rhinitis and rhinosinusitis. Facial Plast Surg Clin North Am 2012;20:61–71.

Cox L, Compalati E, Canonica W. Will sublingual immunotherapy become an approved treatment method in the United States? Curr Allergy Asthma Rep 2011;11:4–6.

Dykewicz M. Management of rhinitis: guidelines, evidence basis, and systematic clinical approach for what we do. Immunol Allergy Clin North Am 2011;31:619–34.

Greiner A, Meltzer E. Overview of the treatment of allergic rhinitis and nonallergic rhinopathy. Proc Am Thorac Soc 2011;8:121–31.

Rondon C, Campo P, Galindo L, et al. Prevalence and clinic relevance of local allergic rhinitis. Allergy 2012;67:1282–8. http://dx.doi.org/10.1111/all.12002.

Settipane R, Charnock D. Epidemiology of rhinitis: allergic and nonallergic. Clin Allergy Immunol 2007;19:23–34.

Sin B, Togias A. Pathophysiology of allergic and nonallergic rhinitis. Proc Am Thorac Soc 2011;8:106–14.

van Cauwenberge P, Bachert C, Passalacqua G, et al. Consensus statement on the treatment of allergic rhinitis. European Academy of Allergology and Clinical Immunology. Allergy 2000;55:116–34.

Wallace D, Dykewicz M. The diagnosis and management of rhinitis: an updated practice parameter. J Allergy Clin Immunol 2008;122:S1–S84.

Young-Yuen Wu A. Immunotherapy: vaccines for allergic disease. J Thorac Dis 2012;4:198–202.

SPINE PAIN

Method of
David Borenstein, MD; and Federico Balagué, MD

CURRENT DIAGNOSIS

- Most spine pain is mechanical in origin in 95% or more of patients.
- Symptoms of mechanical acute spine pain resolve in most patients in 1 to 8 weeks.
- Most patients with spine pain do not require laboratory tests or radiographs to achieve resolution of their symptom of spine pain.

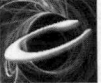

CURRENT THERAPY

- Localized neck or low back pain
  - Encouragement to remain active out of bed
  - Patient education about the natural history to improvement
  - Reassurance about the incidence of resolution
  - Effective oral drug therapy: NSAIDs, analgesics, muscle relaxants
  - Physical therapy with exercise program
- Radicular pain
  - Encouragement to remain active out of bed
  - Patient education about the potential for improvement
  - Efficacy of oral drug therapy: NSAIDs, analgesics, muscle relaxants, corticosteroids, antiseizure medication, epidural corticosteroid injections
  - Physical therapy: Mackenzie exercises for disk herniation
  - Surgical decompression for cauda equina, motor weakness, or intractable pain

Abbreviation: NSAID = nonsteroidal antiinflammatory drug.

Spine pain is a common symptom that is diagnosed and treated by a wide variety of health care professionals. The interest in this medical problem is not limited to its incidence as a patient problem but also stems from the likelihood of spine pain being experienced by the treating physician as well. The good news about spine pain is that the vast majority of patients (about 90%) improve over 2 months with minimal intervention. The bad news is that the smaller number of patients who develop chronic spine pain utilize more than the majority of health resources expended on this expensive medical problem. The goal of therapy is to relieve spine pain while it is acute so that chronic pain does not develop.

The axial skeleton may be divided into cervical, thoracic, lumbar, sacral, and coccygeal locations. The lumbar and cervical areas are the most mobile and at greatest risk for damage. These two areas will be the primary subjects of this article.

Epidemiology

Spine pain is the most common musculoskeletal complaint worldwide and produces direct and indirect costs of hundreds of billions of dollars each year in the United States. More than 80% of the world's population at some time during their lives will have an episode of low back pain. An estimated 20% of the U.S. population has back pain every year. Neck pain occurs at a variable rate ranging from 0.055/1000 person-years (disk herniation with radiculopathy) to 213/1000 person-years (self-reported neck pain). Thoracic spine pain is relatively rare compared to the incidence of pain in the other two locations in the axial skeleton.

Persons of all ages develop spine pain. Younger people are at risk for developmental problems (idiopathic scoliosis, spondylolysis, spondylolisthesis), and older patients develop disorders associated with degeneration of spinal structures (osteoarthritis, spinal stenosis).

Risk Factors

Psychosocial factors are stronger predictors of incident low back pain than mechanical factors in adolescent populations. In adults, psychosocial difficulties are risk factors for chronicity more strongly related to outcome than any clinical or mechanical variables. Previous episodes of spine pain are strong predictors of future ones.

Studies of cohorts of twins have shown that nonspecific low back pain is more than 60% genetically determined, and work and leisure-time physical activities play a minor role. Other environmental factors, such as smoking and obesity, have not been shown to be a predictor of the development of spine pain on a consistent basis.

Pathophysiology

Most of the structures of the axial skeleton receive sensory input. The presence of anatomic alterations in these structures is not sufficient to predict the presence of pain. In general, spine pain is referred to as nonspecific because no definite pain generator can be identified. The nociceptive inputs generated by musculoskeletal structures is referred to as somatic pain.

In the first few decades of life, muscular sprains and strains of the paraspinous muscles in the lumbar and cervical regions are the most likely source of spinal pain. These muscular injuries occur when lifting in a position that places stress on paraspinous structures. Often the spine is in an awkward position and is mechanically disadvantaged. The subsequent muscle injury results in reflexive muscular contraction that can recruit muscles in the same myotome. Tonic contraction approximates the damaged components of the muscle but results in relative anoxia that causes the production of anaerobic metabolites that stimulate nociceptors. The number of recruited muscles may be extensive, manifested by severe spinal stiffness and limitation of motion. Most of these soft-tissue injuries to the muscle heal spontaneously without any long-term structural alterations.

Simultaneously, as people age, intervertebral disks become flatter as the nucleus pulposus loses its absorbency and the annulus fibrosus fissures and degenerates. The process results in the loss of disk integrity. Degeneration of normal biomechanical and biochemical disk properties results. Biomechanical insufficiency inevitably results in a transfer of stresses posterior to the facet joints and ligaments that are ill suited to assume compressive, tensile, and shear loads. Osteophytes form in response to these abnormal pressures, compromising the space for the neural elements. Disk degeneration itself might not be a painful process until alterations in facet joint alignment result in the onset of articular pain.

Spondylolysis is a developmental abnormality associated with a stress fracture in the growth plate of the pars interarticularis. This abnormality may be discovered as a radiographic abnormality in an asymptomatic patient. An increased risk of low back pain occurs with spondylolisthesis, the abnormality associated with instability of spinal elements in the setting of spondylolysis.

Pain generation in the axial skeleton may be somatic or neuropathic in origin. The joints, ligaments, muscles, fascia, blood vessels, and disks can be the source of localized somatic spine pain. Somatic pain, when it does radiate, tends to be less focused in distribution and exacerbated by specific positions of the spine.

Neuropathic or radicular pain is the sensation generated by damage of neural elements. Intervertebral disk herniation with compression of spinal nerve roots causes neural inflammation resulting in neuropathic and radicular pain. Radicular pain follows the path of the corresponding spinal nerve root. In addition to pain, sensory deficits and muscle weakness can occur, depending on the intensity of the nerve compression. In the setting of chronic low back pain, the role of the central nervous system in mediating persistent symptoms has been highlighted increasingly in the medical literature.

Prevention

Since the turn of the century, adolescents have reported nonspecific spine pain at an incidence similar to that in adult populations. This finding suggests that primary prevention must be given at a very early age to have any chance of efficacy.

Among papers reporting on primary prevention, only exercise has shown effectiveness, with effect sizes ranging from 0.39 to 0.69. Other techniques, such as stress management, shoe inserts, back supports, education, and reduced lifting, were found ineffective.

Clinical Manifestations

The most common symptoms of spinal disorders are regional pain and decreased range of motion associated in a minority of patients with radiating pain. For the majority of patients, pain has mechanical characteristics: Its intensity increases with physical activity, movements, or some postures and decreases with rest. However, it has been demonstrated that nocturnal pain is not uncommon in the absence of serious, specific spinal disorders. The precise topography of pain is often difficult for the patient to describe, and its interpretation is difficult owing to the overlap of the cutaneous projections between adjacent spinal levels and the similarities between dermatomes, myotomes, and sclerotomes.

Diagnosis

The diagnosis of spine pain is based upon the patient's history and physical examination. The history and physical examination should include a description of the pain that is as detailed as possible (e.g., past episodes, precise location, beginning of symptoms, factors increasing or decreasing pain intensity, radiating pain, neurologic symptoms, systemic symptoms), patient's medical history (e.g., past spinal surgery, neoplasia, corticosteroid treatments), and a limited physical examination focused on the posture of the spine, range of motion, muscle contraction, pain on palpation or percussion, and a brief neurologic examination.

Besides the high rate of false positives and financial costs, imaging studies have a negative effect on a patient's quality of life. Therefore, unless there is a clear-cut surgical indication or a suspicion of an underlying life-threatening disorder, no imaging studies should be ordered on the first encounter for a patient with acute nonspecific low back or neck pain. Similarly, laboratory testing is not required unless a patient presents with clinical symptoms that suggest a systemic illness (e.g., fever, weight loss).

Differential Diagnosis

A number of guidelines are available in the literature to help a clinician in the diagnosis and treatment of patients with spine pain. The purpose of these approaches is to differentiate the vast majority of patients with mechanical disorders who will improve with noninvasive therapy without the need for radiographic or laboratory investigation from the small minority with a specific cause of spinal pain.

Traditionally, red flags have been used to identify patients with a systemic disorder causing spine pain. The red flags have included questions regarding prior history of cancer, weight loss, prolonged morning stiffness, bladder dysfunction, and bowel dysfunction. The presence of these findings suggests a diagnosis of malignancy, infection, spondyloarthropathy, or cauda equina syndrome, respectively. A study has reported that red-flag disorders occur so infrequently and have so many false positive findings as not to be helpful in the primary care setting at the initial visit. The one exception was spine pain associated with osteoporotic vertebral compression fractures.

Despite the findings of this one report, clinicians need to be mindful of patients who would be harmed to a significant degree by delayed therapy. The disorders that require expeditious evaluation and treatment are intraabdominal vascular disorders with tearing pain and hemodynamic instability (expanding aortic aneurysm); cauda equina syndrome with bilateral sciatica; saddle anesthesia; bladder or bowel incontinence (lumbar space-occupying compressive lesions); and cervical myelopathy with balance difficulties, autonomic dysfunction, and hyperreflexia with spasticity and Babinski's sign (cervical space-occupying compressive lesions). These disorders require expeditious vessel repair or decompression surgery.

The differential diagnosis of mechanical low back pain (Table 1) and mechanical neck pain (Table 2) includes disorders ranging from muscle strain and herniated disk to scoliosis and whiplash injuries. The age of patients, pain pattern with exacerbating and mitigating factors, tension signs, and findings of plain radiographs can help differentiate among these common causes of spine pain.

Nonspecific is a term used commonly to describe the pain associated with mechanical disorders. On occasion, physicians have confused the use of "nonspecific" as meaning an absence of pathology causing pain associated with mechanical disorders. The "nonspecific" designation refers to the inability to identify the specific pain-generating anatomic structure, not the absence of somatic pain.

Therapy

Many mechanical disorders of the spine are self-limited in duration, with a vast majority of patients improving gradually over time (Box 1). This progression to "natural healing" makes placebo look efficacious in many clinical trials investigating therapies for spine pain. This situation results in evidence-based reviews of spine pain therapies revealing very few categories that have a clinically significant impact on improvement. Nonetheless, physicians need to make therapeutic choices for their patients despite this relative paucity of evidence. Therapy for spine pain includes controlled physical activity, nonsteroidal antiinflammatory drugs (NSAIDs), skeletal muscle relaxants, local and epidural corticosteroid injections, and long-term pain therapy. Surgical intervention is reserved for patients who have

TABLE 1 Mechanical Low Back Pain

FEATURE	MUSCLE STRAIN	HERNIATED NUCLEUS PULPOSUS	OSTEOARTHRITIS	SPINAL STENOSIS	SPONDYLOLISTHESIS	SCOLIOSIS
Age (yr)	20–40	30–50	>50	>60	20	30
Pain Pattern						
Location	Back (unilateral)	Back/leg (unilateral)	Back (unilateral)	Leg (bilateral)	Back	Back
Onset	Acute	Acute (previous episodes)	Insidious	Insidious	Insidious	Insidious
Standing	↑	↓	↑	↑	↑	↑
Sitting	↓	↑	↓	↓	↓	↓
Bending	↑	↑	↓	↓	↑	↑
Straight leg	−	+	−	+ (stress)	−	−
Plain radiograph*	−	−	+	+	+	+

Reprinted with permission from Mechanical low back pain. In Borenstein DG, Wiesel SW, Boden SD (eds): Low back and neck pain, 3rd ed. Philadelphia, WB Saunders, 2004.
*Possibility of seeing the abnormality, not a recommendation to get radiographs.
↑, increased; ↓, decreased; +, present; −, absent.

TABLE 2 Mechanical Neck Pain

FEATURE	NECK STRAIN	HERNIATED NUCLEUS PULPOSUS	OSTEOARTHRITIS	MYELOPATHY	WHIPLASH
Age (yr)	20–40	30–50	>50	>60	30–40
Pain Pattern					
Location	Neck	Neck/arm	Neck	Arm/leg	Neck
Onset	Acute	Acute	Insidious	Insidious	Acute
Flexion	+	+	−	−	+
Extension	−	+/−	+	+	+
Plain radiograph*	−	−	+	+	−

Reprinted with permission from Mechanical neck pain. In Borenstein DG, Wiesel SW, Boden SD (eds): Low back and neck pain, 3rd ed. Philadelphia, WB Saunders, 2004.
*Possibility of seeing the abnormality, not a recommendation to get radiographs.
+, present; −, absent.

Box 1 Management of Low Back Pain

Acute (<6 weeks)

First consultation: gather information on core outcome domains

Rule out pain of nonspinal origin

Rule out specific causes (red flags)

No routine imaging

Inform and reassure the patient. Advise to stay active and continue daily activities, if possible, including work

Prescribe analgesia, if necessary. First choice: acetaminophen; second choice: NSAIDs

Consider adding muscle relaxants (short course) or referring for spinal manipulation

Avoid overmedicalizing, especially in patients with favorable outcome

Be aware of yellow flags: inappropriate attitudes and beliefs about back pain, inappropriate pain behavior, emotional problems

Subacute (6–12 weeks)

Reassessment

Bear in mind minimum clinically important difference of core outcome tools

Consider patients' expectations

Consider yellow flags if outcome is not favorable

Reassess regularly by valid outcome tools to evaluate response to treatment

Focus on function

Give priority to active treatments

Consider multidisciplinary program in occupational setting for workers with subacute low back pain and sick leave (>4–8 weeks)

Chronic (>12 weeks)

Repeat thorough clinical examination

In cases of low impairment and disability, simple evidence-based therapies (e.g., exercises, medication, brief interventions) might be sufficient

In cases of more-severe disability or chronicity, give priority to multidisciplinary approaches (biopsychosocial)

Abbreviation: NSAID = nonsteroidal antiinflammatory drug.

From Balagué F, Mannion AF, Pellisé F, Cedraschi C. Clinical update: low back pain. Lancet 2007;369(9563):726–8.

---

surgically correctable abnormalities and who have cauda equina syndrome, increasing motor weakness, spasticity, or intractable pain.

The treatment of an individual patient has to be tailored based on the patient's expectations and preferences. Goals of the treatment should be clearly defined, and the patient should be informed about the expected benefits and side effects of the treatment at the first encounter. A short trial limited to a few days may be a good start.

Self-management with education of the patient about maintaining physical activities as tolerated has been encouraged for neck and low back pain. Information on nonpharmacologic pain-management strategies and daily life activities may be provided by health care providers, but patients adhere more to the former than to the latter.

Exercises are slightly effective for pain and function in patients with chronic low back pain. No specific form of exercise is clearly better than others.

The use of manipulative physical techniques in the care of spine pain patients remains controversial. The absence of clear-cut distinctions between manipulative techniques with or without thrust adds to the confusion when one analyzes the efficacy of manual therapy treatments. Overall there is some clinical trial evidence in favor of spinal manipulation for acute low back pain.

NSAIDs have short-term efficacy for both acute and chronic low back pain; however, the effect sizes are not very large. The efficacy of these drugs for patients with radicular pain has not been evaluated well enough to make general recommendations. No single class of NSAIDs has superiority to another. Cyclooxygenase 2 (COX-2) inhibitors have a better gastrointestinal (GI) safety profile but no greater efficacy. A patient's response cannot be predicted, and a trial-and-error approach is often necessary.

Opiates have not demonstrated any favorable influence in the outcome of low back pain patients. Side effects are quite common and the risk of addiction is real. When these kinds of drugs are effective, the improvement is more important in pain intensity than in terms of function. Muscle relaxants do have some efficacy for acute and chronic low back pain, but the effect size is limited.

Antidepressants are not generally prescribed owing to an inconsistent improvement of patients. For patients with chronic low back pain and depression, an optimized antidepressant treatment shows a better effect on depression than on pain and functional capacity. Duloxetine, a serotonin and norepinephrine reuptake inhibitor, is approved by the U.S. Food and Drug Administration for the indication of chronic low back pain.

Evidence is lacking to support the prescription of systemic corticosteroids. However, corticosteroids have the advantage of not being toxic to the kidneys. Oral corticosteroids may be considered in patients with radicular pain from a herniated disk or spinal stenosis where epidural injections are relatively contraindicated (chronic warfarin therapy).

Some patients will have persistent neuropathic pain despite surgical decompression or as a result of postsurgical fibrosis. Opioid therapy is ineffective in many patients with chronic neuropathic pain. Antiseizure medicines, such as gabapentin (Neurontin)[1] and pregabalin (Lyrica), have efficacy in peripheral neuropathic pain. These same medicines are prescribed in patients with chronic neuropathic radicular pain[1] with the hope that the mechanisms that work with peripheral neuropathy will also work for spine pain patients. Other medicines including antidepressants (duloxetine [Cymbalta],[1] tricyclic antidepressants) have been tried when other drugs have been ineffective.

Epidural, selective nerve root, or facet joint injections have not shown adequate efficacy to be recommended on a regular basis. However, a limited number (2 or 3) of spinal injections may be attempted for patients with radicular pain who do not improve with oral medication.

Spinal surgery is indicated for disk herniation with radicular compromise, cervical or lumbar spinal stenosis with myelopathy or neurogenic claudication, and unstable spondylolisthesis. Controversy remains, however, concerning the relative benefit of surgical versus medical therapy for radiculopathy. Diskectomy significantly shortens (by about 8 weeks) the acute phase of pain associated with radiculopathy. However, studies with longer follow-up periods have never shown a clear difference between conservative and surgical therapies. Some studies have shown that intensive, multidisciplinary, conservative programs can be compared with surgical fusion procedures for patients with spinal instability.

For the most chronically disabled spine pain patients only, intensive multidisciplinary programs including, among others, physical reconditioning and cognitive-behavioral methods, have shown effectiveness.

---

[1]Not FDA approved for this indication.

Spine Pain

55

Monitoring

From the standpoint of monitoring the efficacy of the treatment, five main dimensions have been recommended to evaluate the outcome of patients with spine pain. The intensity of pain is relevant, but so is the perceived functional capacity, generic health status, work disability, and satisfaction with treatment. Many tools are available for the evaluation of each specific dimension. The clinician who decides to start using any specific tool needs to know, among other information, the minimal clinically meaningful changes for each tool, because differences that may be statistically significant when comparing two groups of patients may be irrelevant at the individual patient level. For example, in terms of intensity of pain, the threshold usually accepted is 3.5 to 4.7 and 2.5 to 4.5 for patients with acute and chronic pain, respectively.

Precisely evaluating several domains with specific tools is rather time consuming. However, for busy clinicians, there are brief instruments (core set of measures) with roughly 7 or 8 questions that include all the previously mentioned dimensions and that have been properly validated.

Complications

The clinician should inform the patient about the possible side effects of therapies as they are initiated. At subsequent visits, specific questions regarding the potential side effects are asked. For example, the presence of hypertension, peripheral edema, and hepatic and renal dysfunction need to be evaluated in patients who are taking chronic NSAID therapy.

In addition, a majority of NSAIDs have potential GI toxicity including mild mucosal irritation, ulcers, and perforations. Hematologic and neurologic toxicity are quite variable depending on the prescribed drug. Cardiovascular toxicity may clearly be an issue, particularly for long-term treatments. The benefit of persistent use of NSAIDs for patients with chronic spine pain needs to be weighed against the increased risk of toxicities.

The use of opiates induces constipation and urinary retention that may be a serious problem for some patients. These drugs can also produce drowsiness, headache, nausea, or vomiting.

Antidepressants also produce drowsiness and anticholinergic symptoms during the first couple of weeks of use. These drugs have specific side effects including tachycardia, weight gain, or sexual problems.

References

Balagué F, Mannion AF, Pellisé F, Cedraschi C. Clinical update: Low back pain. Lancet 2007;369(9563):726–8.

Balagué F, Mannion AF, Pellisé F, Cedraschi C. Seminar on nonspecific low back pain. Lancet 2012;379(9814):482–91.

Bigos SJ, Holland J, Holland C, et al. High-quality controlled trials on preventing episodes of back problems: Systematic literature review in working-age adults. Spine J 2009;9(2):147–68.

Borenstein D. Mechanical low back pain - a rheumatologist's view. Nat Rev Rheumatol 2013;9:643–53.

Borenstein DG. Chronic neck pain: How to approach treatment. Curr Pain Headache Rep 2007;11(6):436–9.

Briggs AM, Smith AJ, Straker LM, Bragge P. Thoracic spine pain in the general population: Prevalence, incidence and associated factors in children, adolescents and adults. A systematic review. BMC Musculoskelet Disord 2009;10:77.

Choi BK, Verbeek JH, Tamm WW, Jiang JY. Exercises for prevention of recurrences of low-back pain. Cochrane Database Syst Rev 2010;20(1) CD006555.

Chou R, Qaseem A, Snow V, et al. Diagnosis and treatment of low back pain: A joint clinical practice guideline from the American College of Physicians and the American Pain Society. Ann Intern Med 2007;147:478–91.

Chou R, Huffman LH. Medications for acute and chronic low back pain: A review of the evidence for an American Pain Society/American College of Physicians clinical practice guideline. Ann Intern Med 2007;147:505–614.

Chou R, Fu R, Carrino JA, Deyo RA. Imaging strategies for low-back pain: systematic review and meta-analysis. Lancet 2009;373(9662):463–72.

Chou R, Atlas SJ, Stanos SP, Rosenquist RW. Nonsurgical interventional therapies for low back pain: A review of the evidence for an American Pain Society clinical practice guideline. Spine 2009;34(10):1078–93.

Chou R, Baisden J, Carragee EJ, et al. Surgery for low back pain: A review of the evidence for an American Pain Society Clinical Practice Guideline. Spine 2009;34 (10):1094–109.

Costa Lda C, Maher CG, et al. Prognosis for patients with chronic low back pain: Inception cohort study. BMJ 2009;339:b3829.

Deyo RA, Mirza SK, Turner JA, Martin BI. Overtreating chronic back pain: Time to back off? J Am Board Fam Med 2009;22(1):62–8.

Deyo RA, Von Korff M, Duhrkoop D. Opioids for low back pain. BMJ 2015;350: g380. http://dx.doi.org/10.1136/bmj.g6380.

Friedly JL, Comstock BA, Turner JA, et al. A randomized trial of epidural glucocorticoid injections for spinal stenosis. N Engl J Med 2014;371:11–21.

Henschke N, Maher CG, Refshauge KM, et al. Prevalence of and screening for serious spinal pathology in patients presenting to primary care settings with acute low back pain. Arthritis Rheum 2009;60(10):3072–80.

TINNITUS

Method of
Richard W. Crummer, MD; and Richard Sadovsky, MD

CURRENT DIAGNOSIS

- Tinnitus is common among those exposed to loud noise, among veterans, and among older adults.
- Tinnitus severity can range from very mild occasional noise awareness to a disruptive sound that can result in depression, cognitive impairment, and even suicide.
- Many people who complain of tinnitus also have a moderate to severe hearing loss.
- Pulsatile and/or unilateral tinnitus may be a sign of cardiovascular disease.
- Children also can have tinnitus, but are even less likely than adults to complain.

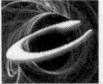

CURRENT THERAPY

- No cure exists for tinnitus, although proper diagnosis and management using a team approach can result in some relief.
- Tinnitus intensity and bother are affected by many individual factors beyond the actual volume and frequency of noise, such as patient affect and mental state.
- Cognitive-behavioral therapy and a hearing aid or masking device are the most common successful management tools for tinnitus, although combined treatment including medication offers the best success for patients with severe idiopathic tinnitus.
- Protection should be worn when exposed to loud noise.
- Successful management of troublesome complications, including insomnia, anxiety, and depression, will decrease tinnitus-associated symptom severity in most patients.

Definition and Epidemiology

Tinnitus is a symptom defined as perception of an internally generated sound that usually cannot be heard by others. Modern definitions include the dynamic advances in underlying neurophysiology noting a clinically conscious awareness of aberrant activity in synaptic circuitry that can manifest as an aberrant auditory perception that may increase with time, causing severe disabling symptoms. Perception can be a tonal sensation or ringing or noise-like sound, but can also include more complex sounds (crickets buzzing, pulsing noise), may fluctuate over time, and can be perceived in one or both ears or heard diffusely in the head. Thirty million people in the United States, or 10% of the entire population, note the presence of tinnitus at some time during their lives, with the incidence as high as 26.7% for people 65 to 84 years of age and a peak from ages 60 to 69. There appears to be no gender difference in tinnitus prevalence, although a few studies report a higher incidence among men. Some estimates of tinnitus incidence among older adults are even higher because fear of serious causes of tinnitus can discourage them from mentioning it. Wartime veterans often suffer from tinnitus, making it one of the major causes of disability among veterans. The incidence of tinnitus among children is 13%, with a higher rate among those who have had severe hearing loss.

Half of sufferers are bothered whereas others report no impact on life. Nearly 40% experience tinnitus more than 80% of the time. There is a wide variety of loudness, pitch, temporal variability, and family history of tinnitus among sufferers.

Some experts believe that the severity of tinnitus appears to be correlated with exposure to noise. Forty-four percent report no hearing loss, although it is agreed that most people with tinnitus have hearing loss. Among some, the hearing loss is mild and not noticed, but others report moderate and even profound hearing loss. Most tinnitus is *subjective*, heard only by the patient. *Objective tinnitus* can be heard by the examiner, by a careful stethoscope examination near the patient's ear, head, and/or neck.

Risk Factors/Etiologies (Subjective and Objective Tinnitus)

The most common risk factors for subjective tinnitus include (1) older age and/or hearing loss (presbycusis) and (2) exposure to loud noises (e.g., wartime veterans). Others include the following:

1. Conductive local causes of hearing loss such as cerumen impaction, obstruction of the external auditory canal, middle ear effusion, otosclerosis
2. Sensorineural and neurovascular causes/associated disorders such as loud sounds, Menicre's disease, acoustic neuroma, multiple sclerosis, head trauma, cerebral infarctions, seizures
3. Cardiovascular and hematologic disorders, including hypertension and blood pressure fluctuations, heart disease, arrhythmias, anemia
4. Metabolic disorders, including diabetes, dyslipidemia, hypertriglyceridemia, hypothyroidism or hyperthyroidism, obesity, vitamin B_{12} or zinc deficiency
5. Ototoxic medications such as salicylates, NSAIDs, aminoglycosides, erythromycin, methotrexate, loop diuretics, chloroquine (Aralen), quinine (Qualaquin)
6. Temporomandibular joint disorder
7. Trigger factors, including anxiety, bad news, upper respiratory infections, and any other activities/disorders causing increased arousal mediated by the autonomic nervous system

The most common risk factors for objective tinnitus include (1) vascular abnormalities (e.g., arterial bruits, venous hums, heart murmurs), (2) neurologic disease, and (3) eustachian tube dysfunction (e.g., patulous eustachian tube causing blowing sounds with breathing). Others include glomus tumor and palatomyoclonus (stapedial muscle spasm).

Pathophysiology

The mechanism that produces tinnitus remains unclear. Subjective tinnitus is considered to be sensorineurophysiologic in origin, whereas objective tinnitus is thought to arise from vascular, muscular, or respiratory origins, as well as the temporomandibular joint. Tinnitus may originate peripherally or centrally at any location along the auditory pathway from the cochlear nucleus to the auditory cortex, as well as from other nonauditory central brain structures. Leading theories for auditory pathway tinnitus include the following: (1) sequential injury to outer, then inner cochlear hair cells; (2) repetitive discharge in auditory nerve fibers in the dorsal cochlear nucleus that are stimulated in a continuous cycle; (3) hyperactive spontaneous activity in the auditory nuclei in the inferior colliculus of the brainstem; and (4) less than the usual suppressive activity of the central auditory cortex on peripheral auditory nerve activity. Pathologic changes in neural patterns create a subjective perception of sounds that resembles the pattern of actual sounds. Recent research is demonstrating a common pathway involving three separate neuroanatomic substrates in the central nervous system that are activated in severe idiopathic tinnitus, including sensory, affective (emotion and behavior), and psychomotor centers, meaning that multiple symptoms may occur at the same time.

The reorganization of edge frequencies in the cortical tonotropic map, in which cortical neurons begin to respond preferentially to sound frequencies at the edge of normal hearing, has recently been detected in tinnitus sufferers by neuromagnetic brain imaging. Other researchers using functional magnetic resonance imaging have recently implicated auditory-limbic interactions to explain the etiology of chronic tinnitus. They found moderate hyperactivity on MRI in the primary and posterior auditory cortices of tinnitus patients. However, the greatest degree of hyperactivity was noted in two limbic structures, the nucleus accumbens and the ventromedial prefrontal cortex.

Positron emission tomography (PET) studies predominantly show increased blood flow in several auditory structures, including the medial geniculate nucleus, the primary and secondary auditory cortex, the auditory brainstem, and temporal-parietal association areas. Brain changes can also be seen in nonauditory areas, including the hippocampus, amygdala, and cingulate gyrus.

Prevention

- Limit or avoid exposure to loud noises.
- Wear earplugs or ear defenders. (Tissues and cotton balls are not sufficient, because they may become lodged in the ear canal).
- Cut back on alcohol and caffeine.
- Do not smoke (nicotine reduces blood flow to the ear structures).
- Exercise regularly to improve blood flow.
- Maintain healthy weight (tinnitus is more common in obese people).
- Take care of cardiovascular health.
- Avoid ototoxic medications (see Risk Factors above), especially among patients predisposed to ototoxicity such as advanced or very young age, pregnancy, renal or hepatic disease, or history of hearing loss. Monitor hearing when these medications must be used.

Clinical Manifestations

Patients with the symptom of tinnitus may complain of a mild inconsequential ringing, buzzing, hissing, roaring, clicking, or rough sounds, heard from time to time and for short periods of time, to an unbearable, constant noise, which can seriously degrade the patient's ability to function and enjoy life. Tinnitus can be acute or chronic in nature, unilateral or bilateral, nonpulsatile or pulsatile: arterial, venous, or nonvascular. The great majority of patients experience tinnitus without significant associated symptoms, but more than one fourth of persons with tinnitus are distressed by it. Associated anxiety or depression often leads to more severe tinnitus-associated symptoms and to a greater negative impact on the patient's life. Various questionnaires, including the Tinnitus Handicap Questionnaire and the Tinnitus Severity Index, quantify the effect that tinnitus has on multiple areas in a patient's life.

The potential adverse effects of tinnitus are noted under Complications.

Diagnosis

The primary care office is an appropriate place to initiate the management of tinnitus.

History
Complete medical and psychological history
Tinnitus components
    Sensory
    Affect
    Psychomotor
Any factors that worsen or relieve symptoms
Prior treatment history

Complete physical examination
Concentrate on the following:
    Audiologic
    Neurologic
    Cardiovascular
    Metabolic
    Psychological

Laboratory tests
Thyroid function tests
Vitamin B_{12}
Complete blood count
Fasting glucose
Lipids, including triglycerides
Zinc

The evaluation of the patient with tinnitus begins with a thorough patient history, which involves an attempt to determine the etiologic and/or contributing factors causing ear noise. Certain parameters of the sounds heard can help to identify potential etiologies and to determine the need for further evaluation and treatment as seen in Box 1. Besides identifying the (sensation) of tinnitus, a review of the patient's affect and psychomotor functioning is an important part of strategizing the total management plan.

In the primary care office, the tinnitus patient should undergo a thorough physical examination with special attention to audiologic (including vertigo), cardiovascular, neurologic, and metabolic systems. A basic otologic examination includes (1) using a stethoscope to identify objective tinnitus, (2) examination of the external canal, (3) basic hearing testing, and (4) specific testing for sensorineural or conductive hearing loss using the Weber and Rinne tests. Thyroid studies, a hematocrit determination, complete blood chemistry, vitamin B_{12}, and lipid profile should be obtained if the patient has any suggestion of a metabolic abnormality. Primary care clinicians can identify many of the parameters that will determine further evaluation and management plans (see Box 1).

The management team evaluation continues with diagnostic audiologic testing, including audio testing, speech discrimination testing, and tympanometry. Other audiologic measurements of tinnitus may include pitch masking, loudness masking, minimum masking level, and residual inhibition.

Further investigation should be dictated by team discussion of potential etiologic/exacerbating factors for the individual patient. Patients with unilateral or pulsatile tinnitus are more likely to have serious underlying disease, such as vascular middle ear tumors,

and should be evaluated by an otolaryngologist and possibly a cardiologist or neurologist. Many of these patients also require accompanying computed tomography (CT) angiogram, magnetic resonance imaging (MRI), carotid ultrasound, and perhaps standard angiography.

Differential Diagnosis

Not all sounds of internal origin perceived by the patient are those defined as tinnitus. Patients can also have ear noise caused by auditory hallucinations, as well as benign "transient noise."

Auditory hallucinations can occur in both psychotic and nonpsychotic patients. In a patient who by appropriate evaluation is considered to be psychotic, and more likely schizophrenic, hearing voices or other sounds may be auditory hallucinations. Stress or sleep deprivation can also cause auditory hallucinations in nonpsychotic patients. In a patient who is not sleep deprived or stressed, or drinking large amounts of caffeine-containing beverages, ear noise is more likely to be tinnitus.

Transient noise is defined as a whistling sound accompanied by a sensation of sudden temporary hearing loss. These episodes generally disappear in seconds and occur rarely, whereas tinnitus is generally defined as lasting over 5 minutes and occurring at least twice weekly. They are usually not related to any specific event or activity, often unilateral, and sometimes accompanied by a feeling of ear blockage. Usually, no treatment is necessary beyond patient education.

Management

There is no cure for tinnitus, although a multidisciplinary approach (tinnitus-targeted therapy) with a medico-audiologic approach can partially alleviate associated symptoms. The goal is "control" rather than "treatment." In expert hands, a majority of severely disabled tinnitus patients can get long-term relief with targeted medication and instrumentation.

Tinnitus management includes the following:
1. Eliminate potentially ototoxic medications and/or any precipitating active diseases/disorders (see Risk Factors/Etiologies above).
2. Administer targeted medication based on contributory medical conditions, severity of distress, tinnitus type (cochlear-peripheral or central), and tinnitus components involved (sensory, affective, and/or psychomotor).
3. Use instrumentation such as hearing aids, tinnitus masks, tinnitus retraining including low noise generators, and/or relaxing external sound stimulation with silence avoidance.
4. Provide mental health support, including stress management, biofeedback, reassurance, and relaxation techniques.

No medications have been found to consistently reduce tinnitus symptoms, probably because of the heterogeneity of clinical tinnitus types. Pharmacologic treatment should deal specifically with the component(s) of severe tinnitus being targeted and uses drugs for their FDA-approved purposes to logically manage an individual's tinnitus presentation. The sensory component symptoms among patients with predominantly cochlear-type severe tinnitus (peripheral) can be treated with pentoxifylline (Trental),[1] which can enhance the oxygen-carrying capacity of the blood. If response is poor, intratympanic drug therapy with a steroid and/or instrumentation can be considered. Sensory symptoms among patients with predominantly central-type severe tinnitus can be offered trial instrumentation or brain scanning. If scanning is positive, neuroprotection using medications such as gabapentin (Neurontin)[1] and clonazepam (Klonopin)[1] may be helpful. The affective component of tinnitus can be pharmacologically managed with psychiatric consultation and may also include gabapentin and/or clonazepam (useful for anxiolytic and antiepileptic effects) or some other anxiolytic. The psychomotor component can sometimes be improved with medications such as papaverine[1] or clopidogrel (Plavix)[1] for cerebrovascular insufficiency and antiseizure

---

[1] Not FDA approved for this indication.

> **Box 1**   Useful Tinnitus Parameters for Primary Care Clinicians
>
> 1. Sensory perception—directs evaluation
>   Subjective
>   Objective
> 2. Level of distress—directs degree of evaluation and management
>   Mild (not bothersome)
>   Moderate (noticeable)
>   Severe (bothersome)
> 3. Etiology/contributors—directs precision vs general management choices
>   Identifiable
>   Idiopathic
> 4. Tinnitus origin (pathways)—directs evaluation and management
>   Central (nonauditory system)
>   Peripheral (auditory system)
> 5. Components of tinnitus sensation—directs priority and types of management strategies
>   Sensory
>   Affective (emotion and behavior)
>   Psychomotor
> 6. Sensory characteristics requiring early consultation with an appropriate specialist
>   Unilateral
>   Objective
>   Sudden onset
>   Pulsatile

drugs for epilepsy. Medications can be used continuously or as needed. There are no set regimens for the pharmacologic management of tinnitus. Because anxiolytics and antidepressants can sometimes cause or worsen tinnitus, close follow-up is important for treatment success. Other potentially contributing conditions and/or distressing symptoms should be appropriately treated.

Patients with severe tinnitus not responding to initial therapies or who are in significant distress should be referred to audiology, dentistry, neurology, physical therapy, and a mental health expert. Audiologist recommendations about masking devices to cover up the constant ringing may be helpful. Pleasant sounds such as TVs, radios, or fans can provide distractions. Sound generators can be worn in the ear to produce stable signal (white noise) and is most effective alone in patients with normal or near-normal hearing. This therapy can be combined with a hearing aid, which is most effective when done by a professional hearing expert with strict protocols. The amplification of ambient sound may also reduce tinnitus. Surgical cochlear implant in the profoundly hard of hearing patient can help with hearing issues but can also cause tinnitus for the first time.

Dentists can be helpful by evaluating for temporomandibular joint problems and other habits, and recommending dental orthotics and home exercises to reduce clenching and grinding when appropriate. Neurologists can evaluate for vestibular symptoms, pain syndromes, and other cranial disorders. Physical therapists can evaluate the head and neck for biomechanical and posture problems, and teach useful exercise techniques. Psychological counseling can improve levels of distress with greater improvement shown in combined cognitive strategies/education interventions. Patients can be taught to pay less attention to symptoms, overcome fear, accept tinnitus as part of life, and keep busy with happy activities. Acceptance and commitment therapy to better understand tinnitus and to look at it more objectively than emotionally may be useful. Careful choices and titrations of anxiolytic, antidepressant, and hypnotic medications reduce some of the affective components of tinnitus. Herbs and dietary supplements are commonly used, but there is no evidence to support their efficacy.

Experimental treatments include transcranial magnetic stimulation, low-level laser therapy, phase-out treatment (individualized sound developed to cancel out tinnitus), neuronomics (customized sound therapy), and tinnitus retraining therapy (remove perception from consciousness). The relationship between the auditory and limbic systems may offer a route of management via limbic stimulation and/or external limbic activation associated with emotional stress or depression. These areas are all under active study.

Monitoring

Patients with tinnitus should be monitored for (1) distress symptoms, (2) adverse effects of symptoms, (3) effectiveness of management plan, and (4) hearing. This can be done using direct questions and annual hearing tests. Scales that have been shown to be particularly useful in monitoring patients with tinnitus include the Tinnitus Handicap Inventory—Screening Version (THI-S), the Patient Health Questionnaire (PHQ-9), the Tinnitus Treatment Monitoring Interview (TOMI), and the Generalized Anxiety Disorder 7 (GAD-7). Although the causal relationship is unclear,

Box 2   Complications and/or Comorbid Conditions

Affective

Stress

Sleep problems/insomnia—trouble falling asleep, waking up in the middle of the night, worries about getting enough sleep

Depression—restlessness, lack of energy, change in appetite

Anxiety and irritability—worrying, muscle tension and headaches, shortness of breath, rapid pulse, difficulty concentrating

Headaches

Psychomotor

Fatigue

    Trouble concentrating, memory problems

    Major negative effect on work performance

suicide risk must be monitored, especially among persons who were at high suicide risk before they developed tinnitus.

Recent data using nuclear imaging hint that patients with severe subjective idiopathic tinnitus may be at high risk for brain ischemia and neurodegenerative central nervous system disease consistent with senile dementia of the Alzheimer's type. Monitoring mental status in chronic severe tinnitus sufferers may be useful.

Complications

Different people are affected by tinnitus in different ways. For some, it may be simply irritating. For others, it may be more disruptive. Tinnitus primarily affects the ability to concentrate and sleep. Newer theories pointing out the central nervous substrate activation with tinnitus of sensory, affect, and psychomotor centers help explain the complexity and variability of tinnitus comorbidities (Box 2).

References

Baguley D, McFerran D, Hall D. Tinnitus. Lancet 2013;382:1600–7.

Crummer RW, Hassan GA. Diagnostic approach to tinnitus. Am Fam Physician 2004;69:120–6.

Fioretti A, Eibenstein A, Fusetti M. New trends in tinnitus management. Open Neurol J 2011;5:12–7.

Folmer RL, Martin WH, Shi Y. Tinnitus: questions to reveal the cause, answers to provide relief. J Fam Pract 2004;53:532–40.

Henry JA, Zaugg TL, Myers PJ, et al. A triage guide for tinnitus. J Fam Pract 2010;59:389–94.

Langguth B, Kreuzer PM, Kleinjung T, De Ridder D. Tinnitus: causes and clinical management. Lancet Neurol 2013;12:920–30.

Newman CW, Sandridge SA, Bea SM, et al. Tinnitus: patients do not have to "just live with it." Cleve Clin J Med 2011;78:312–9.

Roberts LE, Eggermont JJ, Caspary DM, et al. Ringing ears: the neuroscience of tinnitus. J Neurosci 2010;30:14972–9.

Shulman A, Goldstein B. Principles of tinnitology: tinnitus diagnosis and treatment a tinnitus-targeted therapy. Int Tinnitus J 2010;16:73–85.

Shulman A, Goldstein B. Subjective idiopathic tinnitus and palliative care: a plan for diagnosis and treatment. Otolaryngol Clin North Am 2009;42:15–37.

Shulman A, Goldstein B, Strashun A. Central nervous system neurodegeneration and tinnitus: a clinical experience. Part 1: diagnosis. Int Tinnitus J 2007;13:118–31.

Sismanis A. Pulsatile tinnitus. Otolaryngol Clin North Am 2003;36:389–402.

Yew KS. Diagnostic approach to patients with tinnitus. Am Fam Physician 2014;89:106–13.

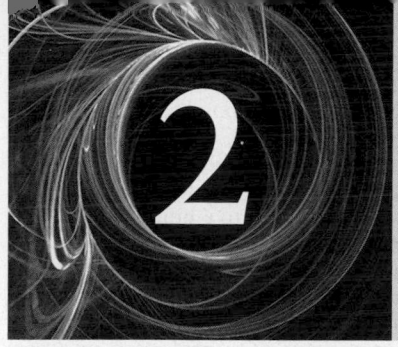

2 Diseases of Allergy

ALLERGIC REACTIONS TO INSECT STINGS

Method of
Theodore M. Freeman, MD

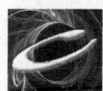

CURRENT DIAGNOSIS

- Determine the insect involved by recording circumstances of sting event.
- Determine the type of reaction: usual (expected), large local, or systemic (anaphylaxis).

CURRENT THERAPY

- Treatment for usual reactions
  - H₁-antihistamines, analgesics, cold compresses
  - Discussion of avoidance measures
- Treatment of large local reactions
  - H₁-antihistamines, analgesics, cold compresses
  - Discussion of avoidance measures and possible prescription of epinephrine autoinjectors (e.g., Auvi-Q, EpiPen)
- Treatment of systemic reactions
  - Epinephrine
  - Supplemental therapy, including antihistamines, β-adrenergics, oxygen, intravenous fluids, and perhaps vasopressors
  - Patients on β-blockers may require glucagon (e.g., Glucagon Emergency Kit, GlucaGen HypoKit)
  - Discussion of avoidance measures, medical alert accessories, prescription for epinephrine autoinjectors
  - Referral to allergist-immunologist to evaluate for specific IgE and possible institution of immunotherapy

Most stinging insects belong to the order Hymenoptera. They include species of bees (genus *Apis*, including honey bees and bumblebees), wasps (genus *Polistes*), yellow jackets (genus *Vespula*), hornets (genus *Dolichovespula*), and fire ants (genus *Solenopsis*).

Diagnosis

There are two important historical points to ascertain when seeing a patient with an allergic reaction to a stinging insect. The first is the type of insect that caused the sting. The physician may not rely on the patient's identification. Clues about the type of insect can be obtained from the circumstances of the sting.

Bees are herbivores and not aggressive. Stings from these insects often occur in fields with flowering plants when a barefoot patient steps or accidently sits on them. Bees have a barbed stinger and attached venom sac, which may be left in place after a sting. These should be removed immediately with a scraping motion; any pinching of the sac may inject additional venom.

Yellow jackets are aggressive scavengers and are found wherever food is left in the open. Stings from these insects usually occur in picnic areas or around open garbage containers. Like bees, yellow jackets occasionally leave a stinger in place, so this historical feature is not definitive. Wasps usually are not aggressive, except in defense of their nests. However, they tend to build these nests under the eaves and overhangs of our homes, and people stung by wasps are usually entering or exiting their homes.

Hornets are not as aggressive, except in defense of their nest. Because the nests are built in trees, stings by these insects are rarer.

Fire ants are very aggressive in defense of their nests, which are low mounds built above ground with extensive tunnels beneath the surface. In endemic areas (mostly the southeastern United States), they swarm and attack as a group when disturbed. Patients stung by fire ants are usually outdoors and accidently stand in a mound or disturb a mound while working or playing in their yard or garden. Fire ant workers do not fly. They bite only to get a grip and then sting from the abdomen and inject a toxic alkaloid venom. Because they attack as a group, they are usually seen and clearly identified by the patient. The size of the fire ants means their venom is injected less deeply than that of other hymenoptera, which leads to the usual development of a pseudopustule about 24 hours after a sting. These pseudopustules contain necrotic cellular material but are sterile because fire ant venom has antibiotic properties that can kill bacteria and fungi. The pseudopustules should be left alone; opening and draining them only increases the risk of secondary infection.

The second historical point is the type of reaction by the patient to the sting. The active venom components produce immediate swelling, redness, and tenderness with fairly intense pain at the site of the sting that slowly resolves over several hours. Sometimes, the immediate reaction progresses, and swelling (>10 cm) continues for 1 to 2 days and extends across several contiguous joints away from the site of the sting. This large local reaction may take 5 to 10 days to fully resolve, and it may be difficult to differentiate this from a secondary infection. Large local reactions peak in 1 to 2 days and then slowly recede, whereas secondary infections continue to get worse. Large local reactions do not cause systemic fever or lymphangitis, which should be treated with antibiotics if they occur.

The reaction of most concern is anaphylaxis. Unfortunately, many of the symptoms are similar to those of anxiety, which also may occur in a concerned patient: feelings of impending doom, a rapid heartbeat, shortness of breath, and nausea. Other symptoms that should not be seen in anxiety include a metallic taste, pruritus, and abdominal or uterine cramping. Signs of anaphylaxis include flushing, urticaria, angioedema, vomiting, diarrhea, bronchospasm, hypotension, and shock. Involvement of the upper airway and cardiopulmonary systems is associated with death, and hymenoptera stings are the cause of about 40 deaths per year in the United States. Documentation of the type of reaction is essential for future risk assessment and determination of whether prophylactic therapy should be offered.

The risk for a systemic reaction after hymenoptera sting in the general population is estimated to be 3% to 5%. In patients who have a documented large local reaction to an insect sting, the risk of systemic reactions increases slightly to about 10%. Patients suffering large local reactions may be referred to a specialist for specific IgE testing. For patients who have suffered anaphylaxis, the risk of systemic reactions after a sting is 50% to 60%. However, children (<16 years old) who have only cutaneous signs and symptoms of anaphylaxis (e.g., pruritus, flushing, urticaria, angioedema) do not seem to have a tendency for life-threatening anaphylaxis, and their risk for more than cutaneous anaphylaxis is only about 10%. If a patient has suffered an anaphylactic event after a hymenoptera sting and has specific IgE to that hymenoptera as determined by in vivo (skin testing) or in vitro methods and is then placed on immunotherapy for that insect, the risk of systemic reaction after another sting is only 2% to 3%. Immunotherapy entails the use of specific venom products for each species, with the exception of fire ants. Because of the difficulty in extracting venom from fire ants, the only commercially available product for fire ants is the whole-body extract. Although whole-body extract is not effective therapy for other hymenoptera, it has been shown to be effective for fire ants.

Treatment

Immediate therapy for insect stings depends on the type of reaction. For the expected short-duration local reaction, treatment includes cold compresses; antihistamines, such as diphenhydramine (Benadryl 25–50 mg for adults; 1 mg/kg [up to 50 mg] for children) or cetirizine (Zyrtec 10 mg for adults and children older than 6 years; 5 mg for children younger than 6 years); and analgesics, such as acetaminophen (Tylenol) or ibuprofen (Motrin). Avoidance of future stings may be discussed with the patient. Recommendations include the following:

- Remove wasps' nests from around the home, especially near doorways.
- Avoid areas near open garbage.
- Do not leave open food or drinks during outdoor eating.
- Wear shoes, socks, and work gloves when working in the yard or garden.

Large local reactions may be treated as described for short-duration local reactions, with the addition of a short course (5–7 days) of oral steroids (e.g., Medrol dose pack), especially if there is significant morbidity associated with the site of the reaction. For instance, if a hand or foot is involved, a patient may not be able to write, work, or walk for up to a week. Avoidance measures should be discussed. Epinephrine autoinjectors (e.g., EpiPen, EpiPen Jr, Adrenaclick, Auvi-Q) may be given, depending on the patient's anxiety about future stings. Epinephrine autoinjectors are simple devices with instructions clearly printed on them, but mistakes in usage do occur. The most common include "bouncing" the injector off the leg, which ejects the epinephrine onto the leg instead of delivering it intramuscularly, and putting the thumb over the end of the injector, which if the injector is reversed leads to no delivery of epinephrine and thumb trauma. The auto-injector Auvi-Q provides audible instructions to the user. Demonstration pens and videos of proper technique may be obtained from the manufacturers (e.g., Dey, Shionogi, Sanofi).

The primary treatment of anaphylaxis is epinephrine (1:1000 concentration), with 0.3 to 0.5 mL given intramuscularly in adults or 0.01 mL/kg in children every 5 to 15 minutes as needed. The patient should be placed in a recumbent position with the feet elevated. Supplemental therapy includes antihistamines (i.e., H_1-receptor antagonists); H_2-blockers (e.g., ranitidine [Zantac[1]] 150 mg PO) for cutaneous signs and symptoms; β-adrenergics (e.g., albuterol [Proventil, AccuNeb]) administered by metered-dose inhaler or nebulizer for bronchoconstriction; oxygen for hypoxia; intravenous fluids and possibly vasopressors for hypotension; and intubation for compromise of the upper airway.

Physicians must avoid the tendency to treat cutaneous-only anaphylaxis with antihistamines alone, because cutaneous signs and symptoms often develop rapidly into life-threatening events.

The appropriate therapy, even for only cutaneous signs and symptoms, is epinephrine. Most anaphylaxis responds quickly to a single dose of epinephrine, although up to 30% of anaphylaxis cases require two or more doses. Because anaphylaxis may be prolonged and last hours and epinephrine has a short duration of action (1 hour), patients should be observed for 4 to 6 hours after the last epinephrine dose. They should remain symptom free during that time before being released from the clinic or emergency department. In 3% to 20% of patients, a biphasic reaction occurs with recurrence of signs and symptoms 4–6 hours (range, 1–72 hours) after the initial reaction. For patients with prolonged or severe reactions, which are more often associated with a recurrence, overnight admission for observation should be considered.

Oral (prednisone 1 mg/kg up to 50 mg daily) or intravenous (methylprednisolone [Solu-Medrol] 1–2 mg/kg every 6 hours) steroids are sometimes given to minimize recurrences. Many patients are on β-blocking agents, which may make patients suffering anaphylaxis refractory to treatment with epinephrine. In this case, glucagon (e.g., GlucaGen HypoKit, Glucagon Emergency Kit[1]) at a dose of 1 to 5 mg (20–30 μg/kg [maximum 1 mg] in children)[3] may be tried intravenously over 5 minutes, followed by infusions (5–15 μg/min)[3] titrated to clinical response. Patients who have suffered anaphylaxis must be given instructions on avoidance of future stings, epinephrine pen autoinjectors (EpiPen), and information on medical alert accessories (e.g., necklaces, bracelets). They should also be referred to an allergist-immunologist to evaluate them for the presence of specific IgE, counseling, and consideration of immunotherapy, which may significantly reduce their future risk.

---

[1]Not FDA approved for this indication.
[3]Exceeds dosage recommended by the manufacturer.

References

Freeman TM. Hypersensitivity to hymenoptera stings. N Engl J Med 2004;351: 1978–84.

Freeman TM, Hylander RD, Ortiz AA, Martin MF. Imported fire ant immunotherapy: Effectiveness of whole body extracts. J Allergy Clin Immunol 1992;90:210–5.

Golden DBK, Moffitt J, Nicklas RA, et al. Stinging insect hypersensitivity: A practice parameter update 2011. J Allergy Clin Immunol 2011;127:852–4.

Hunt KJ, Valentine MD, Sobotka AK, et al. A controlled trial of immunotherapy in insect hypersensitivity. N Engl J Med 1978;299:157–61.

Sampson HA, Munoz-Furlong A, Campbell RL, et al. Second symposium on the definition and management of anaphylaxis: Summary report—Second National Institute of Allergy and Infectious Disease/Food Allergy and Anaphylaxis Network symposium. J Allergy Clin Immunol 2006;117:391–7.

Schuberth KC, Lichtenstein LM, Kagey-Sobotka A, et al. Epidemiologic study of insect allergy in children. II. Effects of accidental stings in allergic children. J Pediatr 1983;102:361–5.

ANAPHYLAXIS AND SERUM SICKNESS

Method of
Stephen F. Kemp, MD

CURRENT DIAGNOSIS

- Cutaneous: urticaria, angioedema, diffuse erythema, generalized pruritus
- Respiratory: tachypnea, bronchospasm, laryngeal or tongue edema, dysphonia
- Cardiovascular: tachycardia, bradycardia, hypotension, angina, cardiac arrhythmias
- Gastrointestinal: nausea, emesis, diarrhea, abdominal cramps, dysphagia
- Other: rhinitis, conjunctivitis, uterine cramps, headache, dizziness, syncope, blurred vision, seizure

---

[1]Not FDA approved for this indication.

Anaphylaxis

Anaphylaxis, an acute and potentially lethal multisystem allergic reaction, is virtually unavoidable in medical practice. Health care professionals must be able to recognize the signs of anaphylaxis, treat an episode promptly and appropriately, and be able to provide preventive recommendations. Epinephrine, which should be administered immediately, is the drug of choice for acute anaphylaxis.

Anaphylaxis is not a reportable disease, and both its morbidity and mortality are probably underestimated. A variety of statistics on the epidemiology of anaphylaxis have been published, but the lifetime risk per person in the United States is presumed to be 1% to 3%, with a mortality rate of 1%.

There is no universally accepted definition of anaphylaxis. An international and interdisciplinary group of representatives and experts from thirteen professional, governmental, and lay organizations proposed the following working definition: "Anaphylaxis is a serious allergic reaction that is rapid in onset and may cause death." Clinically, anaphylaxis is considered likely to be present if any one of the following three criteria is satisfied within minutes to hours:

- Acute onset of illness with involvement of skin, mucosal surface, or both, and at least one of the following: respiratory compromise, hypotension, or end-organ dysfunction;
- Two or more of the following occurring rapidly after exposure to a likely allergen: involvement of skin or mucosal surface, respiratory compromise, hypotension, or persistent gastrointestinal symptoms;
- Hypotension develops after exposure to a known allergen for that patient: age-specific low blood pressure or decline of systolic blood pressure of greater than 30% compared with baseline.

In clinical practice, however, waiting until the development of multiorgan symptoms is risky because the ultimate severity of anaphylactic reaction is difficult to predict from the outset.

Anaphylaxis has varied clinical presentations, but respiratory compromise and cardiovascular collapse cause the most concern because they are the most frequent causes of fatalities. Urticaria and angioedema are the most common manifestations (more than 90% in retrospective series) but may be delayed or absent in rapidly progressive anaphylaxis. The previous severity of anaphylaxis is not predictive of the severity of a future reaction. The more rapidly anaphylaxis occurs after exposure to an offending stimulus, the more likely the reaction is to be severe and potentially life threatening. Anaphylaxis often produces signs and symptoms within 5 to 30 minutes, but reactions sometimes may not develop for several hours.

Pathophysiology

The chemical mediators that cause anaphylaxis are preformed and released from granules (histamine, tryptase, and others) or are generated from membrane lipids (prostaglandin D_2, leukotrienes, and platelet-activating factor) by the activated mast cell or basophil.

Tryptase is concentrated selectively in the secretory granules of all human mast cells. Its plasma levels during mast cell degranulation correlate with the clinical severity of anaphylaxis but need not be elevated in all forms of anaphylaxis (e.g., food-associated anaphylaxis).

Histamine exerts its pathophysiologic effects via both H_1 and H_2 receptors. Erythema (flushing), hypotension, and headache are mediated by both H_1 and H_2 receptors, whereas tachycardia, pruritus, bronchospasm, and rhinorrhea are associated with H_1 receptors alone.

PAF and PAF acetylhydrolase, the enzyme that inactivates PAF, appear to be important in human anaphylaxis. Serum PAF levels directly correlate with anaphylaxis severity, more so than tryptase or histamine levels. PAF acetylhydrolase levels inversely correlate with anaphylaxis severity.

Increased vascular permeability during anaphylaxis can produce a shift of 35% of intravascular fluid to the extravascular space within 10 minutes. This shift of effective blood volume causes compensatory catecholamine release, activates the renin-angiotensin-aldosterone system, and stimulates production of endothelin-1.

Mast cells accumulate at sites of coronary plaque erosion and rupture, and they may contribute to coronary artery thrombosis. Because antibodies attached to mast cells can trigger mast cell degranulation, some investigators suggest that anaphylaxis may promote plaque rupture.

Agents That Cause Anaphylaxis

Cause and effect often is confirmed historically in subjects who experience recurrent, objective findings of anaphylaxis upon inadvertent reexposure to the offending agent. Diagnostic testing, where appropriate, may confirm the presence of specific IgE and/or the degranulation of mast cells and basophils.

Virtually any agent capable of activating mast cells or basophils may potentially precipitate anaphylactic or anaphylactoid reactions. Table 1 lists common causes of anaphylaxis classified by pathophysiologic mechanism. Idiopathic anaphylaxis, anaphylaxis with no identifiable cause, has accounted for approximately a third of cases in most retrospective studies of anaphylaxis. However, of 601 patients evaluated for more than two decades in a university-affiliated practice (the largest retrospective series), 59% of subjects were deemed to have idiopathic anaphylaxis.

Idiopathic anaphylaxis remains a diagnosis of exclusion, however. Serial histories and diagnostic tests for foods, spices, and vegetable gums occasionally identify a specific culprit in subjects previously presumed to have idiopathic anaphylaxis. The most common identifiable causes of anaphylaxis are foods, medications, insect stings, and immunotherapy injections. Anaphylaxis to peanuts and/or tree nuts causes the greatest concern because of its life-threatening severity, especially in subjects with asthma, and the tendency for subjects to develop lifelong allergic responsiveness to these foods.

TABLE 1	Representative Agents That Cause Anaphylaxis

IgE dependent:
- Foods (such as peanuts, tree nuts, and crustaceans)
- Medications (such as antibiotics)
- Venoms (fire ants, yellow jackets, others)
- Allergen extracts
- Latex
- Exercise (where food or medication dependent)
- Hormones

IgE independent:
- Nonspecific degranulation of mast cells and basophils
  - Opioids
  - Muscle relaxants
  - Idiopathic
- Physical factors
  - Exercise
  - Cold, heat
- Disturbance of arachidonic acid metabolism
  - Aspirin and other nonsteroidal anti-inflammatory drugs (NSAIDs)
- Immune aggregates
  - Intravenous immunoglobulin
- Cytotoxic
  - Transfusion reactions to cellular elements (IgM, IgG)
- Multimediator complement activation/activation of contact system
  - Radiocontrast media
  - Angiotensin-converting enzyme (ACE) inhibitor administered during renal dialysis with selected dialysis membranes
  - Protamine (possibly)
- Other
  - c-kit mutation (D816V)

Modified and updated from Kemp SF, Lockey RF. Anaphylaxis: A review of causes and mechanisms. J Allergy Clin Immunol 2002;110:341–8.

Recurrent Anaphylaxis

Depending on the report, recurrent (biphasic) anaphylaxis occurs in 1% to 20% of subjects who experience anaphylaxis. Signs and symptoms experienced during the recurrent phase of anaphylaxis may be equivalent to or worse than those observed in the initial reaction and may occur 1 to 72 hours (most within 8 hours) after apparent remission. Thus, it may be necessary to monitor subjects up to 24 hours after apparent recovery from the initial phase. Observation periods after apparent recovery from the initial phase should be individualized and based on such factors as comorbid conditions and distance from the patient's home to the closest emergency facility, particularly because there are no reliable predictors of biphasic anaphylaxis.

Differential Diagnosis

Several systemic disorders share clinical features with anaphylaxis. The vasodepressor (vasovagal) reaction probably is the condition most commonly confused with anaphylactic reactions. In vasodepressor reactions, however, urticaria is absent, dyspnea is generally absent, the blood pressure is usually normal or elevated, and the skin is typically cool and pale. Tachycardia is the rule in anaphylaxis. Bradycardia may be underrecognized in anaphylaxis, however. Brown and others conducted sting challenges in 19 subjects known to be allergic to jack jumper ants (*Myrmecia*). All eight subjects who became hypotensive developed bradycardia after an initial tachycardia.

Systemic mastocytosis, a disease characterized by mast cell proliferation in multiple organs, usually features urticaria pigmentosa (brownish macules that transform into wheals upon stroking them) and recurrent episodes of pruritus, flushing, tachycardia, abdominal pain, diarrhea, syncope, or headache. Other diagnostic considerations include myocardial dysfunction, pulmonary embolism, foreign body aspiration, acute poisoning, seizure disorder, and psychogenic manifestations (no objective findings observed or documented).

Management of Anaphylaxis

Systematic reviews have noted the lack of optimal, randomized controlled trials of epinephrine, antihistamines, and corticosteroids in anaphylaxis. Pending a stronger evidence base for the treatment of anaphylaxis, current practice parameters and consensus emergency management guidelines afford the best options. Table 2 outlines a sequential approach to management. Assessment and maintenance of airway, breathing, circulation, and mentation are necessary before proceeding to other management steps. Subjects are monitored continuously to facilitate prompt detection of any treatment complications. The recumbent position is strongly recommended. In a retrospective review of prehospital anaphylactic fatalities in the United Kingdom, the postural history was known for 10 individuals. Four of the 10 were associated with assumption of an upright or sitting posture and postmortem findings consistent with "empty heart" and pulseless electrical activity.

Epinephrine is the treatment of choice for acute anaphylaxis. Aqueous epinephrine 1:1000 dilution, 0.2 to 0.5 mL (0.01 mg/kg in children; maximum dose, 0.3 mg) administered intramuscularly every 5 minutes, as necessary, should be used to control symptoms and sustain or increase blood pressure. Comparisons of intramuscular injections to subcutaneous injections during acute anaphylaxis are not available. However, absorption is more rapid and plasma levels are higher in asymptomatic individuals who receive epinephrine intramuscularly in the anterolateral thigh.

All subsequent therapeutic interventions depend on the initial response to epinephrine and the severity of the reaction. Development of toxicity or inadequate response to epinephrine injections indicates that additional therapeutic modalities are necessary.

The α-adrenergic effect of epinephrine reverses peripheral vasodilation, which alleviates hypotension and also reduces angioedema and urticaria. It may also minimize further absorption of antigen from a sting or injection. The β-adrenergic properties of epinephrine increase myocardial output and contractility, cause bronchodilation, and suppress further mediator release from mast cells and basophils.

TABLE 2   Management of Anaphylaxis

Immediate intervention:
- Assess airway, breathing, circulation, and adequacy of mentation.
- Administer aqueous epinephrine 1:1000 dilution, 0.2–0.5 mL (0.01 mg/kg in children; maximum dose, 0.3 mg) intramuscularly q5 min, as necessary, to control symptoms and blood pressure.
- Place subject in recumbent position and elevate lower extremities.

Possibly appropriate, subsequent measures depending on response to epinephrine:
- Consider call for assistance and transportation to an emergency department or intensive care facility. Establish and maintain airway.
- Administer oxygen.
- Establish venous access.
- Use crystalloid (e.g., lactated Ringer's or normal saline) IV (IO) for fluid replacement.

Specific measures to consider after epinephrine injections, where appropriate:
- An epinephrine infusion might be prepared. Continuous hemodynamic monitoring is essential (see reference for specific details).
- Diphenhydramine (Benadryl). Note: In the management of anaphylaxis, a combination of diphenhydramine and ranitidine (Zantac)[1] is superior to diphenhydramine alone in urticarial suppression.
- For bronchospasm resistant to epinephrine, use nebulized albuterol (Proventil).
- For refractory hypotension, consider dopamine (Intropin), 400 mg in 500 mL D_5W, or normal saline administered IV (IO)[1] at 2–20 µg/kg/min titrated to maintain adequate blood pressure. Continuous hemodynamic monitoring is essential.
- Where use of β-blockers complicates therapy, consider glucagon,[1] 1–5 mg (20–30 µg/kg; maximum: 1 mg in children), administered IV (IO)[1] over 5 min followed by an infusion of 5–15 µg/min. Aspiration precautions should be observed.
- For patients with a history of asthma and for those who experience severe or prolonged anaphylaxis, consider methylprednisolone (Solu-Medrol) (1.0–2.0 mg/kg/d).

Observation and subsequent outpatient follow-up:
- Observation periods after apparent resolution must be individualized and based on such factors as the clinical scenario, comorbid conditions, and distance from the patient's home to the closest emergency department. After recovery from the acute episode, patients should receive epinephrine auto-injectors (EpiPen, AuviQ or Adrenaclick) and be instructed in proper technique. Everyone post-anaphylaxis requires a careful diagnostic evaluation in consultation with an allergist-immunologist.

[1]Not FDA approved for this indication.
Modified from Lieberman P, Nicklas RA, Oppenheimer J, Kemp SF, Lang DM (chief eds). Joint Task Force on Practice Parameters. The diagnosis and management of anaphylaxis parameter: 2010 update. J Allergy Clin Immunol 2010;126:477–80. e42.
Abbreviations: IV = intravenous, IO = intraosseous.

Fatalities during witnessed anaphylaxis usually result from delayed administration of epinephrine and from severe respiratory and/or cardiovascular complications. *There is no absolute contraindication to epinephrine administration in anaphylaxis.*

Oxygen should be administered to subjects with anaphylaxis who require multiple doses of epinephrine, receive inhaled $β_2$ agonists, have protracted anaphylaxis, or have preexisting hypoxemia or myocardial dysfunction.

Antihistamines (H_1 and H_2 antagonists) might support the treatment of anaphylaxis. However, these agents act much slower than epinephrine and should never be administered alone as treatment for anaphylaxis. They do, however, attenuate cutaneous symptoms (e.g., urticaria or pruritus). Authors of systematic reviews have concluded they were unable to make any evidence-based recommendations for use of H1 or H2 antihistamines in the treatment of anaphylaxis. Antihistamines thus should be considered as *second-line* treatment.

Systemic corticosteroids have no role in the acute management of anaphylaxis because even intravenous administration of these agents may have no effect for 4 to 6 hours after administration. Although corticosteroids traditionally are used in the management of anaphylaxis, their effect has never been evaluated in placebo-controlled trials. Corticosteroids administered during anaphylaxis might provide additional benefit for patients with asthma or other conditions recently treated with corticosteroids. However, no definite recommendations can be made because the data concerning possible preventive benefits are conflicting and limited.

Numerous cases of unusually severe or refractory anaphylaxis are reported in subjects receiving β-blocking agents. Greater severity of anaphylaxis observed in usual doses of epinephrine administered during anaphylaxis to subjects taking β-blockers may not produce the desired clinical response. In such situations, both isotonic volume expansion and glucagon[1] administration are recommended. Glucagon may potentially reverse refractory hypotension and bronchospasm because it bypasses the β-adrenergic receptor and directly activates adenyl cyclase.

Persistent hypotension despite epinephrine injections should first be treated with intravenous crystalloid solutions (e.g., lactated Ringer's or normal saline). One to 2 L of crystalloid might need to be administered to adults at a rate of 5 to 10 mL/kg in the first 5 minutes. Children should receive up to 30 mL/kg in the first hour. Large volumes (e.g., 7 L) are often required.

Vasopressors should be administered if epinephrine injections and volume expansion fail to alleviate hypotension. Dopamine (Intropin) frequently increases blood pressure while maintaining or enhancing renal and splanchnic perfusion. These agents would not be expected to work as well in patients already maximally vasoconstricted by their internal compensatory response to anaphylaxis.

Prevention of Anaphylaxis

Table 3 outlines the basic principles for the prevention of future anaphylactic episodes in high-risk individuals. An allergist-immunologist can provide comprehensive professional advice on these matters.

All subjects at high risk for recurrent anaphylaxis should carry epinephrine delivery devices and know how to administer them. An EpiPen (Mylan Specialty US) is a spring-loaded, pressure-activated syringe (auto-injector) with a single 0.3 mg dose (1:1000 dilution) of epinephrine. It is easy to use and injects through clothing. An EpiPen Jr, which delivers 0.15 mg (1:2000 dilution) epinephrine, is appropriate for children weighing less

---

[1]Not FDA approved for this indication.

TABLE 3 Preventive Measures for Subjects with Anaphylaxis

General measures:
- Obtain thorough history to diagnose life-threatening food or drug allergy.
- Identify cause of anaphylaxis and those individuals at risk for future attacks.
- Provide instruction on proper reading of food and medication labels, where appropriate.
- Patient should avoid exposure to antigens and cross-reactive substances.
- Manage asthma and coronary artery disease optimally.
- Employ a waiting period of 30 minutes after injections.
- Consider office waiting period of 2 hours for oral medication patient has not taken previously.

Specific measures for high-risk subjects:
- Individuals at high risk for anaphylaxis should carry self-injectable epinephrine (EpiPen, Adrenaclick, or Auvi-Q) at all times and receive instruction in proper use with placebo trainer.
- Individuals should wear a Medic Alert bracelet or chain.
- Other agents for β-adrenergic antagonists, angiotensin-converting enzyme (ACE) inhibitors, tricyclic antidepressants, and monoamine oxidase inhibitors should be substituted whenever possible.
- Agents suspected of causing anaphylaxis should be administered slowly, under supervision, and orally if possible.
- Where appropriate, use specific preventive strategies, including pharmacologic prophylaxis, short-term challenge and desensitization and long-term desensitization.

Modified from Kemp SF. Office approach to anaphylaxis: sooner better than later. Am J Med 2007;120:664–8.

---

than 30 kg. Adrenaclick (Amedra) is available as a single-dose auto-injector of either 0.15 mg or 0.3 mg. Auvi-Q (Sanofi US) is an autoinjector device that is available in either 0.15 mg or 0.3 mg single-dose. Approximately the size of a credit card, it is equipped with blinking lights at the needle end and a voice recording that guides the user throughout administration.

Serum Sickness

Serum sickness is a clinical syndrome of fever, malaise, and urticarial and/or morbilliform cutaneous eruption that is often preceded by generalized erythema and pruritus. Arthralgias or arthritis (mainly large joints), neuropathy, lymphadenopathy, nephritis, abdominal pain (emesis or melena are possible), or vasculitis (cutaneous or systemic) may occur in some cases. Cutaneous vasculitis, also known as hypersensitivity vasculitis, is often manifested by palpable purpura, which most commonly are found on the lower extremities of ambulatory individuals or on the sacral or gluteal region of patients with restricted mobility. These purpura reflect vascular leakage from inflamed postcapillary venules. Systemic vasculitis may occur in association with autoimmune diseases, infection, or malignancy.

Many agents may produce serum sickness or serum sickness–like reactions (Table 4). *Serum sickness* classically refers to the immune complex syndrome caused by immunization with heterologous serum proteins (often equine or murine). The most frequent cause is immune complex–mediated drug hypersensitivity. A serum sickness–like drug reaction generally develops 6 to 21 days after the culprit medication is started, but it can occur within 12 to 48 hours in previously sensitized individuals.

Pathogenesis and Laboratory Abnormalities

Healthy individuals regularly generate low levels of circulating immune complexes, which are either excreted by the kidneys or extracted in the liver and spleen by monocytes and macrophages. It is hypothesized that serum sickness results when a drug (hapten) binds to plasma protein and antibodies are generated in response to the drug-protein complex. Complement activation occurs when large quantities of soluble antigen-antibody (immune) complexes fix to vascular endothelial receptors. Complement fragments attract and activate neutrophils, which release proteases that induce tissue injury. The urticaria in serum sickness probably results from immune complex necrotizing vasculitis and complement activation that induces mast cell degranulation. IgE-dependent mechanisms likely are also contributory in some individuals. Laboratory abnormalities include elevated erythrocyte sedimentation rate, leukopenia (acute phase), occasional plasmacytosis, and decreased total hemolytic complement (CH50), C3, and C4. Slight albuminuria, hyaline casts, and microscopic hematuria may also occur.

Treatment

Stoppage of the culprit agent, when identified, is recommended. Serum sickness is usually self-limited and rarely life threatening when the offending drug or protein is stopped or removed.

TABLE 4 Representative Agents That Cause Serum Sickness

Medications: β-lactam antibiotics, sulfonamides, ciprofloxacin (Cipro), metronidazole (Flagyl), rifampin (Rifadin), allopurinol (Zyloprim), carbamazepine (Tegretol), phenytoin (Dilantin), fluoxetine (Prozac), bupropion (Wellbutrin), methimazole (Tapazole), propylthiouracil, thiazide diuretics, captopril (Capoten), propranolol (Inderal), verapamil (Calan), streptokinase (Streptase), others.
Heterologous (animal-derived) antisera:
- Horse: snake and spider venom, tetanus, botulism, diphtheria
- Horse or rabbit: anti-lymphocyte globulin
- Mouse: monoclonal antibodies (muromonab-CD3 [Orthoclone OKT3])
- Mouse/human monoclonal antibody chimerisms: rituximab (Rituxan), infliximab (Remicade)
Homologous (human-derived) antisera: cytomegalovirus, hepatitis B, rabies, tetanus, perinatal $RH_0(D)$

Symptoms generally improve over 2 to 4 weeks as patients clear their immune complexes, although rarely symptoms can last as long as two to three months. Evidence-based treatment recommendations for serum sickness are very limited. Long-acting, less-sedating H_1 antihistamines such as cetirizine (Zyrtec), desloratadine (Clarinex), fexofenadine (Allegra), or loratadine (Claritin) generally control urticaria. Systemic corticosteroids (e.g., prednisone, 0.5 to 1.0 mg/kg/day) may help severe symptoms (e.g., temperature > 38.5° C, severe arthralgias, or extensive dermatitis). Fever and arthralgias typically resolve within 48 to 72 hours of treatment, and the formation of new cutaneous eruptions usually ceases within the same time frame. Antihistamine therapy is continued for 1 week after apparent resolution of symptoms and then slowly discontinued. Corticosteroids often can be stopped in less than one week.

Diagnostic testing is presently unable to predict future episodes of serum sickness. If no therapeutic alternative is available and repeat treatment with a culprit drug is considered essential, concurrent treatment with antihistamines and possibly corticosteroids might help to prevent a future episode of serum sickness due to the drug.

References

Brown SGA, Kemp SF, Lieberman PL. Anaphylaxis. In: Adkinson Jr NF, Bochner BS, Burks AW, et al., editors. Middleton's allergy: principles and practice. 8th ed. Philadelphia: Mosby Elsevier; 2014. p. 1237–59.

Kemp AM, Kemp SF. Pharmacotherapy in refractory anaphylaxis: when intramuscular epinephrine fails. Curr Opin Allergy Clin Immunol 2014;14:371–8.

Kemp SF, Lockey RF, Simons FE. World Allergy Organization Ad Hoc Committee on Epinephrine in Anaphylaxis. Epinephrine: The Drug of Choice for Anaphylaxis. A statement of the World Allergy Organization. Allergy 2008;63:1061–70.

Lieberman P, Nicklas RA, Oppenheimer J, Kemp SF, Lang DM. Joint Task Force on Practice Parameters. The diagnosis and management of anaphylaxis parameter: 2010 update. J Allergy Clin Immunol 2010;126:477–80. e42.

Pumphrey RSH. Fatal posture in anaphylactic shock. J Allergy Clin Immunol 2003;112:451–2.

Pumphrey RSH. Fatal anaphylaxis in the UK, 1992–2001. Novartis Found Symp 2004;257:116–28.

Sampson HA, Muñoz-Furlong A, Campbell RL, et al. Second symposium on the definition and management of anaphylaxis: Summary report—second National Institute of Allergy and Infectious Disease/Food Allergy and Anaphylaxis Network symposium. J Allergy Clin Immunol 2006;117:391–7.

Simons FER, Ardusso LRF, Bilò MB, et al. World Allergy Organization guidelines for the assessment and management of anaphylaxis. J Allergy Clin Immunol 2011;127:587–93e.1–e.22.

Soar J, Perkins JD, Abbas G, et al. European Resuscitation Council Guidelines for Resuscitation 2010 Section 8. Cardiac arrest in special circumstances: Electrolyte abnormalities, poisoning, drowning, accidental hypothermia, hyperthermia, asthma, anaphylaxis, cardiac surgery, trauma, pregnancy, electrocution. Resuscitation 2010;81:1400–33.

Vadas P, Gold M, Perelman B, Liss GM, et al. Platelet-activating factor, PAF acetylhydrolase, and severe anaphylaxis. N Engl J Med 2008;358:28–35.

Vadas P, Perelman B, Liss G. Platelet-activating factor, histamine, and tryptase levels in human anaphylaxis. J Allergy Clin Immunol 2013;131:144–9.

Wener MH. Serum sickness and serum sickness-like reactions. In: UpToDate, Post TW, editor. UpToDate. Waltham, MA. [accessed February 27, 2015].

DRUG HYPERSENSITIVITY REACTIONS

Method of
Miriam Chan, BSc Pharm, PharmD; and Kristen Rundell, MD

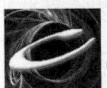

CURRENT DIAGNOSIS

- Detailed history should include past medical history; current diagnosis; previous and current medication use, including over-the-counter drugs and herbals; duration of the medication use; any similar reactions in the past.
- Physical examination should include vitals, temperature, and skin examination for rash.
- Laboratory testing should be conducted based on symptoms that may include complete blood count (CBC) with differential, including eosinophils, sedimentation rate, liver enzymes, international normalized ratio (INR), diagnostic skin biopsy, or testing.

CURRENT THERAPY

- For life-threatening anaphylaxis reaction, start ACB and give epinephrine immediately.
- Discontinue the offending drug if medically possible. Try drug substitution if warranted.
- An alternative option is to reduce the dose or frequency of the drug.
- Start symptomatic treatment based on the type of reaction and the offending medication.
- Some reactions may respond to treatment with antihistamines, H2 blockers, or steroids.

Epidemiology

Drug hypersensitivity reactions are one of the many different types of adverse drug reactions (ADRs). ADRs are common, yet the more severe reactions have been estimated to cause 3% to 6% of hospital admissions. More than 100,000 deaths annually are caused by serious ADRs, making these reactions one of the leading cause of death in the United States. Early detection of all ADRs can potentially improve patient outcomes and lower health care costs.

Classifications

An ADR is a broad term that refers to any predictable or unpredictable reaction to a medication. A predictable (type A) reaction is dose dependent and is related to the known pharmacologic properties of the drug. Predictable reactions account for about 80% of all ADRs. An example of a type A reaction is gastritis that results from taking nonsteroidal antiinflammatory drugs (NSAIDs). The remaining 20% of ADRs are caused by unpredictable (type B) reactions. Type B reactions occur in susceptible individuals. These are hypersensitivity reactions that are different from the pharmacologic actions of the drug; they are results of interactions between the drug and the individual human immune system. Type B reactions can be further divided into drug intolerance, drug idiosyncrasy, drug allergy (immunologically medicated), and pseudoallergic reactions (anaphylactoid reactions). This chapter will focus on these type B drug hypersensitivity reactions.

Pathophysiology

Several mechanisms may play a role in the underlying etiology of immunologic drug reactions. The Gell and Coombs classification system was the original system to describe four predominant immune mechanisms. These four reaction types are listed as: Type I reactions (IgE-medicated), Type II reactions (cytotoxic), Type III reactions (immune complex), and Type IV reactions (delayed, cell mediated). Table 1 provides a detailed description of this classification. Type I and IV reactions are more common than type II and III reactions. Most drugs cause one type of reaction, while certain drugs, such as penicillin, can induce all four types of reactions.

The Gell and Coombs classification has recently been revised to reflect the functional heterogeneity of T cells. Under the new system, type IV reactions is further subclassified into four categories: IVa (macrophage activation), IVb (eosinophils), IVc (CD4$^+$ or CD8$^+$ T cells), and IVd (neutrophils). Nevertheless, many common hypersensitivity reactions cannot be classified in this system because of the lack of knowledge of their immune mechanism or a mixed mechanism.

A new concept of drug interaction with immune receptors has recently been developed by Pichler and colleagues. It is called the p-i concept (pharmacologic interaction with immune receptors). In this concept, a drug binds noncovalently to a T-cell receptor and stimulates an immune response, which can cause inflammatory reactions of different types. The simulation of the T cell is enhanced by the additional interaction with the major histocompatibility complex molecule. This is direct stimulation of memory and

TABLE 1 Classification of Drug Hypersensitivity Reactions

TYPE	MECHANISM	CLINICAL FEATURES	TIMING OF REACTIONS	EXAMPLES
Type 1 (IgE mediated)	Drug-IgE complex bind to mast cells	Urticaria, angioedema, bronchospasm, pruritus, GI symptoms, anaphylaxis	Immediate (minutes to hours after drug exposure, depending on the route of administration)	β-lactam antibiotic
Type II (cytotoxic)	Specific IgG or IgM antibodies directed at drug-hapten-coated cells	Hemolytic anemia, neutropenia, thrombocytopenia	Variable	Penicillin (hemolytic anemia), heparin (thrombocytopenia)
Type III (immune complex)	Antigen-antibody complexes	Serum sickness, vasculitis, drug fever	1–3 wks after drug exposure	Penicillin (serum sickness), sulfonamides (vasculitis), azathioprine (drug fever)
Type IV (delayed, cell mediated)	Activation and expansion of drug-specific T cell	Prominent skin findings: Contact dermatitis, morbilliform eruptions	2–7 days after exposure	Topical antihistamine, penicillin, sulfonamides

effector T cells and no sensitization is required. The skin has a high concentration of effector memory T cells, which can be rapidly stimulated by antigen penetration. The skin also possesses a dense network of dendritic cells that act as antigen-presenting cells and increase hypersensitivity reactions. As a result, clinical symptoms by p-i drugs may appear more rapidly. Some severe reactions—such as Stevens-Johnson syndrome (SJS), toxic epidermal necrolysis (TEN), the drug rash with eosinophilia and systemic symptoms (DRESS) syndrome, or hypersensitivity syndrome—are thought to be p-i related. Examples are abacavir (Ziagen) hypersensitivity syndrome and SJS/TEN from carbamazepine (Tegretol).

Risk Factors for Hypersensitivity Drug Reactions

The chemical structure and molecular weight of the drug may help predict the type of hypersensitivity reaction. Larger drugs with greater structural complexity are more likely to be immunogenic. However, drugs with small molecular weight (<1000 Da) can elicit hypersensitivity reactions by coupling with carrier proteins to form hapten-carrier complexes. Other drug-related factors include the dose, route of administration, duration of treatment, repetitive exposure to the drug, and concurrent illness. Topical and intravenous drug administrations are more likely to cause hypersensitivity reactions than are oral medications.

Patient risk factors include age, female gender, infection with human immunodeficiency virus, atopy, specific genetic polymorphisms, previous drug hypersensitivity reactions, and inherent predisposition to react to multiple unrelated drugs.

Clinical Manifestations

Drug hypersensitivity reactions can manifest in a great variety of clinical symptoms and diseases. While some reactions are mild and often unnoticed, others, such as anaphylaxis, can be severe and even fatal. Dermatologic symptoms are the most common physical manifestation of allergic drug reactions. Drug hypersensitivity reactions can also affect various internal organs, causing diseases such as hepatitis, nephritis, and pneumonitis. The noncutaneous physical findings are generally nonspecific and may not be helpful and even delay the diagnosis and management decisions.

Dermatologic Symptoms

The most common allergic drug reactions affect the skin and can cause a variety of different exanthems. The most common skin reaction is the classic "drug rash," which is a morbilliform eruption originating on the trunk. Other dermatologic symptoms include urticaria, angioedema, acne, bullous eruptions, fixed drug eruptions, erythema multiforme, lupus erythematosus, photosensitivity, psoriasis, purpura, vasculitis, and pruritus. The most severe form of cutaneous drug reactions are SJS, TEN, and DRESS syndrome.

Stevens-Johnson Syndrome

SJS is a systemic disorder that has cutaneous manifestation. SJS was previously thought to be synonymous with erythema multiforme major. There are now criteria that separate the two disorders. In contrast to erythema multiform, the target lesions associated with SJS have only two rings. The inner ring may have urticaria, pustules, or necrotic lesions surrounded by macular erythema. It is a T-cell-mediated toxic reaction to the basement membrane of the epidermal cells. There is massive and widespread apoptosis, for which there are several associated cytokines. The recent theories suggest that there are two pathways, one that consists of granule medicated exocytosis (perforin and granzyme B), and one that the Fas-Fas ligand interaction associated apoptosis for the kerotinocytes. More recent data suggest that granulysin, which is a cationic cytolytic protein released by T lymphocytes, may play a role as well.

Interestingly, HLA genotype may predispose patients to SJS or TEN. Those patients with the HLA-B1502 found among the Han Chinese population may be associated with increased risk of developing SJS/TEN and use of carbamazepine.

SJS and TEN are on the same continuum. The definition of epidermal detachment and desquamation of epidermal cells is less than 10% of the body surface area for SJS and more than 30% for TEN. There is an overlapping diagnosis of SJS/TEN for the 10% to 30% category. To help differentiate from other ADRs, there is often a prodromal period in which a patient may have a cough and a fever. The lesions may occur up to 4 weeks after exposure of the drug. In addition, the lesions may be limited to the trunk; however, they more commonly involve the palmar surface of the hands and the dorsum of the feet as well as the mucous membranes.

The most common drugs associated with SJS and TENs are sulfonamides, cephalosporins, imidazole agents, and oxicam derivatives. Drugs such as carbamazepine, phenytoin (Dilantin), valproic acid (Depakote), lamotrigine (Lamictal), allopurinol (Zyloprim), nevirapine (Viramune), peramivir (Rapivab), and quinolones have been reported to cause SJS/TEN. Recently, the FDA issued a safety alert stating that acetaminophen has been associated with SJS, TEN, and AGEP. The evidence supporting causality primarily comes from a small number of cases reported in the medical literature.

The treatment is immediate cessation of the culprit drug and symptomatic treatment. Glucocorticoids are controversial and depend on the course and extent of the disease.

Toxic Epidermal Necrolysis

As previously stated, TEN is the cell-mediated disorder that involves more than 30% of the body surface. This is the more severe form of the ADR: the mortality rates may be as high as 50%, mostly from sepsis. Patients are usually admitted to the burn unit for electrolyte and infection management. Glucocorticoids are contraindicated. There have been mixed results using IV immunoglobulin (IVIG)[1] in these patients. The IVIG is believed to inhibit the Fas-Fas ligand, which is the underlying mechanism for the basement membrane separation.

Drug Rash with Eosinophilia and Systemic Symptoms

DRESS or DIHS (drug-induced hypersensitivity syndrome) is a rare, life-threatening drug-induced reaction with a mortality rate of 10%. Therefore, it is important to recognize the signs and symptoms early to initiate treatment. Most patients will have fever, lymphadenopathy (75%), eosinophilia, and an erythematous morbilliform rash on the face and body in addition to liver and multiorgan damage. The symptoms can occur 2 to 6 weeks after the drug administration. There are many drugs that can cause DRESS syndrome but carbamazepine is the most frequently reported. The treatment is drug withdrawal, systemic corticosteroids, topical treatment for lesions, and supportive care often in the ICU or burn unit.

Acute Generalized Exanthematous Pustulosis

Acute generalized exanthematous pustulosis (AGEP) is a rare ADR that presents as a fever and small nonfollicular pustules on a widespread erythematous background. AGEP may closely mimic pustular psoriasis clinically. The presence of acanthuses and papillomatosis and a personal or family history of psoriasis favor a diagnosis of pustular psoriasis. Exposure to medication, especially antibiotics with a short latency from the initiation of the drug, favor AGEP. The eruption usually occurs within 24 hours of the initiation of the drug, and healing occurs quickly after the discontinuation of the drug. Lesions heal within 2 weeks of discontinuation without scarring. The exact mechanism of drug-specific T lymphocytes is unknown, yet IL-3 and IL-8 may be the trigger for neutrophil-activating cytokines in the skin.

Evaluation

As the history is essential for determining if a patient is experiencing a drug hypersensitivity reaction, it is important to review all medications and the timeline of exposure. This includes any over-the-counter medications, herbal supplements, or occasional-use medications. Occasional-use medications may include NSAIDs, acetaminophen, cold medications, etc. It is important to establish a temporal relationship to the onset of the medication and the initiation of the symptoms. Oftentimes, the medication may have been discontinued before the appearance of the first symptom, so a review of medications from several weeks before the symptoms is also important. In addition, as the host immune response plays a role in some of the IgE-mediated reactions, it is important to review any immunocompromising chronic or acute illnesses or states that the patient may have or currently experiencing. This includes HIV, COPD, asthma, chemotherapy, and pregnancy. For some ADRs, HLA type may be important. A patient's known genetic predisposition needs to be taken into account as well. A thorough history will also need to include any organ system or symptom that may be related to the suspected ADR.

A physical examination should augment and help to establish the working diagnosis of the type of ADR and the potentially offending drug. This should include vital signs of temperature, respiratory, and hydration status. The skin examination is important as well as appropriate evaluation and documentation of the type of lesion or lesions present. An examination of the oral mucosa and the conjunctiva of the eye are included in the examination. Any lymphadenopathy, petechiae, or pallor should be noted.

Laboratory testing may be obtained to confirm or rule out a diagnosis. This may include a chest x-ray, CBC with differential, possible skin biopsy, liver function testing, creatinine, and electrolyte testing. A sedimentation rate and CRP testing may also be useful. While additional autoimmune or antibody testing may be done, caution is suggested. There may not be a high yield on these tests and they can be quite costly for patients.

Management

Anaphylaxis

Anaphylaxis can be a fatal drug hypersensitivity reaction because of its rapid onset. It is often underrecognized and undertreated because it can mimic other conditions and is variable in its presentation. However, respiratory compromise and cardiovascular collapse are of greatest concern, because they are the most common cause of death. Urticaria and angioedema are the most common manifestations, but may be delayed or absent. The more quickly anaphylaxis occurs after exposure to the offending agent, the more likely the reaction is to be severe and potentially life threatening.

Most anaphylaxis episodes are IgE-mediated reactions resulting in a sudden mast cell and basophil degranulation. This sudden release of mediators affects the cutaneous, pulmonary, cardiac, GI, vascular, and neurologic systems. Medications are a common trigger of anaphylaxis in adults. Most cases of IgE-mediated drug anaphylaxis in the United States are due to penicillins and cephalosporins. Antibiotics are also the most common cause of perioperative anaphylaxis because skin eruptions may be missed in patients who are draped during surgery. Some anaphylaxis reactions involve other immunologic mechanisms. Administration of blood products (e.g., IVIG, animal antiserum) can cause an anaphylactoid reaction due, at least in part, to complement activation. Activation of the complement cascade can cause mast cell/basophil degranulation. Anaphylaxis episodes can also occur independently of any immunologic mechanism. Certain drugs, such as opioid, dextrans, and protamine, can cause a direct release of histamine and other mediators from mast cells and basophils. Finally, there are acute systemic reactions without any obvious trigger or mechanism (idiopathic anaphylaxis).

Anaphylaxis is a clinical diagnosis with a short window of treatment time available. Therefore, laboratory testing is limited and may not be of much value. Initially, the patient will describe flushing, pruritus, and a sense of impending doom. Some patients will have dyspnea, dizziness, syncope, and/or GI symptoms of diarrhea and abdominal cramping. Most of the patients will have cutaneous symptoms of flushing, urticaria, or angioedema. Some patients will progress to respiratory or cardiovascular complications.

The goal of therapy should be early recognition and treatment with epinephrine to prevent a progression to life-threatening respiratory and/or cardiovascular failure. The immediate intervention should include stopping the offending drug if possible, epinephrine injection, basic life support, high-flow oxygen, cardiac monitoring, and IV access. Epinephrine is the drug of choice for anaphylaxis. The therapeutic actions of epinephrine include: alpha-1 adrenergic vasoconstrictor effects (decreases mucosal edema, thereby relieving upper airway obstruction, and increases blood pressure to prevent shock), beta-1 adrenergic effects (increases rate and force of cardiac contractions), and beta-2 effects (increases bronchodilation and decreases the release of mediators of inflammation from mast cell/basophils). Delayed epinephrine administration has been associated with fatalities. Intramuscular epinephrine in the thigh results in high-plasma concentrations and is preferred in the setting of anaphylaxis. The recommended dose of epinephrine is 0.3 mg (1 mg/mL) IM every 5 minutes. Typically, only one or two additional doses are needed. Patients in shock should receive epinephrine by slow IV infusion at 2 to 10 mcg/min with the rate titrated according to response and the presence of continuous hemodynamic monitoring. Patients taking beta blockers may be resistant to treatment with epinephrine. In this case, glucagon[1] 1 to 5 mg IV over 5 minutes should be administered because its cardiac effects are not mediated through beta receptors.

---

[1]Not FDA approved for this indication.

[1]Not FDA approved for this indication.

Adjunctive therapies for the treatment of anaphylaxis include antihistamines and corticosteroids. Consider an inhaled beta-agonist if wheezing. Diphenhydramine (Benadryl), a H1 antihistamine, may be given intravenously at the dose of 25 to 50 mg. If an H2 blocker is considered, give ranitidine (Zantac)[1] 50 mg/20 mL as an IV infusion over 5 minutes. Use of both diphenhydramine and ranitidine is superior to diphenhydramine alone. Corticosteroids are used to prevent a potential late-phase reaction that may occur in up to 23% of adults with anaphylaxis. There is no proven best dose or route of steroid therapy. The most common dosage is prednisone 20 to 60 mg daily for 3 to 5 days.

Angioedema

Angioedema is characterized by a deep dermal, subcutaneous, and/or mucosal swelling. Many patients present with both urticaria and angioedema. Angioedema can progress rapidly from a mild swelling of the oral mucosal to a life-threatening laryngeal edema. With this rapid sequence of events, the most important part of treatment is obtaining and maintaining a patent airway. Epinephrine 0.3 mg IM every 10 minutes should be administered to patients who present with anaphylaxis, respiratory distress, or severe laryngeal edema. Once the airway is patent, the patient should be treated with H1 antihistamines, H2 blockers, and steroids. The milder cases may be treated similarly to other allergic reactions. H1 antihistamines such as diphenhydramine and hydroxyzine (Atarax) are effective in relieving pruritus but can cause significant sedation. Therefore, second-generation H1 antihistamines (loratadine [Claritin][1], cetirizine [Zyrtec][1], desloratadine [Clarinex][1], fexofenadine [Allegra][1]) are often chosen for outpatient therapy. Doxepin (Sinequan)[1], a tricyclic antidepressant with potent H1 and H2 blocker activities, can be used as an alternative to H1 antihistamine. However, it should not be used as first line treatment for acute urticaria and angioedema due to its significant side effects of severe sedation, dry mouth, and weight gain. Corticosteroids are used in patients who are not responsive to antihistamines. For most patients, a short course of oral prednisone is adequate.

In drug-induced angioedema, the offending drug should be stopped and avoided. Further trial of the medication is not recommended, as the patient will respond more quickly and with more severe symptoms upon reintroduction. The patient should be counseled, and epinephrine 0.3 mg in an auto-injectable device (EpiPen) may be prescribed in case of recurrence in the future.

Specific Drugs

Almost all drugs can cause a drug hypersensitivity reaction. However, certain drugs are more frequently associated with specific types of reactions. Some of the more commonly used drugs are discussed here in more detail.

Antibiotics

Penicillin

Penicillin allergy is the most well-known drug allergy and also the most costly ADR. Although most drugs usually have type I and type IV reactions, penicillin may cause all four types of allergic drug reactions. The rate of penicillin-induced anaphylaxis after intravenous administration is approximately 1 to 2 per 10,000 treated patients.

Only about 10% of patients who report a penicillin drug allergy actually have a true immunologic response. The other 90% are actually able to tolerate penicillin or a cephalosporin. Because of this overreporting, there are several patient safety concerns. These include the antibiotic coverage of an organism not being optimal and an increase in drug resistance, which results in higher health care costs. Therefore, it is important to evaluate a patient for true penicillin allergy.

---

[1]Not FDA approved for this indication.

Penicillin skin testing is the best method for diagnosing an IgE-mediated penicillin allergy. A commercially available product, Pre-Pen, contains benzylpenicilloyl polylysine (PPL), which is a major antigenic determinant of penicillin. Minor determinants are metabolic derivatives of penicillin that may also produce an immune response. The current recommendations for penicillin skin testing are to administer both the major determinant (PPL) and the minor determinants (penicillin G). These two tests identify approximately 90% to 97% of the currently allergic patients. Patients with a history of penicillin allergy but negative skin testing to PPL and the minor determinants rarely experience allergic reactions on reexposure. If they should occur, the reactions are mild and self-limiting.

In general, patients who report symptoms consistent with an immediate or type I reaction or are skin-test positive to penicillin should not receive penicillin. Desensitization should be considered if penicillin is the treatment of choice for an infection and no acceptable nonpenicillin alternatives are available. Patients should be desensitized in a hospital setting. Desensitization involves administering incremental doses of oral penicillin every 15 minutes for a total of 4 to 12 hours, after which time the first dose of penicillin is given. An example of a penicillin desensitization protocol is available in the Morbidity and Mortality Weekly Report at http://www.cdc.gov/std/treatment/2010/STD-Treatment-2010-RR5912.pdf.

Penicillin and Cephalosporin Cross-Reactivity

The rate of cross-reactivity between penicillin and cephalosporins has been historically cited to be as high as 10%. Recent data suggest that the rate may be much lower. The degree of cross-reactivity is highest between penicillins and first-generation cephalosporins, which have identical R-group side chains. In this case amoxicillin would be cross-reactive with cefadroxil (Duricef) and cefprozil (Cefzil), while ampicillin would be with cefaclor and cephalexin. Because of the differences in the chemical structures, second- and third-generation cephalosporins (cefdinir [Omnicef], cefuroxime [Ceftin], cefpodoxime [Vantin], and ceftriaxone [Rocephin]) are unlikely to be associated with cross-reactivity with penicillin. According to the new guidelines for acute otitis media from the American Academy of Pediatrics and American Academy of Family Physicians, alternative initial antibiotics in patients with penicillin allergy include cefdinir, cefuroxime, cefpodoxime, or ceftriazone.

Patients with penicillin allergy who have a negative skin-test result to penicillin (major and minor determinants) may safely receive cephalosporins. Cephalosporin treatment of patients with penicillin allergy who did not have a severe or recent penicillin reaction history shows a reaction rate of 0.1%. Use cephalosporin with caution in patients who report an immediate or accelerated penicillin allergy or those with a positive skin test to penicillin.

Sulfonamides (Sulfa Drugs)

Beside penicillins, sulfonamide antibiotics are the second-most common cause of drug-induced allergic reactions. They commonly cause a delayed maculopapular/morbilliform eruption. Acute urticarial reactions (IgE mediated) to sulfamethoxazole (SMX) or trimethoprim (TMP) are relatively infrequent; the incidence of skin rash resulting from SMX-TMP (Bactrim) in healthy subjects is estimated to be 3%. Sulfonamides are also the most common cause of SJS and TEN.

Patients with HIV have the greatest risk of sulfonamide-induced allergic reactions. The typical reaction to SMX-TMP in HIV patients is a generalized maculopapular eruption that occurs during the second week of treatment and is usually accompanied by pruritus and fever. Because SMX-TMP is the drug of choice for a number of HIV-associated infections such as *Pneumocystis carinii* pneumonia and spontaneous bacterial peritonitis, several methods of desensitization have been devised to administer SMX-TMP to HIV patients with a history of allergic reaction to the drug.

| TABLE 2 | Classification of Sulfonamides Based on Chemical Structure |

DRUG

Sulfonylarylamines

Antibiotics:	*Antiinflammatory:*
Sulfadiazine	Sulfasalazine (Azulfidine)
Sulfamethoxazole	*Protease Inhibitors:*
Sulfisoxazole	Darunavir (Prezista)
Sulfapyridine	Fosamprenavir (Lexiva)

Nonsulfonylarylamines

Carbonic Anhydrase Inhibitors:	*Sulfonylureas:*
Acetazolamide (Diamox)	Chlorpropamide
Brinzolamide (Azopt)	Glimepiride (Amaryl)
Dorzolamide (Trusopt)	Glipizide (Glucotrol)
Methazolamide (Neptazane)	Glyburide (Diabeta)
Cyclooxygenase 2 (COX-2)	Tolbutamide
Inhibitors:	Tolazamide (Tolinase)
Celecoxib (Celebrex)	*Other Agents:*
Loop Diuretics:	Mafenide (Sulfamylon)
Bumetanide (Bumex)	Probenecid
Furosemide (Lasix)	Tamsulosin (Flomax)
Torsemide (Demadex)	Tipranavir (Aptivus)
Thiazides Diuretics:	
Chlorothiazide (Diuril)	
Chlorthalidone	
Hydrochlorothiazide	
Indapamide (Lozol)	
Metolazone (Zaroxolyn)	

Sulfonamide Moiety-Containing Drugs

5-HT Agonists:	*Other Agents:*
Naratriptan (Amerge)	Ibutilide (Corvert)
Sumatriptan (Imitrex)	Simeprevir (Olysio)
	Sotalol (Betapace)
	Topiramate (Topamax)
	Zonisamide (Zonegran)

There are three classes of sulfonamides based on chemical structure: sulfonylarylamines (includes sulfa antibiotics), nonsulfonylarylamines, and sulfonamide-moiety-containing drugs. A sulfonylarylamine has a sulfonamide moiety directly attached to a benzene ring with an amine ($-NH_2$) moiety at the N4 position. A nonsulfonylarylamine also has a sulfonamide moiety attached to a benzene ring, but it does not have an amine group at the N4 position. A sulfonamide-moiety-containing drug has a sulfonamide group that is not connected to a benzene ring. Table 2 presents a list of sulfonamide-containing drugs based on their chemical structure.

The N4 amine is critical for the development of delayed reactions to sulfa antibiotics. Given the important chemical differences between drugs containing sulfa antibiotics and sulfa in nonantibiotics, the risk of cross-reactivity is extremely unlikely. A retrospective cohort study by Strom and colleagues showed that approximately 90% of patients with sulfa antibiotic allergy did not have a reaction to a sulfonamide nonantibiotic. Patients with allergic reactions to sulfa antibiotics are also more likely to experience allergic reactions to the other types of sulfonamides, but this is not because of cross-sensitivity. There is no reliable skin test to rule out or confirm sulfa allergy. Some experts recommend avoiding all classes of sulfonamides in patients with serious reactions such as SJS, TEN, and/or anaphylaxis to any one sulfonamide.

Most diuretics are sulfonamide derivatives. The only diuretics that are not in this group are the potassium-sparing diuretics (triamterene [Dyrenium], spironolactone [Aldactone], amiloride [Midamor]), and ethacrynic acid (Edecrin). Dapsone is a sulfone that is chemically unrelated to sulfonamides. *It should also be noted that sulfates, sulfur, and sulfites are chemically unrelated to sulfonamides and do not cross-react.*

Angiotensin-Converting Enzyme Inhibitors

Angiotensin-converting enzyme inhibitors (ACEIs) have two major adverse effects: cough and angioedema. The cough is typically dry and nonproductive. The incidence of ACEI-induced cough has been reported to be 5% to 35%. Cough occurs more commonly in women, African-Americans, and Asians. The onset of cough ranges from within hours of the first dose to months after the initiation of therapy. The diagnosis is confirmed by the resolution of cough, usually within 1 to 4 weeks after discontinuation of the ACEI; however, the cough can linger for up to 3 months. The cause for ACEI-induced cough is unclear but might be related to bradykinin, substance P, or another mechanism. Angiotensin II receptor blockers (ARBs) are not associated with an increased incidence of cough and can be used as an alternative to ACEIs. As the cough may persist for several months after stopping the ACEI, starting the ARB is not a contraindication at this time, yet the cough may persist through the initiation of the new drug.

The incidence of angioedema with ACEIs is approximately 0.1% to 0.7%. With the widespread use of ACEIs, angioedema has become a growing problem. ACEI-induced angioedema is more common in patients who are over age 65, black, or female. Angioedema frequently involves the swelling of the face or upper airway and can be life threatening or fatal. It can occur within days, months, or even years after the start of treatment. However, nearly 60% of cases occur within the first week of therapy. ACEIs cause angioedema by direct interference with the degradation of bradykinin, thereby increasing bradykinin levels and leading to increased vascular permeability, inflammation, and activation of nociceptors. Bradykinin is also a prominent mediator in hereditary angioedema. Therefore, ACEIs are contraindicated in patients with hereditary angioedema.

ARBs directly inhibit the angiotensin receptor and do not interfere with bradykinin degradation. Theoretically, they can be relatively safe alternatives for patients with a previous history of ACEI-associated angioedema. However, some reports of ARB-induced angioedema have recently been published. The mechanism of how ARBs cause angioedema is unclear. A meta-analysis suggests that for patients who developed angioedema when taking an ACEI, the risk of persistent angioedema when subsequently switched to an ARB is less than 10%. Therefore, ARBs may be an alternative only for patients with a high therapeutic need for angiotensin inhibition. ARB treatment should be started with observation. Patients should be educated on the signs of angioedema and provided with proper emergency instructions on how to proceed if angioedema should occur.

The direct renin inhibitor aliskiren (Tekturna) does not alter local or circulating bradykinin and is thought to be an alternative in patients with ACEI and ARB-related angioedema. However, cases of angioedema have been reported with aliskiren. As with ARBs, rennin inhibitors should be used with caution in patients who previously experienced angioedema to ACEIs.

Aspirin and NSAIDs

Aspirin (ASA) and NSAIDs can cause several types of hypersensitivity reactions. The four most common types of reactions are based on the drug pathways. Aspirin-exacerbated respiratory disease (AERD) is a serious reaction induced by ASA and NSAIDs in patients with asthma and chronic rhinosinusitis. AERD does not fit precisely into a specific type of ADRs and is often referred to as a type of psuedoallergic reaction. AERD affects up to 20% of adults with asthma. It is more common in women. The usual age of onset is around 30 years. The pathophysiology of AERD is related to aberrant arachidonic acid metabolism. Patients with AERD also have increased respiratory tract expression of cysteinyl leuckotriene 1 receptor and heightened responsiveness to inhaled leukotriene E4. Administration of aspirin or an NSAID to these patients leads to inhibition of cyclooxygenase 1 (COX-1), resulting in a decrease in prostaglandin E2 levels. Prostaglandin E2 normally inhibits 5-lipooxygenase. As a result of decreased prostaglandin E2 levels, arachidonic acid is preferentially metabolized in the 5-lipooxygenase pathway, leading to increased production of cysteinyl leukotrienes.

Patients with AERD typically have both rhinoconjunctivitis and bronchospasm within minutes of ingestion of a dose of ASA or NSAID. The bronchospasm can be severe and result in respiratory failure, which may need intubation and mechanical ventilation. Management of patients with AERD involves treatment of the patient's asthma and chronic rhinosinusitis and avoidance of aspirin and NSAIDs. Desensitization is available in cases when the patient has a specific therapeutic need for regular ASA or NSAID therapy. Selective COX-2 inhibitors very rarely cause reactions in patients with AERD and can be taken safely.

The second type of ASA and NSAID-drug hypersensitivity reactions is an exacerbation of urticaria or angioedema in patients with chronic idiopathic urticara. Approximate 20% to 40% of patients with chronic urticara may have this drug-induced reaction. The mechanism of this reaction is related to COX-1 inhibition. The exacerbating effects are usually dose dependent. All drugs that inhibit COX-1 cross-react to cause this reaction. Selective COX-2 inhibitors are generally considered safe to take in patients with chronic idiopathic urticaria.

The third type of hypersensitivity reactions is an anaphylactic or immediate urticarial reaction or angioedema appearing soon after the intake of a specific NSAID. Other NSAIDs from other groups or even a NSAID from the same group with a slightly different chemical structure are tolerated by the patient. IgE-mediated mechanism is implicated only in some instances. The diagnosis is made mainly by exclusion. Further research is needed in this topic.

The fourth type of hypersensitivity reactions is urticaria or angioedema caused by ASA or any NSAID that inhibits COX-1 in patients without chronic urticaria. These reactions may be either drug specific or cross-reactive to other NSAIDs. Rarely, patients may have combined respiratory and cutaneous reactions that cannot be classified into one of the four reaction types described.

Corticosteroids

Corticosteroids are the most frequently used drugs for the treatment of allergic conditions, yet they can also induce hypersensitivity reactions. Most hypersensitivity reactions to steroids can be classified into Type I (immediate, IgE-mediated) and Type IV (delayed, cell-mediated) mechanisms. Type I reactions are characterized by the presence of urticaria and anaphylaxis. Type IV reactions can be presented as maculopapular exanthema and delayed urticaria.

Allergic contact dermatitis (type IV reaction) caused by topical administration of steroids is the most common type of allergic reaction induced by this class of drugs, occurring in the rate of 3% to 6%. Usually this is seen as a failure to improve or a worsening of an existing dermatitis that is being treated with topical steroid. Keep in mind that the reaction can also be due to other constituents of the creams, such as neomycin or cetylsteryl alcohol. The diagnosis can be done using patch testing, which detects more than 90% of allergic patients. The topical steroids most frequently involved are nonfluorinated, such as hydrocortisone and budesonide.

Inhaled and intranasal steroids can induce both local and systemic reactions. Local reactions include contact dermatitis, pruritus, nasal congestion, erythema, and dry cough and are quite often irritant in nature. Systemic reactions include eczematous lesions, particularly on the face, exanthema, and urticaria. The most frequently involved steroid is budesonide. The actual mechanism of this reaction is not clear, but it may be a T-cell-mediated reaction.

Hypersensitivity reactions to systemically administered steroids seldom occur. Most of the data come from case reports. Both immediate and delayed reactions have been described, ranging from urticaria to sudden cardiovascular collapse and death. Most immediate reactions are caused by intravenous methylprednisolone and hydrocortisone. In a few cases, the reactions can be induced by salts, such as succinate, or rarely by certain diluents such as carboxymethylcellulose or metabisulfite. Nonimmediate reactions are mainly mild, such as delayed urticaria or maculopapular exanthema. The drug involved most often is betamethasone.

Cross-reactivity between steroids is difficult to assess. Based on corticosteroid patch test results and their chemical structure, Coopman and colleagues divided the steroids into four groups: A (hydrocortisone type), B (triamcinolone acetonide type), C (betamethasone type), and D (hydrocortisone-17-butyrate type). Group D can be subdivided into D1 and D2 depending on the presence or absence of a C16 methyl substitution and/or halogenations on the C9 of the B ring. Table 3 provides the listing of the four groups. High cross-reactivity exists between corticosteroid in each group as well as between Group D2 and Group A and B, with Group D1 exhibiting quite low cross-reactivity with the other groups.

Local Anesthetics

The most common immunologic reaction to local anesthetic is allergic contact dermatitis (type IV). IgE-mediated reactions (type I) to local anesthetics are very rare. Most adverse reactions are due to nonallergic factors such as vasovagal response, anxiety, dysrhythmias, and toxic reactions resulting from inadvertent IV epinephrine effects.

Any patient who presents with a history of an allergic reaction to local anesthetics should be carefully evaluated. Skin testing and graded challenge can be performed in patients who present with a history suggestive of a possible IgE-mediated allergic reaction to these drugs. A local anesthetic that does not contain epinephrine

TABLE 3	Coopman Classification of Cross-Reactivity in Corticosteroids	
GROUP	**TYPE**	**DRUGS**
A	Hydrocortisone	Hydrocortisone (acetate, succinate, phosphate) Methylprednisolone (acetate, succinate, phosphate) Prednisolone, prednisolone acetate Tixocortol pivalate[1]
B	Triamcinolone acetonide	Amcinonide (Cyclocort) Budesonide (Pulmicort, Rhinocort, Entocort) Desonide (Desonate, DesOwen) Flunisolide Flucocinolone acetonide (Synalar) Flucocinolone Halcinonide (Halog) Triamcinolone Triamcinolone acetonide (Kenalog)
C	Betamethasone	Betamethasone (Celestone) Desoxymethasone Dexamethasone Paramethasone[1] Flucortolone[1]
D1	Hydrocortisone-17-butyrate	Beclomethasone dipropionate (Qvar) Betamethasone valerate Betamethasone dipropionate Clobetasone 17-butyrate[1] Clobetasol 17-propyonate (Clobex)
D2	Hydrocortisone-17-butyrate	Fluticasone (Flonase) Mometasone Prednicarbate (Dermatop) Hydrocortisone 17-butyrate (Locoid) Hydrocortisone 17-propionate[1] Methylprednisolone aceponate[1]

[1]Not available in the United States.
From Torres and Canto (2010).

or other additives, such as parabens or sulfites, is preferred in this situation.

It is necessary to identify the type of local anesthetics to be used. Local anesthetics are classified as esters or amides based on their chemical structure. Drugs in the esters group include benzocaine (Americaine, Dermoplast, Lanacaine, Hurricaine), chloroprocaine, cocaine, procaine (Novocaine), proparacaine (Alcaine, Opthaine), and tetracaine (Tetcaine). Most allergic reactions reported in the literature have been caused by agents in the esters group, which are derivatives of para-amino (PABA), a known allergen. Cross-reactivity occurs among members of the ester group, but the esters do not cross-react with the amides. Agents in the amides group include bupivacaine (Marcaine), lidocaine, mepivacaine (Polocaine), prilocaine (Citanest), and ropivacaine (Naropin). Amide local anesthetics generally do not cross react with other amides or with the esters.

Radiocontrast Media

There are two types of radiocontrast media (RCM): ionic high osmolality and nonionic low osmolality. Both of these agents contain iodine. The nonionic RCMs are much more widely used today than the ionic agents.

Allergic reactions to RCM are common and can range from mild to life threatening. Anaphylactoid reactions and severe life-threatening reactions occur in 1% to 3% and 0.22% of patients who receive ionic RCM respectively. Less than 0.5% and 0.04% of patients who receive nonionic agents have anaphylactoid reactions and severe reactions, respectively. The fatality rate is approximately 1 to 2 per 100,000 procedures, and it is similar for both ionic and nonionic agents. RCM reactions are typically not mediated by IgE antibodies. RCM acts directly on mast cells and basophils, resulting in the release of histamine and other systemic mediators, which cause the anaphylactoid reactions. Patients at greater risk for more serious anaphylactoid reactions include females; those with asthma, heart disease, and a history of previous anaphylactoid reaction to RCM; and those taking beta blockers. People who have seafood allergy are not at increased risk for reactions to RCM compared to the general population. The pathogenesis of anaphylactoid reactions is also not related to iodine.

Management of patients with previous RCM reactions include the use of a nonionic, low-osmolarity agent and a pretreatment regimen. One common regimen consists of prednisone (50 mg PO at 13, 7, and 1 hour before the procedure), diphenhydramine (50 mg at 1 hour before the procedure), and a histamine H2-receptor antagonist (1 hour before the procedure). This will significantly reduce the risk for anaphylactoid reaction with re-exposure to RCM.

Delayed reactions to RCM occur 1 hour to 1 week after RCM administration. Approximately 2% of patients have delayed reactions to RCM. These reactions are generally mild, self-limited cutaneous eruptions. The mechanism is usually T-cell mediated. Rarely, more serious and life-threatening delayed reactions such as SJS, TEN, and DRESS have been reported.

Herbal Supplements

There is a perception that herbal supplements are "natural" and therefore safe. In fact, severe allergic reactions including asthma and anaphylaxis have been well documented in patients using bee pollen products and echinacea. Echinacea is an herb belonging to a group of flowering plants known as Asteraceae. Asteraceae-derived pollens are an important cause of hay fever and asthma. Asteraceae may cause contact allergic dermatitis. Cross-reactivity exits between members of the Asteraceae family, such as ragweed, dandelion, daisy, chamomile, echinacea, feverfew, and milk thistle.

A lack of quality control has been a major concern in the herbal supplement industry. Chinese herbal products may be adulterated with synthetic medications not listed on the label. Contaminated supplements may be a potential risk for systemic contact dermatitis in nickel and mercury allergic patients. Because of the widespread use of herbal supplements and the underreporting of adverse events to herbs, all patients should be questioned about the use of herbal supplements when evaluating for hypersensitivity reactions.

Conclusion

Drug hypersensitivity reactions are common; fortunately, severe and often fatal reactions are not. It is important for the clinician to have a working knowledge of common drug-induced hypersensitive reactions as well as the ability to identify and document common dermatologic findings. With that background knowledge, a thorough history and physical examination should enable the clinician to diagnose the majority of these types of reactions. A timely and appropriate management plan can then be implemented. As always, it is important to educate patients in regard with their drug hypersensitivity history and the potential for future reactions.

References

American Academy of Pediatrics. Clinical practice guideline. The diagnosis and management of acute otitis media. Pediatrics 2013;131:e964–9.

CDC. Sexually transmitted disease treatment guidelines 2010. MMWR 2010;59:1–110.

Fernando SL. Acute generalized exanthematous pustulosis. Australas J Dermatol 2012;53:87–92.

Harr T, French L. Toxic epidermal necrolysis and Stevens-Johnson syndrome, Orphanet J Rare Dis 2010;5:39. Available at, http://www.ojrd.com/content/5/1/39 [accessed March 6, 2014].

Haymore BR, Yoon J, Mikita CP, et al. Risk of angioedema with angiotensin receptor blockers in patients with prior angioedema associated with angiotensin-converting enzyme inhibitors: A meta-analysis. Ann Allergy Asthma Immunol 2008;101:495–9.

Husain Z, Reddy BY, Schwartz RA. DRESS syndrome, part I. Clinical perspectives. J Am Acad Dermatol 2013;68:693.e1–693.e14.

Inomata N. Recent advances in drug-induced angioedema. Allergol Int 2012;61:545–57.

Joint Task Force on Practice Parameters, AAAAI, ACAAI. Drug allergy: An updated practice parameter. Ann Allergy Asthma Immunol 2010;105:259–73.

Khan DA, Solensky R. Drug allergy. J Allergy Clin Immunol 2010;125:S126–S137.

Lieberman P, Nicklas RA, Opperheimer J, et al. The diagnosis and management of anaphylaxis practice parameter: 2010 update. J Allergy Clin Immunol 2010;126:477–80.

Murata J, Abe R. Soluble Fas ligand: Is it a critical mediator of toxic epidermal necrolysis and Stevens-Johnson syndrome? J Invest Dermatol 2007;127:744–5.

Philips JF, Yates AB, Deshazo RD. Approach to patients with suspected hypersensitivity to local anesthetics. Am J Med Sci 2007;334:190–6.

Pichler WJ. Consequences of drug binding to immune receptors: Immune stimulation following pharmacological interaction with immune receptors (T-cell receptor for antigen or human leukocyte antigen) with altered peptide-human leukocyte antigen or peptide. Dermatol Sin 2013;31:181–90.

Ponka D. Approach to managing patients with sulfa allergy. Use of antibiotic and nonantibiotic sulfonamides. Can Fam Physician 2006;52:1434–8.

Sharma P, Nagarajan V. Can an ARB be given to patients who have had angioedema on an ACE inhibitor? Cleve Clin J Med 2013;80:755–7.

Torres MJ, Canto G. Hypersensitivity reactions to corticorsteroids. Curr Opin Allergy Clin Immunol 2010;10:273–9.

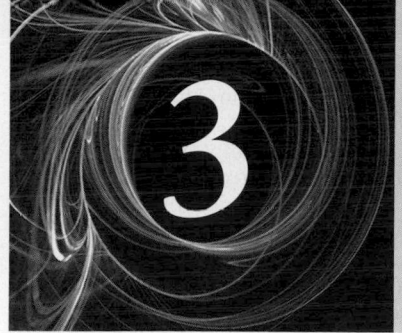

3 The Infectious Diseases

AMEBIASIS

Method of
Guenevere V. Burke, MD; and Sean O. Henderson, MD

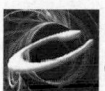

CURRENT DIAGNOSIS

- Amebiasis is infection with *Entamoeba histolytica* and begins with the ingestion of *E. histolytica* cysts, usually via fecally contaminated water or food.
- Amebic colitis is the most common disease presentation. Gradual-onset watery or bloody diarrhea is typical and can last several weeks.
- Diagnosis of amebic colitis is supported by appropriate clinical history, including travel to an endemic area, indolent-onset diarrhea, and positive fecal occult blood testing.
- Noninvasive diagnostic tests include serum antibody titers, stool and serum antigen detection, and stool microscopy (least sensitive).
- Extraintestinal manifestations are rare but can be life threatening. Amebic liver abscess is the most common.

CURRENT THERAPY

- Asymptomatic carriers require treatment with a luminal agent, such as iodoquinol (Yodoxin), to limit transmission and prevent outbreaks.
- Mild to severe colitis and extraintestinal disease require initial treatment with a tissue-active agent, such as metronidazole (Flagyl), followed by a luminal agent to eradicate remaining intestinal cysts and prevent recurrence.

Epidemiology

Amebiasis, human infection with *Entamoeba histolytica*, was originally thought to affect up to 10% of the world's population. However, it was later discovered that the presence of morphologically identical *Entamoeba* species, specifically *Entamoeba dispar* and *Entamoeba moshkovskii*, had confounded this estimate. Indistinguishable on microscopy, the latter organisms are a few of the many commensal *Entamoeba* species that inhabit the human intestinal tract. This has important implications for modern diagnosis, which no longer relies on microscopy (stool ova and parasite test).

The burden of disease lies primarily in Central and South America, South Asia, and Africa. In these areas, serologic testing indicates up to 40% of the population has been exposed. In the United States, recent studies have described amebiasis as the third most common intestinal parasite, affecting approximately 4% of the population. Most cases were reported in California and Texas, with mortality highest among men, Latin Americans, Asians, Pacific Islanders, and the elderly (older than 75 years).

Risk Factors

The risk of developing symptomatic infection with *E. histolytica* depends on a number of host and pathogen factors. Travel to a known endemic area with exposure to contaminated water or food remains an important risk factor. However, even after exposure, a minority of those colonized develop symptoms of infection. Currently, known risk factors for the development of serious complications include male sex, malnourishment, and an immunocompromised state, including extremes of age, pregnancy, and the use of corticosteroids.

Pathophysiology

E. histolytica infection begins with ingestion of the cyst form of the protozoan. Transmission is fecal-oral, and contaminated water, food, and anal-oral sexual practices have been implicated. The cyst form is notable for its environmental stability, demonstrating considerable resistance to chlorination and desiccation.

Once cysts are ingested, excystation occurs in the large intestine, forming the motile trophozoite. It is the trophozoite that is responsible for locally invasive and extraintestinal disease. It binds to mucins and epithelial cells within the large intestine, causing cell death directly through secretion of proteases and contact-dependent apoptosis, and indirectly through the host inflammatory response. These processes are responsible for the findings on colonoscopy of mucosal ulceration, most commonly in the cecum and ascending colon but occurring anywhere from the large intestine to the anus. Invasion into a vessel enables hematogenous spread via the portal circulation, causing amebic liver abscess and other remote sites of disease. Studies have demonstrated differences in genotype between intestine and liver amebic isolates, suggesting tropism.

Clinical Manifestations and Differential Diagnosis

The most common clinical manifestation of disease is amebic colitis, characterized by cramping abdominal pain with a few weeks of diarrhea, which may or may not be grossly bloody, but is almost always positive for occult blood. The differential diagnosis includes other infectious causes of bloody diarrhea, bacterial and parasitic, such as *Salmonella* spp., *Shigella* spp., *Escherichia coli*, *Campylobacter* spp., and *Giardia* spp. Noninfectious causes include inflammatory bowel disease, diverticulitis, and ischemic colitis.

In adults, amebic colitis affects men and women with similar frequency, but amebic liver abscess is much more commonly reported in men. It is the most common extraintestinal manifestation of disease. The presentation is highly variable, often leading to a delay in diagnosis. Many patients with amebic liver abscess do not have concurrent colitis and present with symptoms of relatively short duration (less than 2 weeks). Fever and abdominal pain (usually in the right upper quadrant) are common. Cough and chest pain are less commonly reported symptoms. Laboratory findings are usually nonspecific, including an elevated white blood cell count with normal or mildly elevated liver function tests. The diagnosis is most often facilitated by ultrasound or computed tomography, but confirmatory testing by antigen detection or serology is a necessary adjunct.

Although reported in the literature, additional disease manifestations such as necrotizing colitis, thoracic disease, and cerebral disease are fortunately rare. Necrotizing colitis, reported to occur in less than 0.5% of infections, carries a high mortality risk. It is exacerbated by the use of corticosteroids, creating potentially devastating consequences if amebic colitis is misdiagnosed as inflammatory bowel disease. Extraintestinal disease can occur by local extension from liver to thorax (e.g., empyema, pericarditis) and from hematogenous spread to the central nervous system (e.g., cerebral abscess, encephalitis).

Diagnosis

Traditionally, diagnosis relied upon the identification of the characteristic trophozoite in stool by microscopy. However, this method has poor sensitivity and cannot distinguish the morphologically identical commensal *Entamoeba* organisms, *E. dispar* and *E. moshkovskii*.

Additional noninvasive tests with much greater sensitivity and specificity include antigen and antibody detection methods. Serum antibodies are highly sensitive, but they remain positive for years, limiting their diagnostic utility for acute infection in travelers frequenting endemic regions. Conversely, as with all serologic testing, results may be falsely negative in immune-naive patients with early infection.

Antigen detection tests in both serum and stool are available. The diagnostic sensitivity of each varies according to the presenting clinical entity, but with appropriate selection, greater than 90% sensitivity has been reported. In suspected amebic colitis, stool antigen detection is preferred, but serum testing is superior in suspected amebic liver abscess.

Colonoscopy is useful in ruling out other causes of disease, and biopsy specimens should be examined for characteristic trophozoites.

Treatment

The appropriate therapeutic regimen is dictated by the severity of clinical symptoms, including the treatment of asymptomatic colonized patients (Box 1).

Box 1 — Treatment Recommendations for Amebiasis in Adults

Asymptomatic
Iodoquinol (Yodoxin) 650 mg PO tid × 20 days
or
Paromomycin (Humatin) 25–35 mg/kg/day PO divided tid × 7 days

Mild to Moderate Intestinal Disease
First Line
Metronidazole (Flagyl) 500–750 mg PO tid × 7–10 days
or
Tinidazole (Tindamax) 2 g once PO daily × 3 days

Followed by
Iodoquinol (Yodoxin) 650 mg PO tid × 20 days
or
Paromomycin (Humatin) 25–35 mg/kg/day PO divided tid × 7 days

Severe Intestinal and Extraintestinal Disease
First Line
Metronidazole (Flagyl) 750 mg PO tid × 7–10 days
or
Tinidazole (Tindamax) 2 g once PO daily × 5 days

Followed by
Iodoquinol (Yodoxin) 650 mg PO tid × 20 days
or
Paromomycin (Humatin) 25–35 mg/kg/day PO divided tid × 7 days

Adapted from The Medical Letter Treatment Guidelines 8(Suppl), 2010. Available at www.medicalletter.org.

Asymptomatic carriers require treatment with a luminal active agent, iodoquinol (Yodoxin) or paromomycin (Humatin), to eradicate cysts and limit transmission.

Patients with mild to moderate colitis symptoms often have an excellent response to treatment with the nitroimidazoles metronidazole (Flagyl) or tinidazole (Tindamax). Tinidazole is reported to have similar or superior efficacy to metronidazole and a better side-effect profile. Regardless of symptomatic improvement after initial nitroimidazole therapy, many patients remain colonized with cysts and can suffer disease recurrence unless subsequent treatment with a luminal agent is initiated. Concurrent therapy is poorly tolerated owing to side effects, including diarrhea, which also limits clinical evaluation of treatment response.

Severe disease, such as large abscesses or necrotizing infections, can require imaging-guided drainage, surgical intervention, and additional prophylactic antibiotic therapy, depending on the clinical presentation.

References

Ali IK, Solaymani-Mohammadi S, Akhter J, et al. Tissue invasion by *Entamoeba histolytica*: Evidence of genetic selection and/or DNA reorganization events in organ tropism. PLoS Negl Trop Dis 2008;2:e219.

Gonzales ML, Dans LF, Martinez EG. Antiamoebic drugs for treating amoebic colitis. Cochrane Database Syst Rev 2009;(2), CD006085.

Gunther J, Shafir S, Bristow B, Sorvillo F. Short report: Amebiasis-related mortality among United States residents, 1990–2007. Am J Trop Med Hyg 2011;85:1038–40.

Haque R, Mollah NU, Ali IKM, et al. Diagnosis of amebic liver abscess and intestinal infection with the TechLab *Entamoeba histolytica* II antigen detection and antibody tests. J Clin Microbiol 2000;38:3235–9.

Hoffner RJ, Kilaghbian T, Esekogwu VI, Henderson SO. Common presentations of amebic liver abscess. Ann Emerg Med 1999;34:351–5.

Huston CD, Boettner DR, Miller-Sims V, et al. Apoptotic killing and phagocytosis of host cells by the parasite *Entamoeba histolytica*. Infect Immun 2003;71:964–72.

Petri WA, Haque R. *Entamoeba* species, including amebiasis. In: Mandell GL, Bennett JE, Dolin R, editors. Mandell, Douglas, and Bennet's Principles & Practice of Infectious Diseases. 7th ed. Philadelphia: Churchill Livingstone; 2009. p. 3411–25.

Pritt BS, Clark CG. Amebiasis. Mayo Clin Proc 2008;83:1154–9.

Stanley Jr SL. Amoebiasis. Lancet 2003;361:1025–34.

ANTHRAX

Method of
Shingo Chihara, MD

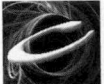

CURRENT DIAGNOSIS

Cutaneous Anthrax
- Incubation period of 1 to 7 days from exposure to cattle
- Painless or pruritic lesion progresses to ulcer and eschar
- Significant swelling
- Gram stain and culture of lesion

Gastrointestinal
- Incubation period of 1 to 6 days after consumption of raw or undercooked meat
- Nonspecific symptoms followed by abdominal pain, ascites
- Diarrhea uncommon
- Obtain blood culture and ascitic fluid for culture and Gram stain

Inhalational
- Incubation period of 1 to 7 days (up to 43 days)
- Biphasic: fever, malaise, myalgia followed by dyspnea
- Widened mediastinum seen on chest x-ray and computed tomography (CT) of chest
- Blood cultures turn positive in most

Injection
- Injection drug use
- Significant swelling seen; eschar rare

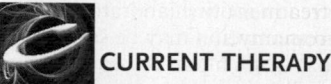
Systemic Anthrax With Possible/Confirmed Meningitis

- Ciprofloxacin (Cipro) 400 mg IV every 8 hours or levofloxacin (Levaquin) 750 mg IV every 24 hours or moxifloxacin (Avelox)[1] 400 mg IV every 24 hours

  plus
- Meropenem (Merrem)[1] 2 g IV every 8 hours or imipenem/cilastatin (Primaxin)[1] 1 g IV every 6 hours or doripenem (Doribax)[1] 500 mg IV every 8 hours
- If penicillin-susceptible strains, then penicillin G 4 million units IV every 4 hours or ampicillin[1] 3 g IV every 6 hours could be an alternative to carbapenems

  plus
- Linezolid (Zyvox)[1] 600 mg IV every 12 hours or clindamycin (Cleocin) 900 mg IV every 8 hours or rifampin (Rifadin) 600 mg IV every 12 hours or chloramphenicol 1 g every 6 to 8 hours

Systemic Anthrax When Meningitis Has Been Excluded

- Ciprofloxacin 400 mg IV every 8 hours or levofloxacin 750 mg IV every 24 hours or moxifloxacin[1] 400 mg IV every 24 hours

  or
- Meropenem[1] 2 g IV every 8 hours or imipenem/cilastatin[1] 1 g IV every 6 hours or doripenem[1] 500 mg IV every 8 hours

  or
- Vancomycin (Vancocin)[1] 60 mg/kg/day IV divided every 8 hours (goal trough 15–20 µg/mL)

  or
- If penicillin-susceptible strains, then penicillin G 4 million units IV every 4 hours or ampicillin[1] 3 g IV every 6 hours

  plus
- Clindamycin[1] 900 mg IV every 8 hours or linezolid[1] 600 mg IV every 12 hours

  or
- Doxycycline 200 mg IV × 1, then 100 mg IV every 12 hours, or rifampin[1] 600 mg IV every 12 hours

Oral Treatment for Cutaneous Anthrax Without Systemic Involvement

- One of the agents below for 7 to 10 days in naturally-acquired cases and for 60 days in bioterrorism-associated cases
- Ciprofloxacin 500 mg PO every 12 hours
- Doxycycline 100 mg PO every 12 hours
- Levofloxacin 750 mg PO daily
- Moxifloxacin[1] 400 mg PO daily
- Clindamycin[1] 600 mg PO every 8 hours
- If penicillin-susceptible strain
- Amoxicillin[1] 1 g PO every 8 hours
- Penicillin VK 500 mg PO every 6 hours

[1]Not FDA approved for this indication.

Anthrax has been described for centuries and the name is derived from Greek for "burnt coal" owing to eschar formation from cutaneous anthrax. Anthrax is rarely seen in developed countries, including the United States, but it is important to be aware of this condition because of its potential as a bioterrorism agent. When anthrax is suspected, the clinician needs to contact the local or state health department immediately. Anthrax has historical significance because it was the agent utilized in Koch's postulate during the 19th century when Koch proved that *Bacillus anthracis* is responsible for anthrax in cattle.

Background

B. anthracis is the bacterium responsible for anthrax. It forms spores which can survive in soil for years. It is hyperendemic in the Middle East and in sub-Saharan Africa. Systemic anthrax is primarily a disease of grazing animals. In naturally-acquired anthrax, humans are accidentally infected from exposure to the animal or its products.

Epidemiology

Since the mid-20th century, there has been a precipitous decline in anthrax owing to animal and human vaccines, improvement in factory hygiene, sterilization procedures for imported animal products, and increased use of alternatives to animal hides or hair. Cutaneous anthrax comprises over 95% of naturally-acquired human anthrax and there are an estimated 2000 cases annually. Between 1900 and 2001 there were 18 cases of inhalational anthrax in the United States, of which 16 were fatal. Over the last decade, there have been several cases of inhalational and cutaneous anthrax related to African drum makers. In late 2001, there were 22 cases of anthrax in the United States from spores delivered in the mail, of which five were fatal. In 1979, accidental release of dried anthrax spores from a biologic weapons facility in Sverdlovsk in the former Soviet Union resulted in 68 deaths from inhalation anthrax.

Pathophysiology

B. anthracis is a gram positive, encapsulated, spore forming, non-hemolytic, nonmotile rod shaped bacterium. Infection with anthrax requires three components: the edema factor, the lethal factor, and protective antigen. The edema factor combines with protective antigen and becomes edema toxin, which causes edema and impairment of the immune system. The lethal factor combines with protective antigen and becomes lethal toxin, which causes lysis of macrophages. For cutaneous anthrax, these exotoxins result in extensive edema and tissue necrosis locally. In inhalation anthrax, spores that reach the alveoli or alveolar ducts are phagocytized by the alveolar macrophage and transported to the mediastinal lymph nodes where they replicate and cause hemorrhagic mediastinitis. With gastrointestinal tract infection, *B. anthracis* is transported from the gastrointestinal tract to mesenteric lymph nodes where they multiply and cause mesenteric lymphadenitis, ascites, and sepsis.

Clinical Manifestations

There are four distinct clinical presentations: cutaneous, inhalation, gastrointestinal tract, and injection anthrax, depending on the site of entry. Meningitis is a devastating complication which could occur with any of the four infections.

Cutaneous Anthrax

Cutaneous anthrax is the most common form and seen in developing countries as a result of contact with infected animals or animal products such as wool, hair, or hides. Spores invade through either skin abrasions or hair follicles. Subsequently, they germinate and multiply. The incubation period is commonly 5 to 7 days with range of 1 to 19 days. The lesions appear in exposed areas such as head, neck, forearms, and hands and begin as a small, painless papule. They are pruritic at times and form blisters. Subsequently, they evolve into painless necrotic ulcers with a black, depressed eschar with extensive edema and lymphadenopathy.

Inhalation Anthrax

Inhalation anthrax occurs when spores are aerosolized while working with contaminated animal products or when they are released intentionally in bioterrorism. The incubation period is 1 to 7 days, but could be as long as 43 days. The course of disease is usually biphasic. Initially, nonspecific symptoms such as fever, malaise, and myalgia are present, resembling influenza. These symptoms last for several days before the bacteremic phase starts. The manifestations include rapidly, fulminant progressive respiratory symptoms such as severe dyspnea, as well as hypoxemia and shock. Once in this phase, the patient dies within a few days despite support in the intensive care unit. Therefore, it is important to suspect anthrax in the prodromal phase which is difficult owing to its rarity and lack of specific symptoms. Widening of the mediastinum on a chest x-ray may be helpful in establishing the diagnosis. This finding was seen in 7 out of 10 cases of inhalation anthrax from 2001. Hilar abnormalities, pulmonary infiltrates, or consolidation and pleural effusion may be seen.

Gastrointestinal Tract Anthrax
Gastrointestinal tract anthrax occurs after ingestion of raw or undercooked meat from an animal infected with anthrax. Gastrointestinal infection is relatively common and has been reported from mouth to ascending colon. The incubation period is 1 to 6 days. Initially, nonspecific symptoms such as asthenia, headache, low grade fever, facial flushing and conjunctival injection occur. They are followed by abdominal pain, abdominal distention from ascites, nausea, and vomiting. Diarrhea occurs less frequently. As the disease progresses, abdominal pain becomes severe and findings of hypotension and intravascular depletion are seen. When the infection occurs in the oropharynx, necrotic ulcers with pseudomembranes cause pain and edema.

Injection Anthrax
An outbreak of injection anthrax was described in 2009. It was reported in Scotland among injection heroin users. Among the 47 confirmed cases, typical eschar formation seen in cutaneous anthrax was not seen in all but one case. Prominent edema was seen in most patients and some developed compartment syndrome.

Meningitis
Meningitis is a complication seen with all forms of anthrax. About half of patients with inhalation anthrax develop hemorrhagic meningitis. Symptoms such as altered mental status, seizures, cranial nerve palsies, and myoclonus may be seen. When anthrax is suspected, lumbar puncture should be done on presentation unless there are contraindications.

Diagnosis
When diagnosis of anthrax is suspected, the provider must notify the local department of health and the clinical microbiology lab. There has been reported transmission of anthrax to laboratory personnel handling *B. anthracis* and specimen handling in biosafety level 3 facilities is recommended. As the genus *Bacillus* is part of the normal skin flora, it is crucial for the microbiology laboratory to distinguish *B. anthracis* from other non-*anthracis* species of *Bacillus*. Conventional culture and staining are used for distinction. *B. anthracis* is nonmotile and nonhemolytic and those characteristics are used to distinguish it from non-*anthracis* species of *Bacillus*. Most microbiology laboratories have the ability to make a presumptive identification of an organism, and the identification is confirmed by a reference laboratory.

Specimen Collection
When collecting clinical specimens for suspected anthrax, proper personal protective equipment such as disposable gloves, disposable aprons, and boots, should be used. When there is any potential of aerosolization of spores, then face shields and respirators are recommended. Hand washing with soap and water will reduce the endospore contamination of the skin but alcohol handrubs are not effective against these endospores. For cutaneous anthrax, the edge of the eschar should be lifted and two specimens of vesicular fluid should be collected by rotating a swab. One swab will be used for culture and Gram stain while the other would be used for polymerase chain reaction (PCR). Punch biopsy of the cutaneous lesion is an alternative. When inhalational anthrax is suspected, blood cultures must be obtained prior to use of antibiotics. If pleural fluid is present, then thoracentesis should be performed for Gram stain, culture and PCR. For alimentary tract anthrax, blood cultures must be obtained. If there are oral lesions, then specimens could be collected with swabs similar to a cutaneous lesion. If ascites is present, then paracentesis should be performed for Gram stain, culture and PCR. For meningitis, cerebrospinal fluid (CSF) should be collected for culture, Gram stain and PCR.

There are unique findings observed in routine laboratories with systemic anthrax. Marked hemoconcentration may be seen in the complete blood count and the initial white blood cell count is frequently within normal limits. In chemistry, decreased sodium, increased blood urea nitrogen, mild transaminitis and hypoalbuminemia are seen. Inflammatory markers such as erythrocyte sedimentation rate and C-reactive protein are elevated in most cases except in cases of injection anthrax, when C-reactive protein is low.

Treatment
Supportive Care
Hospitalization is required for all patients with systemic infections. Only uncomplicated cutaneous anthrax could be treated on an outpatient basis. Close monitoring is warranted because the patient status may deteriorate rapidly. Hemodynamic support should be given, including fluids, vasopressors, blood products, and invasive hemodynamic monitoring. Mechanical ventilation may be needed because of respiratory distress, airway protection for altered mental status, or for airway edema. Adjunctive corticosteroids may be indicated in four situations: patients with history of endocrine or corticosteroid therapy; edema of head or neck; anthrax meningitis; or vasopressor-resistant shock. Pleural fluid and ascites should be drained aggressively. Surgery is indicated in certain situations. Surgery for cutaneous anthrax has led to dissemination and poor outcome. Therefore, in cutaneous anthrax, indication for surgery is limited to tracheotomy for airway obstruction and surgery for compartment syndrome. In gastrointestinal anthrax, surgery might be considered for complications such as bowel ischemia or infarct and perforation. In injection anthrax, removal of necrotic nidus would help reduce the toxin and spore reservoir.

Antimicrobial Treatment for Systemic Disease with Possible Meningitis
At least three intravenous antibiotics with good penetration to the central nervous system are recommended. At least one drug should have bactericidal activity and at least one drug should inhibit protein synthesis. These should be continued for at least 2 weeks or until clinically stable, whichever is longer. The fluoroquinolone class is bactericidal, has good penetration to the central nervous system, and has no reported resistance by *B. anthracis*. Intravenous ciprofloxacin (Cipro) is the primary bactericidal component in the treatment of systemic disease. Levofloxacin (Levaquin) and moxifloxacin (Avelox)[1] are considered to be alternatives. The carbapenem class has good central nervous system penetration and meropenem (Merrem)[1] is the preferred second antibiotic in treatment of systemic disease with possible meningitis. Imipenem/cilastatin (Primaxin)[1] and doripenem (Doribax)[1] are considered alternatives. Penicillin G or ampicillin[1] could be used in place of carbapenems when the isolate is known to have a minimum inhibitory concentration (MIC) of less than 0.125 µg/mL. As for protein synthesis inhibitor, linezolid (Zyvox)[1] is preferred because it provides good central nervous system penetration. If there is contraindication to linezolid use such as drug–drug interaction or myelosuppression, then clindamycin (Cleocin)[1] is the alternative. When both linezolid and clindamycin cannot be used, rifampin (Rifadin)[1] could be used for synergistic effect in combination with the bactericidal drugs. Chloramphenicol is another antibiotic which is a protein synthesis inhibitor. It could be used if linezolid, clindamycin, and rifampin are unavailable. Doxycycline (Vibramycin) is an inhibitor of protein synthesis but does not adequately penetrate the central nervous system. Therefore, doxycycline should not be used when meningitis is not ruled out. If the patient had been exposed to aerosolized spores, then the patient should be transitioned to oral antibiotics after completion of initial intravenous combination therapy to prevent relapse from spores.

---

[1]Not FDA approved for this indication.

Antimicrobial Treatment for Systemic Disease when Meningitis is Ruled Out

At least two antimicrobial agents are recommended for systemic anthrax without meningitis. At least one should be bactericidal and at least one should be a protein synthesis inhibitor. This combination should be administered intravenously for at least 2 weeks or until clinically stable, whichever is longer. For penicillin-susceptible strains, penicillin G is considered equivalent to ciprofloxacin. Vancomycin (Vancocin)[1] is an acceptable alternative bactericidal agent. Clindamycin[1] and linezolid[1] are equivalent first choices for protein synthesis inhibitors. Doxycycline is an alternative agent. If the patient had been exposed to aerosolized spores, then the patient should be transitioned to oral antibiotics after completion of initial intravenous combination therapy to prevent relapse from spores.

Treatment for Cutaneous Anthrax without Systemic Involvement

A single oral antibiotic is adequate to treat cutaneous anthrax without systemic involvement. Fluoroquinolones and doxycycline are considered first-line agents. Clindamycin[1] is a second line agent when first-line agents are unavailable or contraindicated. Penicillin or amoxicillin[1] may be used if the isolate is found to be sensitive in vitro. It is important to give an adequate dose because resistance may develop when underdosed.

Antitoxins

There are two antitoxins in the Centers for Disease Control and Prevention (CDC) Strategic National stockpile: raxibacumab and anthrax immune globulin intravenous (AIGIV). These agents are not readily available to the public. They inhibit binding of protective antigen to the anthrax toxin receptor and translocation of lethal factor and edema factor into cells. There are human and animal data from the pre-antibiotic era which suggest that there is lower mortality in those who received the antitoxin in cutaneous anthrax compared with those who did not. Whether this agent should be given for systemic anthrax is controversial owing to lack of data. Because the mortality rate with systemic anthrax is high while the complication of antitoxin treatment is low, the potential benefit from antitoxins outweighs the potential risk from the antitoxins in systemic anthrax. This agent should be given in addition to appropriate antibiotics when systemic anthrax is suspected.

Pregnancy

Overall management is similar to the nonpregnant patient. In pregnancy, ciprofloxacin is preferred over doxycycline for both treatment and prevention. Newer fluoroquinolones such as levofloxacin and moxifloxacin[1] are not preferred because embryo toxicity has been observed in animal studies. This was not seen with ciprofloxacin. Transplacental transmission of anthrax is known to occur. Ciprofloxacin, levofloxacin, meropenem,[1] ampicillin,[1] penicillin, clindamycin,[1] and rifampin[1] are known to have adequate concentration in the placenta and at least one agent should be used with treatment.

Prognosis

Uncomplicated cutaneous anthrax has a mortality rate of less than 2% with treatment. Injection anthrax has a mortality rate of 28% and gastrointestinal anthrax has a mortality rate of 40%. Inhalational anthrax has mortality of 45% despite antibiotics and modern intensive care. Meningitis from anthrax is almost always fatal.

Prevention

Postexposure prophylaxis should be started as soon as possible after exposure. Sixty days of antibiotics for immediate protection and a three-dose series of Anthrax Vaccine Adsorbed (AVA, BioThrax) for long-term protection are recommended by the United States Advisory Committee on Immunization Practices. Ciprofloxacin and doxycycline are recommended as first-line antibiotic therapy for postexposure prophylaxis and are FDA-approved for this indication. Alternative agents include levofloxacin, moxifloxacin, amoxicillin, or penicillin VK (if sensitive); and clindamycin. AVA should be administered at diagnosis and at 2 and 4 weeks. AVA is not FDA-approved for postexposure prophylaxis.

References

Anthrax. Available at http://www.cdc.gov/anthrax/ [accessed 31.01.15].

Hendricks KA, Wright ME, Shadomy SV, et al. Centers for disease control and prevention expert panel meetings on prevention and treatment of anthrax in adults. Emerg Infect Dis 2014;20. http://dx.doi.org/10.3201/eid2002.130687.

Knox D, Murray G, Millar M, et al. Subcutaneous anthrax in three intravenous drug users. J Bone Joint Surg 2011;93:414–7.

Logan NA, Hoffmaster AR, Shadomy SV, Stauffer KE. In: Versalovic J, editor. Manual of clinical microbiology. 10th ed. Washington DC: ASM Press; 2011. p. 381–402.

Meaney-Delman D, Zotti ME, Creanga AA, et al. Special considerations for prophylaxis for and treatment of anthrax in pregnant and postpartum women. Emerg Infect Dis 2014;20. http://dx.doi.org/10.3201/eid2002.130611.

Ruoff KL, Clarridge J, Bernard K. In: Garcia LS, editor. Clinical microbiology procedures handbook. 3rd ed. Washington DC; ASM Press; 2010, 3.18.1.

Singh K. Laboratory-acquired infections. Clin Infect Dis 2009;49:142–7.

BACTERIAL MENINGITIS

Method of
Gary D. Overturf, MD

CURRENT DIAGNOSIS

- Patient age and epidemiology:
  - Clinical symptoms: Fever, headache, meningeal signs
  - CSF examination: High opening pressure (>300 mm Hg)
  - Elevated white blood cell count (>10–>5000)
  - >60% polymorphonuclear cells
- Low CSF glucose (<40 mg/dL or <50% serum glucose)
- High CSF protein (>50 ->1.0 g/dL)
- Bacteria present on Gram stain of CSF

Abbreviation: CSF = cerebrospinal fluid.

CURRENT THERAPY

- Neonates <2 mo
  - Group B streptococcal infection: cefotaxime (Claforan) or ampicillin
  - Gram-negative rods, other than *Pseudomonas:* cefotaxime
  - *Pseudomonas:* cefepime (Maxipime), ceftazidime (Fortaz), or meropenem (Merrem)
  - *Listeria:* Ampicillin + gentamicin (Garamycin)
- Children >2 mo
  - Empirical for unknown etiology: cefotaxime or ceftriaxone (Rocephin)
  - *Streptococcus pneumoniae:* cefotaxime or ceftriaxone
  - *Haemophilus influenzae:* cefotaxime or ceftriaxone
  - *Neisseria meningitidis:* ampicillin or cefotaxime
- Older children and adults
  - Empirical for unknown etiology: cefotaxime or ceftriaxone
  - *S. pneumoniae:* cefotaxime or ceftriaxone
  - *N. meningitidis:* ampicillin or cefotaxime
  - Gram negative, postoperative, or *Staphylococcus aureus* (see Tables 1–4)
  - Add vancomycin if at risk for infection with resistant pneumococcus

---

[1]Not FDA approved for this indication.

Acute bacterial meningitis occurs in all age groups, but predominantly in children younger than 2 years and the elderly (older than 60 years). With the introduction of effective protein conjugate vaccines for *Haemophilus* and pneumococcal infection, the incidence of bacterial meningitis is rapidly declining in children, and adults are now the major population affected. Bacterial meningitis is a medical emergency requiring rapid and decisive action to prevent death or neurologic sequelae. Since the introduction of chloramphenicol (Chloromycetin) in the early 1950s, the mortality rate has remained between 5% and 40%, depending on the age of the patient and the etiology. Of the survivors, 10% to 30% suffer permanent neurologic deficits. Prognosis is affected by the timeliness of therapy, the age of the patient, and the etiology. Presumptive diagnosis and administration of therapy are critical.

Diagnosis

Acute bacterial meningitis must be considered in the differential diagnosis of persons of any age presenting with fever and headache or signs of meningeal irritation or acute central nervous system dysfunction. Presentations can be subtle at the extremes of age or in patients who have received partially effective antibiotic therapy. The diagnosis of bacterial meningitis requires the examination of the cerebrospinal fluid (CSF), which must be performed as expeditiously as possible. Studies indicate that lumbar puncture may be safely performed on patients who have normal mental status or are without focal neurologic signs or papilledema; clinical impressions are predictive of the computed tomography (CT) findings. If there are signs or symptoms suggesting the presence of an intracranial mass (e.g., tumor, cerebral hematoma, or brain abscess), blood cultures should be obtained and empirical antibiotics should be administered prior to the performance of a CT scan.

Characteristically, the CSF findings in bacterial meningitis include a cell count of greater than 500 to 5000 white blood cells (WBCs) per mm^3 with a predominance of neutrophils, a protein concentration of greater than 150 mg/mL, and a low glucose (e.g., less than 35–40 mg/dL). No single value is absolute, and a single value may be normal in up to a third of the cases. The Gram-stained sediment of centrifuged CSF is the critical examination leading to a specific diagnosis. In patients who have not received antibiotics capable of reaching the CSF, the Gram stain is positive in 80% to 90% of culture-confirmed cases. In persons previously treated with antibiotics (e.g., β-lactam antibiotics, tetracycline, fluoroquinolones), the frequency of positive Gram stains is much reduced (e.g., 60% to 70%), but the cells, cell type, protein, and glucose concentrations are not significantly affected. CSF antigen tests are not reliable, and variable negative and positive predictive values direct against relying on the use of such tests. Clinical judgment is paramount, and antibiotics should be given in situations of ambiguous results of the CSF examination.

Antibiotic Selection

The outcome of bacterial meningitis is closely related to the timely use of antibiotics. Hypotension, seizures, an altered mental status, and hypoglycorrhachia at the time of initial antibiotic administration are predictive of higher case fatality and neurologic sequelae. Because prompt administration of antibiotics is critical, the choice of antibiotics must be made before results of the CSF cultures are known. If organisms are seen on Gram stain, therapy may be directed by the probable bacterial etiology (Table 1). In the event the CSF Gram stain fails to reveal a possible pathogen, empirical antibiotic therapy should be begun based on the age of the patient for those persons who have acquired their infection in the community (Table 2). For those persons who are members of special risk groups, empirical therapy should be based on the likely etiology (Table 3). Once the CSF cultures are completed, therapy can be modified according to results of the culture and sensitivity data.

Antibiotics used in bacterial meningitis should be rapidly bactericidal and achieve high concentrations in the CSF. Antibiotics should be given in maximal doses (Table 4). Because the bactericidal activity of antibiotics in CSF is dose dependent, the fractional CSF-to-serum ratio is very small. Finally, the use of combinations of antibiotics should be minimized to avoid antagonizing the bactericidal activity.

TABLE 1   Cerebrospinal Fluid Gram Stain Morphology and Antibiotic Recommendations

MORPHOLOGY	POSSIBLE OR PROBABLE PATHOGENS	TREATMENT OPTIONS	ALTERNATIVE THERAPIES
Gram-positive cocci, short chains or pairs	*Streptococcus pneumoniae*, *Streptococcus agalactiae* (group B streptococci)	Ceftriaxone (Rocephin) or cefotaxime (Claforan) plus vancomycin (Vancocin)	Chloramphenicol (Chloromycetin)
Gram-positive cocci, clusters; or gram-positive bacilli	*Staphylococcus aureus*, *Listeria monocytogenes*	Vancomycin, ampicillin plus gentamicin (Garamycin)	Nafcillin (Unipen) or Oxacillin, trimethoprim-sulfamethoxazole (Bactrim)
Gram-negative diplococci	*Neisseria meningitidis*	Ceftriaxone or cefotaxime	Ampicillin, Penicillin G, or chloramphenicol
Gram-negative coccobacilli	*Haemophilus influenzae*	Ceftriaxone or cefotaxime	Chloramphenicol
Gram-negative bacilli	*Escherichia coli*, *Klebsiella* species, *Pseudomonas aeruginosa*	Cefepime (Maxipime) or ceftazidime (Fortaz)	Imipenem (Primaxin) or meropenem (Merrem)

TABLE 2   Antibiotic Recommendations for Bacterial Meningitis Acquired in the Community, by Age Group and Probable Pathogen

AGE GROUP	PROBABLE PATHOGENS	EMPIRICAL THERAPY
Neonate <1 mo	Group B streptococcus; *E. coli*, or other gram-negative enteric rod; occasionally *L. monocytogenes*	Ampicillin plus cefotaxime (Claforan)
Infants 1–3 mo	*H. influenzae*, *N. meningitidis*, *S. pneumoniae*, Group B streptococci	Ceftriaxone (Rocephin) or cefotaxime (Claforan)
Children 3 mo–7 y and older children and adults 7–50 y	*H. influenzae*, *S. pneumoniae*, *N. meningitidis*	Ceftriaxone or cefotaxime plus vancomycin (Vancocin)
Older adults >50 y	*S. pneumoniae*, *N. meningitidis*, *L. monocytogenes*	Ceftriaxone plus ampicillin

CONDITION OR RISK FACTOR	COMMON PATHOGENS	ANTIBIOTIC RECOMMENDATIONS
Impaired immunity (e.g., HIV, early complement deficiency, agammaglobulinemia)	*L. monocytogenes, S. pneumoniae, H. influenzae*	Ampicillin plus ceftriaxone (Rocephin) or cefotaxime (Claforan)
Closed head trauma with CSF leak	*S. pneumoniae, H. influenzae*	Ceftriaxone or cefotaxime plus vancomycin (Vancocin)
Asplenia	*S. pneumoniae, H. influenzae*	Ceftriaxone or cefotaxime plus vancomycin
Terminal complement deficiency	*N. meningitidis*	Ceftriaxone or cefotaxime
Neurosurgical procedures	*S. aureus*	Vancomycin plus ceftriaxone or cefotaxime
CSF shunt infections	Coagulase-negative staphylococci, Gram-negative bacilli	
Elderly patients (>65 y)	*S. pneumoniae, L. monocytogenes*	Ceftriaxone or cefotaxime plus vancomycin
Recurrent bacterial meningitis (see CSF leak)	*S. pneumoniae*	Ceftriaxone or cefotaxime plus vancomycin
Alcoholic patients	*S. pneumoniae* and Gram-negative bacilli	Ceftriaxone or cefotaxime plus vancomycin

Abbreviation: CSF = cerebrospinal fluid.

TABLE 4 Antibiotic Doses for Adults and Children for Treatment of Bacterial Meningitis

ANTIBIOTIC	DAILY ADULT DOSE	DAILY PEDIATRIC DOSE	DOSE INTERVAL
Ampicillin	12 g	200–400 mg/kg	4–6 h
Cefotaxime (Claforan)	12 g	200–300 mg/kg	4–6 h
Ceftriaxone (Rocephin)	4 g	100 mg/kg	12 h
Ceftazidime (Fortaz)	6 g	150–200 mg/kg	8 h
Cefepime (Maxipime)	6 g	100–150 mg/kg	8 h
Meropenem (Merrem)	6 g	120 mg/kg	8 h
Nafcillin (Unipen)	12 g	200 mg/kg	4–6 h
Penicillin G	24 million U	250,000 units/kg	4 h
Vancomycin (Vancocin)	2 g	60 mg/kg	12 h

Adapted from Bradley JS, Nelson JD: 2002 2003 Nelson's Pocket Book of Pediatric Antimicrobial Therapy, 15th ed. Philadelphia, Lippincott Williams & Wilkins, 2002; Gilbert DN, Moellering RC, Sande MA. The Sanford Guide to Antimicrobial Therapy 2005. Hyde Park, Antimicrobial Therapy Inc., 2005.

Special Considerations for Antibiotic Therapy

During the past two decades, resistance to penicillin and some third-generation cephalosporins (e.g., ceftriaxone [Rocephin], cefotaxime [Claforan]) has steadily increased among strains of *Streptococcus pneumoniae*. Currently, approximately 30% to 50% of isolates are either intermediately (inhibitory concentration, 0.1–1.0 μg/mL) or fully (inhibitory concentration more than 2.0 μg/mL) resistant to Penicillin G and ampicillin. Resistance to ceftriaxone (Rocephin) and cefotaxime (Claforan) may occur as well in 10% to 15% of strains. Vancomycin (Vancocin) is recommended in those regimens for meningitis when pneumococci are considered. However, higher maximal doses are required for vancomycin because of its relatively poor penetration into the CSF. In general, lumbar puncture with CSF culture should be repeated in 48 hours in those cases where vancomycin therapy is the primary drug because of demonstrated penicillin or cephalosporin resistance.

Meningitis caused by gram-negative bacilli such as *Pseudomonas aeruginosa, Escherichia coli*, or *Enterobacter cloacae* should be treated with a cephalosporin with an extended spectrum of Gram-negative activity, such as ceftazidime (Fortaz) or cefepime (Maxipime). A carbapenem, such as imipenem (Primaxin) or meropenem (Merrem), can also be used for antibiotic-resistant gram-negative enteric and pseudomonas meningitis. Meropenem is associated with less risk of drug-induced seizures and may be a better choice for bacterial meningitis.

Patients with ventriculoatrial and ventriculoperitoneal shunt–associated meningitis and ventriculitis usually require removal of the shunt for cure, as well as the administration of antibiotics to clear the infection. Certain patients with infections caused by organisms of reduced virulence, such as coagulase-negative staphylococci, or those with exquisitely antibiotic-susceptible infections, can be treated with a trial of antibiotics alone.

Because of the extreme sensitivity of *Neisseria meningitidis* to antibiotics, uncomplicated meningitis may be treated with as little as 5 to 7 days of antibiotics. Pneumococcal meningitis may be treated with 10 to 14 days of antibiotics, and haemophilus infections are treated successfully with 7 to 10 days of antibiotics. Gram-negative meningitis was treated in the past with 3 weeks of aminoglycosides, but current experience with newer extended-spectrum cephalosporins (ceftriaxone, cefotaxime, carbapenems) suggests that 2 weeks of therapy is often sufficient in neonates as well as in some elderly patients and postoperative infections.

All patients with bacterial meningitis should be monitored carefully throughout the treatment period. Infectious disease consultation is recommended for most infections of the central nervous system. Repeated lumbar punctures are not routinely recommended for patients with fully susceptible bacterial isolates or in those who show good response to therapy. Repeated sampling of the CSF with lumbar puncture or, when appropriate, shunt or ventricular reservoir puncture should be performed in those with known resistant bacterial isolates, in patients who have an inadequate response, in those patients who deteriorate on therapy, or in those for whom clinical response may correlate poorly with the microbiologic response (shunt infections, neonates, and elderly patients).

Adjunctive Therapy

Corticosteroids reduce the incidence of permanent neurologic sequelae in children with bacterial meningitis, particularly when caused by *Haemophilus influenza* type b. Data in support of steroids in either pneumococcal or meningococcal infections are less robust. Dexamethasone (Decadron[1]), 0.15 mg/kg every 6 hours for the first 2 to 4 days of treatment, was evaluated in children older than 2 months with bacterial meningitis. The first dose of dexamethasone should be given before, at the start, or no later than 12 hours after beginning antibiotics.

Use of corticosteroids in adults is more controversial. Although doses of dexamethasone are recommended by some experts for adults with bacterial meningitis, its efficacy in adult meningitis has not been evaluated in a well-designed prospective trial. A recent study in adults found that corticosteroids significantly reduced the risk for unfavorable outcomes, particularly in patients with pneumococcal meningitis. There has been concern that the anti-inflammatory properties of dexamethasone may decrease the penetration of antibiotics, especially vancomycin, into the CSF. One study in children did not show this to be the case. Dexamethasone[1] should be administered in adults with proven or suspected pneumococcal meningitis, but only if it can be given prior to the first dose of antibiotics in a dose of 10 mg every 6 hours for 4 days. In patients with meningitis caused by *S. pneumoniae* highly resistant to penicillin (minimum inhibitory concentration [MIC] >2.0 µg/mL) or cephalosporins (MIC >4.0 µg/mL), vancomycin should not be used as a single agent if corticosteroids are used. The addition of rifampin (Rifadin[1]) is often recommended in these situations.

Chemoprophylaxis for Bacterial Meningitis

Prophylactic antibiotics are recommended in case of meningitis caused by *Neisseria meningitidis* and *H. influenzae* type b. Prophylaxis is provided to eliminate the carriage of organisms among contacts and prevent spread to hosts susceptible to invasive disease. In cases of meningococcal meningitis, prophylaxis is indicated only for those with household or intimate contact with the index case. Administration of prophylaxis to large groups (e.g., college students, schoolchildren, or preschool classes) requires a special assessment and a recommendation of local or regional health departments. Chemoprophylaxis is not necessary for casual contacts or medical personnel unless there is a direct exposure to respiratory secretions. The recommended dose of rifampin (Rifadin) is 10 mg/kg (600 maximal, adults) twice a day for 2 days; ciprofloxacin (Cipro[1]), 500 mg as single dose, is also effective for adults. Third-generation cephalosporins used in treatment of the index case of meningitis are sufficient to eliminate carriage of the organism.

Chemoprophylaxis for *H. influenzae* type b is recommended for all household contacts of an index case if one of the contacts is an unvaccinated child younger than 4 years. If the index case is treated with ceftriaxone (Rocephin) or cefotaxime (Claforan), prophylaxis is not required, but if treated with ampicillin or chloramphenicol (Chloromycetin), prophylaxis is recommended to eliminate carriage. The recommended regimen for prophylaxis is rifampin,[1] 20 mg/kg (or 600 mg in adults) once a day for 4 days. With the near elimination of invasive infections caused by *H. influenzae* type b with the use of routine immunization of children with conjugate haemophilus vaccines, *H. influenzae* types A, F, and (rarely) other serotypes have emerged, and the use of prophylaxis is not recommended in these situations because sufficient data are not available to support its efficacy, nor has spread within contacts been documented.

Vaccines for Bacterial Meningitis

The universal recommendation for the use of protein-polysaccharide conjugate *H. influenzae* type b (HIB) vaccines in 1987 reduced the incidence of bacterial meningitis by this organism by greater than 97%. Three HIB vaccines (PedvaxHIB, ActHIB, HibTITER), licensed in the United States, are routinely given to children in dosage schedules employing three to four doses by 12 to 18 months of age (see www.cdc.gov).

A pneumococcal protein-polysaccharide conjugate vaccine (Prevnar) licensed in 2000 is routinely recommended for children and has markedly reduced the incidence of invasive infections with seven serotypes of pneumococci in children. This vaccine is also recommended for children at high risk of pneumococcal infections (e.g., HIV infection, asplenia, sickle cell disease, and others). A new Prevnar 13 with thirteen serotypes is now recommended to replace Prevnar 7 for routine use and is also recommended for persons over 50 years of age with high-risk conditions. The full recommendations for the use of this vaccine alone and in combination with the polysaccharide vaccine (Pneumovax 23) are available from the CDC. A pneumococcal polysaccharide vaccine (Pneumovax 23) is recommended for adults older than 65 years or for those over 50 years with risk factors (e.g., alcoholism, diabetes or other metabolic or renal disease, chronic pulmonary or cardiac disease). A polysaccharide conjugate vaccine (Prevnar) has been recently approved for limited adult use in high-risk patients; please see recommendations for use in adults and children at www.vaccines.gov. Although clear evidence for prevention of bacterial meningitis is lacking, evidence supports its efficacy against invasive pneumococcal diseases, many of which are the preceding infections leading to bacteremia and meningitis.

Three vaccines are available in the United States for prevention of meningococcal disease. All available vaccines provide protection against four serotypes: A, C, Y, and 1-135. Either of two protein-conjugate vaccines (Menactra and Menveo) are currently recommended for routine administration to all children at 11 to 12 years of age with a repeated dose at 5 years after the first dose. These vaccines are also recommended for persons at high risk for meningococcal disease (e.g., those with complement deficiencies, or asplenia, as well as microbiology technologists or travelers and workers in endemic areas) as early as 9 months of age, to be repeated at 12 months (Menactra) or equal to those who are 2 years of age or older (Menactra and Menveo) up to 55 years of age. It is recommended that younger patients at high risk be given a two-dose primary series and that all high-risk persons be given a second dose at 3 to 5 years depending upon risk and age at first dose (see the package inserts for dosing details). In addition, a single polysaccharide vaccine (Menomune) remains available for high-risk persons over 55 years of age.

References

Anderson EJ, Yogev LR. A rational approach to the management of ventricular shunt infections. Pediatric Infect Dis J 2005;24:557–8.

Andes DR, Craig WA. Pharmacokinetics and pharmacodynamics of antibiotics in meningitis. Infect Dis Clin North Am 1999;13(2):595–618.

Centers for Disease Control and Prevention. Use of 13-valent pneumococcal conjugate vaccine and 23 valent pneumococcal polysaccharide vaccine among children aged 6–18 years with immunocompromising conditions. MMWR 2012;61:816–9.

Centers for Disease Control and Prevention. Use of 13-valent pneumococcal conjugate vaccine and 23 valent pneumococcal polysaccharide vaccine for adults with immunocompromising conditions. Recommendations of the Advisory Committee on Immunization Practices (ACIP). MMWR 2013;62:521–4.

De Gans J, van de Beek. Dexamethasone in adults with bacterial meningitis. N Engl J Med 2002;347:1549–64.

Gray LD, Fedorko DP. Laboratory diagnosis of bacterial meningitis. Clin Microbiol Rev 1992;5:130–45.

Hussein AS, Shafran SD. Acute bacterial meningitis in adults: A 12-year review. Medicine (Baltimore) 2000;79:360–8.

Klein JO. Bacterial sepsis and meningitis. In: Remington JS, Klein JO, editors. Infectious Diseases of the Fetus and Newborn Infant. 5th ed. Philadelphia: WB Saunders; 2002. p. 943–98.

Klinger G, Chin C-Y, Beyene J, et al. Predicting the outcome of neonatal bacterial meningitis. Pediatrics 2000;106:477–82.

Odio CM, Faingezicht I, Paris M, et al. The beneficial effects of early dexamethasone administration in infants and children with bacterial meningitis. N Engl J Med 1991;324:1525–31.

Ronan A, Hogg GG, Klug CL. Cerebrospinal fluid shunt infections in children. Pediatr Infect Dis J 1995;14:782–6.

Schuchat A, Robinson K, Wenger JD, et al. Bacterial meningitis in the United States in 1995. N Engl J Med 1997;337:970–6.

Unhanand M, Mustapha MM, McCracken GH, et al. Gram-negative enteric bacillary meningitis: A twenty-one year experience. J Pediatr 1993;122:15-7.

Van de Beek D, de Gans J, Spanjaard L, et al. Clinical features and prognostic factors in adults with bacterial meningitis. N Engl J Med 2004;351:1849–58.

[1]Not FDA approved for this indication.

BRUCELLOSIS

Method of
Xinghong Yang, PhD

CURRENT DIAGNOSIS

- The diagnosis of brucellosis relies on the serologic reaction of antibodies to *Brucella's* lipopolysaccharide (LPS) located on the cell surface of smooth *Brucella melitensis, Brucella abortus,* and *Brucella suis.*
- Although the rough species, *Brucella canis,* does not have an intact LPS layer, its detection requires the antigens specifically prepared from *B. canis.*
- Rose Bengal test is regularly used to diagnose infection with smooth *Brucella* spp.
- When patients with brucellosis symptoms test negative by Rose Bengal test, the microagglutination test and 2-mercaptoethanol rapid slide agglutination test are used to determine whether the patient is infected with rough *Brucella* spp.

CURRENT THERAPY

- Three aspects of therapy are critical when using antibiotics to treat brucellosis:
  - The antibiotics must be able to penetrate macrophages to take effect because *Brucella* spp. are intracellular pathogens and normally reside within professional and nonprofessional phagocytes.
  - Multiple antibiotics are typically used to minimize relapses commonly seen when only a single antibiotic is used.
  - In complicated cases, in addition to antibiotic treatment, surgical intervention may be required to remove infected tissues.

Brucellosis is an ancient disease recorded by the Romans more than 2000 years ago. Since *Brucella* was identified as the cause of brucellosis in sick soldiers in 1887 by Sir David Bruce, brucellosis has been defined as an emerging disease. *Brucella* is a zoonotic bacterial pathogen, causing approximately 500,000 new cases annually worldwide. Although rarely fatal (<5% mortality rate), it causes an undulating fever leading to a dramatic decrease in the quality of life. Its incubation time can vary between 1 and 8 weeks, and often infection is asymptomatic; however, serious complications can lead to disability or death. Because no human vaccine is available, antibiotic therapy is the only option for treatment.

A total of ten *Brucella* species have been identified to date (Table 1). Four of these—*Brucella melitensis, Brucella abortus, Brucella suis,* and *Brucella canis*—commonly cause human brucellosis, and their genomes have been sequenced.

Epidemiology

Wildlife and domesticated animals can serve as natural reservoirs for *Brucella* spp. Humans acquire brucellae by exposure to contaminated foods or aerosols or by direct contact. Often contaminated or unpasteurized animal products, such as milk, soft cheese, and butter are consumed, causing oral exposure. *Brucella* spp. can spread via contaminated aerosols or by aerosolization of contaminated animal by-products, resulting in lung infection. *Brucella* can also infect by direct contact of skin cuts or abrasions with sick animals or their products and enter into the blood or lymphatic system and, regardless of route, produce infection, causing a bacteremia. Among the three routes, food ingestion and aerosol

TABLE 1 *Brucella* Species, Preferred Animal Hosts, and Human Infection Potential

SPECIES	HOST ANIMALS OR RESERVOIR	HUMAN INFECTION?*
B. melitensis	Goats, sheep, camels	Yes
B. abortus	Cows, bison, camels, yaks	Yes
B. suis	Pigs, wild hares, caribou, reindeer, wild rodents	Yes
B. canis	Dogs	Yes
B. cetaceae	Seals, harbor porpoises	Yes
B. inopinata	Unknown	Yes
B. microti	Common voles, red foxes, soil	Unknown
B. neotomae	Rodents	No
B. ovis	Sheep	No
B. pinnipedialis	Minke whales, dolphins	No

*"Yes" and "no" mean *Brucella* spp. are able or unable to infect humans, respectively; "unknown" indicates that it is not confirmed whether *Brucella* spp. are able to infect humans.

inhalation can result in brucellosis. Aerosolized brucellae can be used as a bioweapon because the dosage required for infecting 50% of the population is as little as 1885 colony forming units (CFUs).

Currently, brucellosis is endemic to Latin America, Africa, the Mediterranean rim, the Middle East, and Central Asia. To prevent human infection, animal immunization campaigns were adopted by many countries, including the United States and the former Soviet Union. The campaigns successfully curbed animal infection and consequently reduced human infection in these areas. When the programs were stopped, the incidence of brucellosis rapidly increased. Thus, maintenance of animal immunization programs is essential for protecting humans from infection.

Although transmission of brucellae among humans occurs rarely, several cases have been reported. It may be disseminated via sexual contact, milking, and organ transplantation. *B. melitensis* is the most commonly isolated species from brucellosis patients, followed in descending order by *B. abortus, B. suis,* and *B. canis. B. melitensis* and *B. abortus* can cause acute brucellosis and display the most severe symptoms, which can lead to complications. *B. suis* can cause extended duration of illness and results in suppurating lesions in infected tissues. Patients with *B. canis* infections display mild to moderate illness and rarely develop complications.

Risk Factors

The susceptible population includes those who live or travel in the endemic areas, particularly veterinarians, microbiologists, and those who work with or process livestock. The current animal vaccines are all infectious to human, and consequently veterinarians who administer these vaccines are at high risk for being infected. Microbiologists or laboratory workers also can acquire brucellosis through close contact, and indeed laboratory outbreaks are frequently reported. Thus, *Brucella* is also considered an occupational disease or a laboratory-acquired disease.

Pathophysiology

Brucella can be phagocytized by nonprofessional and professional phagocytic cells to establish an intracellular replication niche. Once inside host cells, brucellae stay in early-formed phagosomes, where they prevent phagosomes from fusing with late-formed endosomes and lysosomes and survive intracellularly. Antibiotics must be able to penetrate the host cell membrane to kill brucellae or inhibit their growth.

Brucella employs numerous mechanisms to evade detection by the immune system. Unlike LPS from other gram-negative bacteria, *Brucella* LPS does not trigger an inflammatory response or activate the alternative complement system, so it helps brucellae avoid recognition. *Brucella*'s LPS endows brucellae with a phenotype highly resistant to cationic bactericidal peptides. The intracellular brucellae do not cause cell death in macrophages or apoptosis in respiratory epithelial cells. Thus, the LPS reduces the chances of exposure to the immune system, which aids brucellae survival and meanwhile diminishes the stimulation of the host immune system. *Brucella* inhibits the macrophage response to interferon-γ (IFN-γ), a critical cytokine for stimulating innate and adaptive immunity. Additionally, to maintain vigorous intracellular survival and replication, brucellae equip their outer membranes with phosphatidylcholine and synthesize cyclic β-1,2-glucans to preclude fusion between phagosome and lysosome.

Diagnosis

Accurate diagnosis of brucellosis is always a challenge because brucellosis exhibits symptoms similar to numerous other febrile illnesses (Table 2). In many patients, the symptoms are mild and moderate; thus, in a number of cases the diagnosis might not be even considered.

Isolation of brucellae from blood, bone marrow, urine, cerebrospinal fluid, or joint aspirate serves as the gold standard for diagnosing brucellosis. However, under many circumstances, brucellae cannot be cultured from patients' samples. The rate of blood culture positivity ranges from 16% to 90%. Hence, other indices are used to identify brucellosis. Testing for antibodies against *Brucella* is commonly used. *Brucella* agglutination titer of 1:160 is considered a clear diagnostic index as long as the patient presents signs and symptoms of the disease. Recommended tests are the Rose Bengal test, the serum agglutination test alone or with 2-mercaptoethanol or dithiothreitol reduction, Coombs' antiglobulin, the complement-fixation test, and the enzyme-linked immunosorbent assay (ELISA). The results of a combination of tests such as the serum agglutination test and Coombs' antiglobulin can be used to assess the stage of evolution of the disease at the time of diagnosis. In the blood sample, infection may also be associated with low levels of red and white blood cells, low platelets, and elevated liver function. A biopsy of body tissues can also assist in making the diagnosis because patients can experience bone marrow hypoplasia and/or liver fibrosis and cirrhosis.

Depending on the patient's symptoms and severity of the illness, an investigation may be undertaken. Examinations may include computed tomography (CT) scan or magnetic resonance imaging (MRI) to identify signs of inflammation or abscesses in the brain or other tissues. Electrocardiogram (ECG) may be performed to investigate heart infection or damage, and x-rays can show bone and joint deformations.

TABLE 2 Symptom Pattern of Human Brucellosis

SYMPTOMS	PERCENT*
Fever	93
Chills	82
Sweats	87
Aches	91
Lack of energy	95
Joint and back pain	86
Arthritis	40
Spinal tenderness	48
Headache	81
Loss of appetite	78
Weight loss	65
Constipation	47
Abdominal pain	45
Diarrhea	7
Cough	24
Testicular pain, epididymoorchitis	21[†]
Rash	14
Sleep disturbance	37
Ill appearance	25
Pallor	22
Lymphadenopathy	32
Splenomegaly	25
Hepatomegaly	19
Jaundice	1
Central nervous system disorder	4
Cardiac murmur	3
Pneumonia	1

Data from Corbel MJ: Brucellosis in humans and animals. Geneva, World Health Organization, 2006.
*Percentage based on 500 patients.
[†]Percentage based on 290 male patients.

Differential Diagnosis

Because human brucellosis mimics the symptoms of many other diseases, disease complications vary from patient to patient, and the latency time between exposure and the occurrence of symptoms is irregular and relatively long, making the differential diagnosis tedious and difficult. Therefore, prior to diagnosis, answers to three questions can help narrow the focus to brucellosis:
- Did the patient have direct contact with large or small ruminants, their carcasses, or their products?
- Did the patient consume unpasteurized dairy products?
- Does the patient live in or travel to areas where brucellae are endemic in humans or epidemic in animals?

In spite of the difficulties in diagnosing brucellosis, some clinical features can still be used to distinguish brucellosis from other infectious diseases. If left untreated, fever of brucellosis displays an undulating pattern. In about 50% of patients, the fever of brucellosis is associated with musculoskeletal symptoms; however, these symptoms are rarely observed in typhoid and malaria fevers.

In patients with hepatosplenomegaly or lymphadenopathy, the differential diagnosis includes glandular fever–like illnesses, such as cytomegalovirus (CMV) infection, Epstein-Barr virus (EBV) infection, HIV infection, toxoplasmosis, and tuberculosis (TB). CMV patients can develop antibodies to the virus. Also, in the active infection phase, CMV can be detected from the blood, saliva, urine, or other body tissues. These indices can be used to differentiate CMV infection from the brucellosis. EBV patients have an elevated white blood cell count, an increased total number of lymphocytes, and greater than 10% atypical lymphocytes, but brucellosis patients usually show a decrease in the white blood cell count.

HIV infection can induce antibodies against HIV, and virologic tests can detect HIV antigens or RNA. HIV infection can be further confirmed by a supplemental antibody test, such as Western blot and indirect immunofluorescence assay. Brucellosis patients' sera do not display any reaction in these tests. For toxoplasmosis patients, serum immunoglobulin (Ig)G and IgM titers can be used to detect whether the patient is infected by *Toxoplasma*.

For TB patients, a skin test or a special TB blood test can be used for diagnosis, and other tests such as chest x-ray and a sample of sputum coughed up from deep in the lungs may be used for confirmation. In patients with osteomyelitis or septic arthritis, the most important alternative diagnosis is TB.

In patients with acute epididymoorchitis, the differential diagnosis includes mumps and surgical problems, such as torsion.

For mumps patients, buccal swab specimens are collected for viral detection via culturing virus in cell lines or using real-time polymerase chain reaction (RT-PCR) to detect mumps viral RNA. For testicular torsion in men, an ultrasound examination of the spermatic cord can provide valuable information regarding whether the patient requires emergency surgery.

Treatment

To date, the only option for treating brucellosis is by means of antibiotics. However, in cases of complications, such as heart brucellosis and spinal brucellosis, antibiotic treatment in combination with surgical intervention may be needed. Antibiotics commonly used are doxycycline (Vibramycin), rifampin (Rifadin),[1] streptomycin, cotrimoxazole (TMP-SMX [Bactrim]),[1] and gentamicin (Garamycin)[1] (Table 3). Regimens of a combination of 2 or 3 antibiotics are recommended to reduce the unacceptably high relapse rates with monotherapy. Antibiotic regimens vary and depend on the patient's age, the severity of the disease, pregnancy, cost of the medicine, and availability of the medicine.

Doxycycline combined with rifampin[1] for a full 6-week course is a commonly used therapy recommended by the World Health Organization. It is considered the most effective regimen, particularly when combined with an aminoglycoside. In patients with spondylitis or sacroiliitis, doxycycline plus streptomycin is an effective combination. For pediatric patients older than 8 years, doxycycline plus gentamicin[1] is the recommended therapy. For children younger than 8 years, trimethoprim-sulfamethoxazole (TMP-SMX) therapy for 3 weeks followed by a 5-day course of gentamicin[1] is most effective. TMP-SMX[1] is also effective in treating pregnant women, either as a single agent or in combination with rifampin[1] or gentamicin[1] (see Table 3).

Once brucellosis is diagnosed, immediate therapy is critical because it can alleviate symptoms and also prevent the development of complications. Nevertheless, even when treatment is executed according to the doctor's prescription, rates of relapse can still reach up to 5% to 10%. Depending on the severity or complications of the illness and the treatment time applied, the recovery time can last from several weeks to several months.

Monitoring

After antibiotic therapy is initiated, patients are periodically monitored by doctors to evaluate whether the therapeutic regimen is effective and whether relapse occurs. Because relapse is indicated by the recurrence of a positive blood culture result during the post-therapy period and/or signs and symptoms of brucellosis infection, routine examination of the patient includes serum culture for *Brucella* organism and assessment for brucellosis symptoms after treatment phase. In addition to monitoring brucellosis symptoms, both doctors and patients should monitor any adverse effects of medication. For instance, adverse reactions to TMP-SMX occur in 50% to 100% of patients with AIDS compared to about 14% of patients without AIDS. Up to 57% of AIDS patients treated with TMP-SMX[1] require a change in therapy owing to the adverse effects.

Generally, brucellosis patients should be followed clinically for up to 2 years to detect relapse. Patients should be monitored for regaining of body weight. IgG antibody should be checked by serum agglutination test for levels that remain in the diagnostic range for more than 2 years. Complement fixation titers should fall to normal within 1 year of treatment. Relapse should respond to a prolonged course of the same therapy originally used.

Complications

Brucellae are transported into the lymphatic system and can replicate in spleen, liver, kidney, breast tissue, and joints to cause both localized and systemic infections. Infection of the reproductive system can cause fetal abortion. Owing to the low virulence, low toxicity, and multiple mechanisms to protect them from the immune system, brucellae can survive and reproduce in nearly any tissues or organs. At one year following infection, the disease can develop into chronic brucellosis that can further cause one or multiple complications in one organ or the whole body.

There are seven major types of complications from *Brucella* infection.

- Endocarditis: Brucellae can infect the heart's inner lining, which can destroy the heart valves and, if left untreated, will lead to death of the patient.

[1]Not FDA approved for this indication.

[1]Not FDA approved for this indication.

Brucellosis

TABLE 3   Treatment for Brucellosis

MEDICATION	ADULT DOSAGE	DOSAGE ADJUSTMENT			ADVERSE EFFECTS
		PEDIATRIC DOSAGE	RENAL FAILURE	HEPATIC INSUFFICIENCY	
Doxycycline (Vibramycin)	100 mg PO q12h	2.2–4.4 mg/kg[3] PO div q12h (>8 y)	No change	No change	Dizziness, headache, photosensitivity, nausea, diarrhea, hemolytic anemia, hepatotoxicity
Rifampin (Rifadin)[1]	600–900 mg PO qd	20 mg/kg PO qd (do not exceed 600 mg qd)	No change	Moderate: caution Severe: avoid	Heartburn, epigastric distress, anorexia, nausea, flatulence, cramps, liver dysfunction, jaundice
Streptomycin	15 mg/kg IM q24h *or* 1 g IM qd × 2–3 wk	20–40 mg/kg IM qd (do not exceed 1 g/d)	Necessary	No change	Nausea, vomiting, vertigo, face paresthesias, rash, fever, urticaria, angioedema, eosinophilia
Trimethoprim-sulfamethoxazole (TMP-SMX) (Bactrim)[1]	1 DS tab PO q12h (160 mg TMP/ 800 mg SMX)	8–12 mg/kg TMP PO given in divided doses q12h	Necessary Avoid use in CrCl <15 mL/min	No change	Nausea, vomiting, anorexia, rash, urticaria
Gentamicin (Garamycin)[1]	2 mg/kg[3] IM/IV q8h *or* 5 mg/kg IM/IV q24h[1] *or* 240 mg q24h	2.5 mg/kg q8–12h IM/IV	Necessary	No change	Nephrotoxicity, dizziness, vertigo, tinnitus, hearing loss, numbness, skin tingling, muscle twitching, convulsions

[1]Not FDA approved for this indication.
[3]Exceeds dosage recommended by the manufacturer.
Abbreviations: CrCl = creatinine clearance; DS = double strength.

- Meningitis and encephalitis: Brucellae can infect the central nervous system to cause an inflammation of the brain, the membranes surrounding the brain, and the spinal cord. This is fatal if the patient is not treated in time.
- Arthritis: Osteoarthritis caused by *Brucella* infection is typically associated with pain, stiffness, and swelling of the joints, such as the knees, hips, ankles, wrists, spine, shoulder, elbow, sternoclavicular, and small joints. Spondylitis caused by brucellae is characterized by joint inflammation between the vertebrae bones of the spine or between the spine and pelvis. Spondylitis is difficult to treat and can cause lasting damage. These osteoarticular complications are the clinical forms most commonly observed.
- Epididymitis and epididymoorchitis: Brucellae can infect the epididymis to cause swelling and pain of the testicle.
- Cutaneous complications: Brucellae can infect skin to cause lesions, rashes, nodules, erythema nodosum, papules, petechiae, and purpura.
- Respiratory complications: Inhalation of brucellae can result in lung infection, which can lead to pneumonia, bronchopneumonia, pleural effusion with a predominance of monocytic or lymphocytic infiltrates, and paroxysmal dry cough.
- Hematologic complications: Aspartate aminotransferase (AST) or alanine aminotransferase (ALT) levels can be elevated and are associated with pain in the right upper quadrant or jaundice.

Complications are common in brucellosis patients. Young patients tend to have cutaneous, hematologic, and respiratory complications. Adult patients tend toward osteoarticular and cardiac complications. Middle-aged patients tend to develop genitourinary, neurologic, and gastrointestinal complications.

Prevention

Maintaining hygienic habits is very important for avoiding *Brucella* infection. These include consuming only pasteurized milk and cheese. Meat must be cooked thoroughly before consumption. In these regards, education is beneficial for preventing infection by this pathogen. People who handle animals or animal products should wear personal protective equipment, including glasses, rubber gloves, and clothing to protect skin and eyes from exposure or direct contact. Laboratory workers should use a Biosafety Level 3 (BSL-3) facility to handle the *Brucella* organisms and work according to the laboratory's standard operating procedures. Animal immunization programs must be maintained all over the world to cut off the transmission chain from livestock to humans. In addition, primary care physicians should be familiar with the clinical and laboratory findings of brucellosis symptoms and complications.

References

Centers for Disease Control and Prevention. Sexually Transmitted Diseases Treatment Guidelines, 2010: Epididymitis, Available at http://www.cdc.gov/std/treatment/2010/epididymitis.htm [accessed 07.09.15].

Corbel MJ. Brucellosis in humans and animals. Geneva: World Health Organization; 2006.

Dokuzoguz B, Nurcan Baykam N. Brucellosis. In: Bope ET, Kellerman RD, Rakel RE, editors. Conn's Current Therapy 2011. Philadelphia: Saunders; 2011. p. 74–8.

Gür A, Geyik MF, Dikici B, et al. Complications of brucellosis in different age groups: A study of 283 cases in southeastern Anatolia of Turkey. Yonsei Med J 2003;44:33–44.

Harrison's Practice. Answers on Demand. Brucellosis, Available at http://www.harrisonspractice.com/practice/ub/view/Harrisons%20Practice/141056/all/Brucellosis; 2012 [accessed 07.05.12].

Joint WHO/FAO Expert Committee on Brucellosis. Sixth report. World Health Organ Tech Rep Ser 1986;740:1–132.

Mayo Clinic. Brucellosis: Complications, Available at http://www.mayoclinic.com/health/brucellosis/DS00837/DSECTION=complications; 2012 [accessed 07.09.15].

Pappas G, Akritidis N, Bosilkovski M, et al. Brucellosis. N Engl J Med 2005;352:2325–36.

Pappas G, Bosilkovski M, Akritidis N, et al. Brucellosis and the respiratory system. Clin Infect Dis 2003;37:e95–399.

Skalsky K, Yahav D, Bishara J, et al. Treatment of human brucellosis: Systematic review and meta-analysis of randomised controlled trials. BMJ 2008;336:701–4.

Yang X, Skyberg JA, Cao L, et al. Progress in Brucella vaccine development. Front Biol 2013;8:60–77. doi:10.1007/s11515-012-1196-0.

CAMPYLOBACTER

Method of
Gregory Juckett, MD, MPH

CURRENT DIAGNOSIS

- *Campylobacter jejuni* and *Campylobacter coli* are the leading causes of childhood and traveler's diarrhea worldwide.
- Raw or undercooked poultry (or cross-contamination with poultry juices) is the best-known source of infection.
- Infection is characterized by abrupt onset of crampy abdominal pain, nausea, and profuse diarrhea or dysentery.
- A prodrome of high fever and myalgias precedes diarrheal illness in one third of cases.
- *Campylobacter* gastroenteritis can mimic acute appendicitis and inflammatory bowel disease.
- Late complications of *Campylobacter* infection include reactive arthritis and Guillain-Barré syndrome 1 to 2 weeks after diarrhea.

CURRENT THERAPY

- Antibiotics are not essential for most healthy patients because the illness is self-limited.
- Azithromycin (Zithromax)[1] 500 mg daily × 3 days (pediatric dosage, 10 mg/kg/day) is effective if given early in the course (less than 5% resistance).
- Quinolone antibiotics have been effective, but resistance is developing, particularly in South and Southeast Asia owing to the use of quinolones in poultry feed.
- Prevention entails reducing *Campylobacter* colonization of poultry and using proper food-handling techniques. Vaccination may be possible in the future.

[1]Not FDA approved for this indication.

Epidemiology

Campylobacter enteritis is one of the most common forms of bacterial diarrhea in the world and the most common food-related illness in North America. Most cases (95%) are caused by *Campylobacter jejuni*, a commensal Gram-negative bacteria found in the gut of animals, particularly poultry. The related *Campylobacter coli* causes a clinically identical but much less common (5%) infection. Children in developing countries are usually infected before age 2 years.

Foodborne outbreaks affect adults in developed counties as well as travelers to developing nations. *Campylobacter* is a common cause of traveler's diarrhea, and 13% of U.S. *Campylobacter* infections are acquired abroad. Most infections are due to cross-contamination of food with raw poultry (unwashed cutting boards) or from drinking unpasteurized milk or contaminated water. Infections increase in spring and peak during the summer months. The typical incubation period is 3 to 4 days (range, 1–8 days), with the illness lasting up to a week. After recovery, the bacteria are excreted in the feces for several weeks and may be transmitted by improper hand washing, although person-to-person transmission is unusual.

Risk Factors

Anyone exposed to improperly prepared food, unpasteurized milk, or unchlorinated water is at risk. Improperly cooked poultry or food contaminated by raw poultry is the most common source.

[1]Not FDA approved for this indication.

Contact with infected pets is a common cause of childhood exposure. Elderly, immunocompromised, or very young patients are at additional risk for prolonged symptoms, invasive disease, and hospitalization. Proton-pump inhibitors, by reducing protective stomach acid, appear to increase the risk of campylobacteriosis and other bacterial enteritides.

Pathophysiology

Campylobacter infection starts in the small intestine (jejunum, ileum) and spreads to the colon. Symptoms can begin with enteritis (profuse watery stools) or with frank colitis (bloody stools). Colitis thus can mimic inflammatory bowel disease or appendicitis. Inflammatory bowel disease may be excluded by colon biopsies, which demonstrate acute but not chronic inflammatory change.

Prevention

Proper food-handling techniques are the best means of prevention. Poultry products should be cooked until an internal temperature of 165 °F is reached and all juices run clear. Hands must be washed with soap after contact with raw poultry or animal feces and after using the rest room. Cross-contamination should be avoided by careful disinfection of countertops and utensils after preparing meats or, better yet, using entirely separate surfaces. Only one drop of poultry juice (<500 organisms) is sufficient to cause disease. Although not currently feasible, *Campylobacter* vaccination has been proposed for prevention.

Clinical Manifestations

Campylobacter enteritis typically manifests as sudden onset of cramping, nausea, vomiting, and diarrhea, often indistinguishable from other bacterial diarrheas. Most cases are self-limited, with recovery in 3 to 4 days. About a third of patients experience a febrile prodrome with myalgias occurring for about a day before onset of diarrheal illness. Dysenteric (bloody) stools are common (15%) and imply more-invasive disease. Like *Yersinia*, *Campylobacter* infection can mimic acute appendicitis (ileocecitis), especially if this occurs in the absence of significant diarrhea. Computed tomography or ultrasound in bacterial pseudoappendicitis usually documents mesenteric adenitis, and surgery can be avoided. In young children, seizures can occur before the onset of diarrhea and fever, and dysenteric illness (50%) is more common.

Diagnosis

Most cases are diagnosed by stool culture in the setting of acute diarrhea and crampy abdominal pain. On microscopic examination, *C. jejuni* is a Gram-negative, spiral-shaped rod with a single polar flagellum at one or both ends. It can be isolated in culture media containing cephalothin, to which it is usually resistant. Darkfield microscopic stool examination is occasionally attempted for early diagnosis, but this is not very sensitive. Polymerase chain reaction analysis of stool samples is a very promising diagnostic approach, although it is not yet available in many laboratories. Later diagnosis, subsequent to resolution of diarrhea, requires serologic testing.

Differential Diagnosis

Campylobacter infections are clinically indistinguishable from other bacterial enteritides such as salmonellosis and shigellosis. All of these produce fever, cramps, diarrhea, and dysentery. However, *Campylobacter* colitis is more likely to mimic inflammatory bowel disease and appendicitis and to later cause Guillain-Barré syndrome.

Treatment

Most cases of *Campylobacter* infection are mild and self-limited, and antibiotics are not required. If antibiotics are to be used, they are most effective if given early to high-risk patients, because delayed treatment (e.g., after positive stool culture results) is less likely to affect outcome. First-line choices include macrolides,

such as azithromycin (<5% resistance), or fluoroquinolones, such as ciprofloxacin (Cipro). Azithromycin (Zithromax)[1] is preferred for traveler's diarrhea acquired in South and Southeast Asia, where quinolone-resistant *Campylobacter* is common. Azithromycin has supplanted erythromycin (Ery-Tab)[1] because it is better tolerated and has fewer GI side effects. Rarely, intravenous aminoglycosides or carbapenems are necessary in very ill patients unable to take oral medication.

Unfortunately, quinolone resistance is not limited to Asia. Resistance has also increased in the United States. The widespread practice of using antibiotics, especially fluoroquinolones (enrofloxacin [Baytril]),[2] as additives to chicken feed has resulted in increasing quinolone resistance in *Campylobacter* strains found in poultry, the major source of infection. The Foodborne Diseases Active Surveillance Network (FoodNet) of the Centers for Disease Control and Prevention (CDC) found that 40% of U.S. poultry products were contaminated with *Campylobacter*, and 10% of these strains were ciprofloxacin resistant. Although fluoroquinolones were removed from U.S. animal feed in 2005, they continue to be used overseas. A newer strategy involves supplementing poultry feed with bacteriocins, nontoxic antimicrobial peptides, to reduce *Campylobacter* colonization. Irradiation of poultry meat might also be effective.

Empiric self-treatment of traveler's diarrhea is intended to shorten the duration of symptoms and involves immediate ciprofloxacin (Cipro) or azithromycin (Zithromax)[1] at the onset of diarrheal illness. One or two doses of antibiotics are usually sufficient to abort symptoms, and prolonged treatment is usually unnecessary. Loperamide (Imodium) might help control diarrhea in adults, but it should be avoided in dysenteric illness and in young children.

Complications

Campylobacter complications can occur either acutely or following the illness. Acute complications include cholecystitis, pseudoappendicitis, peritonitis, sepsis, and chest pain (pericarditis) (Box 1). Rashes, such as vasculitis or erythema nodosum, can occur. Rarely, focal extraintestinal infections such as septic arthritis or osteitis develop. Childhood complications include meningitis and encephalopathy, and dysenteric illness in infants occasionally mimics intussusception. *Campylobacter* can provoke postinfectious irritable bowel syndrome and is suspected of contributing to inflammatory bowel disease by damaging the intestinal epithelium, leading to chronic inflammation.

Late-term complications include Guillain-Barré syndrome and reactive arthritis. About one in a thousand *Campylobacter* infections is complicated by Guillain-Barré syndrome, which occurs several weeks after infection and carries a worse prognosis when associated with *Campylobacter*. As much as 30% to 40% of all Guillain-Barré syndrome has been attributed to *Campylobacter*

---

[1]Not FDA approved for this indication.
[2]Not available in the United States.

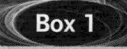
Box 1   Acute and Chronic *Campylobacter* Complications

Acute Complications
Acute colitis, dysentery
Cholecystitis
Pseudoappendicitis (mesenteric adenitis)
Peritonitis
Pericarditis (chest pain)
Postinfectious irritable bowel syndrome

Chronic Complications
Inflammatory bowel disease (possible contributor)
Guillain-Barré syndrome (1:1000 cases)
Reactive arthritis

infection, and even subclinical cases have been associated by later serologic testing.

Reactive arthritis following *Campylobacter* infection is common and also appears unrelated to the severity of the preceding diarrhea. Swelling and arthralgia in the hands, wrists, knees, or ankles develops 1 to 2 weeks following diarrhea and can persist for weeks to months. Nonsteroidal antiinflammatory drugs are usually helpful, and complete recovery is the rule.

References

Centers for Disease Control and Prevention. Campylobacter: General information, Available at http://www.cdc.gov/nczved/divisions/dfbmd/diseases/campylobacter/; 2014 [accessed July 9, 2015].

Gupta A, Nelson JM, Barrett TJ, et al. Antimicrobial resistance among *Campylobacter* strains, United States, 1997–2001. Emerg Infect Dis 2004;10:1102–9.

Kalischuk L, Buret A. A role for *Campylobacter jejuni*–induced enteritis in inflammatory bowel disease? Am J Physiol Gastrointest Liver Physiol 2010;298:G1–9.

Nachamkin I, Allos BM, Ho T. *Campylobacter* species and Guillain-Barré syndrome. Clin Microbiol Rev 1998;11:555–67.

Neal KR, Scott HM, Slack RC, Logan RF. Omeprazole as a risk factor for *Campylobacter* gastroenteritis: Case control study. BMJ 1996;312:414–5.

Neal KR, Wright JM. Reactive arthritis–like symptoms following gastroenteritis—an increased risk with severe *Campylobacter* infection. Int J Med Microbiol 2001;291:110.

Nelson JM, Chiller TM, Powers JH, Angulo FJ. Fluoroquinolone-resistant *Campylobacter* species and the withdrawal of fluoroquinolones from use in poultry: A public health success story. Clin Infect Dis 2007;44:977–80.

Nelson JM, Smith KE, Vugia DJ, et al. Prolonged diarrhea due to ciprofloxacin-resistant *Campylobacter* infection. J Infect Dis 2004;190:1150–7.

Skirrow MB, Blaser MJ. Campylobacter jejuni. In: Blaser MJ, Smith PD, Radin JI, et al., Infections of the Gastrointestinal Tract. 2nd ed Philadelphia: Lippincott Willians & Wilkins; 2002 p. 719–739.

Svetich E, Stern N. Bacteriocins to control *Campylobacter* spp. in poultry—a review. Poult Sci 2010;89:1763–8.

Ternhag A, Asikainen T, Giesecke J, Ekdahl K. A meta-analysis on the effects of antibiotic treatment on duration of symptoms caused by infection with *Campylobacter* species. Clin Infect Dis 2007;44:696–700.

Tribble DR, Sanders JW, Pang LW, et al. Traveler's diarrhea in Thailand: Randomized, double-blind trial comparing single-dose and 3-day azithromycin-based regimens with a 3-day levofloxacin regimen. Clin Infect Dis 2007;44:338–46.

CAT SCRATCH DISEASE

Method of
Ronen Ben-Ami, MD

CURRENT DIAGNOSIS

- The combination of a compatible clinical syndrome of regional lymphadenopathy with a primary inoculation lesion and cat contact is highly suggestive of cat scratch disease.
- Results of *Bartonella henselae* serology are helpful in confirming the diagnosis; however, up to 20% of patients remain seronegative throughout their disease.
- Detection of *B. henselae* DNA by polymerase chain reaction from pus obtained by needle aspiration or lymph node biopsy is a highly sensitive diagnostic modality and may be particularly useful in seronegative patients.

CURRENT THERAPY

- Typical cat scratch disease is a self-limited disease; therefore, systemic antimicrobials are not routinely indicated in immunocompetent patients with uncomplicated cat scratch disease.
- Indications for antimicrobial therapy include an immunocompromised host, endocarditis, retinitis, and other atypical syndromes.

- Treatment may also be considered for patients who have typical cat scratch disease and who have extensive or bulky lymphadenopathy and are highly symptomatic.
- Suppurative lymph nodes should be drained by large-bore needle aspiration.

Cat scratch disease is a worldwide zoonotic infection caused by *Bartonella henselae*, an intracellular, pleomorphic, Gram-negative bacillus. Other *Bartonella* species have rarely been implicated. The disease typically manifests as benign regional lymphadenopathy, but atypical disease can involve almost any organ system and is associated with significant morbidity.

Epidemiology

B. henselae infection is widespread among domestic cats and other felids worldwide, and serologic studies indicate a higher prevalence in warm, humid climates. Transmission among cats occurs via an arthropod vector, the cat flea *Ctenocephalides felis*. *B. henselae* bacteremia is detected at higher rates in feral than in domesticated cats and in kittens as compared to adult cats, explaining the higher infectivity of these animals. Cats infected with *B. henselae* are asymptomatic. Transmission to humans occurs via a scratch, bite, or lick; arthropod vectors have not been shown to play a role in human infection.

Cat scratch disease has been estimated to occur in the United States at a rate approaching 10 per 100,000 population. There is some seasonality, with incidence peaking between September and January. Although traditionally considered a disease of childhood, epidemiologic surveys have found a similar incidence of cat scratch disease in adults, and 6% of patients are aged 60 years or older. Cat contact is the most important risk factor: Almost all patients are cat owners or were otherwise exposed to cats, and about half can recall a recent bite or scratch, most commonly by a kitten.

Clinical Manifestations

Cat scratch disease is divided into two clinical syndromes. Typical cat scratch disease is a subacute, self-limited regional lymphadenopathy and constitutes 80% to 90% of cases. Atypical cat scratch disease encompasses Parinaud's oculoglandular syndrome and other clinical entities with systemic extranodal involvement. Bacillary angiomatosis and bacillary peliosis are manifestations of *B. henselae* infection in immunocompromised persons and are not discussed here.

Typical Cat Scratch Disease

A primary skin lesion, usually a papule or pustule, appears at the site of inoculation 3 to 10 days after cat contact and persists for 1 to 3 weeks. Regional lymphadenopathy develops within 1 to 7 weeks and resolves spontaneously after 2 to 4 months. The primary lesion is still present in about two thirds of patients when they present for evaluation of lymphadenopathy. The most commonly involved lymph nodes are, in descending order of frequency, axillary and epitrochlear nodes, head and neck nodes, and femoral and inguinal nodes. One third of patients develop lymphadenopathy at multiple sites. Lymph nodes are often painful and red; suppuration occurs in 10% of nodes. Mild constitutional symptoms, including low-grade fever and malaise, are noted in about half the cases. Rash, night sweats, anorexia, and weight loss are uncommon. Infection results in lifelong immunity.

Atypical Cat Scratch Disease

Parinaud's oculoglandular syndrome, the most common form of atypical cat scratch disease, is a specific type of regional lymphadenopathy that occurs following conjunctival inoculation of *B. henselae*. The syndrome includes granulomatous conjunctivitis and preauricular lymphadenopathy. Endocarditis and encephalitis represent severe forms of *B. henselae* infection and are more common in elderly patients. Encephalitis manifests with various degrees of altered mental status, agitation, headache, and seizures.

TABLE 1	Antibiotic Treatment Regimens for Cat Scratch Disease			
CLINICAL SYNDROME	**FIRST CHOICE**	**SECOND CHOICE**	**COMMENTS**	
Typical cat scratch disease	Not indicated*	Azithromycin (Zithromax)[1] 500 mg PO on day 1, then 250 mg PO × 4 days	Drain suppurative nodes using large-bore aspiration	
Endocarditis	Gentamicin (Garamycin)[1] 1 mg/kg IV q8h × >14 days plus doxycycline (Vibramycin) 100 mg IV/PO bid × 6 wk	Doxycycline 100 mg PO bid plus rifampicin (Rifadin)[1] 300 mg PO bid × 6 wk	Some experts recommend extending oral doxycycline treatment × 3–6 mo Surgical valve excision may be required	
Neuroretinitis	Doxycycline 100 mg PO bid plus rifampicin[1] 300 mg PO bid × 4–6 wk	NA	Spontaneous resolution is the rule; the utility of treatment remains unproven	
Other atypical cat scratch disease	As for neuroretinitis	NA	Treatment duration should be individualized	

[1]Not FDA approved for this indication.
*Treatment may be considered for patients with bulky or extensive lymphadenopathy and for immunocompromised patients.
Abbreviation: NA = not available.

Cerebrospinal fluid lymphocytic pleocytosis occurs in only one third of cases, and brain-imaging studies usually fail to show any abnormalities. Neuroretinitis manifests as sudden unilateral loss of visual acuity. The diagnosis is suspected on the basis of typical findings on fundoscopic examination: papilledema and macular exudates in a starlike configuration. However, these findings are not pathognomonic of cat scratch disease. Other infrequent manifestations are self-limited granulomatous hepatitis and splenitis and osteoarticular disease. Prolonged fever of unknown origin has been described in children and adolescents.

Diagnosis

A compatible clinical syndrome in a person with a positive history of cat exposure suggests cat scratch disease. The diagnosis is most commonly confirmed with specific serologic assays. Immunofluorescence and enzyme immunoassays are comparably sensitive, although cross-reactivity can occur with other organisms such as *Chlamydia* species, *Coxiella burnetii*, and non-*henselae Bartonella* species. A single elevated titer of immunoglobulin (Ig)M or IgG in the acute phase or a fourfold increase of IgG in convalescent serum supports the diagnosis.

Biopsy and histopathologic examination of lymph nodes are usually only performed when malignancy is suspected. Necrotizing granulomas are typically observed. The Warthin-Starry stain can demonstrate pleomorphic gram-negative bacilli; however, the sensitivity of this method is too low to be clinically useful. Similarly, culture lacks sensitivity and requires prolonged incubation, making it impractical for routine use.

Polymerase chain reaction assays for the detection of *B. henselae* in pus aspirated from suppurative lymph nodes or primary skin lesions is highly sensitive and specific, and it can be performed with a rapid turnaround time. However, these assays are not widely available in most clinical microbiology laboratories.

Differential Diagnosis

Cat scratch disease should be differentiated from other infectious and noninfectious causes of regional lymphadenopathy. Importantly, lymphoma and solid tumors with metastases to lymph nodes may be confused with cat scratch disease. Malignancy should be suspected in patients who have marked constitutional symptoms, who are seronegative, or whose lymphadenopathy fails to resolve spontaneously after more than 6 months. Unlike cat scratch disease, pyogenic lymphadenitis manifests with rapid progression, high-grade fever, and a septic-appearing patient. Mycobacterial infection, syphilis, bubonic plague, tularemia, histoplasmosis, and sporotrichosis should be considered based on the presence of specific risk factors and endemic exposures. *Bartonella* endocarditis must be differentiated from other causes of culture-negative endocarditis, specifically Q fever and brucellosis.

Treatment

Because of the self-limiting course of typical cat scratch disease, patients usually only require observation and reassurance of its benign nature. The goals of therapy are alleviation of symptoms in patients with bulky lymphadenopathy and drainage of suppurating lymph nodes to prevent spontaneous formation of chronic sinus tracts. If drug treatment is initiated, azithromycin (Zithromax)[1] is the agent of choice based on a small randomized placebo-controlled study that showed more-rapid resolution of lymphadenopathy in the azithromycin arm as determined by ultrasound. Suppurative nodes should be drained by large-bore needle aspiration. Incisional drainage is best avoided because it can promote sinus tract formation.

Atypical cat scratch disease syndromes usually require treatment, but there are scant data to support specific regimens, and treatment duration is not well defined. For patients with endocarditis, treatment with an aminoglycoside for at least 14 days is associated with a higher likelihood of recovery and survival (Table 1).

Prevention

Flea control in domestic cats can reduce the likelihood of *Bartonella* bacteremia and transmission to humans. Bites and scratches should be promptly rinsed. HIV-infected patients and other immunocompromised persons should be cautioned about the risks of cat exposure because they are susceptible to disseminated visceral *B. henselae* infection, as well as other zoonotic infections such as toxoplasmosis.

[1]Not FDA approved for this indication.

References

Ben-Ami R, Ephros M, Avidor B, et al. Cat-scratch disease in elderly patients. Clin Infect Dis 2005;41:969–74.

Giladi M, Kletter Y, Avidor B, et al. Enzyme immunoassay for the diagnosis of cat-scratch disease defined by polymerase chain reaction. Clin Infect Dis 2001;33:1852–8.

Hansmann Y, DeMartino S, Piemont Y, et al. Diagnosis of cat scratch disease with detection of *Bartonella henselae* by PCR: A study of patients with lymph node enlargement. J Clin Microbiol 2005;43:3800–6.

Jackson LA, Perkins BA, Wenger JD. Cat scratch disease in the United States: An analysis of three national databases. Am J Public Health 1993;83:1707–11.

Jacobs RF, Schutze GE. *Bartonella henselae* as a cause of prolonged fever and fever of unknown origin in children. Clin Infect Dis 1998;26:80–4.

Raoult D, Fournier PE, Vandenesch F, et al. Outcome and treatment of *Bartonella* endocarditis. Arch Intern Med 2003;163:226–30.

Rolain JM, Brouqui P, Koehler JE, et al. Recommendations for treatment of human infections caused by *Bartonella* species. Antimicrob Agents Chemother 2004;48:1921–33.

Zangwill KM, Hamilton DH, Perkins BA, et al. Cat scratch disease in Connecticut. Epidemiology, risk factors, and evaluation of a new diagnostic test. N Engl J Med 1993;329:8–13.

CHIKUNGUNYA

Method of
Scott Kellermann, MD; and Rick D. Kellerman, MD

The word "chikungunya" is a derivation of the Kimakonde (a Mozambique dialect) word "kungunyala" meaning "to become desiccated or contorted". In the Democratic Republic of the Congo it is called "buka-buka", translated as "broken-broken", reflecting the incapacitating arthralgias that are common manifestations of Chikungunya fever

Epidemiology

Chikungunya, first diagnosed in Tanganyika in 1952, is found in a large percentage of countries in Africa, Southeast Asia and is prevalent in India. Outbreaks occur periodically and in 2013 it was identified for the first time in the Caribbean.

Chikungunya has been diagnosed in nearly all of the states of the United States. Until the summer of 2014, all of the cases of Chikungunya detected in the U.S. were imported, occurring in individuals returning from endemic countries. During the summer of 2014, several locally transmitted cases were diagnosed in Florida non-travelers, indicating that the disease was now borne by the *Aedes* mosquitoes of mainland U.S.

Some believe the Chikungunya virus originated in Africa and migrated to Asia 200 years ago. Evidence derived from molecular genetics suggests it evolved around 1700; the first recorded outbreak of this disease was probably in 1779.

Interestingly, some medical historians believe that a pandemic of Chikungunya occurred in the western hemisphere in the 1800's but was diagnosed as dengue fever. The 21st century researchers who have examined the accounts of this pandemic now speculate that it was caused by Chikungunya because the cases exhibited severe joint arthritis which is more indicative of Chikungunya than dengue. The virus then disappeared from the Americas until it re-emerged during the last decade.

Chikungunya epidemics appear suddenly and unpredictably and proceed explosively.

Risk factors

Individuals at the highest risk of contracting Chikungunya or enduring more severe symptoms are those who have chronic arthritis, underlying chronic medical conditions, those over the age of 65, and pregnant women. Travelers who spend extended periods of time in endemic areas are at greater risk. These include missionaries, humanitarian aid workers and those who frequently work outdoors.

Pathophysiology

Chikungunya is an arthropod transmitted disease caused by a single-stranded RNA arbovirus. As with dengue fever and yellow fever, Chikungunya cycles from mosquito to human to mosquito. The mosquito *Aedes aegypti* is the usual vector for transmission of Chikungunya. *Aedes albopictus*, the Asian tiger mosquito, is also a vector. Both species are found in the southeastern United States and limited parts of the southwest. The *Aedes albopictus* species survives further north into the Mid-Atlantic states and into the lower Midwest. Birds, cattle, monkeys and other vertebrates may serve as reservoirs. The incubation period is 3 – 7 days (range 1–12 days). Between 72% and 97% of those infected will develop symptoms. Chikungunya can be transmitted during childbirth but there are no reported cases of transmission during breastfeeding. Theoretically, Chikungunya can be transferred via blood transfusion but there have been no reported cases. Previous infection is believed to convey long lasting immunity.

Prevention

There is no current vaccine. The best preventive measures are wearing permethrin treated, bite-proof long sleeves and trousers, and using a mosquito repellant such as DEET. Screening windows and doors has only a limited effect, since most contacts between the *Aedes* mosquitoes and humans occur outside.

Standing water, a breeding ground for mosquitoes, should be drained. *Aedes aegypti* breeding sites are associated with human habitation and are seemingly innocuous (i.e. flower vases, water storage vessels and birdbaths).

Standard blood handling procedures are recommended.

If a Chikungunya epidemic were to occur in the U.S., the standard public health measures of avoidance and mosquito control would be major lines of defense.

Clinical Manifestations

Clinical onset is abrupt. The hallmark of chikungunya is erratic, relapsing, and incapacitating arthralgia. High fever, headache, back pain, myalgia, and arthralgia predominate. Arthralgias can be intense, affecting mainly the extremities (ankles, wrists, phalanges) but also the large joints. Typically, the fever lasts for two days and then ends abruptly. Headache and an extreme degree of prostration may persist for a variable period, usually about five to seven days.

Rare symptoms include uveitis, retinitis, myocarditis, hepatitis, nephritis, hemorrhage, and neurologic problems such as myelitis, meningoencephalitis, Guillain-Barré syndrome and cranial nerve palsies.

In 40–50% of cases skin involvement is present consisting of a pruritic maculopapular rash predominating on the thorax, facial edema and localize petechia. Although rarely affecting children, they may exhibit a bullous rash with pronounced sloughing.

The case fatality ratio is approximates 1 per 1000, with most deaths occurring in newborns, the elderly, and the infirm.

Diagnosis

The instructions for serum diagnostic testing are found on the CDC website. (http://www.cdc.gov/chikungunya/hc/diagnostic.html). Blood should be collected in a tiger/speckled-top serum separator tube or a red-top tube. Serum may be sent to the CDC; some state laboratories have testing capabilities. Green-top heparin and purple top EDTA tubes are not appropriate tubes for testing. The virus may be cultured within the first 3 days of illness. Virus isolation provides the most definitive diagnosis, but requires one to two weeks for completion and must be carried out in biosafety level III laboratories. Chikungunya viral RNA may be identifiable in the serum during the first 8 days of illness as Chikungunya virus antibodies usually develop by the end of the first week of illness. IgM antibody levels peak three to five weeks after the onset of illness and persist for approximately two months. In some cases, paired acute-phase and convalescent-phase antibody sampling may be required for accurate diagnosis. False positive results may occur due to infection from closely related viruses.

A complete blood count (CBC) may show lymphopenia. Liver enzymes may elevate and the serum creatinine might also increase. Radiological findings are normal and biological markers of inflammation are normal or modestly elevated.

In many parts of the world, Chikungunya is a clinical diagnosis of exclusion, particularly when laboratory testing is not readily available. The probability of disease depends on the epidemiology of endemic diseases and the patient's clinical symptoms.

Differential Diagnosis

The differential diagnosis for Chikungunya includes influenza, a multitude of viruses (particularly dengue fever), malaria and rickettsia. Dengue and Chikungunya viruses are transmitted by the same mosquitoes and have similar features. The two viruses can occasionally co-infect the same individual. Clinically differentiating Chikungunya from dengue fever may be difficult but in Chikungunya the onset of fever is typically more abrupt, shorter lived and rash and arthralgia more prevalent.

Seasonally, Chikungunya is more likely to be seen in the summer months when *Aedes* mosquitos proliferate.

Treatment

Medical treatment is primarily supportive. The use of antiviral agents is unproven. Though it is generally recommended that acetaminophen, NSAIDs and corticosteroids be used for treatment of joint pain, some experts suggest that typical anti-inflammatory agents may paradoxically make symptoms worse because the arthritis of Chikungunya arises from the virus itself, not an inflammatory response. Typical anti-inflammatory agents may actually inhibit the immune response required to suppress the Chikungunya virus.

Monitoring

Suspected chikungunya cases should be reported immediately to state or local health departments to facilitate diagnosis and mitigate the risk of local transmission.

Complications

Twenty percent of infected patients have severe recurrent joint pains for a year or more after acute illness. During the La Reunion outbreak in 2006, more than 50% of subjects over the age of 45 reporting prolonged painful joints for up to three years following initial infection.

Some patients may have relapses of underlying rheumatologic disorders in the months following acute infection. Others may suffer long-term asthenia.

Chikungunya is one of the agents researched as a potential biological weapon.

References:

Morens DM, Fauci AS. Perspective: Chikungunya at the door — Déjà vu all over again? N Engl J Med 2014;371:885–7.
Staples JE, Fischer M. Perspective: Chikungunya virus in the Americas — what a vectorborne pathogen can do. N Engl J Med 2014;371:887–9.
Pialoux G, Gaüzère B-A, Jauréguiberry S, Strobel M. Chikungunya, an epidemic arbovirus. Lancet Infect Dis 2007;7:319–27.
Mohan A, Kiran DHN, Manohar IC, Kumar DP. Epidemiology, clinical manifestations, and diagnosis of chikungunya fever: lessons learned from the re-emerging epidemic. Indian J Dermatol 2010;55(1):54–63.
Centers for Disease Control and Prevention. Chikungunya virus. November 4, 2014. http://www.cdc.gov/chikungunya/
Centers for Disease Control and Prevention. Chikungunya: atypical and severe disease manifestations. http://www.cdc.gov/chikungunya/pdfs/Chikungunya-atypical-severe-disease_Healthcare-provider-factsheet-10-07-2014.pdf.
World Health Organization. Chikungunya. http://www.who.int/mediacentre/factsheets/fs327/en/.

CHOLERA

Method of
Mark Pietroni, MD

Cholera can kill within hours of the onset of symptoms, and even today the impact of an outbreak of cholera can be catastrophic in locations in which the water and sanitation infrastructure are weak, especially in crisis or war situations. The 21st century has already seen large-scale cholera epidemics in Haiti, Zimbabwe, and Pakistan, as well as many smaller outbreaks in countries and areas in which cholera is endemic. When cholera is untreated, mortality can be as high as 60% to 70%, but even in epidemics, with appropriate management and well-run diarrhea treatment centers, mortality can be reduced to well below 1%.

Oral rehydration therapy (ORT) is now the mainstay of treatment (Table 1). Developed in the 1960s in Dhaka, Bangladesh, ORT was used to great effect during the Bangladesh Liberation War of 1971. Cholera broke out in the refugee camps outside Calcutta, and the medical services ran out of intravenous fluid. ORT was not accepted as routine therapy by the medical profession at that time. The courageous decision to treat people with ORT saved thousands of lives and convinced the world of the effectiveness of ORT in the management of cholera.

Pathophysiology

Cholera is caused by a gram-negative, comma-shaped bacterium called *Vibrio cholerae*. Clinical disease is caused by two serogroups: *V. cholerae* O1 (which has two biotypes: classical and El Tor) and *V. cholerae* O139. Humans are the only known natural host, and asymptomatic human carriage is rare. *V. cholerae* is rapidly killed by boiling water, but it can lie dormant for months in blue-green algae, crustaceans, and copepods in brackish water, especially in estuaries. The Ganges delta provides an ideal habitat and is believed to be the place cholera first emerged.

Human infection is caused by ingestion of contaminated food or drink or from poor hand hygiene in epidemic situations. Relative or absolute achlorhydria facilitates passage through the stomach. Proliferation occurs in the small intestine, where a number of toxins are released. This results in massive secretion of isotonic fluid into the gut. The fluid passes out of the anus full of vibrios to perpetuate the cycle of transmission. Killing the host does not appear to interrupt this cycle!

The cholera toxin is secreted only by the O1 and O139 serogroups. It has two subunits: A (active) and B (binding). Subunit B binds to receptors in the small intestine and subunit A activates adenylate cyclase. This causes the active secretion of a number of ions into the gut, which drags water by osmosis and also blocks the reabsorption of sodium from the gut. The net result is a massive loss of water, sodium chloride, and bicarbonate. This cannot be replaced by drinking a sodium solution because sodium reabsorption is blocked. However, the addition of glucose to a solution of sodium activates a sodium-glucose co-transporter; sodium is absorbed and water follows by osmosis. This is the basis of oral rehydration therapy for diarrhea today.

Clinical Presentation and Diagnosis

Cholera manifests as an acute watery diarrhea without blood in the stool or (usually) abdominal cramps. The majority of cases are clinically indistinguishable from other causes of watery diarrhea and require only oral rehydration fluid as treatment. However, some progress to classic or severe cholera.

TABLE 1	Composition (mEq/L) of Common Solutions Used for Rehydration						
SOLUTION	**NA⁺**	**K⁺**	**CL⁻**	**HCO₃⁻**	**CITRATE**	**CA²⁺**	**GLUCOSE OR CARBOHYDRATE**
Intravenous Solution							
Normal saline	154	—	154	—	—	—	—
Ringer's lactate	130	4	111	28	—	3	—
Ringer's lactate +D₅	130	4	109	28	—	3	278
Cholera saline (Dhaka solution)	133	13	98	48	—	—	140
Oral Solution							
Standard ORS	90	20	80	—	10	—	75
Hypo-osmolar ORS	75	20	65	—	10	—	75
ReSoMal*	45	40	76	—	7	—	125

Abbreviations: $D_5 = 5\%$ dextrose; ORS = oral rehydration solution; ReSoMal = reduced osmolarity ORS for malnourished children.
Reprinted with permission from Harris JB, Pietroni M: Approach to the child with acute diarrhea in developing countries. UpToDate. Available at http://www.uptodate.com/contents/approach-to-the-child-with-acute-diarrhea-in-developing-countries (accessed May 14, 2012).
*Also contains Mg 6 mmol/L, Zn 300 µmol/L, Cu 45 µmol/L.

The classic picture is of the rapid onset of profuse watery diarrhea (rice-water stool) and vomiting, which is painless and can result in circulatory collapse within hours without effective treatment. The history is usually less than 24 hours, although it may be longer if the patient is taking oral rehydration solution. Abdominal cramps can occur. Fever is absent. Patients usually remain alert, but severe electrolyte abnormalities such as hypoglycemia and hyponatremia can cause a reduced level of consciousness or convulsions, especially in children. Acidosis is often severe and commonly results in tachypnea, which is commonly misdiagnosed as pneumonia. Patients should be reassessed for the presence or absence of pneumonia 1 to 2 hours after adequate rehydration. The diagnosis of cholera can be confirmed by the presence of rapidly motile vibrios detected by dark-field microscopy or by stool or rectal swab culture.

However, the classic history, appearance of the stool, and rapid presentation mean that the diagnosis is usually clinical.

Treatment

A clinical syndrome of acute watery diarrhea (three or more watery stools in the last 24 hours) of short duration (24–48 hours) with or without vomiting associated with dehydration in anyone older than 2 years in an endemic or epidemic situation should be treated as cholera. Children younger than 2 years may be managed in the same way, but other diagnoses such as rotavirus should be considered. The mainstay of management (whatever the causative organism) is appropriate early rehydration, and time should not be wasted worrying about investigations or which antibiotic to use (Figure 1).

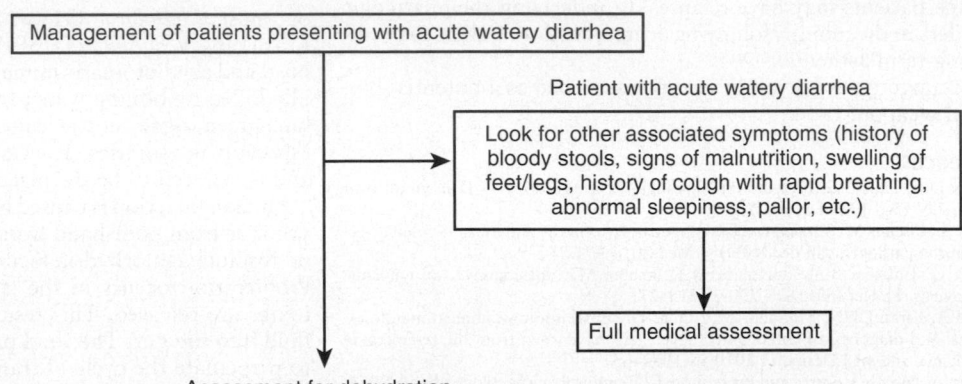

| Management of patients presenting with acute watery diarrhea | | | |

Patient with acute watery diarrhea

Look for other associated symptoms (history of bloody stools, signs of malnutrition, swelling of feet/legs, history of cough with rapid breathing, abnormal sleepiness, pallor, etc.)

Full medical assessment

Assessment for dehydration

Assess	Condition	Normal	Irritable/less active*	Lethargic/comatose*
	Eyes	Normal	Sunken	Sunken
	Tongue	Normal	Dry	Dry
	Thirst	Normal	Thirsty (drinks eagerly)	Unable to drink*
	Skin pinch	Normal	Goes back slowly*	Goes back very slowly*
	Radial pulse	Normal	Reduced*	Uncountable or absent*
Diagnosis		No sign of dehydration	If at least 2 signs, including one (*) sign, are present, diagnose *some dehydration*	If some dehydration plus one of the (*) signs are present, diagnose *severe dehydration*
Management		A	B	C

A. No sign of dehydration—ORS
- 50 mL ORS per kg body weight *plus* ongoing losses
- Send patient home with 4 packets of ORS
- Continue feeding, including breastmilk for infants and young children

B. Some dehydration—ORS
- 80 mL ORS per kg body weight over 4–6 hours plus ongoing losses
- Observe patient for 6–12 hours
- Continue feeding, including breastmilk for infants and young children
- Reassess patient and dehydration status hourly.
- In case of frequent vomiting (>3 times in 1 hour): Treat with IV fluid

C. Severe dehydration—Start IV fluid immediately (100 mL/kg)

IV solution containing sodium, potassium, chloride and bicarbonate (e.g., Ringer's Lactate)

Children <1 year or malnourished
30 mL/kg in first 1 hour
70 mL/kg in next 5 hours

Adults and children >1 year
30 mL/kg in first 1/2 hour
70 mL/kg in next 2 1/2 hours

- Encourage the patient to take ORS as soon as he/she is able to drink
- Antibiotic, if needed, after rehydration
- Zinc 20 mg/day for 10 days in children 6 months to 5 years old

Figure 1. Quick identification of cholera cases can be made using a standard case definition. During an outbreak, cholera should be suspected in any patient who is older than 2 years, is attending a health facility, and has a history of acute watery diarrhea (passage of at least three stools in the last 24 hours) of a short duration (less than 24 hours), with or without vomiting, and with signs of dehydration. (Flow chart modified from International Centre for Diarrhoeal Disease Research, Bangladesh (ICDDR,B) internal treatment protocol.)
Abbreviation: ORS = oral rehydration solution.

Box 1   Fluids for Patients without Signs of Dehydration

Acceptable

Oral rehydration solution (optimal for both repletion and maintenance)

Salted drinks (salted rice water or salted yogurt drink)

Broth or soup (salted vegetable or meat soup)

Water

Rice water

Coconut water (unsweetened)

Weak tea (unsweetened)

Fresh fruit juice (unsweetened)

Unacceptable

Carbonated beverages

Sweetened juices

Coffee

Medicinal teas or infusions

Fluids containing salt should be encouraged. Unacceptable fluids include carbonated beverages and sweetened juices; the sugar in these fluids may worsen diarrhea. Coffee and medicinal teas or infusions are also unacceptable since they can have diuretic and purgative effects.

Reprinted with permission from Harris JB, Pietroni M: Approach to the child with acute diarrhea in developing countries. UpToDate. Available at http://www.uptodate.com/contents/approach-to-the-child-with-acute-diarrhea-in-developing-countries (accessed May 14, 2012).

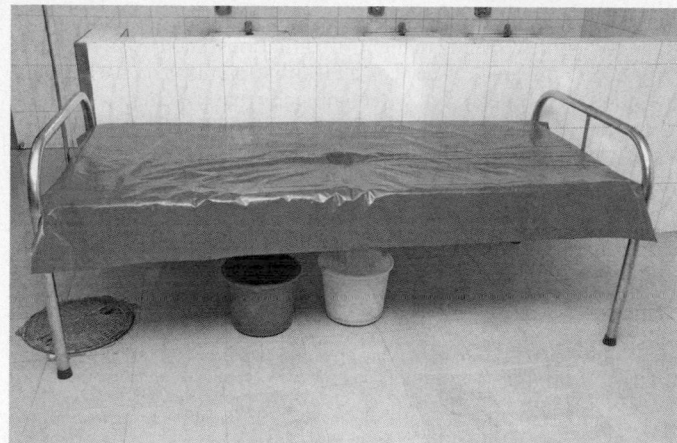

Figure 2. Cholera cot.

Box 2   Antibiotics in Cholera

Antibiotics should be given to all patients with severe dehydration. Choice of antibiotic depends on local sensitivity pattern.

First-Line Drug (If Susceptibility Report Is Not Available)

Adults

Azithromycin (Zithromax)[1] 1 g (500 mg × 2) PO as a single dose after correcting severe dehydration

Children

Azithromycin 20 mg/kg PO as a single dose after correction of dehydration and cessation of vomiting (if any)

Second-Line Drug (Not Recommended for Children <5 Years or Pregnant Women)

Adults

Ciprofloxacin (Cipro)[1] 1 g (500 mg × 2) PO as a single dose after correction of severe dehydration

Children

Ciprofloxacin 20 mg/kg PO as a single dose after correction of dehydration and cessation of vomiting (if any)

Third-Line Drugs

Doxycycline (Vibramycin) 300 mg as a single dose after food (not in children or pregnant women)

---

[1]Not FDA approved for this indication.

The initial assessment should be brief but must:

- Confirm the diagnosis of acute watery diarrhea
- Assess the level of dehydration
- Assess the presence or absence of malnutrition
- Recognize any other comorbidities

Accurate assessment and rapid, appropriate treatment of dehydration is critical to the management of cholera. A simple scoring system based on five clinical signs is sufficient and can accurately predict patients with 5% to 10% (some) dehydration and greater than 10% (severe) dehydration. Common mistakes include overreliance on individual clinical signs and giving too little intravenous fluid during the initial phase and too much during the recovery phase. Patients with less than 5% (no) dehydration and 5% to 10% (some) dehydration can be managed with oral rehydration alone (Box 1) unless there is a reduced level of consciousness or inability to take fluids by mouth. Those with 5% to 10% (some) dehydration must be reassessed every 1 to 2 hours to make sure that hydration is improving.

Patients with severe dehydration require an immediate intravenous fluid bolus of 100 mL/kg given over 3 hours with one third in the first 30 minutes (double the duration in children who are younger than 1 year and have malnutrition). If possible, the intravenous fluid should contain sodium, potassium, and bicarbonate—Ringer's lactate or cholera saline—but normal saline with 5 to 10 mmol/L of potassium may also be used. Oral rehydration should start at the same time. Once the intravenous fluid bolus has finished, further intravenous fluids are usually not required.

Patients are best managed using a cholera cot, especially in an epidemic situation. The cholera cot is a bed (or sometimes a chair) covered with a nonabsorbent sheet with a hole that allows the passage of stool and urine directly to a bucket under the bed (Figure 2). The sheets and bucket should be replaced three times a day and between patients. They may be washed, sterilized, and reused. Patients do not need to use a toilet (which can be several times an hour), linen is not soiled, and body fluids are prevented from running on the floor. This system enables adequate infection control to be maintained with limited resources.

After an initial assessment has been made and fluids started, a fuller clinical assessment can take place. Patients with significant comorbidities can require individually tailored treatment plans.

Antibiotics reduce the length of stay and fluid requirement in patients with severe dehydration due to cholera (Box 2). A single dose is sufficient, but this should be repeated if the dose is vomited back. The choice of antibiotic should be guided by local sensitivities where these are available. If not, a single dose of azithromycin (Zithromax)[1] 1 g in adults and 20 mg/kg in children is recommended. All children between 6 months and 5 years of age should receive zinc[1] 20 mg/day for 10 days because this reduces subsequent mortality and further episodes of diarrhea.

Recovery from cholera is rapid, and mortality is extremely low if the dehydration is treated appropriately. The Cholera Hospital run by the International Centre for Diarrhoeal Disease Research, Bangladesh (ICDDR,B), in Dhaka treats around 120,000 patients a year. The average length of stay is 16 hours, and the mortality rate is zero.

Prevention

Because the transmission of cholera is feco-oral, cholera can be prevented by good hand hygiene and by providing safe drinking water and appropriate sanitation. Standard food and hygiene precautions should be followed by people travelling in endemic areas (e.g., eat only boiled or fried foods; drink only boiled or bottled water). Two cholera vaccines are available (not in the United States) and provide around 60% to 80% efficacy for 6 months. They are

---

[1]Not FDA approved for this indication.

not recommended for the occasional traveler or tourist but may be given to people working in high-risk situations, such as aid workers in a cholera outbreak. The World Health Organization has recently amended its advice and now recommends that vaccination be used in an outbreak to break the transmission cycle. Studies are underway to see if it is effective in endemic settings.

References

Alam NH, Ashraf H. Treatment of infectious diarrhea in children. Paediatr Drugs 2003;5:151–65.

Harris JB, Pietroni M. Approach to the child with acute diarrhea in developing countries, UpToDate 2012;Available athttp://www.uptodate.com/contents/approach-to-the-child-with-acute-diarrhea-in-developing-countries; 2012 [accessed 14.05.12].

Roy SK, Tomkins AM, Akramuzzaman SM, et al. Randomised controlled trial of zinc supplementation in malnourished Bangladeshi children with acute diarrhea. Arch Dis Child 1997;77:196–200.

Saha D, Karim MM, Khan WA, et al. Single-dose azithromycin for the treatment of cholera in adults. N Engl J Med 2006;354:2452–62.

World Health Organization. The treatment of diarrhoea, a manual for physicians and other senior health workers, 4th revision. WHO/FCH/CAH/05.1.Geneva: World Health Organization; 2005. http://whqlibdoc.who.int/publications/2005/9241593180.pdf; [accessed 05.04.12].

CHRONIC FATIGUE SYNDROME

Method of
Stephen J. Gluckman, MD

Chronic fatigue syndrome (CFS) is an often-misunderstood syndrome that should not be confused with malingering or hypochondriasis. Patients with CFS are truly suffering from their often-disabling symptoms. It is impossible to successfully treat a patient with CFS unless the clinician believes the patient is genuinely symptomatic. CFS should also not be confused with the isolated symptom of fatigue. Fatigue is a common patient complaint, whereas CFS has a much lower prevalence.

Definition

CFS is not a new disease; the syndrome has been described since at least the mid-1700s. However, since that time it has been mistakenly ascribed to a number of incorrect pathologic and infectious causes. In the past it has been called febricula, neurasthenia, effort syndrome, DeCosta's syndrome, myalgic encephalitis, chronic brucellosis, chronic Lyme disease, chronic Epstein-Barr syndrome, total allergy syndrome, chronic candidiasis, and multiple chemical sensitivity syndrome. Most recently it has been falsely attributed to infection with xenotropic murine leukemia virus–related virus (XMRV) and related retroviruses, such as murine leukemia virus (MLV). None of these possible causes has proved to be correct.

In 1988, in an attempt to be descriptive rather than attribute an incorrect etiology to the disease, the term *chronic fatigue syndrome* was coined. Therefore, the name is relatively new but the syndrome is not. The disease is chronic and fatigue is a cardinal feature, but it is more than being chronically tired. It is a syndrome that includes a number of additional symptoms as noted in Box 1, the working case definition as published by the CDC and then modified in 1992 by the National Institute of Allergy and Infectious Diseases. One note of caution: This case definition is an epidemiologic tool and not a strict clinical tool. It is useful for studying the disease. However, some patients do not completely fit this definition but CFS can nonetheless be diagnosed by a knowledgeable clinician.

Because some immune abnormalities are often seen in these patients, some people have called this "chronic fatigue and immune dysregulation syndrome." The immune abnormalities seen in CFS patients are mild and differ from patient to patient. Most significantly, these patients are not immunosuppressed.

It has been noted that many of the symptoms of fibromyalgia overlap with CFS, and some clinicians consider fibromyalgia and CFS to be different aspects of the same disease because both often include pain and fatigue. These different names for the same syndrome can be confusing to patients and clinicians, and when managing patients with CFS it is important to explain this to them.

Box 1 International Consensus Definition of Chronic Fatigue Syndrome

Chronic fatigue syndrome is a clinically evaluated, unexplained, persistent or relapsing chronic fatigue (lasting more than 6 months) that is of new or definite onset (has not been lifelong); is not the result of ongoing exertion; is not substantially alleviated by rest; and results in substantial reduction in previous levels of occupational, educational, social, or personal activities.

Four or more of the following symptoms are concurrently present for more than 6 months:
- Impaired memory or concentration
- Multijoint pain
- Muscle pain
- New headaches
- Postexertional malaise
- Sore throat
- Tender cervical or axillary lymph nodes
- Unrefreshing sleep

Exclusionary Clinical Diagnoses
- Any active medical condition that could explain the chronic fatigue
- Any previously diagnosed medical condition whose resolution has not been documented beyond reasonable clinical doubt and whose continued activity can explain the chronic fatiguing illness
- Psychotic major depression, bipolar affective disorder, schizophrenia, delusional disorders, dementias, anorexia nervosa, bulimia nervosa
- Alcohol or other substance abuse within 2 years prior to the onset of the chronic fatigue and at any time afterward

Adapted from Fukuda K, Straus SE, Hickie I, et al. The chronic fatigue syndrome: A comprehensive approach to its definition and study. Ann Intern Med 1994;121:953–9.

Epidemiology

Though chronic fatigue is an extremely common symptom, CFS is not. The former has been noted to have a prevalence of 10% to 25% in a number of studies. However, the point prevalence of CFS has been estimated to be in the range of 0.1%. CFS is overrepresented in young and middle-aged women, but it has been described in men and women and in all age groups.

Pathophysiology

The cause of CFS is unknown. Much effort has gone into trying to discern an infectious, endocrine, immune, or psychiatric cause, but to date none has been proved. Studies have shown a link between CFS and the presence of certain genes that mediate immune and stress responses. The findings suggest that difficulty managing stress may be linked to the development of CFS. They also suggest that there is not a single cause of CFS, but that there may be a number of stress-related triggers (physical or emotional) in those with a genetic predisposition. This is consistent with the typical course, in which a previously healthy person develops an acute illness that resolves but initiates CFS.

In March 2015 the Institute of Medicine (IOM) issued a 300-page review of the topic. As a result of this review they proposed a name change to Systemic Exertion Intolerance Disease (SEID). This comprehensive report has three major themes: 1. CFS has acquired a great deal of negative connotation with associated misunderstanding and prejudice. The name change to SEID is an attempt to disconnect this disease from past misunderstandings. 2. The criteria for diagnosis were greatly simplified with emphasis on the major features. (Box 2) 3. By using the term "disease" and with the ample reference support in the document the IOM unequivocally underscores the very real nature of this malady. The IOM report is too recent to know at this time whether it will be universally adopted, but it by far the most thorough examination of the topic.

Box 2 New Proposed Criteria for CFS/SEID

Diagnosis requires that the patient have the following three symptoms:
- A substantial reduction or impairment in the ability to engage in pre-illness levels of occupational, educational, social, or personal activities that persists for more than 6 months and is accompanied by fatigue, which is often profound, is of new or definite onset (not lifelong), is not the result of ongoing excessive exertion, and is not substantially alleviated by rest.
- Post-exertional malaise
- Unrefreshing sleep

At least one of the two following manifestations is also required:
- Cognitive impairment
- Orthostatic intolerance

Box 4 Diagnostic Testing

Tests to Perform
- Complete blood count
- Comprehensive chemistry screen
- Thyroid-stimulating hormone
- Additional testing *only* with specific clinical indications

Do Not Routinely Do
- ANA
- Serology for CMV, EBV, *Bartonella, Babesia, Ehrlichia, Anaplasma*
- MRI, SPECT or PET scans
- Tilt table testing

Abbreviations: ANA = antinuclear antibody test; CMV = cytomegalovirus; EBV = Epstein–Barr virus; MRI = magnetic resonance imaging; PET = positron-emission tomography; SPECT = single-photon–emission computed tomography.

Clinical Features and Diagnosis

Though there is, as yet, no diagnostic test, the history, physical examination, and laboratory testing are generally very characteristic and allow a clinician to confidently make the diagnosis. The typical story is one of a previously highly functioning person who develops an acute illness or other stressor. The acute problem resolves, but from that time on symptoms of CFS are triggered. Despite often profound symptoms, physical examination is persistently normal, as is laboratory testing. Symptoms are exacerbated by physical activity. The pre-CFS medical history of the patient is not one of multiple medical problems. Affected patients are typically highly functioning persons who are struck down with this disease. Diagnostic features to emphasize in addition to the case definition noted in Box 1 include those noted in Box 3.

In a patient with a typical story and examination, laboratory testing should be limited (Box 4). Testing for diseases with a low pretest likelihood runs the serious risk of false-positive results. This can result in further testing, diagnostic confusion, and unnecessary treatments. Specifically, the signs and symptoms of CFS are not those of systemic lupus, Lyme disease, cytomegalovirus, bartonellosis, ehrlichiosis, or babesiosis. Serologic testing for these diagnoses is not helpful and can be harmful if the presence of antibodies results in the initiation of unwarranted medications. For similar reasons, neuroimaging without objective clinical findings is not indicated. Though abnormalities can be found, they are nonspecific and of no clinical utility. Tilt-table testing seems to be abnormal in many patients with CFS; however, testing is expensive and uncomfortable, and abnormal results do not alter management. Of course, if history,

physical examination, and initial laboratory testing do reveal abnormalities, further laboratory evaluation should be undertaken to elucidate the cause of the aberration(s).

Treatment

There is no established cure for CFS, but patients should be counseled that a number of things can be done to manage this often disabling illness (Box 5). These can be divided into things the clinician should do and things the patient should do.

Things the Clinician Should Do

To successfully manage CFS, a clinician must believe that the patient is truly symptomatic. Patients with CFS are not malingering. Because they often appear well and have consistently normal objective testing, they often become very defensive about their limitations. They are sensitive to the validity of their symptoms. Not only are they suffering but also they are blamed for it. Many patients with CFS are partially or totally disabled. Their outward healthy appearance belies the internal sense of ill health. It is common for relatives and colleagues to believe they are malingering. A vicious cycle of frustration, anger, and depression commonly ensues.

As part of establishing the validity of the diagnosis a clinician should review the history of CFS, emphasizing that this is not a new disease but was originally described centuries ago.

For successful management a clinician should give the patient enough time, specifically inquire about other diagnoses the patient is concerned about, and explain why they are not correct. The clinician should see the patient at regular intervals.

Make sure that the patient has reasonable expectations. Most patients with CFS have not had previous chronic illnesses or significant prolonged limitations. It is often necessary review the information about CFS with the patient's family and to emphasize that this disabling illness is not volitional.

Though it is generally wise to avoid a discussion about whether the origin of CFS is psychiatric or organic, depression is an

Box 3 Frequent features of Chronic Fatigue Syndrome

- Sudden onset of fatigue after a relatively common illness or other stressor
- Previously active and healthy person
- Symptoms very sensitive to exacerbation by physical activity
- Normal physical examination and laboratory testing
- Altered sleep
- "Foggy" thought processes
- Lack of progression to organ failure or any significant objective organ abnormality
- Joint and muscle aching without physical evidence of inflammation
- Feverish feeling (sustained elevated temperatures [>37.4°C] should prompt a search for an alternative diagnosis, because the CFS patient is not truly febrile)
- Diffuse aching that is not well localized to joints or muscles, but without erythema, effusion, or limitation of motion
- Muscles that are easily fatigued (however, strength is normal, and biopsies and electromyograms are also normal)
- Occasional mild cervical and/or axillary lymphadenitis (painful lymph nodes [lymphadenia] are a common complaint, but this is not a true lymphadenopathy)

Box 5 Therapy of Chronic Fatigue Syndrome

Educate the patient and his or her support system about the diagnosis of chronic fatigue syndrome. Emphasize the validity of the diagnosis and of the patient's symptoms. Make sure that there is an understanding about expectations.
- Aggressively manage specific symptoms of sleep disturbance, pain, and depression.
- Consider cognitive behavioral therapy.
- Emphasize the need for gradual, graded exercise. Give the patient a specific "prescription" for this.
- Avoid the temptation to prescribe antimicrobials, corticosteroids, or other medications with no proven benefit and the potential to do harm.
- Discuss the pros and cons of using unstudied, expensive, or potentially dangerous "alternative therapies."

expected consequence of any chronic illness. Depression has specific treatments, and it should be aggressively diagnosed and treated. The patient should be told that successful management of depression will help him or her cope with CFS.

If a sleep disturbance exists that should also be aggressively managed, if necessary by a sleep specialist. Sleep deprivation makes other symptoms more difficult to deal with.

Chronic pain is very enervating. If pain is prominent, that should also be aggressively managed, often by a pain specialist.

It is important for the clinician to be cautious about ascribing all of a patient's symptoms to CFS. Such patients are, of course, not protected from getting additional illnesses. Each symptom should be considered on its own before defaulting it to CFS.

Complementary therapies must be discussed or the patient might get the impression that the clinician is not comfortable in considering them; that can partially undermine the clinician–patient relationship. Though all are of unproved benefit or risk, "complementary" therapies that are not dangerous, such as acupuncture, or expensive are reasonable to consider.

Things the Patient Should Do

Of the 350 studies that have looked at treatment options for CFS only cognitive behavioral therapy and graded exercise therapy have been shown to be of benefit. In cognitive behavioral therapy, the patient undergoes a series of 1-hour sessions designed to alter beliefs and behaviors that might delay recovery. Although exercise can exacerbate symptoms, deconditioning will also do so. Limiting activity can worsen weakness and depression. Thus, increased rest is not recommended and should be strongly discouraged. The risk of exacerbating symptoms can be reduced by cautiously setting less-ambitious exercise goals. Because many patients with CFS were particularly active before the onset of their illness and are impatient to get their former lives back, they often need strict guidelines to try to prevent overdoing exercise while at the same time getting a clear prescription to exercise. The exercise prescription should be individualized based on the degree of impairment, but it is wise to initially set goals on the low side to avoid exacerbating symptoms.

As part of the management of CFS patients, their families and, when appropriate, their employers need to reframe their expectations. CFS patients have a chronic, disabling illness. Families and others need to come to some understanding that patients cannot do all that they were able to do before the onset of CFS and that patients cannot "will" the disease away any more than they could will away a more visible disability.

Things that Should Not Be Done

There are many suggested remedies for CFS. Most are either unstudied or disproved. In particular, treatments that are expensive or potentially harmful should be avoided. There is no role for antimicrobial therapy. There is no role for antiviral therapy, including treatment for retroviruses. There is no role for intravenous immunoglobulin, corticosteroids, special diets, or vitamin treatments.

Prognosis

The likelihood for complete recovery from CFS is only fair. The disease tends to wax and wane over time, but in only a minority of patients does it completely resolve. If sustained improvement occurs it is generally over several years. Several features have been associated with a poorer prognosis, including age older than 38 years, more than eight symptoms, duration over 1.5 years, less than 16 years of formal education, a history of a dysthymic disorder, and a sustained belief that the disease is due to a physical cause.

Monitoring

Despite the lack of very effective treatment, many patients benefit from regular monitoring of their condition. Knowing they have scheduled visits minimizes the number of crises and emergency visits and allows the patient to reconnect with a validating physician. Follow-up on a quarterly basis is a reasonable interval.

References

Aronowitz RA. From myalgic encephalitis to yuppie flu: A history of chronic fatigue syndromes. In: Rosenberg CE, Golden J, editors. Framing Disease. New Brunswick, NJ: Rutgers University Press; 1992.

Clark MR, Katon W, Russo J, et al. Chronic fatigue: Risk factors for symptom persistence in a 2{1/2}-year follow-up study. Am J Med 1995;98:187–95.
Fulcher KY, White PD. Randomised controlled trial of graded exercise in patients with the chronic fatigue syndrome. BMJ 1997;314:1647–52.
Goertzel BN, Pennachin C, de Souza Coelho L, et al. Combinations of single nucleotide polymorphisms in neuroendocrine effector and receptor genes predict chronic fatigue syndrome. Pharmacogenomics 2006;7:475–83.
Goldenberg DL, Simms RW, Geiger A, et al. High frequency of fibromyalgia in patients with chronic fatigue seen in a primary care practice. Arthritis Rheum 1990;33:381–7.
Institute of Medicine. Beyond myalgic encephalitis/chronic fatigue syndrome: redefining an illness. Washington D.C.: National Acdemies Press 2015.
Lightfoot Jr RW, Luft BJ, Rahn DW, et al. Empiric parenteral antibiotic treatment of patients with fibromyalgia and fatigue and a positive serologic result for Lyme disease. A cost-effectiveness analysis. Ann Intern Med 1993;119:503–9.
Schluederberg A, Straus SE, Peterson P, et al. NIH conference. Chronic fatigue syndrome research. Definition and medical outcome assessment. Ann Intern Med 1992;117:325–31.
Schwartz RB, Garada BM, Komaroff AL, et al. Detection of intracranial abnormalities in patients with chronic fatigue syndrome: Comparison of MR imaging and SPECT. Am J Roentgenol 1994;162:935–41.
Simmons G, Glynn SA, Komaroff AL, et al. Failure to confirm XMRV/MLVs in the blood of patients with chronic fatigue syndrome: A multi-laboratory study. Science 2011;334:814–7.
Wessely S, Chalder T, Hirsch S, et al. The prevalence and morbidity of chronic fatigue and chronic fatigue syndrome: A prospective primary care study. Am J Public Health 1997;87:1449–55.
White PD, Goldsmith KA, Johnson AL, et al. Comparison of adaptive pacing therapy, cognitive behaviour therapy, graded exercise therapy, and specialist medical care for chronic fatigue syndrome (PACE): A randomised trial. Lancet 2011;377:823–36.

EBOLA VIRUS DISEASE

Method of
Uma Malhotra, MD

CURRENT DIAGNOSIS

- Detection of viral RNA in the blood by reverse transcriptase-polymerase chain reaction (RT-PCR) beginning 3 days after the onset of symptoms.
- Repeat testing may be necessary for patients with illness duration shorter than 3 days.
- Details on specimen collection and handling can be found on the Centers for Disease Control and Prevention (CDC), and World Health Organization (WHO) websites.

CURRENT THERAPY

- Intensive fluid management to correct volume losses and electrolyte abnormalities.
- Aggressive use of antiemetics, antidiarrheals, and rehydration solutions.
- Respiratory and hemodynamic support.
- Blood products for management of coagulopathy.
- Evaluate and treat any concomitant infections.
- There are no approved antiviral therapies. However, a number of experimental treatments, including monoclonal antibodies, convalescent serum, small-molecule antivirals, and short interfering RNAs are available.
- Strict infection control measures, with contact and droplet precautions, must be used.
- Personnel trained in the correct use of personal protective equipment (PPE) should care for the patients.

Filoviridae, derived from the Latin word "filum," meaning thread-like, is a family of viruses with a filamentous structure that can cause severe hemorrhagic fever and fulminant septic shock. Filoviruses have been divided into two genera: Ebola-like viruses with five species—*Zaire, Sudan, Ivory Coast, Bundibugyo,* and *Reston*; and Marburg-like viruses with a single species—*Marburg,* which has caused outbreaks in Central Africa. Using paleoviruses (genomic fossils) found in mammals, we can extrapolate that the viruses probably diverged several thousand years ago, and that the family itself is at least tens of millions of years old.

Epidemiology

Of the five Ebola virus species only four—*Zaire, Sudan, Ivory Coast, Bundibugyo*—cause disease in humans. Since its first recognition in 1976, *Zaire ebolavirus* has caused multiple outbreaks in Central Africa. It is the causative agent of the 2014 West African epidemic, with an initial estimated case fatality rate as high as 70%, although as the epidemic evolved, lower fatality rates in the range of 30% to 40% were observed. The 2014 epidemic began in Guinea, when a 2-year-old child became infected in late 2013, and *Zaire ebolavirus* subsequently spread to Liberia, Sierra Leone, Nigeria, Senegal, and Mali. *Sudan* virus has been associated with a case-fatality rate of approximately 50% in four epidemics, which occurred in Sudan and Uganda between 1970 and 2004. *Ivory Coast* virus has been identified as the cause of illness in one person following exposure during a necropsy on a chimpanzee found dead in the Tai Forest. *Bundibugyo* virus, most closely related to the Ivory Coast species, emerged in Uganda in 2007, causing an outbreak with a case fatality rate of approximately 30%. *Reston* virus, discovered after an outbreak of lethal infection in macaques imported into the United States in 1989, is maintained in animal reservoirs in the Philippines.

Risk Factors/Transmission

Outbreaks generally begin when an individual becomes infected through contact with the tissue or body fluids of an infected animal. The virus then spreads to others who come into contact with the infected individual's blood, skin, or other body fluids. Prior to the 2014 epidemic in West Africa, outbreaks occurred in remote regions with low population density and were controlled within short periods. However, the recent epidemic has shown that movement of infected individuals facilitates the extensive and rapid spread of the virus.

Transmission occurs most commonly through direct contact of broken skin or mucous membranes with virus-containing body fluids from an infected person, the most infectious being blood, feces, and vomit. During the early phase of illness, the level of virus in the blood is typically quite low, but then increases rapidly to very high levels in advanced stages of the illness, when patients become highly infectious. In fact, corpses of persons who die from Ebola are highly infectious, and ritual washing of bodies at funerals has played a significant role in the spread of infection. The virus has also been detected in urine, semen, saliva, breast milk, tears, and sweat, and can persist in some of these fluids much longer than in blood. To prevent sexual transmission the WHO recommends that men either abstain from sex, or use condoms for three months after onset of symptoms. Ebola virus may also be transmitted though contact with contaminated surfaces where the virus can remain infectious from hours to days.

Transmission to health care workers may occur when appropriate PPE is not used, especially when caring for severely ill patients in advanced stages of illness. During the 2014 outbreak in West Africa, a large number of health care workers became infected. In Sierra Leone, the incidence of confirmed cases at the peak of the epidemic was about 100-fold higher in health care workers than in the general population. Several factors have contributed to the high rates of infections among health providers, including failure to recognize infection among patients and corpses, limited availability and training in the use of appropriate PPE, and inadequate management of contaminated waste and burial of corpses. Although there is no evidence of respiratory transmission, the virus is highly infectious when released in laboratory experiments as a small-particle aerosol, and therefore health care workers may be at risk if exposed to aerosols generated during procedures.

Human infection can occur through contact with infected wild animals during hunting, butchering, and preparing meat, with several episodes having occurred following contact with infected gorillas or chimpanzees. To prevent infection, food products should be properly cooked to inactivate the virus, and basic hygiene measures should be followed. Direct transmission of virus infection from bats to wild primates or humans has not been proven, although Ebola RNA sequences and antibodies have been detected in bats in Central Africa. Bats likely form a major reservoir.

Pathophysiology

Ebolavirus is a negative-sense, single-stranded RNA virus resembling rhabdoviruses and paramyxoviruses in its genome organization and replication mechanisms. The tubular virions contain the nucleocapsid surrounded by an outer envelope, which is derived from the host cell membrane and studded with viral glycoprotein spikes. The virions attach to host cell receptors through the spikes and are then endocytosed into vesicles. Initially, productive infection occurs primarily in dendritic cells, monocytes, and macrophages, resulting in impaired interferon production and release of proinflammatory cytokines, which have secondary effects on innate and adaptive immune responses, inflammation, and vascular integrity. Neutrophils are activated, with resultant degranulation, and lymphocytes undergo apoptosis. The virus then spreads to regional lymph nodes resulting in further rounds of replication, followed by dissemination to the liver, spleen, thymus, and other lymphoid tissues.

When the virus infects cells, it hijacks the cell and forces it to become a virus-producing factory, churning out new copies of the virus, which results in a loss of cellular function and eventual cell death by apoptosis. As the disease progresses, there is extensive tissue necrosis accompanied by a systemic inflammatory response induced by the release of various cytokines, chemokines, and proinflammatory mediators; and a severe coagulopathy triggered by the release of tissue factors. This systemic inflammatory response may contribute to gastrointestinal dysfunction, and ultimately there is a multisystem failure caused by the damage to vascular and coagulation systems.

Clinical Manifestations and Laboratory Findings

Patients with Ebola virus disease (EVD) typically have an abrupt onset of symptoms 5 to 10 days after exposure, with a range of 2 to 21 days. The first phase of the illness is characterized by high fever, chills, headaches, myalgia, and malaise. The second phase is marked by gastrointestinal symptoms, which develop by day 3 to 5, and includes watery diarrhea, nausea, vomiting, and abdominal pain. Patients may also develop chest pain, hiccups, shortness of breath, conjunctival injection, and rash. The rash is usually diffuse erythematous, maculopapular, involving the face, neck, trunk, and arms. Respiratory symptoms such as cough are rare. Common neurologic symptoms include delirium—manifested by confusion, slowed cognition, or agitation, and less frequently, seizures.

The final phase, beginning in the second week, is marked by either progression to shock and death, or gradual recovery. Fatal disease is characterized by development of multisystem failure usually as a consequence of massive fluid losses that lead to shock, loss of consciousness, and renal failure. Major bleeding, typically hemorrhage from the gastrointestinal tract, is infrequent and seen in less than 5% during the terminal phase of illness. Patients who survive begin to improve during the second week of illness, with a prolonged convalescence marked by weakness and fatigue. About half of the survivors are plagued by chronic debilitating joint pain and a quarter experience eye problems. The virus can persist in the eye for months, leading to uveitis, cataracts, and sometimes blindness.

During acute illness patients typically develop leukopenia, lymphopenia, thrombocytopenia, serum transaminase elevations, and proteinuria. They may develop renal insufficiency and electrolyte disturbances as a result of the gastrointestinal losses. Severe cases develop coagulation abnormalities with prolonged prothrombin and partial thromboplastin times, and elevated fibrin degradation products, consistent with disseminated intravascular coagulation.

Diagnosis

The approach to evaluating patients depends upon whether or not appropriate signs and symptoms are evident, and if an exposure occurred within 21 days prior to the onset of symptoms. Infection control precautions must be used for all symptomatic patients with an identifiable risk for EVD. All symptomatic patients should be isolated in a single room with a private bathroom, and implementation of contact and droplet precautions. Only essential personnel who are well-trained in the use of PPE should interact with the patient. Phlebotomy and laboratory testing should be limited to essential tests. Both the CDC and the WHO have provided detailed recommendations for approach to the evaluation of persons who may have been exposed to the virus.

Rapid diagnostic tests are the most commonly used tests for diagnosis. Viral RNA is generally detectable by RT-PCR in the blood 3 days after the onset of symptoms. Repeat testing may be necessary for patients with illness duration shorter than 3 days. A negative RT-PCR test greater than or equal to 72 hours after the onset of symptoms rules out EVD. Details on specimen collection and handling can be found on the CDC website. For clinicians outside the United States, the WHO has issued guidance for the collection and shipment of specimens from patients with suspected disease.

Differential Diagnosis

Acute onset of febrile illness in a person who lives in, or has recently been in West or Central Africa may be caused by a variety of local infectious diseases, which must be considered in the differential diagnosis. **Malaria** may have similar findings and might occur concurrently. Examination of blood smears and rapid antigen tests are typically used to diagnose malaria. **Typhoid** is characterized by fever and abdominal pain, and diagnosed by blood cultures.

Patients with **Lassa fever** may develop a severe clinical syndrome resembling EVD and progress to fatal shock. The illness is restricted to West Africa, where it is transmitted through exposure to the aerosolized excretions of rodents, and diagnosed by RT-PCR testing and/or serology. Clinical manifestations of **Marburg virus disease** are similar to EVD, and cases have been identified in Central Africa. The diagnosis is made by RT-PCR. Patients with **influenza** may have a similar initial presentation, but respiratory signs and symptoms are prominent.

Therapy

Good supportive care can significantly improve the chances of recovery from EVD. Large volumes of intravenous fluids and electrolytes are often needed to correct dehydration and electrolyte abnormalities resulting from gastrointestinal losses. Supportive care is required for complications such as shock, hypoxia, hemorrhage, and multiorgan failure. Patients may develop secondary bacterial infections, which may require concurrent management with antimicrobials. Infection prevention and control measures are critical; all bodily fluids and tissues must be considered potentially infectious.

No FDA-approved antiviral drugs or therapeutic vaccines are available, although several are currently in development. Two antiviral nucleoside agents, favipiravir (T-705, Avigan)[5] and brincidofovir (CMX001)[5] have been used in patients with EVD. Favipiravir inhibits the replication of a wide range of RNA viruses, including influenza, and is currently being evaluated in Ebola-infected macaques. Brincidofovir is being developed for the treatment of poxvirus, cytomegalovirus, and other DNA virus infections, but has also demonstrated *in vitro* activity against Ebola virus.

Ebola-specific agents in development include ZMapp (a combination of humanized monoclonal antibodies),[5] TKM-Ebola (a short interfering RNA molecule [siRNA]),[5] phosphorodiamidate morpholino oligomers (PMO, a type of antisense oligonucleotide),[5] and BCX4430 (a nucleoside analog).[5] Plasma from patients who have recovered from the disease was used to treat patients during the 2014 outbreak, but no clinical trials have been conducted to date. Clinicians may contact the CDC's Emergency Operations Center for additional information on use of experimental therapeutics for treatment of EVD.

Prevention

There is no FDA-approved vaccine available for Ebola, although several vaccines are in various stages of development, and some have shown efficacy against virus challenge in laboratory primates. A vesicular stomatitis virus-based vaccine expressing a surface glycoprotein of *Zaire Ebolavirus* (rVSV-ZEBOV) is a promising candidate that was rapidly escalated into efficacy trials in Africa. In August 2015 the Lancet published an interim analysis showing that rVSV-ZEBOV appears to provide 100% protection

against the virus. The trial was carried out in Guinea and used a 'ring' design in which contacts of infected people are vaccinated, as are any subsequent contacts of those people.

Recommendations for travelers to an area affected by an Ebola outbreak or those residing in such an area are as follows:

- Practice careful hand hygiene and avoid contact with an infected person's blood or body fluids, including personal items that may have come in contact with blood and body fluids.
- Avoid unprotected contact with the body of a deceased person who was infected with EVD.
- Avoid contact with bats and nonhuman primates, including blood, bodily fluids, and tissues from these animals.
- Monitor health for 21 days after return from an Ebola endemic region, and seek medical care immediately if any symptoms develop.

Health care workers at risk for exposure to Ebola must wear PPE and notify appropriate health officials at their institutions if they have unprotected contact with the blood or bodily fluids of a person infected with EVD. Finally institutions must have proper infection control and sterilization measures in place for handling of biohazardous materials. Clinicians may contact the CDC for additional information on use of experimental therapeutics and vaccines for prophylaxis following a high-risk occupational exposure to Ebola virus.

Monitoring

Local authorities may have specific regulations for management of asymptomatic individuals with Ebola virus exposure. This includes self-monitoring versus direct observation by a health official, and the need for quarantine. In general, asymptomatic persons who have had an exposure should be monitored for 21 days after the last known exposure, and should immediately report the development of fever or other clinical manifestations suggestive of EVD to the health authorities.

References

Bah EI, Lamah MC, Fletcher T, et al. Clinical presentation of patients with Ebola virus disease in Conakry, Guinea. N Engl J Med 2015;372:40–7.

Chertow DS, Kleine C, Edwards JK, et al. Ebola virus disease in West Africa—clinical manifestations and management. N Engl J Med 2014;371:2054–7.

Henao-Restrepo AM, Longini IM, Egger M, et al. Efficacy and effectiveness of an rVSV-vectored vaccine expressing Ebola surface glycoprotein: interim results from the Guinea ring vaccination cluster-randomised trial. Lancet 2015;S0140–6736 (15):61117–25.

Schieffelin JS, Shaffer JG, Goba A, et al. Clinical illness and outcomes in patients with Ebola in Sierra Leone. N Engl J Med 2014;371:2092–100.

United States Centers for Disease Control and Prevention (CDC). Ebola (Ebola virus disease). Available at http://www.cdc.gov/vhf/ebola/.

WHO Ebola Response Team. Ebola virus disease in West Africa—the first 9 months of the epidemic and forward projections. N Engl J Med 2014;371:1481–95.

World Health Organization (WHO). Ebola. Available at http://www.who.int/csr/disease/ebola/en/.

FOODBORNE ILLNESSES

Method of
Anita Devi K. Ravindran, MD; and K.N. Viswanathan, MD

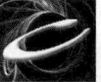

CURRENT DIAGNOSIS

- Infective foodborne illnesses are innumerable and are caused by various microorganisms. Some microorganisms are established agents, several others are emerging pathogens, and the pathogenicity of the remainder is still under speculation.
- Classification of these illnesses is best done according to their incubation periods, the symptoms they produce, or both.
- Nausea and vomiting predominate in illnesses with short incubation periods caused by preformed toxins, whereas diarrhea predominates in those with long incubation periods caused by toxins produced in the intestine.
- Undercooked charcuterie, meat, poultry, and seafood account for a majority of foodborne illness, but dairy products, salads, pastries, fruits, and vegetables can also cause illness.
- Contaminated water acts as a vehicle in almost all instances.

3 The Infectious Diseases

[5]Investigational drug in the United States.

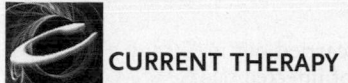

CURRENT THERAPY

- The majority of infective foodborne illnesses with symptoms confined to the gastrointestinal tract, although apparently alarming, are self-limiting and need only supportive measures including replacement of water and electrolytes.
- Antimicrobial agents are indicated only in certain patients, including those with systemic illnesses, extremes of age, immunocompromised and malnourished states, and severe life-threatening illness.
- Antitoxin is useful in botulism poisoning.
- Vaccines are available against *Vibrio cholerae*, *Salmonella typhi*, hepatitis A virus, and rotavirus, but their effectiveness and cost-effectiveness are debatable.

The Centers for Disease Control and Prevention (CDC) estimates that each year roughly one in six Americans (about 48 million people) gets sick from foodborne illnesses; 128,000 are hospitalized, and 3000 die. These figures are higher in developing nations, and many cases are not brought to light because they occur in remote villages. The 2011 estimates provide the most accurate picture of infective foodborne illnesses, of which bacteria, viruses, and parasites account for the majority. Processing of ready-to-eat foods increases the risk of acquiring foodborne illness because of increased food handling, leading to introduction and growth of pathogens. Increased international travel and migration have also resulted in a greater risk because travelers are at high risk for developing foodborne gastroenteritis caused by pathogens to which they have not been exposed at home.

Classification of Foodborne Illnesses

Agents causing foodborne diseases may be classified in several ways. The most common scheme is a taxonomic combined with a classification based on mode of action (Tables 1 to 3).

Bacteria

Aeromonas Species

Species of *Aeromonas* are ubiquitous and autochthonous in aquatic environments, more so after the tsunami that followed

TABLE 1	Classification of Foodborne Illnesses
SIGNS AND SYMPTOMS OR MECHANISM	**PATHOGENS**
Based on Symptoms and Duration of Onset	
Nausea and vomiting within 6 h	*Staphylococcus aureus, Bacillus cereus*
Abdominal cramps and diarrhea within 8–16 h	*Clostridium perfringens, Bacillus cereus*
Fever, abdominal cramps, and diarrhea within 16–48 h	*Salmonella, Shigella, Vibrio parahemolyticus,* enteroinvasive *Escherichia coli, Campylobacter jejuni*
Abdominal cramps and watery diarrhea within 16–72 h	Enterotoxigenic *E. coli, Vibrio cholerae* O1, O139 Bengal, *Vibrio parahemolyticus,* NAG (nonagglutinable) vibrios, *Norovirus*
Fever and abdominal cramps within 16–48 h	*Yersinia enterocolitica*
Bloody diarrhea without fever within 72–120 h	Enterohemorrhagic *E. coli* O157:H7
Nausea, vomiting, diarrhea, and paralysis within 18–36 h	*Clostridium botulinum*
Based on Pathogenesis	
Food intoxications resulting from the ingestion of preformed bacterial toxins	*Staphylococcus aureus, Bacillus cereus, Clostridium botulinum, Clostridium perfringens*
Food intoxications caused by noninvasive bacteria that secrete toxins while adhering to the intestinal wall	Enterotoxigenic *E. coli, Vibrio cholerae, Campylobacter jejuni*
Food intoxications that follow an intracellular invasion of intestinal epithelial cells	*Shigella, Salmonella*
Diseases caused by bacteria that enter the bloodstream via the intestinal tract	*Salmonella typhi, Listeria monocytogenes*
Based on Toxin Production	
The organisms responsible produce two major types of toxins, or they may be invasive, with no toxin production.	
Secretory toxins are enterotoxins produced by microbes that colonize the intestines in large numbers by attaching to the mucosal epithelial cells without invasion of mucosa, and hence there is no fever or other systemic symptoms as a result of lack of inflammatory response. Massive quantities of fluid and electrolytes are lost into the large bowel as its reabsorbing capacity is exceeded by the hypersecretion of isotonic fluid produced by the enterotoxins.	*Vibrio cholerae,* enterotoxigenic *E. coli, Shigella dysenteriae, Salmonella typhimurium*
Cytotoxins are those that destroy the epithelial cells of the mucosa.	*Shigella dysenteriae* elaborating Shiga toxin, causing destructive colitis, enterohemorrhagic *E. coli,* producing a similar toxin causing hemorrhagic colitis and hemolytic uremic syndrome (HUS), and *Vibrio parahemolyticus*) *Clostridium perfringens,* which produces a secretory enterotoxin, also has a cytotoxic action.
Secretory toxins, cytotoxins, and/or neurotoxins that are preformed are ingested directly in food.	*Bacillus cereus, Staphylococcus aureus, Clostridium botulinum*
Certain invasive microbes produce systemic symptoms such as fever, headache, and myalgia, in addition to gastrointestinal symptoms.	Salmonellosis typhoid fever, shigellosis, and brucellosis

97

| TABLE 2 | Common Organisms Implicated in Infective Foodborne Illness |

ETIOLOGIC AGENT	USUAL INCUBATION PERIOD	SYMPTOMS	DURATION OF SYMPTOMS	COMMON VEHICLES
Upper Gastrointestinal Tract Symptoms (Nausea, Vomiting) Occur First or Predominate				
Staphylococcus aureus (preformed toxin)	1–6 h	Sudden onset of severe nausea and vomiting Abdominal cramps, diarrhea, and fever may be present	24–48 h	Unrefrigerated or improperly refrigerated meat, potato and egg salads, cream pastries
Bacillus cereus (preformed toxin)	1–6 h	Sudden onset of severe nausea and vomiting Diarrhea may be present	24 h	Improperly refrigerated cooked or fried rice, meat
Lower Gastrointestinal Tract Symptoms (Abdominal Cramps, Diarrhea) Occur First or Predominate				
Bacillus cereus (diarrheal toxin)	10–16 h	Abdominal cramps, watery diarrhea, nausea	24–48 h	Meat, stew, gravy, vanilla sauce
Clostridium perfringens (toxin)	8–16 h	Watery diarrhea, nausea, abdominal cramps; fever is rare	24–48 h	Meat, poultry, gravy, dried or precooked foods, time- and/or temperature-abused food
Vibrio cholerae	2 h to 5 d	Rice-water purging diarrhea leading to dehydration, shock, acidosis, renal failure, abdominal pain Cholera sicca is a severe form; patient dies before diarrhea is manifest; ileus and abdominal bloating result	2–7 d	Sewage-contaminated water Seafood: fish, shellfish, crabs, oysters, clams Contaminated rice, millet gruel, vegetables
Vibrio parahaemolyticus	12–24 h	Watery diarrhea, abdominal cramps, nausea, vomiting Neurologic symptoms can occur, as with *Clostridium botulinum* and *Trichinella spiralis*	2–5 d	Raw or undercooked seafood
Shigella	1–4 d	Abdominal cramps, fever, diarrhea Stool might contain blood and mucus	4–7 d	Food or water contaminated with fecal matter Ready-to-eat food touched by infected food worker
Salmonella (not *typhi*)	1–3 d	Diarrhea, fever, abdominal cramps, vomiting	4–7 d	Contaminated eggs, unpasteurized milk or juice, cheese, contaminated raw fruits and vegetables
Enterotoxigenic *Escherichia coli*	1–3 d	Watery diarrhea, abdominal cramps, some vomiting	3–7 d (or longer)	Food or water contaminated with human feces
Shiga toxin–producing *E. coli*, including *E. coli* O157:H7	2–6 d	Severe diarrhea that is often bloody; abdominal pain and vomiting Usually little or no fever	5–10 d	Undercooked beef, especially hamburger, unpasteurized milk and juice, raw fruit and vegetables (e.g., sprouts), salami (rarely), contaminated water
Campylobacter jejuni	2–5 d	Diarrhea, cramps, fever, vomiting Diarrhea may be bloody	2–10 d	Raw and undercooked poultry, unpasteurized milk, contaminated milk
Vibrio vulnificus	1–7 d	Vomiting, diarrhea, abdominal pain Fever, bleeding within the skin, ulcers requiring surgical removal Can be fatal to people with liver disease or weakened immune systems	2–8 d	Undercooked or raw seafood, especially oysters
Yersinia enterocolitica	3–7 d	Appendicitis-like symptoms: diarrhea, vomiting, fever, abdominal pain	Can remit and relapse over weeks to 1 mo	Drinking water, food contaminated with human fecal matter
Cyclospora	7–10 d	Diarrhea (usually watery), loss of appetite, weight loss, stomach cramps, nausea, vomiting, fatigue	Can remit and relapse over weeks to 1 mo	Fresh herbs and produce (e.g., raspberries, basil, lettuce)
Giardia lamblia (beaver fever)	7–10 d	Diarrhea (acute or chronic), stomach cramps, flatulence, weight loss, malabsorption, developmental delay	Days to weeks	Drinking water, food contaminated with human fecal matter
Entamoeba histolytica	1–4 wk	Intestinal: diarrhea, fever, abdominal pain, dysentery, colitis, bowel perforation, ameboma Extraintestinal amebiasis: liver abscess with anchovy-sauce pus, spread to viscera, lungs, and brain	Days to weeks	Drinking water Food contaminated with human fecal matter

ETIOLOGIC AGENT	USUAL INCUBATION PERIOD	SYMPTOMS	DURATION OF SYMPTOMS	COMMON VEHICLES
Both Upper and Lower Gastrointestinal Tract Symptoms				
Rotavirus	18–36 h	Acute onset of fever and vomiting followed 12–24 h later by frequent watery stools	3–7 d	Contaminated drinking water, food, fomites
Norovirus and other caliciviruses	12–48 h	Nausea, vomiting, cramping, diarrhea, fever, myalgia, some headache Diarrhea is more prevalent in adults; vomiting is more prevalent in children	12–60 h	Food (including shellfish) or water contaminated with human fecal matter Ready-to-eat food touched by an infected food worker
Generalized Symptoms				
Listeria monocytogenes	9–48 h or GI symptoms; 2–6 wk for invasive disease	Fever, muscle aches, nausea or diarrhea Pregnant women can have mild flulike illness, and infection can lead to premature delivery or stillbirth Elderly and immunocompromised patients can have bacteremia or meningitis	Variable	Fresh soft cheese, unpasteurized milk, ready-to-eat deli meat, hot dogs
Balatidium coli	4–5 d	Mostly asymptomatic Chronic diarrhea, occasional dysentery, nausea, foul breath, colitis, abdominal pain, weight loss, deep intestinal ulcerations, possible perforation of the intestine, pneumonia-like illness	Variable	Water contaminated with pig feces
Salmonella typhi	8–14 d	Fever, anorexia, lethargy, malaise, headache, rose spots, constipation or diarrhea, hepatosplenomegaly	4–6 wk	Contaminated water, contaminated food, mainly via food handlers; shellfish from polluted water
Ascaris lumbricoides	4–16 d	Nausea, abdominal pain, intestinal obstruction, malnutrition, Loeffler's syndrome (cough, pneumonitis, eosinophilia), biliary colic, cholangitis, pancreatitis, appendicitis	Variable (chronic)	Soil-contaminated raw food, food handlers, water
Trichinella spiralis	1–2 wk	Asymptomatic or chronic diarrhea, abdominal pain Allergy leading to rash, periorbital edema, vasculitis, intramural thrombi Weakness of jaw, biceps, diaphragm, intercostals Eosinophilia, subconjunctival, splinter hemorrhages Muscle penetration: myalgia, orbital pain, diplopia Chronic phase: neurologic symptoms	Variable Acute phase: 1–3 wk	Raw or undercooked meat of pig, horse, wild boar, bush pig, warthog, bear
Infective cysticerci of *Taenia solium* (pork tape worm)	2 months on average	Seizures, vasculitis, focal neurologic deficits, intracranial hypertension, hydrocephalus, mental changes, encephalitis and Brun's syndrome (intermittent obstruction of cerebral aqueduct), myositis, vasculitis	Highly variable	Undercooked charcuterie (pork), contaminated raw vegetables, salads, water
Hepatitis A	15–50 d	Diarrhea, dark urine, jaundice, flulike symptoms, fever, headache, nausea, aversion to food, vomiting, abdominal pain; distaste for cigarettes	Variable: 2 wk to 3 mo	Food (including shellfish) or water contaminated with human fecal matter Inadequately cooked clams, oysters, mussels, cockles Contaminated lettuce, slush beverages, frozen strawberries and salad items Ready-to-eat foods touched by an infected food worker

Continued

ETIOLOGIC AGENT	USUAL INCUBATION PERIOD	SYMPTOMS	DURATION OF SYMPTOMS	COMMON VEHICLES
Brucella species	1–8 wk	Flulike illness; undulating fever, malaise, arthralgia, anorexia, hepatosplenomegaly, pleurisy, nausea, vomiting, diarrhea, new onset of increased desire to sleep after lunch	Variable	Unpasteurized dairy products, undercooked meat, bone marrow Contact with laboratory cultures and tissue samples Accidental injection of live brucellosis vaccine
Hepatitis E	3–8 wk	Prodrome: anorexia, nausea, vomiting, arthralgia, myalgia, weight loss, dehydration, abdominal pain Icteric phase: jaundice, pruritus, light-colored stool Urticaria, diarrhea, malaise	Variable (several weeks)	Fecally contaminated drinking water and food Raw and undercooked shellfish incriminated in sporadic outbreaks Possibly zoonotic spread
Microsporidium: *Encephalitozoon, Pleistophora, Nosema, Vittaforma, Trachipleistophora, Brachiola, Microsporidium, Enterocytozoon*	Unknown	Watery or bloody or unspecified diarrhea, abdominal discomfort, cramps, flatulence, weight loss, loss of appetite, wasting syndrome, subfebrile temperatures Extraintestinal: pneumonitis, myositis, keratoconjunctivitis, seizures, nephritis, cholangiopathy	Variable; self-limiting (1–2 wk) in immunocompetent patients	Contaminated water, food, or inhalation

Abbreviation: GI = gastrointestinal.

the Indonesian earthquake in December 2004. These aeromonads share many biochemical characteristics with members of the Enterobacteriaceae. The mesophilic species *Aeromonas caviae, Aeromonas hydrophila,* and *Aeromonas veronii* are principally associated with gastroenteritis; *A. caviae* particularly infects children younger than 3 years.

Transmission is documented as occurring from a contaminated piped water source, as seen in community-based outbreaks, especially among children. The probability of occurrence of *Aeromonas* infection increased significantly when the mean seasonal temperature exceeded 14 °C (57°F), and this was exacerbated where the mean free chlorine concentration fell below 0.1 mg/L.

Aeromonas species are potential food-poisoning agents. *A. hydrophila* is psychrotrophic and has been associated with spoilage of refrigerated animal products including chicken, beef, pork, lamb, fish, oysters, crab, and milk.

The incubation period for *Aeromonas*-associated traveler's diarrhea is 1 to 2 days. It usually causes a sporadic illness. Usually a mild to moderate but self-limiting diarrhea occurs, but it can be severe enough in children to require hospitalization. *Aeromonas* gastroenteritis can occur as a nondescript enteritis, as a more-severe form accompanied by bloody stools, as the etiologic agent of a subacute or chronic intestinal syndrome, as an extremely rare cause of cholera-like disease, or in association with episodic traveler's diarrhea. By far the most common presentation of *Aeromonas* gastroenteritis is watery enteritis. The most serious complication resulting from *Aeromonas* gastroenteritis is hemolytic uremic syndrome.

Pathogenesis

Mesophilic *Aeromonas* spp. can express a range of virulence factors, including attachment mechanisms and production of a number of toxins. Toxins include aerolysin (a pore-forming cytolysin that attaches to cell membrane, leading to leakage of cytoplasmic contents) and a cytotonic enterotoxin with activity similar to that of cholera toxin. Strains of *A. hydrophila* produce lectins and adhesins, which enable adherence to epithelial surfaces and gut mucosa.

Laboratory Diagnosis

Samples are best transported using Cary-Blair medium. *Aeromonas* forms a bull's-eye–like colony on the selective medium cefsulodin irgasan novobiocin (CIN) agar owing to fermentation of D-mannitol. Ampicillin blood agar has an advantage over CIN agar in that hemolytic colonies can readily be tested for oxidase. *Aeromonas* species produce hemolysis on sheep blood agar.

Treatment

In *Aeromonas* infections, ciprofloxacin (Cipro)[1] 500 mg PO or 400 mg IV twice daily is the antimicrobial treatment of choice. Piperacillin-tazobactam (Zosyn)[1] 4.5 g IV three times daily or ceftazidime (Fortaz)[1] 2 g IV daily may be added in severe infections. The organism is also susceptible to aminoglycosides and carbapenems. Resistance is now becoming a problem because *Aeromonas* can produce β-lactamases and carbapenemases. Therefore, it is preferable to initiate therapy with a fluoroquinolone when the organism is isolated.

Bacillus cereus

Bacillus cereus is found abundantly in the environment and vegetation. It is known to produce two forms of food poisoning, emetic and diarrheal. The emetic (short-incubation) type of illness is associated with contaminated fried rice that is not refrigerated. The organism is present in uncooked rice, and the spores survive boiling. The illness is usually self-limiting, with recovery in a day. It is mediated by a heat-stable, preformed enterotoxin resembling that of *Staphylococcus aureus*. The first major outbreak of *Bacillus cereus* food poisoning was in 1971 in England. The diarrheal (long-incubation) type of illness is produced by a heat-labile diarrheal enterotoxin formed in the intestine, which activates adenylate cyclase, causing intestinal fluid secretion, similar to *Escherichia coli* LT toxin and the toxin of *Clostridium perfringens*.

---

[1]Not FDA approved for this indication.

TABLE 3 Rare and Emerging Infections

ETIOLOGIC AGENT	USUAL INCUBATION PERIOD	SYMPTOMS	DURATION OF SYMPTOMS	COMMON VEHICLES
Bacillus subtilis	10 min to 14 h (average, 2.5 h)	Vomiting, diarrhea, abdominal cramps, nausea, headache, flushing, sweating	1.5–8 h	Sausage rolls, meat pasties, turkey stuffing, chicken stuffing, pizza, whole-grain bread, steak pie, pork sandwiches
Cyanobacteria: *Microcystic aeuroginosa, Anabaena circinalis, Anabaena flosaquae, Aphanizomenon flosaquae, Cylindrospermopsis racibarskii*	3–6 h	Diarrhea, vomiting, allergic reactions, breathing difficulty, dizziness, tingling and numbness, liver and kidney toxicity	8–16 h	Drinking water from untreated surface sources, inhaling aerosols from jet-skis and boats, consuming dietary supplements contaminated by microcystin
Anisakis	Few hours to days	Gastric: abdominal pain, nausea, vomiting. Allergic: urticaria, anaphylaxis. Intestinal: ileus, perforation, peritonitis, stenosis	2 wk	Raw, lightly pickled, or salted marine fish: Mackerel, squid, horse mackerel, salmon, bonito Squid, cuttlefish Sushi, sashimi
Astrovirus	1–4 d	Watery diarrhea (especially in children), vomiting, fever, anorexia, abdominal pain	3–4 d	Sewage-polluted water and food
Pleisomonas shigelloides	5 d	Diarrhea with blood and mucus, abdominal pain, headache, nausea, chills, fever, vomiting	1–7 d	Contaminated water used for drinking or rinsing foods to be eaten raw Contaminated raw shellfish, salted fish, crabs, oysters
Cyclospora	7 d	Frequent watery diarrhea, weight loss, abdominal pain, bloating, flatulence, vomiting, nausea, low-grade fever, fatigue, malabsorption, cholecystitis	1–4 wk Relapse is common	Fecally contaminated fresh raspberries, snow peas, mesclun
Iosospora belli	8–11 d	Diarrhea, steatorrhea, headache, fever, malaise, abdominal pain, vomiting, dehydration, weight loss Mesenteric lymph node, liver, spleen involvement	Variable; runs a chronic course in immunocompromised patients	Contaminated food and water
Edwardisella tarda	Not defined	Nausea, vomiting, diarrhea, dysentery, colitis, wound infections, septicemia	Variable: 1–2 wk or longer	Fecal contamination of food, water, raw fish
Citrobacter species	Not defined	Diarrhea, hemolytic uremic syndrome, thrombocytopenic purpura		Meat and milk Parsley (in green butter) from organic gardens using pig manure
Arizona	Not defined	Diarrhea		Cream pie, chocolate eclairs, custard, eggs, chicken, turkey
Achromobacter xylosoxidans	Not defined	Abdominal pain, diarrhea, headache, vomiting		Raw milk, spoiled canned food, contaminated well water

Pathogenesis

During the slow cooling of cooked rice, spores germinate and vegetative bacteria multiply; then they sporulate again. Sporulation is also associated with toxin production. The toxin is heat stable and can easily withstand the temperatures used to cook fried rice.

Laboratory Diagnosis

The disease is diagnosed by the isolation of *B. cereus* from the incriminated food (emetic type) or from stool and food (diarrheal type). Isolation from stools alone is not sufficient because gastrointestinal colonization with *B. cereus* occurs in many persons.

Treatment

B. cereus food poisoning may be symptomatically managed with replacement of fluids and electrolytes. Antimicrobials have no role in treatment. *B. cereus* is also known to produce a variety of ocular and systemic infections such as meningitis, osteomyelitis, pneumonia, and endocarditis. These are usually not foodborne, and it is in this situation that vancomycin (Vancocin)[1] becomes the drug of choice, with clindamycin (Cleocin)[1] and carbapenems being the alternative drugs, both being used along with aminoglycosides for synergistic action.

---

[1]Not FDA approved for this indication.

Campylobacter jejuni

Campylobacter jejuni are harbored in the reproductive and alimentary tracts of some animals. Other than gastrointestinal symptoms, the patient has malaise and headache. The organism may be shed in the patient's stool for up to 2 months. Bacteremia is observed in a small minority of cases. The disease is usually self-limiting. Guillain-Barré syndrome and Reiter's syndrome are recognized sequelae.

Pathogenesis

As few as 500 organisms can cause enteritis. The organism is invasive but generally less so than *Shigella*. *Campylobacter* produces adenylate cyclase–activating toxins resembling *E. coli* LT and cholera toxin.

Laboratory Diagnosis

The feces may be inoculated in enrichment medium or on selective media such as Campy-BAP or Skirrow's medium.

Treatment

Indications for antibiotic therapy in *C. jejuni* infections are prolonged fever, severe diarrhea, dysentery, and persistent symptoms for more than a week. Therapy of *Campylobacter* infection with ciprofloxacin (Cipro 500 mg orally twice daily for 7 days) early in the course of the illness shortens its duration. Unfortunately, this has led to the emergence of fluoroquinolone-resistant *Campylobacter* infections. Erythromycin eradicates carriage of susceptible *C. jejuni* and might shorten the duration of illness if given early in the disease. Erythromycin (Ery-Tab)[1] 250 mg PO four times daily is the drug of choice in *Campylobacter* enteritis. Azithromycin (Zithromax)[1] is also useful and has the advantage of shorter duration of therapy.

Gentamicin (Garamycin), carbapenems, amoxicillin-clavulanate (Augmentin),[1] and chloramphenicol[1] are useful in systemic infections. The usual duration of treatment is 2 weeks. The therapy is prolonged in immunocompromised persons and in patients with endovascular infections.

Clostridium botulinum

Clostridum botulinum is widely distributed in soil, in sediments of lakes and ponds, and in decaying vegetation. *C. botulinum* elaborates the most potent toxin known in humans. When the toxin is ingested, paralysis occurs, often requiring prolonged artificial ventilation. Common signs and symptoms include vomiting, thirst, dry mouth, constipation, ocular palsies, dysphagia, dysarthria, bulbar paralysis, and death due to respiratory paralysis. Coma or delirium occurs in some. Infants present with lethargy, poor feeding, loss of head control, and sometimes sudden infant death syndrome (SIDS).

The incriminated foods are corn syrup, home-canned or bottled meat, fruits, fish, vegetables, herb-infused oils, and cheese sauce. Infant botulism is associated with consumption of honey; honey should not be given to infants younger than 1 year.

Pathogenesis

Not all strains of *C. botulinum* produce botulinum toxin. Toxigenic types of the organism, designated A, B, C1, D, E, F, and G, produce immunologically distinct forms of botulinum toxin. Lysogenic phages encode toxin C and D serotypes.

Foodborne botulism is not an infection but an intoxication because it results from the ingestion of foods that contain the preformed clostridial toxin. If contaminated food has been insufficiently heated or canned improperly, the spores can germinate and produce botulinum toxin. The toxin is released only after cell lysis and death. The toxin resists digestion and is absorbed by the upper gastrointestinal tract and enters the blood. The toxin blocks release of acetylcholine by binding to receptors at synapses and neuromuscular junctions and causes flaccid paralysis.

Laboratory Diagnosis

Spoilage of food or swelling of cans or presence of bubbles inside the can indicate growth of *C. botulinum*. Food is homogenized in broth and inoculated in Robertson cooked meat medium and blood agar or egg-yolk agar, which is incubated anaerobically for 3 to 5 days at 37°C. The toxin can be demonstrated by injecting the extract of food or culture into mice or guinea pigs intraperitoneally.

Treatment

Hospitalization in an intensive care unit with immediate administration of botulinum antitoxin is vital in the management of botulism. The antitoxin neutralizes only toxin molecules unbound to nerve endings and does not reverse the paralysis. It should be given within 24 hours after the diagnosis is made. Penicillin is the antimicrobial of choice. Intubation and mechanical ventilation are needed for respiratory failure. If swallowing difficulty persists, intravenous fluids or alimentation should be given through a nasogastric tube.

Clostridium perfringens

C. perfringens is heat resistant and elaborates two toxins that can induce specific pathology in the human intestinal tract. It is the third leading cause of foodborne illnesses in United States, after norovirus and *B. cereus*. It is present abundantly in the environment, vegetation, sewage, and animal feces.

Human diseases caused by this organism are the more common *C. perfringens* type A food poisoning and the less common, but more serious, *C. perfringens* type C food poisoning producing necrotic enteritis. Necrotic enteritis is characterized by vomiting, severe abdominal pain, and bloody diarrhea. The incubation period is 2 to 5 days. Progression to necrosis of the jejunum and death occur.

Pathogenesis

Spores in food can survive cooking and then germinate when the food is improperly stored. When these vegetative cells form endospores in the intestine, they release enterotoxins. Food poisoning is mainly caused by type A strains, which produce alpha and theta toxins. The toxins result in excessive fluid accumulation in the intestinal lumen.

Laboratory Diagnosis

Because the bacterium is present normally in intestines, isolation from feces might not be sufficient to implicate it as the cause of the illness. Similarly, isolation from food, except in large numbers ($>10^9$/g), might not be significant. The homogenized food is diluted and plated on selective medium as well as Robertson cooked meat medium and subjected to anaerobic incubation. The isolated bacteria must be shown to produce enterotoxin.

Treatment

Food poisoning due to *Clostridium perfringens* is managed conservatively with hydration and replacement of electrolytes. *C. perfringens* is susceptible to benzylpenicillin (penicillin G), which may be useful in managing severe infections (1 mU IV every 4 hours). Vancomycin,[1] clindamycin,[1] cefoxitin (Mefoxin), and metronidazole (Flagyl) are alternatives. *C. perfringens* type C toxoid vaccine[2] (two doses, 4 months apart) is preventive in pigbel.

Cronobacter sakazakii

Cronobacter sakazakii causes neonatal meningitis or necrotizing enterocolitis and bacteremia, which results in an alarming mortality rate. Surviving patients sometimes develop ventriculitis and cerebral abscess. *C. sakazakii* has been isolated from infant formulas.

Enterobacter species are generally resistant to the cephalosporins, except cefepime (Maxipime),[1] but are responsive to carbenicillin (Geocillin),[1] piperacillin (Pipracil),[1] ticarcillin (Ticar),[1] amikacin (Amikin),[1] and tigecycline (Tygacil).[1]

---

[1]Not FDA approved for this indication.

[1]Not FDA approved for this indication.
[2]Not available in the United States.

Enterohemorrhagic *Escherichia coli*

Many serogroups of *E. coli*, including O4, O26, O45, O91, O111, O145, and O157, are pathogenic, but the most common pathogenic serotype is O157:H7. Cattle are the main sources of infection; most cases are associated with the consumption of undercooked beef burgers and similar foods from restaurants and delicatessens.

Pathogenesis

Enterohemorrhagic *E. coli* (EHEC) strains can produce one or more types of cytotoxins, which are collectively referred to as Shiga-like toxins because they are antigenically and functionally similar to Shiga toxin produced by *Shigella dysenteriae*. (Shiga-like toxins were previously known as verotoxins.) The toxins provoke cell secretion and kill colonic epithelial cells, causing hemorrhagic colitis and hemolytic-uremic syndrome (HUS), leading occasionally to disseminated intravascular coagulation (DIC). A fibrin layer forms in the glomerular capillary bed, and acute renal failure occurs due to DIC. These are most likely to occur in children, elderly patients, and pregnant women. The young recover fully, but at times dialysis is warranted.

Laboratory Diagnosis

Laboratory diagnosis is performed by culturing the feces on McConkey's agar or sorbitol McConkey's agar. Strains can then be identified by serotyping using specific antisera. Shiga-like toxins can be detected by enzyme-linked immunosorbent assay (ELISA), and genes coding for them can be detected by DNA hybridization techniques.

Treatment

Hydration with electrolyte replacement is the mainstay of treatment in *E. coli* O157:H7 infection, and patients should be monitored closely and constantly for the development of HUS, which requires management in an intensive care setting with blood transfusion and dialysis. Although dysentery is self-limiting, the use of rifaximin (Xifaxan), a nonabsorbable agent, is recommended in those who are increasingly susceptible to infections. In the absence of dysentery, early institution of drugs like ciprofloxacin (Cipro) or azithromycin (Zithromax),[1] especially in traveler's diarrhea, decreases the duration of illness.

Enterotoxigenic *Escherichia Coli*

Enterotoxigenic *E. coli* (ETEC) is now ubiquitous in nature. Wild animals and cattle act as reservoirs of the organism. *E. coli* is carried normally in the intestine of humans and animals. Some specific serotypes harbor plasmids that code for toxin production. This bacterium is responsible for a majority of traveler's diarrhea. The disease is self-limiting and resolves in few days.

Pathogenesis

The bacteria colonize the gastrointestinal tract by means of fimbriae, attaching to specific receptors on enterocytes of the proximal small intestine. Enterotoxins produced by ETEC include the LT (heat-labile) toxin and the ST (heat-stable) toxins. LTs are similar to cholera toxin in structure and mode of action, consisting of A and B subunits. The B (binding) subunit of LTs binds to specific ganglioside receptors (GM1) on the epithelial cells of the small intestine and facilitates the entry of the A (activating) subunit, which activates adenylate cyclase. Stimulation of adenylate cyclase causes an increased production of cyclic adenosine monophosphate (cAMP), which leads to hypersecretion of water and electrolytes into the lumen and inhibition of sodium reabsorption.

Laboratory Diagnosis

The sample of feces is cultured on McConkey's agar. The ETEC stains are indistinguishable from the resident *E. coli* by biochemical tests. These strains are differentiated from nontoxigenic *E. coli* present in the bowel by a variety of in vitro immunochemical, tissue culture, or DNA hybridization tests designed to detect either the toxins or the genes that encode for these toxins. With the availability of a gene probe method, foods can be analyzed directly for the presence of ETEC in about 3 days. LTs can be detected by ligated rabbit ileal loop test and by observing morphological changes in Chinese hamster ovary cells and Y1 adrenal cells. ELISA, immunodiffusion, and coagglutination are also used in diagnosis.

Listeria monocytogenes

Listeria monocytogenes is quite hardy and resists the deleterious effects of freezing, drying, and heat remarkably well for a bacterium that does not form spores. It is capable of growing at 3 °C and multiplies in refrigerated foods.

Pathogenesis

L. monocytogenes invades the gastrointestinal epithelium. Once the bacterium enters the host's monocytes, macrophages, or neutrophils, it is bloodborne and can grow. Its presence in phagocytes also permits access to the brain and transplacental migration to the fetus in pregnant women. Granulomatosis infantisepticum is a feature of listeriosis. The pathogenesis of *L. monocytogenes* centers on its ability to survive and multiply in phagocytic host cells.

Laboratory Diagnosis

The diagnosis of listeriosis is most commonly made by isolation of *L. monocytogenes* from a normally sterile site. β-Hemolytic colonies, which test negative for catalase, hydrolyze hippurate, and have a positive cAMP reaction, form on blood agar. Serologic testing is not useful in diagnosing acute invasive disease, but it can be useful in detecting asymptomatic disease and gastroenteritis in an outbreak or in other epidemiologic investigations. Stool testing is not commercially available.

Treatment

Ampicillin[1] (2 g IV every 4 hours) is the drug of choice in *Listeria monocytogenes* infections. Aminoglycosides are added for synergistic effect. Trimethoprim-sulfamethoxazole (TMP-SMX)[1] (Bactrim, 20 mg of trimethoprim/day IV every 6 hours) is an alternative for patients allergic to penicillin. Ampicillin and TMP-SMX may be used in combination. Vancomycin (Vancocin),[1] linezolid (Zyvox),[1] carbapenems, macrolides, and tetracyclines are also effective. Cephalosporins are ineffective in the treatment of listeriosis and should not be used. The duration of therapy is highly variable depending on the clinical situation and is 14 days for bacteremia, 21 days for meningitis, 42 days for endocarditis, and 56 days for neurologic infections. Patients whose disease is promptly diagnosed and treated recover fully, but permanent neurologic sequelae are common in patients with cerebral illnesses. Consuming only pasteurized dairy products and fully cooked meats, meticulously cleaning utensils, and thoroughly washing fresh vegetables before cooking will prevent foodborne listerial infections. Pregnant women and others at risk should avoid soft cheeses and thoroughly reheated ready-to-serve and charcuterie foods.

Nontyphoidal Salmonellosis

Nontyphoidal salmonellosis consists of several causative organisms classified under the family Enterobacteriaceae; one such organism is *Salmonella enteritidis*. It does not occur normally in humans, but several animals act as reservoirs.

The diarrhea may be watery, with greenish, foul-smelling stools. This may be preceded by headache and chills. Other findings include prostration, muscle weakness, and moderate fever.

---

[1]Not FDA approved for this indication.

[1]Not FDA approved for this indication.

Pathogenesis

The organism penetrates and passes through the epithelial cells lining the terminal ileum. Multiplication of bacteria in lamina propria produces inflammatory mediators, recruits neutrophils, and triggers inflammation. Release of lipopolysaccharides and prostaglandins causes fever and also loss of water and electrolytes into the lumen of the intestine, resulting in diarrhea.

Laboratory Diagnosis

Culture in selenite F broth and then subculture on deoxycholate citrate agar isolates the organisms. Plates are incubated at 37°C overnight, and growth is identified by biochemical and slide agglutination tests.

Treatment

The antibiotics recommended for gastroenteritis due to nontyphoidal salmonellosis are ciprofloxacin (Cipro)[1] 500 mg PO twice daily, and ceftriaxone (Rosephin) 2 g IV daily, for 3 to 7 days. Amoxicillin (Amoxil)[1] and TMP-SMX[1] are also effective. Therapy is prolonged in bacteremia, endocarditis, or meningitis.

Shigella Species

Shigella species belong to the family Enterobacteriaceae. Bacillary dysentery is caused by *Shigella flexneri*, *Shigella boydii*, *Shigella dysenteriae*, and *Shigella sonnei*. *S. flexneri* is most common in developing countries where hygiene is poor and clean drinking water is unavailable; *S. sonnei* is most common in developed countries. The watery diarrhea that is present initially becomes bloody after a day or two owing to spread of infection from the ileum to the colon. The illness is caused by exotoxin acting in the small bowel.

Extraintestinal manifestations are recognized, including HUS, Reiter's syndrome, meningitis, Ekiri syndrome (reported in Japanese children and consisting of a triad of encephalopathy due to cerebral edema, bizarre posturing, and fatty degeneration of liver), vaginitis, lung infections, and keratoconjunctivitis. Toxic megacolon, pneumatosis coli, perforation, and rectal prolapse are recognized complications.

Tossed salads, chicken, and shellfish are the commonly incriminated foods. Person-to-person spread by anal intercourse or oral sex also occurs. Prepared food acts as vehicle of transmission. Spread of infection is also linked to flies.

Children are at high risk during the weaning period, and increasing age is associated with decreased prevalence and severity. Children in daycare centers, persons in custodial institutions, migrant workers, and travelers to developing countries are also at high risk.

Pathogenesis

The virulence factor is a smooth lipopolysaccharide cell wall antigen, which is responsible for the invasive features, and the Shiga toxin, which is both cytotoxic and neurotoxic. Shigellae survive the gastric acidity and invade and multiply within the colonic epithelial cells, causing cell death and mucosal ulcers, and spread laterally to involve adjacent cells but rarely invade the bloodstream.

Laboratory Diagnosis

Shigellosis can be correctly diagnosed in most patients on the basis of fresh blood in stool. Neutrophils in fecal smears strongly suggest infection. Any clinical diagnosis should be confirmed by cultivation of the etiologic agent from stools. Cary-Blair medium is the transport medium of choice, and MacConkey agar or deoxycholate citrate agar (DCA) as well as a highly selective medium such as xylose-lysin deoxycholate (XLD), Hektoen enteric (HE), or Salmonella-Shigella (SS) agar are also used.

Treatment

Ciprofloxacin (Cipro, 500 mg PO twice daily for 3 days) is the antibiotic of choice for shigellosis. Alternative agents are pivmecillinam (Selexid),[2] ceftriaxone (Rocephin),[1] and azithromycin (Zithromax).[1]

---

[1]Not FDA approved for this indication.
[2]Not available in the United States.

Staphylococcus aureus

A notable incident of staphylococcal food poisoning occurred in February 1975 when 196 of 344 passengers and one flight attendant aboard a jet from Tokyo to Copenhagen via Anchorage contacted a gastrointestinal illness characterized by nausea, vomiting, and abdominal cramps. The flight attendant and 142 passengers were hospitalized. Symptoms developed shortly after a ham and omelet breakfast had been served. *S. aureus* was incriminated as the offending agent and ham as the vehicle of the outbreak. The source was traced to a cook with pustules on his fingers.

S. aureus is ubiquitous in environment. Only strains that produce enterotoxin cause food poisoning. Food is usually contaminated by infected food handlers.

Pathogenesis

If food is stored for some time at room temperature, the organism can multiply in the food and produce enterotoxin. Most food poisonings are caused by enterotoxin A, and the isolates commonly belong to phage type III. These are heat stable, and ingestion of as little as 23 µg of enterotoxin can induce symptoms. The toxin acts on the receptors in the gut, and sensory stimulus is carried to the vomiting center in the brain by vagus and sympathetic nerves.

Because the ingested food contains preformed toxin, the incubation period is very short. In severe illness, profound hypotension occurs. Death is known to occur at extremes of age and in the malnourished.

Laboratory Diagnosis

The presence of a large number of *S. aureus* in food can indicate poor handling or sanitation; however, it is not sufficient evidence to incriminate the food as the cause of food poisoning.

Staphylococcal food poisoning can be diagnosed if staphylococci are isolated in large numbers from the food and their toxins are demonstrated in the food or if the isolated *S. aureus* is shown to produce enterotoxins. Dilutions of food may be plated on Baird-Parker agar or mannitol salt agar. Enterotoxin may be detected and identified by gel diffusion.

Treatment

Therapy is mainly supportive. Antibiotics have no role in the treatment because they are not antitoxins. Intravenous fluids and electrolyte replacement are imperative in the severely dehydrated patient.

Yersinia Species

The *Yersinia* species that cause food poisoning are commonly *Yersinia enterocolitica* and rarely *Yersinia pseudotuberculosis*. Pigs and other wild or domestic animals are the hosts, and humans are usually infected by the oral route. Serogroups that predominate in human illness are O:3, O:5, O:8, and O:9.

Yersiniosis is common in children and occurs most often in winter. *Y. enterocolitica* is associated with terminal ileitis and *Y. pseudotuberculosis* with mesenteric adenitis, but both organisms can cause mesenteric adenitis and symptoms that cause a clinical picture resembling appendicitis, resulting in surgical removal of a normal appendix. Rarer strains of *Y. enterocolitica* are likely to cause systemic infections, especially in patients with diabetes or in iron overload states. In Japan, a form of vasculitis, called Izumi fever, occurs, and in Russia a scarlet fever–like illness has been reported.

Pathogenesis

Yersinia organisms can survive and grow during refrigerated storage. Strains that cause human yersiniosis carry a plasmid that is associated with a number of virulence traits. Ingested bacteria adhere and invade M cells or epithelial cells.

Laboratory Diagnosis

Suspect food is homogenized in phosphate-buffered saline and inoculated into selenite F broth and held at 4°C for 6 weeks. The broth is subcultured at weekly intervals on deoxycholate citrate (DCA) or *Yersinia*-selective agar plates. This is termed *cold-enrichment technique*.

Treatment

Antibiotics are not recommended for gastroenteritis caused by *Yersinia enterocolitica* and the less-common *Yersinia pseudotuberculosis,* but bacteremia and extraintestinal infections require treatment with ciprofloxacin[1] (500 mg PO or 400 mg IV twice daily for 2 weeks). Third-generation cephalosporins (cefotaxime[1] [Claforan]), amoxicillin[1] (Amoxil), TMP-SMX[1] (Bactrim), amoxicillin-clavulanate[1] (Augmentin), carbapenems, and gentamicin (Garamycin) are also effective agents in therapy.

Viruses

Noroviruses

Noroviruses (formerly called Norwalk or Norwalk-like viruses and small round structured viruses [SRSV]) and sapoviruses belong to the family Caliciviridae and are the most common cause of gastroenteritis. They account for about 90% of epidemic nonbacterial outbreaks of gastroenteritis around the world. Norovirus infection often affects people during the winter months and is therefore sometimes called winter vomiting disease; however, people may be affected at any time of the year. After a norovirus infection, immunity lasts only for 14 weeks and is incomplete. Persons with blood group O are more susceptible to infection, whereas those with groups B and AB are partially protected. Norovirus infection outbreaks more commonly occur in closed or semiclosed communities, such as prisons, dormitories, cruise ships, schools, long-term care facilities, and overnight camps—places where infection can spread rapidly from human to human or through tainted food and surfaces. Infection outbreaks can also result from food handled by an infected person.

Outbreaks have often been linked to consumption of cold foods, including salads, sandwiches, and bakery products. Salad dressing, cake icing, and oysters from contaminated waters have also been implicated in gastroenteritis outbreaks. Weight loss, lethargy, low-grade fever, headache, and (rarely) ageusia occur. Vomiting is more likely with infections caused by norovirus than sapovirus.

Pathogenesis

Norovirus strains that infect humans are found in genogroups I, II, and IV. GII.4 strains are more commonly associated with person-to-person transmission, and GI strains are identified more commonly in shellfish associated outbreaks.

Noroviruses were shown to differentially bind to histo-blood group antigens, and the binding pattern correlates with susceptibility to infection and illness. A number of enzymes are important in the synthesis of histo-blood group antigens, including fucosyl transferase-2 (FUT-2, secretor enzyme), FUT-3 (Lewis enzyme), and the A and B enzymes. The glycan produced by FUT-2 H type 1, serves as a viral receptor for noroviruses.

Laboratory Diagnosis

The virus can be recovered from the infected person's stool and vomitus during illness for about 2 weeks. Electron microscopy and reverse-transcriptase polymerase chain reaction (RT-PCR) antigen-detection assays are performed on stool samples. Serologic assays are not available for clinical use. However, infection can be diagnosed by identifying a fourfold or greater increase in antibody titer between acute and convalescent sera using norovirus virus-like particles as antigen.

Treatment

There is no specific treatment for norovirus infection. Hydration is generally adequate for most patients. In developing countries, oral rehydration therapy is the treatment of choice. Effective hand washing, careful food processing, and education of food handlers along with chlorination of water are important preventive measures. A vaccine for norovirus is in clinical trials.

Rotavirus

Among the seven rotavirus species (A to G), rotavirus A, B, and C can cause disease in humans. Rotavirus A is the most common and is the major cause of waterborne outbreaks in humans. Infections are referred to as infantile diarrhea, winter diarrhea, or acute viral gastroenteritis. Children 6 months to 2 years of age, premature infants, the elderly, and the immunocompromised are particularly prone to more-severe symptoms caused by infection with group A rotavirus. Rotavirus can survive in water for days to weeks, depending on water quality and temperature. Waterborne outbreaks are most common, followed by spread by fomites. Rotaviruses infect intestinal enterocytes; diarrhea may be caused by malabsorption secondary to the destruction of enterocytes, villus ischemia and activation of the enteric nervous system, and intestinal secretion stimulated by the action of rotavirus nonstructural protein 4 (NSP4), a novel enterotoxin and secretory agonist with pleiotropic properties.

Outbreaks caused by group B rotavirus, also called adult diarrhea rotavirus, have also been reported in the elderly and adults. Such infections are rare and usually subclinical. Group C rotavirus has been associated with rare and sporadic cases of diarrhea in children in many countries. Subclinical infection to severe gastroenteritis leading to life-threatening dehydration can occur. The illness has an abrupt onset, with vomiting often preceding the onset of diarrhea. Up to one third of patients have fever of about 39 °C. The stools are characteristically watery and only occasionally contain red or white cells. Symptoms generally resolve in a week.

Respiratory and neurologic features in children have been reported. Rotavirus infection has been associated with other clinical conditions including sudden infant death syndrome (SIDS), necrotizing enterocolitis, Kawasaki's disease, and type 1 diabetes.

Laboratory Diagnosis

Electron microscopy, direct antigen detection assays (ELISA, immunochromatography, latex agglutination), and nucleic acid detection (e.g., RT-PCR, polyacrylamide gel electrophoresis [PAGE]), are used mainly in epidemiologic studies during outbreaks.

Treatment

Dehydration due to group A rotavirus infection is treated with early institution of oral and intravenous fluids. The role of probiotics,[7] bismuth subsalicylate (Pepto Bismol),[1] inhibitors of enkephalinase, and nitazoxanide (Alinia)[1] are not clearly defined. Antimicrobials and antimotility agents should be avoided. A marked fall in deaths from childhood diarrhea following introduction of rotavirus vaccines (Rotarix, RotaTeq) has been reported from various parts of the world, and surveillance information has not revealed an association of any serious adverse reactions with the vaccine.

Other Pathogens

Cryptosporidium

Transmission of *Cryptosporidium* is usually by the fecal-oral route, often through food and water contaminated by livestock mammal feces. Persons most likely to be infected by *Cryptosporidium parvum* are infants and young children in daycare centers; those whose drinking water is unfiltered and untreated; those involved in farming practices such as lambing, calving, and muck-spreading; people engaging in anal sexual practices; patients in a hospital setting (from other infected patients or health care workers); veterinarians; and travelers.

Pathogenesis

Cryptosporidium spp. are believed to be noninvasive. Malabsorption resulting from the intestinal damage caused by prolonged protozoal infection can be fatal. Although host cells are damaged in cryptosporidiosis, the means by which the organism causes damage is not known. Mechanical destruction and the effects of toxins, enzymes, or immune-mediated mechanisms, working alone or

---

[1]Not FDA approved for this indication.

[1]Not FDA approved for this indication.
[7]Available as dietary supplement.

together, may be instrumental. In the immunocompromised, the illness is much more debilitating, with cholera-like diarrhea.

Laboratory Diagnosis
Traditionally, cryptosporidiosis is diagnosed by microscopic observation of developmental stages of the organism in an intestinal biopsy specimen. Oocysts can be recovered from stool samples by formalin-concentration techniques, staining with a modified Ziehl-Neelsen acid-fast stain. Serologic tests (ELISA, immunofluorescence antibody, PCR) are of added value.

Treatment
Nitazoxanide (Alinia, 500 mg PO twice daily for 3 days) is recommended with antiretrovirals for HIV-positive patients. Fluid replacement and antidiarrheal agents are also given.

Trichinosis
Trichinosis is due to *Trichinella spiralis* infection, commonly as a result of consuming improperly cooked pork. The parasite lodges in the extraocular muscles, deltoid, biceps, intercostals, diaphragm, tongue, or masseter and produces severe weakness with pain, fever, and cough along with splinter hemorrhages and eosinophilia.

Moderate *T. spiralis* infection is treated with mebendazole (Vermox 200–400 mg PO three times daily for 3 days) or albendazole[1] (Albenza 400 mg PO twice daily for 7–14 days). For severe infections, prednisone is added in a dose of 1 mg/kg/day for 5 days.

Neurocysticosis
Neurocysticercosis is caused by *Taenia saginata* infection, commonly as a result of consuming improperly cooked pork or contaminated raw vegetables and water. The parasite lodges in the central nervous system and skeletal muscle and presents as intracranial calcifications and ring-enhancing lesions on radioimaging studies. Other than leukocytosis, eosinophilia, and raised erythrocyte sedimentation rate, antibodies to species-specific antigens of *T. solium* can be detected by immunosorbent assay and complement fixation-tests. Treatment is aimed at controlling seizures and relief of hydrocephalus. Albendazole (15 mg/kg/day for 8–28 days) or praziquantel (50–100 mg/kg/day in three divided doses for a month) are given for parenchymal cysticerci with glucocorticoids to suppress the inflammatory response around the dying parasites. Surgery may be required to reduce intracranial pressure.

Miscellaneous
Many other organisms are implicated in foodborne and waterborne illnesses (Box 1). Some are discussed elsewhere in this book. Amebiasis, brucellosis, cholera, hepatitis A and E, giardiasis, typhoid fever, and other foodborne intestinal nematodes and cestodes are covered in the infectious diseases section of this text and are not covered in this section.

---

[1]Not FDA approved for this indication.

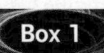

Box 1   Miscellaneous Organisms Implicated in Foodborne and Waterborne Illnesses

Adenovirus 40, 41
Bacillus anthracis
Bacillus mycoides
Burkholderia cepacia
Burkholderia pseudomallei
Clostridium bifermentans
Corynebacterium diphtheriae
Coxiella burnetii
Dientamoeba fragilis
Enterococcus faecalis, E. faecium
Erysipelothrix rhusiopathiae

Francicella tularensis
Klebsiella spp.
Leptospira spp.
Mycobacterium bovis
Parvovirus B
Pediococcus
Pestivirus
Picobirnavirus
Proteus spp.
Pseudomonas aeruginosa
Pseudomonas cocovenanans
Reovirus
Streptobacillus moniliformis
Taenia solium, T. saginata
Torovirus
Toxoplasma gondii

References
Baker AC, Goddard VJ, Davy J, et al. The identification of a diagnostic marker to detect freshwater cyanophages of filamentous cyanobacteria. Appl Environ Microbiol 2003;72:5713–9.
Centers for Disease Control and Prevention. A–Z index for foodborne illness. http://www.cdc.gov/foodsafety/diseases/; 2012 [accessed 16.05.12].
Centers for Disease Control and Prevention. Available at:CDC Estimates of Foodborne Illness in the United States, Available at:http://www.cdc.gov/foodborneburden/PDFs/FACTSHEET_A_FINDINGS.pdf; 2012 [accessed 16.05.12].
Hajmeer MN, Fung DYC. Other bacteria. In: Riemann H, Cliver DO, editors. Foodborne Infections and Intoxications. 3rd ed New York: Academic Press; 2006. p. 341–63.
Hale TL, Keusch GT. Shigella, In: Baron S, editor. Medical Microbiology. 4th ed Galveston: TX: University of Texas Medical Branch at Galveston; 1996 PMID: 21413252 (PubMed). Available at:http://www.ncbi.nlm.nih.gov/books/NBK7627[accessed October 12, 2012].
Hedberg CW, Osterholm MT. Outbreaks of food-borne and waterborne viral gastroenteritis. Clin Microbio Rev 1993;6:199–210.
Janda JM, Abbott SL. The genus *Aeromonas*: Taxonomy, pathogenicity, and infection. Clin Microbiol Rev 2010;23:35–73.
Juranek DD. Cryptosporidiosis: Sources of infection and guidelines for prevention. Clin Infect Dis 1995;21:S57–61.
Nataro JP, Kaper JB. Diarrheagenic *Escherichia coli*. Clin Microbiol Rev 1998;11:142–201.
Niyogi SK. Shigellosis. J Microbiol 2005;43:133–43.
Ortega YR, Sanchez R. Update on *Cyclospora cayetanensis*, a food-borne and waterborne parasite. Clin Microbiol Rev 2010;23:218–34.
Parashar UD, Bresee JS, Gentsch JR, Glass RI. Synopses: Rotavirus. Emerg Infect Dis 1998;4:561–70.
Sodha SV, Griffin PM, Hughes JM. Foodborne disease. In: Mandell GL, Bennett JE, Dolin R, editors. Principles and Practice of Infectious Diseases. 7th ed Philadelphia: Churchill Livingstone; 2009. p. 1413–27.

GIARDIASIS

Method of
Rodney D. Adam, MD

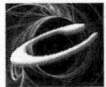

CURRENT DIAGNOSIS

- Giardiasis is the most common intestinal protozoan infection worldwide.
- Most cases result from exposure to contaminated drinking or recreational water.
- The clinical manifestations range from asymptomatic to chronic diarrhea with malabsorption and weight loss.
- The diagnosis can be established by stool microscopy or by immunoassays of fecal specimens.
- Occasionally, the trophozoites can be found in duodenal specimens when fecal assays are negative.
- Serologic testing plays no role in the diagnosis.
- Irritable bowel symptoms are very common after successful treatment of giardiasis.

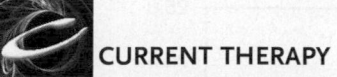

CURRENT THERAPY

- The treatment of choice is metronidazole (Flagyl)[1] or tinidazole (Tindamax); tinidazole can be given as a single dose.
- Albendazole (Albenza)[1] and nitazoxanide (Alinia) are alternative agents.
- Paromomycin,[1] a poorly absorbed aminoglycoside, is commonly recommended during early pregnancy when other agents are avoided.
- True drug resistance has not been documented, but refractory or recurrent cases can be treated by two drugs: a nitroimidazole combined with quinacrine (Atabrine)[2] or albendazole.[1]

[1]Not FDA approved for this indication.
[2]Not available in the United States.

Background

Giardia lamblia (syn. *Giardia intestinalis, Giardia duodenalis*) was initially described by Leuwenhoek in the seventeenth century while doing a microscopic examination of his own diarrheal feces. However, *G. lamblia* was not widely accepted as a human pathogen until the 1960s, when a number of outbreaks were reported in travelers to endemic areas. The presumed source of infection in these cases was contaminated drinking water. Subsequently, *Giardia* has become the most commonly identified parasitic cause of diarrhea, and along with *Cryptosporidium* species is among the most commonly identified parasitic causes of water-borne diarrheal disease.

Organism

Giardia species are members of the diplomonad (two bodies) group of flagellated protozoans. The life cycle consists of the environmentally resistant cyst, which infects its host upon ingestion. It is oval in shape, is about 8 microns × 12 microns in size and contains four nuclei. It excysts into pear-shaped trophozoites in the proximal small intestine that are about 10 to 12 microns by 5 × 7 microns in size. Two symmetrically placed nuclei are in the body of the trophozoites and four pairs of flagella aid with motility. A ventral concave disk uses primarily mechanical means to attach to the intestinal wall of the host. While still in the small intestine, some of the trophozoites then encyst into the cyst form, which is passed in the feces to continue the cycle of infection. The *Giardia* species are all parasitic and were initially assigned to species on the basis of host of origin. However, in 1952, they were divided into three species [*Giardia agilis*, amphibians; *Giardia muris*, rodents; *G. duodenalis* (*G. lamblia*), mammals and birds] that could easily be distinguished on the basis of morphologic appearance of the trophozoites. Subsequently, the *G. lamblia* morphologic group has been divided into additional species based on differences that can be seen at the ultrastructural or molecular level. Of the organisms that remain assigned to *G. lamblia*, all are found in mammals, but are divided into eight genotypes or assemblages (A through H) on the basis of molecular differences with varying host specificities. Only Genotypes A and B have been found in humans. It is likely that at least some of these eight genotypes will eventually be assigned to separate species.

Epidemiology

Giardiasis is the most commonly diagnosed human protozoan infection and is one of the most commonly identified forms of gastroenteritis. The majority of cases occur from ingestion of contaminated water or by human-to-human transmission through the fecal–oral route. Thus, the epidemiology of human infections can be understood by examining these mechanisms of transmission. In the United States, the majority of cases are sporadic and

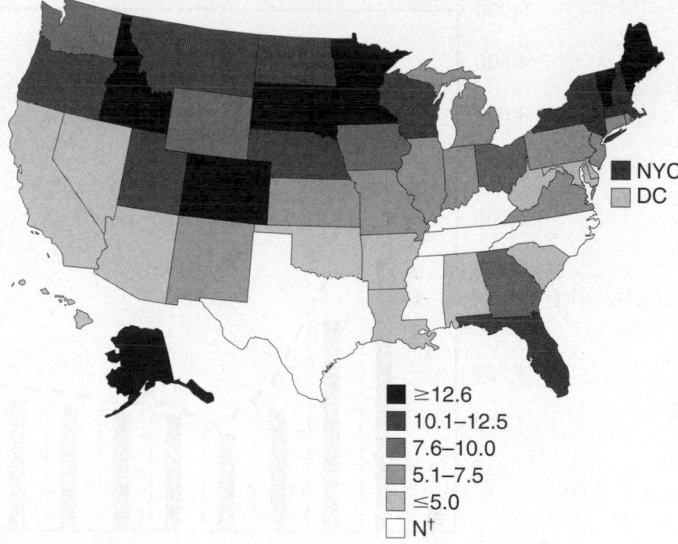

Figure 1. Incidence of giardiasis in the United States, 2010. Information is collected through the National Notifiable Diseases Surveillance System (NNDSS). Rates are per 100,000 population. (From Yoder JS, Gargano JW, Wallace RM, Beach MJ, Centers for Disease Control and Prevention. Giardiasis surveillance—United States, 2009–2010. Morb Mortal Wkly Rep Surveill Summ 2012;61:13–23.)
[†]Not a reportable disease in these states.

occur more often in the summer, probably reflecting infection from recreational water exposure. Infections were more commonly reported in children from ages 1 to 9 years, especially those under 4 years of age. In general, the incidence is higher in the northern states, perhaps because cysts survive longer in cool, moist environments (Figures 1 and 2).

Direct human-to-human transmission by the fecal oral route also occurs, leading to the higher prevalence found in children in daycare centers. The occasional reports of food-borne transmission most likely occurred because of food being contaminated by infected food handlers.

The greater incidence in children could reflect an increased use of recreational water facilities, daycare exposure, or increased susceptibility to symptomatic disease. The epidemiology of giardiasis in the United States is similar to that found in other developed countries located in temperate regions. However, in developing regions with inadequate availability of purified water, the epidemiology is very different. For example, in a shantytown near Lima, Peru, children were almost universally infected by the age of 2 years, and when treated, they were rapidly reinfected, but there were no symptoms that could clearly be correlated with their infections. Perhaps an outbreak at a ski resort town in the United States can explain these different epidemiologic patterns. In this water-borne outbreak, tourists were disproportionately affected despite drinking from the same water source as the local residents. The conclusion was that the local residents had repeatedly been exposed to water contaminated by *Giardia* cysts and were less susceptible to symptomatic disease.

The degree of zoonotic transmission of giardiasis remains controversial. Human acquisition of infection from dogs or cats has not been well documented, and usually the *Giardia* genotypes found in cats or dogs are distinct from those found in humans (A and B), even in regions where both are endemic. However, Genotypes A and B have sometimes been identified in dogs or other animals, so the question is not totally resolved. On the other hand, beavers have been implicated as a source of contaminated water leading to human infections.

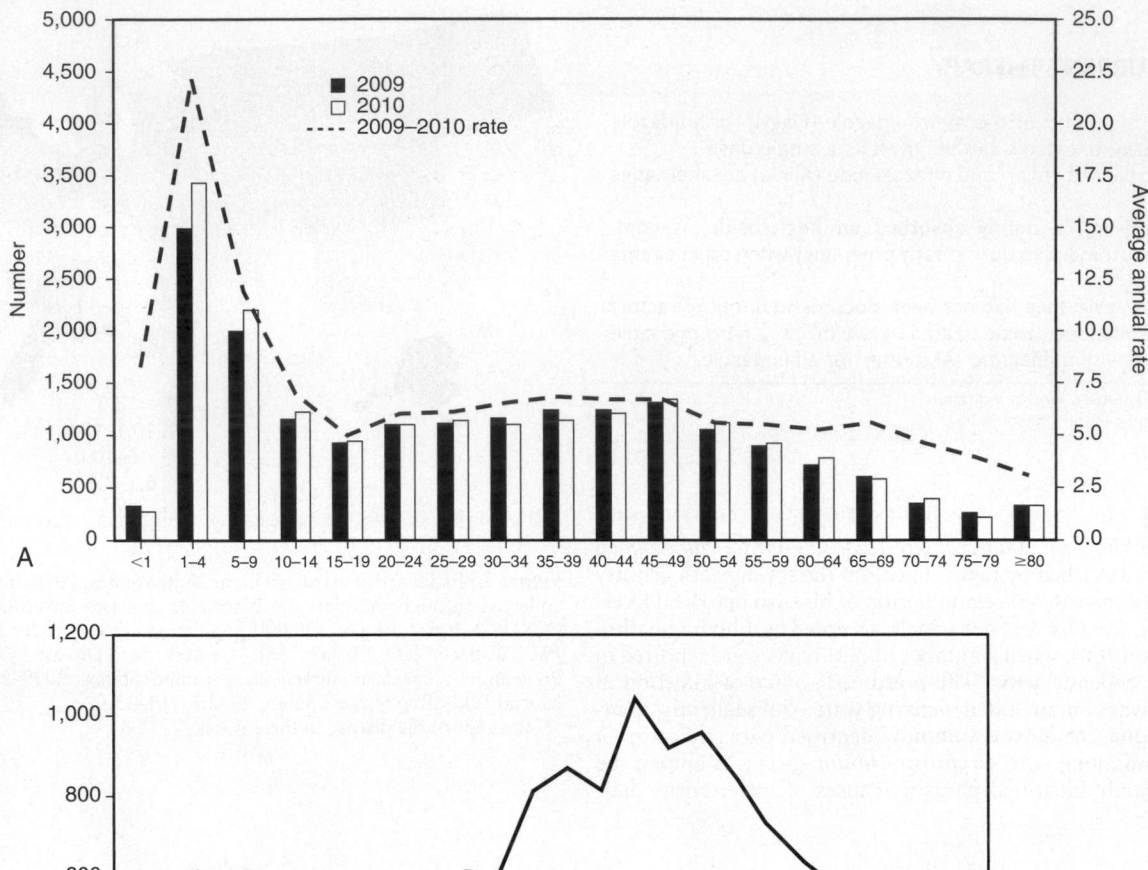

Figure 2. Incidence of giardiasis in the United States (NNDSS). **A,** Incidence by age group from 2009 and 2010. **B,** Incidence by month in 2010. Rates are per 100,000 population. (From Yoder, JS, Gargano, JW, Wallace, RM, Beach, MJ. Centers for Disease Control and Prevention. Giardiasis surveillance—United States, 2009–2010. Morb Mortal Wkly Rep Surveill Summ 2012;61:13–23.)

Risk Factors

People with hypogammaglobulinemia, and possibly those with IgA deficiency, are at increased risk for prolonged giardiasis. In animal models, deficiency in cell mediated immunity (CMI) has been associated with increased risk, but in humans the increased risk has not been associated with defects in CMI.

Pathogenesis

Infection is initiated by the ingestion of as few as 10 cysts. After passage through the acidic environment of the stomach, each cyst excysts into two trophozoites in the proximal small intestine. However, gastric acidity is not required, and people with achlorhydria or who are treated with suppressors of gastric acid remain vulnerable to giardiasis. The trophozoites replicate in the proximal small intestine, where they attach to the intestinal mucosa by their ventral disks. The attachment appears to occur by mechanical means facilitated by the suction generated by the ventral disk and the four pairs of flagella as they provide motility. Although the trophozoites attach to the intestinal wall and leave imprints after separating from the wall, there is no well-documented

evidence of invasion, either of the intestinal wall or at extraintestinal sites. Toxins have not been identified as causes of diarrhea. Thus, the current evidence suggests that the symptoms result from the immune response to the trophozoite. The host–parasite interaction leads to enterocyte apoptosis, epithelial barrier disruption, and CD8 lymphocyte activation that leads to microvillous shortening, leading to the malabsorption that is a hallmark of the infection. The trophozoites are coated with a cysteine-rich protein encoded by one of a family of related genes, and expression can be switched from one to another, perhaps contributing to the chronicity of the infection.

Prevention

The strategies for prevention should be determined by the most prevalent risk factors in specific situations. For travelers to endemic regions, the major risk is from the ingestion of contaminated water. Therefore, drinking water should be purified by boiling for one minute or by filtration through a pore size of <1 micron. Halogenization with iodine or chlorine requires a prolonged contact time (hours) to inactivate cysts and is not

TABLE 1	Symptoms of Giardiasis*
SYMPTOM	**AVERAGE (%)**
Diarrhea	95
Abdominal cramps	70
Weakness or malaise	70
Nausea	60
Weight loss	50
Anorexia (decreased appetite)	50
Abdominal distention (bloating/distension)	50
Flatulence	50
Vomiting	30
Fever	20

(From Hunter 2012; Giardiasis by R. Adam).

*The table includes the approximate frequency of the signs and symptoms reported in six studies of symptomatic giardiasis, but it is important to note that there is substantial variability of symptoms among studies.

recommended. In daycare centers and for food handlers, the best preventive measure is effective hand washing. In addition, children or workers who are infected should be treated.

Clinical Features

The majority of people with giardiasis are asymptomatic, but the percentages range from rates of diarrhea no higher than background among children in some highly endemic regions to attack rates of nearly 100% in visitors to endemic regions. Symptomatic patients typically present for evaluation only after several days or even weeks of illness because of the subacute onset. The symptoms of giardiasis typically develop after an incubation period of 1 to 2 weeks and consist of diarrhea that is characterized by loose, foul-smelling stools and abdominal discomfort described as cramping or bloating (Table 1). Fatigue is very common, but fever is unusual and when present, is mild and occurs only within the first few days. Malabsorption and weight loss are often present. The majority of cases resolve within several weeks, but occasionally the symptoms will last for months in the absence of treatment. Relapse is relatively uncommon after effective treatment.

Diagnosis

The gold standard of diagnosis has been the microscopic evaluation of three separate fecal samples, including concentrated specimens for cysts or, less commonly, trophozoites. The identification of trophozoites is nearly always associated with symptomatic infection, but cysts may be found in asymptomatic persons. Because of the challenges in obtaining three fecal specimens and the interobserver variability in skill at identifying *Giardia* cysts, antigen detection tests have come into widespread use. The enzyme immunoassays are more commonly used and have high degrees of sensitivity and specificity. A direct fluorescent assay is slightly more sensitive than the enzyme immunoassays and can also detect *Cryptosporidium* species, but it requires the availability of fluorescent microscopy. PCR tests have also been described, but are not widely available. Some patients have negative workups of stool samples, but *Giardia* trophozoites can be detected in duodenal contents with the string test. The patient swallows a capsule on a string, which is left in situ for four hours to overnight. The string is then removed and examined microscopically for trophozoites. Alternatively, endoscopy with sampling of duodenal contents and duodenal biopsy can be used. Endoscopy has the added advantage of being able to detect other possible diagnoses, such as Celiac disease or tropical sprue.

Differential Diagnosis

The diagnosis of giardiasis should be suspected in patients presenting with prolonged (>5–7 days) diarrhea without blood in the stools and no fever. In patients presenting relatively early in the course of illness, the major considerations in the differential diagnosis are other infectious etiologies of diarrhea, particularly *Campylobacter jejuni*, *Salmonella*, *Cryptosporidium*, and *Cyclospora cayetanensis*. Thus, patients presenting with compatible symptoms should have stool samples submitted for culture and for microscopic examination for ova and parasites (O and P). Watery diarrhea is uncommon, and bloody stools are not seen with giardiasis; thus, these findings should prompt the search for other etiologies.

For patients presenting with more prolonged symptoms, a number of noninfectious illnesses should be added to the differential diagnosis. Irritable bowel syndrome and lactose intolerance are among the more common etiologies and should be considered in patients presenting with diarrhea but no weight loss. Gluten enteropathy, tropical sprue, and, rarely, Whipple's disease are among the noninfectious etiologies of diarrhea accompanied by weight loss.

Treatment

Patients with symptomatic giardiasis should be treated. The criteria for treatment of patients with asymptomatic giardiasis are not well defined, but in general, patients in regions with low prevalence or linked with outbreaks should be treated. On the other hand, in settings where the prevalence is high and recurrence rates are high, there is probably no value to treating asymptomatic infection.

The most commonly used agents for treatment of giardiasis are the nitroimidazoles. Metronidazole (Flagyl)[1] and tinidazole (Tindamax) are available in the United States, and others, including secnidazole (Secnil)[2] and ornidazole (Tiberal),[2] are available in other countries (Table 2). These agents are completely absorbed from the gastrointestinal tract and are inactivated primarily by hepatic metabolism. Metronidazole has been available in the United States for decades and has generally been considered the drug of choice for treatment of giardiasis in most situations. More recently, tinidazole has become available and is the only agent available in the United States with a high degree of efficacy when given as a single dose. Metronidazole is mutagenic in bacterial assays and showed some carcinogenic activity in an animal model. However, carcinogenicity in humans has not been documented. Serious adverse reactions to the nitroimidazoles are rare, but nausea and a metallic taste are common and may decrease the compliance of patients with metronidazole. The problem with noncompliance can be addressed by the use of tinidazole or the other agents that can be given as a single dose.

Albendazole (Albenza)[1] is a tubulin inhibitor that was introduced as a broad-spectrum antihelminthic, but it also has good activity against *Giardia* trophozoites. It is generally well tolerated and in areas with endemic helminth infections has the added advantage of antihelminthic activity.

The first trimester of pregnancy poses a special problem because none of the agents have been adequately studied or approved for use during this time. Paromomycin[1] is a nonabsorbed aminoglycoside and is expected to be safe during pregnancy. Therefore, it is usually the preferred choice in that setting; however, it is somewhat less effective than other agents. Specialty consultation should be considered for treatment of patients in their first trimester. Metronidazole is used extensively during the second and third trimesters for other indications; thus, it can be considered the drug of choice for those patients. Albendazole is known to be teratogenic and should be avoided during pregnancy.

[1]Not FDA approved for this indication.
[2]Not available in the United States.

DRUG	DOSE		FREQUENCY	DURATION	EFFICACY (%)
	ADULT	PEDIATRIC*			
Metronidazole[2] (Flagyl)	250 mg	5 mg/kg	tid	5–7 days	90–100
Tinidazole (Tindamax)	2 gm	50 mg/kg	Single dose	Single dose	90–100
Quinacrine[†, ‡] (Atabrine)	100 mg	2 mg/kg	tid	5–7 days	80–100
Furazolidone[†, ‡] (Furoxone)	100 mg	1.5 mg/kg	qid	10 days	80–94
Paromomycin[†] (Humatin)	500 mg	8-10 mg/kg	tid	10 days	55–90
Albendazole[†] (Albenza)	400 mg qd	15 mg/kg	Daily	5 days	90–100
Nitazoxanide (Alinia)	500 mg bid	7.5 mg/kg	bid	3 days	70–80

TABLE 2 Treatment of Giardiasis

*The adult dose is the maximum pediatric dose.
[†]Not approved by the FDA specifically for giardiasis.
[‡]Not available commercially in the United States, but available at a compounding pharmacy.

Nitazoxanide (Alinia) has been approved in the United States for treatment of giardiasis (and cryptosporidiosis) and is very well tolerated. However, the somewhat lower efficacy compared to nitroimidazoles and albendazole, along with the requirement for twice daily dosing, limits its role.

Quinacrine (Atabrine)[2] was one of the first effective treatments for giardiasis, but has fallen into disfavor because of toxicity. Nausea and vomiting are common, and toxic psychosis is occasionally seen.

Treatment failures are not uncommon, but may or may not be due to true drug resistance since in vitro cultures are not routinely performed and in vitro testing is not standardized. When treatment failure occurs, the patient may respond to the same or an alternative drug. Treatment-refractory cases have been treated successfully with a combination of metronidazole[1] plus quinacrine[2] or albendazole.[1] The most common reason for persistence of symptoms after treatment is due to post-giardiasis irritable bowel syndrome, which can occur in up to 25% of patients. Thus, it is important to re-evaluate stool specimens from patients with symptoms that persist after therapy.

Diet

Lactose intolerance is quite common while patients have giardiasis and potentially for months thereafter, so lactose ingestion should be moderated or eliminated as needed.

---

[1]Not FDA approved for this indication.
[2]Not available in the United States.

References

Adam RD. Biology of *Giardia lamblia*. Clin Microbiol Rev 2001;14:447–75.

Adam RD. Giardiasis. In: Magill AJ, Ryan ET, Hill D, Solomon T, editors. Hunter's Tropical Medicine and Emerging Infectious Disease. Philadelphia: Elsevier; 2013. p. 668–72.

Cooper MA, Sterling CR, Gilman RH, et al. Molecular analysis of household transmission of *Giardia lamblia* in a region of high endemicity in Peru. J Infect Dis 2010;202:1713–21.

Cotton JA, Beatty JK, Buret AG. Host parasite interactions and pathophysiology in *Giardia* infections. Int J Parasitol 2011;41:925–33.

Hanevik K, Dizdar V, Langeland N, Hausken T. Development of functional gastrointestinal disorders after *Giardia lamblia* infection. BMC Gastroenterol 2009;9:27.

Lengerich EJ, Addiss DG, Juranek DD. Severe giardiasis in the United States. Clin Infect Dis 1994;18:760–3.

Morrison HG, McArthur AG, Gillin FD, et al. Genomic minimalism in the early diverging intestinal parasite *Giardia lamblia*. Science 2007;317:1921–6.

Nash TE, Ohl CA, Thomas E, et al. Treatment of patients with refractory giardiasis. Clin Infect Dis 2001;33:22–8.

Rossignol JF. *Cryptosporidium* and *Giardia*: treatment options and prospects for new drugs. Exp Parasitol 2010;124:45–53.

Yoder JS, Gargano JW, Wallace RM, Beach MJ. Centers for Disease Control and Prevention. Giardiasis surveillance—United States, 2009–2010. Morb Mortal Wkly Rep Surveill Summ 2012;61:13–23.

HIV DISEASE

Method of
Jyoti S. Mathad, MD, MSc; Ryan Westergaard, MD, MPH; and Amita Gupta, MD, MHS

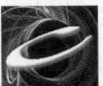

CURRENT DIAGNOSIS

- Revised national guidelines recommend universal screening for HIV infection for patients aged 13 to 64 years in all settings after notification that testing will be done, unless the patient specifically declines (opt-out testing). Patients with behavioral risk factors, sexually transmitted diseases, or tuberculosis should be screened annually.
- Acute HIV infection is recognized as a variable syndrome including fever, pharyngitis, rash, and arthralgias.
- As antiretroviral therapy has prolonged survival for patients living with HIV, non–HIV-related outcomes such as cardiovascular, liver, and renal disease have gained importance as preventable causes of morbidity and mortality.

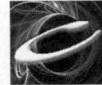

CURRENT THERAPY

- Accumulating evidence suggests that earlier initiation of antiretroviral therapy improves clinical outcomes and reduces HIV transmission risk.
- Several classes and an increasing number of different fixed-dose combinations of antiretroviral medications give treatment-naive and treatment-experienced patients several therapeutic options.
- New guidelines for HIV treatment (including management of special situations such as HIV/TB co-infection) and pre-exposure prophylaxis for persons at high risk of incident HIV infection were released in 2012.
- At least one HIV-infected patient, who underwent a bone marrow transplant for leukemia, has been cured of HIV. Active research to identify the mechanisms underlying this cure is ongoing with the hope of identifying a strategy to cure all people living with HIV.
- The addition of Hepatitis C protease inhibitors has revolutionized treatment of Hepatitis C (HCV), a common co-infection, but caution is advised when treating HIV and HCV simultaneously because of drug-drug interactions.
- At least 16 patients have now been deemed "cured" of HIV. One underwent a bone marrow transplant for leukemia; the others, including a baby diagnosed at birth, achieved a functional cure after receiving combination drug therapy within weeks of acquiring HIV and are now able to maintain an undetectable viral load off of antiretrovirals.

Since its first description in the early 1980s, the acquired immuno-deficiency syndrome (AIDS) has become one of the most devastating epidemics in human history. Millions of new infections occur every year, predominantly in resource-poor settings where access to diagnosis and treatment of human immunodeficiency virus (HIV) infection remains inadequate. The natural history of HIV infection remains one of progressive immune system dysfunction with inevitable acute and chronic infectious complications. With few exceptions, the inexorable decline in T-lymphocyte function eventually leads to the death of untreated patients. Remarkable advances in therapeutics, leading to the development of highly active antiretroviral therapy (HAART), have transformed HIV infection from an almost universally fatal illness to a chronic disease that can be managed over decades with an enlarging repertoire of treatment options. This chapter provides an overview of the current understanding of HIV pathogenesis and epidemiology and reviews guidelines for the initial evaluation and long-term management of HIV infection in adult patients.

Epidemiology

According to the Joint United Nations Programme on HIV/AIDS, an estimated 34 million people were living with HIV at the end of 2010; roughly half of them were women, and more than 2 million were children. Of the estimated 7400 new infections that occur daily, 96% occur in low- and middle-income countries, and approximately 1000 of those infected are children younger than 15 years of age. The prevalence of HIV infection in populations varies widely across the world, with the highest documented rates occurring in southern Africa, where prevalence rates derived from surveillance of asymptomatic pregnant women have exceeded 30% in some settings. AIDS is now the leading cause of death worldwide for persons aged 15 to 59 years, and this trend is associated with particularly dire social and economic consequences in sub-Saharan Africa, where more than half of global AIDS deaths occur. In some sub-Saharan countries such as Swaziland, Botswana, and Lesotho, life expectancy has been reduced by more than 20 years. However, with a rapid and significant increase in funding and commitment from the U.S. government (President's Emergency Plan for AIDS Relief [PEPFAR]) and many multilateral agencies such as the Global Fund, a dramatic increase in prevention, care, and treatment services is now underway. A stabilization and initial trend illustrating a global decrease in AIDS deaths is being observed.

North America has experienced a striking decline in AIDS deaths since the advent of HAART, although a sizeable reduction in the annual number of new HIV infections has not yet been achieved. In the United States, an estimated 1.2 million people are living with HIV. The Centers for Disease Control and Prevention (CDC) estimates that 20% of these individuals are unaware of their HIV status. The CDC estimates that approximately 47,100 people were newly infected with HIV in 2010. Ethnic minorities, particularly African Americans, are disproportionately represented among those with new infections. As is the case worldwide, sexual contact accounts for the majority of HIV transmission for both men and women. In the United States, male-to-male sexual contact represents the mode of acquisition for the majority (61%) of new cases among men, whereas most women are infected via heterosexual contact. Injection drug use accounts for roughly 20% of new HIV infections in both men and women.

The risk of HIV transmission per exposure has been estimated from studies of discordant couples and cohort studies. The average risk of HIV transmission per coital act in serodiscordant heterosexual couples is approximately 0.1%. The presence of other sexually transmitted infections and higher viral load (VL) increase the risk of transmission; condom use and male circumcision considerably reduce the risk. Female-to-male transmission is less effective than male-to-female transmission. Receptive anal intercourse is associated with a higher risk of transmission compared with vaginal intercourse. Even though the risk of transmission by oral sex is very low, it should not be considered completely safe.

Mother-to-child transmission can occur in utero, in the peripartum period, and during breast-feeding. The probability of transmission is most influenced by maternal plasma VL. Other risk factors include maternal CD4$^+$ T-cell count (discussed later), hepatitis C infection, premature rupture of membranes, preterm birth, and duration of breast-feeding. In the United States, mother-to-child transmission has been markedly reduced (from 20%–25% to <1%) through routine HIV testing and effective interventions. These interventions include HAART, elective cesarean delivery if the VL is greater than 1000 copies per milliliter at week 38, and recommendation to avoid breast-feeding. The risk of HIV transmission with breast-feeding is 10% to 16% in the absence of intervention and is thought to be highest during the first 2 to 4 months. Factors that increase transmission include inflammatory or ulcerative conditions of the breast, mastitis, and breast abscess. Infants with thrush are more likely to acquire HIV from an infected mother via breast-feeding. In many low-income countries where breast-feeding is critical for infant nutrition and survival, the issue is complex and is the subject of ongoing investigation.

Pathophysiology

HIV is an enveloped, single-stranded RNA virus belonging to the family Retroviridae. It was recognized as the causative agent of AIDS within 3 years after the initial description of the syndrome in 1981, and ongoing characterization of its molecular biology has provided the identification of multiple targets for drug development. Two human immunodeficiency viruses exist: HIV-1 and HIV-2. HIV-1 has worldwide distribution, accounts for most infections outside western Africa, and is the focus of this chapter.

HIV-2 infection causes a similar clinical syndrome but is less efficiently transmitted and results in lower levels of viremia and slower progression to AIDS. A key difference in terms of management between HIV-1 and HIV-2 is that HIV-2 is naturally resistant to non-nucleoside reverse transcriptase inhibitors (see later discussion). For this reason, it is important to assess for HIV-2 by Western blot in persons who are from regions of the world where HIV-2 is present or coexists with HIV-1.

Genetic heterogeneity of HIV-1 is reflected in categorization of the virus into three groups (M, O, and N) and several clades (e.g., B, C, D, AE, CRF01_AE), some of which have overlapping geographic distribution around the world. Subtype C is prevalent in southern and eastern Africa, China, India, South Asia, and Brazil and accounts for 50% of HIV subtypes, whereas subtype B, the most common subtype in the United States, accounts for 12%.

The HIV viral genome is encoded in single-stranded RNA, packaged in core protein structures, and surrounded by a lipid bilayer envelope that is derived from the cell membrane of the host cell as the virus buds from the cell surface after replication. This outer viral membrane contains HIV-specific glycoproteins, including gp120 and gp41, which facilitate attachment and entry into host cells through interaction with the cell surface receptor, CD4, and coreceptors CCR5 and CXCR4. CD4$^+$ helper T lymphocytes are the predominant host cell affected by HIV; this molecular tropism explains the immune system destruction manifested in chronic HIV infection and provides the rationale for clinical staging of HIV infection using CD4$^+$ T-cell counts. The interaction of HIV with the coreceptor CCR5 led to the development of coreceptor antagonist drugs such as maraviroc. People with genetic mutations of the CCR5 receptor are resistant to HIV infection. This helps explain how the "Berlin" patient, the man with HIV and leukemia who received a bone marrow transplant from a donor with a CCR5 mutation, was cured of HIV.

After host cell entry, the key enzyme responsible for viral replication is reverse transcriptase, an RNA-dependent DNA polymerase that is packaged within the virion core. This enzyme facilitates conversion of the HIV genome into a double-stranded DNA intermediate molecule. The second key enzymatic step is integration of this intermediate nucleic acid product into the host genome, which is facilitated by the viral protein integrase. Protein synthesis with packaging of new viral particles ensues, utilizing an HIV-specific protease. The integrase inhibitor class of drugs acts by blocking this step of integration.

Natural History

The natural history of HIV infection reflects the progressive depletion of circulating CD4$^+$ cells, in addition to diverse effects on other immune cells and tissues that are incompletely understood. Within 1 to 4 weeks after the initial HIV infection, seroconversion may be accompanied by a nonspecific, self-limited illness, often referred to as the acute retroviral syndrome. This illness has variable manifestations but may include fever, malaise, myalgias, arthralgias, generalized lymphadenopathy, pharyngitis, and rash. The associated rash has been described as maculopapular, urticarial, or roseola-like. An illness resembling acute infectious mononucleosis syndrome, similar to that caused by Epstein-Barr virus or cytomegalovirus (CMV), and aseptic meningitis have been described. Very rarely has an acute opportunistic infection (OI) been reported in the setting of acute seroconversion. The proportion of patients experiencing such an illness is not precisely known, because many do not present to medical facilities, and for those who do, HIV infection is commonly not considered. Diagnosis of acute HIV infection requires a high index of suspicion, which does not commonly occur unless the patient reports a recent history of a high-risk exposure.

During the acute phase of infection, high levels of viremia are present (often exceeding 10 million copies per milliliter) as HIV becomes widely disseminated throughout the body and the host defenses are just beginning to counteract circulating virus through cell-mediated and humoral (antibody-mediated) immune mechanisms. Antibodies against HIV usually become detectable between 2 and 4 months after infection. The initial, high-level viremia becomes attenuated as neutralizing antibodies are established and equilibrium is reached whereby ongoing replication is partially controlled by the immune response, resulting in a steady-state level of viremia. This so-called virologic set point differs from patient to patient and is one of the determinants of the rate of disease progression. A small number of HIV-infected persons are able to control viral replication to levels below the limit of detection, and they tend to have a more benign course of disease. In these patients, designated elite suppressors by researchers, HIV replication continues to occur, and HIV RNA can be isolated from latently infected cells by means of specialized laboratory techniques.

After the establishment of HIV infection and seroconversion, a period of asymptomatic infection ensues, during which patients are free of evidence of immune suppression and OIs are uncommon. This phase of clinical latency lasts a median of 8 to 10 years, based on observational studies in the West from the pre-HAART era. Ongoing viral replication leads to gradual decline in the CD4 count.

The symptomatic stage of HIV infection can begin at any time after infection, but clinical manifestations become more likely as the CD4 count falls farther below the normal range of 800 to 1200 cells/mm^3. Both the absolute CD4 count and the percentage of CD4$^+$ T cells correlate with the risk of developing OIs and should be monitored longitudinally to assess patients' candidacy for prophylactic interventions and initiation of HAART. For example, *Pneumocystis jirovecii* (formerly *Pneumocystis carinii*) pneumonia (PCP) usually occurs in patients with a CD4 count of less than 200 cells/mm^3 or a percentage of less than 10%. CMV retinitis occurs almost exclusively in patients with a CD4 count of less than 50 cells/mm^3 or a percentage of less than 5%. Mucocutaneous candidiasis (oral thrush), herpes zoster, HIV-associated nephropathy, peripheral neuropathy, tuberculosis, and community-acquired bacterial pneumonia occur with increased frequency at earlier stages of infection and are less reliably predicted by CD4$^+$ cell measurement.

Diagnosis

Diagnosis of HIV infection during the acute retroviral syndrome requires detection of circulating HIV RNA because of the absence of HIV-specific antibodies at this stage. Other laboratory findings that can raise the suspicion for acute HIV infection include a decreased total lymphocyte count; the T-cell count characteristically decreases during the first several weeks after infection and

later often returns to preinfection levels, after the initial spike in viremia is brought under control by immune defenses. The erythrocyte sedimentation rate and hepatic transaminases may also be elevated. Cerebrospinal fluid pleocytosis has been documented in patients undergoing lumbar puncture in the setting of acute HIV infection.

HIV RNA can be detected by reverse transcriptase polymerase chain reaction (RT-PCR) or branched-chain DNA testing. In the acute retroviral syndrome, the VL is usually very high, and ultrasensitive RT-PCR is not generally needed. Although commercially available PCR and branched DNA tests are licensed for disease monitoring and not for diagnosis of HIV infection, their specificity is sufficiently high that finding high levels of HIV RNA in a patient with suspected acute HIV infection provides convincing evidence for infection. In all such cases, close follow-up with repeat HIV antibody testing to confirm seroconversion within 2 to 4 months is essential.

Diagnosis of HIV at all other stages of disease relies on commercially available assays for detecting HIV-specific antibodies. A standard protocol involves screening with the highly sensitive enzyme immunoassay (EIA) that detects antigens of both HIV-1 and HIV-2. Negative EIA is sufficient to rule out HIV infection, except in cases where acute HIV infection is suspected, as just described. Positive EIA tests require further confirmation with the more specific Western blot test. The CDC has established criteria for Western blot positivity, which include the presence of at least two of the HIV-specific bands p24, gp41, and gp160/120. The Western blot is considered negative if no bands are present and indeterminate if an HIV band is present but the criteria for positivity are not met. Indeterminate Western blot results usually include a single p24 band and can occur during early infection, while seroconversion is in progress, or in advanced AIDS when antibody production is impaired. Causes of indeterminate Western blot results that are unrelated to HIV include pregnancy, autoimmune disease, and cross-reacting antibodies resulting from blood transfusion or organ transplantation.

Other HIV antibody kits have been developed for ease of administration or achievement of rapid results, and they have utility in settings such as community-based screening programs, emergency departments, and even patient-initiated home testing. OraSure, an office-based test that employs a special swab for collecting oral fluid specimens rather than blood, was licensed in 1996. Specimens are collected at the point of care and sent to a central laboratory, where antibodies are detected; the sensitivity and specificity are similar to those of traditional blood-based methods. OraQuick Advance, a rapid HIV test that can utilize whole blood, plasma, or oral fluid, was approved in 2004; OraQuick In-Home, the first over-the-counter home-use version of this test, was approved in 2012. These tests can provide results comparable in accuracy to EIA within about 20 minutes. An advantage of this technique is the ability to provide reliable negative results at the point of care or in the comfort of a patient's home. Positive results still need to be confirmed with standard EIA and Western blot serologic testing.

Screening

The traditional paradigm for screening of asymptomatic patients for HIV has included targeting patients with behavioral risk factors for HIV transmission and patients seeking care for sexually transmitted diseases. Documentation of separate, written consent and administration of formal pretest and posttest counseling has been recommended and is still required by statute in many U.S. states.

In response to the consistent observations that many people are not diagnosed with HIV until late in the course of disease and that transmission rates for infected persons who are unaware of their serostatus are several times higher than for persons who are aware that they are infected, the CDC issued new guidelines in September 2006 to make HIV testing a routine part of medical care. Voluntary (opt-out) screening is now recommended in health care settings for all persons aged 13 to 64 years, regardless of risk.

Screening should be repeated annually for persons with behavioral risk factors for HIV and should be repeated each time a person seeks treatment for symptoms related to sexually transmitted disease. The CDC advocates that requirements for separate, written consent for HIV testing are no longer needed; instead, general consent to receive medical care can be considered sufficient.

Approach to the Patient with HIV Infection

HIV care is a continuously evolving field, and new drugs and classes of drugs have been introduced in recent years. Professional guidelines for antiretroviral therapy (ART) are updated frequently as data from clinical trials are published and accumulating clinical evidence influences beliefs about best practices in HIV care. For these reasons, the receipt of appropriate care by HIV+ patients is determined in large part by the experience of the care provider. The volume of HIV+ patients seen in one's practice is known to correlate with measures of quality care. A U.S. Department of Health and Human Services panel recommends that HIV patients receive care from a health care provider who routinely cares for at least 20 and preferably 50 HIV-infected patients. Referral to a specialist is warranted in cases of treatment failure due to drug resistance or for management of complications of HIV or antiretroviral drugs. Because of the multifaceted nature of the longitudinal care of HIV-infected patients, an interdisciplinary approach, integrated and coordinated by an experienced primary care provider, is optimal.

The initial history and physical examination of HIV-infected patients should be systematic and comprehensive, owing to the multiorgan system nature of diagnoses associated with HIV infection. A thorough review of current and recent symptoms should assess for presence of OIs and malignant or premalignant conditions. Symptoms such as unexplained weight loss, fever, chronic diarrhea, recurrent oral or genital ulcers, dysphagia, dyspnea, or gastrointestinal bleeding should prompt further investigation for the presence of undiagnosed manifestations of HIV-related complications. Because patients with HIV infection have a higher incidence of cognitive impairment, mental illness, and substance abuse than the general population, symptoms of neurocognitive impairment (e.g., impaired memory), depression, suicidality, and unhealthy alcohol and drug use should also be carefully assessed.

The past medical and surgical history should focus on conditions that may follow a more malignant course in the setting of HIV infection, such as chronic viral hepatitis, and conditions that can be exacerbated by HIV or by ART, such as cardiovascular or renal disease and metabolic abnormalities such as dyslipidemia or impaired glucose tolerance. The circumstances surrounding the patient's HIV acquisition should be formally assessed. The provider should understand previous and current patterns of risk behaviors for the purpose of counseling regarding transmission prevention (positive prevention) and to assess the patient's risk of acquisition of drug-resistant virus and current risk for concomitant sexually transmitted infections.

A complete physical examination should be performed at the time of initial evaluation and at subsequent visits. Signs such as temporal wasting, lymphadenopathy, and hepatomegaly or splenomegaly can provide clues to the stage of disease and alert the provider to the presence of OIs or AIDS-related malignancies. The oral cavity should be examined for the presence of thrush, oral hairy leukoplakia, and mucosal lesions of Kaposi sarcoma. A complete skin examination is important on initial evaluation and longitudinally, because many OIs and medication toxicities have cutaneous manifestations. A funduscopic examination should be done, and, in those patients with a CD4 count of less than 50 to 100 cells/mm^3, referral to an ophthalmologist is necessary to screen for evidence of CMV retinitis. Close examination of the anogenital area may identify treatable sexually transmitted infections and premalignant lesions associated with human papillomavirus infection. Recommended laboratory evaluations are presented in Table 1.

TABLE 1	Initial Laboratory Evaluation	
TEST	**FREQUENCY**	**COMMENTS**
HIV antibody testing	At initial visit	If prior documentation is not reliable or if HIV RNA is undetectable
CD4+ T-cell count	At initial visit, then every 3–6 mo	Levels may be falsely elevated in splenectomized patients and with concurrent HTLV-1 infection.
Plasma HIV RNA (viral load)	At initial visit, before ART initiation, every 3 mo while on ART	Ultrasensitive viral load assay detects levels as low as 20 copies/mL and should be used to monitor response while on treatment.
Resistance testing	At initial visit, and with treatment failure before change in ART regimen	Genotype and phenotype tests are available, genotypes are more commonly used.
HLA-B*5701 testing	Before treatment initiation if considering abacavir (Ziagen)	—
Coreceptor tropism assay	Before treatment initiation if considering CCR5 antagonist (maraviroc [Selzentry])	—
Complete blood count	At initial visit, then every 3–6 mo	AZT can cause bone marrow suppression and macrocytosis.
Serum chemistry panel	At initial visit	Up to 75% of HIV-infected patients have elevated hepatic transaminases at diagnosis.
Fasting lipid profile and blood glucose level	At initial visit	Every 3–6 mo
Hepatitis screen (anti-HCV, anti-HAV, anti-HBsAg, anti-HBcAg)	At initial visit	HAV, HBV vaccinations are indicated for nonimmune patients.
Syphilis serology	At initial visit and annually in sexually active patients	Confirm with FTA-ABS test if positive; up to 6% of HIV-infected patients have biologic false-positive RPR result.
Urine NAAT for gonorrhea and *Chlamydia**	Consider at initial visit and annually in sexually active patients	Testing every 3–6 mo is recommended for very-high-risk patients.
Toxoplasma gondii serology	At initial visit and if CD4+ count is <100 cells/mm^3	Most cases of toxoplasmosis represent reactivation of latent infection.

Continued

| TABLE 1 | Initial Laboratory Evaluation—cont'd

TEST	FREQUENCY	COMMENTS
Tuberculin skin test (PPD)	At initial visit, then annually in high-risk persons (e.g., homeless, injection drug users) if initial test is negative	Cutoff of >5 mm of induration is indication for treatment of LTBI.
PAP smear†	At initial visit	Annually
G6PD screen	At initial visit	Identifies patients at risk for hemolysis induced by dapsone or primaquine
Chest radiograph	If patient has pulmonary symptoms or a positive PPD result	Not recommended routinely

*Consider rectal and oral screening.
†Consider anal PAP smear, particularly in MSM.
Abbreviations: ART = antiretroviral therapy; AZT = azidothymidine (zidovudine); FTA-ABS = fluorescent treponemal antibody, absorbed; G6PD = glucose-6-phosphate dehydrogenase; HAV = hepatitis A virus; HBcAg = hepatitis B core antigen; HBsAg = hepatitis B surface antigen; HCV = hepatitis C virus; HLA = human leukocyte antigen; HTLV-1 = human T-lymphotropic virus 1; LTBI = latent tuberculosis infection; NAAT = nucleic acid amplification test; PAP smear = Papanicolaou test; PPD = purified protein derivative; RPR = rapid plasma reagin test.

Antiretroviral Therapy

Antiretroviral drugs that are currently approved for the treatment of HIV fall into six classes: nucleoside reverse transcriptase inhibitors (NRTIs), non-nucleoside reverse transcriptase inhibitors (NNRTIs), protease inhibitors (PIs), fusion inhibitors, integrase inhibitors, and chemokine (CC) receptor 5 (CCR5) antagonists (Table 2). The goals of therapy are to increase disease-free survival, achieve maximal and sustained suppression of viral replication to undetectable levels (<48 copies), preserve immunologic function, and improve quality of life.

When to Initiate Antiretroviral Therapy

In the mid-1990s, when combination HAART became available, the treatment paradigm was to "hit early and hit hard," because it was believed that the virus could be eradicated with treatment and rapid immune restoration could be achieved. However, as

| TABLE 2 | Approved Antiretroviral Medications |

GENERIC NAME (TRADE NAME)	ABBREVIATION	FORMULATIONS AND COFORMULATIONS	RECOMMENDED ADULT DOSING	IMPORTANT POINTS
Nucleoside Analogue Reverse Transcriptase Inhibitors (NRTIs)				
Abacavir (Ziagen)	ABC	300 mg tablets; 20 mg/mL oral solution *Coformulations:* Trizivir (ABC 300 mg + ZDV 300 mg + 3TC 150 mg) Epzicom (ABC 600 mg + 3TC 300 mg)	300 mg bid or 600 mg qd Trizivir 1 tablet bid Epzicom 1 tablet qd	Hypersensitivity reaction (FDA black box warning); screen patients for the HLA-B*5701 haplotype Possible increase in acute MI No food restrictions
Didanosine (Videx)	ddI	125, 200, 250, 400 mg capsules; 2, 4 g powder for oral solution	Body weight ≥60 kg: 400 mg (with TDF 250 mg) qd Body weight <60 kg: 250 mg (with TDF 200 mg) qd	Pancreatitis, peripheral neuropathy, nausea, lactic acidosis; concurrent use of TDF causes increased ddI levels and higher rate of toxicity Take on an empty stomach Must be swallowed whole
Emtricitabine (Emtriva)	FTC	200 mg capsule; 10 mg/mL oral solution *Coformulations:* Atripla (EFV 600 mg + FTC 200 mg + TDF 300 mg) Truvada (FTC 200 mg + TDF 300 mg)	200 mg capsule qd or 240 mg (24 mL) oral solution qd Atripla 1 tablet qd Truvada 1 tablet qd	Skin discoloration, rare nausea and vomiting No food restrictions
Lamivudine (Epivir)	3TC	150, 300 mg tablets; 10 mg/mL oral solution *Coformulations:* Combivir (3TC 150 mg + ZDV 300 mg) Epzicom (see ABC) Trizivir (see ABC)	150 mg bid or 300 mg qd Combivir 1 tablet bid	Minimal toxicity Requires dosage adjustment in renal insufficiency No food restrictions
Stavudine (Zerit)	d4T	15, 20, 30, 40 mg capsules; 1 mg/mL oral solution	30 mg bid (weight-based dosing is no longer recommended)	Peripheral neuropathy, lipodystrophy, pancreatitis, lactic acidosis, dyslipidemia No food restrictions
Tenofovir (Viread)	TDF	300 mg tablet *Coformulations:* Atripla (see FTC) Truvada (see FTC)	1 tablet qd	Renal insufficiency, Fanconi's syndrome, headache, nausea, vomiting, diarrhea No food restrictions

TABLE 2 Approved Antiretroviral Medications—cont'd

GENERIC NAME (TRADE NAME)	ABBREVIATION	FORMULATIONS AND COFORMULATIONS	RECOMMENDED ADULT DOSING	IMPORTANT POINTS
Zidovudine (Retrovir)	AZT, ZDV	100 mg capsules; 300 mg tablets; 10 mg/mL IV solution; 10 mg/mL oral solution *Coformulations:* Combivir (see 3TC) Trizivir (see ABC)	300 mg bid or 200 mg tid	Bone marrow suppression (macrocytic anemia, neutropenia), GI disturbance, lactic acidosis with hepatic steatosis (rare) No food restrictions

Non-nucleoside Analogue Reverse Transcriptase Inhibitors (NNRTIs)

GENERIC NAME (TRADE NAME)	ABBREVIATION	FORMULATIONS AND COFORMULATIONS	RECOMMENDED ADULT DOSING	IMPORTANT POINTS
Delavirdine (Rescriptor)	DLV	100, 200 mg tablets	400 mg tid (four 100-mg tablets may be dispersed in >3 oz water to produce a slurry; 200-mg tablets should be taken as intact tablets)	Rash, elevated hepatic transaminases, headache No food restrictions
Efavirenz (Sustiva)	EFV	50, 200 mg capsules; 600 mg tablets *Coformulation:* Atripla (see FTC)	600 mg qd on an empty stomach at or before bedtime	Rash, CNS symptoms (vivid dreams, impaired concentration, dizziness), hyperlipidemia, false-positive cannabinoid test Take on an empty stomach, preferably at bedtime
Etravirine (Intelence)	ETR	100 mg tablets	200 mg bid after a meal	Rash, nausea Take after a meal Tablets may be dispersed in water
Nevirapine (Viramune)	NVP	200 mg tablets; 50 mg/5 mL oral suspension	200 mg qd for 14 d, then 200 mg PO bid	Hepatotoxicity, rash, lipodystrophy No food restrictions
Rilipivirine (Edurant)	RVP	25-mg capsule	25 mg qd with a meal	Depression, insomnia, headaches, rash; patients with viral load >100,000 at treatment initiation had a higher rate of virologic failure; take with a meal; cannot take with PPI

Protease Inhibitors (PIs)

GENERIC NAME (TRADE NAME)	ABBREVIATION	FORMULATIONS AND COFORMULATIONS	RECOMMENDED ADULT DOSING	IMPORTANT POINTS
Atazanavir (Reyataz)	ATV	100, 150, 200, 300 mg capsules	PI-naive patients only: ATV 400 mg qd PI-experienced patients: 300 mg (with RTV 100 mg) qd (when given with TDF, EFV, NVP)	Indirect hyperbilirubinemia, first-degree atrioventricular block, hyperglycemia, fat maldistribution, nephrolithiasis Avoid taking simultaneously with antacids Take with food
Darunavir (Prezista)	DRV	75, 300, 400, 600 mg tablets	PI-naive patients only: 800 mg (with RTV 100 mg) qd PI-experienced patients: 600 mg (with RTV 100 mg) bid	Rash (contains sulfa moiety), hepatotoxicity, diarrhea, nausea, headache, hyperlipidemia, hyperglycemia, fat maldistribution Take with food
Fosamprenavir (Lexiva)	FPV	700 mg tablet or 50 mg/mL oral suspension	PI-naive patients only: 1400 mg bid *OR* 1400 mg (with RTV 100-200 mg) qd *OR* 700 mg (with RTV 100 mg) bid PI-experienced patients: 700 mg (with RTV 100 mg) bid (once-daily dosing not recommended)	Rash, GI intolerance, headache, hyperlipidemia, hepatotoxicity, fat maldistribution No food restrictions
Indinavir (Crixivan)	IDV	100, 200, 333, 400 mg capsules	800 mg q8h *OR* 800 mg (with RTV 100–200 mg) bid	Nephrolithiasis, GI intolerance, indirect hyperbilirubinemia, hyperlipidemia, headache, blurred vision, alopecia Should be administered without food but with water 1 h before or 2 h after a meal for optimal absorption

Continued

TABLE 2	Approved Antiretroviral Medications—cont'd			
GENERIC NAME (TRADE NAME)	**ABBREVIATION**	**FORMULATIONS AND COFORMULATIONS**	**RECOMMENDED ADULT DOSING**	**IMPORTANT POINTS**
Lopinavir/ritonavir (Kaletra)	LPV/r	100 mg (+RTV 25 mg), 200 mg (+RTV 50 mg) tablets; 400 mg (+RTV 100 mg)/5 mL oral solution	PI-naive patients only: 4 × 200/50 mg tablets or 10 mL qd PI-experienced patients: 2 × 200/50 mg tablets or 5 mL bid	GI intolerance, diarrhea, hyperlipidemia, elevated hepatic transaminases, hyperlipidemia, fat maldistribution No food restrictions
Nelfinavir (Viracept)	NFV	250, 625 mg tablets; 50 mg/g oral powder	1250 mg bid OR 750 mg tid	Diarrhea, hyperlipidemia, hyperglycemia, fat maldistribution, elevated hepatic transaminases Take with food May be dispersed in water
Ritonavir (Norvir)	RTV	100 mg capsules; 80 mg/mL oral solution	Refer to other PIs for dosing recommendations	GI intolerance, headache, hyperlipidemia, hyperglycemia, dysgeusia, paresthesias Take with food
Saquinavir (Invirase)	SQV	200 mg hard gel capsules; 500 mg tablets	1000 mg (with RTV 100 mg) PO bid	GI intolerance, headache, elevated hepatic transaminaes, hyperlipidemia, hyperglycemia, fat maldistribution Take within 2 h after a meal
Tipranavir (Aptivus)	TPV	250 mg capsules	500 mg (with RTV 200 mg) PO bid	Hepatotoxicity, rash (contains sulfa moiety), rare cases of intracranial hemorrhage have been reported Take with food
Fusion Inhibitor				
Enfuvirtide (Fuzeon)	T20	90 mg/1 mL powder for injection	90 mg SQ bid	Injection site reactions (erythema, pain, induration), increased risk of bacterial pneumonia, hypersensitivity reaction
Coreceptor (CCR5) Antagonist				
Maraviroc (Selzentry)	MVC	150, 300 mg tablets	150 mg bid when given with strong CYP3A inhibitors (± CYP3A inducers) including PIs (except TPV/RTV) OR 300 mg bid when given with NRTIs, T20, TPV/RTV, NVP, and other drugs that are not strong CYP3A inhibitors OR 600 mg bid when given with CYP3A inducers (e.g., EFV, ETR, rifampin) without a CYP3A inhibitor	Abdominal pain, cough, dizziness, musculoskeletal symptoms, pyrexia, rash, upper respiratory tract infections, hepatotoxicity, orthostatic hypotension No food restrictions
Integrase Inhibitor[*,†]				
Raltegravir (Isentress)	RAL	400 mg tablets	400 mg bid	Nausea, headache, diarrhea, fever, CPK elevation No food restrictions

*Newer integrase inhibitors, such as Elvitegravir and Dolutegravir, are in the process of FDA approval.
†A new fixed-dose combination pill known as the Quad pill, which contains cobicistat, a novel pharmacologic booster that has no anti-HIV activity, along with tenofovir, emtricitabine, and a novel integrase inhibitor elvitegravir, has been approved for use in the United States.
Abbreviations: ART = antiretroviral therapy; CNS = central nervous system; CPK = creatine phosphokinase; CYP3A = cytochrome P-450 isoenzyme 3A; GI = gastrointestinal; HLA = human leukocyte antigen; MI = myocardial infarction; PPI = proton pump inhibitor.

more data accumulated, there was recognition that the virus establishes itself within hours after infection and cannot be eradicated with HAART. In addition, during this early HAART era, it was observed that several of the regimens used were complicated, were associated with several toxicities and reduced quality of life, and, importantly, were not associated with marked clinical benefits.

Therefore, between 1996 and 2006, the recommended CD4 count threshold for starting therapy steadily declined, with 2006 recommendations of the U.S. Department of Health and Human Services (DHHS), the International AIDS Society–USA, and the British HIV Society all generally indicating a threshold of 200 cells/mm³ for initiation of treatment in asymptomatic patients.

More recently, however, accumulating evidence of the beneficial effects of earlier versus later treatment has resulted in a shift toward earlier initiation of HAART. There are now several classes of drugs, and many of the newer ART regimens are more potent, better tolerated, and less complex than before (i.e., low pill burden and once-daily dosing). The newer regimens, such as PIs boosted with ritonavir (Norvir) and NNRTIs used in triple-drug combinations, are more effective at achieving and sustaining virologic suppression (HIV-1 RNA <20–400 copies, depending on the assay used) than the older regimens that used unboosted PIs and NRTIs. Most cases of virologic failure now occur when patients are lost to follow-up, are nonadherent, or discontinue their treatment. Furthermore, there is mounting evidence from several cohorts with long-term follow-up of HIV-infected patients that demonstrates a benefit of starting ART earlier. Consistently, persons starting treatment at a CD4 count threshold below 200 cells/mm^3 have a two to four times greater risk of AIDS or death than patients who start when their CD4 count is between 201 and 350 cells/mm^3.

There is also increasing recognition of the importance of non–AIDS-defining illnesses, such as cardiovascular, renal, and liver disease, at higher CD4 counts (>350 cells/mm^3). Cohort data (e.g., North American AIDS Cohort Collaboration on Research and Design [NA-ACCORD], ART-Collaborative) and one large trial (Strategies for Management of Anti-Retroviral Therapy [SMART]) reported significant benefits in reducing these complications when ART was initiated at higher CD4 thresholds (>350 or >500 cells/mm^3). Earlier initiation of HAART also appears to be associated with reduced risk of transmission, greater preservation of the R5-tropic virus, and improved immune restoration (including CD4 counts); it also may be cost-effective.

Current Recommendations for Antiretroviral Therapy

Current guidelines for HIV treatment in the United States are shown in Tables 3 and 4. Current U.S. guidelines advocate offering ART to all patients with HIV, regardless of CD4 count. The strength of the recommendation, however, is still stratified by CD4 count, as shown in Table 2. ART has also been shown to reduce the risk of HIV transmission to uninfected partners and may be offered in this scenario as well. Current guidelines recommend considering individualized treatment for specific scenarios such as active hepatitis B co-infection or pregnancy. Critical to all these recommendations, however, is ensuring that the patient is ready to start therapy and understands the regimen, the importance of adherence to it, and the need to continue therapy for life.

Selection of an Antiretroviral Regimen

Table 5 presents the regimens recommended for ART initiation in treatment-naive HIV-1–infected adults residing in the United States and other high-income countries. Current ART strategies that represent the standard of care are based on combining at least three potent antiretroviral agents. Therapy is individualized in high-income settings and takes into account several factors such as comorbidities, concomitant medications, possible drug interactions, pill burden, dosing schedule, adherence issues, risk for side effects, and pregnancy. Triple-NRTI regimens are inferior to PI- and NNRTI-containing regimens and therefore are not recommended.

Efavirenz (Sustiva) is the preferred NNRTI because it has the best long-term treatment response to date, based on clinical trial data. It is available with tenofovir (Viread) and emtricitabine (Emtriva) in a coformulation, called Atripla (efavirenz 600 mg + tenofovir 300 mg + emtricitabine 200 mg), that can be taken once a day. Nevirapine (Viramune) is an alternative NNRTI; it should not be used in women with a CD4 count of less than 250 cells/mm^3 or in men with less than 400 cells/mm^3, because it is associated with increased risk of severe hepatotoxicity in such patients. Newer NNRTIs include etravirine (2007) and rilpivirine (2011). Rilpivirine (Edurant) is also available in a daily coformulation with tenofovir and emtricitabine called Complera (rilpivirine 25 mg + tenofovir 300 mg + emtricitabine 200 mg). Some but not all resistance mutations that develop on efavirenz and nevirapine can confer resistance to the newer NNRTIs. Therefore it is important to review the specific genotypic mutations and consult HIV experts/resources before deciding if an antiretroviral combination can be expected to be effective. Furthermore, patients initiating treatment with rilpivirine at viral loads greater than 100,000 have a higher risk of virologic failure. Efavirenz-based regimens are equivalent to boosted-PI regimens in terms of efficacy and durability but have the advantages of low pill burden and limited long-term toxicity. The main drawback to NNRTI-containing regimens is their low barrier to resistance; for this reason, NNRTIs are less favored in patients for whom adherence is likely to be a problem.

The preferred PIs are the newer ones: atazanavir (Reyataz) boosted with ritonavir, and darunavir (Prezista) boosted with ritonavir. They are potent, have a high genetic barrier to resistance, and can be dosed once daily in many treatment-naive patients. The main drawbacks with PIs as a class are their interactions with other drugs, gastrointestinal intolerance, and metabolic complications (for most members of the class). The relative advantages and disadvantages of initial ART regimens are shown in Table 6. Note that while RAL is

---

TABLE 3   U.S. DHHS Guidelines for Initiation of HIV Treatment, 2012

CLINICAL CONDITION OR CD4 COUNT (CELLS/mm^3)	RECOMMENDATION	STRENGTH OF RECOMMENDATION AND QUALITY OF EVIDENCE*
Clinical Condition		
History of an AIDS-defining illness	Initiation of ART strongly recommended	AI
Pregnant women	Initiation of ART strongly recommended	AI
HIV-associated nephropathy (HIVAN)	Initiation of ART strongly recommended	AII
HIV/hepatitis B virus (HBV) coinfection	Initiation of ART strongly recommended	AII
Patients who are at risk of transmitting HIV to sexual partners—heterosexual or other modes of sexual transmission	ART should be offered†	AI/AIII
By CD4 Count		
CD4 count <350	Initiation of ART recommended	AI
CD4 count 350–500	Initiation of ART recommended	AII
CD4 count >500	Initiation of ART is recommended†	BIII

From U.S. DHHS Guidelines, 2012. Available at http://www.aidsinfo.nih.gov/Guidelines/ (accessed July 9, 2015).
Strength of Recommendations: A = strong evidence to support the recommendation; B = moderate evidence to support the recommendation. *Quality of Evidence:* I = randomized trials with either clinical or validated laboratory outcomes (e.g., viral load); II = nonrandomized trials or well-designed observational cohort studies with long-term clinical outcomes; III = recommendation based on expert opinion.
†Patient should be willing to commit to treatment and should understand the benefits and risks of therapy and the importance of adherence.

TABLE 4 International AIDS Society (IAS)-USA Guidelines for Initiation of HIV Treatment, 2012

MEASURE	RECOMMENDATION	STRENGTH OF RECOMMENDATION AND QUALITY OF EVIDENCE*
Specific Conditions		
Pregnancy	ART should be initiated	AIa
Opportunistic infections	ART should be initiated	AIa
—Tuberculosis with CD4 count <50	ART should be initiated within 2 weeks of tuberculosis treatment	AIa
—Tuberculosis with CD4 count >50	ART should be initiated within 8–12 weeks of tuberculosis treatment	AIa
—Tuberculosis meningitis	ART should be initiated within 2–8 weeks of tuberculosis diagnosis in consultation with experts	BIII
—Cryptococcal meningitis	ART initiation in consultation with experts	BIII
Chronic hepatitis B virus (HBV) coinfection	ART should be initiated	AIIa
HIV-associated nephropathy (HIVAN)	ART should be initiated	AIIa
Age >60 years	ART should be initiated	BIIa
Acute primary HIV infection, regardless of symptoms	ART should be initiated	BIII
Hepatitis C virus (HCV) coinfection	ART should be initiated[†]	CIII
By CD4 Cell Count		
CD4 count ≤500	ART is recommended	AIa
CD4 count >500	ART is recommended	BIII

From Thompson MA, Aberg JA, Hoy J, et al. Antiretroviral treatment of adult HIV infection: 2012 Recommendations of the International AIDS Society-USA Panel. JAMA 2012;308:387–402.
*Strength of Recommendations: A = strong evidence to support the recommendation; B = moderate evidence to support the recommendation; C = limited support for the recommendation. Quality of evidence: Ia = evidence from one or more randomized controlled clinical trials published in the peer-reviewed literature; Ib = evidence from one or more randomized clinical trials presented in abstract form at peer-reviewed scientific meetings; IIa = evidence from nonrandomized clinical trials or cohort or case-control studies published in peer-reviewed literature; IIb = evidence from nonrandomized clinical trials or cohort or case-control studies presented in abstract form at peer-reviewed scientific meetings; III = recommendation based on the panel's analysis of the accumulated available evidence.
[†]May delay ART initiation until after completion of HCV treatment if CD4 >500.

TABLE 5 Starting Regimens for Antiretroviral Naive Patients*

	COLUMN A	COLUMN B		
	DUAL NRTI BACKBONE	NNRTI	PI	INSTI
Preferred	TDF/FTC	EFV	ATV/r DRV/r	RAL
—Pregnant	ZDV/(3TC or FTC)[†]		LPV/r[†]	
Alternative	ABC/(3TC or FTC) TDF/(3TC or FTC)	EFV RPV	ATV/r DRV/r FPV/r LPV/r	RAL

From U.S. DHHS Guidelines, 2012. Available at http://www.aidsinfo.nih.gov/Guidelines/ (accessed July 9, 2015).
*Select one component from Column A (dual NRTI combination) and one from Column B (NNRTI, PI, or INSTI).
[†]ZDV/3TC plus LPV/r is the preferred regimen for pregnant women only (double LPV/r dose in pregnancy).
Abbreviations: 3TC = lamivudine (Epivir); ABC = abacavir (Ziagen); ABC/3TC = abacavir/lamivudine (Epzicom); ATV = atazanavir (Reyataz); DRV = darunavir (Prezista); EFV = efavirenz (Sustiva); FPV = fosamprenavir (Lexiva); FTC = emtricitabine (Emtriva); INSTI = integrase strand transfer inhibitor; LPV/r = lopinavir/ritonavir (Kaletra); NNRTI = non-nucleoside reverse transcriptase inhibitor; NRTI = nucleoside reverse transcriptase inhibitor; PI = protease inhibitor; r = ritonavir (Norvir); RAL = raltegravir (Isentress); RPV = rilpivirine (Edurant); TDF = tenofovir (Viread); TDF/FTC = tenofovir/emtricitabine (Truvada); ZDV = zidovudine (Retrovir); ZDV/3TC = zidovudine/lamivudine (Combivir).

the only integrase inhibitor recommended in initial ARV regimens, there is a daily quadruple combination pill (Stribild), which includes elvitegravir, a newer integrase inhibitor, along with cobicistat, emtricitabine, and tenofovir.

Monitoring Response to Antiretroviral Therapy

After ART is initiated, the CD4 count usually increases within a few weeks, largely because of redistribution of cells. Subsequently, the CD4 count improves over years of therapy, at an average rate of 100 cells/mm³ per year, and then reaches a plateau. The starting CD4 count appears to influence the plateau

reached (i.e., people starting at a lower count also plateau at a lower count than do those whose baseline count was higher). In approximately 5% to 10% of individuals, the CD4 response is less than this or does not increase from baseline. This is not evidence of treatment failure if the VL is undetectable. The plasma HIV VL rapidly decreases after initiation of HAART, and by 4 weeks most patients have at least a 1 log₁₀ drop in VL. In most individuals, it should become undetectable (<50 copies/mL) by 24 weeks.

The CD4 count should be assessed at 3 months after ART initiation and then every 3 to 6 months thereafter. The VL should be

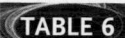

TABLE 6 Advantages and Disadvantages of Initial Antiretroviral Regimens

DRUGS	ADVANTAGES	DISADVANTAGES
Non-Nucleoside Reverse Transcriptase Inhibitors		
Class	• Extensive experience • Saves PI option • Fewer drug interactions than PIs	• Low genetic barrier to resistance • Class resistance with single mutation • Drug interactions, especially with methadone • ADRs: skin rash, especially NVP
EFV	• Potent and never beaten in a clinical trial • Low pill burden (coformulated with TDF and FTC), once-daily dosing	• Teratogenic (avoid use in pregnancy or with potential for pregnancy) • Compared to LPV/r: lower CD4 response, more resistance mutations, and increased lipoatrophy
RPV	• Low pill burden • ART potency comparable to EFV • Higher barrier to resistance than EFV and NVP	• Use with caution in patients with HIV viral load >100,000 • Cannot be used with PPIs
Protease Inhibitors		
Class	• Extensive experience • Saves NNRTI option • Higher genetic barrier to resistance	• ADRs: metabolic complications • Multiple drug interactions • GI intolerance
ATV/r	• High genetic barrier to resistance with boosting • Potency • Once-daily dosing • Low pill burden • No hyperlipidemia • Less GI intolerance	• ADRs: jaundice (harmless) and PR interval prolongation (usually inconsequential) • Drug interaction with TDF and ATV (can be overcome by ATV/r 400/100 mg qd with EFV) • Absorption requires food and gastric acid
DRV/r	• Once-daily dosing • High potency	• ADRs: skin rash • Food requirement
LPV/r	• Potency • Coformulated with RTV • No significant food effect • Option for once-daily therapy in treatment-naïve patients • Preferred in pregnancy	• ADRs: GI intolerance • RTV boosting required (coformulated) • Hyperlipidemia
FPV/r	• Potency • No significant food effect • Option for once-daily dosing • RTV boosting not required in treatment-naïve patients (preferred) • Appears equivalent to LPV/r	• ADRs: skin rash (has sulfa moiety) • Cross-resistance with DRV/r
Integrase Inhibitor		
RAL	• Virologic response noninferior to EFV when used with TDF/FTC • Well tolerated • No food effect • Minimal drug interactions	• Twice-daily dosing • Few data comparing RAL with boosted PI in treatment-naïve patients • Lower genetic barrier to resistance than PI-based regimens
Nucleoside Reverse Transcriptase Inhibitor Combinations		
ZDV/3TC/ABC	• Coformulated • Minimal drug interactions • Low pill burden • ABC may be associated with risk of cardiovascular disease and higher rate of viral failure in patients with baseline VL >100,000 copies/mL	• ADRs: ABC hypersensitivity and AZT marrow suppression, GI intolerance • HBV flare† • Requires twice daily dosing
ZDV/3TC	• Extensive experience • Coformulated • No food effect	• ADRs: GI intolerance and marrow suppression (ZDV) • HBV flare† • Requires twice-daily dosing (ZDV) • HBV flare†
TDF/FTC*	• Well tolerated • Coformulated • Long half-life of each drug may give pharmacologic barrier to resistance. • No thymidine analog mutations • Extensive experience	• Rare cases of nephrotoxicity (ddI/3TC or FTC) • Once-daily dosing • HBV flare† • Food effect

HIV Disease

119

Continued

TABLE 6	Advantages and Disadvantages of Initial Antiretroviral Regimens—cont'd		
DRUGS	**ADVANTAGES**		**DISADVANTAGES**
ABC/3TC*	• Coformulated • Once-daily dosing • No food effect		• ADRs: ABC hypersensitivity • HBV flare[†] • Risk of cardiovascular disease
Nucleoside Combinations to Avoid			
d4T/ddI	—		ADRs: peripheral neuropathy, lipoatrophy, pancreatitis, lactic acidosis.
ABC/TDF/3TC TDF/ddI/3TC	—		High rate of virologic failure
NNRTI/ddI/TDF	—		High rate of virologic failure
d4T/AZT	—		Antagonistic effects
TDF/ddI	—		Drug interaction requiring dose adjustment; avoid with NNRTI

*FTC and 3TC are similar except for convenience of coformulations; FTC has longer intracellular half-life and less extensive experience.
[†]In hepatitis B virus (HBV) co-infection (HBV surface antigen positive), hepatitis B flare may be caused by discontinuation of agent or by HBV resistance to NRTI (3TC, FTC, TDF).
Abbreviations: 3TC = lamivudine (Epivir); ABC = abacavir (Ziagen); ADR = adverse drug reaction; ATV = atazanavir (Reyataz); ddI = didanosine (Videx); d4t = stavudine (Zerit); DRV = darunavir (Prezista); EFV =efavirenz (Sustiva); FPV = fosamprenavir (Lexiva); FTC = emtricitabine (Emtriva); INSTI = integrase strand transfer inhibitor; LPV/r = lopinavir/ritonavir (Kaletra); NNRTI = non-nucleoside reverse transcriptase inhibitor; NRTI = nucleoside reverse transcriptase inhibitor; NVP = nevirapine (Viramune); PI = protease inhibitor; r = ritonavir (Norvir); RAL = raltegravir; RPV = rilpivirine; TDF = tenofovir (Viread); VL = viral load; ZDV = zidovudine (Retrovir).

measured 2 to 8 weeks after ART initiation, every 1 to 2 months until undetectable, and thereafter every 3 to 4 months. If a patient has been on a long-term stable suppressive regimen, visits can be reduced to every 6 months, with VL and CD4 testing performed at that interval. If a change in ART is motivated by drug toxicity or regimen simplification, it is recommended that VL be measured 2 to 8 weeks afterward, to confirm potency of the new regimen.

Other laboratory tests and their frequency of monitoring are shown in Table 1.

Treatment Failure

Treatment failure can be virologic, immunologic, or clinical. Virologic failure is defined as failure to achieve a VL of less than 400 copies/mL by 24 weeks or less than 50 copies/mL by 48 weeks, or a consistent finding (two consecutive measurements) of more than 50 copies/mL after a fall to less than 20–50 copies/mL at 48 weeks. Most patients should have a decrease of at least 1 $\log_{10}$ in VL within 4 weeks. Immunologic failure is the failure to increase the CD4 count by 25 to 50 cells/mm^3 during the first year. In treatment-naive patients, current regimens are associated with an average increase of 150 cells/mm^3 in the first year. Clinical failure is the occurrence or recurrence of HIV-related events 3 months or longer after HAART initiation; this is not to be confused with immune reconstitution syndromes (discussed later).

Today, with the use of appropriate combinations, newer fixed-dose formulations, and more tolerable regimens, treatment failure in patients on their first-line therapy usually occurs because of inadequate adherence or treatment discontinuation (e.g., loss to follow-up, intolerance) rather than regimen inefficacy. Occasionally, pharmacokinetic issues such as a reduced drug level due to genetic polymorphism or a drug interaction (e.g., omeprazole [Prilosec] with atazanavir [Reyataz]) or transmitted resistance can be causes of treatment failure. In the United States, the CDC recently reported that 16% of newly diagnosed HIV-positive people without prior ART use had evidence of ART resistance.

Drug Resistance and Resistance Testing

A patient may be infected with a drug-resistant HIV virus to begin with (primary resistance), or, more commonly, resistance can emerge as a result of treatment (secondary resistance).

Several NNRTI-associated resistance mutations confer resistance to other NNRTIs, including Y181C. However, K103N and 106M mutations, which cause resistance to efavirenz and nevirapine, do not confer resistance to newer-generation NNRTIs such as etravirine and rilpivirine.

Among NRTIs, the resistance mutation most commonly detected when regimens containing lamivudine (Epivir) or emtricitabine are used is M184V. This mutation also makes the virus hypersusceptible to tenofovir or zidovudine (Retrovir), so in many situations lamivudine or emtricitabine may be kept in the regimen if tenofovir or zidovudine is being used. Other NRTIs can be associated with thymidine analogue mutations, or TAMS (e.g., 41L, 210W, 215Y); accumulation of TAMS or presence of multinucleoside mutations (e.g., Q151M, T69 insertion) confers cross-resistance to other NRTIs.

With PIs, accumulation of mutations generally leads to significant cross-resistance. Ritonavir-boosted PIs, particularly lopinavir (i.e., Kaletra) and darunavir, have high barriers to resistance, so development of resistance does not occur as easily as with the NNRTI class. Indications for resistance testing include the baseline resistance (prior to initial therapy), acute HIV infection, suboptimal viral suppression (VL >1000 copies/mL), and virologic failure with VL greater than 1000 copies/mL. Resistance testing should be performed while the patient is on therapy or within 1 month after discontinuation, because, after that point, the wild-type virus may reemerge and predominate.

Current standard methods of genotyping do not detect minority variants (resistant virus populations accounting for <10% to 20% of plasma virus). Resistance testing is usually a genotypic test and should be performed early in cases of virologic failure. The phenotypic resistance assay is more expensive and is typically used in patients who have multiple resistance mutations after multiple virologic failures. Interpretation of resistance testing should include adherence assessment, prior history of antiretroviral agents, and prior resistance testing results, because a history of resistance mutations remains relevant even if they are not detected on the current resistance test. Because resistance testing interpretation is complex, special expertise should be sought.

Adverse Drug Reactions and Drug-Drug Interactions

Adverse drug reactions (ADRs) are common with ART and are a reason for patient nonadherence or treatment discontinuation. ADRs can be idiosyncratic, dose related, time related (delayed), or dose and time related (cumulative). A particular ADR may be drug specific (e.g., hypersensitivity to abacavir [Ziagen]) or class related (e.g., hyperlipidemia because of PIs). It is important to inform patients of potential common or serious ADRs associated with their therapy. Often, the challenge in managing ADRs is that the patient is taking several concomitant medications that may have overlapping toxicities and ADR profiles. A symptom-based approach is often most practical (Table 7). Although many of the ADRs can be managed conservatively, some, such as symptomatic lactic acidosis, systemic hypersensitivity reactions, Stevens-Johnson syndrome, acute pancreatitis, and severe hepatotoxicity,

ADVERSE EFFECT	MANIFESTATIONS	CAUSATIVE DRUGS		STEPWISE ACTION
		ANTIRETROVIRALS	*OTHER DRUGS*	
SJS/TEN[†]	Usually in first few weeks, with rash, mucosal ulcerations (± blistering), fever, hepatic dysfunction	NVP (0.5%–1%); less common with EFV (0.1%), ETR (<1%); rare with FPV, DRV, TPV, LPV/r, ATV, IDV, ABC, ZDV, ddI	Cotrimoxazole (Bactrim), sulfadiazine, dapsone, atovaquone (Mepron), voriconazole (Vfend)	Discontinue all antiretroviral agents and any other possible drug; manage like severe burns; do not rechallenge with offending drug
Hypersensitivity reaction[‡]	In rank order: high fever, diffuse rash, nausea, headache, abdominal pain, diarrhea, arthralgias, pharyngitis, dyspnea. Almost all have two or more systems involved. Always progresses with ABC, 90% present within first 6 wk	ABC (6%–7%); very rare if HLA-B*5701 is negative. Less common in African Americans	Cotrimoxazole, sulfadiazine, dapsone	Discontinue ABC and any other possible drug; rule out other causes; do not rechallenge with ABC. Symptoms resolve 48 h after ABC is stopped
Skin rash	Maculopapular rash ± pruritus	NVP, EFV, FPV > TPV >> ABC, DRV/r[§]	Cotrimoxazole, sulfadiazine, dapsone, atovaquone, voriconazole	Rule out SJS/TEN and hypersensitivity. Antihistamines; continue offending drug; watch for progression of rash (if so, discontinue)
GI intolerance[¶]	Anorexia, nausea, vomiting, epigastric pain; begins with first dose	PIs, ddI, ZDV; common	Isoniazid (Nydrazid), rifamycins, pyrazinamide	Administer with food (not for ddI or unboosted IDV); antiemetics; switch to less emetogenic antiretroviral agent
	Diarrhea; usually begins with first dose	PIs, especially NFV, LPV/r, and buffered ddI formulations	Clindamycin (Cleocin), atovaquone	Antimotility agents, calcium salts, bulk-forming agents; rehydration (if needed)
Hepatotoxicity[#]	Abrupt onset of GI symptoms, fever, rash, jaundice, eosinophilia, hepatic necrosis; encephalopathy can occur	NVP (usually ≤6 wk but up to 18 wk reported). Increased risk for baseline CD4 >250 (women) or CD4 >400 (men)	Isoniazid, rifamycins, pyrazinamide	Discontinue all antiretroviral agents and any other possible drug; rule out viral hepatitis; supportive management; do not rechallenge with NVP
	Symptomatic or subclinical hepatic enzyme elevations	NNRTIs, especially d4T, ddI, ZDV. PIs, especially TPV, MVC. 3TC, FTC, TDF can cause this with HBV co-infection and NRTI withdrawal or HBV resistance	Isoniazid, rifamycins, pyrazinamide, azithromycin (Zithromax), clarithromycin (Biaxin), all azole antifungals	If symptomatic, discontinue all antiretroviral agents and switch to nonhepatotoxic antiretrovirals after normalization; if asymptomatic, monitor closely. May discontinue drugs if ALT >5–10 × upper limit of normal
Lactic acidosis, fatty liver**	Nonspecific GI symptoms, wasting, fatigue, tachypnea, tachycardia, hepatomegaly, pancreatitis, hyperlactatemia, respiratory or multiorgan failure	d4T + ddI > d4T > ddI > ZDV (rare or never with other NRTIs); associated with long duration of use, female gender, obesity	Metformin (Glucophage)	Discontinue all antiretroviral agents; hydration; supportive care; roles of intravenous thiamine[1]/riboflavin,[1] steroids, carnitine,[2] plasmapheresis are unclear; switch to ABC/3TC/TDF or NRTI-sparing regimen
Pancreatitis**	Epigastric pain (postprandial), vomiting, fever, elevated amylase, lipase	ddI, d4T, high-dose RTV; concurrent d4T, ddI, and TDF without ddI dose adjustment; ddI + ribavirin contraindicated	Alcohol, cotrimoxazole, pentamidine (Pentam)	Discontinue offending drugs; manage like acute pancreatitis related to any other cause; do not rechallenge

HIV Disease

121

Continued

ADVERSE EFFECT	MANIFESTATIONS	CAUSATIVE DRUGS		STEPWISE ACTION
		ANTIRETROVIRALS	*OTHER DRUGS*	
Peripheral neuropathy**	Numbness, paresthesia (often painful after weeks to months); depressed ankle jerks; recovery possibly incomplete	ddI, d4T (10%–30% or higher based on duration)	Isoniazid	Switch to ABC/3TC/TDF; gabapentin (Neurontin), tricyclic antidepressants, narcotic analgesics
Myopathy**	Myalgia, muscle tenderness, proximal weakness, elevated creatine kinase	ZDV (uncommon with current doses)	Statins, fibrates, steroids	Switch to another NRTI; improves in 3–4 wk after discontinuation; roles of coenzyme Q10,[7] L-carnitine[7] are unproven
Nephrolithiasis, crystalluria††	Flank pain, nondescript abdominal pain, dysuria, hematuria, renal dysfunction	IDV; ATV (uncommon)	Cotrimoxazole, sulfadiazine, acyclovir (Zovirax)	Discontinue IDV; hydration and analgesics; IDV can be resumed with plenty of oral fluids; if symptoms recur, consider switching
Nephrotoxicity	Renal dysfunction; nephrogenic diabetes insipidus; Fanconi's syndrome	IDV, TDF Occurs primarily in patients with inadequate dose adjustment, baseline renal dysfunction, or concurrent nephrotoxic drugs Risk for Fanconi's with TDF associated with older age, low BMI, low CD4	Acyclovir, amphotericin B (Fungizone), cotrimoxazole, pentamidine	Discontinue offending drug; hydration; generally reversible
Hematologic	Anemia, neutropenia usually after weeks to months‡‡	ZDV	Cotrimoxazole, dapsone, sulfadiazine, pyrimethamine (Daraprim), flucytosine (Ancobon), trimetrexate (Neutrexin), amphotericin B, ganciclovir (Cytovene), valganciclovir (Valcyte), rifabutin (Mycobutin)	Discontinue concomitant marrow suppressant, if any; exclude marrow involvement by opportunistic infections/malignancy; erythropoietin (Procrit) or filgrastim (Neupogen); switch to another NRTI
	Bleeding tendency in hemophiliacs	PIs	—	Factor VIII infusion (Advate); consider NNRTI-based regimens
	Eosinophilia	Enfuvirtide (Fuzeon)	Cotrimoxazole, dapsone, sulfadiazine	Exclude disseminated strongyloidiasis, malignancy; watch for hypersensitivity
Central nervous system symptoms§§	Drowsiness, insomnia, vivid dreams, nightmares, hallucination, impaired concentration/attention Usually resolves in 2–3 wk Worsening of psychiatric disorders, suicidal ideation	EFV; effects can begin with first dose	Isoniazid, dapsone, steroids	Usually resolves in 2–4 wk; consider discontinuation if symptoms are persistent or psychiatric illness is exacerbated
Fat atrophy	Loss of subcutaneous fat (face, buttocks, extremities) Associated with long-term use	d4T > ZDV, ddI; less common with EFV	Steroids	Discontinue d4T, ZDV early if possible; either slow reversal or irreversible changes
Fat accumulation	Increase in abdominal girth, breast size, buffalo hump	PIs, EFV	—	Consider change in regimen for cosmetic reasons; restorative surgery

ADVERSE EFFECT	MANIFESTATIONS	CAUSATIVE DRUGS		STEPWISE ACTION
		ANTIRETROVIRALS	*OTHER DRUGS*	
Hyperlipidemia	Increase in total and low-density lipoproteins, triglycerides; begins within weeks	PIs, except ATV (rank: TPV/r > LPV/r, FPV/r > IDV/r > SQV/r), EFV, d4T	—	Follow NCEP guidelines, statins (preferably pravastatin, atorvastatin, rosuvastatin [Crestor] but may need dose adjustment)¶¶
Insulin resistance	Fasting blood sugar >126 mg/dL, abnormal glucose tolerance test, DM symptoms More likely with family history of DM	PIs, except ATV	—	Diet, exercise, if indicated: metformin, rosiglitazone (Avandia), insulin (no major drug interactions with antiretroviral agents); consider switch to other non-PI regimens

Based on Guidelines for the Use of Antiretroviral Agents in HIV-1-Infected Adults and Adolescents, U.S. Department of Health and Human Services, March 2012.

[1]Not FDA approved for this indication.
[2]Not available in the United States.
[7]Available as dietary supplement.
*Only common and serious side effects are dealt with; side effects such as osteoporosis, avascular osteonecrosis (PIs), unconjugated hyperbilirubinemia, retinoid-like effects (IDV), and cranial malformations (EFV) are also known to occur.
†Approximately 0.3%–1% with NVP; a low dose lead-in period for NVP may decrease the risk; less common (0.1%) with EFV; occurs in the initial weeks after initiation; safety of replacing NVP with another NNRTI is unknown.
‡Approximately 5% with ABC; once-daily dosing possibly increases the risk; if ABC-related, symptoms resolve within 48 h after discontinuation of ABC.
§FPV and TPV are sulfonamide derivatives; potential cross hypersensitivity with sulfonamides.
¶Symptoms begin with first doses; may abate with time.
#Low-dose lead-in period for NVP may reduce the risk; onset within the first few weeks with NNRTIs, after weeks to months with PIs, and after months to years with NRTIs; discontinuation of 3TC, FTC, or TDF in HBV co-infected patients may cause acute flare-up of hepatitis; safety of replacing NVP with another NNRTI is unknown.
**Class-specific adverse effect of NRTIs, because of mitochondrial toxicity; do not combine ddI/d4T/ddC; ABC, 3TC, and TDF are less prone; all four syndromes can occur in variable combinations; symptomatic lactic acidosis is rare but is associated with high mortality.
††Approximately 10% of patients taking IDV experience at least one episode of colic; occurrence is seen in only 50%, if fluid intake is improved (at least 1.5–2 L of non-caffeinated fluid, preferably water).
‡‡Almost all ZDV-treated patients have isolated macrocytosis; anemia and neutropenia occur in approximately 1%–4% and 2%–8%, respectively.
§§Occurs during initial weeks of treatment; patients are to be warned to restrict risky activities.
¶¶Only atorvastatin (Lipitor) and pravastatin (Pravachol) among statins, and gemfibrozil (Lopid) and fenofibrate (Triglide) among fibrates, can be coadministered with PIs.
Abbreviations: 3TC = lamivudine (Epivir); ABC = abacavir (Ziagen); ALT = alanine aminotransferase; ATV = atazanavir (Reyataz); BMI = body mass index; CD4 = CD4+ T-cell count (in cells/mm³); d4T = stavudine (Zerit); ddC = zalcitabine (Hivid)²; ddI = didanosine (Videx); DM = diabetes mellitus; DRV = darunavir (Prezista); EFV = efavirenz (Sustiva); ETR = etravirine (Intelence); FPV = fosamprenavir (Lexiva); FTC = emtricitabine (Emtriva); GI = gastrointestinal; HBV = hepatitis B virus; HLA = human leukocyte antigen; IDV = indinavir (Crixivan); LPV/r = lopinavir/ritonavir (Kaletra); MVC = maraviroc (Selzentry); NARTI = nucleoside reverse transcriptase inhibitor; NCEP = National Cholesterol Education Program; NFV = nelfinavir (Viracept); NNRTI = non-nucleoside reverse transcriptase inhibitor; NVP = nevirapine (Viramune); PI = protease inhibitor; r = RTV as a booster; RTV = ritonavir (Norvir); SJS = Stevens-Johnson syndrome; SQV = saquinavir (Invirase); TDF = tenofovir (Viread); TEN = toxic epidermal necrolysis; TPV = tipranavir (Aptivus); ZDV = zidovudine (Retrovir).

HIV Disease

123

are potentially life threatening. Serious ADRs necessitate withdrawal of the offending drug, and rechallenge with the drug should not be attempted in these situations.

Numerous important drug-drug interactions exist among antiretroviral agents and other medications of various classes. Familiarity with common interactions and ready access to reliable HIV pharmacology reference materials or a clinical pharmacologist with expertise in ART is essential for the clinician prescribing ART. Table 8, although not exhaustive, lists important drug-drug interactions, including combinations that are contraindicated and those that require adjustments to prescribe dosages. Tables 9 and 10 show dose adjustments that must be made with coadministration of certain antiretroviral drugs.

Hepatitis C Co-infection

As shown in Table 1, screening for Hepatitis C virus (HCV) is recommended in all HIV-positive patients. Co-infected individuals, especially those with low CD4 counts (≤350 cells/mm³), are three times more likely to progress to cirrhosis and liver failure than those with HCV mono-infection. Treatment of HCV can slow the progression of liver disease. Until recently, however, the combination of peginterferon and ribavirin (PegIFN/RBV) was the only available treatment option for HCV, but it was poorly tolerated because of adverse drug effects. Now there are new HCV protease inhibitors such as boceprevir (BOC) and telaprevir (TVR)

that have revolutionized treatment of HCV. These newer medications, however, can interact with antiretrovirals.

Clinicians may defer HCV treatment in HIV positive patients with no or minimal liver fibrosis. In that case, the recommended initial antiretroviral therapy for co-infected patients is the same as those with HIV alone (see Table 5). If treatment for both HCV and HIV is to be done simultaneously, careful consideration should be paid to potential drug–drug interactions. If a patient is receiving a RAL-based ARV regimen, either BOC or TVR can be used. If using an ATV/r or EFV-based regimen, TVR can be used, but the TVR dose must be increased to 1125 mg every 7 to 9 hours if prescribed with EFV. Neither BOC nor TVR is safe to use with DRV/r. The treatment of HCV is evolving rapidly, so management of HIV-HCV co-infected patients is likely to change markedly in the coming years.

Complications

Diagnosis and Management of Opportunistic Infections

OIs are the most common cause of disability and death in patients who are not receiving ART. Clinical experience from the pre-HAART era demonstrated that the risk of OIs increases proportionately with the severity of immune system dysfunction and can be roughly predicted by the CD4 count in patients receiving and not receiving HAART. Guidelines for initiating and

TABLE 8	Drug Interactions with Antiretroviral Agents*		
CLASS	**AGENT**	**ANTIRETROVIRAL AGENT**	**COMMENTS**
α-Adrenergic blockers	Alfuzosin (Uroxatral)	RTV, All PIs	Consider tamsulosin (Flomax) or doxazosin (Cardura)
Antianginals	Ranolazine (Ranexa)	All PIs	—
Antiarrhythmics	Flecainide (Tambocor), propafenone (Rythmol), amiodarone (Cordarone), quinidine	All PIs	—
Antihistamines	Astemizole (Hismanal),[2] terfenadine (Seldane)[2]	All PIs, EFV	Loratadine (Claritin), fexofenadine (Allegra), cetirizine (Zyrtec), or desloratadine (Clarinex)
Antimycobacterials	Rifampin (Rifadin) Rifapentine (Priftin)	All PIs, NVP All PIs, NNRTIs	Use rifabutin (Mycobutin) with PIs Rifabutin
Antineoplastics	Irinotecan (Camptosar)	ATV, caution with other PIs	—
Calcium channel blockers	Bepridil (Vascor)	All PIs	—
Ergot alkaloids	Ergotamine (Cafergot)	All PIs, EFV	Sumatriptan (Imitrex)
Gastrointestinal agents	Cisapride (Propulsid)[2] Proton pump inhibitors	All PIs, EFV ATV, NFV	Metoclopramide (Reglan)
Herbs	St. John's wort[7]	All PIs, NNRTIs	Other antidepressants
Intranasal steroids	Fluticasone (Flonase)	All PIs	Beclomethasone (Beconase AQ)
Lipid-lowering drugs	Simvastatin (Zocor), lovastatin (Mevacor)	All PIs	Pravastatin (Pravachol), fluvastatin (Lescol), possibly atorvastatin (Lipitor), rosuvastatin (Crestor)
Neurotropics	Pimozide (Orap)	All PIs	—
Psychotropics	Midazolam (Versed), triazolam (Halcion)	All PIs	Temazepam (Restoril), lorazepam (Ativan)

Adapted from John G. Bartlett's Pocket Guide to Adult HIV/AIDS Treatment 2008-2009. Fairfax, VA, Johns Hopkins HIV Care Program, 2008.
[2]Not available in the United States.
[7]Available as dietary supplement.
*Delavirdine (Rescriptor) drug interactions are not shown as this drug is no longer used in clinical practice. Detailed information about drug interactions and searchable drug interaction databases are available at http://www.hopkins-aids.edu/, http://www.hiv-druginteractions.org/, http://hivinsite.ucsf.edu.
Abbreviations: ATV = atazanavir (Reyataz); EFV = efavirenz (Sustiva); NFV = nelfinavir (Viracept); NRTI = nucleoside reverse transcriptase inhibitor; NNRTI = non-nucleoside reverse transcriptase inhibitor; NVP = nevirapine (Viramune); PI = protease inhibitor; RTV = ritonavir (Norvir).

discontinuing antimicrobial prophylaxis against OIs are based on the CD4 count, as summarized in Table 11.

Diagnosis of OIs requires that clinicians recognize that a diverse array of bacterial, fungal, viral, and parasitic pathogens can cause overlapping clinical syndromes. A broad differential diagnosis must be considered when evaluating an HIV-infected patient with specific or generalized symptoms. Aside from infectious complications, symptoms may arise from toxicities inherent to antiretroviral or other medications. Patients infected with HIV have increased rates of cardiovascular, renal, and hematologic abnormalities, which may also cause nonspecific symptoms. A syndromic approach to recognizing complications of HIV infection is described in the following paragraphs. Recommended treatment regimens for the most common OIs are presented in Table 12. Detailed treatment guidelines that are periodically updated are available from the CDC and the HIV Medicine Association of the Infectious Diseases Society of America (http://aidsinfo.nih.gov/contentfiles/Adult_OI.pdf [accessed July 9, 2015]).

Neurologic Complications

Both central nervous system disease and peripheral nerve abnormalities are common in advanced AIDS. Peripheral neuropathy has been associated with some NRTI medications, most commonly stavudine (d4T, Zerit), as a result of the mitochondrial toxicity inherent to these drugs. HIV infection can directly cause distal sensory neuropathy, which may manifest as dysesthesia or hypersensitivity, decreased reflexes, and chronic neuropathic pain. Inflammatory demyelinating polyneuropathy (e.g., Guillain-Barré syndrome), which has known associations with some enteric pathogens, causes ascending motor weakness, typically without

sensory involvement. CMV infection may cause polyradiculopathy, transverse myelitis, and encephalitis/ventriculitis in patients with CD4 counts lower than 50 cells/mm[3]. CMV end-organ disease, including retinitis (a vision-threatening condition), requires prompt diagnosis and initiation of appropriate anti-CMV therapy.

Focal central nervous system lesions may be caused by infectious and malignant conditions. Cerebral toxoplasmosis usually occurs in patients with prior exposure to *Toxoplasma gondii* who develop reactivation disease when the CD4 count is lower than 100 cells/mm[3]. The main differential diagnosis for one or several enhancing brain lesions includes toxoplasmosis and primary central nervous system lymphoma (PCNSL). PCNSL is almost always associated with Epstein-Barr virus, and detection of nucleic acid for Epstein-Barr virus in cerebrospinal fluid carries a high specificity for this condition in the proper radiographic context. Progressive multifocal leukoencephalopathy, a rare and potentially devastating demyelinating condition, is caused by reactivation of JC virus and can manifest as focal neurologic deficit, seizures, or cognitive dysfunction. *Cryptococcus neoformans* is a common cause of meningitis in AIDS patients and can also manifest with central nervous system mass lesions, pulmonary disease, or gastrointestinal disease. Worldwide, tuberculosis accounts for a large proportion of HIV-associated meningitis; less commonly, it can manifest as single or multiple focal lesions (tuberculomas). Neurosyphilis should be considered in patients with unexplained neurologic disease and sexual risk factors.

Respiratory Complications

Respiratory illnesses are among the most common causes of morbidity in HIV patients. Community-acquired bacterial pneumonia

TABLE 9 Combinations Requiring Dose Adjustments: NRTIs

DRUG	ZIDOVUDINE (RETROVIR, AZT)	STAVUDINE (ZERIT, d4T)	DIDANOSINE (VIDEX, ddI)	TENOFOVIR (VIREAD, TDF)
Methadone (Dolophine)	AZT AUC increase 40%; no dose change Monitor CBC	d4T decreased 27%; no dose change	ddI EC: no interaction	No change in methadone or TDF levels
Didanosine (Videx, ddI)	—	Increased toxicity: pancreatitis, peripheral neuropathy lactic acidosis Avoid	—	ddI increases 44% >60 kg: 250 mg/d ddI EC <60 kg: 200 mg/d ddI EC
Ribavirin (Rebetol)	Monitor for severe anemia In vitro inhibition of AZT activation; not shown in vivo	No data	Magnifies ddI toxicity; contraindicated	Ribavirin unchanged; no data on TDF level
Atazanavir (Reyataz, ATV)	AZT AUC unchanged but C_{min} decrease 30%; significance unknown	No data	Buffered ddI: take ATV 2 h before or 1 h after ddI or use ddI EC (separate dosing due to food restrictions)	ATV AUC decreases 25%; TDF AUC increases 24% Avoid concomitant use unless ATV is combined with RTV (ATV/r)
Indinavir (Crixivan, IDV)	—	No data	Buffered ddI: take 1 h apart	IDV C_{max} increases 14%; clinical significance unknown
Cidofovir (Vistide), ganciclovir (Cytovene), valganciclovir (Valcyte)	Ganciclovir + AZT increases marrow toxicity Monitor CBC	No data	ddI and oral ganciclovir: ddI AUC increased 111% (PO) and 50%–70% (IV); use with caution or avoid	Combination may increase levels of both drugs; monitor for toxicity
Lopinavir/ritonavir (Kaletra, LPV/r)	No pharmacokinetics data but interaction unlikely due to favorable clinical data	No data	No data	TDF AUC increases 34% Use standard doses and monitor for TDF toxicity
Tipranavir (Aptivus, TPV)	AZT decreased 33%–43%; clinical significance unknown	No interaction	Separate dose of ddI EC by >2 h	TPV AUC decreases 9%–18%; clinical significance unknown

Adapted from John G. Bartlett's Pocket Guide to Adult HIV/AIDS Treatment 2008–2009. Fairfax, VA, Johns Hopkins HIV Care Program, 2008.
Abbreviations: AUC = area under the concentration-versus-time curve; CBC = complete blood count; C_{max} = maximum plasma concentration; C_{min} = minimum plasma concentration; EC = enteric coated; NRTI = nucleoside reverse transcriptase inhibitor.

TABLE 10 Combinations Requiring Dose Adjustments: PIs and NNRTIs

DRUG	EFAVIRENZ (SUSTIVA, EFV)	NEVIRAPINE (VIRAMUNE, NVP)	ETRAVIRINE (INTELENCE, ETR)
Atazanavir (Reyataz)/ritonavir (Norvir, RTV) combination (ATV/r)	ATV 400 mg + RTV 100 mg (with food) + EFV SD (avoid coadministration in PI-experienced patients)	Avoid	Avoid
Darunavir (Prezista)/ritonavir combination (DRV/r)	DRV/r SD + EFV SD (dose not established; consider TDM)	DRV/r SD + NVP SD (dose not established; consider TDM)	DRV/r-SD + ETR-SD
Fosamprenavir (Lexiva, FPV)	FPV 1400 mg qd + RTV 300 mg qd + EFV SD FPV 700 mg bid + RTV 100 mg bid + EFV SD	FPV 700 mg + RTV 100 mg bid + NVP SD	Avoid
Indinavir (Crixivan, IDV)	IDV 1000 mg q8h + EFV SD IDV 800 mg q12h + RTV 200 mg bid + EFV SD	IDV 1000 mg q8h + NVP SD IDV 800 mg q12h + RTV 200 mg q12h + NVP SD	Avoid
Lopinavir/ritonavir coformulation (Kaletra, LPV/r)	LPV/r 600/150 mg bid + EFV SD	LPV/r 600/150 mg bid + NVP SD	ETR: SD LPV/r: SD
Nelfinavir (Viracept, NFV)	NFV SD + EFV SD	NVP SD + NFV SD	Avoid
Saquinavir Invirase, SQV)	SQV/r 1000/100 mg bid + EFV SD	SQV 1000 mg bid + RTV 100 mg bid + NVP SD	SQV/r 1000/100 mg bid + ETR SD
Tipranavir (Aptivus)/ritonavir combination (TPV/r)	TPV 500 mg bid + RTV 200 mg bid + EFV SD	Inadequate data; NVP may decrease TPV	Avoid

Adapted from John G. Bartlett's Pocket Guide to Adult HIV/AIDS Treatment 2008–2009. Fairfax, VA, Johns Hopkins HIV Care Program, 2008.
Abbreviations: NNRTI = non-nucleoside reverse transcriptase inhibitor; PI = protease inhibitor; SD = standard dose; TDM = therapeutic drug monitoring.

TABLE 11	Antimicrobial Prophylaxis for Opportunistic Infections			
INFECTION	**INDICATIONS FOR INITIATING PROPHYLAXIS**	**PREFERRED REGIMEN**	**ALTERNATIVE REGIMEN**	**INDICATIONS FOR DISCONTINUING PROPHYLAXIS**
Pneumocystis jirovecii pneumonia (PCP)	CD4 <200	TMP-SMX (Bactrim DS) 1 DS tablet PO qd, or TMP-SMX (Bactrim SS) 1 SS tablet PO qd	TMP-SMX (Bactrim DS) 1 DS tablet PO three times weekly[3] Dapsone[1] 100 mg PO qd or 50 mg PO bid Dapsone 50 mg PO qd + pyrimethamine (Daraprim)[1] 50 mg PO weekly + leucovorin[1] 25 mg PO weekly Aerosolized pentamidine (NebuPent) 300 mg via Respirgard II nebulizer monthly Atovaquone (Mepron) 1500 mg/d Atovaquone 1500 mg/d + pyrimethamine 25 mg/d + leucovorin 10 mg/d	CD4 >200 for 3 mo in response to HAART
Toxoplasma gondii encephalitis	CD4 <100 and *toxoplasma* IgG positive	TMP-SMX[1] 1 DS tablet PO qd	TMP-SMX 1 DS tablet PO three times weekly TMP-SMX 1 SS tablet PO qd Dapsone[1] 50 mg PO qd + pyrimethamine 50 mg PO weekly + leucovorin[1] 25 mg PO weekly Dapsone 200 mg + pyrimethamine 75 mg + leucovorin 25 mg, all PO weekly Atovaquone[1] 1500 mg ± pyrimethamine 25 mg + leucovorin 10 mg, all PO qd	CD4 >200 for 3 mo in response to HAART
Mycobacterium avium-intracellulare (MAI)	CD4 <50	Azithromycin (Zithromax) 1200 mg PO once weekly Clarithromycin (Biaxin) 500 mg PO bid Azithromycin 600 mg PO twice weekly	Rifabutin (Mycobutin) 300 mg PO qd	CD4 >100/mm³ for 3–6 mo and undetectable viral load in response to HAART
Mycobacterium tuberculosis	Positive diagnostic test for LTBI	Isoniazid (INH) 300 mg PO qd (or 900 mg PO twice weekly for 9 mo) + pyridoxine 50 mg PO qd	Rifampin (Rifadin) 600 mg PO qd × 4 mo	Completion of treatment for LTBI

[1]Not FDA approved for this indication.
[3]Exceeds dosage recommended by manufacturer.
Abbreviations: CD4 = CD4⁺ T-cell count (in cells/mm³); DS = double-strength; HAART = highly active antiretroviral therapy; IgG = immunoglobulin G; LTBI = latent tuberculosis infection; SS = single-strength; TMP-SMX = trimethoprim-sulfamethoxazole.

occurs at a significantly higher rate in HIV-infected compared with HIV-noninfected hosts, regardless of CD4 count, and is one of the most common reasons for hospitalization. *Pneumocystis jirovecii* (formerly *Pneumocystis carinii*) pneumonia (PCP) manifests with fever, cough, and dyspnea. Findings on physical examination and chest radiography can be variable, making the diagnosis difficult in the absence of high clinical suspicion. Elevated lactate dehydrogenase and oxygen desaturation with ambulation can be diagnostic clues. More than 90% of cases occur among patients with CD4 counts lower than 200 cells/mm³. The diagnosis is established by visualization of organisms in induced sputum (sensitivity, 50%–90%) or in bronchoalveolar lavage specimens (sensitivity, 90%–99%), most commonly with the use of immunofluorescent staining. Slight worsening of clinical symptoms after initiation of treatment for PCP is common, particularly when adjunctive corticosteroids are not administered.

The risk of reactivation of latent TB is increased 100-fold in patients with HIV infection. HIV⁺ persons who are latently infected have a 10% annual risk of developing symptomatic tuberculosis, compared with a 10% lifetime risk among the general population. The risk of reactivation increases with decreasing CD4 count, and patients with counts lower than 350 cells/mm³ are more likely to have atypical radiographic presentations, including middle- and lower-lobe infiltrates without cavitation. Patients with very low CD4 counts are more likely to have extrapulmonary tuberculosis. Diagnostic approaches to tuberculosis are similar in HIV⁺ and HIV⁻ patients. Tuberculin skin testing can still be used to diagnose latent tuberculosis infection, although the recommended cutoff for a positive test is 5 mm of induration. Treatment of co-infection with *Mycobacterium tuberculosis* and HIV requires consultation with experienced clinicians and pharmacists because of extensive drug-drug interactions among antiretroviral drugs and rifamycins.

TABLE 12	Recommended Treatment for Opportunistic Infections			

INFECTION	PREFERRED REGIMEN	ALTERNATIVE REGIMEN	MAINTENANCE THERAPY	IMPORTANT POINTS
Pneumocystis jirovecii pneumonia (PCP)	TMP-SMX (Bactrim) (15–20 mg TMP and 75–100 mg SMX)/kg/day IV divided q6h or q8h May switch to PO after clinical improvement Duration of therapy: 21 d	Pentamidine (Pentam) 4 mg/kg IV q24h infused over ≥60 min, or Primaquine[1] 15–30 mg PO q24h + clindamycin[1] (Cleocin) 600–900 mg IV q6–8h or 300–450 mg PO q6–8h	Drug regimens for secondary prophylaxis same as for primary prophylaxis	Indications for corticosteroids: PaO_2 <70 mm Hg on room air, A-a gradient >35 mm Hg Prednisone[1] doses: 40 mg PO bid on days 1–5, 40 mg PO qd on days 6–10, 20 mg PO qd on days 11–21
Toxoplasma gondii encephalitis	Pyrimethamine (Daraprim) 200 mg PO × 1, then 50 mg (weight <60 kg) or 75 mg (≥60 kg) PO qd + sulfadiazine 1000 mg (<60 kg) or 1500 mg (≥60 kg) PO q6h + leucovorin[1] 10–25 mg PO qd	Pyrimethamine + leucovorin in same doses as for preferred regimen + clindamycin[1] 600 mg IV or PO q6h, or TMP-SMX[1] (5 mg/kg TMP and 25 mg/kg SMX) IV or PO bid	Pyrimethamine 25–50 mg PO qd + sulfadiazine 2000–4000 mg PO qd (in two to four divided doses) + leucovorin 10–25 mg PO qd	Duration of acute therapy: at least 6 wk; longer if clinical or radiographic response is incomplete at 6 wk
Mycobacterium avium-intracellulare (MAI)	At least two drugs as initial therapy with clarithromycin 500 mg PO bid + ethambutol (Myambutol)[1] 15 mg/kg PO qd Optional third drug in severe disease: rifabutin (Mycobutin)[1] 300 mg PO qd (dosage adjustment may be necessary based on drug-drug interactions)	Azithromycin (Zithromax) 500–600 mg + ethambutol 15 mg/kg PO qd Alternative third drugs include fluoroquinolones: levofloxacin (Levaquin),[1] ciprofloxacin (Cipro),[1] moxifloxacin (Avelox),[1] amikacin (Amikin)[1]	Same as initial treatment	Criteria for discontinuing therapy: CD4 >100 × 6 mo as a result of ART, symptoms have resolved, and at least 12 mo of therapy has been received
Cryptococcus neoformans meningitis	Induction therapy: amphotericin B deoxycholate 0.7 mg/kg IV qd + flucytosine 100 mg/kg PO qd in 4 divided doses for at least 2 wk	Lipid formulation amphotericin B 4–6 mg/kg IV qd + flucytosine 100 mg/kg PO qd in 4 divided doses for at least 2 wk, or Amphotericin B (without flucytosine) at same dose, or Fluconazole 400–800 mg PO once daily for 10–12 wk	Consolidation therapy: Fluconazole 400 mg PO qd for 8–10 wk after induction therapy Maintenance therapy: Fluconazole 200 mg PO qd lifelong or until CD4 ≥200 for >6 mo as a result of ART	Managing elevated intracranial pressure is key to preventing morbidity and mortality; serial lumbar puncture and lumbar drainage is indicated in some cases
Cytomegalovirus (CMV) retinitis	Sight-threatening lesions: Ganciclovir intraocular implant + valganciclovir 900 mg PO (bid for 14–21 d, then once daily) Small or peripheral lesions: Valganciclovir 900 mg PO bid for 14–21 d, then 900 mg PO qd	Ganciclovir 5 mg/kg IV q12h for 14–21 d, then valganciclovir 900 mg PO qd, or Foscarnet 60 mg/kg IV q8h or 90 mg/kg IV q12h for 14–21 d, then 90–120 mg/kg IV q24h, or Cidofovir 5 mg/kg/wk IV for 2 wk, then 5 mg/kg every other week	Valganciclovir 900 mg PO qd, or Ganciclovir implant (may be replaced q6–8mo) + valganciclovir 900 mg PO qd until immune recovery	Maintenance therapy for CMV retinitis can be safely discontinued in patients with inactive disease and sustained CD4 >100 for ≥3–6 mo; consultation with ophthalmologist is advised
CMV esophagitis or colitis	Ganciclovir 5 mg/kg IV q12h for 21–28 d or until symptoms resolve Oral valganciclovir may be used if symptoms are not severe enough to interfere with oral absorption	Foscarnet 60 mg/kg IV q8h or 90 mg/kg IV q12h for 21–28 d	Maintenance therapy is usually not necessary but should be considered after relapses	Patients with CMV gastrointestinal disease should undergo ophthalmologic screening
Esophageal candidiasis	Fluconazole 100 mg (up to 400 mg) PO or IV qd for 14–21 d	Itraconazole oral solution 200 mg PO qd Voriconazole 200 mg PO or IV bid Posaconazole 400 mg PO bid Caspofungin 50 mg IV qd Micafungin 150 mg IV qd Anidulafungin 100 mg IV × 1, then 50 mg IV qd Amphotericin B deoxycholate 0.6 mg/kg IV qd	Not routinely recommended	Patients with fluconazole-refractory oropharyngeal or esophageal candidiasis with response to echinocandin should be started on voriconazole or posaconazole for secondary prophylaxis until ART produces immune reconstitution

[1]Not FDA approved for this indication.
Abbreviations: A-a gradient = alveolar-arterial difference in partial pressure of oxygen (PaO_2 − PaO_2); ART = antiretroviral therapy; CD4 = CD4[+] T-cell count (in cells/mm[3]); PaO_2 = arterial partial pressure of oxygen.

Gastrointestinal Complications

Diagnosis of OIs affecting the gastrointestinal tract is made difficult by the numerous infections and complications of therapies that can result in nonspecific syndromes such as nausea, vomiting, abdominal pain, and diarrhea. Oropharyngeal candidiasis (thrush) commonly manifests as white plaques on the tongue, palate, or buccal mucosa that are painless and can easily be scraped off. Although thrush is typically uncomplicated and easily treatable with topical preparations such as nystatin (Mycostatin) and clotrimazole (Mycelex troches), in the proper clinical setting it can alert the clinician to the presence of esophageal candidiasis. Esophageal involvement should be suspected in patients with dysphagia and odynophagia; retrosternal chest pain may also be present. Thrush is usually present but is not required for the diagnosis, which is often made on clinical grounds rather than being confirmed with endoscopy. Patients with esophageal candidiasis typically respond after several days of treatment, and 7 to 14 days of antifungal therapy is usually sufficient. For cases not responsive to empiric treatment for candidiasis, referral for endoscopy should be considered. Esophagitis caused by CMV or herpes simplex virus requires a histopathologic diagnosis.

Acute diarrhea, defined as three or more loose or watery stools per day for 3 to 10 days, is common among HIV+ patients, and more than 1000 different enteric pathogens have been described. Data from a large cohort indicate that the most common pathogens isolated are *Clostridium difficile*, *Shigella* spp., *Campylobacter jejuni*, *Salmonella* spp., *Staphylococcus aureus*, and *Mycobacterium avium-intracellulare* (MAI). Culture of the stool can yield a microbiologic diagnosis in many cases, particularly for acute diarrheal illnesses caused by *Campylobacter*, *Yersinia*, *Salmonella*, and *Shigella* species. Infection with *C. difficile*, the most common bacterial enteric pathogen in the United States for both HIV-infected and HIV-uninfected persons, is diagnosed in most settings by detection of cytotoxin in the stool by EIA or PCR, although the more laborious tissue culture is considered the gold standard. Enteric viruses are present in 15% to 30% of HIV-infected persons with acute diarrhea. Definitive diagnosis is not feasible in most clinical laboratories; viral enteritis should be suspected in the setting of community outbreaks, because of the high transmissibility of viral pathogens. Treatment is supportive with fluid resuscitation and antimotility agents.

Chronic diarrhea (duration >30 days) was a common manifestation of advanced-stage AIDS in the pre-HAART era and is still considered an AIDS-defining condition. Most pathogens that cause acute gastroenteritis can also cause chronic symptoms. Pathogens that should be suspected in cases of chronic watery diarrhea include protozoa such as *Cryptosporidium parvum*, *Isospora belli*, and *Microsporidia* spp. These entities are self-limited in the absence of severe immunosuppression. In advanced HIV, pathogen-specific antimicrobial therapy is infrequently effective, and symptoms commonly do not improve without immune reconstitution in response to ART. *Giardia lamblia* causes watery diarrhea, abdominal bloating, and occasionally malabsorption syndrome and can occur at any CD4 count. CMV infection can affect any segment of the gastrointestinal tract and is a common cause of chronic diarrhea. Diagnosis of gastrointestinal CMV disease is difficult without biopsy. Detection of CMV viremia with PCR does not correlate well with presence of CMV disease in HIV-infected patients, and CMV can be undetectable in serum in patients with extensive gastrointestinal disease.

Other Conditions

Mycobacterium avium and *Mycobacterium intracellulare* are closely related mycobacteria that are ubiquitous in the environment. They are discussed as a single pathologic entity and referred to as MAI or *Mycobacterium avium* complex (MAC). MAI is a common cause of chronic pulmonary disease in patients with structurally abnormal airways. In advanced HIV infection, it can cause a multiorgan system disease characterized by fever, night sweats, diarrhea, and abdominal pain. Infiltration of the bone marrow and liver may occur, leading to hematologic abnormalities and abnormal liver function tests, which can be a clue to the diagnosis. Biopsy of a lymph node or of bone marrow is sometimes necessary to diagnose disseminated MAI, but it is most often diagnosed by means of blood culture using specialized culture media.

Immune Reconstitution Inflammatory Syndrome

Recovery of cellular and humoral immune system function in response to ART is occasionally associated with severe symptoms resulting from inflammatory responses directed against opportunistic pathogens. Risk factors for this immune reconstitution inflammatory syndrome (IRIS) include a low nadir CD4 count, a high baseline VL, and PI-containing HAART regimens. Most cases of IRIS occur within the first 2 months after initiation of HAART, and onset can occur as early as within the first week. Disseminated MAI accounts for up to one third of the cases of IRIS in the United States. Other important causes of IRIS are tuberculosis, CMV infection, viral hepatitis, and candidal infections. It may be possible to decrease the risk of IRIS by delaying initiation of HAART by several weeks, until therapy for OIs has been instituted, but the risks of other complications of untreated AIDS often outweigh any potential benefit of this strategy. When it occurs, IRIS usually can be managed with nonsteroidal antiinflammatory drugs or corticosteroids. HAART should not be interrupted except in life-threatening illnesses.

Management of HIV in Pregnant Women

Periodically updated guidelines for the treatment of HIV in pregnancy are available on the U.S. Department of Health and Human Services AIDSinfo website (http://www.aidsinfo.nih.gov [accessed July 9, 2015]). Pregnancy is not known to have an effect on HIV progression. HIV progression has been shown to increase rates of preterm delivery and low birth weight in developing countries, but this link has not been established in resource-rich settings. All pregnant women should be offered HAART to reduce perinatal transmission and improve maternal health, regardless of CD4 count or VL. Guidelines for ART are otherwise similar for pregnant and nonpregnant patients, with the important exception that drugs with unacceptable or inadequately studied safety profiles should be avoided. Didanosine (Videx) and stavudine should be avoided. Earlier, efavirenz use during pregnancy was not recommended. Recent guidance, however, suggests that efavirenz can be continued safely in women already on efavirenz-based regimens, as long as the patient is virologically suppressed on that regimen. In fact, as of 2012, the British HIV association's guidelines no longer prohibit the use of efavirenz in pregnancy. If possible, preferred regimens should include zidovudine and lamivudine with lopinavir/ritonavir (Kaletra). Data suggest that nevirapine (Viramune) should be avoided in women who have CD4 counts higher than 250 cells/mm^3 at the time of initiation of therapy. This recommendation does not pertain to the practice of giving a single dose of nevirapine in the intrapartum period in resource-poor settings to prevent perinatal transmission. Elective cesarean should be offered at 38 weeks' gestation to women who are likely to have VLs greater than 1000 copies/mL at the time of delivery. After delivery, infants born to HIV-infected mothers who were not on antepartum ARVs should receive zidovudine for 6 weeks and 3 doses of nevirapine (at birth, at 48 hours, and 96 hours after the second dose).

Pre-exposure Prophylaxis (PrEP) of HIV Infection

Despite community and behavioral interventions, new HIV infections continue to occur, with the highest rates among MSM and Black/African men and women. In 2010, the iPrEx trial showed that daily oral tenofovir disoproxil fumarate 300 mg (TDF) with emtricitabine 200 mg (FTC) was both safe and efficacious in the prevention of incident HIV infections in MSM. Now, several trials have substantiated the findings of the iPREX trial in other high risk populations, including IVDUs and high-risk heterosexual people. The FDA approved TDF/FTC for the prevention of HIV infection among all adults in July 2012. The CDC has issued interim guidance for clinicians while formal guidelines are in process. Before initiating PrEP, a patient should (1) have a documented HIV-negative status; (2) have a substantial ongoing risk of becoming infected with HIV, either through sexual contact or IDU; (3) have a creatinine clearance of greater than 60 mL/min, and (4) have been screened and treated for other sexually transmitted infections (STI). Women of reproductive age requesting PrEP should also have a documented pregnancy test before initiating therapy. If a woman is pregnant or becomes pregnant while taking PrEP, providers should discuss the risks and benefits of continuing therapy. Providers are encouraged to anonymously submit outcome information to the ARV Use in Pregnancy Registry for women who choose to stay on PrEP while pregnant. Repeat HIV and STI testing should be done every 2 to 3 months in addition to renal function tests. No more than a 90-day supply of TDF/FTC should be provided at one time, although prescription renewals can be given if the above criteria remain fulfilled. As always, patients should be counseled on other mechanisms of risk reduction and adherence. Long-term safety and outcomes of HIV-negative adults and following fetal exposure remain unknown. Any serious adverse events that occur as a result of taking TDF/FTC for PrEP should be reported to the FDA's MedWatch (http://www.fda.safety/medwatch).

Postexposure Prophylaxis of HIV Infection

The scarcity of data describing occupationally acquired HIV infection makes it difficult to quantify the risk of transmission associated with exposure of health care workers to an HIV-infected source. Pooled data from multiple studies demonstrated HIV transmission in 20 health care workers out of more than 6000 workers who sustained a needlestick injury from an HIV-infected patient, yielding a transmission rate of 0.33%. HIV transmission due to mucosal exposure was even more uncommon (0.09%), and transmission from exposure of intact skin has not been described.

Despite poorly characterized risks and benefits, postexposure prophylaxis with ART is recommended for health care workers sustaining percutaneous, mucus membrane, or nonintact skin exposure to an HIV-infected source. HIV antibody testing of the worker should be done at the time of exposure and repeated at 6 weeks, 12 weeks, and 6 months after exposure. If given, prophylaxis should be administered as soon as possible, preferably within hours after the exposure. Recommended prophylactic regimens typically contain a two-drug combination of NRTIs; coformulations of zidovudine plus lamivudine (Combivir) and emtricitabine plus tenofovir (Truvada) are used extensively and have good tolerability. Three-drug HAART regimens including a PI are recommended for more severe exposures. The duration of postexposure prophylaxes is typically 4 weeks. The recommendations for prophylaxis have been expanded to include nonoccupational exposures such as unanticipated sexual or needle-sharing behavior.

References

Adult Prevention and Treatment of Opportunistic Infections Guidelines Working Group. Guidelines for prevention and treatment of opportunistic infections in HIV-infected adults and adolescents [draft], Available at http://aidsinfo.nih.gov/contentfiles/Adult_OI.pdf; [accessed July 9, 2015].

Branson B. Current HIV epidemiology and revised recommendations for HIV testing in health care settings. J Med Virol 2007;79(Suppl. 1):S6–10.

Centers for Disease Control and Prevention. Interim guidance for clinicians considering the use of preexposure prophylaxis for the prevention of HIV infection in heterosexually active adults. MMWR Morb Mortal Wkly Rep 2012;61:586–9.

Centers for Disease Control and Prevention. Interim guidance: preexposure prophylaxis for the prevention of HIV infection in men who have sex with men. MMWR Morb Mortal Wkly Rep 2011;60:65–8.

Hirsch MS. Initiating therapy: What to start, what to use. J Infect Dis 2008;197 (Suppl. 3):S252–S260.

Joint United Nations Programme on HIV/AIDS. UNAIDS World AIDS Day Report, Available at http://www.unaids.org/en/media/unaids/contentassets/documents/unaidspublication/2011/JC2216_WorldAIDSday_report_2011_en.pdf [Accessed August 15, 2012].

Landon BE, Wilson IB, McInnes K, et al. Physician specialization and the quality of care for human immunodeficiency virus infection. Arch Intern Med 2005;165(10):1133–9.

Panel on Antiretroviral Guidelines for Adults and Adolescents. Guidelines for the use of antiretroviral agents in HIV-1-infected adults and adolescents, Department of Health and Human Services; 2012. Available at: http://aidsinfo.nih.gov/Guidelines/HTML/1/adult-and-adolescent-treatment-guideline/0 [accessed August 15, 2012].

Thompson MA, Aberg JA, Hoy J, et al. Antiretroviral treatment of adult HIV infection: 2012 Recommendations of the International AIDS Society-USA Panel. JAMA 2012; 308:387–402.

INFECTIOUS MONONUCLEOSIS

Method of
Ben Z. Katz, MD

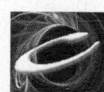

CURRENT DIAGNOSIS

- The classic triad of acute infectious mononucleosis consists of fever, lymphadenopathy, and pharyngitis.
- The diagnosis of infectious mononucleosis is usually based on the clinical picture, the presence of at least 10% atypical lymphocytes in the peripheral blood, and positive heterophil serology.

CURRENT THERAPY

- In most patients, infectious mononucleosis is self-limited and requires only symptomatic treatment.
- Steroids and antiviral therapy have no place in the therapy of uncomplicated acute infectious mononucleosis in healthy persons.

Epidemiology and Risk Factors

One must distinguish between the epidemiology of Epstein-Barr virus (EBV) infection and that of infectious mononucleosis (IM), the most common symptomatic manifestation of primary EBV infection. Almost all adults have been infected with EBV. The symptomatology of primary EBV infection varies with the infected person's age at the time, with younger children usually having inapparent or mild infections. In developing countries and in lower socioeconomic groups in industrialized nations, up to 90% of children acquire primary EBV infection by 6 years of age, and IM almost never develops. In contrast, in higher socioeconomic groups, only 40% to 50% of adolescents have previously experienced EBV infection. From 10% to 20% of susceptible adolescents and adults contract EBV every year thereafter, with IM developing in a significant fraction of these patients.

Pathophysiology

Saliva is the main vehicle for transmission of EBV, a double-stranded DNA herpesvirus. Transmission usually requires direct and prolonged contact with infected oropharyngeal secretions, with salivary exchange being the main mode of transmission. The infection begins with viral replication in oropharyngeal epithelial cells and then spreads to local B lymphocytes, which then disseminate throughout the reticuloendothelial system and induce vigorous T- and NK-cell responses and neutralizing antibodies. The atypical lymphocytes that are produced are mainly suppressor T cells directed against EBV-infected B cells.

It is thought that most of the clinical manifestations of IM are due to these T- and NK-cell responses, which might explain why young children, whose immune responses are incompletely developed, are usually asymptomatic with primary EBV infection. All EBV-seropositive persons shed virus intermittently throughout their lives. EBV may rarely be spread via blood transfusion or transplantation.

Clinical Manifestations

IM is usually an acute, self-limited, benign lymphoproliferative disease. EBV is responsible for nearly all heterophil-positive and most heterophil-negative cases. Other causes of heterophil-negative mononucleosis include cytomegalovirus, toxoplasmosis, hepatitis A and B, adenovirus, HIV, rubella, and human herpesvirus 6.

The classic triad of IM consists of fever, lymphadenopathy, and pharyngitis. Other typical findings include lymphocytosis with atypical lymphocytes and the presence of heterophil antibodies. After a 4- to 6-week incubation period, the illness begins with a 3- to 5-day prodrome of malaise, headache, and fatigue, typically followed in about half of all cases by onset of the triad. Additional symptoms can include anorexia, nausea, vomiting, periorbital or facial edema, and generalized lymphadenopathy, which is usually symmetrical. Splenomegaly occurs by the second or third week of illness in about half of all cases; rarely, splenic rupture can occur and may be fatal. Hepatomegaly occurs in 10% to 15%, with hepatitis occurring in about 5% of cases. Up to 20% of patients have a rash that may be erythematous, maculopapular, morbilliform, scarlatiniform, or urticarial, especially if ampicillin or one of its derivatives has been given. Other symptoms can include arthritis and jaundice.

IM is a self-limited disease in nearly all patients. Median illness duration is 16 days.

Diagnosis

The diagnosis is usually based on the clinical picture, atypical lymphocytosis, and positive heterophil serology. Most adolescents and young adults with IM have most or all of these features, as well as an abnormal white blood cell count with a relative lymphocytosis. Atypical lymphocytes generally represent more than 9% to 10% of the white blood cell count. Many infected persons also have mild thrombocytopenia and elevated hepatocellular enzymes. Heterophil antibody positivity is usually measured as a positive monospot test. If IM is suspected and heterophil antibodies are negative, specific titers for EBV, including viral capsid antigen (VCA), early antigen (EA), and Epstein–Barr nuclear antigen (EBNA), should be obtained, as well as serologic testing for cytomegalovirus (CMV) and toxoplasmosis. Acute EBV infection is characterized by the presence of IgM and IgG VCA antibodies and EA antibodies and the absence of EBNA antibodies.

Differential Diagnosis

If liver chemistries are markedly elevated and antibodies against EBV, CMV, and toxoplasmosis are unrevealing, serology for hepatitis A, B, and C should be measured. If risk factors are present, HIV antibodies should be checked. A throat culture is indicated in patients with pharyngitis or tonsillitis because the tonsillitis of acute IM can be indistinguishable from that of group A streptococcal pharyngitis.

Treatment

In most patients, IM is self-limited and requires only symptomatic treatment, including bed rest, acetaminophen (Tylenol, 10–15 mg/kg every 4–6 hours), aspirin (10–15 mg/kg every 4–6 hours), or nonsteroidal antiinflammatory agents such as ibuprofen (Advil, 5–10 mg/kg every 6–8 hours). Saline gargles can be useful in treating a sore throat. In severe cases, meperidine (Demerol, 1–1.5 mg/kg every 3–4 hours) may be required.

Although a short, tapering course of corticosteroid therapy (e.g., 2 mg/kg of prednisone[1] for 5 days, 1 mg/kg for 5 days, and then 0.5 mg/kg for 5 days) is often prescribed, there is little evidence for its clinical efficacy, and caution is warranted. Infection is ultimately self-limited in nearly all cases, and rare reports of neurologic or septicemic complications after steroid use have

appeared. Long-term immune responses following steroid use appear to be normal. Corticosteroid therapy should, however, be considered for the treatment of severe cases of IM associated with hemolysis, respiratory embarrassment, or thrombocytopenic purpura. The use of corticosteroids in atypical or antibody-negative cases is inappropriate because the diagnosis of lymphoma can then be confounded.

Parenteral administration of acyclovir[1] (Zovirax, 10–20 mg/kg IV every 8 hours) to patients with acute IM secondary to EBV reduces the level of oropharyngeal viral replication; however, replication returns to the previously high levels after cessation of treatment, little or no reduction is seen in the number of EBV-infected B cells in the peripheral circulation, and the drug has little or no effect on the clinical course. Acyclovir administered in high doses orally[1] (20 mg/kg, maximum dose of 800 mg qid for 5 days) is also ineffective. Antiviral therapy is therefore not recommended for acute IM in a normal host.

In immunosuppressed or severely ill patients, however, specific therapy has a role in many cases. For example, etoposide (VePesid),[1] a drug that reduces macrophage activation, is often used in cases of infection-associated hemophagocytic syndrome. In posttransplant lymphoproliferative disorders, first-line therapy is often a reduction in immunosuppression; other options include rituximab[1] (Rituxan, 375 mg/m^2 IV weekly for 4 weeks). Oral leukoplakia in patients with AIDS responds to oral acyclovir[1] (20 mg/kg, maximum dose of 800 mg qid for 20 days), whereas a tapering course of steroids (as recommended earlier) may be used for lymphocytic interstitial pneumonitis (see below).

Monitoring

Quarantine is not indicated. Ampicillin and related drugs should be avoided when treating secondary bacterial complications because of their association with rash in persons with IM. Contact sports should be avoided as long as splenomegaly is still evident because of the rare possibility of splenic rupture, which usually occurs within 3 weeks of onset of IM but has been reported as late as 7 weeks into the illness.

Complications

Complications of acute IM can be neurologic (seizures, cranial nerve palsies, aseptic meningitis, encephalitis, optic neuritis, transverse myelitis, infectious polyneuritis [Guillain-Barré syndrome], psychosis, Alice in Wonderland syndrome, or acute cerebellar ataxia), hematologic (hemolytic or aplastic anemia, thrombocytopenic purpura, agranulocytosis, or agammaglobulinemia), cardiac (pericarditis or myocarditis), pulmonary (cough or atypical pneumonia), renal (glomerulonephritis, acute kidney failure, or acute interstitial nephritis), or ophthalmologic (conjunctivitis) in nature. In about 10% of adolescents and young adults, fatigue can persist for 6 months or longer, and many of these patients meet the criteria for chronic fatigue syndrome.

Rare patients have very high titers of EBV antibodies, and a chronic active EBV infection associated with unusual clinical manifestations such as uveitis or lymphoma can occur. EBV is also associated with lymphoproliferative disorders in persons with underlying abnormal immune responses. These include X-linked lymphoproliferative syndrome, in which affected males usually die of acute EBV infection, and the related infection-associated hemophagocytic syndrome, which is most commonly (about 75% of the time) triggered by EBV and seems to be due to an overly exuberant macrophage response to EBV-infected lymphocytes. Transplant recipients can acquire EBV-associated lymphoproliferative disease that can range from an asymptomatic infection to fatal IM or lymphoma. Patients with AIDS are susceptible to several serious complications of EBV infection, including lymphocytic interstitial pneumonitis, oral leukoplakia, leiomyosarcoma, and lymphoma.

---

[1]Not FDA approved for this indication.

[1]Not FDA approved for this indication.

References

Candy B, Hotopf M. Steroids for symptom control in infectious mononucleosis. Cochrane Database Syst Rev 2006;(3): CD004402.

Cohen JI, Jaffe ES, Dale JK, et al. Characterization and treatment of chronic active Epstein–Barr virus disease: A 28-year experience in the United States. Blood 2011;117:5835–49.

Katz BZ. Commentary on "Steroids for symptom control in infectious mononucleosis (Review)" by B Candy and M Hotopf. Evid Based Child Health 2012;7:447–9.

Katz BZ, Shiraishi Y, Mears CJ, et al. Chronic fatigue syndrome following infectious mononucleosis in adolescents. Pediatrics 2009;124:189–93.

Odumade OA, Hogquist KA, Balfour Jr HH. Progress and problems in understanding and managing primary Epstein-Barr virus infections. Clin Microbiol Rev 2011;24(1):193–209.

Rouphael N, Talati NJ, Vaughan C, et al. Infections associated with haemophagocytic syndrome. Lancet Infect Dis 2007;7:814–22.

Soltys K, Green M. Posttransplant lymphoproliferative disease. Pediatr Infect Dis J 2005;24:1107–8.

INFLUENZA

Method of
Jeffrey A. Linder, MD, MPH, FACP

CURRENT DIAGNOSIS

- Influenza should be considered in any patient with respiratory symptoms between October and May in North America.
- The single most important piece of information when considering a diagnosis of influenza is the community prevalence of influenza.
- During outbreaks, sudden onset of fever and cough has a positive predictive value of about 85%.
- Rapid testing should be used when the community prevalence of influenza among patients with influenza-like illness is between 10% and 30%.

CURRENT THERAPY

- The influenza vaccine is the best means of preventing influenza. The inactivated influenza vaccine is recommended for all persons age 6 months and older.
- The antivirals zanamivir (Relenza) and oseltamivir (Tamiflu) can be used for prophylaxis of influenza in unimmunized patients, in close contacts of infected patients, and during institutional outbreaks of influenza.
- Early antiviral treatment should be used for patients who are hospitalized; have severe, complicated, or progressive illness; or are at higher risk for complications.
- Antivirals may be prescribed within 48 hours of symptom onset for outpatients not at higher risk for influenza complications.

Influenza is a highly contagious viral infection that should be considered in any patient with respiratory symptoms between October and May in North America. Influenza infects 5% to 20% of the population of the United States in a typical year, and is responsible for up to 431,000 hospitalizations and 51,000 deaths per year. Influenza can range in severity from mild illness to life-threatening disease. Those at highest risk of hospitalization, death, or complications from influenza are children younger than 5 years, adults older than 65 years, people of any age who have underlying medical conditions, those infected with HIV, and pregnant women.

Information about influenza changes rapidly. To care optimally for patients with influenza-like illness during the influenza season, clinicians need to keep abreast of updated recommendations and the current prevalence of influenza in their community. The

---

| Box 1 | Influenza Vaccine Recommendations |

- All persons aged ≥6 months should be vaccinated annually
- Vaccination efforts should prioritize people at higher risk of influenza complications:
  - 6 months to 5 years old, especially 6 months to 2 years old
  - ≥50 years old, especially ≥65 years old
  - Chronic pulmonary (including asthma), cardiovascular (except hypertension), renal, hepatic, neurologic, neurodevelopmental, hematologic, or metabolic (including diabetes mellitus) disorders
  - Immunosuppressed
  - Pregnant during the influenza season
  - 6 months to 18 years old receiving long-term aspirin therapy and who therefore might be at risk for Reye syndrome
  - Residents of nursing homes and other chronic-care facilities
  - American Indians/Alaska Natives
  - Morbidly obese (body mass index ≥40)
- Vaccination efforts should also prioritize those likely to transmit influenza to higher risk people:
  - Health care personnel
  - Household contacts and caregivers of children aged <5 years and adults aged ≥50 years, with particular emphasis on vaccinating contacts of children aged <6 months
  - Household contacts and caregivers of persons with medical conditions that put them at higher risk for severe complications from influenza

---

influenza vaccine remains the best means of reducing the incidence, severity, and complications from influenza, but antiviral medications and symptomatic treatments have an important role in the prevention and treatment of influenza (Box 1).

Microbiology

There are two types of influenza viruses, A and B. Influenza A is separated into subtypes based on two surface antigens: hemagglutinin (H) and neuraminidase (N). The predominant circulating strains of influenza in recent decades have been influenza A (H1N1), influenza A (H3N2), and influenza B. Influenza A (H3N2) subtypes generally cause more severe influenza and are associated with higher mortality than other types. Influenza viruses undergo slight genetic changes from year to year, termed *antigenic drift*. Major changes in surface glycoproteins are termed *antigenic shift* and can result in severe pandemic influenza in a nonimmune population, which happened with an antigenically novel influenza A (H1N1) virus in 2009. Because of antigenic drift, and because immunity to a given type or subtype of influenza provides limited cross-immunity to other types and subtypes, the influenza vaccine needs to be reformulated and administered most years.

Patients contract influenza by being exposed to large-sized respiratory droplets from an infected person or contact with surfaces harboring influenza virus. Influenza has a latency of 1 to 4 days before the onset of symptoms. Adults are infectious from the day before symptom onset through about day 7 of illness, but immunosuppressed adults and children shed the virus for longer periods. Symptoms generally last from 7 to 14 days.

Several novel, highly-pathogenic respiratory viruses—avian influenza A (H5N1), avian influenza A (H7N9), and Middle East Respiratory Syndrome Coronavirus (MERS-CoV)—have mortality rates ranging from 30% to 60%. Collectively there have been more than 2200 cases. These pathogens, if they acquire the ability to be highly transmissible between humans, have the potential to cause pandemic respiratory disease.

Prevention

Influenza vaccination is between 20% and 90% effective in preventing influenza or complications of influenza. Influenza vaccination is highly cost-effective and can even be cost-saving in high-risk groups. Influenza vaccination is less effective in younger children, in adults older than 65 years, in adults with comorbid conditions, and when there is a poor match between the influenza vaccine and circulating influenza. The Centers for Disease Control and Prevention's (CDC) Advisory Committee on Immunization Practices (ACIP) puts out annual recommendations and supplementary updates on the prevention and treatment of influenza (www.cdc.gov/flu). Beginning in the 2010 to 2011 influenza season, the ACIP recommended vaccinating all persons 6 months old and older.

At present there are three commonly-administered types of influenza vaccine: trivalent inactivated influenza vaccine (IIV3), quadrivalent inactivated influenza vaccine (IIV4), and quadrivalent live attenuated influenza vaccine (LAIV4).

The IIV4 (Fluarix Quadrivalent, FluLaval Quadrivalent, Fluzone Quadrivalent) and IIV3 (Afluria, Fluarix, Flucelvax, FluLaval, Fluvirin, Fluzone) are administered as an intramuscular injection. Different products are approved for administration in different lower age limits. In particular, Afluria should not be administered to children younger than 9 years old because of an increased risk of febrile seizures. A high-dose IIV3 (Fluzone High-Dose) is available for patients aged 65 years and older, who are less likely to respond immunologically to the traditional dose of inactivated influenza vaccine (IIV). An intradermal IIV3 (Fluzone Intradermal) is available for use in patients 18 to 64 years old. The main adverse effect of the IIV is soreness at the injection site. Patients often report a mild immune response of fever, malaise, myalgia, and headache that can last for 1 to 2 days, but rates of most of these symptoms are no different from those in patients who receive placebo injection. Allergic reactions to egg proteins or other vaccine components (e.g., antibiotics and inactivating compounds) include hives, angioedema, asthma, and anaphylaxis. For patients with egg allergy who have only hives, IIV can be administered, but patients should be observed for 30 minutes by providers familiar with manifestations of egg allergy. Patients aged 18 to 49 years with more severe reactions to egg can receive the recombinant influenza vaccine (RIV3; FluBlok), or cell culture-based IIV (ccIIV3; Flucelvax), which are manufactured without the use of eggs. Vaccination should be deferred in patients with acute febrile illness, but patients with more moderate illness can be vaccinated. Guillain-Barré syndrome was associated with the 1976 swine flu vaccine, but there is no consistent evidence that modern influenza vaccines are associated with Guillain-Barré syndrome.

The LAIV4 (FluMist Quadrivalent) is administered as a nasal spray, is approved for patients ages 2 to 49 years, and preferred to the IIV for use in children aged 2 to 8 years. The LAIV4 is contraindicated in children aged 2 to 4 years with recurrent wheezing or asthma; children who are receiving aspirin or aspirin-containing products; in patients with comorbid conditions or egg allergy; in pregnant women; and in family members or close contacts of severely immunosuppressed patients, who require a protected environment (e.g., hematopoietic stem cell transplant recipients). The LAIV4 should not be administered to those with severe nasal congestion. Adverse effects of the LAIV4 include runny nose, nasal congestion, headache, sore throat, chills, and tiredness, although these are only slightly more common than in patients receiving placebo. Those receiving the LAIV4 should avoid contact with severely immunosuppressed persons for 7 days.

Patients should be vaccinated in the fall when the seasonal vaccine becomes available, even as early as August. In the event of vaccine shortages, higher-risk patients should receive priority. Patients should continue to be vaccinated until February and beyond because in the majority of recent influenza seasons the peak has been February or later. Children 6 months to 8 years of age, who have not been previously immunized against influenza, should be given two doses separated by at least 4 weeks.

Evaluation

Community Prevalence of Influenza

In caring for a patient with suspected influenza, the single most important piece of data is the community prevalence of influenza among patients with influenza-like illness. This ranges from near 0% during summer months to about 30% during a typical influenza seasonal peak. The prevalence may be higher during a particularly severe outbreak. Clinicians can check the local prevalence of influenza among patients with influenza-like illness through the CDC (www.cdc.gov/flu) and their state department of public health.

History and Physical Examination

Beyond the local prevalence of influenza, the diagnosis of influenza rests on the patient's history. All methods of diagnosing influenza—symptom complexes, clinician judgment, and testing—generally are highly specific, but have poor sensitivity. Thus it is important to consider a diagnosis of influenza in any patient with respiratory symptoms during influenza season. Influenza is classically described as the very sudden onset of fever, headache, sore throat, myalgias, cough, and nasal symptoms. Children can also have otitis media, nausea, and vomiting. In differentiating influenza from nonspecific upper respiratory tract infections, it is most useful to consider the circulating prevalence of influenza, the abruptness of onset, and the severity of symptoms.

Certain symptom complexes have been shown in trials of antiviral treatment to strongly suggest influenza. For example, in an area with circulating influenza, the acute onset of cough and fever can have a positive predictive value as high as 85%. One rule assigned 2 points for fever plus cough, 2 points for myalgias, 1 point for duration less than 48 hours, and 1 point for chills or sweats. The prevalence of influenza for patients with 0 to 2 points, 3 points, or 4 to 6 points was 8%, 30%, and 59%, respectively. Other studies have shown that clinician judgment performed as well as or better than hard-and-fast symptom complexes or rapid testing.

The physical examination in influenza primarily serves to identify the severity of influenza, complications, and worsening of underlying medical conditions. Clinicians should record vital signs and perform examinations of the ears, nose, sinuses, throat, neck, lungs, and heart for all patients suspected of having influenza.

Testing

Rapid influenza diagnostic test kits, some of which can distinguish influenza A from influenza B, can provide a point-of-care result in about 15 minutes. Specimens (nasopharyngeal swab, nasal swab, nasal wash, or nasal aspirate, depending on the particular test) should ideally be collected within 3 days of symptom onset. Rapid tests have sensitivities that range from 50% to 70%, but are more than 90% specific. Testing is most useful when there is an intermediate probability of influenza (e.g., a community prevalence of influenza among patients with influenza-like illness of 10% to 30%), and patients have an intermediate probability of complications from influenza. If circulating prevalence of influenza is low (e.g., <10%), testing is unlikely to be positive and is not necessary. If the circulating prevalence of influenza is high (e.g., >30%), the relatively low sensitivity of rapid tests makes the risk of a false-negative test unacceptably high. In the event of a high prevalence of influenza or a high risk of complications from influenza, empiric antiviral treatment is indicated. Testing may be particularly helpful for hospitalized patients to rule out a need for antibiotics, but given the low sensitivities anti-influenza treatment should not be withheld based solely on a negative rapid influenza detection test.

Reverse transcriptase polymerase chain reaction (RT-PCR) testing and viral culture have higher sensitivities than rapid influenza diagnostic tests. RT-PCR should be considered for hospitalized patients, institutional outbreaks, or other situations when clinicians are concerned about false-negative rapid test results. RT-PCR assays return results in under 8 hours. Availability of

RT-PCR in recent years has expanded. Some RT-PCR assays can detect influenza type and subtypes. Other nucleic acid amplification tests, which can differentiate influenza from other respiratory pathogens, are becoming more available.

Chest radiography, cultures, and blood tests are not routinely indicated, but they should be obtained for patients with suspected pneumonia or to identify other suspected complications.

Complications

Complications of influenza include primary complications, suppurative complications, and worsening of comorbid conditions. Primary complications of influenza include viral pneumonia, which is a feared complication and is likely a main cause of mortality in pandemic influenza. Other, less common primary complications of influenza include myositis and rhabdomyolysis, Reye syndrome, myocarditis, pericarditis, toxic shock syndrome, and central nervous system disease (e.g., encephalitis, transverse myelitis, and aseptic meningitis). Children can have a severe course with influenza, including signs and symptoms of sepsis along with febrile seizures. Suppurative complications of influenza include bacterial pneumonia, otitis media, and sinusitis. Influenza can cause worsening of comorbid conditions such as asthma, chronic obstructive pulmonary disease, congestive heart failure, and chronic kidney disease.

Chemoprophylaxis

Antiviral medications can be used to prevent influenza in patients who did not receive the influenza vaccine, cannot receive the influenza vaccine, received the vaccine in the prior 2 weeks (before reliable immunity develops), or in the event of poor matching between vaccine and circulating influenza strains (Table 1). Chemoprophylaxis should also be considered for close contacts of patients with confirmed influenza or for patients with immune deficiency who are unlikely to respond to the influenza vaccine but who are at high risk for having complications from influenza.

Amantadine (Symmetrel) and rimantadine (Flumadine) are not recommended for chemoprophylaxis or treatment because of a high prevalence of resistant influenza A strains. The neuraminidase inhibitors oseltamivir (Tamiflu), and zanamivir (Relenza) are about 80% effective in preventing influenza in household contacts of persons with influenza, and more than 90% effective in preventing influenza in institutional settings. Chemoprophylaxis should be taken for 10 days after a household exposure, 7 days after a nonhousehold exposure, and for a minimum of 2 weeks or until 1 week after the end of long-term care facility or hospital outbreak. For patients allergic to or unable to respond to the vaccine, chemoprophylaxis should be used for the duration of circulating influenza. The IIV can be given to patients receiving chemoprophylaxis. The LAIV should not be given from 2 days before to 14 days after taking an antiviral medication. Patients who receive the LAIV in this window should be revaccinated at a later date.

Treatment

The influenza vaccine is the best means of reducing influenza-related morbidity and mortality, but its limitations include production problems, low vaccination rates, and the variable effectiveness of the vaccine itself. Given these limitations, there is an important role in management for influenza-specific antiviral medications (see Table 1). Antiviral medications reduce the duration of influenza symptoms by about 1 day, reduce complications requiring antibiotics by 30% to 50%, might decrease hospitalizations and mortality, and are cost-effective. Early antiviral treatment starting up to 5 days after symptom onset can reduce complications for patients who are hospitalized; have severe, complicated, or progressive illness; or are at higher risk for complications (see Box 1). For outpatients not at higher risk for complications, antiviral treatment must be started within 48 hours of symptom onset.

Amantadine and rimantadine are not recommended for the treatment of influenza because of a high prevalence of resistant influenza A strains. Zanamivir is taken as an oral inhaled powder and is not recommended for patients with underlying lung or heart disease. Adverse effects of zanamivir include worsening of underlying lung disease and allergic reactions. Oseltamivir is taken as a

ANTIVIRAL AGENT	TREATMENT*		PROPHYLAXIS†		COMMENTS
	CHILDREN	ADULTS	CHILDREN	ADULTS	
Oseltamivir (Tamiflu)	Any age‡ Dose for 5 days bid: <1 yr: 3 mg/kg per dose; <15 kg: 30 mg; 16–23 kg: 45 mg; 24–40 kg: 60 mg; >40 kg: 75 mg	75 mg PO bid for 5 days	Children ≥3 mo‡ Dose qd: ≤15 kg: 30 mg; 16–23 kg: 45 mg; 24–40 kg: 60 mg; >40 kg: 75 mg	75 mg PO qd	For patients with creatinine clearance <30 mL/min, oseltamivir adult dosing should be reduced to 30 mg qd for treatment and to 30 mg qid for prophylaxis
Zanamivir (Relenza)	Approved for children ≥7 yr; 10 mg (2 inhalations) bid for 5 days	10 mg (2 inhalations) bid for 5 days	Approved for children ≥5 yr; 10 mg (2 inhalations) qid	10 mg (2 inhalations) qd	Avoid in patients with chronic lung disease (e.g., asthma, COPD)
Peramivir (Rapivab)	NA§	600 mg IV × 1 over 15 to 30 min	NA§	NA§	For patients with creatinine clearance 30–49 mL/min, the dose should be reduced to 200 mg; For patients with creatinine clearance 10–29 mL/min, the dose should be reduced to 100 mg

TABLE 1 Antiviral Agents for the Treatment and Prophylaxis of Influenza

Adapted from Centers for Disease Control and Prevention. Influenza Antiviral Medications: Summary for Clinicians. Available at http://www.cdc.gov/flu/professionals/antivirals/ [accessed February 4, 2015].

*Suspected or confirmed influenza among persons with severe influenza or for persons at higher risk for influenza complications up to 5 days after symptom onset. For outpatients not at higher risk for influenza complications, treatment should be started within 48 hours of symptom onset.

†Prophylaxis should be given 10 days for household exposure, 7 days for other exposures and for outbreaks, at least 2 weeks or until 1 week after the end of the outbreak.

‡Oseltamivir is approved by the FDA for treatment in children 14 days and older and prophylaxis in children 1 year and older. Treatment in children <14 days old and prophylaxis in children <1 year old is recommended by the Centers for Disease Control and Prevention and the American Academy of Pediatrics.

§NA = not approved.

capsule or oral suspension. The dose of oseltamivir should be reduced in patients with renal disease. Adverse effects of oseltamivir include nausea, vomiting, and, perhaps behavioral changes.

Peramivir (Rapivab), an intravenous neuraminidase inhibitor, was approved in the United State in December 2014 for patients within 48 hours of symptom onset. Peramivir has been associated with diarrhea, rashes including Stevens-Johnson syndrome, and neuropsychiatric changes.

Antibiotics are generally not necessary, but they should be prescribed to treat suppurative complications of influenza. Antitussives such as guaifenesin with codeine (Robitussin AC) help coughing patients sleep at night. Beta-agonists, such as albuterol (Proventil),[1] can help patients with cough, especially if there is wheezing on examination. Analgesics and antipyretics like acetaminophen (Tylenol) and ibuprofen (Motrin) reduce fever and generally help patients feel better. Patients should be encouraged to rest and drink plenty of fluids.

Patients with suspected influenza should minimize contact with others to avoid spreading the infection. Use of face masks and hand hygiene can reduce the transmission of influenza.

---

[1]Not FDA approved for this indication.

References

Centers for Disease Control and Prevention. Influenza (Flu): information for health professionals. http://www.cdc.gov/flu/professionals/index.htm [accessed 20.11.14].

Ebell MH, Afonso AM, Gonzales R, et al. Development and validation of a clinical decision rule for the diagnosis of influenza. J Am Board Fam Med 2012;25:55–62.

Falsey AR, Murata Y, Walsh EE. Impact of rapid diagnosis on management of adults hospitalized with influenza. Arch Intern Med 2007;167:354–60.

Grohskopf LA, Olsen SJ, Sokolow LZ, Bresee JS, et al. Centers for Disease Control and Prevention. Prevention and control of seasonal influenza with vaccines: recommendations of the Advisory Committee on Immunization Practices (ACIP)—United States, 2014–2015 influenza season. MMWR Morb Mortal Wkly Rep 2014;63:691–7.

Rothberg MB, Bellantonio S, Rose DN. Management of influenza in adults older than 65 years of age: Cost-effectiveness of rapid testing and antiviral therapy. *Ann Intern Med* 2003;139:321–9.

LEISHMANIASIS

Method of
Luigi Gradoni, PhD

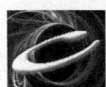

CURRENT DIAGNOSIS

- Infected tissues must be sampled for microscopy demonstration of *Leishmania* organisms in Giemsa-stained impression smears or cultures. Polymerase chain reaction (PCR) detection of *Leishmania* DNA increases diagnostic sensitivity.
- Different tissue samplings are performed depending on the clinical form of leishmaniasis: For visceral leishmaniasis, aspirate or biopsy specimens are obtained from spleen, bone marrow, the liver, or enlarged lymph nodes. For cutaneous and mucocutaneous leishmaniasis the material is obtained by skin lesion scraping or biopsy.
- Serology is useful when the diagnosis of visceral leishmaniasis proves difficult with other methods.

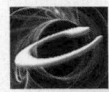

CURRENT THERAPY

- The therapy of leishmaniasis relies on a limited number of drugs, most of which are old and relatively toxic. Systemic drug administration requires hospitalization and monitoring of the patient.

- The pentavalent antimony (Sb) drugs sodium stibogluconate (Pentostam)[10] and meglumine antimoniate (Glucantime)[2] are equivalent and used in all clinical forms of leishmaniasis. Dosage is Sb 20 mg/kg/day IM for 21 to 28 days. In cases of uncomplicated cutaneous leishmaniasis, use intralesional administration intermittently over 20 to 30 days.
- Liposomal amphotericin B (Ambisome) is the gold standard for treating visceral leishmaniasis. Dosage: Total dose of 18 to 21 mg/kg IV using one of the following schedules: 3 mg/kg/day on days 1 to 5 and 10; 3 mg/kg on days 1 to 5, day 14, and day 21; 10 mg/kg/day for 2 days.
- Amphotericin B desoxycholate (Fungizone) is used in visceral leishmanaisis[1] and mucocutaneous leishmaniasis. Dosage is 0.5 mg/kg IV every other day for 14 days.
- Other parenteral drugs: Pentamidine isethionate (Pentam 300)[1] is used to treat some forms of New World cutaneous leishmaniasis; dosage is 2 mg/kg IM every other day for 7 days. Paromomycin (aminosidine) sulfate[2] is used for Indian visceral leishmanaisis; dosage is 11 mg/kg/day IM for 21 days.
- Miltefosine (Impavido)[5] is recommended for visceral leishmaniasis therapy in India and Ethiopia and for cutaneous leishmaniasis therapy in Colombia and Bolivia. Dosage is 2.5 mg/kg/day (not exceeding 100 mg/day) PO for 28 days.

---

[1]Not FDA approved for this indication.
[2]Not available in the United States.
[5]Investigational drug in the United States.
[10]Available in the United States from the Centers for Disease Control and Prevention.

Epidemiology

Leishmaniases are diseases caused by members of the genus *Leishmania*, protozoan parasites infecting numerous mammal species, including humans. The flagellated forms (promastigotes) are transmitted by the bite of phlebotomine sand flies and multiply as aflagellated forms (amastigotes) within cells of the mononuclear phagocyte system. The diseases range over the intertropical zones of America and Africa and extend into temperate regions of Latin America, Southern Europe, and Asia. About 20 named *Leishmania* species and subspecies are pathogenic for humans, and 30 sand fly species are proven vectors. Each parasite species circulates in natural foci of infection where susceptible phlebotomines and mammals coexist. The epidemiology and clinical manifestations of the diseases are largely diverse, being usually grouped into two main entities: zoonotic leishmaniases, where domestic or wild animal reservoirs are involved in the transmission cycle and humans play a role of an accidental host, and anthroponotic leishmaniases, where humans are the sole reservoir and source of the vector's infection.

Visceral leishmaniasis (VL) is caused by *Leishmania donovani* in the Indian subcontinent and East Africa (anthroponotic entity) and by *L. infantum (L. chagasi)* in the Mediterranan basin, parts of Central Asia, and Latin America (a zoonotic entity with domestic dogs acting as the main reservoir host). Several species of *Leishmania* cause cutaneous leishmaniasis (CL) or mucocutaneous (MCL) leishmaniasis. The most common are *L. major* (rural zoonotic entity) and *L. tropica* (urban anthroponotic entity) in the Old World and *L. mexicana, L. braziliensis, L. amazonensis, L. panamensis, L. guyanensis,* and *L. peruviana* (sylvatic zoonotic entities) in the New World.

Globally, 66 Old World and 22 New World countries are endemic for human leishmaniasis, with an estimated yearly incidence of 1 million to 1.5 million cases of CL forms and 500,000 cases of VL forms. Overall estimated prevalence is 12 million people with a disability-adjusted life years burden of 860,000 for men and 1.2 million for women. The disease affects the poorest people in the poorest countries: 72 are developing countries, of which 13 are among the least developed. The incidence is not uniformly distributed in endemic areas: 90% of CL cases are found in only seven countries (Afghanistan, Algeria, Brazil, Iran, Peru, Saudi Arabia, and Syria), whereas 90% of VL cases occur in rural and suburban areas of five countries (Bangladesh, India, Nepal, Sudan, and Brazil). These figures, however, must be regarded as underestimates; currently, it appears that the global incidence of human leishmaniases is higher than before, owing to environmental and human behavioral factors contributing to the changing landscape of these diseases.

Risk Factors

Risk factors for leishmaniasis are primarily associated with geographically and temporally defined human exposure to phlebotomine vectors. In the Old World, colonization and urbanization of desert areas have been identified as the major risk factor for outbreaks of zoonotic CL. Tourists and military personnel are often exposed to *L. major* or *L. tropica* infections in rural or urban endemic settings of North African and Middle Eastern countries. In the New World, the colonization of the primary forest associated with activities of deforestation, road building, mining, and tourism is responsible for the domestication of sylvatic cycles of CL and MCL agents. Increase in density and geographic range of phlebotomine vectors resulting from climate changes, together with the increased mobility of infected pet dogs, has been identified as a cause of northward spreading of zoonotic VL in Europe.

Individual risk factors play a major role in VL disease. Most of the *L. donovani* and *L. infantum* infections are asymptomatic or subclinical in well-nourished immunocompetent persons. Malnourished persons, infants younger than 2 years, and severely immunosuppressed adults are at high risk for acute VL when exposed to infection. Before the era of HAART (highly active antiretroviral therapy), the AIDS epidemics in southern Europe caused more than 2000 HIV and VL co-infection cases among men aged 39 years on average. Other conditions have been reported that influence the clinical outcome of VL, such as immunosuppressive therapies following organ transplantation, corticosteroid and anti–tumor necrosis factor α (TNF-α) treatments for immunologic disorders, hematologic neoplasia, and chronic conditions of hepatic cirrhosis. However, most acute VL episodes in adults remain unexplained. Other factors associated with impaired immune response to *Leishmania* (e.g., genetic factors) are probably involved.

Pathophysiology

Ingestion of metacyclic promastigotes inoculated by the vector in the skin is mediated by several types of receptors found in resident macrophages, monocytes, neutrophils, and dendritic cells. *Leishmania* lipophosphoglycan, the most abundant surface glycoconjugate, is the main factor of virulence. Once in the cell phagolysosome, amastigotes survive from hydrolase activity through pH acidification while selectively inhibiting production of reactive oxygen species. Multiplication of parasites, infection of new cells, and dissemination to tissues are contrasted by the host's inflammatory and specific immune responses. Even in most susceptible natural mammal hosts, the majority of infections are efficiently controlled, giving rise to asymptomatic latent infections. Leishmaniases have typical immunological polarity: Cure or control are associated with robust cellular immune responses driven by production of interleukin (IL) 12, whereas acute or chronic diseases are characterized by the absence of such responses and the presence of high levels of nonprotective serum antibodies, a condition often associated with high levels of IL-10 production. In spite of this polarity, analysis of cytokine patterns in tissues reveals a less-polar situation, as both T_H1 and T_H2 cytokines were found to be secreted in specimens from tissues infected with CL, MCL, and VL.

Prevention

There are no human vaccines available for the immune protection against leishmaniasis. Promising data on safety and immunogenicity have been provided for the only *Leishmania* candidate vaccine under development, consisting of the recombinant polyprotein antigen LEISH-F1 with MPL-SE as adjuvant. Preventive measures are thus limited to the individual protection from sand fly bites or to community protection through reservoir control. Individual protection is through the use of repellents or insecticide-impregnated nets. Reservoir control measures are largely diverse, depending on the epidemiologic entity of leishmaniasis. Examples related to zoonotic entities with synanthropic reservoir hosts are the destruction of rodent populations around human dwellings (e.g., to control zoonotic CL due to *L. major*) and the fight against canine infections through the mass use of topical insecticides or drug treatments (e.g., to control zoonotic VL due to *L. infantum*). Early diagnosis and treatment of human cases is the main control measure against anthroponotic entities of VL (*L. donovani*) and CL (*L. tropica*).

Clinical Manifestations
Visceral Disease

VL, also known as kala-azar, results from the multiplication of *Leishmania* in the phagocytes of the reticuloendothelial system. In endemic settings, the ratio of incident asymptomatic infections to incident clinical cases varies from 4:1 to 50:1 depending on the epidemiologic type (anthroponotic VL is normally more virulent) and the poverty of the affected country. Classic VL manifests as pallor, fever, and hard splenomegaly; hepatomegaly is less common. Laboratory findings document pancytopenia and hypergammaglobulinemia. The clinical incubation period ranges from 3 weeks (exceptional) to more than 2 years, but 4 to 6 months is average. Patients report a history of fever resistant to antibiotics; on physical examination, the spleen is typically appreciated 5 to 15 cm below the left costal margin. Symptomatic VL is 100% fatal when left untreated.

Cutaneous Disease

CL results from multiplication of *Leishmania* in the phagocytes of the skin. In the classic course of the disease, lesions appear first as papules, advance slowly to nodules or ulcers, and then spontaneously heal with scarring over months to years. The clinical incubation period ranges from 1 week (exceptional) to several months; lesions caused by *L. major* and *L. mexicana* tend to evolve and resolve quickly, whereas those caused by *L. braziliensis*, *L. tropica*, and dermotropic strains of *L. infantum* can have longer periods of incubation and spontaneous healing.

Mucosal Disease

MCL results from parasitic metastasis in the nasal mucosal that eventually extends to the oropharynx and larynx. It can develop from CL lesions caused by *L. braziliensis* and *L. panamensis*. Typically, MCL evolves slowly (3 years on average) and does not heal spontaneously.

Diagnosis

The standard diagnosis method for all forms of leishmaniasis is still the microscopy demonstration of *Leishmania* organisms in Giemsa-stained impression smears or cultures from samples of infected tissues. In general, sensitivity increases when both staining and culture are performed. Polymerase chain reaction (PCR) detection of *Leishmania* DNA on samples further increases the diagnostic sensitivity and also might allow species identification by target DNA sequencing or restriction fragment length polymorphism analysis.

Different tissue samplings must be performed depending on the clinical form of leishmaniasis. For VL, aspirate or biopsy specimens are obtained from the spleen, bone marrow, the liver, or enlarged lymph nodes. Higher diagnostic yields are obtained with spleen aspirates (more than 98%), although bone marrow aspirates (80% to 98% of yield) are usually preferred. For CL and MCL, material is obtained by scraping tissue juice from a nodular lesion or from the edge of an ulcer or by taking punch biopsies of inflamed tissue. Diagnostic yields of about 80% are obtained with impression smears and cultures during the first half of the natural course of the lesion. After that, standard parasitologic diagnosis becomes more difficult and PCR remains the only reliable method.

Serology is useful when the diagnosis of VL proves difficult with other methods. Commercially available dipstick tests using recombinant antigen K39 can be employed in decisions for or against treatment. Negative serology results are common in CL and MCL, as well as in VL when patients are severely immunosuppressed.

Differential Diagnosis

Visceral Disease
The differential diagnosis depends on the local disease pattern associated with endemic areas. In many of them it includes chronic malaria, disseminated histoplasmosis, hepatosplenic schistosomiasis, typhoid fever, brucellosis, tuberculosis, endocarditis, relapsing fever, and African trypanosomiasis. Other cosmopolitan diseases include syphilis, lymphomas, chronic myeloid leukemia, sarcoidosis, malignant histiocytosis, and liver cirrhosis.

Cutaneous Disease
A typical history of CL—an inflammatory, slowly developing, and painless skin lesion associated with recent exposure to sand fly bites—can strongly support a clinical diagnosis of disease. However, there is an extensive differential diagnosis, which includes acute or chronic forms of CL. For the former, insect bites, furuncular myiasis, and bacterial tropical ulcers are the most common; for the latter, keloid, lupus vulgaris, discoid lupus erythematosus, and sarcoidosis.

Treatment
The therapy of leishmaniasis relies on a limited number of drugs, most of which are old and relatively toxic compounds. Systemic drug administration requires hospitalizing and monitoring the patient.

Pentavalent Antimonials
Organic salts of pentavalent antimony (Sb) are still the mainstay therapy for all clinical forms of leishmaniasis. Two preparations are available that are equal in efficacy and toxicity when used in equivalent Sb doses: sodium stibogluconate (Pentostam),[10] available in English-speaking countries, and meglumine antimoniate (Glucantime),[2] available in Southern Europe and Latin America. The recommended dosage of Sb is 20 mg/kg/day for 21 to 28 days, given intramuscularly or intravenously. Treatment should be prolonged for 40 to 60 days in areas with documented Sb-resistant VL (e.g., in Bihar State, India). The drugs can be administered intralesionally in cases of uncomplicated CL, intermittently over 20 to 30 days. Systemic toxicity caused by the antimonials relates to the total dose administered and includes anorexia, pancreatitis, and changes on electrocardiography (e.g., prolongation of the QT interval), which can precede dangerous arrhythmias.

Amphotericin B Drugs
Liposomal amphotericin B (Ambisome) is the current gold standard for VL treatment, being highly effective and nontoxic. However, the high cost of the drug precludes its use in developing countries where leishmaniasis is endemic. Liposomal amphotericin B is given intravenously at the total dose of 18 to 21 mg/kg, with various treatment schedules similarly effective: 3 mg/kg/day on days 1 to 5 and 10; 3 mg/kg on days 1 to 5, 14, and 21; or 10 mg/kg/day for 2 days.

Amphotericin B desoxycholate (Fungizone) is a relatively toxic compound used in Sb-resistant VL[1] and MCL, administered intravenously at the low dosage of 0.5 mg/kg every other day for

---

[1]Not FDA approved for this indication.
[2]Not available in the United States.
[10]Available in the United States from the Centers for Disease Control and Prevention.

14 days. Doses in excess of 1 mg/kg/day commonly result in severe infusion-related side effects (fever, chills, and bone pain) and delayed side effects (toxic renal effects).

Other Parenteral Drugs
Other parenteral drugs include old second-line drugs whose use is limited. Pentamidine isethionate (Pentam 300)[1] is a toxic compound used to treat some forms of New World CL resistant to Sb therapy and is given intramuscularly at the low dose of 2 mg/kg every other day for 7 days. Treatment in excess of this dosage can result in common side effects such as myalgias, nausea, headache, and hypoglycemia. Paromomycin (aminosidine) sulfate injection[2] (manufactured by Gland Pharma, India, on behalf of Institute of One World Health) is an old aminoglycoside that is being reevaluated as a first-line drug for Indian VL. It is given intramuscularly at the dose of 11 mg base per kg per day for 21 days. Elevation of alanine aminotranferease (ALT) and aspartate aminotransferase (AST) liver enzymes is usually seen during therapy.

Miltefosine, the First Oral Drug for Leishmaniasis
Miltefosine (Impavido)[5] is a hexadecylphosphocholine originally developed as an anticancer agent. It is the first recognized oral treatment for leishmaniasis and is available in Germany and India. So far, it is recommended for VL therapy in India and Ethiopia and for CL therapy in Colombia and Bolivia. The drug is administered at 2.5 mg/kg/day (not exceeding 100 mg/day) for 28 days. Miltefosine administration does not require the patient to be hospitalized for monitoring. Mild gastrointestinal toxicity may be common. The drug is contraindicated in pregnancy.

Monitoring
In VL patients, fever recedes by day 3 to 5 of treatment, and well-being returns by the first week. Hematologic indices start to improve during the second week. Hemoglobin, serum albumin, and body weight are the most useful indicators of progress. The spleen tends to normalize 1 to 2 months after the end of therapy, although it can take up to 1 year to regress completely. Parasitologic assessment of cure is not normally necessary. Relapses can occur after apparent clinical cure from 2 to 8 months after treatment has been discontinued.

In CL patients, clinical response to drugs is rapid, but complete reepithelialization of lesions is observed in only one third of patients by the end of 3- to 4-week treatment courses.

---

[1]Not FDA approved for this indication.
[2]Not available in the United States.
[5]Investigational drug in the United States.

References

Alvar J, Aparicio P, Aseffa A, et al. The relationship between leishmaniasis and AIDS: The second 10 years. Clin Microbiol Rev 2008;21:334–59.

Berman JJ. Treatment of leishmaniasis with miltefosine: 2008 status. Expert Opin Drug Metab Toxicol 2008;4:1209–16.

Bern C, Adler-Moore J, Berenguer J, et al. Liposomal amphotericin B for the treatment of visceral leishmaniasis. Clin Infect Dis 2006;43:917–24.

Bhattacharya SK, Sinha PK, Sundar S, et al. Phase 4 trial of miltefosine for the treatment of Indian visceral leishmaniasis. J Infect Dis 2007;196:591–668.

Chappuis F, Sundar S, Hailu A, et al. Visceral leishmaniasis: what are the needs for diagnosis, treatment and control? Nat Rev Microbiol 2007;5:873–82.

González U, Pinart M, Rengifo-Pardo M, et al. Interventions for cutaneous and mucocutaneous leishmaniasis. Cochrane Database Syst Rev 2009;(2), CD004834.

Gradoni L, Soteriadou K, Louzir H, et al. Drug regimens for visceral leishmaniasis in Mediterranean countries. Trop Med Int Health 2008;13:1272.

Gramiccia M, Gradoni L. The current status of zoonotic leishmaniases and approaches to disease control. Int J Parasitol 2005;35:1169–80.

Sundar S, Agrawal N, Arora R, et al. Short-course paromomycin treatment of visceral leishmaniasis in India: 14-day vs 21-day treatment. Clin Infect Dis 2009;49:914–8.

LEPROSY

Method of
Gerson O. Penna, MD, PhD; and Maria Lucia Penna, MD, PhD

CURRENT DIAGNOSIS

- Contact with other leprosy cases; travel to or residence in a leprosy-endemic country.
- Skin lesion(s) with altered sensation.
- Thickened or enlarged peripheral nerve, with sensory loss and/or weakness in the muscles supplied by the nerve.
- Presence of acid-fast bacilli in a slit skin smear.
- Skin biopsy with the presence of acid-fast bacilli or typical lesions, thereby aiding disease classification.

CURRENT THERAPY

Paucibacillary Leprosy (6 months)
- ADULT (50–70 kg)
  - Dapsone: 100 mg daily
  - Rifampin (Rifadin)[1]: 600 mg once a month under supervision
- CHILD (under 10 years)
  - Dapsone: 1 mg/kg per day
  - Rifampin[1]: 10 mg/kg once a month under supervision

Multibacillary Leprosy (12 months)
- ADULT (50–70 kg)
  - Dapsone: 100 mg daily
  - Rifampin[1]: 600 mg once a month under supervision
  - Clofazimine (Lamprene)[5]: 50 mg daily and 300 mg once a month under supervision
- CHILD (under 10 years)
  - Dapsone: 1 mg/kg per day
  - Rifampin[1]: 10 mg/kg once a month under supervision
  - Clofazimine: 1 mg/kg per day

[1]Not FDA approved for this indication.
[5]Investigational drug in the United States.

Epidemiology

Leprosy is a chronic disease caused by *Mycobacterium leprae* that affects skin and nerves, often resulting in physical disabilities. The disease has been found around the world, showing that transmission occurs regardless of climate. However, several studies have associated higher transmission with more humid regions.

Nevertheless, disease transmission has ceased in nearly all developed nations, most likely as a consequence of better nutrition and socioeconomic development. Currently, new autochthonous cases are found in all tropical countries, with India and Brazil having the highest number of cases annually. Some insular countries located in the Pacific and Indian Oceans have the highest rates of new case detection, indicating a high risk of transmission.

In the Gulf region of the United States, mostly in the states of Louisiana and Texas, native cases are still diagnosed. There are armadillos (*Dasypus novemcinctus*) in the area that have been infected with strains of *M. leprae* found also in autochthonous human cases. This suggests that leprosy might be a regional zoonosis, even though *M. leprae* was introduced into the Americas by Europeans and Africans. There are also records of *M. leprae* infection in armadillos in Central and South America.

Furthermore, cases in African chimpanzees raise the possibility that these animals could be helping to maintain leprosy transmission in Africa.

The mechanisms of leprosy transmission are not well known due to the fact that there is no easy way to diagnose infection. It is presumed that in endemic areas infection is much more frequent than actual disease onset. The incubation period can vary from a few months to 20 years.

It is known that multibacillary cases excrete a large number of viable bacilli through nasal mucus, suggesting that transmission may be by respiratory route and, in fact, this is believed to be the main source of transmission. Because *M. leprae* can also remain viable in the environment for many days, especially in humid climates, the hypothesis of indirect transmission by means of small skin lesions remains. It is possible to theorize the existence of many different forms of transmission.

Leprosy cases are not uniformly distributed in a community, tending to form clusters within different geographic regions, villages, or groups of domiciles. In the majority of countries, cases are more common among men, and the 15- to 29-year-old age group tends to present the highest risk of disease. In areas where transmission is declining, the incidence tends to be higher among the elderly, affecting those who have lived during a period with a higher risk of infection.

Following the treatment of all new leprosy cases with multidrug therapy (MDT), the backlog of known cases, which had been the main problem faced by leprosy control programs in the 1980s and early 1990s, largely disappeared. Currently, control efforts target new cases so as to not only interrupt transmission but also reduce the disabilities caused by the disease. In more endemic areas, the proportion of cases diagnosed with visible disabilities (grade 2) indicates access to timely diagnosis.

Risk Factors

In endemic areas, the main risk factors are a history of household contact with leprosy cases and low socioeconomic standing. Among infected women, pregnancy is a period of greater risk for developing the disease due to immunologic modulation.

Susceptibility to leprosy is genetically mediated by a group of genes. The low frequency of genetically determined susceptibility may be the cause of the wide difference between infection and disease that is believed to exist.

Even before the highly effective application of antiretroviral treatment, there was no observed association between HIV infection and leprosy. However, in areas of high endemicity, there are accounts of leprosy cases associated with the immunologic reconstitution resulting from antiretroviral treatment. In developed countries, the main risk factor is originating from or having lived in a leprosy-endemic area.

Prevention

Vaccination with bacille Calmette Guérin (BCG)[1] reduces the risk of leprosy, with studies showing a variable efficacy of 20% to 80%. The revaccination of household contacts also provides protection, especially against the multibacillary forms of the disease.

Chemoprophylaxis of contacts or high-risk groups with a single dose of rifampin (Rifadin)[1] has been shown to be effective for a period of 2 years.

Improving socioeconomic conditions in the general population in endemic areas is also a very effective strategy for disease control. This can be seen when comparing the current epidemiologic situation in the Hawaiian Islands with Micronesia or the Marshall Islands, where leprosy continues with a high incidence rate.

Pathophysiology

M. leprae is an intercellular microorganism with a particular tropism for skin and peripheral nerve cells. It cannot be cultivated in vitro, but can be inoculated in mouse foot pads and armadillos, although growth is quite slow.

Active *M. leprae* infection is characterized by a wide clinical range, varying from a disease in which few bacilli are present in

[1]Not FDA approved for this indication.

the body to one in which a high bacterial load is found in skin lesions.

Upon entering the organism, *M. leprae* can be eliminated with a local inflammatory response. When this natural resistance fails, the bacilli multiply within macrophages, enter the lymph stream and bloodstream, reach the regional lymph nodes, and from there move on to the organs of the mononuclear phagocyte system. The mycobacterial antigens are then processed and presented by antigen-presenting cells that can be Langerhans cells, dendritic cells, or others from the monocyte-macrophage system that induce the hapten-protein conjugates to link the HLA-DR class II molecules to the CD4+ lymphocytes. In those individuals where there is stimulation of the T-helper 1 cell response, these lymphocytes will produce interferon (IFN)–gamma cytokines, β–tumor necrosis factor (β-TNF), interleukin-2 (IL2) and IL12 that will promote the differentiation of macrophages in epithelioid cells that will undergo a fusion process resulting in giant cells. This inflammatory response will be sufficient to reduce the *M. leprae* in the tuberculoid form of leprosy.

On the other hand, in the absence of stimulation of the T_H2 subpopulation of T lymphocytes (TLs), these will produce IL4, IL5, IL6, IL8, IL10, and TNF-alpha cytokines. The IL4 and IL10 interleukins are suppressors of macrophage activation, leading to an insufficient immune cell response to combat the level of *M. leprae* proliferation within the macrophages. This characterizes the more infectious forms of the disease at the lepromatous end of the spectrum.

M. leprae uses adult Schwann cells as primary nonimmune cells for colonization. Nerve damage is attributed either to bacterial proliferation or to the immune response of the host to relatively few bacilli in peripheral nerves and adjacent areas of skin.

In this disease spectrum, cell-mediated immunity protects against the disease and limits bacterial dissemination at the tuberculoid pole, whereas this is suppressed at the lepromatous end. Humoral immunity is present only at the lepromatous pole where high levels of specific antibodies to *M. leprae* are found. These immune responses, whether cell mediated or humoral, are dynamic and present spontaneous variations of reactivity that are responsible for leprosy reaction episodes.

Clinical Manifestations

Due to the complexity of the parasite-host relation and the variable efficacy of the host's cellular immune response, the clinical manifestations of the disease cross a wide spectrum. This can vary from an isolated nerve lesion or a single skin patch to a systemic disease that affects several organs beyond just skin and nerves, including eyes, testicles, and kidneys.

Ridley and Jopling, in 1966, proposed a case classification system that takes into consideration clinical, histopathologic, and immunologic parameters: tuberculoid, borderline-tuberculoid, borderline-borderline, borderline-lepromatous, and lepromatous.

Indeterminate leprosy can be considered to be the first clinical manifestation of the disease. It can be cured spontaneously or evolve into one of the other clinical forms.

Indeterminate Leprosy

This is characterized by one or more hypochromic macules with imprecise borders and reduced thermal sensitivity, although pain and tactile sensation may be preserved (Figure 1). These occur as areas of sensory disturbance with no alteration in skin color, sweat glands, or hair growth. Any alteration in nerve function is preliminary and, therefore, there are no physical disabilities described with this classification. Bacilloscopic readings are negative.

Tuberculoid Leprosy

This type is characterized by erythematous or hypochromic skin lesions with clear, raised borders (Figure 2). These are limited in number with an asymmetrical distribution and altered thermal, pain, and tactile sensation. Reduced perspiration and restricted partial or full alopecia may also be seen. Nerves can be affected

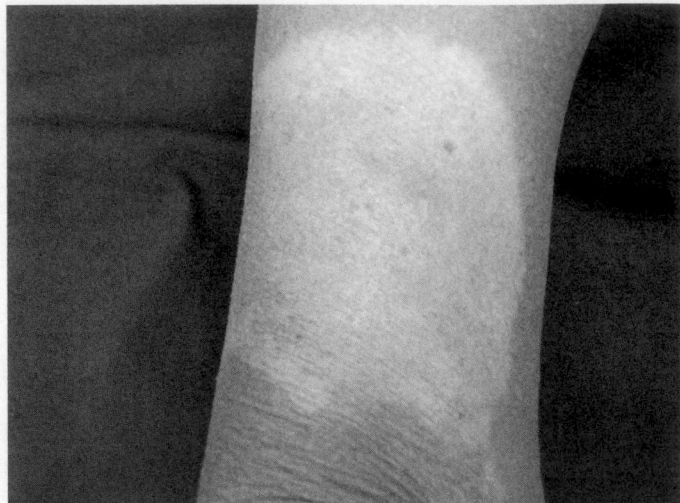

Figure 1. Indeterminate leprosy.

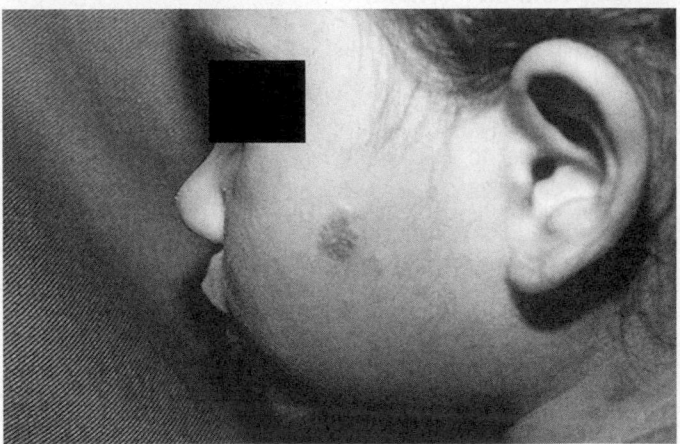

Figure 2. Tuberculoid leprosy in child.

intensively but this usually only happens to a few. Slit skin smear results are negative.

Among children, tuberculoid leprosy lesions have the appearance of nodules or tubercles, generally only on the face. Although these lesions tend to regress spontaneously, treatment should continue as per standard ethical practice.

Borderline-Tuberculoid Leprosy

This form is characterized by lesions similar to those seen at the tuberculoid end of the spectrum, although they will be more numerous. In general, there are more than five lesions with a diameter of 10 cm or more, less clearly defined borders, and containing possible satellite lesions (Figure 3). These lesions tend to be more symmetrical and several nerves may be affected. However, the majority of patients with this disease type will still have a negative bacilloscopy.

Borderline-Borderline Leprosy

This is a relatively rare variation, given that it commonly evolves quickly toward the Virchowian pole, often spurred on by reaction episodes. There are usually many foveal lesions (infiltrated plaques with expanding outer borders and well-defined inner borders with apparently normal skin in the middle) (Figure 4). Generally, nerves are intensively affected and skin smears are almost always positive.

Borderline-Lepromatous (Virchowian) Leprosy

A wide number of lesions are present with a range of possible clinical manifestations (infiltrations, papules, plaques, foveae, and

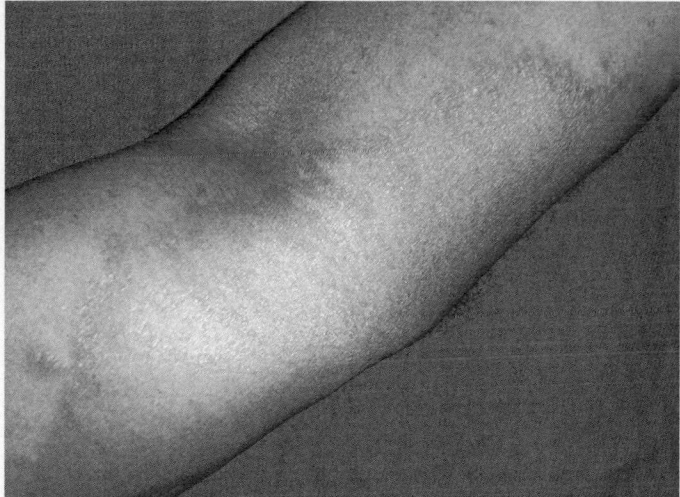

Figure 3. Borderline-tuberculoid leprosy.

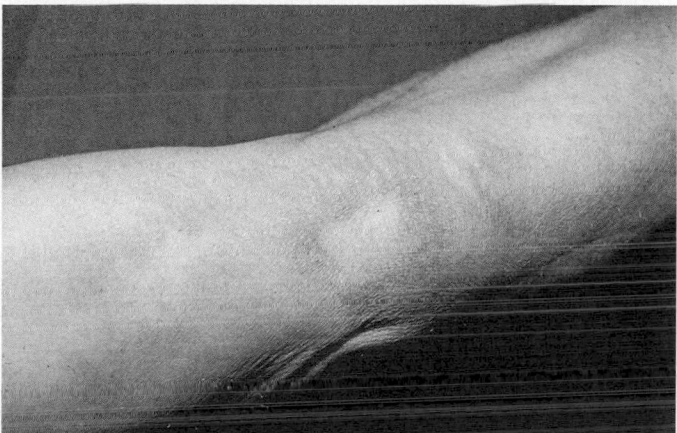

Figure 4. Borderline-borderline leprosy.

nodules) that are common to the Virchowian form. However, with this type there is a tendency to see some delimitation between the lesions and areas of healthy skin. Bacilloscopy is positive with a high bacterial load.

Lepromatous (Virchowian) Leprosy

Lepromatous leprosy (LL) has the highest bacterial burden of human bacterial infections. Extensive lesions tend to be symmetrical, erythematous or hypochromic, infiltrated, and without clear delineation from normal skin areas. Simple lesions evolve to become papules, tubercles, and nodules that can eventually ulcerate and that are especially full of bacilli (Figure 5). There is diffuse infiltration of the face, with auricular appendages affected in the vast majority of cases and bilateral madarosis also common. Hands and feet may also be infiltrated or showing signs of xerodermia.

LL is a systemic disease that can affect the liver, spleen, adrenal glands, lymph nodes, eyes, and nose. Nasal obstruction can be present with little or no response to vasoconstrictors. Often the nasal cavities will be affected and the oropharynges will be full of nasal secretion highly abundant in bacilli. Subsequent nasal dryness can lead to secondary ulceration and infection with possible perforation and destruction of the nasal septum, resulting in what is commonly referred to as saddle nose. With olfactory bulb dysfunction, anosmia will often be the outcome.

Lesions to the palate, lips, gum, and uvula can further compromise the pharynx, nasopharynx, and tonsils. The eyes may show

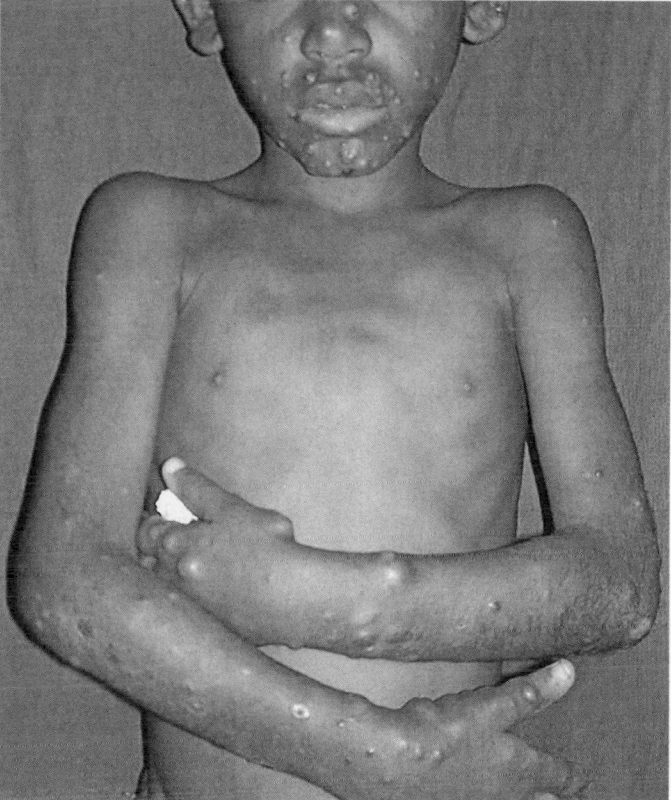

Figure 5. Lepromatous (Virchowian) leprosy (LL).

erythema, dryness, dacryocystitis, lagophthalmos, and/or diminished sensation in the cornea. Likewise, iritis and iridocyclitis may be present, so proper intervention is necessary to ensure prevention of early onset of blindness.

The testes may also be directly affected by bacilli, as witnessed by atrophy of the testicular parenchyma and diffuse fibrosis with eventual sterility and alteration of sexual function. When secondary amyloidosis is present, renal insufficiency may result.

Variations of LL

Histoid Lepromatous Leprosy (or Wade's Lepromatous). Nodular lesions are present, well defined, and of varying sizes. These may be round or oval with a reddish or pink color. These lesions contain a large number of bacilli and are normally associated with sulfone resistance. Histiocytes with a spongy appearance are present under histologic analysis.

Diffuse Lepromatous Leprosy (DLL). Described by Lucio, Alvarado, and Latapi, this is a diffuse form of LL, also called "beautiful" leprosy because this form confers a pinkish and healthy appearance to the skin. It is more frequently seen in Mexico and is characterized by the diffuse infiltration of the skin, altered sensation that starts in the hands and feet, loss of eyebrows, and telangiectasias in the face and torso. Recently a mycobacterium was isolated in cases of DLL whose DNA cannot be amplified using usual *M. leprae* primers. As a result, a new species has been proposed under the name *Mycobacterium lepromatosis*, but many specialists do not yet accept that this is a separate microorganism.

Pure Neural Leprosy. This type presents only nerve lesions without any cutaneous patches. The most common nerves affected are the ulnar, tibial, and fibular. The radial, median, facial, trigeminal, and auricular nerves, among others, may also be damaged.

Neuropathic pain is often present spontaneously or when the nerve is palpated, either with or without thickening of the nerve. This can evolve to sensory loss, paresthesia, or muscular atrophy in the corresponding area, in addition to autonomic dysfunction and nerve abscess.

Leprosy Diagnosis

The patient is examined to locate any possible skin lesions with diminished sensation and/or areas of sensory alteration that may be due to compromised peripheral nerves. Lighting must be adequate, and it is important to observe the entire body surface moving from head to toe. Where there are possible signs of disease, thermal, pain, and tactile sensation testing should be done, also looking for areas of alopecia and/or anhidrosis. It must be noted if there is any type of physical disability.

Bacilloscopy consists of the collection and examination of skin smears taken from a suspected lesion, both earlobes, and both elbows, and helps to classify a patient as paucibacillary (PB) with a negative examination result or multibacillary (MB) when positive.

The bacilloscopic results will generally be negative in the indeterminate, tuberculoid, and borderline-tuberculoid forms, which are considered to be PB forms. Similarly, they tend to be positive for the lepromatous (Virchowian), borderline-lepromatous, and borderline-borderline, which are MB forms.

Ideally, the bacilloscopic reading should be expressed quantitatively as a bacteriologic index (BI) so that it is possible to monitor the patient's progress during treatment. The histologic examination of a skin biopsy also helps to provide a more precise disease classification and can help to confirm diagnosis in cases that are bacilloscopy negative.

In regions with limited access to laboratory resources, clinical diagnosis is sufficient to warrant the beginning of the standard leprosy treatment regimen, keeping in mind that this is the only dermatologic disease with altered sensation in lesions. The World Health Organisation (WHO) suggests the classification of cases as either PB or MB based on the number of skin lesions, with MB cases having five or more such patches.

Available serologic testing does not show sufficient accuracy for disease diagnosis or infection. Real-time polymerase chain reaction is available for leprosy and can act as a means of confirmation for diagnosis of PB cases.

Differential Diagnosis

Differential diagnoses of leprosy include a variety of dermatologic conditions, given the wide range of clinical manifestations in leprosy. The sensory loss symptomatic of leprosy can also be difficult to determine in children and in other diseases that produce changes in the normal skin characteristics (Table 1).

Treatment

Leprosy treatment, like tuberculosis treatment, has to deal with bacillar resistance and persistence. Single-drug therapy selects drug-resistant bacilli and should be avoided. Therapy duration has, as a target, the reduction of the number of persistent bacilli that could lead to relapses.

Standard MDT with dapsone, rifampin (Rifadin),[1] and clofazimine[5] for 12 months for MB cases and 6-month MDT with dapsone and rifampin for PB cases has dramatically changed the prognosis for leprosy patients. However, the evidence is rather weak on the efficacy of this drug regimen, especially regarding the necessary length of time for treatment, both in terms of the proportion of relapse cases and other outcomes, such as physical disability. The use of rifampin once a month was determined for financial reasons, and there is no study comparing this schedule with daily use. For this reason, research on new drugs and treatment regimens continues.

Shorter regimens were used but had shown high relapses rate: daily doses of rifampin and ofloxacin (Floxin)[1] for 4 weeks; single-dose course of rifampin, ofloxacin and minocycline (Minocin)[1] for single-lesion patients.

Fluoroquinolones (pefloxacin,[2] ofloxacin, and moxifloxacin [Avelox][1]), macrolides (clarithromycin [Biaxin][1]), and tetracycline (minocycline) are effective against *M. leprae*. Only rifampin, its derivative rifapentine (Priftin),[1] and moxifloxacin are bactericidal drugs; all others are bacteriostatic.

In cases of intolerance or resistance to dapsone, this can be removed from the drug regimen. Where similar intolerance or resistance is related to rifampin, this should be substituted with a daily dose of 400 mg of ofloxacin. This alternate course lasts 6 months for PB cases and 24 months for MB.

For those who cannot take either dapsone or rifampin, PB patients can be treated with ofloxacin (400 mg/day), minocycline (100 mg/day), and clofazimine (50 mg/day) in self-administered doses for 6 months. Similarly, MB patients can use this regimen during the first 6 months of treatment (intensive phase), followed by 18 months with daily doses of ofloxacin or combined daily doses of minocycline and clofazimine (maintenance phase).

Leprosy Reactions and Control

Over the course of this chronic disease, it is common to experience acute inflammatory episodes called leprosy reactions. These reactions can take place before diagnosis, as well as during or after MDT treatment. They are commonly grouped into (a) type 1 (reversal) reactions (T1Rs) resulting from vigorous cell-mediated immune response; and (b) type 2 reactions (T2Rs), the clinical manifestation of which is frequently erythematous nodosum leprosum (ENL) that comes about mainly from immunocomplex

---

[1]Not FDA approved for this indication.
[2]Not available in the United States.
[5]Investigational drug in the United States.

TABLE 1   Main Differential Diagnosis by Leprosy Forms

INDETERMINATE LEPROSY	TUBERCULOID LEPROSY	BORDERLINE, BORDERLINE-BORDERLINE, BORDERLINE-LEPROMATOUS, AND LEPROMATOUS LEPROSY
Seborrheic dermatitis or seborrheic eczema	Seborrheic dermatitis	Erythema nodosum
Eczema	Dermatofitosis	Diffuse (anergic) cutaneous leishmaniasis
Localized scleroderma (morphea)	Granuloma annulare	Cutaneous and mucosal leishmaniasis
Residual hypochromia and achromia	Cutaneous leishmaniasis	Systemic lupus erythematous and other rheumatologic diseases
Pityriasis versicolor	Discoid lupus erythematous	Neurofibromatosis (von Recklinghausen disease)
Vitiligo	Pityriasis rosea Gibert	Pityriasis rosea Gibert
	Psoriasis	Congenital syphilis, secondary syphilis, tertiary syphilis
	Sarcoidosis	
	Secondary syphilis	
	Cutaneous tuberculosis	

deposits. In patients with borderline-lepromatous leprosy, it is possible to have both reaction types simultaneously. There is also Lucio's phenomenon, which is an immune system response with important clinical manifestations. Its physiopathology is not well understood, with abundant infection of *M. leprae* in endothelium, which can lead to thrombosis in the most superficial vases from immunocomplex deposits with hemorrhaging and cutaneous infarction.

In the literature, a robust positive association has been demonstrated between bacterial load and the frequency of leprosy reactions. A reaction can be set off by various factors, such as pregnancy, childbirth, vaccinations, puberty, intercurrent infections, stress (physical, psychological, or surgical), use of potassium iodate/iodide (SSKI), and immune reconstruction inflammatory syndrome (IRIS) linked to anti-retroviral and/or immune-based therapies.

Those patients who experience leprosy reactions during MDT treatment should continue taking their regimen without modification while also beginning a specific and concurrent treatment for the appropriate reaction type.

Type 1 Reaction or Reversal Reaction

Clinically speaking, lesions become more erythematous and infiltrated, and those with previously diminished sensation can become more sensitive to touch. Desquamation may occur and some lesions may even ulcerate. New lesions can erupt along with edema in the hands, feet, and face, as well as general systemic symptoms. These reactions can last for years in some patients. It is important to begin an immediate intervention given that neuritis is the most common, serious, and potentially disabling clinical manifestation of T1R.

The drug of choice for T1R treatment is prednisone (or prednisolone [Millipred]) with a dosage of 1 to 2 mg/kg/day for at least 12 weeks, at which point it can be tapered off until discontinuing medication around the 24th week.

Type 2 Reaction

This occurs in multibacillary patients, and ENL is the most frequent clinical manifestation of T2Rs. Other variations of T2R are polymorphic erythema and vasculitis.

Clinically, ENL is a systemic condition with the eruption of painful and often symmetrical erythematous nodules on the arms and legs. When deeper, these nodules are more easily palpated than the more visible ones, but will often ulcerate. Neuritis is frequent, although it is less aggressive than seen in T1Rs. The systemic impact can produce edema, myalgia, fever, malaise, asthenia, weight loss, cephalalgia, iritis, episcleritis, iridocyclitis, glaucoma, epistaxis, arthralgia, orchiepididymitis with testicular atrophy, glomerulonephritis, chronic renal insufficiency, hepatosplenomegaly, and amyloidosis.

The most common medication used for ENL is thalidomide (Thalomid) in variable dosage, from 100 to 400 mg/day, depending on the severity of the reaction. The distribution of thalidomide is restricted in some countries due to its teratogenic effects. For this reason, it should be given under strict supervision with proper medical, ethical, and legal measures in place.

For ENL associated with neuritis, iritis, orchitis, and/or handfoot reactions, or in women of childbearing age, a course of corticosteroids should be given (prednisone at 1–2 mg/kg/day).

In chronic cases and those that are nonresponsive to treatment, it is possible to administer clofazimine along with steroids, at the initial dosage of 100 mg three times per day for a maximum of 12 weeks. This should be reduced to 100 mg twice daily for another 12 weeks and finally 100 mg/day for 12 to 24 weeks.

Cyclosporine (Neoral, Sandimmune)[1] may also offer some benefit to the patient with serious ENL, as can the association of azathioprine (Imuran),[1] methotrexate,[1] and corticosteroids.

Lucio's Phenomenon

Lucio's phenomenon can occur in forms of lepromatous leprosy. The skin lesions can be discreet and limited in number, pinkish or cyanotic, often very painful, and potentially necrotizing and ulcerative. This condition can lead to death. Treatment is based on a course of corticosteroid therapy appropriate for each patient.

Differential Diagnosis between Relapse and Reaction

Relapse rates are very low whereas reactions are quite frequent, even after completing treatment. Table 2 shows the main differences between reaction type 1 and relapse.

Complications

Leprosy complications are the result of permanent nerve damage. Lesions to the large nerve trunks, such as the ulnar, median, and tibial, cause motor and sensory loss leading to disabilities such as claw hand and footdrop.

The absence of sensation in the hands, soles of the feet, and cornea leaves these areas predisposed to common wounds and pressure ulcers. This reality demands that patients take specific care to avoid ulcers and detect them as soon as possible to prevent secondary infection. In addition, corneal ulcers can result in blindness.

---

[1]Not FDA approved for this indication.

Leprosy

141

TABLE 2	Differences between Reaction Type 1 and Relapse

REVERSAL REACTION	RELAPSE
Generally occurs during course of MDT or within 6 months of treatment completion	Normally takes place well after the end of MDT, at least a year after treatment completion
Sudden and unexpected onset	Slow and insidious onset
Can be accompanied by fever and malaise	In general, no systemic symptoms present
Old lesions become erythematous, shiny, and infiltrated	Old lesions may present erythematous edges
In general, many new lesions	Few new lesions
There may be ulceration of the reaction lesions	Ulceration may occur on arms and legs in addition to the lesions
Regression with desquamation	No desquamation present
Can quickly affect several nerve trunks, with presence of pain, sensory alteration, and decreased motor function	May affect a single nerve and functional alterations often take place very slowly
Excellent response to corticosteroid therapy	Does not respond well to corticosteroid therapy
Bacteriologic index stable or falls	Bacteriologic index rises

Abbreviation: MDT = multidrug therapy.

Acknowledgment

We thank Dr. Anna Maria Salles for the patient's pictures.

References

Becx-Bleumink M. Relapses among leprosy patients treated with multidrug therapy: experience in the leprosy control program of the All Africa Leprosy and Rehabilitation Training Center (ALERT) in Ethiopia; practical difficulties with diagnosing relapses; operational procedures and criteria for diagnosing relapses. Int J Lepr Other Mycobact Dis 1992;60:421–35.

Fine PE. Leprosy: the epidemiology of a slow bacterium. Epidemiol Rev 1982;4:161–88.

Gelber RH, Grosset J. The chemotherapy of leprosy: an interpretive history. Lepr Rev 2012;83:221–40.

Gillis TP, Scollard DM, Lockwood DN. What is the evidence that the putative *Mycobacterium lepromatosis* species causes diffuse lepromatous leprosy? Lepr Rev 2011;82:205–9.

International Federation of Anti-Leprosy Associations. Available at http://www.ilep.org.uk/about-ilep/; [accessed July 9, 2015].

Penna ML, Penna GO. Leprosy frequency in the world, 1999–2010. Mem Inst Oswaldo Cruz 2012;107(Suppl. 1):3–12.

Talhari S, Neves RG, Penna GO, Oliveira MLWR. Hanseníase. 4th ed. Gráfica Tropical: Manaus; 2006.

Truman RW, Singh P, Sharma R, et al. Probable zoonotic leprosy in the southern United States. N Engl J Med 2011;364:1626–33.

van Brakel W, Cross H, Declercq E, et al. Review of leprosy research evidence (2002–2009) and implications for current policy and practice. Lepr Rev 2010;81:228–75.

Van Veen NH, Lockwood DN, Van Brakel WH, et al. Interventions for Erythema Nodosum Leprosum (Review), Cochrane Collaboration. Hoboken, NJ, John Wiley & Sons; 2012, p. 53.

WHO Expert Committee on Leprosy. World Health Organ Tech Rep Ser., 968:1–61.

LYME DISEASE

Method of
William F. Wright, DO

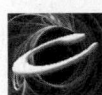

CURRENT DIAGNOSIS

- Lyme disease is a spirochete tick-borne illness of public health importance in temperate regions of North America, Europe, and Asia.
- Evidence suggests that an infected tick must remain attached for at least 36 to 48 hours in order to produce Lyme disease.
- The most common objective manifestation of early localized disease is the characteristic erythema migrans rash.
- Erythema migrans is classically reported as a single uniform erythematous oval to circular lesion that expands for days to weeks and that may or may not produce central clearing of erythema on expansion (known as the "bull's-eye" rash).
- The most common laboratory method endorsed by national guidelines recommends a two-tier serology testing protocol using an enzyme-linked immunosorbent assay (ELISA) as an initial screen, followed by the more specific Western immunoblot to confirm the diagnosis when the ELISA result is equivocal or positive.
- Intrathecal antibody synthesis and polymerase chain reaction (PCR) assays are important diagnostic methods for neuroborreliosis.
- PCR assays are an important diagnostic method for late Lyme arthritis.
- Antibodies produced in response to *Borrelia* species may persist for years following standard antimicrobial therapy; these persistently elevated levels should not be interpreted as an indication of ineffective treatment or chronic infection.

CURRENT THERAPY

- Highly effective oral antibiotics such as doxycycline (Vibramycin),[1] amoxicillin (Amoxil),[1] and cefuroxime axetil (Ceftin) are considered first-line agents.
- Experts recommend doxycycline (Vibramycin) as the preferred agent for oral treatment due to its activity against other tick-borne illnesses such as human granulocytic anaplasmosis (*Anaplasma phagocytophilum*), which may occur in as many as 10% of patients with Lyme disease.
- Doxycycline (Vibramycin) is contraindicated in pregnant and breastfeeding women and in children younger than 8 years.
- Intravenous regimens, such as cefotaxime (Claforan)[1] or ceftriaxone (Rocephin),[1] are reserved for patients with neurologic symptoms (e.g., meningitis with or without facial palsy), symptoms of cardiac disease and/or significant conduction abnormality (e.g., first-degree atrioventricular block and PR interval greater than 30 milliseconds, as well as second- or third-degree atrioventricular block), or, in a few cases, refractory Lyme arthritis.
- Patients with early Lyme disease characterized as a solitary erythema migrans lesion can be treated effectively with a 10-day course of doxycycline (Vibramycin).[1]
- Patients with early disseminated or late disease can be successfully treated with 10 to 28 days of therapy.
- Vaccination for Lyme disease is currently unavailable as a preventive measure for humans.
- The best preventive measures are represented by avoidance of areas with high tick burden (e.g., wooded or grassy areas with a large deer population) and personal protective measures (e.g., bathing following outdoor activities, frequent body checks for ticks, and wearing light-colored protective clothing and tick repellants [diethyltoluamide, DEET]).
- Randomized clinical trials found no evidence that prolonged antibiotic therapy provided benefit in patients with chronic Lyme disease.

[1]Not FDA approved for this indication.

Epidemiology

Lyme disease, also known as Lyme borreliosis, is a spirochete tick-borne illness of public health importance in temperate regions of North America, Europe, and Asia. Among the spirochete genus *Borrelia*, the most common species associated with this illness is *Borrelia burgdorferi* sensu lato. This species is further classified into many different genospecies of which at least three are pathogenic to humans: *B. afzelii*, *B. garinii*, and *B. burgdorferi* sensu lato. All pathogenic spirochetes are transmitted to humans by the hard-bodied ticks of the *Ixodes ricinus* complex. *B. afzelii*, transmitted most commonly by *Ixodes ricinus*, and *B. garinii*, transmitted most commonly by *Ixodes persulcatus*, account for the majority of cases in Europe and Asia, respectively. In the United States, *B. burgdorferi* sensu lato, transmitted by the black-legged deer tick *Ixodes scapularis* (*Ixodes pacificus* on the West Coast), is the sole species to cause infection.

Hard-bodied Ixodid ticks typically have a 2- to 6-year life cycle with four stages of development: egg, larval stage, nymphal stage, and adult stage. Nymph ticks are most active during the period from late spring (May) to early autumn (September) and predominantly obtain blood meals from mice or voles, such as the white-footed mouse (*Peromyscus leucopus*), which serve as a natural reservoir for *B. burgdorferi* sensu lato. Although deer are not considered competent reservoirs for *Borrelia* spirochetes, they are important for the life cycle because they represent a sufficient source of blood meal for adult ticks to maintain the tick population. Although ticks may become infected at any active stage of the life cycle, nymphs and adult females are more likely to harbor the spirochete for further transmission to humans.

The occurrence of a tick bite and the duration of tick attachment are critical factors affecting the risk of spirochete transmission and onset of illness. Evidence suggests that an infected tick must remain attached for at least 36 to 48 hours during a blood meal in order for *B. burgdorferi* sensu lato to migrate from the tick mid-gut through the salivary glands and into the host to produce Lyme disease. Although nymphs and adult Ixodid tick species can transmit the bacterium, it is more likely to occur with nymphs.

As reported by the Centers for Disease Control and Prevention (CDC) for the surveillance of Lyme disease from 1992 through 2006, 93% of cases in the United States occurred within the following states: Connecticut, Delaware, Maine, Maryland, Massachusetts, Minnesota, New Hampshire, New Jersey, New York, Pennsylvania, Rhode Island, and Wisconsin. Lyme disease is associated with a distinct seasonality with the highest number of cases occurring between June and August each year, coinciding with increased nymph activity and outdoor human recreational events. Additionally, the disease is also associated with a slight male predominance and with greater incidence among persons age 5 to 9 years and 55 to 59 years.

Risk Factors

In the United States, the risk of Lyme disease is highest among persons, particularly males, who reside within those 12 states considered as having high endemic rates. Outdoor occupational activities, such as forestry, agricultural farming, and landscaping, with increased exposure to tick-infested areas are considered strong risk factors. Leisure outdoor activities, such as camping, hunting, fishing, and gardening, also place persons at risk for infection.

Clinical Manifestations

In general, the clinical manifestations of Lyme disease are similar among the three pathogenic species and follow three well-recognized clinical stages: early localized disease, early disseminated disease, and late disease.

Early Localized Disease

Lyme disease typically begins within 7 to 14 days (range of 3 to 30 days) following a tick bite that is associated with prolonged tick attachment (at least 36 hours in the United States). The most common objective manifestation of early localized disease, the characteristic erythema migrans rash, may develop in as many as 80% of patients. This characteristic finding is classically reported to begin as a single uniform erythematous oval to circular lesion that expands for days to weeks with a median diameter of 16 cm (range of 5 to 70 cm). Approximately 19% of erythema migrans rashes produce central clearing of erythema on expansion (known as the "bull's-eye" rash). The skin lesion caused by *B. afzelii* often expands, or migrates, more slowly and persists for a longer period of time; therefore, it was initially known as erythema chronicum migrans. The CDC has defined erythema migrans as an expanding red macule or papule, with or without central clearing, which must reach at least 5 cm in size. Lesions most often occur at anatomic sites such as the abdomen, axilla, back, groin or inguinal region, and popliteal fossa and may be associated with nonspecific symptoms that often include chills, fatigue, fever, headache, or myalgia.

Early Disseminated Disease

Multiple erythema migrans lesions, which usually present from 3 to 5 weeks following an initial tick bite, may occur in up to 10% to 20% of patients and is the most common manifestation of early disseminated disease. Borrelia lymphocytoma, characterized as a painless red to blue nodule commonly located on the ear, breast, or scrotum, is an additional cutaneous manifestation of early

disseminated disease that is more frequent in children and seen almost exclusively in Europe. Each of the three pathogenic *Borrelia* species disseminates systemically via the lymphatic system or blood to primarily cause infection of the central nervous system, cardiovascular system, and musculoskeletal system; however, certain species may have a higher frequency to localize to certain areas. For example, whereas *B. burgdorferi* sensu lato often disseminates widely and tends to be more arthritogenic, *B. garinii* often disseminates less widely and is more neurotropic. Musculoskeletal symptoms, such as transient oligoarticular arthralgia or myalgia that may also include joint swelling, are the most common extracutaneous manifestations of early disseminated disease. Approximately 15% of patients may experience neurologic manifestations that may include altered mental status, headache, and neck pain and stiffness (indicating possible Lyme-associated lymphocytic meningitis), as well as motor or sensory radiculoneuropathy, mononeuritis multiplex, cerebellar ataxia, and myelitis. Lyme disease must be included in the differential diagnosis of a seventh cranial nerve palsy (known as Bell's palsy), which is commonly unilateral but may rarely be bilateral. *B. garinii* is associated with a particular meningoradiculoneuritis called Bannwarth's syndrome, which is characterized as painful motor and sensory peripheral radiculopathies, mostly of the cervical and lumbar region, in association with a cerebrospinal fluid lymphocytic pleocytosis. Finally, approximately 4% to 10% of patients may experience Lyme carditis, usually occurring within 1 to 2 months after a tick bite, which may present with dyspnea on exertion, fatigue, nonspecific chest pain, palpitations, or syncope. Evidence suggests that 49% of patients with Lyme carditis may have third-degree atrioventricular block, 28% may have some form of second- or first-degree atrioventricular block, and 23% may have no conduction abnormalities.

Late Lyme Disease

In the United States, the most common manifestation of late Lyme disease, which occurs in as many as 60% of patients, is arthritis. Patients typically present approximately 6 months after an initial tick bite with joint pain and swelling and synovial fluid findings that suggest an inflammatory process. Late Lyme disease arthritis primarily involves the knees. Chronic antibiotic-refractory arthritis may develop in patients who are infected with *B. burgdorferi* sensu lato and also carry the *HLA-DR4* alloantigen. Alternatively, a common late manifestation in Europe, associated with *B. afzelii* infection, is acrodermatitis chronica atrophicans (ACA), which is characterized initially as a progressive painless red to blue fibrous nodule, usually located on the extensor surfaces of the extremities, that eventually becomes atrophic. Rarely, late disease may present with an encephalomyelitis, an axonal polyneuropathy, or a subtle, subacute encephalopathy that typically manifests with cognitive impairment.

Diagnosis

According to the Infectious Diseases Society of America (IDSA) guidelines, the erythema migrans skin lesion is the only clinical manifestation sufficiently distinctive to make the diagnosis of Lyme disease in the absence of laboratory confirmation. Without an erythema migrans skin lesion, serology is the most common laboratory method endorsed by both the CDC and IDSA to confirm the diagnosis (Table 1). Currently, the CDC recommends a two-tier serology testing protocol using an ELISA as an initial screen, followed by the more specific Western immunoblot to confirm the diagnosis when the ELISA result is equivocal or positive. A positive IgM Western immunoblot requires at least two of three significant bands (23, 39, 41 kDa) to be present within 4 weeks' duration of illness because these antibodies typically appear 2 to 4 weeks after the onset of an erythema migrans rash (IgM antibody production peaks at 6 to 8 weeks). A positive IgG Western immunoblot requires at least 5 of 10 significant bands (18, 23, 28, 30, 39, 41, 45, 58, 66, 93 kDa) because these antibodies typically appear after 4 to 6 weeks from the onset of an erythema migrans

TABLE 1

TABLE 1 Estimated Accuracy of Two-tier Serology by Stage and Manifestations of Lyme Disease

STAGE	MANIFESTATIONS	SENSITIVITY	SPECIFICITY	PPV	NPV
Early localized disease	Erythema migrans (EM) rash	17%–53%	98%	75%–90%	26%
Early disseminated disease	Multiple EM lesions, Bell's palsy, Borrelia lymphocytoma, Lyme carditis, neurologic and musculoskeletal Lyme	43%–100%	98%	87%–89%	100%*
Late disease	Lyme arthritis and acrodermatitis chronica atrophicans	100%	98%	94%	100%

*Data calculated from Branda JA et al: Clin Infect Dis 2010;50:20–6; however, the negative predictive value at this stage may more accurately be between 98% and 100%.
Abbreviations: PPV = positive predictive value; NPV = negative predictive value.

skin lesion (IgG antibody production peaks at 4 to 6 months and may remain positive for many years). Antibodies produced in response to *Borrelia* species may persist for years following standard antimicrobial therapy; these persistently elevated levels should not be interpreted as an indication of ineffective treatment or chronic infection. Evidence suggests that a new ELISA called the C6 peptide assay has comparable sensitivity and specificity to the standard two-tier protocol, but further evaluation is needed to determine the optimal use of this assay. Finally, PCR testing may be an option for selected patients with late Lyme arthritis or neurologic disease, and it has the highest sensitivity for Lyme disease using synovial fluid or tissue samples from patients with untreated late Lyme arthritis.

Treatment

Lyme disease treatment recommendations have been published by the IDSA and are guided mainly by the clinical manifestations and stage of the disease (Table 2). Although erythema migrans resolves without antimicrobial therapy, the goals of early treatment are to prevent dissemination and development of further clinical manifestations. Evidence has demonstrated that most *Borrelia* species remain susceptible to many macrolides, most penicillins, many second- and third-generation cephalosporins, and tetracyclines. In general, highly effective oral antibiotics such as doxycycline

(Vibramycin),[1] amoxicillin (Amoxil),[1] and cefuroxime axetil (Ceftin) are considered first-line agents. Many experts recommend doxycycline (Vibramycin) as the preferred agent for oral treatment due to its activity against other tick-borne illnesses such as human granulocytic anaplasmosis (*Anaplasma phagocytophilum*), which may occur in as many as 10% of patients with Lyme disease. Doxycycline (Vibramycin) is contraindicated in pregnant and breastfeeding women and in children younger than 8 years. Intravenous regimens, such as cefotaxime (Claforan)[1] or ceftriaxone (Rocephin),[1] are reserved for patients with neurologic symptoms (e.g., meningitis with or without facial palsy), symptoms of cardiac disease and/or significant conduction abnormality (e.g., first-degree atrioventricular block and PR interval greater than 30 milliseconds, as well as second- or third-degree atrioventricular block), or, in a few cases, refractory Lyme arthritis. In general, patients with early Lyme disease characterized as a solitary erythema migrans lesion can be treated effectively with a 10-day course of doxycycline (Vibramycin).[1] Although the duration of treatment for early Lyme disease can range from 10 to 21 days, patients with early disseminated or late disease can be successfully treated with 10 to 28 days of therapy (duration depends on the choice of agent).

---

[1]Not FDA approved for this indication.

TABLE 2 Recommended Antibiotics* for the Treatment of Lyme Disease

STAGE	FIRST-LINE AGENT(S)	SECOND-LINE AGENT(S)	DURATION
Single or multiple EM skin lesions	Doxycycline (Vibramycin)[1] 100 mg PO twice daily; dosing for children >8 y: 4 mg/kg/day twice daily (maximum of 100 mg/dose) Amoxicillin (Amoxil)[1] 500 mg PO 3 times daily; dosing for children is 50 mg/kg 3 times daily (maximum of 500 mg/dose) Cefuroxime axetil (Ceftin) 500 mg PO twice daily; dosing for children is 30 mg/kg PO twice daily (maximum of 500 mg/dose)	Azithromycin (Zithromax)[1] 500 mg PO daily; dosing for children is 10 mg/kg daily (maximum of 500 mg/day)	7–10 days for azithromycin 10–21 days for doxycycline 14–21 days for amoxicillin or cefuroxime
Early disseminated disease aside from multiple EM skin lesions†	Ceftriaxone (Rocephin)[1] 2 g IV daily; dosing for children is 50–75 mg IV daily (maximum of 500 mg/day)	Cefotaxime (Claforan)[1] 2 g IV every 8 hours; dosing in children is 150–200 mg/kg IV every 6–8 hours (maximum dose of 6 g/day)	14–21 days for ceftriaxone or cefotaxime
Late disease	Late Lyme arthritis‡ without neurologic involvement can be treated the same as early localized disease Late neurologic Lyme is treated the same as early disseminated disease		28 days for late Lyme arthritis without neurologic involvement 14–28 days for late neurologic Lyme

[1]Not FDA approved for this indication.
*All listed antibiotics other than doxycycline (Vibramycin) are classified as pregnancy class B (low pregnancy risk).
†Patients with Bell's palsy and a normal cerebrospinal fluid examination can be treated with a 14-day course of the same antibiotics used to treat early localized disease. Additionally, patients with Lyme meningitis and an allergy or listed intolerance to beta-lactam antibiotics may be treated with doxycycline (Vibramycin) 200–400 mg in two divided doses daily for 10–28 days.
‡Patients with persistent joint pain and swelling following initial therapy may undergo another course of oral antibiotics or a 2- to 4-week course of intravenous antibiotics.
Abbreviation: EM = erythema migrans.

Lyme Disease Relapse versus Reinfection

Patients with untreated early Lyme infection who have not developed further cardiac or neurologic complications may occasionally experience recurrent erythema migrans lesions in association with episodes of arthritis that most often are due to relapse of the original infection. In contrast, patients who have been successfully treated for early Lyme disease with recommended antibiotic therapy may experience reinfection as the result of a new tick-transmitted spirochete characterized as recurrent erythema migrans lesions, with new anatomic locations, during subsequent Lyme transmission seasons (e.g., late spring and early summer). Recent evidence provides further support that recurrent erythema migrans in patients who have successfully completed recommended antibiotic therapy were associated with reinfection due to a new *B. burgdorferi* genotype (based on the evaluation of outer-surface protein C [OspC] genotypes).

Persistent Lyme Arthritis and Post–Lyme Disease Syndrome

In the United States, approximately 10% of patients who have objective evidence of Lyme and have completed treatment for *B. burgdorferi* sensu lato experience an antibiotic-refractory Lyme arthritis that is defined as persistent synovitis for greater than 1 month (following a 60-day course of oral doxycycline) or 2 months (following a standard course of intravenous ceftriaxone) duration despite negative PCR testing on synovial fluid. Persistent Lyme arthritis is a distinct entity from the post–Lyme disease syndrome (also referred as chronic Lyme disease) in which patients may experience nonspecific symptoms (e.g., arthralgia, concentration difficulties, fatigue, headache, memory deficits, or myalgia) with or without clinical or laboratory evidence of Lyme disease. Whereas advocates of the term *chronic Lyme disease* suggest a latent intracellular infection that may require months to years of antimicrobial therapy for eradication, critics suggest that continued symptoms are explained by an autoimmune response that is triggered by an association between Lyme disease and certain human leukocyte antigen (HLA) haplotypes (e.g., *HLA-DR4*). Recent evidence from a mouse model of Lyme disease proposes that the persistence of inflammatory spirochete antigens, but not infectious live bacteria, in close association with cartilage may also provide an explanation of the nonspecific musculoskeletal symptoms associated with antibiotic-refractory Lyme arthritis. Although controversy exists regarding the pathogenesis and treatment of post–Lyme disease syndrome, or chronic Lyme disease, four randomized clinical trials found no evidence that prolonged antibiotic therapy provided benefit in long-term symptom remission. Currently, the American Academy of Pediatrics, American Academy of Neurology, American College of Rheumatology, and IDSA do not recommend prolonged antibiotic therapy for chronic Lyme disease.

Prevention

Vaccination for Lyme disease is currently unavailable as a preventive measure for humans. LYMErix (SmithKline Beecham Biologicals, Philadelphia, PA), a recombinant lipoprotein outer-surface protein A vaccine, was removed from the market in 2002 due to limited demand; therefore, vaccination for Lyme disease is unavailable as a preventive measure for humans. Currently, the best preventive measures are represented by avoidance of areas with high tick burden (e.g., wooded or grassy areas with a large deer population) and personal protective measures (e.g., bathing following outdoor activities, frequent body checks for ticks, and wearing light-colored protective clothing and tick repellants [diethyltoluamide, DEET]). Removal of ticks within 24 hours of attachment using fine-tipped forceps (with care taken to grasp the tick as close to the skin as possible without compressing the body) can also prevent the acquisition of Lyme disease. Antibiotic prophylaxis, using a single 200-mg dose of doxycycline (Vibramycin)[1] within 72 hours of tick removal, in adults and children 8 years or older has been recommended in the United States for engorged ticks that have been attached for 36 hours or longer. Amoxicillin (Amoxil)[1] prophylaxis is not recommended in persons in whom doxycycline is contraindicated (e.g., pregnant and breastfeeding women, and children younger than 8 years) due to insufficient data on dose, duration, and efficacy.

---

[1]Not FDA approved for this indication.

References

Bacon RM, Kugeler KJ, Mead PS. Centers for Disease Control and Prevention (CDC). Surveillance for Lyme disease—United States, 1992–2006. MMWR Surveill Summ 2008;57:1–9.

Bockenstedt LK, Gonzalez DG, Haberman AM, et al. Spirochete antigens persist near cartilage after murine Lyme borreliosis therapy. J Clin Invest 2012;122:2652–60.

Branda JA, Aguero-Rosenfeld ME, Ferraro MJ, et al. 2-Tiered antibody testing for early and late Lyme disease using only an immunoglobulin G blot with the addition of the VlsE band as the second tier test. Clin Infect Dis 2010;50:20–6.

Coulter P, Lema C, Flayhart D, et al. Two-year evaluation of *Borrelia burgdorferi* culture and supplemental tests for definitive diagnosis of Lyme disease. J Clin Microbiol 2005;43:5080–4 [Erratum: J Clin Microbiol 2007;45:277].

Fallon BA, Keilp JG, Corbera KM, et al. A randomized, placebo-controlled trial of repeated IV antibiotic therapy for Lyme encephalopathy. Neurology 2008;70:992–1003.

Klempner MS, Hu LT, Evans J, et al. Two controlled trials of antibiotic treatment in patients with persistent symptoms and a history of Lyme disease. N Engl J Med 2001;345:85–92.

Krupp LB, Hyman LG, Grimson R, et al. Study and treatment of post Lyme disease (STOP-LD): a randomized double masked clinical trial. Neurology 2003;60:1923–30.

Nadelman RB, Hanincova K, Mukherjee P, et al. Differentiation of reinfection from relapse in recurrent Lyme disease. N Engl J Med 2012;367:1883–90.

Nadelman RB, Nowakowski J, Fish D, et al. Tick Bite Study Group. Prophylaxis with a single-dose doxycycline for the prevention of Lyme disease after an *Ixodes scapularis* tick bite. N Engl J Med 2001;345:79–84.

Stupica D, Lusa L, Ruzic-Sabljic E, et al. Treatment of erythema migrans with doxycycline for 10 days versus 15 days. Clin Infect Dis 2012;55:1343–50.

Wormser GP, Dattwyler RJ, Shapiro ED, et al. The clinical assessment, treatment, and prevention of Lyme disease, human granulocytic anaplasmosis, and babesiosis: clinical practice guidelines by the Infectious Diseases Society of America. Clin Infect Dis 2006;43:1089–134 [Erratum: Clin Infect Dis 2007;45:941].

Wormser GP, Ramanathan R, Nowakowski J, et al. Duration of antibiotic therapy for early Lyme disease: a randomized, double-blind, placebo-controlled trial. Ann Intern Med 2003;138:697–704.

Wright WF, Riedel DJ, Talwani R, et al. Diagnosis and management of Lyme disease. Am Fam Physician 2012;85:1086–93.

MALARIA

Method of
Kimberly E. Mace, PhD; and Michael F. Lynch, MD*

CURRENT DIAGNOSIS

History
- Does the patient have fever (with or without other flulike symptoms)?
- Did the patient travel to a malaria-endemic area?
  - When did the travel occur? What was the date of symptom onset?
  - Where was the infection acquired? What are the prevalent parasite species and drug-resistance patterns from this region?
- Did the patient take prophylaxis during travel to a malaria-endemic region?
  - Was prophylaxis properly prescribed for the region?
  - Was the patient compliant with the regimen?

Diagnostic Confirmation
- Thick blood smear for parasite detection

---

*The findings and conclusions in this chapter are those of the authors and do not necessarily represent the views of the Centers for Disease Control and Prevention.

- Thin blood smear to determine *Plasmodium* species and parasite density
- An alternative is to use rapid diagnostic test (RDT) for faster parasite detection followed by blood smear to determine species and parasite density
- Signs of severe malaria: Parasite density >5%; altered consciousness, seizures, or coma; severe anemia; hypoglycemia; respiratory distress/acute respiratory distress syndrome (ARDS); hypotension; acute renal failure; acidosis; hyperbilirubinemia

CURRENT THERAPY

- Promptly diagnose and initiate treatment to avert severe manifestations or death.
- Determine where the patient acquired the infection to assess local drug resistance patterns and develop a treatment strategy.
- Distinguish between uncomplicated and severe malaria:
  - Severe malaria: Treat with parenteral therapy (quinidine or artesunate[10]) in an intensive care setting.
  - Uncomplicated malaria: Distinguish between *P. falciparum* and non-*P. falciparum*.
    - *P. falciparum* malaria: Strongly consider admitting to hospital.
    - *P. vivax* or *P. ovale*: Assess G6PD status and prevent relapsing infections by prescribing primaquine.

[10]Available in the United States from the Centers for Disease Control and Prevention.

Malaria is an intraerythrocytic infection caused by protozoa of the genus *Plasmodium*. It is transmitted by the bite of an infective female *Anopheles* mosquito, which serves as the vector and definitive host.

Malaria is one of the most significant parasitic diseases in the world, with an unacceptably high global burden. There were an estimated million clinical cases with 627,000 deaths in 2012, mostly in children younger than 5 years living in sub-Saharan Africa, making malaria one of the world's leading killers. World Malaria Report 2013 describes 104 countries and territories with areas at risk for malaria transmission, meaning that nearly half the world's population is at risk for malaria infection. Each year, approximately 1500 cases of malaria are reported in the United States. The overwhelming majority of these illnesses occur among travelers to malaria-endemic areas, but rare instances of local mosquito-borne transmission in the United States have occurred.

Malaria should always be considered in the differential diagnosis of fever in a traveler returning from a malarious area or in those with fever of unknown origin regardless of travel history. Prompt diagnosis and treatment are imperative because untreated *Plasmodium* infections can progress to coma, kidney failure, pulmonary edema, and death. Appropriate chemoprophylaxis and the use of personal protective measures are important in preventing malaria infection.

Risk Factors for Transmission

Malaria is a vector-borne disease most commonly transmitted through infective mosquitoes. Rarely, it can be transmitted through exposure to infected blood and blood products, organ transplantation, or contaminated needles (induced malaria) or by vertical transmission (congenital malaria). Most cases of malaria among persons from countries where it is not endemic are acquired while traveling in an endemic area (imported malaria). Imported malaria poses a potential for reintroduction of malaria into a nonendemic country. If a competent mosquito vector exists, a local mosquito could acquire the parasite by biting an infected person and then could transmit that infection to

another person. In the United States, 63 outbreaks due to locally acquired mosquito-borne malaria transmission (introduced malaria) were identified from 1957 to 2003.

Etiology and the Parasite's Life Cycle

Infection with protozoa of the genus *Plasmodium* causes malaria. Typically, four species of *Plasmodium* cause clinical disease in humans: *P. falciparum*, *P. vivax*, *P. ovale*, and *P. malariae*; however, data from Southeast Asia describe an increasing number of human infections caused by *P. knowlesi*, a simian species.

The life cycle of malaria starts with inoculation of sporozoites into the human bloodstream from the bite of a female *Anopheles* mosquito. Sporozoites travel rapidly to the liver, where asexual replication occurs (exo-erythrocytic phase, tissue schizogony). Thousands of merozoites are released from the infected liver cells to invade red blood cells (RBCs), where they multiply every 24 to 72 hours (erythrocytic cycle, blood schizogony), depending on the species. Some parasites differentiate into gametocytes (sexual erythrocytic stage), which can subsequently be ingested by a female *Anopheles* mosquito, develop into sporozoites in the mosquito's midgut, and eventually migrate into the salivary glands, continuing the malaria transmission cycle with the mosquito's next blood meal (Figure 1).

In *P. vivax* and *P. ovale* infections, some sporozoites do not enter the exo-erythrocytic cycle but instead develop into latent hepatic forms, or hypnozoites. These forms can reactivate later and cause acute illness. The resulting infection, a relapse, can occur months to years after the initial infection and can occur repeatedly. If *P. vivax* or *P. ovale* infections are acquired congenitally or through exposure to blood or blood products, there is no liver phase, and therefore relapses cannot occur. Neither *P. falciparum* nor *P. malariae* have latent hepatic forms and therefore do not cause relapse. However, subsequent illness, called *recrudescence*, can occur in all species if the parasite is not cleared after suboptimal therapy. For example, if *P. malariae* infection is not treated, symptomatic recrudescences, often associated with immunosuppression, can occur decades after the primary infection.

The incubation period, or the period from infection to the appearance of symptoms, is species-dependent. The incubation period is usually 9 to 14 days for *P. falciparum*, 12 to 17 days for *P. vivax*, 16 to 18 days for *P. ovale*, and 18 to 40 days (or longer) for *P. malariae*. Persons taking chemoprophylaxis and those who have acquired partial immunity from repeated exposure to malaria infection can experience a prolonged incubation period.

Epidemiology

Malaria is endemic to much of Africa, Asia, and parts of Central Asia, Oceania, Central America, South America, the Caribbean, and the Middle East (Figure 2). *P. falciparum* is the most common species in the tropics and subtropics. *P. malariae*, although less common, follows a similar geographic distribution. *P. vivax* is prevalent in many temperate zones as well as in the tropics and subtropics and has the widest geographic distribution. *P. ovale* is found mainly in West Africa. *P. knowlesi*, a simian strain, has been reported to infect humans in Southeast Asia. Together, *P. falciparum* and *P. vivax* account for more than 90% of clinical malaria illnesses worldwide.

The development of resistance to antimalarial drugs has complicated malaria prophylaxis and treatment. Chloroquine-resistant *P. falciparum* is widespread with few exceptions, and chloroquine-resistant *P. vivax* is an issue in Papua New Guinea, Indonesia, and East Timor. *P. falciparum* resistance to sulfadoxine-pyrimethamine (Fansidar) is widespread in the Amazon River Basin areas and much of Southeast Asia and Africa, whereas mefloquine resistance is so far limited to Southeast Asia. Perhaps most troubling, there have been reports from Southeast Asia of artemisinin resistance manifesting as failure to clear parasites by day 3 of treatment. Knowledge of species-specific resistance patterns is essential to making appropriate decisions about chemoprophylaxis and treatment. Up-to-date information regarding areas

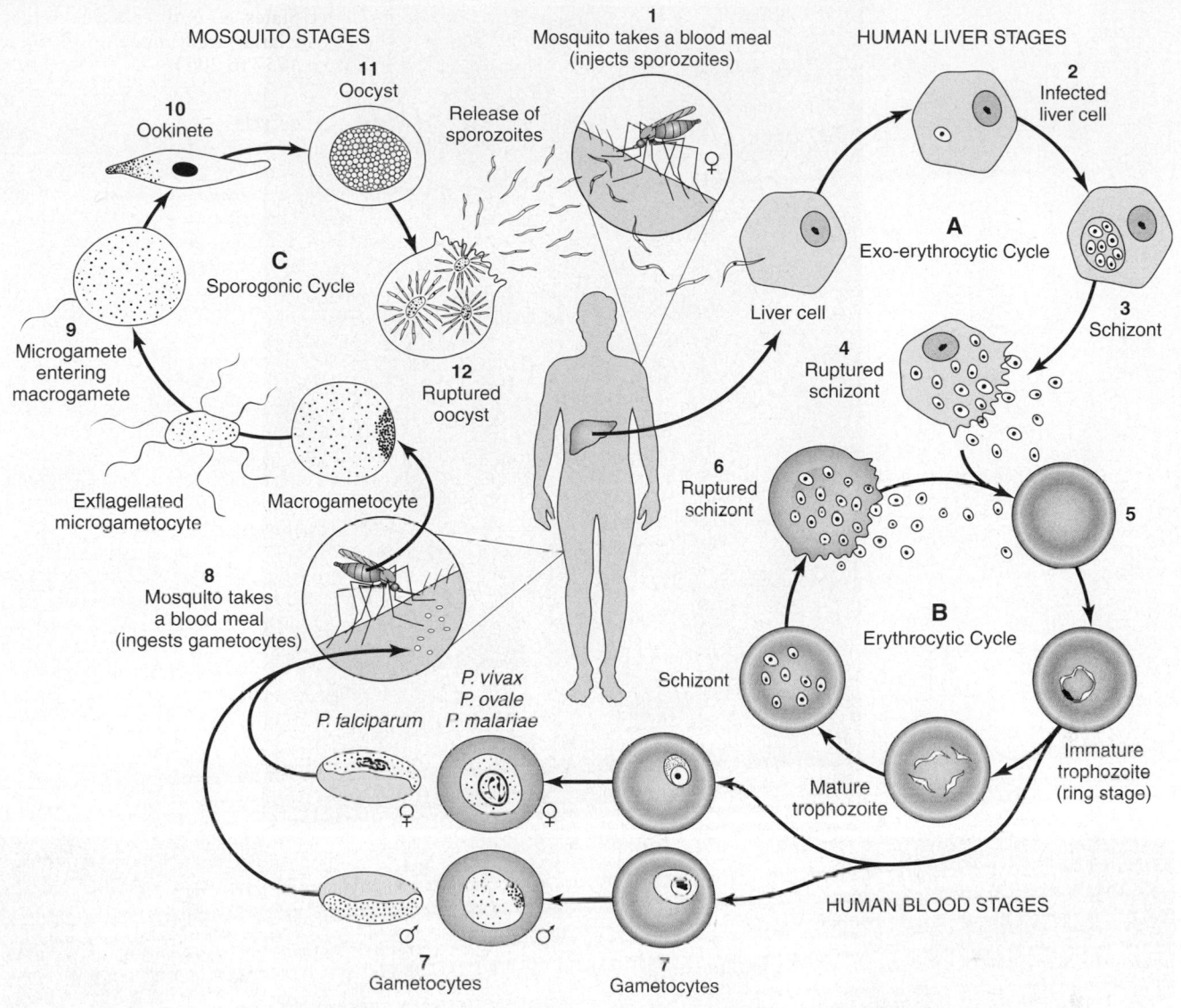

MOSQUITO STAGES

1 Mosquito takes a blood meal (injects sporozoites)

HUMAN LIVER STAGES

11 Oocyst

10 Ookinete

Release of sporozoites

C Sporogonic Cycle

9 Microgamete entering macrogamete

Exflagellated microgametocyte

12 Ruptured oocyst

Macrogametocyte

8 Mosquito takes a blood meal (ingests gametocytes)

P. vivax
P. ovale
P. malariae

P. falciparum

♀

♀

♂

♂

7 Gametocytes

7 Gametocytes

Schizont

Mature trophozoite

2 Infected liver cell

A Exo-erythrocytic Cycle

Liver cell

3 Schizont

4 Ruptured schizont

6 Ruptured schizont

5

B Erythrocytic Cycle

Immature trophozoite (ring stage)

HUMAN BLOOD STAGES

Figure 1. The malaria parasite life cycle involves two hosts. During a blood meal, a malaria-infected female *Anopheles* mosquito inoculates sporozoites into the human host (**1**). Sporozoites infect liver cells (**2**) and mature into schizonts (**3**), which rupture and release merozoites (**4**). (In *Plasmodium vivax* and *Plasmodium ovale,* a dormant stage [hypnozoites] can persist in the liver and cause relapses by invading the bloodstream weeks or even years later.) After this initial replication in the liver (exo-erythrocytic cycle or tissue schizogony (**A**)), the parasites undergo asexual multiplication in the erythrocytes (erythrocytic cycle or blood schizogony (**B**)). Merozoites infect red blood cells (**5**). The ring stage trophozoites mature into schizonts, which rupture, releasing merozoites (**6**). Some parasites differentiate into sexual erythrocytic stages (gametocytes) (**7**). Blood stage parasites are responsible for the clinical manifestations of the disease. The gametocytes, male (microgametocytes) and female (macrogametocytes), are ingested by an *Anopheles* mosquito during a blood meal (**8**). The parasites' multiplication in the mosquito is known as the sporogonic cycle (**C**). While in the mosquito's stomach, the microgametes penetrate the macrogametes, generating zygotes (**9**). The zygotes in turn become motile and elongated (ookinetes) (**10**) and invade the midgut wall of the mosquito, where they develop into oocysts (**11**). The oocysts grow, rupture, and release sporozoites (**12**), which make their way to the mosquito's salivary glands. Inoculation of the sporozoites (**1**) into a new human host perpetuates the malaria life cycle.

where malaria transmission occurs and local patterns of drug resistance can be found on websites of the Centers for Disease Control and Prevention (CDC): http://www.cdc.gov/malaria/map/ or http://www.cdc.gov/travel/default.aspx.

Clinical Manifestations

The clinical presentation of malaria is nonspecific, though it invariably includes fever. Therefore, clinicians must routinely obtain a travel history from febrile patients and maintain a high index of suspicion for malaria among febrile patients returning from malarious areas. The clinical presentation of malaria can vary substantially, depending on the infecting species, the level of parasitemia, and the immune status of the patient. The initial clinical symptoms usually include a flulike prodrome with headache, malaise, and myalgias that is followed by fever.

Malaria paroxysms of chills, high fevers, and then sweats are produced when infected red blood cells rupture and release merozoites. After a number of cycles of erythrocytic schizogony, the release of merozoites may become synchronized, resulting in classic cyclic fevers. With *P. falciparum, P. vivax,* and *P. ovale* infections, the paroxysms can occur in 48-hour cycles (tertian malaria); *P. malariae* infections have 72-hour cycles (quartan malaria) and *P. knowlesi* infections have 24-hour cycles (quotidian malaria). However, many patients, particularly those with *P. falciparum,* do not develop cyclic paroxysms at all, and so a lack of cyclic fevers should not rule out a diagnosis of malaria. Other symptoms include headache, febrile seizures, rigors, cough, chest pain, diarrhea, nausea, vomiting, myalgias, and abdominal pain. On physical examination, a patient can appear well without physical findings or might have signs of jaundice, tachycardia, hypotension (usually secondary to volume depletion), mild hepatomegaly,

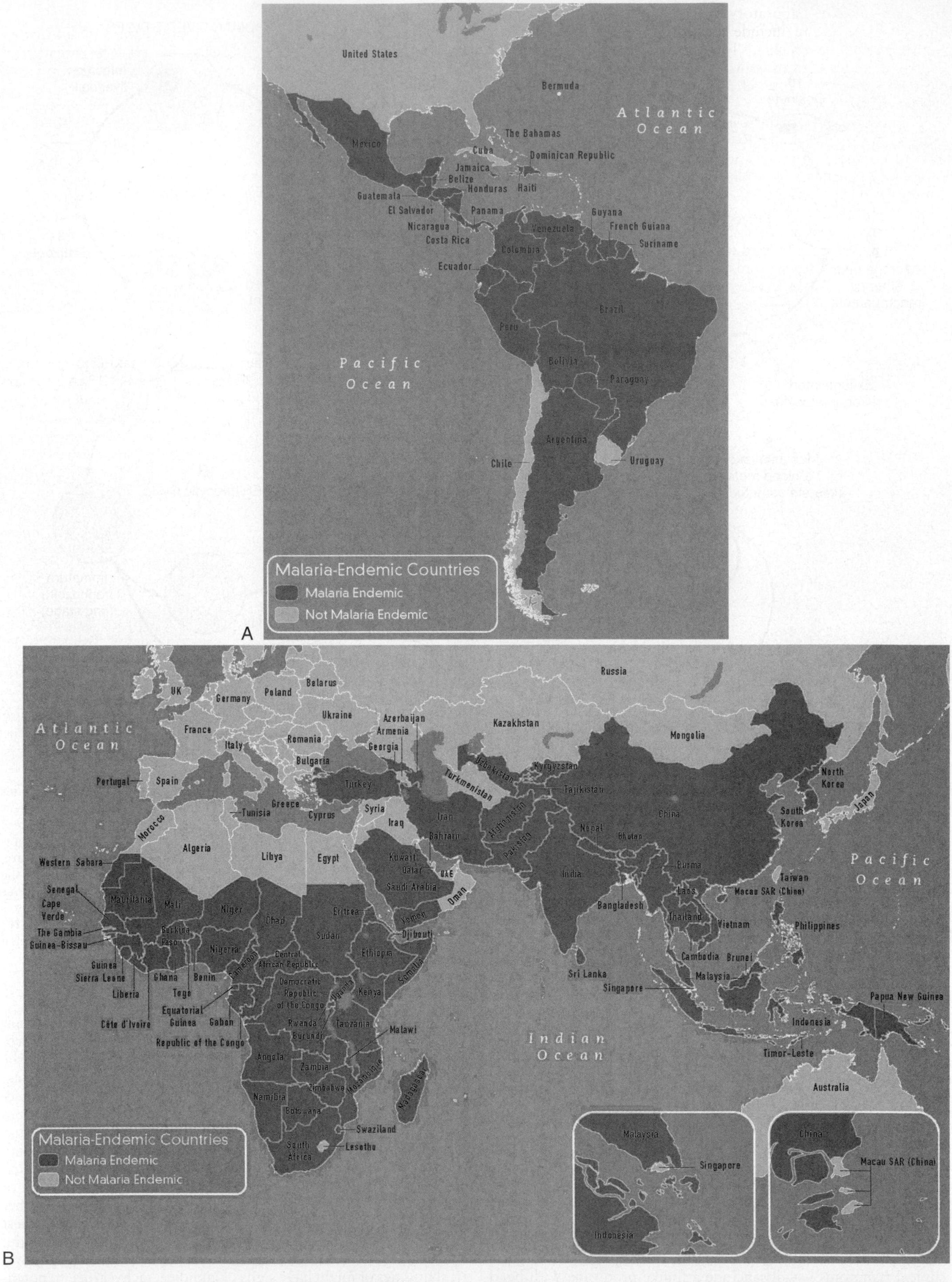

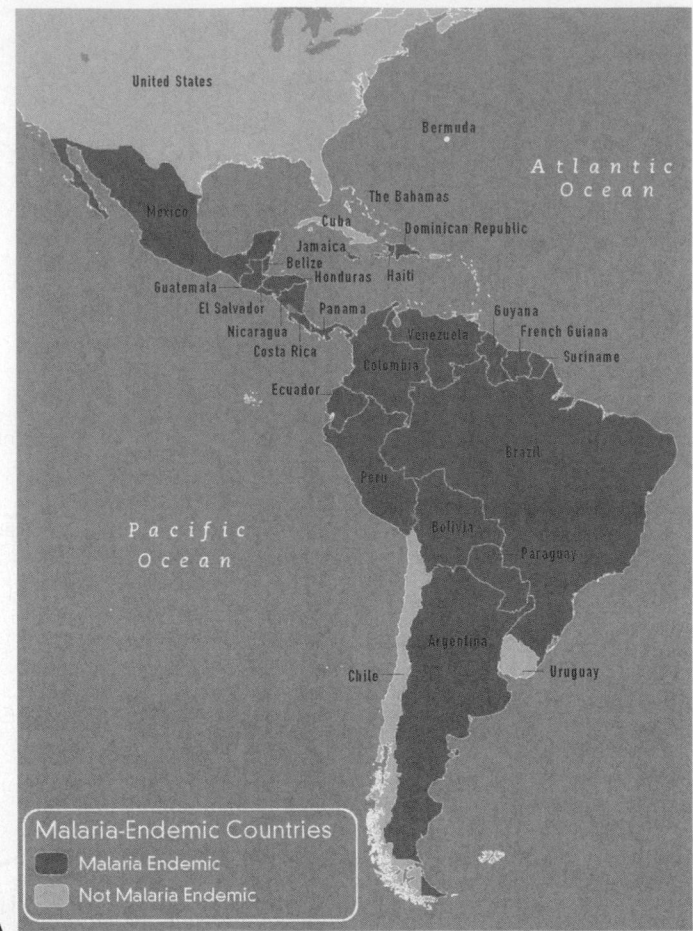

Figure 2. Malaria-endemic countries in the (**A**) Western and (**B**) Eastern Hemispheres. Malaria transmission occurs in large areas of Central and South America, parts of the Caribbean, Africa, Asia (including South Asia, Southeast Asia, and the Middle East), Eastern Europe, and the South Pacific. (Reprinted with permission from Brunette GW, editor. CDC Health Information for International Travel 2012. Atlanta, Georgia.)

and splenomegaly. Laboratory abnormalities in cases of uncomplicated malaria can include anemia, an elevated reticulocyte count, thrombocytopenia, lymphopenia, hyperbilirubinemia, and mildly elevated transaminases. Appropriately treated, uncomplicated malaria has a good prognosis with a case fatality rate around 0.1%.

An uncomplicated malaria infection can progress to severe disease or death within hours. Risk factors for severe malaria include lack of acquired immunity and inadequate, inappropriate, or delayed treatment, a high parasite burden, and age older than 50 years. *P. falciparum*, more than any other species of *Plasmodium*, is responsible for severe disease and death associated with malaria. This severity is attributed to several factors unique to this species. The tissue and blood schizonts release a larger number of merozoites when they rupture, resulting in a rapid rise in parasitemia, and they can also invade red blood cells of all developmental stages, producing more-profound anemia. In addition, the processes of cytoadherence of *P. falciparum*–infected erythrocytes to the vascular endothelium, rosetting of infected erythrocytes with uninfected erythrocytes, and agglutination of infected erythrocytes with other infected erythrocytes contribute to tissue hypoxia and end-organ dysfunction. Even the immune response itself can contribute to many of the cellular and humoral processes that manifest in severe malaria illness. Pro-inflammatory cytokines including TNF-α and IFN-γ likely contribute to endothelial dysfunction, which manifests in cerebral malaria or in acute respiratory distress syndrome (ARDS) secondary to malaria. The complex balance of proinflammatory versus antiinflammatory immune responses might determine if one is protected or predisposed to severe disease.

Severe malaria due to *P. falciparum* is associated with a 15% to 20% mortality rate. Clinical indicators of severe malaria include impaired consciousness, coma, generalized seizures, severe anemia, acute renal failure, ARDS, circulatory collapse, disseminated intravascular coagulation, abnormal bleeding, metabolic (lactic) acidosis, hypoglycemia, hemoglobinuria, jaundice, or a parasitemia greater than 5%.

Cerebral malaria, an ominous complication with an estimated 10% to 40% mortality rate, is characterized by diffuse symmetric encephalopathy. Coma or impaired mental status caused by malaria has to be distinguished from other causes of altered mental status, including hyperpyrexia, hypoglycemia, and concurrent infections such as meningitis. The clinical spectrum of cerebral malaria ranges from odd behavior to delirium, generalized seizures, and coma with extensor posturing (opisthotonos). Children, more commonly than adults, can suffer from cerebral malaria and its residual neurologic sequelae. On the other hand, ARDS, jaundice, and renal impairment occur more often in adults. ARDS can occur as a secondary manifestation of malaria, and it often ensues after initial clinical improvement or clearance of peripheral parasitemia. Severe anemia and hypoglycemia, more common in children and pregnant women, are important features of severe malaria and predict poor prognosis. Acidosis due to an increase in lactate levels and its associated acidotic breathing are also poor prognostic factors.

Non–*P. falciparum* infections are not without risk of severe disease. Severe manifestations of *P. vivax*, in particular, are not uncommon. Notably, *P. vivax* accounted for three of 34 deaths (9%) that occurred in the United States between 2002 and 2008. *P. falciparum* caused 24 deaths (71%) and *P. malariae* infections, mixed *P. falciparum*, and unknown species contributed to the remaining seven deaths (21%). Severe manifestations of *P. vivax*, in adults and children, are often pulmonary. However, jaundice, kidney failure, and acidosis have also been associated with *P. vivax*. Splenic rupture has been described in patients with persistent, untreated *P. vivax* infection who have developed massive splenomegaly. Chronic complications of malarial infections include hyperreactive malarial syndrome (tropical splenomegaly syndrome), nephrotic syndrome (a rare complication of persistent *P. malariae* infection), and possibly Burkitt's lymphoma.

Diagnosis

Malaria should be considered in any febrile patient with a history of travel to an area of malaria transmission even if the patient gives a history of taking appropriate prophylactic therapy. Information on the location and duration of the trip, the date of return, the history of prophylaxis choice and adherence, and the date of symptom onset enables the physician to assess the risk of malaria and, if necessary, choose an appropriate course of treatment.

To provide appropriate therapy, it is essential to identify the infecting malaria species, determine where the infection was acquired, and determine the parasite density. Health care providers evaluating patients for possible malaria must obtain thick and thin blood smears, the most valid diagnostic test, to demonstrate asexual forms of the parasite. Malaria smears should be read without delays; sending specimens to offsite laboratories can delay results. In rare instances, if the patient is extremely ill with symptoms consistent with severe malaria and has a history of malaria exposure, treatment should be started immediately, before results are available. Initial blood smears may be negative, particularly in symptomatic, semi-immune persons and those taking prophylaxis. Therefore, blood smears should be repeated every 12 to 24 hours for a total of three sets before the diagnosis of malaria can be excluded. Initial laboratory evaluation of patients with suspected malaria should include a complete blood count, electrolytes, creatinine, urea, glucose, and bilirubin. In patients with severe disease or respiratory symptoms, lactate level, arterial blood gas, and additional coagulation studies should also be obtained.

Blood smears should be prepared with Giemsa stain (pH 7.2) and examined under light microscopy. Both thick and thin smears should be scanned at low magnification and then examined under oil immersion (1000× magnification). The thick smear concentrates the parasites, resulting in a higher diagnostic sensitivity than the thin smear. The easiest way to determine the percentage of parasitemia using the thin smear is to count the parasitized erythrocytes among 500 to 2000 erythrocytes, divide the number of parasitized erythrocytes by the total number of erythrocytes counted, and multiply by 100. To avoid missing low-density infections, at least 200 high-power fields should be examined before a slide is considered negative. Further details about preparation and diagnostic assistance on digital photographs of blood smears can be found at the CDC's Division of Parasitic Diseases diagnostic Internet site: http://www.dpd.cdc.gov/dpdx.

The relationship between parasitemia and clinical severity is complex. Although severe malaria can occur even with apparently low parasitemia, persons with greater than 5% parasitemia are at higher risk of death from malaria. Thus it is essential to determine the parasite burden at the time of diagnosis as an indicator of disease severity. Although gametocytes can persist much longer, blood smears should be negative for asexual parasites within 48 to 72 hours following the completion of therapy.

Alternative diagnostic tests for malaria include rapid diagnostic tests (RDTs), polymerase chain reaction (PCR), and serology. RDTs identify *P. falciparum*–specific antigens such as histidine-rich protein-2 (HRP-2) or common enzymes such as aldolase and lactate dehydrogenase (pLDH) that are present in all *Plasmodium* species infecting humans. Determination of parasite density is not possible with RDTs, and therefore they do not eliminate the need for thin and thick blood smears. BinaxNOW supplies an RDT to hospitals and commercial laboratories in the United States that detects two different malaria antigens: HRP-2 and aldolase. Therefore, this test identifies *P. falciparum* infections but does not differentiate *P. vivax, P. ovale, P. malariae,* or mixed infections. All malaria RDTs must be performed with proper controls.

PCR may be more sensitive for detecting parasites than microscopy. PCR is particularly valuable for identifying the species of a parasite when that cannot be determined by morphology or RDT alone. Currently, PCR is used mostly as a research tool and is available only in reference laboratories. As access to quality PCR increases, routine species confirmation by PCR might become the standard of care. Malaria serology can detect antibodies to any of the four major species but cannot be used to diagnose acute infections. However, it may be useful for identifying an infective donor in cases of transfusion-related malaria, investigating congenital cases, assessing the validity of clinical malaria diagnoses in empirically treated nonimmune travelers, and diagnosing hyperreactive malarial syndrome.

Antimalarial Drugs

Because of the emergence and spread of drug-resistance, the slow rate of development of new antimalarial drugs, and the infrequency with which newly developed drugs are submitted for United States. Food and Drug Administration (FDA) approval, relatively few drugs are available for the prophylaxis and treatment of malaria infections in the United States. The choice of antimalarial drugs used for treatment should be guided by several factors: local availability of the drug, the infecting species, where it was likely acquired (according to travel history) and drug resistance patterns in that area, severity of symptoms, and percent parasitemia.

Antimalarial drugs can be categorized by their ability to kill the organism at various stages in its life cycle (see Figure 1). Drugs that kill malaria parasites infecting liver cells during the exo-erythrocytic cycle are referred to as tissue schizonticides, whereas blood schizonticides kill malaria parasites that have been released into the bloodstream and are asexually replicating in the erythrocytic cycle. Rapidly acting blood schizonticides are the essential components of acute malaria treatment regimens, and tissue schizonticides targeted toward latent forms can prevent relapse in certain species. Certain drugs can also have activity against gametocytes. Gametocidal activity does not affect a patient's clinical response but can decrease the probability that infection is transmitted to another person. Currently no medications are available that have activity against malaria sporozoites.

Chloroquine phosphate (Aralen) and hydroxychloroquine sulfate (Plaquenil) are used to prevent and treat malaria. They are blood schizonticides that are active against the erythrocytic stages of all *Plasmodium* species and have gametocytocidal activity against *P. vivax, P. ovale,* and *P. malariae.* Chloroquine is the treatment of choice for susceptible strains of all *Plasmodium* species, although the widespread prevalence of chloroquine-resistant forms of *P. falciparum* and *P. vivax* have limited its use in most malaria-endemic areas. Chloroquine can be taken safely by pregnant women and children. Side effects include gastrointestinal disturbance, dizziness, blurred vision, insomnia, headache, and pruritus. Although extremely rare, long-term administration of chloroquine, usually associated with its use in the treatment of rheumatologic conditions, can lead to retinopathy, ototoxicity, and peripheral neuropathy.

Atovaquone-proguanil (Malarone), a fixed-combination antimalarial drug that is both a blood and tissue schizonticide, can be used for chemoprophylaxis and for treatment of chloroquine-resistant *P. falciparum.* Though it has tissue schizonticidal activity, it does not prevent relapses of *P. vivax* and *P. ovale.* Side effects are rare, but abdominal pain, nausea, vomiting, and headache have been reported. Treatment efficacy, safety, and pharmacokinetic data in children weighing 5 to 11 kg have been extrapolated, allowing prophylaxis doses in these children.[1] Providers should note that this prophylactic dosing for children weighing less than 11 kg constitutes off-label use in the United States. Atovaquone-proguanil is contraindicated in children who weigh less than 5 kg, pregnant women, women who are breast-feeding infants who weigh less than 5 kg, and persons with severe renal impairment.

Derivatives of artemisinin (such as artesunate,[10] artemether,[2] and dihydroartemisinin[2]) are compounds derived from the Chinese medicinal plant quinghaosu (*Artemisia annua*) that are active against blood schizonts and gametocytes. Artemisinin and its derivatives are short-acting, highly effective antimalarial drugs for the treatment of uncomplicated multidrug-resistant *P. falciparum* and severe *P. falciparum* infection. These drugs are available in oral, rectal, and intravenous formulations. Although they may be used alone to initiate therapy in severe malaria, artemisinin derivatives should be used in combination with another antimalarial with a different mode of action in order to more effectively cure infections, decrease the length of treatment, and safeguard against selecting for drug-resistant parasites.

Common artemisinin-based combination therapies (ACTs) used worldwide include artesunate copackaged with mefloquine (Artequin)[2] and artemether coformulated with lumefantrine (Coartem or Riamet). Coartem (Novartis Pharmaceuticals) has been FDA approved for use in the United States. This lipid-soluble drug should be taken with fatty food or whole milk to improve absorption. Adverse drug reactions are not common but include abdominal pain, headache, anorexia, dizziness, physical weakness, joint pain, and muscle pain. Additionally, parenteral artesunate, an investigational new drug, is available through the CDC for the treatment of severe malaria if quinidine is not available or is not well tolerated. Inquiries regarding artesunate treatment should be directed to the CDC malaria hotline: 770-488-7788 Monday through Friday 9 AM to 5 PM Eastern time or 770-488-7100 after hours, on weekends, and on holidays.

Quinine sulfate (Qualaquin) (oral) and its dextro isomer, quinidine gluconate (parenteral), are commonly used for the treatment of malaria in the United States, and are particularly useful for chloroquine-resistant malaria. They are blood schizonticides that are effective against the erythrocytic stages of all species of plasmodia and are also active against the gametocytes of *P. vivax, P. ovale,* and *P. malariae.* Parenteral quinidine is currently the only FDA-approved treatment for severe malaria in the United States, whereas intravenous or intramuscular formulations of quinine are used in other countries. Owing to potential cardiac toxicity, intravenous quinidine should be administered with telemetry monitoring. Common side effects include cinchonism (a syndrome of tinnitus, hearing loss, headache, nausea, and visual disturbance) and hyperinsulinemic hypoglycemia. As the duration of therapy increases, so does the risk for adverse events. To shorten the course of therapy (from 7 to 3 days), quinine and intravenous quinidine are combined with doxycycline (Vibramycin),[1] tetracycline,[1] or clindamycin (Cleocin)[1] (see Table 1 for details). Malaria acquired in Southeast Asia exhibits decreased responsiveness to quinine and quinidine; therefore, the treatment regimen for cases acquired there should not be shortened.

Tetracyclines are blood schizonticides that are effective against the erythrocytic stages of all species of *Plasmodium.* Because of their relatively slow onset of action, tetracyclines should never be used alone for treatment. Combined with quinine or quinidine, they are effective against chloroquine-resistant *P. falciparum* and *P. vivax.* Doxycycline[1] alone is effective as prophylaxis against chloroquine-resistant and mefloquine-resistant *P. falciparum.* Side effects include gastrointestinal symptoms, *Candida* vaginitis or stomatitis, and idiosyncratic photosensitivity reactions. Tetracyclines should not be used in pregnant women or in children younger than 8 years old.

Clindamycin[1] is active against blood schizonts of all species of *Plasmodium.* Like the tetracyclines, clindamycin should never be used alone to treat malaria. Clindamycin can be used in combination with quinine to treat chloroquine-resistant *P. falciparum* infections in people who are not able to take tetracyclines. Side effects include diarrhea, nausea, and skin rashes.

Mefloquine (formerly Lariam, now only available in generic) is a long-acting blood schizonticide that is used for both prevention and treatment of malaria. It is effective against the erythrocytic stages of all species. Side effects include nausea, vomiting, diarrhea, abdominal pain, myalgia, a mild skin rash, fatigue, and mild neuropsychiatric complaints (dizziness, headache, somnolence,

[1]Not FDA approved for this indication.
[2]Not available in the United States.
[10]Available in the United States from the Centers for Disease Control and Prevention.

[1]Not FDA approved for this indication.
[2]Not available in the United States.

TABLE 1 Recommended Drugs for Treatment of Specific Types of Malaria	
DIAGNOSIS	**RECOMMENDED DRUG**
Uncomplicated chloroquine-sensitive P. falciparum	Chloroquine phosphate (Aralen)
Uncomplicated chloroquine-resistant P. falciparum or Resistance unknown or Species unknown	Atovaquone/proguanil (Malarone) or Artemether-lumefantrine (Coartem) or Quinine sulfate* (Qualaquin) **plus one of the following:** Doxycycline[1,†] or Tetracycline[1,†] or Clindamycin (Cleocin)[1] or Mefloquine[‡]
Uncomplicated P. malariae	Chloroquine phosphate (Aralen)
Uncomplicated P. vivax or P. ovale (except chloroquine-resistant P. vivax)	Chloroquine phosphate (Aralen) **plus** Primaquine phosphate[§]
Uncomplicated chloroquine-resistant P. vivax	Atovaquone/proguanil **plus** primaquine phosphate[§] or Artemether-lumefantrine (Coartem), plus primaquine phosphate or Quinine sulfate* (Qualaquin) **plus one of the following:** Doxycycline[1,†] or Tetracycline[1,†] **plus** Primaquine phosphate[§] or Mefloquine[‡] **plus** primaquine phosphate[§]
Chloroquine sensitive malaria during pregnancy	Chloroquine phosphate (Aralen), or Mefloquine**
Chloroquine-resistant P. falciparum during pregnancy	Quinine sulfate* (Qualaquin) **plus** Clindamycin,[1] or Mefloquine**
Chloroquine-resistant P. vivax during pregnancy	Quinine sulfate* (Qualaquin), or Mefloquine**
Severe malaria	Parenteral quinidine gluconate **plus one of the following:** Doxycycline[1,†] or Tetracycline[1,†] or Clindamycin[1] or Parenteral artesunate[¶] followed by another oral treatment

[1] Not FDA approved for this indication.
*Quinidine/quinine course = 7 d if infection was acquired in Southeast Asia; = 3 d if infection was acquired in Africa or South America.
[†] Not indicated for use in children younger than 8 y.
[‡] Because of resistant strains, treatment with mefloquine is not recommended in persons who have acquired infections in parts of Thailand, Burma, Cambodia, Laos, China, and Vietnam.
[§] All persons who take primaquine should have a documented normal glucose 6 phosphate dehydrogenase level before starting the medication.
[¶] Investigational new drug; contact Centers for Disease Control and Prevention for information.
**FDA changed the mefloquine pregnancy category from C to B, and CDC now recommends mefloquine for pregnant women as an option for both malaria treatment and to prevent malaria infection in all trimesters.

sleep disorders, fuzzy thinking). Mefloquine has also been associated with rare, serious adverse reactions such as seizures and psychoses at prophylactic doses. Although mefloquine can be used to treat chloroquine-resistant P. falciparum, adverse reactions are more common at the higher doses used for treatment than at prophylactic doses. Any traveler receiving a prescription for mefloquine must receive a copy of the FDA Medication Guide (http://www.fda.gov/downloads/Drugs/DrugSafety/ucm088616.pdf).

Because other options that have fewer adverse events are available for treatment, mefloquine normally is not recommended. Mefloquine is contraindicated for use in patients with known hypersensitivity to the drug and persons with a history of psychiatric disease. Mefloquine is also contraindicated in persons with a history of seizures (not including febrile seizures in childhood). It should be avoided in patients with cardiac conduction disorders because it prolongs the QTc interval, and it should be used with caution in persons taking β-blockers. Concomitant administration of mefloquine and quinine or quinidine should be avoided because it can produce arrhythmias and increase the risk of seizures.

Mefloquine prophylaxis in the second and third trimesters is not associated with an adverse fetal or pregnancy outcome. More limited data suggest that though it is rarely used, it is probably safe in the first trimester.

Primaquine phosphate, a tissue schizonticide with gametocytocidal activity, is the only drug available to prevent relapse of P. vivax and P. ovale infections. Primaquine (up to 30 mg/day)[3] has the following uses: primary prophylaxis for destinations where P. vivax is the main species[1]; presumptive antirelapse therapy (PART) to treat the liver stages (hypnozoites) of P. vivax and P. ovale for persons who have had prolonged exposure in malaria-endemic areas such as missionaries, Peace Corps volunteers, and the military[1]; and radical cure of acute P. vivax and P. ovale infection to prevent relapses. Primary prophylaxis with primaquine eliminates the need for PART. The duration of therapy for PART and radical cure is 14 days, given after the patient has left the malarious area and in conjunction with a blood schizonticide.

[1] Not FDA approved for this indication.
[3] Exceeds dosage recommended by the manufacturer.

Primaquine can cause hemolysis and methemoglobinemia in glucose-6-phosphate dehydrogenase (G6PD)-deficient persons. Before primaquine is used the first time, G6PD deficiency must be ruled out by appropriate laboratory testing. The most common side effects are abdominal pain and headache. Primaquine is contraindicated in pregnant women because of the unknown G6PD status of the fetus and in breast-feeding women if the G6PD status of the infant is unknown.

Other antimalarials often encountered in malaria-endemic countries, such as sulfadoxine-pyrimethamine (Fansidar), amodiaquine (Camoquin),[2] proguanil (Paludrine),[2] or halofantrine (Halfan),[2] are not recommended for use in the United States either because of limited efficacy or the side-effect profile.

Treatment

Ideally, treatment for malaria should not be initiated until the diagnosis has been confirmed by laboratory investigations. However, health care providers should not delay treatment when malaria is strongly suspected and smear results are not available in a timely manner. Once the diagnosis is confirmed, appropriate antimalarial therapy must be initiated immediately. The choice of treatment should be guided by the species of *Plasmodium* found, the level of parasitemia, the clinical status of the patient, and the likely drug susceptibility of the infecting species as determined by where the infection was acquired. All species require treatment with a rapidly acting blood schizonticide; patients with *P. vivax* or *P. ovale* also require treatment with primaquine phosphate to decrease the likelihood of a relapse.

Species identification is necessary to distinguish *P. falciparum* malaria from non–*P. falciparum* malaria. *P. falciparum* can cause rapid progression of disease and death; therefore, patients with *P. falciparum*, mixed infections with *P. falciparum*, or infections in which the species cannot be identified immediately should be hospitalized and monitored closely to assess for the development of severe malaria and subsequent complications. Although uncommon, *P. knowlesi* infections also have the capacity to rapidly result in high parasitemia and progress to a potentially fatal outcome. If the infecting species or probable origin of infection cannot be determined, patients should be treated for multidrug-resistant *P. falciparum* until another pathogen is identified. Using available clinical and laboratory data, physicians must determine whether a patient has uncomplicated or severe malaria. Patients with uncomplicated malaria typically can be treated with oral therapy but might need parenteral therapy if they are unable to tolerate oral medications. Patients with severe malaria should be immediately started on parenteral malaria therapy and monitored in an intensive care setting.

After initiating treatment, when clinically indicated, patients should have repeat blood smears to assess appropriate response. Due to the release of sequestered *P. falciparum*-parasitized RBCs from vascular capillary beds, it is not uncommon for parasite density to increase within the first 24 hours after treatment. In such instances, if the patient is improving clinically, the treatment regimen should be continued with monitoring, until blood smears are negative. If the patient does not improve or blood smears remain positive after 7 days, then the clinician should consider drug failure and initiate an alternative treatment regimen.

For detailed treatment information, including doses and frequency of therapy, refer to Tables 1 and 2.

Chloroquine-Sensitive *P. falciparum*, *P. vivax*, *P. ovale*, *P. malariae*, and *P. knowlesi*

For *P. malariae*, *P. ovale*, *P. knowlesi*, chloroquine-sensitive *P. vivax*, and chloroquine-sensitive *P. falciparum* infection, prompt treatment with oral chloroquine phosphate (Aralen) is recommended. If chloroquine is not available, then other treatments can be used. In addition, infections with *P. vivax* and *P. ovale* require primaquine to reduce the likelihood of a relapse, if patients have a documented normal level of G6PD activity.

Drug-Resistant *P. falciparum*

For *P. falciparum* infections acquired in chloroquine-resistant areas, there are four treatment options: atovaquoneproguanil-lumefantrine; artemether-lumafantrine; quinine sulfate (Qualaquin) plus doxycycline,[1] tetracycline,[1] or clindamycin[1]; and mefloquine Because mefloquine has a higher rate of severe neuropsychiatric reactions at treatment doses, it is recommended only when the other options are not available. Mefloquine is also not recommended for the treatment of falciparum malaria in persons who acquired the infection in Southeast Asia, especially Thailand, Cambodia, Burma (Myanmar), Laos, and Vietnam, because of the potential that the infection results from a mefloquine-resistant strain. Because artemisinin-tolerant strains have been limited to patients in Southeast Asia, and artemether-lumafantrine has only recently been released in the United States, the impact of artemisinin-tolerant strains on clinical managxement of U.S. patients with malaria remains to be seen.

Drug-Resistant *P. vivax*

P. vivax infections acquired in areas with chloroquine resistance can be treated with either of three treatment options: quinine sulfate plus doxycycline[1] or tetracycline,[1] atovaquone-proguanil, or mefloquine alone. As noted earlier, its use is limited by the preponderance of severe neuropsychiatric adverse effects when mefloquine is administered at the treatment dosage. In addition to either of those regimens, persons who have a normal level of G6PD activity and who are infected with *P. vivax* should be treated with primaquine phosphate to prevent relapse.

Severe Malaria

Patients with severe malaria, regardless of species, and those who are unable to take oral medications should be treated with parenteral antimalarial therapy. Severe malaria is a medical emergency, and treatment with intravenous medication should be initiated immediately (see Tables 1 and 2). In the United States, quinidine gluconate is the only parenteral rapidly acting blood schizonticide approved by the FDA. Under an investigational new drug protocol, artesunate, a parenteral drug for the treatment of severe malaria, is available now through the CDC in the United States. Health care providers caring for patients with severe malaria should contact the CDC to assess the need for artesunate (CDC Malaria Hotline: 770-488-7788, Monday through Friday, 9 AM to 5 PM Eastern time; emergency consultation: 770-488-7100 after hours). In addition to antimalarial therapy, patients should receive the necessary supportive care.

The patient should be admitted to an intensive care unit with continuous cardiac monitoring (to assess the QTc interval) and regular measurements of blood pressure and blood glucose. Fluid status, level of consciousness, and vital signs should be monitored closely. Because these patients are at risk for hypoglycemia, severe anemia, renal failure, and acidosis, regular assessment of blood glucose, hemoglobin and hematocrit, creatinine, urea, electrolytes, and acid-base status also is required. Severe anemia requires blood transfusion with packed red blood cells. Hemodialysis or hemofiltration is usually needed in patients with acute renal failure. Oxygen and other respiratory support may be required in patients with ARDS. Thrombocytopenia is common with malaria and should be managed appropriately, but it is not an indicator of severe malaria. One should consider exchange transfusion if parasitemia is greater than 10% or if the patient has altered mental status, ARDS, or renal complications. Blood smears should be initially repeated every 12 hours to monitor response. Once parasite density is lower than 1% and the patient is able to eat and drink, the treatment course should be completed with oral medications.

Various adjunctive therapies for malaria have been shown to be ineffective and sometimes even harmful. These include corticosteroids[1] for the treatment of cerebral malaria, phenobarbital for seizure prophylaxis, heparin for coagulation abnormalities, iron

---

[2]Not available in the United States.

[1]Not FDA approved for this indication.

TABLE 2 Treatment Dosages of Antimalarial Drugs		
DRUG	**ADULT DOSAGE**	**PEDIATRIC DOSAGE***
Artesunate[†]	2.4 mg/kg IV push at 0, 12, 24, and 48 h	2.4 mg/kg IV push at 0, 12, 24, and 48 h
Atovaquone-proguanil (Malarone)	4 adult tabs (each adult tab contains 250 mg atovaquone and 100 mg proguanil) PO as a single daily dose for 3 consecutive days	Dosage is based on weight Each ped tab contains 62.5 mg atovaquone and 25 mg proguanil Daily dose to be taken for 3 consecutive days: 5–8 kg: 2 ped tabs 9–10 kg: 3 ped tabs 11–20 kg: 1 adult tab 21–30 kg: 2 adult tabs 31–40 kg: 3 adult tabs ≥41 kg: 4 adult tabs
Artemether-lumefantrine (Coartem)	1 tab = 20 mg artemether and 120 mg lumefantrine A 3-d treatment schedule with a total of 6 oral doses is recommended for both adult and pediatric patients based on weight The patient should receive the initial dose, followed by the second dose 8 h later, then 1 dose PO bid for the following 2 d. Medication should be taken with food or whole milk to improve absorption. 5 to <15 kg: 1 tab per dose 15 to <25 kg: 2 tabs per dose 25 to <35 kg: 3 tabs per dose ≥35 kg: 4 tabs per dose	
Chloroquine phosphate (Aralen)	600 mg base (=1 g salt) PO, then 300 mg base (=500 mg salt) at 6, 24 and 48 h	10 mg base/kg PO, then 5 mg base/kg at 6, 24 and 48 h
Clindamycin, oral (Cleocin)[1]	20 mg base/kg/d PO divided tid × 7 d	20 mg base/kg/d PO divided tid × 7 d
Clindamycin, parenteral[1]	10 mg base/kg IV followed by 5 mg base/kg IV q8h Switch to oral clindamycin as soon as patient is able to complete 7 d course	10 mg base/kg IV followed by 5 mg base/kg IV q8h Switch to oral clindamycin as soon as patient is able to complete 7-d course
Doxycycline (Vibramycin)[1,‡]	100 mg PO or IV bid × 7 d	2.2 mg/kg PO or IV bid × 7 d[‡]
Mefloquine**	750 mg salt (=684 mg base) PO followed by 500 mg salt (=456 mg base) PO 6–12 h after the initial dose	15 mg salt/kg (=13.7 mg base/kg) PO followed by 10 mg salt/kg (=9.1 mg base/kg) PO 6–12 h after the initial dose
Primaquine phosphate[¶]	30 mg base PO qd × 14 d[3]	0.5 mg base/kg PO qd × 14 d[3]
Quinidine gluconate	6.25 mg base/kg (=10 mg salt/kg) loading dose[§] IV over 1–2 h, then 0.0125 mg base/kg/min (=0.02 mg salt/kg/min) continuous infusion for at least 24 h Alternative regimen: 15 mg base/kg (=24 mg salt/kg) loading dose IV infused over 4 h, followed by 7.5 mg base/kg (=12 mg salt/kg) infused over 4 h q8h, starting 8 h after the loading dose Once parasite density <1% and patient can take oral medication, complete treatment with oral quinine	6.25 mg base/kg (=10 mg salt/kg) loading dose[§] IV over 1–2 h, then 0.0125 mg base/kg/min (=0.02 mg salt/kg/min) continuous infusion for at least 24 h Alternative regimen: 15 mg base/kg (=24 mg salt/kg) loading dose IV infused over 4 h, followed by 7.5 mg base/kg (=12 mg salt/kg) infused over 4 h q8h, starting 8 h after the loading dose Once parasite density <1% and patient can take oral medication, complete treatment with oral quinine
Quinine sulfate (Qualaquin)	650 mg salt (=542 mg base) PO tid × 3 or 7 d (×7 d if acquired in Southeast Asia)	10 mg salt/kg (=8.3 mg base/kg) PO tid × 3 d (×7 d if acquired in Southeast Asia)
Tetracycline[1,‡]	250 mg PO qid × 7 d	25 mg/kg/d PO divided qid × 7 d[‡]

[1]Not FDA approved for this indication.
[3]Exceeds dosage recommended by the manufacturer.
*Pediatric dose should *never* exceed adult dose.
[†]Available only through the Centers for Disease Control and Prevention in the United States.
[‡]Doxycycline and tetracycline are not indicated for use in children younger than 8 years.
[§]Patients should be given a loading dose of quinidine unless they have received >40 mg/kg of quinine in the preceding 48 h or if they received mefloquine treatment within the preceding 12 h.
[¶]All persons who take primaquine should have a documented normal glucose 6 phosphate dehydrogenase level prior to starting the medication.
**FDA changed the mefloquine pregnancy category from C to B and CDC now recommends mefloquine for pregnant women as an option for both malaria treatment and to prevent malaria infection in all trimesters.

chelators[1] to reduce parasite clearance time, pentoxifylline (Trental)[1] to inhibit tumor necrosis system, and dichloroacetate[1] for treatment of metabolic acidosis.

Congenital and Pregnancy-Associated Malaria

Malaria in pregnancy affects both the mother and her fetus. Infection with *P. falciparum* during pregnancy can increase the mother's risk of developing severe disease and anemia as well as increasing the risk of stillbirth, prematurity, and low birth weight, especially for women in their first or second pregnancies and those who are immunocompromised. Babies born to nonimmune mothers with acute malaria are at risk for congenital malaria, but empiric treatment is not recommended. Congenital malaria often manifests as fever, anemia, or failure to thrive at 1 to 2 months of age and can be difficult for an unsuspecting clinician to detect. If the child is asymptomatic at the time of the delivery, blood smears are not recommended. Instead, health care providers should remain alert for the development of signs and symptoms consistent with malaria and initiate a prompt diagnostic evaluation. Treating physicians should judge each case individually, considering such

[1]Not FDA approved for this indication.

factors as reliability of follow-up and access to medical care. Educating the mother about the risk of congenital malaria and instructing her to seek medical care if the infant develops symptoms of malaria may be appropriate in most cases, while presumptive treatment of the newborn may be warranted in others. Primaquine treatment of infants is unnecessary because there is no liver phase with congenitally acquired infections.

For pregnant women with uncomplicated malaria caused by *P. malariae*, *P. ovale*, chloroquine-sensitive *P. vivax*, and chloroquine-sensitive *P. falciparum*, prompt treatment with chloroquine (Aralen) is recommended. For pregnant women who acquired *P. vivax* in a region of chloroquine-resistance, treatment with quinine (Qualaquin) for 7 days is recommended. After treatment, all pregnant women with *P. vivax* and *P. ovale* should be given chloroquine prophylaxis for the duration of the pregnancy to avoid relapses; women may be treated with primaquine after delivery if they (and their infant, if breastfeeding) have a normal G6PD screening test. For pregnant women with uncomplicated chloroquine-resistant *P. falciparum* malaria, prompt treatment with quinine plus clindamycin[1] or mefloquine is recommended. (In 2011, the FDA changed the mefloquine pregnancy category from C to B, and therefore CDC now recommends mefloquine for pregnant women as an option for both malaria treatment and to prevent malaria infection in all trimesters.)

Malaria in Children

For pediatric patients, treatment options are the same as those for adults except that the drug dosage is adjusted by the patient's weight. The pediatric dosage should never exceed the recommended adult dosage. For treatment of chloroquine-resistant *P. falciparum* in children younger than 8 years, doxycycline and tetracycline should not be used. Quinine sulfate (if appropriately dosed) or quinidine may be given in combination with clindamycin[1] to children. Alternatively, children weighing >5 kg can be treated with atovaquone-proguanil or artemether-lumefantrine. Mefloquine can be considered if these options are not available.

In rare instances, doxycycline[1] or tetracycline[1] can be used in combination with quinine in children younger than 8 years if other treatment options are not available or are not tolerated and the benefit of adding doxycycline or tetracycline is judged to outweigh the risk.

Prevention

A combination of personal protective measures and chemoprophylaxis can be highly effective in preventing malaria in travelers and those living in malaria-endemic areas. Malaria-endemic countries have focused on delivering person- and household-level protection through insecticide-treated nets and indoor residual spraying with insecticides. Chemoprophylaxis in the form of intermittent preventive treatment of high-risk groups, pregnant women, and infants has been adopted by several malaria-endemic countries.

Other protective measures include mosquito avoidance (indoors and outdoors) during the peak *Anopheles* biting period between dusk and dawn by wearing clothing that minimizes the amount of exposed skin and applying insect repellents that contain DEET (diethylmethyl-toluamide). DEET may be used on adults, children, and infants older than 2 months. Higher concentrations of DEET can have a longer repellent effect; however, concentrations over 50% provide no added protection. Alternatively, repellents that contain picaridin (e.g., Cutter Advanced Insect Repellent) and IR3535 (e.g., Skin So Soft Bug Guard Plus) are also recommended by the CDC. Travelers who are not staying in well-screened or air-conditioned rooms should sleep under insecticide-treated bed nets.

For travelers to malaria-endemic areas, chemoprophylaxis with an appropriate antimalarial drug is effective in preventing malaria infection. The choice of prophylactic medication should be made in light of the traveler's destination, length of stay, the presence of resistant strains, age, drug allergies, other medications, and medical history. Often, potential side effects, convenience of the dosing regimen, and cost affect patients' choices of medications. Detailed prophylaxis recommendations are presented in Table 3.

---

[1]Not FDA approved for this indication.

	DRUG	**USE**	**ADULT DOSAGE**	**PEDIATRIC DOSAGE**	**COMMENTS**
TABLE 3	Malaria Chemoprophylaxis Recommendations				
	Atovaquone/ proguanil (Malarone)	Prophylaxis in all malaria risk areas	Adult tabs contain 250 mg atovaquone and 100 mg proguanil HCl 1 adult tab PO qd	Ped tabs contain 62.5 mg atovaquone and 25 mg proguanil HCl 5–8 kg[1]: 2 ped tabs PO qd 9–10 kg[1]: 3 ped tab PO qd 11–20 kg: 1 adult tab PO qd 21–30 kg: 2 adult tabs PO qd >31–40 kg: 3 adult tabs PO qd >40 kg: 4 adult tabs PO qd	Begin 1–2 d before travel to malarious areas Take daily at the same time each day while in the malarious area and for 7 d after leaving such areas Contraindicated in persons with severe renal impairment (creatinine clearance <30 mL/min) Atovaquone/proguanil should be taken with food Not recommended for prophylaxis for children <5 kg or pregnant women Partial tab dosages may need to be prepared by a pharmacist and dispensed in individual caps
	Chloroquine phosphate* (Aralen and generic)	Prophylaxis only in areas with chloroquine-sensitive *P. falciparum*	300 mg base (500 mg salt) PO 1×/wk	5 mg/kg base (8.3 mg/ kg salt) PO 1×/wk, up to maximum adult dose of 300 mg base	Begin 1–2 wk before travel to malarious areas Take weekly on the same day of the week while in the malarious area and for 4 wk after leaving such areas Can exacerbate psoriasis
	Doxycycline†	Prophylaxis in all malaria risk areas	100 mg PO qd	≥8 yr of age: 2 mg/kg up to adult dose of 100 mg/d*	Begin 1–2 d before travel to malarious areas Take daily at the same time each day while in the malarious area and for 4 wk after leaving such areas Contraindicated in children <8 yr of age and pregnant women

TABLE 3   Malaria Chemoprophylaxis Recommendations—cont'd

DRUG	USE	ADULT DOSAGE	PEDIATRIC DOSAGE	COMMENTS
Hydroxychloroquine sulfate (Plaquenil)	An alternative to chloroquine for prophylaxis only in areas with chloroquine-sensitive *P. falciparum*	310 mg base (400 mg salt) PO 1×/wk	5 mg/kg base (6.5 mg/kg salt) PO 1×/wk, up to max adult dose of 310 mg base	Begin 1–2 wk before travel to malarious areas Take weekly on the same day of the week while in the malarious area and for 4 wk after leaving such areas
Mefloquine§	Prophylaxis in areas with mefloquine-sensitive *P. falciparum*	228 mg base (250 mg salt) PO 1×/wk	≤9 kg: 4.6 mg/kg base (5 mg/kg salt) PO 1×/wk 10–19 kg: ¼ tab PO 1×/wk 20–30 kg: ½ tab PO 1×/wk 31–45 kg: ¾ tab PO 1×/wk ≥46 kg: 1 tab PO 1×/wk	Begin 1–2 wk before travel to malarious areas Take weekly on the same day of the week while in the malarious area and for 4 wk after leaving such areas Contraindicated in persons allergic to mefloquine or related compounds (e.g., quinine and quinidine) and in persons with active depression, a recent history of depression, generalized anxiety disorder, psychosis, schizophrenia, other major psychiatric disorders, or seizures Use with caution in persons with psychiatric disturbances or a previous history of depression Not recommended for persons with cardiac conduction abnormalities
Primaquine phosphate[1],‡	Prophylaxis in areas with mainly *P. vivax*	30 mg base (52.6 mg salt) PO qd[3]	0.6 mg/kg base (1.0 mg/kg salt) up to adult dose PO qd[3]	Begin 1–2 d before travel to malarious areas Take daily at the same time each day while in the malarious area and for 7 ds after leaving such areas Contraindicated in persons with G6PD† deficiency Contraindicated during pregnancy and lactation unless the infant being breast-fed has a documented normal G6PD level
Primaquine phosphate†	Used for presumptive antirelapse therapy (terminal prophylaxis) to decrease the risk of relapses of *P. vivax* and *P. ovale*	30 mg base (52.6 mg salt) PO qd × 14 d after departure from the malarious area[3]	0.6 mg/kg base (1.0 mg/kg salt) up to adult dose PO qd × 14 d after departure from the malarious area[3]	Indicated for persons who have had prolonged exposure to *P. vivax* or *P. ovale* or both Contraindicated in persons with G6PD‡ deficiency Contraindicated during pregnancy and lactation unless the infant being breast-fed has a documented normal G6PD level

[1]Not FDA approved for this indication.
[3]Exceeds dosage recommended by the manufacturer.
*All pregnant women with *P. vivax* and *P. ovale* should be given chloroquine prophylaxis for the duration of pregnancy to avoid relapses and can be treated with primaquine after delivery.
†Doxycycline and tetracycline are not indicated for use in children younger than 8 y.
§FDA changed the mefloquine pregnancy category from C to B, and CDC now recommends mefloquine for pregnant women as an option for both malaria treatment and to prevent malaria infection in all trimesters.
‡All persons who take primaquine should have a documented normal G6PD level before starting the medication.
Abbreviations: cap = capsule; G6PD = glucose 6 phosphate dehydrogenase; max = maximum; ped = pediatric; tab = tablet.

Malaria infection in pregnant women can be more severe than it is in nonpregnant women. Women who are pregnant or likely to become pregnant should be advised to avoid travel to malaria-risk areas. However, pregnant women who choose to travel to these areas should take appropriate antimalarial prophylaxis and use personal protective measures. Mefloquine can be used for prophylaxis in all trimesters of pregnancy.

Travelers should be advised that they can contract malaria despite the use of prophylaxis and personal protective measures. Travelers should be aware of the signs and symptoms of malaria and should urgently seek medical care if they develop fever or experience flulike symptoms. Because many health care providers do not always ask about a history of recent travel, travelers should be advised to specifically inform providers of their recent travel to a malaria-endemic area so that the appropriate diagnostic evaluation and treatment can be initiated.

A malaria vaccine to protect against the development of illness or to dampen the severity of disease has been elusive despite the development of more than 45 vaccine candidates from 1990 to 2008. The Malaria Vaccine Initiative, partnered with GlaxoSmithKline, has brought a vaccine candidate, RTS,S/AS01, to phase III clinical trials, the first in recent years to progress to such levels. RTS,S is a pre-erythrocytic vaccine designed to promote antibody and T_H1 cell-mediated responses to the circumsporozoite protein expressed on the surface of *P. falciparum* sporozoites. This strategy aims to prevent clinical malaria illness by interfering with parasite progression to blood-stage disease. Studies to date show RTS,S to be of promising efficacy in children and infants living in endemic areas. Though a vaccine is not currently available for travelers or the military, RTS,S is a prospective future tool to decrease malaria burden in endemic areas and in the most vulnerable populations.

References

Baird JK. Effectiveness of antimalarial drugs. N Engl J Med 2005;352(15):1565–77.

Centers for Disease Control and Prevention. Guidelines for Treatment of Malaria in the United States. PDF available at: http://www.cdc.gov/malaria/resources/pdf/treatmenttable.pdf [accessed July 9, 2015].

Food and Drug Administration. FDA Approves Coartem Tablets to Treat Malaria. PDF available at: http://www.fda.gov/NewsEvents/Newsroom/PressAnnouncements/2009/ucm149559.htm [accessed July 9, 2015].

Griffith KS, Lewis LS, Mali S, Parise ME, et al. Treatment of malaria in the United States: A systematic review. JAMA 2007;297(20):2264–77.

Lalloo DG, Hill DR. Preventing malaria in travellers. BMJ 2008;336(7657):1362–6.

Mali S, Kachur SP, Arguin PM. Centers for Disease Control and Prevention (CDC): Malaria Surveillance - United States, 2010. MMWR Surveillance Summaries March 2, 2012;61(SSO2):1–17.

Newman RD, Parise ME, Barber AM, Steketee RW. Malaria-related deaths among U.S. travelers, 1963–2001. Ann Intern Med 2004;141(7):547–55.

Price RN, Douglas NM, Anstey NM. New developments in *Plasmodium vivax* malaria: Severe disease and the rise of chloroquine resistance. Curr Opin Infect Dis 2009;22(5):430–5.

Rosenthal PJ. Artesunate for the treatment of severe falciparum malaria. N Engl J Med 2008;358(17):1829–36.

Targett GA, Greenwood BM. Malaria vaccines and their potential role in the elimination of malaria. Malar J 2008;7(Suppl. 1):S10.

World Health Organization. Severe falciparum malaria. World Health Organization, Communicable Diseases Cluster. Trans R Soc Trop Med Hyg 2000;94(Suppl. 1):S1–90.

World Health Organization. World Malaria Report 2013. Geneva: World Health Organization; 2013.

MEASLES

Method of
Laurie Hommema, MD

CURRENT DIAGNOSIS

Viral prodrome including fever, cough, coryza, conjunctivitis, and Koplik spots.

Generalized, macular-popular rash develops 2 to 4 days after viral prodrome.

History of exposure; travel to endemic area or region affected by outbreak.

Nonvaccinated or incomplete vaccination status.

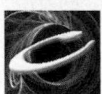

CURRENT THERAPY

Vaccination is the key for prevention of disease.

Supportive Care
- Fluid hydration, oral or IV
- Antipyretics
- Rest
- Antibiotics for secondary bacterial infection

Epidemiology

Also known as rubeola, measles was declared eliminated in the United States in 2000, but has unfortunately returned in multistate outbreaks. Prior to the introduction of the national vaccination program in 1963, approximately 3 to 4 million cases of measles occurred each year, with 500,000 reported. Each year during this time, 500 deaths, 48,000 hospitalizations, and 1000 cases of permanent brain damage were attributed to measles. Cases dropped dramatically from 25,000 to 75,000 per year in the 1970s, to 3750 per year in the mid 1980s. At that time a two vaccine regimen was introduced, and by 2000 measles was considered eliminated in the United States. However, over 2 million cases of measles occur worldwide each year. More recently a decline in vaccinations rates

in the United States for various reasons has led to a resurgence of measles outbreaks when an infected individual is introduced to the population. In 2014 alone, 644 cases from 27 states were reported, which is the largest number of cases since 2000.

Risk factors

Unvaccinated status and contact with infected persons are the largest risk factors in the United States. Contact with infected individuals can occur in a multitude of locations. Careful social and travel history must be obtained for suspected cases. Travel to an international location where measles is still endemic or there is a local outbreak is an essential factor in making the diagnosis in the United States.

Pathophysiology

A member of the genus *Morbillivirus* in the family *Paramyxoviridae,* measles is considered one of the most infectious viral pathogens. The disease is contracted by contact with respiratory droplets of an infected individual. Up to 90% of susceptible individuals develop measles after exposure. An infected individual is considered contagious 4 days prior to the appearance of a rash and 4 days after it is gone. The virus itself remains viable both on surfaces and in the air for 2 hours after a cough or sneeze. Case reports demonstrate that aerosol transmission across large spaces is possible, such as a gymnasium. Average incubation period of the disease is 10 to 14 days.

Prevention

The best way to prevent contracting measles is through individual and herd immunity with vaccination. The MMR (measles, mumps, and rubella) vaccine series is recommended for all individuals born after 1957, with few exceptions. Exceptions include individuals with primary or acquired immunodeficiency, individuals with blood dyscrasias, those with a family history of a first degree relative with hereditary or congenital immunodeficiency, individuals receiving systemic immunosuppressive therapy, and pregnant women. The MMR vaccine is given in children over 1 year of age, and adults in two doses separated by at least 28 days. One dose of vaccine has been shown to provided 95% immunity, and up to 99% immunity after two doses.

The majority of people who have recently contracted measles in the United States have been unvaccinated. Isolation of infected individuals is also recommended, and all suspected cases must be reported to local health departments. There are currently no clear guidelines on the isolation of measles patients. The majority of cases do not need to be hospitalized, but often visit their primary care physician for diagnosis. Masks should be placed on the patient, family, and staff. All health care workers should have documented immunity, and if not, it is recommended they do not treat suspected cases. Measles can remain airborne for up to 2 hours, therefore if possible, keep rooms closed after use, and exits separate for infected individuals.

Postexposure prophylaxis for those exposed to measles is an option for prevention of disease. MMR vaccine may alter the clinical course and offer protection if it is given within 72 hours of initial exposure. Immune globulin (IGIM) can be considered to reduce the risk for infection and complications if given within 6 days of exposure, and is usually reserved for those immunocompromised or who can otherwise not receive the vaccine.

Clinical Manifestations

Symptoms of measles present in two stages. The first stage starts with a viral prodrome of coryza, cough, fever (>38.3 ° C), Koplik spots, conjunctivitis and photophobia. The second stage consists of a generalized, macular popular, erythematous exanthem. Described as 1 to 3 mm white elevations on an erythematous base, Koplik spots can also be seen on the palate and labial mucosa. Koplik spots develop in the buccal mucosa a few days prior to exanthem, and fade and slough during exanthem progression. The exanthem typically begins behind the ears and along the hairline, then proceeds downward to the trunk and extremities. Often the exanthem become confluent, with possible petechiae, and eventually darkens to a brown color. The rash lasts for a total of 6 to 7 days, eventually fading with a fine desquamation.

Diagnosis

Diagnosis is based primarily on clinical presentation, vaccination, travel, and exposure history. Blood counts may show leukopenia, T cell cytopenia, and thrombocytopenia. Histologic evaluation may show giant cells with inclusions in conjunctival, nasopharyngeal, or buccal epithelial cells.

Confirmation can be made by enzyme-linked immunosorbent assay (ELISA) detection of measles specific antibodies. Immunoglobulin M (IgM) is detectable three days after the appearance of the rash, and for up to 30 days after. Immunoglobulin G (IgG) peaks around 14 days after rash. Viral cultures can be obtained from blood, respiratory secretions, conjunctival swabs, or urine. If suspected, obtain specimens for confirmation and genotyping. Local health departments will assist in choosing and submitting specimens for testing.

Differential Diagnosis

In the early stages of disease, measles can appear similar to any viral upper respiratory infection. The viral prodrome is similar to that of the rhinovirus, parainfluenza, adenovirus, respiratory syncytial virus, and influenza. Koplik spots are pathognomonic, but often subtle and overlooked. When the viral exanthema appears, it can be confused with roseola, rubella, scarlet fever, drug eruption, parvovirus B19 infection, and Kawasaki disease.

Therapy

There is currently no specific therapy for measles. Supportive care including fluids, antipyretics, and treatment of secondary bacterial infections are the mainstay of therapy. Avoidance of light for those with photosensitivity is recommended. There is a role for vitamin A[1] in developing countries, but it is not routinely recommended in the United States. Ribavirin (Rebetol)[1] has been shown to be effective in vitro; limited case reports are available.

Monitoring

Follow up visits for confirmed measles are not required unless the patient develops complications. Dehydration from diarrhea, ear pain from otitis media, and difficulty breathing, or prolonged and productive cough are reasons to seek further care. Most cases are self-limiting, and resolve at home with supportive care.

If a patient requires hospitalization, respiratory isolation should be initiated. Rooms should be under negative pressure ventilation and masks (N95) used at all time. Only health care workers with documented immunity should care for these patients. Providers should work closely with their local health departments to determine length of monitoring for contacts, and isolation for confirmed cases.

Complications

Measles can cause many complications, some self-limiting, and others life threatening. Common complications include otitis media (3% to 9%), bronchitis, or bronchopneumonia (1% to 6%). 1 in 1000 infections is complicated by encephalitis. A rare, often fatal neurologic degenerative disease, known as subacute sclerosing panencephalitis can develop 7 to 10 years after acute measles. A higher risk is seen in individuals who are less than 2 years of age when measles is contracted, but averages 4 to 11 per 100,000 cases. Secondary bacterial infections are common because of immunosuppression by the virus, and are responsible for most measles deaths. Overall the risk for death is higher in infants, young children, and adults. Worldwide the death rate can be as high as 25%, particularly in areas where malnutrition is prevalent.

---

[1]Not FDA approved for this indication.

References

Centers for Disease Control and Prevention. Prevention of measles, rubella, congenital rubella syndrome, and mumps, 2013: summary recommendations of the Advisory Committee on Immunization Practices. MMWR Recomm Rep 2013;62:1–34.

Cherry JD. Measles virus. In: Feigin RD, Cherry JD, Demmler-Harrison GJ, et al., editors. Textbook of Pediatric Infectious Diseases. 6th ed. Philadelphia: Elsevier; 2009. p. 2427.

Griffin DE, Bellini WJ. Measles virus. In: Fields BN, Knipe DM, Howley PM, editors. Fields' Virology. Philadelphia: Lippincott-Raven; 1996. p. 1267.

Helmecke MR, Elmendorf SL, Kent DL, et al. Measles investigation: a moving target. Am J Infect Control 2014;42:911–5.

Infectious Disease Society of America: U.S. Multi-state measles outbreak. December 2014–January 2015. Available at: http://www.idsociety.org/Breaking_News_and_Alerts/CDC_IIAN/U_S__Multi-state_Measles_Outbreak,_December_2014-January_2015_(content)/ [accessed 07.05.15].

McLean HQ, Fiebelkorn AP, Temte JL, Wallace GS. Centers for Disease Control and Prevention. Prevention of measles, rubella, congenital rubella syndrome, and mumps, 2013. Summary recommendations of the Advisory Committee on Immunization Practices. MMWR Recomm Rep 2013;62:1–34.

Measles cases and outbreaks. Available at: http://www.cdc.gov/measles/cases-outbreaks.html [accessed 01.02.15].

Treating measles in children. Geneva: World Health Organization; 2004 updated. http://www.measlesinitiative.org/mi-files/Reports/Treatment/Treating%20Measles%20in%20Children.pdf. [accessed 20.01.15].

METHICILLIN-RESISTANT *STAPHYLOCOCCUS AUREUS* (MRSA)

Method of
John M. Conly, MD

CURRENT DIAGNOSIS

- Health care–associated methicillin-resistant *Staphylococcus aureus* (HA-MRSA) is endemic in many hospital settings. The strains are polyclonal, resistant to many non β lactam antimicrobials, and typically cause pneumonia, line-related infection, surgical site infection, bacteremia, and infrequently skin and soft tissue infections.
- Community-associated strains of MRSA (CA-MRSA) have risen exponentially over the past decade. The strains are clonal, sensitive to many non–β-lactam antimicrobials, harbor multiple virulence factors, and typically cause pyogenic skin and soft tissue infections and occasionally severe necrotizing pneumonia, fasciitis, and multifocal osteomyelitis.
- HA-MRSA infections typically affect patients with multiple comorbidities in the health care setting, but CA-MRSA typically affects previously healthy persons.
- It can be difficult to differentiate infectious syndromes due to β-hemolytic streptococci versus CA-MRSA

CURRENT THERAPY

- MRSA strains harbor resistance to the β-lactam antimicrobials, including oxacillin, dicloxacillin, cloxacillin,[2] nafcillin, methicillin,[2] and first-, second-, and third-generation cephalosporins.
- HA-MRSA strains are typically resistant to macrolides, clindamycin (Cleocin), aminoglycosides, and quinolones and are variably resistant to tetracycline and trimethoprim-sulfamethoxazole (Bactrim). They are sensitive to vancomycin (Vancocin), fusidic acid,[2] rifampin (Rifadin),[1] linezolid (Zyvox), and daptomycin (Cubicin).
- CA-MRSA strains are resistant to macrolides and quinolones but usually sensitive to aminoglycosides such as gentamicin (Garamycin), clindamycin, and trimethoprim-sulfamethoxazole.
- Empiric antimicrobial therapy should be guided by the clinical presentation, and when full sensitivities are available, the antimicrobials may be tailored accordingly.

---

[1]Not FDA approved for this indication.
[2]Not available in the United States.

Epidemiology

Staphylococcus aureus is one of the most frequently encountered bacteria causing human infections and may be considered as either methicillin-sensitive *S. aureus* (MSSA) or methicillin-resistant *S. aureus* (MRSA). MRSA was first described in 1961 and is not only resistant to the traditional antistaphylococcal β-lactam antibiotics (methicillin,[2] nafcillin, oxacillin, cloxacillin,[2] dicloxacillin) but also other important β-lactam antibiotics, including the first- to fourth-generation cephalosporins and the carbapenem family, thus eliminating an important class of antibiotics from the clinician's armamentarium. The only β-lactam that has activity against MRSA is the recently approved advanced-generation cephalosporin agent ceftaroline (Teflaro).

MRSA strains acquired in the hospital or other health care settings have traditionally been referred to as health care–associated MRSA (HA-MRSA) whereas community-associated MRSA (CA-MRSA) has referred to isolates acquired in the community setting and in the absence of traditional hospital or health care exposures for at least 1 year (overnight stays in an acute care or long-term care facility, surgery, dialysis, or presence of a central venous catheter). Recently the term *community-onset HA-MRSA* has been used to describe the occurrence of MRSA infection in the setting of the presence of a health care exposure within the past year. MRSA has been recognized as a health care–associated pathogen since the 1970s, and became endemic in hospitals in many countries, including the United States, United Kingdom, and many European countries over the next two decades with exceptions being Denmark, the Netherlands, Scandinavia, and Canada. For several decades, MRSA was typically considered a hospital pathogen. Novel and virulent MRSA strains arising in the community and not associated with any traditional health care exposure risks were first encountered in the late 1990s in the United States, Australia, and some European countries and have since risen explosively on a global basis to become the predominant clone of *S. aureus* associated with community infections. Methicillin resistance among community isolates of *S. aureus* has been reported as high as 75% in some U.S. communities. More recently livestock-associated MRSA (LA-MRSA) has been reported on a global basis and transmission of these strains from swine, cattle and horses has been implicated as a source of human infections, particularly in farmers, abattoir workers and veterinarians.

[2]Not available in the United States.

Specific genetic and molecular distinctions initially distinguished the HA- and CA-MRSA strains (Table 1) and have been used to characterize MRSA strains as likely of community or health care origin. The HA-MRSA strains were found to harbor large staphylococcal cassette chromosome (SCC*mec*) types known as SCC*mec* types I, II, or III; to have multidrug resistance to non–β-lactam antimicrobials; to have the absence of specific virulence characteristics such as carriage of the Panton-Valentine Leukocidin (PVL) gene; and to have varying multilocus sequence types (ST5, ST239, ST 247, ST250). On the other hand, the CA-MRSA strains have been found to harbor SCC*mec* types IV, V, and more recently VI to XI have been described; to have paucidrug resistance to non–β-lactam antimicrobials; to have the presence of specific virulence characteristics such as carriage of the Panton-Valentine Leukocidin gene, and to have multilocus sequence types ST1, ST8, ST80. LA-MRSA strains often are non-typeable or harbor SCC*mec* V, have high rates of tetracycline resistance, carry multiple virulence factors. and are most often multilocus sequence types ST398 or ST9. However, over the last few years, health care–associated strains have moved into the community and likewise community strains have spread rapidly within hospitals, and the original distinctions between CA-MRSA and HA-MRSA from an epidemiologic perspective has become increasingly blurred. The point of transmission of MRSA is not always possible to identify with certainty, making the classification of CA and HA strains increasingly imprecise.

Risk Factors

The risk factors for HA-MRSA may be viewed from the perspective of the health care environment and patient-specific risk factors. A major risk factor for acquiring HA-MRSA is exposure to a health care setting and particularly in hospital or other institutional settings where the prevalence of carriage of MRSA among patients is high. Additional risk factors in the health care environment include poor hand hygiene practices among hospital employees, contaminated bedside equipment and surfaces, overcrowding, and reduced health care worker–to–patient ratios. Patient risk factors (see Table 1) include aging, multiple comorbidities, receipt of antibiotics within the preceding 3 months, prolonged duration of hospital stay, admission to a long-term care facility or hospital in the previous year, invasive procedures, and the presence of indwelling catheters or other devices. Initial risk groups for CA-MRSA were injection drug users, homeless populations, incarcerated persons, and indigenous peoples, and the

---

TABLE 1 General Features Differentiating HA- and CA-MRSA*

CHARACTERISTIC	HA-MRSA	CA-MRSA
SCC*mec* types	I, II, III	IV, V (VI–X1)
Drug resistance to non–β-lactams	Multiresistance	Pauciresistance
Presence of PVL	—	+
Pathogenicity islands	Few	Multiple
MLST	5, 45, 239, 247, 250	1, 8, 80, 398†
Pulsotype	USA100, 200, 600, 800	USA 300, 400
Age predilection	Older	Younger
Comorbidities	Multiple	None
Traditional risk factors	Health care contact, prolonged hospital stay, poor hand hygiene, contaminated equipment, invasive procedures, medical devices, recent antibiotic use	Crowded community environment, lack of cleanliness, loss of skin integrity, intravenous drug user, homelessness, incarceration, aboriginal, HIV+, contact sports, athletes, military, chronic skin disorder, veterinary worker

*Features are generalizations only given the appearance of community strains replacing traditional hospital strains in the health care setting and the appearance of typical HA strains in the community setting.
†ST 398 = untypable "swine-associated" strains.
Abbreviations: SCC*mec* = staphylococcal cassette chromosome; MLST = multilocus sequence type; pulsotype = pulsed field electrophoretic type; PVL = Panton-Valentine Leukocidin.

The "5 Cs" for Transmission of CA-MRSA
• **C**rowding • **C**ontact with skin • **C**ompromised skin • **C**ontaminated personal care items • **C**leanliness lack

Figure 1. The five Cs implicated in transmission of CA-MRSA. (Adapted from the U.S. Centers for Disease Control and Prevention.)

Centers for Disease Control and Prevention suggested the five Cs (Figure 1, Table 2) as contributing factors implicated in the transmission among these groups. The initial risk groups have expanded (Table 3) to include men who have sex with men (MSM), athletes (especially those involved in team and contact sports), military personnel, those with a prior history of abscesses, individuals with chronic skin disorders, individuals with recent antibiotic receipt, underserved urban populations, contact with colonized pets or livestock, and veterinary workers. In the

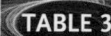

TABLE 3 Principles of Empiric Treatment of Minor Skin and Soft Tissue Infections (Folliculitis, Furuncles, Small Abscesses without Cellulitis, Impetigo, Secondarily Infected Lesions Such as Eczema, Ulcers, or Wounds) Where the Etiology Is Unknown but May Include MRSA as a Possibility

Recommendations

• One or more of the following measures may be employed:
  • Local therapy using hot soaks, elevation, and dressings as appropriate
  • Incision and drainage of furuncles or small abscesses without antimicrobial therapy
  • Topical 2% mupirocin ointment (Bactroban) or fusidic acid[2] for impetigo and secondarily infected lesions if local strains are likely sensitive
  • Topical antiseptics may be considered
• Antimicrobial therapy is recommended in addition to local measures if one or more of the following is present: multiple sites of infection, evidence of progression, clinical evidence of systemic symptoms and signs, presence of comorbidities, extremes of age, immunosuppression, septic phlebitis, or difficult site for incision and drainage.
• In follow-up, routine screening for colonization of the nares or other body sites is not recommended

[2]Not available in the United States.

159

TABLE 2 Risk Factor Associations Reported for CA-MRSA Infections

RISK CATEGORIES	FACTOR	DETAILS FROM REPORTS
High-risk populations	Younger and older age	Age distribution in CA-MRSA younger than HA-MRSA High rate of CA-MRSA in children under 2 years CA-MRSA more common in children compared to adults Outbreaks in hospital nurseries Outbreaks in nursing homes with elderly residents
	Indigenous populations: Native or Aboriginal	Aboriginal communities in midwestern United States, Canada, and Australia
	African American	Alaskan natives More common in African Americans
	Athletes (predominantly contact sports)	Outbreaks on football teams Outbreak on wrestling team Other competitive sports
	Injection (intravenous) drug users (IVDUs)	San Francisco IVDUs Canadian report of USA300 strain outbreak
	Men who have sex with men (MSM)	CA-MRSA described in HIV-positive population of MSM
	HIV+individuals	Risk associated with overlapping social networks Intravenous drug use, hemodialysis, and CD4 counts <200 reported as independent risks
	Military personnel	3% of U.S. Army soldiers colonized
	Inmates of correctional facilities	Reports of outbreaks in U.S. prisons Two outbreaks (total 10 inmates) in Canada
	Students in elementary schools and college dormitories	Reports of outbreaks in schools and college dormitories
Previous positive MRSA cultures	MRSA carriage	Colonized soldiers more likely to get CA-MRSA disease
	Past MRSA infection	Prior abscess risk factor for CA-MRSA
Medical history	Chronic skin disorder	Dermatologic condition most common underlying medical disorder for CA-MRSA infection Classroom contact of index CA-MRSA case had chronic dermatitis
	Recurrent or recent antibiotic use	Antibiotic use associated with CA-MRSA infection in rural Alaska
Environmental	Homelessness and living in shelters	Medically underserved populations at higher risk of CA-MRSA Reports of USA300 strain outbreak involving individuals living in shelters or homeless
	Overcrowding	Close contact implicated in jail outbreaks Neonatal intensive care unit transmission
	Contact with colonized pet	Family dog source of recurrent infection
	Veterinary workers and family members	Veterinarians working with horses and livestock Family members of animal care workers Small animal veterinarians Swine farmers

Adapted from Barton-Forbes et al. (2006).

drug-using and underserved urban populations, prevalence and social networking studies have identified hospices, shooting galleries, and crack houses as key sites in which CA-MRSA transmission may occur. Recent outbreaks have been reported in hospital nurseries, daycare settings, nursing home workers, schools, and college dormitories. Sexual transmission has been reported, but it may reflect close skin-to-skin genital contact rather than a true sexually transmitted pathogen. CA-MRSA has now become endemic in the general population in many communities and the elderly and the very young seem to have a predilection for infection, especially if other risk factors are present. Risk groups for LA-MRSA include farmers, their family members and farm hands who are engaged in livestock production, especially swine and cattle, abattoir workers and veterinarians and veterinary assistants. Recent transmission of strains of LA-MRSA has been reported in the hospital setting as well.

Pathophysiology

The resistance to the antistaphylococcal β-lactam antibiotics in MRSA strains is imparted by the presence of an altered configuration for a specific penicillin-binding protein (PBP) known as PBP2a in the cell wall of staphylococci. Normally the PBPs would act as a site for the attachment of the active moieties of the β-lactam agent, which then would inhibit further cell wall assembly. The alteration in the configuration of PBP2a occurs as the result of the presence of the SCCmec gene in S. aureus which confers resistance to the β-lactam antibiotics. The origins of the mec gene and its insertion into the SCCmec element are not known with certainty. Once the MRSA strains acquired resistance to the antistaphylococcal β-lactam antibiotics in the health care setting, it is not difficult to appreciate how it emerged as a predominant pathogen in the hospital setting over the years, with increasing acuity of illness in the patient populations and increased use of broad-spectrum antimicrobials.

The appearance and rapid spread of CA-MRSA with the clinical impression of more virulent and lethal infections than what had been seen with traditional HA-MRSA strains may be explained by several factors. The SCCmec IV genetic element is very widely distributed among S. aureus isolates, which may explain its appearance in multiple settings globally, and these strains appear to have more rapid growth rates than typical HA-MRSA strains, larger numbers of virulence factors, pathogenicity islands, and higher levels of expression of the virulence factors produced. Recently α-type phenol-soluble modulins were described in strains of CA-MRSA, which are produced at very high levels and are potent lysins of neutrophils. High levels of α-toxin production by these strains, which act as pore-forming toxins for multiple cell types, may also contribute to their virulence. The vast majority of CA-MRSA strains also produce the genes for PVL and it functions as a dermonecrotic factor in skin lesions, a potent cell lysin in high concentrations, and a potent inflammatory mediator in lower concentrations. However, there is controversy about the role of PVL as a single predominant virulence factor, because strains of CA-MRSA that have this gene knocked out have demonstrated no difference in pathogenicity in both vertebrate and invertebrate animal models and in human settings when the PVL is not present.

Prevention

Controlling the spread of either HA-, CA- or LA-MRSA, from an infected or colonized person to others in the hospital, family, or community is a key goal of prevention. In the hospital setting, strict adherence to hand hygiene, application of barrier precautions (gloves, gowns, and private rooms) for patients colonized or infected with MRSA, environmental and equipment cleaning, and antimicrobial stewardship are the key preventive strategies. Active surveillance cultures to identify colonized patients and decolonization may be effective in selected settings but its general application is controversial. In the community setting, practicing hygienic measures including good personal hygiene, consistent hand hygiene, ensuring all draining skin and soft tissue lesions have adequate dressings, not sharing potentially contaminated personal articles, and keeping the household environment hygienic are important. Public health organizations may also contribute to the prevention of CA-MRSA by instituting education programs targeting health care providers and individuals in high-risk groups in the community and by promoting appropriate antimicrobial use. In sports settings, in addition to the basic hygienic measures mentioned previously, avoidance of sharing of towels and other personal items, showering after every practice or tournament, cleaning of communal showering and bathing areas, and cleaning or laundering of equipment after each use are also important.

Clinical Manifestations

The specific clinical infections associated with MRSA parallel those associated with MSSA. Almost any body site, organ, or appendage may be affected by infections due to S. aureus, but there are specific predilections associated with HA- and CA-MRSA. In the hospital or other health care setting, the most commonly encountered sites of infection include pneumonia, line-related infection, surgical site infection, bacteremia, and less often skin and soft tissue infections, whereas in the community setting, the most common sites (>80%) are skin and soft tissue infections (furuncles, cellulitis, and soft tissue abscesses) and less commonly severely invasive infections such as necrotizing pneumonia, necrotizing fasciitis, multifocal osteomyelitis/septic arthritis, epidural abscess, pelvic septic thrombophlebitis, and bacteremia with toxic shock syndrome. The skin and soft tissue infections often affect young previously healthy patients and are characteristically very painful and pyogenic with an initial black eschar that patients presume was a "spider bite" as the initiating process.

Diagnosis

The diagnosis of MRSA infections is based on the clinical presentation and the isolation of the causative organism from purulent discharge, sputum, or urine or from specimens obtained from normally sterile body fluids (joint fluid, abscess or tissue aspirates, blood). The organism appears on Gram stain as a Gram-positive organism in clusters and is usually seen in association with neutrophils and may be either intracellular or extracellular. The organism is very hardy and grows readily on typical media in the microbiology laboratory within 24 to 48 hours. Some laboratories are using rapid agglutination tests to detect the PBP2a protein or polymerase chain reaction (PCR)–based techniques to provide same-day or next-day identification. In settings where no cultures have been obtained or in the setting of toxic shock syndrome where cultures are often negative, the diagnosis may be difficult and only suspected based on a typical clinical presentation.

Treatment

MRSA strains harbor resistance to the β-lactam antimicrobials, including oxacillin, dicloxacillin, cloxacillin,[2] nafcillin, methicillin,[2] and first-, second-, and third-generation cephalosporins. The new advanced-generation cephalosporin antimicrobial ceftaroline (Teflaro) has activity against MRSA strains. The majority of HA-MRSA strains are resistant to macrolides, clindamycin (Cleocin), aminoglycosides, and quinolones and are variably resistant to tetracycline and trimethoprim-sulfamethoxazole (Bactrim), depending on local epidemiologic patterns. They are sensitive to vancomycin (Vancocin) and other glycopeptides such as dalbavancin (Dalvance) and telavancin (Vibativ) and usually sensitive to fusidic acid,[2] rifampin (Rifadin), linezolid (Zyvox) and daptomycin (Cubicin). For hospitalized patients where S. aureus is considered a possible etiology of any major infectious syndrome, it should be considered as methicillin resistant until proven otherwise and empiric choices of vancomycin or other glycopeptides such as dalbavancin (Dalvance) or telavancin (Vibativ), linezolid, or daptomycin (Cubicin) considered as appropriate to the presenting syndrome. CA-MRSA strains are resistant to macrolides and quinolones but

---

[2]Not available in the United States.

usually sensitive to aminoglycosides such as gentamicin (Garamycin), clindamycin, and trimethoprim-sulfamethoxazole, but the resistance patterns vary depending on local resistance patterns. LA-MRSA strains are almost always resistant to tetracyclines, often resistant to quinolones, macrolides, clindamycin and variably resistant to aminoglycosides and trimethoprim-sulfamethoxazole. Treatment guidelines for MRSA with a focus on the ambulatory setting have been published in Canada, the United Kingdom, and the United States and provide both empiric choices for common infectious presentations of unknown etiology and definitive treatment once an etiology of MRSA is known. The treatment options for both empiric and definitive use where MRSA is considered or proven are presented in Tables 3 through 6 and represent a constellation of the various guidelines that have been published.

TABLE 4 Principles of Empiric Treatment of Non–Life-Threatening Skin and Soft Tissue Infections Other Than Minor Skin Infections Where the Etiology Is Unknown but May Include MRSA as a Possibility

Recommendations

- Antibiotic choice should be based on the severity of illness at presentation, clinical judgment, and regional susceptibility patterns of strains
- Empiric therapy for CA-MRSA and β-hemolytic streptococci is recommended*

*The IDSA guideline suggests to differentiate purulent and nonpurulent cellulitis and reserve empiric therapy for β-hemolytic streptococci only in nonpurulent cellulitis but acknowledges it is an area of controversy. The U.K. and Canadian guidelines explicitly recommend coverage for β-hemolytic streptococci and do not differentiate cellulitis into different types.
Abbreviation: IDSA = Infectious Diseases Society of America.

TABLE 5 Principles of Empiric Treatment of Life-Threatening Infections Where the Etiology Is Unknown but May Include MRSA as a Possibility

Recommendations

- Include MRSA coverage, regardless of prevalence rates of CA-MRSA in the community
- Include an agent effective against MSSA until susceptibility results become available

TABLE 6 Guidelines for the Management of MRSA Infections

CLINICAL DISEASE	KEY FEATURES	MANAGEMENT PRINCIPLES	ANTIMICROBIAL CHOICES AND COMMENTS[§]
Skin and Soft Tissue Infection (SSTI)			
Localized lesion	Infected scratches and minor wounds Insect bites Furuncles Small abscesses Absence of systemic illness	Culture selectively* No antibiotic therapy recommended *Exceptions: multiple sites of infection, evidence of progression, systemic symptoms and signs, presence of comorbidities, extremes of age, immunosuppression, septic phlebitis, or difficult site for incision and drainage: antimicrobial therapy is recommended in addition to local measures* Cover draining lesions Emphasize personal hygiene Close follow-up Return if worsening	Generally not indicated Topical antibacterial (e.g., mupirocin [Bactroban] or fusidic ointment[2]) therapy may be considered Systemic antimicrobial therapy indicated if one or more of the following: multiple sites of infection, evidence of progression, systemic symptoms and signs, presence of comorbidities, extremes of age, immunosuppression, septic phlebitis, or difficult site for incision and drainage
Cellulitis (not extensive) or multiple abscesses with minimal or no associated systemic features for oral treatment consideration	Classic features of rubor, dolor, calor, and swelling suggesting cellulitis with or without associated drainage or exudate	Culture site (if purulent or drainage) Drainage of abscess or needle aspiration Oral therapy in older child and adult Appropriate infection control measures Imaging for extent and complications as appropriate Close follow-up Return if worsening	*Empiric:* Include coverage for β-hemolytic streptococci[†] Clindamycin (Cleocin) 300–450 mg tid-qid PO for adults and 30–40 mg/kg/d[3] ÷ q6–8h PO for children TMP-SMX (Bactrim)[1] 1–2 DS tab bid PO for adults and 8–12 mg/kg/d (of TMP) ÷ q12h PO for children PLUS coverage for β-hemolytic streptococci (e.g., amoxicillin, cephalexin [Keflex]) Doxycycline (Vibramycin)100 mg bid PO for adults and 4 mg/kg/d ÷ q12h PO for children[‡] PLUS coverage for β-hemolytic streptococci (e.g., amoxicillin, cephalexin) Linezolid (Zyvox) 600 mg bid PO for adults and 30 mg/kg/d ÷ q8h PO for children, not to exceed 600 mg/ dose; for children >12 years of age 600 mg bid PO *Comment:* Linezolid is more expensive than the other options and may not always be readily available depending on the setting *Comment:* If parenteral therapy considered, see choices for severe SSTI *Proven MRSA:* As above, based on sensitivity testing If parenteral therapy necessary, see choices for SSTI with systemic features

Continued

TABLE 6 Guidelines for the Management of MRSA Infections—cont'd

CLINICAL DISEASE	KEY FEATURES	MANAGEMENT PRINCIPLES	ANTIMICROBIAL CHOICES AND COMMENTS
Cellulitis (severe or rapidly spreading or extensive) or complicated SSTI (deep soft tissue infection, surgical or traumatic wound infection, large or multiple abscesses, or infected ulcers and burns) and/or associated systemic features for parenteral treatment consideration	Classic features of rubor, dolor, calor, and swelling suggesting cellulitis with or without associated drainage or exudate with systemic features of fever, chills, malaise, prostration	Culture (blood if febrile, site if purulent) Hospitalize as appropriate Drainage of abscess or needle aspiration Parenteral therapy Imaging for extent and complications as appropriate Appropriate infection control measures Consultation as indicated	*Empiric:* Include coverage for β-hemolytic streptococci[†] Vancomycin (Vancocin) 15–20 mg/kg/dose q8-12 h IV for adults and 40–60[3] mg/kg/d ÷ q6h IV for children *Proven MRSA:* Based on sensitivity testing Vancomycin 15–20 mg/kg/dose q8-12 h IV for adults and 40–60[3] mg/kg/d ÷ q6h IV for children Clindamycin 600–900 mg q8h IV/IM for adults and 30–40 mg/kg/d[3] ÷ q6–8h IV for children Linezolid 600 mg q12h PO/IV for adults and 30 mg/kg/d ÷ q8h PO/IV for children, not to exceed 600 mg/dose; for children >12 years of age 600 mg bid PO/IV Daptomycin (Cubicin) 4 mg/kg/dose once daily IV for adults and under investigation in children Dalbavancin (Dalvance) 1000 mg IV followed by 500 mg IV 1 week later for adults; safety and efficacy not established in children Telavancin (Vibativ) 10 mg/kg/dose IV once daily *Comment:* Linezolid, daptomycin, dalbavancin, and telavancin are more expensive than the other options and may not always be readily available depending on the setting
Necrotizing fasciitis (NF)	Clinically indistinguishable from group A streptococcus NF disease Extreme toxicity High complication rate	Cultures (blood, tissue) Imaging for extent and complications Surgical débridement Consultation as indicated Parenteral therapy Infection control measures	*Empiric:* Include coverage for β-hemolytic streptococci Vancomycin 15–20 mg/kg/dose q8–12h IV for adults and 40–60[3] mg/kg/d ÷ q6h IV for children Clindamycin 600–900 mg q8h IV/IM for adults and 30–40 mg/kg/d[3] ÷ q6–8h IV for children *Proven MRSA:* Based on sensitivity testing Vancomycin 15–20 mg/kg/dose q8–12h IV for adults and 40–60[3] mg/kg/d ÷ q6h IV for children Clindamycin 600–900 mg q8h IV/IM for adults and 30–40 mg/kg/d[3] ÷ q6–8h IV for children Linezolid 600 mg q12h PO/IV for adults and 30 mg/kg/d ÷ q8h PO/IV for children, not to exceed 600 mg/dose; for children >12 years of age 600 mg bid PO/IV TMP/SMX[1] 8–12 mg/kg/d (of TMP) ÷ q8–12h IV for adults and 8–12 mg/kg/d (of TMP) ÷ q6h IV for children *Comments:* Adjuncts such as IVIG (Gamunex)[1] may be considered in severe cases with septic shock Few data available for the use of TMP-SMX in this indication

Musculoskeletal Infection (MSI)

CLINICAL DISEASE	KEY FEATURES	MANAGEMENT PRINCIPLES	ANTIMICROBIAL CHOICES AND COMMENTS
Osteomyelitis/septic arthritis	Preceding trauma Tendency for multifocal involvement Disease in adjacent muscle not uncommon Progression to chronic osteomyelitis possible May be complicated by deep venous thrombosis	Cultures (blood, bone, and tissue) Imaging for extent and complications Involve surgical team (early débridement and drainage) Consultation as indicated Parenteral therapy Consider combination therapy for severe cases or if slow to respond Infection control measures Look for other infected sites (imaging)	*Empiric:* Vancomycin 15–20 mg/kg/dose q8–12h IV for adults and 40–60[3] mg/kg/d ÷ q6h IV for children Clindamycin 600–900 mg q8h IV/IM for adults and 30–40 mg/kg/d[3] ÷ q6–8h IV for children Linezolid[1] 600 mg q12h PO/IV for adults and 30 mg/kg/d ÷ q8h PO/IV for children, not to exceed 600 mg/dose; for children >12 years of age 600 mg bid PO/IV Daptomycin[1] 6 mg/kg/dose once daily IV for adults and 6–10 mg/kg once daily for children TMP/SMX[1] 8–12 mg/kg/d (of TMP) ÷ q8–12h IV for adults and 8–12 mg/kg/d (of TMP) ÷ q6h IV for children *Comments:* Linezolid and daptomycin are more expensive than the other options and may not always be readily available depending on the setting Few data available for the use of TMP-SMX in these indications for children
Pyomyositis	May be extensive Tendency for multifocal involvement	Cultures (blood, tissue) Imaging for extent and complications Surgical drainage Consultation as indicated Parenteral therapy Infection control measures	*Proven MRSA:* As above, based on sensitivity testing Addition of rifampin (Rifadin)[1] may be considered for osteomyelitis

Respiratory Tract Infection (RTI)

CLINICAL DISEASE	KEY FEATURES	MANAGEMENT PRINCIPLES	ANTIMICROBIAL CHOICES AND COMMENTS
Pneumonia	Influenza-like prodrome, hemoptysis, fever, shock, leukopenia, pneumatoceles, multifocal abscesses, consolidation,	Cultures (blood, pleural fluid, sputum) Imaging for extent and complications Consultation as indicated Intensive care unit as appropriate Infection control measures Combination parenteral therapy Chest tube drainage for empyema	*Empiric:* Vancomycin 15–20 mg/kg/dose q8–12h IV for adults and 40–60[3] mg/kg/d ÷ q6h IV for children Linezolid 600 mg q12h PO/IV for adults and 30 mg/kg/d ÷ q8h PO/IV for children, not to exceed 600 mg/dose; for children >12 years of age 600 mg bid PO/IV Clindamycin 600–900 mg q8h IV/IM for adults and 30–40 mg/kg/d[3] ÷ q6–8h IV for children

TABLE 6 Guidelines for the Management of MRSA Infections—cont'd

CLINICAL DISEASE	KEY FEATURES	MANAGEMENT PRINCIPLES	ANTIMICROBIAL CHOICES AND COMMENTS
	frequent empyema, respiratory failure, high mortality		TMP/SMX[1] 8–12 mg/kg/d (of TMP) ÷ q8–12h IV for adults and 8–12 mg/kg/d (of TMP) ÷ q6h IV for children Telavancin (Vibativ) 10 mg/kg/dose IV once daily for adults for hospital or ventilator acquired pneumonia *Comment:* Daptomycin not indicated because it is inactivated by lung surfactant *Proven MRSA:* As above, based on sensitivity testing

Other

Sepsis syndrome Bacteremia Native valve endocarditis	Shock Multiple-organ failure May have purpura fulminans Associated SSTI, MSI, RTI May be complicated by Waterhouse-Friedrichsen syndrome High mortality	Blood cultures Culture any pus or fluid collection Look for primary or secondary focus Imaging for identification of source including echocardiography Consultation as indicated ICU care Imaging: look for occult abscesses, bone infection, or endocarditis Involve surgery and other specialists as needed Infection control measures Parenteral, multidrug therapy Prolonged therapy for endovascular source infections	*Empiric:* Vancomycin 15–20 mg/kg/dose q8–12h IV for adults and 40–60[3] mg/kg/d ÷ q6h IV for children Daptomycin 6 mg/kg/dose once daily IV for adults and 4–10[3] mg/kg/dose once daily for children[1] *Comments:* Doses of daptomycin of up to 10 mg/kg/dose[3] once daily have been used in adults in this indication Some recommendations have included linezolid in this setting at the doses described above *Proven MRSA:* As above, based on sensitivity testing.

[1]Not FDA approved for this indication. Dosing has varied in published reports and specific dosing guidelines are not available.
[2]Not available in the United States.
[3]Exceeds dosage recommended by the manufacturer.
*Patients with risk factors, as a part of an outbreak investigation, patients with slowly responding or recurrent lesions.
†The IDSA guideline suggests to differentiate purulent and nonpurulent cellulitis and reserve empiric therapy for β-hemolytic streptococci only in nonpurulent cellulitis but acknowledges it is an area of controversy. The U.K. and Canadian guidelines explicitly recommend empiric coverage for β-hemolytic streptococci and do not differentiate cellulitis into different types.
§Choice of antimicrobial therapy depends on local susceptibility patterns.
‡Not recommended for pediatric patients under 8 years of age or in pregnancy.
Abbreviations: ICU = intensive care unit; IVIG = intravenous immunoglobulin, MRSA = methicillin-resistant *Staphylococcus aureus*; TMP-SMX = trimethoprim-sulfamethoxazole.

References

Barton-Forbes M, Hawkes M, Moore D, et al. Guidelines for the prevention and management of community associated methicillin resistant *Staphylococcus aureus* (CA-MRSA): a perspective for Canadian Health Care Practitioners. Can J Infect Dis Med Microbiol 2006;17(Suppl. C):1B–24B.

Chambers HF, Deleo FR. Waves of resistance: *Staphylococcus aureus* in the antibiotic era. Nat Rev Microbiol 2009;7:629–41. http://dx.doi.org/10.1038/nrmicro2200.

David MZ, Daum RS. Community-associated methicillin resistant *Staphylococcus aureus*: epidemiology and clinical consequences of an emerging epidemic. Clin Microbiol Rev 2010;23:616–87. http://dx.doi.org/10.1128/CMR.00081-09.

Fluit AC. Livestock associated *Staphylococcus aureus*. Clin Microbiol Infect 2012;18:735–44. http://dx.doi.org/10.1111/j.1469-0691.2012.03846.x.

Gorwitz RJ, Jernigan DB, Powers JH, et al. Strategies for clinical management of MRSA in the community: summary of an experts' meeting convened by the Centers for Disease Control and Prevention, 2006. Available at, www.cdc.gov/ncidod/dhqp/pdf/ar/CAMRSA_ExpMtgStrategies.pdf [accessed 02.01.13].

Gould FK, Brindle R, Chadwick PR, et al. Guidelines (2008) for the prophylaxis and treatment of methicillin resistant *Staphylococcus aureus* (MRSA) infections in the United Kingdom. J Antimicrob Chemother 2009;63:849–61. http://dx.doi.org/10.1093/jac/dkp065.

Kaplan SL, Hulten KG, Gonzalez BE, et al. Three-year surveillance of community-acquired *Staphylococcus aureus* infections in children. Clin Infect Dis 2005;40:1785–91.

Klevens RM, Morrison MA, Nadle J, et al. Invasive methicillin resistant *Staphylococcus aureus* infections in the United States. JAMA 2007;298:1763–71.

Köck R, Becker K, Cookson B, et al. Methicillin resistant *Staphylococcus aureus* (MRSA): burden of disease and control challenges in Europe. Euro Surveill 2010;15:19688.

Liu C, Bayer A, Cosgrove SE, et al. Clinical practice guidelines by the Infectious Diseases Society of America for the treatment of methicillin resistant *staphylococcus aureus* infections in adults and children: executive summary. Clin Infect Dis 2011;52:285–92. http://dx.doi.org/10.1093/cid/cir034.

Muto CA, Jernigan JA, Ostrowsky BE, et al. SHEA guideline for preventing nosocomial transmission of multidrug-resistant strains of *Staphylococcus aureus* and enterococcus. Infect Control Hosp Epidemiol 2003;24:362–86.

Nathwani D, Morgan M, Masterton RG, et al. Guidelines for UK practice for the diagnosis and management of methicillin resistant *Staphylococcus aureus* (MRSA) infections presenting in the community. J Antimicrob Chemother 2008;61:976–94. http://dx.doi.org/10.1093/jac/dkn096.

MUMPS

Method of
Kristen Rundell, MS, MD

CURRENT DIAGNOSIS

- Parotitis (swelling of the parotid salivary glands): unilateral or bilateral
- Fever
- Headache
- Malaise
- Myalgias
- Anorexia
- Increased serum amylase

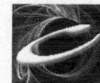

CURRENT THERAPY

- Supportive care
- Warm or cold packs on the parotid
- Analgesics and/or antipyretics (such as acetaminophen [Tylenol] or ibuprofen [Motrin])
- IV fluids or hospitalization for cases of pancreatitis, meningitis, or severe orchitis

Epidemiology

Mumps is an extremely contagious, self-limiting virus that had disease rates of 99% until the vaccine was introduced in 1967. Since that time, the yearly disease rate is less than 1 percent. For the United States and Finland, mumps is almost eradicated. For the rest of the world, mumps is still endemic as a result of a vaccination rate of only 61%.

Pathophysiology

Mumps is a single-stranded RNA virus and a member of the *Paramyxovirus* genus. It is transmitted through respiratory secretions, saliva, and contact with contaminated fomites.

Prevention

With the high rate of transmission and no antiviral therapy, prevention for mumps relies on community immunity as a result of high vaccine rates. There are two formulations of the mumps vaccine currently available in the United States: the measles-mumps-rubella vaccine (MMR) and the measles-mumps-rubella-varicella vaccine (MMRV, ProQuad). The dosing schedule for children calls for the first dose at age greater than 12 months to 15 months, and the second dose for children greater than 4 years to 6 years of age. For infants aged 6 through 11 months who are traveling internationally, a single MMR vaccine is recommended. These children should be revaccinated with 2 doses of MMR vaccine with the first dose at ages 12 months to 15 months and the second dose at ages 4 years to 6 years. During an epidemic, a single dose for adults born before 1957 is recommended and may be required by some health care professionals. The first dose gives approximately 80% immunity. Persons receiving both doses may still get the mumps virus if there is outbreak or if they travel to an endemic area. To avoid exposure or contraction of the disease during travel, it is suggested that travelers wash hands frequently and use alcohol-based sanitizers to decrease the contraction or spread of disease.

The vaccine is contraindicated for patients who are pregnant or planning to conceive in the 28 days after vaccination. Vaccine administration is also contraindicated for those who have a severe anaphylactic reaction to the vaccine or one of the components, and those individuals who are severely immunocompromised.

Clinical Manifestations

The incubation period for the mumps virus is 16 to 18 days. At the onset of the illness, patients may develop acute viral infection symptoms of fever, headache, and malaise. The parotitis, swelling of the parotid gland, is the diagnostic hallmark of the mumps virus. This is caused by the infection and inflammation of the parotid ductal epithelium. The swelling may last up to 10 days. Close to 30% of persons may not have this symptom and may be only mildly symptomatic.

Diagnosis

Diagnosis is made by the history and the constellation of symptoms and physical findings. It is difficult to use IgM to determine active infection, because the response may be short in duration, delayed, or even absent. PCR testing is available and requires early sampling.

Differential Diagnosis

Viral infections such as parainfluenza (also in the paramyxovirus genus) coxsackievirus, influenza A, Epstein-Barr, adenovirus, HIV, and cytomegalovirus may present with similar symptoms as mumps. There are also noninfectious etiologies of parotitis, which include salivary stones or tumors, sarcoid, Sjogren's syndrome, and thiazide diuretics.

Therapy (or Treatment)

Treatment for mumps virus is largely supportive. For complicated cases of pancreatitis, meningitis, encephalitis, and orchitis, patient may need to be hospitalized for additional care. The additional care usually includes fever reduction, analgesia, fluid resuscitation, and treatment of secondary bacterial infections.

Monitoring

For persons with active mumps, it is suggested that they be isolated from school or work for 5 days after the onset of symptoms. Shedding of virus usually occurs 4 days prior to the onset of symptoms. For this reason, it is difficult to slow down outbreaks of the disease. The last outbreak in the United States was in 2010.

Complications

Complications from mumps are rare. In children, pancreatitis and hearing loss are the sensorineural complications most often diagnosed. For adolescents and adults the complications are more common and usually more severe. These include aseptic meningitis; orchitis in males, which rarely leads to sterility; oophoritis in females; pancreatitis; and arthritis. Even more uncommon are Guillain–Barré/ascending polyradiculitis, transverse myelitis, facial palsy, interstitial nephritis, and myocardial involvement.

Mumps in pregnancy has been associated with increased fetal loss. There are no known teratogenic effects.

References

American Academy of Pediatrics. Mumps. In: Pickering LK, Baker CJ, Kimberlin DW, Long SS, editors. Red Book: 2009 Report of the committee on Infectious Diseases. 28th ed. Elk Gove Village IL: American Academy of Pediatrics; 2009. p. 468–72.

Centers for Disease Control and Prevention (CDC). Exposure to mumps during air travel—United States, April 2006. MMWR Morb Mortal Wkly Rep 2006;55(401).

Dayan GH, Rubin S. Mumps outbreaks in vaccinated population: are available mumps vaccines effective enough to prevent an outbreak? Clin Infect Dis 2008;47:1458.

Kleiman MB. Mumps virus. In: Lenette EH, editor. Laboratory Diagnosis of Viral Infections. 2nd ed New York: Marcel Dekker; 1992. p. 549.

Kutty PK, Barskey AE, Gallagher KM. Mumps. Infectious Diseases Related to Travel. CDC Yellowbook; 2012 [chapter 3].

Wharton M, Cochi SLK, William S. Measles, mumps and rubella vaccines. Infect Dis Clin North Am 1990;4:47.

www.cdc.gov/travel/yellowbook.

NECROTIZING SKIN AND SOFT TISSUE INFECTIONS

Method of
Debra Tristram, MD

CURRENT DIAGNOSIS

- Prompt surgical intervention confirms the diagnosis and can be life and limb saving.
- Empiric antibiotic coverage should target organisms obtained from the details of injury.
- Physical examination of the affected area should focus on the following:
  - Exquisite pain and tenderness out of proportion to the visible physical signs of infection
  - Presence of hemorrhagic bullae, skin sloughing, skin anesthesia
  - Palpable gas in the tissue (uncommon)

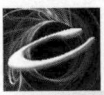

CURRENT THERAPY

- Necrotizing skin and soft tissue infections are rapidly progressive infections capable of breaking down and crossing anatomic barriers quickly, causing extensive destruction of the subcutaneous, fascial, or muscle layers of the integument with little surface evidence of infection.
- Unrecognized or seemingly minor breaks in the skin or mucosa initiate the process in more than 80% of cases.
- A high index of suspicion is needed for prompt, aggressive surgical débridement and treatment with antibiotics to prevent significant morbidity, limb loss, and mortality.

Epidemiology

Necrotizing skin and soft tissue infections (nSSTIs) are uncommon; an annual incidence of approximately 1000 cases/year is estimated for the United States. The microorganisms responsible for nSSTIs are numerous (Table 1); they can be mixtures of aerobic and anaerobic organisms acting synergistically to produce infection or can be a single, highly virulent pathogen.

Polymicrobial infections with 4 or 5 different organisms present the most common form of the disease (55%–75% of all nSSTIs). These infections involve the trunk and perineal areas and are more common in immunocompromised patients. In contrast, monomicrobial infections occur much more often in young, healthy persons. Involvement of the extremities is common, resulting from seemingly minor trauma in more than 75% of cases. A subgroup of nSSTIs is associated with exposure to contaminated water or fish, especially in warmer waters. *Vibrio vulnificus* is the primary pathogen in this scenario, but nSSTIs have also been increasingly reported secondary to other gram-negative waterborne organisms (see Table 1).

Fungal pathogens are also emerging as important causes of nSSTIs. Usually these infections are caused by septated molds, but aseptated zygomyces are reported with increasing frequency (see Table 1).

Risk Factors

Risk factors for the development of skin and soft tissue infections are numerous and are outlined in Table 1. Loss of skin integrity through trauma and immunocompromised states are the most common antecedent risk factors.

Pathophysiology

Necrotizing SSTIs are capable of breaking down and crossing anatomic barriers rapidly by direct spread, causing extensive destruction of the subcutaneous, fascial, or muscle layers of the integument, with little surface evidence of infection. Trivial injuries from cuts, abrasions, scratches, or insect bites provide a portal of entry through direct inoculation. Thrombosis of cutaneous vessels, vasculitis, and necrosis follows microbial and leukocytic invasion of the deep dermal tissue and fascial layer. A smaller percentage of patients have no visible portal of entry; systemic spread from an unrecognized focus through the vasculature or lymphatics might play a role in these cases.

Prevention

Maintenance of skin integrity is the cornerstone of prevention. Cleaning of traumatized skin with antibacterial soaps and removal of all foreign material can reduce the risk for infection. Use of proper skin preparation, perioperative antibiotics, and sterile surgical technique can cut the risk of postoperative infections to nearly zero. Education of patients who have risk factors regarding when to seek medical attention can aid in decreasing serious consequences for compromised hosts.

Clinical Manifestations

Necrotizing SSTIs in the earliest stages can appear like a cellulitis or erysipelas. Localized warmth, erythema, induration, and swelling are characteristic of early nSSTIs. As the disease process progresses, violaceous or darker maroon areas can appear within the

---

TABLE 1   Most Common Pathogens Involved in Necrotizing Skin and Soft Tissue Infections

RISK FACTORS	ORGANISMS	LOCATION	SPECIAL TYPES BY ANATOMIC LOCATION
Polymicrobial			
Immunosuppression Diabetes mellitus Peripheral vascular disease Obesity Chronic renal disease, dialysis HIV Ethanol abuse Bites Blunt or penetrating trauma Surgical incisions Varicella Perforation of the GI tract Malnutrition, cachexia Chronic dermatosis Diabetes mellitus Iron overload and deferoxamine therapy Immunocompromised states (particularly prolonged neutropenia) Soft tissue trauma, especially with soil contamination	Mixture of aerobes, anaerobes, and facultative organisms: *Bacteroides* spp., *Clostridium* spp., *Eikenella corrodens*, *Enterobacter* spp., *Escherichia coli*, *Fusobacter* spp., *Haemophilus influenzae* type B, *Klebsiella* spp., *Peptococcus* spp., *Peptostreptococcus* spp, *Prevotella* spp., *Porphyromonas* spp., *Proteus* spp., *Pseudomonas* spp., *Staphylococcus aureus* (MSSA and MRSA), *Streptococcus* spp. Fungal: *Absidia* spp., *Aspergillus* spp., *Fusarium* spp., *Mucor* spp., *Rhizopus* spp., and others	Perineal area and trunk	Fournier's gangrene: perineal and scrotal necrosis Lemierre's disease: deep neck-space infections with dissemination (*Fusobacter necrophorum* and other oral flora) Malignant otitis externa: *Pseudomonas aeruginosa*, *Staphylococcus aureus*, invasive fungi, especially *Aspergillus* spp. Meleney's synergistic gangrene (MRSA and anaerobic streptococci) Rhinocerebral infections: Invasive fungal pathogens in persons with diabetes mellitus or in profoundly neutropenic patients
Monomicrobial			
Otherwise young, healthy persons Occasionally, recent trauma, surgery, or IV drug use	*S. pyogenes*, *S. aureus*, and anaerobic streptococci (i.e., *Peptostreptococcus*)	Extremities, occasionally trunk	
Exposure to contaminated water or fish, especially seawater; skin break due to fish finning, trauma in water, or handling seafood	*Vibrio vulnificus* and other *Vibrio* spp.: warm seawater Fresh or brackish water: *Aeromonas hydrophia*, *Edwardisella tarda*, *Pseudomonas* spp., and other enterics; *Schewanella putrificiens*; *Streptococcus iniae*	Extremities	

Abbreviations: GI = gastrointestinal; HIV = human immunodeficiency virus; MRSA = methicillin-resistant *Staphylococcus aureus*; MSSA = methicillin-susceptible *Staphylococcus aureus*.

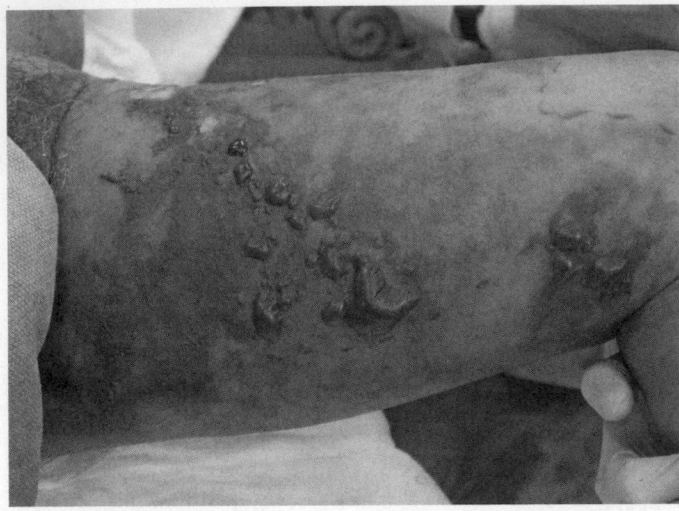

Figure 1. Necrotizing skin and soft tissue infection in an otherwise healthy male patient who sustained an abrasion to his shin several days before presentation. Violaceous patches within the initial area of cellulitis and development of hemorrhagic bullae and skin sloughing are demonstrated. Group A streptococci were recovered from surgery.

margins of initial erythema, and bullae can form, initially filled with clear fluid but progressively filled with hemorrhagic fluid (Figure 1). A peau d'orange appearance to the skin is a late finding. The skin can have a wooden or hardened feel in contrast to the palpable soft tissue structures underlying simple cellulitis. Crepitus in the tissue (common in *Clostridium* infection) is not seen if the responsible organisms are not gas producing (e.g., group A streptococci). Examination of the affected area can reveal pain out of proportion to the observed clinical appearance due to involvement of the cutaneous nerve roots; anesthesia of the area is a more ominous sign, indicating further spread of the infection and destruction of the nerve tissue. Systemic toxicity with high fever, muscle aches, fatigue, and anorexia can usher in more-severe toxic shock–like features with vascular collapse, altered mental status, and respiratory distress.

Diagnosis

Diagnosis of nSSTIs depends on a strong clinical suspicion and is confirmed only by surgical exploration. Laboratory findings are nonspecific and do not differentiate between cellulitis and deeper tissue infections. Muscle enzymes may be elevated if there is muscle necrosis either from direct infection or by compression from edema causing a compartment syndrome. Imaging with computed tomography (CT) or magnetic resonance imaging (MRI) might reveal underlying edema extending along fascial planes, but the sensitivity and specificity of these procedures is unknown. Absence of gas in the tissues does not eliminate nSSTI; other pathogens that cause nSSTIs might not form gas (e.g., group A streptococci).

Imaging should not delay surgical intervention. At the time of surgery, the underlying tissue is swollen, the fascia is grey, and a brownish exudate may ooze from the area. The exudate is replete with microorganisms and provides an early clue to the pathogen(s) on Gram stain. If nSSTI is suspected but not certain, a small incision can be made by the surgeon in the suspect area for inspection, biopsy, and cultures.

Differential Diagnosis

There are multiple other infectious and noninfectious conditions in the differential diagnosis of nSSTIs; these are outlined in Box 1. Many can be eliminated from the differential by a careful history.

Therapy

Necrotizing infection is a surgical emergency; all patients with suspected nSSTI should be seen by a surgeon immediately. Because most nSSTIs begin as cellulitis, administration of empiric

---

Box 1 — Differential Diagnosis of Necrotizing Skin and Soft Tissue Infections

Burns, especially chemical burns due to acids
Buruli ulcer (chronic necrotizing skin ulceration due to *Mycobacterium ulcerans*)
Calciphylaxis
Envenomation
Eosinophilic fasciitis
Hidradenitis suppurativa
Intravenous infiltration, especially with calcium infusion
Jellyfish, scorpion, snake, spider (brown recluse) bites
Langerhans cell histiocytosis
Leukemia, especially cutis leukemia
Lymphedema
Lymphoma
Myxedema
Necrobiosis lipoidica diabeticorum
Nodular fasciitis
Panniculitis
Polyarteritis nodosa
Purpura fulminans
Pyoderma gangrenosum
Stevens-Johnson syndrome
Subcutaneous gas: esophageal perforation, peribronchial dissection, traumatic cutaneous installation of air, wound irrigation with H_2O_2
Superficial or deep thrombophlebitis
Sweet's syndrome (acute febrile neutrophilic dermatosis)
Toxic epidermal necrolysis
Wegener's granulomatosis

---

antibiotics should not be withheld while awaiting full evaluation; if treated early enough, some patients might avoid more extensive, disfiguring surgical débridement. Cultures of drainage and of tissue obtained from the surgical procedure should be sent for aerobic, anaerobic, and fungal stains and cultures. Pus or exudate samples sent in sterile cups or syringes in addition to tissue samples are preferable to swab specimens because the recovery of anaerobes is inhibited by exposure to air. Gram stains done at the time of surgery may be helpful to guide therapy in cases where antibiotic pretreatment inhibits bacterial growth. Empiric antibiotics can be tailored to target the specific organisms isolated from cultures when susceptibilities are available.

Empiric antibiotic coverage of *all* potential pathogens that cause nSSTIs is difficult to achieve. Consultation with an infectious disease specialist for antibiotic management is strongly recommended. Careful attention to the details surrounding the onset and circumstances of infection can give clues to the potential cause(s), but empiric antibiotics should include coverage for gram-positive organisms (especially methicillin-resistant *Staphylococcus aureus* [MRSA]) and anaerobes as well as gram-negative organisms. Certain clinical scenarios noted in Table 1 can give added guidance to the organisms requiring coverage, but nothing can replace cultures for the exact drug(s) of choice for the given infection. All nSSTIs should be suspected to be polymicrobial until proved otherwise; initial empiric therapy for mixed infections should contain an extended-spectrum β-lactam such as ampicillin-sulbactam (Unasyn) or pipercillin-tazobactam (Zosyn) *and* clindamycin (Cleocin) *and* ciprofloxacin (Cipro) or other fluoroquinolone. In areas with a high incidence of MRSA isolates with inducible clindamycin resistance, vancomycin (Vancocin) or daptomycin (Cubicin) should be used instead of clindamycin until culture results are available.

Adjunctive therapies such as hyperbaric oxygen and intravenous immunoglobulin (IVIg, Gammagard)[1] have been used in some

---

[1]Not FDA approved for this indication.

cases. Neither has been evaluated in a controlled fashion, and neither is considered standard therapy but may be useful for certain cases. Nonrandomized observational studies suggest that IVIg infusions reduce morbidity and mortality, but further studies are warranted.

Monitoring

Patients with nSSTIs can have severe systemic reactions, leading to shock, acute respiratory distress syndrome (ARDS), and multiorgan failure. Such patients are best managed in an intensive care setting. Second-look surgery is often beneficial to further assess the extent of the infection and to reculture and débride as needed.

Complications

Necrotizing infections nearly always cause skin scarring as well as the potential for disfigurement and limb loss. Survivors can require multiple revisions of the débrided area to provide satisfactory coverage with grafting and flaps. Despite great improvements in medical care, mortality associated with nSSTIs remains 25% to 35%; mortality is directly proportional to the interval between time of onset and the time of intervention. Mortality rates can be even higher in patients with underlying conditions.

References

Anaya DA, Dellinger EP. Necrotizing soft-tissue infection: Diagnosis and management. Clin Infect Dis 2007;44:705–10.
Miller LG, Perdreau-Remington F, Rieg G, et al. Necrotizing fasciitis caused by community-associated methicillin-resistant *Staphylococcus aureus* in Los Angeles. N Engl J Med 2005;352:1445–53.
Napolitano LM. Severe soft tissue infections. Infect Dis Clin North Am 2009;3:571–91.
Saranti B, Strong M, Pascual J, Scwab CW. Necrotizing fasciitis: Current concepts and review of the literature. J Am Coll Surg 2009;208:279–88.
Stevens DL, Bisno AL, Chambers HF, et al. Practice guidelines for the diagnosis and management of skin and soft-tissue infections. Clin Infect Dis 2005;41:1373–406.

OSTEOMYELITIS

Method of
Brian K. Albertson, MD; and George D. Harris, MD, MS

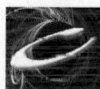

CURRENT DIAGNOSIS (FIGURE 1)

- A bone biopsy remains the gold standard when diagnosing osteomyelitis.
- All patients should have blood cultures performed.
- No one imaging modality is routinely recommended to diagnose osteomyelitis.
- Plain film radiography should always be the initial study and can be diagnostic if positive.
- Magnetic resonance imaging (MRI) can detect acute osteomyelitis as early as 3 days.

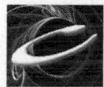

CURRENT THERAPY

- The most important factor in any treatment is identification of the organism.
- The optimal duration of antibiotic therapy remains undefined, with most authorities recommending treatment for about 6 weeks.
- Hematogenous osteomyelitis is usually monomicrobial, whereas contiguous infections are usually polymicrobial.

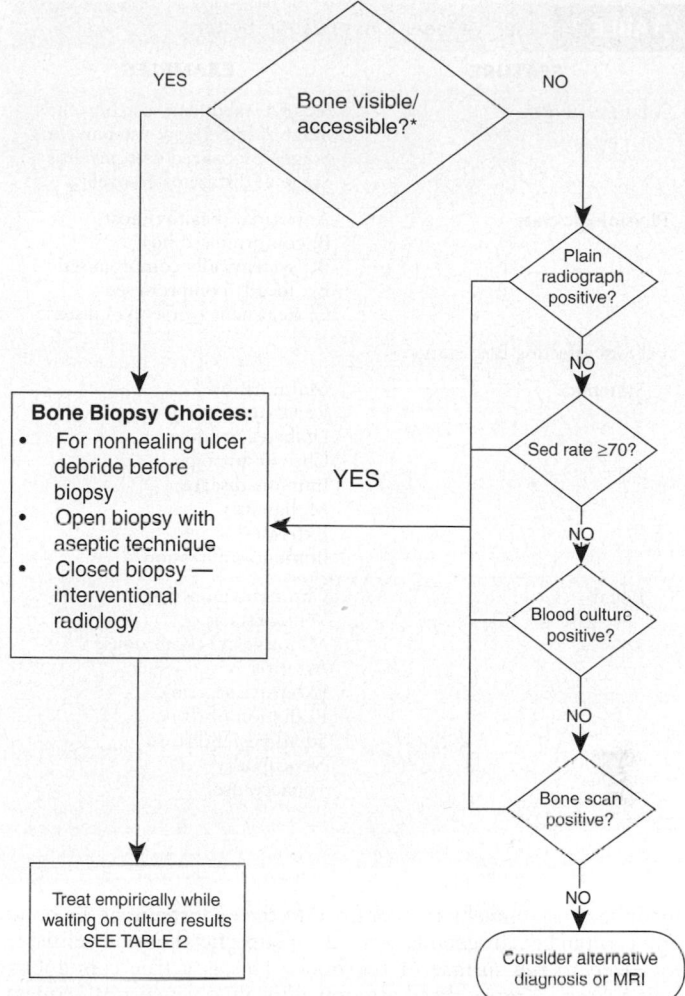

Figure 1. Algorithm for treatment of suspected osteomyelitis. (Courtesy Edward T. Bope.)

Osteomyelitis is a disease of the bone that has changed over the years from a primarily hematogenous disease with high mortality to one of high morbidity. Since the introduction of antibiotics, the incidence of hematogenous osteomyelitis has declined, whereas infection from direct inoculation has increased, especially in those with diabetes. Several methods are used to classify osteomyelitis; most separate the illness into acute or chronic types and hematogenous or contiguous types. Local extension may occur from spread from adjacent structures, or direct implantation of organisms may occur, as seen in cases of trauma or surgical procedures.

The Cierny-Mader system assigns the patient to one of several groups based on the anatomy of the infection and health of the host, including the increased risk for patients who have peripheral arterial obstructive disease or diabetes mellitus. Patients are further separated according to systemic and local factors that may influence disease progression or healing, such as diabetes, extremes of age, and tobacco use. In diabetic patients, osteomyelitis is most commonly caused by overlying lower limb cellulitis. In the nondiabetic adult patient, vertebral osteomyelitis is most common.

The Cierny-Mader classification allows the clinician to use tested treatment protocols, including chemotherapy, surgery, and adjunctive therapies, that are most effective for a specific class of disease and for the host status. The Cierny-Mader system divides the patients into four anatomic groups. Stage 1, or

TABLE 1	Cierny-Mader Classification System	
FEATURE	**EXAMPLES**	
Anatomic type	Stage 1: medullary osteomyelitis Stage 2: superficial osteomyelitis Stage 3: localized osteomyelitis Stage 4: diffuse osteomyelitis	
Physiologic class	A: normal (healthy) host B: compromised host B_S: systemically compromised B_L: locally compromised C: treatment worse than disease	
Factors affecting host status		
Systemic	Malnutrition Renal and hepatic failure Diabetes mellitus Chronic hypoxia Immune disease Malignancy Extremes of age Immunosuppression	
Local	Chronic lymphedema Venous stasis Major vessel compromise Arteritis Extensive scarring Radiation fibrosis Small-vessel disease Neuropathy Tobacco use	

medullary osteomyelitis, is confined to the endosteum of the bone and is often hematogenous. State 2, or superficial osteomyelitis, is localized to the surface of the bone. This is a true contiguous lesion. Stage 3, or localized osteomyelitis, involves cortical sequestration or cavitation, or both, and is a full-thickness lesion that extends into the medullary region. Stage 4, or diffuse osteomyelitis, involves the hard and soft tissues ("through and through"), and it requires surgical débridement of the affected bone to remove all the infected tissue.

For treatment to be successful, the patient must be physiologically able to heal any wounds, defend against contamination or infection, and tolerate the stress of treatment. The hosts are classified as A, B, or C, depending on the ability to resist infections. Those with good immunity are classified as an A host, whereas a B host is compromised locally (B_L) or systemically (B_S); Table 1 shows the physiologic classifications. The final class assigns a C rating to patients whose treatment is more detrimental than the disability from the disease. These patients may require suppressive or no treatment. The clinical stages are adjusted during the course of therapy as conditions change, allowing adjustment of the treatment protocol to optimize therapy.

A much simpler system described by Waldvogel classifies the patient by duration (i.e., acute or chronic) and the mechanism of inoculation (i.e., hematogenous or contiguous). Contiguous infections are further classified as those with or without vascular insufficiency. However, this classification does not provide guidance for specific surgical or antibiotic therapy.

Epidemiology

Acute hematogenous osteomyelitis is usually seen in male children of lower socioeconomic class before the age of 2 years or between 8 and 12 years. There may be some genetic influences. Aboriginal children in Western Australia are known to suffer from acute hematogenous osteomyelitis at a rate nearly four times that of Western European children living in the same neighborhood. An acute infection will progress to chronic osteomyelitis if it is not treated.

Chronic osteomyelitis is usually the result of direct inoculation (e.g., trauma, surgery). Its epidemiology is less clearly described, except in diabetic foot infections. It is estimated that 11 million people in the United States suffer from diabetes. Annually, more than 300,000 of them develop a foot ulcer, and nearly one third of those require amputations. In 2002, osteomyelitis was estimated to cost the citizens of the United States more than $2.3 billion dollars. This major public health problem is expected to increase as the incidence of adults with diabetes increases. Because chronic infection can persist for life, it is important to have early identification and treatment to ensure the best possible outcome.

Pathogenesis

The presence of bacteria in an open wound is not sufficient to cause infection. It is the compromised blood supply of traumatized tissue leading to necrosis and subsequent bacterial adherence that promotes the infection. Trauma can delay the inflammatory response to bacteria, depress cell-mediated immunity, and impair chemotaxis, superoxide production, and the microbial killing capacity of polymorphonuclear neutrophils (PMNs). Osteomyelitis usually involves the metaphysis, which is well vascularized and has significant bone growth.

In acute osteomyelitis, signs or symptoms are usually abrupt. Local infection is characterized by edema, vascular congestion, and small-vessel thrombosis. This leads to increased pressure within the intramedullary canal, allowing extravasation through the Havers and Volkmann canals to the periosteum. In children, the periosteum is usually more flexible and easier to detect radiographically; in adults, the bone matrix is more firmly attached to the periosteum. Untreated, the suppurative infection can reach adjacent soft tissue, leading to a cellulitis. The presence of a Brodie or intraosseous abscess without extravasation into surrounding tissue is classified as subacute pyogenic osteomyelitis. The resulting infection can lead to sequestration involving large areas of bone destruction and dead bone, with reactive bone formation leading ultimately to chronic osteomyelitis.

Chronic osteomyelitis is usually polymicrobial and is characterized by the presence of necrotic bone, new bone growth, and exudation of polymorphonuclear leukocytes, plasma cells, and other infection-fighting cells. The involucrum (i.e., layer of reactive competent bone that covers dead bone) is often dotted with tracts that allow pus to pass into surrounding tissue or to form a sinus tract to the skin surface. These sinus tracts are often contaminated with numerous organisms that do not reflect those found with direct sampling. This repetitive process of bone loss and growth and the involucrum explains why chronic osteomyelitis is difficult to eradicate with antibiotics alone. The antibiotics cannot penetrate avascular areas.

Etiology
Children

In children of all ages, the most common bacterial pathogen is *Staphylococcus aureus*, followed by *Streptococcus pneumoniae* and *Kingella kingae*. However, age and chronic illness allow other organisms to flourish; *Salmonella* and pneumococcal disease (*S. pneumoniae*) are common in patients with sickle cell disease. *Pasteurella multocida*, *Streptococcus* species, and anaerobes often are identified after animal or human bites. In children, most cases arise hematogenously and are characteristically seen in the metaphysis of long bones (i.e., femur, tibia, and humerus), accounting for 68% of childhood infections.

The exact mechanism is unclear, but it is thought that the extensive branching of the nutrient-rich arteries at the metaphyses of the long bones leads to sluggish blood flow and ultimate bacterial seeding. Possible routes include the formation of small hematomas in the metaphysis, allowing microbial seeding after transient bacteremia; penetrating injuries or surgical manipulation, causing direct inoculation of bacteria into bone; and local invasion from a contiguous focus of infection.

Adults

Most infections in adults arise by direct inoculation from sources such as trauma, prosthetic joints, open fractures, and diabetic foot infections. The most common organism remains *S. aureus*. Other organisms to consider include *Staphylococcus epidermis*, *Pseudomonas aeruginosa*, *Escherichia coli*, and *Serratia marcescens*. Most contiguous, related infections are polymicrobial.

Clinical Manifestations

The severity of the signs and symptoms depends on the location of the infection, the patient's age, and any comorbidities. Patients may experience many, few, or no symptoms. Classically, there are marked pain, tenderness, and swelling. Fever and leukocytosis are also common.

Vertebral osteomyelitis often causes severe pain, fever, and disability, whereas osteomyelitis of the foot rarely causes pain. An epidural abscess causes pain and neurologic deficits, whereas vertebral osteomyelitis without abscess formation has no neurologic deficits.

Children often present with systemic symptoms (e.g., fever, weight loss, pain). Pseudoparalysis may be the only sign in a newborn, but toddlers often exhibit pain, fever, erythema, edema, or warmth, or they may suddenly stop walking. In contrast, patients with chronic osteomyelitis may exhibit localized signs and symptoms, including nonhealing ulcers, purulence from sinus tracts, soft tissue edema and pain, abscesses, erythema, pain, and fatigue. Generalized signs and symptoms may be seen early in the disease, but they are unlikely in the later or chronic stages.

Diagnosis
Laboratory tests

A bone biopsy remains the gold standard when diagnosing osteomyelitis. However, there is a high false-negative rate, and the negative predictive value is close to 65%, mainly due to the organism's patchy distribution. No specific laboratory test can be recommended. However, testing acute-phase reactants (e.g., erythrocyte sedimentation rate [ESR], C-reactive protein [CRP], leukocyte count with a differential count) can strongly suggest (positive predictive value of 100%) osteomyelitis if the ESR value is greater than 70 mm/hour in the absence of an inflamed ulcer. However, these tests lack specificity, and it may take several days to demonstrate significantly elevated levels. All patients should have blood cultures performed. A positive blood culture with a suspicious physical finding can suggest a bone infection, but only one half of the cases have a positive test result. Blood cultures, like bone biopsies, can be affected by recent antibiotic exposure.

Radiology

There is no one imaging modality routinely recommended to diagnose osteomyelitis, so diagnosis often requires more than one technique. Plain film radiography should always be the initial study, and the result can be diagnostic if positive. However, changes (usually along the metaphysis) typically require at least 1 to 2 weeks to be seen radiographically.

Positron emission tomography (PET) is the most specific and sensitive of imaging techniques, but its high cost and lack of availability makes it impractical for most clinicians. The best choice for imaging depends on the age of the patient, duration of symptoms, suspected location of infection (if known), and concurrent or previous medical conditions.

Plain radiographs are the most available, least expensive, and easiest to obtain, but they lack sensitivity (43%–75%), and a negative result does not exclude the diagnosis. However, they have reasonable specificity (75%–83%), and a positive finding can confirm the diagnosis or provide clues to alternative pathology, such as a tumor. Bony changes can take between 10 and 21 days to become visible on plain films; however, soft tissue changes can be seen in as little as 3 days. The soft tissue changes are especially important in neonates and children because focal soft tissue swelling around the bony metaphysis may be the first sign of bone involvement.

Radionuclide imaging (i.e., triple-phase bone scan, leukocyte scintigraphy, and PET) is a preferred method of advanced imaging,

and it has several advantages compared with other techniques. Young children often complete the examination without sedation, and prosthetic joints do not produce the artifact commonly seen on magnetic resonance imaging (MRI) and computed tomography (CT) scans. Positive results can be seen 24 to 48 hours after onset of symptoms, and a negative examination result effectively rules out osteomyelitis.

The triple-phase bone scan (technetium 99m diphosphonate) is often the examination of choice (sensitivity of 73%–100%), and it can distinguish between cellulitis and osteomyelitis when complications are absent. However, the sensitivity decreases dramatically when other conditions are present (i.e., trauma, diabetes, or recent surgery), and it has been reported to be as low as 38%. Bone scans usually lack the specificity (25%–90%) of other modalities, fail to provide detailed pictures of complex anatomy, and can be influenced by poor circulation. The examination may take up to 24 hours to complete and often requires the patient to make many trips to the facility. In the early phase, uptake is greatest in areas of acute inflammation. In the next phase, uptake occurs in areas of soft tissue inflammation, and in the late (delayed) phase, uptake remains in the presence of osteomyelitis.

Leukocyte scintigraphy using gallium 67 has a higher specificity (80%–90%) than triple-phase scanning (67%) in the peripheral skeleton, but it decreases to 25% when looking at the axial skeleton. Leukocyte scintigraphy is the preferred method when evaluating patients with previous joint replacements, diabetes, or trauma.

MRI can detect acute osteomyelitis as early as 3 days. It is nearly as sensitive (82%–100%) and specific (75%–96%) as radionuclide studies. MRI allows tracking of disease progress and response to treatment. MRI can be used to date osteomyelitis. Some patients with osteomyelitis are treated and later develop another episode. The MRI can distinguish whether the second episode is a new infection or a recurrence of the previous infection. It also provides detailed visualization of complex anatomy and critical structures, allowing surgeons to map any planned surgical intervention.

CT is rarely used for osteomyelitis, except when sequestered bone is suspected or for interventional procedures. Sinography can be used to map sinus tracts with fluoroscopy or combined with CT. Ultrasound is sometimes used in children and can be helpful in differentiating acute from chronic infections. It provides guidance during drainage, aspirations, or biopsies of the affected bone, and it is a noninvasive method to monitor soft tissue involvement in chronic illness.

Treatment

Older methods, such as closed suction drains, are no longer commonly used because of long hospital stays and the risk of contamination, and newer modalities, such as hyperbaric oxygen therapy, have failed to live up to expectations. The Cierny-Mader classification system provides a straightforward algorithm for treatment. However, the most important factor in any treatment is the identification of the causative organism.

Antibiotic Therapy

Unlike chronic infections, acute infections require hospitalization for initiation of therapy and supportive care. Serial examinations should be undertaken to assess the success of treatment and monitor for systemic signs or symptoms. Cultures of blood and bone should be obtained to guide therapy. Laboratory studies can be followed, but other than CRP levels, they fail to provide significant data. The CRP value can be expected to decrease 24 to 48 hours after initiation of appropriate antibiotic therapy. A lack of response may indicate inappropriate therapy or an occult abscess, and the physician should reconsider surgery if previously delayed.

The medical literature remains inconclusive about the antibiotic treatment of osteomyelitis, especially when trying to determine the best agents, route, or duration of antibiotic therapy. Although the optimal duration of antibiotic therapy remains undefined, most authorities recommend treatment for about 6 weeks (Table 2).

TABLE 2 Antibiotics for Osteomyelitis

ORGANISM	PREFERRED DRUG	ALTERNATIVE DRUGS
Staphylococcus aureus	Nafcillin (Unipen) 1–2 g IV or IM q4h	Cefazolin, vancomycin, clindamycin
Methicillin-resistant *S. aureus*	Vancomycin (Vancocin) 1 g q8h	Trimethoprim-sulfamethoxazole (Bactrim)[1] plus rifampin (Rifadin)[1]
Streptococcus pneumoniae, group A β-hemolytic streptococci	Penicillin G (Pfizerpen)[1] 2 million units IV q4h	Cefazolin, vancomycin, clindamycin
Enterococci, *Haemophilus influenzae* β-lactamase negative	Cefotaxime (Claforan) 2 g q6h	Trimethoprim-sulfamethoxazole, ceftriaxone
H. influenzae β-lactamase positive, *Klebsiella pneumoniae*	Ceftriaxone (Rocephin) 2 g q24h	Trimethoprim-sulfamethoxazole, ciprofloxacin, piperacillin (Pipracil), imipenem (Primaxin)
Escherichia coli	Cefazolin (Ancef) 2 g q8h	Ciprofloxacin, ceftriaxone, imipenem
Pseudomonas aeruginosa	Ciprofloxacin (Cipro) 400 mg q12h	Piperacillin plus aminoglycoside, aztreonam (Azactam)[1]
Salmonella	Choose ampicillin, ceftriaxone, imipenem (Primaxin), or ciprofloxacin, depending on sensitivities	
Bacteroides spp.	Clindamycin (Cleocin) 600 mg q6h	Imipenem, metronidazole (Flagyl)
Serratia marcescens	Ceftriaxone (Rocephin) 2 g q24h	Imipenem, trimethoprim-sulfamethoxazole, ciprofloxacin

Modified from Cohen J, Powderly WG, editors: Infectious Diseases, 2nd ed. St Louis, Mosby, 2003.
[1]Not FDA approved for this indication.

After the infection is under control, the physician may switch the patient to an oral antibiotic for 3 to 12 months (i.e., a fluoroquinolone with or without rifampin [Rifadin][1]). However, treatment can be as short as 3 weeks for uncomplicated, acute, hematogenous osteomyelitis. Management can include oral preparations after a short parenteral course, provided the drug has high bioavailability and the organism is susceptible. A microbiologic diagnosis (preferably by bone biopsy) is essential so that the choice of antibiotic accounts for the specific organism, the host status, and the least toxic medication for the individual. Hematogenous osteomyelitis is usually monomicrobial, whereas contiguous infections are usually polymicrobial and may include *Pseudomonas* in certain populations.

For methicillin-sensitive *S. aureus*, nafcillin (Unipen) or a first- or second-generation cephalosporin can be implemented. For methicillin-resistant *S. aureus*, vancomycin (Vancocin) is recommended. For an anaerobic infection, clindamycin (Cleocin) is a good choice.

Surgery

Bones can heal in the presence of active infection. However, in the presence of obvious signs of infection, such as an abscess or Cierny-Mader stage 3 or 4 disease, acute surgical débridement and irrigation are warranted. The goals of surgery include drainage, débridement, and stabilization. After successful débridement and stabilization, antibiotic therapy is initiated and continued until adequate healing has occurred, usually in 6 weeks. If débridement is unsuccessful, inert substances must be completely removed and tissue débrided. Antibiotics should be placed in contact with the bone using a polymethylmethacrylate antibiotic (PMMA) bead chain or other biodegradable delivery systems to achieve higher local antibiotic concentrations. The site needs to be stabilized with an external fixator, and staged reconstruction should be initiated.

[1]Not FDA approved for this indication.

References

Berendt A, Norden C. Acute and chronic osteomyelitis. In: Cohen J, Powderly WG, editors. Infectious Diseases. 2nd ed St Louis: Mosby; 2003.
Cierny III G, Mader JT, Pennick JJ. A clinical staging system for adult osteomyelitis. Contemp Orthop 1985;10:17–37.
Kaplan SL. Osteomyelitis in children. Infect Dis Clin North Am 2005;19:787–97.
Krogstad P. Osteomyelitis and septic arthritis. In: Feigin RD, Cherry JD, Demmler GJ, et al., Textbook of Pediatric Infectious Diseases. 5th ed Philadelphia: Saunders; 2004. p. 713–36.
Lampe RM. Osteomyelitis. In: Behrman RE, Kliegman RM, Jenson HB, Stanton BF, editors. Nelson Textbook of Pediatrics. 18th ed Philadelphia: Saunders; 2007.
Lazzarini L, Lipsky BA, Mader JT. Antibiotic treatment of osteomyelitis: What have we learned from 30 years of clinical trials? Int J Infect Dis 2005;9:127–38.
Lipsky B, Weigelt J, Gupta V, et al. Skin, soft tissue, bone, and joint infections in hospitalized patients: Epidemiology and microbiological, clinical, and economic outcomes. Infect Control Hosp Epidemiol 2007;28:1290–8.
Pineda C, Vargas A, Rodriguez A. Imaging of osteomyelitis: Current concepts. Infect Dis Clin North Am 2006;20:789–825.
Waldvogel FA, Medoff G, Swartz MN. Osteomyelitis: A review of clinical features, therapeutic considerations and unusual aspects. N Engl J Med 1970;282:198–206.
White LM, Schweitzer ME, Deely DM, Gannon F. Study of osteomyelitis: Utility of combined histologic and microbiologic evaluation of percutaneous biopsy samples. Radiology 1995;197:840–2.
Ziran BH. Osteomyelitis. J Trauma 2007;62(Suppl.):S59–S60.

PLAGUE

Method of
Douglas A. Drevets, MD; and Janice C. Te, MD

CURRENT DIAGNOSIS

- Travel to a plague endemic area or contact with a case of animal or human plague.
- Abrupt onset of fever and prostration.
- Bubo in groin, axillae, or cervical areas.
- Gram-negative coccobacilli with bipolar staining identified in aspirate from bubo, on blood smear, or from blood-tinged sputum.

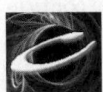

CURRENT THERAPY

- Prompt administration of gentamicin or ciprofloxacin.
- Aggressive supportive care.
- Respiratory isolation of hospitalized cases.
- Postexposure prophylaxis to close contacts.

Historical descriptions indicate that *Yersinia pestis* probably caused Justinian's Plague (AD 541), which led into the first plague pandemic. The second plague pandemic, also known as the Black Death, began in Central Asia in 1347 and then spread to Europe, Asia, and Africa. It killed an estimated 50 million persons. The current (third) plague pandemic began in China and then spread worldwide along shipping routes in 1899–1900. *Y. pestis* is a gram-negative, nonmotile, facultatively anaerobic, non-spore-forming coccobacillus that is approximately 0.5 to 0.8 μm in diameter and 1 to 3 μm in length. Genomic sequencing shows that *Y. pestis* is a recently emerged clone of *Y. pseudotuberculosis*.

Epidemiology

Plague is a zoonosis for which urban and sylvatic rodents (e.g., rats, prairie dogs, and marmots) are the most important enzootic reservoirs. Additionally, domestic cats and dogs have been linked to human disease. Human plague occurs in North and South America, Asia, and Africa. Recent outbreaks reported to the World Health Organization (WHO) have occurred in the Democratic Republic of Congo (2005, 2006), China (2009), and Peru (2010). There were two U.S. cases on Oregon (2010). An average of 2577 (range 876–5419) cases of human plague were reported yearly to the WHO between 1989 and 2003, 80.3% of which were from Africa, with an overall average case fatality rate of 8.14%. In North America, 82% of 295 indigenous cases were from Arizona, Colorado, and New Mexico. Between 1900 and 2010, 999 confirmed or probable cases have occurred in the U.S. with over 80% of these attributable to bubonic plague.

Modes of Transmission

Most human infections are transmitted from rodent to humans via the bite of an infected flea. Infection also can be acquired by contact with body fluids from infected animals, such as during field dressing of game or by inhalation of respiratory droplets from animals, particularly cats, or humans with pneumonic plague.

Bioterrorism Threat

Plague was used as an agent of biowarfare by the Japanese in World War II and was a focus of intensive research and development in the former Soviet Union during the Cold War. Primary pneumonic plague is the most likely form of exposure because of biowarfare or bioterrorism. Recent increases in terrorism worldwide have increased the focus of public health management groups to develop comprehensive statements regarding plague as a biological weapon.

Pathogenesis and Clinical Syndromes

Transdermal inoculation of bacilli from the bite of an infected flea ultimately leads to infection of the regional lymph nodes in which massive replication of bacteria creates the bubo (derived from the Greek *bubon* or "groin"), a swollen, erythematous, and painful lymph node in the groin, axilla, or cervical region. Bacteremia and septicemia frequently develop and lead to secondary infection of other organs including the lungs, spleen, and central nervous system. Primary pneumonic plague is a rare natural occurrence and results from the inhalation of respiratory droplets containing *Y. pestis* bacilli from another case of pneumonic plague, usually in humans or in cats. Secondary pneumonic plague results from seeding of the lungs by blood-borne bacteria in the setting of either bubonic or septicemic plague. Septicemic plague also begins with transdermal exposure but manifests as primary bacteremia/septicemia without the bubo. Less common manifestations include meningitis, pharyngitis, and gastroenteritis.

Bubonic plague is an acute febrile lymphadenitis that develops 2 to 8 days after inoculation. Inflamed lymph nodes are usually 1 to 6 cm in diameter and painful. Abrupt onset of fever is an almost universal finding and occurs simultaneously with, or up to 24 hours before, the appearance of the bubo. Headache, malaise, and chills are frequent, along with nausea, vomiting, and diarrhea. Most patients are tachycardic, hypotensive, and appear prostrate and lethargic with episodic restlessness. Leukocytosis with a left shift is typical. Complications include pneumonia, shock, disseminated intravascular coagulation, purpuric skin lesions, acral cyanosis, and gangrene. The differential diagnosis of bubonic plague includes tularemia and Group A β-hemolytic streptococcal adenitis with bacteremia.

Symptoms of septicemic plague are similar to those caused by other gram-negative bacteria, and are very similar to those of bubonic plague except that abdominal pain is more common in septicemic plague. Septicemic plague must be differentiated from fulminating septicemia caused by other gram-negative bacteria. Primary pneumonic plague has an abrupt onset of fever and influenza-like symptoms 1 to 5 days after inhalation exposure. Symptoms include shortness of breath, cough, chest pain, and bloody sputum with rapid progression to fulminating pneumonia and respiratory failure. Patients with secondary pneumonic infection show respiratory symptoms in addition to those attributed to the bubo or sepsis. Radiographic findings include patchy bronchopneumonia, multilobar consolidations, cavitations, and alveolar hemorrhage and are not pathognomonic of *Y. pestis*. Plague pneumonia must be differentiated from severe influenza, inhalation anthrax, and overwhelming community-acquired pneumonia.

Diagnosis

Plague is diagnosed by demonstrating *Y. pestis* in blood or body fluids such as a lymph node aspirate, sputum, or cerebrospinal fluid. A tentative diagnosis of bubonic plague can be made rapidly with fluid aspirated from a bubo showing gram-negative coccobacilli with bipolar staining. Serology showing a fourfold rise in antibody titers to F1 antigen or a single titer of more than 1:128 is also diagnostic. Rapid tests using monoclonal antibodies to detect *Y. pestis* F1 antigen in bubo aspirates and sputum have been developed and field tested. The use of mass spectrometry as a more rapid and cost-effective diagnostic tool has also been studied.

Treatment

The aminoglycosides (gentamicin and streptomycin), the fluoroquinolones ciprofloxacin (Cipro) and levofloxacin (Levaquin), and doxycycline (Vibramycin) are the first-, second-, and third-line classes of antibiotics, respectively. Typical minimal inhibitory concentrations for 90% (MIC_{90}) of tested strains for the fluoroquinolones are less than 0.03 to 0.25 μg/mL compared with less than 1.0 μg/mL and less than 1.0 μg/mL to 4.0 μg/mL for gentamicin and streptomycin, respectively, and less than 1.0 μg/mL for doxycycline. Streptomycin (15 mg/kg up to 1 g intramuscularly [IM] every 12 hours) and gentamicin (5 to 7 mg/kg/day intravenously [IV]/IM in one or two doses daily) are the drugs of choice for severe infection. Standard fluoroquinolone dosing includes ciprofloxacin 400 mg IV/500 mg orally every 12 hours; levofloxacin 500 mg IV/orally daily; and ofloxacin 400 mg IV/orally every 12 hours. Doxycycline is administered at 100 mg IV/orally every 12 hours. Chloramphenicol (25 mg/kg IV/orally every 6 hours) can be used in select circumstances. Antibiotic therapy should be continued for a total of 10 days.

Prevention and Control

Standard infection control procedures should include a disposable surgical mask, latex gloves, devices to protect mucous membranes, and good hand washing. Hospitalized patients with known or suspected pneumonic plague should be isolated for at least 48 hours after appropriate antibiotics are initiated. Postexposure prophylaxis should be given to individuals with close contact (less than 2 meters) with an infectious case or who have had a potential respiratory exposure. The recommended adult antibiotics for prophylaxis are doxycycline or ciprofloxacin in the same doses used for treatment. Postexposure prophylaxis can be given orally and should be continued for 7 days following exposure. Currently, there is no licensed plague vaccine. An encapsulated *Y. pseudotuberculosis*, strain V674pF1,[5] is an efficient live oral vaccine against pneumonic plague in mice. Recently, flea resistance to insecticides such as DDT and Deltamethrin in Madagascar has prompted an immediate need for alternative insecticides to prevent future plague outbreaks.

References

Boulanger LL, Ettestad P, Fogarty JD, et al. Gentamicin and tetracyclines for the treatment of human plague: review of 75 cases in New Mexico, 1985–1999. Clin Infect Dis 2004;38:663–9.

Boyer S, et al. Xenopsylla cheopis (Siphonaptera: Pulicidae) susceptibility to deltamethrin in Madagascar. PLoS One 2014;9(11):e111998.

Butler T. A clinical study of bubonic plague. Observations of the 1970 Vietnam epidemic with emphasis on coagulation studies, skin histology and electrocardiograms. Am J Med 1972;53:268–76.

Butler T. Plague gives surprises in the first decade of the 21st century in the United States and worldwide. Am J Trop Med Hyg 2013; 89(4):788–93.

CDC. Two cases of human plague—Oregon, 2010. MMWR 2011;60:214.

CDC. Maps and Statistics. http://www.cdc.gov/plague/maps/index.html.

Cler DJ, Vernaleo JR, Lombardi LJ, et al. Plague pneumonia disease caused by Yersinia pestis. Semin Respir Infect 1997;12:12–23.

Derbise A, Cerdà Marín A, et al. An encapsulated Yersinia pseudotuberculosis is a highly efficient vaccine against pneumonic plague. PLoS Negl Trop Dis 2012; Feb;6(2):e1528.

Gage KL, Dennis DT, Orloski KA, et al. Cases of cat-associated human plague in the Western US, 1977–1998. Clin Infect Dis 2000;30:893–900.

Inglesby TV, Dennis DT, Henderson DA, et al. Plague as a biological weapon: Medical and public health management. Working Group on Civilian Biodefense. JAMA 2000;283:2281–90.

Perry RD, Fetherston JD. Yersinia pestis—etiologic agent of plague. Clin Microbiol Rev 1997;10:35–66.

Prentice MB, Rahalison L. Plague. Lancet 2007;369:1196–207.

Wong JD, Barash JR, Sandfort RF, Janda JM. Susceptibilities of Yersinia pestis strains to 12 antimicrobial agents. Antimicrob Agents Chemother 2000;44:1995–6.

World Health Organization. Global Alert and Response. http://www.who.int/csr/disease/plague/en/index.html

PSEUDOMEMBRANOUS COLITIS

Method of
Jennie H. Kwon, DO; and Jeffery D. Semel, MD

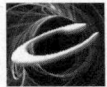

CURRENT DIAGNOSIS

- *Clostridium difficile* infection is diagnosed by a combination of clinical and laboratory findings.
- Diagnosis requires a positive test for the presence of *C. difficile* toxins.
- *C. difficile* cytotoxin assay is the most sensitive and specific test but requires 72 to 96 hours to complete.
- Enzyme immunoassay testing for toxin A and or B has a variable sensitivity and specificity and a turnaround time of about 24 hours.
- Polymerase chain reaction testing has a high sensitivity and specificity and a turnaround time of less than 4 hours.
- Laboratory testing for *C. difficile* toxins should only be performed on unformed stool, and performance on more than one specimen per week is not helpful.
- Pathologic findings can help to confirm diagnosis.

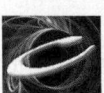

CURRENT THERAPY

- If possible, the clinician should first consider discontinuing concurrent antibacterial therapy.
- Antimotility agents should be avoided because they can decrease gut motility and increase the risk of toxic megacolon.
- Treatment should be initiated only after a positive test result for *C. difficile* toxin unless the patient is at high risk for *C. difficile* infection or is severely ill, in which case empirical therapy is justified.
- Antimicrobials may be administered orally, intravenously, or rectally. Oral therapies are preferred.

- Treatment recommendations depend on the severity of the disease and whether the patient has a first-time diagnosis or recurrence.
- Clinical parameters that guide treatment include increasing age, leukocytosis, elevation of serum creatinine, and presence of hypotension, shock, ileus, or megacolon.
- Antimicrobials used are oral or intravenous metronidazole (Flagyl),[1] oral vancomycin (Vancocin), and rectal vancomycin.[1,6]
- Fidaxomicin (Dificid) was approved for treatment of *C. difficile* infection in 2011. Fidaxomicin was found to be noninferior to vancomycin in a trial and associated with a statistically smaller rate of recurrence of *C. difficile* infection.
- Other agents that have been studied, but for which few high quality studies exist, include fusidic acid (Fucidin),[2] teicoplanin (Targocid),[5] rifaximin (Xifaxan),[1] nitazoxanide (Alinia),[1] and tigecycline (Tygacil).[1]

[1]Not FDA approved for this indication.
[2]Not available in the United States.
[5]Investigational drug in the United States.
[6]May be compounded by pharmacists.

Pseudomembranous colitis is an inflammatory disease of the colon that is almost always associated with the toxin-producing bacteria *Clostridium difficile*. In very rare cases, other organisms can be responsible. In this article we discuss *C. difficile* as an important cause of pseudomembranous colitis.

Epidemiology and Risk Factors

C. difficile is the most common infectious cause of health care–associated diarrhea. Both the incidence and the attributable mortality of *C. difficile* infection appear to be increasing. Studies in U.S. hospitals showed that mortality due to *C. difficile* infection nearly quadrupled from 1999 through 2004. An active population and laboratory based study done by the U.S Center for Disease Control in 2011 suggested that 453,000 new cases occur in the U.S. annually; with a 30 day mortality of 6.4%. Higher rates of infection were found in whites, females, and those > 65 years of age. A Canadian study in 2011 prospectively followed 5422 hospitalized patients and showed that 7.4% had asymptomatic colonization only (60% of these were positive at the time of admission); 2.8% developed *C. difficile* infection during hospitalization. Other studies have found the prevalence of colonization to be as high as 18%.

Additional risk factors for the development of *C. difficile* infection include antimicrobial or chemotherapeutic drug exposure, severe underlying illness, prior hospitalization (acute or long-term care), use of feeding tubes, recent gastrointestinal surgery, and use of proton pump inhibitors. Exposure to antibiotics, which alter the normal intestinal flora, is the main modifiable risk factor. Most antibiotics have been associated with *C. difficile* infection. Increased antimicrobial duration and dosage appear to be associated with higher risk of *C. difficile* infection.

Epidemic strains have been described by pulsed-field gel electrophoresis, (NAP1,4,7,11 etc.), that are associated with decreased regulatory gene function and increased toxin production. The risk and severity of infection are increased following exposure to the NAP1 strains. Failure of standard first-line therapy for *C. difficile* infection has may increase to 10% to 35% during infection with this NAP strains.

C. difficile infection occurs rarely without prior antibiotic exposure. Healthy peripartum women, children, and postsurgical patients rarely develop *C. difficile* infection after a single dose of antibiotics. Newborns have a higher rate of colonization, but generally a low rate of *C. difficile* infection.

Microbiology and Pathophysiology

C. difficile is a Gram-positive, spore-forming, anaerobic rod. The name "difficile" was given because it was historically difficult to grow in culture. *C. difficile* can exist as either a spore or vegetative form. The vegetative form is highly oxygen sensitive; slight exposure can kill the bacteria. The spore form is highly heat-stable and can survive harsh conditions such as the high acidity of the stomach. Spores have been shown to resist many commercial disinfectants. *C. difficile* reproduces in intestinal crypts and releases exotoxins A and B, leading to severe inflammation. Toxin A (enterotoxin) attracts neutrophils and monocytes, and toxin B (cytotoxin) degrades colonic epithelial cells. Most strains of *C. difficile* produce both toxin A and B. Toxins disrupt cell membranes and cause shallow ulcerations on the intestine mucosal surface. Ulcer formation leads to the release of proteins, mucus, and inflammation manifesting as a pseudomembrane. A pseudomembrane is virtually pathognomonic for *C. difficile* infection.

Transmission occurs via the fecal–oral route, person to person, or via fomites. Following exposure to antibiotics, the normal gut flora is altered, allowing *C. difficile* to become more dominant. Exposure to *C. difficile* spores can result in no acquisition, asymptomatic colonization, mild diarrhea, or infection. The incidence of colonization increases at a steady rate during hospitalization, suggesting ongoing exposure to spores. Patients who are colonized at the time of admission to an acute care facility have a much lower risk for *C. difficile* infection than those who acquire it following admission.

Evidence suggests that the host immune response to spore exposure is important in determining the clinical outcome. Approximately 60% of people have detectable levels of antibodies to toxin A and B. It is likely that prior exposure to *C. difficile* spores or related clostridial species and subsequent colonization stimulates antibody production and immunity. Various studies are attempting to define the role of active or passive immunotherapy, including vaccination with nontoxigenic *C. difficile*, to prevent *C. difficile* infection.

Clinical Features

C. difficile infection is diagnosed by a combination of clinical and laboratory findings. Diarrhea is defined as the passage of three or more unformed stools in a 24-hour period. Symptoms include fever, diarrhea, and cramplike abdominal pain. Patients can have nausea, vomiting, or hematochezia. In severe cases, abdominal tenderness and distention are present. Signs of septic shock can develop. The white blood cell count (WBC) is often elevated, as high as 30,000 to 50,000 cells/μL. The extent of leukocytosis correlates with disease severity. Plain abdominal radiographs might show distended loops of bowel or, in severe cases, toxic megacolon. Computed tomography (CT) image findings include colonic wall thickening and dilatation, mesenteric edema, and, rarely, perforation. Endoscopy can reveal pseudomembranes. However, sigmoidoscopy or colonoscopy may be complicated by perforation in severely ill patients and should be performed with caution.

Differential Diagnosis

The differential diagnosis includes bacterial causes such as *Shigella*, *Salmonella*, or *Campylobacter* species, protozoan infections such as *Entamoeba histolytica* or *Strongyloides stercoralis* (immunosuppressed patients), inflammatory disorders such as ulcerative colitis or Crohn's disease, drug toxicity (e.g. chemotherapeutic agents), and vascular disorders such as ischemic bowel disease.

Diagnosis

Confirmation of the diagnosis of *C. difficile* infection requires a positive test for the presence of *C. difficile* toxins. Pathologic findings can help to confirm the diagnosis. *C. difficile* infection should be considered in any patient who develops diarrhea during or after exposure to antibacterial or antineoplastic agents. Laboratory testing should only be performed on unformed stools in patients who meet the definition of diarrhea. A single specimen at the onset of illness is recommended, because additional specimens have not been found to increase the yield. Various methods are available to detect *C. difficile* infection.

Cytotoxin assay for toxin B is highly sensitive and specific but requires a tissue culture facility and is therefore more labor intensive. Enzyme immunoassay (EIA) testing for toxin A or toxin A

and B is currently the most widely used test for *C. difficile* infection and has a sensitivity of 63% to 94% and specificity of 75% to 100%. The turnaround time for EIA is usually 24 hours.

EIA testing is also available for glutamate dehydrogenase (GDH), a "common" *C. difficile* antigen. This test is rapid, is easy to perform, and has a high sensitivity of 85% to 95% and specificity of 89% to 99%. It, too, does not differentiate between nontoxigenic and toxigenic strains. It may be useful to rule out *C. difficile* infection, but would require a second test for toxin assay if positive.

More recently, polymerase chain reaction (PCR) testing has been developed and can be performed in less than 4 hours. The sensitivity is approximately 93% and specificity 97%. Testing costs might initially exceed costs for other methods but are expected to yield savings based upon greater accuracy and from lower costs of barrier precautions.

Treatment

If possible, the clinician should first consider discontinuing concurrent antibacterial therapy, unless there is a compelling clinical indication to continue. Antimotility agents should be avoided because decreased gut motility can increase the potential for tissue toxin exposure and toxic megacolon. Treatment for *C. difficile* infection should be initiated only after a positive test result unless the patient is at high risk for *C. difficile* infection or is severely ill, in which case empirical therapy is reasonable even with negative test results.

Antibacterials used to treat *C. difficile* infection can be administered orally, intravenously, or rectally. Oral therapies are preferred. Oral metronidazole (Flagyl), a nitroimidazole antibiotic, is eliminated primarily in the urine, although 6% to 15% is eliminated in the feces. Oral vancomycin (Vancocin) is not absorbed in the gastrointestinal tract and is eliminated in the feces.

The Society for Healthcare Epidemiology of America (SHEA) and the Infectious Diseases Society of America (IDSA) published treatment guidelines in 2010. Recommendations for the treatment of *C. difficile* infection depend on the severity of the disease. Clinical parameters that correlate with severity include increasing age, leukocytosis, and elevation of the serum creatinine.

For patients with a first episode of *C. difficile* infection that is mild to moderate, metronidazole (Flagyl)[1] 500 mg PO three times per day for 10 to 14 days is recommended. Supportive clinical data in mild to moderate disease includes a WBC count less than 15,000 cells/μL and a serum creatinine less than 1.5 times the premorbid level.

For patients with a first episode that is severe, vancomycin (Vancocin) 125 mg PO for 10 to 14 days is recommended. A WBC count of at least 15,000 cells/μL or a serum creatinine at least 1.5 times the premorbid level suggests a severe infection.

Patients with an initial episode that is complicated by hypotension, shock, ileus, or megacolon should be treated with vancomycin 500 mg PO 4 times per day,[3] plus metronidazole[1] 500 mg IV every 8 hours. If the patient has a complete ileus, the clinician may consider adding a rectal instillation of vancomycin[1,6] 500 mg every 6 hours.

Monitoring

The response to therapy should be monitored clinically. Reversal of hemodynamic instability, decreasing stool frequency, and a declining WBC count are objective measures of response. Stool tests for *C. difficile* toxin are not valuable for monitoring disease elimination, because these tests can remain positive following improvement.

Complications and Recurrence

Another challenging problem in *C. difficile* infection is recurrence. Recurrence is defined as another episode that occurs within eight weeks of the initial episode. Recurrence occurs in approximately 20% to 30% of cases following resolution of the initial episode. Continued use of antibacterials (other than treating agents), increased age, longer hospitalization, severe underlying disease,

[1]Not FDA approved for this indication.
[3]Exceeds dosage recommended by the manufacturer.
[6]May be compounded by pharmacists.

and inadequate antitoxin antibody response are risk factors for relapse. Even though treatment failure and relapse are common, resistance to metronidazole or vancomycin is uncommon.

Treatment is the same for the first recurrence as for a primary episode. For additional recurrent episodes, consider an infectious diseases consult and a vancomycin taper with a pulsed dose regimen.[3] This consists of vancomycin 125 mg PO 4 times per day for 2 weeks, followed by 125 mg PO 2 times per day for 1 week, followed by vancomycin 125 mg PO once daily for 1 week, followed by 125 mg PO once every 2 to 3 days for 2 to 8 weeks.

Other agents that have been studied, but for which few high-quality studies exist, include fusidic acid (Fucidin),[2] teicoplanin (Targocid),[5] rifaximin (Xifaxan),[1] nitazoxanide (Alinia),[1] and tigecycline (Tygacil).[1] Fidaxomicin (Dificid) was approved for treatment of C. difficile infection in 2011. Fidaxomicin, a macrocyclic antibacterial, has greater in vitro activity against C. difficile than vancomycin does, and it is also nonabsorbed. Fidaxomicin, 200 mg PO twice daily was compared to vancomycin 125 mg PO four times daily in patients with C. difficile infection. Fidaxomicin was found to be noninferior to vancomycin in this trial and associated with a statistically smaller rate of recurrence of C. difficile infection.

Another option for recurrent C. difficile infection is fecal reconstitution or fecal microbiota therapy (FMT). The goal is to restore normal colonic flora. Healthy donor stool from a related or unrelated donor is infused. A randomized study of patients with recurrent C. difficile infection compared duodenal FMT to vancomycin alone or vancomycin and bowel lavage and found FMT to be superior. A review of 536 patients with recurrent C. difficile infection showed a 81% to 93% response rate regardless of whether the stool was infused into the stomach, duodenum, cecum, or distal colon. Frozen FMT has also been used successfully. Donor stool must be screened for infectious agents prior to installation. An IND (investigational new drug) application is suggested for physicians or programs wishing to employ FMT. A written consent should be obtained stating the potential risks and that FMT is an investigational procedure.

Probiotics[7] are live organisms that seek to restore the normal gastrointestinal microflora. Most studies have employed Lactobacillus species or Saccharomyces boulardii in an effort to prevent, or treat C. difficile infection. A few small studies have shown benefit, but none are able to demonstrate adequate statistical power for efficacy. Occasional cases of fungemia or bacteremia have been reported in immunocompromised patients and those with central venous catheters treated with probiotics. Probiotics should be avoided in these patients.

Total colectomy is often considered as a last measure for patients who remain critically ill despite standard therapy. The exact indications for surgery are not clear, though refractory shock, signs of peritonitis, megacolon, and multiorgan failure are most often cited. As expected, the mortality rate for total colectomy is high, ranging from 35% to 80%. Neal and colleagues reported that in a series of 42 patients, performance of a diverting loop ileostomy and intraoperative colonic lavage with polyethylene glycol, followed by postoperative antegrade vancomycin flushes, resulted in 19% mortality and 93% colon preservation.

Prevention

Given the current difficulties in controlling the spread of C. difficile, prevention is critical. C. difficile spores resist desiccation and can survive in the hospital environment for months. Environmental contamination is highest in and around the rooms of patients with C. difficile infection. Items that have been found to harbor C. difficile spores include clothing, blood pressure cuffs, telephones, toilets, doorknobs, oral and rectal thermometers, and

other medical equipment. In addition, the hands of health care workers have been found to be a vehicle of transmission.

Current recommendations for prevention of transmission of C. difficile include the following. Careful hand hygiene with soap and water is essential. Programs to monitor the compliance and technique of hand hygiene are recommended. Alcohol-based hand rubs, which are widely used, have been shown to be less effective at removing spores than conventional hand washing. Thus alcohol-based hand rubs should not be used for C. difficile isolation. Barrier precautions with gowns and gloves should be used. Programs to ensure adequate and effective cleaning of health care facilities following use are recommended. Disposable electronic thermometers are recommended. Antimicrobial stewardship programs aimed at promoting the judicious use of antibacterial therapy have been found to be effective in reducing C difficile infection rates should be employed.

References

Aichinger E, Schleck CD, Harmsen WS, et al. Nonutility of repeat laboratory testing for detection of clostridium difficile by use of PCR or enzyme immunoassay. J Clin Microbiol 2008;46:3795–7.

Bignardi GE. Risk factors for Clostridium difficile infection. J Hosp Infect 1998;40:1–15.

Cammarota G, Ianiro G, Gasbarrini A. Fecal microbiota transplantation for the treatment of Clostridium difficile infection: a systematic review. J Clin Gastroenterol 2014 Jan 16 (Epub ahead of print).

Cohen SH, Gerding DN, Johnson S, et al. Clinical practice guidelines for Clostridium difficile infection in adults: 2010 update by the Society for Healthcare epidemiology of America (SHEA) and the Infectious diseases Society of America (IDSA). Infect Control Hosp Epidemiol 2010;31:431–55.

Feazel L, Malhotra A, Perencevich E, et al. Effect of antibiotic stewardship programmes on Clostridium difficile incidence: a systematic review and meta-analysis. J Antimicrob Chemother 2014;69:1748–54.

Hsu J, Abad C, Dinh M, et al. Prevention of endemic healthcare-associated Clostridium difficile infection: reviewing the evidence. Am J Gastroenterol 2010;105:2327–39.

Johnson S. Recurrent Clostridium difficile infection: A review of risk factors, treatments, and outcomes. J Infection 2009;58:403–10.

Lessa E, Mu Y, Bamberg W, et al. Burden of Clostridium difficile infection in the United States. N Engl J Med 2015;372:825–34.

Loo VG, Bourgalt A, Poirier L, et al. Host and pathogen factors for Clostridium difficile infection and colonization. N Engl J Med 2011;365:1693–703.

Louie TJ, Miller MA, Mullane KM, et al. Fidaxomicin versus vancomycin for Clostridium difficile infection. N Engl J Med 2011;364:422–31.

Neal M, Alverdy JC, Hall DE, et al. Diverting loop ileostomy and colonic lavage: An alternative to total abdominal colectomy for treatment of severe, complicated Clostridium difficile associated disease. Ann Surg 2011;254:423–7.

Peterson LR, Manson RU, Paule SM, et al. Detection of toxigenic Clostridium difficile in stool samples by real-time polymerase chain reaction for the diagnosis of C. difficile–associated diarrhea. Clin Inf Dis 2007;45:1152–60.

Stevens V, Dumyati G, Fine LS, et al. Cumulative antibiotic exposures over time and the risk of Clostridium difficile infection. Clin Infect Dis 2011;53:42–8.

Van Nood E, Vrieze A, Nieuwdorp M, et al. Duodenal Infusion of Donor Feces for Recurrent Clostridium difficile. N Engl J Med 2014;368:407–15.

PSITTACOSIS

Method of
Christopher C. McGuigan, MBChB, MPH

CURRENT DIAGNOSIS

- The key to successful management of psittacosis is to consider this diagnosis, particularly in cases of community-acquired pneumonia (CAP), especially given a history of bird contact.
- The typical clinical pictures are of CAP, influenza-like illness, or fever of unknown origin. Onset is usually sudden with fever, chills and a prominent headache. Consider this diagnosis in a patient with CAP unresponsive to β-lactam antibiotics.
- Investigation will typically reveal a normal or slightly elevated white blood cell count with a left shift or toxic changes, increase in C-reactive protein (CRP) or erythrocyte sedimentation rate (ESR), mildly abnormal liver function tests, hyponatremia, and mild renal impairment. Chest x-ray may be more abnormal than examination alone would predict.

---

[1]Not FDA approved for this indication.
[2]Not available in the United States.
[3]Exceeds dosage recommended by the manufacturer.
[5]Investigational drug in the United States.
[7]Available as a dietary supplement.

- Diagnosis can be confirmed with (ideally) paired serum samples: using either the complement fixation test (widely used but unable to differentiate between *Chamydophila* species), or the microimmunofuorescence test, which is specific for individual *Chamydophila* species. Either a single high titer or a fourfold rise in titer using samples collected at least 14 days apart are interpreted as positive. More recently, real-time polymerase chain reaction (rt-PCR) tests have been used to detect specific DNA and can provide a more rapid diagnosis as well as sub-specific genotype.

CURRENT THERAPY

- Therapy should commence when the diagnosis is suspected on clinical presentation and initial investigation.
- Tetracyclines are the drugs of choice; for example, doxycycline (Vibramycin) 100 mg bid for 10 to 14 days.
- Macrolides are suitable (but probably less effective) alternatives in those intolerant of tetracyclines (e.g., children and pregnant women).
- Notification to health authorities facilitates public health investigation and interventions to reduce transmission and control outbreaks.

Psittacosis is caused by infection with the bacterium *Chlamydopila psittaci* (formerly *Chlamydia psittaci*). It is twice as common in men than in women, and mainly affects adults typically aged 40 to 50 years. The main reservoir for psittacosis is birds, particularly psittacine birds (parrots, parakeets, budgerigars and cockatoos), but other bird species and mammals can be infected.

Risk Factors

The most common etiological factor is exposure to infected birds—especially a new, sick, or dead bird—typically a pet or via occupational exposure (e.g., work as a veterinarian, zoo keeper, or poultry-worker). Most cases are sporadic, but outbreaks have occurred associated with pet shops, aviaries, and poultry-processing plants and with mowing lawns in areas with large numbers of psittacine birds. Person-to-person transmission is rare. Ingestion of poultry products is *not* a risk factor.

Pathophysiology

C. psittaci infection is via the respiratory tract, and is typically thought to be by inhalation of an aerosol of dried faeces or other avian secretion. It then either travels via the blood to the liver and spleen (where it replicates, causing a secondary bacteremia) or directly infects respiratory epithelial cells.

Prevention

Prevention is aimed at controlling disease and/or colonization in susceptible host species: usually birds. This is facilitated by import restrictions including quarantine and treatment of suspected infections with tetracycline-impregnated feeds. Notification of health authorities is important for initiating public health investigations and interventions to reduce transmission and control of outbreaks.

Clinical Manifestations

The incubation period varies from 4 to 14 or more days. The typical presentation of psittacosis is of an influenza-like illness with sudden onset of fever, chills, and prominent headache, with or without rigors. A more gradual onset is also seen. A typically mild, dry cough usually starts later. There may also be diarrhea, pharyngitis, altered mental state, or shortness of breath. Chest examination is usually abnormal, but the findings are often minimal and

less prominent than symptoms or x-ray findings would suggest. Pleural effusion is rare.

Patients might present with a fever of unknown origin without obvious respiratory involvement, or the disease can be misdiagnosed as meningitis due to prominent headache, sometimes with photophobia.

The white cell count is usually normal or slightly raised, but there is often a left shift or toxic changes. Increases in the C-reactive protein (CRP) and erythrocyte sedimentation rate (ESR) are common. Mildly abnormal liver function tests, hyponatraemia, and mild renal impairment are also common. The cerebrospinal fluid sometimes contains a few mononuclear cells but is otherwise normal. The chest x-ray usually shows more (nonspecific) abnormality than examination findings might predict. The most common finding is lobar consolidation, but bilateral consolidation and interstitial opacities are also common.

Confirmation of diagnosis is more commonly performed using serology. The complement fixation (CF) test is widely used, but it cannot differentiate between *Chlamydophila* species. A fourfold rise in titer, using samples collected at least 14 days apart, or a single titer of 1:128 or higher, is interpreted as positive, but this test is not widely available. Culture of *C. psittaci* is difficult and hazardous. Polymerase chain reaction (PCR) assays have been developed, but are not yet widely available for routine clinical use.

Diagnosis

Diagnosis is facilitated by eliciting a history of recent bird contact from a patient with a compatible clinical syndrome, most commonly an influenza-like presentation, community acquired pneumonia (CAP), or a fever of unknown origin. The diagnosis should be considered in a patient with CAP and prominent headache, splenomegaly, or failure to respond to β-lactam antibiotics.

Differential Diagnosis

Differential diagnosis of an atypical CAP, includes infection with *Legionella* species, *Mycoplasma pneumoniae*, or *Chlamydophila pneumoniae*.

Treatment

When the diagnosis is suspected on clinical presentation and initial investigations, empiric therapy should be commenced. Tetracyclines are the drugs of choice, for example doxycycline (Vibramycin) 100 mg bid for 10 to 14 days. Tetracycline treatment usually leads to improvement in symptoms (including fever) within 24 to 48 hours. Macrolides are usually recommended for pregnant women, children, and other patients intolerant of tetracyclines. However, erythromycin (Erythrocin)[1] has been shown to fail in situations where a tetracycline was effective, and there are few clinical data on the efficacy of the other agents in this class. Some data suggest that quinolones may be effective. Tetracycline hydrochloride[2] or doxycycline (4.4 mg/kg/d divided into two infusions) may be given intravenously for critically ill patients.

Monitoring

Symptomatic improvement usually occurs within 24 to 28 hours of starting a tetracycline; typically including reduction of fever.

Complications

The degree of illness varies from asymptomatic to life threatening. Given appropriate antimicrobial therapy, subsequent mortality is less than 1%. Elderly persons and pregnant women are susceptible to more severe illness. Neurologic sequelae (e.g., meningoencephalitis) are recognized but rare complications. Other less-common findings include hemoptysis, proteinuria, hepatosplenomegaly, and encephalitis. Cardiac manifestations include relative bradycardia and, rarely, myocarditis, culture-negative endocarditis, and pericarditis. Erythema nodosum and other skin

---

[1]Not FDA approved for this indication.
[2]Not available in the United States.

manifestations have also been described. *C. psittaci* has been demonstrated by PCR to be present in ocular adnexal lymphoma (OAL) in parts of Eurasia, with up to one half of cases responding to antibiotic treatment. However, studies elsewhere suggest that this organism might not play a ubiquitous role in OAL. Recovery with minimal residual deficit is normal.

References

Contini C, Seraceni S, Carradori S, et al. Identification of *Chlamydia trachomatis* in a patient with ocular lymphoma. Am J Hematol 2009;84:597–9.

Grayston JT, Thom DH. The chlamydial pneumonias. Curr Clin Top Infect Dis 1991;11:1–18.

Heddema ER, Beld MG, De Wever B, et al. Development of an internally controlled real-time PCR assay for detection of *Chlamydophila psittaci* in the LightCycler 2.0 system. Clin Microbiol Infect 2006;12:571–5.

Hughes P, Chidley K, Cowie J. Neurological complications in psittacosis: a case report and literature review. Respir Med 1995;89:637–8.

National Association of State Public Health Veterinarians. Compendium of measures to control *Chlamydophila psittaci* infection among humans (psittacosis) and pet birds (avian chlamydiosis), 2010. Available at: http://www.nasphv.org/Documents/Psittacosis.pdf [accessed July 9, 2015].

Richards M. Psittacosis, Up to date 2006; Available at http://www.uptodate.com/physicians/pulmonology_toclist.asp [accessed 31.12.12; subscription required].

Williams J, Tallis G, Dalton C, et al. Community outbreak of psittacosis in a rural Australian town. Lancet 1998;351:1697–9.

Yung AP, Grayson ML. Psittacosis: a review of 135 cases. Med J Aust 1988;148:228–33.

Q FEVER

Method of
Didier Raoult, MD, PhD

Q fever is a widespread zoonosis caused by *Coxiella burnetii*, a small, coccoid, strict intracellular gram-negative bacterium. It lives within the phagolysosome of its eukaryotic host cell at very low pH (4.5-4.8). It had previously been classified in the rickettsial family; however, recent phylogenic data based on study of the 16S rRNA gene sequence have shown that it belongs to *Legionellales* with the *Legionella* species and *Francisella tularensis*.

The bacterium has a sporelike life cycle, which explains its marked resistance to physicochemical agents. In cultures, *C. burnetii* exhibits a phase variation (from virulent phase I to avirulent phase II) caused by a spontaneous chromosome deletion. The avirulent form paradoxically generates high antibody levels in patients, but only patients with chronic infection have high antiphase I immunoglobulin G (IgG) and IgA antibody titers.

The reservoir of *C. burnetii* is wide, and nearly all tested mammals, birds, and ticks can be infected. Outbreaks have also been reported in association with the birth products of mammals (including ungulates and pets), raw milk, slaughterhouses, and farm work. Laboratory outbreaks have been reported. The disease is prevalent everywhere in the world but in New Zealand and South Pacific Islands, but because its clinical spectrum is wide and nonspecific, the observed incidence is directly related to physician interest in Q fever.

Clinical Features

Q fever is a reportable disease in the United States. In humans, infection is symptomatic in only 50% of patients. Most symptomatic patients experience a flulike syndrome lasting 2 to 7 days and consisting of severe headaches and cough; 5% to 10% of infected patients may be sick enough to be investigated. They initially have high fever and one or several of pneumonia, hepatitis, meningoencephalitis, rash, myocarditis, and pericarditis. Routine laboratory investigation commonly shows mildly elevated transaminase levels and mild thrombocytopenia.

In special hosts such as immunocompromised patients (specifically those with lymphoma or splenectomy), *C. burnetii* can cause endocarditis. In pregnant women it can lead to recurrent miscarriage, low-birth-weight offspring, and prematurity.

In patients with valvular heart disease and those with arterial aneurysms or a vascular prosthesis, it can cause chronic endocarditis or vascular infection in patients in the 2 years following primary infection. The clinical picture is that of a chronic blood culture–negative endocarditis; the modified Duke criteria are of diagnostic value in such cases. It is spontaneously fatal in most cases.

Diagnosis

Because Q fever is pleomorphic, the diagnosis is based mainly on comprehensive serum testing in patients with an unexplained infectious syndrome. Liver biopsy may be of diagnostic value because the typical doughnut granuloma is quasispecific to acute Q fever. Valves obtained at surgery or autopsy can be used for culture, direct immunostaining, and polymerase chain reaction (PCR).

Three serologic techniques are used. Complement fixation lacks sensitivity, and one third of patients with acute Q fever do not exhibit complement-fixing antibodies within 1 month after onset of the disease. However, a fourfold increase in antibodies to phase II antigen indicates acute Q fever, and antibody levels against phase I that are higher than 1:200 indicate chronic Q fever. Indirect immunofluorescence assay is the reference method. A single titer of 1:200 for IgG antiphase II associated with a titer of 1:50 for IgM is diagnostic of acute infection. IgG antibody levels against phase I that are greater than 1:800 and IgA antibody levels greater than 1:50 are highly predictive of endocarditis or vascular infection. Enzyme-linked immunosorbent assay (ELISA) is useful for diagnosing acute infection in detecting IgM antiphase II.

PCR has recently been developed to detect *C. burnetii* DNA in the sera of patients with Q fever. Real-time PCR using multicopy gene *IS1111* is the more-sensitive technique. It is positive in the sera of patients with acute Q fever before IgG antibodies to *C. burnetii* become apparent. It is also positive in patients with untreated chronic Q fever. Contamination of PCR can occur, and many unconfirmed results are reported in the literature. Detection of patients at risk for endocarditis may be provided by systematic echocardiography in patients with acute Q fever specifically seeking for aortic bicuspidy and serologic follow-up at 3 and 6 months after acute infection.

Use of a positron emission tomography (PET) scanner may help in the diagnosis of endocarditis (and may reveal mycotic aneurysms), vascular infection, and joint infection.

Treatment

To be active against Q fever, an antibiotic compound has to enter the cell, be effective at an acidic pH (where *C. burnetii* multiplies), and have activity against *C. burnetii*. No antibiotic is bactericidal, but bactericidal activity can be achieved by the addition of hydroxychloroquine (Plaquenil)[1] to doxycycline (Vibramycin).

For acute Q fever, the reference treatment is doxycycline 100 mg orally twice daily for 2 to 3 weeks. Other compounds have been reported to be effective, such as trimethoprim-sulfamethoxazole (TMP-SMX) (Bactrim),[1] Rifampin (Rifadin)[1] 300 mg twice daily, and ofloxacin (Floxin)[1] 200 mg twice daily. In the case of Q fever in pregnant women, one double-strength TMP-SMX tablet (trimethoprim 160 mg, sulfamethoxazole 800 mg)[1] twice daily until delivery prevents fetal death (Table 1).

Chronic endocarditis should be treated for 18 months to 2 years, and antibody levels should be monitored. Patients with prosthetic valves may be treated for 2 years. Two protocols have been evaluated: doxycycline 200 mg daily combined with ofloxacin[1] 400 mg daily for 4 years to lifetime, and doxycycline combined with hydroxychloroquine[1] for 1.5 to 2 years in an amount to achieve a 1 ± 0.20 µg/mL plasma concentration. Doxycycline serum levels greater than 4.5 µg/mL of serum are associated with a more rapidly favorable outcome. This last regimen is apparently more efficacious in terms of relapse. However, regular

---

[1]Not FDA approved for this indication.

TABLE 1	Treatment		
Q FEVER	**RECOMMENDED TREATMENT**	**ALTERNATIVE TREATMENT**	
Acute	Doxycycline (Vibramicyn) 100 mg PO q12h × 14 d	Ofloxacin (Floxin)[1] 200 mg PO q8h[3] × 14 d Cotrimoxazole (Bactrim)[1] 160/800 mg/PO q12h × 14 d	
Endocarditis	Doxycycline 100 mg PO q12h *plus* hydroxychloroquine (Plaquenil)[1] 200 mg PO q8h[3] × 18–24 mo	Doxycycline 100 mg PO q12h *plus* ofloxacin[1] 200 mg PO q8h[3] for 3 y to lifetime	
Acute in a patient with a valvular lesion	Same as chronic Q fever for 12 mo		
In pregnancy	Cotrimoxazole (Bactrim)[1] 160/800 mg PO q12h until term		

[1]Not FDA approved for this indication.
[3]Exceeds dosage recommended by the manufacturer.

ophthalmologic surveillance is critical to detect the accumulation of chloroquine in the retina. Both regimens expose the patient to a major risk of photosensitization.

The combination of doxycycline and hydroxychloroquine for 1 year has demonstrated efficacy in preventing endocarditis.

Prevention

Prevention depends on avoiding exposure, particularly by pregnant women and patients with valvulopathy. No vaccine is currently available outside Australia.

References

Klee SR, et al. Highly sensitive real-time PCR for specific detection and quantification of Coxiella burnetii. BMC Microbiol 2006;19:2.

Maurin M, Raoult D. Q fever. Clin Microbiol Rev 1999;12:518–53.

Merhej V, Cammilleri S, Piquet P, et al. Relevance of the positron emission tomography in the diagnosis of vascular graft infection with *Coxiella burnetii*. Comp Immunol Microbiol Infect Dis 2012;35(1):45–9.

Million M, Roblot F, Carles D, D'Amato F, Protopopescu C, Carrieri MP, et al. Reevaluation of the risk of fetal death and malformation after q fever. Clin Infect Dis 2014;59(2):256–60.

Million M, Thuny F, Richet H, Raoult D. Long-term outcome of Q fever endocarditis: a 26-year personal survey. Lancet Infect Dis 2010;10:527–35.

Million M, Walter G, Thuny F, Habib G, Raoult D. Evolution from acute Q fever to endocarditis is associated with underlying valvulopathy and age and can be prevented by prolonged antibiotic treatment. Clin Infect Dis 2013;57(6):836–44.

Raoult D. Chronic Q fever: expert opinion versus literature analysis and consensus. J Infect. 2012 April 23 (Epub ahead of print).

Rolain JM, Maurin M, Raoult D. Bacteriostatic and bactericidal activities of moxifloxacin against Coxiella burnetii. Antimicrob Agents Chemother 2001;45:301–2.

RABIES

Method of
Alan C. Jackson, MD

CURRENT DIAGNOSIS

- A history of animal bite or exposure is often absent in North America.
- Pain, paresthesias, and pruritus are early neurologic symptoms of rabies, probably reflecting infection in local sensory ganglia.
- Autonomic features are common.

- Hydrophobia is a highly specific feature of rabies.
- Paralytic features may be prominent, and the clinical presentation can resemble that of Guillain-Barré syndrome.
- Saliva samples for reverse transcription polymerase chain reaction (RT-PCR) and a skin biopsy should be obtained to detect rabies virus antigen in order to make a laboratory diagnosis of rabies.

CURRENT THERAPY

- Details of an exposure determine whether postexposure rabies prophylaxis should be initiated.
- Wound cleansing is important after potential rabies exposure.
- Active immunization with a schedule of four doses of rabies vaccine (RabVert or Imovax) at intervals is recommended. Four doses is a new Centers for Disease Control and Prevention (CDC) recommendation and is not yet reflected in the package insert, which calls for five doses.
- Passive immunization (if previously the patient was not immunized) consists of infiltrating human rabies immune globulin (HyperRAB, Imogam Rabies) into the wound, with the remainder of the 20 IU/kg dosage given intramuscularly.

Rabies is an acute infection of the nervous system caused by rabies virus, which is a member of the family Rhabdoviridae in the genus *Lyssavirus*. Other lyssaviruses have only very rarely caused rabies in locations outside of the Americas.

Pathogenesis

Rabies virus is usually transmitted by bites from rabid animals. Transmission has rarely occurred through an aerosol route (in a laboratory accident or bat cave containing millions of bats) or by transplantation of infected organs or tissues (e.g., corneas). The virus is in the saliva of the rabid animal and is inoculated into subcutaneous tissues or muscles via a bite.

During most of the long incubation period (lasting 20–90 days or longer), the virus is close to the site of inoculation. The virus binds to the nicotinic acetylcholine receptor at the postsynaptic neuromuscular junction and travels toward the central nervous system (CNS) in peripheral nerves by retrograde fast axonal transport. There is rapid dissemination throughout the CNS by fast axonal transport. Under natural conditions, degenerative neuronal changes are not prominent, and it is thought that the rabies virus induces neuronal dysfunction by mechanisms that are not well understood. In rabies vectors, the encephalitis is associated with behavioral changes that lead to transmission by biting. After the CNS infection is established, the virus spreads by autonomic and sensory nerves to multiple organs, including the salivary glands of rabies vectors in which the virus is secreted in saliva.

Clinical Features

In North America, where the bat is the most common rabies vector, a history of an animal bite is usually absent, and there may be no known contact with animals. The incubation period is usually between 20 and 90 days, but it occasionally lasts 1 year or longer. Prodromal features are nonspecific and include malaise, headache, and fever, and patients can also have anxiety or agitation. Approximately half of patients experience pain, paresthesias, or pruritus at the site of the wound, which has often healed, and these symptoms likely reflect infection and inflammation involving local sensory ganglia. Approximately 80% of patients with rabies have encephalitic rabies; approximately 20% have paralytic rabies.

In encephalitic rabies, there are characteristic periods of generalized arousal or hyperexcitability separated by lucid periods. Autonomic dysfunction is common and includes hypersalivation, gooseflesh, cardiac arrhythmias, and priapism. Hydrophobia is the most characteristic feature of rabies and occurs in 50% to 80% of patients; contractions of the diaphragm and other inspiratory muscles occur on swallowing. This can become a conditioned reflex, and even the sight or thought of water can precipitate the muscle contractions. Hydrophobia is thought to be caused by inhibition of inspiratory neurons near the nucleus ambiguus.

In paralytic rabies, prominent muscle weakness usually begins in the bitten extremity and progresses to quadriparesis; typically there is sphincter involvement. Patients have a longer clinical course than in encephalitic rabies. Paralytic rabies is often misdiagnosed as Guillain-Barré syndrome.

Coma subsequently develops in both clinical forms. With aggressive medical therapy, a variety of medical complications develop, and multiple organ failure is common. Survival is very rare and has usually occurred in the context of incomplete postexposure rabies prophylaxis that included administration of some rabies vaccine.

Epidemiology

Worldwide more than 55,000 human deaths per year are attributed to rabies. The impact is particularly significant in terms of years of life lost because children are commonly the victims. Most human rabies cases occur through transmission from dogs in developing countries with endemic dog rabies, particularly in Asia and Africa. In the United States and Canada, transmission of rabies virus occurs most commonly in human cases from insect-eating bats, and often there is no known history of a bat bite or exposure to bats. A bat bite might not be recognized. The rabies virus variant responsible for most human cases is found in silver-haired bats and tricolored bats. These are small bats not often in contact with humans. Other rabies vectors in North American wildlife include skunks, raccoons, and foxes, but these species are rarely responsible for transmission to humans. This is likely because of effective postexposure rabies prophylaxis.

Diagnosis

Most cases of rabies can be diagnosed clinically or the diagnosis will be strongly suspected, which is particularly important so that appropriate barrier nursing techniques can be initiated in order to prevent exposures of many health care workers. Some patients are candidates for an aggressive therapeutic approach. A serum-neutralizing titer can be useful for diagnosis in a previously unimmunized person, but a positive titer might not develop until the second week of clinical illness, and the result of the test might not be readily available. Detection of rabies virus antigen in a skin biopsy obtained from the nape of the neck using a fluorescent antibody technique is a useful diagnostic test. Detection of rabies virus ribonucleic acid (RNA) in saliva or in skin biopsies using RT-PCR amplification is an important recent advance for rapid rabies diagnosis. Rabies virus antigen can be detected in brain tissue obtained by brain biopsy or postmortem.

Prevention

After a rabies exposure is recognized, rabies can be prevented with initiation of appropriate steps, including wound cleansing and active and passive immunization. After a human is bitten by a dog, cat, or ferret, the animal should be captured, confined, and observed for a period of at least 10 days; initiation of postexposure rabies prophylaxis is not necessary if the animal remains healthy. The animal should also be examined by a veterinarian prior to its release. If the animal is a stray, unwanted, shows signs of rabies, or develops signs of rabies during the observation period, the animal should be killed immediately, and its head should be transported under refrigeration for a laboratory examination. The brain should be examined via an antigen-detection method using the fluorescent antibody technique and viral isolation using cell culture or mouse inoculation.

The incubation period for animals other than dogs, cats, and ferrets is uncertain; these animals should be killed immediately after an exposure, and the head should be submitted for examination. If the result is negative, one may safely conclude that the animal's saliva did not contain rabies virus; if immunization has been initiated, it should be discontinued. If an animal escapes after an exposure, it should be considered rabid unless information from public health officials indicates this is unlikely, and rabies prophylaxis should be initiated. The physical presence of a bat might warrant postexposure prophylaxis when a person (such as a small child or sleeping adult) is unable to reliably report contact that could have resulted in a bite.

Local wound care should be given as soon as possible after all exposures, even if immunization is delayed, pending the results of an observation period. All bite wounds and scratches should be washed thoroughly with soap and water. Devitalized tissues should be débrided.

Purified chick embryo cell culture vaccine (RabAvert) and human diploid cell vaccine (Imovax) are licensed rabies vaccines in the United States and Canada. Other vaccines grown in either primary cell lines (hamster or dog kidney) or continuous cell lines (Vero cells) are also satisfactory and available in other countries. A regimen of four 1-mL doses of rabies vaccine should be given IM in the deltoid area (anterolateral aspect of the thigh is also acceptable in children). Four doses is a recent CDC recommendation and is an update from the five doses recommended in the current package insert. Ideally, the first dose should be given as soon as possible after exposure, but failing that, it should be given regardless of the length of a delay. Three additional doses should be given on days 3, 7, and 14. Pregnancy is not a contraindication for immunization. Live vaccines should not be given for 1 month after rabies immunization.

Local and mild systemic reactions are common. Systemic allergic reactions are uncommon, and anaphylactic reactions may be treated with epinephrine and antihistamines. Corticosteroids can interfere with the development of active immunity. Immunosuppressive medications should not be administered during postexposure therapy unless they are essential. The risk of developing rabies should be carefully considered before deciding to discontinue vaccination because of an adverse reaction. A serum-neutralizing antibody determination is necessary only after immunization of immunocompromised patients. Less-expensive vaccines derived from neural tissues are still used in some developing countries; these vaccines are associated with serious neuroparalytic complications.

Human rabies immune globulin (Imogam Rabies or Hyper-RAB) should also be administered as passive immunization for protection before the development of immunity from the vaccine. It should be given at the same time as the first dose of vaccine and no later than 7 days after the first dose. Rabies vaccine and human rabies immune globulin should never be administered at the same site or in the same syringe. The recommended dose of human rabies immune globulin is 20 IU/kg; larger doses should not be given because they can suppress active immunity from the vaccine. After wounds are washed, they should be infiltrated with human rabies immune globulin (if anatomically feasible), and the remainder of the dose should be given IM in the gluteal area. If the exposure involves a mucous membrane, the entire dose should be administered IM. With multiple or large wounds, the human rabies immune globulin might need to be diluted for adequate infiltration of all of the wounds. Adverse effects of human rabies immune globulin include local pain and low-grade fever.

After an exposure, a previously immunized patient should receive two 1-mL doses of rabies vaccine on days 0 and 3, but the patient should not receive human rabies immune globulin.

Management of Human Rabies

Only 11 people have survived rabies, and 10 received rabies vaccine prior to the onset of their disease. The possibilities for an aggressive approach were reviewed (see Jackson et al., 2003). There was one survivor in Wisconsin in 2004 who did not receive rabies vaccine. It is now doubtful whether the therapy she received played a significant role in her favorable outcome because a similar approach has failed in many cases (see Jackson, 2013). Palliation is an alternative approach and may be appropriate for many patients who develop rabies.

References

Fooks AR, Banyard AC, Horton DL, et al. Current status of rabies and prospects for elimination. Lancet 2014;384:1389–99.

Jackson AC. Human disease. In: Jackson AC, editor. Rabies: scientific basis of the disease and its management. 3rd ed. Oxford, UK: Elsevier Academic Press; 2013. p. 269–98.

Jackson AC. Update on rabies diagnosis and treatment. Curr Infect Dis Rep 2009;11:196–201.

Jackson AC. Current and future approaches to the therapy of human rabies. Antiviral Res 2013;99:61–7.

Jackson AC, Warrell MJ, Rupprecht CE, et al. Management of rabies in humans. Clin Infect Dis 2003;36:60–3.

Jackson AC. Rabies: scientific basis of the disease and its management. 3rd ed. Oxford, UK: Elsevier Academic Press; 2013.

Manning SE, Rupprecht CE, Fishbein D, et al. Human rabies prevention—United States, 2008: Recommendations of the Advisory Committee on Immunization Practices. MMWR Recomm Rep 2008;57(RR-3):1–28.

World Health Organization. WHO expert consultation on rabies. Second report, WHO Technical Report Series 982. Geneva: WHO; 2013.

RAT-BITE FEVER

Method of
Jatin M. Vyas, MD, PhD

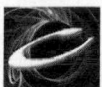

CURRENT DIAGNOSIS

- Exposure to rats is the major risk factor. Transmission can occur with simple contact with infected animals or excreta.
- A maculopapular rash and septic arthritis following initial symptoms of fever and/or sepsis should raise the suspicion of rat-bite fever.
- Clinicians must maintain a high index of suspicion for this diagnosis.
- Notify microbiology laboratory of clinical suspicion (slow growth, 5% 10% CO_2 microaerophilic conditions, 20% normal rabbit serum media supplementation, and avoidance of sodium polyanethol sulfonate when collecting blood cultures from the patient).

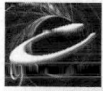

CURRENT THERAPY

Bite Site
- Clean and disinfect the bite site.
- Administer tetanus toxoid (tetanus-diphtheria toxoids, Td), if indicated.
- Postexposure rabies prophylaxis (Imovax Rabies) for animal bites should be considered in consultation with local public health authorities, though there are no reports of rat-to-human transmission of the rabies virus.

Established and Suspected Cases
- Give intravenous penicillin G at a dose of 1.2 million U/day for 5 to 7 days, followed by oral penicillin (PenVK)[1] or ampicillin (Omnipen)[1] 500 mg qid for an additional 7 days.
- For penicillin-allergic patients, consider doxycycline (Vibramycin)[1] 100 mg IV/PO twice daily or tetracycline (Achromycin)[1] 500 mg PO four times daily.
- *S. moniliformis* can be resistant to gentamicin (Garamycin),[1] tobramycin (Nebcin),[1] ciprofloxacin (Cipro),[1] and levofloxacin (Levaquin).[1]

[1]Not FDA approved for this indication.

Rat-bite fever (RBF) is a systemic, febrile disease caused by infection with *Streptobacillus moniliformis* or *Spirillum minus*. As the name implies, this infection is transmitted by a rat bite. However, the bacteria can also be transmitted by simple contact with infected rats or even through ingestion of food contaminated with rat excreta. Diagnosis can be difficult, and a high degree of suspicion is necessary to make a correct diagnosis. Recognition and early treatment are crucial, because case fatality is as high as 25% in untreated cases.

Epidemiology

S. moniliformis is part of the normal respiratory flora of the rat. From 50% to 100% of healthy wild, laboratory, and pet rats harbor *S. moniliformis* in the nasopharynx. *S. moniliformis* is also excreted in the urine. *S. minus* causes rat-bite fever mostly in Asia, but this organism is found worldwide. *S. minus* has been demonstrated in rat conjunctival secretions and blood. Thus, rat-bite fever can be transmitted not only from a bite but also through scratches, handling of dead rats, handling litter material, or by contamination of rat excreta.

Although the rat is the natural reservoir and major vector of the disease, *S. moniliformis* has also been found in other rodents such as mice, squirrels, gerbils, and weasels. No precise data are available on the true incidence of rat-bite fever because it is not a reportable disease. It appears to be unusual in Western countries, a rarity that might reflect failed diagnosis, empiric treatment of infected bites and scratches caused by animals, or spontaneous recovery.

Risk Factors

The major risk factor is exposure to rats, either as an occupational hazard for persons such as laboratory workers, veterinarians, or pet shop employees, or for persons who have rats for pets or feed rats to snakes, especially children. Classically, homelessness and lower socioeconomic status were described as major factors, but most cases reported in the last few years have involved pet rats. Thirty percent of patients with rat-bite fever do not report any exposure to rats or other rodents. Therefore, the lack of documented exposure does not exclude this diagnosis.

Pathophysiology

Very little is known about the pathophysiology of *S. moniliformis* infections. Presumably, the failure of local control by dendritic cells, tissue macrophages, neutrophils, and other components of the innate immune system results in deeper infection, leading to bacteremia. Studies using histologic analysis have revealed intravascular thrombosis near the port of entry.

Prevention

The role of prophylactic antibiotics is unknown, but some authors recommend the use of oral penicillin V (PenVK)[1] after documented exposure to rats and a break in the skin. Penicillin V should be given for 3 days at a dose of 2 g per day for adults. Primary prevention should be encouraged for patients with occupational risk by using protective gloves to handle animals or cages.

Clinical Manifestations

Rat-bite fever is a systemic febrile disease. Classically, following a rat bite and a short incubation of 2 to 10 days, systemic dissemination of the organism is associated with an abrupt onset with intermittent relapsing fever, rigors, myalgias, arthralgias, headache, sore throat, malaise, and vomiting. These symptoms are followed within the first week by the development of a maculopapular rash in 75% of patients. The rash can be pustular, purpuric, or petechial, and it typically involves the extremities, in particular the palms and soles. The bite site typically heals promptly, with minimal inflammation and no significant regional lymphadenopathy.

Following the rash, approximately 50% of infected patients develop an asymmetric migrating polyarthritis, which appears to be exceedingly painful and affects large and middle-sized joints.

[1]Not FDA approved for this indication.

Joint effusion appears more common in adults. Infection can occur in any tissue. Although most cases of rat-bite fever resolve spontaneously, there have been reports of complications. These include meningitis, endocarditis (including prosthetic valve endocarditis), myocarditis, pericarditis, pneumonia, brain abscess, septic arthritis, DIC (disseminated intravascular coagulation), and infarcts of the spleen and kidneys. The mortality rate in untreated cases is around 10% to 15%, and it rises to more than 50% in the rare cases with cardiac involvement.

Two closely related variants have been described. In Havervill fever, the organism is transmitted by ingestion of contaminated food. Havervill fever tends to occur in epidemics and also causes rashes and arthritis, but upper respiratory tract symptoms and vomiting appear more prominent. It is important to note that these patients do not provide a history of exposure to rodents. Sodoku is a rat-bite fever caused by *S. minus*; it is common in Japan. The course is more subacute, arthritic symptoms are rare, and if the bite initially heals, it then ulcerates and is associated with regional lymphadenopathy and a distinctive rash. *S. minus* cannot be grown using synthetic media, and thus microbiologic diagnosis rests on visualization of these organisms in infected tissues.

Diagnosis

Diagnosis is difficult and requires a high clinical index of suspicion. The initial symptoms of rat-bite fever are nonspecific, triggering a broad differential diagnosis. Additionally, the fastidious nature of this organism makes isolation from blood cultures difficult. Clinicians should ask about rodent exposure when compatible symptoms are seen in patients. Rat-bite fever should not be ruled out in the absence of bite history, because transmission can occur without a bite, and pet owners or laboratory workers can minimize the significance of the bite, especially in the absence of a local reaction.

No reliable serologic test is available, and the definitive diagnosis requires isolation of *S. moniliformis* from the wound, blood, or synovial fluid in patients with septic arthritis. The microbiology laboratory should be specifically notified of any clinical suspicion to enhance the chances of recovering the pathogen.

S. moniliformis is a highly pleomorphic, nonencapsulated, nonmotile, gram-negative rod, which can stain positively on Gram stain (Figure 1). It is often dismissed as proteinaceous debris because of its numerous bulbous swellings with occasional clumping (*moniliformis* = "necklace-like"). It grows slowly and requires a microaerophilic environment with 5% to 10% CO_2 or anaerobic

conditions and media supplementation with 20% normal rabbit serum. Cultures can take up to 7 days to turn positive. Some experts recommend holding blood cultures for 21 days to permit sufficient time to grow this organism. *S. moniliformis* is also inhibited by sodium polyanethol sulfonate, a common adjunct in most commercial blood culture media at a concentration as low as 0.0125%. *S. moniliformis* has been identified using polymerase chain reaction amplification and gene sequencing, which shows great promise though it is not routinely used in clinical microbiology laboratories. Fatty acid profiles obtained by gas-liquid chromatography can also be used for identification.

S. minus, the other etiologic agent of rat-bite fever, is a short, thick, gram negative, tightly coiled spiral rod that measures 0.2 to 0.5 µm and has two to six helical turns.

Differential Diagnosis

Differential diagnosis for fever, rash, and polyarthritis is broad. Malaria, typhoid fever, and neoplastic disease can cause relapsing fevers, and the presence of a rash and polyarthritis might suggest viral and rickettsial diseases including Rocky Mountain spotted fever. An asymmetric oligoarthritis suggests disseminated gonococcal and meningococcal diseases in the context of cutaneous lesions on the palms and soles. Lyme disease, leptospirosis, or secondary syphilis can have a similar clinical presentation. Finally, when classic infectious symptoms such as fever or rash are missing, any causes of polyarthritis, from crystal-induced arthropathies to rheumatoid arthritis, should be considered.

Treatment

All established cases of rat-bite fever should be treated with antibiotics because of the associated mortality and potential for complications. Intravenous penicillin G at a dose of 1.2 million units per day should be initiated as soon as the clinical diagnosis is made. Empiric therapy is necessary and should not be delayed for laboratory confirmation of this bacterial infection. The intravenous treatment should continue for 5 to 7 days. After treatment with IV penicillin and suitable clinical response, therapy should be continued with oral penicillin (PenVK)[1] or ampicillin (Omnipen)[1] at a dose of 500 mg qid for an additional 7 days. For patients allergic to penicillin, intravenous doxycycline (Vibramycin)[1] at a dose of 100 mg every 12 hours or oral tetracycline (Achromycin)[1] at a dose of 500 mg four times a day can be used.

Streptomycin[1] and cephalosporins including cefotamxine (Claforan)[1] have been reported to be potentially useful. Other antibiotics including azithromycin (Zithromax),[1] erythromycin,[1] carbapenems,[1] aztreonam (Azactam),[1] clindamycin (Cleocin),[1] vancomycin (Vancocin),[1] and nitrofurantoin (Macrodantin)[1] have shown efficacy in vitro, but they lack good clinical correlation to recommend them for routine use. Erythromycin has been associated with treatment failures. Trimethoprim-sulfamethoxazole (Bactrim),[1] polymyxin B,[1] gentamicin (Garamycin),[1] tobramycin (Nebcin),[1] ciprofloxacin (Cipro),[1] and levofloxacin (Levaquin)[1] should not be used because in vitro resistance has been demonstrated.

Typically, the bite site heals promptly. It should be cleaned and disinfected, as is typical for management of other wounds. Tetanus prophylaxis (tetanus-diphtheria toxoids, Td) administration is indicated as required by the patient's immunization record. Rabies prophylaxis (Imovax Rabies) is usually not required for rodent bite, but consultation with local public health authorities is encouraged. There are no reports of transmission of the rabies virus from rats to humans.

---

[1]Not FDA approved for this indication.

References

Adam JK, et al. Notes from the field: fatal rat-bite Fever in a child - San Diego County, California, 2013. MMWR Morb Mortal Wkly Rep 2014;63(50):1210–1.

Chen PL, Lee NY, Yan JJ, et al. Prosthetic valve endocarditis caused by *Streptobacillus moniliformis*: A case of rat bite fever. J Clin Microbiol 2007;45:3125–6.

Crews JD, Palazzi DL, Starke JR. A teenager with fever, rash, and arthralgia. *Streptobacillus moniliformis* infection. JAMA Pediatr 2014;168(12):1165–6.

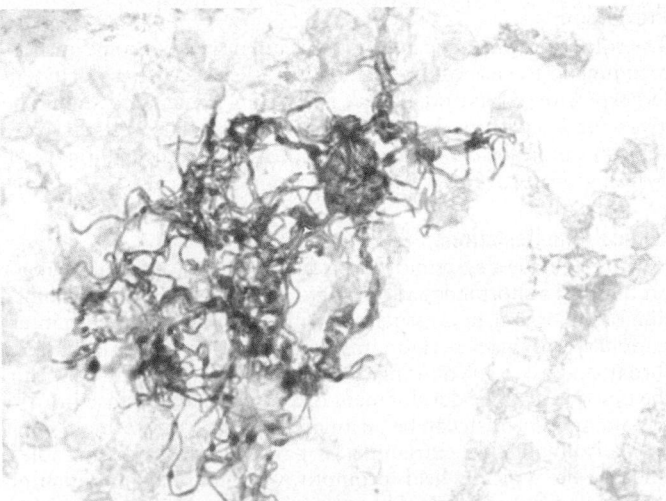

Figure 1. Gram stain of *Streptobacillus moniliformis*. Gram stain of growth from anaerobic bottle, ×100 magnification [microphotography]. (Reprinted with permission from Partners' Infectious Disease Images; accessed on February 14, 2012, from http://www.idimages.org/images/detail/?imageid=373.)

Elliott SP. Rat bite fever and *Streptobacillus moniliformis*. Clin Microbiol Rev 2007;20:13–22.

Fenn DW, et al. An unusual tale of rat-bite fever endocarditis. BMJ Case Rep 2014. 2014.

Gaastra W, Boot R, Ho HT, Lipman LJ. Rat bite fever. Vet Microbiol 2009;133:211–28.

Graves MH, Janda JM. Rat-bite fever (*Streptobacillus moniliformis*): A potential emerging disease. Int J Infect Dis 2001;5:151–5.

Holroyd KJ, Reiner AP, Dick JD. *Streptobacillus moniliformis* polyarthritis mimicking rheumatoid arthritis: An urban case of rat bite fever. Am J Med 1988;85:711–4.

Lambe Jr DW, McPhedran AM, Mertz JA, Stewart P. *Streptobacillus moniliformis* isolated from a case of Haverhill fever: Biochemical characterization and inhibitory effect of sodium polyanethol sulfonate. Am J Clin Pathol 1973;60:854–60.

Schachter ME, Wilcox L, Rau N, et al. Rat-bite fever, Canada. Emerg Infect Dis 2006;12:1301–2.

Stehle P, Dubuis O, So A, Dudler J. Rat bite fever without fever. Ann Rheum Dis 2003;62:894–6.

Trucksis M. Rat Bite Fever. UpToDate. http://www.uptodate.com/contents/rat-bite-fever; [accessed July 9, 2015].

Washburn RG. Streptobacillus moniliformis (rat–bite fever). In: Mandell GL, Bennett JE, Dolin R, editors. Principles and Practice of Infectious Diseases, vol 2. 6th ed. Philadelphia: Elsevier; 2005. p. 2708–10.

RELAPSING FEVER

Method of
Diego Cadavid, MD

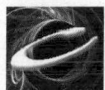

CURRENT DIAGNOSIS

- There are two forms of relapsing fever: epidemic and endemic.
- Epidemic relapsing fever is transmitted from person to person by the body louse *Pediculus humanus*.
- Endemic relapsing fever is transmitted from rodent reservoirs to humans exposed to endemic areas by soft-bodied ticks of the genus *Ornithodoros*.
- The hallmark of relapsing fever is two or more febrile episodes separated by periods of relative well-being.
- The diagnosis is confirmed by visualization of the etiologic spirochetes in thin peripheral blood smears prepared at times of febrile peaks by phase-contrast or darkfield microscopy or light microscopy after Wright or Giemsa staining.

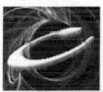

CURRENT THERAPY

- The antibiotic of choice for treatment of relapsing fever is doxycycline (Doryx) except in children or pregnant women. In children <8 y, erythromycin (E-Mycin)[1] or oral penicillin[1] is used instead of tetracycline (Table 3).
- Relapsing fever, if severe or complicated with neuroborreliosis, requires treatment with the intravenous antibiotics ceftriaxone (Rocephin) or penicillin G (Table 3).
- The louse-borne epidemic form is treated with a single dose, whereas the endemic tick-borne form is treated with multiple doses for at least 1 week (Table 3).
- Antibiotic treatment of relapsing fever results in the Jarisch-Herxheimer reaction (JHR) in as many as 60% of cases, more often in the epidemic than in the endemic form. It is characterized by the sudden onset of tachycardia, hypotension, chills, rigors, diaphoresis, and high fever. To reduce the risk of JHR, antibiotics should be started between but not at times of febrile peaks.

[1]Not FDA approved for this indication.

Relapsing fever is one of several diseases caused by spirochetes. Other human spirochetal diseases are syphilis, Lyme disease, and leptospirosis. Notable features of spirochetes are wavy and helical shapes, length-to-diameter ratios of as much as 100 to 1, and flagella that lie between the inner and outer cell membranes. The spirochetes that cause relapsing fever are in the genus *Borrelia*. Other *Borrelia* species cause Lyme disease, avian spirochetosis, and epidemic bovine abortion. Table 1 shows the main *Borrelia* species of relapsing fever, their vectors, and an estimate of their geographic ranges. In the United States, relapsing fever was considered a disease endemic only in the West. However, the recent finding of relapsing fever–like *Borrelia* in ticks and dogs in the eastern United States suggests that the risk of relapsing fever may extend into the East.

Epidemiology

There are two forms of relapsing fever: epidemic transmitted to humans by the body louse *Pediculus humanus* (louse-borne relapsing fever, LBRF) and endemic transmitted to humans by soft-bodied ticks of the genus *Ornithodoros* (tick-borne relapsing fever, TBRF). In LBRF, itching caused by skin infestation with lice leads to scratching, which may result in crushing of lice and release of infected hemolymph into areas of skin abrasion. Louse infestation is associated with cold weather and a lack of hygiene. Migrant workers and soldiers at war are particularly susceptible to this infection. Historically, massive outbreaks of LBRF occurred in Eurasia, Africa, and Latin America, but currently the disease is found only in Ethiopia and neighboring countries. However, immigrants can spread LBRF to other parts of the world.

The main risk factor for TBRF is exposure to endemic areas (Table 1). The risk of infection increases with outdoor activities in areas where rodents nest, like entering caves or sleeping in rustic cabins. *Ornithodoros* ticks are soft-bodied and feed for short periods of time (minutes), usually at night. They can live many years between blood meals and may transmit spirochetes to their offspring transovarially. Infection is produced by regurgitation of infected tick saliva into the skin wound during tick feeding. There are several natural vertebrate reservoirs for TBRF, but most common are rodents (deer mice, chipmunks, squirrels, and rats). In contrast, the body louse *Pediculus humanus* is a strict human parasite, living and multiplying in clothing.

Clinical Diagnosis

Relapsing fever should be suspected in any patient presenting with two or more episodes of high fever and constitutional symptoms spaced by periods of relative well-being. The index of suspicion increases if the patient has been exposed to endemic areas for TBRF or to countries where LBRF still occurs (Table 1). Whereas LBRF is usually associated with a single febrile relapse, TBRF usually has multiple relapses (up to 13). In LBRF the second episode of fever is typically milder than the first; in TBRF the multiple febrile periods are usually of equal severity. The febrile periods last from 1 to 3 days, and the intervals between fevers last from 3 to 10 days. During the febrile periods, numerous spirochetes are circulating in the blood. This is called *spirochetemia* and is sometimes unexpectedly detected during routine blood smear examinations. Between fevers, spirochetemia is not observed because the numbers are low. The fever pattern and recurrent spirochetemia are the consequences of antigenic variation of abundant outer membrane lipoproteins of relapsing fever *Borrelia* species that are the target for serotype-specific antibodies.

The mean latency between exposure to ticks in the endemic form or to lice in the epidemic form and onset of symptoms is 6 days (range, 3–18 days). Because *Ornithodoros* ticks feed briefly and painlessly at night, patients with TBRF may not be able to recall having been bitten by a tick. The clinical manifestations of TBRF and LBRF are similar, although some differences do exist. Table 2 lists the frequency of the most common manifestations of TBRF. The usual initial presentation is sudden onset of chills followed by high fever, tachycardia, severe headache, vomiting, myalgia and arthralgia, and often delirium. In the early stages, a reddish rash may be seen over the trunk, arms, or legs. The fever remains high for 3 to 5 days, and then it clears abruptly. After an

TABLE 1	Relapsing Fever *Borrelia* Species Pathogenic to Humans		
RELAPSING FEVER	**BORRELIA SPECIES**	**ARTHROPOD VECTOR**	**DISTRIBUTION OF DISEASE**
Endemic	*B. hermsii*	*Ornithodoros hermsi*	Western North America
	B. turicatae	*O. turicata*	Southwestern North America and northern Mexico
	B. venezuelensis	*O. rudis*	Central America and northern South America
	B. hispanica	*O. marocanus*	Iberian peninsula and northwestern Africa
	B. crocidurae	*O. erraticus*	North and East Africa, Middle East, southern Europe
	B. duttoni	*O. moubata*	Sub-Saharan Africa
	B. persica	*O. tholozani*	Middle East, Greece, Central Asia
	B. uzbekistan	*O. pappilipes*	Tajikistan, Uzbekistan
Epidemic	*B. recurrentis*	*Pediculus humanus*	Worldwide (recently only in East Africa including immigrants to Europe)

TABLE 2	Frequent Clinical Manifestations of Tick-Borne Relapsing Fever
SIGN OR SYMPTOM	**FREQUENCY (%)**
Headache	94
Myalgia	92
Chills	88
Nausea	76
Arthralgia	73
Vomiting	71
Abdominal pain	44
Confusion	38
Dry cough	27
Ocular pain	26
Diarrhea	25
Dizziness	25
Photophobia	25
Neck pain	24
Rash	18
Dysuria	13
Jaundice	10
Hepatomegaly	10
Splenomegaly	6

asymptomatic period of 7 to 10 days, the fever and other constitutional symptoms can reappear suddenly. The febrile episodes gradually become less severe, and the person eventually recovers completely. As the disease progresses, fever, jaundice, hepatosplenomegaly, cardiac arrhythmias, and cardiac failure may occur, especially with LBRF. Jaundice is more common at times of relapses. Patients with LBRF are more likely to develop petechiae on the trunk, extremities, and mucous membranes; epistaxis; and blood-tinged sputum. Rupture of the spleen may rarely occur. Multiple neurologic complications can occur as a result of disseminated intravascular coagulation in LBRF and as a result of infection of the meninges and cranial and spinal nerve roots by spirochetes in TBRF. The most common neurologic complications of TBRF are aseptic meningitis and facial palsy. Relapsing fever in pregnant women can cause abortion, premature birth, and neonatal death. Sometimes patients can have nonfebrile relapses, consisting of periods of severe headache, backache, weakness, and other constitutional symptoms without fever that occur at the time of expected relapses. Delirium may persist for weeks after the fever resolves, and, rarely, symptoms may be protracted.

Relapsing fever may be confused with many diseases that are relapsing or cause high fevers. These include typhoid fever, yellow fever, dengue, African hemorrhagic fevers, African trypanosomiasis, brucellosis, malaria, leptospirosis, rat-bite fever, intermittent cholangitis, cat-scratch disease, and echovirus 9 infection, among others. Relapsing fever *Borrelia* spp. have antigens that are cross reactive with Lyme disease *Borrelia* spp. and inasmuch as the endemic areas of relapsing fever and Lyme disease overlap to some extent, confusion between the two infections can be expected.

Laboratory Diagnosis

Although the pattern of recurring fever is the clue to diagnosing relapsing fever, confirmation of the diagnosis requires demonstration of spirochetes in peripheral blood taken during an episode of fever. The comparatively large number of spirochetes in the blood during relapsing fever provides the opportunity for the simplest method for laboratory diagnosis of the infection, light microscopy of Wright- or Giemsa-stained thin blood smears or darkfield or phase-contrast microscopy of a wet mount of plasma. The blood should be obtained during or just before peaks of body temperature. Between fever peaks, spirochetes often can be demonstrated by inoculation of blood or cerebrospinal fluid (CSF) into special culture medium (BSK-H with 6% rabbit serum available from Sigma) or experimental animals. Enrichment for spirochetes is achieved by using the platelet-rich fraction of plasma or the buffy coat of sedimented blood. In the United States the most common causes of relapsing fever are *Borrelia hermsii* and *Borrelia turicatae;* both grow in BSK-H medium and in young mice or rats. Whereas direct visual detection of organisms in the blood is the most common method for laboratory confirmation of relapsing fever, immunoassays for antibodies are the most common means of laboratory confirmation for Lyme disease. Although serologic assays have been developed for the agents of relapsing fever, these are not widely available and of dubious utility. The antigenic variation displayed by the relapsing fever species means there are hundreds of different "serotypes." If a different serotype or species is used for preparing the antigen, only antibodies to conserved antigens may be detected. For this reason, a standardized enzyme-linked immunosorbent assay (ELISA) with Lyme disease *Borrelia* as antigen may be the best available serologic assay for relapsing fever. ELISA for *Borrelia burgdorferi* antibodies is routinely done across the United States and Europe. If a positive result for IgM or IgG antibodies is obtained, the Western blot for antibodies to *B. burgdorferi* antigens would be expected to discriminate current or past Lyme disease from relapsing fever, as well as from syphilis, another cause of false-positive Lyme disease ELISA results. Other frequent laboratory abnormalities can occur in relapsing fever but are not diagnostic. These include elevated white blood cell count with increased neutrophils, thrombocytopenia, increased serum

TABLE 3 Treatment Options for Tick-Borne Relapsing Fever*

Adults

Nonsevere forms

1. Doxycycline (Doryx oral), 100 mg PO bid for 1–2 wk[†]

2. Tetracycline (Sumycin), 500 mg PO qid for 1–2 wk

3. Erythromycin (Erythrocin),[1] 500 mg PO tid for 1–2 wk

Severe forms

1. Ceftriaxone (Rocephin),[1] 2 g IV qd for 1–2 wk

2. Penicillin G parenteral aqueous (Pfizerpen),[1] 4 million U IV q4h for 1–2 wk

Children (≤8 y)

Nonsevere forms

1. Erythromycin suspension oral (EryPed),[1] 30–50 mg/kg/d divided tid for 1–2 wk

2. Azithromycin oral suspension (Zithromax),[1] 20 mg/kg on the first day followed by 10 mg/kg/d for 4 more days

3. Penicillin V (Pen-Vee K),[1] 25–50 mg/kg/d divided qid for 1–2 wk

4. Amoxicillin (Amoxil),[1] 50 mg/kg/d divided tid for 1–2 wk

Severe forms

1. Ceftriaxone (Rocephin),[1] 75–100 mg/kg/d IV for 1–2 wk

2. Penicillin G parenteral aqueous (Pfizerpen),[1] 300,000 U/kg/d given IV in divided doses q4h for 1–2 wk

[1]Not FDA approved for this indication.
*The same oral agents are used for treatment of louse-borne (epidemic) relapsing fever but given as a single dose.
[†]In general, treatment for 1 wk is recommended in early/milder cases and for up to 2 wk for more severe cases.
Abbreviations: IV = intravenous; PO = orally.

bilirubin, proteinuria, microhematuria, prolongation of the prothrombin time (PT) and partial thromboplastin time (PTT), and elevation of fibrin degradation products.

Treatment

Relapsing fever *Borrelias* are very sensitive to several antibiotics, and antimicrobial resistance is rare. Table 3 summarizes the treatment options for adults and children younger than 8 years. Children older than 8 years can be treated with the same antibiotics as adults, but the doses should be adjusted by weight. Before antibiotics are given, the possibility of causing the Jarisch-Herxheimer reaction (JHR) should be considered (see later). The tetracycline antibiotics are most commonly used for treatment of LBRF and TBRF. The first antibiotic of choice in adults and children older than 8 years is doxycycline (Doryx). In general, shorter treatments are needed for LBRF than for TBRF. Single-dose therapy is usually recommended for LBRF. In contrast, in TBRF even multiple doses of tetracyclines for up to 10 days may fail to prevent relapses, and retreatment can be required.

Alternative oral antibiotics to the tetracyclines are erythromycin (E-Mycin),[1] azithromycin (Zithromax),[1] amoxicillin (Amoxil),[1] penicillin,[1] and chloramphenicol (Chloromycetin).[1] However, oral chloramphenicol is no longer available in the United States. Erythromycin, azithromycin, and penicillin do not appear as effective as the tetracyclines; however, they are recommended for children younger than 8 years and for pregnant women. Amoxicillin is another alternative for young children with early Lyme disease; however, it is ineffective for human granulocytic ehrlichiosis, which sometimes occurs as a co-infection with Lyme disease.

Although treatment with antibiotics is usually given orally, they may need to be given intravenously if severe vomiting makes swallowing impractical. If there are symptoms and signs of meningitis

[1]Not FDA approved for this indication.

or encephalitis without clinical and/or radiologic signs of increased intracranial pressure, the CSF should be examined to rule out central nervous system (CNS) infection. The finding of elevation of CSF cells and protein demands the use of parenteral antibiotics, such as penicillin G or ceftriaxone (Rocephin). Optimally, antibiotic treatment should be started during afebrile periods when the spirochetemia is low. Starting therapy near the peak of a febrile period may induce JHR, in which high fever and a rise and subsequent fall in blood pressure, sometimes to dangerously low levels, may occur. Dehydration should be treated with fluids given intravenously. Severe headache can be treated with pain relievers such as codeine, and nausea or vomiting can be treated with prochlorperazine.

Jarisch-Herxheimer Reaction

Antibiotic treatment of relapsing fever causes JHR in as many as 60% of cases. JHR is more common in LBRF than in TBRF. It is characterized by the sudden onset of tachycardia, hypotension, chills, rigors, diaphoresis, and high fever. Patients with JHR have said that they felt as if they were going to die. JHR is caused by the rapid killing of circulating spirochetes 1 to 4 hours after the first dose of antibiotic, which results in the release of large amounts of *Borrelia* lipoproteins in the circulation followed by massive release of tumor necrosis factor and other cytokines. If possible, patients with JHR should be transferred to an intensive care unit for close monitoring and treatment. Over several hours, the temperature declines and the patient feels better. Large amounts of intravenous fluids (0.9% sodium chloride solution) may be required to treat hypotension. Steroids and nonsteroidal antiinflammatory agents have no effect on the frequency or severity of the JHR. One study found that pretreatment with anti-TNF-alpha monoclonal antibody (Humira)[1] suppressed JHR after penicillin treatment for LBRF and reduced the associated increases in plasma cytokines. Death can occur as a result of JHR secondary to cardiovascular collapse in up to 5% of patients with treated LBRF and much less frequently in TBRF.

Outcome

Complete recovery occurs in 95% or more of adequately treated patients. The prognosis for untreated cases or if treatment is delayed varies. Mortality as high as 40% is reported in untreated epidemics of LBRF. Relapsing fever also has a high mortality in neonates. Some neurologic sequelae can occur in patients with TBRF complicated with neuroborreliosis.

Prevention

Prevention of TBRF involves avoidance of rodent- and tick-infested dwellings such as animal burrows, caves, and abandoned cabins. Wearing clothing that protects skin from tick access (e.g., long pants and long-sleeved shirts) is also helpful. Repellents and acaricides provide additional protection. Diethyltoluamide (DEET) repels ticks when applied to clothing or skin, but it must be used with caution. It loses its effectiveness within 1 to several hours when applied to skin and must be reapplied; it is absorbed through the skin and may cause CNS toxicity if used excessively. Picaridin (KBR 3023), which has been used as an insect repellent for years in Europe and Australia, is now available in the United States in 7% solution as Cutter Advanced Repellent (Spectrum Brands). The U.S. Centers for Disease Control and Prevention (CDC) is recommending it as an alternative to DEET. Permethrin Insect Repellent, an acaricide, is more effective than DEET but should not be applied directly to skin. When applied to clothing, it provides good protection for 1 day or more. In LBRF, prevention can be achieved by promoting personal hygiene and by dusting undergarments and the inside of clothing with malathion[1,2] or lindane powder[2] when available. Widespread antibiotic use may be necessary to control epidemics of LBRF, using one or two doses of 100 mg doxycycline given within 1 week of exposure.

[1]Not FDA approved for this indication.
[2]Not available in the United States.

References

Barbour AG, Hayes SF. Biology of *Borrelia* species. Microbiol Rev 1986;50:381–400.

Bryceson AD, Parry EH, Perine PL, et al. Louse-borne relapsing fever. Q J Med 1970;39:129–70.

Cadavid D, Barbour AG. Neuroborreliosis during relapsing fever: Review of the clinical manifestations, pathology, and treatment of infections in humans and experimental animals. Clin Infect Dis 1998;26:151–64.

Fekade D, Knox K, Hussein K, et al. Prevention of Jarisch-Herxheimer reactions by treatment with antibodies against tumor necrosis factor alpha. N Engl J Med 1996;335:311–5.

Kazragis RJ, Dever LL, Jorgensen JH, Barbour AG. In vivo activities of ceftriaxone and vancomycin against *Borrelia* spp. in the mouse brain and other sites. Antimicrob Agents Chemother 1996;40:2632–6.

Melkert PW. Fatal Jarisch-Herxheimer reaction in a case of relapsing fever misdiagnosed as lobar pneumonia. Trop Geogr Med 1987;39:92–3.

Southern P, Sanford J. Relapsing fever. Medicine 1969;48:129–49.

Taft W, Pike J. Relapsing fever. Report of a sporadic outbreak including treatment with penicillin. JAMA 1945;129:1002–5.

RICKETTSIAL AND EHRLICHIAL INFECTIONS (ROCKY MOUNTAIN SPOTTED FEVER AND TYPHUS)

Method of
Stephen Waller, MD

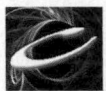

CURRENT DIAGNOSIS

- The diagnosis of Rocky Mountain spotted fever (RMSF) is typically made clinically. RMSF should be considered in the setting of fever, headache, rash, and a history of probable tick exposure. Thrombocytopenia, hyponatremia, and elevated serum hepatic transaminases are common. A rash is typically present by days 3–5.
- RMSF is usually confirmed by demonstrating a fourfold increase between acute and convalescent serum antibody titers.
- Early evaluation of peripheral blood leukocytes for morulae can confirm the diagnosis of human monocytic ehrlichiosis (HME) or human granulocytic anaplasmosis (HGA). However, this method lacks sensitivity.
- PCR analysis performed within the first 48 hours of presentation and convalescent antibody titers are often required to confirm a diagnosis of HME or HGA.
- Typical findings of HME and HGA include fever, headache, malaise, leukopenia, thrombocytopenia, elevated serum transaminases, and potential exposure to ticks.

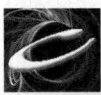

CURRENT THERAPY

- Given the potential for rapid clinical decline in patients with RMSF, HME, and HGA, initiation of therapy should be based on clinical suspicion and one should not await laboratory confirmation of illness.
- Treatment of choice for RMSF, HME, and HGA is doxycycline (Vibramycin) 100 mg PO or via IV twice daily.
- For children ≤45 kg,[1] the recommended doxycycline dose is 2.2 mg/kg given via IV or orally every 12 hours.
- Though optimal duration of therapy has not been well studied, a common treatment course for RMSF is at least 3 days after the patient defervesces (typically 5–7 days of therapy).
- HME and HGA are commonly treated for 5–10 days, or at least 3 days after defervescence.

- Chloramphenicol (Chloromycetin) is the treatment of preference for RMSF in pregnant women and those with adverse reactions to tetracyclines.
- Potential treatment alternatives for HME and HGA include rifampin (Rifadin)[2] and chloramphenicol, although patient experience is limited.

[1]Not FDA approved for this indication.
[2]Not available in the United States.

Rickettsial Infections

RMSF

Rocky Mountain spotted fever (RMSF) is the most serious of the Rickettsial infections found in the United States. If not promptly treated, death can ensue.

Epidemiology

RMSF is caused by *Rickettsia rickettsii*, a small, gram-negative coccobacillus. The name RMSF can be misleading. Though first described in the Snake River Valley of Idaho in 1896, the greatest density of illness can be found in the south central and southeastern United States (see Figure 1). RMSF can also be found in Canada, Mexico, Central America, and northern portions of South America.

In the United States, *R. rickettsii* is transmitted primarily by three species of ticks: *Dermacentor variabilis* (the American dog tick, most common vector in the central and eastern United States), *D. andersoni* (the Rocky Mountain wood tick, primary vector in the western United States), and *Rhipicephalus sanguineus* (the brown dog tick, found throughout the United States). *R. sanguineus* also serves as a vector in Mexico, while *Amblyomma cajennense* has been found to transmit *R. rickettsii* in Central and South America. These ticks, and the mammals on which they feed, serve as reservoirs. Therefore, these tickborne infections occur more commonly in the warmer months, when tick activity is greater. *R. rickettsii* can have a lethal effect on most of its tick vectors, limiting the number that survive to transmit infection to humans. Less than 1% of *D. andersoni* ticks harbor *R. rickettsii*.

Pathogenesis

R. rickettsii is transmitted from the tick to humans via a painless bite, which often goes unrecognized. The organism resides in the salivary gland of the tick and is passed during acquisition of a blood meal. *R. rickettsii* can be transmitted as early as 10 to 24 hours after tick attachment. Tick saliva results in local host immune modulation, assisting bacterial survival. Once injected, the bacteria invade vascular endothelial cells. This obligate intracellular pathogen utilizes the nutrients of the cytosol for proliferation and host cell actin elements to propel the organism through the cytosol, to the surface membrane, and onto adjacent endothelial cells. Small and medium-sized blood vessels are most heavily invaded by this pathogen, with invasion of macrophages, monocytes, and hepatocytes to a lesser degree. Invasion of the endothelium results in a local cell injury resulting from oxidative stress. This endothelial injury results in increased vascular permeability and stimulation of inflammatory cytokines, which can progress to multiorgan failure.

Clinical Manifestations and Diagnosis

Up to 40% of patients will be unaware of a tick bite at the time of presentation. RMSF must be considered given the appropriate clinical and laboratory picture. The median incubation period is 7 days, with a range of 2 to 14 days. Classically, one would consider this diagnosis in the setting of fever, headache, rash, and a history of probable tick exposure. However, these clinical findings are often variably present early in the course of the illness. Within the first 3 days, a temperature of >100 °F occurs in 73%, headache in 71%, and rash in 49%. A rash usually develops within 3 to 5 days of fever onset. As the disease progresses, 99% of those infected will develop a temperature of >100°F, 91% will develop a

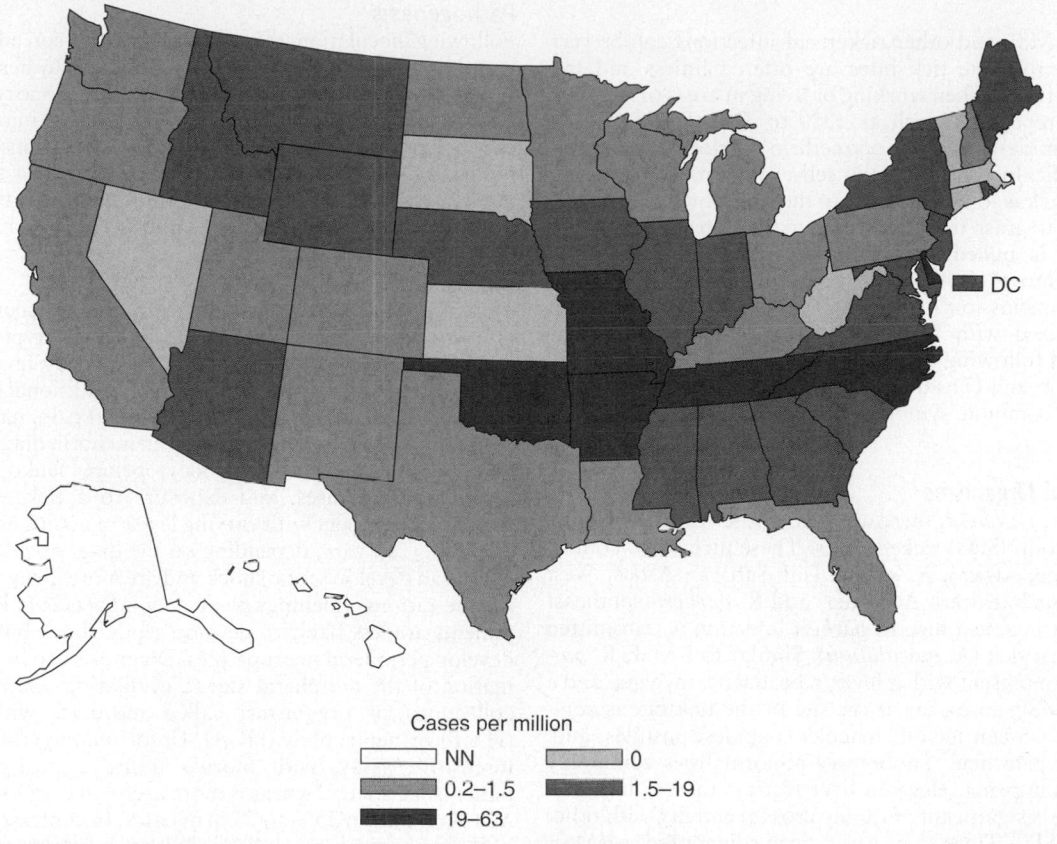

Cases per million

NN   0
0.2–1.5   1.5–19
19–63

Figure 1. Annual reported incidence (per million population) for RMSF in the United States for 2010 http://www.cdc.gov/rmsf/stats/ (accessed January 4, 2014).

headache, and 88% will develop a rash. The rash often presents as maculopapular, but can transition to a petechial exanthem. Gangrenous changes occur much less commonly. Traditionally, many have considered rash involvement of the palms and soles and the "centripetal" rash, progression of rash from wrists and ankles toward the trunk, to be pathognomonic of this infection. However, disregarding the diagnosis of RMSF in the absence of these findings could prove problematic. Rash involvement of the palms and soles is commonly not present in the first few days of illness, but may appear as the disease progresses in a majority of patients. Similarly, the centripetal rash occurs in a minority of patients. Other common manifestations include malaise, anorexia, generalized myalgia, arthralgia, abdominal pain, nausea, vomiting, and, less commonly, diarrhea. Common laboratory abnormalities include hyponatremia, thrombocytopenia, and elevated serum transaminases.

Diagnosis

When appropriate clinical features and history of tick exposure are present, the diagnosis of RMSF should be considered. Initiation of treatment should not be delayed, awaiting laboratory confirmation. Currently available tests include serologic tests and skin biopsy. Indirect immunofluorescent antibody tests are the most widely available. Other serologic tests include latex agglutination, complement fixation, and enzyme-linked immunosorbent assays. These assays typically measure both IgM and IgG levels. A single IgM level ≥1:64 is considered evidence of recent or current infection. However, false negative tests can occur during the first 5 days of the illness. For more accurate results, convalescent titers should also be performed 2 to 4 weeks after illness onset. A fourfold increase between acute and convalescent IgG levels would suggest recent illness. IgM levels wane after 3 to 4 months. IgG levels may also diminish after 7 to 8 months, but can remain detectable for many years. These persistently elevated IgG levels can cause some confusion as cross-reactivity to other rickettsia, e.g., *R. parkeri* (an organism of lesser virulence), can occur.

At the time of presentation, a biopsy of rash-involved skin can be performed with immunohistochemical staining of the specimen. Test specificity is 100%; however, the sensitivity is approximately 70%. The sensitivity also declines quickly following the initiation of therapy. The sensitivity of the assay and lack of its wide availability limits the usefulness of this test.

Differential Diagnosis

Differential diagnosis could include meningococcemia, leptospirosis, measles, mononucleosis, and certain streptococcal and staphylococcal infections.

Treatment

Given the high mortality rate associated with RMSF, treatment should be initiated early based on clinical suspicion. The drug of choice for nonpregnant individuals is doxycycline (Vibramycin). The recommended dose for patients >45 kg (adults and children >8 years of age) is doxycycline 100 mg intravenously (IV) or orally every 12 hours. For patients ≤45 kg, the recommended doxycycline dose is 2.2 mg/kg given IV or orally every 12 hours. Chloramphenicol (Chloromycetin) has been used successfully in treating RMSF and is the preferred agent during pregnancy, given the known effects of tetracyclines on fetal bones and teeth.

The optimal duration of therapy is not well defined. It's recommended to continue therapy at least 3 days after the patient defervesces. Unless suffering from multiorgan injury, most patients will defervesce 2 to 3 days after the initiation of treatment, resulting in a typical treatment course of 5 to 7 days of antibiotics. Short courses of doxycycline in young children (<8 years of age),[1] as outlined above, have not been associated with discoloration of permanent teeth.

---

[1]Not FDA approved for this indication.

Prevention

Prevention of RMSF and other rickettsial infections can be very challenging, because the tick bites are often painless and frequently go unnoticed. When working or living in areas of high tick density, use of repellants, such as 20% to 30% DEET (N, N-diethyl-m-toluamide) on skin or permethrin on clothing, can provide some benefit. In addition, daily self-examination for ticks is important. If a tick is found attached to the skin, fine-tipped tweezers can be used to grasp the tick as close to the skin surface as possible. The tick is pulled upward with steady pressure. Early detection and removal within the first several hours of attachment may prevent transmission of the pathogen. Given that <1% of ticks are colonized with *R. rickettsii*, prophylactic antibiotics are not required following a tick bite. However, one should seek medical attention and consider therapy for RMSF if fever, headache, or other common symptoms develop within 2 weeks of the tick bite.

Other Rickettsial Organisms

In addition to *R. rickettsii*, there are many other members of the spotted fever group (SFG) rickettsioses. These include *R. conorii* (southern Europe, Africa), *R. africae* (sub-Saharan Africa, West Indies), *R. australis* (eastern Australia) and *R. parkeri* (southeast United States), to name a few. *R. parkeri* infection is transmitted by the Gulf Coast tick (*A. maculatum*). Similar to RMSF, *R. parkeri* infection can present with a fever, a headache, myalgia, and a rash. Unlike RMSF, an eschar at the site of the tick bite is commonly noted. Rash can include macules, papules, pustules, and, less commonly, petechiae. Laboratory abnormalities commonly include mild leukopenia, elevated liver transaminases, and total bilirubin. There is significant antibody cross-reactivity with other members of the SFG. Thus, some cases are misdiagnosed as RMSF. Typhus group rickettsial infections include *R. prowazekii* and *R. typhi*. *R. prowazekii* is louseborne infection most commonly encountered in Africa. *R. typhi*, the cause of "murine typhus," is transmitted by the oriental rat flea. This infection is seen uncommonly in the United States, but is more common in Asia, Africa, and southern Europe.

Ehrlichial Infections

Ehrlichiosis is a term to define infections caused by bacteria in the family *Anaplasmatacea*, primarily comprised of the genera *Ehrlichia* and *Anaplasma*. The genus *Ehrlichia* was named after the German-born physician Paul Ehrlich in 1937. However, human ehrlichiosis was not identified until 1986. Since then, many additional species have been identified. In total, three species from the genus *Ehrlichia* and one species in the genus *Anaplasma* have been found to cause human disease in the United States. These include *A. phagocytophilum*, *E. chafeensis*, *E. ewingii*, and *E. muris-like*. Our focus will remain on the two most prevalent diseases, human monocytic ehrlichiosis (HME), caused by *E.chafeensis*, and human granulocytic anaplasmosis (HGA), caused by *A. phagocytophilum*.

Epidemiology

Ehrlichia and *Anaplasma* are small (0.5–1.5 μm) gram-negative organisms. *E. chaffeensis* is primarily transmitted by *A. americanum* (lone star tick), but has been identified in *Ixodes pacficus* and *D. variabilis*. Consistent with the location of *A. americanum* ticks, HME is commonly found in the Midwest, southeastern, and Atlantic states. *E. chaffeensis* has been detected in 2.6% and 9.8% of lone star ticks in Tennessee and Missouri, respectively. *A. phagocytophilum*, the cause of HGA, is transmitted by *I. scapularis* ticks in the northern Midwest and eastern United States and by *I. pacificus* in the western United States. These *Ixodes* ticks are vectors for pathogens that cause Lyme disease and babesiosis, thus making co-infection a concern in those diagnosed with HGA. As with other tickborne zoonoses, HME and HGA are more commonly acquired during warmer months, when ticks are more active. Vertebrates, such as the white-tailed deer, are reservoirs for both *E. chaffeensis* and *A. phagocytophilum*.

Pathogenesis

Following inoculation, these small organisms spread initially via the lymphatic system to regional nodes, followed by hematogenous dissemination. *E. chaffeensis* invade primarily monocytes and macrophages, and less commonly lymphocytes. These infected monocytes can be found within the peripheral blood, bone marrow, CSF, lymphatic system, and most major organs. In a similar fashion, *A. phagocytophilum* disseminate throughout the body, eventually invading neutrophils, band cells, and possibly endothelial cells.

Clinical Manifestations and Diagnosis

The onset of symptoms of HGA and HME occurs 5 to 21 days after inoculation from an infected tick. Both typically present as an undifferentiated febrile illness, marked by fever, chills, headache, malaise, myalgia, and arthralgia. Additional symptoms, particularly in HME, may include abdominal pain, nausea, vomiting, cough, and a nonspecific rash. Key elements in diagnosing HME or HGA include fever, thrombocytopenia, leukopenia, elevated serum transaminases, and exposure to a tick endemic region. Patients can present with varying levels of acuity, and rates of complications can vary, depending on the diagnosis. Individuals with HME can develop septic shock and are more likely to develop CNS manifestations (meningitis or meningoencephalitis). In HGA, patients are less likely to develop septic shock but more likely to develop peripheral neuropathies. Diagnosis can be made by examination of the peripheral smear, evaluating for intracytoplasmic collections of organisms, called morulae, within monocytes (HME) or neutrophils (HGA). Unfortunately, this is a relatively insensitive assay, with morula found typically in <10% of patients. Peripheral smear is more useful in diagnosing HGA, with morula visible in 25% to 75% of cases. In contrast, PCR detection of the pathogen is much better, with sensitivities ranging between 60% to 85% (HME) and 67% to 90% (HGA). However, in both the peripheral smear and PCR assay, the sensitivity of the test will quickly decline following initiation of therapy. The diagnosis can also be made by the demonstration of a fourfold change in antibody titers during convalescence; with repeat antibody titers acquired 2 to 4 weeks after symptom onset. A single elevated titer ≥1:64 may represent an acute infection. However, IgG antibodies may persist for months to years after an infection, thus complicating the interpretation of the assay. Therefore, acute and convalescent titers are recommended in making a diagnosis.

Treatment

As the severity of illness in both HME and HGA can progress quite quickly, initiation of treatment should not be delayed while awaiting laboratory confirmation. The treatment of choice for ehrlichiosis is doxycycline (Vibramycin).[2] The recommended dose for patients >45 kg (adults and children >8 years of age) is doxycycline 100 mg IV or orally every 12 hours. For those ≤45 kg,[1] the recommended doxycycline dose is 2.2 mg/kg given IV or orally every 12 hours. Following treatment with doxycycline, a prompt response usually ensues, with marked clinical improvement typically noted within 24 to 48 hours. Absence of such response should lend to consideration of other diagnoses. There is little data to support the routine use of alternative antibiotics. Limited numbers of pediatric and pregnant HGA patients have been treated successfully with rifampin (Rifadin).[2] *In vitro* data does not support the use of chloramphenicol, β-lactams, cephalosporins, macrolides, and aminoglycosides. Though levofloxacin (Levaquin)[2] has shown some *in vitro* activity against *A. phagocytophilum*, one case report demonstrated a failure of this antibiotic to treat HGA. In addition, fluoroquinolones appear to have poor *in vitro* activity against *E. chaffeensis*. The optimal duration of therapy is unknown. A typical course of doxycycline is 5 to 10 days, given at least 3 days after defervescence, which typically occurs within 48 hours of initiation of therapy.

---

[1]Not FDA approved for this indication.
[2]Not available in the United States.

References

Belman AL. Tick-borne diseases. Semin Pediatr Neurol 1999;6:249–66.

Chen LF, Sexton DJ. What's new in Rocky Mountain spotted fever? Infect Dis Clin North Am 2008;22:415–32.

Dantas-Torres F. Biology and ecology of the brown dog tick, Rhipicephalus sanguineus. Parasit Vectors 2010;3:1–11.

Dumler JS, Madigan JE, Pusterla N, et al. Ehrlichioses in humans: Epidemiology, clinical presentation, diagnosis, and treatment. Clin Infect Dis 2007;45(Suppl. 1): S45–S51.

Helmick CG, Bernard KW, D'Angelo LJ. Rocky Mountain spotted fever: Clinical, laboratory, and epidemiological features of 262 cases. J Infect Dis 1984;150:480–8.

Mansueto P, Vitale G, Cascio A, et al. New insight into immunity and immunopathology of Rickettsial diseases. Clin Dev Immunol 2012;2012:1–26.

Niebylski ML, Peacock MG, Schwan TG. Lethal effect of Rickettsia rickettsii on its tick vector (Dermacentor andersoni). Appl Environ Microbiol 1999;65:773–8.

Paddock CD, Finley RW, Wright CS, et al. Rickettsia parkeri rickettsiosis and its clinical distinction from Rocky Mountain spotted fever. Clin Infect Dis 2008;47:1188–96.

Salinas LJ, Greenfield RA, Little SE, et al. Tickborne infections in the southern United States. Am J Med Sci 2010;340:194–201.

Thomas RJ, Dumler JS, Carlyon JA. Current management of human granulocytic anaplasmosis, human monocytic ehrlichiosis and Ehrlichia ewingii ehrlichiosis. Expert Rev Anti Infect Ther 2009;7:709–22.

Woodward TE. Rocky Mountain spotted fever: Epidemiological and early clinical signs are keys to treatment and reduced mortality. J Infect Dis 1984;150:465–8.

Woods CR. Rocky Mountain spotted fever in children. Pediatr Clin North Am 2013;60:455–70.

RUBELLA AND CONGENITAL RUBELLA

Method of
Judith M. Hübschen, PhD; and Claude P. Muller, MD

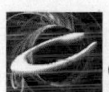

CURRENT DIAGNOSIS

- Laboratory confirmation of rubella is necessary to exclude other diseases with similar clinical symptoms.
- Laboratory diagnosis is normally done by serologic testing and increasingly also by molecular diagnostic methods, including reverse-transcriptase polymerase chain reaction.

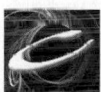

CURRENT THERAPY

- There is no specific therapy for the treatment of acute rubella or congenital rubella syndrome.
- Rubella in pregnant women requires a careful diagnosis and counseling based on thorough risk assessment.
- Patients with congenital rubella syndrome should be referred to specialists depending on their congenital defects.
- Protection against rubella and congenital rubella syndrome relies on vaccination.

Rubella is normally a mild, self-limiting rash-fever illness. Infection during pregnancy, however, can result in fetal death or congenital defects known as congenital rubella syndrome (CRS). Rubella virus is a single-stranded RNA virus (family Togaviridae) of which only one serotype but several genotypes are known.

Epidemiology

Humans are the only known natural host for rubella virus, and before the first licensed vaccine was introduced in 1969, the virus circulated worldwide, causing epidemics every few years.

Rubella spreads mainly via aerosols, but in contrast to measles, a close and prolonged contact is usually required for transmission. Children with CRS can shed large quantities of virus for many months after birth. In unvaccinated populations, approximately 15% to 20% of women of childbearing age are susceptible to the disease and can become infected during pregnancy.

Effective vaccination programs have already led to the elimination of rubella and CRS in some countries (e.g., the United States and Finland). However, routine rubella vaccination has not yet been introduced in many developing countries in Africa and Asia, and endemic virus continues to circulate in many countries worldwide. Insufficient vaccination rates in industrialized countries and the refusal to be vaccinated for religious and other reasons represent a considerable threat to control and elimination goals of the World Health Organization (WHO).

Reinfections with rubella virus are possible and have been reported more often after vaccination than after natural primary infection. Normally, reinfections are asymptomatic and congenital malformations seem to be very rare.

Clinical Manifestations

Rubella virus normally causes only a mild disease, and it is estimated that depending on the cohort, between 20% and 50% of infections are subclinical. The incubation period lasts about 2 weeks (range, 12–23 days), at the end of which a maculopapular rash can appear, which spreads from the face to the trunk and limbs. Lymphadenopathy can develop before the rash and can persist for up to 2 weeks after rash. Especially in adults, a prodromal phase may be observed with fever, malaise, and other uncharacteristic symptoms. Viremia occurs for about 1 week before onset of rash, and virus can be transmitted from around 1 week before, until up to nearly 2 weeks (and exceptionally longer) after onset of rash.

Complications

Rubella infection acquired after birth is rarely associated with complications other than arthralgia and arthritis in post-pubertal women. Male patients and prepubertal girls only rarely have these symptoms. Joint symptoms normally last a few days, but they sometimes persist for up to 1 month. Encephalopathy and thrombocytopenia are other rare complications associated with rubella.

Infection during pregnancy can lead to miscarriage and, especially if acquired in the first trimester, is likely to result in congenital defects. The range and severity of the damages is related to the developmental stage of the fetus at the time of infection. The most common manifestations of CRS include defects of the eyes (e.g., cataracts, glaucoma, pigmentary retinopathy), ears (e.g., deafness), heart (e.g., patent ductus arteriosus, pulmonary artery stenosis, ventricular septal defect, neonatal myocarditis) and the central nervous system (e.g., microcephaly, meningoencephalitis, mental and motor retardation, speech, behavior and psychiatric disorders). Most of the clinical features are permanent, but some are transient (e.g., intrauterine growth retardation, hepatosplenomegaly, thrombocytopenic purpura, haemolytic anemia, bone lesions). Not all manifestations are apparent at birth; some appear only later in life (e.g., type 1 diabetes mellitus, thyroid dysfunction).

Diagnosis and Differential Diagnosis

A rubella diagnosis based on clinical symptoms alone is unreliable. Laboratory confirmation is necessary to exclude other rash-fever diseases such as infections caused by measles virus, parvovirus B19, human herpesvirus 6, dengue virus, enteroviruses, and group A *Streptococcus*. Rubella-specific immunoglobulin (Ig) M, which normally persists for 2 to 3 months but occasionally much longer, points to a current or recent infection. False-positive IgM results occur more often with indirect serologic assays than with antibody-capture assays and are sometimes linked to rheumatoid factor or cross-reacting non-rubella IgM antibodies. During pregnancy, false-positive IgM tests are of particular concern. A significant increase in rubella-specific IgG antibody titer between acute and convalescent phase sera also indicates a recent infection with rubella virus. IgG avidity testing can also differentiate between old and recent infections. The virus can also be detected by reverse transcription polymerase chain reaction (RT-PCR) or virus isolation in cell culture.

Fetal infections are usually diagnosed either by rubella-specific IgM in fetal blood or by rubella virus in amniotic fluid. However, the time point for testing is critical. After birth, laboratory confirmation of CRS is normally done by detecting rubella-specific IgM, which is almost always detectable during the first 3 months of life but only very rarely after the age of 18 months. Detection of rubella-specific IgG antibodies at a time when maternal antibodies have normally disappeared also suggests a congenital infection. In addition, detecting rubella virus by isolation in cell culture or by RT-PCR in respiratory secretions, oral fluid, urine, cerebrospinal fluid, or lens aspirates of infants with CRS may be possible for up to 1 year and sometimes even longer.

Treatment

No specific therapy exists, either for acute cases of rubella or for CRS cases, and emphasis must therefore be on prevention. Rubella infection during pregnancy requires a careful laboratory diagnosis, comprehensive risk assessment, and counseling. Depending on the defects, children with CRS should be referred to specialists as early as possible.

Prevention

The first rubella vaccine was licensed in 1969 in the United States and contained a live-attenuated strain obtained after serial passaging of a wild-type isolate. Since then, several other vaccine strains have been prepared, and strain RA 27/3, which was licensed in 1979, is currently the most widely used worldwide. Rubella vaccine is available in combination with measles and mumps vaccines (MMR) and as a quadrivalent vaccine containing additionally a varicella component (MMRV) (ProQuad). About 95% of all vaccinees develop an immune response; occasional failures may be due to inappropriate storage and handling of the vaccine, coexisting infections, or the presence of passively acquired antibodies. Antibodies induced by vaccination are thought to be long-lasting (>20 years) and to provide lifelong protection in most vaccinees.

Immunity against rubella infection is usually assumed if a rubella-specific IgG titer of at least 10 IU/mL is present. The immune status of women should be checked before pregnancy, and, if necessary, vaccination should be offered. Health care workers in contact with pregnant women should also be immune.

Vaccination is contraindicated in pregnancy, although inadvertent vaccination is no indication for therapeutic abortion. Although some studies reported cases of congenital infection after vaccination during pregnancy, cases of CRS due to rubella vaccine strains do not seem to occur or must be very rare. Other contraindications include severe immunosuppression and severe allergic reactions to components of the vaccine. Only very few and rare side effects are known following rubella vaccination, but lymphadenopathy, joint symptoms, and rash are sometimes observed.

References

Banatvala JE, Brown DW. Rubella. Lancet 2004;363(9415):1127–37.

Best JM. Rubella. Semin Fetal Neonatal Med 2007;12(3):182–92.

Best JM, Castillo-Solorzano C, Spika JS, et al. Reducing the global burden of congenital rubella syndrome: Report of the World Health Organization Steering Committee on research related to measles and rubella vaccines and vaccination, June 2004. J Infect Dis 2005;192(11):1890–7.

Cooper LZ, Alford Jr. CA. Rubella. In: Remington, Klein, Wilson, Baker, editors. Infectious Diseases of the Fetus and Newborn Infant. 6th ed Philadelphia: Elsevier Saunders; 2006. p. 893–926.

da Silva e Sá GR, Camacho LA, Siqueira MM, et al. Seroepidemiological profile of pregnant women after inadvertent rubella vaccination in the state of Rio de Janeiro, Brazil, 2001–2002. Rev Panam Salud Publica 2006;19(6):371–8.

Reef SE, Redd SB, Abernathy E, et al. The epidemiological profile of rubella and congenital rubella syndrome in the United States, 1998–2004: The evidence for absence of endemic transmission. Clin Infect Dis 2006;43(Suppl. 3): S126–S132.

SALMONELLOSIS

Method of
Arvid E. Underman, MD

CURRENT DIAGNOSIS

- More than 95% of nontyphoid salmonellosis presents as uncomplicated acute gastroenteritis.
- The clinical presentation of different causes of gastroenteritis and diarrhea overlaps significantly.
- The physician should be familiar with groups of patients at risk for complicated salmonellosis.
- Specific diagnosis requires culture of the stool or blood.
- Focal complications are always suspect in high-risk patients who are blood culture positive for nontyphoid *Salmonellae* (e.g., aortitis or mycotic aneurysm in patients older than age 60 years with atherosclerosis).

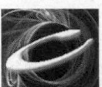

CURRENT THERAPY

- Fluid and electrolyte replacement is of paramount importance.
- The physician should avoid routine empiric antibiotic in acute uncomplicated patients.
- The physician should avoid antimotility agents for diarrhea presenting with fever or with mucus and blood present.
- More than 95% of patients with nontyphoid salmonellosis *will get better* on their own.
- Fluoroquinolone antibiotics should be reserved for when they are truly indicated clinically.
- Increasing resistance mandates sensitivity testing (including tests for ESBL) to guide therapy of bacteremia and its complications.
- Do not prescribe *prophylactic* antibiotics to prevent diarrhea in travelers.
- Stress personal hygiene and prudent food choice with proper preparation.

Abbreviation: ESBL = extended spectrum beta lactamases.

Salmonellosis refers to a group of infections caused by members of the genus *Salmonella*. This genus is named after Salmon, a pathologist who first isolated the organism, later designated as *Salmonella choleraesuis*, from the intestine of pigs with diarrhea. *Salmonellae* are widely distributed throughout nature and are adapted to a myriad of warm and cold-blooded hosts. In humans there are four main clinical presentations:
1. Acute gastroenteritis
2. Bacteremia
3. Focal extraintestinal infection
4. Chronic carriage (Table 1)

Microbiology

Salmonellae are motile, gram-negative, nonspore-forming bacilli that are differentiated from other *Enterobacteriaceae* by inability to ferment lactose and sucrose while producing acid, hydrogen sulfide, and gas (except *Salmonella typhi*). Members of the genus were more accurately classified into serotypes using the Kauffman-White schema, which differentiated and grouped them serologically dependent on their lipopolysaccharide somatic (O) and flagellar (H) antigens.

More recently, DNA analysis has divided the genus into two species. Initially the first of the two species was named *Salmonella choleraesuis* and was divided into six subspecies, each of which was then divided into more than 2400 serotypes (serovars) by

TABLE 1	Clinical Presentations of Salmonellosis

Acute gastroenteritis (90%–95% of cases)

Bacteremia (< 5% of cases)
- Transient during acute gastroenteritis
- Enteric fever (nontyphoid)
- Persistent or recurrent (especially HIV)

Focal complications following bacteremia
- Bronchopneumonia, empyema, chest wall abscess
- Aortitis with mycotic aneurysm
- Prosthetic graft or valve infection
- Endocarditis, endarteritis
- Osteomyelitis (especially with sickle cell anemia)
- Septic arthritis
- Soft tissue abscess
- Hepatic or splenic abscess
- Meningitis or brain abscess
- Suppurative urogenital disease

Carriage (asymptomatic)
- Convalescent excretors (<2 mo)
- Convalescent carriers (2–12 mo)
- Chronic carriers (>12 mo)

TABLE 2	Predisposing Factors for Salmonellosis

Gastrointestinal
- Achlorhydria
- Gastric surgery
- Inflammatory bowel disease

Immune or structural compromise
- Age (<6 mo, >60 y)
- Lymphoma
- Splenectomy
- Cirrhosis with portal hypertension
- Diabetes mellitus
- Chronic uremia
- Hemolytic anemia (iron overload)
- Sickle cell (bone infarct, autosplenectomy)
- Systemic lupus
- Atheromata, aortic aneurysm

Infections
- HIV/AIDS (decreased T-cells)
- Malaria
- Bartonellosis
- Schistosomiasis

Drugs
- H_2-blockers, H^+ proton pump inhibitors
- Antibiotic administration
- Antimotility agents
- Chemotherapy
- Corticosteroids
- Transplant antirejection agents

Kauffman-White methodology. The second species, *Salmonella bongori*, is inconsequential. Serotypes were named historically from the host or the geographic locale of the first isolate, such as *Salmonella typhimurium* or *Salmonella dublin*. However, under the new DNA division, *choleraesuis* was both a species and a serotype. To avoid confusion the name *Salmonella enterica* has been widely adopted. The first of the six subspecies (Group I) is also named *enterica*. It contains the more than 1400 serotypes that occur in warm-blooded animals. Using nomenclature employed by the United States Centers for Disease Control (CDC) and the World Health Organization (WHO), the species and subspecies name is understood and the serotype is capitalized. Thus, the formal *S. enterica* subspecies *enterica* serotype *typhimurium* becomes simply *S. Typhimurium*, which except for the capital *T* is where we started!

Epidemiology

In the last 25 years, the incidence of nontyphoid salmonellosis has increased two- to threefold, with approximately 1.5 million cases occurring annually in the United States. This is an underestimate because most cases are sporadic (endemic) and go unreported. Children younger than 5 years of age have the highest incidence of gastroenteritis and constitute the greatest number of cases.

Animals are the source of nontyphoid salmonella infection in humans. Infection occurs from food of animal origin such as meat, poultry, eggs, and dairy products. Contamination may occur during the production, slaughter, processing, or distribution of these products. Outbreaks have been associated with eggs, ice cream, and processed meats. Increasingly there have been outbreaks associated with raw vegetables (e.g., scallions) that are crosscontaminated during growth and distribution. Restaurant or home outbreaks occur in the context of improper preparation, cooking, and refrigeration. Most of the outbreaks can be attributed to centralized mass production and preparation of food along with globalization of the food trade. Novel sources of human salmonella include pet turtles, lizards, iguanas, African hedgehogs, rattlesnakes, and even marijuana contaminated by manure.

Emergence of antibiotic resistant species is a formidable problem. It is believed that resistance is driven worldwide by improper antibiotics use. However, in developed countries it is attributable to widespread use in animal feeds. Large numbers of transferable-resistance plasmids have been described. Resistance rates of more than 50% to ampicillin, chloramphenicol (Chloromycetin), and trimethoprim-sulfamethoxazole (TMP-SMZ) (Bactrim) occur in parts of Asia, Africa, and Latin America. One strain of *S. Typhimurium* (DT104) is resistant to five antimicrobials; the three

mentioned previously plus tetracycline and streptomycin. This organism has spread widely in livestock throughout the United States, Canada, the United Kingdom, Europe, and the Middle East. Likewise, resistance to third-generation cephalosporins is increasing and is mediated by plasmids producing both regular and extended-spectrum beta-lactamases (ESBLs). Even more disturbing is fluoroquinolone resistance caused by mutated DNA gyrase, topoisomerase IV, or efflux pumps. The latter literally expel the quinolone from the bacterium before it can act on its target. Fluoroquinolone resistance is most pronounced in Southeast Asia, Europe, and the Middle East.

Pathogenesis

Human infection usually requires 10^6 organisms. Fewer organisms may cause disease in patients who have hypochlorhydria or achlorhydria, have impaired cellular immunity, are at the extremes of age, or are taking certain drugs (Table 2). *Salmonellae* predominately infect the terminal ileum and proximal colon through attachment. Initially, host response is by neutrophils followed by lymphocytes and macrophages. Strains vary genetically in their virulence and invasiveness. The organisms can survive intracellularly, thus avoiding antibiotic agents that lack intracellular penetration. Bacteria that are not contained regionally in the gut or lymph nodes may enter the blood. There are many predisposing factors associated with this and subsequent focal complications (see Table 2).

Clinical Presentation

Gastoenteritis

Acute gastroenteritis is by far the most common clinical presentation of salmonellosis. It should be emphasized that there is considerable overlap in its presentation with other infectious intestinal pathogens such as *Campylobacter* species. Given this, the incubation ranges from 6 to 96 hours but most commonly occurs between 12 and 48 hours. Initial symptoms include nausea and vomiting, followed by headaches, myalgias, malaise, chills, low-grade fever, abdominal cramps, and diarrhea. High temperatures (40°C [104° F]) should alert the clinician to invasive disease. Stools may be merely loose or profuse and watery. On direct examination, they may or may not contain polymorphonuclear leukocytes or occult blood. The presence of mucus or gross blood in the absence of hemorrhoids or fissures should alert the clinician to organisms causing dysentery such as *Shigella* species. The white blood cell count is most often normal or slightly elevated, with a left shift containing 10 to 15 bands. Low white blood cell counts with greater numbers of bands should alert the clinician to possible bacteremia or enteric fever. The diagnosis can be confirmed only by stool or blood culture. Serum serology examinations are not helpful. Most healthy adults have a self-limited, uncomplicated course, with resolution of symptoms without treatment within 48 to 72 hours.

Treatment
Fluid and Electrolyte Replacement
The sine qua non in the treatment of diarrhea is fluid and electrolyte replacement. In most cases increased oral intake of bland juices coupled with clear broth and temporary elimination of lactose-containing foods will suffice. Commercial electrolyte solutions (Pedialyte) may be useful. Although not readily available in the United States, rehydration salts are widely employed in many developing countries. WHO distributes packets containing its recommended formula of 90 mmol sodium, 20 mmol potassium, 80 mmol chloride, 30 mmol bicarbonate, along with 111 mmol glucose to dissolve in 1 L sterile or boiled water. This mixture should be consumed at a rate sufficient to compensate for diarrheal losses while maintaining an adequate output of dilute-appearing urine. Within 24 to 48 hours, the diet can be supplemented with bland, soft foods given in small, frequent feedings. If the patient has profuse vomiting or severe dehydration as determined by orthostatic changes in blood pressure, parenteral rehydration should be used. Frequently, this can be accomplished as an outpatient in an infusion room or with a home agency rather than through admission to hospital. When there is persistent emesis, profuse diarrhea, systemic toxicity, or abnormalities in serum electrolytes, parenteral rehydration in hospital is prudent.

Antimotility and Antinausea Agents
The use of agents such as atropine-diphenoxylate (Lomotil) or loperamide (Imodium) should be discouraged. Although they may result in symptomatic improvement in cramps and diarrhea, they can increase complications and even predispose to bacteremia. In general, if the patient has a fever and the diarrhea contains blood or mucus, their use should be eschewed. Most pediatricians feel they should never be used in children younger than 5 years of age. An alternative is bismuth subsalicylate (Pepto-Bismol). The adult dose is 1 ounce (2 tablespoons) or 2 tablets (262.5 mg) every 30 minutes for 8 hours. The pediatric dose is 1.1 mL/kg at 4-hour intervals for up to 5 days. Although nausea and vomiting are occasional presenting symptoms with enterocolitis, they rarely persist. Prochlorperazine (Compazine) or trimethobenzamide (Tigan) may be helpful. Both are available in oral, suppository, or parenteral form, even though injectable prochlorperazine (Compazine) has been in short supply. Suppositories usually stimulate further diarrhea. Vomiting may preclude oral administration. A singular muscular injection of prochlorperazine (Compazine) 5 to 10 mg, is often all that is needed. This may be repeated every 4 to 6 hours as needed. Promethazine hydrochloride (Phenergan) is more frequently used in children and may be used orally (0.5 mg/pound or 1 mg/kg every 6 hours) or intramuscularly in the same doses. A 5-HT$_3$ receptor antagonist such as ondansetron (Zofran)[1] is expensive and inefficacious.

Antibiotics
The routine empiric use of antibiotics, especially fluoroquinolones, for any and all cases of diarrhea is not only unjustifiable but should be decried. Certainly antibiotics are not needed in the treatment of uncomplicated *Salmonella* gastroenteritis in otherwise healthy children or adults. Studies have shown that they neither shorten the course nor improve symptoms. No doubt some of this usage is patient driven. However, overuse is contributing to the emergence of resistance, and may increase risk of symptomatic and bacteriologic relapse. Indeed, antibiotic use may actually prolong the convalescent excretion or contribute to chronic carriage of the organism. Postponing antibiotic therapy until the return of a stool culture often provides the physician with a way to avert the frequent demand for antibiotic therapy. Often patients are better by the time results become available. Nevertheless, high-risk patients, as previously identified (see Table 2), should receive treatment to prevent potential complications from bacteremia. Additionally, if patients are sick enough to require hospitalization, antibiotic therapy should be considered.

Appropriate antibiotic therapy should be guided by susceptibility testing. Initially, TMP-SMZ (cotrimoxazole, Bactrim, or Septra)[1] may be administered to the nonsulfonamide-sensitive patient. The dose is 5 to 8 mg/kg trimethoprim every 12 hours for children or 1 double-strength tablet (160 mg trimethoprim/800 mg sulfamethoxazole) every 12 hours for adults. Although widely used, trimethoprim-sulfamethoxazole has not yet received FDA approval. If the organism is susceptible, ampicillin, 50 mg/kg orally to 100 mg/kg/day intravenously, each in four divided doses for children, or 2 to 4 g/day in four divided doses for adults, may be administered. Amoxicillin (Amoxil)[1] in equivalent oral dosage may be substituted. The duration of therapy is generally 5 days.

Newer fluoroquinolone antibiotics, such as ciprofloxacin,[1] ofloxacin,[1] and norfloxacin,[1] are among the most effective agents, with excellent oral bioavailability and intracellular concentration. They are contraindicated in prepubertal children and pregnant women. Adult doses are ciprofloxacin (Cipro), 500 mg twice daily; ofloxacin (Floxin), 400 mg twice daily; or norfloxacin (Noroxin), 400 mg twice daily. It must be emphasized that the trend in the United States to use these agents empirically for all suspected bacterial diarrhea should be vigorously resisted by the thoughtful clinician.

Bacteremia and Focal Infection
Bacteremia in acute uncomplicated *Salmonella* gastroenteritis is infrequent. Therefore, blood cultures are not routinely necessary except for patients who are in high-risk categories. Shaking chills or high fever (40°C [104°F]) should alert the clinician to possible bacteremia. Focal suppurative infection following bacteremia is also infrequent but may occur at any site. Thus, *Salmonella* has been associated with bronchopneumonia, soft tissue infection, aortic mycotic aneurysms, endocarditis, septic arthritis, splenic or hepatic abscesses, meningitis, and osteomyelitis. The clinician should suspect an endovascular mycotic aneurysm in all blood culture–positive patients older than 50 years of age. *Salmonella* should always be suspected in individuals with sickle cell disease in whom bone and joint infection is the most frequent cause of extraintestinal infection. Meningitis occurs primarily in infants younger than 5 months of age. The diagnosis of a *Salmonella* bacteremia in HIV patients will almost always be accompanied by recurrent episodes.

Treatment
Antibiotics
Bacteremia and localized suppurative infection require antibiotic therapy. The choice of effective treatment is less predictable with the emergence of resistance. Therapy must be altered according to the results of susceptibility testing. Therefore the recovery of the organism is extremely important, and adequate cultures of blood or infected material must be obtained before initiation of therapy.

Parenteral ampicillin, 100 to 200 mg/kg/day divided into four doses, or TMP/SMZ,[1] 8 to 10 mg/kg of trimethoprim per day in three divided doses, may be used. In the case of resistance or allergy to the foregoing, third-generation cephalosporins such as

---

[1]Not FDA approved for this indication.

---

[1]Not FDA approved for this indication.

cefotaxime (Claforan) or ceftriaxone (Rocephin) have reasonable activity, but intracellular concentrations are not optimal. Cefotaxime, 1 to 2 grams every 6 to 8 hours for adults, or 100 to 200 mg/kg/day in three or four divided doses for children, has been found effective in bacteremia, osteomyelitis, septic arthritis, and a variety of other focal Salmonella infections. The use of chloramphenicol (Chloromycetin) is not recommended, but a preparation of it in oil (Typhomycine)[2] is in use in developing countries. Ciprofloxacin (Cipro)[1] 7.5 mg/kg intravenously twice daily is becoming a favored agent; not only is it effective, but oral bioequivalence facilitates the change to 500 to 750 mg by mouth twice daily. If fluoroquinolone resistance is encountered, imipenem (Primaxin)[1] may be tried. Efficacy data for it or other agents such as azithromycin (Zithromax)[1] are scant.

Surgery

Focal infection often requires surgery. Often this is as simple as the drainage of localized suppuration or lavage of a septic joint. However, in the case of infected aortic aneurysms, extensive resection and vascular reconstruction are required. Infected prosthetic grafts must be removed in nearly all cases, with courses of antibiotics before and after surgery.

The duration of therapy for simple bacteremia is 10 to 14 days. Septic arthritis is usually treated for 4 weeks whereas osteomyelitis and endovascular infections require 6 weeks. Oral fluoroquinolones such as ciprofloxacin (Cipro), 500 mg twice daily, may be helpful in treating osteomyelitis. TMP-SMZ (Bactrim)[1] can also be used in this manner. Both have adequate blood levels after oral administration. I have had to use continuous prophylaxis of either TMP-SMZ or ciprofloxacin in several HIV patients to prevent recurrent bacteremia. Because prophylactic TMP-SMZ is used chronically for Pneumocystis, it may be preferred.

Enteric Fever

The clinical picture of nontyphoid Salmonella enteric fever is indistinguishable from that of typhoid fever, which is discussed elsewhere in this publication. However, the following discussion also applies to enteric fever caused by nontyphoid Salmonellae.

Treatment

The adjunct and antibiotic therapy of nontyphoid enteric fever parallels that of the treatment of typhoid. Antibiotics should be adjusted and altered once the results of susceptibility testing are available. Acceptable regimens include ampicillin, amoxicillin,[1] and TMP-SMZ (Bactrim),[1] along with third-generation cephalosporins and fluoroquinolone antibiotics. My preference was cefotaxime (Claforan)[1] in the same doses as for bacteremic salmonellosis. The duration is 10 to 14 days. Relapse rates are low, and relapse is seen within 2 to 6 weeks. Relapse requires an equivalent course of therapy in both dose and duration. Currently, I prefer ciprofloxacin (Cipro)[1] intravenously 7.5 mg/kg every 12 hours continued until the patient is afebrile and clinically able to start taking it orally. Comparative studies are ongoing, using both third-generation cephalosporins, such as ceftriaxone (Rocephin)[1] or cefixime (Suprax),[1] and oral fluoroquinolones in short-course therapy of typhoid as well as nontyphoid enteric fever. Although these show some promise, they are currently not the standard of practice in the United States. Nevertheless, a strong case can be made for oral fluoroquinolones use, with obvious cost saving. Otherwise healthy young adults may be treated orally as outpatients. This advantage, if for no other reason, should prevent the physician from prescribing quinolones for uncomplicated gastroenteritis or other self-limited diarrheas of bacterial origin.

Adjunctive measures are of importance, including attention to fluid and electrolyte balance and nutrition. As in typhoid, the routine use of corticosteroids is controversial. Use in patients who are steroid dependent or believed to be hypoadrenal is indicated. In those who are delirious, obtunded, comatose, or in shock it may be warranted, but there are little supportive data. It has been my overall impression that nontyphoid enteric fever is somewhat milder than typhoid itself, and complications such as gastrointestinal bleeding or ileal perforation are exceedingly rare.

Carrier State

Asymptomatic excretion of organisms invariably occurs following clinical Salmonella gastroenteritis. It exceeds 8 weeks in 5% to 10% of patients. Chronic carriage, either in the stool or urine, is defined as excretion of the organism for more than 1 year. Its incidence is stated to be 1% in adults and 5% in children younger than 5 years of age. This is somewhat less than that seen with S. typhi. Convalescent excreters need only maintain strict personal hygiene to prevent transmission of the organism. Those involved in food preparation or in child care and health care should be kept off work until three successive cultures are negative at intervals required by the public health department. It goes without saying that all positive cases of salmonellosis are reportable by law to local public health authorities.

Recently, oral quinolones have been used (ciprofloxacin [Cipro],[1] 500 to 750 mg twice daily for 5 to 14 days) to curtail institutional outbreaks, as in nursing homes or psychiatric facilities. Although this may be expeditious, eliminating or preventing the source of the outbreak in a prospective fashion is preferable. In the case of food handlers and health care or child care workers, some feel that quinolone therapy eliminates the problem of convalescent excretion, hence individuals may return to work without delay. The data are debatable and the successive negative stool requirement will not be obviated.

The management of the chronic carriage of nontyphoidal salmonellosis is the same as that of S. typhi, which is discussed in detail elsewhere. A 4- to 6-week course of oral antibiotics may be tried when no evidence of gallbladder disease exists. However, if chronic cholecystitis and/or cholelithiasis are present, cholecystectomy is almost always necessary. Despite cholecystectomy, a certain number of individuals will continue to excrete organisms thought to be of hepatobiliary origin. Chronic carriage is seen, albeit rarely, in the United States with either Schistosoma mansoni or Schistosoma haematobium. When these parasites are treated, subsequent therapy of the Salmonella results in termination of the stool or urinary carrier state.

Prevention

Prevention of salmonellosis has both personal and public health dimensions. Food and leftovers should be rapidly refrigerated. I recommend separate plastic (not wood) cutting boards for meats and vegetables and washing them after each use. Spillage of raw animal juices should be immediately cleaned. All preparation surfaces should be washed and dried after each meal. Detergent rather than antibacterial cleaners should be used; bleach is beautiful.

Public health surveillance is essential via regular inspection of restaurants, food retailers, and industrial food processors. National efforts to coordinate and computerize surveillance systems such as FoodNet should be expanded and fully funded so as to guarantee our food supply. Preservation technologies, including irradiation, need study.

Finally, the practicing physician should take the time to reiterate to patients with HIV or malignancies or other immune-compromised patients (see Table 2) how they can avoid food-borne pathogens.

---

[1]Not FDA approved for this indication.

References

Brenner FW, Villar RG, Angulo FJ, et al. Salmonella nomenclature. J Clin Microbiol 2000;38:2465.

Fierer J, Swancutt M. Non-typhoid Salmonella: A review. In: Remington JS, Swartz MN, editors. Current Clinical Topics in Infectious Diseases 20. Boston: Blackwell Science; 2000. p. 134–57.

Herikstad H, Hayes P, Mokhtar M, et al. Emerging quinolone-resistant Salmonella in the United States. Emerg Infect Dis 1997;3:371–2.

---

[1]Not FDA approved for this indication.
[2]Not available in the United States.

Molbak K. Human health consequences of antimicrobial drug resistant *Salmonella* and other foodborne pathogens. Clin Infect Dis 2005;41:1613–20.

Sirinivan S, Garner P. Antibiotics for treating Salmonella gut infections. Cochrane Database Sys Rev 2000;93: CD001167.

Su LH, Chiu CH, Chu CS, et al. Antimicrobial resistance in nontyphoid *Salmonella*: A global challenge. Clin Infect Dis 2004;39:546–51.

Voetsch AC, Van Gilder TJ, Angulo FJ, et al. FoodNet estimate of the burden of illness caused by nontyphoidal Salmonella infections in the United States. Clin Infect Dis 2004;38(Suppl. 3):S127–S134.

SEVERE SEPSIS

Method of
Jerome Larkin, MD; and Marisa Holubar, MD

CURRENT DIAGNOSIS

Systemic Inflammatory Response Syndrome (SIRS)
- Diagnosis is based on the presence of two or more of the following:
  - Temperature >38°C or <36°C
  - Pulse >90 beats/min
  - Respirations >20 breaths/min or arterial partial pressure of carbon dioxide ($Paco_2$) <32 mm Hg
  - White blood cell count >12,000 or <4000 cells/mm³ or >10% bands

Sepsis
- Diagnosis is based on a finding of SIRS plus proven or suspected infection as the cause.

Severe Sepsis
- Diagnosis is based on a finding of sepsis plus organ dysfunction of one or more major systems (typically kidney, lung, or heart; less often, central nervous system).

Septic Shock
- Diagnosis is based on a finding of severe sepsis plus persistent hypotension despite aggressive fluid resuscitation (i.e., vasopressors are required to maintain mean arterial pressure >65 mm Hg).

Supportive Laboratory Findings
- Hyperglycemia
- Lactic acidosis
- Hyperbilirubinemia
- Acute renal failure
- Thrombocytopenia
- Coagulopathy
- Leukocytosis or leukopenia
- Elevated erythrocyte sedimentation rate or C-reactive protein

Supportive Physical Findings
- Decreased capillary refill or mottling of skin
- Mental status changes or obtundation
- Tachypnea or respiratory failure
- Tachycardia
- Anuria or oliguria
- Edema

CURRENT THERAPY

Initial Six Hours
- Initiate fluid resuscitation with crystalloid or colloid to achieve central venous pressure of 12 mm Hg (or 15 mm Hg if intubated).
- Add dopamine (Intropin) or norepinephrine (Levophed) for persistent hypotension (mean arterial pressure <65 mm Hg).

- Obtain blood, urine, and other appropriate cultures (cerebrospinal fluid, abscess drainage, catheter tip, tissue, sputum).
- Administer empiric antimicrobial therapy.
- Perform appropriate imaging studies with urgent source control as indicated and allowed by clinical status; remove potentially infected foreign bodies.
- All interventions should be undertaken simultaneously and initiated within 1 hour after making a presumptive diagnosis of sepsis.

Subsequent Interventions
- Maintain glycemic control with a target blood glucose level of less than 150 mg/dL.
- Use unfractionated or low-molecular-weight heparin for prophylaxis against deep venous thrombosis.
- Use a histamine 2 (H_2) blocker or proton pump inhibitor for gastric ulcer prophylaxis.
- Initiate therapy with dobutamine (Dobutrex) for low cardiac output in the face of adequate filling pressures.
- Consider therapy with activated protein C (drotrecogin alfa [Xigris]) for patients with an Acute Physiology and Chronic Health Evaluation (APACHE) II score of 25 or greater.
- Consider therapy with hydrocortisone (Solu-Cortef)[1] for patients with continued hypotension despite adequate fluid resuscitation and vasopressors.
- Achieve adequate sedation.

---

[1]Not FDA approved for this indication.

Epidemiology

The true prevalence and incidence of sepsis remain unknown. A study by Martin and colleagues in 2003 analyzed data from the National Hospital Discharge Survey from 1979 to 2000. Although some limitations apply, particularly shifts in the understanding of and use of coding, their findings have the advantage of assessing a large sample size over a prolonged period of observation. The most striking finding was a rise in the incidence of sepsis in the United States over this period, from an annual occurrence of 164,000 cases in 1979 to 660,000 cases in 2000. This reflects an average annual increase of 8.7% for more than 20 years. Coincident with this increase was a rise in the percentage of patients with a diagnosis of sepsis due to fungal organisms (4.6% in 2000). Gram-positive organisms supplanted gram-negative organisms as the largest group of pathogens after 1987 (52% versus 37%).

Mortality was highest among African American men and was associated with failure of three or more organs. Men were more likely to become septic than women (relative risk, 1.90). In-hospital mortality fell from 27.8% to 17.9% between 1995 and 2000. Total mortality increased, most likely as a result of the increase in the total burden of disease. This increase, although perhaps in part attributable to greater use of the diagnostic code for sepsis, is thought to have resulted from a combination of aging of the population, greater numbers of immunosuppressed individuals surviving longer, greater use of prosthetic devices, and greater numbers of and more invasive medical interventions. Diabetes, hypertension, chronic obstructive pulmonary disease, congestive heart failure, and HIV infection all increased as a proportion of medical conditions contributing to sepsis, whereas the proportion of patients with cancer and that of pregnant patients declined. The percentage of patients with one or more organs failing (i.e., severe sepsis) increased from 17% to 35% of all patients with a diagnosis of sepsis.

A study by Dombrovskiy and associates described an even greater increase in the proportion of severe sepsis, from 25.6% in 1993 to 43.8% in 2003. They also found an absolute increase in the number of cases of sepsis, as well as an increase in total mortality, again likely due to increased incidence. Case-fatality rates fell from 45.8% to 37.8%, but mortality was substantially higher at both the beginning and the end of their study period than was described by Martin. These findings suggest acceleration in both severity and incidence of severe sepsis and septic shock.

Sepsis is the tenth most common cause of death in the United States. The incidence is highest during the winter, most likely reflecting increased respiratory viral infections that precede the development of community-acquired pneumonia, which is itself a medical condition with increased risk of developing severe sepsis.

A remarkable aspect of sepsis, severe sepsis, and septic shock is the relatively small number of associated pathogens out of the more than 1000 microorganisms known to cause human disease. *Staphylococcus aureus,* streptococci, enterococci, and gram-negative rods are the most commonly isolated species. *Escherichia coli, Klebsiella, Pseudomonas, Serratia, Acinetobacter, Enterobacter, Citrobacter,* and *Neisseria meningitidis* (a gram-negative coccus) constitute the most common gram-negative pathogens. This relative paucity of etiologic bacterial pathogens has implications for empiric antimicrobial therapy. The emergence of resistant organisms, particularly methicillin-resistant *S. aureus* (MRSA) and gram-negative bacteria harboring extended-spectrum β-lactamases, increases the risk of antibiotic failure and attendant mortality. Fungal pathogens, particularly non-candidal species, continue to increase in incidence. This is most likely the result of better empiric management of gram-negative and candidal sepsis in patients with hematologic malignancies.

Although sepsis is most typically a disease of the elderly, the immune suppressed, and those with chronic medical problems, otherwise young and healthy individuals can also be stricken with no clear cause or known risk factor, such as in meningococcemia, toxic shock syndrome, and necrotizing fasciitis.

Definitions

The term *sepsis* derives from a Greek word that generally implies putrefaction. It also has a colloquial meaning, understood by most laypeople to mean a serious, potentially overwhelming infection. Historically, it has been intuitively understood by physicians to mean an infection, once localized, that has now disseminated and is life threatening. Bacteremia is implied if not always proven. Sepsis was usually fatal in the preantibiotic era, and its morbidity and mortality remain substantial.

In 2001, a consensus conference, sponsored by the American College of Chest Physicians and the Society of Critical Care Medicine and involving the European Society of Intensive Care Medicine, the Surgical Infection Society, and the American Thoracic Society, was convened to arrive at a specific definition of sepsis. Achieving such a definition is critically important to ongoing research on interventions aimed at improving mortality. Their deliberations, building on the work of a previous conference and published in 2003, elaborated several key concepts. They defined systemic inflammatory response syndrome (SIRS) as a state of immune activation characterized by the findings of fever with tachycardia, tachypnea, and/or leukocytosis or leukopenia. Although sensitive, this definition is so overly broad as to be rather unhelpful to an experienced clinician who would not need to resort to such terms to understand that a patient is seriously ill. Nonetheless, it provides a useful construct in beginning to arrive at a specific definition of sepsis. Both infectious and noninfectious processes—severe burn and pancreatitis being the most notable examples of the latter—can cause SIRS.

Sepsis is defined as the finding of SIRS in the presence of known or suspected invasion by a microbe into a normally sterile body site. Severe sepsis is sepsis that has become more generalized. The cardinal finding is organ dysfunction that is unrelated to the primary site of infection. Other typical findings include hyperglycemia, thrombocytopenia, hyperbilirubinemia, acidosis, coagulopathy, edema, oliguria, hypotension, ileus, hypoxia, and poor perfusion. Heart, kidney, and respiratory failure are the most common forms of organ dysfunction. Altered sensorium is also common. Septic shock refers to the presence of hypotension with systolic blood pressure lower than 90 mm Hg or mean arterial pressure lower than 60 mm Hg despite adequate fluid resuscitation. These terms (sepsis, severe sepsis, and septic shock) are all part of a continuum, implying a progressively graver degree of illness with associated increasing mortality. No single symptom, physical finding, organ dysfunction, or laboratory abnormality serves to make or exclude the diagnosis, although isolation of a microorganism in the setting of such findings is highly suggestive. Increasing numbers of physical findings and other abnormalities correlate with an increasing likelihood of the diagnosis of sepsis.

The consensus conference put forward a staging system for sepsis based on host predisposition, nature of infection, host response, and organ dysfunction (mnemonic: PIRO). By this, it is understood that a given patient may be predisposed to infection based on medical conditions such as diabetes, vascular disease, sickle cell anemia, or inherited or acquired immunodeficiencies. Additionally, there are likely to be more subtle genetic predispositions to the development of sepsis, as well as age-related factors. The nature of infection in terms of the site, inoculum, and virulence of the infecting organism clearly plays a role in determining the development of sepsis. The host response—ranging from localization and clearing of the infection without deleterious effect on the host to a state of immunologic dissonance whereby the inflammatory response is itself the driver of pathology—is signaled by the development of organ dysfunction. This staging system allows patients to be stratified at different points and serves as a template for evaluating the efficacy of various interventions as the characterization of sepsis and research into novel therapies progresses.

Pathophysiology

Infection of the immunocompetent host by a microorganism typically leads to immune activation. This serves to isolate the site and source of infection. Local tissue is often damaged, but eventually the infection is cleared, and repair and regeneration occur. This process is highly regulated, with a number of different cell types and mediators involved, all in delicate balance between proinflammatory and antiinflammatory effects. The patient may have few or no symptoms, or there may be systemic evidence of infection (i.e., SIRS). Sepsis is the failure of localization such that the process becomes generalized and leads to tissue destruction remote from the site of infection. Why the immune system enters this state of dysregulation remains unknown, although an enormous amount of research over the last 4 decades has elucidated many of the pathways and mediators involved. Tumor necrosis factor, platelet-activating factor, interleukins, eicosanoids, interferons, and nitric oxide are among the biologically active molecules characterized to date. Particular microbes also contribute to this process through the elaboration of toxins (typically by gram-positive organisms) and endotoxins (gram-negative–derived lipopolysaccharide). These events lead to tissue destruction as a result of ischemic insult, direct cytotoxicity, and accelerated apoptosis. The characterization of inflammatory mediators has led to attempts to modify the immune response through the use of novel therapies such as monoclonal antibodies directed against tumor necrosis factor. To date such attempts have not met with success, and investigation continues.

Diagnosis

The diagnosis of sepsis ultimately relies on the clinical suspicion of infection in the setting of SIRS. A constellation of other supportive evidence establishes a greater or lesser likelihood of the presence of sepsis (see the Current Diagnosis box). It is rare that specific microbiologic evidence for infection is available in a manner timely enough to determine that sepsis is present or to help guide the initial, typically urgent, therapy. When it is available, it usually is a Gram stain or other type of specialized microbiology stain that confirms the presence of a potential pathogen in a site where none should be (e.g., gram-positive cocci in cerebrospinal fluid). Early therapy therefore relies on aggressive resuscitative measures and the administration of empiric antibiotics.

Treatment

Early Goal-Directed Resuscitation: The First Six Hours

Initial treatment of sepsis should focus on correction of hemodynamic parameters, early administration of antibiotics, and source control of potential sites of infection. The 2008 guidelines from the Surviving Sepsis Campaign, an international initiative to improve sepsis outcomes, emphasized the importance of aggressive fluid resuscitation. Therapy should be implemented according to a protocol directed at achieving the following specific goals:

- Central venous pressure 8 to 12 mm Hg, or 12 to 15 mm Hg in those who are mechanically ventilated or have decreased left ventricular compliance
- Central venous or mixed venous oxygen saturation 70% or greater
- Mean arterial pressure (MAP) 65 mm Hg or greater
- Urine output 0.5 mL/kg/hour or greater

Administration of fluid boluses of 1000 mL or more of crystalloids or 300 to 500 mL of colloids over 30 minutes should begin as soon as hypoperfusion is recognized. There is no evidence that one type of fluid is superior to the other, although crystalloid is substantially cheaper. In cases of profound intravascular volume depletion, more rapid and more frequent fluid administration may be needed. Hemodynamic improvement (decreased heart rate, increased blood pressure, increased urine output) and the goal of optimizing central venous pressure should direct the need for continued infusion of fluid while avoiding the development of volume overload and pulmonary edema. Transfusion of packed red blood cells should be considered if anemia is present, with a goal of achieving a hemoglobin level of 7.0 to 9.0 g/dL. If tissue hypoperfusion or hypoxia persists (central mixed venus oxygen saturation <70%) despite achieving a central venous pressure of 12 mm Hg, therapy with dopamine (Intropin) or norepinephrine (Levophed) should be initiated with a goal of achieving a MAP of 65 mm Hg. There is no role for the use of low-dose dopamine for renal protection. An arterial line for more precise and continuous measurement of blood pressure should be inserted as soon as possible after the initiation of vasopressor therapy. Ideally, vasopressors should not be introduced to increase MAP until after the fluid deficit has been corrected. However, in cases of severe shock, vasopressor therapy may be needed early in the resuscitation effort to improve perfusion to the peripheral vascular beds. If there is no response to dopamine and norepinephrine, the patient should be treated with epinephrine (Adrenalin).[1]

Appropriate antibiotics should be administered within 1 hour after diagnosis of severe sepsis or septic shock, because mortality increases in a linear fashion with each hour of delay. All efforts should be made to obtain appropriate cultures, in particular at least two sets of blood cultures. At least one of these should be peripheral, with the second from any long-term (>48 hours) vascular device. Cultures of urine, sputum, wounds, abscesses, and cerebrospinal fluid should also be obtained as appropriate and before the administration of antibiotics, assuming that such specimens can be obtained during the first hour. Specific antibiotic choices are discussed later.

Source Control

A survey for potential sources of infection should be performed, and early resuscitation efforts should occur concomitantly. Elimination of the source of infection is critical to reversing septic shock. Conditions that require emergent intervention, such as necrotizing fasciitis, cholangitis, and intestinal infarction, should be ruled out within the first 6 hours after presentation. Potentially infected indwelling devices should be removed as soon as possible. Necrotic tissue should be débrided and abscesses drained if either condition is detected. Practitioners must consider the risks and benefits of the specific invasive procedures and the timing of such interventions for each patient individually. Every effort should be made to limit the invasiveness of necessary procedures, to avoid further stress in patients with an already hemodynamically fragile state. Imaging studies such as computed tomography of the head, chest, abdomen, and pelvis are necessary to identify or rule out potential sources of infection. An exception to the mandate to drain or débride infected collections is the presence of infected pancreatic necrosis, in which case surgical intervention should be delayed.

Other Interventions

After hemodynamic parameters have been stabilized with fluid and vasopressors, cultures have been obtained, antibiotics have been administered, and initial source control of infected foci has been achieved, other interventions may be appropriate. Many of these are typical components of good critical care.

Cardiac Dysfunction. Patients who have adequate left ventricular filling pressures (as determined by a central venous pressure ≥12 mm Hg) but low cardiac output may benefit from therapy with dobutamine (Dobutrex) to increase cardiac output and improve tissue perfusion.

Corticosteroid Therapy. Activation of the hypothalamic-pituitary axis and the consequent increase in serum cortisol levels are vital aspects of the body's acute stress response to shock. Recent data suggest that critical illness–related corticosteroid insufficiency is more prevalent in septic shock than previously thought, with rates as high as 60%. Therapy with corticosteroids is indicated only for those patients who have continued hypotension in the face of adequate fluid resuscitation and vasopressor support. Hydrocortisone (Solu-Cortef)[1] should be administered intravenously 200–300 mg/day for seven days, either divided every 6 hours or as a continuous infusion. Dexamethasone (Decadron)[1] should not be used unless hydrocortisone is not available. Because of the unclear long-term benefits and the known immunosuppressive side effects of corticosteroids, patients should be weaned from hydrocortisone as soon as vasopressors are no longer necessary. If another form of corticosteroid other than hydrocortisone is used, then fludrocortisone (Florinef)[1] at a dose of 50 mcg/day should be added for mineralocorticoid effect.

Activated Protein C. Patients who are at increased risk of death with Acute Physiology and Chronic Health Evaluation (APACHE) II scores of 25 or higher and those with multiple organ dysfunction may benefit from infusion of activated protein C (drotrecogin alfa [Xigris]). This drug has numerous contraindications, including current active bleeding, recent (within 3 months) hemorrhagic stroke, recent (within 2 months) severe head trauma or intracranial or intraspinal surgery, trauma with a risk of life-threatening bleeding, presence of an epidural catheter, and intracranial neoplasm or mass lesion or evidence of herniation. It is not recommended for use in children. It is given as a 96-hour continuous infusion.

Glycemic Control. Maintenance of the blood glucose concentration lower than 150 mg/dL is associated with decreased mortality and length of stay in the intensive care unit. Control should be achieved with intravenous insulin, paying close attention to serum glucose levels every 1 to 2 hours until stable, with adjustments made on the basis of a validated protocol. Patients receiving intravenous insulin should simultaneously receive some form of glucose as a calorie source to minimize the risk of hypoglycemia.

Sedation and Paralytics. Sedation and treatment of pain should be aggressively managed according to validated protocols. Daily interruption of sedation allows for more accurate titration of drug and decreases the total time of mechanical ventilation. Paralytics should be avoided or used only briefly if required.

Anticoagulation. Patients should receive prophylaxis for deep venous thrombosis with either low-molecular-weight heparin or unfractionated heparin unless contraindicated by severe thrombocytopenia, recent intracranial bleeding, or coagulopathy. Those patients who cannot receive heparin should receive prophylaxis with graduated compression stockings or intermittent

---

[1]Not FDA approved for this indication.

[1]Not FDA approved for this indication.

TABLE 1	Empiric Antibiotic Choices for Severe Sepsis*	
SOURCE	**ANTIBIOTIC AND DOSE**	**COMMENTS**
Community-acquired pneumonia	Ceftriaxone (Rocephin) 2 g q24h *plus* azithromycin (Zithromax) 500 mg q24h	Should include atypical coverage; alternative is moxifloxacin (Avelox)
Health care–associated pneumonia	Piperacillin/tazobactam (Zosyn) 4.5 g q6h *or* meropenem (Merrem)[1] 2 g q8h[3] *plus* vancomycin (Vancocin)[1] 1 g q12h	Should cover for *Pseudomonas* and other resistant gram-negative rods
Neutropenia/fever	Piperacillin/tazobactam[1] 4.5 g q6h *or* meropenem[1] 2 g q8h[3]	Consider empiric fungal coverage for prolonged neutropenia
Abdominal sepsis	Ampicillin/sulbactam (Unasyn) 3 g q6h *or* piperacillin/tazobactam 4.5 g q6h	Consider coverage for yeast, MRSA
Urosepsis	Ampicillin/sulbactam[1] 3 g q6h *or* piperacillin/tazobactam[1] 4.5 g q6h	Obtain imaging and decompression as appropriate
Foreign body/vascular catheter–related sepsis	Piperacillin/tazobactam[1] 4.5 g q6h *or* meropenem[1] 2 g q8h[3] *plus* vancomycin 1 g q12h	Vascular catheters or other foreign bodies should be removed urgently
Meningitis	Ceftriaxone 2 g q12h *plus* vancomycin[1] 750 mg q8h *plus* rifampin (Rifadin)[1] 600 mg q24h	Consider steroid therapy before or simultaneously with administration of antibiotics
Soft-tissue infection	Cefazolin (Ancef) 2 g q8h *plus* vancomycin 1 g q12h	Image for abscess with débridement as appropriate
Necrotizing fasciitis	Ampicillin/sulbactam 3 g q6h *plus* vancomycin 1 g q12h *plus* clindamycin (Cleocin) 900 mg q8h	Obtain urgent surgical consultation
Unknown	Piperacillin/tazobactam 4.5 g q6h *or* meropenem 2 g q8h[3] *plus* vancomycin 1 g q12h *plus* tobramycin (Tobrex) 7 mg/kg q24h	Obtain appropriate imaging studies, especially of abdomen, pelvis, central nervous system

[1]Not FDA approved for this indication.
[3]Exceeds dosage recommended by the manufacturer.
*In all cases, prior antimicrobial therapy, kidney and liver dysfunction, and the probable source of sepsis should be carefully considered. Always consider coverage for methicillin-resistant *Staphylococcus aureus* (MRSA) in areas where incidence in bloodstream isolates is >10%.

compression devices. Patients who are at especially high risk for deep venous thrombosis (e.g., prior history of clot, orthopedic surgery, trauma) should receive both pharmacologic and mechanical prophylaxis. Low-molecular-weight heparin is preferred to unfractionated heparin in high-risk patients.

Ulcer Prophylaxis. Patients should receive prophylaxis with a proton pump inhibitor or a histamine 2 (H_2) blocker to prevent upper gastrointestinal bleeding.

Bicarbonate Therapy. There is no role for the administration of bicarbonate to correct acidosis or improve hemodynamic status.

Antibiotics

Antibiotic choices should take into account the most likely pathogens for the suspected site or process. In general, initial empiric therapy (Table 1) should be broad, with an intention to narrow therapy once a microorganism has been isolated or a more precise clinical diagnosis has been made. Such a reevaluation should take place approximately 72 hours after the initiation of therapy. Numerous studies have documented the mortality associated with initial therapy that did not include agents active against the pathogen eventually isolated. In general, drugs from the β-lactam and related classes of antibiotics should be preferred for at least a part of most empiric regimens.

Special considerations include patients with neutropenia and fever, who should always be treated with at least one agent active against *Pseudomonas*. Some debate continues regarding the use of two anti-pseudomonal drugs as part of the initial antibiotic regimen. Given the possibility of resistance on the part of this pathogen, it would seem reasonable to use two drugs initially, until *Pseudomonas* has been isolated (if present) and its susceptibilities are known, allowing coverage to be narrowed. The Surviving Sepsis Campaign guidelines advocate this approach. There is no benefit in treating with two drugs known to be active in an attempt to achieve a supposed synergy.

Patients with hematologic malignancies are at increased risk for sepsis from fungal organisms. Severe sepsis or septic shock in such patients warrants empiric treatment with an echinocandin, a broad-spectrum azole such as voriconazole (Vfend) or posaconazole (Noxafil), or amphotericin (Fungizone).

MRSA continues to increase in incidence nationally and is now common as a community-acquired pathogen. It is also to be suspected as a cause of postinfluenza bacterial pneumonia. Empiric treatment with an antibiotic active against this bacterium, such as vancomycin (Vancocin), linezolid (Zyvox), or daptomycin (Cubicin), should be strongly considered in septic patients in communities where the rate of MRSA in bloodstream infections exceeds 10%. This pathogen should always be considered in a patient with a long-term intravenous catheter, prosthetic device, or other indwelling foreign body. Although vancomycin-resistant *S. aureus* is extremely rare, caution should be taken when using daptomycin and linezolid as empiric therapy, because resistance has been reported.

Prior administration of antibiotics and the attendant risk of infection by a pathogen resistant to the previous therapy should be considered in arriving at a course of empiric therapy. A typical scenario is a patient who presents with a catheter-related bloodstream infection while taking vancomycin. One would expect a gram-negative bacterium, a fungal organism, or, potentially, a vancomycin-resistant enterococcus as the pathogen. Recent hospitalization or residence in a nursing home places patients at risk for colonization and subsequent infection with resistant gram-negative rods.

Prognosis and Limits of Care

Patients who present with severe sepsis or septic shock often have substantial prior medical morbidity, decreasing their chance of survival. The overall mortality rate remains between 20% and 40%. Patients often have expressed wishes regarding limits of care to family members or others close to them before becoming ill. It is always appropriate to discuss goals of therapy, possible and probable outcomes, and plans for further evaluation and treatment with patients (if possible) and their proxies in all instances. Decisions to proceed with or limit care should be made within the context of a patient's expressed or expected wishes and should take into account unfolding clinical data and circumstances. Time spent in this endeavor can substantially decrease the amount of futile care rendered to a patient and lead to care that more truly reflects the patient's wishes regarding life-prolonging measures. The stress and anxiety experienced by family members may also be reduced.

Substantial progress has been made in the last 3 decades in decreasing the mortality associated with severe sepsis and septic shock. Nevertheless, the mortality rate remains unacceptably high, and the overall incidence and severity of disease appear to be increasing, by as much as 1.5% annually by some estimates. The risk of death for an individual patient appears to stabilize approximately 6 months after the original illness. Many patients who do survive remain with the same risk factors (e.g., diabetes, vascular disease, prosthetic devices, immunosuppression) that contributed to their infection and therefore are at risk for recurrence. Moreover, certain organisms, such as MRSA, resistant gram-negative rods, and fungi, remain difficult to treat, and success rates are relatively low despite aggressive, timely, and prolonged therapy.

There is some cause for optimism. The Surviving Sepsis Campaign has now entered phase III. This is a program in which a core set of recommendations, described in the guidelines, is being implemented with opportunities to measure outcomes, assess physician behavior, and provide feedback to improve survival through evidence-based interventions. This effort involves more than 12,000 patients in 239 hospitals in 17 countries and will undoubtedly change the future course of this lethal disease.

References

Bone RC. Immunologic dissonance: A continuing evolution in our understanding of the systemic inflammatory response syndrome (SIRS) and the multiple organ dysfunction syndrome (MODS). Ann Intern Med 1996;125:680–7.

Delinger RP, Levy MM, Carlet JM, et al. Surviving Sepsis Campaign: Internatonal guidelines for management of severe sepsis and septic shock—2008. Crit Care Med 2008;36:296–327.

Dombrovskiy VY, Martin AA, Sunderram J, Paz HL. Rapid increase in hospitalization and mortality rates for severe sepsis in the United States: A trend analysis from 1993 to 2003. Crit Care Med 2007;35:1244–50.

Ibrahim EH, Sherman G, Ward S, et al. The influence of inadequate antimicrobial treatment of bloodstream infections on patient outcomes in the ICU setting. Chest 2000;118:146–55.

Jimenez MF, Marshall JC. Source control in the management of sepsis. Intensive Care Med 2001;27(Suppl. 1):S49–62.

Kumar A, Roberts D, Wood KE, et al. Duration of hypotension before initiation of effective antimicrobial therapy is the critical determinant of survival in human septic shock. Crit Care Med 2006;34:1589–96.

Leibovici L, Shraga I, Drucker M, et al. The benefit of appropriate empirical antibiotic treatment in patients with bloodstream infection. J Intern Med 1998;244:379–86.

Levy MM, Fink MP, Marshall JC, et al. 2001 SCCM/ESICM/ACCP/ATS/SIS International Sepsis Definitions Conference. Intensive Care Med 2003;29:530–8.

Martin GS, Mannino DM, Easton S, et al. The epidemiology of sepsis in the United States from 1979 through 2000. N Engl J Med 2003;348:1546–54.

McDonald JR, Friedman ND, Stout JE, et al. Risk factors for ineffective therapy in patients with bloodstream infection. Arch Intern Med 2005;165:308–13.

Miller PJ, Wenzel RP. Etiologic organisms as independent predictors of death and morbidity associated with bloodstream infection. J Infect Dis 1987;156:471–7.

Sasse KC, Nauenberg E, Long A, et al. Long-term survival after intensive care unit admission with sepsis. Crit Care Med 1995;23:1040–7.

SMALLPOX

Method of
Raul Davaro, MD

Smallpox, a disease unique to humans, is one of the oldest recorded infections affecting humankind. In endemic forms and in epidemic waves, smallpox killed and disfigured millions of people throughout history. This viral infection, spread by respiratory droplets, continued to have worldwide distribution at the beginning of the 20th century. Because smallpox confers immunity in the survivors of an attack, its persistence depends on contact of nonimmune persons with infected persons in the initial 2 weeks of acquiring the infection.

Centuries ago, physicians realized that inoculating smallpox matter into nonimmune persons conferred partial or total immunity against smallpox. This practice was known in India and China

as *variolation*. Variolation was introduced in England in 1721 by the wife of Ambassador Montagu, Lady Montagu, who herself was disfigured by smallpox. The practice spread rapidly in England despite skepticism from the scientific community and resistance from the Church. Variolation was risky and sometimes fatal. In 1783 Octavius, the son of King George III, died as a result of complications from variolation. Benjamin Franklin was an ardent supporter of variolation in the American colonies.

In 1778, Edward Jenner, an English physician, reported that milkmaids infected with cowpox were immune to smallpox during epidemics. In 1796 he decided to test his hypothesis by injecting cowpox material into James Phipps. Phipps developed no signs or symptoms of smallpox 2 months after the inoculation, when he had variolation. This experiment was the birth of vaccination (Latin *vacca*, "cow") against smallpox. With the support of King George IV, vaccination was implemented in England, and variolation was slowly abandoned and finally declared illegal in 1840. Vaccination was introduced in the United States in 1800 by Dr. Benjamin Waterhouse, a Harvard physician, and supported by President Thomas Jefferson, who immunized members of his household. The last-documented natural case of smallpox in the United States was documented 1947.

The World Health Organization (WHO) designed an Intensified Eradication Program based on a ring vaccination strategy that began in 1966 and eradicated smallpox from humans in an unprecedented effort in less than 10 years. The last natural case was documented in Somalia in 1977. Routine immunization against smallpox ceased in the United States in 1972 and worldwide in 1980. It was thought that without a human reservoir, reemergence of this infection would not occur.

Smallpox virus stocks are still available in the United States at the CDC in Atlanta, Georgia, and in Russia at the State Center for Virology and Biotechnology in Novosibirk, Siberia. These stocks are maintained under strict bio-containment measures. In the aftermath of the terrorist attacks on September 11, 2001 and the deliberate distribution of *Bacillus anthracis* afterwards, President Bush announced plans to immunize health care workers and first responders against smallpox by 2003. Although the plan fell short of it goals, 40,000 first responders and health care workers were vaccinated by the end of 2003.

The Agent

Smallpox is a single, linear double-stranded DNA virus that belongs to the *Orthopoxvirus* genus, family Poxviridae. The poxviruses replicate in cell cytoplasm. They are brick-shaped and measure about 300 by 250 by 200 nm.

Epidemiology

The natural reservoir of smallpox is the patient suffering from the disease. Smallpox spreads from person to person through droplet nuclei or fine-particle aerosols released from the pharynx of infected persons. Smallpox can also be transmitted by fomites such as clothing and bedding. Smallpox patients are not infectious until the third day of the clinical disease, typically 1 day before the skin eruption. The secondary attack rate of smallpox is 37% to 88% among unvaccinated contacts, depending on many variables.

Clinical Presentation

Smallpox occurs as either variola major or variola minor (Alastrim). Variola major had a mortality rate of 30% compared with 1% for variola minor.

After an incubation period of 10 to 14 days, the illness begins with intense prostration and high fever lasting 4 to 6 days (Figure 1). Headache, photophobia, and vomiting are noted. During the prodrome phase most patients are bedridden. Around the fourth day the fever breaks and the patient feels better.

The eruptive phase is signaled by an enanthem involving the buccal mucosa and pharynx and a centrifugal exanthem that begins on the face and forearms. The initial rash is macular

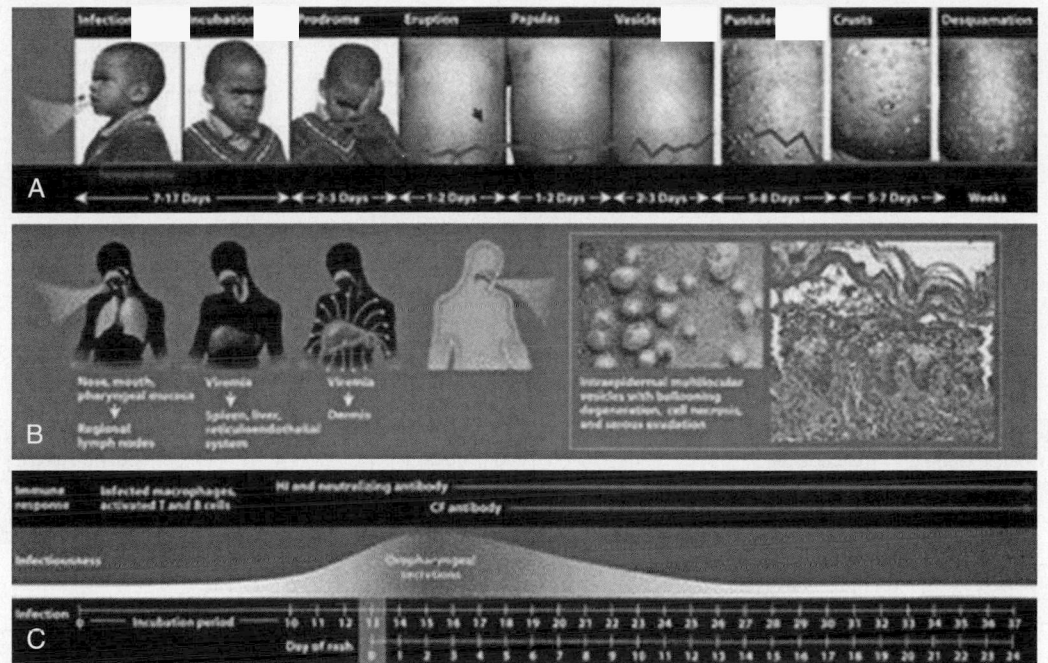

Figure 1. Clinical manifestations and pathogenesis of smallpox and the immune response. **A,** The initial phases of infection and the clinical manifestations include temperature spikes and progressive skin lesions (photographs of lesions courtesy of Dr. David Heymann, World Health Organization). **B,** The pathogenesis of the infection. The photographs on the *right* show the characteristic features of the vesicles caused by smallpox (H&E, ×90). **C,** The immune response to smallpox and the period of infectiousness.
Abbreviations: CF = complement fixation; HI = hemagglutination inhibition. (Reprinted with permission from Breman JG, Henderson DA. Diagnosis and management of smallpox. N Eng J Med 2002;346:1300–8.)

and turns pustular in 1 to 2 days. Within 2 days the papules evolve into vesicles that become cloudy and pustular. Most patients exhibit lesions on their soles and palms. A typical feature of variola is that the exanthem everywhere is in the same state of evolution, unlike the exanthem of chickenpox, in which lesions exhibit all stages of evolution. At the end of day 8 to 10 the skin rash crusts and dries; it takes 3 to 4 weeks from the onset of the disease for all the scabs to fall off. The period of contagiousness ends when the last scab falls off. Scarring and pitting of the skin are common sequelae.

Patients with hemorrhagic disease develop severe prostration, high fever, abdominal pain, petechiae, and extensive cutaneous ecchymoses. In the malignant or flat form, the lesions fail to progress to the pustular stage. In the hemorrhagic and the malignant forms, death invariably occurs within 1 week.

History of smallpox vaccination modifies the course of the disease. Vaccinated persons who contract smallpox have fewer skin lesions and an accelerated clinical course.

Complications

Bacterial infections of the skin and other organs are common. Ocular involvement may result in blindness. Encephalitis (one in 500 cases of variola major) is a devastating complication.

Differential Diagnosis (Figure 2)

Many rashes can be confused with smallpox, especially at the outset of the eruption, when the rash is maculopapular. Herpes zoster, chickenpox, herpes simplex, impetigo, scabies, erythema multiforme, and syphilis are some of the conditions that can be confused with smallpox (Box 1). When smallpox was endemic, chickenpox was the most common condition confused with smallpox. The most useful clinical points of smallpox are the following:

- Centrifugal distribution of the lesions
- All the lesions in the same stage of development
- Progression of the rash from the face to the arms, trunk and legs
- A severe prodrome phase that lasts 4 days
- In an epidemic, known contact with an active case

Diagnosis

The identification of a suspected case of smallpox should be treated as an international health emergency. Clinical samples may be collected from vesicular or pustular fluid, blood, tonsillar swabs, and skin biopsy and must be transported to a Biosafety level 4 facility for processing and testing, with real-time polymerase chain reaction (PCR) assays to detect virus DNA.

Lesions of varicella zoster virus (chickenpox, herpes zoster) demonstrate multinucleated giant cells on Tzanck smears; lesions of smallpox do not. Serology or electronic microscopy are not recommended for the diagnosis of smallpox because these modalities cannot distinguish among different Orthopoxviruses.

Treatment

A suspected case of smallpox should be placed in a negative-pressure room with strict respiratory and contact isolation precautions. Ideally to minimize the risk of contagion in health care personnel, patient with smallpox should be assisted by providers documented to have been immunized against this condition. Patients with smallpox require careful care of their eyes to avoid complications and this is accomplished with daily eye rinsing. Patients must receive adequate nutrition and hydration. Skin and soft issue infections must be treated with an antistaphylococcal β-lactams, and initially pending results of cultures, with an antimicrobial with activity against methicillin-resistant Staphylococcus aureus. There is no antiviral drug with demonstrated activity against smallpox.

Vaccines and Vaccination

Sanofi's U.S.-licensed ACAM2000, a second-generation vaccine, was made from cell culture-derived vaccinia virus found in Dryvax, a first-generation vaccine that is no longer produced. ACAM2000 is indicated for active immunization of people who are determined to be at high risk for smallpox. A two-pronged stainless steel (or bifurcated) needle is dipped into the vaccine solution and the skin is pricked several times in the upper arm with a droplet of the vaccine. The virus begins growing at the injection site causing a localized infection or "pock" to form. A red, itchy

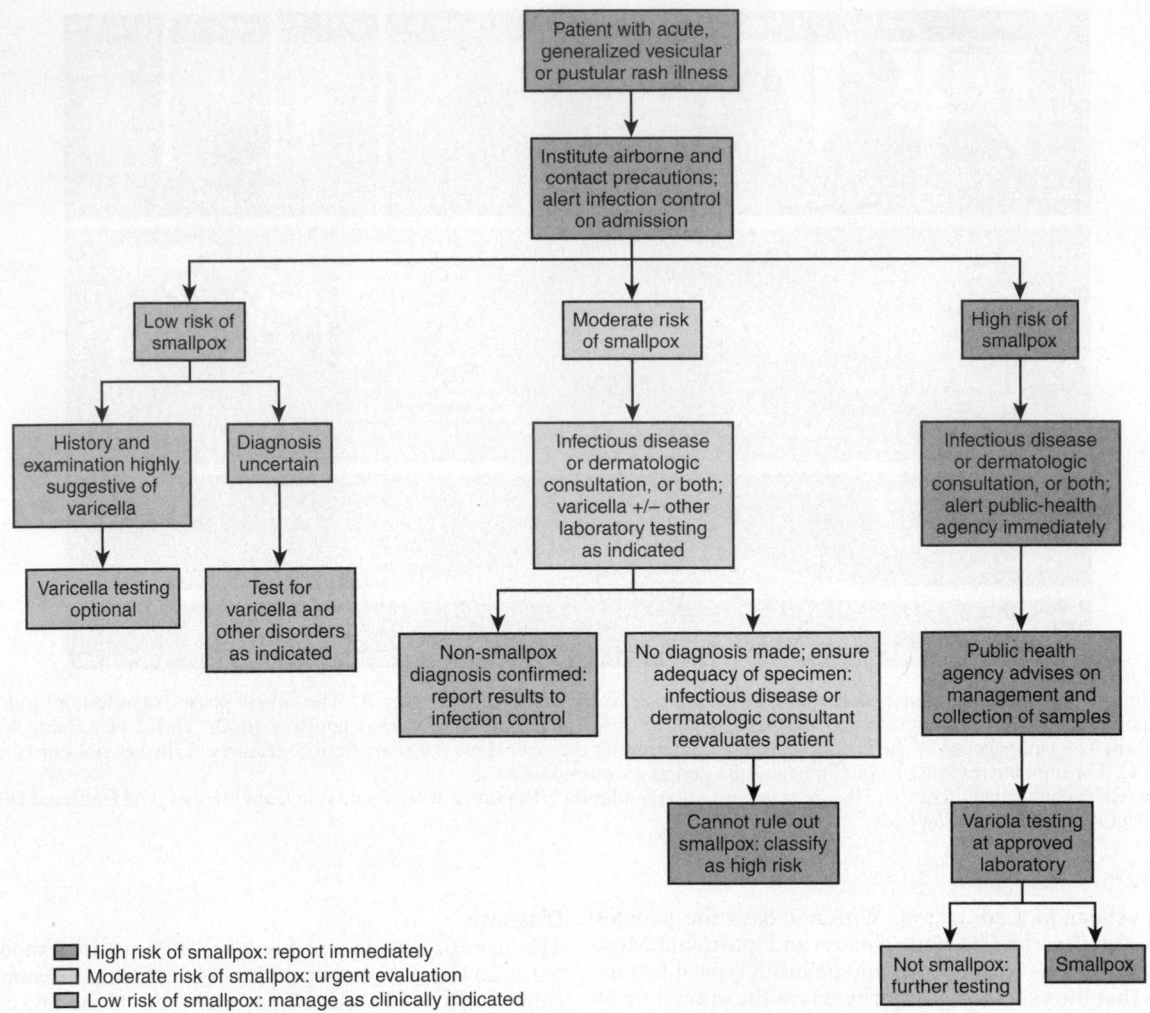

High risk of smallpox: report immediately
Moderate risk of smallpox: urgent evaluation
Low risk of smallpox: manage as clinically indicated

Figure 2. Algorithm for assessing patients for smallpox. (Reprinted with permission from Moore ZS, Seward JF, Lane JM: Smallpox. Lancet 2006;367:425–35.)

Box 1	Conditions that Might Be Confused with Smallpox

Maculopapular Stage
Measles
Rubella
Drug eruptions
Secondary syphilis
Erythema multiforme
Scabies, insect bites
Acne
Scarlet fever

Vesicular/Pustular Stage
Chickenpox
Disseminated herpes zoster
Disseminated herpes simplex virus
Drug eruptions
Contact dermatitis
Erythema multiforme (including Stevens-Johnson syndrome)
Enteroviral infections
Secondary syphilis
Acne
Generalized vaccinia
Monkeypox
Impetigo
Scabies, insect bites
Disseminated molluscum contagiosum

sore spot at the site of the vaccination within 3-4 days is an indicator that the vaccination was successful; that is, there is "a take." A blister develops at the vaccination site and then dries up forming a scab that falls off in the third week, leaving a small scar. If no evidence of vaccine take is apparent after 7 days, the person can be vaccinated again.

The vaccine causes local and systemic symptoms. There is an eruption at the injection site with redness and pain, systemic symptoms such as fever, and headaches. Swelling and tenderness of regional lymph nodes begin 3 to 10 days after vaccination and can last up to a month.

Complications
Adverse events of vaccinia have been reviewed extensively and include postvaccinial encephalitis, progressive vaccinia, eczema vaccinatum, and generalized vaccinia (Table 1). The most common complication is inadvertent autoinoculation causing self-limited satellite lesions. Generalized vaccinia results from viremia and may be life threatening in immunocompromised patients. Progressive vaccinia is characterized by necrosis at the inoculation site and distal sites such as bones and internal organs. Progressive vaccinia is often a fatal complication. Myopericarditis was observed with the use of adult vaccines in the United States in 2002 (Table 1).

Contraindications to Vaccination
Persons who are immune compromised or who have severe eczema or who are pregnant should not receive Post-exposure vaccination against smallpox. However, in the event of exposure to a patient with smallpox, no absolute contraindication is applicable.

TABLE 1 Rates of Complications from Vaccinia, According to Vaccination Status and Age*

COMPLICATIONS	PRIMARY VACCINATION (N = 650,000)				REVACCINATION (N = 996,000)			
	0–4 YR	5–19 YR	>20 YR	ALL AGES	1–4 YR†	5–19 YR	>20 YR	ALL AGES
Accidental infection	564	371	606	529	198	48	25	42
Generalized vaccinia	263	140	212	242	0	10	9	9
Erythema multiforme	299	87	30	165	73	2	9	10
Eczema vaccinatum	39	35	30	39	0	2	5	3
Postvaccinal encephalitis	15	9	0	12	0	0	5	2
Progressive vaccinia	3	0	0	2	0	0	7	3
Other	222	214	6636	266	18	24	55	39

*Data are from a 1968 survey of 10 states. No deaths occurred.
†No children younger than 1 year were revaccinated.
Reprinted with permission from Breman JG, Henderson DA: Diagnosis and management of smallpox. N Engl J Med 2002;346:1300–8.

Control of Outbreaks

As soon as a diagnosis of smallpox is considered, suspected persons should be isolated and close contacts should be immunized. Post-exposure vaccination within the first 4 days can greatly mitigate subsequent illness. Contact isolation and ring vaccination are the strategies of choice to contain an outbreak of smallpox.

Use in Warfare

During the 15th century, variola-laden clothing and blankets were distributed by Europeans among Native Americans to spread smallpox in the local population. British soldiers used variola-contaminated blankets among the natives supporting the French during the French and Indian wars. The use of infectious agents in warfare is not new, and the potential use of smallpox as a weapon increased when routine immunization against smallpox ceased and worldwide immunity waned.

Because natural smallpox has been eradicated, the only possibility of a smallpox outbreak is the deliberate release of smallpox in a population by a nation or a terrorist group to inflict casualties in a civilian population. Preemptive vaccination of first responders and ring immunization of those exposed are the means available to avoid massive propagation of smallpox.

References

Behbehani A. The smallpox story: Life and death of an old disease. Microbiol Rev 1983;47:455–509.
Breman JG, Henderson DA. Diagnosis and management of smallpox. N Engl J Med 2002;346:1300–8.
Bronze MS, Huycke MM, Machado LJ, et al. Viral agents as biological weapons and agents of bioterrorism. Am J Med Sci 2002;323:316–25.
Centers for Disease Control and Prevention. Smallpox vaccination. Information for Health Care professionals Available from http://www.bt.cdc.gov/agent/smallpox/vaccination/ [accessed 05.05.15].
Cleri DJ, Porwancher RB, Ricketti AJ, et al. Smallpox as a bioterrorist weapon: Myth or menace? Infectious Dis Clin North Am 2006;20:329–58.
Kempe HC. Variola. In: Beeson PB, McDermott W, editors. Textbook of Medicine. 12th ed. Philadelphia: WB Saunders; 1967. p. 44–6.
Lofquist J, Weimert NA, Hayney MS. Smallpox: A review of clinical disease and vaccination. Am J Health Syst Pharm 2003;60:749–58.
Moore ZS, Seward JF, Lane JM. Smallpox. Lancet 2006;367:425–35.
Weiss MM, Weiss PD, Mathisen G, et al. Rethinking smallpox. Clin Infect Dis 2004;29:1668–73.
Whitley RJ. Smallpox: A potential agent of bioterrorism. Antiviral Res 2003;57:7–12.

TETANUS

Method of
Dilip R. Karnad, MD

Tetanus is a potentially fatal illness caused by the neurotoxin produced by the spore-bearing anaerobic bacterium *Clostridium tetani*. As the causative organism and its spores are ubiquitous, nonimmune individuals in any part of the world may get tetanus unless they are protected by the highly effective vaccine.

Epidemiology

As a result of effective universal immunization, tetanus is rare in the developed world. Twenty to 40 cases of tetanus occur annually in the United States and 12 to 15 cases per year have been reported from the United Kingdom in the last 10 years. Although progressively declining in the developing world due to improved immunization coverage, according to WHO figures, more than 500 cases were reported in 2012 from each of these nations: Angola, Bangladesh, Congo, India, and Uganda. While tetanus may affect individuals of all ages, a significant number of cases in developed countries are elderly people who did not receive a primary immunization or lacked the booster dosage needed to maintain protective immunity. In developing countries, most cases are neonates (*tetanus neonatorum*), children who are born to nonimmunized mothers and thus lack transplacentally acquired passive immunity. Infection of the umbilical stump due to poor hygiene results in severe tetanus that has mortality in excess of 60%.

The infection is caused by the gram-positive, spore-bearing bacterium C. *tetani*, the spores of which exist in the soil, in animal feces, and even in the human gastrointestinal tract. Spores remain dormant and viable for several months and are destroyed by autoclaving at 1 atmosphere pressure at 120°C for 15 minutes. When inoculated into human or animal tissues, they transform into motile bacilli in an anerobic environment that produce a potent exotoxin, tetanospasmin, which produces the manifestations of tetanus. It must be emphasized that tetanus is not transmitted from human to human, and patients do not require isolation.

Risk Factors

Elderly individuals are at increased risk, as they may not have received adequate immunization or may have waning immunity. Other predisposed groups include immigrants from countries with an unreliable immunization program, immunosuppressed individuals (with HIV infection or receiving immunosuppressive drugs), and intravenous drug addicts. Local factors include wounds with crushed, devitalized tissue or contaminated by dirt or rust, such as open fractures, punctures, and abscesses. However, even scratches, chronic ulcers, or tattooing may cause tetanus. In developing countries, unsafe practices related to termination of pregnancy may cause maternal tetanus; newborn babies born outside of medical facilities are at risk of neonatal tetanus.

Pathophysiology

Tetanospasmin is a highly toxic protein released by C. *tetani*. It is absorbed into the circulation and reaches the ends of motor axons all over the body, from where it is transported proximally along the axonal cytoplasm to motor nuclei in the brainstem and spinal cord at a rate of 3 to 13 mm/hour. A fragment of the toxin then binds inhibitory interneurons that produce gamma-amino butyric acid (GABA) and glycine and inactivates synaptobrevin, a protein that is essential for the release of these neurotransmitters from pre-synaptic vesicles.

The loss of normal inhibition at motor and autonomic neurons results in spontaneous discharge of nerve impulses as well as exaggerated responses to stimuli manifesting as tonic muscle contraction with superadded intermittent muscle spasms. As tetanospasmin reaches the motor nuclei of the shortest motor axons first, muscles innervated by motor cranial nerves are affected first, followed by trunk muscles, and finally the extremities. Autonomic overactivity results in severe tachycardia, swings in blood pressure, profuse sweating, and (rarely) ileus. An exaggerated startle-like response to stimuli with motor and autonomic components is also typical. Generalized spasms may mimic tonic seizures.

Clinical Manifestations

An attempt should be made to locate the predisposing wound, such as cuts, abrasions, burns, puncture wounds, and other skin lesions. Uncommon causes include needle-sticks in intravenous drug abusers, ulcerated malignant tumors, and chronic middle-ear infection in children (otogenic tetanus). In up to 30% of patients, no site of infection is discovered. The incubation period is the interval between the injury and the onset of symptoms and can range from a few days to a few months (usually 3–21 days). A short incubation period (<7 days) suggests the likelihood of developing severe tetanus; however, a long incubation period does not necessarily indicate a milder disease. The period of onset (the interval between the first symptom and first paroxysmal muscle spasm) is a better predictor of severity: early elective tracheal intubation and mechanical ventilation are usually required if the interval is <48 hours.

Generalized Tetanus

Initial symptoms include an inability to open the mouth (lockjaw or trismus), difficulty in chewing and swallowing, and stiffness of neck muscles. The contraction of facial muscles produces the characteristic sneering smile (*risus sardonicus*) (Figure 1). In severe cases, intermittent spasms are provoked by attempts to speak or swallow. Pooled saliva from hypersalivation and dysphagia may trigger cough and laryngeal spasms; if prolonged, these may prove fatal. Rigidity of paraspinal muscles follows, and hyperextension of the spine results in opisthotonus (Figure 2). Finally, proximal muscles of the extremity are also affected. Deep tendon reflexes are always exaggerated and ankle clonus is common. Tonic muscle spasms may affect head and neck muscles and laryngeal muscles, or may be generalized. Paroxysmal spasms occur spontaneously or in response to loud noise, bright lights, or attempts to speak or swallow. Prolonged spasms may compromise breathing.

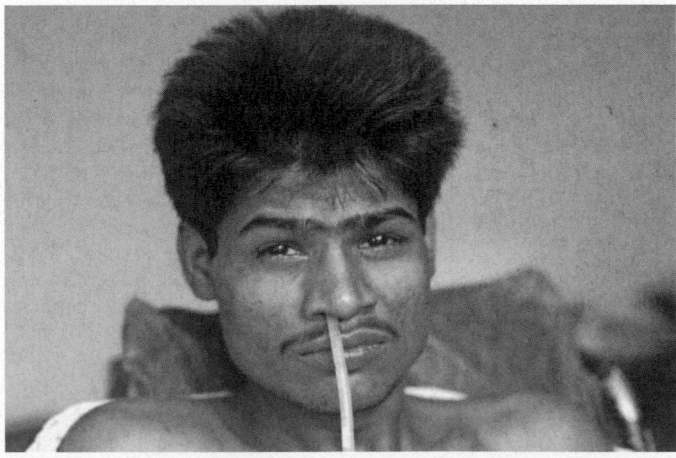

Figure 1. Typical facial expression with the sneering smile (risus sardonicus), wrinkled forehead, narrow palpebral fissures, and "crow's feet" at the lateral palpebral margins from the tonic contraction of muscles of facial expression in moderate tetanus.

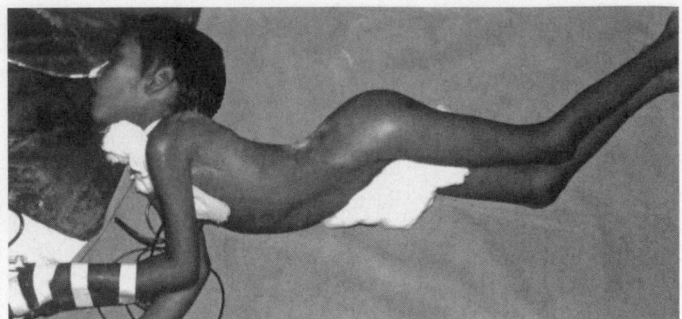

Figure 2. Spasm of paraspinal muscles, producing the hyperextended opisthotonic posture in severe tetanus.

The Ablett classification is commonly used to grade the severity of tetanus. Grade I (mild) tetanus is characterized by moderate trismus and general spasticity without spasms, dysphagia, or respiratory distress. Grade II (moderate) tetanus has severe trismus, intermittent short spasms, mild tachypnea, and dysphagia. Grade III (severe) tetanus is associated with severe rigidity, prolonged spasms, severe dysphagia, tachypnea, apneic spells, and tachycardia. The presence of additional violent autonomic disturbances with persistent or intermittent episodes of severe hypertension and tachycardia alternating with hypotension and bradycardia is classified as Grade IV (very severe) tetanus. Cardiac arrhythmias, peripheral vasoconstriction, and sudden asystole may also occur in very severe tetanus.

Despite the use of antitetanus immune globulin (HyperTET) to neutralize circulating tetanus toxin, the disease may progress for up to 2 weeks as more intraaxonal toxin continues to reach the central nervous system. Manifestations persist for another 2 to 3 weeks before gradually subsiding. During this period, an apparently stable patient is at risk of developing sudden asphyxia due to severe generalized or laryngeal spasms. Patients may develop fever, rhabdomyolysis, and hyperthermia due to excessive muscular activity.

Cephalic Tetanus

Following injuries to the head or face, in some patients, the toxin reaches the local motor nuclei earlier and produces a combination of partial paralysis and overactivity—more severely affected motor neurons stop functioning while the remaining fibers are overactive and cause muscle spasm (Figure 3).

Localized Tetanus

In this rare form of tetanus, manifestations are restricted to muscles in the region of the wound. These patients have a good prognosis.

Diagnosis

C. tetani can be isolated from the wound in <30% of cases, and microbiological and other laboratory tests do not help in confirming the diagnosis. The diagnosis is entirely clinical. In an individual with a predisposing injury, the presence of trismus, rigidity of neck, abdominal and paraspinal muscles, and severe hyperreflexia are suggestive. The spatula test is a useful bedside test: A spatula (tongue depressor) is inserted into the mouth to touch the posterior pharyngeal wall. Normally, a gag reflex is activated in an attempt to expel the spatula. In tetanus, severe spasms of the masseters results in the patient biting on the spatula, making it difficult to withdraw—a positive test. In one study, the spatula test was positive in 94% of patients with tetanus and in none without tetanus. The electromyogram shows the continuous discharge of motor units in moderate tetanus and the absence of the normal silent period.

Differential Diagnosis

While the diagnosis of tetanus is easy in severe tetanus, it may be mistaken for other conditions in its initial stages (Table 1). The spatula test is negative in other conditions causing trismus. Abdominal muscles usually relax after adequate sedation. As in

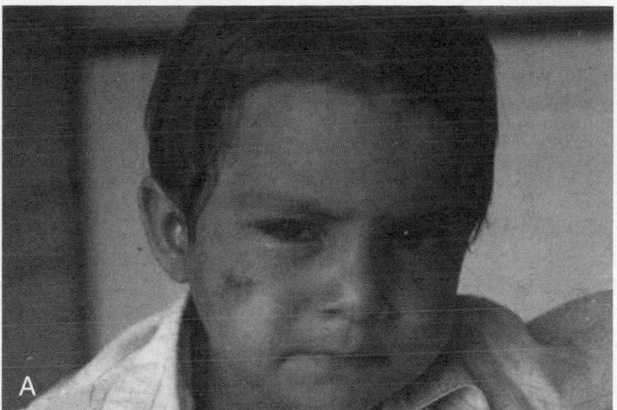

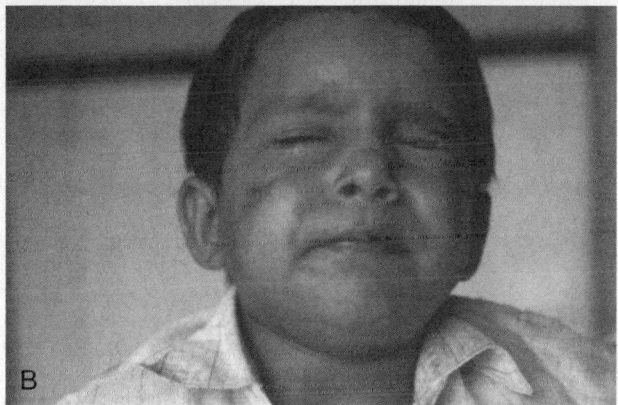

Figure 3. Cephalic tetanus: This 6-year-old child developed mild tetanus 3 weeks after a wound on his right cheek was sutured. He had cephalic tetanus characterized by partial paralysis of the right facial nerve along with overactivity of the unaffected nerve fibers. **A,** Note the overactivity of the facial muscles with a narrow palpebral and prominent nasolabial fold on the same side as the injury. On asking him to shut his eyes tight **(B)**, weakness of the orbicularis oculi and other facial muscles on the right side become manifest.

TABLE 1	Conditions that Mimic Clinical Manifestations of Tetanus
CLINICAL FEATURE	**DIFFERENTIAL DIAGNOSIS**
Trismus	Acute tonsillar abscess, temporomandibular joint disease, extrapyramidal reaction to drugs, dental pathology
Neck stiffness	Cervical spine disease; extrapyramidal reaction to drugs such as antipsychotics, antiemetics, or metoclopramide; meningitis; subarachnoid hemorrhage
Abdominal rigidity	Acute abdomen
Dysphagia	Myasthenia gravis, acute bulbar paralysis, rabies
Muscle spasms	Seizures, spasticity due to spinal cord disease, stiff man syndrome

spasticity due to cord compression, deep reflexes are exaggerated; however, the plantar response, which is extensor in spinal cord disorders, is always flexor with tetanus. Unlike seizures or other intracranial diseases, the patient with tetanus is always fully alert and awake.

Treatment

In patients with life-threatening spasms, prompt, adequate sedation is the first step in management. Patients must be observed in an intensive care unit because the disease may rapidly worsen. They should be nursed in a quiet, dimly lit room in order to keep external stimuli to a minimum—this is difficult in modern intensive care units.

Neutralization of Toxin

Although unsupported by randomized studies, human tetanus immune globulin (HyperTET) (3000–6000 units) is administered intramuscularly to neutralize the circulating toxin. This does not bind to the toxin that has already entered neurons. There is insufficient evidence favoring intrathecal administration[1] of tetanus immune globulin over the usual intramuscular route, although one randomized study showed a shortening of the course of tetanus. Equine antiserum[2] (10,000–20,000 units) may be administered after skin testing for hypersensitivity. Though rarely used today due to the risk of anaphylaxis or serum sickness, it has the advantage of being administered intravenously.

Control of Clostridial Infection

Benzylpenicillin (Penicillin G) in a dose of 10 to 12 million units per day is given intravenously for 10 days. In one study, metronidazole (Flagyl) (500 mg every 6 hour for 10 days) was superior to procaine penicillin (Wycillin),[1] presumably because procaine and penicillin are GABA antagonists and may worsen manifestations of tetanus. However, a more recent study showed that a single intramuscular injection of 1.2 million units of benzathine penicillin (Bicillin LA)[1] was as effective as benzylpenicillin or metronidazole. Fortunately, resistance to these antibiotics has not been reported. Debridement of the infected wound and abscess drainage should be performed after spasms have been adequately controlled.

Control of Muscle Spasms

Benzodiazepines (diazepam [Valium] or lorazepam [Ativan][1]) are the preferred drugs and act by enhancing the effect of GABA on its receptor on the postsynaptic membrane, thus potentially antagonizing the effect of tetanospasmin. However, as very little GABA is released in tetanus, large doses (up to 1000 mg/day[3]) of diazepam may be required to achieve adequate sedation and muscle relaxation. Diazepam may be administered intravenously (10–30 mg in 5 mg boluses every 5 minutes)[3] or through a nasogastric tube (10–40 mg every 1 to 2 hours).[3] Barbiturates and chlorpromazine (Thorazine)[1] are alternative agents. Other sedative hypnotic agents such as midazolam (Versed)[1] and propofol (Diprivan)[1] have also been used with good effect. In mild to moderate tetanus, drug doses can be titrated to achieve moderate sedation and control rigidity and spasms without causing respiratory depression. In severe cases, however, spasms may not be controlled despite large doses, increasing the risk of severe central nervous system (CNS) depression. In these patients, heavy sedation combined with neuromuscular blockade and mechanical ventilation is required. In about 10% of cases, benzodiazepines may produce paradoxical excitation instead of sedation; increasing doses make the patient more wakeful, agitated, and delirious, with increased spasms. Discontinuation of diazepam and the use of barbiturates and chlorpromazine may prevent the need for paralysis and mechanical ventilation. Pancuronium (Pavulon),[1] vecuronium (Norcuron),[1] and rocuronium (Zemuron)[1] are often used for neuromuscular blockade. Atracurium (Tracrium)[1] could also be used but may have unfavorable cardiovascular effects. Intravenous and intrathecal baclofen (Lioresal Intrathecal)[1] have been used in some case.

Airway Management

Tracheostomy or endotracheal intubation is required in moderate and severe tetanus to prevent respiratory failure due to laryngeal spasm and aspiration of oropharyngeal secretions. In most developing countries, elective tracheostomy is performed early in severe

---

[1]Not FDA approved for this indication.
[2]Not available in the United States.
[3]Exceeds dosage recommended by the manufacturer.

tetanus. In countries with superior intensive care facilities, heavy sedation, neuromuscular blockade, endotracheal intubation, and mechanical ventilation are preferred, with tracheostomy being reserved for those who need prolonged ventilation.

Control of Autonomic Disturbances

With good intensive care, mortality due to respiratory failure has been drastically reduced. Autonomic dysfunction is now the major challenge in patients with severe tetanus; it is common even in sedated and paralyzed patients. Various measures to control autonomic fluctuations include intravenous fluid loading, oral and parenteral beta-blockers, alpha-blockers, centrally acting sympatholytics such as clonidine (Catapres)[1] or dexmedetomidine (Precedex),[1] and epidural or spinal bupivacaine (Marcaine).[1] More recently, infusion of dexmedetomidine has been used by some authors. Many patients may develop sudden asystole, possibly due to sudden parasympathetic discharge, catecholamine-induced myocardial damage, or sudden loss of sympathetic drive. Consequently, the use of long-acting antiadrenergic drugs should be avoided. Increasing the level of sedation itself is also effective, to a significant extent.

The agent most frequently used for autonomic dysfunction is intravenous magnesium sulfate.[1] A randomized controlled trial in Vietnamese patients showed that magnesium sulfate did not decrease mortality, ICU stay, or the need for mechanical ventilation but did reduce the dose of sedatives and neuromuscular blocking drugs required. This study used a loading dose of 40 mg/kg over 30 minutes, followed by intravenous infusion of 2 g/hour in patients >45 kg and 1 to 5 g/hour in patients ≤45 kg. Infusion was titrated to maintain serum magnesium levels between 2 and 4 mmol/L.

Other Measures

Continuous muscle hyperactivity and spasms greatly increase caloric requirements. Most patients require nasogastric tube feeding because of trismus and dysphagia. A catabolic state similar to sepsis may develop in very severe tetanus. Consequently, patients lose up to 15% of their body weight during the illness. Good nursing care is essential to prevent pressure sores, deep vein thrombosis, stress ulcers, and aspiration pneumonia. Urinary catheterization is required in most patients as urinary retention is common and distension of the urinary bladder may provoke spasms and autonomic overactivity. All patients should be started on a primary immunization schedule against tetanus.

Complications

Respiratory failure may occur due to laryngeal obstruction, prolonged spasm of respiratory muscles, aspiration pneumonia, or sedative drugs. Severe spasms may result in tongue-bite, compression fractures of midthoracic vertebrae, rhabdomyolysis, myoglobinuria, and renal failure. Rarely, patients may develop acute respiratory distress syndrome (ARDS) either due to tetanus itself or as a result of secondary bacterial sepsis. Cardiac arrhythmias and sudden asystole are common in patients with autonomic dysfunction. Acute myocardial infarction may occur in elderly patients with underlying coronary artery disease due to sympathetic overactivity. Deep vein thrombosis and pressure sores are preventable complications. The overall mortality ranges from 40% to 60% in countries with inadequate health care facilities. With good intensive care, mortality as low as 10% is reported in some series. Mortality is higher in neonates, the elderly, and patients with a short incubation period and period of onset.

Prevention

Adsorbed tetanus toxoid (Tt), derived from formaldehyde-treated tetanus toxin, is extremely effective in inducing active immunity. It is available as a single-antigen preparation or in combination with diphtheria toxoid as pediatric diphtheria-tetanus toxoid (DT) or adult tetanus-diphtheria (Td), and with both diphtheria toxoid

---

[1]Not FDA approved for this indication.

and acellular pertussis vaccine as DTaP (Infanrix, Tripedia) or Tdap (Adacel, Boostrix) (lower-case alphabets indicate lower doses of antigens). Pediatric vaccines (DT and DTaP) contain identical amounts of tetanus toxoid as adult vaccines, but three to four times as much diphtheria toxoid. The usual schedule for primary immunization in children <7 years consists of four doses of DTaP or DT at age 2, 4, 6, and 15 to 18 months. A booster dose is recommended at 4 to 6 years of age. In individuals aged 7 years or older, three doses of the adult formulation are administered; the second dose is given 4 to 8 weeks after the first, and the third dose after another 4 to 6 months. Further booster doses are needed every 10 years to maintain antibody titers above the protective level of 0.1 IU/mL.

After administration of Tt to individuals with wounds, protective titers of antibody are achieved after at least 2 weeks. Consequently, passive immunization with 250 units of human tetanus immune globulin (HyperTET) or 1500 units of equine antitetanus serum[2] administered intramuscularly is needed to confer protection during these initial few weeks. This is especially required in individuals with tetanus-prone wounds who have not received at least three doses of tetanus toxoid in the past. Previously unimmunized individuals with clean, minor, nontetanus prone wounds do not need any passive immunization, but should receive active immunization. Passive immunization is not necessary in those who have received three or more doses of the toxoid. These individuals should receive a dose of Tt (or Td) if more than 10 years have elapsed since the last booster dose and they have nontetanus prone wounds or if >5 years have elapsed after the booster dose and they have a tetanus-prone wound. In countries where neonatal tetanus is common, primary immunization of women during pregnancy has been advocated as a public health program to prevent neonatal tetanus.

---

[2]Not available in the United States.

References

Apte NM, Karnad DR. The spatula test: A simple bedside test to diagnose tetanus. Am J Trop Med Hyg 1995;53:386–7.

Centers for Disease Control and Prevention. In: Atkinson W, Wolfe S, Hamborsky J, editors. Epidemiology and Prevention of Vaccine-Preventable Diseases. 12th ed. Washington, DC: Department of Health and Human Services, Centers for Disease Control and Prevention; 2011. p. 291–9.

Farrar JJ, Yen LM, Cook T, et al. Tetanus. J Neurol Neurosurg Psychiatry 2000;69:292–301.

Gibson K, Uwineza JB, Kiviri W, Parlow J. Tetanus in developing countries: A case series and review. Can J Anaesth 2009;56:307–15.

Lisboa T, Ho YL, Filho GTH, et al. Guidelines for the management of accidental tetanus in adult patients. Rev Bras Ter Intensiva 2011;23:394–409.

Rodrigo C, Samarakoon L, Fernando SD, Rajapakse S. A meta-analysis of magnesium for tetanus. Anaesthesia 2012;67:1370–4.

Roper MH, Vandelaer JH, Gasse FL. Maternal and neonatal tetanus. Lancet 2007;370:1947–59.

Thwaites CL, Yen LM, Loan HT, et al. Magnesium sulphate for treatment of severe tetanus: A randomized controlled trial. Lancet 2006;368:1436–43.

Trujillo MH, Castillo A, Espana J, et al. Impact of intensive care management on the prognosis of tetanus. Analysis of 641 cases. Chest 1987;92:63–5.

TOXIC SHOCK SYNDROME

Method of
Julius Larioza, MD; and Richard B. Brown, MD

 CURRENT DIAGNOSIS

- Toxic shock syndrome (TSS) and toxic shock-like syndrome (TSLS) are rapid-onset illnesses causing fever, hypotension, rash, vomiting, diarrhea, and the potential for multiorgan failure.
- TSS and TSLS are associated with elaboration of bacterial toxins, which results in a vigorous cytokine cascade, rather than direct bacterial invasion.

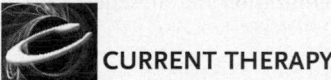

CURRENT THERAPY

Toxic shock syndrome (TSS) is an acute illness caused by the production of local exotoxins capable of diffusing into the mucosa and exerting an exaggerated immunologic response resulting in the development of multisystem disease. These substances are superantigens belonging to a family of pyrogenic toxins produced by bacteria that include *Staphylococcus aureus* and *Streptococcus pyogenes*. The former produces classic TSS, whereas the latter causes a modified form of TSS known as toxic shock-like syndrome (TSLS). A high burden (colonization or infection) with these organisms in the setting of certain parameters allows for the production of superantigens and the subsequent development of the syndrome.

Epidemiology

TSS was first described in 1978 and is now recognized in both menstrual and nonmenstrual forms. The former, as initially described, was typically noted after several days of menstruation and was commonly related to use of high-absorbency tampons, such as the Rely brand, which have since been taken off the market. Currently, nonmenstrual TSS has become almost as common as menstrual TSS, with most cases reported after surgical procedures (e.g., sinonasal manipulation with packing). It has also been linked with use of contraceptive diaphragms, chronic peritoneal dialysis catheters, viral influenza, sinusitis, intravenous drug use, and burn wounds.

TSLS was first described in 1987. Similar in clinical appearance to TSS, it was associated with *S. pyogenes* and was initially labeled as streptococcal toxic shock syndrome. Most commonly, organisms produce streptococcal pyrogenic exotoxin type A. However, other toxins and other streptococci have been occasionally implicated. Although those at the extremes of life and persons with underlying comorbidities appear to be at risk, most cases of TSLS occur in otherwise healthy persons between the ages of 20 and 50 years. It may be a result of the absence of protective immunity.

Clinical Manifestations

TSS is a rapid-onset illness that causes fever, hypotension, rash, vomiting, diarrhea, and, eventually, multiple organ failure. If not treated promptly, it can be lethal. TSLS displays many of the typical TSS symptoms with the addition of severe soft tissue necrosis. Menstrual and nonmenstrual TSS share similar features. The rash is most commonly a diffuse erythema that may resemble severe sunburn. However, a rash mimicking that of scarlet fever may also be seen. Hyperemia of conjunctiva and mucous membranes and strawberry tongue may also be present. Desquamation of the palms and soles, as noted in many bacterial toxin-mediated disorders, often appears during convalescence. When it occurs after surgery, the classic signs of localized infection, such as erythema, tenderness, and purulence, may be absent, making diagnosis more difficult. Multiple organ involvement may include the gastrointestinal, hepatic, renal, musculoskeletal, hematologic, or central nervous systems.

There are several notable differences between TSS and TSLS. The skin is often the portal of entry in TSLS, with soft tissue infections developing in 80% of patients. Cutaneous signs may include localized erythema and edema, a bullous or hemorrhagic cellulitis, necrotizing fasciitis, myositis, or gangrene. Soft tissue involvement of this nature is uncommonly encountered in TSS. Bacteremia is present in more than 50% of patients with TSLS, compared to 15% of those with TSS. Perhaps as a result of this fact, the mortality rate is as much as five times greater with TSLS, reaching 25%.

Pathogenesis

Production of toxic shock syndrome toxin type 1 (TSST-1) has been associated with the majority of menstrual TSS cases (90%); non-menstrual cases are mediated by TSST-1 or by staphylococcal enterotoxins B and C. The dependence of menstrual TSS on TSST-1 may be related to the ability of this protein, but not other pyrogenic toxins, to cross vaginal mucosa. Toxin production is regulated by the *agr* gene, which is expressed under conditions that include high protein levels, relatively neutral pH, and high partial pressures of CO_2 and O_2. All of these conditions are met when menstruation occurs in the setting of high-absorbency tampon use.

Most TSS-susceptible patients lack specific antibodies capable of blocking the responsible superantigens. Nonmenstrual onset of TSS is most likely related to clinically trivial *S. aureus* infections in the vagina and elsewhere (e.g., sinonasal passages). A major subclass of nonmenstrual TSS is viral influenza–associated *S. aureus*, which can infect nasopharyngeal tissues damaged by influenza infection and cause TSS by secreting TSST-1 or staphylococcal enterotoxins.

S. pyogenes causes TSLS by secreting streptococcal pyrogenic exotoxins of three serotypes: A, B, and C. Infection usually occurs after minor injury or surgery, although a portal of entry may never be identified.

Diagnosis

The diagnosis of TSS or TSLS is based on identification of a constellation of clinical and laboratory data proposed by the Centers for Disease Control and Prevention (Table 1).

Differential diagnosis for patients presenting with components of this syndrome includes sepsis caused by other bacteria, staphylococcal scalded skin syndrome, Rocky Mountain spotted fever, meningococcemia, exanthematous viral syndromes, and leptospirosis. Noninfectious causes include severe hyperthermia, drug reactions, and insect-related allergic reactions.

Additional laboratory data that are helpful in diagnosis include complete blood count (CBC) with differential, serum electrolytes, assessment of muscle enzymes, and renal and liver function studies. Urinalysis, chest radiography, and electrocardiography may also help in identification of end-organ complications. Blood, wound, urine, and respiratory cultures should always be performed before initiation of antibiotic therapy. If menstrual TSS is suspected, vaginal cultures for *S. aureus* should be obtained. Testing for TSST-1 should be undertaken if the test is available.

Treatment

Treatment strategies for TSS and TSLS are similar. Initial management should include cleaning of any obvious wounds, removal of foreign bodies (e.g. tampons, nasal packing), and drainage or débridement of affected tissues. Such strategies result in decreased bioburden and toxin production.

Antibiotics active against offending pathogens should be employed parenterally and in the highest dose appropriate for the patient's circumstances. With the emergence of methicillin-resistant *Staphylococcus aureus* (MRSA), vancomycin (Vancocin) and daptomycin (Cubicin) are agents likely to be effective against typical pathogens, even if associated with bacteremia. The former is often monitored by measuring trough levels and maintaining them at 15 to 20 µg/mL. The latter has the additional potential

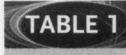

TABLE 1 Diagnostic Criteria for Toxic Shock Syndrome (Staphylococcal) and Toxic Shock-Like Syndrome (Streptococcal)

TSS*	TSLS
Fever	Isolation of group A streptococci
Hypotension	from a sterile site (definite case)
Diffuse macular rash with	or from a nonsterile site
subsequent desquamation	(probable case)
Plus involvement of three of the	Hypotension
following organ systems:	Plus two of the following:
Liver	Renal dysfunction
Blood	Liver dysfunction
Renal	Erythematous macular rash
Mucous membrane	Coagulopathy
Gastrointestinal	Soft tissue necrosis
Muscular	Adult respiratory distress
Central nervous system	syndrome
Negative serologic tests for	
measles, leptospirosis, Rocky	
Mountain spotted fever	
Negative cultures from blood or	
cerebrospinal fluid for	
organisms other than	
Staphylococcus aureus	

Adapted from McCormick JK, Yarwood JM, Schlievert PM. Toxic Shock syndrome and bacterial superantigens: An update. Annu Rev Microbiol 2001; 55:77–104.
*Proposed revision of diagnostic criteria for TSS secondary to *Staphylococcus aureus* includes isolation of *S. aureus* from a mucosal or normally sterile site, production of TSS-associated superantigen by the isolate, lack of antibody to the implicated toxin at the time of acute illness, and development of antibody to the toxin during convalescence.
Abbreviations: TSLS = toxic shock-like syndrome; TSS = toxic shock syndrome.

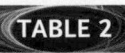

TABLE 2 Recommended Doses of Selected Antibiotics Useful in the Management of Toxic Shock Syndrome and Toxic Shock-Like Syndrome

AGENT	DOSE
Vancomycin* (Vancocin)	15 mg/kg q12h
Daptomycin* (Cubicin)	6 mg/kg q24h
Clindamycin (Cleocin)	900 mg q8h

*Adjust for renal dysfunction.

advantage of killing organisms without major cell lysis, which may spare cytokine release and elaboration of sepsis cascades. Clindamycin (Cleocin) should be employed as a second agent because of its activity against likely pathogens and because it may terminate toxin production at a cellular level. Table 2 depicts usual doses. Because of their potential for affecting renal function, agents such as vancomycin and daptomycin need to be assessed carefully for optimal dosing during the period of illness. Duration of therapy is typically 7 days, although bacteremic patients may be treated for more extended periods.

As appropriate, local wound management may include use of topical agents. in vitro studies of silver sulfadiazine (Silvadene)[1] cream suggest that sublethal concentrations may actually increase toxin production by *S. aureus*. For that reason, mupirocin (Bactroban) or povidine iodine (Betadine) may be a better choice. Management and monitoring of end organs and treatment of shock are mandatory, and severely ill patients are best managed in the critical care unit. Corticosteroids and specialized forms of intravenous gamma globulin[1] have been employed but are not considered standard care.

[1]Not FDA approved for this indication.

Prevention

Awareness of these syndromes may help with prevention. Patients who have developed menstrual TSS should be encouraged to avoid tampon use for at least three cycles, and to then employ the lowest-absorbency tampon feasible. Careful cleansing of skin wounds, drainage of abscesses, and judicious use of topical antimicrobials for injuries may help to prevent colonization and subsequent toxin production.

References

Davies HD, McGeer A, Schwartz B, et al. Invasive group A streptococcal infections in Ontario, Canada. Ontario Group A Streptococcal Study Group [see comment and author reply]. N Engl J Med 1996;335:547–54.
Edwards-Jones V, Foster HA. The effect of topical antimicrobial agents on the production of toxic shock syndrome toxin-1. J Med Microbiol 1994;41:408–13.
Jamart S, Denis O, Deplano A, et al. Methicillin-resistant *Staphylococcus aureus* toxic shock syndrome. Emerg Infect Dis 2005;11(4):636–7.
Manders SM. Toxin-mediated streptococcal and staphylococcal disease. J Am Acad Dermatol 1998;39:383–98.
McCormick J, Yarwood JM, Schlievert PM, et al. Toxic shock syndrome and bacterial superantigens: An update. Ann Rev Microbiol 2001;55:77–104.
Parsonnet J, Hansmann MA, Delaney ML, et al. Prevalence of toxic shock syndrome toxin 1-producing *Staphylococcus aureus* and the presence of antibodies to this superantigen in menstruating women. J Clin Microbiol 2005;43 (9):4628–34.
Schlievert PM. Staphylococcal toxic shock syndrome: Still a problem. Med J Aust 2005;182(12):651–2.
Stevens DL. The toxic shock syndromes. Infect Dis Clin North Am 1996;10 (4):727–46.
Tierno Jr PM. Reemergence of staphylococcal toxic shock syndrome in the United States since 2000. J Clin Microbiol 2005;43(4):2032author reply 2032–3.
Wood TF, Potter MA, Jonasson O. Streptococcal toxic shock-like syndrome: The importance of surgical intervention. Ann Surg 1993;217:109–14.

TOXOPLASMOSIS

Method of
Carlo Contini, MD

CURRENT DIAGNOSIS

- The diagnosis of *Toxoplasma gondii* infection relies on serologic detection of specific IgM and IgG antibodies.
- Specific IgM antibodies with low IgG (IgG-avidity testing) are consistent with recent infection in immunocompetent persons. Positive IgG antibodies in the absence of IgM in healthy persons indicate past infection and resistance to reinfection.
- Amniocentesis and polymerase chain reaction (PCR)-based analysis (past 18 weeks of gestation) are useful to establish a certain or presumed seroconversion in pregnancy and to determine whether the infection was transmitted to the offspring.
- IgM and/or IgA at birth indicate probable connatal infection.
- Serologic testing is not useful for the diagnosis of toxoplasmic encephalitis in AIDS patients, who should instead have CT or MRI imaging, cerebrospinal fluid (CSF)-PCR testing, or demonstration of tachyzoites by histology.

CURRENT THERAPY

- Pyrimethamine (Daraprim) plus sulfadiazine[1] plus folinic acid (Leucovorin)[1] is the standard and preferred regimen against toxoplasmosis. It is recommended for acute *T. gondii* infection in immunocompetent adults with acute illness; pregnant women who acquire the infection after 18 weeks of gestation or in whom fetal infection is documented (positive PCR-AF); and immunosuppressed patients, including AIDS patients. Patients who do not tolerate the standard regimen should be given alternative drugs such as clarithromycin (Biaxin),[1] azithromycin (Zithromax),[1] atovaquone (Mepron),[1] and dapsone.[1]

- Oral spiramycin (Rovamycine)[2] is the drug most often used in the prenatal therapy of congenital toxoplasmosis (before 18 weeks of gestation) because of its relative lack of toxicity compared to the teratogenic effects of pyrimethamine. Spiramycin is more efficacious when administered early after maternal seroconversion.
- Trimethoprim-sulfamethoxazole (TMP-SMX; Bactrim)[1] should be given as a prophylaxis to HIV-positive patients who have $CD4^+$ cell counts that are less than $100/mm^3$ and IgG T. gondii antibodies and who are not already receiving a PCP prevention regimen as well as to patients with active toxoplasmosis, transplant patients, and workers following accidental laboratory exposure.

[1]Not FDA approved for this indication.
[2]Not available in the United States.

Toxoplasma gondii is a ubiquitous protozoan parasite that is extremely widespread and of great medical importance, infecting all mammalian cells and responsible for human and veterinary diseases. It was initially described in Tunis by Nicolle and Manceaux (1908) in the tissues of the gundi (*Ctenodoactylus gundi*) and later in Brazil by the microbiologist Alfonso Splendore (1908) in the rabbit. Its identification was rapidly followed by the recognition that it was a human pathogen. In this regard, the Italian bacteriologist Castellani (1914) was probably the first to describe a *T. gondii*-like parasite in smears of blood and spleen from a 14-year-old Singhalese boy who died from a disease characterized by severe anemia, fever, and splenomegaly. However, it was not until the 1960s and 1970s that the parasite was identified as a coccidian and the cat recognized as the definite host.

Toxoplasma belongs to the phylum *Apicomplexa*, which contains many other protozoan pathogens of human and veterinary importance, such as *Plasmodium* spp. (malaria), *Cryptosporidium* spp. (cryptosporidiosis), and *Eimeria* spp. (poultry coccidiosis).

Disease can occur through acute infection after recent contact with *T. gondii* cysts or oocysts or through endogenous reactivation. Primary infection is usually subclinical, but in some patients cervical or occipital lymphadenopathy or ocular disease is present. Infection acquired during pregnancy can cause severe damage to the fetus if *Toxoplasma* crosses the placental barrier, and it causes abortion or congenital birth defects if the mother becomes infected for the first time shortly before or during pregnancy.

In AIDS patients and others who are immunocompromised persons, reactivation of latent disease can cause life threatening encephalitis. Ocular infection by *Toxoplasma* is a major cause of retinochoroiditis in several geographic areas in both immunocompetent and immunocompromised persons.

Epidemiology and Risk Factors

Toxoplasmosis is a cosmopolitan zoonotic disease that has important implications for public health because it affects one-third of the world's population. It is also a significant veterinary pathogen that can infect many species of warm-blooded animals.

The incidence of positive serology for *Toxoplasma* varies greatly around the world and is influenced by different cultures. In Colombia, approximately half of the women of child bearing age have T. gondii antibodies, and the clinical disease in congenitally infected children is more severe than in Europe. In humans, seroprevalence of *T. gondii* infection rises with age; does not vary greatly between sexes; and is lower in cold regions, hot and arid areas, and at high elevations. Prevalence rates are thought to depend on food production and harvesting practices, water treatment, environment, climate, and exposure to soil or sand. In the United States, the seroprevalence of *T. gondii* appears to be declining. Seroprevalence in Europe is high, up to 54% in southern European countries; it decreases with increasing latitude to 5% and 10% in northern Sweden and Norway, respectively. In Brazil, there is a higher prevalence of *T. gondii* infection among male patients (79.0%) than among female patients (63.4%), according

to data obtained from a blood bank. In general, *Toxoplasma* infections are especially prevalent in Europe, South America, and Africa.

The sexual cycle of *T. gondii* occurs in felines. The estimated seroprevalence for *T. gondii* in domestic cats (*Felis catus*), worldwide, is 30% to 40%. Most feline infections occur postnatally through ingestion of infected tissue cysts or rarely oocysts, although congenital infections occur. Tens of millions of unsporulated oocysts may be released in the feces of a single cat in a day, depending on the stage of *T. gondii* ingested. These sporulate in 1 to 21 days and are highly infectious to the parasite's intermediate hosts (asexual cycle), which include almost any warm-blooded animal, such as birds, humans, and sea otters.

Sporulated oocysts are very resistant to environmental conditions and to disinfectants; however, they are killed within 1 to 2 minutes by heating to 55°C to 60°C, and the risk of infection is reduced by deep-freezing meat (−12°C or lower) before cooking.

Feline infections are typically subclinical. Common symptoms of *T. gondii* infection in cats can include fever, ocular inflammation, anorexia, lethargy, abdominal discomfort, and neurologic abnormalities. Occasionally, pneumonia, liver damage, and loss of vision develop. Why only some cats show symptoms is not known.

Identification of locally prevalent risk factors is critical for health education, and it is generally important for policy. The most important recognized factors influencing the risk of *T. gondii* infection are having a cat or a dog, doing household work, having a lower education level, having poor hygiene habits, eating raw vegetables, and working in contact with soil.

Most people are infected inadvertently, and thus the specific route of transmission usually cannot be established. The contact with this obligate intracellular protozoan can occur through the ingestion of oocysts containing sporozoites or cysts containing bradyzoites in contaminated food or water. The major risk factors for *T. gondii* exposure are directly related to exposure to cats and more specifically to cat feces, which represent the source of ingestion of sporozoites from the environment. Because cats are the primary host for *T. gondii*, cats in the house or stray cats in and around the house or property are considered a primary risk factor for acquiring this parasite during pregnancy. Moreover, any job or activity that puts a pregnant woman in direct contact with soil, sand, or materials such as fruit, vegetables, or drinking water that could have been contaminated by cat feces puts her at risk for being infected. In this setting, rain and surface water can transport infectious oocysts into drinking water supplies and irrigation waters. Coprophagous insects that can contaminate food and fertilizer also contribute to the spread of oocysts. Climate plays an indirect role in allowing better (in the case of moist and hot climate) or worse (in the case of dry and cold climate) survival of oocysts in the environment.

Consumption of undercooked meat of secondary hosts such as pig and sheep is also a major route of transmission of the disease to humans. The ingestion of undercooked or raw meat during pregnancy is also an important risk factor because the tissue can contain *T. gondii* cysts that, unless destroyed by cooking or by food-preparation practices, could infect a pregnant woman. Heating at 60°C to 100°C for 10 minutes, freezing at either −10°C for 3 days or −20°C for 2 days, or irradiation at doses of 75 to 100 krad is sufficient to kill tissue cysts. Tissue cysts are also killed by gamma irradiation at a dose of 1.0 kGy, but irradiation of meat has not been approved in the European Union (EU). Neither cooking in a microwave oven nor chilling at 5°C for 5 days is sufficient to kill tissue cysts.

Pork was previously identified as a main risk factor in some EU countries such as Norway and Italy, but its importance as a route for infection is now reduced, possibly because pregnant women are most aware of this specific risk. In this regard, it was found that the risk of infection rises in women who taste meat when preparing meals or who eat raw or undercooked beef, lamb, or other meats, but not pork. Eating raw horsemeat imported from non-EU countries can expose consumers to high inocula of highly virulent atypical *T. gondii* strains, which can cause a life-threatening primary infection or severe congenital toxoplasmosis with atypical outcome. Transmission during breast-feeding or direct human-to-human transmission other than from mother to fetus (discussed later in the chapter) has not been recorded. Drinking unpasteurized milk and consuming milk products also correlates with increased risk of infections. Other routes are transplacental infection of the fetus, transfusion of white blood cells, and organ transplantation from a seropositive donor to a seronegative recipient.

It is not uncommon for health care professionals, laboratory workers, pet lovers (especially cat owners), butchers, cooks (those handling raw meat), veterinarians, and farmers to acquire acute toxoplasmosis.

Dogs can also have a role in the transmission of toxoplasmosis as a mechanical vector by rolling in foul-smelling substances and by ingesting fecal material. Unlike in cats, T. gondii does not replicate in the dog's gut and no cysts are shed. In areas where dogs and cats are plentiful, immunocompromised persons and pregnant women should be warned of the possibility of acquiring T. gondii from dogs as well as from soil contaminated by cats. People should be encouraged to wash their hands after contact with soil, dogs, or cats as well as before eating.

T. gondii infection has important veterinary implications because it causes disease, miscarriage, and congenital malformations in the definitive and intermediate host. Cats, sheep, pigs, and goats are the domestic animal species most seriously affected by the protozoan. In sheep, T. gondii is an important agent of abortion and neonatal mortality in lambs.

Pathophysiology

Disease can occur through acute infection after recent contact with T. gondii cysts or oocysts or through endogenous reactivation. Following ingestion, the sporozoites or bradyzoites invade the intestinal epithelium and differentiate to tachyzoites, which disseminate and replicate within the new host. Transport of the parasite via the bloodstream can occur intracellularly within dendritic cells or monocytes or as a free tachyzoite. Certain Toxoplasma surface antigens aid in the interaction between the tachyzoite and the host cell. One of this is the Perforin-like Protein 1 (PLP-1) forming pores in the host-cell membrane after binding as well as playing a role in egress. The success of Toxoplasma as a widespread pathogen is due to the effortlessness with which it can be transmitted among the intermediate hosts. Once inside a host, the parasite develops powerful tools to modulate its host cell and to develop into a chronic infection, undergoing bradyzoite development that can evade the host's immune system as well as, in contrast with acute toxoplasmosis, all known antitoxoplasmic drugs.

Host protection from T. gondii results from a complex cell-mediated immune response involving inflammatory cells, lymphocytes and macrophages, and cytokines. Inoculum size, parasite virulence (strain), genetic background, time of infection (congenital versus postnatal contamination), and sex also contribute to affect the course of infection in human beings and animal models of toxoplasmosis. In particular, the T. gondii genotype affects its replication rate, migration, and tendency to differentiate to bradyzoites, virulence, and epidemiologic pattern of occurrence. Type II genotypes (most strains isolated from AIDS patients and newborns with congenital disease) and type III genotypes (mostly isolated from animals) are generally less virulent and more cystogenic compared to type I genotypes (also found in congenital disease). Ocular toxoplasmosis in humans is associated with type I but not type II or III genotypes.

Genetic background also plays a significant role in increased susceptibility to T. gondii in humans; HLA-DQ3 appears to be a genetic marker associated with susceptibility to developing toxoplasmic encephalitis in AIDS patients. The mechanisms by which T. gondii invades host cells and forms an intracellular niche have been extensively reviewed, and several aspects of this process are directly relevant to immunity and pathogenesis. During invasion, three successive waves of proteins are secreted from parasite organelles, (the micronemes, dense granules, and rhoptries) into the host cell. Rhoptry proteins are the major virulence factors of Toxoplasma gondii and are located in different parts of the host cells. Blocking the cell intrinsic defense mechanisms of the host, let T. gondii invade, parasitize and proliferate in the host successfully. These proteins can alter host cell function and inhibit the immune response directed toward the parasite.

During infection in the intermediate host, T. gondii undergoes stage conversion between the rapidly dividing tachyzoite that is responsible for acute toxoplasmosis and the slowly replicating, encysted bradyzoite stage. This process of tachyzoite-bradyzoite interconversion is central to the pathogenesis and longevity of infection. In normal conditions, the tachyzoite stage is thwarted by the prompt and efficient interferon (IFN)-γ-dependent cell-mediated immune response, which eventually kills off the majority of the disseminating tachyzoites before eventually entering the persistent form, the bradyzoite. Bradyzoites are encysted within various tissues, most notably the brain but also muscle, eye, and lung, and are infectious to another intermediate host or the cat if eaten. Cell-mediated immune mechanisms thus play a major role in the control of T. gondii infection because the parasite is exclusively localized intracellularly.

Following infection, T. gondii evokes a powerful and persistent T-helper-1 (Th1) response (dendritic cell activated) together with neutrophils, inflammatory monocytes, and macrophages. The response is characterized by production of proinflammatory cytokines, including interleukin (IL)-12, INF-α and tumor necrosis factor (TNF)-α, which, together with other immunologic mechanisms, protect the host against rapid replication of tachyzoites and subsequent pathologic changes. The outcome of toxoplasmic infection depends on a balance between proinflammatory (IL-12, TNF-α) and downregulatory (IL-10, IL-27) cytokines that suppress parasite proliferation and control the inflammatory response, respectively.

INF-γ, produced by both CD4 and CD8 cells in response to Toxoplasma is the major cytokine involved with acute and chronic resistance to T. gondii infection in immunocompetent hosts because it controls tachyzoite growth and subsequent pathologic changes. Macrophages activated by INF-γ inhibit parasite replication through a number of potent microbicidal systems, including oxidative and nonoxidative mechanisms as well as the induction of indoleamine 2-3-dioxygenase that degrades tryptophan, which is required for T. gondii replication.

The toll-like receptor (TLR) is another critical pathway in initiating defense against this opportunistic protozoan, which can also be a mediator of pathology during immune dysfunction. In fact, the innate production of IL-12 requires that the parasite first be sensed by the host; innate TLRs, particularly 2, 4, 9, and 11, have an important role in this process. TLR4 plays important roles in the recognition and stimulation of immune responses against T. gondii. To combat the host immune system, the parasite targets TLR4 and its intracellular signaling. TLR4 also participates in the pathogenesis of Toxoplasmosis. A therapeutic strategy using the TLR4 pathway to treat T. gondii would be possible, but treatment would need to be followed carefully to avoid the detrimental consequences associated with this pathway.

Clinical Presentation in the Immunocompetent

Acute acquired toxoplasmosis has traditionally been considered an oligosymptomatic and self-limited infection in previously healthy patients. The typical clinical presentation of acute T. gondii infection is a short flu-like or mononucleosis-like illness that includes prolonged fever, headache, persistent enlarged but firm lymph nodes (rarely painful, but initially tender) unattached to the overlying skin, and, occasionally, myalgia and gastrointestinal symptoms that rarely need treatment. Special consideration must be given to other infectious or noninfectious diseases that cause similar symptoms and should always be included in the differential diagnosis: mononucleosis, cat scratch disease, tuberculosis, primary HIV infection, sarcoidosis, metastatic cancer, and lymphoma. In these cases, serologic testing is the initial and primary method of diagnosis.

Lymph node biopsy should be reserved for when *Toxoplasma* serology is uncertain and all other infectious serologic investigations are negative. A form of the disease characterized by chronic lymphadenopathy has been described, and lymph node enlargement can fluctuate for months. Hepatomegaly and hepatitis with a moderate increase in liver enzyme levels (a 5- to 10-fold elevation) are common. The incidence of hepatitis in persons with *Toxoplasma* infection varies between 11% and 89%. Lymphocytosis and atypical lymphocytes are other laboratory hallmarks of toxoplasmosis. The spleen appears to be involved early in toxoplasmosis, but palpable splenomegaly is uncommon.

Clinical pulmonary involvement is rarely described in immunocompetent hosts, in whom it usually manifests as atypical pneumonia. Myocarditis, polymyositis, or encephalitis can be observed very infrequently in otherwise healthy persons. Acute *Toxoplasma* infection during pregnancy is asymptomatic in most women.

Latent toxoplasmosis is characterized by the lifelong presence of cysts of the parasite in different host tissues, including the nervous system, and by the presence of anamnestic *Toxoplasma* immunoglobulin (Ig)G antibodies in the serum. Long considered asymptomatic, latent toxoplasmosis might increase the risk of schizophrenia and Parkinson's disease; influence human personality and behavior; impair psychomotor performance; and increase the risk of suicide, traffic accidents, and the probability of the birth of male offspring. Toxoplasmosis should also be regarded as an epilepsy risk factor. Epileptogenic mechanisms are probably multifactorial (direct lodgment of parasite, direct modulation of neuronal functions, abnormalities in GABA, role of calcium, etc). etc. Recently, it was suggested that chronic latent neuroinflammation caused by the parasite may be responsible for the development of several neurodegenerative diseases manifesting with the loss of smell. Olfactory dysfunction reported in Alzheimer's disease, multiple sclerosis, and schizophrenia was frequently associated with the significantly increased serum anti-T gondii immunoglobulin G antibody levels. Higher rates of *T. gondii* seropositivity have been reported for several psychiatric conditions in multiple parts of the world. A series of studies comparing the prevalence rates of the parasite with the national suicide rates in 20 European countries found that suicide rates were higher in countries with greater *T. gondii* prevalence, regardless of national wealth or gross domestic product. Many of the observed behavioral effects of toxoplasmosis might be a result of the impairment of the immune system and of increased level of dopamine in the brain tissue in response to IL-2 produced by immune cells in the sites of local inflammation in the infected brain. However, RhD phenotype also plays an important role in the strength and direction of association between latent toxoplasmosis and personality and intelligence. Another recent finding is that people seropositive for both *Helicobacter pylori* and latent toxoplasmosis – both of which appear to be common in the general population – appear to be more susceptible to cognitive deficits than are people seropositive for either *Helicobacter pylori* and or latent toxoplasmosis alone, suggesting a synergistic effect between these two infectious diseases on cognition in young to middle-aged adults.

Finally, a very important aspect that has emerged in recent years concerns the possible occurrence of toxoplasmosis in patients receiving biotherapies, particularly anti-TNF-α agents for the treatment of rheumatologic diseases and other conditions. In this setting, rituximab (Rituxan) induces B-cell depletion and influences T-cell immunity, which could consequently predispose patients to serious infectious complications, including cerebral toxoplasmosis. *Toxoplasma* serology should be performed in patients before treatment with TNF-α antagonists is initiated, and patients should be advised to avoid situations that increase risk of exposure to *Toxoplasma*.

Clinical Presentation in Immunocompromised Patients

The presence of latent bradyzoite cysts, along with the ability of bradyzoites to reconvert into the active and rapidly growing tachyzoites that can result in often-fatal injury, explains the high incidence of acute toxoplasmosis often observed in immunocompromised persons. In immunocompromised hosts and in AIDS patients, the central nervous system (CNS) is the site most typically affected by infection, and toxoplasmic encephalitis is the most common manifestation. This is also the third most common condition associated with AIDS in Brazil, still accounting for high mortality and morbidity despite free access to Antiretroviral therapy (ART).

However, as in transplant patients or those with malignant hemolymphopathies or solid tumors, other organs such as the lungs or eyes may be involved. Most of these cases result from reactivation of latent infection, although reinfection with a different *T. gondii* strain in the transplanted organs can also occur.

Although the mortality of pulmonary toxoplasmosis was high before the advent of ART, AIDS patients and recipients of bone marrow transplants are also at risk for developing pulmonary toxoplasmosis, especially patients with very low CD4 cell counts. The clinical manifestations are nonspecific and are similar to those of *Pneumocystis jirovecii*.

The predictive value of elevated blood levels of lactate dehydrogenase (LDH) is of uncertain value. Patients with toxoplasmic encephalitis typically present with headache, confusion, altered mental status, and motor weakness. Focal neurologic deficits or seizures, weakness, sensory abnormalities, cerebellar signs, and neuropsychiatric manifestations are also common. Fever is usually, but not reliably, present. Accompanying nausea or vomiting usually indicates elevated intracranial pressure. Computed tomography (CT) scan or magnetic resonance imaging (MRI) of the brain typically shows multiple contrast-enhancing lesions, often with associated edema. These should be distinguished from other infectious or noninfectious CNS diseases in the course of AIDS.

In immunocompromised patients, the infection can disseminate rapidly and manifests with nonspecific symptoms such as fever and malaise. It can affect a number of organs, including the brain, cerebellum (an uncommon presentation) eye, liver, and lungs as well as skeletal muscle, bone marrow, bladder, and spinal cord. Cardiac toxoplasmosis can occur during the course of multivisceral dissemination. However, in patients with AIDS, it is usually asymptomatic and found only at autopsy, typically in the setting of widely disseminated infection. Acquired toxoplasmosis with cutaneous involvement can also occur in the pediatric population, particularly in immunocompromised patients after stem cell transplantation. Early diagnosis and treatment of this life-threatening opportunistic infection may improve patient outcomes.

Toxoplasmosis of the Eye

Toxoplasmosis can affect the retina and the underlying choroid, causing retinochoroiditis, the most common manifestation of ocular toxoplasmosis. Ocular toxoplasmosis is the major cause of visual impairment in high *T. gondii* endemic regions of the United States and Europe, where it accounts for 30% to 50% of the posterior uveitis. Ocular involvement can be a result of acquired infection or, more commonly, a recurrence of the congenital form of the disease.

Ocular toxoplasmosis is a progressive and recurrent disease with vision-threatening complications, including retinal detachment, chorioretinal anastomosis, and choroidal neovascularization, which can occur any time in the clinical course of the disease, even after treatment. Periodic follow-up is therefore necessary to reduce the occurrence of late complications. Many lesions are self-limiting and heal, forming characteristic unilateral or bilateral pigmented scars in the retina, where *Toxoplasma* cysts are found. Ocular lesions can recur in adolescence and adulthood, even after treatment in infancy. The severity of the disease is mainly a function of the parasite genotype and the host's immune status.

In clinical practice, diagnosis in immunocompetent patients is based on the findings of typical ocular manifestations, including eye pain and decreased visual acuity, and may be confirmed by biological tools applied to ocular fluids. The value of serology is limited. However, there are many asymptomatic seropositive persons in areas where the parasite is endemic, and they have atypical lesions that are similar to other necrotizing forms of retinitis, specifically acute retinal necrosis and cytomegalovirus retinitis.

Atypical lesions also occur and are seen especially in elderly persons and in those with underlying immunodeficiency. In these cases, the toxoplasmic origin can be demonstrated only by laboratory testing or by a positive response to treatment.

Symptoms and signs in immunocompromised patients do not distinguish ocular toxoplasmosis from other ocular infections in HIV, including tuberculosis, *P. jirovecii* pneumonia, and cytomegalovirus (CMV) retinitis. Toxoplasmic chorioretinitis appears as raised yellow-white, cottony lesions in a nonvascular distribution, unlike the perivascular exudates of CMV retinitis. Vitreal inflammation is usually present, in contrast to ocular toxoplasmosis in immunocompetent patients. Up to 63% of AIDS patients with *Toxoplasma* chorioretinitis have concurrent CNS lesions.

Maternal Infection and Congenital Toxoplasmosis

Infection with *T. gondii* is particularly dangerous for pregnant women because it can lead to the transplacental passage of the parasite from the circulation of the primarily infected mother. During pregnancy, the prevalence of toxoplasmosis increases throughout the second and third quarter of gestation, simultaneously progesterone and 17!-estradiol also increase. Thus, it has been suggested that these hormones can aggravate or reduce parasite reproduction. Infection of the placenta is a prerequisite for congenital transmission. More than 60% of infected pregnant women do not experience any symptoms or signs, and the clinical features, when present, are the same as in other immunocompetent persons.

Currently, congenital toxoplasmosis is the second most common intrauterine infection and remains a public health problem throughout the world. The global annual incidence of congenital toxoplasmosis has been estimated to be 190,100 cases (95% credible interval, CI: 179,300–206,300). This is equivalent to a burden of 1.20 million DALYs (95% CI: 0.76–1.90). High burdens are seen in South America and in some Middle Eastern and low-income countries. The risk of transmission of *T. gondii* to the fetus ranges from 0.6 to 1.7 per 1,000 pregnant women. In France, about 300 cases are reported each year to the National Reference Center. The frequency of transmission and severity of disease are inversely related.

The development of possible consequences depends on many factors, including the degree of parasitemia in the mother, the maturity of the placenta, the age of the fetus, and immunologic maturity. Early maternal infection (first trimester) can cause severe congenital toxoplasmosis and can result in death of the fetus in utero and spontaneous abortion. By contrast, late maternal infection (acquired during the third trimester) usually results in a normal-appearing newborn who may be at high risk for seizures, mental retardation, and chorioretinitis. Infection during the second trimester also can result in symptomatic infection, but the clinical manifestations vary from mild to severe and depend on individual factors. Nevertheless, most neonates (70%–90%) with congenital toxoplasmosis are asymptomatic or have subclinical infection; overall, incidence is as high as 85%. Infection initially goes unnoticed, but if it is not treated, these children can later develop chorioretinitis or experience a delay in growth in the second or third decade of life.

Clinical manifestations of congenital toxoplasmosis observed in infancy or later in life are numerous and include jaundice, rash, hepatosplenomegaly, anemia, thrombocytopenia, hydrocephalus, microcephalus, intracranial calcifications, convulsions, psychomotor and mental retardation, chorioretinitis, microphthalmia, blindness, and strabismus. All these signs and symptoms are included in the general work-up of suspected congenital TORCH infections: *toxoplasmosis, other* (syphilis, varicella-zoster, parvovirus B19, HIV infection, listeriosis, hepatitis B), *rubella, cytomegalovirus*, and *herpes*. The classic triad of bilateral chorioretinitis, hydrocephalus, and cerebral calcifications is exceptional.

A significant correlation has been found between toxoplasmosis cases and the number of pregnancies in a woman. In multiparous women, the risk of infections was twice as high as in nulliparas.

The clinical course of the disease in a child with congenital toxoplasmosis is not influenced by whether the mother showed any clinical symptoms of the disease or was entirely asymptomatic. Infants born to women infected simultaneously with HIV and *T. gondii* should be evaluated for congenital toxoplasmosis, considering the increased risk of reactivation of parasitemia and disease in these mothers. Severely immunocompromised mothers chronically infected with *T. gondii* can transmit the disease to the fetus as a result of reactivation. However, the rate of vertical transmission in this setting seems to be moderately low.

Diagnosis

In immunocompetent persons, confirmation of acute infection can exclude other potentially more serious etiologies. In other clinical settings where *Toxoplasma* infection can result in severe sequelae, the interpretation of laboratory findings poses significant challenges. The parasite can in fact be present in acute, chronic, latent, or reactivated form. Thus, discrimination of these forms is often crucial in understanding clinical relevance. A schematic diagnostic pathway that can be followed for the diagnosis of toxoplasmosis is shown in Figure 1. Methodical serologic screening for *T. gondii* IgG and IgM antibodies in adult symptomatic immunocompetent persons, in pregnant women as early in gestation as possible (preferably in first trimester), and in seronegative women each month or trimester thereafter is optimal. Such screening allows detection of seroconversion and early initiation of treatment.

The laboratory tests used most commonly for initial investigation are serologic, targeting detection of IgG, IgM, and IgA specific for *T. gondii* by available commercial kit. In addition to confirming infection, these tests can aid in determining prognosis, influence management, and assist in monitoring response to treatment. Typically, acute-phase IgM appears first about 1 to 2 weeks after infection, closely followed by IgA and IgE. Generally, IgM peaks at about 2 months. The time at which immunoglobulins can no longer be detected is highly variable depending on the test employed, usually about 6 to 9 months. In a small minority of cases IgM can persist at high levels for up to 18 months or for years, leading to an inaccurate assessment of when the exposure occurred. This circumstance can be problematic because congenital toxoplasmosis can occur if the mother was infected during her pregnancy, and it is thus important to ascertain in which trimester of pregnancy the infection occurred. IgA antibodies are considered to be a marker of acute toxoplasmosis as their kinetics are faster than those of IgM antibodies; however, they can also persist for more than a year, and their detection, together with IgM detection, strongly suggests neonatal infection. IgE serology is highly specific in pregnant women but has low sensitivity, remaining detectable for less than 4 months after infection; moreover, it is not useful in samples from newborns.

To date, an IgM test is still used by most laboratories to determine if a patient has been infected recently or in the distant past, but confirmatory testing (double sandwich or capture IgM-ELISA [enzyme-linked immunosorbent assay] kits and the immunosorbent agglutination assay [IgM-ISAGA]) should always be performed owing to the difficulties in interpreting a positive IgM test result for the relatively high incidence of false-positive results (due to the rheumatoid factor and antinuclear antibodies in some IgM-IFA tests). Thus, a positive IgM test result in a single serum sample can be interpreted as a true-positive result in the setting of a recently acquired infection, a true-positive result in the setting of an infection acquired in the distant past, or a false-positive result. IgM levels decline more rapidly than IgG antibodies, which typically reach maximal levels at about 4 months, then decline to a lower level over the next 12 to 24 months but persist for decades. Elevated IgG levels confirm if a patient has been exposed to the parasite, but they do not differentiate between a recent or past exposure, because IgG persists at a low level throughout the life of the patient. The absence of IgG antibodies in early pregnancy indicates that women are at risk for acquiring toxoplasmosis.

The most commonly used tests for the measurement of IgG antibody are the Sabin-Feldman dye test (still considered the gold standard diagnostic test; it measures primarily IgG antibodies to *T. gondii*, but it requires viable *Toxoplasma* organisms), the ELISA, the IFA, and the modified direct agglutination test.

All Persons with Suspected Toxoplasmosis, Including Pregnant Women: First Visit

First-level T. gondii Diagnostic Test

Detection of serum anti–T. gondii IgM and IgG in first trimester
- If IgM and IgG negative: absence of specific immunity; mother prophylaxis, monthly serologic control[*]
- If only IgG is detected: infection likely took place 6–12 months before or before pregnancy; immunity
- If only IgM is detected: initial phase seroconversion of false IgM positivity[†]
- If IgM and IgG are detected: possible recent infection; consider a more thorough workup (reference laboratory) to try to determine the time of infection in the mother[‡]

↓

Second-level Diagnostic Test

IgG avidity assay
- If negative (high avidity): infection occurred 3–5 months before testing
- If positive (low avidity): probable recent T. gondii infection; repeat serology 3 weeks after the first sample; start spiramycin, ecographic surveillance
Try to establish a certain or presumed seroconversion in pregnancy and to determine whether the infection was transmitted to the product of conception.

↓

Third-level Diagnostic Tests (further maternal and fetal assessment)

In the mother

Detection of T. gondii-specific DNA by PCR-AF at 18 weeks of gestation[§]
- If positive: the fetus has been infected; consider starting treatment and monthly fetal ultrasound examination to detect abnormalities; start pyrimethamine-sulfadiazine[||]
- If negative: fetus unaffected; T. gondii has not crossed the placental barrier; continue spiramycin[¶]
- Parasite isolation on tissue culture: mouse inoculation[**]

In the newborn

Detection of serum anti-T. gondii IgM and IgA[††]
- If IgM and/or IgA are present at birth: probable connatal infection
- If IgM and/or IgA are not present at birth: monthly control

Western blot assay of serum IgG and IgM from mother-baby pairs[‡‡]
- If positive: confirmation of early postnatal diagnosis; therapy and serological control[§§]
- If negative: monthly control for the first 3 months

Figure 1. A schematic diagnostic pathway for the diagnosis of toxoplasmosis. [*]No treatment is required. [†]Repeat the tests weekly to detect the appearance of IgG antibodies to confirm the seroconversion. [‡]Given that IgM may persist for several months, try to date the beginning of infection through education and counselling to guide the prenatal diagnosis of the patient. [§]PCR sensitivity is significantly higher for infections occurred between the 17th and 21st week of gestation. [||]If ecographic abnormalities, consider abortion. [¶]A negative PCR cannot completely rule out congenital infection; consider follow-up through ultrasounds and continue prophylaxis with spiramycin (Rovamycine)[2] until delivery and neonatal testing. [**]For confirmation of PCR results; however, they are complex, expensive, and relatively insensitive. [††]Limitations because IgA antibodies may persist for several months and are not always produced. [‡‡]This test is not widely used mainly because of its technical complexity and high price. [§§]Administer pyrimethamine (Daraprim)-sulfadiazine[1] therapy and serologic controls after cessation of therapy and every 6 months for the first 2 years.

In recent years, significant progress has been made toward improving the ability to diagnose recently acquired T. gondii infection. In this setting, the introduction of IgG avidity testing based on the increase in functional affinity (avidity) between T. gondii-specific IgG and the antigen over time, as the host immune response (and specific B-cell selection) evolves, represents an irreplaceable test. The utility of the avidity test is based on the observation that Toxoplasma IgG antibodies from patients with a recently acquired T. gondii infection bind antigens weakly (low avidity), whereas IgG antibodies from chronically infected patients have stronger binding capacity (high avidity).

Depending on the method used, the avidity tests currently available are helpful primarily to rule out that a patient's infection occurred within the prior 4 to 5 months and that the fetus is not at risk for congenital toxoplasmosis. The avidity test is most important when only a single serum sample is available at the time when critical decisions must be made. A major problem with this test is that the maturation of the IgG response after a primary Toxoplasma infection varies considerably among patients; in fact, low-avidity results can persist for as long as 1 year, and substantial numbers of patients have borderline or equivocal results. These equivocal cases require that in addition to a more careful interpretation of all laboratory test results in conjunction with other clinical findings, other serologic methods should then be undertaken in serology reference laboratories.

Interesting diagnostic approaches that rely on antigens produced by recombinant DNA technologies and specifically expressed during either the primary phase (granule dense proteins [GRA-7, GRA-4]) or the latent phase (GRA-1) of infection can lead to a more informative serologic diagnosis, even based on a single serum sample.

The employment of polymerase chain reaction (PCR) to identify T. gondii DNA in amniotic fluid (AF) obtained by amniocentesis at 18 weeks and later represents a milestone in the early diagnosis of intrauterine T. gondii infection, thereby avoiding the use of more-invasive procedures on the fetus. Sensitivity and specificity of PCR may even increase when performed on AF samples obtained from the sixteenth week of pregnancy onwards. The specificity and positive predictive value of PCR on AF samples is close to 100%, although different protocols influence its sensitivity and specificity. PCR is generally carried out with various gene targets, of which the most widely used is the 35-fold repetitive gene *B1*. With the recent employment of sensitive and specific real-time PCR techniques, which use as target regions of the gene *AF146527* repeated 300 times in the genome of *T. gondii*, it is possible to perform a quantitative study and follow the parasite load, allowing determination of parasite count and its correlation with clinical symptoms and impact of treatment.

However, a definitive correlation between the number of *Toxoplasma* organisms in AF and the severity of congenital infection has not yet been demonstrated. PCR should be considered for pregnant women (without a contraindication for the procedure) with positive diagnostic serology or highly suggestive of an infection because of ultrasonographic abnormalities in the fetus acquired during gestation or shortly before conception. If the PCR-AF test result is negative, the fetus should be unaffected, presumably because *T. gondii* has not yet crossed the placental barrier even if there is the theoretical possibility that fetal infection can occur later in pregnancy from a placenta that was infected earlier in gestation. Samples obtained by cordocentesis, funipuncture, or periumbilical fetal blood sampling should not be used because fetal risk of contamination with maternal blood is higher than with amniocentesis, and cordocentesis is less sensitive.

In the newborn, diagnosis of infection is based on detection of serum anti-*Toxoplasma* IgM and IgA antibodies that do not cross the placenta, unlike maternal IgG antibodies. Better results are obtained if the ISAGA method is used. Maternal IgG antibodies present in the newborn can reflect either past or recent infection in the mother and require serologic follow-up of the newborn for the 1st year of life until the complete disappearance of these antibodies. A negative *T. gondii*-specific IgG test result at 1 year of age essentially rules out congenital toxoplasmosis. Detection of IgG in oral fluid appears to be a promising tool for monitoring infants with suspected congenital toxoplasmosis.

Detection of specific IgA antibodies appears to be more sensitive than detection of IgM antibodies for establishing infection in the newborn, because these antibodies may be present when there is no *T. gondii*-specific IgM, and the converse can also occur. However, transmission of maternal IgM or IgA antibodies can occur during the birth process. Because of the relatively brief half-life of IgM and IgA, positive tests for these antibodies usually must be confirmed by repeat testing at 2 to 4 days of life in the case of IgM antibodies and at 10 days of life for IgA antibodies.

The suspected infection can be verified by a mother and child comparative immunologic profile analysis using the Western blot assay and two-dimensional immunoblot of serum from mother-baby pairs. This technique, although laborious and expensive, permits early postnatal diagnosis irrespective of the time of maternal infection and can identify newborns who have congenital infection with a sensitivity that reaches 85% within the 3 months of life.

Although complex and expensive, other methods that may be successfully employed to diagnose the infection in infants include direct demonstration of the organism by isolation of the parasite (e.g., inoculation in tissue cultures of placental tissue or mouse inoculation) and amplification of *T. gondii*-specific DNA.

Evaluation of infants with suspected congenital toxoplasmosis should always include ophthalmologic examination, electroencephalogram, hearing test, blood tests, noncontrast CT scanning or ultrasound of the brain, and examination of CSF. Although CT scanning is the first-line diagnostic method used in the United States to detect CNS abnormalities caused by toxoplasmosis, ultrasound can be used as an alternative diagnostic method to avoid the effects of radiation in the neonatal period. Ultrasound is recommended for women with suspected or diagnosed acute infection acquired during or shortly before gestation. This technique can reveal fetal abnormalities, including hydrocephalus, brain or hepatic calcifications, splenomegaly, and ascites. Because most infants do not show signs of toxoplasmosis at birth, a negative ultrasound does not rule out the possibility of infection and might need to be followed by a CT scan for confirmation because ultrasound results can vary depending on the examiner and technology used. Newborns thus need a thorough examination after birth and follow-up blood tests during the first year of life.

Diagnosis in Immunocompromised Patients

In immunocompromised persons and AIDS patients with toxoplasmic encephalitis, indirect serologic methods widely used in immunocompetent patients are unreliable because they fail to produce significant titers of specific antibodies. Although incidence of toxoplasmic encephalitis among HIV-infected persons directly correlates with the prevalence of anti-*T. gondii* antibodies, the absence of IgG antibody makes a diagnosis of toxoplasmosis unlikely, but not impossible. Anti-*Toxoplasma* IgM antibodies are usually absent. CSF findings are normal or show nonspecific alterations such as lymphocytic pleocytosis and discrete CSF hyperproteinorrachia.

In clinical practice, the diagnosis of toxoplasmic encephalitis is presumptive and mainly based on clinical presentation, imaging, and laboratory test results. Imaging includes CT or MRI, preferably with gadolinium contrast, and shows isodense or hypodense single or multiple lesions with a mass effect, taking up the contrast dye in a ringlike or nodular manner in more than 90% of cases. However, as neither CT nor MRI can reliably distinguish CNS infections, such as toxoplasmosis, from lymphoma in HIV-1-positive patients, the use of FDG-PET has been shown to offer better sensitivity to noninvasively differentiate cerebral toxoplasmosis and other infectious diseases from primary CNS lymphoma. Laboratory results include the presence of serum-specific *T. gondii* IgG antibodies. Diagnosis is also made from an objective response, on the basis of clinical and radiographic improvement, to specific anti-*T. gondii* therapy in the absence of a likely alternative diagnosis. In general, the occurrence of low $CD4^+$ T-cell count (less than $150–200/mm^3$) and the presence of *T. gondii* IgG antibody is habitually accepted as being a good predictor of toxoplasmic encephalitis reactivation, although less than 6% of toxoplasmic encephalitis patients show negative tests. If the suspected diagnosis of toxoplasmosis is correct, clinical or radiographic improvement should become evident by more than 50% within 7 to 14 days. If symptoms persist, a brain biopsy should be performed. This should be considered in immunocompromised patients with presumed CNS toxoplasmosis with a single MRI lesion, absence of IgG antibodies, or an unsatisfactory clinical response to specific anti-*T. gondii* treatment.

Diagnosis of toxoplasmic encephalitis is crucial because other brain diseases—such as CNS lymphoma, bacterial abscess, progressive multifocal leukoencephalopathy, viral or fungal encephalitis, neurotuberculosis, cytomegalovirus encephalitis, and focal lesions caused by fungi (*Cryptococcus neoformans*, *Aspergillus* spp., and *Nocardia* spp.)—could share similar clinical and CT scan signs. In general, no imaging technique is completely specific. Thallium single-photon emission computed tomography (SPECT) and positron emission tomography (PET) can be useful in distinguishing toxoplasmosis or other infections from CNS lymphoma. CNS lymphoma has greater thallium uptake on SPECT and greater glucose and methionine metabolism on PET than neurotoxoplasmosis or other infections.

Definitive diagnosis of toxoplasmic encephalitis is made by pathologic examination of brain tissue obtained by open or stereotactic CT-guided brain biopsy, although there is morbidity and even mortality associated with the biopsy procedure. Tachyzoites are demonstrated on hematoxylin and eosin stains or immunoperoxidase staining, which can increase diagnostic sensitivity, or by Giemsa on cytocentrifuged CSF samples. Toxoplasma organisms must be distinguished from other intracellular organisms such as *Histoplasma*, *Trypanosoma cruzi*, and *Leishmania*.

Since the turn of the twenty-first century, molecular techniques have allowed significant improvement and have been shown to be an important diagnostic tool in laboratory diagnosis of toxoplasmic encephalitis. Their use is principally appropriate for immunocompromised patients, because these techniques are not affected by the immunologic status of the host. PCR-based assays, in particular, have been shown to be rapid, sensitive, and specific enough to be used as a front-line test for detecting CSF *T. gondii* DNA in most patients with CNS infection, thus avoiding invasive and expensive brain biopsy procedures. However, results usually are negative once specific anti-*Toxoplasma* therapy has been started.

Moreover, parasite levels in blood and CSF may be very poor in some patients and cause difficulties in interpreting the PCR product. For this reason, a number of quantitative real-time PCRs with specific *T. gondii* genome sequence have been developed and employed in patients with AIDS and CNS damage with different rates of sensitivity and specificity.

PCR testing for other pathogens (e.g., Epstein-Barr virus [EBV], JC virus, *Mycobacterium tuberculosis*, *C. neoformans*) can be considered in patients who have focal brain lesions and who are already taking prophylactic antibiotics for toxoplasmosis or are seronegative.

In general, PCR enables detection of *T. gondii* DNA in vitreous and aqueous fluids, bronchoalveolar lavage (BAL) fluid, and blood and in patients with AIDS with other toxoplasmic localizations, and thus it is useful in the diagnosis and assessment of this disease. Currently, the search for parasites in clinical specimens by PCR has overtaken direct inoculation into mice.

Diagnosis of toxoplasmic encephalitis in AIDS patients can also be supported by demonstration of intrathecal antibody production based on detection of oligoclonal bands in CSF with antibody-specific index (ASI) and affinity-mediated immunoblot (AMI) techniques. This approach has also been shown to discriminate toxoplasmic encephalitis from other opportunistic CNS infections in AIDS. In non-AIDS immunocompromised patients, regular PCR follow-up of allogeneic hematopoietic stem-cell transplant (allo-HSCT) patients could guide pre-emptive treatment and improve outcome.

Treatment

The main goal of treatment is to interrupt the replication of the parasite and prevent further damage to the organs involved. Non-pregnant immunocompetent patients with acute toxoplasmosis plus lymphadenitis generally do not require antimicrobial therapy because the infection is self-limited and usually subclinical. Chronic lymphadenopathy accompanied by fever and marked weakness can be cured with specific therapy. Patients whose *T. gondii* infection occurred during laboratory accidents or blood transfusions need specific treatment. Pregnant women must be treated to reduce the risk and severity of congenital infection. Immunocompromised patients, including AIDS patients and transplant recipients, should always be treated with antitoxoplasmic agents. For eye disease, treatment usually includes anti-*Toxoplasma* agents plus systemic corticosteroids. The most important treatment and prophylactic regimens for the therapy of toxoplasmosis are shown in Tables 1 and 2.

The standard treatment for acquired toxoplasmosis in both immunocompetent and immunodeficient patients is the synergistic combination of pyrimethamine (Daraprim) (the most effective anti-*Toxoplasma* agent available) and sulfonamides. Pyrimethamine plus sulfadiazine[1] plus folinic acid (Leucovorin)[1] is the preferred regimen. Azithromycin (Zithromax)[1] and atovaquone (Mepron)[1] have been shown to be partially effective against tissue cysts in experimental studies.

Treatment during Pregnancy

Management of maternal and fetal infection of *T. gondii* varies considerably between different countries and even centers in the same country. According to the European Multicentre Study on Congenital Toxoplasmosis (EMSCOT) data, which suffer from the lack of a large-scale controlled clinical trial, treatment for

---

[1]Not FDA approved for this indication.

TABLE 1 Treatment Regimens for Toxoplasmosis

PATIENTS	DRUG OF CHOICE	RECOMMENDED DOSAGE	LENGTH OF ADMINISTRATION	ADVERSE EFFECTS
Acute infection in *T. gondii* seropositive pregnant patients (with undocumented fetal infection)	Spiramycin (Rovamycine)[1]	1,000 mg PO q8h (without food)	Throughout pregnancy or until fetal infection is documented	Mild GI disturbances, possible skin eruptions
Acute infection in a pregnant patient with documented fetal infection (positive PCR-AF)	Pyrimethamine (Daraprim) * plus	Loading dose, 50 mg PO q12h × 2 d, then 50 mg PO daily	Throughout pregnancy; avoid before 18th wk of gestation because of high risk of teratogenesis	Pyrimethamine is a potential teratogen (kidney and heart malformation) and should be used only after the first trimester
	Sulfadiazine[2] plus	Loading dose 75 mg/kg PO, then 50 mg/kg q12h (max 4 g daily)	Throughout pregnancy; do not administer before 18th wk of gestation[†]	Sulfadiazine can cause crystal-induced nephropathy[†]
	Folinic acid (Leucovorin)[2]	10–20 mg PO daily	During and for 1 wk after pyrimethamine use	Complete regimen: rash, fever and dose-dependent myelosuppression; weekly monitoring of blood cell counts
Congenital infection in the infant	Pyrimethamine plus	Loading dose 2 mg/kg PO daily × 2 d; then 1 mg/kg PO daily × 2–6 mo; then 1 mg/kg tiw	1 y	Same as above
	Sulfadiazine[2] plus	50 mg/kg PO q12h	1 y	
	Folinic acid[2]	10 mg/kg PO tiw	During and for 1 wk after pyrimethamine use	
Acute *T. gondii* infection in adult immunocompetent patients and in pregnant patients infected >6 mo before conception	Treatment not recommended or, if acutely ill: Pyrimethamine plus	Loading dose 200 mg PO daily in 2 divided doses, then 0.5–1 mg/kg/d (max 50 mg/d; 75 mg (if >60 kg)	4–6 wk, or 1–2 wk after resolution of symptoms	Same as above
	Sulfadiazine[2] plus	1,000–1,500 mg PO q6h	During and 1 wk after pyrimethamine use	
	Folinic acid[2]	5–20 mg PO tiw		

Continued

TABLE 1 Treatment Regimens for Toxoplasmosis—cont'd

PATIENTS	DRUG OF CHOICE	RECOMMENDED DOSAGE	LENGTH OF ADMINISTRATION	ADVERSE EFFECTS
Chorioretinitis in immunocompetent patients	Pyrimethamine[§,2] *plus*	200 mg loading dose, then 50–75 mg PO daily	1–2 wk after resolution of symptoms	
	Sulfadiazine[§,2] *plus*	1,000–1,500 mg PO q6h	1–2 wk after resolution of symptoms	
	Folinic acid[2] *plus*	5–20 mg PO tiw	During and for 1 wk after pyrimethamine use	
	Prednisone	1 mg/kg daily in 2 divided doses	Until resolution of signs and symptoms	
Alternatives	TMP-SMX (Bactrim)[2] *or*	160–800 mg q12h	6 wk	Skin rash, fever, leukopenia, thrombocytopenia, hepatotoxicity; also available as an IV formulation
	Azithromycin (Zithromax)[2] alone or associated with pyrimethamine *or*	500 mg/d	5 wk	Not reported
	Intravitreal clindamycin (Cleocin)[2]-dexamethasone (Decadron)	One injection 1–400 mcg	Not reported	Not reported
For untreatable cases only	Photocoagulation	Not usually done	Not reported	Not reported
Immunocompromised patients and patients with toxoplasmic encephalitis[∥]	Pyrimethamine *plus*	Loading dose 200 mg PO, then 50–75 mg PO daily	At least 4–6 wk after signs and symptoms resolve	Same as above
	Folinic acid[2] *plus either*	10–20 mg PO or IV or IM daily (max 50 mg daily)		
	Sulfadiazine *or*	1,000–1,500 mg PO q6h	During and for 1 wk after pyrimethamine use	Rash, fever, diarrhea, hepatotoxicity
	Clindamycin[2,¶] *plus*	600 mg PO or IV q6h (max 1,200 mg q6h)	At least 4–6 wk after signs and symptoms resolve	Fever, rash, diarrhea, hepatotoxicity
	Prednisone	1 mg/kg daily in 2 divided doses	Until improvement of edema or mass effect related to focal lesion	
	Alternatives TMP-SMX[2] alone *or*	5 mg/kg TMP PO or IV q12h (max 15–20 mg/kg/d)	Same as above	Same as above
	Pyrimethamine *plus* folinic acid[2] *plus one of the following*:	Same as above pyrimethamine and folinic acid doses 500 mg PO q12h	Same as above	Same as above
	Clarithromycin (Biaxin)[2]	750 mg PO q6h	At least 4–8 wk after resolution of signs and symptoms	
	Atovaquone (Mepron)[1]	1,200–1,500 mg PO daily	Not reported	Atovaquone can increase LFTs and skin rash Take with a meal to enhance absorption
	Azithromycin[2]	100 mg PO daily	Not reported	
	Dapsone[2]	750 mg PO q6h	Not reported	
	Atovaquone (Mepron)[2] alone or with sulfadiazine	1,000–1,500 mg PO q6h	Not reported	
Acute infection in patients with *T. gondii* and HIV infection**	Spiramycin[1] (as for immunocompetent pregnant women)	1,000 mg PO q8h (without food)	Throughout pregnancy or until fetal infection is documented	

[1]Investigational drug in the United States.
[2]Not FDA approved for this indication.
*Take with food to minimize gastrointestinal adverse effects.
[†]This might change in some European countries.
[‡]Should be taken on an empty stomach with adequate water.
[§]Take both for 3 weeks followed by 1-week off; repeat for three or four cycles.
[∥]After initial phase of therapy, maintenance therapy must be continued as long as the patient remains immunocompromised.
[¶]Clindamycin can be used instead of sulfadiazine in patients intolerant to sulfonamides.
**Amniocentesis should be avoided because of the risk of transmitting HIV infection to the fetus.
Abbreviations: GI, gastrointestinal; LFT, liver function test; PCR-AF, polymerase chain reaction testing of amniotic fluid; TMP-SMX, trimethoprim-sulfamethoxazole.

3 The Infectious Diseases

TABLE 2 Prophylaxis Regimens for Toxoplasmosis

PATIENTS WHO SHOULD RECEIVE PROPHYLAXIS	DRUG OF CHOICE*	RECOMMENDED DOSAGE	LENGTH OF ADMINISTRATION
Primary prophylaxis for immunocompromised patients, including advanced pregnant HIV-positive women (CD4+ count <100 cells/mm[3] and *T. gondii* IgG positive)	First choice: TMP-SMX (Bactrim)[1]	1 DS tab 160–800 mg PO daily	For life or until immunoreconstitution has occurred[†]
	Alternatives		
	Pyrimethamyne (Daraprim)[1]	50–75 mg/wk	
	plus		
	Dapsone[1]	50 mg/d	
	plus		
	Folinic acid (Leucovorin)[1]	25 mg/wk	
	or		
	Pyrimethamine-sulfadoxine (Fansidar)[1]	1 tab twice weekly	Same as above
	plus		
	Folinic acid[1]	25 mg/wk	Same as above
	or		
	Atovaquone (Mepron)[1]	1,500 mg PO daily	Same as above
Secondary prophylaxis for immunocompromised patients after primary or induction treatment	Same regimen used in the acute phase: TMP-SMX[1]	Half doses of those used in the acute phase 2.5 mg/kg TMP PO or IV q12h, max 15–20 mg/kg/d	For life or until immunoreconstitution has occurred[1]
Prophylaxis in adults receiving heart, lung, or liver transplant, especially in the case of a seropositive donor (D+) and seronegative recipient (R−)[‡]	First choice: TMP-SMX[1]	80 mg TMP/400 mg SMX (1 tab single-strength Bactrim) twice daily	For 6 wk after transplant
	Alternative		
	Pyrimethamine[1]	50–75 mg PO daily	Same as above
	plus		
	Folinic acid[1]	5–10 mg PO daily	During and for 1 wk after pyrimethamine use
Prophylaxis in adults receiving bone marrow and allogeneic stem cell transplants[§]	First choice: TMP-SMX[1]	Same as above[‖]	For more than 6 mo
	Alternatives[¶]:		
Prophylaxis for accidental laboratory exposure and blood transfusions	Pyrimethamine[1]	Not standardized	Not reported
	plus		
	Clindamycin (Cleocin)[1]		
	plus		
	Folinic acid[1]		
	Pyrimethamine[1]	Same as for acute infection**	2 wk
	plus		
	Sulfadiazine[1]		
	plus		
	Folinic acid[1]		

[1]Not FDA approved for this indication
*For side effects, see Table 1.
[†]In patients with AIDS, primary and secondary prophylaxis are generally discontinued when the patient's CD4[1] cell count has returned to more than 200 cells/µL and HIV PCR peripheral blood viral load has been reasonably controlled for at least 6 months following ART.
[‡]Preemptive antiparasite treatment should be considered for all symptomatic, seropositive, immunocompromised patients in whom toxoplasmosis is suspected.
[§]There are no clear recommendation for anti *T. gondii* prophylaxis in allogeneic stem cell transplantation because the optimal regimen has not yet been determined.
[‖]Not specifically codified.
[¶]Alternative regimen in sulfonamide-allergic patients.
**Presumptive therapy should be given with the same dosages as for acute infection and monitored serologically for several months after the exposure or until seroconversion is noted; that is, testing immediately after the exposure, weekly for at least 1 month, and at least monthly thereafter. Seroconversion can occur despite presumptive therapy. Although presumptive therapy typically prevents disease or at least substantial morbidity, it does not necessarily prevent infection.
Abbreviations: ART, highly active retroviral therapy; PCR, polymerase chain reaction; TMP-SMX, trimethoprim-sulfamethoxazole.

the fetus should be started immediately (within 3 weeks of infection) after diagnosis of recently acquired maternal infection. This has been shown to significantly reduce sequelae and to have a beneficial effect when therapy is begun soon after birth. Later treatment has been shown to have no effect.

The macrolide antibiotic spiramycin (Rovamycine)[2] is prescribed immediately after diagnosis of maternal infection in most centers in Europe and the United States, and there has been no evidence that this drug is teratogenic. Because Spiramycin does not cross the placenta but is concentrated within with placenta, it has been estimated to reduce the incidence of vertical transmission of *T. gondii* by about 60%. It is used 1 g every 8 hours in many EU countries, especially France, and in Asia and South America and does not seem to have any fetal effects, although a small percentage of women develop gastrointestinal side effects.

Spiramycin is theoretically most beneficial for patients with negative PCR-AF testing; it should be continued as prophylaxis until delivery, along with periodic ultrasound examination, because the placenta could have been infected earlier in gestation.

In the case of positive PCR-AF at, or immediately after, 18 weeks of gestation, or with high probability of fetal infection acquired late in the second trimester (after 18 weeks) or during the third trimester of gestation (because of ultrasound abnormalities), and in women who cannot undergo amniocentesis, the spiramycin regimen should be replaced with the drug combination of sulfadiazine[1] and pyrimethamine plus leucovorin.[1] This treatment strategy varies in some U.S. and European centers.

Throughout the pregnancy, therapy with pyrimethamine in conjunction with leucovorin should be continued to prevent hematologic toxicities, along with monitoring of blood cell counts and rigorous periodic ultrasound examination. Because spiramycin

[2]Not available in the United States.

[1]Not FDA approved for this indication.

does not readily cross the placenta, it is not reliable for the treatment of infection in the fetus. In the absence of clinical and laboratory signs suggestive of congenital toxoplasmosis, therapy is not indicated in infants, but it is necessary to inform the specialist and to plan, with the specialist, periodic clinical and serologic controls. In symptomatic infants, the combination of pyrimethamine plus sulfadiazine[1] plus folinic acid (leucovorin)[1] is recommended. The duration of this treatment is not specifically defined, but it must be continued for up to a year, possibly alternating cycles of antifolate for 4 weeks with spiramycin cycles of equal duration.

Ocular Toxoplasmosis

Although no treatment regimen seems to decrease the rate of chorioretinitis, pyrimethamine, sulfadiazine[1] plus folinic acid (leucovorin),[1] and corticosteroids form the most common drug combination currently used to treat ocular toxoplasmosis. Patients may also be treated with TMP-SMX (Bactrim),[1] which appears to be a safe and effective substitute for pyrimethamine, sulfadiazine, and folinic acid, or with azithromycin (Zithromax)[1] or intravitreal clindamycin (Cleocin)[1] and prednisone for 4 to 6 weeks. Pyrimethamine plus azithromycin is another drug combination that is similar to the standard treatment and can be considered an acceptable alternative treatment for sight-threatening ocular toxoplasmosis.

Recurrent toxoplasmic retinochoroiditis, probably related to the rupture of the dormant retinal cyst or Toxoplasma circulating in peripheral blood, remains a major health crisis and can be associated with severe morbidity if the disease extends to structures critical for vision, including the macula and optic disk. Severe morbidity can also occur if there is damage to the eye from inflammation or if there are complications such as retinal detachment or neovascularization. In patients with frequent recurrences, the rate of recurrent toxoplasmic retinochoroiditis can be significantly reduced by long-term intermittent treatment with TMP-SMX 160 mg/800 mg (Bactrim DS),[1] with one tablet administered three times a week as a prophylactic regimen. Intravitreal clindamycin injection[1] and possibly steroids may be an acceptable alternative to the classic treatment in ocular toxoplasmosis. It can offer the patient more convenience, a safer systemic side-effect profile, greater availability, and fewer follow-up visits and hematologic evaluations. Although research has identified wide variation in practices regarding the use of corticosteroids, a recent Cochrane review did not identify evidence from randomized controlled trials for the role of corticosteroids in the management of ocular toxoplasmosis. The question of foremost importance, however, is whether they should be used as adjunct therapy (that is, in addition) to antiparasitic agents. There is no evidence to support that one antibiotic regimen is superior to another so choice needs to be informed by the safety profile. Intravitreous clindamycin with dexamethasone[1] seems to be as effective as systemic treatments. There is currently level I evidence that intermittent trimethoprim-sulfamethoxazole prevents recurrence of the disease.

Toxoplasmosis in Immunosuppressed Patients

With the advent of the ART, the natural course of HIV infection has markedly changed, and opportunistic infections including toxoplasmosis have declined and changed in presentation, outcome, and incidence. However, toxoplasmic encephalitis is a major cause of morbidity and mortality, especially in resource-poor settings, and it is a common neurologic complication in some countries despite the availability of ART and effective prophylaxis.

The initial therapy of choice in toxoplasmic encephalitis patients consists of the combination of pyrimethamine, which is able to penetrate the brain parenchyma efficiently even in the absence of inflammation, plus sulfadiazine or clindamycin[1] plus leucovorin.[1]

Adjunctive corticosteroids should be administered when clinically indicated only for treatment of a mass effect associated with focal lesions or associated edema. Because of the potential immunosuppressive effects of corticosteroids, they should be discontinued as soon as clinically feasible. Patients receiving corticosteroids

should be closely monitored for the development of other effects, including CMV retinitis and tuberculosis. Anticonvulsants should be administered to patients with a history of seizures, but should not be administered prophylactically to all patients. Drug interactions between anticonvulsants and antiretroviral agents should be carefully evaluated, and doses should be adjusted according to established guidelines. The preferred alternative regimen for patients unable to tolerate or who fail to respond to first-line therapy is pyrimethamine plus clindamycin plus leucovorin.

Common clindamycin toxicities include fever, rash, nausea, diarrhea (including pseudomembranous colitis or diarrhea related to Clostridium difficile toxin), and hepatotoxicity. Other alternative regimens shown in Table 1 are active in the treatment of toxoplasmic encephalitis and may be used in sulfa-intolerant patients or those who have not responded to treatment, although their relative efficacy compared with the previous regimens is unknown.

The combination of atovaquone (Mepron)[1] with either pyrimethamine or sulfadiazine has demonstrated utility for the treatment of acute toxoplasmic encephalitis in patients with a Karnofsky Performance Status Score greater than 30, which combines the ability to work, to undertake normal activities without external assistance, and to take care of personal needs. Acute therapy should be continued for at least 6 weeks, if there is clinical and radiologic improvement. This should be followed by maintenance therapy (lifelong secondary prophylaxis), usually with the same regimen that was used in the acute phase but at half doses (see Table 2).

Currently, maintenance treatment should be continued for the life of the patient or until underlying immunosuppression has ceased (immune reconstitution resulting from ART). Adult and adolescent patients appear to be at low risk for recurrence of toxoplasmic encephalitis when they have successfully completed initial therapy, remain asymptomatic with respect to signs and symptoms, and have a sustained (i.e., more than 6 months) increase in their $CD4^+$ T-lymphocyte counts to greater than 200 cells/μL on ART. AIDS patients with $CD4^+$ T cell counts less than 100/μL and IgG Toxoplasma antibody should receive primary prophylaxis for toxoplasmosis. Fortunately, the same daily regimen of one double-strength tablet of TMP/SMX (Bactrim DS)[1] used for Pneumocystis jirovecii prophylaxis provides adequate primary protection against toxoplasmosis. Secondary prophylaxis for toxoplasmosis may be discontinued in the setting of effective ART and when $CD4^+$ T-cell counts increase to more than 200/μL for 6 months.

Prophylaxis and treatment measures of disease in bone marrow transplant recipients as well as in those receiving organ transplantation are shown in Table 2.

Toxoplasma gondii Infection during Pregnancy in HIV-Positive Women

Immunocompromised women with chronic infection do rarely transmit the parasite to the fetus, resulting in congenital infection. This includes women with AIDS as well as those on immunosuppressive treatment. Vertical transmission occurs in up to 4% of cases, particularly when the $CD4^+$ count is less than 100/mm³. The risk of transmission is low when the $CD4^+$ count is greater than 200/mm³ (see Table 2).

Consideration should be given to screening all immunosuppressed women for evidence of maternal T. gondii serologic status to establish an early diagnosis of reactivation. Seropositive women with low CD4 counts should receive TMP-SMX (Bactrim)[1] to prevent reactivation of Toxoplasma. Because of reports of congenital toxoplasmosis in mildly or moderately immunosuppressed women, it is recommended that immunocompromised women not infected with HIV and women who are infected with HIV and who have CD4 counts less than 200/mm³ be treated with spiramycin (Rovamycine)[2] for the duration of the pregnancy. A nonpregnant woman who has been diagnosed with an acute T. gondii infection should be counseled

---

[1]Not FDA approved for this indication.

[1]Not FDA approved for this indication.
[2]Not available in the United States.

to wait 6 months before attempting to become pregnant. Each case should be considered separately in consultation with an expert.

Detailed ultrasound examination of the fetus specifically evaluating for hydrocephalus, cerebral calcifications, and growth restriction should be done for HIV-1-infected women with suspected primary or symptomatic reactivation of *T. gondii* during pregnancy.

Prevention

Strategies for the primary prevention of toxoplasmosis in pregnant women and in immunosuppressed patients with negative serology are shown in Box 1.

All the primary measures for preventing congenital toxoplasmosis concern mainly agricultural areas, veterinary practices, zoological shops, and gastronomy. Efforts toward health education are focused on avoiding personal exposure to the parasite (hygienic and culinary practices during pregnancy). Although *T. gondii* can be avoided by implementing relatively simple strategies in daily life, the majority of pregnant women are unaware of how to prevent exposure.

Most women are aware that toxoplasmosis is associated with cat litter. Contact with cat litter should be avoided if possible; if not, gloves should be worn while changing the litter box and hands should be washed thoroughly afterward. Litter should be changed frequently because it takes several days for oocysts to become infectious, and the box should be thoroughly cleaned with disinfecting agents. Preventing a cat from hunting outdoors or eating raw meat also can prevent the feline from being infected with *T. gondii*. Practitioners should encourage pregnant women to keep indoor-only cats and to feed them only canned or dry food that has been bought in a store. Contact with any utensils that might have been contaminated with cat feces and cat litter should be strictly avoided. Hands should be washed after contact with soil, dogs, and cats, and before meals.

Women should also devote particular attention to environmental exposure. Sporulated oocysts can be found in dirt, sand, or soil and on the skins of raw fruits and vegetables grown in these substrates. Limiting contact with dirt, sand, or soil can help prevent the ingestion of oocysts from the environment, and if contact occurs, an expectant mother should be taught to thoroughly wash her hands to avoid ingesting the parasite. Wearing gloves while gardening, for example, also can limit the contact a pregnant woman might have with these environmental hazards. The skins of all raw fruits and vegetables should be washed and then peeled away because oocysts may be attached to these parts of the food and could be ingested. Hand washing should be strongly emphasized after handling any raw food including fruits, vegetables, and meat products. Other exposure risks include eating raw oysters, clams, or mussels. *T. gondii* cysts can reside in the meat of many different types of mammals, including imported horse meat containing *T. gondii* atypical strains, or birds. In the United States, it is estimated that 8% of beef and 20% of lamb and pork contains *T. gondii* tissue cysts. All pregnant women should be taught to never ingest raw meat and to cook all meat to an internal temperature of at least 80°C (175°F) to destroy the tissue cysts.

Secondary prevention by serologic monitoring of seronegative pregnant women should be closely connected with detailed primary prevention. Routine toxoplasmosis screening programs for pregnant women have been established in France, Austria, and Brazil. In France, guidelines recommend that nonimmune pregnant women be tested every month throughout pregnancy to detect seroconversion to *Toxoplasma* infection. In the United States, routine serologic screening is not performed. In Italy, serologic screening is recommended to prevent congenital toxoplasmosis as part of the antenatal care protocol. Serologic screening of women should begin before conception, with follow-up monthly tests during pregnancy to detect seroconversion. This is the basis for the French screening program and the Austrian Toxoplasmosis Prevention Program, which recommend routine serologic testing. Treatment is recommended if one of the tests suggests definite or probable primary maternal infection.

Vaccination is one of the most efficient strategies to prevent and control the spread of toxoplasmosis by immunization of humans and animals (the source of infection). To date, there is much debate about whether a human vaccine is feasible. Costs, target population, method for testing the vaccine, and risks associated with the vaccine are important factors affecting development of the vaccine. Much of the work has been focused on SAG1, a surface antigen expressed on tachyzoites, in attempts to induce protective immune response (mainly T-helper response) when introduced to the host with various adjuvants. SAG1 is primarily involved in adhesion, signal transduction, invasion, material transport and host immune responses. Thus, this protein may be crucial for both the diagnosis of *T. gondii* infection and the ability to immunize against this parasite. This exciting progress on SAG1 will lay a solid foundation to combat toxoplasmosis.

In general, a simpler route to prevent human disease would be to vaccinate animals (cats and intermediate hosts) that are responsible for transmission to humans, as demonstrated using a live attenuated vaccine developed for the prevention of chronic infection in sheep. However, it cannot be used in humans because of the risk of reversion to a pathogenic form. Vaccine development to prevent feline oocyst shedding is ongoing, mostly involving live vaccines. More recently, *T. gondii* dense granule proteins including GRA-6, a secretory vesicular organelle that produces proteins that participate in the modification of the parasitophorous vacuole, have been shown to be suitable as possible DNA vaccines for immunity against toxoplasmosis. Aspartic protease 1 (Asp 1) has also shown to play an essential role in the *T. gondii* lifecycle. This could be a novel vaccine candidate against toxoplasmosis.

Box 1 Strategies for the Primary Prevention of Toxoplasmosis in Pregnant Women and in Immunosuppressed Patients with Negative Serology

- Check immunity to toxoplasmosis. If the patient has no protection (absence of anti *Toxoplasma* IgG), take direct or indirect prophylactic measures against cats, food, and water.
- Avoid contact with food (including unwashed fruit or vegetables) or water potentially contaminated with cat feces. Wash before consuming.
- Avoid any job or activity that requires contact with dirt, soil, or other material potentially contaminated with cat feces (e.g., gardening or handling cat litter). Wear gloves when gardening or handling cat litter.
- Keep cats inside. Do not adopt or handle stray cats. Do not feed cats raw or undercooked meat but only canned or dried commercial food or well-cooked food. Do not obtain a new kitten or cat during pregnancy.
- Disinfect the cat litter box with near-boiling water for 5 min before handling.
- Wash hands thoroughly after contact with raw meat.
- Kitchen surfaces and utensils that have come in contact with raw meat should be washed.
- Avoid ingesting raw or dried meat, raw eggs, or unpasteurized milk.
- Avoid eating raw oysters, clams, or mussels.
- Protect foods from flies, cockroaches, and other insects.
- Avoid touching the eyes or face or any mucous membrane during or immediately after preparing food.
- Cook meat thoroughly. Pork, lamb, beef, veal, and poultry should be cooked until the meat reaches 80°C in the center.
- Refrain from skinning animals.
- Avoid children's sandboxes.
- Avoid contact with stray dogs (xenosmophilia); if this is not possible, wash your hands after contact.

References

Boothroyd JC. Toxoplasma gondii: 25 years and 25 major advances for the field. Int J Parasitol 2009;39:935–46.

Contini C, Seraceni S, Cultrera R, et al. Evaluation of a Real-time PCR-based assay using the lightcycler system for detection of Toxoplasma gondii bradyzoite genes in blood specimens from patients with toxoplasmic retinochoroiditis. Int J Parasitol 2005;35:275–83, Epub 2005 Jan 18.

Contini C. Clinical and diagnostic management of toxoplasmosis in the immunocompromised patient. Parassitologia 2008;50:45–50.

Jasper S, Vedula SS, John SS, et al. Corticosteroids for ocular toxoplasmosis. Cochrane Database Syst Rev 2013;30:4, CD007417.

Derouin F, Pelloux H. ESCMID study group on clinical parasitology: Prevention of toxoplasmosis in transplant patients. Clin Microbiol Infect 2008;14:1089–101.

Elmore SA, Jones JL, Conrad PA, et al. Toxoplasma gondii: Epidemiology, feline clinical aspects, and prevention. Trends Parasitol 2010;26:190–6.

Flegr J, Preiss M, Klose J. Toxoplasmosis-associated difference in intelligence and personality in men depends on their Rhesus blood group but not ABO blood group. PLoS One 2013;8:e61272.

Dupont CD, Christian DA, Hunter CA. Immune response and immunopathology during toxoplasmosis. Semin Immunopathol 2012;34:793–813, Epub 2012 Sep 7.

Seeber F, Cooke BM. 12th International Congress on Toxoplasmosis. Int J Parasitol 2014;44:83–4. http://dx.doi.org/10.1016/j.ijpara.2014.01.001.

Safa G, Darrieux L. Cerebral toxoplasmosis after rituximab therapy. JAMA Intern Med 2013;173:924–6.

Maenz M, Schlüter D, Liesenfeld O, et al. Ocular toxoplasmosis past, present and new aspects of an old disease. Prog Retin Eye Res 2014;39C:77–106. http://dx.doi.org/10.1016/j.preteyeres.2013.12.005, Epub 2014 Jan 9.

Montoya JG, Liesenfeld O. Toxoplasmosis. Lancet 2004;363:1965–76.

Ngoungou EB, Bhalla D, Nzoghe A, Dardé ML, Preux PM. Toxoplasmosis and epilepsy–systematic review and meta analysis. PLoS Negl Trop Dis 2015;9(2):e0003525.

Petersen E. Toxoplasmosis. Semin Fetal Neonatal Med 2007;12:214–23.

Remington JS, McLeod R, Thulliez P, et al. Toxoplasmosis. In: Remington JS, Klein J, Wilson CB, Baker MD, editors. Infectious Disease of the Fetus and Newborn Infant. Philadelphia: Saunders; 2006. p. 946–1091.

Sathekge M, Maes A, Van de Wiele C. FDG-PET imaging in HIV infection and tuberculosis. Semin Nucl Med 2013;43(5):349–66.

Sullivan Jr WJ, Jeffers V. Mechanisms of Toxoplasma gondii persistence and latency. FEMS Microbiol Rev 2012;36:717–33.

TYPHOID FEVER

Method of
Tamilarasu Kadhiravan, MD

CURRENT DIAGNOSIS

- Typhoid fever typically manifests as an undifferentiated acute febrile illness.
- Soft splenomegaly, normal or low white cell count, and elevated liver enzymes are subtle diagnostic pointers.
- Blood culture, drawn before antibiotic administration, is the most useful investigation.
- Consider presumptive treatment in appropriate epidemiologic settings.

CURRENT THERAPY

- Decreased susceptibility to fluoroquinolones is widespread among *Salmonella enterica* serovar Typhi.
- High-dose fluoroquinolones are suboptimal for treating such infections.
- Azithromycin (Zithromax)[1] is the preferred drug for uncomplicated typhoid fever.
- Ceftriaxone (Rocephin)[1] is preferred for treating hospitalized and seriously ill patients.

[1]Not FDA approved for this indication.

Typhoid fever is a bacteremic infection caused by the gram-negative bacillus *Salmonella enterica* serovar Typhi. S. Paratyphi also causes an illness clinically indistinguishable from typhoid fever. Humans are the only known host of S. Typhi, and it is transmitted by ingestion of contaminated food or water. Improvement in sanitation and hygiene led to the elimination of typhoid fever from the developed world long before the advent of antibiotics. On the other hand, in parts of the world lacking sanitation, it continues to be an important cause of febrile illness despite the availability of effective antibiotics.

Epidemiology

Typhoid fever is endemic in the developing world, especially the South and South East Asian countries of India, Nepal, Pakistan, Bangladesh, Vietnam, and Indonesia. Annual incidence in endemic settings is typically more than 100 cases per 100,000 population, and it predominantly affects children and young adults. Apart from sick persons with typhoid fever, convalescent carriers and asymptomatically infected food handlers (long-term carriers) are the sources of infection. Potential vehicles of infection include food or water consumed from roadside eateries, ice cubes and ice cream made from contaminated water, and raw vegetables and fruits. In contrast, most cases of typhoid fever in developed countries are imported by travel, especially to the Indian subcontinent.

Pathogenesis and Clinical Features

Following ingestion, the bacilli invade and multiply in the small-intestinal lymphoid tissue before entering the bloodstream. This primary bacteremia leads to widespread seeding of the reticuloendothelial system and intestinal lymphoid tissue, where the infection is amplified and spills over into the circulation. Onset of symptoms usually coincides with this secondary bacteremia. Interestingly, unlike other Gram-negative bacteremic infections, septic shock develops relatively late in the course of illness, and the infection can be eminently cured by oral antibiotic therapy. Nonetheless, it should be emphasized that any delay in initiating antibiotic therapy increases the risk of complications (Box 1).

During the first week, temperature gradually increases in a step-ladder fashion. Localizing symptoms are usually minimal. Anorexia, lassitude, and malaise are often marked. Headache and vomiting are common; however, a supple neck helps rule out meningitis. Abdominal symptoms such as constipation, loose stools, and abdominal pain are not infrequent, but they are nonspecific and often overlooked. Soft, tender enlargement of liver or

Box 1	Complications of Typhoid Fever

Abdominal
Paralytic ileus
Intestinal hemorrhage
Intestinal perforation
Secondary peritonitis
Symptomatic liver dysfunction
Acalculous cholecystitis

Extra-abdominal
Encephalopathy
Cerebellar dysfunction
Myocarditis
Osteomyelitis and soft tissue abscesses
Multiorgan dysfunction syndrome
Hemophagocytic syndrome
Hemolysis
Glomerulonephritis

Long-term
Gallbladder cancer

spleen is seen in about half the patients. Rose spots and relative bradycardia, though classic, are rare. When the infection goes untreated, hypertrophied lymphoid tissue of the Peyer's patches can ulcerate toward the end of the second week, resulting in torrential gastrointestinal bleeding, small intestinal perforation, and secondary bacterial peritonitis. Patients with severe illness can present with a muttering delirium described as *coma vigil*. Untreated typhoid fever often resolves spontaneously in about 4 to 6 weeks. However, the risk of death is high (>10%), and relapses are frequent. Many patients excrete S. Typhi in feces and urine during convalescence (convalescent carriers), and some of them continue to excrete beyond 1 year (long-term carriers).

Current Pattern of Antimicrobial Susceptibility

Since 1990, a sea change has occurred in the antimicrobial susceptibility of S. Typhi in endemic countries and elsewhere. Unregulated use of fluoroquinolones has resulted in emergence of S. Typhi strains with decreased susceptibility. These strains have a subthreshold increase in minimal inhibitory concentration (MIC) that is not detected by conventional disk-diffusion testing. Hence, determination of MIC is recommended at present. Resistance to nalidixic acid (NegGram) (a quinolone) is often used as a surrogate marker for such strains. In fact, most infections in the community are now caused by nalidixic acid-resistant S. Typhi (NARST). Not surprisingly, this change is reflected in far-away geographic locales such as the United States and the United Kingdom.

Diagnosis

Clinical features are nonspecific, and laboratory testing is essential to confirm a diagnosis of typhoid fever. A soft splenomegaly, absence of leukocytosis, mild leukopenia, and modest elevation of transaminases are subtle pointers to a diagnosis of typhoid fever. Blood culture drawn early in the illness before initiation of antibiotics is often fruitful and is the gold standard for the diagnosis of typhoid fever. The time-honored Widal test, which detects agglutinating antibodies to somatic and flagellar antigens of S. Typhi, adds little to decision making. Initial enthusiasm about rapid serologic tests such as Typhidot and Tubex TF has not been confirmed in community-based studies. None of these tests are sensitive enough to rule out typhoid. In a patient who has nonlocalizing acute febrile illness lasting more than 5 to 7 days in a suggestive epidemiologic setting (residence in or travel to endemic area; outbreaks), it is prudent to treat presumptively for typhoid fever, after reasonably ruling out competing diagnoses such as malaria, dengue, leptospirosis, and rickettsial infection.

Treatment

Fluoroquinolones (ciprofloxacin [Cipro] or ofloxacin [Floxin][1] 7.5 mg/kg twice a day for 5–7 days) are unparalleled in efficacy for treating fully susceptible S. Typhi strains. However, their use is associated with frequent treatment failures, prolonged defervescence, and higher rates of complications in NARST infections. Given the widespread emergence of NARST, fluoroquinolones are no longer to be considered the drug of choice. Several alternatives have been evaluated in randomized, controlled trials for treating uncomplicated typhoid fever caused by NARST (Table 1). Ease of oral administration, proven efficacy, and safety (under FDA review) make azithromycin (Zithromax)[1] a reasonable first choice for uncomplicated typhoid fever. In hospitalized seriously ill patients and treatment failures, parenteral ceftriaxone (Rocephin)[1] is preferred. Usually, it takes about 4 to 7 days for defervescence after the initiation of antibiotics. Antipyretics should be used for symptom relief; ibuprofen (Motrin; 10 mg/kg every 6 hours) is superior to acetaminophen (Tylenol; 12 mg/kg every 6 hours). However, ibuprofen should be avoided when dengue fever is a possibility. A soft, low-residue diet is traditionally advised to prevent intestinal perforation. Such a practice, however, is not founded on scientific evidence. Treatment of S. Paratyphi infection is identical to that of S. Typhi infection.

Prevention

Sustained improvement in sanitation and access to safe drinking water are essential to control typhoid fever in endemic areas. Avoiding potentially contaminated food and beverages and being vaccinated before travel decrease the risk of typhoid fever among travelers (see the article on travel medicine). Recently, mass administration of the Vi polysaccharide vaccine (Typhim Vi, Typherix [outside United States]) has been found to confer herd immunity and is a potential tool for the control of typhoid fever in endemic settings.

---

[1]Not FDA approved for this indication.

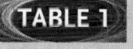

TABLE 1 Outcomes of Alternative Treatments for Nalidixic Acid–Resistant S. Typhi (NARST) Infection Evaluated in Randomized, Controlled Trials

DRUG	DOSAGE	FEVER CLEARANCE TIME (MEDIAN OR MEAN)	RATE OF TREATMENT FAILURE	RELAPSE RATE	COMMENTS
High-dose ofloxacin (Floxin)[1]	10 mg/kg[3] bid × 7 d	8.2 d	36%	<1%; insufficient data	Not recommended
Gatifloxacin (Tequin)[2]	10 mg/kg qd × 7 d	4.4 d	9%	3%	Serious concerns about dysglycemia
Azithromycin (Zithromax)[1]	10–20[3] mg/kg qd × 7 d	4.4 d	9%	<1%; insufficient data	Unproven in complicated typhoid fever
Cefixime (Suprax)[1]	10 mg/kg[3] bid × 7 d	5.8 d	27%	9%	High cost; not recommended
Ceftriaxone* (Rocephin)[1]	60–75 mg/kg qd × 10–14 d	6.1 d	9%	5%	High relapse rate (14%) with 7-day regimen

Data from Dolecek C, Tran TP, Nguyen NR, et al: A multi-center randomised controlled trial of gatifloxacin versus azithromycin for the treatment of uncomplicated typhoid fever in children and adults in Vietnam. PLoS One 2008;3:e2188; Pandit A, Arjyal A, Day JN, et al: An open randomized comparison of gatifloxacin versus cefixime for the treatment of uncomplicated enteric fever. PLoS One 2007;2:e542; and Parry CM, Ho VA, Phuong le T, et al: Randomized controlled comparison of ofloxacin, azithromycin, and an ofloxacin-azithromycin combination for treatment of multidrug-resistant and nalidixic acid-resistant typhoid fever. Antimicrob Agents Chemother 2007;51:819.
[1]Not FDA approved for this indication.
[2]Not available in the United States.
[3]Exceeds dosage recommended by the manufacturer.
*No trials on treatment of NARST infection; extrapolated data from Parry CM, et al: Typhoid fever. N Engl J Med 2002;347:1770–82.

References

Bhutta ZA. Current concepts in the diagnosis and treatment of typhoid fever. BMJ 2006;333:78.

Dolecek C, Tran TP, Nguyen NR, et al. A multi-center randomised controlled trial of gatifloxacin versus azithromycin for the treatment of uncomplicated typhoid fever in children and adults in Vietnam. PLoS ONE 2008;3:e2188.

Dutta S, Sur D, Manna B, et al. Evaluation of new-generation serologic tests for the diagnosis of typhoid fever: data from a community-based surveillance in Calcutta, India. Diagn Microbiol Infect Dis 2006;56:359.

Effa EE, Bukirwa H. Azithromycin for treating uncomplicated typhoid and paratyphoid fever (enteric fever). Cochrane Database Syst Rev 2008;(4)CD006083.

Lynch MF, Blanton EM, Bulens S, et al. Typhoid fever in the United States, 1999–2006. JAMA 2009;302:859.

Ochiai RL, Acosta CJ, Danovaro-Holliday MC, et al. A study of typhoid fever in five Asian countries: Disease burden and implications for controls. Bull World Health Organ 2008;86:260.

Pandit A, Arjyal A, Day JN, et al. An open randomized comparison of gatifloxacin versus cefixime for the treatment of uncomplicated enteric fever. PLoS ONE 2007;2:e542.

Parry CM, Ho VA, Phuong le T, et al. Randomized controlled comparison of ofloxacin, azithromycin, and an ofloxacin-azithromycin combination for treatment of multidrug-resistant and nalidixic acid-resistant typhoid fever. Antimicrob Agents Chemother 2007;51:819.

Vinh H, Parry CM, Hanh VT, et al. Double blind comparison of ibuprofen and paracetamol for adjunctive treatment of uncomplicated typhoid fever. Pediatr Infect Dis J 2004;23:226.

VARICELLA (CHICKENPOX)

Method of
Laura Mayans, MD

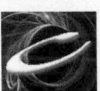

CURRENT DIAGNOSIS

- Clinical diagnosis is based on the characteristic pruritic rash. It is generalized but concentrated on the head, scalp, and trunk, with fewer lesions on the extremities.
- The rash progresses from maculopapular to vesicular, to pustular, and finally scabs. Often all stages of the rash are present at the same time.
- In uncertain cases, the polymerase chain reaction (PCR) test can be used to detect VZV in vesicular fluid, scabs, throat swabs, cerebrospinal fluid (CSF), blood, or saliva.

CURRENT THERAPY

- Uncomplicated cases in healthy children over 1 year and under 12 years can be treated symptomatically with antipyretics and antipruritics. Do not use aspirin because of the risk of Reye's syndrome.
- Disease is more severe in infants, adolescents, and adults. Antiviral treatment is recommended in these age groups.
- Acyclovir is available in a liquid suspension. Infant dosing is 20 mg/kg (max 800 mg) every 6 hours for 7–10 days.
- In adolescents and adults, Valacyclovir (Valtrex) is preferred because of better bioavailability. It is dosed 1000 mg twice daily for 7 days.
- For disease in the immunocompromised, IV acyclovir is indicated. The recommended dosage is 10–15 mg/kg every 8 hours.

Epidemiology

Varicella is a benign, self-limited disease in healthy children but can cause severe morbidity and mortality in infants, adolescents, adults, and the immunocompromised. Before routine vaccination beginning in 1995, varicella was an extremely common disease of childhood. In temperate climates, over 90% of people were infected before adolescence. Incidence peaked in late winter to early spring with epidemics occurring every 2 to 5 years. In tropical climates, infection was much less common and often occurred later in life.

Risk Factors and Prevention

Before the vaccine, varicella was a ubiquitous disease affecting both sexes and all races in similar climates equally. In 1995, a live attenuated varicella vaccine was licensed for use in the United States. It is now routinely used in many other countries. Initially a single 0.5 mL dose was given subcutaneously to children under 12 years of age; however, outbreaks among the vaccinated were often seen. In 2006, the Centers for Disease Control and Prevention (CDC) recommended a two-dose regimen. The first dose is given between 12 and 15 months of age, and the second between 4 and 6 years of age. It is unclear if the vaccine failures seen after only one dose were due to incomplete seroconversion or waning immunity. Though the ideal timing of the two doses is unknown, the regimen was chosen to coincide with the already established measles-mumps-rubella (MMR) vaccination schedule. In those under 12 years, doses need only be separated by 3 months. In those over 12 years, two doses given at least 4 weeks apart is advised. Most adults in the United States are immune even if they have never had the disease or vaccine. This is due to the widespread presence of the disease in the prevaccine years. It is believed they likely had a mild case that was attributed to another viral illness of childhood. However, adults who immigrated from warmer climates may not be immune and vaccination is advised. The vaccine has decreased primary varicella cases by 85% and moderate to severe cases by over 95%. The vaccine does not prevent herpes zoster.

Pathophysiology

The varicella zoster virus (VZV) is host specific, with humans being the only natural reservoir. It is a member of the herpes virus family. The virus is transmitted by aerosolized respiratory droplets or by contact with varicella or herpes zoster skin lesions. It infects a new host through inoculation of respiratory or conjunctival mucosal cells. There, the virus infects local immune cells and lymph tissues. These cells carry the virus to epithelial cells where the virus replicates, causing cutaneous lesions and viremia. The incubation period can range from 10 to 21 days, and patients are infectious up to 48 hours before the appearance of cutaneous lesions. The lesions first appear as small, erythematous papules and over 12 to 24 hours become vesicles, leading to the characteristic "dewdrop on a rose petal" appearance (Figure 1). They are highly pruritic and often first appear on the head and scalp or trunk (Figure 2). The virus can also produce ulcers in the mucous membranes of the oropharynx and vagina. Over the next 48 hours, vesicular fluid becomes cloudy and then crusts over. The virus can no longer be detected in the fluid after 72 to 96 hours. The highest contagion period is during the vesicular phase, and one is generally considered no longer contagious after all lesions have crusted over. New skin lesions can continue to develop for an average of 3 to 5 days with a range of 1 to 7, leading to another characteristic feature of varicella: all stages of skin lesions are often present at the same time. Later crops of lesions tend to develop on the extremities. The lesions are usually superficial and do not scar except possibly at the earliest sites, often the hairline or eyebrows. The varicella zoster virus remains latent in neurons of the dorsal root ganglia, cranial root ganglia, or autonomic ganglia. This occurs after disease or vaccination. If reactivated later in life, it causes herpes zoster (shingles).

Clinical Manifestations

The disease often begins with fever, malaise, headache, and anorexia, followed by the appearance of the distinctive rash. The rash is pruritic, and after 24 to 48 hours, papules, vesicles, pustules, and scabs are all present on the body at the same time. The rash is more heavily concentrated on the head, scalp, and trunk and lesions can be tender. Lesions on mucous membranes are possible. The rash may also be accompanied by mild abdominal pain.

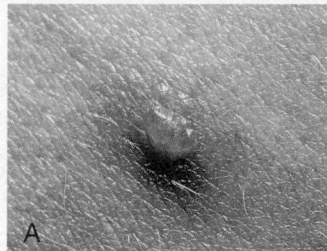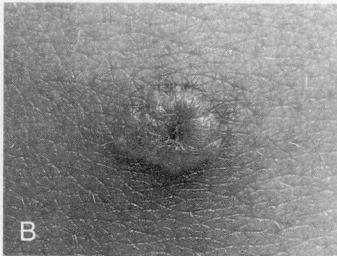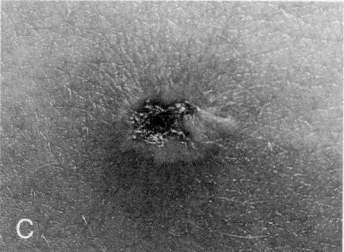

Figure 1. **A**, "Dewdrop on a rose petal"; a thick-walled vesicle with clear fluid forms on a red base. **B**, The vesicle becomes cloudy and depressed in the center (umbilicated), the border is irregular (scalloped). **C**, A crust forms in the center and eventually replaces the remaining portion of the vesicle at the periphery.

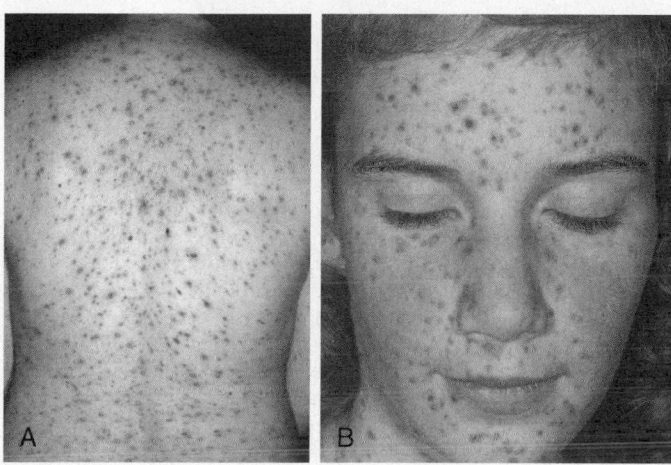

Figure 2. The disease starts with lesions on the trunk and then spreads to the face and extremities.

Diagnosis

The diagnosis has historically been clinical, based upon the distinctive rash, associated symptoms, and possible exposures. However, because the incidence of varicella has dramatically decreased with the use of the vaccine, many newer physicians may have a difficult time recognizing varicella. Diagnosis can also be difficult in the immunocompromised, who can have a severe and atypical presentation. In the past, the gold standard for diagnosis was viral culture of vesicular or bodily fluids. However, this was time-consuming and expensive. Today, PCR is used to amplify and detect viral DNA in vesicular fluid, scabs, skin or throat swabs, blood, CSF, saliva, and even tissue biopsies.

Differential Diagnosis

Historically, smallpox was the most serious possibility. There have been no documented cases of smallpox since 1949, and it retains only minimal concern today as a result of the threat of bioterrorism. The main differentiating feature is that smallpox lesions are larger and present in the same stage of evolution. Other conditions similar to varicella include impetigo, eczema herpeticum, herpes simplex infection, hand-foot-mouth disease, herpes zoster, insect bites, drug reactions, and atypical measles. Coxsackievirus and echovirus also cause similar viral exanthems. Hemorrhagic varicella can appear similar to meningococcemia. Stevens-Johnson syndrome and toxic shock syndrome could also present similarly. The main differentiating features are the distribution of rash, simultaneous presence of multiple stages of skin lesion evolution, associated symptoms, and exposures.

Treatment

The decision to treat depends on the age and health status of the patient and the time since the development of the rash. Studies have shown that, if acyclovir therapy is initiated within 24 hours of the onset of rash, a shorter duration of fever and a modest decrease in skin lesions are seen. Overall, the duration of illness may be shortened up to 24 hours. Improvement in clinical course is relatively small and the window for treatment is short; therefore antiviral therapy is still considered optional in otherwise healthy children. Often, supportive treatment with acetaminophen and antipruritics is all that is needed. Aspirin should be avoided, however, because of the risk of Reye's syndrome. Infants, adolescents (over age 12), and adults are at a much higher risk of complications and often have more severe disease. Treatment of these groups with antiviral medication is advised. Studies have shown treatment with antiviral medication to be of benefit for up to 48 hours, possibly even longer, after the appearance of the rash. Both acyclovir and valacyclovir (Valtrex) can be used. Valacyclovir is preferred because of better bioavailability and is dosed 20 mg/kg up to 1000 mg twice daily for 7 days. Acyclovir is dosed 800 mg 5 times daily for 5 days. For infants and children who require liquid suspension, acyclovir is the only option. Liquid acyclovir is dosed 20 mg/kg every 6 hours for 7 to 10 days. Pregnant women appear to be particularly vulnerable to pulmonary complications, and any pregnant woman with varicella and evidence of pulmonary involvement (cough, shortness of breath, or abnormal chest X-ray) should be treated. Though not specifically approved for varicella in pregnancy, both acyclovir and valacyclovir have been used in pregnancy for treatment of herpes simplex without evidence of maternal or fetal toxicity. Immunocompromised people, such as those with HIV, cancer, organ transplant recipients, or those on immunocompromising drugs are very vulnerable to severe complications and should receive IV treatment as soon as the disease is diagnosed. IV acyclovir is given at 10 to 15 mg/kg twice daily for 7 to 10 days. A switch to orals can be considered when the patient is afebrile and no new lesions appear for at least 24 hours. If acyclovir or valacyclovir cannot be used, either because of resistance or allergy, IV foscarnet (Foscavir) is available. This is not first line, however, given the much lower safety profile, most notably nephrotoxicity, hypocalcemia, and other electrolyte disturbances. Foscarnet can be given at a dose of 40 mg/kg every 8 hours or 100 mg/kg every 12 hours. To prevent adverse effects, it must be infused over at least 1 hour. Currently, famciclovir (Famvir) is primarily used in herpes simplex and herpes zoster outbreaks and not routinely used in varicella infections.

Complications

The most common complication in healthy children is secondary bacterial infection from scratching the skin lesions. Keeping nails trimmed can be helpful. The most common infecting agents are *Staph. aureus* and *Strep. pyogenes*. If this occurs, antibiotics may be needed. Serious complications are more likely to occur in adolescents, adults, or the immunocompromised. Pneumonitis or viral pneumonia is the most common, followed by subclinical hepatitis. Neurologic complications are estimated to occur in 1 to 3 per 10,000 cases and include encephalitis, meningitis, cerebellar ataxia, and transverse myelitis. Stroke syndromes, hemorrhagic rashes, and Guillain-Barré syndrome are rarer, but also possible. Infection during the first or second trimester of pregnancy can result in severe congenital malformations. Infection in the third trimester can lead to disseminated severe disease in the newborn.

A common long-term consequence of varicella zoster infection is reactivation later in life, manifesting as herpes zoster, or shingles. Zoster affects over 1 million people in the United States each year, and most are over age 60. It begins with a prodromal phase that includes pain, paresthesias, and dysesthesia in a dermatomal distribution. Within a few days, a unilateral, dermatomal maculopapular rash appears. The rash evolves into vesicles, which usually scab over in 10 days. Complete resolution of the rash and accompanying pain and dysesthesias generally occurs over 4 to 6 weeks. If pain persists after resolution of the rash, this is called postherpetic neuralgia. Postherpetic neuralgia can be severe, difficult to treat, and last from months to years. In 2006, the FDA approved a zoster vaccine for VZV-seropositive adults over age 60. It is the same live, attenuated vaccine given to children, but at a higher dosage. It increases cell-mediated immunity to the varicella virus. Initial studies showed that the zoster vaccine resulted in a 61% decrease in illness among the vaccinated compared to placebo groups. In those who still developed shingles after receiving the vaccine, there was a shortened severity and duration of the illness as well as a twofold reduction in the occurrence of postherpetic neuralgia. Herpes zoster does recur in 3% to 5% of affected individuals, and those with a history of herpes zoster can still be vaccinated and benefit from the further boost in immunity. The vaccine is generally well tolerated, with minor injection site reactions and headache being the most common adverse effects. The vaccine is contraindicated in pregnant women and those with severe immunodeficiency.

References

Bonanni P, Gershon A, Gershon M, et al. Primary versus secondary failure after varicella vaccination: Implications for interval between 2 doses. Pediatr Infect Dis J 2013;32:e305–e313.

Gershon A, Gershon M. Pathogenesis and current approaches to control of varicella-zoster virus infections. Clin Microbiol Rev 2013;26:728–43.

Gnann J. Varicella-zoster virus: Atypical presentations and unusual complications. J Infect Dis 2002;186(Suppl. 1):S91–98.

Gnann J. Antiviral therapy of varicella-zoster virus infections, In: Arvin A, Campadelli-Fiume G, Mocarski E, et al., editors. Human Herpesviruses: Biology, Therapy, and Immunoprophylaxis. Cambridge: Cambridge University Press; 2007. Chapter 65. Available from, http://www.ncbi.nlm.nih.gov//books/NBK47401/?report.

Izikson L, Lilly E. Primary varicella in an immunocompetent adult. J Clin Aesthet Dermatol 2009;2:36–8.

Moffat J, Ku C, Zerboni L, et al. VZV: Pathogenesis and the disease consequences of primary infection, In: Arvin A, Campadelli-Fiume G, Mocarski E, et al., editors. Human Herpesviruses: Biology, Therapy, and Immunoprophylaxis. Cambridge: Cambridge University Press; 2007. Chapter 37. Available from, http://www.ncbi.nlm.nih.gov//books/NBK47382/?report.

Mueller NH, Gilden DH, Cohrs RJ, et al. Varicella zoster virus infection: Clinical features, molecular pathogenesis of disease, and latency. Neurol Clin 2008;26:675–97.

Sanford M, Keating GM. Zoster vaccine: A review of its use in preventing herpes zoster and postherpetic neuralgia in older adults. Drugs & Aging 2010;27:159–76.

WHOOPING COUGH (PERTUSSIS)

Method of
Michael E. Pichichero, MD

CURRENT DIAGNOSIS

- An illness marked by a staccato cough lasting >7 d in the absence of fever in an adolescent or adult may be pertussis.

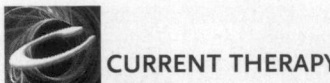

CURRENT THERAPY

- Early treatment of pertussis not only eliminates contagion, it also shortens the illness.
- Macrolides are the treatment of choice; azithromycin (Zithromax) is preferred for ease of dosing, tolerability, and short duration of treatment.

Pertussis, or whooping cough, is a highly contagious acute respiratory tract infection caused by *Bordetella pertussis*. It causes prolonged cough illness, without associated fever, characterized by paroxysms of coughing, inspiratory "whoops," and post-tussive vomiting in severe cases and persistent intermittent staccato cough episodes in teenagers and adults. The incidence of pertussis is rising in the United States despite record-high vaccination coverage. In 2004, more cases occurred in adolescents and in adults than children.

Microbiology and Pathophysiology

B. pertussis is a gram-negative coccobacillus that is difficult to grow with standard media. *B. pertussis* does not invade the human host; bacteremia does not occur. The systemic effects of illness are produced by the organism's toxins, especially pertussis toxin. *B. pertussis* attaches to the nasopharynx and tracheobronchial tree with adhesins such as fimbriae, filamentous hemagglutinin, and pertactin. Once attached it produces toxins such as pertussis toxin, adenylate cyclase toxin, and tracheal cytotoxin that paralyze the respiratory cilia, resulting in inflammation of the respiratory tract.

Epidemiology

B. pertussis is a human pathogen transmitted from person to person via aerosolized droplets. Pertussis is highly contagious, similar to varicella, infecting 80% to 90% of susceptible contacts. Persons with pertussis are most contagious in the 2 weeks before cough onset and during the first 2 weeks of cough, typically a time frame before medical care is sought or clinicians consider the possibility of the diagnosis.

In 2004, approximately 20,000 cases of pertussis were reported to the Centers for Disease Control and Prevention (CDC); because substantial underreporting is a recognized problem, current estimates of true pertussis incidence per year in the United States probably is in the range of 1 to 3 million cases. A new development is the recognition that pertussis is a disease of adolescents and adults as well as children. Several studies showed that among teenagers and adults who seek care for cough illness of more than 1 week duration, approximately 20% have pertussis.

Immunity

It has been known for decades that immunity to tetanus wanes over time and boosters are needed approximately every 10 years to sustain protective antibody levels. The phenomenon of waning immunity to pertussis is a newer observation and one of the explanations of the rising incidence of pertussis in the United States. Apparently, boosters of pertussis vaccines are also needed, perhaps, like tetanus, approximately every 10 years. Two new adolescent/adult pertussis vaccine formulations that are combined with tetanus and diphtheria vaccines (Boostrix, Adacel) were licensed and recommended for universal use in 2005 to address this problem.

Clinical Symptoms

Classic pertussis is a 30- to 90-day illness that presents in three stages: catarrhal, paroxysmal, and convalescent. The stages may be shorter in immunized children, adolescents, and adults. Pertussis is most severe when it occurs during the first 6 months of life.

In the catarrhal stage, nonspecific symptoms similar to the common cold predominate. The paroxysmal stage is characterized by a persistent cough, sometimes with bursts of numerous rapid coughs. A long inspiratory effort sometimes causes a high-pitched whoop. Typically, the patient is afebrile and, between coughing attacks, usually appears normal. The paroxysmal stage usually lasts 6 weeks. The cough gradually lessens over 2 to 3 weeks during the convalescent period. Milder paroxysms may recur with subsequent respiratory infections for many months following a pertussis infection. Infants may appear very ill and distressed during the paroxysmal stage and require close observation and supportive care. Older children, adolescents, and adults have a prolonged cough with paroxysms but no whoop.

Complications

Complications occur most commonly among young infants with pertussis. The most common complication is secondary bacterial pneumonia. Hypoxia or effects of pertussis toxin may contribute to neurologic complications including seizures and encephalopathy. In the United States, 90% of deaths occur in children younger than 6 months. Complications from pertussis in adolescents and adults are not uncommon (Table 1).

Diagnosis

A clinical diagnosis of pertussis is typically made based on the characteristic cough, although patients are often seen several times before the correct diagnosis is considered. Absolute lymphocytosis ($>$10,000 lymphcytes/mm^3) may be seen during the late catarrhal and paroxysmal stages but is less common among adults and immunized children. Chest radiographs may show peribronchial consolidation, interstitial edema, or variable atelectasis. The presence of fever and consolidation with pertussis suggests a secondary bacterial pneumonia.

Isolation of *B. pertussis* from a culture of nasal secretions remains the gold standard for laboratory diagnosis. A nasopharyngeal specimen is obtained by inserting a small flexible Dacron or calcium alginate swab through the nose to the posterior nasopharynx (attempting to touch the adenoids), where it is held for a few seconds, perhaps inducing a cough. The specimen is transferred to *Bordetella*-specific transport media and subsequently plated on Regan-Lowe charcoal agar or Stainer-Scholte agar. Cultures are usually positive if obtained in the catarrhal or early paroxysmal stage of disease. Success in isolating *B. pertussis* diminishes if patients have received pertussis vaccine or recent antimicrobials or if specimens are obtained beyond the first 2 weeks of cough.

Polymerase chain reaction (PCR) is more sensitive among persons with mild or atypical symptoms and those who have received prior antimicrobial therapy. The CDC recommends using PCR as a presumptive assay in conjunction with culture. Direct fluorescent antibody (DFA) testing has a low sensitivity and variable specificity, requiring experienced laboratory personnel for consistent results. DFA testing should only be performed as a adjunct to culture or PCR. Serologic testing methods have recently emerged as a very valuable diagnostic tool. Single samples of 100 μL of blood can be used to measure pertussis antibodies that are compared to age-specific standards to confirm a clinical diagnosis. These methods are not widely available in hospitals or private laboratories, but state laboratories often can provide this testing.

TABLE 1 Complications From Pertussis in Adolescents and Adults

SYMPTOMS/SIGNS	MINNESOTA	MASSACHUSETTS	
		ADOLESCENTS	*ADULTS*
Paroxysmal cough	100%	85%	87%
Whooping	26%	30%	35%
Post-tussive emesis	56%	45%	41%
Apnea	—	19%	37%
Cyanosis	—	6%	9%
Hospitalization	0%	1.4%	3.5%

TABLE 2 Licensed Vaccines for the Prevention of Pertussis in Infants, Children, Adolescents, and Adults

INDICATED AGE GROUP	SANOFI PASTEUR TRIPEDIA INFANTS/CHILDREN[†]	GLAXO SMITHKLINE INFANRIX* INFANTS/CHILDREN[†]	SANOFI PASTEUR DAPTACEL INFANTS/CHILDREN[†]	GLAXO SMITHKLINE BOOSTRIX ADULTS/ADOLESCENTS	SANOFI PASTEUR ADACEL ADULTS/ADOLESCENTS
Antigens					
PT (μg)	23.4	25	10	8	2.5
FHA (μg)	23.4	25	5	8	5
PRN (μg)	—	8	3	2.5	3
FIM 2 + 3 (μg)	—	—	5	—	5
D (Lf)	6.7	25	15	2.5	2
T (Lf)	5	10	5	5	5

*PEDIARIX also contains these DTaP components.
[†]6 wk to <7 y.
Abbreviations: D = diphtheria toxoid; FHA = filamentous hemagglutinin; FIM 2 + 3 = fimbrial agglutinogen 2 and 3; PRN = pertactin; PT = pertussis toxoid; T = tetanus toxoid.

Treatment

Infants and children with severe cough paroxysms associated with cyanosis or apnea require hospitalization and intensive care. Infants younger than 3 months should be admitted routinely for observation of their paroxysmal episodes, their need for supportive interventions, and their ability to feed appropriately. Continuous monitoring of heart rate, respiratory rate, and oxygen saturation is indicated.

All patients should receive antibiotics. Macrolides are the treatment of choice: erythromycin, clarithromycin (Biaxin),[1] azithromycin (Zithromax),[1] or telithromycin (Ketek).[1] Fluoroquinolones are also effective therapy for pertussis. Trimethoprimsulfamethoxazole (Bactrim)[1] is an alternative choice, although less effective.

Prevention

Pertussis can be prevented by vaccination. Vaccines are available and recommended for universal use in infants, children, adolescents, and selected adult populations (health care workers,

_____

[1]Not FDA approved for this indication.

adults caring for infants younger than 6 months, and those with chronic respiratory conditions, e.g., chronic obstructive pulmonary disease). Table 2 lists the vaccines licensed in the United States.

References

Farizo KM, Cochi SL, Zell ER, et al. Epidemiological features of pertussis in the United States, 1980–1989. Clin Infect Dis 1992;14(3):708–19.

Lee LH, Pichichero ME. Costs of illness due to *Bordetella pertussis* in families. Arch Fam Med 2000;9(10):989–96.

Pichichero ME, Rennels MB, Edwards KM, et al. Combined tetanus, diphtheria, and 5-component pertussis vaccine for use in adolescents and adults. JAMA 2005;293 (24):3003–11.

Purdy KW, Hay JW, Botteman MF, et al. Evaluation of strategies for use of acellular pertussis vaccine in adolescents and adults: A cost-benefit analysis. Clin Infect Dis 2004;39:20–8.

Skowronski DM, De Serres G, MacDonald D, et al. The changing age and seasonal profile of pertussis in Canada. J Infect Dis 2002;185(10):1448–53 [Epub 2002 Apr 22].

Strebel P, Nordin J, Edwards K, et al. Population-based incidence of pertussis among adolescents and adults, Minnesota, 1995–1996. J Infect Dis 2001;183(9):1353–9 [Epub 2001 Mar 30].

Yih WK, Lett SM, des Vignes FN, et al. The increasing incidence of pertussis in Massachusetts adolescents and adults, 1989–1998. J Infect Dis 2000;182(5):1409–16 [Epub 2000 Oct 09].

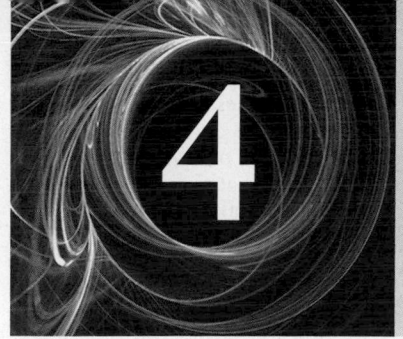

4 Diseases of the Skin

ACNE VULGARIS

Method of
Daniel J. Van Durme, MD; and Lisa M. Johnson, MD

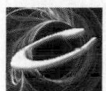

CURRENT DIAGNOSIS

- Acne vulgaris is primarily found in teenagers and young adults and is characterized by microcomedones that develop into open and closed comedones (blackheads and whiteheads) as well as inflammatory papules and pustules, or nodules and cysts.
- Acne vulgaris lesions are primarily on the face, neck, upper arms, back, and chest.
- Acneiform lesions are typically found in various stages, with many patients having a predominant type.

CURRENT THERAPY

- Acne therapy targets abnormal hyperkeratinization, excess sebum production, colonization by *Propionibacterium acnes*, and inflammation. Therapy involves prevention of new lesions and control over a long period of time with response generally seen in 6 to 8 weeks.
- Numerous topical and oral medications have demonstrated efficacy for patients with acne; there is little evidence for which is best.
- Benzoyl peroxide is an excellent starting agent owing to extensive safety and efficacy studies, its demonstrated benefit in controlling *P. acnes*, and some benefits in controlling abnormal keratinization and inflammation.
- Topical retinoids should also be considered as starting agents owing to their demonstrated benefits in controlling abnormal keratinization leading to microcomedones, a primary lesion in acne.
- Topical antibiotics such as clindamycin (Cleocin-T) and erythromycin (Akne-Mycin) should be used in combination with topical retinoids for more efficacy or with benzoyl peroxide to decrease the likelihood of bacterial resistance.
- Oral antibiotics such as doxycycline (Vibramycin) should be used if acne is widespread or unresponsive to topical agents.
- Oral contraceptives have proven benefits for most types of acne.
- Oral isotretinoin (Accutane, Claravis) can be very effective and even cures many patients, but the teratogenic and other side effects are profound and mandate use with extreme caution.

Acne (or acne vulgaris) and rosacea (previously called acne rosacea and sometimes adult acne) are often thought of together. However, they actually represent different pathophysiologic processes and require different therapeutic approaches.

Epidemiology

Acne is a chronic inflammatory dermatosis that is most common in adolescents, affecting approximately 85% of teenagers with the average age of onset being 11 to 12 years of age, peaking at ages 15 to 17, and decreasing with age. It is typically worse in male patients. The severity varies widely. Although significant physical scarring is uncommon, the psychological burden may be severe and includes depression, anxiety, social withdrawal, and suicidal ideation. More severe forms of acne are found in those with a genetic predisposition and those with earlier onset.

Prevention

Cigarette smoking raises acne risk, and the severity increases in a dose-dependent fashion. There are many myths, anecdotes, and limited (flawed) studies regarding acne and its triggers, but there is no good evidence to date to support the roles of chocolate, greasy foods, or other dietary factors in causing acne. There is some evidence that dairy products (particularly milk) might contribute to acne, but others have questioned the strength of these studies.

Pathophysiology

The pathophysiology of acne involves androgens as a major contributing factor, and thus acne starts with puberty. Four intersecting pathophysiologic processes are involved in acne, and the sequence and degree of contribution of each factor is still under study. The lesions begin with abnormal keratinization of the pilosebaceous glands that are more concentrated on the face, neck, and trunk. The keratin that lines the opening of the glands becomes more cohesive; this blocks the gland from being able to adequately excrete the sebum, and the plugged opening dilates. This leads to a closed comedone (whitehead) or open comedone (blackhead). Additional factors include the proliferation of the gram-positive *Propionibacterium acnes* (*P. acnes*) and an increase in inflammatory mediators, such as cytokines, leukotrienes, lymphocytes, and macrophages, which lead to the papules and pustules of inflammatory acne. Finally, the abnormal and excess production of sebum, particularly triggered by androgens, can play a key role as well, notably in nodulocystic acne.

Diagnosis

Diagnosis is generally straightforward, especially in teenagers. Dermatologic lesions include open and closed comedones, pustules, inflammatory papules, nodules, and cysts. Lesions are primarily found on the face, neck, upper arms, back, and chest. They are typically found in various stages, and many patients have a predominant type.

Clinical Manifestations

Clinical manifestations include open and closed comedones (blackheads and whiteheads), inflammatory papules and pustules, and in severe cases, nodules and cysts. There are several proposed classification schemes to help identify the numbers and types of lesions. Perhaps the most useful combines an estimate of the numbers of lesions with a descriptor of the lesions and location. Thus, a patient can have mild (few lesions) papulopustular acne of the face and severe (many lesions) comedonal acne on the back and shoulders. This classification helps to identify optimal treatment and provide a better description to assess response to therapy.

Differential Diagnosis

Differential diagnosis should include drug-induced acne (especially from steroids), which can be identified by seeing all lesions at nearly the same stage of development. Rosacea should also be considered in the differential diagnosis of acne vulgaris, though the age of onset and symptomatology are usually distinguishing.

Treatment

Treatment of acne begins with careful patient education and often involves a negotiation of management with teenagers who are taking responsibility for their health for the first time. It is increasingly important to address myths and misperceptions that they might hear from others or find on the Internet (such as the use of toothpaste for acne as seen on YouTube). Additionally, it is key to set realistic expectations about how acne can be controlled with the regular use of a variety of agents and how it can take 6 to 8 weeks to see improvement. If these issues are not addressed, the likelihood of adherence and long-term improvement are low.

Medical treatment should begin with a benzoyl peroxide agent because these are available over the counter and have an extensive history of safety and efficacy. They are available in a wide range of vehicles (soaps, lotions, gels); strengths vary from 2.5% to 10%. Many patients go straight to the maximum strength and report significant irritation, so it is important to educate that higher strengths dry the skin but are otherwise no more effective against *P. acnes* than the lower strengths. Patients should be advised that this reflects the base of treatment upon which other agents are added. Benzoyl peroxide plays a key role as a combination with both topical and oral antibiotics in preventing the development of bacterial resistance. If necessary, the patient can use it every other day to develop a tolerance to any irritation and gradually work up to once- or twice-daily dosing.

Topical retinoids (tretinoin [Retin-A, Renova, Avita], adapalene [Differin], or tazarotene [Tazorac]) are all extremely effective for abnormal keratinization and comedone development and thus treat existing lesion and prevent the development of new lesions. These can be irritating and come in a variety of strengths. Patients might need to start at the lowest strength with every-other-day dosing and work up to the highest strength needed and tolerated. All are contraindicated in pregnancy.

Salicylic acid preparations are comedolytic and can be used for patients who cannot tolerate either benzoyl peroxide or topical retinoids, although salicylic acid preparations have not been shown to be as effective.

For patients with moderate inflammatory and comedonal lesions, it can be appropriate to start both benzoyl peroxide and topical retinoids at the initial visit; however, the applications should be separated in time because the benzoyl peroxide will inactivate the retinoid. An effective regimen (if tolerated) is a benzoyl peroxide wash in the morning and topical retinoid at bedtime.

Antibiotics should be added if response to topical benzoyl peroxide and retinoids is inadequate at the 6- to 8-week follow-up visit. Topical clindamycin (Cleocin-T) and erythromycin (Akne-Mycin) have demonstrated efficacy and can be used twice a day at the same time as the benzoyl peroxide. There are also combination agents that conveniently add the two agents into a single preparation: clindamycin 1% plus benzoyl peroxide 5% gel (BenzaClin, Duac) and erythromycin 3% plus benzoyl peroxide 5% gel (Benzamycin). They are more expensive, however.

Oral antibiotics should be started if the acne is moderate to severe, if it is too widespread to reasonably cover with topical antibiotics, or if there is an inadequate response after 6 to 8 weeks of topical antibiotics. Effective oral agents include the tetracyclines, macrolides, and trimethoprim-sulfamethoxazole (TMP-SMX [Bactrim])[1]; however, side effects of each must be considered, and bacterial resistance is an increasing issue.

Doxycycline (Vibramycin) at 100 mg/day is generally considered the optimal antibiotic despite some issues with photosensitivity. Minocycline (Minocin) at 100 mg twice daily has side effects that include pigment deposition in skin, mucous membranes, and teeth (as well as rare autoimmune hepatitis and other problems). TMP-SMX (Bactrim, Septra DS)[1] taken twice daily also has side effects to consider but can be useful when other agents are not tolerated. Macrolides, particularly erythromycin (Ery-Tab),[1] have had the most problems with bacterial resistance. For this reason, they should be reserved for pregnant patients or when other agents cannot be used and should always be used with benzoyl peroxide to minimize that resistance. All oral agents should be used in combination with benzoyl peroxide and/or a topical retinoid but not in combination with topical antibiotics. If significant improvement is noted, oral agents should be decreased after 3 to 4 months and stopped in order to attempt maintenance control with topical agents.

Oral contraceptives can be very helpful in female patients with moderate acne owing to their antiandrogenic effects, which decrease sebum production. Several oral contraceptives have won FDA approval for acne, including Ortho Tri-Cyclen, Estrostep Fe, and Beyaz, although many others have also shown significant improvement in acne.

Several other topical agents have shown benefit for acne, including azelaic acid (Azelex, Finacea) used twice a day. It seems less effective than other agents, but can be useful when multiple types of lesions are present. It can also cause gradual hypopigmentation, which may be helpful in those with inflammatory hyperpigmentation. Topical sulfacetamide 10% (Klaron)[1] applied twice daily has also shown benefit.

Oral isotretinoin (Accutane, Claravis) has demonstrated marked benefit for patients with severe recalcitrant acne, even inducing a full remission. It is a potent teratogen and has a host of other significant side effects, including cheilitis, epistaxis, photosensitivity, and many others. Prescribed at 0.5 to 2 mg/kg per day over 20 weeks, it is like chemotherapy for acne. It is extremely tightly regulated, and both prescribers and patients must register with the iPledge program in order to write for the medicine and to receive the prescriptions. See www.ipledgeprogram.com. When all the precautions are managed, it can be an extremely effective option for the patients with the worst cases of acne.

[1]Not FDA approved for this indication.

References

Gannon M, Underhill M, Wellik KE. Which oral antibiotics are best for acne? J Fam Pract 2011;60:290–2.

Strauss JS, Krowchuk DP, Leyden JJ, et al. Guidelines of care for acne vulgaris management. J Am Acad Dermatol 2007;56:651–63.

Titus S, Hodge J. Diagnosis and treatment of acne. Am Fam Physician 2012;86:734–40.

Knutsen-Larson S, Dawson AL, Dunnick CA, et al. Acne vulgaris: Pathogenesis, treatment, and needs assessment. Dermatol Clin 2012;30:99–106.

ATOPIC DERMATITIS

Method of
Peck Y. Ong, MD

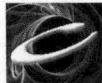

CURRENT DIAGNOSIS

- Itch must be present for the diagnosis of atopic dermatitis. In addition, the diagnosis must include three or more of the following criteria (U.K. Working Party's Diagnostic Criteria for Atopic Dermatitis):
  - History of generalized dry skin

[1]Not FDA approved for this indication.

- Visible flexural dermatitis
- Onset of the skin condition before 2 years (not used for patients younger than 4 years)
- History of itchy skin involving the following areas: elbows, behind knees, front of ankles, or around the neck
- History of asthma or allergic rhinitis (or for children younger than 4 years, history of atopic disease in a first-degree relative)

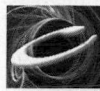

CURRENT THERAPY

- Bathe or shower for 10 to 20 minutes daily and pat dry gently.
- Follow immediately by applying an emollient on unaffected areas and an antiinflammatory medication on affected areas.
- Use topical corticosteroids as a first-line antiinflammatory medication; alternative medications are topical calcineurin inhibitors or barrier creams.
- Avoid environmental triggers such as extreme heat, humidity, or dryness.
- Avoid food allergens that may cause anaphylaxis. Consult an allergist regarding the interpretation of serum-specific IgE tests or food challenge.
- Treat skin infection only when clinical signs are present (e.g., oozing, impetigo).
- Severe, generalized infection or vesicular lesions may indicate herpes simplex virus infection; persistent fever may indicate invasive *S. aureus* infection.

Atopic dermatitis (AD) is a chronic inflammatory skin disease that is characterized by itch and a predilection of eczema on extensor areas in young infants or flexural areas in older children and adults. In the United States, AD affects about 15% of children and 2% of adults. For more than 85% of patients, AD begins during the first 5 years, but 50% of the children with AD improve significantly or outgrow the disease by age 7. The persistence of AD depends on various factors: early onset, severity, family history of AD, personal history of asthma, and food or inhalant allergies.

The itch associated with AD causes significant discomfort in these patients and often leads to sleep loss and to poor school or work performance. The quality of life of children with generalized AD is worse than that for children with diabetes, epilepsy, asthma, cystic fibrosis, or renal disease. The maternal stress in taking care of children with moderate to severe AD is equivalent to that associated with care of children with diabetes, Rett syndrome, profound deafness, or the need for enteral feeding.

Pathophysiology

AD is caused by a combination of genetic and environmental factors. Patients with AD have a defective skin barrier. This leads to a loss of skin hydration and susceptibility to environmental triggers. There is evidence that the skin barrier defects of AD are caused by genetic mutations. Studies have shown that many AD patients carry a genetic mutation in filaggrin, a protein with important barrier function.

Potential external triggers of AD include microbial pathogens and environmental allergens. Almost 100% of AD skin lesions are colonized by *Staphylococcus aureus*, which may produce toxins that trigger immune response in the skin. As a result, AD patients produce an increased amount of pro-allergic cytokines, such as interleukin-4 (IL-4), IL-5, and IL-13, in their skin. These cytokines lead to an increased infiltration of inflammatory T cells and eosinophils. IL-4 and IL-13 also are important for the production of serum IgE, the level of which is elevated in AD patients.

Diagnosis and Clinical Assessment

Most AD patients can be diagnosed by clinical history and physical examination. Typical presentation includes itch, dryness, flexural

TABLE 1	Differential Diagnoses of Atopic Dermatitis
DISEASE CATEGORY	**DIFFERENTIAL DIAGNOSES**
Dermatologic diseases	Contact dermatitis, seborrheic dermatitis, psoriasis, dyshidrotic eczema, eosinophilic pustular folliculitis, ichthyosis vulgaris
Neoplastic diseases	Cutaneous T-cell lymphoma, Langerhans cell histiocytosis
Immunodeficiencies	Hyper-IgE syndrome, severe combined immunodeficiency, Omenn syndrome, IPEX (immune dysregulation, polyendocrinopathy, enteropathy X-linked) syndrome
Infectious diseases	Scabies, cutaneous candidiasis, tinea versicolor
Nutritional deficiencies	Acrodermatitis enteropathica (zinc deficiency), essential fatty acid deficiency, biotin deficiency
Multisystemic disorders	Netherton syndrome, dermatitis herpetiformis

dermatitis, early age of onset, and atopy such as multiple food allergies. Patients with generalized eczema or adult-onset eczema can present as a diagnostic challenge. The differential diagnosis includes immunodeficiency (e.g., hyper-IgE syndrome, Omenn syndrome), malignancy (e.g., cutaneous T-cell lymphoma), zinc deficiency (i.e., acrodermatitis enteropathica), and celiac-associated dermatitis (i.e., dermatitis herpetiformis) (Table 1). AD children seldom present with failure to thrive, unless they are under severe dietary restriction. Failure to thrive should therefore prompt further investigation. Punch skin biopsies may be needed when the diagnosis is still unclear.

The prevalence of mild, moderate, and severe AD is 80%, 18%, and 2%, respectively. Most patients with mild to moderate disease have flexural, extensor, or facial involvement, whereas patients with severe disease often present with total-body involvement with or without erythroderma (Figure 1). Validated scales for assessing the severity of AD include Scoring of Atopic Dermatitis (SCORAD) and Eczema Area and Severity Index (EASI). These scoring systems or a simplified diagram documenting the extent of dermatitis are useful for more objective follow-up of the patient's progress.

Management of Atopic Dermatitis and Associated Conditions

Daily Maintenance Care

Changes in humidity can adversely affect AD symptoms. Dry conditions lead to increased transepidermal water loss and dry AD skin. Extreme heat, humidity, and sweating may lead to irritation of AD skin. AD patients are at increased risk for contact or irritant dermatitis, which may occur with over-the-counter topical skin medications that contain multiple ingredients. Wool or synthetic acrylic fabrics may also be irritating to AD skin.

To improve barrier function, AD patients should bathe or shower for 10 to 20 minutes once or twice daily, followed immediately by gently drying the skin and applying an emollient on the unaffected areas and a topical antiinflammatory medication on the affected areas. A petrolatum-based emollient is recommended in infants and young children because of its occlusive property. In older children and adults, the ointment may not be tolerated well because of its greasy feel, and another emollient or moisturizer may be chosen based on the patient's preference or experience.

Itch may continue to be a problem even if the rash has improved. The mechanisms of itch in AD are not fully understood but do not appear to be mediated solely by histamine. The use of first-generation antihistamines (diphenhydramine [Benadryl] and hydroxyzine [Vistaril]) in AD largely depend on their sedative

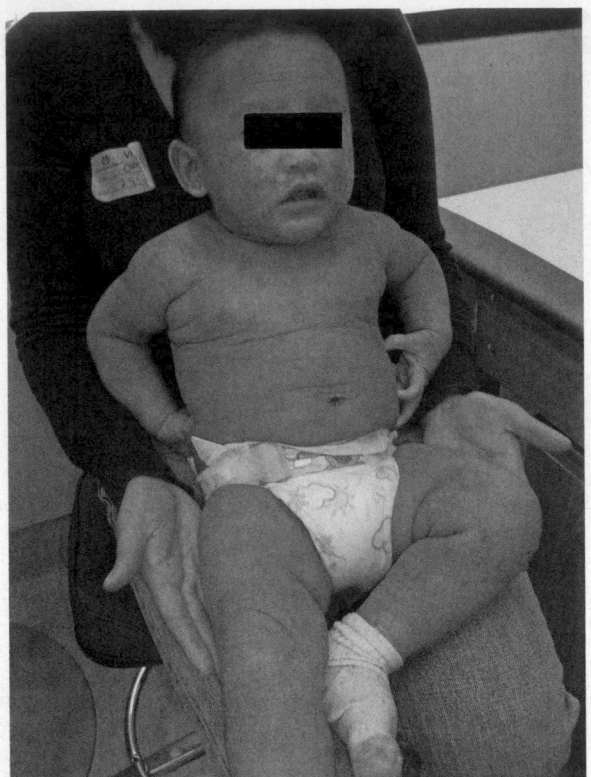

Figure 1. Generalized atopic dermatitis.

effects and are best used at bedtime. The second-generation, nonsedating antihistamines such as loratadine (Claritin)[1] and cetirizine (Zyrtec)[1] have not proved helpful in treating AD. Low-dose Doxepin has been used anecdotally to treat itching in AD.

Topical and Systemic Medications

The first-line medication for AD is a topical corticosteroid (TCS). For mild AD, a TCS with group VI and VII potency (Table 2) may suffice. However, for moderate to severe AD, a TCS with at least group III to V potency is chosen to increase efficacy and to shorten the duration of need for these medications.

The use of TCS is confronted with various obstacles, including rare side effects such as skin atrophy, but mostly patients' or parents' misunderstanding of TCS. Studies have shown that twice-daily use of fluticasone propionate (Cutivate) 0.05% cream (group V) and desonide (DesOwen, Tridesilon) 0.05% ointment or aqueous gel (group V and VI, respectively) continuously up to 1 month in young children with AD results in no significant adverse effect. It is therefore important to clarify for patients or parents the safety and side effects based on the potency of the TCS.

Topical calcineurin inhibitors (TCI) (pimecrolimus [Elidel] 1% cream and Protopic/tacrolimus ointment) are alternative nonsteroidal antiinflammatory medications for AD. Elidel is indicated for mild to moderate AD in patients older than 2 years, whereas 0.03% and 0.1% Protopic are indicated for moderate to severe AD in patients 2 to 15 years old and in patients 16 years old or older, respectively. Both Elidel and Protopic have an FDA black box warning saying that their long-term use may be associated with cancer risk. However, a recent large longitudinal study has failed to confirm this risk. These medications continue to be useful alternatives for skin areas that are prone to atrophy, including the face, axillae, and groins.

A third class of topical medications (so-called barrier creams) emphasize skin barrier repair. These medications include Atopiclair, MimyX, Eletone, and EpiCeram. Only a few studies have compared barrier creams to TCS in AD. Further studies are needed. Barrier creams have no age limitations, but they require a prescription because they have been approved as a medical device by the FDA.

Wet-wrap treatment, phototherapy, and systemic immunosuppressive therapies (e.g., cyclosporine [Sandimmune, Neoral],[1] azathioprine [Imuran],[1] methotrexate [Trexall],[1] and mycophenolate mofetil [CellCept][1]) are reserved for severe AD patients. Because of the potential serious adverse effects associated with these treatments, referral to an allergist or dermatologist is recommended before their initiation.

Systemic corticosteroids usually are not recommended for AD because of their known adverse effects, including stunted growth in children, adrenal suppression, osteoporosis, and cataracts. A rebound of AD symptoms is common after the medication is stopped. If a systemic corticosteroid is used, it should be tapered over a short period (e.g., a week) while topical antiinflammatory treatment is intensified.

The efficacy and side effects of the following medications have not been established in AD: intravenous immunoglobulin (IVIG), anti-IgE (omalizumab [Xolair][1]), probiotics,[7] montelukast (Singulair),[1] Chinese medicinal herbs,[7] and fish oils.[1]

---

[1]Not FDA approved for this indication.

[1]Not FDA approved for this indication.
[7]Available as a dietary supplement.

TABLE 2	Classification of Topical Corticosteroids Based on Potency
GROUP	**TOPICAL CORTICOSTEROIDS**
I (most potent)	Clobetasol propionate 0.05% (Temovate) (cream, ointment, gel), betamethasone dipropionate, augmented 0.05% (Diprolene) (cream, ointment), diflorasone diacetate 0.05% (Psorcon) (ointment)
II	Amcinonide 0.1% (Cyclocort) (ointment), betamethasone dipropionate 0.05% (Diprosone) (ointment), mometasone furoate 0.1% (Elocon) (ointment), halcinonide 0.1% (Halog) (cream), fluocinonide 0.05% (Lidex) (gel, cream, ointment), desoximetasone (Topicort) (0.05% gel, 0.25% cream, 0.25% ointment)
III	Fluticasone propionate 0.005% (Cutivate) (ointment), amcinonide 0.1% (Cyclocort) (lotion, cream), diflorasone diacetate 0.05% (Florone) (cream), betamethasone valerate 0.1% (Valisone) (ointment)
IV	Flurandrenolide 0.05% (Cordran) (ointment), mometasone furoate 0.1% (Elocon) (cream), triamcinolone acetonide 0.1% (Kenalog) (cream), fluocinolone acetonide 0.025% (Synalar) (ointment), hydrocortisone valerate 0.2% (Westcort) (ointment)
V	Flurandrenolide 0.05% (Cordran) (cream), fluticasone propionate 0.05% (Cutivate) (cream), hydrocortisone butyrate 0.1% (Locoid) (cream), fluocinolone acetonide 0.025% (Synalar) (cream), desonide 0.05% (Tridesilon) (ointment), betamethasone valerate 0.1% (Valisone) (cream), hydrocortisone valerate 0.2% (Westcort) (cream), prednicarbate 0.1% (Dermatop) (cream)
VI	Alclometasone dipropionate 0.05% (Aclovate) (cream, ointment), fluocinolone acetonide 0.01% (Synalar) (solution, cream) (Derma-Smoothe/FS Oil), Desonide 0.05% (Tridesilon) (cream and aqueous gel)
VII (least potent)	Hydrocortisone 1%/2.5% (lotion, cream, ointment).

Data from Stoughton RB. Vasoconstrictor assay—specific applications. In Maibach HI, Surber C, editors. Topical Corticosteroids. Basel, Switzerland: Karger, 1992, p 42–53.

Food Allergies

At least 30% of children with moderate to severe AD have one or more food allergies, compared with 4% to 6% of the general population. Accurate diagnosis of food allergies in AD patients is crucial, because it can prevent life-threatening anaphylaxis or unnecessary food restriction.

The diagnosis of food allergy involves one or more of the following: history taking, skin tests, serum-specific IgE tests, and food challenge. History taking is helpful in the diagnosis of food allergy in most patients. It is often useful to begin by asking the patients whether they have any problems or reactions with any of the seven food allergens: milk, egg, peanut, wheat, soybean, seafood, and tree nuts. These foods account for more than 90% of food allergies. Almost all food allergic reactions occur in the first hour. AD patients may complain of immediate worsening of itching after ingestion. Symptoms of anaphylactic reactions include throat-clearing, cough, shortness of breath, vomiting, dizziness, fainting, and headache, which may be attributed to hypotension. Most food allergic reactions also manifest with skin symptoms, including hives, swelling, or generalized itching.

Skin tests are useful in the context of negative test results because they have a negative predictive value of more than 95%. A positive test result has only a 50% positive predictive value.

Quantitative serum-specific IgE antibodies (ImmunoCAP, Phadia) have become useful in the diagnosis of food allergies because of their high positive predictive values (Table 3). These tests are also useful for deciding whether a food challenge is necessary to confirm the diagnosis.

Although history, skin tests, and serum-specific IgE values are useful in the diagnosis of food allergy, a double-blind, placebo-controlled food challenge remains the gold standard in diagnosing food allergy. Food challenge should be done in consultation with an allergist because of the risk of anaphylaxis.

Patients with confirmed food allergy should avoid any amount of the food allergen. Parents or patients should be instructed to read food allergen labels carefully. All packaged foods in the United States are required to label the contents of milk, eggs, peanuts, wheat, soybeans, fish, shellfish, or tree nuts. Organizations, such as the Food Allergy Research & Education, can provide patients and parents with useful information on potential hidden food allergens and alternative food sources.

AD children often have multiple food allergies, including cow's milk and soy, and the use of a hydrolyzed or amino acid–based formula can provide an alternative source of nutrition. For these patients, consultation with a dietitian can be helpful in managing food avoidance and nutrition needs.

Patients or parents of children with anaphylactic reactions should be prescribed and instructed on the use of an epinephrine autoinjector (EpiPen or Auvi-Q 0.15 mg for patients who weigh more than 15 kg but less than 30 kg; 0.3 mg for patients who weigh 30 kg or more).

Withholding highly allergenic foods in early childhood remains controversial. However, a recent study showed that early introduction of peanut in infants with AD and a moderate risk for developing peanut allergy (i.e. peanut prick skin test wheal of equal or less than 4 mm) may decrease the risk of peanut allergy development in these infants.

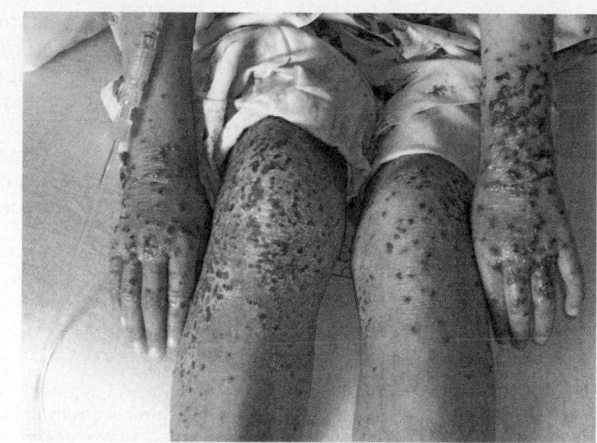

Figure 2. Eczema herpeticum.

Infections

Most AD patients are colonized by *S. aureus* on their skin lesions or in their nostrils. The frequency of colonization increases with AD severity. Exacerbation of AD is frequently associated with secondary *S. aureus* skin infections. Other common skin pathogens in AD include group A β-hemolytic *Streptococcus* and herpes simplex virus (HSV), which causes eczema herpeticum (Figure 2). Many reports have documented invasive *S. aureus* infections such as bacteremia, septic arthritis, osteomyelitis, and endocarditis in AD patients. Persistent fever or focal limb pain should alert the physician to the possibility of these infections.

The reasons for the high rate of bacterial colonization and skin infections in AD are not completely understood. A defective skin barrier and decreased cutaneous innate immunity (i.e., deficiency in natural skin antibiotics) likely contribute to the frequency of skin infections in patients with AD.

Because of the concern about increasing bacterial resistance, antibiotics are not recommended for treating *S. aureus* colonization in patients with AD. Treating AD patients with methicillin-resistant *S. aureus* (MRSA) can be challenging, due to possibly re-colonization from family contacts. Decolonization may be effective but controversial.

Inhalant Allergies and Asthma

Eighty-five percent of AD infants have concurrent respiratory allergies or are at risk for allergic rhinitis or asthma. However, whether inhalant allergens lead to a worsening of AD remains controversial. Randomized, double blind, placebo-controlled studies have shown positive and negative effects of house dust mites (HDM) as a trigger for AD symptoms. Because there is no serious side effect associated with the use of HDM-proof bed and pillow encasings, unless cost is an issue, these encasings are recommended for AD patients with HDM sensitization. Further research is needed to confirm the role of inhalant allergens, including furry pets and pollens, as triggers for AD.

Investigational Treatments for Atopic Dermatitis

Because of the concern about potential side effects associated with existing therapies of AD, several agents are being investigated for the treatment of AD. They include a topical nuclear factor-κB

TABLE 3	Predictability of ImmunoCAP-Specific IgE						
REACTION*	**MILK**	**SOY**	**EGG**	**WHEAT**	**PEANUT**	**FISH**	**TREE NUTS**
Reaction highly probable	>15 kU/L	>60 kU/L	>7 kU/L	>80 kU/L	>14 kU/L	>20 kU/L	>15 kU/L
Reaction highly probable (young children)	>5 kU/L (<1 y)		>2 kU/L (<2 y)				

*Because of their high positive predictive values, quantitative serum-specific IgE antibodies are used in the diagnosis of food allergies.

decoy, phosphodiesterase 4 inhibitors, urocanic acid oxidation products, vitamin B$_{12}$,[1] rose bengal disodium,[1] *Vitreoscilla filiformis*, alefacept (Amevive),[1] and anti-IL-4 receptor antibody (dupilumab).[5] Subcutaneous and sublingual allergen immunotherapy may also be helpful in a subgroup of patients with HDM sensitization. Topical opioid receptor antagonists, systemic chymase inhibitors, and cannabinoid receptor agonists are potential anti-itch medications for AD. Topical capsaicin may be effective in controlling local itching in select AD patients.

---

[1]Not FDA approved for this indication.
[5]Investigational drug in the United States.

References

Beattie PE, Lewis-Jones MS. A comparative study of impairment of quality of life in children with skin disease and children with other chronic childhood diseases. Br J Dermatol 2006;155:145–51.

Du Toit G, Roberts G, Sayre PH, et al. Randomized trial of peanut consumption in infants at risk for peanut allergy. N Engl J Med 2015;372:803–13.

Eichenfield LF, Basu S, Calvarese B, et al. Effect of desonide hydrogel 0.05% on the hypothalamic-pituitary-adrenal axis in pediatric subjects with moderate to severe atopic dermatitis. Pediatr Dermatol 2007;24:289–95.

Elias PM. Barrier-repair therapy for atopic dermatitis: Corrective lipid biochemical therapy. Expert Rev Dermatol 2008;3:441–52.

Faught J, Bierl C, Barton B, Kemp A. Stress in mothers of young children with eczema. Arch Dis Child 2007;92:683–6.

Friedlander SF, Hebert AA, Allen DB. for the Fluticasone Pediatrics Safety Study Group: Safety of fluticasone propionate cream 0.05% for the treatment of severe and extensive atopic dermatitis in children as young as 3 months. J Am Acad Dermatol 2002;46:387–93.

Margolis DJ, Abuabara K, Hoffstad OJ, et al. Association between malignancy and topical use of pimecrolimus. JAMA Dermatol 2015; Epub ahead of print.

Ong PY. New insights in the pathogenesis of atopic dermatitis. Pediatr Res 2014;75:171–5.

Ong PY. Recurrent MRSA infections in atopic dermatitis. J Allergy Clin Immunol Pract 2014;2:396–9.

Ong PY, Leung DYM. Immune dysregulation in atopic dermatitis. Curr Allergy Asthma Rep 2006;6:384–9.

Sampson HA. The evaluation and management of food allergy in atopic dermatitis. Clin Dermatol 2003;21:183–92.

BACTERIAL DISEASES OF THE SKIN

Method of
Dennis L. Stevens, MD, PhD

CURRENT DIAGNOSIS

- Most infections are superficial and local and not associated with systemic toxicity.
- Deeper infections may involve many layers of the soft tissues, including fascia and muscle.
- Systemic toxicity is always present in deeper infections.
- Rapid advancement of the local infection with areas of necrosis indicates more serious infections, including necrotizing and gangrenous processes.
- Streptococci and clostridial microorganisms are the cause of most gangrenous infections.
- Mixed aerobic and anaerobic microflora cause most necrotizing infections.

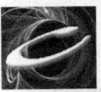

CURRENT THERAPY

- Local care and oral antibiotics chosen for the suspected or culture-proven pathogens are the usual treatment for most limited skin infections.

- Infections that show evidence of rapid advancement associated with bullae, blebs, crepitus, or necrosis require parenterally administered antibiotics and prompt surgical débridement.
- Morbidity and mortality rates associated with the deeper infections increase with delays in antibiotic therapy and surgical débridement.
- Antibiotic therapy should be guided by clinical presentation and changed if necessary when culture and sensitivity studies are available.

The spectrum of bacterial diseases of the skin ranges from superficial, localized, easily recognized, and treated skin eruptions to deep, aggressive, gangrenous, or necrotizing infections that may appear innocuous at first but quickly become life threatening. The prompt recognition and treatment of these infections are paramount in limiting morbidity and mortality. A healthy respect for the aggressiveness of gangrenous and necrotizing infections of the skin and soft tissues is developed by first harboring a high index of suspicion to provide early recognition and appropriate treatment before overwhelming clinical infection occurs.

Common Infections

Impetigo

Impetigo is the most common bacterial infection of the skin. It is highly contagious and can occur at any age from infancy to adulthood, but it is most common in preschool-age children. There are two classic forms of impetigo: nonbullous and bullous. Both forms have a predominantly staphylococcal cause, but they manifest with different morphologic characteristics.

Nonbullous (crusted) impetigo can be recognized by the development of a serous, yellow-brown exudate, which dries into a golden crust. Lesions rarely elicit pain but can be associated with erythema and pruritus. They are most common on exposed areas such as the hands, feet, face, and legs and are often associated with a minor traumatic event such as an insect bite, abrasion, or laceration. Crusted impetigo is usually caused by a heavy mixed flora of staphylococci and streptococci. Streptococcal impetigo has been associated with the postinfectious sequelae of post-streptococcal glomerulonephritis.

The bullous variety usually manifests as a rapidly spreading papule, which may progress to a thin-walled vesicle if the lesion is infected with *Staphylococcus aureus*, an organism that produces an exfoliative toxin. These lesions occur most often in warm, moist areas of the body. Predisposing factors include warm ambient temperatures, humidity, poor hygiene, and crowded living conditions.

Treatment of impetigo begins with eradication or with the environmental factors thought to be influential in its development. Aggressive lesion débridement with mesh gauze sponges or brushes and antibacterial soap is encouraged. Special attention to hygiene and disinfection of towels and bedding are also necessary. Topical antibiotic treatment with mupirocin (Bactroban) or bacitracin[1] has been effective in mild to moderate cases. In more extensive cases, oral antibiotic therapy with a penicillinase-resistant synthetic penicillin (oxacillin) is the treatment of choice (Table 1). However, a high percentage of methicillin-resistant strains of *S. aureus* (MRSA) are isolated in institutional and community settings. Patients should be treated for at least 5 to 7 days. If no improvement is seen, lesions should be cultured and antibiotics adjusted appropriately.

Systemic complications from impetigo are very uncommon. Cellulitis has occurred but is usually susceptible to systemic antibiotic therapy. Septicemia and staphylococcal scaled skin syndrome are rare complications of impetigo. When they occur, systemic therapy is indicated.

---

[1]Not FDA approved for this indication.

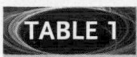 **TABLE 1**	Suggested Antibiotic Therapy for Gram-Positive Bacterial Isolates	

ISZOLATE	ORAL	PARENTERAL
GABHS	Penicillin G or V Erythromycin First-generation cephalosporin	Penicillin G Ampicillin/sulbactam (Unasyn) First-generation cephalosporin
Staphylococcus aureus (methicillin sensitive)	Penicillinase-resistant synthetic penicillin (Oxacillin)	First-generation cephalosporin Clindamycin (Cleocin) Oxacillin
Staphylococcus aureus (methicillin resistant)	Linezolid (Zyvox)	Vancomycin (Vancocin) Daptomycin (Cubicin) Linezolid (Zyvox) Ceftaroline (Teflaro)
Clostridial species	Penicillin G or V Clindamycin (Cleocin) Metronidazole (Flagyl)	Penicillin G Clindamycin Metronidazole

Abbreviation: GABHS — group A β-hemolytic *Streptococcus*.

Folliculitis

Folliculitis is a pyoderma that arises within a hair follicle. The process is known as a furuncle (boil) when the infection extends beyond the hair follicle. These lesions occur most frequently in the moist areas of the body and in areas subject to friction and perspiration. Host factors known to predispose one to folliculitis include obesity, blood dyscrasias, defects in neutrophil function, immune deficiency states (e.g., diabetes, transplantation-related immunosuppression, acquired immunodeficiency syndrome [AIDS]), and treatment with corticosteroids or cytotoxic agents. The offending organism in most immunocompetent patients is *S. aureus*; however, when immunosuppression impairs host defenses, gram-negative organisms (*Klebsiella*, *Enterobacter*, and *Proteus* species) can be involved. *Pseudomonas* species such as *aeruginosa* or *cepacia* are associated with hot-tub folliculitis, which involves numerous hair follicles. It is usually self-limited, resolving in 7 to 10 days.

Successful treatment of folliculitis depends on correcting the predisposing factors that promote the development of this condition. For patients with localized disease, topical wound care including antibiotics such as mupirocin (Bactroban) is effective. Patients with furunculosis or multiple lesions with surrounding erythema of more than 2.5 cm should be treated with orally administered systemic antibiotics that are effective against *S. aureus*. Any fluctuant nodules or abscesses should be incised and drained. Patients with recurrent furunculosis should have their nares cultured for methicillin-susceptible *Staphylococcus aureus* (MSSA) or MRSA because nose rubbing and self-inoculation are the usual means of developing infection. This not only determines which type of *Staphylococcus* is causing the infection, but illustrates to the patient the importance of self-inoculation. Intranasal bacitracin or mupirocin (Bactroban) and daily baths with chlorhexidine (Hibiclens) or hexachlorophene (PHisoHex) (adults only) may break the cycle of nasal colonization and reinfection.

Cellulitis

Cellulitis is an acute infection of the skin and underlying soft tissues. It commonly begins as a hot, red, edematous, sharply defined eruption and may progress to lymphangitis, lymphadenitis, or in severe cases, necrotizing fasciitis and gangrene. Cellulitis usually occurs in local skin trauma caused by insect bites, abrasions, surgical wounds, contusions, or other cutaneous lacerations. Immunosuppressed patients are particularly susceptible to the progression of cellulitis to regional or systemic infections, and these patients should be treated aggressively with systemic antibiotics, drainage, and débridement when indicated. Cellulitis is 20-fold more common in patients with chronic venous stasis or lymphedema. Recurrent cellulitis may occur in patients at the exact site of saphenous donor site surgery.

Initial presentation is that of a rapidly expanding, tender, erythematous, indurated area of skin. An ascending lymphangitis may be present, especially in cellulitis involving an extremity often associated with regional lymphadenopathy. Systemic signs and symptoms can eventually evolve and when present, mandate hospitalization and treatment with systemic antibiotics. Offending organisms are most commonly group A β-hemolytic *Streptococcus* (GABHS) species and *S. aureus*. Cellulitis caused by *S. aureus* usually is associated with localized abscess, furuncles, or carbuncles. In diabetic patients, cellulitis can be caused by group B *Streptococcus*.

Localized processes are treated with oral antibiotics (see Table 1). If fever, septicemia, or other signs of advancement to deeper tissues are present, the patient should be admitted to the hospital for blood and wound cultures, parenteral antibiotics (see Table 1), and observation. If a prompt response is not observed after parenteral antibiotic treatment, surgical exploration of the involved area may be indicated to establish an etiologic diagnosis and rule out the presence of necrotic or gangrenous tissue. Immunosuppressed patients or patients with recurrent cellulitis should be extensively examined to exclude chronic sources of infection, and these patients should be treated with parenteral antibiotics until the cellulitis resolves, followed by 5 to 7 days of oral antibiotics.

Abscess

Local skin signs and symptoms such as pain (dolor), redness (rubor), warmth (calor), and swelling (tumor) often denote an abscess. Loss of function associated with fluctuation may also indicate abscess formation. Localization of purulent fluid necessitates surgical drainage and local wound care. The administration of oral or parenteral antibiotic therapy should not be used routinely after incision and drainage of localized abscesses. They should be administered only when clinically indicated, and antibiotic therapy should be based on culture and sensitivity testing.

Life-Threatening Infections

Group A β-Hemolytic Streptococcal Gangrene

Group A β-hemolytic streptococcal gangrene is an extremely rapidly progressing skin and soft tissue infection commonly caused by *Streptococcus pyogenes*. These organisms secrete hemolysins and streptolysins O and S, which are cardiotoxic, leukocytic, and responsible for the characteristic hemolysis. Gangrene results when the cutaneous blood vessels thrombose, a finding that is often associated with intense local pain. The involved skin is initially erythematous and indurated and quickly evolves to hemorrhagic blebs with focal necrotic zones. The potential for extensive tissue loss and mortality exists, especially if treatment is delayed. Prompt, aggressive tissue débridement and antibiotic therapy are necessary for a favorable outcome (see Table 1).

Synergistic Necrotizing Cellulitis

Synergistic necrotizing cellulitis (SNC) is an extremely aggressive, often lethal, polymicrobial infection of the skin and soft tissues that exhibits progressive invasion superficial to fascial planes. This condition may initially begin as a benign process with scant indication of its impending severity. The initial lesion is typically an erythematous, tender pustule or abscess with a small area of necrosis. The benign appearance of this lesion belies the widespread and aggressive tissue destruction that has occurred beneath it.

Direct inspection through skin incisions reveals extensive gangrene of the superficial tissues and fat that rarely involves the underlying fascia and muscles. These lesions characteristically exude a thin, brown, malodorous discharge, which manifests mixed flora with abundant polymorphonuclear leukocytes with a Gram stain. Crepitus, which is caused by the accumulation of gas in the tissue produced by facultative or obligate anaerobes, can be palpated in 25% of patients, and it mandates immediate surgical attention.

The most common site of involvement is the perineum, which is involved in 50% of patients with SNC. Predisposing factors include perirectal abscess and ischiorectal abscess, both of which may track to the deeper structures of the pelvis, leading to abscess formation and subsequent septicemia. The thigh and leg are involved in approximately 40% of patients. This infection can occur after amputation and is usually associated with diabetes mellitus (75% of cases) or peripheral vascular disease (50% of cases). The relative immunosuppression and poor circulation that accompany these significant causes of morbidity are also responsible for upper extremity and neck SNC, which account for the remaining 10% of cases.

Synergistic necrotizing cellulitis is commonly caused by mixed flora originating in the gastrointestinal tract. Coliforms are the most prevalent aerobes (*Escherichia coli*, *Klebsiella*, *Proteus*), and anaerobic flora include *Bacteroides*, *Peptostreptococcus*, *Clostridium*, and *Fusobacterium*. The primary treatment modality is aggressive débridement of nonviable skin and subcutaneous tissues. This may involve several operations and dressing changes under general anesthesia, which should be performed until all necrotic tissue is removed. Rotation or free myocutaneous flaps and split-thickness skin grafting may cover areas of tissue loss when necessary. If the perineum is involved, fecal diversion by colostomy may be necessary to facilitate healing. Empiric parenteral antibiotics effective against polymicrobial gram-positive and gram-negative aerobic and anaerobic flora are also a mainstay of therapy. However, antibiotic coverage must be modified as soon as culture and susceptibility testing reveal specific offending organisms (Table 2) to reduce the emergence of resistant organisms.

Clostridial Myonecrosis

Clostridial myonecrosis (i.e., gas gangrene) is a destructive infectious process of muscle associated with infections of the skin and soft tissues. It is often associated with local crepitus and systemic signs of toxemia, which are caused by the anaerobic, gas-forming bacilli of the *Clostridium* species. This infection most often occurs after abdominal operations on the gastrointestinal tract; penetrating trauma, such as gunshot wounds, and frostbite can also expose muscle, fascia, and subcutaneous tissues to these organisms. Common to all these conditions is an environment containing tissue necrosis, low oxygen tension, and sufficient amounts of amino acids and calcium to allow germination of clostridial spores and production of the lethal α toxin.

Clostridia are gram-positive, spore-forming, obligate anaerobes that are widely found in soil contaminated with animal excreta. They have also been isolated in the human gastrointestinal tract and skin, most importantly in the perineum and oropharynx. *Clostridium perfringens* is the most common isolate (in 80% of cases) and is among the fastest growing clostridial species, having a generation time under ideal conditions of approximately 16 minutes. This organism produces collagenases and proteases that cause widespread tissue destruction and produces α toxin, which is associated with the high mortality rate of clostridial myonecrosis. The α toxin, a phospholipase C, causes platelet-neutrophil complexes, vascular obstruction, and extensive compromised vascular perfusion, leading to necrosis of the muscle and overlying fascia, skin, and subcutaneous tissues.

Historically, clostridial myonecrosis was a disease associated with battle injuries, but 60% of current cases occur after trauma: 50% after automobile accidents and the remainder after crush injuries, industrial accidents, and gunshot wounds. Mortality can be the result of a failure to recognize that clostridial infection is underway, which leads to a delay in the débridement of devitalized tissues. Patients often complain of a sudden onset of pain at the site of trauma or surgical wound, which increases rapidly in severity and extends beyond the original borders of the wound. The skin initially exhibits tense edema, but its pale appearance progresses to a magenta hue. Hemorrhagic bullae and a thin, watery, foul-smelling discharge are common. A Gram stain examination of wound discharge reveals abundant gram-positive rods with a paucity of leukocytes.

The diagnosis of gas gangrene is based on the appearance of the muscle on direct visualization by surgical exposure, because many changes are not apparent when inspected through a small traumatic wound. Initially, the muscle is pale, edematous, and unresponsive to stimulation. As the disease process continues, the muscle becomes frankly gangrenous, black, and extremely friable. This occurs as a late event and is often accompanied by septicemia and shock. Despite profound hypotension and impending organ failure, these patients may be remarkably alert and extremely sensitive to their surroundings. They feel their impending doom and often panic just before slipping into toxic delirium and eventually into coma.

The clinical features should arouse suspicion early in the course, so the disease can be recognized and treated with aggressive surgical débridement. Gas in the wound is a relatively late finding, and by the time crepitation is observed, the patient may be near death. Approximately 15% of blood cultures are positive, but this is also a late finding. Serum creatinine kinase levels, although relatively nonspecific, are always elevated in cases with muscle involvement.

The mortality rate for gas gangrene is as high as 60%. It is highest in cases involving the abdominal wall and lowest in those affecting the extremities. Among the signs that prognosticate a poor outcome are leukopenia, thrombocytopenia, hemolysis, and severe renal failure. Myoglobinuria is common and can contribute significantly to worsening renal function. Frank hemorrhage may also be present and indicates disseminated intravascular coagulation.

Successful treatment of this life-threatening infection depends on early recognition and débridement of devitalized and infected tissues. Hyperbaric oxygen and systemic antibiotics are important adjuncts. Surgical intervention should include wide débridement of all necrotic tissue and amputation if extremities are involved. Hyperbaric oxygen (100% O_2 at 3 atm) has been reported to reduce associated tissue loss and mortality; however, core treatment is surgical débridement, and it should never be delayed to arrange for hyperbaric oxygen treatments. In animal studies of gas gangrene, hyperbaric oxygen was not efficacious, whereas clindamycin (Cleocin) treatment had dramatic effects in reducing mortality. A parenteral antibiotic is directed toward the offending organism (see Table 1). Clindamycin is the treatment of choice because of its ability to suppress toxin production. Cardiovascular collapse mandates careful monitoring of intravenous fluid resuscitation, which may require large volumes. Failure to adequately

TABLE 2	Suggested Parenteral Antibiotic Therapy for Mixed Infections
ORGANISMS	**PRIMARY CHOICE**
Aerobic (must include an agent effective against anaerobic organisms)	Amikacin (Amikin) Aztreonam (Azactam) Ceftriaxone (Rocephin) Ciprofloxacin (Cipro) Gentamicin (Garamycin) Levofloxacin (Levaquin) Tobramycin (Nebcin)
Anaerobic (must include an agent effective against aerobic organisms)	Clindamycin (Cleocin) Metronidazole (Flagyl)
Aerobic and anaerobic	Ampicillin/sulbactam (Unasyn) Imipenem/cilastatin (Primaxin) Meropenem (Merrem) Piperacillin/tazobactam (Zosyn) Tigecycline (Tygacil)

resuscitate these patients compromises therapy by limiting oxygen delivery and antibiotic distribution to the affected tissues and may promote progression to multisystem organ failure.

A less life-threatening form of this disease is known as clostridial cellulitis. In this process, the bacterial tissue invasion is primarily superficial, extending to the fascial layer without muscle involvement. Prompt recognition and treatment can reduce morbidity and mortality. Spontaneous gas gangrene caused by *Clostridium septicum* can occur in the absence of trauma in patients with gastrointestinal lesions such as carcinoma of the colon.

Necrotizing Fasciitis

Necrotizing fasciitis is an aggressive soft tissue infection involving the fascia with extensive undermining and tracking along anatomic planes. This process usually occurs in patients with significant comorbidity, such as diabetes mellitus or peripheral vascular disease, but it is also seen in obese or malnourished patients and intravenous drug abusers. Cellulitis is a frequent occurrence, and progressive necrosis to subcutaneous tissue results from thrombosis of the perforating vessels. Necrotizing fasciitis can be caused by single organisms such as GABHS and staphylococci (MRSA), *Vibrio vulnificus* or *Aeromonas hydrophila*, or a combination of a variety of organisms, including aerobic streptococci, staphylococci, and coliforms, as well as anaerobic *Peptostreptococcus* and *Bacteroides*. Ninety percent of these infections have a polymicrobial cause, and it is common to culture up to five organisms from the fascial planes involved with this infection.

Polymicrobial necrotizing fasciitis most commonly evolves from a benign-appearing skin lesion (80% of cases). Minor abrasions, insect bites, injection sites, and perirectal abscesses have been implicated. Rare cases have been reported in women with Bartholin's gland abscess, from which the infection has spread to fascial planes of the perineum and thigh. The remaining 20% of patients have no visible skin lesion. Surgical procedures, especially bowel resections, and penetrating trauma can be complicated by superficial wound infections that evolve into necrotizing fasciitis. The infection commonly involves the buttocks and perineum, which results from untreated perirectal abscesses or decubitus ulcers; intravenous drug abusers commonly participate in "skin popping," which leads to infections of the upper extremities.

Fifty percent of group A streptococcal necrotizing fasciitis patients have a portal of entry such as an insect bite, slivers, surgical procedures, or burns, whereas the other 50% have no portal of entry, and the infection begins at the exact site of nonpenetrating trauma, such as a muscle strain or bruise. This idiopathic form, commonly known as spontaneous necrotizing fasciitis, is particularly dangerous because of the frequent delay in diagnosis.

For those with a portal of entry, the initial presentation is a slowly advancing cellulitis that progresses to a firm, tense, woody feel of the subcutaneous tissues. This entity may be distinguished from other aggressive anaerobic soft tissue infections (e.g., SNC) by the brawny, pale, erythematous appearance of the skin overlying subcutaneous tissues that are unyielding, making fascial planes and muscle groups indistinguishable during palpation. Often, a broad, erythematous tract along the route of the underlying fascial plane can be discerned through the skin. If an open wound exists, probing the edges with a blunt instrument permits ready dissection of the superficial fascia well beyond the wound margins, and this is the most important diagnostic feature of necrotizing fasciitis. On direct inspection, the fascia is swollen and dully gray in appearance, with stringy areas of fat necrosis. A thin, brown exudate can be expressed from the wound, but frank purulent drainage is rare. These wounds are remarkably insensate when found and mandate immediate débridement.

As with other gangrenous soft tissue infections, the most important component of the treatment plan is aggressive, total débridement of all devitalized and necrotic tissue. This often necessitates frequent operations and dressing changes. Wide débridement and parenteral antibiotics have a profound effect on survival, and limited or staged débridement has no place in the treatment of this very aggressive, life-threatening infection. Parenteral antibiotics

(see Table 2) should be directed against the polymicrobial aerobic and anaerobic microorganisms isolated from these infections. Every effort should be made to quickly identify the offending organisms, and antibiotic therapy should be changed accordingly.

In patients with no defined portal of entry, severe pain at the site of previous nonpenetrating trauma is common. Early in the course, there may be no cutaneous evidence of infection. Severe pain and fever may be the only presenting symptoms. These patients usually have a slightly elevated white blood cell count with a left shift and an elevated pulse. Later, erythema, induration, and warmth occur and may rapidly progress to violaceous skin, ecchymosis, and blister formation. A markedly elevated creatine phosphokinase level in a patients with any erythematous rash may suggest a necrotizing process. By the time these late cutaneous findings are present, most patients have evidence of shock and organ failure. Misdiagnosis and delay in diagnosis are common and associated with significant morbidity and mortality. Surgical exploration with débridement of infected and necrotic tissue in addition to systemic antibiotic therapy directed toward the aerobic *Streptococcus* organism can result in decreased morbidity and mortality (see Table 1).

Special Circumstances
Fournier's Gangrene

Fournier's gangrene is a necrotizing fasciitis that originates as a necrotic black area on the scrotum of male patients or the labia of female patients, and it most often has a cryptogenic origin. In my experience, Fournier's gangrene occurs more commonly without a predisposing event or after routine, uncomplicated hemorrhoidectomy. Less commonly, this condition has occurred after urologic manipulation or as a late complication of deep anorectal suppuration.

Fournier's gangrene is characterized by necrosis of the skin and soft tissues of the scrotum or perineum and is associated with a fulminant, painful, and severely toxic infection. Definitive diagnosis is made by identification of a necrotic black area on the scrotum associated with local and systemic signs of infection. Left untreated, death ensues from uncontrolled, severe systemic sepsis and multiple-organ failure. Prompt recognition and treatment can minimize tissue loss, especially the skin and soft tissues of the scrotum, labia, and perineum, and may prevent complete loss of genitalia.

The infection is often polymicrobial, as with necrotizing fasciitis, with several species of aerobic and anaerobic bacteria predominating. Successful treatment is based on early recognition and vigorous surgical débridement, occasionally including diversion of the fecal stream. Empiric treatment is appropriate until results of culture and susceptibility testing are available (see Table 2). The therapeutic benefit of hyperbaric oxygen treatments has not been proved, and it should be used only as an adjunct to surgical débridement.

Ecthyma Gangrenosum

Occasionally, hospitalized patients with overwhelming pseudomonal septicemia develop a patchy dermal and subcutaneous necrosis. Although sepsis caused by *Pseudomonas aeruginosa* is often indistinguishable from other types of gram-negative sepsis, a characteristic skin lesion may develop with erythematous macular eruptions that quickly become bullous with central ulceration and necrosis. This lesion may resemble a decubitus ulcer with the characteristic black eschar. There are usually multiple lesions occurring in different stages of development. They may concentrate on the extremities or the gluteal region. These lesions may be distinguished from the lesions of pyoderma gangrenosum (a noninfectious dermatosis) by their association with clinical signs of infection (i.e., fever and leukocytosis) in addition to the isolation of *P. aeruginosa* from culture of the lesion.

Treatment is primarily administration of antimicrobial therapy effective against the *Pseudomonas* organism and by débridement of the multiple lesions. This may lessen the bacterial burden, perhaps allowing greater antibiotic efficacy.

Sea and Freshwater Infections

Infections caused by *V. vulnificus* and *A. hydrophilia* can be extremely aggressive, with necrosis often occurring within hours and necessitating rapid, wide débridement. Although infections caused by these organisms cannot be differentiated from those caused by mixed infections, a history of exposure to sea water (*V. vulnificus*) or fresh water (*A. hydrophila*) and the rapidity with which the infection spreads often suggest the cause of the infection. The antibiotics of choice for *V. vulnificus* infection are doxycycline (Vibramycin) or tetracycline and an aminoglycoside. In patients with impaired renal function, chloramphenicol (Chloromycetin) may be used. *A. hydrophila* is susceptible to cephalosporins such as ceftazidime (Fortaz), cefuroxime (Ceftin), and fluoroquinolones such as levofloxacin (Levaquin) and ciprofloxacin (Cipro).

Conclusions

The many types of soft tissue infections caused by bacteria may be distinguished by their presenting signs, symptoms, and body location and by the time course of the pathologic processes unique to each. Early recognition is of paramount importance to an effective treatment plan, which most often includes aggressive surgical débridement and specific antimicrobial therapy. This approach can often minimize tissue damage and promote recovery.

References

Adinolfi MF, Voros DC, Moustoukas NM, et al. Severe systemic sepsis resulting from neglected perineal infections. South Med J 1983;76:746–9.
Craig ML, Hardin Jr WD, Fox LS, et al. Ecthyma gangrenosum: A deadly complication. Hosp Physician 1987;23:65–71.
Moustoukas NM, Nichols RL, Voros D. Clostridial sepsis: Usual clinical presentations. South Med J 1985;78:440–5.
Nichols RL, Florman S. Clinical presentations of soft-tissue infections and surgical site infections. Clin Infect Dis 2001;33(Suppl. 2):84–93.
Nichols RL. Postoperative infection in the age of drug-resistant gram-positive bacteria [review]. Am J Med 1998;104(Suppl. 5A):11S–16S.
Stevens DL, Bisno DL, Chambers HF, et al. Practice Guidelines for the Diagnosis and Management of Skin and Soft Tissue Infections: 2014 Update by the Infectious Diseases Society of America. Clin Infect Dis 2014;50(2):e10–e52.

BULLOUS DISEASES

Method of
Diya F. Mutasim, MD

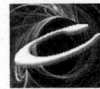

CURRENT DIAGNOSIS

- Clinical
- Histology (always required)
- Direct immunofluorescence (always required)
- Indirect immunofluorescence (sometimes required)
- Antibody specificity for the antigen by enzyme-linked immunosorbent assay (ELISA) (rarely required)

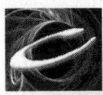

CURRENT THERAPY

- Topical steroids
- Systemic glucocorticoids
- Steroid-sparing (adjuvant) immunosuppressive agents
  - Azathioprine (Imuran)[1]
  - Mycophenolate mofetil (Cellcept)[1]
  - Methotrexate (Trexall)[1]
  - Cyclosporine (Neoral)[1]
  - Cyclophosphamide (Cytoxan)[1]

- Dapsone
- Tetracycline (Sumycin)[1]
- Other
  - Niacinamide, nicotinamide[1]
  - High-dose intravenous immunoglobulin (IVIg) (Gammagard)[1]
  - Rituximab (Rituxan)[1]
  - Plasmapheresis, immunoapheresis

[1]Not FDA approved for this indication.

Epidemiology

The primary lesion in bullous diseases is a vesicle or a bulla. Autoimmune bullous diseases result from immune dysregulation that increases with age, hence the incidence of autoimmune bullous diseases is higher in the elderly. This group of disorders is heterogeneous, and generalizations about the epidemiology cannot be made.

Risk Factors

In general, predisposition to autoimmune bullous diseases is genetic and manifests as loss of tolerance toward self antigens followed by a T-cell and B-cell response resulting in antibody production. Age may be a risk factor in the development of bullous pemphigoid and mucous membrane pemphigoid. Pemphigus vulgaris has a higher incidence among persons of Jewish ancestry.

Pathophysiology

Autoimmune bullous diseases result from an immune response against proteins of desmosomes or the epidermal (or other epithelial) basement membrane. The pemphigus group of diseases is associated with antibodies to different desmosomal proteins. There is strong direct experimental evidence that these antibodies cause acantholysis and blister formation directly without significant participation of cellular components of the immune system. The subepidermal autoimmune bullous diseases, however, result from antibodies against one or more components of the basement membrane that activate the complement system. The latter results in chemoattraction of inflammatory cells, particularly eosinophils and neutrophils, to the basement membrane, as well as activation of local mast cells with degranulation of their cytoplasmic granules, resulting in the release of mediators that further attract inflammatory cells. Both complement and inflammatory cells are required for blister formation. Experimental animals that lack complement or leukocytes fail to develop lesions when injected with patients' serum antibodies.

Prevention

There are no methods for preventing autoimmune bullous diseases. These disorders result from genetically controlled immune dysregulation.

Clinical Manifestations

Clinical manifestations are described for each disease separately under the section on therapy.

Complications

Severe blistering can lead to extensive erosions that heal slowly, especially in the elderly and in those with nutritional deficiencies or systemic disease. Slow healing of extensive erosions predisposes patients to considerable loss of fluids and electrolytes as well as secondary bacterial infection and sepsis. Superficial erosions can become ulcers owing to increased local pressure in immobile and bedridden patients. Temperature regulation can also be compromised following loss of large areas of epidermis. Over the past several decades, mortality from bullous disease has decreased significantly. At present, the common causes of death are complications of the pharmacologic agents used in the treatment.

Diagnosis

The diagnosis of autoimmune bullous diseases requires clinical evaluation, histopathology, direct immunofluorescence, and indirect immunofluorescence. The ideal specimen for direct immunofluorescence should be from normal-appearing skin immediately adjacent to a lesion (perilesional skin). Immunofluorescence tests are usually performed in specialized immunopathology laboratories and are best interpreted by a dermatopathologist with special expertise in the area of immunofluorescence and autoimmune bullous diseases.

Differential Diagnosis

An accurate diagnosis is essential for predicting the course and prognosis of a disease as well as for choosing therapy. Autoimmune bullous diseases overlap clinically and histologically, hence the need for immunofluorescence studies. For example, epidermolysis bullosa acquisita can have clinical and histologic overlap with both bullous pemphigoid and linear IgA disease. The three diseases, however, have different courses and therapeutic responses and may be easily differentiated on the basis of immunofluorescence tests.

Treatment

Principles

Because autoimmune bullous disorders result from immune dysregulation, the principle of treatment is immune modulation. Immune modulation can be accomplished by several methods: blocking antibody production by B cells and plasma cells, eliminating antibodies from the circulation, suppressing inflammation, or inducing resistance of target epithelial cells to separation and blister formation. Antibody production by B cells and plasma cells may be blocked by destroying the B cell lineage or suppressing activation of T or B cells. The former is accomplished by the drug rituximab (Rituxan) and, to a lesser degree, cyclophosphamide (Cytoxan), and the latter may be accomplished by many immunosuppressive agents including corticosteroids, azathioprine (Imuran), cyclosporine (Neoral), cyclophosphamide, methotrexate (Trexall), and mycophenolate mofetil (Cellcept). Antibodies may be eliminated from circulation by plasmapheresis, high-dose intravenous immunoglobulin (IVIg, Gammagard), and immunoadsorption.

Inflammation that is required for blister formation, especially in subepidermal bullous diseases, may be suppressed by several agents. These include systemic and topical corticosteroids, dapsone, tetracyclines, erythromycin, nicotinamide, and etanercept (Enbrel). Although not yet available, agents that experimentally inhibit signal transduction and agents that inhibit apoptosis can induce resistance of the target epidermal or epithelial cell to separation (acantholysis) and blister formation.

The choice of agents in therapy of bullous diseases requires evaluation of both disease-specific parameters and patient-specific parameters. Disease-specific parameters include the pathophysiology of the disease and its severity; patient-specific parameters include age and concomitant illness such as diabetes, hypertension, active infection, or cancer. There are very few controlled studies that provide high-quality evidence for bullous disease therapy. This is primarily a result of the rarity of many of these disorders. Because of the relative frequency of bullous pemphigoid, some controlled studies have been performed on the disease in Europe. Most of the evidence for bullous disease therapy is available from case reports, case series, and personal experience.

Pharmacologic Treatment

Glucocorticoids

Glucocorticoids (prednisone, prednisolone) have both antiinflammatory and immunosuppressive effects. Long-term use of glucocorticoids is associated with well-known adverse effects.

Azathioprine

Azathioprine (Imuran)[1] interferes with de novo purine synthesis and hence DNA synthesis. This results in suppression of T-cell function and a decrease in B-cell antibody production. In low doses (1–2 mg/kg/day), azathioprine is usually well tolerated. In higher doses (2–4 mg/kg/day), bone marrow may be suppressed, resulting in leukopenia (most commonly) and, less commonly, thrombocytopenia and anemia. Severe bone marrow suppression can occur in patients who are homozygous deficient for the enzyme thiopurine methyltransferase. Other adverse effects include hepatotoxicity and gastrointestinal toxicity as well as pancreatitis and are all dose related. Allopurinol (Zyloprim) is contraindicated in patients receiving azathioprine because it results in an increase in the blood level of azathioprine.

Mycophenolate Mofetil

Mycophenolate mofetil[1] is a purine analogue antimetabolite that inhibits inosine monophosphate dehydrogenase, resulting in suppression of purine and DNA synthesis and hence suppression of both T and B cell function. Mycophenolate mofetil is usually well tolerated.

Methotrexate

Methotrexate[1] is an antimetabolite and a folic acid analogue. Its metabolites inhibit folate-dependent enzymes of de novo purine and thymidylate synthesis. This results in the suppression of DNA and RNA synthesis, which causes decreased lymphocyte function and hence immune modulation.

Cyclophosphamide

Cyclophosphamide[1] is an alkylating agent that binds DNA, resulting in cell cycle arrest, DNA repair, and cell death. The most susceptible cells reside in rapidly proliferating tissues. The toxicity of cyclophosphamide is significantly higher than that of azathioprine, mycophenolate mofetil, and methotrexate. Acute myelosuppression is common, with a nadir at 6 to 10 days and recovery in 2 to 3 weeks. Both cellular and humoral immunity are suppressed.

Cyclosporine

Cyclosporine[1] significantly suppresses cellular immunity and preferentially inhibits antigen-triggered signal transduction in T lymphocytes, which results in decreased expression of several lymphokines. Cyclosporine forms complexes with the receptor protein cyclophilin in the cytoplasm. The complex binds and inhibits calcineurin, resulting in failure of T cells to respond to antigenic stimulation.

Several drugs can interact with cyclosporine and influence its blood level. Agents that can increase cyclosporine blood level include calcium channel antagonists (diltiazem [Cardizem], nicardipine [Cardene], and verapamil [Calan]), systemic antifungal agents (fluconazole [Diflucan], itraconazole [Sporanox], and ketoconazole [Nizoral]), antibacterials (clarithromycin [Biaxin], erythromycin), methylprednisolone (Medrol), other drugs (allopurinol [Zyloprim], bromocriptine [Parlodel], danazol [Danocrine], metoclopramide [Reglan], colchicine [Colcrys], and amiodarone [Cordarone]), and grapefruit juice.

Dapsone

Dapsone is highly effective in neutrophil-mediated conditions. The mechanism of action of dapsone is not well understood. Its clinical benefit in inflammatory conditions probably results from inhibition of neutrophil chemotaxis. Dapsone is associated with multiple potential adverse effects that include dose-related hemolysis, methemoglobulinemia (which is common and may be severe in patients who are genetically predisposed), and agranulocytosis (not dose-related and usually occurs in the first 3 months of therapy).

Tetracycline

Tetracycline (Sumycin),[1] doxycycline (Vibramycin),[1] and minocycline (Minocin)[1] have been used interchangeably for the treatment

---

[1]Not FDA approved for this indication.

of subepidermal, inflammation-mediated, bullous diseases. Their mechanism of action is not clear.

Niacinamide (Nicotinamide)
Niacinamide[1] is a vitamin whose mechanism of action in cutaneous disorders including autoimmune bullous diseases is not known.

High-Dose Intravenous Immunoglobulin
IVIg[1] is a purified human source of immunoglobulin that is given as a slow infusion over 6 to 8 hours. Treatment is repeated every 3 to 4 weeks. IVIg is highly expensive.

Rituximab
Rituximab[1] is a chimeric monoclonal antibody against CD20 on the surface of pre-B, mature B, and malignant B cells and is not expressed on stem, pro-B or plasma cells. B cells are depleted primarily by antibody-dependent cellular cytotoxicity and, to a lesser degree, by complement-dependent cytotoxicity or apoptosis. Rituximab is given in different regimens, including 375 mg/m^2/week (approximately 500 mg for an average-size adult) for 4 consecutive weeks, or 1000 mg once or on two occasions 2 weeks apart.

Plasmapheresis and Immunoapheresis
Plasmapheresis and immunoapheresis are procedures that aim to physically remove pathogenic antibodies. Plasmapheresis consists of withdrawing the patient's blood, filtering cellular elements from the plasma, and returning the cellular components to the patient. Immunoapheresis consists of exposing the patient's plasma to an immunoglobulin-binding matrix that contains the disease-specific antigen. Plasmapheresis and immunoapheresis are usually used in patients who are resistant to other therapies. Plasmapheresis or immunoapheresis is accompanied by immunosuppressive drugs to prevent the rebound phenomenon of excessive antibody production.

Treatment of Individual Disorders
Pemphigoid
There are three forms of pemphigoid: bullous pemphigoid (primary skin involvement); mucous membrane pemphigoid (primary mucosal disease), previously referred to as cicatricial pemphigoid; and pemphigoid gestationis (bullous pemphigoid in pregnant women), previously called herpes gestationis. The pemphigoid group of diseases shares the histology of a subepithelial vesicle with usually eosinophil-rich infiltrate, skin-bound IgG and C3 along the basement membrane, and circulating IgG antibodies against two hemidesmosomal proteins of the basement membrane.

Bullous Pemphigoid. Bullous pemphigoid affects primarily persons older than 60 years and is rarely reported in children. Lesions have a predilection for the inner thighs, groin, axillae, neck, and abdomen. The course of bullous pemphigoid is variable. The disease is self-limited within 5 years, and the mortality from the disease is low.

Because blisters in bullous pemphigoid result from an abnormal immune response that is mediated by inflammatory cells, therapy for bullous pemphigoid should suppress inflammation or the immune response. Potent topical steroids may be considered for patients with localized disease. Although potent topical steroids lead to rapid resolution of a lesion at its earliest manifestation, they are impractical for patients with generalized disease because they do not prevent new lesions. Patients with generalized bullous pemphigoid require systemic therapy. Glucocorticoids are the most commonly used agents. Prednisone (or methylprednisolone) is sufficient as the only therapy in most cases. The dose varies between 0.2 and 0.5 mg/kg/day depending on the severity of the

disease, the age of the patient, and the patient's general health status. A clinical response is usually obtained within 1 to 2 weeks and is manifested by healing of existing lesions and cessation of new blister formation. The dose is then gradually decreased by relatively large amounts initially (approximately 10 mg) and smaller amounts (2.5–5 mg) subsequently. If the patient develops a flare of lesions during the tapering phase, the dose may be increased to the previous level or higher and maintained longer before further, slower tapering. In many patients, prednisone may be decreased to 5 mg every day or completely discontinued after 6 months.

For patients who require a high dose of steroid for either clearing or maintenance, adjuvant therapy with another agent should be considered in order to avoid the long-term adverse effects of corticosteroids. These drugs include azathioprine[1] (1–3 mg/kg/day in two equally divided doses), mycophenolate mofetil[1] (1000–3000 mg/day or 40 mg/kg/day in two divided doses), and methotrexate[1] (10–15 mg/week). The dose of the second drug may be decreased a few months after clinical remission, slowly tapered, and ultimately discontinued. Dapsone[1] and sulfapyridine[1] are used less commonly and may be effective. Dapsone may be commenced at 25 to 50 mg/day and increased as needed by 25 mg every week until a beneficial effect is obtained. The maximum dose of dapsone is 250 mg/day.

Plasmapheresis and high-dose IVIg[1] are reserved for more resistant cases. Antibiotics of the tetracycline family as well as erythromycin[1] have been used alone or in combination with niacinamide[1] and have been shown to have some benefit. The dose of tetracycline[1] is 500 mg four times daily and niacinamide 500 mg three times daily. Minocycline[1] or doxycycline[1] in a dose of 100 mg twice daily may be substituted for patients who do not tolerate tetracycline. In my view, a tetracycline with niacinamide is indicated in two situations. In mild cases, the combination alone can lead to a clinical remission. In patients with extensive disease, the addition of this combination to prednisone can have a corticosteroid-sparing effect.

Mucous Membrane Pemphigoid. Therapy for mucous membrane pemphigoid varies with the disease location, extent, and severity. In limited oral disease, local therapy with topical anesthetic agents and topical glucocorticoids in addition to oral hygiene can suffice. The steroid may be applied under occlusion with a prosthetic device or may be injected intralesionally. Patients with extensive oral involvement can require systemic therapy.

Dapsone[1] is effective in some patients with oral mucous membrane pemphigoid. The drug may be started at 50 mg daily and increased gradually. Tetracyclines,[1] with or without niacinamide,[1] may be effective. In patients with severe oral disease and in patients with ocular, pharyngeal, or laryngeal involvement, systemic glucocorticoids, in combination with cyclophosphamide[1] are indicated. In my experience, most patients have an excellent response, with a prolonged remission after treatment with the combination of prednisone (1 mg/kg/day for 6 months) and cyclophosphamide (1–2 mg/kg/day for 18–24 months).

Azathioprine[1] and mycophenolate mofetil[1] are generally less effective but may be used if there are contraindications to steroid or cyclophosphamide use. High-dose IVIg[1] may be used for patients who are refractory to other therapy.

Patients with severe ocular scarring might benefit from cryotherapy ablation of eyelashes. Ocular surgery is contraindicated when the disease is active. Surgical intervention may cause severe flares of the disease.

Epidermolysis Bullosa Acquisita
Unlike bullous pemphigoid and other subepidermal autoimmune bullous diseases, epidermolysis bullosa acquisita is generally resistant to therapy. The disease waxes and wanes, with periods of exacerbation and remission. Trauma contributes to blister formation, especially in the classic form of epidermolysis bullosa

234

---

[1]Not FDA approved for this indication.

---

[1]Not FDA approved for this indication.

acquisita. The inflammatory form of epidermolysis bullosa acquisita responds more easily to therapy than the classic form.

Because of the neutrophil predominance in the inflammatory form, patients might respond to dapsone.[1] The drug may be started at a dose of 50 mg daily and increased by 50 mg every week until clinical remission (usually 100–250 mg). The dose is maintained for several months. If the patient remains in remission, the dose may be decreased slowly and ultimately discontinued. Colchicine[1] 0.6 mg two or three times daily is variably effective. Patients who do not tolerate or do not respond to colchicine and dapsone may be treated with oral glucocorticoids such as prednisone in a dose of 0.5–1 mg/kg/day in divided doses. The response is variable. If there is no response to glucocorticoids or the patient develops adverse effects, cyclosporine[1] 4–6 mg/kg/day may be initiated and is usually associated with a rapid response. Once disease activity is controlled, the dose may be slowly decreased. Cyclosporine should be discontinued if there is no response in a few weeks.

The duration of treatment varies with the course of the disease. The same agents used for the inflammatory form may be used for the classic form. The latter is generally more resistant to treatment. Patients who fail to respond may be treated with immunosuppressive agents such as azathioprine,[1] cyclophosphamide,[1] mycophenolate,[1] or methotrexate[1] in a manner similar to pemphigus vulgaris, bullous pemphigoid, or mucous membrane pemphigoid. Patients who are resistant to these agents may be treated with extracorporeal photochemotherapy or with IVIg[1] alone or in conjunction with plasmapheresis.

Dermatitis Herpetiformis

Dermatitis herpetiformis results from an immune response to gluten and manifests as pruritic papulovesicles over the elbows, knees, buttocks, and scalp. A gluten-free diet is extremely helpful and is often associated with a marked decrease in the requirement for pharmacologic therapy. A strict gluten-free diet can result in complete remission of the disease without requiring dapsone. Reinstitution of gluten-containing diet results in rapid recurrence of the disease.

Many patients find a strict gluten-free diet too restrictive and instead choose pharmacologic therapy. The drug of choice is dapsone. Treatment is initiated with dapsone 50 mg daily and is increased by 25 to 50 mg every week as needed and as tolerated. The average daily maintenance dose is 100 mg. Some patients require slowly increasing doses several years later, likely secondary to increased deposition of IgA in the skin that results in increased disease activity.

In patients who are intolerant or allergic to dapsone, therapy with sulfapyridine may be considered. The initial dose is 500 mg three times daily and may be increased slowly to 2 g three times daily. The response to sulfapyridine is not as predictable as that to dapsone. Patients who are allergic to dapsone often tolerate sulfapyridine.

Patients who are intolerant or allergic to dapsone and sulfapyridine may be treated with colchicine,[1] cholestyramine (Questran),[1] heparin,[1] tetracycline,[1] or nicotinamide.[1] These agents are much less effective than dapsone and sulfapyridine. Topical steroids are only minimally effective.

Linear Immunoglobulin A Disease

Linear IgA disease is mediated by neutrophils and clinically mimics bullous pemphigoid and dermatitis herpetiformis. Dapsone[1] is the first-line agent. The drug may be started at 25 to 50 mg daily and increased by 25 to 50 mg every 1 to 2 weeks until an effective dose is reached. Patients with early disease tend to respond to lower doses of dapsone.

Sulfapyridine[1] is an alternative agent for patients who cannot tolerate dapsone. The starting dose is 500 mg twice daily and may be increased by 1000 mg every 1 to 2 weeks until the disease is adequately controlled. Colchicine[1] 0.6 mg 2–3 times daily may also be used if a patient is allergic to dapsone. Glucocorticoids may be added if patients do not respond completely to these agents.

Tetracyclines in combination with niacinamide[1] have been reported to be effective. The dose of tetracycline[1] is 500 mg 4 times daily. Alternatively, doxycycline[1] or minocycline[1] 100 mg twice daily may be used. The dose of niacinamide is 500 mg three times daily. Cyclosporine[1] or high-dose IVIg[1] may be used in resistant cases.

Pemphigus

Pemphigus Vulgaris. Pemphigus vulgaris often manifests with erosions in the oral cavity that may be followed by skin blisters. Successful therapy suppresses the production of pathogenic autoantibodies. Therefore immunosuppressive drugs are used. A positive clinical response is associated with a decrease in or absence of pathogenic circulating autoantibodies in the serum and then absence of bound autoantibodies in the skin. There has been a dramatic decrease in the mortality of pemphigus vulgaris owing to the increasing availability of immunosuppressive drugs and glucocorticoids, as well as earlier diagnosis and treatment.

Unless there is an absolute contraindication, the initial therapy of pemphigus vulgaris is systemic glucocorticoid. Prednisone is the most commonly used agent. The initial dose is 1 mg/kg/day divided into two or three doses. Most patients obtain remission within 4 to 12 weeks. The dosage is maintained for 6 to 10 weeks, then decreased by 10 to 20 mg every 2 to 4 weeks. If there is no recurrence, the patient is maintained on 5 mg daily or every other day for several years. Pulsed-steroid therapy with intravenous methylprednisolone, 1 g daily for 3 consecutive days, is reserved for severe cases. The goal of this approach is to quickly achieve the immunosuppressive effects of glucocorticoids while avoiding the long-term side effects.

If prednisone fails to induce a remission, or if the patient develops serious adverse effects, adjuvant immunosuppressive drugs should be instituted. My practice is to initiate adjuvant therapy concomitant with steroid therapy to decrease the total dose of glucocorticoid used. The glucocorticoid is tapered rapidly and the patient is maintained on the steroid-sparing agent for 24 to 36 months. The most commonly used steroid-sparing immunosuppressive drugs are azathioprine[1] and mycophenolate mofetil.[1] Cyclophosphamide[1] is used for resistant cases at a dose of 2 to 3 mg/kg/day, azathioprine at a dose of 3 to 5 mg/kg/day, and mycophenolate at a dose of 2 to 3 g daily (or 40 mg/kg/day in two divided doses). Methotrexate[1] may also be used, but it is generally less effective than other treatments.

The response of pemphigus vulgaris to cyclosporine[1] is controversial. High-dose IVIg[1] has a rapid onset of action and appears most effective when used as an adjuvant to conventional therapy, especially as a steroid-sparing agent. Plasmapheresis is used in refractory cases. To avoid the rebound phenomenon (increased production of autoantibodies), immune suppression (usually with cyclophosphamide) is used concomitantly with plasmapheresis. Rituximab[1] has been used successfully in several cases of pemphigus vulgaris and other autoimmune bullous diseases. For resistant cases, extracorporeal photochemotherapy may be considered.

Pemphigus Foliaceous. The principles and practice of managing pemphigus foliaceous are similar to those for pemphigus vulgaris.

Paraneoplastic Pemphigus. Paraneoplastic pemphigus is a unique intraepidermal blistering disease associated with antibodies against a unique set of skin and internal organ antigens. The most common associated neoplasms are lymphoproliferative. The management of paraneoplastic pemphigus consists of the treatment of the underlying neoplasm as well as immune suppression. Surgical excision of benign neoplasms such as thymoma and Castleman's disease can result in clinical and serologic improvement. In patients with malignant neoplasms, treatment of the associated neoplasm might not result in remission. Generally, skin lesions respond more rapidly than mucosal lesions.

Systemic glucocorticoids are often used as the first-line agent in a dose of 1 to 2 mg/kg/day. Patients usually have a partial response

---

[1]Not FDA approved for this indication.

---

[1]Not FDA approved for this indication.

and rarely have complete resolution of lesions. Other immunosuppressive drugs have been used with variable success. These include mycophenolate mofetil,[1] azathioprine,[1] and cyclosporine.[1]

Rituximab[1] has been reported to be effective in a case of paraneoplastic pemphigus associated with CD20-positive follicular lymphoma and in a case of paraneoplastic pemphigus associated with follicular non-Hodgkin's lymphoma. Immunoapheresis has been used successfully occasionally.

---

[1]Not FDA approved for this indication.

References

Bystryn JC, Jiao D, Natow S. Treatment of pemphigus with intravenous immunoglobulin. J Am Acad Dermatol 2002;47:358–63.

Herron MD, Zone JJ. Treatment of dermatitis herpetiformis and linear IgA bullous dermatosis. Dermatol Ther 2002;15:374–81.

Kirtschig G, Middleton P, Hollis S, et al. Interventions for bullous pemphigoid. Cochrane Database Syst Rev 2005;(3):CD002292.

Kirtschig G, Murrell D, Wojnarowska F, Khumalo N. Interventions for mucous membrane pemphigoid and epidermolysis bullosa acquisita. Cochrane Database Syst Rev 2003;(1):CD004056.

Mutasim DF. Treatment considerations while awaiting the ideal bullous pemphigoid trial. Arch Dermatol 2002;138:404.

Mutasim DF. Management of autoimmune bullous diseases: Pharmacology and therapeutics. J Am Acad Dermatol 2004;51:859–77.

Mutasim DF. Autoimmune bullous dermatoses in the elderly: An update on pathophysiology, diagnosis and management. Drugs Aging 2010;7:1–19.

Nousari HC, Sragovich A, Kimyai-Asadi A, et al. Mycophenolate mofetil in autoimmune and inflammatory skin disorders. J Am Acad Dermatol 1999;40:265–8.

Rogers 3rd. RS, Seehafer JR, Perry HO. Treatment of cicatricial (benign mucous membrane) pemphigoid with dapsone. J Am Acad Dermatol 1982;6:215–23.

Wojnarowska F, Kirtschig G, Highet AS, et al. Guidelines for the management of bullous pemphigoid. Br J Dermatol 2002;147:214–21.

CANCER OF THE SKIN

Method of
Bernhard Ortel, MD; and Diana Bolotin, MD, PhD

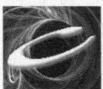

CURRENT DIAGNOSIS

- Skin cancers are polymorphous in appearance, ranging from small papules and plaques to nodules and tumors of different colors, sizes, and consistencies.
- The surface may be smooth, scaly, ulcerated, or crusted.
- A common feature is that all of these skin neoplasms grow continuously and relapse when superficially treated.
- The distinction between skin cancers and benign neoplasms or inflammatory dermatoses may be difficult for the nondermatologist to make.

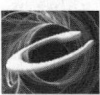

CURRENT THERAPY

- For the majority of nonmelanoma skin cancers, localized treatments are sufficient and include cryotherapy, immunotherapy, topical chemotherapy, and photodynamic therapy.
- Surgical techniques include electrodesiccation and curettage, simple excision, and Mohs' micrographic surgery, which offers intraoperative confirmation of complete tumor removal and maximal cure rates.
- The Mohs procedure is indicated for more-aggressive tumors, for tumors in certain anatomic locations, and in immunosuppressed patients.
- Rarely, sentinel lymph node dissection and adjuvant therapies, such as radiation and chemotherapy, are warranted.

Nonmelanoma skin cancer (NMSC) is a heterogeneous group of skin malignancies that includes basal cell cancer (BCC) and squamous cell cancer (SCC). These are the most common skin cancers and NMSC in the stricter sense of the definition (Figure 1). The more-inclusive use of the term NMSC also includes malignant neoplasms of adnexal, fibrohistiocytic, and vascular origin, as well as Merkel cell carcinoma and metastatic tumors. The vast majority of NMSCs are slowly growing and locally invasive neoplasms that are often diagnosed and treated by dermatologists. Management of the more aggressive tumors often requires a team approach to diagnosis, treatment, and clinical follow-up (Table 1).

Basal Cell Carcinoma

BCC accounts for the majority of NMSC seen in the United States and is increasingly diagnosed in younger patients. Light skin complexion and history of ultraviolet (UV) light exposure are the predominant risk factors for BCC in the majority of the population. Intermittent intense UV light exposures early in life, but not cumulative UV light exposure, pose the highest risk factor for developing BCC later in life. Other risk factors for BCC include exposure to ionizing radiation, psoralen photochemotherapy, arsenic, and smoking. A history of BCC also increases one's risk for developing a subsequent BCC. Immunosuppression, especially in recipients of solid-organ transplants, presents a significant risk factor for BCC. Inherited genodermatoses such as Gorlin's, Bazex's, and Rombo's syndromes, xeroderma pigmentosum, and some forms of albinism are predisposing factors for BCC as well. Mutations in *PTCH1* that are found in Gorlin's syndrome have been shown to be an early event underlying BCC pathogenesis.

Clinically, BCC is most commonly found on the head and neck region, though any part of the body can develop this tumor. The presentation varies depending on the histologic subtype of the tumor. Although many histologic variants of BCC exist, the most common subtypes are superficial, nodular and micronodular, morpheaform, and metatypic. The histologic heterogeneity results in variable clinical findings. Superficial BCC typically forms an erythematous scaly patch or plaque. Nodular BCC is the more classic-appearing lesion, a pink pearly nodule with or without central crust or ulcer. Unlike these subtypes, morpheaform BCC clinically resembles an ill-defined scar; it is the most histologically aggressive variant with a tendency for deep local invasion. Metatypic BCC is also known as basosquamous carcinoma, because it has histologic features of both BCC and SCC, though it is distinguished from the latter by molecular markers. This subtype also has a tendency for more-aggressive growth.

Although it is potentially locally destructive, BCC rarely metastasizes. Successful treatment of this tumor involves its local eradication. A number of treatment options exist and depend on the histologic subtype of the tumor. For small, superficial tumors, a nonsurgical approach can suffice, though nonsurgical treatment often carries a higher risk of recurrence than surgical treatment. Nonsurgical options include topical 5-fluorouracil (Efudex 5%), topical imiquimod (Aldara), liquid nitrogen cryotherapy, photodynamic therapy, and local radiation therapy.

Electrodesiccation and curettage (ED&C) is an option that has a high cure rate for small and superficial tumors (95%–98%). Standard excision with adequate margins is an appropriate surgical treatment providing good cure rates, especially for tumors with nonaggressive histologic pattern. Mohs micrographic surgery (MMS) offers the advantage of precise margin examination during excision and therefore carries the lowest overall rate of recurrence. This tissue-sparing procedure is also advantageous in terms of reconstruction on cosmetically sensitive regions. MMS is indicated to treat recurrent tumors, those in immunosuppressed patients, aggressive histologic variants, and BCCs located on certain areas of the face known to carry a higher risk of recurrence.

Figure 1. Clinical images of skin cancers. **A,** Squamous cell carcinoma in sun-exposed skin of a 102-year-old African American woman. **B,** Depressed scarlike appearance of a morpheiform basal cell carcinoma on the nose. **C,** This firm tumor on the abdomen is a dermatofibrosarcoma protuberans. **D,** Violaceous plaques on the instep in an elderly Greek man typical for endemic Kaposi's sarcoma.

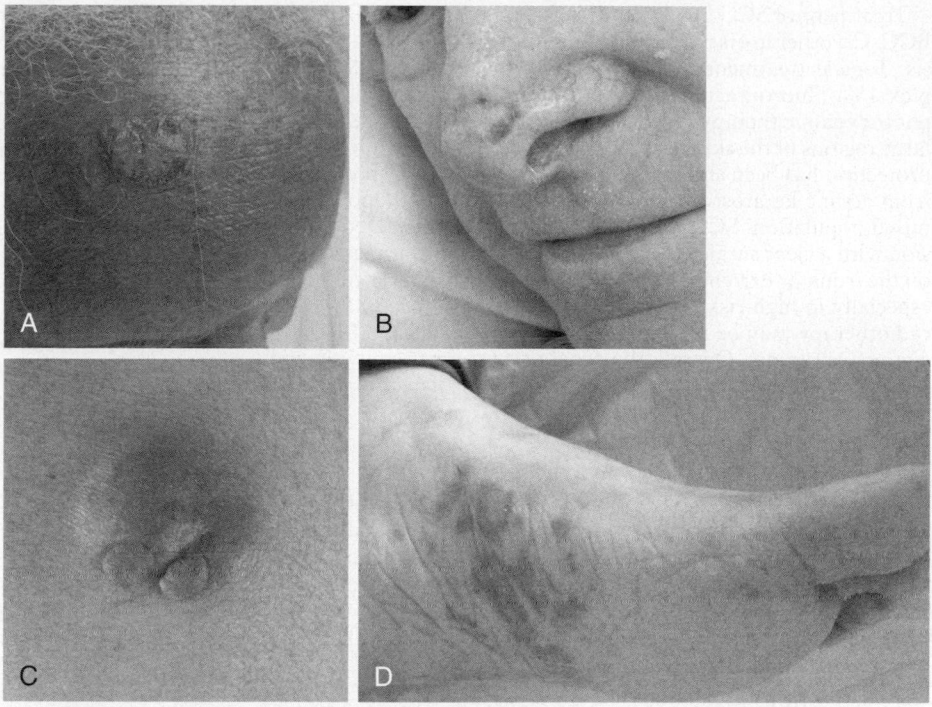

TABLE 1	Overview of Therapeutic Modalities for the Management of Skin Cancers	
THERAPEUTIC MODALITY	**NEOPLASM**	**COMMENT**
Cryotherapy	AK, SCC in situ Superficial BCC Kaposi's sarcoma	Versatile, but operator dependent
Topical 5-fluorouracil (Efudex)	AK, SCC in situ Superficial BCC	Will treat preclinical AK
Topical imiquimod (Aldara)	AK Superficial BCC	Flulike adverse effects can occur
Photodynamic therapy	AK, SCC in situ Superficial BCC	SCC and BCC are off-label uses
Electrodesiccation and curettage	AK, SCC BCC	
Excision	All	
Mohs micrographic surgery	BCC, SCC MAC, sebaceous carcinoma DFSP, AFX Angiosarcoma EMPD, MCC	Preferred for certain types of invasive tumors (e.g., morpheaform BCC), on high-risk regions (e.g., nose, lip), and settings (e.g., recurrence, immunosuppressed patient)
Radiation therapy	BCC, SCC Kaposi's sarcoma, angiosarcoma MCC Inoperable tumors	Careful risk-to-benefit evaluation

Abbreviations: AFX = atypical fibroxanthoma; AK = actinic keratosis; BCC = basal cell carcinoma; DFSP = dermatofibrosarcoma protuberans; EMPD = extramammary Paget's disease; MAC = microcystic adnexal carcinoma; MCC = Merkel cell carcinoma; SCC = squamous cell carcinoma.

Squamous Cell Carcinoma

Cutaneous squamous cell carcinoma (SCC) is the second most common skin malignancy. Its incidence is rising among both men and women in the United States. Development of SCC is intimately linked to the cumulative ultraviolet radiation exposure of the patient via a mechanism that combines DNA damage with immunosuppression. History of ionizing radiation exposure is a risk factor as well. Similar to BCC, occupational exposures such as arsenic can also predispose one to SCC. Patients with xeroderma pigmentosum or oculocutaneous albinism also are at higher risk for SCC.

Chronic inflammation or injury can predispose to epidermal malignant transformation. Examples of this phenomenon are SCC developing within scars from burns, in chronic ulcers and skin overlying osteomyelitis, and in persistent lichen sclerosus or lichen planus. These tumors have a more-aggressive behavior and higher rates of metastasis.

Human papilloma virus (HPV) predisposes to SCC. Verrucous carcinoma, a well-differentiated subtype of SCC, has a well-documented association with HPV types 6 and 11.

Transplant patients are at high risk for SCC that correlates with the degree of immunosuppression. In fact, SCC development is up to 250 times greater in the immunosuppressed compared to the general population, whereas BCC increases to a lesser extent with immunocompromise. A more common association between HPV and SCC has been noted in the immunocompromised population and might account for the disproportional increase of SCC over BCC in this population.

As with BCC, history of previous SCC has been found to be a risk factor for developing a subsequent SCC. This risk appears especially pronounced in smokers.

Unlike BCC, SCC often has a precursor lesion: actinic keratosis. Histologically, actinic keratosis demonstrates partial thickness atypia of the epidermis, and patients often describe it as waxing and waning. Full-thickness histologic atypia is seen in SCC in situ (Bowen's disease), whereas invasive SCC penetrates the basement membrane to invade underlying dermis. Histologically, the degree of differentiation of SCC tends to correlate with its clinical behavior. Well-differentiated lesions tend toward local invasion, as opposed to poorly differentiated SCC, which more commonly is infiltrative.

The typical clinical presentation of SCC is that of a hyperkeratotic pink plaque. More-advanced lesions may be nodular and can ulcerate. In most cases, SCC shows only local invasion; however, perineural invasion and rarely metastasis are more likely with SCC than BCC. The central face, temples, and scalp present high-risk zones for recurrence and metastasis.

Treatment of SCC involves modalities similar to those used for BCC. Cryotherapy is the mainstay of treatment for actinic keratosis. Topical treatment with 5-fluorouracil (Carac 0.5%, Fluoroplex 1%, Fluorouracil 2%, Efudex 5%), imiquimod (Aldara) or photodynamic therapy is often used as field therapy to depopulate large regions of the skin of actinic keratosis lesions. Continued sun protection has been shown to be of benefit to prevent progression from actinic keratosis to SCC, especially in the immunocompromised population. SCC in situ may be treated with ED&C. Excision with a clear surgical margin is often used in treatment of SCC on the trunk or extremities, but MMS yields the highest cure rates, especially in high-risk areas such as the face and scalp. Adjuvant radiotherapy may be used along with surgical excision for more-aggressive tumors. Overall, the prognosis for a patient with cutaneous SCC depends heavily on location, degree of histologic differentiation, invasion, and metastasis.

Neoplasms of Adnexal Origin

The adnexal structures of the skin include the pilosebaceous unit as well as apocrine and eccrine glands and ducts. A great number of benign and malignant tumors of adnexal origin occur in the skin. Most of the adnexal malignancies are rare. Sebaceous carcinoma and microcystic adnexal carcinoma (MAC) are two of the more common adnexal carcinomas that have an aggressive nature and may be subtle at presentation.

Sebaceous Carcinoma

Sebaceous carcinoma is an aggressive malignancy that is most commonly found on the head and neck region. More specifically, it is one of the more common tumors of the eyelid and periocular area. Due to its nonspecific clinical presentation it is often treated as chalazion before biopsy and diagnosis. Population-based risk factors associated with development of sebaceous carcinoma include older age and European ethnicity. History of irradiation and immunosuppression predisposes to sebaceous carcinoma development, similar to BCC and SCC. Sebaceous carcinoma is one of the cutaneous neoplasms characteristic of Muir-Torre syndrome, which results from mutations in DNA mismatch repair genes and is associated with multiple sebaceous neoplasms and internal malignancy.

Clinical diagnosis of sebaceous carcinoma is difficult, and therefore progressive or nonresolving eyelid lesions require biopsy. Treatment of sebaceous carcinoma is primarily surgical. Wide local excision with 5- to 6-mm margins or MMS is indicated. A lower rate of recurrence with MMS (11.1%) has been shown as compared to local excision (32%). Close follow-up is indicated to monitor for recurrence and metastasis.

Microcystic Adnexal Carcinoma

MAC is another adnexal malignancy with predilection for the head and neck. In the United States it is most prevalent in the white population and on the left side of the body, suggesting UV irradiation as a risk factor. Although it can be seen in a wide age range of patients, older patients have a higher risk of developing MAC. The low incidence of this tumor makes it difficult to evaluate other risk factors, though cases have been reported in immunosuppressed patients and those with a history of radiation therapy.

Clinically, MAC occurs as a slowly growing, pink to flesh-colored ill-defined plaque. Paresthesia and/or numbness are common complaints and have been attributed to the high degree of perineural invasion by this tumor. MAC is a locally aggressive tumor with an unpredictable pattern of infiltrative growth. Histologically, MAC exhibits both pilar and sweat duct differentiation, deep invasion with a desmoplastic stromal response, and perineural invasion.

Surgical excision is the standard of care treatment for MAC, and radiation as an adjunct therapy is reported in a few cases. Because this tumor can extend for centimeters subclinically, MMS is favored as the first-line surgical treatment because it allows complete examination of the surgical margins intraoperatively and has been reported to have a lower recurrence rate than standard excision.

Fibrohistiocytic Malignancies

Fibrohistiocytic tumors of the skin are derived from the mesenchymal tissue and range from those of intermediate malignant potential to aggressive pleomorphic sarcomas. Of these overall rare malignancies, dermatofibrosarcoma protuberans (DFSP) and atypical fibroxanthoma are more frequently encountered.

Dermatofibrosarcoma Protuberans

DFSP is the most common fibrohistiocytic malignancy of the skin. It occurs at various ages ranging from infancy to older adulthood. The pathogenesis of DFSP involves a translocation between chromosomes 17 and 22 that fuses the collagen type 1 α1 gene (COL1A1) with the platelet-derived growth factor B-chain gene (PDGFB). This fusion gene results in overexpression of PDGFB, which acts as a potent growth stimulant for mesenchymal cells. In general slowly growing, DFSPs are locally invasive and infiltrative rather than metastatic. Therefore, treatment of this tumor is primarily surgical.

A high recurrence rate has been noted in a number of studies and is attributed to the infiltrative growth of the tumor. MMS reduces recurrence rates, and is often recommended. DFSP is thought to be a radiosensitive tumor, and adjunctive radiation therapy has been successful used both pre- and postoperatively. The discovery of COL1A1-PDGFB fusion has led to trials of imatinib (Gleevec) therapy as an adjunct to surgery for DFSP. So far, a limited number of clinical reports have demonstrated regression of DFSPs during treatment with imatinib. Larger studies and long-term follow-up are needed to determine whether this warrants a change to the current treatment recommendations.

Atypical Fibroxanthoma

Atypical fibroxanthoma is a low-grade sarcoma of the skin. This locally invasive tumor favors sun-damaged skin of the head and neck region in older adults. Patients with xeroderma pigmentosum have a higher risk for developing atypical fibroxanthoma. It has a nonspecific clinical presentation, and a biopsy with histopathology is needed for diagnosis. Histologically, this tumor often exhibits marked pleomorphism and frequent mitoses. Often immunohistochemical staining is necessary for definitive diagnosis. Surgery is the treatment of choice for atypical fibroxanthoma. Either wide local excision or MMS may be used, though lower recurrence rates have been reported with MMS. Despite the pleomorphic microscopic appearance, this tumor rarely metastasizes, and the prognosis with appropriate treatment is favorable.

Vascular Malignancies

Vascular neoplasms of the skin are rare. Kaposi's sarcoma (KS) and angiosarcoma, both increasingly encountered in healthy older adults as well as immunosuppressed patients, are discussed here.

Kaposi's Sarcoma

Controversy exists regarding the nature of cell proliferation seen in KS. Some regard it as a true malignancy, and others view it as a reactive proliferation. Four types of KS exist: KS of elderly men of Jewish and Mediterranean origin, African endemic KS, immunosuppression-associated KS, and AIDS-associated KS. Infection with human herpesvirus 8 (HHV 8) is involved in the pathogenesis of all types of KS. Clinical findings include nonblanching purpuric patches and plaques that can progress to nodules with ulceration. KS can be isolated to the skin or can become disseminated to the lymph nodes and viscera. Diagnosis is established with histopathology and immunostaining. Management of KS is complex owing to the varied clinical course of the four subtypes. In cases of localized lesions, surgery, cryotherapy, or laser treatment may be useful. Radiotherapy can also be used for localized disease. Patients with disseminated KS are generally treated with chemotherapy. In AIDS-associated KS, institution of HIV medications has been shown to effect resolution of KS.

Angiosarcoma

Angiosarcoma is a more rare but aggressive vascular cutaneous malignancy that tends to metastasize and carries a poor prognosis. Clinically, angiosarcoma favors the head and neck area of elderly men; it can also arise within sites of previous radiation therapy or chronic lymphedema. No association between angiosarcoma and HHV 8 has been found. Patients present with an asymptomatic enlarging purpuric plaque that can eventually develop a nodular component. Angiosarcoma may have multifocal involvement that is often not appreciated clinically. The treatment for angiosarcoma involves wide local excision and postoperative radiation. The overall prognosis is poor, and distant metastasis-free 5-year survival rates range between 20% and 37%.

Other Nonmelanoma Skin Cancers

Merkel Cell Carcinoma

Merkel cell carcinoma (MCC) is a rare but often fatal NMSC that derives from cutaneous neuroendocrine cells. Fair skin and a history of exposure to UV light are risk factors for developing MCC. Like many other NMSCs, MCC favors the head and neck and is much more common in the elderly. Immunosuppression appears to be a risk factor for MCC development because its incidence is significantly increased in patients with AIDS and recipients of organ transplants. Polyomavirus has been implicated in the pathogenesis of MCC.

This malignancy is often metastatic upon presentation. Clinically, it occurs as a nonspecific, red asymptomatic papule or nodule. A biopsy with immunohistochemical analysis is diagnostic. The therapy for MCC involves surgery with wide local excision or MMS. Sentinel lymph node biopsy can be performed for staging purposes but should be considered on a case-by-case basis. MCC is sensitive to radiation therapy, which is a recommended adjuvant treatment for patients with lymph node involvement. Palliative chemotherapy often produces a response; however, recurrence is common. Prognosis is poor for metastatic disease or lymph node involvement.

Paget's Disease

Paget's disease refers to intraepidermal spread of adenocarcinoma. Two types are seen in the skin: mammary Paget's disease and extramammary Paget's disease. Mammary Paget's disease is most commonly seen in women and has a strict association with adenocarcinoma of the breast. The lesions are usually unilateral scaly red plaques that favor the nipple. Often the underlying tumor is not clinically present but is detected through imaging. Other dermatoses of the nipple can resemble mammary Paget's disease, and therefore definitive diagnosis requires biopsy and immunohistochemistry. Surgical excision along with appropriate treatment of the breast cancer is the recommended treatment. Prognosis depends on the extent of breast cancer at diagnosis, though it appears to be worse for breast cancer patients with mammary Paget's disease than those without.

Extramammary Paget's disease consists of two types of disease: type I disease, which is associated with distant adenocarcinoma, and type II, primary cutaneous EMPD. Both are very rare but, like mammary Paget's disease, have a female predominance. Most commonly extramammary Paget's disease is found in the genital or perianal region; however, other areas of the skin can be affected less frequently. Clinically, extramammary Paget's disease manifests as a well-demarcated red plaque that can become erosive. Long-standing disease can spread from the groin to the trunk, mimicking an inflammatory dermatosis. Definitive diagnosis is based on biopsy findings, and further work-up includes extensive screening for associated internal malignancy. Treatment relies on surgical excision with wide margins. MMS can be used to examine margins intraoperatively. Prognosis for type I extramammary Paget's disease depends on the extent of underlying tumor, but that for type II is favorable.

Cutaneous Metastases

Metastasis to the skin often heralds the systemic spread of an internal malignancy. Primary malignancy underlying the skin metastasis tends to differ by sex and age. In men, lung cancer is the most common source of skin metastasis, whereas breast cancer is the more common primary tumor in women. The head and neck are favored as sites of skin metastasis in men but the trunk is favored in women.

The clinical presentation of skin metastasis is varied and often nonspecific. A new, asymptomatic cutaneous or subcutaneous nodule may be the reason for a biopsy that reveals metastasis of an unknown primary tumor. Diagnosis is made by histopathology and appropriate molecular staining. Specific clinical patterns of metastasis may be encountered. Inflammatory carcinoma can be seen with cutaneous breast cancer metastases. Occasionally, neoplastic infiltration leads to localized areas of alopecia. Zosteriform distribution of skin metastasis has been reported with breast, colon, or squamous cell cancer.

Leukemia cutis refers to skin involvement with acute myelogenous leukemia, chronic myelogenous leukemia, myelodysplastic syndromes, chronic lymphocytic leukemia, or adult T-cell lymphoproliferative diseases. In rare cases, skin involvement precedes bone marrow disease and is termed *aleukemic leukemia cutis*. In chronic leukemias, skin involvement tends to predict disease progression into the acute phase. Children appear to have a higher incidence of leukemia cutis as compared to adults but have a better overall prognosis.

Metastatic skin tumors are distinguished from primary cutaneous malignancies histologically. Treatment is always geared toward the primary malignancy. Regardless of type of neoplasm or site of metastasis, spread of an internal malignancy to the skin carries a poor prognosis.

References

Alam M, Ratner D. Cutaneous squamous-cell carcinoma. N Engl J Med 2001;344 (13):975–83.

Billings SD, Folpe AL. Cutaneous and subcutaneous fibrohistiocytic tumors of intermediate malignancy: An update. Am J Dermatopathol 2004;26(2):141–55.

Buitrago W, Joseph AK. Sebaceous carcinoma: The great masquerader: Emerging concepts in diagnosis and treatment. Dermatol Ther 2008;21(6):459–66.

Cho-Vega JH, Medeiros LJ, Prieto VG, Vega F. Leukemia cutis. Am J Clin Pathol 2008;129(1):130–42.

Christenson LJ, Borrowman TA, Vachon CM, et al. Incidence of basal cell and squamous cell carcinomas in a population younger than 40 years. JAMA 2005;294 (6):681–90.

Cumberland L, Dana A, Liegeois N. Mohs micrographic surgery for the management of nonmelanoma skin cancers. Facial Plast Surg Clin North Am 2009;17 (3):325–35.

Dasgupta T, Wilson LD, Yu JB. A retrospective review of 1349 cases of sebaceous carcinoma. Cancer 2009;115(1):158–65.

Dubina M, Goldenberg G. Viral-associated nonmelanoma skin cancers: A review. Am J Dermatopathol 2009;31(6):561–73.

Eisen DB, Michael DJ. Sebaceous lesions and their associated syndromes: Part I. J Am Acad Dermatol 2009;61(4):549–60.

Fan H, Oro AE, Scott MP, Khavari PA. Induction of basal cell carcinoma features in transgenic human skin expressing Sonic Hedgehog. Nat Med 1997;3(7):788–92.

Feng H, Shuda M, Chang Y, Moore PS. Clonal integration of a polyomavirus in human Merkel cell carcinoma. Science 2008;319(5866):1096–100.

Hussein MR. Skin metastasis: A pathologist's perspective. J Cutan Pathol 2010;37(9): e1–320.

Kamino H, Jacobson M. Dermatofibroma extending into the subcutaneous tissue. Differential diagnosis from dermatofibrosarcoma protuberans. Am J Surg Pathol 1990;14(12):1156–64.

Kanitakis J. Mammary and extramammary Paget's disease. J Eur Acad Dermatol Venereol 2007;21(5):581–90.

Karagas MR, Stukel TA, Greenberg ER, et al. Risk of subsequent basal cell carcinoma and squamous cell carcinoma of the skin among patients with prior skin cancer. Skin Cancer Prevention Study Group. JAMA 1992;267(24):3305–10.

Lee DA, Miller SJ. Nonmelanoma skin cancer. Facial Plast Surg Clin North Am 2009;17(3):309–24.

Lehmann P. Methyl aminolaevulinate-photodynamic therapy: a review of clinical trials in the treatment of actinic keratoses and nonmelanoma skin cancer. Br J Dermatol 2007;156(5):793–801.

Lemm D, Mugge LO, Mentzel T, Hoffken K. Current treatment options in dermatofibrosarcoma protuberans. J Cancer Res Clin Oncol 2009;135(5):653–65.

Maddox JS, Soltani K. Risk of nonmelanoma skin cancer with azathioprine use. Inflamm Bowel Dis 2008;14(10):1425–31.

Marcet S. Atypical fibroxanthoma/malignant fibrous histiocytoma. Dermatol Ther 2008;21(6):424–7.

McGuire JF, Ge NN, Dyson S. Nonmelanoma skin cancer of the head and neck. I: Histopathology and clinical behavior. Am J Otolaryngol 2009;30(2):121–33.

Mendenhall WM, Mendenhall CM, Werning JW, et al. Cutaneous angiosarcoma. Am J Clin Oncol 2006;29(5):524–8.

Prieto VG, Shea CR. Selected cutaneous vascular neoplasms. A review. Dermatol Clin 1999;17(3):507–20, viii.

Rockville Merkel Cell Carcinoma Group. Merkel cell carcinoma: Recent progress and current priorities on etiology, pathogenesis, and clinical management. J Clin Oncol 2009;27(24):4021–6.

Rubin AI, Chen EH, Ratner D. Basal-cell carcinoma. N Engl J Med 2005;353 (21):2262–9.

Schwartz RA, Micali G, Nasca MR, Scuderi L. Kaposi sarcoma: a continuing conundrum. J Am Acad Dermatol 2008;59(2):179–206.

Smeets NW, Krekels GA, Ostertag JU, et al. Surgical excision vs Mohs' micrographic surgery for basal-cell carcinoma of the face: Randomised controlled trial. Lancet 2004;364(9447):1766–72.

Spencer JM, Nossa R, Tse DT, Sequeira M. Sebaceous carcinoma of the eyelid treated with Mohs micrographic surgery. J Am Acad Dermatol 2001;44(6):1004–9.

Ulrich C, Jurgensen JS, Degen A, et al. Prevention of non-melanoma skin cancer in organ transplant patients by regular use of a sunscreen: A 24 months, prospective, case-control study. Br J Dermatol 2009;161(Suppl. 3):78–84.

Wetter R, Goldstein GD. Microcystic adnexal carcinoma: a diagnostic and therapeutic challenge. Dermatol Ther 2008;21(6):452–8.

Yu JB, Blitzblau RC, Patel SC, et al. Surveillance, Epidemiology, and End Results (SEER) Database analysis of microcystic adnexal carcinoma (sclerosing sweat duct carcinoma) of the skin. Am J Clin Oncol 2010;33(2):125–7.

CONTACT DERMATITIS

Method of
James A. Yiannias, MD; and Genevieve L. Egnatios, MD

CURRENT DIAGNOSIS

- Gather a Detailed History on Skin Exposures, Including the Use of These Items:
  - Irritants
  - Alkalis: soaps, detergents, cleansers
  - Acids
  - Hydrocarbons: petroleum, oils
  - Solvents
  - Allergens
  - Nickel sulfate
  - Balsam of Peru (fragrance)
  - Fragrance mix
  - Quaternium-15 (formaldehyde-releasing preservative)
  - Neomycin
  - Bacitracin
  - Formaldehyde
  - Cobalt chloride (metals, personal products)
- Examine the Skin for the Location and Pattern of Eruption:
  - Eyelid: nail polish
  - Postauricular scalp: perfume
  - Perioral area: chewing gum, toothpaste
  - Trunk: dyes, clothing finish
  - Wrist: nickel, chrome
  - Waistline: rubber
  - Feet: shoes
  - Wounds: topical antibiotic ointment
- Perform Patch Testing:
  - TRUE test with 35 allergens (note: one common allergen, benzalkonium chloride, is not included in this panel)
  - Customized series with 70 or more allergens

CURRENT THERAPY

- Avoid irritants and allergens, using the prepared patient handout.
- Consult the SkinSAFE shopping list of skin-care products free of top 10 most common allergens (if patch testing is not performed).

- Consult a customized SkinSAFE shopping list of skin-care products free of the patient's contact allergens, based on patch test results.
- Topical corticosteroids can be applied.
- Hydrocortisone 2.5% (Hytone) can be applied twice daily on the face, neck, axillae, groin, and intertriginous areas.
- Triamcinolone 0.1% (Kenalog) can be applied twice daily on the body.
- For severe reactions, short-term, higher-potency steroids can be taken (e.g., clobetasol [Clobex] 0.05% twice daily).
- Sedating antihistamines can be taken: doxepin (Sinequan)[1] 10 to 20 mg nightly 2 hours before bed.
- Steroid-sparing topical agents can be applied: tacrolimus 0.1% (Protopic), pimecrolimus 1% (Elidel).
- For severe, acute episodes, systemic corticosteroids can be taken in a several-week, tapering course (e.g., prednisone 60 mg for 5 days, 40 mg for 5 days, and 20 mg for 5 days).
- Longer-term systemic therapy is possible for severe or recalcitrant disease.
- Phototherapy is suggested, with narrowband ultraviolet B.
- Azathioprine (Imuran)[1] can be taken 1 to 3 mg/kg daily.
- Mycophenolate mofetil (CellCept)[1] can be taken 2 to 3 g daily.
- Methotrexate[1] can be taken 10 to 25 mg weekly.
- Cyclosporine (Neoral)[1] can be taken 2.5 to 5 mg/kg daily.

[1]Not FDA approved for this indication.

Dermatitis typically manifests as papules and vesicles with weeping and oozing that can become lichenified and scaly when chronic. When this clinical picture is secondary to an exogenous substance coming into contact with the skin, it is termed *contact dermatitis*. Further delineation leads to irritant versus allergic contact dermatitis, although in practice these often overlap.

Irritant contact dermatitis is not an allergic process. It represents damage to the skin from repeated and cumulative exposure to an agent. Irritants do not require prior sensitization. A decreased barrier function of the skin—for example, with frequent hand washing—can predispose or exacerbate the condition. Examples include alkalis (in soaps, detergents, and cleansers), acids (in germicides, dyes, and pigments), hydrocarbons (in petroleum and oils), and solvents.

Allergic contact dermatitis is an immunologic process classified as a type IV cell-mediated delayed hypersensitivity reaction. Poison ivy is a classic example. It requires an initial exposure to the contactant in which sensitization occurs but without outward physical effect. Subsequent exposure can elicit a striking response that is independent of the amount of the contactant.

From 1994 to 2010, the most common contact allergens have changed very little. Based on studies performed by the North American Contact Dermatitis Group (NACDG) and the Mayo Clinic Contact Dermatitis Group (MCCDG), the allergens most consistently in the top 10 were nickel sulfate, balsam of Peru, fragrance mix, quaternium-15, neomycin, bacitracin, formaldehyde, and cobalt chloride (Box 1). Common sources of exposure to nickel include costume jewelry, snaps, zippers, and other metal objects. Balsam of Peru and fragrance mix are markers for fragrance sensitivity. Sources of exposure to formaldehyde include skin-care products, household products, and the resins in plastics and clothing. Quaternium-15 is a formaldehyde-releasing preservative and may be found in items such as skin-care products, paper, inks, and photocopier toner. Neomycin and bacitracin are topical antibiotics available alone and in combination with polymyxin (Neosporin), antifungals, and corticosteroids. Cobalt is found with other metals, including zinc, and in items such as jewelry, crayons, hair dye, and antiperspirants.

Others less consistently in the top 10 during that period were methyldibromo glutaronitrile, gold sodium thiosulfate, potassium dichromate, benzalkonium chloride, p-phenylenediamine, and thiuram mix. Methyldibromo glutaronitrile is a preservative and

Box 1 Top 10 Most Common Allergens

North American Contact Dermatitis Group
- Nickel sulfate
- Neomycin
- Fragrance mix I
- Bacitracin
- Balsam of Peru
- Cobalt chloride
- Formaldehyde
- Quaternium-15
- p-Phenylenediamine
- Fragrance mix II

Mayo Clinic Contact Dermatitis Group
- Gold sodium thiosulfate
- Nickel sulfate
- Balsam of Peru
- Cobalt
- Fragrance mix
- Quaternium-15
- Benzalkonium chloride
- Formaldehyde
- Potassium dichromate

From Warshaw and colleagues (2013) and Wentworth and colleagues (2014).

can be found in health-care and personal products. Clinically relevant sources of gold may be found in jewelry and dental appliances. Potassium dichromate is used in cement, leather, and steel surfaces. Benzalkonium chloride is commonly used in the health-care field as a cleanser, antiseptic, and preservative but is also found in personal-care products such as wipes and medications. Permanent hair dyes are the usual source of p-phenylenediamine. Thiuram mix is in rubber and some personal products.

Each year since 2000, the American Contact Dermatitis Society has designated an allergen of the year, designed to spotlight allergens, common or not, that are rising in significance. In 2015, formaldehyde was chosen. Benzophenones, such as oxybenzone, are chemical ultraviolet light filters that are found in sunscreens and personal-care products. Other designated allergens of the year have been benzophenones, methylisothiazolinone (MI), acrylates, dimethyl fumarate, neomycin, mixed dialkyl thioureas, nickel, fragrance, p-phenylenediamine, corticosteroids, cocamidopropyl betaine, bacitracin, thimerosal, gold, and disperse blue. MI is a common preservative found in personal-care products often in combination with methylchloroisothiazolinone (MCI/MI), although more recently it has become prevalent as a sole agent. Artificial nails, dentures, and bone cement contain acrylates, but these substances are only allergenic when in the liquid, powder, or paste forms. Dimethyl fumarate is a biocide in furniture, shoes, and textiles. It is often placed in little paper packets with these items. Rubber products and shoe glue are common sources of mixed dialkyl thioureas. Shampoos often contain cocamidopropyl betaine as a lathering agent. Thimerosal is a preservative for medications and personal-care products, including contact lens solution. Disperse blue is a fabric dye. Patients with an allergy to disperse dyes may also react to p-phenylenediamine.

Diagnosis

The evaluation of a patient with suspected contact dermatitis begins with the history. Specific questions directed at the patient's occupation, hobbies, and home routine will be helpful. Examination should note the location and pattern of the eruption. Although eyelid dermatitis may be seen in the atopic patient, nail polish may be the source of the offending allergen. Dyshidrotic eczema occurs as vesicles along the lateral aspects of the fingers, whereas eczematous changes along the dorsal hands are more commonly due to an allergen. Other distributions as clues include postauricular scalp (perfume), perioral area (chewing gum, toothpaste), trunk (dyes or clothing finish), wrist (nickel or chrome), waistline (rubber), feet (shoes), and history or presence of wounds (topical antibiotic ointment).

Patch testing can confirm or reveal a contact allergy. It involves placement of allergens against the skin of the patient's back for 48 hours. An initial reading is then done, with follow-up readings typically at 96 hours. Prepared series include the thin-layer, rapid-use epicutaneous test (TRUE test), which consists of 35 allergens and 1 negative control (www.truetest.com); customized series, such as the NACDG Standard Series with 70 allergens and the Mayo Clinic's Standard Series with 73 allergens, must be manually assembled. The majority of dermatologists performing patch testing use the TRUE test. Note that benzalkonium chloride is not included in that panel.

In addition to ascertaining degree of positivity, relevance must be determined. This involves collaborating with patients to assess the likelihood that they are currently exposed to the positive antigen.

Treatment

Ideally, the allergen(s) will be identified and avoided. Realistically, compliance is a challenge. To assist patients in avoiding antigens in skin-care products, SkinSafe (formerly known as Contact Allergen Replacement Database [CARD] was created in 1999. It includes approximately 11,997 ingredients and 5177 individual over-the-counter and prescription skin-care products. Once the patient's allergens have been identified with patch testing, they can be entered into the database, and a list of products free of those substances is generated. The patient should be reminded that even small and infrequent exposures can perpetuate the eczema.

Topical corticosteroids applied twice daily are helpful in hastening resolution and may also be used for disease control when the allergen is unknown. Low-potency corticosteroids such as 2.5% hydrocortisone (Hytone) are recommended for the thinner skin of the face, neck, axillae, groin, and intertriginous areas. Mid-potency steroids such as triamcinolone 0.1% (Kenalog, Kenonel) are appropriate for the thicker skin of the body. Short-term use of higher-potency steroids may be necessary if the reaction is severe. If there is significant pruritus, sedating antihistamines such as doxepin (Sinequan)[1] 10 to 20 mg taken nightly 2 hours before bedtime can provide relief. Steroid-sparing topical immunosuppressants such as tacrolimus (Protopic) and pimecrolimus (Elidel) may be helpful adjuncts. Treatment for severe acute episodes can entail a several-week tapering course of systemic corticosteroids, especially if the eruption is widespread. Other longer-term systemic therapies for severe or resistant disease include phototherapy or systemic immunosuppressants such as azathioprine (Imuran),[1] mycophenolate mofetil (Cellcept),[1] methotrexate,[1] or cyclosporine (Neoral).[1]

It may take many weeks before the skin reverts to a normal appearance despite successful avoidance of antigens. A prepared handout with concrete recommendations for the patient on truly hypoallergenic skin care is beneficial. A sample of that used at Mayo Clinic Arizona is shown in Figure 1.

If patch testing is not performed, an initial approach may be to instruct the patient on avoiding the most common contact allergens via such a handout and prescribing symptomatic treatment including topical and oral therapies. SkinSAFE can generate a shopping list of products free of the top 10 allergens as identified by the NACDG and the MCCDG. Patients may access SkinSAFE independently (at www.SkinSAFE.com or at Apple's App Store under "SkinSAFE") to generate this list or build customized lists free of fragrances and common preservatives. In 35% of patients, only using products free of the top 10 allergens can prompt clearance. Some physicians follow these measures for several months, especially if the eruption is mild, before pursuing formal patch testing.

An excellent primer for the physician interested in learning more about contact allergy diagnosis and management is *Contact and Occupational Dermatology.*

---

[1]Not FDA approved for this indication.

Introduction

Eczema, also known as dermatitis, is an inflammation of the skin due to dryness, irritation, or possible external allergy. Eczema/dermatitis is not contagious.

Some skin care products contain fragrance even though the package says "fragrance free" or "unscented." Therefore, please choose the skin care products as listed below by their *exact brand name*.

Suggestions

Soaps/Cleansing

- Vanicream® cleansing bar
- Free and Clear® liquid cleanser
- Aveeno® moisturizing bar for dry skin fragrance Free or Aveeno® advanced care body wash
- Oilatum® unscented soap
- Neutrogena® original formula fragrance-free (bar or liquid)
- *Any of the shampoos listed in this brochure may be used as your hand or body soap.*
- Vanicream® shave cream for sensitive skin

Moisturizers

- Vanicream®, Vanicream® Lite
- Aveeno® daily moisturizing lotion fragrance Free
- Plain Vaseline®, Vaniply®
- DML® unscented
- Use moisturizers twice daily.
- All of the above are OK to use on the face.
- After showering, blot excess water with hands and apply cream. Do not use a towel to dry.
- Robathol® bath oil

Deodorants

- Almay® unscented antiperspirants
- Plain cornstarch from the grocer can be used.

Shampoo

- Free and Clear® shampoo and conditioner
- DHS® clear shampoo and DHS® conditioner
- If you have dandruff, use DHS® sal shampoo or Neutrogena® T-SAL shampoo (not T-Gel).
- Conditioners can be used as "leave on" hair gel.

Hairspray

- Fragrance-free hairspray such as Free and Clear® hairspray
- Caution: Hairsprays labeled as "unscented" may not be fragrance free.

Laundry and Home Care

- Unscented laundry detergents (Tide® free, Cheer® free and gentle, All ® free clear, Arm & Hammer® unscented, Wisk ® free, Purex ® unscented)
- Wash all new clothes and linens five times before using.
- Old clothes and fabrics are preferred.
- Use white vinegar in rinse cycle to help remove soap.

Hand, Nail, and General Skin Care Tips

- Wear cotton gloves under rubber/vinyl gloves for any activities where hand-wetting is expected.
- Trim nails short. Long nails are dangerous to skin, especially when sleeping.

Sunscreens

- Vanicream® sunscreen #30 or #60

Make-ups/cosmetics

- If you would like a list of make-ups and cosmetics that are free of the most common allergy-causing ingredients, ask your provider about a "virtual patch testing" printout from our Mayo CARD program.

Avoid

Soaps/Cleansing

- No hot water (use lukewarm).
- Avoid hot tubs.
- No rubbing alcohol.

Moisturizers

- No creams, lotions, oils or powders other than those recommended in this brochure.
- No Neosporin®, triple antibiotic, or bacitracin antibiotic ointments.

Fragrances

- No perfumes, colognes, after shave, or pre-shave on any part of body/clothing.

Laundry and Home Care

- No fabric softener in washer.
- Bounce® unscented fabric softener sheets in dryer if desired.
- No washing machine water softener such as Calgon® (in-house water softeners are acceptable).
- White vinegar may be used as a general household cleaner.

Hand, Nail, and General Skin Care Tips

- No wetting of hands more than five times a day.
- Avoid tight-fitting clothes unless your doctor has advised you to wear a pressure garment such as support hose.
- No scrubbing! No loofah! No pumice stone!
- Do not pull off dead skin. Snip with scissors instead.

Figure 1. Sample of prepared handout (used at Mayo Clinic Arizona) with recommendations for the patient on hypoallergenic skin-care products.

References

Bruze M, Zimerson E. Dimethyl fumarate. Dermatitis 2011;22:3–7.

Castanedo-Tardana MP, Zug KA. Methylisothiazolinone. Dermatitis 2013;24:2–6. http://dx.doi.org/10.1097/DER.0b013e31827edc73.

Heurung AR, Raju SI, Warshaw EM. Benzophenones. Dermatitis 2014;25:3–10. http://dx.doi.org/10.1097/DER.0000000000000025.

Macneil JS: Henna tattoo ingredient is allergen of the year. Skin & Allergy News. March 1, 2006. Available at http://www.skinandallergynews.com/index.php?id=372&cHash=071010&tx_ttnews%5Btt_news%5D=559 (accessed February 12, 2014).

Marks JG, Elsner P, DeLeo VA. Contact and Occupational Dermatology. 3rd ed. St. Louis: Mosby; 2002.

Nelson SA, Yiannias JA. Relevance and avoidance of skin-care product allergens: Pearls and pitfalls. Dermatol Clin 2009;27:329–36.

Sasseville D. Acrylates. Dermatitis 2012;23:3–5. http://dx.doi.org/10.1097/DER.0b013e31823d5cd8.

Thin-layer rapid-use epicutaneous test (TRUE-test). Available at http://www.truetest.com/9.1%20TT%20QandA_FNL_2013.pdf (accessed May 02, 2014).

Warshaw EM, Belsito DV, Taylor JS, et al. North American Contact Dermatitis Group patch test results: 2009 to 2010. Dermatitis 2013;24:50–9.

Wentworth AB, Yiannias JA, Keeling JH, et al. Trends in patch test results and allergen changes in the standard series: A Mayo Clinic 5-year retrospective review. January 1, 2006, through December 31, 2010, J Am Acad Dermatol 2014;70:269–275.e4. http://dx.doi.org/10.1016/j.jaad.2013.09.047.

Yiannias J. Virtual patch testing: Data driven empiric contact allergen avoidance, In: American College of Allergy, Asthma and Immunology Annual Scientific Meeting, November 11, 2013, Baltimore, MD; 2013.

CUTANEOUS T-CELL LYMPHOMAS, INCLUDING MYCOSIS FUNGOIDES AND SÉZARY SYNDROME

Method of
Gary S. Wood, MD

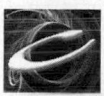

CURRENT DIAGNOSIS

For Cutaneous T-cell Lymphomas, obtain the following:
- History: duration and pace of lesion development
- Skin examination: extent of patches, plaques, tumors, and ulcers
- Extracutaneous examination: status of lymph nodes, liver, and spleen
- Laboratory: complete blood cell count, differential, and lesional biopsy results
- Imaging: CT or fused PET/CT scans of the chest, abdomen, and pelvis (not needed for early stage mycosis fungoides)

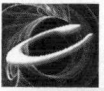

CURRENT THERAPY

Guidelines Are Primarily for Mycosis Fungoides and Sézary Syndrome:
- Stages IA–IIA: skin-directed therapy with potent topical corticosteroids, topical mechlorethamine (Mustargen),[1] or phototherapy; radiation therapy or topical bexarotene (Targretin) in selected cases
- Stages IIB–IVB: skin-directed therapy plus one or more systemic therapies, such as interferon alfa-2b (Intron A),[1] bexarotene (Targretin), vorinostat (Zolinza), denileukin diftitox (Ontak), or methotrexate; photopheresis for erythrodermic cases
- Combination therapies are often used in intermediate- and advanced-stage disease.
- Multiagent chemotherapy is usually not an effective long-term treatment strategy.

[1]Not FDA approved for this indication.

Cutaneous T-Cell Lymphomas

Classification

Virtually every subtype of T-cell lymphoma involves the skin primarily or secondarily. The principal types of primary cutaneous T-cell lymphomas (CTCLs) recognized in the World Health Organization and European Organization for Research and Treatment of Cancer classification include mycosis fungoides (MF) and its leukemic variant, the Sézary syndrome (SS); CD30$^+$ large cell lymphoma; CD30$^-$ large cell lymphoma; and pleomorphic CD4$^+$ small or medium cell variants (Table 1). All other primary CTCLs comprise only a few percent of the total. This discussion focuses on MF and SS because they account for up to 75% of primary cutaneous cases.

Standard Diagnosis and Staging Methods

The evaluation of CTCL patients begins with a thorough clinical history and physical examination. Key elements of the history include the pace and nature of disease development, the presence or absence of spontaneous regression of lesions, prior therapy, and ingestion of drugs (e.g., anticonvulsants, antihistamines, other agents with antihistaminic properties) that have been associated with pseudolymphomatous skin eruptions that can mimic CTCLs. The review of systems should establish the presence of lymphoma-associated constitutional symptoms (e.g., fever of unknown origin, night sweats, weight loss, fatigue). In addition to general aspects, the physical examination should document the type and distribution of skin lesions and whether there is lymphadenopathy, hepatosplenomegaly, or edema of extremities (i.e., potential sign of lymphatic obstruction).

Histopathologic analysis of representative lesional skin biopsy specimens is the primary means of confirming the clinical diagnosis. Biopsy specimens should be deep enough to include the deepest portions of the cutaneous lymphoid infiltrates because these areas often exhibit the most diagnostic features. Putative extracutaneous involvement should be confirmed by biopsy if it is relevant to clinical management.

Routine blood tests include a complete blood cell count, differential review, and general chemistry panel. A "Sézary prep" is used to assess peripheral blood involvement.

Internal nodal and visceral involvement by lymphoma usually is assessed with chest radiography, computed tomography (CT), or combined positron emission tomography and CT (PET/CT) scans of the chest, abdomen, and pelvis. These radiologic studies usually are not needed for patients with early forms of MF (i.e., nontumorous skin lesions without evidence of extracutaneous involvement assessed by physical examination); however, they are usually obtained during the work-up of other types of CTCLs. The role of immunopathologic and molecular biologic assays in the diagnosis and staging of CTCLs is discussed later.

TABLE 1	Classification of Primary Cutaneous T-Cell Lymphomas	
CTCL TYPE	**PROPORTION OF PRIMARY CTCL (%)**	**5-YEAR SURVIVAL RATE (%)**
MF and variants	70	85
SS	<5	<50*
CD30$^+$ large cell	13	90
CD30$^-$ large cell	7	15
Pleomorphic small/ medium cell	4	60
Miscellaneous	<1	Variable

*The 5-year survival rate depends on the criteria used to define SS, and it may be as low as 10%.

Abbreviations: CTCL = cutaneous T-cell lymphoma; MF = mycosis fungoides; SS = Sézary syndrome.

An algorithm for the diagnosis of early MF has been proposed by the International Society for Cutaneous Lymphomas (ISCL) (see Pimpinelli et al. in References). It relies on a combination of clinical, histopathologic, immunopathologic, and clonality criteria. This differs from former approaches that have been based primarily on histopathologic criteria.

Mycosis Fungoides, Sézary Syndrome, and Variants
Clinical Features
MF classically manifests as erythematous, scaly, variably pruritic, flat patches or indurated plaques, often favoring the most sun-protected areas. The patches or plaques may progress to cutaneous tumors and involvement of lymph nodes or viscera, although this usually does not occur as long as the skin lesions are reasonably well controlled by therapy. SS manifests as total-body erythema and scaling (i.e., erythroderma), generalized lymphadenopathy, hepatosplenomegaly, and leukemia. Large-plaque parapsoriasis is essentially the prediagnostic patch phase of MF. Lesions may exhibit poikiloderma (i.e., atrophy, telangiectasia, and mottled hyperpigmentation and hypopigmentation) and have then been referred to as *poikiloderma atrophicans vasculare*.

Follicular mucinosis refers to a papulonodular eruption in which hair follicles are infiltrated by T cells and contain pools of mucin. In hairy areas, this may result in alopecia. Follicular mucinosis may exist as a lesional variant of MF (i.e., follicular MF) or as a clinically benign entity (i.e., alone or associated with other lymphomas).

Granulomatous slack skin is a variant of MF that manifests with pendulous skin folds in intertriginous areas. Lesional skin biopsy specimens contain atypical T cells in a granulomatous background.

Pagetoid reticulosis manifests as a solitary or localized, often hyperkeratotic plaque containing atypical T cells that are frequently confined to a hyperplastic epidermis. Some authorities regard it as a variant of unilesional MF, whereas others think it is a distinct entity.

Other variants of MF include hypopigmented, palmoplantar, bullous, and pigmented purpuric forms. The latter form shows clinicopathologic overlap with the pigmented purpuric dermatoses. *Tumor d'emblée* MF is an outmoded concept used in the past to refer to supposed cases of MF that manifested as cutaneous tumors in the absence of patches or plaques. Most experts now prefer to classify such cases as other forms of CTCL, depending on their histopathologic features.

Histopathologic and Cytologic Features
A well-developed plaque of MF contains a bandlike, cytologically atypical lymphoid infiltrate in the upper dermis that infiltrates the epidermis as single cells and cell clusters known as Pautrier's microabscesses. The atypical lymphoid cells exhibit dense, hyperchromatic nuclei with convoluted, cerebriform nuclear contours and scant cytoplasm. The term *cerebriform* comes from the brain-like ultrastructural appearance of these nuclei. In more advanced cutaneous tumors, the infiltrate extends diffusely throughout the upper and lower dermis and may lose its epidermotropism. In the earlier patch phase of the disease, the infiltrate is sparser, and lymphoid atypia may be less pronounced. In some cases, it may be difficult to distinguish early patch-type MF from various types of chronic dermatitis. The presence of lymphoid atypia and absence of significant epidermal intercellular edema (i.e., spongiosis) help to establish the diagnosis of early MF.

Involvement of lymph nodes by MF begins in the paracortical T-cell domain and may progress to complete effacement of nodal architecture by the same types of atypical lymphoid cells that infiltrate the skin. These cells can be seen in low numbers in the peripheral blood of many MF patients; however, those with SS develop gross leukemic involvement, usually defined as at least 1000 tumor cells/mm[3]. These cells are known as Sézary cells, and they are traditionally detected by manual review of the peripheral blood smear (the so-called Sézary prep). They may also be defined by various immunophenotypic criteria.

---

[3]Exceeds dosage recommended by the manufacturer.

Immunophenotyping
Cellular antigen expression is usually assessed by immunoperoxidase methods for tissue biopsy specimens and by flow cytometry for blood specimens. Almost all cases of MF or SS begin as phenotypically and functionally mature CD4+ T-cell neoplasms of skin-associated lymphoid tissue (SALT). MF and SS express homing markers consistent with "effector memory" and "central memory" T cells, respectively. They express the SALT-associated homing molecule cutaneous lymphocyte antigen (CLA) and most mature T-cell surface antigens, with the exceptions of CD7 and CD26, which are often absent. As disease progresses, the tumor cells often dedifferentiate and lose one or more mature T-cell markers, such as CD2, CD3, or CD5.

Cases typically express the α/β form of the T-cell receptor. At least in advanced cases, the cytokine profile is consistent with the T_H2 subset of CD4+ T cells (i.e., production of interleukin [IL]-4, IL-5, and IL-10 rather than T_H1 cytokines such as IL-2 and interferon-γ). Expression of the high-affinity IL-2 receptor (CD25, TAC) ranges widely, with most cases showing a variable minority of lesional CD25+ cells. Tumor cells can be induced to express a regulatory T-cell phenotype (Treg) in vitro. MF cases that express CD8+ or other aberrant phenotypes occur occasionally but behave like conventional cases. They should not be confused with rare aggressive CTCLs exhibiting cytotoxic T-cell differentiation.

In addition to tumor cells, MF and SS lesions contain a minor component of immune accessory cells (i.e., Langerhans cells and macrophages) and CD8+ T cells with a cytolytic phenotype. This presumed host response correlates positively with survival and tends to decrease as lesions progress. A favorable response to therapy such as photopheresis appears to correlate with normal levels of circulating CD8+ cells.

Molecular Biology
Well-developed MF or SS is a monoclonal T-cell lymphoproliferative disorder. Southern blotting or polymerase chain reaction (PCR) assays demonstrate monoclonal T-cell receptor gene rearrangements. The greater sensitivity of PCR assays allows the demonstration of dominant clonality in many early patch-type lesions of MF. These assays sometimes detect dominant clonality in lesional skin showing only chronic dermatitis histopathologically. These cases are called *clonal dermatitis* and may represent the earliest manifestation of MF because several have progressed to histologically recognizable MF within a few years. However, some cases of clinicopathologically defined early-phase MF lack a detectable monoclonal T-cell population until later in their clinical course. Next generation high throughput T-cell receptor sequencing is emerging as a more sensitive and quantitative alternative to other molecular assays of T-cell clonality.

In addition to aiding initial diagnosis, gene rearrangement analysis has facilitated staging and prognosis. Because some patients without MF or SS can have low levels of circulating Sézary-like cells and because not all cases of peripheral blood involvement in MF or SS exhibit morphologically recognizable tumor cells, the demonstration of dominant clonality that matches the clone in lesional skin has proved to be a useful diagnostic adjunct. The same holds true for assessing lymph node involvement. T-cell receptor gene rearrangement analysis of MF and SS lymph nodes is more sensitive than histopathology and possesses at least some prognostic relevance.

TNMB Staging
Although several proposed methods have used a weighted extent approach to more accurately determine the MF or SS tumor burden, the preferred approach is the tumor–node–metastasis–blood (TNMB) system, which is detailed in Tables 2 and 3. The original tumor (skin), lymph nodes, and metastasis (visceral organs) version of this system has been modified by the ISCL to incorporate the extent of blood involvement (B classification) into the staging process. Table 2 shows the TNMB classification relevant to MF and SS, and Table 3 shows how this information is used to determine the stage of disease. The prognostic relevance of this staging

TABLE 2 TNMB Classification of Mycosis Fungoides and Sézary Syndrome

Skin (T)

T1	Patches and/or plaques; <10% body surface area
T2	Patches and/or plaques; ≥10% body surface area
T3	Tumors with/without other skin lesions
T4	Generalized erythroderma

Lymph Nodes (N)

N0	Not clinically enlarged; histopathology not required
N1	Clinically enlarged; histopathologically negative
N2	Clinically enlarged; histopathologically equivocal
N3	Clinically enlarged; histopathologically positive

Visceral Organs (M)

M0	No involvement
M1	Involvement

Peripheral Blood (B)

B0	Atypical cells ≤5% of leukocytes
B1	Atypical cells >5% of leukocytes
B2	Atypical cells ≥1000/mm^3

TABLE 3 TNMB Staging System for Mycosis Fungoides and Sézary Syndrome

STAGE	SKIN	LYMPH NODES	VISCERA	BLOOD
IA	T1	N0	M0	B0–1
IB	T2	N0	M0	B0–1
IIA	T1–2	N1–2	M0	B0–1
IIB	T3	N0–2	M0	B0–1
IIIA	T4	N0–2	M0	B0
IIIB	T4	N0–2	M0	B1
IVA-1	T1–4	N0–2	M0	B2
IVA-2	T1–4	N3	M0	B0–2
IVB	T1–4	N0–3	M1	B0–2

Modified from Olsen E, Vonderheid E, et al: Revisions to the staging and classification of mycosis fungoides and Sézary syndrome: A proposal of the International Society for Cutaneous Lymphomas (ISCL) and the cutaneous lymphoma task force of the European Organization of Research and Treatment of Cancer (EORTC). Blood 2007;110(6):1713–22.

system has been supported by numerous studies, and use of the TNMB helps to guide the selection of therapies. For example, early-stage MF is the most amenable to control with topically directed treatments, whereas advanced MF or SS with extracutaneous involvement usually requires systemic therapies or topical plus systemic combinations.

Treatment

Treatment guidelines for CTCL published by the National Comprehensive Cancer Network can be found at www.nccn.org. Rather than cure, which is attained in less than 10% of cases, the goal of MF and SS therapy is to reduce the impact of the skin disease on quality of life. For most patients, this is achieved by reducing pain, itch, and infection and improving clinical appearance. Appearance is affected by the disfigurement of the eruption and by the profound degree of scale shedding in some patients. Because the natural history of early-stage MF predicts a virtually normal life span, the goal of treatment must be directed at quality of life. For more advanced stages, prolongation of life expectancy may be a reasonable treatment goal.

Regardless of presentation, relief of symptoms should be addressed early. For dryness and scaling, the use of emollient ointments is indicated. These include petrolatum, Aquaphor, and commercially available shortening such as Crisco (an inexpensive alternative).[1] For modest dryness, creams (e.g., Nivea, Cetaphil, Eucerin) can be adequate and more acceptable to patients. Mild superfatted soaps such as Dove and Oil of Olay are recommended. Soap substitutes such as Cetaphil are also acceptable. Pruritus can be addressed with oral agents such as hydroxyzine (Atarax) or diphenhydramine (Benadryl)[1] 2 to 5 mg/kg/day and divided into four daily doses. Antipruritics work better when used on a regular basis rather than on an as-needed basis. Nonsedating antihistamines tend to be less effective. Measures to reduce dryness also help to reduce pruritus. Secondary infection needs to be treated with appropriate antibiotics. Their selection is guided by results of skin cultures but usually involves coverage of gram-positive organisms.

Phototherapy

Two main phototherapeutic regimens are used to treat CTCLs. Ultraviolet B radiation (290–320-nm broad band or 311-nm narrow band) can be used for patients with patches but not those with well-developed plaques or tumors. Seventy percent of patients achieve total clinical remission, usually within about 3 to 5 months. Another 15% achieve partial remission. Narrow-band UVB usually is more effective than broadband UVB and achieves maximal responses more rapidly.

Psoralen–ultraviolet A (PUVA) photochemotherapy uses oral 8-methoxypsoralen (8-MOP)[1] 0.6 mg/kg as a photosensitizer before UVA (320–400 nm) exposure. Sixty-five percent of patients with patch or plaque disease achieve complete remissions, and 30% have partial responses to this modality. For most patients, maximal responses are achieved within 3 months, and after 5 months, it is unlikely that further improvement will be gained. Limitations of these modalities include actinic damage, photocarcinogenesis, retinal damage (if eyes are not protected), and the inconvenience of getting to phototherapy centers. PUVA also has the risk of nausea and a theoretical risk of cataract induction without proper eye protection.

During the clearing phase of treatment, phototherapy treatments usually are administered three times per week. After resolution of skin lesions, treatment frequency is usually tapered gradually to once weekly for UVB and once every 4 to 6 weeks for PUVA. These maintenance regimens are often continued for months to years because abrupt cessation of phototherapy is commonly associated with rapid relapse, which is probably related to the persistence of microscopic disease after clinical clearing.

Topical Therapy

Like phototherapeutic regimens, topical therapies are appropriate for disease confined to the skin (stage I). Topical corticosteroids are frequently used for CTCLs, often before diagnosis. Low-potency formulations are useful on the face and skin folds. Medium-potency preparations are appropriate for the trunk and extremities. High-potency formulations are useful for recalcitrant lesions; however, prolonged use of such potent agents can cause local atrophy and adrenal suppression. Roughly half of patients achieve complete remissions, and most others have partial remissions. Response duration varies widely with the individual pace of disease and patient compliance. Topical corticosteroids are particularly useful as a means to relatively quickly ameliorate severe signs and symptoms and as an adjuvant therapy in combination with other primary treatments.

Mechlorethamine (nitrogen mustard, HN_2, Mustargen) is applied topically in an aqueous solution or in an ointment, such as Aquaphor. Although these forms are not FDA approved for this indication, a 0.016% gel formulation (Valchlor) is now commercially available and FDA approved. The aqueous form is prepared at home and involves a daily dose totaling 10 mg in 60 mL water.

---

[1]Not FDA approved for this indication.

245

The ointment form is prepared by a pharmacist in 1-pound lots at a concentration of 10 mg mechlorethamine per 100 g ointment. Only the amount of ointment needed to apply a thin layer is used. Either formulation is usually applied at bedtime to lesional skin for limited disease or to the entire skin surface (excluding the head unless it is also involved) for more extensive disease. It is then showered off every morning using soap and water. Results are similar to those from PUVA. Advantages include therapy at home and availability in all regions of the country. Disadvantages are daily preparation (aqueous form only), daily application, and possible allergic contact dermatitis (more common with the aqueous preparation). Maximal efficacy is expected within 6 months. Mild flare-ups of disease may occur during the first few months of treatment and probably represent inflammation of subclinical skin lesions, analogous to the clinical accentuation of actinic damage during topical therapy with 5-fluorouracil (Efudex). As with phototherapy, topical mechlorethamine is tapered gradually after remission is achieved in an effort to delay clinical relapse.

Carmustine (BCNU, BiCNU)[1] is applied to the total skin surface as an alcohol/aqueous solution (10–20 mg in 60 mL).[6] Complete responses are seen in 85% of patients with stage IA disease (<10% involvement) and 50% of patients with stage IB disease (>10% involvement). Another 10% of patients obtain partial responses. Advantages include those described for nitrogen mustard and reports of success with application only to lesional skin. Disadvantages include skin irritation followed by telangiectasia formation and possible bone marrow suppression necessitating blood monitoring.

A topical gel formulation of the retinoid X receptor (RXR)–specific retinoid, bexarotene (Targretin), is useful for localized or limited skin lesions. The principal side effect is local irritation.

Radiotherapy

Conventional radiotherapy for mycosis fungoides therapy has been used for approximately 100 years. It is useful in the treatment of isolated, particularly problematic lesions such as recalcitrant tumors or ulcerated plaques. In addition to benefit from the photons delivered by radiotherapy, electron beam therapy (0.4 Gy per week for 8–9 weeks) is also useful for CTCL therapy. An approximately 85% complete response rate of skin disease with a median duration of 16 months is expected with electron beam therapy. An advantage is an excellent rate of complete response. Disadvantages include limited access to required equipment and expertise and cutaneous toxic effects, such as alopecia, sweat gland loss, radiation dermatitis, and skin cancers. As with other skin-directed therapy, the benefit for internal disease is limited. Cumulative toxicity also limits the number of courses a patient may receive. Localized electron beam therapy is also useful for treating cases of limited-extent MF and in treating selected problematic MF lesions in patients who are otherwise responding to therapy. After completion of total-skin electron beam therapy, patients require maintenance therapy such as topical mechlorethamine[6] or phototherapy to prolong remission. Low dose radiotherapy is emerging as an effective alternative to conventional regimens.

Apheresis-Based Therapy

Leukapheresis and particularly lymphocytapheresis (6000–7000 mL of blood treated three times per week initially, then according to response) have been used in the treatment of SS patients. Benefit has been reported in several case reports and small case series; however, response rates are not possible to determine. Photopheresis (i.e., extracorporeal photochemotherapy) describes an apheresis-based therapy in which circulating lymphocytes are first exposed to a psoralen (orally or extracorporeally) and then exposed to UVA extracorporeally. In contrast to leukapheresis, in which leukocytes are discarded, all cells are returned to the patient's circulation during photopheresis. Response rates in erythrodermic patients are 33% to 50%, and median survival for SS patients is prolonged from 30 months to more than 60 months. In recent years, extracorporeal photochemotherapy has been used increasingly in conjunction with one or more systemic therapies to enhance efficacy. The toxicity of the systemic agents is diminished because they are often used in combination at reduced doses.

Cytokine Therapy

Interferon alfa-2a (Roferon-A) or alfa-2b (Intron-A)[1] (1 to 100 × 10^6 units) is given subcutaneously or intralesionally every other day to once weekly. A standard starting dose is 3×10^6 units three times per week. Response rates are approximately 55%, with complete responses occurring in 17% of patients. Advantages include the relative ease of delivery. Disadvantages include anorexia, fever, malaise, leukopenia, and risk of cardiac dysrhythmia. Interferon alfa-2a or alfa-2b combined with narrow-band UVB or PUVA is effective for many patients with generalized skin lesions unresponsive to phototherapy alone.

Tumor-Associated Antigen-Directed Therapies

Various specific tumor-associated antigens have been targeted with antibody-based therapy. The response rate typically is low, and response durations are short. Less specific targets are CD4, CD5, and IL-2 receptors. Of this class of agent, the most promising is denileukin diftitox (Ontak, DAB389 IL-2) (9–18 μg per/kg/day IV on 5 consecutive days, every 3 weeks). This agent is a fusion protein combining IL-2 and diphtheria toxin. Cells bearing the IL-2 receptor (in the lesions of at least one half of MF patients) bind and internalize the drug. The drug also may destroy Treg cells that are CD25$^+$ and suppress immune responses. Inside the cell, the toxin portion of the molecule disrupts protein synthesis, leading to cell death. Approximately 10% of patients achieve complete responses, and total response rates of near 40% have been reported. Half of responders and 20% of nonresponders experienced decreased pruritus. Adverse events include capillary leak syndrome, flulike symptoms, and allergic reactions. Combination therapy with denileukin diftitox and multiagent chemotherapy is being explored for advanced disease. Alemtuzumab (Campath)[1] is an antibody directed against CD52. It has shown benefit in advanced-stage disease. This agent can be used alone or in conjunction with multiagent chemotherapy. Brentuximab vedotin (Adcetris)[1] is an anti-CD30 antibody linked to the microtubule toxin monomethyl auristatin E. It can be effective in those cases of MF that express sufficient CD30.

Systemic Chemotherapy

Various regimens of single-agent and multiagent chemotherapy have been used in the treatment of MF and SS. Oral methotrexate, chlorambucil (Leukeran)[1] with or without prednisone,[1] and etoposide (VePesid)[1] have shown therapeutic activity. The best response has been in erythrodermic patients treated with methotrexate (5 to 125 mg weekly),[3] who have shown a 58% response rate. The combination of low-dose methotrexate and interferon alfa has been reported to yield a high response rate in advanced-stage MF and SS.

The use of multiagent regimens is controversial because of the small number of patients treated with any given regimen. There is even some evidence that for some populations of CTCL patients, survival may be reduced. For individual patients with advanced disease, however, cyclophosphamide (Cytoxan),[1] doxorubicin (Adriamycin),[1] vincristine (Oncovin),[1] and prednisone[1] (CHOP regimen) can provide some short-term palliation. In some cases, CHOP has successfully eradicated large cell transformation of MF and returned patients to their more clinically indolent patch or plaque baseline disease. Idarubicin (Idamycin)[1] in association with etoposide, cyclophosphamide, vincristine, prednisone, and bleomycin (Blenoxane)[1] (VICOP-B regimen) has demonstrated response rates of 80% (36% complete response rate) for patients with stage II through IV disease and 84% for MF patients, with a

---

[1]Not FDA approved for this indication.
[6]May be compounded by pharmacists.

[1]Not FDA approved for this indication.
[3]Exceeds dosage recommended by the manufacturer.

median duration of response longer than 8 months. Other regimens have been used with more modest success.

Several purine nucleoside analogues have been used for CTCL treatment, including erythrodermic variants. These include 2-chlorodeoxyadenosine (cladribine [Leustatin],[1] with a response rate of 28%), 2-deoxycoformycin (pentostatin [Nipent],[1] with a response rate of 39%), and fludarabine (Fludara).[1] Toxicities include pulmonary edema, bone marrow and immune suppression, and neurotoxicity.

Retinoids

Retinoids have therapeutic activity against MF and SS alone and in combination with other therapies, such as interferon alfa or PUVA (the latter combination is called Re-PUVA). Arotinoid,[5] acitretin (Soriatane),[1] and 13-cis-retinoic acid (isotretinoin [Accutane])[1] have various degrees of efficacy, and they typically are used in conjunction with other modalities. A newer RXR-specific retinoid, bexarotene, has an overall response rate of about 40% and can be used alone or in combination with phototherapy and other systemic agents such as interferon alfa-2. Disadvantages of bexarotene therapy include signs of hypothyroidism and vitamin A toxicity, particularly hyperlipidemia.

Enzyme Inhibitors

Vorinostat (Zolinza) is the first histone deacetylase inhibitor to be FDA approved for MF and SS. The overall response rate approaches 40% using a standard oral dose of 400 mg/day. Side effects include gastrointestinal symptoms, thrombocytopenia, and cardiac conduction abnormalities. Rhomidepsin (Isotodax) is an intravenously administered histone deacetylase inhibitor recently approved by the FDA for MF and SS. Forodesine[5] is a purine nucleoside phosphorylase inhibitor that preferentially affects T cells because they contain relatively high concentrations of this enzyme. Forodesine is undergoing clinical trials for MF and SS in the United States and appears to have a response rate of about 40%.

Miscellaneous Therapies

Various other therapies have been tried for MF and SS with modest success. Nonmyeloablative allogeneic stem cell transplantation has led to favorable responses in some patients; however, the total number treated is small. Cyclosporine (Sandimmune)[1] has been used for MF and SS. Transient improvement is followed by worsened survival due to immunosuppression, and it is not a recommended therapy. Thymopentin[5] has given excellent results in SS patients (i.e., 40% complete response rate and 35% partial response rate, with a median duration of response of 22 months). The lack of follow-up reports in recent decades leaves the status of this therapy in question.

Selection of Therapy

Initial choices among conventional treatments for MF and SS depend on the types of lesions and the stage of disease. Disease subsets are followed by recommended initial treatments in parentheses: unilesional or localized MF (local radiation therapy), patch MF (broad- and narrow-band UVB, PUVA, mechlorethamine), patch/plaque MF (PUVA, mechlorethamine), thick plaque/tumor MF (electron beam radiation therapy, interferon alfa-2, bexarotene, histone deacetylase inhibitors), erythrodermic MF/SS (photopheresis), and nodal or visceral MF or SS (interferon alfa-2, bexarotene, histone deacetylase inhibitors, denileukin diftitox, experimental systemic therapies, systemic chemotherapy).

Second-line therapeutic choices often involve interferons, retinoids, or histone deacetylase inhibitors, usually in combination with primary modalities. Multimodality combinations, often at reduced doses, are used commonly to treat patients with stage IIB or more advanced disease. Medium-potency topical corticosteroids, such as 0.1% triamcinolone cream or ointment (Kenalog),[1] are useful adjuncts to many different therapies. The optimal use of

newer therapeutic agents in various subtypes and stages of MF and SS is still being established. Evidence-based guidelines for MF and SS therapy have been developed by the National Comprehensive Cancer Network (NCCN) (www.nccn.org).

Lymphoproliferative Disorders Associated with Mycosis Fungoides and Sézary Syndrome

Types and Clinical Features

Patients with MF or SS are at increased risk for large T-cell lymphomas, lymphomatoid papulosis, and Hodgkin's disease. Molecular biologic analysis has shown that these disorders and MF often share the same clonal T-cell receptor gene rearrangement when they arise in the same individual. As a consequence, they are considered to be subclones of the original MF tumor clone. The development of large T-cell lymphoma in a patient with MF or SS is referred to as *large cell transformation of MF*. This occurs in up to 20% of cases in some series and is associated with a median survival of only 1 to 2 years. One half of these large T-cell lymphomas are CD30[+]; however, the generally favorable prognosis of primary cutaneous CD30[+] anaplastic large cell lymphoma does not extend to these secondary forms of CD30[+] lymphoma. These patients are usually treated with systemic chemotherapy such as CHOP or with experimental systemic therapies appropriate for advanced-stage CTCL.

Lymphomatoid papulosis manifests as recurrent, usually generalized crops of spontaneously regressing, erythematous papules that can exhibit crusting or vesiculation before resolution. It is the clinically benign end of a disease continuum that has primary cutaneous CD30[+] anaplastic large cell lymphoma at its other extreme. Intermediate forms of disease can occur. Histopathologically, lesions contain a mixed-cell infiltrate, including large, atypical T cells that resemble Reed-Sternberg cells and their mononuclear variants (so-called type A) or large MF-type cells (so-called type B). Type A cells are CD30[+]. A type C form is also recognized. It has sheets of type A cells histologically mimicking CD30[+] large T-cell lymphoma but is different from it clinically. A type D variant containing CD8[+] CD30[+] large atypical cells has also been described recently. All types of lymphomatoid papulosis behave similarly. Patients with lymphomatoid papulosis sometimes respond to tetracycline or erythromycin (500 mg PO bid), presumably on the basis of antiinflammatory activity. Most cases improve within 1 month with low-dose methotrexate (10–20 mg PO every week). PUVA and narrow-band UVB given three times per week are other therapeutic options.

Treatment

In most cases, non-MF/SS CTCLs are treated with radiation therapy (with or without complete surgical excision) if they are localized or with various multiagent systemic chemotherapy regimens if they are generalized. The roles of other agents remain to be defined, except that studies have proved that methotrexate (10–40 mg PO every week) is effective therapy for most cases of primary cutaneous CD30[+] anaplastic large cell lymphoma. Therapies being investigated for this lymphoma include anti-CD30 antibodies, alone or conjugated to toxins. One of these antibody conjugates (brentuximab vedotin) is FDA approved for systemic CD30[+] lymphomas and Hodgkin's disease. Denileukin diftitox has been reported to be effective against some subcutaneous panniculitic T-cell lymphomas.

References

Olsen E, Vonderheid E, et al. Revisions to the staging and classification of mycosis fungoides and Sézary syndrome: A proposal of the International Society for Cutaneous Lymphomas (ISCL) and the cutaneous lymphoma task force of the European Organization of Research and Treatment of Cancer (EORTC). Blood 2007;110(6):1713–22.

Pimpinelli N, Olsen EA, Santucci M, et al. Defining early mycosis fungoides. J Am Acad Dermatol 2005;53(6):1053–63.

Richardson SK, Lin JH, Vittorio CC, et al. High clinical response rate with multimodality immunomodulatory therapy for Sézary syndrome. Clin Lymphoma Myeloma 2006;7(3):226–32.

Vonderheid EC, Bernengo MG, Burg G, et al. Update on erythrodermic cutaneous T-cell lymphoma: Report of the International Society for Cutaneous Lymphomas. J Am Acad Dermatol 2002;46(1):95–106.

---

[1]Not FDA approved for this indication.

[5]Investigational drug in the United States.

Willemze R, Jaffe ES, Burg G, et al. WHO-EORTC classification for cutaneous lymphomas. Blood 2005;105(10):3768–85.

Wood GS, Greenberg HL. Diagnosis, staging, and monitoring of cutaneous T-cell lymphoma. Dermatol Ther 2003;16(4):269–75.

CUTANEOUS VASCULITIS

Method of
Molly Hinshaw, MD; and Susan Lawrence-Hylland, MD

CURRENT DIAGNOSIS

- Cutaneous vasculitis can be limited to skin (leukocytoclastic vasculitis) or associated with systemic disease.
- Perform punch biopsy of intact, nonulcerated skin lesion.
- "Vasculitis" on skin biopsy describes vessel appearance and is not a clinical diagnosis.
- Thorough review of systems and physical examination are necessary to evaluate for systemic vasculitis.

CURRENT THERAPY

Leukocytoclastic Vasculitis
- First identify instigating factors: infection, medications.
- Care is symptomatic. Lesions typically remit without treatment.
- If needed, short course of prednisone may be given and tapered over 3 to 6 weeks.

All Forms of Vasculitis
- Treat underlying systemic vasculitis.

Vasculitis is an inflammatory-mediated destruction of blood vessels. The systemic vasculitides have historically been differentiated by their involvement of small, medium, or large blood vessels. Names used to describe isolated cutaneous vasculitis have included hypersensitivity vasculitis and leukocytoclastic vasculitis (LCV). In 1990, the American College of Rheumatology proposed five criteria for the classification of hypersensitivity vasculitis: age older than 16 years, possible drug trigger, palpable purpura, maculopapular rash, and skin biopsy showing neutrophils around vessel. At least three out of five criteria yield a sensitivity of 71% and specificity of 84%. In 1994, a new nomenclature proposed at the Chapel Hill International Consensus Conference in North Carolina further classified vasculitis (Box 1). The term

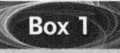 **Box 1** Chapel Hill Consensus 1994 Classification of Vasculitis

Large-Vessel Vasculitis
Giant cell arteritis
Takayasu's arteritis

Medium-Vessel Vasculitis
Classic polyarteritis nodosa
Kawasaki's disease

Small-Vessel Vasculitis
Churg-Strauss syndrome
Cutaneous leukocytoclastic vasculitis
Essential cryoglobulinemia
Henoch-Schönlein purpura
Microscopic polyangiitis (polyarteritis)
Wegener's granulomatosis

"hypersensitivity vasculitis" was not used, because most vasculitides that would have previously been in this category fall into either microscopic polyangiitis or cutaneous LCV. LCV is vasculitis restricted to the skin without involvement of vessels in other organs. Cutaneous vasculitis may be a clue to systemic vasculitis and guides the clinician to a comprehensive evaluation (Table 1).

Vasculitis can affect almost any organ, and once affected, end organs can become dysfunctional. Such dysfunction may be as innocuous as cutaneous, tender, transient papules or as devastating as a stroke. A thorough evaluation of the patient with a complete review of systems, physical examination, laboratory evaluation, and clinical follow-up allows a distinction to be made between the different forms of vasculitis.

Leukocytoclastic Vasculitis

Epidemiology
LCV is common. The incidence and prevalence are unknown. Mean age of onset ranges from 34 to 49 years of age. The female-to-male ratio ranges from approximately 2:1 to 3:1.

Risk Factors
LCV is often secondary to a known trigger including infection, drug ingestion, or malignancy. LCV can also be a presenting feature of autoimmune disease.

Pathophysiology
LCV is best characterized as immune complex–mediated inflammatory destruction of the postcapillary venules of any organ. The exact mechanisms of vascular destruction is unknown.

Clinical Manifestations
LCV typically manifests as nonblanchable macules that evolve to papules or, less commonly, pustules and ulcers (Figure 1). Clues to the diagnosis include a monomorphous, ruddy-brown appearance owing to leakage of hemosiderin pigment from vessels. Lesions measure a few millimeters to a few centimeters in diameter. LCV is often localized to the lower extremities but may be diffuse. Pruritus, pain, or burning of the skin lesions are indicators that the patient might have a vasculitis extending beyond LCV.

Diagnosis
To confirm a clinical impression of LCV, perform a punch biopsy in the center of a nonulcerated cutaneous lesion that is less than 24 to 48 hours old and submit the sample in 10% formalin (standard medium). It is important to biopsy an intact, nonulcerated active lesion (Figure 2) because ulcers can show histologic features simulating vasculitis regardless of whether the patient has true vasculitis or not.

Pathology reveals a mononuclear or polymorphonuclear inflammation of the small blood vessels (called LCV), most prominent in the postcapillary venules. The appearance may be necrotizing or non-necrotizing.

Differential Diagnosis
LCV manifests as erythematous papules or occasionally as papulopustules that can simulate a variety of entities (see Table 1). The review of systems and physical examination should be directed to evaluate for diseases that have cutaneous vasculitis as a component of their presentation (see Table 1). All patients with LCV should have a urinalysis to evaluate for hematuria as a sign of kidney involvement, with subsequent evaluation and management if identified.

Treatment
The primary goal in the management of LCV is to identify and treat instigating factors, including infection and medications. Supportive treatment includes resting, elevating legs, and wearing support hose. When review of systems, physical examination, and urinalysis do not reveal associated systemic diseases, treatment of LCV is generally not necessary. Lesions typically remit without

TABLE 1 Diseases with Cutaneous Vasculitis as a Component of Their Presentation

DISEASE	SKIN LESIONS	CLUES AND CONFIRMATION
Urticarial vasculitis	Individual lesions look like urticaria but last >24 h; typical urticaria last a few hours, always <24 h Pruritus, burning of skin lesions	May be associated with connective tissue disease, medications, low complement, viral infections (e.g., hep B, hep C, EBV) Skin biopsy
Henoch-Schönlein purpura	Wheals progress to petechia, ecchymoses and palpable purpura Lesions are in gravity-dependent or pressure-dependent areas such as legs or the buttocks in toddlers	Arthralgia or arthritis, hematuria, abdominal pain, melena Skin biopsy and DIF for IgA
Essential mixed cryoglobulinemia	Palpable purpura	Peripheral neuropathy, GN Hep C positive Serum cryoglobulins
Wegener's granulomatosis	Palpable purpura, hemorrhagic lesions, petechiae, skin ulcers	c-ANCA >80% Pulmonary hemorrhage, GN Biopsy affected organ
Churg-Strauss syndrome	Maculopapular rash, palpable purpura, hemorrhagic lesions, subcutaneous nodules, livedo reticularis or Raynaud's disease	ANCA (50%) Asthma, allergic rhinitis Eosinophilia >1.5 × 10⁹/L Pulmonary infiltrates, pulmonary neuropathy Biopsy affected organ
Microscopic polyangiitis	Palpable purpura, hemorrhagic lesions, petechiae, skin ulcers, splinter hemorrhages	p-ANCA >60% Pulmonary hemorrhage, GN Biopsy affected organ
Polyarteritis nodosa	Livedo reticularis, tender nodules, skin ulcers, bullae or vesicles	Hypertension, elevated creatinine, abdominal pain, constitutional symptoms (fever) Abnormal angiogram Biopsy affected organ

Abbreviations: c-ANCA = classic antineutrophil cytoplasmic antibody; DIF = direct immunofluorescence; EBV = Epstein-Barr virus; GN = glomerulonephritis; hep = hepatitis; Ig = immunoglobulin; p-ANCA = protoplasmic-staining antineutrophil cytoplasmic antibody.

Figure 1. Leukocytoclastic vasculitis: palpable, purpuric, nonblanching, erythematous to ruddy-brown thin papules. Additional secondary changes include small pustules (pustular vasculitis) or shallow, small ulcerations.

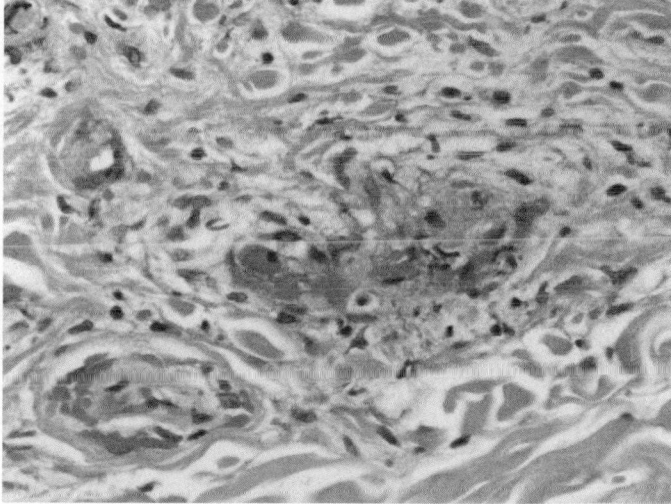

Figure 2. Biopsy of intact clinical lesion of leukocytoclastic vasculitis. Histology shows destruction of postcapillary venules with fibrin deposition, degenerate inflammatory cells, and extravasated erythrocytes.

treatment. In rare patients with symptomatic, extensively pustular, or progressive lesions, a short course of prednisone[1] dosed at 1 mg/kg/day initially and tapered over 3 to 6 weeks may be used, although no controlled trials have been performed using oral corticosteroids for isolated LCV. Rapid steroid taper can lead to rebound. Systematic evaluation of the use of other medications, such as colchicine[1] or dapsone,[1] to treat isolated LCV has not been performed.

Monitoring
Patients with LCV are at risk for recurrent or chronic vasculitis. In addition, apparent LCV can occur as a systemic disease that is not recognizable at the first episode. Patients with persistent or recurrent LCV require follow-up to ensure disease clearance, to monitor for medication side effects, and to evaluate for evolving disorders known to be associated with cutaneous vasculitis (see Table 1).

Complications
Isolated LCV generally resolves without sequelae. However, pustular or ulcerative LCV may be complicated by local sequelae such as cutaneous ulcerations and scars.

Cutaneous Vasculitis Associated with Systemic Vasculitis
Cutaneous vasculitis may be a component of the presentation of multiple diseases (see Table 1). When a clinician reads a pathology report from a biopsy of a skin lesion that states "vasculitis," it is

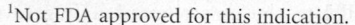

[1]Not FDA approved for this indication.

important to realize that this term is a descriptor of the histopathology. It is the clinician's challenge to determine whether "vasculitis" is as potentially innocuous as LCV or part of a more severe systemic disease. Symptoms that are clues to a systemic process can include fever, arthralgias, myalgias, anorexia, abdominal pain, pulmonary abnormalities, or neurologic symptoms.

Skin biopsy may aid in the diagnosis of a systemic vasculitis (Henoch-Schönlein purpura), but biopsy of an affected end organ may be necessary to confirm a diagnosis. Pathology focuses on the confirmation of vasculitis in a small, medium, or large vessel.

Aside from Henoch-Schönlein purpura, treatment of systemic vasculitis is typically much more aggressive than treatment of LCV and should be pursued in conjunction with involvement of a rheumatologist, nephrologist, or pulmonologist. Systemic disease leads to severe complications including renal failure, pulmonary damage, permanent vascular disease, or neurologic insult depending on the viscera affected.

References

Gayraud M, Guillevin L, le Toumelin P, et al. Long-term followup of polyarteritis nodosa, microscopic polyangiitis, and Churg-Strauss syndrome: Analysis of four prospective trials including 278 patients. Arthritis Rheum 2001;44:666–75.

Hannon CW, Swerlick RA. Vasculitis. In: Bolognia J, Jorizzo J, Rapini R, editors. Dermatology, vol 1. St Louis: Mosby; 2003. p. 381–402.

Hoffman GS, Kerr GS, Leavitt RY, et al. Wegener granulomatosis: An analysis of 158 patients. Ann Intern Med 1992;116:488–98.

Jennette JC, Thomas DB, Falk RJ. Microscopic polyangiitis (microscopic polyarteritis). Semin Diagn Pathol 2001;18:3–13.

Jenette JC, Falk RF, Andrassy K, et al. Nomenclature of systemic vasculitides. Proposal of an international consensus conference. Arthritis Rheum 1994;37(2):187–92.

DISEASES OF THE HAIR

Method of
Dirk M. Elston, MD

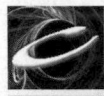

CURRENT DIAGNOSIS

- A sudden increase in shedding most commonly represents telogen effluvium.
- Hair thinning is more likely to represent pattern alopecia.
- Scarring alopecia generally requires a biopsy for diagnosis.
- Most medically significant hirsutism results from polycystic ovarian syndrome.
- New-onset virilization suggests the possibility of a tumor.

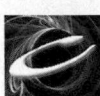

CURRENT THERAPY

- Pattern alopecia in men is treated with oral finasteride (Propecia), topical minoxidil (Rogaine), or both.
- Pattern alopecia in women is treated with antiandrogens (such as spironolactone [Aldactone][1]), topical minoxidil, or both.
- Alopecia areata can require intralesional corticosteroid injections, topical immunotherapy, or systemic therapy with agents such as methotrexate (Trexall).[1]
- A scalp biopsy is critical to guide therapy in scarring alopecia.
- Hirsutism may be treated with laser epilation or systemic antiandrogens. Topical eflornithine (Vaniqa) can slow regrowth of hair.

[1]Not FDA approved for this indication.

Epidemiology

Hair disorders are common, with more than half of the population affected by pattern alopecia and the prevalence of hirsutism varying significantly by ethnicity.

Risk Factors

Most causes of alopecia and hirsutism are genetically determined.

Pathophysiology

Pattern alopecia relates to increased sensitivity to dihydrotestosterone. Telogen effluvium relates to an alteration in the normal hair cycle, with many hairs shedding synchronously. Alopecia areata represents an inflammatory insult directed against melanocytes in the hair bulb. There is strong evidence that the disease is mediated by T_H1 lymphocytes. Polycycstic ovarian syndrome is an insulin-resistance syndrome resulting in excess production of androgens.

Prevention

Little can be done to prevent hair disorders, so the focus is generally on diagnosis and treatment.

Clinical Manifestations

Pattern alopecia manifests with apical scalp thinning. In men, receding of the hairline at the temples is typical, whereas women demonstrate widening of the part but retain the anterior hairline. Telogen effluvium manifests with diffuse shedding of telogen hairs (hairs with a nonpigmented bulb). Alopecia areata typically occurs with patchy hair loss. Shed hairs demonstrate tapered fracture at the base. Syphilitic alopecia resembles alopecia areata but often affects smaller areas, with only partial hair loss, resulting in a moth-eaten appearance. Scarring alopecia shows permanent areas of smooth alopecia lacking follicular openings.

Polycystic ovarian syndrome manifests with evidence of anovulation and excess androgen production. Signs of virilization suggesting a possible tumor include new onset of hirsutism, deepening of the voice, change in body habitus, and clitoromegaly.

Diagnosis

Alopecia

The first step is to determine if a hair shaft abnormality exists (Box 1). This is particularly important in black patients, in whom trichorrhexis nodosa is a common cause of hair loss. Trichorrhexis nodosa results from overprocessing of the hair. Hair density is normal at the level of the scalp, but hairs break off, leaving patches of short hair.

The next step is to determine if telogen effluvium exists. Telogen effluvium manifests with increased shedding of hairs with a blunt nonpigmented bulb (Figure 1), and it commonly follows an illness, surgery, delivery, or crash diet by 3 to 5 months. Hairs can often be easily extracted with a gentle hair pull or 1 minute of combing. The presence of tapered fracture suggests alopecia areata, syphilis, or heavy metal poisoning. Alopecia areata can result in diffuse hair loss, but it more commonly manifests with well-defined round patches of hair loss. The skin is either normal or salmon pink. Syphilis more often shows a moth-eaten pattern of alopecia (Figure 2).

Most patients with hair loss need only limited laboratory testing or none at all. Thyroid disorders and iron deficiency are common, and testing for them is relatively inexpensive. I recommend them when telogen effluvium is present. Their presence can also accelerate the course of pattern alopecia, and it is reasonable to test for them in women with this disorder. Thyroid-stimulating hormone is the best screen for thyroid disorders. The role of iron deficiency in telogen hair loss is controversial, but iron deficiency is common, easily established, and inexpensive to correct. Iron status also serves as an indicator of overall nutritional status. Although a low ferritin level proves iron deficiency, ferritin behaves as an acute phase reactant and a normal level does not rule out iron deficiency. Therefore, I recommend measurement of ferritin, serum iron, iron binding capacity, and saturation.

A scalp biopsy is required in any patient with scarring alopecia. It may also be necessary in other patients if history and physical examination do not establish a diagnosis and the alopecia is progressive. The scalp biopsy should be performed with a 4-mm biopsy punch oriented parallel to the direction of hair growth.

Box 1   Diagnosis of Alopecia

Trichodystrophy
Types
Trichorrhexis nodosa
Inherited trichodystrophies
Fractures

Causes
- Alopecia areata
- Chemotherapy
- Heavy metal

Determine Type
Anagen Effluvium
Tapered fractures can be caused by
- Alopecia areata
- Chemotherapy
- Heavy metal
Loose anagen can be caused by
- Loose anagen syndrome
- Easily extractable anagen in scarring alopecia

Telogen Effluvium
Increased shedding of club hairs can be caused by
- Diet, illness
- Pregnancy
- Medication
- Papulosquamous disorders
- Pattern alopecia

Diagnosis
Laboratory Studies
Iron
Thyroid stimulating hormone
Endocrine studies in virilized women

Biopsy
Nonscarring types
- Telogen effluvium
- Pattern alopecia
- Alopecia areata
Scarring types
- Lupus erythematosus
- Lichen planopilaris
- Folliculitis decalvans

Other Permanent Alopecia
Idiopathic pseudopelade
Morphea

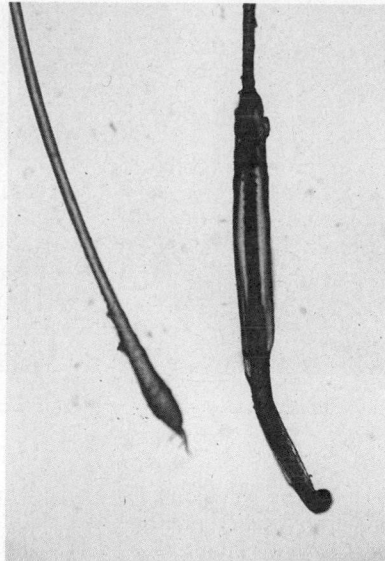

Figure 1. Telogen hair on *left*, anagen hair on *right* for comparison.

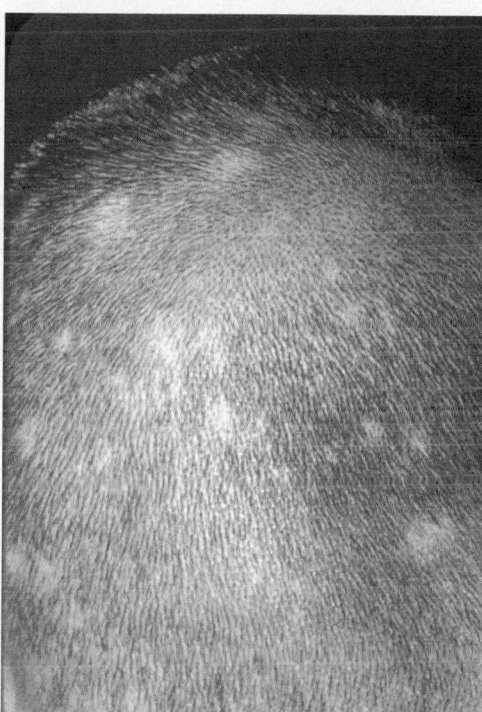

Figure 2. Moth-eaten syphilitic alopecia.

Gelfoam can be placed into the resulting hole to stop bleeding and eliminate the need for sutures. The biopsy should be done in a well-established but still active area of inflammation if one can be identified. A combination of vertical and transverse sections increases the diagnostic yield and is usually recommended. In patients with scarring alopecia, half of the vertically bisected specimen should be sent for direct immunofluorescence. An additional biopsy of an end-stage scarred area can demonstrate characteristic patterns of scarring with an elastic tissue stain. This can help distinguish among causes of scarring alopecia such as lupus erythematosus (Figure 3), lichen planopilaris, pseudopelade, and folliculitis decalvans.

Hirsutism

Patients with *new-onset* virilization should be evaluated to rule out an ovarian or adrenal tumor. Ovarian and adrenal imaging studies and a total testosterone level are the best screens. A total testosterone more than 200 ng/dL or dehydroepiandrostenedione sulfate (DHEAS) more than 8000 ng/dL suggests tumor. In patients with physical signs of Cushing's disease, a 24-hour urine cortisol should be obtained. Most patients with *chronic* medically significant hirsutism have polycystic ovarian syndrome (PCOS). The diagnosis is established by means of history and physical examination, and the most important laboratory tests are serum lipids and fasting glucose to establish associated cardiac risk factors. A clinical diagnosis of PCOS requires the presence of hirsutism, acne or pattern alopecia, and evidence of anovulation (fewer than 9 periods per year or cycles longer than 40 days). Ratios of luteinizing hormone (LH) to follicle-stimulating hormone (FSH) have poor sensitivity and specificity for diagnosing PCOS. Imaging for ovarian cysts seldom affects management.

Differential Diagnosis

Syphilis can mimic alopecia areata, and serologic testing should be performed in any sexually active patient with a new diagnosis of alopecia areata. Correct diagnosis of scarring alopecia depends of a thorough examination for other cutaneous signs of lupus erythematosus or lichen planus as well as the results of a skin biopsy.

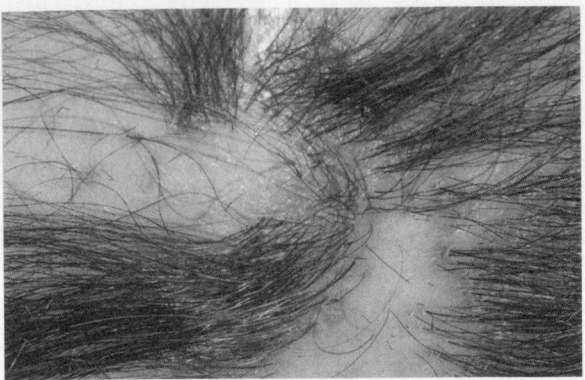

Figure 3. Scarring alopecia secondary to chronic cutaneous lupus erythematosus.

Tinea capitis can occur as inflammatory boggy areas with hair loss (kerion) or with subtle seborrheic-type scale and black-dot areas of hair loss. A potassium hydroxide (KOH) examination can be performed by rubbing the affected area with moist gauze and examining broken hairs that cling to the gauze.

Hirsutism should be distinguished from hypertrichosis. Hirsutism is a male pattern of hair growth occurring in a woman and is hormonal in nature. Hypertrichosis is excess hair growth that occurs outside of an androgen-dependent distribution. It can be found in metabolic disorders such as porphyria or may be a sign of internal malignancy (Figure 4).

Nonclassic 21-hydroxylase deficiency accounts for up to 10% of patients with medically significant hirsutism. Screening with a baseline morning 17-OH-progesterone is associated with many false positive results. A stimulated 17-OH- progesterone is more specific, but the results of testing seldom affect management because outcomes with dexamethasone (Decadron)[1] are no better than with spironolactone (Aldactone).[1]

Treatment
Alopecia
Telogen effluvium commonly resolves spontaneously once the cause has been eliminated. Poor diet and papulosquamous diseases of the scalp such as seborrheic dermatitis and psoriasis can perpetuate a telogen effluvium and should be treated. Seborrheic dermatitis responds to topical corticosteroids. Medicated shampoos containing selenium sulfide (Selsun Blue) or zinc pyrithione (T-gel Daily Control) can be helpful. Scalp psoriasis can require more potent topical steroids such as fluocinonide solution (Lidex) and calcipotriene (Dovonex) applied on weekends or daily. Systemic agents such as

---

[1]Not FDA approved for this indication.

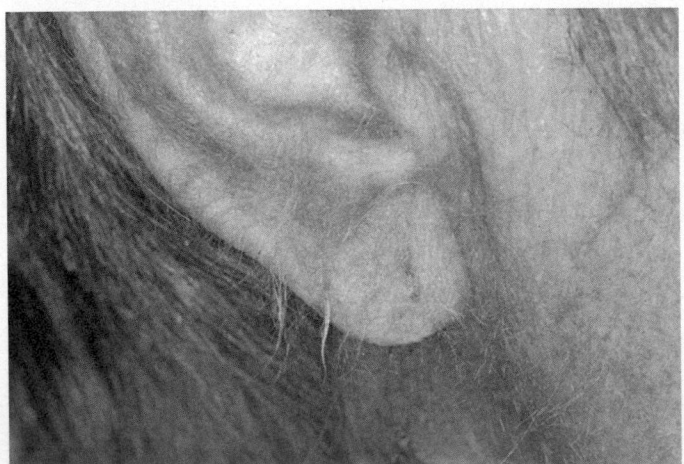

Figure 4. Malignant hypertrichosis secondary to ovarian cancer.

methotrexate (Trexall) at doses of 7.5 to 20 mg once weekly may be required to control severe scalp psoriasis.

Pattern alopecia in men is mediated by dihydrotestosterone (DHT). Men with pattern alopecia may be treated with daily topical minoxidil 2% to 5% (Rogaine) or oral finasteride (Propecia) at a dose of 1 mg daily. In women, the pathogenesis is complex, and adrenal androgens may play a larger role. Finasteride[1] is of little benefit in the majority of women with pattern alopecia. Spironolactone[1] 100 mg twice daily can be helpful. In women of childbearing potential, spironolactone should always be used in conjunction with an oral contraceptive. Side effects are uncommon but can include urinary frequency, irregular periods, dyspareunia, and nausea. Most patients demonstrate a minor increase in serum potassium. Those with kidney failure are at risk for life-threatening potassium retention. Topical 2% minoxidil can also be of benefit, an some women derive added benefit from the 5% formulation. All patients with pattern alopecia should be evaluated for superimposed causes of telogen effluvium such as inadequate diet and seborrheic dermatitis.

Tinea capitis is often overlooked in adults and black children, in whom the manifestations of inflammation can be subtle. Black dot and seborrheic tinea are common in black children. Patchy hair loss is an important clue to the diagnosis. Treatment is summarized in Table 1.

Localized patches of alopecia areata respond to intralesional injections of triamcinolone hexacetonide (Aristospan) (2.5–5 mg/mL) given once per month. Approximately 0.1 mL/cm^2 is injected to a maximum of 3 mL during any one session. Minoxidil[1] solution produces slow regrowth in some patients who cannot tolerate other treatments. Anthralin (Dritho-Scalp 0.5%)[1] is sometimes used in children. It is applied 30 minutes before showering. It can stain skin and anything else it touches.

Topical immunotherapy with dinitrochlorobenzene (DNCB),[1] squaric acid dibutylester (SADBE)[1] or diphenylcyclopropenone (DPCP)[1] is more effective than either minoxidil or anthralin. DNCB is mutagenic in the Ames assay and none of the topical immunotherapies are currently approved for human use. A 2% solution of the sensitizer is applied to the arm in acetone to induce initial sensitization. Subsequently, diluted solutions, starting at about 0.001%, are applied weekly to the scalp with a cotton-tipped applicator. Roughly 20% to 60% of patients have responded to this regimen in various studies.

Biologic agents have been disappointing, but methotrexate[1] in psoriatic doses (7.5–20 mg weekly for an adult) can be effective. Sulfasalazine (Azulfidine)[1] is sometimes effective in doses ranging from 500 to 1500 mg three times a day.[3] Patients should be encouraged to read about new therapies on the National Alopecia Areata Foundation website (www.naaf.org).

---

[1]Not FDA approved for this indication.

TABLE 1	Treatment of Tinea Capitis	
ANTIFUNGAL AGENT	**DOSAGE**	**USUAL DURATION OF THERAPY**
Griseofulvin (Fulvicin U/F)	Required dosages are often higher than reflected in the product label; 4–10 mg/kg/d is a good starting dosage	1 mo or more
Fluconazole (Diflucan)[1]	5–6 mg/kg/d	1 mo or more
Itraconazole (Sporanox)[1]	3–5 mg/kg/d	1 wk, repeated monthly until cured
Terbinafine (Lamisil)	Patient <20 kg: 62.5 mg/d Patient 20–40 kg: 125 mg/d Patient >40 kg: 250 mg/d	1 mo or more

[1]Not FDA approved for this indication.

Early, aggressive therapy for discoid lupus erythematosus is recommended to prevent permanent scarring. Topical corticosteroids are rarely sufficient. Intralesional injections are performed in a manner similar to that described above. Initial control of severe disease can be achieved with a single 3-week tapered course of oral prednisone at a dose of 60 mg daily for the first week, 40 mg daily for the second week, and 20 mg daily for the third week. Intralesional steroid injections or a systemic steroid-sparing agent are required for maintenance therapy. Systemic agents that can be effective include antimalarials, dapsone,[1] methotrexate,[1] mycophenolate mofetil (CellCept),[1] and thalidomide (Thalomid).[1] I generally begin treatment with hydroxychloroquine (Plaquenil) at a dose of 400 mg daily for an adult. Dapsone is used at a dose of 100 mg daily for an adult. Thalidomide has been used effectively at doses of 50 to 100 mg daily, but peripheral neuropathy and teratogenicity limit its use. Mycophenolate mofetil is used at a dose of 1 gram twice daily, and methotrexate is used at doses of 7.5 to 20 mg weekly.

End-stage cicatricial alopecia is best treated by scalp reduction and hair transplantation. The disease can flare up in response to surgery, and it is best to plan a 3-week tapered course of prednisone[1] as described to help prevent the flare.

Lichen planopilaris is treated in a manner similar to lupus, except that hydroxychloroquine[1] is of less benefit and oral retinoids (Soriatane[1] at doses of 25 to 50 mg daily) are more likely to be successful. Pioglitazone (Actos)[1] can induce remission in a subset of patients and the frontal fibrosing alopecia variant can respond to dutasteride (Avodart).[1] Mycophenylate mofetil 1 g twice daily is often effective when other treatments fail.

Folliculitis decalvans manifests with crops of pustules that result in permanent scarring. Patients respond to weekend applications of clobetasol (Clobex, Olux) together with prolonged use of anti-staphylococcal antibiotics such as doxycycline (Doryx)[1] 100 mg twice daily.

Hirsutism

Treatment options include laser epilation, eflornithine (Vaniqa) cream to reduce the rate of hair growth, or spironolactone[1] at a starting dose of 100 mg twice daily as described for pattern alopecia. Cyproterone acetate is used in some countries but is not available in the United States. Other options that are less commonly used include insulin sensitizers, flutamide (Eulexin),[1] metformin (Glucophage),[1] and leuprolide (Lupron)[1] plus estrogen.

Monitoring

Patients treated with topical or intralesional corticosteroids should be monitored for cutaneous atrophy. Those on hydroxychloroquine should be monitored for ocular toxicity, including corneal deposits and retinal damage, although these are very rare at usual doses. They should also be monitored periodically for thrombocytopenia, agranulocytosis, and hepatitis. Patients beginning dapsone therapy should be screened for G6PD deficiency. Potential side effects include hemolysis, methemoglobinemia, and neuropathy. Monitoring includes periodic blood count assessment and measurement of strength and sensation. Mycophenolate mofetil can produce pancytopenia, and blood counts should be monitored. Methotrexate is cleared by the kidneys, and kidney function should be assessed at baseline. Periodic assessment of liver-function tests and blood count is warranted, as is a yearly chest radiograph. I also monitor procollagen 3 terminal peptide levels quarterly to assess the risk of hepatic fibrosis. Patients on antiandrogen therapy should be monitored for dyspareunia resulting from vulvar atrophy.

Complications

Patients with pattern alopecia and polycystic ovarian syndrome have a greater risk of metabolic syndrome with cardiac complications. They should be evaluated for lipid abnormalities and glucose intolerance and treated appropriately.

---

[1]Not FDA approved for this indication.
[3]Exceeds dosage recommended by the manufacturer.

References

Brown J, Farquhar C, Lee O, et al. Spironolactone versus placebo or in combination with steroids for hirsutism and/or acne. Cochrane Database Syst Rev 2009;(2): CD000194.

Buzney E, Sheu J, Buzney C, Reynolds RV. Polycystic ovary syndrome: a review for dermatologists: Part II. Treatment. J Am Acad Dermatol 2014 Nov;71(5):859. e1–859.e15.

Durdu M, Özcan D, Baba M, Seçkin D. Efficacy and safety of diphenylcyclopropenone alone or in combination with anthralin in the treatment of chronic extensive alopecia areata: A retrospective case series. J Am Acad Dermatol 2015.

Elston DM, Ferringer T, Dalton S, et al. A comparison of vertical versus transverse sections in the evaluation of alopecia biopsy specimens. J Am Acad Dermatol 2005;53(2):267–72.

Housman E, Reynolds RV. Polycystic ovary syndrome: a review for dermatologists: Part I. Diagnosis and manifestations. J Am Acad Dermatol 2014 Nov;71(5): 847.e1–847.e10.

Jayasena CN, Franks S. The management of patients with polycystic ovary syndrome. Nat Rev Endocrinol 2014 Oct;10(10):624–36.

Johnson NP. Metformin use in women with polycystic ovary syndrome. Ann Transl Med 2014 Jun;2(6):56.

Setji TL, Brown AJ. Polycystic ovary syndrome: update on diagnosis and treatment. Am J Med 2014 Oct;127(10):912–9.

Somani N, Turvy D. Hirsutism: an evidence-based treatment update. Am J Clin Dermatol 2014 Jul;15(3):247–66.

Tsuboi R, Arano O, Nishikawa T, et al. Randomized clinical trial comparing 5% and 1% topical minoxidil for the treatment of androgenetic alopecia in Japanese men. J Dermatol 2009;36(8):437–46.

DISEASES OF THE MOUTH

Method of
Wendy S. Hupp, DMD

CURRENT DIAGNOSIS

High-Risk Conditions
- Obvious soft tissue enlargement that could lead to trismus or airway compromise: acute exacerbation of odontogenic infections; rapid onset, swelling, purulence, broken or decayed teeth.
- Suspicion of oral cancer: mucosal surface color change, slowly progressing enlargement, asymptomatic or with nonhealing ulcer, incidental finding, use of tobacco and alcohol.

Opportunistic Infections
- Necrotizing ulcerative gingivitis (trench mouth): compromised host resistance, generalized dental pain, usually acute onset, bleeding gums, fetid odor.
- Oral candidiasis: compromised host resistance, chronic or recurring course, bad taste, generalized burning sensation, superficial change in mucosal appearance (white or red).

Dry Mouth
- Salivary dysfunction (xerostomia): patient's perception of dry mouth, difficulty swallowing or speaking, tooth sensitivity as a result of new decay or receding gums; related to medication use or autoimmune gland dysfunction.

Acute-Onset Oral Ulcers
- Aphthous stomatitis: recurring episodes, formation of one or more superficial oral ulcers, located on nonbound mucosa, healing in approximately 7 to 10 days.
- Primary herpetic gingivostomatitis: acute onset of systemic viral infection features, including fever, and multiple oral vesicles, degenerating into ulcers; resolution in 7 to 10 days.
- Recurrent herpes: recurring episodes, acute formation of vesicles collapsing to ulcers, located on exposed lip, or bound mucosa; healing in 7 to 10 days.
- Erythema multiforme: acute onset of oral ulcers, triggering event, mild systemic features such as fever, characteristic skin lesions; resolution in 2 to 4 weeks.

Chronic Oral Ulcers
- Erosive lichen planus and lichenoid reaction: reticular appearance at periphery of ulcers, buccal mucosa affected, may cause desquamative gingivitis, skin lesions possible.

- Mucous membrane pemphigoid: typically desquamative gingivitis presentation, possible eye and genital ulcers, skin lesions unlikely.
- Pemphigus vulgaris: ulcers of irregular shape and jagged peripheral contour, possible skin lesions.

Osteonecrosis of the Jaw
- Radiation related: resulting from treatment of oral or head and neck cancer.
- Medication related: secondary to antiresorptives used to treat osteoporosis or bone metastases in cancer patients; bisphosphonates, antiangiogenics, receptor activator of nuclear factor kappa-B ligand (RANKL) inhibitors.
- More common in the mandible: exposed bone that persists for more than 8 weeks; may be asymptomatic with localized soft tissue irritation, rough edges of necrotic bone may be irritating; can progress to osteomyelitis and physiologic fractures.

CURRENT THERAPY

Topical Management of Oral Ulcerations
- Ice chips as needed to help with pain.
- Diphenhydramine (Benadryl)[1] liquid 12.5 mg/5 mL (50/50 mix) with liquid antacid[1] (Maalox, Kaopectate, etc.), rinse with 1 to 2 teaspoons every 2 hours then spit; for pain.
- Triamcinolone acetonide 0.1% in oral paste (Oralone): dab a small amount on the lesion to provide a protective film, 2 to 4 times a day until ulcers are healed.
- Dexamethasone (Decadron)[1] elixir 0.5 mg/5 mL: rinse with 1 teaspoon for 2 minutes and spit out after meals and at bedtime until ulcers are healed.

Management of Resistant Ulcers with Topical Ultrapotent Corticosteroid Preparations
- Clobetasol propionate (Temovate)[1] 0.05%: apply a thin film to affected area after meals and at bedtime until healed.
- Halobetasol propionate (Ultravate)[1] 0.05%.

Management of Ulcers That Cannot Be Controlled with Topical Preparations
- Prednisone[1] 5- to 20-mg tablets; take 60 mg per day by mouth as needed to control ulcers; no taper indicated if less than 2 weeks of daily use; topical corticosteroid should be titrated to maintain control of ulcers.
- Methylprednisolone 4 mg tablets (Medrol Pak)[1] are used to control ulcers, taken with tapered doses, then topical corticosteroid should be titrated to maintain control of ulcers.

Management of Osteonecrosis of the Jaw
- Antibiotics if purulent exudate is present.
- Pain medication as needed.
- Conservative resection of hard tissue may be necessary (referred to Oral Surgeon).

Management of Dry Mouth
- Saliva substitute, sugarless mints or gum, ice chips as needed.
- Cholinergic agonist e.g., pilocarpine (Salagen) 5 to 10 mg by mouth 30 minutes before meals, not to exceed 30 mg per day.

[1]Not FDA approved for this indication.

Patients often consult the physician with problems in the orofacial region, including those that are clearly dental in nature. For these problems, the intervention may simply be to treat the pain and/or infection until definitive treatment can be provided by a dentist. These problems may include a broken tooth or restoration with sharp edges that causes soft tissue injury; infected or traumatized nerves with spontaneous pain; or focal infections that cause

swelling (likely to be less painful) or acute pain when the pressure of the purulent exudate is trapped within the bone at the apex of the root of the tooth.

Oral manifestations of systemic disease, such as pyostomatitis vegetans (Crohn disease), or mucosal petechiae (idiopathic thrombocytopenic purpura) are uncommon, and can pose difficult diagnostic challenges. Similarly, adverse oral reactions to therapeutic medications are inconsistent and may be unavoidable, for example, xerostomia, dysgeusia, and gingival overgrowth. These issues may best be handled in concert with the patient's dentist. Regional conditions, such as headache, cranial neuralgia, or sinusitis may cause oral complaints, and vice versa. The diagnosis and treatment of these conditions is not discussed in this chapter.

Nevertheless, there are a few orofacial conditions that have serious implications and should be addressed by the physician rather than referred to the dentist. These conditions are addressed in the Current Diagnosis box. The Current Therapy box includes recommended treatment; if resolution does not occur in a reasonable amount of time, for example 2 weeks, the diagnosis must be questioned. For biopsy confirmation of potential oral neoplasms and autoimmune disorders, an oral pathologist is preferred.

Odontogenic Infection
With few exceptions, disseminated bacterial infections of odontogenic origin represent a dramatic, acute exacerbation of a chronic, asymptomatic infection. A variety of dental conditions are possible causes, such as a periodontal abscess, an abscess within the supportive bone resulting from the pulpal necrosis of a carious tooth, or an infection of the gingiva surrounding a partially erupted third molar. The patient often describes a history of one or more prior acute episodes of bacterial infection symptoms from the site, followed by resolution. The degree of swelling, lymphadenopathy, pain, and fever is proportional to the risk of potential complications such as septicemia. Of particular concern is evidence of the rapid progression of diffuse swelling into the floor of the mouth and neck because of the risk of respiratory distress (i.e., Ludwig angina), or superiorly from the anterior portion of the maxilla because of the possibility of cavernous sinus thrombosis.

Definitive dental treatment to eliminate the underlying infectious source is the treatment goal after the acute, disseminated infection has been controlled. Penicillin is still considered the empiric antibiotic choice for disseminated odontogenic bacterial infections in individuals with no history of adverse reaction, and clindamycin (Cleocin) is used for those hypersensitive to penicillin. Many patients mistakenly assume that empiric antibiotic treatment can eliminate the infection in the same sense that antibiotic treatment can cure bacterial sinusitis or pharyngitis. The patient should be informed that improvement of an acute odontogenic infection after antibiotic treatment is not curative and that dental care to eliminate the underlying cause is necessary. One or more courses of antibiotics without elimination of the source increase the probability of the emergence of more virulent, antibiotic-resistant pathogens. More aggressive treatment, including intravenous antibiotics and surgical drainage in a hospital setting, must be considered in cases of rapid progression or extensive swelling, particularly if the anterior maxilla or submandibular areas are involved and in instances of compromised host resistance.

Suspicion of Oral Cancer
About 90% of oral cancers are squamous cell carcinoma (SCC), but sarcoma, adenoma, and metastatic tumors of solid organs are also found. Although the 5-year survival rate of oral SCC has improved over the past decade, it still hovers about 50%. Many patients deny the presence of a lump or mass until it becomes painful, and even then first seek care from a physician instead of a dentist or oral surgeon. Routine oral examination is still the best weapon against morbidity and mortality as there are no diagnostic tests that are satisfactory.

Oral cancer has been called the great imitator, for it can appear as many different oral conditions. It can be red, white or pigmented, exophytic, nodular, or ulcerative, smooth-surface or verrucous, and occur in any location of the oral cavity. The greatest suspicion is associated with an older patient, likely male, who uses tobacco and alcohol. The most common sites are the floor of the mouth and the lateral borders of the tongue, with the great majority being unilateral. Recently an increase in younger patients (less than 40 years old) has been tied to the presence of human papilloma virus, although no etiology has been confirmed.

Biopsy is indicated for lesions that show induration, are tied to underlying structures, are nontender, slow-growing, and especially if simple treatment of ulceration or infection has not eliminated the problem. The decision to obtain a biopsy of an oral lesion should be made with consideration of the substantial positive impact that early detection has on a disease with an otherwise unfavorable prognosis.

Necrotizing Ulcerative Gingivitis

Necrotizing ulcerative gingivitis (NUG) is a characteristic, potentially destructive infection of the dental supportive tissues caused by a predominance of fusiform bacteria and spirochetes. Some combination of psychologic stress, compromised immune function, malnutrition, or other condition of diminished host resistance dramatically increases the risk of NUG. This is suggested by the colloquial phrase *trench mouth* used to refer to this infection, because it was frequently observed among debilitated soldiers during World War I. It has also been called Vincent infection and acute NUG (ANUG).

Acute onset of poorly localized, severe dental pain, and a putrid taste are typically the patient's chief complaints. Onset usually corresponds with a significant alteration in the general health or emotional status, although a more chronic course of variably pronounced symptoms can be expected with protracted conditions, such as acquired immunodeficiency syndrome (AIDS). Visual features of NUG include necrotic deterioration of the gingiva with pronounced peripheral erythema and a superficial pseudomembrane. The tissue around the mandibular anterior teeth is most severely affected in most cases, and the gingiva often appears "punched out" from between the teeth. The gingival necrosis produces the characteristic fetid breath that is far more pungent than that caused by typical gingivitis. The putrid odor in combination with the acute onset and poor localization of pain is usually a more reliable basis for diagnosis than visual findings. Additional features, such as fever and cervical lymphadenopathy, are proportional to the severity of the oral findings.

Treatment of NUG consists of the combination of supportive care, antimicrobial measures, and improvement in the underlying compromising health conditions. Supportive care is nonspecific and includes rest, fluid intake, and a soft but nutritious diet. Warm saline, dilute hydrogen peroxide, and chlorhexidine gluconate (Peridex) are effective antimicrobial rinses. Penicillin and metronidazole (Flagyl) are the empiric systemic antibiotics of choice. Ultimately the most effective antimicrobial treatment is the combination of thorough dental cleaning of the teeth, with debridement of the necrotic soft tissue, and improved oral hygiene. Resolution of NUG, including complete healing of the gingival tissue, is strikingly rapid in most instances if this is accomplished, and underlying health status improves. Persistence or recurrence of NUG after debridement suggests the possibility of human immunodeficiency virus (HIV) infection or another undiagnosed compromising condition.

Oral Candidiasis

Oral candidiasis is a superficial fungal infection of the oral mucosa that is clinically similar to vaginal candidiasis in many respects. With isolated exceptions, the infection is caused by the fungus *Candida albicans,* which can be identified in the mouths of approximately 50% of healthy adults. The risk of oral candidiasis is increased by one or more factors of compromised host resistance: decreased local resistance, compromised immune function, or uncontrolled systemic disease. Frequently encountered examples of decreased local resistance include poor oral hygiene, xerostomia, wearing dentures that provide an organism reservoir or

limit hygiene, and recent antibiotic therapy that has altered the normally competitive oral bacteria. The combination of one or more of these local factors with a systemic condition that causes compromised immune status or constitutional compromise, dramatically increases the risk of clinical apparent infection. Common examples include AIDS, corticosteroid therapy, severe anemia, and poorly controlled diabetes mellitus.

Oral candidiasis lesions can have four distinct appearances. The most characteristic form is the pseudomembranous, curdlike, plaques of thrush that wipe off with cotton gauze leaving a sore, erythematous mucosal surface. The erythematous or atrophic form of oral candidiasis produces a thin, "beefy" appearance often affecting the dorsum of the tongue, or mucosa that supports a denture. The third type of lesion is the formation of fissures similar to those of tinea pedis that usually are at the corners of the mouth and are referred to as angular cheilitis. The fourth is a hyperplastic form that produces a patchy, white thickening of the surface epithelium that does not rub off and that appears similar to the hyperkeratosis of chronic frictional irritation. Oral candidiasis often produces more than one lesion form simultaneously in different areas of the mouth, which may be a confirmational finding. Patients often describe only a little discomfort or a mild burning sensation from affected sites, and also bad taste.

The clinical course of the infection may be acute, chronic, or cyclic in severity, depending on the nature of the underlying causes. The combination of clinical appearance, suspected compromised host status, and improvement after empiric treatment provides an adequate basis for the diagnosis. Exfoliative cytology provides definitive evidence of the infection in more equivocal situations.

Antifungal treatment eliminates oral candidiasis in most instances, but recurrences or a chronic, subclinical course can be expected if the predisposing condition remains unchanged. This implies that treatment of superficial oral candidiasis may not be justified in such instances, if the affected individual is asymptomatic, because the only realistic treatment goal is elimination of symptoms. That decision must be weighed against the possibility of spread to the esophagus.

Options for routine topical treatment of oral candidiasis include clotrimazole (Mycelex) troches, or nystatin (Mycostatin pastilles),[6] and use should continue for 1 week after resolution of symptoms. Several considerations can complicate effectiveness. Patients with xerostomia have difficulty dissolving the troches or pastilles and prefer a nystatin rinse. Concurrent management of the dry mouth (discussed later) increases the effectiveness of topical antifungal treatment for candidiasis. Limiting the *Candida* organism reservoir in the denture acrylic can be accomplished for those who wear dentures, by soaking them overnight in most commercial denture soaking solutions, mouthwashes such as Listerine, or chlorhexidine gluconate (Peridex). These products are adequately fungicidal, and keeping the denture out overnight disrupts adherence and colonization of candidal organisms. Some patients are more compliant about managing the denture problem by applying a thin layer of nystatin ointment[1] or clotrimazole cream (Lotrimin)[1] to the denture before wearing. Direct application of these preparations also promotes rapid resolution of angular cheilitis. Systemic administration of ketoconazole (Nizoral)[1] or fluconazole (Diflucan) is an alternative for patients who cannot manage topical treatment, or for severely immunocompromised individuals in the interest of controlling oral symptoms and minimizing the risk of spread to the esophagus.

Xerostomia

Xerostomia is defined by the patient's subjective perception of "dry mouth" rather than by any objective parameter. The amount of saliva is decreased, and its character typically is altered to a more viscous, ropey consistency. The condition is common because salivary function is adversely affected by so many

---

[1]Not FDA approved for this indication.
[6]May be compounded by pharmacists.

routinely encountered influences, including many frequently prescribed medications, smoking, methamphetamine abuse, several common systemic diseases, and radiation exposure for cancer treatment in the orofacial region. In addition to these influences, primary Sjögren syndrome is characterized by chronic dry eyes and dry mouth caused by autoimmune-mediated acinar degeneration. Secondary Sjögren syndrome is defined as oral and ocular dryness concurrent with an autoimmune connective tissue disorder such as rheumatoid arthritis.

The subjective response of different individuals to a mild or moderate degree of oral dryness varies considerably. Many patients who appear to produce adequate saliva complain of dryness, whereas others who seem unusually dry during oral examination have no complaints. Most patients with an advanced degree of dryness find the continual "cotton mouth" sensation and other consequences to be a significant quality-of-life issue. Decreased saliva production causes difficulty speaking, chewing, and swallowing, in addition to painful abrasion of the mucosa by coarse foods. Beyond the physical irritation, limited saliva alters the sense of taste and the enjoyment of food. Saliva contributes to oral health by providing antimicrobial components such as lactoperoxidase and IgE antibodies, and it has a significant flushing and cleansing function. Xerostomia causes a rampant and rapidly progressive pattern of dental decay that is particularly destructive, even for previously caries-resistant individuals. This is compounded if the patient compensates for the dryness by drinking sucrose-rich soft drinks or sucking on hard candy. Similarly, periodontitis tends to progress rapidly, despite normally effective treatment, if saliva production is limited. Xerostomia is also associated with complaints of generalized soreness of the mouth caused by frequent and persistent episodes of oral candidiasis.

Management of xerostomia is challenging and often frustrating for the patient and the clinician. The treatment for severe, irreversible xerostomia, as in cases of head and neck radiotherapy, is essentially symptomatic. Different patients prefer different combinations of compensation methods. Sipping water throughout the day is the single most effective and simplest way to counter loss of saliva. Some patients report additional improvement with the use of commercially available saliva substitutes, although many do as well with water and ice chips. Most patients soon learn to avoid abrasive foods, irritating commercial mouth rinses that contain alcohol, and highly flavored toothpastes in favor of less irritating alternatives. Use of a humidifier at night is often beneficial. Comprehensive dental treatment should be recommended to limit the progression and severity of dental caries and periodontitis. Smoking and compensation by drinking sucrose-rich soft drinks, sports drinks, drinks that contain caffeine, and highly acidic citric juices should be discouraged.

Additional options beyond the previous recommendations are available for those who have some residual salivary function. Drinking ample water moistens the mucosa and maintains general hydration, which maximizes the residual saliva production. Sugar-free gum or hard candy significantly stimulates saliva flow. Alternative medications that are equally effective therapeutically but less likely to cause xerostomia may be substituted in some cases to treat conditions such as hypertension.

Several cholinergic agonists are available, including cevimeline (Evoxac), pilocarpine (Salagen), and bethanechol (Urecholine).[1] Titration of dosage is usually necessary to optimize saliva flow, while minimizing frequent adverse effects such as excessive sweating and gastritis. Many patients discontinue treatment because of these and less common side effects that become more troublesome than the xerostomia. Contraindications such as glaucoma and the risk of serious complications such as arrhythmia must also be considered.

Aphthous Stomatitis

Recurrent aphthous stomatitis, colloquially known as *canker sores,* is a common condition of complex immune-mediated pathogenesis. Patients describe recurring episodes of painful ulcers that often follow triggering events such as minor tissue abrasion, eating certain foods, or episodes of emotional stress. The phrase *minor aphthous stomatitis* differentiates the most common, mild form of the disease from the more severe major and herpetiform variations. Most authorities believe these categorizations are somewhat artificial distinctions within a continuum of a single process. Similar ulcers are a feature of Behçet syndrome, but are of minor diagnostic and treatment significance compared with the other manifestations of this rare, multisystem condition.

The clinical features of minor recurrent aphthous stomatitis are characteristic. One or more painful ulcers develop soon after a short prodromal period of burning or itching at the affected site. The round or oval superficial ulcers exhibit a uniform, yellowish white, pseudomembranous surface with an erythematous peripheral halo at the sharply delineated ulcer margin. Typical size is less than 10 mm in diameter, and lesions affect only unbound oral mucosal surfaces of the lips, cheeks, floor of the mouth, or soft palate. This distribution specifically excludes the bound surfaces of the gingiva, hard palate, and the dorsum of the tongue. This feature is valuable for differentiating aphthous stomatitis from the intraoral recurrent herpetic lesions (discussed later) that affect only bound surfaces.

Aphthous lesions typically heal within 7 to 10 days, and most patients describe a long clinical course of symptom-free periods of various durations interrupted by episodes of ulcer formation. Lesion-free periods of weeks, months, or even years typically distinguish recurrent aphthous stomatitis from autoimmune conditions such as erosive lichen planus (discussed later) that produce a continuous course of oral ulcers.

The major form of recurrent aphthous stomatitis produces ulcers of similar appearance, but the lesions are larger, require a longer healing time, often heal with scarring, and form so frequently that at least one ulcer is usually present. The herpetiform variant is characterized by a cluster of numerous smaller (1 to 3 mm) ulcers that often coalesce into a single, large lesion, and the ulcers are described as exceptionally painful.[1] The clustering distribution explains the somewhat misleading herpetiform designation for this nonviral condition. This form of aphthous stomatitis may affect keratinized and nonkeratinized surfaces, which in addition to the clustering distribution may lead to confusion with recurrent herpes simplex lesions.

Minor recurrent aphthous stomatitis is more irritating than serious, and treatment beyond symptomatic management is usually not justified. Patients soon learn to avoid their particular trigger event as much as possible, and many find relief during outbreaks from over-the-counter preparations such as Orabase with benzocaine 20%, or by rinsing with soothing, coating products such as bismuth subsalicylate (Kaopectate).[1] Rinses containing a variety of ingredients, such as diphenhydramine,[1] tetracycline,[1] aloe,[7] and chlorhexidine gluconate (Peridex),[1] have been reported to promote ulcer healing in some cases. Treatment with corticosteroids (see Current Therapy box), however, is more consistently effective, and is justified for major and herpetiform variants, as well as for particularly severe or frequent outbreaks of minor aphthous lesions.

Orofacial Herpes Simplex Infection

Most herpes simplex infections of the oral mucosa are caused by herpes simplex virus type 1 (HSV-1). A much smaller proportion of oral cases results from the type 2 herpes simplex virus that typically causes genital lesions. Transmission occurs by direct contact or contaminated saliva, and serologic studies demonstrate that as much as 90% of the population has been infected by age 50.

The initial infection, referred to as acute herpetic gingivostomatitis or primary herpes, usually affects children and causes acute onset of cervical lymphadenopathy, chills, and fever similar to

---

[1]Not FDA approved for this indication.

[1]Not FDA approved for this indication.
[7]Available as a dietary supplement.

many acute viral infections. The distinguishing manifestation is the formation of multiple, painful oral vesicles that rapidly rupture. The resulting ulcers most prominently affect the gingiva, lips, and tongue but may occur on any oral surface. Primary herpes in adults is more likely to cause complaints of pharyngitis rather than oral ulcers, which makes distinguishing it from other systemic viral infections unlikely. The severity of primary herpes varies from virtually subclinical or indistinguishable from nonspecific viral infections, to debilitating. The distinguishing oral lesions are probably seen only in severe cases, because relatively few seropositive individuals recall the oral ulcers of the primary infection when questioned. Symptoms resolve within 5 days to 2 weeks, depending on the severity of the manifestations, and significant complications such as encephalitis or keratoconjunctivitis are rare.

The HSV-1 virus becomes latent within the sensory neurons that supply the primary infection site. Episodes of recurrent lesions may develop after the primary infection, a pattern similar to the recurring genital lesions caused by HSV-2. The frequency, severity, and course of these outbreaks vary widely among individuals, and at least one half of HSV-1 seropositive individuals, rarely or never suffer recurrent lesions. Those who do often associate occurrence with causative events, such as sun exposure of the exposed lip, abrasion of the surface, or an illness such as a nonspecific viral infection. This explains the colloquial terms *cold sore* and *fever blister* used to describe the most common presentation affecting the exposed lip, which is referred to as herpes labialis.

The typical episode begins with a prodromal sensation of burning or itching at the site near the vermillion border, followed by formation of one or more vesicles within 24 hours. The vesicles soon rupture, forming a coalesced crust that heals after 7 to 10 days. A few individuals suffer similar recurrent herpes lesions of the intraoral mucosa. Intraoral herpes lesions produce features of pain, onset, recurrent course, and healing time that are similar to those for aphthous stomatitis, which may present some differential diagnostic uncertainty. The diagnosis can be made in most cases based on the affected surface. Aphthous lesions are usually limited to the unbound mucosa of the lips, cheeks, soft palate, and floor of the mouth, whereas the intraoral ulcers of recurrent herpes simplex infection are limited to the bound mucosa of the gingiva and hard palate.

Treatment of primary herpes simplex infection for immunocompetent individuals is supportive and symptomatic, as for any acute systemic viral infection. In cases of significant oral discomfort, a rinse consisting of a 1:1 mixture of diphenhydramine (Benadryl)[1] elixir 12.5 mg/5 mL and a liquid antacid, or bismuth subsalicylate (Kaopectate)[1] used as needed, provides some relief by coating the ulcers. The use of systemic antiviral medication such as acyclovir (Zovirax) and valacyclovir (Valtrex) is not recommended for primary infections, except for immunocompromised patients to reduce the risk of systemic dissemination.

Most individuals affected by secondary herpes lesions suffer relatively few episodes, and no treatment is warranted. Patients prone to frequent lip lesions after sun exposure soon learn the preventive value of sunscreen lip balms, but the advice may be helpful to those who have not made the association. For patients who experience numerous secondary herpetic episodes, the systemic administration of valacyclovir (Valtrex) can be used therapeutically during the prodromal stage or prophylactically. The one-day dosing is 2 g by mouth 12 hours apart. For immunocompromised patients, valacyclovir 1 g twice a day[1] or famciclovir (Famvir) 500 mg twice a day are recommended for 10 days.

Erythema Multiforme

Erythema multiforme, which is discussed in greater detail elsewhere in this textbook, is characterized by shallow oral ulcers and characteristic "target" skin lesions. Outbreaks of secondary herpetic lesions have been implicated as a frequent trigger for erythema multiforme. A prodrome of mild fever, malaise, sore throat, and headache may precede the appearance of the oral ulcers and skin lesions. The shallow oral ulcers usually affect the lips, tongue, or soft palate, and are less likely to develop on the gingiva or hard palate. Ulcers gradually heal after 2 to 4 weeks, and approximately 20% of affected individuals experience multiple episodes. Certain medications, especially antibiotics, have also been implicated as triggers for erythema multiforme. Medication exposure is the typical stimulus for the onset of Stevens-Johnson syndrome and toxic epidermal necrolysis, which by similar allergic mechanisms produce much more extensive, generalized epithelial sloughing.

Treatment of the oral lesions of erythema multiforme is somewhat controversial. Topical and systemic corticosteroids have been recommended in the past based largely on the presumed pathogenesis of the lesions. However, little evidence exists to demonstrate the effectiveness of this approach. Supportive care usually is adequate and includes a less abrasive diet, maintaining hydration, use of analgesics, and use of a soothing, coating rinse (1:1 mixture of Benadryl[1] elixir and Kaopectate[1]).[6] Patients who experience recurring episodes may benefit from herpes simplex virus suppression with acyclovir or valacyclovir. More extensive epithelial sloughing or rapid progression suggesting Stevens-Johnson syndrome or toxic epidermal necrolysis requires hospitalization and systemic corticosteroids.

Erosive Lichen Planus and Similar Autoimmune Ulcerative Conditions of the Oral Mucosa

Several diseases cause oral ulcers by autoimmune-mediated degeneration at or near the epithelial–connective tissue interface. In some patients, painful oral ulceration is the only presenting feature of the disease. For other patients, the oral pain is only an occasional or secondary complaint. However, with few exceptions a chronic course of oral pain for months or years without complete remission is described by the patient. The location and severity may change over time with cyclic formation of new ulcers and concurrent healing of others, but the dominant trend is a chronic, protracted, or progressive course with little or no complete relief. This continuous course distinguishes the ulcers caused by autoimmune diseases from those of other conditions, such as aphthous stomatitis, which characteristically have an episodic pattern of occurrence. As with autoimmune diseases in general, the demographic pattern tends toward middle-aged women. Definitive diagnosis typically relies on biopsy results, but the differential diagnosis is often narrowed by the appreciation of additional findings, such as lesions of the skin or other mucous membranes, and by laboratory tests, such as obtaining an antinuclear antibody (ANA) titer. Lichenoid drug reactions can occur in any patient at anytime during the administration of a medication, although onset of ulcers associated with a new prescription is often indicative of a causative agent.

Distinguishing between chronic oral ulcers from four conditions, erosive lichen planus (ELP), lichenoid drug reaction, mucous membrane pemphigoid (MMP), or pemphigus vulgaris (PV), can be assisted by reviewing the location and appearance of the ulcers, and the history of the condition.

ELP is relatively common and oral lesions may occur before the characteristic skin lesions in many patients. In the mouth, the nonerosive lichen planus is characterized by a reticular white lacy expression on the buccal mucosa that may be visualized more easily by drying the tissue with a gauze. Erosions may be related to stressful experiences, or exposure to certain foods or dental materials. The erosive lesions of ELP and the lichenoid drug reaction are indistinguishable, so history is helpful relating the chronologic onset of a medication. Many medications are implicated in the etiology of lichenoid drug reactions, including commonly prescribed thiazide diuretics, nonsteroidal anti-inflammatory drugs, and penicillins.

Mucous membrane pemphigoid (MMP) has also been referred to as *cicatricial pemphigoid* and *benign MMP*. The typical presentation of MMP is a chronic course of primarily gingival vesicles and bullae that rapidly degenerate into ulcers, usually occurring on the gingival tissue, although any intraoral area may be affected. The patient may also have genital and conjunctival mucous membrane lesions. The incidence of the eye lesions approaches nearly 25% of affected individuals during the protracted disease course, and these lesions may cause blindness in severe cases.

Of the four characteristic forms of pemphigus, only PV causes oral lesions to any clinically significant degree. Approximately one half of patients develop oral ulcers before the appearance of skin lesions. Most PV oral lesions are found on the marginal gingiva in the upper and lower premolar regions. They appear as bands of beefy red ulceration about 2 mm wide that bleed very easily and are painful when the patient attempts to brush or floss. Initial vesicle or bulla formation is unusual with oral PV, in contrast to MMP, and the peripheral striations described with ELP are absent. The oral ulcers caused by PV tend to show slow progression without healing over time, in contrast to the cyclic variation of concurrent healing and lesion formation characteristic of ELP and MMP.

The oral ulcers caused by all of the conditions in this group respond to corticosteroid medications in the recommended therapeutic approach as described in the Current Therapy box. Several pivotal issues about these conditions and treatment with corticosteroids are important for successful management:

- Ulcers from infectious diseases (fungal or viral) should not be treated with corticosteroids as this may worsen the condition.
- Most patients will not be cured, but the erosive nature of these ulcers will be controlled and therefore the pain will be reduced.
- Oral candidiasis is a frequent complication of corticosteroid treatment, and this risk is increased with any concurrent condition such as xerostomia. Candidiasis can be detected early with periodic recall evaluation and by exfoliative cytology in suspected situations. Understanding the typical oral candidiasis symptoms increases the patient's awareness of the need to return for treatment.
- Empiric topical corticosteroid treatment should be discontinued for 2 weeks if a biopsy becomes necessary for a definitive diagnosis.

Every effort should be made to identify and discontinue use of causative or irritating agents. Examples such as the link of acidic foods with aphthous ulcers are obvious to the patient, but many are more subtle. One example is cinnamon flavoring agents in many foods, mouthwashes, and toothpastes. Others are irritating to the mucosa but are mistakenly perceived as beneficial. Hydrogen peroxide, phenol preparations, and alcohol-based mouth rinses that "seem to be doing some good" because they are painful and consequently assumed to be killing bacteria are examples that should be avoided by patients with oral ulcers.

Corticosteroid Treatment of Immune-Mediated Oral Ulcers

Corticosteroid management of oral ulcers is similar to the approach for immune-mediated skin lesions. The therapeutic goal is lesion and symptom control, because disease cure or spontaneous remission is unlikely. This should be understood by the patient to avoid unreasonable expectations. Healing of ulcers should be achieved with as little corticosteroid medication as possible. Topical corticosteroids should be tried first, limiting systemic administration to "bursts" as needed to control outbreaks of refractory ulcers followed by maintenance with topical treatment. Long-term systemic corticosteroid administration should be considered only as a last resort. The severity of lesions in these conditions typically varies with time, which means that the need for treatment beyond topical control also varies. Understanding several issues unique to the oral cavity can increase treatment effectiveness:

- Application of the topical corticosteroid after eating and at bedtime and avoiding frequent snacks promote adherence, absorption, and effectiveness.
- Low- and intermediate-potency topical corticosteroid preparations such as triamcinolone (Kenalog), and dexamethasone (Decadron) tend to be less than optimally effective in the oral environment. Initial trial with a higher-potency preparation is justifiable because significant systemic absorption through the oral mucosa is minimal. The use of ultrapotent topical corticosteroids is reserved for persistent ulcers if some systemic absorption is acceptable.
- Titration of a topical steroid should be explained to the patient so that the least amount of steroid to keep the lesions from recurring is found by experimenting with the interval of use.

Osteonecrosis of the Jaw

Due to the limited blood supply in the mandible, there is a greater risk of osteonecrosis of the jaw (ONJ) than in the maxilla. Many patients who have received radiation to treat head and neck or oral cancer may have an increased risk of ONJ due to the proximity of the mandible to the field of treatment. Secondary to the use of bisphosphonates and other antiresorptive drugs such as denosumab (Prolia), a small number of patients will develop an area of necrotic bone that persists for 8 weeks or more. Often the patient will first complain of an area that feels rough to the tongue on the medial side of the mandible. This is difficult to see because the tongue is in the way, but physicians who prescribe the medications for osteoporosis or metastatic tumors to the bone should be aware of the risk and use a tongue depressor to better visualize the area during examination. Some patients on these medications will have spontaneous development of the condition due to the forces put on the bone during each bite. Others will need dental surgery and the nonhealing area will appear after a tooth is extracted.

While some studies show that a drug holiday from these medications reduces the risk, there appears to be no way to evaluate this. The blood tests that show bone turnover by measuring c-telopeptide (CTX) activity are not specific, and although these tests correlate to improvement in osteoporosis, there has not been any evidence that predicts which patient will develop ONJ.

Treatment is to prescribe systemic antibiotics when there is purulent exudate, with the use of pain medication as needed. Antimicrobial mouthwash such as chlorhexidine gluconate (Peridex) is helpful to eliminate plaque when it is uncomfortable to brush. For extensive areas of necrotic bone, the oral surgeon should be consulted for conservative resection of the affected bone.

References

American Association of Oral and Maxillofacial Surgeons. Medication-Related Osteonecrosis of the Jaw—2014 Update. Available at www.aaoms.org/docs/position_papers/mronj_position_paper.pdf?pdf=MRONJ-Position-Paper [accessed January 25, 2015].

Glick M. Burket's Oral Medicine: Diagnosis and Treatment. 12th ed. Shelton Conn.: People's Medical Publishing House-USA; 2015.

Hupp WS, Migliorati CA, Brennan MT, editors. AAOM Clinician's Guide "The Dentist's Role in the Management of the Cancer Patient." Seattle, Wash.: American Academy of Oral Medicine; 2011.

Neville BW, Damm DD, Allen CM, Bouquot JE. Oral and Maxillofacial Pathology. 3rd ed. St Louis: Saunders Elsevier; 2009.

Ruggiero SL, Dodson TB, Fantasia J. American Association of Oral and Maxillofacial Surgeons position paper on medication-related osteonecrosis of the jaw—2014 update. J Oral Maxillofac Surg 2014;72:1938–56.

U.S. Preventive Services Task Force. Screening for Oral Cancer. Updated November 2013. Available at http://www.uspreventiveservciestaskforce.org/Home/GetFileBy ID/1081 [accessed January 15, 2015].

DISEASES OF THE NAILS

Method of
David de Berker, MRCP

Anatomy

The nail plate arises from the nail matrix and grows out attached to the nail bed (Figure 1). The plate is inert and physiologically comparable to the stratum corneum as a structure composed of modified corneocytes containing a high proportion of keratins specific to the hair and nail differentiation that provide the hard and flexible characteristics of the appendage. The matrix is clinically

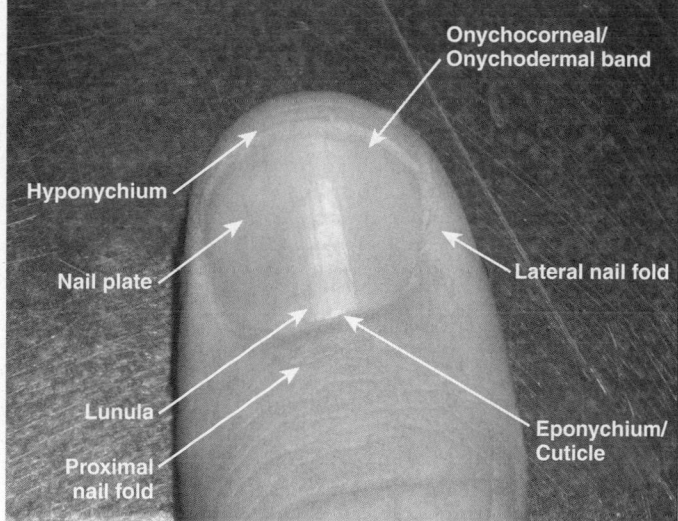

Figure 1. Surface anatomy of the nail.

visible as the lunula or half moon in the radial digits, particularly in the thumb. It usually is concealed by the proximal nail fold in digits further round to the little finger and in the toes. The proximal nail fold is a flap of skin that provides a cover to the base of the nail and is adherent to it, with a seal at the distal edge of the nail fold in the form of the cuticle. The lateral nail folds provide a soft tissue boundary to the nail sides. Distally, the nail is firmly attached to the nail bed, with a specialized configuration of epidermis that serves the purpose of minimizing the risk of separation of the nail from the nail bed. Such lifting is called *onycholysis* and is seen in a range of inflammatory and traumatic diseases. Once established, onycholysis can result in pain and loss of function of the digit.

Physiology

Fingernails grow at approximately 3 mm a month, with a faster rate on the dominant hand, on larger digits, in men, in pregnant women, and possibly in warmer weather. The rate diminishes with age from about 45 years. It is slower in toenails, with a rate of approximately 1 mm a month, which can mean that it takes 12 months or more for a big toenail to grow out fully. This has significance for the assessment of the outcome of treatment interventions. It can take several months before a result can be assessed, and in the instance of treatment of onychomycosis it can mean that the treatment has been stopped before the benefits have been fully appreciated.

Function

Fine manipulation, picking up small objects, or scratching an itch or a sticky label are all common uses of a nail. All these functions can be lost in nail disease. Where many nail diseases are associated with soft tissue inflammation of the digit tip or nail fold, there can also be pain that limits function further.

Diseases

Onychomycosis

Onychomycosis is the infection of the nail plate and nail bed with fungus. Pathogenic fungi can damage the nail plate and its attachments. Fungus can also be present in an altered nail but not be the cause of the altered appearance in that it is biologically normal for fungus to occupy cracks in a damp space where there is organic material. Dermatophyte fungi (e.g., *Trichophyton* sp.) are more likely to be pathogenic than nondermatophytes, also referred to as molds (e.g., *Fusarium* sp.). *Candida* sp. also commonly colonizes rather than gives rise to an active onychomycosis with nail changes. However, when a nondermatophyte becomes established as a pathogen, it is often more difficult to eradicate than a dermatophyte and may well manifest with associated biological or occupational factors in the patient (e.g., working with soil, wet work).

CURRENT DIAGNOSIS: ONYCHOMYCOSIS

- Make an objective diagnosis with KOH, culture, or clipping for periodic acid–Schiff.
- Onychomycosis is much more common on the toenails than the fingernails.
- The most common organisms are *Trichophyton rubrum* and *Trichophyton mentagrophytes*.
- *Candida* only rarely causes onychomycosis. It is primarily a colonizer where the local environment is conducive.
- Nondermatophyte molds (e.g., *Aspergillus* and *Fusarium* spp.) are unusual causes of onychomycosis in the United States. Repeat tests showing the same organisms and ruling out other causes are required before initiating treatment.

Clinical Features and Diagnosis

Fungal invasion of nail alters the color and integrity of the nail. It may also alter attachment to the nail bed and the shape of the nail. The main color change is the development of shades of yellow or cream that are not transparent, in contrast with the normal color of the nail. Patterns of onychomycosis are described according to the dominant aspect of the infection.

Distal or distolateral onychomycosis is the most common, with the patient's history revealing the progress of a yellow discoloration that has extended gradually over many months or years from the free edge proximally up the nail bed or up one margin. This is usually associated with debris beneath the nail: subungual hyperkeratosis. Diagnosis relies on laboratory confirmation by obtaining a sample of nail and subungual debris for microscopy and mycological culture to provide the identity of the fungus, from which its role and likely sensitivities can be determined. Nail plate histology and polymerase chain reaction assay can be used as second-line tests.

Superficial white onychomycosis can manifest as small white powdery islands within the surface of the nail plate or as larger confluent areas. Scraping with a semisharp blade can demonstrate that it is limited to the dorsal aspect of the nail, and this sample can be sent to mycology for confirmation of the pathogen. It is a form of onychomycosis more common in children, who as a rule do not often suffer onychomycosis.

Proximal white subungual onychomysis is a variant of onychomycosis seen relatively more often on the fingernails and in people with immunosuppression, either through medication or as part of disease such as HIV. The infection manifests as a white appearance arising proximal to the rim of the proximal nail fold and beneath the nail plate. With time, as the nail grows out, there may be disturbance of the dorsal nail plate, and disease may progress to the distal free edge with nail destruction.

All three forms of infection can combine or progress to result in a nail that is almost or entirely overtaken with fungal infection, creating a variant known as *total dystrophic onychomycosis*.

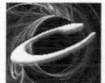

CURRENT THERAPY: ONYCHOMYCOSIS

- Oral treatment should be reserved for patients with mycological confirmation, with emphasis on those at risk for complications (diabetics, immunosuppressed patients, those at risk for secondary bacterial cellulitis).
- Topical treatment is disappointing when used in isolation, except in cases of superficial white onychomycosis. When used in combination with oral therapy, it can increase the cure rate by about 10%.
- Oral treatment is more successful than topical treatment. Terbinafine (Lamisil) 250 mg PO once a day for 6 weeks for a fingernail and 3 months for a toenail in adults is the first-line treatment. Itraconazole (Sporanox), dosed 200 mg daily or

Treatment

All national guidelines on the management of onychomycosis require that the clinical diagnosis be confirmed by microscopy of the nail for fungi and preferably also by mycological culture before commencing systemic treatment. It is common to see patients who have been treated for nonfungal disease with antifungal treatment, which wastes patients' time and money and puts them at needless risk of serious adverse effects if they take oral therapy. Polymerase chain reaction assays are available as an alternative to routine mycology but remain unable to determine the difference between a pathogenic and saprophytic role.

The main oral treatment for dermatophyte fungi is terbinafine (Lamisil). Itraconazole (Sporanox) is the main alternative. The concomitant treatment with a topical antifungal agent such as amorolfine 5% (Curanail, Loceryl)[1] or ciclopirox 8% (Penlac) can increase the rate of success, which in a trial environment is between 50% and 80% depending on accepted end points. There is a significant relapse or reinfection rate in the following 5 years, and some patients choose to use a topical therapy intermittently on the nail to attempt to avoid this. Ongoing intermittent treatment of tinea pedis is also likely to help prevent relapse.

Topical therapy alone has a smaller chance of success in dermatophytes, but it can be effective, especially if combined with thorough debridement by the dermatologist or with the help of a podiatrist with a nail Burr and curette. Topical therapy can also be undertaken in combination with surgical or chemical avulsion (50% urea paste in yellow soft paraffin), and this is of value in nondermatophytes, where the fungi are less susceptible to common oral treatments. Voriconazole (Vfend)[1] and other emerging systemic antifungals might have a place in complex nondermatophyte onychomycosis, and normally they would be used in collaboration with a clinical microbiologist. Laser therapy remains under evaluation.

Candidal onychomycosis responds to both of the main oral agents, but it is very prone to relapse if the circumstances that gave rise to the infection remain in place.

Psoriasis

Nail involvement in psoriasis is seen in 80% of psoriasis patients at some point in the course of their disease. In those with significant involvement, it results in pain and loss of function in more than 50%. Nail disease usually is in tandem with skin involvement and in particular with arthropathy of the distal interphalangeal joint, where the inflammation of the joint contributes to a zone of disease that alters matrix function.

Clinical Features and Diagnosis

A personal or family history of psoriasis assists in interpretation of the signs. Sometimes, nail psoriasis occurs in isolation, and clinical signs alone provide the diagnosis or may be supported by a nail unit biopsy. The presence of fungus does not rule out an underlying diagnosis of psoriasis, especially on a big toenail, where fungus has been noted in 27% of psoriatic nails. Nail psoriasis has features that reflect the focus of disease within the nail unit.

Treatment

Treatment requires close attention to hand care, which entails avoiding manicure or work practices that are likely to exacerbate the problem. Typical issues are the clearance of debris from

beneath the nail with a sharp instrument that elicits the isomorphic reaction with further psoriasis. Manipulation of the cuticle does the same, and having long nails results in leverage on the nail plate with minor trauma to exacerbate onycholysis. So the rules are:
- No clearance of debris except with a gentle soft nail brush
- No trimming or manipulation of the cuticle
- All nails to be as short as possible.
- General hand care with protection from solvents and wet work and use of plenty of emollient

Where potent topical steroid is to be used (Table 1), it is best applied at night only and for 2 to 3 months. Nail steroid injections have the theoretical risk of rupture of the tendon of the distal interphalangeal joint if undertaken frequently and so are usually done up to several months apart; my practice is to provide a ceiling of four injections per digit. As a rule, all systemic agents work, including biologicals, but their use is rarely justified by nail disease alone. It can be argued that cyclosporine (Sandimmune) in 3-month pulses is good for younger people with no kidney problems, methotrexate (Trexall) might suit older people, and acitretin (Soriatane) may suit those with hypertrophic nail disease. But most choices will be determined by the additional characteristics of the patient and the psoriasis elsewhere.

Idiopathic Onycholysis

Onycholysis is the separation of the nail from the nail bed, with a cleavage that commences at the free edge and progresses proximally.

CURRENT DIAGNOSIS: ONYCHOLYSIS

- Primary onycholysis and chronic paronychia are diagnoses of exclusion.
- Onychomycosis, psoriasis, lichen planus, and drug reactions all must be ruled out before diagnosis.
- Primary onycholysis and chronic paronychia are more common on the fingernails than the toenails, in women, in adults, in those who use nail cosmetics, and in those who have recurrent exposure to moisture or chemicals.
- Both primary onycholysis and chronic paronychia represent breakdown in the normal barrier of the nail apparatus.
- Onycholysis results from breakdown of the onychocorneal band or nail bed–nail plate connection. Chronic paronychia results from breakdown of the cuticle and nail folds.
- In both scenarios, moisture, contact irritants, contact allergens, colonizing yeast, and bacteria invade the exposed nail apparatus and contribute to a cycle of inflammation.

Clinical Features and Diagnosis

Most patients with onycholysis also have psoriasis. However, for some with problems of nail attachment, the cause is multifactorial and it might not be possible to provide a unifying diagnosis. A subtype of onycholysis occurs in people who undertake manicure vigorously and have long nails. Such people are troubled by the debris beneath a nail and significantly damage the area by scraping material out with a sharp object. This then creates more pathology, a bigger split, and the accumulation of more debris managed by physical manipulation. It is common for people with such cosmetic sensibilities to have long nails, which then exacerbates the onycholysis further through the mechanics of creating a large lever represented by the overhanging margin of the nail. The principle is shared with the wrench in your tool set: The longer the arm on the wrench, the easier it is to exert a torsion force on the point of contact. In this instance the contact is the margin of attachment with the nail bed.

Clipping for mycology is usually undertaken and sometimes reveals *Candida* sp. This is not causal, but is a colonizing microbe in the warm onycholytic space.

---

[1]Not FDA approved for this indication.

TABLE 1 Nail Psoriasis: Clinical Features and Diagnosis

CLINICAL FEATURE	FOCUS OF DISEASE	TREATMENT MODALITY	OPTIONS
Pitting	Proximal matrix	Potent topical steroid to nail fold	Clobetosone dipropionate[2]
		Tazarotene to nail fold	
		Steroid injection	Triamcinolone acetonide (Kenalog)
Onycholysis	Nail bed	Clip back and treat topically	Steroid and or vitamin D analogues
		Antiseptic finger soaks for secondary infection e.g., *Candida* and *Pseudomonas*	
		Systemic therapy	Cyclosporine (Sandimmune), methotrexate (Trexall), fumaric acid esters,[2] acitretin (Soriatane), biologicals
Salmon patch or oily patch		No topical therapy	
Transverse ridging and undulations	Proximal nail fold	Potent topical steroid, vitamin D analogues	See pitting
		Steroid injection	Triamcinolone acetonide
Subungual hyperkeratosis	Nail bed	Steroid injection	Triamcinolone acetonide
		Systemic therapy	Cyclosporine, methotrexate, fumaric acid esters, acitretin, biologicals
Nail shedding	Matrix and nail bed	Systemic therapy	Cyclosporine, methotrexate, fumaric acid esters, acitretin, biologicals

[2]Not available in the United States.

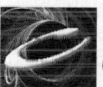

CURRENT THERAPY: ONYCHOLYSIS

- It is important not to misdiagnose the presence of yeast (especially *Candida*) as a primary infection or pathogen.
- It almost always represents a colonizer. Treatment of the yeast is therefore secondary.
- Avoidance is the mainstay of treatment. Avoid all wet work and exposure to acids, bases, and chemicals by wearing cotton gloves under heavy-duty vinyl gloves.
- Avoid all nail cosmetics and nail manipulation except for regular plate trimming. No nail salon. Keep the plate trimmed to its proximal-most attachment point. Avoid obvious triggers and traumas to the nail apparatus.
- Use a potent topical steroid, sometimes under occlusion for paronychia in the first month.
- It can take up to 6 months for the nail apparatus to normalize.

Treatment

Treatment principles are shared with psoriasis (see earlier). The presence of *Candida* sp. on mycology might tempt the clinician to try itraconazole (Sporanox)[1] systemically. However, it rarely helps, although the removal of one factor in the pathology can help other treatments to improve the situation. Success mainly requires avoidance of all physical exacerbating factors and clipping back the separated nail to treat the exposed nail bed with moderate-potency topical steroid. Antiseptic soaks can help if clipping back is not an option or there is significant microbial colonization.

Lichen planus

Lichen planus of the nail has features in common with psoriasis in that it can involve all the different structures of the nail unit and give rise to a range of features accordingly. The area of greatest concern is when it manifests with features of scarring, which can cause permanent loss or splits in nails, with considerable cosmetic and physical handicap.

Clinical Features and Diagnosis

In common with its presentation on the skin, nail lichen planus can be hypertrophic, with thickened nails, or it can be atrophic, with patterns of pronounced pitting that coalesce and eventually fragment the nail. In some instances the disease is very focal and the matrix pathology results in complete loss of nail production, with scarring sequelae. If this occurs with normal matrix remaining on either side, a pterygium may be the outcome, with a scar and nail split being bordered by viable nail spurs like wings. This is normally irreversible, and any suggestion of this pattern of disease should prompt rapid and usually systemic treatment. The potential for side effects with systemic therapy, which may be prolonged, means that I favor a diagnostic biopsy when there is any doubt or when presentation is with nail disease alone. Sometimes, clinical corroboration with mucosal, skin, or scalp disease allows certainty without a biopsy. Biopsy is best taken of nail bed, matrix, and nail fold to ensure it is representative and does not miss the diagnosis.

Treatment

The general protective and topical steroid therapies used in psoriasis can apply in lichen planus. If systemic therapy is needed, oral or intramuscular steroid injection can be used and represent flexible and effective therapy. The duration of the treatment means that monitoring of blood pressure, glucose, and weight may be indicated and bone protection might be needed. Regimens vary, but oral prednisolone 0.25 to 0.5 mg/kg for 4 to 6 weeks, tapering in the 2 weeks following, normally reverses active disease. It also allows assessment of what may be the irreversible scarred element, although nail growth rate means that this judgment should wait until a further 4 to 6 weeks after the end of treatment. Acitretin (Soriatane)[1] and cyclosporine (Sandimmune)[1] also can be used in lichen planus and may be better where patient morbidity does not allow prolonged or repeated oral steroids. Injected steroids may be used to address areas of focal scaring but seldom result in full cure.

---

[1]Not FDA approved for this indication.

[1]Not FDA approved for this indication.

Eczema

Eczema of the nail folds or nail bed may be associated with eczema elsewhere on the hand or foot and can cause nail unit disturbance in a manner similar to psoriasis. Special patterns of eczema can be relevant for allergic contact sensitivity.

Clinical Features and Diagnosis

The most common pattern of nail changes in eczema is where the nail fold is inflamed as part of an irritant hand eczema or as part of atopic eczema. This acts as a focus of inflammation that in turn disturbs matrix function owing to their adjacency. The nail then suffers transverse ridges and alterations of color, which reflect the fluctuating inflammation. Where the eczema is more directed at the digit tip, the nail bed is more likely to be involved, which in turn results in onycholysis. Both patterns often manifest most in the dominant hand because trauma, or simply use, increases the likelihood of pathology.

Occupational factors can be important both for analysis of the cause and for helping patients manage the global situation because they can suffer degrees of incapacitation. Where the occupation plays a part in the pathology, such as irritants in a health care or food-preparation worker, it may be necessary to review career choices. Hairdressers, beauticians, and engineers in certain fields come into contact with a wide range of contact sensitizers. The use of nail cosmetics alone can be relevant. Consider patch testing.

Treatment

Treatment is as for eczema elsewhere and shares many of the points made for managing psoriasis of the nail unit:
- Avoidance of irritants, trauma, nail manipulation, and frequent wetting
- Use of copious thick emollient
- Topical steroid tailored to severity
- Hand protection

Infective and chronic paronychia can be a complicating factor in nail unit eczema and requires additional systemic antibiotics in some instances.

Paronychia

Paronychia means inflammation of the proximal or lateral nail folds. There can be an infective component, and there is often a traumatic or eczematous background pathology.

Clinical Features and Diagnosis

An acute paronychia manifests as a focus of redness, pain, and sometimes a point of purulent collection and discharge in the nail fold. There may be a history of preceding trauma or, in children, of nail biting.

Chronic paronychia is seen with a raised, bolstered proximal nail fold, loss of cuticle, and transverse ridges in the nail extending up the nail plate, indicating many months of fluctuating inflammation. There is an account of episodic pain and sometimes discharge of pus. Antibiotics or antifungals alone do not settle the pathology.

Treatment

Acute paronychia is primarily infective and will subside after management of the bacterial infection and the associated wound or inflamed focus. Chronic paronychia has substantial crossover with an irritant hand eczema, and management is as for hand eczema. The low level of infection is secondary to the loss of cuticle and loss of barrier function in a digit that has substantial exposure to microbes. Where wet work is a factor, *Candida* sp. may be found, but short-term eradication with systemic therapy does not resolve the chronic problem. Management is with potent steroid, sometimes under tape occlusion. Evening (10 minutes) antiseptic soaks can help diminish the risk of infective exacerbation, but once a cuticle has re-formed and the nail fold is flat, the risk has passed.

If there is a failure to respond to this regimen, the diagnosis might need challenging. Periungual squamous cell carcinoma can manifest in this manner and requires lateral longitudinal biopsy for assessment.

Ingrown Toenail

An ingrown nail represents a conflict between the shape of the nail and the soft tissues surrounding it. This conflict can be highlighted by an episode or period of trauma such as sport or new shoes, or may be a sustained anatomical state. It is compounded by cutting the nail short at the distolateral corner such that the nail fold overlaps the end of the nail. Symptoms arise through the soft tissue inflammation, which can sometimes be complicated by bleeding or infection. Treatment is directed at the acute inflammation and subsequently at the anatomy if needed.

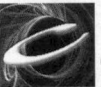

CURRENT DIAGNOSIS: INGROWN TOENAIL

- Common risk factors include incorrect nail cutting, wide feet, narrow-toed shoes, lateral plate malalignment, and lateral nail fold hypertrophy.
- Neonates and infants demonstrate distal nail ingrowing, which is separate in pathogenesis and treatment from the disease in adolescents and adults.
- Ingrown nails can be graded on a scale from I to III, with I being erythema and swelling with drainage from the nail fold and III being associated with exuberant overgrowth of granulation tissue over and around the ingrown nail plate.

Clinical Features and Diagnosis

Ingrowing can occur at any nail margin, with the most common site being the lateral nail fold in the big toe of someone in the second or third decade of life. At this site, it is the angle of the distal and lateral nail that becomes embedded in the lateral nail fold to create a puncture wound. The inflammation that follows creates a more bulky lateral nail fold and a positive feedback loop such that resolution typically requires medical intervention.

In a newborn or in a nail regrowing after loss, ingrowing can occur at the free edge as it meets the distal digit pulp. Proximally, an incompletely shed nail may be displaced upwards to embed into the ventral aspect of the proximal nail fold, with a pattern of pain and inflammation that matches ingrowing at other sites. This is called *retronychia*. All variants can evolve to create a mass resembling a pyogenic granuloma coupled with ooze and potential for secondary infection and local cellulitis.

CURRENT THERAPY: INGROWN TOENAIL

- Infantile disease should be treated with warm soaks with antiseptic followed by massage of the nail and distal phalangeal tuft.
- Adolescent and adult disease should be addressed with correct nail plate cutting and shoes. For mild disease, twice daily antiseptic soaks, topical steroids, 20% to 40% topical urea cream (Keralac, Carmol), and cotton wisps or dental floss under the aggravating part of the lateral nail plate will decrease inflammation, improve symptoms, and normalize the nail plate without surgery.
- For more advanced cases, use twice-daily warm soaks and oral antibiotics (with signs of infection), followed by lateral plate avulsion and lateral matricectomy (either chemical or surgical).

Treatment

Mild acute ingrowing can be treated with antiseptic soaks, potent topical steroid, and oral antibiotic if infection is suspected.

Causal footwear or activities should be avoided and shoes with a high toe box to accommodate the tips of the toes should be worn. It may be possible to insert a pledget of cotton, wool or similar between the embedding edge of nail and the damaged soft tissue. Advice on square end nail cutting to avoid an overshort nail is important.

If this conservative approach does not work, surgery is indicated. This is normally ablation of the lateral 3 to 4 mm of nail matrix and can be done with 85% aqueous phenol to create a chemical burn or with excision. The latter requires considerable skill for a reliable outcome because the apex of the horn of the matrix is difficult to access, and a remnant, if left, results in a spicule of nail regrowth that will continue to cause problems. Phenol, however, tends to find the entire exposed matrix because it is a liquid flowing into a crevice and does not need precise placement.

Distal embedding normally settles with conservative measures, and proximal ingrowing with retronychia requires avulsion. Avulsion is not the treatment for lateral or distal ingrowing because it results in recurrence of the problem as the nail regrows in most instances.

Single Digit Dystrophy
Dystrophy of a single nail is relatively common.

CURRENT DIAGNOSIS: SINGLE DIGIT DYSTROPHY

- Nail dystrophy on a single digit represents a risk factor for squamous cell carcinoma or melanoma of the nail unit.
- This is more common on a finger than a toe, where trauma is more often the explanation on a toe.
- When history, examination, and investigations do not provide a clear diagnosis, then a nail unit biopsy is indicated to exclude neoplasm and direct definitive treatment.

Clinical Features and Diagnosis
Dystrophy in a single digit can have any appearance, but the important thing for the clinician is that single-digit dystrophies include the uncommon but significant category of skin cancer. The most common of these is in situ squamous cell carcinoma (SCC), but the main other diagnosis is melanoma, either with a longitudinal melanonychia or as amelanotic melanoma with a lesion resembling a pyogenic granuloma. Both SCC and melanoma are infamous for having a late diagnosis in the digit, and the reason for this is lack of awareness shared by patient and clinician.

Following exclusion of inflammatory dermatoses by history and body examination and of onychomycosis by multiple clippings, the area should be biopsied for histology of matrix and nail bed. The classic biopsy is the lateral longitudinal biopsy, although this should be tailored to the perceived focus of pathology. It is best undertaken by someone familiar with nail pathology and the procedure, because there is a further risk of false reassurance of a negative biopsy if the sample is too small or directed at the wrong area of the nail unit.

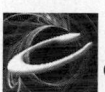

CURRENT THERAPY: SINGLE DIGIT DYSTROPHY

- Once a biopsy has been obtained it is possible to pursue one of the three avenues of definitive treatment: antimicrobial, immunosuppressive, or surgical. Each option is directed at infection, inflammation or neoplasm, respectively, and each is counterproductive for management of either of the other two diagnostic groupings.

Treatment
Where malignancy is detected, treatment is normally surgery. Topical therapy for in situ SCC does not work well owing to obstruction of the involved surfaces beneath the nail. The crevices created by the nail folds make photodynamic therapy ineffective.

References
Dalle S, Depape L, Phan A, et al. Squamous cell carcinoma of the nail apparatus: Clinicopathological study of 35 cases. Br J Dermatol 2007;156:871–4.
de Berker D. Clinical practice. Fungal nail disease N Engl J Med 2009;360:2108–16.
de Berker DA, Lawrence CM. A simplified protocol of steroid injection for psoriatic nail dystrophy. Br J Dermatol 1998;138:90–5.
Jiaravuthisan MM, Sasseville D, Vender RB, et al. Psoriasis of the nail: Anatomy, pathology, clinical presentation, and a review of the literature on therapy. J Am Acad Dermatol 2007;57:1–27.
Piraccini BM, Saccani E, Starace M, et al. Nail lichen planus: response to treatment and long term follow-up. Eur J Dermatol 2010;20:489–96.
Sánchez-Regaña M, Sola-Ortigosa J, Alsina-Gibert M, et al. Nail psoriasis: A retrospective study on the effectiveness of systemic treatments (classical and biological therapy). J Eur Acad Dermatol Venereol 2011;25:579–86.

ERYTHEMA MULTIFORME

Method of
Gabriel P. Currie, MD; and Jose A. Plaza, MD

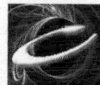

CURRENT DIAGNOSIS

- Acute, symmetrical, primarily extensor surfaces of acral surfaces.
- Target-like papules, plaques, and bullae.
- Mucosal lesions can be present.
- Young adults, female preponderance.
- Often preceded by herpes simplex infection.

CURRENT THERAPY

- First episode: symptomatic care (oral antihistamines, topical corticosteroids).
- Recurrent episodes: prophylaxis with antivirals.
- Persistent: cyclosporine (Neoral, Sandimmune),[1] prednisone, azathioprine (Imuran),[1] dapsone,[1] and antimalarials.

[1]Not FDA approved for this indication.

Epidemiology
Erythema multiforme (EM) is an uncommon, acute, self-limited immune-mediated mucocutaneous disorder. The exact incidence of EM is unknown, but estimated to be far less than 1% but possibly greater than 0.01%. The disorder occurs predominantly in young adults between ages 20 and 40, but as many as 20% may be seen in children and adolescents. There is a slight female predominance and the disease affects all races equally.

Risk Factors
EM has been associated with infections, medication use, malignancy, autoimmune disease, radiation, immunization, and menstruation. However, of these, infection represents approximately 90% of cases, the most common of which is herpes simplex virus (HSV) infection. Other infectious associations include mycoplasma, histoplasmosis, *Yersinia*, and tuberculosis. Approximately 10% of cases are drug associated, most often sulfonamide induced.

Pathophysiology

Studies of the pathophysiology of EM have been based on the study of herpes-associated EM. It has been postulated that peripheral blood mononuclear cells transport HSV DNA to lesional skin, where a subsequent virus-specific response occurs. CD4 + T helper type 1 (TH1) cells release interferon-gamma (IFN-gamma), leading to a nonspecific inflammatory amplification through autoreactive T cells and subsequent keratinocyte destruction. In drug-induced EM, tumor necrosis factor–alpha, perforin, and granzyme B cause the epidermal destruction.

Prevention

To date, there is no known preventive strategy. However, as the fields of pharmacogenomics advance, new human leukocyte polymorphisms that predispose to EM may be identified.

Clinical Manifestations and Diagnosis

Erythema multiforme is generally a self-limited illness that lasts 1 to 4 weeks. In approximately one-third of cases, the cutaneous lesions are preceded by a prodrome of fever, headache, sore throat, cough, rhinorrhea, and malaise. Although the skin lesions may vary between individual patients, the earliest lesions are usually round, erythematous, edematous papules surrounded by areas of blanching. The lesions evolve to target-like papules and plaques with a central portion of epidermal necrosis that appear dusky and can form central bullae (Figures 1 and 2). The lesions are symmetrically distributed on extensor surfaces of the extremities.

Differential Diagnosis

The clinician must consider urticaria, fixed drug eruption, bullous pemphigoid, paraneoplastic pemphigus (PNP), Sweet's syndrome, Rowell's syndrome, and polymorphous light eruption (PMLE), as well as the more serious Stevens-Johnson syndrome (SJS)/toxic epidermal necrolysis (TEN) spectrum of disorders.

Treatment

Although generally EM is a self-limited condition, the recurrent or persistent nature of the disease in some patients has led to a variety of potential treatments. Of utmost importance is discontinuation of all provocative factors, including potential medications. Although HSV induces the majority of cases, anti-HSV treatments do not alter the clinical course. However, in recurrent HSV-associated disease, suppressive therapy can provide relief. With mild disease, symptomatic treatment with oral antihistamines (diphenhydramine [Benadryl] 25–50 mg PO every 6 hours as needed, hydroxyzine [Atarax, Vistaril] 25–100 mg PO every

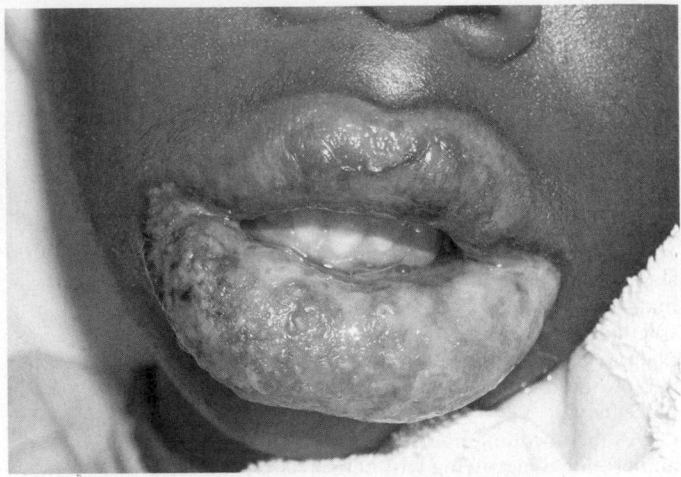

Figure 2. Erosions with extensive crusting on the vermilion and mucosal lip. (Photo courtesy of Sheila Galbraith, MD.)

6 hours as needed) and midpotency topical corticosteroids (triamcinolone 0.1% ointment [Triderm] applied to affected skin twice daily) will suffice. In more problematic mucosal disease, as well as recurrent EM, cyclosporine (Neoral, Sandimmune),[1] prednisone, azathioprine (Imuran),[1] dapsone,[1] and antimalarials have all been used with varying degrees of success.

Monitoring and Complications

EM is a self-limiting disease. As a rule, lesions do not lead to scarring. However, postinflammatory hyperpigmentation may take months to resolve. Patients with ocular involvement can develop scarring without ophthalmologic intervention.

---

[1]Not FDA approved for this indication.

References

Aurelian L, Ono F, Burnett J. Herpes simplex virus (HSV)–associated erythema multiforme (HAEM): a viral disease with an autoimmune component. Dermatol Online J 2003;9:I.

Howland WW, Golitz LE, Weston WL, Huff JC. Erythema multiforme: clinical, histopathologic, and immunologic study. J Am Acad Dermatol 1984;10:438–46.

Huff JC, Weston WL, Tonneson MG. Erythema multiforme: a critical review of characteristics, diagnostic criteria, and causes. J Am Acad Dermatol 1983;8:763–75.

Ono F, Sharma BK, Smith CC, et al. CD34 + Cells in the peripheral blood transport herpes simplex virus DNA fragments to the skin of patients with erythema multiforme (HAEM). J Invest Dermatol 2005;124:1215–24.

Schofield JK, Tatnall F, Leigh IM. Recurrent erythema multiforme: clinical features and treatment in a large series of patients. Br J Dermatol 1993;128:542–5.

Sokumbi O, Wetter DA. Clinical features, diagnosis, and treatment of erythema multiforme: a review for the practicing dermatologist. Int J Dermatol 2012;51:889–902.

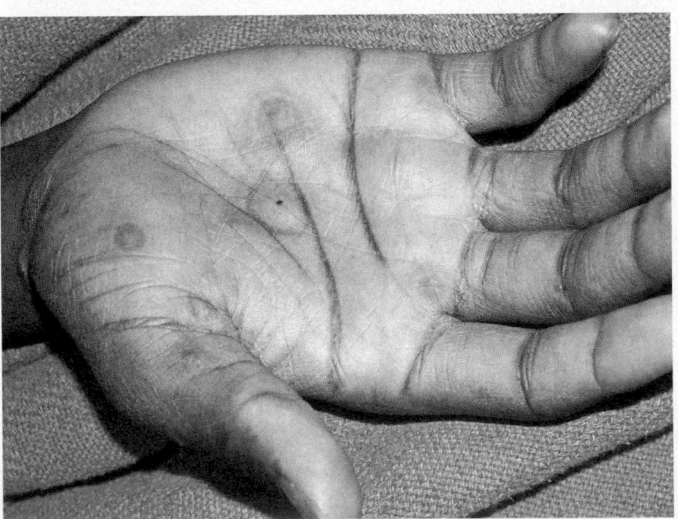

Figure 1. Typical target lesions with three zones of coloration and one central bulla on the palm. (Photo courtesy of Sheila Galbraith, MD.)

FUNGAL DISEASES OF THE SKIN

Method of
Robert Grossberg, MD

Fungal infections of the skin, hair, and nails are some of the most common infections worldwide, with special prominence among children, the elderly, men, and immunocompromised hosts such as those with diabetes, cancer, or HIV infection. Fungal infections of the skin can be divided into four general categories. Superficial fungal infections are caused by dermatophytes such as those from the *Trichophyton*, *Microsporum*, and *Epidermophyton* genera.

Cutaneous infections include tinea corporis, candidiasis, and onychomycosis. Subcutaneous (e.g., mycetoma, sporotrichosis) and systemic fungal infections (cryptococcosis, blastomycosis) that manifest in the skin are less common.

Diagnosing superficial fungal infections is generally based on clinical characteristics and response to empiric treatment. In unclear or recalcitrant cases, confirmation of diagnosis can be attempted by potassium hydroxide (KOH) preparation or histologic examination of scrapings, examination of scrapings under Wood's light, or culture. Fungal elements, however, are sometimes difficult to detect by microscopy, and tinea species grow poorly on routine culture media. Growth of dermatophytes is best performed on specific mycologic media at laboratories experienced in fungal isolation. However, depending on the specific fungal disease, the optimal site to obtain scrapings varies and affects the yield on culture.

Differential diagnosis depends on the location of the suspected fungal infection and specific clinical characteristics. Most commonly, discrimination must be made from eczema, contact dermatitis, acneiform eruptions, folliculitis of other cause, skin maceration, psoriasis, lichen planus, or trauma.

Tinea Pedis
Tinea pedis (also called athlete's foot) is most commonly caused by *Trichophyton rubrum*. It is spread by contact with infected desquamated skin and is more prevalent among men than women or children. Infection may be asymptomatic or cause various degrees of interdigital itching and cracking, erythema, scaling, and, rarely, blisters. The scaling occasionally causes an extensive moccasin sole appearance, one manifestation of dry-type tinea pedis. The disease can become extensive in immunocompromised patients, especially those with AIDS.

Tinea Cruris
Tinea cruris (also called "jock itch") is most commonly caused by *T. rubrum* or *Epidermophyton floccosum*. Occurring more commonly during summer months, tinea cruris manifests with unilateral or bilateral medial thigh and/or scrotal redness, itching, and scaling, generally with a sharp border and occasionally with papules and pustules near the leading edge. There are no satellite lesions as with candidiasis of the skin.

Tinea Corporis
Also called ringworm, tinea corporis is now relatively uncommon in the United States, being seen more commonly in tropical parts of the world. However, cases still occur in this country, especially among the homeless, HIV-infected persons, and inner city children and their caregivers. Clusters have also occurred among athletes who have skin-to-skin contact, such as wrestlers. Typical cases are caused by *T. rubrum* and appear ringlike, well demarcated, and scaly, with central clearing and little inflammation. Lesions may be hyperpigmented in darker-skinned persons. Less commonly, infection derives from animal sources such as cows, dogs, and cats and is caused by *Trichophyton verrucosum* or *Microsporum canis*. Animal-associated species tend to cause a more nodular and inflammatory form of tinea corporis that is especially seen in children. Kerions are characteristic large pustular lesions caused by these dermatophytes.

Tinea Manuum
Tinea infection of the hand usually involves only a single palm, and concurrent foot infection is typical. The appearance is of a diffuse, dry, scaly eruption, similar to the moccasin-sole form of tinea pedis. *T. rubrum* is the most common cause.

Tinea Faciei and Tinea Barbae
Tinea infections of the face (tinea faciei) are typically caused by *T. rubrum* but appear different from infections by this organism at other sites. Lesions may be follicular, pruritic, and mildly red, with inexact margins. Highly inflamed and pustular lesions of the neck and beard (tinea barbae) are caused by the animal dermatophytes *T. verrucosum* or *Trichophyton mentagrophytes*, thereby being similar to tinea corporis lesions caused by these dermatophytes, and are mainly an occupational illness.

Tinea Capitis
Tinea capitis (scalp ringworm) is principally a disease of young children. After puberty, changes in fatty acid content of sebum are believed to inhibit dermatophyte growth and lead to a dramatic decline in disease incidence. Large geographic variation occurs in overall incidence as well as causative genera and species, but most infections are due to *Trichophyton* species. Characteristic features of tinea capitis include mild to severe scaling, itching, hair loss, erythema, and sometimes pustules or kerions. Ectothrix infections have dermatophyte arthrospores forming on the outside of the hair shaft and cause hair breakage just above the surface of the scalp. In endothrix infections, arthrospores form within the hair shaft, so hair breakage occurs at the skin surface. Favus is a particularly severe form of tinea capitis caused by *T. schoenleinii*, in which a thick inflammatory crust forms on the scalp and hair follicles. This can lead to scarring and permanent alopecia if untreated.

Onychomycosis
Onychomycosis, fungal infection of the nails (also called tinea unguum), usually occurs in the setting of chronic dermatophyte infection of adjacent skin. The disease is common in elderly, diabetic, and immunocompromised persons, but it also occurs commonly in those without predisposing conditions. Various forms of onychomycosis can occur, but the most common begins at the distal and lateral subungual margins of the nail, can extend to involve the whole nail, and is caused by *T. rubrum*. Affected nails are typically thickened and raised, with white or yellow discoloration and various degrees of cracking. Nail growth may be impaired, and at times the nail dislodges spontaneously or with minor pressure. Candidiasis of the nails almost exclusively involves the fingernails, sometimes inoculated by nail biting, and is usually less extensive than typical dermatophytic infection.

Tinea (Pityriasis) Versicolor
Tinea versicolor is not a true tinea infection as it caused by lipophilic skin commensals of the *Malassezia* family, most commonly *Malassezia furfur*. This common infection is characterized by hypo- or hyperpigmented macules of the trunk or proximal extremities, sometimes with scaling. Diagnosis is usually clinical, but it can be confirmed by a scraping that demonstrates numerous round yeasts with short hyphae. After treatment, pigmentation changes can persist for weeks or months, often until the area receives sun exposure.

Candidiasis
Candida species are normal flora of the mouth and vagina, especially in settings such as antibiotic exposure, dry mouth, excessive skin moisture, and extremes of age and in immunocompromised hosts, and can cause disease on skin and mucosal surfaces. In the mouth or vagina, candidiasis is suggested by white plaques, cheesy exudates, and erythema. Candidiasis of the mouth can also occur in other forms such as erythematous plaques, angular cheilitis, acute or chronic atrophic lesions (the latter in the setting of dentures), or chronic hypertrophic plaques. Candidiasis of the skin most commonly occurs in moist or occluded areas such as the groin, buttocks (especially under diapers), and axillae, but it can involve any area including the nails (described earlier). Satellite lesions help to differentiate skin candidiasis from tinea or other conditions.

Treatment
Treatments for fungal infections are shown in Table 1.

TABLE 1. Treatments of Choice for Fungal Infections of the Skin, Hair, and Nails

INFECTION	PREFERRED AGENTS AND REGIMENS	ALTERNATIVE AGENTS/REGIMENS	ADJUNCTIVE TREATMENTS/COMMENTS
Tinea pedis	Topical terbinafine (Lamisil AT) or naftifine (Naftin)	Oral azole,[†] oral terbinafine (Lamisil),[1] griseofulvin (Grifulvin V)	Improve foot hygiene; Whitfield's ointment (benzoic acid/salicylic acid) may be applied for extensive disease; oral agents may be more effective for dry-type disease
Tinea cruris	Topical azole*	Oral azole,[†] terbinafine[1]	
Tinea corporis	Topical* or oral[†] azole	Terbinafine	Minimum 4–6 wk of treatment; oral if >1–2 lesions or large areas of skin involvement
Tinea manuum	Topical* or oral[†] azole	Terbinafine	
Tinea faciei	Oral azole[†] or terbinafine[1]		
Tinea barbae	Oral azole[†] or terbinafine[1]		
Tinea capitis	Griseofulvin (children), oral itraconazole (Sporanox),[1] oral terbinafine, fluconazole (Diflucan)[1]		Selenium sulfide shampoo (Selsun)[1] or ketoconazole shampoo (Nizoral)[1] is used only as an adjunct to oral therapy
Onychomycosis	Oral terbinafine or itraconazole	Pulse itraconazole: 200 mg PO bid for 1 wk of the mo, repeated 3–4 consecutive mo Ciclopirox nail lacquer (Penlac)	Prolonged therapy needed (3–6 mo); topical therapy is usually ineffective alone, though success has been shown with some regimens including combined oral plus topical treatments Fingernails respond better than toenails Culture of deep specimens can help guide therapy Débridement or nail removal may be needed
Tinea versicolor	Oral azole,[†] selenium sulfide shampoo or lotion, ketoconazole shampoo	Topical azole* or terbinafine	Recurrence is common; hypopigmentation might persist despite treatment
Candidiasis	Topical azole* or nystatin (Mycostatin)	Oral[†] or IV azole, amphotericin B (Fungizone)	Improve underlying cause such as moisture, diabetes, etc.

[1] Not FDA approved for this indication.
*Topical azoles include clotrimazole (Lotrimin), econazole (Spectazole), ketoconazole (Nizoral), miconazole (Micatin), oxiconazole (Oxistat), and tioconazole (Vagistat).
[†] Oral azoles include ketoconazole (Nizoral), fluconazole (Diflucan), and itraconazole (Sporanox).

References

Crissey JT, Lang H, Parish LC. Manual of Medical Mycology. Cambridge: Blackwell Science; 1995.

Havlickova B, Friedrich M. The advantages of topical combination therapy in the treatment of inflammatory dermatomycoses. Mycoses 2008;51(Suppl. 4):16–26. Erratum in: Mycoses 2009;52(1):96.

Schwartz RA. Superficial fungal infections. Lancet 2004;364(9440):1173–82.

Smith ES, Fleischer AB, Feldman SR, Williford PM. Characteristics of office-based physician visits for cutaneous fungal infections. An analysis of 1990 to 1994 National Ambulatory Medical Care Survey Data. Cutis 2002;69(3):191–8, 201–2.

KELOIDS

Method of
Leslie A. Greenberg, MD

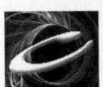

CURRENT DIAGNOSIS

- Clinical characteristics: firm, raised, papular, plaque-like, nodular, and tumorous scar tissue that extends beyond the initial wound borders. May be painful or pruritic and disfiguring.
- Location: more commonly found on ears, upper back and chest, and upper arms.
- Cause: results from an abnormal healing process after skin trauma or inflammation.

- Histologic characteristics: abnormally functioning dermal fibroblasts and overproduction of extracellular matrix result in markedly thickened bundles of hyalinized collagen arranged in a haphazard fashion.

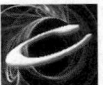

CURRENT THERAPY

Medical Therapies
- Intralesional corticosteroids (triamcinolone acetonide [Kenalog])
- Interferon alfa (IFN-alfa2b [Intron A])[1]
- Intralesional fluorouracil (5-FU, Adrucil)[1]

Surgical Therapies
- Cryosurgery
- Primary excision

Physical Modalities
- Pressure earrings
- Radiation therapy
- Laser therapy

Miscellaneous Therapies
- Silicone gel sheeting

[1] Not FDA approved for this indication.

Keloids are common, benign fibroproliferative lesions resulting from altered wound healing caused by abnormalities of fibroblast function and extracellular matrix overproduction. Lesions may be painful and severely disfiguring—at times limiting range of motion. Histologically, keloids are foci of brightly eosinophilic-staining collagen bundles laid haphazardly.

Keloids may be papular, plaque-like, nodular, or tumorous. The term *keloid* is derived from the Greek word meaning "tumor-like." A keloid extends beyond the site of injury. Keloids tend to shrink over time, but rarely resolve.

Epidemiology

Keloids occur more commonly in people of African and Asian descent. There may be a familial or genetic contribution to keloid development. Studies show that varied modes of inheritance may influence keloid formation. Keloids may be intentionally induced for cosmetic purposes. For example, the ancient Olmec of Mexico in pre-Columbian times are one ethnic group which has used keloid scarification as an intentional means of decoration.

Pathophysiology

Unlike scars, keloids are made up of markedly thickened bundles of collagen that are arranged in a haphazard fashion. Normal scar tissue formation, in contrast, consists of fibrillary bundles of collagen that are aligned parallel to the skin surface.

The pathogenesis of keloid formation is unknown. Fibroblast proliferation and increased collagen synthesis are due to overexpression of growth factors. Growth factor production fails to self-regulate and does not turn off once the wound is well healed. Alteration of programmed fibroblast apoptosis has been implicated. It has been suggested that keloid fibroblasts fail to undergo physiologically programmed cell death and thereby produce extra connective tissue. Genetic factors are likely involved, and studies have identified four susceptibility loci.

Keloids represent the end stage of an inflammatory process that starts after a traumatic disruption of skin integrity. Over a period of weeks, abnormally functioning fibroblasts replace the granulation tissue associated with the early stages of healing. At that point, a distinctive morphologic scar or keloid may be noticeable. After a keloid is fully formed it may look the same for years, though it may eventually shrink.

Risk Factors

Certain populations are at higher risk to develop keloids. Dark-skinned individuals such as those of Asian, African, and Hispanic descent have a 15-fold increased risk to develop keloids compared to light-skinned individuals. Skin insults such as lacerations, secondarily infected skin lesions, surgery, or ear piercings challenge the body's healing processes and may result in keloids. Keloids are more commonly found on the ears, upper back and chest, and upper arms. Ongoing tension or movement across the wound healing site may predispose to keloid formation. Genetics are a factor as there are reports of familial cases with varied modes of inheritance, indicating multiple genetic disorders that may influence keloid formation. Age affects propensity to make a keloid with the highest incidence in individuals age 10 to 20 years. Keloids are rarely found in newborns or the elderly.

Prevention

The best treatment is prevention of unnecessary trauma or surgery, including ear piercing and elective mole removal. Early treatment of acne helps decrease inflamed pustules and papule formation, which when located at the posterior neck may become acne keloidalis nuchae. Patients with acne keloidalis nuchae should avoid shaving the neck region and instead should use scissors to trim hair no shorter than one-eighth of an inch. Consider varicella vaccination (Varivax)[1] to decrease keloid risk of chickenpox lesions. Lack

---

[1]Not FDA approved for this indication.

of ultraviolet (UV) B light may increase risk of keloid formation. In fact, using UV A1 phototherapy may be a promising treatment of keloids.

Clinical Manifestations

Keloids are firm, rubbery, raised, papular, plaque-like, nodular, and tumorous scar tissue that extends beyond the initial wound borders. Frequently lesions are pruritic, are tender to palpation, and may be the source of sharp, shooting pains. Location is more often on the ears, jaw, neck, shoulders, upper back, and presternal chest. Keloids may be disfiguring and, in rare instances (e.g., location over a joint), may impair function.

Diagnosis

The clinical diagnosis of a keloid is usually apparent. Rarely is histologic confirmation necessary. Lesions may continue to grow for weeks to months. Keloids on the ears, neck, and abdomen tend to be pedunculated whereas those on the central chest and extremities are usually raised with a flat surface. Most keloids are round, oval, or oblong with regular margins; however, some have a claw-like configuration with irregular borders.

Differential Diagnosis

Hypertrophic scars appear different than keloids because the wound healing is linear, stays within the boundaries of the original wound site, and may be transiently indurated or tender to palpation. Hypertrophic scars are as prevalent in light- or dark-skinned individuals and as a rule tend to flatten significantly over time without treatment.

Morphea (otherwise known as localized scleroderma) begins as an inflammatory, erythematous patch that usually is not associated with an injury. Itching or pain may be present with morphea.

Lichen sclerosus et atrophicus is a chronic and sometimes pruritic inflammatory disorder that may involve the female genitals. Unlike keloids, this appears as a porcelain white atrophic plaque.

Dermatofibrosarcoma protuberans is an uncommon, locally aggressive cutaneous soft tissue sarcoma that may present as a plaque-like area of cutaneous thickening that may be violet-red or blue at the margins. Rarely, this may arise within a preexisting scar or tattoo. Definitive diagnosis usually requires a core needle or incisional biopsy.

Treatment

Intralesional Corticosteroid. Injections of intralesional corticosteroids are considered first-line therapy for keloids. A systematic review showed that up to 70% of cases respond with flattening of lesions, though the recurrence rate is up to 50% at 5 years. For local anesthesia, apply liquid nitrogen for 10 to 15 seconds or lidocaine-prilocaine cream (EMLA) under occlusion for 1.5 hours before injection. Do not use liquid nitrogen for more than 30 seconds or permanent hypopigmentation may result. Use triamcinolone acetonide (Kenalog) 10 mg/mL. Space injections approximately 0.5 to 1.0 cm apart. Use a ½-inch, 30-gauge Luer-Lok (twist-on) needle with bevel directed up toward the skin and a tuberculin syringe to allow injection under pressure. Wear a face shield to avoid contact with back-pressure spray. Inject within the bulk of the lesion with enough triamcinolone to make the keloid blanch, usually 0.1 to 0.5 mL. Multiple injections may be needed. Injections may be given monthly until the desired degree of involution and/or symptomatic relief is achieved. If no change occurs after one injection with triamcinolone acetonide 10 mg/mL, increase the strength to 40 mg/mL (Figure 1). If no change occurs after three or four injections, consider referral to a plastic surgeon or dermatologist for surgical excision.

Surgical Excision. Surgical excision of a keloid may help aesthetically and symptomatically, though lesions tend to recur and may result in more extensive scarring. After excision, immediately inject the base of the surgical site in multiple sites with triamcinolone acetonide 20 mg/mL. Use a 30-gauge needle and then occlude the excision site with a pressure dressing such as

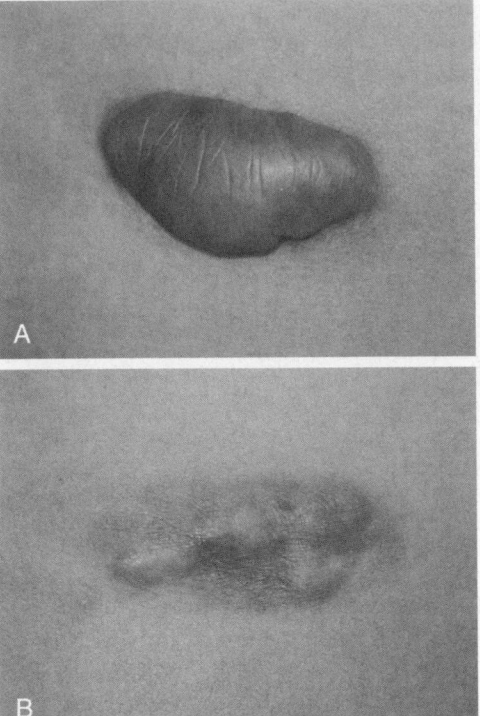

Figure 1. A, A keloid on the back. **B,** The scar after four intralesional injections of corticosteroid 10 mg/mL at 4 weeks apart. Note side effects of skin atrophy and hypopigmentation. (Reprinted with permission from Manuskiatti W: Current management of hypertrophic scars and keloids. Siriraj Hosp Gaz 2003;55:249–58.)

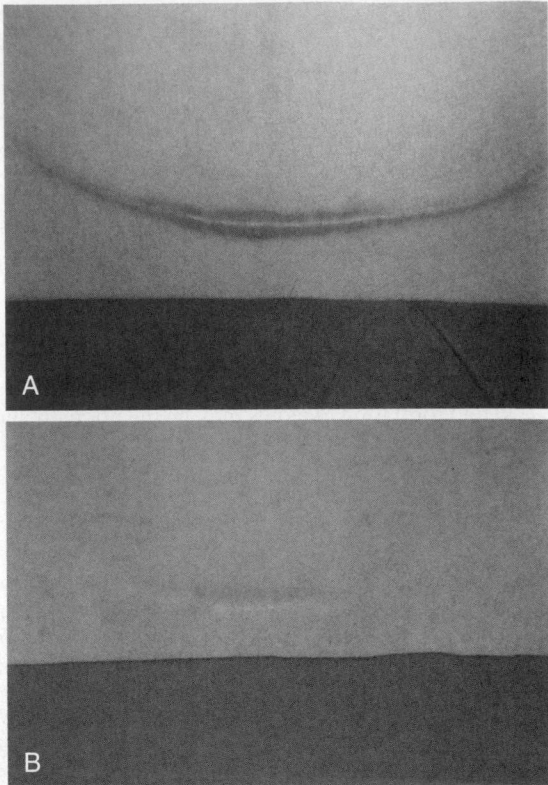

Figure 2. A, A scar developing after cesarean section. **B,** The scar after two pulsed dye laser treatments 8 weeks apart.

Elastoplast. Corticosteroid injections should then be repeated at 2-week intervals over a course of 3 to 4 months.

Silicon Sheeting. The use of silicon sheeting may be effective for treatment of symptoms such as pain and itching for established keloids. It may also be used early in wound healing to prevent keloids at the site of new injuries. In some trials, silicone sheeting was effective in 70% to 80% of cases to avoid keloid formation. Sheeting is placed on top of the keloid, taped into place, and left on for 12 to 24 hours per day. The sheet is washed daily and replaced every 10 to 14 days. Consider effectiveness after 2 to 6 months of therapy. Self-drying silicone gels shows less efficacy than the sheeting.

Cryosurgery. Cryotherapy can be used in conjunction with intralesional corticosteroids. This is widely available, is effective, and has an excellent safety profile. A 10- to 30-second freeze-thaw cycle can be repeated up to three times per treatment session. One major permanent side effect is hypopigmentation, which limits its use in darker-skinned patients.

Pressure Earrings. Zimmer splints are inexpensive, molded earring-like pressure therapy that may be effective treatment for keloids following ear piercing. One online source for these is Delasco (www.delasco.com).

Radiation Therapy. Radiation therapy is effective in reducing keloid recurrence with improvement rates of 70% to 90% when used after surgical excision. Recurrence rates of keloids after radiation therapy are 13% to 33%. There are concerns about potential long-term risks such as malignancy when used for an essentially benign condition.

Intralesional 5-Fluorouracil (5-FU). A commonly used schedule is weekly intralesional injections of 5-FU (Adrucil)[1] 50 mg/mL with a volume of 0.5 to 2.0 mL per session for up to 12 weeks. Intralesional 5-FU has been shown to improve keloids by 50% and is considered to work best on small keloids. Injections may be painful, and one study revealed a 21% rate of ulceration. 5-FU is frequently

mixed with triamcinolone acetonide: 0.1 mL of triamcinolone acetonide 40 mg/mL can be mixed with 0.9 mL of 5-FU 50 mg/mL and injected weekly for 8 weeks. Pulsed dye laser has been used in combination with intralesional injection of a mixture of 5-FU and steroid with cumulative beneficial effect.

Pulsed Dye Laser. Pulsed dye laser therapy may minimize the erythema and telangiectasias of keloids. One study showed effectiveness of treatment with a combination of pulsed dye laser and intralesional steroid on recalcitrant keloid scars (Figure 2). These patients noted a 60% decrease in height of keloid, 40% improvement in erythema, and 75% decrease in pain and itching. Presternal scars did not benefit. It is speculated that the laser helped make the scar edematous and softer so that the intralesional steroid could work better.

A combination of triamcinolone acetonide 0.1 mL of 40 mg/mL with 0.9 mL of 5-FU (50 mg/mL) injected weekly for 8 weeks with pulsed dye laser treatments at the first, fourth, and eighth week has been studied. This combination showed statistically significant benefit with regard to itch and erythema reduction compared to injected therapeutic components alone. Side effects include pain at the injection site, burning sensation, atrophy, telangiectasias, or ulceration.

Other. Retinoic acid, a topical form of isotretinoin (Accutane),[1] has been shown to be beneficial in two small clinical trials but may cause contact dermatitis. Intradermal injection of tacrolimus (Prograf)[1] has been used experimentally on rabbits and was shown to decrease scar height by 50%. Onion extract (Mederma) has not been found to decrease scar height or itching when used alone, but has helped with normalizing keloid skin color. Onion extract may be considered a useful adjunct when used with occlusive silicon dressing to help decrease keloid scar height and normalize color. UV A1 phototherapy has shown some promise in the treatment of keloids. Use of intralesional verapamil (Isoptin),[1] topical imiquimod (Aldara),[1] and vitamin E–containing oils[1] is not supported by scientific evidence.

---

[1]Not FDA approved for this indication.

[1]Not FDA approved for this indication.

Monitoring

Surveillance of scars during wound healing is important to alert the provider that keloids may be forming. Appropriate, focused, and timed treatment can then be performed. In a patient with keloid history, using prophylactic therapy may be instituted when a new wound is incurred. Close follow-up monitoring is vital during immediate and aggressive treatment.

Complications

Patients should be advised that keloids can be recalcitrant to all types of therapy. If a keloid recurs (especially if ablative methods such as electrosurgery are used), it may be more disfiguring than the original lesion. Trauma to the keloid may predispose the lesion to erosion and localized bacterial infection.

References

Asilian A, Darougheh A, Shariati F. New combination of triamcinolone, 5-fluorouracil, and pulsed-dye laser for treatment of keloids and hypertrophic scars. Dermatol Surg 2006;32:907.

Derm101.com. Scars, keloids, and anetodermas. Available at http://www.derm101.com/content/8553; [accessed 27.09.12].

Gisquet H, Liu H, Blondel WC, et al. Intradermal tacrolimus prevent scar hypertrophy in a rabbit ear model: A clinical, histological and spectroscopical analysis. Skin Res Technol 2011;17:160–6.

Hosnuter M, Payasli C, Isikdemic A, et al. The effects of onion extract on hypertrophic and keloid scars. J Wound Care 2007;16:251–4.

Kelly AP. Update on the management of keloids. Semin Cutan Med Surg 2009;28:71–6.

Kontochristopoulos G, Stefanaki C, Panagiotopoulos A, et al. Intralesional 5-fluorouracil in the treatment of keloids: an open clinical and histopathologic study. J Am Acad Dermatol 2005;52(3 Pt 1):474.

Medscape.com. Keloid and hypertrophic scar differential diagnosis. Available at http://emedicine.medscape.com/article/1057599-differential; [accessed 04.10.12].

Nakashima M, Chung S, Takahashi A, et al. A genome-wide association study identifies four susceptibility loci for keloid in the Japanese population. Nat Genet 2010;42:768.

Shaffer JJ, Taylor SC, Cook-Bolden F. Keloidal scars: a review with a critical look at therapeutic options. J Am Acad Dermatol 2002;46:63.

MELANOMA

Method of
Vesna Petronic-Rosic, MD, MSc

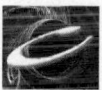

CURRENT DIAGNOSIS

- ABCDEs:
  - **A**symmetry of lesion.
  - **B**order irregularity, bleeding, or crusting.
  - **C**olor change or variegation.
  - **D**iameter larger than 6 mm or growing lesion.
  - **E**volving. Surface changes or symptomatic.
- The "ugly duckling" sign: A mole that looks or feels different compared to surrounding moles.
- Total-body photography and dermoscopy.
- Excisional biopsy with narrow margins.
- Interpretation by physician experienced in the microscopic diagnosis of pigmented lesions.
- Molecular analyses (rarely).
- Appropriate staging work-up.
- Genetic testing when appropriate (rarely).

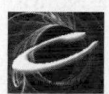

CURRENT THERAPY

- Early diagnosis and appropriate surgical therapy is the gold standard.
- Complete excision must be achieved with appropriate margins based on tumor thickness.

- Sentinel lymph node biopsy may be offered to patients with melanoma 1 to 4 mm thick, with clinically unaffected regional nodes, and without distant metastases.
- Dissection of the lymph node basin may be offered to patients with micronodal or macronodal metastases.
- Adjuvant therapy may be considered for stage III disease.
- Stage IV treatment depends on location and extent of metastatic disease and may include surgical resection, chemotherapy, biological therapy, or radiation therapy.

Melanoma is a malignancy of pigment-producing cells (melanocytes). Melanocytes are located predominantly in the skin but are also found in the eyes, ears, gastrointestinal tract, leptomeninges, and oral and genital mucous membranes.

Epidemiology

Even though melanoma accounts for less than 5% of skin cancer cases, it causes most skin cancer deaths. U.S. incidence figures estimate that there were about 108,230 new cases of melanoma in 2007: 48,290 in situ (noninvasive) and 59,940 invasive (33,910 in men and 26,030 in women). The American Cancer Society's most recent estimates for melanoma in the United States for 2009 are 68,720 new cases with 8650 deaths. Overall, the lifetime risk for developing melanoma is about 1 in 50 for whites, 1 in 1000 for blacks, and 1 in 200 for Latin Americans. At current rates, 1 in 63 Americans will develop an invasive melanoma over a lifetime.

Risk Factors

A large number of nevi is the strongest risk factor for melanoma in persons of European ancestry. Atypical mole syndrome is another risk factor. Exposure to ultraviolet light is a major risk factor, especially in persons who have fair hair and skin, who have solar damage, who had sunburns and short sharp bursts of sun exposure in childhood, and who used tanning beds. Tanning beds appear more detrimental when used before the age of 20 years. Familial risk factors include mutations in *CDKN2A*(p16INK4a), which are associated with increased risks for both melanoma and pancreatic cancer; they are transmitted in an autosomal dominant fashion and account for approximately 20% to 50% of familial melanoma cases. Organ transplant recipients have an increased risk for melanoma. Genodermatoses with a defect in DNA repair (such as xeroderma pigmentosum) increase risk for melanoma.

Pathophysiology

Transformation of normal melanocytes into melanoma cells likely involves a multistep process of progressive genetic mutations that alter cell proliferation, differentiation, and death and affect susceptibility to the carcinogenic effects of ultraviolet radiation. Primary cutaneous melanoma can develop in preexisting melanocytic nevi, but more than 60% of cases likely appear de novo.

Melanomas arising in skin that is chronically sun damaged show molecular features that distinguish them from melanomas arising in skin that is not sun damaged. These features might determine tumor behavior and potential response to new targeted drugs. About 70% of melanomas arising in skin that is not sun damaged carry *BRAF* mutations. Genetic studies have shown that 50% of familial melanomas and 25% of sporadic melanomas may be due to mutations in the tumor suppressor gene *p16*. Linkage studies have identified chromosome 9p21 as the site of the familial melanoma gene.

Prevention

Early detection of thin cutaneous melanoma is the best means of reducing mortality. Patients with a history of melanoma should be educated regarding sun protective clothing and sunscreens, skin self-examinations for new primary melanoma, possible recurrence within the surgical scar, and screening of first-degree relatives, particularly if they have a history of atypical moles.

Clinical Manifestations

Early signs of melanoma include the ABCDEs:

- Asymmetry of lesion
- Border irregularity, bleeding, or crusting
- Color change or variegation
- Diameter larger than 6 mm or growing lesion
- Evolving: Surface changes or symptomatic

The "ugly duckling" sign is also useful to recognize lesions that look or feel different compared to surrounding moles.

Lentigo maligna (melanoma in situ) begins as an irregular tan-brown macule that slowly expands on sun-damaged skin of elderly persons. Long-term cumulative sun exposure confers the greatest risk. Progression to invasive lentigo maligna melanoma is estimated to be 30% to 50%.

Superficial spreading melanoma, the most common type in light skin, represents approximately 70% of all melanomas. Peak incidence is in the fourth and fifth decade. Superficial spreading melanoma can arise in a preexisting melanocytic nevus that slowly changes over several years; it most commonly affects intermittently sun-exposed areas with the greatest nevus density (upper backs of men and women and lower legs of women). Pigment varies from black and blue-gray to pink or gray-white, and the borders are irregular. Absence of pigmentation often represents regression.

Nodular melanoma represents 15% of all melanomas. The median age at onset is 53 years. Clinically, a uniform blue-black, blue-red, or red nodule usually begins de novo and grows rapidly. About 5% are amelanotic. The most common sites are the trunk, head, and neck. Acral lentiginous melanoma accounts for 10% of melanomas overall but is the most common type among Japanese, African Americans, Latin Americans, and Native Americans. The median age is 65 years, with equal gender distribution. It occurs on the palms or soles or under the nails and is on average 3 cm in diameter at diagnosis. Clinically, the lesion is a tan, brown-to-black, flat macule with color variegation and irregular borders. It does not appear to be linked to sun exposure.

Diagnosis

Excisional biopsy with narrow margins is recommended for diagnosis. Incisional biopsy is acceptable when suspicion for melanoma is low, the lesion is large, or it is impractical to perform a complete excision. It is believed not to be detrimental if subsequent therapeutic surgery is performed within 4 to 6 weeks. Dermoscopy and total body photography are adjunctive noninvasive diagnostic techniques. Routine laboratory tests and imaging studies are not required for asymptomatic patients with primary cutaneous melanoma 4 mm or less in thickness for initial staging or routine follow-up. Indications for such studies are directed by a thorough medical history and complete physical examination.

Histologic interpretation should be performed by a physician experienced in the microscopic diagnosis of pigmented lesions. Molecular analyses for evidence of gene mutations, DNA copy-number abnormalities, or changed protein expression are useful adjunctive tools in the assessment of histologically ambiguous primary melanocytic tumors. It is now known that melanomas from sun-damaged skin, non-sun-damaged skin, or mucosal or acral surfaces harbor distinct molecular phenotypes. Specifically, activating mutations in BRAF are present in approximately 40% to 60% of advanced melanomas, especially those arising from non-sun-damaged skin, and result in activation of the RAS/RAF/MEK/ERK pathway, providing a constitutive growth signal.

The new revised American Joint Committee on Cancer (AJCC) staging system (Tables 1 and 2) includes simplified tumor-thickness thresholds of 1.0, 2.0, and 4.0 mm. Although tumor thickness and ulceration continue to define T2, T3, and T4 categories, T1b melanomas are defined by a tumor mitotic rate of 1/mm^2 or greater or ulceration, rather than Clark level of invasion. N1 and N2 categories remain for microscopic and macroscopic nodal disease respectively, with sentinel node biopsy recommended for pathologic staging. M staging continues to be

TABLE 1 Tumor, Node, and Metastasis (TNM) Staging Categories for Cutaneous Melanoma

Tumor (T)

CLASSIFICATION	THICKNESS (mm)	ULCERATION STATUS/MITOSES
Tis	NA	NA
T1	≤1.00	a: Without ulceration and mitosis <1/mm^2 b: With ulceration or mitoses <1/mm^2
T2	1.01–2.00	a: Without ulceration b: With ulceration
T3	2.01–3.00	a: Without ulceration b: With ulceration
T4	≥4.00	a: Without ulceration b: With ulceration

Nodes (N)

CLASSIFICATION	NUMBER OF METASTATIC NODES	NODAL METASTATIC BURDEN
N0	0	NA
N1	1	a: Micrometastasis b: Macrometastasis
N2	3	a: Micrometastasis b: Macrometastasis
N3	4+ metastatic nodes or matted nodes or in transit metastases/satellites with metastatic nodes	c: In transit metastases/satellites without metastatic nodes

Metastases (M)

CLASSIFICATION	SITE	SERUM LDH
M0	No distant metastasis	NA
M1a	Distal skin, subcutaneous, or nodal metastasis	Normal
M1b	Lung metastasis	Normal
M1c	All other visceral metastasis	Normal
	Any distant metastasis	Elevated

Note: Micrometastases are diagnosed after sentinel lymph node biopsy. Macrometastases are defined as clinically detectable nodal metastases confirmed pathologically.

Abbreviations: is, in situ; LDH, lactate dehydrogenase; NA, not applicable.

determined both by site of distant metastasis and serum concentration of lactate dehydrogenase, but in patients with regionally isolated metastases from an unknown primary site, disease will be categorized as stage III rather than stage IV, because the prognosis corresponds to that of stage III disease from a known primary site.

Five-year and 10-year survival rates based on the TNM classification range from 97% and 93% for patients with T1a N0 M0 melanomas to 53% and 39%, respectively, for patients with T4b N0 M0 melanomas.

Differential Diagnosis

The differential diagnosis includes melanocytic nevus, angioma, pigmented basal cell carcinoma, pyogenic granuloma, seborrheic keratosis, Kaposi's sarcoma, and hematoma (especially for acral lentiginous melanoma).

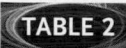

TABLE 2	Pathology Staging for Cutaneous Melanoma and Survival Rates				
PATHOLOGY STAGING				**5-YEAR SURVIVAL**	**10-YEAR SURVIVAL**
STAGE	**T**	**N**	**M**		
0	Tis	N0	M0		
IA	T1a	N0	M0	97%	95%
IB	T1b	N0	M0		88%
	T2a	N0	M0		
IIA	T2b	N0	M0	82%	
	T3a	N0	M0	79%	
IIB	T3b	N0	M0	68%	
	T4a	N0	M0	71%	
IIC	T4b	N0	M0	53%	39%
IIIA	T1-4a	N1a	M0		
	T1-4a	N2a	M0		
IIIB	T1-4b	N1a	M0		
	T1-4b	N2a	M0		
	T1-4a	N1b	M0		
	T1-4a	N2b	M0		
	T1-4a	N2c	M0		
IIIC	T1-4b	N1b	M0		
	T1-4b	N2b	M0		
	T1-4b	N2c	M0		
	Any T	N3	M0		
IV	Any T	AnyN	M1		

Adapted from Balch et al. (2009).
Pathology staging includes microstaging of the primary melanoma and pathologic information about the regional lymph nodes after partial (i.e., sentinel node biopsy) or complete lymphadenectomy. Pathologic stage 0 or stage IA patients are the exception; they do not require pathologic evaluation of their lymph nodes.

Treatment

Early diagnosis combined with appropriate surgical therapy is currently the only curative treatment. The recommended margins are

- Melanoma in situ: 0.5 cm
- Melanoma less than 1 mm: 1 cm
- Melanoma 1 to 2 mm: 1 to 2 cm
- Melanoma greater than 2 mm: 2 cm

The recommended deep margin is muscle fascia. Wider margins and Mohs' micrographic surgery can reduce the risk of contiguous subclinical spread for the desmoplastic variant of melanoma.

Sentinel lymph node biopsy (SLNB) provides accurate staging information for patients with clinically unaffected regional nodes and without distant metastases. Candidates for SLNB include patients with newly diagnosed primary cutaneous melanoma who are clinically node-negative and, based on primary tumor characteristics, are predicted to be at intermediate-risk or high-risk of harboring occult nodal disease. In cases of positive SLNB or clinically detected regional nodal metastases (palpable, positive cytology, or histopathology), radical removal of lymph nodes of the involved basin is indicated. There is clinical trial evidence suggesting that the survival outcome for patients who are sentinel node-positive is improved if an immediate regional lymphadenectomy is done.

For resectable local or in-transit recurrences, excision with a clear margin is recommended. For numerous or unresectable in-transit metastases of the extremities, isolated limb perfusion or infusion with melphalan may be considered.

Radiotherapy is indicated in select patients with lentigo maligna melanoma, as an adjuvant in select patients with regional metastatic disease, and for palliation, especially in bone and brain metastases.

Numerous adjuvant therapies have been investigated for the treatment of localized cutaneous melanoma following complete surgical removal. Adjuvant interferon (IFN) alfa-2b (Intron A) is the only adjuvant therapy approved by the FDA for high-risk melanoma that affects outcome after surgery. No survival benefit has been demonstrated for adjuvant chemotherapy, nonspecific (passive) immunotherapy, radiation therapy, retinoid therapy, vitamin therapy, or biologic therapy.

Various experimental melanoma vaccines show promise in the adjuvant setting, although caution is needed because four phase III trials (E1694, MMAIT-III [Canvaxin], MMAIT-IV, and EORTC 18961) showed a deleterious effect of the experimental vaccine compared with control intervention. Considerable effort is now being focused on selecting patients on the basis of molecular profiling and on combining agents targeting melanoma-specific aberrations in signaling and apoptotic pathways to overcome the many resistance mechanisms in melanoma cells.

Metastatic melanoma is an aggressive, immunogenic and molecularly heterogeneous disease. Recently, significant clinical breakthroughs of gene-mutation-based therapies with signaling pathway inhibitors and immune modulators have revolutionized the treatment of advanced melanoma, leading to the licensing of ipilimumab (Yervoy), a monoclonal antibody targeting cytotoxic T-lymphocyte-associated antigen 4, and vemurafenib (Zelboraf), a BRAF inhibitor used in patients whose tumors contain a V600 mutation in the BRAF gene. Compared with intravenous dacarbazine (DTIC), vemurafenib significantly improved overall survival and progression-free survival in patients with unresectable, previously untreated, BRAF(V600E) mutation-positive, stage IIIC or IV melanoma. Oral vemurafenib was generally well tolerated, with cutaneous adverse events among the most commonly occurring adverse events. Phase III trials with ipilimumab also demonstrated an overall survival benefit with its use when compared with standard treatments and other investigational therapies. However, the drug poses a notable challenge, given its propensity for toxicity, and requires close surveillance when administered in clinical practice. Both of these strategies prolong patients' survival but still have specific limitations, either in the duration of response (selective BRAF inhibitors) or the proportion of responding patients (ipilimumab), demanding the identification of additional genetic and immunologic biomarkers as predictors of treatment response and prognosis.

Although melanoma has traditionally been regarded as a uniformly fatal malignancy, personalized treatment of this cancer relies on the recognition of its genetic heterogeneity and our ability to pharmacologically target these specific and recurrent changes. Recent advances in the treatment of melanoma have come from the understanding that melanoma is a large family of molecularly distinct diseases. Emerging evidence suggests that different melanoma subtypes may each be driven by diverse mechanisms of progression, associated with differing mechanisms of tumor escape and specific immunosuppression, innate immune cell activation, and altered T-cell trafficking into tumor sites that in turn modulate response to immunotherapies.

Monitoring

Most metastases occur in the first 1 to 3 years after treatment of the primary tumor, and an estimated 4% to 8% of patients with a history of melanoma develop another primary melanoma, usually within the first 3 to 5 years following diagnosis. The risk of new primary melanoma increases in the presence of multiple dysplastic nevi and family history of melanoma. Consider cancer genetics consultation in patients with three or more melanomas in aggregate in first-degree or second-degree relatives on the same side of the family, families with three or more cases of melanoma or pancreatic cancer on the same side of the family, and (in low-incidence countries) patients with three or more primary melanomas.

The frequency of monitoring is as follows: For patients with melanoma smaller than 1 mm: every 3 months for 1 year, then every 6 to 12 months for 4 years, then annual examinations thereafter. For patients with melanoma larger than 1 mm: every 3 months for 1 to 2 years, then every 6 months until the fifth year, then annual examinations thereafter.

Followup visits for all patients should include a thorough history, review of systems, complete skin examination, and examination of lymph nodes. In patients at high risk for metastatic disease or with an abnormal examination, appropriate imaging studies, laboratory studies, or biopsies may be indicated. Evidence to support the use of routine imaging and laboratory studies in asymptomatic patients with a normal physical examination remains controversial and is left to the discretion of the physician.

Complications

Metastasis may occur locally in the regional lymph node basins, or it can occur distally in the skin (away from the melanoma scar), the remote lymph node(s), the viscera, and skeletal and central nervous system sites.

References

Abbasi NR, Shaw HM, Rigel DS, et al. Early diagnosis of cutaneous melanoma: Revisiting the ABCD criteria. JAMA 2004;292:2771–6.

American Cancer Society. Overview: Skin cancer: Melanoma, Available at: http://www.cancer.org/%20cancer/skincancer-melanoma/index (accessed 6-24-15).

Balch CM, Gershenwald JE, Soong SJ, et al. Final version of 2009 AJCC melanoma staging and classification. J Clin Oncol 2009;27:6199–206.

Curtin JA, Fridlyand J, Kageshita T, et al. Distinct sets of genetic alterations in melanoma. N Engl J Med 2005;353:2135–47.

Eggermont AM. Vaccine trials in melanoma—time for reflection. Nat Rev Clin Oncol 2009;6:256–8.

Griewank KG, Ugurel S, Schadendorf D, et al. New developments in biomarkers for melanoma. Curr Opin Oncol 2013;25:145–51.

Leachman SA, Carucci J, Kohlmann W, et al. Selection criteria for genetic assessment of patients with familial melanoma. J Am Acad Dermatol 2009;61:677e1–677e4.

Sladden MJ, Balch C, Barzilai DA, et al. Surgical excision margins for primary cutaneous melanoma. Cochrane Database Syst Rev 2009, CD004835.

Thompson JF, Scolyer RA, Kefford RF. Cutaneous melanoma in the era of molecular profiling. Lancet 2009;374:362–5.

Ross MI, Gershenwald JE. Sentinel lymph node biopsy for melanoma: A critical update for dermatologists after two decades of experience. Clin Dermatol 2013;31:298–310. http://dx.doi.org/10.1016/j.clindermatol.2012.08.004, Review. PubMed PMID: 23608449.

Davar D, Tarhini AA, Kirkwood JM. Adjuvant immunotherapy of melanoma and development of new approaches using the neoadjuvant approach. Clin Dermatol 2013;31:237–50. http://dx.doi.org/10.1016/j.clindermatol.2012.08.012, Review. Erratum in: Clin Dermatol 2013;31:501. PubMed PMID: 23608443; PubMed Central PMCID: PMC3654101.

Dean E, Lorigan P. Advances in the management of melanoma: Targeted therapy, immunotherapy and future directions. Expert Rev Anticancer Ther 2012;12:1437–48. http://dx.doi.org/10.1586/era.12.124, Review. PubMed PMID: 23249108.

Bis S, Tsao H. Melanoma genetics: The other side. Clin Dermatol 2013;31:148–55. http://dx.doi.org/10.1016/j.clindermatol.2012.08.003, Review. PubMed PMID: 23438378.

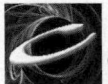

NEVI

Method of
Jane M. Grant-Kels, MD; and Michael Murphy, MD

CURRENT DIAGNOSIS

Benign Melanocytic Lesions
- Symmetrical
- Sharply demarcated border
- Uniform color
- Diameter usually 6 mm or less and stable

Malignant Melanocytic Lesions
- Asymmetrical
- Poorly circumscribed border
- Variegated in color
- Diameter often >6 mm and increasing (changing or evolving)

CURRENT THERAPY

- Acquired melanocytic nevus: No treatment is required unless the lesion is asymmetrical or has an irregular border, change or variegation in color, or change in diameter. Symptomatic lesions should be biopsied.
- Recurrent melanocytic nevus: No treatment required if the original biopsy was benign.
- Halo melanocytic nevus: No treatment, but excision is recommended if atypical clinical features are identified.
- Congenital melanocytic nevus: Removal based on melanoma risk, cosmetics, and functional outcome. If not excised, routine follow-up with the use of photography, dermoscopy, and computer assistance is recommended.
- Blue nevus: No treatment, but excision is recommended if atypical clinical features are identified.
- Spitz nevus: If clinically unusual, a complete excisional biopsy is recommended.
- Dysplastic nevus: If only one lesion is present, excision may be considered. Patients with many dysplastic nevi require close surveillance with removal of any lesion suspicious for melanoma.

Melanocytic nevi, or moles, are benign neoplasms composed of melanocytes. Melanocytic nevus cells are derived from melanocytes. Compared with melanocytes, nevus cells are not dendritic, are larger, and contain more abundant cytoplasm, often with coarse melanin granules. Nevus cells tend to aggregate into groups or nests. Melanocytic nevi are extremely common and can be found on almost everyone, anywhere on the cutaneous surface. This article discusses the most common types of melanocytic nevi: acquired melanocytic nevi, recurrent melanocytic nevi, halo melanocytic nevi, congenital melanocytic nevi (CMN), blue nevi, Spitz nevi, and dysplastic melanocytic nevi.

Acquired Melanocytic Nevi

Acquired melanocytic nevi are subdivided into junctional, compound, and intradermal types based on the location of the nevus cells. By definition, these lesions are not present at birth but can begin to appear in early childhood, usually after 6 to 12 months of age. Peak ages of appearance of melanocytic nevi are 2 to 3 years of age in children and 11 to 18 years in adolescents. Although nevi can appear at any age, it is relatively unusual for new melanocytic nevi to develop in middle-aged or older adults. With time, nevi can spontaneously regress. Consequently, patients in their ninth decade of life usually demonstrate few melanocytic nevi. An average white adult has 10 to 40 melanocytic nevi, but African Americans have far fewer, averaging only 2 to 8.

The number and location of melanocytic nevi have been shown to be associated with sun exposure, immunologic factors, and genetics. Consequently, melanocytic nevi are most numerous on the sun-exposed skin of the head, neck, trunk, and extremities, but they are only rarely found on covered areas such as the buttocks, female breasts, and scalp. Evidence suggests that patients with an increased number of melanocytic nevi (>50) might have an increased risk of melanoma.

Melanocytic nevi appear in a sequential fashion. Junctional melanocytic nevi arise during childhood as flat, dark macules. Histologically, an increase in single or nests of melanocytes are located at the dermoepidermal junction. With time, some of the junctional nests of melanocytes migrate into the dermis (compound melanocytic nevi). Clinically, compound melanocytic nevi are elevated and less heavily pigmented than junctional melanocytic nevi. Ultimately, all of the nevus cells migrate into the dermis (intradermal melanocytic nevi), resulting in the development of a tan or skin-colored dome-shaped papule. Melanocytic nevi can be flat or elevated and even polypoid, papillomatous, or verrucous and can demonstrate a range of color from skin-tone to black, but they are characteristically uniform in color, symmetrical, well marginated, and usually smaller than 6 mm in diameter.

All melanocytic lesions of clinical concern should be examined with a dermatoscope, a hand-held instrument with a magnified lens and a light source similar to an ophthalmoscope. This instrument allows evaluation of colors and microstructures not visible to the naked eye, helps distinguish whether pigmented lesions are melanocytic or nonmelanocytic, and helps distinguish whether melanocytic pigmented lesions are likely to be malignant. Used by an experienced dermatologist with proper training, the dermatoscope improves diagnostic accuracy by 20% to 30%.

It is unnecessary to surgically remove all melanocytic nevi because they are benign neoplasms of melanocytes. However, indications for removal include ABCD (asymmetry, irregular border, variegation or change in color, or change in diameter), symptoms (e.g., pruritus), evidence of inflammation or irritation, cosmetic issues, and patient anxiety. Melanocytic nevi on acral, genital, or scalp skin that appear benign do not require surgical removal. Shave biopsies are appropriate therapy for lesions considered clinically benign. However, if a lesion is being removed because of concern regarding the possibility of malignancy, an excisional biopsy (biopsy of choice) or incisional biopsy (including a deep scoop) that extends to the subcutaneous tissue is indicated. All melanocytic lesions should be submitted to a dermatopathologist for histologic review. A history of recent sun exposure or trauma should be conveyed to the dermatopathologist because such external trauma can induce reactive atypical histologic findings.

Recurrent Melanocytic Nevi

Recurrent melanocytic nevi are melanocytic nevi that have previously been incompletely removed (either iatrogenically or traumatically) and have recurred weeks to months later. Irregular brown pigmentation is clinically noted within the scar site. If the original biopsy demonstrated a benign melanocytic nevus, re-treatment is unnecessary unless the aforementioned indications are present. However, these nevi can demonstrate pseudomelanomatous histologic features. Therefore, if the repigmented area is excised, the dermatopathologist should be notified of the clinical history and, if possible, the slides from the original biopsy should be obtained and reviewed to ensure that the lesion is not histologically misdiagnosed.

Halo (Melanocytic) Nevi

Halo (melanocytic) nevi are melanocytic nevi in which a white rim or halo has developed. This phenomenon most commonly occurs around compound or intradermal nevi and is histologically associated with a dense, bandlike inflammatory infiltrate. The white halo area is histologically characterized by diminished or absent melanocytes and melanin. Approximately 20% of patients with halo nevi also exhibit vitiligo.

Although a halo can develop around many lesions in the skin, the most important differential diagnosis is between a halo nevus and melanoma with a halo. The halo and the central melanocytic nevus of halo nevi are symmetrical, round or oval, and sharply demarcated. Halo nevi most commonly occur in adolescence as an isolated event, but approximately 25% to 50% of affected persons have two or more.

The clinical course of halo nevi is variable. With time, the halo can repigment while the central nevus persists. Alternatively, the melanocytic nevus can regress completely and leave a depigmented macule that can persist or repigment over months or years.

Halo nevi do not require surgical excision unless atypical clinical features suggest the possibility of an atypical melanocytic lesion. It is advisable (particularly in adults, in whom halo nevi are less common) to perform a complete cutaneous examination with and without the aid of a Wood's lamp to rule out any associated atypical pigmented or regressed lesions. All patients should be warned to use sunscreens or protective clothing because of the increased risk of sunburn in the depigmented halo region.

Congenital Melanocytic Nevi

By definition, CMN are present at birth. Arbitrarily, they have been classified into small (<1.5 cm), medium (1.5–20 cm) and large (>20 cm) lesions. Terms such as *bathing trunk* or *garment-type* nevi refer to CMN that cover a significant portion of the cutaneous surface.

The approximate incidence of small congenital nevi is 1% of all live births. Large congenital nevi are rare and reported in only 1 in 20,000 births. Histologically, some congenital nevi have distinguishing histologic features (melanocytic nevus cells that extend into the deeper dermis as well as the subcutis and melanocytic nevus cells arranged periadnexally, angiocentrically, within nerves, and interposed between collagen bundles). However, these features have been identified in some acquired melanocytic nevi and are absent in some congenital nevi (especially small ones). In addition, the history obtained from the patient or their parents is often inaccurate. Consequently, it can be very difficult in some cases to distinguish a small congenital nevus from an acquired nevus.

Congenital nevi can give rise to dermal or subcutaneous nodular melanocytic proliferations. The vast majority of these lesions, particularly in the neonatal period, are biologically benign, despite a worrisome clinical presentation and atypical histologic features. Genetic analysis has shown that benign melanocytic proliferations within congenital nevi harbor aberrations qualitatively and quantitatively different from those seen in melanoma.

The primary significance of congenital nevi is related to the potential risk for progression to melanoma. Essentially, the larger the nevus, the greater the risk of progression to melanoma. Historically, even small nevi were estimated to exhibit a lifetime melanoma risk of 5%. However, recent prospective studies suggest that small and medium congenital nevi are associated with a low risk that may approximate the risk of acquired nevi. Conversely, large congenital nevi have a lifetime risk of melanomatous progression of approximately 6.3%. Up to two thirds of melanomas that arise in these giant congenital nevi have a nonepidermal origin, thus making clinical observation for malignant change difficult. Approximately 50% of these melanomas occur in the first 5 years of life, 60% in the first decade, and 70% before 20 years of age. Patients with large congenital nevi, especially those that involve posterior axial locations (head, neck, back, or buttocks) and are associated with satellite congenital nevi, are at increased risk for neurocutaneous melanosis (melanosis of the leptomeninges).

For large congenital nevi that involve a posterior axial location, magnetic resonance imaging (MRI) is indicated. If clinical symptoms or MRI indicate neurocutaneous melanosis, excision of the large nevus should be postponed until 2 years of age (the median age of neurologic symptoms). Patients with neurocutaneous melanosis have a greater than 50% mortality rate within 3 years. The risk and morbidity of multiple, staged excisions of a large CMN is not appropriate in patients with symptomatic neurocutaneous melanosis. All other large CMN are candidates for excision as soon as general anesthesia is considered a relatively safe risk. Other issues that need to be considered before undertaking staged excisions include cosmetic issues, functional outcome, and psychosocial issues. The staged excisions are usually started after 6 months of age for nevi on the trunk and extremities and later for those on the scalp to allow closure of the fontanelle. If removal is not undertaken, follow-up with monthly self-examination, photography, dermoscopy, confocal laser microscopy, and computer assistance are recommended.

For small congenital nevi, routine excision is not always recommended because the risk of melanoma is lower, and if it occurs, it usually arises within the epidermis after puberty. If the lesions are not excised, follow-up by alternating visits to a dermatologist and primary care physician along with serial photography are indicated. Inasmuch as small congenital nevi typically enlarge with the growth of the child and can change in appearance with time, educating families on benign, predictable changes in contradistinction to potentially alarming changes is extremely important.

If a lesion enlarges or changes suddenly or if parental anxiety or cosmetic issues arise, excision should then be contemplated for even small congenital nevi. Elective excision is best done when the patient is approximately 8 years old. With the use of topical anesthetic cream EMLA (eutectic mixture of local anesthetics: 2.5% lidocaine plus 2.5% prilocaine) or topical 4% lidocaine (ELA-Max), children of this age are usually cooperative and unscathed by the procedure.

Blue Nevi

Blue nevi occur primarily on the face and scalp, in addition to the dorsal surfaces of the hands and feet, as well-circumscribed, slightly raised or dome-shaped bluish papules that are usually less than 1 cm in diameter. Although these lesions are usually acquired in childhood and adolescence, rare congenital lesions have been reported. Histologically, blue nevi demonstrate a combination of intradermal spindle or dendritic melanin-pigmented melanocytes and melanophages with dermal fibrosis. The blue appearance of these lesions is a function of both the depth of the melanin in the dermis and the Tyndall phenomenon: longer wavelengths of light penetrate the deep dermis and are absorbed by the lesional melanin, and shorter wavelengths (e.g., blue) are reflected back. Blue nevi that are clinically stable and that do not demonstrate atypical features do not require removal.

Spitz Nevi

Nevi of large spindle and epithelioid cells (Spitz nevi) are relatively uncommon. In Australia, an annual incidence of 1.4 per 100,000 people has been recorded. Most Spitz nevi are noted in children and adolescents: One third occur before the age of 10 years, one third between the ages 10 to 20 years, and one third past the age of 20 years. Rarely, lesions can occur in patients older than 40 years. Seven percent of Spitz nevi have been reported as congenital.

Four clinical types of Spitz nevi are recognized: light-colored soft Spitz nevi that can resemble a pyogenic granuloma; light-colored hard Spitz nevi that can resemble a dermatofibroma; dark Spitz nevi that must be distinguished from other melanocytic lesions, including melanoma; and disseminated or agminated Spitz nevi. Spitz nevi are typically smaller than 6 mm in diameter and dome shaped, with a smooth pink or tan surface and sharp borders. Although they can occur anywhere on the cutaneous surface except mucosal or palmoplantar areas, they are most commonly seen on the face (especially in children) and legs (especially in women). Spitz nevi in adults are usually more heavily melanized than those in children.

Dermatoscopy or epiluminescent microscopy (examination of lesions with enhanced light and a dermatoscope) helps magnify the images in vivo and can assist in establishing the clinical diagnosis of some Spitz nevi. Histologically, the lesion can demonstrate features similar to those of melanoma, which earned the lesion its original designation by Sophie Spitz as a melanoma of childhood. Because Spitz nevi can be histologically difficult to distinguish from melanoma, if a biopsy is performed on a lesion because of parental, cosmetic, or transitional concern, complete excision with clear margins is recommended. Spitz nevi show fundamental genomic differences compared with MM, consistent with the generally benign behavior of these lesions. Spitz nevi typically demonstrate no or only a very restricted set of chromosomal aberrations (i.e., 11p gain in a subset of Spitz nevi). A distinct subset of atypical Spitz tumors is characterized by BRAF mutation and loss of BAP1 expression.

Dysplastic Melanocytic Nevi

Dysplastic melanocytic nevi, or Clark's nevi, or nevi with architectural disorder and cytologic atypia can occur sporadically as an isolated lesion or lesions or as part of a familial autosomal dominant syndrome. When such lesions occur sporadically, they are considered a marker for a patient who is at increased risk of melanoma (6% risk versus an approximate 0.6% risk in the normal white population in the United States). In association with a family history or personal past medical history of melanoma, patients with dysplastic melanocytic nevi should be considered to have a significant risk of melanoma. One first-degree family member with melanoma is associated with a lifetime risk of melanoma of 15% for the patient with dysplastic melanocytic nevi. Two or more first-degree family members with melanoma place a patient with dysplastic melanocytic nevi at a lifetime risk of developing melanoma that approaches 100%. Less commonly, dysplastic melanocytic nevi can progress to melanoma. Such progression has been documented by serial photography. However, these data are confounded by the fact that clinically and histologically, dysplastic melanocytic nevi may be difficult to distinguish from an early melanoma.

Dysplastic melanocytic nevi are clinically distinguished from common acquired melanocytic nevi by a diameter usually larger than 6 mm, irregular border, asymmetry, and variable color with possible shades of brown, red, pink and black; dysplastic melanocytic nevi can be flat with or without a raised center (fried egg appearance). The lesions begin to appear in mid-childhood and early adolescence. New lesions can appear throughout the patient's life. In addition to the back and extremities, these lesions can occur on sun-protected areas, including the scalp, buttocks, and female breasts. Dysplastic melanocytic nevi can be few or numerous, with hundreds of lesions.

Histologically, dysplastic melanocytic nevi show both architectural disorder: extension of the junctional component beyond the dermal component (shouldering); bridging of nests between adjacent rete ridges; papillary dermal concentric and lamellar fibroplasia; and a variable lymphocytic infiltrate with vascular ectasias. They also show cytologic atypia of melanocytes: increased nuclear size, hyperchromasia, dispersion or variation of nuclear chromatin patterns, and presence of nucleoli. Although there is some discordance in the histologic grading of dysplastic melanocytic nevi among expert dermatopathologists, there is some evidence to support the use in clinical practice of a two-tier grading system: Grade A are dysplastic melanocytic nevi with mild or moderate cytologic atypia and grade B are dysplastic melanocytic nevi with severe cytologic atypia. The probability of having a personal history of melanoma in any given dysplastic melanocytic nevi patient correlates with the grade of cytologic atypia in dysplastic melanocytic nevi. In addition, the presence of severe cytologic atypia in dysplastic melanocytic nevi correlates with a significantly greater risk of melanoma development (19.7%) compared with moderate (8.1%) or mild (5.7%) cytologic atypia.

Management of these patients is difficult. Dysplastic melanocytic nevi are not uncommon. Reportedly, as many as 4.6 million people in the United States have one or more sporadic dysplastic melanocytic nevi. Familial dysplastic melanocytic nevi are estimated to involve 50,000 patients in the United States. The risk of melanoma for these patients is probably on a continuum and correlated with their family history of melanoma or dysplastic melanocytic nevi, personal history of melanoma, number of acquired melanocytic and dysplastic lesions, and history of sun exposure. Removal of all dysplastic melanocytic nevi is inappropriate inasmuch as the chance of any single lesion becoming malignant is small and, in addition, the melanoma can arise de novo.

Management includes patient education and total body photography for comparison at future skin examinations. Patients should avoid the sun and use sunscreens and protective clothing. These patients should have regular biannual or quarterly examinations of the entire integument, including the oral, genital, and perianal mucosa, the scalp, and an ophthalmologic examination. Comparison with the previous total body photographs and use of the dermatoscope can be helpful. Any lesions that are suspicious for melanoma should be excised. Examination of first-degree family members (parents, siblings, and children) of patients with melanoma or dysplastic melanocytic nevi is recommended to identify other persons at high risk.

References

Argenziano G, Catricala C, Ardigo M, et al. Dermoscopy of patients with multiple nevi. Arch Dermatol 2011;147:46–9.

Arumi-Uria M, McNutt BS, Finnerty B. Grading of atypia in nevi: Correlation with melanoma risk. Mod Pathol 2003;16:764–71.

Bauer J, Bastian BC. Distinguishing melanocytic nevi from melanomas by DNA copy number changes: Comparative genomic hybridization as a research and diagnostic tool. Dermatol Ther 2006;19:40–9.

de Snoo FA, Kroon MW, Bergman W, et al. From sporadic atypical nevi to familial melanoma: risk analysis for melanoma in sporadic atypical nevus patients. J Am Acad Dermatol 2007;56:748–52.

Ferrara G, Soyer HP, Malvehy J, et al. The many faces of blue nevus: A clinicopathologic study. J Cutan Pathol 2007;34:543–51.

Gelbard AN, Tripp JM, Marghoob AA, et al. Management of Spitz nevi: A survey of dermatologists in the United States. J Am Acad Dermatol 2002;47:224–330.

Goodson AG, Florell SR, Boucher KM, et al. Low rates of clinical recurrence after biopsy of benign to moderatively dysplastic melanocytic nevi. J Am Acad Dermatol 2010;62:591–6.

King R, Hayzen BA, Page RN, et al. Recurrent nevus phenomenon: a clinicopathologic study of 357 cases and histologic comparison with melanoma with regression. Mod Pathol 2009;22:611–9.

Massi D, Cesinaro AM, Tomasini C, et al. Atypical spitzoid melanocytic tumors: A morphological, mutational, and FISH analysis. J Am Acad Dermatol 2011;64:919–35.

Naeyaert JM, Brochez L. Dysplastic nevi. N Engl J Med 2003;349:2233.

Price HN, Schaffer JV. Congenital melanocytic nevi: when to worry and how to treat: Facts and controversies. Clin Dermatol 2010;28:283–302.

Sommer LL, Barcia SM, Clarke LE, Helm KF. Persistent melanocytic nevi: a review and analysis of 205 cases. J Cutan Pathol 2011;38:503–7.

PAPULOSQUAMOUS ERUPTIONS

Method of
Tam T. Nguyen, MD

CURRENT DIAGNOSIS

- Psoriasis can be clinically described as erythematous plaques with silvery white scales.
- Severity is rated as mild (<5% body surface area [BSA]), moderate (5%–10% BSA), or severe (>10% BSA).
- Most cases are mild chronic plaques involving the extensor surfaces.
- Involvement of scalp and palmar and plantar surfaces is classified as severe.
- Psoriasis is commonly comorbid with several conditions, including cardiovascular disease, depression, and metabolic disorders.

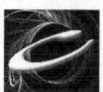

CURRENT THERAPY

- Class I/II (super-potent) topical steroid is the mainstream treatment of mild to moderate psoriasis.
- For moderate- to severe cases, systemic treatment with methotrexate is the gold standard.
- Narrowband ultraviolet B (UVB) remains a safe treatment option for all patients including children and pregnant women.
- Several immunomodulators or biologicals including etanercept have been proved very effective therapy. Biologicals can be given as monotherapy or in combination with other modalities for very recalcitrant cases.
- Treatment of comorbid conditions is paramount.

Epidemiology

Psoriasis, a common chronic idiopathic inflammatory disorder, affects 2% to 3% of Americans. The number of persons affected by this condition has more than doubled from 1970 to 2000. It is a chronic disorder that can involve many organ systems including skin, mucosa, the gastrointestinal tract, and joints. Although the onset of psoriasis can occur at any age, there is a bimodal distribution peaking in young adults in their early 20s and again in persons in their 50s. There is an equal prevalence among male and female patients, but the incidence is higher in men among younger adult populations.

Risk Factors

There is a strong family history and association with HLA-Cw6, HLA-B13, and HLA-B27. Psoriatic genes appear to be located on four key genes called pSOR1-4, which show an autosomal dominant pattern. The genome-wide association study (GWAS) showed that the genes STAT3 and STAT5 regulate the cytokines associated with psoriasis. In addition to the genetic etiology, environmental triggers, such as drugs, infection, and stress, also have a role in the pathogenesis of the psoriasis. Psychogenic stress from home and school is especially common in pediatric cases. Lithium and β-blockers are two well-known triggers of psoriasis. Certain conditions, such as Crohn's disease and multiple sclerosis, predispose patients to developing psoriasis.

Pathophysiology

Even though the exact mechanism is unknown, psoriasis is a disease of T cells that leads to abnormal epidermal differentiation and hyperproliferation. Normal skin has epidermal turnover of about 21 to 28 days, but psoriatic skin turns over every 3 to 4 days. Several cytokines, including IL-12 and IL-23, are part of the immune-mediated disease.

Diagnosis

Although most psoriatic lesions have characteristic scaly and silvery plaques, the lesions can be misleading. Refer to Box 1 for the differential diagnosis. Psoriasis has several subtypes including erythrodermic, pustular, and vulgaris. Psoriasis vulgaris has several subtypes including chronic plaque, guttate (Figure 1), and inverse psoriasis. More than 80% to 90% of psoriasis cases are the chronic plaque psoriasis. Therefore, this chapter focuses on this subtype.

Severity of psoriasis is classified based on the body surface area (BSA) involved. There are several severity instruments, such as Koo-Menter Psoriasis, for assessing the severity. One of the best validated tools is the Psoriasis Area Severity Index (PASI). These instruments are used to classify the condition according to coverage of body surface area (BSA) as either mild (<5% of BSA), moderate (5%–10% of BSA), or severe (>10% of BSA). BSA can be

---

| Box 1 | Differential Diagnosis of Psoriasis |

Plaque-like
Eczema
Fungal infection
Squamous cell carcinoma
Subacute cutaneous lupus erythematous

Guttate
Secondary syphilis
Pityriasis rosea

Erythrodermic
Pityriasis rubra pilaris
Drug eruptions

Pustular
Candidiasis
Acute generalized exanthematic pustulosis

Inverse
Intertrigo
Cutaneous T-cell lymphoma

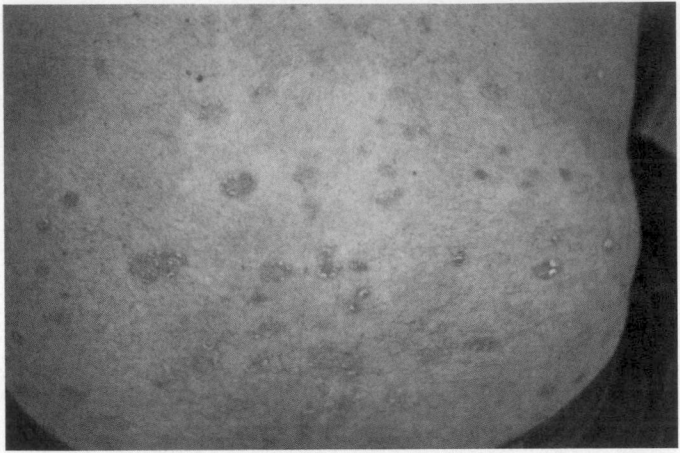

Figure 1. Guttate psoriasis with droplike, discrete papules and small plaques with scales.

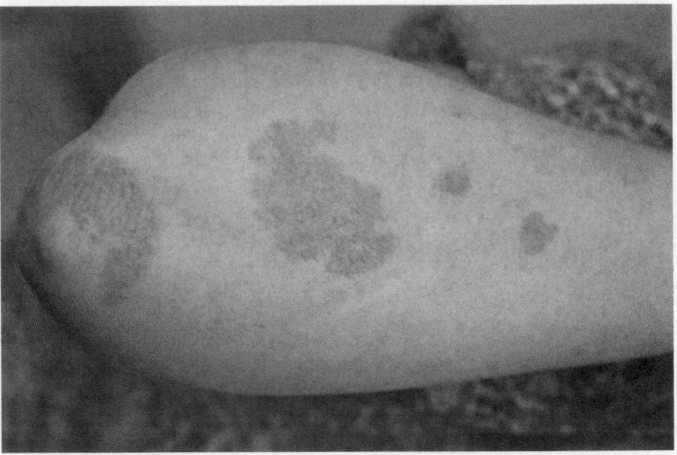

Figure 2. Chronic plaque psoriasis on the extensor surfaces.

estimated using the rule of 9s. Each upper extremity and the head is 9%, and the chest, back, and each lower extremity are 18%. For children, similar rules apply, except that each lower extremity is 13.5%. When the lesions involve difficult regions such as hands, feet, face, scalp, and genitalia, they are treated as severe regardless of the amount of BSA they cover.

Fortunately, more than 70% to 75% of cases are classified as mild to moderate, and there is no need for blood work. However, when psoriasis is associated with comorbidities, such as depression and heart disease, or when systemic medications cause serious side effects, it may be reasonable to get basic laboratory tests such as a complete blood count with platelet (CBC), chemistry, liver function tests (LFTs), cholesterol panel, hepatitis B and C, uric acid, and erythrocyte sedimentation rate (ESR). For patients at high risk, consider HIV testing. Also, consider evaluating for tuberculosis with a PPD test. These laboratory tests are even more crucial when considering treating with immunosuppressants like methotrexate (Trexall) and biological agents. Liver biopsy should be done if methotrexate is used at a cumulative dose of 3.5 to 4 g. Equally important, patients' quality of life needs to be assessed, which can be done with an instrument called the Dermatology Life Quality Index (DLQI).

Differential Diagnosis
The differential diagnosis of psoriasis is lengthy and can be tricky. Box 1 lists the differential diagnosis of psoriasis.

Clinical Manifestations
Most presentations of psoriasis are asymptomatic. When symptomatic, the most common clinical manifestation is pruritus. Other possible symptoms include fever and malaise, especially for more extensive disease. When psoriasis involves the joints, patients can have pain and stiffness in the involved joints; many of these cases involve the distal interphalangeal joints. On physical examination, the lesions are well-circumscribed dark pink to red plaques with silvery to white scales (Figures 2 and 3). Scales can be absent in certain locations, such as the intertriginous area (gluteal folds) (Figures 4 and 5). The margins are sharp and distinct, especially over extensor surfaces such as the elbows and knees (see Figure 2). Lesions also can involve the sacral area, nails, scalp, and the genitalia. If psoriasis forms under a nail, onycholysis (lifting of the nail plate) can occur with pitting and subungual keratosis.

When the scales are removed, several distinctive minute blood droplets appear; called the Auspitz sign. Use caution when removing the scales because it can be painful. When new lesions form at a site of trauma, it is called the Koebner phenomenon. Diagnosis can be made clinically. However, when in doubt, biopsy the lesion, which will show a thickened epidermis with an absent granular cell layer. The stratum corneum is hyperkeratotic, with classic infiltration of neutrophils.

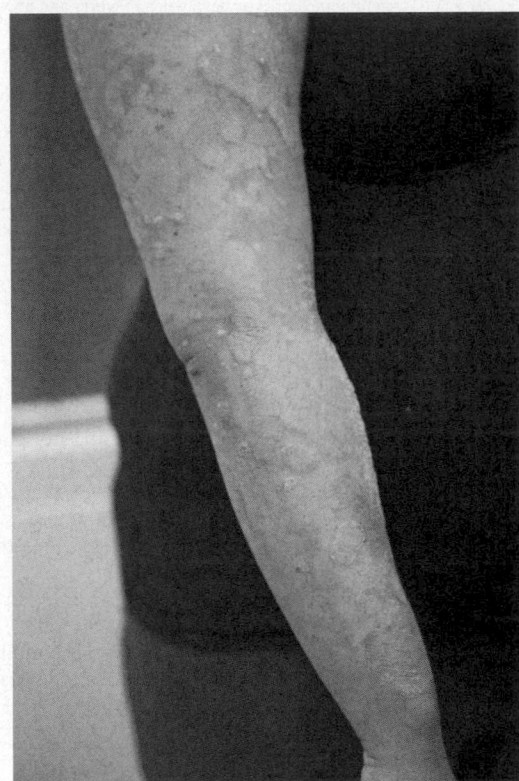

Figure 3. Chronic plaque psoriasis with classic silvery scales.

If this inflammatory process affects the joints, psoriatic arthritis ensues. Although this article does not discuss psoriatric arthritis, it is important to recognize when it occurs. Unlike rheumatoid arthritis, the distal interphalangeal (DIP) joints are regularly involved, but it can affect any joints. Psoriatric arthritis only occurs in 4% to 42% of patients with psoriasis. Diagnosis can be made with the CASPAR criteria, which evaluates five possible presentations, including having psoriasis, nail dystrophy, negative rheumatoid factor, dactylitis, and radiographic evidence.

Treatment
Corticosteroids remain the mainstay for psoriasis therapy; they reduce inflammation, decrease mitosis, and reduce erythema. Because most cases are mild to moderate, the first-line therapy to consider is topical corticosteroids. Even for severe cases that require systemic treatment, topical steroids should still be considered as a first-line adjuvant therapy. Because psoriatic lesions are

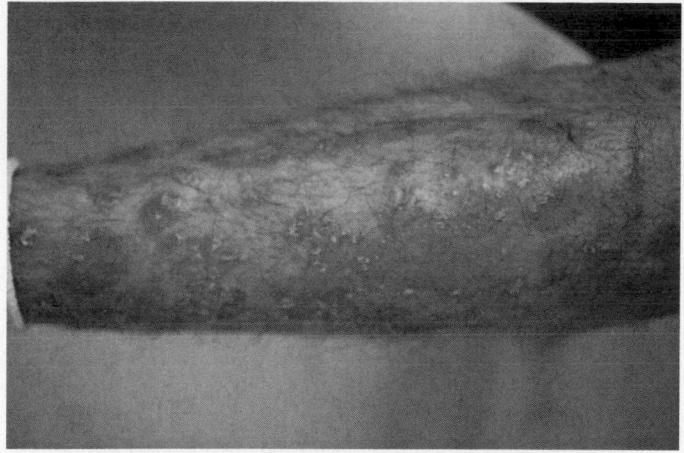

Figure 4. Chronic plaque psoriasis with limited scales.

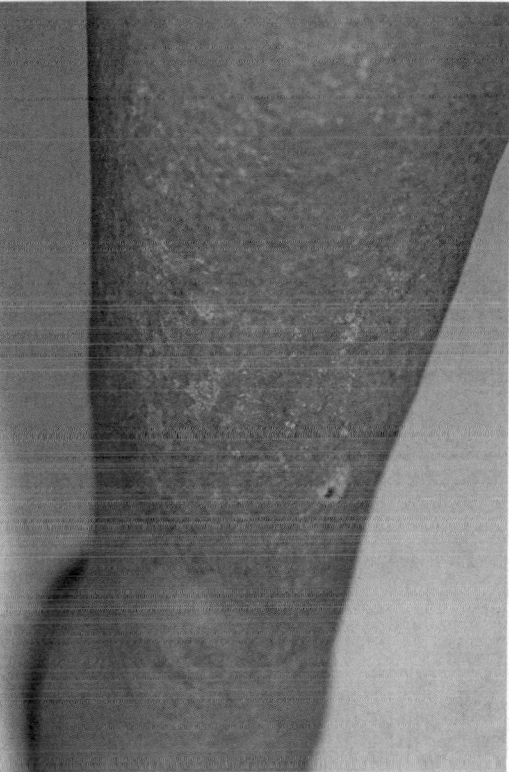

Figure 5. Chronic plaque psoriasis without scales.

> **Box 2** Classification of Topical Steroids, with a Few Samples from Each Class
>
> **Class 1: Super Potent**
> Clobex lotion 0.05%, clobetasol propionate
> Cormax cream or solution, 0.05%, clobetasol propionate
> Diprolene gel or ointment, 0.05%, bethamethasone dipropionate
> Olux foam, 0.05%, clobetasol propionate
>
> **Class 2: Potent**
> Elocon ointment, 0.1%, mometasone furoate
> Florone ointment, 0.05%, diflorasone diacetate
> Halog ointment/cream, 0.1%, halcinonide
> Lidex cream, gel, ointment, 0.05%, fluocinonide
>
> **Class 3: Upper Mid-Strength**
> Cutivate ointment, 0.005%, fluticasone propionate
> Cyclocort cream/lotion, 0.1%, amcinonide
> Lidex-E cream, 0.05%, fluocinonide
> Maxivate cream/lotion, 0.05%, betamethasone dipropionate
> Valisone ointment, 0.1%, betamethasone valerate
>
> **Class 4: Mid-Strength**
> Aristocort cream, 0.1%, triamcinolone acetonide
> Cordran ointment, 0.05%, flurandrenolide
> Elocon cream, 0.1%, mometasone furoate
> Kenalog cream, ointment, spray, 0.1%, triamcinolone acetonide
>
> **Class 5: Lower Mid-Strength**
> DesOwen ointment, 0.05%, desonide
> Diprosone lotion, 0.1%, betamethasone dipropionate
> Kenalog lotion, 0.1%, triamcinolone acetonide
> Synalar cream, 0.025%, fluocinolone acetonide
>
> **Class 6: Mild**
> Derma-Smoothe/FS Oil, 0.01%, fluocinolone acetonide
> DesOwen cream, 0.05%, desonide
> Synalar cream/solution, 0.01%, fluocinolone acetonide
> Tridesilon cream, 0.05%, desonide
>
> **Class 7: Least Potent**
> Topicals with hydrocortisone, dexamethsone,[6] methylprednisolone,[6] and prednisolone[6]
>
> ——————————————————————
> [6]May be compounded by pharmacists.

thickened, it is critical to go directly to super-potent steroids (class I), such as clobetasol (Clobex) (refer to Box 2 for steroid potency). When the localized lesions are lichenified and do not respond to potent topical corticosteroids, using steroid-impregnated tapes (flurandrenolide tape [Cordran]), which function as an occlusive wrap, can help. However, for areas of thinner skin, such as mucosa and lesions on the face, use less-potent topical steroids. Use caution when using class 1 steroids owing to all the potential side effects, including skin atrophy, hypopigmentation, telangiectasis, striae, and potential systemic absorption. In addition to the possible side effects, tachyphylaxis (reduced efficacy with prolonged use) can occur. Therefore, it is crucial to limit the use of potent topical steroids to less than 12 weeks.

One way to reduce the use of topical steroids is by using the vitamin D_3 analogue class, such as calcipotriene (Dovonex). This class of drugs inhibits epidermal proliferation and stimulates cellular differentiation. It is considered as effective as medium-potency corticosteroids, without the side effects. However, one drawback is that it takes about 8 weeks to be effective. Therefore, it should not be used for acute psoriatic eruptions. More often it is used in combination with topical steroids. It is generally well tolerated topically, but about 10% of patients experience burning and itching or hypercalcemia.

Other topical applications include tazarotene (Tazorac) and anthralin (Dritho-Crème HP 1%, Dritho-Scalp 0.5%). Tazarotene is an acetylenic retinoid and can be as effective as high-potency topical corticosteroids. However, its use is limited owing to the side effects of erythema, burning, pruritus, and peeling. Therefore, it is best to combine it with corticosteroids to reduce the irritation. In addition, tazarotene can stain clothing, and it is less popular owing to the side effects (redness and irritation on skin as well as staining) and the feel and smell of the solutions. However, it is a good alternative to topical corticosteroids.

For a limited number of thickened lesions, consider intralesional steroid injections, such as a single intralesional injection of a mid-potency steroid (e.g., triamcinolone acetonide or Kenalog-10, 5–10 mg/mL). Most injected plaques clear completely and remain in remission for months. However, as with other steroid injections, side effects of skin atrophy and telangiectasis can occur. Therefore, the face and intertriginous areas should not be injected because of the increased risk of side effects.

For severe and recalcitrant cases, systematic medications are needed. One of the gold standards in the United States and many other countries is methotrexate (Trexall) because it is available as a generic. Its exact mechanism is unknown; initially it was believed to inhibit proliferation, but more-recent studies describe an antiinflammatory property. The most common serious side effect of this drug is hepatotoxicity (as many as 33% of patients show some liver disease). Therefore, it is crucial to screen for alcohol dependency, liver disease, and obesity. Standard practice is to check baseline CBC and liver function enzymes, and then repeat these laboratory tests after 1 month of therapy. Methotrexate is highly teratogenic; hence it is absolutely contraindicated in pregnancy. After stopping the medication, men should wait at least 3 months and women should wait one ovulatory cycle before attempting to conceive.

There are two methods for initiating methotrexate. Most patients start at an initial dose of 7.5 mg (3 tabs of 2.5 mg) weekly; in pediatric cases dosage[1] is 0.2 to 0.7 mg/kg weekly. Others start at a higher dosage of 0.4 to 0.5 mg/kg weekly. Unfortunately, there is no current study to compare the two methods. With either dosing regimen, do not exceed 30 mg per week. Methotrexate depletes the body's storage of folic acid, so it is important to supplement folic acid 1 mg daily except the day when methotrexate is taken. The methotrexate can be titrated upward every 2 to 4 weeks.

Unlike methotrexate, which can take several weeks before it becomes effective, cyclosporine (Sandimmune),[1] a calcineruin inhibitor, is rapidly effective for severe cases. It is dosed at a low dose of 2 to 5 mg/kg/day divided into two doses and increased slowly every 2 to 4 weeks. Maintenance dosage is about 3 to 5 mg/kg/day. A main concern for this drug is nephrotoxicity. As long as the use of cyclosporine is limited to 1 year, it is generally safe. However, kidney function still needs to be monitored regularly. Cyclosporine has been associated with an increased risk of squamous cell carcinoma, especially when the patient has a history of psoralen plus ultraviolet A (PUVA) therapy.

Although not FDA-approved, azathioprine (Imuran)[1] has been a successful systemic medication for psoriasis. Generally, it is initially dosed at 0.5 mg/kg. If there is cytopenia, then the dosage can be increased by 0.5 mg/kg/day every 4 to 6 weeks as needed. Another dosing method is based on thiopurine methyltransferase (TPMT) levels. If the TPMT is less than 5.0 U, do not use azathioprine. If the level is between 5 and 13.7 U, the maximum daily dose should be 0.5 mg/kg/daily. If the TMPT level is between 13.7 and 19.0 U, then the maximum daily dose may be increased to 1.5 mg/kg.

Acitretin (Soriatane) and isotretinoin (Claravis)[1] are retinoids, which are vitamin A derivatives. Although acitretin is more commonly used, either may be used and requires a period of 3 to 6 months to achieve results. However, these retinoids are generally less effective than methotrexate and cyclosporine. Though they are less effective and a longer time is required for this class of agents to work, their main benefits include no malignancy potential and no immunosuppression. Therefore, these drugs are safe in patients with HIV and other immunosuppressive conditions. Unfortunately, acitretin and isotretinoin are highly teratogenic. Both male and female patients need to be drug free for 1 year for isotretinoin and 3 years for acitretin before they conceive. For other possible treatment agents, refer to Box 3.

In recent years, immunomodulators or biologicals have revolutionized the treatment course of psoriasis. Generally, criteria for this class of therapy are PASI greater than 10 and failure of other therapies or a contraindication to other therapies such as methotrexate. Most agents are limited to 1 to 2 years of use because most studies have not been evaluated beyond 2 years. Tuberculosis should be evaluated (PPD and possibly chest x-ray) before starting these biologics. All the medications in this class should be avoided in pregnancy. Alefacept (Amevive) and efalizumab (Raptiva) are T-cell inhibitors. Efalizumab (Raptiva) was withdrawn from the market in 2009 owing to reported cases of progressive multifocal leukoencephalopathy. Etanercept (Enbrel) is a tumor nerosis factor (TNF) inhibitor and should not be used in patients with multiple sclerosis. The three monoclonal antibodies include inflixmab

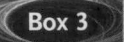 **Box 3** Other Treatment Modalities for Moderate to Severe Psoriasis

Fumaric acid esters[2]: First-line therapy in a couple of European countries

Hydroxyurea (Hydrea)[1]: A good option because there is no liver or kidney toxicity; however, be cautious of bone marrow suppression

Leflunomide (Arava)[1]

Mycophenolate mofetil (Cellcept)[1]: good choice for HIV patients and patients with immunobullous disorders

Retinoic acid metabolism–blocking agents: liarozole[5] and talarozole (Rombozale)[5]

Alitretinoin topical (Panretin)[1]

Sulfasalazine (Azulfidine)[1]

Tacrolimus (Prograf)[1]

6 thioguanine (Tabloid)[1]

[1]Not FDA approved for this indication.
[2]Not available in the United States.
[5]Investigational drug in the United States.

(Remicade), adalimumab (Humira), and golimumab (Simponi). A new drug in the class is ustekinumab (Stelara), which inhibits interleukin (IL)-12 and IL-23. Secukinumab (Cosentyx), a new biological for plaque psoriasis is a recombinant, high-affinity, fully humanized IgG monoclonal antibody that selectively binds and neutralizes interleukin-17A (IL-17A).

Etanercept (Enbrel) blocks TNF-α. It is generally dosed at 50 mg SC twice weekly for 12 weeks and then 50 mg weekly. Patients can self-administer the drug; laboratory monitoring is not required. There are limited data beyond 2 years. Etanercept[1] is the preferred drug for children. Infliximab (Remicade) blocks both soluble and bound TNF-α. Its dosage is 3 to 5 mg/kg IV on weeks 0, 2, and 6, and then every 6 to 8 weeks. Medication generally is infused over 2 hours. It is crucial to have a PPD (but not chest x-ray) before treatment. It is approved for 1 year. In a comparative study, infliximab was found to be superior to methotrexate.

Adalimumab (Humira) blocks both soluble and bound TNF-α. Initiate the dose at 40 mg SC every 2 weeks, although some patients require dosing every 7 to 10 days. Alternatively, the initial dose may be 80 mg followed by 40 mg. Patients may self-administer the injections. As with infliximab, before initiating treatment, obtain a PPD (and consider chest x-ray as well). Antibodies can develop within the first 28 weeks, which will decrease the efficacy of the drug. Both infliximab, which has been in use for many years, and adalimumab have limited long-term safety data beyond 1 year. Some data suggest an increase in cancer risk beyond 1 year.

The fourth biological is alefacept (Amevive) which is dosed at 15 mg IM or IV once a week for 12 weeks. Its efficacy follows the rule of thirds: It works well in about one third of cases, does not work at all in one third of cases, and the rest fall in between. After a cycle of 12 weeks, the courses may be repeated as needed. However, it is crucial initially to monitor T-cell counts biweekly. The newest agent is ustekinumab (Stelara), which has been shown to improve lesions in 66% to 76% of cases. It is initially dosed at 45 to 90 mg SC at weeks 0 and 4, depending on body weight. Maintenance is every 12 weeks.

When these therapies are contraindicated, one alternative is phototherapy. This is the reason many patients report decreased symptom severity during the summer months due to the natural UV light. Phototherapy started with photochemotherapy with oral or topical psoralens combined with UVA light (PUVA). Although phototherapy is very effective for psoriasis, even in very thick lesions, recent studies have shown an increased risk of skin cancer. Therefore, PUVA has become less popular since the advent of UVB radiation treatment, especially with narrow band UVB (NB-UVB).

TABLE 1	Methods for Initiating Narrow-Band Ultraviolet B (NB-UVB) Therapy and Subsequent Dosing of Phototherapy						

MED NB-UVB PROTOCOL

THERAPY	TYPE 1	TYPE 2	TYPE 3	TYPE 4	TYPE 5	TYPE 6	MED NB-UVB PROTOCOL
Initial dose	130 mJ/cm^2	220 mJ/cm^2	260 mJ/cm^2	330 mJ/cm^2	350 mJ/cm^2	400 mJ/cm^2	Start with 50%–70% MED The starting dose should be based on the provider's comfort and the patient's history of response to light; e.g., start closer to 70% if the patient has a history of tanning and start closer to 50% if the patient has a history of burning; most centers start at 70%

Subsequent Doses

Severe erythema	No treatment. When burn resolves, decrease by 50% of last dose and then increase dose by 10%						
Mild erythema	Same dose	Same dose	Same dose	Same dose	Same dose	Same dose	Decrease dose by 20%
Barely perceptible erythema	—	—	—	—	—	—	Same (erythmogenic) or slight decrease (suberythmogenic)
No erythema: increase dose by	15 mJ/cm^2	25 mJ/cm^2	40 mJ/cm^2	45 mJ/cm^2	60 mJ/cm^2	65 mJ/cm^2	20%

Dosing Schedule

Optimal schedule	3 ×/wk (M, W, F) is the optimal schedule because less is not as effective and more does not improve the resolution. Subsequent treatments should not be less than 24 hours from the last treatment. For the treatment of eczema, no clear guideline to the frequency. Some use 5 ×/wk.

Dose Adjustments for Missed Days

MISSED DAYS	DOSE ADJUSTMENT
1–7	Increase doses per skin type
8–11	Same dose
12–14	Decrease by 2 treatments' worth
15–20	Decrease by 25%
21–27	Decrease by 50%
28+	Start over

NB-UVB is equally effective as PUVA and does not have the risk of skin cancer. The exact mechanism is unknown, but it is believed to affect DNA and to suppress IL-17 and IL-23, creating photoproducts that interfere with cell cycle progression. NB-UVB is first-line course of therapy for pregnant and pediatric patients. There are two methods for initiating NB-UVB phototherapy: the skin type protocol, which is easier to execute, and the minimum erythema dose (MED), which is more detailed but more accurate. Refer to Table 1 for treatment protocols. Both protocols generally require 30 to 35 treatments with the optimal frequency of three times a week.

Given all the treatment options (refer to Box 4), the choice of the treatment regimen depends on several factors. First, the severity of the psoriasis must be determined as well as the social and emotional impact of the condition. Another consideration is financial, including the insurance coverage, copayment, and deductibles. The lowest-cost treatment is methotrexate, and alefacept is the highest. The patient's conveniences and preferences should be discussed. If the severity is only mild to moderate without much emotional impact, topical steroid and vitamin D analogue should be considered the first options. Other topicals include tar (Medotar, Balnetar, Psorent), anthralin (Dritho-Crème HP, Dritho-Scalp), and tretinoin (Retin-A).[1] If the degree is severe and/or the patient

has emotional impact, systemic medications should be used. Most insurance plans will probably require that the patient try at least one oral medication before employing the biologicals. If systemic therapy is used, consider combining it with phototherapy (if possible). If there is no improvement within 2 to 4 months, the regimen should be changed to biologicals. Other combinations may be employed for better resolution.

For healthy patients, any of these therapies may be tried. Unfortunately, there are limitations with children, pregnant women, and patients trying to conceive. For pediatric patients, topical agents should be tried first, followed by UVB monotherapy. If the plaques are still recalcitrant, add either methotrexate (Trexall)[1] or phototherapy. If phototherapy is not available and topical agents have failed, consider using methotrexate or cyclosporine (Sandimmune).[1] Other options for pediatric patients include adalimumab (Humira)[1] and etanercept (Enbrel).[1] For pregnant women and patients trying to conceive, first try topical agents followed by UVB (ideally narrowband). This combination remains the safest option. If stronger options are needed, the only class B drugs are systemic steroids, adalimumab, alefacept (Amevive), infliximab (Remicade), and ustekinumab (Stelara). An absolute contraindication in this population is the retinoid class, such as isotretinoin (Claravis)[1] and acitretin (Soriatane).

---

[1]Not FDA approved for this indication.

[1]Not FDA approved for this indication.

Box 4 Treatment Options for Psoriasis

Topical
Steroid
Tar (e.g., Medotar, Balnetar, Psorent)
Anthralin (Dritho-Crème Hp, Dritho-Scalp)
Calcipotriene (Dovonex)
Calcitriol (Rocaltrol)[1]
Adapalene (Differin)[1]
Tazarotene (Tazorac)
Tretinoin (Retin-A)[1]
Calcineurin inhibitors (pimecrolimus [Elidel],[1] tacrolimus [Protopic][1])

Oral or Systemic
Methotrexate (Trexall)
Acitretin (Soriatane)/Isotretinoin (Claravis)[1]
Cyclosporine (Sandimmune)[1]
Mycophenolate mofetil (Cellcept)[1]

Immunomodulators
Alefacept (Amevive)
Etanercept (Enbrel)
Infliximab (Remicade)
Adalimumab (Humira)
Ustekinumab (Stelara)
Secukinumab (Cosentyx)

Phototherapy
UVA
UVB

[1]Not FDA approved for this indication.

Complications

Patients suffering from psoriasis cope with the physical appearance of their lesions as well as the associated mental anguish associated with many other chronic ailments. Furthermore, psoriasis is associated with other chronic diseases, such as abdominal obesity, metabolic syndrome, and atherogenic dyslipidemia. Weight loss can improve the apperance of psoriatic plaques. Patients with psoriasis are more likely to have coronary artery disease, elevated blood pressure, obesity, and insulin resistance. Treating psoriasis decreases the cardiovascular risks. There is an increased risk of malignancy, such as lymphoma. Substance abuse and smoking are common among these patients as well.

References

Ahlehoff O, et al. Cardiovascular disease event rates in patients with severe psoriasis treated with systemic anti-inflammatory drugs: a Danish real-world cohort study. J Intern Med 2012;273:197–204.

American Academy of Dermatology Work Group. Menter A, Korman NJ, Elmets CA, et al. Guidelines of care for the management of psoriasis and psoriatic arthritis: Section 6. Guidelines of care for the treatment of psoriasis and psoriatic arthritis: Case-based presentations and evidence-based conclusions. J Am Acad Dermatol 2011;65(1):137–74.

Callen JP, Krueger GG, Lebwohl M, et al. AAD. AAD consensus statement on psoriasis therapies. J Am Acad Dermatol 2003;49(5):897–9.

Dubertret L. Retinoids, methotrexate and cyclosporine. Curr Probl Dermatol 2009;38:79–94.

Foulkes AC, Grindlay DJ, Griffiths CE, Warren RB. What's new in psoriasis? An analysis of guidelines and systematic reviews published in 2009–2010. Clin Exp Dermatol 2011 Aug;36(6):585–9, quiz 588–9.

Gottlieb A, Korman NJ, Gordon KB, et al. Guidelines of care for the management of psoriasis and psoriatic arthritis: Section 2. Psoriatic arthritis: overview and guidelines of care for treatment with an emphasis on the biologics J Am Acad Dermatol 2008;58(5):851–64.

Herrier RN. Advances in the treatment of moderate-to-severe plaque psoriasis. Am J Health Syst Pharm 2011;68(9):795–806.

Jensen P, Zachariae C, Christensen R, et al. Effect of weight loss on the severity of psoriasis: a randomized clinical study. JAMA Dermatol 2013;149:795–801.

Johnson-Huang LM, Suárez-Fariñas M, Sullivan-Whalen M, et al. Effective narrowband UVB radiation therapy suppresses the IL-23/IL-17 axis in normalized psoriasis plaques. J Invest Dermatol 2010;130(11):2654–63.

Kalb RE, Strober B, Weinstein G, Lebwohl M. Methotrexate and psoriasis: 2009 National Psoriasis Foundation Consensus Conference. J Am Acad Dermatol 2009;60:824–37.

Kimball AB, Gladman D, Gelfand JM, et al. National Psoriasis Foundation. National Psoriasis Foundation clinical consensus on psoriasis comorbidities and recommendations for screening. J Am Acad Dermatol 2008;58:1031–142.

Kuhn A, Patsinakidis N, Luger T. Alitretinoin for cutaneous lupus erythematosus. J Am Acad Dermatol 2012;67(3):e123–6.

Menter A, Gottlieb A, Feldman SR, et al. Guidelines of care for the management of psoriasis and psoriatic arthritis: Section 1. Overview of psoriasis and guidelines of care for the treatment of psoriasis with biologics. J Am Acad Dermatol 2008;58:826–50.

Ormerod AD, Campalani E, Goodfield MJ. BAD Clinical Standards Unit. British Association of Dermatologists guidelines on the efficacy and use of acitretin in dermatology. Br J Dermatol 2010;162:952–63.

Trueb RM. Therapies for childhood psoriasis. Curr Probl Dermatol 2009;38:137–59.

Tsoi LC, et al. Identification of 15 new psoriasis susceptibility loci highlights the role of innate immunity. Nat Genet 2012;44:1341–8.

PARASITIC DISEASES OF THE SKIN

Method of
Andreas Katsambas, MD, PhD; and Clio Dessinioti, MD, MSc

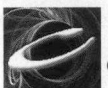

CURRENT DIAGNOSIS

Cutaneous Amebiasis
- Purulent, foul-smelling nodules, ulcers, cysts, sinuses
- Microscopic identification of *Entamoeba histolytica* in stool or biopsy samples
- Molecular methods

Cutaneous Leishmaniasis
- Ulcerated nodule (i.e., volcano sign)
- Identification of *Leishmania* parasites by direct examination or culture from the lesion aspirate or biopsy
- Montenegro skin test
- In vitro lymphocyte proliferation assay
- Polymerase chain reaction

Trypanosomiasis
Chagas' Disease
- Chagoma: painful erythematous nodule
- Regional adenopathy
- Cardiomyopathy, megaesophagus, megacolon
- Microscopic examination of *Trypanosoma cruzi* in blood, lymph node biopsy, or skin biopsy or culture

African Sleeping Sickness
- Trypanosome chancre: painful, inflammatory nodule
- Regional adenopathy
- Fever, generalized pruritic eruption with erythematous annular plaques
- Central nervous system involvement
- Microscopic identification of *Trypanosoma brucei* in chancre fluid, lymph node aspirates, blood, bone marrow, cerebrospinal fluid

Cutaneous Toxoplasmosis
- Roseola, urticaria, prurigo-like nodules
- Isolation of *Toxoplasma gondii* in the skin

Ascariasis
- Urticaria
- Identification of adult worm or eggs in stool

Cutaneous Larva Migrans
- Creeping eruption
- Intense pruritus

Cysticercosis
- Subcutaneous nodules
- Isolation of *Taenia solium* in skin lesion
- Serologic tests

Dracunculiasis
- Ruptured blister with prolapsing worm

Filariasis

Lymphatic Filariasis
- Fever with lymphangitis and lymphadenitis
- Chronic pulmonary infection
- Progressive lymphedema leading to massive tissue thickening, especially of the legs and scrotum (i.e., elephantiasis)
- Microscopic identification of microfilariae in blood

Onchocerciasis (River Blindness)
- Subcutaneous nodules, dermatitis, "leopard skin," "lizard skin," lymphedema
- Identification of microfilariae in skin snips
- Blindness

Loiasis (Calabar Swellings)
- Pruritus, localized subcutaneous swellings
- Serpiginous lesion on the conjunctivae
- Microscopic identification of microfilariae in blood

Schistosomiasis (Snail Fever)
- Pruritic papules, edema
- Fever, lymphadenopathy, diarrhea
- Bilharziasis cutanea tarda: pruritic, grouped papules
- Identification of the eggs in stool, urine, biopsy of affected tissues
- Enzyme-linked immunosorbent assay (ELISA) tests

Cercarial Dermatitis (Swimmer's Itch)
- Extremely pruritic erythematous macules, papules, vesicles on body areas exposed to infested water

Human Scabies
- Pruritus worsening at night
- Papules, excoriations, nodules, burrows on genitals, interdigital spaces, axillae, wrists
- Microscopic identification of mites or eggs or feces from burrows or papules

Pediculosis

Pediculosis Capitis
- Intense pruritus of the scalp
- Nape dermatitis
- Identification of lice and nits on the hair

Pediculosis Corporis (Vagabond's Itch)
- Intense pruritus, erythema, urticarial lesions, papules, nodules, and excoriations
- Identification of lice and nits on clothing

Pediculosis Pubis
- Pruritus
- Blue macules
- Identification of lice and nits on pubic hair

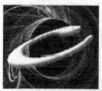

CURRENT THERAPY

Cutaneous Amebiasis
- Metronidazole (Flagyl) 750 mg PO three times daily for 7 to 10 days, or
- Tinidazole (Tindamax) 2 g once PO daily for 5 days, followed by iodoquinol (Yodoxin) 650 mg PO three times daily for 20 days or paromomycin (Humatin) 25 to 35 mg/kg/day PO in three doses for 7 days

Cutaneous Leishmaniasis
- Sodium stibogluconate (Pentostam)[10] 20 mg/kg/day IV or IM for 20 days, or
- Meglumine antimoniate (Glucantime)[2] 20 mg/kg/day IV or IM for 20 days, or
- Miltefosine (Impavido) 2.5 mg/kg/day PO (up to 150 mg/day) for 28 days, or

- Topical paromomycin, a formulation of 15% paromomycin and 12% methylbenzethonium chloride in soft white paraffin (Lesheutan)[1,6] applied twice daily for 10 days or
- Pentamidine (Pentam 300)[1] 2 to 3 mg/kg IV or IM daily or every second day for four to seven doses

Trypanosomiasis

Chagas' Disease (American Trypanosomiasis)
- Nifurtimox (Lampit)[10] 8 to 10 mg/kg/day PO in three or four doses for 90 to 120 days, or
- Benznidazole (Radanil, Rochagan)[2] 5 to 7 mg/kg/day PO in two doses for 60 to 120 days

East African Sleeping Sickness
- Suramin (Germanin)[10] 100 to 200 mg (test dose) IV, then 1 g IV on days 1, 3, 7, 14, 21
- For late disease with involvement of the central nervous system, melarsoprol (Mel-B)[10] 2 to 3.6 mg/kg/day IV for 3 days; after 7 days, 3.6 mg/kg/day for 3 days; repeat after 7 days

West African Sleeping Sickness
- Pentamidine (Pentam 300)[1] 4 mg/kg/day IM for 10 days,[1] or
- Suramin (Germanin)[10] 100 to 200 mg (test dose) IV, then 1 g IV on days 1, 3, 7, 14, 21
- For late disease with involvement of the central nervous system, melarsoprol (Mel-B)[10] 2.2 mg/kg/day IV for 10 days, or
- For late disease with involvement of the central nervous system, eflornithine (Ornidyl)[2] 400 mg/kg/day IV in four doses for 14 days

Cutaneous Toxoplasmosis
- Self-limited disease; treatment not needed in healthy, nonpregnant persons
- For pregnant women or immunocompromised patients: pyrimethamine (Daraprim) 25 to 100 mg/day PO for 3 to 4 weeks (plus leucovorin 10–25 mg with each dose of pyrimethamine) and sulfadiazine[1] 1 to 1.5 g PO four times daily for 3 to 4 weeks

Ascariasis
- Albendazole (Albenza)[1] 400 mg PO once, or
- Mebendazole (Vermox) 100 mg PO twice daily for 3 days or 500 mg once, or
- Ivermectin (Stromectol)[1] 150 to 200 μg/kg PO once

Cutaneous Larva Migrans
- Ivermectin (Stromectol)[1] 200 μg/kg PO once; a second dose may be needed, or
- Albendazole (Albenza)[1] 400 mg daily PO for 3 days
- Topical thiabendazole[6] 10% to 15% applied three times daily for 5 to 7 days for a limited number of lesions

Dracunculiasis
- Slow extraction of the worm, which is facilitated by metronidazole (Flagyl)[1] 250 mg PO three times daily for 10 days

Filariasis

Lymphatic Filariasis
- Diethylcarbamazine (DEC, Hetrazan)[10] 6 mg/kg/day PO in three doses for 12 days, or
- Ivermectin (Stromectol)[1] 200 μg/kg PO once together with albendazole (Albenza)[1] 400 mg PO once; kills only the microfilaria, not the adult worms
- For patients with microfilaria in the blood, DEC as follows: day 1: 50 mg; day 2: 50 mg three times daily; day 3: 100 mg three times daily; days 4 through 14: 6 mg/kg in three doses

Onchocerciasis
- Ivermectin (Stromectol) 150 μg/kg PO once for 6 to 12 months, until asymptomatic
- DEC: contraindicated because it may lead to blindness

Loiasis
- DEC[10] 6 mg/kg/day PO in three doses for 12 days

- For patients with microfilaria in the blood, DEC as follows: day 1: 50 mg; day 2: 50 mg three times daily; day 3: 100 mg three times daily; days 4 through 14: 9 mg/kg in three doses

Schistosomiasis
- Praziquantel (Biltricide) 40 mg/kg/day[3] in two doses for 1 day (*S. haematobium* and *S. mansoni*) and 60 mg/kg/day[3] in three doses for 1 day (*S. japonicum, S. mekongi*)

Human Scabies
- Permethrin (Acticin, Elimite) 5% cream rinse, applied for 10 hours; a second application 7 to 10 days later, or
- Benzyl benzoate 25% solution[6] applied topically; second application 7 to 10 days later, or
- Crotamiton 10% (Eurax) applied twice daily for 2 days; second application 7 to 10 days later
- Sulfur 6% to 10% ointment in petrolatum[6]
- Ivermectin (Stromectol)[1] 200 µg/kg PO once: treatment of choice for crusted scabies

Pediculosis
Pediculosis Capitis
- Malathion (Ovide) 0.5% lotion, applied for 8 to 12 hours before being washed off; approved for children older than 6 years, or
- Permethrin (Nix) 1% lotion, applied to shampooed hair and washed off after 10 minutes; second application 7 to 10 days later; approved for children older than 2 years
- Pyrethrins with piperidyl butoxide (RID) applied for 10 minutes
- Benzyl benzoate 25% solution[6]
- Lindane shampoo: for recalcitrant disease, not to be used in children
- Ivermectin 0.5% lotion (Sklice), apply to dry hair and scalp then rinse off after 10 minutes

Pediculosis Corporis
- Disinfection of clothes

Pediculosis Pubis
- Same treatment as pediculosis capitis: three times daily

---

[1]Not FDA approved for this indication.
[2]Not available in the United States.
[3]Exceeds dosage recommended by the manufacturer.
[6]May be compounded by pharmacists.
[10]Available in the United States from the Centers for Disease Control and Prevention.

Parasitic diseases are a common cause of morbidity and mortality, particularly in tropical and developing countries. They may be caused by protozoa, helminths, or arthropods. Because of the immigration of persons from tropical and subtropical countries worldwide and the travel of people from industrialized to tropical regions, parasitic diseases may be found in temperate climates. Skin lesions may provide important diagnostic clues for parasitic infections, and they are reviewed in the following sections, along with updated treatment guidelines.

Diseases Caused by Protozoa
Cutaneous Amebiasis
Intestinal amebiasis is caused by *Entamoeba histolytica,* which may rarely invade the skin and cause cutaneous amebiasis. The disease is transmitted by ingestion of food or water contaminated with cyst forms of the parasite and through fecal exposure during sexual contact.

Cutaneous amebiasis develops at the site of the invasion of the parasites into the skin from an underlying amebic abscess, usually at the perianal area or the abdominal wall. Cutaneous findings include purulent, foul-smelling nodules, cysts, and sinuses, which are associated with regional adenopathy and dysentery. Skin lesions grow rapidly and may lead to death if left untreated.

Diagnosis of cutaneous amebiasis is confirmed by microscopic identification of *E. histolytica* in the stool and in aspirates or biopsy samples obtained during colonoscopy, during surgery, or from the border of an ulcer. Treatment of choice for extraintestinal amebiasis is oral metronidazole (Flagyl) 750 mg PO three times daily for 7 to 10 days or tinidazole (Tindamax). Tinidazole was FDA approved in 2004 for the treatment of intestinal amebiasis in adults (2 g/day for 3 days) and children older than 3 years, and it appears to be as effective as and better tolerated than metronidazole. Either treatment should be followed by iodoquinol (Yodoxin) 650 mg PO three times daily for 20 days or paromomycin 25 to 35 mg/kg/day PO divided in three doses for 7 days.

Leishmaniasis
Leishmaniasis results from the infection with intracellular protozoan parasites belonging to the genus *Leishmania*. Leishmania parasites are transmitted to humans and other mammalian hosts (e.g., dogs, rodents) during feeding by infected female phlebotomine sandflies that serve as vectors. The parasites exist as promastigotes in the midgut of sandflies and as amastigotes (i.e., Leishman-Donovan bodies) within macrophages of humans and other mammals. Based on the extent and the severity of involvement in the human host, leishmaniasis may be clinically classified as cutaneous leishmaniasis, diffuse cutaneous leishmaniasis, mucocutaneous leishmaniasis, and visceral leishmaniasis.

Cutaneous leishmaniasis (New World or Old World form) begins as a small erythematous papule at the site of the bite of the sandfly, which evolves into an ulcerated nodule with a raised and indurated border (i.e., volcano sign) (Figure 1). The lesions gradually heal with a depressed scar. Diffuse cutaneous leishmaniasis is characterized by widespread cutaneous involvement without visceralization. Mucocutaneous leishmaniasis (known as espundia in South America) affects the skin, the mucosa, and the cartilages of the upper respiratory tract (especially the nose and the larynx) and may result in severe disfigurement. Visceral leishmaniasis results from the involvement of the bone marrow, spleen, and the liver, and it may lead to death if left untreated. It manifests with fever, splenomegaly, pancytopenia, and wasting. Post–kala azar dermal leishmaniasis may appear within a year after visceral disease independent of treatment, and it is characterized by macules, papules, and nodules, which are usually hypopigmented.

Diagnosis of leishmaniasis is based on finding the parasites in the skin from the lesion aspirate or biopsy by direct examination or culture. The leishmanin (Montenegro) skin test shows past and current infections, and it detects the inflammatory response in the skin after injection of phenol-killed parasites into the dermis. A past or current infection is also documented by an in vitro lymphocyte proliferation assay that requires a drop of blood from a finger prick. Polymerase chain reaction (PCR) techniques may be used to identify different *Leishmania* species. Circulating antibody levels are not considered a useful diagnostic sign.

Cutaneous leishmaniasis is usually self-limited and may not require treatment. Treatment of cutaneous leishmaniasis is indicated in case of numerous lesions or when lesions affect the face to avoid scarring. Therapies include sodium stibogluconate

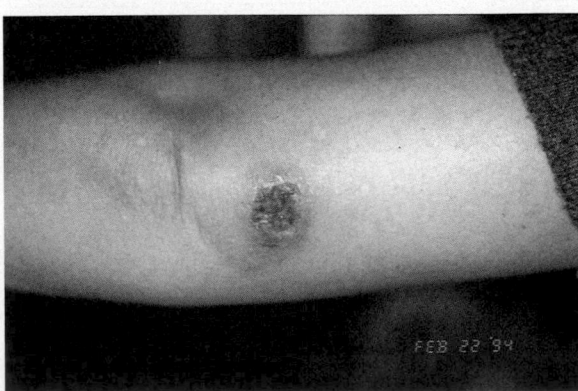

Figure 1. Cutaneous leishmaniasis is characterized by an ulcerated nodule with a raised and indurated border (i.e., volcano sign).

(Pentostam)[10] 20 mg/kg/day IV or IM for 20 days. Meglumine antimoniate (Glucantime)[2] 20 mg/kg/day IV or IM for 20 days or miltefosine (Impavido) for 28 days may be used. In 2014, FDA approved oral miltefosine for the treatment of cutaneous leishmaniasis caused by *L. braziliensis, L. paramensis*, and *L. guyanensis* in adults and adolescents who are not pregnant or breastfeeding. The FDA-approved treatment regimen for persons who weigh from 30 to 44 kg is one 50-mg oral capsule of miltefosine twice a day (total of 100 mg per day) for 28 consecutive days. The approved regimen for persons who weigh at least 45 kg (99 pounds) is one 50-mg capsule three times a day (total of 150 mg per day) for 28 consecutive days. Miltefosine is contraindicated in pregnant women during treatment and for 5 months thereafter. Alternatively, intralesional injections of antimonials 1 mg/kg once weekly, cryotherapy, local heat, oral ketoconazole (Nizoral),[1] topical amphotericin B,[2] pentamidine (Pentam)[1] 2 to 3 mg/kg IV or IM daily or every second day for four to seven doses, or topical paromomycin[6] (applied twice daily for 10–20 days) may be used.

The production of antileishmanial antibodies does not correlate with resolution of the disease. Infection and recovery are associated with lifelong immunity to reinfection by the same species of *Leishmania*, although interspecies immunity may also exist.

Trypanosomiasis
There are three types of trypanosomiasis:
- American trypanosomiasis or Chagas' diseases, caused by *Trypanosoma cruzi*
- East African sleeping sickness, caused by *Trypanosoma brucei rhodesiense*
- West African sleeping sickness, caused by *Trypanosoma brucei gambiense*

American trypanosomiasis (i.e., Chagas' disease) is caused by the parasite *T. cruzi*, and it is endemic in Central and South America. The disease is transmitted by the bite of infected "cone-nosed" insects, by transfusion of infected blood, by organ transplantation, and across the placenta. During the acute stage, Chagas' disease manifests with a painful erythematous nodule, known as chagoma, which is associated with regional adenopathy. The chronic stage manifests with cardiomyopathy, megaesophagus, and megacolon. Diagnosis is confirmed by microscopic identification of the parasite in fresh anticoagulated blood, in blood smears, by lymph node biopsy or skin biopsy, or by culture. Treatment includes benznidazole (Radanil, Rochagan)[2] 5 to 7 mg/kg/day PO in two doses for 60 to 90 days or nifurtimox (Lampit)[10] 8 to 10 mg/kg/day PO in three or four doses for 90 to 120 days.

African trypanosomiasis (i.e., East and West African sleeping sickness) occurs in Africa and is transmitted by the bite of infected male and female tsetse flies. It manifests with a highly inflammatory, painful, red or violaceous, indurated nodule surrounded by an erythematous halo, called trypanosome chancre, at the site of the inoculation of the parasites. There is regional adenopathy. Later, the chancre resolves spontaneously, and the patient has fever, malaise, a generalized pruritic eruption with erythematous annular plaques or urticarial lesions, and central nervous system (CNS) involvement with personality changes, apathy, somnolence, coma, and death. Diagnosis is based on the identification of trypanosomes by microscopic examination in chancre fluid, affected lymph node aspirates, blood, bone marrow, or in the late stages of infection, cerebrospinal fluid.

Treatment of East African sleeping sickness consists of suramin (naphthylamine sulfonic acid, Germanin)[10] 100 to 200 mg (test dose) IV and then 1 g IV on days 1, 3, 7, 14, and 21. For late disease with CNS involvement, melarsoprol B (a trivalent organic arsenical, Mel-B)[10] is used in the following dosage regimen: 2 to 3.6 mg/kg/day IV for 3 days; after 7 days, 3.6 mg/kg/day for 3 days; and the latter repeated after 7 days. For West African sleeping sickness, treatment of choice is pentamidine isethionate (Pentam 300)[1] 4 mg/kg/day IM for 10 days or suramin (Germanin) as used for East African sleeping sickness. For late disease with involvement of the CNS, eflornithine (Ornidyl)[2] 400 mg/kg/day IV in four doses for 14 days is used.

Cutaneous Toxoplasmosis
Systemic toxoplasmosis (congenital or acquired) is caused by the parasite *Toxoplasma gondii*, and it usually is transmitted from contact with infected cats. The disease may also be acquired by eating raw or undercooked meats from infected animals. Cutaneous involvement is rare. It manifests with punctate macules or ecchymoses in the congenital form, and the acquired form manifests with roseola and erythema multiforme lesions, urticaria, prurigo-like nodules, and maculopapular lesions. Diagnosis of cutaneous toxoplasmosis is confirmed by isolation of the parasite in the skin. Treatment is not needed for healthy nonpregnant patients because symptoms resolve in a few weeks. Treatment for pregnant women or immunocompromised patients includes pyrimethamine (Daraprim) 25–100 mg/d PO for 3–6 wks together with sulfadiazine[1] 1–15 g PO qid for 3–6 wks. Leucovorin should be taken with each dose of pyrimethamine.

Diseases Caused by Helminths
Ascariasis
Ascariasis is caused by *Ascaris* species, mainly *Ascaris lumbricoides*. It is transmitted by the ingestion of eggs in soil contaminated with human feces. Skin involvement of ascariasis manifests with urticaria. Diagnosis is based on finding the adult worm or eggs in the feces. Treatment includes albendazole (Albenza)[1] 400 mg PO once or mebendazole (Vermox) 100 mg PO twice daily for 3 days (or 500 mg once) or ivermectin (Stromectol)[1] 150 to 200 µg/kg PO once.

Cutaneous Larva Migrans
Cutaneous larva migrans is also known as creeping eruption, with the first term describing a syndrome and the second a clinical sign found in various conditions. The syndrome cutaneous larva migrans is caused when various nematode larvae (i.e., hookworms, such as *Ancylostoma braziliense, Ancylostoma caninum, Bunostomum phlebotomum*) of dogs, cats, and other mammals penetrate and migrate through the skin. Cutaneous larva migrans is transmitted by skin contact to soil contaminated with animal feces. In humans, larvae are unable to reach internal organs and eventually die. Cutaneous larva migrans manifests with intensely pruritic, papular lesions, which evolve as the larvae migrate to a characteristic linear, minimally elevated, serpiginous tract that moves forward in an irregular pattern. Diagnosis is easily made clinically and is supported by a travel history or by possible exposure in an endemic area.

Treatment of choice consists of ivermectin (Stromectol)[1] at a single dose of 200 µg/kg. In case of treatment failure, a second dose usually suffices. Ivermectin has an excellent safety profile, without any notable adverse events, and it has been used in millions of individuals in developing countries during onchocerciasis and filariasis control operations. It is contraindicated in children who weigh less than 15 kg (or are younger than 5 years) and in pregnant or breastfeeding women. Alternatively, repeated courses of oral albendazole (Albenza)[1] 400 mg daily for 3 days may be used. Treatment with oral thiabendazole (Mintezol) 50 mg/kg daily for 2 to 4 days has been associated with adverse events such as dizziness, nausea, vomiting, and intestinal cramps, and it is therefore not recommended. In the absence of multiple or widespread lesions, topical treatments may be considered, such as topical thiabendazole[6] 10% to 15%, applied three times daily for 5 to 7 days, which has similar efficacy with oral ivermectin and no adverse events.

Cysticercosis
Cysticercosis is caused by the larval stage (i.e., cysticerci) of the pork tapeworm *Taenia solium*, and it is the most common helminthic infection of the CNS. It is transmitted by ingesting eggs in

---

[1]Not FDA approved for this indication.
[2]Not available in the United States.
[6]May be compounded by pharmacists.
[10]Available in the United States from the Centers for Disease Control and Prevention.

---

[1]Not FDA approved for this indication.
[2]Not available in the United States.
[6]May be compounded by pharmacists.

food, in water, or on hands contaminated with human feces. Cutaneous manifestations are subcutaneous nodules that occur mainly on the extremities and trunk. There may be involvement of the CNS (i.e., seizures), eye, intestines, skeletal muscle, heart, kidneys, lung, and liver. Diagnosis is confirmed by isolation of the parasite in a nodule and by serologic tests.

Treatment options include surgery, albendazole (Albenza) 400 mg PO twice daily for 8 to 30 days, or praziquantel (Biltricide)[1] 100 mg/kg/day PO in three doses for 1 day and then 50 mg/kg/day in three doses for 29 days. Any cysticercocidal drug may cause irreparable damage when used in the presence of ocular or spinal cysts.

Dracunculiasis

Dracunculiasis is caused by the nematode *Dracunculus medinensis*. It is transmitted by drinking water with copepods (i.e., tiny aquatic arthropods) infected with the larvae of *D. medinensis*. In the human stomach, copepods release the larvae that mature and migrate to the skin, causing an erythematous papule or blister. The blister ruptures, and the female worm can often be seen prolapsing through the skin. Treatment includes extraction of the worm combined with wound care. Metronidazole (Flagyl)[1] 250 mg PO three times daily for 10 days may be efficacious and facilitates removal of the worm.

Filariasis

Filariasis is caused by nematodes (i.e., roundworms) that inhabit the lymphatics and subcutaneous tissues. The most common filarial infections include lymphatic filariasis, onchocerciasis, and loiasis.

Lymphatic Filariasis

Lymphatic filariasis is caused by *Wuchereria bancrofti, Brugia malayi,* and *Brugia timori,* and it is transmitted by mosquitoes. Adult worms result in a chronic inflammatory cell infiltrate around lymphatic vessels, causing their dilatation, hypertrophy, and obstruction. Many patients are asymptomatic, but some may develop fever with lymphangitis and lymphadenitis, chronic pulmonary infection, and progressive lymphedema leading to massive tissue thickening, especially of the legs and scrotum (i.e., elephantiasis). The overlying skin is thickened. Diagnosis is based on microscopic identification of the microfilariae in the blood and affected tissues.

Treatment consists of diethylcarbamazine (DEC, Hetrazan)[10] in the following regimen: 50 mg on day 1, 50 mg three times daily on day 2, 100 mg three times daily on day 3, and 6 mg/kg in three doses on days 4 through 14. Prophylaxis with DEC 500 mg/day for 2 days each month is effective against *W. bancrofti* infection for travelers in endemic areas.

Onchocerciasis

Onchocerciasis (i.e., blinding filariasis) is caused by the filarial nematode *Onchocerca volvulus,* which is transmitted by the blackflies *Simulium*. It may manifest with subcutaneous onchocercid nodules, acute or chronic dermatitis, depigmentation (i.e., leopard skin), and skin atrophy (i.e., lizard skin), and in later stages, it may manifest with lymphadenopathy and lymphedema. The microfilariae have a predilection for the eyes, and the infection can lead to blindness (i.e., river blindness). Diagnosis is based on identification of microfilariae in skin snips.

Treatment consists of ivermectin (Stromectol) 150 µg/kg PO every 6 to 12 months until asymptomatic. DEC is contraindicated as it may lead to blindness.

Loiasis

Loiasis (i.e., Calabar swellings) is caused by the parasite *Loa loa,* which is transmitted by deerflies (*Chrysops*). Cutaneous manifestations include pruritus, urticaria, and Calabar swellings, which are erythematous, warm, subcutaneous swellings associated with the migration of the worm through the subcutaneous tissues. Occasionally, there is subconjunctival migration of the adult worm, producing a migrating serpiginous lesion on the conjunctivae. Diagnosis is confirmed by identification of microfilariae in the blood by microscopic examination.

DEC[10] is the treatment of choice in the following regimen: 50 mg on day 1, 50 mg three times daily on day 2, 100 mg three times daily on day 3, and 9 mg/kg/day in three doses on days 4 through 14. Ivermectin (Stromectol)[1] may cause encephalopathy in patients with a heavy *L. loa* infection. Prophylaxis with DEC is effective for *L. loa* in adults who travel in endemic areas.

Schistosomiasis

Schistosomiasis (i.e., snail fever) in humans is caused mainly by the trematodes *Schistosoma haematobium, Schistosoma japonicum,* and *Schistosoma mansoni*. All trematodes have a life cycle that involves the snail as an intermediate host. The infective cercariae leave the snail, swim, and penetrate the human skin, causing a pruritic papular dermatosis. The disease is transmitted by exposure to contaminated water with live cercariae or by drinking infested water. Skin findings of acute schistosomiasis include pruritic schistosomal dermatitis due to a hypersensitivity response to the cercariae and edema of the face, extremities, genitals, and trunk. Schistosomal fever (i.e., Katayama fever), lymphadenopathy, and diarrhea may also develop. Late skin findings (i.e., bilharziasis cutanea tarda) appear in patients with visceral disease and include firm, pruritic, grouped papules. Secondary infection, ulceration, and development of squamous cell carcinoma may follow. Diagnosis is confirmed by identification of the eggs in the urine or stool, by biopsy of affected tissues, or by enzyme-linked immunosorbent assay (ELISA).

Treatment includes praziquantel (Biltricide)[3] 40 mg/kg/day in two doses for 1 day (for *S. haematobium* and *S. mansoni*) or 60 mg/kg/day in three doses for 1 day (for *S. japonicum*).

Cercarial Dermatitis

Cercarial dermatitis (i.e., swimmer's itch) is caused by cercariae (i.e., larvae) of nonhuman schistosomes that penetrate the skin and die without invading other tissues. It is transmitted by contact with fresh or salt water contaminated with cercariae. It manifests with extremely pruritic, erythematous macules of sudden onset, which evolve into papules, vesicles, and urticarial lesions located on parts of the body directly exposed to the water, while sparing clothed areas. Cercarial dermatitis is a self-limited disease, and treatment is symptomatic with topical steroids and oral antihistamines.

Diseases Caused by Arthropoda

Human Scabies

Scabies is a common skin infestation caused by the mite *Sarcoptes scabiei,* which is an obligate human parasite. Scabies is transmitted by direct contact with an infested individual or by contact with bedding and clothing. The incubation period for scabies is about 3 weeks, and reinfestation results in symptoms within 1 to 3 days. Scabies is characterized by pruritus that usually worsens at night. Papules, nodules, excoriations, and burrows may be found. Lesions are usually located on interdigital spaces, wrists, ankles, axillae, waist, and genitals. Scabies manifests as red-brown nodules that represent a hypersensitivity response. In adults, the head is usually spared, whereas the involvement of the scalp, palms, and soles is common in infants.

Crusted or Norwegian scabies manifests with hyperkeratotic papules or plaques of the hands and feet (often with nail involvement) and an erythematous scaly eruption on the face, neck, scalp, and trunk. Because pruritus is often absent, this disease can be misdiagnosed as psoriasis, eczema, or an adverse drug reaction. Lesions contain thousands of mites and are highly contagious.

---

[1]Not FDA approved for this indication.

[10]Available in the United States from the Centers for Disease Control and Prevention.

---

[1]Not FDA approved for this indication.

[3]Exceeds dosage recommended by the manufacturer.

[10]Available in the United States from the Centers for Disease Control and Prevention.

Crusted scabies mainly affects immunocompromised patients (e.g., patients with human immunodeficiency virus infection), mentally retarded persons, or debilitated patients.

Diagnosis is based on the microscopic identification of mites or their eggs or feces from burrows or papules. Treatment should be applied from the neck down in adults, and in infants, application should include the scalp and face (avoiding the eyes and mouth).

Treatment includes 5% permethrin (Elimite) applied for 10 hours and repeated after 1 week. A 25% benzyl benzoate solution[6] is also efficacious in adults, and because of low toxicity, it is recommended in a lower concentration (10%) for children older than 4 months and for women during pregnancy. Sulfur ointments in petrolatum[6] at concentrations of 6% to 10% may be used for scabies in children and pregnant women. Alternative treatments for scabies include crotamiton 10% (Eurax) applied once daily for 2 days, or ivermectin (Stromectol)[1] as a single- or two-dose regimen of 200 μg/kg/dose can be used. Aggressive treatment with ivermectin at a single dose of 200 μg/kg, repeated after 2 weeks with or without topical 5% permethrin cream (two applications, 1 week apart) and keratolytics (5% salicylic acid ointment[1] applied twice daily) is the treatment of choice for crusted scabies. All sexual and close personal and household contacts within the preceding 6 weeks should be treated simultaneously. Bedding and clothing should be decontaminated (i.e., machine washed and dried using the hot cycle or dry cleaned) or removed from body contact for at least 3 days, because the mite dies when separated from the human host.

Pediculosis

Pediculosis (i.e., lice) is a contagious dermatosis, caused by lice, which are blood-sucking, wingless insects and are obligate human parasites. Two species of lice infest humans causing three clinical forms of infestation: *Pediculus humanus capitis* (i.e., head louse), *Pediculus humanus corporis* (i.e., body louse), and *Phthirus pubis* (i.e., pubic louse). The body louse is the only louse that can carry human disease, including rickettsioses and epidemic typhus.

Pediculosis Capitis

Pediculosis capitis is caused by *P. humanus capitis*, and it is transmitted by close contact or by fomites with combs, brushes, towels, and hats. It manifests with pruritus (due to the saliva of the louse), excoriations, nape dermatitis, secondary bacterial infection, and cervical and suboccipital lymphadenopathy. Diagnosis is based on identification of lice and eggs or nits on the hair and on fluorescence of nits with Wood's light. Visible nits are deposited on the hair shaft, close to the scalp. After adequate treatment, nits found at 1.0 to 1.5 cm from the scalp are not alive.

Treatment includes malathion (Ovide) 0.5% lotion applied for 8 to 12 hours or permethrin (Nix) 1% cream rinse applied to shampooed hair for 10 minutes. A second application with permethrin is recommended 1 week later to kill hatching progeny. Alternatively, pyrethrins with piperidyl butoxide (RID) can be applied and washed off after 10 minutes. Benzyl benzoate 25% solution[6] is mainly a scabicide, but it may also be used as a pediculicide. Ivermectin lotion 0.5% (Sklice) was approved by the FDA in 2012 for treatment of head lice in persons 6 months of age and older, using a fine-toothed comb. Bedding, clothing, and headgear should be decontaminated (as for scabies) or removed from body contact for 2 weeks. Information for managing head lice can be found at the National Pediculosis Association web site (http://www.headlice.org).

Pediculosis Corporis

Pediculosis corporis (i.e., vagabond's itch) is caused by *P. humanus corporis*, which lives and reproduces in the lining of clothes and leaves the clothing only for feeding from the skin. This disease is usually found among vagabonds. Transmission occurs mainly through contact with contaminated clothing or bedding. Clinical manifestations include pruritus, excoriations, and small, red macules that usually occur on the back. Clothes should be examined carefully for lice.

---

[1]Not FDA approved for this indication.
[6]May be compounded by pharmacists.

Treatment is the same as for pediculosis capitis. Dry heat or washing in hot water followed by ironing is effective in killing the lice and their ova in clothing. Items that cannot be washed should be removed from body contact for 2 weeks.

Pediculosis Pubis

Pediculosis pubis is caused by *P. pubis* and affects the pubic hair. However, if left untreated, it may also affect very hairy regions of the chest, abdomen, axillary region, and especially in children, the eyelashes, edge of the scalp, and eyebrows. Patients present with pruritus. Useful diagnostic signs include small, blue-gray macules on the trunk, thighs, and axillae (i.e., taches bleuâtres or maculae ceruleae) due to conversion of bilirubin to biliverdin by the saliva of the louse and a brown "dust" found on underclothing due to the excreta of the insects. *P. pubis* is transmitted mainly by sexual contact, but it also may be transmitted by clothing or from parents to children.

Patients with pubic lice should be evaluated for other sexually transmitted diseases. Treatment of pediculosis pubis is the same as for pediculosis capitis. Bedding and clothing should be decontaminated (as for scabies) or removed from body contact for 2 weeks. Attention should be paid to treating sexual partners within the previous month because they are a common cause of reinfestation. For infested eyelashes and eyebrows, ophthalmic-grade petrolatum ointment may be used two to four times daily for 10 days, and lice and nits should be carefully removed from the eyelashes with forceps.

References

Centers for Disease Control (CDC). Disease exposure while traveling. Available at: http://www.cdc.gov/travel/ [accessed August 15, 2014].

Centers for Disease Control (CDC). Leishmaniasis. Available at: http://www.cdc.gov/parasites/leishmaniasis/health_professionals/index.html#tx. [accessed March 1, 2015].

Centers for Disease Control. Malathion. Available at: http://www.cdc.gov/parasites/lice/head/gen_info/faqs_malathion.html. [accessed March 1, 2015].

Gorkiewicz-Petkow A. Scabicides and pediculicides. In: Katsambas AD, Lotti TM, editors. European Handbook of Dermatological Treatments. 2nd ed. Berlin: Springer; 2003. p. 775–9.

Goyal NN, Wong GA. Psoriasis or crusted scabies. Clin Exp Dermatol 2008;33:211–2.

Heukelbach J, Feldmeier H. Epidemiological and clinical characteristics of hookworm-related cutaneous larva migrans. Lancet Infect Dis 2008;8:302–9.

Klaus SN, Frankenburg S, Dhar AD. Leishmaniasis and other protozoan infections. In: Freedeberg IM, Eisen AZ, Wolff K, et al., editors. Fitzpatrick's Dermatology in General Medicine. 6th ed. New York: McGraw-Hill; 2003. p. 2215–24.

Lucchina LC, Wilson ME. Cysticercosis and other helminthic infections. In: Freedeberg IM, Eisen AZ, Wolff K, et al., editors. Fitzpatrick's Dermatology in General Medicine. 6th ed. New York: McGraw-Hill; 2003. p. 2225–59.

Paller AS, Mancini AJ. Bites and infestations. In: Hurwitz Clinical Pediatric Dermatology. 3rd ed. Philadelphia: WB Saunders; 2006. p. 479–501.

Stone SP. Scabies and pediculosis. In: Freedeberg IM, Eisen AZ, Wolff K, et al., editors. Fitzpatrick's Dermatology in General Medicine. 6th ed. New York: McGraw-Hill; 2003. p. 2283–9.

Tsourdi-Nikita E, Campanile G, Hautmann G, et al. Pediculosis. In: Katsambas AD, Lotti TM, editors. European Handbook of Dermatological Treatments. 2nd ed. Berlin: Springer; 2003. p. 775–9.

PIGMENTARY DISORDERS

Method of
Rebat M. Halder, MD; and Ahmad Reza Hossani-Madani, MD

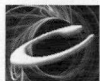

CURRENT DIAGNOSIS

Hyperpigmentation
- Ephelides: Multiple, small (1–4 mm), light to dark brown macules with poorly defined margins that occur on sun-exposed areas of the body
- Solar lentigines: Light brown to dark brown macular hyperpigmented lesions that are induced by natural or artificial sources of radiation and that can coalesce; they are located on face, neck, forearms, and hands

- Melasma: Arcuate or polycyclic brown to blue macules that coalesce into patches on face, neck, or forearms
- Postinflammatory hyperpigmentation: Dark patches or macules with indistinct margins at the location of an inciting inflammatory event

Hypopigmentation

- Pityriasis alba: 2 to 3 round, well-defined, paler macules with overlying powdery white scales, ranging in size from 0.5 to 5 cm in diameter, that transition to smooth, hypopigmented macules
- Vitiligo: Sharply demarcated, depigmented, milky white macules in a localized or generalized distribution
- Idiopathic guttate hypomelanosis: Multiple circular, smooth, small macules that are porcelain white, with occasional black dots, found on sun-exposed areas of upper and lower extremities
- Postinflammatory hypopigmentation: Off-white or tan macules, with ill-defined borders at the site of an inciting inflammatory event

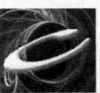

CURRENT THERAPY

Hyperpigmentation

- Ephelides: Hydroquinone 4% (Claripel) or glycolic plus kojic acid combination (Brown Spot Night Gel) plus maximum UVA-blocking sunscreen in the morning and tretinoin 0.1% cream (Retin-A)[1] in the evening
- Solar lentigines: Hydroxyanisole (mequinol) 2% plus tretinoin 0.01% (Solage) applied twice daily; cryotherapy; laser therapy
- Melasma: Monotherapy with hydroquinone 4% twice daily or tretinoin 0.1%[1] once daily; double therapy with hydroquinone 4% twice daily plus tretinoin[1] 0.05% once daily; triple therapy with fluocinolone acetonide 0.01% plus hydroquinone 4% plus tretinoin[1] 0.05% (Tri-Luma) once daily
- Postinflammatory hyperpigmentation: Treat inciting event; hydroquinone 4% alone or in combination with topical steroid; mequinol 2% plus tretinoin 0.01% combination[1] twice daily; fluocinolone acetonide 0.01% plus hydroquinone 4% plus tretinoin 0.05% combination[1] once daily

Hypopigmentation

- Pityriasis alba: Emollients, lubricants, sunscreen; tacrolimus 0.1% ointment (Protopic)[1] twice daily or mild nonhalogenated steroid for face and medium potency steroid for body; phototherapy (PUVA or UVB) for extensive disease
- Vitiligo: In patients with less than 20% body surface area (BSA) involvement, treat with cosmetics, topical (potent or very potent steroid or calcineurin inhibitor trial for less than 2 months), topical PUVA, or excimer laser. If local treatment fails, the surgical approach may be used if the patient has less than 20% BSA involvement. For patients with more than 20% BSA involvement, UVB is preferred over oral PUVA. For patients with more than 50% BSA or disfiguring facial involvement, treat with monobenzyl ether of hydroquinone (monobenzone 20%), 4-methoxyphenol or Q-switched ruby laser (694 nm).
- Idiopathic guttate hypomelanosis: Cryotherapy; dermabrasion; surgical minigrafting; intralesional steroids
- Postinflammatory hypopigmentation: Cosmetics; topical corticosteroids; topical PUVA

[1]Not FDA approved for this indication.

Definition

The word *chromophore* is defined as elements that impart color to the skin. Hyperchromias describe abnormally darker skin, and hypochromias describe abnormally lighter skin. Pigmentation refers to melanotic causes of skin color change, differentiating it from skin color changes due to blood, carotene, bilirubin, or other causes. Hyperpigmentation refers to an increase in melanin production, melanocyte number, or both in the skin. Hypopigmentation refers to decrease of melanin, melanocytes, or both in the skin. Depigmentation refers to the absence of both melanin and melanocytes. Deposition of melanin in the epidermal layers visibly appears as a yellow to brownish hue. Dermal deposition appears as blue or blue-gray, with mixed epidermal and dermal melanin deposition appearing gray or blue-brown.

Evaluation

A thorough history and visual inspection of the pigmentary disorder can provide useful clues to the diagnosis, particularly recognition of pigmentary patterns (diffuse, circumscribed, linear, or reticulated). Further examination may be achieved by using the Wood's lamp to differentiate epidermal from dermal melanin.

General Recommendations for All Pigmentary Disorders

Broad-spectrum sunscreen with an SPF of 30 is recommended, in addition to wearing protective clothing. Avoiding prolonged sun exposure is also desired, if possible.

Hyperpigmentation
Ephelides
Description

Ephelides (freckles) are multiple, small (1–4 mm), light to dark brown macules with poorly defined margins that occur on sun-exposed areas of the body (face, upper back, arms). They are more commonly found in children (fading with age), fair-skinned persons, and those with red or blonde hair (especially those of Celtic ancestry). A relationship has been shown between painful sunburns in youth and development of ephelides, and the macules become darker with greater UV exposure. They are thought to be genetic in origin, following an autosomal dominant pattern, and are strongly associated with variants in the melanocortin-1-receptor (MC1R). Ephelides are significant because they are associated with an increased risk of melanoma and nonmelanoma skin cancer, perhaps serving as a marker for sun susceptibility.

Treatment

Although treatment is not necessary, modalities include either hydroquinone 4% (Claripel, Eldopaque Forte) or glycolic plus kojic acid combination (Brown Spot Night Gel) plus maximum ultraviolet A (UVA)-blocking sunscreen in the morning and tretinoin 0.1% cream (Retin-A)[1] in the evening. Other therapies have included cryotherapy, lasers, and chemical peels.

Solar Lentigo (Lentigo Senilis Et Actinicus)
Description

Solar lentigines are pigmented spots that share morphologic similarities with ephelides, making differentiation difficult. They are defined as light brown to dark brown macular hyperpigmented lesions induced by natural or artificial sources of radiation, which can coalesce. The incidence increases with age, and more than 90% of white persons older than 50 years demonstrate lesions. They appear most often on the face, neck, forearms, and hands. They can occur on nonclassic locations in those receiving phototherapy (such as the penis). Histologically, they differ from ephelides by the presence of epidermal hyperplasia, increased melanocyte number, and elongation of the rete ridges.

Treatment

Although treatment is not necessary, two different modalities have been used: physical therapies and topical therapies. Physical therapies include cryotherapy and lasers, and topical treatments include retinoids or combinations of agents. Liquid nitrogen may be used

[1]Not FDA approved for this indication.

with a cotton swab for 5 to 10 seconds to induce lightening. Recurrence rates may be as high as 55% at 6 months. Side effects include atrophy with longer cryoprobe application, postinflammatory hyper- or hypopigmentation, and pain. The Q-switched Nd:YAG (532 nm), among others, has been used with success. An effective combination topical treatment includes hydroxyanisole (mequinol) 2% plus tretinoin 0.01% (Solage) applied twice daily. Side effects include erythema and burning or stinging.

Melasma
Description
Melasma is a hypermelanosis of the face, neck, and forearms that occurs with a higher incidence in women of African American, Latin American, and Asian descent. It appears on sun-exposed areas as arcuate or polycyclic macules that coalesce into patches. Epidermal melanin deposition causes a brownish appearance, and dermal melanin appears bluish. Combined epidermal and dermal melanin deposition appears gray. It is distributed in a central facial (65%), malar (20%), or mandibular (15%) pattern. It is more commonly seen in women and those with darker skin, but it can also be found in men. Contributing factors include a genetic predisposition, pregnancy, oral contraceptive use, endocrine dysfunction, hormonal treatment, UV light exposure, cosmetics, and phototoxic drugs.

Treatment
First-line treatment for melasma consists of broad-spectrum sunscreen with greater than SPF 30 coverage in addition to monotherapy with hydroquinone 4% twice daily or tretinoin 0.1%[1] once daily. Double therapy with hydroquinone 4% twice daily plus tretinoin 0.05% may prove efficacious after an unsuccessful trial of monotherapy. If that fails, triple therapy may be attempted, with fluocinolone acetonide 0.01%, hydroquinone 4%, and tretinoin 0.05% (Tri-Luma) once daily being effective. Side effects of triple therapy include erythema, desquamation, burning, dryness, and pruritus at the site of application; telangiectasia; perioral dermatitis; acne breakouts; and hyperpigmentation. Chemical peels, superficial and medium depth, and erbium:YAG laser may also be used for patients whose topical treatments have failed.

Postinflammatory Hyperpigmentation
Description
Postinflammatory hyperpigmentation is a very common condition that occurs as a result of a previous or ongoing inflammatory process, most commonly acne vulgaris, atopic dermatitis, infections, and phototoxic reactions and as a result of treatment with topical medications, chemical peels, and lasers. Postinflammatory hyperpigmentation occurs more commonly in persons with darker skin pigmentation and appears as dark patches or macules with indistinct margins at the location of the inciting inflammatory event.

Treatment
Primary treatment is aimed at treating the inciting cause of the hyperpigmentation. Additional effective therapies include 4% hydroquinone alone or in combination with a topical steroid. Other combination treatments include mequinol 2% plus tretinoin 0.01% combination[1] twice daily or fluocinolone acetonide 0.01%, hydroquinone 4%, tretinoin 0.05%[1] once daily. Treatment must be temporarily stopped if irritation occurs. Broad-spectrum sunscreen should also be employed.

Hypopigmenation or Depigmentation
Pityriasis Alba
Description
Pityriasis alba is a childhood or adolescent condition that affects all races. It begins as an erythematous macule with ill-defined borders. The erythema fades after a few weeks, leaving two or three round, well-defined, paler macules with overlying powdery white scale,

ranging in size from 0.5 cm to 5 cm in diameter. These eventually transition to smooth, hypopigmented lesions, which are generally located on the face. The pathogenesis of this disorder is unknown.

Treatment
Pityriasis alba is thought to be a self-limited skin disease. However, general treatment guidelines include use of emollients and lubricant, use of sunscreen, and decreasing sun exposure. Lesions limited to the face may be treated with hydrocortisone 1% (Lanacort 10 Crème)[1] or other mild, nonfluorinated steroid. More-potent steroids may be used for lesions on the body, including hydrocortisone valerate 0.2% (Westcort)[1] or alclometasone dipropionate 0.05% (Aclovate).[1] However, these can lead to atrophy if used over an extended period. Newer, safer, effective alternatives include tacrolimus 0.1% ointment (Protopic)[1] twice daily. Side effects include a burning sensation that fades over time. Extensive disease that is not amenable to topical therapy might benefit from photochemotherapy (psoralen plus UVA [PUVA] or UVB alone).

Vitiligo
Description
Persons with vitiligo acquire sharply demarcated, depigmented macules in a localized or generalized distribution. These macules appear milky white as compared with the surrounding normally pigmented skin. Lesions can increase in size. There is no predilection for race or sex, and three quarters of patients generally present before the age of 30 years.

Treatment
General recommendations include the use of sunscreen, avoidance of the sun, and use of protective clothing. Treatments for localized vitiligo (<20% of body surface area) include cosmetics, a 2-month trial of topical treatment (potent or very potent corticosteroid or calcineurin inhibitor), excimer laser, or topical PUVA. Adults who have failed treatments for localized vitiligo may be considered for narrow-band UVB, oral PUVA, or surgical treatment, which includes split-skin grafting, transfer of suction blisters, or autologous epidermal suspensions added to dermabraded skin (followed by UVB). Surgical candidates should have localized, limited involvement and should not demonstrate lesion enlargement or Koebner phenomenon for 12 months prior to treatment. Patients with more than 20% body involvement may be considered for narrow-band UVB (311 nm) or oral PUVA. Those with greater than 50% body involvement or disfiguring facial involvement may be considered for complete depigmentation with monobenzyl ether of hydroquinone (Benoquin 20%), 4-methoxyphenol, or the Q-switched ruby laser (694 nm). Children are generally not offered surgical treatment, and oral PUVA is relatively contraindicated in children younger than 10 years.

Idiopathic Guttate Hypomelanosis
Description
This is an acquired, asymptomatic leukoderma with multiple, circular, smooth, small macules that have a porcelain white color. Black dots are occasionally observed within the macules. The macules increase in number with age, but they generally do not increase in size. They are most commonly located on sun-exposed areas of the upper and lower extremities.

Treatment
Treatments have included cryotherapy, dermabrasion, surgical minigrafting, and intralesional steroids; however, none of these have shown consistent acceptable results. Phototherapy has not been shown to be effective.

Postinflammatory Hypopigmentation
Description
Postinflammatory hypopigmentation is the result of an inciting inflammatory event leading to lesions that are off-white or tan,

---
[1]Not FDA approved for this indication.

---
[1]Not FDA approved for this indication.

with ill-defined borders. This entity is noticed more commonly in those with darker skin.

Treatment

Hypopigmentation resolves with treatment of the underlying condition. Topical cosmetics may be useful. Topical corticosteroids and topical PUVA therapy may also be used in patients who have lesions in cosmetically distressing areas.

References

Cestari T, Arellano I, Hexsel D, Ortonne JP. Melasma in Latin America: Option for therapy and treatment algorithm. J Eur Acad Dermatol Venereol 2009;23:760–72.

Gupta AK, Gover MD, Nouri K, Taylor S. The treatment of melasma: A review of clinical trials. J Am Acad Dermatol 2006;55:1048–65.

Halder RM, Richards GM. Management of dyschromias in ethnic skin. Dermatol Ther 2004;17:151–7.

Halder RM, Richards GM. Topical agents used in the management of hyperpigmentation. Skin Therapy Lett 2004;9:1–3.

Hexsel DM. Treatment of idiopathic guttate hypomelanosis by localized superficial dermabrasion. Dermatol Surg 1999;25:917–8.

Lin RL, Janniger CK. Pityriasis alba. Cutis 2005;76:21–4.

Nordlund JJ, Boissy RE, Hearing VJ, et al., editors. The Pigmentary System: Physiology and Pathophysiology. 2nd ed. Malden, Mass: Blackwell Publishing; 2007.

Nordlund JJ, Cestari TF, Chan F, Westerhof W. Confusions about color: A classification of discolorations of the skin. Br J Dermatol 2007;156(Suppl. 1):S3–S6.

Ortonne JP, Pandya AG, Lui H, Hexsel D. Treatment of solar lentigines. J Am Acad Dermatol 2006;54:S262–S271.

Ploysangam T, Dee-Ananlap S, Suvanprakorn P. Treatment of idiopathic guttate hypolemanosis with iquid nitrogen: Light and electron microscopic studies. J Am Acad Dermatol 1990;23:681–4.

Rigopoulos D, Gregoriou S, Charissi C, et al. Tacrolimus ointment 0.1% in pityriasis alba: An open-label randomized, placebo-controlled study. Br J Dermatol 2006;155:152–5.

Taylor SC, Burgess CM, Callender VD, et al. Postinflammatory hyperpigmentation: evolving combination treatment strategies. Cutis 2006;78:S6–S19.

PREMALIGNANT LESIONS

Method of
Juliet Aylward, MD

CURRENT DIAGNOSIS

Actinic Keratoses or Cheilitis
- Flesh-colored, red, or pigmented lesions with thick or delicate keratotic scale
- Swelling, fissures, and scaling on lower lip
- Sun-exposed sites

Arsenical Keratoses
- Punctate, hyperkeratotic lesions of palms and soles
- Exposure to contaminated well water or medications

Porokeratoses
- Lesions with atrophic center and peripheral grooved ridge of hyperkeratosis
- Large and solitary; diffuse, small, and annular on sun-exposed sites; linear, segmental, or generalized; punctate on palms and soles without ridge

Human Papillomavirus Disease
- Verrucous, hyperkeratotic lesions on palms and soles
- Fleshy, hyperkeratotic lesions or shiny, atrophic lesions or erosions in the anogenital region
- White, adherent, keratotic lesions on mucosal surfaces; may become verrucous and exophytic

Atypia in Melanocytic Nevi
- "Fried egg" appearance with a papular center on a macular base
- Asymmetry, ill-defined borders, variegated color, diameter larger than 6 mm, ulceration, bleeding, pain, or pruritus in a new or previously stable pigmented lesion

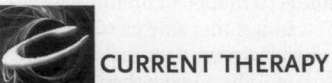

CURRENT THERAPY

Actinic Keratoses or Cheilitis
- Physical methods: curettage, liquid nitrogen, dermabrasion, ablative laser resurfacing
- Nonselective topical chemical agents: glycol acid 20%,[1] trichloroacetic acid 10% to 30%[1]
- Selective topical chemical agents: 5-fluorouracil (Carac, Efudex), diclofenac sodium (Solaraze), ingenol mebulate gel (Picato), imiquimod (Aldara, Zyclara), 5-aminolevulinic acid (Levulan Kerastick) or methyl aminolevulinate (Matvix) activated by a light source, and retinoids, including tretinoin (Retin-A),[1] adapalene (Differin),[1] and tazarotene (Tazorac)[1]
- Oral agents: retinoids[1]

Arsenical Keratoses
- Surgery and modalities used for actinic keratoses

Porokeratoses
- Surgery and modlities for actinic keratoses

Human Papillomavirus Disease
- Blistering agents: liquid nitrogen, Cantharone (0.7% cantharidin),[1,6] podophyllin 25% in tincture of benzoin (Podocon-25), purified podophyllotoxin 0.5% solution or gel (Condylox)
- Keratolytics: topical salicylic acid products (e.g., Compound W, Wart-Off, Dr. Scholl's, Duofilm, Salactic, Mediplast, Sal-Acid), topical retinoids,[1] and topical urea 10% to 40% (Carmol, Gordon's)
- Physical methods: curettage, liquid nitrogen, surgery, ablative laser, electrofulguration, occlusive tapes such as duct tape
- Immunotherapy: imiquimod (Aldara), intralesional candida or mumps antigen injections[1]
- Oral agents: cimetidine (Tagamet)[1]
- Other: sinecatechins (Veregen and Polyphenon E)

Atypia in Melanocytic Nevi
- Close clinical observation and mole mapping
- Surgery, curettage, ablative laser

[1]Not FDA approved for this indication.
[6]May be compounded by pharmacists.

Identification and clinical monitoring of premalignant skin lesions can reduce the morbidity and mortality of skin cancer for many patients with diverse histories and exposures. The link between precancerous and cancerous lesions and ultraviolet (UV) light exposure has been studied extensively. Some patients do not understand the importance of or choose not to adhere to sun-protection precautions and the prudent use of sunscreens. The cause of premalignant lesions also includes human papillomavirus (HPV) disease, arsenic exposures, and degeneration of benign nevi, birthmarks, and neoplasms.

Although certain exposures and conditions are associated with premalignant lesions, some groups of patients are at higher risk for precancerous and cancerous lesions. In many cases, these cancers are rapidly progressive, high grade, and aggressive. Patients who are at high risk are immunocompromised due to human immunodeficiency virus infection or acquired immunodeficiency syndrome, have heritable immunodeficiencies, have had effective immunosuppression of chronic lymphocytic leukemia, have undergone organ transplantation, or are on immunosuppressive medications. An increased susceptibility to infection with oncogenic HPV types may be important in the pathogenesis of malignancies in these patients. Genodermatoses associated with a higher risk of skin cancer include xeroderma pigmentosa, oculocutaneous albinism, Bazex syndrome, and nevoid basal cell carcinoma syndrome. A history of UV exposure and cigarette smoking further compounds the risk for many of these patients.

A variety of dermatoses and neoplasms have a demonstrated association with development of malignancies, although these benign conditions or lesions are not necessarily precancerous. In certain long-standing skin diseases, persistence or progression of characteristic lesions despite apparent appropriate treatment may herald development of skin cancer. Similarly, atypical appearance of or change in the classic lesion of a skin condition or in a previously stable neoplasm is suspicious. These conditions include Zoon balanitis or vulvitis, discoid lupus erythematosus, lichen planus, lichen sclerosus, lymphedema, and chronic radiodermatitis. The neoplasms include nevus sebaceus, plexiform neurofibromas, and leukoplakia or erythroplakia. Scars, epitomized by the persistent scarring seen in dystrophic epidermolysis bullosa, and non-healing wounds (e.g., burns, chronic ulcers) also may provide sites for malignant growth.

By recognizing these risk factors, predispositions, special populations, and associations, the practitioner can identify premalignant lesions in at-risk patients and recommend appropriate follow-up evaluation and treatment. This approach is essential for prevention and early detection of various types of cancers of cutaneous and mucosal surfaces. Lesions that progress, become symptomatic, become locally destructive or disfiguring, do not respond to appropriate treatment, or change their clinical appearance or behavior should be evaluated for malignancy. Biopsy and referral to a dermatologist are recommended.

Actinic Keratoses or Cheilitis
Clinical Manifestations
Precursors to squamous cell carcinoma in situ (SCCIS) and squamous cell carcinoma (SCC) can develop on cutaneous and mucosal surfaces subjected to intense, intermittent, or frequent sun exposure. They manifest as flesh-colored, red, or pigmented papules and plaques. Some are rather firm and indurated with a hard scale; others are thin and friable, with a more delicate scale or without scale, appearing shiny and atrophic.

Clinical diagnosis is facilitated by light palpation of sun-exposed sites with the fingertips because the characteristic, gritty, sandpaper-like scale can be very prominent. Involvement can range from multiple or few discrete lesions to an ill-defined zone or field. Occurrence on the lip, often exclusively the lower lip, may be associated with pain, swelling, and fissures. Most lesions remain stable for years without progression or degeneration. The absolute risk is not known but is estimated at 0.1% to 10% per year. Lesions that persist after treatment or show rapid progression should raise suspicion for malignant degeneration. Suspicion should be elevated if mucosal lesions are ulcerated, and biopsy is recommended.

Treatment
Limited mechanical removal of discrete lesions is possible with curettage. Liquid nitrogen applied with a cotton-tipped applicator or spraying device is a common and effective treatment for cutaneous and mucosal lesions. Lesions can be treated until they appear white or frozen; treatment is for 8 to 10 seconds on the lip and other delicate tissues. Thicker skin and thicker lesions require freeze times of 20 seconds or to the patient's tolerance. After this, a second cycle may be used immediately. Some lesions may require two or three such treatments separated by 4 to 12 weeks before resolution. Posttreatment pain, swelling, and blistering can be limiting. Because this modality is nonselective, normal and atypical cells are affected equally.

Other destructive modalities may be beneficial for discrete lesions; these include dermabrasion and ablative lasers such as carbon dioxide (CO_2) and erbium:yttrium–yttrium–aluminum–garnet (Er:YAG) lasers.

Treatment of individual lesions with chemical peeling agents such as glycolic acid 20% (e.g., Biomedic MicroPeel Solution)[1] and trichloroacetic acid 10% to 30%[1] can be effective and repeated as

needed. These nonselective agents can also be applied to a wider field of involvement for broader effect (i.e., field treatment).

Field treatment also is available as a patient-delivered topical chemotherapy. Topical 5-fluorouracil (available as 0.5% [Carac], 1% [Fluoroplex], and 5% cream [Efudex] for cutaneous surfaces and 1% [Fluoroplex], 2% [Efudex], and 5% solution [Efudex] for mucosal surfaces) can be applied in various regimens, once or twice daily for 2 to 6 weeks as the patient tolerates. More delicate mucosal tissues should be treated once or twice daily for 1 to 3 weeks. Use is limited by development of irritation, pain, and skin breakdown. Because this is a selective chemical treatment, affected cells are targeted, and a more vigorous response should lead to more significant improvement. Inflammatory response is individual, and for patients who are not tolerating treatment well, application can be reduced to once to three times weekly. Breaks or time off during a treatment course can be introduced. The treatment course can be abbreviated if needed. An effective treatment course also may treat early or in situ lesions of SCC or basal cell carcinoma (BCC) in the field.

Other topical chemotherapeutic field treatments include diclofenac sodium 3% gel (Solaraze) applied once or twice daily for 8 to 12 weeks. The inflammatory response is attenuated and therefore may be better tolerated by patients. Concomitantly, improvement is less dramatic. A shorter course may be preferred, so ingenol mebutate (Picato) as 0.015% gel can be applied to the face and scalp for 3 consecutive days or can be applied as 0.05% gel to the trunk and extremities for 2 consecutive days. Imiquimod 5% cream (Aldara) may be applied daily for 3 to 6 weeks or twice daily for 3 days per week for 4 to 8 weeks. Another regimen is application once or twice per week for 4 to 8 months, used continuously or in alternating 1-month cycles. The daily dosing schedule and treatment course should be decreased by about one half for mucosal surfaces. The disadvantage is unpredictability of response. Imiquimod 2.5% and 3.75% cream (Zyclara) can be used each night for two 2-week treatment cycles separated by a 2-week no-treatment period for the face and scalp. Imiquimod also may treat early or in situ lesions of SCC and BCC in the field.

Photodynamic treatment is another selective treatment for individual lesions or field treatment. Application of 20% 5-aminolevulinic acid (ALA [Levulan Kerastick]) or 16% methyl-aminolevulate (MAL [Metvix]) to affected areas is followed by activation by a light source. Treatment can be completed by the practitioner in 1 day. Before application, scale should be removed with acetone, chemical peel, or microdermabrasion. Alternatively, the patient can apply 5-fluorouracil cream or solution for 5 days or any topical retinoid (tretinoin [Retin-A],[1] adapalene [Differin],[1] or tazarotene [Tazorac][1]) for 1 month. ALA is available as a stick or swablike applicator, and application is challenging on larger areas. After ALA application, absorption or incubation is required. 1 to 2 hours for the face and lips, 3 to 4 hours for the chest and upper extremities, and 5 to 24 hours for the lower extremities. MAL is available as a cream and requires occlusion for 3 hours. To achieve the best response, two treatments should be given at 1-week intervals. The light source for activation of ALA is blue light (412–422 nm) and for activation of MAL is red light (570–670 nm). To treat discrete lesions with ALA or MAL, laser (585 or 595 nm) or intense pulsed light (560–1200 nm) may be used. Like 5-fluorouracil and imiquimod, photodynamic therapy may treat early or in situ lesions of BCC or SCC in the field.

Topical (tretinoin, adapalene, or tazarotene) and oral (acitretin [Soriatane][1]) retinoids can decrease development of actinic keratoses and nonmelanoma skin cancer in at-risk individuals. Efficacy is relatively mild, but any topical retinoid can be used each night indefinitely as tolerated by the patient. Acne and early signs of aging improve with this regimen. Oral retinoids can be used daily or every other day at the lowest dose (acitretin 10 mg) producing clinical improvement. The dose should be titrated up (to 50 mg maximum) as needed and as tolerated. Benefits are conferred only with maintenance of retinoid therapy.

---

[1]Not FDA approved for this indication.

---

[1]Not FDA approved for this indication.

Arsenical Keratoses

Clinical Manifestations

The small, punctate, hyperkeratotic lesions of arsenical keratoses are seen on the palms and soles of patients exposed to arsenic through contaminated well water and various medications. Carcinoma may develop after 10 to 20 years and evolve from precancerous keratoses or on any skin surface.

Treatment

Although acute toxicity can be treated with chelation, it has little value in chronic exposure. As for actinic keratoses, treatment of arsenical keratoses includes cryotherapy, topical chemotherapy, photodynamic therapy, and retinoids.[1] Discrete lesions can be treated with surgery or curettage.

Porokeratoses

Clinical Manifestations

The classic porokeratosis has a smooth, atrophic center surrounded by a grooved ridge of hyperkeratosis called a *cornoid lamella*. The plaque form (i.e., Mibelli's porokeratosis) is large and progressive, often appearing early in life. The disseminated superficial type favors sun-exposed sites and manifests as numerous, small, annular papules. The linear type may be generalized or segmental and often manifests very early in life. Only the punctate keratotic papules seen in *porokeratosis palmaris, plantaris et disseminate* have no clinically evident cornoid lamellae. Malignant transformation occurs mostly commonly in the linear type, followed by the Mibelli type. It is rare in the disseminated type and has not been reported in the punctate type.

Treatment

Treatment modalities include those described for actinic keratoses and surgical excision may be beneficial.

Human Papillomavirus Disease

Clinical Manifestations

The clinical manifestations of precancerous HPV infection on cutaneous and mucosal surfaces are diverse. The initial appearance and clinical behavior of verrucous carcinoma (i.e., Buschke-Lowenstein tumor on the genitals and oral florid papillomatosis) is as plantar, genital, and mucosal HPV disease; verrucous hyperkeratotic papules and plaques on the plantar surface; fleshy or hyperkeratotic papules in the anogenital region; and white, adherent keratotic plaques or leukoplakia of the mucosal surfaces. The clinically benign appearance and behavior change may signal malignant degeneration. Lower-risk types HPV-6 and -11 or high-risk HPV-16 may be implicated.

HPV-8, -16, -31, and -33 may be the causative agents in premalignant anogenital squamous intraepithelial lesions. The preferred terms *vulvar intraepithelial lesions/neoplasia* (VIL/N), *anal intraepithelial lesions/neoplasia* (AIL/N), and *penile intraepithelial lesions/neoplasia* (PIL/N) have replaced the confusing terminology Bowen's disease, erythroplasia of Queyrat, and bowenoid papulosis for these anogenital lesions. Dermatologists reserve the term *bowenoid papulosis* for discrete, fleshy, red-brown papules with a better prognosis that are seen in younger patients. Clinical appearance includes verrucous keratotic plaques, erosions, bowenoid-papulosis–type lesions, erosions, and erythematous, well-demarcated plaques, which may be shiny on the glans penis.

Progressive verrucous leukoplakia may appear as benign leukoplakia early—hyperplastic, thin, white plaques of the mucosal surface. These slowly progress to verrucous exophytic masses, many of which degenerate to SCC. HPV-16 infection has been associated with this multifocal premalignant condition.

Epidermodysplasia verruciformis (EDV) is a rare, inherited condition that predisposes to infection with the less common viral types of HPV-5, -8, -9, -12, -14, -15, -17, -19, -25 through -36, and -38 and with the more common types of HPV-3 and -10. This leads to flat verrucous papules on the extremities, face, and neck, which may be numerous and may coalesce. Lesions similar to tinea versicolor may develop over the trunk. SCC develops in 30% to 60% of these patients, and HPV-5, -8, and -47 are identified in 90% of the lesions.

Treatment

Eradication of HPV infection is challenging and often requires months of treatment. Observation may be reasonable for certain lesions with clinically benign appearance and behavior, and spontaneous resolution may occur.

Lesions of nonmucosal sites, including the plantar feet, can be treated by freezing with liquid nitrogen for 10 to 30 seconds for two cycles. This may need to be repeated every 3 to 6 weeks until resolution. Another blistering agent, Cantharone (0.7% cantharidin [Canthacur][1,6]), can be applied under occlusion for 6 to 24 hours. The advantage is painless application, but individual responses are unpredictable. Hyperkeratotic lesions, such as those on the plantar surface, require more aggressive use of these modalities. Imiquimod (Aldara)[1] applied daily can be beneficial, but it may require 6 months of treatment. Constant use of occlusive tapes such as duct tape has demonstrated efficacy and may be combined with any treatments. Between liquid nitrogen treatments or as adjunctive therapy, use of keratolytics such as topical salicylic acid products (e.g., liquid [Compound W, Wart-Off, Dr. Scholl's, Duofilm], film [Salactic], plaster [Mediplast, Duofilm, Sal-Acid], compounded in ointment), topical retinoids, and topical urea 10% to 40% (Carmol, Gordon's), as well as mechanical paring, can reduce the size of the lesion. This approach is rarely effective as monotherapy. Oral cimetidine (Tagamet)[1] 30 to 40 mg/kg/day may be a helpful adjunctive therapy. In those demonstrating sensitivity, cure rates of 60% to 80% can be achieved with intralesional candidal (*Candida albicans* skin test antigen [Candin])[1] or mumps antigen (mumps skin test antigen)[1] injections. Surgical treatment, including excision, curettage, and ablative CO_2 laser, have relatively low efficacy and may result in painful scars.

For treatment of lesions in the anogenital region, liquid nitrogen may be used less aggressively. Imiquimod 5% cream (Aldara) applied twice daily for 3 days of the week for 10 to 16 weeks is about 50% effective. Imiquimod 3.75% cream (Zyclara) can be applied daily until total clearance up to 8 weeks with 28.3% efficacy. Adjunctive treatment with cimetidine (Tagamet)[1] has a role as described earlier. Physician-applied podophyllin 25% in a tincture of benzoin (Podocon-25) is placed for 4 to 8 hours each week for 6 weeks. Alternatively, purified podophyllotoxin 0.5% solution or gel (podofilox [Condylox]) is applied by the patient over 3 consecutive days for 4 to 6 weeks. Sinecatechins 15% ointment (Veregen and Polyphenon E) is a botanical drug product derived from green tea leaves. With application three times per week for up to 16 weeks, 53% to 58% of patients reported total clearance. Electrofulguration may be the most effective treatment, with a cure rate of 70% at 3 months. Surgical treatments, including excision, curettage, and ablative CO_2 laser, have relatively low efficacy and may result in painful scars.

Lesions of the oral mucosa are best treated with cryotherapy as for anogenital lesions, curettage, surgical excision, electrofulguration, and ablative CO_2 laser.

Treatment recommendations for lesions of EDV include those for lesions on nonmucosal surfaces as described earlier. Although there is no particular treatment for patients with EDV, prevention (i.e., UV protection and smoking cessation) is important, as it is for all patients.

Atypia in Melanocytic Nevi

Clinical Manifestations

Because almost one half of melanomas arise in benign, preexisting melanocytic nevi, these nevi can be considered premalignant

---

[1]Not FDA approved for this indication.

[1]Not FDA approved for this indication.
[6]May be compounded by pharmacists.

lesions. Nevi manifest as acquired pigmented macules and papules in the first 3 decades of life. Dysplastic nevi are clinically and histologically atypical and therefore likely represent a higher risk. They have a "fried egg" appearance, with a papular center on a macular base, and they are 5 to 12 mm in diameter, larger than common nevi. Their shape is often irregular with indistinct borders and variegated tan, brown, and pink coloration.

The incidence of melanoma arising in a giant congenital melanocytic nevus (CMN) is 2% to 15%. Other associated sarcomas are rare. Giant CMN are pigmented plaques larger than 20 cm in diameter in adults. They often cover most of an extremity, the trunk, the scalp, or even the entire dorsal surface in the neonate. They grow with the individual but do not spread. Often, satellites or smaller nevi are seen beyond the border of the primary lesion.

Treatment

Pigmented lesions should be monitored for changes such as development of asymmetry, irregular borders, change or variegation in color, and growth, especially greater than 6 mm. Ulceration, bleeding, pain, or pruritus can signal malignant degeneration. On a given individual, identification of the pigmented lesion clinically dissimilar to the others is known as the ugly duckling sign. Changes in a giant CMN or a satellite such as nodularity are worrisome. In these cases, biopsy or very close monitoring, including use of clinical photographs called mole mapping, is essential. For giant CMNs, in theory, decreasing the number of nevus cells should decrease the risk of malignant degeneration, and partial or serial excision using tissue expanders, curettage, and ablative laser treatment may be beneficial.

References

Bolognia JL, Jorizzo J, Schaffer JV, editors. Dermatology. New York: Elsevier; 2012.
James WD, Berger TG, Elston DM, editors. Andrews' Diseases of the Skin—Clinical Dermatology. 11th ed. Philadelphia: WB Saunders; 2011.
Morton CA, McKenna KE, Rhodes LE, et al. Guidelines for topical photodynamic therapy: Update. Br J Dermatol 2008;159:1245–66.
Robinson JK, Hanke CW, Sengelman RD, Siegel DM, editors. Surgery of the Skin—Procedural Dermatology. New York: Elsevier; 2010.
Wood GS, Gunkel J, Stewart D, et al. Nonmelanoma skin cancers. In: Abeloff MD, Armitage JO, Niederhuber JE, Kastan MB, editors. Abeloff's Clinical Oncology, 4th ed. Philadelphia, Churchill Livingstone; 2008.

PRESSURE ULCERS

Method of
David R. Thomas, MD

CURRENT DIAGNOSIS

- Differentiate among pressure, diabetic, venous stasis, and arterial ulcers.

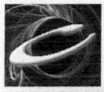

CURRENT THERAPY

Seven Principles of Pressure Ulcer Therapy
- Relieve pressure.
- Assess pain.
- Assess nutrition and hydration.
- Remove necrotic debris.
- Maintain a moist wound environment.
- Encourage granulation and epithelial tissue formation.
- Control infection.

A pressure ulcer is the visible evidence of pathologic changes in blood supply to the dermal and underlying tissues, usually because of compression of the tissue over a bony prominence.

A differential diagnosis of ulcer type is critical to treatment. Chronic ulcers of the skin include arterial ulcers, venous stasis ulcers, diabetic ulcers, and pressure ulcers. Pressure ulcers generally appear in soft tissue over a bony prominence. A classic presentation aids the diagnosis. For example, arterial ulcers occur in the distal digits or over a bony prominence, diabetic ulcers occur in regions of callus formation, and venous stasis ulcers occur on the lateral aspect of the lower leg. However, atypical presentations may occasionally obscure the etiology. The treatment of these various etiologies differs considerably. This discussion is limited to the treatment of pressure ulcers and should not be used to treat other types of ulcers.

Seven principles of management guide treatment of pressure ulcers. The chief cause of these ulcers is pressure applied to the tissues that compromises blood flow. Therefore, the first treatment principle is to relieve pressure. Pressure relief can be obtained by positioning the patient frequently at a fixed interval to relieve pressure over the compromised area. Turning and positioning may be difficult to achieve because of a patient's self-positioning or medical treatments that interfere with the ability to position the patient. Because of this difficulty, a number of medical devices are designed in an attempt to relieve pressure. These devices can be classified as static or dynamic. Static devices include air-, gel-, or water-filled containers that reduce the tissue–surface interface. Dynamic devices use a power source to inflate compartments that support the patient's weight or alternate the pressure on different areas of the body. Choose a static device when the patient has good bed mobility. Choose a dynamic device when the patient cannot self-position in bed.

At the present time, results of reported clinical trials do not favor one device over another. The choice should be based on durability, ease of use, and patient comfort. A simple check for so-called bottoming out should be done for all devices. Your hand should be inserted palm upward under the patient's sacrum between the device and the bed surface. If there is not an air column between the patient and the bed surface, the device is ineffective and should be changed. No device is effective in reducing heel pressure, the second most common site for pressure ulcers. Bridging with pillows is effective in reducing heel pressure in immobile patients; patients with high bed mobility may require boot devices to elevate the heel off the bed surface. Patients who fail to improve or who have multiple pressure ulcers should be considered for a dynamic-type device, such as a low-air-loss bed or air-fluidized bed.

Studies in turning and positioning suggest an optimum interval of 4 hours while on a pressure reducing device. More frequent turning schedules, including the often-suggested 2-hour interval, have not been demonstrated to prevent pressure ulcers. Recent prevention studies after hip fracture have failed to demonstrate effectiveness of turning or pressure reduction on ulcer incidence.

The second principle of pressure ulcer therapy is to assess pain. Pressure ulcers do not always result in pain, particularly in insensate patients. However, some pressure ulcers do result in pain and should be treated aggressively. Oral or parenteral pain medications should be used to control symptoms.

The third principle of ulcer therapy is to assess nutrition and hydration. Pressure ulcers occur in sicker individuals in whom nutrient intake may be reduced by coexisting illness. Increased intake of protein (1.2 to 1.5 g/kg/day) is associated with higher healing rates. Achievement of high protein intake may be difficult because of anorexia of aging or anorexia associated with coexisting diseases. Adequate calories, adjusted for stress (30 to 3 kcal/kg/day), should be prescribed. Adequate dietary intake should provide adequate vitamins and minerals. No difference in healing rates is associated with supertherapeutic doses of vitamin C or zinc. If adequate dietary intake is compromised, a supplemental vitamin/mineral prescription at RDA (recommended daily allowance) doses should be considered. Adequate hydration can be maintained by 30 mL/kg/day of water. The decision to institute enteral feeding in patients with pressure ulcers who are unable to maintain adequate oral intake should not be undertaken lightly. The decision to use enteral feeding must consider the patient's wishes, overall goal of care, and the complications of enteral feeding. Recent studies surprisingly observed that the use of percutaneous gastroscopy feedings increased the incidence of pressure ulcers and was associated with poorer healing, perhaps because of adverse patient selection.

The fourth principle of pressure ulcer management requires removing necrotic debris. Phagocytosis removes necrotic debris naturally. Accelerating the rate of removal may shorten healing time. Options include sharp surgical débridement, mechanical débridement with gauze dressings, application of exogenous enzymes, or autolytic débridement under occlusive dressings. Choose surgical débridement if the ulcer is infected. Surgical débridement is the fastest method but may remove some viable tissue, may cause discomfort, and is the most expensive method, especially if done in an operating room. Applying moist gauze that is allowed to adhere to the ulcer bed by drying is a form of débridement. When the dry dressing is removed, nonselective tissue removal occurs. This method can be associated with discomfort, may delay healing while débridement is in progress, and is often defeated when the dressing is remoistened before removal. Enzymatic débridement can digest necrotic material. Only one enzymatic preparation is currently available in the United States: collagenase. Enzyme preparations are nonselective, possibly resulting in some damage to fibroblasts, epithelial cells, or granulation tissue. Enzymatic débridement is slower, can be associated with discomfort, and should be limited in duration until a clean wound bed is obtained. Autolytic débridement is achieved by allowing autolysis under an occlusive dressing. Both enzymatic and autolytic débridement may require 2 to 6 weeks to achieve a clean wound bed. A total of five clinical trials did not show that enzymatic agents increased the rate of complete healing in chronic wounds compared to control treatment. Unless clinically infected, heel ulcers are better left undébrided because they occur in poorly vascularized tissues.

The fifth principle of pressure ulcer management is to maintain a moist wound environment. Maintaining a moist wound environment is associated with more rapid healing rates compared to dressings that are allowed to dry. Continuously moist saline gauze is the historical standard dressing for stage II through IV pressure ulcers. Care must be taken to change the gauze frequently to prevent drying because this may delay healing. Newer wound dressings provide a low moisture vapor transmission rate (MVTR), a measure of how quickly the dressing allows drying. A MVTR of less than 35 g of water vapor per square meter per hour is required to maintain a moist wound environment. Woven gauze has a MVTR of 68 g/m^2/hour, and impregnated gauze has a MVTR of 57 g/m^2/hour. By comparison, hydrocolloid dressings have a MVTR of 8 g/m^2/hour. Dressings with low MVTR provide a healing environment that encourages granulation tissue formation and epithelialization.

The use of occlusive-type dressings is more cost effective than gauze dressings primarily because of a decrease in nursing time for dressing changes. A meta-analysis of five clinical trials comparing a hydrocolloid dressing with a dry dressing demonstrated that treatment with a hydrocolloid dressing resulted in a statistically significant improvement in the rate of pressure ulcer healing (odds ratio: 2:6).

Occlusive dressings can be divided into broad categories of polymer films, polymer foams, hydrogels, hydrocolloids, alginates, and biomembranes. Each has advantages and disadvantages. No single agent is perfect. The choice of a particular agent depends on the clinical circumstances. Nonpermeable polymers can be macerating to normal skin. Polymer films are not absorptive and may leak, particularly when the wound is highly exudative. Most films have an adhesive backing that may remove epithelial cells when the dressing is changed. Hydrogels are hydrophilic polymers that are insoluble in water but absorb aqueous solutions and are available in amorphous gels or sheet dressings. They are poor bacterial barriers and are nonadherent to the wound. Because of their high specific heat, these dressings are cooling to the skin, aiding in pain control and reducing inflammation. Most of these dressings require a secondary dressing to secure them to the wound. Hydrocolloid dressings are complex dressings similar to ostomy barrier products. They are impermeable to moisture and bacteria and highly adherent to the skin. Hydrocolloid dressings have an accelerated healing of 40% compared to moist gauze dressings. Hydrocolloid dressings are particularly suited for areas subject to urinary and fecal incontinence. Their adhesiveness to surrounding skin is higher than some surgical tapes, but they are nonadherent to wound tissue and do not damage epithelial tissue in the wound. The adhesive barrier is frequently overcome in highly exudative wounds. Hydrocolloid dressings should be used cautiously over tendons or on wounds with eschar formation. Alginates are complex polysaccharide dressings that are highly absorbent in exudative wounds. This high absorbency is particularly suited to exudative wounds. Alginates are nonadherent to the wound, but if the wound is allowed to dry, damage to the epithelial tissue may occur with removal. Alginates may be used under other dressings to absorb exudate. The biomembranes are very expensive and not readily available.

Stages I and II pressure ulcers can be managed with a polymer film or hydrocolloid dressing. Stages III and IV pressure ulcers may be treated with a film or hydrocolloid dressing. In addition, some stage III and IV wounds with dead space or tunneling may require a wound filler, such as a calcium alginate or an amorphous hydrogel, to obliterate dead space and decrease potential for anaerobic colonization.

Vacuum-assisted closure is used in both acute and chronic wounds. Only two randomized, controlled trials in pressure ulcers are reported. In both trials, vacuum-assisted closure was not superior (despite a higher cost) to treatment with a hydrogel or moistened gauze.

Electrotherapy is used for stages III and IV pressure ulcers unresponsive to conventional therapy. Several clinical trials suggest that electrotherapy is likely to be marginally effective. Hyperbaric oxygen, ultrasound, infrared, ultraviolet, and low-energy laser irradiation have insufficient data to recommend their use currently. No data support the use of a systemic vasodilator, hemorheologics, serotonin inhibitors, or fibrolytic agents in the treatment of pressure ulcers. Topical agents such as zinc, phenytoin,[1] aluminum hydroxide,[1] sugar, yeast, aloe vera gel, or gold[1] were not effective in clinical trials.

Because the theory of augmenting ulcer healing under the newer dressings suggests that wound fluid contains favorable healing factors, it is important not to change the dressings too frequently. Unless the wound fluid seeps from under the dressing, it should not be changed more often than every 3 to 7 days.

The sixth principle of pressure ulcer treatment is to encourage granulation tissue formation and promote reepithelialization. Growth factors show promising early results, but the data do not suggest accelerated healing of pressure ulcers. It is important not to affect granulation and epithelial tissue negatively. A number of wound cleaners and antiseptics are toxic to fibroblasts and epithelial tissues, including benzalkonium chloride, povidone-iodine solution (Betadine), Dakin's solution, hydrogen peroxide, Granulex, Hibiclens, and pHisoHex. The use of these agents in a pressure ulcer should be limited to use in infected ulcers and strictly limited in duration.

The seventh principle of pressure ulcer management is to control infection. Quantitative microbiology alone is a poor predictor of clinical infection in chronic wounds. All pressure ulcers are colonized with bacteria, usually from skin or fecal flora. The presence of microorganisms alone (colonization) does not indicate an infection in pressure ulcers. The diagnosis of infection in chronic wounds must be based on clinical signs. Consensus panels on diagnosis of infection in pressure ulcers suggest that advancing cellulitis is the most reliable sign. Edema, odor, and purulent exudate are much more nonspecific. In the presence of clinical signs of

---

[1]Not FDA approved for this indication.

infection, enteral or parenteral antibiotics should be used. In ulcers that are not progressing toward healing, an empirical trial of topical antimicrobials may be considered, although the data are inconclusive.

References

Thomas DR. The role of nutrition in prevention and healing of pressure ulcers. Geriatr Clin North Am 1997;13:497–512.

Thomas DR. Are all pressure ulcers avoidable? J Am Med Dir Assoc 2001;2:297–301.

Thomas DR. Improving the outcome of pressure ulcers with nutritional intervention: A review of the evidence. Nutrition 2001;17:121–5.

Thomas DR. Issues and dilemmas in managing pressure ulcers. J Gerontol Med Sci 2001;56:M238–340.

Thomas DR. Prevention and management of pressure ulcers. Rev Clin Gerontol 2001;11:115–30.

Thomas DR. The promise of topical nerve growth factors in the healing of pressure ulcers. Ann Intern Med 2003;139:694–5.

Thomas DR. Management of pressure ulcers. J Am Med Dir Assoc 2006;7:46–59.

Thomas DR. Managing pressure ulcers: Learning to give up cherished dogma. J Am Med Dir Assoc 2007;8:347–8.

Thomas DR. Prevention and management of pressure ulcers. Clin Rev Gerontol 2008;17:1–17.

Thomas DR. Does pressure cause pressure ulcers? An inquiry into the etiology of pressure ulcers. J Am Med Dir Assoc 2010;11:397–405.

Thomas DR. Clinical management of pressure ulcers. Clin Geriatr Med 2013;29:397–413.

PRURITUS ANI AND VULVAE

Method of
Muhammad A. Ghazi, MD

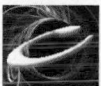

CURRENT DIAGNOSIS

- Anogenital pruritis is primarily idiopathic; most secondary etiologies can be divided into dermatologic, anogenital conditions, and systemic causes.
- Good history and physical examination are important for accurate diagnosis.
- Laboratory tests and procedures to diagnose the cause of pruritis ani and vulvae should be tailored to individual patients based on their presentation.

CURRENT THERAPY

- Initial treatment is usually conservative, and clinicians should focus on reassurance, education about hygienic practices, regular bowel movements, avoidance of moisture and irritants, and a trial of topical corticosteroids.
- Anogenital conditions such as hemorrhoids, fissures, skin tags, and fistulas—if present—must be treated first.
- Pruritus vulvae secondary to lichen planus, lichen sclerosus, and lichen simplex chronicus usually require superpotent topical steroid treatment.
- Refractory cases of pruritus ani may benefit from injectable treatments of methylene blue.[1]
- Suspicious lesions of vulva and perineum that are resistant to initial treatment must be biopsied to rule out malignancy.

[1]Not FDA approved for this indication.

Pruritus ani and vulvae is not a disease per se; rather, it is a symptom or manifestation of an underlying disease or the result of poor personal hygienic practices. Pruritus is derived from the Latin *prurire*, which means "to itch." Pruritis ani is literally an unpleasant sensation leading to scratching the skin around the anal opening. Anogenital pruritus is a commonly ignored skin condition. Symptoms range from mild to severe and can be complicated by sleep disturbances, anxiety, depression, and social embarrassment. Pruritus ani and vulvae can be primary, in which case there is no identifiable cause, or be secondary to an underlying condition. Most of the secondary causes are anorectal, including hemorrhoids, fistulas, and fissures. Psoriasis, lichen sclerosus, and lichen simplex chronicus are common secondary dermatological causes of pruritus in the vulvar region.

Epidemiology

Pruritus ani is a common condition with an estimated prevalence of 1% to 5% of the population. It affects all ages and both genders. Male to female prevalence of pruritus ani is about 4:1. Symptoms are worse at night and in warm, moist climates. Pruritus vulvae is seen in women of all ages. Young females usually present with an infectious etiology while the primary disease is more common in postmenopausal women. Genital pruritus in men is rare and usually presents with balanitis.

Risk Factors

Poor personal hygiene, chronic diarrhea, obesity, high-risk sexual behaviors, and immunodeficiency states predispose a person to pruritus in the anogenital area. Heat, sweating, and tight undergarments may exacerbate the condition. A proposed list of causative factors is included in Boxes 1 and 2.

Pathophysiology

The itching sensations of pruritus ani and vulvae are mediated by unmyelinated C fibers, which are distributed densely in the perineal region at the dermal-epidermical junction of the skin. Irritants

Box 1	Common Causes of Pruritus Ani
Acute	**Chronic**
Idiopathic up to 25% of cases	Dermatoses:
Fecal contamination:	Allergic or contact dermatitis,
Poor hygiene	psoriasis, lichen planus,
Fecal incontinence	lichen simplex chronicus,
Anal sphincter dysfunction	lichen sclerosis, Hailey-
Anorectal pathology: 10% to	Hailey disease
50% of cases	Inflammatory:
Hemorrhoids, perianal	Inflammatory bowel disease
fissures, pilonidal sinus,	(ulcerative colitis and
perianal abscess, rectal	Crohn's disease)
prolapse, polyps, and	Malignant:
papilloma	Anal squamous cell cancer
Mechanical factors:	Extramammary Paget's
Excessive washing, rubbing,	disease
synthetic undergarments	Lymphoma/leukemia
Infectious:	Metabolic:
Erythrasma (corynebacterium	Diabetes mellitus, chronic
infection), Candida,	liver disease and chronic
dermatophytosis, herpes	kidney disease, celiac
simplex, human papilloma	disease, iron deficiency
virus, HIV, syphilis	anemia, hypovitaminosis
Parasitic:	A, B, D, E
Scabies, pinworm	Miscellaneous:
Dermatoses:	Hyperhidrosis
Allergic or contact dermatitis,	Neuropathic pruritus
psoriasis, drug eruptions	Psychogenic (anxiety related)
Dietary factors:	
Tomatoes, chilis, coffee, beer,	
soda, dairy, chocolate, tea,	
citrus fruits	

| Box 2 | Common Causes of Pruritus Vulvae in Women |

PREPUBERTAL AGE
Poor hygiene
Sensitization of vulvar skin: soaps, deodorants
Contact dermatitis
Parasitic infestations: Pinworms (*Enterobius vermicularis*), pediculosis, scabies
Bacterial infections (Group A beta hemolytic infections and *Escherichia coli*)
Vaginal candidiasis (rare in this age group)
Lichen sclerosis
Suspected child sexual abuse (based on evidence of genital trauma)

REPRODUCTIVE AGE
Vaginitis
Trichomonas
Bacterial vaginosis
Candidiasis
Rarely tinea cruris
Herpes simplex type II
HIV, syphilis
Dermatitis
Atopic dermatitis
Contact dermatitis
Psoriasis
Lichen planus
Lichen simplex chronicus
Lichen sclerosis
Seborrheic dermatitis
Pregnancy
  Vulvar itching is worsened because of vulvar engorgement; pregnancy also predisposes women to vaginal discharge and candidiasis
Systemic diseases:
Diabetes, renal and liver diseases
Miscellaneous
Vulvar intraepithelial neoplasia (HPV)
Mechanical trauma
Idiopathic

POSTMENOPAUSAL AGE
Urinary or fecal incontinence
Menopause: Lack of estrogen leads to loss of skin elasticity and makes it prone to itching
Atrophic vaginitis
Lichen sclerosis
Paget's disease of vulva
Vaginal malignancy (squamous cell cancer)
*May include the causes in reproductive age group

in stool (exotoxins, intestinal lysosymes, endopeptidase, trypsins) and increased alkalinity of certain foods such as tomatoes, chocolate, and caffeine contribute to the perianal itching that precedes scratching. The itch-scratch cycle is mediated by several mechanical and inflammatory mediators, including histamine, kallikrein, bradykinin, trypsin, serotonin, and neuropeptides. The resulting nerve impulse is carried via spinothalamic tract to the thalamus, where the itching sensation is perceived. Intestinal transit time and altered anal sphincter pressure are influenced by certain foods that predispose people to perianal seepage and pruritus.

Pruritus vulvae is the result of increased permeability of the dermis resulting from a structurally thin strateum corneum as compared to the rest of the vulvar skin. Factors aggravating the pruritus include constant friction, rubbing, anatomic location, occlusion, moistness, fear of uncleanliness in women, and excessive washing. The most common cause of pruritus vulvae is vulvar dermatitis or eczema, which affects one-third to half of all women presenting with this complaint. Dermatitis or eczema can be endogenous and the result of familial disposition, and it manifests as atopic dermatitis. Exogenous dermatitis such as contact dermatitis can be allergic, given that a trigger (allergen) might induce an immune response or contact irritant dermatitis. Common irritants include soaps, shampoos, vaginal creams, alcohol, tea tree oil,[2] douches, vaginal hygiene products, vaginal contraceptives, sanitary pads, nylon underwear, and toilet paper. Chemical allergens contributing to contact dermatitis in the genital area include benzocaine, neomycin, ethylenediamide, propylene glycol, latex dyes, nickels, semen, lanolin, perfumes, and tampons.

Clinical Manifestations
Perianal and vulvar itching, erythema, excoriations, fissures, hemorrhoids, pinworms, and fecal incontinence may be noticed on inspection of the perineal area. In the acute phase, skin redness of varying degrees is visible. Excoriations from the skin from itching may be present. Fissures in the labial folds may be present. Superinfection with yeast or bacteria may complicate the presentation.

Chronic anogenital dermatitis usually presents as erythema of varying degrees, and papillae appear in the labial folds. Hypo-

[2]Not available in the United States.

or hyperpigmentation of the skin or thickening of the labial skin might develop over time, causing "lichenification," which leads to lichen simplex chronicus.

Diagnosis of Pruritus Ani and Vulvae
A detailed history of bowel habits and personal hygiene (including products used, such as perfumes); dietary habits (e.g., caffeine consumption); and previous medical, psychiatric, and surgical history help elucidate the cause of pruritus ani. The patient should be asked about personal or family history of hives, asthma, conjunctivitis, or atopy when allergic dermatitis is suspected. Other relevant questions of history include recent use of antibiotics, clothing preferences, family history of cancers, other family members with similar symptoms (pinworms and scabies), rectal bleeding, change in bowel habits, or sexual preference (anal receptive intercourse). For pruritus vulvae, the patient should be asked about any history of itching, burning sensation, vaginal discharge, postcoital bleeding, or dysperunia.

Physical Examination
Inspection with a bright light and a chaperone is recommended. Palpation includes a digital rectal exam and a female pelvic examination in case of pruritus vulvae. Wet preparation of vaginal secretions for Candida, bacterial vaginosis, potassium hydroxide testing, and cultures for *Neisseria gonorrhoeae* and chlamydia are recommended. Microscopic examination of scrapings will help to differentiate the parasitic and fungal infections.

Laboratory Tests
Laboratory tests should not be done routinely in all cases and should be tailored to the patient's history and physical examination. Below is a list of laboratory tests that should be considered when diagnosing possible causes of anogenital pruritus:
1. CBC (complete blood count) helps to differentiate between parasitic and infectious cases and diagnoses anemia (a possible cause of chronic pruritus ani)
2. Chemistry profile (to identify systemic causes such as hepatic and kidney diseases)

3. Urinalysis to screen for infection and systemic diseases such as diabetes
4. DNA polymerase chain reaction probe for gonorrhea and chlamydia
5. Cellophane tape test to look for pinworms
6. Stool for ova and parasites
7. Test for diabetes mellitus and HIV if suspected
8. Anal Pap smear for HPV is indicated if there is a history of anal receptive intercourse

Procedures

Anoscopy and proctoscopy are indicated to diagnose hemorrhoids and perianal fistulae. Colposcopic examination of the perineum may provide a detailed view of local pathology.

Colonoscopy is indicated for patients over 40 with a family history of colon cancers. Patch testing should be performed to diagnose allergic contact dermatitis. A skin biopsy is indicated in case of ulcerated skin lesions, refractory cases, and suspicious lesions to rule out malignancy. A 3 to 6 mm punch biopsy is recommended.

Differential Diagnosis

A broad range of clinical problems can be enumerated in the differential diagnosis, including (but not limited to) allergic skin reactions, infections, parasitic infestations, chronic liver disease, diabetes, and neoplasms; chronic conditions such as psoriasis or dermatitis; infections such as condylomata accuminata; and skin cancers such as Bowen's disease, squamous cell cancer, Paget's disease, or melanoma.

Prevention and Treatment

General Principles of Treatment

The goal of treatment should be the resolution of symptoms, restoration of skin anatomy, and prevention of recurrence. The most important step in the management of pruritus ani and vulvae is reassurance and patient education (Figure 1). An informed and educated patient tends to deal with symptom-related anxiety better. To identify and treat the cause, it should be understood that pruritus ani and vulvae are commonly idiopathic, and conservative measures are usually sufficient to treat the condition. However, secondary causes need to be identified and treated.

Anorectal conditions such as hemorrhoids, fistulas, and fissures may require surgical treatment and consultation. Antidiarrheals should be used in cases of loose stool. A high-fiber diet should be started.

Women presenting with vulvar pruritus should be screened and treated for vaginal infection (e.g., one dose of oral fluconazole [Diflucan] 150 mg for vulvovaginal candidiasis; metronidazole [Flagyl] 500 mg oral twice daily for 7 days for bacterial vaginosis). Dermatological conditions such as psoriasis and dermatitis are treated with topical steroids. Hormone replacement therapy can be used in cases of menopause. Topical estrogen creams are better alternatives for symptomatic relief.

Patients should be instructed to gently cleanse the perianal area twice daily and after each bowel movement. Sitz baths with plain warm water are recommended for perianal pruritus. The perianal area should be patted dry after washing. Patients with vulvar pruritus should avoid tight undergarments, jeans, and panty hose. The use of laundry detergents, bubble baths, feminine douches, or sprays containing protease should be discouraged. Women with a predisposition to vulvar dermatitis should wear loose pants. Panty liners should be avoided and replaced with tampons or cotton cloth. Vulvae should be washed gently; women should avoid vigorous rubbing or cleaning. Patients with vulvar pruritus should use a bland moisturizer as a soap substitute to avoid irritation resulting from chemicals. The vulva should be dried before wearing underwear, and excessive perspiration should be controlled with talcum powder. Patients should be encouraged to manage incontinence and maintain an ideal body weight. Cornstarch should be avoided, as it can lead to bacterial colonization and exacerbation of symptoms.

Dietary modifications (for anal pruritus) are imperative, including limitations on the consumption of chocolate, tea, coffee, citrus fruits, and alcoholic beverages. Eating yogurt is recommended, especially while on antibiotics, to prevent diarrhea and worsening of perianal seepage.

Emollients such as aqueous creams or petrolatum or emulsifying ointments treat itching and dry skin, which can prevent erosion and ulcer formation. These agents can be used irrespective of the etiology of pruritus. Zinc oxide (Desitin) cream is used topically to prevent excoriations in cases of perianal and vulvar pruritus. Combination products such as zinc oxide/bacitracin (rash relief antibacterial), zinc oxide/menthol (Calmoseptine), and zinc oxide/miconazole (Vusion) are available and can be used for symptomatic relief. Topical anesthetics (lidocaine 5% [L-M-X5 Anorectal, Topicaine 5]) may be used twice a day to help with acute symptoms. Topical benzocaine (Vagisil Anti-Itch Creme) should be avoided, as it is a strong irritant and allergen. Cool compresses and gel packs can help. Ice should not be used, as it can cause frostbite.

Antihistamines should be used to improve sleep, and patients should wear cotton gloves at night to prevent itching while asleep. Nails should be cut short, and nail varnish should be avoided. Sedating antihistamines might help (e.g., hydroxyzine [Vistaril] 50 mg PO at bedtime; doxepin [Sinequan][1] 10 to 100 mg at bedtime; citalopram [Celexa][1] 20 to 40 mg during the daytime). Citalopram can also help with underlying anxiety symptoms, but caution is advised in the elderly and patients at risk of arrhythmias, because citalopram can cause QT interval prolongation. Any suspicious lesions of the vulvae and perineum should be biopsied to rule out underlying malignancy.

Pharmacologic Treatments

For mild pruritus ani, 1% to 2.5% hydrocortisone (Hydrocort) topical ointment is effective. Pramoxine (Prax, Senna Sensitive) can also be used alone or in combination with topical hydrocortisone cream (Analpram-HC, Pramosone). 1% Hydrocortisone/1% iodoquinol (Vytone) can be used as an antiinflammatory treatment for external use in the anal and vulvar area. Topical capsaicin cream 0.006%[3] has been used in cases of refractory itching and can be combined with topical hydrocortisone cream[3] to avoid hypersensitivity. This strength of capsaicin cream is not commercially available. Mild topical corticosteroid ointments are sufficient to treat the perianal pruritus, and superpotent steroids should be avoided, as the skin is thin and there is a risk of ulcer formation. Methylene blue[1] injections are reserved for long-standing, intractable pruritus ani. Methylene blue 0.5% to 1% 5 to 30 mL mixed with normal saline and local anesthetics is injected intradermally, subcutaneously, and intracutaneously in the perianal skin to produce hypoesthesia. This treatment may be repeated, and studies report a success rate of 80% to 90%.

For moderate vulvar disease, 0.1% triamcinolone (Kenalog) ointment is recommended. For severe cases and thickened skin, the superpotent steroid topical clobetasol (Temovate) or halobetasol (Ultravate) 0.05% ointments can be used. The use of these superpotent steroid creams should be limited and reserved for the resistant cases of pruritus vulvae, lichens simplex chronicus, lichen sclerosus, or resistant lichen planus. Vulvar lichen and lichen planus should be treated over the long term with superpotent steroids for adequate response and treatment. A very thin layer of steroid cream should be used, and patients should be educated about the side effects of the medication before starting the treatment. For vulvar lichen planus and lichen sclerosus, superpotent steroids are used topically once or twice daily for 2 to 3 months; three times a week for 1 month; then once or twice per week for the long term. For lichen simplex chronicus, treatment is twice daily for 2 weeks and then once daily for 2 weeks. It then moves to three times per week.

Topical calcineurin inhibitors 1% pimecrolimus cream (Elidel)[1] or 0.03% to 1% tacrolimus ointment (Protopic)[1] may be used for

---

[1]Not FDA approved for this indication.
[3]Exceeds dosage recommended by the manufacturer.

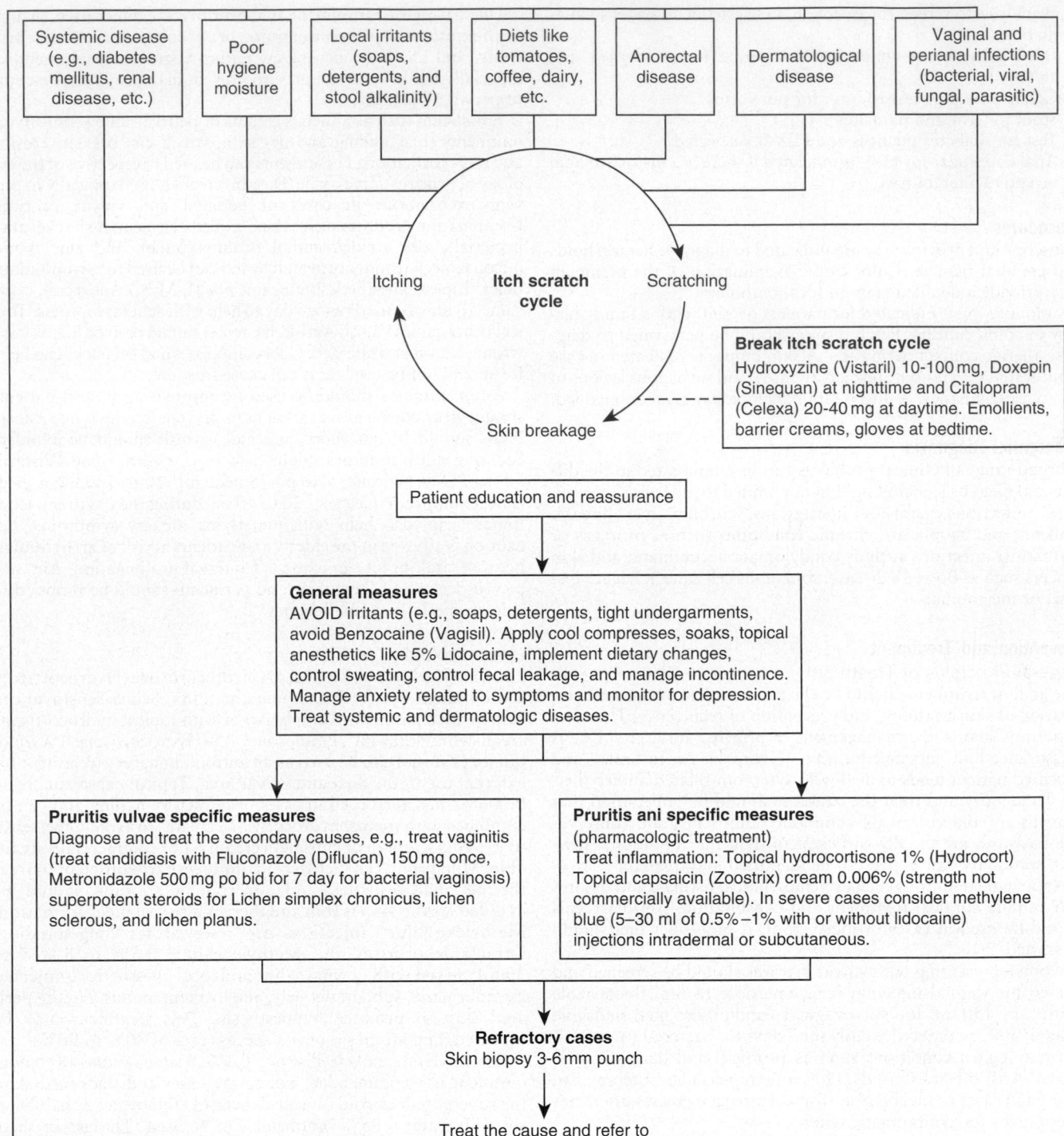

Figure 1. Pathogenesis and management of pruritus ani and vulvae.

refractory cases as steroid-sparing agents. A common side effect of these agents is a burning sensation, so their use is controversial in cases of lichen sclerosis and lichen planus.

In cases of neuropathic pruritus ani and vulvae, amitriptyline (Elavil)[1] 10 to 150 mg at bedtime is suggested. Other options are gabapentin (Neurontin)[1] 300 to 3600 mg three times a day[4]; pregabalin (Lyrica)[1] 75 to 400 mg/day; and mirtazapine (Remeron)[1] 7.5 to 15 mg at bedtime. In resistant and rare cases in which none of the above mentioned treatments is effective, radiation treatment may be indicated to destroy nerve endings. Several experimental treatments, such as laser phototherapy, alcohol injection therapy, radiation, and surgery, have not been studied and are not recommended routinely.

Complications

Pruritus ani and vulvae can lead to myriad complications, including lichenification, skin excoriations, ulcers, secondary bacterial infections, and abscess formation.

Referral

For undiagnosed and resistant skin conditions, patients should be referred to a dermatologist. Persistent anal itching, a change in bowel habits, and rectal bleeding should prompt a referral to a gastroenterologist and colorectal specialist. Pruritus vulvae with

[1]Not FDA approved for this indication.
[4]Not yet approved for use in the United States.

vaginal bleeding and weight loss are indications for referral to a gynecologist.

Monitoring and Prognosis

Most cases of pruritus ani and vulvae are treated with general measures that lead to a full recovery. Long-term use of corticosteroids should be discouraged, and periodic monitoring for side effects, including skin erosions and bleeding, is advisable based on reported symptoms. The idiopathic disease usually persists and depicts a relapsing remitting course.

References

Al-Ghnaniem R, Short A, Pullen A. 1% Hydrocortisone ointment is an effective treatment of pruritus ani: A pilot randomized controlled crossover trial. Int J Colorectal Dis 2007;22:1463–7.

Family Practice Notebook. Pruritus vulvae, Available at: http://www.fpnotebook.com/gyn/vulva/vlvrprts.htm; 2013 (accessed December 14, 2013).

Jones DJ. ABC of colorectal disease. Pruritus ani. BMJ 1992;1305:575–7.

Margesson LJ. Overview of treatment of vulvovaginal disease. Skin Therapy Lett 2011;16:5–7.

Margesson L, Danby WF. Pruritus ani and vulvae. In: Conn's Current Therapy 2013: Expert Consult. Philadelphia: Elsevier; 2012. p. 276–8.

Markell KW, Billingham RP. Pruritus ani: Etiology and management. Surg Clin North Am 2010;90:125–35.

Mentes BB. Intradermal methylene blue injection for the treatment of intractable idiopathic pruritus ani: Results of 30 cases. Tech Coloproctol 2004;8:11–4.

Reidy T, Rafferty JF. Management of pruritus ani. In: Current Surgical Therapy. Philadelphia: Elsevier Mosby; 2011. p. 243–6.

Siddiqi S, Vijay V, Ward M, et al. Pruritus ani. Ann R Coll Surg Engl 2008;90:457–63.

Stermer E, Sukhotnic I, Shoul R. Pruritus ani: An approach to an itching condition. J Pediatr Gastroenterol Nutr 2009;48:513–6.

Weichert GE. An approach to the treatment of anogenital pruritus. Dermatol Ther 2004;17:129–33.

PSYCHOCUTANEOUS MEDICINE

Method of
Ladan Mostaghimi, MD

Psychocutaneous medicine explores the interactions between mind and skin. The spectrum of patients ranges from those who are delusional and refuse to see a psychiatrist to those who are depressed because of chronic disfiguring skin problems. The relationship between chronic skin diseases and psychological factors has been known for many years. In the first reference to psychocutaneous medicine from 1200 BC, the physician to the Prince of Persia speculated that his patient's skin disease (possibly psoriasis based on the description) was related to his anxiety about succeeding his father. Research in psychoneuroimmunology has better defined the relationship between skin and mind. This chapter discusses common psychodermatologic disorders and their treatment.

Classification

The five general categories encountered in psychocutaneous medicine are as follows:

- Psychophysiological disorders: Emotional factors can exacerbate a skin disorder, such as psoriasis.
- Primary psychiatric disorders: Patients have no primary skin disorder, and the cutaneous signs are self-induced such as delusions of parasitosis. This category includes primary psychiatric disorders such as delusions of dysmorphosis, a variant of body dysmorphic disorder, and pathological skin grooming behaviors (i.e., trichotillomania, onychotillomania [Figures 1 and 2], pathological skin picking (Figure 3), and nail biting).
- Secondary psychiatric disorders: A chronic, disfiguring skin disorder causes psychological problems.
- Cutaneous sensory disorders: Patients have purely sensory complaints, such as pruritus, burning, stinging, and biting, without visible primary skin disease or an underlying medical condition.
- Use of psychotropic medications for dermatologic conditions such as urticaria or postherpetic neuralgia.

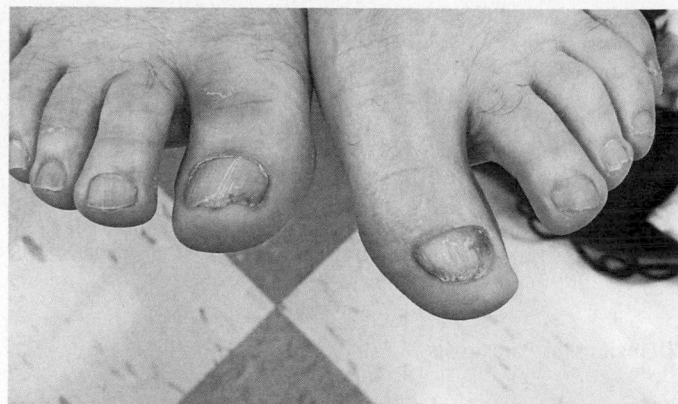

Figure 1. Onychotillomania of toenails.

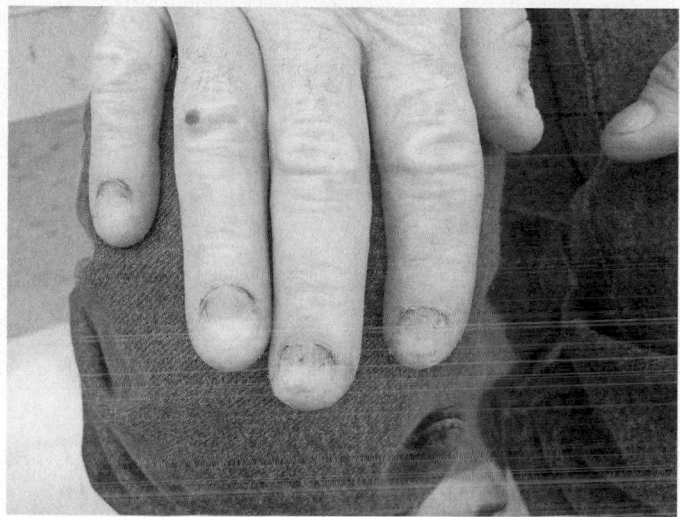

Figure 2. Onychotillomania of fingernails.

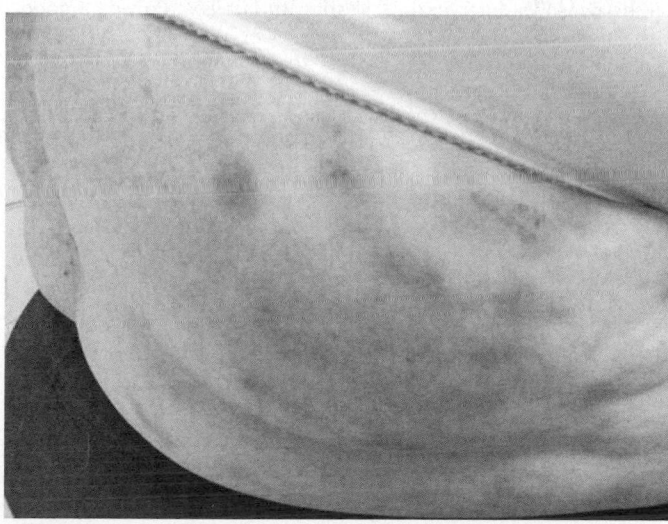

Figure 3. Bruising of skin due to severe scratching in atopic dermatitis.

Another, more practical classification of psychocutaneous conditions is based on the underlying psychopathology such as depression, anxiety, obsessive-compulsive disorder (OCD), delusional disorders, body dysmorphic disorder, and impulse control disorders. Standardized self-rating questionnaires are available for different conditions. These questionnaires can be administered and rated by office staff before the visit with the physician. This classification system can also help with treatment choices and follow-up plans.

An important area of psychocutaneous medicine's contribution to dermatology is assessing quality of life of patients with and without treatments. Research in this area guides clinicians on their treatment choices and risks/cost benefits of medications.

Finally, for psychocutaneous research to be successful, the use of needs assessment surveys is important. The first sample of these surveys was published in the *International Journal of Dermatology* in 2009.

Delusions of Parasitosis

CURRENT DIAGNOSIS

- The patient has false fixed beliefs about being infested.
- Look for the matchbox sign: samples of excoriated pieces of skin, scabs, clothing lint, or other debris are kept in bags, in plastic wrap, on adhesive tape, or in matchboxes by the patient and brought to the physician for examination to detect suspected parasites.
- Determine the type of delusional disorder: primary or secondary such as mood disorder with delusional features.
- For secondary delusions determine the possible causes and contributing factors, such as substance abuse, organic brain pathology, pernicious anemia, hypothyroidism or hyperthyroidism, and systemic lupus erythematosus (SLE).
- Determine the extent of damage to the skin and history of skin infections.

CURRENT THERAPY

- In secondary delusional disorders, treatment of the main disorder will help to clear the delusions.
- Psychosocial intervention. Work with families. Provide a good support system.
- Evaluate and monitor safety for the patient, family members, and health care providers.
- Some patients may try to get rid of parasites by burning their belongings or their body, or by using toxic substances, damaging their skin and causing serious toxicity.
- Treatment may include psychoeducation and cognitive-behavioral therapy (CBT).
- Neuroleptics/antipsychotic medications:
  - Pimozide (Orap)[1] is a first-generation antipsychotic frequently used by dermatologists.
  - There are case reports of second-generation antipsychotics working well in these situations.
- The treatment needs to be customized based on each patient's profile and medication side effects.

[1]Not FDA approved for this indication.

Delusions of parasitosis falls under the *Diagnostic and Statistical Manual of Mental Disorders, Fifth Edition* (DSM-5) category of *delusional disorder somatic type*.

These patients have false fixed beliefs that they are infested by parasites. To meet the diagnostic criteria the problem should last at least a month and should not be part of schizophrenia manifestations. Apart from the impact of the delusions, the patient's functioning is not markedly impaired and behavior is not always odd or bizarre.

Besides delusions about infestation patients may have delusions of having foreign material in their skin (e.g., strings coming out of skin, materials getting crystalized under skin). Tactile and olfactory hallucinations, if present, are related to the main delusional theme.

Other delusional disorders for which a patient would seek dermatology advice are delusion of bromhidrosis (i.e., patients are convinced they have a foul odor that no one else can perceive) and the delusion of dysmorphosis (i.e., patients are convinced that they have a defect in their appearance that no one else can appreciate). The delusion of dysmorphosis is part of body dysmorphic disorder—delusional variant and it is differentiated in DSM-5 from other somatic delusions because it responds to the same treatments as the nondelusional variant of body dysmorphic disorder.

Another group of patients with delusions of parasitosis are patients with psychotic mood disorders such as depression or bipolar disorder and false fixed somatic beliefs. If the patient has mood symptoms in addition to delusional symptoms, treatment of the mood problem may correct the delusional beliefs. For about 12% of patients, the delusion of parasitosis is shared by a family member or significant other. This condition is called folie à deux (i.e., madness of two) or folie partagé (i.e., shared delusions).

The *Diagnostic and Statistical Manual of Mental Disorders, Fifth Edition,* published in May 2013, recommends eliminating the requirement that the delusion must be nonbizarre. APA also decided to change the "shared delusions." Instead if the criteria is met for delusional disorder that diagnosis is used. If shared beliefs are present but the criteria is not met then the term "other specified schizophrenia spectrum and other psychotic disorder" is used.

The patient with delusions of parasitosis usually has multiple superficial excoriations or deep wounds due to manipulating the skin to try to remove the parasites. Physicians should be alert to the matchbox sign. In the matchbox sign, many samples of excoriated pieces of skin, scabs, clothing lint, or other debris are kept in bags, in plastic wrap, on adhesive tape, or in matchboxes by the patient and brought to physician's office for examination to detect suspected parasites. The patient can become very agitated when the physician denies the presence of any infestation after physical examination or assessment of the samples collected and brought in.

The physician should rule out substance abuse disorders. Some substances, especially amphetamines, cocaine, and phencyclidine (PCP), can cause formication and organic delusional syndrome in some patients. Organic reasons such as temporal lobe epilepsy or other brain pathology, neurosyphilis, pernicious anemia, hypothyroidism or hyperthyroidism, and SLE should be investigated, especially in older patients and if any neurologic symptoms are identified during the physical examination.

Treatment consists of antipsychotic or neuroleptic medications. For patients with psychotic mood disorder, treatment of the mood disorder usually improves the delusional symptoms. Depending on the amount of distress that the delusions are causing, treatment may start with combination of a neuroleptic medication and an antidepressant, with subsequent tapering off the neuroleptic and continuation of the antidepressant alone. Second-generation neuroleptics have problems with weight gain and metabolic syndrome and require regular monitoring during treatment (Table 1). To facilitate acceptance of the treatment, it is important for the physician to have a good rapport with patients and address their concerns; at the same time, the physician must not accept or feed into the patient's delusions by giving the impression that the delusion is believed to be real. Statements such as the following may encourage patients to accept treatment: "I'll be very honest with you; what you are telling me is very unusual. In most cases of infectious diseases, the doctors are able to easily identify the culprit. In your case, we have not found anything. Although we will keep looking to find the culprit, if any, I know it is difficult to live with this condition and we have medications that can help alleviate the symptoms you are experiencing."

If the patient refuses psychotropic medications, he or she should be monitored for safety. If, at any point, the safety of the patient, family, or physician is threatened due to dangerous behaviors related to delusional beliefs, local mental health providers should

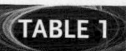

TABLE 1 Recommended Monitoring for Patients on Atypical Antipsychotics According to the American Diabetic Association Consensus Statement on Diabetes Care 2004

	BASELINE	4 WEEKS	8 WEEKS	12 WEEKS	QUARTERLY	ANNUALLY	EVERY 5 YEARS
Personal/family history	+					+	
Weight (body mass index [BMI])	+	+	+	+	+		
Waist circumference	+					+	
Blood pressure	+			+		+	
Fasting plasma glucose	+			+		+	
Fasting lipid profile	+			+			+

Modified with permission from the American Diabetes Association: Diabetic Care 2004;27:596–601. Copyright 2004 American Diabetes Association.

be consulted regarding institution of a court order for involuntary commitment for treatment.

Pimozide (Orap)[1] is a first-generation antipsychotic that dermatologists have traditionally used for delusions of parasitosis. However, most antipsychotic medications can help this condition. Physicians should be familiar with the first- and second-generation antipsychotics (Tables 2 and 3) and their side effect profile and select the treatment that is best tailored to each patient. Notice the FDA warning on increased risk of stroke with the use of neuroleptics in elderly patients with Alzheimer's disease.

A detailed, step-by-step approach to treating patients with delusions of parasitosis is discussed in *Cutis* (see References).

In recent years the Internet has been helpful in contributing to medical education and multiple other aspects of the physician's

life. At the same time, the Internet has served as a medium to attract patients who feel their concerns are not validated by the medical community. Doctors are confronted with patients visiting their office with a self-diagnosis of diseases that do not exist in the medical literature.

One example of these "Internet-borne diseases" is "Morgellons disease" or, as the Centers for Disease Control and Prevention (CDC) named it, "unexplained dermopathy." In 2001 a former medical research laboratory technician believed that a nonhealing wound on her 2-year-old son's lip was due to an unknown parasite, called the disease "Morgellons," and started a foundation and website under that name. Very soon multiple patients self-identified with the symptoms, which included different-color fibers coming out of one's skin. The campaign spread rapidly. Both the Internet and mainstream media were involved in publicity for the new disease. The advocacy led to

[1]Not FDA approved for this indication.

TABLE 2 Medications Used in Psychocutaneous Disorders

CLASS	NAME	DOSAGE RANGE	SIDE EFFECTS TO MONITOR
First-generation neuroleptics	Pimozide (Orap)[1]	1 mg daily in divided doses, gradually increase up to 0.2 mg/kg/day or maximum dose of 10 mg/day. Perform CYP2D6 genotyping when the daily dose in adults is >4 mg	Multiple drug-drug interactions due to metabolism through CYP 450 1A2 and CYP 3A4; prolonged QT interval; torsades de pointes; GI, hematologic, hepatic, neurologic (tardive dyskinesia, neuroleptic malignant syndrome, extrapyramidal symptoms, akathesia); drug-induced SLE and priapism
	Haloperidol[1]	0.5–3 mg two to three times daily	Neurologic side effects, QT prolongation, drug-drug interactions
Second-generation neuroleptics	Olanzapine (Zyprexa)[1]	2.5–max 20 mg/d	Common side effects of second-generation neuroleptics include QT prolongation; neurologic side effects (extrapyramidal symptoms, tardive dyskinesia, neuroleptic malignant syndrome); risk of neurologic side effects is less with second-generation neuroleptics (least for quetiapine), but still exists; metabolic syndrome (needs regular monitoring; see Table 1); drug-drug interactions; blood dyscrasias (periodically assess and consider D/C if ANC <1000 or if unexplained decrease of WBC count)
	Risperidone (Risperdal)[1]	1–4 mg/d max 8 mg/d. Age >65 keep max daily dose at 4 mg/d. Doses above max recommended are rarely more effective and have more side effects	
	Aripiprazole (Abilify)[1]	2–max 30 mg/d	
	Quetiapine (Seroquel)[1]	25–max 800 mg/d in divided doses	
	Ziprasidone (Geodon)[1]	20–80 mg bid	
Antidepressants/ antianxiety SSRIs	Sertraline (Zoloft)[1]	50–200 mg/d	Each SSRI has its own side-effect profile (e.g., fluoxetine may prolong QT interval; citalopram has dose depending QT interval prolongation with FDA warning on recommended dosage; fluvoxamine may cause Stevens-Johnson syndrome). Overall watch for sweating, GI symptoms, sexual side effects, myalgia, sleep problems, tremor, dizziness, bleeding tendencies, hyponatremia (rare), seizure (rare), manic episode, suicidal ideation and suicide (rare); watch for drug-drug interactions
	Citalopram (Celexa)[1]	20–40 mg/d. Do not exceed 20 mg for adults over age 60 or poor CYP2C19 metabolizers.	
	Escitalopram (Lexapro)[1]	10–20 mg/d. 10 mg/d in geriatric patients	
	Fluoxetine (Prozac)[1]	20–60 mg/d	
	Paroxetine (Paxil)[1]	20–50 mg/d, max 40 mg/d if age >60	
	Fluvoxamine,[1] works best in OCD	50–300 mg/d in divided doses (bid)	

Continued

TABLE 2 Medications Used in Psychocutaneous Disorders—cont'd

CLASS	NAME	DOSAGE RANGE	SIDE EFFECTS TO MONITOR
Antidepressants/ antianxiety SNRIs Helpful in peripheral neuropathies	Venlafaxine,[1] extended-release form available (Effexor XR)	37.5–225 mg/d	Hypertension, sweating, GI symptoms, blurred vision, sexual side effects, hyponatremia, bleeding tendencies, neuroleptic malignant syndrome, serotonin syndrome, hepatitis (rare), drug-drug interactions
	Duloxetine (Cymbalta)[1] Also for treatment of fibromyalgia	30–60 mg/d, may increase to 120 mg/d but rarely more effective	Sweating, GI symptoms, sleep problems, bleeding tendencies, hepatotoxicity, fatigue, drug-drug interactions
Antidepressants/ antianxiety other	Trazodone,[1] helps insomnia and sometimes itching	50–400 mg/d	Sweating, weight change, GI symptoms, neurologic symptoms, blurred vision, hypertension, hypotension (rare), cardiac dysrhythmia (rare), priapism, seizure, drug-drug interactions
	Mirtazapine (Remeron),[1] helps insomnia and itching with higher affinity for histamine receptors than doxepin	15–45 mg/d	Increased appetite, hyperlipidemia, somnolence, neurologic disorders, agranulocytosis and neutropenia (rare), seizure, drug-drug interactions
	Bupropion (Wellbutrin),[1] sustained release and extended release forms available	100–450 mg/d divided doses	Hypertension, tachycardia, arrhythmia, pruritus, urticaria, GI symptoms, arthralgia, myalgia, neurologic symptoms, agitation, anger outbursts, menstrual problems, Stevens-Johnson syndrome, anaphylaxis, drug-drug interactions
	Buspirone (Buspar)[1] works for anxiety problems	5–60 mg/d in divided doses	Nausea, blurred vision, nervousness, angry behavior, neurologic symptom, congestive heart failure (rare), myocardial infarction (MI) (rare), cerebrovascular accident (CVA) (rare), drug-drug interactions
Tricyclic antidepressants for pruritus and hives	Doxepin[1] Topical 5% doxepin cream (Zonalon) has FDA approval for pruritus (for atopic dermatitis and lichen simplex chronicus)	25–300 mg/d single and divided doses for depression, 10–25 mg/d for pruritus Topical: every 3–4 h max for 8 days; do not use under occlusion	Weight gain, GI symptoms, neurologic symptoms, blurred vision, urinary retention, arrhythmia (rare), blood pressure changes, bleeding tendencies, hematologic changes, drug-drug interactions
Tricyclic antidepressant for trichotillomania	Clomipramine (Anafranil)[1]	25–250 mg/d	Weight gain or loss, GI symptoms, blurred vision, neurologic symptoms, urinary retention, MI, orthostatic hypotension, hematologic side effects, hepatotoxicity
Neuropathic pain treatments Tricyclic antidepressant	Amitriptyline[1]	10–150 mg/d	Weight gain, GI symptoms, neurologic symptoms, blurred vision, cardiac dysrhythmia, hematologic symptoms, hepatic symptoms, CVA, drug-drug interactions
Antiepileptic medications	Gabapentin (Neurontin) FDA approved for neuropathic pain and postherpetic neuralgia	100 mg at night gradually increase to up to 1800 mg daily in divided doses if needed	Myalgia, peripheral edema, neurologic symptoms, angry behavior, mood swings, problems with thinking, Stevens-Johnson syndrome, seizure, drug-drug interactions
	Pregabalin (Lyrica) Also treatment of fibromyalgia	50 mg tid with gradual increase up to 600 mg/d in divided doses	Peripheral edema, weight gain, GI symptoms, ataxia, somnolence, blurred vision, euphoria, problems with thinking, angioedema
	Carbamazepine (Tegretol)[1]	50–1200 mg/d in divided doses for blood levels of 4–12 mcg/mL	Hyponatremia, severe blood dyscrasias (rare but needs regular CBC monitoring), toxicity over therapeutic ranges, atrioventricular block, cardiac dysrhythmia, congestive heart failure, syncope, hypertension or hypotension, GI symptoms, hepatitis, SLE, skin rash, Stevens-Johnson syndrome, toxic epidermal necrolysis (TEN), psoriasis, acne, angioedema, nephrotoxicity, drug-drug interactions
	Lamotrigine (Lamictal)[1] helps impulsive behavior and neuropathic pain	25–200 mg/d in divided doses; do not increase >50 mg/every two weeks	Headaches, sleep problems, diplopia, ataxia, GI symptoms, rhinitis, photosensitivity, rash, Stevens-Johnson syndrome, TEN, angioedema, hypersensitivity reactions, neutropenia, DIC, hematologic problems, hepatic failure, pancreatitis, rhabdomyolysis, teratogenicity, drug-drug interactions

TABLE 2 Medications Used in Psychocutaneous Disorders—cont'd

CLASS	NAME	DOSAGE RANGE	SIDE EFFECTS TO MONITOR
Miscellaneous treatments for intractable pruritus	Thalidomide (Thalomid)[1] (also used in Behcet's syndrome)	50–200 mg/d	Severe birth defects in pregnancy, edema, skin rash, GI symptoms, leukopenia, thrombotic disorder, peripheral neuropathy, Stevens-Johnson syndrome, TEN, seizure, pulmonary embolism, hypocalcemia, tremor, somnolence, drug-drug interactions
	Naltrexone (ReVia)[1] Vivitrol (IM Naltrexone)[1]	50 mg/d 380 mg/mo IM usually used for alcohol dependence and not in dermatology	GI symptoms, headaches, anxiety, hepatic damage, opioid withdrawal (rare), drug-drug interactions
	Cyclosporine (Sandimmune)[1] Monitor drug level	4–5 mg/kg/d	Hirsutism, pruritus in some patients, GI symptoms, neurologic symptoms (headaches, tremor, seizures, progressive multifocal encephalopathy [rare], coma [rare]), hepatotoxicity, nephrotoxicity, infections, hyperkalemia, hypomagnesemia, hypertension, anaphylaxis, lymphoproliferative disorder, drug-drug interactions
Benzodiazepines (sometimes used for burning mouth syndrome)	Clonazepam (Klonopin)[1]	0.25 mg at night with gradual increase. Usual dosage for neuralgia is 2–4 mg/d	Sialorrhea, ataxia, dizziness, somnolence, impaired cognition, aggravation of seizure, depression, behavioral problems, respiratory depression

[1]Not FDA approved for psychocutaneous disorders.

Abbreviations: ANC = absolute neutrophil count; bid = twice a day; CBC = complete blood count; D/C = discontinuation; DIC = disseminated intravascular coagulopathy; GI = gastrointestinal; IM = intramuscular; SLE = systemic lupus erythematosus; WBC = white blood cell.

TABLE 3 New Medications with Potential Use in Psychocutaneous Medicine but no FDA Approval for Any of the Psychocutaneous Ailments

CLASS	NAME	DOSAGE RANGE	SIDE EFFECTS TO MONITOR
Antidepressants /antianxiety Other	Vilazodone hydrochloride (Viibryd)[1] Serotonin reuptake inhibitor (SRI) plus 5-HT1A partial agonist; like buspirone	10 mg/day × 7 d Then 20 mg/d × 7 d Then 40 mg/d Not tested in children	GI side effects: most frequent, diarrhea and nausea, occasionally vomiting; dry mouth; dizziness; insomnia; rare but serious: palpitation, ventricular premature beats, suicidal thoughts and serotonin syndrome.
	Desvenlafaxine (Pristiq)[1]; Serotonin norepinephrine reuptake inhibitor (SNRI)	50 mg/d Not to exceed 100 mg/d Needs to be tapered gradually at discontinuation by increasing the dosage interval Dose adjustment needed for renal impairment	Increased sweating in 10% to 20% of patients. May cause increase in triglycerides and cholesterol. Also watch for GI side effects, fatigue, blurred vision, proteinuria, anxiety. Rare but serious side effects including hypertension in 1%–2% and other cardiac effects to monitor, hyponatremia, GI hemorrhage, hypersensitivity reactions, seizure, mania, suicidal thoughts, withdrawal symptoms.
	Milnacipran (Savella)[1]; SNRI, pain reliever	Start 12.5 mg daily Maximum dose 100 mg bid daily Dose adjustment needed for renal impairment FDA application is for fibromyalgia	Increased blood pressure (2%–19.5%), tachycardia, palpitations, increased sweating (9%), hot sweats (12%), GI side effects, headache. Rare but serious: abnormal bleeding, serotonin syndrome, worsening of depression and suicidality, withdrawal symptoms. Need to have low-tyramine diet.
	Selegiline transdermal (Emsam)[1]; Monoamine oxidase inhibitor (MAOI)	6, 9, 12 mg patch/24 h May increase 3 mg/24 h every 2 weeks not to exceed 12 mg/24 h FDA label for major depressive disorder	Decreased systolic pressure, orthostatic hypotension, application site reaction (24%), weight loss, diarrhea, indigestion, headache, insomnia, dry mouth. Rare but serious: atrial fibrillation, hypertensive crisis (with tyramine-containing food), suicidal thoughts.

Continued

CLASS	NAME	DOSAGE RANGE	SIDE EFFECTS TO MONITOR
New second-generation neuroleptics	Paliperidone (Invega)[1] A major active metabolite of risperidone IM form: Invega Sustenna	Start with extended-release tablets 6 mg/d and gradually increase to maximum of 12 mg/d Adjust dose for renal impairment FDA approved for schizophrenia and schizoaffective disorder For injectable Sustenna form dosage range is 39–234 mg IM once a month after initial titration	Tachycardia (up to 16%), hyperprolactinemia (45%–49%), weight gain (2%–19%), GI side effects, akathesia, dyskinesia, dystonia, EPS and parkinsonism, somnolence, tremor, anxiety, nasopharyngitis (up to 5%). Rare but serious: Prolonged QT interval (7%), agranulocytosis, leukopenia, priapism, dysphagia, and TD.
	Asenapine (Saphris)[1]	Sublingual medication No titration is needed 5–10 mg bid FDA indications: bipolar I, acute mixed or manic episodes, and schizophrenia	Weight gain (3%–5%), oral hypoesthesia (5%), akathisia, dizziness, EPS, somnolence. Rare but serious: QT prolongation, hypersensitivity reactions, angioedema, neuroleptic malignant syndrome. TD is not listed but is always a possibility.
	Lurasidone (Latuda)[1]	Initial dose titration not required 40 to maximum of 160 mg/d take with food (350 calories), needs dose adjustment in renal and hepatic impairment	Nausea, akathisia, EPS, parkinsonism, somnolence. Rare but serious: orthostatic hypotension, syncope, agranulocytosis, CVA, seizure, TD, transient ischemic attack, suicidal thoughts, neuroleptic malignant syndrome.
	Iloperidone (Fanapt)[1]	1 mg bid on day 1 and titrate to maximum of 12 mg bid Do not use in patients with hepatic impairment FDA approval: schizophrenia	Weight gain (1%–18%), orthostatic hypotension (3%–5%), tachycardia, dizziness, somnolence, GI problems, nasal congestion, fatigue, hyperprolactinemia (26%). Rare but serious: prolonged QT interval, syncope (0.4%), hyperglycemia, CVA, transient ischemic attack, suicidal intent. TD is a risk in all neuroleptics. Risk differs per medication.
Miscellaneous For pathological grooming behaviors (trichotillomania, skin picking, nail biting)	N-acetylcysteine (NAC)[1]	1200–2400 mg/d	GI (nausea, indigestion), abdominal pain, headache, worsening of asthma. In long-term treatment needs to be taken with a multivitamin plus vitamin C.

[1]Not FDA approved for this indication.
Abbreviations: CVA=cerebrovascular accident; EPS=extrapyramidal symptoms; FDA=U.S. Food and Drug Administration; GI=gastrointestinal; IM=intramuscular; TD=tardive dyskinesia.

Congress requesting that the CDC investigate the cause of the disease. The CDC started the investigation but avoided calling the disease by its Internet name and named it "unexplained dermopathy." In January 2012, the CDC published the results of its investigation in the Public Library of Science online journal *PLOS ONE*, stating that "no common underlying medical condition or infectious source was identified, similar to more commonly recognized conditions such as delusional infestation." The prevalence reported in the CDC report was 3.65 per 100,000 enrollees.

Even after the CDC report, many patients continue to advocate for an infectious cause and argue against a noninfectious cause. Even though the Morgellons research foundation site has closed, many other sites are still active. Unfortunately these sites even have some physicians working with them, advising patients on how to talk to their physicians so they are not labeled as delusional and push for more testing. The online advice includes instructions on avoiding the matchbox sign at the first visit.

Our clinical approach is to do a complete physical examination and necessary laboratory testing. If we do not find a culprit and we believe the patient has somatic delusions, we give the patient the correct diagnosis and work closely with the patient and his or her family to treat the delusions. In the long run this will decrease individual and family suffering. It will also reduce unnecessary health care costs and doctor shopping.

Dermatitis Artefacta (Factitious Dermatitis), Neurotic Excoriation, and Acne Excoriée

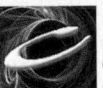

CURRENT DIAGNOSIS

- Determine the type of problem: patient need to assume sick role, or secondary gain, or impulsive skin picking (neurotic excoriation and acne excoriée).
- Assess the severity and degree of scarring, which may require intensive treatment.

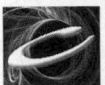

CURRENT THERAPY

- For dermatitis artefacta, the patient should be confronted in a nonjudgmental, empathetic way. Provide supportive dermatologic care for the skin and refer the patient for appropriate psychological interventions.

- For acne excoriée and neurotic excoriation, rule out underlying psychopathology and use a combination of therapy (CBT or behavioral therapy) and medications that help impulsive behavior such as selective serotonin reuptake inhibitors (SSRIs),[1] serotonin-norepinephrine reuptake inhibitors (SNRIs),[1] buspirone (Buspar),[1] anticonvulsants,[1] naltrexone (ReVia),[1] N-acetylcysteine (NAC),[1] and neuroleptics,[1] depending on the extent of the problem and scarring.
- There are no FDA-approved medications for this type of impulse control problem, and use of suggested medications should be based on the risk-benefit assessment for each patient.

[1]Not FDA approved for this indication.

Dermatitis Artefacta or Factitious Dermatitis

Dermatitis artefacta (i.e., factitious dermatitis) refers to intentional production of skin lesions to satisfy a psychological need. This could be achieved by different methods, such as excoriation, burning, or injection of toxic substances. Patients usually deny the self-induced nature of the problem. Clinically the lesions are located in reachable areas of the skin and can mimic any skin disease.

The DSM-5 has two subtypes of factitious disorder:
- Factitious disorder imposed on self
- Factitious disorder imposed on another (previously, Factious disorder by proxy)

DSM-5 proposes the grouping of the Factitious disorders with the Somatic symptom disorders to facilitate research on the broad spectrum of symptom reporting by patients, from feigning symptoms to experiencing symptoms with no clinical findings.

Factitious dermatitis usually occurs in patients with underlying psychopathology. After a diagnosis is made, the physician needs to discuss it with the patient in a nonjudgmental, empathetic way. Supportive dermatologic care should be provided for wounds, and the patient should be referred for psychological evaluation. Antidepressant and antianxiety medications can help to treat underlying depression and anxiety. Supplementary therapies include biofeedback, relaxation, acupuncture, hypnosis, CBT, behavioral therapy, and family therapy if the family members are involved in care.

Neurotic Excoriation and Acne Excoriée

Patients with acne excoriée create excoriations by repetitive scratching or skin picking. Women are affected more than men. Patients scratch and pick at their acne, an insect bite, dermatitis, or other bumps or rough spots of the skin (Figure 4). Any part of the skin that is not smooth or is pruritic (Figures 4 and 5) can be a target. However, patients may inflict excoriations without the

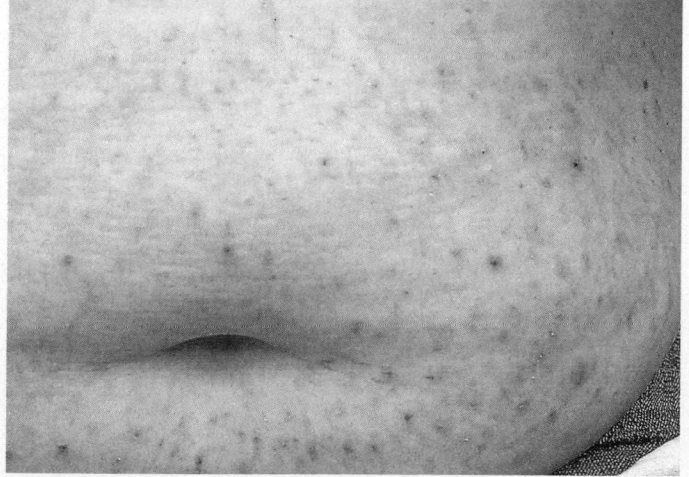

Figure 4. Skin picking at rough spots of skin.

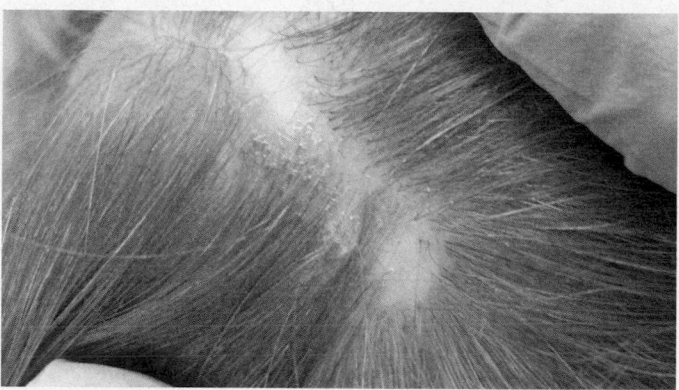

Figure 5. Scarring alopecia from chronic picking and new onset of lichen planopilaris around the scar on the scalp.

trigger of any skin pathology because the condition is a psychological process with dermatologic manifestations. Patients usually have ritualistic picking habits and report building of tension before picking and release of tension afterward.

Often patients with neurotic excoriations complain of pruritus. In this case a pruritus workup to rule out causes such as iron deficiency and gluten sensitivity is important.

The DSM-5 has recognized that pathologic skin picking is a prevalent and disabling condition. The DSM-5 (as opposed to the DSM-IV, where skin picking was classified under impulse control disorders NOS) has the skin picking classification under the chapter of "Obsessive-Compulsive and Related Disorders."

For any self-injurious behavior, patients must be screened for underlying psychopathologies such as personality disorders. However, in many patients, the behavior results from an impulse control problem.

In addition to the treatment of underlying psychopathology, treatment includes a combination of behavioral therapy and medications that help with impulsive behavior. The success of treatment depends on the patient's motivation to avoid scarring and to replace the self-injurious behavior with better behavior, including gentle skin care. Motivational interviewing could help patients explore and resolve their ambivalence and participate fully in treatment. Patients need to replace picking with other relaxing behaviors that are not harmful to skin, such as breathing relaxation, using a stress ball, Chinese exercise balls, Greek worry beads, stuffed animals, or Silly Putty. In finding appropriate replacement behavior, the physician should remember that tactile stimulation is important in these patients' anxiety relief.

Another therapy model for skin pickers is to consider chronic picking as an addiction and apply addiction therapy models to picking. Self-help groups and websites such as Pickers Anonymous (www.stoppickingonme.com) could help with treatment.

There is no FDA-approved medication for this condition. The use of different classes of medications is mostly based on case reports. The first step is to use an SSRI,[1] such as fluoxetine (Prozac),[1] sertraline (Zoloft),[1] paroxetine (Paxil),[1] or citalopram (Celexa),[1] or an SNRI, such as venlafaxine (EffexorXR)[1] or duloxetine (Cymbalta).[1] Dosage and side-effect profiles are provided in Table 2. If this is insufficient, the physician can add antianxiety medications, such as buspirone (Buspar),[1] and some of the newer anticonvulsant medications, such as lamotrigine (Lamictal).[1] In the case of severe picking, such as in patients with Prader-Willi syndrome, multiple infections and scarring can occur. Naltrexone (ReVia),[1] as well as the occasional use of neuroleptics such as aripiprazole (Abilify)[1] and quetiapine (Seroquel),[1] can help to break the cycle of scratching and give time for behavioral treatments to take effect. Once the patient has improved, medications can be tapered and discontinued, but he or she may need to stay on a maintenance dose of medications.

[1]Not FDA approved for this indication.

Prurigo Nodularis and Lichen Simplex Chronicus

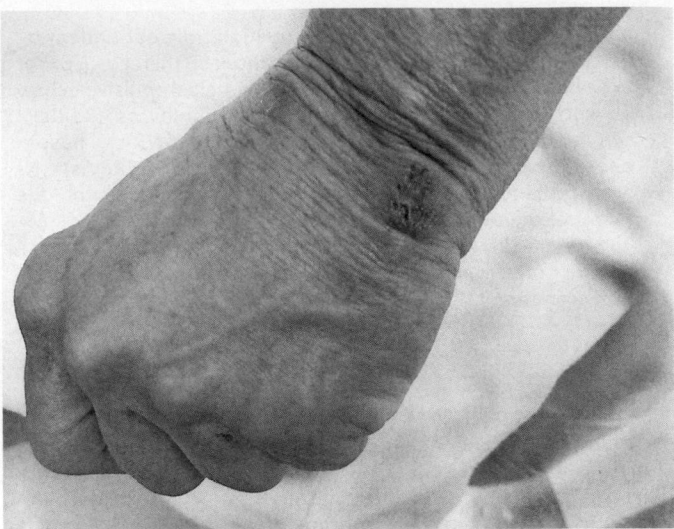

Figure 6. Prurigo nodularis.

CURRENT DIAGNOSIS

- Prurigo nodularis (Figure 6): hard nodules that are 1 to 5 cm in diameter with hyperpigmentation and warty or excoriated surface.
- Lichen simplex chronicus: lichenification (thickening) of the skin.
- Different histopathology for prurigo nodularis and lichen simplex chronicus.
- Drug history to rule out pruritus induced by medications or drugs of abuse.
- Complete blood cell count to rule out lymphoma and polycythemia rubra vera.
- Iron studies.
- Renal function tests (blood urea nitrogen [BUN], creatinine, and electrolytes) to rule out renal failure.
- Liver function tests to rule out chronic obstructive biliary disease.
- Serology for hepatitis.
- Test for diabetes mellitus.
- Thyroid and parathyroid hormone levels.
- Total serum immunoglobulin E (IgE) levels for atopy.
- Patch test if allergies are suspected.
- HIV test and purified protein derivative (PPD) (if indicated).
- Rapid plasma reagen (RPR) test.
- Skin biopsy and direct and indirect immunofluorescence assays to rule out immunobullous and autoimmune diseases.
- Stool check for parasites.
- Gastrointestinal and serum testing to rule out malabsorption and gluten sensitivity.
- Psychological evaluation.
- Chest x-ray and computed tomography (CT) scan if lymphoma is suspected.

CURRENT THERAPY

- Topical antipruritic creams such as topical doxepine (Zonalon), Sarna Anti-Itch, Eucerin Calming Cream.
- Topical steroids or intralesional steroid injection.
- Topical capsaicin (Zostrix).[1]
- Topical vitamin D₃ derivative (calcipotriene).[1]
- Cryosurgical treatment for a small number of prurigo nodularis lesions.
- For lichen simplex chronicus, some reports of efficacy of tacrolimus (Protopic).[1]
- Narrowband or broadband ultraviolet B (UVB) light is more effective than UVA.
- Psychosocial and therapy interventions to break the itch/scratch cycle.
- Psychotropic medications to help with itching and sleep: mirtazapine (Remeron),[1] doxepine,[1] or trazodone.[1]
- In resistant cases, other treatments such as naltrexone (ReVia),[1] cyclopsorine (Sandimmune),[1] thalidomide (Thalomid),[1] and lenalidomide (Revlimid).[1]

[1]Not FDA approved for this indication.

Clinically, prurigo nodularis (i.e., chronic circumscribed nodular lichenification, Picker's nodules) is a chronic, severe itch accompanied by 1 to 5 cm hard nodules with smooth or warty surfaces and a hyperpigmented periphery (Figure 6). The new lesions are usually red and inflamed, whereas the old lesions are pigmented. The lesions may also be excoriated. Lesions are mostly located on extensor surface of limbs, but they can also be located on the face, scalp, and trunk. Histopathology evaluation shows lichenification, a dense infiltrate in dermis and neural hyperplasia, and proliferation of Schwann cells.

A good history and physical examination should include a medications history because pruritus is a side effect of many classes of medications (e.g., diuretics, angiotensin-converting enzyme [ACE] inhibitors, beta blockers, antidepressants).

Laboratory testing (see Current Diagnosis box) is required before treatment. CT scans and chest radiographs are obtained if lymphoma is suspected.

Topical treatments with antipruritic creams are not very helpful. Potent topical steroids such as betamethasone dipropionate (Diprosone)[1] ointment under occlusion or intralesional injection of steroids such as triamcinolone acetonide (Kenalog-10)[1] may be successful, but they have the risk of skin atrophy. Topical capsaicin (0.025%–0.1% Zostrix),[1] a component of red pepper, can help in early stages. In some cases topical vitamin D₃ derivative (calcipotriene)[1] may help.

For diffuse and resistant forms of prurigo nodularis, broadband and narrowband UVB and UVA can be effective. Narrowband UVB is more effective and has fewer side effects than UVA.

Also for resistant forms, cyclosporine (Sandimmune)[1] 4 mg/kg/day can help. It should be continued for at least 6 months (see Table 2).

Thalidomide (Thalomid)[1] 200 to 400 mg in different studies has been an effective treatment for prurigo nodularis. Thalidomide is difficult to obtain because of its teratogenicity and it does have serious side effects such as irreversible peripheral neuropathies. A similar compound, lenalidomide (Revlimid)[1] 5 mg/day with less potential for peripheral neuropathy, was effective in one case of a patient resistant to all the other treatment (see References).

Naltrexone (ReVia),[1] an opioid antagonist, 50 mg/day is effective in some cases. It has a Food and Drug Administration (FDA) black box warning on hepatotoxicity.

Another treatment that has had some success was the synthetic retinoid, etretinate (Tegison),[2] but it was removed from the U.S. market because of the high risk of birth defects. Other synthetic retinoids such as acitretin (Soriatane)[1] may be considered in severe resistant cases. They all have serious teratogenicity risk.

Psychological intervention is important in breaking the itch/scratch cycle. Help can be obtained with techniques such as biofeedback, in which subjects learn how to consciously control their autoimmune responses; hypnosis; CBT; and supportive counseling.

[1]Not FDA approved for this indication.
[2]Not available in the United States.

Some psychotropic medications can help with excessive itching and compulsive scratching, including doxepine (10 mg at bedtime; can be increased up to 25 mg). The recommended dose for pruritus is lower than the dose for the treatment of depression, anxiety, or alcoholism (where it can be increased up to a maximum of 300 mg daily in divided doses), mirtazapine (Remeron) (15–45 mg at night), and trazodone (50–400 mg in divided doses). Doxepine is a tricyclic medication and because it has the potential to cause cardiac arrhythmias, it should not be used in patients with a recent myocardial infarction (MI). Patients need to have periodic cardiovascular evaluation if they use tricyclic medications long term. Antidepressants should not be used in patients with bipolar disorder without a mood stabilizer, due to the risk of triggering a manic episode. All antidepressants have an FDA black box warning for increased risk of suicidality in children, adolescents, and young adults under age 25. Patients need to be closely monitored.

Lichen Simplex Chronicus

Lichen simplex chronicus (i.e., circumscribed neurodermatitis) is characterized by lichenification of skin due to chronic excessive scratching or rubbing. Clinically, it appears as plaques of thickened skin with hyperpigmentation and accentuated skin lines. The most commonly affected areas are the occipital scalp, sides of the neck, ankles, genital areas, and extensor forearms. Itch is the main symptom. The histopathologic pattern in lichen simplex chronicus is different from that of prurigo nodularis and does not show the neural hyperplasia.

The physician must rule out the underlying diseases that may cause pruritus. The treatment for lichen simplex chronicus is similar to that for prurigo nodularis. In addition to other treatments, topical tacrolimus (Protopic) has shown efficacy in some cases of lichen simplex chronicus. Short-term topical 5% doxepin cream (Zonalon) can be used for lichen simplex chronicus (see Table 2).

Trichotillomania

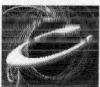

CURRENT DIAGNOSIS

- Hair loss is caused by repeated hair pulling, producing oddly shaped patches of alopecia with broken hair and no signs of inflammation.
- Other areas beside the scalp may be affected.
- The age of onset and underlying psychopathology should be determined.
- If patient denies hair pulling, rule out other causes of alopecia.

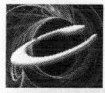

CURRENT THERAPY

- In children, trichotillomania is usually self-limited and parents should be reassured. Psychotherapeutic interventions are helpful.
- In adolescents and adults, first-line treatment is psychotherapy: CBT or behavioral therapy and habit reversal. Improving coping mechanisms with stress is helpful.
- Case reports and small double-blind studies have shown the efficacy of clomipramine (Anafranil)[1] and SSRIs.[1]
- Depending on the extent of the problem, augmentation with neuroleptics[1] can be considered, but because of the important side-effect profiles of these medications their risks and benefits should be carefully considered.
- Before using antidepressants, patients should be screened for a family history of bipolar disorder or personal history of previous manic episodes.

[1]Not FDA approved for this indication.

Trichotillomania is partial hair loss caused by repeated hair pulling. Clinically, the patient has patches of alopecia with broken hair. The broken hairs are of different lengths and there is no inflammation of the scalp. The affected area has an unusual shape. A hair pull test is negative. The hair pull test consists of grasping between 40 and 60 hairs between thumb and index finger and pulling them with moderate traction while moving fingers toward the distal shaft. If less than 10% of the hair is pulled off the test is negative. Trichotillomania can involve areas other than the scalp, and patients may pull hair in many sites. Trichotillomania can occur in any age group. In children it is usually benign and self-limited, but in adults it usually accompanies other psychopathologies and requires psychological intervention. Lifetime prevalence rate is about 0.5% to 3.5%, and the prevalence in some reports is as high as 4.4%.

Trichotillomania was classified with impulse control disorders in DSM-IV TR. If a patient denies hair pulling, other causes of alopecia, especially alopecia areata, need to be ruled out. In DSM-5, trichotillomania is classified with obsessive-compulsive and related disorders.

In children trichotillomania may occur during periods of increased stress, such as arrival of a new sibling, parent's divorce/separation, or stressful events at school. It is usually self-limited, and parents should be reassured. In preadolescents and young adults the diagnosis needs to be established first, followed by psychotherapeutic interventions; behavioral modification usually works well. Psychopharmacologic treatments should be reserved for last. Because of the FDA black box warning about the increased risk of suicide and suicidal behavior with use of antidepressants in children, adolescents, and young adults, these patients should be referred to a psychiatrist, if needed.

In adults, trichotillomania often accompanies other psychopathology and the treatment of the underlying illness helps to resolve the condition. Habit reversal therapy usually works better than negative feedback. Habit reversal therapy teaches the patient to monitor the behavior and the triggering factors and to replace the harmful habit with another habit. Working on increasing coping skills for stress is also helpful. Relaxation and other stress-relief techniques are helpful, especially in patients with underlying anxiety. The Trichotillomania Learning Center (www.trich.org) is a good source of information for patients.

Psychotropic medications can be used if psychotherapy alone is not enough. Most reports of effective medications are based on open-label studies. In a small, double-blind comparison, clomipramine (Anafranil)[1] 180 mg to 250 mg/day showed greater efficacy than desipramine (Norpramin).[1] There have been some open-label studies showing efficacy of fluoxetine (Prozac),[1] but these results were not reproduced in double-blind placebo-controlled trials. Other SSRIs, such as sertraline (Zoloft),[1] fluvoxamine (Luvox),[1] and paroxetine (Paxil),[1] have shown efficacy in case reports and open-label studies. In some augmentation trials adding haloperidol (Haldol),[1] pimozide (Orap),[1] or olanzapine (Zyprexa)[1] has been beneficial for patients taking fluoxetine or clomipramine. Small studies using haloperidol or lithium[1] have shown some efficacy. Because of important side effects such as tardive dyskinesia with haloperidol and the narrow therapeutic window with lithium, it is best to use these medications judiciously. Olanzepine has been tested as monotherapy in a double-blind study and was effective. Note that before antidepressants are prescribed for these patients, it is important to screen them for bipolar disorder.

In 2009 Grant et al evaluated N-acetylcysteine (NAC),[1] a glutamatergic agent that restores extracellular glutamate concentration in the nucleus accumbens and blocks compulsive behavior, 1200 to 2400 mg/day in a double-blind placebo-controlled trial for trichotillomania for a 12-week period. Fifty-six percent of patients were much or very much improved compared to 16% for placebo. Side effects were mild and short term, mostly affecting the gastrointestinal system (e.g., nausea, indigestion, abdominal pain) and causing headache. NAC may worsen asthma and should not be used in patients with asthma. If taken for an

[1]Not FDA approved for this indication.

extended period of time, the authors recommend taking supplemental zinc, copper, and other trace minerals, as well as two to three times the typical amount of vitamin C. It is recommended to take NAC with a multivitamin plus vitamin C. In a small case series, NAC has shown efficacy in pathological skin picking and nail biting as well.

Trichotillomania, skin picking, and nail biting can be considered as pathologic grooming behaviors. A review of available literature shows probable sufficient evidence from randomized controlled trials for the use of naltrexone (ReVia),[1] NAC, and olanzepine for trichotillomania; the SSRIs fluoxetine and citalopram for pathologic skin picking; and clomipramine for nail biting.

Cutaneous Sensory Disorders

CURRENT DIAGNOSIS

- Patients have a sensation of burning and itching in different areas of skin and mucous membranes, with no signs and symptoms of inflammation.

CURRENT THERAPY

- Rule out possible causes of abnormal sensations: infection, allergic reactions (e.g., dental fillings), vitamin and mineral deficiencies, iron deficiency or overload, diabetes, Sjögren's syndrome, nerve injuries, medications, and neoplasia.
- Treat the primary cause of the abnormal sensation if found.
- In cases of idiopathic abnormal sensations, some medications may help: tricyclic antidepressants,[1] gabapentin (Neurontin),[1] pregabalin (Lyrica),[1] SNRIs,[1] and SSRIs.[1]

[1]Not FDA approved for this indication.

Cutaneous sensory disorders are part of chronic pain syndromes, with pain occurring in different parts of the skin or mucous membranes. Disorders include burning mouth syndrome and vulvodynia (i.e., burning and itching of the vagina).

Burning mouth syndrome is a burning sensation that happens more frequently in middle-aged women. It affects the tongue more frequently, but other parts of the mouth may be affected. It can be associated with dry mouth and a metallic taste in the mouth.

The physician should rule out local problems (e.g., dental disorders, allergic reactions, infection) and systemic problems, such as vitamin B, folate, iron, and zinc deficiencies; diabetes; autoimmune problems such as Sjögren's syndrome; nerve injury; side effects of medications, including antivirals, antiretrovirals, antiepileptics, hormones, and ACE inhibitors; and medications causing dysgeusia, such as asenapine (Saphris) and eszopiclone (Lunesta).

The workup needs a thorough physical examination, medication history, and laboratory workup, as well as screening for depression and anxiety. Mood problems may result from chronic pain issues.

The primary cause needs to be treated. In idiopathic cases, therapy to help relaxation, coping skills training, and biofeedback may help. There is no FDA-approved medication for this condition, but medications used to treat neuropathies may help. These include gabapentin (Neurontin),[1] which can be started at 100 mg at night for 3 days and gradually increased to 100 mg three times a day. The dosage can be adjusted to 300 to 600 mg three times a day as tolerated up to a maximum of 1800 mg. Tricyclics such as amitriptyline[1] (10–25 mg orally at bedtime, may be increased every week to a maximum dosage of 150 mg/day) can be given. SNRIs such as venlafaxine extended-release form (Effexor XR)[1] can be given as 37.5 mg in the morning with a gradual weekly increase to the maximum of 225 mg daily, and duloxetine (Cymbalta)[1] can be given as 30 mg

[1]Not FDA approved for this indication.

daily and increased to 60 mg in 1 week dosages over 60 mg per day are rarely more effective. Clonazepam (Klonopin)[1] [2] 2 to 4 mg at night may help in some cases. Up to two thirds of patients report spontaneous partial recovery within 6 to 7 years of onset.

Vulvodynia is burning and pain in the vulvar area. Infectious, neoplastic, and inflammatory causes need to be ruled out. Depression and the impact on quality of life should be evaluated. Biofeedback and gabapentin[1] or amitriptyline[1] have been helpful in some cases.

Depression and anxiety lower the pain threshold, and their treatment can help patients with chronic pain syndromes to better cope with their pain and have a higher pain threshold.

Medications for Pain and Itching

Some of the psychotropic medications can be used for various dermatologic conditions, such as urticaria or postherpetic neuralgia. The older tricyclic medications have specific effects on pain or itching.

When itching is the main symptom, doxepin[1] has a much higher affinity for histamine receptors than do conventional antihistamines. It has a long half-life, and taking it once at night can control the daytime itching. The effective antipruritic dosage is usually 10 to 25 mg at night, but it could be increased at weekly intervals as needed. Amitriptyline[1] works best for disorders with pain as their main symptoms, such as burning mouth syndrome or postherpetic neuralgia. The usual dosage is 10 to 25 mg orally at bedtime, but may increase every week to a maximum dosage of 150 mg/day. Because tricyclic medications can affect cardiac conduction, patients need to have stable cardiovascular status. Periodic testing is required during long-term treatment. These drugs should not be used with other medications that prolong the QT interval, such as cisapride (Propulsid).[2] They should not be prescribed during the immediate recovery period after an MI, and they should not be used at the same time as monoamine oxidase inhibitors. Patients need to be instructed to avoid driving due to the drowsiness side effect of tricyclics.

Other medications that could help with pain symptoms include the following:

- Gabapentin (Neurontin) is started at 100 mg at night, increased every 3 days to 300 mg at night, and then increased weekly to 900 to 1800 mg daily in three to four divided doses as tolerated.
- Pregabalin (Lyrica) is started with 50 mg taken orally three times daily and increased to 100 mg three times daily within 1 week based on efficacy and tolerability. If patients with postherpetic neuralgia do not experience sufficient pain relief in 2 to 4 weeks and are tolerating the medication well, the dosage can be increased to 300 mg twice daily or 200 mg three times daily (600 mg/day).
- SNRIs such as duloxetine (Cymbalta) 60 mg daily have FDA approval for diabetic neuropathy and fibromyalgia. Venlafaxine extended-release capsule (Effexor XR),[1] which has a mechanism of action similar to that of duloxetine, can be started at 37.5 mg in the morning, with a gradual weekly increase to a maximum of 225 mg daily, for pain symptoms, though it is not FDA approved for pain treatment.
- There are some reports that SSRIs can help pain symptoms.
- Recent research has focused attention on the interaction between the pain and itch neurobiologic pathways. The potential to block variant opioid receptors may lead to new therapies such as novel uses of butorphanol (Stadol),[1] a kappa agonist that comes in the form of nasal spray.
- The substance P/neurokinin 1 (NK1) antagonist aprepitant (Emend)[1] can potentially be used for the treatment of pain.
- Another potential treatment for pruritus, nalfurafine (Remitch),[5] is under testing. This is a novel derivative of the opioid receptor antagonist naltrexone. It is a selective kappa-opioid receptor agonist and has a potent antipruritic effect in different types of pruritus.

[1]Not FDA approved for this indication.
[2]Not available in the United States.
[5]Investigational drug in the United States.

- In our experience for resistant cases of postherpetic neuralgia applications of small amount of the following compound cream a couple of times a day on the painful area is helpful: Amitriptyline 2% and Ketamine 0.5% in Vanicream base.[1,6]

Body Dysmorphic Disorder in Dermatology

 CURRENT DIAGNOSIS

- Patients have excessive preoccupation with an imagined defect or a slight flaw in their appearance. The problem is not perceived by, or appears slight to, others.
- Patients have rituals and repetitive behaviors in response to the appearance concern.
- Preoccupation causes clinically significant impairment in functioning and is not better accounted for by another mental illness.

 CURRENT THERAPY

- Rule out other mental illnesses or causes (e.g., severe depression with bodily focus, delusional disorder, substance abuse).
- CBT and high-dose SSRIs[1] have been shown to be effective.
- Clomipramine (Anafranil)[1] is more effective than desipramine (Norpramin).[1]
- In severe cases, augmentation with an antipsychotic such as ziprasidone (Geodon)[1] has been effective in case series.

[1]Not FDA approved for this indication.

Body dysmorphic disorder (BDD) is an excessive preoccupation with an imagined defect or a slight flaw in appearance. It is a severe, underrecognized problem. Patients are unwilling to discuss the symptoms due to sense of shame. Concerns about physical appearance vary across cultures and affect the presentation of BDD. Patients most commonly focus on hair, skin, and nose, but they may focus on other areas of the body as well. These patients usually seek dermatology or plastic surgery help. There is a high rate of depression and suicidal ideation. More than 50% of patients experience suicidal ideation.

BDD usually starts early in the teenage years and rarely starts after age 55. Patients could be between ages 6 and 80 but they are mostly in their thirties. Prevalence in dermatology is about 9% to 12%. Correct diagnosis and treatment is important because dermatology or surgical interventions usually are not effective. Patients are often unhappy with the results, and this may lead to litigation and suicidal ideation. Retrospective studies have shown that even when patients are satisfied with the intervention results, they focus their attention on other parts of their body.

Feusner performed interesting neuroimaging studies with functional magnetic resonance imaging (fMRI) in patients with BDD compared to normal controls. Researchers studied subjects' processing of images using fMRI and showed that patients with BDD had an abnormal focus on details and tiny abnormalities and failed to process the images holistically. Studies also showed that compared to controls, patients with BDD had an activation of the amygdala, a structure that is involved in the processing of many emotions, including fear, while viewing faces. Patients usually demonstrate ritualistic grooming behavior, excessive mirror checking, and reassurance seeking. They try to camouflage the perceived defect. Some may have skin picking in an effort to get rid of a perceived imperfection. They may also compulsively tan to cover acne or pale skin.

Patients with acne and BDD usually have mild acne and often doctor shop in hopes of receiving aggressive treatments such as isotretinoin (Accutane). They also seek laser and other cosmetic treatments to treat the perceived acne scars.

Once the diagnosis is suspected use screening questionnaires, and a visual analogue scale should be used by both the patient and physician to rate the perceived defect. This could help clarify the diagnosis by showing the discrepancy between the two ratings. Treatment consists of a combination of pharmacotherapy and CBT.

Therapy should be tailored to BDD and is different from OCD or social anxiety. It is important to show sympathy for the patient's suffering, but do not try to reassure the patient that the perceived defect does not exist. This approach will only reinforce patients' reassurance-seeking behavior and will not change their perception.

SSRIs[1] are effective in treatment, but usually high doses for at least 12 to 14 weeks are necessary to have results. Clinical follow-up of ritualistic behaviors helps to assess the response to treatment. For resistant cases, augmentation with antipsychotics[1] may be helpful, but these medications do not have FDA approval for this indication.

[1]Not FDA approved for this indication.

References

Bjornsson AS, Didie ER, Phillips KA. Body dysmorphic disorder. Dialogues Clin Neurosci 2010;12:221–32.

Epcrates database. Available at http://www.epocrates.com; [accessed 04.11.2012].

Feusner JD, Townsend J, Bystritsky A, Bookheimer S. Visual information processing of faces in body dysmorphic disorder. Arch Gen Psychiatry 2007;64:1417.

Grant JE, Odlaug BL, Kim SW. Lamotrigine treatment of pathologic skin picking: an open-label study. J Clin Psychiatry 2007;68:1384.

Grant JE, Stein DJ, Woods DW, et al. Trichotillomania, skin picking, and other body-focused repetitive behaviors. Washington, DC: American Psychiatric Publishing; 2011.

Harth W, Gieler U, Kusnir D, Tausk FA. Clinical management in psychodermatology. Berlin: Springer; 2010.

Kanavy H, Bahner J, Korman NJ. Treatment of refractory prurigo nodularis with lenalidomide. Arch Dermatol 2012;148:794–6.

Koo JY. Psychotropic agents in dermatology. Dermatol Clin 1993;11:215.

Koo JY, Lee CS. Psychocutaneous medicine. New York: Marcel Dekker; 2003.

Koo JY, Lee CS. Psychocutaneous diseases. In: Bolognia JL, Jorizzo JL, Rapini RP, editors. Dermatology. Philadelphia: Elsevier; 2008.

Kowahara T, Henry L, Mostaghimi L. Needs assessment survey of psychocutaneous medicine. Int J Dermatol 2009;48:1066–70.

Lotti T, Buggiani G, Prignano F. Prurigo nodularis and lichen simplex chronicus. Dermatol Ther 2008;21:42.

Madhavi S. Burning mouth syndrome. Philadelphia, Elsevier Mosby: In Ferri's Clinical Advisor; 2009.

Micromedex database. Available at http://www.micromedex.com/products/; [accessed 04.11.12].

Mostaghimi L. Treating patients with delusions of parasitosis: a blueprint for clinicians. Cutis 2010;86:65–8.

Odlaug BL, Grant JE. N-acetyl cysteine in the treatment of grooming disorders. J Clin Psychopharmacol 2007;27:227–9.

Pearson ML, Selby JV, Katz KA, et al. Clinical, epidemiologic, histopathologic and molecular features of an unexplained dermopathy. PLoS One 2012;7:e29908. http://dx.doi.org/10.1371/journal.pone.0029908.

ROSACEA

Method of
Daniel J. Van Durme, MD; and Lisa M. Johnson, MD

 CURRENT DIAGNOSIS

- Rosacea is most common in adults aged 30 to 50 years and can have any of four overlapping presentation types: facial flushing and erythema with telangiectasias, inflammatory papules and pustules, ocular dryness and irritation, and nasal sebaceous gland hypertrophy leading to fibrotic changes and rhinophyma.
- Common exacerbating factors include alcohol, heat, spicy foods, and sunlight.

[1]Not FDA approved for this indication.
[6]May be compounded by pharmacists.

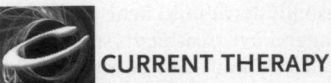

CURRENT THERAPY

- Therapy is best chosen on the basis of severity and predominant manifestation(s).
- Avoidance of known triggers is key for all four types, especially the erythematotelangiectatic type.
- Topical antibiotics (metronidazole [Metrogel], azelaic acid [Finacea], sodium sulfacetamide, and sulfur [Sulfacet-R]) are appropriate for milder forms of papulopustular rosacea. Oral antibiotics (doxycycline [Oracea], minocycline [Minocin],[1] erythromycin [Ery-Tab],[1] azithromycin [Zithromax],[1] or metronidazole [Flagyl][1]) are used for more severe cases. Isotretinoin (Accutane, Claravis)[1] can be effective in treating very severe and refractory rosacea.
- Ocular rosacea can be treated with increased eyelid hygiene, adding topical or oral antibiotics if needed.
- Rhinophyma (sebaceous gland hypertrophy and fibrosis) needs surgical management.

[1]Not FDA approved for this indication.

Rosacea is a common facial dermatosis found primarily in adults aged 30 to 50 years, particularly those of northern European or Celtic descent.

Diagnosis

Rosacea can have any of four primary manifestations, and although these overlap, most patients tend toward one predominant type. Facial erythema and flushing that also has telangiectasia is called erythematotelangiectatic type. The papulopustular type has inflammatory papules, small pustules, and occasionally small nodules. The presentation of papulopustular rosacea differs from acne vulgaris because the onset is in the 30- to 50-year-old age group instead of adolescence, and comedones are not present in papulopustular rosacea. When the sebaceous glands get markedly hypertrophic and fibrotic, this is called *phymatous type* and can lead to profound disfigurement of the nose, called rhinophyma. The ocular type involves dryness of the eyes with decreased tear production, blepharitis, and conjunctivitis.

Treatment

One key aspect of management is to have the patient maintain a careful diary for the purpose of determining and then avoiding his or her own triggers. Common triggers include alcohol, heat, certain foods, sunlight, stress, and menstruation, among others. Broad-spectrum sunblock (UVA and UVB) should be used daily. Cosmetics with a red-neutralizing green pigment can help appearance.

The erythematotelangiectatic type of rosacea is the most difficult to treat, although benefit can be found with topical antibiotics such as metronidazole 0.75% to 1% cream, lotion, or gel (Metrogel, Noritate) or azelaic acid cream (Azelex)[1] or gel (Finacea) applied once or twice daily. Sodium sulfacetamide with sulfur is made by several manufacturers, and some brands (Sulfacet-R) include a pigmenting agent to help hide the erythema. The sulfur component can also help in cases of coexisting seborrheic dermatitis. Persistent telangiectasias can be effectively treated with laser ablation.

Papulopustular rosacea can respond to topical antibiotics, but when it is moderate to severe, oral antibiotics are indicated. Doxycycline (Adoxa)[1] 50 to 100 mg taken once or twice a day for 2 to 3 months can markedly decrease symptoms, and then the patient can switch to topical agents for long-term maintenance as needed. Minocycline (Minocin)[1] 50 to 100 mg, erythromycin[1] 250 to 500 mg, and lower-dose metronidazole (Flagyl)[1] 250 mg can each be taken once or twice a day as alternatives. Resistant cases can be treated with azithromycin (Zithromax)[1]

[1]Not FDA approved for this indication.

500 mg three times weekly in the first month; 250 mg three times weekly in the second month; and 250 mg twice weekly in the third month. Side effects can limit longer-term use of these agents, especially metronidazole.

Patients resistant to conventional treatment can be treated with oral isotretinoin (Claravis)[1] (at low dose 0.1–0.3 or "classic" dose of 0.5–1.0 mg/kg/day) for 16 weeks. Isotretinoin has many severe side effects and is tightly regulated. Both prescribers and patients must register with the iPledge program in order to prescribe and to receive the prescriptions. See www.ipledgeprogram.com.

Ocular rosacea can often be controlled with increased eyelid hygiene, washing with warm water and baby (no-tears) shampoo twice a day along with artificial tears. If severe, it can be treated with topical erythromycin ointment (Ilotycin)[1] or oral antibiotics. If it still persists, ophthalmology referral is necessary.

The disfigurement of rhinophyma is often of concern to patients with rosacea. They can be reassured that this is uncommon; women can be further reassured that it is much more common in men. Unfortunately, the only effective treatments involve surgery, often laser surgery.

[1]Not FDA approved for this indication.

References

Goldgar C, Keahey DJ, Houchins J. Treatment options for acne rosacea. Am Fam Physician 2009;80:461–8.
Powell FC. Clinical practice: Rosacea. N Engl J Med 2005;352:793–803.
Wollina U. Rosacea and rhinophyma in the elderly. Clin Dermatol 2011;29:61–8.

STEVENS-JOHNSON SYNDROME AND TOXIC EPIDERMAL NECROLYSIS

Method of
Gabriel P. Currie, MD; and Jose A. Plaza, MD

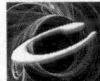

CURRENT DIAGNOSIS

- Serious, potentially fatal hypersensitivity reaction.
- Erythematous to purpuric or dusky macules, patches, and/or bullae on skin and mucous membranes.
- Associated prodrome and systemic illness in overwhelming majority of cases.

CURRENT THERAPY

- Rapid discontinuation of offending agent (usually a drug—see Box 1).
- Supportive care in a dedicated burn unit.
- Meticulous wound care with avoidance of manipulation and shearing force.
- Fluid, electrolyte, and nutrition management.
- Pain control.
- Consider intravenous immunoglobulin (IVIG),[1] high-dose corticosteroids, plasmapheresis, and/or cyclosporine (Neoral, Sandimmune).[1]

[1]Not FDA approved for this indication.

Epidemiology

The incidence of Stevens-Johnson syndrome (SJS) is estimated at 1 to 7 cases per million person-years and for toxic epidermal necrolysis (TEN) it is 0.4 to 1.5 cases per million person-years. TEN occurs equally frequently in male and female children.

However, in adults, women are more frequently affected by a ratio of 3:2 to 2:1. Those over 60 years seem to be more likely to develop TEN.

Risk Factors
It has been shown that SJS/TEN has a genetic predisposition based on the human leukocyte antigen (HLA) genotype. With this predisposition, medications are thought to cause approximately 80% of SJS/TEN cases. Other implicated etiologies include chemical exposures, mycoplasma pneumonia, viral infections, and immunizations.

Pathophysiology
The precise pathophysiology of SJS and TEN has yet to be definitively elucidated. However, it is believed that there is interplay between an inciting drug in susceptible individuals and reactive oxygen species (ROS) within keratinocytes. One theory involves the activation of cytotoxic T cells, ultimately leading to the release of granzyme B and perforin and activation the caspase cascade. Another posits that Fas-Fas ligand binding activates caspase 8, which results in nuclease activation and the widespread skin blistering that defines this disease.

Prevention
There is no known way to prevent SJS or TEN. However, the continual advances in the field of pharmacogenomics have led to the association of drug-specific associations with individual HLA antigens. For example, the strongest known HLA-disease association is carbamazepine (Tegretol)–induced SJS/TEN with the HLA-B*1502 allele among Han Chinese. Allopurinol (Zyloprim) has also been associated with HLA-B*5801.

Clinical Manifestations and Diagnosis
SJS, SJS-TEN overlap, and TEN are infrequent but severe and potentially life-threatening diseases, with some estimates of mortality rate in TEN at 30%. They tend to present with fever and flu-like symptoms 1 to 3 weeks after the use of the inciting factor. One to three days later, mucous membrane involvement develops in 90% of patients, including eyes, mouth, nose, and genitalia. The typical skin lesions appear as generalized macules with purpuric centers, ultimately progressing to large confluent bulla with epidermal detachment (Figure 1). The Nikolsky sign, which is defined as the induction of a dermal-epidermal cleavage plane when tangential pressure is applied to a blister, is generally positive. In the subsequent 3 to 5 days, separation of the epidermis yields large denuded areas with extreme pain (Figure 2). SJS, SJS-TEN overlap, and TEN are defined by the extent of epidermal involvement. At least two mucosal sites are involved. SJS is defined by less than 10% loss of epidermis, TEN is defined by greater than 30%

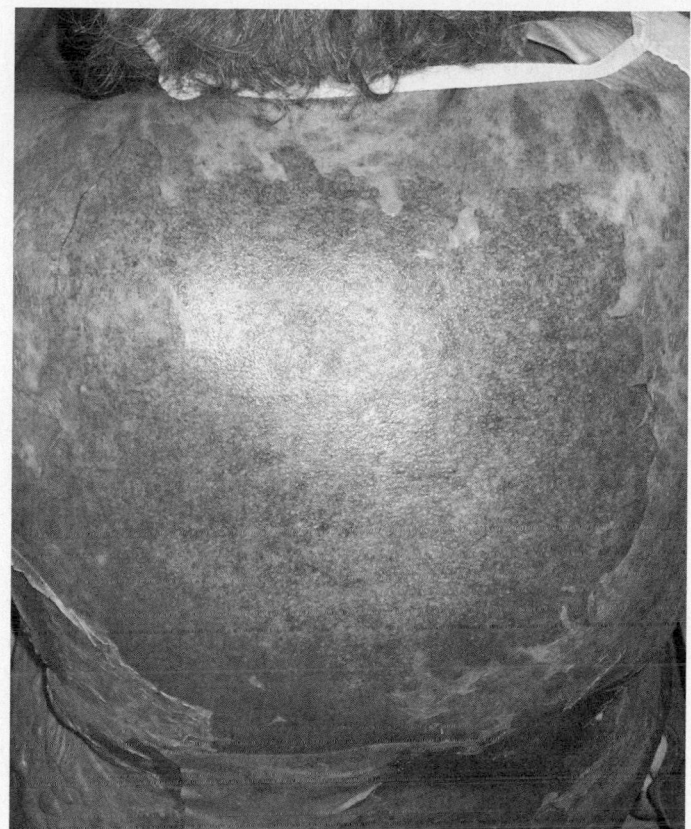

Figure 2. Confluent bright red erythema with near-complete loss of the epidermis on the back.

involvement, and SJS-TEN overlap is defined by 10% to 30% involvement.

SJS, SJS-TEN overlap, and TEN are clinically different from erythema multiforme (EM) in terms of demographic characteristics, recent exposure to drugs, and association with risk factors other than drugs, such as immunosuppression (especially HIV infection), collagen vascular diseases, and cancer.

Differential Diagnosis
It is important for the clinician to consider possible alternative diagnoses. These include autoimmune blistering diseases (i.e., pemphigus, pemphigoid, paraneoplastic pemphigus, linear IgA bullous dermatosis), EM, EM-like reactions, urticaria, staphylococcus scalded skin syndrome, graft-versus-host disease, and acute generalized exanthematous pustulosis.

Treatment
The two most important steps in initial management of SJS and TEN are immediate cessation of any potential causative drug (Box 1) and early referral to a burn unit. Meticulous attention to fluids and electrolyte balances, infection risk, nutrition, and pain control are also of utmost importance. Because all epidermal and mucosal surfaces can be affected, enteral or parental feeding should be established early. Individual areas of necrotic epidermis should be gently removed and covered with a nonadherent dressing with avoidance of frequent dressing changes because they can inhibit reepithelialization. Vaseline gauze and/or mupirocin ointment (Bactroban) to open areas should be utilized. Application of a silicone dressing with silver-impregnated gauze overtop can be beneficial.

Data on the use of systemic corticosteroids are conflicting. There is concern of increased risk of sepsis and poorer wound healing with the use of corticosteroids, but there is some evidence that institution of methylprednisolone (Solu-Medrol) within the first

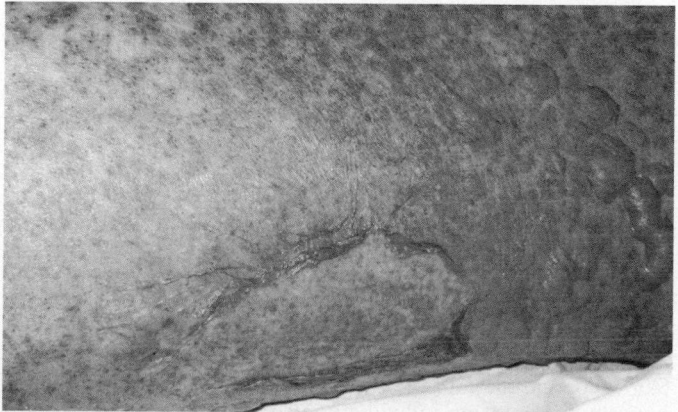

Figure 1. Deep red macules and patches, tense and flaccid bullae, and a denuded patch on the leg.

Trimethoprim-sulfamethoxazole (Bactrim) and other sulfonamide antibiotics
Allopurinol (Zyloprim)
Sertraline (Zoloft)
Aminopenicillins
Cephalosporins
Quinolones
Acetaminophen (Tylenol)
Carbamazepine (Tegretol), phenytoin (Dilantin), phenobarbital, and valproic acid (Depakene)

Oxicam—nonsteroidal antiinflammatory drugs
Corticosteroids
Nevirapine (Viramune)
Tramadol (Ultram)
Pantoprazole (Protonix)
Lamotrigine (Lamictal)

References

Auquier-Dunant A, Mockenhaupt M, Naldi L, et al. Correlations between clinical patterns and causes of erythema multiforme majus, Stevens-Johnson syndrome, and toxic epidermal necrolysis. Arch Dermatol 2002;138:1019.

Downey A, Jackson C, Harun N, et al. Toxic epidermal necrolysis: review of pathogenesis and management. J Am Acad Dermatol 2012;66:995.

Gerull R, Nelle M, Schaible T. Toxic epidermal necrolysis and Stevens-Johnson syndrome: a review. Crit Care Med 2011;39:1521.

Hughey LC. Approach to the hospitalized patient with targetoid lesions. Dermatol Ther 2011;24:196.

Somkrua R, Eickman EE, Saokaew S, et al. Association of HLA-B*5801 allele and allopurinol-induced Stevens-Johnson syndrome and toxic epidermal necrolysis: a systematic review and meta-analysis. BMC Med Genet 2011;12:118.

Worswick S, Cotliar J. Stevens-Johnson syndrome and toxic epidermal necrolysis. A review of treatment options. Dermatol Ther 2011;24:207.

48 hours, before epidermal detachment, may be beneficial. There is also conflicting evidence for the use of IVIG.[1] Numerous case series have reported a decrease in mortality. If instituted, it should be instituted as early as possible at a dose of 2 to 3 g/kg over 48 to 72 hours. Other reported treatments include plasma exchange. Most analyses advocate a survival benefit using one to four sessions. Cyclosporine (Neoral, Sandimmune)[1] and cyclophosphamide (Cytoxan)[1] have been used in limited circumstances and reported to be beneficial. Several case reports describe the use of tumor necrosis factor–α (TNF-α) inhibitors in the treatment of SJS/TEN. A single dose of infliximab (Remicade)[1] 5 mg/kg can be instituted if other options prove unsuccessful.

Monitoring and Complications

A severity-of-illness score for TEN has been proposed called the SCORTEN (Box 2). SCORTEN stands for "SCORe of Toxic Epidermal Necrosis." It assigns points based on one of seven criteria, predicting mortality with increasing criteria met. This is applied on initial evaluation and the patient is not rescored.

Management in a burn unit is of critical importance. Judicious attention to fluids and electrolytes, as well as infectious risk, is mandatory. Ophthalmology and gynecology or urology should be consulted in order to prevent potential scarring and/or adhesions of the respective organ systems. Sepsis and severe fluid and electrolyte imbalances are the most common causes of death.

[1]Not FDA approved for this indication.

Box 2 SCORTEN

Prognostic Factors	Points
Age >40 years	1
Heart rate >120 beats/min	1
Cancer or hematologic malignancy	1
Body surface area involved on day 1 above 10%	1
Serum urea level (>10 mmol/L)	1
Serum bicarbonate level (<20 mmol/L)	1
Serum glucose level (>14 mmol/L)	1

Scorten	Mortality Rate
0–1	3.2%
2	12.1%
3	35.8%
4	58.3%
5	90%

SUNBURN

Method of
Warwick L. Morison, MD

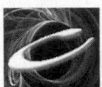

CURRENT DIAGNOSIS

- Sunburn appears 3 to 4 hours after exposure to sunlight or an artificial source of UV radiation such as a sunlamp.
- The redness of skin is diffuse and continuous, unlike rashes, which are often discontinuous.
- Sunburns are graded as pink, red, and blistering.

CURRENT THERAPY

- Prevention is the best approach to management and consists of a package of measures: avoiding over-exposure, using sunscreens, and wearing protective clothing.
- Treatment of a sunburn consists of cool baths and use of moisturizing creams.
- Topical and systemic corticosteroids do not alter the course of a sunburn.

Sunburn is a common problem, particularly in fair-skinned white persons, caused by excessive exposure to ultraviolet (UV) radiation from sunlight or artificial sources such as sunlamps. When induced by sunlight, it is mainly due to UVB (280–320 nm) radiation plus a smaller contribution from UVA (320–400 nm) radiation. Sunburn is also described as erythema, and it appears 3 to 4 hours after exposure, reaches a maximum at 12 to 18 hours, and usually settles after 72 to 96 hours. In severe reactions with blistering, complete resolution can take a week or more.

Sunburns are graded as pink, red, and blistering. In contrast, thermal burns are graded by degree (first, second, and third), but this classification should not be applied to sunburns because thermal burns have quite different sequelae, such as scarring and death, which are extremely rare consequences of a sunburn. Keratoconjunctivitis, or ocular sunburn, can also be caused by UV radiation and it follows a similar time course.

There are two facets to management of sunburn: prevention and treatment. Because there is no effective treatment for an established sunburn, most emphasis should be placed on prevention.

Prevention

Skin color and the capacity of a person to tan will determine how important it is for an individual person to take preventive measures. However, even dark-skinned people can sunburn provided the exposure dose is sufficiently high. Skin color, past history of sunburn, and likely exposure should therefore be used as a guide in advising people about protection. Protection from sunlight is often equated with use of sunscreens, but this approach is too narrow, and protection should consist of a package of measures: avoiding overexposure to sunlight, using sunscreens, and wearing protective clothing.

Avoidance of Exposure

Simple avoidance of excessive exposure to a threshold dose of UV radiation is often the best advice for fair-skinned people. Scheduling outdoor activities for before 10 am and after 4 pm will avoid the peak UV irradiance period and still permit enjoyment of the outdoors. This advice should be accompanied by several warnings. Sitting in the shade or under a beach umbrella only reduces exposure by about 70%. A cloudy day is often the setting for the worst sunburns because even complete white cloud cover reduces UV exposure by only about 50%.

Clothing is not always an effective protector. If it is possible to see through a fabric, UV radiation can also penetrate to a significant extent. The geographic location of exposure must also be considered because UV radiation may be twice as intense at the equator as compared with much of continental North America.

Sunscreens

There are now a great number of sunscreens on the market, and they contain numerous active ingredients. If this is not enough to cause confusion, some are not even labeled as sunscreens: sunblocks and tanning lotions are other terms. However, the informed physician need only know four properties of a sunscreen: the sun protection factor (SPF), the spectrum of protection, the base, and whether or not it is water resistant.

The SPF is an index of the amount of protection provided by the sunscreen. For example, a fair-skinned person who normally begins to sunburn after a 10-minute exposure to sunlight should be able to tolerate up to 150 minutes of exposure after application of an SPF 15 sunscreen.

There are several provisos for this statement. To provide the stated protection, a sunscreen must be applied 10 minutes before exposure to allow binding to skin proteins to occur, and it must be applied in an adequate amount. Several studies have shown that under ideal circumstances in which sunscreen is supplied freely and the subject is observed while making the application, most people only use one half the required amount. Ordinary use probably provides much less protection. As a rough guide, one ounce of sunscreen is necessary to cover a 70-kg adult in a bathing suit; in other words, a four ounce bottle of sunscreen only provides four applications.

Sunscreens vary in the amount of the solar spectrum for which they provide protection. All sunscreens provide protection against UVB radiation and the shorter end of UVA radiation. Some sunscreens claim to provide broad-spectrum protection against UVB and UVA radiation and contain avobenzone or titanium dioxide to protect against the longer wavelengths in the UVA spectrum. Ecamsule (Mexoryl SX), a recently approved sunscreen active, provides good absorption in the middle of the UVA spectrum; a sunscreen containing this, avobenzone, and octocrylene—an absorber of UVB radiation—provides very good broad-spectrum protection.

The base of a sunscreen is also important because it often determines whether or not a sunscreen will be used. Men usually prefer alcohol-based lotions because they dry quickly and leave a dry and nongreasy film. Women usually prefer lotions or creams because they give a moisturizing feel to the skin.

Finally, a sunscreen may be labeled water resistant or very water resistant. Because almost all outdoor pastimes involve perspiring or contact with water, a very water-resistant sunscreen should be selected.

A fair-skinned person should always use a sunscreen with an SPF 15 or higher. People who tan well and never burn are probably adequately protected with an SPF of 8 to 10. People with black or brown skin probably do not need sunscreens except for extreme occupational or social exposure.

A few myths should be dismissed. There is no effective oral sunscreen. Many have been tested and all have failed. Self-tanning preparations are not sunscreens. They do provide the appearance of a tan and are safe to use but they provide no significant protection against UV radiation.

Protective Clothing

There has been significant progress in recent years in the development, testing, and classification of UV-protective clothing. Akin to the SPF for sunscreens, such clothing is labeled with an ultraviolet protective factor (UPF), and a fabric with a UPF of 50 blocks transmission of 98% of UV radiation. A hat with a 3-inch brim all around completes the package of protection.

Protective Tanning

The proliferation of suntan parlors has generated a lot of interest in protective tanning, with much misinformation provided by the commercial interests involved. Little scientific information is available to provide a guide as to whether protective tanning is of any value in preventing the long-term hazards of excessive exposure to sunlight, namely skin cancer and premature aging of the skin. Certainly, preventive tanning using multiple suberythemal doses of UV radiation can prevent sunburn, but the cost in terms of chronic damage is unknown.

Most tanning salons claim to use only UVA radiation in their tanning beds, but this claim is false. All so-called UVA tanning beds emit some UVB radiation, the most damaging wavelengths, and in addition, UVA radiation, especially in large doses, can produce the same damaging effect as UVB radiation. Furthermore, a UVA-induced tan is not very protective and at most has an SPF of 6 to 8.

A person who tans well and never burns might gain some protection from sunlight by preventive tanning without incurring too much damage. However, the risk-to-benefit ratio for people who do sunburn is probably very unfavorable.

Treatment

When a person has a sunburn, general supportive measures are the only approach to treatment. Cold compresses and cool baths with bath oil provide some relief. Frequent application of moisturizing creams help alleviate dryness. Blistering of the skin can lead to secondary infection and require use of an antibiotic cream. Rarely, an extremely severe sunburn necessitates hospitalization and management as a thermal burn.

Topical corticosteroids reduce erythema by causing vasoconstriction, but this effect is temporary and does not reduce epidermal damage. Systemic corticosteroids, even in very large doses, do not alter the course of a sunburn. Nonsteroidal antiinflammatory drugs, if given at the time of exposure or beforehand, reduce the degree of erythema over the first 24 hours but do not change epidermal damage. Of course, few people lying on the beach anticipate an excessive exposure, so they are unlikely to embark on such preventive measures.

URTICARIA AND ANGIOEDEMA

Method of
Joyce M.C. Teng, MD, PhD

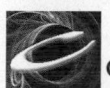 **CURRENT DIAGNOSIS**

- Acute and chronic urticaria have the same features, including erythematous, edematous papules or wheals with central pallor that last less than 24 to 48 hours.
- Laboratory assessments are not recommended for acute urticaria in the absence of evidence suggesting underlying systemic illness.
- Limited laboratory studies are indicated for chronic urticaria.

- Serum measurements of C4 and C1-esterase inhibitor are the recommended initial tests if hereditary or acquired angioedema are suspected.
- Skin biopsy should be considered to rule out urticarial vasculitis if an individual lesion is painful and persists for more than 2 to 3 days with accompanying ecchymosis or petechiae.

CURRENT THERAPY

- Primary treatment of urticaria and angioedema is removal of triggering factors and initiation of therapy for symptomatic relief.
- Oral antihistamines are the cornerstones of therapy. The application of first-generation H_1-antihistamines may be limited by central nervous system and anticholinergic side effects.
- Nonsedating second generation antihistamine are often used as first line therapy.
- Systemic corticosteroids and immunosuppressive therapy, especially cyclosporine (Neoral),[1] have been used successfully in cases that are refractory to the maximum dose of antihistamines.
- Fresh-frozen plasma infusions along with standard airway precautions have been recommended for angioedema patients with laryngeal edema.

Urticaria, or hives, is a common cutaneous eruption that occurs in up to 25% of the general population sometime during their lives.[1] It is characterized by transient, circumscribed, pruritic, erythematous papules or plaques, often with central pallor. Individual lesions often coalesce into large wheals on the trunk and extremities that may resolve over a few hours without leaving any residual skin changes. The process is mediated by mast cells in the superficial dermis.

Angioedema is a similar process occurring in deep dermis or subcutaneous tissue. Angioedema may occur independently, accompanied by urticaria, or as a component of anaphylaxis. It is characterized by localized swelling that develops over minutes to hours and resolves within 24 to 48 hours. Common locations of angioedema include the mucosa and areas with loose connective tissue, such as the face, eyes, lips, tongue, and genitalia. Patients usually do not have pruritus, but they may have pain and a sensation of warmth. Angioedema is usually a benign process that resolves without sequelae unless it involves the larynx. African Americans are disproportionately affected, representing up to 40% of the hospital admissions for angioedema.[2]

Classification

Urticaria can be classified as acute or chronic, depending on the duration. Acute urticaria usually lasts for less than 6 weeks and is commonly triggered by infection, medication, insect bite, and food (Table 1). The chronic form, lasting more than 6 weeks, accounts for approximately 30% of cases of urticaria, and no clear causes can be identified in more than 80% of these cases. Stress however has been identified as a trigger in some of the cases. A significant number of patients with chronic urticaria may have persistent symptoms for more than 10 years.[3] Approximately 40% of patients with chronic urticaria have associated angioedema, although the incidence of laryngeal edema is low.

Diagnosis

Urticaria is diagnosed clinically in most cases. A detailed history, physical examination, and complete review of systems are essential for diagnosing patients with urticaria and angioedema. The

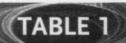

TABLE 1 Mechanisms in Urticaria and Angioedema

DISORDER	CAUSES
Immunoglobulin-mediated urticaria	Ig-E mediated: food, medication, insect bites, contact allergen, aeroallergens, other causes Urticaria associated with autoimmunity: antinuclear antibodies (ANAs), thyroid autoantibodies, other causes
Direct activation of mast cell degranulation	Physical stimuli: exercise, heat, cold, pressure, aquagenic, solar radiation, etc. Other agents: opiates, antibiotics (e.g., vancomycin [Vancocin]), radiocontrast, ACTH (Cortrosyn), muscle relaxants
Complement-mediated	Viral infections, parasites, blood transfusion
C1-esterase inhibitor deficiency	Genetic and acquired angioedema, paraproteinemia
Reduced kinin metabolism	Angiotensin-converting enzyme (ACE) inhibitors
Reduced arachidonic acid metabolism	Aspirin

history should include the distribution and characteristics of lesions (e.g., pain, pruritus), duration of skin eruption, accompanying angioedema, airway involvement and other associated systemic symptoms (e.g., fever, arthralgia, swelling joints, refusal to walk by children). Patients should also be questioned about changes in dietary habits, stress, recent exposures, infection, and newly administered medications, including antibiotics, over-the-counter analgesia, and hormones.

Laboratory assessment is usually not helpful in diagnosing patients with acute urticaria who lack any history or clinical findings to suggest an underlying disease process. A limited number of diagnostic tests are indicated in the evaluation of patients with chronic urticaria, such as a complete blood cell count with differential white blood cell count, an erythrocyte sedimentation rate (ESR) or C-reactive protein (CRP) determination, a thyroid-stimulating hormone (TSH) level, antithyroglobulin and antimicrosomal antibodies, antinuclear antibodies (ANA), folate, B12, ferritin, liver function test, and hepatitis B and C serologies. A detailed review of systems may help to narrow the focus of the screening test.

A skin biopsy of an early lesion should be performed to rule out urticarial vasculitis if the affected individual has skin lesions that are painful and last for more than 2 to 3 days with residual ecchymosis or petechiae. In patients with angioedema, prominent edema of the interstitial tissue may be demonstrated by biopsy. It is associated with antibodies against C1q, which leads to persistent complement activation and low serum C3, C4. Serum measurements of C4 and C1-esterase inhibitor are recommended initial tests if hereditary or acquired angioedema is suspected. A C1q level should be obtained to screen for the acquired form of angioedema if the affected individual is middle-aged.[3]

Treatment

More than two thirds of cases of urticaria are self-limited. Spontaneous remission of chronic urticaria and angioedema is also common. The primary objective of management is to identify and discontinue the offending trigger. A patient presenting with angioedema must first be assessed for signs of airway compromise. Medical therapy is indicated for those who are symptomatic.

Antihistamines remain the first-line therapy for most patients with urticaria, because the primary complaint of pruritus is predominantly mediated by histamine released from mast cells.[5,6] First-generation antihistamines such as hydroxyzine (Atarax or Vistaril 25–50 mg every 6 hours), diphenhydramine (Benadryl 25–50 mg

---

[1]Not FDA approved for this indication.
[2]Not available in the United States.
[3]Exceeds dosage recommended by the manufacturer.

[3]Exceeds dosage recommended by the manufacturer.
[5]Investigational drug in the United States.
[6]May be compounded by pharmacists.

every 6 hours), cyproheptadine (Periactin 4 mg three times daily), and chlorpheniramine (Chlor-Trimeton 4 mg every 6 hours) are potent and have the quickest onset of action. However, the treatments are often limited by their sedating and anticholinergic side effects. Many first-generation antihistamines are available over the counter, providing accessible first-line therapy for patients. Patients with urticaria that lasts for several days should be considered for treatment using second-generation antihistamines such as loratadine (Claritin[1] 10 mg twice daily[3]), desloratadine (Clarinex 5 mg twice daily[3]), cetirizine (Zyrtec 10 mg twice daily[3]), levocetirizine (Xyzal 5 mg daily), and fexofenadine (Allegra 180 mg twice daily[3]). Doxepin (Sinequan),[1] an H_1- and H_2-receptor antagonist, is seven times more potent than hydroxyzine in suppression of wheal and flare responses. Because of its central nervous system side effects, combined use of doxepin with a first-generation antihistamine should be restricted. Topical 5% doxepin cream (Zonalon)[1] may help to suppress pruritus in patients with localized urticaria.

Systemic prednisone at 30 to 40 mg in a single morning dose is sufficient to suppress acute urticaria in adults. Tapering should be gradual over a 3- to 4-week period by decreasing the dosage 5 mg every 3 to 5 days to minimize rebound. Alternate-morning dosing when reaching 20 mg daily may help to minimize the steroid side effects. Methylprednisolone (Solu-Medrol 40 mg) should be given intravenously as initial therapy to patients with angioedema. Chronic therapy is to be avoided. This may be followed by a tapering oral course. Chronic therapy is to be avoided. Three months of treatment with cyclosporine (Neoral)[1] at 3 to 5 mg/kg can be given safely to patients who are refractory to corticosteroid therapy or have difficulty tapering their therapy. Close monitoring for hypertension and renal insufficiency is necessary during the treatment.

Leukotriene inhibitors such as zileuton (Zyflo[1] 600 mg four times daily), zafirlukast (Accolate[1] 20 mg twice daily), and montelukast (Singulair[1] 10 mg once daily) may be effective for patients with autoimmune urticaria. Successful treatment of chronic urticaria with anti-IgE (omalizumab [Xolair][1]) has been reported but the medication is approved by the FDA for moderate to severe allergic asthma only for patients above 12 years of age.

Proper management of underlying autoimmune thyroid disease or autoimmune collagen vascular diseases has been beneficial for patients with associated urticaria. Life-threatening angioedema triggered by angiotensin-converting enzyme (ACE) inhibitors has been successfully treated with infusion of fresh-frozen plasma. Hereditary angioedema can be prevented with tranexamic aid or modified androgens. Intravenous C1 esterase inhibitor or icatibant, a bradykinin B2 antagonist, can be administered to prevent acute attacks. Treatments with methotrexate, warfarin (Coumadin),[1] plasmapheresis, and intravenous immunoglobulin (Baygam)[1] have been reported for severe, refractory[1] urticaria. These treatments are administered only by specialists on an individual basis.

---

[1]Not FDA approved for this indication.
[3]Exceeds dosage recommended by the manufacturer.

References

Bailey E, Shaker M. An update on childhood urticaria and angioedema. Curr Opin Pediatr 2008;20(4):425–30.

Champion RH, Roberts SO, Carpenter RG, Roger JH. Urticaria and angio-oedema. A review of 554 patients. Br J Dermatol 1969;81(8):588–97.

Joint Task Force on Practice Parameters. The diagnosis and management of urticaria: A practice parameter. Part II. Chronic urticaria/angioedema. Ann Allergy Asthma Immunol 2000;85(2):521–44.

Kaplan AP, Joseph K, Maykut RJ, et al. Treatment of chronic autoimmune urticaria with omalizumab. J Allergy Clin Immunol 2008;122(3):569–73.

Lin RY, Cannon AG, Teitel AD. Pattern of hospitalizations for angioedema in New York between 1990 and 2003. Ann Allergy Asthma Immunol 2005;95(2):159–66.

Maurer M, Rosen K, Shieh HJ. Omalizumab for chronic urticaria. N Engl J Med 2013;386:2530. http://dx.doi.org/10.1056/JEJMc1305687.

Nizami RM, Baboo MT. Office management of patients with urticaria: An analysis of 215 patients. Ann Allergy 1974;33(2):78–85.

Powell RJ, Du Toit GL, Siddique N, et al. BSACI guidelines for the management of chronic urticaria and angio-oedema. Clin Exp Allergy 2007;37 (5):631–50.

VENOUS ULCERS

Method of
Zuleika L. Bonilla-Martinez, MD; and Robert S. Kirsner, MD, PhD

CURRENT DIAGNOSIS

- Venous ulcers are the most common cause of lower-extremity ulceration.
- Valvular incompetence, vein distention, muscular weakness, or a decrease in the range of motion of the ankle may lead to calf muscle pump failure.
- The mechanism of cutaneous ulceration resulting from venous insufficiency remains unknown.
- The typical location for a venous ulcer is around the medial malleolus.
- Complications of chronic venous ulcers are cellulitis and less often squamous cell carcinoma.
- Compression is the gold standard of treatment of venous disease.

CURRENT THERAPY

- Compression therapy is used to deliver a graded compression of 30 to 40 mm Hg at the ankle. Exclude arterial disease before using compression.
- Systemic medications as adjuvant therapy to compression bandages include aspirin,[1] pentoxifylline (Trental), or micronized purified flavonoid fraction (Daflon 500).[2]
- Other treatments, along with compression, include engineered skin, skin graft, electrical stimulation, locally derived growth factors, and venous surgery.
- The lifelong use of elastic compression stockings (30–40 mm Hg) is the mainstay of prevention.

[1]Not FDA approved for this indication.
[2]Not available in the United States.

Ulcers resulting from venous insufficiency are the most common cause of leg ulceration. Many definitions exist for a chronic wound, which ultimately reflect the demographics, incidence, and prevalence data available. For example, although sometimes referred to as stasis ulcers, patients actually have increased blood flow locally. The Wound Healing Society classifies wounds as *acute* if they sustain restoration of anatomic and functional integrity in an orderly and timely process and *chronic* if they do not. Some of the biologic events that affect the "orderly" process include inflammation, angiogenesis (i.e., new blood vessel formation), matrix regeneration, and remodeling. The "timely" process is affected by the environment, age, pathologic process, wound location, and other factors.

Epidemiology

Venous disease affects approximately 5% of the world's population and about 2% of the American population. It was once thought to be a disease affecting solely the elderly. The incidence increases from middle age onward. Seventy percent of all leg ulcers result solely from venous disease, and an additional 20% of patients have mixed arterial and venous disease. The other 10% of leg ulcers result from a variety of causes, including neuropathy, prolonged pressure, infectious, malignant, and inflammatory causes.

The high prevalence of venous disease directly affects patients' quality of life. Family history of venous disease, obesity, smoking, high cost of treatment, time off work, prolonged standing, and hypertension are among the factors that contribute to a strong socioeconomic impact of a country's health care. A retrospective study from Cleveland Clinic Foundation showed the average cost per month of care was approximately $2400, and the mean total cost per patient was between $9685 and $14,136 U.S. dollars.

Pathophysiology

In the lower extremities, the venous system comprises the deep and superficial veins, which are connected by the perforating venous system. Blood flows from the superficial to the deep veins through the communicating veins to ultimately reach the heart. Veins contain valves that prevent blood reflux and allow the unidirectional flow. When a healthy individual contracts the calf muscles, a high pressure develops in the deep vein system, allowing blood flow to go from the deep to the superficial veins. During calf muscle relaxation, the pressure difference (high pressure in the superficial veins) allows blood flow from the superficial to deep veins. Venous ulcers are associated with venous hypertension, which is defined as sustained elevated venous pressures during ambulation. Venous hypertension results from failure of the calf muscle pump, which normally assists in venous return. Blood reflux from the deep to superficial veins creates the sustained high pressure in the superficial vein system and therefore increased cutaneous blood flow. Valvular incompetence, vein distention, muscular weakness, and a decreased in the range of motion of the ankle may lead to calf muscle pump failure. Alterations in the microcirculation because of calf muscle pump failure ultimately lead to ulceration.

How does the skin ulcerate in patients with venous insufficiency? The mechanism of cutaneous ulceration as a consequence of venous insufficiency remains unknown. Several hypotheses have been reported since the beginning of the 20th century. In the early 1980s, Browse and Burnard suggested that venous hypertension could lead to endothelial distention, causing extravasation of fibrinogen into the interstitial fluid, which results in "pericapillary fibrin cuff" formation around the capillary vessels. Fibrin cuffs act as a barrier to diffusion of oxygen and nutrients, causing ischemia and ulcer formation. A few years later, Coleridge and colleagues suggested that venous hypertension could lead to decreased capillary perfusion, resulting in leukocyte trapping. The trapped leukocytes release proteolytic enzymes, which result in free radical formation and capillary damage. The increased capillary permeability causes extravasation of fibrinogen and other metabolites, which leads to formation of a fibrin cuff around the capillaries and ultimately ischemia.

Further studies supported the presence of increased levels of monocyte aggregation. Claudy and colleagues showed that leukocyte activation caused release of tumor necrosis factor alpha (TNF-α), ultimately leading to pericapillary fibrin cuff formation. In 1993, Falanga and Eaglstein observed that fibrin cuffs were discontinuous around capillaries and therefore did not form a barrier to oxygen and nutrients causing ischemia. They also postulated the "trap" hypothesis, which suggests that venous hypertension causes endothelial cell distention leading to extravasation of macromolecules (i.e., α2-macroglobulin and fibrinogen) into the dermis. Moreover, α2-macroglobulin can bind to growth factors, such as TNF-α and transforming growth factor beta (TGF-β), making them unavailable for wound repair. Patients with venous disease may have other factors that contribute to venous ulcer formation, such as systemic alteration in fibrinolysis and arteriovenous shunting. Despite all previously conducted studies and hypotheses, further research is needed to explain the mechanism of cutaneous ulceration resulting from venous insufficiency.

Evaluation and Diagnosis

The typical location for a venous ulcer is around the medial aspect of the lower extremity near the ankle (medial malleolus) or the gaiter area. The ulcer usually begins as a blister or erosion on the skin. Ulcer borders are irregular and usually smooth. The base of the ulcer may be covered with granulation tissue or yellow slough, or both.

Venous ulcers are associated with presence of pigmentation, erythema, dermatitis, edema, and induration (i.e., lipodermatosclerosis) of the surrounding skin and with varicose veins in the lower leg. Hemosiderin deposition resulting from red blood cell extravasation causes the surrounding hyperpigmentation. Lipodermatosclerosis, commonly known as an inverted bottle shape, is caused by sclerosis of the dermis and subcutaneous tissue. The presence of lipodermatosclerosis has been associated with a greater impairment of fibrinolysis in patients with venous ulcers and may be a poor prognostic factor for restriction of leg movement. Other known prognostic factors are duration and size of the ulcer and history of venous surgery. Ulcers present for longer than 6 months and larger than 5 cm^2 in diameter tend to be more refractory to therapy.

A diagnosis of venous ulcers may be based on clinical presentation. The findings of a lower leg ulcer associated with lipodermatosclerosis or varicose veins, or both, suggest a venous ulcer. Other common findings include atrophie blanche (i.e., porcelain white scars with telangiectasia and dyspigmentation) and dermatitis. Venous dermatitis is associated with erythema, eczema, pruritus, and scaling of the skin. Contact dermatitis surrounding the ulcer may result from the use of topical agents.

Venous disease can be confirmed by a variety of techniques, including duplex ultrasound or plethysmography. However, it is critical that arterial disease be excluded because treatment with compression bandages is the mainstay of therapy and should be used cautiously in patients with arterial disease. A simple, noninvasive measurement to assess peripheral vascular disease is the ankle brachial index (ABI). This value is calculated by dividing the systolic pressure in the ankle by the systolic pressure in the arm. An ABI of less than 0.9 indicates peripheral vascular disease and represents an independent risk factor for vascular disease in other vascular beds, such as the coronary arteries. Care must be taken with diabetic or elderly patients who may have a falsely negative ABI value. All patients with an abnormal ABI value should be further evaluated. Consider a vascular consultation, magnetic resonance angiography (MRA), angioplasty, and stent bypass.

To aid in the exclusion of any underlying disease (e.g., hematologic disease, diabetes), initial laboratory tests should include complete blood cell (CBC) count with a differential count, chemistry panel, hemoglobin A$_{1C}$, prealbumin and albumin determinations, liver function tests, and levels of homocysteine, protein C and S, antithrombin III, and factor V Leiden.

Several vascular studies help in the diagnosis and severity of venous disease. Color duplex ultrasound is usually the initial study done to assess venous reflux in the lower extremities. Continuous-wave Doppler studies may yield false-negative results because it may be difficult to differentiate between the superficial and deep venous system. Air plethysmography and photoplethysmography are helpful in evaluating venous reflux and calf muscle dysfunction. Invasive venography is the gold standard to assess venous reflux, but it is used only as a last resort because of its invasive properties.

The CEAP classification was developed in 1994 by the American Venous Forum (AVF) to standardize the diagnosis and treatment of venous disease. It was based on clinical manifestations (C), etiologic factors (E), anatomic distribution of disease (A), and underlying pathophysiologic findings (P).

Complications

Main complications of long-term or chronic venous ulcers are cellulitis, osteomyelitis, and squamous cell carcinoma. A finding of exposed tendon or bone, in addition to suggesting an underlying osteomyelitis, suggests an ulcer with a nonvenous cause.

Radiographs and biopsy for histology and culture are appropriate first steps in evaluation. Consult an orthopedic surgeon for further analysis and treatment, which may include a bone biopsy and bone débridement.

Treatment

Compression is the gold standard of treatment of venous disease. After arterial disease has been excluded, reversal of the effects of venous hypertension through compression bandages and leg elevation is the cornerstone of therapy.

The goal of compression therapy is to deliver sustained graded compression with 30 to 40 mm Hg at the ankle. These bandages are applied circumferentially from the toes to the knees (involving the heel) with the foot dorsiflexed. The optimal method to deliver this pressure is through multilayered elastic compression dressings. Elastic compression dressings deliver compression during ambulation (i.e., walking) and at rest, accommodate to reduction in edema, and are superior to single-layered dressings. Inelastic compression (short-stretch compression) may deliver similar results but appear to require greater sophistication by those applying them to accomplish this. Inelastic bandages, which do not deliver compression at rest, may be advantageous in patients with arterial disease or patients who do not tolerate full compression (e.g., elderly). Patients with associated lymphatic damage may also benefit from pneumatic compression.

Systemic medication as adjuvant therapy to compression bandages, such as pentoxifylline (Trental 400–800 mg three times daily[3]), aspirin,[1] or micronized purified flavonoid fraction (MPFF, Daflon 500[2] [diosmin[7] 90% and hesperidin[7] 10%]) may be superior to compression bandages alone with regard to the rate of healing. The use of pentoxifylline as adjuvant therapy to compression in venous ulcers has been shown to be very beneficial.

Wound bed preparation was proposed as a way to help the healing process. It is a multistep process that improves the wound bed by removing necrotic and fibrinous wound tissue, increasing the amount of granulation tissue, and decreasing edema, chronic wound fluid (i.e., exudate), and bacterial burden.

Local care is best accomplished with occlusive dressings. Occlusive dressings provide a moist environment for healing. A variety of types of occlusions may be used, and the choice depends on several factors, including the location of the wound and the amount of fibrinous slough and exudate present. A fear of excessive infection with the use of occlusive dressings is unfounded. Topical antiseptics and cleansing agents should be used with caution because they may increase the time required for healing. Topical agents such as cadexomer iodine (Iodosorb), silver-impregnated dressings, and topical anesthetics are alternatives that do not prolong healing, but they should be applied directly to the wound because they may lead to skin sensitization.

Up to 50% of venous ulcers may be refractory to compression therapy alone. This refractory subset may be predicted by baseline characteristics (size and duration) and by a decrease in size with 2 to 4 weeks of treatment (Figure 1). Other available treatments include tissue-engineered skin, autologous skin, electrical stimulation, treatment with locally delivered growth factors, and venous surgery. Three categories exist for skin grafts: autograft, allogeneic (cultured), and artificial (tissue-engineered skin). Two types of autografts are full-thickness (FTSG) and split-thickness (STSG) skin grafts. The latter is commonly used by expanding it with a meshing technique.

Apligraf, a bilayered engineered living skin composed of keratinocytes and fibroblasts from neonatal foreskin, is approved by the FDA for treatment of venous leg and diabetic neuropathic foot ulcers. Surgical treatment of incompetent superficial and perforator veins along with standard of care (i.e., compression) reduce the risk of recurrence.

After healing occurs, patients with venous insufficiency are at risk for recurrence. The lifelong use of elastic compression stockings (30–40 mm Hg) is the mainstay of therapy, but early intervention after recurrence is critical. Health professionals need to understand the importance of further research to ultimately minimize the psychological, physical, and socioeconomic impact that ulcers caused by venous insufficiency have on patients and society.

---

[1]Not FDA approved for this indication.
[2]Not available in the United States.
[3]Exceeds dosage recommended by the manufacturer.
[7]Available as a dietary supplement.

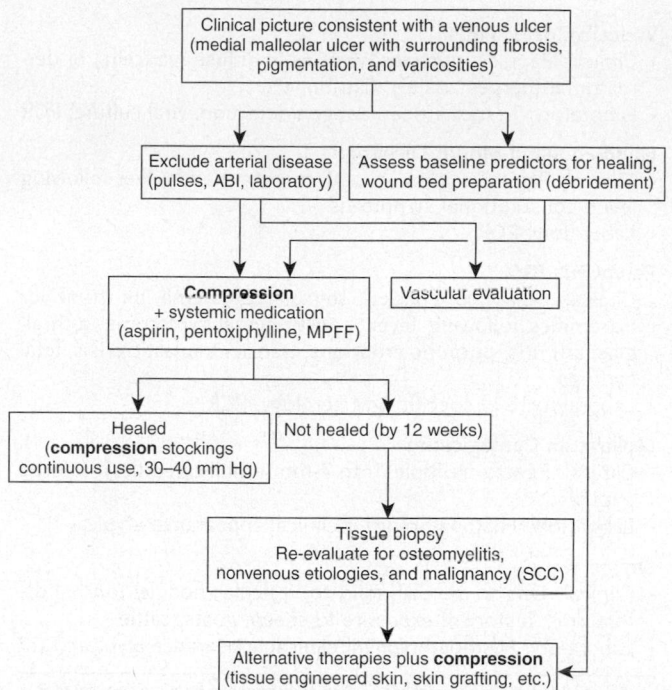

Figure 1. Simplified algorithm for the diagnosis and treatment of patients with venous ulcers. *Abbreviations:* ABI = ankle-brachial index; MPFF = micronized purified flavonoid fraction; SCC = squamous cell carcinoma.

References

Abbade LP, Lastória S. Venous ulcer: Epidemiology, physiopathology, diagnosis and treatment. Int J Dermatol 2005;44.449–56.

Browse NL, Burnand KG. The cause of venous ulceration. Lancet 1982;2:243–5.

Claudy AL, Mirshahi M, Soria C, et al. Detection of undegraded fibrin and tumor necrosis factor alpha in venous leg ulcers. J Am Acad Dermatol 1991;25:623–7.

Coleridge-Smith PD, Thomas P, Scurr JH, et al. Causes of venous ulceration: A new hypothesis? Br Med J 1988;296:1726–7.

Falanga V, Eaglstein WH. The trap hypothesis of venous ulceration. Lancet 1993;341:1006–8.

Jull A, Arroll B, Parag V, Waters J. Pentoxyphilline for treating venous leg ulcers. Cochrane Database Syst Rev 2007;(3)CD001733.

Kirsner R. Wound bed preparation. Ostomy Wound Manage 2003;(Feb, Suppl.):2–3.

Kirsner RS, Falanga V. Techniques of split-thickness skin grafting for lower extremity ulcerations. J Dermatol Surg Oncol 1993;19:779–83.

Kirsner RS, Pardes JB, Eaglstein WH, Falanga V. The clinical spectrum of lipodermatosclerosis. J Am Acad Dermatol 1993;28:623–7.

Lazarus GS, Cooper DM, Knighton DR, et al. Definitions and guidelines for assessment of wounds and evaluation of healing. Arch Dermatol 1994;130:489–93.

Olin JW, Beusterien KM, Childs MB, et al. Medical costs of treating venous stasis ulcers: Evidence from a retrospective cohort study. Vasc Med 1999;4:1–7.

Phillips TJ, Machado F, Trout R, et al. Prognostic indicators in venous ulcers. J Am Acad Dermatol 2000;43:627–30.

Trent JT, Falabella A, Eaglstein WH, Kirsner RS. Venous ulcers: Pathophysiology and treatment options. Ostomy Wound Manage 2005;51:38–54.

VIRAL DISEASES OF THE SKIN

Method of
Sylvia L. Brice, MD

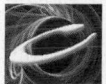

CURRENT DIAGNOSIS

Herpes Simplex Viruses 1 and 2
- Clinical: Grouped vesicles or erosions, especially in perioral or anogenital location
- Laboratory: Tzanck smear, viral culture, antigen detection, PCR, gG-based type-specific serology

Varicella-Zoster Virus
- Clinical: Papules, pustules, vesicles in diffuse (varicella) or dermatomal (herpes zoster) distribution
- Laboratory: Tzanck smear, antigen detection, viral culture, PCR

Hand-Foot-and-Mouth Disease
- Clinical: Papulovesicles on oral mucosa, hands, feet following fever, constitutional symptoms
- Laboratory: PCR

Parvovirus B19
- Clinical: "Slapped cheeks" reticular erythema on trunk or extremities following fever, constitutional symptoms; arthralgias, arthritis, purpuric eruptions; transient aplastic crisis, fetal hydrops
- Laboratory: B19 specific IgM serology, PCR

Molluscum Contagiosum
- Clinical: Few to multiple 1- to 4-mm umbilicated flesh-colored papules
- Laboratory: Histopathology if clinical appearance atypical

Orf
- Clinical: One to several solid to vesicular nodules on hands, forearms; history of exposure to sheep, goats, cattle
- Laboratory: Histopathology if clinical appearance atypical; PCR

Abbreviations: gG = glycoprotein G; IVIg = intravenous immunoglobulin; PCR = polymerase chain reaction.

 CURRENT THERAPY

Herpes Simplex Viruses 1 and 2
- Acyclovir (Zovirax), valacyclovir (Valtrex), famciclovir (Famvir)
- For acyclovir resistance: foscarnet (Foscavir),[1] cidofovir (Vistide)[1]

Varicella-Zoster Virus
- Acyclovir, valacyclovir, famciclovir
- For acyclovir resistance: foscarnet,[1] cidofovir (Vistide)[1]

Hand-Foot-and-Mouth Disease
- Supportive care

Parvovirus B19
- Supportive care, IVIg (Gammagard)[1]

Molluscum Contagiosum
- Surgical or chemical methods of destruction
- Immunomodulators (imiquimod [Aldara],[1] cimetidine [Tagamet][1])

Orf
- Self-limited

---

[1]Not FDA approved for this indication.
Abbreviations: HSV = herpes simplex virus; IVIg = intravenous immunoglobulin.

Herpes Simplex Viruses 1 and 2

Herpes simplex virus types 1 and 2 (HSV-1 and HSV-2) are the most closely related members of the human herpesvirus family, and the skin lesions they produce are clinically indistinguishable. Clusters of tense blisters on an erythematous base often quickly evolve into erosions or ulcerations with associated crusting. Lesions can develop at any mucocutaneous site but are typically found in the perioral or anogenital regions. Both HSV-1 and HSV-2 are transmitted by direct mucocutaneous contact with an infected host. Following viral replication in the skin or mucosa, intact viral nucleocapsids travel via sensory neurons to the corresponding dorsal root ganglia to establish latency. Later, a variety of stimuli can trigger reactivation. The virus travels back along the

sensory neurons to the mucocutaneous surface to replicate and induce active or subclinical infection. In the case of subclinical infection, no active skin lesions are evident, but infectious particles are present, a state known as asymptomatic shedding. Although the viral titer is much lower than during clinically active disease, asymptomatic shedding of the virus in oral and genital secretions is thought to be responsible for the majority of cases of HSV transmission.

Primary, initial nonprimary (also known as first episode), and recurrent are terms used to further define the nature of the HSV infection. A *primary* infection refers to a patient's first infection with either type of HSV at any site. These patients are seronegative initially but subsequently develop HSV type-specific antibodies. A patient who is already infected with one HSV type and then develops an infection with the alternate type experiences an *initial nonprimary* or first-episode infection (e.g., the first episode of genital herpes in a patient with a prior history of orofacial herpes). These patients are seropositive for one type-specific HSV antibody (e.g., HSV-1) and later develop antibodies specific for the alternate HSV type (e.g., HSV-2). A *recurrent* infection is one that occurs at a site of prior infection. These patients are seropositive for HSV-1 or HSV-2, or both. Because most primary infections, whether oral or genital, are asymptomatic, the first evidence of disease often represents a recurrent or initial nonprimary infection.

Orofacial Herpes Simplex Virus Infection

Orofacial HSV, also known as herpes labialis, fever blisters, or cold sores, is commonly acquired during childhood or adolescence. Symptomatic primary disease usually takes the form of gingivostomatitis with or without additional lesions on the cutaneous perioral surfaces. Fever, malaise, and tender lymphadenopathy may also be present. In recurrent episodes, clusters of blisters erupt along the vermillion border of the lips, and subsequent erosions and crusting persist for several days up to 2 weeks. Lesions can develop anywhere in the perioral area, especially on the cheeks. In men, a viral folliculitis of the beard area (herpetic sycosis) may be mistaken for a bacterial process because it is often pustular. The presence of a prodrome and recurrence in the same site are clues to the correct diagnosis. Although recurrent intraoral lesions of HSV can occur, they are uncommon in immunocompetent persons. Exposure to ultraviolet light is a common trigger factor for herpes labialis, as is fever or intercurrent infection.

Genital Herpes Simplex Virus Infection

When symptomatic, primary genital herpes often involves bilaterally distributed lesions in the anogenital area with associated fever, inguinal adenopathy, and dysuria or urinary retention. Aseptic meningitis can also occur. The lesions often persist for 2 to 3 weeks or longer. Nonprimary infections are usually less severe and have fewer constitutional symptoms. Recurrent episodes tend to be milder and shorter in duration. Often, there is a prodrome of tingling or burning followed by the development of localized vesicles that can quickly rupture, leaving nonspecific erosions or ulcerations. The lesions may be anywhere within the anogenital region but tend to recur close to the same area in subsequent episodes. The time between exposure and development of primary disease is estimated to be from 3 to 14 days. However, more often the first clinical indication of disease is a recurrence, which can occur weeks to years after the initial infection. Prior infection with HSV-1 provides some protection against acquisition of HSV-2.

Based on seroepidemiologic evidence, it is estimated that approximately 17% of the United States population aged 14 to 49 years is infected with HSV-2. In most of these persons, this disease has not been officially diagnosed and they are unaware that they are infected. Nevertheless, they experience asymptomatic shedding and unknowingly transmit the disease to sexual partners. Interrupting this cycle of transmission has become a major focus among health care providers who work with these patients. A combination of patient education and appropriate use of systemic antiviral agents may be gradually having some impact on this epidemic. Recommendations for patients with genital herpes include avoiding sex with uninfected partners when active lesions or prodromal symptoms are present and routinely using latex condoms to minimize transmission during periods of asymptomatic shedding. Chronic suppressive doses of oral antiviral agents (Table 1), including acyclovir (Zovirax), valacyclovir (Valtrex), and famciclovir (Famvir), significantly reduce the frequency of clinical recurrences as well as the rate of asymptomatic shedding and may be recommended together with these other practices to reduce the risk of transmission.

Although HSV-2 is the etiologic agent in a majority of cases of genital herpes infections, an increasing number of genital herpes infections are caused by HSV-1. Symptomatic recurrences and asymptomatic shedding are less frequent with genital HSV-1 infection than with genital HSV-2 infection, and this distinction becomes important for patient counseling and prognosis.

Other Mucocutaneous Herpes Simplex Virus Infections
Eczema herpeticum, also known as Kaposi's varicelliform eruption, represents a cutaneous dissemination of HSV usually seen in patients with atopic dermatitis or other underlying skin disease.

Herpetic vesicles develop over an extensive mucocutaneous surface, most often the face, neck, and upper trunk, presumably spreading from a recurrent oral HSV infection or asymptomatic shedding from the oral mucosa. Eczema herpeticum can also develop in the presence of genital HSV. As with other HSV infections, eczema herpeticum may be recurrent. In addition, patients can develop localized, recurrent HSV in previously involved areas. Because of the extensive and inflammatory nature of the process and the possible secondary bacterial infection, the underlying viral etiology may be obscured. A history of eczema and recurrent HSV in the patient and careful observation for the grouped vesicles or erosions can be key to the correct diagnosis.

Herpetic whitlow refers to HSV infection of the hand, usually one or more distal digits. Previously thought to be limited to health care professionals with exposure to oral secretions of their patients, it is now recognized that autoinoculation from orolabial or genital HSV contributes to a significant number of cases.

Herpes gladiatorum is a problem seen most commonly in athletes who participate in close contact sports such as wrestling. Typically transmitted from active herpes labialis or asymptomatic shedding in oral secretions of an infected opponent, herpes gladiatorum often affects the head, neck, or shoulders and may be recurrent. In the wrestler with frequent outbreaks, chronic suppressive therapy may be recommended.

Diagnosis
Viral culture remains a common and acceptable method for diagnosing HSV infection. This method is sensitive when specimens are obtained from lesions that have not yet become too dry or crusted, usually during the first 2 to 3 days after onset. An adequate sample, obtained by unroofing the blister and swabbing the base, increases the likelihood of an accurate result. Antigen detection tests can remain positive even after lesions have dried, as long as the specimen includes epithelial cells and not just debris. For this method, a scraping from the lesion is usually smeared on a glass slide to be sent to the laboratory. Not all antigen detection methods are designed to distinguish HSV-1 from HSV-2.

Polymerase chain reaction (PCR) is highly sensitive and has become routinely available for diagnosis of mucocutaneous HSV infections.

The Tzanck smear (cytologic detection) is both insensitive and nonspecific but may be of use in some clinical settings. It does not differentiate HSV types or HSV from varicella-zoster virus (VZV).

Serologic testing for HSV was previously of limited use because it could not reliably differentiate HSV-1 from HSV-2. Because they share significant genetic homology, HSV-1 and HSV-2 code for a number of common proteins that are not antigenically distinct. However, they also code for type-specific proteins that can be used to differentiate them. Current tests based on detecting type-specific viral glycoprotein G (gG-based, type-specific assays) are accurate and should be requested for this purpose. A positive HSV-2 serology may be useful in confirming the diagnosis of genital herpes in a patient with a negative viral culture or with unrecognized or asymptomatic disease. Alternatively, a negative serology can help exclude the diagnosis of HSV in a patient with chronic, nonspecific oral or genital symptoms.

Varicella-Zoster Virus
VZV, another member of the human herpesvirus family, produces two specific patterns of disease in the skin. The primary infection results in varicella, also known as chickenpox, a widespread vesicular eruption usually seen in the pediatric population. Following the primary infection, VZV establishes latency in the dorsal root ganglia until some later point, when reactivation can occur. The ensuing unilateral dermatomal distribution of blisters, often preceded by neuralgic pain, is known as herpes zoster or shingles. Herpes zoster is especially common in patients older than 50 years, but it may be seen at any age. It is also seen more commonly in immunocompromised patients, such as organ-transplant recipients or patients infected with HIV. Herpes zoster is no longer

---

TABLE 1	Recommendations for Systemic Antiviral Treatment of Mucocutaneous Herpes Simplex Virus Infection	
EPISODE	**DRUG**	**DOSAGE**
Genital Herpes Simplex Virus		
Primary or first episode	Acyclovir	Mild to moderate: 400 mg PO tid[3] or 200 mg PO 5 ×/d × 7–10 d Severe: 5 mg/kg IV q8h × 5 d
	Valacyclovir	1 g PO bid × 7–10 d
	Famciclovir[1]	250 mg PO tid × 10 d
Recurrent episode (start at prodrome)	Acyclovir	400 mg PO tid × 5 d[3] or 800 mg PO bid × 5 d[3] or 800 mg PO tid × 2 d[3]
	Valacyclovir	500 mg PO bid × 3 d or 1 g daily × 5 d
	Famciclovir	1 g PO bid × 1 d or 125 mg PO bid × 5 d
Chronic suppression	Acyclovir	>6 outbreaks per year: 400 mg PO bid or 200 mg PO tid Adjust up or down according to response
	Valacyclovir	6–10 outbreaks per year: 500 mg PO qd ≥10 outbreaks/year: 1 g PO qd
	Famciclovir	≥6 outbreaks/year: 250 mg PO bid
Orofacial Herpes Simplex Virus		
Primary or first episode	Acyclovir[1] Valacyclovir[1] Famciclovir[1]	15 mg/kg 5 ×/d × 7 d 1 g bid × 7 d 500 mg bid × 7 d
Recurrent episode (start at prodrome)	Acyclovir[1] Valacyclovir[1] Famciclovir	400 mg PO 5 ×/d × 5 d 2 g PO bid × 1 d 1500 mg in 1 dose
Chronic suppression	Acyclovir[1] Valacyclovir[1]	400 mg PO bid-tid 500 mg–1 g PO qd
Orolabial or Genital Herpes Simplex Virus in Immunosuppressed Patients		
Recurrent or suppressive	Acyclovir[1]	400 mg PO tid or 5–10 mg/kg IV q8h
	Valacyclovir	500 mg–1 g PO bid
	Famciclovir	500 mg PO bid

[1]Not FDA approved for this indication.
[3]Exceeds dosage recommended by the manufacturer.

considered a marker for underlying cancer, and evaluation for occult malignancy in an otherwise asymptomatic patient is not indicated. A single recurrence of herpes zoster, usually in the same dermatome, may occur but this is uncommon in immunocompetent individuals. Additional recurrences, however, suggest a dermatomal form of HSV, and laboratory assessment for this possibility may be indicated.

The most common dermatomes involved with herpes zoster are in the thoracolumbar (T3-L2) and trigeminal (V1) regions. Skin lesions typically evolve from papules to vesicles and pustules, and then to crusted erosions, before healing approximately 2 to 4 weeks after onset. The associated neuropathic pain commonly persists after the lesions have healed. Pain that continues for more than 3 months after the skin lesions resolve is referred to as postherpetic neuralgia, one of the most common and debilitating complications of this infection.

Several clinical presentations of herpes zoster deserve additional attention. Ophthalmic zoster, with lesions along the tip, side, or base of the nose indicating involvement of the nasociliary branch of the trigeminal nerve (Hutchinson's sign), may be associated with increased risk for ocular complications. Prompt initiation of a systemic antiviral agent (Table 2) and evaluation by an ophthalmologist are recommended. Disseminated zoster, with more than a few lesions outside the primary and immediately adjacent dermatomes, can indicate visceral involvement and its associated complications. The term "zoster sine herpete" describes patients with neuropathic pain resembling zoster but without any skin lesions. The diagnosis can be supported by demonstration of increased IgG antibody titers between the acute and convalescent phases. Chronic zoster is seen predominantly in HIV-infected persons. Single or multiple warty growths can persist for weeks or months in areas of skin previously involved by typical lesions of varicella or herpes zoster. Chronic zoster is often resistant to acyclovir. Tissue biopsy and viral cultures, with further testing for antiviral resistance, may aid in assessment.

Herpes Zoster

Diagnosis

Diagnosis of herpes zoster is often made on clinical grounds alone. A Tzanck smear can provide additional support of the viral etiology. With atypical presentations, however, the diagnosis is best confirmed by either an antigen detection method or viral culture. Both differentiate VZV from HSV. Samples submitted for viral culture should be obtained from vesicular fluid because dried or crusted lesions are unlikely to yield positive results. Viral cultures are required if there is a need to assess possible antiviral resistance. PCR can be useful for detecting VZV in bodily fluids such as cerebrospinal fluid. Basic VZV serology is rarely useful for diagnosis, because a majority of the population is seropositive.

Treatment

There are three systemic antiviral agents routinely used for the treatment of HSV and VZV infections: acyclovir, valacyclovir, and famciclovir. All three are highly effective and generally well tolerated. Because they inhibit only actively replicating viral DNA, they have no impact on latent infection. Recommendations for antiviral treatment of mucocutaneous HSV infections and herpes zoster, localized topical measures, and available formulations are outlined in Tables 1 to 5. Optimal antiviral dosage schedules for less-common HSV infections, such as herpetic whitlow, have not been determined. The doses outlined in Table 1 for either episodic or chronic suppressive therapy can be used as a guideline in these cases.

Acyclovir became available more than 25 years ago and continues to be widely used. Inside an infected host cell, acyclovir must be phosphorylated—first by a virally encoded enzyme (thymidine kinase) and then by host-cell enzymes—to the active form of the drug, acyclovir triphosphate. As a nucleotide analogue, acyclovir triphosphate is incorporated into replicating viral DNA, abruptly terminating further synthesis of that viral DNA chain. Acyclovir triphosphate also interferes with viral DNA replication by directly inhibiting viral DNA polymerase. Valacyclovir is an oral prodrug of acyclovir and has a much higher bioavailability. After ingestion, valacyclovir is rapidly metabolized to acyclovir, and the subsequent mechanism of action is as just described. Famciclovir is an oral prodrug of penciclovir (Denavir), designed for greater bioavailability. Similar to acyclovir, penciclovir must first be phosphorylated by viral thymidine kinase and then by cellular

---

TABLE 2 Recommendations for Systemic Antiviral Treatment of Herpes Zoster

	DOSAGE	
DRUG	**IMMUNO-COMPETENT PATIENTS**	**IMMUNO-SUPPRESSED PATIENTS**
Acyclovir	800 mg PO 5 × per d × 7–10 d	800 mg PO 5 × per d × 10 d* 10 mg/kg/dose IV q8h × 7–10 d*
Valacyclovir	1 g PO tid × 7 d	1 g PO tid × 10 d*
Famciclovir	500 mg PO tid × 7 d	500 mg PO tid × 10 d*

*Continue until there are no new lesions for 48 h.

TABLE 3 Topical Treatment Options for Mucocutaneous Herpes Simplex Virus and Varicella-Zoster Virus Infections

TREATMENT	COMMENT
Cool, moist compresses using tap water or aluminum acetate 1:20 to 1:40 (Burow's solution, Domeboro, Bluboro)	Good for moist, oozing lesions to accelerate drying. Apply wet dressing to involved skin and cover with a dry cloth to allow evaporation
Calamine lotion or similar shake lotion containing alcohol, menthol, and/or phenol; Aveeno colloidal oatmeal	Useful as drying and antipruritic agent. May be applied after wet dressing
Bacitracin,[1] Polysporin, mupirocin[1] (Bactroban)	Use if there is concern for localized secondary bacterial infection
2% Viscous lidocaine, compounded suspensions[1,6] (e.g., Kaopectate[1] or Maalox,[1] diphenhydramine,[1] lidocaine)	Useful for temporary pain relief of oral or genital mucosal involvement
Acyclovir ointment	Used together with systemic antiviral agents, may be of benefit to immunocompromised individuals for localized HSV
Penciclovir (Denavir) cream	Can decrease the duration of lesions in herpes labialis by half a day if applied every 2 h while awake for 4 days beginning at the first sign of disease
Acyclovir buccal tablet (Sitavig) 50 mg	Can decrease the duration of herpes labialis by 0.8 days if single tablet is applied within 1 hour of prodromal symptons

[1] Not FDA approved for this indication.
[6] May be compounded by pharmacists.
Abbreviation: HSV = herpes simplex virus.

TABLE 4 Formulations of Acyclovir, Valacyclovir, and Famciclovir

DRUG	ORAL	TOPICAL	INTRAVENOUS
Acyclovir	200, 400, 800 mg 50 mg buccal tablet	5% Ointment (5g, 15g, 30g) 5% cream (5 g)	Yes
Valacyclovir	500 mg, 1 g	No	No
Famciclovir	125, 250, 500 mg	No	No
Penciclovir (Denavir)	No	1% cream (1.5 g, 5 g)	No

TABLE 5 Recommended Antiviral Dose Modification in Patients with Impaired Renal Function

CREATININE CLEARANCE (ml/min)	GENITAL HERPES SIMPLEX VIRUS			HERPES ZOSTER	HERPES LABIALIS
	INITIAL	RECURRENT	SUPPRESSION		
Acyclovir (Zovirax)					
>25	200 mg 5 ×/d	200 mg 5 ×/d	400 mg q12h	800 mg 5×/d	
10–24	200 mg 5 ×/d	200 mg 5 ×/d	400 mg q12h	800 mg q8h	
<10	200 mg q12h	200 mg q12h	200 mg q12h	800 mg q12h	
Valacyclovir (Valtrex)					
>50	1 g q12h	500 mg q12h	500 mg-1 g q24h	1 g q8h	2 g PO bid for 1 d
30–49	1 g q12h	500 mg q12h	500 mg-1 g q24h	1 g q12h	1 g PO bid for 1 d
10–29	1 g q24h	500 mg q24h	500 mg q24-48h	1 g q24h	500 mg bid for 1 d
<10	500 mg q24h	500 mg q24h	500 mg q24-48h	500 mg q24h	500 mg single dose
Famciclovir (Famvir)					
>60		125 mg q12h	250 mg q12h	500 mg q8h	
40–59		125 mg q12h	250 mg q12h	500 mg q12h	
20–39		125 mg q24h	125 mg q12h	500 mg q24h	
<20		125 mg q24h	125 mg q24h	250 mg q24h	
>60	1 g bid × 1 d				1500 mg single dose
40–59	500 mg bid × 1 d				750 mg single dose
20–39	500 mg single dose				500 mg single dose
<20	250 mg single dose				250 mg single dose

enzymes to penciclovir triphosphate. In this active form, penciclovir triphosphate interferes with viral DNA synthesis and replication by inhibiting viral DNA polymerase. Famciclovir has greater bioavailability and a longer intracellular half-life than acyclovir. For all three agents, the required activation by viral thymidine kinase and the preferential inhibition of viral DNA synthesis contribute to the highly specific antiviral activity.

If taken as recommended, acyclovir, valacyclovir, and famciclovir are generally comparable in their safety and effectiveness. Valacyclovir and famciclovir offer the convenience of less-frequent dosing. Dosing for all three should be adjusted in the presence of renal insufficiency (see Table 5).

Although antiviral therapy does not decrease the incidence of postherpetic neuralgia, all three agents decrease the time for lesion healing and shorten the overall duration of pain if initiated within 48 to 72 hours after the onset of herpes zoster. Valacyclovir and famciclovir appear to be more effective than acyclovir for this purpose, presumably because of easier dosing. An otherwise healthy person younger than 50 years who has discrete involvement on the trunk and mild to moderate pain might benefit minimally or not at all from this intervention, especially if it is initiated after 72 hours of lesion onset. However, patients who are older than 50 years, are immunosuppressed, have involvement in the ophthalmic distribution, or have more-extensive lesions or severe pain should receive systemic antiviral therapy, even if the 72-hour deadline has expired. Adequate pain control, often requiring opiates, is also important.

The addition of systemic corticosteroids to the antiviral regimen remains controversial. There is evidence to suggest this can lessen the severity of the acute episode but does not decrease the incidence or duration of postherpetic neuralgia. Corticosteroids may be of benefit in herpes zoster complicated by facial paralysis or cranial polyneuropathy. Corticosteroids should not be used without concomitant systemic antiviral therapy.

In patients 60 years of age or older, the live-attenuated herpes zoster vaccine (Zostavax) was shown to substantially reduce the incidence of both herpes zoster and postherpetic neuralgia. It is recommended that this option be discussed with immunocompetent patients in this older age group.

Despite widespread use of these antiviral agents, antiviral resistance is rarely a problem in the immunocompetent population. However, it does arise in the setting of immunosuppression. The basis for the resistance is most commonly a mutation in the gene coding for thymidine kinase. Less often there is a mutation in the viral DNA polymerase. In either case, all three standard drugs become ineffective. Alternative antiviral agents available for treatment of acyclovir-resistant HSV and VZV infections include foscarnet (Foscavir)[1] and cidofovir (Vistide).[1]

---

[1]Not FDA approved for this indication.

Hand-Foot-and-Mouth Disease

Hand-foot-and-mouth disease is typically a disease of childhood. The most common etiologic agent is a nonpolio enterovirus, Coxsackie A16, and transmission is via the oral–oral or fecal–oral route. It is highly contagious. Several days after exposure, a prodrome of low-grade fever, malaise, abdominal pain, or respiratory symptoms can develop, followed by the appearance of papulovesicles on the palate, tongue, or buccal mucosa. Similar lesions can subsequently develop on the feet and hands. The eruption persists for 7 to 10 days and then resolves. Treatment is symptomatic. Nail dystrophies including onychomadesis (separation of the proximal portion of the nail plate from the nail bed) and Beau's lines (horizontal grooves in the nail plate) may be seen 2-4 weeks later.

Since 1997, outbreaks of hand-foot-and-mouth disease caused by enterovirus 71 have been reported in Asia and Australia. Although hand-foot-and-mouth disease associated with Coxsackie A16 infection is typically a mild illness, hand-foot-and-mouth disease caused by enterovirus 71 has shown a higher incidence of neurologic involvement, including fatal cases of encephalitis.

An atypical hand-foot-and-mouth disease with more widespread cutaneous involvement has been reported as associated with coxsackievirus A6. There is a predilection for areas commonly involved in atopic dermatitis, such as the antecubital and popliteal fossae and this presentation may be confused with eczema herpeticum or VZV infection. Diagnosis of these more atypical cases may require laboratory assessment. This could include antigen detection or PCR to exclude HSV and VZV. Reverse Transcription PCR (RT-PCR) of vesicle fluid, oropharyngeal swab or stool specimen may be used to confirm the enterovirus infection.

Parvovirus B19

Cutaneous manifestations of parvovirus B19 infection include the childhood exanthem known as erythema infectiosum (fifth disease) and, less commonly, petechial or purpuric eruptions. The virus is transmitted primarily via respiratory secretions and, to a much lesser extent, through blood or blood products. The host cells for viral replication are erythroid progenitor cells, which subsequently undergo cell lysis.

A child with erythema infectiosum typically develops a low-grade fever and nonspecific upper respiratory symptoms approximately 2 days before the onset of rash. The rash has been described as having a slapped-cheeks appearance, with prominent redness over the malar eminences. This is followed by a pink-to-red lacy or reticular eruption over the trunk and extensor surfaces of the arms and legs. The rash usually lasts a week to 10 days but can transiently recur over months in response to precipitating factors such as sunlight, exercise, and bathing. Diagnosis of erythema infectiosum is usually made on clinical grounds, and treatment is symptomatic. By the time the rash appears and the diagnosis has been made, the child is no longer infectious. Much less commonly parvovirus B19 infection may manifest as a papular-purpuric eruption with edema, erythema, and patecchiae in a "gloves and socks" distribution on the hands and feet.

Infection with parvovirus B19 in older adolescents and adults often manifests with arthralgias or arthritis rather than a rash. In certain patient populations, parvovirus B19 infections may be associated with complications including transient aplastic crisis, chronic anemia, and hydrops fetalis. In these less-typical presentations, serology (anti-B19 IgM or documented seroconversion) may be needed for diagnosis. Intravenous immunoglobulin (IVIg [Gamimune N][1]) is used successfully for treatment of chronic or persistent infection in immunosuppressed patients.

Molluscum Contagiosum

Molluscum contagiosum are benign umbilicated papules caused by infection with the *Molluscipoxvirus,* a member of the poxvirus family. Lesions are limited to the mucocutaneous surface and typically appear in clusters on the face, trunk, and skin fold areas in

---

[1]Not FDA approved for this indication.

TABLE 6	Treatment Options for Molluscum Contagiosum
TREATMENT	**COMMENT**
Cryotherapy (liquid nitrogen)	Freeze individual lesions for 5–10 sec Repeat PRN in 2–3 wk
Curettage	Entire lesion may be removed using a curette; this results in bleeding Removal of central core with toothpick or other pointed instrument is also effective
Cantharidin (Cantharone)[1]	Blister-inducing agent: Apply to lesion with toothpick, air dry Cover with tape or adhesive bandage Patient to wash area after 24 h (or sooner if significant pain)
Podophyllin (25% in tincture of benzoin)[1]	Cytotoxic agent: Apply to lesion with toothpick Patient to wash off after 4–6 h Contraindicated in pregnancy
Podofilox (Condylox 0.5% gel or solution)[1]	Done by patient: Apply bid for 3 consecutive d/wk × 2–4 wk Contraindicated in pregnancy
Salicylic acid/lactic acid (Occlusal, Duofilm)[1]	Done by patient: Apply daily
Imiquimod (Aldara) 5% cream[1]	Done by patient: Apply daily 5 consecutive d/wk Leave on overnight Continue for 8–12 wk
Cimetidine (Tagamet)[1]	30 mg/kg/d PO × 6–12 wk Can boost cell-mediated immunity
Candida antigen (Candin)[1]	Intralesional injection 0.3 mL[3]

[1]Not FDA approved for this indication.
[3]Exceeds dosage recommended by the manufacturer.

children and on thighs, lower abdomen, and suprapubic areas in sexually active adults. Large numbers of lesions in an extensive distribution may be seen in the immunosuppressed population.

Transmission routinely occurs by skin-to-skin contact with an infected host, but transmission from contaminated fomites has been reported. Autoinoculation commonly occurs. Diagnosis is usually based on clinical examination, but histopathology of atypical lesions may be used for confirmation.

Because molluscum contagiosum tends to be self-limited, treatment is not always required, but it can reduce the risk of autoinoculation and transmission to others. Treatment modalities are primarily aimed at destroying the lesions, similar to those used for verruca vulgaris (Table 6). In the case of sexual transmission, evaluation for other sexually transmitted diseases may be indicated.

Orf and Milker's Nodules

Orf (also known as ecthyma contagiosum) and milker's nodules are caused by the closely related *Parapoxvirus,* a member of the poxvirus family. The virus responsible for orf is widespread in sheep and goats, whereas the virus causing milker's nodules is found in cattle. Transmission to humans is by direct contact with infected animals or recently vaccinated animals and is usually seen several days and up to 2 weeks after exposure. Preexisting skin trauma or other disruption of the normal cutaneous barrier enhances the risk of transmission. Barrier precautions and proper hand hygiene are important preventive measures.

Orf and milker's nodules most commonly appear as one to several nodules on the dorsal aspect of the hands or forearms. Lesions evolve through several clinical stages over a period of 3 to 5 weeks, ranging from solid red nodules to vesicular, exudative, or wartlike tumors. As with other poxvirus infections, lesions of orf often demonstrate central umbilication. Regional lymphadenopathy and lymphangitis are commonly seen.

Diagnosis is based on a history of exposure and clinical examination. Tissue biopsy for histopathology or electron microscopy may also be used. Orf virus infection can resemble skin lesions associated with potentially life-threatening zoonotic infections such as tularemia, cutaneous anthrax, and erysipeloid. Should this be a concern, definitive diagnostic testing using PCR is available through the Centers for Disease Control and Prevention (CDC).

In general, the lesions of orf are self-limited, resolving within 4 to 6 weeks, and treatment is not routinely required. However, immunocompromised persons can develop more progressive and destructive lesions requiring therapeutic intervention such as topical cidofovir[1,6] or imiquimod (Aldara).[1]

---

[1]Not FDA approved for this indication.
[6]May be compounded by pharmacists.

References

Centers for Disease Control and Prevention. Sexually Transmitted Diseases Treatment Guidelines, 2010. MMWR 2010:59(RR-12). Available from URL: http://www.cdc.gov/STD/treatment/2010/.

Cernik C, Gallina K, Brodell RT. The treatment of herpes simplex infections: an evidence-based review. Arch Intern Med 2008;168(11):1137–44. http://dx.doi.org/10.1001/archinte.168.11.1137.

Chen X, Anstey AV, Bugert JJ. Molluscum contagiosum virus infection. Lancet Infect Dis 2013;13(10):877–88.

Downing C, Ramirez-Fort MK, Doan HQ, et al. Coxsackievirus A6 associated hand, foot and mouth disease in adults: Clinical presentation and review of the literature. J Clin Virol 2014;60(4):381–6.

Fang Y, Wang S, Zhang L, et al. Risk factors of severe hand, foot and mouth disease: A meta-analysis. Scand J Infect Dis 2014;46(7):515–22.

Human Orf virus infection from household exposures - United States, 2009–2011. Centers for Disease Control and Prevention (CDC). MMWR Morb Mortal Wkly Rep 2012;61(14):245–8.

Kim SR, Khan F, Ramirez-Fort MK, Downing C, Tyring SK. Varicella zoster: an update on current treatment options and future perspectives. Expert Opin Pharmacother 2014;15(1):61–71.

Sabanathan S, Tan le V, Thwaites L, Wills B, Qui PT, Rogier van Doorn H. Enterovirus 71 related severe hand, foot and mouth disease outbreaks in South-East Asia: current situation and ongoing challenges.

Valentin MN, Cohen PJ. Pediatric parvovirus B19: spectrum of clinical manifestations. Cutis 2013;92(4):179–84.

Westhoff GL, Little SE, Caughey AB. Herpes simplex virus and pregnancy: a review of the management of antenatal and peripartum herpes infections. Obstet Gynecol Surv 2011;66(10):629–38.

WARTS (VERRUCAE)

Method of
M. Chantel Long, MD

CURRENT DIAGNOSIS

- Common warts: rough, hyperkeratotic, firm papules usually found on the extremities.
- Flat warts: small, flat, pink or flesh-colored papules on the face, arms, or legs.
- Plantar and palmar warts: callus-like lesions that disrupt skin lines on the soles or palms.
- Mosaic warts: large clusters of warts.
- Filiform warts: small, finger-like lesions on the face.
- Genital warts: flesh to brown colored, flat or exophytic, found in the anogenital region.
- Differential diagnoses: seborrheic keratoses, molluscum contagiosum, keratoacanthoma, squamous cell carcinoma, acrochordon, amelanocytic melanoma, calluses, and corns.

CURRENT THERAPY

- Approximately 20% of warts spontaneously resolve within 3 months and 60% within 2 years in a healthy person.
- Salicylic acid and dimethyl ether.
- Cryotherapy.
- Cantharidin (Cantharone).[1,6]
- Surgical removal.
- Pulsed-dye laser.
- Immunotherapy: topical imiquimod (Aldara),[1] intralesional *Candida* antigen (Candin).[1]
- Photodynamic therapy.

---

[1]Not FDA approved for this indication.
[6]May be compounded by pharmacists.
Note: Cantharidin and Candin are not FDA approved. Aldara is approved for genital and perianal warts only.

Verrucae, commonly known as cutaneous warts, are benign skin growths caused by the human papillomavirus (HPV). Cutaneous warts are divided into common warts, plantar warts, flat warts, and genital warts. Common warts account for 70% of all cutaneous warts. Two-thirds of untreated common warts spontaneously regress within 2 years, but previously infected individuals have a higher rate of developing new warts than those who were never infected.

Epidemiology

It is estimated that 10% of the general population has cutaneous warts, and warts are one of the most common reasons for dermatologic visits. Transmission occurs through direct contact with an infected person or indirectly through fomites. As a result, warts are seen with greater frequency among groups of people in close contact, such as schoolchildren. Thus, warts are more common in adolescents with a frequency estimated as high as 20%. Since the extent of infection is determined by the immune response, warts are also more common in immunocompromised patients. Autoinoculation is possible by scratching the lesions, often leading to a linear pattern.

Pathophysiology

Warts are caused by HPV. More than 100 genotypes of HPV have been identified, and the virus is prevalent. HPV causes both clinical and subclinical infections and plays a role in certain cutaneous malignancies, including squamous cell carcinoma. It is found in the basal layer of the epidermis but replicates in the superficial, well-differentiated layer of the skin. The cellular proliferation gives rise to thick, hyperkeratotic lesions generally known as warts. The warts can occur anywhere on the skin or mucous membranes.

Clinical Manifestations

Most warts are asymptomatic, though patients often present with complaints of a "bump." Usually, the warts appear flesh-colored, brown, or gray and can be flat to exophytic, giving them the classic "cauliflower" appearance. The lesions may be single or multiple and may range in size from miniscule to several centimeters in diameter. Localized irritation, pruritus, pain, or bleeding may occur. Symptoms vary based on the location and size of the lesions.

Several types of warts occur with variations in appearance, site of infection, and the specific type of HPV involved. Common warts (verrucae vulgaris) are white to flesh-colored, rough, hyperkeratotic, raised, and firm, usually found on the extremities. They disrupt normal skin lines on the fingers and toes and are most associated with HPV types 1, 2, and 4. Flat warts (verrucae plana) are caused by HPV types 3, 10, or 28 and are tan to flesh colored. They are small, 1 to 3 mm in diameter, flat, sharply demarcated growths that appear in large numbers on the face, arms, or legs. They usually occur in a linear arrangement related to local trauma, such as shaving. Butcher warts are associated with HPV type 7 and have a thick, raised, exophytic appearance. They are most common in workers who regularly handle raw meat or fish. Plantar and palmar warts (verrucae plantaris and verrucae palmaris) are hard, thickened, callus-like lesions that disrupt skin lines on the soles or palms. They are associated with HPV types 1, 2, 4, 27, and 57. They are usually flesh colored, covered with callus, and can be painful, especially when located on pressure points. If warts coalesce into a plaque, this is termed a *mosaic* wart. Filiform warts are slender, finger-like growths most commonly seen on the face, especially around the eyelids, nose, and mouth. Periungual warts are common warts impinging on and growing under toenails or fingernails. Genital warts (condyloma acuminatum) are flesh colored to brown, flat or exophytic lesions, occurring in anogenital regions. Mucosal papillomas are warts that occur on mucous membranes, usually in the mouth or vagina, and tend to be white in color.

Epidermodysplasia verruciformis is a rare, autosomal recessive disorder that leads to widespread reddish brown, flat papules on the trunk, hands, face, and extremities. These warts have malignant potential, especially on sun-exposed areas. It is estimated that one-third may become malignant. These patients present in childhood. Chronically infected with multiple types of HPV, including types 3, 5, 8, 9, 12, 14, 15, 17, 19 to 25, 36 to 38, 47, 49, and 50, the warts have lifelong persistence. Another related disease is verrucous carcinoma. This is a slow-growing variant of squamous cell carcinoma that occurs in the oral mucosa, anogenital region, or plantar surface. These warts are associated with HPV types 6 and 11.

Risk Factors

Risk factors most associated with verrucae include immunosuppression and close contact. Due to their decreased immune response, immunocompromised hosts are at increased risk not only for infection, but also for malignant transformation of the warts. Pregnancy, previous wart infection, and handling raw meat or fish are also known risk factors.

Differential Diagnosis

The differential diagnosis of warts includes seborrheic keratoses, molluscum contagiosum, keratoacanthoma, squamous cell carcinoma, acrochordon, amelanocytic melanoma, porokeratosis, calluses, and corns.

Diagnosis is based on clinical findings. When the clinical appearance of the lesion is typical, no other confirmatory tests are usually necessary. Paring down the stratum corneum, or outer layer of skin, may reveal black dots, which are thrombosed or bleeding capillaries, and helps confirm the diagnosis. If needed, tissue biopsy can provide histopathologic confirmation. In immunocompromised patients, biopsy is recommended to rule out squamous cell carcinoma in any suspicious lesions, which includes large or rapidly growing, pigmented, atypical, friable, bleeding, or ulcerated lesions.

Treatment

Approximately 20% of warts spontaneously resolve within 3 months and 60% within 2 years in a healthy person. Therefore, treatment is not always necessary. Current treatments do not eradicate the virus and do not guarantee resolution. Most patients seek treatment because of the physical appearance, discomfort, or interference with daily and social functioning, especially if located on the palms, digits, or soles. The American Academy of Dermatology established reasoning for wart treatment, including the desire of the patient; for symptoms of pain, bleeding, itching, or burning; for disabling or disfiguring lesions; for large numbers or large size of lesions; for a desire to prevent spread to unblemished skin; and because of a concomitant immunocompromised condition. Immunosuppressed patients are at higher risk for developing numerous

warts and require treatment to prevent progression to squamous cell carcinoma. It is often more difficult to eradicate warts in an immunosuppressed host.

Many therapeutic modalities are available for the treatment of warts. No single therapy is universally effective. Warts can resolve, recur, shrink, or grow despite therapy. It is likely that all wart therapies work by triggering an immune response to the presence of papillomavirus in the skin. Treatment of warts must be individualized and often more than one modality is needed to achieve resolution. Conservative, less painful, and less expensive treatments are preferred.

Treatment methods are divided into the categories of home remedies, over-the-counter treatments, and office-based therapies. Office-based treatments include destructive methods, surgical or laser procedures, immunologic intervention, and combination therapy.

Home Remedies

Home remedies include applications of tea tree oil,[7] garlic extract,[7] duct tape,[1] and hyperthermic therapy. One study comparing cryotherapy with duct tape occlusion of common warts showed resolution in 85% of the children treated by occlusion, compared with 60% in the liquid nitrogen group. Proper protocol involves covering the wart with duct tape, which is left in place for 6 days. Then the site should be soaked, pared down with an emery board, and left uncovered overnight. This is repeated for a total of eight cycles. Another common home remedy is hyperthermic therapy. This involves immersing the affected area in a 45°C water bath for 30 minutes three times per week. It is a safe and inexpensive option.

Over-the-Counter Treatment

The most common over-the-counter option used by patients is one of the salicylic acid products, such as Compound W, Duofilm, Occlusal-HP, and Mediplast. These keratolytic products are offered as a solution, gel, cream, or pad in concentrations from 10% to 60%. They can be quite successful when used consistently and as directed in motivated patients. Repeated application, with pumice stone or callus file use, results in cure rates of 60% to 80%, but takes several weeks to work.

More recently, several over-the-counter wart-freezing therapies have become available. One such option is dimethyl ether, marketed as Compound W Freeze Off or Dr. Scholl's Freeze Away. These are available in aerosol form for wart treatment, which can be repeated every 2 weeks. Dimethyl ether achieves a temperature of −57°C, which is markedly higher than the −196°C temperature obtained with liquid nitrogen. This results in a more shallow depth of destruction. Because salicylic acid and dimethyl ether treatments destroy the infected epidermis and cause an immune reaction, they can be irritating and tedious, prompting many patients to seek medical care.

Office-based Treatment

Office-based treatments are largely destructive, immunomodulating, or both. Destructive treatments include cryosurgery, surgical excision, laser therapy, or repeated application of topical chemotherapy agents, such as salicylic acid, cantharidin (Cantharone),[1,6] podophyllin (Podocon),[1] or 5-fluorouracil (Efudex).[1] The most commonly used physician office-based treatment is cryotherapy with liquid nitrogen. It can be applied by a cotton-tipped applicator or cryogun. The wart and a 1 to 2 mm margin are frozen for 10 to 30 seconds. The freeze should be repeated once after a thaw of 20 seconds. If the warts are thick, they can initially be pared down. The patient is told that a blister will result and should be left intact if possible. Treatment should be repeated every 3 to 4 weeks until normal skin markings return. Cryotherapy has demonstrated a

---

[1]Not FDA approved for this indication.
[6]May be compounded by pharmacists.
[7]Available as a dietary supplement.

60% to 80% cure rate. If warts persist beyond 3 months of therapy, another method of treatment should be selected.

Another option is cantharidin (Cantharone) in a 0.7% colloidal solution. It is a chemical derived from blister beetles that is painless on application and well tolerated by children. It causes epidermal necrosis with blistering after application and occlusion for 8 hours. It is applied in the office and repeated every 4 weeks. Although not Food and Drug Administration (FDA) approved, it is a commonly used technique and can be compounded by a pharmacist. It is useful for treatment of common, periungual, and plantar warts in children, and the cure rate approaches 80%. Unfortunately, an occasional "donut wart," a ring of new warts surrounding the cleared original site, occurs.

Surgery is used for large, solitary warts, and is more direct. Large common warts of the hands or extremities are more easily treated if they are debulked surgically. This method is not recommended for plantar warts because of scarring. Surgical removal followed by electrodesiccation and curettage is effective but requires local anesthesia and can result in scarring.

Other destructive methods of wart removal usually are reserved for resistant, multiple lesions, or recalcitrant warts in immunosuppressed patients. This often requires specialty referral. Acids, including bichloroacetic and trichloroacetic acid (Tri-Chlor),[1] should be applied by a skilled practitioner because they are known to cause pain on application, ulceration, and even scarring. Laser therapy, most often with a pulsed-dye laser (PDL) or carbon dioxide (CO_2) laser, provides selective photothermolysis of blood vessels within the wart, which compromises blood supply and results in necrosis. The PDL method is less aggressive and less painful than CO_2 vaporization. These treatments cause minimal damage to normal skin. Overall, both therapies are generally well tolerated, but local anesthesia may be necessary. Although more expensive, these methods have cure rates ranging from 45% to 90%. Photodynamic therapy (PDT) is useful for patients with multiple recalcitrant warts, especially patients who are immunosuppressed. PDT involves a topical photosensitizer applied by a trained provider. It is activated by visible light, resulting in tissue destruction. Studies of this method have been promising.

Immune modulation alone or in combination with destructive methods is helpful in treating resistant warts. The self-applied immunomodulator imiquimod (Aldara) was initially approved for treatment of genital warts. It is also used anecdotally to treat flat and common warts by inducing cytokines, including interferon production, at the site of application. A thin coat is applied at bedtime and then washed off after 6 to 10 hours. It is usually applied three times weekly and combined with cryotherapy or salicylic acid.

Intralesional immunotherapy, which includes *Candida* antigen (Candin),[1] interferon alfa-2b (Intron A),[1] bleomycin,[1] and MMR vaccine,[1] is an effective option for treatment in some patients. *Candida* antigen injection (Candin) is considered a first-line therapy in children with large or multiple warts and a second-line therapy for patients with resistant warts. It is well tolerated. *Candida* antigen is commercially available as a 1:1000 dilution. Using a 30-gauge needle and tuberculin syringe, one can inject 0.2 to 0.3 mL directly into the wart. Pretesting is unnecessary, side effects are minimal, and more than 75% of patients treated with a series of three injections have clearing of the injected and distant warts. Intralesional interferon alfa-2b (Intron A) has been used successfully to treat genital warts and warts that have not responded to conventional therapies. The clearance rate varies from 36% to 62%, but it requires multiple injections in a physician's office, is expensive, and can cause systemic adverse effects such as flu-like symptoms. Intralesional bleomycin is effective but expensive and causes severe pain. The MMR vaccine is used off-label for intralesional injection and often combined with lidocaine for comfort.

Other topical immunomodulators, such as squaric acid dibutylester (SADBE)[1,6] or diphencyprone,[1,6] are contact sensitizers that induce an allergic dermatitis through type IV hypersensitivity reactions. Although time consuming, treatment with SADBE is well tolerated and a good choice for recalcitrant warts in children. Other topical products available for off-label treatment include retinoids, formaldehyde compounds, and 5-fluorouracil (Efudex).[1] These agents interfere with epidermal proliferation, effect a nonspecific antiviral action, or inhibit mitosis, leading to keratinocyte and viral death. All of these choices usually require specialty referral.

Oral immunomodulation with high-dose cimetidine (Tagamet)[1] has been proposed. It is postulated to enhance cell-mediated immune response. Evidence has been anecdotal. Daily doses of 30 to 40 mg/kg have been used divided twice a day to four times a day for 8 to 12 weeks.

---

[1]Not FDA approved for this indication.

[1]Not FDA approved for this indication.
[6]May be compounded by pharmacists.

TABLE 1 Treatment Regimens

DRUG	AVAILABLE AS	MECHANISM OF ACTION	DISADVANTAGES	INSTRUCTIONS
Patient Applied				
Salicylic acid (Compound W, Duofilm, Occlusol-HP, or Mediplast)	Solution, gel, lotion, cream, plaster, pad 10%–60% concentration	Keratolytic that destroys the infected epidermis while irritation stimulates an immune response	Local irritation Requires multiple applications Requires compliance Wart may need to be pared down to increase penetration	Apply nightly until clear, usually for weeks to months
Dimethyl ether (Compound W, Freeze Off, Dr. Scholl's Freeze Away)	OTC in spray canister	As above	Local irritation Requires compliance Blistering may occur	May treat every 2 weeks Total of four treatments per wart advised
Retinoids (Accutane, Retin-A, Soriatane)[1]	Soriatane (10 and 25 mg tabs), Accutane (10, 20, and 40 mg tabs), Retin-A cream/gel	Antimitotic that interferes with epidermal proliferation	Systemic with mucocutaneous dryness, elevated triglycerides, abnormal liver enzymes Avoid use in pregnancy Local irritation and dryness	Take PO daily If topical form, apply nightly

Continued

TABLE 1 Treatment Regimens—cont'd

DRUG	AVAILABLE AS	MECHANISM OF ACTION	DISADVANTAGES	INSTRUCTIONS
Imiquimod (Aldara)[1]	Cream 5%	Immunomodulator that mediates cytokines	Irritation, erythema, pruritus, scarring, hyperpigmentation	Apply 3 times/wk on mucosal skin Apply daily on keratinized skin
Cimetidine (Tagamet)[1]	Tablets (200, 300, 400 mg) Liquid (300 mg/5 mL)	Immunomodulator that may enhance immune response	Unclear efficacy Diarrhea Many drug-drug interactions	30–40 mg/kg daily, divided bid–qid for 8–12 weeks
Provider Applied				
Cryotherapy	Cryogun or cotton-tip application	Destroys infected dermis, induces inflammation, and leads to stimulated immune response	Pain, erythema, blistering, hypopigmentation, scarring Onychodystrophy if not careful with periungual warts	Freeze for 10–30 seconds with a 1–2 mm border, allow to thaw, then repeat May offer/need local anesthesia May repeat every 3–4 weeks
Candida antigen injections (Candin)[1]	1:1000 dilution	Immunomodulator	Discomfort	Intralesional injection of 0.2–0.3 mL
Trichloroacetic acid (TCA)[1]	Solution, up to 50%	Destroys infected epidermis; best for mucosal surfaces	Pain	Apply sparingly with cotton tip, air dry Repeat weekly to every other week Do not allow to "run" on normal skin Neutralize with soap or sodium bicarbonate
Cantharidin (Cantharone)[1]	Colloidal solution 0.7%, compounded	Destroys epidermis, leads to blister formation Is painless, good for kids	Avoid on face Blistering will occur	Apply with fine applicator to wart only and have patient wash off after 6–8 hr
Surgery		Surgical removal	Avoid if bleeding disorder Often requires anesthesia Scarring	Surgical excision followed by curettage and cauterization
Interferon alpha-2b (Intron A)[1] injections		Immunomodulator	Expensive Flu-like side effects	Multiple intralesional injections several times a week Often requires specialty referral
Laser vaporization		Destroys epidermis	Expensive Requires local anesthesia	Requires specialty referral

[1]Not FDA approved for this indication.
Abbreviations: bid = twice a day; OTC = over-the-counter; PO = orally; qid = four times a day.

To ensure resolution and no recurrence of warts, the patient and practitioner must often make compromises in regard to convenience, discomfort, and scarring. The factors to consider when deciding on treatment include wart location and size, patient tolerance and preference, cost, convenience, and clinician preference. Patient-applied options allow the patient greater control; however, this requires good compliance and the warts must be accessible by the patient or caregiver. Provider-applied treatments are good choices for large treatment areas. Data regarding the efficacy of using more than one modality at a time are lacking. It is common practice for health care providers to combine treatment modalities. Table 1 outlines current therapy regimens.

Patient Education
Counseling of patients regarding the goal and length of treatment is necessary. Patients should be educated that current treatments do not eradicate HPV, and therefore the objective of therapy is elimination of symptoms. They also need to understand that a repeated course of therapy is often required and it may take weeks to months to achieve desired results. Each treatment should be reviewed in detail, including risks and benefits. Subsequently, the management should be tailored depending on the wart, patient, and practitioner.

References
Cockayne S, Hewitt C, Hicks K, et al. Cryotherapy versus salicylic acid for the treatment of plantar warts: a randomized controlled trial. BMJ 2011;342:d3271.
Kwok CS, Holland R, Gibbs S. Efficacy of topical treatments for cutaneous warts: a meta-analysis and pooled analysis of randomized controlled trials. Br J Dermatol 2011;65:233–46.
Leung L. Recalcitrant nongenital warts. Aust Fam Physician 2011;40–2.
Simonart T, De Maertelaer V. Systemic treatments for cutaneous warts: a systematic review. J Dermatolog Treat 2012;23:72–7.
Yelverton CB. Warts. In: Manual of dermatologic therapeutics. 7th ed. Philadelphia: Lippincott Williams & Wilkins; 2007. p. 233–40.

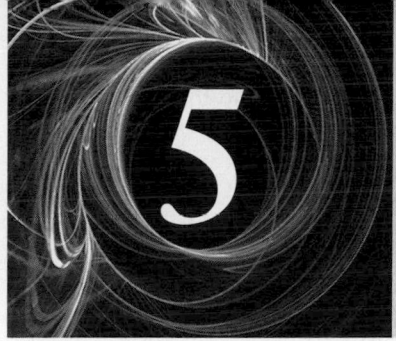

5 Diseases of the Head and Neck

DRY EYE SYNDROME

Method of
John N. Dorsch, MD

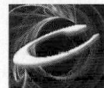

CURRENT DIAGNOSIS

- Signs and symptoms of dry eye syndrome are nonspecific.
- There are many potential causes of dry eye syndrome. There is no definitive diagnostic test for dry eye syndrome.

CURRENT THERAPY

- Artificial tears may help to palliate symptoms, but preservatives in artificial tears may complicate dry eye syndrome.
- Cyclosporine (Restasis) topical medication should be administered under the care of an ophthalmologist.
- Patients with severe symptoms (especially visual disturbance or eye pain) should be referred to an ophthalmologist.

Introduction

Dry eye syndrome, also known as *dry eye, chronic dry eye, dry eye disease,* and *keratoconjunctivitis sicca,* is a condition in which reduced tear secretion and/or increased evaporation of tears causes inflammation of the corneal and conjunctival (ocular) surface.

Epidemiology

An estimated 15% to 20% of patients over 65 years of age have dry eye syndrome, with a higher prevalence in females. Dry eye syndrome is common in a mild form in many patients over the age of 40.[1] The prevalence of dry eye syndrome is believed to be rising as patients live longer and a greater proportion of the population is over 65.

Risk factors

Aging is believed to be the most common cause of dry eye syndrome. Decreases in sex hormone concentration, particularly androgens, play a significant role in lacrimal dysfunction. As patients age, they tend to lose function of many of the accessory lacrimal glands, and experience relatively less secretion from the major lacrimal glands.[1] In many cases, the cause of tear deficiency is not apparent. Box 1 lists many of the common causes of dry eye syndrome.

Pathophysiology

Desiccation of the ocular surface results in symptoms of discomfort, blurry vision, and instability of tear film. Tears are vital for the protection of the ocular surface, which is constantly challenged by the shearing force of blinking, various microbes, and environmental factors such as dust, smoke, wind, and low humidity.

In order to maintain a healthy film of tears, the patient must have synergistic interaction of lacrimal glands, eyelids, ocular surface, afferent and efferent neural pathways, and meibomian glands. Each component works together with all other components; not in isolation. If there is dysfunction of any of these components or any combination of them, the patient is likely to develop dry eye syndrome.

Healthy tear film consists of an outer oily (lipid) layer, a middle aqueous layer, and an inner mucin layer. The oily layer is secreted by meibomian glands in the posterior portion of the upper and lower eyelids. The aqueous portion of tear film is secreted by the exocrine lacrimal gland located superior and slightly lateral to the eye, as well as smaller accessory lacrimal glands (Figure 1). The mucinous layer of tears is secreted by goblet cells on the corneal surface as well as the conjunctivae. The oily outer surface of tear film functions to prevent evaporation of tears. The inner mucin layer of tear film helps to lubricate the ocular surface as it constantly undergoes healing. In dry eye syndrome, tears become hyperosmolar as a result of water evaporation from the exposed ocular surface. Hyperosmolarity stimulates a cascade of inflammatory events in corneal epithelial cells resulting in mast cell release of cytokines, leading to damage. When normal ocular surface defense mechanisms are compromised, the cornea is more susceptible to infections.

Prevention

There is no known prevention for dry eye syndrome.

Clinical Manifestations

Symptoms of dry eye syndrome are listed in Box 2. Excessive tearing is a paradoxical sign of dry eye syndrome. Ocular surface damage or irritation activates the neural reflex that stimulates the lacrimal gland to secrete more aqueous tears. As time goes on, this compensatory ability is often gradually lost. Signs of dry eye from examination are listed in Box 3.

Diagnosis

The presence of symptoms alone is not sufficient to make a diagnosis of dry eye syndrome, because they are often nonspecific and may not be accompanied by ocular changes.

Diagnostic tests for dry eye syndrome include (1) testing for abnormally rapid corneal tear film break up time (TFBUT), the Schirmer test (can give quite variable results), and fluorescein or rose Bengal staining of the cornea and conjunctiva (usually positive in more advanced cases). There is no single definitive test in the identification of dry eye syndrome or to measure the severity of disease. Several validated patient questionnaires have been developed that may also be useful.

Differential Diagnosis

The differential diagnosis of dry eye includes blepharitis[3] (which may co-exist with dry eye), ocular allergies, viral conjunctivitis (usually a shorter course), and other infections.

Treatment

Treatment of dry eye syndrome is aimed at increasing tear production, decreasing tear evaporation, or reducing tear resorption. Patients usually need to treat dry eye indefinitely. If patients are

---

[1]Not FDA approved for this indication.

[3]Exceeds dosage recommended by the manufacturer.

Box 1 Causes of Dry Eye Syndrome

Aging
Congenital disorders (e.g., congenital alacrima and familial dysautonomia)
Evaporative dry eye:
  Meibomian gland dysfunction: posterior blepharitis
  Entropion and ectropion
  Low blink rate: Parkinson disease, prolonged computer or microscope use
  Low-humidity environment
  Smoking (direct irritant)
High estrogen levels
Lacrimal duct obstruction: trachoma, pemphigoid, erythema multiforme, chemical and thermal burns
Lacrimal gland denervation
Lacrimal gland infiltration: sarcoidosis, lymphoma, AIDS, graft-vs-host disease
Low androgen levels
Ocular surface disorders: topical anesthetic drops, vitamin A deficiency, preservatives in artificial tears and other ophthalmic medications, contact lens wear, allergic conjunctivitis
Other autoimmune disorders (rheumatoid arthritis [RA], scleritis, episcleritis)
Reflex hyposecretion:
Reflex motor block: damage to the VII nerve, systemic drugs (antihistamines, beta-blockers, antispasmodics, diuretics, tricyclic antidepressants, selective serotonin reuptake inhibitors (SSRIs), psychotropic medications, isotretinoin
Reflex sensory block: topical anesthetic drops, contact lens wear, laser-assisted in situ keratomileusis (LASIK) surgery, diabetes, keratitis from herpes zoster or ulcerative colitis
Pregnancy
Sjogren syndrome

Box 2 Symptoms of Dry Eye Syndrome

- Dryness
- Redness
- General irritation of eyes
- Gritty sensation in eyes (especially later in the day)
- Burning sensation in eyes
- Foreign body sensation in eyes
- Excessive tearing
- Light sensitivity
- Blurred vision

Box 3 Signs from Physical Examination suggesting Dry Eye Syndrome

- Conjunctival injection, usually symmetric
- Excessive tearing
- Blepharitis (erythematous or irritated eyelid edges)
- Malposition of eyelids (entropion/ectropion)
- Reduced blink rate
- Visual impairment
- Scant, white, stringy discharge

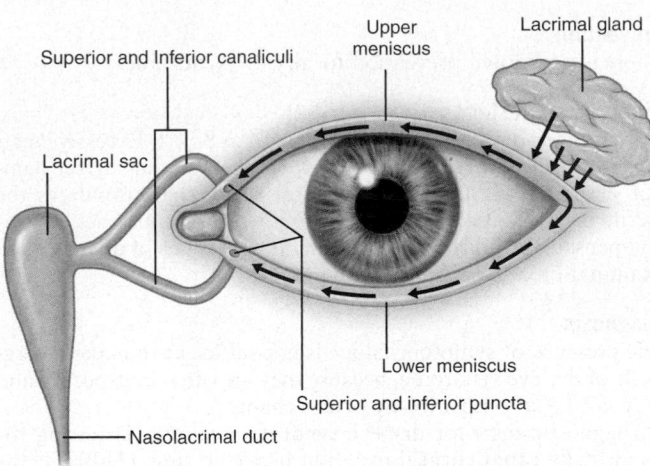

Figure 1. Anatomy of the major lacrimal gland and drainage system.

taking medications (see Box 1) that cause dry eye, they should stop them if at all possible.

Many forms of artificial tears are available commercially over the counter. Most preparations of artificial tears contain cellulose to increase viscosity, polyethylene glycol or polyvinyl alcohol to help spread the tears across the ocular surface, and a preservative (benzalkonium chloride or cetrimide). Some patients develop sensitivity to preservatives in artificial tears, especially with more frequent or prolonged use. The usual starting dose for artificial tears is one drop in both eyes four times a day. If artificial tears are needed more than four to six times per day, it is best to use preparations without preservatives. Preservative-free artificial tear preparations often range in price from $16 to $22 per month, compared to $4 to $10 per month for preparations containing preservatives.

Examples of preservative-free products include Refresh (Allergan), TheraTears, Soothe (Bausch and Lomb), and Systane (Alcon).

Environmental factors can increase the rate of evaporation of tears. People who do not blink frequently enough (e.g., reading, microscope, and computer use) may need to make a conscious effort to blink more. Patients who work very close to heating and air conditioning ducts need to distance themselves from ducts when possible, and should use a humidifier in areas with low humidity. Swim goggles and moisture chambers for glasses may be helpful as well to conserve moisture around the eyes. Lowering computer screens below eye level will decrease exposure of the ocular surface between eyelids. Patients who work at computer terminals should take periodic breaks.[6]

Ophthalmologists may insert silicone plugs to obstruct the puncta and decrease resorption of tears from the surface of the eye.

Sodium hyaluronate (over the counter product) is a lipid-like substance that slows the evaporation of tears.

Topical cyclosporine (Restasis) is a second line agent used in moderate-to-severe disease.[2] It is expensive (about $400 per month) and should not be used if infection is present since cyclosporine is an immunosuppressive agent. It is probably judicious to leave the decision to use cyclosporine to an ophthalmologist primarily because of cost and possibility of adverse effects. Cyclosporine is usually administered one drop in both eyes twice daily, and may take several weeks for symptom reduction. It may cause a temporary burning sensation in the eyes.

Topical glucocorticoids may cause symptom reduction in the short term, but are not a good option for long term use as they can cause cataracts and glaucoma.

Dietary supplements containing omega-3 and omega-6 fatty acids are under investigation.[5]

Surgical correction of eyelid abnormalities such as entropion and ectropion may be helpful to prevent or lessen ocular surface damage.

Complications

Inflammation and damage to the ocular surface can lead to visual disturbance.

Monitoring

Patients using cyclosporine drops should be under the care of an ophthalmologist.

---

[2]Not available in the United States.
[5]Investigational drug in the United States.
[6]May be compounded by pharmacists.

Conclusions

Dry eye syndrome is a multifactorial disease of tears and the ocular surface that can result in discomfort and visual impairment. There is considerable variability in patient-reported symptoms over time.

There is no single definitive diagnostic test for dry eye syndrome. Artificial tears should be used for initial management, but this treatment is only palliative. Environmental strategies should also be considered.

References

Harper RA. Basic Ophthalmology. 9th ed., American Academy of Ophthalmology: 2010.

Management and therapy of dry eye disease: report of the Management and Therapy Subcommittee of the International Dry Eye WorkShop (2007). Ocul Surf 2007;5:163–78.

O'Brien PD, Collum L. Dry eye: diagnosis and current treatment strategies. Curr Allergy Asthma Rep 2004;4:314–9.

The definition and classification of dry eye disease: report of the definition and Classification Subcommittee of the International Dry Eye Workshop (2007). Ocul Surf 2007;5:75–92.

Trobe JD. The physician's guide to eye care. 4th ed. The Foundation of the American Academy of Ophthalmology; 2012.

Wojtowicz JC, Butovich I, Uchiyama E, et al. Pilot, prospective, randomized, double-masked, placebo-controlled clinical trial of an omega-3 supplement for dry eye. Cornea 2011;39:308–14.

GLAUCOMA

Method of
Albert P. Lin, MD; and Kristin Schmid Biggerstaff, MD

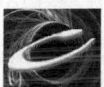

CURRENT DIAGNOSIS

Primary Open Angle Glaucoma

- Primary open angle glaucoma is an irreversible optic neuropathy typically associated with elevated intraocular pressure.
- Primary open angle glaucoma is the most common form of glaucoma and is projected to affect more than 3 million Americans in 2020. It is more common in African-Americans (6%–7%), Asians (2%–3%), and Hispanics (2%) and less common in whites (1%). It is more common in older adults: 1%–2% in 50-year-olds compared to 6%–12% in 80-year-olds.
- Primary open angle glaucoma is diagnosed by a complete ophthalmic examination, including dilated stereoscopic optic nerve examination and formal visual field.
- Untreated primary open angle glaucoma can lead to slow irreversible loss of vision and blindness. Other common causes of slow and progressive vision loss in older adults include cataracts, macular degeneration, and diabetic retinopathy.

Acute Angle Closure Glaucoma

- Pupillary block in susceptible patients leads to block of aqueous drainage and sudden and extreme rise of intraocular pressure. Acute angle closure can damage the optic nerve, resulting in acute angle closure glaucoma.
- About 0.5% to 1.0% of U.S. adults are at risk for acute angle closure. It is more common in Inuits and Asians and rare in African-Americans. The risk of acute angle closure increases with age. It is also more common in hyperopes.
- Patients can present with blurry vision, red eye, pain, headache, nausea, or vomiting. Acute angle closure is sometimes misdiagnosed as migraines or gastrointestinal illnesses. Patients with conjunctivitis, keratitis, uveitis, and corneal abrasion can also present with the same symptoms.
- Peripheral iridotomy prevents acute angle closure in susceptible patients. High intraocular pressure can result in irreversible damage of the optic nerve within hours, making acute angle closure one of the true ophthalmic emergencies.

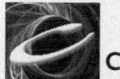

CURRENT THERAPY

Primary Open Angle Glaucoma

- Topical eye drops, including β-blockers, selective α_2 agonists, carbonic anhydrase inhibitors, and prostaglandin analogues can be used to reduce intraocular pressure.
- Oral carbonic anhydrase inhibitors are typically used in recalcitrant cases until surgery can be performed.
- Laser trabeculoplasty may be used as first-line or adjunct therapy.
- Glaucoma surgery, including trabeculectomy, tube shunt, and cyclodestruction, may be performed if goal intraocular pressure cannot be reached with medical therapy or in nonadherent patients.

Acute Angle Glaucoma

- All glaucoma eye drops are used to reduce intraocular pressure.
- Oral and intravenous medications are added sequentially to reduce intraocular pressure as needed.
- Laser iridotomy can be performed as prophylactic treatment or acutely to break the pupillary block if the patient is unresponsive to medical intervention.
- Emergent glaucoma incisional surgery is performed if the patient is unresponsive to all other treatments.

Glaucoma is an optic neuropathy with characteristic optic nerve head appearance: narrowing of the neuroretinal rim. The optic nerve is a collection of more than 1 million axons from the retinal ganglion cells. The anterior 1-mm portion of the optic nerve within the globe is referred to as the *optic disk* or simply the disk. When the disk is examined with direct or indirect ophthalmoscopy, a cup, or a physiologic empty space, is observed centrally. The remainder of the disk, which has a yellow-orange appearance, contains the axons and is referred to as the *neuroretinal rim*. The area of the cup compared to the entire disk is the cup-to-disk ratio, which is normally less than 0.4 (Figure 1A). When patients develop glaucoma, axons are lost from the neuroretinal rim and the size of the cup increases in relation to the disk. Narrowing of the neuroretinal rim and increased cup-to-disk ratio are the hallmarks of glaucomatous optic neuropathy (Figure 1B).

Glaucoma can result in significant and irreversible loss of vision and is one of the leading causes of blindness in the United States. Early in the disease state, glaucoma is asymptomatic; it is sometimes called "the sneak thief of sight." As the disease progresses, the patient develops decreased peripheral vision and eventually loss of the central vision.

Glaucoma is typically associated with increased intraocular pressure (IOP), but it is possible to have normal-tension or low-tension glaucoma. Glaucoma treatment is focused on the reduction of IOP to prevent or slow optic nerve damage and preserve visual function.

Glaucoma is classified in many ways, and it is most useful to approach it clinically based on the status of the angle, the area between the cornea and iris where aqueous exits the globe through the trabecular network. We further discuss primary open angle glaucoma, the most common form of glaucoma in the United States, and the management of acute angle closure, one of the true ophthalmic emergencies.

Primary Open Angle Glaucoma

Glaucoma is one of the leading causes of blindness in older adults, especially in patients of African-American descent. Vision loss from glaucoma is irreversible, and the treatment goal is to reduce IOP, slow disease progression, and preserve visual function during the patient's lifetime. Glaucoma is a slowly progressive disease, and progression to blindness often takes more than 10 years, even in untreated patients. Given its slow progression and the fact that

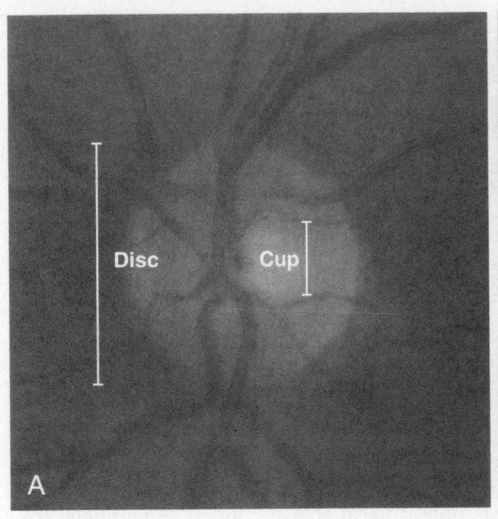
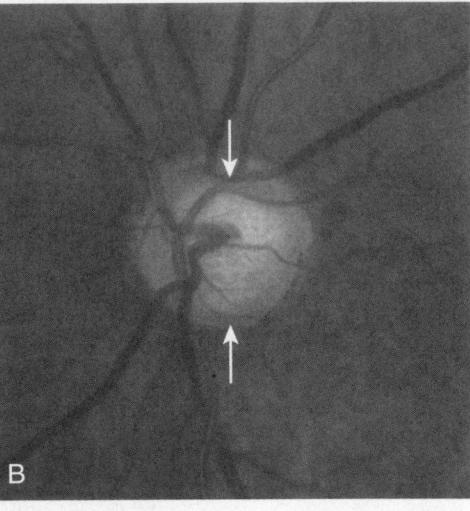

central vision loss occurs in late disease, most patients do well with early diagnosis and treatment. Treatment is more difficult in late disease because the rate of disease progression and visual deterioration is accelerated, sometimes despite good control of IOP.

Due to the early asymptomatic nature of the disease, the patient's adherence to and persistence with treatment is often less than optimal. Studies have shown patients who obtain glaucoma information from physicians other than their ophthalmologists have a higher rate of medication adherence. Ophthalmologists have the options to use treatment modalities such as laser and surgery to obtain pressure control and decrease or eliminate the need for medication use.

The American Academy of Ophthalmology recommends asymptomatic patients older than 40 years be referred for ophthalmic evaluation once every several years for early detection of glaucoma and other chronic eye diseases. However, the U.S. Preventive Services Task Force found insufficient evidence to recommend for or against screening for glaucoma in adults. Risks, benefits, and cost effectiveness of screening are beyond the scope of this chapter, but symptomatic patients or patients at high risk for glaucoma (African American ethnicity and family history) might benefit from ophthalmology consultation. It is possible to diagnose glaucoma by direct ophthalmoscopy, but this is not a substitute for binocular assessment of the disk through dilated pupils and formal visual field testing. If glaucoma is suspected or diagnosed, primary care visits should include inquiries regarding glaucoma medication use, medication side effects, and the time of last eye examination. Primary care physicians can improve glaucoma outcome by promoting adherence to medication and follow-up. Glaucoma

patients need to follow up with their ophthalmologists at least annually, and in severe cases every 3 months, for intraocular pressure checks.

Treatment

Topical Glaucoma Medications

Topical glaucoma medications are administered once or twice daily. Patients should look up, pull down their lower eye lid, drop the medication on the inferior conjunctival cul-de-sac, and keep their eyes closed for 5 minutes. Applying gentle pressure next to the bridge of the nose to occlude the puncta can improve absorption of the medication. Medication bottle caps are color-coded by their class, and patients can usually identify their eye drops by color. Glaucoma medications are not subject to first-pass effect through the liver and can sometimes have significant systemic side effects, especially the β-blockers. Topical glaucoma medications are described later and summarized in Table 1.

Prostaglandin Analogues. Latanoprost (Xalatan), travoprost (Travatan), and bimatoprost (Lumigan) are prostaglandin analogues and are color-coded by teal caps. They are administered once at bedtime but may be administered once at any time during the day to promote adherence. They decrease IOP by increasing aqueous outflow. Side effects are primarily local and include increased conjunctival hyperemia, increased lash growth, and possible irreversible increase in periocular and iris pigmentation.

β-Blockers. Timolol (Betimol, Istalol, Timoptic), levobunolol (Betagan), and betaxolol (Betoptic) are color-coded by yellow caps. They are administered once or twice daily and decrease IOP by decreasing aqueous production. Side effects include bradycardia, exacerbation of chronic obstructive pulmonary disease (COPD) and

| TABLE 1 | Topical Glaucoma Medications: Carbonic Anhydrase Inhibitors |

CLASS	β-BLOCKER	SELECTIVE α₂ AGONIST	CARBONIC ANHYDRASE INHIBITOR	PROSTAGLANDIN ANALOGUE	COMBINATION
Medication	Timolol (Timoptic) Betaxolol (Betoptic) Levobunolol (Betagan)	Brimonidine (Alphagan)	Dorzolamide (Trusopt) Brinzolamide (Azopt)	Latanoprost (Xalatan) Travoprost (Travatan) Bimatoprost (Lumigan)	Timolol/Dorzolamide (Cosopt) Timolol/Brimonidine (Combigan)
Dosing	bid or qd	bid	bid	qhs	bid
Cap color	Yellow	Purple	Orange	Teal	Blue
Side effects	Bradycardia, COPD, and asthma exacerbation	Allergic conjunctivitis, dry mouth, fatigue in elderly	Stinging, bitter taste	Hyperemia, lash growth, increased pigmentation	See individual components

Abbreviation: COPD = chronic obstructive pulmonary disease.

asthma, impotence, and decreased serum high-density lipoprotein (HDL) cholesterol. Physicians need to be aware that a topical β-blocker is a potential cause of acute changes in cardiovascular or pulmonary status. There are several reported incidents of death following the use of topical β-blockers mostly due to exacerbation of asthma.

Selective α₂ Agonists. Brimonidine (Alphagan) and apraclonidine (Iopidine) belong to the class of selective α₂ receptor agonists, and brimonidine is more commonly prescribed; it is color-coded by purple caps. It is administered twice daily and decreases IOP by decreasing aqueous production. Allergic conjunctivitis has been reported in up to 25% of patients. Rarely, it causes dry mouth and chronic fatigue and drowsiness in the elderly.

Carbonic Anhydrase Inhibitors. Dorzolamide (Trusopt) and brinzolamide (Azopt) are color-coded by orange caps and are sulfa-based medications. They are administered twice daily and decrease IOP by decreasing aqueous production. This class of medication has minimal systemic side effects. However, some patients complain about transient stinging and a bitter taste in the mouth after administration. These side effects, if tolerable, are not indications for discontinuing therapy.

Combined Topical Medications. Timolol and dorzolamide (Cosopt) and timolol and brimonidine (Combigan) are color-coded by blue caps. Combined medications decrease exposure to preservatives and can decrease irritation and problems with dry eyes. Adherence might also be improved.

Oral Carbonic Anhydrase Inhibitors

Oral carbonic anhydrase inhibitors include acetazolamide (Diamox), 250 mg or 500 mg given twice daily, and methazolamide (Neptazane), 25 mg or 50 mg given twice daily. They are sulfa-based medications and decrease IOP by decreasing aqueous production. Oral carbonic anhydrase inhibitors are not commonly used today because effective topical medications are available. They are typically used on a short-term basis to achieve IOP control in acute or refractory cases. Side effects can include aplastic anemia, kidney stones, bitter taste, indigestion, paresthesia of the extremities, tinnitus, and polyuria. Clinicians need to consider the possibility of hypokalemia when patients take other diuretics to control blood pressure (Table 2). Acetazolamide may also be given intravenously.

Laser Trabeculoplasty

Argon or selective laser trabeculoplasty can be used to increase aqueous outflow. Laser trabeculoplasty is noninvasive and safe, and it can be performed in the office in less than 10 minutes. Compared to surgery, IOP reduction is limited, up to 25% as primary treatment, but less as an adjunct modality. It is ineffective or less effective in some patients with light trabecular meshwork pigmentation. The effect of laser decreases over time but may be repeated in the case of selective laser trabeculoplasty.

Surgery

The most commonly performed glaucoma surgeries are trabeculectomy, tube shunt, and cyclodestruction. Trabeculectomy and tube shunt are procedures that create an opening in the sclera to increase aqueous outflow. Cyclodestruction destroys the ciliary body and decreases aqueous production. The procedure can be transscleral or endoscopic; the endoscopic method is typically done at the time of cataract surgery. Alternative surgical methods, such as deep sclerectomy, Trabectome, canaloplasty, and iStent, are being developed and performed to minimize the invasiveness and potential complications associated with traditional glaucoma surgery.

Visual Impairment and Blindness

Patients who are visually impaired (Snellen vision of less than 20/40) or legally blind (Snellen vision of less than 20/200 or visual field of less than 20 degrees) may have significantly decreased mobility and ability to function. Continued glaucoma treatment is still important in these patients because even maintenance of count-finger vision can allow the patients some degree of independence. Low-vision devices and services, including high-contrast video magnifiers, audiobooks, eccentric viewers, and mobility training, can allow patients maximal use of their residual vision and improve their confidence and quality of life.

Acute Angle Closure Glaucoma

Pupillary block in susceptible patients blocks aqueous drainage and leads to sudden and extreme rise of intraocular pressure. Acute angle closure can damage the optic nerve, resulting in acute angle closure glaucoma.

About 0.5% to 1.0% of U.S. adults is at risk for acute angle closure. It is more common in Inuits and Asians and rare in African Americans. The risk of acute angle closure increases with age. It is also more common in hyperopes (farsightedness).

Mechanism of Acute Angle Closure: Pupillary Block

After aqueous is produced in the ciliary body in the posterior chamber, it travels through the pupil and exits the anterior chamber through the trabecular meshwork located between the iris and the cornea. Pupillary block occurs when the iris comes in contact with the lens and obstructs the flow of aqueous through the pupil. Increased posterior chamber pressure displaces the iris anteriorly against the trabecular meshwork and stops aqueous outflow.

Patients at risk for acute angle closure have narrow occludable angles. These patients have smaller eyes, allowing the lens to contact the iris to initiate papillary block. The distance between the iris and the lens is the shortest when the pupil is mid-dilated. Therefore, patients who present with acute angle closure might have a history of dim light exposure (movies) or use of medications with anticholinergic properties (antihistamines, decongestants, antispasmodics). High IOP causes iris and corneal endothelial cell dysfunction, resulting in nonreactive pupil and hazy cornea, respectively. High IOP also results in inflammation and red eye as well as severe pain, nausea, and vomiting (Figure 2). Elevated IOP can damage the optic nerve within hours, and acute angle closure needs to be treated emergently to prevent permanent loss of vision.

TABLE 2	Oral and Intravenous Glaucoma Medications			
	ACETAZOLAMIDE (DIAMOX)	**METHAZOLAMIDE (NEPTAZANE)**	**MANNITOL (OSMITROL)**	**GLYCERIN 50% (OSMOGLYN)**
Class	CAI	CAI	Hyperosomtic	Hyperosmotic
Dosage	250 or 500 mg bid	25 mg or 50 mg bid	1 g/kg in 30 min	1 g/kg once
Route	PO or IV	PO	IV	PO
Side effects	Bitter taste, indigestion, paresthesia, tinnitus, polyuria, kidney stones, hypokalemia, aplastic anemia, sulfa allergy		Polyuria, dehydration Exacerbate CHF and diabetes (glycerin)	

Abbreviations: CAI = carbonic anhydrase inhibitor; CHF = congestive heart failure.

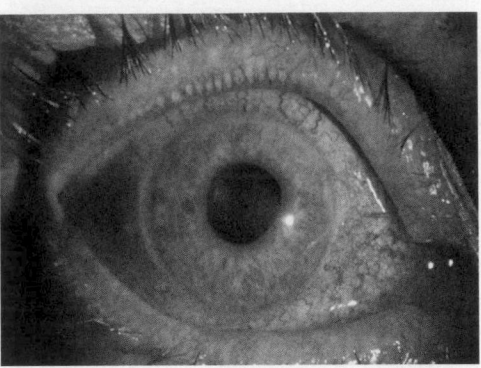

Figure 2. Acute angle closure patient with red eye and mid-dilated and nonreactive pupil.

Diagnosis

Patients with acute angle closure can present with blurry vision, red eye, pain, headache, nausea, or vomiting. History can include hyperopia, onset after exposure to a dim environment, or taking anticholinergic medications. Examination findings include decreased vision, conjunctival hyperemia, mid-dilated, nonreactive pupil with or without an afferent papillary defect, and increased IOP (by palpation or tonometry). Acute angle closure is sometimes misdiagnosed as migraines or gastrointestinal illness. Patients with conjunctivitis, keratitis, uveitis, and corneal abrasion can also present with the same symptoms.

Treatment

If acute angle closure is suspected, an emergent referral to ophthalmology is indicated. If an ophthalmologist is not immediately available, the goal will be to medically control the IOP as soon as possible. One drop of topical aqueous suppressant—β-blocker, selective α2 agonist, or carbonic anhydrase inhibitor—should be administered (timolol, brimonidine, dorzolamide) (see Table 1). The maximum dose of oral or intravenous carbonic anhydrase inhibitor is given: acetazolamide 500 mg or methazolamide 50 mg (see Table 2). The patient is placed in the supine position to allow the lens and iris to fall posteriorly. The patient is reassessed in 30 minutes, and if the condition is not improved, topical drops are repeated. If there is no improvement after another 30 minutes, a hyperosmotic, oral glycerin (Osmoglyn) 1 g/kg or intravenous mannitol (Osmitrol) 1 g/kg over 30 minutes, is administered. Hyperosmotics may be contraindicated in patients with congestive heart failure, and glycerin can cause severe hyperglycemia in diabetic patients.

An ophthalmologist can break the papillary block by medically lowering the IOP or by performing anterior chamber paracentesis, compression gonioscopy, laser peripheral iridotomy, and, in recalcitrant cases, emergent trabeculectomy. Once the pressure is controlled, it is important to perform an iridotomy in both eyes to prevent future episodes. Patients with patent iridotomies may safely take anticholinergic medications.

References

Allingham RR, Damji KF, Freedman S, et al., editors. Shield's Textbook of Glaucoma. 5th ed. Philadelphia: Lippincott Williams & Wilkins; 2005. pp. 155–90.

American Academy of Ophthalmology. Practice guidelines. Preferred practice patterns. Primary angle closure, Available at: http://www.aao.org/preferred-practice-pattern/primary-angle-closure-ppp–october-2010; October 2010 [accessed July 10, 2015].

American Academy of Ophthalmology. Practice guidelines. Preferred practice patterns. Primary open-angle glaucoma, Available at: http://www.aao.org/preferred-practice-pattern/primary-openangle-glaucoma-ppp–october-2010; October 2010 [accessed July 10, 2105].

Congdon N, O'Colmain B, Klaver CC, et al. Eye Diseases Prevalence Research Group; Causes and prevalence of visual impairment among adults in the United States. Arch Ophthalmol 2004;122:477–85.

Friedman DS, Wolfs RC, O'Colmain BJ, et al. Eye Diseases Prevalence Research Group: Prevalence of open-angle glaucoma among adults in the United States. Arch Ophthalmol 2004;122(4):532–8.

Lin AP, Orengo-Nania S, Braun UK. PCP's role in chronic open-angle glaucoma. Geriatrics 2009;64:20–8.

Nordstrom BL, Friedman DS, Mozaffari E, et al. Persistence and adherence with topical glaucoma therapy. Am J Ophthalmol 2005;140:598–606.

Schwartz GF, Quigley HA. Adherence and persistence with glaucoma therapy. Surv Ophthalmol 2008;54:S57–68.

US Preventive Services Task Force. Screening for glaucoma, Available at: http://www.uspreventiveservicestaskforce.org/Page/Topic/recommendation-summary/glaucoma-screening; October 2013 [accessed July 10, 2015].

MÉNIÈRE'S DISEASE

Method of
Terry D. Fife, MD

CURRENT DIAGNOSIS

- Ménière's disease is characterized by recurrent attacks of severe vertigo, nausea, and vomiting typically lasting 1 to 6 hours.
- Ménière's disease causes tinnitus on the side of the affected ear; the tinnitus can change in pitch and loudness during attacks of vertigo.
- Attacks of vertigo are associated with reduced or muffled hearing on the side of the affected ear.
- Fluctuating unilateral hearing loss and low-frequency hearing loss on the side of the affected ear is characteristic.

CURRENT THERAPY

- Initial therapy includes a sodium-restricted diet (preferably <1500 mg of sodium daily) and a diuretic agent (e.g., thiazide diuretics).
- Betahistine,[1] a medication widely used in Europe that may be obtained at compounding pharmacies in the United States, may be helpful in selected patients at a dosage of 8 to 16 mg three times daily.
- Transtympanic infusion of gentamicin[1] or corticosteroids and endolymphatic sac surgery may be considered as minimally invasive options in patients with serviceable hearing because these procedures have a reasonably low risk of inducing hearing loss.
- Vestibular nerve sectioning is highly effective in stopping vertigo attacks with a reasonably low risk of causing further hearing loss, but it is a more invasive procedure.
- Labyrinthectomy is highly effective in stopping vertigo attacks but causes complete hearing loss, so it is only an option for patients who have already lost all useful hearing.

Patients who have undergone procedures that cause acute loss of vestibular function often have vertigo for a while after the surgery; the vertigo improves more quickly with vestibular rehabilitative therapy.[1]

[1]Not FDA approved for this indication.

Ménière's disease is a disorder of the inner ear that results in recurrent, spontaneous episodes of vertigo, hearing loss, ear fullness, and tinnitus affecting the same ear. The hearing loss often fluctuates early in Ménière's disease, but fluctuating hearing is not always present. Eventually permanent hearing loss occurs, affecting the low frequencies initially but ultimately affecting all frequencies.

Epidemiology

The reported prevalence of Ménière's disease varies from about 50 to 200 per 100,000. Both sexes are equally affected.

Risk Factors

Possible risk factors for later development of Ménière's syndrome include syphilitic otitis and viral infection of the inner ear, head trauma, and a family history of Ménière's disease.

Pathophysiology

The underlying mechanism is generally thought to be due to endolymphatic hydrops, a type of swelling of the endolymphatic compartment that ultimately leads to permanent damage of the inner ear structures. Possible reasons for this periodic swelling of the endolymph compartment include mechanical obstruction of endolymph flow or at least dysregulation of the electrochemical membrane potential between endolymph and perilymph compartments.

Endolymphatic hydrops appears to be the mechanism for a number of conditions that can lead to Ménière's syndrome. When no primary cause is identified, the idiopathic form of the syndrome is called Ménière's disease. When an underlying cause is found, it is referred to as Ménière's syndrome or secondary Ménière's or secondary endolymphatic hydrops. Secondary Ménière's syndrome can result from delayed endolymphatic hydrops in which symptoms come on years after a prior disorder or viral injury of the labyrinth, syphilitic otitis, autoimmune inner ear disease, and trauma.

Prevention

There is no known way of preventing the development of Ménière's disease because it occurs in many people with no risk factors.

Clinical Manifestations

Ménière's can manifest with periodic unilateral (or, less commonly, bilateral) hearing loss or isolated attacks of vertigo. Not uncommonly, Ménière's has both elements present at its onset, but the vertigo is usually the symptom that gets the most attention. Vertigo usually lasts 1 to 6 hours but can last as little at 30 minutes or as long as all day. Patients prone to motion sickness often report that their dizziness lasts longer because the aftereffect of vertigo lingers longer in those who are motion sensitive. Vertigo attacks in Ménière's disease are often quite severe and generally render patients unable to move around owing to the vertigo, nausea, and recurrent vomiting.

The hearing loss is usually unilateral, and patients might notice fluctuation in hearing accompanied by ear fullness and a low-pitched roaring tinnitus either before or coincident with the vertigo. If audiometry can be performed during this time, low-frequency (250–1000 Hz) hearing loss may be documented and might improve after the attack ceases. This signature fluctuating low-frequency sensorineural hearing loss is very helpful (Figure 1) when found, but getting patients with vertigo attacks in for testing while they are in the acute stage of vertigo is usually not feasible.

Occasionally, patients with Ménière's have sudden random drop attacks in which they abruptly fall without loss of consciousness. These spells, referred to as otolithic crises of Tumarkin, can lead to serious injury and should prompt aggressive treatment. The mechanism is presumed to be related to sudden mechanical deformation or sudden neural discharges related to the otolith structures of the inner ear. Because there is no specific treatment for Tumarkin crises, treatment entails the standard treatments for Ménière's disease in general.

As Ménière's disease progresses, usually over months to years, permanent low-frequency hearing loss develops that gives way to hearing loss at all frequencies. Eventually, the patient can lose all or most hearing on the affected side. Meanwhile, with each vertigo attack, some vestibular function is lost, and so as vertigo attacks continue, vestibular loss ensues, often paralleling the hearing loss. Ménière's occasionally burns out, meaning that enough vestibular function has been lost that acute hydrops no longer produces vertigo. Patients might report less severe dizziness or just a vague feeling of unsteadiness. This usually indicates advanced Ménière's, and unilateral hearing and vestibular loss should be expected.

Bilateral Ménière's has treatment implications because treating one side alone will be unlikely to stop the vertigo attacks, which could be emanating from the untreated side. Surgical treatment of both sides is also problematic because it could leave the patient with bilateral hearing loss, vestibular loss, or both.

Diagnosis

The diagnosis of Ménière's disease is made clinically based on unilateral hearing loss, tinnitus, ear fullness, and episodic vertigo typically lasting 1 to 6 hours. The criteria for definite, probable, and possible Ménière's are listed in Box 1.

Differential Diagnosis

Vestibular neuritis causes a single attack of vertigo, sometimes with acute hearing loss (labyrinthitis), but it can usually be

Figure 1. Audiogram showing typical low frequency hearing trough of Ménière's disease affecting the right ear.

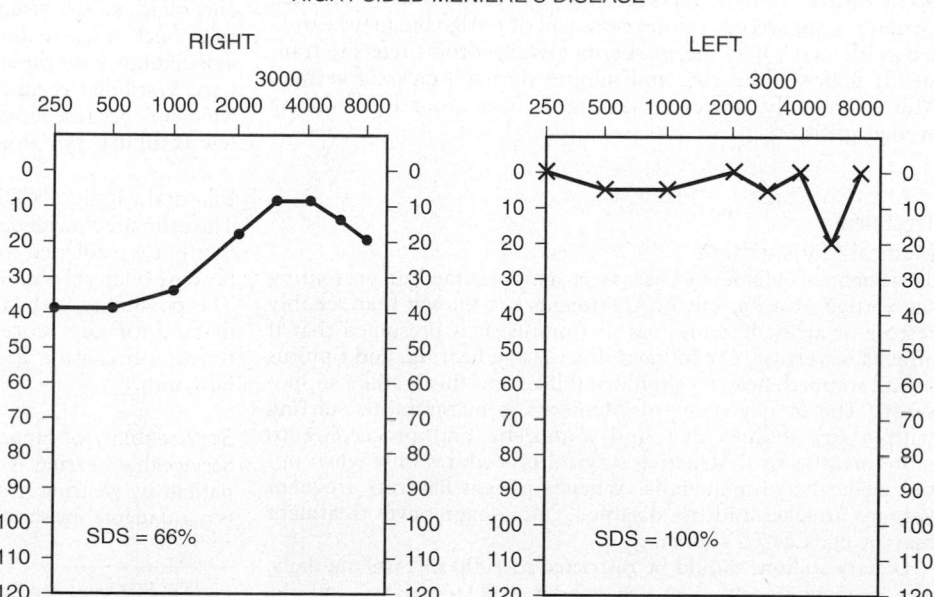

RIGHT-SIDED MÉNIÈRE'S DISEASE

distinguished from Ménière's because vestibular neuritis has a lifetime recurrence rate of only 2%, whereas Ménière's vertigo attacks recur multiple times and cause fluctuating and gradual decline in hearing.

When a patient reports episodic vertigo attacks in the absence of unilateral tinnitus, ear fullness, and hearing loss, one must be cautious in diagnosing Ménière's disease because vestibular migraine (basilar-type migraine) can produce a similar pattern. Diagnostic criteria have been published for vestibular migraine (see Lempert).

Benign paroxysmal positional vertigo causes brief recurrent spells of spinning without hearing loss, so it is rarely confused with Ménière's disease.

Vertebrobasilar insufficiency can cause isolated vertigo, but the duration is usually only several minutes and without hearing loss, whereas Ménière's attacks last hours and are associated with unilateral auditory symptoms.

Acoustic neuroma (vestibular schwannoma) typically leads to slowly progressive unilateral sensorineural hearing loss, but vertigo is infrequently a prominent feature because patients compensate gradually as their vestibular function wanes due to compressive effects of the tumor.

Fluctuating unilateral hearing loss, ear fullness, and tinnitus can occur without vertigo and is referred to as cochlear hydrops. Such symptoms can precede the development of vertigo but may be treated as Ménière's nonetheless. Lermoyez's syndrome refers to transiently improved hearing and tinnitus during attacks of vertigo. More commonly, however, hearing declines around and during vertigo spells.

Treatment
Medical Management
Treatment of Ménière's disease is mainly aimed at preventing the vertigo attacks, but no treatments are known that reliably restore or arrest hearing loss or tinnitus. It is presumed that if attacks of vertigo, ear fullness, fluctuating hearing, and tinnitus are all stopped, hearing should stabilize, but this is still a supposition. The management of Ménière's is hierarchical, starting with a low-sodium diet and a diuretic and proceeding to more-invasive or destructive surgical procedures only when initial medical treatment fails. When a patient has very frequent vertigo attacks and is disabled, more-aggressive treatment may be considered sooner.

Dietary sodium should be restricted to 1000 to 1500 mg daily. The average person consumes about 4000 mg daily, and the maximum recommended daily intake of sodium is 2300 mg. Because more than 70% of the daily sodium comes from processed foods, this dietary restriction generally requires more than simply stopping the use of table salt, which generally accounts for only about 10% of daily sodium intake for most people.

A diuretic is usually added to the sodium restriction. The most commonly prescribed diuretic is hydrochlorothiazide 25 mg combined with triamterene 37.5 mg (Dyazide)[1] because this combination usually obviates the need for potassium supplementation. Acetazolamide (Diamox)[1] 125 to 250 mg bid or furosemide (Lasix)[1] 10 to 20 mg daily are also options. Patients with severe sulfa allergy can use low-dose ethacrynic acid (Edecrin)[1] 12.5 to 25 mg daily.

An acute attack of vertigo from Ménière's disease can be managed with vestibular suppressants such as dimenhydrinate (Dramamine)[1] 50 mg, meclizine (Antivert) 25 to 50 mg, diazepam (Valium)[1] 2 to 5 mg, or promethazine (Phenergen)[1] 12.5 to 50 mg. Scopolamine in patch form (Transderm-Scōp)[1] is too slow to be useful because it takes hours to be absorbed transdermally; oral scopolamine tablets (Scopace)[1] 0.4 mg may be effective. Nausea can additionally be managed with prochlorperazine (Compazine) 10 mg orally or 25 mg by suppository, with oral or sublingual ondansetron (Zofran)[1] 4 to 8 mg, or with other antiemetics. Generally the vertigo attacks subside in several hours even without treatment.

Betahistine (Serc)[1] may also be helpful in Ménière's, though it is not commonly used in the United States. The role of betahistine is not firmly established, although it is widely prescribed for vertigo throughout the world. Betahistine may be helpful when successful medical management with diet and diuretics has helped but is inadequate to stop attacks. Betahistine is a vasodilator, a modest H_1 histamine agonist, and a powerful H_3 histamine receptor antagonist. Its method of action in Ménière's is unknown, though it increases blood flow and might also influence endolymphatic fluid regulation and receptors in the endolymphatic sac. Doses of betahistine may start at 8 mg PO three times daily and may be increased to 16 mg three times daily. It is available outside the United States in the form of Serc (Solvay Pharmaceuticals, Belgium). Betahistine may be made within the United States at compounding pharmacies with a physician prescription and may also be imported from outside the United States for individual use. Side effects are few, though occasionally patients report some headache. Betahistine is not histamine, and we have not found it to cause or aggravate urticaria.

Oral corticosteroids are often used but rarely seem effective except in cases of bilateral Ménière's resulting from autoimmune inner ear disease (AIED). Oral corticosteroids rarely seem to be effective in typical Ménière's disease.

Ménière's attacks have been said to be triggered by caffeine, chocolate, stress, visual stimuli, and dropping barometric pressure. Such triggers should be avoided when possible, but strong associations with these triggers can also occur in migrainous vertigo. Vestibular rehabilitative therapy is not generally helpful in Ménière's because most vertigo attacks remit and the patients have few vestibular symptoms between attacks.

Bilateral Ménière's Disease
The estimated incidence of bilateral Ménière's varies in the literature but is estimated to occur in about 15% of cases and tends to become bilateral within the first few years of onset in most cases. The possibility of bilateral involvement weighs on the decision making for any procedures that sacrifice hearing or vestibular function because it leaves the patient with only one functioning labyrinth.

Serviceability of Hearing
Serviceable hearing is residual hearing that can be useful to the patient by wearing hearing aids. In general, because hearing loss is permanent, one should avoid sacrificing any serviceable hearing.

---

[1]Not FDA approved for this indication.

Injections and Surgical Treatments

Patients who continue to have disabling vertigo despite a low-salt diet, diuretics, and possibly betahistine are considered to have failed conservative medical therapy. The next step in treatment depends on the age, health status, and residual hearing and vestibular function of the patient and also on the surgeon's opinion and experience with the various options. If spells are infrequent, symptomatic management of vertigo attacks may be the best option. Table 1 outlines some of the additional interventional options.

Intratympanic Gentamicin

Transtympanic gentamicin (Garamycin)[1] administration has become increasingly used as an effective treatment of Ménière's. This is partly due to the ease of administration of gentamicin and its relative safety. Gentamicin is a commonly used aminoglycoside antimicrobial agent with activity against gram-negative bacteria that also happens to be ototoxic. It damages hair cells of the labyrinth and preferentially affects hair cells of the vestibular neuroepithelium over that of the cochlea. Even so, transtympanic administration still has some risk of causing hearing loss. Gentamicin is administered by injecting a small amount (usually about 0.5 mL) of gentamicin sulfate (80 mg/2 mL) solution through the tympanic membrane into the middle ear space. To avoid rapid drainage through the eustachian tube, the injection is done with the patient supine and kept in that position for an hour or so to allow the gentamicin to absorb through the round window into the inner ear. There are many protocols, but commonly an injection is given once, and additional injections can be considered every 3 to 4 weeks until improvement in vertigo attacks is realized. Studies suggest that intratympanic gentamicin is an effective treatment for vertigo complaints in Ménière's disease but there is some risk of hearing loss.

Endolymphatic Sac Surgery

Another option for patients with residual functional hearing is endolymphatic sac shunt or decompression. This procedure eliminates vertigo in 50% to 75% of those treated. Nevertheless, its

[1] Not FDA approved for this indication.

effectiveness compared to placebo has remained a point of contention based on a number of studies. It has been suggested that the procedure's effectiveness depends on the operative technique and experience of the surgeon.

Intratympanic Steroids

Sometimes, a trial of intratympanic corticosteroids may be tried, though its effectiveness in controlled trials is still not compelling. Even so, a trial of corticosteroids administered in this manner poses little risk.

Vestibular Neurectomy

The most definitive procedure for stopping vertigo attacks in Ménière's when the goal is to preserve hearing is vestibular neurectomy. This procedure involves craniotomy and severing the vestibular nerve while preserving the cochlear nerve. This procedure requires overnight hospitalization and general anesthesia, and it does pose some risk to facial nerve function and hearing on the affected side.

Labyrinthectomy

For patients who have unilateral Ménière's and no serviceable hearing, labyrinthectomy is a commonly used procedure. This procedure entails the removal of the membranous labyrinth and is highly effective in stopping recurrent vertigo attacks from that ear. In elderly patients or those who are poor surgical candidates, a more limited transtympanic cochleosacculotomy may be performed.

Meniett Treatment

The Meniett device is a portable low-frequency pressure-wave delivery system that administers a wave of pressure of about 12 cm H_2O to the middle ear via a tympanostomy tube for about 0.6 seconds pulsed at 6 Hz for 5 minutes about three to five times daily. Quality randomized trials demonstrating the effectiveness of this treatment are very limited, however. This method has few risks and only requires myringotomy and a pressure equalization tube. A practical limitation is the cost of the device, which is not often paid for by many health insurance companies.

TABLE 1 Procedures Used in the Management of Ménière's Disease

METHOD	TECHNIQUE	ADVANTAGES	DISADVANTAGES
Procedures Intended to Spare Serviceable Hearing			
Meniett device	Applies repetitive low pressure pulses of air with the aim of enhancing endolymph drainage	Minimally invasive, no significant side effects and no risk of hearing loss	Requires tympanostomy tube placement; usually not covered by insurance; rate of effectiveness still unclear
Intratympatic corticosteroids	Injection of steroid through the tympanic membrane to the middle ear to be absorbed in the inner ear	Minimally invasive, few side effects	Effectiveness unclear when compared to placebo
Transtympanic gentamicin (Garamycin)[1]	Injection of gentamicin through the tympanic membrane to the middle ear to be absorbed in the inner ear	Simple office-based procedure, low risk profile	Number of injections is unpredictable; some risk of hearing loss
Endolymphatic mastoid shunt	Placing a shunt from the endolymphatic sac to the mastoid air cells	Effective in 50%–75% of cases; low risk of hearing loss; day procedure	Vertigo can recur; effectiveness depends on surgical experience and technique
Vestibular neurectomy	Surgical sectioning of the vestibular part of cranial nerve VIII, sparing the auditory part of the nerve	Highly effective in eliminating vertigo attacks	Requires general anesthesia; risk of facial weakness, hearing loss
Procedures Expected to Eliminate Residual Hearing			
Labyrinthectomy or cochleosacculotomy	Several methods of removing all or part of the labyrinth	Highly effective in stopping vertigo attacks	Inevitable complete hearing loss

[1] Not FDA approved for this indication.

Monitoring

Following patients with Ménière's disease should include monitoring of the frequency and severity of vertigo spells and the fluctuation in hearing, ear fullness, and tinnitus. Periodic audiometry is probably the most sensitive measure of stabilization of the condition. Vestibular testing may be considered when changes might alter the treatment strategy. Brain imaging is only helpful in excluding other disorders, but it has no role in the management of Ménière's disease.

Complications

Known complications include the progression of unilateral and occasionally bilateral hearing and vestibular function. There may also be complications associated with some of the treatments as described earlier. Owing to the unpredictability of the vertigo attacks, many patients avoid certain activities and might even develop agoraphobic features because the attacks are so severe and disruptive. In most cases, these avoidance behaviors improve if Ménière's can be controlled.

Conclusion

The management of Ménière's disease is still part art and part science. Treatment options are many, but patients should be reassured that, in most cases, something can be offered to help improve their vertigo and quality of life.

References

Ahsan SF, Standring R, Wang Y. Systematic review and meta-analysis of Meniett therapy for Meniere's disease. Laryngoscope 2014 Jun 10. http://dx.doi.org/10.1002/lary.24773. [Epub ahead of print].

Kaylie DM, Jackson CG, Gardner EK. Surgical management of Ménière's disease in the era of gentamicin. Otolaryngol Head Neck Surg 2005;132(3):443–50.

Lempert T. Vestibular migraine. Semin Neurol 2013;33:212–8.

Lopez-Escamez JA, et al. Diagnostic criteria for Ménière's disease. J Vestib Res 2015;25(1):1–7.

Phillips JS, Westerberg B. Intratympanic steroids for Ménière's disease or syndrome. Cochrane Database Syst Rev 2011;(7):CD008514. http://dx.doi.org/10.1002/14651858.CD008514.pub2.

Pullens B, van Benthem PP. Intratympanic gentamicin for Ménière's disease or syndrome. Cochrane Database Syst Rev 2011;(3):CD008234. http://dx.doi.org/10.1002/14651858.CD008234.pub2.

Rosenberg SI. Vestibular surgery for Ménière's disease in the elderly: A review of techniques and indications. Ear Nose Throat J 1999;78(6):443–6.

OTITIS EXTERNA

Method of
David Larrabee, MD, MPH

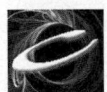

CURRENT DIAGNOSIS

- Ear pain or itching
- External ear tenderness
- Clear or purulent discharge (otorrhea), and debris in ear canal
- Possible ear canal edema

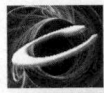

CURRENT THERAPY

- Topical antibiotic therapy, with or without topical corticosteroid
- Topical acetic acid (VoSol) less effective than topical antibiotics
- Oral antibiotics usually unnecessary
- Analgesic therapy

Epidemiology

Otitis externa is inflammation of the external auditory canal, usually caused by bacterial infection. It is a common problem in primary care, with an annual incidence of about 1% and lifetime incidence of about 10%. It affects both adults and children and is commonly known as "swimmer's ear."

Risk Factors

Increased moisture in the ear canal, often caused by swimming, hearing aids, or a humid environment, increases the risk of developing otitis externa. Trauma to the external canal (such as self-inflicted injury with a cotton swab) is also a risk factor. Genetic factors may play a role, and people with narrow external canals or absence of ear wax are at increased risk. Ear wax, which is acidic, is protective except when it causes total occlusion and a moist environment behind the occlusion.

Pathophysiology

Otitis externa is usually (98%) caused by bacteria: the most common culture results are *Pseudomonas aeruginosa, Staphylococcus aureus,* or polymicrobial. Fungi are an occasional cause. In most cases the infection is superficial, but infection can cause edema of the auditory canal and spread locally, causing cellulitis and even osteomyelitis.

Prevention

Topical acetic acid (VoSol),[1] topical corticosteroids, water exclusion (wearing ear plugs while swimming), and aural toilet have not been evaluated in clinical trials. However, people who have recurrent otitis externa should be advised that water in the ear canal increases risk of developing otitis externa. If they swim, ear plugs may be helpful in preventing water from entering the ear canal. After swimming, the canal can be dried with a hair dryer on the lowest setting. Also, acetic acid 2% (VoSol)[1] 2 to 5 drops could be applied after swimming to reacidify the ear canal.

Clinical Manifestations

The main symptom of acute otitis externa is pain. Mild cases can present with only itching or ear fullness. Often there is otorrhea and debris in the external canal, which can obscure the tympanic membrane and cause hearing loss. There can be preauricular lymphadenopathy. Fever, if present, may indicate local cellulitis.

Diagnosis

Acute otitis externa is diagnosed clinically. It presents with pain, itching or fullness in the ear, appearing within a period of 48 hours, with duration of less than 3 weeks. Tenderness of the tragus or movement of the pinna is a key symptom. Otorrhea and canal erythema and edema may be present but are not necessary for diagnosis (Figure 1). If possible, debris should be cleared from the canal to allow visualization of the tympanic membrane to assess if it is intact.

Granulation tissue at the bone-cartilage junction of the external canal (Figure 2), fever >39 °C, and severe pain are signs of malignant otitis externa.

Differential Diagnosis

Though the diagnosis of otitis externa is usually clear-cut, a differential diagnosis should be considered when symptoms do not resolve with usual treatment or the symptoms are particularly severe (Table 1).

Treatment

Topical antibiotics (Table 2) with or without steroid are effective in treating otitis externa. Fluoroquinolones have not been shown to be clearly superior to other antibiotics. Topical 2% acetic acid (VoSol) is also effective, though significantly less effective when compared with antibiotic/steroid drops in terms of cure rate at 2 and 3 weeks (OR 0.29). Oral antibiotics are not helpful unless there are signs of local cellulitis, in which case an antibiotic effective against *Pseudomonas* and *Staphylococcus* should be chosen.

---

[1]Not FDA approved for this indication.

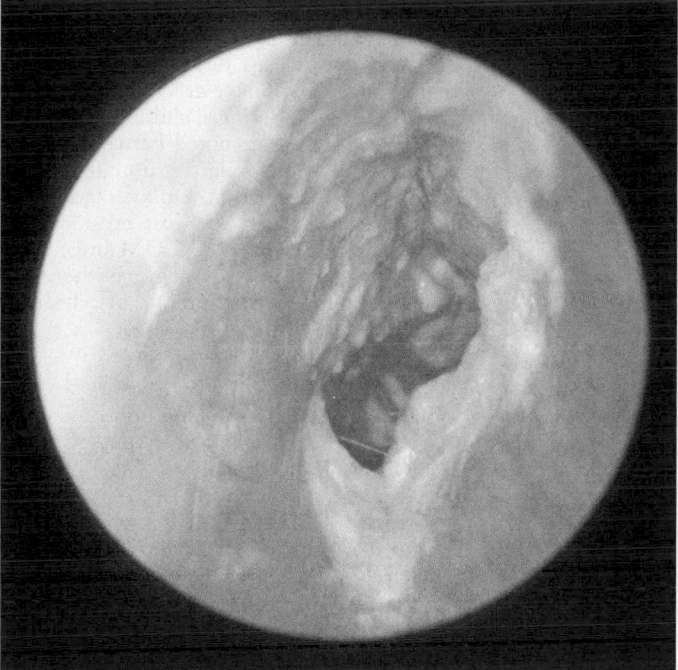

Figure 1. Chronic otitis externa with debris in canal.

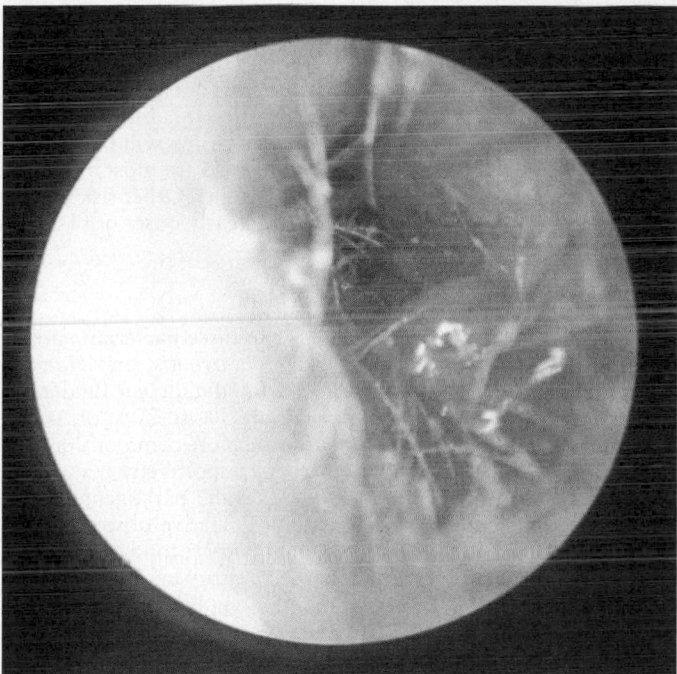

Figure 2. Necrotizing otitis with granulation tissue at junction.

To improve the penetrance of antibiotic drops, cotton ear wicks are often used when there is significant canal edema, but there have been no randomized controlled trials comparing this with antibiotic drops without ear wicks. Aural toilet by suctioning is recommended by specialists, but this option is often not available in primary care, and there have been no randomized controlled trials showing efficacy. If debris needs to be removed and suction is unavailable, gentle use of cotton-tipped swabs, ear cerumen curette or ear cerumen spoon is safer than irrigation, which is dangerous if the tympanic membrane is ruptured. If the tympanic membrane is perforated or cannot be visualized, topical ofloxacin (Floxin Otic) and ciprofloxacin/dexamethasone (Ciprodex, but not Cipro HC) are nonototixic and FDA approved for treatment.

TABLE 1	Differential Diagnosis of Otitis Externa
Otitis media with perforated tympanic membrane	
Malignant otitis externa	
Contact dermatitis	
Eczema	
Psoriasis	
Seborrhea	
Ramsey-Hunt Syndrome (otic herpes zoster)	
Cellulitis	

TABLE 2 Topical Antibiotics

MEDICATION	DOSING AND FREQUENCY	NOTES
Ofloxacin 0.3% solution (Floxin Otic)	10 drops in ear 1 × /day × 7 days	Approved for cases of perforated tympanic membrane
Ciprofloxacin/ dexamethasone (Ciprodex) Ciprofloxacin/ hydrocortisone (Cipro HC)	4 drops bid × 7 days	Ciprodex approved for cases of perforated tympanic membrane
Neomycin/ polymyxin B/ hydrocortisone (Cortisporin Otic)	4 drops tid/ qid × 7 days	Neomycin can cause hypersensitivity reaction
Acetic acid 2% (Vosol Otic)	5 drops tid/ qid × 7–14 days	Less effective; can cause stinging when applied
Clotrimazole 1% otic[6]	4 drops qid × 7 days	When a fungal cause is suspected

[6]May be compounded by pharmacists.

Ciprofloxacin (Ciloxan), tobramycin (Tobrex) or gentamicin (Garamycin) ophthalmic drops are sometimes used off-label to treat otitis externa.

Pain can usually be controlled with nonsteroidal anti-inflammatory drugs or acetaminophen. Opioids can be considered when pain is severe.

Monitoring

Symptoms should improve significantly within the first 24 hours of treatment. The average time to complete resolution of symptoms is 6 days. If a patient is not improving by 48 to 72 hours, he or she should be reassessed and possibly referred to an otolaryngology specialist. Patients at high risk for complications include those with diabetes, immunocompromised patients (such as in HIV), and the elderly.

Complications

Hypersensitivity reactions to otic antibiotics are possible, with neomycin being the most common agent. There will be pruritus and erythema, which can spread from the canal to the external ear. The causative antibiotic should be stopped and a preparation with another topic antibiotic and topical steroid should be used.

The most serious complication is malignant otitis externa, which is an extension of bacterial infection into local tissues and the mastoid or temporal bones, and can be life-threatening. It should be considered if there is fever (>39 °C), disproportionate pain, and facial or other cranial nerve palsies. The causative organisms are similar to acute otitis externa (*P. aeruginosa* and *S. aureus* are most common). It occurs mostly in immunocompromised individuals, such as those with diabetes or HIV, or who are undergoing chemotherapy. Patients should be given parenteral antibiotics and managed in a hospital with ENT consultation. Culture with sensitivity and CT scanning are usually necessary for accurate diagnosis and management.

References

Kaushik V, Malik T, Saeed SR. Interventions for acute otitis externa. Cochrane Database Syst Rev 2010;(1). http://dx.doi.org/10.1002/14651858.CD004740.pub2, CD004740.

Rosenfeld RM, et al. Clinical practice guideline: acute otitis externa. Otolaryngol Head Neck Surg 2006 Apr;134(Suppl. 4):S4–S23

Schaefer P, Baugh R. Acute otitis externa: an update. Am Fam Physician December 1, 2012.

OTITIS MEDIA

Method of
Gretchen M. Dickson, MD, MBA

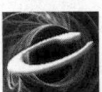

CURRENT DIAGNOSIS

- History of acute onset of symptoms
- Middle ear effusion
  - Bulging tympanic membrane
  - Limited mobility of tympanic membrane or air fluid level visible behind tympanic membrane
- Middle ear inflammation
  - Erythema of tympanic membrane or distinct otalgia

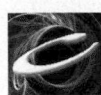

CURRENT THERAPY

- Watchful Waiting—appropriate for children:
  i. Greater than 2 years of age with nonsevere illness
  ii. Greater than 6 months of age with uncertain diagnosis and nonsevere illness
  iii. Greater than 2 years of age with severe illness, but uncertain diagnosis
  - Need close follow-up in 48 hours
  - Consider delayed prescription
- Antibiotics
  - First line should be amoxicillin (Amoxil) 80 to 90 mg/kg/day[3]
  - Treat 10 days if child less than 6 years of age, 5 to 7 days if greater than 6 years of age
  - Follow-up if not improving in 48 hours
- Analgesia
  - Acetaminophen (Tylenol), ibuprofen (Motrin, Advil)
  - Benzocaine in combination with antipyrine (Allergen, Auroguard), benzocaine with antipyrine and acetic acid (Auralgan)
- Antihistamines and decongestants are of no benefit
- Surgery—consider tympanostomy tubes when:
  i. First AOM episode at less than 6 months of age and child with 2 or more episodes in 6 months or 3 in 24 months
  ii. First AOM episode at more than 12 months of age and child with 3 episodes in 6 months, 5 episodes in 12 months or 7 episodes in 24 months

[3]Exceeds dosage recommended by the manufacturer.

Epidemiology

Acute otitis media (AOM) is a common condition of childhood, with one in four children having at least one episode of AOM by age 10. In fact, 86% of children will have at least one episode of AOM within the first year of life. Younger children are more likely to be affected, with peak incidence noted between ages 6 and 20 months likely because of the relative immaturity of immune system and eustachian tube function. On average, 5 billion dollars are spent per year on office visits, lost productivity, and diminished parental quality of life due to AOM infections. As a result, research has focused on effective strategies both to prevent episodes of AOM and also to efficiently treat episodes that do occur.

Risk Factors

Identifying children at risk for AOM has been an important strategy to attempt to limit instances of AOM. Unfortunately, many of the risk factors associated with AOM are not modifiable, including male gender, Native American ethnicity, presence of siblings within the home, and a family history of recurrent AOM. Additional risk factors include low socioeconomic status, premature birth, attendance at out-of-home daycare, lack of breastfeeding, and history of poor maternal health during pregnancy. Limited studies have suggested that interventions such as avoiding supine feeding or bottle propping, reducing pacifier use after the first 6 months of life, and eliminating passive tobacco exposure can help to reduce incidence; however, the evidence in which these interventions demonstrate clear impact is limited. Public health programs that encourage breastfeeding and optimal maternal health during pregnancy, as well as those focused on reducing tobacco use, have perhaps the best opportunity to impact AOM incidence rates.

Not only are these identified risk factors for any episode of AOM, but children with these characteristics are also more likely to have recurrent AOM. Although many children will be affected in their lifetimes, those with recurrent disease are most at risk of complications leading to morbidity or mortality. Other risk factors specifically for recurrent AOM include an early onset of first episode and low parental education.

Pathophysiology

AOM has classically been associated with three bacteria; namely, *Streptococcus pneumoniae*, *Moraxalla catarrhalis*, and *Haemophillus influenzae*. Using data derived from middle-ear fluid analysis, *M. catarrhalis* is responsible for only 3% to 20% of AOM, while *S. pneumoniae* and *H. influenzae* are more common contributors at 25% to 50% and 15% to 30%, respectively.

The bacteria responsible for AOM become pathogenic in the setting of eustachian tube dysfunction. A relative obstruction of the eustachian tube develops most commonly secondary to secretions from an antecedent viral upper respiratory infection or allergies, but may result from neuromuscular conditions or abnormal anatomy. Such relative obstruction creates a negative pressure within the middle ear leading to serous effusion and secondary infection of this collection of interstitial fluid. Thus, prevention of AOM is aimed at both reducing the presence of pathogenic bacteria and preventing upper respiratory infections that may create eustachian tube dysfunction.

Prevention

The successes of immunization programs in virtually eliminating childhood illnesses such as measles, polio, and varicella have led to great interest in the development of vaccines capable of eradicating the causative agents of AOM. Immunizations targeting the specific bacteria most commonly associated with AOM have had mixed success, however.

For example, although the serotypes contained in the 7-valent pneumococcal conjugate vaccine (PCV, Prevnar) are responsible for approximately 66% of pneumococcal-related AOM, only moderate effectiveness has been noted in reducing AOM incidence among vaccinated children. After the introduction of the 7-valent

PCV into practice in February of 2000, AOM incidence decreased only 6% to 7% among vaccinated children. The 9-valent and 11-valent PCVs[2] have been shown to result in a risk reduction of *S. pneumoniae* isolates in children with AOM of 17% and 34%, respectively. An increase in serotype 19A has been noted that is not covered in the 7-, 9- or 11- valent PCVs[2], but is included in the new 13-valent PCV (Prevnar 13). The 13-valent PCV was incorporated into the recommended childhood immunization schedule in February 2010. The effect of this change on AOM rates will be interesting to observe.

While the ability of the vaccine to prevent AOM episodes may be relatively small, recurrent disease has decreased 23% whereas the need for tympanostomy tubes has decreased nearly 25% in vaccinated children. Hence, the power of the vaccine may be in preventing recurrent disease requiring surgical intervention rather than in prevention of any AOM episodes.

Similar vaccines are in development for *H. influenzae* and *M. catarrhalis* as causative agents of AOM. The current *H. influenzae* b vaccine, or Hib, has had little impact on AOM, because less than 5% of episodes are caused by the type b strain of *Haemophilus*. Rather, non-typeable *Haemophillus influenzae* is a much more common cause of AOM.

Although the vaccines targeting specific bacteria that have been shown to cause AOM have been successful, so too has the influenza vaccine been shown to impact the course of AOM. In several studies, children who received seasonal influenza vaccine (Fluzone) were found to have fewer episodes of AOM than unvaccinated children. Furthermore, those who did have an AOM episode were found to use fewer antibiotics and have shorter duration of middle-ear effusion compared with unvaccinated counterparts.

With evidence that reducing incidence of viral influenza may reduce the occurrence of secondary AOM, several other interventions aimed at reducing viral upper respiratory infection incidence have been studied for their impact on AOM rates. The use of zinc[7] and propolis[7] as agents to prevent viral upper respiratory infections, for instance, has been shown to have mixed benefit in reducing AOM in children. In multiple studies, zinc has been well tolerated with no contraindications to use identified. Zinc as a single agent has been shown to prevent AOM only when used in children under age five who are also malnourished. However, when combined with propolis, zinc was shown to be effective at reducing AOM episodes for children with a history of recurrent AOM. Of note, in several trials zinc did not reduce upper respiratory infection rates; rather, rates of secondary AOM alone were decreased. While not necessarily effective as a preventive measure for all children, zinc and propolis may be an option for children with recurrent infection.

Similarly, probiotics[7] added to infant formula have been shown to be beneficial for some children. Although breastfeeding as compared to formula supplementation has been shown to be most beneficial in preventing AOM, infant formulas supplemented with *Lactobacillus rhamnosus* GG and *Bifidobacterium lactis* Bb-12 (Enfamil Premium, Nestle Good Start) were shown to reduce incidence of AOM over the first 7 months and the first 1 year. Children who received placebo formula had an incidence of AOM of 50% in the first 7 months, whereas children who received the probiotic-supplemented formula had an incidence of only 22%.

Dietary supplementation to limit AOM is not limited to infant formulas, however. Xylitol[7], a polyol sugar alcohol found in birch plants, plums, strawberries, and raspberries, has been demonstrated in several studies to be effective at preventing both dental caries and AOM, though its dosage forms make administration difficult. Xylitol is available as a chewing gum, which raises concern as a choking hazard in young children. Similarly, in its oral syrup form, xylitol must be administered five times daily to be effective. Studies of thrice daily dosing have not been able to demonstrate the same preventive effect as dosing five times daily

despite a consistent total daily dose of 10 grams per day. Furthermore, emerging evidence suggests that xylitol must be given daily to remain effective at reducing AOM episodes, as prophylaxis only during winter months or use only during upper respiratory tract infections is ineffective. Of note, children who have already received tympanostomy tubes receive no prevention benefit from xylitol administration. Research is ongoing to increase physician awareness of xylitol as a possible prophylactic measure as current studies suggest less than one half of United States physicians are aware of xylitol and less than one fourth discuss or recommend its use to patients.

Echinacea[7] and osteopathic manipulation have also been cited as potential prophylactic treatments, particularly for children at high risk of recurrence. However, little evidence exists that either are effective. In fact, one large study demonstrated an increased risk of AOM with Echinacea use during an upper respiratory tract infection episode and no benefit to manipulation treatment. Ongoing studies are examining the use of these modalities.

Clinical Manifestations

AOM presents with a rapid onset of symptoms that may include fever, chills, ear pain, or ear pulling. In fact, ear pulling and ear rubbing have been demonstrated to be quite sensitive for the diagnosis of AOM in the setting of a history consistent with AOM and middle ear effusion. Often, symptoms may be preceded by upper respiratory symptoms such as rhinorrhea, cough, or congestion. Children who have had tympanostomy tubes placed will likely have a far different presentation, with fever and pain being quite unlikely; rather, a thin, yellow or milky discharge may be the only sign that AOM is present.

Diagnosis

The 2013 update of the guidelines of the American Academy of Pediatrics for the diagnosis and treatment of AOM acknowledged that no gold standard exists for the clinical diagnosis of AOM. History and physical examination should be consistent with rapid onset of inflammation in the middle ear. Both pneumatic otoscopy and tympanometry may be useful in the diagnosis of AOM. Tympanic membranes should be evaluated for position, mobility, color, and degree of translucency using pneumatic otoscopy to assess for presence of middle ear effusion and/or inflammation. Moderate to severe bulging of the tympanic membrane, new onset of otorrhea without other cause, or mild bulging of the tympanic membrane with intense erythema or ear pain should prompt diagnosis of AOM. Furthermore, tympanomtry may be useful in determining if an effusion is present if the diagnosis is otherwise unclear.

One concern of physicians has been accurately diagnosing middle ear inflammation after a child has been vigorously crying. A study of 125 healthy children, age less than 30 months, assessed the impact of crying on tympanic membrane color by performing otoscopy both before and after administering at least two immunizations. While crying can cause a pinkening of the tympanic membrane, it should disappear when the child quiets and should be less intense than what is observed with inflammation. True middle ear inflammation results in an angry, red eardrum, not the milder, pink flush seen with vigorous crying. The presence of effusion should also help to support a diagnosis of inflammation.

Differential Diagnosis

Otitis media with effusion is often misdiagnosed as an episode of AOM. Like AOM, OME is common, with 2.2 million episodes annually representing an estimated cost of 4 billion dollars. OME can also occur with a viral upper respiratory infection and may follow or precede an episode of AOM. OME differs from AOM, however, as fluid may be present in the middle ear with OME, but there are no signs of acute infection.

Although OME is not associated with acute infection, it is nonetheless critical to diagnose, as research has demonstrated that

---

[2]Not available in the United States.
[7]Available as a dietary supplement.

---

[7]Available as a dietary supplement.

chronic OME is associated with hearing loss and subsequent developmental delay. In fact, OME in infancy has been shown to be associated with, on average, a 7-point reduction in IQ at age 7.

The cornerstone of treatment for OME is observation for 2 to 3 months to allow the effusion to clear. Avoidance of allergens and tobacco exposure that may worsen eustachian tube dysfunction is also important. Decongestants and antihistamines are not effective. If an effusion does not clear within 2 months, a single course of amoxicillin (Amoxil) or penicillin may be given.

Audiometry should be performed in all children with OME for greater than 3 months or, in the setting of language delay, learning problems or suspected hearing loss in a child with OME. If the effusion persists, or if a child has multiple episodes of OME or has hearing or learning difficulties as a result of OME, surgical intervention should be considered.

Initial surgical intervention for children with persistent OME should be myringotomy with placement of tympanostomy tubes. Tonsillectomy and myringotomy alone are not indicated for treatment of OME. However, adenoidectomy may have a role, particularly in children ages 4 to 8 years. Current recommendations include adenoidectomy only if repeat surgery for OME is needed. However, emerging evidence suggests adenoidectomy may decrease need for surgical retreatment, reduce ongoing hearing loss, and be of benefit during initial surgery for older children.

Treatment

The treatment of AOM has been controversial in recent years. As it is the most common childhood bacterial infection for which antibiotics are prescribed worldwide, debate continues about both the most effective regimen and appropriate time to treat AOM. On average, 2.8 billion dollars are spent per year on antibiotics for episodes of AOM, yet emerging evidence suggests that watchful waiting is appropriate for some children. Judicious use of antibiotic therapy remains key in the prevention of morbidity and mortality associated with otitis media, but is not an appropriate therapy for every child. All children require analgesia of some type as well as close, scheduled follow-up, but use of observation or antibiotic varies with severity of illness and age of the child. Treatment options are summarized in Table 1.

Treatment Options: Observation

For some children with AOM, observation has been shown to be an appropriate therapy that avoids the possible side effects of antibiotics with low risk of complications developing from an untreated otitis media. Evidence suggests that 78% of AOM episodes will spontaneously resolve within the first few days of infection. In fact, for every 100 otherwise healthy at-risk children with AOM, 80 will improve within 3 days without antibiotic therapy. If the same 100 children were all treated with amoxicillin or ampicillin, 92 would improve, though 3 to 10 would develop a rash and 5 to 10 would develop diarrhea. Thus, in a typical family medicine practice 16 children with AOM would need to be treated with antibiotics to prevent 1 child from experiencing ongoing otalgia, while 1 of every 24 children treated will experience harm related to therapy. Hence, the use of antibiotics is not without risk. Multiple studies have demonstrated that even in children as young as 2 months of age, many will improve without antibiotic therapy and delaying antibiotics may prevent undesirable side effects without exposing the child to undue risk. No studies have demonstrated a resurgence of either mastoiditis or meningitis with implementation of watchful waiting for AOM.

If observation is chosen as a management strategy for acute otitis media, it is important to re-evaluate the child in 48 to 72 hours to ensure that they are improving and that a rescue antibiotic is prescribed if symptoms are not resolving. Delayed prescriptions are one strategy that has been effective at reducing antibiotic use, maintaining parental satisfaction, and improving healthcare efficiency.

Physicians are often concerned that parental satisfaction will decrease if watchful waiting for an episode of AOM is recommended. Interestingly, satisfaction has been tied to the receipt of an antibiotic prescription, though not necessarily the administration of antibiotics to the child. Declines in satisfaction are noted when parents are advised to return to care in 2 to 3 days if the child is not improving while undergoing watchful waiting. By offering a delayed prescription, the parent can avoid the difficulties associated with needing to be re-seen if the child fails to improve and parental satisfaction is maintained even if the child never receives any medication. Parents should be educated that up to one third of children who initially are treated with observation will eventually need antibiotic therapy. While this suggests up to two thirds of children can avoid unnecessary antibiotics, parents should be aware that many children will go on to need antibiotic therapy. Clearly, however, not every child is a candidate for observation therapy.

Treatment Options: Antibiotic Therapy

Antibiotic therapy may be associated with less duration of pain, less analgesic use, and less absence for both children and parents from school and work, respectively. The American Academy of Pediatrics and the American Academy of Family Physicians in a joint position statement have recommended that, when a decision is made to use antibiotics, amoxicillin (Amoxil) be given as a first-line agent at a dose of 80 to 90 mg/kg/day.[3] For penicillin-allergic children, cefdinir (Omnicef), cefpodoxime (Vantin), or cefuroxime (Ceftin) may be used. Although the cross reactivity of cephalosporins and penicillins is likely lower than previously believed, if concern exists about treating a child with a cephalosporin, clindamycin (30–40mg/kg/day) may be used. Macrolide antibiotics may have limited efficacy. Ceftriaxone (Rocephin) may be used as a single dose for a child unable to tolerate oral medications.

While amoxicillin continues to be the preferred first-line agent, 30% to 70% of strep pneumoniae strains have become penicillin and macrolide resistant while 20% to 40% of *H. influenzae* has beta-lacatamase–producing capabilities. Given the various resistance patterns of organisms, a child who fails to improve on amoxicillin should receive amoxicillin with clavulanate (Augmentin) or ceftriaxone as second-line therapy. Clindamycin (Cleocin) or tympanocentesis to identify a causative organism may also be considered.

Current evidence continues to suggest that a 10-day course is optimal for children under the age of 2 years. Less benefit to longer duration therapy is noted in older children, and therefore a shorter 5- to 7-day course is recommended for those older than 2 years.

---

[3]Exceeds dosage recommended by the manufacturer.

TABLE 1	Treatment Options for Acute Otitis Media					
	AOM WITH OTORRHEA		**AOM WITHOUT OTORRHEA**		**AOM WITH SEVERE SYMPTOMS***	
AGE OF CHILD	UNILATERAL	BILATERAL	UNILATERAL	BILATERAL	UNILATERAL	BILATERAL
6 months to 2 years	Antibiotics	Antibiotics	Antibiotics or observation	Antibiotics	Antibiotics	Antibiotics
>2 years	Antibiotics	Antibiotics	Antibiotics or observation	Antibiotics or observation	Antibiotics	Antibiotics

*Severe symptoms include: toxic-appearing child, persistent otalgia for >48 hours, temperature >39 °C in past 48 hours, or uncertain access to follow-up.

TABLE 2 — Antibiotic Selection for Specific Patient Populations

	ANTIBIOTIC OF CHOICE	DOSE (mg/kg/day)	ROUTE	DURATION OF THERAPY
AOM in child older than 2 years	Amoxicillin (Amoxil)	80–90[3]	PO	5–7 days
AOM in child less than 2 years	Amoxicillin	80–90[3]	PO	10 days
AOM in child with allergy to penicillin	Cefdinir (Omnicef)	14	PO	10 days
	Cefpodoxime (Vantin)	10	PO	5 days
	Cefuroxime (Ceftin)	30	PO	10 days
AOM with inability to tolerate oral medications	Ceftriaxone (Rocephin)	50	IV/IM	1 day
AOM with amoxicillin failure	Amoxicillin with clavulanate (Augmentin)	90 of amoxicillin and 6.4 of clavulanate[3]	PO	10 days
	Ceftriaxone (Rocephin)	50	IV/IM	3 days[3]
AOM with amoxicillin/clavulanate failure	Ceftriaxone (Rocephin)	50	IV/IM	3 days[3]
AOM with ceftriaxone failure and tympanocentesis not available	Clindamycin (Cleocin)[1]	30–40[3]	PO	10 days
Perforated tympanic membrane	Amoxicillin	80–90[3]	PO	10 days
Tympanostomy tube in place	Amoxicillin AND topical 0.3% ciprofloxacin/0.1% dexamethasone (Ciprodex Otic)	80–90 / 8 drops	PO / Topical BID	10 days / 7 days

[1]Not FDA approved for this indication.
[3]Exceeds dosage recommended by the manufacturer.
Abbreviation: AOM = acute otitis media.

If a child has a perforation of the tympanic membrane, treatment considerations may be slightly different. Oral antibiotics continue to be recommended if perforation is a result of the AOM episode; however, if a child has an episode of AOM with tympanostomy tubes in place topical 0.3% ciprofloxacin/0.1% dexamethasone (Ciprodex Otic) should be added to oral amoxicillin. See Table 2 for antibiotic dosing recommendations.

Regardless of the decision to implement watchful waiting or antibiotic therapy, any child with AOM should be expected to improve within 48 to 72 hours. If improvement is not occurring, the child should be re-evaluated.

Treatment Options: Surgery

For some children, AOM will not be an isolated event. Rather, they will have recurrent infections and require multiple antibiotic courses throughout a year, prompting consideration of tympanostomy tube placement. Currently, referral for evaluation for tympanostomy tubes is recommended when a child has had three or more episodes of AOM within a 6-month period or more than four episodes within a 12 month period. Some have argued, however, that this recommendation should be considered within the context of the child's age at first presentation. A child who has the first episode of AOM prior to 6 months of age is likely to go on to have many more episodes. Ultimately, they will likely meet the criteria for myringotomy and thus may warrant a more aggressive approach from the outset. Conversely, a child who presents with a first episode of AOM as an older child is less likely to have recurrent episodes and can therefore be treated in a more conservative manner.

Using an age-stratified approach, children who experience a first episode of AOM prior to 6 months of age should receive tympanostomy tubes if they have two episodes in a 6- or 12-month time period or three episodes in 24 months. Similarly, children who have a first episode of AOM after 1 year of age should receive tympanostomy tubes only if they have three episodes within 6 months, five within 12 months, or seven within 24 months.

Referral may also occur if a child has a history of AOM associated with meningitis, facial nerve paralysis, coalescent mastoiditis, or brain abscess. Tympanostomy tubes are also often placed due to prolonged OME resulting in hearing loss and language delay. Myringotomy without tube placement may be considered for either diagnosis of an infection that has not responded to numerous antibiotics or for relief of severe otalgia.

AOM episodes will continue to occur despite tympanostomy tube placement. However, episodes will likely be less severe, of shorter duration, and less frequent. In addition to ongoing AOM episodes, tympanostomy tubes can be problematic if they become clogged. New studies in animal models suggest that applying colchicine[1] in the external ear may prevent this complication.

Treatment Options: Analgesia

Regardless of a decision to pursue watchful waiting or antibiotics, analgesics are an important component in the treatment of AOM. Multiple homeopathic interventions and home remedies including application of heat, ice, or mineral oil (Min-O-Ear)[1] have been used for pain control, though no studies exist to verify their effectiveness. Acetaminophen (Tylenol), ibuprofen (Motrin), narcotics, and tympanostomy have all been demonstrated to be effective at reducing pain. However, the side effects of altered mental status, gastrointestinal upset, and respiratory depression with narcotics as well as the skill needed to perform tympanostomy limit the usefulness of these interventions in primary care practice. Topical medications may help avoid the systemic effects of oral medication. Antipyrine and benzocaine are the only topical analgesics available in the United States. Topical benzocaine has been demonstrated to have minimal side effects and in patients over 5 years of age may offer more relief than acetaminophen alone. Benzocaine is available in combination with antipyrine (Allergen Ear Drops, Auroguard Otic). Benzocaine is also available with antipyrine and acetic acid (Auralgan) but may be expensive. In other countries, antipyrine, also known as phenazone, is available in combination with procaine and is effective.

Antihistamines have often been prescribed, as have decongestants, in an attempt to reduce the fluid volume in the middle ear and hence provide relief. Unfortunately, use of antihistamines and decongestants has been shown to result in a fivefold to eightfold increase in the risk of side effects with no benefits, including no decreased time to cure, no prevention of surgery or complications, and no increased symptom resolution. Therefore, antihistamines and decongestants have not been routinely recommended.

Conclusion

AOM continues to be one of the most costly and common childhood illnesses in developed nations throughout the world.

[1]Not FDA approved for this indication.

Otitis Media

339

Successful management of this condition requires much more than choosing amoxicillin at an appropriate dose and duration or appropriately timing a surgical referral. Vigilant attention to modifying risk factors when possible, promoting immunization, and limiting the spread of viral illnesses has been shown to prevent AOM instances. Furthermore, adherence to diagnostic criteria to attempt to accurately distinguish between AOM and OME, as well as implementing observation when appropriate, can significantly reduce antibiotic usage, thereby minimizing side effects for patients and opportunity to develop resistance in pathogens.

RED EYE

Method of
John N. Dorsch, MD

CURRENT DIAGNOSIS

- Patients with traumatic injury to the eye, loss of vision, extreme pain not explained by pathology, keratitis, suspected uveitis or glaucoma, chemical injury, or nonhealing corneal abrasion should be referred to an ophthalmologist.
- Bacterial, viral, and allergic conjunctivitis can often be distinguished by the type of ocular discharge present.
- Subconjunctival hemorrhage can occur from trauma, from increased intrathoracic pressure, from anticoagulants, or idiopathically.

CURRENT THERAPY

- Do not use eye patches in patients with corneal abrasions.
- Do not use topical anesthetics for the eye outside a clinic or hospital setting, because corneal toxicity can occur.
- Patients with corneal abrasions should be reexamined the following day.
- Patients with corneal abrasions from extended-wear contact lenses often become colonized with *Pseudomonas aeruginosa* and should be treated with appropriate antibiotics (quinolones).

In the primary care office, the most common causes of red eye are conjunctivitis, subconjunctival hemorrhage, and foreign body causing corneal abrasions. Other common causes of red eye include blepharitis and hordeolum. Less common but serious causes of red eye include viral keratitis, uveitis, scleritis, and angle-closure glaucoma. Other usually less serious causes of red eye include episcleritis, pingueculum, and pterygium. All primary care physicians should have expertise in recognizing and treating the common causes of red eye, and should recognize and refer patients with higher-stakes diagnoses (Boxes 1 and 2).

Physical Examination

Always check visual acuity in any patient with an eye complaint. Fluorescein strips (Flu-Glo, Fluorets), topical anesthetic drops, and cobalt blue light are used to examine the cornea for abrasions, keratitis, and ulceration. Cotton-tipped applicators are used to evert the upper eyelid and look for a foreign body.

Pupillary reaction is often affected by angle closure glaucoma and uveitis, but it is rarely affected by conjunctivitis, blepharitis, and corneal disorders. The pupil may be irregular in the patient with uveitis.

Patients with uveitis often have pain in the closed affected eye when a bright light is shined in the normal eye or with convergence of the eyes. This is due to consensual reflex of the pupils to light and accommodation.

Box 1   Approach to the Patient with Red Eye

The following questions are often helpful in making the diagnosis in patients with red eyes.

- *Is one eye or are both eyes involved?* Infections, allergy, and systemic illness are more likely to cause bilateral eye involvement.
- *Does the patient have intense eye pain?* If yes, likely diagnoses include acute angle closure glaucoma, uveitis, scleritis, keratitis, foreign body, or corneal abrasion.
- *Does the patient have a foreign body sensation?* If so, consider corneal abrasion, trauma, dry eye, keratitis, and other corneal disorders.
- *Is there a discharge?* If it is *very* copious and purulent, consider gonococcal conjunctivitis. If it is discolored and purulent, consider bacterial conjunctivitis. Copious watery discharge is typical of viral conjunctivitis. Stringy, mucoid discharge is typical of allergic or chlamydial conjunctivitis.
- *Do the eyes itch?* If so, consider blepharitis or allergy in the differential.
- *Are the eyelids swollen?* Consider allergy or infection.
- *Do the eyelids have lumps?* Hordeolum and chalazion should be considered.
- *Do the eyes burn?* Consider blepharitis or dry eye.
- *Is the eye redness recurrent?* Consider herpes keratitis, uveitis, and allergic conjunctivitis.
- *Does the patient have photophobia?* Corneal problems (abrasions, keratitis) and uveitis should be considered.
- *Is there loss of vision?* Consider corneal ulcer, uveitis, and angle closure glaucoma.
- *Is the patient using ocular medications?* Prolonged use of neomycin and sulfa ophthalmic medications can cause sensitization and redness of the eyes.

Box 2   Red Eye

Common Causes
- Conjunctivitis: bacterial, viral, allergic
- Subconjunctival hemorrhage
- Corneal abrasion
- Blepharitis

Less Common Causes
Less Serious
- Episcleritis

- Pingueculum
- Pterygium

More Serious
- Viral keratitis
- Uveitis
- Scleritis
- Angle closure glaucoma

The diagnosis of conjunctivitis is made by pulling the lower eyelid down with the examiner's finger. If the bulbar or palpebral conjunctivae are inflamed (i.e., hyperemic, edematous, discharge), conjunctivitis is present. Palpable preauricular nodes may be present with viral conjunctivitis and chlamydial conjunctivitis.

Conjunctivitis

Conjunctivitis is the most common cause of red eye encountered by primary care providers. Among the etiologies of conjunctivitis, viral conjunctivitis is the most common. Although patients with conjunctivitis might have some minor irritation of the eyes, they usually do not complain of pain in the eye or loss of vision. Ocular discharge is generally considered to be an important diagnostic feature of conjunctivitis (Table 1). Although much has been written about characterizing conjunctivitis by the nature of the discharge, one meta-analysis failed to find evidence of the diagnostic

TABLE 1	Conjunctivitis		
TYPE	**COURSE**	**CHARACTERISTICS**	**DISCHARGE**
Bacterial	Starts in one eye, often spreads to other eye		Purulent
Allergic	Accompanies allergic rhinitis	Itchy eyes	Mucus
Viral	Usually bilateral	Very red eyes	Watery

usefulness of clinical signs and/or symptoms in distinguishing bacterial conjunctivitis from viral conjunctivitis.

Viral Conjunctivitis

Viral conjunctivitis is often seen in epidemics and is most commonly caused by members of the Adenovirus family. Typically, viral conjunctivitis starts in one eye and spreads to the other eye a few days later. The conjunctivae appear red and swollen, with copious watery discharge (Figure 1). The natural course of viral conjunctivitis is self-limiting, lasting 10 to 14 days. Tender preauricular lymph nodes, when present, indicate the presence of viral or chlamydial conjunctivitis. Management should be directed at scrupulous hygiene. Patients must be informed that their infection is highly contagious. They should avoid close contact with other persons (e.g., towels, direct contact, swimming pools) for 2 weeks and wash hands frequently to prevent the spread of their infection. Topical antibiotics have been prescribed to try to prevent bacterial superinfection, but there is no good evidence that they have any significant impact. Symptomatic treatment with cold compresses and topical vasoconstrictors may be helpful.

Bacterial Conjunctivitis

Bacterial conjunctivitis typically starts abruptly in one eye and spreads to the other eye in 1 to 2 days. Usually a purulent discharge is present that persists throughout the day. A variety of gram-positive and gram-negative organisms cause bacterial conjunctivitis, but the most common etiologies are *Staphylococcus aureus*, *Streptococcus pneumoniae*, and *Haemophilus pneumoniae*. Treatment of bacterial conjunctivitis is usually empiric, but conjunctival scraping for smears and cultures should be done in infants, immunocompromised patients, and patients with hyperacute conjunctivitis in which *Neisseria gonorrhoeae* or *Chlamydia trachomatis* infection is suspected. Treatment of bacterial conjunctivitis (excluding gonococcal or chlamydial conjunctivitis) usually consists of a topical antibiotic used four times a day (Table 2). Topical antibiotics are usually prescribed for 5 to 7 days, and resolution of conjunctivitis is expected within that time.

Hyperacute bacterial conjunctivitis has an abrupt onset, copious purulent discharge, and rapid progression, and it is usually associated with gonococcal infection in a sexually active patient. Chemosis (edema of the conjunctivae) may be present.

Chlamydial conjunctivitis is acquired through exposure to infected secretions from the genital tract, either direct or indirect. The infection is usually unilateral (at least initially), and often

TABLE 2	Topical Antibiotics Used to Treat Bacterial Conjunctivitis	
DRUG	**DOSAGE**
Bacitracin (Ak-Tracin, Bacticin) ointment	Apply 0.5 inch in eye q3–4h
Ciprofloxacin (Ciloxan) 0.3% ophthalmic solution	1–2 gtt in eye q15min × 6h, then q30min × 18h, then q1h × 1 d, then q4h × 12 d[3]
Gatifloxacin (Zymar) 0.3% ophthalmic solution	1 gt in eye q2h up to 8 ×/day × 2 days, then 1 gt qid × 5 d
Gentamicin (Gentak, Gentasol) 0.3% ophthalmic solution or ointment	Ointment: 0.5 inch applied to eye 2–3 times per day Solution: 1–2 gtt in eye q4h
Levofloxacin (Quixin) 0.5% ophthalmic solution	1–2 gtt in eye q2h × 2 d while awake, then q4h while awake × 5 d
Moxifloxacin (Vigamox) 0.5% ophthalmic solution	1 gt in eye tid × 7 d
Neomycin/polymyxin B/ gramicidin (Neosporin) ophthalmic solution	1–2 gtt in eye q4h × 7–10 d
Ofloxacin (Ocuflox) 0.3% ophthalmic solution	1–2 gtt in eye q2–4h × 2 d, then 1–2 gtt in eye qid × 5 d
Polymyxin B and trimethoprim (Polytrim) ophthalmic solution	1 gt in eye q3h × 7–10 d
Sulfacetamide (Isopto Cetamide, Ocusulf-10, Sodium Sulamyd, Sulf-10, AK-Sulf) 10% ophthalmic solution, ointment	Ointment: 0.5-inch ribbon in eye q3–4h and qhs × 7 d Solution: 1–2 gtt in eye q2–3h × 7–10 d
Tobramycin (AK-Tob, Tobrex) 0.3% ophthalmic solution	1–2 gtt in eye q4h

[3]Exceeds dosage recommended by the manufacturer.

there is involvement of the preauricular node on the ipsilateral side. Gonococcal and chlamydial infections are treated systemically (Box 3).

Conjunctivitis of the Newborn

Chlamydial conjunctivitis is the most common cause of infectious conjunctivitis of the newborn in the United States. Onset of conjunctivitis is 3 to 10 days after birth, but it has been reported as

Box 3	Treatment of Chlamydial and Gonococcal Conjunctivitis

Chlamydial Conjunctivitis
- Erythromycin (Ery-Tab)[1] 250 mg PO qid × 14 d

or
- Doxycycline (Vibramycin) 100 mg PO bid × 14 d
- Treat partners

Gonococcal Conjunctivitis
- Ceftriaxone (Recephin 1 g IM)

[1]Not FDA approved for this indication.

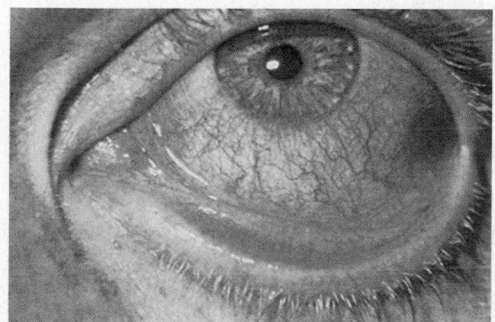

Figure 1. Viral conjunctivitis. (Reproduced with permission from the University of Michigan Kellogg Eye Center, http://www.kellogg.umich.edu.)

late as 2 months after birth. *Chlamydia trachomatis* infection can also cause pneumonia, otitis media, proctitis, and vulvovaginitis in infants. Treatment consists of erythromycin (EryPed Drops) orally 50 mg/kg/day in four divided doses for 14 days. Erythromycin ointment (Ilotycin 0.5%) or tetracycline ointment[2] given shortly after delivery is effective in preventing chlamydial conjunctivitis but not systemic chlamydial infections.

Gonococcal conjunctivitis of the newborn is a hyperacute infection that occurs 2 to 4 days after birth. It can cause corneal ulceration and loss of vision. Gonococcal conjunctivitis can be prevented with silver nitrate drops[2] or erythromycin (Ilotycin) or tetracycline ointment[2] administered shortly after delivery. Silver nitrate commonly causes a self-limited chemical conjunctivitis, which can delay visual bonding of the infant to the parents in the first few hours of life. Therapy of gonococcal conjunctivitis of the newborn consists of IV penicillin G[1] given four times a day for 7 days or ceftriaxone (Rocephin) IV or IM once a day for 7 days or gentamicin (Garamycin)[1] IM given twice a day for 7 days.

Conjunctivitis–Otitis Media Syndrome

Conjunctivitis–otitis media syndrome is a common condition in which children with otitis media also have purulent bilateral ocular discharge. It responds to treatment of otitis media; no topical treatment of conjunctivitis is required.

Methicillin-Resistant *Staphylococcus Aureus* Conjunctivitis

Increasing numbers of cases of bacterial conjunctivitis are caused by methicillin-resistant *S. aureus* (MRSA). MRSA conjunctivitis manifests as bacterial conjunctivitis resistant to conventional therapy and is treated with the same drugs used to treat MRSA in other parts of the body (Doxycycline [Vibramycin],[1] vancomycin [Vancocin], sulfamethoxazole-trimethoprim [Bactrim][1]). Cultures should be obtained when MRSA is suspected.

Allergic Conjunctivitis

Allergic conjunctivitis is an immunoglobulin E (IgE)-mediated condition characterized by bilateral eye involvement, itchy eyes, and mucoid discharge. *Seasonal* conjunctivitis is caused by exposure to common allergens (e.g., pollens, dander) and usually accompanies allergic rhinitis. *Perennial* allergic conjunctivitis is similar to seasonal allergic conjunctivitis, but the symptoms are usually less severe. Patients are usually treated with a systemic antihistamine. Ophthalmic (topical) medications include antihistamine or decongestants, mast cell inhibitors, nonsteroidal antiinflammatory drugs (NSAIDs), H_1-antagonists, and various combinations of these (Table 3). Milder cases can be treated with a decongestant-antihistamine combination for about 2 weeks. Moderate to more severe cases can require longer use of these medications or the addition of systemic antihistamines or mast cell inhibitors. Some patients require topical corticosteroids or cyclosporine (Restasis)[1] for severe allergic conjunctivitis, but these should be evaluated by an ophthalmologist because of potential complications of therapy.

Subconjunctival Hemorrhage

In subconjunctival hemorrhage, the redness of the eye is localized and sharply circumscribed, and the underlying sclera is not visible (Figure 2). Conjunctivitis is not present, and there is no discharge. There is typically no pain or visual change. Subconjunctival hemorrhage may be spontaneous, but it can also result from trauma, hypertension, bleeding disorders, or increased intrathoracic pressure (e.g., straining, coughing, retching). No treatment is necessary, but investigation may be warranted if the etiology is in question or the hemorrhage is recurrent. Referral to an ophthalmologist should be considered if the subconjunctival hemorrhage is from trauma or has not resolved within 2 to 3 weeks.

Corneal Abrasion

Corneal abrasions typically result from scratching of the corneal epithelium due to trauma, but they can also occur from extended-wear contact lenses. Patients with corneal abrasions present with pain, excessive tearing from the involved eye, photophobia, a foreign-body sensation (like having sand in the eye), and blurry vision.

Corneal abrasions are identified by staining the cornea with fluorescein and examining under cobalt blue light (Figure 3). The eye should also be examined carefully to check for foreign bodies. Topical anesthetic is administered to make the patient

[3]Exceeds dosage recommended by the manufacturer.
[2]Not available in the United States.

[1]Not FDA approved for this indication.

TABLE 3 Topical Medications for Allergic Conjunctivitis

GENERIC NAME	BRAND NAME(S)	DOSING	MODE OF ACTION
Azelastine 0.05% solution	Optivar	1 gt in eye(s) bid	H_1-antagonist, mast cell inhibitor
Cromolyn 4% solution	Crolom, generic	1–2 gtt in eye(s) 4–6 times per day	Mast cell inhibitor
Emedastine 0.05% solution	Emadine	1 gt in eye(s) qid	H_1-antagonist
Epinastine 0.05% solution	Elestat	1 gt in eye(s) bid	H_1- and H_2-antagonist, mast cell inhibitor
Ketorolac 0.5% solution	Acular	1 gt in eye(s) qid up to 1 wk	NSAID
Diclofenac 0.1% solution[1]	Voltaren ophthalmic	1 gt in eye(s) qid × 2 wk	NSAID
Lodoxamide 0.1% solution	Alomide	1–2 gtt in eye(s) qid up to 3 mo	Mast cell inhibitor
Loteprednol 0.2% susp.	Alrex	1 gt in eye(s) qd	Corticosteroid
Naphazoline/pheniramine (solution)	Naphcon-A (OTC) Opcon-A (OTC) Visine-A (OTC)	1–2 gtt in eye(s) qd-qid prn	Antihistamine, decongestant
Nedrocomil 2% solution	Alocril	1–2 gtt in eye(s) bid	H_1-antagonist, mast cell inhibitor
Olopatadine 0.1% solution	Patanol	1 gt in eye(s) bid	H_1-antagonist, mast cell inhibitor
Olopatadine 0.2% solution	Pataday	1 gt in eye(s) qd	Mast cell inhibitor

[1]Not FDA approved for this indication.
Abbreviation: NSAID = nonsteroidal antiinflammatory drug.

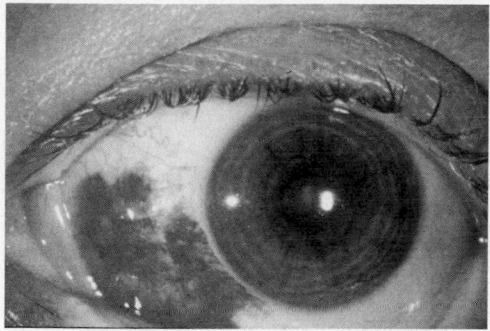

Figure 2. Subconjunctival hemorrhage. (Reprinted with permission from American Academy of Ophthalmology: Managing the Red Eye. Eye Care Skills for the Primary Care Physician Series. San Francisco: American Academy of Ophthalmology, 2001.)

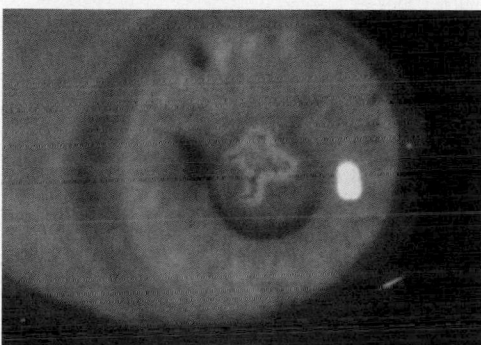

Figure 3. Corneal abrasion with fluorescein stain with cobalt blue light. (Reprinted with permission from American Academy of Ophthalmology: Managing the Red Eye. Eye Care Skills for the Primary Care Physician Series. San Francisco: American Academy of Ophthalmology, 2001.)

comfortable during the examination, but continued use can cause corneal damage.

Management of corneal abrasions consists of pain relief and prevention of infection. Pain can be relieved with topical NSAIDs such as ketorolac (Acular)[1] and Diclofenac (Voltaren),[1] oral over-the-counter analgesics, and occasionally oral narcotics. Topical antibiotics are usually prescribed to prevent infection. Antibiotic ointments are lubricating and soothing to the eye, making them a good option for traumatic corneal abrasions. Topical ophthalmic antibiotic ointments commonly used are bacitracin (Bacticin), erythromycin (Ilotycin), and gentamicin (Gentak).

In patients who have corneal abrasions from contact lens over-wear, eyes are commonly colonized with *Pseudomonas aeruginosa*. These patients should be treated with topical antibiotics such as ciprofloxacin (Ciloxan) or ofloxacin (Ocuflux) solutions.

Patching of the eye, though a common practice of the past, has not shown evidence of benefit in recent studies. It was found that eye patching can actually cause harm, so this practice is no longer recommended.

Infrequently, patients have traumatic uveitis accompanying corneal abrasion. Traumatic uveitis usually causes significantly more

---

[1]Not FDA approved for this indication.

pain than a corneal abrasion, and, if uveitis is suspected, the patient should be evaluated by an ophthalmologist.

Patients with corneal abrasions should be reexamined in 24 hours. Corneal abrasions typically should be healed or greatly improved in 24 hours. If the abrasion is not completely healed after 24 hours, the patient should be examined again in 2 or 3 days. Referral should be considered if any worsening occurs or if the abrasion does not heal within 5 days. Corneal abrasions can be prevented by using protective eyewear.

Other Causes of Red Eye

Other causes of red eye are somewhat less common.

Blepharitis

Blepharitides are inflammatory conditions of the eyelid caused by infection or obstruction of eyelid glands (Table 4). Blepharitis may be accompanied by conjunctivitis. Staphylococcal blepharitis arises from the accessory glands to the eyelashes and causes discharge from the eyelid, often associated with erythema, induration, loss of eyelashes, and crusting of the eyelid (Figure 4). This is treated with hot, moist packs to the eyes, baby shampoo scrubs (3 oz. water and 3 drops baby shampoo used on a washcloth BID), and erythromycin ointment (Ilotycin) at bedtime. Seborrheic blepharitis, a more chronic form of blepharitis, arises from the meibomian glands and causes scaling of the eyelids (Figure 5). Seborrheic blepharitis is often associated with skin disorders such as rosacea, eczema, and seborrheic dermatitis. This is treated with hot, moist packs and baby shampoo scrubs. Resistant cases are treated with oral tetracycline (Sumycin) (or one of its derivatives).

Hordeolum (Stye)

A hordeolum is an acute, painful mass of the eyelid that is caused by inflammation of the glands (Figure 6). It does not usually cause the eye to become red as well. Warm compresses to the eyelid four times a day for 3 to 5 minutes typically causes resolution within 1 week. Because they arise from the same glands, hordeola and blepharitis commonly occur together.

Episcleritis

Episcleritis is a self-limited inflammation of the episcleral vessels and is believed to be autoimmune. It has a rapid onset and usually minimal discomfort. Redness is most often confined to a sector of the eye. Episcleritis usually resolves in 7 to 10 days. Recurrence is not uncommon. Oral NSAID drugs may be prescribed, but treatment is usually not necessary.

Scleritis

Scleritis is, fortunately, much less common than episcleritis. Patients with scleritis experience intense inflammation and deep eye pain. Scleritis is commonly associated with rheumatoid arthritis and inflammatory bowel disease. The patient should be promptly referred to an ophthalmologist if scleritis is suspected.

Acute Angle Closure Glaucoma

Acute angle closure glaucoma is characterized by acute ocular pain and is often accompanied by vomiting, blurred vision, acute photophobia, pupils unreactive to light, and circumcorneal redness (ciliary flush). Treatment of glaucoma with pilocarpine (Isopto Carpine), topical timolol (Timoptic), and acetazolamide (Diamox) should be started, and the patient should be given an urgent referral to an ophthalmologist.

TABLE 4	Blepharitis		
TYPE	**SITE OF ORIGIN**	**CLINICAL CHARACTERISTICS**	**TREATMENT**
Staphylococcal	Accessory glands of eyelids	Erythema and induration of eyelid; crusting; discharge; loss of eyelashes	Warm compresses Baby shampoo scrubs Erythromycin ointment (Ilotycin)
Seborrheic	Meibomian glands	More chronic, scaling	Warm compresses Baby shampoo scrubs Oral tetracycline for resistant cases

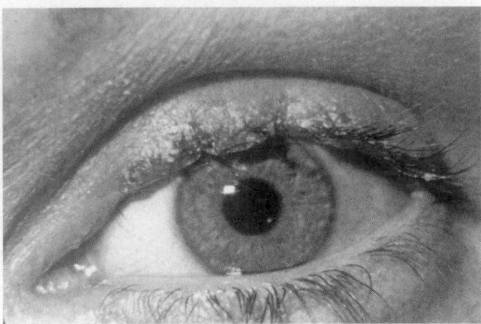

Figure 4. Staphylococcal blepharitis. (Reprinted with permission from American Academy of Ophthalmology: Managing the Red Eye. Eye Care Skills for the Primary Care Physician Series. San Francisco: American Academy of Ophthalmology, 2001.)

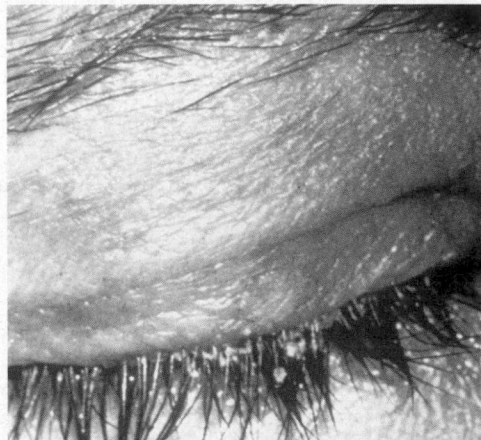

Figure 5. Seborrheic blepharitis. (Reprinted with permission from American Academy of Ophthalmology: Managing the Red Eye. Eye Care Skills for the Primary Care Physician Series. San Francisco: American Academy of Ophthalmology, 2001.)

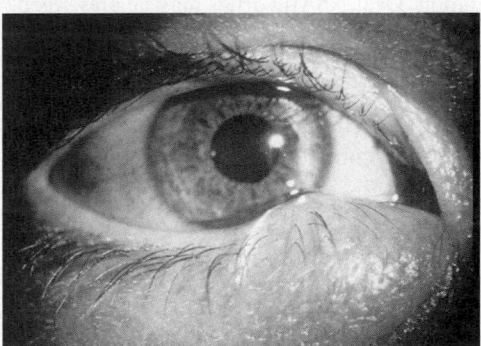

Figure 6. Hordeolum. (Reprinted with permission from American Academy of Ophthalmology: Managing the Red Eye. Eye Care Skills for the Primary Care Physician Series. San Francisco: American Academy of Ophthalmology, 2001.)

Anterior Uveitis

Uveitis is the inflammation of the iris and ciliary muscle, often associated with autoimmune disease. Trauma can also cause uveitis. Signs of uveitis include ocular pain, ciliary flush, and occasionally irregularity of the pupil. Prompt referral should be arranged for a patient in whom uveitis is suspected.

In general, referral to an ophthalmologist should strongly be considered for:

- Traumatic injury to the eye
- Loss of vision
- Extreme eye pain not explained by pathology
- Keratitis
- Suspected uveitis or glaucoma
- Chemical injury (especially alkali)
- Corneal abrasion not healing

References

American Optometric Association. Optometric clinical practice guideline: Care of the patient with anterior uveitis, Revised March 1999. PDF available at www.aoa.org/documents/CPG-7.pdf; June 23, 1994 [accessed July 10, 2015].

Arbour JD, Brunette I, Boisjoly HM, et al. Should we patch corneal abrasions? Arch Ophthalmol 1997;115(3):313–7.

Au YK, Henkind P. Pain elicited by consensual pupillary reflex: a diagnostic test for acute iritis. Lancet 1981;2:1254–5.

Avdic E, Cosgrove SE. Management and control strategies for community-associated methicillin-resistant *Staphylococcus aureus*. Expert Opin Pharmacother 2008;9 (9):1463–79.

Boder F, Marchant C, et al. Bacterial etiology of conjunctivitis-otitis media syndrome. Pediatrics 1985;76:26–8.

Bradford CA. Basic Ophthalmology. 8th ed. San Francisco: American Academy of Ophthalmology; 2004.

De Toledo AR, Chandler JW. Conjunctivitis of the newborn. Infect Dis Clin North Am 1992;6(4):807–13.

Frith P, Gray R, MacLennan S, et al. The Eye in Clinical Practice. Oxford: Blackwell Scientific; 1994.

Jackson WB. Blepharitis: Current strategies for diagnosis and treatment. Can J Ophthalmol 2008;43(2):170–9.

Liebowitz HM. The red eye. N Engl J Med 2000;343(5):345–51.

Patterson J, Fetzer D, Krall J, et al. Eye patch treatment for the pain of corneal abrasion. South Med J 1996;89(2):227–9.

Prochazka AV. Diagnosis and treatment of red eye. Primary Care Case Reviews 2001;4:23–31.

Rietveld RP, van Weert H, Riet G, Bindels P. Diagnostic impact of signs and symptoms in acute infectious conjunctivitis: Systematic literature search. BMJ 2003;327 (4):789.

Tarabishy A, Jeng B. Bacterial conjunctivitis: A review for internists. Cleve Clin J Med 2008;75(7):507–12.

Talbot EM. A simple test to diagnose iritis. BMJ 1987;295:812–3.

Trobe JD. The Physician's Guide to Eye Care. 2nd ed. San Francisco: Foundation of the American Academy of Ophthalmology; 2001.

Wilson SA, Last A. Management of corneal abrasion. Am Fam Physician 2004;70:123–30.

Wong AH, Barg SS, Leung AK. Seasonal and perennial allergic conjunctivitis. Recent Pat Inflamm Allergy Drug Disc 2009;3(2):118–27.

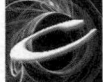

RHINOSINUSITIS

Method of
Ann M. Aring, MD

CURRENT DIAGNOSIS

- Given that inflammation of the sinuses rarely occurs without concurrent inflammation of the nasal mucosa, rhinosinusitis is a more accurate term for what is commonly called sinusitis.
- Most cases of sinusitis are caused by viral infections associated with the common cold. Viral rhinosinusitis improves in 7–10 days.
- Diagnosis of acute bacterial rhinosinusitis requires that symptoms persist for longer than 10 days or worsen after 5–7 days.
- Diagnostic criterion for acute rhinosinusitis include symptoms following upper respiratory tract infection; facial pain, pressure, or fullness; purulent rhinorrhea; maxillary toothache; and biphasic history with worsening symptoms after initial improvement.
- Acute rhinosinusitis lasts up to 4 weeks, subacute rhinosinusitis lasts from 4 to 12 weeks, and chronic rhinosinusitis lasts 12 weeks or longer. Recurrent acute rhinosinusitis is defined as four or more episodes per year with complete resolution between episodes.
- Radiographic imaging in a patient with acute rhinosinusitis is not recommended unless a complication or an alternative diagnosis is suspected.

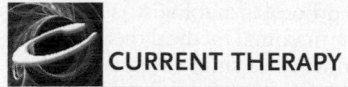

- Mild rhinosinusitis symptoms less than 7 days duration can be managed with supportive care, including analgesics, short-term decongestants, saline nasal irrigation, and intranasal corticosteroids.
- Antibiotic therapy is recommended for patients with sinusitis symptoms that do not improve within 7–10 days or that worsen at any time; those with moderate illness (moderate to severe pain or temperature $\geq$101 °F [38.3 °C]); or those who are immunocompromised.
- Amoxicillin-clavulanate (Augmentin) is recommended as the first-line antibiotic in adults with acute bacterial rhinosinusitis.
- "High-dose" amoxicillin-clavulanate (Augmentin XR) (2 g orally twice daily) is recommended for adults with ABRS from geographic regions with high endemic rates ($\geq$10%) of invasive penicillin-nonsusceptible *Streptococcus pneumoniae*, those with severe infection with fever of 102 °F (39 °C) or higher, those age >65 years, those who have had a recent hospitalization, those who have had antibiotic use within the past month, or those who are immunocompromised.
- Macrolides and trimethoprim-sulfamethoxazole (Bactrim) are not recommended for empiric therapy because of high rates of resistance among *S. pneumoniae* and *Hemophilus influenza*.
- For adults allergic to penicillin, doxycycline (Vibramycin)[1] or a respiratory fluoroquinolone (levofloxacin [Levaquin] or moxifloxacin [Avelox]) may be used as an alternative regimen for initial empiric therapy for bacterial rhinosinusitis.
- In adults with confirmed acute rhinosinusitis, more than 70% will clinically improve after 7 days with or without antibiotic therapy.
- Antibiotic use increased the absolute cure rate by 15% compared with a placebo at 7–12 days (NNT = 7).

[1]Not FDA approved for this indication.

Epidemiology of Acute Rhinosinusitis and Predisposing Factors

Each year in the United States, rhinosinusitis affects one in seven adults and is diagnosed in 31 million patients. Rhinosinusitis is the fifth most common diagnosis for which antibiotics are prescribed. Rhinosinusitis has a higher frequency in the winter months and lower frequency in the summer and autumn months. Acute sinusitis is diagnosed more often in women; two-thirds of patients with sinusitis are women.

Predisposing Factors

Predisposing factors for acute rhinosinusitis include viral upper respiratory infections and allergic rhinitis. Anatomic malformations including polyps, deviated nasal septum, foreign bodies, and tumors can also predispose to acute rhinosinusitis. In addition, rhinosinusitis can also be caused by upper tooth infections that spread directly to the maxillary sinus.

Pathogenesis and Etiology of Rhinosinusitis

Most cases of acute rhinosinusitis are caused by viral infections associated with the common cold. The most common viruses in acute viral rhinosinusitis are rhinovirus, adenovirus, influenza virus, and parainfluenza virus. Mucosal edema occurs with the viral infection with subsequent obstruction of the sinus ostia. In addition, viral and bacterial infections impair the cilia that help transport the mucus. The ostia obstruction and slowed mucus transport cause stagnation of secretions and lowered oxygen tension within the sinuses. This environment is an excellent culture medium for both viruses and bacteria and the infectious particles grow rapidly. The body responds with an inflammatory reaction. Polymorphonuclear leukocytes are mobilized, which results in pus formation. The most common bacteria found in acute community-acquired bacterial rhinosinusitis are *S. pneumoniae*, *H. influenza*,

Staphylococcus aureus, and *Moraxella catarrhalis*. Acute adult rhinosinusitis most commonly involves the maxillary and ethmoid sinuses. More than one of the paranasal sinuses can be affected.

Diagnosis of Acute Rhinosinusitis

Diagnosis of acute bacterial rhinosinusitis requires that symptoms persist for longer than 10 days or worsen after 5 to 7 days. Diagnostic criterion for acute bacterial rhinosinusitis include symptoms following upper respiratory tract infection; facial pain, pressure, or fullness; purulent rhinorrhea; maxillary toothache; and biphasic history with worsening symptoms after initial improvement. The American College of Physicians has proposed diagnostic criteria for acute rhinosinusitis. The diagnostic criteria were endorsed by the Infectious Disease Society of America, the Centers for Disease Control and Prevention (CDC), and the American Academy of Family Physicians. Table 1 lists the sensitivity, specificity, positive predictive value (PPV), and negative predictive value (NPV) of criteria used to diagnose acute rhinosinusitis. If resistant pathogens are suspected or if the patient is immunocompromised, a bacterial culture of the secretions may be used.

Imaging

For uncomplicated acute rhinosinusitis, radiographic imaging is not recommended. Plain sinus radiography shows air-fluid levels in patients with both viral and bacterial rhinosinusitis. Sinus computed tomography should not be used for the routine evaluation of acute bacterial rhinosinusitis. However, sinus computed tomography can be used to identify suspected complications and define anatomic abnormalities.

Differential Diagnosis

The signs and symptoms of acute bacterial rhinosinusitis and prolonged viral upper respiratory infection are similar, which can lead to the overdiagnosis of acute bacterial rhinosinusitis. Other conditions that mimic bacterial rhinosinusitis are migraine headache, tension headache, trigeminal neuralgia, and temporomandibular joint disorders.

Treatment of Acute Rhinosinusitis

Symptomatic Treatment

Mild rhinosinusitis symptoms less than 7 days in duration can be managed with supportive care, including analgesics, short-term decongestants, saline nasal irrigation, and intranasal corticosteroids. There are no RCTs that evaluate the effectiveness of decongestants in a patient with sinusitis. In a systematic review of seven studies, nasal decongestants were found to be modestly effective for short-term relief of congestion in adults with the common cold. Nasal saline is used to soften viscous secretions and improve mucociliary clearance. The mechanical cleansing of the nasal cavity with saline has been shown to benefit patients with rhinosinusitis. Most studies of intranasal corticosteroids are industry sponsored. A Cochrane review of four RCTs with 1943 patients supported intranasal corticosteroids as monotherapy or as adjuvant therapy to antibiotics. According to another Cochrane

345

TABLE 1	Signs and Symptoms Used to Predict Acute Sinusitis			
	SENSITIVITY %	**SPECIFICITY %**	**PPV %**	**NPV %**
Purulent rhinorrhea	35	78	62	78
Nasal obstruction	60	22	53	15
Facial pain, pressure, or fullness	75	77	78	73
Maxillary toothache	66	49	59	56
Symptoms after URI	89	79	83	87

Reprinted with permission from Aring and Chan (2011).

review, antihistamines do not significantly alleviate nasal congestion, rhinorrhea, or sneezing in persons with the common cold. In addition, antihistamines can overdry the nasal mucosa, causing problems with sinus drainage and further discomfort. Antihistamines should not be used for symptomatic relief of acute rhinosinusitis except in patients with a history of allergic rhinitis.

Antibiotic Treatment

Antibiotic therapy is recommended for patients with sinusitis symptoms that do not improve within 7 to 10 days or that worsen at any time; those with moderate illness (moderate to severe pain or temperature ≥101 °F [38.3 °C]); or those who are immunocompromised. Amoxicillin-clavulanate (Augmentin) is recommended as the first-line antibiotic in adults with acute bacterial rhinosinusitis. "High-dose" amoxicillin-clavulanate (Augmentin XR) (2 g orally twice daily) is recommended for adults with ABRS from geographic regions with high endemic rates (≥10%) of invasive penicillin-nonsusceptible *S. pneumonia*, those with severe infection with fever of 102 °F (39 °C) or higher, those age >65 years, those who have had a recent hospitalization, those who have had antibiotic use within the past month, or those who are immunocompromised.

Macrolides and trimethoprim-sulfamethoxazole (Bactrim) are not recommended for empiric therapy because of high rates of resistance among *S. pneumonia* and *H. influenza*. For adults allergic to penicillin, doxycycline (Vibramycin)[1] or a respiratory fluoroquinolone (levofloxacin [Levaquin] or moxifloxacin [Avelox]) may be used as an alternative regimen for initial empiric therapy for bacterial rhinosinusitis. In adults with confirmed acute rhinosinusitis, more than 70% will clinically improve after 7 days with or without antibiotic therapy. Antibiotic use increased the absolute cure rate by 15% compared with a placebo at 7 to 12 days (NNT = 7).

Complications and Referral

Complications of acute bacterial rhinosinusitis are estimated to occur in 1 in 1000 cases. Patients with acute bacterial rhinosinusitis who present with visual symptoms (diplopia, decreased visual acuity, disconjugate gaze, difficulty opening the eye), severe headache, somnolence, or high fever should be evaluated with emergent computed tomography with contrast. Sinonasal cancers are uncommon in the United States, with an annual incidence of less than 1 in 100,000 patients. However, cancer should be included in the differential diagnosis. Table 2 summarizes the complications of

---

[1]Not FDA approved for this indication.

TABLE 2	Complications of Acute Sinusitis
Bony	
Osteomyelitis	
Pott's puffy tumor	
Intracranial	
Cavernous sinus thrombosis	
Epidural abscess	
Intracranial abscess	
Meningitis	
Subdural abscess	
Superior sagittal sinus thrombosis	
Orbital	
Cavernous sinus thrombosis	
Inflammatory edema and erythema (preseptal cellulitis)	
Orbital cellulitis and abscess	
Subperiosteal abscess	

Reprinted with permission from Aring and Chan (2011).

acute rhinosinusitis. Referral to an otolaryngologist is needed if symptoms persist or progress after maximal medical therapy when computed tomography shows evidence of sinus disease.

References

Ahovuo-Saloranta A, Rautakorpi U, Borisenko OV, et al. Antibiotics for acute maxillary sinusitis. Cochrane Database Syst Rev 2008, CD000243.

Aring AM, Chan MM. Acute rhinosinusitis in adults. Am Fam Physician 2011;83:1057–63.

Chow AW, Benninger MS, Brook I, et al. IDSA clinical practice guideline for acute bacterial rhinosinusitis in children and adults. Clin Infect Dis 2012;54:e72–e112.

Cornelius R, Wippold II FJ, Brunberg JA, et al. ACR Appropriateness Criteria—Sinonasal Disease Expert Panel on Neurologic Imaging, Reston, VA: American College of Radiology; 2009. [Online Publication]. Available at, http://www.acr.org/~/media/8172B4DE503149248E64856857674BB5.pdf, pp. 1-5 (accessed January 1, 2014).

DeSutter AI, Lemiengre M, Campbell H. Antihistamines for the common cold. Cochrane Database Syst Rev 2003, CD001267.

Kassel JC, King D, Spurling GK. Saline nasal irrigation for acute upper respiratory tract infections. Cochrane Database Syst Rev 2010, CD006821.

Rosenfeld RM, Andes D, Bhattacharyya N, et al. Clinical practice guideline: Adult sinusitis. Otolaryngol Head Neck Surg 2007;137(3suppl):S1–S31.

Taverner D, Latte GJ. Nasal decongestants for the common cold. Cochrane Database Syst Rev 2007, CD001267.

Young J, De Sutter A, Merenstein D, et al. Antibiotics for adults with clinically diagnosed acute rhinosinusitis: A meta-analysis of individual patient data. Lancet 2008;371:908–14.

Zalmanovici A, Yaphe J. Intranasal steroids for acute sinusitis. Cochrane Database Syst Rev 2009, CD005149.

TEMPOROMANDIBULAR DISORDERS

Method of
Jeffrey P. Okeson, DMD

Temporomandibular disorder (TMD) is a collective term that includes a number of clinical complaints involving the muscles of mastication, the temporomandibular joints (TMJs) and associated orofacial structures. Other commonly used terms are Costen's syndrome, TMJ dysfunction, and craniomandibular disorders. TMDs are a major cause of nondental pain in the orofacial region and are considered a subclassification of musculoskeletal disorders. In many TMD patients the most common complaint is not with the TMJs but rather the muscles of mastication. Therefore, the terms TMJ dysfunction or TMJ disorder are actually inappropriate for many of these complaints. It is for this reason that the American Dental Association adopted the term *temporomandibular disorder.*

Signs and symptoms associated with TMDs are a common source of pain complaints in the head and orofacial structures. These complaints can be associated with general joint problems and somatization. Approximately 50% of patients suffering with TMDs do not first consult with a dentist but seek advice for the problem from a physician. The family physician should be able to appropriately diagnose many TMDs. In many instances the physician can provide valuable information and simple therapies that will reduce the patient's TMD symptoms. In other instances, it is appropriate to refer the patient to a dentist for additional evaluation and treatment.

Epidemiology

Cross-sectional population-based studies reveal that 40% to 75% of adult populations have at least one sign of TMJ dysfunction (e.g., jaw movement abnormalities, joint noise, tenderness on palpation), and approximately 33% have at least one symptom (e.g., face pain, joint pain). Many of these signs and symptoms are not troublesome for the patient, and only 3% to 7% of the population seeks any advice or care. Although in the general population women seem to have only a slightly greater incidence of TMD symptoms, women seek care for TMD more often than men at a ratio ranging from 3:1 to 9:1. For many patients TMDs are self-limiting, or are associated with symptoms that fluctuate over time without evidence of progression. Even though many of these

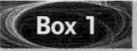

Box 1   Common Primary and Secondary Symptoms Associated with Temporomandibular Disorders

Primary Symptoms
Facial muscle pain
Preauricular (TMJ) pain
TMJ sounds: jaw clicking, popping, catching, locking
Limited mouth opening
Increased pain associated with chewing

Secondary Symptoms
Earache
Headache
Neckache

Abbreviation: TMJ = temporomandibular joint.

---

disorders are self-limiting, the health care provider can provide conservative therapies that will minimize the patient's painful experience.

Signs and Symptoms

The primary signs and symptoms associated with TMD originate from the masticatory structures and are associated with jaw function (Box 1). Pain during opening of the mouth or during chewing is common. Some persons even report difficulty speaking or singing. Patients often report pain in the preauricular areas, face, or temples. TMJ sounds are often described as clicking, popping, grating, or crepitus and can produce locking of the jaw during opening or closing. Patients commonly report painful jaw muscles, and, on occasion, they even report a sudden change in their bite coincident with the onset of the painful condition.

It is important to appreciate that pain associated with most TMDs is increased with jaw function. Because this is a condition of the musculoskeletal structures, function of these structures generally increases the pain. When a patient's pain complaint is not influenced by jaw function, other sources of orofacial pain should be suspected.

The spectrum of TMD often includes commonly associated complaints such as headache, neckache, or earache. These associated complaints are often referred pains and must be differentiated from primary pains. As a general rule, referred pains associated with TMDs are increased with any activity that provokes the TMD pain. Therefore, if the patient reports that the headache is aggravated by jaw function, it could very well represent a secondary pain related to the TMD. Likewise, if the secondary symptom is unaffected by jaw use, one should question its relationship to the TMD and suspect two separate pain conditions. Pain or dysfunction due to nonmusculoskeletal causes such as otolaryngologic, neurologic, vascular, neoplastic, or infectious disease in the orofacial region is not considered a primary TMD even though musculoskeletal pain may be present. However, TMDs often coexist with other craniofacial and orofacial pain disorders.

Anatomy and Pathophysiology

The TMJ is formed by the mandibular condyle fitting into the mandibular fossa of the temporal bone. The movement of this joint is quite complex as it allows hinging movement in one plane and at the same time allows gliding movements in another plane.

Separating these two bones from direct articulation is the articular disk. The articular disk is composed of dense fibrous connective tissue devoid of any blood vessels or nerve fibers. The articular disk is attached posteriorly to a region of loose connective tissue that is highly vascularized and well innervated, known as the retrodiskal tissue. The anterior region of the disk is attached to the superior lateral pterygoid muscle.

The movement of the mandible is accomplished by four pairs of muscles called the muscles of mastication: the masseter, temporalis, medial pterygoid, and lateral pterygoid. Although not considered to be muscles of mastication, the digastric muscles also play an important role in mandibular function. The masseter, temporalis, and medial pterygoid muscles elevate the mandible and therefore provide the major forces used for chewing and other jaw functions. The inferior lateral pterygoid muscles provide protrusive movement of the mandible, and the digastric muscles serve to depress the mandible (open the mouth).

When discussing the pathophysiology of TMD one needs to consider two main categories: joint pathophysiology and muscle pathophysiology. Because etiologic considerations and treatment strategies are different for these conditions, they are presented separately.

Pathophysiology of Intracapsular TMJ Pain Disorders

Several common arthritic conditions such as rheumatoid arthritis, traumatic arthritis, hyperuricemia, and psoriatic arthritis can affect the TMJ. These conditions, however, are not nearly as common as local osteoarthritis. As with most other joints, osteoarthritis results from overloading the articular surface of the joint, thus breaking down the dense fibrous articular surface and ultimately affecting the subarticular bone. In the TMJ, this overloading commonly occurs as a result of an alteration in the morphology and position of the articular disk. In the healthy TMJ, the disk maintains its position on the condyle during movement because of its morphology (i.e., the thicker anterior and posterior borders) and interarticular pressure maintained by the elevator muscles. If, however, the morphology of the disk is altered and the diskal ligaments become elongated, the disk can be displaced from its normal position between the condyle and fossa. If the disk is displaced, normal opening and closing of the mouth can result in an unusual translatory movement between the condyle and the disk, which is felt as click or pop. Disk displacements that result in joint sounds might or might not be painful. When pain is present it is thought to be related to either loading forces applied to the highly vascularized retrodiskal tissues or a general inflammatory response of the surrounding soft tissues (capsulitis or synovitis).

Pathophysiology of Masticatory Muscle Pain Disorders

The muscles of mastication are a very common source of TMD pain. Understanding the pathophysiology of muscle pain, however, is very complex and still not well understood. The simple explanation of muscle spasm does not account for most TMD muscle pain complaints. It appears that a better explanation would include a central nervous system affect on the muscle that results in an increase in peripheral nociceptive activity originating from the muscle tissue itself. This explanation more accurately accounts for the high levels of emotional stress that are commonly associated with TMD muscle pain complaints. In other words, an increase in emotional stress activates the autonomic nervous system, which in turn seems to be associated with changes in muscle nociception.

These masticatory muscle pain conditions are further complicated when one considers the unique masticatory muscle activity known as bruxism. Bruxism is the subconscious, often rhythmic, grinding or gnashing of the teeth. This type of muscle activity is considered to be parafunctional and can also occur as a simple static loading of the teeth known as clenching. This activity commonly occurs while sleeping but can also be present during the day. These parafunctional activities alone can represent a significant source of masticatory muscle pain, and certainly bruxism in the presence of central nervous system–induced muscle pain can further accentuate the patient's muscle pain complaints.

Etiology

Because TMD represents a group of disorders, any of several etiologies may be associated. Problems arising from intracapsular conditions (clicking, popping, catching, locking) may be associated with various types of trauma. Gross trauma, such as a blow to the chin, can immediately alter ligamentous structures of the joint, leading to joint sounds. Trauma can also be associated with a subtler injury such as stretching, twisting or compressing forces during eating, yawning, yelling, or prolonged mouth opening.

When the patient's chief complaint is muscle pain, etiologic factors other than trauma should be considered. Masticatory muscle pain disorders have etiologic considerations similar to other muscle pain disorders of the neck and back. Emotional stress seems to play a significant role for many patients. This can explain why patients often report that their painful symptoms fluctuate greatly over time.

Although most TMD patients do not have a major psychiatric disorder, psychological factors can certainly enhance the pain condition. The clinician needs to consider such factors as anxiety, depression, secondary gain, somatization, and hypochondriasis. Psychosocial factors can predispose certain person to TMD and can also perpetuate TMD once symptoms have become established. A careful consideration of psychosocial factors is therefore important in the evaluation and treatment of every TMD patient.

TMDs have a few unique etiologic factors that differentiate them from other musculoskeletal disorders. One such factor is the occlusal relationship of the teeth. Traditionally it was thought that malocclusion was the primary etiologic factor responsible for TMD. Recent investigations, however, do not support this concept. Still, in certain instances occlusal instability of the teeth can contribute to a TMD. This may be true in patients with or without teeth. Poorly fitting dental prostheses can also contribute to occlusal instability. The occlusal condition should especially be suspected if the pain problem began with a change in the patient's occlusion (e.g., following a dental appointment).

History and Examination

All patients reporting pain in the orofacial structures should be screened for TMD. This can be accomplished with a brief history and physical examination. The screening questions and examination are performed to rule in or out the possibility of a TMD. If a positive response is found, a more extensive history and examination is indicated. Box 2 lists questions that should be asked during a screening assessment for TMD. Any positive response should be followed by additional clarifying questions.

Patients experiencing orofacial pain should also be briefly examined for any clinical signs associated with TMD. The clinician can easily palpate a few sites to assess tenderness or pain as well as assess for jaw mobility. The masseter muscles can be

---

Box 2 Recommended Screening Questionnaire for Temporomandibular Disorder

All patients reporting pain in the orofacial region should be screened for TMD with a questionnaire that includes these questions. The decision to complete a comprehensive history and clinical examination depends on the number of positive responses and the apparent seriousness of the problem for the patient. A positive response to any question may be sufficient to warrant a comprehensive examination if it is of concern to the patient or viewed as clinically significant by the physician.

1. Do you have difficulty, pain, or both when opening your mouth, for instance when yawning?
2. Does your jaw get stuck or locked or go out?
3. Do you have difficulty, pain, or both when chewing, talking, or using your jaws?
4. Are you aware of noises in the jaw joints?
5. Do your jaws regularly feel stiff, tight, or tired?
6. Do you have pain in or about the ears, temples, or cheeks?
7. Do you have frequent headaches, neckaches, or toothaches?
8. Have you had a recent injury to your head, neck, or jaw?
9. Have you been aware of any recent changes in your bite?
10. Have you been previously treated for unexplained facial pain or a jaw joint problem?

Abbreviation: TMD = temporomandibular disorder.

Box 3 Recommended Screening Examination Procedures for Temporomandibular Disorder

All patients with face pain should be briefly screened for TMD using this or a similar cursory clinical examination. The need for a comprehensive history and clinical examination depends on the number of positive findings and the clinical significance of each finding.

1. Palpate for pain or tenderness in the masseter and temporalis muscles.
2. Palpate for pain or tenderness in the preauricular (TMJ) areas.
3. Measure the range of mouth opening. Note any incoordination in the movements.
4. Auscultate and palpate for TMJ sounds (i.e., clicking or crepitus).
5. Note excessive occlusal wear, excessive tooth mobility, buccal mucosal ridging, or lateral tongue scalloping.
6. Inspect symmetry and alignment of the face, jaws, and dental arches.

Abbreviation: TMJ = temporomandibular joint.

---

palpated bilaterally while asking the patient to report any pain or tenderness. The same assessment should be made for the temporal regions as well as the preauricular (TMJ) areas. While the examiner's hands are over the preauricular areas, the patient should repeatedly open and close the mouth. The presence of joint sounds should be noted along with whether these sounds are associated with joint pain.

A simple measurement of mouth opening should be made. This can be accomplished by placing a millimeter ruler on the lower anterior teeth and asking the patient to open as wide as possible. The distance should be measured between the maxillary and mandibular anterior teeth. It is generally accepted that less than 40 mm is a restricted mouth opening.

It is also helpful to inspect the teeth for significant wear, mobility, or decay that may be related to the pain condition. The clinician should examine the buccal mucosa for ridging and the lateral aspect of the tongue for scalloping. These are often signs of clenching and bruxism. A general inspection for symmetry and alignment of the face, jaws, and dental arches may also be helpful. A summary of this screening examination is shown in Box 3.

Treatment

Most recent studies suggest that TMDs are generally self-limiting and symptoms often fluctuate over time. Understanding this natural course does not mean these conditions should be ignored. TMD can be a very painful condition leading to a significant decrease in the patient's quality of life. Understanding the natural course of TMD does suggest, however, that therapy might not need to be very aggressive. In general, initial therapy should begin very conservatively and only escalate when therapy fails to relieve the symptoms.

When the physician identifies a patient with a TMD, he or she has two options. The physician can elect to treat the patient or refer the patient to a dentist who specializes in TMD for further evaluation and treatment. The decision to refer the patient should be based on whether the patient needs any unique care provided only in a dental office. The following are some indications for referral to a dentist:

- History of trauma to the face related to the onset of the pain condition
- The presence of significant TMJ sounds during function
- A feeling of jaw catching or locking during mouth opening
- The report of a sudden change in the occlusal contacts of the teeth
- The presence of significant occlusal instability

- Significant findings related to the teeth (e.g., tooth mobility, tooth sensitivity, tooth decay, tooth wear)
- Significant pain in the jaws or masticatory muscles upon awakening
- The presence of an orofacial pain condition that is aggravated by jaw function and has been present for more than several months

The specific therapy for a TMD varies according to the precise type of disorder identified. In other words, masticatory muscle pain is managed somewhat differently than intracapsular pain. Generally, however, the initial therapy for any type of TMD should be directed toward the relief of pain and the improvement of function. This initial conservative therapy can be divided into three general types: patient education, pharmacologic therapy, and physical therapy.

Patient Education

It is very important that patients have an appreciation for the factors that may be associated with their disorder, as well as the natural course of the disorder. Patients should be reassured, and if necessary, convinced by appropriate tests, that they are not suffering from a malignancy. Properly educated patients can contribute greatly to their own treatment. For example, knowing that emotional stress is an influencing factor in many TMDs can help the patient understand the reason for daily fluctuations of pain intensity. Attention should be directed toward changing the patient's response to stress or, when possible, reducing exposure to stressful conditions. Patients with pain during chewing should be told to begin a softer diet, chew slower, and eat smaller bites. As a general rule the patient should be told "if it hurts, don't do it." Continued pain can contribute to the cycling of pain and should always be avoided. The patient should be instructed to let the jaw muscles relax, maintaining the teeth apart. This will discourage clenching activities and minimize loading of the teeth and joints.

When pain is associated with a clicking TM joint, the patient should be informed of the biomechanics of the joint. This information often allows the patient to select functional activities that are less traumatic to the joint structures. For example, some patients may report that the pain and clicking are less when they chew on a particular side of the mouth. When this occurs, they should be encouraged to continue this type of chewing.

Pharmacologic Therapy

Pharmacologic therapy can be an effective adjunct in managing symptoms associated with TMDs. Patients should be aware that medication alone will not likely solve or cure the problem. Medication, however, in conjunction with appropriate physical therapy and definitive treatment, does offer the most complete approach to many TMD problems. Mild analgesics are often helpful for many TMDs. Control of pain is not only appreciated by the patient but also reduces the likelihood of other complicating pain disorders such as muscle co-contraction, referred pain, and central sensitization.

Nonsteroidal antiinflammatory drugs (NSAIDs) are very helpful with many TMDs. Included in this category are aspirin, acetaminophen (Tylenol), and ibuprofen. Ibuprofen (Motrin, Advil, Nuprin) is often very effective in reducing musculoskeletal pains. A dosage of 600 to 800 mg three times a day for 3 to 5 days commonly reduces pain and stops the cyclic effects of the deep pain input. For patients with gastrointestinal issues, short-term use of a cyclooxygenase-2 (COX-2) inhibitor such as celecoxib (Celebrex) can also be useful.

Physical Therapy

In many patients with TMD, symptoms are relieved with very simple physical therapy methods. Simple instructions for the use of moist heat or cold can be very helpful. Surface heat can be applied by laying a hot, moist towel over the symptomatic area. A hot water bottle wrapped inside the towel will help maintain the heat. This combination should remain in place for 10 to 15 minutes, not to exceed 30 minutes. An electric heating pad may be used, but care should be taken not to leave it on the face too long. Patients should be discouraged from using the heating pad while sleeping because prolonged use is likely.

Like thermotherapy, coolant therapy can provide a simple and often effective method of reducing pain. Ice should be applied directly to the symptomatic joint or muscles and moved in a circular motion without pressure to the tissues. The patient will initially experience an uncomfortable feeling that will quickly turn into a burning sensation. Continued icing will result in a mild aching and then numbness. When numbness begins the ice should be removed. The ice should not be left on the tissues for longer than 5 minutes. After a period of warming a second cold application may be desirable.

The physician should be aware that many TMDs respond to the use of orthopedic appliances such as occlusal appliances, bite guards, and splints. These appliances are made by the dentist and are custom fabricated for each patient. Several types of appliances are available. Each is specific for the type of TMD present. The dentist should be consulted for this type of therapy.

Other Therapeutic Considerations

Sometimes TMDs become chronic and, as with other chronic pain conditions, might then be best managed by a multidisciplinary approach. If the patient reports a long history of TMD complaints, the physician should consider referring the patient to a dentist associated with a team of therapists, such as a psychologist, a physical therapist, and even a chronic pain physician. Generally, patients with chronic TMD are not managed well by the simple initial therapies discussed in this chapter. Often other factors, such as mechanical conditions within the TMJs or psychological factors, need to be addressed. The physician who attempts to manage these conditions in the private practice setting can become very frustrated with the results. It is therefore recommended that if the patient's history suggests chronicity or if initial therapy fails to reduce the patient's symptoms, referral is indicated.

References

de Leeuw RF. Orofacial Pain: Guidelines for Assessment, Diagnosis, and Management. 5th ed. Chicago: Quintessence; 2013.
Okeson JP. Management of Temporomandibular Disorders and Occlusion. 7th ed. St. Louis: Elsevier; 2013.
Okeson JP. Bell's Orofacial Pains. 7th ed. Chicago: Quintessence; 2014.
Scrivani SJ, Keith DA, Kaban LB. Temporomandibular Disorders. N Engl J Med 2008;359(25):2693–705.

UVEITIS

Method of
Petros E. Carvounis, MD

CURRENT DIAGNOSIS

- The most common form of uveitis is anterior uveitis.
- Anterior uveitis is commonly idiopathic.
- Posterior uveitis is most likely infectious.
- In any form of uveitis, syphilis, tuberculosis, and Lyme disease need to be ruled out.
- In immunosuppressed individuals, the uveitis is most likely infectious: the patient's HIV status needs to be determined, because a positive status completely changes the diagnostic approach.
- The key to correct diagnosis is a good history, including a thorough review of systems and a careful ophthalmologic examination as well as dilated funduscopy; laboratory and radiographic

- investigations, sometimes including aqueous or vitreous polymerase chain reaction or cytologic studies, are frequently necessary.
- Involvement of an ophthalmologist with expertise in the diagnosis and treatment of uveitis is mandatory.

CURRENT THERAPY

- Uveitis resulting from a systemic infection (e.g., syphilis, Lyme disease, tuberculosis) needs to be treated as a central nervous system infection.
- Idiopathic anterior uveitis or anterior uveitis related to an autoimmune disease responds to topical corticosteroids (e.g., prednisolone acetate [Pred Forte] 1% 1 drop every 2 hours while awake[3]) and cycloplegia (e.g., homatropine [Isopto Homatropine][1] 2% 1 drop three times daily).
- Periocular steroids (posterior or anterior sub-Tenon's steroid injection) is useful in the management of severe anterior uveitis and in intermediate uveitis.
- Intraocular triamcinolone acetonide injection (Kenalog)[1] or implantation of a sustained-release dexamethasone implant (Ozurdex) or fluocinolone acetonide implant (Retisert) is reserved for cases of severe uveitis.
- Oral steroids (prednisone 1–2 mg/kg PO) can be effective in cases of severe uveitis that is unresponsive to topical, periocular, and intraocular steroids.
- Systemic immunosuppressants can control uveitis unresponsive to steroids or be used as steroid-sparing agents. Some specific uveitides mandate systemic immunosuppression as first-line treatment.
- Commonly used immunosuppressants are azathioprine (Imuran),[1] methotrexate (Trexall),[1] cyclosporine (Neoral),[1] and mycophenolate mofetil (CellCept).[1]
- Anti-tumor necrosis factor-α agents are increasingly being used for the treatment of severe uveitis unresponsive to steroids or requiring steroid-sparing agents.

[1]Not FDA approved for this indication.
[3]Exceeds dosage recommended by the manufacturer.

Uveitis refers to intraocular inflammation: it comprises multiple disease entities, some of which are caused by infectious agents and some of which are immune mediated. Uveitis can be classified by the predominant anatomic location of the inflammation: if it is in the anterior chamber, it is an anterior uveitis (previously known as iritis or iridocyclitis); if it is in the vitreous, it is an intermediate uveitis; and if it is in the retina or choroid, it is a posterior uveitis. In panuveitis, inflammation involves all of these sites. Uveitis is said to be limited if it lasts less than 3 months or persistent if it lasts longer than 3 months.

Clinical Features and Diagnosis

Anterior Uveitis

Anterior uveitis is the most commonly encountered type. It typically manifests with sudden-onset severe photosensitivity, pain, blurred vision, and red eye. Clinical examination documents decreased vision, limbal injection, keratic precipitates (cells and protein on the corneal endothelium), and an anterior chamber reaction (white cells and flare-increased light scatter in the anterior chamber caused by the increased protein concentration resulting from inflammation-induced vascular permeability). The anterior uveitis associated with juvenile idiopathic arthritis in children may be asymptomatic.

Anterior uveitis is commonly idiopathic but may be associated with human leukocyte antigen (HLA) B27; other HLA-B27 conditions, such as ankylosing spondylitis, Achilles tendonitis, plantar fasciitis, and dactylitis, should be sought. Anterior uveitis may also be associated with psoriatic arthropathy, Reiter's syndrome (although conjunctivitis is its most common feature), inflammatory bowel disease (which is also associated with intermediate uveitis), or sarcoidosis. Rheumatoid arthritis does not cause uveitis, although it may cause scleritis. In a patient with prior intraocular surgery or recent trauma, postoperative infectious endophthalmitis is a possibility. Infectious causes such as tuberculosis, syphilis, and Lyme disease need to be excluded, because they are curable. Viral infections (e.g., herpes simplex virus, varicella-zoster virus) can lead to an anterior uveitis, but they more frequently cause keratitis. Other rare associations are possible.

A good history, including a very thorough systems review combined with a good clinical examination including dilated funduscopy (to rule out retina or choroid involvement) by an ophthalmologist with expertise and interest in uveitis is mandatory for appropriate diagnosis and management.

A first occurrence of anterior uveitis that readily responds to topical corticosteroids (see later discussion) does not require further investigation unless there is strong suggestion of an associated systemic disorder based on the history and general physical examination. Investigation for anterior uveitis that is recurrent or is unresponsive to topical corticosteroids should be tailored based on the clinical examination findings but should not neglect to rule out syphilis, tuberculosis, Lyme disease, and HIV.

Intermediate Uveitis

Intermediate uveitis typically manifests in a young or middle-aged adult with pain, photosensitivity, blurred vision, and floaters. The most important finding on clinical examination is a vitreitis (white cells in the vitreous and vitreous haze).

Intermediate uveitis is commonly idiopathic (pars planitis) or may be associated with tuberculosis, sarcoidosis, Lyme disease, syphilis, inflammatory bowel disease, or, rarely, multiple sclerosis. Intraocular lymphoma should be considered in patients older than 50 years of age who have vitreitis. Investigation of intermediate uveitis is mandatory, because it is usually unresponsive to topical corticosteroid drops.

Posterior Uveitis

Posterior uveitis is commonly infectious. Patients complain of visual loss and floaters. Clinical signs include decreased visual acuity, vitreous cells and haze, and some of the following: retinal infiltrates, serous retinal detachment, retinal hemorrhage, chorioretinal scars, choroidal granulomas, venular sheathing, or arteriolar sheathing.

The most common cause of posterior uveitis is *Toxoplasma* retinochoroiditis. Viral infections such as varicella-zoster or herpes simplex can uncommonly cause acute retinal necrosis, and cytomegalovirus retinitis can be devastating in immunocompromised individuals. Tuberculosis, Lyme disease, and syphilis are bacterial causes of posterior uveitis. *Pneumocystis jiroveci*, (formerly called *Pneumocystis carinii*) and *Cryptococcus* can cause a choroiditis in the immunocompromised individual. Sarcoidosis can also cause posterior uveitis. There is a plethora of well-defined posterior uveitides without associated systemic findings (e.g., serpiginous chorioretinitis). Intraocular lymphoma can masquerade as posterior uveitis and needs be considered in older patients.

Unless a clinical diagnosis is possible (e.g., in *Toxoplasma* chorioretinitis), further investigations are required. If a rapid plasma reagin test is negative, a diagnostic vitrectomy should be considered in all patients and is mandatory in immunocompromised patients; otherwise, tailored laboratory and radiographic investigations need to be performed.

Panuveitis

Panuveitis combines the signs and symptoms of anterior and posterior uveitis, although early in the course one location may predominate. Bacterial or fungal endophthalmitis needs be considered. Vogt-Koyanagi-Harada syndrome is a common cause in the Far East and in patients of Native American ancestry. Adamantiades-Behçet syndrome, sympathetic ophthalmia, tuberculosis, syphilis, and, rarely, Lyme disease need be considered, among others.

Sequelae and Complications of Uveitis

Uncontrolled uveitis can be a blinding condition. Visual loss results commonly from cystoid macular edema or from cataracts, glaucoma, band keratopathy, hypotony maculopathy, macular scar, macular necrosis, or retinal detachment.

Current Treatment

Almost all of the medications employed in the treatment of uveitis are used off-label (FDA approved for an indication other than the treatment of uveitis).

Anterior Uveitis

If photosensitivity is a prominent complaint, topical cycloplegia affords considerable relief. Homatropine (Isopto Homatropine) 2% or 5%, scopolamine (Isopto Hyoscine) 0.25%, or tropicamide (Mydriacyl) 1% may be used. Cyclopentolate (Cyclogyl) should be avoided, because it has chemoattractant properties in vitro. Topical cycloplegia is also necessary with severe anterior uveitis to prevent posterior synechiae.

Topical corticosteroid drops are the first line of treatment for anterior uveitis (e.g., prednisolone acetate [Pred Forte] 1% 1 drop every 2 hours while awake).[3] Patient education to ensure compliance is of paramount importance. Difluprednate 0.05% (Durezol) is also being used with increasing frequency.

After 1 to 2 weeks, a slow taper of the drops is commenced (administer four times daily for 7–10 days, then taper by 1 drop every 7–10 days), provided that the anterior chamber cells have resolved. If there is an increase in activity during the taper, an increase in the dosing frequency to re-achieve a complete response, followed by a slower taper, is performed. Occasionally, patients have to be maintained for the long term on topical prednisolone; this is acceptable, provided that no adverse side effects occur.

If there is incomplete response to prednisolone acetate 1% given every 2 hours or if the drops cannot be tapered without recurrence and investigations are negative, the next step to be considered could be a sub-Tenon's (under the conjunctiva) injection of 0.5 to 1.0 mL triamcinolone acetonide 40 mg/mL (Kenalog),[1,6,*] which forms a depot providing continuous steroid release for up to 6 months; alternatively, oral corticosteroids (usually prednisone) may be used in patients with especially severe bilateral uveitis, although this is uncommon. For the rare severe anterior uveitis that is unresponsive to these treatments or to decreases in the steroid dose, immunosuppressant medications such as methotrexate,[1] cyclosporine,[1] or mycophenolate mofetil[1] or an anti-tumor necrosis factor-α (anti-TNF-α) agent such as infliximab[1] may be given (see later discussion for recommended doses).

It cannot be overemphasized that a severe "anterior uveitis," especially with a hypopyon, occurring after recent intraocular surgery or trauma should alert the physician to the possibility of endophthalmitis. Emergent anterior chamber and vitreous cultures need to be obtained, and intravitreous nonpreserved vancomycin (Vancocin) 1.0 mg/0.1 mL[6] and ceftazidime (Fortaz) 2.25 mg/0.1 mL[6] must be injected.

The main side effects of topical steroid use are cataract formation and ocular hypertension, which can lead to glaucoma. Untreated uveitis can cause the same side effects; therefore, inflammation needs be controlled promptly, and then the corticosteroids need to be tapered off as soon as possible without precipitating a recurrence. Topical steroid use also predisposes to cornea

infection, including reactivation of herpes simplex or varicella-zoster keratitis.

Intermediate Uveitis, Posterior Uveitis, and Panuveitis

Uveitis associated with systemic infection (e.g. syphilis, Lyme disease) is treated in consultation with an infectious disease specialist, because intraocular involvement is considered central nervous system involvement. Adjuvant topical corticosteroids and mydriatics can afford relief without jeopardizing cure in most cases (as for anterior uveitis).

Ocular toxoplasmosis, the most common posterior uveitis, is self-limited. Treatment is required in cases in which the optic nerve or macula is threatened or the vitreitis is particularly severe. Treatment consists of pyrimethamine (Daraprim) (loading dose 50 mg, then 25 mg twice daily), sulfadiazine (1 g four times daily), and folinic acid (Leucovorin)[1] 5 mg three times weekly. More recently, clindamycin (Cleocin)[1] 150 to 300 mg PO four times daily or trimethoprim-sulfamethoxazole[1] (Bactrim DS 800 mg sulfamethoxazole/160 mg trimethoprim twice daily) have been found to be equally efficacious and are more widely used. Prednisone 40 mg/day is added 24 to 48 hours later. Treatment duration is usually 30 to 40 days, with a prednisone taper guided by the clinical response.

For intermediate uveitis, posterior uveitis, or panuveitis not associated with systemic infection, treatment options are to be considered in the following order:

1. Periocular steroids (posterior sub-Tenon's injection of triamcinolone acetonide)[1] are commonly efficacious for intermediate uveitis.
2. Oral corticosteroids are very efficacious but have ocular as well as systemic side effects. If the uveitis cannot be controlled with less than prednisone 10 mg after 6 months of treatment, one of the other options needs to be considered.
3. In severe cases of intermediate, posterior, or panuveitis, intravitreous triamcinolone acetonide (Kenalog or Triessence 4 mg[1,*]), an injectable dexamethasone implane (Ozurdex), or a fluocinolone implant (Retisert) can be used; intravitreous long-acting steroid treatment has similar efficacy to systemic immunosuppression; the former has ocular complications (cataract formation, glaucoma), and the latter carries the risk of systemic side effects.
4. Systemic immunosuppression with azathioprine (Imuran)[1] up to 2.5 to 4 mg/kg/day, cyclosporine (Neoral)[1] 2.5 to 5.0 mg/kg/day in 2 divided doses, tacrolimus (Prograf)[1] 0.15 to 0.30 mg/kg/day, mycophenolate mofetil (CellCept)[1] 500 to 1000 mg twice daily, methotrexate (Trexall)[1] (12.5 to 25 mg weekly), or an anti-TNF-α agent (e.g., infliximab [Remicade])[1] have all been used with success as steroid-sparing agents or to control uveitis that is poorly responsive to corticosteroids alone.

There are specific uveitis entities that mandate the use of immunosuppression as first-line treatment (together with steroids initially). These include Wegener's retinal vasculitis, Adamantiades-Behçet's syndrome, sympathetic ophthalmia, and possibly birdshot choroidopathy, uveitis related to Vogt-Koyanagi-Harada syndrome, and serpiginous chorioretinitis.

---

[1]Not FDA approved for this indication.
[*]Kenalog is commercially available as 40 mg/mL. Special compounding is needed for the concentration of 4 mg/mL.

References

Harper SL, Chorich LJ, Foster CS. Diagnosis of uveitis. In: Foster CS, Vitale A, editors. Diagnosis and Treatment of Uveitis. Philadelphia: WB Saunders; 2002. p. 79–97.

Jabs DA, Rosenbaum JT, Foster CS, et al. Guidelines for the use of immunosuppressive drugs in patients with ocular inflammatory disorders: Recommendations of an expert panel. Am J Ophthalmol 2000;130:492–513.

Nussenblatt RB. Philosophy, goals and approaches to medical therapy. In: Nussenblatt SM, Whitcup SM, editors. Uveitis, Fundamentals and Clinical Practice. 3rd ed. Philadelphia: Mosby; 2004. p. 95–136.

The Standardization of Uveitis Nomenclature (SUN) working group. Standardization of uveitis nomenclature for reporting clinical data: Results of the first international workshop. Am J Ophthalmol 2005;140:509–16.

---

[1]Not FDA approved for this indication.
[3]Exceeds dosage recommended by the manufacturer.
[6]May be compounded by pharmacists.
[*]Kenalog is commercially available as 40 mg/mL. Special compounding is needed for the concentration of 4 mg/mL.

VISION CORRECTION PROCEDURES

Method of
Elizabeth Yeu, MD

CURRENT DIAGNOSIS

- Refractive errors are an extremely common cause for blurred vision.
- Refractive errors include myopia (nearsightedness), hyperopia (farsightedness), astigmatism, and presbyopia, which is the age-related loss of near vision.
- Medical management includes the use of spectacles, contact lenses, or both.
- Both corneal and intraocular surgical options exist to successfully and permanently correct refractive errors.
- Corneal refractive surgery options include excimer laser, such as laser in situ keratomileusis (LASIK) and photorefractive keratectomy (PRK), and corneal relaxing incisions for the management of astigmatism.
- In eyes that are not candidates for corneal refractive surgery, intraocular surgery with phakic intraocular lens implants or refractive lens exchange can be considered.
- Increasing advancements now offer, and continue to expand, the various surgical options available to correct myopia, hyperopia, astigmatism, and presbyopia.

CURRENT THERAPY

- Laser in situ keratomileusis (LASIK) and photorefractive keratectomy (PRK) use an excimer laser to reshape the anterior surface of the cornea and permanently correct the eye's refractive error. LASIK and PRK can correct myopia, hyperopia, and astigmatism and help reduce presbyopia.
- In LASIK, a corneal flap is created and lifted before the excimer laser is applied to correct the refractive error. In contrast, the PRK procedure requires no lamellar flap. In PRK, the laser treatment is applied directly to the anterior stromal surface after the surface epithelium is removed.
- Radial keratotomy (RK) was the first modern form of corneal refractive surgery to correct myopia. In RK, spokelike corneal incisions were created to flatten the central cornea and reduce myopia. Although RK surgery is effective, the results were often unpredictable and unstable and led to overcorrection, with progressive hyperopia.
- Astigmatic keratotomy (AK) incisions are a modification of RK surgery and are used to reduce corneal astigmatism. The two forms of corneal relaxing incisions, AK and limbal relaxing incisions (LRI)—or, more accurately, peripheral corneal relaxing incisions (PCRIs)—are differentiated by their location on the cornea.
- A refractive lens exchange (RLE) is a surgical option that can correct refractive errors by removing and replacing the crystalline lens. In essence, RLE is cataract surgery performed before a visually significant cataract forms; a visually significant cataract is the clouding or opacification of the natural lens. RLE is a viable option for high myopes and hyperopes, where laser vision correction is not an option, and to correct presbyopia.
- Presbyopia correction is a very dynamic field in refractive surgery. Surgical correction options include surgical monovision, which is popularly used with presbyopic contact lens wearers, where one eye is corrected for distance vision and the other eye for near vision. Monovision can be produced through excimer laser, RLE, or cataract surgery. Also, various intraocular lenses (IOLs) can correct presbyopia.

- Surgically implanted lenses, or phakic intraocular lens implants, can be used to treat myopia only in the United States. Phakic IOLs are an alternative to laser vision correction and can successfully correct myopia in patients for whom keratorefractive surgery is not an option.
- No surgery is without its potential for complications. The more devastating complications of corneal refractive surgery include flap-related complications in LASIK, corneal weakening and ectasias, and vision-limiting haze in PRK. Endophthalmitis is a sight-threatening infection that can occur with any intraocular surgery such as RLE, phakic intraocular lenses, and cataract surgery.

The term *refractive error* describes any condition where light is poorly focused within the eye, resulting in blurred vision. This is the most common eye problem encountered in the United States and includes such conditions as nearsightedness (myopia), farsightedness (hyperopia), astigmatism, and age-related loss of near vision (presbyopia). A person who is able to see without the aid of spectacles or contact lenses has minimal to no refractive error. A wide variety of techniques are available for correcting refractive errors and restoring visual function. The most common methods employ corrective eyewear, such as eyeglasses and contact lenses. In addition to these noninvasive modalities, several surgical procedures can also be used to treat these conditions. These surgical techniques range from minimally invasive procedures, such as laser vision can be divided to corneal and intraocular procedures.

Whichever method is selected, the primary goal of every vision-correcting procedure should be to choose the technique that is most appropriate for each patient. The chosen method should not only correct the patient's visual deficit but also satisfy the patient's goals for visual function. This chapter focuses on the various surgical options that are available for vision correction. To set the groundwork for this discussion, we begin with some background information on ocular anatomy, refractive errors, and the clinical assessment of visual function.

Pathophysiology
Background
Although the human eye is a complex structure, from a conceptual standpoint, it can be thought to function much like a simple camera. In general, light enters the eye and needs to be focused on the center of the retina, or the fovea, to generate images. Light first enters through the cornea, a convex transparent window that performs approximately 66% to 75% of the focusing for the eye. After passing through the cornea, the light encounters the iris and pupil. The pupil is an aperture centered within the iris, a muscular diaphragm that controls the diameter of the pupil and thus the amount of light that continues into the eye.

The crystalline lens sits behind the pupil and provides the remaining 25% to 34% of the eye's focusing ability (Figure 1). The lens is suspended by a network of hundreds of supporting cables called zonular fibers. These zonules insert into the ciliary body, a muscular ring that is a peripheral extension of the iris. The refractive power of the lens is somewhat adjustable and can be increased to move the focal point of the eye from distance to close range, a process known as *accommodation* (Figure 2). Accommodation results from contraction of the ciliary muscle, which results in a decreased diameter of the ciliary ring, similar to a lens aperture of a camera. This loosens the zonules, which simultaneously reduces zonular tension on the lens, thereby causing the thickness and anterior curvature to increase, along with its amplified refractive power.

After being focused by the lens, light passes through the transparent vitreous humor until it reaches the retina, which lines the inside of the back of the eye. The retina functions like the film in a camera, converting the focused image into an electrical signal that is transmitted to the brain via the optic nerve.

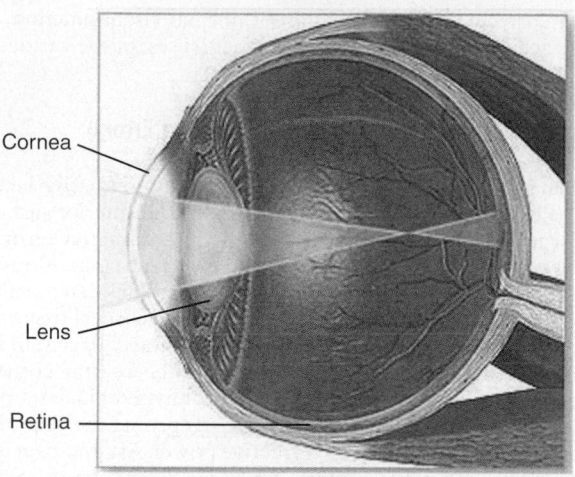

Figure 1. The refraction, or bending, of light in the eye occurs through the cornea and the crystalline lens. Refractive errors result when the light is not perfectly focused onto the retina. (Illustration courtesy A.D.A.M, Inc.)

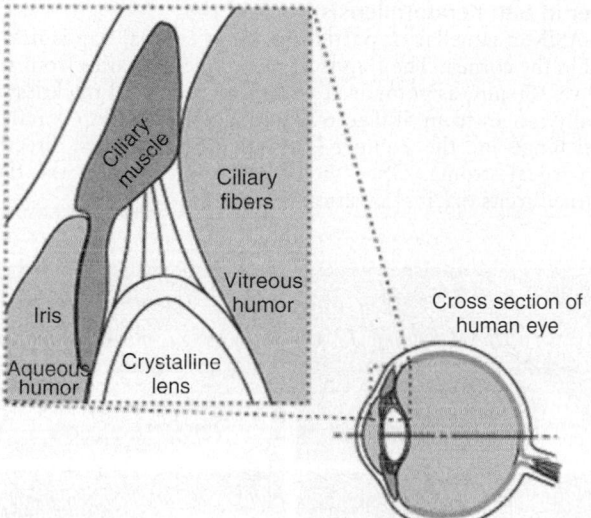

Figure 2. The lens is suspended in place by the zonular fibers. These zonules insert into the ciliary body. Accommodation, or the ability to focus at close range, occurs as the result of the contraction of the zonules and a change in shape to the crystalline lens.

Refractive Errors

Emmetropia is the condition where the eye has essentially no refractive error and requires no correction for distance vision. Refractive errors result when the cornea and lens inadequately focus incoming light, resulting in blurred images projected onto the retina. The unit of measure for refractive error is the diopter (D), which for a thin lens (in air) is defined as the reciprocal of the lens focal length. Most refractive errors refer to the patient's visual status when viewing objects in the distance. For example, a lens that focuses light over a distance of 0.5 m has a refractive power of +2.0 D.

In myopia, or nearsightedness, the focusing powers of the cornea are too strong or the axial length of the eye is too long, or both. The resulting image comes into focus anterior to the retina and is out of focus by the time it reaches the back of the eye. As a result, myopic eyes can see better at close range than at a distance. To correct a myopic eye, its refractive power must be decreased by using a lens with negative refractive power, which weakens the focusing of light and redirects it toward the retina.

Hyperopes, or farsighted persons, are the opposite of myopes. The cornea is flatter and focuses too weakly or the axial length

is too short (or both) in the hyperopic eye. The images from objects viewed at a distance are not yet in focus by the time they reach the retina. To see clearly, a hyperopic eye must accommodate to increase its lenticular power to bring distant objects into sharp focus. Because this requires contraction of the ciliary muscle, the farsighted eye is never at rest and must work even harder to see near objects clearly. Because of this, hyperopic refractive corrections must add positive focusing power to the eye (Figure 3).

In astigmatism, the eye has different refractive powers along different meridians; light entering in the vertical direction gets focused differently than light in the horizontal direction. Conceptually, it is easier to think of the astigmatic cornea or lens as shaped like a football rather than a basketball, with the meridian of steeper curvature having greater refractive power. The astigmatic eye produces a blurred image because essentially two focal points of images are being produced. This requires different corrections along each of these meridians to produce a single focused image on the retina (Figure 4).

Presbyopia describes the normal age-related loss of near vision. To see near objects clearly, young distance-corrected eyes must accommodate to increase their refractive power. However, this ability progressively declines with age, usually reaching clinical significance in the 5th decade. Several factors have been implicated

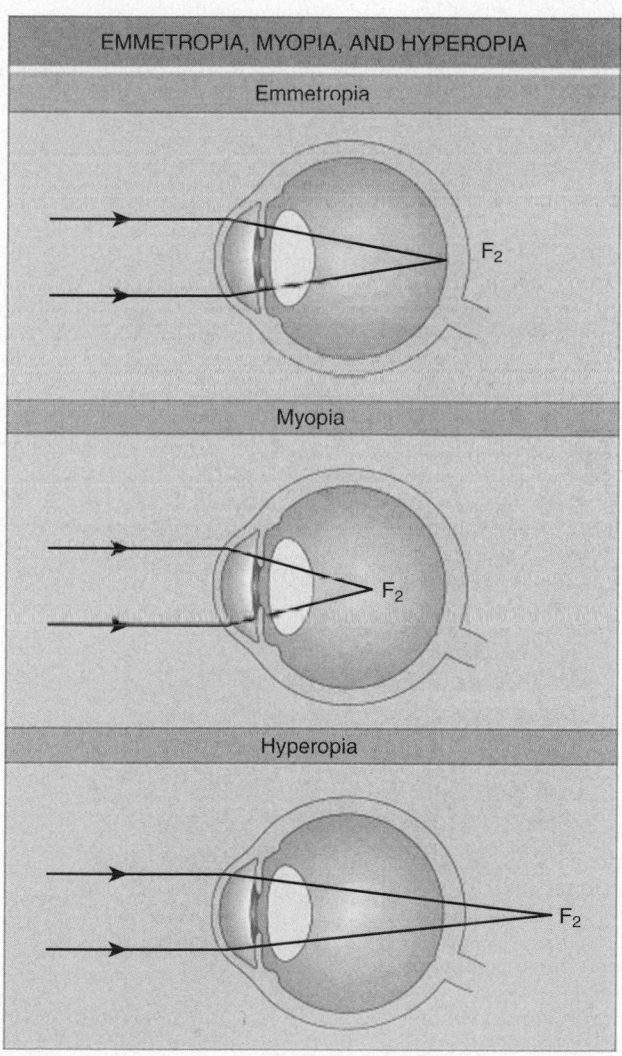

Figure 3. Emmetropia, myopia, and hyperopia. In emmetropia, the secondary focal point (F_2) is at the retina. In myopia, the secondary focal point (F_2) is in the vitreous. In hyperopia, the secondary focal point (F_2) is behind the eye. (Reprinted with permission from Mimura T, Azar DT: Part 3: Refractive Surgery. In Yanoff M, Duker JS (eds): Ophthalmology, 3rd ed. St. Louis, Mosby, 2008.)

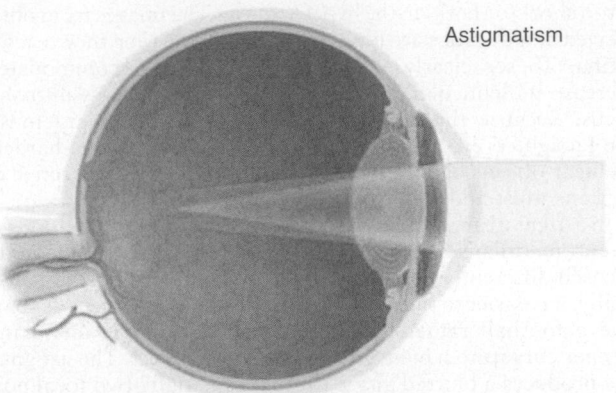

Figure 4. Astigmatism occurs when the refractive power of the eye is not symmetrical. The focusing poser of one axis is stronger than the other axis. This effectively leads to multiple focal points of light, which results in blurred images. (Reprinted with permission from Haw WW, Manche EE: Vision correction procedures. In Bope ET, Rakel RE, Kellerman R (eds): Conn's Current Therapy 2010. Philadelphia, Saunders, 2010, 193–197.)

in this process, including loss of lens elasticity, decreased zonular tension, and altered ciliary muscle function. Although there is currently no way to reverse this natural consequence of aging, several vision-correction options are available to improve near vision in presbyopic persons.

Epidemiology

Population-based studies indicate that approximately 25% to 40% of people in their 40s have myopia, and 10% to 20% have hyperopia. Myopia is the most common refractive error and affects about 35% of whites and 13% to 30% of African Americans. Approximately three-quarters of the American population older than 40 years have refractive errors greater than 0.5 D. Astigmatism of more than 0.5 D is common in adults, and the prevalence increases to approximately 28% in persons in their forties. In general, a higher prevalence of hyperopia and less myopia is observed with increasing age from about 45 to 65 years. This levels off with older age and is eventually followed by an increase in myopia at older ages, which is thought to largely be from cataract formation. Regarding the correction of refractive errors, about 150 million Americans currently use some form of eyewear to correct refractive errors at a cost of approximately $150 billion annually, including 36 million who use contact lenses.

Diagnosis (Assessment of Vision)

There are many aspects of vision, including visual acuity, contrast sensitivity, color perception, and peripheral vision. The most common assessment of visual function is to test the central vision through visual acuity. Visual acuity testing determines a patient's ability to read high-contrast symbols (usually black letters on a white background) of varying sizes at a standard testing distance. This reference distance approximates optical infinity and is typically 20 feet in the United States and 6 meters in Europe. A 20/20 letter on the standard eye chart devised by Snellen is approximately three-eighths of an inch tall at a distance of 20 feet (subtending a visual angle of 5 minutes of arc). Twenty-twenty vision is considered normal visual acuity.

Visual acuities less than 20/20 are represented by ratios whose denominator is greater than 20. For example, a visual acuity of 20/60 means that the smallest letter the eye can read is three times larger than a 20/20-size letter.

Refractive errors can result in *uncorrected* visual acuities that fall below 20/20. However, in the absence of other disease, the conditions of myopia, hyperopia, astigmatism, and presbyopia

can be corrected with restoration of normal visual function. This can be achieved with spectacles, contact lenses, or the various surgical procedures discussed next.

Treatment (Surgical Correction of Refractive Errors)

Laser Vision Correction

Laser in situ keratomileusis (LASIK) and photorefractive keratectomy (PRK) use an excimer laser to reshape the anterior surface of the cornea and permanently correct the eye's refractive error. The excimer laser was developed in the 1970s and emits ultraviolet light at a wavelength of 193 nm. This particular wavelength has been found to accurately and efficiently ablate corneal tissue without causing thermal damage to the surrounding collagen. In myopia, the excimer laser treatment flattens the central cornea to decrease its focusing power. Conversely, for hyperopia, laser pulses are applied to the periphery, indirectly steepening the central cornea and thereby increasing its refractive power. Astigmatism is corrected by combining central and peripheral treatments to differentially steepen the flattest corneal meridian and flatten the steepest meridian. Since the first excimer treatment in the late 1980s, LASIK and PRK have been used to treat refractive errors in millions of patients.

Laser in Situ Keratomileusis

In LASIK, a lamellar or partial-thickness corneal flap is first created in the cornea. The flap thickness typically varies from about 100 to 180 μm, as compared with a total corneal thickness that usually ranges from 500 to 600 μm. The LASIK flap is reflected at its hinge and the excimer laser ablation is applied directly to the corneal stroma. Once the ablation is complete, the flap is returned to its original position (Figure 5).

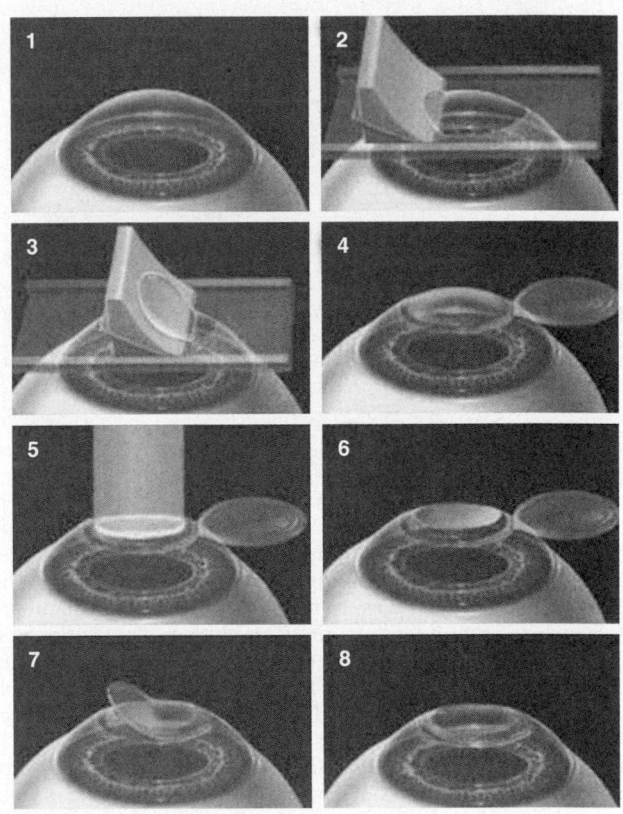

Figure 5. LASIK procedure. 1, The normal cornea. 2 and 3, A microkeratome (or laser) is used to create a partial-thickness corneal flap attached at a hinge. 4, The corneal flap is lifted. 5, The excimer laser ablates the corneal stroma. 6, The corneal stroma is reshaped. 7 and 8, The corneal flap is repositioned. (Reprinted with permission from Haw WW, Manche EE: Vision correction procedures. In Bope ET, Rakel RE, Kellerman R (eds): Conn's Current Therapy 2010. Philadelphia, Saunders, 2010, 193–197.)

The LASIK flap is created by either a microkeratome, a device containing a motorized oscillating blade connected to a suction ring, or via a femtosecond laser. The femtosecond laser uses ultra-short microscopic pulses of infrared light to define the lamellar flap. The femtosecond laser has allowed greater accuracy with the flap thickness. Also, there are significantly less flap-related complications, such as free (without flap hinge), partial, or button-hole (doughnut-shaped) flaps.

Recovery of vision usually takes a few days; some patients note gradual improvement over a few weeks. Postoperative medications usually include topical antibiotic and steroid eye drops for approximately 5 to 7 days.

Complications with laser vision correction in general are extremely low. Most intraoperative complications associated with LASIK involve the flap. If during the surgery the patient moves the eye (fixation loss), the laser can focus on the wrong part of the eye (decentration of the laser treatment), which can degrade the postoperative vision creating a chromatic aberration called coma.

LASIK carries the postoperative risks of flap displacement or induction of flap striae. Most of these cases require a lifting and repositioning of the flap. However, more severe or refractory cases can require further intervention, such as suturing.

On rare occasions, epithelial cells from the corneal surface can migrate underneath the LASIK flap and proliferate in the interface. Usually, the peripheral nests of epithelial cells are small and insignificant visually, thus requiring no intervention. Larger collections of cells can compromise vision or cause corneal necrosis and scarring, so they need to be removed. Epithelial ingrowth requires lifting the flap and manually débriding the cells. This treatment might need to be supplemented with alcohol or suturing, or both, to prevent recurrence.

Corneal weakening and subsequent distortion are other potential sequelae of laser vision correction. Certain preoperative corneal shapes suggest a predisposition toward weakening, especially those with steeper curvature in the inferior region as compared with the superior region. Preoperative corneal thicknesses less than 500 μm or post LASIK residual stromal bed thicknesses less than 250 μm can also be associated with corneal weakening.

As with any surgery, LASIK and PRK are also associated with a risk of infection. The incidence varies, but published rates have been about 0.03%. Staphylococcal and streptococcal species are most common, but atypical organisms such as mycobacteria and fungi have also been reported. Sterile inflammation can also occur in the flap interface and is known as *diffuse lamellar keratitis*. Diffuse lamellar keratitis has been associated with bacterial endotoxin, cleaning solutions, corneal abrasions, and excessive femtosecond laser energy levels. Treatment primarily relies on topical steroid eyedrops, but it may also include oral steroids and irrigation of the flap interface.

Photorefractive Keratectomy

PRK also uses the excimer laser to reshape the cornea, but this procedure requires no lamellar flap. In this method, the laser treatment is applied directly to the anterior stromal surface after the surface epithelium is removed. Several techniques are available to remove the corneal epithelium. Mechanical débridement with a spatula or rotating brush is very common. *Advanced surface ablation* has replaced other techniques used to manipulate the surface epithelium, including a devitalizing 20% alcohol solution, followed by gentle débridement with a blunt spatula or an epikeratome (similar to a LASIK microkeratome) to separate a flap of epithelium at the level of the basement membrane.

Laser-assisted subepithelial keratomileusis (LASEK) was another modification of PRK but has now fallen largely out of use. In LASEK, a flap consisting of only epithelium is created and replaced onto the cornea, which some surgeons believed provided greater postoperative comfort and expedited re-epithelialization of the corneal surface.

Each of these methods has certain advantages and disadvantages, but all do an effective job of preparing the corneal surface for laser ablation.

Once the laser treatment is complete, a soft contact lens is placed on the cornea. The corneal epithelium typically heals in 4 to 7 days, after which the contact lens is removed. Once the contact lens is removed, recovery of vision can take a few more weeks, although some patients experience improvement in vision that continues over several months. Antibiotic eye drops are used until the contact lens is removed, and steroid eye drops may be tapered over several months.

Regarding complications, PRK has fewer intraoperative risks than LASIK because no lamellar flap is being created. Postoperatively, there is a higher risk of subepithelial haze. Fibroblastic transformation of keratinocytes can cause the deposition of disorganized collagen that decreases the smoothness and clarity of the post-PRK cornea. This development is usually associated with higher myopic corrections and may be reversed by increased application of topical steroid eyedrops. Short-duration intraoperative use of low-concentration topical mitomycin-C (Mitosol)[1] (0.02%) appears to decrease the risk of haze formation. As discussed with LASIK, postoperative infectious or sterile inflammation is a rare but potential risk with PRK as well.

Both PRK and LASIK damage corneal nerves, which appears to have a secondary effect on the ocular hydration status. Postoperative dry eye is greater in LASIK than PRK owing to its greater depth of penetration into the cornea. The increased dryness appears to be temporary, and most patients return to baseline by 6 to 9 months, but a subset of patients experience chronic dry eyes following the procedure. A careful preoperative assessment of dry eye risk factors is recommended, and those at risk may be steered toward PRK or toward no surgery at all.

Radial Keratotomy

Modern keratorefractive surgery can attribute some of its origins to a flurry of research produced by Sato of Japan in the 1940s that led to radial keratotomy (RK) and astigmatic keratotomy (AK) surgeries. Russian ophthalmologist Fyodorov is credited with advancing keratorefractive surgery in the 1970s through RK surgery. He created up to 16 spoke-like cuts radiating from the central cornea at 90% to 95% corneal depth to balloon the peripheral cornea. This would, in turn, flatten the central cornea and reduce myopia. The combination of RK and AK surgeries were very popular procedures that effectively reduced myopia and astigmatism throughout the 1970s and 1980s. Although RK surgery was effective, the results were often unpredictable and unstable and led to overcorrection, with progressive hyperopia. RK surgery was quickly replaced by laser vision correction with the introduction of PRK in the late 1980s (Figure 6).

Astigmatic Keratotomy

Astigmatic keratotomy incisions are a modification of RK surgery and are used to reduce corneal astigmatism. The two forms of corneal relaxing incisions, astigmatic keratotomy (AK) and limbal relaxing incisions (LRI), or more accurately peripheral corneal relaxing incisions (PCRI), are differentiated by their location on the cornea (Figure 7).

Several nomograms exist for AK and PCRIs that consider the age of the patient and the amount and meridian of the steep axis of astigmatism in order to calculate the length of the incisions. In both procedures, incisions are made to a 90% to 95% depth in the cornea to flatten the steep meridian. The basic principles of astigmatism correction hold true for both types of keratotomy surgeries: a greater effect is achieved with longer incisions, with smaller optical zones, with deeper incisions, and in older patients. Hence, the more central AK incisions have a greater effect and can correct upwards of 6 to 7 diopters of astigmatism.

---

[1]Not FDA approved for this indication.

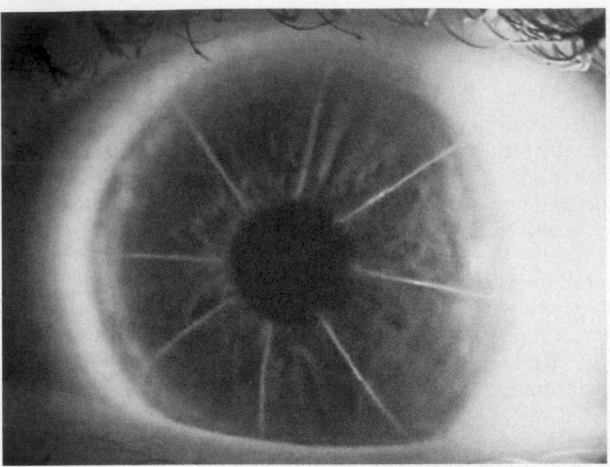

Figure 6. Radial keratotomy was the first modern form of refractive surgery for the correction of myopia. Up to 16 spokelike cuts radiating from the central cornea at 90% to 95% of corneal depth can be created to flatten the central cornea and balloon the peripheral cornea to correct myopia.

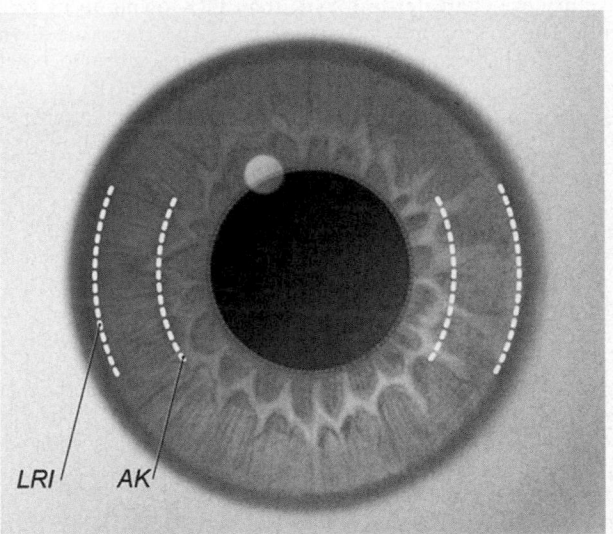

Figure 7. Incisions can be placed on the cornea to reduce astigmatism. The more central astigmatic keratotomy (AK) incisions have a greater effect than their peripheral limbal relaxing incision (LRI) counterparts. (Reprinted with permission from Yeu E, Rubenstein JB: Management of astigmatism during lens-based surgery. In American Academy of Ophthalmologists: Focal Points, Clinical Modules for Ophthalmologists, February, 2008.)

PCRIs have a weaker effect because of their more peripheral location and generally can correct 2 to 3 diopters of astigmatism. Because the incisions are made closer to the limbus, they heal faster, and thus the refractive effect stabilizes more quickly. Given their peripheral location, the ratio of flattening in meridian of incision-to-steepening ratio in the opposite meridian, or *coupling ratio*, is usually 1:1. Patients experience less irregular astigmatism, flare, and foreign body sensation as compared to their more central counterparts. Technically, PCRIs are easier to perform and more forgiving as well.

Corneal relaxing incisions are most commonly performed intraoperatively, at the time of cataract surgery, but are also performed as a separate procedure to treat corneal astigmatism. The procedure is fairly quick to perform and the patient experiences little discomfort. Postoperatively, a topical antibiotic is used for 4 to 7 days, and a topical analgesic is used as needed.

Regarding complications of corneal relaxing incisions, patients commonly experience a foreign body sensation during the first few days. Less-common complications include glare, undercorrection or overcorrection, irregular astigmatism from the incisions, wound gape or perforation, decreased corneal sensation, and dry eye syndrome.

Intraocular Procedures
Refractive Lens Exchange
Unlike the corneal procedures that have been discussed, refractive lens exchange (RLE) is a surgical option that can correct refractive errors by removing and replacing the crystalline lens. In essence, RLE is cataract surgery without a visually significant cataract, which is the clouding or opacification of the natural lens. RLE is a viable option for high myopes and hyperopes, where laser vision correction is not an option, and for correcting presbyopia.

The natural crystalline lens is removed via emulsification with ultrasound energy. This lens is then replaced by an acrylic or silicone intraocular lens (IOL) implant that can effectively and accurately correct refractive errors. Preoperative biometric measurements, including the corneal curvature and axial length, are used in different formulas to calculate the proper intraocular lens power.

Since the turn of the century, a variety of IOLs has been brought forth to address presbyopia correction. There are different designs, including multifocal designs and accommodating IOLs. Monovision, popularly used with presbyopic contact lens wearers (one eye is corrected for distance vision and the other eye for near), can also be reproduced permanently with RLE and cataract surgery.

Although currently available presbyopia-correcting IOL technology is effective in providing a greater range of vision and freedom from spectacle use, the IOLs are not without their faults. Although improved, the multifocal IOL can cause glare and halos from its inherent concentric ring design, and diminished contrast sensitivity can result from the light's being "split" for distance and near vision. The only currently FDA-approved accommodating IOL has neither of these disadvantages of the multifocal IOLs, but it does not provide UV light protection and also provides less predictable near vision (Figure 8).

Because RLE is intraocular, it is much more invasive than the previous extraocular corneal procedures. Hence, although both eyes can undergo corneal procedures simultaneously, elective intraocular procedures should always be performed as two separate staged surgeries. Being intraocular, RLE procedures likely have a similar risk of endophthalmitis (severe postoperative intraocular infection) as modern cataract surgeries do, which is between 0.05% to 0.10%. Other postoperative complications of RLE include retinal detachment in high myopes (1.85%-8%) and a likely need for a laser capsulotomy procedure to treat capsular haze that commonly occurs behind the IOL after surgery.

In addition to the postoperative risks of RLE, other common obstacles can be encountered intraoperatively because operating on soft lenses, very long eyes (high myopes), and very short eyes (high hyperopes) has its own set of potential complications. Preoperative surgical planning and strategy are key to a successful RLE.

Phakic Intraocular Lens Implant
Surgically implanted lenses, or phakic intraocular lens implants, may be used only to treat myopia in the United States. Phakic IOLs are an alternative to laser vision correction and can successfully correct myopia in patients for whom keratorefractive surgery is not an option. As compared to laser vision correction for myopia, some studies suggest that the quality of vision with a phakic IOL is superior. Phakic IOLs function very similarly to contact lenses that are permanently implanted inside the eye. Regarding the two FDA-approved phakic IOLs available today, a phakic IOL can be implanted to sit in front of and attached to the iris (see Figure 8) or just behind the iris. As in RLE, the implantation of a phakic IOL is intraocular, and surgery should be performed

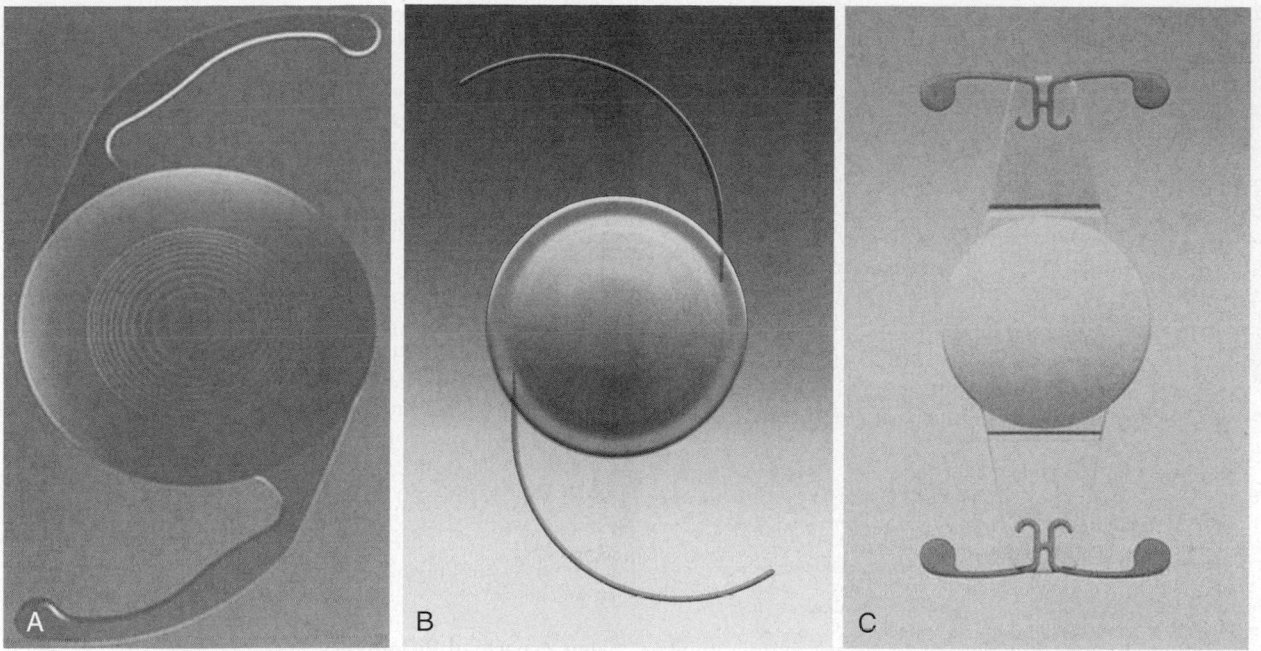

Figure 8. Examples of currently FDA-approved intraocular lens implants. **A** and **B,** Multifocal. **C,** Accommodating. (**A,** From Alcon Labs, Fort Worth, TX. **B,** From Abbott, Abbott Park, IL. **C,** From Bausch and Lomb, Rochester, NY.)

on only one eye at a time to respect the risks involved in the more-invasive procedure. Unlike RLE, all structures inside the eye, including the crystalline lens, are left untouched when a phakic IOL is implanted.

As do all surgical procedures, phakic IOLs are subject to various complications, of which cataract formation is a more common one (up to 9%). Other surgical complications include infection, retinal detachment, acute glaucoma, and loss of corneal endothelial cells, which are the nonregenerating cells on the back surface of the cornea that are responsible for maintaining corneal clarity.

Future Outlook

Refractive surgery technology continues to evolve. Regarding corneal refractive surgery, there has been a lot of focus on procedures that involve removing an intracorneal lenticule of stromal corneal tissue to create refractive correction. One of these procedures, Femtosecond lenticule extraction (FLEx), creates and lifts a corneal flap to then remove the lenticule. Another, small incision lenticular extraction (SMILE), removes the lenticule through a small incision without the creation of a corneal flap. SMILE has so far offered better corneal biomechanics stability than the flap created procedures and has raised the possibility of correcting higher refractive myopic errors. In addition, SMILE appears to cause less dry eye syndrome in a statistically significant manner. In a recent study by Sekundo, et al., 1.1% of subjects after the SMILE procedure had superficial punctate keratitis at 1 week follow-up with none having subjective complaints of dry eye syndrome while 13.9% of subjects had superficial punctate keratitis and 8.3% had dry eye symptoms after FLEx. This disparity has been attributed to the severing of corneal nerves that occurs on any flap creating procedure. There are also several options on the horizon for the correction of presbyopia. Various corneal inlays have been used outside the US, with promising outcomes, that provide greater near vision while only minimally sacrificing the distance vision. (Figure 9, Figure 10).

For intraocular refractive surgery options, phakic lens technology, which is currently only approved in the United States for the correction of myopia, may be available for hyperopic correction, as it is in Europe.

Lastly, options for presbyopia-correcting lens technology to replace the crystalline lens during a refractive lens exchange or

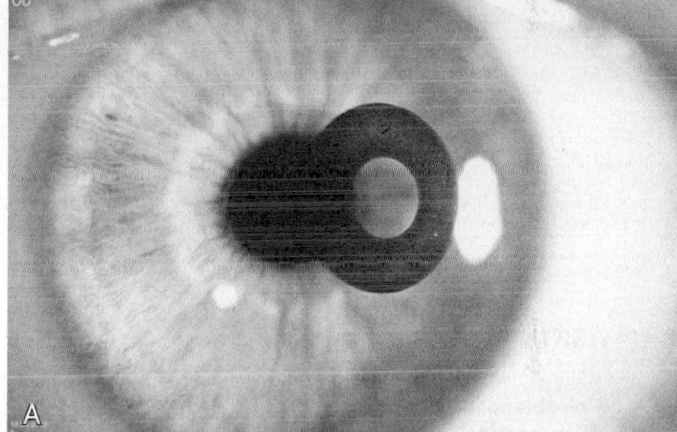

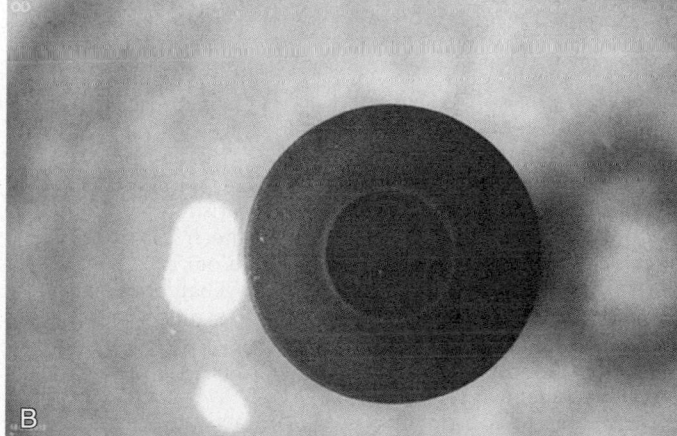

Figure 9. Kamra inlay. Uses pinhole effect to increase depth of field.

cataract surgery are ever-expanding. There are numerous platforms, including greater multi-focal designs, true accommodating IOLs, and a new family of lenses to increase the range of vision, called "extended depth of focus" lenses, will likely be available domestically in the foreseeable future.

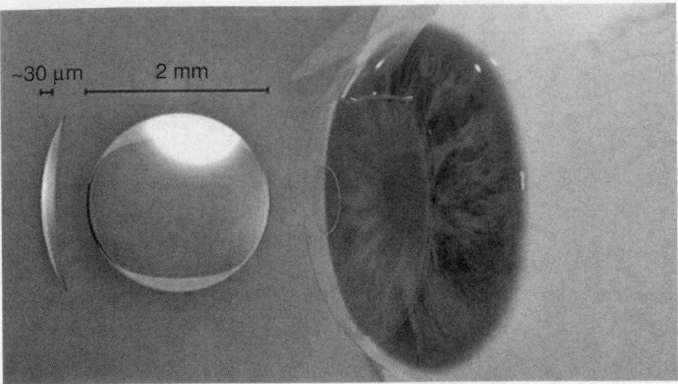

Figure 10. Raindrop inlay. Reshapes cornea to a hyperprolate state.

References

Buratto L. Phakic IOLs: Which approaches are likely to be effective and safe? In Program and abstracts of the 2006 Joint Meeting of the American Academy of Ophthalmology and Asia Pacific Academy of Ophthalmology, Las Vegas Nevada. Refractive Surgery Subspecialty Day. November 2006.

Cowden JW, Bores LD. A clinical investigation of the surgical correction of myopia by the method of Fyodorov. Ophthalmology 1981;88(8):737–41.

Donders RC, Moore WD. On the anomalies of accommodation and refraction of the eye. London: New Sydenham Society; 1864.

Langenbucher A, Goebels S, Szentmáry N, Seitz B. Eppig T. Vignetting and field of view with the KAMRA corneal inlay. Biomed Res Int; 2013.

Packard R. Refractive lens exchange for myopia: A new perspective? Curr Opin Ophthalmol 2005;16(1):53–6.

Price FW, Grene RB, Marks RG, Gonzales JS. Astigmatism reduction clinical trial: A multicenter prospective evaluation of the predictability of arcuate keratotomy. Evaluation of surgical nomogram predictability. ARC-T Study Group. Arch Ophthalmol 1995;113(3):277–82.

Raindrop Inlay. ReVision Optics. 2014. Sekundo, W, Kunert, K, Blum, M. Small incision corneal refractive surgery using the small incision lenticule extraction (SMILE) procedure for the correction of myopia and myopic astigmatism: results of a 6 month prospective study. Br J Ophthalmol 2011;95:335–339.

Stulting RD, Carr JD, Thompson KP, et al. Complications of laser in situ keratomileusis for the correction of myopia. Ophthalmology 1999;106(1):13–20.

Vitale S, Ellwein L, Cotch MF, et al. Prevalence of refractive error in the United States, 1999–2004. Arch Ophthalmol 2008;126(8):1111–9.

VISION REHABILITATION

Method of
August Colenbrander, MD; Donald C. Fletcher, MD; and Kim Schoessow, OTD, OTR/L

Vision rehabilitation refers to the multidisciplinary effort of assisting those with various degrees of vision loss in coping with the *consequences* of that loss. To describe vision rehabilitation, the nature of vision itself must be understood.

Vision is the major source of information about our environment. The eyes alone contribute as much information to the brain as all other organs combined. It is not surprising, therefore, that many people fear loss of vision almost as much as loss of life.

Most people will state that "We see with our eyes." On closer examination, this is not true. An isolated eyeball cannot produce any vision; our brain, however, can produce exquisite visual imagery in our dreams, without any input from the eyes.

The visual process goes through three distinct stages. Each stage comes with its own specific problems.

- First is the *optical stage*, where the refractive media of the eye deliver an image to the retina. Familiar problems in this area include refractive errors and cataracts.
- Second is the *receptor stage*, where the optical image is translated into neural impulses. Age-related macular degeneration (AMD) is a significant problem of the receptor stage, which is becoming increasingly common as the population ages.
- Third are various stages of *neural processing*, initially in the inner retina, then in the visual cortex, and finally in higher cortical centers, where the visual input gives rise to visual perception and to visually guided behaviors, actions, and interactions.

The most common visual problems vary for different ages. Today, brain-damage-related vision problems (cerebral visual impairment or CVI) are the most prevalent cause of visual impairment in *infants and young children*. Given that vision is so important for normal development, vision loss in infants constitutes a developmental emergency and should be detected and addressed as early as possible. When a child does not smile back at the mother, the mother may be inclined to leave the baby in its crib instead of holding him or her to provide extra tactile stimulation to compensate for missing visual stimulation.

At *school age* and later, visual health is critical because reading becomes important for academic development. For *adults*, vision is important for maintaining independence in activities of daily living (ADL) and development of vocational skills. For *seniors*, vision loss may exacerbate other age-related dysfunctions. Studies of the elderly have shown correlations between visual impairment and depression, falls, and reduced longevity. In all of these instances, early detection and early intervention are essential; the primary care physician plays a crucial role in this respect.

Four Aspects of Vision Loss

Vision is a complex phenomenon.

A convenient framework for discussing the various impacts of vision loss is to consider four aspects of visual functioning (Figure 1). First to consider is how various external causes may result in *structural changes* to the eyes and the visual pathways. For this aspect, the focus is on the tissue; an ocular pathologist is needed to describe the pathologic condition. However, structural changes alone do not determine how well the eyes actually function. Clinicians need to measure *organ function*, such as visual acuity, visual field, and contrast sensitivity.

Yet even knowing how the eyes function does not tell us how the person functions. In other words, the *abilities* of the person to perform tasks, such as reading, mobility, face recognition, and ADL, must be considered. Occupational therapists (OTs) and other rehabilitation professionals work with patients to teach them how residual vision can be used most effectively. OTs also assess the person in a societal context. For example, do the visual changes have an impact on the person's *participation* in society, on his or her ability to perform necessary tasks, and on general satisfaction with one's quality of life? It is clear that to cover all aspects of vision rehabilitation, a team approach is necessary, and that the patient must be part of that team.

A single activity of daily living may cover several of the above aspects. When reading, the aspect of minimum print size falls under organ function (retinal resolution). Reading speed (words/minute) and reading endurance (hours/day) define abilities of the person; reading endurance may be poor, even if reading acuity is adequate. Reading enjoyment, finally, falls under the aspect of quality of life.

It is helpful to draw a line between the organ side of Figure 1 on the left and the person side on the right. On the left side of the diagram, we discuss *visual functions*, which describe how the eyes function. On the right side, we speak of *functional vision*, which describes how the person functions in vision-related activities. Medical specialists are well versed in dealing with the left side of the diagram. Yet, the ultimate goal of all interventions is to improve the patient's quality of life. It is the function of vision rehabilitation to make sure that "eye" doctors become "people" doctors by extending their interest to the right side of the diagram as well.

Comprehensive Vision Rehabilitation

Considering all of these aspects, comprehensive vision rehabilitation involves much more than the patient's performance on a letter chart and requires teamwork between different professionals who

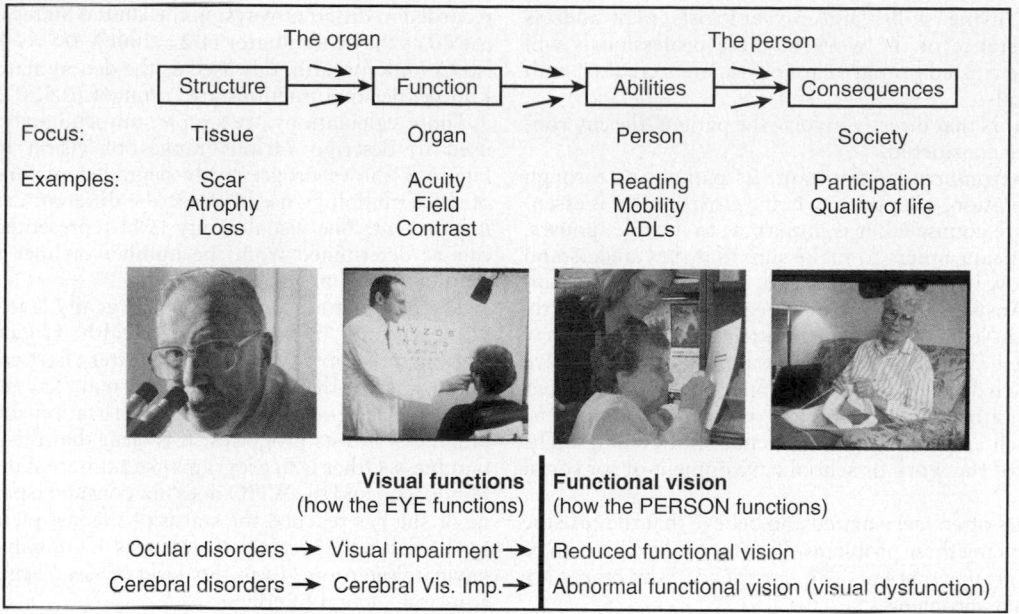

The organ		The person	
Structure →	Function →	Abilities →	Consequences

Focus:	Tissue	Organ	Person	Society
Examples:	Scar Atrophy Loss	Acuity Field Contrast	Reading Mobility ADLs	Participation Quality of life

Visual functions
(how the EYE functions)

Functional vision
(how the PERSON functions)

Ocular disorders → Visual impairment → Reduced functional vision

Cerebral disorders → Cerebral Vis. Imp. → Abnormal functional vision (visual dysfunction)

Figure 1. Aspects of vision loss.

specialize in different aspects of vision loss. All vision loss starts with some medical condition. So, primary care physicians are well positioned to coordinate team activities. Primary care physicians need to be aware of what other team members can contribute and should know where to locate vision rehabilitation resources and to make appropriate referrals.

Figure 2 illustrates that comprehensive vision rehabilitation involves much more than does the traditional low vision care offered in the past.

Low vision is a term used to describe individuals who suffer from a visual impairment that cannot be eliminated with refractive correction, yet are not blind. Individuals who suffer from visual impairment from low vision may benefit from vision enhancement, vision substitution, and vision assistance as well as from honing of coping skills.

Low vision is distinct from blindness (i.e., no vision). Blindness differs from low vision in that in blindness, the emphasis of rehabilitation is entirely on vision substitution. Patients with severe or profound low vision may combine the use of some blindness rehabilitation skills with some low vision rehabilitation skills.

Vision enhancement, which is the traditional focus of low vision care, is primarily oriented at improving residual visual function through visual aids, including a wide range of magnification devices. Additionally, enhancement of contrast, illumination, and filters need to be explored.

Vision substitution expands the options for rehabilitation by optimizing the use of other senses. This can range from using simple tactile markings to sense the position of a stove dial, to devices such as talking books, a long cane for travel, and Braille for reading. Vision enhancement and vision substitution are not mutually exclusive. A patient may use a magnifier to read price tags and may prefer talking books for recreational reading. A patient with retinitis pigmentosa, which causes reduced night vision, may have normal mobility in the daytime and need a cane at night. Digital audio books may have Braille labels.

Vision assistance. A special form of vision substitution involves using the eyes of others. Family members, caregivers, and office personnel should be familiar with *sighted guide* techniques to effectively assist visually impaired patients with minimal embarrassment. *Guide dogs* are also a possibility. Using a guide dog requires training of the patient as well as of the dog, so that they can work as a team. Dog users must also demonstrate mastery of long cane travel skills.

Coping skills. How different patients will accept visual aids may differ greatly. It is important to recognize that vision loss often causes a reactive depression. On the one hand, a depressed patient will be less receptive to rehabilitative suggestions. On the other hand, demonstration of rehabilitative success can be a powerful tool to lift a reactive depression and to motivate the patient for further success. It has been shown that the teaching of problem-solving skills may improve the effectiveness of vision rehabilitation.

Many professionals may be involved in vision rehabilitation. Technicians may prescribe magnifiers, rehabilitation workers

Figure 2. Comprehensive vision rehabilitation.

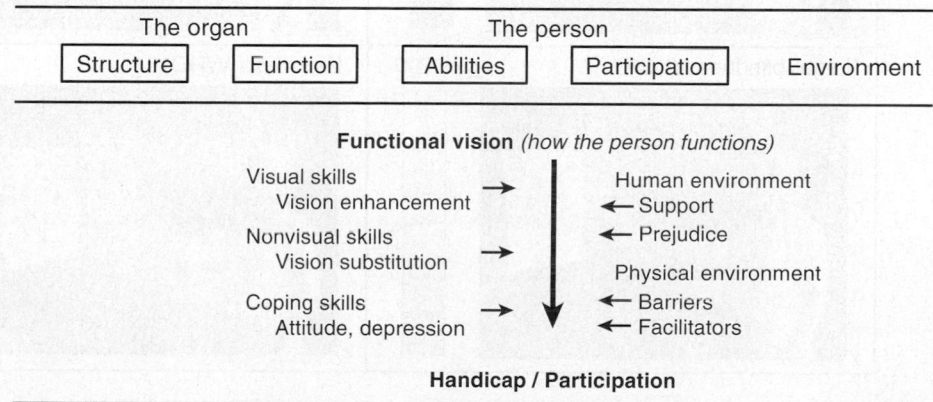

The organ		The person		
Structure	Function	Abilities	Participation	Environment

Functional vision *(how the person functions)*

Visual skills Vision enhancement	→	Human environment ← Support
Nonvisual skills Vision substitution	→	← Prejudice
Coping skills Attitude, depression	→	Physical environment ← Barriers ← Facilitators

Handicap / Participation

may teach daily living skills, and psychologists may address depression. Acceptance of the work of these professionals will be improved if the trusted primary care physician is credited with making the referrals.

Beyond the factors that directly involve the patient, the environment must also be considered.

The *human environment* is important. As patients go through the stages of adaptation, a supportive home environment is essential. As patients are counseled, it is important to include spouses, children, or significant others to make sure that they understand the condition, know what can be expected, and know how to support the patient. Answering family and caregiver questions directly is often better than leaving this to the patient, who initially may not have absorbed everything that was said. An overprotective environment, which deprives patients of opportunities to do things for themselves, can be as detrimental as an overdemanding one that puts too much emphasis on the patient's shortcomings. The same holds true for the work or school environment or for social groups.

Initially, patients often feel isolated and believe that they are the only ones experiencing these problems. *Peer support groups* can be helpful; in these groups, patients can experience how others are dealing with similar problems.

Finally, the *physical environment* needs to be considered. An uncluttered environment, where things have a defined, fixed place is helpful because it reduces the need for searching. Good general illumination and task lighting often help, because at higher illumination levels retinal cells that are damaged but not dead can still contribute to vision. Good contrast is important: do not serve milk in a white Styrofoam cup; mark the edges of steps and stairs. The triangles and circles on men's and women's bathrooms are designed to be visible for those with very low vision; Braille labels in elevators are useful for people who are totally blind.

How Blind Is Blind?

The most common visual function test is the letter chart, developed by Snellen in 1862. That test determines how large a letter, or other symbol, must be to be recognized by the patient. That size is then compared to the size recognized by a standard observer. If the magnification requirement is $2\times$, visual acuity is said to be 1/2; if it is $5\times$, visual acuity is said to be 1/5, etc. That fraction can be recorded in different ways; in the United States, it is customary to use 20 as the denominator ($1/2 = 20/40$, $1/5 = 20/100$); in the British Commonwealth, 6 is used as the denominator (6/12, 6/30); in Europe, decimal fractions are common (0.5, 0.2).

Those calculations are simple; unfortunately, the terminology used to describe various ranges of vision loss is confusing. Figure 3 shows progressively degraded pictures with examples of the terminology used to describe different definitions of visual impairment. The visual acuity level represented by each picture can be determined from the number of lines that are readable on the low vision letter chart.

The first picture shows the visual acuity level that is labeled as "low vision" by the World Health Organization (WHO). Although the bottom lines of the letter chart cannot be read, the appearance of the room is near normal. The next picture shows what the U.S. Social Security Administration considers "statutory blindness" for its programs. It is clear that this is far from actual blindness. Other U.S. programs use a different definition for "legal blindness," and the WHO does not consider a person "blind" until he or she has reached the status of the last picture. At that level, reading even the special letter chart is not possible, but one can still navigate the room. Even this level of visual impairment does not constitute actual blindness.

The widespread use of the word "blindness" is unfortunate, because it cannot be used with modifiers. One is either blind or sighted; one cannot be "a little bit blind." This black-and-white thinking has hampered the acceptance of vision rehabilitation. Terms such as vision loss or visual impairment are preferred because they can be used with modifiers, including mild, moderate, severe, profound, and total vision loss. Although "legal blindness" and "severe vision loss" (ICD-9-CM) have the same definition, there is a big difference between telling a patient *You are legally blind* and *You have a severe visual impairment*. The first statement might be followed by *I am sorry, there is nothing more we can do for your eyes*; the second statement leads to the question *What can be done to help you cope with this problem?*

Vision Rehabilitation Techniques and Devices

Having considered the general outlines of vision rehabilitation, some details of rehabilitative interventions can be discussed.

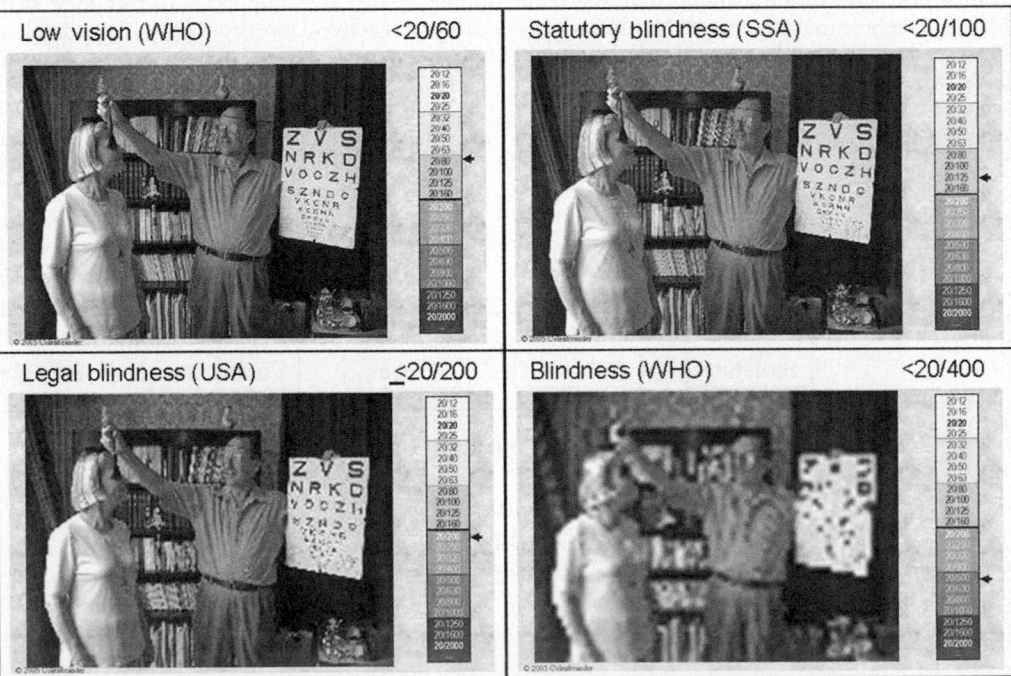

Figure 3. Ranges of vision loss.

Primary care physicians should know what vision rehabilitation techniques are available.

Optical Problems

The most commonly encountered visual problems are those involving the optical system of the eye.

Refractive errors are the easiest visual problems to deal with. Refractive errors can be corrected with glasses or contact lenses, and for those who hate glasses, by refractive surgery. Even if there are other causes of vision loss, determining the best refractive correction is still important.

Uncorrected refractive error is a major cause of visual impairment worldwide. In developed countries, the question may be why people do not avail themselves of the solutions that are available. In developing countries, availability of and accessibility to eye care and to the means for correcting refractive errors often do not exist. Providing these is a matter of infrastructure, not of individual health care.

Opacities disrupt visual image formation. Cataracts are the most familiar opacity; they can be removed by surgery. Other opacities of a temporary or permanent nature may occur in the cornea, in the anterior chamber, or in the vitreous cavity. Corneal and conjunctival infections may cause corneal scarring, as is the case in trachoma; this condition does not exist in the developed world anymore but is a major cause of blindness worldwide.

Letter chart acuity is a good way to measure optical problems. It should be understood, however, that letter chart acuity only measures the function of the retina where the letter read is projected. Even for a patient with 20/200 acuity, this area of the retina is less than 1° in diameter. For optical problems this does not matter, because foveal defocus predicts equal defocus in all other areas of the retina.

Magnification is the primary way to compensate for reduced acuity. One way to provide magnification is to bring print closer to the eye. For the elderly, this requires reading glasses with extra power. Alternatively, large print may be helpful. Larger print on medicine labels, as required in several states, can reduce medication errors by the elderly, who often take several medications. Handheld magnifiers are another option; many have built-in LED illumination that provides more light. Video-magnifiers with a table mounted large screen are ideal for prolonged reading; they can enhance contrast and brightness, while some devices can even read the text out loud. Tablets and smartphone apps can provide similar advantages in a portable form and are increasingly popular as visual aids.

Retinal Problems

While primitive forms of cataract surgery have existed for centuries, the study of retinal disorders has only been possible since the invention of the ophthalmoscope in 1851. The ability to effectively treat some retinal disorders is even more recent. Important retinal disorders include the following.

AMD is the most frequent diagnosis encountered in any low vision rehabilitation service. Because the condition is age related, its frequency will increase in the future as our population ages. This has caused profound changes in the nature of low vision care. Until the mid-20th century, most low vision care was provided by special education teachers serving young students in schools for the blind. Today, the majority of low vision patients are seniors. This has resulted in a significant influx of OTs into the field with skills in addressing multiple geriatric impairments. Yet, the needs of seniors to be served still outstrip the available services.

Given that macular degeneration affects central vision and the ability to read, most patients will ultimately seek rehabilitation help. However, if only one eye is affected, AMD may go unnoticed. The patient may only complain when the second eye starts to deteriorate; at that point, the damage in the first eye may be beyond repair. Therefore, it is useful to ask patients to alternately cover one eye to see whether there is any vision difference between the eyes. If there is, this is a reason for referral.

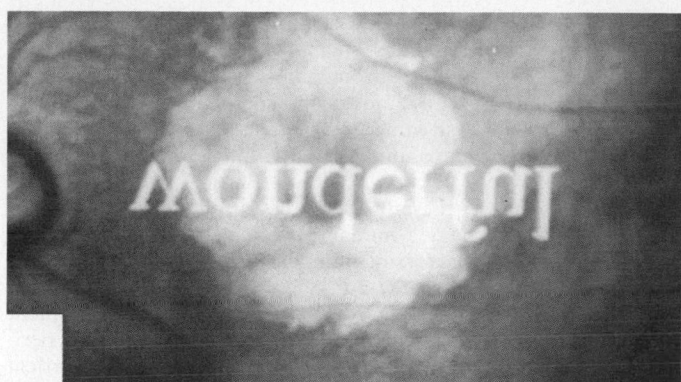

Figure 4. Ring scotoma.

Glaucoma is another age-related condition. Glaucoma often goes undetected because it causes loss of peripheral vision and affects central vision only in the late stages. Therefore, glaucoma must be sought out, primarily by measuring the intraocular pressure.

Diabetic retinopathy is not limited to seniors. As the incidence of diabetes is rising worldwide, so is the incidence of diabetic retinopathy. Even if treated with photocoagulation, it will cause scattered blind spots throughout the visual field.

There are many other hereditary and nonhereditary retinal conditions that may cause vision loss, but they occur in small numbers. They all require the help of vision rehabilitation professionals to help patients cope effectively.

Scotomata. Whatever the cause, retinal conditions will generally cause localized blind spots (scotomata). Therefore, when retinal damage is suspected, visual acuity alone is no longer a sufficient descriptor of visual impairment, because the retinal area where the chart letter is projected does not predict anything about other retinal areas. In addition to letter chart acuity, the condition of the visual field and the presence of blind spots (scotomata) must be considered. (Figure 4)

Figure 4 shows a retinal image, where a word is projected across a ring scotoma that leaves only a small central island of vision. This patient will be able to recognize the central letter, but will not be able to read the word. Clinicians must be careful when providing such patients with magnification, because too much magnification will mean that fewer letters fit into the central area. This example also makes it clear that when retinal involvement is suspected, a reading test may be more informative than a letter chart test, given that reading requires a larger retinal area.

Neural Processing Problems

As stated earlier, the most important stages of the visual process take place after the retinal receptors have translated the optical image into neural impulses.

The first transformations take place in the *inner retina*. Here, the input from 100 M receptors in each eye is preprocessed and compressed for transmission through 1 M nerve fibers in each optic nerve. The optic nerve fibers do not simply transmit a pixel-by-pixel image, as does a digital camera. Different retinal ganglion cells probably transmit different aspects of the image, such as edges (contrast enhancement), movement, color, brightness, etc. These separate "movies" are transmitted in parallel. At a later stage of neural processing, the different aspects of the image are combined again into a single visual perception.

In the *visual cortex*, the visual information is further analyzed for shapes and contours. Interestingly, at the first synaptic station in the lateral geniculate nucleus, only 20% of the incoming connections come from the optic nerves; the other 80% come from other cortical centers and probably contribute to filtering based on attention and other factors.

In *higher cortical centers*, the visual information is further processed. Here, the flow of information is no longer strictly visual, because it is combined with information from other senses. This results in identification and recognition of objects through comparison to stored concepts (through the ventral stream to the temporal lobe of the brain) and in spatial location of an object (through the dorsal stream to the parietal lobe of the brain), which then result in voluntary or involuntary visually guided action.

Our knowledge of these processes is still relatively new. It has been greatly helped by new modalities for neural and retinal imaging. Today, neural processing problems are increasingly recognized in all age groups.

In young children, CVI is now recognized as the most frequent cause of visual perceptual problems. CVI is often caused by perinatal ischemia, which may cause cortical as well as subcortical changes (periventricular leucomalacia). Because this ischemia is not localized, impairments are often not limited to the visual system. Schools for the blind have increasingly developed into schools for the multiply handicapped.

In contact sports, the results of repeated subclinical injuries are now recognized.

In veterans, traumatic brain injuries may cause problems that may be hard to define. Often visual interpretation and decision making are impaired; oculomotor system problems are often found. Traffic accidents may cause similar damage.

In the elderly, strokes may cause more localized problems and agnosias for specific tasks. In all of these cases, the term *visual impairment* may be used when visual acuity and/or visual field are impaired. The term *visual dysfunction* may be more appropriate when the visual input to the brain is normal, but the processing of this information is not.

Patient-Centered Functional Priorities

Vision problems affect all aspects of a patient's life. It is no longer sufficient for clinicians to determine that *nothing more can be done* about the *causes* of vision loss, because *much more can be done* about the *consequences* of vision impairment.

To determine the range of services that may be appropriate for an individual with vision impairment, the American Academy of Ophthalmology recommends consideration of the following functional priority areas:

- *Reading*—for many patients, this is their foremost concern.
- *Activities of Daily Living (ADL)*—even though reading may be the most prominent complaint, most people spend the larger part of their day performing a variety of other vision dependent activities for self-care and home management.
- *Safety*—are people at risk for falls? How do they cross the street? Do they drive?

- *Community participation*—can the individual still participate in community events, including religious gatherings?
- *Physical, cognitive, and psychosocial well-being*—because many patients with vision loss are elderly, this is an important aspect that should not be overlooked. If cognitive problems exist, it may affect the recommendations to be made.

Based on these considerations, patient-centered priorities can be set and specific rehabilitation goals formulated that reflect the patient's needs and desires.

References

Colenbrander A. Measuring vision and vision loss. In Tasman W, Jaeger EA, editors. Duane's Ophthalmology Vol. 5. Philadelphia, PA: Lippincott Williams & Wilkins; 2013 Chapter 51 (2001, updated and expanded: 2010 and later editions).

Schoessow KA. Shifting from compensation to participation: A model for occupational therapy in low vision. Br J Occup Ther 2010;73:160–9.

Cimarolli VR, Boerner K. Social support and well-being in adults who are visually impaired. J Vis Impair Blind 2005;99:521–34.

Cimarolli VR, Reinhardt JP, Horowitz A. Perceived overprotection: Support gone bad? J Gerontol B Psychol Sci Soc Sci 2006;61:S18–S23.

Moore JE, Giesen JM, Weber JM, Crews JE. Functional outcomes reported by consumers of the independent living program for older individuals who are blind. J Visual Impair Blind 2001;95:403–17.

Brunnstrom G, Sorensen S, Alsterstad K, Sjostrand J. Quality of light and quality of life—the effect of lighting adaptation among people with low vision. Ophthalmic Physiol Opt 2004;24:274–80.

Haymes SA, Lee SA. Effects of task lighting on visual function in age-related macular degeneration. Ophthalmic Physiol Opt 2006;26:169–79.

Resnikoff S, Pascolini D, Mariotti SP, Pokharel GP. Global magnitude of visual impairment caused by uncorrected refractive errors in 2004. Bull World Health Organ 2008;86:63–70.

Fletcher DC, Schuchard RA. Preferred retinal loci relationship to macular scotomas in a low-vision population. Ophthalmology 1997;104:632–8.

Fletcher DC, Schuchard RA, Watson G. Relative locations of macular scotomas near the PRL: Effect on low vision reading. J Rehabil Res Dev 1999;36:356–64.

Colenbrander A. Towards the development of a classification of vision-related functioning—A potential framework. Chapter 20, In Dutton GH, Bax M, editors. Visual Impairment in Children Due to Damage to the Brain. London: Mac Keith Press; 2010.

Faul MD, Xu L, Wald MM, et al. Traumatic brain injury in the United States; emergency department visits, hospitalizations, and deaths, 2002-2006. Atlanta (GA): Centers for Disease Control and Prevention, National Center for Injury Prevention and Control; 2010.

American Academy of Ophthalmology (2013). Preferred practice pattern for vision rehabilitation. Available at http://one.aao.org/preferred-practice-pattern/vision-rehabilitation-ppp-2013.

Additional Website Sources

The AFB Senior Site (www.AFB.org/seniorsitehome.asp) contains resources for seniors.

The MDsupport website (www.MDsupport.org) specializes in support and documentation for AMD patients and care givers.

The Lighthouse Guild International in New York (www.lighthouse.org) offers extensive resources for all forms of vision loss.

These websites contain links to many more websites with additional information and often can provide information about local resources.

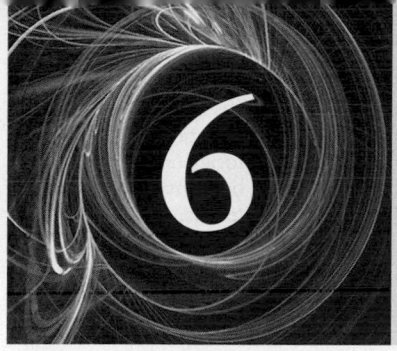

6 The Respiratory System

ACUTE BRONCHITIS

Method of
Susan Davids, MD, MPH; and Ralph M. Schapira, MD

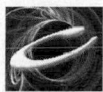

CURRENT DIAGNOSIS

- Normal healthy adult with cough
- Predominance of cough
- Lasts 1 to 3 weeks
- With or without sputum
- Can be accompanied by other respiratory and constitutional symptoms
- Absence of abnormal vital signs and physical examination suggesting pneumonia, particularly
  - Heart rate >100 beats per minute
  - Respiratory rate >24 breaths per minute
  - Temperature >100.4°F (38°C)
  - Lung findings suggest a consolidation process

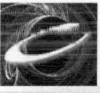

CURRENT THERAPY

- Antibiotics not routinely recommended
- If influenza is highly probable and patient is presenting within the first 48 hours, consider treatment with
  - Oseltamivir (Tamiflu) 75 mg PO bid with food for 5 days (influenza A/B)
  - Zanamivir (Relenza) 10 mg bid by inhalation for 5 days (influenza A/B)
  - *Amantadine (Symmetrel) 100 mg bid or 200 mg once daily for 5 days (influenza A)
  - *Rimantadine (Flumadine) 100 mg bid for 5 days (influenza A)
- In patients with evidence of bronchial hyperresponsiveness, consider treatment with
  - β_2-agonists for 1 to 2 weeks
  - Antitussives in those with cough for 2 to 3 weeks
  - Antipyretics and analgesics as needed
  - Smoking cessation
- Education: cough likely to last 3 weeks or more.

*Due to antiviral medication resistance, the choice of agent to treat influenza should be based on recommendations from the CDC and local health departments.

Acute bronchitis is one of the most common diagnoses made by primary care physicians in the United States and accounts for nearly 10 million office visits per year. Acute bronchitis is a transient, self-limited inflammatory process of the upper respiratory tract, specifically the trachea and bronchi. Antibiotics are overprescribed to patients with acute bronchitis; this practice has raised significant concern related to the worldwide rise of antibiotic resistance, which is viewed as one of the world's most pressing public health problems.

Acute bronchitis manifests as an acute respiratory illness of less than 3 weeks' duration, with or without sputum production. Acute bronchitis is a clinical diagnosis and must be distinguished from other respiratory diseases, such as pneumonia, acute exacerbation of chronic bronchitis (episode of worsening of symptoms and expiratory airflow obstruction in patients with chronic obstructive pulmonary disease), and the onset of asthma. Most cases of acute bronchitis occur in the fall and winter. The etiology of acute bronchitis is infectious, and viruses appear to be the cause of most cases. Influenzas A and B are the most common viruses isolated, although a wide variety of infectious agents have been identified, such as adenovirus, coronavirus, parainfluenza virus, respiratory syncytial virus, coxsackievirus, *Mycoplasma pneumoniae*, *Bordetella pertussis*, and *Chlamydia pneumoniae*.

Diagnosis of acute bronchitis is based on findings of a prominent cough that may be accompanied by wheezing and sputum production. Most patients are otherwise healthy and without pre-existing respiratory disease. Nonspecific constitutional symptoms may also be part of acute bronchitis. Appropriate management of acute bronchitis is essential because it is one of the most common illnesses that present to physicians in the outpatient setting. Antibiotics are often prescribed unnecessarily for acute bronchitis and other respiratory tract illnesses; these prescriptions may potentially lead to adverse events (i.e., allergic reactions and gastrointestinal side effects) and bacterial resistance. Other medications, such as inhaled bronchodilators and antitussives, are often prescribed for acute bronchitis despite questionable evidence to support their routine use.

Pathophysiology of acute bronchitis involves an acute inflammatory response involving the mucosa of the trachea and bronchi, resulting in injury to the respiratory tract epithelium. Sputum production is increased and bronchoconstriction (potentially resulting in airflow obstruction and wheezing) can occur. Positron emission tomography (PET) of a patient with acute bronchitis confirms that the primary inflammatory changes occur in the trachea and bronchi and not the remainder of the lower respiratory track.

Diagnosis
Cough, phlegm (which may be purulent, as both bacteria and viruses can cause purulent sputum), and wheezing help differentiate acute bronchitis from upper respiratory infections such as pharyngitis and sinusitis. Acute bronchitis must be differentiated from acute bacterial pneumonia. The absence of abnormalities in vital signs (heart rate >100 bpm, respiratory rate >24 breath/min, oral temperature >100.4°F [38°C]) and physical examination of the chest support the diagnosis of acute bronchitis and make the need for chest radiography unnecessary in most cases. The treatment and outcome of acute bronchitis and pneumonia are very different; a chest radiograph should always be obtained if there is uncertainty about the diagnosis. Chest radiography will demonstrate no lung infiltrates in a patient with acute bronchitis. In contrast, lung infiltrates are present in pneumonia. Pertussis or whooping cough should be considered in adults with cough in the

setting of what appears to be an upper respiratory infection, even in those previously immunized. Typically, the cough of pertussis, unlike acute bronchitis, lasts for longer than 3 weeks. Other respiratory diseases, such as previously undiagnosed asthma, can also mimic acute bronchitis, although several features differentiate asthma from acute bronchitis (see Section 12). Rapid testing to diagnose influenza viruses A and B (the most common causes of acute bronchitis) as a cause of acute bronchitis should be considered given the availability of effective treatment if initiated in the first 48 hours.

Treatment

Antibiotics, Inhaled Bronchodilators, and Antitussives

Existing evidence does not support the routine use of antibiotics for uncomplicated cases of acute bronchitis. Although most cases of acute bronchitis are caused by viral infections, upwards of 60% of patients are prescribed antibiotic therapy, which is contributing to the rise of bacterial resistance to commonly used antibiotics. Meta-analyses examining the effectiveness of antibiotic therapy in patients without underlying lung disease suggest no consistent effect of antibiotics on the severity or duration of acute bronchitis. A recent study evaluated children and patients with colored sputum and found that they also did not benefit from antibiotics. This study also found that compared to other populations, the elderly were less likely to benefit from antibiotics. Smokers with acute bronchitis are even more likely to be prescribed antibiotics. Their response to antibiotics was either equal to or worse than that of nonsmokers.

One possible reason for overuse of antibiotics is the concern by physicians about patient satisfaction. Studies show that patients presenting to the doctor expecting antibiotics were more likely to be prescribed antibiotics; studies also suggest that satisfaction is more related to appropriate patient education than to receiving antibiotics. Patient education should include information regarding the duration of symptoms associated with acute bronchitis. It was found that patients presented on average after 9 days of cough and that the cough persisted for an additional 12 days after the physician visit. This information can impart a realistic expectation of illness duration to the patient.

If influenza is highly suspected and the patient presents within 48 hours of the onset of symptoms, rapid diagnostic testing and treatment should be considered. Both amantadine (Symmetrel) and rimantadine (Flumadine) are effective for influenza A, and neuraminidase inhibitors, inhaled zanamivir (Relenza), and oral oseltamivir (Tamiflu) are effective for influenzas A and B. If these medications are initiated within the first 48 hours of symptoms (and ideally within 30 hours), the duration of illness can be shortened.

The evidence supporting the use of inhaled bronchodilators for the treatment of the symptoms has been variable. Two small trials reported a shorter duration of cough with the use of inhaled β-agonists; another study reported benefit in those with evidence of bronchial hyperresponsiveness. Current recommendations support the use of β-agonists only in patients with evidence of bronchial hyperresponsiveness (wheezing or spirometry demonstrating a forced expiration volume in 1 second [FEV_1] <80% of predicted).

Antitussive agents have not been shown to improve the acute or early cough but did show some improvements in cough lasting longer than 3 weeks. The current recommendations are to use antitussives, namely dextromethorphan (Benylin) or codeine, in patients with cough of 2 to 3 weeks' duration.

Acute uncomplicated bronchitis is most often a viral illness in which antibiotics are not routinely indicated. Patients presenting with an acute respiratory illness, who are younger than 65 years old without existing pulmonary disease or other significant comorbid illness, should have a thorough physical examination, including vital signs. If the vital signs are normal and physical examination of the chest is clear, pneumonia can most likely be ruled out. In patients who present within 48 hours of onset of symptoms, influenza should be considered, as effective therapy is available for acute bronchitis caused by influenzas A or B. Otherwise, the evidence for treatment with antibiotics does not support their routine use. Bronchodilators should be considered in those with evidence of bronchial hyperresponsiveness; cough suppressants should be considered in those with 2 to 3 weeks of cough. Patient education is an integral part of the treatment, and patients should receive information that provides realistic expectations regarding the duration of cough.

References

Aagaard E, Gonzales R. Management of acute bronchitis in healthy adults. Infect Dis Clin North Am 2004;18:919–37.

Ebell MH. Antibiotic prescribing for cough and symptoms of respiratory tract infection. JAMA 2005;294(3):3062–4.

Fahey T, Smucny J, Becker L, Glazier R. Antibiotics for acute bronchitis. Cochrane Database Syst Rev 2004;(4):CD000245.

Gonzales R, Sande M. Uncomplicated acute bronchitis. Ann Intern Med 2000; 133:981–91.

Kicska G, Zhuang H, Alavi A. Acute bronchitis imaged with F-18 FDG positron emission tomography. Clin Nucl Med 2003;28(6):511–2.

Linder JA, Sim I. Antibiotic treatment of acute bronchitis in smokers. J Gen Intern Med 2002;17:230–4.

Little R, Rumsby K, Kelly J, et al. Information leaflet and antibiotic prescribing strategies for acute lower respiratory tract infection. JAMA 2005;293(24):3029–35.

Martinez FJ. Acute bronchitis: State of the art diagnosis and therapy. Compr Ther 2004;30(1):55–9.

Smucny J, Flynn C, Becker L, Glazier R. Beta$_2$-agonists for acute bronchitis. Cochrane Database Syst Rev 2004;(1):CD001726.

ACUTE RESPIRATORY FAILURE

Method of
Scott K. Epstein, MD

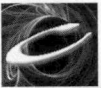

CURRENT DIAGNOSIS

- History and physical examination can give insight into the etiology of hypoxic and hypercapneic respiratory failure but may be insufficient to make a definitive diagnosis and guide therapy.
- An arterial blood gas is mandatory to define severity and whether hypoxic or hypercapneic (or both) respiratory failure is present.
- Additional diagnostic modalities, including chest radiograph, electrocardiogram, cardiac laboratory tests (troponin, brain natriuretic peptide), echocardiography, and selected use of a pulmonary artery catheter, can help identify a specific etiology.

CURRENT THERAPY

- Treatment of acute respiratory failure often begins with nonspecific approaches such as oxygen and mechanical ventilation (noninvasive or invasive).
- The goal of mechanical ventilation is to improve gas exchange and rest the respiratory muscles while waiting for the beneficial effects of specific therapy aimed at the underlying cause (e.g., bronchodilators, antibiotics, and corticosteroids in acute exacerbations of chronic obstructive pulmonary disease [COPD]).
- Noninvasive ventilation avoids many complications associated with invasive ventilation and improves outcomes for patients with acute cardiogenic pulmonary edema and acute exacerbations of COPD.
- Invasive mechanical ventilation can be lifesaving but can cause clinical deterioration if not properly administered.

- Using low tidal volumes (6 mL/kg ideal body weight) can help avoid dangerous dynamic hyperinflation in acute exacerbations of COPD and further lung injury in acute lung injury (e.g., volutrauma, barotrauma).
- Once signs of improvement are evident, focus rapidly shifts to liberating the patient from the ventilator using spontaneous breathing trials to assess the need for ventilatory support followed by airway assessment to determine readiness for extubation.

The respiratory system serves many complex physiologic functions, the most important of which is gas exchange. Using the interface between the alveolar space and capillaries, O_2 is taken up and CO_2 is eliminated. Acute respiratory failure, a life-threatening entity, is present when this system fails, over the course of minutes to hours, resulting in hypoxemia (type I) or hypercapnia (type II), or both. Most patients with acute respiratory failure present with dyspnea, although the correlation with disease severity is poor. Indeed, dyspnea might seem mild in those with baseline chronic respiratory failure, and it might be absent in those with an underlying neurologic process (e.g., drug overdose). Other symptoms and signs such as cough, chest pain, orthopnea, fever, tachypnea, rales, and wheezing are insensitive and nonspecific.

This chapter outlines the general pathophysiology and therapeutic approach to acute respiratory failure by using the examples of three common entities: acute lung injury (ALI), cardiogenic pulmonary edema (congestive heart failure [CHF]), and acute exacerbation of chronic obstructive pulmonary disease (COPD).

Definitions and Pathophysiology

Acute Hypoxic Respiratory Failure

Hypoxic respiratory failure is conventionally defined as an arterial oxygen tension (Pao_2) of less than 60 mm Hg. Because this definition ignores the inspired fraction of oxygen (Fio_2), some favor a Pao_2/Fio_2 ratio of less than 300. To account for the arterial CO_2 tension ($Paco_2$), others favor an alveolar–arterial (A–a) O_2 gradient greater than 250 mm Hg, using the equation

$$A–a\ O_2\ gradient = PAo_2 – Pao_2$$
$$= (713 \times Fio_2) – (PAo_2 + Paco_2/0.8)$$

where 713 is the barometric pressure (760) minus the water vapor pressure. A normal A–a O_2 is less than 10 mm Hg, but this threshold value increases with age. The determination of Pao_2 requires an invasive test, an arterial blood gas. Oxygenation can be continuously monitored noninvasively by pulse oximetry, which provides an estimate of arterial oxygen saturation (Sao_2). In general, an Sao_2 of 0.90 corresponds to a Pao_2 of 60 mm Hg, but the relation depends on temperature, pH, $Paco_2$, and 2,3-diphosphoglycerate (2,3-DPG). Accuracy is adversely affected by low perfusion states,

dark skin pigmentation, nail polish, dyshemoglobins (e.g., carboxyhemoglobin, methemoglobin), intravascular dyes, motion, and ambient light.

Clinicians tend to focus on Pao_2 and Sao_2, but the real parameter of interest is O_2 delivery (Do_2) to organs and tissues. Do_2 depends on cardiac output and O_2 carrying capacity of arterialized blood (Cao_2):

$$Do_2 = CO \times Cao_2$$

where

$$Cao_2 = k(Hb \times Sao_2) + 0.003\ Pao_2$$

where k is a constant. Do_2 decreases when cardiac output or hemoglobin is reduced despite a normal Pao_2 and Sao_2. The peripheral response to reduced Do_2 is an increased O_2 extraction ratio (O_2ER), allowing oxygen uptake ($\dot{V}o_2$), an indicator of metabolic demand, to remain constant. Cellular and organ dysfunction occurs when Do_2 and O_2ER are outstripped by metabolic demand. The balance between Do_2 and demand can be estimated by examining the mixed venous O_2 saturation (Mvo_2) using the rearranged Fick equation:

$$Mvo_2 = Sao_2 – (\dot{V}o_2/CO \times Hb)$$

When Mvo_2 falls below 65% to 75%, imbalance is present.

When cellular injury is present, extraction capabilities are limited and cellular hypoxia occurs despite "adequate" Do_2. Under these circumstances, the Mvo_2 can be paradoxically normal. These parameters can be determined using a pulmonary artery catheter. The data obtained may be useful in individual patients, but randomized, controlled trials show no benefit when the pulmonary artery catheter is used routinely to guide therapy.

The pathophysiologic mechanisms of type I respiratory failure are listed in Table 1. The most common mechanism is ventilation–perfusion ($\dot{V}/\dot{Q}$) mismatch, characterized by a widened A–a O_2 gradient, a dramatic increase in Pao_2 in response to supplemental O_2, and a variable $Paco_2$. When areas of low $\dot{V}/\dot{Q}$ predominate (e.g., reduced ventilation with normal perfusion), the $Paco_2$ may be low as the patient hyperventilates in an effort (only partially effective) to increase the Pao_2. When areas of high $\dot{V}/\dot{Q}$ predominate, much ventilation is wasted, and hypercapnia is also present. Areas of lung that are perfused but not ventilated characterize shunt. The resulting fall in Pao_2 depends on the percentage of cardiac output circulating through the shunt and the O_2 content of that blood. Supplemental O_2 has minimal or small effect on Pao_2 because the shunted blood is not exposed to the increased Fio_2. Therefore, treatment is aimed at decreasing shunt by improving ventilation to the affected area or reducing perfusion to that area. When shunt results from a unilateral process (e.g., pneumonia, atelectasis), placing the good lung down decreases shunt perfusion, and oxygenation improves.

TABLE 1 Pathophysiologic Mechanisms of Acute Hypoxic Respiratory Failure

MECHANISM	A–a O_2 GRADIENT	$Paco_2$	RESPONSE TO 100% O_2	CAUSE
Diffusion abnormality	↑	↑ normal	↑↑	Severe interstitial lung disease
Hypoventilation	Normal	↑	↑↑↑	Narcotic overdose, obesity hypoventilation syndrome, respiratory muscle weakness
↓ Fio_2	Normal	Usually ↓	↑↑↑	High altitude, smoke inhalation
↓ Mvo_2	↑	Usually ↓	↑	ALI, shock, CHF, PE
Shunt	↑	Usually ↓	None or ↑	ALI, CHF, atelectasis, PE
$\dot{V}/\dot{Q}$ mismatch	↑	↑, normal, ↓	↑↑↑	Acute exacerbation of COPD, asthma, PE

Abbreviations: ↑ = increased; ↓ = decreased; A–a O_2 = alveolar–arterial O_2; ALI = acute lung injury; CHF = cardiogenic pulmonary edema; COPD = chronic obstructive pulmonary disease; Fio_2 = fraction of inspired oxygen; Mvo_2 = mixed venous oxygen saturation; $Paco_2$ = partial pressure of arterial CO_2; PE = pulmonary embolism; $\dot{V}/\dot{Q}$ = ventilation–perfusion ratio.

Acute Hypercapneic Respiratory Failure

Hypercapneic respiratory failure is defined as a $Paco_2$ greater than 45 mm Hg. The equation used to determine $Paco_2$ provides insight into the three basic mechanisms underlying hypercapnia:

$$Paco_2 = k(\dot{V}Co_2)/V_E(1 - V_D/V_T)$$

where k is a constant, V_E is total minute ventilation (respiratory rate times tidal volume) and V_D/V_T is the dead space. Therefore, hypercapnia can result from increased CO_2 production ($\dot{V}Co_2$), increased physiologic dead space (V_D/V_T), and decreased minute ventilation (Box 1). Increased $\dot{V}Co_2$ alone is usually insufficient to cause hypercapnia because the respiratory system responds by increasing minute ventilation to keep $Paco_2$ normal (37–43 mm Hg). Conversely, with abnormalities of respiratory muscle function or respiratory drive or with increased dead space (and diminished reserve), the respiratory response to increased $\dot{V}Co_2$ may be insufficient, and hypercapnia results.

Treatment

Treatment of acute hypoxemic and hypercapneic respiratory failure combines nonspecific (e.g., supplemental O_2, mechanical ventilation) and specific therapy (Boxes 2 and 3).

Oxygen Therapy

In the hospital, 100% O_2 is supplied from a wall source with a regulator determining flow rate in liters per minute. The final delivered oxygen concentration (Fio_2) depends on this flow rate and the amount of room air breathed by the patient. The O_2 flow rate is almost never sufficient to meet all of the patient's ventilatory demands, so varying amounts of room air are entrained to meet these needs. The final inspired oxygen concentration depends on the relative fraction of each gas, total minute ventilation, and the pattern of breathing (including the inspiratory-to-expiratory ratio). O_2 may be administered using nasal prongs, a facial mask, or high-flow devices designed to deliver higher Fio_2 (Table 2).

In hypercapneic patients (e.g., with acute exacerbation of COPD), high-flow O_2 can lead to worsening hypercapnia and acute respiratory acidosis. The mechanisms are multifactorial: worsening $\dot{V}/\dot{Q}$ matching (increased dead space), decreased intracellular binding of CO_2, and minute ventilation inadequate for the amount of CO_2 produced. Therefore, the goal in these patients is to achieve a Pao_2 of 55 to 60 mm Hg (Sao_2 88%–90%) with low-flow oxygen (~24%–28% O_2). If this (often delicate) balance between maintaining tissue oxygenation and avoiding significant respiratory acidosis cannot be achieved, short-term mechanical ventilation may be required. In most nonhypercapneic patients, high flow of oxygen (50%–100%) can be administered safely for 24 hours with a goal Pao_2 of between 65 and 80 mm Hg.

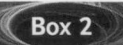

Box 1   Pathophysiologic Mechanisms of Hypercapnia

Increased Carbon Dioxide Production ($\dot{V}Co_2$)
Fever
Overfeeding
Seizure
Sepsis
Thyrotoxicosis

Decreased Ventilation (V_E)
Depressed respiratory drive
Phrenic nerve injury
Respiratory muscle weakness

Increased Dead Space (V_D/V_T)
Acute exacerbation of chronic obstructive pulmonary disease
Interstitial lung disease
Pulmonary vascular disease

Box 2   Causes of and Treatments for Acute Hypoxemic Respiratory Failure

Acute Exacerbation of Chronic Obstructive Pulmonary Disease
Antibiotics
Bronchodilators
Systemic steroids

Acute Lung Injury or Acute Respiratory Distress Syndrome
Efforts to decrease lung water
Lung-protective mechanical ventilation

Congestive Heart Failure
Afterload reduction
Diuretics
Inotropes

Lobar Collapse or Atelectasis
Bronchoscopy
Pulmonary toilet (airway suctioning to improve clearance of secretions)

Pneumonia
Antibiotics
Chest physiotherapy

Pneumothorax
Tube thoracostomy to drain pleural air and facilitate lung re-expansion

Pulmonary Embolism
Anticoagulation
Thrombolytic therapy

Status Asthmaticus
Bronchodilators
Systemic steroids

Box 3   Causes of and Treatments for Acute Hypercapneic Respiratory Failure

Acute Exacerbation of Chronic Obstructive Pulmonary Disease
Antibiotics
Bronchodilators
Systemic steroids

Acute Respiratory Muscle Weakness (e.g., myasthenic crisis)
Acetylcholinesterase therapy

Drug Overdose
Flumazenil (Romazicon)
Naloxone (Narcan)
Other antidotes

Guillain-Barré Syndrome
Immunoglobulin
Plasmapheresis

Spinal Cord Injury
Intravenous methylprednisolone

Status Asthmaticus
Bronchodilators
Systemic steroids

Toxin (e.g., botulinum toxin)
Antitoxin

TABLE 2 Short-Term Oxygen Delivery Systems

DELIVERY SYSTEM	O₂ FLOW RATE (L/min)	Fio₂ RANGE	COMMENTS
Basic Systems			
Nasal cannula (prongs)	1–6	0.22–0.40	Comfortable Facilitates communication and oral intake Humidification required at high flow rates
Simple masks	5–6	0.30–0.50	Mask acts as reservoir to increase Fio₂ High flow combats CO_2 rebreathing Less comfortable Must be removed to facilitate communication and oral intake Easily displaced with movement
Reservoir Masks			
Nonrebreathing	4–10	0.60–1.00	One-way valve between the mask and the reservoir bag Inspired O₂ from wall source and reservoir bag
Partial rebreathing	5–10	0.35–0.90	Lacks one-way valve
Venturi masks	4–10	0.24–0.40	Uses Bernoulli principle (fixed amount of entrained room air added to O₂) Maximum delivered Fio₂ can be controlled Often used in COPD to avoid excessive Fio₂ and risk for hypercapnia

Abbreviations: COPD = chronic obstructive pulmonary disease; Fio₂ = fraction of inspired oxygen.

Mechanical Ventilation

Mechanical ventilation can be delivered noninvasively through a tight-fitting face mask or invasively via an endotracheal tube. The goals of mechanical ventilation are to correct severe arterial blood gas abnormalities, provide respiratory support while specific therapy is used, and unload and rest the respiratory muscles. The ventilator should be set to optimize patient–ventilator interaction and avoid dynamic hyperinflation and intrinsic positive end-expiratory pressure (PEEPi). PEEPi can worsen gas exchange, predispose to barotrauma, and cause hypotension.

Noninvasive Ventilation

Noninvasive ventilation is most commonly applied as continuous positive airway pressure (CPAP), when airway pressure is kept constant throughout the respiratory cycle, or by bilevel positive airway pressure (BiPAP), when inspiratory pressure support actively assists each inspiration. Noninvasive ventilation offers numerous advantages over invasive ventilation, including increased comfort; maintenance of normal swallowing, speech, and cough; less need for sedation; and avoiding the trauma of intubation.

The effective application of noninvasive ventilation starts with carefully explaining the procedure to the patient, followed by selection of a proper-fitting face mask. The mask is placed close to the face to acclimate the patient to high inspiratory flow. The mask is then secured using straps (but not too tightly), and ventilator settings are adjusted to minimize leaks and ensure comfort. The patient is reassessed frequently. Failure to improve within 2 to 4 hours (e.g., reduction in dyspnea, respiratory rate, accessory muscle use, and hypercapnia) signals noninvasive ventilation failure and need for intubation.

Noninvasive ventilation improves outcome (avoids intubation, decreases length of stay, improves survival) in a number of conditions (Table 3). Although randomized, controlled trials show dramatic benefit in acute exacerbation of COPD (AECOPD), other studies show no or uncertain benefit in community acquired pneumonia, acute respiratory distress syndrome (ARDS), pulmonary fibrosis, and routinely after planned extubation. One mechanism for improved outcome is the reduction in infection (pneumonia, sepsis) seen with noninvasive ventilation compared with intubated patients. Noninvasive ventilation should not be used in the presence of respiratory arrest, shock, excessive secretions, inability to protect the airway, an agitated or uncooperative patient, and facial abnormalities that preclude proper application of the mask.

Invasive Ventilation

Invasive mechanical ventilation is delivered via an endotracheal tube. The set parameters include Fio₂ and positive end-expiratory pressure (PEEP). For volume-assist control, the clinician chooses respiratory rate and tidal volume. For pressure support, the clinician chooses the inspiratory pressure level above PEEP, and the patient determines respiratory rate. The resulting tidal volume depends on inspiratory pressure level and patient factors including respiratory muscle strength and respiratory system mechanics. Initially the ventilator is set to meet most of the patient's minute ventilation, allowing respiratory muscle rest. Such full support should not be prolonged because diaphragmatic dysfunction can result. Most patients require sedation, but excessive sedation levels are associated with worse outcomes. Therefore, strategies to minimize continuous intravenous sedation using a sedation protocol or once-daily interruption of sedation are recommended.

Invasive mechanical ventilation, especially when prolonged, is associated with numerous complications including ventilator-associated pneumonia, sinusitis, airway injury, thromboembolism, and gastrointestinal bleeding. Therefore, once significant clinical improvement occurs, efforts should focus on rapidly removing the patient from the ventilator. This is achieved by daily screening for readiness (Box 4) followed by a 30- to 120-minute spontaneous breathing trial on minimal or no ventilator support. Patients tolerating the spontaneous breathing trial are extubated if they have a good cough, manageable respiratory secretions, and an adequate mental status to protect the airway. Approximately 25% of patients do not tolerate the spontaneous breathing trial; they should be returned to full ventilator support for 24 hours and undergo careful evaluation for reversible causes. The clinician should consider a more gradual approach to weaning these patients.

Specific Causes of Acute Respiratory Failure

Acute Exacerbation of Chronic Obstructive Pulmonary Disease

Patients with COPD can experience two or three exacerbations per year, especially if they are actively smoking; this results in 500,000 hospitalizations every year in the United States. Hospital mortality ranges from 2% to 11%, rising to 25% for those requiring critical care.

AECOPD is defined by increased sputum volume, purulence, and dyspnea. Physical examination is notable for tachypnea, use of accessory respiratory muscles, diminished breath sounds, prolonged expiratory phase with wheezing, thoraco-abdominal

TABLE 3 Efficacy of Noninvasive Ventilation in Various Conditions

CONDITION	QUALITY OF EVIDENCE	COMMENT
AECOPD	Strong	↓ Need for intubation ↑ Survival
Acute cardiogenic pulmonary edema	Strong	↓ Need for intubation ↑ Survival
Hypoxemic respiratory in ICH with diffuse pulmonary infiltrates	Strong	↓ Need for intubation ↑ Survival
Facilitating weaning in select patients	Strong	↓ Duration of intubation Most effective in AECOPD
High risk for extubation failure	Strong	↓ Need for reintubation
Extubation failure in heterogeneous patient population	Moderate	Not effective, two RCTs
Routinely after extubation	Moderate	Not effective, single RCT
Extubation failure in AECOPD	Moderate	Single case-control study
Type I RF, diffuse infiltrates, not ICH	Moderate	↓ Need for intubation
Asthma	No RCTs	Probably effective in ↓ need for intubation
Obesity hypoventilation	No RCTs	Probably effective in ↓ need for intubation
Postoperative respiratory failure	Small RCTs	Probably effective in ↓ need for reintubation
Do not intubate patients	Observational studies	Most effective with CHF, COPD
Pulmonary fibrosis	Observational studies	Not effective

Abbreviations: AECOPD = acute exacerbation of chronic obstructive pulmonary disease; CHF = cardiogenic pulmonary edema; COPD = chronic obstructive pulmonary disease; Fio_2 = fraction of inspired oxygen; ICH = immunocompromised host; RCT = randomized, controlled trial; RF = respiratory failure.

Box 4 Screening Criteria to Assess Readiness to Undergo a Trial of Spontaneous Breathing

Required Criteria
Pao_2/Fio_2 ≥150 *or* Sao_2 ≥90% *or* Fio_2 ≤40% *and* PEEP ≤5 cm H_2O
Absence of hypotension

Additional Criteria (optional criteria)
Weaning parameters*
- Negative inspiratory force < −20 to −25 cm H_2O
- Respiratory rate (f) ≤35 breaths/min
- Spontaneous tidal volume (V_T) >5 mL/kg
- f/V_T <105 breaths/L/min
Absence of significant anemia (e.g., Hb ≥8–10 mg/dL)
Absence of fever (e.g., core temperature ≤38.5°C)
Adequate mental status: patient awake and alert or easily aroused

*Recent studies indicate that these parameters are often unnecessary in deciding whether to initiate trials of spontaneous breathing.
Abbreviations: Hb = hemoglobin; PEEP = positive end-expiratory pressure.

---

paradox (inward inspiratory abdominal motion), and Hoover's sign (inward inspiratory motion of the lower rib cage). The latter two physical signs indicate the presence of dynamic hyperinflation and diaphragmatic dysfunction. AECOPD is further characterized by hypoxemia (resulting from $\dot{V}/\dot{Q}$ mismatch) and hypercapnia. Patients with more severe underlying disease might demonstrate evidence of acute and chronic respiratory acidosis.

Etiology and Diagnosis

Approximately 50% of AECOPDs result from bacterial infection (e.g., *Pneumococcus* species, *Haemophilus influenzae*, *Moraxella catarrhalis*, and *Pseudomonas* species). The remainder result from viral infection and air pollution. In many cases a cause cannot be identified, although there is increasing appreciation that acute myocardial infarction and pulmonary embolism may be present in up to 25%. Pulmonary embolism may be suggested by a $Paco_2$ lower than baseline and the need for a higher than expected Fio_2 to maintain the Sao_2 at greater than 90%. Computed tomographic pulmonary arteriogram is recommended to make the diagnosis, because $\dot{V}/\dot{Q}$ scanning is nondiagnostic in nearly half of COPD patients, and false-positive high-probability scans occur.

Treatment

Treatment for AECOPD is based on high-quality evidence consisting of numerous randomized, controlled trials and well-performed meta-analyses. Bronchodilator therapy is essential. Nebulized combination therapy (albuterol and ipratropium [DuoNeb]) is effective, but it is not demonstrably superior to single-agent therapy delivered via a metered-dose inhaler. Theophylline should generally be avoided because toxicity outweighs benefits.

Antibiotics improve outcome, especially in the presence of fever and increased sputum purulence and volume. Older agents, such as amoxicillin and tetracycline, appear to be less effective than newer macrolides and fluoroquinolones.

Corticosteroids enhance β-agonist activity and counteract the inflammatory state seen in AECOPD. Oral prednisone at a dose of 30 to 40 mg is recommended. Intravenous therapy (methylprednisolone [SoluMedrol] 125 mg every 6 hours for 72 hours followed by oral prednisone) should be used in the critically ill patient or when response to oral therapy is suboptimal.

There is no role for mucolytic agents or chest physiotherapy.

Admission to the intensive care unit (ICU) is indicated for patients with hemodynamic instability, confusion, lethargy and coma, severe dyspnea unresponsive to emergency management, or severely abnormal gas exchange despite initial therapy (Pao_2 <40 mm Hg, $Paco_2$ >60 mm Hg, pH <7.25).

Randomized, controlled trials demonstrate that noninvasive ventilation decreases the risk for intubation and improves survival in AECOPD when there are severe dyspnea, hypoxemia, tachypnea, and significant respiratory acidosis ($Paco_2$ >45 mm Hg and pH <7.35). Patients who fail noninvasive ventilation or who are not candidates require intubation and mechanical ventilation.

A major risk is the development of dynamic hyperinflation (PEEPi), which can worsen gas exchange, predispose to barotrauma (e.g., pneumothorax), and cause hypotension. PEEPi is minimized by keeping delivered minute ventilation at 5 L/min or less; this is achieved by lowering tidal volume (e.g., 6 mL/kg ideal body weight) or respiratory rate (8–10 breaths/min), or by increasing inspiratory flow rate, allowing more time for expiration. PEEPi is suggested by an elevated plateau pressure or persistent expiratory flow at the time of the next ventilator breath. PEEPi can also increase work of breathing by increasing the patient's inspiratory effort to trigger the ventilator. When extrinsic PEEP is at or just below the PEEPi level, the patient triggers more easily and work of breathing is reduced.

The approach to weaning and extubation in AECOPD is similar to that for other conditions, although the risk of failing a spontaneous breathing trial is increased.

Acute Lung Injury and Acute Respiratory Distress Syndrome

ALI is the result of an acute process and is characterized by hypoxemia ($Pao_2/Fio_2 <300$), bilateral diffuse alveolar infiltrates, and no evidence of cardiac etiology. When the Pao_2/Fio_2 is less than 200, the patient is said to have ARDS. ALI results from pulmonary and extrapulmonary etiologies. Pulmonary causes include pneumonia, gastric aspiration, near drowning, toxic gas inhalation, and lung contusion. Extrapulmonary causes include sepsis, pancreatitis, fat embolism, drug overdose, nonthoracic trauma, and massive transfusion. Conditions that can mimic the clinical findings of ALI include CHF, diffuse alveolar hemorrhage (DAH), acute cryptogenic organizing pneumonia (COP), and acute eosinophilic pneumonia (AEP). These latter three entities can be diagnosed by bronchoscopy (DAH, AEP) or by open lung biopsy (COP), all are treated with high doses of corticosteroids. Studies indicate that corticosteroids do not improve the outcome of ALI/ARDS.

Differentiating cardiogenic pulmonary edema from ALI can be challenging, especially because these conditions can coexist. Physical findings of jugular venous distention and a positive third heart sound, abnormal electrocardiogram (ECG), elevated brain natriuretic peptide (BNP), and positive cardiac enzymes (troponin) point to a cardiac etiology. A chest radiograph showing cardiomegaly, vascular redistribution, widened vascular pedicle, perihilar alveolar infiltrates, and pleural effusions also suggests a cardiac cause. Bedside echocardiography can demonstrate reduced left ventricular function. A pulmonary artery catheter provides definitive evidence of an elevated pulmonary capillary wedge pressure and reduced cardiac output. That said, recent randomized, controlled trials demonstrate no improvement in survival with routine use of the pulmonary artery catheter in ALI.

ALI causes heterogeneous effects in the lung, resulting in poorly ventilated, atelectatic, dependent regions of lung. Traditional tidal volumes of 10 to 15 mL/kg can cause lung injury by creating significant shear stress by repeatedly opening these atelectatic areas (atelectrauma) and overdistending less affected areas (volutrauma, barotrauma). Indeed, experimental and clinical studies demonstrate that a lung-protective strategy, using a tidal volume of 6 mL/kg ideal body weight, improves survival in ALI. Using small tidal volumes often results in significant hypercapnia, which can have an independent protective effect (permissive hypercapnia). The application of PEEP recruits and opens atelectatic lung, thereby reducing harmful shear forces. The optimal level of PEEP remains uncertain: Recent multicenter studies found no difference in mortality in patients randomized to high ($\sim$14 cm H_2O) or low ($\sim$8 cm H_2O) PEEP when all patients received a tidal volume of 6 mL/kg ideal body weight.

Cardiogenic Pulmonary Edema

CHF occurs in patients with cardiomyopathy or acutely when ischemia is present. Diagnosis is suggested by jugular venous distension, a third heart sound, diffuse rales, abnormal ECG, and a chest radiograph showing cardiomegaly, diffuse alveolar infiltrates, and bilateral pleural effusion. A markedly elevated BNP or pro-BNP further suggests a cardiac etiology.

Therapy consists of oxygen, nitrates, diuretics, afterload reduction, and anti-ischemic therapy if the history or ECG is suggestive. Mechanical ventilation produces positive intrathoracic pressure, which improves cardiac function by decreasing both left ventricular preload and afterload, reversing hypoxemia, and decreasing work of breathing. In hemodynamically stable patients without active ischemia, CPAP at levels of 8 to 12 cm H_2O should be used. A meta-analysis of 15 randomized, controlled trials showed that noninvasive ventilation decreased the need for intubation and improved survival. CPAP and BiPAP appear to be equivalent, although many prefer BiPAP when hypercapnia is present.

Because cardiogenic pulmonary edema is rapidly reversible, intubated patients can often be extubated within 24 hours. That said, the transition from positive pressure ventilation to negative ventilation (e.g., T-piece or extubation) can precipitate pulmonary edema.

References

Acute Respiratory Distress Syndrome Network. Ventilation with lower tidal volumes as compared with traditional tidal volumes for acute lung injury and the acute respiratory distress syndrome. N Engl J Med 2000;342:1301–8.

Bach PB, Brown C, Gelfand SE, et al. Management of acute exacerbations of chronic obstructive pulmonary disease: A summary and appraisal of published evidence. Ann Intern Med 2001;134:600–20.

Brower RG, Lanken PN, MacIntyre N, et al. Higher versus lower positive end-expiratory pressures in patients with the acute respiratory distress syndrome. N Engl J Med 2004;51:327–36.

Ely EW, Baker AM, Dunagan DP, et al. Effect on the duration of mechanical ventilation of identifying patients capable of breathing spontaneously. N Engl J Med 1996;335:1864–9.

Epstein SK. Complications in ventilator supported patients. In: Tobin M, editor. Principles and Practice of Mechanical Ventilation. New York: McGraw Hill; 2006. p. 877–902.

Kress JP, Pohlman AS, O'Connor MF, et al. Daily interruption of sedative infusions in critically ill patients undergoing mechanical ventilation. N Engl J Med 2000;342:1471–7.

MacIntyre NR, Cook DJ, Ely Jr EW, et al. Evidence-based guidelines for weaning and discontinuing ventilatory support: A collective task force facilitated by the American College of Chest Physicians, the American Association for Respiratory Care, and the American College of Critical Care Medicine. Chest 2001;120: 375S–395S.

Majid A, Hill NS. Noninvasive ventilation for acute respiratory failure. Curr Opin Crit Care 2005;11:77–81.

Masip J, Orque M, Sanchez B, et al. Noninvasive ventilation in acute cardiogenic pulmonary edema: Systematic review and meta-analysis. JAMA 2005;294: 3124–30.

Schumaker G, Epstein SK. Management of acute respiratory failure in acute exacerbations of COPD. Resp Care 2004;49:766–82.

ASTHMA IN ADOLESCENTS AND ADULTS

Method of
Michael Schatz, MD, MS

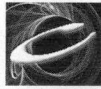

CURRENT DIAGNOSIS

- Confirm the diagnosis by demonstrating an increase in FEV_1 by 12% or more after asthma therapy.
- Assess past severity by a history of exacerbations requiring hospitalization, intubation, or oral corticosteroids.
- Identify environmental exposures, allergic sensitization, and comorbidities that may be aggravating asthma.
- Assess current *severity* in patients not taking long-term control medications and assess *control* in patients who are taking long-term control medications based on symptom frequency, nocturnal awakenings, rescue therapy use, activity limitation, spirometry, and recent exacerbation history.

Abbreviation: FEV_1 = forced expiratory volume in 1 second.

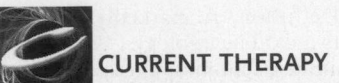

CURRENT THERAPY

- Nonpharmacologic therapy includes asthma education (especially regarding inhaler technique, self-monitoring, and self-management), reduction in environmental triggers, addressing any relevant psychosocial issues, and immunotherapy for select patients.
- Preferred step therapy for long-term asthma management is (in order): low-dose inhaled corticosteroids; medium-dose inhaled corticosteroids or low-dose inhaled corticosteroids plus long-acting β-agonists; medium-dose inhaled corticosteroids plus long-acting β-agonists; high-dose inhaled corticosteroids plus long-acting β-agonists; and oral prednisone.
- Asthma exacerbations should be treated with high-dose inhaled β-agonists and early use of systemic corticosteroids.

Asthma is an extremely common chronic medical condition that causes substantial morbidity among its sufferers. In addition to discomfort, asthma can cause sleep disruption, missed school and work, limitations of recreational activities, and acute episodes requiring emergency hospital care. Although the past 30 years have seen the introduction of increasingly effective and convenient medications, recent surveys continue to suggest that asthma remains suboptimally controlled in a substantial proportion of patients. The purpose of this article is to describe an approach to assessment and therapy that leads to optimal asthma control. It is based on the National Asthma Education and Prevention Program (NAEPP) Expert Panel Report 3: Guidelines for the Management of Asthma (http://www.nhlbi.nih.gov/guidelines/asthma/asthgdln.pdf).

Diagnosis

The first step in evaluating a patient with asthma is to confirm the diagnosis. This is particularly important in patients with atypical symptoms or a poor response to asthma therapy. Asthma is confirmed by the demonstration of reversible airways obstruction, which most commonly is an increase in forced expiratory volume in 1 second (FEV_1) by 12% or more and at least 200 cc after an inhaled bronchodilator. For some patients, 2 to 4 weeks of chronic inhaled asthma therapy or 2 weeks of oral corticosteroid therapy is necessary to demonstrate reversibility. The latter is particularly important in adults with a history of smoking in whom chronic obstructive pulmonary disease (COPD) is a diagnostic consideration. In patients with normal pulmonary function, asthma can also be confirmed by means of methacholine (Provocholine) or exercise challenge. In addition, an elevated fractional exhaled nitric oxide (FENO >25 ppb) is consistent with a diagnosis of asthma.

Particularly important masqueraders of asthma include vocal cord dysfunction, panic attacks, hyperventilation, and cough due to postnasal drip, reflux, or angiotensin-converting enzyme (ACE) inhibitor therapy. All of these can also coexist with asthma, so their presence does not exclude asthma. Even when these conditions coexist with asthma, their diagnosis and appropriate therapy usually reduce the patient's respiratory symptoms.

Assessment

Assessment of asthmatic patients involves assessment of past severity, identification of aggravating factors, and definition of current status regarding treatment and clinical severity or control.

Past Severity

Asthma can be a mild, infrequent illness or a daily severe one. Certain severity markers identify patients who are more likely to experience severe exacerbations or to have symptoms that are more difficult to control and who thus require more careful surveillance. These include histories of asthma hospitalization, especially requiring intensive care or intubation, past requirement for oral corticosteroids, and exacerbation by aspirin or other NSAIDs.

In patients with prior severe exacerbations, the rapidity of the onset of the exacerbation should be ascertained.

Aggravating Factors

Factors that appear to trigger asthma symptoms should be assessed because they may be targets for avoidance therapy. Certain aspects of the patient's environment that can contribute to asthma triggering should be specifically ascertained, including occupational exposures, age of the home, pets, carpeting, visible mold, passive smoke, and cockroach exposure. Patients with persistent asthma should have in vitro or skin tests to identify allergic sensitization to pollens, house dust mites, mold spores, animal dander, and cockroaches that can contribute to the maintenance of asthma inflammation or can trigger episodes. The presence of comorbidities that can aggravate asthma, including cigarette smoking, obesity, rhinitis, sinusitis, reflux, and COPD, should be identified and treated. Finally, psychosocial factors to assess include a history or symptoms of anxiety or depression, attitudes toward asthma and asthma therapy, adherence to therapy, and social support. These may be targets for therapy or may be necessary to understand in order to create an effective therapeutic plan and therapeutic alliance.

Current Status

Assessment of the current therapy the patient is actually taking is necessary for understanding the asthma's severity and to appropriately initiate or change therapy. It is particularly important to determine if the patient is taking long-term control medications, such as inhaled corticosteroids, long-acting β-agonists, leukotriene modifiers, theophylline, or tiotropium. If the patient is not taking controllers, severity should be assessed, as described in Table 1, based on symptom frequency, nocturnal awakenings, rescue therapy use, activity limitation, spirometry, and exacerbation history. If the patient is already taking controllers, control should be assessed (Table 2). Normal FEV_1/FVC (forced vital capacity) by age is shown in Table 3.

Long-Term Management

The goals of long-term management are to achieve and maintain well-controlled asthma. Both nonpharmacologic and pharmacologic therapy must be considered.

Nonpharmacologic Therapy

The first tenet of nonpharmacologic therapy in the long-term management of asthma is education. Patients need to understand the inflammatory pathophysiology of asthma and the relationships among airway inflammation, bronchospasm, and symptoms. Patients should be informed that the cause of asthma is unknown and there is no cure, but that triggers can be identified and asthma can be controlled. They should receive education regarding self-assessment, either based on symptoms or peak flow monitoring, and regarding the recognition of early signs of an impending exacerbation.

The next step is to discuss and agree on the goals of therapy. The NAEPP has defined the following goals:
- Prevent chronic and troublesome daytime and nighttime symptoms.
- Maintain optimal pulmonary function for that patient.
- Maintain normal activity, including work, school, leisure activity, and exercise.
- Prevent recurrent exacerbations, especially those requiring urgent medical visits.
- Provide pharmacotherapy with minimal or no adverse effects.
- Achieve patient and family satisfaction with asthma care.

The physician should let the patient know that these are the expectations of optimal management and confirm that those are the patient's goals as well.

A very important component of nonpharmacologic therapy is reduction of relevant environmental triggers. Information should be given regarding environmental control of pollen, mite, mold,

COMPONENTS OF SEVERITY	CLASSIFICATION OF SEVERITY*			
		PERSISTENT		
	INTERMITTENT	MILD	MODERATE	SEVERE
Impairment				
Symptoms	≤2 d/wk	>2 d/wk but not daily	Daily	Throughout the d
Nighttime awakenings	≤2 ×/mo	3–4 ×/mo	>1 ×/wk but not nightly	Often 7 ×/wk
Short-acting β₂-agonist use for symptom control (not prevention of EIB)	≤2 d/wk	>2 d/wk but not daily, and not more than 1 time on any d	Daily	Several times per d
Interference with normal activity	None	Minor limitation	Some limitation	Extremely limited
Lung function†	Normal FEV₁ between exacerbations FEV₁ >80% predicted FEV₁/FVC normal	FEV₁ >80% predicted FEV₁/FVC normal	FEV₁ >60% but <80% predicted FEV₁/FVC reduced 5%	FEV₁ <60% predicted FEV₁/FVC reduced >5%
Risk				
Exacerbations requiring oral systemic corticosteroids	0–1/y‡	≥2/y‡		

Consider severity and interval since last exacerbation. Frequency and severity may fluctuate over time for patients in any severity category. Relative annual risk of exacerbation may be related to FEV₁.

Recommended Steps for Initiating Treatment§

Initiation	Step 1	Step 2	Step 3¶	Step 4 or 5¶
Follow-up	In 2–6 wk, evaluate level of asthma control and adjust therapy accordingly.			

Abbreviations: EIB = exercise-induced bronchospasm; FEV₁ = forced expiratory volume in one second; FVC = forced vital capacity; ICU = intensive care unit.
Data from the National Asthma Education and Prevention Program (NAEPP) Expert Panel Report 3: Guidelines for the Management of Asthma.
*Level of severity is determined by assessment of both impairment and risk. Assess impairment domain by patient's/caregiver's recall of previous 2–4 weeks and spirometry. Assign severity to the most severe category in which any feature occurs.
†See Table 3 for normal FEV₁/FVC.
‡At present, there are inadequate data to correlate frequencies of exacerbations with different levels of asthma severity. In general, more frequent and intense exacerbations (e.g., requiring urgent, unscheduled care, hospitalization, or ICU admission) indicate greater underlying disease severity. For treatment purposes, patients who had ≥2 exacerbations requiring oral systemic corticosteroids in the past year may be considered the same as patients who have persistent asthma, even in the absence of impairment levels consistent with persistent asthma.
§See Table 6 for treatment steps. The stepwise approach is meant to assist, not replace, the clinical decision making required to meet individual patient needs.
¶And consider short course of oral systemic corticosteroids.

animal dander, and cockroach antigens (Box 1) that appear to be relevant based on the history and results of skin or in vitro specific IgE tests. Inhalant allergen immunotherapy should be considered for patients who have persistent asthma when there is clear evidence of a relationship between symptoms and exposure to an allergen to which the patient is sensitive.

Finally, psychosocial issues should be considered and addressed. For many patients, the education and therapeutic alliance described earlier adequately addresses psychosocial concerns. For other patients, poor past adherence requires identifying the barriers to adherence and finding solutions together. Resources for patients with poor social support should be identified. Clinically significant anxiety or depression that can make asthma harder to control should be treated.

Pharmacologic Step Therapy

The main principle of asthma pharmacologic step therapy is to add therapy in steps until control is achieved (step up) and decrease therapy in reverse steps (step down) to established the lowest effective dose necessary to maintain control.

There are two types of asthma medications: quick-relief medications (Table 4) and long-term control medications (Table 5). Systemic corticosteroids can be used either short-term to treat an exacerbation (see Table 4) or as long-term maintenance therapy for patients with severe disease (see Table 5). The generally recommended steps of pharmacologic therapy are shown in Table 6. Definitions of low, medium, and high dose inhaled

corticosteroids for each of the available preparations are given in Table 7. At each therapeutic step level, the NAEPP Expert Panel has indicated preferred medications, which generally identify medications with the best balance of efficacy and safety in clinical trials for patients at that level of severity. However, these recommendations are based on population data and must be tailored to individual patient needs, circumstances, and responsiveness to therapy.

All patients with asthma should have an action plan that describes their pharmacologic self-management. Aspects of pharmacologic self-management include the maintenance medication schedule, rescue therapy doses for increased symptoms, when and how to increase controller medication therapy, when and how to use prednisone, how to recognize a severe exacerbation, and when and how to seek urgent or emergency care. Controller medications should be increased with an upper respiratory infection or with symptoms requiring more than two doses of rescue therapy in 12 hours. Although doubling the dose of inhaled corticosteroids does not appear to generally be sufficient to provide clinical benefit under these circumstances, greater increases may be effective (e.g., three- or fourfold increases). The increased dose of controller medications should be maintained at least until increased symptoms resolve. Prednisone is usually needed for patients with incomplete or temporary responses to adequate doses of β-agonists (4 puffs with a spacer, waiting at least 1 minute between puffs), substantial interference with sleep every night, requirement for 12 or more puffs of β-agonist in a 24-hour period,

| TABLE 2 | Assessing Asthma Control and Adjusting Therapy in Patients 12 Years and Older |

COMPONENTS OF CONTROL	CLASSIFICATION OF CONTROL*		
	WELL CONTROLLED	NOT WELL CONTROLLED	VERY POORLY CONTROLLED
Impairment			
Symptoms	≤2 d/wk	>2 d/wk	Throughout the d
Nighttime awakenings	≤2 ×/mo	1–3 ×/wk	≥4 ×/wk
Short-acting β₂-agonist use for symptom control (not prevention of EIB)	≤2 d/wk	>2 d/wk	Several times per d
Interference with normal activity	None	Some limitation	Extremely limited
FEV₁ or peak flow	>80% predicted or personal best	60%–80% predicted or personal best	<60% predicted or personal best
Validated Questionnaires†			
ACQ	≤0.75‡	≥1.5	N/A
ACT	≥20	16–19	≤15
ATAQ	0	1–2	3–4
Risk			
Exacerbations requiring oral systemic corticosteroids	0–1/y	≥2/y§ ⟶	
Progressive loss of lung function	Evaluation requires long-term follow-up care.		
Treatment-related adverse effects	Medication side effects can vary in intensity from none to very troublesome and worrisome. The level of intensity does not correlate to specific levels of control, but it should be considered in the overall assessment of risk.		
Recommended action for treatment‖	Maintain current step Regular follow-up at every 1–6 mo to maintain control Consider step down if well controlled for ≥3 mo	Step up 1 step and reevaluate in 2–6 wk For side effects, consider alternative treatment options	Consider short course of systemic oral corticosteroids Step up 1–2 steps and reevaluate in 2 wk For side effects, consider alternative treatment options

FEV_1 or peak flow uses subscript.

Abbreviations: ACQ = Asthma Control Questionnaire; ACT = Asthma Control Test; ATAQ = Asthma Therapy Assessment Questionnaire; EIB = exercise-induced bronchospasm; FEV_1 = forced expiratory volume in one second; N/A = not applicable.
Data from the National Asthma Education and Prevention Program (NAEPP) Expert Panel Report 3: Guidelines for the Management of Asthma.
*The level of control is based on the most severe impairment or risk category. Assess impairment domain by patient's recall of previous 2–4 weeks and by spirometry or peak flow measures. Symptom assessment for longer periods should reflect a global assessment, such as inquiring whether the patient's asthma is better or worse since the last visit.
†Validated questionnaires for the impairment domain (the questionnaires do not assess the risk domain). Minimal important difference. 0.5 for the ACQ, 1.0 for the ATAQ and 3.0 for the ACT.
‡ACQ values of 0.76–1.4 are indeterminate regarding well-controlled asthma.
§At present, there are inadequate data to correlate frequencies of exacerbations with different levels of asthma control. In general, more frequent and intense exacerbations (e.g., requiring urgent, unscheduled care, hospitalization, or ICU admission) indicate poorer disease control. For treatment purposes, patients who had ≥2 exacerbations requiring oral systemic corticosteroids in the past year may be considered the same as patients who have not-well-controlled asthma, even in the absence of impairment levels consistent with not-well-controlled asthma.
‖See Table 6 for treatment steps. The stepwise approach is meant to assist, not replace, the clinical decision making required to meet individual patient needs. Before a step up in therapy, review adherence, inhaler technique, environmental control, and comorbid conditions. If an alternative treatment option was used in a step, discontinue it and use the preferred treatment for that step.

| TABLE 3 | Normal FEV₁/FVC by Age |

AGE RANGE (y)	NORMAL FEV₁/FVC (%)
8–19	85
20–39	80
40–59	75
60–80	70

Abbreviations: FEV_1 = forced expiratory volume in one second; FVC = forced vital capacity.
Data from the National Asthma Education and Prevention Program (NAEPP) Expert Panel Report 3: Guidelines for the Management of Asthma.

or a peak flow less than 60% predicted. Home treatment of exacerbations is further discussed later.

For patients not on long-term control medications, assess severity and select the level of treatment that corresponds to the patient's level of severity (see Table 1). Persistent asthma is most effectively controlled with daily long-term control medications, specifically anti-inflammatory therapy. For patients receiving long-term control medications, identify their current step of therapy, based on what they are actually taking (see Table 6), and their level of control (see Table 2). In general, step up one step for patients whose asthma is not well controlled. For patients with very poorly controlled asthma, consider increasing by two steps, a course of oral corticosteroids, or both. Before increasing pharmacologic therapy, consider adverse environmental exposures, poor adherence, or comorbidities as targets for intervention. For patients with troublesome or debilitating side effects from asthma therapy, explore a change in therapy.

Follow-up

Patients whose asthma is not controlled should be seen every 2 to 6 weeks (depending on their initial level of severity or control) until control is achieved. Once control is achieved, follow-up contact at 1- to 6-month intervals is recommended. These checkups should

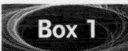

Allergens
Reduce or eliminate exposure to the allergen(s) the patient is sensitive to:

Animal Dander
- Remove animal from house or, at a minimum, keep animal out of the patient's bedroom and keep the bedroom door closed.

Dust Mites
- Recommended
  - Encase mattress in a special dust-proof cover
  - Encase pillow in a special dust-proof cover or wash it weekly in hot water.
  - Wash sheets and blankets on the patient's bed in hot water weekly. Water must be hotter than 130°F to kill the mites. Cooler water used with detergent and bleach can also be effective.
- Desirable
  - Reduce indoor humidity to 60% or less.
  - Remove carpets from the bedroom.
  - Avoid sleeping or lying on cloth-covered cushions or furniture.
  - Remove carpets that are laid on concrete.

Cockroaches
- Keep all food out of the bedroom.
- Keep food and garbage in closed containers.
- Use poison baits, powders, gels or paste (e.g., boric acid). Traps can also be used.
- If a spray is used to kill cockroaches, stay out of the room until the odor goes away.

Pollens (from Trees, Grass, or Weeds) and Outdoor Molds
- Try to keep windows closed
- If possible, stay indoors, with windows closed, during periods of peak pollen exposure, which are usually during the midday and afternoon.

Indoor Mold
- Fix all leaks and eliminate water sources associated with mold growth.
- Clean moldy surfaces.
- Dehumidify basements if possible.

Tobacco smoke
- Advise patients and others in the home who smoke to stop smoking or to smoke outside the home
- Discuss ways to reduce exposure to other sources of tobacco smoke, such as from daycare providers and the workplace.

Indoor and Outdoor Pollutants and Irritants
- If possible, do not use a wood-burning stove, kerosene heater, fireplace, unvented gas stove, or heater
- Try to stay away from strong odors and sprays, such as perfume, talcum powder, hair spray, paints, new carpet, or particle board.

Data from the National Asthma Education and Prevention Program (NAEPP) Expert Panel Report 3: Guidelines for the Management of Asthma.

---

ensure continued control, identify other changes in the patient's status, and update the patient's action plan.

When well-controlled asthma has been maintained for at least 3 months, a step down in therapy can be considered to determine the minimum amount of medication required to maintain control or reduce the risk of side effects. Reduction in therapy should be gradual because asthma can deteriorate at a highly variable rate

---

and intensity. Doses of inhaled corticosteroids may be reduced about 25% to 50% every 3 months to the lowest dose possible to maintain control. Most patients with persistent asthma relapse if inhaled corticosteroids are totally discontinued.

Patients should be encouraged to contact their asthma physician for signs of loss of asthma control, such as nocturnal symptoms, increasing β-agonist use, or activity limitation. The Expert Panel recommends consultation with an asthma specialist if the patient has difficulties achieving or maintaining control of asthma, immunotherapy or omalizumab (Xolair) is being considered, the patient requires step 4 care or higher, or the patient has had an exacerbation requiring hospitalization.

Treatment of Exacerbations
Asthma exacerbations are acute or subacute episodes of progressively worsening shortness of breath, cough, wheezing, or chest tightness associated with decreases in expiratory airflow.

Home Management
Patients' action plans should direct their home therapy of asthma exacerbations according to the following recommendations.

Initial therapy should be with inhaled short-acting β-agonists (2–6 puffs by metered-dose inhaler [MDI] or nebulizer). This may be repeated in 20 minutes. With a good response (minimal or no symptoms and peak expiratory flow (PEF) ≥80% predicted or personal best), the patient may continue β-agonists every 3 to 4 hours for 24 to 48 hours. If repeated β-agonists are needed, a short course of oral corticosteroids should be considered.

With an incomplete response to initial therapy (persistent wheezing and dyspnea and PEF 50% to 79% predicted or personal best), oral corticosteroids should be added, β-agonists should be repeated, and the clinician should be contacted that day.

With a poor response (marked wheezing and dyspnea at rest, PEF <50% predicted or personal best), oral corticosteroids should be added, the β-agonist should be repeated immediately, and the patient should call the clinician and usually proceed to the emergency department. For signs of severe distress (e.g., difficulty talking in full sentences, diaphoresis, drowsiness, confusion, or cyanosis), 911 should be called. Patients with histories of rapid-onset severe exacerbations should have self-injectable epinephrine (EpiPen)[1] at home to use at the onset of increased symptoms.

Emergency Department and Hospital Management
Assessment should rapidly determine the severity of the exacerbation based on intensity of symptoms, signs (heart rate, respiratory rate, use of accessory muscles, chest auscultation), peak flow (unless the patient is too dyspneic to perform), and pulse oximetry. Treatment should begin immediately following recognition of an exacerbation severe enough to cause dyspnea at rest, peak flow less than 70% predicted or personal best, or pulse oximetry oxygen saturation less than 95%. While treatment is being given, a brief, focused history and physical examination pertinent to the exacerbation can be obtained.

In patients with mild to moderate exacerbations (PEF >40% predicted), initial therapy is oxygen to achieve oxygen saturation greater than 90% and inhaled short-acting β-agonist by nebulizer or MDI (4–8 puffs) with holding chamber, which may be repeated up to three times in the first hour. Oral corticosteroids (prednisone 40–80 mg) are recommended if there is no immediate response to therapy or if the patient had been recently treated with oral corticosteroids.

In patients with severe exacerbations (PEF <40% predicted), initial therapy is oxygen as above, inhaled high-dose short-acting β-agonist (e.g., albuterol 5 mg) and ipratropium (0.5 mg) by nebulizer, and oral or intravenous corticosteroids (prednisone or methylprednisolone 80 mg). The albuterol may be repeated every 20 minutes or used continuously for 1 hour.

---

[1]Not FDA approved for this indication.

MEDICATION	DOSAGE FORM	ADULT DOSE	COMMENTS
Inhaled Short-Acting β₂-Agonists (SABA)			
Metered-Dose Inhaler			*Applies to all three SABAS*
Albuterol HFA (Proventil, Ventolin)	90 µg/puff, 200 puffs/canister	2 puffs 5 min before exercise	An increasing use or lack of expected effect indicates diminished control of asthma.
Pirbuterol CFC (Maxair) Levalbuterol HFA (Xopenox)	200 µg/puff, 400 puffs/canister 45 µg/puff, 200 puffs/canister	*or* 2 puffs q4–6h prn	Not recommended for long-term daily treatment. Regular use exceeding 2 d/wk for symptom control (not prevention of EIB) indicates the need for additional long-term control therapy. Differences in potencies exist, but all products are essentially comparable on a per-puff basis. May double usual dose for mild exacerbations. For levalbuterol, should prime the inhaler by releasing 4 actuations prior to use. For HFA, periodically clean HFA activator, as drug may block/plug orifice. Nonselective agents (epinephrine [Primatene Mist], isoproterenol [Isopro Aerometer], metaproterenol [Alupent]) are not recommended due to their potential for excessive cardiac stimulation, especially in high doses.
Nebulizer Solutions			
Albuterol (Accuneb, Proventil)	0.63 mg/3 mL 1.25 mg/3 mL 2.5 mg/3 mL 5 mg/mL (0.5%)	1.25–5 mg in 3 mL saline q4–8h prn	May mix with budesonide (Pulmicort) inhalant suspension, cromolyn (Intal) or ipratropium (Atrovent) nebulizer solutions. May double the dose for severe exacerbation.
Levalbuterol (R-albuterol) (Xopenex)	0.31 mg/3 mL 0.63 mg/3 mL 1.25 mg/0.5 mL 1.25 mg/3 mL	0.63 mg–1.25 mg q8h prn	Compatible with budesonide (Pulmicort) inhalant suspension. The product is a sterile-filled, preservative-free, unit-dose vial.
Anticholinergics			
Metered-Dose Inhalers			
Ipratropium HFA (Atrovent)	17 µg/puff, 200 puffs/canister	2–3 puffs q6h	Multiple doses in the emergency department (not hospital) setting provide additive benefit to short-acting beta agonists. Treatment of choice for bronchospasm due to β-blocker. Does not block EIB. Reverses only cholinergically mediated bronchospasm; does not modify reaction to antigen. May be alternative for patients who do not tolerate short-acting beta-agonist. Evidence is lacking for ipratropium producing added benefit to β₂ agonists in long-term control asthma therapy.
Ipratropium with albuterol (Combivent)[1]	18 µg/puff of ipratropium bromide and 90 µg/puff of albuterol, 200 puffs/canister	2–3 puffs q6h	
Nebulizer Solutions			
Ipratropium bromide	0.2 mg/mL (0.2%)	0.5 mg q6h	
Ipratropium bromide with albuterol (DuoNeb)[1]	0.5 mg/3 mL ipratropium bromide and 2.5 mg/3 mL albuterol	3 mL q4–6h	Contains EDTA to prevent discoloration of the solution. This additive does not induce bronchospasm.
Systemic Corticosteroids			
Methylprednisolone (Medrol) Prednisolone (Delta-Cortef, Prelone) Prednisone (Deltasone, Orasone)	2, 4, 6, 8, 16, 32 mg tab 5 mg tabs; 5 mg/5 mL, 15 mg/5 mL 1, 2.5, 5, 10, 20, 50 mg tabs; 5 mg/mL, 5 mg/5 mL	Short course (burst): 40–60 mg/d as single or 2 divided doses for 3–10 d	Short courses (bursts) are effective for establishing control when initiating therapy or during a period of gradual deterioration. Action may be begin within an hour. The burst should be continued until symptoms resolve. This usually requires 3–10 d but can require longer. There is no evidence that tapering the dose following improvement prevents relapse in asthma exacerbations.
Repository Injection			
Methylprednisolone acetate (Depo-Medrol)	40 mg/mL 80 mg/mL	240 mg[3,*] IM once	May be used in place of a short burst of oral steroids in patients who are vomiting or if adherence is a problem.

Abbreviations: CFC = chlorofluorocarbon; EDTA = edetic acid; EIB = exercise-induced bronchospasm; HFA = hydrofluoroalkane; PEF = peak expiratory flow; tab = tablet.
Data from the National Asthma Education and Prevention Program (NAEPP) Expert Panel Report 3: Guidelines for the Management of Asthma.
[1]Not FDA approved for this indication.
[3]Exceeds dosage recommended by the manufacturer.
*80–120 mg per package insert.

TABLE 5 Usual Dosages for Long-Term Control Medications for Patients 12 Years and Older

MEDICATION	DOSAGE FORM*	ADULT DOSE	COMMENTS
Systemic Corticosteroids			
Methylprednisolone (Medrol)	2, 4, 8, 16, 32 mg tab	7.5–60 mg qd in a single dose in AM or qod as needed for control	For long-term treatment of severe persistent asthma, administer single dose in AM either daily or on alternate days (alternate-day therapy may produce less adrenal suppression).
Prednisolone (Delta-Cortef, Prelone)	5 mg tab 5 mg/5 mL, 15 mg/5 mL	Short-course (burst) to achieve control, 40–60 mg/d as single or 2 divided doses for 3–10 d	Short courses (bursts) are effective for establishing control when initiating therapy or during a period of gradual deterioration. There is no evidence that tapering the dose following improvement in symptom control and pulmonary function prevents relapse.
Prednisone (Deltasone, Orasone)	1, 2.5, 5, 10, 20, 50 mg tab 5 mg/mL, 5 mg/5 mL		
Inhaled Long-Acting β₂-Agonists			Should not be used for relief of acute symptoms or exacerbations. Use only with ICS.
Salmeterol (Serevent)	DPI 50 µg/blister	1 blister q12h	Decreased duration of protection against EIB may occur with regular use.
Formoterol (Foradil)	DPI 12 µg/single-use capsule	1 cap q12h	Each cap is for single use only; additional doses should not be administered for at least 12 h. Caps should be used only with the Aerolizor inhaler and should not be taken orally.
Inhaled Combined Medications			
Fluticasone and salmeterol (Advair)	DPI 100 µg/50 µg, 250 µg/50 µg, or 500 µg/50 µg	1 inhalation bid†	100/50 DPI or 45/21 HFA for patients not controlled on low-to-medium dose ICS.
	HFA 45 µg/21 µg 115 µg/21 µg 230 µg/21 µg	2 puffs bid†	250/50 DPI or 115/21 HFA for patients not controlled on medium-to-high dose ICS.
Budesonide and formoterol (Symbicort)	HFA MDI 80 µg/4.5 µg 160 µg/4.5 µg	2 inhalations bid†	80/4.5 for patients not controlled on low-to-medium dose ICS. 160/4.5 for patients not controlled on medium-to-high dose ICS.
Mometazone and formoterol (Dulera)	100 µg/5 µg 200 µg/5 µg	2 inhalations bid†	100/5 for patients not controlled on low-to-medium dose ICS 200/5 for patients not controlled on medium-to-high dose ICS
Inhaled Long-acting Anticholinergic			
Tiotripium	18 mg capsule	Inhale contents of 1 cap qd	Not FDA approved for this indication. May be as effective as LABA as add-on therapy to ICS.
Leukotriene Modifiers			
Leukotriene Receptor Antagonists			
Montelukast (Singulair)	4 mg or 5 mg chewable tab 10 mg tab	10 mg qhs	Montelukast exhibits a flat dose-response curve. Doses >10 mg do not produce a greater response in adults.
Zafirlukast (Accolate)	10 or 20 mg tab	40 mg/d (20 mg tab bid)	For zafirlukast: Administration with meals decreases bioavailability; take at least 1 h before or 2 h after meals. Zafirlukast is a microsomal p450 enzyme inhibitor that can inhibit the metabolism of warfarin. Doses of this drug should be monitored accordingly. Monitor for signs and symptoms of hepatic dysfunction.
5-Lipoxygenase Inhibitor			
Zileuton (Zyflo)	600 mg tab	2400 mg daily (600 mg qid)	Monitor hepatic enzymes (ALT). Zileuton is a microsomal p450 enzyme inhibitor that can inhibit the metabolism of warfarin and theophylline. Doses of these drugs should be monitored accordingly.

Continued

TABLE 5 Usual Dosages for Long-Term Control Medications for Patients 12 Years and Older—cont'd

MEDICATION	DOSAGE FORM	ADULT DOSE	COMMENTS
Methylxanthines			
Theophylline (Slophyllin, Theobid, TheoDur)	Liquids, sustained-release tab, cap	Starting dose 10 mg/kg/d up to 300 mg max Usual max 800 mg/d	Adjust dosage to achieve serum concentration of 5–15 µg/mL at steady-state ($\geq$48 h on same dosage). Due to wide interpatient variability in theophylline metabolic clearance, routine serum theophylline level monitoring is essential. Patient should be told to discontinue if they experience symptoms of toxicity. Various factors (diet, food, febrile illness, age, smoking, and other medications) can affect serum concentration.
Immunomodulators			
Omalizumab (Anti-IgE)	Subcutaneous (SQ) injection 150 mg/ 1.2 mL following reconstitution with 1.4 mL sterile water for injection	150–375 mg SQ every 2–4 wk, depending on body weight and pretreatment serum IgE level	Do not administer more than 150 mg per injection site. Monitor patient following injections; be prepared and equipped to indentify and treat anaphylaxis that may occur. Whether patients will develop significant antibody titers to the drug with long-term administration is unknown.

Abbreviations: ALT = alanine aminotransferase; amp = ampule; cap = capsule; DPI = dry powder inhaler; EIB = exercise-induced bronchospasm; HFA = hydrofluoroalkane; ICS = inhaled corticosteroid; LABA = long-acting β_2-agonist; max = maximum; MDI = metered-dose inhaler; SABA = short-acting β_2-agonist; tab = tablet.
Data from the National Asthma Education and Prevention Program (NAEPP) Expert Panel Report 3: Guidelines for the Management of Asthma.
*See Table 7 for estimated comparative daily dosages for inhaled corticosteroids.
†Dose depends on level of severity or control.

TABLE 6 Stepwise Approach for Managing Asthma in Patients 12 Years and Older*

STEP	PREFERRED THERAPY	ALTERNATIVE THERAPY
1	Short-acting β-agonist prn	—
2	Low-dose ICS	LTRA, theophylline
3	Low-dose ICS *plus* LABA *or* Medium-dose ICS	Low-dose ICS *plus* LTRA *or* theophylline *or* zileuton (Zyflo) *or* tiotropium (Spiriva)[1]
4	Medium-dose ICS *plus* LABA	Medium-dose ICS *plus* LTRA *or* theophylline *or* zileuton (Zyflo) *or* tiotropium (Spiriva)[1]
5	High-dose ICS *plus* LABA Consider omalizumab (Xolair) for patients who have allergies	—
6	High-dose ICS *plus* LABA *plus* oral corticosteroid† Consider omalizumab for patients who have allergies	—

Abbreviations: ICS = inhaled corticosteroid; LABA = long-acting β agonist; LTRA = leukotriene receptor antagonist.
Data updated from the National Asthma Education and Prevention Program (NAEPP) Expert Panel Report 3: Guidelines for the Management of Asthma.
[1]Not FDA approved for this indication.
*The stepwise approach is meant to assist, not replace, the clinical decision making required to meet individual patient needs.
†In step 6, before oral corticosteroids are introduced, a trial of high-dose ICS + LABA + either LTRA, theophylline, zileuton, or tiotropium may be considered, although this approach has not been studied in clinical trials.

TABLE 7 Estimated Comparative Daily Dosages for Inhaled Corticosteroids for Patients 12 Years and Older

DRUG	DOSAGE FORM	DAILY DOSE		
		LOW (µg)	MEDIUM (µg)	HIGH (µg)
Beclomethasone HFA (QVAR)	40 or 80 µg/puff	80–240	>240–480	>480
Budesonide DPI (Pulmicort)	90 or 180 µg/inhalation	180–540	>540–1080	>1080
Ciclesonide (Alvesco)	80 or 160 µg/actuation	160–320	>320–640	>640
Flunisolide HFA (AeroSpan)	80 µg/puff	320	>320–640	>640
Fluticasone-HFA (Flovent HFA) (Flovent Diskus)	MDI: 44, 110, 220 µg/puff DPI: 50, 100, 250 µg/inhalation	88–264 100–300	>264–440 >300–500	>440 >500
Mometasone DPI (Asmanex)	110 or 220 mcg/actuation	110–220	>220–440	>440

Abbreviations: DPI = dry powder inhaler; HFA = hydrofluoroalkane; MDI = metered-dose inhaler.
Data from the National Asthma Education and Prevention Program (NAEPP) Expert Panel Report 3: Guidelines for the Management of Asthma and *Ann Pharm* 2009;43:519.

Repeated assessments of symptoms, signs, PEF, and oxygen saturation determine the responsiveness of the exacerbation to therapy. Such assessments should be made in patients presenting with severe exacerbations after the initial bronchodilator treatment and in all patients after three doses of bronchodilator therapy (60–90 min after initial treatment). In patients who are improving, short-acting β-agonists may be repeated every hour until a good response is achieved (no distress, PEF >70%). When this response is sustained at least 60 minutes after the last treatment, the patient may usually be discharged on a course of oral corticosteroids (generally prednisone 40–60 mg for 5–10 days), initiation or continuation of medium-dose inhaled corticosteroids, and arrangement for outpatient follow-up.

In patients who are not improving with the above therapy, adjunctive therapy, such as with intravenous magnesium sulfate[1] (2 g) or heliox, may be considered. Intubation and mechanical ventilation may be required for patients with respiratory failure in spite of treatment.

Summary

Asthma is a very common problem with the potential to cause substantial interference with quality of life. Although there is no cure for asthma, asthma can be well controlled in the majority of patients with proper management and an effective patient-physician relationship. I hope that the method described herein for assessing and managing asthma will help physicians help their patients to achieve well-controlled asthma.

---

[1]Not FDA approved for this indication.

ATELECTASIS

Method of
Alykhan S. Nagji, MD; Joshua S. Jolissaint, BA; and Christine L. Lau, MD

CURRENT DIAGNOSIS

- Hypoxia
- Tachypnea
- Diminished breath sounds
- Wheezing
- Radiologic signs of atelectasis

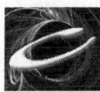

CURRENT THERAPY

- Chest percussion or vibration
- Nasotracheal or bronchoscopic suctioning
- Incentive spirometry
- Positive-pressure ventilation
- Ambulation
- Postoperative pain control

Atelectasis refers to the collapse of alveoli that affects segmental or lobar regions of the lung or the entire lung and results in hypoventilation. However, recent studies have suggested that the alveoli are not collapsed but are filled with fluid and foam. These hypotheses are not mutually exclusive; collapsed alveoli and fluid- and foam-filled alveoli may be present concurrently in an atelectatic lung. Although atelectasis is considered a benign condition, early treatment, reversal, and prevention are essential to an overall improved outcome.

Etiology

Compression Atelectasis
Compression atelectasis occurs when the transmural pressure distending the alveolus is reduced to a level that allows the alveolus to collapse. To best illustrate this mechanism, consider the patient who has undergone induction of anesthesia. The diaphragm is relaxed and is displaced cephalad. In the supine position, the pleural pressures increase to the greatest extent in the dependent lung regions and can compress the adjacent lung tissue.

Surfactant Impairment
Surfactant serves to reduce the alveolar surface tension, thereby stabilizing the alveoli and preventing collapse. Reduction in surfactant occurs with certain types of anesthesia. Studies have shown that hyperinflation by means of increased tidal volume, sequential air inflations to the total lung capacity, or even a single cycle of increased tidal volume can increase the release of surfactant, aiding in recruitment and stabilization of alveoli.

Gas Resorption
One mechanism by which gas resorption results in atelectasis involves the patent airway. In regions of the lung with increased ventilation compared to perfusion, which produces a ventilation/perfusion ($\dot{V}/\dot{Q}$) mismatch, there is low alveolar oxygen tension. Increasing the fraction of inspired oxygen (FIO_2) initiates a cascade of events that increases alveolar oxygen tension (PAO_2) and decreases alveolar nitrogen tension (PAN_2), which results in loss of alveolar volume secondary to increased absorption of oxygen.

Another mechanism by which gas resorption leads to atelectasis occurs after complete airway occlusion. In such cases, gas is trapped distal to the obstruction. Gas uptake by the proximal blood flow continues without additional gas inflow. This causes the alveoli to collapse.

Pathophysiology
The trapping of air and hyperinflation of the alveoli are produced from the aforementioned mechanisms. The gases that are trapped are absorbed by the blood perfusing through that region of the lung, which eventually causes collapse of the alveoli. The atelectasis produces alveolar hypoxia and pulmonary vasoconstriction to prevent $\dot{V}/\dot{Q}$ mismatching and to minimize arterial hypoxia. This vascular response is effective only if a large part of the lung is not collapsed; otherwise, intrapulmonary shunting occurs.

Clinical Presentation
The signs and symptoms of atelectasis are often nonspecific. The natural course of atelectasis may lead to fever, cough, tachypnea, wheezing, rhonchi, and chest pain. On physical examination, atelectasis may manifest as an area of localized reduced breath sounds with constant wheeze or reduced chest wall expansion or both.

Diagnosis
Chest radiographs aid in the diagnosis of atelectasis. They provide both direct and indirect signs that may indicate an atelectatic etiology for the patient's symptoms.
Direct signs include:
- Displaced pulmonary vessels
- Air bronchograms
- Displacement of intralobar fissures (most reliable sign)
Indirect signs include:
- Pulmonary opacification
- Diaphragmatic elevation
- Hyperexpansion of unaffected lung
- Tracheal, heart, and mediastinal shift toward atelectatic side
- Shift of the hilum toward the collapsed lobe
- Segmental ipsilateral rib approximation

Treatment

Treatment of atelectasis is geared toward the underlying cause. It is important to recognize respiratory distress and to intubate the patient if appropriate.

If the etiology is that of an obstructive atelectasis, chest percussion or vibration and nasotracheal or bronchoscopic suctioning may help in the clearing of secretions. With regard to lung re-expansion, incentive spirometry, continuous or intermittent positive-pressure ventilation, and early ambulation may be used.

Those patients who have a nonobstructive atelectasis caused by a pneumothorax or pleural effusion benefit from tube thoracostomy or thoracentesis. Additionally, appropriate pain management in the postoperative setting allows for proper ventilation.

References

Duggan M, Kavanagh BP. Pulmonary atelectasis: A pathogenic perioperative entity. Anesthesiology 2005;102:838–54.

Duggan M, Kavanagh BP. Atelectasis in the perioperative patient. Curr Opin Anaesthesiol 2007;20:37–42.

Hubmayr RD. Perspective on lung injury and recruitment: A skeptical look at the opening and collapse story. Am J Respir Crit Care Med 2002;165:1647–53.

Peroni DG, Boner AL. Atelectasis: Mechanisms, diagnosis and management. Paediatr Respir Rev 2000;1:274–8.

Wagner PD, Laravuso RB, Uhl RR, West JB. Continuous distributions of ventilation-perfusion ratios in normal subjects breathing air and 100 per cent O_2. J Clin Invest 1974;54:54–68.

BACTERIAL PNEUMONIA

Method of
Edward Septimus, MD

Pneumonia occurs in about 3 to 4 million patients per year in the United States, with approximately 1 million patients requiring hospitalization. The symptoms of pneumonia include cough, shortness of breath, sputum production, and chest pain. Physical examination includes fever in most, with crackles and bronchial breath sounds on auscultation in about 80% of cases. Pneumonia is classified by where it was acquired: community-acquired pneumonia (CAP) and health care–acquired pneumonia (HAP, sometimes called *hospital-acquired pneumonia*). This chapter focuses on adult patients with CAP or HAP.

Community-Acquired Pneumonia

CAP remains a leading cause of death in the United States. One study estimated that more than 900,000 cases of CAP occur in persons older than 65 years each year. The emergence of drug-resistant *Streptococcus pneumoniae* (DRSP) and less common pathogens including methicillin-resistant *Staphylococcus aureus* (MRSA) is well documented. Pneumonia in long-term care institutions usually resembles HAP and is discussed later.

Diagnostic Testing

Symptoms plus an infiltrate by chest radiograph or other imaging studies are required for the diagnosis. Clinical features and physical findings may be absent in the elderly. All patients should be screened by pulse oximetry. Arterial blood gases should be reserved for patients with suspected CO_2 retention. Routine diagnostic studies to determine the etiology for outpatients with CAP are optional. For patients requiring admission, diagnostic studies to determine the etiology of CAP should be attempted. Increased mortality is more common with inappropriate initial empiric therapy. De-escalation of antimicrobial therapy based on pathogen-specific treatment has been shown to decrease adverse drug effects including C. diff and selection of antimicrobial resistance.

Blood cultures and sputum for Gram stain and culture (in patients with a productive cough) should be obtained in most patients who are admitted to the hospital. Pretreatment blood cultures have a 5% to 14% yield in patients hospitalized with CAP. The most common positive blood culture to be considered a pathogen is *S. pneumoniae*. In some series, false-positive blood cultures (contaminants) exceed positive blood culture with true pathogens.

Box 1   Criteria for Severe Community-Acquired Pneumonia

Minor Criteria
Confusion or disorientation
Hypotension requiring fluid resuscitation
Hypothermia ($<36°C$)
Leukopenia (WBC <4000 cell/mm^3)
Multilobar infiltrates
Pao$_2$/Fio$_2$ ≤250
Respiratory rate ≥30
Thrombocytopenia (platelet count $<100,000$ cells/mm^3)
Uremia (BUN ≥20 mg/dL)

Major Criteria
Invasive mechanical ventilation
Septic shock requiring vasopressors

Abbreviations: BUN = blood urea nitrogen; Fio$_2$ = fraction of inspired oxygen; Pao$_2$ = partial pressure of arterial oxygen; WBC = white blood cell count.
Adapted from Mandell LA, Wunderink RG, Anzueto A, et al: Infectious Diseases Society of America/American Thoracic Society Consensus Guidelines on the Management of Community-Acquired Pneumonia in Adults. Clin Infect Dis 2007;44: S27–S72.

A false-positive blood culture can lead to extra days in the hospital and unnecessary use of antibiotics, especially vancomycin (Vancocin). The highest yield has been demonstrated with severe CAP (Box 1). Pretreatment Gram stain and culture should be performed only if a good quality specimen can be obtained. A Gram stain can direct initial empiric therapy, especially with less common pathogens such as *S. aureus* or gram-negative bacteria.

Patients with pleural effusions greater than 5 cm on a lateral upright chest radiograph or greater than 1 cm on a lateral decubitus film should undergo a thoracentesis for Gram stain and culture. Urinary antigen tests are available for *S. pneumoniae* and *Legionella pneumophila*. These tests are rapid and specific in adults. For pneumococcal pneumonia, studies in adults show a sensitivity of 50% to 80% and a specificity of greater than 90%. False-positives are seen in children colonized with *S. pneumoniae*; therefore, this test is not recommended in children. For *L. pneumophila*, the urinary antigen can only detect *L. pneumophila* serogroup 1, which accounts for 80% to 90% of legionnaires' disease cases in the United States. The urinary antigen has a sensitivity of 70% to 90% and a specificity of greater than 95%. The disadvantage of urinary antigen assay for the diagnosis of pneumococcal pneumonia include lower sensitivity without bacteremia and no organism is available for sensitivity testing. A new polymerase chain reaction (PCR) test can detect all serotypes of *L. pneumophila* in sputum; however, clinical experience is currently limited.

The diagnosis of atypical pneumonia such as *Chlamydophila pneumoniae*, *Mycoplasma pneumoniae*, and *Legionella* species other than *L. pneumophila* rely on acute and convalescent serologies. In general, management on a single acute serology is unreliable; therefore, serologies are often retrospective and usually do not affect initial antimicrobial therapy. Newer tests approved by the FDA include PCR for detecting Chlamydophila and Mycoplasma. These tests are rapid, sensitive, and specific.

Admission Criteria

The initial decision of the treatment of CAP often revolves around severity of illness and if the patient requires hospitalization. Two severity-of-illness scores are commonly used, CURB-65 and the pneumonia severity index (PSI). CURB-65 stands for *c*onfusion, *u*remia (blood urea nitrogen >20 mg/dL), *r*espiratory rate greater than 30 breaths/minute, systolic *b*lood pressure less than 90 mm Hg, and age older than 64 years. The PSI score is based primarily on history of underlying diseases and age that increase the risk of mortality, whereas CURB-65 does not rely on underlying diseases.

With CURB-65, mortality was higher when three (14.5%), four (40%), or five (57%) factors were present. Patients with a score of 0 or 1 can be treated on an outpatient basis, patients with a score of

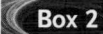

TABLE 1	Pneumonia Severity Index	
	RISK FACTORS	**POINTS**
Demographic Factors		
Age for men		Age (yr)
Age for women		Age (yr) −10
Nursing home resident		+10
Coexisting Illnesses		
Active neoplastic disease		+30
Chronic liver disease		+20
CHF		+10
Cerebrovascular disease		+10
Chronic renal disease		+10
Physical Examination		
Altered mental status		+20
Respiratory rate >30		+20
Blood pressure <90 mm Hg		+20
Temperature <35°C or ≥40°C		+15
Pulse ≥125		+10
Laboratory and Radiographic Findings		
Arterial pH <7.35		+30
BUN ≥30 mg/dL		+20
Sodium <130 mmo/L		+20
Glucose ≥250 mg/dL		+10
Hematocrit <30%		+10
Pao_2 <60 mm Hg		+10
Pleural effusion		+10

Abbreviations: BUN = blood urea nitrogen; CHF = congestive heart failure; Pao_2 = partial pressure of arterial oxygen.
Adapted from Fine MJ, Auble TE, Yealy DM, et al. A predictive rule to identify low-risk patients with community-acquired pneumonia. N Engl J Med 1997; 336:243–50.
Risk classes: I = 0; II <70 (low risk); III = 71–90 (low risk); IV = 91–130 (moderate risk); V = >130 (high risk).

2 can be admitted to the floor, and patients with scores higher than 3 often require admission to the intensive care unit (ICU). PSI uses 20 different variables and places patients into five risk groups (Table 1). Risk classes I and II patients can be treated as outpatients, risk class III patients can be treated on a short hospitalization or observational unit, and risk classes IV and V patients should be treated as inpatients.

Etiology

CAP may be caused by a number of pathogens, but only a few account for the majority of cases. Box 2 lists the more common pathogens divided by site of care and severity. According to most studies, an etiology is established in only about 40% of patients with CAP. In confirmed cases, *S. pneumoniae* is the most common bacterial pathogen identified. Atypical pathogens are the most common in mild to moderate CAP; *S. aureus*, Gram-negative bacilli, and *L. pneumophila* are more common in severe CAP. Nontypable *Haemophilus influenzae* can be seen in patients with underlying chronic lung disease. *S. aureus* is often associated with preceding influenza. Gram-negative bacilli, including *Pseudomonas aeruginosa*, can be seen in patients who are taking steroids or chemotherapy, who have previously used antibiotics, are alcoholics, or who have underlying pulmonary disease.

Box 2	Community-Acquired Pneumonia Pathogens by Site

Outpatient Setting
Chlamydophlia pneumoniae
Haemophilus influenzae
Mycoplasma pneumoniae
Respiratory viruses: adenovirus, influenza, parainfluenza, respiratory syncytial virus
Streptococcus pneumoniae

Inpatient outside Intensive Care Unit
Aspiration
Chlamydophlia pneumoniae
Haemophilus influenzae
Legionella species
Mycoplasma pneumoniae
Respiratory viruses
Streptococcus pneumoniae

Inpatient in Intensive Care Unit
Gram-negative bacilli
Haemophilus influenzae
Legionella species
Staphylococcus aureus
Streptococcus pneumoniae

Adapted from File TM: Community-acquired pneumonia. Lancet 2003;362: 1991–2001.

Treatment

Antimicrobial therapy remains the mainstay of treatment. Until better diagnostic tests are available, initial treatment remains largely empiric. Box 3 reviews the most recent recommended empiric antibiotics. Anaerobic coverage should be considered with a history of loss of consciousness in patients with gingival or esophageal disease. Antibiotics should be modified based on local epidemiology and susceptibilities.

Current levels of penicillin and cephalosporin resistance in *S. pneumoniae* do not usually result in failure when appropriate doses are administered. However, recent studies indicate that resistance to macrolides and older fluoroquinolones (levofloxacin [Levaquin] and ciprofloxacin [Cipro]) have resulted in clinical failures in patients with CAP caused by *S. pneumoniae*. Pneumonia caused by community-acquired MRSA may be increasing, especially associated with influenza. Many of these cases are genotypically and phenotypically different from hospital-acquired MRSA. Community-acquired MRSA isolates are less antibiotic resistant and often contain the gene for Panton Valentine leukocidin (PVL), a toxin associated with necrotizing pneumonia. Recent studies have not always correlated presence of PVL with severity and outcome. It is possible other toxins may play a role. Anecdotal and in vitro studies suggest clindamycin (Cleocin) (if susceptible) or linezolid (Zyvox) can affect toxin production and improve outcome. More studies are needed to determine the most effective treatment for CAP caused by community-acquired MRSA. Several studies have reported that combination therapy with the combination of a macrolide and a β-lactam for bacteremic pneumococcal pneumonia is associated with lower mortality compared with a single effective drug. A possible explanation might relate to the fact that macrolides have immunomodulatory effects, including cytokine production.

Time to first antibiotic dose for CAP has been studied in two retrospective studies in Medicare patients. These studies demonstrated lower mortality in patients who received timely antimicrobial treatment. The first study showed that if the first dose was given within 8 hours of arrival, mortality was reduced. The second study demonstrated that a 4-hour interval was associated with better outcomes. Treatment should be given for a minimum of 5 days; the patient should be afebrile for 48 to 72 hours and clinically stable. Longer treatment may be needed for CAP caused by *S. aureus*, *L. pneumophila*, or *P. aeruginosa* and in patients with evidence of associated endocarditis, septic arthritis, or meningitis.

Box 3 — Empiric Antimicrobial Choice for Community-Acquired Pneumonia

Outpatient Treatment

Healthy patient, no prior antibiotics within the previous 3 months
- Macrolide (azithromycin [Zithromax], clarithromycin [Biaxin], or erythromycin) *or*
- Doxycycline (Vibramycin) (weak recommendation)

Patient with comorbidity (e.g., chronic heart, lung, liver, or renal disease; malignancies; alcoholism; asplenia; diabetes mellitus; immunosuppression) or use of antibiotics in previous 3 months
- Respiratory fluoroquinolone (moxifloxacin [Avelox], gemifloxacin [Factive], or levofloxacin [Levaquin] (750 mg) *or*
- β-Lactam (high-dose amoxicillin or amoxicillin-clavulanate [Augmentin]); alternatives are ceftriaxone (Rocephin), cefpodoxime (Vantin), or cefuroxime (Ceftin) plus a macrolide

In regions with a high rate (>25%) of infection with high-level (MIC ≥16 μg/mL) macrolide-resistant *Streptococcus pneumoniae*
- Use a fluoroquinolone or a β-lactam plus either a macrolide or doxycycline

Inpatients Not in Intensive Care
- Fluroquinolone alone *or*
- β-Lactam (e.g., ceftriaxone, cefotaxime [Claforan], ampicillin, ertapenem [Invanz]) plus a macrolide

Intensive Care Unit Patients
- β-Lactam (e.g., ceftriaxone, cefotaxime, or ampicillin-sulbactam [Unasyn]) *plus* either azithromycin or a fluoroquinolone

For *Pseudomonas* infection
- Antipneumococcal, antipseudomonal β-lactam (piperacillin-tazobactam [Zosyn], cefepime [Maxipime], imipenem [Primaxin], meropenem [Merrem]), or doripenem plus either ciprofloxacin (Cipro) or levofloxacin (750 mg) *or*
- Antipneumococcal, antipseudomonal β-lactam *plus* an aminoglycoside and azithromycin

Community-Acquired MRSA
- Add vancomycin (Vancocin) or linezolid (Zyvox)

Abbreviations: MIC = minimum inhibitory concentration; MRSA = methicillin-resistant *Streptococcus aureus*.
Adapted from Mandell LA, Wunderink RG, Anzueto A, et al: Infectious Diseases Society of America/American Thoracic Society Consensus Guidelines on the Management of Community-Acquired Pneumonia in Adults. Clin Infect Dis 2007;44: S27–S72.

Prevention

Yearly influenza vaccination is now recommended for all patients older than 6 months. Several reviews have demonstrated that influenza vaccination not only prevents pneumonia but also decreases hospitalizations, decreases cerebrovascular events, and decreases deaths from all causes.

Pneumococcal polysaccharide vaccine (Pneumovax 23) is recommended for all persons older than 65 years and persons with certain underlying illnesses (e.g., functional and anatomic asplenia, cardiopulmonary disease, diabetes). Studies have documented moderate effectiveness for preventing invasive pneumococcal disease (bacteremia and meningitis). The overall efficacy in patients older than 65 years is reported to be between 44% and 75%. Pneumococcal conjugated vaccine (PCV13) is now recommended for adult patients 19 years or older with compromised immune systems (e.g., HIV, chronic renal failure or nephrotic syndrome, underlying hematologic or solid tumor malignancies, systemic steroids). If patient has not been previously immunized, PCV13 should be given first followed by pneumococcal polysaccharide at least 8 weeks later. If patient has received a dose of polysaccharide vaccine, PCV13 should be administered no sooner than 1 year after the last dose.

Vaccination status should be determined in all patients admitted to the hospital. Vaccination should be offered year-round for pneumococcal vaccine and during the fall and winter months for influenza vaccine.

Health Care–Acquired Pneumonia

HAP is defined as a pneumonia that occurred more than 48 hours after admission and that was not incubating at the time of admission. Ventilator-associated pneumonia (VAP) is defined as pneumonia that develops 48 to 72 hours after intubation. Health care–associated pneumonia (HCAP) is a new category; HCAP occurs in a patient who attended a hospital or hemodialysis clinic, who was hospitalized in an acute-care hospital for more than 2 days within the prior 90 days, or who resided in a long-term care facility or nursing home. The remaining comments are directed at HAP and VAP.

HAP is the second or third most common health care–associated infection in the United States and is associated with significant morbidity and mortality, resulting in increased length of stay and costs. HAP accounts for about 25% of all ICU infections. VAP occurs in 9% to 27% of intubated patients, and the mortality is double that of similar patients without VAP. The risk of VAP is highest in the first 1 to 2 weeks. Some investigators consider time of onset an important factor in terms of outcomes and pathogens. Early-onset HAP and VAP are pneumonia occurring within 4 to 7 days of hospitalization. Early-onset HAP and VAP usually carry a better prognosis and are more likely to be caused by more sensitive pathogens. Late-onset HAP and VAP are more likely to be caused by multidrug-resistant organisms (MDRO) with a higher mortality.

Aspiration of oropharyngeal secretions or leakage of bacteria around the endotracheal tube is the primary source of bacteria causing HAP or VAP. The stomach and sinuses, blood, and contaminated aerosols are much less common sources. Contaminated biofilm in the endotracheal tube, with subsequent embolization into the lower airway, may be an important factor in the pathogenesis of VAP.

Diagnosis

Unfortunately, there is no universally accepted gold standard for the diagnosis of HAP or VAP. The diagnosis is suspected if a patient has a new or progressive infiltrate along with new-onset fever, purulent sputum (>25 neutrophils per low-power field), leukocytosis, and decreased oxygenation.

Unfortunately, the clinical parameters are overly sensitive; therefore, other diagnostic tests are desirable. For a start, blood and lower respiratory secretions should be collected for culture in all patients with suspected HAP or VAP. A thoracentesis should be performed if a large pleural effusion is present. The microbiological approach favors quantitation or semiquantitation of lower respiratory secretions. The diagnostic threshold used to differentiate colonization versus true infection varies by specimen collection. The proposed diagnostic threshold for endotracheal aspirate is greater than 10^5 colony-forming units (CFU)/mL; for bronchoalveolar lavage, greater than 10^4 CFU/mL; and for protected-specimen brush, greater than 10^3 CFU/mL. A major reservation to this approach is the possibility of false-negative results, which can result if a patient has been started on an antimicrobial agent before the specimens are collected.

Treatment

For patients with suspected HAP or VAP, appropriate broad-spectrum antimicrobial therapy should be ordered to cover anticipated pathogens. Consider a Gram stain to guide initial therapy. Whenever possible, select antimicrobial therapy based on local microbiology and epidemiology. Use combination therapy in patients whenever an MDRO is suspected until culture results are available. Risk factors include prolonged hospitalization (>5–7 days), admission from another health care facility, and recent antibiotic therapy. Table 2 summarizes suggested empiric

TABLE 2	Initial Empiric Therapy for Suspected Health Care–Acquired Pneumonia or Ventilator-Associated Pneumonia	
SUSPECTED PATHOGEN	**RECOMMENDED THERAPY**	
Patients with No Known Risk Factors for MDRO and Early Onset		

Streptococcus pneumoniae
Haemophilus influenzae
Methicillin-sensitive
  Streptococcus aureus
Antibiotic-sensitive enteric
  gram-negative *Escherichia*
  coli
Klebsiella pneumoniae
Enterobacter species
Proteus species
Serratia marcescens
	One of the following:
	Ceftriaxone (Rocephin) or
	Fluoroquinolone (levofloxacin
	  [Levaquin], moxifloxacin [Avelox],
	  or ciprofloxacin [Cipro])
	or
	Ertapenem (Invanz)
	or
	Piperacillin-tazobactam (Zosyn)	

Patients with Risk Factors for MDRO or Late Onset		

Pathogens listed above and
  MDRO
Pseudomonas aeruginosa
K. pneumoniae (ESBL)*
Acinetobacter species
MRSA
Legionella species†
	Antipseudomonal cephalosporin
	  (e.g., cefepime [Maxipime] or
	  ceftazidime [Fortaz])
	or
	Antipseudomonal carbepenem
	  (e.g., imipenem [Primaxin] or
	  meropenem [Merrem])
	or
	Piperacillin-tazobactam (Zosyn) or
	  doripenem
	plus
	Aminoglycoside
	or
	Antipseudomonal fluoroquinolone
	  (e.g., ciprofloxacin [Cipro] or
	  levofloxacin [Levaquin])
	plus
	Vancomycin (Vancocin) or linezolid
	  (Zyvox)	

Abbreviations: ESBL = extended-spectrum β-lactamase; MDRO = multidrug-resistant organisms; MRSA = methicillin-resistant *Staphylococcus aureus*.
Modified from American Thoracic Society; Infectious Diseases Society of America. Guidelines for the management of adults with hospital-acquired, ventilator-associated, and healthcare-associated pneumonia. Am J Respir Crit Care Med 171:388–416, 2005.
*If an ESBL strain, a carbepenem is preferred.
†If *Legionella* suspected, the combination regimen should include either a macrolide (e.g., azithromycin) or a fluoroquinolone.

therapy. De-escalation of therapy is strongly recommended when culture results become available. Discontinue antimicrobial therapy if results of cultures and other clinical parameters do not confirm pneumonia. Based on recent studies, a shorter duration of therapy (7–8 days) is now recommended in patients with uncomplicated HAP or VAP who received initial appropriate therapy and have had a good clinical response. *P. aeruginosa, Acinetobacter* species, and MRSA can require longer durations of therapy.

Prevention

The incidence of HAP and VAP can be reduced by following certain proved measures. An effective infection control program, which includes education, hand-washing compliance, surveillance of ICU infections, and isolation of patients with MDRO to reduce cross-infection should be followed. Noninvasive ventilation should be used whenever possible. If intubation is required, the orotracheal route is preferred to reduce health care–associated infections due to sinusitis and VAP. Consider continuous aspiration of subglottic secretions, if available. Follow a protocol for using sedation with daily interruptions. Perform daily assessment for extubation. For patients on a ventilator, keep the head of the bed at 30 to 45 degrees to prevent aspiration (except when contraindicated). Use agents such as oral chlorhexidine (Peridex) to reduce oropharyngeal colonization. Glucose control to maintain level lower than 180 mg/dL results in lower mortality without increasing the risk of severe hypoglycemia.

References

American Thoracic Society; Infectious Diseases Society of America. Guidelines for the management of adults with hospital-acquired, ventilator-associated, and healthcare-associated pneumonia. Am J Respir Crit Care Med 2005;171:388–416.

Chastre J, Wolff M, Fagon JY, et al. Comparison of 8 vs 15 days of antibiotic therapy for ventilator-associated pneumonia in adults: A randomized trial. JAMA 2003;290:2588–98.

Fagon JY, Chastre J, Wolff M, et al. Invasive and noninvasive strategies for management of suspected ventilator-associated pneumonia: A randomized trial. Ann Intern Med 2000;132:621–30.

File TM. Community-acquired pneumonia. Lancet 2003;362:1991–2001.

Fine MJ, Auble TE, Yealy DM, et al. A predictive rule to identify low-risk patients with community-acquired pneumonia. N Engl J Med 1997;336:243–50.

Houck PM, Bratzler DW, Nsa W, et al. Timing of antibiotic administration and outcomes for Medicare patients hospitalized with community-acquired pneumonia. Arch Intern Med 2004;164:637–44.

Lim WS, van der Eerden MM, Laing R, et al. Defining community acquired pneumonia severity on presentation to hospital: An international derivation and validation study. Thorax 2003;58:377–82.

Mandell LA, Wunderink RG, Anzueto A, et al. Infectious Diseases Society of America/American Thoracic Society Consensus Guidelines on the Management of Community-Acquired Pneumonia in Adults. Clin Infect Dis 2007;44:S27–72.

Metersky ML, Ma A, Houck PM, Bratzler DW. Antibiotics for bacteremic pneumonia: Improved outcomes with macrolides but not fluoroquinolones. Chest 2007;131:466–73.

NICE-SUGAR Study Investigators. Intensive versus conventional glucose control in critically ill patients. N Engl J Med 2009;360:1283–97.

Richards MJ, Edwards JR, Culver DH, Gaynes RP. Nosocomial infections in medical ICUs in the United States: National Nosocomial Infections Surveillance System. Crit Care Med 1999;27:887–92.

van den Berghe G, Wilmer A, Hermans G, et al. Intensive insulin therapy in the medical ICU. N Engl J Med 2006;354:449–61.

BLASTOMYCOSIS

Method of
John M. Embil, MD; and Donald C. Vinh, MD

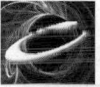

CURRENT DIAGNOSIS

- Blastomycosis is caused by the thermally dimorphic fungus *Blastomyces dermatitidis*.
- *B. dermatitidis* is endemic to the United States (southeastern and south central states bordering Mississippi and Ohio rivers; upper Midwestern states bordering the Great Lakes) and to Canada (Manitoba and Ontario bordering the Great Lakes; Quebec adjacent to St. Lawrence River).
- Blastomycosis should be suspected in the appropriate clinical context in patients who have resided or traveled to an endemic area.
- Blastomycosis has a broad range of manifestations, mimicking other infectious (e.g., bacteria, mycobacteria) and neoplastic processes.
- Blastomycosis may be asymptomatic, or it can manifest with disease involving the lung, skin, bone and joints, genito-urinary system, or central nervous system.
- Diagnosis requires microscopic examination and/or culture of clinical specimens. Blastomyces antigen detection is also useful. Serology has no diagnostic value.

CURRENT THERAPY

- Treatment varies with the severity of disease.
- Long-term suppressive therapy may be required for those who are immunosuppressed.

Blastomyces dermatitidis is the thermally dimorphic fungus that causes blastomycosis. The mycelial form of *B. dermatitidis* exists in the environment but grows as a yeast at body temperature. Although *B. dermatitidis* is endemic to certain specific regions within North America, numerous cases have been reported from areas where it is not considered endemic. It is presumed that those patients acquired infection in the endemic areas and subsequently presented outside of these geographic locations. The clinical manifestations of blastomycosis can be diverse, and therefore this infection should be suspected within the appropriate clinical context in persons with a history of residence or travel to such endemic areas.

Epidemiology

Our knowledge of the exact geographic distribution of B. dermatitidis is limited by the fact that the fungus cannot be readily recovered from nature; thus, identification of the endemic area has been largely derived from outbreak investigations and small case series. Most epidemiologic studies have depended upon recovery of B. dermatitidis in culture from clinical specimens or histologic visualization to establish the diagnosis. In addition, the incidence and prevalence of blastomycosis has been difficult to establish because suitable serologic or skin-prick assays (demonstrating acceptable sensitivity and/or specificity) to confirm infection are lacking. The geographic niche of B. dermatitidis may therefore be greater than is currently believed.

The currently known areas of endemicity for B. dermatitidis are the south central and upper midwestern United States, including areas surrounding the Great Lakes. B. dermatitidis is also endemic in Wisconsin (1.3 cases per 100,000 population) and Mississippi (1.4 cases per 100,000 population), as well as parts of Missouri, Kentucky, Tennessee, Arkansas, and Alabama. In Canada, the major areas of endemicity include the province of Manitoba (0.62 cases per 100,000 population), the southern region of Québec (0.46–0.79 cases per 100,000 population), and the Kenora region of the province of Ontario (7.11 cases per 100,000 population). Although most cases of blastomycosis are concentrated in these regions, it should be remembered that persons can acquire infection with B. dermatitidis in these areas but present at a later time to health care providers in locations where blastomycosis is not usually observed. Inquiring about residence or travel to these areas is important to help establish the diagnosis.

Risk factors for acquiring blastomycosis have been defined by case reports, case series, and a small number of case-control studies and have not been conclusively established. Exposure while in endemic regions to soil, decaying wood, or to dust clouds generated by soil disruption is important; however, specific outdoor occupations or activities have not been confirmed. The fungus may also be associated with exposure to river waterways.

Race may be a contributing factor to disease. In one study from Mississippi, African-American race and prior history of pneumonia were independent risk factors for blastomycosis; however, neither environmental nor socioeconomic risk factors were detected. These findings were in contrast to previously noted studies where race and gender were not identified as specific risk factors for acquisition of blastomycosis. One study in Canada noted an increased incidence among the aboriginal population of Manitoba. Thus, it remains unclear if certain ethnic groups are at increased risk for disease or simply reflect differences in exposure.

Immunosuppression may also be an important risk factor, particularly for the tendency to develop severe disease. Blastomycosis has been reported in pregnant women, persons with diabetes mellitus, organ transplant recipients, and persons infected with HIV.

Dogs and humans are the species most commonly affected by B. dermatitidis. Anecdotally, dogs can serve as a sentinel marker for human disease (i.e., dogs present with systemic infection before their owners), leading to early suspicion of human infections by astute veterinarians. In such cases, it is speculated that humans and their pet dogs have a simultaneous exposure to the same source of fungus and therefore develop synchronous infection. This hypothesis, however, remains to be confirmed, and in a more recent study, canine blastomycosis was not deemed to predict human disease among the human owners. Additional studies are required to establish the relationship between blastomycosis in humans and disease in their pet dogs.

The most common mode of transmission is presumed to be by inhalation of aerosolized conidia from the environment. There are, however, reports of cutaneous blastomycosis occuring after accidental cutaneous inoculation, for example in the laboratory setting during autopsy or after dog bites. The median incubation period, established by reviewing the results of point-source outbreaks, ranges from 30 to 45 days.

Pathophysiology

Following inhalation of conidia into the lungs, the fungus is phagocytosed by alveolar macrophages. The human body temperature allows the fungus to transform to the yeast phase. It is speculated that a process similar to infection with Mycobacterium tuberculosis then occurs. The fungus might spread to other organs via the bloodstream and lymphatics. The primary defense against B. dermatitidis is through a suppurative response initially with neutrophils, followed by influx of monocytes with establishment of cell mediated immunity, resulting in noncaseating granuloma. The patient with intact immunologic responses can contain the process without progression to clinical disease. Alternatively, the patient can develop a symptomatic pneumonia and then mount a suitable immunologic response and recover. Impaired immunity favors the development of progressive pulmonary disease with or without extrapulmonary manifestations. It has also been suggested that reactivation of disease can occur at pulmonary or extrapulmonary sites. A vaccine that protects humans against infection with B. dermatitidis is unavailable.

Clinical Manifestations

After inhalation of the conidia, an initial infection can occur. Most primary infections (at least 50%) are asymptomatic or mild and usually go unrecognized, resolving spontaneously. In others, a symptomatic pneumonia can develop; recovery can occur either spontaneously or with therapy, without further progression. Some persons develop progressive pneumonia or extrapulmonary manifestations. The type of clinical manifestations (localized, extrapulmonary or disseminated disease) can have a seasonal variation: Persons with manifestations occurring early after exposure (1–6 months) developed localized pneumonia, whereas those who presented later after exposure (4–9 months) tended to have isolated extrapulmonary or disseminated disease. Blastomycosis has been termed "the great mimic," because its clinical manifestations are nonspecific and can be similar to those of many different clinical entities. The most common organ systems involved in blastomycosis, in descending order of frequency, include lung, skin, bone, genitourinary, and central nervous systems (CNS). Box 1 summarizes the key clinical manifestations of blastomycosis.

Blastomycosis in Special Populations

Children account for a small percentage of the cases of blastomycosis, ranging from 2% to 11%. Children demonstrate a similar spectrum of manifestations as in adults (excluding prostatic disease). The most common symptoms include cough, headache, chest pain, weight loss, fever, abdominal pain, and night sweats. It is postulated that children experience disseminated infection more frequently than do adults.

Although there are few published reports of blastomycosis in pregnancy, disease has been observed in pregnant women, with presumed subsequent intrauterine and perinatal transmission.

Blastomycosis has been reported in persons with advanced HIV and among those who have undergone solid organ transplants. In immunocompromised hosts, it appears that a significant percentage developed rapidly progressive pulmonary disease, leading to respiratory failure and death. For those who are immunocompromised, the reported mortality rate range is 30% to 40%, with death occurring within the first few weeks of disease onset.

Diagnosis

The most reliable technique for confirming the diagnosis of blastomycosis is recovery of the fungus in culture. Alternatively, direct observation of the pathogen by light microscopy or with calcofluor white stain or in histopathologic examination of tissue

| Box 1 | Clinical Manifestations of Blastomycosis

Lung

Acute Pneumonia

Acute pneumonia is clinically indistinguishable from bacterial pneumonia.

Patients may present with fevers, chills, dyspnea, and cough, which initially might not be productive but, with time, may be accompanied by sputum production.

Radiographic findings can also be difficult to discern from those due to a bacterial pneumonia.

The radiographic pattern of pulmonary blastomycosis includes the following:

- Lobar infiltrates that mimic bacterial pneumonias
- Cavitary lung lesions and miliary patterns, which can mimic tuberculosis
- Mass lesions that may be mistaken for neoplasms
- Cystic lesions that resemble abscesses

There is no definitive plain radiograph or computed tomographic scan findings characteristic of pulmonary blastomycosis.

The spectrum of clinical pulmonary disease ranges from spontaneous resolution to pneumonia, with or without the acute respiratory distress syndrome; the latter is accompanied by high (50%–89%) mortality rates.

Chronic Pneumonia

A nonresolving pneumonia is one of the hallmarks of pulmonary blastomycosis.

Chronic pneumonia may be associated with fever, chills, weight loss, sputum-producing cough, and hemoptysis.

There is no characteristic radiographic appearance to help establish the diagnosis.

Skin

Cutaneous lesions are the most common extrapulmonary manifestations of blastomycosis. Lesions usually result from dissemination of a primary pulmonary lesion or rarely from direct inoculation.

Lesions can have a number of different appearances, with verrucae (wartlike lesions) and ulcers being the most common

manifestations. The verrucous lesions have a heaped-up appearance with a raw excoriated center. These lesions can mimic squamous cell carcinomas. Cutaneous abscesses may be associated with these lesions.

Ulcerative lesions initially manifest as pustules that eventually erode, producing a bed of granulation tissue that is friable and bleeds when traumatized. Other skin lesions include subcutaneous nodules and isolated abscesses.

Bone and Joint

The most common manifestation of extrapulmonary blastomycosis, after cutaneous disease, is involvement of bones and joints.

Any bone may be involved, although the long bones and axial skeleton are the most commonly affected.

The radiographic findings are indistinguishable from bacterial osteomyelitis and arthritis.

Genitourinary Tract

In the genitourinary tract, the prostate has been reported to be commonly affected by blastomycosis.

Symptoms can mimic prostatitis, and patients can present with obstructive uropathy.

Central Nervous System

The CNS is infrequently affected by B. dermatitidis. Infection may occur in isolation or with concomitant non-CNS infection.

CNS blastomycosis can occur in immunocompromised patients (e.g., HIV, solid organ transplant), as well as in patients with little/no risk factors (e.g., diabetes mellitus alone; persons with no underlying co-morbidities).

Clinical manifestations depend on the area of involvement and range from focal neurologic findings (e.g., due to mass lesions in the brain parenchyma) to symptoms of meningitis due to involvement of the meninges.

Radiographically, the findings may be indistinguishable from bacterial processes. Other sites of involvement have been described but are infrequent compared to those summarized above.

---

establishes a presumptive diagnosis. *B. dermatitidis* is characteristically observed as a thick-walled, broad-based budding yeast. Because colonization does not occur, identification of *B. dermatitidis* should never be considered a contaminant. Serologic assays are extremely variable in their sensitivity and specificity and do not play a role in confirming or excluding the diagnosis, thus limiting their value in therapeutic decision making. A reliable skin test is unavailable, but a urinary antigen detection assay exists that may aid in diagnosis and may be of benefit to follow the efficacy of treatment in established infections. Box 2 summarizes techniques for establishing the diagnosis of blastomycosis.

Treatment

The treatment recommendations for blastomycosis from the Infectious Diseases Society of America (IDSA) are summarized in Table 1. Amphotericin B deoxycholate (Fungizone) is the agent with which there is the greatest experience, particularly for the treatment of patients with severe blastomycosis or for those who have CNS involvement. Lipid preparations of amphotericin B (Abelect, Amphotec, AmBisome)[1] have been shown to be effective in animal models, although clinical trial data are unavailable for these agents in humans. Clinical experience suggests that the lipid formulations are as effective but less toxic than the deoxycholate preparation.

It is generally accepted that in patients with severe disease or CNS involvement, amphotericin B-based products should be used to initiate therapy until the patient is stable, followed by step-down to an azole, specifically itraconazole (Sporanox), to complete the total duration of therapy. Patients on itraconazole should have serum

levels of the antifungal drug measured after at least 2 weeks of therapy, targeting a level >1.0 mcg/mL and <10.0 mcg/mL. Ketoconazole (Nizoral), although once recommended as the agent of choice, is less effective and more toxic than itraconazole. Experience with fluconazole (Diflucan)[1] for the treatment of blastomycosis is limited, although *in vitro* studies have demonstrated that fluconazole is effective against *B. dermatitidis*. Fluconazole does, however, have excellent penetration into the CNS; therefore, fluconazole may be considered as an alternative treatment of CNS blastomycosis. There are also a number of reports of voriconazole (Vfend)[1] being used for the successful treatment of CNS blastomycosis, as well as in persons with refractory blastomycosis. A case series of patients with CNS blastomycosis suggested that voriconazole may be the most desirable azole for the management of CNS disease. The echinocandins (caspofungin [Cancidas],[1] micafungin [Mycamine],[1] and anidulafungin [Eraxis][1]) have limited activity against *B. dermatitidis* and are not considered appropriate choices.

Box 2 summarizes the therapeutic options for treatment of various types of blastomycosis. Amphotericin B-based therapy is usually the treatment option of choice in persons who have severe disease. Whenever the patient is clinically stable, it is desirable to switch from the potentially toxic amphotericin B to a less-toxic agent (usually an azole). It is important to note that amphotericin B in cumulative doses of 1.5 to 2.5 grams for persons with disseminated blastomycosis, with life-threatening disease, or in those who are immunocompromised or pregnant, can lead to cure without relapses.

In patients with overwhelming pulmonary disease, amphotericin B-based products are the therapeutic agents of choice. Although

Blastomycosis

---

[1]Not FDA approved for this indication.

[1]Not FDA approved for this indication.

Box 2 — Establishing the Diagnosis of Blastomycosis

Direct Examination
A wet preparation of respiratory secretions or a touch preparation of tissues examined under high magnification by light microscopy can reveal the characteristic thick-walled, broad-based budding yeast form. However, this method has a low diagnostic yield: 36% for a single specimen and 46% for multiple specimens.

Calcofluor white stains can help in identifying the pathogen but require fluorescence microscopy.

Histopathologic Examination
The fungus may be difficult to identify with hematoxylin and eosin stain.

If there is a high index of suspicion, the Gomori methenamine-silver stain should be used to optimize detection of thick-walled, broad-based budding yeast forms compatible with *B. dermatitidis*.

Culture
Diagnostic yield ranges from approximately 86% from sputum to 92% from specimens obtained by bronchoscopy.

Culture is the gold standard for diagnosis. However, the fungus can take several weeks to be isolated in culture.

Confirmation of identity traditionally requires demonstration of thermal-dimorphism (mycelial-to-yeast conversion), which can further delay diagnosis.

Isolation of *B. dermatitidis* should not be considered a contaminant.

Serology
Current serologic assays are neither sensitive nor specific, and they should not be used to establish or refute a diagnosis or in therapeutic decision making.

Nucleic Acid Detection
This method permits genetic-based identification of *B. dermatitidis* from culture of clinical specimens, rather than relying on thermal-dimorphism to confirm identity of the fungus, thus reducing the time required for its identification.

Antigen Detection
The only currently available antigen detection assay has its greatest sensitivity in urine, although antigens can be detected in serum and other body fluids.

Cross reaction with antigens from other fungi (e.g., *Histoplasma* spp.) can occur.

The greatest benefit of the antigen detection assay may be to follow efficacy of treatment in patients with established disease (antigen levels decrease with successful treatment or rise with recurrence).

Skin Testing
A commercially available standardized reagent for skin testing is not available.

Modified from Chapman SW, Bradsher RW, Campbell GD, et al: Practice guidelines for the management of patients with blastomycosis. Cin Infect Dis 2000;30:679–83; and Martynowicz MA, Prakash UBS: Pulmonary blastomycosis: An appraisal of diagnostic techniques. Chest 2002;121:768–73.

TABLE 1 — Treatment Suggestions for Infections Caused by *Blastomycosis dermatitidis*

TREATMENT RECOMMENDATIONS

MANIFESTATION	PRIMARY RECOMMENDATION	ALTERNATIVE RECOMMENDATION	COMMENTS
Pulmonary Infection			
Mild to moderate	Itraconazole (Sporanox) 200 mg PO tid × 3 days, then QD or BID × 6–12 mo	Fluconazole (Diflucan)[1] 400–800[3] mg/day or ketoconazole (Nizoral) 400–800 mg/kg × 6–12 mo	For Itraconazole, measure serum levels after at least 2 weeks, to ensure adequate drug exposure. Target level: >1.0 mcg/mL and <10.0 mcg/mL
Moderate to severe	Lipid formulation of amphotericin B (AmBisome, Abelect, Amphotec)[1] 3–5 mg/kg/day OR Amphotericin B deoxycholate (Fungizone) 0.7–1 mg/kg/d for 1–2 wk or until improvement, followed by itraconazole 200 mg PO tid × 3 days then 200 mg PO bid × 6–12 mo		Amphotericin B toxicity can be attenuated by minimizing the duration of therapy and switching to oral therapy when the patient is stable. For Itraconazole, measure serum levels after at least 2 weeks, to ensure adequate drug exposure. Target level: >1.0 mcg/mL and <10.0 mcg/mL
Disseminated Infection Not Involving the Central Nervous System			
Mild to moderate	Itraconazole 200 mg PO tid × 3 days then QD or BID × 6–12 mo		
Moderate to severe	Lipid formulation of amphotericin B 3–5 mg/kg/d OR Amphotericin B deoxycholate 0.7–1 mg/kg/d for 1–2 wk or until improvement, followed by Itraconazole 200 mg PO tid × 3 days then 200 mg PO BID to complete at least 12 mo		To minimize toxicity, switching to oral therapy once the patient is stable should be considered. Bone and joint infections are usually treated for at least 12 mo with itraconazole. For Itraconazole, measure serum levels after at least 2 weeks, to ensure adequate drug exposure. Target level: >1.0 mcg/mL and <10.0 mcg/mL
Central Nervous System Involvement (with or without other manifestations)			
	Lipid preparations of amphotericin B[1] 5 mg/kg/d × 4–6 wk followed by an oral azole for ≥12 mo		It has been suggested that liposomal amphotericin B achieves higher CNS levels than other lipid formulations. When switching to oral azole, options include fluconazole[1] 800 mg PO qd,[3] itraconazole 200 mg PO bid or tid,[3] or voriconazole (Vfend)[1] 200–400[3] mg PO bid. Longer durations of therapy may be necessary in the immunocompromised host

Continued

TABLE 1	Treatment Suggestions for Infections Caused by *Blastomycosis dermatitidis*—cont'd		
	TREATMENT RECOMMENDATIONS		
MANIFESTATION	**PRIMARY RECOMMENDATION**	**ALTERNATIVE RECOMMENDATION**	**COMMENTS**
Special Populations			
Immunocompromised	Lipid formulation of amphotericin B 3–5 mg/kg/d OR Amphotericin B deoxycholate 0.7–1 mg/kg/d for 1–2 wk or until improvement, followed by Itraconazole 200 mg PO tid × 3 days then 200 mg PO BID to complete at least 12 mo		Lifelong suppression with itraconazole 200 mg PO qd may be required for those in whom immunosuppression cannot be reversed
Pregnant patients	Lipid formulation of amphotericin B 3–5 mg/kg/d		No duration of lipid formulation amphotericin B treatment provided; continue until clinical cure During pregnancy, azoles should be avoided because of potential teratogenicity If the placenta or newborn demonstrates evidence of infection, give amphotericin B deoxycholate 1.0 mg/kg/d
Children: mild to moderate	Itraconazole[1] 10 mg/kg/d for 6–12 mo		Maximum dose of itraconazole should be 400 mg/d
Children: moderate to severe	Amphotericin B deoxycholate 0.7–10.0 mg/kg/d OR Lipid formulation amphotericin B 3–5 mg/kg/d × 1–2 wk followed by itraconazole 10 mg/kg/d × 12 mo		

Modified from Chapman SW, Bradsher RW, Campbell GD, et al: Practice guidelines for the management of patients with blastomycosis. Clin Infect Dis 2000;30:679; and Chapman SW, Dismukes WE, Proia LA, et al: Clinical practice guidelines for the management of blastomycosis: 2008 update by the Infectious Diseases Society of America. Clin Infect Dis 2008;46:1801–12.
[1]Not FDA approved for this indication.
[3]Exceeds dosage recommended by the manufacturer.

acute respiratory distress syndrome (ARDS) can complicate the management of these patients, data on the beneficial role of corticosteroids in the management of patients with overwhelming pulmonary disease or ARDS are limited to few case reports. For patients with less-severe pulmonary disease, an alternative to amphotericin B is a 6- to 12-month course of oral itraconazole. A similarly prolonged course of oral itraconazole is also appropriate for persons with bone and joint disease. The precise duration of therapy, however, is unknown and should be individualized. The same is true for cutaneous blastomycosis. For persons with CNS blastomycosis, an initial treatment course of 4 to 6 weeks with intravenous lipid formulation of amphotericin B should be followed with an oral azole to complete at least 12 months of therapy. For those who are immunocompromised, prolonged therapy is also necessary. Patients who are immunosuppressed and in whom the immunosuppression cannot be reversed can require lifelong suppressive itraconazole therapy at 200 mg per day. Additional details for the management of the various stages of blastomycosis should be sought from the most current version of the IDSA guidelines.

References

Bariola JR, Perry P, Pappas PG, et al. Blastomycosis of the central nervous system: a multicenter review of diagnosis and treatment in the modern era. Clin Infect Dis 2010;50:797–804.

Bush JW, Wuerz T, Embil JM, Del Bigio MR, McDonald PJ, Krawitz S. Outcomes of persons with blastomycosis involving the central nervous system. Diagn Microbiol Infect Dis 2013;76(2):175–81.

Chapman SW, Sullivan DC. Blastomyces dermatitidis. In: Mandell GL, Bennett JE, Dolin R, editors. Mandell, Douglas, and Bennett's Principles and Practice of Infectious Diseases. 7th ed. Philadelphia: Elsevier; 2010. p. 3319–32.

Chapman SW, Lin AC, Hendricks KA, et al. Endemic blastomycosis in Mississippi: Epidemiological and clinical studies. Semin Respir Infect 1997;12:219–28.

Chapman SW, Dismukes WE, Proia LA, et al. Clinical practice guidelines for the management of blastomycosis: 2008 update by the Infectious Diseases Society of America. Clin Infect Dis 2008;46:1801–12.

Choptiany M, Wiebe L, Limerick B, et al. Risk factors for acquisition of endemic blastomycosis. Can J Infect Dis Med Microbiol 2009;20:117–21.

Crampton TL, Light RB, Berg GM, et al. Epidemiology and clinical spectrum of blastomycosis diagnosed at Manitoba hospitals. Clin Infect Dis 2002;34:1310–6.

Litvinov IV, St-Germain G, Pelletier R, Paradis M, Sheppard DC. Endemic human blastomycosis in Quebec, Canada, 1988–2011. Epidemiol Infect 2013;141 (6):1143–7.

Martynowicz MA, Prakash UBS. Pulmonary blastomycosis: An appraisal of diagnostic techniques. Chest 2002;121:768–73.

Meyer KC, McManus EJ, Maki DG. Overwhelming pulmonary blastomycosis associated with the adult respiratory distress syndrome. N Engl J Med 1993;329:1231–6.

Oppenheimer M, Cheang M, Trepman E, et al. Orthopedic manifestations of blastomycosis. South Med J 2007;100:570–8.

Pappas PG. Blastomycosis in the immunocompromised patient. Semin Respir Infect 1997;12:243–51.

Ward BA, Parent AD, Raila F. Indications for the surgical management of central nervous system blastomycosis. Surg Neurol 1995;43:379–88.

CHRONIC OBSTRUCTIVE PULMONARY DISEASE

Method of
Nicola A. Hanania, MD, MS; and Amir Sharafkhaneh, MD, PhD

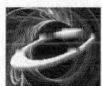

CURRENT DIAGNOSIS

- COPD is a preventable disease most commonly caused by cigarette smoke exposure.
- COPD is not diagnosed in approximately 50% of patients suffering from it.
- COPD should be ruled out in any smoker 40 years or older presenting with respiratory symptoms (cough, dyspnea, sputum production or activity limitation).
- The diagnosis of COPD is confirmed by spirometry.
- A post-bronchodilator FEV_1/FVC less than 70% is diagnostic of COPD.
- Staging of severity of this disease is based on percentage of predicted FEV_1: mild is greater than 80%, moderate is 50% to 80%, severe is between 30% and 50%, and very severe less than 30% (or less than 50% in the presence of signs of chronic respiratory failure).
- The course of COPD may be complicated by multiple extrapulmonary comorbidities such as cardiac disease, depression, osteoporosis, and muscle wasting.

Abbreviations: COPD = chronic obstructive pulmonary disease; FEV_1 = forced expiratory volume in 1 second; FVC = forced vital capacity.

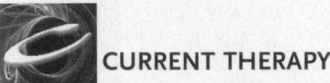

- COPD is a treatable disease.
- The goals for treatment of COPD are to reduce symptoms, exacerbations, complications, progression of the disease, and mortality and improve lung function, exercise tolerance, and health status (quality of life).
- Several pharmacologic and nonpharmacologic interventions are available.
- Smoking cessation is the most important intervention in the management of COPD.
- Nonpharmacologic interventions include influenza vaccination, exercise, and pulmonary rehabilitation.
- All symptomatic patients with COPD should be treated with medications.
- Pharmacologic agents available include bronchodilators (short-acting and long-acting) and inhaled corticosteroids in combination with long-acting β_2-agonists.
- Short-acting bronchodilators should be considered for rescue of symptoms, and long-acting bronchodilators (β_2-agonists and anticholinergics) should be considered for maintenance therapy in all stages of severity.
- Inhaled corticosteroids should be considered in patients with recurrent exacerbations and those with severe disease (FEV_1 <50% predicted).
- Oxygen therapy should be considered in stable patients who on optimal therapy have documented hypoxemia on room air (Po_2 <55 mm Hg).
- Surgical interventions in COPD are limited to some patients with severe emphysema.

Abbreviations: COPD = chronic obstructive pulmonary disease; FEV_1 = forced expiratory volume in 1 second; FVC = forced vital capacity.

Epidemiology

Chronic obstructive pulmonary disease (COPD) is the sixth most prevalent chronic medical condition in the United States, affecting more than 5% of the population. It is estimated that COPD is not diagnosed in 50% of patients suffering from it, probably because symptoms early in the disease are very subtle, causing delay in seeking medical attention, and because spirometry testing is underutilized. For many years, COPD was thought to be a disease of "old men"; however, its incidence has dramatically increased in women, and middle-aged (45–65 years) persons are also at risk. COPD causes more than 700,000 hospitalizations every year. COPD is the fourth leading cause of death in the United States, leading to more than 120,000 deaths every year. COPD-related mortality in women has now surpassed that of men in the United States. The annual cost of COPD in the United States exceeds $42 billion, with the majority of costs being secondary to issues related to COPD exacerbations.

Risk Factors

Cigarette smoking is the most common cause of COPD, and most patients report a smoking history of more than 20 pack-years upon diagnosis. Genetic susceptibility is important in this disease because only 20% to 30% of smokers develop the disease. α_1-Antripsyn deficiency is currently the only known genetic risk factor, but it is a rare cause of the disease and several other genes remain to be identified. In addition to cigarette smoke, other environmental exposures can lead to COPD; these include environmental tobacco smoke, occupational exposures, and exposures to air pollution. The role of recurrent respiratory infections in causing COPD is still debatable.

Pathophysiology

COPD is a multicomponent disease caused by exposure to noxious agents including cigarette smoke. The increased exposure to oxidative stress is believed to be the most important trigger for this disease in susceptible persons. COPD manifests with impaired lung function (including expiratory airflow limitation, hyperinflation, and abnormalities of gas exchange), which leads to respiratory symptoms including dyspnea, exercise limitation, and deconditioning. Airflow limitation in this disease is caused by airway inflammation, mucociliary dysfunction, and structural changes in the lung parenchyma (destruction and loss of elastic recoil), small airways (airway remodeling), and pulmonary vasculature (pulmonary hypertension). Large airways show hypertrophy of mucous glands and infiltration of the airway walls with inflammatory cells.

Clinically, chronic bronchitis with cough and sputum production occurring in the majority of patients is a manifestation of large airways involvement; however, physiologically, this large airways involvement does not contribute markedly to the airflow limitation. Small airways involvement includes airway inflammation which occurs in all stages of severity and is characterized by infiltration with neutrophils, macrophages, and T-lymphocytes (particularly $CD8^+$), luminal obstruction with inflammatory mucus, airway wall thickening, and hypertrophy of airway smooth muscles.

Lung parenchymal involvement in COPD manifests with destruction of alveolar walls and enlargement of alveolar spaces beyond terminal bronchioles (emphysema). With disease advancement, the airspace enlargement creates large empty spaces called *bullae*. Loss of lung tissue results in reduced alveolar-capillary membrane that is needed for gas exchange and reduced lung elastic recoil. These changes cause impaired gas exchange, increased lung volume and hyperinflation, airflow limitation, and exercise impairment. Involvement of vasculature includes thickening of the vessel wall and endothelial dysfunction. Loss of capillaries due to emphysema and associated hypoxemia in advanced COPD results in pulmonary hypertension.

Prevention

COPD is a preventable disease. Because more than 90% of patients with the disease are smokers, smoking cessation is an important intervention to prevent this disease. In patients with the disease, smoking cessation was shown to slow the decline in lung function and mortality. Other preventive measures should include avoiding exposure to respiratory irritants such as environmental tobacco smoke (secondhand smoke) and respiratory infections (by receiving vaccinations). None of the pharmacologic interventions available for treating COPD can diminish the deterioration in lung function that occurs with this disease.

Clinical Manifestations

COPD is a slowly progressive disease that ultimately causes severe limitation of physical activity, deterioration of quality of life, and ultimately premature death. COPD commonly occurs in patients who are 40 years of age and older. In most instances, the smoking history is very prominent (>20 pack-years). Cough and sputum production (chronic bronchitis) are present in the majority of patients. Early in the disease, symptoms may be subtle, and many patients relate them to the aging process. Fatigue and activity limitation are very common. Dyspnea on exertion is common, although many patients limit their activity and might not report dyspnea until late in the disease. Dyspnea is usually progressive and leads to exercise intolerance.

The course of COPD is often complicated with repeated exacerbations, which are the first presenting symptoms in some cases. Several extrapulmonary morbidities can complicate its course, including cardiac disease, depression, osteoporosis, and muscle wasting. Several clinical phenotypes for COPD that can have therapeutic implications have been described, although these need to be further explored.

Diagnosis

The diagnosis of COPD should be considered in any smoker who is 40 years of age or older who presents with respiratory symptoms such as smoker's cough, sputum production, dyspnea, or activity limitation. Many patients with COPD do not perceive symptoms, and therefore thorough questioning by clinicians is of paramount importance.

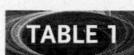

TABLE 1 Stepwise Approach to the Pharmacologic Management of COPD

SEVERITY	SPIROMETRIC FINDINGS	INTERVENTION
Stage I: mild	$FEV_1/FVC < 70\%$ $FEV_1 \geq 80\%$	Add a short-acting bronchodilator to be used when needed; anticholinergic or β_2-adrenoceptor agonist
Stage II: moderate	$FEV_1/FVC < 70\%$ $50\% \leq FEV_1 < 80\%$	Add one or more long-acting bronchodilators on a scheduled basis Consider pulmonary rehabilitation.
Stage III: severe	$FEV_1/FVC < 70\%$ $30\% \leq FEV_1 < 50\%$	Add inhaled steroids if repeated exacerbations
Stage IV: very severe	$FEV_1/FVC < 70\%$ $FEV_1 < 30\%$	Evaluate for adding oxygen Consider surgical options

Abbreviations: FEV_1 = forced expiratory volume in 1 sec; FVC = forced vital capacity.

Physical examination of the COPD patient may be normal, and the classic "blue bloater" and "pink puffer" phenotypes are rarely seen early in the disease process. Patients with advanced emphysema may have evidence of hyperinflation on chest examination (barrel-shaped chest and hyperresonance), use of accessory muscles, and muscle wasting (cachexia). Spirometry should be performed on patients who report symptoms. The diagnosis of COPD is made based on the demonstration airway obstruction following bronchodilator administration: forced expiratory volume in 1 second per forced vital capacity (FEV_1/FVC) less than 70%. The severity of the disease is based on the percentage of predicted FEV_1 and is classified into four stages (Table 1).

Lung volume measurements as well as measurement of the diffusion capacity (DLCO) of the lung can aid in assessing the presence of hyperinflation (increased lung volume) and lung destruction (low DLCO). A 6-minute walk test can help in assessing exercise tolerance and to rule out exercise-induced hypoxemia, although it is not routinely needed in patients with mild disease. Although the role of the chest radiograph in diagnosing COPD is limited, it is usually needed during the initial evaluation to rule out other pathologies such as lung cancer. Screening for α_1-antitrypsin deficiency is also recommended in all patients with COPD. Routine use of computed tomography (CT) has no utility in the routine diagnosis of COPD, although it may be helpful in detecting early emphysema.

Differential Diagnosis

Several diseases can manifest with symptoms and signs of COPD. Asthma and COPD have similar symptoms and signs. Asthma usually has an early onset as opposed to COPD, which rarely occurs before the fourth decade. The presence of allergy history, family history, and the absence of smoking history favors the diagnosis of asthma. Spirometry can show complete reversibility in asthma, and partial reversibility is usually observed in COPD. Another lung disease that can mimic COPD is bronchiectasis. Dyspnea may be a presenting symptom in diseases other than COPD in the elderly population; these include congestive heart failure and coronary insufficiency.

Treatment
Goals of Therapy

The main goals of therapy of COPD are focused on relieving symptoms, improving health status, preserving lung function from decline, improving exercise performance, preventing exacerbations, and decreasing mortality. These goals should be reached with minimal side effects from treatment. Traditional COPD therapies have focused on controlling symptoms and aim to alleviate the problems of reduced airflow and declining lung function. However, with our improved knowledge about the multicomponent nature of the disease, therapeutic approaches aim to target both the symptoms and the inflammation that underlies and drives COPD.

Nonpharmacologic Interventions
Vaccination

Reducing further damage to lung tissue is a main goal of therapy in any chronic lung disease. With that in mind, yearly influenza vaccination (killed [Fluzone, Fluarix] or live inactive [FluMist] viruses) can reduce more-severe forms of influenza and acute exacerbations of COPD (by 60%). Pneumococcal vaccination (Pneumovax 23) reduces invasive pneumococcal disease and is recommended in COPD patients with more-severe lung disease ($FEV_1 < 40\%$) and elderly patients.

Smoking Cessation

Smoking cessation is the single most effective and cost-effective intervention to reduce the progression of COPD and should be attempted in all patients. Unfortunately, even with the best intervention strategies, less than a third of smokers become sustained quitters. Once patients develop demonstrable airflow obstruction, their symptoms and airway inflammation can persist even after smoking cessation. Several effective therapies for tobacco dependence are available and should be considered in patients interested in quitting smoking. These include behavioral techniques, support groups, and pharmacotherapy (Table 2) including nicotine supplements, bupropion (Zyban), and nicotine-receptor partial agonists like varenicline (Chantix).

Exercise and Pulmonary Rehabilitation

Pulmonary rehabilitation is currently recommended to be considered in the management of patients with moderate or worse COPD. Pulmonary rehabilitation is an individualized multidisciplinary program that aims to optimize patients' performance and self-control. The program includes upper and lower body and breathing exercises; nutritional, psychological, and behavioral interventions; and education. Pulmonary rehabilitation

TABLE 2 Pharmacologic Therapies for Smoking Cessation

DRUG	DOSE	FREQUENCY
Oral		
Nicotine polacrilex (Nicotine gum, Nicorette)	2 mg, 4 mg	10–20 mg/d, q1–2h
Nicotine lozenges/ tablets (Commit)	2 mg, 4 mg	10–20 mg/d 1 piece every h
Bupropion sustained-release (Zyban)	150 mg	150 mg × 3 d, then 300 mg qd
Varenicline (Chantix)	1 mg	Initial 1-week dose titration, then 1 mg bid × 12 wk
Patch		
Nicotine Transdermal System Step 1, 2, 3	21, 14, 7 mg	Over 24 h
Nicoderm CQ Step 1, 2, 3 Nicotrol Step 1, 2, 3	15, 10, 5 mg	Over 16 h
Prostep	22, 11 mg	Over 24 h
Inhaled		
Nicotine nasal spray (Nicotrol NS)	0.5 mg/inhalation	10–40 mg/d in hourly or prn dosing
Nicotine inhaler (Nicotrol Inhaler)	10 mg/ampule	6–10 ampules/d

produces significant improvement in respiratory symptoms, exercise capacity, quality of life, and health care utilization.

Surgical Therapies

Lung volume reduction surgery (LVERS) includes resection of severely emphysematous areas of the lungs. The procedure can be performed through thoracoscopy or median sternotomy. In the National Emphysema Treatment Trial (NETT), LVRS improved spirometry, lung volumes, exercise tolerance, dyspnea, and quality of life. Subjects with upper lobe disease and low baseline exercise capacity had improved longevity when compared to optimal medical therapy. In contrast, NETT showed that patients with very advanced COPD including FEV_1 of 20% or less, diffusing capacity of 20% or less, or diffuse emphysema had shorter longevity with LVRS. LVRS can help COPD patients with severe lung disease as long as it is performed in centers with experience in this type of surgery.

COPD patients with giant bulla (>1/3 hemithorax) might benefit from bullectomy with improvement in symptoms (dyspnea), lung function, oxygenation and ventilation, exercise capacity, and quality of life.

In selected patients with advanced COPD, lung transplant can improve pulmonary function, exercise capacity, and quality of life.

Pharmacologic Interventions

Evidence-based guidelines for COPD emphasize the comprehensive and stepwise approach to the management of COPD and stipulate that all patients who are symptomatic merit a trial of pharmacologic intervention (see Table 1). Short-acting bronchodilators given when needed are recommended for patients with intermittent symptoms such as cough, wheeze, or exertional dyspnea. However, maintenance therapy should be initiated in patients who have persistent symptoms such as dyspnea or nighttime awakenings, despite use of as-needed short-acting agents. In this setting, maintenance treatment should be initiated with a long-acting bronchodilator or, alternatively, a short-acting agent given four times per day. Rescue therapy with albuterol (Proventil, Ventolin) should be continued as needed. If the benefit of treatment is limited, then a bronchodilator from another drug class or a combination of two drug classes (e.g., long-acting bronchodilator plus inhaled corticosteroids [ICS]) should be attempted. The addition of regular ICS therapy should be considered in patients with FEV_1 less than 50% of predicted who had disease exacerbations requiring a course of oral steroids or antibiotics at least once in the preceding year.

Bronchodilators

Bronchodilators work through their direct relaxation effect on airway smooth muscle cells, although many have non-bronchodilator activities that might contribute to their beneficial effects in COPD. Three classes of bronchodilators—β_2-agonists, anticholinergics, and theophylline—are currently available and can be used individually or in combination (Box 1).

Several issues need to be considered when assessing the response to bronchodilator therapy. First, the lack of acute response to one class of bronchodilator does not necessarily imply nonresponsiveness to another. One further consideration is that a patient's FEV_1 response to acute bronchodilator therapy does not predict long-term response to bronchodilator therapy and can vary from day to day. The clinical efficacy of bronchodilators has traditionally been assessed by the degree of improvement in FEV_1. However, other physiologic measures, such as the change in inspiratory capacity (IC), correlate better with change in symptoms, such as dyspnea and exercise tolerance. This suggests that assessment of bronchodilator treatment using indices of hyperinflation or air trapping might provide a better indicator of efficacy. Although changes in lung volumes are independent of changes in FEV_1, several studies have demonstrated that the more-sustained airway patency offered by long-acting bronchodilators reduces air trapping.

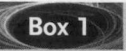 Box 1   Commonly Used Pharmacologic Agents for COPD

Short-Acting Agents
β_2-Adrenoceptor Agonists
Albuterol (Ventolin, Proventil, ProAir, AccuNeb) (MDI, NS)
Levalbuterol (Xopenex) (MDI, NS)
Pirbuterol (Maxair) (MDI)

Anticholinergic
Ipratropium bromide (Atrovent) (MDI, NS)

Fixed Combination
Albuterol-ipratropium (Combivent, DuoNeb) (MDI, NS)

Long-Acting Agents
β_2-Adrenoceptor Agonists
Salmeterol (Serevent Diskus) (DPI)
Formoterol (Foradil, Perforomist) (DPI, NS)
Arformoterol (Brovana) (NS)

Anticholinergic
Tiotropium bromide (Spiriva) (DPI)

Fixed Combination
Salmeterol-fluticasone (Advair Diskus, Advair HFA)* (DPI, MDI)
Formoterol/Budesonide (Symbicort)† (MDI)

Methylxanthines
Theophylline (Uniphyl, Theo-24) (PO)

---

*Only one dose formulation (250/50) is approved for COPD in the United States.
†Only one dose formulation (160/4.5) approved for COPD in the United States.
Abbreviations: COPD = chronic obstructive pulmonary disease; DPI = dry powder inhaler; MDI = metered dose inhaler; NS = nebulized solution; PO = oral preparation.

Several other outcome measures are now used to assess response to bronchodilator therapy. COPD exacerbation is an important but occasionally overlooked parameter. The use of long-acting β_2-adrenoceptor agonists and long-acting anticholinergic agents reduces the frequency of exacerbation and severity of individual exacerbations. The effects of long-acting bronchodilators on health status have been well documented in several clinical trials. The long-term effects of tiotropium (Spiriva) on the decline in postbronchodilator FEV_1 over 4 years was investigated in the Understanding of Potential Long-term Impact on Function with Tiotropium trial (UPLIFT). Although tiotropium failed to slow the decline in lung function over the 4 years of the study, it had a significant effect on improving health status and reducing exacerbations.

To achieve maximal benefit, a bronchodilator must be correctly delivered to the airway using a proper technique. Inhaled bronchodilators have traditionally been delivered to the lung using a metered dose inhaler (MDI). However, a significant number of patients with COPD cannot effectively coordinate their breathing using an MDI. This problem may be remedied by the use of a dry-powder device (DPI), an MDI with a spacer device, or a nebulizer.

Inhaled Corticosteroids

Given the prominence of airway inflammation in COPD, highly potent but nonspecific antiinflammatory agents such as corticosteroids could be expected to have some effects on lung function and health outcomes of COPD patients. Although these agents appear to have minimal significant effects on key inflammatory chemoattractants, there are data to suggest an association with reduced neutrophil chemotaxis. Current guidelines recommend the use of regular treatment with ICS for symptomatic patients who suffer frequent exacerbations and whose FEV_1 is less than 50% of predicted. Several large, 3-year randomized trials have failed to show a significant effect of ICS on the rate of decline of FEV_1, compared with placebo.

Although both ICS and long-acting β_2-agonists (LABAs) are effective by themselves in improving lung function and reducing exacerbations, their beneficial effects are amplified when they are given together. There is a large and growing body of experimental and clinical evidence supporting the use of combination therapy with inhaled corticosteroids and LABAs for the long-term treatment of COPD patients with moderate to severe disease. The use of ICS and LABA combination products has been shown to improve lung function, symptoms, and health status and reduce exacerbations in patients with moderate to severe COPD. More recently, a large ($N = 6112$) 3-year study, TORCH, demonstrated a significant effect of therapy with salmeterol-fluticasone combination (SFC) (Advair) over 3 years on several COPD outcomes. SFC had a 2.6% absolute risk reduction in all-cause mortality compared to placebo ($P = 0.052$) and was significantly superior to placebo and both component drugs in reducing moderate-to-severe exacerbations and improving health status ($P < 0.001$). Over the 3-year treatment period, patients taking SFC experienced a 25% reduction in the annual rate of moderate-to-severe exacerbations compared with placebo ($P < 0.001$).

Oropharyngeal candidiasis was reported as the most common adverse event for the use of LABA-ICS combination relative to placebo over a period of 24 to 52 weeks, with headache, upper respiratory tract infection, and musculoskeletal pain reported less frequently. Data from TORCH showed that neither SFC, salmeterol alone (Serevent) or fluticasone alone (Flovent) led to increased cardiac disorders, ophthalmic adverse events, or increased probability of bone fractures over the 3-year treatment period. However, an unexpected safety finding was an increased incidence of pneumonia reported in patients taking fluticasone and SFC.

Oxygen

Supplemental long-term oxygen therapy (LTOT) has been associated with a variety of beneficial effects in patients with severe COPD who are hypoxemic in room air. These include prolonged survival, reduced secondary polycythemia, improved cardiac function during rest and exercise, reduction in the oxygen cost of ventilation, and improved exercise tolerance. Patients with Pao_2 less than 55 mm Hg (Sao_2 <88%) whose disease is stable despite receiving otherwise comprehensive medical treatment are candidates to receive LTOT. Patients whose Pao_2 is 55 to 59 mm Hg (Sao_2 89%) are eligible to receive LTOT if they show signs of pulmonary hypertension, cor pulmonale, erythrocytosis, edema from right heart failure, or impaired mental state. If oxygen desaturation only occurs during exercise or sleep, then oxygen therapy should be considered specifically under those conditions.

Mucolytics

Mucus impaction contributes to worsening of symptoms of patients with COPD. A number of studies investigating the role of mucolytics such as potassium iodide (SSKI, Pima)[1] and guaifenesin (Mucinex)[1] failed to demonstrate significant clinical efficacy of these agents in the management of patients with COPD, although some have shown some decrease in COPD exacerbations. A variety of new agents addressing mucociliary clearance and mucus production are under investigation.

Antibiotics

Although empiric treatment with antibiotics has been shown to be of benefit in COPD exacerbations (see later), their role in chronic management is not well defined and their use is currently not recommended. The role of chronic macrolide therapy in COPD is under investigation.

Augmentation Therapy for α_1-Antitrypsin Deficiency

Replacement therapy with α_1-proteinase inhibitor (Prolastin) has been approved for patients with emphysema due to the α_1-antiprotease deficiency. Given in weekly infusions to patients with ZZ or null AAT phenotypes, therapy can increase serum levels above the target threshold of 11 μM and can provide protective levels within the epithelial lining of the lung. Although AAT augmentation therapy has a sound theoretical basis, proof of its efficacy has been difficult to document. However, available evidence supports the use of this therapy in patients with AAT serum levels less than 11 μM and FEV_1 between 30% and 65% predicted, but it might not be useful in other subsets of patients with COPD.

Complications
COPD Exacerbations

AECOPD is defined as worsening of respiratory symptoms including dyspnea, cough, and sputum production beyond daily variations that warrant change in therapy. AECOPD is associated with worsening quality of life and faster decline of lung function. AECOPD has a 10% in-hospital mortality rate and up to 25% mortality in patients admitted to an ICU. Although AECOPD is usually caused by bacterial or viral infections, environmental pollution, and lack of compliance with medications, in many cases the cause is not clear. Differential diagnosis of AECOPD includes pneumonia, myocardial ischemia, congestive heart failure, pneumothorax, pleural effusion, pulmonary embolism, cardiac arrhythmias, and noncompliance with medications.

For treatment purposes, AECOPD severity is divided into level I (ambulatory), level II (requiring hospitalization), and level III (acute respiratory failure). The evaluation of patients during AECOPD should include the severity of COPD, comorbid medical conditions, and history of prior AECOPD and its outcomes, including hospitalization and intubation. Effect of AECOPD on respiratory and hemodynamic function should be evaluated and considered for severity classifications. Initial diagnostic procedures, depending on the severity of AECOPD, include saturation of oxygen, chest radiography, electrocardiogram (ECG), and routine blood tests, including complete blood count (CBC) and basic metabolic panel. Other diagnostic tests may be indicated to rule out other diagnoses.

Early treatment of AECOPD is associated with faster recovery. Main pharmacotherapy includes increased short-acting bronchodilators, antibiotics, and systemic steroids. Short-acting β-agonists (albuterol [Proventil, Ventolin]) and anticholinergics (ipratropium [Atrovent]) offer similar benefits. Several studies have shown reduction in treatment failure and mortality (especially for in-patient treatment) with the use of antibiotics for AECOPD. Systemic corticosteroids reduce treatment failure and length of hospital stay and improve FEV_1 but are associated with increased side effects, particularly hyperglycemia. Nonpharmacotherapeutic interventions include supplemental oxygen and ventilatory support.

Outpatient therapy for AECOPD includes educating the patient and reviewing how to use various inhalational agents. Optimization of short-acting bronchodilator use with a spacer or in the form of nebulized therapy is the mainstay of therapy in mild AECOPD. Systemic steroids at a dose of 40 to 60 mg daily for 10 to 14 days and oral antibiotics (in patients with altered sputum characteristics) may be indicated. First-line antibiotic therapy includes macrolides, doxycycline, and cephalosporins. In case of treatment failure, respiratory fluoroquinolones or amoxicillin-clavulanate (Augmentin) are recommended.

For patients with level II AECOPD or hospitalized patients, in addition to optimization of short-acting bronchodilator therapy and systemic steroids, antibiotics should be started in patients with changed sputum characteristics. Antibiotic should be chosen on

---

[1]Not FDA approved for this indication.

the basis of the local bacterial resistance patterns. In level III AECOPD, special attention should be given to more resistant bacteria, such as *Pseudomonas* spp. In such cases, combination antibiotics should be considered.

Patients with more severe AECOPD (levels II and III) need supplemental oxygen if oxygen saturation is less than 90%. In case of respiratory failure, noninvasive or invasive ventilator support may be needed. Noninvasive ventilatory support reduces the risk of intubation, in-hospital mortality, and the length of hospitalization.

References

Agusti AG. COPD, a multicomponent disease: implications for management. Respir Med 2005;99:670–82.

American Thoracic Society/European Respiratory Society. Statement: Standards for the diagnosis and management of individuals with alpha-1 antitrypsin deficiency. Am J Respir Crit Care Med 2003;168:818–900.

Calverley PM, Anderson JA, Celli B, et al. Salmeterol and fluticasone propionate and survival in chronic obstructive pulmonary disease. N Engl J Med 2007;356:775–89.

Carlin BW. Pulmonary rehabilitation: A focus on COPD in primary care. Postgrad Med 2009;121(6):140–7.

Cazzola M, Hanania NA, Jones PW, et al. It's about time—directing our attention toward modifying the course of COPD. Respir Med 2008;102(Suppl. 1):S37–48.

Celli BR, Barnes PJ. Exacerbations of chronic obstructive pulmonary disease. Eur Respir J 2007;29:1224–38.

Celli BR, Macnee W. Standards for the diagnosis and treatment of patients with COPD: A summary of the ATS/ERS position paper. Eur Respir J 2004;23: 932–46.

Edwards MA, Hazelrigg S, Naunheim KS. The National Emphysema Treatment Trial: Summary and update. Thorac Surg Clin 2009;19(2):169–85.

Fiore MC. US public health service clinical practice guideline: treating tobacco use and dependence. Respir Care 2000;45:1200–62.

Hanania NA. Optimizing maintenance therapy for chronic obstructive pulmonary disease: Strategies for improving patient-centered outcomes. Clin Ther 2007;29 (10):2121–33.

Hanania NA, Donohue JF. Pharmacologic interventions in chronic obstructive pulmonary disease: Bronchodilators. Proc Am Thorac Soc 2007;4(7):526–34.

Hanania NA, Sharafkhaneh A. Update on the pharmacologic therapy for chronic obstructive pulmonary disease. Clin Chest Med 2007;28(3):589–607.

Mundey K. An appraisal of smoking cessation aids. Curr Opin Pulm Med 2009;15 (2):105–12.

Nocturnal Oxygen Therapy Trial Group. Continuous or nocturnal oxygen therapy in hypoxemic chronic obstructive lung disease: A clinical trial. Ann Intern Med 1980;93:391–8.

Quon BS, Gan WQ, Sin DD. Contemporary management of acute exacerbations of COPD: a systematic review and metaanalysis. Chest 2008;133(3):756–66.

Rabe KF, Hurd S, Anzueto A, et al. Global strategy for the diagnosis, management, and prevention of COPD—2006 update. Am J Respir Crit Care Med 2007;176 (6):532–55.

Tashkin DP, Celli B, Senn S, et al. UPLIFT Study Investigators. A 4-year trial of tiotropium in chronic obstructive pulmonary disease. N Engl J Med 2008;359 (15):1543–54.

Varkey JB, Varkey AB, Varkey B. Prophylactic vaccinations in chronic obstructive pulmonary disease: Current status. Curr Opin Pulm Med 2009;15(2):90–9.

COCCIDIOIDOMYCOSIS

Method of
Gregory M. Anstead, MD

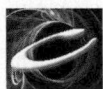

CURRENT DIAGNOSIS

- Maintain a high index of suspicion in patients from endemic areas and travelers.
- Diagnostic tests include:
  - Serologic detection of immunoglobulin M and immunoglobulin G antibodies by immunodiffusion, complement fixation, and enzyme immunoassay
  - Culture of sputum, exudates, cerebrospinal fluid, and tissue
  - Direct observation of *Coccidioides* spherules in histopathologic and cytologic specimens
  - Urine antigen enzyme immunoassay

CURRENT THERAPY

Pulmonary Infection

- No risk factors for dissemination; not severe disease—observe
- Risk factors; prolonged symptoms—fluconazole (Diflucan)[1] 400 mg/day or itraconazole (Sporanox)[1] 200 mg twice a day for 3 to 6 months
- Diffuse or severe pneumonia—amphotericin B (Fungizone) 1 mg/kg/day or lipid formulation of amphotericin (Abelcet, AmBisome)[1] 5 mg/kg/day; after improvement, switch to azole; treat for 1 year
- Chronic fibrocavitary disease—azole therapy for at least 1 year; resection in selected cases

Disseminated Disease

- Nonmeningeal, severe disease—amphotericin B 1 mg/kg/day or lipid formulation of amphotericin[1] 5 mg/kg/day; after improvement, switch to azole for 1 to 2 years; consider posaconazole (Noxafil)[1] 200 mg four times daily in refractory cases
- Nonmeningeal, slowly progressive—azole therapy for 1 to 2 years; itraconazole[1] preferred for bony involvement; consider posaconazole[1] 200 mg four times daily in refractory cases
- Meningeal, central nervous system involvement—fluconazole 800 to 2000 mg/day[3]; intrathecal amphotericin B[1] or voriconazole (Vfend)[1] 200 mg twice daily in refractory cases; shunting for hydrocephalus; consider corticosteroids if vasculitis is present

[1]Not FDA approved for this indication.
[3]Exceeds dosage recommended by the manufacturer.

Coccidioidomycosis is caused by soil fungi of the genus *Coccidioides*, divided genetically into *Coccidioides immitis* (California isolates) and *Coccidioides posadasii* (isolates outside California). There are no distinct clinical differences between the two species. *Coccidioides* occurs only in the Western hemisphere, primarily in the southwestern United States (Arizona and parts of California, New Mexico, Utah, Nevada, and Texas) and in northern Mexico, areas characterized by arid to semiarid climates, hot summers, low altitude, alkaline soil, and sparse vegetation. Hyperendemic areas include the San Joaquin Valley of California and Pima, Pinal, and Maricopa Counties in Arizona. *Coccidioides* is also found in parts of Latin America (Guatemala, Honduras, Nicaragua, Argentina, Paraguay, Venezuela, and Colombia). Cases may be observed in nonendemic areas because of travel or reactivation of prior infection. In the United States, an estimated 150,000 cases of coccidioidomycosis occur annually, with the clinical presentation ranging from a self-limited respiratory infection to devastating disseminated disease. Persons with occupations involving exposure to soil are at risk for coccidioidomycosis. Immunocompromised persons are also at high risk, including patients with AIDS, transplant recipients (especially those who received *Coccidioides*-infected organs), patients receiving tumor necrosis factor-α antagonists, pregnant women, and cancer patients. Filipinos, African Americans, and persons with blood group B are also at increased risk for disseminated disease. Outbreaks may occur after dust storms, earthquakes, droughts, and activities causing soil disruption, such as construction and archeological digs.

Coccidioides is dimorphic; in the soil, the organism exists in its mycelial form, which produces barrel-shaped arthroconidia. The usual means of infection is the inhalation of arthroconidia; uncommon routes include direct cutaneous inoculation and organ transplantation. Arthroconidia germinate to produce spherules filled with endospores, the characteristic tissue phase. Spherules rupture to release endospores, which form additional spherules. The spherules become surrounded by neutrophils and macrophages, which leads to granuloma formation. Both B and T lymphocytes are essential for host defense against this pathogen.

Clinical Manifestations

Coccidioidomycosis is asymptomatic in 60% of infected individuals. In the remaining 40% a self-limited, flu-like illness, with dry cough, pleuritic chest pain, myalgias, arthralgia, fever, sweats, anorexia, and weakness, develops 1 to 3 weeks after exposure. Primary infection may be accompanied by immune complex–mediated complications, including an erythematous macular rash, erythema multiforme, and erythema nodosum. Acute infection usually resolves without therapy, although symptoms may persist for weeks. In 5% of these patients, asymptomatic pulmonary residua persist, including pulmonary nodules and cavitation. Immunocompromised patients may develop chronic progressive pulmonary infection, with the evolution of thin-walled cavities that may rupture, leading to bronchopleural fistula and empyema formation.

Extrapulmonary disease develops in 1 of every 200 patients and can involve the skin, soft tissues, bones, joints, and meninges. The most common cutaneous lesions are verrucous papules, ulcers, or plaques. The spine is the most frequent site of osseous dissemination, although the typical lytic lesions may also occur in the skull, hands, feet, and tibia. Joint involvement is usually monoarticular and most commonly involves the ankle and knee. Fungemia may occur in immunocompromised patients and carries a poor prognosis.

In coccidioidal meningitis, the basilar meninges are usually affected. Cerebrospinal fluid findings include lymphocytic pleocytosis (often with eosinophilia), hypoglycorrachia, and elevated protein levels. The mortality rate is greater than 90% at 1 year without therapy, and chronic infection is the rule. Hydrocephalus or hydrocephalus coexisting with brain infarction is associated with a higher mortality rate.

Coccidioidomycosis is a great imitator and has many diverse clinical presentations, including immune thrombocytopenia, ocular involvement, massive cervical lymphadenopathy, laryngeal and retropharyngeal abscesses, endocarditis, pericarditis, peritonitis, hepatitis, and lesions of the male and female genitals and urogenital tracts.

Diagnosis

Coccidioidomycosis may be diagnosed by direct observation of spherules in tissues or in wet mounts of sputa or exudates. The growth of Coccidioides in culture usually occurs in 3 to 5 days, with sporulation after 5 to 10 days. Definitive identification is made by DNA probe or exoantigen testing. Laboratory personnel should exercise extreme caution when handling cultures of Coccidioides.

Serologic methods are quite useful in establishing the diagnosis and for monitoring the course of the infection. Immunoglobulin M (IgM) antibodies are present soon after infection or relapse but then wane; quantification does not correlate with disease severity. The IgG antibody appears later and remains positive for months. Rising titers of IgG are associated with progressive disease, and declining titers are associated with resolution. The IgG antibodies are able to fix complement when combined with coccidioidal antigen, and can be detected by immunodiffusion for complement fixation (IDCF); titers of 1:16 or greater suggest disseminated disease. In the cerebrospinal fluid, a positive IDCF of any titer is considered diagnostic of meningitis and is much more sensitive than culture in making the diagnosis. An enzyme immunoassay is also available, but it is less specific. Recently, a specific urinary antigen test became available for the diagnosis of coccidioidomycosis; this assay has a sensitivity of 71% in moderate-to-severe disease, compared with 84% for culture, 29% for histopathologic examination, and 75% for serologic testing.

Treatment

In most patients, primary pulmonary infection resolves spontaneously without treatment. However, all patients require observation for at least 2 years to document resolution of infection and to identify any complications as soon as possible. For patients who have risk factors for disseminated disease (listed earlier), treatment is necessary. Other indications for treatment are severe disease (infiltrates involving both lungs or more than half of one lung; significant hilar or mediastinal lymphadenopathy; complement fixation titers

>1:16) and highly symptomatic disease (weight loss >10%; night sweats present for >3 weeks; symptoms present for >2 months).

For diffuse or severe pneumonia, therapy with amphotericin B deoxycholate (Fungizone) 0.5 to 1.5 mg/kg/day, or a lipid formulation of amphotericin B (Abelcet or AmBisome)[1] 2 to 5 mg/kg/day should be given for several weeks, followed by an oral azole, such as itraconazole (Sporanox)[1] 200 mg twice daily or fluconazole (Diflucan)[1] 400 to 800 mg/day). The total duration of therapy should be at least 1 year; for immunosuppressed patients, oral azole therapy should be maintained as secondary prophylaxis. In HIV patients with CD4-positive T-cell counts greater than 250 cells/mm^3 who had focal pneumonias that responded to azoles, antifungals may be discontinued. Azole therapy may be used initially for less severe disease. During pregnancy, amphotericin B is the preferred drug, because of the teratogenicity of azoles.

An asymptomatic patient with a solitary nodule or pulmonary cavitation due to C. immitis does not require specific antifungal therapy or resection. However, the development of complications from the cavitation, such as hemoptysis or bacterial or fungal superinfection, necessitates initiation of azole therapy. Resection of the cavities is an alternative to antifungal therapy. Rupture of a cavity into the pleural space requires surgical intervention with closure by lobectomy with decortication, in addition to antifungal therapy. For chronic pneumonia, the initial treatment should be an oral azole for at least 1 year. If the disease persists, one may switch to another oral azole, increase the dose if fluconazole was initially selected, or switch to amphotericin B. Resection should be performed for patients with refractory focal lesions or severe hemoptysis.

The treatment of disseminated infection without central nervous system involvement is based on oral azole therapy, such as itraconazole or fluconazole (400 mg/day, or higher in case of fluconazole). If there is little or no improvement or if there is vertebral involvement, treatment with amphotericin B is recommended (dosage as for diffuse pneumonia). Concomitant surgical débridement or stabilization is also recommended. In patients with refractory coccidioidomycosis that has failed to respond to fluconazole, itraconazole, and amphotericin B and its lipid formulations, treatment with posaconazole (Noxafil)[1] 200 mg four times daily has been successful.

For coccidioidal meningitis, lifetime treatment with azoles is indicated. Fluconazole, at doses of 800 mg/day or higher,[3] is recommended. There have been a few reports of successful treatment of coccidioidal meningitis with voriconazole (Vfend)[1] 200 mg orally twice daily after a loading dose. Itraconazole is not recommended because of its irregular oral absorption. Obstructive hydrocephalus requires shunting. Intrathecal amphotericin B[1] was previously used for meningeal coccidioidomycosis, but it is now strictly reserved for infections that are refractory to high-dose azoles.

---

[1]Not FDA approved for this indication.
[3]Exceeds dosage recommended by the manufacturer.

References

Ampel NM. New perspectives on coccidioidomycosis. Proc Am Thorac Soc 2010;7:181–5.

Anstead GM, Graybill JR. Coccidioidomycosis. Infect Dis Clin North Am 2006;20:621–43.

Blair JE. State-of-the art treatment of coccidioidomycosis skeletal infections. Ann N Y Acad Sci 2007;1111:422–33.

Blair JE. State-of-the-art treatment of coccidiodomycosis skin and soft tissue infections. Ann N Y Acad Sci 2007;1111:411–21.

Crum NF, Lederman ER, Stafford CM, et al. Coccidioidomycosis: A descriptive survey of a reemerging disease—Clinical characteristics and emerging controversies. Medicine (Baltimore) 2004;83:149–75.

Crum-Cianflone NF, Truett AA, Teneza-Mora N, et al. Unusual presentations of coccidioidomycosis: A case series and review of the literature. Medicine (Baltimore) 2006;85:263–77.

Johnson L, Gaab EM, Sanchez J, et al. Valley fever: danger lurking in a dust cloud. Microbes Infect 2014;16:591–600.

Parish JM, Blair JE. Coccidioidomycosis. Mayo Clin Proc 2008;83:343–8;quiz 348–349.

Saubolle MA, McKellar PP, Sussland D. Epidemiologic, clinical, and diagnostic aspects of coccidioidomycosis. J Clin Microbiol 2007;45:26–30.

Williams PL. Coccidioidal meningitis. Ann N Y Acad Sci 2007;1111:377–84.

CYSTIC FIBROSIS

Method of
Robert Giusti, MD

Cystic fibrosis (CF), an autosomal recessive disease, is the most common lethal inherited disease in the white population. In this population the carrier rate is approximately 1 in 30, with an incidence of 1 in 3200 births. CF also occurs in African Americans (1 in 15,000), Hispanic Americans (1 in 8000) and Asian Americans (1 in 31,000), but diagnosis may be delayed because of a low index of suspicion in these ethnic groups. Lung disease is the primary cause of morbidity and mortality in CF. Progressive fibrosis and destruction of lung tissue from chronic cycles of infection and inflammation lead to respiratory failure. The median predicted age of survival for people with CF has risen steadily over the last 25 years. Since 2002, the median predicted survival age has increased almost 10 years from age 31.3 in 2002 to 41.1 in 2012.

Pathophysiology

The defect that results in CF is an abnormal gene located on the long arm of chromosome 7 that codes for a protein known as the cystic fibrosis transmembrane regulator (CFTR). This protein becomes incorporated into the lipid bilayer of the epithelial surface of the cell and functions as a chloride channel. Defective cyclic adenosine monophosphate (cAMP)-regulated chloride secretion through a mutated CFTR protein results in dehydrated airway surface fluid, which impedes the normal ciliary function, resulting in chronic infection and atelectasis. In addition, CFTR also down-regulates an epithelial sodium channel (ENaC). When CFTR is defective, this down-regulation is diminished, resulting in increased sodium reabsorption and a further reduction in airway surface fluid. The *CFTR* gene is expressed in the biliary ducts, vas deferens, pancreatic ducts, sweat glands, and the mucous glands of the lung.

Researchers have identified more than 1,800 mutations in the cystic fibrosis (CF) gene (http://www.genet.sickkids.on.ca/Home. html) The functional consequences of mutations at the cellular level have been classified based on the way the mutations affect the CFTR protein production (http://www.CFTR2.org). These genetic changes can be grouped into different types, based on how confident scientists are that the change actually causes the CF disease:

- **Confirmed CF-causing mutations.** These mutations are seen in people with CF. When a person inherits two of these mutations (one from each parent) that person will always have CF.
- **Suspected CF-causing mutations.** These are mutations that have been reported in people with CF, but have not been confirmed to always cause CF.
- **Variants of uncertain clinical impact.** We do not know if these mutations cause CF.
  - Mutations that sometimes cause CF, but sometimes do not.
  - Mutations that have not been found often enough through genetic testing to know for sure if they do or do not cause CF.
- **Mutations linked with having one or more symptoms related with CF.** When people who had one or two of the clinical signs of CF (for example, chronic pancreatitis, sinus disease or male infertility) but not full CF disease were examined, certain CF mutations were found. They can be called CF-related mutations and often overlap with the "variants of uncertain clinical impact" group.
- **Neutral variants.** These are genetic changes that do not cause CF.

There is excitement concerning possible new treatments for CF patients who have 2 copies of Delta 508 mutation. A Phase 3 Combination Studies of Ivacaftor (Kalydeco™) and Lumacaftor (VX-809) show that all four 24–week treatment arms achieved primary endpoint of mean absolute improvement in FEV_1 compared to placebo, with a range of 2.6 to 4.0 percentage points (p≤0.0004); mean relative improvement of 4.3% to 6.7% (p≤0.0007). In addition, Pooled analysis of Phase 3 studies showed statistically significant reductions of 30 and 39 percent in rate of pulmonary exacerbations for those who received the combination regimens compared to those who received placebo (p≤0.0014). Based on these results, Vertex plans to submit a New Drug

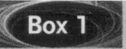 **Box 1** Differentiating Between Criteria of CFTR Genotypes

Pancreatic Insufficient
Class I, II, or III mutation
1% CFTR activity
Absent or minimal chloride channel function
Elevated sweat chloride >60 mmol/L
Classic early presentation (50% diagnosed by 6 months of age)
Median survival is 37.4 years
Patients require pancreatic enzymes
Fecal pancreatic elastase-1 <100 µg/g
Atrophic scarred pancreas
Risk of diabetes mellitus increases with age

Pancreatic Sufficient
Class IV or V mutation
5% CFTR activity
Some chloride channel function
Borderline or mildly elevated sweat chloride (40–60 mmol/L)
Atypical late presentation (sometimes in adulthood)
Survival to 50 years is not uncommon
No pancreatic enzyme supplement required
Fecal pancreatic elastase-1 >250 µg/g
Adequate functional pancreatic tissue to develop recurrent pancreatitis
Lower risk of diabetes mellitus

Abbreviation: CFTR = cystic fibrosis transmembrane regulator (protein).
Class I, II and III mutations result from abnormal protein production, trafficking through the cell and regulation at the cell surface. These mutations result in 1% CFTR activity and are associated with more severe disease., worse pulmonary function and pancreatic insufficient phenotype.

Application (NDA) by the end of 2014 to the U.S. Food and Drug Administration (FDA) for review, with possible approval in 2015.

In Classes IV and V mutations, CFTR is present on the apical surface but chloride channel conduction is defective, resulting in 5% residual CFTR activity and the pancreatic sufficient (PS) phenotype. In the PS phenotype, respiratory symptoms might not present until adulthood, and sufficient pancreatic function is maintained to prevent malabsorption. Because PS patients have residual pancreatic function, there is adequate pancreatic tissue to become inflamed, and these patients might present with recurrent pancreatitis. Residual CFTR function is also manifested in the sweat gland, with sweat tests in the borderline range (40–60 mEq/L). The presence of a class IV or V mutation with a Δ508 mutation results in a PS phenotype.

There is another polymorphism found on intron 8, a noncoding region of the CFTR gene, which affects the amount of normal CFTR transcripts produced. The length of the poly T sequence (5T, 7T, or 9T) is significant in the presence of variable mutation R117H. A lower number of thymidine units results in less efficient splicing of CFTR transcripts and therefore a lower amount of functional CFTR protein. The 5T allele has been classified as a mutation causing mild disease with partial penetrance. The 5T polymorphism is found on about 21% of the *CFTR* genes derived from patients with congenital bilateral absence of the vas deferens (CBAVD). In CBAVD there is 10% CFTR activity, which is sufficient to have obstructive azoospermia as the only clinical manifestation (Box 1).

Clinical Presentation

Gastrointestinal

About 15% of infants present with meconium ileus, obstruction of the distal ileum with thickened viscid meconium. Prenatal ultrasound might detect echogenic bowel, which suggests CF. Infants present shortly after birth with feeding intolerance and a distended abdomen that requires surgical intervention. Colostomies are placed to permit irrigation to dilate the underdeveloped microcolon, and resection of the terminal ileum is sometimes required.

In utero perforation of the bowel can occur, manifesting with calcifications on abdominal x-ray.

The distal intestinal obstruction syndrome (DIOS) is an intestinal obstruction seen in older CF patients. It manifests with abdominal pain, constipation, and a palpable mass in the right lower quadrant consisting of viscous mucus and undigested fecal material that causes obstruction at the ileocecal valve. This can predispose to intussusception. The obstruction is treated by oral or nasogastric administration of polyethylene glycol and electrolytes (GoLY-TELY),[1] an osmotic agent, which causes water to be retained in the intestine, inducing diarrhea. If the obstruction persists, a therapeutic gastrograffin enema with reflux past the iliocecal valve may be necessary. Rectal prolapse and the meconium plug syndrome, in which there is delayed passage of meconium in the newborn period, are additional reasons for referring a child for a sweat test.

Infants might also present with prolonged obstructive jaundice, which can progress to hepatic steatosis, complete biliary obstruction, and acholic stools. In the biliary tree, sludging of bile due to inadequate chloride and fluid transfer into the bile canaliculus can result in focal biliary cirrhosis and cholethiasis. Approximately 2% of patients progress to multilobular cirrhosis with portal hypertension, hypersplenism, and esophageal varices. Progression to liver failure and the need for transplantation is a possibility. Ursodeoxycholic acid (Actigall),[1] a cholorectic bile acid that increases the flow of bile, has been shown to lower hepatic enzymes and delay the progression of liver disease.

Chloride channel dysfunction in the pancreas results in thickened secretions within the pancreatic ducts and obstruction to the flow of pancreatic chyle. Approximately 85% of patients with CF develop exocrine pancreatic insufficiency. The inadequate production of pancreatic lipase and amylase results in fat and protein malabsorption, steatorrhea, failure to thrive, hypoalbuminemia, and edema. The buffering capacity of pancreatic chyle is diminished, resulting in decreased effectiveness of pancreatic enzyme replacement therapy, which is optimally effective at a neutral pH.

The 72-hour recording of dietary intake and stool collection for quantitative determination of fecal fat content is inconvenient and prone to collection errors in the nonresearch setting. The pancreatic enzyme elastase-1 is stable during intestinal transit and is not affected by porcine pancreatic replacement therapy. The measurement of fecal elastase-1 in stool has been found to be a less cumbersome and a sensitive assay to assess pancreatic function. This can be performed on a small specimen and does not require a timed collection.

Treatment with pancreatic enzyme replacement (pancrelipase [Creon, Pancrease]) improves linear growth and weight gain. The recommended dose per meal is 1000 to 2500 U/kg/dose. A high-fat diet is recommended to increase caloric intake to 150 kcal/kg of body weight, which is necessary to ensure optimal growth. The report of the Cystic Fibrosis Foundation Patient Registry indicates that 14% of CF patients are below the 5th percentile for height and 22% are below the 10th percentile for weight. Because nutritional failure as measured by body mass index (BMI) has been shown to be a predictor of progressive pulmonary deterioration, aggressive use of nutritional supplementation and nighttime gastrostomy feeds are advocated to improve the quality of life and lung function. Supplementation of fat-soluble vitamins is necessary to prevent nutritional deficiency.

Because CF patients are living longer, progressive fibrosis of the pancreas results in an increased incidence of diabetes, which is seen in 15% of CF patients. Annual glucose tolerance testing has become the standard of care in adolescents and adults to diagnose glucose intolerance before the onset of diabetes, which has been found to result in deterioration of lung function. Respiratory infection and steroid therapy can result in hyperglycemia, leading to a need for insulin before the patient develops frank diabetes. Because there are reductions of both insulin and glucagon, ketoacidosis is rare.

Infants with CF lose a great deal of salt in their sweat and can develop hyponatremic dehydration, heat prostration, and hypochloremic alkalosis. Salt supplementation is the norm, especially during warm summer months.

---

[1]Not FDA approved for this indication.

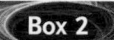

Box 2 Clinical Presentation of Cystic Fibrosis

Gastrointesinal
Failure to thrive
Malabsorption
Meconium ileus
Meconium plug syndrome
Rectal prolapse
Recurrent pancreatitis
Steatorrhea

Pulmonary
Bronchiectasis
Chronic cough
Chronic sinusitis
Digital clubbing
Nasal polyps
Purulent bronchitis
Recurrent and persistent pneumonia

Other
Growth failure
Hyponatremia and dehydration
Male infertility

Pulmonary

The lungs in CF are normal at birth. In young CF patients *Staphylococcus aureus* and *Haemophilus influenzae* are common early colonizers, but as patients age, *Pseudomonas aeruginosa* becomes the predominant organism and is present in the sputum of 80% of adults. *P. aeruginosa* undergoes a mucoid transformation, which interferes with the effectiveness of antibiotic therapy. Because the acquisition of *P. aeruginosa* has been correlated with a more rapid deterioration of lung function and decreased survival, aggressive antibiotic therapy is initiated when this organism is isolated to prevent chronic colonization of the airway.

Burkholderia cepacia, an organism that is intrinsically resistant to a broad range of antibiotics, has been associated with poorer lung function. Nine genetically distinct species, known as genomovars, make up the *B. cepacia* complex. *Burkholderia cenocepacia* and *Burkholderia multivorans* are most commonly isolated from CF patients. The transmission of these organisms and other multiply resistant gram-negative bacteria from person to person in CF clinics and summer camps has resulted in strict infection-control guidelines.

A chronic cough, recurrent chest infections, purulent sputum, digital clubbing, chronic sinusitis, and nasal polyps are common presenting symptoms in CF. The incidence of recurrent pneumothorax is increased in CF, and chemical pleurodesis or pleurectomy are often required. Massive hemoptysis and recurrent episodes of hemoptysis are often a result of collateral bronchial arteries that can require embolization. CF patients often have opacification of the sinuses and nasal polyposis (Box 2).

Diagnosis

Sweat testing remains the standard for making the diagnosis of CF. The elevation of the chloride results from CFTR chloride channel dysfunction in the sweat ducts, where reabsorption of chloride occurs. Pilocarpine is iontophoresized into the skin to stimulate sweating. A chloride level greater than 60 mEq/L is consistent with the diagnosis of CF, but the result must be interpreted in the context of the clinical picture. The borderline range for sweat chloride is 40 to 60 mEq/L. Additional testing is necessary to confirm the diagnosis when the sweat test is in the borderline range. False-positive sweat test results can occur with malnutrition, Addison's disease, and ectodermal dysplasia, so it is essential to confirm the diagnosis with a confirmatory sweat test or a genetic analysis, or both. Sweat tests can be performed after 2 weeks of age, at which time a sufficient quantity of sweat can be collected to ensure a proper analysis.

Genetic analysis for mutations known to cause CF symptoms is an alternative diagnostic approach. The presence of two abnormal CFTR mutations known to cause CF disease predicts with a high degree of certainty that a patient has CF. Prenatal screening is recommended by the American College of Obstetrics and Gynecology for pregnant women. When both parents are found to be carriers, amniocentesis and chorionic villous sampling can be used to assess the 25% chance of having an infant affected by CF.

The active transport of ions generates a transepithelial electrical potential difference (PD). Abnormalities of chloride ion transport in patients with CF are associated with a different pattern of PD compared with normal epithelium. This assay thus provides a direct view of the physiology at the ion channel level. Nasal PD measurements help to resolve diagnostic dilemmas in atypical patients and a change of PD measurement toward normal is an outcome measure of therapeutic interventions that correct the chloride channel dysfunction.

Three features distinguish the nasal PD in a patient with CF. A high basal PD reflects enhanced sodium transport across a relatively chloride impermeable membrane. A larger inhibition of PD after nasal perfusion with the sodium channel inhibitor amiloride reflects inhibition of accelerated sodium transport. Little or no change in PD in response to perfusion of the nasal epithelial surface with a chloride-free solution in conjunction with isoproterenol reflects an absence of CFTR-mediated chloride secretion.

Newborn screening for CF has been shown to improve nutritional and neurodevelopmental outcomes. Trypsinogen, a precursor of trypsin, is commonly elevated in the serum of newborns with CF. Infants with CF have elevated immunoreactive trypsinogen (IRT) levels for 2 to 3 weeks after birth. When the IRT is elevated in a blood specimen collected shortly after birth, then an analysis for the presence of CF mutations on the same blood specimen or a persistent elevation of IRT at 2 to 3 weeks of age in a repeat blood specimen are two different methods to determine which infants should be referred for sweat testing. Mutation analysis performed during newborn screening detects carriers of CF mutations, and genetic counseling for these families is warranted to permit informed decisions concerning future pregnancies.

Treatment
Therapeutic interventions are shown in Figure 1.

Gene Therapy
The goal of gene therapy is to correct the basic defect by inserting a normal functioning gene into the ciliated cells in the submucous glands that express abnormal CFTR function. Initial attempts using the adenovirus as the vehicle for transporting the gene into the cells lining the airway appeared promising; however, the host immune response to the virus has limited the effectiveness of this approach. The ideal vector would efficiently deliver the gene to the appropriate target cell without causing toxicity or an inflammatory response. Although gene therapy offers the potential to correct the basic defect of CF, many technical barriers to effective gene therapy need to be addressed to permit this form of therapy to become an effective treatment. Liposomes are being evaluated as an alternate delivery system for administering the normal gene into epithelial cells.

CFTR Potentiator
Kalydeco (ivacaftor), a CFTR potentiator, is the first treatment to the underlying cause of CF in patients with the G551D mutation (approximately 4% of CF patients in U.S. Cystic Fibrosis Foundation Registry). Ivacaftor facilitates increased chloride transport by potentiating the channel-open probability (or gating) of the G551D-CFTR protein. It improves lung function, reduces pulmonary exacerbations, decreases the length of time needed to treat a pulmonary exacerbation with intravenous antibiotics, and improves weight gain. In clinical trials in patients with the G551D mutation, Kalydeco led to statistically significant reductions in sweat chloride concentration. FDA approval has also been provided for 9 additional class III CF mutations.

Hydration of Airway Surface Fluid
Hypertonic saline (Hyper-sal), at a 7% concentration, has been shown to increase the hydration of the airway surface fluid and reduce the frequency of pulmonary exacerbations. This recent addition to the therapeutic treatment regimen has been shown to facilitate the clearance of airway mucus, resulting in improved pulmonary function, and to decrease the frequency of pulmonary exacerbations. Hypertonic saline induces coughing and bronchospasm and is administered following bronchodilator therapy. An inhaled dry powder preparation of mannitol (Bronchitol) has also been developed to increase hydration of the airway surface fluid.

Physical Therapy
Airway clearance can be performed using various techniques, including conventional percussion therapy, pneumatically inflated chest vest percussion device, oscillating positive pressure devices such as the Flutter or Acapella, autogenic drainage, and exercise. These techniques are recommended on a daily basis to help mobilize secretions and prevent the complications related to persistent accumulation of airway mucus.

Bronchodilators
Airway hyperreactivity is present in 50% to 60% of CF patients. β-Agonists keep airways open and facilitate airway clearance by increasing ciliary beat frequency and smooth muscle relaxation. The spirometric response to β-agonists should be monitored because with worsening bronchiectasis and the development of floppy airways, airflow may be impaired. Because anticholinergics alter viscosity of mucus and can have an adverse effect on gastrointestinal motility, this class of bronchodilator has not been recommended for routine use in CF by a consensus conference of the Cystic Fibrosis Foundation.

Antibiotics
Aggressive use of antibiotics for the chronic bacterial colonization of the airways in CF has resulted in improving longevity and quality of life. Prophylactic inhaled antibiotics have been effective in CF patients to decrease the bacterial burden in the CF airway. Alternate-month therapy with a 300-mg aerosol preparation of tobramycin (TOBI) in a nebulized or powder preparation used with a podhaler device improves lung function, delays the time to the onset of pulmonary exacerbation, and decreases the need for hospitalization. A preparation of aztreonam (Cayston) for inhalation, which is administered by a very efficient portable nebulizer (Altera nebulizer system), is also approved by the FDA.

Pulmonary exacerbations are characterized by an increased cough, copious purulent sputum, decreased appetite, weight loss, and decreased exercise tolerance. Quinolone antibiotics are effective for treating *P. aeruginosa* in an oral preparation, but the development of resistance to this class of drug is a limiting factor. Ciprofloxacin (Cipro) is not approved by the FDA for use in children, but there is considerable experience with this drug in children with CF. When oral and inhaled antibiotics are not effective, hospitalization for aggressive airway clearance and a 10- to 14-day course of IV antibiotics is indicated. A combination of two drugs

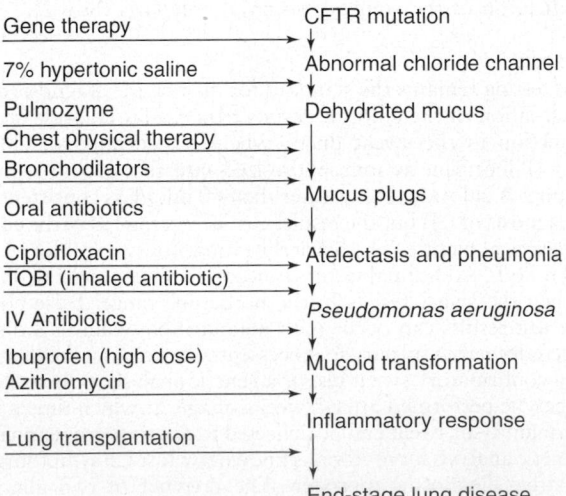

Gene therapy →	CFTR mutation ↓
7% hypertonic saline →	Abnormal chloride channel ↓
Pulmozyme →	Dehydrated mucus
Chest physical therapy →	↓
Bronchodilators →	
Oral antibiotics →	Mucus plugs ↓
Ciprofloxacin →	Atelectasis and pneumonia
TOBI (inhaled antibiotic) →	↓
IV Antibiotics →	*Pseudomonas aeruginosa* ↓
Ibuprofen (high dose) →	Mucoid transformation
Azithromycin →	↓
Lung transplantation →	Inflammatory response ↓
	End-stage lung disease

Figure 1. Therapeutic interventions for cystic fibrosis lung disease.

(usually an aminoglycoside and a β-lactam semisynthetic penicillin or a cephalosporin) is selected based on susceptibility of the organism recovered by culture of sputum or a deep throat swab. In young children who are not able to produce sputum, bronchoscopy may be performed to obtain a specimen for culture and sensitivity and to assess the amount of airway inflammation.

Mucolytic Therapy

DNase (Pulmozyme) is a nebulized mucolytic agent that cleaves neutrophil-derived DNA that contributes to the thick airway secretions that clog the CF airways. Daily inhalation therapy (2.5 mg) reduces sputum viscosity, facilitating airway clearance and resulting in a 5% improvement in lung function. This therapy has largely replaced treatment with N-acetylcysteine (Mucomyst),[1] which causes bronchial irritation.

Antiinflammatory Therapy

There has been growing awareness of the role of the host inflammatory responses in the progression of CF lung disease. Chronic endobronchial colonization with bacteria results in the release of proinflammatory mediators interleukin (IL)-8 and nuclear factor (NF)-κB. These mediators recruit neutrophils into the airway; the neutrophils release elastase, protease, superoxide ions, and hydroxyl radicals, which damage lung tissue and contribute to the development of bronchiectasis.

Corticosteroids

Alternate-day systemic steroids were studied in a multicenter placebo-controlled study as a therapeutic intervention to decrease the inflammatory response in the CF airway. Significant risks of growth impairment, diabetes, and cataracts were found. Although inhaled steroids are commonly prescribed for CF patients, there is no double-blind study to demonstrate the benefit of long-term therapy in CF patients who do not have a component of asthma.

Nonsteroidal Antiinflammatory Drugs

Oral administration of twice-daily high-dose ibuprofen[1] (20–30 mg/kg)[3] to achieve peak plasma concentration of 50 to 100 µg/mL interferes with neutrophil migration and inhibits the activation of NF-κB. Konstan studied 85 CF patients and found that ibuprofen therapy results in less decline in lung function, fewer hospitalizations, and improved weight gain. This effect is most pronounced in patients who are younger than 13 years and have minimal lung disease. Although prolonged use of this therapy has been shown to have ongoing benefit, the risk of GI side effects has limited the implementation of this therapy by most CF patients.

Macrolide antibiotics (azithromycin [Zithromax])[1] are not considered effective in the treatment of infection with *P. aeruginosa*, but a number of clinical trials have demonstrated a modest improvement in lung function and a decrease in the frequency of infectious exacerbations and need for antibiotic therapy in CF patients chronically colonized with *P. aeruginosa*. The mechanisms of action are not well understood but are believed to be related to a number of antiinflammatory and immunomodulatory effects of this class of antibiotic. The expression of *P. aeruginosa* pathogenicity factors and neutrophil recruitment appear to be altered by chronic macrolide therapy.

Oxygen therapy to correct alveolar hypoxia is effective to prevent pulmonary hypertension in CF patients with severe lung disease. Pulmonary hypertension results from pulmonary vascular remodeling, which results in increased pulmonary vascular resistance. Cor pulmonale contributes to the morbidity of CF with right heart failure, progressive exercise intolerance, and risk of syncope.

---

[1]Not FDA approved for this indication.
[3]Exceeds dosage recommended by the manufacturer.

Lung Transplantation

Approximately 150 patients receive bilateral cadaveric lung transplants per year. Evaluation at a lung transplant center is considered when progressive deterioration in lung function results in a forced expiratory volume in one second (FEV$_1$) less than 30% predicted. Survival rates in CF lung-transplant recipients are comparable with other groups of patients. The availability of donor organs continues to be a limiting factor, and the disparity between donor availability and a growing recipient pool has progressively lengthened the waiting time for organs and has increased the mortality for patients awaiting lung transplantation. Living-donor lobar transplantation, which involves removal of both diseased lungs from the recipient and the implantation of two lower lobes donated by two donors, is an alternative for CF patients awaiting lung transplantation.

References

Cystic Fibrosis Foundation. Cystic Fibrosis Foundation Patient Registry, 2005 Annual Data Report to the Center Directors. Bethesda Md: Cystic Fibrosis Foundation; 2006.

http://www.genet.sickkids.on.ca/cftr/app.

Konstan MW, Byard PJ, Hoppel CL, Davis PB. Effect of high-dose ibuprofen in patients with cystic fibrosis. N Engl J Med 1995;332(13):848–54.

Solomon MP, Wilson DC, Corey M, et al. Glucose intolerance in children with cystic fibrosis. J Pediatr 2003;142:128–32.

HISTOPLASMOSIS

Method of
David van Duin, MD, PhD

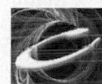

CURRENT DIAGNOSIS

- The most common symptomatic manifestation of histoplasmosis is acute pulmonary histoplasmosis, which is generally characterized by nonspecific symptoms including fevers, chills, malaise, a nonproductive cough, and chest pain.
- Other presentations of histoplasmosis include chronic pulmonary histoplasmosis, disseminated histoplasmosis in immunocompromised hosts, and extrapulmonary disease such as mediastinal histoplasmosis.
- A multimodality approach to diagnosis, which may include serology, histopathology, antigen testing, and culture, should be considered in the appropriate setting.

CURRENT THERAPY

- Oral itraconazole is the treatment of choice for most forms of histoplasmosis.
- Serum levels of itraconazole are unpredictable and should be monitored during treatment.
- Depending on localization and severity of disease, induction with amphotericin B formulations may be required.
- Careful monitoring of patients during and after treatment is recommended, because relapses are observed in a subset of patients.

Mycology and Pathogenesis

Histoplasma capsulatum var. *capsulatum* and *H. capsulatum* var. *duboisii* are the two varieties of *H. capsulatum* that cause human histoplasmosis. *H. capsulatum* var. *duboisii* is the causative agent of African histoplasmosis, which is characterized by skin, bone, lymph node, and subcutaneous tissue involvement. This chapter focuses solely on the manifestations and treatment of *H. capsulatum* var. *capsulatum*, hereafter referred to as *H. capsulatum*.

H. capsulatum is a thermally dimorphic fungal pathogen, which grows as a mold in the environment, and converts to a yeast at 37°C during infection. During mold growth, *H. capsulatum* forms macroconidia, which are 8 to 15 μm and have thick walls and protuberances, as well as microconidia, which are 2 to 4 μm and have a smooth surface.

Disruption of soil containing *H. capsulatum*, such as during a construction project, results in the aerosolization of microconidia, which are the infectious particles. Inhaled microconidia are phagocytized but are able to survive and convert to yeast phase inside pulmonary macrophages. The resulting dissemination through the reticuloendothelial system is usually quickly contained in immunocompetent hosts, but it can lead to severe disease in the absence of normal immunity. Microconidia can be carried for several miles by air currents. Therefore, persons who are not in the direct vicinity of the disrupted soil are also at risk for developing histoplasmosis.

In tissues, *H. capsulatum* is recognized as 2- to 4-μm oval yeast forms with narrow-based budding. *H. capsulatum* does not have a capsule; the name is derived from the erroneous interpretation by Samuel Darling of an apparent clearing surrounding these yeasts in tissues as a capsule.

Epidemiology

Histoplasmosis is most common in North and Central America, but cases occur worldwide, some in microfoci of infection. Areas of high prevalence include the Mississippi and Ohio River valleys in the United States and Rio de Janeiro State in Brazil. *H. capsulatum* thrives in soil that is enriched with bird or bat guano, and it can be found in high quantities near bird roosts, chicken coops, abandoned old buildings, and bat-infested caves. Because *H. capsulatum* can enter a state of latency and reactivate years later, cases have been described in patients who have a remote history of living in or visiting endemic areas. A complete geographic history and a high index of suspicion are required for the correct diagnosis of such cases in nonendemic areas.

Clinical Manifestations

Most *H. capsulatum* infections are asymptomatic; it is estimated that less than 5% of infections lead to clinical symptoms. The occurrence and severity of a clinical syndrome are thought to be related to the immune status of the host, as well as the size of the infectious inoculum. The most common clinical scenario is acute pulmonary histoplasmosis, but a variety of other symptomatic histoplasmosis syndromes have been described. Also, a substantial number of cases come to clinical attention years after the initial infection during the course of a pulmonary nodule work-up, when malignancy is suspected. Although they are asymptomatic, these cases can lead to anxiety, as well as the morbidity and health care costs associated with radiographic exposures and biopsy procedures.

Acute Pulmonary Histoplasmosis

Most commonly, acute pulmonary histoplasmosis is a self-limited flulike illness. Symptoms are generally nonspecific and include fevers, chills, malaise, a nonproductive cough, and chest pain. Chest radiographs can show diffuse infiltrates in one or more lobes, often with hilar lymphadenopathy. The differential diagnosis includes more common infections such as bacterial and viral pneumonias. Symptoms usually resolve without treatment in 2 to 3 weeks. However, more-severe cases do occur, even in seemingly immunocompetent hosts. In these cases, severe respiratory distress, prolonged symptoms, and even death can occur in the absence of adequate treatment. This highlights the importance of timely diagnosis and treatment when indicated.

Chronic Pulmonary Histoplasmosis

Some patients with acute pulmonary histoplasmosis fail to clear their infection and go on to develop a chronic pulmonary infection. A subset of these patients has chronic cavitary disease.

Chronic pulmonary histoplasmosis may be arbitrarily defined when the duration of symptoms from pulmonary histoplasmosis exceeds 6 weeks. The classic patient is a white middle-aged to elderly man with chronic obstructive pulmonary disease (COPD).

Although these are clearly risk factors for the development of chronic disease, case series have illustrated that even never-smokers without preexisting lung disease are at risk for developing this complication.

A combination of systemic and pulmonary signs and symptoms is usually found in chronic pulmonary histoplasmosis. Fevers, night sweats, weight loss, lack of appetite, subjective loss of energy, and malaise are common systemic symptoms, and pulmonary symptoms include cough, sometimes with minimal hemoptysis, dyspnea, and sputum production. In patients with preexisting lung disease it may be difficult to distinguish these symptoms from baseline symptomatology. Radiology studies classically show cavitary disease without hilar lymphadenopathy. However, nodules, infiltrates, and lymphadenopathy are also seen, especially in nonsmoking women.

Untreated, this form of histoplasmosis can lead to death secondary to respiratory failure. With treatment, prognosis depends on coexisting pulmonary disease, and is generally favorable with regard to microbiological cure. However, relapses occur in up to 20% of cases even after prolonged treatment.

Disseminated Histoplasmosis

Most, if not all, episodes of histoplasmosis have a period of dissemination, during which infected macrophages spread throughout the body via the reticuloendothelial system. In the majority of cases this is a self-limited event, which is quickly contained upon activation of the immune system. However, about 1 in 2000 infections results in progressive disseminated disease. Almost invariably, these cases occur in immunocompromised hosts. Patients at risk for progressive disseminated disease include those with advanced HIV infection, solid organ transplant recipients, patients with hematologic malignancies, and those treated with immunomodulating agents, most notably corticosteroids or tumor necrosis factor α (TNF-α) inhibitors. Infants are also at risk.

Recognition of disseminated histoplasmosis can be challenging. Symptoms include fevers, malaise, anorexia, respiratory symptoms, and weight loss. Laboratory investigations often reveal elevated acute phase reactants, abnormal liver function tests, and pancytopenia. Hepatosplenomegaly and lymphadenopathy occur in about half of cases. Severe cases can be clinically indistinguishable from bacterial sepsis, and patients present with hypotension and multiorgan failure. A potential diagnostic clue to the diagnosis is the presence of mucosal ulcerations, which are generally painful and can occur anywhere in the oral, pharyngeal, or laryngeal mucosa. Various morphologies may be seen, ranging from superficial to verrucous. Adrenal involvement resulting in adrenal insufficiency can occur. These patients present with enlarged adrenals on imaging and clinical symptoms of Addison's disease.

Although survival without antifungal therapy has been described, disseminated histoplasmosis is generally fatal if left untreated.

Mediastinal Manifestations of Histoplasmosis

Mediastinal disease can manifest itself as mediastinal fibrosis or granulomatous mediastinitis. Mediastinal fibrosis or fibrosing mediastinitis is an uncommon complication of pulmonary disease, in which extensive fibrotic tissue develops in the mediastinum in response to infection. Men between ages of 20 and 40 years are at the highest risk for this complication. The fibrosis consists of mature collagen, rather than granulomatous tissue, which encases the structures of the mediastinum and can have a progressive course eventually leading to death. The prognosis depends on the extent of involvement of mediastinal structures. Bilateral disease in which the pulmonary veins are involved is especially associated with poor outcomes. No satisfactory treatment is available.

In contrast, granulomatous mediastinitis, also known as mediastinal granuloma, is characterized by a caseous inflammatory mass of mediastinal lymph nodes. Most patients remain asymptomatic, and cases are often recognized only as an incidental imaging finding. However, a subset of patients develops symptoms related to compromise of mediastinal structures. The prognosis is more benign; usually the process resolves and the involved lymph nodes calcify. The role of treatment in this entity remains unclear.

Central Nervous System Histoplasmosis

Central nervous system (CNS) involvement during *H. capsulatum* infection occurs infrequently. Like other extrapulmonary disease, CNS disease may be seen as a part of progressive disseminated histoplasmosis in about 5% to 10% of disseminated histoplasmosis cases. Additionally, isolated cases in which no other signs of dissemination are found have been reported. CNS histoplasmosis typically results in chronic lymphocytic meningitis, but parenchymal lesions can also be found. Symptoms are similar to those of other chronic infectious meningitides. The typical presentation is a combination of systemic symptoms including fevers, weight loss, and night sweats and localizing symptoms of headache, focal neurologic deficits, or behavioral changes. Treatment failures and relapses are common. Prognosis in the context of adequate treatment is dependent on the degree and the reversibility of immunosuppression.

Other Manifestations of Histoplasmosis

Involvement of all organ systems with *H. capsulatum* has been reported, either in the setting of clinical disseminated histoplasmosis or as an isolated extrapulmonary site of infection.

H. capsulatum as a cause of endovascular and cardiac infections is well established. In endocarditis cases, native and prosthetic valves may be involved. Pericarditis is found in around 5% of patients with pulmonary histoplasmosis, and it appears to represent an immunologic reaction. Consistent with this, symptoms usually resolve with nonsteroidal antiinflammatory drugs (NSAIDs) or corticosteroids. Bone, joint, and skin infections can also occur and can present diagnostic difficulty.

Urogenital involvement is often documented in autopsy series, but it infrequently results in clinical symptoms. Few cases of *H. capsulatum* causing symptomatic prostatitis, nephritis, epididymitis, vaginal and penile ulcers, and ovarian involvement have been reported. Similarly, although autopsy series report gastrointestinal involvement in disseminated histoplasmosis in up to 70% to 90% of cases, specific symptoms attributable to the gastrointestinal tract are much less common. Diarrhea, gastrointestinal bleeding, bowel perforation, or bowel obstruction can result from gastrointestinal histoplasmosis.

Diagnosis

Diagnosing histoplasmosis can be complicated, and the available specific diagnostic tests each have their limitations. If the diagnosis is suspected, using available modalities in combination is generally the right approach. Turn-around time can vary depending on circumstances, and in severe or disseminated cases, empiric therapy may be warranted. Obtaining tissue, when it is feasible to do so, is essential for a pathologic diagnosis.

Histopathology

One of the most useful modalities in reaching a diagnosis is histopathology. Necrotizing or non-necrotizing granulomas are often seen. An experienced pathologist can recognize the specific pattern of yeast forms, mostly inside but also outside of macrophages. The yeast forms are best visualized by a methamine silver stain, such as the Gomori-Grocott methenamine silver stain (GMS). Alternatively, periodic acid–Schiff (PAS) staining may be used. Confusion with other pathogens or, more commonly, staining artifacts can occur, and expert consultation is required in such cases. Obtaining tissue for histopathology is usually the real challenge, and a careful evaluation of the risk-to-benefit ratio for each individual patient needs to be made.

Cultures

Culture confirmation of histoplasmosis is desirable, but often the yield of cultures is limited. In addition, cultures may be subject to a substantial time delay of several weeks. In disseminated histoplasmosis, cultures are often positive from several sites, including blood and bone marrow. In acute pulmonary histoplasmosis, the yield of respiratory cultures is estimated to be between 9% and 40%, depending on the degree of lung involvement. In mild to moderate cases, cultures are rarely positive. In chronic cavitary lung disease, the yield of culture improves, probably as a reflection of the increased fungal burden in these patients, and cultures can grow *H. capsulatum* in as many as 85% of cases. A positive fungal culture, with microscopic characteristics suggesting *H. capsulatum*, should be confirmed by specific testing. This is usually accomplished by DNA probing.

Serology

Antibody testing can be helpful when used in conjunction with the clinical scenario and other specific testing. The presence of antibodies to *H. capsulatum* may be determined by complement fixation (CF) or immunodiffusion (ID). Immunodiffusion methods evaluate the presence of M and H precipitin bands. Mild acute infections may be characterized by presence of an M band in isolation. Presence of an H band generally indicates more severe or chronic infection and is usually found in combination with an M band. Complement fixation determines the level of antibodies directed against mycelial and yeast antigens separately. For diagnosis, a fourfold rise in either mycelial or yeast CF antibody titer is required.

The incidence of detectable antibodies in persons in endemic areas is much lower than the incidence of positive skin testing, which suggests that detectable antibodies probably wane after exposure to undetectable levels. Therefore, although an isolated antibody titer of 1:32 or greater is not diagnostic, it is very suggestive of histoplasmosis in a patient with a consistent clinical presentation. In addition, any positive titer should lead to additional work-up because a substantial number of patients with confirmed histoplasmosis have antibody titers that are in the low positive range. Antibodies take 2 to 6 weeks to appear, which limits their use in acute cases. Immunosuppressed states clearly diminish the sensitivity of serology, but positive serologies are found in around 50% of disseminated histoplasmosis in immunocompromised patients. Antibody testing may be particularly helpful in CNS histoplasmosis, where cerebrospinal fluid (CSF) cultures are often negative. The finding of detectable anti–*H. capsulatum* antibodies in the CSF is diagnostic in the right clinical setting.

Antigen Detection

A commercial assay is available to determine the presence of polysaccharide antigens shed by *H. capsulatum* in urine or serum. Previously, urine assays appeared to outperform serum assays, but the most recent generation of antigen assays seems to be equivalent in urine and serum. Measuring antigen shedding in bronchoalveolar lavage (BAL) fluid is a new and promising development. Preliminary data indicate that yields from BAL may be increased in pulmonary disease. In general, antigen detection assays are a valuable adjunct to diagnosis and should be obtained in any case in which histoplasmosis is suspected. Because direct shedding is measured, the yield of this test is not diminished in immunocompromised hosts. In limited disease with a minimal fungal burden, antigens are unlikely to be detected.

Treatment

In 2007, the Infectious Diseases Society of America (IDSA) published updated management guidelines for the treatment of histoplasmosis (Table 1). The IDSA emphasizes that all of its guidelines "cannot always account for individual variation among patients. They are not intended to supplant physician judgment with respect to particular patients or special clinical situations." Regarding acute pulmonary histoplasmosis, no evidence from clinical trials is available to guide treatment decisions, and the IDSA guidelines are relatively conservative, reserving treatment only for "moderately severe to severe" cases. No explicit definition of severity is provided. Also, when mild to moderate symptoms persist, treatment is not recommended until the patient has been symptomatic for more than 4 weeks. Here, careful clinical judgment is warranted. Although poor long-term outcomes are uncommon in these patients, symptom resolution upon antifungal treatment is the rule. Therefore, some experts treat even mild to moderate acute pulmonary disease with a symptom duration of less than 4 weeks, in contrast to IDSA guideline recommendations.

TABLE 1 2007 IDSA Guidelines for Treating Histoplasmosis				
CLINICAL MANIFESTATION	**INDUCTION**	**DURATION**	**MAINTENANCE**	**TOTAL DURATION**
Acute Pulmonary				
Mild to moderate <4 weeks	None			
Mild to moderate >4 weeks	None		Itra*	6–12 wk
Moderately severe to severe	AmB[†]	1–2 wk	Itra*	12 wk
Chronic Pulmonary				
	Itra*	3 day	Itra*	1–2 yr
Disseminated				
Mild to moderate	Itra*	3 day	Itra*	1 yr
Moderately severe to severe	AmB[†]	1–2 wk	Itra*	1 yr
Granulomatous mediastinitis	Itra*	3 day	Itra*	6–12 wk
CNS	AmB[†]	4–6 wk	Itra*	1 yr

Abbreviations: AmB = amphotericin B; CNS = central nervous system; ISDA = Infectious Diseases Society of America; Itra = itraconazole.
[1]Not FDA approved for this indication.
*Itraconazole (Sporanox) dosing for mild to moderate disease is 200 mg qd or bid; for all other indications a loading dose of 200 mg tid × 3 d is recommended followed by 200 mg qd or bid, guided by blood levels.
[†]Amphotericin B, in general liposomal (AmBisome)[1] or lipid formulations (Abelcet)[1] are preferred, but deoxycholate formulation of amphotericin B (Fungizone) may be used as an alternative in the treatment of acute pulmonary histoplasmosis. In CNS histoplasmosis, liposomal amphotericin B[1] is preferred.

Recommended induction treatment for the first 1 to 2 weeks in moderately severe to severe acute pulmonary histoplasmosis is a lipid formulation of amphotericin B (AmBisome, Abelcet)[1] 3 to 5 mg/kg IV daily. During induction therapy, methylprednisolone (Solu-Medrol) may be used as needed for respiratory complications. After that, oral itraconazole (Sporanox) can be used (200 mg three times daily for 3 days and then 200 mg twice daily) for a total duration of treatment of 12 weeks. Oral itraconazole for 6 to 12 weeks is the treatment of choice when the decision is made to treat mild to moderate acute pulmonary histoplasmosis.

When itraconazole is used, careful instructions should be given to ensure optimal oral absorption. Using the solution results generally in higher blood levels, but the unpleasant taste can be an issue for patients. To optimize absorption of the capsules, encourage patients to take them with a cola beverage. Because of substantial interpersonal variability in itraconazole metabolism, blood levels remain unpredictable. As a result, levels should be monitored on all patients whose treatment exceeds 2 weeks. In general, blood levels between 1.0 and 10.0 µg/mL are recommended, even though strong evidence for these cutoffs is lacking.

Chronic pulmonary histoplasmosis requires oral itraconazole therapy for 1 to 2 years. As noted earlier, relapses can occur even with prolonged therapy, and some patients require lifelong suppressive therapy. When an asymptomatic pulmonary nodule is found to be a histoplasmoma in the course of a malignancy work-up, no treatment is generally indicated.

In disseminated histoplasmosis with moderately severe to severe symptoms, induction treatment with liposomal amphotericin B[1] (3 mg/kg IV daily) is recommended for the first 1 to 2 weeks. This is followed by oral itraconazole for a total of at least 1 year. When symptoms of disseminated histoplasmosis are mild to moderate, the induction phase can be omitted, and treatment with oral itraconazole for 1 year should suffice. The role of treatment in mediastinal complications of histoplasmosis depends on the etiology. If symptomatic and inflammatory findings predominate, as in granulomatous mediastinitis, treatment with oral itraconazole is warranted. In mediastinal fibrosis, antifungal treatment generally does not improve the prognosis. CNS histoplasmosis should be aggressively treated with liposomal amphotericin B (5 mg/kg daily intravenously) for 4 to 6 weeks, followed by oral itraconazole for at least 1 year.

References

Ashbee HR, Evans EG, Viviani MA, et al. Histoplasmosis in Europe: Report on an epidemiological survey from the European Confederation of Medical Mycology Working Group. Med Mycol 2008;46(1):57–65.

Assi MA, Sandid MS, Baddour LM, et al. Systemic histoplasmosis: A 15-year retrospective institutional review of 111 patients. Medicine (Baltimore) 2007;86(3):162–9.

Cuellar-Rodriguez J, Avery RK, Lard M, et al. Histoplasmosis in solid organ transplant recipients: 10 years of experience at a large transplant center in an endemic area. Clin Infect Dis 2009;49(5):710–6.

Deepe Jr GS. Immune response to early and late *Histoplasma capsulatum* infections. Curr Opin Microbiol 2000;3(4):359–62.

Gugnani HC. Histoplasmosis in Africa: A review. Indian J Chest Dis Allied Sci 2000;42(4):271–7.

Hage CA, Bowyer S, Tarvin SE, et al. Recognition, diagnosis, and treatment of histoplasmosis complicating tumor necrosis factor blocker therapy. Clin Infect Dis 2010;50(1):85–92.

Hage CA, Davis TE, Fuller D, et al. Diagnosis of histoplasmosis by antigen detection in bronchoalveolar fluid. Chest 2010;137(3):623–8.

Hage CA, Wheat LJ, Loyd J, et al. Pulmonary histoplasmosis. Semin Respir Crit Care Med 2008;29(2):151–65.

Kahi CJ, Wheat LJ, Allen SD, Sarosi GA. Gastrointestinal histoplasmosis. Am J Gastroenterol 2005;100(1):220–31.

Kauffman CA. Histoplasmosis: A clinical and laboratory update. Clin Microbiol Rev 2007;20(1):115–32.

Kauffman CA. Diagnosis of histoplasmosis in immunosuppressed patients. Curr Opin Infect Dis 2008;21(4):421–5.

Kauffman CA. Histoplasmosis. Clin Chest Med 2009;30(2):217–25.

Kennedy CC, Limper AH. Redefining the clinical spectrum of chronic pulmonary histoplasmosis: A retrospective case series of 46 patients. Medicine (Baltimore) 2007;86(4):252–8.

Mata-Essayag S, Colella MT, Rosello A, et al. Histoplasmosis: A study of 158 cases in Venezuela, 2000-2005. Medicine (Baltimore) 2008;87(4):193–202.

Nosanchuk JD, Gacser A. *Histoplasma capsulatum* at the host–pathogen interface. Microbes Infect 2008;10(9):973–7.

Pasqualotto AC, Oliveira FM, Severo LC. *Histoplasma capsulatum* recovery from the urine and a short review of genitourinary histoplasmosis. Mycopathologia 2009;167(6):315–23.

Thompson GR 3rd, Cadena J, Patterson TF. Overview of antifungal agents. Clin Chest Med 2009;30(2):203–15.

Wheat LJ. Approach to the diagnosis of the endemic mycoses. Clin Chest Med 2009;30(2):379–89, viii.

Wheat LJ, Freifeld AG, Kleiman MB, et al. Clinical practice guidelines for the management of patients with histoplasmosis: 2007 update by the Infectious Diseases Society of America. Clin Infect Dis 2007;45(7):807–25.

Wheat LJ, Kauffman CA. Histoplasmosis. Infect Dis Clin North Am 2003;17(1):1–19, vii.

Wheat LJ, Musial CE, Jenny-Avital E. Diagnosis and management of central nervous system histoplasmosis. Clin Infect Dis 2005;40(6):844–52.

[1]Not FDA approved for this indication.

HYPERSENSITIVITY PNEUMONITIS

Method of
David I. Bernstein, MD; and Haejin Kim, MD

CURRENT DIAGNOSIS

- Objective evidence of parenchymal and/or interstitial infiltrative disease by physical examination, spirometry, and radiography associated with exposure to a causative agent
- Improvement in symptoms, lung function, and radiographic abnormalities with avoidance of the causative agent

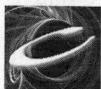

CURRENT THERAPY

- Avoidance of contact with the offending antigen is essential and is often curative if performed early in the course of the disease.
- Systemic corticosteroids are often required during the acute phase of hypersensitivity pneumonitis.

Hypersensitivity pneumonitis, also known as extrinsic allergic alveolitis, is an inflammatory disorder of the lungs that is mediated by immunologic hypersensitivity to a specific antigen, usually organic in nature. Table 1 lists causative agents in hypersensitivity pneumonitis.

Pathophysiology

Hypersensitivity pneumonitis is thought to involve primarily type IV (cell-mediated) hypersensitivity. Bronchoalveolar fluid obtained from patients with hypersensitivity pneumonitis shows a predominant $CD8^+$ lymphocytosis supporting T cell–mediated disease. Viruses are thought to play a role in the development of hypersensitivity pneumonitis through upregulation of costimulatory molecules on alveolar macrophages and dendritic cells, leading to increased activation of type 1 helper T cells. Adoptive transfer models in animals have shown that $CD4^+$ T cells and cytotoxic T cells are the most important effector cells in experimental hypersensitivity pneumonitis, rather than cytokines, antibodies, or complement alone. Genetic susceptibility to this disorder could be associated with presence of specific MHC class II alleles.

Clinical Presentation and Diagnosis

The main clinical features for hypersensitivity pneumonitis are listed in Table 2. Hypersensitivity pneumonitis is most likely to be diagnosed if the history, physical findings, high-resolution chest CT, and pulmonary function tests indicate infiltrative and restrictive lung disease; exposure is documented to a recognized or new causative agent; and there is significant improvement in symptoms, lung function, and radiographic findings with avoidance of the offending cause. Antibody to the offending antigen may be demonstrated but is not required for diagnosis. These are the most widely accepted criteria, but evidence-based diagnostic

TABLE 1 Hypersensitivity Pneumonitis: Representative Sources and Causative Agents

CONDITION OR PERSONS AT RISK	SOURCE	CAUSATIVE ANTIGENS
Dairy farmers	Hay, grains, silage	Thermophilic actinomycetes
Bird fancier's or pigeon breeder's disease	Avian droppings or feathers	Avian proteins
Humidifier lung	Contaminated water	Thermophilic actinomycetes or other microorganisms
Chemical workers	Polyurethane foam, varnishes, lacquers	Isocyanates
Machine workers	Metalworking fluid	*Pseudomonas fluorescens, Aspergillus niger, Staphylococcus capitis, Rhodococcus* spp., *Bacillus pumilus*
Familial hypersensitivity pneumonitis	Contaminated wood dust in walls	*Bacillus subtilis*
Hot tub lung	Mold on ceiling	*Cladosporium* spp., *Mycobacterium avium*

Modified from Richerson HB, Bernstein IL, Fink JN, et al: Guidelines for the clinical evaluation of hypersensitivity pneumonitis: Report of the subcommittee on hypersensitivity pneumonitis. J Allergy Clin Immunol 1989;84:839–44; and Hanak V, Golbin JM, Hartman TE, et al: High-resolution CT findings of parenchymal fibrosis correlate with prognosis in hypersensitivity pneumonitis. Chest 2008;134:133–38.

TABLE 2 Clinical Features of Hypersensitivity Pneumonitis

FEATURE	ACUTE	SUBACUTE	CHRONIC
Exposure to antigen	Hours to days	Days to weeks	Months
Symptoms	Influenza-like illness ± cough/dyspnea	Cough and dyspnea with severe cyanosis	Increasing cough and exertional dyspnea; fatigue, weight loss
Physical findings	Fever; lungs normal or bibasilar crackles	Cyanosis; lungs normal or bibasilar crackles	Cyanosis; right-sided heart failure; lungs normal or bibasilar crackles
High-resolution computed tomography	Diffuse ground-glass infiltrates	Reticulation; small centrilobular nodules; air trapping on expiration	Honeycombing, traction bronchiectasis
Pulmonary function testing	↓ FEV_1 and FVC (restrictive pattern); ↓ TLC; ↓ PaO_2 on exercise challenge; ↓ D_{LCO}		
Other findings supportive of a diagnosis of HP	• Positive natural challenge or increase in signs and symptoms on reexposure • Positive precipitating antibodies to HP antigens or antigens cultured directly from the causative environment • Improvement with avoidance • Surgical lung biopsy: interstitial lymphocytic or plasma cell infiltrates and/or noncaseating granulomas; pulmonary fibrosis in advanced cases • BAL lymphocytosis with reduced CD4/CD8 ratio		

Abbreviations: BAL = bronchoalveolar lavage; D_{LCO} = carbon monoxide diffusion in the lungs; FEV_1 = forced expiratory volume in 1 second; FVC = forced vital capacity; HP = hypersensitivity pneumonitis; PaO_2 = arterial partial pressure of oxygen; TLC = total lung capacity.
From Richerson HB, Bernstein IL, Fink JN, et al: Guidelines for the clinical evaluation of hypersensitivity pneumonitis: Report of the subcommittee on hypersensitivity pneumonitis. J Allergy Clin Immunol 1989;84:839–44; and Bernstein D, Lummus Z, Santilli G, et al: Machine operator's lung: A hypersensitivity pneumonitis disorder associated with exposure to metalworking fluid aerosols. Chest 2006;108:636–41.

guidelines have not been established. A careful home, environmental, and occupational history is essential to identify one or more causative antigens.

Treatment

The primary treatment is cessation of exposure to the sources of offending antigens at home or in the workplace. Effective environmental control measures may include modification of work habits, improvement in ventilation, or change in manufacturing procedures. Systemic corticosteroids are often required and aid in recovery during the acute or subacute phases, but there are no long-term studies of their impact on disease progression or survival rates. Referral to a specialist in occupational lung diseases is recommended for proper diagnosis and identification of the sources of causative antigens.

References

Bernstein D, Lummus Z, Santilli G, et al. Machine operator's lung: A hypersensitivity pneumonitis disorder associated with exposure to metalworking fluid aerosols. Chest 2006;108:636–41.

Girard M, Lacasse Y, Cormier Y. Hypersensitivity pneumonitis. Allergy 2009;65:322–34.

Hanak V, Golbin JM, Hartman TE, et al. High-resolution CT findings of parenchymal fibrosis correlate with prognosis in hypersensitivity pneumonitis. Chest 2008;134:133–8.

Jacobs RL, Andrews CP, Coalson JJ. Hypersensitivity pneumonitis: Beyond classic occupation disease: Changing concepts of diagnosis and management. Ann Allergy Asthma Immunol 2005;95:115–28.

Lacasse Y, Assayag E, Cormier Y. Myths and controversies in hypersensitivity pneumonitis. Semin Respir Crit Care Med 2008;29:631–42.

Richerson HB, Bernstein IL, Fink JN, et al. Guidelines for the clinical evaluation of hypersensitivity pneumonitis: Report of the subcommittee on hypersensitivity pneumonitis. J Allergy Clin Immunol 1989;84:839–44.

Schuyler M, Gott K, French V. The role of MIP-1alpha in experimental hypersensitivity pneumonitis. Lung 2004;182:135–49.

LEGIONELLOSIS (LEGIONNAIRES' DISEASE AND PONTIAC FEVER)

Method of
Julio A. Ramirez, MD

In the summer of 1976, an outbreak of approximately 182 cases of pneumonia occurred in persons attending the American Legion convention in Philadelphia. One year later, Dr. McDade reported the identification of *Legionella pneumophila*, the bacterium responsible for the infection. Today, the family of Legionellaceae is composed of more than 40 species, with some species having different serogroups. *L pneumophila* causes approximately 85% of all *Legionella* infections. *L. pneumophila* serogroup 1 is the single most common member of the family causing clinical infections.

Epidemiology

Legionella is an intracellular organism that lives in natural water. In the aquatic environment, the bacteria live and multiply within freshwater amebae. The number of *Legionella* organisms in the water can increase significantly with appropriate local conditions such as warm temperature, lack of biocides, stagnant water, and presence of amebae and other nutrients. These special conditions can be present in artificial water systems such as cooling towers, whirlpools, decorative fountains, and respiratory therapy devices.

The susceptible host acquires the bacteria from water containing the organism. Infection can be acquired by inhaling aerosols containing *Legionella* organisms or by microaspiration of water contaminated with *Legionella*. The hospitalized patient with *Legionella* pneumonia does not require respiratory isolation because legionellosis is not transmitted from person to person.

Clinical Features

Once *Legionella* organisms reach the respiratory tract, based on the interactions of the organism with the host immune system, the patient can have four possible clinical outcomes: asymptomatic infection, Pontiac fever, Legionnaires' disease, or extrapulmonary disease involving the liver, heart, brain, or other organs. Pontiac fever is a nonpneumonic form of disease characterized by fever, headaches, myalgias, and malaise. The patient has an influenza-like illness, with resolution of disease in a few days without specific antimicrobial therapy. Patients with Legionnaires' disease present with community-acquired pneumonia associated with high fever, gastrointestinal complaints such as diarrhea, and central nervous system complaints such as headaches or mental status changes. Hospital-acquired pneumonia can occur if *Legionella* is present in the hospital water supply.

Diagnosis

The currently available laboratory tests for diagnosis of *Legionella* infections include the direct fluorescent antibody stain (DFA), culture, antigen detection in the urine, antibody detection in serum by indirect fluorescent antibody testing (IFA), and DNA amplification using the polymerase chain reaction (PCR). The DFA stain can detect all *L. pneumophila* serogroups, but a large number of bacteria need to be present in sputum for a positive result. *Legionella* can be cultured from respiratory specimens on selective media composed of buffered charcoal–yeast extract agar. The urinary antigen detection has a specificity greater than 95%; the disadvantage is that the test detects only the antigen of *L. pneumophila* serogroup 1. Clinical specimens that have been used to detect *Legionella* by PCR include throat swabs, sputum, tracheal suction, bronchoalveolar lavage fluid, pleural fluid, and lung tissue.

Treatment

In the pulmonary parenchyma, *Legionella* can infect and multiply inside alveolar macrophages, alveolar epithelial cells, and capillary endothelial cells. The poor clinical outcome with β-lactam antibiotics is due to their lack of penetration into cells. Antibiotics with good intracellular penetration that can be used as monotherapy for *Legionella* infections include macrolides, ketolides, tetracyclines, and quinolones (Table 1). Rifampin (Rifadin)[1] is not used as monotherapy because resistance can rapidly emerge when it is used alone.

---

[1]Not FDA approved for this indication.

TABLE 1 Antibiotic Therapy for *Legionella* Infections

ANTIBIOTIC	ORAL DOSE	INTRAVENOUS DOSE
Ketolides		
Telithromycin (Ketek)[1]	800 mg qd	—
Macrolides		
Azithromycin (Zithromax)[1]	500 mg qd	500 mg qd
Clarithromycin (Biaxin)[1]	500 mg bid	—
Erythromycin (Ery-Tab)	500 mg q6h	1 g q6h
Quinolones		
Ciprofloxacin (Cipro)[1]	750 mg bid	400 mg bid
Levofloxacin (Levaquin)	750 mg qd	750 mg qd
Moxifloxacin (Avelox)[1]	400 mg qd	400 mg qd
Rifamycins		
Rifampin (Rifadin)[1]	300 mg bid	300 mg bid
Tetracyclines		
Doxycycline (Vibramycin)[1]	100 mg bid	100 mg bid

[1]Not FDA approved for this indication.

Therapy of the patient with severe disease is initiated with intravenous antibiotics. Once the patient reaches clinical stability, the intravenous therapy can be switched to oral therapy. Doses for the most common antibiotics for intravenous and oral therapy are depicted in Table 1. In the nonimmunocompromised patient, the recommended duration of therapy is 7 to 10 days. In immunocompromised patients, because they are at risk for relapsing infection, the recommended duration of therapy is 14 to 21 days.

Several antibiotics have demonstrated clinical efficacy in legionnaires' disease. Data with several in vitro and animal studies comparing different anti-*Legionella* antibiotics indicate that erythromycin (Ery-Tab) is a weak anti-*Legionella* agent. If erythromycin is selected for therapy, it is important to add rifampin to the regimen to increase intracellular killing. From the family of macrolides, azithromycin (Zithromax)[1] is the most active. The best bactericidal activity in the laboratory is achieved with quinolones. Retrospective observational studies indicate that patients treated with levofloxacin (Levaquin) have a shorter time to reach clinical stability and shorter duration of hospital stay. These antibiotics are considered primary anti-*Legionella* agents.

In clinical practice, I treat immunocompromised patients who have severe Legionnaires' disease with a combination of an intravenous quinolone plus an intravenous macrolide (e.g., levofloxacin plus azithromycin). This regimen is based only on the theoretical consideration that synergistic killing may be obtained using a quinolone to alter DNA synthesis and a macrolide to alter protein synthesis.

---

[1]Not FDA approved for this indication.

OBSTRUCTIVE SLEEP APNEA

Method of
Melinda V. Davis-Malesevich, MD; and Masayoshi Takashima, MD

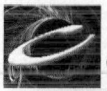

CURRENT DIAGNOSIS

Symptoms
- Excessive daytime fatigue and somnolence
- Morning headaches
- Loud snoring and gasping for air
- Witnessed apneic episodes following loud snoring
- Frequent nocturia with no other underlying etiology
- Hypertension

Clinical Signs and Risk Factors
- Central obesity with body mass index (BMI) >30 kg/m²
- Large neck circumference (>17 inches in men, >16 inches in women)
- Being male or a postmenopausal woman
- Use of sedatives or alcohol before going to bed
- Family history of sleep apnea
- Craniofacial abnormalities: retrognathia, micrognathia, congenital malformations

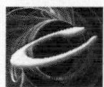

CURRENT THERAPY

- Gold standard for treatment is positive airway pressure
- Weight loss, smoking cessation, avoidance of sedatives
- Improvement of sleep hygiene and sleep schedule
- Minimally invasive procedures (oral appliances, palatal stents, radiofrequency turbinate reductions) may be beneficial for a select patient population

- Surgical therapy is usually reserved for patients not tolerating or unable to use CPAP or BiPAP
- Initial procedures are focused on decreasing upper airway resistance to improve compliance with CPAP or BiPAP
- Identification of anatomic sites of obstruction is critical to successful surgical outcomes

---

Abbreviations: BiPAP = bilevel positive airway pressure; CPAP = continuous positive airway pressure.

Sleep-disordered breathing encompasses the spectrum from upper airway resistance syndrome to obstructive sleep apnea (OSA). OSA is characterized by episodes of partial or complete upper airway collapse leading to cessation or reduction of airflow. Such events lead to oxygen desaturation and sleep fragmentation, causing excessive daytime sleepiness, morning headaches, depression, memory loss, impaired alertness, decreased libido, and reduced cognitive function. Nighttime symptoms are often more telling, and obtaining a sleep history from a bed partner is exceptionally helpful. The most common symptoms include loud snoring, restless sleep, choking or gasping episodes, and awakenings during sleep. Nocturnal perspiration, nocturia, and symptoms of nocturnal gastroesophageal reflux are also commonly associated with severe OSA.

As the severity of OSA typically increases with age, nightly hypoventilation and activation of the sympathetic nervous system lead to pathophysiologic derangements, such as hypertension, ischemic heart disease, myocardial infarction, stroke, arrhythmia, and premature death. An apnea–hypopnea index (AHI) of greater than 5 has been shown to be associated with increased risk of cerebrovascular accident, AHI greater than 20 is associated with increased mortality, and patients with oxygen desaturation below 90% have an elevated incidence of cardiac arrhythmias. These potentially severe consequences, along with a patient's decreased quality of life, substantiate the need for early recognition and treatment.

Definitions of terms related to sleep apnea are listed in Box 1.

Box 1 Definitions of Sleep Medicine Terms

Apnea–hypopnea index (AHI): Sum of apneas and hypopneas per hour of sleep.
Obstructive apnea: Cessation of airflow for ≥10 seconds associated with ongoing ventilatory effort.
Obstructive hypopnea: 1. Decreased airflow by >30% which is ≥10 seconds and a ≥3% oxygen desaturation and or associated with an arousal. 2. Decreased airflow ≥30% which is ≥10 seconds which is associated with a ≥4% oxygen desaturation
Obstructive sleep apnea (OSA): AHI >5 events per hour of sleep, often associated with oxygen desaturation <90%. Mild OSA is defined by an AHI of 5 to 15. Moderate OSA is an AHI 15 to 30, and severe OSA is an AHI >30.
Obstructive sleep apnea syndrome: OSA in association with daytime symptoms of excessive sleepiness or other neurobehavioral symptoms.
Primary snoring: Snoring with an AHI <5 and no complaints of excessive daytime sleepiness.
Respiratory effort–related arousals: Sleep fragmentation that is caused by arousals from increasing respiratory effort but that does not meet criteria for an apnea or hypopnea. The event lasts longer than 10 seconds.
Respiratory disturbance index: Sum of apneas, hypopneas, and respiratory effort–related arousals per hour of sleep.
Upper airway resistance syndrome (UARS): Snoring in association with AHI <5, frequent arousals, and abnormally negative midesophageal pressure (less than −10 cm H₂O) or increased diaphragmatic electromyogram activity.

Epidemiology

Based on available population-based studies, the prevalence of OSA among adults between 30 and 60 years of age is estimated to be 9% for women and 24% for men, and approximately 9% of men and 4% of women have at least moderate disease (AHI 15–30). OSA remains undiagnosed in 70% to 80% of patients because their symptoms are often vague, and OSA must be diagnosed with polysomnography.

Risk Factors

Elderly persons 65 years and older have a higher prevalence of obstructive sleep apnea secondary to decreased muscle tone.

Obesity (body mass index [BMI] greater than 30 kg/m^2) is a risk factor for OSA. A 10% increase in weight is associated with a six-fold increase in risk for development of OSA, and a 10% weight loss is associated with 26% decrease in AHI. There is evidence of a potential link between OSA and insulin resistance.

Approximately 30% of hypertensive persons have OSA. Patients with moderate to severe OSA have a 2.9 odds ratio of developing hypertension. Up to 50% of patients with cardiovascular disease have OSA, even after adjusting for hypertension and other comorbid conditions.

Male patients are nearly twice as likely to have OSA as female patients. Estrogen and progesterone might have a protective role because population-based studies have demonstrated that postmenopausal women have a two- to threefold increased risk of OSA compared to premenopausal women.

African Americans and Asians are at greater risk for OSA than whites. Being African American is an independent risk factor for severe sleep-disordered breathing, with an odds ratio of 2.55 compared with whites. Asians have a narrower cranial base, a higher Mallampati score, smaller thyromental distance, and steeper thyromental plane than whites, which might account for their increased risk.

Pathophysiology

Airway obstruction leading to OSA can occur anywhere along the pathway from the nostrils, soft palate, hypopharynx, base of tongue, and the epiglottis. The airway lacks skeletal structure and is vulnerable to influences such as muscle tone, fat deposition, and tissue redundancy.

Prevention

Lifestyle modification can prevent OSA. Patients should adopt a healthy and athletic lifestyle to develop good muscle tone and weight loss, avoid sedatives and alcohol at bedtime, establish regular sleeping patterns, avoid the supine sleeping position, and elevate the head when sleeping.

Diagnosis

Definitive diagnosis of OSA is made by polysomnography. Mild OSA is defined as an AHI of 5 to 15 per hour, moderate OSA is an AHI of 15 to 30 per hour, and severe OSA is an AHI greater than 30 per hour. Patients spend the night in a sleep laboratory during which multiple physiologic variables are continuously monitored. These include electroencephalogram (EEG), electrooculogram (EOG), electromyogram (EMG), oronasal airflow, chest wall effort, body position, snore volume, electrocardiogram (ECG), and oxyhemoglobin saturation. Laboratory testing also includes a complete accounting of sleep variables, monitoring of cardiac rhythm, and assessment of possible restless legs syndrome (RLS) or periodic limb movements (PLMs) during sleep. This information enables the clinician to determine the severity of the condition and identifies potentially relevant comorbidities.

A thorough diagnostic study requires at least 6 hours of sleep, allowing assessment of variability related to sleep stages. If there are sufficient apneas or hypopneas during the first half of the study (ideally 4 hours of diagnostic testing, with a minimum of 2 hours if an AHI >40 is confirmed), a split-night study may be performed, in which the second half of the night (minimum of 3 hours of sleep) is devoted to titration of continuous positive airway pressure (CPAP) therapy. If the criteria for a split-night sleep study are not achieved during the night, a second night for titration study is ordered. The split-night protocol is a cost-effective use of laboratory resources that is particularly well suited for patients with severe OSA.

According to the Institute for Clinical Systems Improvement (ICSI), polysomnography should be performed in patients with symptoms of OSA and one or more of the following: cardiovascular disease, hypertension, coronary artery disease, obesity, sleep complaint, type 2 diabetes mellitus, recurrent atrial fibrillation, and large neck circumference.

Treatment

Initially, patients should be counseled to avoid practices that can potentially worsen the severity of OSA. Relaxation caused by the use of CNS depressants before sleep (alcohol, sleep medications, pain medications) can worsen upper airway collapse during sleep and should be discouraged. In some patients with positional OSA, avoiding the supine position during sleep might suffice in helping normalize ventilation during sleep. Sewing a tennis ball onto the backs of pajamas or wearing a knapsack filled with polystyrene foam (Styrofoam) has been useful in promoting non-supine sleep. If significant upper airway pathology is identified (nasal septum deviation, enlarged tonsils, craniofacial abnormalities), surgical consultation should be pursued. Weight loss and maintenance should always play a role in the treatment of these patients.

Continuous Positive Airway Pressure Therapy

CPAP remains the therapeutic mainstay for primary treatment of OSA. It serves as a pneumatic stent for the upper airway and is effective in reducing the physiologic abnormalities measured on polysomnography. Additionally, CPAP is thought to augment lung volumes and elicit a reflex that increases tone in the upper airway musculature. Overall, it has been shown to reduce AHI, improve quality of life, and reduce cardiovascular risk.

There are many manufacturers of CPAP devices and many interfaces that help maximize comfort with treatment. Expiratory pressure release (EPR) is available through a couple of CPAP manufacturers. EPR does not seem to compromise the effectiveness of CPAP therapy and improves the patient's sense of comfort with therapy, but it does not seem to systematically improve the level of adherence.

Bi-level respiratory-assist devices deliver alternating levels of positive airway pressure and might be considered an alternative therapeutic option when standard CPAP is not tolerated or when oxygen saturation is not raised sufficiently with standard CPAP. In some cases of severe OSA (in particular among patients with underlying pulmonary conditions), supplemental oxygen can be used in conjunction with CPAP therapy.

The main disadvantage with positive airway pressure treatment is poor compliance. Short-term adherence data reveal compliance with CPAP therapy is variable, with 29% to 83% of patients using CPAP for less than 4 hours per night. Treatment is effective as long as the patient uses the device for the entire night, every night. The use of integrated heated humidifiers has minimized issues of upper airway dryness and has helped improve adherence to therapy.

Oral Appliances

Prostheses worn in the mouth during sleep can help maintain a patent airway, especially in patients who sleep on their back and experience airway collapse secondary to the tongue. In general, there are two types of appliances, mandibular-advancement appliances and tongue-retaining devices. The mandibular-advancement appliances are currently used more often and have been more widely studied. They require viable dentition for retention. They are fitted to the maxillary and mandibular dentition to enable the protrusion of the mandible and therefore increase oropharyngeal patency. The most common side effect is drooling. Temporomandibular joint pain might limit the viability of this therapy. Chronic use of the appliance can result in a change of the dental occlusion.

A dentist with expertise in sleep medicine should ideally implement and monitor this type of treatment.

Surgical Procedures
Patients with an identifiable anatomic upper airway obstruction or craniofacial abnormality might benefit from surgery. A variety of procedures help stabilize the retropalatal region, and others are intended to stabilize the retrolingual airway (Box 2). Sleep surgery has been shown to be most effective when addressing multiple levels of obstruction. Procedures are often combined for maximum effectiveness, such as septoplasty, turbinate reduction, tonsillectomy, uvulopalatopharyngoplasty and genial tubercle advancement. With the advent of transoral robotic surgery, surgeons are now able to access the posterior oropharynx, base of tongue and hypopharynx more easily, and procedures to address these areas are more common. A substantially more invasive procedure, the maxillomandiublar advancement, has been shown very effective in a number of case series. Of course, a tracheostomy completely bypasses the upper airway, curing sleep apnea, but it is not without its comorbidities.

It is hard to predict which patients are likely to have a successful surgical outcome. Part of the reason is the difficulty associated with accurately identifying the site(s) of obstruction. Sleep endoscopy, a relatively new technique, helps define this better. Patients are examined in a drug-induced sleep-resembling relaxed state. As the patient snores and obstructs while sleeping, a flexible fiberoptic scope is passed through the nose to evaluate the upper airway to reveal the site of obstruction. The data on the validity of this procedure are scant yet promising.

Monitoring
The patient's response to therapy needs to be monitored. In the case of CPAP therapy, monitoring of CPAP adherence is critical, because subjective reports are inaccurate. Resolution of excessive sleepiness is the desired outcome for patients who are symptomatic at baseline. If excessive sleepiness remains problematic despite documentation of desirable CPAP adherence, treatment with modafinil (Provigil) 100 to 400 mg in the morning might be considered. Other potential conditions affecting sleep need to be monitored and, if necessary, treated. Often, other conditions such as poor sleep hygiene, restless legs syndrome, periodic limb movements, or psychophysiologic insomnia interfere with adequate response to therapy.

For patients who undergo surgery, retesting is indicated. The interval at which retesting should be done depends on the type of surgery that was performed. Retesting 3 months following the surgical intervention is adequate in most cases.

Box 2　Treatments for Obstructive Sleep Apnea

Nasal Obstruction
Septoplasty
Rhinoplasty or nasal valve surgery
Turbinate reduction
Adenoidectomy

Retropalatal Obstruction
Tonsillectomy
Uvulopalatopharyngoplasty
Z-palatoplasty
Lateral pharyngoplasty
Palatal stents
Radiofrequency soft palate surgery

Retrolingual Obstruction
Transoral robotic-assisted base of tongue reduction
Lingual tonsillectomy
Genioglossus advancement
Hyoid suspension
Tongue base suspension
Maxillomandibular advancement

References
Al Lawati NM, Patel SR, Ayas NT. Epidemiology, risk factors, and consequences of obstructive sleep apnea and short sleep duration. Prog Cardiovasc Dis 2009;51:285–93.
Ancoli-Israel S, Klauber MR, Stepnowsky C, et al. Sleep-disordered breathing in African-American elderly. Am J Respir Crit Care Med 1995;52:1946–9.
Caples SM, Rowley JA, Prinsell JR, et al. Surgical modifications of the upper airway for obstructive sleep apnea in adults: a systematic review and meta-analysis. Sleep 2010;33(10):1396–407.
Fujita S, Conway W, Zorick F, Roth T. Surgical correction of anatomic abnormalities in obstructive sleep apnea syndrome; Uvulopalatopharyngoplasty. Otolaryngol Head Neck Surg 1981;89(6):923–34.
Hsin-Ching L, Friedman M, Hsueh-Wen C, et al. The efficacy of multilevel surgery of the upper airway in adults with obstructive sleep apnea/hypopnea syndrome. The Laryngoscope 2008;118:902–8.
Institute for Clinical Systems Improvement (ICSI). Diagnosis and Treatment of Obstructive Sleep Apnea in Adults. Bloomington, MN: Institute for Clinical Systems Improvement; 2008.
Li KK, Powell NB, Kushida C, et al. A comparison of Asian and white patients with obstructive sleep apnea syndrome. Laryngoscope 1999;109:1937–40.
Peppard PE, Young T, Palta M, et al. Prospective study of the association between sleep-disordered breathing and hypertension. N Engl J Med 2000;342:1378–84.
Peppard PE, Young T, Palta M, et al. Longitudinal study of moderate weight change and sleep-disordered breathing. JAMA 2000;284:3015–21.
Punjabi NM. The epidemiology of adult obstructive sleep apnea. Proc Am Thorac Soc 2008;5:136–43.
Quan SF, Howard BV, Iber C, et al. The Sleep Heart Health Study: Design, rationale, and methods. Sleep 1997;20:1077–85.
Sher AF, Schechtman KB, Piccirillo JF. The efficacy of surgical modifications of the upper airway in adults with obstructive sleep apnea syndrome. Sleep 1996;19(2):156–77.
Vilaseca I, Morello A, Montserrat JM, et al. Usefulness of uvulopalatopharyngoplasty with genioglossus and hyoid advancement in the treatment of obstructive sleep apnea. Arch Otolaryngol Head Neck Surg 2002;128:435–40.

PLEURAL EFFUSIONS AND EMPYEMA THORACIS

Method of
David J. Finley, MD; and Raja Flores, MD

Pleural effusions have multiple etiologies, making the diagnosis and management a common clinical issue. Though the amount of fluid produced varies significantly, an average 0.1 to 0.2 mL/kg is maintained within the pleural space. Production of fluid is matched with removal during normal physiologic states, but aberrations of this homeostasis with local or systemic diseases lead to the formation of an effusion. Symptoms are related to the volume of fluid and the etiology of the fluid accumulation, including both benign and malignant processes. Secondary infection of a pleural effusion, known as an empyema, is a significant complication necessitating aggressive treatment of both the underlying cause and the empyema itself.

Symptoms are variable and include dyspnea, shortness of breath, cough, and chest discomfort, though patients can be asymptomatic, even with very large effusions. Dullness to percussion and decreased breath sounds are often hallmarks of effusions, but these signs are also seen with lung masses and consolidative pneumonias. A clinical history, physical examination, and imaging studies are often needed in combination to diagnose an effusion.

Etiology
Many local and systemic illnesses are associated with the formation of a pleural effusion. Systemic symptoms can indicate the most common cause of the effusion, but diagnostic procedures are often necessary to delineate the etiology. Determination of an exudative or transudative effusion can point out possible disease that may be the cause (Box 1).

Fluid that is low in total protein is a transudative effusion, which is most commonly caused by decreased oncotic pressure or increased capillary hydrostatic pressure. Transudative effusions can also be caused by fluid traversing the diaphragm, as seen in patients with ascites.

Exudative effusions are high in total protein (pleural fluid-to-serum ratio >0.5) and often have an elevated cell count. Increased capillary permeability and decreased lymphatic clearance, usually due to a local or systemic inflammatory illness, produce exudative effusions. The causes are varied, but the most common causes are malignancy, infection, and pulmonary emboli.

<table>
<tr><td>

Box 1 — Etiologies of Transudative and Exudative Effusions

Transudative
Congestive heart failure
Cirrhosis
Pulmonary emboli
Peritoneal dialysis
Renal disorders
Myxedema
Sarcoidosis

Exudative
Malignancy
Infection
Drugs (e.g., nitrofurantoin [Marcodantin, Macrobid], methotrexate [Trexall])
Chylothorax
Pulmonary emboli
Gastrointestinal diseases (e.g., pancreatitis)
Collagen vascular disease (e.g., rheumatoid arthritis)
Asbestos exposure
Trauma (e.g., hemothorax, chest surgery)
Postpericardiectomy or postmyocardial infarction syndrome
Pleuropericarditis

</td></tr>
</table>

Diagnosis

Imaging

Approximately 200 to 500 mL of pleural fluid is necessary before it can be visualized on a posteroanterior upright chest x-ray, usually as blunting of the costophrenic angle. A lateral chest x-ray is more sensitive, often discerning fluid with as little as 100 mL present; layering of the fluid confirms that it is free flowing. Loculations can be seen on x-ray but may be mistaken for lung or pleural masses. Large effusion can completely opacify the hemithorax where the effusion is located. Ultrasound is useful in defining the location and extent of an effusion and can also identify loculated effusions, pleural thickening, and masses. When used to help guide thoracentesis, it can increase diagnostic accuracy and yield and decrease complications.

Chest computed tomography (CT) has distinct advantages over x-ray and ultrasound, though its utility is significantly decreased when there is a large effusion. Imaging with CT after initial drainage of a large effusion is recommended to obtain the most information regarding the possible etiologies of the effusion and aid in operative planning for treatment of an empyema. It also delineates pleural masses and helps differentiate pleural disease from lung pathology (e.g., loculated effusion vs. lung abscess).

Thoracentesis

Often it is difficult to discern the cause of an effusion solely based on the patient's clinical presentation and image studies. Also, when concerned about a malignant process or an infected effusion, these studies do not give enough information to make a definitive diagnosis. Thoracentesis is the diagnostic procedure of choice, allowing drainage of the fluid to relieve symptoms for the patient and provide a specimen for evaluation. Ultrasound should be employed to help guide thoracentesis, especially if the effusion is small or loculated. Care must be taken when draining a large amount of fluid in one setting due to the risk of reexpansion pulmonary edema. If a patient becomes symptomatic during the procedure (persistent cough, significant pleuritic pain, or shortness of breath) no more fluid should be remove at that time. Coagulopathy is a contraindication to thoracentesis due to the risk of intrathoracic bleeding.

Pleural Fluid

The initial evaluation of pleural fluid is done at the bedside by determining the nature of the fluid: clear, cloudy, bloody, or milky. One should also evaluate the fluid for odor and cellularity. These simple steps can point the clinician toward the correct diagnosis. In addition to bedside evaluation, the fluid should be sent for the

<table>
<tr><td>

Box 2 — Light's Criteria for an Exudative Effusion

Pleural fluid-to-serum ratio of protein >0.5
Pleural fluid-to-serum ration of LDH >0.6
Absolute pleural fluid LDH >2/3 of upper limit of normal serum levels

Abbreviation: LDH = lactate dehydrogenase.

</td></tr>
</table>

following laboratory studies: pH, glucose, lactate dehydrogenase (LDH), protein, cytology, Gram stain, and culture (including fungal and viral). Serum pH, protein, LDH and glucose should be sent at the same time.

Light's criteria are helpful in differentiating between an exudative and transudative effusion (Box 2). The sensitivity and specificity of Light's criteria is 82% to 90%.

Transudative effusions rarely need any further intervention, and the goal of treatment is directed at the underlying condition (see Box 1). For exudative effusions, the cause of the effusion dictates the treatment. Incorporating the clinical picture and radiographs with the pleural fluid chemistry studies, cytology, and cultures, the diagnosis is often obtained. Malignant effusions can have positive cytology, but they are more likely to have a pleural fluid glucose level less than 60 mg/dL and to be bloody. An elevated amylase level is seen in esophageal perforation, pancreatitis, and malignant effusions. Chylothorax can be definitively diagnosed if the triglyceride level is more than 110 mg/dL within the pleural fluid. Finally, pH, glucose, and cultures are useful in the treatment of patients with a presumed infected pleural effusion (empyema).

Up to 25% of patients will not have a definitive diagnosis based on the clinical scenario and pleural fluid evaluation. These patients can require further diagnostic testing, including repeat thoracentesis or evaluation of the chest cavity via video-assisted thoracoscopic surgery (VATS) with pleural biopsies.

Treatment

After initial evacuation of the effusion, treatment is directed at controlling the underlying disease that caused the effusion. Malignant effusions are best managed with pleurodesis, usually employing talc (Sterile Talc), if lung re-expansion can be obtained. This is best performed via VATS, which allows biopsies to be performed, confirming the diagnosis and visually confirming lung re-expansion. Though it can be done via tube thoracostomy at the bedside, VATS pleurodesis has been shown to reduce hospital stay and the risk of recurrence. If the lung cannot expand fully, then the fluid is often best managed with an indwelling long-term silicone-elastic catheter for palliation. In patients with benign disease, pleurodesis is rarely done because of the high complication and failure rates.

Infected Pleural Space and Empyema

A parapneumonic effusion (exudative effusion in the setting of pulmonary infection) is seen in 20% to 40% of patients admitted for pneumonia, of whom 10% to 20% will develop a complicated parapneumonic effusion or empyema (pus in the pleural space). Progression to empyema is most often due to delay in treatment and leads to longer hospital stays and increased morbidity and mortality. Other causes of infected effusions are trauma, thoracic surgical procedures, perforated esophagus, systemic infection, and transdiaphragmatic spread.

Parapneumonic effusions can be separated into three stages: exudative (stage I), fibropurulent (stage II), and organizational (stage III). Though thoracentesis is indicated in each stage, it is usually sufficient for stage I effusions when coupled with appropriate antibiotics. These effusions are free flowing, have negative cultures, and often do not reaccumulate.

Complicated parapneumonic, or stage II, effusions require drainage beyond the initial thoracentesis. The fluid is more viscous and has positive bacterial cultures, a low glucose level, and low pH. Progression to frank pus, or empyema, occurs in this stage, with the formation of loculations as fibrin deposition increases.

Complete evacuation of the effusion is required, and initial tube thoracostomy is indicated. If the patient does not improve over the next 24 hours or the space is not completely drained (residual loculations), then surgery is recommended. Randomized, placebo-controlled trials showed no improved outcomes with the use of fibrinolytics as compared to standard tube thoracostomy drainage. The introduction of DNase (Pulmozyme)[1] may be of benefit, but data are insufficient to recommend this treatment. We strongly recommend early intervention with VATS, which has been shown to reduce hospital stay and offers definitive treatment as compared to tube thoracostomy with fibrinolytic therapy.

Delayed or inadequate treatment causes the patient to progress to the organizational stage. This is characterized by heavy fibrin deposit with the formation of a thick peel throughout the pleura with loculations, trapping, and retarding lung re-expansion. Classic CT findings include thickened pleura with multiple loculations and inability of the lung to expand after tube thoracostomy. Decortication, either via VATS or thoracotomy, is required to completely remove the peel off the parietal and visceral pleura. Without obliteration of the empyema space it is very unlikely that the infection can be cleared. In these situations an open thoracostomy, or Eloesser flap, may be required to eradicate the infection.

---

[1]Not FDA approved for this indication.

References

Cameron R, Davies HR. Intra-pleural fibrinolytic therapy versus conservative management in the treatment of adult parapneumonic effusions and empyema. Cochrane Database Syst Rev 2008;(2):CD002312.

de Campos JR, Vargas FS, de Campos Werebe E, et al. Thoracoscopy talc poudrage: A 15-year experience. Chest 2001;119:801–6.

Light R. Clinical practice. Pleural effusion. N Engl J Med 2002;346:1971–7.

Light RW. Parapneumonic effusions and empyema. Proc Am Thorac Soc 2006; 3:75–80.

Luh SP, Chen CY, Tzao CY. Malignant pleural effusion treatment outcomes: Pleurodesis via video-assisted thoracic surgery (VATS) versus tube thoracostomy. Thorac Cardiovasc Surg 2006;54:332–6.

Luh SP, Hsu GJ, Cheng-Ren C. Complicated parapneumonic effusion and empyema: Pleural decortication and video-assisted thoracic surgery. Curr Infect Dis Rep 2008;10:236–40.

Rahman NM, Chapman SJ, Davies RJ. Diagnosis and management of infectious pleural effusion. Treat Respir Med 2006;5:295–304.

Tokuda Y, Matsushima D, Stein GH, et al. Intrapleural fibrinolytic agents for empyema and complicated parapneumonic effusions: A meta-analysis. Chest 2006;129:783–90.

PNEUMOCONIOSIS: ASBESTOSIS AND SILICOSIS

Method of
David N. Weissman, MD

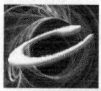

CURRENT DIAGNOSIS

- History of inhalation of mineral or metal dust
- Respiratory symptoms such as cough and dyspnea
- Spirometry and lung volumes show restriction in advanced disease
- Interstitial lung disease can usually be demonstrated by chest imaging. Biopsy is usually unnecessary
- No other likely cause of interstitial lung disease is present

The pneumoconioses are a group of interstitial fibrotic lung diseases predominantly associated with occupational exposures. They are caused by inhalation of particulate matter in the respirable size range (0.3–5 μm mean aerodynamic diameter), especially mineral or metallic dusts (Table 1). These agents interact with pulmonary target cells, including alveolar macrophages and alveolar epithelial cells, to activate a cascade of inflammatory mediators including growth factors. Although exposure to these dusts can induce other types of respiratory disease as well, the final common pathway leading to pneumoconiosis is alveolar epithelial cell damage and interstitial fibrosis. This chapter focuses on silicosis and asbestosis, two common forms of pneumoconiosis.

Asbestosis

Asbestos is composed of strong, heat-resistant fibers of hydrated magnesium silicate classified morphologically as serpentine (chrysotile) or amphibole (crocidolite [riebeckite asbestos]), amosite (cummingtonite-grunerite asbestos), anthophyllite asbestos, actinolite asbestos, and tremolite asbestos. In addition, certain asbestiform fibers (winchite, richterite, erionite) can cause adverse health effects identical to those of asbestos. Fiber dimensions and persistence in tissues are key determinants of toxicity. There is a dose–response effect between the quantity of asbestos inhaled and the severity of fibrotic lung disease. Asbestos is also a carcinogen, and increasing exposure is associated with increased risk, for lung cancer, mesothelioma, ovarian cancer, and laryngeal cancer.

Although asbestos is no longer mined in the United States, importation of asbestos-containing products continues. Exposures also continue to occur, especially in construction and renovation (due to reservoirs of asbestos that are still present in many older buildings), the heating trades (where asbestos is often encountered), and with exposure to older or imported asbestos-containing automotive friction products such as brake linings and clutch facings. Workers exposed to asbestos can carry it home on their clothing, resulting in exposure of family members. Living near geological formations prone to asbestos formation in California has been implicated as a risk factor for mesothelioma.

The Occupational Safety and Health Administration (OSHA) permissible exposure limit (PEL) for asbestos is 0.1 fiber per cc air. This limit was affected in part by the limits of the analytical methodology used in exposure assessment. Exposure to the PEL every day over a 45-year working lifetime has been estimated to be associated with an increased risk of cancer (lung, mesothelioma, and gastrointestinal) of 336 cases per 100,000 exposed persons and an increased risk of asbestosis of 250 cases per 100,000 exposed persons.

Asbestosis causes symptoms of dyspnea and cough. Latency between initial exposure and disease onset is related to exposure intensity. In the United States, this period is generally about two decades. The disease can lead to chronic respiratory failure. Effects of smoking add to the severity of the disease and can cause obstructive findings in addition to the expected decreased lung volume and diffusion capacity associated with fibrotic lung diseases. Bibasilar rubs and inspiratory crackles on auscultation, finger clubbing, and diffuse, bilateral, small, irregular parenchymal opacities and linear streaking at the lung bases on chest x-ray are characteristic.

The International Labour Organization (ILO) has established a system for classification (grading) of radiographs for the presence of radiographic abnormalities in lung parenchyma and pleura that are associated with pneumoconiosis, as well as their severity. The ILO classification system is widely used in epidemiology, surveillance, administrative, and legal settings. The small opacity profusion grades of 0/1 and 1/0 are often considered as defining the boundary between normal and abnormal lung parenchyma.

High-resolution computed tomography (CT) is the most sensitive imaging method for suspected asbestosis. It detects a range of parenchymal abnormalities related to the fibrotic process, such as ground glass and honeycombing, and pleural abnormalities, such as pleural plaques and diffuse pleural thickening. The presence of pleural plaques on radiography (particularly bilateral calcified pleural plaques); uncoated asbestos fibers or fibers coated with an iron-rich proteinaceous material (asbestos bodies) in sputum, bronchoalveolar lavage, or lung biopsy; and the slower progression of symptoms help differentiate asbestosis from idiopathic pulmonary fibrosis.

TABLE 1 Representative Pneumoconioses

SOURCE	MAIN CLINICAL FEATURES	OCCUPATION	DUST
Crystalline silica	Silicosis, increased susceptibility to TB, airways obstruction, lung cancer	Mining, stone cutting, pottery, foundry work	Free crystalline silica (SiO_2)
Asbestiform fibers	Asbestosis, bronchogenic carcinoma, mesothelioma, various forms of benign pleural disease	Insulation, shipbuilding, construction, some mining (e.g., vermiculite mining in Libby, Mont)	Various asbestiform fibers
Coal	Coal workers' pneumoconiosis, COPD	Coal mining	Coal mine dust
Hard metal	Hard metal lung disease (cobalt lung), asthma	Machinists, metal workers	Hard metal, composed primarily of tungsten carbide and cobalt

Abbreviations: COPD = chronic obstructive pulmonary disease; TB = tuberculosis.

Criteria for Diagnosis

Diagnosis is supported by radiographic chest imaging or lung biopsy findings of interstitial lung disease compatible with asbestosis; documentation of exposure to asbestos by history, the presence of pleural plaques (bilateral pleural plaques are essentially pathognomonic for asbestos exposure), or the presence of asbestos bodies or an excessive burden of uncoated asbestos fibers in lung biopsy tissue or possibly via bronchoalveolar lavage or sputum; and no other likely explanation for the diffuse fibrotic lung disease.

Asbestos-Related Benign Pleural Disease

Pleural plaques are characteristic forms of localized parietal pleural thickening that are usually bilateral and asymmetrical, involve the lower lung fields or the diaphragm, and spare the costophrenic angles and apices. Pleural plaques are a marker for exposure to asbestos and are often associated with other asbestos-related conditions. Pleural plaques generally result in minimal reductions in forced vital capacity and do not degenerate into malignant lesions.

In contrast, diffuse visceral pleural thickening can result in adhesions between the visceral and parietal pleura with major decreases in forced vital capacity, respiratory insufficiency, and the requirement for decortication.

Benign pleural effusions can occur in the first decade after asbestos exposure and contain erythrocytes and a mixed inflammatory cell infiltrate of lymphocytes, neutrophils, and eosinophils. The thickened visceral pleura and adjacent atelectatic lung tissue can result in a pleural-based area of rounded atelectasis, simulating a lung mass on chest radiography. CT can reveal the comet sign, a pleural band connecting the apparent mass to an area of thickened pleura.

Lung Cancer and Malignant Mesothelioma

Exposure to all forms of asbestos increases the risk of lung cancer. The peak risk occurs at about 30 to 35 years after the onset of exposure. Tobacco smoking increases this risk in a supra-additive fashion, increasing risk to a level greater than for asbestos or smoking alone. In contrast, smoking does not further increase the asbestos-associated risk for malignant mesothelioma. Asbestos-associated malignant mesothelioma can also affect the peritoneum (and sometimes the pericardium), but when it affects the pleura, this disease manifests with dyspnea, chest pain, and bloody pleural effusion (most often unilateral). A latency period of 30 years or longer after initial exposure is common. Special immunochemical stains and electron microscopy of pleural fluid or pleural biopsies may be necessary to differentiate mesothelioma from adenocarcinoma. It is currently unclear when to screen asbestos-exposed individuals at increased risk for lung cancer with low-dose chest computed tomography.

Treatment

Treatment of asbestosis is symptomatic and similar to that for other patients with chronic lung disease (Box 1). Lung transplantation should be considered in the setting of end-stage lung disease.

Box 1 Recommendations for Managing Patients with Silicosis or Asbestos-Related Lung Disease

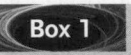

Patients

Stop further exposure to silica or asbestos.

Stop smoking, avoid exposure to tobacco products.

Physicians

Provide early treatment of respiratory infections with antibiotics.

Give pneumococcal and influenza vaccinations.

Maintain a high index of suspicion and provide early evaluation of symptoms for lung, laryngeal, and ovarian cancers and mesothelioma in asbestos-exposed patients.

Maintain a high index of suspicion for pulmonary infection with *Mycobacterium tuberculosis*, nontuberculous mycobacteria, and fungi in silica-exposed patients.

Screen silica-exposed patients for latent tuberculosis infection. Treat latent infections with one of the currently-approved drug protocols.

Provide empiric treatment with short- and long-acting inhaled bronchodilators and inhaled corticosteroids when they are found to provide symptomatic relief.

Give supplemental oxygen therapy if pulmonary hypertension is present or to prevent pulmonary hypertension if O_2 saturation is less than 85% at rest, with exercise, or with sleep.

Consider lung transplantation in the setting of end-stage lung disease.

Treatment of benign pleural disease is also symptomatic; as already noted, decortication is sometimes required for managing diffuse visceral pleural thickening. Depending on extent of disease, mesothelioma may be treated with surgery, radiation, chemotherapy, or some combination of these. In general, prognosis is poor. Mesothelioma-associated malignant pleural effusion can require palliation through procedures such as pleurodesis, pleurectomy, and decortication. Asbestos-associated lung cancer is managed in the same fashion as lung cancer occurring without a history of exposure to asbestos.

Silicosis

Silicosis is a fibrosing interstitial lung disease resulting from the inhalation of crystalline silicon dioxide (silica) in dust of respirable size. The commonest form of crystalline silica is quartz, which is the main component of sand and is present in most rocks. Noncrystalline (amorphous) silica, like that in diatomaceous earth or glass, does not cause silicosis. However, heating amorphous silica, as occurs in foundries when molten metal is poured into clay castings, can convert amorphous silica into cristobalite, a hazardous form of crystalline silica. Mining, stone cutting, sandblasting, and foundry work are all examples of trades associated with exposure to respirable dust containing crystalline silica. The International Agency for Research on Cancer (IARC) has designated crystalline silica from occupational sources as a Group 1 human lung carcinogen.

The current OSHA PEL for respirable crystalline silica is approximately 0.1 mg/m^3.

A number of studies have suggested that this PEL is not fully protective for exposures over an entire working lifetime. The National Institute for Occupational Safety and Health (NIOSH) recommended exposure limit (REL) for respirable crystalline silica is lower than the PEL, at 0.05 mg/m^3 and OSHA has proposed to lower its PEL to this level. Reporting of silicosis cases to public health authorities is required in some states.

Radiographic Patterns of Silicosis

Three main radiographic patterns of silicosis have been described. Two are nodular interstitial patterns and one is an alveolar-filling pattern. The *simple* pattern is associated with nodules that are smaller than 10 mm and that are predominantly rounded and in the upper lung zones. *Progressive massive fibrosis* (PMF) is found in more advanced interstitial disease. It is associated with multiple coalescent larger nodules, upper lobe fibrosis, upward retraction of the hila, and compensatory hyperinflation of the lower lobes. The large upper-zone opacities can cavitate, sometimes in the setting of superimposed mycobacterial infection. Hilar adenopathy can occur, sometimes with an egg-shell pattern of hilar node calcification. A third radiographic pattern is an alveolar-filling process. Overwhelming silica exposure over a short period can cause a pathologic response called *silicoproteinosis*, in which alveoli become flooded with proteinaceous fluid. The condition resembles idiopathic pulmonary alveolar proteinosis. The radiographic alveolar filling pattern favors the lower lung zones and is not associated with the changes of simple silicosis or PMF.

Silicosis Syndromes

Three syndromes of silicosis can be defined based on clinical course and radiographic pattern. Chronic silicosis develops slowly, usually 10 to 30 years after first exposure. It most often has the simple radiographic pattern, but it can be associated with PMF.

Accelerated silicosis develops more rapidly, within 10 years after first exposure. It is associated with higher intensity exposures and can be associated with either the simple or PMF radiographic patterns. Accelerated silicosis is differentiated from chronic silicosis by its more rapid course. Patients with accelerated courses are at greater risk for developing PMF. The clinical presentations of chronic and accelerated silicosis are variable but include cough, dyspnea, and a variety of chest findings ranging from a normal chest examination to crackles, rhonchi, or wheezing. PMF is associated with more severe symptoms and respiratory impairment. Findings compatible with both restrictive and obstructive lung disease (decreased forced vital capacity [FVC], forced expiratory volume at 1 sec [FEV$_1$], FEV$_1$/FVC, diffusion capacity) can occur, potentially leading to cor pulmonale and respiratory failure.

Acute silicosis is associated with very intense exposures to silica, leading to symptoms within a few weeks to a few years after exposure. Intense exposure results in lung injury caused by flooding of alveoli with proteinaceous material, or silicoproteinosis. As already noted, the radiographic appearance is that of an alveolar-filling pattern favoring the lower lung zones. Patients present weeks to a few years after exposure with cough, weight loss, fatigue, and occasional pleuritic chest pain, crackles on auscultation, and progression to respiratory failure often complicated by mycobacterial infection.

Criteria for Diagnosis

The diagnosis of silicosis is predicated on a history of exposure to respirable crystalline silica, typical chest x-ray findings, and the lack of a more likely diagnosis. There is no consensus on the use of high-resolution CT, and lung biopsy is seldom required for diagnosis.

Treatment

Treatment is symptomatic and similar to that for other patients with chronic lung disease (see Box 1). Experimental therapies such as oral corticosteroid therapy and whole-lung lavage have been reported, but clinical benefit is unclear. Lung transplantation should be considered for patients with end-stage lung disease.

All forms of silicosis, as well as substantial exposure to crystalline silica in the absence of silicosis, are associated with an increased risk of pulmonary tuberculosis and fungal infections. Patients should be evaluated for latent tuberculosis infection by tuberculin skin testing or with an interferon gamma release assay. A positive tuberculin skin test in a patient with a history of substantial silica exposure of at least 10 mm of induration should be considered evidence of tuberculosis infection, regardless of previous immunization with bacille Calmette-Guérin. If testing for latent tuberculosis infection is positive, an evaluation for active tuberculosis should be performed and active disease treated. If active tuberculosis is not present, treat for latent infection. As in other settings, treatment for active or latent infection should be provided using one of the drug treatment protocols recommended by the Centers for Disease Control and Prevention. Vaccination for influenza should be provided annually. Adults up to 64 years old with silicosis should be vaccinated with 23-valent pneumococcal polysaccharide vaccine (PPSV23, Pneumovax 23). Adults 65 years or older who have not previously been vaccinated should receive 13-valent pneumococcal conjugate vaccine (PCV13, Prevnar 13) followed by PPSV23 in 6 to 12 months. Adults 65 years or older who received PPSV23 before age 65 should receive PCV13 at least 1 year after the most recent dose of PPSV23. Also, a dose of PPSV23 6 to 12 months after PCV13 (or as soon as possible if this time window has passed), and at least 5 years after the most recent dose of PPSV23.

Disclaimer

The findings and conclusions in this report are those of the authors and do not necessarily represent the views of the National Institute for Occupational Safety and Health or the Centers for Disease Control and Prevention.

References

American Thoracic Society. Diagnosis and initial management of nonmalignant diseases related to asbestos. Am J Respir Crit Care Med 2004;170(6):691–715.

Department of Labor. Mine Safety and Health Administration: 30 CFR Parts 56, 57, and 71. Asbestos exposure limit; proposed rule. Fed Reg 2005;70: 43950–89

Leung CC, Yu IT, Chen W. Silicosis. Lancet 2012;379(9830):2008–18.

Miller A. Radiographic readings for asbestosis: Misuse of science—validation of the ILO classification. Am J Ind Med 2007;50:63–7.

Oksa P, Wolff H, Vehmas T, Pallasaho P, Frilander H, editors. Asbestos, Asbestosis, and Cancer–Helsinki Criteria for Diagnosis and Attribution 2014. Tampere: Juvenes Print; 2014.

Petsonk EL, Rose C, Cohen R. Coal mine dust lung disease. New lessons from old exposure. Am J Respir Crit Care Med 2013;187(11):1178–85.

PRIMARY LUNG ABSCESS

Method of
Dan Schuller, MD

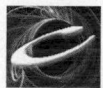

CURRENT DIAGNOSIS

- Lung abscess is usually a complication of aspiration in patients with gingivitis or periodontal disease.
- Mixed aerobic-anaerobic copathogens are common, but sputum cultures are not reliable.
- Lung abscesses are rare in edentulous patients and should prompt evaluation for bronchial obstruction.
- CT scan of the chest is very useful in the diagnostic evaluation.

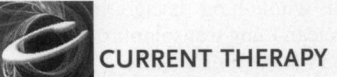
- Prolonged antimicrobial therapy (6–8 weeks) and postural drainage are the cornerstones of therapy.
- Clindamycin (Cleocin) or alternative anaerobic coverage is required even if sputum cultures grow only aerobic bacteria (colonizers or copathogens).
- Percutaneous or bronchoscopic drainage is reserved for selected cases refractory to medical management or at a high risk for complications.
- Surgical resection is seldom needed because of the success of medical therapy.
- Evaluation and management of underlying predisposing conditions should not be neglected.

Definition and Classification

Lung abscess is defined as a focal area of necrosis of the lung parenchyma resulting from microbial infection and usually measuring more than 2 cm in diameter. Smaller or multiple areas of necrosis in contiguous areas are referred to as *necrotizing pneumonia*. Primary lung abscess (80%) is due to direct infection or aspiration. Secondary lung abscess (20%) is secondary to bronchial obstruction, immunodeficiency, pulmonary infarction, trauma, or complications from surgery. Lung abscesses can also be classified according to pathogen (e.g., mixed anaerobic, *Pseudomonas*, mycobacterial, fungal) or duration of symptoms (e.g., chronic with symptoms for more than a month before presentation).

Epidemiology and Risk Factors

Most lung abscesses result from aspiration of oral secretions in patients who harbor high bacterial concentrations in the gingival crevices. Periodontal disease, especially gingivitis, is a major predisposing condition, particularly in hosts impaired by altered sensorium due to alcoholism, anesthesia, coma, drug overdose, seizures, or stroke. Because edentulous persons rarely develop lung abscesses, other causes such as malignancy should be carefully sought. Patients with dysphagia, esophageal disease, poor airway protection, or weak cough and respiratory clearance mechanisms are also at risk for developing lung abscess.

Patients whose immune systems are compromised by malignancy, HIV infection, malnutrition, diabetes, chronic use of corticosteroids, or previous organ transplantation are more likely to be infected with aerobic bacteria, mycobacterial or fungal pathogens. These patients are more likely to have multiple abscesses, less response to treatment, and a worse prognosis.

In children, consider secondary causes including foreign body aspiration, congenital cystic adenomatoid malformation, pulmonary sequestration, cystic fibrosis, bronchiectasis, bronchogenic cyst, congenital immunodeficiency, or severe underlying neurologic abnormality.

Lemierre's disease or jugular vein suppurative thrombophlebitis, usually caused by *Fusobacterium necrophorum*, is a rare infection that begins in the pharynx as a tonsillar or peritonsillar abscess and spreads to involve the internal jugular vein, with septic emboli to the lung with secondary cavitations.

Pathophysiology

The development of a lung abscess usually starts when an insult (e.g., inoculum of highly contaminated oral secretions) overcomes the pulmonary mechanisms of defense and begins a process of pneumonitis in the dependent areas affected by aspiration. Depending on the microbiology and the intensity of the inflammatory response, the acute pneumonitis evolves to tissue necrosis after 7 to 14 days and subsequent cavitation. At first, the enclosing wall is poorly defined, but with time and progressive fibrosis it becomes more discrete. When a communication with the airway exists, the suppurative debris from the abscess can partially drain,

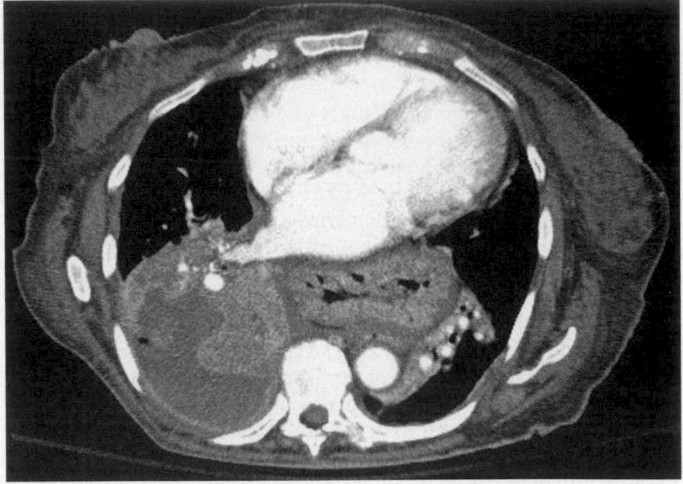

Figure 1. Primary lung abscess in the right lower lobe with rupture into the pleural space causing an empyema.

leaving an air-containing cavity with a radiographic air-fluid level. Occasionally, abscesses rupture into the pleural cavity yielding an empyema or a bronchopleural fistula (Figure 1). Primary abscesses due to aspiration are much more common on the right side than the left and are most often single. The most common locations include the superior segments of the lower lobes and the posterior segment of the right upper lobe.

Clinical Manifestations

Most patients present with insidious symptoms that evolve over a period of weeks to months. Cough productive of copious amounts of putrid, foul-smelling sputum that occurs in paroxysms after changing position are characteristic. Fevers, chills, night sweats, chest pain, dyspnea, general malaise, and fatigue are common. Hemoptysis can vary from blood-streaked sputum to life-threatening hemorrhage. Physical findings can include fever, tachycardia, periodontal disease, halitosis, signs of lung consolidation or pleural effusion, amphoric breath sounds, and occasionally clubbing of the fingers and toes can appear within a few weeks after the onset of an abscess.

Diagnosis

Lung abscess is easily diagnosed when there is a classic clinical presentation with indolent symptoms lasting more than 2 weeks in a host with predisposing risk factors and a chest radiograph revealing a cavitary infiltrate or an air-fluid level. However, numerous pathogens are associated with this syndrome, and attempts to establish microbiological diagnosis and exclude other conditions are warranted.

Computed tomography (CT) scans can be useful for better anatomic definition, to evaluate possible associated conditions such as malignancy, and to rule out pleural involvement. Distinguishing between a lung abscess and an empyema with an associated bronchopleural fistula leading to an air-fluid level can sometimes be challenging, but it is crucial because the management of these conditions is very different. Features that suggest empyema include a lenticular shape or a larger diameter of the air-fluid level on the lateral view of the chest film, an obtuse angle of the cavity with the chest wall, and a split pleural sign with contrast enhancement of the pleura.

Most lung abscesses are caused by anaerobic or mixed aerobic and anaerobic infections. Anaerobic bacteria include *Peptostreptococcus*, *Prevotella*, *Bacteroides* spp., and *Fusobacterium* spp. and are difficult to isolate owing to technical issues and contamination by upper airway flora. Other pathogens, including *Staphylococcus aureus*, *Klebsiella pneumonia*, *Pseudomonas*, *Burkholderia pseudomallei*, *Nocardia*, *Actinomyces*, and mycobacterial or fungal organisms, are more likely to occur in secondary lung abscesses.

Sputum Gram stains and culture should be performed in all patients but interpreted with caution because prior antimicrobial therapy can inhibit growth, and contaminant strains can be misleading. Even when there is abundant growth of a species of aerobic bacteria, treatment should still be directed at covering anaerobes.

In the absence of positive blood or pleural fluid cultures, microbiological confirmation of a lung abscess requires other invasive methods such as a transthoracic needle aspirates (TTNA) or bronchoscopy with bronchoalveolar lavage (BAL) or protected specimen brush (PSB). The best timing for bronchoscopy is controversial because early intervention has the highest diagnostic yield but at the risk of provoking spillage of a relatively contained abscess into additional lobes or the contralateral lung. In patients who are edentulous or in whom there is a high suspicion for malignancy, the indication for bronchoscopic evaluation is almost universal but should be scheduled when the risk for clinical deterioration (e.g., spillage with resultant respiratory failure) has been minimized.

Differential Diagnosis

In addition to the multiple necrotizing infections or an empyema with a bronchopleural fistula (see earlier), there are many noninfectious diseases that can cause cavitary lung lesions and mimic a lung abscess. The differential diagnosis includes neoplasm (primary or metastatic), bullae or cyst with air-fluid level, bronchiectasis, necrotizing vasculitis, or pulmonary infarction. In patients with multiple cavitary lesions, consider septic emboli.

Treatment

Lung abscess is best treated with a prolonged course of adequate antimicrobials and postural drainage. Percutaneous or bronchoscopic drainage and surgery are considered only for selected patients whose disease is refractory to standard care.

Initial empiric antibiotic treatment for a typical community-acquired lung abscess should consist of intravenous clindamycin (Cleocin) 600 to 900 mg every 6 to 8 hours, which has been shown to be superior to penicillin. For patients with a nosocomial or health care–associated lung abscess, additional coverage for enteric gram-negative pathogens including *Pseudomonas aeruginosa* and *Staphylococcus aureus* is appropriate.

Alternative antimicrobial options include ampicillin–sulbactam (Unasyn)[1] 1.5 to 3.0 g IV every 6 hours, piperacillin–tazobactam (Zosyn)[1] 3.35 g IV every 6 hours, cefoxitin (Mefoxin) 2 to 3 g every 6 to 8 hours, or a combination of moxifloxacin (Avelox)[1] 400 mg IV daily and metronidazole (Flagyl) 500 mg IV every 6 to 8 hours. The use of metronidazole as single agent has been associated with a high therapeutic failure rate.

After defervescence and radiographic improvement, parenteral antibiotics can be switched to oral bioequivalent therapy for 6 to 8 weeks or longer depending on the course. Shorter antimicrobial courses are associated with a high rate of relapse. Most experts suggest continuing therapy until there is radiographic resolution or a small stable lesion.

Indications for percutaneous or bronchoscopic drainage include persistent sepsis after 5 to 7 days of antimicrobial therapy, abscesses larger than 4 cm that are under tension or enlarging, and need for mechanical ventilator support. Percutaneous drainage should only be considered when there is a reasonable abscess–pleura symphysis and no associated coagulopathy.

Postural drainage and chest physiotherapy facilitate removal of pus, relieving symptoms and improving gas exchange. Surgical resection is required in less than 10% of patients whose disease is refractory to medical management.

Finally, evaluation and management of the predisposing conditions leading to aspiration should take place after the patient is stabilized. This can include swallowing assessment, dental work, or oral surgery.

---

[1]Not FDA approved for this indication.

Prognosis

Primary lung abscesses in nonimmunocompromised hosts have cure rates of 90% to 95% with antimicrobial therapy and postural drainage alone. However, in immunocompromised patients and those with bronchial obstruction due to cancer, the mortality has been reported between 20% and 75%.

References

Bartlett JG. Anaerobic bacterial pleuropulmonary infections. Semin Respir Med 1992;13:159–64.

Bartlett JG. The role of anaerobic bacteria in lung abscess. Clin Infect Dis 2005;40:923–5.

Gudiol F, Manresa F, Pallares R, et al. Clindamycin vs. penicillin for anaerobic lung infections. Arch Intern Med 1990;150:2525–9.

Hammer DL, Aranda CP, Galati V, Adams FV. Massive intrabronchial aspiration of contents of pulmonary abscess after fiberoptic bronchoscopy. Chest 1978;7:306–7.

Herth F, Ernst A, Becker HD. Endoscopic drainage of lung abscesses. Technique and outcome. Chest 2005;127:1378–81.

Levinson ME, Mangura CT, Lorber B, et al. Clindamycin compared with penicillin for the treatment of anaerobic lung abscess. Ann Intern Med 1983;98:466 71.

Mandell LA, Wunderink RG, Anzueto A, et al. Infectious Diseases Society of America/American Thoracic Society consensus guidelines on the management of community-acquired pneumonia in adults. Clin Infect Dis 2007;44:S27–72.

Mueller PR, Berlin L. Complications of lung abscess aspiration and drainage. AJR Am J Roentgenol 2002;178:1083–6.

PRIMARY LUNG CANCER

Method of
Robert A. Kratzke, MD; and Manish R. Patel, DO

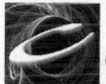

CURRENT DIAGNOSIS

- A history of cigarette smoking is the greatest risk factor.
- Cough, dyspnea, and chest pain are the most common presenting symptoms.
- Diagnosis is made by needle biopsy or pleural fluid cytology.
- The initial staging evaluation should include
  - Positron-emission tomography/computed tomography to evaluate for distant metastasis
  - Magnetic resonance imaging of the brain for small cell lung cancer
- Patients with resectable cancers should have an additional evaluation of mediastinum before resection (i.e., mediastinoscopy or endoscopic ultrasonography)

CURRENT THERAPY

Non–small cell lung cancer
- Stage I: Surgical resection
- Stage II: Surgery + adjuvant chemotherapy
- Stage IIIA: Induction chemotherapy
  - Responders: Surgery with or without XRT
  - Nonresponders: Concurrent chemotherapy + XRT
- Stage IIIB: Concurrent chemotherapy and XRT
- Stage IV: Chemotherapy and drugs targeting the epidermal growth factor receptor
  - 1st line: Platinum doublet chemotherapy with bevacizumab (Avastin) or cetuximab (Erbitux)
  - 2nd line: Pemetrexed (Alimta), docetaxel (Taxotere), or erlotinib (Tarceva) as a single agent

---

Small cell lung cancer

- Limited stage: Concurrent chemotherapy + XRT; PCI for responders
- Extensive stage:
  - 1st line: Carboplatin (Paraplatin)/etoposide (VePesid) or cisplatinum (Platinol)/irinotecan (Camptosar) for four cycles; PCI for responders; supportive care
  - 2nd line: Topotecan (Hycamtin)

Abbreviations: PCI = prophylactic cranial irradiation; XRT = radiation therapy.

Lung cancer is the leading cause of cancer-related death in North America for both men and women. It is not the most common cancer, but most patients with lung cancer are diagnosed at a late stage, accounting for the excess mortality. In the United States, lung cancer accounts for only 13% of new cancer cases but almost one third of cancer-related deaths. Although approximately one third of patients are diagnosed at an early stage, the 5-year survival rate for all patients with lung cancer is less than 20%.

Lung cancer is broadly divided into two groups, small cell lung cancer (SCLC) and non–small cell lung cancer (NSCLC). Approximately 80% of lung cancers are NSCLC, and most of those are squamous carcinomas, adenocarcinomas, or bronchoalveolar carcinomas. Carcinoid tumors and other neuroendocrine tumors are less common, and adenoid cystic carcinomas are rare. Although there is increasing awareness of the importance of histologic subtype in determining responses to newer therapies, the concept of histology-targeted therapy is still evolving, and the standard treatments for NSCLC are generally the same regardless of the histologic subtype.

Epidemiology

Lung cancer occurs most commonly in middle-aged and elderly people. The peak incidence occurs in those aged 65 to 85 years. It is extremely rare in people younger than 30 years of age, and the incidence decreases after 85 years. Before the 1960s, lung cancer was rare among women. However, in North America, the current incidence of lung cancer is almost equal between men and women.

The incidence is decreasing among men and has leveled off in women over the past decade. Lung cancer occurs at a higher frequency in African Americans. This most likely reflects socioeconomic status more than genetic risk, because cigarette smoking remains more common among African Americans. However, there is some evidence that African Americans are more vulnerable to the effects of tobacco-related carcinogens.

Etiology

Cigarette smoking is the established cause of the lung cancer in general. In particular, there is a positive smoking history in 95% of all cases of SCLC. Eighty percent of newly diagnosed lung cancers are in patients who are current or former smokers. Current smokers with a greater than 20-pack-year smoking history have a 2000-fold greater risk of developing lung cancer compared with nonsmokers. Smoking cessation decreases the risk but does not eliminate it. The risk of developing lung cancer in former smokers remains increased by 2- to 10-fold over that in nonsmokers even decades after smoking cessation. There is also clearly a dose-response relationship in tobacco smoke–induced lung cancer in that the risk is highest among those with the greatest prior cigarette exposure. Pipe and cigar smoke also increase the risk of lung cancer. Among nonsmokers, there is a twofold increased risk of developing lung cancer that is clearly associated with inhalation of second-hand smoke.

Other environmental factors have been associated with the development of lung cancer. Up to 20% of lung cancer cases occur among nonsmokers, and this population of patients appears to be rising. Certainly, some of this increase is a result of second-hand exposure to cigarette smoke, but this is difficult to quantify. Asbestos exposure has been associated with the development of lung cancer, and the risk is particularly accentuated by combination with cigarette smoke. Radon exposure has also been associated with the development of lung cancer, particularly in uranium mine workers, in whom the risk approaches 10 times that of the general population. Several other environmental exposures, including chromium, arsenic, and polyvinyl chloride, have been implicated in the development of lung cancers; however, a clear causal link is less well established. Although a patient with a family history of lung cancer has an approximately twofold higher risk, the genetic basis of this finding is not well understood.

Clinical Presentation

The location of tumors and the appearance of paraneoplastic syndromes often determine the clinical presentation of patients with lung cancer (Table 1). Many patients with early-stage disease are asymptomatic and have a mass discovered incidentally on chest radiography or computed tomography (CT) scanning done for some other reason. Centrally located tumors often cause symptoms associated with local effects of the tumor, such as cough, hemoptysis, wheezing, or stridor. Obstruction of the bronchi can lead to postobstructive pneumonia (i.e., pneumonia distal to the obstruction) as the presenting sign, and obstruction of the superior vena cava can lead to the superior vena cava syndrome, with facial edema, bluish discoloration of the upper chest, and shortness of breath. Mediastinal lymph node involvement can cause disruption of the recurrent laryngeal nerve, leading to hoarseness. Tumors arising in the superior sulcus (Pancoast tumors) can lead to a lower brachial plexopathy and Horner's syndrome. Peripheral tumors tend to manifest later as pain when they involve the chest wall or pleura. Pleural effusion may also be the presenting sign for lung cancer.

Lung cancer frequently metastasizes early, and symptoms caused by metastatic lesions may be the first sign of malignancy.

TABLE 1 Clinical Manifestations of Lung Cancer

TUMOR LOCAL EFFECTS	DISTANT METASTASES	PARANEOPLASTIC SYNDROMES
Cough	Bone pain	Hypercalcemia
Dyspnea	Neurologic symptoms	SIADH
Hemoptysis	Headache	Lambert-Eaton syndrome
Chest pain	Nausea and vomiting	Cerebellar ataxia
Hoarseness	Weight loss	Encephalitis
Horner's syndrome	Fatigue	Cachexia/anorexia
SVC syndrome	Abdominal pain	Cushing's syndrome
Postobstructive pneumonia	Spinal cord compression	
Pericardial effusion	Pathologic fracture	

Abbreviations: SIADH = syndrome of inappropriate antidiuretic hormone; SVC = superior vena cava.

Brain metastases are a common presentation, particularly in patients with SCLC, but also in NSCLC. Symptoms such as seizures, nausea and vomiting, headache, and focal neurologic signs may be the initial presentation in such patients. Bony metastases are common in all types of lung cancer and can manifest with pain, pathologic fracture, or spinal cord compression. Liver metastases can cause biliary obstruction and jaundice, but this is not particularly common.

Lung cancers are notable for ectopic production of hormones leading to several paraneoplastic syndromes. These are most commonly described in SCLC but also occur in NSCLC. Probably the most common paraneoplastic syndromes in NSCLC are tumor cachexia and hypercalcemia. Although the causes of tumor cachexia are not well characterized, hyperkalemia is mediated by the production of parathyroid hormone–related peptide. This leads to release of calcium from bones and elevation of calcium in the blood. This syndrome is effectively treated with bisphosphonate therapy. Hypertrophic pulmonary arthropathy can occur with NSCLC or SCLC and is characterized by digital clubbing and periostitis of the long bones demonstrable on plain radiographs. SCLC frequently manifests with paraneoplastic syndromes, the most common being the Lambert-Eaton myasthenic syndrome. Approximately 50% of patients who present with this syndrome have an underlying malignancy, and 95% of those are SCLCs. Other paraneoplastic syndromes related to SCLC are the syndrome of inappropriate antidiuretic hormone, Cushing's syndrome caused by ectopic production of corticotropin, and cerebellar degeneration associated with the elaboration of anti-Yo autoantibodies.

Diagnosis and Evaluation

Once lung cancer is suspected, tissue biopsy is required to make a definitive diagnosis. Several methods can be used to obtain tissue, depending on the location of the tumor. Mediastinal involvement can be assessed by mediastinoscopy; endoscopic ultrasonography is also being increasingly used. Transbronchial biopsy can be performed for centrally located tumors, and the yield may be increased by using endobronchial ultrasonography techniques. For peripheral lesions, CT-guided needle biopsy is usually recommended. If equivocal results are obtained, open procedures using video-assisted thoracoscopic surgery (VATS) are occasionally required. For patients presenting with pleural effusion, cytologic examination of pleural fluid can establish the diagnosis.

Once the diagnosis is confirmed, accurate staging of disease is important to determine the prognosis and appropriate therapy. The first step is to rule out metastatic disease. For NSCLC, fusion positron-emission tomography (PET)-CT scanning is often the best test. Although SCLC tumors are PET-avid tumors, the added

benefit of PET-CT over the CT scan is not clear for this disease. For NSCLC, additional imaging of the brain or the bones is not necessary unless symptoms warrant additional evaluation. In SCLC, the frequency of metastasis to these sites warrants a baseline evaluation with bone scanning and magnetic resonance imaging of the brain at the time of diagnosis.

In patients that are potentially resectable, accurate staging of the mediastinum becomes paramount. Abnormal lymphadenopathy on CT is not adequate to determine lymph node involvement for NSCLC. PET-CT scans have higher sensitivity and specificity, but these tests do not replace direct sampling of the lymph nodes by mediastinoscopy. Endoscopic and endobronchial ultrasonography techniques are less invasive, can be combined with lymph node sampling, and are emerging as an appropriate method of staging the mediastinum in experienced hands.

All patients should be evaluated with baseline blood work including a complete blood count, liver function tests, and assessment of renal function. Assessment of the patient's performance status has important prognostic and therapeutic implications and should be documented for all patients. Furthermore, for patients who are considered surgically resectable, it is important to assess the tolerability of lobectomy or pneumonectomy. A forced expiratory volume in 1 second (FEV_1) greater than 2 L generally predicts the ability to tolerate pneumonectomy, whereas an FEV_1 of less than 1 L predicts worse outcome with lobectomy. The diffusion capacity of carbon monoxide (DL_{CO}) can also be a useful measurement in borderline cases.

Treatment

Non Small Cell Lung Cancer

For NSCLC, the stage at diagnosis is the best predictor of overall survival and the most appropriate therapy (Tables 2 and 3).

Stage I

In the tumor-node-metastasis (TNM) staging system, stage I comprises T1 (stage IA) and T2 (stage IB) tumors that do not have any nodal involvement (N0) and no evidence of distant metastasis (M0). The primary mode of therapy for these patients is surgical resection, which results in 5-year survival rates of approximately 70%. Whenever possible, lobectomy with complete mediastinal lymph node dissection is recommended for accurate pathologic staging. Occasionally, pneumonectomy is required based on the location of the primary tumor; however, the morbidity and mortality of this procedure are much higher than with lobectomy. Video-assisted thoracoscopy approaches, if possible, are often desirable and may result in lower surgical morbidity. Surgical resection may not be feasible for all patients, particularly those with poor

---

TABLE 2 Tumor-Node-Metastasis (TNM) Staging*

PRIMARY TUMOR (T)		REGIONAL LYMPH NODES (N)	
T0	No demonstrable tumor	N0	No regional lymph node disease
T$_{is}$	Carcinoma in situ	N1	Ipsilateral involvement of hilar, peribronchial, or interlobar nodes including by direct extension of the primary tumor
T1	Tumor <3 cm	N2	Involvement of ipsilateral mediastinal nodes
T1a	Tumor <2 cm	N3	Involvement of contralateral mediastinal or hilar nodes or involvement of ipsilateral or contralateral scalene or supraclavicular nodes
T1b	Tumor >2 cm and <3 cm		
T2	Tumor >3 cm but <7 cm		
T2a	Tumor >3 cm but <5 cm	**Distant Metastasis (M)**	
T2b	Tumor >5 cm but <7 cm	M0	No metastasis identified
T3	Tumor >7 cm or any of the following:	M1	Distant metastasis
	• Directly invades the chest wall, diaphragm, phrenic nerve, mediastinal pleura, pericardium, or main bronchus <2 cm from carina	M1a	Separate tumor nodule in contralateral lobe, tumor with pleural nodules, or malignant pleural or pericardial effusion
	• Atelectasis or obstructive pneumonitis of the entire lung	M1b	Distant metastasis
	• Separate tumor nodules within the same lobe		
T4	Tumor of any size that invades the mediastinum, heart, great vessels, esophagus, trachea, recurrent laryngeal nerve, vertebral body, or carina or separate tumor nodule in a different ipsilateral lobe		

*For staging groups, see Table 3.

TABLE 3 Staging Groups*

STAGE	T	N	M
IA	T1	N0	M0
IB	T2	N0	M0
IIA	T1–2a	N0	M0
	T2b	N0	M0
IIB	T2b	N1	M0
	T3	N0	M0
IIIA	T1–2	N2	M0
	T3	N1	M0
	T4	N0–1	M0
IIIB	T4	N2	M0
	Tx	N3	M0
IV	Tx	NX	M1

*For staging of tumors (T), nodes (N), and metastases (M), see Table 2.

pulmonary function or poor performance status. For such patients, primary radiotherapy may be considered. Traditional external-beam radiation therapy results in much poorer outcomes than surgery, although newer techniques are emerging; for example, stereotactic radiosurgery is becoming an effective method of providing local control for stage I tumors.

Several studies have evaluated the role of adjuvant chemotherapy in this group of patients, but no clear survival benefit has emerged. The Cancer and Leukemia Group B (CALGB) 9633 study randomized 344 patients with stage IB tumors to receive either surgery alone or surgery followed by carboplatin (Paraplatin)[1] and paclitaxel (Taxol). A survival benefit was demonstrated only for patients with tumors larger than 4 cm. The JBR.10 study, conducted by the National Cancer Institute of Canada, showed a survival benefit for carboplatin and vinorelbine (Navelbine) adjuvant therapy; however, this study included patients with stage IB, II, and III disease. Additional studies from Europe and Asia have also demonstrated advantages to adjuvant chemotherapy in resected NSCLC, but typically not in tumors smaller than 4 cm. The LACE (Lung Adjuvant Cisplatin Evaluation) meta-analysis incorporated data from five large, randomized trials and also found no significant benefit for adjuvant chemotherapy in stage I patients. In light of these findings, adjuvant therapy in NSCLC is not routinely recommended for small stage I tumors (<4 cm) except as part of a clinical trial. Larger stage I tumors may benefit from adjuvant chemotherapy, and this decision is largely left to the practicing oncologist and patient.

There does not appear to be any added benefit for the use of radiation therapy after surgical resection of stage I tumors. If the surgical margins are positive, adjuvant radiation therapy is routinely recommended, but this occurs infrequently. As discussed later, some patients with a clinical stage I NSCLC are upstaged by the finding of malignant disease in the mediastinum, and in this group postoperative radiation therapy improves local control and, potentially, survival when combined with adjuvant chemotherapy.

Stage II

The approach to treating stage II NSCLC is largely the same as for stage I, with surgical resection as the primary modality of treatment. Again, lobectomy using a minimally invasive video-assisted thoracoscopic approach is preferred whenever possible. Adjuvant chemotherapy offers a more clear survival advantage in patients with stage II disease. All of the aforementioned studies and the meta-analysis showed a benefit for adjuvant chemotherapy in stage II patients.

---

[1]Not FDA approved for this indication.

Stage III

Stage III NSCLC denotes metastasis to mediastinal lymph nodes. The hallmark of treatment in stage III patients is a multimodal approach in which surgery, radiation, and chemotherapy all may play a significant role. The division of this stage into IIIA and IIIB denotes ipsilateral and contralateral nodal involvement, respectively. Whereas the overall prognosis in this group of patients is poor, treatment with curative intent results in long-term survival in 10% to 30% of cases. This also represents the stage with the most heterogeneity, so the approach should be individualized, taking into consideration the patient's performance status, resectability, and extent of disease.

Whether patients with stage III disease should undergo resection of the tumor is still open to some debate. The Intergroup 0139 trial randomized stage IIIA and selected stage IIIB patients to receive concurrent chemoradiation with cisplatin (Platinol)[1] and etoposide (VePesid)[1] plus 45 Gy of radiation followed by surgical resection, or the same chemoradiation with 61 Gy of radiation therapy. Patients in the surgical arm who experienced progression while receiving the chemotherapy were given additional radiation therapy to 61 Gy. There was no difference in overall survival between the two groups (23.6 versus 22.2 months for trimodality and chemoradiation therapy, respectively). Recurrence rates and progression-free survival were much more favorable for the surgery arm. Much of the excess mortality in the surgery arm occurred among those patients who required a pneumonectomy for complete resection. Forty-six percent of patients were downstaged by induction chemotherapy to N0 disease at the time of resection. Among those patients, the 5-year survival rate was 40%, suggesting that good response to induction chemoradiotherapy may predict a benefit for surgical resection. Therefore, for patients with stage IIIA, two cycles of induction chemotherapy with or without irradiation should be offered, followed by restaging. Those with a good response to chemotherapy could be considered for complete resection followed by consolidation chemotherapy. Radiation therapy to the mediastinum should be offered to patients who have residual mediastinal disease at the time of resection. Pneumonectomy for complete resection should be undertaken only in patients who have an excellent performance status and after careful discussion of the risks of this procedure.

In general, stage IIIB disease is inoperable. Patients who have satellite tumors within the same lobe may be considered for resection provided that they do not have disease in the mediastinum and that resection can be accomplished with no more than a lobectomy. For patients with inoperable stage III disease, chemotherapy with irradiation is clearly superior to irradiation alone and can lead to long-term survival, with a 3-year survival rate as high as 30%. The optimal strategy is not known, but a commonly used regimen is the combination of cisplatin[1] and etoposide[1] given concurrently with radiation therapy to 66 Gy for 6 weeks. The use of induction chemotherapy followed by chemoradiation has been evaluated, as has the use of consolidation chemotherapy, but neither regimen has clearly been proven to be superior. For patients with poor performance status, a sequential chemotherapy followed by irradiation might be preferred; for those deemed unfit for chemotherapy, palliative irradiation might be the most appropriate therapy.

Stage IV

For patients with metastatic NSCLC, the treatment is mainly palliative; however, prolongation of survival is a reasonable goal. Despite best therapy, however, median survival time remains less than a year. Several platinum combinations have efficacy in NSCLC. Schiller and colleagues randomized 1207 patients to receive either cisplatin[1] in combination with paclitaxel, docetaxel (Taxotere), or gemcitabine (Gemzar), or a combination of carboplatin[1] and paclitaxel, with survival as the primary endpoint. Response rates were highest with the cisplatin/gemcitabine combination;

---

[1]Not FDA approved for this indication.

however, overall survival was not significantly different for any of the groups. Based on tolerability, carboplatin-containing regimens have largely replaced cisplatin doublets for patients with metastatic disease. Carboplatin can be combined with one of the previously mentioned drugs or with newer agents such as pemetrexed (Alimta) and irinotecan (Camptosar).[1] All have demonstrated efficacy, but no single regimen has emerged with clear superiority. Recently, the addition of bevacizumab (Avastin), a monoclonal antibody against vascular endothelial growth factor, to carboplatin and paclitaxel was shown to prolong median survival to 12.3 months, compared with 10.3 months for chemotherapy alone. This study excluded patients with squamous histology and brain metastasis because of the risk of bleeding complications in those subgroups. Therefore, in patients with nonsquamous NSCLC, this regimen is standard of care. It remains to be seen whether the addition of bevacizumab to other platinum doublets results in similar improvements in survival. In one trial, the combination of cisplatin, gemcitabine, and bevacizumab did not provide any additional benefit to cisplatin and gemcitabine alone.

There has also been interest in the use of drugs targeting the epidermal growth factor receptor (EGFR). Data presented at the 2008 American Society of Clinical Oncology annual meeting demonstrated a modest benefit for the addition of cetuximab (Erbitux),[1] a monoclonal antibody against EGFR, to a regimen of cisplatin[1] and vinorelbine, compared with the chemotherapy regimen alone, in patients whose tumors expressed EGFR. Targeting of EGFR in combination with chemotherapy has not extended to the oral EGFR tyrosine kinase inhibitors, erlotinib (Tarceva) and gefitinib (Iressa). Four phase III randomized trials, two with gefitinib and two with erlotinib, failed to show a survival benefit for EGFR tyrosine kinase inhibitors in combination with platinum doublet chemotherapy in unselected NSCLC patients, although subgroup analysis did demonstrate a benefit for never-smokers, patients with bronchioalveolar histology, and patients with somatic mutations in EGFR. Therefore, cetuximab with cisplatin and vinorelbine can be considered for first-line therapy, but this should be limited to patients with squamous histology and those who have brain metastases, because such patients are not eligible for bevacizumab therapy.

Patients are commonly evaluated for response after two cycles of treatment and continued for four cycles if they have responsive or stable disease. There has been controversy as to whether additional chemotherapy after four cycles of treatment offers any benefit, and the general trend among North American oncologists is to limit the first-line chemotherapy to four cycles. Thus far, no clear benefit to maintenance chemotherapy or extended chemotherapy beyond six cycles has been demonstrated. It should be noted that in the bevacizumab trial and the cetuximab trial, these agents were maintained after completion of four cycles of chemotherapy, until progression or unacceptable toxicity developed. Maintenance pemetrexed resulted in an improvement in progression-free survival, without a clear improvement in overall survival; but it was not clear whether this strategy was better than simply using second-line pemetrexed at the time of progression.

When relapse occurs, there continues to be a survival and quality-of-life benefit associated with salvage therapy. Single-agent regimens should be used to avoid excess toxicity in this poor-prognosis population. Approved second-line treatments include docetaxel and erlotinib, based on improved survival compared with best supportive care. Pemetrexed has also been approved based on non-inferiority to docetaxel in the second-line setting and is better tolerated than docetaxel. If these therapies fail, salvage therapy can be attempted with several active chemotherapy agents, although none of these has demonstrated a clear survival benefit in this population. Chemotherapy should be considered only for patients who have good performance status, and careful emphasis should be placed on palliation of symptoms.

Supportive care is an important adjunct to chemotherapy in the treatment of stage IV lung cancer. Palliative irradiation can be applied to tumors that are causing significant pain or symptoms. Palliative response is seen in more than 50% of patients. Patients with superior vena cava syndrome benefit from the addition of palliative irradiation, as do patients with obstructive pneumonia. One or a few metastases to the brain should be treated with surgical resection followed by whole-brain radiotherapy whenever possible. Stereotactic radiosurgery is an alternative if surgery is not feasible.

Small Cell Lung Cancer

SCLC is hallmarked by aggressive growth and early metastasis. If it is left untreated, median survival time is only 2 to 4 months. However, these tumors are highly sensitive to chemotherapy, and response rates of 60% to 80% are expected. These tumors are also highly radiosensitive, but radiation therapy is limited by the extent of metastatic disease. Although the TNM staging system for NSCLC is applicable, in practical terms SCLC is usually referred to being of limited stage (if the disease is limited to one radiation field) or extensive stage (if not so limited). Surgery is not usually a viable treatment option except in those with very small tumors and no evidence of metastasis to the mediastinum or distant sites.

Patients with limited-stage disease should be treated with four cycles of cisplatin[1] and etoposide with concurrent radiotherapy to the involved field. With this approach approximately 20% of patients are disease free at 3 years. Extensive-stage SCLC is incurable, and median survival is in the range of 8 to 12 months. Chemotherapy can result in dramatic improvements in performance status, and this is one of the few situations in which chemotherapy should be offered even to very moribund patients. The standard of care is carboplatin[1] plus etoposide. Despite numerous trials of multiagent chemotherapy and novel targeted agents, no other regimen has surpassed the results of the standard of care. The combination of carboplatin and irinotecan[1] was shown to be superior to the standard of care in a large, randomized, phase III trial in Japan, but an American trial showed no benefit for this approach. Therefore, cisplatin and irinotecan could be considered an acceptable alternative to the standard of care. The toxicity profile is similar, with the irinotecan regimen causing significant gastrointestinal toxicity and the etoposide regimen having mainly hematologic toxicity. If first-line therapy fails, topotecan (Hycamtin) has been shown to improve quality of life and overall survival when used as second-line therapy. There are no other second- or third-line agents with proven survival or palliative benefit, and, given the dismal prognosis, patients should be considered for a clinical trial whenever possible.

For both limited- and extensive-stage disease, relapse in the brain is a significant cause of morbidity and mortality and has prompted the use of prophylactic cranial irradiation. This approach has consistently proved to be of benefit for patients who have a good response to primary therapy. The benefit has been seen to prevent symptomatic brain metastasis and also to improve overall survival. Cognitive dysfunction after prophylactic cranial irradiation can occur, particularly if it is given concurrently with chemotherapy. Therefore, whenever possible, it should be given only after chemotherapy is completed.

---

[1]Not FDA approved for this indication.

References

Arriagada R, Bergman B, Dunant A, et al. Cisplatin-based adjuvant chemotherapy in patients with completely resected non-small-cell lung cancer. N Engl J Med 2004;350:351–60.

DeVita VT, Hellman S, Rosenberg SA, editors. Cancer: Principles and Practice of Oncology. 4th ed. Philadelphia: Lippincott; 1993.

Noda K, Nishiwaki Y, Kawahara M, et al. Irinotecan plus cisplatin compared with etoposide plus cisplatin for extensive small-cell lung cancer. N Engl J Med 2002;346:85–91.

Pignon JP, Tribodet H, Scagliotti GV, et al. Lung adjuvant cisplatin evaluation: A pooled analysis by the LACE Collaborative Group. J Clin Oncol 2008;26:3552–9.

Sandler A, Gray R, Perry MC, et al. Paclitaxel-carboplatin alone or with bevacizumab for non-small-cell lung cancer. N Engl J Med 2006;355:2542–50.

Schiller JH, Harrington D, Belani CP, et al. Comparison of four chemotherapy regimens for advanced non-small-cell lung cancer. N Engl J Med 2002;346:92–8.

---

[1]Not FDA approved for this indication.

Shepherd FA, Rodrigues Pereira J, Ciuleanu T, et al. Erlotinib in previously treated non-small-cell lung cancer. N Engl J Med 2005;353:123–32.

Slotman B, Faivre-Finn C, Kramer G, et al. Prophylactic cranial irradiation in extensive small-cell lung cancer. N Engl J Med 2007;357:664–72.

Strauss GM, Herndon 2nd JE, Maddaus MA, et al. Adjuvant paclitaxel plus carboplatin compared with observation in stage IB non-small-cell lung cancer: CALGB 9633 with the Cancer and Leukemia Group B, Radiation Therapy Oncology Group, and North Central Cancer Treatment Group Study Groups. J Clin Oncol 2008;26:5043–51.

van Meerbeeck JP, Kramer GW, Van Schil PE, et al. Randomized controlled trial of resection versus radiotherapy after induction chemotherapy in stage IIIA-N2 non-small-cell lung cancer. J Natl Cancer Inst 2007;99:442–50.

Winton T, Livingston R, Johnson D, et al. Vinorelbine plus cisplatin vs. observation in resected non-small-cell lung cancer. N Engl J Med 2005;352:2589–97.

SARCOIDOSIS

Method of
Marc A. Judson, MD

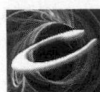

CURRENT DIAGNOSIS

- The diagnosis of sarcoidosis is one of exclusion.
- Tissue biopsy, confirming noncaseating granulomatous inflammation, is required in most cases.
- Efforts should be made to search for the least invasive biopsy site.

CURRENT THERAPY

- Many cases of sarcoidosis do not require treatment.
- All patients should be evaluated for possible pulmonary, eye, and cardiac disease.
- When therapy is indicated, corticosteroids are most commonly used.
- Topical corticosteroids should be given whenever possible.

Sarcoidosis is a multisystem granulomatous disease of unknown cause. The lung is most commonly affected, but any organ may be involved. The clinical presentation of sarcoidosis is variable for two main reasons. First, the manifestations of pulmonary sarcoidosis are variable and can range from an asymptomatic state to significant pulmonary dysfunction. Second, extrapulmonary manifestations of sarcoidosis are common and can cause the prominent symptoms of the disease. This variability in disease presentation often makes the diagnosis of sarcoidosis problematic.

Epidemiology

Sarcoidosis occurs worldwide and affects all races and ages. Although the disease shows a predilection for the third decade of life, a smaller second peak in diagnosis occurs in women older than 50 years. There is a slightly higher disease rate in women at younger ages as well. The highest prevalence of sarcoidosis is found in whites in Scandinavia and in persons of African descent in the United States. In the United States, the lifetime risk of sarcoidosis is 0.85% in whites and 2.4% in African Americans, with an age-adjusted incidence rate of 10.9 per 100,000 persons for the white population and 35.5 per 100,000 persons for African Americans. The relative risk for having sarcoidosis increases significantly if a family member has it as well. In the United States, nearly 20% of African Americans with sarcoidosis have an affected first-degree relative, compared with 5% in whites.

The clinical presentation and severity of sarcoidosis vary among racial and ethnic groups. The disease tends to be more severe in African Americans, whereas whites are more likely to be asymptomatic at presentation. Extrathoracic manifestations are more common in certain populations, such as ocular and cardiac

sarcoidosis in Japanese populations, chronic uveitis in African Americans, and erythema nodosum in Europeans. There is increasing evidence that genetic polymorphisms affect the risks and manifestations of the disease. This is consistent with the current theory that sarcoidosis does not have a single cause but is the result of an abnormal host (granulomatous) response to one of many potential antigens in a genetically susceptible person.

Immunopathogenesis

The exact immunopathogenesis of sarcoidosis is unknown, but it is thought to be similar to that of other granulomatous diseases. That is, antigen-presenting cells (APCs), usually either macrophages or dendritic cells, process and present an antigen via a human leukocyte antigen (HLA) class II molecule to T lymphocytes and their receptors. These T lymphocytes are usually of the CD4 T-helper 1 (T_H1) class. The antigen involved in this reaction is unknown, and there may be many antigens that are each associated with a specific HLA class II molecule and T-cell receptor. This could explain the inability to determine one specific cause of sarcoidosis and the varied phenotypic expressions of the disease.

The interaction of APCs and T lymphocytes activates the APCs to produce tumor necrosis factor α (TNF-α), and other cytokines. A proliferation of CD4 T_H1 lymphocytes also ensues that results in the secretion of interferon-γ (IFN-γ), interleukin (IL)-2, IL-12, and other cytokines. These cytokines activate and recruit monocytes and macrophages and transform them into giant cells, which are important building blocks of the granuloma. Recent evidence suggests that an additional factor leading to this series of immunologic events is persistence of antigen, possibly related to production of soluble AA amyloid fibrils, that prevents antigen degradation.

The typical sarcoidosis lesion is a noncaseating (non-necrotic) granuloma. The sarcoid granuloma consists of a compact core of macrophage-derived epithelioid and multinucleated giant cells surrounded by a perimeter of monocytes, lymphocytes, and fibroblasts. Granulomas can resolve spontaneously or with therapy; however, they can also persist and lead to persistent hyalinization and fibrosis. The development of such fibrosis can cause permanent organ damage and in large part determines the prognosis.

Clinical Features and Clinical Course
Pulmonary Sarcoidosis

Between 30% and 60% of patients with pulmonary sarcoidosis are asymptomatic, and the disease is detected incidentally on chest x-ray. Some patients present with nonspecific pulmonary symptoms, such as dyspnea, cough, wheezing, and chest pain. Respiratory failure from sarcoidosis is extremely rare at presentation. Unlike in many other interstitial lung diseases, crackles are rarely heard on chest auscultation. Abnormalities on the chest radiograph occur in more than 90% of patients with pulmonary sarcoidosis. Bilateral hilar adenopathy occurs in 50% to 85% at disease presentation, and 25% to 50% have parenchymal infiltrates. Sarcoid granulomas have a predilection for the bronchovascular bundles, subpleural locations, intralobular septa, and the airways.

A radiographic staging system was developed several decades ago (Table 1). Groups of patients with higher radiographic stages have more-severe pulmonary dysfunction, lower remission rates,

TABLE 1	Chest Radiograph Stages of Sarcoidosis	
RADIOGRAPHIC STAGE	**BILATERAL HILAR LYMPH NODE ENLARGEMENT**	**PARENCHYMAL DISEASE**
I	Yes	No
II	Yes	Nonfibrotic
III	No	Nonfibrotic
IV	No or yes	Fibrotic

Adapted from Judson MA, Baughman RP: Sarcoidosis. In Baughman RP, du Bois RM, Lynch JP, Wells AU (eds): Diffuse Lung Disease: A Practical Approach. London, Arnold, 2004, p 109–29.

and greater mortality. However, there is significant overlap among these groups, and predictions concerning individual patients based on stage are highly inaccurate.

Advanced pulmonary stage IV sarcoidosis displays destruction of the lung architecture, with upward traction of the hila, lung distortion, upper-lobe volume loss, fibrocystic disease, honeycombed cysts, and decreased lung volumes. Aspergillomas can develop in these large cystic lesions and may be associated with life-threatening hemoptysis. Bronchiectasis from airway distortion also can occur and is an additional potential cause of hemoptysis.

The majority of patients with pulmonary sarcoidosis have a vital capacity of greater than 70% of predicted at diagnosis. Pulmonary function and the chest radiographic findings are often discordant. In pulmonary sarcoidosis patients with a normal lung parenchyma (stage I), the vital capacity, diffusing capacity, partial pressure of arterial oxygen (Pao_2) at rest, Pao_2 with exercise, and lung compliance are abnormal in 20% to 40% of cases. Patients with abnormal lung parenchyma have abnormal pulmonary function tests 50% to 70% of the time. Patients with stage IV fibrocystic sarcoidosis tend to have the most severe pulmonary dysfunction.

Sarcoidosis is an interstitial lung disease with a restrictive ventilatory defect often found on spirometry. It is underappreciated, however, that endobronchial involvement is common in sarcoidosis, and therefore airflow obstruction may be the major abnormality found on pulmonary function testing. Wheezing may be the prominent presenting symptom of sarcoidosis, and many cases of sarcoidosis are misdiagnosed as asthma. Airflow obstruction is also common in chronic pulmonary sarcoidosis, where it is caused by airway distortion from fibrosis. The cause of dyspnea in pulmonary sarcoidosis is multifactorial. It may be the result of abnormalities of gas exchange or lung mechanics, weakness of the respiratory muscles, obesity from corticosteroid therapy, pulmonary hypertension, or sarcoidosis involvement of the heart.

Only 3% to 5% of patients die of sarcoidosis. In the United States, 75% of these deaths are the result of pulmonary involvement. Death from pulmonary involvement is rarely acute but normally is an insidious process that develops over 5 to 25 years with the development of progressive pulmonary fibrosis. Several studies have suggested that pulmonary hypertension is a major risk factor for death from pulmonary sarcoidosis. Patients with aspergillomas are also at risk for death from episodes of life-threatening hemoptysis. Both pulmonary hypertension and aspergillosis are most comonly found in the sarcoidosis patients with stage IV fibrocystic disease. Other organs that result in fatalities from sarcoidosis are the heart and the central nervous system. In Japan, death from sarcoidosis is more commonly caused by cardiac than pulmonary involvement.

Extrapulmonary Sarcoidosis

Sarcoidosis is a multisystem disease that can affect any organ in the body. The extrapulmonary manifestations of sarcoidosis can predominate in many patients. Extrapulmonary disease can affect the prognosis and treatment options for sarcoidosis.

The eyes and skin are the most common extrapulmonary organs involved with sarcoidosis. Ocular manifestations occur in 25% to 50% of patients; anterior uveitis is the most common manifestation. Symptoms of anterior uveitis include red eyes, painful eyes, and photophobia. However, in one third of patients with anterior uveitis from sarcoidosis, the eye is quiet and without symptoms. In addition, an intermediate or posterior uveitis can cause vision problems or can be asymptomatic. For these reasons, all patients with sarcoidosis should undergo an eye examination by an ophthalmologist. Other ocular manifestations of sarcoidosis include conjunctivitis, keratoconjunctivitis sicca (dry eyes), scleritis, and optic neuritis.

Skin lesions in sarcoidosis can be classified into two categories: specific lesions that demonstrate noncaseating granulomas on biopsy and nonspecific lesions that do not. The specific skin lesions are often papular and have a predilection for areas of previous scars and tattoos. Lupus pernio is a type of specific skin lesion causing disfiguring lesions on the face, often with erythema and significant induration. These lesions have a predilection for the nose, cheeks, medial and lateral sides of the eyes, and lateral sides of the mouth. Lupus pernio lesions are relatively recalcitrant to therapy and often respond only partially to corticosteroids. The most common nonspecific skin lesion is erythema nodosum, which is often seen with an acute sarcoidosis presentation of fever, arthritis (especially in the ankles), pulmonary symptoms, and bilateral hilar adenopathy on chest radiograph. This syndrome is known as *Löfgren's syndrome* and tends to have a good long-term prognosis.

Cardiac and neurologic sarcoidosis can be life threatening and are therefore important to recognize. Cardiac involvement is detected clinically in 5% of sarcoidosis patients during life but in 25% at autopsy. Cardiac sarcoidosis can cause left ventricular dysfunction and cardiac arrhythmias, possibly resulting in sudden death. All patients with sarcoidosis should be screened for cardiac sarcoidosis. Such screenings should include eliciting symptoms of left ventricular dysfunction (e.g., orthopnea, peripheral edema) and cardiac arrhythmia (e.g., palpitations, sensation of skipped heartbeats, syncope). Echocardiography and Holter monitoring have been recomended by some as appropriate additional screening tests. The diagnosis of cardiac sarcoidosis is problematic, because the disease is patchy and diagnosed less than 25% of the time by endomyocardial biopsy because of sampling error. Often the diagnosis is made noninvasively, if a typical clinical presentation is coupled with detection of abnormalities on echocardiography, gallium scanning, thallium scanning, cardiac magnetic resonance imaging (MRI), or positron emission tomography (PET).

Clinically apparent neurosarcoidosis occurs in less than 10% of sarcoidosis patients. Palsy of the seventh cranial nerve is the most common manifestation of neurosarcoidosis, and it often predates the diagnosis of the disease. Sarcoidosis can affect any part of the peripheral nervous system and central nervous system and can cause a cranial nerve palsy, mononeuropathy or polyneuropathy, aseptic meningitis, seizures, mass lesions in the brain and spinal cord, and encephalopathy.

Sarcoidosis causes clinically apparent peripheral lymphadenopathy in more than 10% of patients. The spleen may be involved in up to 50% of patients, but it is usually asymptomatic and rarely causes hypersplenism.

Bone involvement is occasional, usually occurring as small cysts or cortical defects found in the small bones of the hands and feet. An acute sarcoid arthritis often is present at disease onset and has a good prognosis. This is commonly found in the ankles of patients who present with Löfgren's syndrome. Chronic sarcoid arthritis is rare. It is usually a nondestructive arthropathy of the shoulders, wrists, knees, ankles, and small joints of the hands and feet.

Sarcoidosis of the sinuses is underappreciated. It can occur in the nasopharynx, hypopharynx, larynx, or any of the sinuses and is known as *sarcoidosis of the upper respiratory tract*. Sarcoidosis of the upper respiratory tract is often relatively recalcitrant to therapy.

Histologic evidence of hepatic sarcoidosis is present in 50% to 80% of sarcoidosis patients, although most of these patients are asymptomatic and have normal liver function tests. Hepatomegaly, abdominal pain, and pruritus are the most common symptoms associated with hepatic sarcoidosis but are present only in 15% to 25% of patients with hepatic involvement. Elevation of the serum alkaline phosphatase is the most common liver function test abnormality.

Hypercalcemia or hypercalciuria leading to nephrolithiasis and renal dysfunction can occur with sarcoidosis. These phenomena are the result of the enzyme 1α-hydroxylase in activated macrophages that convert 25-hydroxyvitamin D to 1,25-dihydroxyvitamin D, the active form of the vitamin. This results in increased gut absorption and increased renal excretion of calcium that can cause nephrolithiasis.

Sarcoidosis rarely involves the thyroid, kidney, breast, renal parenchyma, GU tract, and GI tract.

Box 1 — Factors Associated with a Poor Prognosis in Sarcoidosis

African American race
Extrathoracic disease
Stage II to III versus stage I on chest x-ray
Age >40 years
Splenic involvement
Lupus pernio
Disease duration >2 years
Forced vital capacity <1.5 L
Stage IV chest x-ray or aspergilloma
Pulmonary hypertension

Data from Judson MA, Baughman RP: Sarcoidosis. In Baughman RP, du Bois RM, Lynch JP, Wells AU (eds): Diffuse Lung Disease: A Practical Approach. London, Arnold, 2004, p 109–29.

Patients can have constitutional symptoms such as fever, night sweats, weight loss, malaise, and fatigue at presentation. These symptoms occasionally are associated with hepatic sarcoid involvement but together may be a sign of the systemic nature of the disease, presumably from cytokine release, rather than specific organ involvement. A small fiber neuropathy may occur with sarcoidosis and cause pain or autonomic dysfunction. Patients who present with Löfgren's syndrome or with asymptomatic bilateral hilar adenopathy on chest radiograph have a good prognosis. African Americans tend to have a worse prognosis than whites, with lower forced vital capacity and more new organ involvement within 2 years of diagnosis. Box 1 lists risk factors associated with a poor prognosis.

Diagnosis and Initial Work-up
The diagnosis of sarcoidosis requires a compatible clinical picture, histologic demonstration of noncaseating granulomas, and exclusion of other diseases capable of producing a similar histologic and clinical picture. Mycobacterial and fungal diseases always must be considered as alternative diagnoses. Therefore, stains and cultures of tissue specimens for mycobacteria and fungi always should be obtained when the diagnosis of sarcoidosis is considered. Because sarcoidosis is a diagnosis of exclusion (granulomatous inflammation of unknown cause), bear a healthy degree of skepticism in the diagnosis and follow the patient closely for additional clues supporting an alternative diagnosis.

Sarcoidosis is a systemic disease, so the signs or symptoms of extrathoracic disease such as uveitis, skin lesions, or an elevated serum alkaline phosphatase should be sought. The diagnosis in a patient who has granulomas on lung biopsy and interstitial infiltrates without adenopathy on radiographic studies is suspect. In this situation, granulomatous infections and bioaerosol exposure causing hypersensitivity pneumonitis should be strongly considered. Because of the varied clinical presentation of sarcoidosis, there is no single diagnostic algorithm.

It is prudent to select a biopsy site associated with less morbidity, such as the skin if a lesion is present. Transbronchial lung biopsy has a diagnostic yield of 40% to more than 90% in pulmonary sarcoidosis. It is recommended that at least four lung biopsy specimens be collected to maximize the diagnostic yield. Endobronchial biopsy has a 40% to 60% sensitivity and adds to the yield of transbronchial biopsy.

Bronchoalveolar lavage (BAL) with examination of lymphocyte populations has been used in the evaluation of possible pulmonary sarcoidosis. In sarcoidosis, there is an increased number of BAL lymphocytes, and these are predominantly $CD4^+$. It has been proposed that an increase in BAL lymphocytes and a BAL CD4/CD8 ratio greater than 3.5 make the diagnosis of sarcoidosis highly likely.

Although serum angiotensin-converting enzyme (ACE) often is elevated in active sarcoidosis, the specificity and sensitivity of this test are inadequate for it to be used diagnostically. Serum ACE may be used as supportive evidence for the diagnosis, and it also may be used in some instances to follow disease activity.

Gallium-67 (^{67}Ga) scanning is cumbersome because it takes several days to complete and is infrequently used as a diagnostic test. However, bilateral hilar uptake and right paratracheal uptake (lambda sign) coupled with lacrimal and parotid uptake (panda sign) with ^{67}Ga strongly suggest a diagnosis of sarcoidosis.

Gadolinium enhancement on MRI and fluorodeoxyglucose PET scanning may replace ^{67}Ga scanning for detecting sarcoidosis activity because evidence suggests that they may be more sensitive in detecting sarcoidosis activity and they can be performed in one sitting.

Ideally, the diagnosis of sarcoidosis requires demonstration of noncaseating granulomas in at least one organ. However, certain clinical presentations are so specific for the diagnosis of sarcoidosis that the diagnosis may be accepted without tissue biopsy. Extreme caution must be used in these situations to ensure that there is no clinical information that would suggest an alternative diagnosis that should prompt a tissue biopsy. Clinical or laboratory findings that strongly support the diagnosis of sarcoidosis without a tissue biopsy are listed in Box 2.

Treatment
Therapy is not mandated for sarcoidosis because the disease can remit spontaneously. Therapy is indicated for potentially dangerous disease that includes neurosarcoidosis, cardiac sarcoidosis, hypercalcemia that does not respond to dietary measures, ocular sarcoidosis that does not respond to topical (eyedrop) therapy, and other life- or organ-threatening disease. Therapy also should be considered when the disease is progressive. Relative indications for therapy include arthritis that fails to respond to nonsteroidal anti-inflammatory drugs (NSAIDs); a systemic inflammatory response syndrome of fever, night sweats, fatigue, and arthralgias; and symptomatic hepatic disease. In general, treatment is discouraged for asymptomatic elevations of serum liver function tests, specific levels of ACE, or asymptomatic uptake on ^{67}Ga scan (with the possible exceptions of the heart or brain).

The decision to treat sarcoidosis can be problematic, because the disease has a variable prognosis that must be weighed against the potential side effects of therapy. It is often most prudent to monitor patients without therapy if they are asymptomatic or have only mild organ dysfunction. For pulmonary sarcoidosis, asymptomatic patients and those with mild disease that might spontaneously remit usually are not treated. For patients with clinical findings that predict spontaneous remission (e.g., erythema nodosum), the benefits of treatment often are offset by the toxicity of therapy. Often these patients can be managed with palliative therapy such as NSAIDs for arthralgias and fever and bronchodilators and inhaled corticosteroids for wheezing and cough.

It is recommended that patients with mild to moderate pulmonary sarcoidosis be observed for 2 to 6 months, if possible. Patients who improve will have avoided the toxicity of corticosteroids, and patients who deteriorate over this period should be considered for treatment. Patients with pulmonary dysfunction who neither improve nor deteriorate during the observation period may be given a corticosteroid trial, or they may be observed further. Patients with severe pulmonary dysfunction or pulmonary symptoms causing significant impairment should be treated.

Corticosteroids often are used to treat sarcoidosis, but the dose, duration of therapy, and method by which one can assess effectiveness have not been standardized. Topical corticosteroid therapy

Box 2 — Clinical or Laboratory Findings that Strongly Support a Diagnosis of Sarcoidosis without a Tissue Biopsy

Löfgren's syndrome
Heerfordt's syndrome (uveoparotid fever)
Asymptomatic bilateral hilar adenopathy on chest x-ray
^{67}Ga scan showing a lambda sign and a panda sign

should be used whenever possible in an attempt to minimize systemic complications. This includes corticosteroid eye drops for anterior sarcoid uveitis and corticosteroid creams and injections for localized skin lesions. Pulmonary sarcoidosis usually is treated initially with 20 to 40 mg/day of prednisone or its equivalent. Higher doses may be required for neurosarcoidosis and cardiac sarcoidosis. The patient usually is evaluated within 2 to 12 weeks for a response. Patients failing to respond to therapy within 3 months are unlikely to respond to a more protracted course of therapy or a higher dose. Among the responders, the corticosteroid dose is tapered to 5 to 10 mg/day of a prednisone equivalent or an every-other-day regimen. Treatment is usually continued for 12 months.

The relapse rate after corticosteroid therapy is withdrawn may be as high as 70%, and therefore patients need to be followed closely as the corticosteroid dose is tapered and discontinued. In some patients, there may be recurrent relapses requiring long-term low-dose therapy. On occasion, the chronic prednisone dose needed to prevent relapse is less than 5 mg/day. Patients who relapse after corticosteroids have been withdrawn should be re-treated with corticosteroids. Alternative agents, such as corticosteroid-sparing agents, to control the disease in a patient on a chronic low dose of prednisone should be considered. On occasion, alternative agents may completely replace corticosteroid therapy. In general, corticosteroid-sparing agents should not be considered unless the patient requires more than 7.5 mg/day of prednisone to control the disease.

Methotrexate (Rheumatrex)[1] and hydroxychloroquine (Plaquenil)[1] are the most-studied alternative sarcoidosis medications. They are usually used as corticosteroid-sparing agents but at times can be used as replacement therapy. Methotrexate is most useful for pulmonary, skin, joint, and eye sarcoidosis. Hydroxychloroquine is often used for sarcoidosis of the skin, joints, and nerves and for hypercalcemia from sarcoidosis. Azathioprine (Imuran)[1] may be useful for sarcoid uveitis, but usually it is added to corticosteroid plus methotrexate in this instance. Monocycline (Minocin)[1] and doxycycline (Vibramycin)[1] may be useful for skin sarcoidosis. Cyclophosphamide (Cytoxan)[1] is used occasionally and seems to have a potential role in neurosarcoidosis. Leflunimide has also been shown to be useful in the treatment of pulmonary and extrapulmonary sarcoidosis. Recently anti–TNF-α therapies have shown promise in the treatment of sarcoidosis. Such agents include pentoxifylline (Trental),[1] thalidomide (Thalomid),[1] and monoclonal antibodies against TNF-α, such as infliximab (Remicade)[1] and adalimumab (Humira).[1]

---

[1]Not FDA approved for this indication.

References

Baughman RP, Culver DA, Judson MA. A concise review of pulmonary sarcoidosis. Am J Respir Crit Care Med 2011;183:573–891.

Baughman RP, Nunes H, Sweiss NJ, et al. Established and experimental medical therapy of pulmonary sarcoidosis. Eur Respir J 2013;41(6):1424–38.

Baughman RP, Teirstein AS, Judson MA, et al. Clinical characteristics of patients in a case control study of sarcoidosis. Am J Respir Crit Care Med 2001;164:1885–9.

Chen ES, Song Z, Willett MH, et al. Serum amyloid A regulates granulomatous inflammation in sarcoidosis through Toll-like receptor-2. Am J Respir Crit Care Med 2010;181:360–73.

Hunninghake GW, Costabel U, Ando M, et al. ATS/ERS/WASOG statement on sarcoidosis. Am J Respir Crit Care Med 1999;160:736–55.

Iannuzzi MC, Rybicki BA, Teirstein AS. Sarcoidosis. N Engl J Med 2007;357: 2153–65.

Judson MA. An approach to the treatment of pulmonary sarcoidosis with corticosteroids. Chest 1999;111:623–31.

Judson MA. The diagnosis of sarcoidosis. Clinics Chest Med 2008;29:415–27.

Judson MA. Sarcoidosis: Clinical presentation, diagnosis, and approach to treatment. Am J Med Sci 2008;335:26–33.

Judson MA, Costabel U, Drent M, et al. The WASOG Sarcoidosis Organ Assessment Investigators. The WASOG Sarcoidosis Organ Assessment Instrument: An update of a previous clinical tool. Sarcoidosis Vasc Diff Lung Dis 2014;31:19–27.

Lower EE, Baughman RP. Prolonged use of methotrexate in refractory sarcoidosis. Arch Intern Med 1995;155:846–51.

Lynch JP, Kazerooni EA, Gay SE. Pulmonary sarcoidosis. Clin Chest Med 1997;755–85.

Sahoo DH, Bandyopadhyay D, Xu M, et al. Effectiveness and safety of leflunomide for pulmonary and extrapulmonary sarcoidosis. Eur Respir J. 2011;38:1145–50.

TUBERCULOSIS AND OTHER MYCOBACTERIAL DISEASES

Method of

Jotam Pasipanodya, MD; Ronald Hall II, PharmD, MSCS; and Tawanda Gumbo, MD

Mycobacterial diseases are some of the oldest documented infectious diseases in humans, and they still cause significant morbidity and mortality. *Mycobacterium tuberculosis* complex, *Mycobacterium avium* complex (MAC), and *Mycobacterium leprae* are slow-growing, acid-fast bacilli that belong to the family Mycobacteriaceae of the order Actinomycetales. This chapter deals with management of diseases caused by *M. tuberculosis*, MAC, and *M. leprae*. A summary of diseases caused by other, less common mycobacteria is presented in Table 1.

Recent evidence suggests that the mycobacteria causing tuberculosis (TB) might have co-evolved with humans. Clues attesting to the success of mycobacteria as human pathogens include the prolonged period of latency and the ability to cause extensive disease in only a narrow host range. DNA evidence suggests that the *M. tuberculosis* strains causing the current waves of TB epidemics most likely evolved from a common ancestor. *Mycobacterium canetti* and the other strains that form the *M. tuberculosis* complex (i.e., *Mycobacterium africanum*, *Mycobacterium microti*, and *Mycobacterium bovis* strains) also evolved from the ancestral strain through successive loss of DNA. This is contrary to the belief that the *M. tuberculosis* complex evolved from *M. bovis*.

Tuberculosis

Epidemiology

TB remains a global pandemic, with 9.3 million new cases and 1.4 million deaths reported worldwide in 2007. Approximately 1 of every 7 patients who has TB is co-infected with the human immunodeficiency virus (HIV). Whereas global TB incidence trends are stabilizing after reaching a peak in 2004, rates in countries with a low TB burden have been declining gradually. An explanation could be the similar plateau and declines in HIV prevalence observed in the year 2000. On the other hand, this could merely reflect the natural ebbs and increases inherent to epidemic cycles.

Global estimates show that one third of humankind has been infected with *M. tuberculosis*, the TB disease-causing bacillus. About 80% of global TB is accounted for by the 22 high-burden countries. The top five countries in rank order are India, China, Indonesia, Nigeria, and South Africa. TB program priorities and approaches to combating the disease differ among and within countries. These differences are based on the availability of resources and the prevalence of HIV within communities. For example, program goals in areas of low TB incidence, such as the United States, are aimed at TB elimination. Therefore, in the United States, treatment of latent TB is a priority. Reducing TB transmission through increased diagnosis of patients with active TB disease is the primary goal in high-incidence areas.

In 2007, a total of 13,299 TB cases (case rate, 4.4 per 100,000 population) were reported to the Centers for Disease Control and Prevention (CDC) from the 50 U.S. states and the District of Columbia. Foreign-born persons accounted for 58% of the national case total. This means that a high degree of suspicion is needed for the diagnosis of TB when recent immigrants are seen in the clinic. The top five countries of origin for foreign-born persons with TB in the United States were Mexico, the Philippines, India, Vietnam, and China. Since the 1992 TB resurgence peak, the number of cases reported annually in the United States has decreased by 50%.

Natural History

Susceptibility to *M. tuberculosis* infection and the subsequent progression of that infection to active TB disease is influenced by the complex interaction of host, pathogen, and environmental factors. Between 20% and 30% of people exposed to a person with active

TABLE 1	Species of Mycobacteria	
MICROBE	**RESERVOIR**	**CLINICAL MANIFESTATION**
Always Pathogenic in Humans		
M. tuberculosis	Humans	Pulmonary and disseminated tuberculosis
M. bovis	Cattle, humans	TB-like disease
M. africanum	Humans, monkeys	Rarely, TB-like pulmonary disease
M. leprae	Humans	Leprosy
M. canetti	Humans, possibly others	Rarely, TB-like pulmonary disease
Potentially Pathogenic in Humans		
M. avium complex	Soil, water, birds, swine, cattle, environment	Disseminated and pulmonary TB-like disease
M. microti	Rodents, llamas, cats, ferrets, and possibly humans	Rarely, TB-like pulmonary disease
M. kansasii	Water, cattle	TB-like disease
Uncommon or Rarely Pathogenic in Humans		
M. flavescens	Humans, environment	TB-like disease
M. genavense	Humans, birds	Blood-borne disease with AIDS
M. haemophilum	Unknown	Skin, joint, bone, and pulmonary infections in immunocompromised individuals; lymphadenitis in children
M. malmoense	Environment, possibly others	TB-like pulmonary disease in adults; lymphadenitis in children
M. marinum	Fish, water	Skin infections
M. scrofulaceum	Soil, water	Cervical lymphadenitis
M. simiae	Monkeys, water	TB-like pulmonary disease and disseminated disease with AIDS
M. szulgai	Water, environment	TB-like pulmonary disease
M. ulcerans	Humans, environment	Skin infections (Buruli ulcer)
M. xenopi	Water, birds	TB-like pulmonary disease

Abbreviations: M. = genus *Mycobacterium*; TB = tuberculosis.
Adapted from Coberly JS, Chaisson RE: Tuberculosis. In Nelson KE, Williams CM (eds): Infectious Disease Epidemiology: Theory and Practice, 2nd ed. Boston, Jones and Bartlett, 2007.

TB become infected. Animal models, twin studies, segregation studies, and candidate gene analysis studies provide insight into the role of host genetic factors in susceptibility to TB.

The immune system contains the infection in more than 90% to 95% of persons infected. Protective immunity mediated by subsets of T lymphocytes produces soluble lymphokines that enable macrophages to kill intracellular bacilli. The bacilli are often not completely eradicated and remain dormant in macrophages or other cells, with the potential to reactivate to active disease when the immune system wanes. This is termed latent TB infection (LTBI). The lifetime risk of reactivation to active TB disease is 5% to 10%. This risk of reactivation increases with several factors, including development of the acquired immunodeficiency syndrome (AIDS), renal failure, immunomodulatory therapy, and poorly controlled diabetes mellitus.

In a small subgroup of patients, *M. tuberculosis* infection is not brought under control during primary infection and quickly progresses to disseminated disease. TB that follows such a course is called progressive primary TB. Primary TB is associated with a higher mortality rate, and death typically occurs within 2 years after infection. The risk of developing TB disease after being infected is higher in males from infancy to 6 years of age. Males older than 45 years of age are also at an increased risk compared to females of the same age.

Diagnosis of Active Tuberculosis

In immunocompetent persons, pulmonary involvement is the most common presentation, followed by isolated extrapulmonary disease. Involvement of only extrapulmonary sites is rare, and most immunocompromised patients present with both pulmonary and extrapulmonary involvement. The presenting signs and symptoms of active TB disease are site specific. However, constitutional symptoms such as fever, night sweats, and fatigue are common and gradually evolve over many weeks. Patients should be specifically asked about constitutional symptoms, because these symptoms raise the index of suspicion. Atypical presentations are common in patients who are immunosuppressed and can delay diagnosis.

Definitive diagnosis is made on the basis of a positive culture. Therefore, all patients with suspected TB must have the appropriate specimens collected for microscopic and, if appropriate, histologic examination. Mycobacterial culture and sensitivity testing should also be performed, if available. Acid-fast bacillus (AFB) staining and microscopy is limited by poor sensitivity (45%–80% with culture-confirmed TB cases) and poor positive predictive value (50%–80%) for TB in settings where nontuberculous mycobacteria are commonly isolated. TB culture results are available only after 2 to 6 weeks. Nucleic acid amplification (NAA) testing can also be used to confirm a TB diagnosis in 24 to 48 hours, even when the specimen sample is limited. NAA tests can detect the presence of *M. tuberculosis* in 50% to 80% of AFB-negative and culture-positive specimens. The CDC now recommends that evaluation of at least the first diagnostic specimen include NAA testing.

Serial radiologic images can be used to exclude active TB and assess clinical improvement.

Principles of Treatment

The goal of anti-TB therapy is cure. A secondary objective is minimizing the transmission of *M. tuberculosis* to others by curing the patient. Treatment outcomes are best when patient-centered treatments and care are offered, regardless of whether the treatment facility is private or public. Patient management and supervision plans should be tailored to the patient's clinical and social circumstances. Directly observed therapy (DOT) is recommended by regulatory bodies to help ensure adherence to treatment and is regarded as central to current case management. However, the efficacy of DOT compared with self-administration has been questioned in recent studies. There are three types of anti-TB therapy: prophylaxis, definitive TB therapy for drug-susceptible infection, and therapy for drug-resistant TB.

Chemoprophylaxis

The confusing terms preventive therapy and chemoprophylaxis are sometimes used to describe treatment of LTBI. Preventive therapy, in this context, does not actually prevent infection; rather, it prevents development of active TB in those already infected. Therefore, the better descriptive term, treatment of LTBI, is preferred. Treatment of minimal or latent TB infection prevents subsequent evolution to active disease. A series of double-blind, placebo-controlled clinical trials done in the 1950s and 1960s provided evidence demonstrating the effectiveness of treatment of LTBI. Priority is usually given to those patients with the highest risk for reactivation.

Treatment of LTBI, particularly when it is targeted toward persons with higher risks of reactivation, is one of the major strategies for elimination of TB in the United States. Targets include people who have been recently infected and those who were remotely infected but have concurrent disease that puts them at higher risk for developing reactivation disease. There are more than 11 million people with LTBI in the United States, each with a 5% to 10% lifetime risk of developing TB disease.

The Mantoux method of tuberculin skin testing is commonly used to diagnose LTBI as well as active disease. Use of tuberculin skin testing is hampered by low sensitivity in immunocompromised patients, low specificity in persons who have received the bacille Calmette-Guérin (BCG) vaccine, and the requirement to return to a trained person to have the test read after 48 to 72 hours. Results are interpreted based on the patient scenario (Box 1).

Recently, various blood-testing methods that are based on detection of the interferon γ (IFN-γ) released by T lymphocytes in response to *M. tuberculosis*–specific antigens have become available as an alternative to skin testing. These tests may be more specific than the tuberculin skin test in BCG-vaccinated and immunocompromised populations. However, IFN-γ release assays do not differentiate LTBI from active TB disease. Currently available IFN-γ release assays are QuantiFERON, QuantiFERON-Gold, and ELISPOT. The CDC recommends these tests for LTBI screening of health care workers, recent immigrants, injection drug users, prison and jail inmates and workers, and contacts of TB cases within schools, workplaces, and the military. Prohibitive costs limit the use of these assays in resource-limited places.

Table 2 summarizes the regimens currently recommended by the American Thoracic Society (ATS), CDC, and Infectious Diseases Society of America (IDSA) for treatment of LTBI. Because of high rates of hospitalization and death from liver injury, the ATS and the CDC no longer recommend the 2-month regimen of daily or twice-weekly rifampin (Rifadin) plus pyrazinamide for LTBI. Directly observed 12-dose once-weekly regimen of isoniazid (INH; Nydrazid) and rifapentine (RPT; Priftin) is recommended as an option equal to the standard INH 9-month daily regimen for treating LTBI in otherwise healthy people 12 years of age and older who were recently in contact with infectious TB, or who had tuberculin skin test or blood test for TB infection conversions, or those with radiologic findings consistent with healed pulmonary TB. In recent large clinical trials of mostly adults without HIV, this regimen was associated with fewer serious adverse events, higher completion rates, and equal efficacy, as compared with isoniazid for 9 months. Rifampin or rifabutin (Mycobutin)[1]

---

[1]Not FDA approved for this indication.

may be used to treat LTBI in HIV-infected persons exposed to TB that is resistant to isoniazid (INH; Nydrazid) and susceptible to rifampin, with dose adjustments and diligence taken to prevent cytochrome P-450–derived drug interactions with antiretroviral agents.

Definitive Therapy

The decision to initiate therapy is made based on local epidemiologic information; the patient's clinical, pathologic, and radiologic data; and the results of microscopic and culture examination. Therapy may be started immediately if the index of suspicion is high or if the patient is gravely ill. However, in general, clinicians should still collect initial specimens for microscopic evaluation and culture before starting treatment. HIV testing and baseline liver function testing, serum creatinine levels, and platelet counts should be conducted as part of standard medical care for patients with suspected or documented TB disease.

Achieving microbiologic cure by killing all bacilli and preventing emergence of clinically significant drug-resistant mutants are the primary goals of definitive TB therapy. Therapy is prolonged despite sputum conversion and resolution of symptoms, because

TABLE 2 CDC-Recommended Treatment for Latent Tuberculosis Infection

DRUG	INTERVAL*	ORAL DOSE (mg/kg)		MONITORING
		CHILDREN	ADULTS	
Isoniazid (INH, Nydrazid)	Daily Twice weekly	10–20[3] 20–40	5 15	Monthly, LFTs[†] at baseline, repeat in selected patients if initial results are abnormal; hepatitis risk increases with age and alcohol consumption; pyridoxine[1] 10–25 mg/d may prevent peripheral neuropathy and CNS effects
Rifampin (Rifadin)	Daily Twice weekly	10–20 —	10 10	Weeks 2, 4, and 8 with pyrazinamide; contraindicated in patients receiving antiretroviral drugs; baseline LFTs[†] and CBC and platelets
Rifabutin (Mycobutin)[1]	Daily Twice weekly	— —	5 5	Weeks 2, 4, and 8; baseline LFTs[†] and CBC and platelets; use adjusted daily doses of rifabutin and monitor for decreased antiretroviral activity and rifabutin toxicity if PIs or NNRTIs are taken concurrently; contraindicated with saquinavir (Invirase) or delavirdine (Rescriptor)
Pyrazinamide[‡]	Daily Twice weekly	— —	15–20 50	Weeks 2, 4, and 8; LFTs[†] at baseline; avoid in first trimester of pregnancy
Rifapentine (Priftin)[§]	Weekly	—	10–14 kg: 300 mg 14.1–25 kg: 450 mg 25.1–32.0 kg: 600 mg 32.1–49.9 kg: 750 mg ≥50.0 kg: 900 mg	Monthly, LFTs[†] at baseline, repeat in selected patients if initial results are abnormal; hepatitis risk increases with age and alcohol consumption

Abbreviations: CBC = complete blood count; CDC = Centers for Disease Control and Prevention; CNS = central nervous system; LFT = liver function test; NNRTI = nonnucleoside reverse transcriptase inhibitor; PI = protease inhibitor.
Adapted from American Thoracic Society: Treatment of tuberculosis. Am J Respir Crit Care Med 2003;167:603–62.
[1]Not FDA approved for this indication.
[3]Exceeds dosage recommended by the manufacturer.
*All intermittent dosing should be given by directly observed therapy (DOT).
[†]LFTs include aspartate aminotransferase (AST), alanine aminotransferase (ALT), and serum albumin.
[‡]Used with either rifampin or rifabutin in combination therapy for 2–4 mo.
[§]Rifapentine (RPT) is formulated as 150-mg tablets in blister packs that should be kept sealed until usage, as shown above. Combined wih INH.

some organisms persist in some tissues. DOT is generally recommended to ensure compliance with prescribed medications.

The four ATS/CDC/IDSA-recommended regimens used for treating TB caused by drug-susceptible organisms are shown in Table 3. Each regimen has an initial phase of 2 months followed by a choice of several options for the continuation phase of 4 or 7 months. Treatment of previously untreated TB consists of 2 months of an initial phase of four drugs: isoniazid, rifampin, pyrazinamide, and ethambutol (Myambutol) or streptomycin (generally not used in the United States). The newer rifamycins are also first-line drugs used under certain circumstances. Rifabutin[1] is used if rifampin is contraindicated, as in patients taking certain antiretroviral drugs; rifapentine (Priftin) is used in the once-weekly continuation phase with isoniazid in selected patients (see Table 3). If the organisms are later demonstrated to be susceptible to isoniazid and rifampin, ethambutol is discontinued. The continuation phase is usually 4 months of daily or intermittent isoniazid and rifampin or rifapentine. The 7-month continuation phase is recommended only for those patients with cavitary TB caused by susceptible organisms that remains sputum positive after 2 months of DOT, patients whose initial treatment phase did not include pyrazinamide, and patients on weekly isoniazid and rifapentine whose sputum smear was still positive at the end of the intensive phase. There is evidence from many clinical trials done worldwide that demonstrates the efficacy of supervised intermittent therapy is similar to daily dosing in terms of various clinical outcomes. Routine follow-up to monitor adverse events and adherence to the treatment regimen should occur at least monthly.

Approximately 80% of patients who take the four-drug therapy for susceptible organisms are expected to convert from culture positive to negative after 2 months, and 90% to 95% after 3 months. Failure of treatment is defined by positive culture or, at times, positive smears after 4 months of supervised therapy. Relapse is defined by recurrent TB at any time after completion of treatment or apparent cure. Relapses most commonly occur during the first 6 to 12 months after the end of therapy. Treatment of initially susceptible disease can fail for many reasons, including extensive cavitary disease, drug resistance, malabsorption of drugs, laboratory error, and biologic variation in response. In any case, positive smears or cultures after 2 months of supervised therapy should be carefully evaluated to determine the cause. In addition, a full course of therapy is determined by the number of doses completed. Hence, a 6-month daily regimen (including both initiation and continuation phases) consists of at least 182 doses of isoniazid and rifampin and 56 doses of pyrazinamide (see Table 3). All missed doses should be taken. Patients interrupting therapy by more than 14 days during the initial phase or more than 3 months during continuation phase should be restarted on therapy from the beginning.

Treatment of Tuberculosis in Resource-Poor Settings
Direct observation of patients taking therapy is just one of five elements of DOTS recommended by the World Health Organization and the International Union Against Tuberculosis and Lung Disease for TB treatment programs in resource-poor settings. The five elements of DOTS are:
- Government commitment to sustained TB control activities
- Case detection by sputum microscopy in symptomatic patients self-reporting to health centers
- Standardized treatment regimen of 6 to 9 months for at least all confirmed sputum smear-positive cases, with DOT for at least the intensive phase
- Regular, uninterrupted supply of essential anti-TB drugs
- Standardized recording and reporting system that allows for patient and program assessments

Smear microscopy for AFB is emphasized because of cost concerns and because access to culture facilities is limited in most countries. Three AFB stains that include early-morning sputum smears are recommended for a diagnosis. However, some recent data refute the need for three sputum samples by suggesting that no significant benefit is derived from the third smear when performed in high-burden countries. A new molecular diagnostic test called Xpert MTB/RIF assay detects *M. tuberculosis* complex within 2 hours with an assay sensitivity that is much higher than that of smear

---

[1]Not FDA approved for this indication.

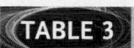

TABLE 3 Drug Regimen for Culture-Positive Pulmonary Tuberculosis Caused by Drug-Susceptible Organisms

REGIMEN	DRUGS	INTERVAL AND MINIMUM DURATION*	DOSE (MAXIMUM DOSE IN 24 h OR MAXIMUM DURATION)	
			CHILDREN	ADULTS
Initial Phase				
1	Isoniazid (INH, Nydrazid) Rifampin (Rifadin) Pyrazinamide Ethambutol (Myambutol)	Once daily on 7 d/wk for 56 doses (8 wk), or Once daily on 5 d/wk for 40 doses (8 wk)	10–20 mg/kg/d[3] (300 mg) 10–20 mg/kg/d (600 mg) 15–30 mg/kg/d (2000 mg) 15–25 mg/kg/d	5 mg/kg/d (300 mg) 10 mg/kg/d (600 mg) 15–30 mg/kg/d (2000 mg) 15–25 mg/kg/d
2	Isoniazid Rifampin Pyrazinamide Ethambutol	Once daily on 7 d/wk for 14 doses (2 wk), then twice weekly for 12 doses (6 wk), or Once daily on 5 d/wk for 10 doses (2 wk), then twice weekly for 12 doses (6 wk)	20–40 mg/kg/d (900 mg) 10–20 mg/kg/d (600 mg) 50–70 mg/kg/d (4000 mg) 50 mg/kg/d[3]	15 mg/kg/d (900 mg) 10 mg/kg/d (900 mg)[3] 50–70 mg/kg/d (4000 mg) 50 mg/kg/d[3]
3	Isoniazid Rifampin Pyrazinamide Ethambutol	Three times weekly for 24 doses (8 wk)	20–40 mg/kg/d (900 mg) 10–20 mg/kg/d (600 mg) 50–70 mg/kg/d (3000 mg) 50 mg/kg/d[3]	15 mg/kg/d (900 mg) 10 mg/kg/d (900 mg)[3] 50–70 mg/kg/d (3000 mg) 50 mg/kg/d[3]
4	Isoniazid Rifampin Ethambutol	Once daily on 7 d/wk for 56 doses (8 wk), or Once daily on 5 d/wk for 40 doses (8 wk)		
Continuation Phase[†]				
1a	Isoniazid Rifampin	Once daily on 7 d/wk for 126 doses (18 wk), or Once daily on 5 d/wk for 90 doses (18 wk)	182–130 doses (max. 26 wk)	
1b[‡]	Isoniazid Rifampin	Twice weekly for 36 doses (18 wk)	92–76 doses (max. 26 wk)	
1c[§]	Isoniazid Rifapentine	Once weekly for 18 doses (18 wk)	74–58 doses (max. 26 wk)	
2a[‡]	Isoniazid Rifampin	Twice weekly for 36 doses (18 wk)	62–58 doses (max. 26 wk)	
2b[§]	Isoniazid Rifapentine (Priftin)	Once weekly for 18 doses (18 wk)	44–40 doses (max. 26 wk)	
3a	Isoniazid Rifampin	Three times weekly for 54 doses (18 wk)	78 doses (max. 26 wk)	
4a	Isoniazid Rifampin	Once daily on 7 d/wk for 217 doses (31 wk), or Once daily on 5 d/wk for 155 doses (31 wk)	273–195 doses (max. 39 wk)	
4b	Isoniazid Rifampin	Twice weekly for 62 doses (31 wk)	118–102 doses (max. 39 wk)	

Adapted from the American Thoracic Society: Treatment of tuberculosis. Am J Respir Crit Care Med 2003;167:603–62.
[3]Exceeds dosage recommended by the manufacturer.
*When directly observed therapy (DOT) is used, drugs may be given on 5 d/wk, with the necessary number of doses adjusted accordingly; therapy administered on 5 d/wk should always be given by DOT.
[†]Patients with cavitation on initial chest radiography and positive cultures at 2 mo should receive a 7-mo (31-wk) regimen of either 217 (daily) or 62 (twice weekly) doses in the continuation phase
[‡]Not recommended for HIV-infected patients with CD4+ T-cell count <100 cells/mm[3].
[§]Use only in HIV-negative patients who have negative smears at 2 mo and no cavitation on chest radiography.

microscopy, and detects multidrug-resistant tuberculosis at the same time. In HIV infected patients, the test has a rate of case detection that is increased by 45%, as compared to smear microscopy.

Susceptibility testing is strongly recommended for patients who fail to convert to smear-negative status after 2 months of treatment. The prevalence of drug resistance in areas of high TB burden is unknown because of limited laboratory capacity.

Individualized TB care in resource-limited areas is difficult to implement because most decisions are made based solely on clinical judgment or limited radiologic findings. These challenges result in the use of standardized treatments that emphasize cost-effectiveness for utilitarian returns. This "one size fits all" approach is likely to worsen the financial and clinical outcomes of some patients.

Treatment of Tuberculosis in Special Circumstances
Multidrug-Resistant Tuberculosis
In resource-poor settings, where susceptibility testing facilities usually are not available, the surrogate terms "retreatment" and "chronic" are used to define various forms of drug-resistant strains. In the United States, about 1.1% of TB cases reported in 2007 had

primary multidrug resistance, which is defined as resistance to at least isoniazid and rifampin in a patient with no previous history of TB treatment. Combination therapy including first- and second-line drugs is used to treat multidrug-resistant TB, and at least one of the drugs must be an injectable agent. Some of the second-line TB drugs are levofloxacin (Levaquin),[1] cycloserine (Seromycin), ethionamide (Trecator), p-aminosalicylic-acid (Paser), capreomycin (Capastat), kanamycin (Kantrex),[1] and amikacin (Amikin).[1]

Therapy takes several years to complete. Treatment failure, costs, and drug-related side-effects are higher with the second-line drugs. Patients with suspected treatment failure should be managed at specialized facilities with necessary expertise where the full range of drug susceptibilities can be performed. As a general rule, single drugs should never be added to failing regimens because this leads to acquired resistance to each new drug. Drug resistance in mycobacteria occurs through random genetic mutations, with minimal lateral transfer of genetic material. Chances of detecting primary

[1]Not FDA approved for this indication.

resistance are greater when the bacillary load is high, for example in patients with multiple cavitary disease. In addition, selective pressure can induce the emergence of drug-resistant mutants.

Extrapulmonary and Sputum-Negative Tuberculosis

TB can involve any organ or tissue in the body. Therefore, histologic examination or smear microscopy with AFB staining of specimens from appropriate sites is necessary to confirm extrapulmonary TB. The specimens may include cerebrospinal, pleural, pericardial, or ascitic fluids and lymph node tissue, bone, bone marrow, or brain biopsy specimens. The yield of bacilli in staining or culture from body fluids is usually very low (<50% for pericardial fluid). A diagnosis of extrapulmonary TB can also be made based on clinical and radiologic improvement on empiric therapy if it is not possible to obtain a specimen.

The same four drugs and dosing regimens used to treat pulmonary TB are also used for extrapulmonary disease. Use of adjunct corticosteroids in patients with pericardial or meningeal TB was associated with lower mortality in some prospective and retrospective studies. Bone and joint TB is treated for 6 to 9 months, and central nervous system TB (including meningitis) for 9 to 12 months. Duration of treatment for TB in all other sites is 6 months if pyrazinamide is given during the first 2 months; otherwise, the continuation phase is prolonged to 7 months. The ATS/CDC/IDSA guidelines also recommend intermittent therapy. Once-weekly administration of isoniazid and rifapentine should be avoided in the continuation phase, because data to support the efficacy of this regimen in patients with extrapulmonary TB is lacking. However, recent data report poor long-term outcomes despite adequate therapy in patients successfully treated for pericardial and meningeal TB. These and other studies question the wisdom of using the same drug exposures to target organisms in different physiologic spaces, given that drug penetration, and therefore drug concentrations, in these spaces differs.

A diagnosis of sputum-negative TB is made in patients for whom the clinical and radiologic findings strongly suggest TB but the culture and AFB smears are negative. In addition, there is clinical and/or radiologic improvements at the end of 2 months of therapy. A 2-month continuation phase of isoniazid and rifampin is used for these patients, rather than the 4 months used for sputum-positive patients.

Mycobacterium avium *Complex Infection*

In patients with advanced AIDS and other causes of severe cell-mediated immune deficiency, MAC causes disseminated infections. In others with ill-defined immunologic disorders, and in those who are immunocompetent, MAC causes chronic pulmonary disease. Therapy for these patients is long and complicated, with many adverse effects. The same regimens are used for all patients regardless of their HIV/AIDS status. Drug resistance is frequent.

Culture from blood or other sites (e.g., lymph node, bone marrow) is required to demonstrate invasive or disseminated disease. Bacteriologic diagnosis should be based on positive cultures or smears (or both) from sputum or bronchial wash specimens. If sputum specimens are used to diagnose pulmonary disease, at least three positive sputum smears are needed for diagnosis. Clinical and radiologic findings must also be consistent with MAC.

Combination therapy is used to prevent selection of drug-resistant mutants and to capitalize on the additive and synergistic effects of antimycobacterial drugs. Clarithromycin (Biaxin) or azithromycin (Zithromax) together with ethambutol is now the cornerstone of MAC therapy. Three- or four-drug combinations that included ethambutol, a rifamycin (rifampin[1] or rifabutin), clofazimine (Lamprene),[1] isoniazid,[1] or ciprofloxacin (Cipro)[1] were shown to clear bacteremia better in some AIDS patients, especially those with a bacillary burden of greater than 2 $\log_{10}$ colony-forming units per milliliter. However, adherence to therapy was poor because of toxicity. Two-way interactions between

antiretroviral medications (e.g. protease inhibitors, nonnucleoside reverse transcriptase inhibitors) and the rifamycins as well as clarithromycin and rifabutin can make patient management complicated. AIDS patients with CD4-positive T-cell counts lower than 50 cells/mm^3 should be offered prophylactic therapy to protect against disseminated MAC. Azithromycin has greater efficacy, has fewer drug interactions, and can be given once weekly. Resistance has been observed in 16% of patients treated with azithromycin and in 29% to 58% of those treated with clarithromycin. Resistance of MAC to rifamycin is rare.

Mycobacterium leprae

Leprosy is a legendary disease that has been stigmatized throughout many societies and eras of human history. The causative organism is *M. leprae*. The global incidence of this disease has been on the decline. Fewer than 200 cases are diagnosed each year in the United States, almost exclusively in immigrants. Most practitioners in the United States will not encounter patients with this disease.

The important clinical features of leprosy are skin lesions, nerve involvement, disfigurement of the face, and reversal reactions. Skin lesions are hypopigmented anesthetic macules and papules. Peripheral nerve enlargement can also occur, as can disfigurement of parts of the face (e.g., leonine faces). Leprosy has a spectrum of manifestations. Some patients have multibacillary leprosy associated with poor cell-mediated immunity. Others have paucibacillary leprosy resulting in a few skin patches with a robust cell-mediated immunity. Skin reactions encountered in paucibacillary leprosy due to delayed hypersensitivity to *M. leprae* antigens are called reversal reactions. These may also occur when massive numbers of bacilli are killed by chemotherapy.

Diagnosis is established on the basis of a compatible clinical picture and demonstration of *M. leprae* in smears or on histologic analysis of skin and nerve biopsy specimens. The lepromin skin test is nonreactive in multibacillary disease but reactive in paucibacillary disease. Unlike other mycobacteria, *M. leprae* has stringent growth requirements; it can only grow when injected into foot pads of some animals and does not grow on artificial laboratory media.

The aim of leprosy treatment is total cure. As with other slow-growing mycobacteria, multidrug therapy is administered. Therapy consists of rifampin,[1] clofazimine (Lamprene), and dapsone. Recently, fluoroquinolones have been investigated for a role in the treatment of leprosy. In the United States, the therapy for paucibacillary leprosy is oral rifampin 600 mg/day and dapsone 100 mg/day for 6 months, followed by dapsone monotherapy for at least 3 years. The treatment of multibacillary leprosy is similar to that of paucibacillary leprosy, with dual therapy being continued for 3 years. Clofazimine is added for reverse reactions and if there is dapsone resistance. After 3 years of dual or even triple therapy, dapsone monotherapy is continued for 10 years. These regimens differ from those recommended by the World Health Organization, which are utilized elsewhere.

Mycobacteria Other Than Tuberculosis

Mycobacteria other than tuberculosis (MOTT) are mycobacterial species that may cause human disease but do not cause TB (see Table 1). The incidence of infection is reported to be about 2 in 100,000, but this may be an underestimate. The common mycobacteria identified in the United States are *M. avium, Mycobacterium gordonae, Mycobacterium fortuitum, Mycobacterium kansasii,* and *Mycobacterium chelonae.* MOTT infections are not contagious, but some produce signs and symptoms similar to those of TB, whereas others cause suppurative-like disease. MOTT primarily affect the lungs, and disease progression is slow. MOTT cause reportable disease.

Diagnosis is based on clinical presentation, radiologic findings, examination of histologic specimens, culture, and smear staining for microscopy of sputa or bronchial washings. The diagnostic criteria for MOTT in AIDS and non-AIDS patients are

- Chest radiographs showing infiltrates or nodular or cavitary disease or computed tomographic scans consistent with bronchiectasis or small nodules
- Three positive cultures with negative AFB smears or two positive cultures and one positive AFB smear from three sputum or bronchial washing specimens obtained within the previous 12 months
- Positive culture from bronchial wash with AFB smear or growth on solid media greater than 2+
- Transbronchial or lung biopsy consistent with mycobacterium histologic features and sputum or bronchial washings that are nondiagnostic of another disease.
- For mycobacteria other than tuberculosis such as *M. abscessus/ chelonae* therapy is more with standard antibiotics like ceftriaxone. However, all these patients should be reported to specialist centers.

References

Agins BD, Berman DS, Spicehandler D, et al. Effect of combined therapy with ansamycin, clofazimine, ethambutol, and isoniazid for *Mycobacterium avium* infection in patients with AIDS. J Infect Dis 1989;159:784–7.

American Thoracic Society. Centers for Disease Control and Prevention, Council of the Infectious Diseases Society of America. Diagnostic standards and classification of tuberculosis in adults and children. Am J Respir Crit Care Med 2000; 161:1376–95.

Bach MC. Treating disseminated *Mycobacterium avium-intracellulare* infection. Ann Intern Med 1989;110:169–70.

Bellamy R, Beyers N, McAdam KP, et al. Genetic susceptibility to tuberculosis in Africans: A genome-wide scan. Proc Natl Acad Sci U S A 2000;97:8005–9.

Blumberg HM, Burman WJ, Chaisson RE, et al. American Thoracic Society/Centers for Disease Control and Prevention/Infectious Diseases Society of America: Treatment of tuberculosis. Am J Respir Crit Care Med 2003;167: 603–62.

Brosch R, Gordon SV, Marmiesse M, et al. A new evolutionary scenario for the *Mycobacterium tuberculosis* complex. Proc Natl Acad Sci U S A 2002;99:3684–9.

Cegielski JP, Devlin BH, Morris AJ, et al. Comparison of PCR, culture, and histopathology for diagnosis of tuberculous pericarditis. J Clin Microbiol 1997; 35:3254–7.

Centers for Disease Control and Prevention. Reported Tuberculosis in the United States, 2007. Atlanta: U.S. Department of Health and Human Services, CDC; 2007.

Comstock GW. Frost revisited: The modern epidemiology of tuberculosis. Am J Epidemiol 1975;101:363–82.

Comstock GW. Tuberculosis in twins: A re-analysis of the Prophit survey. Am Rev Respir Dis 1978;117:621–4.

Comstock GW, Livesay VT, Woolpert SF. Evaluation of BCG vaccination among Puerto Rican children. Am J Public Health 1974;64:283–91.

Dannenberg Jr AM. Delayed-type hypersensitivity and cell-mediated immunity in the pathogenesis of tuberculosis. Immunol Today 1991;12:228–33.

Engel ME, Matchaba PT, Volmink J. Corticosteroids for tuberculous pleurisy. Cochrane Database Syst Rev 2007;(4):CD001876.

Guerra RL, Hooper NM, Baker JF, et al. Use of the amplified *Mycobacterium tuberculosis* direct test in a public health laboratory: Test performance and impact on clinical care. Chest 2007;132:946–51.

Guerra RL, Hooper NM, Baker JF, et al. Cost effectiveness of different strategies for amplified *Mycobacterium tuberculosis* direct testing for cases of pulmonary tuberculosis. J Clin Microbiol 2008;46:3811–2.

Gumbo T, Louie A, Deziel MR, et al. Concentration-dependent *Mycobacterium tuberculosis* killing and prevention of resistance by rifampin. Antimicrob Agents Chemother 2007;51:3781–8.

Gumbo T, Louie A, Liu W, et al. Isoniazid bactericidal activity and resistance emergence: Integrating pharmacodynamics and pharmacogenomics to predict efficacy in different ethnic populations. Antimicrob Agents Chemother 2007;51: 2329–36.

Haas CJ, Zink A, Palfi G, et al. Detection of leprosy in ancient human skeletal remains by molecular identification of *Mycobacterium leprae*. Am J Clin Pathol 2000;114:428–36.

Iseman MD. A Clinician's Guide to Tuberculosis. Philadelphia: Lippincott Williams & Wilkins; 2000.

Kallmann FJ, Reisner D. Twin studies on the significance of genetic factors in tuberculosis. Am Rev Tuberculosis 1943;47:549–74.

Kramnik I, Demant P, Bloom BB. Susceptibility to tuberculosis as a complex genetic trait: Analysis using recombinant congenic strains of mice. Novartis Found Symp 1998;217:120–31.

Kramnik I, Dietrich WF, Demant P, Bloom BR. Genetic control of resistance to experimental infection with virulent *Mycobacterium tuberculosis*. Proc Natl Acad Sci U S A 2000;97:8560–5.

Mabaera B, Lauritsen JM, Katamba A, et al. Sputum smear-positive tuberculosis: Empiric evidence challenges the need for confirmatory smears. Int J Tuberc Lung Dis 2007;11:959–64.

Mabaera B, Lauritsen JM, Katamba A, et al. Making pragmatic sense of data in the tuberculosis laboratory register. Int J Tuberc Lung Dis 2008;12:294–300.

Mayosi BM, Wiysonge CS, Ntsekhe M, et al. Clinical characteristics and initial management of patients with tuberculous pericarditis in the HIV era: The Investigation of the Management of Pericarditis in Africa (IMPI Africa) registry. BMC Infect Dis 2006;6:2.

Mayosi BM, Wiysonge CS, Ntsekhe M, et al. Mortality in patients treated for tuberculous pericarditis in sub-Saharan Africa. S Afr Med J 2008;98:36–40.

Moonan PK, Weis SE. Assessing the impact of targeted tuberculosis interventions. Am J Respir Crit Care Med 2008;177:557–8.

Moore DF, Guzman JA, Mikhail LT. Reduction in turnaround time for laboratory diagnosis of pulmonary tuberculosis by routine use of a nucleic acid amplification test. Diagn Microbiol Infect Dis 2005;52:247–54.

Nerlich AG, Haas CJ, Zink A, et al. Molecular evidence for tuberculosis in an ancient Egyptian mummy. Lancet 1997;350:1404.

Nuermberger E, Grosset J. Pharmacokinetic and pharmacodynamic issues in the treatment of mycobacterial infections. Eur J Clin Microbiol Infect Dis 2004; 23:243–55.

Prasad K, Singh MB. Corticosteroids for managing tuberculous meningitis. Cochrane Database Syst Rev 2008;(1):CD002244.

Stein CM, Nshuti L, Chiunda AB, et al. Evidence for a major gene influence on tumor necrosis factor-alpha expression in tuberculosis: Path and segregation analysis. Hum Hered 2005;60:109–18.

Stein CM, Zalwango S, Malone LL, et al. Genome scan of *M. tuberculosis* infection and disease in Ugandans. PLoS ONE 2008;3:e4094.

Volmink J, Garner P. Directly observed therapy for treating tuberculosis. Cochrane Database Syst Rev 2007;(4):CD003343.

Weis SE, Miller TL, Hilsenrath PE, Moonan PK. Comprehensive cost description of tuberculosis care. Int J Tuberc Lung Dis 2005;9:467–8.

World Health Organisation. Global leprosy situation. Wkly Epidemiol Rec 2005;80:289–95.

World Health Organization. Global Tuberculosis Control: Epidemiology, Strategy, Financing: WHO Report 2009. Geneva: WHO; 2009.

Zink A, Haas CJ, Reischl U, et al. Molecular analysis of skeletal tuberculosis in an ancient Egyptian population. J Med Microbiol 2001;50:355–66.

VENOUS THROMBOEMBOLISM

Method of

Sarah Takach Lapner, MD; and Clive Kearon, PhD

Venous thromboembolism (VTE), which includes deep venous thrombosis (DVT) and pulmonary embolism (PE), is the third most common cause of vascular death (after myocardial infarction and stroke) and the leading cause of preventable death among hospitalized patients. Thrombosis starts in the deep veins, and PE occurs when such thrombi break free and lodge in the pulmonary arteries, where they obstruct blood flow and can cause lung damage (i.e., pulmonary infarction). About 90% of the instances of DVT involve the legs, about 5% involve the upper extremities (axillary, subclavian, or jugular veins), and the remaining 5% involve other veins of the body (e.g., internal iliac, renal, ovarian). DVT that is confined to the deep veins of the calf, without involvement of the popliteal vein, is termed isolated distal DVT, whereas that involving the popliteal or a more proximal vein is termed proximal DVT (most proximal DVT also involves the distal veins). Thrombosis of the subcutaneous veins is referred to as superficial vein thrombosis or superficial thrombophlebitis. Superficial vein thrombosis mostly occurs in the legs (e.g., long or short saphenous veins, often in association with varicosities), and its main importance is that it causes pain and swelling and may extend to cause DVT. This chapter focuses on DVT of the legs and PE.

Pathogenesis and Risk Factors

Virchow is credited with identifying stasis, vessel wall injury, and hypercoagulability as the pathogenic triad responsible for thrombosis. This classification of risk factors for VTE remains valuable. Most patients who develop VTE have more than one, and often multiple, risk factors.

Venous Stasis

The importance of venous stasis as a risk factor for VTE is demonstrated by the fact that most DVT associated with stroke affects the paralyzed leg, and most DVT associated with pregnancy affects the left leg, due to extrinsic compression of the left common iliac vein by the pregnant uterus and the right common iliac artery. General immobilization, such as in hospitalized patients and in patients with leg injuries or other chronic illness, is also an important risk factor. Venous stasis is thought to predispose to thrombosis by causing local hypoxia (e.g., in venous valve cusps), which attracts inflammatory cells and causes endothelial dysfunction, leading to an increase in the local concentration of clotting factors and tissue factor and an increase in interactions between circulating cells and the venous endothelium.

Vessel Damage

Venous endothelial damage, usually as a consequence of accidental injury, manipulation during surgery, or iatrogenic injury, is an important risk factor for VTE. Three quarters of proximal DVT that complicates hip surgery occurs in the operated leg, and thrombosis is common with indwelling venous catheters. Venous injury is thought to predispose to thrombosis by exposing blood to subendothelial tissue factor and to collagen, which binds von Willebrand's factor.

Hypercoagulability

A complex balance between naturally occurring coagulation and fibrinolytic factors and their inhibitors serves to maintain blood fluidity and hemostasis. Inherited or acquired changes in this balance can predispose to thrombosis. The most important inherited biochemical disorders associated with VTE are defects of the naturally occurring inhibitors of coagulation (i.e., deficiencies of antithrombin, protein C, or protein S and resistance to activated protein C caused by factor V Leiden) and the G20210A prothrombin gene mutation, which is associated with elevated levels of prothrombin. The first three coagulation deficiencies listed are rare in the normal population (combined prevalence, <1%), have a combined prevalence of approximately 5% in patients with a first episode of VTE, and are associated with a 10- to 40-fold increase in the risk of VTE. The factor V Leiden mutation is common, occurring in approximately 5% of Caucasians and 20% of patients with a first episode of VTE (i.e., a fourfold increase in VTE risk). The G20210A prothrombin gene occurs in approximately 2% of Caucasians and 5% of patients with a first episode of VTE (i.e., a 2.5-fold increase in VTE risk).

Elevated levels of a number of coagulation factors (I, II, VIII, IX, XI) are also associated with thrombosis in a dose-dependent manner. It is probable that such elevations are often inherited, and there is strong evidence for this supposition for factor VIII and factor II; for example, the G20210A prothrombin gene is associated with an increase of approximately 25% in factor II (prothrombin). Abnormalities of the fibrinolytic system have a questionable association with VTE.

Acquired hypercoagulable states include estrogen therapy (threefold increase in VTE, highest during the first 6 months), antiphospholipid antibodies (anticardiolipin antibodies or lupus anticoagulants or both), systemic lupus erythematosus, malignancy, chemotherapy for cancer, and surgery. Patients who develop immunologically related heparin-induced thrombocytopenia also have a very high risk for arterial and venous thromboembolism. Unlike the congenital abnormalities, acquired risk factors are often transient, and this fact has important implications for the duration of anticoagulant prophylaxis and treatment.

Combinations of Risk Factors and Risk Stratification

The risk of developing VTE depends on the prevalence and severity of risk factors (Box 1). By assessment of these factors, hospitalized patients can be categorized as having a low, moderate, or high risk of VTE (Table 1). Patients with active cancer are among those with the highest risk of thrombosis, because they often have a large number of major risk factors, such as the hypercoagulable state associated with cancer, recent surgery, chemotherapy, generalized immobility from weakness, localized stasis associated with venous obstruction by tumor, and the presence of indwelling venous catheters.

Epidemiology and Natural History of Venous Thromboembolism

The overall incidence of VTE is about 1.5 per 1000 persons per year in adults, with about two thirds of these episodes being symptomatic DVT and about one third being symptomatic PE (with or

---

Box 1	Risk Factors for Venous Thromboembolism (VTE)*

Patient Factors
- Previous VTE[†]
- Age older than 40 years, and particularly older than 70 years[†]
- Pregnancy, puerperium
- Marked obesity
- Inherited hypercoagulable state

Underlying Condition and Acquired Factors
- Malignancy[†]
- Estrogen therapy
- Cancer chemotherapy
- Paralysis[†]
- Prolonged immobility
- Major trauma[†]
- Lower limb injuries[†]
- Heparin-induced thrombocytopenia
- Antiphospholipid antibodies

Type of Surgery
- Lower limb orthopedic surgery[†]
- General anesthesia >30 min

*Combinations of factors have an at least an additive effect on the risk of VTE.
[†]Common major risk factors for VTE.

---

without symptoms of DVT). However, the incidence of VTE is highly influenced by age. Before the age of 16 years, most likely because the immature coagulation system is resistant to thrombosis, VTE is very rare and is largely confined to children with major provoking factors such as indwelling venous lines. The risk of VTE increases exponentially with advancing age, with an almost twofold increase every decade, from an annual incidence of 0.3 per 1000 at 40 years to 1 per 1000 at 60 years and 4 per 1000 at 80 years of age.

VTE occurs slightly more frequently in men than in women, although this pattern is reversed before 40 years of age because of the association of VTE with estrogen-containing contraceptives and pregnancy. The relative frequency of PE to DVT is somewhat higher in the elderly.

About 50% of the cases of VTE are associated with hospitalization (about half before and half after discharge), which emphasizes the importance of using appropriate prophylaxis to prevent VTE in high-risk patients. Among hospital-associated VTE cases, about half occur in surgical and half in medical patients. About one quarter of VTE cases are associated with cancer; one quarter are associated with minor illnesses, injuries, or estrogen therapy; and one quarter are not associated with any apparent clinical risk factor (referred to as unprovoked or idiopathic VTE). There is overlap among these categories; for example, there is a particularly high risk of VTE among patients with cancer who are hospitalized.

Of all episodes of VTE, about three quarters are first episodes and one quarter are recurrent episodes. Clinically important components of the natural history of VTE are summarized in Box 2.

Diagnosis of Deep Venous Thrombosis

Clinical Features

The clinical features of DVT, such as localized swelling, redness, tenderness, and distal edema, are nonspecific, and the diagnosis should always be confirmed by objective tests. About 85% of ambulatory patients with clinically suspected DVT have another cause for their symptoms. The conditions that are most likely to simulate DVT are a ruptured Baker's cyst, cellulitis, muscle tears, muscle cramp, muscle hematoma, external venous compression, superficial thrombophlebitis, and the postthrombotic syndrome. Of patients with symptomatic DVT, about 75% have proximal

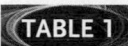

TABLE 1 Risk Stratification for VTE in Hospitalized and Postoperative Patients, Frequency of VTE without Prophylaxis, and Recommended Methods of Prophylaxis*

RISK FACTOR	VENOGRAPHIC DVT[†] (%)		PULMONARY EMBOLISM (%)		RECOMMENDED PROPHYLAXIS
	CALF	PROXIMAL	SYMPTOMATIC	FATAL	
Low Risk: Minor (usually same-day) surgery in a mobile patient Medical patients, fully mobile No additional risk factors	2	0.4	0.2	<0.01	Early mobilization
Moderate Risk: Most general surgery patients Most medical patients	20	5	2	0.5	Low-dose UFH (5000 U SQ preoperatively and bid or tid postoperatively) LMWH (~3000 U/d SQ with a preoperative start)[‡] Fondaparinux (Arixtra)[1] IPC or GC stockings, alone or with pharmacologic methods
High Risk: Most general surgery patients with previous VTE Major knee or hip surgery Major trauma, spinal cord injury (Heparin-induced thrombocytopenia)	50	15	5	2	LMWH (>3000 U/d) Fondaparinux Warfarin (Coumadin)[§], Dabigatran (Pradaxa)[1], Rivaroxaban (Xarelto), Apixaban (Eliquis) IPC devices, alone or with GC stockings or pharmacologic methods or both (Specific nonheparin therapy)

Abbreviations: DVT = deep venous thrombosis; GC = graduated compression; IPC = intermittent pneumatic compression; LMWH = low-molecular-weight heparin; UFH = unfractionated heparin; VTE = venous thromboembolism.

[1]Not FDA approved for this indication.

*New anticoagulants (e.g., oral direct thrombin, anti-factor Xa inhibitors) are becoming available for moderate- and high-risk patients. Additional new anticoagulants are becoming available.

[†]Asymptomatic DVT detected by screening bilateral venography.

[‡]Higher doses are used in high-risk patients (e.g., ~ 4000 U once daily with a preoperative start in Europe; ~3000 U twice daily with a postoperative start in North America).

[§]Usually started postoperatively and adjusted to achieve an international normalized ratio of 2.0–3.0.

Box 2 Natural History of Venous Thromboembolism: Key Points

- Clinical factors can identify high-risk patients.
- VTE starts in the calf veins in >75% of patients.
- Three quarters of asymptomatic DVT detected postoperatively by screening venography are confined to the distal (calf) veins.
- About 20% of symptomatic isolated calf DVT subsequently extends to the proximal veins, usually within 1 week after presentation.
- More than 90% of asymptomatic postoperative DVT resolves without causing symptoms.
- More than 80% of symptomatic DVT involves the popliteal or more proximal veins.
- Symptomatic PE usually arises from proximal DVT.
- Most (70%) patients with symptomatic proximal DVT have asymptomatic PE (high-probability lung scans in 40%), and most patients with symptomatic PE (80%) have DVT.
- Only one quarter of patients with symptomatic PE have symptoms or signs of DVT.
- About 50% of untreated symptomatic proximal DVT is expected to cause symptomatic PE.
- About 10% of symptomatic PE is rapidly fatal.
- Most fatal PE is not diagnosed.
- About 30% of patients with untreated symptomatic nonfatal PE have a fatal recurrence.
- The risk of recurrent VTE after stopping anticoagulant therapy is much lower if VTE was provoked by a reversible risk factor (particularly recent surgery) than if it was unprovoked or provoked by a persistent risk factor.

Abbreviations: DVT = deep venous thrombosis; PE = pulmonary embolism; VTE = venous thromboembolism.

vein thrombosis; in the rest, thrombosis is confined to the calf. Although clinical features cannot unequivocally confirm or exclude a diagnosis of DVT, clinical assessment can stratify the probability of DVT as high (prevalence of thrombosis, ~60%), intermediate (~25%), or low (~5%) based on: the presence or absence of risk factors (e.g., recent immobilization, hospitalization within the past month, malignancy); whether the clinical manifestations at presentation are typical or atypical and their severity; and whether there is an alternative explanation for the symptoms that is at least as likely as DVT (Table 2).

Venography

Venography, which involves the injection of a radiocontrast agent into a distal vein, is the reference standard for the diagnosis of DVT. Venography detects both proximal and isolated distal DVT. However, it is expensive and technically difficult to perform, can be painful, and requires injection of radiographic contrast, which can cause allergic reactions or renal impairment. For these reasons, venography is now rarely performed.

Venous Ultrasonography

Venous ultrasonography is the noninvasive imaging method of choice for diagnosing DVT. It is not painful and is easy to perform. The common femoral vein, the femoral vein (previously called the superficial femoral vein), the popliteal vein, and the calf vein trifurcation (i.e., proximal junction of deep calf veins) are imaged in real time and compressed with the transducer probe (compression ultrasound). Inability to fully compress (i.e., obliterate) the vein lumen with pressure from the ultrasound probe is diagnostic for DVT. Duplex ultrasonography, which combines compression ultrasound with pulsed Doppler or color-coded Doppler technology, facilitates identification of the deep veins (particularly in the calf; see later discussion) and may enable thrombus to be detected if it is not feasible to assess vein compressibility (e.g., iliac or subclavian veins).

TABLE 2 Wells Model for Determining Clinical Suspicion of Deep Venous Thrombosis (DVT)*

VARIABLE	POINTS
Active cancer (treatment ongoing or within previous 6 mo or palliative)	1
Paralysis, paresis, or recent plaster immobilization of the lower extremities	1
Recently bedridden >3 d or major surgery within 4 wk	1
Localized tenderness along the distribution of the deep venous system	1
Entire leg swollen	1
Calf swelling 3 cm greater than on asymptomatic side (measured 10 cm below tibial tuberosity)	1
Pitting edema confined to the symptomatic leg	1
Dilated superficial veins (non-varicose)	1
Previous documented DVT	1
Alternative diagnosis as likely or greater than that of DVT	−2

*Pretest probability of DVT is calculated from the total points: >2 points, high; 1 or 2, moderate; <1, low.

Venous ultrasonography is highly accurate for diagnosis of proximal vein thrombosis, with a sensitivity and specificity approaching 95%. The sensitivity for symptomatic calf vein thrombosis is considerably lower and appears to be highly operator dependent. For this reason, many centers do not examine the deep veins of the calf with ultrasonography. Instead, if examination of the proximal veins excludes proximal DVT in a patient with a moderate or high clinical assessment for DVT, the test is repeated in 7 days to detect the small number of calf vein thrombi (~3%) that subsequently extend into the proximal veins. If the test remains negative after 7 days, the risk that thrombus is present and will extend to the proximal veins is negligible, and it is safe to withhold treatment (Box 3).

If the clinical assessment for DVT is low and the result of an initial proximal venous ultrasound scan is normal, it is not necessary to repeat ultrasonography after 7 days, because the prevalence of DVT is only about 2% (mostly distal). If the calf veins below the level of the calf vein trifurcation are also examined and there is no isolated distal DVT as well as no proximal DVT, then DVT is excluded without the need for repeat ultrasonography after 7 days. However, examination of the calf veins has the disadvantage of resulting in diagnosis and treatment of DVT in substantially more patients than does serial examination of the proximal veins, without further reducing the risk of VTE during follow-up (approximately 1% over 3 months in both groups) in those who are not initially diagnosed with DVT.

Ultrasonography is less accurate when its results are discordant with clinical assessment. Therefore, if the clinical suspicion for DVT is low and the ultrasound study shows a localized abnormality (i.e., less convincing findings), or if clinical suspicion is high and the ultrasound is normal, further diagnostic testing (e.g., venography) should be considered.

D-dimer Blood Testing

D-dimer is formed when cross-linked fibrin in thrombi is broken down by plasmin. Because it is usually increased in patients with acute VTE, low levels of D-dimer can be used to exclude DVT and PE. A variety of D-dimer assays are available, and they vary markedly in their accuracy as diagnostic tests for VTE. All D-dimer assays have a low specificity for DVT; consequently, an abnormal result is associated with a low positive predictive value and cannot be used to diagnose DVT.

D-dimer assays that are used for diagnosis of VTE can be divided into two groups based on their sensitivity and specificity. Very highly sensitive D-dimer assays (e.g., sensitivity >98%; specificity ~40%) have a sufficiently high negative predictive value

Box 3 Test Results That Confirm or Exclude Deep Venous Thrombosis (DVT)

Diagnostic for First DVT
Venography: Intraluminal filling defect in proximal or distal deep veins
Venous ultrasound: Noncompressible popliteal or common femoral vein

Excludes First DVT
Venography: All deep veins seen, and no intraluminal filling defects
D-dimer:
- Normal result on a D-dimer test with a very high sensitivity (i.e., ≥98%) and at least a moderate specificity (i.e., ≥40%)
- Normal result on a D-dimer test with a moderately high sensitivity (i.e., ≥85%) and specificity (i.e., ≥70%), plus low clinical suspicion for DVT at presentation
Venous ultrasound: Fully compressible proximal veins and one or more of the following:
- Low clinical suspicion for DVT
- Normal result on a D-dimer test with a moderately high sensitivity (i.e., ≥85%) and specificity (i.e., ≥70%) at presentation
- Fully compressible distal deep veins (whole leg ultrasound)
- Normal repeat ultrasound of the proximal veins after 7 days

Diagnostic for Recurrent DVT
Venography: Intraluminal filling defect
Venous ultrasound:
- A new, noncompressible common femoral or popliteal vein segment
- A 4.0-mm increase in diameter of the common femoral or popliteal vein compared with a previous test

Excludes Recurrent DVT
Venogram: All deep veins seen, and no intraluminal filling defects
Venous ultrasound: Normal, or ≤1 mm increase in diameter of the common femoral or popliteal veins compared with a previous test, which remains unchanged on repeat testing after 2 and 7 days
D-dimer:
- Normal result on a D-dimer test with a very high sensitivity (i.e., ≥98%) and at least a moderate specificity (i.e., ≥40%)
- Normal result on a D-dimer test with a moderately high sensitivity (i.e., ≥85%) and specificity (i.e., ≥70%), plus low clinical suspicion for DVT

(>98%) that a normal result can be used to exclude VTE without the need to perform additional diagnostic testing. With moderate to highly sensitive D-dimer assays (sensitivity 85%–97%; specificity 50%–70%), a negative result needs to be combined with another assessment that identifies patients as having a lower prevalence of VTE in order to exclude DVT. Management studies have shown that it is safe to consider DVT excluded in patients who have a normal result on a moderately sensitive D-dimer test in combination with either a low clinical suspicion for DVT or no proximal DVT on venous ultrasonography (see Box 3).

Traditionally, a single cut-off has been used to define a negative D-dimer assay. Recently, it has been shown that the efficiency of D-dimer testing can be improved by varying the D-dimer cut-off used to define a negative result according to clinical probability. Because the prevalence of DVT is low in patients with low clinical probability, a more liberal D-dimer threshold of 1000ug/L can be used to exclude DVT in these patients, whereas a cut-off of 500ug/L is required to exclude DVT in patients with moderate clinical probability.

D-dimer testing is much less specific (i.e., fewer negative tests among those without venous thrombosis), and therefore has less clinical utility in postoperative and hospitalized patients and in the elderly (>75 years). Also, D-dimer testing has less clinical utility in patients with a high clinical suspicion of VTE because negative results are rarely obtained, and if a negative test is obtained, its predictive value is lower because of the high prevalence of disease.

Computed Tomographic and Magnetic Resonance Imaging Venography

Computed tomography (CT) and magnetic resonance imaging (MRI) have been reported to have high accuracy (sensitivity and specificity >90%) for the diagnosis of DVT but are rarely used for this purpose, because CT requires the use of radiographic contrast and is associated with high radiation exposure, and both CT and MRI are costly. CT and MRI are expected to be more accurate than ultrasound for DVT that does not involve the limbs, such as that confined to the pelvic veins or the inferior vena cava. Diagnosis of DVT on CT (or, less commonly, on MRI) is most commonly an incidental finding in patients who undergo CT to stage a known malignancy. In this situation, because the clinical suspicion for DVT is low and the examination will not have been designed to diagnose DVT, patients need to be carefully reviewed, often including further testing, before a diagnosis of DVT is accepted.

Diagnosis of Recurrent Deep Venous Thrombosis

The diagnosis of recurrent DVT can be difficult. A negative D-dimer test can exclude recurrent DVT, although the safety of this approach has been less well evaluated than for first episodes of DVT. If D-dimer testing is positive or has not been done, venous ultrasonography is performed. If the result is normal (i.e., full compressibility of the veins), treatment is withheld, and the test should be repeated twice over the next 7 to 10 days. If the result is positive in the popliteal or common femoral vein segments and the result of a previous test was negative at the same site, a recurrence is diagnosed. Recurrence can also be diagnosed if venous ultrasonography shows other convincing evidence of more extensive thrombosis than was seen on a previous examination (e.g., an increase in compressed thrombus diameter of >4 mm in the common femoral or the popliteal segments; unequivocal extension within the femoral vein of the thigh).

If a comparison between current and previous venous ultrasound findings is equivocal, or if no previous ultrasound is available for comparison, venography should be performed; however, many hospitals no longer perform venography. If the venogram shows an intraluminal filling defect, which is seen with acute rather than remote thrombosis, recurrent DVT is diagnosed. If the venogram outlines all of the deep veins and does not show an intraluminal filling defect, recurrent DVT is excluded. If the venogram is nondiagnostic (i.e., nonfilling of segments of the deep veins) or if venography is not performed in a patient with equivocal findings on ultrasound, the patient can be observed with repeat venous ultrasonography to detect extending DVT or, less satisfactorily, recurrent DVT can be diagnosed based on the results of all assessments, including clinical features. Clinical assessment of the probability of recurrent DVT is less well standardized than for a first episode of DVT; however, many of the factors that are predictive of a first episode are also expected to be predictive of recurrent DVT (Box 3).

Diagnosis of Pulmonary Embolism
Clinical Features

Dyspnea is the most common symptom of PE. Chest pain is also common and is usually pleuritic but can be substernal and compressive. Hemoptysis is less frequently present. Tachycardia and tachypnea are common signs. Evidence of right heart failure is less common but of prognostic importance, and a pleural rub may be heard in association with pulmonary infarction. Although most patients with PE also have DVT, fewer than 25% have symptoms or signs. The clinical features of PE, like those of DVT, are nonspecific, and PE is diagnosed in only about 20% of those in whom it is suspected.

Two groups have published explicit criteria for determining the clinical probability of PE. The model by Wells and colleagues incorporates an assessment of symptoms and signs, the presence of an alternative diagnosis that could account for the patient's condition, and the presence of risk factors for VTE. With this model, a

TABLE 3 Wells Model for Determining Clinical Suspicion of Pulmonary Embolism*

VARIABLE	POINTS
Clinical signs and symptoms of DVT (minimum leg swelling and pain with palpation of the deep veins)	3.0
An alternative diagnosis is less likely than PE	3.0
Heart rate >100 beats/min	1.5
Immobilization or surgery in the previous 4 wk	1.5
Previous DVT/PE	1.5
Hemoptysis	1.0
Malignancy (treatment ongoing or within previous 6 months or palliative)	1.0

Abbreviations: DVT = deep venous thrombosis; PE = pulmonary embolism.
*Pretest probability of PE is calculated from the total points: >6 points, high; 4 to 6, moderate; <4, low.

patient's clinical probability of PE can be categorized as low or unlikely (prevalence of PE <10%), moderate (~25%), or high (~60%) (Table 3).

Chest Radiography and Electrocardiography

In patients with PE, chest radiographs show either normal or non-specific findings. However, a chest radiograph is useful for exclusion of pneumothorax and other conditions that can simulate PE (e.g., left ventricular failure). The electrocardiogram also frequently shows normal or nonspecific findings but is valuable for excluding acute myocardial infarction. In the appropriate clinical setting, right ventricular strain can suggest PE and a poorer short-term outcome among those with PE.

Ventilation/Perfusion Lung Scanning

Planar ventilation/perfusion lung scanning was the most important test for diagnosing PE in the past. Computed tomographic pulmonary angiography (CTPA) has now supplanted lung scanning, although the latter is still used, particularly if CTPA is contraindicated because of renal failure or associated radiation exposure to the chest (e.g., in young women). A normal perfusion scan excludes PE but is obtained in only about 25% of patients; a higher proportion of normal scans is obtained in patients who are young, who do not have chronic lung disease, or who have a normal chest radiograph. An abnormal perfusion scan is nonspecific. Ventilation imaging improves the specificity of perfusion scanning. If the ventilation scan is normal at the site of two or more large (>75% of a segment) perfusion defects, the lung scan is associated with a greater than 85% prevalence of PE and is termed a high-probability scan. About half of patients with PE have a high-probability lung scan. Therefore, among consecutive patients who are investigated for PE, about 25% have a normal perfusion scan and can have the diagnosis excluded; about 15% have a high-probability scan and can have PE diagnosed (provided that the clinical probability is moderate or high) (Box 4); and about 60% have a nondiagnostic lung scan that requires further diagnostic testing.

Three-dimensional SPECT (single-photon emission CT) is now used by many centres in place of planar ventilation-perfusion scanning. SPECT may be more accurate than planar ventilation/perfusion scanning and, with current approaches to interpretation of SPECT, a much smaller proportion of ventilation/perfusion scans are reported as non-diagnostic. However, there are no standardized criteria for the interpretation of SPECT scans, and the accuracy and safety of using SPECT in patients with suspected PE have not been evaluated in large prospective studies.

Computed Tomographic Pulmonary Angiography

CTPA is able to directly visualize the pulmonary arteries. Results of the Prospective Investigation of Pulmonary Embolism Diagnosis (PIOPED II) study suggested that CTPA is nondiagnostic

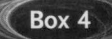

Box 4 Test Results That Confirm or Exclude Pulmonary Embolism (PE)

Diagnostic for PE
Pulmonary angiography: Intraluminal filling defect
Computed tomographic pulmonary angiography (CTPA):
- Intraluminal filling defect in a lobar or main pulmonary artery
- Intraluminal filling defect in a segmental pulmonary artery, plus moderate or high clinical suspicion
Ventilation/perfusion scan: High-probability scan, plus moderate to high clinical suspicion
Positive diagnostic test for deep venous thrombosis: With a nondiagnostic ventilation/perfusion scan or CTPA

Excludes PE
CTPA: Negative good quality scan
Pulmonary angiogram: Normal
Perfusion scan: Normal
D-dimer:
- Normal result on a D-dimer test with a very high sensitivity (i.e., ≥98%) and at least a moderate specificity (i.e., ≥ 40%)
- Normal result on a D-dimer test with a moderately high sensitivity (i.e., ≥85%) and specificity (i.e., ≥70%), plus low clinical suspicion for PE
- In patients over 50 years, D-dimer level less than 10 times the patient's age and a low clinical suspicion for PE
Nondiagnostic ventilation/perfusion scan or suboptimal CTPA, plus normal venous ultrasound of the proximal veins and one or more of the following:
- Low clinical suspicion for PE
- Normal result on a D-dimer test with at least a moderately high sensitivity (i.e., ≥85%) and specificity (i.e., ≥ 70%)
- Normal repeat venous ultrasound of the proximal veins after 7 and 14 days

in 6% of patients and that, among adequate examinations, sensitivity for PE is 83%, specificity is 96%, positive predictive value is 86% and negative predictive value is 95%. Accuracy varies according to the size of the largest pulmonary artery involved: the positive predictive value was 97% for defects in the main or lobar artery, 68% in segmental arteries, and 25% in subsegmental arteries (4% of PE in this study but over 10% with current higher resolution scanners). Predictive values were also influenced by the clinical assessment of PE probability: the positive predictive value of CTPA was 96% in combination with high, 92% with intermediate, and 58% with low clinical probability (8% of patients); likewise, the negative predictive value was 96% with low, 89% with intermediate, and 60% with high clinical probability (3% of patients). Management studies, in which anticoagulant therapy was withheld in patients with a negative CTPA result suggested that fewer than 2% of patients with a negative CTPA for PE will return with symptomatic VTE during 3 months of follow-up. Taken together, these observations suggest the following conclusions (see Box 4).

- An intraluminal filling defect in a segmental or larger pulmonary artery is generally diagnostic for PE. However, if the clinical probability is low and if there are additional findings that undermine a diagnosis of PE (e.g., technically suboptimal study, negative D-dimer test), further diagnostic testing should be considered (e.g., venous ultrasonography, ventilation/perfusion scanning, repeat CTPA), particularly if the most proximal pulmonary artery involved is at the segmental level.
- A good-quality negative CTPA finding excludes PE. If the CTPA does not show PE but is suboptimal, ultrasonography of the proximal deep veins of the legs should be performed to supplement the findings of the CTPA and exclude DVT.
- Abnormalities suggestive of intraluminal defects that are confined to subsegmental pulmonary arteries are generally nondiagnostic and require further investigation.

CTPA exposes patients to chest radiation and potentially nephrotoxic contrast dye, and is costly. CTPA should be avoided in younger women because of the associated increased risk of breast cancer, with ventilation/perfusion scanning often being preferred if imaging is necessary.

MRI is less well evaluated than CTPA for the diagnosis of PE and appears to be less accurate. Both CTPA and MRI have the advantage of identifying alternative pulmonary diagnoses. MRI does not expose the patient to radiation or radiographic contrast media.

D-Dimer Blood Testing

D-dimer testing is a valuable test for the exclusion of PE, either alone (very sensitive D-dimer assay) or in combination with other assessments that are associated with a reduced prevalence of PE (see Box 4 and earlier discussion of D-dimer testing for suspected DVT).

Compression Ultrasonography

Compression ultrasonography, usually evaluating the proximal deep veins of the legs, can aid in the diagnosis of PE. Demonstration of DVT, which occurs in about 5% of patients with nondiagnostic ventilation/perfusion lung scans, serves as indirect evidence of PE. Exclusion of proximal DVT does not rule out PE in a patient with a nondiagnostic ventilation/perfusion scan, although it does reduce that probability somewhat. However, if there is no proximal DVT on the day of presentation and proximal DVT is not detected on two subsequent examinations performed 1 and 2 weeks later (DVT is diagnosed during serial testing in approximately 2% of patients), anticoagulant therapy can be withheld with a very low risk that the patient will return with VTE (<2% during 3 months of follow-up).

As previously noted for patients with a nondiagnostic ventilation/perfusion lung scan, withholding of anticoagulant therapy and performance of serial ultrasonography is a reasonable approach to management in patients who have a CTPA result that is nondiagnostic, including patients with isolated subsegmental abnormalities.

Pulmonary Angiography

Although pulmonary angiography was considered to be the reference standard for PE in the past, it is now very rarely performed, because it is invasive and can usually be replaced by CTPA. Combinations of test results that confirm and exclude PE are shown in Box 4.

Prevention of Venous Thromboembolism

The most effective way to reduce mortality from PE and morbidity from the postthrombotic syndrome is to use primary prophylaxis in patients at risk for VTE, particularly during hospitalization. On the basis of well-defined clinical criteria, patients can be classified as being at low, moderate, or high risk for VTE, and use of prophylaxis can then be tailored to the patient's risk (see Table 1). By reducing the need to diagnose and treat VTE, prophylaxis is cost-saving in many situations, rather than just being cost-effective.

Prophylaxis is achieved by reducing blood coagulability or by preventing venous stasis. Anticoagulants, including subcutaneous heparin, low-molecular-weight-heparin (LMWH), and fondaparinux (Arixtra), as well as oral vitamin K antagonists, oral direct thrombin, and factor Xa inhibitors, reduce coagulability. Mechanical methods, including graduated compression stockings and intermittent pneumatic compression (IPC) devices, prevent venous stasis. Antiplatelet agents, such as aspirin,[1] also prevent VTE, but less effectively than the previously stated methods, and they are not usually recommended for this purpose.

---

[1]Not FDA approved for this indication.

Heparin is given subcutaneously at a dose of 5000 U 2 hours before surgery and 5000 U every 8 or 12 hours after surgery. LMWH, fondaparinux, vitamin K antagonists and the newer non-vitamin K oral anticoagulants are preferred over low dose heparin in patients undergoing major orthopedic surgery as they are more effective and, other than for the vitamin K antagonists, are easier to use.

LMWH is also given subcutaneously, once or twice a day. It is effective in high-risk patients undergoing elective hip surgery, major general surgery, or major knee surgery and in patients with hip fracture, spinal injury, or acute medical illness. LMWH is more effective than vitamin K antagonist therapy at preventing VTE after major orthopedic surgery while patients are in hospital, but it is also associated with more frequent early postoperative bleeding; both of these differences may be related to the more rapid onset of anticoagulation with LMWH than with vitamin K antagonist therapy.

Graduated compression stockings (about 15 mmHg pressure at the ankle) are thought to reduce the risk of venous thrombosis without increasing the risk of bleeding. On their own or in conjunction with IPC, they are indicated in patients who are at high risk for bleeding and in those who are unable to tolerate any bleeding (e.g., neurosurgical patients). In surgical patients, the combined use of graduated compression stockings and pharmacological agents (e.g., low-dose heparin) is more effective than use of either alone. In the absence of a contraindication, pharmacologic prophylaxis is preferred to graduated compression stockings alone, because the evidence of efficacy is greater with the former. A recent controlled trial in 2500 patients with acute stroke found that graduated compression stockings did not reduce VTE; this has added to uncertainty about their efficacy.

IPC of the legs enhances blood flow in the deep veins and may increase blood fibrinolytic activity. IPC is more effective than graduated stockings alone, particularly after major orthopedic surgery. A recent controlled trial in 2900 patients with acute stroke found that IPC reduced VTE by about one-third; this provides direct support for IPC use in stroke patients and indirect support for IPC use in other populations.

Vitamin K antagonist therapy (international normalized ratio [INR], 2.0 to 3.0) is effective for preventing postoperative VTE, including after major orthopedic surgery, but it is difficult to use because of the need for laboratory monitoring.

Fondaparinux, the synthetic pentasaccharide that corresponds to the active component of heparin that binds antithrombin and inhibits factor Xa, has been shown to reduce the frequency of venographically detected DVT by 50%, compared with LMWH, but is associated with an additional risk of bleeding.

Non vitamin K oral anticoagulants (NOACs) can also be used for the prevention of VTE. Dabigatran (Pradaxa)[1] (oral direct thrombin inhibitor) and apixaban (Eliquis) (oral factor Xa inhibitor) are as effective as LMWH in preventing VTE after major orthopedic surgery with a comparable risk of bleeding. Rivaroxaban (Xarelto) (oral factor Xa inhibitor) appears to be more effective than LMWH in preventing VTE after major orthopedic surgery but may be associated with a higher risk of bleeding.

General Surgery and Medicine
Low-dose heparin or LMWH prophylaxis is the method of choice for moderate-risk general surgical and medical patients. It reduces the risk of VTE by 50% to 70% and is simple, inexpensive, convenient, and safe. If anticoagulants are contraindicated because of an unusually high risk of bleeding, graduated compression stockings, IPC of the legs, or both, should be used.

Major Orthopedic Surgery
Dabigatran (Pradaxa),[1] rivaroxaban (Xarelto), apixaban (Eliquis), LMWH, fondaparinux (Arixtra), or vitamin K antagonists provide effective prophylaxis after major orthopedic surgery. If pharmacologic agents are contraindicated because of the risk of

bleeding, IPC (with or without graduated compression stockings) is recommended until it becomes safe to use anticoagulant therapy. Aspirin has also been shown to reduce the frequency of symptomatic VTE and fatal PE after hip fracture; however, because aspirin is expected to be much less effective than anticoagulant therapies, aspirin is not recommended as the sole agent for postoperative prophylaxis.

A minimum of 10 days of prophylaxis is recommended after major orthopedic surgery, which usually includes treatment after discharge from hospital. In addition, extended prophylaxis for another 10 to 30 days is generally recommended, particularly in patients who have had hip surgery or have other risk factors for thrombosis, such as previous VTE or active cancer. Whereas we favour anticoagulants as the primary means of prophylaxis after major orthopaedic surgery, aspirin may be used to extend prophylaxis after the first 10 days of treatment (e.g., for 30 days).

Endoscopic Genitourinary Surgery, Neurosurgery, and Ocular Surgery
Anticoagulant therapies are avoided in patients undergoing endoscopic genitourinary surgery, neurosurgery, or ocular surgery because of the associated risk of bleeding, particularly close to the time of surgery. Graduated stockings may be used, or IPC in patients with additional risk factors for VTE. If hospitalization is prolonged and the risk of bleeding recedes, patients can subsequently be started on an anticoagulant.

Treatment of Venous Thromboembolism
Anticoagulation is the mainstay of therapy for acute DVT of the leg and PE. The main objectives of anticoagulant therapy are to prevent extension of DVT, early PE, and later recurrences of VTE.

Acute Anticoagulant Therapy
Outpatient treatment of DVT is recommended in the absence of very severe symptoms and signs (e.g., impending venous gangrene), severe comorbidity, or marked renal failure. A recent randomized trial and many observational trials have shown that up to 50% of patients with PE—those who are without severe symptoms or cardiorespiratory compromise and have good social supports—can also safely be treated as outpatients.

Parenteral options for acute anticoagulant therapy include unfractionated heparin, LMWH and fondaparinux. Intravenous unfractionated heparin requires laboratory monitoring and admission to hospital and has largely been replaced with other options for acute anticoagulant therapy. Weight-adjusted LWMH (150-200 IU/kg per day) by subcutaneous injection is at least as safe and effective as intravenous heparin. Once-daily fixed-dose subcutaneous fondaparinux (7.5 mg for body weight 50–100 kg; 5 mg for <50 kg; 10 mg for >100 kg) and twice-daily subcutaneous unfractionated heparin (with or without laboratory monitoring) have also been shown to be as safe and as effective as treatment with LMWH. Danaparoid (Orgaran),[2] argatroban, lepirudin (Refludan),[2] or fondaparinux[1] should be used to treat heparin-induced thrombocytopenia with or without associated thrombosis.

Vitamin K antagonist therapy is usually started on the same day as parenteral anticoagulant therapy. If warfarin (e.g., Coumadin) is used, the initial dose is usually 2.5 to 10 mg, with a lower dose being appropriate in older patients, women, and those with impaired nutrition, and a higher dose being appropriate in younger (<60 years), otherwise healthy outpatients. Subsequent doses should be adjusted to maintain the INR at a target of 2.5 (range, 2.0–3.0). Parenteral anticoagulant therapy is continued until it has been given for 5 days and until the INR is at least 2.0 on two consecutive days.

Rivaroxaban and apixaban have been shown to be as effective as heparin-vitamin K antagonist combinations for the acute treatment of VTE, and do not require initial parenteral (e.g., heparin) therapy. Both are given at a higher dose initially (rivaroxaban 15 mg twice daily for 20 days; apixaban 10 mg twice daily for 7 days),

---

[1]Not FDA approved for this indication.

[1]Not FDA approved for this indication.
[2]Not available in the United States.

followed by a lower maintenance dose (rivaroxaban 20 mg daily; apixaban 5 mg twice daily). Dabigatran (150 mg twice daily) and edoxaban (Savaysa) (60 mg daily; 30 mg daily if creatinine clearance 30 to 50 mL/min or ≤60 kg) are also very effective for the acute treatment of VTE but require an initial 5-day course of heparin. All of the NOACs are associated with a lower risk of bleeding, and especially intracranial bleeding, than VKA. All of the NOACs should not be used if the creatinine clearance is <30 mL/min.

Long-Term Anticoagulant Therapy

During the last 2 decades, a series of well-designed studies using vitamin K antagonists have helped to define the optimal duration of anticoagulation for VTE. The findings of these studies can be summarized as follows:

- Shortening the duration of anticoagulation from 3 or 6 months to 4 or 6 weeks results in a doubling of the frequency of recurrent VTE during 1 to 2 years of follow-up.
- Patients with VTE provoked by a transient risk factor have a lower (about one third) risk of recurrence, compared to those with an unprovoked VTE or a persistent risk factor. The greater the provoking transient risk factor (e.g., recent major surgery), the lower the expected risk of recurrence after stopping anticoagulant therapy.
- Three months of anticoagulation is adequate treatment for VTE provoked by a transient risk factor; in the first year after stopping therapy, the risk of recurrence is about 2% if VTE was provoked by a major transient risk factor (e.g., recent surgery) and about 5% if there was a minor risk factor.
- The risk of recurrent VTE is similar if anticoagulant therapy is stopped after 3 months of treatment compared to after 6 or 12 months of treatment; this suggests that 3 months of treatment is sufficient to treat the acute episode of VTE.
- The risk of recurrence is about 10% in the first year, 30% in the first 5 years, and 50% in the first 10 years after stopping anticoagulant therapy in patients with a first unprovoked episode of proximal DVT or PE.
- After 3 months of initial treatment of unprovoked VTE:
  - Vitamin K antagonist therapy targeted to an INR of 2.5 reduces the risk of recurrent VTE by over 90%.
  - NOACs reduce the risk of recurrent VTE by over 80% and may be as effective as a vitamin K antagonist.
  - Aspirin reduces the risk of recurrent VTE by about one third. This reduction in VTE can be considered in the overall risks and benefits of aspirin therapy in patients who are not candidates for indefinite anticoagulation.
- A second episode of VTE suggests a higher risk of recurrence (increased by about 50%). If both episodes of VTE were provoked by a transient risk factor, 3 months of anticoagulant therapy is expected to be adequate, with subsequent aggressive prophylaxis during transient periods of high risk. A second episode of unprovoked proximal DVT or PE is a strong argument for indefinite anticoagulant therapy.
- The risk of recurrence is lower (about half) after an isolated calf (distal) DVT than after proximal DVT or PE. This argues against treating unprovoked isolated calf DVT for longer than 3 months.
- The risk of recurrence is similar after an episode of proximal DVT or PE. However, recurrent VTE is about three times as likely to be a PE after an initial PE (about 60% of episodes) than after an initial DVT (about 20% of episodes). This effect is expected to increase mortality from recurrent VTE about twofold after a PE compared with a DVT.
- The risk of recurrence is about threefold higher in patients with active cancer. The risk is higher in patients with metastatic rather than localized disease, and it is expected to be lower if VTE occurred while the patient was receiving chemotherapy and the chemotherapy was subsequently stopped.
- Long-term treatment with LMWH, particularly for the first 3 or 6 months, is more effective than warfarin in patients with VTE

associated with cancer and is the preferred treatment for such patients.
- NOACs appear to be as effective as vitamin K antagonists in patients with VTE associated with cancer, but have not been well evaluated in this setting.
- Estrogen therapy is a risk factor for first and recurrent episodes of VTE; consequently, the risk of recurrent VTE after stopping anticoagulants is expected to be lower in women who had VTE while on estrogen therapy, provided that they have stopped taking estrogens, and estrogen therapy should be avoided in patients with a previous VTE who are not on anticoagulant therapy.
- The presence of a hereditary predisposition to VTE does not appear to be a clinically important risk factor for recurrence during or after anticoagulant therapy. Consequently, testing for hereditary thrombophilias is not required in selecting the duration of therapy.
- The presence of an antiphospholipid antibody has uncertain significance as a predictor of recurrence independently of clinical presentation (e.g., provoked versus unprovoked). Absence of an antiphospholipid antibody on routine testing is not a good reason to stop anticoagulant therapy at 3 months in a patient with unprovoked proximal DVT or PE, and presence of an antiphospholipid antibody is not a good reason to treat patients with VTE provoked by a transient risk factor for longer than 3 months.
- In patients with a first unprovoked proximal DVT or a PE who have completed 3 months of anticoagulant therapy, both male sex and a positive D-dimer test 1 month after stopping anticoagulant therapy are each associated with about a two-fold increased risk of recurrent VTE. There is emerging evidence that the risk of recurrence in women with unprovoked VTE who have a negative post-treatment D-dimer is low enough to justify not using indefinite anticoagulant therapy.
- The presence of residual DVT on ultrasound may be a marker of a heightened risk of recurrence in patients with unprovoked VTE. However, the strength of this relationship is uncertain, and further studies are needed to determine whether absence of residual DVT on ultrasound justifies stopping anticoagulant therapy in patients who have had an unprovoked proximal DVT.
- The presence of an inferior vena caval filter increases the long-term risk of DVT, decreases the risk of PE, and has no net effect on the risk of recurrent VTE. Consequently, the presence of an inferior vena caval filter need not influence the duration of anticoagulant therapy.
- The risk of anticoagulant-induced bleeding is highest during the first 3 months of treatment and stabilizes after the first year.
- The risk of bleeding differs markedly among patients depending on the prevalence of risk factors such as advanced age (particularly >75 years), previous bleeding or stroke, renal failure, anemia, antiplatelet therapy (avoid unless there is a good indication for dual therapy), malignancy, and poor anticoagulant control.
- The risk of major bleeding in younger patients (<60 years) without risk factors for bleeding who have good anticoagulant control (target INR, 2.0–3.0) is about 1% per year, and in those aged 60 to 75 years it is about 2% per year.

Whether anticoagulant therapy is recommended for 3 months or for an indefinite period (with annual review) depends primarily on the presence of a provoking risk factor for VTE (i.e., major or minor transient risk factor, no risk factor, or cancer), risk factors for bleeding, and patient preference (i.e., burden associated with treatment) (Table 4).

Thrombolytic Therapy

Systemic thrombolytic therapy (e.g., with tissue plasminogen activator) accelerates the rate of resolution of DVT and PE at the cost of an approximately fourfold increase in frequency of major bleeding, and a 10-fold increase in intracranial bleeding, in the short term. Such therapy can be lifesaving for those who have PE with hypotension, and regimens that are administered over 2 hours or less are

TABLE 4 Duration of Anticoagulant Therapy for Venous Thromboembolism

CATEGORIES OF VTE	DURATIONS OF TREATMENT (TARGET INR 2.5, RANGE 2.0–3.0)
Provoked by a transient risk factor*	3 mo
Unprovoked VTE[†]	Minimum 3 mo, then reassess
First unprovoked proximal DVT or PE; no risk factors for bleeding**	Indefinite therapy with annual review
Isolated distal DVT as a first event	3 mo
Second unprovoked VTE	Indefinite therapy (unless high risk of bleeding) with annual review
Cancer-associated VTE	Indefinite treatment[‡]

Abbreviations: DVT = deep venous thrombosis; INR = international normalized ratio; LMWH = low-molecular-weight heparin; VTE = venous thromboembolism.

*Transient risk factors include surgery, hospitalization, or plaster cast immobilization within 3 mo; estrogen therapy; pregnancy; prolonged travel (>8 hr); and lesser leg injuries or immobilizations occurring more recently (≤6 wk). The greater the provoking reversible risk factor (e.g., recent major surgery), the lower the expected risk of recurrence after stopping anticoagulant therapy.

**As noted in text, patient sex, with or without D-dimer testing, may be used to further assess a patient's risk of recurrence. D-dimer testing should not be done unless it has first been established with the patient that the results will influence the patient's decision to stop or to continue treatment. For a man, this would be a decision to stop anticoagulants with a risk of recurrence of 8% in the first year (negative D-dimer) and a decision to remain on therapy indefinitely with a risk of recurrence of 16% in the first year. For a woman, this would be a decision to stop anticoagulants with a risk of recurrence of 5% in the first year (negative Ddimer) and a decision to remain on therapy indefinitely with a risk of recurrence of 10% in the first year.

[†]Absence of a transient risk factor or active cancer.

[‡]Indefinite therapy is suggested if there is a moderate risk of bleeding, and 3 months is suggested if there is a high risk of bleeding; both of these decisions are sensitive to patient preference.

recommended in this situation. Most patients with PE, including those with right ventricular dysfunction or an increase in cardiac biomarkers, do not require thrombolytic therapy in the absence of hypotension. However, thrombolysis should be considered in patients with severe PE and without risk factors for bleeding who fail to improve or deteriorate on anticoagulation therapy.

Catheter-directed therapy, with or without a thrombolytic agent administered in lower doses than are used systemically, may be used in patients with severe PE who have failed or have a contraindication to thrombolysis (i.e. high risk of bleeding). Catheter-directed therapy also has the potential to reduce the risk of postthrombotic syndrome after DVT and, therefore, may be indicated for patients with extensive DVT and severe symptoms who do not have risk factors for bleeding.

Inferior Vena Cava Filters
Inferior vena caval filters reduce the risk of PE at the expense of increasing the risk of DVT. Their use is usually confined to patients with acute DVT or PE, or both, who cannot be anticoagulated because of a high risk of bleeding. Removable filters can be used for patients with acute VTE who have a temporary contraindication to anticoagulation. Patients who have an inferior vena caval filter inserted should receive anticoagulant therapy if it becomes safe to do so.

Graduated Compression Stockings
Routine early use of graduated compression stockings was previously recommended after acute DVT. A large recent trial, however, failed to show that stockings reduced the post thrombotic syndrome. In patients with acute DVT, and in those who have developed the postthrombotic syndrome, stockings may help to reduce symptoms.

Acknowledgment
Dr. Kearon is supported by the Heart and Stroke Foundation of Ontario and holds the Jack Hirsh Professorship in Thromboembolism.

References

Bates SM, Jaeschke R, Stevens SM, Goodacre S, Wells PS, Stevenson MD, et al. Diagnosis of DVT: antithrombotic therapy and prevention of thrombosis, 9th ed: American College of Chest Physicians evidence-based clinical practice guidelines. Chest. 2012;141:e351S–e418S.

Beyer-Westendorf J, Ageno W. Benefit-risk profile of non-vitamin K antagonist oral anticoagulants in the management of venous thromboembolism. Thromb Haemost. 2015;113:231–46.

Castellucci LA, Cameron C, Le Gal G, Rodger MA, Coyle D, Wells P, et al. Efficacy and safety outcomes of oral anticoagulants and antiplatelet drugs in the secondary prevention of venous thromboembolism: a systematic review and meta-analysis. BMJ;2013:347:f5133.

Castellucci LA, Cameron C, Le Gal G, Rodger MA, Coyle D, Wells P, et al. Clinical safety and outcomes associated with treatment of acute venous thromboembolism: a systematic review and meta-analysis. JAMA 2014;312:1122–35.

Chattergee S, Chakraborty A, Weinberg I, et al. Thrombolysis for pulmonary embolism and risk of all-cause mortality, major bleeding, and intracranial hemorrhage. JAMA 2014;311:2414–21.

Falck-Ytter YC, Francis W, Johanson NA, et al. Prevention of VTE in orthopedic surgery patients: antithrombotic therapy and prevention of thrombosis, 9th ed: American College of Chest Physicians evidence-based clinical practice guidelines. Chest 2012;141:e278S–325S.

Gould MK, Garcia DA, Wren SM, et al. P. J. Karanicolas, J. I. Arcelus, J. A. Heit, and C. M. Samama. Prevention of VTE in nonorthopedic surgery patients: antithrombotic therapy and prevention of thrombosis, 9th ed: American College of Chest Physicians evidence-based clinical practice guidelines. Chest 2012;141:e227S–277S.

Kahn SR, Lim W, Dunn AS, et al. Prevention of VTE in nonsurgical patients: antithrombotic therapy and prevention of thrombosis, 9th ed: American College of Chest Physicians evidence-based clinical practice guidelines. Chest 141:e195S–226S.

Kearon C, Akl EA, Comerota AJ, et al. Antithrombotic therapy for VTE disease: antithrombotic therapy and prevention of thrombosis, 9th ed: American College of Chest Physicians evidence-based clinical practice guidelines. Chest 2012;141:e419S–494S.

Konstantinides S, Torbicki A, Agnelli G, Danchin N, Fitzmaurice D, Galie N, et al. 2014 ESC. Guidelines on the diagnosis and management of acute pulmonary embolism. Euro Heart J 2014;35:3033–80.

Maccallum P, Bowles L, Keeling D. Diagnosis and management of heritable thrombophilias. Br Med J 2014;349:g4387.

Takach Lapner S, Kearon C. Diagnosis and management of pulmonary embolism. Br Med J 2013;346:f757.

VIRAL RESPIRATORY INFECTIONS

Method of
Robert C. Welliver, Sr., MD

CURRENT DIAGNOSIS

- Rapid diagnostic kits are available for many common respiratory viruses. These tests are used increasingly to establish that antibiotic therapy is not necessary in many patients with febrile respiratory illnesses or with lower respiratory tract infections.
- The presence of wheezing on physical examination virtually excludes bacterial infection from consideration in subjects with lower respiratory disease.

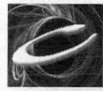

CURRENT THERAPY

- The management of most viral respiratory infections consists of rest, adequate caloric and fluid intake, and management of fever and malaise.
- Corticosteroids are essential in the management of croup.
- Specific antiviral therapy is available only for influenza virus infection, and beneficial effects have been more readily achieved in prevention rather than treatment.

Viral infections of the respiratory tract are among the most common infections in humans, and they account for significant morbidity at all ages. Infants and young children can sustain six to eight such infections annually, and adults have an average of nearly two such infections per year.

Rhinoviruses are the most commonly identified etiologic agents and cause illness year-round. Other common causative agents during winter months include influenza viruses and respiratory syncytial virus, and enteroviruses predominate in summer months. The parainfluenza viruses also commonly cause respiratory infection, particularly in autumn (type 1) and late spring or summer (type 3). Coronaviruses, metapneumoviruses, adenoviruses, and other agents are identified less often.

Although each of these agents can cause a common cold, some viral infections are associated with characteristic patterns of respiratory disease. Most of these viruses can also exacerbate asthma, cystic fibrosis, and chronic obstructive pulmonary disease (COPD).

Common Colds

Colds are the most common of the viral respiratory illnesses. Pharyngitis is usually the earliest sign of a cold, beginning a few days after infection has taken place. Nasal congestion and clear or slightly cloudy rhinorrhea usually follow within 24 to 48 hours. Cough occurs in approximately 30% to 40% of those infected, and fluid can accumulate in middle ear or sinus cavities that have become blocked as a result of mucosal swelling. Ear and sinus cavity infections occur when this fluid is trapped for a week or more. Treatment with antibiotics is ineffective before this time, and they are ineffective especially in the absence of other clinical signs of ear and sinus infections.

Colds are a frequent cause of missed school and work, and even of mild morbidity, but they are rarely serious in otherwise healthy persons. The most appropriate approach to treatment therefore entails rest, with adequate nutrition and hydration. Agents that inhibit the activity of cyclooxygenase probably represent the most effective form of pharmacologic intervention. These compounds include acetaminophen (Tylenol) and the nonsteroidal anti-inflammatory agents (NSAIDs) such as ibuprofen (Motrin). They are effective in reducing fever and, perhaps more importantly in most colds, reducing malaise, headache, and pharyngitis.

Nasal congestion and some rhinorrhea during colds are related to dilation of blood vessels in the nose and sinuses. Vasoconstrictors have therefore been used extensively to attempt to reverse these symptoms. Oral decongestants such as pseudoephedrine (Sudafed) have minimal effect on nasal congestion, and can result in systemic hypertension, anxiety, and difficulty sleeping. The propensity for these compounds to cause cardiac arrhythmias in the very young child has led to recommendations against their use in the first year or two of life. Nasal sprays containing vasoconstricting agents such as oxymetazoline (Afrin) can result in mild temporary relief of nasal obstruction. However, the use of these compounds for more than 3 or 4 days can result in rebound vasodilation and paradoxically increased rhinorrhea.

Numerous investigations have evaluated the role of antihistamines in colds. The release of histamine itself is not associated with fever, cough, or malaise, so effects on these symptoms would not be expected. Furthermore, nasal congestion and discharge may be more related to the release of kinins, and not histamine. Indeed, the administration of antihistamines in adults and, particularly, in children has not demonstrated strikingly positive results. As many as 40% of subjects treated with placebo report beneficial effects. Side effects of histamine use, primarily sedation and dry mouth, are commonly encountered.

Cough can be one of the most irritating symptoms during colds. Cough during colds is principally caused by secretions entering the airway (postnasal drip) and not by inflammation of the airway itself. Therefore, it is not surprising that cough suppressants, especially codeine, have little effect on cough induced by colds. Antihistamines have also been found to be ineffective in relief of cough during colds.

Influenza-Like Illness

The influenza syndrome is defined as the abrupt onset of fever, headache, and striking degrees of malaise and prostration, often with intense myalgia. Respiratory symptoms can occur concurrently, but they might not be prominent features. The principal cause is, of course, influenza virus, although infection with many other viruses can cause similar (although not as intense) symptoms. The illness is generally self-limited, and most symptoms resolve over 4 or 5 days. Lassitude can persist for up to 2 weeks.

Influenza virus infection and influenza-like illness are best treated symptomatically, relying on rest, adequate intake of fluids and calories, and appropriate analgesic therapy. Compounds referred to as *M2 inhibitors* such as amantadine (Symmetrel) and rimantadine (Flumadine) have been approved for therapy. Positive outcomes from therapy with these agents are observed only when therapy is instituted within 48 hours after the onset of symptoms, and benefits are not striking. In recent years, resistance to M2 inhibitors has been commonly observed among circulating epidemic strains of influenza virus.

More recently, inhibitors of the activity of influenza viral neuraminidase have been used in treatment and prevention of influenza virus infection in adults and children. The first such compound released, zanamivir (Relenza), was administered by inhalation but was unpopular because of its irritating effects on the airway. An oral compound, oseltamivir (TamiFlu), has been used to prevent and to treat influenza virus infection. As with M2 inhibitors, it is believed that treatment should be started within the first 48 hours of symptoms and that prophylaxis should be instituted within 48 hours of exposure. Treatment with oseltamivir shortens the duration of subsequent illness by only about 24 hours. Treatment can prevent some of the complications of influenza infection, including pneumonia. The drug may be more effective as a therapeutic agent, because it may be up to 90% effective in preventing culture-positive symptomatic influenza illness. The recommended dose for adults is 75 mg orally every 12 hours for 5 days. In children, the appropriate dose based on body weight is 30 mg twice daily for children weighing less than 15 kg, 45 mg twice daily for children weighing 15 to 23 kg, 60 mg twice daily for children weighing 23 to 40 kg, and 75 mg twice daily for children weighing more than 40 kg. The principal side effect is nausea, which can be reduced by taking the drug with food.

In 2009, a novel H1N1 strain of influenza caused a worldwide pandemic. At the time of this writing, both this epidemic H1N1 strain as well as the seasonal influenza A/H3N2 and type B strains continue to circulate in the world. The considerable majority of these epidemic and seasonal strains continue to show sensitivity to oseltamivir, while most are resistant to M2 inhibitors. All strains continue to show sensitvity to zanamivir.

Croup

Croup is defined by the occurrence of hoarseness or laryngitis, a deep, brassy or barking cough, and inspiratory stridor. Airway obstruction in croup is caused by constriction in the subglottic area, often noted on radiographs by a steeple-shaped narrowing of the air column in this region. Affected children are usually afebrile and nontoxic in appearance.

Parainfluenza virus type 1 is the primary cause of croup, although infection with many different viruses can produce this illness, and influenza virus can cause a particularly severe form of croup. Bacterial secondary infection occurs uncommonly, but it can result in fever and severe obstruction of the airway. Administration of dexamethasone (Decadron)[1] at 0.6 mg/kg either orally or intramuscularly markedly reduces the rate of hospitalization, admission to the intensive care unit, and intubation for croup.

---

[1]Not FDA approved for this indication.

Bronchiolitis

Bronchiolitis represents the most common cause for hospitalization of infants in developed countries. Infants present with a history of several days of upper respiratory symptoms, followed by the rapid onset of wheezing and labored breathing. Respiratory syncytial virus (RSV) is the most common cause and is the agent found in the most severe cases that result in respiratory failure. Contrasting with asthma, obstruction of the airway in bronchiolitis is a result of plugging of bronchioles with detached epithelium and inflammatory cells. Mucus plugging and constriction of smooth muscle are not prominent. Also in contrast with asthma is the absence of a sustained response to bronchodilators and corticosteroids among infants with bronchiolitis.

Therapy of bronchiolitis primarily consists of administration of supplemental oxygen and replacement of fluid deficits as needed. Ribavirin (Virazole)[1] is a compound with antiviral activity against RSV, but controlled studies have not demonstrated meaningful differences in outcomes between treated and untreated subjects. The compound is quite expensive and must be delivered via a special aerosol generator.

Palivizumab (Synagis), a preparation consisting of a monoclonal antibody against the fusion protein of RSV, has proved to be effective in reducing the rate of hospitalization for RSV infection by approximately 50% when given to high-risk infants. Infants who may be considered candidates for therapy include those with chronic lung disease, those born prematurely, and those with hemodynamically significant congenital heart disease. Doses of palivizumab (15 mg/kg) are given on a monthly basis throughout the local RSV season, usually November through March.

---

[1]Not FDA approved for this indication.

References

Akerlund A, Klint T, Olen L, Runderantz H. Nasal decongestant effect of oxymetazoline in the common cold: An objective dose-response study in 106 patients. J Laryngol Otol 1989;103:743–6.

Buckingham SC, Jafri HS, Bush AN, et al. A randomized, double-blind, placebo-controlled trial of dexamethasone in severe respiratory syncytial virus (RSV) infection: Effects on RSV quantity and clinical outcome. J Infect Dis 2002;185:1222–8.

Curley FJ, Irwin RS, Pratter MR, et al. Cough and the common cold. Am J Respir Crit Care Med 1988;138:305–11.

Flores G, Horwitz RI. Efficacy of β2-agonists in bronchiolitis: A reappraisal and meta-analysis. Pediatrics 1997;100:233–9.

Johnson DW, Jacobson S, Edney PC, et al. A comparison of nebulized budesonide, intramuscular dexamethasone, and placebo for moderately severe croup. N Engl J Med 1998;339:498–503.

Muether PS, Gwaltney Jr JM. Variant effect of first- and second-generation antihistamines as clues to their mechanism of action on the sneeze reflex in the common cold. Clin Infect Dis 2001;33:1483–8.

Randolph AG, Wang EL. Ribavirin for respiratory syncytial virus lower respiratory tract infection. Arch Pediatr Adolesc Med 1996;150:942–7.

Tavorner D, Danz C, Economos D. The effects of oral pseudoephedrine on nasal patency in the common cold: A double-blind single-dose placebo-controlled trial. Clin Otolaryngol 1999;24:47–51.

Treanor JJ, Hayden FG, Vrooman PS, et al. Efficacy and safety of the oral neuraminidase inhibitor oseltamivir in treating acute influenza: A randomized controlled trial. US Oral Neuraminnidase Study Group. JAMA 2000;283:1016–24.

Van Voris LP, Betts RF, Hayden FG, et al. Successful treatment of naturally occurring influenza A/USSR/77 H1N1. JAMA 1981;245:1128–31.

VIRAL AND MYCOPLASMAL PNEUMONIAS

Method of
Burke A. Cunha, MD; and Cheston B. Cunha, MD

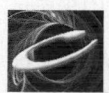

CURRENT DIAGNOSIS

Influenza (human, avian, swine)
- Mild influenza A or B presents acutely with headache, fever, sore throat, plus/minus rhinorrhea.
- Severe influenza A presents with an acute onset (patients often able to name the hour the influenza began) and rapidly become bed bound.
- Headache, myalgias, and prostration may be severe.
- With swine influenza, gastrointestinal symptoms (e.g., nausea/vomiting or diarrhea) may be prominent.
- Auscultation of the lungs is quiet, disproportionate to the degree of respiratory distress. Influenza is an interstitial process and not alveolar, which explains the absence of rales.
- With severe influenza, patients rapidly become hypoxemic. Hypoxemia is accompanied by an A-a gradient >35, which indicates a interstitial oxygen diffusing defect.
- Severe tracheobronchitis is common and manifested by hemoptysis.
- Relative lymphopenia with monocytosis occurs early followed by thrombocytopenia and later leukopenia. Low titer elevations of cold agglutinins are not infrequent (≥1:18).
- Patients may have chest pain exacerbated by breathing mimicking pleuritic chest pain. This is the result of direct intracostal muscle involvement with the influenza virus, which results in myositis and pain on inspiration.
- The chest radiograph in early influenza, in mild to moderate cases, is normal or near normal, with minimal, if any, increase in interstitial markings. The chest radiograph in fulminant cases shows symmetrical bilateral patchy infiltrates without pleural effusion in 48 hours.
- Severe influenza A is accompanied by severe hypoxemia cyanosis, and may be followed by an early fatal outcome.
- Influenza pneumonia most often presents alone without bacterial superinfection, but bacterial infection may accompany (MSSA/CA-MRSA) or follow influenza (S. pneumoniae or H. influenzae).
- Purulent sputum with influenza indicates concurrent bacterial pneumonia usually caused by S. aureus (MSSA/MRSA). Bacterial pneumonia following influenza (after 1–2 weeks), is suggested by leukocytosis, focal or segmental pulmonary infiltrates, and purulent sputum; the pathogens are not S. aureus, but most commonly are S. pneumoniae or H. influenzae.
- A laboratory diagnosis may be made by multiplex PCR of respiratory secretions.

Mycoplasma pneumoniae
- In a patient with CAP and a dry nonproductive cough, without severe headache or myalgias, the most likely diagnosis is M. pneumoniae. M. pneumoniae CAP is commonly accompanied by non-exudative pharyngitis and/or loose stools or watery diarrhea.
- The temperature is usually less than 102°F (38.9°C) and is not accompanied by frank rigors or pleuritic chest pain.
- Relative bradycardia and elevations in the serum transaminases are not features of M. pneumoniae CAP.
- Respiratory viruses are often associated with mild elevations of cold agglutinins (≤1:16) but M. pneumoniae is the only pathogen causing CAP associated with highly elevated cold agglutinin titers (≥1:64). Elevated cold agglutinin titers occur in up to 75% of patients with M. pneumoniae, and occur early and transiently.
- In a patient with CAP, elevated cold agglutinin titers (>1:8) effectively rule out the typical pathogens, as well as Legionella species and C. pneumoniae.
- Elevated M. pneumoniae ELISA IgG titers indicate past exposure/infection and not current infection or co-infection with another pathogen.
- In the absence of an antecedent respiratory tract infection (e.g., nonexudative pharyngitis, otitis, etc., in the preceding 3 months), the presence of an increased M. pneumoniae ELISA IgM titer is diagnostic of acute infection.

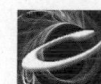

CURRENT THERAPY

Viral Influenza
- The aim of therapy is to inhibit the influenza virus and prevent its attachment/spread to uninfected respiratory epithelial cells.

- The neuramidase inhibitors shorten the course of influenza by 1 to 2 days and have antiviral activity. These agents are active against both influenza A and B.
- Most strains of human and avian, but not swine flu strains, are resistant to amantadine (Symmetrel) or rimantadine (Flumadine).
- Amantadine and rimantadine may have an important therapeutic effect in severe influenza A by increasing distal airway dilation and increasing oxygen action.
- Peramivir (Rapivab) may be useful in those unable to take oral neuraminase inhibitors.

Mycoplasma pneumoniae

- The agents active against M. pneumoniae are macrolides, tetracyclines, quinolones, and ketolides. β-Lactam antibiotics are not active against M. pneumoniae because the organisms do not contain a bacterial cell wall.
- Goals of therapy of M. pneumoniae CAP are to eradicate the infection, decrease the shedding of Mycoplasma in respiratory secretions posttherapy, and to prevent post-treatment asthma.
- Therapy is equally efficacious with macrolides, doxycycline (Vibramycin), or a respiratory quinolone intravenously, orally, or in combination for 1 to 2 weeks.
- The mode of administration is determined by the severity of the CAP and the setting. Outpatients are usually treated orally. Patients hospitalized with severe CAP are initially treated intravenously and then changed to an oral agent.
- Macrolide resistance to M. pneumoniae has been described in children and reported in adults.

Influenza pneumonia is the most important cause of viral pneumonia in adults. Influenza A is the predominant type of influenza found in adults, and influenza B is more common in children. Influenza A has the potential for severe disease, occurs seasonally, and is the predominant type involved in influenza pandemics. *Mycoplasma pneumoniae* community-acquired pneumonia (CAP) was first recognized decades ago as distinctive from bacterial and viral pneumonias. It was originally described by Eaton as "Eaton agent" pneumonia caused by a pleuropneumonia-like organism (PPLO), later shown to be caused by M. pneumoniae. M. pneumoniae is a common cause of pneumonia in all age groups, but the peak incidence of M. pneumoniae CAP is in young adults. M. pneumoniae CAP is a common cause of ambulatory CAP.

The term *atypical pneumonia* was first applied to viral pneumonias because the clinical laboratory and radiologic findings were different from those caused by typical bacterial pulmonary pathogens. In influenza pneumonia, the clinical findings are confined to the trachea, bronchi, lung parenchyma, and central nervous system. M. pneumoniae CAP is a systemic infection with a pulmonary component. Over the years, atypical pneumonia has come to refer to pneumonia caused by systemic nonviral/nonbacterial pathogen agents that have a pulmonary component. Viral pneumonias are no longer considered atypical pneumonias. Atypical pneumonias may be divided into nonzoonotic and zoonotic atypical CAPs. Nonzoonotic CAPs are most commonly caused by M. pneumoniae, Chlamydia pneumoniae, or Legionella species, whereas the three most common zoonotic atypical pneumonias are caused by Chlamydia psittaci (psittacosis), Francisella tularensis (tularemia), or Coxiella burnetii (Q fever). All of the atypical pneumonias are distinct clinical entities that may be differentiated on the basis of their characteristic pattern of extrapulmonary organ involvement. Although some viruses may occasionally have extrapulmonary manifestations (i.e., influenza, adenovirus with viral pneumonias), the primary clinical features are confined to the lungs. M. pneumoniae is a critical cause of nonzoonotic atypical CAP, particularly in the ambulatory setting. M. pneumoniae CAP may be severe in patients with impaired host defenses or those with severe, preexisting cardiopulmonary disease.

Influenza (Human, Avian, and Swine)

Viral influenza pneumonia affects children and adults. Influenza B is the primary type causing mild influenza in children and adults. Influenza A is primarily an infection of adults that may be mild to severe. Influenza A has the potential for pandemic spread (e.g., swine influenza [H_1N_1]).

Influenza occurs during the winter months, usually peaking in February. Influenza is spread by aerosolized droplet infection from person to person and via fomites. Influenza A is classified into subtypes based on hemagglutinin (H) and neuramidase (N) surface proteins. An important characteristic of influenza A virus is antigenic drift, which refers to minor changes in surface protein shift in the neuramidase or hemagglutinin receptors. With influenza A, these surface receptor proteins are important in cellular adherence of the influenza virus and spread of influenza from respiratory epithelial cells. The vaccine for the flu season most often includes the influenza hemagglutinin and neuramidase types seen at the end of the preceding year's season. Prevention of attachment and spread of the virus is helpful to controlling the spread of influenza; vaccine protection conferred by specific antibody response to influenza A is highly protective (approximately 80% in noncompromised hosts).

During the years when influenza B has been prevalent, vaccines for the subsequent year contain an influenza B component.

Clinical manifestations of influenza A in adults varies considerably from mild to fatal infection. Mild infection is usually manifested as an acute febrile illness characterized by headache and myalgias with dry unproductive cough and rhinorrhea. Mild influenza may be due to influenza A or B and usually resolves in a few days without complications in normal hosts who have good cardiopulmonary function.

Severe influenza A (human, avian, swine) occurs in normal healthy adults and may be fatal. The onset of severe influenza A (human, avian, swine) is sudden, and the patient often recalls the exact hour of onset. The patient is febrile with early/extreme prostration rendering the patient bedridden. Fever rapidly rises and may be accompanied by chills. Neck soreness, severe headache, and myalgias are typical. Sore throat, eye pain, conjunctival injection, and hemoptysis are frequently present. Chest pain worsened by deep inspiration is not truly pleuritic but rather reflects influenza A myositis of the intracostal muscles. Shortness of breath is related to the degree of hypoxemia. Severe influenza A causes an oxygen diffusion defect as manifested by an increased A-a gradient (>35). Profound hypoxemia may be accompanied by cyanosis. Hypotension caused by hypoxemia and vascular collapse may follow. The course of fulminant viral influenza A is of short duration.

Physical findings are few in viral influenza (i.e., conjunctival suffusion). Auscultation reveals absolutely quiet lungs because the infectious process is interstitial and not alveolar. Routine blood tests are usually unremarkable except for leukopenia, relative lymphopenia, and thrombocytopenia. Atypical lymphocytes are not present, but low titers of cold agglutinins may be present. Cold agglutinins (if present) have low titers less than or equal to 1:18. In fatal cases, a pale bluelike hue of the skin may be noted, and there may be bleeding from multiple orifices preterminally. The chest radiograph in uncomplicated influenza A is unremarkable or may have minimal perihilar bilateral increased prominence of interstitial markings. In severe influenza A pneumonia, the chest radiograph shows bilateral symmetrical perihilar infiltrates without pleural effusions in <48 hours.

Patients may die from severe influenza A without superimposed bacterial pneumonia. Most deaths during the 1918–1919 pandemic were young military recruits who died early of influenza A pneumonia without bacterial pneumonia. Influenza may be complicated by bacterial pneumonia. Bacterial pneumonias complicating influenza may occur concurrently at presentation or may occur 1 to 2 weeks after an interval of improvement after the presentation of influenza. Influenza A presenting concurrently with bacterial pneumonia is caused by *Staphylococcus aureus*. In contrast to influenza alone, MSSA/CA-MRSA is manifested by an increase in fever, shaking chills, leukocytosis, purulent sputum, localized rales on auscultation, bacteremia, and focal/segmental

TABLE 1 Mimics of Influenza A in Hospitalized Adults Presenting with Influenza-like illnesses (ILIs)

INFLUENZA-LIKE ILLNESSES (ILIS)	CHEST FILM FEATURES	CLINICAL CLUES
MERS (MERS-CoA)	• Ill defined infiltrates (early) • Bilateral dense interstitial nodular infiltrates (late) • Severe cases often develop ARDS	• Recent travel to Middle East or contact with MERS case • Dry cough and sore throat • Hemoptysis (in some) • Diarrhea (common) • WBC count normal, thrombocytopenia • Elevated LDH
RSV	• Clear CXR (early) • Bilateral ill defined infiltrates on CXR(late) • Chest CT : GGO (non-specific)	• Antecedent/concurrent rhinorrhea • Hoarseness • Lymphocyte/monocyte ratio > 2
HPIV-3	• Clear CXR (early) • Bilateral ill defined infiltrates on CXR (late)	• Hoarseness • Prolonged lymphocyte/monocyte ratio < 2 • Monocytosis
EV-D86	• Clear CXR (early) • Bilateral ill defined infiltrates on CXR (late)	• Diarrhea (common) • Flaccid paralysis
Legionnaire's disease	• Rapidly progressive asymmetric ill defined infiltrates on CXR • Consolidation and small pleural effusions (common) • Cavitation (rare)	• High fevers (>102 °F) • Highly elevated ESR (>90 mm/hr) • Ferritin (>2 xn) • Leukocytosis with relative lymphopenia • Elevated CPK (in some) • Mild transient elevated transaminates common (early) • Microscopic hematuria (early)

MERS = Middle East respiratory syndrome, RSV = respiratory syncytial virus, HPIV = human parainfluenza virus, EV = enterovirus, GGO = ground gloss opacity, CXR = chest x-ray, ARDS = acute respiratory distress syndrome.

infiltrates on chest radiograph that rapidly cavitate in less than 72 hours. Alternately, patients with influenza A may develop a secondary bacterial infection 1 to 2 weeks later. Secondary bacterial pneumonia is less severe and is usually caused by *Streptococcus pneumoniae* or *Haemophilus influenzae*.

Viral influenza-like illnesses (ILIs) most often present during the winter months or influenza season. For clinical and therapeutic purposes, it is important to differentiate influenza A from viral ILIs in hospitalized adults. Some clinical features may point to a specific ILI viral etiology, but a specific viral diagnosis can be made by viral respiratory PCR of nasopharyngeal swab specimens. The only viral ILI likely to mimic influenza A presenting with a fulminant severe viral CAP is MERS-CoA. The mimics of ILIs are presented (Table 1). The main non-viral mimic of influenza A in hospitalized adults is Legionnaire's disease (LD). LD may be different from influenza A and other viral ILIs by CXR findings and characteristic non-specific laboratory tests. With LD CAP, the CXR shows one or more non-focal infiltrates. Fever, usually > 102° F, is accompanied by relative bradycardia. With LD, the ESR is highly elevated > 90 mm/hr, the ferritin is highly elevated > 2 xn, and the serum phosphorus is decreased early as is serum sodium. Although an elevated CPK and mild transaminitis often accompany LD, these findings are not uncommon in influenza A and some viral ILIs. There are few infections that may mimic the dry, productive cough of *Mycoplasma pneumoniae* CAP. Pertussis is most likely to mimic mycoplasma. Pertussis, unlike mycoplasma, is not accompanied by watery diarrhea. The distinguishing laboratory feature of mycoplasma CAP is elevated cold agglutinins not found with pertussis. The key non-specific laboratory finding in pertussis is marked lymphocytosis (Table 2).

Anti-Influenza Therapy

Therapy of viral influenza is directed at inhibiting viral replication and preventing further infection of respiratory epithelial cells. The neuramidase inhibitors zanamivir (Relenza), oseltamivir (Tamiflu), and peramivir (Rapivab) have anti-influenza A and B activity. Neuramidase inhibitors decrease the severity and duration of influenza symptoms by 1 to 2 days. Current flu strains are resistant to amantadine and rimantadine, but these drugs may still be useful to increase peripheral airway dilatation and oxygenation, which may be of critical importance in severe influenza A with severe

TABLE 2 Mimics of Mycoplasma pneumoniae in Community Acquired Pneumonia (CAP) Hospitalized Adults

MYCOPLASMA CAP MIMICS	CHEST FILM FEATURES	CLINICAL CLUES
C. pneumoniae	• Ill defined lower lobe infiltrates (often ovoid) • No consolidation, cavitation or effusion	• No seasonal predisposition • Hoarseness • Protracted dry cough • Mycoplasma-like illness that doesn't respond to erythromycin • Wheezing (in some) • No diarrhea • No cold agglutinins • Rhinorrhea proceeds dry cough (1–2 weeks)
Pertussis	• Perihilar ill defined infiltrates ("shaggy heart" sign) • No consolidation, cavitation or effusions	• Protracted dry cough • Persistent cough (without typical "whoop" of children) • Afebrile or minimal fevers • Marked lymphocytes (>60%) • No cold agglutinins

hypoxemia. Mild influenza A/B may be treated with neuramidase inhibitors. Mild cases of influenza A should be treated at the onset of the illness. For severe influenza A, neuramidase inhibitors provide optimal anti-influenza therapy (Table 3). For human and avian influenza (H_5N_1), these antiviral drugs may be ineffective, but are effective against swine influenza.

Mycoplasma pneumoniae

M. pneumoniae is a common cause of ambulatory CAP. It affects all age groups, and in normal hosts with intact cardiopulmonary function, *Mycoplasma* CAP is usually a mild, self-limiting

TABLE 3 Adult Anti-Influenza Antivirals

ANTIVIRAL	TREATMENT DOSE	PROPHYLACTIC DOSE
Mild Influenza A/B		
Zanamivir (Relenza)[†]	2 inhalations (5 mg per inhalation) q12h × 5d	2 inhalations (5 mg per inhalation) q24h × 5d
Influenza A		
Oseltamivir (Tamiflu)[†]	75 mg (PO) q12h × 5d*	75 mg (PO) q24h × 7d
Peramivir (Rapivab)	600 mg (IV) over 30 min × 1 d	None

*For avian (H5N1) influenza, 150 mg (PO) q12h may be effective.
[†]Currently most human and avian influenza strains are resistant.

infection. However, *M. pneumoniae* derives its importance from difficulty in diagnosis, the necessity for non–β-lactam therapy, and because of its effect on peripheral airways.

Mycoplasma CAP is one of the nonzoonotic causes of CAP (the others being *Legionella* and *Chlamydia pneumoniae*). *M. pneumoniae* is an atypical pneumonia that is a systemic infectious disease with a pulmonary component. It may be distinguished from other atypical pneumonias by its characteristic pattern of extrapulmonary organ involvement. *M. pneumoniae* CAP most closely resembles *C. pneumoniae* CAP clinically, but is very different from Legionnaires' disease in terms of its epidemiology, age distribution, pattern of extrapulmonary organ involvement, and severity.

Clinically, *M. pneumoniae* presents as a subacute febrile illness. Temperatures rarely exceed 102°F (38.9°C). Rigors are not a feature of *M. pneumoniae* CAP, but patients may complain of chilly sensations. Mild headache and/or myalgias are not uncommon. The most common presenting symptom in *Mycoplasma* CAP is the prolonged, nonproductive dry cough. Patients with *Mycoplasma* CAP often complain of or have mild nonexudative pharyngitis. Rhinorrhea and conjunctivitis are not features of *M. pneumoniae* CAP. Watery diarrhea is commonly present in *Mycoplasma* CAP, but abdominal pain is not a clinical finding. Other extrapulmonary manifestations are uncommon or rare (e.g., meningoencephalitis, pericarditis, hemolytic anemia, glomerular nephritis, Guillain-Barré syndrome, erythema multiforme). *M. pneumoniae* has a distinctive pattern of extrapulmonary organ involvement that does not include cardiac involvement (relative bradycardia) or hepatic involvement, including normal serum glutamate-oxaloacetate transaminase (SGOT) or serum glutamate-pyruvate transaminase (SGPT). The distinguishing laboratory feature of *M. pneumoniae* CAP is elevated cold agglutinin titers. Although a variety of infectious and noninfectious diseases are associated with cold agglutinin elevations, they are usually of low titer (i.e., <1:16). There are no pulmonary infections presenting as CAP that are associated with high elevations of cold agglutinin titers (i.e., ≥1:64). Although elevated cold agglutinins occur early in up to 75% of patients with *M. pneumoniae* CAP, they are still diagnostically important when present. In a patient with CAP and a cold agglutinin titer greater than or equal to 1:64, the diagnosis of *M. pneumoniae* CAP is very likely.

M. pneumoniae may be differentiated from the typical bacterial pneumonias because of the presence of extrapulmonary findings, including nonexudative pharyngitis, loose stools or watery diarrhea, erythema multiforme, and high cold agglutinin. Patients with typical bacterial CAP usually have a more acute onset of presentation, a productive cough, and temperatures that may exceed 102°F (38.9°C), often accompanied by chills. Patients with typical pneumonia often have pleuritic chest pain, which is not a feature of *M. pneumoniae* CAP. Among the atypical pneumonias, the zoonotic pneumonias (i.e., tularemia, psittacosis, Q fever) may be eliminated from consideration if there is a recent zoonotic contact history with the appropriate vector.

C. pneumoniae resembles closely *M. pneumoniae* CAP. *C. pneumoniae* may be distinguished by the absence of cold agglutinins and the presence of hoarseness, which is a feature of *C. pneumoniae* but not *M. pneumoniae* CAP. Loose stools or watery diarrhea are not usual features of *C. pneumoniae* CAP. The most common clinical problem is differentiating *Legionella* from *Mycoplasma* CAP; this may be done by appreciating the differences in the pattern of extrapulmonary organ involvement with each of these pathogens. *Legionella* may be clinically differentiated from *Mycoplasma* by acuteness of onset or severity, the presence of relative bradycardia, temperatures greater than 102°F (38.9°C), and the presence of abdominal pain. From a laboratory standpoint, highly elevated cold agglutinin titers argue strongly against the diagnosis of *Legionella* and point to *M. pneumoniae*. Nonspecific laboratory tests in a patient with CAP that suggest *Legionella* and argue against *M. pneumoniae* include otherwise unexplained hypophosphatemia, hyponatremia, microscopic hematuria, and increased creatinine. *Legionella* does not affect the upper respiratory tract as does *Mycoplasma* (e.g., nonexudative pharyngitis). Ear findings are not a feature of Legionnaires' disease but are common in *M. pneumoniae* CAP. The finding most likely to cause confusion between *M. pneumoniae* and *Legionella pneumophila* is the presence of loose stools or watery diarrhea, which is found in both.

M. pneumoniae may be cultured from the throat in viral culture media, but the diagnosis is usually made serologically. An elevated enzyme-linked immunosorbent assay (ELISA) or enzyme immunoassay (EIA) IgM titer suggests acute or recent infection, but an elevated IgG titer indicates past exposure but not acute infection. Elevated IgG titers regardless of degree of elevation are not diagnostic of current infection with *M. pneumoniae* and only indicate previous antigenic exposure. *M. pneumoniae* ELISA IgM levels may take up to 3 months to decrease. Therefore, clinicians should take into account recent antecedent respiratory illness in order to properly interpret elevated IgM titers, including patients with nonexudative pharyngitis within 3 months prior to the presentation of CAP. The combination of an increased *M. pneumoniae* IgM titer and highly elevated cold agglutinin titers is virtually diagnostic of acute infection. Cold agglutinin titers are elevated transiently early and rapidly fall; the simultaneously elevated cold agglutinins and IgM titers of *M. pneumoniae* indicate active or current infection. In patients with CAP caused by another organism (e.g., *S. pneumoniae*), the presence of elevated *Mycoplasma* IgG titers does not indicate co-infection but only preexisting serologic exposure to *M. pneumoniae*.

Therapy

M. pneumoniae has a predilection for the respiratory epithelial cells and resides literally on their surface. Mycoplasmas have no definite cell wall like the typical pathogens causing CAP. Their position on the surface of the respiratory epithelium and their absence of a cell wall necessitates the therapeutic approach, which includes non–β-lactam antibiotics with the capacity to penetrate into the *Mycoplasma* organisms. Traditionally, macrolides and tetracyclines have been used successfully to treat *M. pneumoniae*. Both CAP tetracyclines and macrolides are effective against *Mycoplasma* because they interfere with intracellular protein synthesis at the ribosomal level. Tetracyclines penetrate intracellularly better than macrolides, with the exception of penetration into the alveolar macrophage, which is relevant in *Legionella*, but not *M. pneumoniae*, infections. Macrolides and tetracyclines are both active against *Mycoplasma*. Patients treated with macrolides or tetracyclines defervesce rapidly over 24 to 48 hours. Clinical defervescence manifests by an increased feeling of well-being and a decrease in fever. The dry cough persists during and after therapy regardless of the anti-*Mycoplasma* antimicrobial used.

There are important differences in the shedding rates of *Mycoplasma* from respiratory epithelial cells posttherapy when using tetracyclines instead of macrolides. Tetracycline therapy is associated with a more rapid decrease in shedding. Tetracyclines with better ability to penetrate intracellularly, such as doxycycline

TABLE 4	Antibiotics Effective Against *M. pneumoniae*	
ANTIBIOTIC	**DOSE (ADULT)**
Mild/Moderate CAP	
Doxycycline	100 mg (IV/PO) q12h
Erythromycin	500 mg (base, estolate, stearate) (PO) q6h
Erythromycin lactobionate	1 g (IV) q6h
Clarithromycin (Biaxin)	500 mg (PO) q12h
Azithromycin (Zithromax)	500 mg (IV) q24h × 2 doses, followed by 500 mg (PO) q24h
Severe CAP	
Levofloxacin (Levaquin)	500 mg (IV/PO) q24h, or 750 mg IV/PO q24h (may allow for shorter duration of therapy)
Moxifloxacin (Avelox)	400 mg (IV/PO) q24h

(Vibramycin), are the most rapid at decreasing *Mycoplasma* shedding, which is an important public health consideration. Mycoplasmas are transmitted by aerosolized droplet infection. Because patients with *Mycoplasma* have a prolonged cough, organisms not eliminated from respiratory epithelial cells may be aerosolized during coughing for weeks following the acute infection, spreading the infection to susceptible individuals via aerosolized droplets. The aim of therapy is to rapidly treat the patient's pneumonia and extrapulmonary sites of involvement. The secondary goal is to rapidly decrease shedding and aerosolization to prevent the spread of *Mycoplasma* to other individuals. An additional therapeutic goal is to decrease the incidence of post-*Mycoplasma* asthma seen in some patients. *M. pneumoniae* CAP may exacerbate preexisting asthma, but may also cause permanent post-CAP asthma in some individuals.

Until recently, doxycycline was the most active antimicrobial to use against *M. pneumoniae*. Currently, the "respiratory quinolones," levofloxacin (Levaquin) and moxifloxacin (Avelox), are highly active anti–*M. pneumoniae* antimicrobials. The respiratory quinolones and doxycycline penetrate cells efficiently and interfere with intracellular enzymes or protein synthesis of intracellular organisms. Respiratory quinolones and doxycycline are highly effective anti-*Mycoplasma* agents and rapidly decrease shedding of *M. pneumoniae* in respiratory secretions.

Therapy for *M. pneumoniae* is ordinarily 1 to 2 weeks. Patients who have impaired cardiopulmonary disease or compromised host may require 2 full weeks of therapy. In patients with borderline cardiopulmonary function, *M. pneumoniae* as with other relatively low virulence pathogens may present as severe CAP. Antimicrobial therapy for typical or atypical CAP should be directed against the presumed pathogen and not based on co-morbidities. Normal healthy hosts are treated with the same antimicrobial as patients hospitalized with severe CAP. Patients hospitalized with compromised cardiopulmonary function severe *Mycoplasma* CAP are most often initially treated intravenously with doxycycline (Vibramycin), a macrolide, or a respiratory quinolone. Most patients with *M. pneumoniae* CAP present in the ambulatory setting, which permits therapy with oral doxycycline, macrolide, or a respiratory quinolone (Table 4).

References

Ali NJ, Sillis M, Andrews BE, et al. The clinical spectrum and diagnosis of *Mycoplasma pneumoniae* infection. Q J Med 1986;58:241–51.

Cunha BA. Hepatic involvement in *Mycoplasma pneumoniae* community-acquired pneumonia. J Clin Microbiol 2003;3:385–6.

Cunha BA. Influenza: Historical aspects of epidemics and pandemics. Infect Dis Clin North Am 2004;18:141–55.

Cunha BA. The atypical pneumonia: Clinical diagnosis and importance. Clin Microbiol Infect 2006;12:12–24.

Cunha BA. Pneumonia Essentials. 3rd ed. Sudbury, MA: Jones & Bartlett; 2010.

Cunha BA. Antibiotic Essentials. 14th ed. Jaypee Medical Publishers: New Delhi; 2015.

Cunha BA, Corbett M, Mickail N. Human parainfluenza virus type 3 (HPIV-3) viral community-acquired pneumonia (CAP) mimicking swine influenza (H1N1) during the swine flu pandemic. Heart Lung 2011;40:76–80.

Cunha BA, Pherez FM, Strollo S, Syed U, Laguerre M. Severe swine influenza A (H1N1) versus severe human seasonal influenza A (H3N2): clinical comparisons. Heart Lung 2011;40:257–61.

Cunha BA, Raza M. During influenza season: all influenza-like illnesses are not due to influenza: dengue mimicking influenza. J Emerg Med 2015;48:e117–20.

Cunha CB, Opal SM. Middle East respiratory syndrome (MERS): a new zoonotic viral pneumonia. Virulence 2014;5:650–4.

Cunha CB. The first atypical pneumonia: the history of the discovery of Mycoplasma pneumoniae. Infect Dis Clin North Am 2010;24:1–5.

Debré R, Couvreur J. Influenza: Clinical features. In: Debré R, Celers J, editors. Clinical Virology: The Evaluation and Management of Human Viral Infections. Philadelphia: WB Saunders; 1970. p. 507–15.

File TM. Tan JS: *Mycoplasma pneumoniae* pneumonia. In: Marrié TJ, editor. Community-Acquired Pneumonia. New York: Kluwer Academic/Plenum Publishers; 2001. p. 487–500.

Foster CB, Friedman N, Carl J, Piedimonte G. Enterovirus D68: a clinically important respiratory enterovirus. Cleve Clin J Med 2015;82:26–31.

Hammerschlag MR. *Mycoplasma pneumoniae* infections. Curr Opin Infect Dis 2001;14:181–6.

Hurt AC, Selleck P, Komadina N, et al. Susceptibility of highly pathogenic A(H5N1) avian influenza viruses to the neuraminidase inhibitors and adamantanes. Antiviral Res 2007;73:228–31.

Louria DB, Blumenfield HL, Ellis JT. Studies on influenza in the pandemic of 1957–1958. II. Pulmonary complications of influenza. J Clin Invest 1959;38:213–65.

Lu QB, Wo Y, Wang HY, Wei MT, Zhang L, Yang H, et al. Detection of enterovirus 68 as one of the commonest types of enterovirus found in patients with acute respiratory tract infection in China. J Med Microbiol 2014;63:408–14.

Marrie TJ. Empiric treatment of ambulatory community-acquired pneumonia: Always include treatment for atypical agents. Infect Dis Clin North Am 2004;18:829–41.

Murray HW, Masur H, Senterfit LS, Roberts RB. The protean manifestations of *Mycoplasma pneumoniae* infection in adults. Am J Med 1975;58:229–42.

Nisar N, Guleria R, Kumar S, et al. Mycoplasma pneumoniae and its role in asthma. Postgrad Med J 2007;83:100–4.

Yang Y, Guo F, Zhao W, Gu Q, Huang M, Cao Q, Shi Y, et al. Novel avian-origin influenza A (H7N9) in critically ill patients in China. Crit Care Med 2015;43:339–45.

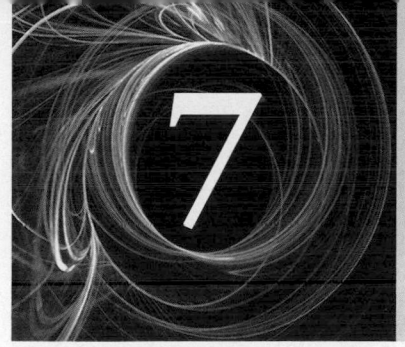

7 The Cardiovascular System

ACUTE MYOCARDIAL INFARCTION

Method of
Stephen Boateng, DO; and Timothy Sanborn, MD

An acute myocardial infarction (MI) is a subset of a spectrum of acute coronary syndromes that includes unstable angina and acute MI with or without ST elevation (Box 1). The diagnosis of acute MI is confirmed by a typical rise and fall in biochemical markers of myocardial necrosis with at least one of the following: ischemic symptoms, electrocardiographic (ECG) changes (ST elevation or depression, pathologic Q waves), or imaging evidence of new myocardial injury.

Epidemiology

There are an estimated 5 million emergency department visits each year in the United States for acute chest pain. Annually, more than 800,000 people experience an acute MI; 27% die, and most do so before reaching the hospital. These statistics, though dismal, represent significant improvement in mortality. There has been a significant decline in cardiovascular deaths since the 1970s owing to advances in diagnosis and management of acute MI. In one estimate, the in-hospital mortality prior to the era of cardiovascular intensive care units was greater than 30%. Today, with percutaneous coronary intervention (PCI) and stenting, antithrombotic therapy, and routine use of adjunctive medical treatment, the in-hospital mortality of ST-segment elevation MI (STEMI) has reached a low of 6% to 7%.

Pathophysiology

An acute MI occurs when there is a reduction in myocardial perfusion sufficient to cause cell necrosis. This is most commonly due to thrombus formation in a coronary artery. The inciting event is rupture or fissuring of an atherosclerotic plaque, which exposes the blood to thrombogenic lipids and leads to activation of platelet and clotting factors. The coronary plaques that are most prone to rupture are those with a rich lipid core and thin fibrous cap. Other rare causes of MI include coronary artery embolism from a valvular vegetation or intracardiac thrombi, cocaine use, coronary artery dissection, hypotension, and anemia.

Risk Factors

Risk factors for an MI fall into three general categories: nonmodifiable, modifiable, and emerging. Nonmodifiable risk factors include age, sex, and family history. Modifiable risk factors include smoking, alcohol intake, physical inactivity, poor diet, hypertension, type 2 diabetes, dyslipidemias, and the metabolic syndrome. Emerging risk factors are C-reactive protein (CRP), fibrinogen, coronary artery calcification (CAC), homocysteine, lipoprotein(a), and small, dense low-density lipoprotein (LDL). The Framingham Heart Study developed a coronary risk estimate using the major risk factors to estimate the 10-year cardiovascular risk of a patient.

Primary Prevention

Primary prevention of an acute MI is aimed at reducing the modifiable risk factors. Goals include lifestyle changes such as regular exercise, a healthy diet, smoking cessation, and a reduction in alcohol intake. Medications aimed at controlling blood pressure and reducing cholesterol are also recommended.

Clinical Manifestations

Patients with acute MI usually present with chest pain due to involvement of a neural reflex pathway via the thoracic and cervical nerves. It is a deep and visceral pain that is usually described as a heavy, squeezing, tightness, crushing, and sometimes stabbing or burning pain. It is typically substernal and can radiate to the corresponding dermatomes (C7-T4) that supply afferent nerves to the same segments of the spinal cord as the heart. These include the epigastrum, shoulders, arms, back (interscapular region), lower jaw, and neck. Radiation to both arms is a stronger predictor of acute MI. About 20% of patients (diabetic, elderly, postoperative, or female) do not have chest pain. These patients might only have atypical symptoms corresponding to the dermatomes C7 to T4. Physical examination findings are usually absent; however, when present, they are of prognostic value (Table 1).

Diagnosis

The initial evaluation of a patient with a suspected acute MI should include a focused clinical history, physical examination, ECG, cardiac markers, and a chest radiograph.

Electrocardiogram

An ECG is especially useful for distinguishing between a non-ST-elevation MI (NSTEMI) and STEMI. It should be performed within 5 to 10 minutes of arrival at an emergency department. Posterior leads (V7-V9) and leads VR3 and VR4 should be used in patients with suspected posterior and right ventricle (RV) infarctions, respectively. ECG findings predictive of adverse outcomes in patients with NSTEMI and unstable angina include ST-segment depression, new ST-segment deviation (≥ 0.05 mV), and new deep T-wave inversions 0.3 mV or greater. Other T wave changes are sensitive for ischemia but are not specific for acute MI.

Diagnosis of STEMI is established by ECG findings revealing elevation greater than 1 mm J point (junction of the ST segment and QRS complex) in two or more contiguous limb leads or precordial leads V4 to V6, or greater than 2 mm in two or more precordial leads V1 to V3. Development of a new left bundle branch block should be considered a STEMI equivalent until proved otherwise. A significant number of patients with acute MI develop Q waves. The diagnosis of acute MI may be difficult in the presence of a left bundle branch block (LBBB) or a pacemaker. In the presence of LBBB, the Sgarbossa criteria may be applied:

- ST-segment elevation at least 1 mm concordant with a predominantly positive QRS complex in at least one lead (5 points)
- ST depression at least 1 mm in leads V1, V2 or V3 (3 points)
- ST elevation at least 5 mm discordant (in the opposite direction) from a predominantly negative QRS complex (2 points)

TABLE 1 Killip Class and Hospital Mortality

KILLIP CLASS	CLINICAL CLASSIFICATION	MORTALITY (%)
I	No heart failure	6
II	Mild heart failure, rales, S3, congestion on chest radiograph	17
III	Pulmonary edema	38
IV	Cardiogenic shock	81

Data from Killip T 3rd, Kimball JT: Treatment of myocardial infarction in a coronary care unit. A two year experience with 250 patients. Am J Cardiol 1967;20(4): 457–64.

If all three criteria are met, the specificity for acute MI is 90%, though the sensitivity is only 20%. The third criterion has been shown to add little diagnostic or prognostic value. Greater than 5 mm elevation in discordant segments has been described in uncomplicated LBBB, particularly in the presence of left ventricular hypertrophy.

Serum Markers
Serum biomarkers of myocardial necrosis include cardiac-specific troponins T and I, creatine kinase (CK), MB isoform of CK (CK-MB), and myoglobin.

Troponins T and I are highly specific for myocardial injury and are preferred for the diagnosis of an acute MI. They are rarely elevated in noncardiac conditions and are only mildly elevated in other cardiac conditions such as tachycardia and heart failure and inflammatory conditions such as myocarditis. They begin to rise 4 to 6 hours after the onset of symptoms. Thus, they should be measured on admission and again 6 to 9 hours later. They peak at 18 to 24 hours after the onset of symptoms, and may remain elevated for 7 to 10 days after a STEMI. These have replaced other biomarkers owing to their higher sensitivity, specificity, and prognostic value.

Levels of CK-MB are less specific for MI than troponins; however, they are considerably more specific than CK. They serve as the next best alternative to cardiac troponins. Cardiac surgery, myocarditis, and electrical cardioversion often result in elevated serum levels of CK-MB. CK-MB levels increase within 4 to 8 hours, peak at 24 hours, and return to normal by 48 to 72 hours. Levels of total CK are generally not very useful for predicting an acute MI because they are not specific for acute MI. However, a ratio of CK-MB to CK activity at least 2.5%, even in the presence of skeletal muscle injury, is usually due to an acute MI. Myoglobin also lacks cardiac specificity; it usually returns to normal within 24 hours of the onset of an acute MI. Other nonspecific but notable reactions include leukocytosis (usually 12,000–15,000/mm³), which can

persist for 3 to 7 days, and elevated erythrocyte sedimentation rate (ESR), which rises slowly, peaks during the first week, and sometimes remains elevated for 1 or 2 weeks.

Imaging
Myocardial injury is diagnosed as wall motion abnormalities on echocardiography. An echocardiogram, however, cannot distinguish between an acute STEMI from an old myocardial scar or from acute, severe ischemia, but ease and safety make it useful as a screening tool to aid management decisions. It is particularly useful for detecting complications of MI such as ventricular septal defects, acute mitral regurgitation, ventricular aneurysms, pericardial effusions, a left ventricle (LV) thrombus, or valvular abnormalities.

Differential Diagnosis
Several other causes of chest pain can masquerade as MI. The most notable include acute pericarditis, pulmonary embolism, acute aortic dissection, costochondritis, and gastroesophageal reflux disease.

Treatment
The goals of initial treatment of an MI are relief of pain, immediate identification of ST changes via 12-lead ECG, initiation of reperfusion (if the patient is a candidate), and assessment and treatment of hemodynamic abnormalities. Pain relief is best achieved with oxygen, nitroglycerin, and morphine sulfate. Patients with ST-segment elevation or a new LBBB with symptoms for 12 hours or less are candidates for reperfusion therapy. Further treatment of an MI may be separated into two pathways, depending on whether the patient has STEMI or NSTEMI (Figure 1).

ST-Elevation Myocardial Infarction
The diagnosis of STEMI mandates immediate reperfusion; however, PCI is not promptly available in many areas. The best choice of reperfusion therapy for particular clinical settings remains controversial. For facilities that can offer PCI, however, current

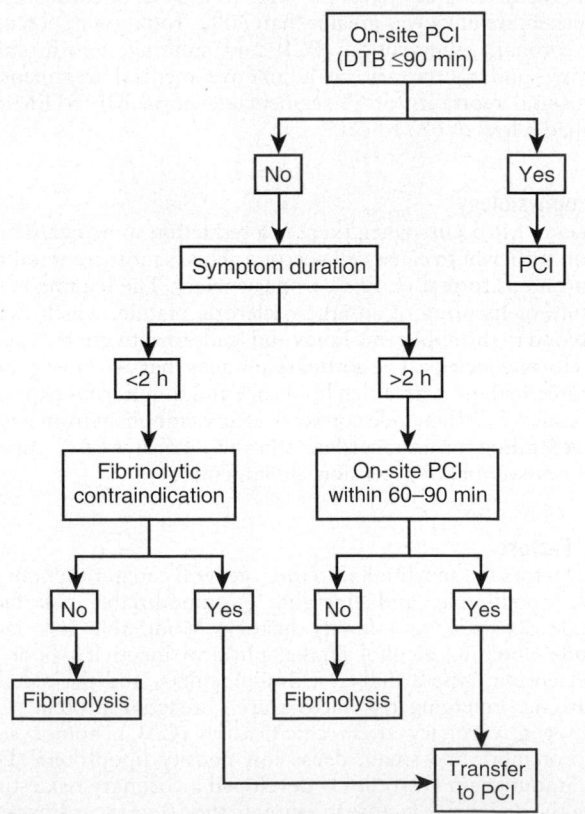

Figure 1. Selection of reperfusion therapy. *Abbreviations:* DTB = door-to-balloon time; PCI = percutaneous coronary intervention.

literature indicates that this approach is superior to pharmacologic reperfusion. The American College of Cardiology and American Heart Association (ACC/AHA) recommend a door-to-needle time of 30 minutes and a door-to-balloon time of 90 minutes. Most interventional cardiologists now aim for a median door-to-balloon time of less than 60 minutes.

Intravenous fibrinolytic therapy is widely available, but it is slightly less effective than PCI in randomized trials and carries a risk of hemorrhagic stroke. Fibrinolytics should be administered within 30 minutes of arrival at the emergency department. The greatest benefit is seen when this is performed within the first 4 hours of onset of pain, resulting in an absolute 3% reduction in mortality, but it is associated with a 0.4% increase in stroke rate. The decision regarding which therapy to employ should be made based on a written institution-specific protocol, which considers symptom duration, availability of PCI locally, time to transfer to a facility, and fibrinolytic contraindications (see Figure 1). In general, patients presenting within 2 hours of symptom onset derive significant benefit from fibrinolytics; if transfer time to a PCI facility results in a door-to-balloon time of longer than 90 minutes, fibrinolytics are preferred.

Primary Percutaneous Coronary Intervention

Although fibrinolytic therapy is easy to administer and widely available, it provides early reperfusion in only 80% of patients and is usually not administered owing to perceived or actual contraindications in a significant number of patients (Box 2). In contrast, primary PCI has only a few contraindications and leads to a higher reperfusion rate (approximately 90%). Randomized trials performed in high volume academic centers comparing fibrinolytic therapy with PCI for acute MI demonstrated a 30% reduction in mortality and reinfarction rates and a significant reduction in cerebrovascular accidents with PCI. Primary PCI should be performed within 60 to 90 minutes of arrival to the hospital.

Box 2 Indications and Contraindications for Fibrinolytic Therapy in Acute Myocardial Infarction

Indications
ST segment elevation ≥1 mV in ≥2 contiguous limb leads or ≥2 mV in contiguous precordial leads
New left bundle branch block
Posterior myocardial infarction: ST segment depression >2 mV in leads V1 and V2 with either imaging evidence of posterior LV wall motion abnormality or ST segment elevation of 1 mV in the posterior leads V7 to V9

Contraindications
Absolute
Active bleeding
Prior intracranial hemorrhage, other strokes or neurologic events within 1 year, intracranial neoplasm
Recent major surgery (<6 wk) or major trauma (<2 wk)
Recent vascular puncture in a noncompressible site (<2 wk)
Suspected aortic dissection

Relative
Active peptic ulcer disease or recent gastrointestinal bleeding (<4 wk)
Severe uncontrolled hypertension on presentation (BP >180/110 mm Hg) or chronic severe hypertension
Cardiopulmonary resuscitation >10 min
Prior nonhemorrhagic stroke
Pregnancy
Bleeding diathesis or INR >2

Abbreviations: BP = blood pressure; INR = international normalized ratio.

Adjunct Therapy

Adjunct therapy has been shown to reduce mortality, facilitate and maintain coronary reperfusion, limit the consequences of myocardial ischemia, and reduce the likelihood of recurrent events.

Relieving Chest Pain

Nitroglycerin. Nitroglycerin 0.4 mg sublingual tablets (Nitrostat) or aerosol sprays (NitroMist) should be given every 5 minutes for up to three doses to relieve chest pain. Nitroglycerin should, however, be avoided in patients who have taken a nitric oxide synthetase inhibitor or phosphodiesterase inhibitors within the past 24 hours to avoid hypotension. Nitroglycerin should also be avoided in the following situations:
- Hypotension: systolic blood pressure less than 90 mm Hg or 30 mm Hg or more below baseline
- Severe bradycardia: less than 50 beats per minute
- Infarct in the distribution of the right coronary artery

Morphine. Morphine is the analgesic of choice in patients with STEMI. The patient may be administered morphine 2 to 4 mg IV push over 5 minutes every 5 to 15 minutes as needed for pain. In rare instances, morphine can depress respiration and reduce myocardial contractility and is a potent venous vasodilator. In hemodynamically unstable patients, the concomitant elevation of the lower extremities (to facilitate venous return) or administration of atropine (0.5–1.5 mg) can overcome hypotension and bradycardia secondary to morphine.

Antiplatelet Therapy

Aspirin. Unless there is a history of allergic reactions, aspirin in a dose of 162 mg to 325 mg should be administered immediately on arrival to the emergency department and continued indefinitely at a dose of at least 75 to 162 mg per day in all patients with STEMI. In patients with severe nausea and vomiting, an aspirin suppository of 300 mg may be administered. Patients with a true aspirin allergy should be administered clopidogrel (Plavix) instead.

Thienopyridine. Thienopyridines block the adenosine diphosphate (ADP) receptor on platelets, resulting in platelet aggregation. Prime examples of these are clopidogrel and prasugrel. Ticagrelor is a new agent also included in this group; however, it is a cyclopentyltriazolopyrimidine. A loading dose of 300 to 600 mg[3] of clopidogrel, 60 mg of prasugrel, or 180mg of Ticagrelor is recommended by the ACC/AHA for administration at the time of PCI, after which a maintenance dose of 75 mg daily for clopidogrel, 10 mg daily for prasugrel, and 90mg twice daily for ticagrelor is initiated. For patients who present with an ACS (for whom PCI is not elective), it is recommended that the duration of thienopyridine therapy should be at least 12 months irrespective of whether the patient received a bare-metal stent (BMS) or a drug-eluting stent (DES). Dual anti-platelet therapy is associated with a lower mortality and morbidity than that seen with aspirin alone.

Glycoprotein IIb/IIIa Antagonists. Glycoprotein IIb/IIIa antagonists inhibit the final common pathway in platelet aggregation by blocking IIb/IIIa receptors, which activate fibrinogen. They are the most potent antiplatelet drugs available. Currently available glycoprotein IIb/IIIa antagonists include the chimeric monoclonal antibody abciximab (Reopro) and the synthetic peptide eptifibatide (Integrilin). Studies investigating the role of glycoprotein IIb/IIIa antagonists in STEMI have demonstrated a reduction in the composite endpoint of death, MI, and target revascularization in patients treated with PCI. Results appear to be better if the drug is initiated at least 6 hours before PCI and continued for 18 to 24 hours thereafter. Glycoprotein IIb/IIIa inhibitors are not recommended for patients receiving fibrinolytics. The adjunctive use of glycoprotein IIb/IIIa therapy in the setting of dual-antiplatelet (aspirin and clopidogrel) therapy with unfractionated heparin or bivalirudin (Angiomax) as the anticoagulant has been shown to be beneficial only at the time of primary PCI. It may also be used in patients with a large thrombus burden or patients who did not receive adequate thienopyridine loading during primary PCI.

---

[3]Exceeds dosage recommended by the manufacturer.

Anticoagulant Medications. Anticoagulant medications such as unfractionated heparin, low-molecular-weight (LMW) heparin, or bivalirudin have been shown to decrease reocclusion and reinfarction following reperfusion therapy. They are given routinely to patients with acute coronary syndrome unless contraindicated. Unfractionated and LMW heparin are considered equivalent in patients who have STEMI and who do not receive reperfusion therapy. In patients who undergo reperfusion either by angioplasty or thrombolytics, unfractionated heparin or bivalirudin are recommended.

Unfractionated Heparin. For patients undergoing primary PCI, 60 to 100 units/kg of UFH, with a target activated clotting time (ACT) of 250 to 350 seconds, is recommended. Patients receiving a glycoprotein IIb/IIIa inhibitor should be administered 50 to 70 units/kg of unfractionated heparin, with a target ACT greater than 200 seconds. The activated partial thromboplastin time (aPTT) should be checked at 4 to 6 hours after initiation of heparin and then every 6 to 8 hours for a target of 1.5 to 2 times control. This makes unfractionated heparin more complicated to use. Anticoagulation with unfractionated heparin may be continued in patients after PCI, for 48 hours, if there is a large anterior MI, known LV thrombus, or atrial fibrillation or if symptoms persist. Otherwise, short-term anticoagulation may be discontinued immediately following PCI. Long-term anticoagulation with warfarin (Coumadin) may be indicated in patients with an intracardiac thrombus, atrial fibrillation, or ejection fraction less than 30% following MI. The effects of heparin are short lived and can be reversed either by stopping heparin or administering protamine sulfate.

Low-Molecular-Weight Heparin. Enoxaparin (Lovenox) is the prototypical LWM heparin and has been studied widely in STEMI and acute coronary syndromes. Compared to unfractionated heparin, LMWH products have better bioavailability, are easier to administer by weight-based regimens, and do not require aPTT monitoring. There is also a lower risk of heparin-induced thrombocytopenia. Enoxaparin is typically administered as a 30-mg IV bolus followed by 1 mg/kg SC every 12 hours until hospital discharge. It should be used with caution in patients with renal insufficiency, and its effects are not immediately reversible.

Alternative to Heparin. For STEMI patients who have a history of heparin-induced thrombocytopenia or patients in whom there is a high risk of bleeding, bivalirudin may be used as an alternative. An initial dose of 0.75 mg/kg IV followed by 1.75 mg/kg per hour is recommended for the duration of PCI. The infusion may be continued for up to 4 hours after the procedure. An IV infusion of 0.2 mg/kg per hour can then be initiated for up to 20 hours if needed.

β-Adrenergic Antagonist Drugs. Early intravenous β-blocker therapy—metoprolol (Lopressor) 5 mg IV every 15 minutes for up to three doses—is indicated in all patients except those with contraindications. This should be followed by oral metoprolol 50 mg every 6 hours for 24 hours, then 100 mg twice per day thereafter. Contraindications to β-blocker administration include bradycardia, heart block, and hypotension. β-Blockers reduce myocardial workload and oxygen demand by reducing contractility, heart rate, and arterial pressure. When given within the first few hours, β-adrenergic antagonist drugs improve prognosis by reducing infarct size, incidence of ventricular arrhythmias, and mortality.

Angiotensin-Converting Enzyme Inhibitors and Angiotensin II Receptor Blockers. Angiotensin-converting enzyme (ACE) inhibitors reduce cardiac workload and decrease post-MI cardiac remodeling. ACE inhibitors have been shown to reduce mortality in MI patients, especially those with anterior infarction, pulmonary congestion, or ejection fraction less than 40%. ACE inhibitors should be administered orally within 24 hours of symptoms (e.g., lisinopril (Prinivil) 5 mg daily). In the ISIS-4 trial, an initial 6.25-mg dose of captopril (Capoten) was given and, if tolerated, was followed by 12.5 mg 2 hours later, 25 mg 10 to 12 hours later, and then 50 mg twice per day. Contraindications include hypotension, kidney failure (creatinine >2.5 mg/dL), and bilateral renal artery stenosis. Angiotensin II receptor blockers may be an effective alternative for patients who cannot tolerate ACE inhibitors.

HMG CoA Reductase Inhibitors. HMG CoA (3-hydroxy-3-methyl-glutaryl coenzyme A) reductase inhibitors (statins) are used to prevent coronary artery disease and acute coronary syndrome, because LDL cholesterol plays a critical role in the pathogenesis of atherosclerosis. There is increasing evidence that they also have short-term benefits in the treatment of acute MI. Treatment with statins in the acute setting can promote plaque stabilization, reverse endothelial dysfunction, and decrease thrombogenicity. A lipid profile should be assessed within 24 hours of the acute MI and, unless contraindicated, statin therapy should be started as soon as possible. Goal LDL levels of 70 to 80 mg/dL are recommended.

Nitrates. Nitroglycerin dilates veins, arteries, and arterioles, reducing preload and afterload. It reduces myocardial oxygen demand, increases perfusion of ischemic zones, and enhances collateral blood flow. IV nitroglycerin should be administered within the first 24 to 48 hours to patients with heart failure, large anterior acute MI, persistent chest discomfort, or hypertension. Nitrates should be used with caution in patients with RV infarction or dehydration (who are preload dependent) to avoid excessive hypotension. Blood pressure should be monitored carefully and kept above 90 mm Hg systolic. Nitroglycerin should be avoided in patients who have taken nitric oxide synthetase inhibitors or phosphodiesterase inhibitors within 24 hours prior to presentation.

Calcium Channel Blockers. Calcium channel blockers have vasodilative, antianginal, and antihypertensive actions. Calcium channel blockers do not reduce mortality in patients with MI and are not recommended for routine therapy or secondary prevention. In patients in whom β-adrenergic antagonists are contraindicated, verapamil (Isoptin)[1] or diltiazem (Cardizem)[1] may be appropriate as an alternative.

Unstable Angina and Non–ST Elevation Myocardial Infarction

An unstable angina and NSTEMI occur when there is an incompletely occluded coronary thrombus or extensive collateral blood supply (or both), resulting in a subendocardial infarction. The presentation may be identical to that of STEMI, except for the absence of acute ST-segment elevation or Q waves. ST-segment depression or T-wave inversion may be present.

Initial Therapy

Management differs from STEMI in that emergent reperfusion therapy is not indicated. Exceptions to this are patients with persistent pain (despite initial medical treatment), or hemodynamic deterioration. The focus of initial therapy is medical stabilization with oxygen to keep saturations above 90%, morphine for pain control, aspirin to prevent clot propagation, nitrates and β-blockers for anti-ischemic effects (if there are no contraindications; see Figure 2) and full-dose anticoagulation for acute coronary syndrome. As part of the initial management of a NSTEMI, it is important to risk-stratify patients into two groups: high or low risk. A useful tool for risk stratification is the TIMI risk score calculator (Table 2). Patients with a score greater than 3, markedly elevated cardiac markers, or persistent symptoms should be considered high risk. Risk stratification is essential in guiding the approach to further therapy (Figure 2). Within the first 24 to 48 hours of hospitalization, patients with unstable angina usually undergo stress testing, then angiography if the stress test is positive for ischemia. Patients with NSTEMI undergo coronary angiography.

A noninterventional approach and a trial of medical management is used for those in whom angiography demonstrates only a small area of myocardium at risk, lesion morphology not amenable to PCI, anatomically insignificant disease (less than 50% coronary stenosis), or significant left main disease in patients who are candidates for coronary artery bypass grafting (CABG). Angiography or PCI should be deferred in favor of medical management for patients with a high risk of procedure-related morbidity or mortality.

---

[1]Not FDA approved for this indication.

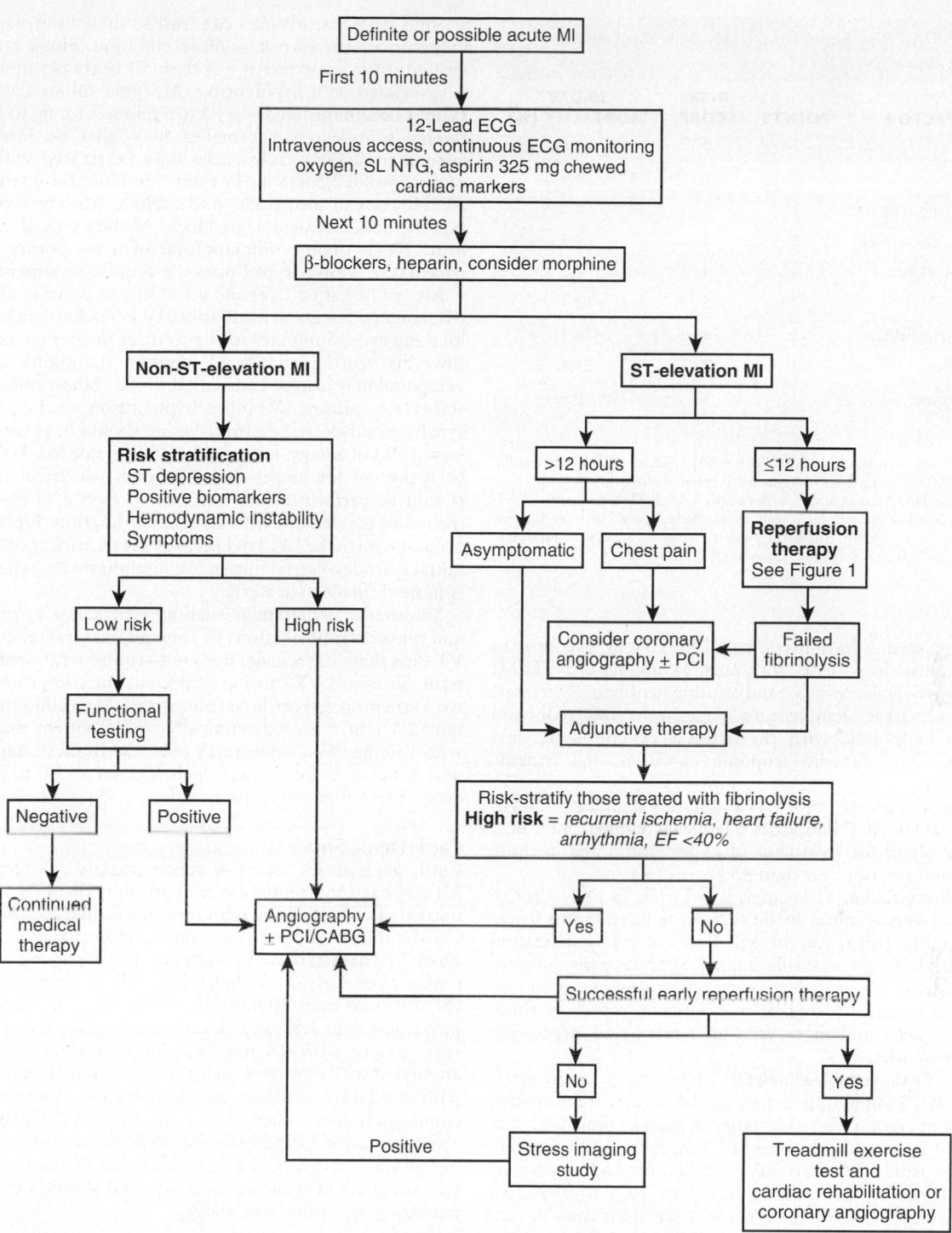

Figure 2. Definite or possible acute myocardial infarction (MI). *Abbreviations:* CABG=coronary artery bypass graft; ECG=electrocardiogram; EF=ejection fraction; PCI=percutaneous coronary intervention; SL NTG=sublingual nitroglycerin.

Adjunct Therapy

Anticoagulants. Anticoagulant medications such as LMW or unfractionated heparin should be started in all high-risk patients. Because its effects can be easily reversed, unfractionated heparin is favored over LMW heparin in patients who require urgent catheterization. Unfractionated heparin is also preferred in patients with creatinine clearance less than 30 or weight greater than 150 kg. Enoxaparin has shown modest outcome benefits over unfractionated heparin in patients with NSTEMI. Bivalirudin, a direct thrombin inhibitor, may be used as an alternative to the heparins in patients with a high risk of bleeding or with a history of heparin-induced thrombocytopenia (HIT). For patients with NSTEMI, an initial dose of bivalirudin is 0.1 mg/kg IV followed by a drip of 0.25 mg/kg per hour is administered.

Antiplatelet Medications. In addition to aspirin, clopidogrel is beneficial in NSTEMI. However, the benefit must outweigh the bleeding risk if CABG surgery is performed within 5 days of drug administration. Generally, clopidogrel administration is avoided until establishment of coronary anatomy and a decision is made regarding the need for a bypass. Clopidrogel is given as a 300 to 600 mg[3] oral load, then 75 mg daily.

---

[3]Exceeds dosage recommended by the manufacturer.

TABLE 2 TIMI Risk Score for ST-Elevation Myocardial Infarction

RISK FACTOR	POINTS	RISK SCORE	30-DAY MORTALITY (%)
Age ≥75 y	3	0	0.8
Age 65–74 y	2	1	1.6
Diabetes or hypertension	1	2	2.2
Systolic BP <100 mm Hg	3	3	4.4
Heart rate >100/min	2	4	7.3
Killip class II–IV	2	5	12.4
Anterior MI or LBBB	1	6	16.1
Weight <67 kg	1	7	23.4
Time to treatment >4 h	1	8	26.8
		>8	35.9

Abbreviations: BP = blood pressure; LBBB = left bundle branch block; MI = myocardial infarction; TIMI = Thombolysis in Myocardial Infarction (trial).
Data from Morrow DA, Antman EM, Charlesworth A, et al: TIMI risk score for ST-elevation myocardial infarction: A convenient, bedside, clinical score for risk assessment at presentation: An intravenous nPA for treatment of infarcting myocardium early II trial substudy. Circulation 2000;102:2031–7.

Several large studies have investigated the role of glycoprotein IIb/IIIa antagonists in patients with unstable angina or NSTEMI with some controversial results. Studies using tirofiban (Aggrastat) and eptifibatide have demonstrated significant risk reduction in composite endpoints, with the greatest benefit in patients with diabetes, patients with troponin elevation, and patients undergoing PCI.

Other Drugs. The use of β-blockers and statins is similar to that in STEMI. The role of ACE inhibitors is less well defined, but it may be selectively useful for treatment of hypertension and in those with LV ejection fraction less than 45%.

Elective Catheterization. Meta-analyses of trials of early elective catheterization versus initial medical therapy have shown lower rates of mortality and recurrent MI. Rates of rehospitalization are lower for recurrent unstable angina after an early invasive approach. Benefits of early elective catheterization are predominantly in intermediate- to higher-risk patients, especially those older than 65 years and those who have resting ST depression or elevated biomarkers.

Implantable Cardioverter-Defibrillator. Implantable cardioverter-defibrillator (ICD) implantation reduces the occurrence of sudden cardiac death in certain high-risk patients, such as those with late (more than 24 hours after the onset of symptoms) sustained ventricular tachycardia and ventricular fibrillation and in patients with ejection fraction persistently less than 30% to 35%. An ICD may also be beneficial in patients with late nonsustained ventricular tachycardia who have an ejection fraction of less than 40% and ventricular tachycardia induced during an electrophysiology study. ICD therapy should be considered when the patient is judged to be at continuous high risk for ventricular arrhythmia after revascularization for significant spontaneous or inducible ischemia.

Complications
Electrical Dysfunction
Arrhythmias and conduction abnormalities occur in greater than 90% of MI patients. These commonly cause death within the first 3 days and include tachycardia, Mobitz type II block or complete atrioventricular (AV) block, ventricular tachycardia, and ventricular fibrillation. Amiodarone (Cordarone) is the drug of choice for treating symptomatic ventricular arrhythmias in the setting of an MI. Lidocaine may also be used for 24 to 48 hours to treat ventricular tachycardia and following resuscitation for ventricular fibrillation.

Sinus node disturbances can lead to sinus bradycardia or sinus tachycardia; the former is more common. Sinus bradycardia is treated if the heart rate is less than 50 beats per minute and if it is associated with hypotension. Atropine sulfate 0.5 mg to 1 mg IV may be administered every 3 to 5 minutes for up to 3 mg. A temporary transvenous pacemaker may also be inserted. When encountered, sinus tachycardia may be treated with low doses of metoprolol 2.5 to 5 mg IV every 5 minutes for up to three doses. AV blocks can also occur and include Mobitz type I, Mobitz type II, or a complete heart block. Mobitz type II and complete heart blocks require implantation of a temporary transvenous pacemaker. Mobitz type I does not require treatment.

Atrial fibrillation (AF) and atrial flutter occur in about 10% of MI patients. For atrial fibrillation, IV β-blockers such as metoprolol 5 mg every 5 minutes for up to three doses may be initiated to slow the ventricular rate. IV digoxin (Lanoxin), diltiazem, or verapamil may also be considered. If AF compromises circulatory status (e.g., causing LV failure, hypotension, or chest pain), urgent synchronized electrical cardioversion should be performed with at least 100 J of energy, followed by 200 J if needed. For AF that has been present for longer than 48 hours, electrical cardioversion should be performed only after the presence of an intracardiac thrombus is ruled out with an echocardiogram. Electrical cardioversion with 50 to 100 J of energy is the treatment of choice for an initial episode of atrial flutter, because pharmacologic rate control is more difficult to achieve.

Ventricular arrhythmias such as ventricular tachycardia (VT) and ventricular fibrillation (VF) are not uncommon. Nonsustained VT (less than 30 seconds) does not require treatment in the short term. Sustained VT causing hemodynamic compromise is treated with synchronized cardioversion with 100 to 200 J of energy. Sustained VT in a hemodynamically stable patient may be treated with 150 mg of amiodarone IV over 10 minutes (may repeat once in 5 minutes) or lidocaine, which is given as 1.0 to 1.5 mg/kg IV every 3 to 5 minutes up to 3 mg/kg.

Cardiogenic Shock
Cardiogenic shock occurs in approximately 7% of patients with MI and has a mortality rate of approximately 80% to 90% when untreated. When treated with early revascularization using PCI or CABG, the 30-day mortality rate is close to 50%. Cardiogenic shock is characterized by systemic hypotension: systolic blood pressure persistently less than 90 mm Hg or mean arterial pressure (MAP) more than 30 mm Hg below baseline, reduced cardiac index (less than 1.8), and elevated pulmonary artery wedge pressure greater than 16 mm Hg. Initial stabilization should be attempted with inotropes such as dobutamine (Dobutex), together with intraaortic balloon counterpulsation. Intraaortic balloon counterpulsation reduces cardiac afterload and improves coronary artery perfusion by increasing systolic blood pressure. Early angiography and revascularization with either PCI or CABG has a significant effect in reducing mortality and should be considered in patients with cardiogenic shock.

Structural Disorders
Structural complications that may result from acute MI include papillary muscle rupture, ventricular aneurysms, interventricular septal rupture, and ventricular free wall rupture. Papillary muscle rupture may be repaired surgically if it causes severe valvular regurgitation. Interventricular septal rupture may be diagnosed with a balloon-tipped catheter revealing a significant drop in PO_2 from the right ventricle. It can be repaired surgically, after a 6-week waiting period to allow healing of the ventricular muscle. Free wall rupture may also be repaired surgically, but it is almost always fatal.

Right Ventricular Infarction
RV infarction occurs in approximately 40% of patients with acute inferior MI; however, hemodynamically significant RV dysfunction is less common. Patients usually present with an elevated

jugular venous pressure without hemodynamic compromise. Some patients present with hypotension, particularly after the administration of vasodilators such as nitrates. On physical examination, patients might have an elevated jugular venous pressure, Kussmaul sign (filling of the jugular vein on inspiration), clear lungs, and a right-sided gallop on cardiac auscultation. The diagnosis is strengthened by demonstrating the presence of at least 1 mm of ST segment elevation in leads V1, V3R, or V4R or RV dysfunction by echocardiography.

The treatment is supportive, with intravenous fluids and inotropic support with dopamine or dobutamine, if needed. These interventions may be tailored using guidance from hemodynamic data obtained from a pulmonary artery catheter. Patients with RV infarction are more likely to have complications with bradycardia or AV block that can require temporary atrial or ventricular pacing. Most patients improve spontaneously after 48 to 72 hours. Patients with shock might benefit from early revascularization with PCI to the right coronary artery.

Cardiac Rehabilitation and Secondary Prevention

Cardiac rehabilitation should be initiated before discharge from the hospital, with the goals of improving quality of life, facilitating return to normal activities, encouraging regular exercise, and promoting secondary prevention. Secondary prevention is aimed at smoking cessation and at aggressive dietary and pharmacologic treatment of hyperlipidemia, hypertension, and diabetes mellitus. Blood pressure goal should be less than 140/90 mm Hg or less than 130/80 mm Hg in patients with diabetes or chronic kidney disease. Lipid management should involve statin use and dietary restrictions. There should be a reduction in intake of saturated fats (to less than 7% of total calories), trans fatty acids, and cholesterol (to less than 200 mg per day). Goal LDL cholesterol should be substantially less than 100 mg/dL. If triglycerides are 200 mg/dL or higher, non–high-density lipoprotein cholesterol should be less than 130 mg/dL. Physical activity should be emphasized with a goal of 30 minutes at a minimum of 5 days per week. Patients with diabetes should have a hemoglobin A1c goal of less than 7%. An annual influenza vaccine is also recommended in all patients with cardiovascular disease. Patients with cardiovascular disease are candidates for pneumococcal vaccination. Weight management is essential, and a goal BMI should be 18.5 to 24.9 kg/m². Men should have a waist circumference of less than 40 inches and women less than 35 inches.

References

Alpert JS, Thygesen K, Antman E, Bassand JP. Myocardial infarction redefined—a consensus document of the Joint European Society of Cardiology/American College of Cardiology Committee for the redefinition of myocardial infarction. J Am Coll Cardiol 2000;36:959–69.

Anderson JL, Adams CD, Antman EM, et al. ACC/AHA 2007 guidelines for the management of patients with unstable angina/non-ST-elevation myocardial infarction. J Am Coll Cardiol 2007;50:e1–e157.

Antman EM, Anbe DT, Armstrong PW, et al. ACC/AHA guidelines for the management of patients with ST-elevation myocardial infarction: A report of the American College of Cardiology/American Heart Association Task Force on Practice Guidelines (Committee to Revise the 1999 Guidelines for the Management of Patients With Acute Myocardial Infarction). J Am Coll Cardiol 2004;44(3):E1–E211.

Antman EM, Cohen M, Bernink PJ, et al. The TIMI risk score for unstable angina/non-ST elevation MI: A method for prognostication and therapeutic decision making. JAMA 2000;284:835–42.

Cannon CP, Hand M. Bahr R, et al. Critical pathways for management of patients with acute coronary syndromes: An assessment by the National Heart Attack Alert Program. Am Heart J 2002;143:777–89.

Krumholz HM, Anderson JL, Brooks NH, et al. ACC/AHA clinical performance measures for adults with ST-elevation and non–ST-elevation myocardial infarction: A report of the ACC/AHA task force on performance measures (ST-Elevation and Non–ST-Elevation Myocardial Infarction Performance Measures Writing Committee). J Am Coll Cardiol 2006;47:236–65.

Mehta SR, Cannon CP, Fox KA, et al. Routine vs selective invasive strategies in patients with acute coronary syndromes: A collaborative meta-analysis of randomized trials. JAMA 2005;293:2908–17.

O'Rourke RA, Walsh RA, Fuster V. Hurst's The Heart. 12th ed. New York: McGraw-Hill Professional Publishing; 2009.

Smith Jr SC, Allen J, Blair SN, et al. AHA/ACC guidelines for secondary prevention for patients with coronary and other atherosclerotic vascular disease: 2006 update endorsed by the National Heart, Lung, and Blood Institute. J Am Coll Cardiol 2006;47:2130–9.

Smith Jr SC, Feldman TE, Hirshfeld Jr JW, et al. ACC/AHA/SCA1 2005 guideline update for percutaneous coronary intervention: A report of the American College of Cardiology/American Heart Association Task Force on Practice Guidelines (ACC/AHA/SCAI Writing Committee to Update the 2001 Guidelines for Percutaneous Coronary Intervention). Circulation 2006;113(7):e166–e286.

Weaver WD, Cerqueira M, Hallstrom AP, et al. Prehospital-initiated vs hospital-initiated thrombolytic therapy. The Myocardial Infarction Triage and Intervention Trial. JAMA 1993;270:1211–6.

Wright R, et al. ACCF/AHA Focused Update of the Guidelines for the Management of Patients With Unstable Angina/Non–ST-Elevation Myocardial Infarction (Updating the 2007 Guideline). A Report of the American College of Cardiology Foundation/American Heart Association Task Force on Practice Guidelines. Circulation 2011;123:2022–60.

Wright RS, Anderson JL, Adams CD, et al. 2007 Focused update of the ACC/AHA 2004 guidelines for the management of patients with ST-elevation myocardial infarction. J Am Coll Cardiol 2008;51:210–47.

ANGINA PECTORIS

Method of
Kenneth Tobin, DO; and Kim Eagle, MD

CURRENT DIAGNOSIS

- The clinical diagnosis of angina depends largely on the accurate assessment of a patient's risk factor profile for coronary artery disease and the typicality of the symptom complex.
- The most common symptom of angina pectoris is left-sided chest pain or pressure, with or without associated radiation of pain or pressure to the jaw or left arm, occurring with exertion and relieved with rest or sublingual nitroglycerin.
- Women may present with atypical symptoms such as sharp, nonexertional chest pain; generalized fatigue; or right-sided chest pain.
- Basic screening tests (e.g., 12-lead electrocardiogram, laboratory data, chest radiograph) are normal in most cases.
- For an initial diagnosis, appropriate noninvasive testing or coronary angiography, or both, is important to define the amount of ischemic myocardium and an overall treatment plan.
- Even when invasive procedures are clinically indicated, aggressive medical therapy with high-dose statins, attainment of appropriate blood pressure levels, smoking cessation, and use of antiplatelet therapy is of paramount importance.
- Patients who have clinical evidence of unstable angina and laboratory evidence of myocardial ischemia most often benefit from early invasive treatment strategies.

CURRENT THERAPY

Stable Angina Pectoris
- Treatment includes β-blockers, nitrates, and calcium channel blockers for symptom control.
- Consider the addition of ranolazine (Ranexa) if symptoms are not adequately controlled.

Aggressive Cholesterol Treatment Based on the ACC-AHA Blood Cholesterol Guidelines
- Blood pressure management
- Antiplatelet therapy
- Lifestyle modifications:
  - Smoking cessation
  - Exercise prescription
  - Dietary guidelines
  - Depression assessment

Unstable Angina

- With positive biomarkers for myocardial ischemia, consider coronary angiography.
- With negative biomarkers for myocardial ischemia, consider noninvasive assessment once symptoms are controlled.
- With a substantial ischemic burden identified, consider coronary angiography.
- With no or minimal ischemia identified, consider increasing medical therapy.
- With persistent symptoms, consider other treatment modalities.

Angina pectoris is defined as cardiac-induced pain that is a direct result of a mismatch between myocardial oxygen supply and demand. The initial presentation of ischemic heart disease is chronic stable angina in approximately 50% of patients; it is estimated that 16.5 million Americans have this diagnosis. Ischemic heart disease is the leading cause of death in the United States.

Stable angina refers to predictable chest discomfort during various levels of exertional activity that is predictably resolved with rest or administration of sublingual nitroglycerin (Nitrostat). Unstable angina is an acute ischemic event; this diagnosis includes patients with new-onset cardiac chest pain, angina at rest, post-myocardial infarction angina, or an accelerating pattern of previously stable angina. The terms unstable angina and non–Q wave myocardial infarction are often used interchangeably and should be further defined on the basis of myocardial necrosis as measured by serum biomarkers.

The clinical sensation of angina pectoris is caused by stimulation of chemosensitive and mechanosensitive receptors of unmyelinated nerve cells found within cardiac muscle fibers and around the coronary vessels. This stimulation cascade is thought to occur when lactate, serotonin, bradykinin, histamine, reactive oxygen species, and adenosine are released into the coronary circulation during periods of lactic acidosis. Nerve stimulation via the sympathetic ganglia occurs most commonly between the seventh cervical and fourth thoracic portions of the spinal cord. This explains from an anatomic standpoint why the most commonly recognized pain patterns for angina pectoris involve discomfort in the chest, neck, jaw, and left arm.

The most common cause of angina pectoris is coronary atherosclerosis. As plaque is initially deposited within a coronary vessel, there may be no significant internal luminal compromise during the early positive remodeling phase. However, at the point at which this compensatory mechanism fails, internal luminal compromise ensues. As long as the coronary artery segment distal to the stenosis retains the ability to vasodilate in response to increasing blood flow demands, coronary homeostasis is maintained. Once the critical threshold is passed, the blood supply cannot accommodate this demand, and angina may occur. The four major factors that determine myocardial oxygen demand are heart rate, systolic blood pressure, myocardial wall tension, and myocardial contractility.

Clinical Features

For patients with documented coronary artery disease (CAD) who have predictable episodes of classic symptoms, the diagnosis of angina pectoris is straightforward. Most patients are aware of the levels of exertion that typically induce angina symptoms. Most describe a pain or heaviness across their middle chest that may or may not radiate to the jaw or left arm. Some patients deny chest pain symptoms altogether and instead complain of exertional dyspnea or diaphoresis. Environmental situations such as cold exposure, emotional stress, or heavy meals can induce angina. The Canadian Cardiovascular Society and the New York Heart Association classification systems are used to define angina severity. Both systems use a I through IV scale, with mild angina (class I) referring to episodes that occur with extreme exertion and severe angina (class IV) to episodes that occur with minimal or no

TABLE 1	Differential Diagnosis of Chest Pain
Cardiac ischemia
Angina
Myocardial infarction
Vasospastic angina
Pericarditis
Aortic dissection (new-onset chest pain and new aortic insufficiency noted on auscultation is an aortic dissection until proven otherwise)
Pulmonary embolism
Esophageal spasm
Gastroesophageal reflux disease
Musculoskeletal pain
Biliary colic
Acute pneumonia

exertion. These classification systems are useful for risk stratification and for assessing medical therapy efficacy.

There are clear gender differences in the clinical presentations of angina. Pleuritic, musculoskeletal-type pain, nonexertional pain, and nocturnal pains have been reported as anginal equivalents in women. Fatigue is one of the most common presenting symptoms for CAD in women. The key to the diagnosis in men and women lies in a thorough history, which should always include the quality, location, provoking activities, and duration of pain and factors that relieve the pain. Based on a detailed clinical history, the many diagnoses that can masquerade as angina may be eliminated (Table 1).

Diagnostic Testing

A baseline electrocardiogram (ECG) is often one of the initial tests obtained in a patient with the complaint of chest pain. A normal tracing does not exclude the diagnosis of ischemic heart disease. More than 50% of patients with diagnosed angina have a normal ECG at rest. The baseline ECG may, however, show evidence of pathologic Q waves or left ventricular hypertrophy, either of which increases the statistical probability of significant CAD. Baseline laboratory data should include a fasting lipid panel to help define the patient's risk factor profile.

Stress testing is an appropriate screening tool for the initial diagnosis of CAD, risk stratification after acute ischemic syndrome, and assessment of treatment efficacy. Whenever feasible, it is more advantageous to obtain an exercise stress test rather than a pharmacologically based study. The additional prognostic data obtained through exercise include blood pressure response, heart rate response, heart rate recovery, metabolic equivalent level attained, and ECG assessment of the ST segment. There are several validated exercise protocols that add additional risk stratification measures to the test results.

The predictive value of exercise treadmill stress testing ranges from 40% for single-vessel disease to 90% for three-vessel disease. A baseline left bundle branch block, paced rhythm, poorly controlled atrial arrhythmia, or left ventricular hypertrophy with secondary ischemic changes often renders the test inconclusive when assessing for ischemic changes. However, if stress testing is being performed for attainment of hemodynamic responses and achievable metabolic equivalent levels, these baseline ECG abnormalities may be overlooked.

Stress test accuracy is markedly improved by the addition of an imaging modality such as echocardiography or nuclear perfusion scanning. The sensitivity and specificity of stress echocardiography and stress nuclear imaging are 85% to 90%. Stress echocardiography is believed to be somewhat more specific, and stress nuclear imaging is thought to be more sensitive. A stress echocardiogram also allows assessment of left ventricular systolic function and valvular function and prediction of right ventricular pressure. In deciding on which stress test to perform, one should rely on the expertise of the testing facility and the individual patient's circumstance.

Risk Factor Management

Hypertension

Hypertension is a commonly occurring, well-established, major cardiovascular risk factor. Initial treatment of hypertension in patients with ischemic heart disease should always include lifestyle management. Appropriate weight loss with a goal of achieving a body mass index <25 kg/m^2 can improve hypertension control. A reduction in dietary salt intake can also have positive effects on a patient's blood pressure.

Discord has resulted from the publication of recent hypertension guidelines by various medical societies as well as the 2014 Evidence-Based Guideline for the Management of High Blood Pressure in Adults Report from the Panel Members Appointed to the Eighth Joint National Committee. It has been shown that cardiovascular risk progressively increases at blood pressures greater than 115/75 mm Hg. A meta-analysis of 61 prospective observational trials of hypertension involving 1 million adults with no known vascular disease at baseline revealed several interesting findings. Patient outcomes were related per decade of age to the usual blood pressure at the start of that decade. For example, from ages 40 to 69, for each increase in 20 mm Hg systolic blood pressure, a twofold increase in cardiovascular death rate occurred. These findings were much more pronounced in patients who were between 80 and 89 years old than in the youngest cohort, 40 and 49 years old. Although the relative risk was much higher in the younger group, the absolute risk was greatest among the octogenarians. These increased cardiovascular risks were not confined to subjects with blood pressures greater than 140/90 mm Hg; rather, there was a threshold of risk shown all the way down to 115/75 mm Hg. Even small reductions in blood pressure can have a significant positive impact on cardiovascular disease. Blood pressure reductions of 4 mm Hg systolic and 3 mm Hg diastolic were shown to reduce cardiovascular events by 15% in a cohort of 20,888 patients.

The Heart Outcomes Prevention Evaluation study asked the question whether all patients with atherosclerosis, regardless of blood pressure, should be treated with an angiotensin-converting enzyme inhibitor. Although many subsequent editorials implied that all patients with CAD could benefit from this therapy, a closer look at the data suggests a different interpretation. The mean blood pressure was 139/79 mm Hg, suggesting that a significant portion of the 9297 participants had a baseline blood pressure higher than this value. Compared with placebo, the treatment group had a 22% reduction in the primary outcome composite of myocardial infarction, stroke, or cardiovascular death. A small substudy using 24 hour ambulatory blood pressure monitoring showed blood pressure differences of 11 mm Hg systolic and 4 mm Hg diastolic in the treatment group compared with the placebo group, which may explain the cardiovascular event reductions reported.

The blood pressure goal for treatment of hypertension in patients with established ischemic heart disease should be $<130/80$ mm Hg. One must be careful with aggressive diastolic blood pressure management, as some studies have shown a J-shaped curve relationship between diastolic blood pressures and coronary events.

Hyperlipidemia

Dyslipidemia is an important risk factor for atherosclerotic cardiovascular disease, and the lowering of LDL-cholesterol has been shown to correlate with reductions in cardiovascular disease event rates. Previously published cholesterol treatment guidelines recommended achieving less than 70 mg/dL LDL-cholesterol levels in CAD patients. The current guidelines published by the ACC-AHA depart from these specific values, and instead recommend using high-intensity 3-hydroxy-3-methylglutaryl coenzyme reductase inhibitors (statins) to reduce the LDL-cholesterol levels by more than 50%. These agents have been shown to be well tolerated and have positive nonlipid pleiotropic effects as well as the ability to dramatically lower LDL levels.

Observational evidence suggests that regardless of how cholesterol is lowered, a reduction in atherosclerotic cardiovascular disease will result. However, to achieve meaningful reductions in cardiovascular mortality, the recommended choice for lowering LDL-cholesterol levels among the currently available pharmacologic are the statins. These agents have been studied exclusively using fixed dose combinations and not dose titrated to achieve various LDL-c levels; therefore, currently available data does not support specific LDL target goals.

The Cholesterol Treatment Trialists' meta-analysis, including 90,056 subjects from 14 trials, showed a 12% reduction in all-cause mortality per 38.6 mg/dL (1 mmol/L) reduction in LDL-cholesterol, with a 19% reduction in coronary mortality, a 24% reduction in need for revascularization, a 17% reduction in stroke incidence, and a 21% reduction in any major vascular event during a mean follow-up period of 5 years. These benefits were observed in different age groups, across genders, at different baseline cholesterol levels, and equally among those with and without prior CAD and cardiovascular risk factors.

The Heart Protection Study showed that in patients with established CAD, other atherosclerotic vascular disease, or diabetes, statin therapy reduced cardiovascular events regardless of the baseline LDL-cholesterol level. The trial, which enrolled 20,536 patients aged 40 to 80 years, showed a 24% reduction in major cardiovascular events, a 25% reduction in stroke, and a 13% reduction in overall mortality with statin therapy.

Patients with a recent acute ischemic syndrome were enrolled in the Pravastatin or Atorvastatin Evaluation and Infection Therapy trial, known as Thrombolysis in Myocardial Infarction 22, which compared 80 mg atorvastatin (Lipitor) with 40 mg of pravastatin (Pravachol). The atorvastatin group achieved a median LDL level of 62 mg/dL, compared with 96 mg/dL in the pravastatin group. The relative risk reduction for this reduced LDL level was 16%. A substudy looking at the LDL-cholesterol levels achieved with atorvastatin showed that those subjects achieving a level of 40 to 60 mg/dL had a 22% reduction in events, compared with those achieving a level of 80 to 100 mg/dL. Therefore, it appears that high-dose statin therapy and aggressive LDL-lowering in this patient population lead to reduced cardiovascular events.

The Treating to New Targets trial was the first to compare a more intensely treated group with a less intensely treated group using the same agent. The design of this 10,000-patient study eliminated concerns that outcome differences were induced by dissimilar statin preparations. The mean LDL level achieved was 101 mg/dL with 10 mg atorvastatin, and 77 mg/dL with the 80 mg dose. This LDL reduction was associated with a relative risk reduction of 27% for the primary endpoint of the first major cardiovascular event.

Data from the recently published Study of the Effectiveness of Additional Reductions in Cholesterol and Homocysteine revealed an increased risk of myopathy and rhabdomyolysis in patients taking 80 mg simvastatin (Zocor). The FDA has subsequently restricted high-dose simvastatin to patients who have been on this dose for longer than 12 months without evidence of myopathy, and the agency has recommended that new patients should not be started on this particular dose.

To effectively achieve a greater than 50% LDL-cholesterol reduction in CAD patients utilizing currently available pharmacologic agents, the most recent treatment guidelines suggest either atorvastatin 40 to 80 mg or rosuvastatin (Crestor) 20 to 40 mg. In other patient populations that require moderate-intensity statin therapy, there are several statin choices. Because there is no currently available evidence to suggest that non–statin lipid-altering agents effectively reduce cardiovascular mortality, these medications should not be routinely prescribed.

It is apparent from both primary and secondary prevention lipid trials that achieving lower LDL levels reduces cardiovascular event rates. Because there is no high-quality clinical evidence to support achieving specific LDL levels in patients with diagnosed CAD, high-dose statin therapy should be the mainstay of pharmacologically based therapy, if tolerated.

Metabolic Syndrome

The combined presence of insulin resistance, hypertension, dyslipidemia, and abdominal obesity define metabolic syndrome. There is debate about whether this is a true syndrome or simply a clustering of cardiovascular risk factors in a particular individual. The key concept is that the concomitant presence of these particular cardiovascular risk factors markedly increases a patient's chances of developing diabetes mellitus and coronary atherosclerosis. The approach to treatment for this syndrome is no different from that for the individual components. Recognition of the components is key to the treatment of this disorder.

Smoking

Cigarette smoking is probably the most important of the identified modifiable cardiovascular risk factors. The incidence of CAD is two to four times higher in smokers than in nonsmokers. The pathophysiologic process that leads to atherosclerosis from smoking stems from induced platelet dysfunction, endothelial dysfunction, smooth muscle cell proliferation, and attenuated high-density lipoprotein-cholesterol levels. Smoking cessation must be sought for every CAD patient.

Diet

Lifestyle changes for patients with CAD must incorporate healthy eating habits. The Mediterranean diet has been shown to positively affect cardiovascular disease, and conversely, a diet high in saturated fats has been shown to negatively influence multiple cardiac risk factors. Patients should be encouraged to incorporate high proportions of fruits and vegetables into their diet, along with olive oil and regular servings of fish coupled with a reduced amount of red meats.

Other Lifestyle Changes

Exercise should be encouraged in patients with stable angina, once all appropriate invasive and noninvasive tests have been completed and a stable medical regimen has been established.

Increasing a patient's aerobic capacity can lower the body's oxygen requirement for a given workload, which can lead to increased exercise tolerance and reduced anginal symptoms. Aerobic exercise can improve endothelial function and positively affect baroreflex sensitivity and heart rate variability in patients with CAD.

Endorphins released during exercise are thought to be mood enhancers as well as effective muscle relaxants. Exercise itself improves sleep patterns. Cortisol levels are reduced with regular exercise, which may attenuate the body's sensation of stress and anxiety. For these reasons, appropriate exercise programs for patients with stable angina have far-reaching positive benefits. Exercise guidelines for CAD patients have been published and should be reviewed before patients begin aggressive secondary prevention efforts.

Major depression affects approximately 25% of people recovering from a myocardial infarction, and another 40% suffer from mild depression. In any given year, one of every three long-term acute ischemic syndrome survivors will develop depression. The Heart and Soul Study examined 1017 patients with stable CAD over a period of 4.8 years. Patients identified with depression were twice as likely to experience recurrent cardiovascular events. Physical inactivity was associated with a 44% greater rate of cardiovascular events. Patients with symptoms of depression were less likely to follow dietary, exercise, and medication recommendations.

Approach to Treatment

Medical Therapy

Medications used to treat angina pectoris and typical dosages are listed in Table 2.

Nitrates

Nitrates provide an exogenous source of nitric oxide, which serves to relax smooth muscle and inhibit platelet aggregation. Nitrates exert their antianginal effect by reducing myocardial oxygen demand through coronary and systemic vasodilatation. Nitrates are strong venodilators, and in higher doses they can also induce

TABLE 2 Medications Used for the Treatment of Angina Pectoris

NAME	DOSAGE
β-Blockers	
Atenolol (Tenormin)	25–200 mg PO qd
Metoprolol tartrate (Lopressor)	25–200 mg bid
Metoprolol succinate (Toprol XL)	25–200 mg qd
Carvedilol (Coreg)[1]	6.25–25 mg PO bid
Carvedilol phosphate (Coreg CR)[1]	20–80 mg PO qd
Propranolol (Inderal)	80–320 mg/d, divided bid or tid
Propranolol (Inderal LA)	80–160 mg PO qd
Labetalol (Trandate, Normodyne)[1]	200–800 mg bid
Nitrates	
Isosorbide dinitrate (Isordil)	10–40 mg PO bid or tid
Isosorbide mononitrate (Imdur)	30–240 mg PO qd
Nitroglycerin (Nitrostat)	0.4 mg SL q5min
Nitroglycerin transdermal (Nitro-Dur)	0.2–0.8 mg/h 12–14 h patch
Calcium Channel Blockers	
Dihydropyridines	
Amlodipine (Norvasc)	2.5–10 mg PO qd
Felodipine (Plendil)[1]	2.5–10 mg PO qd
Nifedipine (Procardia XL)	30–90 mg PO qd
Nondihydropyridines	
Verapamil (Calan)	80–120 mg PO tid
Verapamil (Calan SR)	120–480 mg PO qd
Diltiazem (Cardizem)	360 mg/d PO, divided tid or qid
Diltiazem (Cardizem LA)	180–360 mg PO qd
Other	
Ranexa	500 mg twice daily and increase to 1000 mg twice daily as needed, based on clinical symptoms

[1]Not FDA approved for this indication.

arterial dilatation. Reducing the preload through venodilatation reduces myocardial oxygen demand. Coronary artery dilatation of stenotic vessels and intracoronary collaterals directly increases myocardial oxygen delivery. Through these mechanisms, nitrates have been shown to prevent recurrent episodes of angina and to increase exercise tolerance.

There are several nitrate preparations; they differ mainly in route of administration, onset of action, and effective half-life. Nitrate tolerance can occur with long-term use of any nitrate preparation and can be avoided by providing a 10- to 12-hour nitrate-free interval. "Nitrates should be used with caution in patients with a diagnosis of hypertrophic obstructive cardiomyopathy."

β-Blockers

β-Blockers competitively inhibit catecholamines from binding to β-receptors. Over time, β-blocker therapy leads to an increase in β-receptor density. Because of receptor upregulation, acute β-blocker withdrawal may lead to a transient supersensitivity to catecholamines and subsequent angina or even myocardial infarction. There are three classes of β-receptors. Some β-blockers are receptor specific, and some exert an effect over all three receptors. However, at higher doses, even β-selective agents have cross-reactivity for all β-receptors. β-Blockers reduce myocardial oxygen demand through a negative inotropic effect, a chronotropic effect, and a reduction in left ventricular wall stress.

Several cardioselective β-blockers, including atenolol (Tenormin) and metoprolol (Lopressor), have been shown to be effective antianginals that are fairly well tolerated in patients with underlying bronchospastic disease. Dosing is important for β-blocker efficacy. A study comparing atenolol with placebo showed that all doses from 25 through 200 mg/day were effective in reducing angina, but only the two highest doses led to an increase in exercise tolerance. Certain β-blockers have intrinsic sympathomimetic activity, including pindolol (Visken)[1] and acebutolol (Sectral).[1] Although they may be effective in reducing angina, they should be used with caution in patients with a prior history of myocardial infarction and in those with left ventricular dysfunction, because they may not reduce heart rate or blood pressure at rest.

When β-blockers are used to treat angina, a goal resting heart rate should be between 55 and 60 beats/minute. Caution should be used in patients with resting bradycardia and in those with known reactive airway disease. Atenolol is renally excreted and should be used with caution in the elderly and in those with known renal dysfunction.

Calcium Channel Blockers

Calcium channel blockers are classified as either dihydropyridines or nondihydropyridines. The former group includes amlodipine (Norvasc), felodipine (Plendil),[1] nifedipine (Procardia), and nicardipine (Cardene); the latter includes diltiazem (Cardizem) and verapamil (Calan). There are differences among the two subclasses in regard to chronotropic, dromotropic, and inotropic effects.

Calcium channel blockers positively alter myocardial oxygen supply and demand, mainly through direct arterial vasodilatation. The nondihydropyridines also exhibit negative chronotropic and inotropic effects, thus further lowering myocardial oxygen demands.

One of the early quick-release preparations of a dihydropyridine calcium channel blocker, nifedipine, was reported to potentially induce myocardial infarction when used to treat angina. This was most likely due to a rapid drop in afterload leading to reflex adrenergic activation. Sustained-release preparations of nifedipine (Procardia XL), as well as the other dihydropyridines, have been proven safe and effective in patients with cardiovascular disease. Although amlodipine and felodipine are tolerated in patients with left ventricular systolic dysfunction, other calcium channel blockers should be avoided in this patient subset.

Ranolazine (Ranexa)

Ranolazine (Ranexa) is a new and unique antianginal drug approved for the treatment of stable angina. It is a sustained-release preparation that has been approved for patients who remain symptomatic while on standard angina pharmacotherapy. Its mechanism of action may be through reduction of fatty acid oxidation or effects on sodium shifts and intracellular calcium levels. QT prolongation has been reported, but a significant increase in arrhythmias has not been seen. Side effects include dizziness, constipation, and nausea. Dosing is 500 or 1000 mg twice daily, and the major route of metabolism is the cytochrome P-450 system. Ranolazine should be used cautiously in patients who are taking other pharmacologic agents that have the potential to prolong the QT interval, "and in patients with liver cirrhosis."

Medication Combinations

Many patients with chronic stable angina require more than one antianginal medication to control their symptoms. "Current guidelines recommend β-blockers or calcium channel blockers as initial therapy unless otherwise contraindicated, with the addition of nitrates as symptoms dictate. Further medications may be added and individualized to each patient based on their degree of angina and overall clinical response."

However, it is important to recognize medication side effects when deciding which agents to combine. β-Blockers block the atrioventricular (AV) node and exert a portion of their effectiveness through this mechanism. The nondihydropyridine calcium channel blockers also have AV-nodal blocking properties, and therefore should be used cautiously with β-blockers, especially in patients with preexisting conduction system disease. The dihydropyridine agents do not have AV-nodal blocking effects and may be a safer choice when used in combination with β-blockers. Nitrates do not have a side-effect profile that raises concerns when they are used with β-blockers or with calcium channel blockers.

Antiplatelet Therapy

The common etiology leading to an acute ischemic syndrome is a platelet-rich clot occurring at the site of a significant coronary artery stenosis, often after a plaque rupture. Antiplatelet medications have been shown to consistently decrease morbidity and mortality in a wide array of cardiovascular disease patients. A meta-analysis suggested that for patients with stable cardiovascular disease, low-dose aspirin therapy (50–100 mg daily) is as effective as higher doses (>300 mg). In this patient population, aspirin therapy resulted in a 26% reduction in myocardial infarction; the number of patients needed to treat to prevent a myocardial infarction was 83.

The Antiplatelet Trialists' Collaboration study demonstrated a reduction in myocardial infarction, stroke, and death in high-risk cardiovascular patients treated with antiplatelet therapy. Consensus guidelines recommend indefinite oral aspirin for the secondary prevention of cardiovascular events in all angina patients.

Clopidogrel (Plavix)[1] is an effective alternative to aspirin for the treatment of stable cardiovascular disease in those patients with a true aspirin allergy. However, there are no compelling data to indicate that clopidogrel (or newer agents, such as prasugrel [Effient][1] and ticagrelor [Brilinta][1]) are superior to aspirin in this particular patient population. In patients with unstable angina, dual antiplatelet therapy with aspirin and clopidogrel is recommended.

Invasive Assessment

The decision to pursue an invasive treatment approach differs significantly in patients with chronic stable angina and in those with acute coronary syndromes. Within both groups, accurate risk stratification is the key consideration in choosing who will benefit from coronary angiography and subsequent percutaneous coronary intervention. An invasive strategy in unstable angina patients has been shown to reduce recurrent acute coronary syndrome events consistently in many trials. A routine invasive strategy is recommended for patients with non–ST-segment acute ischemic syndromes who have refractory ischemia, elevated cardiac biomarkers suggesting myocardial necrosis, or new ST-segment depression on ECG monitoring.

In patients with unstable angina, there are significant gender differences in outcomes related to the use of invasive therapy. Both men and women with elevated biomarkers from myocardial necrosis have comparable reductions in rates of death, myocardial infarction, and rehospitalization with invasive treatment strategies. However, in the absence of positive biomarkers, women appear to have potentially negative outcomes with an invasive approach. The current American College of Cardiology and American Heart Association guidelines recommend a conservative approach in such women.

Patients diagnosed with stable angina comprise a vast array of clinical presentations. The two most heated debates in this arena concern the initial choice of medical therapy versus an invasive approach, and when to cross over from a medical treatment plan to an invasive one. The Atorvastatin Versus Revascularization Treatment (AVERT) trial studied the effects of intensive lipid-lowering therapy on ischemic events in a relatively low-risk population of patients with single- or two-vessel disease compared with percutaneous transluminal coronary angioplasty. AVERT randomized 341 patients to medical therapy plus atorvastatin

Angina Pectoris

---

[1]Not FDA approved for this indication.

[1]Not FDA approved for this indication.

80 mg or to angioplasty followed by usual medical care (which included the option of statin therapy at the choice of the treating physician). The medical treatment group experienced a 36% reduction in the composite endpoint of ischemic events compared with the angioplasty group. This difference was due primarily to repeated angioplasty, coronary artery bypass grafting, or hospitalization for worsening angina. The primary outcome of this trial from a practical standpoint was that high-dose statin therapy was safe in this patient population and did not increase cardiovascular events, compared with an angioplasty-based treatment plan.

One of the keys in interpreting the available data is recognizing that by the time many of these trials are published, the percutaneous treatment choices are often outdated. Early trials used mainly balloon angioplasty; later trials used early-generation bare metal stents. Equally as important is to determine what the background medical treatment plans were for any particular trial on this subject. Often, lipid therapy was not aggressive, hypertension management was not confirmed to be adequate, and intravenous glycoprotein IIb/IIIa antagonists were either not available or not used as a standard protocol when indicated.

The Clinical Outcomes Utilizing Revascularization and Aggressive Drug Evaluation (COURAGE) trial was designed to address the potential advantages of current medical therapy over a percutaneous approach in patients with demonstrable ischemia but stable CAD. Of the 35,000 patients screened, only 2287 met the study inclusion criteria. All participants of the COURAGE trial underwent a coronary angiography, and patients with high-risk anatomic findings such as severe left main coronary artery stenosis were excluded. The biggest difference in this trial compared with previous studies was that strict guideline-based medical therapy was followed in both groups. In the entire cohort, 85% of subjects were taking a β-blocker, 93% were taking a statin, and 85% were taking aspirin. The final interpretation of the COURAGE trial results was not that medical therapy is superior for all patients with CAD, but that in selected cohorts, aggressive medical therapy is an appropriate first step in the treatment of ischemic heart disease.

Novel Therapies
Transmyocardial Laser Revascularization
Transmyocardial laser revascularization is an invasive treatment that can be performed as an open-heart procedure or percutaneously. The mechanism was originally thought to be the creation of myocardial channels leading to collateral circulation to ischemic zones, but this concept has been called into question. Current theories suggest cardiac denervation, laser-induced angiogenesis, or placebo effect. Likely selection bias within trials has also limited published outcomes data. In a randomized trial involving patients with class III or IV angina and percutaneously untreatable CAD, there was no reduction in angina, no improvement in exercise tolerance, and no decrease in adverse cardiac events after percutaneous transmyocardial laser revascularization, compared with maximal medical therapy. In this trial, the placebo effect was dramatically reduced through extensive blinding protocols for patients and treating physicians.

Angiogenesis leading to the induction of newly formed coronary vessels has been an active area of research for many years. Three main angiogenic growth factors have been studied: fibroblastic growth factors, vascular endothelial growth factor, and platelet-derived growth factor. Major research limitations for these agents are that they do not act independently, and their biologic properties are poorly understood. Potential complications such as aberrant vascular proliferation, tumor development or proliferation, and proatherogenic effects have made patient enrollment difficult. Although there are some trial results suggesting that the ischemic burden shown on perfusion imaging may be reduced, no firm positive outcome data have yet been published.

External Counterpulsation
External counterpulsation is a noninvasive method of increasing coronary blood flow through diastolic augmentation. Large blood pressure cuffs are placed on both legs and thighs and are inflated

to a pressure of 300 mm Hg in early diastole (triggered by the patient's ECG), promoting venous return to the heart. The mechanism is unclear but may be related to enhanced endothelial function, improved myocardial perfusion, and possibly placebo effect. Several small studies have suggested "a clinical reduction in angina episodes, but no positive mortality benefit has yet been published. A meta-analysis that included 13 observational studies and followed 949 patients' angina class using the CCS classification scheme noted at least a one-class improvement in 86%" of the study population. Contraindications to this treatment include certain aortic valvular diseases, aortic aneurysm, and peripheral vascular disease.

Spinal Cord Stimulation
For patients whose angina is refractory to medical therapy and who are not candidates for revascularization, spinal cord stimulation may be considered. Little intermediate or long-term data are available, but many short-term studies suggest reduced angina episodes. Placement of the device and subsequent stimulation at the C7-T1 level suggests that the mechanism of action is reduced pain sensation.

Acupuncture
Acupuncture has been shown to be of benefit for the relief of both acute and chronic pain in various medical conditions. With respect to patients with documented CAD and symptomatic angina, there is insufficient data currently available to recommend this modality. The difficulty in devising a true blinded study may limit randomized data from being effectively obtained in the future.

Other Causes of Angina
Syndrome X
The cardiac syndrome X refers to patients who have normal or near-normal epicardial coronary arteries and episodic chest pain. This disorder is much more common in women and is often seen in patients younger than 50 years of age. The chest pain episodes may last longer than 30 minutes and may have a variable response to sublingual nitrates. Patients with syndrome X often describe typical stress-induced angina. Risk factors include hypertension, diabetes, and hyperlipidemia. Female patients are typically postmenopausal and frequently have stress-induced symptoms and ischemia on stress imaging. They often respond to standard angina medications and typically have a better prognosis than patients with significant epicardial plaque.

Vasospastic or Prinzmetal's Angina
The classic definition of Prinzmetal's angina is chest pain with documented ST-segment elevation during symptoms or during exercise in the face of angiographically normal or near-normal coronary arteries. Over the years, the definition has expanded to include patients who have classic angina symptoms commonly relieved with nitrates or calcium channel blockers and minimal or no CAD. It has been shown that patients with nonobstructive CAD may be prone to focal artery spasm at the stenosis site; therefore, the previous requirement of normal coronary arteries is not an absolute necessity. Other disease states (e.g., Raynaud's phenomenon) can increase a patient's development of coronary artery spasm, as can illicit drug usage (e.g., cocaine). Vasospasm is more common in active smokers. β-Blockers should be used cautiously in these patients because they may exacerbate coronary spasm. Patients with angiographically documented intramyocardial bridging may be prone to focal coronary spasm and subsequent angina pectoris.

Newer Imaging Techniques
Calcium Scoring
Coronary artery calcium scoring is a well-studied imaging modality used to assess a patient's pretest probability of CAD. With respect to evaluation for angina, one must remember that electron-beam computed tomographic (CT) scanning does not offer physiologic data and therefore does not allow determination of myocardial ischemia. This study is most useful in the work-up of a low-risk patient with an atypical chest pain syndrome. If such a

patient has an elevated calcium score, other studies may be reasonable "and further assessment of the patients cholesterol values should be performed."

CT Coronary Angiography

CT coronary angiography is a noninvasive way to image the coronary arteries. Like electron-beam CT, it does not provide physiologic data regarding coronary artery perfusion, but it does provide anatomic information such as the presence and percentage of coronary artery stenosis. Although selected patients with stable or unstable angina may be considered candidates for CT angiography, its main utility is to evaluate patients for chest pain who are otherwise at low risk and have a low pretest probability. Because of the volume of intravenous contrast required by CT angiography, the risk of contrast nephropathy must be considered when contemplating this study.

Summary

The approach to the patient with angina should be based on a global assessment and intensive treatment of all identified cardiovascular risk factors. "It is recommended that all patients receive the appropriate dose of statin and antiplatelet therapy." Noninvasive testing is helpful for an initial diagnosis and to guide the decision for a more invasive approach. Familiarity and adherence to current treatment guidelines is of paramount importance. There are important gender differences that should not be overlooked in the clinical presentation of angina and in the approach to optimal therapy.

References

Anderson JL, Adams CD, Antman EM, et al. ACC/AHA 2007 guidelines for the management of patients with unstable angina/non-ST-elevation myocardial infarction: A report of the American College of Cardiology/American Heart Association Task Force on Practice Guidelines. J Am Coll Cardiol 2007;5067:e1–e157.

Antithrombotic Trialists Collaboration. Collaborative meta-analysis of randomized trials of antiplatelet therapy for prevention of death, myocardial infarction, and stroke in high risk patients. BMJ 2002;324:71–86.

Berger J, Brown D, Becker R, et al. Low-dose aspirin in patients with stable cardiovascular disease: A meta-analysis. Am J Med 2008;121:43–9.

Blood Pressure Lowering Treatment Trialists Collaboration. Effects of different blood pressure lowering regimens on major cardiovascular events: Results of prospectively-designed overviews of randomized trials. Lancet 2003;362:1527–45.

Boden WE, O'Rourke RA, Teo KK, et al. Optimal medical therapy with or without PCI for stable coronary disease. N Engl J Med 2007;35:1503–16.

Cholesterol Treatment Trialists' Collaborators. Efficacy and safety of cholesterol-lowering treatment: Prospective meta-analysis of data from 90056 participants in 14 trials of statins. Lancet 2005;366:1267–78.

ESC GUIDELINES: Task Force Members. Montalescot G, Sechtem U, Achenbach S, et al. Editor's choice: 2013 ESC guidelines on the management of stable coronary artery disease: The Task Force on the management of stable coronary artery disease of the European Society of Cardiology. Eur Heart J 2013;34:2949–3003.

Fihn SD, Gardin JM, Abrams J, et al. 2012 ACCF/AHA/ACP/AATS/PCNA/SCAI/STS guideline for the diagnosis and management of patients with stable ischemic heart disease: A report of the American College of Cardiology Foundation/American Heart Association Task Force on Practice Guidelines, and the American College of Physicians, American Association for Thoracic Surgery, Preventive Cardiovascular Nurses Association, Society for Cardiovascular Angiography and Interventions, and Society of Thoracic Surgeons. J Am Coll Cardiol 2012;60:e44–e164. http://dx.doi.org/10.1016/j.jacc.2012.07.013.

Gibbons RJ, Abrams J, Chatterjee K, et al. ACC/AHA 2007 guideline update for the management of patients with chronic stable angina: A report of the American College of Cardiology/American Heart Association Task Force on Practice Guidelines (Committee to Update the 2002 Guidelines for the Management of Patients with Chronic Stable Angina), Reston, VA: American College of Cardiology, American Heart Association; 2002. Available at: www.acc.org/qualityandscience/clinical/guidelines/stable/stable_clean.pdf (accessed August 20, 2014).

Grundy SM, Cleeman JI, Merz NB, et al. Implications of recent clinical trials for the National Cholesterol Education Program Adult Treatment Panel III guidelines. Circulation 2004;110:227–39.

Heart Outcomes Prevention Evaluation Study Investigators. Effects of an angiotensin-converting-enzyme inhibitor, ramipril, on cardiovascular events in high-risk patients. N Engl J Med 2000;342:145–53.

James PA, Oparil S, Carter BL, et al. 2014 evidence-based guideline for the management of high blood pressure in adults: Report from the panel members appointed to the eighth Joint National Committee (JNC 8). JAMA 2014;311:507–20. http://dx.doi.org/10.1001/jama.2013.284427.

Mehta SR, Cannon CP, Fox KA, et al. Routine vs selective invasive strategies in patients with acute coronary syndromes: A collaborative meta-analysis of randomized trials. JAMA 2005;293:2908–17.

Messerli FH, Mancia G, Conti CR, et al. Dogma disrupted: Can aggressively lowering blood pressure in hypertensive patients with coronary artery disease be dangerous? Ann Intern Med 2006;144:884–93.

Ray K, Cannon C. Optimal goal for statin therapy use in coronary artery disease. Curr Opin Cardiol 2005;20:525–9.

SEARCH Collaborative Group. Intensive lowering of LDL cholesterol with 80 mg versus 20 mg simvastatin daily in 12,064 survivors of myocardial infarction: A double-blind randomised trial. Lancet 2010;376:1658–69.

Stone G, Teirstein P, Rubenstein R, et al. A prospective, multicenter, randomized trial of percutaneous transmyocardial laser revascularization in patients with nonrecanalizable chronic total occlusions. J Am Coll Cardiol 2002;39:1581–7.

Stone NJ, Robinson J, Lichtenstein AH, et al. 2013 ACC/AHA guideline on the treatment of blood cholesterol to reduce atherosclerotic cardiovascular risk in adults: A report of the American College of Cardiology/American Heart Association Task Force on Practice Guidelines. Circulation 2013;.

Weber MA, Schiffrin EL, White WB, et al. Clinical practice guidelines for the management of hypertension in the community. J Clin Hypertens 2014;16:14–26. http://dx.doi.org/10.1111/jch.12237.

Wenger NK. Cardiac Rehabilitation: A Guide to Practice in the 21st Century. New York: Marcel Dekker; 1999.

Whooley MA, Jonge P, Vittinghoff E, et al. Depressive symptoms, health behaviors, and risk of cardiovascular events in patients with coronary heart disease. JAMA 2008;300:2379–88.

AORTIC DISEASE: ANEURYSM AND DISSECTION

Method of
David G. Neschis, MD

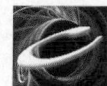

CURRENT DIAGNOSIS

- Because the majority of patients with abdominal aortic aneurysms are asymptomatic, the majority of abdominal aortic aneurysms are detected on imaging studies performed for other indications.
- Patients older than 50 years who present with abdominal or back pain of unclear etiology should be considered for evaluation of possible abdominal aortic aneurysm.
- Asymptomatic men older than 65 years who have ever smoked are eligible for abdominal aortic aneurysm screening.
- All patients older than 60 years who have a strong family history of abdominal aortic aneurysms should be considered for screening.
- Patients presenting with sudden onset of chest or back pain without clear etiology should be evaluated for dissection.
- Dissection can mimic numerous other conditions.

CURRENT THERAPY

Indications for Repair of Aneurysm
- Fusiform abdominal aortic aneurysms greater than 5.5 cm in maximum diameter
- Most saccular aneurysms and pseudoaneurysms
- Thoracic and thoracoabdominal aortic aneurysms of greater than 6 cm in maximal diameter
- Aneurysms that are symptomatic or are rapidly enlarging

Indications for Repair of Aortic Dissection
- Dissections involving the ascending aorta
- Dissections involving only the descending aorta are usually managed medically unless complicated by the following: unrelenting pain, end organ ischemia, or significant aneurysmal degeneration to greater than 6 cm in maximal diameter

Abdominal Aortic Aneurysms
Epidemiology
A ruptured abdominal aortic aneurysm is a devastating event leading to approximately 15,000 deaths per year, and it is the 13th leading cause of death in the United States. It is the 10th leading cause of death in men. Once rupture occurs, there is an 85%

chance of death overall and approximately 50% mortality in the patients who make it to the hospital alive. Clearly, the goal is to identify this life-threatening lesion and repair prior to rupture. Abdominal aortic aneurysms are approximately four times more prevalent in men than in women. The overall incidence in persons older than 60 years is approximately 3% to 4%, with incidence as high as 10% to 12% in an elderly hypertensive population.

Risk Factors

Men are approximately 4 times more likely than women to develop an abdominal aortic aneurysm. Clearly, older persons, particularly those older than 60 years, are higher risk. Tobacco use is probably the strongest preventable risk factor, with tobacco users being approximately eight times more likely to be affected than nonsmokers. Hypertension is present in approximately 40% of patients with abdominal aortic aneurysms. Family history also plays a significant role. In fact, men who have first-degree female relatives who had aneurysms are approximately 18 times more likely than the general population to develop an abdominal aortic aneurysm. There is also a strong correlation between abdominal aortic aneurysms and other peripheral artery aneurysms. Patients with bilateral popliteal artery aneurysms have an approximately 50% to 60% risk of having an abdominal aortic aneurysm.

Pathophysiology

An aneurysm is a dilatation of a blood vessel that could occur in any blood vessel in the body, even in the veins. Most commonly it is defined as a dilatation of approximately 1.5 to 2 times at that diameter of the adjacent normal vessel.

The definition of a pseudoaneurysm is often misunderstood. The attempt to describe a pseudoaneurysm in terms of the number of layers of the artery wall involved does nothing to help resolve this confusion. A pseudoaneurysm is a walled-off defect in the artery wall. A circular shell of adventitial and surrounding connective tissue contains the blood, preventing free hemorrhage. However, there remains continued flow out and back into the artery lumen, resulting in a classic to-and-fro pattern on duplex ultrasound. The most common cause of a pseudoaneurysm is iatrogenic, from needle puncture, but also can be caused by trauma or focal rupture of the artery at the site of an atherosclerotic ulcer.

The etiology of true aneurysms is not clear, although in the past these have been attributed to atherosclerosis. However, it is well known that the majority of patients with abdominal aortic aneurysms do not have associated significant occlusive disease. Biochemical studies have demonstrated decreased quantities of elastin and collagen in the walls of aneurysmal aortas. It is believed that a family of enzymes known as matrix metalloproteinase (MMP), particularly those that have collagenase and elastase activity, are likely involved in development of arterial aneurysms. The propensity for growth and rupture is based on Laplace's law, $T = PR$, where T represents wall tension (or in other words the propensity to rupture), P is the transmitted pressure, and R is the radius. This explains why patients with hypertension and those with larger aneurysms are at higher risk for aortic rupture.

Prevention

Currently the most effective means to prevent aneurysm rupture is early detection and elective repair. Avoidance of smoking and aggressive control of blood pressure would likely be helpful in preventing aneurysmal development and growth. Patients with known abdominal aortic aneurysms that are relatively small and at low risk for rupture are generally serially followed with imaging studies over time. These patients are advised to avoid straining (e.g., heavy lifting), avoid smoking, and keep their blood pressure well controlled.

Investigation is ongoing in efforts to develop a medication that may be helpful in slowing the growth of abdominal aortic aneurysms. It has been known since 1985 that tetracycline antibiotics have activity against MMPs. There had been several animal studies and at least one small human study suggesting that doxycycline (Vibramycin)[1] may be effective at slowing the growth of abdominal aortic aneurysms. Currently, larger human studies are ongoing. At this point, there are no formal recommendations regarding the use of doxycycline for the purpose of slowing aneurysmal growth.

Clinical Manifestations

Approximately 75% of abdominal aortic aneurysms are asymptomatic and discovered incidentally. Unfortunately, physical examination is an unreliable method for detecting aneurysms or determining aneurysm size. In heavier patients it may be simply impossible to adequately palpate the aorta. The majority of aneurysms are incidental findings identified on imaging studies performed for other reasons. Occasionally, an aneurysm is first detected upon operation for another condition.

Unfortunately, when an aneurysm becomes symptomatic, this is usually a sign of impending rupture. Symptoms related to abdominal aortic aneurysms can include abdominal or back pain. The classic triad of findings in the setting of abdominal aortic aneurysm rupture includes abdominal pain, hypotension, and a pulsatile abdominal mass. This triad, however, occurs in only approximately 20% of the patients. Often a high index of suspicion needs to be maintained.

The episode of hypotension associated with aneurysm rupture may be manifested as an episode of syncope or near-syncope before the patient arrives at the hospital. It is quite possible for the patient to have a contained rupture of the abdominal aorta and appear quite stable with a normal blood pressure in the emergency department. Although uncommon, a primary fistula between the aneurysm and gastrointestinal tract can occur and manifest as gastrointestinal bleeding.

Diagnosis

Several imaging modalities are available that can accurately diagnose and measure abdominal aortic aneurysms. Real-time B-mode ultrasound has the advantage of being almost universally available, relatively inexpensive, and essentially risk free. The major disadvantage, however, is that it is technician dependent. Computed tomography (CT) scans can provide a very accurate representation of the aorta in a very short study time (Figures 1 and 2). The use of iodinated contrast is not necessary to obtain a gross size measurement of the aorta. The contrast, however, helps delineate the flow lumen more clearly, and it is quite valuable in planning repair.

---

[1]Not FDA approved for this indication.

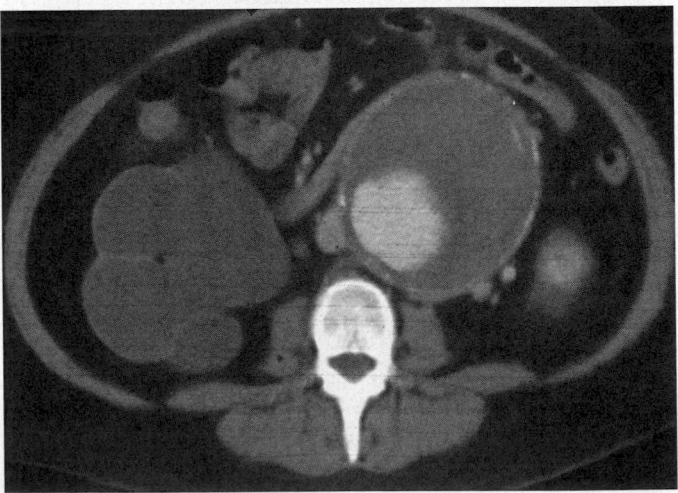

Figure 1. Large abdominal aortic aneurysm. Notice how the majority of this aneurysm is filled with laminated thrombus. The flow lumen is only mildly dilated, and this aneurysm could be missed on angiography alone.

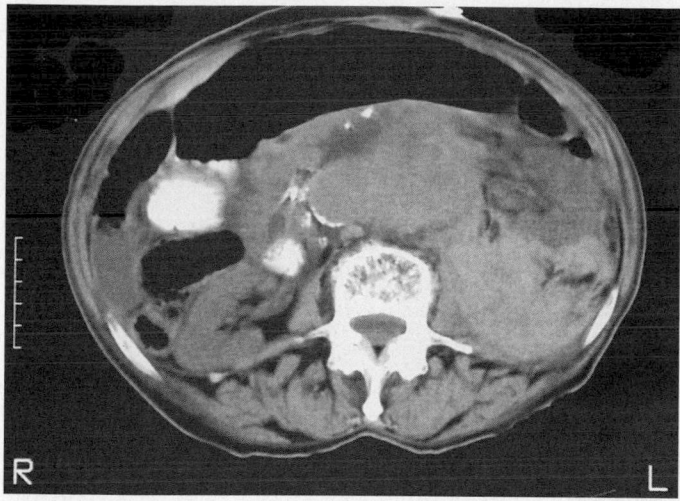

Figure 2. Classic image of a ruptured abdominal aortic aneurysm, which in this case can be seen even without the use of intravascular contrast. Note the lack of symmetry and obliteration of tissue planes in the retroperitoneum on the left.

Disadvantages include the use of ionizing radiation and the use of iodinated contrast material. MRI is also accurate in determining the size of the aneurysm; however, study times are longer, equipment is less widely available, and the expense is considerable. Angiography, while excellent for evaluating the status of important aortic branches and for evaluating occlusive disease, is not an accurate study for the purpose of determining maximal diameter of the aneurysm. Often aneurysms are filled with laminated thrombus, and the flow lumen, which was seen on aortography, is not representative of the true aneurysm size.

Treatment

The decision on when to intervene in an abdominal aortic aneurysm is based on a careful analysis of the patient's risk for rupture versus the risk of operative repair. Historically, open repair can be performed with less than 5% in-hospital mortality. Based on historical studies it was estimated that the risk of rupture for an approximately 5-cm aneurysm was about 1% per year, which increased dramatically to 6.6% for aneurysms between 6 cm and 7 cm. It has been fairly well established for years that aneurysms larger than 5.5 cm are generally recommended for repair and those less than 4 cm are generally observed over time. There remains a gray area for moderate aneurysms in the 4 to 5.5 cm category.

Two large prospective randomized trials were developed to answer this question. These include the United Kingdom Small Aneurysm Trial and the Department of Veterans Affairs Aneurysm Detection and Management (ADAM) trial. Both these studies randomized patients with moderately sized aneurysms to observation versus open repair. Results of both trials were fairly similar. The rupture rate for aneurysms under observation was 0.5% to 1% per year, and neither trial showed a difference in long-term survival. Both studies concluded that it was relatively safe to observe patients with aneurysms less than 5.5 cm in diameter, particularly in men who would be compliant with the follow-up regimen. The diameter of the aneurysm, however, should not be the only data point used for a decision on whether to repair.

Women seem to have a higher rupture rate for a particular aneurysm diameter than men, perhaps because they are starting with smaller aortas to begin with. Patients with COPD may be at higher risk for rupture as well. Saccular or eccentric-shaped aneurysms may also have a higher propensity to rupture and should not be subject to diameter recommendations for fusiform aneurysms (Figures 3 and 4). Additionally, rapidly growing aneurysms—growing at a rate faster than approximately 0.5 cm per year—should be considered for repair.

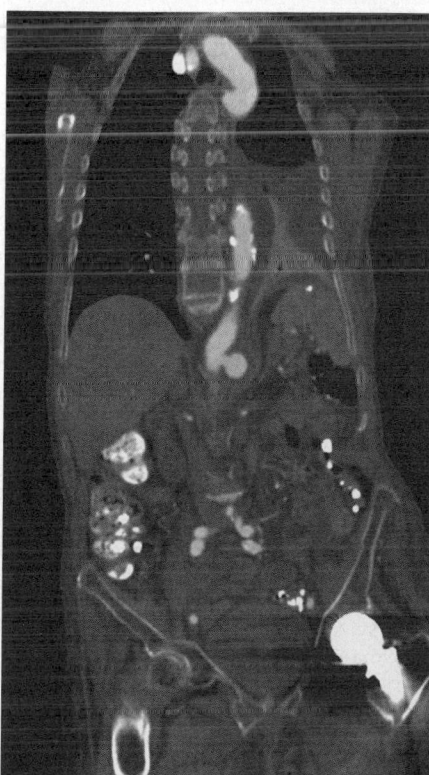
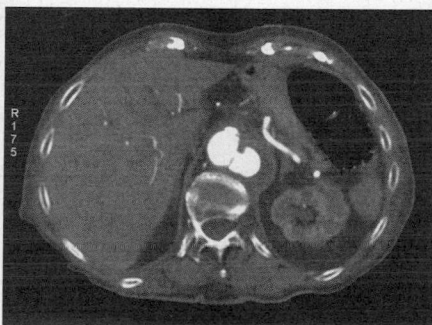
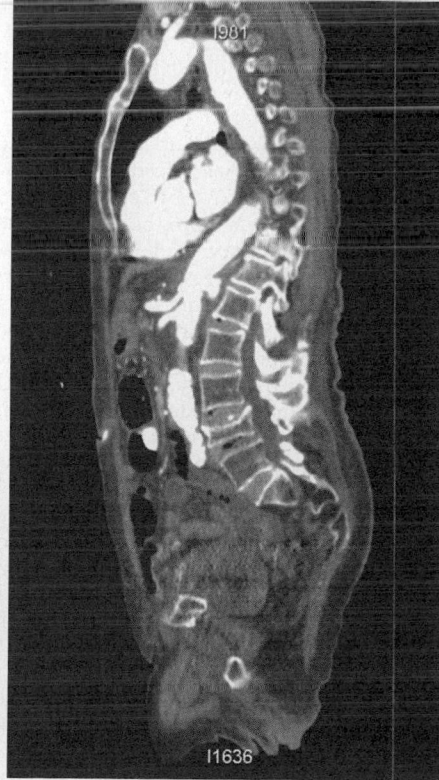

Figure 3. Axial CT slice and reconstructed images of a saccular abdominal aortic aneurysm. This lesion could also be described as a pseudoaneurysm. For these, treatment is recommended because it is thought that the risk of rupture is higher than for a similarly sized fusiform abdominal aortic aneurysm.

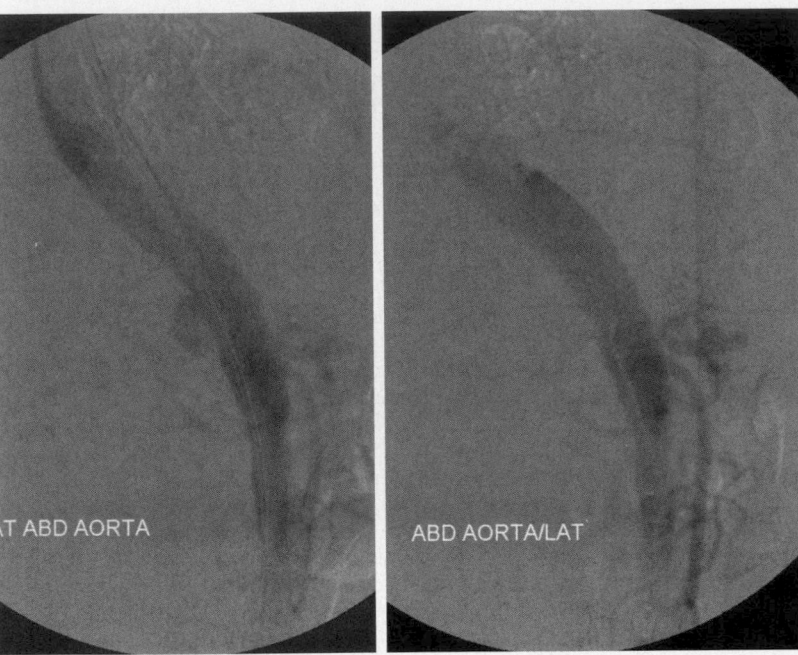

Figure 4. Angiogram of patient in Figure 3, demonstrating aneurysm before and after deployment of an endograft, which successfully excluded the lesion from the circulation.

Once it has been determined that repair is indicated, a number of options are available. Traditional open repair involves a relatively large abdominal incision, cross clamping of the aorta, and replacement of the aneurysmal segment with a graft of polyethylene terephthalate (Dacron) or polytetrafluoroethylene (PTFE; Teflon). Often the iliac arteries are involved, and in these cases a bifurcated graft is placed. Open repair is quite durable and very effective at preventing aneurysm-related deaths. Long-term complications are rare, and patients following open repair generally enjoy 95% freedom from issues related to the repair over the course of their lifetime. Disadvantages, however, include the large incision and an approximate 1-week hospital stay. Recovery to a relatively normal level of function occasionally takes months. In the past, many patients were deemed too old or frail to be expected to undergo open surgery.

Endograft repair has revolutionized the practice of vascular surgery. Using small incisions placed at the groin and performing the procedure under fluoroscopy guidance, devices can now be advanced into the aorta from the femoral artery. Using angiography as a guide, the graft typically is deployed below the renal arteries and effectively excludes the aneurysm from the circulation. Advantages include small incisions and very short hospital stays. Patients are typically discharged on the first or second day following aneurysm repair. Recovery to normal activity is also quite rapid, taking approximately 1 to 2 weeks. Use of this modality has allowed treatment of older and frailer patients who previously denied treatment due to concerns of operative risk.

Endograft repair, however, is clearly not without its disadvantages. Currently, the durability of endograft repair is unknown, and these patients are subject to frequent serial imaging. Also, there is a higher incidence of graft-related complications, which can occur in up to 35% of patients. These include the development of leaks of blood into the aneurysm sac outside the graft device, issues related to graft failure and migration, and graft limb thrombosis. These grafts are also quite expensive.

Two major prospective randomized trials studying traditional open versus endograft repair are often cited. These include the United Kingdom–based EVAR-1 trial (first Endovascular Aneurysm Repair trail) and the Dutch-based DREAM trial (Diabetes REduction Assessment with ramipril and rosiglitazone Medication trial). Both these studies randomized patients who were believed to be good risks for open repair to endograft versus

traditional open repair. The results of both of these studies were relatively similar in that both studies demonstrated a clear early survival benefit for patients in the endograft group. However, this came at a cost of an increased incidence of graft-related complications in the endograft group and a higher cost for the endograft group. Additionally, at 2 to 4 years, there was no clear difference in long-term survival in either group.

Ultimately, the decision on whether to proceed with open or endograft repair is a decision between surgeon and patient based on the patient's aortic anatomy, overall health, and the patient's and physician's preference. It would appear, however, that older and frail patients with good anatomy should be strongly considered for endograft repair.

Monitoring

Patients with abdominal aortic aneurysms should be evaluated for the presence of femoral and popliteal aneurysms (particularly in men) and for thoracic aortic aneurysms. Following open repair, a follow-up CT scan with contrast should be considered approximately 5 years out to evaluate for the integrity of the graft (i.e., pseudoaneurysms) as well as development of new aneurysms. Patients who have undergone endograft repair require more-intensive monitoring. Typical regimens include a contrast-enhanced CT scan approximately 2 weeks following repair, then 6 months after repair, and then based on the perceived stability of the graft, approximately yearly thereafter. Some centers have used duplex ultrasonography for evaluating patients following endograft repair in efforts to reduce the amount of ionizing radiation the patients receive. However, it should be remembered that duplex ultrasound is highly technician dependent, and follow-up of patients with endograft repairs using only duplex ultrasound should be performed in experienced centers.

Thoracic Aortic Aneurysms

Thoracic aortic aneurysms are limited to the chest cavity. Although they are less common than infrarenal abdominal aortic aneurysms, they share similar risk factors. The male-to-female ratio incidence of the TAA is approximately 1:1.

In the past, the threshold for repair was at a diameter greater than 6 cm. This threshold was chosen due to the higher operative risks associated with repair of the thoracic aorta. Now with the availability of endograft, patients with good anatomy are generally recommended for repair at a diameter similar to those for the infrarenal aorta.

Open repair involves performing a thoracotomy and cross clamping the aorta. Repair in this location is often performed with the addition of extracorporeal bypass to maintain perfusion to the viscera and spinal cord drain performance of the repair. Although the risk of paraplegia in the treatment of infrarenal aortic is exceedingly low, the risk of paraplegia from a repair of an isolated thoracic aortic aneurysm is approximately 6%. Endograft devices for repair of thoracic aortic aneurysm are now widely available and have reduced the incidence of paraplegia to approximately 3%.

Thoracoabdominal Aortic Aneurysms

By definition, thoracoabdominal aortic aneurysms require entrance to both the thoracic and abdominal cavity to perform repair. These lesions are usually true aneurysms of the aorta and should not be confused with dissection. Repair of thoracoabdominal aortic aneurysms is quite complex and carry risks of death and paraplegia as high as 20% in some settings. These procedures are generally performed at larger institutions with considerable experience with this condition. Unfortunately, endograft devices for the repair of thoracoabdominal aortic aneurysms are limited to a handful of centers in the United States.

Thoracic Aortic Dissection

Thoracic aortic dissection is the most common aortic emergency, even more common than ruptured abdominal aortic aneurysm. This potentially fatal condition is rare in patients younger than 50 years and is approximately two times more common in men than women. Patients at risk include patients with a history of connective tissue disorders and patients with severe, poorly controlled hypertension.

An aortic dissection occurs when there is loss of integrity of the intima and blood dissects into the media. Once in the media, there is a natural plane through which dissection is quite easy.

Although there are various classification systems for aortic dissection, the Stanford classification is perhaps the most widely used and the most useful. In this classification, any dissection that involves the ascending aorta, whether it involves the ascending aorta alone or both the ascending and descending thoracoabdominal aorta, are classified as type A. Dissections that do not involve the ascending aorta are classified as type B. This classification is useful because type A dissections require urgent surgery. Type B dissections are typically managed medically unless they are associated with complications such as unremitting pain, aneurysmal expansion, and end-organ ischemia. By convention, aortic dissections that are evaluated within 14 days after the onset of symptoms are considered acute, and those evaluated beyond 14 days are considered chronic.

Helical CAT scanners with the use of contrast are excellent at defining the location and extent of aortic dissection. However, being alert to the potential for this diagnosis requires a high index of suspicion. Aortic dissection can mimic a variety of common conditions based on the extent of the dissection and the aortic branches involved (Table 1). Uncomplicated type B dissections are typically managed medically. This is usually performed in an intensive care setting with the use of intravenous medications to control contractility and, if necessary, hypertension.

In the past, due to the friability of dissected aortic tissue, the results of operative repair for type B dissections have been particularly poor. Currently, endograft repair with the purpose of excluding the entry point of dissection and reestablishing flow to the true lumen is gaining popularity in the treatment of complex dissection. This at times may be supplemented by stenting of affected aortic side branches and fenestration to establish a connection between the true and false lumen in order to restore perfusion to certain organs. Once the acute phase has passed and medically treated patients are under good hypertensive control, these patients are then converted to an oral medication regimen and transferred out of the intensive care setting. Patients need to be followed with serial CT imaging following discharge to evaluate for aneurysmal degeneration of the false lumen. This evaluation should occur every 6 months until the patient is stable, and then yearly thereafter.

TABLE 1	Dissection: The Great Mimick
TERRITORY INVOLVED OR AFFECTED BY DISSECTION	**MIMICS**
Rupture into pericardial sac	Cardiac tamponade
Dissection through aortic valve	Acute aortic insufficiency
Dissection occluding coronary arteries	Myocardial infarction
Involvement of cerebral vessels	Stroke
Involvement of subclavians arteries	Upper extremity ischemia (cold arm)
Dissection running down descending thoracic aorta	Severe back pain and paralysis
Mesenteric artery obstruction	Mesenteric ischemia
Renal artery obstruction	Oliguria and acute renal failure
Iliac artery occlusion	Lower extremity ischemia (cold leg)

In cases where the total aortic diameter grows to greater than 6 cm, repair for the purpose of preventing rupture is indicated, although this is often technically more complicated than treating a fusiform aneurysm in the absence of a previous dissection. Patients should strictly adhere to their blood pressure medication regimen for life.

References

Blankensteijn JD, de Jong SE, Prinssen M, et al. Two-year outcomes after conventional or endovascular repair of abdominal aortic aneurysms. N Engl J Med 2005;352(23):2398–405.

Crawford ES, Crawford JL, Safi HJ, et al. Thoracoabdominal aortic aneurysms: Preoperative and intraoperative factors determining immediate and long-term results of operations in 605 patients. J Vasc Surg 1986;3(3):389–404.

Daily PO, Trueblood HW, Stinson EB, et al. Management of acute aortic dissections. Ann Thorac Surg 1970;10(3):237–47.

EVAR Trial Participants. Endovascular aneurysm repair versus open repair in patients with abdominal aortic aneurysm (EVAR trial 1): Randomised controlled trial. Lancet 2005;365(9478):2179–86.

EVAR Trial Participants. Endovascular aneurysm repair and outcome in patients unfit for open repair of abdominal aortic aneurysm (EVAR trial 2): Randomised controlled trial. Lancet 2005;365(9478):2187–92.

Lederle FA, Wilson SE, Johnson GR, et al. Immediate repair compared with surveillance of small abdominal aortic aneurysms. N Engl J Med 2002;346(19):1437–44.

Lee ES, Pickett E, Hedayati N, et al. Implementation of an aortic screening program in clinical practice: Implications for the Screen For Abdominal Aortic Aneurysms Very Efficiently (SAAAVE) Act. J Vasc Surg 2009;49(5):1107–11.

Nevitt MP, Ballard DJ, Hallett Jr JW. Prognosis of abdominal aortic aneurysms. A population-based study. N Engl J Med 1989;321(15):1009–14.

Nienaber CA, Rousseau H, Eggebrecht H, et al. Randomized comparison of strategies for type B aortic dissection: The INvestigation of STEnt Grafts in Aortic Dissection (INSTEAD) trial. Circulation 2009;120(25):2519–28.

Rentschler M, Baxter BT. Pharmacological approaches to prevent abdominal aortic aneurysm enlargement and rupture. Ann N Y Acad Sci 2006;1085:39–46.

ATRIAL FIBRILLATION

Method of
Rahul Wadke, MD

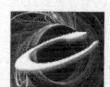

CURRENT DIAGNOSIS

- Detailed history and physical examination are important.
- Symptoms fall on a broad spectrum from asymptomatic to palpitations, chest discomfort, shortness of breath, and decreased exercise tolerance.
- Signs include irregular pulse, irregular jugular venous pulsations, variations in the intensity of the first heart sound, and loss of S4 heard in sinus rhythm.

- Investigation includes 12-lead electrocardiogram (ECG) for confirmation, transthoracic echocardiogram for valvular abnormalities, and blood tests for thyroid, renal, and hepatic function.
- Additional evaluations include Holter monitoring, event recording, electrophysiological studies, and chest radiograph.

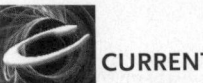 CURRENT THERAPY

Heart Rate Control
- β-Blockers: metoprolol (Lopressor, Toprol XL),[1] propranolol (Inderal)
- Non-dihydropyridine calcium channel blockers: diltiazem (Cardizem), Verapamil (Calan)
- Digoxin (Lanoxin)
- Amiodarone (Cordarone)[1]

Rhythm Control
- Antiarrhythmic drugs: amiodarone,[1] flecainide (Tambocor), propafenone (Rythmol), sotalol (Betapace)
- Pharmacologic and electric cardioversion
- Ablation
- Suppression of AF through pacing

Thromboembolism Prevention
- Aspirin 81 to 325 mg
- Warfarin (Coumadin)
- Dabigatran (Pradaxa)

[1]Not FDA approved for this indication.

Epidemiology

Atrial fibrillation (AF) is the most common arrhythmia in clinical practice. Current prevalence of 1% to 2% of populations is estimated to at least double in next 50 years. It is a very costly public health problem, with $3600 spent annually per patient in the European Union. The prevalence of AF increases with age, from less than 0.5% at age 40 to 50 years up to 8% to 10% in those older than 80 years. The lifetime risk of developing AF in 40-year-olds is about 25%. Men are more often affected than women, with the exception of women 75 years or older. The prevalence and incidence in the nonwhite population is less well studied.

Pathophysiology

Atrial Factors

Any kind of structural heart disease can trigger remodeling of both atria and ventricles. Structural remodeling facilitates initiation and perpetuation of AF. Atrial refractoriness shortens within the first days of new-onset AF. Even in patients with a single episode of AF, fibrosis and inflammatory changes have been documented.

Electrophysiologic Mechanisms

Focal mechanisms of triggered activity and re-entry have attracted much attention. The wavelet hypothesis suggests several independent wavelets propagating AF rather than a single focus. A familial component should be investigated with early-onset AF.

AF reduces left atrial flow velocities, which causes delayed emptying from the atrial appendage and is implicated in thrombus formation.

Causes and Risk Factors

Reversible Causes

AF can be related to temporary causes including alcohol use (holiday heart syndrome), surgery, myocardial infarction, pericarditis, pulmonary embolism, electrocution, hyperthyroidism, and other metabolic syndromes. AF remains a common early postoperative complication of cardiothoracic surgery. Successful treatment of

TABLE 1	Types of Atrial Fibrillation	
TYPE	**DEFINITION**	**DESCRIPTION**
1	First diagnosed AF	First-time diagnosis of AF irrespective of duration of arrhythmia, presence of symptoms, or severity of symptoms
2	Paroxysmal AF	Usually self-terminating within 48 hours After 48 hours, likelihood of spontaneous conversion is low and anticoagulation should be considered
3	Persistent AF	AF episode lasting longer than 7 days or requiring cardioversion (chemical or direct current)
4	Long-standing persistent AF	AF lasting longer than 1 year.
5	Permanent AF	Presence of AF is accepted by patient and physician Rhythm control usually is not pursued in patients with permanent AF
6	Silent AF	Patient presents with AF-related complications (thromboembolic stroke, cardiomyopathy) or incidental finding on ECG in an asymptomatic patient

Abbreviations: AF = atrial fibrillation; ECG = electrocardiogram.

underlying medical problems often causes termination of AF (Table 1).

Obesity is an important risk factor for development of AF. Studies suggest a possible physiologic basis. Increasing left atrial size correlates with increase in weight and regression.

In young adults, 30% to 45% of cases of paroxysmal AF have no demonstrable underlying heart disease.

Cardiovascular conditions associated with AF include mitral valve disease, heart failure, coronary artery disease, and hypertension associated with left ventricular hypertrophy. Other associations include hypertrophic obstructive cardiomyopathy, dilated cardiomyopathy, atrial septal defect, restrictive cardiomyopathies, cardiac tumors, and constrictive pericarditis. AF is commonly found in patients with obstructive sleep apnea.

Clinical Manifestations

Patients might or might not have symptoms with AF. Commonly associated symptoms include palpitations, shortness of breath, fatigue, decreasing exercise tolerance, and chest discomfort. Intermittent episodes of AF can progress in duration and frequency, and over time many patients develop sustained AF.

An irregular pulse should raise the suspicion for AF. Patients might present initially with transient ischemic attack or ischemic stroke. Most patients experience asymptomatic episodes of arrhythmias before the AF is diagnosed. Patients with mitral valve disease and heart failure often have higher incidence of AF. For a patient with newly diagnosed AF, reversible causes such as pulmonary embolism, hyperthyroidism, pericarditis, and myocardial infarction should be investigated.

Diagnosis

An irregular pulse can raise the suspicion for AF, but ECG remains essential in diagnosing AF. AF is defined with the following characteristics:
- Arrhythmia absoluta: Absolutely irregular RR intervals
- No distinct P waves on ECG. Regular atrial activity is occasionally noted on lead V1.
- Atrial cycle length (interval between two atrial activations) is usually variable and less than 200 msec (>300 beats/min).

Numerous options are available to capture AF rhythm depending on the frequency of symptoms. A 12-lead ECG is recommended as a first step (Figure 1). Noncontinuous ECG methods include

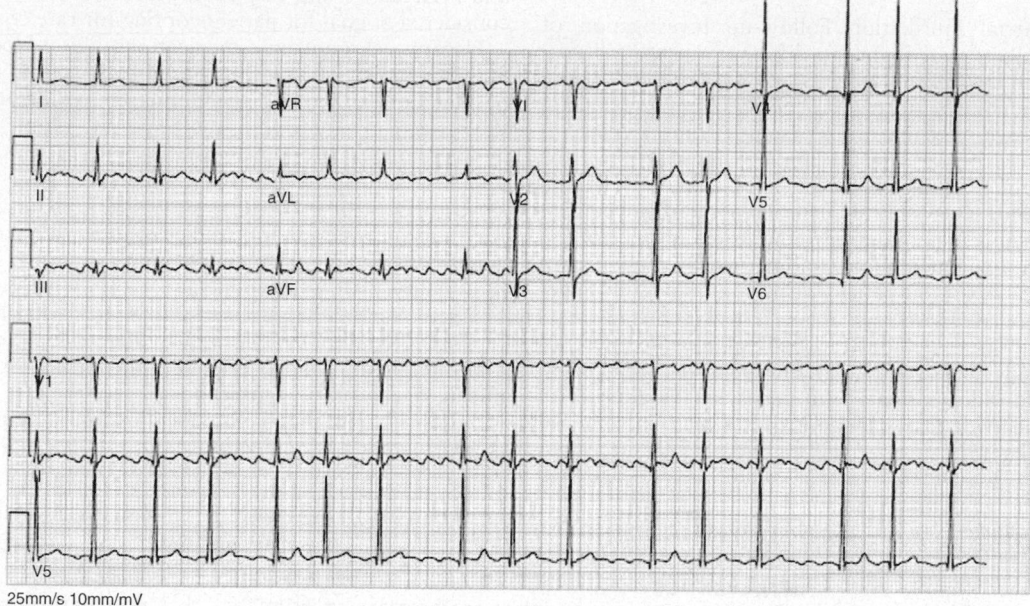

25mm/s 10mm/mV

Figure 1. Atrial fibrillation 12-lead electrocardiogram.

scheduled or symptom-activated ECGs, Holter monitoring (24 hours to 7 days), and an external loop recorder. An implantable loop recorder can be used to monitor over a 2-year period.

Differential Diagnosis

Arrhythmias that can mimic AF include atrial tachycardia, atrial flutter with variable atrioventricular (AV) block, frequent atrial ectopies, and antegrade AV node conduction. Any episode of suspected AF should be recorded by a 12-lead ECG. An ECG recording will help in differentiating AF from rare supraventricular arrhythmias with irregular RR intervals.

Occasionally, use of AV node blocking using the Valsalva maneuver, carotid massage, or intravenous adenosine (Adenocard)[1] may be necessary to establish the diagnosis.

Treatment

Management of patients with AF is aimed at reducing symptoms by rate control or correction of rhythm disturbances and prevention of thromboembolism. Rate control strategy attempts control of ventricular rate without restoration or maintenance of sinus rhythm. Rhythm control strategy attempts restoration and maintenance of sinus rhythm with attention to rate control. Regardless of the strategy chosen, the need for anticoagulation depends upon stroke risk and not on type of rhythm.

Risk Stratification for Stroke and Thromboembolism

The risk factor–based approach for patients with nonvalvular AF is CHA2DS2-VASc (Table 2). This new risk-stratification scheme builds on the original CHADS2 scheme by considering additional risk factors. Major risk factors are prior stroke or TIA or thromboembolism, and older age (≥75 years). Clinically relevant nonmajor risk factors include heart failure, moderate to severe systolic LV dysfunction (LV ejection fraction less than 40%), hypertension, diabetes, female sex, age 65 to 74 years, and vascular disease (myocardial infarction, peripheral artery disease, complex aortic plaque).

There is a clear relationship between the CHA2DS2-VASc score and stroke rate. In patients with a CHA2DS2-VASc score of 2 or more, chronic anticoagulation therapy is recommended unless contraindicated. When using warfarin, the goal international normalized ratio (INR) is in the range of 2.0 to 3.0 (Table 3). An assessment of bleeding risk should be part of the patient

[1]Not FDA approved for this indication.

TABLE 2	CHA2DS2VASc Score	
RISK FACTOR		**SCORE**
Congestive heart failure, LV dysfunction		1
Hypertension		1
Age ≥75 years		2
Diabetes mellitus		1
Stroke, TIA, or thromboembolism		2
Vascular disease (MI, PAD, complex aortic plaque)		1
Age 65–74 years		1
Sex category: female		1
Maximum score		9

Abbreviations: LV = left ventricular; MI = myocardial infarction; PAD = peripheral artery disease; TIA = transient ischemic attack.

TABLE 3	Approach to Thromboprophylaxis
CHA2DS2-VASc SCORE	**RECOMMENDED THERAPY**
2 or more	Anticoagulation
1	Anticoagulation or aspirin 75–325 mg daily
0	Aspirin 75–325 mg daily or no antithrombotic therapy

assessment before starting anticoagulation. It is reasonable to use HAS-BLED (hypertension, abnormal kidney or liver function, stroke, bleeding history or predisposition, labile INR, elderly [more than 65 years old], drugs or alcohol use) to assess the bleeding risk in atrial fibrillation patients. The risk of falls is usually overstated. The patient needs to fall approximately 300 times per year for the risk of intracranial hemorrhage to outweigh the benefits of anticoagulation in the stroke prevention.

Dabigatran has been approved by the FDA for nonvalvular AF. Dabigatran is a prodrug that is rapidly converted to an active direct thrombin inhibitor independent of cytochrome P-450.

Rate Control

The AFFIRM (Atrial Fibrillation Follow-up Investigation of Rhythm Management) trial found no difference in mortality or stroke rate between the patients assigned to either rhythm control or ventricular rate control strategies. The RACE (Rate Control versus Electrical Cardioversion for Persistent Atrial Fibrillation) trial found rate control was not inferior to rhythm control for prevention of death.

The RACE II study shows that lenient ventricular rate control less than 110 beats/min is not inferior to the strict rate control less than 80 beats/min. Lenient rate control is generally more convenient and requires fewer outpatient visits and generally fewer medications.

None of the major trials demonstrated any significant difference in the quality of life with ventricular rate control compared to rhythm control. In older patients with persistent AF along with hypertension or heart disease, rate control is a reasonable initial therapy. Ventricular rates between 60 and 80 beats/min at rest and between 90 and 115 beats/min during moderate exercise is considered at goal for patients opting for rate control.

Negative chronotropic medications like β-blockers, amiodarone,1 digitalis glycosides, or non-dihydropyridine calcium channel antagonists prolong the refractory period of the AV node, thus effectively controlling the heart rate (Table 4). Bradycardia and heart blocks are some of the side effects of these medications.

Rhythm Control

Rhythm control in certain studies resulted in better exercise tolerance than rate control but did not show any improvement in the quality of life. In younger patients with paroxysmal atrial fibrillation, ablation is considered a better approach. For patients remaining symptomatic despite an adequately controlled ventricular rate, rhythm control is an appropriate next step. Antiarrhythmic agents (Table 5) significantly reduce the rate of recurrence of atrial fibrillation; the likelihood of maintaining the sinus rhythm is approximately doubled with the use of antiarrhythmic drugs.

TABLE 4 Medications for Rate Control

DRUG	INTRAVENOUS ADMINISTRATION	ORAL MAINTENANCE DOSE	MAJOR SIDE EFFECTS
β-Blockers			
Metoprolol CR/XL (Toprol XL)[1]	2.5–5 mg IV bolus; up to 3 doses	100–200 mg daily	Bradycardia, hypotension, heart blocks, asthma, heart failure
Bisoprolol (Zebeta)1	N/A	2.5–10 mg daily	
Atenolol (Tenormin)[1]	N/A	25–100 mg daily	
Esmolol (Brevibloc)	50–200 µg/kg/min IV	N/A	
Propranolol (Inderal)	1–3 mg IV	10–40 mg tid	
Carvedilol (Coreg)[1]	N/A	3.125–25 mg bid	
Non-Dihydropyridine Calcium Channel Antagonists			
Verapamil (Calan)	5–10 mg bolus	40 mg bid to 360 mg max daily	Hypotension, heart blocks, heart failure
Diltiazem (Cardizem)	0.25–0.35 mg/kg	60 mg tid to 360 mg XL daily	
Digitalis Glycosides			
Digoxin (Lanoxin)	0.5–1 mg	0.125–0.5 mg daily	Digitalis toxicity, bradycardia, heart blocks
Others			
Amiodarone (Cordarone)[1]	5 mg/kg loading, 50 mg/h IV	100–200 mg daily	Hypotension, heart blocks, bradycardia
Dronedarone (Multaq)	N/A	400 mg bid	

Abbreviation: N/A = not applicable.
[1]Not FDA approved for this indication.

TABLE 5 Medications for Rhythm Control

DRUG	INTRAVENOUS ADMINISTRATION	ORAL MAINTENANCE DOSE	MAJOR SIDE EFFECTS
Flecainide (Tambocor)	1.5–3.0 mg/kg[2]	50–150 mg bid	Hypotension, atrial flutter with high ventricular rate
Flecainide XL[2]	N/A	200 mg daily	
Propafenone (Rythmol)	1.5–2.0 mg/kg[2]	150–300 mg tid	Hypotension, atrial flutter with high ventricular rate
Propafenone SR (Rythmol SR)	N/A	225–425 mg bid	
Sotalol (Betapace)	N/A	80–160 mg bid	Bradycardia, hypotension
Amiodarone (Cordarone)[1]	5 mg/kg loading, then 50 mg/h	100–200 mg daily	Hypotension, bradycardia, QT prolongation, torsades de pointes
Dronedarone (Multaq)	N/A	400 mg bid	

[1]Not FDA approved for this indication.
[2]Not available in the United States.

If one antiarrhythmic drug fails, it is acceptable to try another. QT prolongation and drug-induced torsades de pointes are some of the significant side effects of these medications. Amiodarone,[1] flecainide (Tambocor), propafenone (Rythmol), and sotalol (Betapace) are often used in Western countries.

Cardioversion

Cardioversion may be considered emergently or electively to restore the sinus rhythm in patients with atrial fibrillation. Anticoagulation is considered mandatory before elective cardioversion for atrial fibrillation of more than 48 hours or atrial fibrillation of unknown duration because of the increased risk of thromboembolism following cardioversion. The current data suggest patients need to be anticoagulated for at least 3 weeks before cardioversion. Immediate cardioversion should be performed in hemodynamically unstable patients, and patients should be anticoagulated before cardioversion. Transesophageal echo-guided cardioversion strategy may be applied as an alternative to precardioversion anticoagulation. Cardioversion can be performed with the help of drugs or electrical shocks. Dofetilide (Tikosyn) or flecainide (Tambocor) are usually tried before a direct current cardioversion. Pharmacologic cardioversion is usually most effective within 7 days after the onset of an episode of atrial fibrillation.

Ablation

Patients who are symptomatic or who have tachycardia-mediated cardiomyopathy that is related to the rapid ventricular rate and that cannot be controlled adequately with pharmacologic agents are most likely to benefit from AV node ablation in conjunction with permanent pacemaker implantation. Postablation anticoagulation should be continued for a minimum of 3 months and thereafter depending upon the individual stroke risk.

Prevention

Measures for primary prevention of AF have not been widely studied. Losartan (Cozaar)[1] (LIFE trial) and candesartan (Atacand)[1] (CHARM trial) reduced incidence of AF in hypertensive patients with LV hypertrophy and symptomatic heart failure, respectively. These results suggest a role for an angiotensin-converting enzyme inhibitor or angiotensin-receptor blocker in primary prevention of AF associated with hypertension, myocardial infarction, heart failure, or diabetes. Statins might protect against AF, but this has been inadequately explored. Dietary interventions, pharmacologic interventions, and pacing have insufficient data supporting their utility in preventing AF.

Special Considerations
Elderly Patients

Elderly patients usually have multiple medical problems including cardiovascular comorbidities such as a higher incidence and prevalence rate of AF, higher thromboembolic risk, and higher bleeding risk. The prevalence of AF is as high as 18% in those older than 85 years. The Screening for Atrial Fibrillation in the Elderly (SAFE) trial found that ECG for irregular pulse is an effective screening tool. All patients older than 75 years who have AF should be considered for anticoagulation. In elderly patients, sinus rhythm is often difficult to maintain. For rate control, β-blockers and non-dihydropyridine calcium channel antagonists can be considered.

Postoperative Atrial Fibrillation

Atrial fibrillation is the most common complication after coronary artery bypass graft (CABG) surgery (30%), valvular surgery (40%), and combined CABG and valvular surgery (50%). The peak incidence of AF is during postoperative days 2 and 4. β-Blocker therapy is most effective in preventing postoperative atrial fibrillation. Prophylactic amiodarone[1] decreases the incidence of postoperative AF and significantly shortens the duration

of hospital stay. Hypomagnesaemia is an independent risk factor for postoperative AF. The use of statins is associated with lower risk of postoperative AF. The majority of the postoperative hemodynamically stable patients convert spontaneously to sinus rhythm within 24 hours of initial management, which includes correction of predisposing factors such as pain management, correcting electrolytes and metabolic abnormalities, addressing hypoxia, addressing anemia, and hemodynamic optimization.

References

Camm AJ, Kirchhof P, Lip GYH, et al. Guidelines for the management of atrial fibrillation. The Task Force for the Management of Atrial Fibrillation of the European Society of Cardiology (ESC). Eur Heart J 2010;31:2369–429.

Hagens VE, Crijins HJ, Veldhuisen DJ, et al. Rate control versus rhythm control for patients with persistent atrial fibrillation with mild to moderate heart failure: Results from the Rate Control versus Electrical cardioversion (RACE) study. Am Heart J 2005;149:1106–11.

Lip GYH, Nieuwlaat R, Pisters R, et al. Refining clinical risk stratification for predicting stroke and thromboembolism in atrial fibrillation using a novel risk factor–based approach: The Euro heart survey on atrial fibrillation. Chest 2010;137(2):263–72.

Olshansky B, Rosenfeld LE, Warner AL, et al. The Atrial Fibrillation Follow-up Investigation of Rhythm Management (AFFIRM) study: Approaches to control rate in atrial fibrillation. J Am Coll Cardiol 2004;43:1201–8.

Van Gelder IC, Groenveld HF, et al. Lenient versus strict rate control in patients with atrial fibrillation. N Engl J Med 2010;362:1363–73.

Wann LS, Curtis A, January CT, et al. 2011 ACCF/AHA/HRS focused update on the management of patients with atrial fibrillation (update on dabigatran): American College of Cardiology Foundation/American Heart Association Task Force on Practice Guidelines. J Am Coll Cardiol 2011;57:223–42.

CARDIAC ARREST: SUDDEN CARDIAC DEATH

Method of
Roy M. John, MD, PhD

Cardiac arrest, or sudden cardiac death, accounts for 60% of deaths from cardiac disease. It may be the initial manifestation or a complication of preexisting heart disease. Most cases are the result of potentially correctable arrhythmias, but the rate of successful resuscitation from an out-of-hospital cardiac arrest to neurologically intact survival remains dismally low. Recognition of patients who are at high risk for sudden cardiac arrhythmic death is critical for prevention. The ability to recognize those at risk for sudden death has increased appreciably, such that prophylactic measures can be implemented in a number of cardiac conditions to minimize risk.

Whereas specific antiarrhythmic drugs have proved disappointing in the prevention of sudden death, drugs that block the effects of β-adrenergic stimulation, angiotensin, and aldosterone have consistently led to reduced mortality among patients with cardiac disease and left ventricular (LV) dysfunction, partly through their salutary effects on sudden death. The implantable cardioverter-defibrillator (ICD) has emerged as a dominant therapeutic strategy based on clinical trials of its efficacy. This review addresses the clinical conditions associated with a high risk for sudden death and the current therapeutic options.

Definition and Causes

Sudden cardiac death is defined as abrupt, unexpected natural death occurring within a short time period (generally <1 hour) after onset of acute symptoms. Primary cardiac arrhythmia is responsible for most of the cases, but acute severe myocardial dysfunction, intracardiac obstruction, and acute aortic dissection are other important causes (Table 1). Structural abnormalities of the myocardium resulting from hypertrophy, scarring, and fibrosis serve as substrates for malignant arrhythmias. The majority of patients who die suddenly have atherosclerotic coronary artery disease (CAD). However, only about 20% of those who survive a cardiac arrest demonstrate evidence of an acute myocardial infarction. Instead, a large number have evidence of prior myocardial infarction and LV dysfunction. It is now recognized that

---

[1]Not FDA approved for this indication.

TABLE 1	Causes of Sudden Cardiac Death

Coronary artery disease
  Atherosclerotic disease
  Congenital anomalies
  Spasm
  Arteritis
  Dissection
  Embolism
Primary cardiomyopathies
  Nonischemic dilated cardiomyopathy
  Hypertrophic cardiomyopathy
Myocarditis
Valvular heart disease
Arrhythmogenic right ventricular dysplasia
Electrophysiologic abnormalities
  Conduction system disease involving the His-Purkinje conduction
    system
  Primary ventricular arrhythmia associated with the following
    cardiac conditions:
Abnormalities of the QT interval
Brugada syndrome
Wolff-Parkinson-White syndrome
Catecholaminergic ventricular tachycardia
Idiopathic ventricular fibrillation and early repolarization syndromes
Malignant ventricular arrhythmia resulting from metabolic
  abnormalities
Commotio cordis
Pulmonary hypertension
Hypertensive heart disease
Congenital heart disease
Noncompaction of the left ventricle
Inflammatory and infiltrative diseases of the myocardium
  Sarcoidosis
  Chagas' disease
  Hemochromatosis
  Amyloidosis
  Hydatid cyst
Neuromuscular diseases
  Muscular dystrophy
  Myotonic dystrophy
  Kearns-Sayre syndrome
  Friedreich's ataxia
Intracardiac obstruction
  Primary cardiac tumors (e.g., myxoma)
  Intracardiac thrombus
  Massive pulmonary embolism
Acute aortic dissection

chronic LV dysfunction is the most important predictor of sudden death in ischemic and nonischemic cardiomyopathy.

A significant number (10%) of sudden deaths occur in the absence of obvious structural heart disease. Young, active, and otherwise healthy individuals are often the victims. Inherited or spontaneous mutations in genes coding for ion channels are responsible for most of these cases. A number of specific syndromes have been recognized, allowing for screening of relatives.

Tests to Identify Risk for Sudden Death

Electrocardiography (ECG) and echocardiography can provide several clues. Assessment of ventricular function provides the most information in determining the risk for sudden death.

Several noninvasive tests, including detection of microvolt T-wave alternans, signal-averaged ECG, and heart rate variability, have been developed to predict the future risk of sudden death. These tests have poor generalized applicability because of their low positive predictive value. In addition, most have not been coupled with a therapeutic intervention to show that therapy based on them can reduce the risk of dying. Cardiac MRI showing evidence for myocardial scar is emerging as a useful tool for predicting risk.

Intracardiac electrophysiologic testing has retained some value, especially in patients with CAD. Inducibility of a sustained

arrhythmia can be a marker for arrhythmic events, and therapy based on results of electrophysiologic testing has been shown to reduce mortality.

Treatment

This article summarizes the treatment modalities that have been shown to be effective in the various conditions leading to sudden cardiac death. Data based on randomized clinical trials are limited to common conditions such as CAD and the cardiomyopathies. The rarer diseases lack large clinical experience, and recommendations are based on the current consensus.

Acute Management of Survivors of Cardiac Arrest

Once stabilized with the use of standard advanced cardiac life support guidelines, patients should undergo cardiac evaluation by echocardiography and cardiac catheterization. Electrolyte abnormalities should be sought and corrected. Mild hypokalemia (3.0–3.5 mmol/L) is common after a cardiac arrest and resuscitation and is related to hypotension and transient acidosis. Hence, it is often the result and not the cause of the cardiac arrest. Similarly, in the acute phase after resuscitation, it is not uncommon to find global LV hypokinesis, but this should not be taken as a marker for preexisting heart disease. LV function tends to improve over the next 24 to 48 hours and should then be reassessed.

Ventricular fibrillation that occurs during the acute phase of a myocardial infarction (within the first 24–48 hours) is presumed to be secondary to electrical instability resulting from myocardial ischemia and reperfusion. If treated promptly by defibrillation, this arrhythmia has little prognostic value so long as overall myocardial function is preserved.

If acute ischemia or infarction is the documented cause of a cardiac arrest, revascularization by percutaneous angioplasty or coronary bypass surgery is the best treatment. The risk of recurrence is determined by the residual LV ejection fraction. In the Antiarrhythmic Versus Implantable Defibrillator (AVID) trial and Canadian trial of Implantable Defibrillators (CIDS), ICDs did not offer any survival benefit for patients with preserved LV function (>35%). Therefore, postrevascularization electrophysiologic evaluation is recommended only for patients with impaired ejection fraction or significant LV scarring.

Survivors of a malignant arrhythmia other than that due to a reversible cause such as severe metabolic disturbance, toxic drug effect, or acute myocardial infarction are best treated with an ICD. In the largest prospective, randomized trial of drugs versus an ICD (the AVID trial), the ICD reduced mortality by 39% at 1 year and by 31% at 3 years, compared with amiodarone (Cordarone) or sotalol (Betapace). In the absence of specific contraindication, ICD therapy is currently the standard of care for secondary prevention of life-threatening arrhythmic events.

Primary Prevention of Ventricular Arrhythmias and Sudden Cardiac Death

Coronary Artery Disease

There are considerable data to guide efforts at primary prevention of sudden death in patients with CAD. β-Adrenergic blockers and angiotensin-converting enzyme inhibitors reduce mortality after myocardial infarction and should be routinely prescribed in the absence of major contraindications (Table 2). Part of the benefit on mortality offered by these drugs is achieved through reduction of the incidence of sudden death. There is no role for the use of antiarrhythmic drugs in primary prevention. Amiodarone, sotalol, and dofetilide (Tikosyn) have largely neutral effects, but class 1 antiarrhythmic drugs such flecainide (Tambocor) and propafenone (Rythmol) are clearly harmful and increase mortality in patients with ventricular dysfunction.

Ventricular arrhythmias occurring late (>24 hours) after a myocardial infarction usually indicate a persisting propensity for recurrent arrhythmia and risk of death. Commonly, these patients have impaired LV function and benefit from treatment with an ICD; an intracardiac electrophysiologic study is helpful in determining the

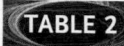

TABLE 2 Drugs That Have Been Shown to Reduce Sudden Cardiac Death

β-Adrenergic blockers: metoprolol (Lopressor), carvedilol (Coreg)

Angiotensin-converting enzyme inhibitors

Angiotensin receptor blockers

Aldosterone antagonists

Antiplatelet drugs

Lipid-lowering agents

Fish oil[1]

[1]Not FDA approved for this indication.

risk of recurrence. Inducibility of ventricular tachycardia (VT) on electrophysiologic study is considered a predictor of sudden death, and treatment of such patients with an ICD lowers mortality.

For the stable patient with CAD, depressed ejection fraction and nonsustained VT are recognized risk factors for sudden death. If severe LV dysfunction is present (ejection fraction <30%), implantation of an ICD will significantly reduce sudden death. In the presence of moderate LV dysfunction (ejection fraction ≤35%), a defibrillator is indicated if patients have New York Heart Association class II or III heart failure symptoms. Nonsustained VT occurring in the context of moderate LV dysfunction warrants an intracardiac electrophysiologic study (Table 3). In all cases ICD should be avoided in patients where meaningful survival is limited to less than a year from non arrhythmic causes.

Idiopathic Dilated Cardiomyopathy

Unlike CAD, nonischemic dilated cardiomyopathy is more variable in its course. This is partly because the etiology is often unclear; the disease process may be progressive in some and self-limited with spontaneous improvement in others. Consequently, benefit from ICD therapy is not as convincing as in patients with CAD. Nonsustained VT, syncope, and heart failure symptoms are predictors of high risk of sudden death in this population. In the Defibrillators in Nonischemic Cardiomyopathy Treatment Evaluation trial (DEFINITE), implantation of an ICD based on the presence of LV dysfunction, symptomatic heart failure, and nonsustained VT resulted in a reduction in arrhythmic mortality. The Sudden Death in Heart Failure trial (SCD Heft) showed that ICDs reduce mortality in the presence of heart failure symptoms and an LV ejection fraction of 35% or less.

Syncope in the presence of cardiomyopathy can be a harbinger of sudden death and merits the use of ICD therapy if another cause of syncope cannot be identified.

Hypertrophic Cardiomyopathy

Hypertrophic cardiomyopathy is a genetically heterogenous disease with an autosomal dominant mode of inheritance caused by mutations in genes coding for sarcomeric proteins. Unrecognized hypertrophic cardiomyopathy is a frequent cause of sudden death in young athletes.

Sudden death in hypertrophic cardiomyopathy is caused by ventricular arrhythmias and can be prevented by implantation of an ICD. A number of risk factors for sudden death have been identified in retrospective studies and are outlined in Table 4. The presence of any one of the major risk factors is an indication for ICD implantation. Electrophysiologic testing has no major value in risk stratification.

Genetic abnormalities do not always correlate with phenotypic expression of disease, and some abnormalities in the troponin gene may have minimal clinical features but high risk for arrhythmias. Genetic testing of the index case is useful in screening of family members.

Arrhythmogenic Right Ventricular Dysplasia

Arrhythmogenic right ventricular dysplasia is characterized by progressive replacement of myocytes with fibrofatty tissue due to an inherited autosomal dominant abnormality in the genes coding for cell-to-cell junction proteins. Typically, the right ventricle is involved, but progressive involvement of the LV has been described. Right bundle branch blockade with late potentials (epsilon wave) and T-wave inversion in the precordial lead may be present on ECG. Ventricular arrhythmia and sudden death are common modes of presentation between the ages of 20 and 40 years, although occasionally heart failure is the presenting symptom.

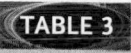

TABLE 3 Indication for ICD Therapy Based on the ACC/AHA 2008 Guidelines

Class I Indication*

1. Cardiac arrest due to VF or VT not due to a transient or reversible cause
2. Spontaneous sustained VT in association with heart disease
3. Recurrent syncope of undetermined origin in the presence of ventricular dysfunction and inducible ventricular arrhythmias on electrophysiologic study
4. NYHA class II or III heart failure and persistent systolic left ventricular dysfunction with LVEF ≤35%
5. Coronary artery disease and systolic left ventricular dysfunction (LVEF ≤30%) persisting >40 days after myocardial infarction or revascularization
6. Nonsustained VT with coronary disease, prior myocardial infarction, left ventricular dysfunction, and inducible VF or sustained VT on electrophysiologic study

Class II Indication†

1. Familial or inherited conditions with a high risk for life-threatening ventricular tachyarrhythmia
2. Unexplained syncope in the presence of left ventricular dysfunction and nonischemic cardiomyopathy
3. Patients with cardiac sarcoid, Chagas' disease, or giant cell myocarditis
4. Adult congenital heart disease with high risk for sudden cardiac death

Abbreviations: ACC/AHA = American College of Cardiology/American Heart Association Task Force; ICD = implantable cardioverter-defibrillator; LVEF = left ventricular ejection fraction; NYHA = New York Heart Association; VF = ventricular fibrillation; VT = ventricular tachycardia.
*There is good clinical evidence and general agreement that ICD is beneficial.
†There is inadequate data or some divergence of opinion regarding ICD benefit.

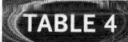

TABLE 4 Clinical Risk Factors for Sudden Death in Hypertrophic Cardiomyopathy

Major Risk Factors

Cardiac arrest

Spontaneous sustained or nonsustained ventricular tachycardia

History of sudden cardiac death in first-degree relatives

Syncope

Left ventricular thickness ≥30 mm

Abnormal blood pressure response to exercise

Possible Risk Factors

Atrial fibrillation

Myocardial ischemia

Left ventricular outflow obstruction

High-risk mutations

Intense (competitive) physical exertion

Patients presenting with stable VT may respond to radiofrequency ablation and antiarrhythmic therapy, but the recurrence rates are high. Consequently, most patients will require ICD therapy. ICD is the first line of treatment for patients with prior cardiac arrest, inducible ventricular arrhythmias on electrophysiologic study, and unexplained syncope.

Sudden Death Associated with Abnormalities of the QT Interval

Congenital long QT (LQT) syndrome is commonly caused by inherited abnormalities of the potassium channel (e.g., LQT1 and LQT2) or of the sodium channel (e.g., LQT3) that result in abnormal cardiac repolarization. These patients carry a risk of developing torsades de pointes VT. Torsades de pointes can lead to syncope but is frequently self-limited. However, the arrhythmia can degenerate to ventricular fibrillation, and sudden death may be the initial manifestation.

The mortality rate is high in untreated patients (approximately 1% per year). Once syncopal episodes begin, the risk of death increases; in one study, 20% of patients had died within 1 year after a syncopal spell. However, ideal management of the congenital LQT syndrome remains controversial. β-Adrenergic blockers and left stellate ganglionectomy, at times in conjunction with cardiac pacing, have been shown to reduce symptoms and mortality. However, the response to beta blockers may vary based on the type of genetic mutations. Because most patients are children or teenagers at the time of diagnosis, there is concern about long-term therapy with implantable devices because of the need for generator changes, potential lead malfunction, and risk of infection. ICD therapy is currently reserved for high-risk patients identified by prior cardiac arrest, recurrent syncope, or VT while on β-blockers, QTc exceeding 500 msec, siblings with sudden death, and symptoms in the patient with LQT3 and possibly LQT2.

One of the major precipitants of torsades in the asymptomatic patient is iatrogenic effects. Numerous drugs have the potential to prolong the QT interval (Table 5). In addition, hypokalemia and hypomagnesemia can induce QT prolongation and torsades de pointes.

In patients without a recognized QT abnormality, drug-induced torsades is treated by discontinuation and avoidance of the offending drug. A number of risk factors have been recognized for drug-induced torsades. They include female gender, hypokalemia and hypomagnesemia, bradycardia, congestive heart failure, baseline QT prolongation, and high drug concentrations (with the

exception of quinidine). Conversion of atrial fibrillation with rapid heart rates to sinus rhythm in the presence of a QT-prolonging drug is a known risk for torsades because of the relative bradycardia interacting with QT prolongation. Administration of class III antiarrhythmic drugs such as sotalol, ibutilide (Corvert), and dofetilide used for conversion and prevention of atrial fibrillation should be commenced under telemetric monitoring. The potential for accumulation of antiarrhythmic drugs in the face of renal dysfunction (e.g., sotalol, dofetilide) should be recognized and dosing adjusted.

A familial form of the short QT syndrome associated with sudden death has been described. A family history of sudden death appears to confer a high risk of sudden arrhythmic death in these patients, warranting ICD therapy.

Brugada Syndrome

Brugada syndrome is characterized by ECG features of incomplete right bundle branch block, J-point elevation with ST-segment elevation in the right precordial leads, normal QT interval, and risk of ventricular fibrillation. The condition has been shown to be caused by an inherited abnormality of the sodium channel involving the same gene (SCN5A) that is responsible for LQT3. The clinical features share similarities with those of LQT3: relative inefficacy of β-blockade, high mortality in symptomatic patients, and sudden death occurring during rest or sleep. Diagnostic criteria are equivocal. ST-segment abnormalities may be transient and dynamic and tend to be augmented by administration of sodium channel blockers.

The general consensus is that symptomatic patients should be treated with an ICD. Asymptomatic patients with a malignant family history should also be considered for ICD therapy. As with the LQT syndromes, drugs have a potential for provoking arrhythmias; sodium channel blockers, including tricyclic antidepressants, have the potential for inducing ventricular arrhythmias and are best avoided in these patients.

Catecholaminergic Ventricular Tachycardia

Inherited defects in genes coding for handling of calcium by the sarcoplasmic reticulum result in ventricular arrhythmia triggered by exercise or emotional stress. The resting ECG is normal. Children are usually affected, but late onset of this condition has been recognized. An autosomal dominant form is caused by mutations in the gene coding for the cardiac ryanodine receptor. The autosomal recessive form is caused by mutation in the gene encoding for calsequestrin, a calcium-buffering protein in the sarcoplasmic reticulum. β-Blockers are the primary form of treatment. However, those patients who have had ventricular fibrillation or continue to have VT or syncope despite β-blocker therapy are considered to be at high risk and should receive ICD therapy.

Wolff-Parkinson-White Syndrome

In the Wolff-Parkinson-White (WPW) syndrome, atrial fibrillation can be conducted rapidly via an accessory pathway with a short refractory period, resulting in ventricular fibrillation and death. The risk of sudden death in patients with WPW syndrome is estimated to be less than 1 in every 1000 patient-years of follow-up. Although the risk is reportedly very low among asymptomatic patients, a potentially lethal arrhythmia can be the initial manifestation in a small number of patients (up to 10%).

The treatment of choice for WPW syndrome is catheter ablation of the accessory pathway; this is successful in 95% of patients. If ablation is ineffective or preferentially avoided because of a high risk of heart block, use of antiarrhythmic drugs such as flecainide or propafenone is an alternative. Rarely, amiodarone may be required to suppress arrhythmias including atrial fibrillation.

Management in the asymptomatic individual who exhibits the WPW pattern on ECG is controversial. Until recently, the consensus was that asymptomatic patients did not require invasive

TABLE 5	Drugs Known to Cause QT Prolongation and Torsades de Pointes

Common

Quinidine

Sotalol (Betapace)

Dofetilide (Tikosyn)

Ibutilide (Corvert)

Disopyramide (Norpace)

Procainamide (Pronestyl)

Less Common

Amiodarone (Cordarone)

Antibiotics: clarithromycin (Biaxin), erythromycin, pentamidine (Pentam), sparfloxacin (Zagam)[2]

Antiemetic agents: domperidone (Motilium),[2] droperidol (Inapsine)

Antipsychotic agents: chlorpromazine (Thorazine), haloperidol (Haldol), mesoridazine (Serentil),[2] thioridazine (Mellaril)

[2]Not available in the United States.

evaluation. Patients with intermittent ventricular preexcitation and those in whom the refractory period of the accessory pathway can be determined to be long are at low risk for sudden death. If a benign nature of the accessory pathway cannot be confirmed by noninvasive evaluation, intracardiac electrophysiologic testing should be considered, with radiofrequency ablation if appropriate. A recent study showed that prophylactic ablation in asymptomatic patients younger than 35 years of age significantly reduced subsequent arrhythmias. Prophylactic ablation should also be considered for individuals in situations in which there is minimal tolerance of a potential for arrhythmias, such as in airline pilots.

Idiopathic Ventricular Fibrillation

A small number of patients who are resuscitated from sudden death episodes have no identifiable structural or electrical abnormalities. The term idiopathic ventricular fibrillation is applied to these patients. Clinically silent focal myocarditis, cardiomyopathy, or unrecognized ionic channel abnormalities may be responsible and may become apparent during subsequent follow-up. The current consensus is that drug therapy is ineffective, and ICD therapy is the safest and most effective secondary prevention strategy. An early repolarization pattern on ECG with >0.1mV J-point elevation in the inferior and lateral leads has recently been associated with vulnerability to VF but the prognostic significance of this pattern in the general population is uncertain.

Adult Congenital Heart Disease

A number of congenital heart diseases can be corrected or palliated by surgery, and survival into adulthood is common. However, sudden arrhythmic cardiac death is a leading cause for late mortality. Unexplained syncope in such patients warrants evaluation by electrophysiologic testing. Intracardiac repair of tetralogy of Fallot has been accomplished since the mid-1950s, with favorable long-term outcome. Risk of late arrhythmic death increases with wide QRS duration, right ventricular dilatation from pulmonary regurgitation, and LV dysfunction. Ventricular arrhythmias or complete heart block may lead to sudden death. Syncope in such patients is an ominous symptom and should be investigated by electrophysiologic evaluation. Pulmonary valve replacement is known to reduce subsequent arrhythmia risk. Inducible VT and evidence for spontaneous ventricular arrhythmias should prompt the consideration of ICD therapy.

A rare condition called noncompaction, caused by an arrest in development of the LV, is known to be associated with sudden death. Prophylactic ICD implantation is recommended.

Neuromuscular Diseases

Some neuromuscular diseases are associated with conduction system disease and ventricular arrhythmias leading to sudden death. Myotonic dystrophy and Kearns-Sayre syndrome are situations in which prophylactic cardiac pacing at the first sign of conduction system disease can be lifesaving. If evidence of cardiac disease precedes the onset of respiratory muscle disease, the risk of cardiac arrhythmia is high, and ICD implantation is often necessary.

Bradyarrhythmia

Bradyarrhythmias resulting from atrioventricular blockade below the atrioventricular node is a cause for sudden death. Most cases of Mobitz type II block or complete heart block below the His bundle are caused by sclerodegenerative changes in the specialized conduction system. Occasionally, cardiac sarcoid or other infiltrative diseases may be responsible. Chagas' disease is a common cause in endemic areas in South America. A familial form of progressive heart block caused by a defect in the *SCN5A* gene has been identified in some families.

Symptomatic bradyarrhythmias and heart block due to disease in the His-Purkinje system are indications for permanent cardiac pacing. In the absence of the other structural heart disease, permanent cardiac pacing can restore longevity to match that of age-matched controls.

References

Antiarrhythmics Versus Implantable Defibrillators (AVID) Investigators. A comparison of antiarrhythmic drug therapy with implantable defibrillators in patients resuscitated from near fatal ventricular arrhythmias. N Engl J Med 1997;337:1576–83.

Ezekowitz JA, Armstrong PW, McAlister FA. Implantable cardioverter defibrillators in primary and secondary prevention: A systematic review of randomized, controlled trials [see comments]. Ann Intern Med 2003;138:445–52.

Goldberg I, Moss AJ, Peterson DR, et al. Risk factors for aborted cardiac arrest and sudden cardiac death in children with the congenital long QT syndrome. Circulation 2008;117:2184–91.

Pappone C, Santinelli V, Manguso F, et al. A randomized study of prophylactic catheter ablation in asymptomatic patients with the Wolff-Parkinson-White syndrome. N Engl J Med 2003;349:1803–11.

Priori SG, Schwartz PJ, Napolitano C, et al. Risk stratification in the long-QT syndrome. N Engl J Med 2003;348:1866–74.

Santinelli V, Radinovic A, Manguso F, et al. The natural history of asymptomatic ventricular pre-excitation: A long-term prospective follow-up study of 184 asymptomatic children. J Am Coll Cardiol 2009;53:275–80.

Zipes DP, Camm AJ, Borggrefe M, et al. ACC/AHA/ESC 2006 Guidelines for management of patients with ventricular arrhythmias and the prevention of sudden cardiac death. Circulation 2006;114(10):e385–484.

CONGENITAL HEART DISEASE

Method of
Richard A. Lange, MD; and L. David Hillis, MD

CURRENT DIAGNOSIS

- Examine blood pressures in arms and legs, pulse oximetry, mucous membranes and nail beds, respiratory rate, and peripheral pulses.
- In addition to listening over the precordium for heart sounds and murmurs, palpate for thrills and evidence of right or left chamber enlargement.
- Ancillary testing should include chest radiography, electrocardiography, and echocardiography.
- Consult a cardiologist if the physical examination or ancillary tests suggest congenital heart disease.

CURRENT THERAPY

- All congenital heart disease patients should have long-term follow-up for possible complications.
- Endocarditis prophylaxis is recommended for subjects with:
  - Unrepaired cyanotic congenital heart disease
  - Recently repaired congenital heart disease (<6 months after surgical or percutaneous repair)
  - Repaired congenital heart disease with residual defects
- Closure of defects with large left-to-right shunts (i.e., atrial septal defect, ventricular septal defect, atrioventricular canal, or patent ductus arteriosus) is recommended unless pulmonary vascular obstructive disease is far advanced.
- Patients with bicuspid aortic valves should be monitored for aortic root dilatation.
- Pregnancy should be avoided in women with cyanotic congenital heart disease because of high maternal and fetal morbidity and mortality.

Congenital heart disease affects 0.4% to 0.9% of live births. Nowadays, most survive to adulthood because of improved diagnosis and treatment. Congenital cardiac defects can be categorized according to the presence or absence of cyanosis (due to right-to-left shunting) and the amount of pulmonary blood flow (Box 1).

Acyanotic Cardiac Defects
Increased pulmonary blood flow
- Atrial septal defect
- Ventricular septal defect
- Atrioventricular canal defect
- Patent ductus arteriosus

Normal pulmonary blood flow
- Aortic stenosis
- Pulmonic stenosis
- Aortic coarctation

Cyanotic Cardiac Defects
Normal pulmonary blood flow
- Ebstein's anomaly

Decreased pulmonary blood flow
- Tetralogy of Fallot
- Eisenmenger's syndrome

Acyanotic Conditions

Atrial Septal Defect

Atrial septal defect (ASD) occurs in female patients two to three times as often as in male patients. Although most result from spontaneous genetic mutations, some are inherited.

The physiologic consequences of ASD result from the shunting of blood from one atrium to the other; the direction and magnitude of shunting are determined by the size of the defect and the relative compliances of the ventricles. A small defect (<0.5 cm in diameter) is associated with a small shunt and no hemodynamic sequelae, whereas a sizable defect (>2 cm in diameter) usually is associated with a large shunt and substantial hemodynamic consequences. In most patients with ASD, the right ventricle is more compliant than the left; as a result, left atrial blood is shunted to the right atrium, causing increased pulmonary blood flow and dilatation of the atria, right ventricle, and pulmonary arteries (Figure 1).

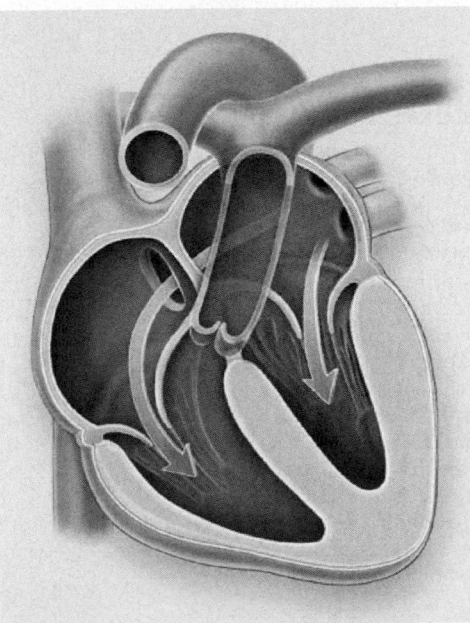

Figure 1. Atrial septal defect. Blood from the pulmonary veins enters the left atrium, after which some of it crosses the atrial septal defect into the right atrium and ventricle *(longer arrow)*. Thus, left-to-right shunting occurs. (Reprinted with permission from Brickner ME, Hillis LD, Lange RA: Congenital heart disease in adults. First of two parts. N Engl J Med 2000;342:256–63.)

Eventually, if the right ventricle fails or its compliance declines, the magnitude of left-to-right shunting diminishes.

In a patient with a large ASD, a right ventricular or pulmonary arterial impulse may be palpable, and wide, fixed splitting of the second heart sound is present. A systolic ejection murmur, audible in the second left intercostal space, is caused by increased blood flow across the pulmonic valve; flow across the ASD itself does not produce a murmur.

Because ASDs initially produce no symptoms or striking physical examination findings, they are often undetected for years. Small defects with minimal left-to-right shunting cause no symptoms or hemodynamic abnormalities, so they do not require closure. Even patients with moderate or large ASDs (characterized by a ratio of pulmonary to systemic blood flow of 1.5 or more) often have no symptoms until the third or fourth decade of life. Over the years, the increased blood volume flowing through the right heart chambers usually causes right ventricular dilatation and failure. Obstructive pulmonary vascular disease (Eisenmenger's syndrome) occurs uncommonly in adults with ASD.

The symptomatic patient with an ASD typically reports fatigue or dyspnea on exertion. Alternatively, the development of supraventricular tachyarrhythmias, right heart failure, paradoxical embolism, or recurrent pulmonary infections might prompt the patient to seek medical attention. Although an occasional patient with an unrepaired ASD survives to an advanced age, those with sizable shunts often die of right ventricular failure or arrhythmias in their 30s or 40s.

Echocardiography can reveal atrial and right ventricular dilatation and identify the ASD's location. The sensitivity of echocardiography may be enhanced by injecting microbubbles in solution into a peripheral vein, after which the movement of some of them across the defect into the left atrium can be visualized.

An ASD with a pulmonary-to-systemic flow ratio of 1.5 or more should be closed (surgically or percutaneously) to prevent worsening right ventricular dysfunction. Prophylaxis against infective endocarditis is not recommended for patients with ASD (repaired or unrepaired) unless a concomitant valvular abnormality is present.

Ventricular Septal Defect

Ventricular septal defect (VSD) is the most common congenital cardiac abnormality, with similar incidence in boys and girls. Approximately 25% to 40% of them close spontaneously by 2 years of age.

The physiologic consequences of a VSD are determined by the size of the defect and the relative resistances in the systemic and pulmonary vascular beds. A small defect causes little or no functional disturbance, because pulmonary blood flow is only minimally increased. In contrast, a large defect causes substantial left-to-right shunting, because systemic vascular resistance exceeds pulmonary vascular resistance (Figure 2). Over time, however, the pulmonary vascular resistance usually increases, and the magnitude of left-to-right shunting declines. Eventually, the pulmonary vascular resistance equals or exceeds the systemic resistance; the shunting of blood from left to right ceases; and right-to-left shunting begins (e.g., Eisenmenger's physiology).

A small, muscular VSD can produce a high-frequency systolic ejection murmur that terminates before the end of systole (when the defect is occluded by contracting heart muscle). With a moderate or large VSD and substantial left-to-right shunting, a holosystolic murmur, loudest at the left sternal border, is audible and is usually accompanied by a palpable thrill. If pulmonary hypertension develops, the holosystolic murmur and thrill diminish in magnitude and eventually disappear as flow through the defect decreases.

Echocardiography is usually performed to confirm the presence and location of the VSD and to delineate the magnitude and direction of shunting. With catheterization, one can determine the magnitude of shunting and the pulmonary vascular resistance.

The natural history of VSD depends on the size of the defect and the pulmonary vascular resistance. Adults with small defects and normal pulmonary arterial pressure are generally asymptomatic,

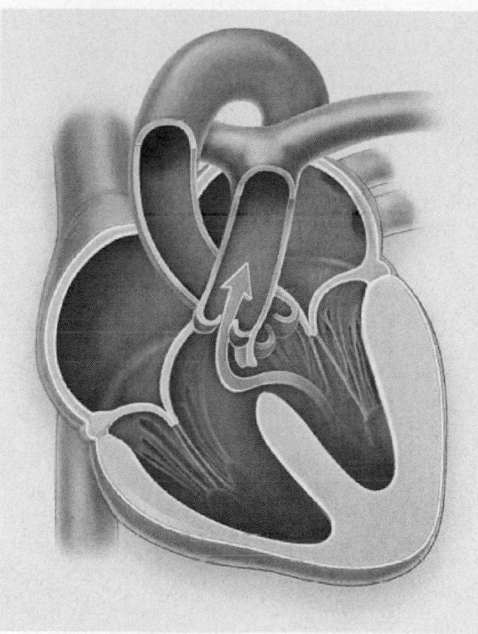

Figure 2. Ventricular septal defect. When the left ventricle contracts, it ejects some blood into the aorta and some across the ventricular septal defect into the right ventricle and pulmonary artery *(arrow)*, resulting in left-to-right shunting. (Reprinted with permission from Brickner ME, Hillis LD, Lange RA: Congenital heart disease in adults. First of two parts. N Engl J Med 2000;342:256–63.)

and pulmonary vascular disease is unlikely to develop. In contrast, patients with large defects who survive to adulthood usually have left ventricular failure or pulmonary hypertension (or both) with associated right ventricular failure.

Closure of VSDs (surgically or percutaneously) is recommended if the pulmonary vascular obstructive disease is not severe. Prophylaxis against infective endocarditis is recommended for patients with unrepaired VSD and those with a residual shunt despite surgical or percutaneous closure.

Atrioventricular Canal Defect

The endocardial cushions normally fuse to form the tricuspid and mitral valves as well as the atrial and ventricular septa. Atrioventricular (AV) canal defects are caused by incomplete fusion of the endocardial cushions during embryonic development. They are the most common congenital cardiac abnormality in patients with Down syndrome. Such cushion defects include a spectrum of abnormalities, ranging from ASD with a cleft anterior mitral valve leaflet to a common AV canal defect in which a single AV valve in association with a large ASD and VSD is present.

A common AV canal defect permits substantial left-to-right shunting at both the atrial and ventricular levels, which leads to excessive pulmonary blood flow and resultant pulmonary congestion within months of birth. Eventually, the excessive pulmonary blood flow leads to irreversible pulmonary vascular obstruction (e.g., Eisenmenger's physiology).

In the patient with an AV canal defect and left-to-right intracardiac shunting, the physical examination reveals a loud holosystolic murmur audible throughout the precordium. As pulmonary vascular resistance increases, the holosystolic murmur diminishes in intensity and duration, eventually disappearing as flow through the defect decreases.

AV canal defects require surgical repair if the magnitude of pulmonary vascular obstructive disease is not prohibitive. Although such patients might initially benefit from medical treatment with diuretics and afterload reduction, the onset of heart failure symptoms is generally the point at which surgery is considered. Prophylaxis against infective endocarditis is recommended for patients with repaired and unrepaired AV canal defects.

Patent Ductus Arteriosus

The ductus arteriosus connects the descending aorta (just distal to the left subclavian artery) and the left pulmonary artery. In the fetus, it permits pulmonary arterial blood to bypass the unexpanded lungs and to enter the descending aorta for oxygenation in the placenta. Although it normally closes spontaneously soon after birth, it fails to do so in some infants, so that continuous flow from the aorta to the pulmonary artery (i.e., left-to-right shunting) occurs (Figure 3). The incidence of patent ductus arteriosus (PDA) is increased in pregnancies complicated by persistent perinatal hypoxemia or maternal rubella infection as well as among infants born prematurely or at high altitude.

A patient with PDA and a moderate or large shunt has bounding peripheral arterial pulses and a widened pulse pressure. A continuous "machinery" murmur, audible in the second left intercostal space, begins shortly after the first heart sound, peaks in intensity at or immediately after the second heart sound (thereby obscuring it), and diminishes in intensity during diastole. If pulmonary vascular obstruction and hypertension develop, the murmur decreases in duration and intensity and eventually disappears.

With echocardiography, the PDA can usually be visualized, and Doppler studies demonstrate continuous flow in the pulmonary trunk. Catheterization and angiography allow one to quantify the magnitude of shunting and the pulmonary vascular resistance and to visualize the PDA.

The subject with a small PDA has no symptoms attributable to it and a normal life expectancy. However, it is associated with an elevated risk of infective endarteritis. A PDA of moderate size might cause no symptoms during infancy; during childhood or adulthood, fatigue, dyspnea, or palpitations can appear. Additionally, the PDA can become aneurysmal and calcified, with subsequent rupture. Larger shunts can precipitate left ventricular failure. Eventually, pulmonary vascular obstruction can develop; when the pulmonary vascular resistance equals or exceeds the systemic vascular resistance, the direction of shunting reverses.

One third of patients with an unrepaired moderate or large PDA die of heart failure, pulmonary hypertension, or endarteritis by 40 years of age, and two thirds die by 60 years of age. Because of the risk of endarteritis associated with unrepaired PDA (about

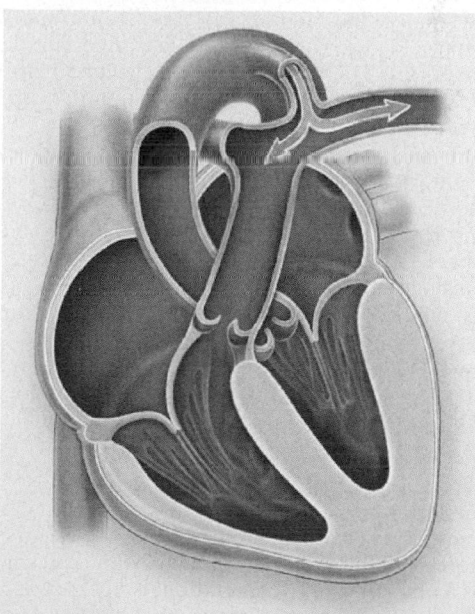

Figure 3. Patent ductus arteriosus. Some of the blood from the aorta crosses the ductus arteriosus into the pulmonary artery *(arrows)*, with resultant left-to-right shunting. (Reprinted with permission from Brickner ME, Hillis LD, Lange RA: Congenital heart disease in adults. First of two parts. N Engl J Med 2000;342:256–63.)

0.45% annually after the second decade of life) and the safety of surgical ligation (generally accomplished without cardiopulmonary bypass) or percutaneous closure, even a small PDA should be ligated surgically or occluded percutaneously. Once severe pulmonary vascular obstructive disease develops, ligation or closure is contraindicated.

Aortic Stenosis

A bicuspid aortic valve is found in 2% to 3% of the population and is four times more common in male than female patients. The bicuspid valve has a single fused commissure and an eccentrically oriented orifice. Although the deformed valve is not typically stenotic at birth, it is subjected to abnormal hemodynamic stress, which can lead to leaflet thickening and calcification. In many patients, an abnormality of the ascending aortic media is present, predisposing the patient to aortic root dilatation. Twenty percent of patients with a bicuspid aortic valve have an associated cardiovascular abnormality, such as PDA or aortic coarctation.

In patients with severe aortic stenosis (AS), the carotid upstroke is usually delayed and diminished. The aortic component of the second heart sound is diminished or absent. A systolic crescendo–decrescendo murmur is audible over the aortic area and often radiates to the neck. As the magnitude of AS worsens, the murmur peaks progressively later in systole.

In most patients, echocardiography with Doppler flow permits an assessment of the severity of AS and of left ventricular systolic function. Cardiac catheterization is performed to assess the severity of AS and to determine if concomitant coronary artery disease is present.

The symptoms of AS are angina pectoris, syncope or near syncope, and those of heart failure (dyspnea). Asymptomatic adults with AS have a normal life expectancy. Once symptoms appear, survival is limited: The median survival is 5 years once angina develops, 3 years once syncope occurs, and 2 years once symptoms of heart failure appear. Therefore, patients with symptomatic AS should undergo valve replacement.

Pulmonic stenosis

Pulmonic stenosis (PS) is the second most common congenital cardiac malformation (after VSD). Although typically an isolated abnormality, it can occur in association with VSD.

The patient with PS is usually asymptomatic, and the condition is identified by auscultation of a loud systolic murmur. When it is severe, dyspnea on exertion or fatigue can occur; less often, patients have retrosternal chest pain or syncope with exertion. Eventually, right ventricular failure can develop, with resultant peripheral edema and abdominal swelling.

In patients with moderate or severe PS, the second heart sound is widely split, with its pulmonic component soft and delayed. A crescendo-decrescendo systolic murmur that increases in intensity with inspiration is audible along the left sternal border. If the valve is pliable, an ejection click often precedes the murmur. On echocardiography, right ventricular hypertrophy is evident; the severity of PS can usually be assessed with measurement of Doppler flow.

Adults with mild PS are usually asymptomatic and do not require a corrective procedure. In contrast, patients with moderate or severe PS should undergo percutaneous balloon dilatation.

Aortic Coarctation

Aortic coarctation typically consists of a diaphragm-like ridge extending into the aortic lumen just distal to the left subclavian artery (Figure 4), resulting in an elevated arterial pressure in both arms. Less commonly, the coarctation is located immediately proximal to the left subclavian artery, in which case a difference in arterial pressure is noted between the arms. Extensive collateral arterial circulation to the lower body through the internal thoracic, intercostal, subclavian, and scapular arteries often develops in patients with aortic coarctation. The condition, which is two to five times as common in male as in female patients, can occur in

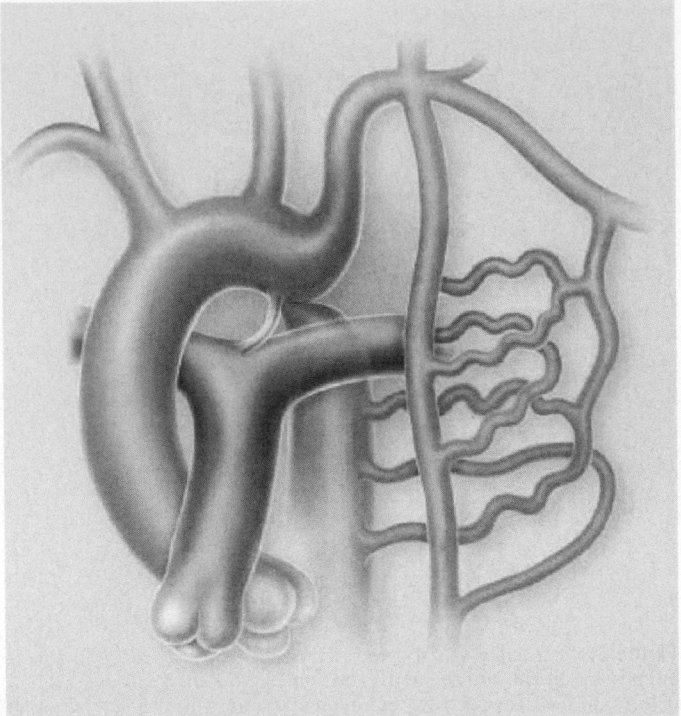

Figure 4. Coarctation of the aorta. Coarctation causes obstruction to blood flow in the descending thoracic aorta; the lower body is perfused by collateral vessels from the axillary and internal thoracic arteries through the intercostal arteries. (Reprinted with permission from Brickner ME, Hillis LD, Lange RA: Congenital heart disease in adults. First of two parts. N Engl J Med 2000;342:256–63.)

conjunction with gonadal dysgenesis (e.g., Turner's syndrome), bicuspid aortic valve, VSD, or PDA.

On physical examination, the arterial pressure is higher in the arms than in the legs, and the femoral arterial pulses are weak and delayed. A harsh systolic ejection murmur may be audible along the left sternal border and in the back, particularly over the coarctation. A systolic murmur, caused by flow through collateral vessels, may be heard in the back.

On chest radiography, increased collateral flow through the intercostal arteries causes notching of the posterior third through eighth ribs. The coarctation may be visible as an indentation of the aorta, and one may see prestenotic and poststenotic aortic dilatation, producing the "reversed E" or "3" sign. Computed tomography, magnetic resonance imaging, and contrast aortography provide precise anatomic delineation of the coarctation's location and length.

Most adults with aortic coarctation are asymptomatic. When symptoms are present, they are usually those of hypertension: headache, epistaxis, dizziness, and palpitations. Complications of aortic coarctation include hypertension, left ventricular failure, aortic dissection, premature coronary artery disease, infective endocarditis, and cerebrovascular accidents (due to rupture of an intracerebral aneurysm). Two thirds of patients older than 40 years who have uncorrected aortic coarctation have symptoms of heart failure. Three fourths die by the age of 50 years and 90% by the age of 60 years.

Surgical repair or intraluminal stenting should be considered for patients with a transcoarctation pressure gradient greater than 30 mm Hg, with the choice of procedure influenced by the age of the patient, anatomic considerations of the coarctation, and the presence of concomitant cardiac abnormalities. Persistent hypertension is common despite surgical or percutaneous intervention, and recurrent coarctation or aneurysm formation at the repair site may occur.

Cyanotic Conditions

Ebstein's Anomaly

With Ebstein's anomaly, the tricuspid valve's septal leaflet and often its posterior leaflet are displaced into the right ventricle, and the anterior leaflet is usually malformed and abnormally attached or adherent to the right ventricular free wall. As a result, a portion of the right ventricle is atrialized, in that it is located on the atrial side of the tricuspid valve, and the remaining functional right ventricle is small (Figure 5). The tricuspid valve is usually regurgitant, but it may be stenotic. Eighty percent of patients with Ebstein's anomaly have an interatrial communication (atrial septal defect or patent foramen ovale) through which right-to-left shunting of blood can occur.

The severity of the hemodynamic derangements in patients with Ebstein's anomaly depends on the magnitude of displacement and the functional status of the tricuspid valve leaflets. On the one extreme, patients with mild apical displacement of the tricuspid valve leaflets have normal valvular function; on the other extreme, those with severe leaflet displacement or abnormal anterior leaflet attachment, with resultant valvular dysfunction, have an elevated right atrial pressure and right-to-left interatrial shunting.

The clinical presentation of subjects with Ebstein's anomaly ranges from severe right heart failure in the neonate to the absence of symptoms in the adult in whom it is discovered incidentally. Older children with Ebstein's anomaly often come to medical attention because of an incidental murmur, whereas adolescents and adults may be identified because of a supraventricular arrhythmia.

On physical examination, the severity of cyanosis depends on the magnitude of right-to-left shunting. The first and second heart sounds are widely split, and a third or fourth heart sound is often present, resulting in triple or even quadruple heart sounds. A systolic murmur caused by tricuspid regurgitation is usually present at the left lower sternal border.

Echocardiography is used to assess the presence and magnitude of right atrial dilatation, anatomic displacement and distortion of the tricuspid valve leaflets, and the severity of tricuspid regurgitation or stenosis.

Prophylaxis against infective endocarditis is recommended. Patients with symptomatic right heart failure should receive diuretics. Tricuspid valve repair or replacement in conjunction with closure of the interatrial communication is recommended for older patients with severe symptoms despite medical therapy and those with less severe symptoms who have cardiac enlargement.

Tetralogy of Fallot

Tetralogy of Fallot is characterized by a large VSD, an aorta that overrides both ventricles, obstruction to right ventricular outflow (subvalvular, valvular, supravalvular, or in the pulmonary arterial branches), and right ventricular hypertrophy (Figure 6).

Most patients with tetralogy of Fallot have substantial right-to-left shunting through the large VSD because of increased resistance to flow in the right ventricular outflow tract; the magnitude of right ventricular outflow tract obstruction determines the magnitude of shunting. Because the resistance to flow across the right ventricular outflow tract is relatively fixed, changes in systemic vascular resistance affect the magnitude of right-to-left shunting: A decrease in systemic vascular resistance increases right-to-left shunting, whereas an increase in systemic resistance decreases it.

Patients with tetralogy of Fallot typically have cyanosis from birth or beginning in the first year of life. In childhood, they might have sudden hypoxic spells, characterized by tachypnea and hyperpnea, followed by worsening cyanosis and, in some cases, loss of consciousness, seizures, cerebrovascular accidents, and even death. Such spells do not occur in adolescents or adults. Without surgical intervention, most patients die in childhood.

On physical examination, patients with tetralogy of Fallot have cyanosis and digital clubbing. A right ventricular lift or tap is palpable. The second heart sound is single, because its pulmonic component is inaudible. A systolic ejection murmur, audible along the left sternal border, is caused by the obstruction to right ventricular outflow. The intensity and duration of the murmur are inversely related to the severity of right ventricular outflow

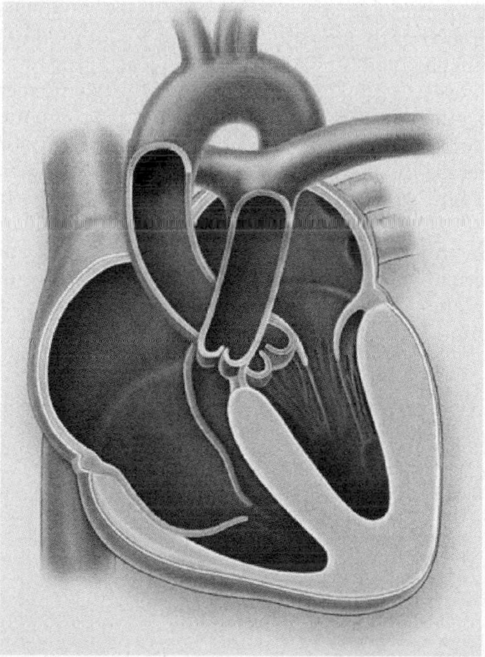

Figure 5. Ebstein's anomaly. With Ebstein's anomaly, the tricuspid valve is displaced apically, a portion of the right ventricle is atrialized (i.e., located on the atrial side of the tricuspid valve), and the functional right ventricle is small. (Reprinted with permission from Brickner ME, Hillis LD, Lange RA: Congenital heart disease in adults. Second of two parts. N Engl J Med 2000;342:334–42.)

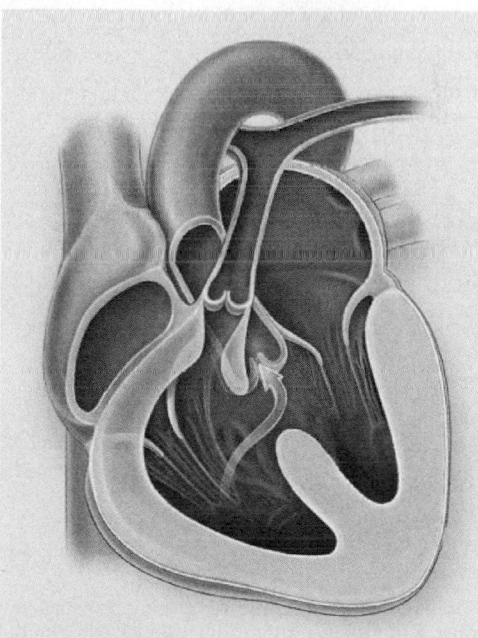

Figure 6. Tetralogy of Fallot. Tetralogy of Fallot is characterized by a large ventricular septal defect, obstruction of the right ventricular outflow tract, right ventricular hypertrophy, and an aorta that overrides the left and right ventricles. With right ventricular outflow tract obstruction, blood is shunted through the ventricular septal defect from right to left *(arrow)*. (Reprinted with permission from Brickner ME, Hillis LD, Lange RA: Congenital heart disease in adults. Second of two parts. N Engl J Med 2000;342:334–42.)

obstruction; a soft, short murmur suggests that severe obstruction is present.

Laboratory examination reveals arterial oxygen desaturation and compensatory erythrocytosis. Echocardiography can be used to establish the diagnosis and to assess the location and severity of right ventricular outflow tract obstruction.

Complete surgical repair (closure of the VSD and relief of right ventricular outflow tract obstruction) is recommended to relieve symptoms and to improve survival; it should be performed when patients are very young. Those with tetralogy of Fallot (repaired or unrepaired) are at risk for endocarditis and therefore should receive antibiotic prophylaxis before dental or elective surgical procedures.

Patients with repaired tetralogy of Fallot require careful follow-up, because they can subsequently develop atrial or ventricular arrhythmias, pulmonic regurgitation, right ventricular dysfunction, or recurrent obstruction of the right ventricular outflow tract.

Eisenmenger's Syndrome

With substantial left-to-right shunting, the pulmonary vasculature is exposed to increased blood flow under increased pressure, often resulting in pulmonary vascular obstructive disease. As the pulmonary vascular resistance approaches or exceeds systemic resistance, the shunt is reversed (right-to-left shunting develops), and cyanosis appears (Figure 7).

Most patients with Eisenmenger's syndrome have impaired exercise tolerance and exertional dyspnea. Palpitations are common and most often result from atrial fibrillation or flutter. As erythrocytosis (due to arterial desaturation) develops, symptoms of hyperviscosity (visual disturbances, fatigue, headache, dizziness,

and paresthesias) can appear. Patients with Eisenmenger's syndrome can experience hemoptysis, bleeding complications, cerebrovascular accidents, brain abscess, syncope, and sudden death.

Eisenmenger's syndrome patients typically have digital clubbing and cyanosis, a right parasternal heave (due to right ventricular hypertrophy), and a prominent pulmonic component of the second heart sound. The murmur caused by a VSD, PDA, or ASD disappears when Eisenmenger's syndrome develops.

The chest x-ray reveals normal heart size, prominent central pulmonary arteries, and diminished vascular markings (pruning) of the peripheral vessels. On transthoracic echocardiography, evidence of right ventricular pressure overload and pulmonary hypertension is present. The underlying cardiac defect can usually be visualized, although shunting across the defect may be difficult to demonstrate by Doppler because of the low jet velocity.

Even though patients with Eisenmenger's syndrome have severe pulmonary hypertension, they have a favorable long-term survival: 80% at 10 years after diagnosis, 77% at 15 years, and 42% at 25 years. Death is usually sudden, presumably caused by arrhythmias, but some patients die of heart failure, hemoptysis, brain abscess, or stroke.

Phlebotomy with isovolumic replacement should be performed in patients with moderate or severe symptoms of hyperviscosity; it should not be performed in asymptomatic or mildly symptomatic patients regardless of the hematocrit. Repeated phlebotomy can result in iron deficiency, which can worsen the symptoms of hyperviscosity, because iron-deficient erythrocytes are less deformable than iron-replete ones. Anticoagulants and antiplatelet agents should be avoided, because they exacerbate the hemorrhagic diathesis.

Patients with Eisenmenger's syndrome should avoid intravascular volume depletion, high altitude, and the use of systemic vasodilators. Because of high maternal and fetal morbidity and mortality, pregnancy should be avoided. Patients with Eisenmenger's syndrome who are undergoing noncardiac surgery require meticulous management of anesthesia, with attention to maintenance of systemic vascular resistance, minimization of blood loss and intravascular volume depletion, and prevention of iatrogenic paradoxical embolization. In preparation for noncardiac surgery, prophylactic phlebotomy (usually of 1 to 2 units of blood, with isovolumic replacement) is recommended for patients with a hematocrit greater than 65% to reduce the likelihood of perioperative hemorrhagic and thrombotic complications.

Lung transplantation with repair of the cardiac defect or combined heart–lung transplantation are options for patients with Eisenmenger's syndrome who are deemed to have a poor prognosis (as reflected by the presence of syncope, refractory right heart failure, a high New York Heart Association (NYHA) functional class, or severe hypoxemia). Because of the somewhat limited success of transplantation and the reasonably good survival among patients treated medically, careful selection of patients for transplantation is imperative. Although pulmonary vasodilators improve exercise capacity, they have not been proved to improve survival.

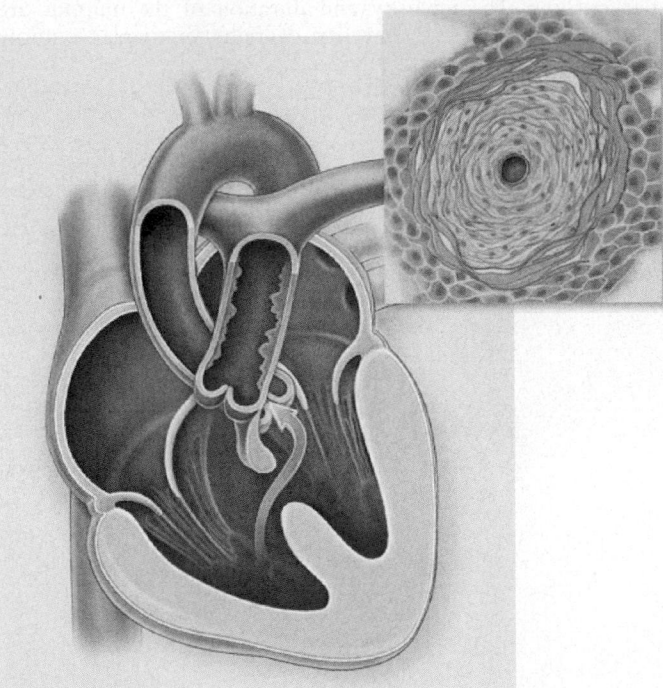

Figure 7. Eisenmenger's syndrome. In response to substantial left-to-right shunting, morphologic alterations occur in the small pulmonary arteries and arterioles *(inset)*, leading to pulmonary hypertension and the resultant reversal of the intracardiac shunt *(arrow)*. In the small pulmonary arteries and arterioles, medial hypertrophy, intimal cellular proliferation, and fibrosis lead to narrowing or closure of the vessel lumina. With sustained pulmonary hypertension, extensive atherosclerosis and calcification often develop in the large pulmonary arteries. (Reprinted with permission from Brickner ME, Hillis LD, Lange RA: Congenital heart disease in adults. Second of two parts. N Engl J Med 2000;342:334–42.)

References

Brickner ME, Hillis LD, Lange RA. Congenital heart disease in adults. First of two parts. N Engl J Med 2000;342:256–63.

Brickner ME, Hillis LD, Lange RA. Congenital heart disease in adults. Second of two parts. N Engl J Med 2000;342:334–42.

Deanfield J, Thaulow E, Warnes C, et al. Management of grown up congenital heart disease. Eur Heart J 2003;24:1035–84.

Lange RA, Hillis LD, Vongpatanasin WP, Brickner ME. The Eisenmenger syndrome in adults. Ann Int Med 1998;128:745–55.

Marelli AJ, Mackie AS, Ionescu-Ittu R, et al. Congenital heart disease in the general population: Changing prevalence and age distribution. Circulation 2007; 115:163–72.

Warnes CS, Williams RG, Bashore TM, et al. ACC/AHA 2008 Guidelines for the management of adults with congenital heart disease: Executive summary. A report of the American College of Cardiology/American Heart Association Task Force on Practice Guidelines (Writing Committee to Develop Guidelines for the Management of Adults With Congenital Heart Disease). Circulation 2008;118:2395–451.

CONGESTIVE HEART FAILURE

Method of
Elaine Winkel, MD; and Walter Kao, MD

CURRENT DIAGNOSIS

- Identify the presence of characteristics associated with left ventricular systolic dysfunction.
- Document the degree of left ventricular dysfunction by imaging.
- Ascertain clinical volume and perfusion status.
- Determine the cause of cardiac dysfunction, if possible, with special attention to coronary artery disease.

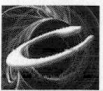

CURRENT THERAPY

- Angiotensin-converting enzyme (ACE) inhibitors, angiotensin receptor blocking agents, β-blockers, and aldosterone receptor antagonists improve survival and are integral to the treatment plan.
- Use nonpharmacologic therapy along with medical therapy. Sodium and fluid restriction, smoking and alcohol cessation, stress reduction and treatment of depression, and exercise and weight loss, all improve symptoms and reduce hospitalization.
- Treat comorbidities that exacerbate the heart failure state (e.g., hypertension, arrhythmias, sleep-disordered breathing).
- Consider interventions to treat concomitant structural heart disease, such as coronary revascularization, mitral valve surgery, arrhythmia treatment, and cardiac resynchronization therapy.
- Refer patients with refractory disease early to an advanced heart failure center for implantation of a ventricular assist device or cardiac transplantation.
- Provide palliative care for patients who are not candidates for advanced heart failure therapy.

Despite the decrease in the incidence of other circulatory conditions, or perhaps rather because of improvements in the management of related circulatory conditions, heart failure represents the major clinical challenge facing all clinicians who manage patients with cardiac disease today. It continues to be the most common cause of hospitalization for patients older than 65 years of age and results in the expenditure of almost 40 billion dollars annually in the United States. Heart failure is a chronic degenerative disease; if left untreated, it will result in progressively deteriorating functional capacity and premature death. For optimal patient outcome, it must be managed aggressively and proactively.

This discussion focuses exclusively on heart failure resulting from systolic dysfunction, the management of which has been most extensively studied. However, it is now recognized that diastolic dysfunction, particularly of the left ventricle (LV), is an increasingly common condition, particularly in the elderly, and can result in similar symptoms. The optimal management of this vexing condition has yet to be determined with certainty, although there are ongoing efforts to establish evidence-based approaches to this disease as well.

Definition

Although heart failure is defined traditionally as a condition in which the heart is unable to pump enough blood to satisfy the metabolic demands of the body, this expression has little direct clinical relevance. On a practical level, heart failure is perhaps better thought of as a condition involving abnormality of cardiac emptying or filling associated with increased intracardiac filling pressures or decreased cardiac output, exercise intolerance, frequent arrhythmias, and early death. The abnormalities in cardiac structure and function typically precede, often by many years, the onset of symptoms. Therefore, to most effectively treat this disease, it is critically important to affirmatively seek out and diagnose cardiac dysfunction before overt symptoms develop.

History and Physical Examination

In the United States, the most common cause of cardiac dysfunction is coronary artery disease due to atherosclerotic cardiovascular disease (ASCVD). Because ASCVD is typically a systemic rather than a localized phenomenon, any suggestion of atherosclerotic disease in any vascular bed should prompt a thorough cardiac evaluation as well.

Exercise intolerance due to dyspnea or fatigue is the most common presenting symptom in patients with heart failure, although other symptoms may also be present, such as orthopnea, paroxysmal nocturnal dyspnea, dependent edema, or palpitations. Many of these symptoms are nonspecific, and a high index of suspicion is necessary to diagnose underlying heart failure. Other historical findings that should heighten the suspicion for underlying heart failure include the presence of predisposing conditions such as hypertension, diabetes mellitus or metabolic syndrome, obesity, prior exposure to known cardiotoxic agents, ASCVD, and a family history of premature ASCVD, documented cardiomyopathy, or unexplained premature death. When such characteristics are present, particularly in concert with other suggestive findings from the history or physical examination, they should prompt a more directed evaluation, including strong consideration of imaging studies to measure cardiac function.

Physical examination findings are often subtle, especially if the underlying disease has been progressing insidiously for an extended period before presentation, as is often the case. The vital signs may be normal, although the heart rate is frequently elevated due to the compensatory hyperadrenergic state associated with untreated cardiac dysfunction. Tachycardia, especially sinus tachycardia, should always be considered a symptom of underlying systemic disease and should spur further investigation. Chronic arterial hypertension is a frequent cause of heart failure, particularly in non-Caucasian populations; it often persists despite substantial degrees of cardiac dysfunction and should prompt additional cardiac evaluation. Increased central venous pressure may manifest as an elevation in measured jugular venous pressure or as systemic edema; however, the latter symptom is frequently nonspecific, being often seen in older individuals with venous insufficiency, obesity, or sedentary lifestyles. In contrast, visceral edema, when detected, is more specifically associated with increased central venous pressure. The carotid impulse is typically normal, although in patients with severe degrees of LV systolic dysfunction the impulse may be less dynamic than normal. Asymmetrical arterial pulses or bruits suggest systemic atherosclerotic disease, including likely coronary artery disease.

The presence of pulmonary rales, although classically described in patients with cardiogenic or noncardiogenic intraalveolar pulmonary edema, is typically seen only with new and rapid onset of cardiac dysfunction, the prototype of which is acute myocardial infarction with associated LV dysfunction. The compensatory potential of pulmonary venous and lymphatic drainage is such that more insidious, slowly developing cardiac dysfunction is most often not associated with intraalveolar fluid; for this reason, the lung fields may be clear on auscultation or even on radiographic examination. In patients with disease of longer standing, in whom one or both ventricular chambers has had a chance to dilate, the apical (LV) impulse may be laterally displaced; in more severe degrees of LV dysfunction, it may not be palpable at all.

The heart sounds are often subtly decreased in intensity due to decreased LV contractile power, but they remain physiologic in the absence of conduction disease. With an acute onset, gallops may be present, particularly an early diastolic sound (S_3); however, a slowly dilating dysfunctional heart may retain a substantial degree of compliance, lessening the chance of an audible filling sound even if LV filling pressures are elevated. In more advanced stages of disease, evidence of impaired peripheral or end-organ perfusion may be present, such as jaundice, cool extremities, delayed capillary refill, or decreased intensity of peripheral pulses. These symptoms are typically accompanied by unequivocal symptoms or other suggestive cardiopulmonary signs of cardiac disease.

Laboratory and Diagnostic Procedures

The chest radiography and 12-lead electrocardiography are simple, rapid, and low-risk procedures that can frequently add to the initial diagnostic impression. Depending on the degree of cardiac chamber dilation, the radiographic cardiac silhouette may be variably affected. The LV silhouette is most often enlarged in patients with slowly progressive disease, because the LV chamber has had an opportunity to dilate significantly, whereas in instances of acute onset (e.g., acute myocardial infarction without antecedent disease), the LV may appear normal sized. Patients with chronic valvular or coronary atherosclerotic disease may also demonstrate calcification that can be detected on plain chest films. The presence of intraalveolar pulmonary edema typically is easily detected on standard chest radiographs, although pulmonary interstitial edema can be much more subtle and difficult to discern. More commonly, in patients with chronic LV dysfunction and resultant secondary postcapillary pulmonary hypertension, the central pulmonary arteries are dilated and more prominent than normal. However, patients with chronically elevated left atrial pressure may not manifest traditional evidence of decompensated hemodynamics (e.g., pulmonary rales on examination or infiltrative changes on chest radiography), due to increased pulmonary lymphatic capacity and thickened alveolar-capillary interface.

Many electrocardiographic abnormalities associated with heart failure are nonspecific. Because the most common cause of heart failure is coronary artery disease, any indication of ongoing myocardial ischemia or pattern of prior infarction or injury should prompt further intensive evaluation. The presence of arrhythmias, especially those of ventricular origin, also suggests underlying organic cardiac disease.

Standard laboratory results are typically nonspecific but in more advanced cases can yield findings of impaired end-organ perfusion, such as elevations in serum urea nitrogen, creatinine, or liver transaminases. Patients with chronic heart failure may also be anemic and may manifest other chemical evidence of malnutrition or chronic disease. However, patients who have progressed to this degree of impairment typically have a host of other symptoms and signs that point unequivocally to a severe heart failure syndrome. More recently, the presence of elevated levels of plasma brain natriuretic peptide has been associated with cardiac disease in patients with dyspnea. This test has gained increasing popularity as an initial diagnostic tool, although its utility in the diagnosis of nondecompensated heart failure remains to be fully elucidated.

Transthoracic echocardiography has emerged as the most common method of definitively diagnosing LV systolic dysfunction. It is typically available at short notice in most clinical settings and can provide a wealth of structural and functional data in a noninvasive fashion. After the history, physical examination, and standard laboratory studies discussed earlier, echocardiography should be the next diagnostic study performed if cardiac dysfunction is suspected. Although a complete review of the echocardiographic findings typically seen in heart failure is beyond the scope of this discussion, standard studies can establish the diagnosis, provide clues to the underlying etiology, and help guide initial therapy. Moreover, an echocardiographic study obtained at initial diagnosis establishes an important baseline data set to which subsequent studies can be compared to gauge the efficacy of therapy and assist in determining prognosis.

Once the diagnosis of LV systolic dysfunction has been established, an effort should be made to determine the underlying etiology, because it may dictate therapy. Cardiac catheterization, including coronary angiography and right heart catheterization for hemodynamic assessment, should be strongly considered in all patients with newly diagnosed LV systolic dysfunction, because

noncontracting or poorly contracting myocardium, if ischemic or hibernating (viable but hypoperfused), may regain contractile strength after proper revascularization. In addition, hemodynamic data obtained during catheterization can assist in guiding medical and surgical therapy for heart failure; moreover, like other initial imaging studies, it can provide valuable baseline information for future comparison. The use of supplemental catheter-based procedures such as endomyocardial biopsy remains controversial, predominantly because of the risk associated with these procedures and the variable sensitivity of routine endomyocardial biopsy in the diagnosis of infiltrative myocardial processes such as myocarditis. In specific cases in which the index of suspicion for certain infiltrative diseases is particularly high, biopsy may be used to confirm the diagnosis. If this procedure is employed, it is important that a sufficient volume and distribution of specimens be collected to optimize diagnostic yield, and that the procedure be performed by an experienced operator to minimize the risk of complications.

Provocative testing (e.g., treadmill exercise testing), with or without supplemental imaging modalities such as radionuclide perfusion imaging, is less useful in patients with already established cardiac dysfunction, although the response to exercise testing in a patient with previously undiagnosed heart failure can be revealing. In addition to the likely finding of decreased exercise performance, the blood pressure and heart rate response to increasing exercise demand may be impaired. Further scrutiny (e.g., cardiac catheterization) should follow the demonstration of inducible or fixed myocardial perfusion defects with exercise or of a decreased left ventricular ejection fraction (LVEF). Resting radionuclide ventriculography can also be employed to determine global LV systolic function (LVEF) in patients in whom effective imaging cannot be achieved with echocardiography. Exercise testing with expired gas analysis may be used to determine peak exercise oxygen consumption and has been demonstrated to correlate with prognosis in patients with chronic heart failure. However, its value when measured before optimization of therapy in patients with newly diagnosed heart failure is uncertain.

Classification

Patients with heart failure are classified according to their self-described degree of functional impairment and assigned a New York Heart Association (NYHA) functional class (Table 1). Although it is subjective on the part of both the patient and the interviewer, this classification has long been used for gross estimation of functional status. The NYHA class has been reported to correlate with mortality risk, but its ability to discriminate among patients and its relevance in an individual patient over time remains questionable.

Heart failure can also be classified by evolutionary stage (Table 2), based predominantly on management strategy (pharmacologic, nonpharmacologic, or surgical).

Management of Heart Failure
Nonpharmacologic Therapy

Nonpharmacologic heart failure therapy reduces symptoms and improves functional capacity and quality of life. It is vital to provide ongoing patient and family education about dietary restrictions, avoidance of unhealthy behaviors, stress reduction, and energy

TABLE 1	New York Heart Association Functional Classification of Chronic Heart Failure
CLASS*	**SYMPTOMS**
I	No perceived limitation of physical activity
II A/B	Symptoms with moderate physical exertion
III A/B	Symptoms with low levels of physical exertion (i.e., activities of daily living)
IV	Resting symptoms

*Abbreviations: A = early stage; B = late stage.

TABLE 2	Stages of Heart Failure	
STAGE	**DESCRIPTION**	**EXAMPLES**
A	High risk for development of HF due to presence of conditions strongly associated with HF development No identified structural or functional abnormalities of the pericardium, myocardium, or cardiac valves No history of signs or symptoms of HF	Systemic hypertension Coronary artery disease Diabetes mellitus Prior cardiac drug therapy Prior alcohol abuse Family history of cardiomyopathy
B	Presence of structural heart disease strongly associated with HF development No history of signs or symptoms of HF	LV hypertrophy or fibrosis LV dilation or dysfunction Asymptomatic valvular heart disease Previous myocardial infarction
C	Current or prior symptoms of HF with underlying structural heart disease	Dyspnea or fatigue from LV systolic dysfunction Asymptomatic patient undergoing treatment for prior symptoms of HF
D	Advanced structural heart disease and marked symptoms of HF at rest despite maximal medical therapy Requirement for specialized interventions	Frequent HF hospitalizations and cannot be discharged In hospital awaiting heart transplantation Home continuous inotropic or mechanical support In hospice setting for HF management

Abbreviations: HF = heart failure; LV = left ventricular.

conservation. Participation in an exercise program to combat deconditioning and promote weight loss improves functional capacity. Close outpatient monitoring, including a heart failure disease management program, improves compliance and reduces hospitalization. Identification and treatment of sleep-disordered breathing, present in as many as 40% of patients with heart failure, can dramatically improve symptoms.

Pharmacologic Therapy

Angiotensin-converting enzyme (ACE) inhibitors and selected β-blockers have been shown in randomized clinical trials to improve symptoms and survival in patients with LV systolic dysfunction and are the cornerstones of medical therapy for heart failure. Angiotensin receptor blocking agents, or the combination of hydralazine (Apresoline)[1] and a nitrate, provide similar (but not superior) benefit in patients with contraindications to use of ACE inhibitors. Digoxin (Lanoxin) provides no survival benefit but improves symptoms and hemodynamics in patients with atrial fibrillation and in those patients who remain symptomatic on optimal doses of vasodilators and may also decrease risk for hospitalization. Diuretics provide symptomatic relief if volume overload is present. Antialdosterone agents should be prescribed for all patients with symptomatic LV dysfunction after acute myocardial infarction. For all other heart failure patients, spironolactone was previously reserved for those who remained symptomatic despite optimal doses of vasodilator and β-blocker therapy, but new data suggests that all symptomatic patients benefit from antialdosterone therapy (NYHA functional class II-IV symptoms). Antiarrhythmics should be used only for symptomatic atrial or ventricular arrhythmias, because they may be proarrhythmic. Table 3 describes the use of various medications in patients with heart failure.

Parenteral agents for heart failure, including dobutamine (Dobutrex), milrinone (Primacor), and nesiritide (Natrecor), are used primarily in the inpatient setting to treat acutely decompensated heart failure and are beyond the scope of this discussion. However, it should be noted that intravenous inotropic agents (dobutamine, milrinone) have been shown in uncontrolled trials to improve symptoms and quality of life but to increase mortality. Therefore, they should be used only for short periods, at the lowest possible doses, and in a monitored setting. Short-term inpatient use of nesiritide also improves symptoms.

Device Therapy

Implantable cardioverter-defibrillators (ICDs) have been shown in randomized clinical trials to improve survival in heart failure patients with ischemic or nonischemic cardiomyopathy. Indications for implantation are an LVEF of less than 30% and mild-to-moderate symptoms of heart failure in a patient whose anticipated survival exceeds 1 year or ischemic cardiomyopathy and an LVEF of less than 35% regardless of symptoms.

Cardiac resynchronization therapy, with or without implantation of a cardioverter-defibrillator, has been shown in randomized clinical trials to improve symptoms and survival in selected heart failure patients when added to optimal medical heart failure therapy. One third of heart failure patients with low LVEF and moderate to severe symptoms have ventricular dyssynchronous contraction, which is associated with increased mortality. Indications for cardiac resynchronization therapy include an LVEF lower than 35%, NYHA functional class II-IV symptoms, and a QRS duration of greater than 120 msec, which is a marker for ventricular dyssynchrony.

Therapy for Advanced Heart Failure

Patients with heart failure that has become refractory to medical and resynchronization therapy should be referred to an advanced heart failure center experienced in the surgical treatment of heart failure. Surgical therapies improve symptoms and survival and are now considered the standard of care for heart failure patients in whom standard medical therapy has failed.

Heart transplantation is the only definitive surgical therapy for advanced heart failure, but alternative surgical approaches include coronary revascularization, valve surgery, LV reconstruction, and the use of ventricular assist devices. In patients with ischemic cardiomyopathy and hibernating myocardium, coronary revascularization improves LV function, functional capacity, and survival, compared with medical therapy. Mitral valve repair or replacement can improve symptoms in selected patients. Ventricular reconstruction may benefit patients with LV aneurysms or recurrent ventricular arrhythmias.

Left ventricular assist devices are implantable pumps that work in parallel with the native heart to provide short-term mechanical circulatory support in patients who are expected to recover heart function (e.g., patients with myocarditis, after acute myocardial infarction, after coronary artery bypass grafting) and in patients awaiting heart transplantation. In addition, these devices are approved as a permanent alternative to transplantation (destination therapy) in patients for whom heart transplantation is not an option. Early identification and referral of patients who might benefit from these therapies is essential for the best surgical outcomes.

---

[1]Not FDA approved for this indication.

TABLE 3	Heart Failure Medications	
DRUG CLASS	**NAME/DOSE**	**COMMENTS**
ACEIs (in enalapril [Vasotec] equivalents)	10–20 mg bid	Likely a class effect, so agent choice depends on duration of action and tolerability. Higher doses decrease hospitalization rates. Hyperkalemia limits use. Reduced doses may be necessary to allow adequate β-blocker dose titration.
Angiotensin receptor blockers	Valsartan (Diovan) 40–160 mg bid Candesartan (Atacand) 4–32 mg/d	The only two agents in this class to show benefit in randomized clinical trials. Good for patients intolerant of ACEIs. Noninferior but not superior to ACEIs, so use second line. Hyperkalemia limits use.
Hydralazine and nitrates	Hydralazine (Apresoline)[1] 25–100 mg qid with isosorbide dinitrate (Isordil Titradose)[1] 20–40 mg qid	Agents of choice in patients with significant renal insufficiency or other contraindications to ACEIs or aldosterone receptor antagonists.
β-Blockers	Metoprolol succinate (Toprol XL) 100–200 mg/d Carvedilol (Coreg) 25–50 mg bid Bisoprolol (Zebeta)[1] 2.5–10 mg/d	The only three agents in this class to show benefit in randomized clinical trials. Dose is based on body size. Some clinical and survival improvement with lower doses, but target dose is recommended.
Loop diuretics (expressed as furosemide [Lasix] equivalents)	40–100 mg qd or bid	Dietary compliance, fluid restriction, and titration of other heart failure drugs affect dose required.
Aldosterone receptor antagonists	Spironolactone (Aldactone) 12.5–25 mg/d Eplerenone (Inspra) 25–50 mg/d	For patients who remain NYHA functional class III despite adequate doses of vasodilators and β-blockers. Hyperkalemia limits use. For patients with left ventricular dysfunction after acute myocardial infarction. Fewer side effects than spironolactone. Hyperkalemia limits use.
Digoxin (Lanoxin)	0.125–0.25 mg/d	Adjust for renal insufficiency. Women need lower doses. Serum level measurement not routinely necessary; only to confirm toxicity.

Abbreviations: ACEI = angiotensin-converting enzyme inhibitor; NYHA = New York Heart Association.
[1]Not FDA approved for this indication.

Common Management Errors

Heart failure management errors result in increased hospitalizations and mortality. ACE inhibitors remain underused, despite evidence from clinical trials in more than 10,000 patients. Although Losartan (Cozaar)[1] is commonly used for the patient who cannot tolerate ACE inhibitors, only two members of the angiotensin receptor blocker class, valsartan (Diovan) and candesartan (Atacand), have been shown in clinical trials to provide benefit. The combination of hydralazine (Apresoline)[1] and isosorbide dinitrate (Isordil Titradose)[1] is also underused, despite evidence that these drugs improve exercise tolerance and survival.

Only three β-blockers, metoprolol succinate (Toprol XL), carvedilol (Coreg), and bisoprolol (Zebeta),[1] have been shown in trials to improve symptoms and survival in heart failure patients. Metoprolol tartrate (Lopressor)[1] and atenolol (Tenormin)[1] are commonly used as substitutes, even though there are no data supporting their use. β-Blockers are commonly started too early in the course of heart failure, when the patient is experiencing decompensation and fluid overload, and lead to further decompensation. Care should be taken to fully optimize volume status and unloading agents (e.g., vasodilators), before initiating and titrating β-blockers.

Patients may receive drugs that worsen the heart failure state, such as first-generation calcium channel blockers, nonsteroidal antiinflammatory drugs, cyclooxygenase 2 inhibitors, and antiarrhythmic drugs. Intravenous inotropic therapy or nesiritide (Natrecor) may be used when the patient would be better served by optimization of his or her oral heart failure regimen. Patients are commonly overdiuresed, which results in symptomatic hypotension and makes initiation and titration of vasodilators and β-blockers difficult.

Many physicians fail to utilize nonpharmacologic therapies as an adjunct to drug therapy. In addition, lack of education and close follow-up can undermine the best medical regimen. Physicians also commonly fail to refer patients who need advanced heart failure therapy, or refer them too late, when end-organ damage is irreversible.

References

Bardy GH, Lee KL, Mark DB, et al. Amiodarone or an implantable cardioverter defibrillator for congestive heart failure. N Engl J Med 2005;352:225–37.

Cleland JG, Daubert JC, Erdmann E, et al. The effect of cardiac resynchronization on morbidity and mortality in heart failure. N Engl J Med 2005;352:1539–49.

Cohn JN, Archibald DG, Ziesche S, et al. Effect of vasodilator therapy on mortality in chronic congestive heart failure: Results of a Veterans Administration Cooperative Study. N Engl J Med 1986;314:1547–52.

Cohn JN, Johnson G, Ziesche S, et al. A comparison of enalapril with hydralazine-isosorbide dinitrate in the treatment of chronic congestive heart failure. N Engl J Med 1991;325:303–10.

The Digitalis Investigation Group. Effect of digoxin on mortality and morbidity in patients with heart failure. N Engl J Med 1997;336:525–33.

Hunt SA, Abraham WT, Chin MH, et al. ACC/AHA 2005 Guideline Update for the Diagnosis and Management of Chronic Heart Failure in the Adult: A report of the American College of Cardiology/American Heart Association Task Force on Practice Guidelines (Writing Committee to Update the 2001 Guidelines for the Evaluation and Management of Heart Failure). Developed in collaboration with the American College of Chest Physicians and the International Society for Heart and Lung Transplantation; endorsed by the Heart Rhythm Society. Circulation 2005;112:e154–235.

International Registry for Heart and Lung Transplantation (ISHLT Registry). Available at: https://www.ishlt.org/registries/heartLungRegistry.asp; July 16, 2015, Accessed.

Metoprolol CR/XL Randomized Intervention Trial in Congestive Heart Failure (MERIT-HF). Effect of metoprolol CR/XL in chronic heart failure. Lancet 1999;353:2001–7.

Moss AJ, et al. Cardic resynchronization therapy for the prevention of heart failure events. N Engl J Med 2009;361:1329–38.

Packer M, Bristow MR, Cohn JN, et al. The effect of carvedilol on morbidity and mortality in patients with chronic heart failure. U.S. Carvedilol Heart Failure Study Group. N Engl J Med 1996;334:1349–55.

[1]Not FDA approved for this indication.

Pitt B, Zannad F, Remme WJ, et al. The effect of spironolactone on morbidity and mortality in patients with severe heart failure. Randomized Aldactone Evaluation Study Investigators. N Engl J Med 1999;341:709–17.

Rose EA, Gelijns AC, Moskowitz AJ, et al. Long-term mechanical left ventricular assistance for end-stage heart failure. N Engl J Med 2001;345:1435–43.

The SOLVD Investigators. Effect of enalapril on mortality and the development of heart failure in asymptomatic patients with reduced left ventricular ejection fractions. N Engl J Med 1992;327:685–91.

Zannad F, et al. Eplerenone in patients with systolic heart failure and mild symptoms. N Engl J Med 2011;364:11–21.

HEART BLOCK

Method of
Kelley P. Anderson, MD

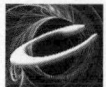

CURRENT DIAGNOSIS

- Assess risk for heart block in the absence of symptoms or heart block on electrocardiogram (ECG).
  - Review cardiac or systemic disorders associated with cardiac conduction disease (CCD), ECG pattern, family history, maternal antibodies, cardiac interventions, and surgery.
- Evaluate documented asystole or bradycardia due to heart block.
  - Classify heart block: transient, recurrent, progressive, permanent.
  - Grade signs and symptoms: none, mild, severe.
- Evaluate signs or symptoms of possible transient heart block with no documentation.
  - Establish temporal pattern: recent versus remote onset, solitary versus recurrent, daily, weekly, monthly, yearly.
  - Grade signs and symptoms: none, mild, severe.
  - Document rhythm during symptoms: telemetry monitoring, Holter monitor, external loop recorder, implantable recorder.

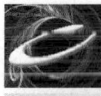

CURRENT THERAPY

- Methods of heart rate support:
  - Immediate: intravenous catecholamines, atropine, or aminophylline[1]; transcutaneous pacing.
  - Short term: transvenous temporary pacing
  - Long term: permanent pacemakers.
- Pacemaker configuration:
  - Number of leads: 1, 2, 3, 4.
  - Lead locations: right atrial appendage, Bachman's bundle, right ventricular apex, outflow tract, left ventricle, coronary sinus.
  - Programming to minimize ventricular pacing: manufacturer dependent.

[1]Not FDA approved for this indication.

Heart block refers to block or delay of electrical propagation between the atria and ventricles. It is a form of cardiac conduction disease (CCD), which applies more generally to disorders of electrical impulse formation or propagation anywhere along the cardiac conduction system from the sinus node to the ventricular myocardium. Heart block or CCD may present as a syndrome, as an electrocardiographic (ECG) pattern, or as a mechanism of serious signs and symptoms such as sudden death or syncope. Pacemaker therapy is an effective treatment, but it is associated with significant short- and long-term complications. This underscores the importance of recognizing preventable and reversible causes of heart block for accurate targeting of permanent pacing. Risk stratification of patients with heart block, assessment of the benefits and risks of the therapeutic options, and patient education and guidance are largely in the domain of heart rhythm specialists. However, heart block may be encountered unexpectedly in any patient during any clinical encounter. Furthermore, some patients may require evaluation in the absence of known cardiac disease because of increased risk of CCD, or increased risk of CCD in family members or future children. A basic understanding of heart block may be useful in order to initiate emergency treatment and to recognize patients who warrant further evaluation or specialist referral.

Epidemiology

The prevalence and incidence of heart block are difficult to establish because they are strongly dependent on the demographic and clinical characteristics of the population sample. The prevalence is higher among the elderly and those with cardiovascular disease. First-degree heart block, defined as prolongation of the PR interval >200 ms on ECG, occurs in the population setting with prevalence of 0.7% to 2% in the young and up to 14% in the elderly. Higher degrees of heart block can be expected to be less common but similarly associated with age and underlying cardiovascular disease. In a study of the Framingham population, the prevalence of first-degree heart block was 1.6% and was associated with an incidence of pacemaker implantation of 59 per 10,000 person-years in persons with a PR interval >200 ms compared to 6 per 10,000 person-years in persons with a PR interval <200 ms. Approximately 36% of the pacemakers were for high-grade atrioventricular (AV) block.

Risk Factors

Patients with genetic or acquired CCD and patients subject to trauma or surgical procedures that can damage the conduction system are at increased risk for developing symptomatic advanced heart block. In the Framingham population, subjects with first-degree AV block had an increased risk of mortality, atrial fibrillation, and pacemaker implantation. However, the vast majority with risk factors never develop symptomatic heart block and have not been shown to benefit from intense monitoring or prophylactic pacemaker placement. The few possible exceptions are discussed below.

Pathophysiology

The function of the cardiac conduction system is to initiate and coordinate cardiac contraction in order to circulate blood according to physiologic needs. Electrical activation is initiated by pacemaker cells of the sinus node regulated by the autonomic nervous system. Unlike conduction in common electrical circuits in which electrons flow along a conductor according to the voltage gradient, electrical activity in cardiac cells propagates from segment to segment of the cell membrane in cardiac myocytes (myocardial cells) and in specialized cardiac conduction cells. Energy-requiring ion pumps maintain an electrochemical gradient across the insulating cell membrane. Electrical activity opens voltage-sensitive ion channels causing regenerative electrical activity as ions shift along their electrochemical gradient. Electrical activity in a single cell excites several adjacent cells via gap junctions. This cascade effect makes it possible for a single cell impulse to spread rapidly throughout the myocardium to enhance synchronous contraction. This also provides a safety mechanism in that each myocardial cell can be activated by many electrical paths. In addition, specialized conduction cells exhibit automaticity (impulse formation). Although normally latent because normal activation inhibits spontaneous discharge, when the normal impulse is blocked, discharges from these subsidiary physiologic pacemakers provide vital heart rate support.

Block of electrical activation can occur due to failure of any step in the process, for example, lack of metabolic energy, electrolyte imbalance, inflammatory disruption of the membrane, block of

| **TABLE 1** | Mechanisms of Conduction Disturbances (Examples) |

- Prolonged refractory period (vagal activity, drugs, ischemia)
- Sarcolemmal ion gradient disturbances (hyperkalemia, hypokalemia)
- Sodium channel dysfunction (SCN5A mutations, sodium channel blocking drugs such as lidocaine, procainamide, flecainide [Tambocor], amiodarone [Cordarone], and imipramine [Tofranil])
- Calcium channel dysfunction (verapamil [Isoptin], diltiazem [Cardizem], mutations)
- Energy deprivation (ischemia, cyanide)
- Cell dysfunction (inflammation, barotrauma, thermal injury)
- Cell death (apoptosis, ischemic necrosis, inflammatory necrosis, surgical trauma, ablation)
- Congenital structural defects (endocardial cushion defects)
- Gap junction disturbances (fibrosis, edema, inflammation, genetic defects)
- Genetic defects (SCN5A and NKX2.5 mutations)

| **TABLE 2** | Etiologies of Heart Block |

- Frequently permanent or progressive (examples)
  - Alcohol septal ablation (acute, delayed)
  - Cardiomyopathies (hypertrophic, idiopathic, mitochondrial)
  - Catheter ablation (atrioventricular nodal reentry, accessory atrioventricular connections)
  - Congenital heart block (neonatal lupus)
  - Congenital heart disease (endocardial cushion defects)
  - Genetic disorders (SCN5A sodium channel mutations, gap junction gene mutations, fatty acid oxidation disorders, PRKAG2 mutations, LMNA gene mutations)
  - Hypertension
  - Idiopathic fibrosis and calcification (Lev's disease, Lenegre's disease)
  - Infectious disorders—destructive (endocarditis)
  - Infiltrative disorders (amyloidosis)
  - Myocardial infarction
  - Neuromyopathic disorders (myotonic dystrophy, Erb's dystrophy, peroneal muscular atrophy)
  - Noninfectious inflammatory disorders (HLA-B27–associated disorder, sarcoidosis)
  - Tumors (mesothelioma, metastatic cancer)
  - Valvular heart disease
- Frequently transient or reversible (examples)
  - Blunt trauma (baseball)
  - Cardiac surgery (valve replacement)
  - Cardiac transplant rejection
  - Central nervous system
  - Drugs (antiarrhythmics, digoxin [Lanoxin], edrophonium [Enlon])
  - Electrolyte disturbances (hyperkalemia)
  - Metabolic disturbances (hypothermia, hypothyroidism)
  - Increased vagal activity
  - Infectious disorders—nondestructive (Lyme disease)
  - Myocardial ischemia
  - Myocarditis (Chagas disease, giant cell myocarditis)
  - Rheumatic fever

ion channels by drugs, or interference with gap junction function due to infiltration of fibrous tissue (Table 1). Because of the extensive redundancy and interconnectivity and because of the capacity to compensate for injury by electrical and anatomic remodeling, there may be extensive damage before signs or symptoms of heart block occur. Regions of the heart where there are fewer alternative paths for electrical activation, such as proximal portions of the His-Purkinje system where all conducting fibers are confined to a relatively small area, are more vulnerable to complete block. Subsidiary pacemakers sometimes fail to provide adequate rate support when heart block occurs because of preexisting injury. If the patient survives an episode of heart block, there is a possibility for recovery due to remodeling. However, remodeling can be maladaptive and result in an adverse long-term outcome by further conduction system damage, by left ventricular dysfunction, and by bradycardia-induced ventricular tachyarrhythmias (VTAs). The mechanisms of bradycardia-induced VTAs are not known, but bradyarrhythmias precipitate torsades de pointes, a specific form of VTA, in the presence of drugs that block potassium channels, electrolyte disturbances, certain genetic abnormalities of ion channel function, heart failure, and myocardial hypertrophy. A comprehensive list of drugs that may account for bradyarrhythmia-related ventricular arrhythmias is available at www.torsades.org.

Although there are many potential causes of heart block, the pathophysiology is not known for the vast majority of cases because there are no tests that allow detailed structural or functional examination in patients. By the time of death, morphologic examination may reveal only nonspecific changes such as fibrosis. Instead, most etiologies are inferred by history of recent or past exposures (e.g., trauma or radiation), concomitant disorders (e.g., muscular dystrophy, cardiac sarcoidosis), abnormal test results (e.g., Lyme disease) or family history (e.g., SCN5A sodium channel mutations) (Table 2). Because most etiologies cannot be verified, the clinician must remain open to alternative explanations and accept the likelihood of multiple contributors.

Some patients, usually young, otherwise healthy individuals, present with prolonged asystole due to heart block but have no other detectable abnormalities and have excellent outcomes in the absence of intervention beyond counseling. This suggests that autonomic influences alone can cause prolonged heart block and suppression of subsidiary pacemakers. It is not known if such responses result from an abnormality or an exaggerated normal reflex. However, the identification of such patients is important because the majority can be managed without pacemakers.

Prevention

Prevention of heart block is a challenge for the future. Some instances can be prevented by treatment of inflammatory disorders that cause heart block, such as Lyme disease or cardiac sarcoid. Other individuals who should be identified are those with conditions that place them, their relatives, or their unborn children at

risk for heart block. This includes patients and family members with genetic disorders associated with heart block. Genetic testing and counseling may be appropriate in some patients with a family history of CCD. Neonatal lupus syndrome is a rare disorder with a high mortality rate and risk of permanent complete heart block in survivors. This occurs in pregnant women with anti-Ro/SSA and/or anti-La/SSB antibodies. Some such women have autoimmune disorders such as systemic lupus erythematosus and Sjögren's syndrome, but many are asymptomatic. Members of this group may benefit from counseling and anticipatory evaluation and treatment of offspring. Although controversial, fetal monitoring of pregnant women with anti-Ro/SSA and/or anti-La/SSB antibodies and treatment of those with signs of fetal conduction system involvement have been recommended. It should be recognized that with current methods the vast majority of heart block events cannot be predicted or prevented and the vast majority of persons with risk factors never develop symptomatic heart block.

Clinical Manifestations

Most of the symptoms experienced by patients with heart block are common and nonspecific, including syncope, lightheadedness, fatigue, and dyspnea. Asystole or profound bradycardia may cause syncope, death, or other manifestations of hypoperfusion. Rarely, first-degree AV block results in significant symptoms (e.g., fatigue, palpitations, chest fullness) probably due to atrial contraction against a partially closed mitral valve.

Diagnosis

Because various arrhythmias and other cardiac and noncardiac disorders may be responsible for similar symptoms, it is important to identify the cause. An ECG recording of asystole or bradycardia due to heart block at the time of symptoms strongly suggests a causal relationship, but this is usually difficult to accomplish as the symptoms are often transient and infrequent. Absence of arrhythmias at the time of symptoms is also helpful in excluding heart block as the cause. Asymptomatic heart block is not infrequent. Cardiac conduction disturbances are classified by the pattern of ECG complexes. A normal 12-lead ECG lessens the probability of conduction disturbances due to structural changes but it does not eliminate the possibility of transient third-degree block due to reversible functional effects such as intense vagal activity or ischemia. Significant disease of the His bundle may be electrocardiographically silent, but more often concomitant distal disease is evident in the form of fascicular or bundle branch block or a nonspecific intraventricular conduction delay. In a patient with syncope, the presence of bifascicular block raises the possibility of transient third-degree block as the mechanism and of progression to permanent complete block. Most patients with conduction disorders are not symptomatic and do not progress to complete block. However, the combination of right bundle branch block (RBBB) and left posterior fascicle block has a greater tendency to progress to complete block than the more common RBBB and left anterior fascicle block. Nevertheless, conduction disturbances of the His-Purkinje system should not be assumed to be responsible for syncope or cardiac arrest because they are relatively common in patients with cardiovascular disorders that cause syncope or cardiac arrest due to other mechanisms. Conduction disturbances can cause dyssynchronous contraction and result in adverse remodeling. In addition, they can mask or mimic the ECG signs of myocardial infarction. Alternating bundle branch block refers to a changing ECG pattern in which both RBBB and left bundle branch block are observed or when the bifascicular block pattern switches between the anterior and posterior fascicle involvement. This pattern is considered a harbinger of complete block and warrants continuous monitoring and evaluation for permanent pacemaker implantation.

Differential Diagnosis

The challenge in second- and transient third-degree AV block is distinguishing between block in the AV node, which is often functional and reversible, and infranodal block, which often progresses to permanent complete heart block. ECG clues that block is in the AV node include normal QRS duration (<100 ms), type I (Wenckebach) pattern, PR prolongation before blocked impulses and PR shortening after pauses, occurrence during enhanced vagal activity (e.g., sleep), narrow QRS escape complexes, and no factors favoring infranodal block. ECG clues for infranodal block include prolonged QRS duration (≥ 120 ms), type II pattern, and escape QRS complexes broader than intrinsic complexes. Type II second degree AV block is almost always due to block in the His-Purkinje system. Other second-degree AV block ECG patterns have poor sensitivity and specificity for site of block.

Unsustained polymorphic ventricular tachycardia is an ominous sign in any context and may result from a variety of cardiac, metabolic, and autonomic abnormalities. However, in the presence of heart block it suggests that heart rate support may be necessary to prevent sustained VTA. QT prolongation and post-pause U-wave accentuation should be sought as other harbingers of bradycardia-related VTA.

The importance and value of ECG documentation of heart block cannot be overemphasized. ECGs are subject to artifact and may be misleading when standards for acquisition and analysis are not followed. Multiple tracings of suspicious events should be obtained in multiple leads when possible. A 12-lead simultaneous rhythm recording mode is available on most modern ECG machines and should be used when continuous recordings are obtained to document arrhythmias.

Clinicians encounter heart block in three general contexts. For the patient with documented heart block, the clinician selects therapy based, in part, on whether or not the arrhythmia is permanent or likely to recur. There are currently no tests that provide direct information about the pathologic state of the AV conduction system. Instead, these outcomes must be inferred from functional assessment, that is, from the ECG or electrophysiologic testing.

Other indirect sources such as coronary angiography, magnetic resonance imaging, nuclear imaging, and myocardial biopsy, as well as a large number of specific laboratory tests, are often helpful for identifying disorders that may be causative or associated with heart block and that may affect the choice of treatment.

Another common context is the patient with symptoms for whom the objective is to verify or exclude heart block as the mechanism by correlating the cardiac rhythm with symptoms. Real-time monitoring (e.g., in-patient telemetry) is used for patients who might require immediate access to drugs or pacing devices to prevent or terminate asystole or bradycardia-dependent VTA. Holter monitoring is useful for patients who have very frequent events (at least 1 every 24 hours), and they are useful for capturing asymptomatic rhythm disturbances. External recorders are applied for a month or longer and are very helpful to associate rhythm abnormalities with symptoms and to rule out a rhythm disorder as the cause of symptoms in patients with at least one event per month. Patients with infrequent events may be candidates for implantable loop recorders, which monitor for greater than a year. Modern monitors will provide a permanent record of arrhythmias on activation by the patient or by a detection algorithm.

Electrophysiologic studies allow precise measurements of AV node and His-Purkinje system function and can provide definitive information regarding the site of block if the conduction disturbance occurs during the study. Additional tests have been developed that "stress" the AV conduction system, including rapid atrial and ventricular pacing and administration of drugs such as procainamide and disopyramide (Norpace). The provocation of heart block is assumed to indicate a propensity for spontaneous AV block. Unfortunately, the sensitivity is low and a negative test does not imply a low risk of future episodes. Electrophysiologic studies have the additional advantage of providing immediate test results, as well as providing the results of programmed stimulation for provocation of supraventricular and VTAs, which may be included in the differential diagnosis.

Therapy

The object of the evaluation and management for heart block is to prevent death and morbidity by (1) heart rate support in patients with poorly tolerated bradycardia; (2) monitoring and standby heart rate support in patients at high risk for asystole or severe bradycardia; (3) identifying and treating reversible causes of heart block; (4) identifying patients at high risk for sudden death, syncope, or recurrent symptoms; and (5) selecting and implanting the appropriate rate support system as soon as safety permits.

Advanced cardiac life-support guidelines apply to the patient who is unresponsive or severely compromised by heart block. However, heart block is rarely the primary problem. Therefore, evaluation and treatment of other disorders should continue while efforts to obtain the appropriate heart rate are underway.

The initial evaluation should include a detailed history and physical examination and review of current and previous ECGs and rhythm strips to determine if heart block is present or occurred in the past and if there were symptoms or other evidence of hemodynamic compromise. Basic laboratory tests (electrolytes, metabolic panel, cardiac biomarkers, thyroid function, blood count, and coagulation studies) and basic imaging (chest x-ray and echocardiography) are usually appropriate. The patient should then be stratified for the appropriate level of care: (1) the unstable patient who requires ongoing evaluation and treatment in an intensive care setting, (2) the stable patient at high risk for asystole or complications who needs temporary transvenous pacing or other invasive procedures, (3) the patient at moderate risk who requires continuous monitoring and standby noninvasive heart rate support measures, (4) the patient at low risk who requires rapid but not immediate access to heart rate support measures that hospital monitoring provides, and (5) the patient at low risk who can be evaluated and managed as an outpatient. Additional testing and procedures may be necessary to determine the etiology of heart block and to determine if there is a significant risk of future adverse events.

Determination of the need for long-term heart rate support, as well as other issues that may affect implantable device selection (e.g., risk for VTAs), should be accomplished as soon as possible because the risk of complications and anxiety associated with temporary heart rate support measures increases over time. Major societies have developed guidelines for implantable rhythm management devices (http://www.cardiosource.org/Science-And-Quality/Practice-Guidelines-and-Quality-Standards.aspx; http://www.escardio.org/guidelines-surveys/esc-guidelines/Pages/GuidelinesList.aspx). The reasons for the selected therapy, including the rationale for any deviation from established guidelines, should be documented and provided to the patient. This will reduce future confusion or misunderstanding about the original rationale for implantation that can affect management of patients with device complications, recalls (safety alerts), and those with a compelling need for device upgrade or explanation.

Patients with acute coronary syndromes require special consideration. The incidence of heart block in patients with myocardial infarction based on creatine phosphokinase as the marker of necrosis is approximately 10%. Although the incidence is probably lower using more sensitive markers such as troponin, heart block is still likely to be associated with increased in-hospital mortality due to larger infarct size. Tachycardia and high blood pressure increase myocardial oxygen consumption. Therefore, overcorrection of heart rate and blood pressure should be avoided and ischemia should be relieved by reperfusion as soon as possible. Studies in the prethrombolytic era did not demonstrate a benefit in mortality with prophylactic temporary transvenous pacing, and complications were frequent. The risks of transvenous insertion may be higher in patients requiring administration of thrombolytics and other anticoagulants. Catheter-based revascularization methods should be given strong consideration because of established effectiveness, the possible avoidance of thrombolytic drugs, and because transvenous temporary pacing, if needed, is readily and safely accomplished during the procedure. Suggestions for standby temporary pacing (Table 3) should take into consideration the risks of transvenous pacing based on local circumstances (experience, fluoroscopic guidance, insertion site, use of anticoagulants, etc.). Most conduction disturbances associated with myocardial ischemia or infarction resolve quickly but can persist for days or weeks. The need for permanent pacemaker implantation as a consequence of myocardial infarction is rare, and prophylactic pacemaker implantation in high-risk subsets has not been shown to reduce mortality. Guidelines for temporary and permanent pacing in acute myocardial infarction have been published (http://www.cardiosource.org/Science-And-Quality/Practice-Guidelines-and-Quality-Standards.aspx; http://www.escardio.org/guidelines-surveys/esc-guidelines/Pages/GuidelinesList.aspx).

Selection of the correct therapeutic approach balances the risks and benefits of therapy against the risks of heart block for both immediate and long-term management. Catecholamines (dobutamine, dopamine, epinephrine, isoproterenol [Isuprel]) are useful for emergency, temporary, and standby heart rate support. The standby mode is accomplished by a prepared infusion at the bedside. To avoid underdoses or overdoses at the time of sudden symptomatic heart block, the optimal dose can be established in advance by test doses starting at low infusion rates. Atropine (0.5 mg every 3–5 minutes, with a maximum dose of 0.04 mg/kg or total of 3 mg) may be useful for treatment or pretreatment of patients who develop heart block at the level of the AV node in the context of elevated vagal tone (e.g., in association with nausea or endotracheal tube suction). Atropine should be avoided in patients with infranodal AV block because prolonged asystole sometimes occurs due to more frequent His-Purkinje system depolarization from increased sinus rate. Vagal activity inhibits sympathetic activity; therefore, reduction of vagal tone by atropine disinhibits sympathetic activity and may account for the unpredictable effects of atropine on heart rate. Elevations in heart rate after atropine can persist for hours and cannot be readily reversed. Aminophylline[1] (2.5–6.3 mg/kg IV) is reported to reverse heart block resistant to atropine and epinephrine by antagonizing adenosine. Stimulation of β-adrenergic receptors increases sinus node and subsidiary pacemaker rates, AV node and His-Purkinje system conduction velocities, and myocardial contractility. The effective refractory period shortens in most tissue but this effect varies with dose and specific tissue type. Dobutamine[1] (2–40 mcg/kg/min) is a useful β-receptor agonist because it increases cardiac output and lowers filling pressures without excessive rise or fall of blood pressure. Dopamine[1] (2–20 mcg/kg/min IV) stimulates β_1-adrenergic receptors and increases heart rate by enhancing impulse formation and conduction, as well as myocardial contractility. At higher doses (10–20 mcg/kg/min) dopamine causes vasoconstriction by α_1-receptor stimulation. Isoproterenol (0.02–0.06 mg IV bolus, 0.5–10.0 mcg/min IV infusion) stimulates β_1- and β_2-adrenergic receptors and enhances vasodilation more than the other catecholamines. This can result in unwanted hypotension in some circumstances but it is also less likely to cause a reflex increase in vagal tone than drugs that cause vasoconstriction. Epinephrine (1 mg IV boluses for cardiac arrest, 0.2–1 mg subcutaneously, 0.5–10 mcg/min IV) stimulates both α- and β-adrenergic receptors. It is recommended for asystolic cardiac arrest in part because it increases myocardial and cerebral flow. However, the increase of systemic vascular resistance may be detrimental by augmenting metabolic acidosis and decreasing cardiac performance in patients with poor left ventricular function. The suggested dose ranges are broad because the response to β-adrenergic stimulants such as improved AV conduction varies widely and may be affected by β-adrenergic receptor downregulation in patients with chronic elevations in sympathetic activity such as patients with long-standing heart failure.

Temporary pacing includes primarily transcutaneous and transvenous approaches. Transthoracic, transesophageal, and transgastric approaches are rarely used. Transcutaneous pacing provides noninvasive heart rate support as well as immediate access to countershock, but it is often so painful that most patients require sedation. For these reasons its principal uses are for short-term pacing during cardiopulmonary resuscitation and standby pacing in patients at risk for bradyarrhythmias. Capture is not achieved in some patients. Therefore, users should be ready to continue mechanical cardiopulmonary support and seek alternative methods. If used in standby applications, ventricular capture should be verified in advance. Capture is often difficult to ascertain because transcutaneous stimuli cause large deflections on the ECG and pectoral muscle stimulation can be confused with a pulse. Capture should be verified by careful ECG analysis at subthreshold and suprathreshold stimulus amplitudes and confirmed by appropriately timed femoral artery pulses, Korotkoff sounds, or arterial pressure waveforms.

TABLE 3   Suggestions for Temporary Pacing in Acute Myocardial Infarction

- Transvenous pacing
  - Asystole or poorly tolerated bradycardia unresponsive to atropine or aminophylline
  - Persistent third-degree AV block
  - Alternating RBBB and LBBB, or RBBB and alternating LAFB and LPFB
  - Bifascicular block, new
  - Second-degree AV block (any type) and QRS >110 ms
  - Any indication listed below at time of cardiac catheterization if performed
- Standby transcutaneous pacing
  - Any indication listed above until transvenous pacing system inserted
  - Transient asystole or poorly tolerated bradycardia
  - Bifascicular block, uncertain time of onset, or old
  - Second-degree AV block (any type) and QRS <110 ms
  - New first-degree AV block

Abbreviations: AV = atrioventricular; LAFB, LPFB = left anterior, left posterior fascicle block; LBBB, RBBB = left, right bundle branch block.

---

[1]Not FDA approved for this indication.

Transvenous insertion of an electrode catheter is the method of choice for most patients who require temporary pacing. This approach is reliable and safe when performed by competent staff with strict aseptic technique, fluoroscopic guidance, and appropriate catheters. Small studies suggest that long-term (>5 days) temporary pacing can be accomplished with active-fixation permanent pacemaker leads attached to an external pulse generator (not approved by the U.S. Food and Drug Administration [FDA]). Tunneling the lead may enhance stability and reduce the risk of infection.

Monitoring

Patients with high-grade or symptomatic heart block require close monitoring until the process is reversed by treatment or a pacemaker is implanted. All patients who receive pacemakers require lifelong follow-up by a trained team of physicians, nurses, and ancillary personnel using standard procedures guided by practice guidelines and manufacturer recommendations.

Complications

Catecholamines used to increase heart rate may precipitate tachyarrhythmias by electrophysiologic effects mediated by adrenergic receptors or by myocardial ischemia, and they may worsen hemodynamic status. The adverse effects of catecholamines increase with duration of exposure. Ischemia and receptor-mediated electrophysiologic effects occur immediately after administration; changes in gene expression of ion channels begin as early as several hours; and long-term changes such as myocardial hypertrophy, apoptosis, and fibrosis occur within 24 hours and may progress over much longer periods. This suggests that the duration and dose of catecholamine infusions should be minimized. Complications of temporary transvenous pacing include inadequate pacing or sensing thresholds, vascular complications, pneumothorax, myocardial perforation, infection, and dislodgment. Permanent pacemakers are highly effective, safe, and cost-effective with few contraindications. Although the complications are rarely life threatening, they should be carefully considered and acknowledged. Septicemia or endocarditis has been reported in 0.5% of patients. In patients with pacemaker-related endocarditis, the in-hospital mortality rate is reported to be over 7% with a 20-month mortality rate over 25%. The rate of significant complications has been reported to be 3.5%. About 10% of pacemakers will become infected or develop some other type of failure that may require extraction. In a recent series the rate of major complications associated with extraction was 1.4%. There is a long-term continuous risk of infection, thrombosis, and erosion. In young persons there is a periodic need to replace generators and leads. Abandoned leads block venous access and extractions are associated with significant risks. Perhaps of greater consequence is the constant inconvenience of lifelong follow-up, electromagnetic interference, and false alarms from electronic surveillance devices, as well as exclusion from important procedures, such as magnetic resonance imaging of the thorax. Conventional pacing, that is, from the right ventricular apex, is now known to be detrimental and may cause adverse ventricular remodeling, atrial fibrillation, heart failure, and premature death. Although it has been shown that patients with reduced left ventricular function are at greater risk for adverse effects, it is not known how to identify other patients at risk. Strategies for reducing the adverse effects of conventional pacing are under study and recommendations are evolving. Because the decision for pacemaker implantation includes selection of lead configuration, lead locations, and pacing mode, patient guidance and education are complex.

Conclusions

Heart block remains a challenge because the cellular mechanisms responsible are poorly understood, prediction of symptomatic heart block (who and when) is unreliable, treatments that restore normal conduction do not exist for most conditions, and pacemaker therapy can have significant long-term adverse consequences. Fortunately, current devices and leads are much more reliable than in the past and remote monitoring has enhanced early detection of problems and has substantially reduced the inconvenience of device monitoring. The newest generation of devices will allow many patients with pacemakers to safely undergo magnetic resonance imaging. Ongoing clinical trials will provide guidance in pacemaker configurations and programming that will minimize adverse effects. In the future, achievements in molecular biology will elucidate mechanisms and produce treatments that will relegate artificial pacemakers to museum pieces.

References

Ackerman MJ, Priori SG, Willems S, et al. HRS/EHRA expert consensus statement on the state of genetic testing for the channelopathies and cardiomyopathies. Europace 2011;13:1077.

Carvalheiras G, Faria R, Braga J, et al. Fetal outcome in autoimmune diseases. Autoimmun Rev 2012;11:A520.

Cheng S, Keyes MJ, Larson MG, et al. Long-term outcomes in individuals with prolonged PR interval or first-degree atrioventricular block. JAMA 2009;301:2571.

Epstein AE, DiMarco JP, Ellenbogen KA, et al. ACC/AHA/HRS 2008 guidelines for device-based therapy of cardiac rhythm abnormalities. J Am Coll Cardiol 2008;51:e1.

Hazinski MF, Samson R, Schexnayder S. Handbook of emergency cardiovascular care for healthcare providers. Dallas, TX: American Heart Association; 2010.

Smits JPP, Velkkamp MW, Wilde AAM. Mechanisms of inherited cardiac conduction disease. Europace 2005;7:122.

Vardas PE, Auriccho A, Blanc JJ, et al. Guidelines for cardiac pacing and cardiac resynchronization therapy. Eur Heart J 2007;28:2256.

HYPERTENSION

Method of
Horacio E. Adrogué, MD

CURRENT DIAGNOSIS

- Blood pressure (BP) should be taken in a seated position, with the right arm supported, the patient at rest for 5 minutes, and without recent smoking or caffeine intake.
- BP should be repeated at least twice on two separate clinic visits before the label of hypertension is given unless stage 2 hypertension is diagnosed on the first visit.
- Every effort should be made to use standard nomenclature when documenting stages of hypertension.
- In those individuals whose hypertension does not manifest or behave like essential hypertension, it is imperative to rule out any secondary, treatable, or reversible causes.

CURRENT THERAPY

- Lifestyle modification should be the first line of treatment for all patients with hypertension, especially when medications are started on the first clinic visit.
- Secondary causes of hypertension should be treated along with an appropriate specialist consultation to ensure the best outcomes for the patient.
- Hypertension should be considered a modifiable risk factor for heart disease, stroke, and chronic kidney disease.
- Cardiovascular risk should be calculated using a published formula to help patients understand how they can affect their own health.
- Every effort should be made to match the drug class used with compelling indications present in each patient.
- Control of hypertension is more important than what medication is used, with the exception of compelling indications.

It has been more than 35 years since the National Heart, Lung, and Blood Institute (NHLBI) published the first Report of the Joint National Committee on Prevention, Detection, Evaluation, and Treatment of High Blood Pressure (JNC 1). The most recent report (JNC 8) was published in December of 2013 in the Journal of the American Medical Association, more than 10 years after JNC 7. It was also announced in June of 2013 that the NHLBI would no longer issue hypertension or any other clinical guidelines "including those in process." The authors of JNC 8 decided to move forward with publication of their completed report based on the original predefined process that had started with invitations sent out by the NHLBI in March 2008. The members of the JNC 8 committee clearly state in their report that it is not sanctioned by the NHLBI and does not reflect NHLBI views.

The comments and controversy about the JNC 8 members' report started with almost no delay from the time the report had been printed. The report has caused much dissention in the hypertension community. The American College of Cardiology and the American Heart Association (AHA) have gone so far as to say that they "continue to recognize JNC 7 as the national standard." The ACA and AHA are now in the process of developing their own new guidelines, which are promised to be released in 2015. So, what are those of us on the front line to do with the patients who sit in our office and ask for advice today? This chapter will compare and contrast the differences between JNC 7 and JNC 8.

Epidemiology

The earth's population was over 7.1 billion people in 2013, and about one out of every four adults has hypertension. As the world gravitates toward a Western diet and lifestyle, the pandemic of obesity will only worsen, adding to the increasing incidence of hypertension worldwide. In the United States, it is estimated that in 2006, 76 million people had hypertension, a tremendous increase from the 50 million with hypertension estimated from 1988 through 1994. The population of the Unites States in 2012 was 314 million: this means that about 24% of our citizens have hypertension.

Systolic blood pressure (BP) progressively rises as we exceed the age of 40 years. Between 27% and 40% of men and 20% and 45% of women between 40 and 59 years old in the United States have hypertension. The total number of affected people increases to nearly 60% to 75% of adults older than 60 years.

Non-Hispanic whites and Mexican Americans have a similar prevalence of hypertension; non-Hispanic blacks have much higher BP values than the other two groups. In fact, non-Hispanic black men have a 15% to 20% higher prevalence than that of the other two groups, and non-Hispanic black women have up to 25% higher prevalence. The combination of a higher prevalence and more difficulty in controlling hypertension in the non-Hispanic black population greatly contributes to the disproportionately high representation of this group of Americans on dialysis.

Risk Factors

Modern Western Diet and Lifestyle

The modern Western diet and lifestyle is one of the most important and potentially modifiable risk factors that most patients and many doctors ignore. It is much easier for both patients and physicians alike to accept a new medication than adopt and implement a healthier life style. Although it takes a lot of work to change our lifestyle, the potential rewards are great. Because most large trials show positive effects of a 2- to 4-mm Hg reduction in systolic BP with the use of antihypertensive medications, it is very important to be aware of similar or better results with lifestyle modification.

As shown in Table 1, improvement in cardiovascular disease (CVD) risk can be attained with modest changes in lifestyle when compared to people who do not make these modifications. Regular aerobic exercise (30 minutes at least three times per week), dietary potassium increase and sodium restriction, moderate alcohol consumption, and low-fat diet have all been shown to improve systolic BP in several studies (Table 2).

TABLE 1 Effect of Diet Modification on Risk of Cardiovascular Disease

FOOD	AMOUNT	REDUCTION IN CVD (%)
Fish	114 g 4 × per wk	14
Fruit and vegetables	400 g/d	21
Wine	150 mL/d (5 oz/d)	32
Garlic	2.7 g/d	25
Dark chocolate	100 g/d	21
Almonds	68 g/d	12

Abbreviation: CVD = cardiovascular disease.

TABLE 2 Effect of Lifestyle and Diet Modification on Systolic Blood Pressure

MODIFICATION	AMOUNT	REDUCTION IN SBP (mm Hg)
Dietary sodium restriction	<30–50 mmol/d	2–8
Moderation of daily alcohol intake	150–200 mL	2–4
Increased physical activity	30 min 3 × per wk	4–9
Reduction in body weight	10 kg or 22 lb	5–10
Adoption of DASH eating plan (high potassium)		8–14

Abbreviations: DASH = dietary approaches to stop hypertension; SBP = systolic blood pressure.

Age

Wish as we might, age is a nonmodifiable risk factor. Between the ages of 18 and 39 years, 10% of American women and 15% of men have hypertension. There is a large increase in the prevalence between the ages of 40 and 59 years, affecting up to 40% of men and 50% of women. Almost 60% of those older than 60 years, 70% of those older than 70 years, and 80% of those older than 80 years have hypertension, with older non-Hispanic blacks having the highest prevalence. This is the trend in the United States; however, it might turn out to be somewhat modifiable if we reverse our "expected" weight gain and sedentary lifestyle as we age.

Sex

In general, men have a higher prevalence of hypertension until the age of 45 years. After that, men and women have the same rates. The Prospective Studies Collaboration found that ischemic heart disease mortality associated with hypertension in women was higher than in men. It does not appear that the female sex is a protective state, as we once thought.

Ethnicity

Non-Hispanic blacks have a higher incidence and prevalence of hypertension in the United States. In addition, the rate of death from CVD among black patients has been shown to be 25% higher than among whites. However, this trend is not present worldwide. Paradoxically, among Hispanics of Mexican origin, there is less hypertension and CVD than in whites and blacks even though there is more obesity and diabetes.

Body Weight

In general, as the population gains weight, its BP rises. In those with hypertension and excess caloric intake, the simple act of decreasing caloric intake can drop BP even before significant weight loss actually occurs. This phenomenon is not completely understood, but insulin might play a role by promoting mild vascular pressor effect and salt retention. In 2008, over 1.4 billion adults were considered overweight (BMI between 25 and 30). Over the next 10 years, this number is expected to exceed 2 billion. This underscores the critical role of weight loss in treatment of both hypertension and diabetes.

Diet

It has now become very clear that the combination of a high sodium chloride diet exceeding 50 to 100 mmol per day and a low potassium intake of less than 30 to 50 mmol is critical in the pathogenesis of hypertension. Daily consumption of more than approximately 400 mL (13 oz) of alcohol has been shown to contribute to essential hypertension. One study found that excess alcohol consumption correlated even better than sodium chloride intake.

Family History

Similar to type 2 diabetes mellitus, essential hypertension clearly runs in families. This accounts for one-third to one-half of the cause of essential hypertension, with the rest due to environmental causes. Monogenic hypertension has been identified in a few select families. This is hypertension caused by mutations in genes that increase the reabsorption of sodium chloride in the renal tubule.

Figure 1. Interaction of the modern Western diet and the kidneys in the pathogenesis of primary hypertension. The modern Western diet interacts with the kidneys to generate excess sodium and cause a deficit of potassium in the body; these changes increase peripheral vascular resistance and establish hypertension. An initial increase in the volume of extracellular fluid is countered by pressure natriuresis. (Reprinted with permission from Adrogué IIJ, Madias NE: Sodium and potassium in the pathogenesis of hypertension. N Engl J Med 2007;356:1966–78.)

Other Factors

Smoking, physical inactivity, higher altitudes, and colder weather have all been linked to acute elevations of BP and chronic hypertension. Recent data point to a link between essential hypertension and hyperuricemia (uric acid levels ≥ 6 mg/dL) in adolescents.

Pathophysiology

The role of excess sodium chloride and inadequate potassium intake is central to the pathogenesis of essential hypertension (Figure 1). The human kidney was designed to conserve sodium and get rid of potassium because our prehistoric diet was high in potassium and low in sodium. Unfortunately for those of us who partake of the typical Western diet, the end result can be hypertension. The deficit of total body potassium (most being intracellular) contributes to vascular smooth-muscle cell contraction, increased peripheral vascular resistance, and hypertension.

Simultaneously, the excess quantity of sodium expands the extracellular fluid volume, releasing digitalis-like factor, which stimulates the Na^+, K^+-ATPase to conserve sodium and waste potassium. This excess cellular sodium increases vascular smooth-muscle cell contraction, increasing peripheral vascular resistance, leading to hypertension.

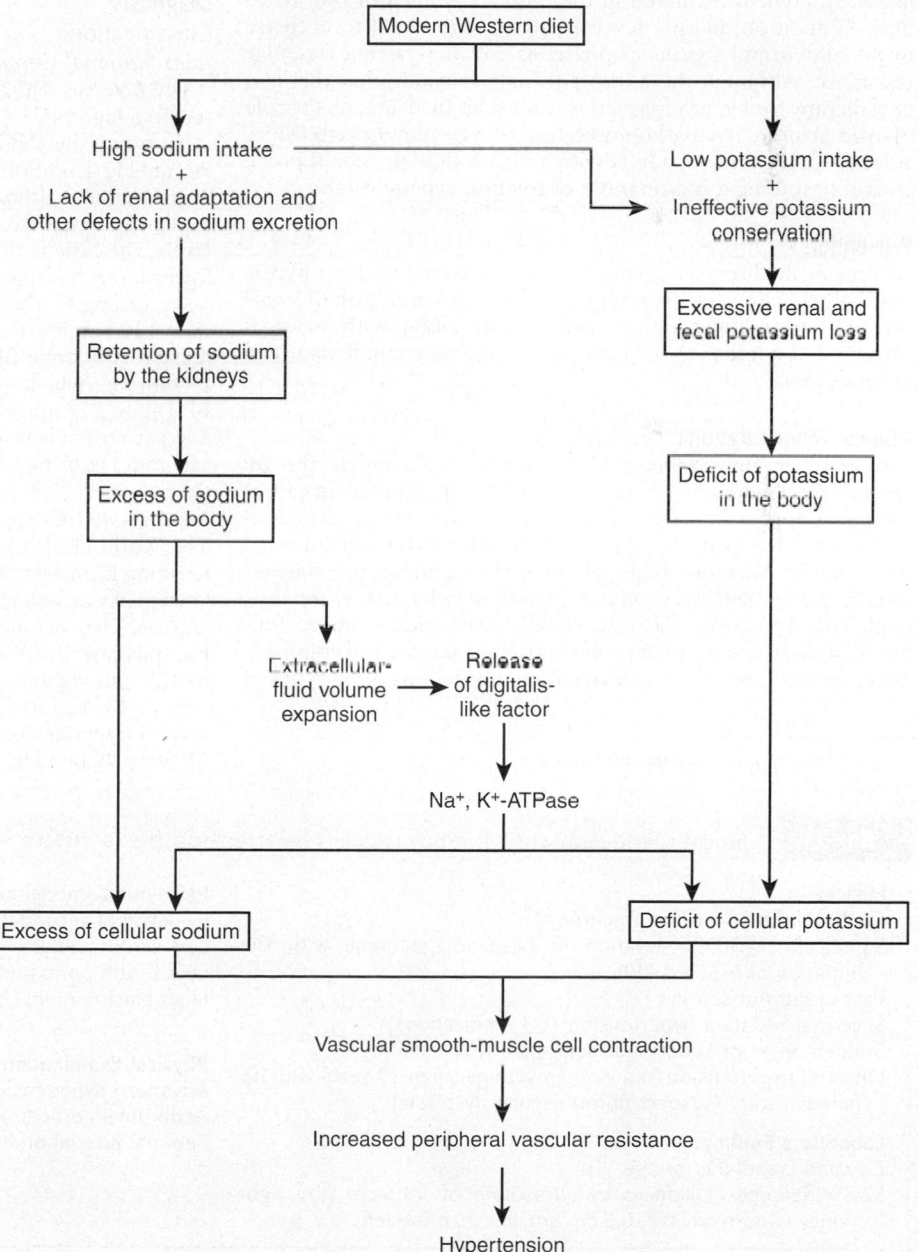

Uricase, an enzyme that degrades uric acid to allantoin, is not expressed by humans, which contributes to higher levels of uric acid in humans than in most other mammals. The role of hyperuricemia (uric acid level ≥ 6 mg/dL) in the pathogenesis of hypertension has been the subject of much debate. JNC 7 does not consider it a true risk factor for hypertension. However, more recent data in children might lead to a change of opinion on the role of hyperuricemia and hypertension.

A randomized, double-blind, placebo-controlled crossover trial of allopurinol (Zyloprim)[1] use was performed in children 11 to 17 years old who had newly diagnosed essential hypertension. The hypothesis was that the treatment of hyperuricemia (≥ 6 mg/dL) with allopurinol would lead to a lowering of BP. Thirty adolescents with stage 1 hypertension and obesity (70%) were enrolled and randomized to allopurinol 200 mg twice per day ($n=15$) or placebo ($n=15$) for 4 weeks, had a 2-week washout, and then crossed over to the opposite group for an additional 4 weeks. Twenty-two of the 30 allopurinol-treated patients achieved a uric acid level of less than 5 mg/dL by the end of the study. Casual systolic BP decreased by 6.9 mm Hg in the allopurinol group but only 2 mm Hg in the placebo group ($P=0.009$). Diastolic BP decreased by 5.1 mm Hg in the allopurinol group but only 2.4 mm Hg in the placebo group ($P=0.05$). An even larger difference was noted in the 24-hour ambulatory BP readings. In addition, plasma levels of renin were noted to decrease in the allopurinol treatment phase, as did the systemic vascular resistance. Although the authors do not conclude that this is a new therapy for hypertension, this study does shed light on the role of uric acid in the pathophysiology of essential hypertension. A larger study, done in adults with longer follow-up, could prove critical in finding a new manner of treating hypertension.

Prevention

As previously discussed, being born into a family without hypertension helps prevent hypertension if you also take care of yourself. A low-sodium, high-potassium diet along with physical activity and avoidance of smoking and excess alcohol also help in prevention.

Clinical Manifestations

Essential hypertension is usually asymptomatic unless the BP reaches very high levels. A mean arterial BP of 150 mm Hg causes lesions to appear in arterial walls and can start the syndrome of accelerated malignant hypertension (AMH). AMH is manifested by diastolic BP more than 140 mm Hg, funduscopic changes (bleeding, papilledema, exudates), neurologic changes (vision loss, confusion, headache, seizures, coma), acute kidney injury (oliguria), and gastrointestinal problems such as nausea and vomiting. An extensive description of clinical manifestations of all types of

---

[1]Not FDA approved for this indication.

---

secondary hypertension is beyond the scope of this chapter, but I will discuss clues to these diseases.

Cushing's syndrome is associated with an approximately four-fold higher mortality than essential hypertension. Because obesity is a growing problem, it is important to be alert for the sign of truncal obesity (50%–90% incidence) in Cushing's. Other important clues include facial plethora (80%), hirsutism (80%), menstrual disorders or impotence (75%), purple striae (50%–70%), easy bruising (50%), weakness from myopathy (30%–90%), glucose intolerance (75%), and kidney stones and hypokalemia (20%).

Primary hyperaldosteronism can account for up to 10% of those with hypertension and 20% of those with resistant hypertension. This new incidence can reach up to 40% of highly selected groups and is very different from the 1% rate that was commonly quoted in recent years. It is very important to detect this disease early because 75% of cases are due to an adenoma, 20% are due to hyperplasia, and 5% are due to carcinoma. Detection and treatment of this disease can be lifesaving.

Renovascular hypertension is another secondary cause of hypertension that can account for up to 7% of those with elevated BP and suggestive clinical signs and symptoms (Box 1). Once properly diagnosed, it can respond to treatment very well.

Diagnosis
Classifications
Joint National Committee Classification
JNC 8 Versus JNC 7. It is important to note that JNC 8 "did not redefine high BP."

To quote the JNC 8 report, "the panel believes that the 140/90 mm Hg definition from JNC 7 remains reasonable." The report also noted that although there is a linear relationship between naturally occurring BP and risk that is maintained to very low-BP levels, the benefit of using antihypertensive drugs to treat BP to lower levels has not been established.

According to JNC 7, normal BP is defined as systolic BP less than 120 mm Hg and diastolic BP less than 80 mm Hg. Prehypertension is systolic BP 120 to 139 mm Hg or diastolic BP 80 to 89 mm Hg (whichever is higher). Stage 1 hypertension is systolic BP 140 to 159 mm Hg or diastolic BP 90 to 99 mm Hg, and stage 2 hypertension is systolic BP 160 mm Hg or higher or diastolic BP 100 mm Hg or higher.

International Classification
The World Health Organization, International Society of Hypertension, European Society of Hypertension, and the European Society of Cardiology have also published a classification of hypertension. They define optimal BP as a systolic BP less than 120 mm Hg and diastolic BP less than 80 mm Hg. Normal is systolic BP 120 to 129 mm Hg and diastolic BP 80 to 84 mm Hg; high-normal is systolic BP 130 to 139 mm Hg or diastolic BP 85 to 89 mm Hg. Stage 1 hypertension is systolic BP 140 to 159 mm Hg or diastolic BP 90 to 99 mm Hg, and stage 2 hypertension is systolic BP 160 to

---

Box 1   Clinical Manifestations of Renovascular Hypertension (Renal Artery Stenosis and Fibromuscular Dysplasia)

History
Flash pulmonary edema (recurrent)
Significant ($\geq 30\%$) elevation in baseline creatinine with the initiation of ACEI or ARB
Past or current smoker
Severe or resistant hypertension (>3 medications)
Sudden onset or sudden worsening of hypertension
Onset of hypertension in a woman younger than 30 years with no family history (suspect fibromuscular dysplasia)

Laboratory Findings
Elevated creatinine for age
Size difference in kidneys by ultrasound of >1.5 cm (the right kidney is normally 0.3–0.5 cm smaller than the left)

Proteinuria (moderate, approximately 1–2 g/day, but is variable)
Evidence of secondary hyperaldosteronism
Low serum sodium
Low serum potassium
High plasma renin

Physical Examination Findings
Advanced hypertensive retinopathy
Abdominal aortic bruits
Femoral arterial bruits

Abbreviations: ACEI = angiotensin-converting enzyme inhibitor; ARB = angiotensin receptor blocker.

179 mm Hg or diastolic BP 100 to 109 mm Hg. The designation of stage 3 hypertension is reserved for those with systolic BP 180 mm Hg or higher or diastolic BP 110 mm Hg or higher.

AHA Classification

The AHA further classifies hypertension into several specific categories.

Isolated systolic hypertension is systolic BP 140 mm Hg or higher and diastolic BP less than 90 mm Hg. Isolated diastolic hypertension is systolic BP less than 140 mm Hg and diastolic BP 90 mm Hg or higher. White coat hypertension is becoming a more recognized diagnosis and is diagnosed when the clinic BP is more than 140/90 mm Hg while the ambulatory BP averages less than 135/85 mm Hg.

Isolated ambulatory hypertension is a clinic BP of less than 135/85 mm Hg and an average ambulatory BP of more than 140/90 mm Hg. The use of 24-hour ambulatory BP monitors has become much more common in the practice of medicine. People who have a personal history of prehypertension or a family history of hypertension and wish to donate a kidney are evaluated via this method to assess their candidacy to donate. Patients with BP that is difficult to control or evaluate benefit greatly from this method. Ambulatory hypertension is a 24-hour average of more than 135/85. In addition, current data show that patients without a normal drop in nighttime BP have an increased cardiovascular morbidity. For this reason, ambulatory nighttime hypertension is defined as an average nighttime BP of >125/75 mm Hg and ambulatory daytime hypertension is average values of more than 140/90 mm Hg.

The last category is accelerated or malignant hypertension, which should be treated as a medical emergency. Diastolic BP is higher than 120 mm Hg and evidence of grade III retinopathy (arteriolar nicking and narrowing, flame-shaped hemorrhages and exudates) or grade IV retinopathy (papilledema) is an indication for hospital admission for careful and monitored treatment of hypertension.

Pseudohypertension

Pseudohypertension is defined as the overestimation of BP when taken by a standard manual sphygmomanometer in certain patients. Hypertension should not be diagnosed in these patients unless the measurements can be verified by the Osler maneuver. It should be suspected in elderly patients and in diabetic patients with known or suspected sclerosis or calcification of radial and brachial arteries. The presence of pseudohypertension can be confirmed in the outpatient setting by the use of the Osler maneuver. The cuff is inflated 30 mm Hg above the auscultated systolic BP and the brachial or radial artery distal to the cuff is palpated and rolled under the examiner's finger. If a pulse is no longer felt but the artery remains palpable like a stiff tube (likely calcified), then the Osler maneuver is positive and pseudohypertension is present.

Other noninvasive clues to the diagnosis include the absence of end-organ damage (left ventricular hypertrophy, retinopathy) and excessive postural hypotension with the use of low doses of antihypertensive agents. An automatic oscillometric recorder or finger BP can also help to detect the patient's true BP. In cases where doubt still remains, intraarterial pressure measurements should be considered, and those values should be compared to the cuff BP to ensure correct classification of the patient's BP. The importance of proper diagnosis cannot be overstated because these patients will suffer from postural hypotension and risk of injury from antihypertensive medications that they do not need.

Treatment

How Do JNC 8 and JNC 7 Differ?

JNC 8 used three critical questions to guide their review of evidence and limited their evidence review to randomized controlled trials (RCT). They asked three things about adults with hypertension. First, does initiation of antihypertensive medication at specific BP thresholds improve health outcomes? Second, does treatment with medications to a specified BP goal lead to improvement in health outcomes? Third, do various antihypertensive drugs or classes differ in comparable benefits and harms on specific health outcomes?

JNC 7 used a nonsystematic literature review by experts that included a range of study designs. JNC 8 methodologists restricted their evidence review to RCTs. JNC 8 did not review observational studies, systematic reviews, or meta-analyses. Conflicts of interest were actively managed by the JNC 8 panel. JNC 7 used separate treatment goals for "uncomplicated" hypertension and disease states such as diabetes and chronic kidney disease (CKD). JNC 8 used similar treatment goals for all hypertensive populations, except when the evidence supported different goals for specific subpopulations.

Both reports support lifestyle modification, with JNC 8 endorsing the evidence-based recommendations of the 2013 Lifestyle Work Group.

As far as drug therapy is concerned, JNC 8 recommends four classes (angiotensin-converting enzyme inhibitor [ACEI], or angiotensin receptor blocker [ARB], calcium-channel blocker [CCB], or thiazide-type diuretics) of drugs based on RCT evidence. A table of drugs and doses used in RCTs is also provided in the JNC 8 report. Table 3 in this chapter lists commonly used antihypertensive agents, and the agents used in RCTs have been bolded, underlined, and italicized. JNC 7 recommends five drug classes as initial therapy, emphasizing the use of thiazide diuretics for most patients who do not have a compelling indication for a specific class (Table 4). β Blockers are recommended in JNC 7, but are not specifically recommended as initial therapy for patients with hypertension in JNC 8. The exclusion of β-blockers from JNC 8 was related to a higher overall rate of death from CVD compared to the other drugs.

The main difference in the scope of topics for JNC 8 versus JNC 7 is that JNC 8 focused on a limited number of questions judged by the panel to be most useful to the practicing health care provider.

The last difference between the two guidelines may be the most controversial. While JNC 7 was reviewed by the National High Blood Pressure Education Program Coordinating Committee, a coalition of 39 major professional organizations and seven federal agencies, JNC 8 was reviewed by multiple experts, including those affiliated with professional, public, and governmental organizations, using an open access process, though JNC 8 does not claim official sponsorship by any organization. JNC 8 was published through the internal and external peer-review process of the Journal of the American Medical Association. JNC 7 was a comprehensive overview of hypertension, and JNC 8 was an evidence-based review of the three questions developed *a priori* by the review panel.

What Are the Recommendations of JNC 8?

The authors of JNC 8 used the evidence-quality rating system produced by the National Heart Lung and Blood Institute Evidence-Based Methodology Lead. The strength of recommendation grading system used was also developed by the National Heart Lung and Blood Institute Evidence-Based Methodology Lead. The JNC 8 panel adhered to the standards set by the Institute of Medicine "Clinical Practice Guidelines We Can Trust" study committee rather than follow the prior practices of other JNC panels.

Recommendation 1

In the general population of 60 years or older, start medication therapy at 150/90 mm Hg and treat to a goal of less than 150/90 mm Hg. This is considered a strong recommendation based on grade A data. The panel noted that there is evidence that setting a goal SBP of 140 mm Hg or less in this age group offers no additional benefit compared with higher goals of 140 to 149 mm Hg. The new recommendation allows physicians, who at times find it difficult to meet the systolic BP goal of 140 mm Hg in older patients, some liberalization in treatment goals. For those patients who need an excessive amount of medications or have near-syncope episodes, it is reasonable to allow them to have the higher goal of the systolic BP 150 mm Hg. Recently, several other guideline documents, such as those from the American Diabetes Association and the European Society of Hypertension, have recommended systolic hypertension goals in older patients that are similar to the JNC 8 recommendation.

The JNC 8 panel was unable to reach a unanimous decision on this recommendation. An article by 5 of the 17 JNC 8 panel

| TABLE 3 | Some Common Oral Antihypertensive Drugs |

DRUG (TRADE NAME)	INITIAL DOSE	MAXIMUM DOSE	HOW SUPPLIED	MAJOR SIDE EFFECTS/ COMMENTS
Angiotensin-Converting Enzyme Inhibitors				
Benazepril (Lotensin, generic)*	10 mg/d	80 mg/d†	Tab: 5, 10, 20, 40 mg	Cough, hypotension, renal failure, hyperkalemia, loss of taste, rash, leukopenia, angioedema (rare)
Captopril (Capoten, generic)	25 mg bid–tid	450 mg/d	Tab: 12.5, 25, 50, 100 mg	
	25 mg bid	_200 mg/d_		
Enalapril (Vasotec, generic)	5 mg/d	40 mg/d†	Tab: 2.5, 5, 10, 20 mg	
	_5 mg/d_	_20 mg/d_		
Fosinopril (Monopril, generic)	10 mg/d	80 mg/d†	Tab: 10, 20, 40 mg	
Lisinopril (Prinivil, Zestril, generic)	10 mg/d	80 mg/d	Tab: 2.5, 5, 10, 20, 40 mg	
	_10 mg/d_	_40 mg/d_		
Moexipril (Univasc, generic)	7.5 mg/d	30 mg/d†	Tab: 7.5, 15 mg	
Perindopril (Aceon)	4 mg/d	16 mg/d	Tab: 2, 4, 8 mg	
Quinapril (Accupril, generic)	10–20 mg/d	80 mg/d†	Tab: 5, 10, 20, 40 mg	
Ramipril (Altace, generic)	2.5 mg/d	20 mg/d†	Cap: 1.25, 2.5, 5, 10 mg	
Trandolapril (Mavik)	1–2 mg/d	8 mg/d†	Tab: 1, 2, 4 mg	
Angiotensin Receptor Blockers				
Candesartan (Atacand)	16 mg/d	32 mg/d†	Tab: 4, 8, 16, 32 mg	Similar to ACEIs, but not significantly associated with cough and have lower incidence of angioedema than ACEIs
	_4 mg/d_	_12–32 mg/d_		
Eprosartan (Teveten)	600 mg/d	800 mg/d	Tab: 400, 600 mg	
	_400 mg/d_	_600–800 mg/d_		
Irbesartan (Avapro)	150 mg/d	300 mg/d	Tab: 75, 150, 300 mg	
	_75 mg/d_	_300 mg/d_		
Losartan (Cozaar)	50 mg/d	100 mg/d†	Tab: 25, 50, 100 mg	
	_50 mg/d_	_100 mg/d_		
Olmesartan (Benicar)	20 mg/d	40 mg/d	Tab: 5, 10, 20 mg	
Telmisartan (Micardis)	40 mg/d	80 mg/d	Tab: 20, 40, 80 mg	
Valsartan (Diovan)	80–160 mg/d	320 mg/d	Tab: 40, 80, 160, 320 mg	
	_40–80 mg/d_	_160–320 mg/d_		
Direct Renin Inhibitors				
Aliskiren (Tekturna)	150 mg/d	300 mg/d	Tab: 150, 300 mg	Same as ARBs, but can have more GI side effects such as diarrhea
β-Adrenergic Blockers				
Cardioselective β-Blockers				
Atenolol (Tenormin, generic)	50 mg/d	100 mg/d	Tab: 25, 50, 100 mg	Bradycardia, heart failure, impaired peripheral circulation, fatigue, decreased exercise tolerance, insomnia; bronchospasm at higher doses; can mask hypoglycemia
	_25-50 mg/d_	_100 mg/d_		
Betaxolol (Kerlone, generic)	10 mg/d	20 mg/d	Tab: 10, 20 mg	
Bisoprolol (Zebeta, generic)	5 mg/d	20 mg/d	Tab: 5, 10 mg	
Metoprolol (Lopressor, generic), extended-release (Toprol XL)	50 mg bid or 100 mg XL/d	400 mg/d	Tab: 50, 100 mg XL tab: 25, 50, 100, 200 mg	
	_50 mg/d_	_100–200 mg/d_		
Noncardioselective β-Blockers				
Nadolol (Corgard, generic)	40 mg/d	320 mg/d	Tab: 20, 40, 80, 120, 160 mg	Bronchospasm, bradycardia, heart failure, impaired peripheral circulation, insomnia, fatigue, decreased exercise tolerance; can mask hypoglycemia
Propranolol (Inderal, generic), long-acting (Inderal LA)	20–40 mg bid or 60–80 mg SR/d	480 mg/d	Tab: 10, 20, 40, 60, 80 mg LA tab: 60, 80, 120, 160 mg	
Timolol (Blocadren, generic)	10 mg bid	60 mg/d	Tab: 5, 10, 20 mg	
Intrinsic Sympathomimetic Agents				
Acebutolol (Sectral, generic)	200 mg bid	600 mg bid	Cap: 200, 400 mg	Same as other β-blockers, except less bradycardia
Carteolol (Cartrol)	2.5 mg/d	10 mg/d	Tab: 2.5, 5 mg	
Penbutolol (Levatol)	20 mg/d	20 mg/d	Tab: 20 mg	
Pindolol (Visken, generic)	5 mg bid	60 mg/d	Tab: 5, 10 mg	
β-Blockers with α-Blocking Activity				
Carvedilol (Coreg, generic)	6.25 mg bid	25 mg bid	Tab: 3.125, 6.25, 12.5, 25 mg	Same as noncardioselective β-blockers
Labetolol (Normodyne, generic)	100 mg bid	600 mg bid	Tab: 100, 200, 300 mg	Same as noncardioselective β-blockers; hepatic toxicity
β-Blockers with Nitric Oxide Activity				
Nebivolol (Bystolic)	5 mg/d	40 mg/d	Tab: 2.5, 5, 10, 20 mg	Similar to other β-blockers; might have lower incidence of side effects

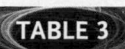 **TABLE 3**   Some Common Oral Antihypertensive Drugs—cont'd

DRUG (TRADE NAME)	INITIAL DOSE	MAXIMUM DOSE	HOW SUPPLIED	MAJOR SIDE EFFECTS/ COMMENTS
Calcium-Channel Blockers				
Dihydropyridines *Amlodipine* (Norvasc, generic)	2.5–5 mg/d *2.5 mg/d*	10 mg/d *10 mg/d*	Tab: 2.5, 5, 10 mg	Ankle edema, flushing, headache, dizziness, palpitations, gingival hypertrophy
Felodipine (Plendil, generic)	2.5–5 mg/d	10 mg/d	Tab: 2.5, 5, 10 mg	
Isradipine (generic, DynaCirc CR)	5 mg/d	20 mg/d	Tab: 5, 10 mg	
Nicardipine, sustained release (Cardene SR, generic)	30 mg bid	60 mg bid	Cap: 30, 45, 60 mg	
Nicardipine extended-release (Adalat CC, generic)	30–60 mg/d	120 mgd	Tab: 30, 60, 90 mg	
Nisoldipine, extended-release (Sular, generic)	20 mg/d	60 mg/d	Tab: 10, 20, 30, 40 mg	
Nondihydropyridines				
Diltiazem, extended-release (Cardizem SR, Cardizem CD, Dilacor XR, Tiazac, generic)	120–180 mg/d *120–180 mg/d*	360–480 mg/d *360 mg/d*	Once daily tab: 60, 90, 120 mg Twice-daily tab: 180, 240, 300, 360, 420 mg	AV block, bradycardia, heart failure, constipation (especially with verapamil), rash (with diltiazem), dizziness, headache, gingival hyperplasia
Verapamil, extended-release (Calan SR, Covera-HS, Isoptin SR, Verelan, generic)	120 mg/d	480 mg/d	Tab: 120, 180, 240 mg Cap: 120, 180, 240 mg Verelan PM: 100, 200, 300 mg	
Diuretics				
Thiazides				
Chlorothiazide (Diuril, generic)	12.5–250 mg qd–bid	1 g/d	Tab: 250, 500 mg Susp: 250 mg/5 mL	Hypokalemia, hypomagnesemia, hyperuricemia, hypercalcemia, hyperlipidemia, hyperglycemia, hyponatremia, impotence, rashes, photosensitivity, pancreatitis
Hydrochlorothiazide (Esidrix, Oretic, generic)	12.5–25 mg/d *12.5–25 mg*	50 mg/d *25–100 mg/d*	Tab: 25, 50, 100 mg Soln: 50 mg/5 mL	
Thiazide Congeners				
Chlorthalidone (Hygroton, generic)	12.5–25 mg/d *12.5 mg/d*	50 mg/d *12.5–25 mg/d*	Tab: 25, 50, 100 mg	Same as thiazides
Indapamide (Lozol, generic)	1.25 mg/d *1.25 mg/d*	5 mg/d *1.25–2.5 mg/d*	Tab: 1.25, 2.5 mg	Same as thiazides, may have fewer metabolic effects
Metolazone (Zaroxolyn, others)	2.5 mg/d	5 mg/d	Tab: 2.5, 5, 10 mg	Same as thiazides
Loop Diuretics				
Bumetamide (Bumex, generic)	0.5 mg bid	4 mg/d	Tab: 0.5, 1, 2 mg	Same as thiazides, no hypercalcemia
Ethacrynic acid (Edecrin)	12.5 mg bid	50 mg bid	Tab: 25, 50 mg	Same as thiazides, ototoxicity
Furosemide (Lasix, generic)	10–20 mg/d	240 mg/d (bid–tid)	Tab: 20, 40, 80 mg Soln: 10 mg/mL, 40 mg/mL	Same as thiazides, more pancreatitis and allergic reactions
Torsemide (Demadex, generic)	5 mg qd	10 mg/d	Tab: 5, 10, 20, 100 mg	Same as thiazides, more potent
Potassium-Sparing Agents				
Amiloride (Midamor, generic)	5 mg/d	10 mg/d	Tab: 5 mg	More hyperkalemia, nausea, flatulence, skin rash
Triamterene (Dyrenium)	25 mg/d–bid	100 mg/d	Tab: 50, 100 mg	Hyperkalemia; nephrolithiasis; folic acid antagonist; contraindicated in pregnancy
Aldosterone Receptor Antagonists				
Eplerenone (Inspra)	50 mg/d	50 mg bid	Tab: 25, 50, 100 mg	Hyperkalemia, hyponatremia, hypertriglyceridemia, dizziness, cough, fatigue, diarrhea, abdominal pain, mastodynia, gynecomastia
Spironolactone (Aldactone, generic)	12.5 mg/d–bid	50 mg bid	Tab: 25, 50, 100 mg	Hyperkalemia, impotence, gynecomastia in men, breast tenderness in women
α_1-Adrenergic Blockers				
Doxazosin (Cardura, generic)	1 mg/d	16 mg/d	Tab: 1, 2, 4, 8 mg	First-dose hypotension (more with prazosin), dizziness, palpitations, GI disturbances
Prazosin (Minipress, generic)	1 mg bid–tid	20 mg/d	Cap: 1, 2, 5 mg	
Terazosin (Hytrin generic)	1 mg qhs	20 mg/d	Tab or cap: 1, 2, 5, 10 mg	
Central α-Adrenergic Agonists				

Continued

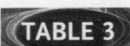

TABLE 3 Some Common Oral Antihypertensive Drugs—cont'd

DRUG (TRADE NAME)	INITIAL DOSE	MAXIMUM DOSE	HOW SUPPLIED	MAJOR SIDE EFFECTS/ COMMENTS
Clonidine (Catapres, generic)	0.1 mg bid	1.2 mg/d	Tab: 0.1, 0.2, 0.3 mg	Sedation, drowsiness, depression, dry mouth, impotence, withdrawal hypertension (more with clonidine, less with guanfacine)
Catapres TTS (patch)	TTS-1 q wk	2 TTS-3 patches per wk	Patch: TTS-1, TTS-2, TTS-3	
Guanabenz (Wytensin, generic)	4 mg bid	32 mg bid	Tab: 4, 8 mg	
Guanfacine (Tenex, generic)	1 mg qhs	3 mg qhs	Tab: 1, 2 mg	
Methyldopa (Aldomet, generic)	250 mg bid	3000 mg/d	Tab: 125, 250, 500 mg Susp: 250 mg/5 mL	Same as other central agonists, plus hepatic and hemolytic anemia
Direct Vasodilators				
Hydralazine (Apresoline, generic)	10 mg qid–25 mg bid	200 mg/d	Tab: 10, 25, 50, 100 mg	Headaches, flushing, tachycardia, fluid retention, lupus-like reaction
Minoxidil (Loniten, generic)	5 mg/d	40 mg/d	Tab: 2.5, 10 mg	ECG changes, tachycardia, edema, pericardial effusion, hirsutism
Peripheral Adrenergic Antagonists				
Reserpine (generic)	0.05 mg/d	0.25 mg/d	Tab: 0.1, 0.25 mg	Depression, nasal stuffiness, activation of peptic ulcer

Abbreviations: ACEI = angiotensin-converting enzyme inhibitor; ARB = angiotensin receptor blocker; cap = capsule; ECG = electrocardiogram; GI = gastrointestinal; soln = solution; susp = suspension; tab = tablet.

Table compiled by Miriam Chan, PharmD, updated by Horacio E. Adrogue, MD (2014).

Please note that medications and doses in *__bold, underlined italics are the medications and doses from JNC 8 evidence-based dosing guidelines.__*

*Reduce diuretic dose before starting ACEI to prevent hypotension; reduce ACEI dosage in renal impairment (except moexipril). Contraindicated in bilateral renal artery stenosis. Pregnancy category C in the first trimester and category D in the second and third trimesters. Nonsteroidal antiinflammatory drugs reduce effect of ACEIs.

†Might require twice-daily dosing for 24-h control of blood pressure.

TABLE 4 Common Combination Products for Hypertension

DRUG COMBINATION	BRAND NAME	DOSAGE FORMS (mg/mg)
Angiotensin-Converting Enzyme Inhibitors and Calcium-Channel Blockers		
Amlodipine/benazepril	Lotrel, generic	2.5/10, 5/10, 5/20, 5/40, 10/20
Amlodipine/valsartan	Exforge	5/160, 5/320, 10/160, 10/320
Enalapril/felodipine	Lexxel	5/5
Trandolapril/verapamil	Tarka	1/240, 2/180, 2/240, 4/240
Angiotensin-Converting Enzyme Inhibitors and Diuretics		
Benazepril/HCTZ	Lotensin HCT, generic	5/6.25, 10/12.5, 20/12.5, 20/25
Captopril/HCTZ	Capozide, generic	25/15, 25/25, 50/15, 50/25
Enalapril/HCTZ	Vaseretic, generic	5/12.5, 10/25
Fosinopril/HCTZ	Monopril HCT, generic	10/12.5, 20/12.5
Lisinopril/HCTZ	Prinzide, Zestoretic, generic	10/12.5, 20/12.5, 20/25
Moexipril/HCTZ	Uniretic, generic	7.5/12.5, 15/12.5, 15/25
Quinapril/HCTZ	Accuretic, generic	10/12.5, 20/12.5, 20/25
Angiotensin Receptor Blocker and Calcium-Channel Blocker		
Telmisartan/amlodipine	Twynsta	40/5, 40/10, 80/5, 80/10
Angiotensin Receptor Blockers and Diuretics		
Candesartan/HCTZ	Atacand HCT	16/12.5, 32/12.5, 32/25
Eprosartan/HCTZ	Teveten-HCT	600/12.5, 600/25
Irbesartan/HCTZ	Avalide	150/12.5, 300/12.5, 300/25
Losartan/HCTZ	Hyzaar, generic	50/12.5, 100/12.5, 100/25
Olmesartan/HCTZ	Benicar HCT	20/12.5, 40/12.5, 40/25
Telmisartan/HCTZ	Micardis HCT	40/12.5, 80/12.5, 80/25
Valsartan/HCTZ	Diovan HCT	80/12.5, 160/12.5, 160/25, 320/12.5, 320/25
β-Blockers and Diuretics		
Atenolol/chlorthalidone	Tenoretic, generic	50/25, 100/25
Bisoprolol/HCTZ	Ziac, generic	2.5/6.25, 5/6.25, 10/6.25
Metoprolol/HCTZ	Lorpressor HCT, generic	50/25, 100/25, 100/50
Nadolol/bendroflumethiazide	Corzide	40/5, 80/5
Propranolol/HCTZ	Inderide LA, generic	40/25, 80/25

	TABLE 4	Common Combination Products for Hypertension—cont'd

DRUG COMBINATION	BRAND NAME	DOSAGE FORMS (mg/mg)
Calcium-Channel Blocker, Angiotensin-Converting Enzyme Inhibitor, and Diuretic		
Amlodipine/valsartan/HCTZ	Exforge HCT	5/160/12.5, 5/160/25, 10/160/12.5, 10/160/25, 10/320/25
Centrally Acting Drug and Diuretic		
Methyldopa/HCTZ	Aldoril, generic	250/15, 250/25, 500/30, 500/50
Clonidine/chlorthalidone	Clorpres	0.1/15, 0.2/15, 0.3/15
Direct Vasodilator and Diuretic		
Hydralazine/HCTZ	HydraZide, generic	25/25, 50/50
Diuretic and Diuretic		
Amiloride/HCTZ	Moduretic, generic	5/50
Spironolactone/HCTZ	Aldactazide, generic	25/25, 50/50
Triamterene/HCTZ	Dyazide, Maxzide, generic	37.5/25, 50/25, 75/50
Renin Inhibitor and Angiotensin Receptor Blocker		
Aliskiren/valsartan	Valturna	150/160, 300/320

Abbreviation: HCTZ = hydrochlorothiazide.
Table compiled by Miriam Chan, PharmD.

members published in the Annals of Internal Medicine disagreed with the recommendation to increase the target SBP from 140 to 150 in people aged 60 or older who did not have diabetes or CKD. This minority opinion noted that the evidence was insufficient and inadequate to reset the optimal SBP goal in this age group. While the majority voted to increase the goal, the minority felt that until RCT data was clearer, the goal should remain at a systolic BP of 140 mm Hg or less. The minority also expressed concern about raising the systolic BP target from lower than 140 to lower than 150 in high risk groups such as African Americans or those with a history of stroke or multiple risk factors. The JNC 8 panel did agree that more research is needed to identify optimal goals for systolic BPs for patients with high BP.

Recommendation 2
In the general population younger than 60 years old, start medications to lower BP at diastolic BP of 90 mm Hg or higher and treat to a goal diastolic BP of lower than 90 mm Hg. For patients aged 30 to 59, the JNC 8 panel considered this a strong recommendation with grade A data. For patients aged 18 through 29, this recommendation is based on expert opinion with grade E data. One way to interpret this recommendation would be that for those patients 18 through 29 years old, the diastolic BP goal could be anywhere between 80 and 90 mm Hg. The panel of JNC 8 concluded that there were no good or fair quality randomized control trials that assessed the benefits of treating elevated diastolic BP on health outcomes in adults younger than 30. Without this data available, the panel's expert opinion was to set the diastolic BP treatment threshold and goal for adults younger than 30 at the same level as adults 30 through 59 years of age.

Recommendation 3
In those patients younger than 60 years of age, medications should be initiated to treat the systolic BP of 140 or higher and treat to goal of lower than 140 mm Hg. This recommendation is based on expert opinion with a grade E strength of recommendation. The main logic for this recommendation was the absence of any randomized control trials that compared the current systolic BP standard of 140 mm Hg with another higher or lower standard in this group; therefore, there were no compelling reasons to change from the JNC 7 recommendation.

Recommendation 4
In patients aged 18 or older with CKD, medication treatment should be started to lower BP at a systolic BP of 140 mm Hg or higher or diastolic BP of 90 mm Hg or higher. The goal of treatment should be a systolic BP of lower than 140 mm Hg and a diastolic BP of lower than 90 mm Hg. This was based on expert opinion with a grade E recommendation. More specifically, in adults below the age of 70 with CKD, there is insufficient data to determine the benefit in mortality or cardiovascular or cerebrovascular health outcomes with a BP therapy goal of less than 130/80 when compared to less than 140/90. Evidence of moderate quality demonstrated no benefit in slowing the progression of CKD using a lower BP goal of less than 130/80 compared with 140/90. In patients with CKD and more than 3 g per 24-hour period of proteinuria, only a *post hoc* analysis of 1 study (the Modification of Diet in Renal Disease study) indicated benefits from treatment to a lower BP goal of less than 130/80, and those outcomes were related only to kidney function outcomes, not mortality or morbidity. The JNC 8 panel conclusion for this category of patients, after weighing the risks and benefits of a BP goal for people aged 70 years or older with an estimated glomerular filtration rate (GFR) of less than 60 mL per minute BP, was that treatment should be individualized and take into consideration the comorbidities of the patient. One important point to remember in patients who have CKD with proteinuria is to avoid combining treatment with both an ACEI and ARB. The combination of these two classes of agents has shown to increase the risk of hyperkalemia and worsen CKD. This represents an important change in commonly accepted practice in the current management of these patients.

Recommendation 5
In patients aged 18 or older with diabetes mellitus, medications should be initiated to treat patients with systolic BPs of 140 or higher or diastolic BP of 90 mm Hg or higher. The treatment goal should be a systolic BP of less than 140 mm Hg and a diastolic BP goal of lower than 90 mm Hg. This recommendation was based on expert opinion with grade E data. The panel did recognize that a systolic BP goal of lower than 130 mm Hg is commonly recommended for adults with diabetes and hypertension. However this was not supported by any randomized control trials that they reviewed. The commonly quoted ACCORD-BP trial was specifically reviewed. The panel did not feel that it provided sufficient evidence to recommend a systolic BP of lower than 120 in adults with diabetes and hypertension. A review of the HOT trial, which is frequently used to support a lower diastolic BP goal, only found a *post hoc* analysis of a small subgroup to support a diastolic BP goal of 80 mm Hg per lower. The UKPDS trial did show that treatment in the lower goal BP group was associated with less stroke, heart failure, and diabetes-related endpoints and death related to

diabetes. However the comparison in this trial was a diastolic BP goal of less than 85 when compared to 105 mm Hg. Based on their review of the data, the JNC 8 recommendation was to treat to a diastolic BP of less than 90 mm Hg.

Recommendation 6

In the nonblack population, including those with diabetes mellitus, high BP treatment should include a thiazide-type diuretic, CCB, ACEI, or ARB. This is a moderate recommendation with grade B data. It is important to note that for this recommendation only, randomized control trials that compared one class of antihypertensive medication to another and assessed the effects on health outcomes were reviewed. Placebo-controlled randomized control trials were not included. Notably, β-blockers are not recommended for initial treatment of hypertension based on the LIFE study showing that their use resulted in a high rate of the primary composite outcome of cardiovascular death, myocardial infarction, or stroke compared to the use of an ARB for initial therapy. This finding was largely driven by an increase in stroke. Similarly, alpha blockers were not recommended as first-line therapy because of the ALLHAT study showing that initial treatment resulted in worse cerebrovascular, heart failure, and combined cardiovascular outcomes when compared to initial treatment with a thiazide diuretic. The other classes of medications may be added to the initial therapy as needed to control BP. An important note was made to clarify that this recommendation is only specific to thiazide diuretics such as chlorthalidone (Hygroton), indapamide (Lozol), and hydrochlorothiazide. Loop or potassium-sparing diuretics are not included in this recommendation. One last important note applies to specific populations who have coronary artery disease or heart failure but do not have hypertension. RCTs for treatment of the population who do not have hypertension were not reviewed for this recommendation. Therefore, recommendation 6 does not apply to those who do not have hypertension.

Recommendation 7

In the black population, including those with diabetes mellitus, initial therapy should include a thiazide-type diuretic or a CCB. For the general black population, this is a moderate recommendation with grade B data. For black patients with diabetes mellitus, this is a weak recommendation with grade C data. This recommendation stems from the ALLHAT study specifically using thiazide-type diuretics and showing improvement in cerebrovascular, heart failure, and combined cardiovascular outcomes compared to an ACE inhibitor in this subgroup. A CCB is recommended over an ACE inhibitor as first-line therapy in black patients because there was a 51% higher rate of stroke in the ALLHAT study with the use of an ACE inhibitor as initial therapy compared with the use of a CCB.

Recommendation 8

In patients age 18 or older with CKD and hypertension, initial or subsequent BP medication treatment should include an ARB or an ACE inhibitor to improve kidney outcomes. This applies to all CKD patients with hypertension with or without diabetes and to blacks and nonblacks. Direct renin inhibitors are not included in this recommendation because there were no randomized controlled studies demonstrating benefit on kidney or cardiovascular outcomes. In patients who are black with CKD and proteinuria, an ACE inhibitor or ARB is recommended as initial therapy because of the high likelihood of progression to end-stage kidney disease when compared to nonblacks. In blacks with CKD but without proteinuria, the choice for initial therapy is not quite as clear but does include thiazide-type diuretics, CCBs, ACE inhibitors, or ARBs. JNC 8 mentions that an ACEI or an ARB can be added as a second-line drug if necessary to a patient not already on an ACEI or an ARB. The combination of an ACE inhibitor and an ARB is potentially very dangerous and has been shown to increase the risk of hyperkalemia and progression of CKD. It is no longer recommended to use both of these agents together. Patients with CKD while on an ACEI or an ARB should be followed very closely for elevations in potassium and worsening of kidney function. Patient with CKD should

also be screened for renal artery stenosis prior to initiating of an ACE inhibitor or an ARB.

Recommendation 9

Once antihypertensive medications have been started, they should be given for at least 1 month to achieve the treatment goal. If the BP goal is not reached within 1 month, the dose of the initial medication could be increased or a second agent could be added from the other recommended classes such as thiazide diuretics, CCBs, ACE inhibitor, or ARB. If the BP goal cannot be reached with two medications, adding a third medication is indicated. Recommendation 9 underscores the importance of not using an ACEI and an ARB together for the same patient. If the goal BP cannot be reached through the use of thiazide diuretics, CCBs, ACE inhibitor, or ARB because of contraindications, side effects, or the need to use more than three drugs, antihypertensive medications from other classes may be used. The JNC 8 panel recommended consideration of referral to a hypertensive expert if the patient cannot be controlled with three medications. This recommendation is based on expert opinion with grade E data. No randomized controlled data could be found to recommend any specific strategy for adding or titrating antihypertensive medications.

The limitations of JNC 8 were clearly noted with these recommendations. The JNC 8 panel clearly stated that these evidence-based guidelines for the management of high BP in adults is limited in scope because of the focused evidence review to address the three specific questions noted above. The evidence reviewed did not include observational studies, systemic reviews, or meta-analysis. The focus of the recommendations was based on RCTs. Randomized control trials including participants with normal BP were excluded from the analysis.

The panel members appointed to JNC 8 were selected from more than 400 nominees based on expertise in hypertension, primary care, geriatrics, cardiology, nephrology, nursing, pharmacology, clinical trials, evidence-based medicine, epidemiology, informatics, and the development and implementation of clinical guidelines and systems of care. The initial literature search dates for the literature review were January 1, 1966, through December 31, 2009. A subsequent search was performed through August 2013; the panel found no additional studies that they felt should change the recommendations.

Diuretics

Agents targeting the distal convoluted tubule (thiazide-type diuretics) are preferred in the treatment of hypertension. Hydrochlorothiazide (HydroDiuril) (12.5 to 25 mg/day) is the most commonly used, and chlorthalidone (12.5 to 100 mg/day) has been used in all the National Institutes of Health trials. Chlorthalidone is a stronger and longer-acting agent than hydrocholothiazide.

It is important to allow up to 4 weeks for the full effect of diuretic agents. Creatinine, magnesium, uric acid, and electrolyte levels should be measured every 1 to 2 weeks when diuretics are being instituted. When the dosage is stable, laboratory values can be checked every 4 to 6 weeks. In patients whose GFR is less than 40 mL/minute/1.73 m^2, thiazide-type agents might not work, and loop diuretics will be a better choice.

Furosemide (Lasix) is best dosed every 6 to 8 hours with doses of 20 to 40 mg. Doses up to 400 mg have been used in severe edema, but such high doses require close monitoring of electrolytes. In patients with heart failure and severe proteinuria (>4 g/day), a better choice may be bumetanide (Bumex)[1] 1 to 10 mg/day, which is up to 40 times more potent and twice as orally bioavailable. If hypokalemia becomes a problem, the use of a potassium-sparing diuretic such as amiloride (Midamor) 5 to 10 mg/day may be indicated. Care must be taken to avoid hyperkalemia, especially in those with a GFR less than 50 mL/min/1.73 m^2.

The aldosterone blocker spironolactone (Aldactone) has been shown to decrease mortality in patients with congestive heart failure (25 mg/day). It has also been found to help control refractory hypertension at much higher doses (1 mg/kg/day) when used in

---

[1]Not FDA approved for this indication.

combination with ACEIs or ARBs. Great care should be taken to watch for life-threatening hyperkalemia that can develop with this combination of medications.

Adrenergic-Inhibiting Drugs

Central α-agonists such as clonidine (Catapres) are often added to diuretics and act centrally on both imidazoline receptors and α_2-receptors. Clonidine can be given 0.1 to 1.4 mg twice per day. Sedation and dry mouth can be dose-limiting side effects, and rebound hypertension will occur with a sudden cessation of clonidine.

β-Adrenergic receptor blockers can cause worsening bradycardia when used in combination with clonidine. Carvedilol (Coreg) has been tested against metoprolol (Toprol XL) and found to provide survival benefit in heart failure. When used for hypertension, carvedilol is best dosed twice a day starting with 6.25 mg twice daily to a maximum of 25 mg twice daily. It is superior to metoprolol because it does not worsen insulin sensitivity and has a limited effect on lipids.

The most notable comparative drug trials for hypertension are ANBP2 (Second Australian National Blood Pressure Study: ACEI superior to thiazide in men only); LIFE (Losartan Intervention for Endpoint reduction: ARB superior to β-blocker) and ACCOMPLISH (Avoiding Cardiovascular Events in Combination Therapy in Patients Living with Systolic Hypertension: ACEI plus calcium-channel

blocker superior to ACEI plus thiazide) and the AASK trial (African American Study of Kidney Disease and Hypertension).

The AASK study enrolled 1094 African Americans with hypertensive kidney disease (GFR 20–65 mL/min/1.73 m^2) and studied two BP goals using three different agents. The normal BP control group (mean arterial pressure [MAP], 102–107 mm Hg; $n = 554$) was compared to the tight control group (MAP $\leq$92 mm Hg; $n = 540$). The groups of patients were divided into groups treated with the β-blocker metoprolol (Lopressor) ($n = 441$) or the ACEI ramipril (Altace) ($n = 436$) or the dihydropyridine CCB amlodipine (Norvasc) ($n = 217$). Other open-label agents were also allowed. The low-BP group reached an average of 128/78 mm Hg and the normal group reached 141/85 mm Hg.

The conclusion in this study was that ramipril appears to be more effective in slowing progression of CKD than metoprolol and amlodipine when followed over 3 to 6 years. Only subjects with more than 1 g of proteinuria showed a trend toward slower progression of CKD in the lower BP group. One last very important point was that the amlodipine group showed a significant *increase* in proteinuria (58%) when compared to the *reduction* in the ramipril group (20%) and the metoprolol group (14%).

One very useful algorithm has been proposed and is depicted in Figure 2. Doses should be titrated every 1 to 2 weeks, and

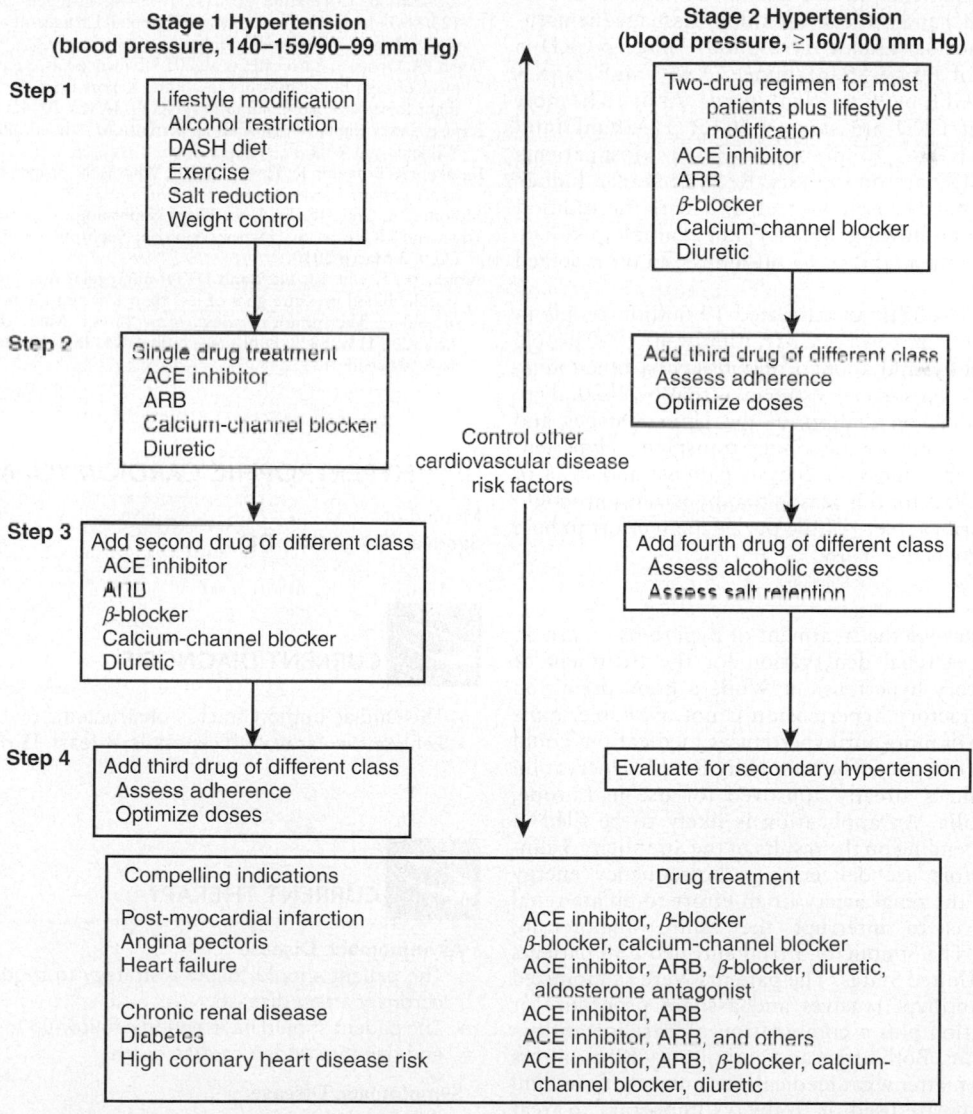

Figure 2. Algorithm for management of hypertension. *Abbreviations*: ACE = angiotensin-converting enzyme; ARB = angiotensin receptor blocker; DASH = dietary approaches to stop hypertension. (Reprinted with permission from Chobanian AV: Shattuck Lecture. The hypertension paradox—More uncontrolled disease despite improved therapy. N Engl J Med 2009;361:878–87.)

great care should be taken to ensure that the physician looks for compelling indications and matches them with appropriate drug therapy.

BP should be monitored every 2 to 4 weeks while medications are increased or added. Laboratory testing should be individualized to the patient's needs, comorbid conditions, and the medications being used to treat the patient's hypertension. If large doses of diuretics, ACEIs, or ARBs are used, weekly laboratory studies may be indicated.

Complications

The most common complications from long-standing hypertension include stroke, heart disease, and CKD. One of the most important points to remember about hypertension is that it is one factor that must be taken into account in the patient's overall risk for heart disease. There are several cardiovascular risk calculators. One such calculator can be found at www.qintervention.org. This calculator estimates the 10-year risk for TIA or stroke and heart disease as well as the 10-year risk of developing type 2 diabetes mellitus. The Framingham score is still considered the gold standard for risk calculation and can be found at http://hp2010.nhlbihin.net/atpiii/calculator.asp?usertype=prof#moreinfo.

CKD is not only a consequence of hypertension but also a newly recognized risk factor for heart disease. CKD is defined as kidney damage for more than 3 months, irrespective of the underlying cause. CKD stage 1 patients have a normal or increased GFR (>90 mL/min/1.73 m^2) and evidence of kidney damage (hematuria, proteinuria, abnormal kidney ultrasound). Stage 2 CKD is defined by a GFR of 60 to 89 mL/min/1.73 m^2, and stage 3 CKD is defined by a GFR of 30 to 59 mL/min/1.73 m^2. The most concerning stages of CKD are stage 4 (GFR 15–29 mL/min/1.73 m^2) and stage 5 (GFR <15 mL/min/1.73 m^2). Most patients who have stage 5 CKD are on dialysis. Recipients of a kidney transplant are CKD-staged based on their GFR with the addition of a "T" for transplant following the stage. For example, a kidney transplant recipient with a GFR of 65 mL/min/1.73 m^2 is staged CKD 2 T.

According to NHANES III, an estimated 19 million people in the United States have some form of CKD. Almost 400,000 people are on dialysis currently, and about 150,000 have a functioning kidney transplant. The most recent estimate is that by 2020, there will be 530,000 people on dialysis in the United Stages and 250,000 people with a functioning kidney transplant. Hypertension continues to affect almost all dialysis patients and 70% of transplant recipients. It is for this reason that hypertension should be managed as one critical piece of the puzzle in an effort to help patients live long, productive lives.

Future Therapy

Many new approaches for the treatment of hypertension are on the way. We may see renal denervation for the treatment of uncontrolled refractory hypertension. While a good definition for uncontrolled refractory hypertension is not available, most patients taking three or more antihypertensive medications could be considered in this category. The Simplicity Renal Denervation system by Medtronic is already approved for use in Europe, Canada, and Australia. An application is likely to be filed in the United States depending on the results of the Simplicity 3 clinical trial. Investigators are delivering radiofrequency energy through the wall of the renal artery in an effort to ablate renal nerves. The goal is to interrupt the renin, angiotensin, aldosterone system. The Simplicity 3 trial enrolled 530 patients in 88 centers in the United States. The patients were randomized either to baseline antihypertensives and a sham procedure or renal nerve denervation plus a combination of baseline antihypertensive medications. Both office and ambulatory BP monitors will be reported. No matter what medications, interventions, and lifestyle modifications are used, it is always important to treat each patient as an individual. RCTs and recommendations are based on ideal circumstances. The lives of humans on this earth are never ideal or strictly controlled. One size certainly does not fit all. The most important component of treatment of any disease is the patient-physician relationship. Without this, there is never success.

References

Adrogué HJ, Madias NE. Sodium and potassium in the pathogenesis of hypertension. N Engl J Med 2007;356:1966–78.

CDC. Vital signs: Awareness and treatment of uncontrolled hypertension among adults—United States, 2003–2010. MMWR Morb Mortal Wkly Rep 2012;61:703–9. http://www.cdc.gov/mmwr/preview/mmwrhtml/mm6135a3.htm.

Chobanian AV. Shattuck Lecture. The hypertension paradox—More uncontrolled disease despite improved therapy. N Engl J Med 2009;361:878–87.

Chobanian AV, Bakris GL, Black HR, et al. Clinician's corner: The seventh report of the Joint National Committee on prevention, detection, evaluation, and treatment of high blood pressure. The JNC 7 report. JAMA 2003;289:2560–71, Special Communication.

Collins AJ, Foley RN, Gilbertson DT, Chen SC. The state of chronic kidney disease, ESRD, and morbidity and mortality in the first year of dialysis. Clin J Am Soc Nephrol 2009;4:S5–S11.

Cooney MT, Dudina AL, Graham IM. Value and limitations of existing scores for the assessment of cardiovascular risk: A review for clinicians. J Am Coll Cardiol 2009;54:1209–27.

Feig DI, Soletsky B, Johnson RJ. Effect of allopurinol on blood pressure of adolescents with newly diagnosed essential hypertension: A randomized trial. JAMA 2008;300:924–32.

Go AS, Mozaffarian D, Roger VL, et al. Heart disease and stroke statistics—2013 update: A report from the American Heart Association. Circulation 2013; 127:e6–e245, http://circ.ahajournals.org/content/127/1/e6http://www.cdc.gov/TemplatePackage/images/icon_out.pnghttp://www.cdc.gov/Other/disclaimer.html.

Heidenreich PA, Trogdon JG, Khavjou OA, et al. Forecasting the future of cardiovascular disease in the United States: A policy statement from the American Heart Association. Circulation 2011;123:933–44, http://circ.ahajournals.org/content/123/8/933.longhttp://www.cdc.gov/TemplatePackage/images/icon_out.pnghttp://www.cdc.gov/Other/disclaimer.html.

James PA, Oparil S, Carter BL, et al. 2014 Evidence-based guidelines for the management of high blood pressure in adults. Report from the panel appointed to the Eight Joint National Committee (JNC 8). JAMA 2014;311:507–20.

Kaplan NM. Kaplan's Clinical Hypertension. 9th ed. Philadelphia: Lippincott Williams and Wilkins; 2006.

Katakam R, Brukamp K, Townsend RR. What is the proper workup of a patient with hypertension? Cleve Clin J Med 2008;75:663–72.

Molony DA, Craig JC. Evidence-Based Nephrology. Oxford: Blackwell; 2009.

Townsend RR, Textor SC. Hypertension. In: Nephrology Self-Assessment Program 9; 2010, 2 March 2010.

Wright Jr JT, Fine LJ, Lackland DT, et al. Special report: Evidence supporting a systolic blood pressure goal of less than 150 mm Hg in patients aged 60 years of older: The minority view, Ann Intern Med 2014; http://dx.doi.org/10.7326/M13-2981. Published online 14 January, http://annals.org/article.aspx?articleid=1813288.

HYPERTROPHIC CARDIOMYOPATHY

Method of
Sandeep Sangodkar, DO

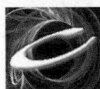

CURRENT DIAGNOSIS

- The cardiac outflow tract is obstructed.
- Left ventricular wall thickness is at least 15 mm.

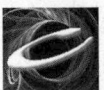

CURRENT THERAPY

Asymptomatic Disease
- The patient should follow a strategy to modify risk factors for coronary artery disease.
- The patient should have periodic follow-up to assess symptoms and risk for sudden cardiac death.

Symptomatic Disease
- β-Blockade or calcium channel blockers are drugs of choice.
- Implantable defibrillator is indicated if the patient has risk factors for sudden cardiac death.

- Surgical myectomy may be undertaken in patients who do not respond to pharmacologic therapy.
- Alcohol ablation may be used in patients who are not candidates for surgery.

Definition

Many names, terms, and acronyms (more than 80) have been used to describe hypertrophic cardiomyopathy (HCM). Common names such as idiopathic hypertrophic subaortic stenosis and hypertrophic obstructive cardiomyopathy, popular in the literature in the 1960s and 1970s, imply that left ventricular outflow tract (LVOT) obstruction is a required component of the disease, whereas one third of patients have no obstruction at rest or exertion. The term *hypertrophic cardiomyopathy,* first used in 1979, encompasses both the obstructive and nonobstructive hemodynamic variants of this disease and is now considered the formal name.

Epidemiology

HCM is a common genetic cardiovascular disease. Epidemiologic studies from various parts of the world report similar prevalence of hypertrophy of the left ventricle (LV) of about 0.2% based on detection of LV wall thickness greater than 15 mm. A true estimate may be higher owing to variable genetic penetrance, but this is offset by the fact that clinical diagnosis is unable to distinguish true HCM from HCM phenocopy conditions.

Risk Factors

HCM is caused by an autosomal-dominant mutation in sarcomere genes, with most evidence indicating that eight genes—those for beta myosin heavy chain, myosin binding protein C, troponin T, troponin I, alpha tropomyosin, actin, regulatory light chain, and essential light chain—are most accountable.

Clinical Manifestations

Most patients with HCM are asymptomatic or only mildly symptomatic, most commonly presenting with dyspnea and chest pain. Initial presentations are seen in every age range, from pediatric to geriatric, and most patients have normal life expectancy without need for major intervention. The major pathways of disease progression are sudden cardiac death due to ventricular tachyarrhythmias in young, asymptomatic patients; heart failure with exertional dyspnea with or without chest pain, with sinus rhythm and preserved systolic function or with systolic dysfunction due to myocardial scarring; and atrial fibrillation with increased risk of thromboembolism.

Pathogenesis

The pathophysiology of HCM is a group of multiple abnormalities including LVOT obstruction, diastolic dysfunction, mitral regurgitation, cardiac ischemia, and arrhythmias. The peak instantaneous LV outflow gradient (rather than the mean) is important in determining treatment options. The obstruction was originally thought to be caused by a hypertrophied basal septum that caused ventricular outflow obstruction during systolic contraction. However, now evidence points toward mitral valve systolic anterior motion and mitral–septal contact (possibly as a result of hypertrophied or anomalous papillary muscles), resulting in drag force on the mitral leaflets, with displacement into the outflow tract. The increased LV systolic pressure in turn results in elevated diastolic pressures, prolonged diastole, mitral regurgitation, and, ultimately, decreased cardiac output.

Diagnosis

Clinically, HCM is defined as maximal LV wall thickness of at least 15 mm based on echocardiography. Patients with thickened LV wall and concurrent presence of HCM genetic substrates (storage disease, mitochondrial disorders, and triplet repeat syndromes) or family members with pathologic sarcomere mutations are considered to have genotype positive–phenotype negative HCM or subclinical HCM. A distinction between HCM and physiologic LV hypertrophy from athletic conditioning must be recognized because the latter may be responsible for enlargement of the left ventricle, right ventricle, left atrium, and aorta and thickening of the septum. The likelihood of clinically significant HCM is determined by identification of sarcomere mutations, marked LV thickness (more than 25 mm), and LV outflow tract obstruction with systolic anterior motion and mitral–septal contact.

Imaging

The mainstay of imaging currently lies with echocardiography. Transthoracic echocardography is recommended in the initial evaluation of all patients with suspected HCM as well as family members of those with diagnosed HCM. Transesophageal echocardiography is used for intraoperative guidance of surgical myectomy and intraprocedural guidance of alcohol septal ablation.

As new imaging modalities such as cardiac magnetic resonance imaging (MRI) are becoming increasingly available, they are indicated for suspected HCM when echocardiography is inconclusive for diagnosis, and they can be used when HCM is known but anatomy cannot be properly visualized via echocardiography.

Treatment

Asymptomatic Disease

Given that a large subset of HCM patients are asymptomatic and will achieve normal life expectancy, it is important to educate patients about the disease process, screening family members, and avoiding strenuous activity. Coronary artery disease has an impact on survival, and thus aggressive modification of risk factors contributing to atherosclerosis (diabetes, hyperlipidemia, obesity) should play a significant role in management. Low-intensity aerobic exercise is reasonable to allow the patient to maintain fitness. Adequate hydration and avoidance of situations leading to vasodilation are encouraged to minimize exacerbation of an existing LVOT obstruction.

Although animal studies suggest renin-angiotensin pathway inhibitors, diltiazem (Cardizem),[1] or statins can prevent hypertrophy in animal models, there are no randomized, controlled trials in humans to indicate human benefit. Septal reduction therapy is not indicated in an asymptomatic patient with any degree of obstruction.

Symptomatic Disease
Pharmacologic Management

β-Blockade is the mainstay of treatment because of its potent negative inotropic effects as well as antagonizing adrenergic tachycardia. β-Blocking agents are recommended for angina and dyspnea in adult patients with either obstructive or nonobstructive HCM, but caution must be observed in the presence of concomitant sinus bradycardia or conduction disease. Verapamil (Calan)[1] (beginning at a low dose and titrating to 480 mg/day) is recommended for those who do not respond or who have contraindications to β-blockade. IV phenylephrine (Neo-Synephrine) is recommended for acute hypotension with obstructive HCM in those who do not respond to fluids.

Nifedipine (Procardia)[1] or other dihydropyridine calcium channel blocking agents are potentially harmful owing to their vasodilative effects, which can worsen LVOT obstruction. Digitalis is potentially harmful in patients without atrial fibrillation. Dopamine, dobutamine, norepinephrine (Levophed), and other positive inotropic agents may be harmful for the treatment of acute hypotension.

Invasive Therapies

The major septal reduction therapies are surgical myectomy and alcohol ablation. Septal reduction therapy should not be performed in asymptomatic adults.

---

[1]Not FDA approved for this indication.

Transaortic septal myectomy is considered the most appropriate therapy for eligible patients unresponsive to optimal medical therapy. The traditional (Morrow procedure) approach involved a 3-cm-long resection. An extended myectomy involves a 7-cm resection that is wider at the mid-ventricular level opposite the lateral portion of the anterior leaflet. The extended myectomy attempts to avoid conduction tissue, chordae, and papillary muscles as well as resection along the left lateral free wall. Eligible patients include those with severe dyspnea, chest pain, or exertional syncope that affect everyday activity even with maximal medical therapy. Hemodynamic considerations that determine eligibility consist of an LVOT gradient of at least 50 mm Hg associated with septal hypertrophy and mitral valve systolic anterior motion. Ultimately, the anatomic septal thickness must be evaluated by the individual operator.

When surgery is contraindicated, alcohol septal ablation can benefit adult patients with HCM and LVOT obstruction. This procedure, first reported in 1995, involves percutaneous access of the coronary arteries and injection of ethanol,[1] with the intent of inducing infarction of the basal septal wall near the anterior leaflet contact point. The effectiveness of alcohol septal ablation is not clear in patients with more than 30 mm of septal hypertrophy, and it should not be performed in patients with concomitant disease (coronary artery disease, mitral valve repair) that would need surgical correction regardless.

Implantable Devices

Dual-chamber pacemaker implantation was originally proposed for severe obstructive symptomatic HCM with the premise that pacing at the RV apex with maintenance of AV synchrony would result in decreased LVOT gradient. Prior trials showed a considerable placebo effect. Current guidelines now state that patients who have a dual-chamber device for non-HCM indications may consider a trial of dual-chamber AV pacing. Permanent pacing may be considered in poor candidates for septal reduction therapy.

All patients with HCM need comprehensive sudden cardiac death risk stratification, with strong consideration for those with personal history of ventricular fibrillation, sustained ventricular tachycardia, family history of sudden cardiac death, unexplained syncope, or documented nonsustained VT greater than 3+ beats equal to 120 beats/min on Holter monitor. Implantable defibrillators are recommended for patients with prior cardiac arrest, ventricular fibrillation, or hemodynamically significant VT (class 1, level of evidence B). ICDs should also be considered in those with relatives who succumbed to sudden cardiac death presumably caused by HCM, maximum LV wall thickness more than 30 mm, or unexplained syncope (class 2a, level of evidence C).

Participation in Competitive Sports

It is reasonable for HCM patients to engage in low-intensity competitive sports (golf, bowling) and recreational sporting activities. They should avoid participation in intense competitive sports regardless of age, sex, LVOT obstruction, prior septal reduction, or ICD.

Monitoring

With a family history of sudden cardiac death, periodic screening by transthoracic echocardiography (every 12 to 18 months) is recommended in children by age 12 years (or younger if the child has signs of early puberty) or if there are plans for intense sports competition. Repeat transthoracic echocardiography is recommended for any change in clinical status or new cardiovascular event. Genetic screening and counseling of all first-degree family members of patients with HCM is now recommended (class I, level of evidence B).

Future Research

Although significant progress has been made in elucidating the etiology and pathophysiology of HCM, there is much room for advancement. In addition, the relationship between genetics and environmental influences as well as the management of family members of genotype positive–phenotype negative patients is still unclear. Further investigation regarding the clinical significance of myocardial fibrosis, therapies to modify HCM pathophysiology, and direct comparison of septal reduction strategies is also needed.

References

Cannan CR, Reeder GS, Bailey KR, et al. Natural history of hypertrophic cardiomyopathy. A population based study, 1976 through 1990. Circulation 1995; 92:2488–95.

Gersh BJ, Maron BJ, Bonow RO, et al. 2011 ACCF/AHA guideline for the diagnosis and treatment of hypertrophic cardiomyopathy. Circulation 2011;124: e783–e831.

Marian AJ. Genetic determinants of cardiac hypertrophy. Curr Opin Cardiol 2008;23:199–205.

Marian AJ. Recent advances in genetics and treatment of hypertrophic cardiomyopathy. Future Cardiol 2005;1:341–53.

Maron BJ. Hypertrophic cardiomyopathy: A systematic review. JAMA 2002;287:1308–20.

INFECTIVE ENDOCARDITIS

Method of
Andrew Wang, MD

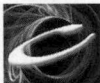

CURRENT DIAGNOSIS

- Infective endocarditis should be considered as a diagnosis in the setting of fever and heart murmur.
- Health care–associated interventions and resulting infections are an increasingly noted cause of IE, changing the epidemiology of this disease.
- Blood cultures show growth in approximately 90% of cases, and multiple sets should be obtained before initiating antibiotics to improve diagnostic yield.
- Echocardiography, particularly transesophageal echocardiography, improves diagnostic sensitivity for infective endocarditis as well as its complications (e.g., intracardiac abscess, fistula).
- The diagnosis of complications, including heart failure, embolic events, and abscess, requires close surveillance, particularly during the first week of therapy, and has adverse prognostic implications.

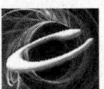

CURRENT THERAPY

- Because of changes in the epidemiology of infective endocarditis (IE), empiric antibiotic therapy for *Staphylococcus aureus* should be considered before results of blood cultures are available.
- Prompt initiation of antibiotic therapy is important, because the rate of complications such as embolization decreases rapidly within several days.
- Multidisciplinary care for the patient with IE should include evaluation by specialists in infectious diseases, cardiology, and cardiothoracic surgery, especially in cases of complicated IE.
- Surgery for IE has not been studied in randomized, controlled trials compared to medical therapy alone. Surgery should be considered for IE complicated by heart failure, embolism, intracardiac abscess, or persistent bacteremia.
- Although stroke due to embolism is not uncommon in IE, data do not suggest a benefit in delaying cardiac surgery after cerebral infarction if surgery is otherwise indicated.

Definition

Infective endocarditis (IE) is a microbial infection of the valves or endocardium of the heart.

---

[1]Not FDA approved for this indication.

Epidemiology and Risk Factors

The incidence of IE varies regionally from 2.6 per 100,000 population reported in France to 11.6 per 100,000 population in urban areas of the United States. This range of incidence has been attributed to differences in predisposing cardiac conditions or risk factors, such as use of injection drugs. The incidence of IE is also affected by age and sex. The incidence of native valve IE increases with age and exceeds 30 per 100,000 after 30 years of age. The average age of the patient with IE has increased over time, likely related to the decreased prevalence of rheumatic heart disease and increased prevalence of degenerative valvular disease in the aging population. IE is more commonly diagnosed in men, with studies showing male-to-female ratios as high as 9:1.

In earlier eras, streptococcal species were the predominant cause of native valve IE. However, changes in the delivery of health care, with increasing exposure to invasive procedures and devices, and the changing demographics of patients and their risk factors for IE have led to major changes in the microbiologic causes of endocarditis. There is an increasing incidence of health care–associated IE, including nosocomial infection and infection related to ambulatory care, which accounts for approximately 25% of IE cases. For example, in one large multinational study, the International Collaboration on Endocarditis (ICE) registry ($N = 2781$ patients with definite native or prosthetic endocarditis), 31% of cases were attributable to *Staphylococcus aureus*, 17% to viridans streptococci, 11% to enterococci, 10% to coagulase-negative staphylococci, 12% to other streptococcal species, 2% to the HACEK (*Haemophilus* spp., *Aggregatibacter* spp., *Cardiobacterium hominis*, *Eikenella corrodens*, *Kingella* spp.) group, 2% to non-HACEK Gram negative bacteria, and 2% to fungi. Among those with *S. aureus* endocarditis, health care–associated infection accounted for 39% of cases.

Predisposing cardiac conditions to the development of IE include degenerative valve disease (in approximately 40% of cases of mitral and 25% of aortic valve IE), presence of prosthetic valve, injection drug use, and rheumatic heart disease.

Pathophysiology

A preexisting valvular or endocardial condition, such as mitral valve prolapse with regurgitation, degenerative aortic valve disease (including bicuspid aortic valve), or congenital heart disease, is a major host factor related to development of IE. Endothelial damage and denudation of the endothelium exposes the underlying basement membrane and fosters platelet and fibrin deposition, a process that occurs spontaneously in persons with valvular heart disease. These deposits are called *nonbacterial thrombotic endocarditis* and form the nidus for vegetation to begin in the setting of bacteremia. The classic lesion of IE, the vegetation, is made up of fibrin, platelets, inflammatory cells, and microorganisms adherent to the endothelium of the heart.

The degree of mechanical stress exerted on the valve might contribute to endothelial denudation and the location of vegetation formation, with left-sided IE more common than right-sided IE. Endocarditis involving the nonvalvular endocardium of the heart similarly occurs at sites of endothelial damage due to mechanical stress, such as the left ventricular outflow tract in patients with hypertrophic obstructive cardiomyopathy and congenital heart defects (ventricular septal defects and patent ductus arteriosus).

The adhesion of bacteria to the denuded endothelium might depend on specific properties of the bacteria. Cell surface characteristics of the organism promote its adherence. For example, the adherence of *S. aureus* to a traumatized animal heart valve has been found to be reduced in the setting of impaired fibronectin binding. Similarly, the ability of bacteria to form biofilm may be associated with their ability to form localized clusters of infections that can make these clusters more resistant to killing by the host immune system and antimicrobial therapy.

With the progressive development of a vegetation, function of the specific heart valve is impaired. Regurgitation or insufficiency of the affected valve most commonly results, leading predominantly to volume overload of the ventricular chamber. In the setting of acute or rapid development of regurgitation, there may be no ventricular adaptation to this volume overload; as a result, acute, severe pulmonary edema and cardiogenic shock may quickly ensue. Less commonly, a large vegetation can result in stenosis of the valve orifice and pressure overload of the proximal or upstream cardiac chamber. As infection extends, destruction of other cardiac tissue, including myocardium and fibrous structures, can occur and result in intracardiac abscess or fistula formation between cardiac chambers.

Prevention

The efficacy of antimicrobial prophylaxis in preventing IE continues to be debated. Current recommendations are generally based on the likelihood of bacteremia occurring as a result of the procedure, the potential for adverse outcome as related to the predisposing cardiac condition, and the level of evidence for antibiotic prophylaxis as effective for the prevention of IE. The American Heart Association has published updated guidelines for IE prophylaxis with a continued trend toward fewer indications for prophylaxis.

Based on an extensive review of published literature and expert consensus, these guidelines have concluded that IE is more likely to result from bacteremia associated with daily activities than with a dental procedure. Antibiotic prophylaxis, even if 100% effective, is estimated to prevent only an extremely small number of cases of IE. These recommendations concluded that antibiotic prophylaxis should not be prescribed solely on the basis of an increased lifetime risk of IE but on the basis of cardiac conditions associated with highest risk of an adverse outcome from IE.

Conditions that warrant IE prophylaxis before dental procedures and procedures on respiratory tract, skin, and musculoskeletal structures are listed in Box 1 and Table 1. The American Heart Association no longer recommends prophylaxis before gastrointestinal or genitourinary procedures solely for the prevention of IE.

Clinical Manifestations and Diagnosis

The diagnosis of IE depends on findings of bacteremia with an organism associated with IE and evidence of endocardial involvement. Because these objective findings may not be sought unless the possibility of IE is considered, careful attention to the patient's history and physical examination is critical to the eventual diagnosis. The clinical presentation of IE is highly variable and can range from chronic fatigue with low-grade fever to acute heart failure due to new, severe valvular regurgitation. Although the virulence of the organism can influence acuity of presentation, the onset of infection is generally followed by the onset of symptoms within 2 weeks of bacteremia. Four processes contribute to the clinical presentation of IE: infection on the valve, including the local intracardiac complications; septic or aseptic embolization to distant organs; continuous bacteremia, often with metastatic foci of

---

Box 1 | Prophylaxis Against Infective Endocarditis

Procedures Warranting Prophylaxis
Dental procedures that involve manipulating gingival tissue or the periapical region of teeth
Dental procedures that involve perforating the oral mucosa

Cardiac Conditions with High Risk of Adverse Outcome
Prosthetic heart valve or prosthetic material used for valve repair
Previous infective endocarditis
Congenital heart disease including unrepaired cyanotic lesions, palliative shunts or conduits, previous repair with residual defect at site of prosthetic patch or device, and recent repair (<6 months) involving prosthetic device or material
Cardiac transplant with valve regurgitation due to structurally abnormal valve

TABLE 1   Regimens for Dental Procedure

REGIMEN	ANTIBIOTIC AGENT	ADULT	CHILDREN
Oral	Amoxicillin	2 g	50 mg/kg
Penicillin allergy	Cephalexin	2 g	50 mg/kg
	or clindamycin	600 mg	20 mg/kg
	or azithromycin or clarithromycin	500 mg	15 mg/kg
Unable to take oral medication	Ampicillin	2 g IM or IV	50 mg/kg IM or IV
Unable to take oral medication plus penicillin allergy	Cefazolin or ceftriaxone	1 g IM or IV	50 mg/kg IM or IV
	or clindamycin	600 mg IM or IV	20 mg/kg IM or IV

Adapted from Bonow RO, Carabello BA, Kanu C, et al: ACC/AHA 2006 guidelines for the management of patients with valvular heart disease: A report of the American College of Cardiology/American Heart Association Task Force on Practice Guidelines (writing committee to revise the 1998 Guidelines for the Management of Patients with Valvular Heart Disease): Developed in collaboration with the Society of Cardiovascular Anesthesiologists: Endorsed by the Society for Cardiovascular Angiography and Interventions and the Society of Thoracic Surgeons. Circulation 2006;114(5):e84–e231.
Note: The antibiotic agent is administered as single dose 30–60 minutes before the procedure.

infection; and circulating immune complexes and other immunopathologic factors.

Approximately 85% of patients present with fever, although this finding might not be present in immunosuppressed states and in patients who have previously been on antibiotic therapy. Nonspecific signs and symptoms such as chills, sweats, anorexia, weight loss, malaise, dyspnea, and cough are common but generally occur in less than half of patients with IE. In addition, predisposing conditions or risk factors for the development of IE, including a history of structural heart disease, injection drug use, or recent invasive procedure, should be sought in the patient's history.

Evidence of a *new or changing* regurgitant murmur in the presence of fever of undetermined origin should prompt additional, timely evaluation for possible IE. Because of the lack of ventricular adaptation to acute volume overload and the resulting hemodynamic changes (tachycardia, hypotension), the murmur in acute aortic insufficiency may be poorly audible. Embolic phenomena, a common extracardiac complication of IE, can manifest with localizing symptoms such as focal neurologic deficit due to stroke or left upper abdominal pain due to splenic infarction. The patient should be carefully examined for any peripheral stigmata of IE such as petechiae, splinter hemorrhages, Janeway lesions, Osler nodes, and Roth spots. Many of these findings are immune-mediated yet infrequently present. Although Janeway lesions, Osler nodes, and Roth spots are more specific abnormalities for IE, they can occur in other conditions and their low incidence in cases of proven IE limits their diagnostic utility.

Blood Cultures

Blood cultures are the definitive microbiologic procedure for the diagnosis of IE. Continuous and low-grade bacteremia makes it unnecessary to await fever spikes or chills to obtain blood cultures, and the first two blood cultures yield an etiologic agent in 90% of cases. In patients who have not received antibiotics recently, it is recommended that at least three blood culture sets from separate venipunctures should be obtained over the first 24 hours, which will increase the yield to more than 95% in cases of untreated IE with continuous bacteremia. Each culture media bottle should be inoculated with at least 10 mL of blood to increase the number of colony-forming units per culture. The results of blood cultures should be interpreted based on the specific microorganisms identified as well as the recognized, constant nature of bacteremia in IE.

Other laboratory data may provide clues to the diagnosis yet lack specificity for IE. Hematologic parameters are often abnormal. A normocytic, normochromic anemia (70%–90%), thrombocytopenia (5%–15%), and leukocytosis (30%) are common findings. The erythrocyte sedimentation rate (ESR) and C-reactive protein concentrations are usually elevated. Similarly, the C-reactive protein concentration is also elevated in IE but is a nonspecific finding. Rheumatoid factor assay is positive in up to half of the cases, especially if the illness is protracted. Urinalysis might demonstrate microscopic hematuria and mild proteinuria. Red blood cell casts and heavy proteinuria can be seen in patients with immune complex glomerulonephritis.

Electrocardiography

Although the electrocardiogram (ECG) lacks sufficient sensitivity and specificity for the diagnosis of IE, ECG abnormalities commonly occur in patients with IE and are associated with invasive infection and increased in-hospital mortality. The presence of atrioventricular heart block in a patient with IE is diagnostic of the presence of a ring abscess, typically of the aortic valve, with invasion posteriorly toward the atrioventricular conduction system. One single-center study found that 53% of patients with invasive infection had ECG changes and about a third of the patients with ECG conduction abnormalities died during hospitalization in their cohort of 137 patients with definite IE.

Echocardiography and Diagnostic Criteria

The diagnosis of IE is based upon clinical suspicion derived from signs and symptoms and, most importantly, the demonstration of associated bacteremia. Given the nonspecific nature of findings from history, physical examination, and even blood cultures, the inclusion of echocardiographic findings has improved the sensitivity of diagnostic criteria for this condition (see modified Duke criteria, Box 2).

ECG findings provide specific evidence of IE that include vegetations, evidence of periannular tissue destruction (abscess), aneurysm, fistula, leaflet perforation, and valvular dehiscence. Box 3 outlines specific definitions of these characteristic findings.

The diagnostic utility of transthoracic echocardiogram (TTE) for suspected IE is highest in patients with intermediate to high likelihood of this disease (e.g., a patient with a new or changed heart murmur and bacteremia). Hence, TTE should be performed in all patients with suspected IE. However, the diagnostic sensitivity of TTE for the visualization of an intracardiac vegetation or abscess is limited, ranging from 40% to 80%, and thus the diagnosis of IE cannot be ruled out on the basis of a negative study. The absence of five clinical criteria has been associated with zero probability of a TTE showing evidence of IE: positive blood cultures, presence of central venous access, recent history of injection drug use, presence of prosthetic valve, and vasculitic or embolic phenomena.

Transesophageal echocardiography (TEE) has greater spatial resolution compared to TTE and so is more sensitive than TTE for detecting intracardiac vegetations (sensitivity, 87%; specificity, 95%). As a result, TEE should be performed in patients with a high likelihood of IE and a negative TTE. Although TTE and TEE have been found to have concordant results in approximately half of patients with suspected IE, TEE provides additional diagnostic information in a high percentage of patients, particularly those with prosthetic valves. Specific subsets of patients in whom TEE should be performed, even as the primary imaging modality (without TTE), include patients with prosthetic heart valves and suspected IE and patients with persistent staphylococcal bacteremia without known source or nosocomial infection. In addition, TEE should be performed in patients with IE when paravalvular abscess is suspected.

Box 2   The Modified Duke Criteria and Case Definitions of Infective Endocarditis

Modified Duke Criteria
Major Criteria
Positive blood cultures

- Typical microbes consistent with IE from two separate blood cultures: viridans streptococci, *Streptococcus bovis*, HACEK group, *Staphylococcus aureus*; community-acquired enterococci in absence of another focus

or

- Microrganisms consistent with IE from persistently positive blood cultures defined as follows: at least 2 blood cultures drawn more than 12 hours apart or all of three or a majority of more than four separate blood cultures
- Single positive blood culture for *Coxiella burnetti* or antiphase IgG antibody titer >1:800

Evidence of endocardial involvement
Echo findings of IE, defined as:

- Oscillating intracardiac mass on valve or supporting structure
- Abscess
- New partial dehiscence of prosthetic valve
- New valvular regurgitation

Minor Criteria
Predisposition: predisposing heart condition or injection drug use
Fever, temperature >38°C
Vascular phenomena, major arterial emboli, septic pulmonary infarcts, mycotic aneurysm, intracranial hemorrhage, conjunctival hemorrhage, and Janeway lesions
Immunologic phenomena: glomerulonephritis, Osler's nodes, Roth's spots, rheumatoid factor
Microbiologic evidence: positive blood cultures but does not meet a major criterion as noted above, or serologic evidence of active infection with organism consistent with causing IE

Case Definitions
Definite Infective Endocarditis
Presence of any pathologic criteria:

- Microorganisms demonstrated by culture or histologic examination of a vegetation, a vegetation that has embolized, or an intracardiac abscess specimen

or

- Pathologic lesions; vegetation or intracardiac abscess confirmed by histologic examination showing active endocarditis

If there are no pathologic criteria, then clinical diagnosis of definite IE:

- Two major criteria

or

- One major and three minor criteria

or

- Five minor criteria

Possible Infective Endocarditis
One major criterion and one minor criterion
or
Three minor criteria

Rejected
Firm alternative diagnosis explaining evidence of IE
or
Resolution of IE syndrome with antibiotic therapy for ≤4 days
or
No pathologic evidence of IE at surgery or autopsy, with antibiotic therapy for <4 days
or
Does not meet criteria for possible IE, as above.

Abbreviations: HACEK = *Haemophilus* spp., *Aggregatibacter* spp., *Cardiobacterium hominis*, *Eikenella corrodens*, *Kingella* spp.; IE = infective endocarditis; Ig = immunoglobulin.
Adapted from Li JS, Sexton DJ, Nettles R, et al. Proposed modifications to the Duke criteria for the diagnosis of infective endocarditis. Clin Infect Dis 2003;30(4):633–8.

Box 3   Echocardiographic Findings in Infective Endocarditis

Vegetation
Irregularly shaped, discrete echogenic mass
Adherent to but distinct from endocardial surface or intracardiac device
Oscillation of mass (supportive, not mandatory)

Abscess
Thickened area or mass within the myocardium or valve annulus
Evidence of flow into region (supportive, not mandatory)

Aneurysm
Echolucent space with thin surrounding tissue

Fistula
Blood flow between two distinct cardiac blood spaces or chambers through an abnormal path or channel

Leaflet perforation
Defect in body of valve leaflet with flow through defect

Valve dehiscence
Prosthetic valve with abnormal rocking motion/excursion >15 degrees in at least one direction

---

Adapted from Sachdev M, Peterson GE, Jollis JG: Imaging techniques for diagnosis of infective endocarditis. Cardiol Clin 2003;21:185–195.

Other Cardiac Imaging Modalities

Cardiac magnetic resonance imaging with contrast appears promising for detecting paravalvular abscesses, thrombus associated with vegetations, valvular complications, and aortocameral fistulas, although temporal resolution might limit its use for detecting vegetation. Cardiac computed tomography has also been used to detect aortic root abscess. However, clinical experience with these techniques in IE patients is limited and their sensitivities and specificities in comparison to echocardiography are not well defined. Positron emission tomography-computed tomography (PET-CT) scans have been used to evaluate prosthetic devices, including cardiac implanted electronic devices, for inflammation localized to these devices, and may help differentiate post-surgical changes from active infection.

Routine coronary angiography is recommended in patients older than 55 years and in those at high risk for coronary artery disease before surgery for IE.

Differential Diagnosis

Given the protean manifestations of IE, the differential diagnosis includes a number of systemic conditions: systemic lupus erythematosus, acute rheumatic fever, atrial myxoma, vasculitis, and renal cell carcinoma.

Treatment, Complications, and Outcome

Antibiotic therapy has improved survival in IE by 70% to 80% and has been shown to reduce the incidence of complications of IE. Detailed descriptions of antibiotic regimens for specific

ORGANISM	SUSCEPTIBILITY	REGIMEN	DOSAGE	DURATION (WK)
Native Valve				
Streptococcus viridans, Streptococcus bovis	Penicillin	Penicillin *or* Ceftriaxone *or* Vancomycin	12–18 MU IV q24h 2 g IV or IM q24h 30 mg/kg IV q24h in 2 divided doses Max: 2 g/24 h	4 4 4
	Penicillin-relative resistance	Penicillin	24 MU IV per 24 h	4
		or Ceftriaxone *plus* Gentamicin *or* Vancomycin	2 g IV/IM per 24 h 3 mg/kg IV/IM per 24 h in 1 dose 30 mg/kg IV per 24 h in 2 divided doses (limit 2 g/24 h)	4 2 4
Enterococcus spp.	Penicillin	Ampicillin *or* Penicillin *plus* Gentamicin *or* Vancomycin *plus* Gentamicin	12 g IV per 24 h in 6 divided doses 18–30 MU IV per 24 h 3 mg/kg IV or IM per 24 h in 3 divided doses 30 mg/kg IV per 24 h in 2 divided doses (limit 2 g/24 h) 3 mg/kg IV or IM per 24 h in 3 divided doses	4–6 4–6 4–6 6 6
Staphylococcus spp.	Oxacillin	Nafcillin or oxacillin *plus* Gentamicin *or* Cefazolin *plus* Gentamicin	12 g IV per 24 h in 4–6 divided doses 3 mg/kg IV/IM per 24 h in 3 divided doses 6 g IV per 24 h in 3 divided doses 3 mg/kg IV or IM per 24 h in 3 divided doses	6 3–5 *days* 6 3–5 *days*
Oxacillin-resistant *Staphylococcus* spp.		Vancomycin	30 mg/kg IV per 24 h in 2 divided doses Goal: 1-h peak concentration 30–45 µg/mL and trough 10–15 µg/mL	6
Prosthetic Valve				
Staphylococcus spp.	Oxacillin	Nafcillin or oxacillin *plus* Gentamicin *plus* Rifampin	12 g IV per 24 h in 4–6 divided doses 3 mg/kg IV or IM per 24 h in 3 divided doses 900 mg IV or PO per 24 h in 3 divided doses	6 6 6
	Oxacillin-resistant	Vancomycin	30 mg/kg IV per 24 h in 2 divided doses Goal: 1-h peak concentration 30–45 µg/mL and trough 10-15 µg/mL	6
		plus Gentamicin *plus* Rifampin	3 mg/kg IV or IM per 24 h in 3 divided doses 900 mg IV or PO per 24 h in 3 divided doses	6 6

Abbreviation: max = maximum.

causative organisms are found in guidelines by the American Heart Association (updated in 2008) and the European Society of Cardiology (new in 2009). Recommended antimicrobial regimens against typical organisms causing IE are outlined in Table 2. Although the choice of antimicrobial therapy is mainly guided by the infecting organism and its antibiotic susceptibilities, there are three basic principles of antibiotic treatment for the eradication of native valve infection.

First, a prolonged course of antibiotic treatment (4 to 6 weeks) is necessary to eradicate infection because bacterial concentration within vegetations is high and organisms deep within vegetations are inaccessible to phagocytic cells. Repeat sets of blood cultures after antibiotic initiation should be obtained every 24 to 48 hours until the resolution of bacteremia is confirmed. If surgery for IE is performed, completion of the 4- to 6-week course of antibiotic therapy is generally favored to reduce the risk of recurrent IE.

Second, parenteral administration of antibiotic therapy is necessary to achieve adequate drug levels required to eradicate infection. Parenteral therapy is typically initiated in the hospital setting, and the patient may receive outpatient parenteral treatment for the remaining duration after an initial period of observation to assess for clinical response to therapy (e.g., clearance of bacteremia and absence of complications).

Third, because of the need for prolonged therapy and rising antimicrobial resistance among organisms, combination therapy typically involving a β-lactam and aminoglycoside antibiotic is recommended. Combination therapy has been shown to reduce the duration of bacteremia in *S. aureus* endocarditis, although this more-rapid resolution of bacteremia was not associated with an improved clinical response or outcome. Both antibiotics should be given temporally close together so that maximum synergistic microcidal effect is obtained. In addition, the dosage

and kidney function should be monitored carefully, because combination therapy has been associated with a higher rate of kidney dysfunction.

IE can progress to the development of various intracardiac and extracardiac complications before or despite effective treatment. Heart failure or pulmonary edema is a common complication, occurring in about one third to one half of patients with IE, and it is the most common indication for urgent surgery. Valvular destruction and ensuing insufficiency can result in volume overload and heart failure; in rare cases of large vegetations, heart failure may be a result of valvular stenosis. Heart failure complicates aortic valve IE more often than mitral or tricuspid IE and can result in the setting of moderate, rather than severe, regurgitation, because the left ventricle is unable to compensate for the acute increase in preload and afterload in this condition.

Medical therapy alone is generally insufficient in managing IE complicated by heart failure, particularly in the setting of severe or progressive valvular regurgitation. Surgery should be prompt, and unnecessary delays should be avoided.

Para-valvular abscess complicates 30% to 40% cases of IE and is a result of invasive infection that spreads generally along contiguous tissue planes, particularly with aortic valve infection. In the International Collaboration on Endocarditis (ICE) cohort, 22% cases of definite aortic valve IE were complicated by a periannular abscess. These patients were more likely to have prosthetic valves and coagulase-negative staphylococcal infection. TEE is the diagnostic test of choice when an abscess is suspected clinically. An abscess is diagnosed by TEE as the visualization of a periannular area of thickening or mass with a heterogeneous echogenic or echolucent appearance. Rarely, antibiotic therapy alone may be used to treat an intracardiac abscess, though this treatment alone is generally reserved for patients who are poor surgical candidates.

The vast majority of patients with an intracardiac abscess require cardiac surgery for débridement. In addition, surgery represents the gold standard for the diagnosis of abscess.

Embolic phenomena often complicate the clinical course in IE. Although clinical signs of embolization occur in approximately one third of patients with IE, at least another third of patients have silent embolism. In the majority of cases, embolic events occur before antibiotic therapy is initiated. The most frequent sites of embolic events were the central nervous system (approximately 40% of embolic events), lungs (approximately 20%), spleen (20%), peripheral artery (approximately 15%), and kidney (10%).

Factors including vegetation size, mobility, and location as well as the causative organism have been associated with the likelihood of embolic event. Vegetations larger than 10 mm in greatest diameter are associated with an increased risk of embolization. Causative organisms such as *S. aureus* and *Streptococcus bovis* confer an independent risk of embolization. Embolism also occurs with greater frequency in IE caused by enterococci, fastidious gram-negative organisms (HACEK), and fungi as compared to streptococcal IE. In addition to causing infarction of distal vascular beds, embolic events can result in metastatic sites of infection.

Cerebral embolization occurs in 10% to 35% of cases and is at times complicated by meningitis, brain abscess, or intracerebral hemorrhage. The risk of stroke dramatically decreases with initiation of antibiotic therapy. Findings from the ICE merged database suggested a 65% reduction in stroke incidence by week 2 of initiating antimicrobial therapy. Given the low incidence of embolic event after initiation of antibiotic therapy, routine screening for emboli in patients with IE is not recommended. However, patients with persistent fever or bacteremia or localizing symptoms of possible infarction should undergo computed tomographic imaging with radiographic contrast for the diagnosis of embolic complications.

Embolic events have been found to be an independent predictor of in-hospital death in IE. In patients who experience recurrent embolic events, particularly if they occur after initiation of antibiotic therapy, surgical treatment is indicated. For the prevention of embolic events, surgery may be considered for patients with IE who have residual large (>10 mm), mobile vegetations involving mitral or aortic valve. A recent, small, randomized trial of early surgery for native, left sided IE has found significant reduction in embolic events in patients treated with earlier surgery.

Surgical intervention for IE may be performed either in the acute or active phase of infection or after the eradication of infection. The optimal timing of surgery in the setting of active IE has not been well evaluated. In patients with serious, life-threatening complications of IE, surgery should be performed emergently. A number of case series have shown that surgery in the active phase of IE can be performed with acceptable risk and without an obvious risk of infecting a prosthetic valve. Surgery during the active phase is generally considered for patients in whom the likelihood of cure of infection with antibiotic therapy alone is low or in whom severe complications have or will likely occur. In contemporary series, surgery is performed in 40% to 50% of patients with IE during the index hospitalization. Surgery after eradication of infection is predominantly performed for adverse hemodynamic effects of valvular regurgitation that results from valve damage.

Indications for surgery in IE are shown in Box 4. A majority of patients with left-sided IE will have an indication for surgery, but may be poor candidates for surgery due to hemodynamic instability or other comorbid conditions. Heart failure is the most common indication for urgent surgical intervention, yet even without overt heart failure symptoms, hemodynamic evidence of severe regurgitation (such as premature closure of the mitral valve in severe aortic regurgitation or pulmonary hypertension in severe mitral regurgitation) should also prompt surgical intervention because valvular regurgitation—or rarely, stenosis—is a mechanical complication of IE that will not improve with antimicrobial therapy alone. For mitral valve regurgitation, surgical repair of the native valve without replacing the valve with a prosthesis has been reported in a number of case series. However, the role

---

---

of repair versus replacement has not been evaluated in controlled studies, and its feasibility will be limited by the extent of infection and valvular damage as well as the experience of the surgeon. Surgery for IE may be performed with an acceptable operative mortality, although urgent or emergent surgery is associated with higher mortality.

Because embolic complications often involve the central nervous system and can worsen neurologic function after cardiopulmonary bypass, the timing of surgery after a cerebral embolic infarct is controversial. One study found that neurologic deterioration did not occur among patients with IE who experienced transient ischemic attacks or asymptomatic emboli, even if surgery was performed acutely. However, patients with recent hemorrhagic strokes may be at risk for extension and deterioration after cardiac surgery.

Regarding persistent bacteremia as an indication for surgery, it is important to recognize that certain microorganisms, particularly *S. aureus*, may be associated with prolonged bacteremia (up to 10 days) after initiation of antibiotic therapy. Because of possible difficulty in eradicating infection from prosthetic materials, all cases of prosthetic valve IE should receive surgical consultation. With valve conservation and improved surgical techniques, the surgical mortality rates have declined over time, with recent reported rates in the range of 7% to 14%. In comparison to therapy alone, surgery appears to confer a survival benefit for those patients with major complications of IE, such as heart failure or intracardiac abscess.

Despite the high rate of surgical intervention in IE, the in-hospital mortality rate for native valve IE in the contemporary era remains high at approximately 15% to 20%, and nearly 25% for prosthetic valve IE. Among host factors, older age, female sex, diabetes mellitus, acute physiology (APACHE II) score, elevated white blood cell count, serum creatinine level greater than 2 mg/dL, and lower serum albumin have been associated with worse outcome. Congestive heart failure, paravalvular complication (e.g., abscess formation), infection with virulent organisms (particularly *S. aureus*), prosthetic valve infection, and absence of surgical intervention are also factors related to higher mortality in IE.

References

Nishimura RA, et al. 2014 AHA/ACC guideline for the management of patients with valvular heart disease: executive summary: a report of the American College of Cardiology/American Heart Association Task Force on Practice Guidelines. Circulation 2014;129(23):2440–92.

Chu VH, Cabell CH, Benjamin Jr DK, et al. Early predictors of in-hospital death in infective endocarditis. Circulation 2004;109(14):1745–9.

Fowler Jr VG, Miro JM, Hoen B, et al. *Staphylococcus aureus* endocarditis: A consequence of medical progress. JAMA 2005;293(24):3012–21.

Gaca JG, Sheng S, Daneshmand MA, et al. Outcomes for endocarditis surgery in North America: a simplified risk scoring system. J Thorac Cardiovasc Surg 2011;141:98–106.

Hasbun R, Vikram HR, Barakat LA, et al. Complicated left-sided native valve endocarditis in adults: Risk classification for mortality. JAMA 2003;289(15):1933–40.

Hoen B, Alla F, Selton-Suty C, et al. Changing profile of infective endocarditis: Results of a 1-year survey in France. JAMA 2002;288(1):75–81.

Kang DH, Kim YJ, Kim SH, et al. Early surgery versus conventional treatment for infective endocarditis. N Engl J Med 2012;366:2466–73.

Kiefer T, Park L, Tribouilloy C, et al. Association between valvular surgery and mortality among patients with infective endocarditis complicated by heart failure. JAMA 2011;306:2239–47.

Li JS, Sexton DJ, Nettles R, et al. Proposed modifications to the Duke criteria for the diagnosis of infective endocarditis. Clin Infect Dis 2000;30(4):633–8.

Moreillon P, Que YA. Infective endocarditis. Lancet 2004;363(9403):139–49.

Nishimura RA, Carabello BA, Faxon DP, et al. ACC/AHA 2008 guideline update on valvular heart disease: Focused update on infective endocarditis: A report of the American College of Cardiology/American Heart Association Task Force on Practice Guidelines endorsed by the Society of Cardiovascular Anesthesiologists, Society for Cardiovascular Angiography and Interventions, and Society of Thoracic Surgeons. Catheter Cardiovasc Interv 2008;72(3):E1–E12.

Task Force on the Prevention, Diagnosis, and Treatment of Infective Endocarditis of the European Society of Cardiology; European Society of Clinical Microbiology and Infectious Diseases; International Society of Chemotherapy for Infection and Cancer; ESC Committee for Practice Guidelines. Guidelines on the prevention, diagnosis, and treatment of infective endocarditis (new version 2009): the Task Force on the Prevention, Diagnosis, and Treatment of Infective Endocarditis of the European Society of Cardiology (ESC). Eur Heart J 2009;30(19):2369–413.

Vikram HR, Buenconsejo J, Hasbun R, et al. Impact of valve surgery on 6-month mortality in adults with complicated, left-sided native valve endocarditis: A propensity analysis. JAMA 2003;290(24):3207–14.

Wang A, Athan E, Pappas PA, et al. Contemporary clinical profile and outcome of prosthetic valve endocarditis. JAMA 2007;297(12):1354–61.

MITRAL VALVE PROLAPSE

Method of
Kurt M. Jacobson, MD; and Peter S. Rahko, MD

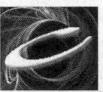

CURRENT DIAGNOSIS

- A midsystolic click with or without a middle- to late-peaking crescendo systolic murmur is the classic auscultatory finding of mitral valve prolapse (MVP).
- Key examination maneuvers can help differentiate MVP from other valvular heart diseases.
- Diagnostic echocardiographic findings of MVP are systolic billowing of the mitral valve leaflets 2 mm above the annulus into the left atrium.
- The presence of significant myxomatous thickening of the valve leaflets (>5 mm) is significant for prognosis.

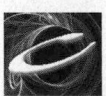

CURRENT THERAPY

- Patients with physical findings of mitral valve prolapse (MVP) should have an echocardiogram to confirm the diagnosis, determine the severity of prolapse, determine the amount of myxomatous thickening, document the severity (if present) of mitral regurgitation, and determine left ventricular size and function.
- Uncomplicated MVP without significant mitral regurgitation can be evaluated clinically every 3 to 5 years.
- Complicated MVP (associated with significant mitral regurgitation, left ventricular structural changes, pulmonary hypertension, atrial fibrillation, or stroke) should be observed closely with serial clinical evaluation and echocardiography.

- Surgery may be required for complicated MVP associated with severe mitral regurgitation. Repair rather than replacement is the procedure of choice and should be performed at surgical centers experienced with mitral valve repair.
- Recommendations for surgery are the same for MVP as for other forms of chronic severe mitral regurgitation.

Mitral valve prolapse (MVP) has been known by many names, including floppy valve syndrome, Barlow's syndrome, click/murmur syndrome, myxomatous mitral valve disease, and billowing mitral cusp syndrome. MVP is a common cardiac valvular abnormality characterized by redundant, floppy mitral valve leaflets; it is often detected initially by characteristic nonejection clicks or a middle- to late-peaking crescendo systolic murmur on physical examination.

Prevalence

MVP is the most common congenital cause of mitral regurgitation (MR) in adults and the most common indication for mitral valve surgery in the United States today. Previously, it was one of the most overdiagnosed conditions within cardiology, with suggested prevalence rates ranging from 5% to 15%. With the use of current diagnostic standards, rates are much lower; the overestimation was a consequence of diverse and nonuniformly accepted two-dimensional echocardiographic diagnostic criteria. Freed and colleagues, using the Framingham study population and applying consistent and more stringent echocardiographic diagnostic criteria, demonstrated a much lower prevalence of MVP (approximately 2.4%). The incidence appeared to be similar among men and women. Gender differences do exist, however. Women tend to have a more benign course, whereas men tend to have more advanced myxomatous disease resulting in a greater chance of more severe MR.

Classification

Primary MVP is characterized by idiopathic myxomatous change of the mitral valve leaflets or the chordal structures or both. Secondary MVP is present when underlying conditions such as Marfan's syndrome, Ehlers-Danlos syndrome, osteogenesis imperfecta, or other collagen vascular disorders are evident. Certain congenital cardiac abnormalities, including Ebstein anomaly, aortic coarctation, hypertrophic cardiomyopathy, and ostium secundum atrial septal defects, are also associated with MVP. Familial variants with an autosomal dominant pattern of inheritance have been identified, and work to identify the genes involved is under way. The reported prevalence of MVP in first-degree relatives is between 30% and 50%.

Pathology

Macroscopic and microscopic changes can involve both the anterior and posterior leaflets as well as the chordal structures of the leaflet apparatus. Macroscopically, the surface area of the leaflet is increased, providing the accentuated, billowing appearance of the valve leaflets. Additional notable changes are thickening of the individual leaflets, increased leaflet length, thinning and stretching of the chordae, and increased circumference of the mitral valve annulus. At the microscopic level (Figure 1), normal mitral valves have three well-defined layers, each containing cells and a characteristic composition and configuration of the extracellular matrix: the fibrosa, composed predominantly of collagen fibers densely packed and arranged parallel to the free edge of the leaflet; the centrally located spongiosa, composed of loosely arranged collagen and proteoglycans; and the atrialis, composed of elastic fibers. In myxomatous mitral valves, the spongiosa layer is expanded by loose, amorphous extracellular matrix that has more proteoglycans but less collagen and more fragmented elastic fibers. What collagen is present appears to be disorganized and fragmented, giving the appearance of a haphazard layering of the spongiosa. It is this thickening that produces the classic

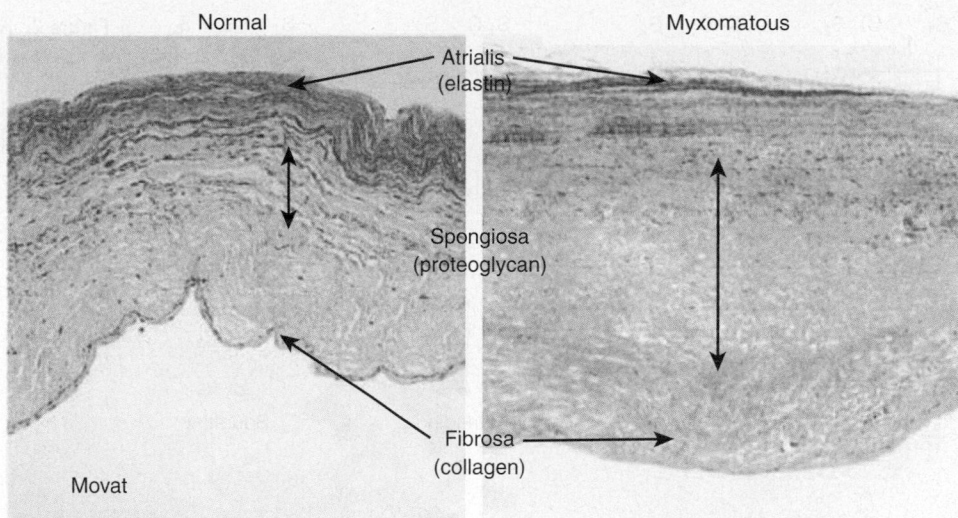

Figure 1. Morphologic features of normal mitral valves *(left)* and valves with myxomatous degeneration *(right)*. Myxomatous valves have an abnormal layered architecture: loose collagen in fibrosa, expanded spongiosa strongly positive for proteoglycans, and disrupted elastin in atrialis *(top)*. Movat pentachrome stain (collagen stains yellow, proteoglycans blue-green, and elastin black). (Modified from Rabkin E, Aikawa M, Stone JR, et al: Activated interstitial myofibroblasts express catabolic enzymes and mediate matrix remodeling in myxomatous heart valves. Circulation 2001;104:2525.)

macroscopic appearance of the myxomatous valve on two-dimensional echocardiography.

Clinical Presentation

Most patients with MVP are asymptomatic and will remain so, testifying to the often benign nature of this disease. Previously, various nonspecific symptoms, including fatigue, dyspnea, palpitations, postural orthostasis, anxiety, and panic attacks, were described as an MVP syndrome when present in association with the characteristic nonejection systolic click or middle- to late-peaking crescendo systolic murmur. Other symptoms, including chest discomfort, near-syncope, and syncope, have also been described by patients with MVP. However, in a community-based study, the prevalence of various clinical complaints including chest pain, dyspnea, and syncope was no higher in patients with MVP than in those without evidence of MVP, making such findings nonspecific. In a controlled study that compared symptomatic MVP patients with first-degree relatives with and without echocardiographic evidence of MVP, there also was no association of MVP with atypical chest pain, dyspnea, panic attacks, or anxiety. There was, however, a significant association of MVP with physical findings of systolic clicks, systolic murmurs, thoracic bony abnormalities, low body weight, and low blood pressure. Congestive heart failure, atrial fibrillation, stroke or transient ischemic attack, hypertension, diabetes, and hypercholesterolemia are no more likely in patients with MVP than in those without MVP. However, previous retrospective studies suggested a higher incidence of cerebral embolic events, infectious endocarditis, severe MR, and need for mitral valve replacement in patients with classic (complicated) versus nonclassic MVP. Symptoms of poor cardiac reserve, such as reduced exercise tolerance, dyspnea on exertion, and fatigue, may reflect the presence of significant MR and warrant clinical concern.

Diagnosis

Symptoms are not predictive of the presence or absence of MVP. Certain physical and auscultatory characteristics on examination do support the diagnosis of MVP. Patients with MVP more often have a lower body mass index, have a lower waist-to-hip ratio, and are taller. Findings of scoliosis, pectus excavatum, and hyperextensibility are also prevalent among patients with MVP. The classic auscultatory findings include a midsystolic click and a middle- to late-peaking crescendo systolic murmur heard best at the apex. The auscultatory findings are best elicited with the diaphragm of the stethoscope, and they change in relation to the first and second heart sounds (S_1 and S_2) in response to changes in left ventricular (LV) volume. Therefore, the patient should be examined in several positions: supine (including lateral decubitus), sitting, standing, and, if possible, squatting. Changes in LV filling and volume affect the degree of prolapse.

The most important and most specific finding on auscultation is the presence of a nonejection midsystolic click or clicks caused by snapping of the valve apparatus as parts of the valve leaflets billow into the atrium during systole. Although these clicks can be heard over the entire precordium, they are best heard at the apex. The click can be misinterpreted as a split S_1, a true S_1 with an S_4, or a true S_1 with an early ejection click from a bicuspid valve. It can be differentiated from an ejection click heard in bicuspid aortic valves by its timing relative to the beginning of the carotid upstroke. Ejection clicks occur as the aortic valve opens and therefore precede the carotid upstroke, whereas the nonejection clicks of MVP occur afterward. Clicks from atrial septal aneurysms are uncommon but can be difficult to distinguish from those of MVP. Ejection clicks and clicks from atrial septal aneurysms are not altered by changes in loading characteristics, allowing them to be differentiated from clicks of MVP. Often, but not always, a middle- to late-peaking crescendo systolic murmur can be appreciated by itself or after a click. The murmur terminates with closure of the aortic valve (A2). This represents MR, and, in general, the duration of the murmur correlates with the severity of the MR. The earlier in systole the murmur is detected, the more severe the MR. Eventually, with more severe MR, the murmur becomes holosystolic. MVP manifestations on examination vary, and they may not always be reproducible, even in the same patient.

Certain maneuvers can aid in more accurately diagnosing MVP on examination (Figure 2). MVP is very sensitive to LV filling, and subtle changes in auscultatory findings elicited by careful examination maneuvers can be instrumental in separating MVP from other valvular abnormalities. Generally, measures that decrease LV volume or increase contractility produce earlier and more prominent systolic prolapse of the mitral leaflets, causing the systolic click and murmur to move closer to S_1. For example, in the transition from squatting to standing, LV volume is reduced, and the onset of the click and murmur is moved closer to S_1. Conversely, anything that increases LV volume, such as leg-raising, squatting, or slowing the heart rate (increased diastolic filling), delays the onset of the click or murmur and usually diminishes its duration and intensity.

Use of Echocardiography

Two-dimensional echocardiography has proved to be the most accurate noninvasive tool for the diagnosis, assessment, and follow-up of clinically suspected MVP. In fact, physical signs of MVP in an asymptomatic patient are an American College of Cardiology/American Heart Association (ACC/AHA) class I indication for use of echocardiography to make the diagnosis of MVP

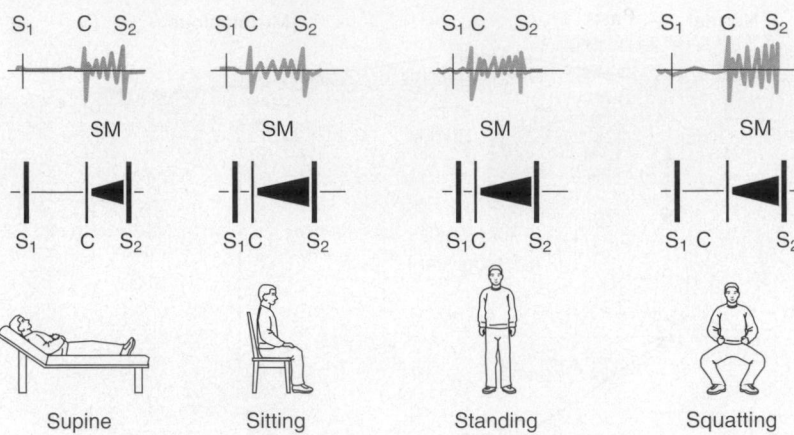

Figure 2. Auscultative findings with changes in position in patients with mitral valve prolapse (MVP). *Abbreviations*: C = click of MVP; S$_1$, mitral valve closure; S$_2$, aortic valve closure. (Modified from Devereux RB, Perloff JK, Reichek N, et al: Mitral valve prolapse. Circulation 1976;54[1]:3–14.)

and assess the severity of MR, leaflet morphology, and ventricular size and function. Once the diagnosis is made, follow-up is determined by the severity of MVP. Routine echocardiographic follow-up of asymptomatic patients with MVP is not recommended unless there are significant findings of MR or LV structural changes. Frequency of follow-up in patients with prolapse and MR is determined by the severity of MR and should be at least annual in patients with severe MR.

Diagnostic criteria for MVP on two-dimensional echocardiography are

- Billowing of one or both mitral valve leaflets or their prolapse superiorly across the mitral annular plane in the parasternal long-axis view by greater than 2 mm during systole
- The degree of thickening of the leaflets

Combined leaflet prolapse of greater than 2 mm and leaflet thickness greater than 5 mm are supportive of classic MVP, whereas prolapse in the absence of increased thickness is considered nonclassic MVP. In addition to more often being associated with the auscultative findings of the click and murmur, the classic form is more commonly associated with increased risk of endocarditis, stroke, progressive MR, and need for mitral valve repair or replacement.

Because the mitral apparatus is saddle-shaped, certain echocardiographic views are more specific than others for determining leaflet prolapse. Most practitioners agree that the parasternal long-axis and apical two-chamber or apical long-axis views are the most accurate for determining prolapse. A finding of prolapse as determined on other views, particularly the apical four-chamber view, is much less specific and frequently leads to a false-positive diagnosis.

Medical Management

Most patients with MVP remain asymptomatic and require no additional management aside from careful observation over time. It is appropriate to provide reassurance that uncomplicated (non-classic) MVP is a non–life-threatening condition and is unlikely to affect longevity. Periodic clinical evaluation every 3 to 5 years is reasonable. Patients who develop palpitations, lightheadedness, dizziness, or syncope should undergo Holter or event monitoring for detection of arrhythmias. Palpitations are frequently controlled with β-blockers or calcium channel blockers, although the presence of specific arrhythmias may mandate additional therapy. Endocarditis prophylaxis is no longer recommended for patients with MVP unless they have a history of endocarditis or valve replacement. Prophylaxis is recommended for patients who have undergone repair if prosthetic material was used (e.g., in ring repairs). Aspirin or warfarin (Coumadin) therapy may be recommended for certain symptomatic patients with neurologic events who have atrial fibrillation, significant MR, hypertension, or heart failure (Table 1).

TABLE 1	ACC/AHA Recommendations for Oral Anticoagulation in Patients with Mitral Valve Prolapse
CLASS	**RECOMMENDATION**
I	ASA therapy (75–325 mg/d) for cerebral TIAs Warfarin (Coumadin) therapy for patients ≥65 years in atrial fibrillation with hypertension, MR, or history of congestive heart failure ASA therapy (75–325 mg/d) for patients <65 years in atrial fibrillation with no history of MR, hypertension, or congestive heart failure Warfarin therapy after stroke for patients with MR, atrial fibrillation, or left atrial thrombus
IIa	ASA therapy is reasonable in patients after stroke who do not have MR, atrial fibrillation, left atrial thrombus, or echocardiographic evidence of thickening >5 mm or redundancy of leaflets Warfarin therapy is reasonable after stroke for patients without MR, atrial fibrillation, or left atrial thrombus who have echocardiographic evidence of thickening >5 mm or redundancy of leaflets Warfarin therapy is reasonable for TIAs that occur despite ASA therapy ASA therapy (75–325 mg/d) can be beneficial for patients with a history of stroke who have contraindications to anticoagulants
IIb	ASA therapy (75–325 mg/d) may be considered for patients in sinus rhythm with echocardiographic evidence of complicated mitral valve prolapse

Abbreviations: ACC/AHA = American College of Cardiology/American Heart Association; ASA = aspirin; MR = mitral regurgitation; TIA = transient ischemic attack.
Adapted from Bonow RO, Carabello BA, Chatterjee K, et al: ACC/AHA 2006 guidelines for the management of patients with valvular heart disease. J Am Coll Cardiol 2006;48(3):e1–e148. [Erratum in J Am Coll Cardiol 2007;49 (9):1014.]

Patients with classic (complicated) MVP deserve regular clinical follow-up, particularly if MR is present. These patients are more likely to develop moderate or severe MR over time. Patients with mild to moderate MR and normal LV function should be clinically evaluated at least annually and should undergo echocardiography every second or third year if stable. Patients with severe MR should have an annual echocardiogram and closer clinical follow-up. Those who have severe MR and develop symptoms or impaired LV systolic function require cardiac catheterization and evaluation for mitral valve surgery. Often the valve can be repaired rather than replaced, with a low operative mortality rate and excellent short- and long-term results when performed at experienced centers. Preservation of the native valve allows for lower risks of thrombosis and endocarditis than does prosthetic valve replacement.

TABLE 2	ACC/AHA Recommendations for Surgery in Patients with Chronic Primary Mitral Valve Regurgitation
CLASS	**RECOMMENDATION**
I	Mitral valve (MV) surgery is recommended for symptomatic patients with chronic severe primary MR (stage D) and left ventricular ejection fraction (LVEF) >30%
	MV surgery is recommended for asymptomatic patients with chronic severe primary MR and left ventricular (LV) dysfunction (LVEF 30%-60% and/or left ventricular end-systolic dimension (LVESD) _40 mm, stage C2)
	MV repair is recommended in preference to mitral valve replacement (MVR) when surgical treatment is indicated for patients with chronic severe primary MR limited to the posterior leaflet
	MV repair is recommended in preference to MVR when surgical treatment is indicated for patients with chronic severe primary MR involving the anterior leaflet or both leaflets when a successful and durable repair can be accomplished
	Concomitant MV repair or replacement is indicated in patients with chronic severe primary MR undergoing cardiac surgery for other indications
IIa	MV repair is reasonable in asymptomatic patients with chronic severe primary MR (stage C1) with preserved LV function (LVEF >60% and LVESD <40 mm) in whom the likelihood of a successful and durable repair without residual MR is >95% with an expected mortality rate of <1% when performed at a Heart Valve Center of Excellence
	MV repair is reasonable for asymptomatic patients with chronic severe nonrheumatic primary MR (stage C1) and preserved LV function in whom there is a high likelihood of a successful and durable repair with 1) new onset of atrial fibrillation or 2) resting pulmonary hypertension (pulmonary artery systolic arterial pressure >50 mm Hg)
	Concomitant MV repair is reasonable in patients with chronic moderate primary MR (stage B) undergoing cardiac surgery for other indications
IIb	MV surgery may be considered in symptomatic patients with chronic severe primary MR and LVEF _30% (stage D)
	MV repair may be considered in patients with rheumatic mitral valve disease when surgical treatment is indicated if a durable and successful repair is likely or if the reliability of long-term anticoagulation management is questionable
	Transcatheter MV repair may be considered for severely symptomatic patients (New York Heart Association class III/IV) with chronic severe primary MR (stage D) who have a reasonable life expectancy but a prohibitive surgical risk because of severe comorbidities
III Harm	MVR should not be performed for treatment of isolated severe primary MR limited to less than one half of the posterior leaflet unless MV repair has been attempted and was unsuccessful

Adapted from ACC/AHA 2014 guidelines for the management of patients with valvular heart disease. J Am Coll Cardiol 2014;63(22), e103.

Surgical Management

MVP is the most common cause of adult MR requiring mitral valve surgery. Symptoms of heart failure, severity of MR, presence or absence of atrial fibrillation, LV systolic function, LV end-diastolic and end-systolic volumes, and pulmonary artery pressure (at rest and with exercise) influence the decision to recommend mitral valve surgery. Indications for surgery in patients with MVP and MR mirror those with other forms of nonischemic severe MR. Patient outcomes after mitral valve repair are typically very good, and the surgical risk is lower than for many other forms of cardiac surgery, including mitral valve replacement.

Based on a Cleveland Clinic review of 1072 patients who underwent primary isolated mitral valve repair for MR due to myxomatous disease, the in-hospital mortality rate was 0.3%. The Mayo Clinic reviewed 1173 patients who underwent mitral valve repair for MVP from 1980 to 1999, observing mortality rates of 0.7%, 11.3%, and 29.4% at 30 days, 5 years, and 10 years, respectively.

Because of the remarkably low mortality rates associated with MVP repair, some experts advocate earlier rather than later repair of MVP in asymptomatic patients with severe MR and no evidence of LV dysfunction, pulmonary hypertension, or atrial fibrillation. AHA/ACC recommendations for surgery in patients with chronic primary mitral valve regurgitation are shown in Table 2.

References

Bonow RO, Carabello BA, Chatterjee K, et al. ACC/AHA 2006 guidelines for the management of patients with valvular heart disease: A report of the American College of Cardiology/American Heart Association Task Force on Practice Guidelines (Writing Committee to Revise the 1998 guidelines for the management of patients with valvular heart disease) developed in collaboration with the Society of Cardiovascular Anesthesiologists endorsed by the Society for Cardiovascular Angiography and Interventions and the Society of Thoracic Surgeons. J Am Coll Cardiol 2006;48(3):e1–148, [Erratium in J Am Coll Cardiol 2007;49(9):1014].

Devereux RB, Kramer-Fox R, Brown WT, et al. Relation between clinical features of the mitral prolapse syndrome and echocardiographically documented mitral valve prolapse. J Am Coll Cardiol 1986;8:763–72.

Flack JM, Kvasnicka JH, Gardin JM, et al. Anthropometric and physiologic correlates of mitral valve prolapse in a biethnic cohort of young adults: The CARDIA study. Am Heart J 1999;138:486.

Freed LA, Benjamin EJ, Levy D, et al. Mitral valve prolapse in the general population: The benign nature of echocardiographic features in the Framingham Heart Study. J Am Coll Cardiol 2002;40:1298–304.

Freed LA, Levy D, Levine RA, et al. Prevalence and clinical outcome of mitral-valve prolapse. N Engl J Med 1999;341:1–7.

Gillinov AM, Cosgrove DM, Blackstone EH, et al. Durability of mitral valve repair for degenerative disease. J Thorac Cardiovasc Surg 1998;116(5):734–43.

Levy D, Savage D. Prevalence and clinical features of mitral valve prolapse. Am Heart J 1987;113:1281–90.

Marks AR, Choong CY, Sanfilippo AJ, et al. Identification of high-risk and low-risk subgroups of patients with mitral-valve prolapse. N Engl J Med 1989;320:1031–6.

Rabkin E, Aikawa M, Stone JR, et al. Activated interstitial myofibroblasts express catabolic enzymes and mediate matrix remodeling in myxomatous heart valves. Circulation 2001;104:2525–32.

Savage DD, Devereux RB, Garrison RJ, et al. Mitral valve prolapse in the general population: 2. Clinical features: The Framingham Study. Am Heart J 1983;106:577–81.

Savage DD, Garrison RJ, Devereux RB, et al. Mitral valve prolapse in the general population: 1. Epidemiologic features: The Framingham Study. Am Heart J 1983;106:571–6.

Suri RM, Schaff HV, Dearani JA, et al. Survival advantage and improved durability of mitral repair for leaflet prolapse subsets in the current era. Ann Thorac Surg 2006;82(3):819–26.

PERICARDITIS

Method of
Miguel A. Leal, MD

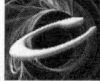

CURRENT DIAGNOSIS

- Pericarditis usually manifests as a pleuritic-type chest pain syndrome, frequently preceded by a nonspecific prodrome (e.g., malaise, fatigue, recent viral infection).
- The physical examination may reveal a pericardial friction rub, pulsus paradoxus, and signs of elevated filling pressures (e.g., jugular venous distention, congestive hepatomegaly, and edema of the extremities).
- Electrocardiography, chest radiography, and transthoracic echocardiography are diagnostic tests that may contribute to establishing the diagnosis and the need for possible intervention, in the case of an associated hemodynamically significant pericardial effusion.
- Laboratory studies may also be helpful, including cultures, erythrocyte sedimentation rate, C-reactive protein, thyroid-stimulating hormone, creatinine, and markers of autoimmune disease.
- Prognosis is usually favorable, except in specific causes such as malignancy, trauma, or aortic dissection.

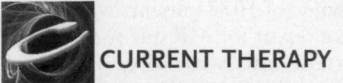

CURRENT THERAPY

- Nonsteroidal antiinflammatory drugs such as ibuprofen (Advil), indomethacin (Indocin),[1] and ketorolac (Toradol) are the usual treatment modality of choice.
- Colchicine[1] may also be used for prevention of disease recurrence.
- Pericardiocentesis and surgical pericardial windows are needed if there is hemodynamic instability (cardiac tamponade).
- Steroids may be used in refractory cases or if autoimmune causes are involved.

[1]Not FDA approved for this indication.

Embryologic Origin of the Pericardium

During the fifth week of embryonic development, lateral structures called the pleuropericardial folds begin to grow toward the midline. As the folds move medially, they bring along the phrenic nerves, and the root of each fold migrates ventrally. At the end of the fifth week, the pleuropericardial folds fuse, partitioning the thoracic cavity into a pericardial cavity and two partially formed pleural cavities.

The pericardium comprises two juxtaposed layers of connective tissue, which form the parietal and the visceral pericardium. The virtual space between the two layers is called the pericardial space. It normally contains a very small amount of transudative fluid (approximately 5 mL). Its function is not well established, but it could conceptually minimize friction and trauma to the epicardium during the cardiac cycle.

Pathologic Processes Involving the Pericardium

The pericardium can be secondarily involved in a large number of systemic disorders, and it can be primarily affected in an isolated disease process. Clinically, most disease processes involving the pericardium manifest with varying degrees of inflammation, constituting the clinical syndrome of pericarditis. In addition, the amount of pericardial fluid may be increased and may result in a pericardial effusion, which can be transudative or exudative and is sometimes hemodynamically significant.

Although pericarditis and pericardial effusions are distinct phenomena, both manifestations are present in a large group of patients. In some cases, the clinical presentation of acute pericardial inflammation predominates, and the presence of excess pericardial fluid has no clinical significance. In other cases, the effusion and its clinical consequences, such as hemodynamic instability, are the main pathologic mechanism.

Classification

Classically, pericardial disease has been categorized as inflammatory, neoplastic, degenerative, vascular, or idiopathic. Some of the major causes of inflammatory disease are infections (viral infections, including HIV, Coxsackie A and B viruses, echoviruses, influenza and adenoviruses; purulent pericarditis; tuberculosis), myocardial infarction (Dressler's syndrome), and collagen vascular diseases. Neoplastic disease may be related to breast, lung, esophagus, lymphoma, melanoma, or renal cell carcinoma. Degenerative disease is related to mediastinal radiation, whether recent or remote.

Miscellaneous causes of pericardial disease include cardiac surgery, aortic dissection, cardiac contusion (with recent or remote sharp or blunt chest trauma), iatrogenic causes (usually after cardiac diagnostic or interventional procedures, such as coronary angiography or placement of a pacemaker or defibrillator), metabolic causes (uremia, myxedematous state), and idiopathic causes.

Most of these causes of pericardial disease can produce both dry pericarditis (i.e., pericarditis with minimal or no effusion) and pericardial effusive disease. Some causes (e.g., HIV infection, hypothyroidism) are primarily associated with effusion without a significant amount of pericardial inflammation.

The frequencies reported for specific causes of pericardial disease vary significantly in the medical literature, depending on the epidemiology, the population at risk, and how the diagnosis was established. The diagnostic yield of pericardiocentesis or pericardial biopsy is typically higher in patients who are found to have a pericardial effusion than in those who present with apparent acute pericarditis without concomitant effusion.

Clinical Manifestations

Acute Pericarditis

The typical clinical manifestations of acute pericarditis are chest pain, which is usually pleuritic in nature (i.e., associated with inspiration and positional changes); a pericardial friction rub; and widespread ST-segment elevation on the 12-lead surface electrocardiogram (ECG). Usually, at least two of these features, with or without an accompanying pericardial effusion, should be present for the clinical diagnosis.

The yield of a full diagnostic evaluation is much lower in patients who present with acute pericarditis than in those presenting with pericardial effusion. In two series with a total of 331 patients, a specific diagnosis was established in only 54 (16%). The most common causes of pericarditis were neoplasia (20 patients), tuberculosis (13 patients), nontuberculous infection (7 patients), and collagen vascular disease (7 patients).

In patients with acute pericarditis for which no cause is identified (idiopathic pericarditis), the etiology is frequently presumed to be viral, but evidence for this is often not pursued, given the expense involved and the time required for the results of viral titers to become available. It is likely that some cases for which an identifiable cause exists are labeled idiopathic as the result of an insufficient diagnostic evaluation. However, complex and exhaustive testing strategies are typically not justified by the limited implications for clinical management. An exception to this recommendation is the absence of a prompt and adequate response to standard treatment.

Pericardial Effusion

Pericardial effusions are typically diagnosed by chest radiography (Figure 1) or transthoracic echocardiography (Figure 2). The latter may reveal a layer of echo-free space between the epicardium and the pericardial sac, sometimes associated with fibrin strands, hematoma, or amorphous material deposited around the heart. The distribution of causes varies with demographics and diagnostic strategies.

In a review of 322 patients with a moderate to large pericardial effusion on echocardiography, the most common causes were idiopathic (20%), iatrogenic (16%), malignancy (13%), chronic idiopathic effusion (9%), acute myocardial infarction (8%), uremia or end-stage renal disease (6%), and collagen vascular disease (5%).

In a different series, including 75 patients presenting to a tertiary care medical center in the United States with a new, unexplained, large pericardial effusion, a diagnosis was made in 53 patients. The most common causes were malignancy (23%), infection (27%), irradiation (14%), collagen vascular disease (12%), uremia or dialysis (12%), and idiopathic (7%). Examination of pericardial fluid yielded a diagnosis in 26%, mostly of malignancy,

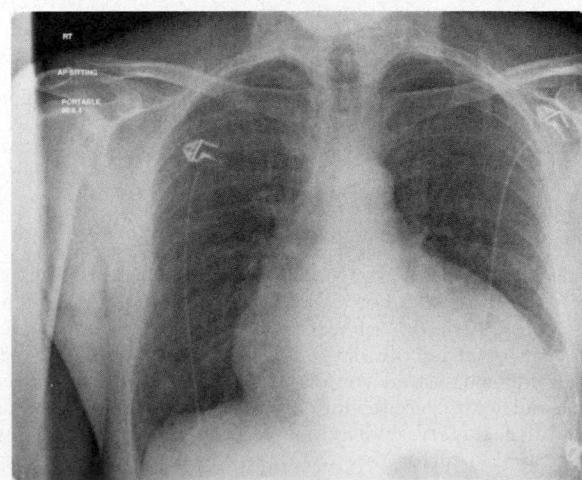

Figure 1. Cardiomegaly is demonstrated on a chest radiograph; the double-shadow pattern suggests a large pericardial effusion.

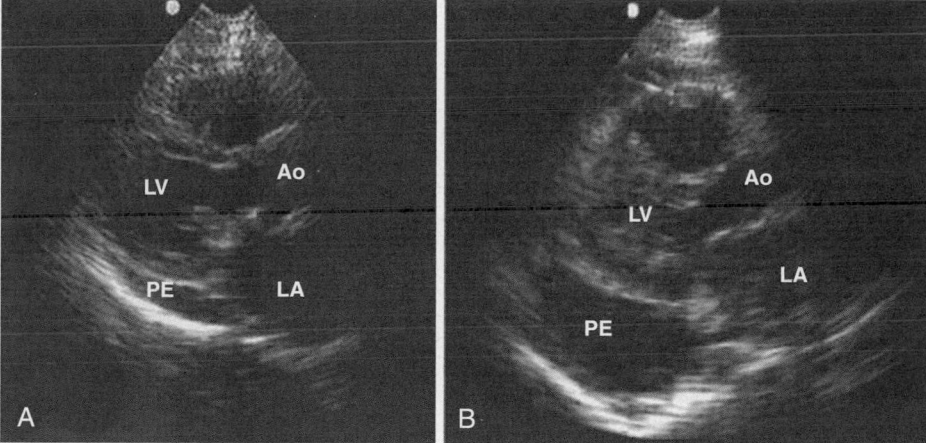

Figure 2. Parasternal long-axis views on transthoracic echocardiography demonstrate a large pericardial effusion (PE), lying predominantly posterior to the heart. *Abbreviations:* Ao = aorta; LA = left atrium; LV = left ventricle.

whereas examination of pericardial tissue was useful for diagnosis in 23%, mostly with infection.

A higher rate of idiopathic disease was found in a review of 204 patients from France; a specific cause was identified in 107 patients (52%). The following distribution was noted: idiopathic (48%), infection (16%), malignancy (15%), collagen vascular disease (10%), hypothyroidism (10%), and renal failure (2%).

Diagnostic Work-up

A careful history and physical examination may reveal a pericardial friction rub, which is usually triphasic (with early diastolic, late diastolic, and systolic components), and the presence of pulsus paradoxus (a drop of 10–12 mm Hg in the systolic blood pressure with inspiration, reflecting enhanced interventricular dependence in the setting of limited pericardial compliance). In addition, laboratory and imaging studies may contribute to establishing the diagnosis.

Laboratory Studies

A complete blood count with differential may show leukocytosis. The erythrocyte sedimentation rate and C-reactive protein level are usually elevated, especially if active inflammation is present. Blood urea nitrogen and creatinine levels should also be checked if uremia is suspected.

Cardiac biomarkers are part of the diagnostic work-up and are abnormal in cases of associated myocarditis or myocardial infarction. In a recent study, an elevated troponin I level was found in 32% of patients with viral or idiopathic pericarditis. This was related to the extent of myocardial inflammation but was not a negative prognostic marker.

Further laboratory work may include blood or viral cultures, tuberculin testing with sputum for acid-fast bacilli, rheumatoid factor, antinuclear antibody, and thyroid function tests.

Other Studies and Procedures
Chest Radiography

Chest radiography may demonstrate an enlarged cardiac silhouette (see Figure 1), which is sometimes the first indication of a large pericardial effusion.

Electrocardiography

Acute pericarditis classically evolves through stages. Initial ECG changes include diffuse, concave upward ST-segment elevation, except in leads aVR and V_1 (where it is usually depressed). T waves are upright in the leads with ST elevation, and the PR segment deviates opposite to P-wave polarity. Several days later, the ST segments return to baseline, followed by flattening of the T waves. The T waves then become inverted, and the ECG eventually returns to baseline weeks to months after the acute episode. The T-wave inversion may persist indefinitely in the chronic inflammation observed with tuberculosis, uremia, or neoplastic processes.

Electrical alternans, the beat-to-beat variability in QRS voltage caused by excessive cardiac mobility, may be seen with a large-size pericardial effusion.

Echocardiography

Universally recommended, echocardiography should be performed urgently if cardiac tamponade is suspected. Cardiac tamponade occurs when the extracardiac pressure from a large effusion causes collapse of the cardiac chambers during diastole. The collapse occurs in a progressive fashion, with right atrial collapse initially, followed by right ventricular collapse and eventual decrement in the cardiac output once the left-sided chambers are affected.

Echocardiograms are particularly helpful if pericardial effusion is suspected on clinical or radiographic grounds, if the illness lasts longer than 1 week, or if myocarditis or purulent pericarditis is suspected. Other causes of pericardial echo-free spaces that must be considered include pleural effusion, pericardial masses, and epicardial fat. Echocardiography can also be used to evaluate for chamber size, tamponade, and ventricular dysfunction (see Figure 2).

Computed Tomography

Effusions are easily detected on computed tomography by virtue of the different x-ray coefficients of fluid and pericardium. The nature of the effusion also may be anticipated, given the different attenuation coefficients for blood, exudates, lipid-rich fluids, and serous fluids. Hemopericardium can be difficult to assess without intravenous contrast, because blood has the same radiodensity as myocardium.

Magnetic Resonance Imaging

Magnetic resonance imaging is a sensitive technique for detecting pericardial effusion and loculated pericardial effusion and thickening.

Cardiac Catheterization

Cardiac catheterization can assist in the differentiation between constrictive and restrictive cardiomyopathy.

Pericardiocentesis

Pericardiocentesis is relatively safe when it is guided by angiography or echocardiography, especially with a large, free anterior effusion. One study reported only 3 minor complications in 117 procedures with ultrasound guidance. Heterogeneous exudates may indicate a potentially difficult pericardiocentesis, especially if the fluid is loculated in pockets—a common finding in autoimmune pericarditis, postsurgical cases, and recurrent disease.

In a large study, diagnostic pericardiocentesis led to a diagnosis in only 6% of cases, compared with 29% diagnosed by therapeutic pericardiocentesis. As such, pericardiocentesis should not be performed unless tamponade or suspected purulent pericarditis is present.

If a pericardiocentesis is performed for drainage, an indwelling catheter should be placed in the pericardial space for continued drainage over several days. If the catheter continues to drain a large amount, a more definitive procedure should be performed.

The pericardial fluid should be analyzed for red cells, total protein level, lactic acid dehydrogenase level, adenosine deaminase activity, and cultures. Cytologic studies are also indicated if malignancy is suspected.

Pericardial Window

In the pericardial window procedure, a small area of the pericardium is resected (usually ≤10 cm^2). In critically ill patients, a balloon catheter may be used to create a pericardial window. In some studies almost 25% of patients who underwent the procedure required repeat operation within 2 years. Constrictive pericarditis may be a long-term complication if pathologic healing affects the pericardium and leads to thickening of the pericardial sac, usually beyond 1.5 cm.

Pericardiectomy

Pericardiectomy is used for constrictive pericarditis, effusive pericarditis, or recurrent pericarditis with multiple attacks; steroid dependence; or intolerance to other medical management. Studies demonstrate that failure rates are proportional to the amount of pericardium removed (i.e., the more pericardium removed, the less likely it is that the procedure will fail). In effusive pericarditis, the higher failure rate associated with a pericardial window or partial pericardiectomy is probably secondary to continued fluid production from the remaining pericardium, with sealing of the remaining pericardium to the heart.

The operative mortality rate was 14% in one series, with a range of 1% for New York Heart Association class I-II, 10% for class III, and 46% for class IV. The 5-year survival rate was 80% for class III-IV and approximately 95% for class I-II.

Treatment

All patients admitted with suspected or established pericarditis, with or without an effusion, should be monitored by telemetry. Other life-threatening causes of chest pain (e.g., myocardial infarction, aortic dissection) should be considered in the differential diagnosis.

In selected cases (young patients with no hemodynamic instability and minor clinical symptoms), pericarditis may be managed on an outpatient basis. In a recent study, fever greater than 38°C, subacute onset, immunosuppression, trauma, oral anticoagulation therapy, failure of therapy with aspirin or nonsteroidal antiinflammatory drugs (NSAIDs), myopericarditis, severe pericardial effusion, and cardiac tamponade were poor prognostic predictors. Patients without these factors were treated on an outpatient basis, without serious complications after a mean follow-up of 38 months.

In another study, the presence of cardiac tamponade and an unfavorable clinical outcome, with persistence of fever, significant pericardial effusion, or general illness lasting longer than 1 week, were highly associated with finding a specific etiology.

If significant clinical activity persists for 3 weeks after admission without an etiologic diagnosis, some authors recommend pericardial biopsy. Complicated cases, such as tuberculous, purulent, or uremic causes, require multidisciplinary involvement, including consultations with a cardiologist, cardiac surgeon, and medical subspecialists (e.g., infectious diseases specialist, nephrologist).

Treatment for specific causes of pericarditis is directed according to the underlying cause. For patients with idiopathic or viral pericarditis, therapy is directed at symptom relief. NSAIDs such as indomethacin[1] (Indocin 50 mg PO every 8 hours), ibuprofen (Motrin or Advil 400–800 mg PO every 6–8 hours), or ketorolac (Toradol 30–90 mg IV/IM every 4 hours[3]) are the mainstay of therapy. These agents have similar efficacies, with relief of chest pain in 85% to 90% of patients within days of treatment. Ibuprofen has the advantage of fewer adverse effects and fewer negative effects on coronary flow. Indomethacin has a poor adverse effect profile and has been shown to reduce coronary flow. Ketorolac is used if the oral route of treatment is not an option. The duration of treatment depends on the clinical course, but common therapeutic courses rarely extend beyond 7 to 10 days.

Aspirin (325 mg PO daily) is recommended for treatment of pericarditis after an ST-elevation myocardial infarction, as part

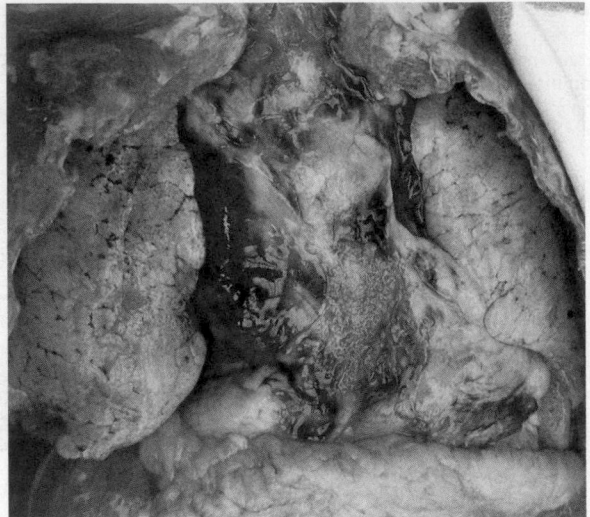

Figure 3. Autopsy findings of a large hemorrhagic pericardial effusion.

of a secondary prevention regimen against recurrent coronary events. Colchicine[1] (1 mg PO daily), in combination with an NSAID, can be considered in the initial treatment to prevent recurrent pericarditis. Colchicine, alone or in combination with an NSAID, can be considered for patients with recurrent or continued symptoms beyond 14 days.

Corticosteroids (prednisone tapering regimens, starting usually at 40–60 mg PO daily and tapered over the course of 10–14 days) should not be used for initial treatment of pericarditis unless indicated for the underlying disease. Corticosteroids also may be used if the patient has had no response to NSAIDs or colchicine, or if these drugs are contraindicated.

Prognosis

The prognosis depends on the etiology. Pericarditis from idiopathic and viral causes usually has a self-limited course. Purulent, tuberculous, hemorrhagic (Figure 3), and neoplastic causes of pericarditis and pericardial effusions result in more complicated courses with worse outcomes.

References

Atar S, Chiu J, Forrester JS, Siegel RJ. Bloody pericardial effusion in patients with cardiac tamponade: Is the cause cancerous, tuberculous, or iatrogenic? Chest 1999;116:1564–9.

Corey GR, Campbell PT, van Trigt P, et al. Etiology of large pericardial effusions. Am J Med 1993;95:209–13.

Galve E, Garcia-del-Castillo H, Evangelista A, et al. Pericardial effusion in the course of myocardial infarction: Incidence, natural history, and clinical relevance. Circulation 1986;73:294–9.

Permanyer-Miralda G, Sagrista-Sauleda J, Soler-Soler J. Primary acute pericardial disease: A prospective series of 231 consecutive patients. Am J Cardiol 1985;56:623–30.

Sagrista-Sauleda J, Merce J, Permanyer-Miralda G, Soler-Soler J. Clinical clues to the causes of large pericardial effusions. Am J Med 2000;109:95–101.

Spodick DH. Pericardial disease. In: Braunwald E, Zipes DP, Libby P, editors. Heart Disease: A Textbook of Cardiovascular Medicine. New York: WB Saunders; 2001. p. 183–202.

Troughton RW, Asher CR, Klein AL. Pericarditis. Lancet 2004;363:717–27.

Zayas R, Anguita M, Torres F, et al. Incidence of specific etiology and role of methods for specific etiologic diagnosis of primary acute pericarditis. Am J Cardiol 1995;75:378–82.

PERIPHERAL ARTERIAL DISEASE

Method of
Wei Zhou, MD; and Marcus Kret, MD

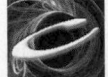 **CURRENT DIAGNOSIS**

Carotid Artery Diseases
- Presentation: transient ischemic attack and stroke
- Physical examination: bruit and lateralized neurologic deficit

---

[1]Not FDA approved for this indication.
[3]Exceeds dosage recommended by the manufacturer.

- Diagnostic modalities: carotid ultrasonography, magnetic resonance angiography (MRA), computed tomographic angiography (CTA), and carotid angiography

Lower Extremity Occlusive Diseases
- Presentation: claudication, rest pain, tissue loss, and numbness
- Physical examination: diminished pulse, hair loss, pallor, cool extremities, tissue wasting, ulcerations, and delayed capillary refill (>3 sec).
- Imaging modalities: ankle-brachial index, segmental pressures with waveforms, CTA, MRA, and lower extremity angiography

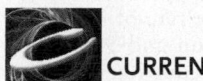

CURRENT THERAPY

Carotid Artery Diseases
- Medical therapy: lifestyle modification and risk factor reduction, lipid-lowering agents, and antiplatelet agents
- Percutaneous carotid stenting procedures
- Carotid artery endarterectomy

Lower Extremity Occlusive Diseases
- Medical management: lifestyle and risk factor modification, and cilostazol (Pletal)
- Exercise regimen
- Percutaneous interventions: angioplasty, stent, and atherectomy
- Surgery: arterial bypass and endarterectomy

Peripheral vascular disease comprises a diverse group of conditions that result in significant morbidity and mortality and offers an opportunity for the astute clinician to recognize common but underdiagnosed problems for which effective interventions exist. Peripheral vascular disease is defined as pathology of the blood vessels outside the brain and heart, and peripheral arterial disease (PAD) involves the subset that affects arteries. Most manifestations of PAD follow logically from the consequences of reduced perfusion of end organs and tissues downstream from sites of flow obstruction. Common forms of PAD include extracranial carotid stenosis, aortoiliac disease, and lower extremity occlusive disease (LEOD). This chapter focuses on extracranial carotid and lower extremity diseases; venous conditions are described in the next chapter.

Epidemiologic data suggest that the prevalence of PAD is 12.2% for American adults older than 60 years of age, increasing to 23.2% for those older than 80 years. Risk factors include increased age, diabetes, past or current tobacco use, renal insufficiency, hypertension, dyslipidemia, and African American or Hispanic ethnicity. More than 95% of patients with PAD have one or more risk factors for cardiovascular disease, and the diagnosis of either condition should raise suspicion for the other. The 10-year risk of death after a diagnosis of PAD is 40%. Alarmingly, an estimated 68% of patients with PAD are undiagnosed by their primary care physicians, although as a group these patients have mainly less advanced cases of atherosclerosis.

The history and physical examination are of paramount importance in detecting peripheral vascular disease and prompting further evaluation. Risk factors for peripheral vascular disease should merit elicitation of common presenting symptoms, including claudication, limb pain at rest, and nonhealing extremity ulcers for LEOD; and amaurosis fugax, transient ischemic attack (TIA), and stroke for carotid occlusive diseases. An appropriate physical examination includes palpation of radial, aortic, femoral, popliteal, and pedal pulses; careful examination of distal extremities for stigmata of arterial insufficiency; cervical and abdominal auscultation for carotid and renal bruits; and a thorough neurologic evaluation.

Carotid Artery Disease

Stroke is the most common cause of permanent disability in the United States, and it remains the third leading cause of death in industrialized countries. Atherosclerotic disease involving the extracranial carotid artery is one of the major causes of all strokes and TIAs. Management of stroke consumes $45 billion annually and is responsible for more than 1 million hospital admissions each year in this country. Neurologic sequelae related to cerebrovascular accidents severely limit a patient's ability to carry out activities of daily living and invariably create an enormous burden on health care costs. As a result, the prevention of cerebrovascular accidents through safe treatment of extracranial carotid occlusive disease remains an important health care goal.

Pathophysiology
The underlying pathophysiology of atherosclerotic plaque formation continues to be an area of active investigation, with explanatory models incorporating elements of flow dynamics, endothelial damage, lipid deposition, and inflammatory mediators. Plaque deposition frequently occurs at sites of bifurcation, and the carotid bifurcation is a common location for plaque formation. The neurologic sequelae from carotid disease mostly result from micro- or macroembolization of disrupted thrombus into the cerebral circulation, with symptoms determined by the vascular territory disrupted and the availability of collateral circulation. Rarely, symptoms can also result from critical flow limitation secondary to severe carotid stenosis, although typically the collateral circulation through the vertebral arteries and the contralateral carotid is adequate to compensate. It is not uncommon to find complete occlusion of a single carotid artery without any perceptible neurologic dysfunction.

Carotid stenosis is categorized as symptomatic or asymptomatic, with divergent therapeutic strategies based on this determination. Most patients are asymptomatic. Symptomatic patients can present with TIA or stroke. Although the classification for neurologic insults is constantly evolving, TIA is defined as a focal neurologic deficit that resolves completely within 24 hours. Symptoms of TIA can include loss of strength or sensation at contralateral upper or lower extremities, and difficulty with speech, vision, or memory. Amaurosis fugax, which presents at painless monocular vision loss as a result of temporary occlusion of a retinal or ophthalmic artery is another possible manifestation of TIA. Patients often describe this as having the appearance of a curtain being drawn down over the eye. Stroke, in contrast, is defined as a neurologic deficit with acute onset that resolves incompletely or not at all after a thromboembolic or hemorrhagic event.

Evaluation
Asymptomatic carotid stenosis may be detected on auscultation of a cervical bruit (although most stenoses are not accompanied by bruits) or on imaging, which includes screening duplex ultrasonography based on risk factors or, increasingly, incidental findings on computed tomography or magnetic resonance scans performed for other indications. The physical examination for a patient with suspected or confirmed carotid stenosis includes a comprehensive neurologic evaluation, auscultation for cervical bruits, and the palpation of peripheral pulses. Vigorous palpation of carotid pulses is discouraged. Important components of the neurologic examination include a thorough evaluation of cranial nerves, strength, sensation, gait, memory, speech, and comprehension. One needs to pay particular attention to lateralized symptoms.

Imaging modalities are important in diagnosing carotid artery stenosis. The most useful screening imaging modality is a carotid duplex examination, which provides information regarding the estimated degree of stenosis, plaque location and characteristics, and flow dynamics (Figure 1). Confirmatory imaging includes computed tomographic or magnetic resonance angiography, which can also be used to evaluate intracerebral circulation and to confirm or detect acute or chronic stroke. Of note, magnetic resonance angiography often overestimates the degree of carotid

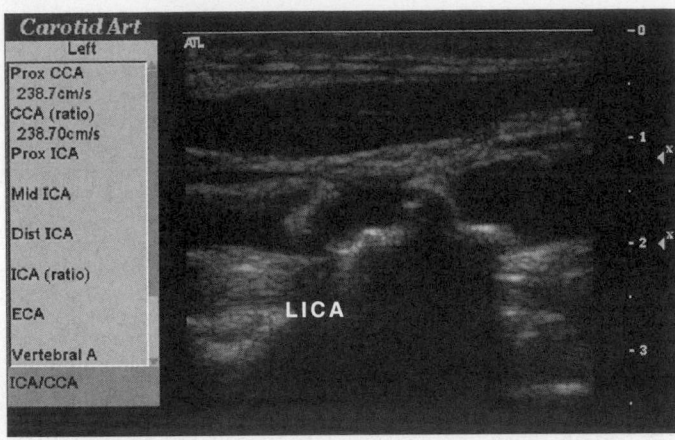

Figure 1. Ultrasound scan of left internal carotid artery (LICA) shows severe carotid stenosis and echogenic calcification at the carotid bulb.

stenosis, particularly for calcified lesions, and should be interpreted in conjunction with duplex results. Carotid and cerebral angiography, historically considered the gold standard, is increasingly being supplanted by these noninvasive imaging modalities. Carotid angiography is now generally reserved for patients who have had conflicting findings on two noninvasive diagnostic tests and patients for whom percutaneous interventions are contemplated.

Management

Management options for carotid stenosis include medical optimization, carotid endarterectomy (CEA), and carotid angioplasty and stenting (CAS) (Figure 2). Medical optimization involves strategies for diet and lifestyle modification, blood pressure control, lipid-lowering agents, antiplatelet therapy, and smoking cessation.

Surgical intervention most commonly involves CEA, in which the carotid artery is exposed, controlled, and opened, and atherosclerotic plaque is removed. A patch angioplasty is performed during closure of the artery to avoid luminal narrowing. An estimated 98,000 CEAs were performed in the United States in 2004. Potential perioperative complications include stroke, cranial nerve injury, hematoma, myocardial infarction, and death. Recommendations for surgical intervention are based on balancing the demonstrated benefits of stroke reduction with the incidence of periprocedural complications; such decisions have been shaped by the results of four large, multicenter trials of carotid endarterectomy published during the 1990s. The North American Symptomatic Carotid Endarterectomy Trial (NASCET) randomly assigned 651 patients with severe (70%–99%) symptomatic carotid stenosis to receive either medical therapy alone or CEA in addition to medical therapy. At 2 years, the rate of ipsilateral stroke was 26% in the medical therapy group and 9% in the CEA group, demonstrating a relative risk reduction of 65%. The European Carotid Surgery Trial (ECST) randomized 3024 patients with symptomatic carotid stenosis to CEA versus initial nonoperative management. Rates of stroke, death, and other adverse events were monitored for 3 years and stratified by degree of stenosis. For patients with stenosis equal to or greater than 80%, the risk of major stroke or death at 3 years was 26.5% in the nonoperative group, compared with 14.9% in the CEA group, for a relative risk reduction of 44%. A large Veterans Affairs trial for symptomatic patients with greater than 70% stenosis demonstrated similar results.

The Asymptomatic Carotid Atherosclerosis Study (ACAS) evaluated the utility of CEA in patients with asymptomatic carotid stenosis. A total of 1662 patients with asymptomatic stenosis of 60% or greater were randomized to CEA or medical treatment. The aggregate risk of ipsilateral stroke and perioperative stroke or death at 5 years was 11.0% for patients treated medically and 5.1% for those treated surgically, with an aggregate risk reduction of 53%. Because this represents an absolute risk reduction of only about 1% per year, considerable controversy still

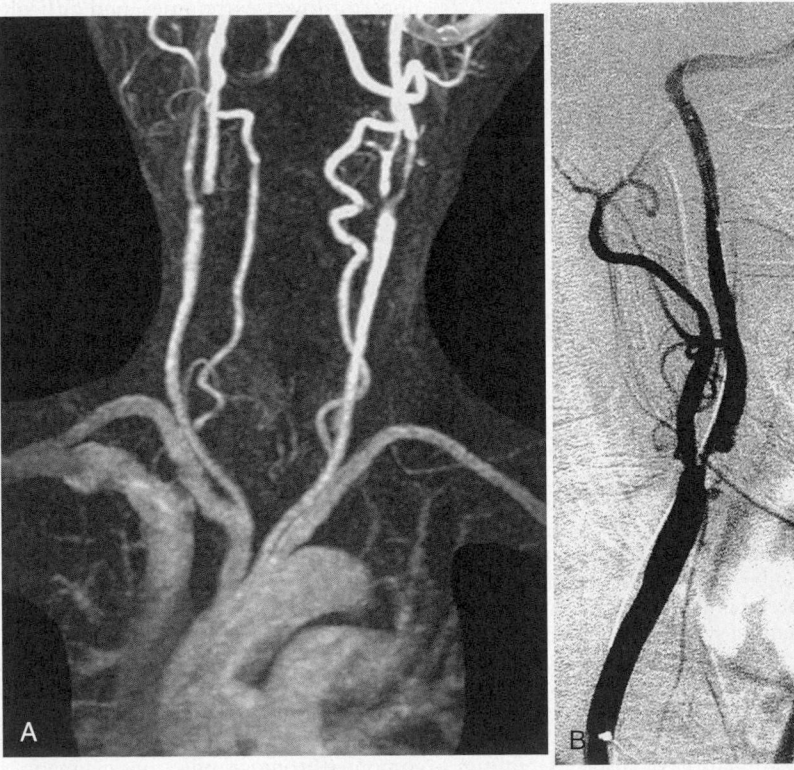

Figure 2. **A,** Time-of-flight magnetic resonance angiogram of the aortic arch and carotid artery demonstrates a severe right carotid artery stenosis. **B,** Carotid angiography confirms a severe stenosis before carotid stenting procedure. A distal protection device is positioned at middle of the internal carotid artery.

exists as to the degree of asymptomatic stenosis that should prompt surgical intervention.

Endovascular techniques represent a recent addition to the arsenal of available treatments for carotid stenosis. CAS, typically with deployment of a distal protection device to minimize the risk of embolization, has emerged as a promising therapeutic option for patients who are considered to be at high surgical risk. Although initial randomized trials demonstrated that CAS was associated with higher perioperative stroke rates, recent studies have suggested that with improved operator experience and appropriate patient selection, CAS can have similar outcomes to CEA. The latest multicenter randomized clinical trial to demonstrate this is the Carotid Revascularization Endarterectomy versus Stenting Trial (CREST), which demonstrated no difference in the composite endpoint of death, stroke, and myocardial infarction between CAS and CEA (5.2% versus 4.5%). However, these findings are interpreted differently by different medical organizations and medical subspecialties. At the core of this argument are the true rates of perioperative stroke in patients who receive carotid revascularization, which, in most studies, including CREST, are higher among patients who receive CAS. Currently, CAS is only FDA approved for patients who are symptomatic and are at high surgical risk for significant medical comorbidities, recurrent stenosis after CEA, prior neck irradiation or dissection, and inaccessible lesions above the C2 level. After CAS, a second antiplatelet agent, such as clopidogrel (Plavix),[1] is recommended for at least 6 weeks in addition to lifelong aspirin.

Postprocedure restenosis is an uncommon but well-recognized long-term complication after CEA or CAS. A severe restenosis can lead to neurologic symptoms and warrants reintervention. For this reason, routine ultrasound surveillance of the carotid arteries is necessary after CEA or CAS. Higher rates of restenosis have been reported after CAS compared with CEA, particularly for patients with prior surgeries.

A recent consensus statement from the Society for Vascular Surgery issued the following recommendations for the management of carotid stenosis:

- Symptomatic patients with less than 50% stenosis: optimal medical therapy
- Symptomatic patients with greater than 50% stenosis: CEA. However, most vascular surgeons accept the intervention threshold of greater than 70% stenosis.
- Asymptomatic patients with less than 60% stenosis: optimal medical therapy
- Asymptomatic patients with greater than 60% stenosis and low perioperative risk: CEA. With improved medical therapy, most vascular surgeons accept greater than 80% stenosis as an indication for CEA in asymptomatic patients.
- Carotid stenting was described as a potential alternative in symptomatic patients with greater than 50% stenosis and high operative risk.

Lower Extremity Occlusive Disease

LEOD is a common form of peripheral vascular disease in which arterial obstruction or stenosis results in inadequate blood flow to meet peripheral tissue demands. Areas of partial or complete occlusion can occur anywhere from the aorta to the pedal vessels, frequently in the iliofemoral, femoropopliteal, or tibial arterial systems. LEOD can best be understood as the peripheral analog to the imbalance between oxygen supply and demand found in coronary artery disease, and it similarly represents a spectrum from mild disease symptomatic only at exertion to severe disease manifesting at rest. The distribution and intensity of symptoms depend on the location and severity of occlusion, the acuteness of onset, and the efficiency of tissue oxygen extraction and utilization. Mild disease can manifest with symptoms of claudication, defined as limb discomfort in specific muscle groups at a reproducible level of exertion. Severe disease can manifest with pain at rest in the affected extremity, tissue loss, or chronic nonhealing wounds.

---

[1]Not FDA approved for this indication.

A distinction should be made between acute and chronic LEOD. Acute LEOD may result from a thrombotic or embolic event and is characterized by an abrupt onset of symptoms. Chronic LEOD is typically less dramatic in presentation and slowly progressive in nature. However, many patients present with acute LEOD. Acute LEOD is a surgical emergency and merits urgent evaluation by a vascular surgeon or specialist.

Evaluation

The presenting symptoms of PAD are myriad and include cramping or pain in the legs or hips, cool extremities, and diminished extremity sensation. Approximately 50% of patients have atypical symptoms, and the classic symptom of claudication has been observed in only 10% of affected patients in some series. It is worth noting that the term *intermittent claudication* is frequently misapplied; this term correctly refers to the reproducible nature of the symptoms after a given level of exertion, not to a sporadic manifestation of discomfort. Several classification systems have been established to create uniform standards for evaluation and reporting of PAD. Among them, the Rutherford classification is one of the most commonly used (Table 1).

After careful elicitation of presenting symptoms, a focused physical examination is critical in the diagnosis of LEOD. Physical findings of PAD include reduced or absent pulses, hair loss, pallor, cool extremities, tissue wasting, ulcerations, and delayed capillary refill (>3 seconds).

A useful and inexpensive test for diagnosing and monitoring LOED is the ankle-brachial index (ABI), which can be readily performed in a clinic. Doppler ultrasonography is used to measure systolic blood pressures in bilateral dorsalis pedis, posterior tibial, and brachial arteries. The highest pedal systolic value in each leg is then divided by the highest arm pressure to calculate the ABI. An ABI of greater than 0.9 is considered normal. Claudicants typically have ABIs between 0.5 and 0.9. A value lower than 0.5 is concern for critical limb ischemia, and a value lower than 0.3 is often associated with tissue loss. Diabetic patients and patients with noncompressible tibial vessels secondary to calcification often have falsely elevated ABIs that are not dependable predictors of arterial disease. The numeric value of an ABI might not correlate precisely with symptoms or with vascular imaging findings, but it can be used to monitor progression of disease and should be interpreted in the clinical context.

A more sophisticated diagnostic screening test includes segmental pressures with evaluation of arterial waveforms. This test is routinely performed in noninvasive vascular laboratories and can provide both anatomic and functional information regarding blood flow without exposing the patient to radiation or nephrotoxic contrast agents. In segmental pressure measurement, systolic blood pressures are recorded at multiple levels, including the upper thigh, lower thigh, upper calf, ankle, and toes. A decrease of 20 mm Hg pressure between segments indicates significant arterial disease within that segment. For example, a pressure difference of

TABLE 1 Rutherford Classification for Peripheral Arterial Occlusive Disease

SYMPTOMS	GRADE	CATEGORY
Asymptomatic	0	0
Claudication		
Mild	I	1
Moderate	I	2
Severe	I	3
Ischemic rest pain	II	4
Tissue loss		
Minor	III	5
Major	III	6

30 mm Hg between the upper and lower thigh suggests severe superficial femoral artery occlusive disease.

After a careful history and physical examination and noninvasive ultrasound evaluations have been performed, other diagnostic modalities may be required to further delineate anatomy, particularly if interventions are intended. Computed tomographic angiography produces a more detailed anatomic description and is useful for both diagnosis and preoperative planning but requires the use of radiation and intravenous contrast. Magnetic resonance angiography is emerging as a complementary modality, but is typically more expensive than computed tomographic angiography and has limited availability outside academic centers. Traditional angiography is performed if noninvasive modalities are unobtainable. Angiography affords the additional advantage of enabling endovascular intervention at the time of evaluation (Figure 3).

Treatment

Treatment options for PAD include medical optimization, exercise training, and surgical or percutaneous interventions. Patients with mild claudication can benefit from risk factor modification, including smoking cessation and medical optimization for hypertension, diabetes, and dyslipidemia. Based on guidelines from the Inter-Society Consensus for the Management of Peripheral Arterial Disease (TASC II), patients with symptomatic PAOD should receive antiplatelet therapy with either aspirin or clopidogrel (Plavix) to decrease the risk of cardiovascular morbidity and mortality. Studies investigating agents such as pentoxifylline (Trental) and cilostazol (Pletal) have shown mixed results, and thus their use in treatment of claudication symptoms remains controversial. Medical management alone can lead to improvement in symptoms in a significant proportion of claudicants (as high as 75% in some series), and there is evidence that multimodality therapy is more effective than any single intervention. It is reasonable to perform a trial of medical optimization before more invasive therapeutic modalities are considered, particularly in patients with mild and moderate symptoms. Supervised exercise regimens have also demonstrated efficacy for some patients with mild and moderate symptoms and should be considered before surgical or percutaneous interventions.

For patients who have not responded to medical optimization, multiple revascularization options exist. As with any surgical intervention, the risks and benefits of the proposed procedure must be carefully weighed against potential improvements in quality of life. Indications for revascularization include critical limb ischemia with rest pain, tissue loss, or nonhealing lesions. Lifestyle-limiting claudication is a relative indication for revascularization. Surgical revascularization options include bypassing the occluded arterial segment with a venous or synthetic graft and removing plaque from an arterial segment (endarterectomy) with local reconstruction. In the acute setting, removal of thromboembolus can be performed by direct exposure, balloon thrombectomy, or purely endovascular techniques. Commonly performed bypass operations that have achieved durable long-term results include aortofemoral bypass for aortoiliac occlusive disease and femoropopliteal and femorotibial bypasses for more distal disease. Perioperative morbidity is not insignificant (2%–6%). In this patient population with substantial comorbidity, complications can include myocardial infarction, wound infection, graft infection, graft thrombosis, limb loss, and death. Long-term surveillance of bypass grafts with regular duplex ultrasonographic evaluations is necessary.

Driven by developments in technology and efforts to decrease periprocedural morbidity and mortality, endovascular interventions are increasingly being performed for the treatment of LEOD. Endovascular options include angioplasty alone, angioplasty with stenting, and atherectomy (a percutaneous analog of endarterectomy). In general, endovascular treatment is effective and durable for treatment of focal lesions with good distal run-off vessels. Patients with distal three-vessel run-off have better long-term outcome than those with one-vessel run-off or no run-off vessel. Lesion characteristics are also important. Long segments of occlusion, diffuse lesions, and calcified lesions are associated with poor long-term outcomes. The decreased invasiveness and shorter convalescence achieved with percutaneous approaches are appealing, but fewer long-term data are available than for traditional surgical

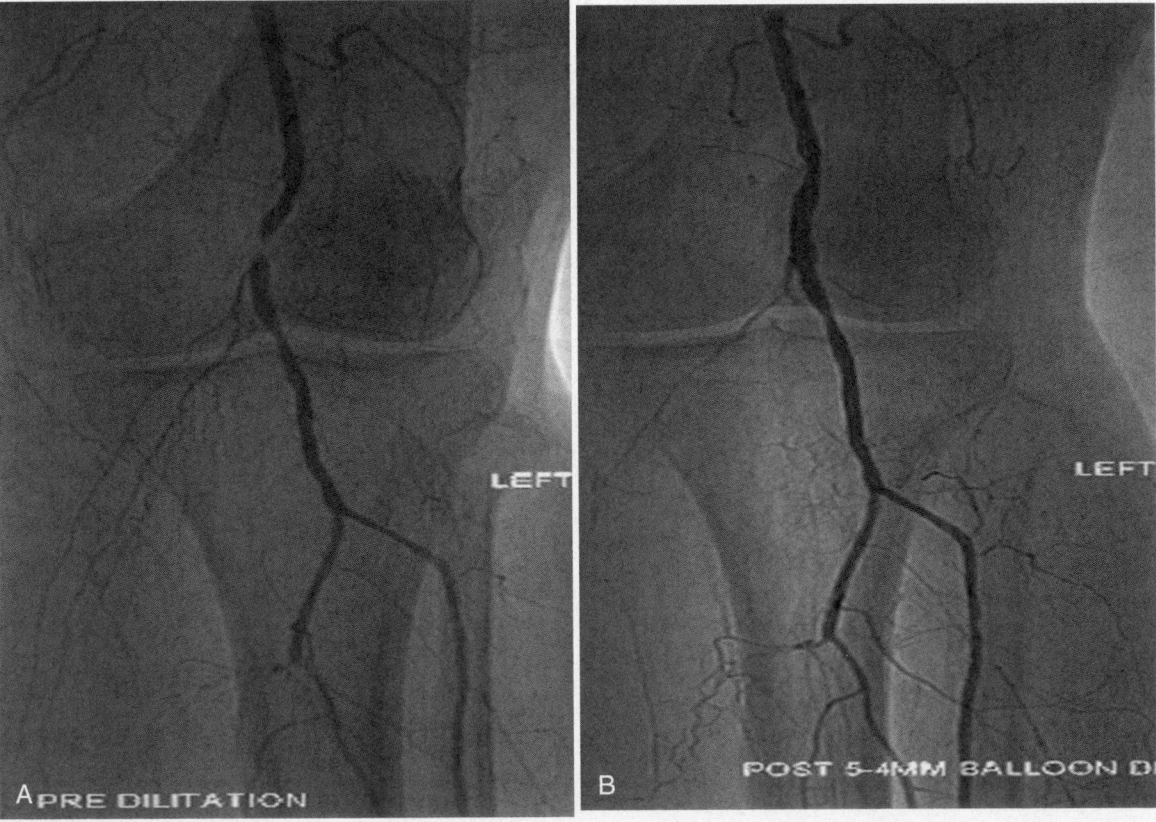

Figure 3. A, Lower extremity angiogram shows a focal occlusive lesion of the popliteal artery. B, Postprocedure angiogram shows complete resolution of the stenosis after balloon angioplasty.

approaches, and complications can be equally devastating. Endovascular technology is an area of active research and development, and improvements may expand the use of endovascular approaches to LEOD in the future. As with open approaches, routine postintervention surveillance is essential to identify severe restenoses that require secondary intervention. Given that percutaneous interventions can limit options for future reconstruction, patients with LEOD are best managed by vascular specialists familiar with the full range of therapeutic techniques as well as the natural history of disease progression.

References

Arain F, Cooper L. Peripheral arterial disease: Diagnosis and management. Mayo Clin Proc 2008;83(8):944–50.

Brott TG, Hobson RW 2nd, Howard G, et al. CREST Investigators. Stenting versus endarterectomy for treatment of carotid-artery stenosis N Engl J Med 2010;363:198.

Donnan G, Fisher M, Macleod M, Davis SM. Stroke. Lancet 2008;371:1612–23.

European Carotid Surgery Trialists Collaborative Group. Randomised trial of endarterectomy for recently symptomatic carotid stenosis: Final results of the MRC European Carotid Surgery Trial (ECST). Lancet 1998;351:1379–87.

Ferguson G, Eliasziw M, Barr HW, et al. The North American Symptomatic Carotid Endarterectomy Trial: Surgical results in 1415 patients. Stroke 1999;30:1751–8.

Hobson 2nd. RW, Mackey WC, Ascher E, et al. Management of atherosclerotic carotid artery disease: Clinical practice guidelines of the Society for Vascular Surgery. J Vasc Surg 2008;48:480–6.

Norgren L, Hiatt WR, Dormandy JA, et al. Inter-Society Consensus for the Management of Peripheral Arterial Disease (TASC II). J Vasc Surg 2007;45(1):S5A–S67A.

Ostchega Y, Paulose-Ram R, Dillon CF, et al. Prevalence of peripheral arterial disease and risk factors in persons aged 60 and older: Data from the National Health and Nutrition Examination Survey 1999–2004. J Am Geriatr Soc 2007;55(4):583–9.

Rosamond W, Flegal K, Friday G, et al. Heart Disease and Stroke Statistics 2007 Update: A Report from the American Heart Association Statistics Committee and Stroke Statistics Subcommittee. Circulation 2007;115:e69–171.

Selvin E, Erlinger T. Prevalence of and risk factors for peripheral arterial disease in the United States: Results from the National Health and Nutrition Examination Survey, 1999–2000. Circulation 2004;110:738–43.

White C. Intermittent claudication. N Engl J Med 2007;356:1241–50.

PREMATURE BEATS

Method of
Prakash C. Deedwania, MD; and Enrique V. Carbajal, MD

CURRENT DIAGNOSIS

- Premature beats are identified by their occurrence at times considerably shorter than the regular sinus rhythm cycles.
- The origin of the premature beats is determined by the presence or absence of P waves, morphology of the P wave (when present), QRS configuration, and the presence or absence of a compensatory period.
- The presence of frequent PVCs (≥10 per hour) during the post-discharge evaluation of survivors of acute MI predicts increased risk of arrhythmic death and overall cardiac mortality.

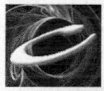

CURRENT THERAPY

- In general, premature beats in patients without evidence of organic heart disease do not require any specific antiarrhythmic therapy because generally there is no significant increased risk of life-threatening arrhythmia.
- Correction of any underlying structural cardiopulmonary disorder and other precipitating factors (e.g., electrolyte or metabolic abnormalities).
- Suppression of PVCs using currently available antiarrhythmic drugs (except for amiodarone) is not advisable for most patients, primarily because of the increased risk of proarrhythmic effects of these drugs.

- In the occasional patient who is disabled by annoying symptoms due to PVCs, a trial of β-blocker therapy should be considered and often Is effective in many patients.

Premature beats are the most common form of cardiac arrhythmia encountered in clinical practice. Premature beats are one of the most common causes of irregular pulse and palpitations. In many instances, premature beats are not associated with any symptoms. They result from electrical depolarization of myocardium that occurs earlier than the sinus impulse. Premature beats have been referred to by a variety of names, including premature contractions, premature complexes, ectopic beats, and early depolarizations. Although no single term is ideal, most electrophysiologists refer to them as premature complexes because although the term *ectopic beat* denotes the abnormal site of origin of the depolarization, it does not necessarily require the beat to be premature, and, in some cases, ectopic rhythm indeed occurs as an escape phenomenon.

Although premature beats generally occur in patients with organic heart disease, they frequently can be seen in the absence of any structural heart disease, especially in elderly patients. Premature beats can be triggered by, or increase in frequency with, myocardial ischemia and heart failure. Premature beats can be provoked by, or occur in association with, a variety of systemic abnormalities, including electrolyte disturbances, acid-base imbalance, toxins from recreational drug and/or alcohol abuse, metabolic perturbations, systemic illnesses such as thyroid disorders, pulmonary disease, infections, and febrile illnesses, and any condition associated with increased catecholamine levels.

Most premature beats occur as a result of enhanced automaticity, but other electrophysiologic mechanisms, including reentry and triggered activity, might play a role. Based on the corresponding site of origin, premature electrical depolarizations are called *premature atrial complexes* (PACs), *premature junctional complexes* (PJCs), and *premature ventricular complexes* (PVCs). Morphologic features and timing of the premature beat on electrocardiographic (ECG) recording(s) help determine the site of origin and the nature of premature complexes. Premature beats can occur in a repetitive fashion as bigeminy (after every other normal beat), trigeminy (after each sequence of two normal beats), or quadrigeminy (after each sequence of three normal beats). They also can occur as two or three successive premature beats, defined as couplets and triplets, respectively. In this article, the primary focus is on single premature beats.

Premature Atrial Complexes

PACs are the most common form of atrial arrhythmias that can originate at any site in the atria. The exact morphology of the atrial activation (P wave) varies depending on the site of origin of the PAC. Careful and systematic examination of the ECG features of PACs usually can distinguish them from PVCs.

Electrocardiographic Features

The cardinal features of PACs include their prematurity with reference to sinus beats, abnormal P wave morphology, and, in most cases, QRS morphology that is similar to that of sinus beats. The P wave morphology of the PAC generally differs from the sinus P wave unless the premature complex originates in the high right atrial area adjacent to the sinus node, in which case distinguishing PACs from sinus arrhythmia may be difficult. Although sinus arrhythmias are generally phasic in nature, being influenced by the respiratory cycle, this feature would be helpful in differentiating from high right atrial PACs only when the PACs are frequent and repetitive. When the PAC occurs quite early in the diastolic phase, the P wave may not be obvious on surface ECG because it is often hidden in the preceding T wave and would be evident only by watching carefully for the notched or peaked T wave.

If the PAC is too premature, it might fail to conduct to the ventricles if the atrioventricular (AV) node is refractory owing to conduction of the preceding sinus impulse. Such nonconducted PACs are called *blocked PACs*, and they are important because they can be confused with instances of AV block. Such erroneous interpretation can be avoided by simply remembering a common rule of thumb that requires normal successive P-P intervals for all sinus beats, including the interval for a blocked P wave, before considering the diagnosis of AV block. Although most PACs have a normal or prolonged PR interval, the relationship of the PAC to the subsequent QRS complex depends on the site of origin of the PAC and the prematurity index. For example, a PAC originating in the lower atrial area near the AV node generally has a shorter PR interval, whereas a PAC that is quite premature and originates in the upper left atrial area might have a longer than usual PR interval. In general, the PR interval of a PAC is inversely related to its prematurity.

Because most PACs are able to depolarize the sinus node, they usually can reset the sinus automaticity; therefore, the subsequent pause following most PACs is generally less than compensatory because the sinus node fires earlier than expected. In this case, measurement of the P-P interval between the sinus P wave preceding the PAC and the P wave following the PAC is generally less than twice the basic sinus cycle length. This is in contrast to the full compensatory pause often observed in conjunction with PVCs. In some cases, the PAC collides with the sinus impulse in the perinodal tissue and thus fails to reset the sinus node, thereby resulting in a full compensatory pause.

In general, electrical depolarization below the AV node is normal with PAC and results in an unchanged (baseline) QRS complex. Aberrant conduction, however, may be encountered when the PAC reaches the infranodal tissue during the period when it is still partially refractory. Most frequently, the aberrant conduction usually occurs when a short coupled PAC follows a long pause in patients with sinus bradycardia (long-short cycle). This usually results in a right bundle-branch block pattern and is commonly referred to as the *Ashman phenomenon*.

Clinical Features

Although PACs can occur in normal individuals of all ages, they are quite infrequent except in the elderly. Their frequency increases with age; as many as 50% to 70% of the elderly may have occasional PACs. Some elderly individuals without organic heart disease have frequent PACs and occasionally atrial bigeminy or two to three PACs in a row. Whether the increased frequency of PACs in these individuals is secondary to senile amyloidosis, myocardial fibrosis, or diastolic dysfunction secondary to aging-related changes in the heart is not known. PACs are extremely common in patients with heart disease and in patients with acute as well as chronic respiratory failure. The frequency of PACs can increase markedly during periods of acute febrile illness, shock states, and metabolic disorders, especially in patients with hyperthyroidism and conditions associated with increased catecholamine levels. Use of excessive caffeine, alcohol, tobacco, and recreational drugs can increase the frequency of PACs. In patients with acute myocardial infarction (MI), frequent PACs usually are precursors of atrial fibrillation and occur in association with ventricular failure. In general, the presence of frequent PACs in the setting of acute MI is an indicator of poor prognosis.

In general, PACs are benign except when they are a marker of an underlying cardiopulmonary disorder(s). The major clinical importance of PACs is related to the increased risk of atrial tachyarrhythmias in patients with an established history of such arrhythmias as well as in the elderly who are generally at high risk for atrial fibrillation. As indicated earlier, in rare instances the blocked PACs may be confused with episodes of AV nodal block; however, careful examination of the ECG features described previously easily establishes the correct diagnosis and avoids unnecessary pacemaker implantation.

Treatment

The correction of an underlying structural cardiopulmonary disorder and other precipitating factors (e.g., electrolyte or metabolic abnormalities) usually is all the treatment that is needed. No specific treatment is generally required in most patients because PACs usually are benign except in patients with a history of recurrent atrial tachyarrhythmias, for example, atrial flutter/fibrillation. In such patients, specific treatment may be indicated and could include a β-blocker or a heart rate-modulating calcium channel blocking agent such as verapamil (Calan) or diltiazem (Cardizem). Recent studies have shown that verapamil is quite effective in patients with frequent PACs and multifocal atrial tachycardia in the setting of acute or chronic ventilatory insufficiency. In patients who are at risk for recurrent atrial fibrillation, treatment with a specific antiarrhythmic agent, such as propafenone (Rythmol) or flecainide (Tambocor), may be beneficial; however, these drugs should be used only when the patient has a history of recurrent atrial flutter/fibrillation because of the increased risk of proarrhythmia, especially in the presence of organic heart disease such as recurrent ischemia or heart failure.

Premature Junctional Complexes

PJCs are rarely seen in normal individuals and are infrequently encountered even in patients with organic heart disease. When present, PJCs can occur due to abnormal automaticity or reentry phenomenon. Although digitalis toxicity is cited as a common etiologic factor, PJCs also can occur in the setting of MI, myocarditis, and electrolyte/metabolic disturbances.

Electrocardiographic Features

The ECG characteristics of PJCs are distinct from those of PACs in that the P wave usually is inverted in the inferior leads (II, III, and aVF) because of retrograde conduction to the atria from the ectopic foci in the junctional area. The second feature of PJCs is that the PR interval almost always is shorter than the normal PR interval because of the proximity of ectopic foci to the AV node and bundle of His. In most cases, the P wave might not even be visible on surface ECGs because it lies hidden within the QRS complex. Rarely, the P wave precedes the QRS complex when the ectopic impulse traverses to the atria before traveling down to depolarize the ventricle. In general, the infranodal conduction of PJCs is normal, and thus the QRS morphology of the conducted PJCs is similar to that noted during sinus rhythm. When the PJC is closely coupled to the preceding sinus beat, aberrant conduction might occur if the impulse traverses down the bundle branch during the relative refractory period (most frequently manifesting as a right bundle-branch block pattern). Because in many instances no obvious P wave accompanies a PJC, aberrantly conducted PJCs may be hard to differentiate from PVCs.

In some instances when PJCs occur during the period when the AV node as well as the infranodal conduction systems both are refractory, the PJC may encounter both retrograde and antegrade blocks for impulse propagation. In such situations, no P wave or QRS complex is related to the PJC. Although the ectopic impulse would be invisible on a surface ECG, it would penetrate a portion of the conduction system and thus make it partially or completely refractory to conduction of the subsequent sinus impulse. This would be manifested as a sudden prolongation of subsequent PR interval in case of partial refractoriness or as an episode of "pseudo AV nodal block" due to the blocked sinus beat if the infranodal tissue were unable to conduct the sinus impulse. Thus, even though some PJCs might not have any surface ECG complexes, their presence can be suspected based on their influence on the conduction of the following sinus beat, owing to the electrophysiologic phenomenon described as "concealed conduction."

Clinical Features

PJCs usually are not seen in normal persons and are rarely encountered in cardiac patients except in the setting of digitalis intoxication and infrequently in the setting of MI or myocarditis. In patients with digitalis toxicity, PJCs may lead to junctional tachycardia, occasionally resulting in palpitation, but are rarely associated with hemodynamic compromise. Because in some cases concealed conduction of PJCs might result in periods of varying degrees of pseudo AV blocks, it is clinically important to recognize their presence in order to prevent undue concern and avoid inappropriate pacemaker implantation.

Premature Ventricular Complexes

PVCs are the most common form of arrhythmia and can be encountered frequently in healthy individuals as well as in patients with a variety of cardiac disorders. PVCs are often triggered by electrolyte abnormalities, acid-base imbalance, metabolic perturbations, hypoxia, and ischemia.

Electrocardiographic Features

PVCs occur as a result of premature depolarization of the ventricles due to ectopic foci in the ventricular myocardium or Purkinje fibers. In general, PVCs result in wide QRS complexes with the T wave axis usually opposite to that of the QRS. In the vast majority of cases, PVCs do not conduct retrogradely and thus do not result in a distinct P wave. The sinus beats may, however, continue uninterrupted and thus manifest as an instance of AV dissociation in conjunction with PVCs. For the same reason, because PVCs usually do not conduct retrogradely and depolarize the atrium and the sinus node, there usually is a full compensatory pause in contrast to the partial compensatory pause generally seen with PACs. In patients with slow sinus rates, however, interpolated PVCs might occur. If the ectopic foci for PVCs are located high in the His-Purkinje system, the resulting premature complexes may have a narrow QRS morphology quite similar to that seen during sinus rhythm. Additionally, if the PVCs occur rather late, in close proximity to the sinus impulse, there may also be a narrow complex QRS because of fusion between the normal depolarization due to sinus impulse and the abnormal activation sequence from the ectopic foci. In the instance of fusion beats, a normal P wave precedes the QRS. The PR interval is shorter, and the QRS morphology may be only partially altered. In some cases, this might give the appearance of an intermittent bundle-branch block or preexcitation (Wolff-Parkinson-White syndrome) pattern.

Based on the morphologic features of PVCs, they have been classified as uniform or multiform; they also have been referred to as unifocal or multifocal. Also recommended is classification of PVCs based on their coupling interval with the preceding sinus beat. PVCs with a short coupling interval near or on the previous T wave have been described as showing R-on-T phenomenon; alternatively PVCs may have long coupling intervals. Based on the underlying electrophysiologic mechanism responsible for PVCs, the coupling interval may be fixed, as in reentrant beats, or variable, as seen with ventricular parasystole. PVCs may have a repetitive pattern, for example, bigeminy or trigeminy, or they may occur in pairs. It is now thought that repetitive PVCs, such as couplets and triplets, are prognostically more important than just the frequency of isolated PVCs.

Clinical Features

PVCs can be recorded frequently in normal individuals, and, similar to PACs, their frequency increases with age. In patients without organic heart disease or without prior evidence of sustained ventricular tachyarrhythmias, the mere presence of frequent PVCs is not considered prognostically important. However, individual exceptions do exist, and the clinician is advised to evaluate each given patient accordingly. In patients with organic heart disease, PVCs are the most common form of arrhythmia and carry significant prognostic importance, especially in survivors of acute MI and patients with recurrent ischemia and advanced heart failure. It has been well established during the past two decades that frequent PVCs occurring during the acute phase of MI are associated with an increased risk of sustained ventricular arrhythmias in the initial 48 hours, but they do not predict long-term outcome or risk of arrhythmic events. More recently, it has been shown in patients receiving thrombolytic therapy that PVCs, particularly episodes of nonsustained ventricular tachycardia, increase in frequency but are generally short-lived and represent a sign of myocardial reperfusion. However, the presence of frequent PVCs during the postdischarge evaluation of survivors of MI is indicative of a poor prognosis.

Although as many as 80% to 90% of patients with chronic heart failure have frequent PVCs, the results of several recent studies have shown that only the presence of nonsustained ventricular tachycardia (defined as three or more PVCs in a row) at a rate greater than 100 bpm is strongly predictive of an increased risk of sudden cardiac death in these patients. This is in clear contrast to the findings of several large clinical trials, which showed that more than 10 PVCs per hour in post-MI patients are predictive of a poor prognosis and an increased risk of arrhythmic death.

Overall, the association between PVCs and an increased risk of ventricular tachyarrhythmias and sudden cardiac death appears to be related not only to the frequency and complexity of PVCs but also to the severity of underlying structural heart disease. For example, a patient with mitral valve prolapse and frequent PVCs would be at relatively low risk for arrhythmic events compared to a patient with advanced heart failure who has repetitive PVCs and episodes of nonsustained ventricular tachycardia. Proper evaluation of the risk of PVCs has become more crucial than ever because most currently available antiarrhythmic drugs have the potential for causing serious adverse reactions, including proarrhythmias, in patients with advanced cardiac disorders.

Treatment

In general, PVCs in patients without evidence of organic heart disease do not require any specific antiarrhythmic therapy because generally there is no significantly increased risk of life-threatening arrhythmia. However, when PVCs are associated with disabling palpitations, reassurance and treatment with β-blockers (atenolol [Tenormin], metoprolol [Toprol-XL]) may help in relieving symptoms. In patients with systemic illness or other provoking factors (e.g., electrolyte abnormalities or acid-base imbalance), immediate correction of the underlying abnormality usually is associated with beneficial effects.

Because of the associated poor prognosis with PVCs in the setting of acute MI, common practice in the past consisted of routine administration of intravenous lidocaine (Xylocaine) in an effort to suppress PVCs during the initial phase of acute MI. However, because recent data suggest that the routine use of lidocaine is not necessary and often can be harmful, lidocaine should be avoided because of the risk of serious adverse reactions, especially central nervous system side effects such as seizures in the elderly. With the ready availability of cardiac monitoring, it now is possible to accurately identify a harbinger of ventricular tachyarrhythmias early in the coronary care unit, so prophylactic use of lidocaine is generally not recommended. Furthermore, results from several studies and their meta-analyses have demonstrated that routine use of prophylactic lidocaine during the acute or healing phase of MI does not alter the overall mortality in patients with acute MI.

In contrast, it is well established that the presence of frequent PVCs (≥ 10 per hour) during the postdischarge evaluation of survivors of acute MI predicts an increased risk of arrhythmic death and overall cardiac mortality. Numerous trials have been conducted with a variety of different antiarrhythmic drugs. Many of the studies demonstrated that suppression of PVCs with most currently available antiarrhythmic drugs is not beneficial in reducing the increased risk associated with PVCs. The Cardiac Arrhythmia Suppression Trials (CAST I and II) clearly demonstrated that, compared to placebo, treatment with class Ic antiarrhythmic drugs (which primarily work by slowing conduction) was associated with an increased risk of arrhythmic death despite adequate suppression of PVCs. The findings from CAST I and II, as well as several other clinical trials, indicate that although frequent PVCs may be a marker for an adverse event, suppression of PVCs with type I antiarrhythmic agents does not favorably influence the associated increased risk of death. Results from the Canadian Amiodarone Myocardial Infarction Arrhythmia Trial (CAMIAT) and the European Myocardial Infarct Amiodarone Trial (EMIAT) suggest that in patients with frequent PVCs in the post-MI setting, use of amiodarone (Cordarone), a complex drug with predominantly class III antiarrhythmic properties, in combination with β-blockers is associated with improved outcome. However, because of the associated drug toxicity with long-term amiodarone use, it is generally considered suitable only for the high-risk cohort (although many patients with low left ventricular ejection fraction now undergo implantation of an automatic internal cardiac defibrillator).

In general, suppression of PVCs using currently available antiarrhythmic drugs (except for amiodarone) is not advisable for most patients, primarily because of the increased risk of proarrhythmic effects of these drugs. In the occasional patient who is disabled by annoying symptoms due to PVCs, an initial trial of β-blocker therapy should be considered and is effective in many patients. Correction of the provoking factors and appropriate management of any underlying heart disease often are beneficial in managing patients with frequent PVCs.

References

Barrett PA, Peter CT, Swan HJ, et al. The frequency and prognostic significance of electrocardiographic abnormalities in clinically normal individuals. Prog Cardiovasc Dis 1981;23:299.

Boutitie F, Boissel J-P, Connolly SJ, et al. EMIAT and CAMIAT Investigators: Amiodarone interaction with β-blockers: Analysis of the merged EMIAT (European Myocardial Infarct Amiodarone Trial) and CAMIAT (Canadian Amiodarone Myocardial Infarction Trial) databases. Circulation 1999;99:2268.

Brodsky M, Wu D, Denes P, et al. Arrhythmias documented by 24 hour continuous electrocardiographic monitoring in 50 male medical students without apparent heart disease. Am J Cardiol 1977;39:390.

Cairns JA, Connolly SJ, Roberts R, et al. Randomised trial of outcome after myocardial infarction in patients with frequent or repetitive ventricular premature depolarisations: CAMIAT. Lancet 1997;349:675.

Echt DS, Liebson PR, Mitchell B, et al. Mortality and morbidity in patients receiving encainide, flecainide, or placebo. N Engl J Med 1991;324:781.

Fleg J, Kennedy H. Cardiac arrhythmias in a healthy elderly population. Chest 1982;81:302.

Julian DG, Camm AJ, Frangin G, et al. Randomised trial of effect of amiodarone on mortality in patients with left-ventricular dysfunction after recent myocardial infarction: EMIAT. Lancet 1997;349:667.

Morganroth J. Premature ventricular complexes. Diagnosis and indications for therapy. JAMA 1984;252:673.

Romhilt D, Chaffin C, Choi S, et al. Arrhythmias on ambulatory electrocardiographic monitoring in women without apparent heart disease. Am J Cardiol 1984;54:582.

Rosen KM, Rahimtoola SH, Gunnar RM. Pseudo A-V block secondary to premature nonpropagated His bundle depolarizations: Documentation by His bundle electrocardiography. Circulation 1970;42:367.

Ruskin JN. Ventricular extrasystoles in healthy subjects. N Engl J Med 1985;312:238.

Simpson Jr RJ, Cascio WE, Schreiner PJ, et al. Prevalence of premature ventricular contractions in a population of African American and white men and women: The Atherosclerosis Risk in Communities (ARIC) study. Am Heart J 2002;143:535.

TACHYCARDIAS

Method of
Stephen Boateng, DO

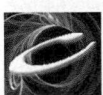

CURRENT DIAGNOSIS

- A hemodynamic assessment and a 12-lead ECG should be obtained on every patient presenting with tachycardia.
- Tachycardia is defined as a cardiac rhythm greater than 100 beats/min.
- Tachycardias may be supraventricular or ventricular in origin.
- SVTs may be narrow complex (QRS duration less than 120 ms) or wide complex (QRS duration greater than 120 ms). VTs are always wide complex.
- History taking is useful in aiding in the diagnosis and definition of tachycardia.
- Patients with tachycardias might complain of palpitations, fatigue, lightheadedness, chest discomfort, dyspnea, presyncope, or syncope.
- A history of syncope is a red flag and should prompt immediate referral to an electrophysiologist.

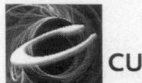

CURRENT THERAPY

- All wide-complex tachycardias should be treated as ventricular in origin unless proved otherwise. The misdiagnosis of SVT when VT is present is associated with worse prognosis.
- Radiofrequency ablation is often successful in curing SVTs and some VTs.
- Wide-QRS complex tachycardias are commonly secondary to VT in the setting of structural heart disease, and effective therapy is accomplished with cardioverter-defibrillator implantation.

Tachycardia

Tachycardia is any cardiac rhythm with a rate greater than 100 beats/min. It may be supraventricular or ventricular in origin. Supraventricular tachycardias (SVTs) almost always manifest as narrow-complex (less than 120 msec) tachycardias on an electrocardiogram (ECG). However, wide-complex (greater than 120 msec) tachycardias occur if there is aberrant conduction or a bundle branch block. Ventricular tachycardias (VTs) occur when there are more than three consecutive ventricular beats at a rate greater than 100 beats per minute. VTs always manifest as wide-complex tachycardias.

Epidemiology

Supraventricular Tachycardias

Though rarely life threatening, SVTs are common, may be persistent, and often reoccur throughout one's lifetime. The etiology of SVTs varies with age, sex, and comorbid conditions. Paroxysmal SVTs (PSVTs) are estimated to have a prevalence of 2.25 per 1000 and an incidence of 35 per 100,000 person-years, according to the Marshfield Epidemiologic Study Area (MESA) conducted in Wisconsin. In this study, the mean age of onset of PSVT was 57 years, and age of onset ranged from infancy to more than 90 years. Female patients were shown to have a twofold risk compared with their male counterparts in the MESA study.

Ventricular Tachycardias

VTs have a prevalence of about 20 per 100,000 persons in the general population and occur more commonly in men. An appreciable percentage (3.5%) of VTs occur after myocardial infarction (MI), and the incidence of post-MI VT increases with age.

Pathophysiology

All tachycardias are produced by one or more mechanisms that include disorders of impulse initiation (automaticity) and abnormalities of impulse conduction (reentrance). Tissues exhibiting abnormal automaticity that underlie SVT can reside in the atria, the AV junction, or vessels that communicate directly with the atria, such as the vena cava or pulmonary veins. Normally, the sinus node contains the dominant pacemaking function and is made of cells with faster rates of phase 4 diastolic depolarization (Figure 1). Cells with abnormal automaticity (enhanced diastolic phase 4 depolarization) can arise in other locations (ectopic foci), and if their firing rate exceeds that of the sinus node, then the ectopic focus becomes the predominant pacemaker of the heart.

Reentry is the most common mechanism by which SVT occurs. It is also the mechanism for atrial flutter, atrioventricular (AV) node reentry tachycardia (AVNRT), some atrial tachycardias, AV reciprocating tachycardia (AVRT), some VTs, and ventricular fibrillation (VF). Initiation and maintenance of a reentrant tachycardia requires a unidirectional block in one limb of the circuit and slow conduction in the other. A unidirectional block can result from acceleration of the heart rate or from a premature impulse that is blocked during the refractory period of the pathway.

As shown in Figure 1A, a normal impulse arriving at Π is propagated down both *a* and *b*. Conduction through pathway *a* is initially faster and unimpeded, while conduction through *b* is slow. A normal sinus beat is produced. A second impulse attempts

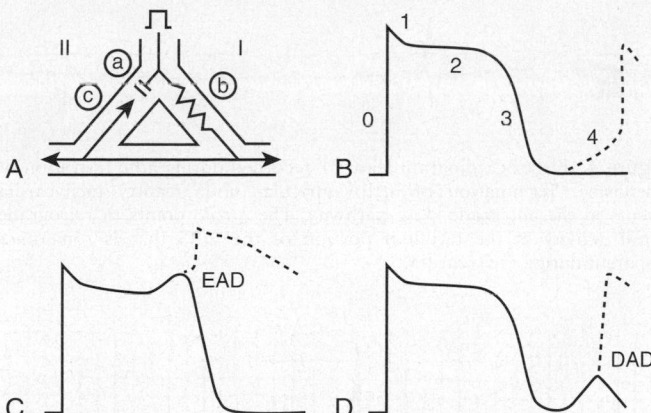

Figure 1. **A,** Diagram of reentry. The impulse is initiated at Π. I and II represent two distinct pathways. *a* represents unidirectional block, *b* represents slow conduction, and *c* shows the propagation of the wavefront reentering the circuit. **B,** A cardiac action potential. The different phases of the action potential are 0–4. Phase 4 demonstrates automaticity, which, when it reaches threshold, will initiate the next cardiac action potential. **C,** A cardiac action potential demonstrating early afterdepolarization (EAD) at the end of phase 2. **D,** A cardiac action potential demonstrating a delayed afterdepolarization (DAD) during phase 4.

to go down *a* and *b;* however, this time finds *a* refractory, and thus no conduction occurs (unidirectional block). Pathway *b,* which is slow conducting and has a shorter refractory period, conducts the impulse. This results in a premature supraventricular beat with a prolonged PR interval. The impulse through *b* may continue in a retrograde pathway *(c)* to *a,* and if *a* is past its refractory period a circuit is created through which the impulse can continue to circle, producing a persistent reentrant tachycardia.

Clinical Manifestations

Patients with paroxysmal arrhythmias are often asymptomatic on presentation. When symptoms are present, they can include palpitations, fatigue, lightheadedness, chest discomfort, dyspnea, presyncope, and syncope. Syncope is observed in about 15% of patients with SVT. Patients with ventricular arrhythmias more often present with presyncope, syncope, or even cardiac arrest. A history of syncope should warrant immediate referral to an electrophysiologist.

Diagnosis

History taking is useful in aiding in the diagnosis and definition of tachycardia. It is important for the clinician to assess whether or not the palpitations are regular or irregular, the number of episodes, possible triggers, and the nature of onset and termination (whether abrupt or gradual). Recurrent episodes with abrupt onset and termination are designated *paroxysmal.* Episodes with a gradual onset and termination are nonparoxysmal (e.g., sinus tachycardia). Irregular palpitations likely are due to premature depolarizations, suggesting atrial fibrillation or multifocal atrial tachycardia. Multifocal atrial tachycardia is often encountered in patients with pulmonary disease. Premature beats are often described by the patient as pauses followed by a sensation of a strong heart beat or as irregularities in heart rhythm.

On physical examination, if irregular cannon A waves are observed in the jugular vein or variation in the intensity of the S1 heart sound is heard, then a ventricular origin is strongly suggested. Termination of the tachycardia with vagal maneuvers strongly suggests a reentrant tachycardia involving AV nodal tissue such as AVNRT or AVRT.

A resting echocardiogram should be recorded. In the absence of symptoms this may be of low diagnostic yield. However, the presence of preexcitation (Figure 2) on the ECG suggests AVRT and is enough to make a presumptive diagnosis. Baseline ECG with

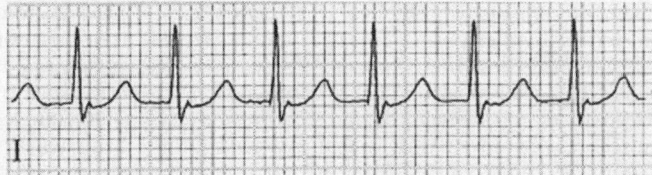

Figure 2. A 12-lead electrocardiogram depicting typical AV node reentry tachycardia. Note the absence of obvious atrial activity or P wave.

preexcitation in combination with a history consistent with paroxysmal palpitations strongly suggests episodic atrial fibrillation and is concerning. These patients are at risk for sudden cardiac death and require immediate electrophysiologic evaluation. Patients without concerning symptoms such as syncope or persistent regular tachycardia may be sent home with an event monitor, with follow-up at a later date. A 24-hour Holter monitor can be used in patients who report daily transient tachycardia. In patients with infrequent arrhythmias, a loop recorder is more useful. An implantable loop recorder may be used in patients who have rare episodes associated with hemodynamic instability.

Differential Diagnosis

Narrow QRS-Complex Tachycardia

Narrow QRS-complex (less than 120 msec) SVTs are differentiated according to the their mechanism and include sinus tachyarrhythmias, AVNRT, focal and nonparoxysmal junctional tachycardias, AVRT, focal atrial tachycardias, and macro-reentrant atrial tachycardia.

Wide QRS-Complex Tachycardia

Wide QRS-complex tachycardias may be supraventricular or ventricular in origin. Examples of wide QRS-complex SVTs include SVT with AV conduction via an accessory pathway, such as in Wolff–Parkinson–White (WPW) syndrome, or any SVT with aberrant conduction or ventricular pacing.

Specific Tachycardias

Supraventricular Tachycardias

Sinus Tachyarrhythmias

Sinus tachycardia can result from physiologic stimulation of the sinus node or sinus node reentry (sinus node reentry tachycardia). The latter results in paroxysmal nonsustained episodes of tachycardia. Normally, sinus tachycardia occurs as an appropriate response to physiologic stimulus such as exercise. Pathologic causes that can induce sinus tachycardia include hyperthyroidism, pyrexia, hypovolemia, infections, or anemia. Drugs that can cause sinus tachycardia include atropine, aminophylline, catecholamines, and anticancer treatments (such as doxorubicin [Adriamycin]). Stimulants such as caffeine, alcohol, and nicotine and recreational drugs such as cocaine, amphetamines, and ecstasy can induce sinus tachycardia. It can also result from an excessive stimulus such as hyperthyroidism. On ECG, a normal axis with upright P waves in I, II, and aVF and a negative P wave in aVR is revealed.

In addition to eliminating the underlying offensive agent such as excessive caffeine use or hyperthyroidism, β-blockers are very effective for terminating and suppressing sinus tachycardia. Nondihydropyridine calcium-channel blockers, such as diltiazem (Cardizem) or verapamil (Isoptin) may also be used. Vagal maneuvers, adenosine (Adenocard), β-blockers, and nondihydropyridine calcium-channel blockers are effective in treating reentry sinus tachycardia. In rare cases where inappropriate sinus tachycardia is refractory, catheter ablation may be performed.

Atrioventricular Nodal Reciprocating Tachycardia

AVNRT is the most common form of PSVT, and it produces rates of tachycardia between 140 and 250 beats per minute. It is more prevalent in female patients. Patients typically report associated palpitations, dizziness, and neck pulsations.

The mechanism of AVNRT is a reentry circuit that is now known to involve perinodal atrial tissue as well, and it is not always confined to the compact AV node as previously believed. In AVNRT, reciprocation occurs between two distinct pathways: The first, fast pathway, is located near the apex of Koch's triangle; the second is a slow pathway that extends from the compact AV-node tissue and stretches along the septal margin of the tricuspid annulus at the level of, or slightly superior to, the coronary sinus. The fast pathway conducts rapidly with a slow recovery time and a longer refractory period, and the second pathway conducts slowly with a short refractory period. AVNRT is initiated when a premature impulse finds the fast pathway refractory and is thus conducted anterogradely through the slow pathway. The impulse continues past the AV node, down the His–Purkinje system, activates the ventricles, and approaches the His bundle. Here, the impulse finds the fast pathway in recovery. The fast pathway then serves as a retrograde pathway for conduction back to the atria (Figure 3). This produces a P wave during or very close to the QRS complex, often with a pseudo-R′ in V1.

Rarely, an atypical AVNRT occurs in which there is anterograde conduction through the fast pathway and retrograde conduction through the slow pathway, producing a long R-P tachycardia. The P wave, negative in III and aVF, is inscribed prior to the QRS. Sometimes, though infrequently, the circuit is composed of slowly conducting tissues in both limbs of the circuit, resulting in a P wave inscribed after the QRS (a retrograde P wave) (Figure 4).

Adenosine 6 mg IV push is administered to terminate the rhythm, and if the initial dose is unsuccessful, two more doses of 12 mg of adenosine may be administered. Adenosine has a half-life of only 9 seconds, and it terminates the circuit by causing transient block in AVN conduction. Long-term therapy with a β-blocker or calcium channel blocker can prevent recurrence. If AVN is recurrent, radiofrequency ablation is the treatment of choice and has a low risk of complication.

Atrioventricular Reciprocating Tachycardia (Extranodal Accessory Pathways)

An accessory pathway is a pathway outside the AV node that connects the myocardium of the atrium and the ventricle. Accessory pathways may be located across the mitral or tricuspid annulus and may be capable of anterograde or retrograde conduction, or both. Accessory pathways that conduct in a retrograde function are referred to as "concealed" because they do not reveal preexcitation on ECG. Those capable of anterograde conduction are referred to as "manifest." WPW syndrome is diagnosed if the patient has both preexcitation on ECG and tachyarrhythmias (Figure 5). AVRT may be orthodromic or antidromic. Orthodromic AVRT occurs when there is anterograde conduction down the AV node and

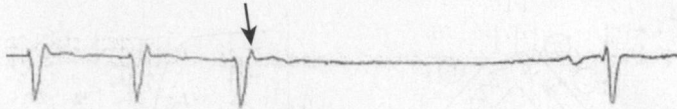

Figure 4. Electrocardiogram lead V1 recorded during administration of adenosine. Termination of atrioventricular node reentry tachycardia occurs in the antegrade slow pathway. The *arrow* points to retrograde atrial activity at the terminal portion of the QRS that is sometimes apparent during tachycardia.

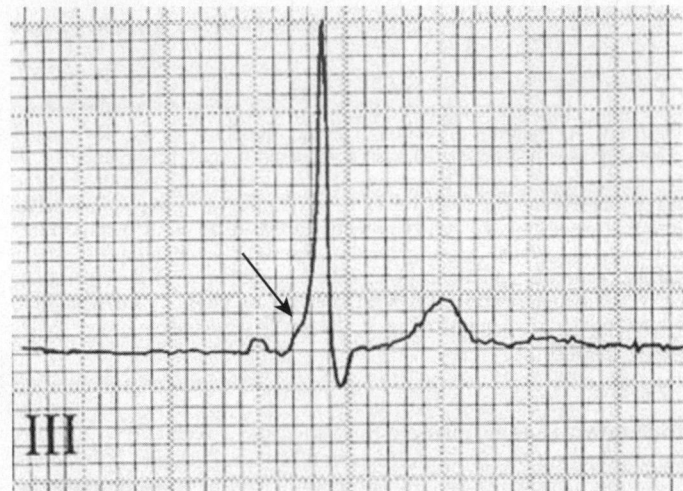

Figure 5. Electrocardiogram lead III recording of a QRS demonstrating ventricular preexcitation *(arrow)*, also called Wolff–Parkinson–White pattern.

retrograde conduction up the accessory pathway (Figure 6). In antidromic AVRT the reverse occurs.

Atrial fibrillation is considered life-threatening in patients with WPW syndrome. This is because rapid repetitive conduction can occur via the accessory pathway (which has a short refractory period), resulting in a rapid ventricular rate that can degenerate into VF.

Administration of adenosine can precipitate atrial fibrillation in 10% to 15% of patients with an extranodal accessory pathway. Therefore, if it is unknown whether or not the patient has an anterogradely conducting accessory pathway, it is good practice to have a defibrillator present at the bedside during administration of adenosine. For patients with known WPW syndrome (or delta

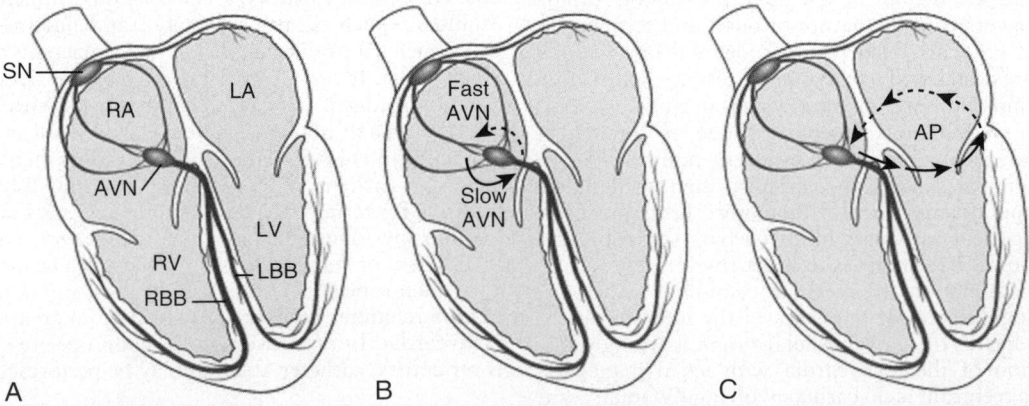

Figure 3. **A,** Normal conduction system. *Abbreviations:* AVN = atrioventricular node; LA = left atrium; LBB = left bundle branch; LV = left ventricle; RA = right atrium; RBB, right bundle branch; RV = right ventricle; SN, sinus node. **B,** Diagram of heart depicting typical atrioventricular node reentry tachycardia (AVNRT) with antegrade conduction via the slow AVN and retrograde conduction via the fast AVN. **C,** Diagram of the heart depicting orthodromic atrioventricular reciprocating tachycardia (o-AVRT), with antegrade conduction via the AVN and retrograde conduction via the accessory pathway (AP).

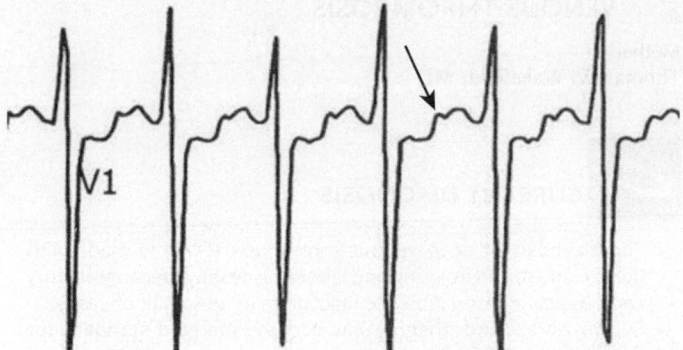

Figure 6. A 12-lead electrocardiogram depicting orthodromic atrioventricular reciprocating tachycardia. The *arrow* highlights the atrial activity, which is occurring well after the QRS complex.

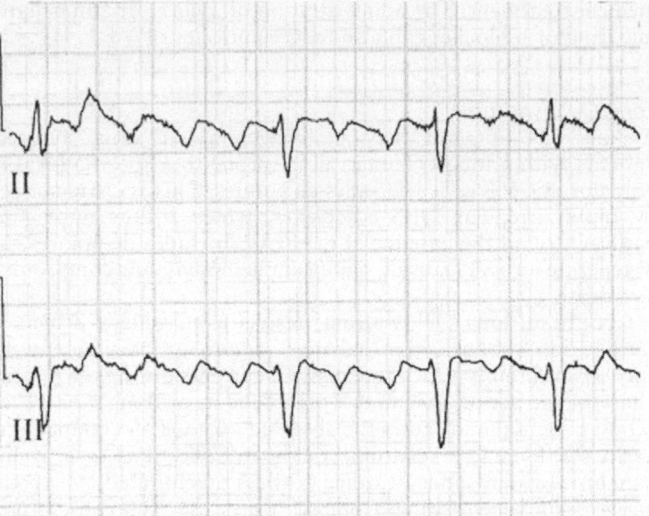

Figure 7. Electrocardiogram of leads II and III depicting typical atrial flutter. Note the sawtooth atrial activity.

wave on baseline ECG), procainamide (Pronestyl)[1] or ibutilide (Corvert), drugs that slow conduction over the accessory pathway, can be administered instead of adenosine.

Focal and Nonparoxysmal Junctional Tachycardia
Focal Junctional Tachycardia
Focal junctional tachycardia is a generally rare phenomenon that can occur by automaticity or reentry mechanisms. By definition, focal junctional tachycardia originates from the AV node or His bundle. On ECG, focal junctional tachycardia may be varied in its features. It often has a rate of 110 to 250 beats/min, with narrow QRS complexes or a bundle branch block (BBB) conduction pattern. AV dissociation often occurs. However, one-to-one retrograde conduction can also occur. Focal junctional tachycardia often occurs in young adulthood and is precipitated by exercise or stress. Patients might respond to β-blockers or flecainide (Tambocor) (which may be administered IV initially to terminate the tachycardia, followed by an oral dose), but drug therapy is not always effective. Catheter ablation is most effective and can be curative, though there is a 5% to 10% risk of AV block.

Nonparoxysmal Junctional Tachycardia
Nonparoxysmal junctional tachycardia is a benign arrythmia that his characterized by narrow QRS complexes at a rate of 70 to 120 beats/min. It occurs via automaticity and can indicate serious underlying pathology such as digitalis toxicity, hypokalemia, hypoxia, or myocardial ischemia. It is treated by correcting the underlying abnormality.

Focal Atrial Tachycardias
Focal atrial tachycardias are usually benign unless they are persistent, when they can cause tachycardia-induced cardiomyopathy. They usually manifest with rates between 100 and 250 beats/min, rarely getting up to 300 beats/min. The mechanism is thought to be via automaticity, and the majority originate along the crista terminalis from the SA node to the AV node. Recommended initial therapy is with calcium channel blockers or β-blockers. If these are unsuccessful, flecainide or propafenone (Rythmol) may be added. If the tachycardia is refractory to drug therapy, catheter ablation may be performed; it had a success rate of up to 86% in one study. Though inadvertent, AV node blockage is of concern.

Multifocal Atrial Tachycardia
Multifocal atrial tachycardia is exemplified by ECG findings of an irregular tachycardia with three or more different P-wave morphologies at different rates. It is commonly associated with underlying pulmonary disease or electrolyte abnormalities. Calcium

channel blockers are a highly successful form of treatment. There is no role for direct-current cardioversion, antiarrythmic drugs, or ablation.

Macro-Reentrant Atrial Tachycardia (Atrial Flutter)
Atrial flutter, also known as macro-reentrant atrial tachycardia, is characterized by an organized atrial rhythm at a rate between 250 and 350 beats/min and occurs via a reentry mechanism. Typical atrial flutter is sometimes called isthmus-dependent flutter (Figure 7), so named because it involves the cavotricuspid isthmus. Patients typically present with a 2:1 AV conduction block producing a ventricular rate of about 150 beats/min. Patients can also present with a variable AV block producing an irregular rhythm. Acute management focuses on ventricular rate control using AVN blocking agents such as β-blockers or calcium channel blockers. Rapid atrial overdrive pacing can also terminate the arrhythmia. Direct current cardioversion is also a very effective mode of therapy for patients who present with hemodynamic collapse. An energy level of 50 J is typically effective. In patients with atrial flutter for more than 48 hours, anticoagulant therapy should be started and an echocardiogram should be obtained to rule out the presence of a intracardiac clot before cardioversion. Anticoagulation is usually achieved with warfarin (Coumadin), with an international normalized ratio (INR) goal of 2 to 3.

Cure of atrial flutter can be achieved with radiofrequency ablation in more than 98% of patients. The macroreentrant circuit in atrial flutter uses the atrial tissue between the tricuspid valve annulus and the inferior vena cava, and radiofrequency energy delivered across the cavotricuspid isthmus prevents atrial flutter from recurring. Radiofrequency ablation is the treatment of choice for patients with recurrent atrial flutter.

Ventricular Tachycardias
Three broad categories of pathologies contribute to the development of VT: structural heart diseases, prolonged QT syndrome, and accelerated idioventricular rhythm.

Structural Heart Disease
VT in patients with structural heart disease is secondary to reentry and is a result of fibrotic tissue or infiltrative disease causing areas of slow conduction. Common causes of structural heart disease include ischemia, congestive heart failure, and infiltrative heart disease (e.g., sarcoidosis, amyloidosis, and Chagas' disease). The mainstay of treatment is implantation of an implantable cardioverter-defibrillator (ICD) to prevent sudden death from VT or VF. An ICD is indicated in congestive heart failure patients with an ejection fraction less than 35% that is refractory to

---

[1]Not FDA approved for this indication.

medical treatment. The administration of a class III antiarrhythmic drug or β-blocker can also reduce episodes of VT.

Long-QT Syndrome

A long QT interval may be congenital or drug induced. Patients with a long QT interval are prone to a specific form of polymorphic VT called torsades de pointes. This is characterized by rapid, irregular QRS complexes, which follow a twisting pattern around the baseline of the ECG. Torsades de pointes can degenerate into VF, causing significant hemodynamic compromise and death.

Congenital long QT syndrome results from genetic defects in cardiac ion channels that enhance sodium or calcium inward currents or inhibit outward potassium currents during the plateau phase of the action potential. This results in prolongation of the action potential and causes the observed long QT. A common scenario for long QT syndrome on board questions is a young patient in whom sudden cardiac death is precipitated by exercising, especially swimming. Common drugs that can cause a prolonged QT include class Ia, Ic, or III antiarrythmic agents, tricyclic antidepressants, phenothiazines, and certain antivirals and antifungals. Torsades de pointes is usually treated with unsynchronized direct-current cardioversion and sometimes defibrillation.

Accelerated Idioventricular Rhythm

Accelerated idioventricular rhythm usually has a heart rate that ranges from 60 to 120 beats per minute. It is characterized by gradual onset and offset. It is typically self-limiting and brief in duration. It is often encountered in the setting of cocaine intoxication, acute myocarditis, and digoxin intoxication and following cardiac surgery.

References

Blomström-Lundqvist C, Scheinman MM, Aliot EM, et al. European Society of Cardiology Committee, NASPE-Heart Rhythm Society. ACC/AHA/ESC guidelines for the management of patients with supraventricular arrhythmias–executive summary. a report of the American College of Cardiology/American Heart Association Task Force on Practice Guidelines and the European Society of Cardiology Committee for Practice Guidelines (writing committee to develop guidelines for the management of patients with supraventricular arrhythmias) developed in collaboration with NASPE-Heart Rhythm Society. J Am Coll Cardiol 2003;42:1493–531.

Cheung DW. Pulmonary vein as an ectopic focus in digitalis-induced arrhythmia. Nature 1981;294:582–4.

Delacretaz E. Supraventricular tachycardia. N Eng J Med 2006;354:1039–51.

Epstein AE, Dimarco JP, Ellenbogen KA, et al. American College of Cardiology/American Heart Association Task Force on Practice; American Association for Thoracic Surgery; Society of Thoracic Surgeons. ACC/AHA/HRS 2008 guidelines for device-based therapy of cardiac rhythm abnormalities: executive summary. Heart Rhythm 2008;5:934–55.

Haqqani HM, Morton JB, Kalman J. Using the 12-lead ECG to localize the origin of atrial and ventricular tachycardias. Part 2: Ventricular tachycardia. J Cardiovasc Electrophysiol 2009;20:825–32.

Luchsinger JA, Steinberg JS. Resolution of cardiomyopathy after ablation of atrial flutter. J Am Coll Cardiol 1998;32:205–10.

Monteforte N, Priori S. The long QT syndrome and catecholaminergic polymorphic ventricular tachycardia. Pacing Clin Electrophysiol 2009;32:S52–S57.

Orejarena LA, Vidaillet Jr H, DeStefano F, et al. Paroxysmal supraventricular tachycardia in the general population. J Am Coll Cardiol 1998;31:150–7.

Pappone C, Santinelli V, Manguso F, et al. A randomized study of prophylactic catheter ablation in asymptomatic patients with the Wolff–Parkinson–White syndrome. N Eng J Med 2003;349:1803–11.

Teh AW, Kistler PM, Kalman JM. Using the 12-lead ECG to localize the origin of ventricular and atrial tachycardias. Part I: Focal atrial tachycardia. J Cardiovasc Electrophysiol 2009;20:706–9.

Vereckei A, Duray G, Szénási G, et al. Application of a new algorithm in the differential diagnosis of a wide QRS complex tachycardia. Eur Heart J 2007;28:589–600.

Zipes DP, Camm AJ, Borggrefe M, et al. European Heart Rhythm Association; Heart Rhythm Society; American College of Cardiology; American Heart Association Task Force; European Society of Cardiology Committee for Practice Guidelines. ACC/AHA/ESC 2006 guidelines for management of patients with ventricular arrhythmias and the prevention of sudden cardiac death: A report of the American College of Cardiology/American Heart Association Task Force and the European Society of Cardiology Committee for Practice Guidelines (Writing Committee to Develop Guidelines for Management of Patients with Ventricular Arrhythmias and the Prevention of Sudden Cardiac Death). J Am Coll Cardiol 2006;48:e247–e346.

VENOUS THROMBOSIS

Method of
Thomas W. Wakefield, MD

CURRENT DIAGNOSIS

- The diagnosis of deep venous thrombosis (DVT) is made with duplex ultrasound imaging and laboratory testing, because history and physical examination are inaccurate in up to half of cases.
- Duplex ultrasound imaging has become the gold standard for the diagnosis of DVT.
- Spiral computed tomographic (CT) scanning is preferred as the initial imaging test to establish the diagnosis of pulmonary embolus, replacing ventilation/perfusion scanning ($\dot{V}/\dot{Q}$).
- Although clinical assessment and D-dimer levels are useful to rule out thrombosis, there is no combination of clinical findings and biomarker testing at this time that can rule in the diagnosis.

CURRENT THERAPY

- Initial therapy includes low-molecular-weight heparin (LMWH), compression garments, and ambulation once anticoagulation is therapeutic.
- LMWH should be administered for at least 5 days, during which time an oral anticoagulant (usually warfarin) is begun. Warfarin should be started after heparinization is therapeutic to prevent warfarin-induced skin necrosis. Therapeutic heparinization with LMWH means an appropriate weight-based dose is administered and allowed to circulate. The international normalized ratio (INR) should be therapeutic for 2 consecutive days before stopping LMWH.
- The goal for warfarin dosing is an INR between 2.0 and 3.0.
- The duration of anticoagulation depends on a number of factors, including the presence of risk factors for thrombosis, the type of thrombosis (idiopathic or provoked), the number of times thrombosis has occurred, venous patency, and the level of D-dimer measured approximately 1 month after stopping warfarin.
- Significant iliofemoral deep venous thrombosis should be treated with aggressive pharmocomechanical thrombolysis, and pulmonary embolism causing hemodynamic deterioration or right heart strain should be treated with thrombolysis.

Epidemiology

Venous thromboembolism (VTE) includes deep venous thrombosis (DVT) and pulmonary embolism (PE). VTE affects up to 900,000 patients per year and results in 300,000 deaths per year. The incidence has remained constant and may actually be increasing since the 1980s and increases with age.

Risk Factors

Risk factors for VTE include acquired and genetic factors. Acquired factors include increasing age, malignancy, surgery, immobilization, trauma, oral contraceptives and hormone replacement therapy, pregnancy and the puerperium, neurologic disease, cardiac disease, obesity, and antiphospholipid antibodies. Genetic factors include antithrombin deficiency, protein C deficiency and protein S deficiency, factor V Leiden, prothrombin 20210A, blood group non-O, abnormalities in fibrinogen and plasminogen, elevated levels of clotting factors (e.g., factors XI, IX, VII, VIII, X, and II), and elevation in plasminogen activator inhibitor-1 (PAI-1). When a patient presents with an idiopathic VTE, family history of thrombosis, recurrent thrombosis, or thrombosis in unusual locations, a work-up for hypercoagulability, including testing for the conditions noted in the previous sentence, may be indicated. Hematologic diseases associated with VTE include heparin-induced thrombocytopenia and thrombosis syndrome (HITTS), disseminated intravascular coagulation (DIC), antiphospholipid antibody syndrome, myeloproliferative disorders, thrombotic thrombocytopenic purpura (TTP), and hemolytic uremic syndrome (HUS).

Pathophysiology

Although Virchow's triad of stasis, vein injury, and hypercoagulability has defined the events that predispose to DVT formation since the mid-19th century, the understanding today of events that occur at the level of the vein wall and thrombus, including the inflammatory response on thrombogenesis, is increasingly becoming appreciated.

Diagnosis

Deep Venous Thrombosis

The diagnosis of DVT must be made with duplex ultrasound imaging and laboratory testing, because history and physical examination is inaccurate in up to half the cases. Patients often complain of a dull ache or pain in the calf or leg. Wells has classified patients into a scoring system that emphasizes physical presentation, and the most common physical finding is edema. Characteristics that score points in the Wells system include active cancer, paralysis or paresis, recent plaster immobilization of the lower extremity, being recently bedridden for 3 days or more, localized tenderness along the distribution of the deep venous system, swelling of the entire leg, calf swelling that is at least 3 cm larger on the involved side than on the noninvolved side, pitting edema in the symptomatic leg, collateral superficial veins (nonvaricose), and a history of previous DVT. With extensive proximal iliofemoral DVT there may be significant swelling, cyanosis, and dilated superficial collateral veins.

Massive iliofemoral DVT can result in phlegmasia alba dolens (white swollen leg) or phlegmasia cerulean dolens (blue swollen leg). If phlegmasia is not aggressively treated, it can lead to venous gangrene when the arterial inflow becomes obstructed owing to venous hypertension. Alternatively, arterial emboli or spasm can occur and contribute to the pathophysiology. Venous gangrene is often associated with underlying malignancy and is always preceded by phlegmasia cerulea dolens. Venous gangrene is associated with significant rates of amputation and pulmonary embolism and with mortality.

Duplex ultrasound imaging has become the gold standard for the diagnosis of DVT. Duplex imaging includes both a B-mode image and Doppler flow pattern. Duplex imaging demonstrates sensitivity and specificity rates greater than 95%. According to the Grade criteria for the strength of medical evidence, duplex ultrasound is given a 1B level of evidence, depending on the pretest probability for DVT. Even at the level of the calf, duplex is an acceptable technique in symptomatic patients. Duplex imaging is painless, requires no contrast, can be repeated, and is safe during pregnancy. Duplex imaging also identifies other causes of a patient's symptoms. Other tests available for making the diagnosis include magnetic resonance imaging (MRI) (especially good for assessing central pelvic vein and inferior vena cava [IVC] thrombosis) and spiral computed tomographic (CT) scanning (especially with chest imaging during examination for PE).

A single complete negative duplex scan is accurate enough to withhold anticoagulation with minimal long-term adverse thromboembolic complications. This requires that all venous segments of the leg have been imaged and evaluated. If the duplex scan is indeterminate owing to technical issues or to edema, treatment may be based on factors such as biomarkers, with the duplex repeated in 24 to 72 hours. Combining clinical characteristics with a D-dimer assay can decrease the number of duplex scans performed. Although clinical characteristics and D-dimer levels are useful to rule out thrombosis, the converse is not true and there is no combination of biomarkers and clinical presentation that

can rule in the diagnosis. Work is ongoing to establish new biomarkers based on the inflammatory response to DVT. We have data suggesting that a combination of soluble P-selectin and the Wells score can rule in the diagnosis of DVT, while D-dimer plus Wells is still the best combination to rule out the diagnosis of DVT.

Conditions that may be confused with DVT include lymphedema, muscle strain, and muscle contusion and systemic problems such as cardiac, renal, or hepatic abnormalities. These systemic problems usually lead to bilateral edema.

Pulmonary Embolism

The diagnosis of PE historically has involved ventilation-perfusion $(\dot{V}/\dot{Q})$ scanning and pulmonary angiography. However, the most current techniques include spiral CT scanning and MRI. CT scanning demonstrates excellent specificity and sensitivity. Emboli down to the subsegmental level can be identified. The sensitivity for isolated chest CT imaging is increased when clinical analysis is added and when adding lower extremity imaging to the chest scan. Results from the PIOPED II study demonstrate that if the clinical presentation and spiral CT scan results are concordant, therapies can be safely recommended. However, if clinical presentation and spiral CT scanning are discordant, other confirmatory tests are necessary. For the diagnosis of PE, spiral CT imaging is given a 1A level of evidence. Useful alternate techniques include MRI and VQ imaging.

Axillary and Subclavian Vein Thrombosis

Thrombosis of the axillary and subclavian veins accounts for less than 5% of all cases of DVT. However, it may be associated with PE in up to 10% to 15% of cases and can be the source of significant disability. Upper extremity DVT may be primary (approximately 20%), such as from thoracic outlet syndrome, effort thrombosis, or idiopathic; or secondary (approximately 80%), such as from catheter-related, cancer-associated, surgery-related, or pregnancy-related events. Primary axillary and subclavian vein thrombosis results from obstruction of the axillary vein in the thoracic outlet from compression by the subclavius muscle and the costoclavicular space, the Paget-Schrötter syndrome, noted especially in muscular athletes. Secondary axillary and subclavian vein thrombosis results from mediastinal tumors, congestive heart failure, and nephrotic syndrome. Patients with axillary and subclavian vein thrombosis present with arm pain, edema, and cyanosis. Superficial venous distention may be apparent over the arm, forearm, shoulder, and anterior chest wall.

Upper extremity venous duplex ultrasound is used to make the diagnosis of axillary and subclavian vein thrombosis. Thrombolysis and phlebography are considered as next interventions. If phlebography is performed, it is important that the patient undergo positional phlebography with arm abducted to 120 degrees to confirm extrinsic subclavian vein compression at the thoracic outlet once the vein has been cleared of thrombus. Because a cervical rib may be the cause of such obstruction, chest x-ray should be obtained to exclude its presence (although its incidence is quite low).

Treatment

Standard Therapy for Venous Thromboembolism

The traditional treatment of VTE is systemic anticoagulation, which reduces the risk of PE, extension of thrombosis, and thrombus recurrence. Because the recurrence rate for VTE is higher if anticoagulation is not therapeutic in the first 24 hours, immediate anticoagulation should be undertaken. For PE, this usually means anticoagulation and then testing. For DVT, since duplex imaging is rapidly obtained, usually testing precedes anticoagulation. Recurrent DVT can still occur in up to one third of patients over an 8-year period, even with appropriate anticoagulant therapy.

Heparin

Unfractionated heparin or low-molecular-weight heparin (LMWH) is given for 5 days, during which time oral anticoagulation with vitamin K antagonists (usually warfarin) is begun as soon as anticoagulation is therapeutic. It is recommended that the international normalized ratio (INR) be therapeutic for 2 consecutive days before stopping heparin or LMWH.

LMWH, derived from the lower molecular weight range of standard heparin, has become the standard for initial treatment. LMWH is preferred because it is administered subcutaneously, it requires no monitoring (except in certain circumstances such as renal insufficiency or morbid obesity), and it is associated with a lower bleeding potential. Additionally, LMWH demonstrates less direct thrombin inhibition and more factor Xa inhibition. Compared to standard unfractionated heparin, LMWH has significantly improved bioavailability, less endothelial cell binding and protein binding, and an improved pharmacokinetic profile. The half-life of LMWH is dose independent. LMWH is administered in a weight-based fashion.

Use of LMWH in outpatient settings usually requires a coordinated effort of multiple health care providers. Certain LMWHs decrease indices of chronic venous insufficiency compared to standard therapy when used over an extended period. This suggests that there are pleotropic effects of the LMWH or that more consistent anticoagulation is accomplished.

Based on all of the available evidence, LMWH is now preferred over standard unfractionated heparin for the initial treatment of VTE with a level of evidence given 2B (according to the 2012 Chest consensus guidelines).

Warfarin

Warfarin (Coumadin) should be started after heparinization is therapeutic to prevent warfarin-induced skin necrosis. For standard unfractionated heparin, this requires a therapeutic activated partial thromboplastin time (aPTT); for LMWH, warfarin is administered after an appropriate weight-based dose of LMWH is administered and allowed to circulate. Warfarin causes inhibition of protein C and S before factors II, IX and X, leading to paradoxical hypercoagulability at the initiation of therapy. The goal for warfarin dosing is an INR between 2.0 and 3.0. The duration of anticoagulation depends on a number of factors, including the presence of continuing risk factors for thrombosis, the type of thrombosis (idiopathic or provoked), the number of times thrombosis has occurred, the status of the veins when stopping anticoagulation, and the level of D-dimer measured approximately 1 month after stopping warfarin. One study demonstrated a statistically significant advantage to resuming warfarin over an average 1.4-year follow-up (odds ratio [OR], 4.26; $P = 0.02$) if the D-dimer is elevated, and a meta-analysis has confirmed this relationship.

Duration of Treatment

The recommended duration of anticoagulation after a first episode of VTE is 3 months for both proximal and distal thrombi. After a second episode of VTE, the usual recommendation is prolonged oral anticoagulation unless the patient is very young at the time of presentation or there are other mitigating factors. VTE recurrence is increased with homozygous factor V Leiden and prothrombin 20210A mutation, protein C or protein S deficiency, antithrombin deficiency, antiphospholipid antibodies, and cancer until resolved. Long-term oral anticoagulation is usually recommended in these situations. However, heterozygous factor V Leiden and prothrombin 20210A do not carry the same risk as their homozygous counterparts, and the length of oral anticoagulation is shortened for these conditions.

Regarding idiopathic DVT, in those with a low bleeding risk, the recommended length of treatment is extended therapy for more than 3 months. One multicenter trial suggested that low-dose warfarin (INR 1.5–2.0) is superior to placebo, with a 64% risk reduction for recurrent DVT after the completion of an initial 6 months of standard therapy. A second study then suggested that full-dose warfarin (INR 2–3) is superior to low-dose warfarin in these patients without a difference in bleeding. Taken together, criteria for discontinuing anticoagulation, including

thrombosis risk, residual thrombus burden, and coagulation system activation, are given a level of evidence of 1B to 2B, depending on the clinical situation. In addition, there is growing evidence that in certain circumstances, such as active cancer, the use of LMWH is superior to LMWH converted to warfarin for long-term treatment.

Complications

Bleeding is the most common complication of anticoagulation. With standard heparin, bleeding occurs over the first 5 days in approximately 10% of patients.

Another complication is heparin-induced thrombocytopenia (HIT), which occurs in 0.6% to 30% of patients. Although historically morbidity and mortality has been high, it has been found that early diagnosis and appropriate treatment have decreased these rates. HIT usually begins 3 to 14 days after heparin is begun, although it can occur earlier if the patient has been exposed to heparin in the past. A heparin-dependent antibody binds to platelets, activates them with the release of procoagulant microparticles leading to an increase in thrombocytopenia, and results in both arterial and venous thrombosis.

Both bovine and porcine unfractionated heparin and LMWH have been associated with HIT, although the incidence and severity of the thrombosis is less with LMWH. Even small exposures to heparin, such as heparin coating on indwelling catheters, can cause the syndrome. The diagnosis should be suspected with a 50% or greater drop in platelet count, when the platelet count falls below 100,000/μL, or when thrombosis occurs during heparin or LMWH therapy.

The enzyme-linked immunosorbent assay (ELISA) detects the antiheparin antibody in the plasma. This test is highly sensitive but poorly specific. The serotonin release assay is another test that can be used, and this test is more specific but less sensitive than the ELISA test.

When the diagnosis is made, heparin must be stopped. Warfarin should not be given until an adequate alternative anticoagulant has been established and until the platelet count has normalized. Because LMWHs demonstrate high cross-reactivity with standard heparin antibodies, they cannot be substituted for standard heparin in patients with HIT. Agents that have been FDA approved as alternatives include the direct thrombin inhibitor argatroban. Fondaparinux (Arixtra)[1] has also been found effective for treatment of HIT in most cases, but it is not FDA approved for this indication. The use of these alternative agents is given either a 2C and 1C level of evidence.

Alternative and Future Medical Treatments for Deep Venous Thrombosis and Pulmonary Embolism

New agents for venous thrombosis treatment include factor Xa inhibitors and direct thrombin inhibitors.

Fondaparinux (Arixtra) a synthetic pentasaccharide that has an antithrombin sequence identical to heparin, targets factor Xa. Fondaparinux has been approved for the treatment of DVT and PE; for thrombosis prophylaxis in patient with total hip replacement, total knee replacement, and hip fracture; in extended prophylaxis in patients with hip fracture; and in patients undergoing abdominal surgery. It is administered subcutaneously and has a 17-hour half-life. Dosage is based on body weight. It exhibits no endothelial or protein binding and does not produce thrombocytopenia. However, no antidote is readily available. In a meta-analysis involving more than 7000 patients, there was more than a 50% risk reduction using fondaparinux as prophylaxis begun 6 hours after surgery compared to LMWH begun 12 to 24 hours after surgery. Major bleeding was increased, but critical bleeding was not. Fondaparinux has also been found effective in prophylaxis of other groups of patients including general medical patients.[1] For the treatment of VTE, fondaparinux was

---

[1]Not FDA approved for this indication.

found equal to LMWH for DVT, and for PE, it was found equal to standard heparin.

Dabigatran targets activated factor II (factor IIa), whereas rivaroxaban, apixaban, and edoxaban target activated factor X (factor Xa). Dabigatran etexilate (Pradaxa) is FDA approved for stroke and systemic embolization prevention in patients with atrial fibrillation and for treating DVT and PE in patients who have been treated with a parenteral anticoagulant for 5–10 days. Rivaroxaban (Xarelto) is FDA approved for VTE prophylaxis in patients undergoing hip or knee replacements, for stroke and systemic embolization prevention in patients with atrial fibrillation, and for VTE treatment. The Einstein trial evaluated rivaroxaban compared to standard anticoagulation in the treatment of acute DVT. As monotherapy, rivaroxaban was found statistically noninferior to standard therapy, without increased bleeding. Additionally, the Einstein group added a continued treatment group compared to placebo for an additional 6 to 12 months. Extended rivaroxaban showed a significant decrease in recurrent VTE without a significant increase in major bleeding. A similar finding with PE has been noted. Apixaban (Eliquis) is currently FDA approved for the prevention of complications of atrial fibrillation, for prophylaxis of DVT following hip or knee replacement surgery, for the treatment of DVT/PE, and for the reduction in risk of recurrence of DVT/PE. Recently, apixaban as extended treatment of VTE was investigated. After initial treatment, an additional 12 months of apixaban therapy was compared to placebo. This study revealed a significant decrease in the rate of VTE without an increase in bleeding risk. Finally, edoxaban (Savaysa) has been approved for prevention of stroke and non-central-nervous system (CNS) systemic embolism in patients with nonvalvular atrial fibrillation and for treating DVT and PE in patients who have been treated with a parenteral anticoagulant for 5 to 10 days. Problems with these new agents include the inability at the present time to reliably reverse their anticoagulant effects and the fact that little data are available on bridging of these agents when other procedures need to be performed.

Nonpharmacologic Treatments

The rate and severity of postthrombotic syndrome after proximal DVT can be decreased by approximately 50% by the use of compression stockings. This measure is often forgotten by clinicians. Discussion with the patient on its importance is also critical to ensure good compliance. Additionally, walking with good compression does not increase the risk of PE, whereas it significantly decreases the incidence and severity of the postthrombotic syndrome. The use of strong compression and early ambulation after DVT treatment can significantly reduce the pain and swelling resulting from the DVT and carries a 1A level of evidence. However, a recent multicenter randomized trial has suggested that stockings do not prevent postthrombotic syndrome after a first proximal DVT. However, new evidence is calling into question the effectiveness of compression stockings and future data is necessary.

Aggressive Therapies for Venous Thromboembolism

For DVT treatment, the goals are to prevent extension or recurrence of DVT, prevent pulmonary embolism, and minimize the late squeal of thrombosis, namely chronic venous insufficiency. Standard anticoagulants accomplish the first two goals but not the third goal. The postthrombotic syndrome (venous insufficiency related to venous thrombosis) occurs in up to 30% of patients after DVT and in an even higher percentage of patients with iliofemoral level DVT. The following evidence suggests more aggressive therapies for extensive thrombosis are indicated.

Experimentally, prolonged contact of the thrombus with the vein wall increases damage. The thrombus initiates an inflammatory response in the vein wall that can lead to vein wall fibrosis and valvular dysfunction. Thus, removing the thrombus should be an excellent solution to decrease this interaction. For example, the longer a thrombus is in contact with a vein valve, the more chance that valve will no longer function.

Venous thrombectomy has proved superior to anticoagulation over 6 months to 10 years as measured by venous patency and prevention of venous reflux. Catheter-directed thrombolysis has been employed in many nonrandomized studies and in small, randomized trials was more effective than standard therapy. Quality of life was improved with thrombus removal, and results appear to be optimized further by combining catheter-directed thrombolysis with mechanical devices. These devices include, but are not limited to, the Trellis balloon occlusion catheter, the Angiojet rheolytic catheter, the EKOS ultrasound accelerated catheter, and new larger bore extraction devices. With these devices, thrombolysis is hastened, the amount of thrombolytic agent is decreased, and bleeding is thus decreased.

Additionally, the use of venous stents for iliac venous obstruction has been shown to decease the incidence of postthrombotic syndrome and chronic venous insufficiency. To more fully elucidate the role of aggressive therapy in proximal iliofemoral venous thrombosis, a study has been approved by the National Institutes of Health (NIH) to compare catheter-directed pharmacomechanical thrombolysis to standard anticoagulation for significant iliofemoral venous thrombosis. This study, the Attract Trial, will evaluate anatomic, physiologic, and quality-of-life endpoints.

For pulmonary embolism, evidence exists that thrombolysis is indicated when there is hemodynamic compromise from the embolism. It is controversial if thrombolysis should be used in situations in which there is no hemodynamic compromise but there is evidence of right heart dysfunction or there are positive biomarkers.

Inferior Vena Cava Filters

Traditional indications for the use of IVC filters include failure of anticoagulation, a contraindication to anticoagulation, or a complication of anticoagulation. Protection from pulmonary embolism is greater than 95% using cone-shaped, wire-based permanent filters in the IVC. With the success of these filters, indications have expanded to the presence of free-floating thrombus tails, prophylactic use when the risk for anticoagulation is excessive, when the risk of pulmonary embolism is thought to be high, and to allow the use of perioperative epidural anesthesia.

IVC filters can be either permanent or optional (retrievable). If a retrievable filter is left, then it becomes a permanent filter; the long-term fate of these filters has yet to be defined adequately in the literature. Most filters are placed in the infrarenal location in the IVC. However, they may be placed in the suprarenal position or in the superior vena cava.

Indications for suprarenal placement include high-lying thrombi, pregnancy or childbearing age, or previous device failure filled with thrombus. Although some have suggested that sepsis is a contraindication to the use of filters, sepsis has not been found to be a contraindication because the trapped material can be sterilized with intravenous antibiotics.

Filters may be inserted under x-ray guidance or using ultrasound techniques, either external ultrasound and intravascular ultrasound. Other than one randomized prospective study on the use of IVC filters as treatment of DVT (which is not how filters are traditionally used), evidence for the use of filters is rated at a 2C grade.

References

Bruinstroop E, Klok FA, Van De Ree MA, et al. Elevated D-dimer levels predict recurrence in patients with idiopathic venous thromboembolism: A meta-analysis. J Thromb Haemost 2009;7:611.

Comerota AJ, Throm RC, Mathias SD, et al. Catheter-directed thrombolysis for iliofemoral deep venous thrombosis improves health-related quality of life. J Vasc Surg 2000;32(1):130.

Elsharawy M, Elzayat E. Early results of thrombolysis vs. anticoagulation in iliofemoral venous thrombosis. A randomised clinical trial. Eur J Vasc Endovasc Surg 2002;24(3):209.

Fowl RJ, Strothman GB, Blebea J, et al. Inappropriate use of venous duplex scans: An analysis of indications and results. J Vasc Surg 1996;23(5):881.

Gross PL, Weitz JI. New anticoagulants for treatment of venous thromboembolism. Arterioscler Thromb Vasc Biol 2008;28:380.

Guyatt GH, Akl EA, Crother M, et al. Executive summary: Antithrombotic therapy and prevention of thrombosis, 9th ed: American College of Chest Physicians' evidence based clinical practice guidelines. Chest 2012;141:7S–47S.

Hull RD, Pineo GF, Brant R, et al. Home therapy of venous thrombosis with long-term LMWH versus usual care: Patient satisfaction and post-thrombotic syndrome. Am J Med 2009;122:762.

Kahn SR, Shapiro S, Wells PS, et al. Compression stockings to prevent post-thrombotic syndrome: A randomized placebo controlled trial. Lancet 2014; 383:880–8.

Kearon C, Akl EA, Comerota AJ, et al. Antithombotic therapy and VTE Disease. Antithombotic therapy and prevention of thrombosis, 9th ed: American College of Chest Physicians Evidence-Based Clinical Practice Guidelines. Chest 2012;141(Suppl):e419S–e494S.

Knepper J, Horne D, Obi A, Wakefield TW. A systematic update on the state of novel anticoagulants and a primer on reversal and bridging. J Vasc Surg 2013;1(4)418–26.

Kucher N. Deep-vein thrombosis of the upper extremity. N Engl J Med 2011;364:861.

Merli G, Spyropoulos AC, Caprini JA. Use of emerging oral anticoagulants in clinical practice: Translating results from clinical trials to orthopedic and general surgical patient populations. Ann Surg 2009;250:219.

Neglen P, Hollis KC, Olivier J, et al. Stenting of the venous outflow in chronic venous disease: Long-term stent-related outcome, clinical, and hemodynamic result. J Vasc Surg 2007;46(5):979.

Palareti G, Cosmi B, Legnani C, et al. D-dimer testing to determine the duration of anticoagulation therapy. N Eng J Med 2006;355:1780.

Schulman S. Advances in the management of venous thromboembolism. Best Prac Res Clin Haematol 2012;25:361–77.

Schulman S, Kearon C, Kakkar AK, et al. Dabigatran versus warfarin in the treatment of acute venous thromboembolism. N Engl J Med 2009;361(24):2342.

Stein PD, Fowler SE, Goodman LR, et al. Multidetector computed tomography for acute pulmonary embolism. N Engl J Med 2006;354(22):2317.

Turpie AG, Bauer KA, Eriksson BI, et al. Fondaparinux vs. enoxaparin for the prevention of venous thromboembolism in major orthopedic surgery: A meta-analysis of 4 randomized double-blind studies. Arch Intern Med 2002;162 (16):1833.

Wakefield TW, Caprini J, Comerota AJ. Thromboembolic diseases. Curr Probl Surg 2008;45(12):844.

Wells PS, Anderson DR, Rodger M, et al. Evaluation of D-dimer in the diagnosis of suspected deep-vein thrombosis. N Engl J Med 2003;349(13):1227.

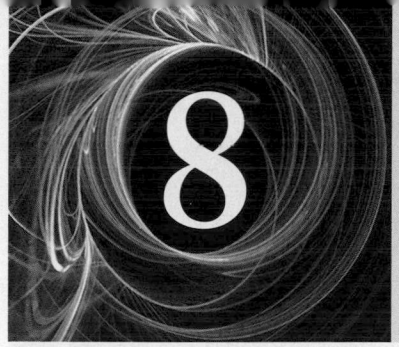

8 The Digestive System

ACUTE AND CHRONIC PANCREATITIS

Method of
George Van Buren, II, MD; and William E. Fisher, MD

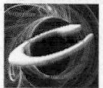

CURRENT DIAGNOSIS

- Acute pancreatitis is usually caused by gallstones, and chronic pancreatitis is usually caused by alcohol abuse.
- Other less-common causes of acute and chronic pancreatitis are considered only when gallstones and alcohol are definitively ruled out.
- Pancreatic cancer and chronic pancreatitis can sometimes be difficult to distinguish.

CURRENT THERAPY

- There has been a recent trend toward conservative medical therapy for acute and chronic pancreatitis, reserving surgery as a last resort.
- In acute pancreatitis, try to avoid necrosectomy except in the setting of infected necrosis with organ failure.
- Asymptomatic pseudocysts can generally be observed.
- Persistent symptomatic pseudocysts can often be addressed endoscopically.
- Medical therapy for chronic pancreatitis includes pain management, nutrition, diabetes control, and cessation of drinking alcohol and smoking.
- Surgical treatment for chronic pancreatitis currently favors strict patient selection and parenchyma-preserving techniques.

Acute Pancreatitis

Acute pancreatitis is an inflammatory disease of the pancreas that is associated with little or no fibrosis of the gland. It can be initiated by several factors including gallstones, alcohol, trauma, and infections, and in some cases it is hereditary (Box 1). Very often, patients with acute pancreatitis develop additional complications such as sepsis, shock, and respiratory and renal failure, resulting in considerable morbidity and mortality.

Epidemiology

The annual incidence is of acute pancreatitis is probably about 50 cases per 100,000 population in the United States. Roughly 3000 of these cases are severe enough to lead to death.

Risk Factors

Biliary tract stone disease accounts for 70% to 80% of the cases of acute pancreatitis. Alcoholism accounts for another 10%, and the remaining 10% to 20% is accounted for either by idiopathic disease or by a variety of iatrogenic and miscellaneous causes including trauma, endoscopy, surgery, drugs, heredity, infection, and toxins.

Pathophysiology

Pancreatitis begins with the activation of digestive zymogens inside acinar cells, which cause acinar cell injury. Digestive zymogens are colocalized with lysosomal hydrolase, and cathepsin-B catalyzed trypsinogen activation occurs, resulting in acinar cell injury and necrosis. This triggers acinar cell inflammatory events with the secretion of inflammatory mediators. Studies suggest that the ultimate severity of the resulting pancreatitis may be determined by the events that occur subsequent to acinar cell injury. These include inflammatory cell recruitment and activation, as well as generation and release of cytokines, reactive oxygen species, and other chemical mediators of inflammation, ultimately leading to ischemia and necrosis. Early mortality in severe acute pancreatitis is caused by a systemic inflammatory response syndrome with multiorgan failure. If the patient survives this critical early period, a septic complication caused by translocated bacteria, mostly Gram-negative microbes from the intestine, leads to infected pancreatic necrosis. Late deaths are caused by infected necrosis, leading to septic shock and multiorgan failure.

Prevention

Gallstones are present in about 15% to 20% of patients older than 60 years, but only a fraction become symptomatic. Although gallstone pancreatitis can rarely be the first symptom of gallstones, most patients have symptoms of cholecystitis before developing pancreatitis. Thus it is important to make early and prompt referral of patients with symptomatic cholelithiasis for laparoscopic cholecystectomy to prevent life-threatening complications such as acute pancreatitis.

Clinical Manifestations

All episodes of acute pancreatitis begin with severe pain, generally following a substantial meal. The pain is usually epigastric, but it can occur anywhere in the abdomen or lower chest. It has been described as penetrating through to the back, and it may be relieved by the patient's leaning forward. It precedes the onset of nausea and vomiting, with retching often continuing after the stomach has emptied. Vomiting does not relieve the pain, which is more intense in necrotizing than in edematous pancreatitis.

On examination the patient may show tachycardia, tachypnea, hypotension, and hyperthermia. The temperature is usually only mildly elevated in uncomplicated pancreatitis. Voluntary and involuntary guarding can be seen over the epigastric region. The bowel sounds are decreased or absent. There are usually no palpable masses. The abdomen may be distended with intraperitoneal fluid. There may be pleural effusion, particularly on the left side. With increasing severity of disease, the intravascular fluid loss may become life-threatening as a result of sequestration of edematous fluid in the retroperitoneum. Hemoconcentration then results in an elevated hematocrit. However, there also may be bleeding into the retroperitoneum or the peritoneal cavity. In some patients (about 1%), the blood from necrotizing pancreatitis can dissect through the soft tissues and manifest as a bluish discoloration around the umbilicus (Cullen's sign) or in the flanks (Grey Turner sign). The severe fluid loss can lead to prerenal azotemia, with elevated blood urea nitrogen and creatinine levels. There also may be hyperglycemia, hypoalbuminemia, and hypocalcemia sufficient in some cases to produce tetany.

Gallstones
Alcoholism
Hereditary
Hypertriglyceridemia
Trauma (including iatrogenic: ERCP or surgery)
Drugs: azathioprine, furosemide, mercaptopurine, opiates, pentamidine, steroids, sulfasalazine, sulindac, tetracycline, trimethoprim-sulfamethoxazole, valproic acid
Tumor
Infection (parasitic and viral)
Idiopathic

Abbreviation: ERCP = endoscopic retrograde cholangiopancreatography.

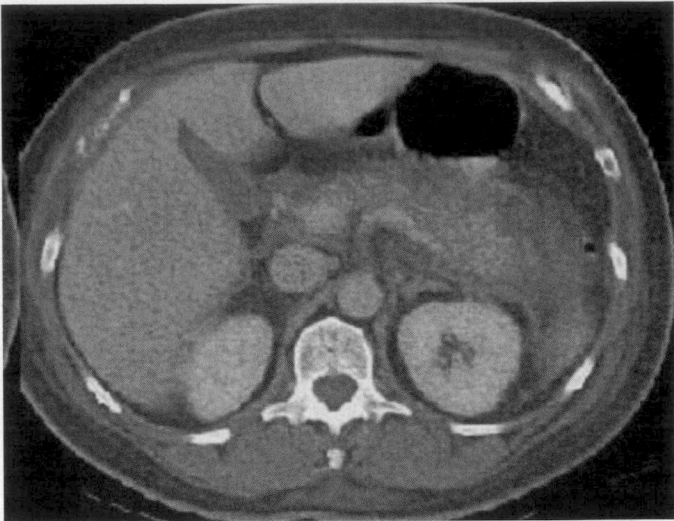

Figure 1. Computed tomographic scan confirming acute edematous pancreatitis.

Diagnosis

Although serum amylase is often elevated in acute pancreatitis, there is no significant correlation between the magnitude of serum amylase elevation and severity of pancreatitis. Other pancreatic enzymes also have been evaluated to improve the diagnostic accuracy of serum measurements. Specificity of these markers ranges from 77% to 96%, the highest being for lipase. Measurements of many digestive enzymes have methodologic limitations and cannot be easily adapted for quantitation in emergency laboratory studies. Because serum levels of lipase remain elevated for a longer time than total or pancreatic amylase, it is the serum indicator of highest probability of the disease.

Abdominal ultrasound examination is the best way to confirm the presence of gallstones in suspected biliary pancreatitis. It also can detect extrapancreatic ductal dilations and reveal pancreatic edema, swelling, and peripancreatic fluid collections. However, in about 20% of patients, the ultrasound examination does not provide satisfactory results because of the presence of bowel gas, which can obscure sonographic imaging of the pancreas.

A computed tomographic (CT) scan of the pancreas is more commonly used to diagnose pancreatitis. CT scanning is used to distinguish milder (nonnecrotic) forms of the disease from more severe necrotizing or infected pancreatitis, in patients whose clinical presentation raises the suspicion of advanced disease (Figures 1 and 2). Pancreatic protocol computed tomography (CT) scan of the abdomen and pelvis is recommended when not limited by renal insufficiency. A tri-phasic thin, multislice CT scan with an arterial, venous, and delayed phase in conjunction with sagital and coronal views. No oral contrast, instead drink 1000cc water to opacify the stomach. The scan asses the degree of pancreatic necrosis, peripancreatic fluid collections, and the surrounding vascular structures.

Magnetic Resonance Cholangiopancreatography (MRCP) is also of value to assess the pancreatic duct and biliary tree. This can often reveal pancreatic ductal disruption.

Differential Diagnosis

The clinical diagnosis of pancreatitis is one of exclusion. Hyperamylasemia can also occur as a result of conditions not involving pancreatitis. The other upper abdominal conditions that can be confused with acute pancreatitis include perforated peptic ulcer and acute colecystitis, and occasionally a gangrenous small bowel obstruction. Because these conditions often have a fatal outcome without surgery, urgent intervention is indicated in the small number of cases in which doubt persists. A tumor should be considered in a nonalcoholic patient with acute pancreatitis who has no demonstrable biliary tract disease. Approximately 1% to 2% of patients with acute pancreatitis have pancreatic carcinoma, and an episode of acute pancreatitis can be the first clinical manifestation of a periampullary tumor.

Treatment

The severity of acute pancreatitis covers a broad spectrum of illness, ranging from the mild and self-limiting to the life-threatening necrotizing variety. Some cases are so mild they can be treated in

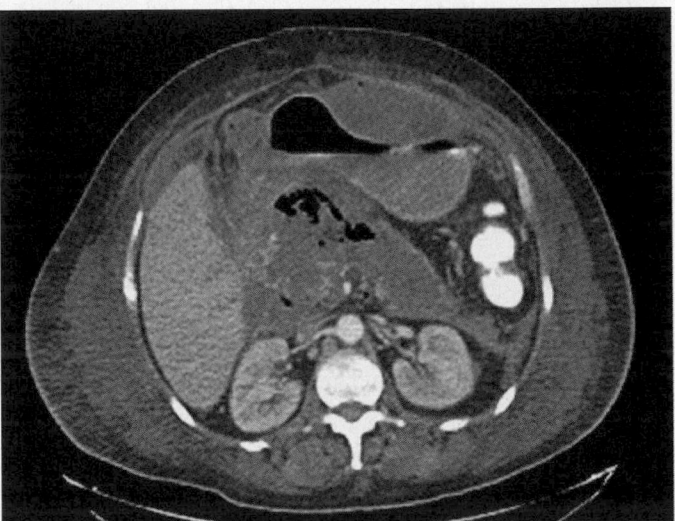

Figure 2. Computed tomographic scan confirming acute necrotizing, emphysematous pancreatitis.

an outpatient setting. However, most cases require hospitalization for observation and diagnostic study. A conservative approach has been advocated in the treatment of acute pancreatitis (Box 2). Severity is assessed with imaging results and clinical parameters and is quantitated with scores such as Ranson's criteria (Box 3), the Atlanta classification, and the APACHE II (Acute Physiology

Assessment of severity
Fluid resuscitation and oxygenation
Early nasojejunal feeding
Avoid prophylactic antibiotics (reserve antibiotic therapy for specific infections)
Avoid or postpone necrosectomy if possible
Options for necrosectomy
• Open anterior approach with closed lavage
• Open anterior approach with packing and reoperation
• Open retroperitoneal approach
• Laparoscopic anterior approach with closed lavage
• Video-assisted retroperitoneal débridement (VARD)

Box 3   Ranson's Criteria

There are 11 Ranson signs. Five of the signs are evaluated when the patient is admitted to the hospital, and the remaining six are evaluated 48 hours after admission. The signs are added to reach a score:
- If the score <3, severe pancreatitis is unlikely.
- If the score ≥3, severe pancreatitis likely.

or
- Score 0-2: 2% mortality
- Score 3-4: 15% mortality
- Score 5-6: 40% mortality
- Score 7-8: 100% mortality

At Admission

Age in years >55 years
White blood cell count >16,000 cells/mm^3
Blood glucose >11 mmol/L (>200 mg/dL)
Serum AST >250 IU/L
Serum LDH >350 IU/L

At 48 Hours

Calcium (serum calcium) <2.0 mmol/L (<8.0 mg/dL)
Hematocrit fall >10%
Oxygen (hypoxemia Po$_2$ <60 mm Hg)
BUN increased by ≥1.8 mmol/L (≥5 mg/dL) after IV fluid hydration
Base deficit (negative base excess) >4 mEq/L
Sequestration of fluids >6 L

Abbreviations: AST = aspartate aminotransferase; BUN = blood urea nitrogen.

And Chronic Health Evaluation) score. Severe acute pancreatitis is defined by associated organ dysfunction. The Atlanta classification is based on an international consensus conference held in Atlanta in 1992 and has been updated. APACHE II was designed to measure the severity of disease for adult patients admitted to intensive care units. Though not specific to pancreatitis, APACHE II can be used in an effort to differentiate patients with mild and severe acute pancreatitis. APACHE II scores of 8 points or more correlate with a mortality rate of 11% to 18%.

Upon confirmation of the diagnosis, patients with severe disease should be transferred to the intensive care unit for observation and maximum support. Adequate fluid resuscitation optimizing organ perfusion and oxygenation is essential. The use of prophylactic intravenous antibiotics in the initial stages of severe acute pancreatitis is not proved to be useful. Two randomized, controlled studies failed to show any benefit from antibiotics. Prophylactic antibiotics did not decrease the incidence of infected pancreatic necrosis or lower mortality. Data from these well-designed trials refutes prior data from less-rigorous studies suggesting prophylactic antibiotics were useful. Additional studies are required, but there is increasing concern that the prolonged use of potent antibiotics might result in an increased prevalence of fungal infections and possibly increased mortality. Currently, antibiotic therapy should be reserved for treatment of specific infections such as positive blood, sputum, and urine cultures or percutaneous or operative cultures of necrotic tissue.

Randomized clinical trials have also shown a benefit from early nasojejunal feeding compared to total parenteral nutrition. Gastric decompression with a nasogastric tube is selectively used in patients with severe ileus and vomiting but is not necessary in a majority of cases.

In biliary pancreatitis, the gallbladder must eventually be removed or recurrent acute pancreatitis will occur in 30% to 60% of cases. The timing of the cholecystectomy depends on the severity of the pancreatitis. Usually laparoscopic cholecystectomy is performed during the index admission as soon as the attack of acute pancreatitis has resolved. In more-severe cases, the cholecystectomy is delayed and often combined with interventions for late complications of acute pancreatitis. In cases with severe comorbidity, endoscopic sphincterotomy has been considered as an alternative to cholecystectomy. However, if the patient has a postinflammatory fluid collection, bacteria can be introduced during endoscopic retrograde cholangiopancreatography (ERCP), and sphincterotomy should be delayed.

Currently, there is no role for routine early laparotomy and necrosectomy or resection in the setting of acute necrotizing pancreatitis. If the necrotic pancreas becomes infected and the patient fails to respond to conservative treatment, then necrosectomy may be warranted. Patients with infected necrosis are rarely managed conservatively without eventual surgical intervention. However, even in the setting of infected necrosis, there has been consideration for antibiotic therapy until the acute inflammatory response has subsided, if possible, with the view that surgery that is deferred for several weeks is more easily accomplished with one intervention. Patients who suffer from infected necrosis without having clinical signs of sepsis or other systemic complications might not need immediate surgical necrosectomy.

A nonsurgical alternative for the treatment of infected necrosis is percutaneous catheter drainage. This is considered a temporary measure to allow stabilization of the patient so that a safer surgical necrosectomy can be done at a later time. Multiple large drains are required, and patients frequently undergo repeat CT and revision of the drains. Current recommendations are to postpone surgery for as long as possible, usually beyond the second or third week of the disease or later, when necrotic tissue can be easily distinguished from viable pancreas and débridement without major blood loss can be performed. When surgery is performed, tissue-preserving digital necrosectomy is the usual technique rather than a classic surgical resection of the pancreas (Figure 3).

Necrosectomy can be performed by an open anterior approach with closed lavage or with leaving the abdomen open and packing. The packing is replaced at intervals of 24 to 72 hours. Sometimes a left lateral retroperitoneal approach is helpful. Newer approaches are the video-assisted retroperitoneal débridement (VARD). This procedure is a combination of percutaneous drainage and the open lateral retroperitoneal approach. An anterior laparoscopic approach has also been described and mimics the open anterior approach using laparoscopic ports. Surgical necrosectomy is indicated in patients with sepsis caused by infected necrosis and in selected patients with extended sterile necrosis causing severe systemic organ dysfunction and sepsis without a septic focus.

In some cases, the acute inflammatory process can lead to erosion into retroperitoneal vessels, and acute hemorrhage occurs. This acute emergent complication is best managed with immediate angiography to determine the exact site of bleeding and can often be treated with embolization rather than surgery (Figure 4).

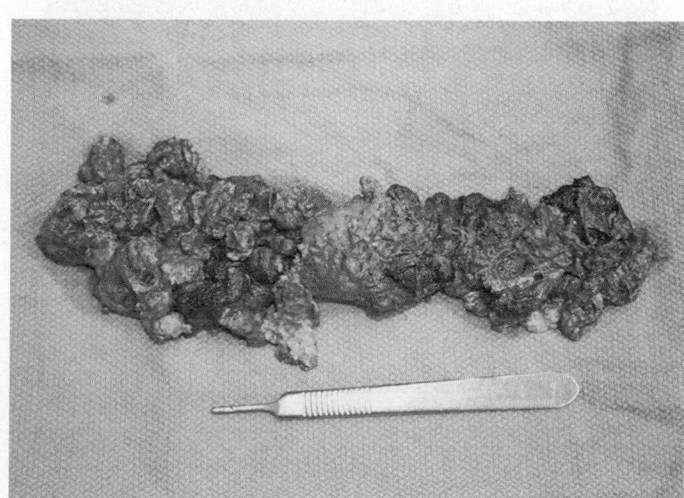

Figure 3. Necrotic material débrided from the retroperitoneum in a case of acute necrotizing pancreatitis.

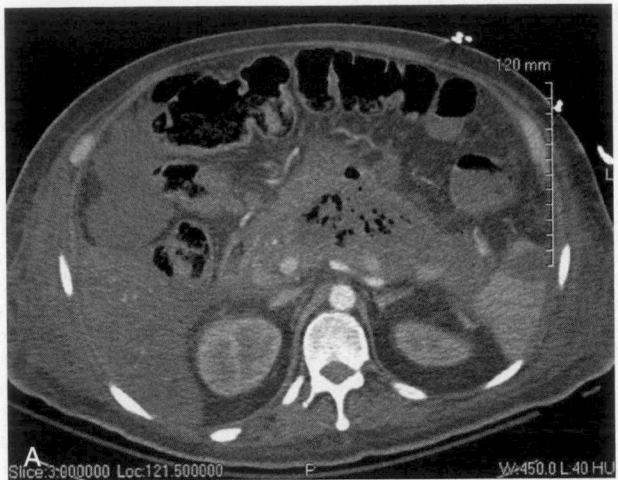
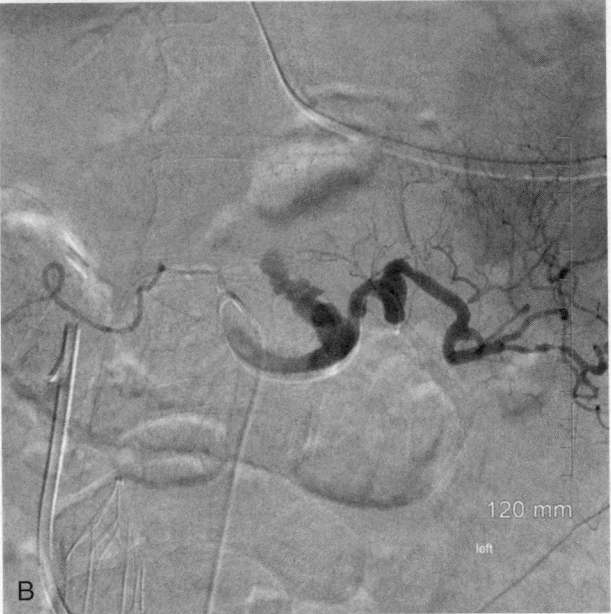
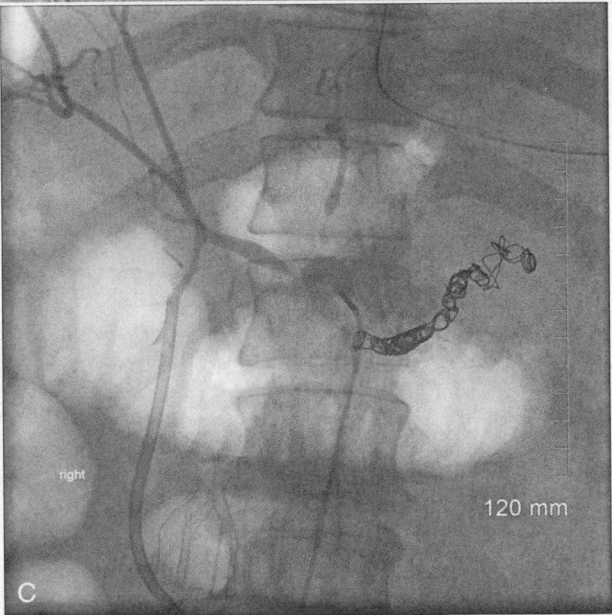

Figure 4. Acute necrotizing pancreatitis. **A,** Erosion into the splenic artery as seen on computed tomography. **B,** Erosion into the splenic artery as seen on angiogram. **C,** This complication of acute pancreatitis is best treated with angiographic embolization.

Although previously frowned upon, there has been a move toward enteric drainage of all necrotic collections (even when infected) when technically feasible.

Monitoring

Despite a conservative operative approach, endocrine and exocrine insufficiency develop in as many as half of the patients and are determined by the extent of pancreatic necrosis. Therefore, patients must be monitored with blood glucose measurements, stabilization of body weight, and proper nutrition.

Complications

The most common complication after successful management of acute pancreatitis is a pseudocyst. The term "pseudocyst" is currently used to broadly categorize most pancreatic and peripancreatic fluid collections (including walled-off pancreatic necrosis [WOPN] and acute peripancreatic fluid collection). The Acute Pancreatitis Classification Working Group recently proposed a revised Atlanta classification refers to collections within 4 weeks of symptom onset as either acute peripancreatic fluid collections (APFC) or postnecrotic pancreatic fluid collections (PNPFC) depending upon the absence or presence of pancreatic/peripancreatic necrosis, respectively. After 4 weeks of the onset of symptoms, persistent collections with discrete walls are referred to as pseudocyst or WOPN, again depending upon the absence or presence of necrosis, respectively. In addition, these collections are further classified as sterile or infected and the term "pancreatic abscess" has been abolished.

The management of pseudo-cysts has followed a minimally invasive trend. Most pseudo-cysts resolve spontaneously, even beyond 6 weeks, so asymptomatic pseudocysts are usually observed. (70% of pseudocysts will resolve without intervention) Endoscopic cystogastrostomy is the approach of choice for symptomatic fluid-predominant pseudocysts when there is minimal necrosis. If there is significant necrotic debris or a solid-predominant pseudocyst, surgical drainage with laparoscopic cystogastrostomy is preferred (Figure 5). This can also be performed with the traditional open technique. Cystjejunostomy (laparoscopic or open) is used in cases in which the site of the pseudocyst precludes drain-age into the posterior aspect of the stomach.

Chronic Pancreatitis

Chronic pancreatitis is a chronic inflammatory disease of the pancreas characterized by irreversible morphologic changes that typically are associated with pain or permanent loss of function, or both.

Epidemiology

Population studies suggest a prevalence of chronic pancreatitis that ranges from 5 to 27 persons per 100,000 population, with considerable geographic variation. Autopsy data are difficult to interpret because a number of changes associated with chronic pancreatitis, such as fibrosis, duct ectasia, and acinar atrophy, are also present in asymptomatic elderly patients. Differences in diagnostic criteria, regional nutrition, alcohol consumption, and medical access account for variations in the frequency of the diagnosis, but the overall incidence of the disease has risen progressively since the 1960s. Chronic pancreatitis in the United States currently results in more than 120,000 outpatient visits and more than 50,000 hospitalizations per year.

Risk factors

Alcohol consumption and alcohol abuse are associated with chronic pancreatitis in up to 70% of cases. Other major causes include tropical (nutritional) and idiopathic disease, as well as hereditary causes. There is a linear relationship between exposure to alcohol and the development of chronic pancreatitis. The incidence is highest in heavy drinkers (15 drinks/day or 150 g/day). However, chronic pancreatitis can occur in patients who drink very little, and it occurs in less than 15% of documented alcoholics. The duration of alcohol consumption is definitely associated with the development of pancreatic disease. The onset of

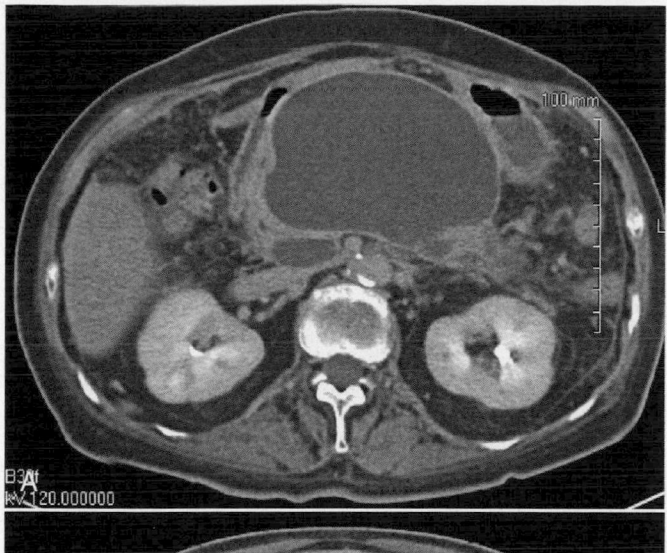

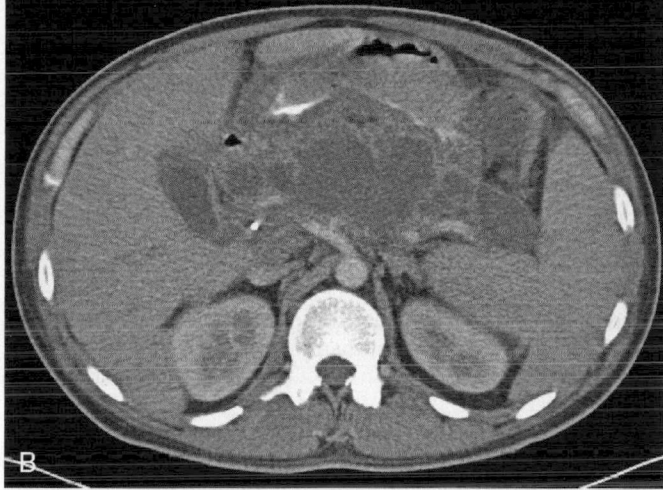

Figure 5. Computed tomographic scan showing fluid-predominant (A) and solid-predominant (B) pseudocysts. The former can be treated with endoscopic cystogastrostomy, and the latter is best treated with laparoscopic cystogastrostomy.

disease typically occurs between ages 35 and 40 years, after 16 to 20 years of heavy alcohol consumption. Recurrent episodes of acute pancreatitis are typically followed by chronic symptoms after 4 or 5 years.

Pathophysiology

Multiple episodes (or a prolonged course) of pancreatic injury ultimately leading to chronic disease is widely accepted as the pathophysiologic sequence. Most investigators believe that alcohol metabolites such as acetaldehyde, combined with oxidant injury, result in local parenchymal injury that is preferentially targeted to the pancreas in predisposed persons. Repeated or severe episodes of toxin-induced injury activate a cascade of cytokines, which in turn induces pancreatic stellate cells to produce collagen and cause fibrosis.

The pain caused by chronic pancreatitis is thought to be due to increased pressure in the pancreatic ducts and tissue. Neural and perineural inflammation is also thought to be important in pathogenesis of pain in chronic pancreatitis. Neuropeptides released from enteric and afferent neurons and their functional interactions with inflammatory cells might play a key role.

Prevention

Because alcohol is the cause of most cases of chronic pancreatitis, cessation of alcohol consumption is recommended to prevent progression to chronic pancreatitis. Unfortunately, the majority of patients are not able to recover from alcoholism, and relapse is common.

Clinical Manifestations

Symptoms of chronic pancreatitis may be identical to those of acute pancreatitis, typically midepigastric pain penetrating through to the back. Patients with chronic pancreatic pain typically flex their abdomen and either sit or lie with their hips flexed, or lie on their side in a fetal position. Unlike ureteral stone pain or biliary colic, the pain causes the patient to be still. Nausea or vomiting can accompany the pain, but anorexia is the most common associated symptom. Patients with continuous pain can have a complication of chronic pancreatitis, such as an inflammatory mass, a cyst, or even pancreatic cancer. Other patients have intermittent attacks of pain with symptoms similar to those of mild to moderate acute pancreatitis. The pain sometimes is severe and lasts for many hours or several days.

As chronic pancreatitis progresses, endocrine and exocrine insufficiency begin to appear. Patients describe a bulky, foul-smelling, loose (but not watery) stool that may be pale and float on the surface of toilet water. Patients often describe a greasy or oily appearance to the stool or describe an "oil slick" on the water's surface. In severe steatorrhea, an orange, oily stool is often reported. As exocrine deficiency increases, symptoms of steatorrhea are often accompanied by weight loss. Patients might describe a good appetite despite weight loss, or they might have diminished food intake due to abdominal pain. The combination of decreased food intake and malabsorption of nutrients usually results in chronic weight loss. As a result, many patients with severe chronic pancreatitis are below ideal body weight. Usually islet cells are spared early in the disease process despite being surrounded by fibrosis, but eventually the insulin-secreting beta cells are also destroyed, gradually leading to diabetes.

Diagnosis

The diagnosis of chronic pancreatitis depends on the clinical presentation, a limited number of indirect measurements that correlate with pancreatic function, and selected imaging studies. Diagnosis is usually simple in the late stages of the disease because of the presence of structural and functional alterations of the pancreas. Early in the disease, the diagnosis is more difficult. Various classification systems have been developed. The Cambridge classification uses imaging tests such as ERCP, CT, and ultrasound to grade severity. The Mayo Clinic system is based on functional as well as imaging results. Tests of pancreatic function include the secretin-cerulein test, Lundh test, fecal excretion of pancreatic enzymes, and quantitation of fecal fat.

Chronic pancreatitis can be classified as calcifying (lithogenic), obstructive, inflammatory, autoimmune, tropical (nutritional), hereditary, or idiopathic. Autoimmune and hereditary pancreatitis have recently been better understood and diagnosed more than before. Autoimmune pancreatitis is associated with fibrosis, a mononuclear cell (lymphocyte, plasma cell, or eosinophil) infiltrate, and an increased titer of one or more autoantibodies. It is usually associated with autoimmune diseases such as Sjögren's syndrome. Increased levels of serum β-globulin or immunoglobulin (Ig)G_4 are often present. This disease can be mistaken for chronic pancreatitis, with an inflammatory mass in the head of the pancreas suspicious for pancreatic cancer (Figure 6). Diagnosis is important because steroid therapy is uniformly successful in ameliorating the disease, including any associated bile duct compression.

Hereditary pancreatitis first occurs in adolescence with abdominal pain; patients develop progressive pancreatic dysfunction, and the risk of cancer is greatly increased. The disease follows an autosomal dominant pattern of inheritance with 80% penetrance and variable expression. Recent mutational analysis has revealed a missense mutation resulting in an Arg to His substitution at position 117 of the cationic trypsinogen gene, or *PRSS1*, one of the primary sites for proteolysis of trypsin. This mutation prevents trypsin from being inactivated by itself or other proteases, and it results in persistent and uncontrolled proteolytic activity and autodestruction within the pancreas. Similarly, *PSTI*, also known as *SPINK1*, has been found to have a role in hereditary pancreatitis and some cases of sporadic chronic pancreatitis. *SPINK1* specifically inhibits trypsin action by competitively blocking the active site of the enzyme.

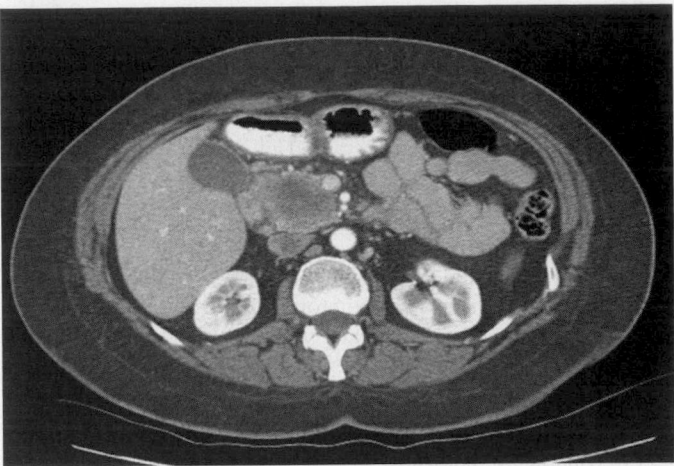

Figure 6. Computed tomographic scan of a patient with autoimmune pancreatitis and an inflammatory mass in the head of the pancreas. Preoperative diagnosis is not always possible, but surgery should be avoided because this disease often responds to steroid therapy.

It is likely that many of the "idiopathic" forms of chronic pancreatitis, as well as some patients with the more common forms of the disease, will be found to have a genetic linkage or predisposition.

Differential Diagnosis

There are several clinical conditions from which chronic pancreatitis needs to be distinguished. Other causes of upper abdominal pain, such as peptic ulcer disease, biliary tract disease, mesenteric vascular disease, or malignancy must be excluded. The major difficulty in the differential diagnosis of chronic pancreatitis is distinguishing it from pancreatic ductal adenocarcinoma. Chronic pancreatitis can closely mimic pancreatic cancer, both clinically and morphologically. In addition, chronic pancreatitis is a risk factor for the development of pancreatic cancer. Although in pancreatic resection specimens this problem may be finally resolved, distinguishing these two diseases preoperatively in small (needle) biopsy specimens is a formidable challenge for the pathologist. Therefore, especially in the setting of an inflammatory mass in the head of the pancreas, consideration of pancreatic cancer and surgical referral is important. Work up of these patients should include a pancreatic protocol CT scan, a MRCP, and an endoscopic ultrasound to evaluate the parenchyma and the ducts of the pancreas.

Treatment

Therapy for chronic pancreatitis is aimed at managing associated digestive dysfunction and relieving pain (Box 4). It is important to first address malabsorption, weight loss, and diabetes. When pancreatic exocrine capacity falls below 10% of normal, diarrhea and steatorrhea develop. Lipase deficiency tends to manifest itself before trypsin deficiency, so the presence of steatorrhea may be the first functional sign of pancreatic insufficiency. As pancreatic exocrine function deteriorates further, the secretion of bicarbonate into the duodenum is reduced, which causes duodenal acidification and further impairs nutrient absorption. Frank diabetes is seen initially in about 20% of patients with chronic pancreatitis,

---

| **Box 4** | Treatment of Chronic Pancreatitis |

Pancreatic enzyme replacement
Proper nutrition and vitamin supplementation
Blood sugar control
Long-acting narcotic analgesics at lowest effective doses
Cessation of alcohol and tobacco
Endotherapy (pancreatic duct stenting and removal of stones)
Parenchymal preserving surgery (Frey, Beger) in carefully selected patients

---

and impaired glucose metabolism can be detected in up to 70% of patients.

The medical treatment of chronic or recurrent pain in chronic pancreatitis requires the use of analgesics, a cessation of alcohol use, oral enzyme therapy, and endoscopic stent thearpy. Administration of pancreatic enzyme (e.g., Pancrease MT, Pancrelipase, Creon) serves to reverse the effects of pancreatic exocrine insufficiency and might also reduce or alleviate the pain[1] experienced by patients. Interventional procedures to block visceral afferent nerve conduction or to treat obstructions of the main pancreatic duct are also an adjunct to medical treatment. It has been taught that the pain of chronic pancreatitis decreases with increasing duration of the disease, the so called burn-out phase, where endocrine and exocrine insufficiency occurs and the pain decreases. However, recent studies have called this concept into question, demonstrating continued pain in patients with chronic pancreatitis despite long-standing disease and pancreatic insufficiency. Cessation of alcohol abuse, if possible, causes the pain to stop in about half of the patients.

Pain relief usually requires the use of narcotics, but these should be titrated to achieve pain relief with the lowest effective dose. Opioid addiction is common, and the use of long-acting analgesics by transdermal patch together with oral agents for pain exacerbations slightly reduces the sedative effects of high-dose oral narcotics. Celiac plexus neurolysis has been an effective form of analgesic treatment in patients with pancreatic carcinoma. However, its use in chronic pancreatitis has been disappointing, with about half of the patients deriving a benefit that lasts 6 months or less.

Pancreatic duct stenting is used for treatment of proximal pancreatic duct stenosis, decompression of a pancreatic duct leak, and drainage of pancreatic pseudocysts that can be catheterized through the main pancreatic duct. Pancreatic duct stones can also be removed endoscopically. Stent therapy in chronic pancreatitis definitely plays a role and can help select patients for successful operative therapy. However, the duration of success with stent therapy for chronic pancreatitis is probably less than with surgical therapy.

Major pancreatic resections for chronic pancreatitis have a high complication rate, both early and late. Patients with large duct disease who can have nutrition restored, are working, are not drinking alcohol, and have a supportive family structure fare better. Failure to carefully select patients leads to disappointing results. The surgical management of pancreatic duct stones and stenoses has been shown to be superior to endoscopic treatment in randomized clinical trials. Beger introduced the duodenum-preserving pancreatic head resection (DPPHR) in the early 1980s. Later in the decade, Frey and Smith described the local resection of the pancreatic head with longitudinal pancreaticojejunostomy, which included excavation of the pancreatic head including the ductal structures in continuity with a long ductotomy of the dorsal duct. This operation is basically a hybrid of the Beger and Puestow (Partington-Rochelle modification) procedures and is more popular in the United States (Figures 7 and 8).

Recent randomized prospective studies have compared the Whipple, Beger, and Frey procedures for chronic pancreatitis. Patients who had a Beger procedure had a shorter hospital stay, greater weight gain, less postoperative diabetes, and less exocrine dysfunction than standard Whipple patients over a 3- to 5-year follow-up. Pain control was similar between the two procedures. In a study comparing the pylorus-preserving Whipple to the Frey procedure, there was a lower postoperative complication rate associated with the Frey procedure (19%) compared to the pylorus-preserving Whipple group (53%), and the global quality-of-life scores were better (71% versus 43%, respectively). Both operations were equally effective in controlling pain over a 2-year follow-up. Operation times, intraoperative blood loss, and transfusion requirements have been shown to be decreased with the Frey and Beger procedures compared to the Whipple procedure. In long-term (>8 years) follow-up, there was no difference between the Beger and Frey procedures in pain relief, pancreatic insufficiency, quality of life, and late mortality. Compared to the Whipple

---

[1]Not FDA approved for this indication.

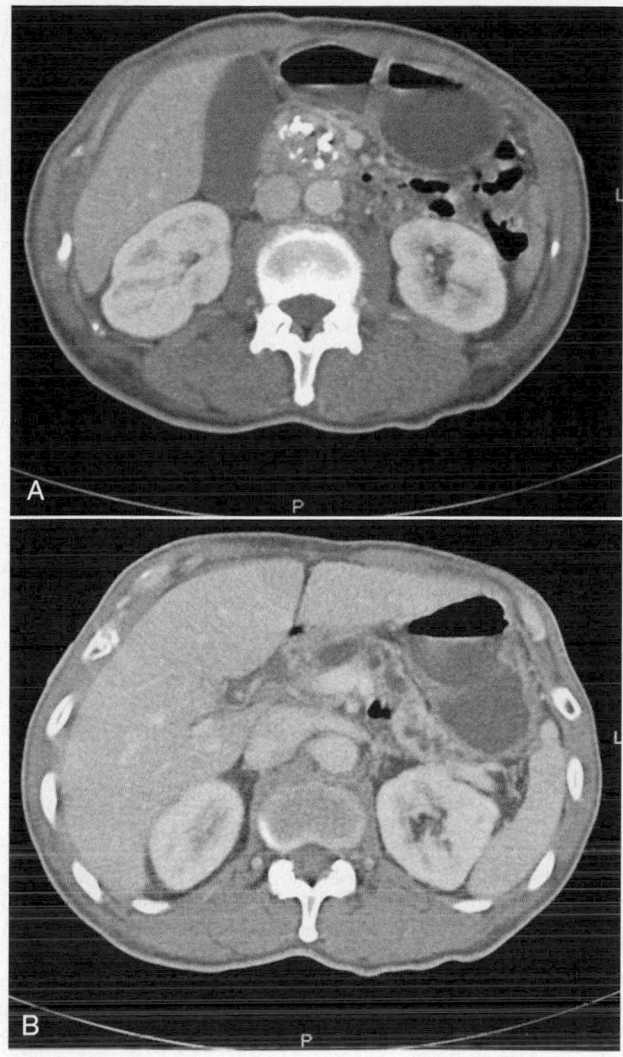

Figure 7. Computed tomographic scan of a patient with chronic calcific pancreatitis and a massively dilated pancreatic duct.

procedure, the Beger and Frey procedures seem to produce a lower incidence of immediate complications and diabetes but no significant differences in pain relief. Although these limited pancreatic procedures have a lower initial rate of endocrine dysfunction, the long-term risk of diabetes is more related to the progression of the underlying disease than to the effects of operation.

Recent refinements in the methods of harvesting and preserving pancreatic islets, and standardization of the methods by which islets are infused into the portal venous circuit for intrahepatic engraftment, have improved the success and rekindled interest in islet autotransplantation for chronic pancreatitis. The ability to recover a sufficient quantity of islets from a sclerotic gland depends on the degree of disease present, so the selection of patients as candidates for autologous islet transplantation is important. As success with autotransplantation increases, patients with nonobstructive, sclerotic pancreatitis may be considered for resection and islet autotransplantation earlier in their course, because end-stage fibrosis bodes poorly for transplant success. As the necessary expertise with islet transplantation becomes more widespread, this therapy could become routine in the treatment of chronic pancreatitis.

Monitoring

Chronic pancreatitis is of course a chronic disease, so continued monitoring and maintenance therapy is essential after an acute exacerbation of chronic pancreatitis. Pain control, proper nutrition, and alcohol and smoking cessation must be maintained as an outpatient. The clinician must also be looking for the development of common complications.

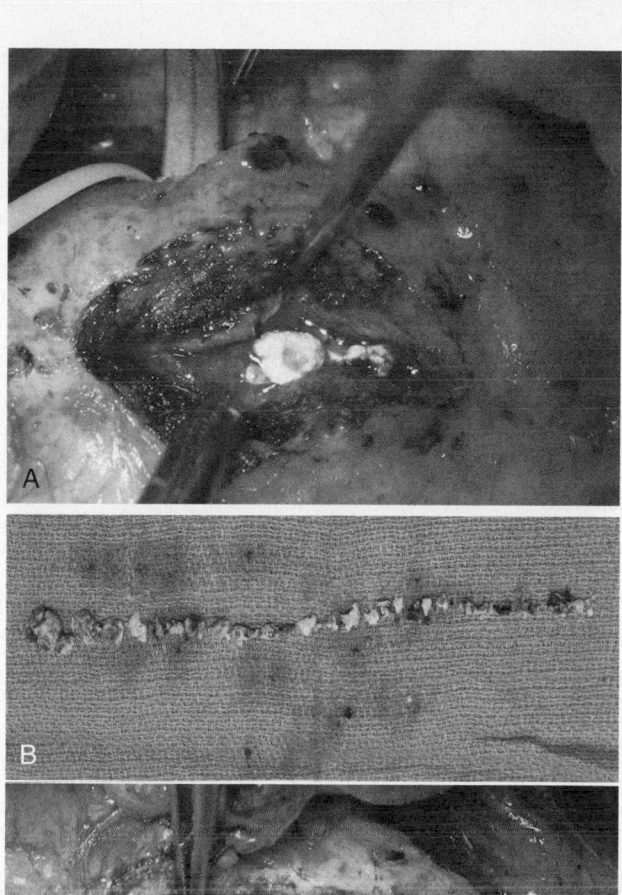

Figure 8. A, The pancreatic duct is opened to reveal a preoperatively placed pancreatic duct stent. B, The residual stones removed from the pancreatic duct. C, In the Frey procedure, the head of the pancreas is cored out in addition to a longitudinal pancreatic ductotomy. The pancreas is drained with a Roux-en-Y limb of jejunum.

Complications

Pseudocysts in the setting of chronic pancreatitis are less likely to resolve without intervention. Often, the pancreatic duct and bile duct are compressed, and the compression might need to be addressed at the same time as the pseudocyst. A trend toward minimally invasive management remains appropriate, with endoscopic drainage preferred over laparoscopic cystogastrostomy unless additional procedures are required. Resection of a pseudocyst is sometimes indicated for cysts located in the pancreatic tail, or when a midpancreatic duct disruption has resulted in a distally located pseudocyst. Distal pancreatectomy for removal of a pseudocyst, with or without splenectomy, can be a challenging procedure in the setting of prior pancreatitis. An internal drainage procedure of the communicating duct, or of the pseudocyst itself, should be considered when distal resection is being contemplated.

Pancreatic ascites results from a disrupted pancreatic duct with extravasation of pancreatic fluid that does not become sequestered as a pseudocyst but drains freely into the peritoneal cavity. Occasionally, the pancreatic fluid tracks superiorly into the thorax, causing a pancreatic pleural effusion. Both complications are seen more often in patients with chronic pancreatitis, rather than after acute pancreatitis. Paracentesis or thoracentesis reveals noninfected fluid with a protein level greater than 25 g/L and a markedly elevated amylase level. Paracentesis is critical to differentiate pancreatic from hepatic ascites.

ERCP is most helpful to delineate the location of the pancreatic duct leak and to elucidate the underlying pancreatic ductal anatomy. Pancreatic duct stenting may be considered at the time of ERCP. Paracentesis and antisecretory therapy with the somatostatin analogue octreotide acetate, together with bowel rest and parenteral nutrition, is successful in more than half of patients. Reapposition of serosal surfaces to facilitate closure of the leak is considered a part of therapy, and this is accomplished by complete paracentesis. For pleural effusions, a period of chest tube drainage can facilitate closure of the internal fistula. Surgical therapy is reserved for those who fail to respond to medical treatment.

References

Acute Pancreatitis Classification Working Group. Revision of the Atlanta Classification of Acute Pancreatitis, PDF available for download at: http://www.pancreasclub.com/resources/AtlantaClassification.pdf [accessed 25.08.14].

Beger HG, Matsuno S, Cameron JL. Diseases of the pancreas: Current surgical therapy. Berlin: Springer-Verlag; 2008.

Beger HG, Warshaw AL, Buchler MW, et al., The pancreas: An integrated textbook of basic science, medicine, and surgery. 2nd ed. Malden, MA: Blackwell Publishing; 2008.

Cunha EF, Rocha Mde S, Pereira FP, et al. Walled-off pancreatic necrosis and other current concepts in the radiological assessment of acute pancreatitis. Radiol Bras 2014;47(3):165–75.

Dellinger EP, Tellado JM, Soto NE, et al. Early antibiotic treatment for severe acute necrotizing pancreatitis: A randomized, double-blind, placebo-controlled study. Ann Surg 2007;245:674–83.

Fisher WE, Anderson DK, Bell RH, et al. Pancreas. In: Brunicardi FC, Andersen DK, Billiar TR, et al, editors: Schwartz's Principles of Surgery. 9th ed. New York: McGraw-Hill; 2010. p. 1167–243.

Isenmann R, Runzi M, Kron M, et al. Prophylactic antibiotic treatment in patients with predicted severe acute pancreatitis: A placebo-controlled, double-blind trial. Gastroenterology 2004;126:997–1004.

Zaheer A, Singh VK, Qureshi RO, Fishman EK. The revised Atlanta classification for acute pancreatitis: updates in imaging terminology and guidelines. Abdom Imaging 2013;38(1):125–36.

ACUTE AND CHRONIC VIRAL HEPATITIS

Method of
John Garber, MD; and Daniel S. Pratt, MD

The progress achieved in understanding viral hepatitis over the past decade has been dramatic. There are better diagnostic tools and rapidly evolving therapies, both for hepatitis B and hepatitis C. This improved therapy has made it critical that physicians effectively screen for chronic hepatitis B and hepatitis C to identify all appropriate candidates for treatment.

Hepatitis A virus

Hepatitis A virus (HAV), a member of the Picornaviridae family, exists as a single positive-stranded RNA virus of 7474 nucleotides, which encodes four structural proteins (capsids V1, V2, V3, and V4) and seven nonstructural proteins (e.g., protease, RNA-dependent polymerase). Four distinct genotypes exist. Despite intergenomic sequence variation of up to 20%, the genotypes are immunologically indistinguishable, so infection with one strain of HAV confers lifelong immunity to all strains.

Epidemiology

The virus is extremely stable in the environment and is shed in the stool of infected persons at a very high titer. It spreads within a population predominantly via the fecal-oral route, most commonly through ingestion of contaminated food or water. In the United States, the likelihood of having serologic evidence of past exposure is associated with age; it is approximately 11% at the age of 5 years and increases to almost 75% in those older than 50 years.

Diagnosis

The presence of anti-HAV antibodies of the immunoglobulin M (IgM) class is diagnostic of acute HAV infection. Positive anti-HAV IgG antibodies along with negative anti-HAV IgM antibodies indicates immunity, from either prior infection or vaccination.

Clinical laboratories often report the total anti-HAV antibodies, which is a mixture of IgG and IgM. To distinguish acute HAV infection from prior exposure, it is important to specifically test for the presence of anti-HAV IgM.

Natural History

HAV causes an acute hepatitis only; it never results in chronic hepatitis, and lifelong immunity is expected in all patients who recover. Once the virus is orally ingested, it reaches the liver via the portal vein. Viral shedding occurs when the replicating virus is excreted from hepatocytes through the bile duct into the intestine. Shedding continues until the prodromic phase and begins to decline once jaundice develops. However, infectious virions can be detected in the feces up to 2 weeks after the onset of jaundice.

The severity of symptoms associated with HAV depends in part on the age of the patient at the time of exposure: 90% of those infected before 5 years of age are asymptomatic, whereas 70% to 80% of those infected as adults have symptoms. HAV has an incubation period of approximately 25 days. This is followed by a prodromal phase of variable severity, characterized by weakness, anorexia, nausea, abdominal pain, and, less often, fevers, arthralgias, and diarrhea. The levels of the serum aminotransferases are elevated during this time, often to values greater than 500 U/L, and their peak usually coincides with intense nausea, vomiting, and anorexia. Jaundice typically occurs 1 to 2 weeks later and is associated with a lessening of the prodromal symptoms. The serum bilirubin level peaks later than the aminotransferases, rarely exceeds 10 mg/dL, and normalizes more slowly than the aminotransferases. In most patients, jaundice lasts less than 2 weeks. Complete normalization of the serum biochemical abnormalities is observed in 60% of patients by 2 months and in almost 100% by 6 months.

Treatment

There is no specific therapy for hepatitis A; treatment is largely supportive. Dehydration is common during the symptomatic phase and requires administration of intravenous fluids. A rare complication of acute HAV is the development of acute liver failure marked by encephalopathy and coagulopathy. The risk of developing acute liver failure is higher in older patients; those infected after the age of 50 years have a case-fatality rate of 2.7%. Patients with coexisting chronic HBV or HCV infection are also at higher risk for a more severe clinical course. Vaccination for HAV should be offered to all patients who have chronic viral hepatitis or cirrhosis and negative HAV antibodies.

Six vaccines containing inactivated HAV are currently licensed for use: HAVRIX (GlaxoSmithKline), VAQTA (Merck), AVAXIM (Sanofi Pasteur),[2] HEALIVE (Sinovac),[2] EPAXAL[2] (Crucell), and TWINRIX (GlaxoSmithKline). All are highly effective at generating antibody responses, with approximately 95% of recipients developing protective levels of anti-HAV antibodies within 1 month after the first dose, and 100% after the second dose. The Advisory Committee on Immunization Practices recommends HAV immunoprophylaxis for all children at the age of 1 year. Vaccination is also recommended for adults who travel to areas of high or intermediate endemicity (Figure 1), men who have sex with men, people with underlying chronic liver disease, and users of injection drugs.

Passive immunization, in the form of pooled human anti-HAV immunoglobulins (IG; IGIM; GamaSTAN), can be given to patients who have been exposed to HAV. HAV IG is 80% effective in preventing HAV infection if given within 2 weeks after exposure, and a single intramuscular dose of 0.02 mL/kg confers protection for 3 to 5 months. Although the concurrent administration of HAV IG with the first dose of anti-HAV vaccine somewhat reduces the immunogenicity of the vaccine, patients develop antibody levels well above those considered to be protective. There are growing data suggesting that vaccination is as effective as HAV IG for postexposure prophylaxis.

Hepatitis E Virus

Hepatitis E virus (HEV) is an enterically transmitted RNA virus that causes an acute, self-limited hepatitis which varies in severity

---

[2]Not available in the United States.

Figure 1. Prevalence of hepatitis A virus, by country, 2006. (From http://wwwn. cdc.gov/travel/yellowBookCh4-HepA.aspx [accessed June 30, 2009].)

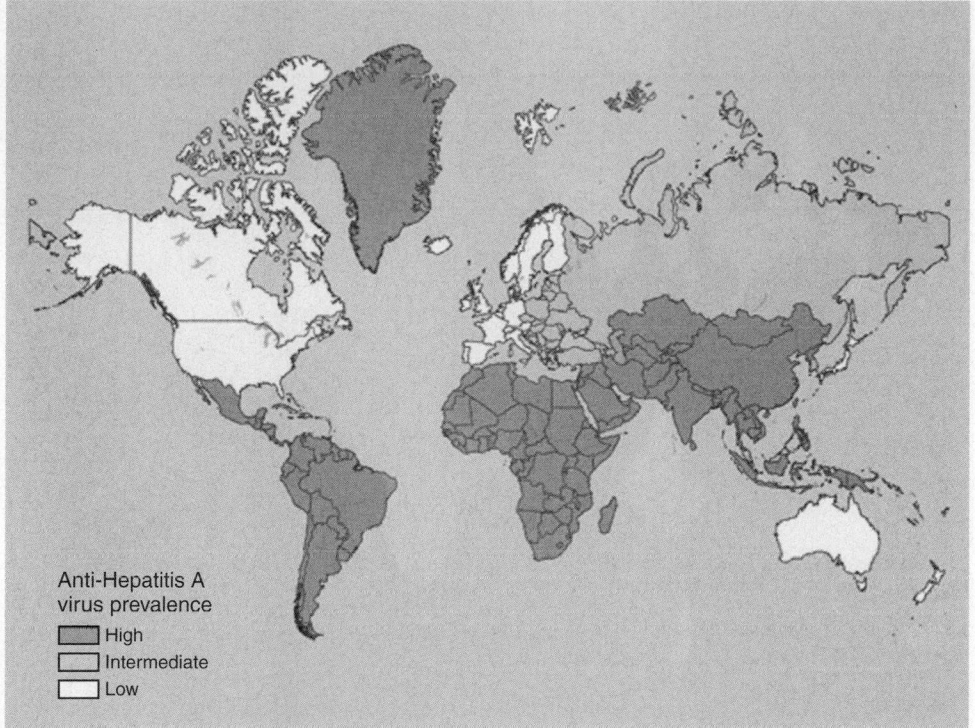

Anti-Hepatitis A virus prevalence

- High
- Intermediate
- Low

from an asymptomatic infection to acute liver failure. Its genome consists of a single, positive-stranded RNA that encodes several structural and nonstructural proteins using overlapping open reading frames. As with HAV, there are multiple genotypes but only one serotype. Major protection epitopes are common to all HEV isolates, and exposure to one strain confers immunity to all strains.

Epidemiology

Geographically, endemic regions of high HEV prevalence include Central America, Africa, the Middle East, Southeast Asia, and India. In nonendemic regions, HEV accounts for fewer than 1% of reported cases of acute viral hepatitis, and most of these occur in patients who have recently traveled to endemic areas.

Diagnosis

The diagnosis of HEV is made by serologic detection of anti-HEV IgM and IgG antibodies. Anti-HEV IgM is the hallmark of acute HEV infection. Anti-HEV IgM is usually undetectable by 6 months after infection. Anti-HEV IgG appears during the convalescent phase and is a serologic marker for past infection.

Natural History

Infection with HEV is typically a self-limited disease, and patients are often anicteric. An incubation period of 2 to 8 weeks is followed by a classic prodromal phase. The symptoms usually resolve within 6 weeks. For reasons that are not well understood, women in the second and third trimesters of pregnancy are at risk for a more severe clinical course. Mortality due to acute liver failure from HEV ranges from 20% to 25% in pregnant woman.

Treatment

There is no specific treatment for HEV infection; therapy is strictly supportive. There are currently no commercially available vaccines for HEV in the United States. China's State Food and Drug Administration approved a hepatitis E vaccine in 2012: HECO-LIN (Xiamen Innovax Biotech).[2] Monoclonal antibodies against HEV have been produced and have proved effective for protecting nonhuman primates from HEV infection, but these preparations are not yet commercially available.

Hepatitis B Virus

Hepatitis B virus (HBV) is a partially double-stranded DNA virus in the Hepadnaviridae family with a 3200 base pair genome that

[2]Not available in the United States.

uses multiple overlapping reading frames to encode surface, core, polymerase, and X proteins. Proteins of clinical importance include hepatitis B surface antigen (HBsAg), hepatitis B core antigen (HBcAg), and hepatitis B e antigen (HBeAg). Serum HBsAg is a marker of HBV infection, and HBeAg is a marker of active viral replication.

Epidemiology and Mode of Transmission

HBV infects an estimated 1.25 million people in the United States and 460 million people globally. Areas with a low prevalence of HBV (<2%) include North America, western and northern Europe, Australia, New Zealand, and southern South America; all other parts of the world have an intermediate prevalence (2%–8%) or high prevalence (>8%) in the general population (Figure 2). Alaska is the only region in the United States considered to have a high prevalence of HBV, with a rate of 6.4% in the native population.

HBV is transmitted more efficiently than either HCV or HIV. The likelihood of transmission increases with the level of HBV DNA in serum. It is transmissible through perinatal, sexual, or percutaneous exposure; close person-to-person contact with open cuts and sores; and sharing of household items such as razors and toothbrushes. In high-prevalence areas, HBV is most often vertically transmitted. In the United States, the route is primarily horizontal; sexual transmission accounts for approximately 30% of cases.

In 2008, the CDC significantly expanded its recommendations for screening for chronic HBV (Box 1) to include all persons from intermediate-prevalence areas in addition to those from areas of high prevalence. Those recommendations also now include patients who require treatment with immunosuppressive medications.

Diagnosis

The presence of HBsAg in serum is the hallmark of infection with hepatitis B. Patients who recover from hepatitis B clear the HBsAg and develop an antibody to it, HBsAb. The presence of HBsAg for longer than 6 months indicates chronic HBV infection. Hepatitis B core antibody (HBcAb) is found in patients with both acute and chronic HBV. The acute illness is marked by the presence of HBcAb of the IgM class, whereas patients with chronic disease have HBcAb of the IgG class.

Appropriate testing for patients with suspected acute hepatitis B includes HBsAg, HBcAb IgM, HBeAg, and HBV DNA. Appropriate testing for patients with suspected chronic HBV includes

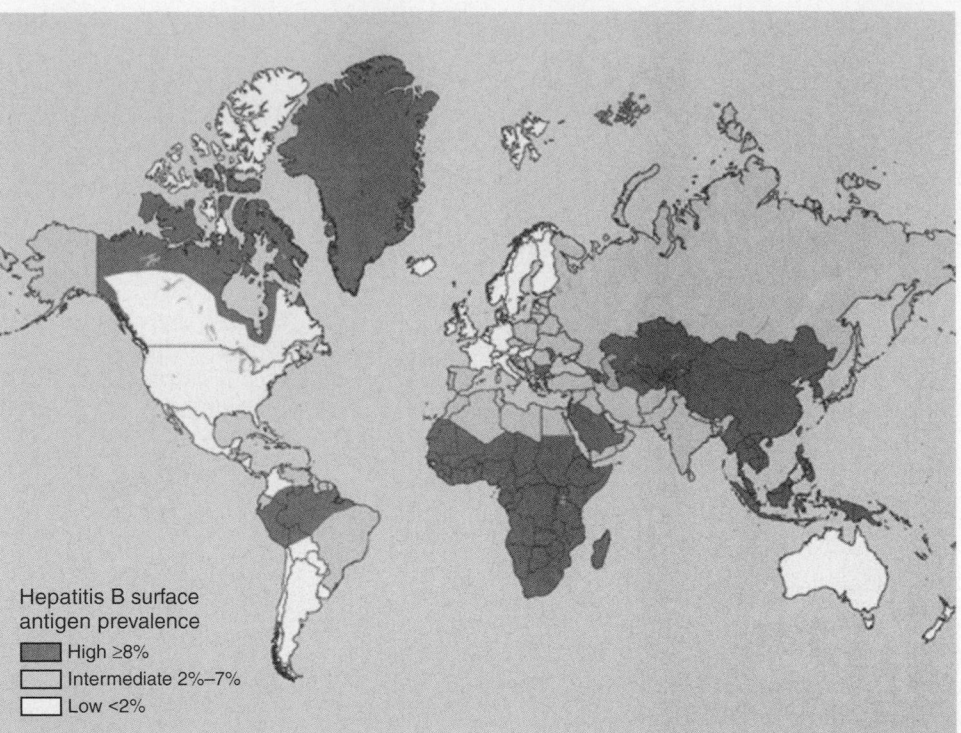

Figure 2. Prevalence of chronic hepatitis B virus infection, by country, 2006. (From http://wwwn.cdc.gov/travel/yellowBook Ch4-HepB.aspx [accessed June 30, 2009].)

Hepatitis B surface antigen prevalence
- ☐ High ≥8%
- ☐ Intermediate 2%–7%
- ☐ Low <2%

Box 1 — Populations for Whom Screening for Chronic Hepatitis B Virus Infection Is Recommended

- Persons born in areas with intermediate or high disease prevalence (>2%)*
- U.S.-born persons who were not vaccinated at birth and have parents from areas of high disease prevalence
- Injection-drug users*
- Men who have sex with men*
- Persons who require immunosuppressive therapy*
- Persons with unexplained elevation of the serum aminotransferases*
- Hemodialysis patients
- Pregnant women
- Infants born to HBsAg-positive mothers
- Household, needle-sharing, or sex contacts of HBsAg-positive persons
- Persons infected with the human immunodeficiency virus
- Persons who are the source of blood or body fluid exposures who might require postexposure prophylaxis

Abbreviation: HBsAg = hepatitis B virus surface antigen.

From Recommendations for identification and public health management of persons with chronic hepatitis B virus infection. MMWR Morb Mortal Wkly Rep 2008;57(RR08):1–20. Available at http://www.cdc.gov/mmwr/preview/mmw rhtml/rr5708a1.htm (accessed June 30, 2009).

*New recommendations.

HBsAg, HBcAb, and HBsAb. Patients found to have chronic HBV should undergo additional testing to assess their viral replication status by checking the levels of HBV DNA, HBeAg, and hepatitis B e antibody (HBeAb). This information allows the physician to determine whether a patient with chronic HBV is a candidate for antiviral therapy.

Natural History

Symptoms of acute HBV infection appear after an incubation period that ranges from 60 to 180 days. The presentation of acute HBV ranges from asymptomatic disease to acute liver failure. Markers of infection and viral replication—HBsAg, HBeAg, and HBV DNA—appear approximately 6 weeks after exposure. Their appearance is followed shortly by a rise in serum aminotransferases;

the serum alanine aminotransferase (ALT) level is greater than the serum aspartate aminotransferase (AST) level, and both are generally higher than 500 U/L. During this time, anti-hepatitis B core antibody (HBcAb) of the IgM class, the only marker of acute infection, appears and may persist for many months.

Aminotransferase levels correspond well with the degree of necroinflammation. The liver injury results from a cytotoxic T lymphocyte–induced apoptosis of virally infected hepatocytes. Acute liver failure occurs when the severity of the injury results in insufficient residual hepatic mass and function. Patients who clear the virus have normalization of aminotransferases by 4 months, followed by a slower resolution of hyperbilirubinemia. The likelihood of progression to chronicity (defined as persistence of HBsAg for >6 months) depends on the age at exposure. Whereas 90% of those perinatally infected progress to chronic infection, this rate decreases to 20% to 50% in those infected between age 1 to 5 years, and is less than 5% in persons infected with HBV as an adult.

It is useful to conceptualize the natural history of chronic HBV infection as a spectrum encompassing an immunotolerant stage, an immunoactive stage, an inactive carrier stage, a resolution stage, and an e antigen–negative chronic hepatitis (Figure 3). This is particularly useful in patients infected via vertical transmission.

In addition to the testing needed to assess viral replication, the serum albumin level and prothrombin time should be checked to assess synthetic function, and a complete blood count should be performed to assess for thrombocytopenia and leukopenia, which are potential indicators of hypersplenism. Careful interpretation of these data allows proper placement of patients with chronic HBV on the natural history continuum and identifies patients who are candidates for therapy.

The immunotolerant stage of disease is characterized by very high HBV DNA levels, normal aminotransferases, and no hepatic necroinflammation. These patients are not currently thought to be candidates for therapy. At an undefined and variable point in time, these immunotolerant patients progress to the immunoactive stage, which is characterized by high serum HBV DNA levels, elevated aminotransferases, and hepatic necroinflammation. They are then at increased risk for disease progression and hepatocellular carcinoma and are candidates for therapy.

The next transition is from the immunoactive stage to the inactive carrier stage; this occurs spontaneously at a rate of 8% to 12% per year. The inactive carrier stage is marked by HBeAg seroconversion (i.e., loss of HBeAg and development of HBeAb). This

Figure 3. Natural history of chronic hepatitis B. *Abbreviations:* ALT = alanine aminotransferase; eAb = hepatitis B e antibody; eAg = hepatitis B e antigen; HBsAb = hepatitis B surface antibody; HBsAg = hepatitis B surface antigen; HBV = hepatitis B virus; HCC = hepatocellular carcinoma. (Adapted from Pratt DS: Evaluation and management of hepatitis B virus infection. J Clin Outcomes Manage 2008;15:147–53.)

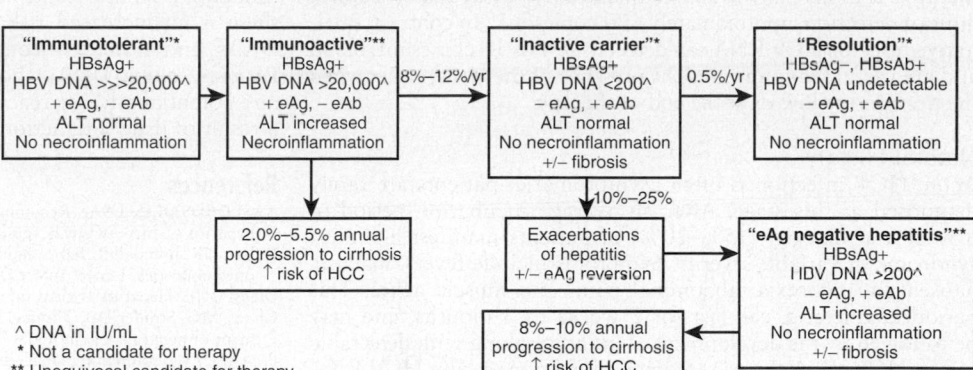

event carries with it a number of beneficial effects, including a significant reduction in serum HBV DNA levels, resolution of necroinflammation, prevention of histologic progression, reduced risk of hepatocellular carcinoma, and decreased mortality.

Patients in the inactive stage require continued attention, because 10% to 25% will have flareups of hepatitis, with or without e-antigen reversion. The rate of reversion for patients who achieve e-antigen seroconversion through treatment is higher than for those who seroconvert spontaneously. Patients in the inactive carrier stage can develop precore or core promoter mutations that allow for viral replication in the absence of e antigen. Like patients in the immunoactive stage, these patients with e-antigen–negative hepatitis have elevated serum aminotransferases levels and necroinflammation on liver biopsy but lower levels of serum HBV DNA, compared with those in the immunoactive stage. They are at increased risk for histologic progression and for hepatocellular carcinoma and are candidates for therapy.

Patients in the inactive stage move into the resolution stage at a rate of 0.5% per year. The resolution stage is marked by surface antigen seroconversion (i.e., loss of surface antigen and development of surface antibody).

Treatment

Seven therapies approved by the U.S. Food and Drug Administration (FDA) for the treatment of HBV:

- Interferon: interferon alfa-2b (Intron A) and pegylated interferon alfa-2a (Pegasys)
- Nucleoside analogues: lamivudine (Epivir-HBV), telbivudine (Tyzeka), and entecavir (Baraclude)
- Nucleotide analogues: adefovir (Hepsera) and tenofovir (Viread)

The interferons are prescribed for a defined period (48 weeks), whereas the nucleoside and nucleotide analogues are continued until a specific end point of therapy is reached. The end point of therapy in immunoactive patients is loss of HbeAg and development of HbeAb, which is generally associated with sustained viral suppression. In HBeAg-negative patients, no such marker of treatment success exists, and there is a high likelihood of relapse when therapy is discontinued. These patients are usually treated indefinitely or until surface antigen seroconversion occurs.

Hepatitis D Virus

The hepatitis D virus (HVD) is a subviral particle composed of a single-stranded RNA genome complexed with hepatitis D antigen (HDAg) and enclosed in an outer lipoprotein envelope derived from HBsAg. It is believed that HDV uses some of the same pathways for attachment and entry into host cells as HBV; HDV infection requires the presence of HBV for infectivity. Immunity to HBV also protects against infection with HDV.

Epidemiology

HDV is a blood-borne pathogen with the same modes of transmission as HBV. Co-infection occurs when an individual is infected with both HBV and HDV at the same time. In contrast, HDV infection of a chronically HBV-infected individual is referred to as superinfection and carries a much higher risk of precipitating

fulminant hepatic failure. Chronic carriers of both HBV and HDV tend to have more rapid progression of liver disease, compared to those infected with HBV alone. It is estimated that 20 million HBV-infected people also have chronic HDV.

Diagnosis

HDV elicits specific IgM and IgG antibody responses. Anti-HDV IgM is the only specific marker of acute HDV infection, although assays for IgM detection are not in clinical use in the United States. High titers of anti-HDV IgG often characterize chronic infections, but can also be seen in patients with prior infection, and therefore are not useful in distinguishing carriers from those who have cleared the virus. HDV RNA detection via polymerase chain reaction is commercially available in the United States and has a lower limit of detection (10 copies per milliliter). The diagnosis of HDV infection also requires evidence of concurrent HBV infection, and the presence of anti-HBV IgM suggests acute co-infection.

Natural History

HDV infection can produce a broad spectrum of liver injury, ranging from an asymptomatic carrier state to acute liver failure.

Treatment

The goal of treatment is suppression of HDV replication. The only drug shown to be of benefit in treating chronic HDV is interferon-alfa.[1] However, although interferon-alfa is capable of suppressing viral replication, its antiviral effect is not sustained after withdrawal of therapy.

Hepatitis C Virus

Hepatitis C virus (HCV) is a single minus-strand RNA virus of 9.6 kb whose genome encodes a core protein, envelope proteins, and several nonstructural proteins.

Epidemiology

Almost 170 million people are chronically infected with HCV worldwide. In the United States, there are an estimated 3.2 million individuals chronically infected, although the number of new cases per year has appreciably declined since 1990. In 2012 the CDC expanded its recommendations for screening for chronic HCV to include a one-time screening test for all individuals born between 1945 and 1965—the so-called Baby Boomers.

Diagnosis

The initial test in diagnosing HCV infection is the presence of anti-HCV antibodies. The current serologic test uses a combination of the core protein and several nonstructural proteins in an immunoassay that can detect reactive antibodies within 4 to 10 weeks of infection. As a screening test, the detection of anti-HCV antibodies is very sensitive, and it is estimated that only 0.5% to 1.0% of cases will be missed in a low-prevalence population. HCV RNA is used to confirm positive serologic testing and to assess the response to therapy. Measurement of HCV RNA can be either quantitative or qualitative. The quantitative assay is best for determining large changes in viral load and is therefore useful for monitoring the response to

[1]Not FDA approved for this indication.

Acute and Chronic Viral Hepatitis

therapy; commercially available quantitative assays have a lower limit of detection, approximately 600 copies/mL. In contrast, qualitative tests for HCV RNA can detect as few as 10 copies/mL blood and are useful for confirming the presence of the virus, either when the titer is very low or at the end of therapy.

Natural History

Acute HCV infection is often asymptomatic; patients are rarely diagnosed at this stage. After an average incubation period of 6 weeks, a minority (15%–20%) of patients manifest a clinical syndrome of variable severity. Symptoms include fevers, malaise, nausea and anorexia, abdominal pain, and muscle aches. This period is anicteric, can last for 2 weeks to 3 months, and may be followed by the development of jaundice along with detectable serum HCV RNA. In asymptomatic infection, serum HCV RNA and aminotransferase elevations are usually detectable within 1 to 3 weeks of infection, and anti-HCV antibody becomes positive 3 weeks to 5 months after acute infection.

In approximately 30% of patients, acute HCV infection is self-limited and is followed by the resolution of aminotransferase elevations and disappearance of serum HCV RNA. Most patients who spontaneously clear HCV do so within 12 weeks after infection. Patients who do not clear the acute infection progress to chronic HCV infection, which is most often characterized by an asymptomatic elevation of serum aminotransferases. Approximately 30% of patients with chronic HCV infection have normal ALT levels.

Treatment

Treatment algorithms for hepatitis C are evolving rapidly with the recent FDA approval of new direct acting antivirals (DAAs). These new drugs are categorized in four classes according to their mechanism of action.
1. NS5B nucleotide polymerase inhibitor- sofosbuvir (Sovaldi)
2. NS5A protein inhibits- Ledipasvir, ombitasvir, daclatasvir (Daklinza)
3. NS3/4A protease inhibits- Simeprevir (Olysio), paritaprevir
4. NS5B non-nucleoside polymerase inhibitor- Dasabuvir

The availability of these highly potent DAAs has resulted in more effective and better tolerated, though expensive, therapy. The treatment algorithms for chronic HCV will continue to evolve as additional DAAs and research become available. The Infectious Diseases Society of America (IDSA) and American Association for the Study of Liver Diseases (AASLD), in collaboration with the International Antiviral Society–USA (IAS–USA), publish Guidance for Hepatitis C Treatment in Adults at their website (www. hcvguidelines.org) which is constantly being updated.

The treatment of patients with chronic HCV is determined by the genotype of the virus. Therapy options for treatment-naïve patients with genotype 1 infection include: 1) Daily combination of sofosbuvir and daclatasvir with or without ribavirin (RBV), 2) Daily fixed-dose combination of ledipasvir/sofosbuvir (Harvoni), 3) Daily fixed-dose combination of paritaprevir/ritonavir/ombitasvir plus twice-daily dasabuvir (Viekira PAK) and RBV (not in genotype 1b infection), 4) Daily simeprevir and sofosbuvir with or without RBV.

Treatment-naïve patients with genotype 2 infection can be treated with: 1) Daily combination of sofosbuvir and daclatasvir, or 2) Daily sofosbuvir and RBV. Treatment options for treatment-naïve patients with genotype 3 infection include: 1) Daily combination of sofosbuvir and daclatasvir with or without RBV, 2) Daily sofosbuvir and RBV plus weekly pegylated interferon alfa-2a (PEG-IFN, Pegasys) if IFN eligible.

Treatment-naïve patients with genotype 4 infection have the following options: 1) Daily fixed-dose combination of ledipasvir/sofosbuvir (Harvoni), 2) Daily fixed-dose combination of paritaprevir/ritonavir/ombitasvir (Technivie) and RBV, 3) Daily sofosbuvir and RBV. An alternative is a daily combination of sofosbuvir and RBV plus weekly pegylated interferon alfa-2a. For treatment-naïve patients with genotype 5 or 6 infection, a daily fixed-dose combination of ledipasvir/sofosbuvir (Harvoni) can be used.

Many of these treatment regimens can also be considered in patients who have failed PEG-INF and RBV treatment. Even though DDAs are well tolerated and effective for most patients, there is an increased risk of significant drug interactions with DAAs and other concomitant medications used by patients. Patients taking DDAs should be monitored regularly to avoid any potential adverse reactions and reduced therapeutic effect as a result of drug interactions.

References
AASLD/IDSA/IAS–USA. Recommendations for testing, managing, and treating hepatitis C. http://www.hcvguidelines.org [accessed 11.09.15].
Dalton HR, Brendall R, Ijaz S, Banks M. Hepatitis E: An emerging infection in developed countries. Lancet Infect Dis 2008;8:698–709.
Dienstag JL. Hepatitis B virus infection. N Engl J Med 2008;359:1486–500.
Ghany MG, Strader DB, Thomas DL, Seeff LB. Diagnosis, management, and treatment of hepatitis C: An update. Hepatology 2009;49:1335–74.
Pratt DS. Evaluation and management of hepatitis B virus infection. J Clin Outcomes Manage 2008;15:147–53.
Wasley A, Fiore A, Bell BP. Hepatitis A in the era of vaccination. Epidemiol Rev 2006;28:101–11.
Wrinbaum CM, Williams I, Mast EE, et al. Recommendations for identification and public health management of persons with chronic hepatitis B virus infection, MMWR Morb Mortal Wkly Rep 2008;57(RR08):1–20. Available at: http://www.cdc.gov/mmwr/preview/mmwrhtml/rr5708a1.htm [accessed June 30, 2009].

ACUTE DIARRHEA

Method of
Tate de Leon, MD

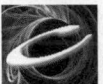

CURRENT DIAGNOSIS

History
- Onset, duration, and frequency of diarrhea
- Related symptoms (fever, abdominal pain, nausea, emesis, bloody stool)
- Current medications, including recent antibiotic use
- Recent sick contacts or hospitalizations
- Recent foreign travel
- Exposure to contaminated water source or undercooked meats and seafood
- Immune status

Physical Examination
- Hydration status
- Abdominal examination

Laboratory Testing
- Acute secretory diarrhea: normally not necessary
- Acute bloody diarrhea: complete blood count, stool culture, consider ova and parasite testing and *Clostridium difficile* evaluation

CURRENT THERAPY

- Symptomatic therapy
- Rehydration: enteral versus parenteral
- Antibiotics (depending on duration, severity, and other risk factors)
  - Emperic therapy
    - Adults
      - Fluoroquinolones
        - Ciprofloxacin (Cipro) 500 mg PO twice daily for 3–7 days
        - Levofloxacin (Levaquin)[1] 500 mg PO four times daily for 3–5 days
    - Children
      - Azithromycin (Zithromax)[1] 5–12 mg/kg PO four times daily for 3–5 days

- **C. difficile**
  - Metronidazole (Flagyl)[1] 500 mg PO every 8 hours for 10–14 days
  - Vancomycin (Vancocin) 125 mg PO every 6 hours for 10 days
- Antidiarrheal medications (if no contraindications such as fever or hematochezia)
  - Loperamide (Imodium) Initial 4 mg PO followed by 2 mg PO with each loose stool. Max 16 mg per day
- Probiotics[2]

---

[1]Not FDA approved for this indication.
[2]Not available in the United States.

Box 1   Clinical History of Acute Infectious Diarrhea

- Description of diarrhea
  - Duration
  - Frequency
  - Presence of blood, pus, in stool
  - Symptoms of fever, tenesmus, dehydration
  - Weight loss
- Other GI symptoms
  - Anorexia
  - Cramping
  - Emesis
  - Nausea
- Previous episodes with similar symptoms
- Ill contacts with similar symptoms
- Recent antibiotic exposure
- Other medication exposure
  - Anticholinergics
  - Antimotility agents
  - Aspirin (ASA)
  - Proton pump inhibitors (PPIs)
- Recent dietary history
  - Shellfish
  - Undercooked meat (chicken)
  - Unsanitary water
  - Animal or reptile contacts
- Travel history
  - Travel to endemic or epidemic areas
- Sexual history
- Vaccination history
- Contact with institutions, e.g., hospitals, nursing homes, day care facilities
- Employment history
- Immune status
  - Presence of HIV
  - Presence of other congenital or acquired immunodeficiencies

Box 2   Physical Examination for Acute Infectious Diarrhea

- Vital signs
- Blood pressure (look for postural changes)
- Heart rate (look for postural changes)
- Respiratory rate
- Temperature
- Weight changes (particularly useful to assess effects of rehydration)
- Cardiovascular examination
  - Volume status
- Respiratory examination
- Rule out hyperventilation (compensatory respiratory alkalosis for metabolic acidosis resulting from dehydration and loss of bicarbonate)
- Abdominal examination
- Focal tenderness
- Guarding
- Hepatosplenomegaly
- Consider rectal examination (look for bloody stool)
- Decreased skin turgor
- Lymphadenopathy
- Rashes

Acute diarrhea in the United States is one of the most common diagnoses in general practice. Acute diarrhea can have a functional definition of a greater number of loose stools from normal lasting less than 14 days. If the episode lasts more than 14 days, it is called persistent diarrhea. If the episode lasts for more than 30 days, it is deemed chronic diarrhea. These episodes may be accompanied by nausea, vomiting, abdominal cramping, other systemic symptoms, and malnutrition. The majority of acute diarrhea cases are self-limited and do not need medical intervention. Most often, these cases are caused by infectious agents such as viruses, bacteria, or parasites. Infection is often spread through contaminated food or drinking water or from person-to-person. Pathogens that cause diarrhea are usually transmitted through a fecal–oral route. The main risk factor for this transmission is poor hand hygiene. Other risk factors include improper food preparation, inadequate food refrigeration, and exposure to contaminated water.

Thorough investigation of a patient with acute diarrhea should include a detailed history, physical examination, and laboratory testing when indicated (Boxes 1 and 2). Acute diarrhea can be classified into two subtypes: secretory diarrhea and inflammatory diarrhea. Determining the subtype of the diarrhea is useful for suggesting the etiology and therefore the management of the diarrhea.

Secretory diarrhea is an electrolyte absorption impairment that leads to profuse, watery diarrhea that contains little or no blood or leukocytes. These episodes can last from a few hours to days. The main concern is dehydration and weight loss if oral intake is not continued. Clinical signs of severe dehydration include lethargy or unconsciousness, dry or sunken eyes, dry mouth, decreased skin turgor, and a history of poor or absent fluid intake.

Inflammatory diarrhea is bloody, usually has leukocytes, and produces less volume. The most common causes are *Salmonella*, *Campylobacter, Shigella, Escherichia coli* O157:H7, and *Entamoeba hystolytica*. The main concerns related to inflammatory diarrhea are intestinal damage, sepsis, and malnutrition. Stool cultures and evaluation for ova and parasite are recommended.

Preventive measures can help reduce the spread of infectious agents. Proper hand hygiene with soap and water, especially after exposure to feces or individuals with acute diarrhea, can help limit the spread of infection. Barrier precautions are an effective adjunct when dealing with the possibility of exposure to feces in a hospital setting. For children, vaccinations have shown to be effective in reducing rotavirus infections. Furthermore, it is imperative to separate diaper-changing areas from food-preparation areas. Proper sanitization with a bleach-based cleaner is recommended. Proper food handling and storage, along with water purification, are important means to help prevent the spread of infectious agents. Probiotics[2] are finding a home in the prevention and treatment of diarrhea. Initial studies have suggested that probiotics are useful in reducing antibiotic-associated diarrhea. Currently, more studies are needed to confirm their usefulness. Prophylactic antibiotics are usually only reserved for possible exposure to traveler's diarrhea.

---

[2]Not available in the United States.

Epidemiology

Worldwide, acute diarrhea still accounts for significant morbidity and mortality. The very young, the very old, and the immunocompromised populations are the most adversely affected. Acute infectious diarrhea is more prevalent in developing countries and among travelers to developing countries. Diarrhea is the second leading cause of death in children under 5 years of age worldwide. The World Health Organization estimates that globally, there are over 1.7 billion cases of acute diarrhea each year and attributes 760,000 deaths to it annually. The majority of these deaths are in children who are younger than age 5 and live in developing countries. In the United States, foodborne infectious diarrhea accounts for approximately 325,000 hospitalizations and 5000 deaths each year.

Etiology and Treatment

The precise cause of acute diarrhea is usually not found. Causes can be both infectious and noninfectious. Noninfectious causes can include medications, food allergies, and other gastrointestinal diseases. In general, clinical investigation of acute infectious diarrhea is more useful in identifying consequences of diarrhea, such as dehydration, than it is in revealing the precise etiology. Most cases of diarrhea are likely viral, as indicated by negative stool culture results in most studies. Severe cases of diarrhea tend to be a result of bacterial infection. The most common pathogens for bacteria-induced diarrhea is discussed below. To date, the optimal strategy for obtaining stool cultures has not been ascertained. It is thus reasonable to treat the patient symptomatically for several days before obtaining a stool culture for mild to moderate cases because most cases of diarrhea are self-limited. The clinician should take into consideration individual comorbidities, immune status, the presence of severe or bloody diarrhea, underlying inflammatory bowel disease, and occupation (food handlers, day care employment, etc.) as possible indications for stool evaluation.

Bacteria
Campylobacter

Campylobacter is a common cause of diarrhea in the United States. The pathogen is often spread by consumption of undercooked meat and poultry. Symptoms may present 2 to 5 days after exposure and last up to 1 week. The patient presents with diarrhea (possibly bloody), abdominal pain, nausea, vomiting, and fever. Stool cultures are needed for a definitive diagnosis. Prevention includes thoroughly cooking all meat products, good hand and utensil hygiene before preparing foods, and avoiding unpasteurized milk. The treatment for severe *Campylobacter* diarrhea includes azithromycin (Zithromax)[1] and ciprofloxacin (Cipro), although resistance to fluoroquinolones is growing. Antimicrobial susceptibility testing is required for specific resistance. Positive stool cultures should be reported to the local health department. *Campylobacter* infections have been linked to both rheumatoid arthritis and also Guillain-Barré syndrome.

Clostridium difficile

C. difficile is the organism of antibiotic-associated colitis. Antibiotics disrupt the normal flora of the GI tract, which in turn provides a window of opportunity for *C. difficile* to produce toxins and flourish. The most frequent antibiotics implicated are clindamycin (Cleocin), fluoroquinolones, and beta-lactam antibiotics. *C. difficile* is treated with oral metronidazole[1] (Flagyl 500 mg PO every 8 hours for 10–14 days) and vancomycin (Vancocin 125 mg PO every 6 hours for 10 days). The diagnosis is confirmed with either polymerase chain reaction (PCR), enzyme immunoassay, or anaerobic culture. Endoscopy and biopsy can also be obtained if there is a high clinical suspicion for *C. difficile* with negative laboratory results, or if the patient failed to respond to antibiotic treatment.

---

[1]Not FDA approved for this indication.

E. coli

E. coli are a large and versatile group of pathogens that can cause widespread disease and affect multiple organ systems. *E. coli* is a normal part of the normal flora of both human and animal digestive tract. Certain *E. coli* strains can cause acute diarrhea. Pathogenic strains include enterotoxigeneic *E. coli* (ETEC), enteropathogenic *E. coli*, enteroaggregative *E. coli*, enteroinvasive *E. coli*, diffusely adherent *E. coli*, and enterohemorrhagic *E. coli* (EHEC may also be referred as Shiga toxin-producing *E. coli* or verocytotoxin-producing *E. coli*). The two most common and notorious strains are ETEC and EHEC. ETEC is a major cause of traveler's diarrhea and diarrhea in children of developing countries. EHEC has led to high-profile outbreaks of diarrhea as a result of contaminated meats.

ETEC is a type of *E. coli* that produces toxins that stimulate the intestines to secrete excessive fluid, thus producing diarrhea. ETEC produces two different toxins: heat-stabile toxin and heat-labile toxin. Both types of toxins produce similar illnesses. Contaminated food and water is the usual source of infection. Although stool culture is needed for definitive diagnosis, ETEC infections are usually diagnosed on history and clinical symptoms. Symptoms usually appear after 1 to 2 days after exposure and may last from 5 to 7 days. Most cases of ETEC diarrhea are treated symptomatically with adequate rehydration alone. Oral rehydration salts may be used and purchased over the counter to help address electrolyte losses. Both bismuth compounds (e.g., Pepto-Bismol) and antimotility agents (e.g. loperamide [Imodium]) can help reduce severity of symptoms; they both may prolong the time the body takes to clear the toxin. Antibiotics are reserved for moderate to severe disease. The most common effective antibiotics include fluoroquinolones. Antibiotics can shorten the duration of symptoms but are usually not required.

EHEC is a strain of *E. coli* that produces a Shiga toxin. The toxin acts on vascular endothelium of small vessels of multiple organ systems. The toxin causes the breakdown and hemorrhage of the endothelium. When the toxin affects the vascular endothelium of the digestive tract, it causes bloody diarrhea. The pathogen often invades the kidney and lungs. Sequelae of EHEC infection include hemorrhagic diarrhea, hemolytic uremic syndrome, and thrombotic thrombocytopenic purpura. *E. coli* O157 is the most common stain of EHEC. The infection is spread via the oral–fecal route, which includes consumption of contaminated food, unpasteurized milk and cheeses, and unsanitary water. Good hand hygiene is imperative. Symptoms usually appear 3 to 4 days after exposure and may last as long as 10 days. Positive stool cultures should be reported to the local health department. Supportive treatment, including rehydration, is the cornerstone of treatment. Antibiotics are contraindicated because of evidence of increased Shiga toxin release and thus increased risk of hemolytic uremic syndrome.

Salmonella

Salmonella is the most common foodborne cause of diarrhea in the United States. It is associated with ingestion of infected poultry, eggs, and milk products. *Salmonella* can also be transmitted from pets, especially reptiles. Stool cultures are required for definitive diagnosis. Fluoroquinolones remain the antibiotic of choice, although sensitivities will guide antibiotic usage.

Shigella

Shigella is the pathogen that causes dysentery and is a major cause of morbidity in developing countries. Dysentery usually presents as high fever, abdominal cramping, and bloody diarrhea. Positive stool cultures usually warrant treatment with fluoroquinolones.

Vibrio

Vibrio cholera is endemic to developing countries. Symptoms usually present 1 to 3 days after exposure. Symptoms usually include profuse watery diarrhea (rice-water stools), abdominal cramping, and vomiting. Fever is infrequent. Rehydration with appropriate electrolyte replacement is paramount. Antibiotics can be an adjunct to rehydration and include fluoroquinolones and tetracycline at 500 mg PO every 8 hours for 3 days.

Yersinia

Yersinia enterocolitica infections are less common. Symptoms include diarrhea, fever, abdominal pain, and vomiting. Stool cultures are needed to confirm the diagnosis.

Viruses

Viral pathogens are likely responsible for the majority of gastroenteritis in the United States. Given the transient nature and characteristic symptoms, the specificity of the exact virus is not usually obtained. The most common viral etiologies tend to be adenovirus, rotavirus, norovirus, and astrovirus. Rotavirus tends to affect infants and children from 3 to 36 months of age, resulting in a spectrum of disease from asymptomatic shedding to severe gastroenteritis. Vaccination has played an important role in decreasing the cases of rotavirus infections.

Norovirus (i.e., Norwalk virus) is responsible for many high-profile outbreaks in daycares, cruise ships, and hospitals. Norovirus can be easily transmitted from person to person, from contact of contaminated surfaces of from exposure to contaminated food or water. Symptoms present 1 to 3 days after exposure. Symptoms include fever, explosive vomiting, and diarrhea. PCR testing can confirm the diagnosis but is not usually necessary unless there seems to be an outbreak.

Parasite

Entamoeba histolytica, Cryptosporidium, Giardia, and *Cyclospora spp.* are the most common parasitic or protozoal infections that cause diarrhea. Protozoa infections are even less common. It is usually not cost-effective to evaluate for ova and parasites unless there are specific indications, such as a history of immunocompromise, exposure to day care centers, or history of exposure to contaminated water. Multiple stool samples are needed if there are concerns of parasite infection resulting from possible intermittent shedding. *E. histolytica* can cause amoebic dysentery and lead to bloody diarrhea. Microscopy, antigen testing, and serology are all possible tests for diagnosis. Parasitic infections are usually treated with metronidazole (Flagyl), tinidazole (Tindamax 2 g PO four times daily for 1–3 days) or albendazole[1] (Albenza 400 mg PO four times daily for 5 days).

Traveler's Diarrhea

Traveler's diarrhea is common to individuals from developed countries traveling to developing countries. Episodes can be caused by bacteria, viruses, and parasites. The most common pathogen is *E. coli* (ETEC). Travelers should choose their food and water sources carefully. Water purification and avoiding foods prepared with contaminated water is useful. Prolonged or other symptoms such as fever or bloody stool should be further investigated.

Treatment

Fluid and electrolyte replacement are the most important therapies for acute diarrhea. The route of administration depends on the severity of the dehydration. For mild cases of diarrhea in a normally healthy individual, adequate oral intake of juices, soups, and electrolyte-infused water can be sufficient. For severe dehydration, IV fluids or oral rehydration therapy with isotonic electrolyte solutions may be needed. Oral hydration is preferred over IV fluids if possible. IV fluids are more expensive and less practical then oral rehydration. The World Health Organization has a lower-osmolarity oral rehydration solution (ORS), which is very effective in reducing stool volume and the need for switching to IV therapy in children. A number of effective ORSs are also available over the counter, including Pedialyte and Rehydralyte. IV fluids, including normal saline and lactated ringers, are indicated in severe dehydration or in patients who cannot tolerate oral fluid intake.

Antimicrobial agents have a secondary role in treatment of acute diarrhea. Given the fact that most cases of diarrhea are mild, self-limited, and caused by nonbacterial pathogens, antibiotics should be used sparingly. Antibiotic treatment should be used in invasive bacterial infections, traveler's diarrhea, or in patients with immunosuppression. Empirical antibiotics can be appropriate as described above for *Campylobacter* or *C. difficile* infections.

Antidiarrheal medications can be useful to help alleviate symptoms in patients with no other contraindications, such as fever or bloody diarrhea. Loperamide (Imodium initial 4 mg PO followed by 2 mg PO with each loose stool, maximum 16 mg per day) decreases intestinal peristalsis and facilitates intestinal absorption. Bismuth (Pepto-Bismol) is less effective. Bismuth produces both antisecretory and antimicrobial effects in the GI tract.

References

Centers for Disease Control and Prevention: Division of Foodborne, Waterborne, and Environmental Diseases (DFWED). Available at: http://www.cdc.gov/ncezid/dfwed/a-z.html. Updated April 2013.

Fontaine O, Griffin P, Henao O, et al. Diarrhea, Acute. In: Heymann DL, editor. Control of Communicable Diseases Manual. 19th ed. Washington, DC: American Public Health Association; 2008. p. 179–94.

Guerrant RL, Van Gilder T, Steiner TS, et al. Practice guidelines for the management of infectious diarrhea. Clin Infect Dis 2001;32:331–51.

Singh SK. Diarrhea. In: Andreoli TE, Benjamin IJ, Griggs RC, Wing EJ, editors. Cecil Essentials of Medicine. 8th ed. Philadelphia, PA: WB Saunders; 2010. p. 396–400.

Theilman NM, Guerrant RL. Clinical practice. Acute infectious diarrhea. N Engl J Med 2004;350:38–47.

World Health Organization. Diarrheal disease, Available at: http://www.who.int/mediacentre/factsheets/fs330/en/; 2013, Updated April.

BLEEDING ESOPHAGEAL VARICES

Method of
Cecilio Azar, MD; and Ala I. Sharara, MD

CURRENT DIAGNOSIS

- Endoscopic screening for esophageal varices is recommended in patients with liver cirrhosis.
- Noninvasive predictors of the presence of large varices, such as splenomegaly and thrombocytopenia, have limited accuracy.
- A combination of clinical and endoscopic findings including the Child-Pugh class, size of varices, and the presence of red wale markings correlates with the risk of first bleeding in patients with cirrhosis.
- Measurement of hepatic venous pressure gradient may be the best indicator of risk and severity of bleeding in patients with varices. It is an invasive test and is not widely available or used routinely in practice.

[1]Not FDA approved for this indication.

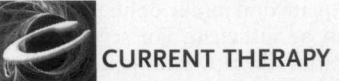

CURRENT THERAPY

- Nonselective β-blockers and endoscopic band ligation are both effective first-line therapy in the primary prophylaxis of esophageal varices.
- The management of acute variceal hemorrhage consists of prompt resuscitation and correction of coagulation abnormalities, followed by endoscopic and pharmacologic therapy with vasoactive agents. Antibiotic prophylaxis is given to decrease the risk of infection and of rebleeding. Transjugular intrahepatic portosystemic shunt (TIPS) is reserved for refractory, uncontrolled, acute variceal bleeding.
- Strategies for secondary prophylaxis of variceal bleeding include endoscopic band ligation, pharmacologic therapy with nonselective β-blockers with or without nitrates, TIPS, and surgical shunts.
- Comparative cost-effectiveness of secondary prophylaxis strategies is unknown but should take into consideration the cost of failed therapy (e.g., rebleeding, shunt revision) and that of treatment related-complications (e.g., encephalopathy, esophageal stricture).

Epidemiology

Bleeding of esophageal varices is a major complication of portal hypertension, usually in the setting of liver cirrhosis, accounting for 10% to 30% of all cases of upper gastrointestinal hemorrhage. More than any other cause of gastrointestinal bleeding, this complication results in considerable morbidity and mortality, prolonged hospitalization, and increased affiliated costs. Variceal bleeding develops in 25% to 35% of patients with cirrhosis and accounts for up to 90% of upper gastrointestinal bleeding episodes in these patients. About 10% to 30% of these episodes are fatal, and as many as 70% of survivors rebleed following an index variceal hemorrhage. Following such events, the 1-year survival is 34% to 80%, being inversely related to the severity of the underlying liver disease.

Treatment of patients with esophageal varices includes preventing the initial bleeding episode (primary prophylaxis), controlling active variceal hemorrhage, and preventing recurrent bleeding after a first episode (secondary prophylaxis). Data on the optimal management of gastric varices are much more limited, and this topic is not covered in this article.

Pathophysiology

Chronic liver disease leading to cirrhosis is the most common cause of portal hypertension. The level of increased resistance to flow varies with the level of circulatory breach and can be divided into prehepatic, hepatic or sinusoidal, and posthepatic. In cirrhosis, several organ systems are involved in the pathophysiology of portal hypertension. At the splanchnic vascular bed level there is marked vasodilatation and increase in angiogenesis, leading to increase in portal blood flow and formation of collateral circulation, such as gastroesophageal varices, along with decrease in response to vasoconstrictors. At the systemic circulation level, there is an increase in cardiac output, decrease in vascular resistance, and hypervolemia. This hyperkinetic syndrome leads to an effective hypovolemia, with a resultant increase in vasoactive factors to maintain a normal arterial blood pressure.

Varices represent portosystemic collaterals derived from dilatation of preexisting embryonic vascular channels, such as those between the coronary and short gastric veins and the intercostal, esophageal, and azygous veins. In the distal esophagus, over an area extending 2 to 5 cm from the gastroesophageal junction, veins are found more superficially in the lamina propria rather than the submucosa. This results in reduced support from surrounding tissues owing to the predominant intraluminal location of these varices and might explain the predilection for bleeding at this site. The opening and dilation of portosystemic collaterals appears to depend on a threshold portal pressure gradient

(measured as hepatic venous pressure gradient [HVPG]) of 12 mm Hg, below which varices do not form. This pressure gradient is necessary but not sufficient for the development of gastroesophageal varices.

Diagnosis

The current consensus states that every patient with liver cirrhosis should undergo an upper endoscopy to detect gastroesophageal varices. The main aim behind screening for gastroesophageal varices is to identify patients requiring prophylactic treatment or further surveillance. Several invasive and noninvasive procedures help in detecting portal hypertension and can, with variable accuracy, predict the presence of gastroesophageal varices. Unfortunately, none are sensitive enough to replace endoscopy. A recent meta-analysis showed that transient elastography may be a useful screening tool for the detection of significant liver fibrosis and associated portal hypertension, but it is not useful at predicting the presence or size of esophageal varices. Endoscopic videocapsule is a new modality introduced for visualizing the esophagus; it allows correct identification of varices in 80% of cases but can have poor accuracy in identifying the presence of hypertensive gastropathy and gastric varices.

Not all esophageal varices bleed; hemorrhage occurs in only 30% to 35% of patients with cirrhosis. Variceal rupture is directly related to physical factors such as the radius, thickness, and elastic properties of the vessel in addition to intravariceal and intraluminal pressure and tension. Endoscopic findings that predict a higher risk of bleeding include larger size of varices and the presence of endoscopic red signs (described as red wale markings) on the variceal wall, indicating dilated intraepithelial and subepithelial superficial veins. A combination of clinical and endoscopic findings, including the Child-Pugh class, size of varices, and the presence or absence of red wale markings, was found to correlate highly with the risk of first bleeding in patients with cirrhosis. Hemodynamic parameters examined as predictors of bleeding include HVPG, azygous blood flow, and direct measurement of intravariceal pressure.

HVPG, calculated by the gradient of wedged and free hepatic vein pressure (normal value, 5 mm Hg), is used most often and provides reliable measurement of portal pressure in patients with cirrhosis. The extent of elevation of HVPG may be the best indicator of risk of bleeding, severity of bleeding, and survival. A rise in pressure in a patient with known varices increases the risk of bleeding, and the extent of portal pressure elevation has an inverse relationship to prognosis after hemorrhage has occurred. In general, however, a linear relationship between the degree of portal hypertension and the risk of variceal hemorrhage or formation of varices does not exist, so this technique cannot be used routinely to identify individual patients at high risk for bleeding.

Treatment

Primary Prophylaxis

The natural evolution of gastroesophageal varices without treatment is characterized by an increase in size from small to large varices, which eventually rupture and bleed. The progression rate ranges from 5% to 30% per year. The incidence of bleeding from small esophageal varices is estimated to be 4% per year, and it is as high as 15% per year for medium to large varices. In a randomized, controlled trial, the nonselective β-blocker timolol (Blocadren)[1] failed to reduce the development of varices or variceal bleeding in patients without varices. Adverse events were more common in the timolol group. Therefore, it is not recommended to start β-blockers in patients who do not yet have esophageal varices.

Based on prospective studies of cirrhotic patients with varices identified at endoscopy and of untreated groups in randomized controlled trials, the risk of bleeding from esophageal varices has been estimated at 25% to 35% at 1 year. Therapy for primary prophylaxis against variceal bleeding (prevention of a first variceal bleeding) is summarized in Table 1.

---

[1]Not FDA approved for this indication.

8 The Digestive System

TABLE 1 Summary of Therapy for Esophageal Varices

	FIRST-LINE THERAPY	COMMENTS	ALTERNATIVE THERAPY	COMMENTS
Primary prophylaxis*	β-Blockers or band ligation	In advanced cirrhosis, the best therapy is unclear (probably band ligation) Transplantation should be considered for these patients		The effectiveness of combined β-blockers and band ligation is unknown Neither TIPS nor sclerotherapy is recommended for primary prophylaxis
Active variceal bleeding	Somatostatin, octreotide (Sandostatin),[1] vapreotide (Octastatin),[5] or terlipressin (Glypressin)[2] *plus* Endoscopic therapy	Vasoconstrictors should be continued for ≥2 days after endoscopic therapy Band ligation is superior to endoscopic sclerotherapy Antibiotic prophylaxis should be initiated	Balloon tamponade TIPS Shunt surgery	Tamponade is indicated primarily as a temporizing measure if first-line treatment fails TIPS is reserved for refractory or recurrent early bleeding but should also be considered when basal HVPG >20 mm Hg Surgery is reserved for patients with compensated liver disease in whom TIPS fails or is not technically feasible
Secondary prophylaxis	β-Blockers ± nitrates *or* Band ligation	The combination of band ligation and β-blockers ± nitrates may be more effective than either alone Nitrates alone are not recommended Patients with advanced liver disease are often intolerant of β-blockers	TIPS Shunt surgery	TIPS is best used after failure of first-line therapy or as a bridge to transplantation in patients with advanced liver disease Shunt surgery is reserved for selected patients with compensated cirrhosis in whom TIPS fails or is not feasible

Abbreviations: HVPG = hepatic venous pressure gradient; TIPS = transjugular intrahepatic portosystemic shunt.
[1]Not FDA approved for this indication.
[2]Not available in the United States.
[5]Investigational drug in the United States.
*Upon documentation of varices, variceal hemorrhage occurs in 25%–30% of patients by 2 years. β-Blockers reduce the risk to 15%–18%, and combination β-blockers plus nitrates reduce the risk to 7.5%–10%.

Pharmacologic Therapy

The general objective of pharmacologic therapy for variceal bleeding is to reduce portal pressure and consequently intravariceal pressure. Drugs that reduce portocollateral venous flow (vasoconstrictors) or intrahepatic vascular resistance (vasodilators) have been used and include β-blockers, nitrates, β_2-adrenergic blockers, spironolactone (Aldactone),[1] pentoxifylline (Trental),[1] molsidomine (Corvaton),[2] and simvastatin (Zocor).[1] Because varices do not bleed at an HVPG less than 12 mm Hg, reduction to this level is ideal, but substantial reductions in HVPG (i.e., by >20%) are also clinically meaningful.

β-Blockers exert their beneficial effect on portal venous pressure by diminishing splanchnic blood flow and consequently gastroesophageal collateral and azygous blood flow. The effectiveness of β-blockers for primary prophylaxis against variceal bleeding has been demonstrated in several controlled trials. Meta-analyses have revealed a 40% to 50% reduction in bleeding and a trend toward improved survival. The estimated overall response rate is 49%, with bleeding rates of 6% in responders and 32% in nonresponders, with a number needed to treat (NNT) of 10.

The nonselective β-blockers, such as propranolol (Inderal)[1] and nadolol (Corgard),[1] are preferred because of the dual benefit of β_1- and β_2-receptor blockade. In the absence of HVPG determination, β-blockers are titrated to achieve a reduction in resting heart rate to 55 beats/min or 25% of baseline. Propranolol is generally given as a long-acting preparation and titrated to a maximum dose of 320 mg/day. Nadolol is initiated at 80 mg daily up to a maximum daily dose of 240 mg. Carvedilol (Coreg)[1] is initiated at 6.25 mg daily and increased if tolerated to 12.5 mg/day. Carvedilol is superior to propranolol at reducing portal hypertension although available data do not allow a satisfactory comparison of adverse events. The portal pressure–reducing effects of β-blockers are not predictable; the resultant reduction in heart rate or the measurement of drug blood levels are not good indicators of response to therapy.

For example, portal venous pressure is reduced in about 60% to 70% of patients who receive propranolol therapy, but only 10% to 30% of these patients show a substantial response (i.e., >20% reduction). Additionally, approximately 20% to 25% of patients have no measurable decline in portal pressure despite increasing dosage of propranolol. Of note, there is increasing evidence that the use of beta-blockers can be deleterious in patients with decompensated liver cirrhosis and refractory ascites (Sersté) or in patients with spontaneous bacterial peritonitis (Mandorfer).

In addition to β-blockers, a number of vasodilators have been investigated in patients with portal hypertension and in animal models of portal hypertension, most notably isosorbide mononitrate (Imdur).[1] Of note, there is increasing evidence that the use of beta-blockers can be deleterious in patients with decompensated liver cirrhosis and refractory ascites or in patients with spontaneous bacterial peritonitis. The exact mechanism of action of nitrates is unclear but is thought to be mediated primarily by reducing intrahepatic resistance and possibly by splanchnic arterial vasoconstriction induced in response to venous pooling and vasodilation in other regional vascular beds. Monotherapy with nitrates is ineffective in primary prophylaxis and can have detrimental effects, particularly in cirrhotic patients with ascites, and should not be used.

The addition of isosorbide mononitrate to β-blockers, however, has been shown to result in an enhanced reduction in portal pressure in humans. In a randomized, controlled trial involving 42 patients with cirrhosis and esophageal varices, a reduction of greater than 20% in HVPG was documented in only 10% in the propranolol group compared to 50% in the combination therapy group. In patients with Child-Pugh class A and B cirrhosis, the addition of isosorbide mononitrate to nadolol has been shown, in a randomized trial, to result in a greater than 50% additional reduction in variceal bleeding rate when compared with nadolol monotherapy (12% versus 29%). However, a large subsequent double-blind, placebo-controlled study failed to confirm these results. Based on the existing

[1]Not FDA approved for this indication.
[2]Not available in the United States.

[1]Not FDA approved for this indication.

evidence, the combination of β-blockers and isosorbide is not recommended in primary prophylaxis.

Endoscopic Therapy

Endoscopic therapies play a prominent role in treatment of esophageal varices. Endoscopic band ligation (EBL) is the endoscopic procedure of choice in the management of esophageal varices. As of 2010, 16 randomized, controlled trials have compared EBL to β-blockers in the primary prevention of variceal bleeding. These studies suffered from significant heterogeneity, and a large number were published in abstract form. Two meta-analyses of these trials showed a slight advantage of EBL over β-blockers in terms of primary prevention of variceal bleeding, but there were no differences in mortality. A recent Cochrane database systematic review found a beneficial effect of band ligation compared to β-blockers in primary prevention of upper gastrointestinal bleeding in adult patients with esophageal varices. Again, there was no difference in mortality.

β-Blockers are cheaper and much easier to administer but are associated with issues of noncompliance and a higher incidence of adverse events (e.g., hypotension, impotence, insomnia) than EBL. However, most of these side effects are easy to manage and none require hospitalization or result in direct mortality. On the other hand, adverse events related to EBL, such as bleeding from band-related ulcers, albeit infrequent, are more significant, often requiring hospitalization and blood transfusion, and may rarely be associated with death.

According to the Baveno consensus conference, nonselective β-blockers should be considered as a first choice for preventing first variceal bleeding in high-risk patients who have not bled, and EBL should be provided for patients with contraindications or intolerance to β-blockers. The recent guidelines by the American College of Gastroenterology (ACG) and American Association for the Study of Liver Diseases (AASLD) recommend using β-blockers in low-risk patients who have medium to large varices but suggest both EBL and β-blockers for high-risk patients as first-line therapy. The optimal primary prophylaxis in patients with decompensated cirrhosis remains unclear and is arguably expedited liver transplantation. The combination of pharmacologic plus endoscopic therapy has been investigated in such patients with conflicting results. In one study, EBL plus β-blockers offered no benefit in terms of prevention of first bleeding when compared to EBL alone. In a more recent study, combination therapy significantly reduced the occurrence of the first episode of variceal bleeding and improved bleeding-related survival in a group of cirrhotic patients with high-risk esophageal varices awaiting liver transplantation.

Management of Acute Variceal Hemorrhage

Variceal hemorrhage is usually an acute clinical event characterized by rapid gastrointestinal blood loss manifesting as hematemesis (which can be massive), with or without melena or hematochezia. Hemodynamic instability (tachycardia, hypotension) is common. Although variceal bleeding is common in patients with cirrhosis presenting with acute upper gastrointestinal hemorrhage, other causes of bleeding, such as ulcer disease, must be considered. Urgent initiation of empiric pharmacologic therapy with vasoactive agents is indicated in situations where variceal hemorrhage is likely. Subsequently, direct endoscopic examination is critical to establish an accurate diagnosis and to provide the rationale for immediate and subsequent therapies. The immediate steps in the management of acute variceal bleeding include: volume resuscitation, prevention of complications, ensuring hemostasis, and initiating measures to prevent early and delayed rebleeding.

Patients with variceal hemorrhage and ascites are at increased risk for bacterial infections, particularly spontaneous bacterial peritonitis. This risk appears to be increased in the setting of uncontrolled hemorrhage or as a result of transient bacteremia following endoscopic sclerotherapy or variceal ligation. Short-term systemic antibiotics (e.g., third-generation cephalosporins or fluoroquinolones for 4–10 days) have been shown to decrease the risk of bacterial infections and to reduce rebleeding as well as mortality in cirrhotic patients with gastrointestinal bleeding.

The role of platelet transfusion or fresh frozen plasma administration has not been assessed appropriately. The use of recombinant activated coagulation factor VII (rFVIIa [Novoseven]),[1] which corrects prothrombin time in cirrhotic patients, has been assessed in two randomized, controlled trials. The first trial showed, in a post hoc analysis, that rFVIIa administration might significantly improve the results of conventional therapy in patients with moderate and advanced liver failure (Child-Pugh B and C) without increasing the incidence of adverse events. A more recent trial tested rVIIa in patients with active bleeding at endoscopy and with a Child-Pugh score 8 points or higher. This trial failed to show a benefit of rVIIa in terms of decreasing the risk of 5-day failure, but it did show improved 6-week mortality. In a small prospective study involving cirrhotic patients with acute variceal bleeding and new portal vein thrombosis identified by positive intra-thrombus enhancement on contrast ultrasonography, the use of low molecular weight heparin after hemostasis is achieved by band ligation was shown to be safe, well tolerated, and effective, with complete recanalization of the portal vein within 2 to 11 days and no recurrence of bleeding.

Pharmacologic Therapy

Pharmacologic therapy can be administered early, requires no special technical expertise, and is thus a desirable first-line option for managing acute variceal hemorrhage. Drugs that reduce portocollateral venous flow (vasoconstrictors) or intrahepatic vascular resistance (vasodilators) or both have been used to achieve this effect. Vasoconstrictors work by decreasing splanchnic arterial flow, and vasodilators are used in combination with vasoconstrictors to reduce their systemic side effects, but they can also exert an added beneficial effect on intrahepatic resistance (see Table 1).

Vasopressin and Terlipressin. Vasopressin (Pitressin)[1] is a nonselective vasoconstricting agent that causes a reduction of splanchnic blood flow and thereby a reduced portal pressure. Vasopressin, which is associated with severe vascular complications, has been largely replaced by other vasoconstrictors such as its synthetic analogue, triglycyl-lysine vasopressin (terlipressin [Glypressin]).[2] Terlipressin has fewer side effects and a longer biological half-life, allowing its use as a bolus intravenous injection (2 mg every 4 hours for the initial 24 hours, then 1 mg every 4 hours for the next 24–48 hours). Terlipressin has been shown in numerous placebo-controlled trials to control bleeding in about 80% of cases and is the only pharmacologic therapy proven, as of 2010, to reduce mortality from acute variceal hemorrhage. In patients with esophageal variceal bleeding, a 24-hour course of terlipressin was shown to be as effective as a 72-hour course when used as adjunct therapy to successful variceal band ligation. Terlipressin is not currently available in the United States.

Somatostatin, Octreotide, and Vapreotide. Somatostatin, a naturally occurring peptide, and its analogues, octreotide (Sandostatin)[1] and vapreotide (Octastatin),[5] stop variceal hemorrhage in up to 80% of patients and are generally considered equivalent to vasopressin (Pitressin), terlipressin (Glypressin), and endoscopic therapy for the control of acute variceal bleeding. Their precise mechanism of action is unclear but might result from an effect on the release of vasoactive peptides or from reduction of postprandial hyperemia. Somatostatin is used as a continuous intravenous infusion of 250 μg/hour following a 250-μg bolus injection. Octreotide is used as a continuous infusion of 50 μg/hour and does not require a bolus injection. Side effects are minor, including hyperglycemia and mild abdominal cramps. The addition of octreotide or vapreotide to endoscopic sclerotherapy or banding improves control of bleeding and reduces transfusion requirements, with no change in overall mortality. A continuous infusion of octreotide or vapreotide is therefore recommended for 2 to 5 days following emergency endoscopic therapy.

---

[1]Not FDA approved for this indication.
[2]Not available in the United States.
[5]Investigational drug in the United States.

Endoscopy

Endoscopic sclerotherapy stops variceal hemorrhage in 80% to 90% of cases. Its drawbacks include a significant risk of local complications including ulceration, bleeding, stricture, and perforation. Rare systemic complications have been reported including bacteremia with endocarditis, formation of splenic or brain abscesses, and portal vein thrombosis. Randomized trials in patients with acute variceal bleeding have shown that EBL is essentially equivalent to endoscopic sclerotherapy in achieving initial hemostasis with lesser complications. These include superficial ulcerations, transient chest discomfort, and, rarely, stricture formation. Erythromycin infusion before endoscopy[1] in patients with acute variceal bleeding has been shown to significantly improve endoscopic visibility and to shorten the duration of the procedure.

Balloon Tamponade

The use of the Sengstaken-Blakemore or Minnesota tube for hemostasis of variceal bleeding is based on the principle of the application of direct pressure on the bleeding varix by an inflatable—esophageal or gastric—balloon fitted on a rubber nasogastric tube. When properly applied, balloon tamponade is successful in achieving immediate hemostasis in almost all cases. However, early rebleeding following balloon decompression is high. Complications of balloon tamponade include esophageal perforation or rupture, aspiration, and asphyxiation from upper airway obstruction. Balloon tamponade is generally not recommended and should largely be reserved for rescue of cases of hemorrhage uncontrolled by pharmacologic and endoscopic methods and as a temporary bridge to more definitive therapy.

Transjugular Intrahepatic Portosystemic Shunt

Treatment with a transjugular intrahepatic portosystemic shunt (TIPS) consists of the vascular placement of an expandable metal stent across a tract created between a hepatic vein and a major intrahepatic branch of the portal system. TIPS can be successfully performed in 90% to 100% of patients, resulting in hemodynamic changes similar to a partially decompressive side-to-side portocaval shunt while avoiding the morbidity and mortality associated with a major surgical procedure. TIPS has been shown to be effective in treating refractory, uncontrolled, acute variceal bleeding. Patients with advanced liver disease and multiorgan failure at the time of TIPS have a 30-day mortality that approaches 100%.

Surgery

Surgery is generally considered in the setting of continued hemorrhage or recurrent early rebleeding—uncontrolled by repeated endoscopic or continued pharmacologic therapy—and when TIPS is not available or is not technically feasible. Surgical options include portosystemic shunting or esophageal staple transection alone or with esophagogastric devascularization and splenectomy (Sugiura procedure). Devascularization procedures may be useful in patients who cannot receive a shunt because of splanchnic venous thrombosis. Regardless of the choice of surgical technique, morbidity is high and the 30-day mortality for emergency surgery approaches 80% in some series. Understandably, rescue liver transplantation is not a practical option in patients with uncontrolled variceal hemorrhage.

Secondary Prophylaxis

Variceal hemorrhage recurs in approximately two thirds of patients, most commonly within the first 6 weeks after the initial episode. Patients with advanced liver disease (MELD [model for end-stage liver disease] score ≥18) have an increased risk of early rebleeding and death. Early rebleeding (within the first 5 days) is reduced by the adjuvant use of octreotide[1] or vapreotide[5]—and possibly terlipressin[2] and somatostatin—after initial endoscopic or pharmacologic control of hemorrhage.

---

[1]Not FDA approved for this indication.
[2]Not available in the United States.
[5]Investigational drug in the United States.

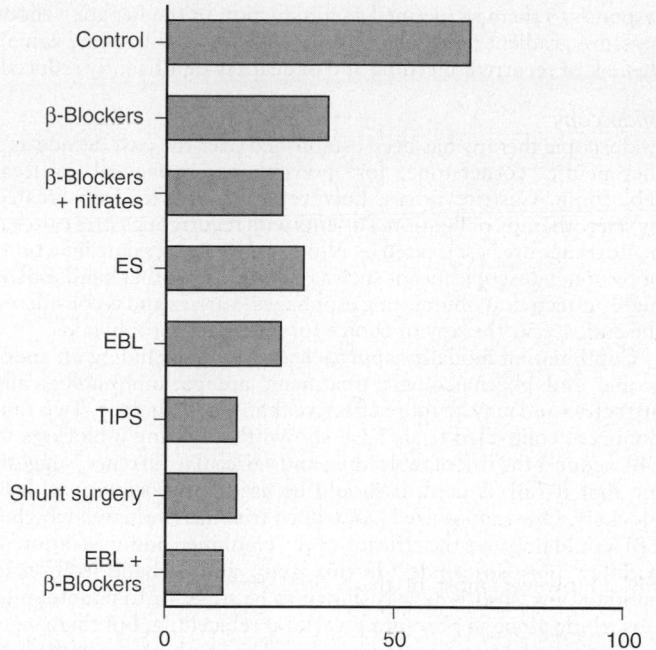

Figure 1. Relative effectiveness of available therapies for preventing recurrent variceal bleeding. The estimates shown are based on the cumulative data available in the literature for recurrent bleeding at 1 year. *Abbreviations:* EBL = endoscopic band ligation; ES = endoscopic sclerotherapy; TIPS = transjugular intrahepatic portosystemic shunt.

The severity of portal hypertension correlates closely with the severity and risk of rebleeding as well as actuarial probability of survival following an index episode. In a cohort of patients presenting with variceal hemorrhage, those with an initial HVPG greater than 20 mm Hg had a 1-year mortality of 64% compared to 20% for patients with lesser elevations in portal pressure. Given the high risk of recurrent hemorrhage and its associated morbidity and mortality, strategies aimed at prevention should be rapidly instituted following the index episode. The choice of preventive therapy should, therefore, take into consideration the efficacy of therapy, the side effects of the selected treatment, the patient's expected survival, and overall cost. Preventive strategies include pharmacologic, endoscopic, and surgical methods and are listed in Table 1. Relative effectiveness of these strategies is shown in Figure 1.

Pharmacologic Therapy

Reducing the portal pressure by more than 20% from the baseline value pharmacologically results in a reduction in the cumulative probability of recurrent bleeding from 28% at 1 year, 39% at 2 years, and 66% at 3 years to 4%, 9%, and 9%, respectively. Although adjustment of medical therapy based on portal pressure measurement would be ideal, HVPG determination might not be readily available, and treatment must be adjusted using empiric clinical parameters. Several randomized, controlled trials, including a meta-analysis, have demonstrated that β-blockers prevent rebleeding and prolong survival. The addition of isosorbide mononitrate[1] to β-blockers appears to enhance the protective effect of β-blockers alone for preventing recurrent variceal bleeding but offers no survival advantage and reduces the tolerability of therapy. A recent randomized controlled trial showed that carvedilol is as effective as the combination of nadolol plus isorsorbide-5 mononitrate in the prevention of gastroesophageal variceal rebleeding, with fewer severe adverse events and similar survival. Compared with either sclerotherapy or endoscopic band ligation, combination medical therapy is superior in reducing the risk of recurrent bleeding in patients with esophageal variceal hemorrhage, primarily in patients with Child-Pugh class A and B cirrhosis. Notably, in patients who show a significant hemodynamic

---

response to therapy (defined as a reduction in the hepatic venous pressure gradient to <12 mm Hg or >20% of the baseline value), the risk of recurrent bleeding and of death is significantly reduced.

Endoscopy

Endoscopic therapy has been established over the past decade as a therapeutic cornerstone for preventing esophageal variceal rebleeding. Gastric varices, however, are not effectively treated by sclerotherapy or ligation. Patients with recurrent gastric variceal hemorrhage are best treated by N-butyl-2-cyanoacrylate injection[1] or by nonendoscopic means such as TIPS. On the other hand, EBL is highly effective at obliterating esophageal varices and is considered the endoscopic therapy of choice for secondary prophylaxis.

Combination modality approaches, usually including an endoscopic and pharmacologic treatment, are pathophysiologically attractive and may be more effective than single therapy. Two randomized, controlled trials have shown that adding β-blockers to EBL reduces the risk of rebleeding and variceal recurrence, suggesting that if EBL is used, it should be used in association with β-blockers. One randomized, controlled trial has evaluated whether EBL could improve the efficacy of the combined administration of nadolol[1] plus isosorbide.[1] In this study, adding band ligation to nadolol plus isosorbide was shown to be superior to nadolol plus isosorbide alone in preventing variceal rebleeding, but there were no significant differences in mortality. The combination of the best endoscopic treatment (EBL) and the best pharmacologic treatment (β-blockers plus isosorbide) may be the best choice in preventing rebleeding but needs further studies for confirmation.

Transjugular Intrahepatic Portosystemic Shunt

Transjugular shunting is more effective than endoscopic therapy for preventing variceal rebleeding but offers no survival benefit. The cumulative risk of rebleeding following TIPS placement is 8% to 18% at 1 year. The trade-off, however, is that TIPS is associated with a higher incidence of clinically significant hepatic encephalopathy (new or worsened portosystemic encephalopathy was noted in about 25% of patients after TIPS). Advanced liver disease is the main determinant of poor outcome following TIPS. Consequently, in patients with advanced liver disease, TIPS is best used as a bridge to liver transplantation.

TIPS, using bare stents, has been compared with surgical shunts in two studies (8 mm portocaval H-graft shunt in one and distal splenorenal shunt in the second). Although the first study showed a significantly lower rebleeding rate in the surgical group, the second and larger trial did not find any differences in rebleeding rates, hepatic encephalopathy, or mortality, but it found a significantly higher reintervention rate in the TIPS group. However, the obstruction and reintervention rates are markedly decreased with the recent use of polytetrafluoroethylene (PTFE)-covered stents. According to these data, TIPS using PTFE-covered stents represents the best rescue therapy for failures of medical and endoscopic treatment.

Surgery

Portosystemic shunt surgery is the most effective means by which to reduce portal pressure. Although effective at eradicating varices and preventing rebleeding, nonselective portocaval shunts are associated with a significant incidence of hepatic encephalopathy, portal vein thrombosis, and occasionally liver failure. Commonly used shunts include the distal splenorenal shunt and the low-diameter (mesocaval or portocaval) interposition shunt. Rates of recurrent bleeding are on the order of 10%, with the highest risk of bleeding occurring in the first month after surgery. Devascularization procedures (i.e., esophageal transection and gastro-esophageal devascularization) are usually considered in patients who cannot receive shunts because of splanchnic venous thrombosis and should be performed only by experienced surgeons. Surgical therapy has been largely supplanted by TIPS.

---

[1]Not FDA approved for this indication.

Cost-Effectiveness of Available Therapies

Data examining the cost of variceal bleeding and the cost-effectiveness of commonly used therapies are limited. The treatment cost of an episode of variceal bleeding has been estimated at $15,000 to $40,000. The cost-effectiveness of diagnostic methods used to guide therapy is unclear. For example, HVPG determination, which can accurately predict pharmacologic response to therapy, is an attractive, although invasive, adjunct in the management of patients with variceal bleeding, but its cost-effectiveness remains in question. Further, screening endoscopy for detecting large varices, while recommended, has not been demonstrated to be cost-effective.

There are areas in which management is controversial and not standardized. For example, given the right expertise, secondary prophylaxis with surgical shunts or TIPS may be more effective than medical or endoscopic therapy in Child-Pugh class A patients. On the other hand, patients with advanced cirrhosis are often intolerant of β-blockers—let alone in combination with nitrates—and therefore the use of combination therapy remains controversial in such patients. Arguably, the preferred treatment for such patients is TIPS as a bridge to early liver transplantation.

Therefore, when choosing a specific treatment plan, the clinician must take into consideration the direct costs of health care utilization, as well as the efficacy and morbidity of therapy. The treatment chosen should be tailored to fit the patient's clinical condition while also taking into account the possibility that the patient's liver disease can progress and thus necessitate transplantation. The cost-effectiveness of various treatment modalities should factor in the cost of failed therapy (e.g., rebleeding, shunt revision) and that of treatment-related complications (e.g., encephalopathy, esophageal stricture).

Summary

Esophageal variceal hemorrhage is a common and devastating complication of portal hypertension and is a leading cause of morbidity and mortality in patients with cirrhosis. Because the clinical outcomes are poor once variceal bleeding has occurred, primary prophylaxis with β-blockers or EBL should be considered in high-risk patients. The treatment of acute variceal hemorrhage is aimed at volume resuscitation and ensuring hemostasis with pharmacologic agents and endoscopic techniques as well as prevention of complications, such as infections by the use of prophylactic antibiotics.

A high risk of rebleeding after an index episode mandates the institution of preventive strategies. Wedge pressure-guided medical therapy may be the preferred mode of secondary prophylaxis in patients with Child Pugh class A or B cirrhosis, but is invasive and not widely available. Patients at high risk for rebleeding, including those with decompensated or advanced liver disease, should be considered for TIPS followed by liver transplantation when applicable. Treatment with a combination of methods is pathophysiologically attractive, but the choice of therapy should ultimately be tailored to fit the patient's clinical condition, risk factors, and prognosis, taking into account issues of risk-to-benefit ratio, compliance, and cost.

References

Azam Z, Hamid S, Jafri W, et al. Short course adjuvant terlipressin in acute variceal bleeding: a randomized double blind dummy controlled trial. J Hepatol 2012;56:819–24.

Bambha K, Kim WR, Pedersen R, et al. Predictors of early rebleeding and mortality after acute variceal haemorrhage in patients with cirrhosis. Gut 2008;57:814–20.

Feu F, Garcia-Pagan JC, Bosch J, et al. Relation between portal pressure response to pharmacotherapy and risk of recurrent variceal haemorrhage in patients with cirrhosis. Lancet 1995;346:1056–9.

Garcia Pagan JC, De Gottardi A, Bosch J. Review article: the modern management of portal hypertension—primary and secondary prophylaxis of variceal bleeding in cirrhotic patients. Aliment Pharmacol Ther 2008;28:178–86.

Garcia-Pagan JC, Feu F, Bosch J, Rodes J. Propranolol compared with propranolol plus isosorbide-5-mononitrate for portal hypertension in cirrhosis. A randomized controlled study. Ann Intern Med 1991;114:869–73.

Gluud LL, Krag A. Banding ligation versus beta-blockers for primary prevention in oesophageal varices in adults. Cochrane Database Syst Rev 2012;8: CD004544.

Laine L, Cook D. Endoscopic ligation compared with sclerotherapy for treatment of esophageal variceal bleeding. A meta-analysis. Ann Intern Med 1995; 123:280–7.

Lo GH, Chen WC, Wang HM, Yu HC. Randomized, controlled trial of carvedilol versus nadolol plus isosorbide mononitrate for the prevention of variceal rebleeding. J Gastroenterol Hepatol 2012;27(11):1681–7.

Mandorfer M, Bota S, Schwabl P, et al. Nonselective b-blockers increase risk for hepatorenal syndrome and death in patients with cirrhosis and spontaneous bacterial peritonitis. Gastroenterology 2014;146:1680–90.

Maruyama H, Takahashi M, Shimada T, Yokosuka O. Emergency anticoagulation treatment for cirrhosis patients with portal vein thrombosis and acute variceal bleeding. Scand J Gastroenterol 2012;47:686–91.

Merkel C, Marin R, Sacerdoti D, et al. Long-term results of a clinical trial of nadolol with or without isosorbide mononitrate for primary prophylaxis of variceal bleeding in cirrhosis. Hepatology 2000;31:324–9.

Moitinho E, Escorsell A, Bandi JC, et al. Prognostic value of early measurements of portal pressure in acute variceal bleeding. Gastroenterology 1999; 117:626–31.

North Italian Endoscopic Club for the Study and Treatment of Esophageal Varices. Prediction of the first variceal hemorrhage in patients with cirrhosis of the liver and esophageal varices: A prospective multicenter study. N Engl J Med 1988;319:983–9.

Polio J, Groszmann RJ. Hemodynamic factors involved in the development and rupture of esophageal varices: a pathophysiologic approach to treatment. Semin Liver Dis 1986;6:318–31.

Poynard T, Cales P, Pasta L, et al. β-Adrenergic-antagonist drugs in the prevention of gastrointestinal bleeding in patients with cirrhosis and esophageal varices. An analysis of data and prognostic factors in 589 patients from four randomized clinical trials. Franco-Italian Multicenter Study Group. N Engl J Med 1991; 324:1532–8.

Sersté T, Melot C, Francoz C, et al. Deleterious effects of beta-blockers on survival in patients with cirrhosis and refractory ascites. Hepatology 2010;52:1017–22.

Sharara AI, Rockey DC. Gastroesophageal variceal hemorrhage. N Engl J Med 2001;345:669–81.

Shi KQ, Fan YC, Pan ZZ, et al. Transient elastography: a meta-analysis of diagnostic accuracy in evaluation of portal hypertension in chronic liver disease. Liver Int 2013;33:62–71.

Sinagra E, Perricone G, D'Amico M, Tiné F, D'Amico G. Systematic review with meta-analysis: the haemodynamic effects of carvedilol compared with propranolol for portal hypertension in cirrhosis. Aliment Pharmacol Ther 2014;39:557–68.

Villanueva C, Minana J, Ortiz J, et al. Endoscopic ligation compared with combined treatment with nadolol and isosorbide mononitrate to prevent recurrent variceal bleeding. N Engl J Med 2001;345:647–55.

CALCULOUS BILIARY DISEASE

Method of
Zachary L. Smith, DO; and Mick S. Meiselman, MD

CURRENT DIAGNOSIS

- True biliary colic is characterized by the abrupt onset and cessation of severe mid-epigastric or, less commonly, right upper quadrant pain.
- Pain commonly starts 1 to 2 hours after eating and can be localized or radiate to the back, right shoulder, or chest.
- The onset of biliary colic commonly occurs during sleep.
- Nausea and vomiting commonly follow the onset of pain.
- Elevations of total and conjugated bilirubin, ALP and GGT with modest elevations in AST and ALT support a suspected diagnosis of choledocholithiasis.
- A normal serum biochemistry profile has a negative predictive value of 97% for ruling out choledocholithiasis.
- Transabdominal ultrasonography is a useful and cost-effective test for diagnosing cholelithiasis; however, it has significantly lower utility for choledocholithiasis.
- For intermediate-risk patients with suspected choledocholithiasis, examination of the common bile duct with magnetic resonance cholangiopancreatography (MRCP) or endoscopic ultrasonography (EUS) is warranted.

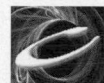

CURRENT THERAPY

- The treatment of choice for symptomatic cholelithiasis is laparoscopic cholecystectomy. Elective laparoscopic cholecystectomy should only be performed for true biliary colic. Vague symptoms such as bloating, dyspepsia, and atypical abdominal pain are not commonly related to gallstone disease and thus are not an indication for gallbladder removal.
- Laparoscopic cholecystectomy should generally take place within 72 hours of presentation for acute cholecystitis in appropriate surgical candidates.
- Laparoscopic cholecystectomy is recommended in pregnant patients with symptomatic cholelithiasis and acute cholecystitis. This is best done by experienced surgeons in the second or early third trimesters.
- Patients who should undergo preoperative ERCP for choledocholithiasis include those with high risk stratification and those deemed intermediate risk in whom a common bile duct stone is identified on MRCP or endoscopic ultrasonography.

Cholelithiasis

Epidemiology

Gallstone disease is common in Western populations, affecting 10% to 15% of adults. It is estimated that 6.3 million men and 14.2 million women United States have gallstones. Although the vast majority of patients remain asymptomatic throughout their lifetime, roughly one third develop symptoms or complications.

Pathophysiology

Gallstones can be categorized based on their composition. Of patients with gallstone disease in the Western world, 80% to 90% have cholesterol stones or cholesterol-predominant stones (mixed stones). Pigment gallstones account for the remaining 5% to 10%. Patients with hemolytic disorders are prone to pigment stone formation, and therefore the correspondence with disorders such as sickle cell anemia, hereditary spherocytosis, and Gilbert's syndrome is high.

Risk Factors

Risk factors for gallstone disease include female gender, age greater than 40 years, white, Latin American, and Native American descent, family history, obesity, rapid weight loss, starvation, total parenteral nutrition, bariatric surgery, diabetes mellitus, and hypertriglyceridemia.

Clinical Manifestations

The typical symptomatic presentation of gallstone disease is biliary colic. This is described as severe pain located in the mid-epigastrium or, less commonly, the right upper quadrant, that begins and ceases abruptly. The pain is typically constant, occurring 1 to 2 hours following a meal, and can either be localized or radiate to the back or right shoulder. Often the onset of pain occurs during sleep. Nausea and vomiting commonly accompany biliary pain, and as with most surgical entities, pain typically precedes the onset of these symptoms. Biliary colic can also manifest as chest pain and is occasionally mistaken for cardiac angina. Prolonged episodes of pain localized to the right upper quadrant often herald cholecystitis rather than biliary colic. A clinical history containing the cardinal features of biliary colic carries a high diagnostic accuracy.

Diagnosis

Transabdominal ultrasonography is the preferred initial imaging test for cholelithiasis. The sensitivity for detecting the presence of gallstones within the gallbladder lumen on ultrasonography is 97%.

Biliary Sludge

Biliary sludge is often diagnosed on transabdominal ultrasonography. It appears as low-amplitude nonshadowing echoes that layer in dependent portions of the gallbladder. The clinical course of biliary sludge varies from patient to patient. Some patients remain asymptomatic and others develop overt biliary colic. A fraction of patients demonstrate resolution of biliary sludge on repeat imaging. Symptomatic biliary sludge should be treated the same as cholelithiasis. Similarly, patients with asymptomatic biliary sludge should be managed expectantly.

Treatment

In patients with symptomatic cholelithiasis, treatment should be aimed at acute pain control and prevention of recurrent episodes. In patients without contraindications, cholecystectomy is the preferred choice for treatment of symptomatic uncomplicated cholelithiasis. This is preferably done via laparoscopy, which offers lower rates of complications and postoperative pain along with better cosmetic results when compared to open cholecystectomy.

Because of the high incidence of cholelithiasis, true biliary colic should be identified before a decision is made to proceed with laparoscopic cholecystectomy. Vague symptoms such as bloating or atypical abdominal pain are not typical of gallstone disease and thus often persist after surgery. In cases of asymptomatic uncomplicated cholelithiasis, elective cholecystectomy is not recommended unless the patient is diabetic or is undergoing an operation such as gastric bypass surgery after which there is an increased risk of gallstone formation.

There is a very limited role for medical management of gallstone disease. Nonoperative management of symptomatic cholelithiasis involves bile dissolution with ursodeoxycholic acid (Actigall). The use of medical therapy is limited based on poor efficacy and high rates of recurrence and thus should be reserved only rarely for nonsurgical candidates.

Analgesia is an important adjunct in the treatment of symptomatic cholelithiasis. In patients with severe symptoms requiring narcotic pain medication, meperidine (Demerol) is preferred over morphine because it has less effect on the sphincter of Oddi. Nonsteroidal antiinflammatory drugs (NSAIDs) are another mainstay of therapy. Parenterally administered ketorolac (Toradol) is perhaps the most commonly used agent for biliary colic in the acute care setting. Studies have shown that NSAIDs are beneficial in the management of pain due to gallstones, and at least one study has suggested that early administration of NSAIDs might decrease the progression to acute cholecystitis.

Complications

Complications that can potentially arise from cholelithiasis include acute cholecystitis, cholangitis, pancreatitis, obstructive jaundice, and, rarely, gallstone ileus.

Choledocholithiasis

Choledocholithiasis often manifests concomitantly with symptomatic gallstone disease and is a finding in 5% to 10% of patients undergoing laparoscopic cholecystectomy for symptomatic cholelithiasis. The work-up for suspected choledocholithiasis combines history, physical examination, laboratory data, and various imaging modalities. If the clinical history and physical examination are suggestive, the clinician should obtain serum liver biochemistry tests including alanine aminotransferase (ALT), aspartate aminotransferase (AST), total and fractionated bilirubin, alkaline phosphatase (ALP), and γ-glutamyl transpetidase (GGT).

The typical pattern of serum biochemistry is one of cholestasis. A conjugated hyperbilirubinemia along with high levels of GGT and ALP are seen often in the setting of modest elevation of the transaminases. ALP is usually elevated out of proportion to the transaminases; however, extreme levels of AST and ALT have been described. Transaminase levels greater than 1000 U/L, although rare in gallstone disease, should not dissuade the clinician from a diagnosis of choledocholithiasis. Serum biochemistries provide

---

Box 1 Proposed Strategy to Assign Risk of Choledocholithiasis in Patients with Symptomatic Cholelithiasis, Based on Clinical Predictors

Predictors of Choledocholithiasis

Very Strong
Common bile duct stone on transabdominal ultrasound
Clinical ascending cholangitis
Total bilirubin > 4 mg/dL

Strong
Dilated common bile duct on transabdominal ultrasound (>6 mm with gallbladder in situ)
Total bilirubin 1.8–4 mg/dL

Moderate
Abnormal liver biochemistry test other than bilirubin
Age older than 55 years
Clinical gallstone pancreatitis

Likelihood of Choledocholithiasis Based on Clinical Predictors
Presence of any very strong predictor: High
Presence of both strong predictors: High
No predictors present: Low
All other patients: Intermediate

From ASGE Standards of Practice Committee, Maple JT, Ben-Menachem T, Anderson MA, et al: The role of endoscopy in the evaluation of suspected choledocholithiasis. Gastrointest Endosc 2010;71:1–9, with permission.

---

the most utility in ruling out common bile duct stones. A normal biochemical profile has a negative predictive value of 97%. Clinical predictors for assessing the likelihood of choledocholithiasis in patients with symptomatic cholelithiasis are listed in Box 1.

Diagnosis

A variety of modalities are available for diagnosing choledocholithiasis. Perhaps the least expensive and most widely available test is transabdominal ultrasound. While the sensitivity for cholelithiasis is quite high with transabdominal ultrasound, identifying stones in the common bile duct (Figure 1) is more difficult. Prospective studies have reported sensitivities ranging from 22% to 55% for detecting common bile duct stones; however, in our clinical experience the sensitivity is much lower. Other indirect

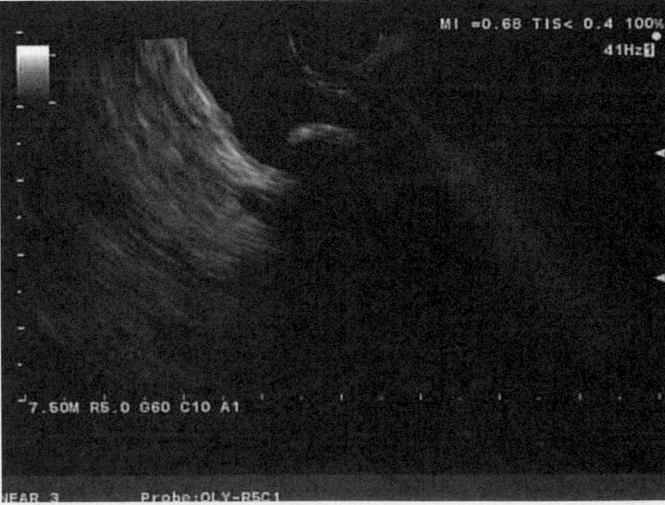

Figure 1. A large gallstone in the common bile duct (CBD) with dilatation of the CBD proximally. The endoscopic ultrasound probe is visualized in the top of the image, and a large cone-shaped shadow is cast distal to the gallstone.

indicators of choledocholithiasis such as common bile duct dilatation (77%–88% sensitivity) can provide additional diagnostic clues. Based on the high false-negative rates for common bile duct stones and dilatation, a negative transabdominal ultrasound cannot rule out choledocholithiasis. CT scan has a higher sensitivity for choledocholithiasis than transabdominal ultrasound. Levels of radiation and cost have limited its use as a first-line diagnostic tool.

Three nonsurgical modalities offer true visualization of the common bile duct with comparable sensitivities: Magnetic resonance cholangiopancreatography (MRCP), endoscopic retrograde cholangiopancreatography (ERCP), and endoscopic ultrasonography (EUS). MRCP has a diagnostic sensitivity of 85% to 92% for detecting choledocholithiasis, and although it is useful for helping determine which intermediate-risk patients would benefit from preoperative ERCP, small and distal common bile duct stones are often missed.

EUS and ERCP are both minimally invasive techniques useful in the diagnosis and management of choledocholithiasis. Owing to the proximity of the extrahepatic bile duct to the proximal duodenum, EUS provides high sensitivity (89%–94%) for detecting common bile duct stones and is especially useful for detecting stones less than 5 mm in diameter. ERCP provides similar diagnostic sensitivity; however, ERCP offers therapeutic capability. Because of the reasonably high risk of complications including pancreatitis (1.3%–15.1%), infection (0.6%–5.0%), gastrointestinal hemorrhage (0.3%–2.0%), and perforation (0.1%–1.1%), ERCP as an initial modality should be reserved for patients who have a high pretest probability for choledocholithiasis and particularly for those with complications such as acute cholangitis or severe pancreatitis.

Research has evaluated the use of ultrasound-guided ERCP with the goal of avoiding unnecessary bile duct cannulation, and reserving its use for therapeutic purposes only. A systematic review from 2009 showed that compared to ERCP alone, the use of EUS avoided unnecessary ERCP in 67.1% of patients in whom no common bile duct stone was identified. As more gastroenterologists become trained in this modality, EUS-guided ERCP might prove to be the preferred diagnostic modality in intermediate-risk patients for the diagnosis and initial therapy of choledocholithiasis.

Treatment

Patients with choledocholithiasis should be treated to avoid recurrent symptoms and development of complications. Stones can be extracted from the common bile duct via ERCP or laparoscopic cholecystectomy with bile duct exploration. Studies have shown similar efficacies without significant differences in morbidity or mortality; however, clinical expertise varies widely with the laparoscopic approach. Ultimately, cholecystectomy should be performed to prevent recurrence in surgical candidates. In patients undergoing laparoscopic cholecystectomy for suspected choledocholithiasis, perioperative management differs based upon the risk stratification of the patient (see Box 1). High risk patients should proceed directly to ERCP before surgery for attempted stone extraction. In intermediate-risk patients, a preoperative MRCP or EUS should be performed, and if the results are positive the patient should undergo ERCP as a prelude to surgery. For suspected choledocholithiasis in low-risk patients, surgery should be performed without further imaging of the common bile duct.

Complications

The two most common adverse complications of choledocholithiasis are gallstone pancreatitis and acute cholangitis. Gallstone pancreatitis develops in 3% to 7% of patients with gallstones and is the most common cause of acute pancreatitis in the United States. The diagnosis and management of acute pancreatitis is discussed in a separate chapter.

Acute cholangitis is caused by obstruction and stasis of the biliary tract with complicating bacterial infection. The syndrome is characterized by fever, jaundice, and abdominal pain, also known as Charcot's triad. Patients who develop hypotension and changes in mental status (Reynold's pentad) have a poorer prognosis.

Elderly patients often do not demonstrate the classic signs of acute cholangitis, but they can develop a delayed-sepsis–like syndrome of which hypotension is the most pronounced feature. High biliary pressures promote the translocation of bacteria from the portal circulation into the biliary tree. The most common bacterial organism seen in acute cholangitis is *Escherichia coli* (25%–50%), followed by *Klebsiella, Enterobacter,* and *Enterococcus* species.

Treatment for acute cholangitis should focus on antimicrobial therapy and biliary drainage. Empiric antibiotic regimens should provide adequate activity against gram-negative and anaerobic organisms. Common regimens include monotherapy with ampicillin and sulbactam (Unasyn) or pipercillin and tazobactam (Zosyn) or combination therapy with a fluoroquinolone plus metronidazole (Flagyl).

Patients without hypotension or mental status changes commonly show initial improvement after empiric antibiotics are administered, and thus biliary drainage can be done nonurgently. In patients demonstrating signs of sepsis or severe infection, emergent biliary drainage via ERCP is warranted. Patients who are not candidates for ERCP may undergo percutaneous transhepatic biliary drainage as an alternative.

Acute Cholecystitis

Acute cholecystitis is a syndrome defined by right upper quadrant pain, fever, and leukocytosis in the setting of gallbladder inflammation. Nausea and vomiting often occur as concurrent symptoms. Patients commonly have a positive Murphy's sign on physical examination, which is defined as abrupt cessation of inspiration upon deep palpation of the gallbladder fossa, just beneath the liver edge. Approximately 95% of patients with acute cholecystitis have gallstones. In these instances, cholecystitis is thought to be precipitated by obstruction of the cystic duct and by local irritation of the gallbladder wall. Local inflammation is followed by release of pro-inflammatory prostaglandins. Superimposed bacterial infection might or might not complicate acute cholecystitis. As with cholangitis, the main bacteria responsible for infections during acute cholecystitis are *E. coli* and *Klebsiella, Enterobacter,* and *Enterococcus* species.

Diagnosis

The diagnosis of acute cholecystitis can often be made on physical examination alone. The most common laboratory finding in acute cholecystitis is leukocytosis. Mild elevations in AST and ALT can also be seen. Elevations of bilirubin and ALP are typical of biliary obstruction and are not commonly seen in acute cholecystitis. These abnormalities, if present, should raise suspicion for other conditions such as choledocholithiasis, cholangitis, or Mirizzi's syndrome. Mirizzi's syndrome is a rare cause of obstructive jaundice characterized by an impacted cystic duct stone that causes mass effect and compression of the common bile duct or common hepatic duct.

The initial imaging study of choice for acute cholecystitis is transabdominal ultrasound. Findings suggestive of cholecystitis include cholelithiasis, pericholecystic fluid (Figure 2) and a sonographic Murphy's sign (Figure 3). Thickening of the gallbladder wall supports a diagnosis of acute cholecystitis, but is a nonspecific finding. Transabdominal ultrasound has a sensitivity of 88% for diagnosing acute cholecystitis. Hepatobiliary cholescintigraphy (HIDA scan) (Figure 4) is recommended if the suspicion of cholecystitis remains after a negative transabdominal ultrasound. MRCP and CT scan are typically not necessary for the diagnosis, although CT scan can be useful if complications from cholecystitis such as perforation are suspected.

Treatment

The treatment for acute cholecystitis involves supportive care, analgesia, antibiotics, and either surgery or percutaneous gallbladder drainage. If treatment is delayed or inadequate, numerous potential complications can result. These include emphysematous or gangrenous cholecystitis and gallbladder perforation.

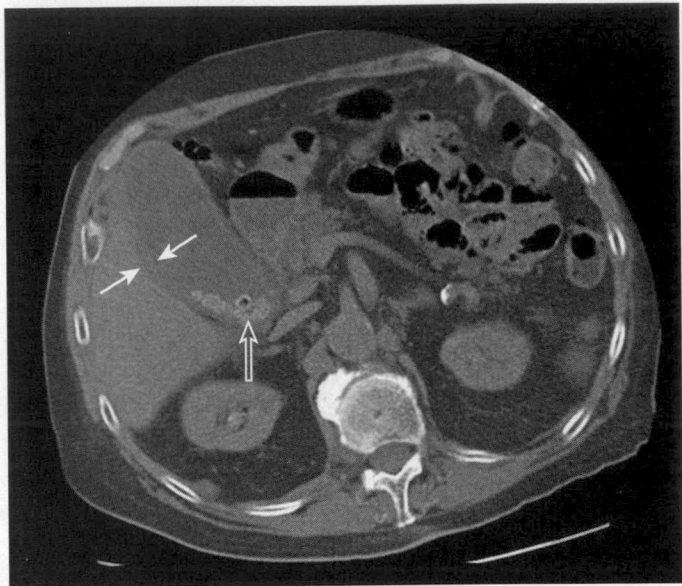

Figure 2. Computed tomography (CT) scan demonstrating acute cholecystitis. The *hollow arrow* indicates gallstones within the gallbladder lumen. The two *solid arrows* highlight mural thickening of the gallbladder wall and small amounts of pericholecystic fluid. (Image courtesy of Richard M. Gore, MD, Department of Radiology, NorthShore University Health System, Evanston, IL.)

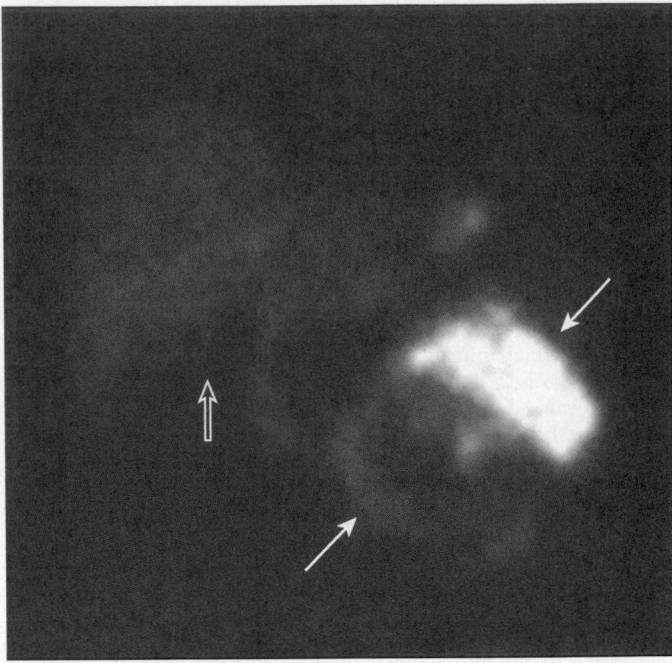

Figure 4. Hepatobiliary iminodiacetic Acid (HIDA) scan demonstrating acute cholecystitis. There is nonfilling of the gallbladder *(hollow arrow)*, with isotope noted in the stomach and duodenum *(solid arrows)*. (Image courtesy of Richard M. Gore, MD, Department of Radiology, NorthShore University Health System, Evanston, IL.)

In patients who are adequate surgical candidates, cholecystectomy should be performed within 72 hours of initial presentation. Numerous prospective trials and a Cochrane Database review have evaluated early versus delayed (6–12 weeks) cholecystectomy. There is overwhelming consensus that early surgery carries no increase in complications or perioperative morbidity and is associated with shorter hospital stays. Furthermore, early laparoscopic cholecystectomy eliminates the risk of recurrent episodes of acute cholecystitis.

Acute Acalculous Cholesystitis

An estimated 5% to 10% of cases of acute cholecystitis develop without the presence of gallstones. Acute acalculous cholecystitis is often seen in the setting of serious medical illness, complicated surgery, severe blunt trauma, and burn injuries. Other conditions such as diabetes mellitus, vasculitis, AIDS, and congestive heart failure have also been implicated as risk factors. Acute acalculous cholecystitis carries major risks of gangrene (50%) and perforation (10%), and mortality ranges from 30% to 50%. Numerous organisms have been associated with acute acalculous cholecystitis, including bacterial, viral, fungal, and parasitic infections.

The diagnosis is difficult. Patients are often critically ill and unable to elicit their symptoms. Transabdominal ultrasound is the best modality to evaluate acute acalculous cholecystitis in the critically ill patient owing to its availability, cost, and ease of performance. Hepatobiliary iminodiacetic acid (HIDA) and computed tomography (CT) scanning can have a role in difficult-to-diagnose acute acalculous cholecystitis and should be considered if ultrasound is nondiagnostic. Whereas false positive tests can occur, a normal HIDA scan has a high negative predictive value in evaluating acute acalculous cholecystitis.

Because of the high rate of gangrene and perforation, early cholecystectomy should be performed in patients who are surgical candidates. In patients too ill to undergo surgery, biliary drainage with percutaneous cholecystostomy should be considered.

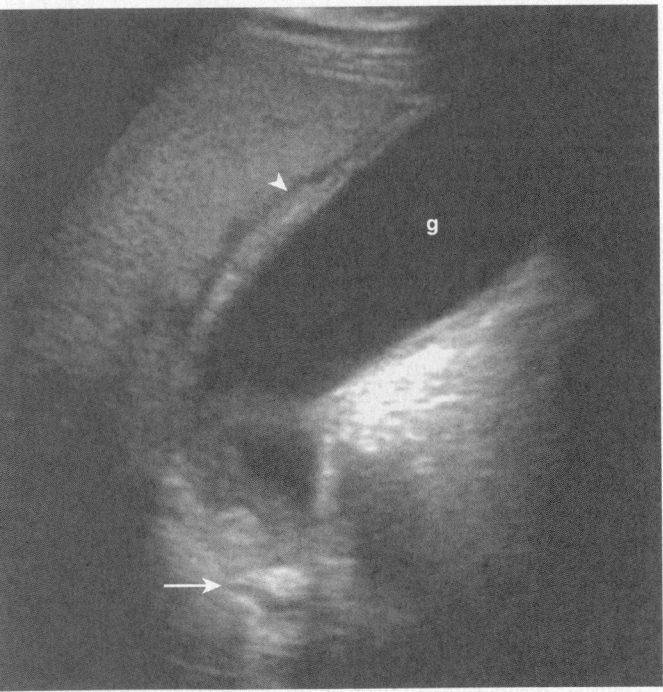

Figure 3. Acute cholecystits: ultrasound. Gallbladder *(g)* is distended, with mural thickening *(arrowhead)* and a stone in the gallbladder neck *(arrow)*. Positive sonographic Murphy sign was present.

All patients with acute cholecystitis should be admitted to the hospital and given supportive care including intravenous fluids. NSAIDs and opioid analgesics are typically used for pain control.

Although bacterial etiologies complicate less than half of all episodes, empiric antibiotics are commonly administered to patients with acute cholecystitis. Appropriate antibiotic regimens are the same as those used in the setting of acute cholangitis (see the discussion of complications of choledocholithiasis).

Gangrenous Cholecystitis, Emphysematous Cholecystitis and Gallbladder Perforation

Gangrenous cholecystitis is most often seen in elderly patients and diabetics along with patients who delay seeking medical treatment for their symptoms. It is the most common complication of acute cholecystitis and carries a high mortality. Emphysematous cholecystitis is caused by gas-forming bacteria that infect the gallbladder. *E coli* and *Clostridium* species are most commonly implicated. Gas in the gallbladder may be seen on imaging, particularly CT or magnetic resonance imaging (MRI). Patients with gangrenous or emphysematous cholecystitis are at an elevated risk for gallbladder perforation. Early empiric antibiotics and cholecystectomy are crucial in the management of these complications to minimize mortality and prevent perforation of the gallbladder, a condition that carries a mortality rate of 42% to 60%.

Gallbladder Disease in Pregnancy

Pregnancy is a major risk factor for cholesterol gallstone formation. Because of anatomic changes secondary to the gravid uterus, biliary colic can be difficult to delineate from other causes of abdominal pain. Pregnant patients often have gallstones on transabdominal ultrasound, and thus a detailed history and physical examination are needed to diagnose a patient's abdominal pain as biliary. Patients with other symptoms including bloating or dyspepsia should be evaluated for other etiologies.

In pregnant patients with recurrent symptomatic cholelithiasis, laparoscopic cholecystectomy remains the treatment of choice. The second and early third trimesters are the best times to perform cholecystectomy owing to ease and lower rates of complications. Nonsurgical management of gallstones is limited in pregnancy. NSAIDs are generally avoided late in pregnancy owing to the risk of premature closure of the ductus arteriosis, especially after 30 to 32 weeks of gestation.

After appendicitis, acute cholecystitis is the second most common nonobstetric surgical emergency during pregnancy. As with nonpregnant patients, pregnant women with acute cholecystitis should be treated with cholecystectomy in addition to medical management. Early surgery for pregnant patients with acute cholecystitis has been found to decrease relapse rates and hospital readmissions. No differences in maternal or fetal morbidity and mortality have been found in patients treated conservatively versus surgically for acute cholecystitis during pregnancy.

References

Abboud PA, Malet PF, Berlin JA, et al. Predictors of common bile duct stones prior to cholecystectomy: A metaanalysis. Gastrointest Endosc 1996;44:450–5.

Akriviadis EA, Hatzigavriel M, Kapnias D, et al. Treatment of biliary colic with diclofenac: a Randomized, double-blind, placebo-controlled study. Gastroenterology 1997;113:225–31.

ASGE Standards of Practice Committee, Maple JT, Ben-Menachem T, Anderson MA, et al. The role of endoscopy in the evaluation of suspected choledocholithiasis. Gastrointest Endosc 2010;71:1–9.

ASGE Standards of Practice Committee, Maple JT, Ikenberry SO, Anderson MA, et al. The role of endoscopy in the management of choledocholithiasis. Gastrointest Endosc 2011;74:731–44.

Barie PS, Eachempati SR. Acute acalculous cholecystitis. Gastroenterol Clin North Am 2010;39:344–57.

Dhupar R, Smaldone GM, Hamad GG. Is there a benefit to delaying cholecystectomy for symptomatic gallbladder disease during pregnancy? Surg Endosc 2010;24:108–12.

Everhart JE, Khare M, Hill M, Maurer KR. Prevalence and ethnic differences in gallbladder disease in the United States. Gastroenterology 1999;117:632–9.

Freitas ML, Bell RL, Duffy AJ. Choledocholithiasis: Evolving standards for diagnosis and management. World J Gastroenterol 2006;12:3162–7.

Gore RM, Thakrar KH, Newmark GM, et al. Gallbladder imaging. Gastroenterol Clin North Am 2010;39:265–7.

Gurusamy KS, Samraj K. Early versus late laparoscopic cholecystectomy for acute cholecystitis. Cochrane Database Syst Rev 2006;18: CD005440.

Papi C, Catarci M, Ambrosio D, et al. Timing of cholecystectomy for acute calculous cholecystitis: A meta-analysis. Am J Gastroenterol 2004;99:147–55.

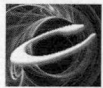

CHRONIC DIARRHEA

Method of
André de Leon, MD

CURRENT DIAGNOSIS

History
- Duration and frequency
- Presence of fever/blood
- Food/medication intake
- Travel history

Physical Examination
- Gastrointestinal examination
- Hydration status
- Digital rectal examination
- Other Systems: endocrine, ophthalmologic, skin

Testing
- Fecal occult blood testing
- Stool for ova/parasites, *C. difficile* and other bacteria
- Stool antigen for cryptosporidium, giardia
- Fecal electrolytes (Na, K, Osm)
- Fecal leukocytes
- Erythrocyte sedimentation rate (ESR)
- Complete blood count (CBC)
- Other: iron panel (celiac sprue), TSH (hyperthyroidism), liver function tests (LFTs)
- Colonoscopy with biopsy

CURRENT THERAPY

- Supportive care and rehydration, if necessary
- Trial of discontinuation of possible offending medication/food (lactose, gluten, sorbitol)
- Dietary modification with increased fiber intake (dietary or supplementation)
- Specific therapy as directed by culture and susceptibilities or biopsy
- Empiric therapy trial with antibiotics
- Empiric trial of probiotics[1] (limited evidence of efficacy in healthy adults with chronic diarrhea)

[1]Not FDA approved for this indication.

Chronic diarrhea has traditionally been defined based on consistency, volume, and frequency of stools. However, recent studies have found that there is considerable variability in definition when using these markers. Therefore, the American Gastroenterological Association has released a consensus statement suggesting that chronic diarrhea should be defined as a decrease in fecal consistency lasting for 4 or more weeks.

Epidemiology

Chronic diarrhea is a common cause of mortality in developing countries as well as the second leading cause of overall mortality in children 1 to 59 months old. The prevalence in the general population in developed nations and economic impact of chronic diarrhea has not been well established. This could be related to the variable nature of the studies that have been performed with regard to definition, population characteristics, and overall study design. Rough estimates based on this limited information suggest that chronic diarrhea can affect up to 5% of the population and can cost up to $350,000,000 annually from work loss alone.

Classification Based on Pathophysiology

Elucidating the exact cause of chronic diarrhea can be very challenging, as there are several hundred conditions that can be related. It is often separated into three basic categories, including watery, fatty (malabsorption), and inflammatory (with blood and pus); however, these should not be strictly adhered to as there is often considerable overlap between the categories. Watery diarrhea can be further subdivided into osmotic, secretory, drug-induced, and functional types. Osmotic diarrhea is related to water retention; secretory diarrhea is due to reduced absorption of water; drug-induced is as stated in its name; and functional diarrhea is due to hypermotility of the gut.

Watery Diarrhea

Watery diarrhea can be subdivided into four categories, including osmotic, secretory, drug-induced, and functional types. Fecal osmotic gap can be calculated, which will help guide further workup and diagnosis. An elevated osmotic gap (>125 mOsm/kg) is suggestive of possible osmotic causes, such as lactose intolerance. A normal osmotic gap can be associated with irritable bowel syndrome or may be indicative of a further workup for possible celiac disease. A decreased osmotic gap (<50 mOsm/kg) points toward secretory causes, including infectious (ova, parasite, bacteria, giardia), endocrine (hyperthyroidism), autoimmune (Addison's), neoplastic (pheochromocytoma), and anatomic defect.

Fatty/Malabsorptive Diarrhea

Malabsorptive diarrhea is, as the name implies, secondary to impaired absorption along the gut. This can be due to structural abnormalities (gastric bypass, short bowel syndrome, celiac sprue, pancreatic insufficiency) or structural abnormalities related to vascular compromise (mesenteric ischemia). Impaired absorption can also occur secondary to infections such as *Tropheryma whipplei* (Whipple's disease), *Giardia*, small bowel bacterial overgrowth, and tropical sprue. Medications such as aminoglycoside antibiotics, orlistat (Alli, Xenical), thyroid supplementation, acarbose (Precose), and ticlopidine (Ticlid) can also cause malabsorptive diarrhea.

Inflammatory Diarrhea

Inflammation leading to diarrhea is often due to autoimmune, infectious, or neoplastic processes or radiation exposure. Autoimmune processes are felt to play a large role in inflammatory bowel disease (IBD), which often manifests as Crohn's disease or ulcerative colitis. Infections such as *Clostridium difficile*, *Mycobacterium tuberculosis*, *Yersinia*, cytomegalovirus, herpes simplex virus, amebiasis, and *Strongyloides* can lead to a diarrhea with associated inflammation of the bowel. Colon cancer (villous adenocarcinoma) and lymphoma can also cause inflammatory diarrhea.

Clinical Manifestations

History. Thorough investigation of a patient complaining of ongoing diarrhea-like features should always include a detailed medical history. A clear understanding of the patient's symptoms is vital: not all complaints may truly be defined as diarrhea but may rather be symptoms related to an interplay between fecal incontinence and stool impaction. A detailed history of travel, food intake, and medication use is essential. This can help direct the early workup and diagnostic testing. Stool frequency, volume, and consistency can aid in categorization; however, they are no longer what define the condition, as noted above.

Physical Examination. The physical examination is very important to the workup and diagnosis of chronic diarrhea. Ophthalmologic findings such as episcleritis or exophthalmia can be related to IBD; skin findings such as dermatitis herpetiformis can be related to celiac sprue (seen in 15–25% of patients with celiac disease). Prominent lymphadenopathy and weight loss can be suggestive of possible infection or malignancy. A thorough abdominal examination should include the evaluation of bowel sounds (hypermotility), skin for scars (surgical cause of diarrhea), tenderness (infection/inflammation), and masses (neoplasia) and should be followed by a digital rectal examination with fecal occult blood

testing. Anoscopy can also be employed to detect for ulcerations or fecal impaction, given that seepage around impacted stools can create a picture similar to diarrhea.

Testing for Diagnosis

Serum testing for chronic diarrhea should include a complete blood count (CBC), serum electrolytes, liver function tests, serum albumin, thyroid-stimulating hormone, and erythrocyte sedimentation rate. An iron panel should be performed if indicated based on the results of the CBC. Serum anti-tissue transglutaminase antibody testing may be helpful if symptoms are suggestive of celiac sprue. Stool evaluation may include fecal occult blood testing, fecal leukocytes, stool ova and parasites, stool culture (including *Salmonella*, *Shigella*, and *Campylobacter*), and stool antigen for *Giardia*. Stool testing for *Cryptosporidium* should be considered, especially in the immunocompromised. Stool pH and electrolytes may be helpful, especially when the patient is lactose intolerant. Stool testing for *C. difficile* should be performed if the patient has recently used antibiotics or been hospitalized. If medication abuse is suspected as a possible cause, a stool laxative screen (i.e., stool phenolphthalein test) may be warranted. Diagnostic testing may include a colonoscopy with biopsy.

Treatment

The exact cause of chronic diarrhea can prove elusive, and treatment trials may be warranted. Specific treatment depends on the specific diagnosis. If there is concern of possible bacterial or protozoa infection, an empiric trial of vancomycin (Vancocin), ciprofloxacin (Cipro), or metronidazole (Flagyl) may be warranted. If there is concern for possible medication (Table 1) or food relation

TABLE 1 Medications Commonly Associated with Diarrhea

Antiarrhythmic medications
- Digoxin
- Quinidine

Antibiotic medications
- Aminoglycosides
- Macrolides

Antihypertensive medications
- ACE inhibitors
- Beta blockers

Anti-inflammatory medications
- 5-aminosalicylates
- Nonsteroidal antiinflammatories (NSAIDs)

Antiretroviral medications (many)

Chemotherapeutic medications (many)

Dermatologic medications
- Isotretinoin (occasionally causes diarrhea)

Endocrine medications
- Alpha-glucosidase inhibitors (cause diarrhea in ≥20% of patients)
- Biguanides (cause diarrhea in ≥20% of patients)
- Thyroid hormones

Gastrointestinal medications
- Acid-reducing medications
  • H2-receptor blocker
  • Proton pump inhibitors
- Antacid medications (magnesium containing)

Parasympathetic nervous system medication
- Cholinergic agonists

Psychiatric medications
- Selective serotonin reuptake inhibitors

Respiratory medications
- Xanthine derivative (Theophylline)

Data from Schiller LR, Sellin JH. Sleisenger and Fordtran's Gastrointestinal and Liver Disease: Pathophysiology/Diagnosis/Management. 9th Edition, Philadelphia, 2010, Elsevier; and Soriano M, Vaziri H. Clinical Gastroenterology, Diarrhea: Diagnostic and Therapeutic Advances, New York, October 2010, Humana Press, Springer.

to diarrhea, a trial of discontinuation of offending substance/food may be reasonable. The effectiveness of probiotics[1] looks favorable; however, large intervention studies and epidemiologic investigations of long-term probiotic effects on healthy adults are largely missing. At this time, probiotics have been found efficacious in treatment of acute diarrhea, prevention of antibiotic-associated diarrhea, and prevention of traveler's diarrhea. Dietary modification continues to be an important starting point for treatment with increased intake in bulk forming agents such as fiber. Treatment of specific disorders such as Crohn's disease and ulcerative colitis are discussed in other chapters.

---

[1]Not FDA approved for this indication.

References

De Vrese M, Marteau PR. Probiotics and prebiotics: Effects on diarrhea. J Nutr 2007;137:803S–115.

Everhart JE, editor. Digestive Disease in the United States: Epidemiology and impact. Washington, DC: National Institutes of Health; 1994, NIH Publication No. 94-1447.

Fine KD, Schiller LR. AGA technical review on the evaluation and management of chronic diarrhea. Gastroenterology 1999;116:1464–86.

Juckett G, Trivedi R. Evaluation of chronic diarrhea. Am Fam Physician 2011;84:1119–26.

Rodrigo L. Celiac disease. World J Gastroenterol 2006;12:6585–93.

Soriano M, Vaziri H. Clinical Gastroenterology, Diarrhea: Diagnostic and Therapeutic Advances. New York: Humana Press, Springer; 2010, October.

Thomas PD, Forbes A, Green J, et al. Guidelines for the investigation of chronic diarrhea, 2nd edition. Gut 2003;52(Suppl. 5):v1–v15.

Whitehead WE, Borrud L, Goode PS, et al. Fecal incontinence in U.S. adults: Epidemiology and risk factor. Gastroenterology 2009;137:512–7, e2.

World Health Organization. Children: Reducing mortality, Fact Sheet #178, Available at http://www.who.int/mediacentre/factsheets/fs178/en/ (accessed October 17, 2013).

CIRRHOSIS

Method of
Harmit Kalia, DO; Priya Grewal, MD; and Paul Martin, MD

Although cirrhosis is the 12th most common cause of death in the United States, it is the fourth most frequent cause in the 45 to 54 year age group. Cirrhosis reflects the consequences of chronic hepatic necroinflammatory activity with an incomplete repair response. This involves collagen deposition and nodule formation, leading to disruption of the normal lobular arrangement of hepatocytes, blood vessels, and lymphatics. Although the definitive diagnosis is based on histology, in the absence of a liver biopsy cirrhosis can be inferred in the appropriate setting by manifestations such as portal hypertension or appearance on imaging consistent with the diagnosis.

Cirrhosis can result from any cause of chronic liver disease (Table 1). Most manifestations of advanced cirrhosis, such as portal hypertension and coagulopathy, reflect the consequences of extensive distortion of the hepatic architecture and impaired hepatocellular function. However, some symptoms also reflect the specific etiology of cirrhosis—most notably, pruritus in patients with cholestasis and malabsorption of fat-soluble vitamins in patients with primary biliary cirrhosis or primary sclerosing cholangitis.

An important distinction is whether the cirrhosis is compensated or decompensated. Cirrhosis that remains compensated implies the absence of an index complication such as onset of ascites or variceal hemorrhage, whereas overt hepatic decompensation indicates that a major complication has supervened and the patient now has evidence of frank hepatic failure. The prognosis of cirrhosis reflects its stage: stage I (compensated without esophageal varices) has a 1% mortality rate per year, and stages 2 (varices), 3 (ascites) and 4 (gastrointestinal bleeding) have annual mortality rates that increase from 3.4% to 20% to 57%, respectively. Thus recognition of cirrhosis per se does not suggest the need for evaluation for liver transplantation, but transplantation needs to be

CAUSE	EXAMPLES
Infection	Hepatitis B Hepatitis C Hepatitis D
Toxins	Alcohol, drugs
Cholestasis	Primary biliary cirrhosis Secondary biliary cirrhosis Primary sclerosing cholangitis
Autoimmune	Autoimmune hepatitis
Vascular	Cardiac cirrhosis Budd–Chiari syndrome Sinusoidal obstruction syndrome
Metabolic	Hemochromatosis Wilson's disease α_1-Antitrypsin deficiency Nonalcoholic steatohepatitis
Cryptogenic	

TABLE 1 Common Causes of Cirrhosis

considered once a major complication such as a variceal hemorrhage, onset of ascites, or hepatic encephalopathy has supervened. Less florid evidence of cirrhosis can include a hyperdynamic circulation reflecting peripheral vasodilation with a resting tachycardia. However, many patients with cirrhosis are completely asymptomatic until a major complication of their liver disease occurs. Clues to underlying cirrhosis are thrombocytopenia or coagulopathy not related to a primary hematologic disorder or biochemical dysfunction with hyperbilirubinemia and elevated serum aminotransferases or alkaline phosphatase.

In a patient with well-compensated cirrhosis, physical signs of liver disease may be subtle. The liver span may be somewhat diminished on percussion, with a firm edge and with splenic dullness due to splenomegaly. Cutaneous signs of cirrhosis other than jaundice include palmar erythema and spider nevi. In cirrhotic male patients, gynecomastia results from altered metabolism of sex hormones with testicular atrophy; it also reflects the antigonadal effects of alcohol in some patients. The catabolic effects of cirrhosis often result in a diminished muscle mass, obvious on physical examination. More florid evidence of cirrhosis on physical examination includes varying degrees of disturbed mentation along with asterixis, indicating hepatic encephalopathy. Other key findings include ascites and peripheral edema. Additional physical findings can provide some clues to the underlying etiology of liver disease. For instance, xanthelasmata are common in patients with cholestatic liver disease, whereas patients with alcoholic cirrhosis can have other end-organ injury such as peripheral neuropathy.

Laboratory findings that suggest portal hypertension are a low platelet count and a low leukocyte count due to hypersplenism. Impaired hepatic synthetic and secretory functions are reflected in a diminished serum albumin, elevated serum bilirubin, and prolonged prothrombin time.

Transition from compensated to decompensated cirrhosis occurs at a rate of 5% to 7% per annum. Various models have been developed to predict the likelihood of hepatic decompensation in individual patients. They typically incorporate a combination of routine blood tests, including the platelet count, which is depressed in portal hypertension mainly because of hypersplenism as well as diminished thrombopoietin. The development of hepatocellular carcinoma (HCC) accelerates the progression of cirrhosis as a result of the tumor mass and vascular invasion, most typically of the portal vein. However, the morbidity and mortality in chronic liver disease are related to a large extent to the severity of portal hypertension. The median survival time in patients with compensated cirrhosis is 12 years, whereas in those with decompensated cirrhosis it is 1.5 years. There is an increasing emphasis on anticipating the complications of cirrhosis, such as variceal hemorrhage (discussed in the chapter on bleeding esophageal varices), HCC, and spontaneous bacterial peritonitis (SBP), in an effort to enhance survival and allow appropriate intervention with liver transplantation.

Cirrhotic patients are immunocompromised and therefore are at increased risk for bacterial infections. Pulmonary complications of cirrhosis include portopulmonary hypertension (PPHTN) and hepatopulmonary syndrome (HPS).

Ascites

Cirrhosis is the underlying cause for ascites in 85% of patients in the Western world. Ascites is the most common complication of cirrhosis, with a 2-year survival rate of only 50% following its onset. The pathogenesis of ascites in cirrhosis mainly reflects increased intrahepatic resistance due to fibrosis, which raises portal pressures. Compensatory mechanisms cause splanchnic vasodilation, resulting in a decrease in effective arterial blood volume. This results in a compensatory activation of the neurohumoral (renin–angiotensin) system and increased retention of sodium by the kidneys. The imbalance of elevated hydrostatic pressure due to portal hypertension and decreased oncotic pressure (low albumin) causes ascites. Therefore, sodium retention is key to the development of ascites. Other mechanisms can include disruption of normal lymphatic drainage in the liver due to extensive fibrosis.

Diagnosis

Physical examination can reveal a bulging abdomen with shifting dullness; this sign is reliable when the volume of ascites is greater than 1500 mL. Ultrasound of the abdomen is helpful in locating smaller amounts of ascites (as little as 100 mL). Once ascites is detected, diagnostic paracentesis should be performed to determine whether it is exudative or transudative, a determination that narrows the differential diagnosis of ascites (Table 2). The fluid is tested for white blood cell count, culture, and albumin to calculate serum–ascites albumin gradient (SAAG). This must be done on initial paracentesis and accurately distinguishes ascites related to portal versus nonportal hypertensive causes. A SAAG of 1.1 g/dL or higher accurately predicts portal hypertension. Once the diagnosis of ascites is made, it is important to mitigate aggravating factors in fluid retention. Dietary indiscretion, noncompliance with diuretics, therapeutic volume expansion after gastrointestinal bleeding, and renal toxicity from use of nonsteroidal antiinflammatory drugs (NSAIDs) are common culprits.

Treatment

The mainstay of management of ascites is sodium restriction and judicious diuresis. Patients should be encouraged to adhere to a sodium-restricted diet of 2 g/day. A sodium-to-potassium concentration ratio greater than 1 on a random urine sample correlates well with a 24-hour sodium excretion greater than 78 mmol/day and implies patient compliance with salt restriction. In reality, dietary restriction of sodium is efficacious in only 10% of patients; more typically, diuretics are needed. Mild to moderate ascites is controlled best by the use of diuretics with different modes of action, such as spironolactone (Aldactone) 100 mg (an aldosterone antagonist) and furosemide (Lasix) 40 mg (a loop diuretic) taken once daily. Serial blood chemistries need to be monitored to avoid electrolyte disturbance or renal insufficiency. Dosages of spironolactone and furosemide can be increased in a 100:40 ratio every 3 to 5 days until an adequate diuresis is achieved. Dosages greater than spironolactone 400 mg and furosemide 160 mg are generally not recommended because of concern about electrolyte imbalance or renal insufficiency.

Fluid restriction is recommended if the serum sodium concentration is less than 120 to 125 mmol/L, because hyponatremia in this circumstance reflects an excess of free water rather than sodium depletion. Hospitalized patients should be weighed daily to help guide management. Ideally, the patient should shed about 1 pound of weight every day; failure to do so implies inadequate diuretic dosing or lack of compliance with fluid restriction. Excessive weight loss should also be avoided, to reduce the risk of hepatorenal syndrome. Diuretic therapy should be withheld if a patient presents with encephalopathy, infection, renal insufficiency, or a serum sodium concentration of 120 mmol/L or less.

Refractory ascites, defined as inability to obtain a diuresis with high-dose diuretics without inducing renal dysfunction, occurs in 10% of cirrhotic patients with ascites; the resultant 1-year survival rate is only 25%. Serial large-volume paracenteses (LVP) of greater than 5 L of fluid is safe and effective in controlling ascites. Continued dietary restriction of sodium is necessary to avoid overly frequent paracenteses. Patients requiring LVP more frequently than every 2 weeks are probably not complying with a sodium-restricted diet. Intravenous albumin is used as colloid replacement to lessen postparacentesis circulatory dysfunction leading to renal insufficiency.

A patient who requires frequent LVP may be a candidate for a transjugular intrahepatic portosystemic shunt (TIPS). This vascular shunt is placed under fluoroscopic guidance and bridges a branch of the hepatic vein with a branch of the portal vein to reduce portal pressure. It is effective in about 90% of patients with refractory ascites. Diuretic therapy, albeit at a lower dosage, needs to be continued in many patients despite TIPS placement. There is a survival advantage for TIPS compared with LVP in cirrhotic patients.

The Model for End-Stage Liver Disease (MELD) score assesses the severity of liver disease and is based on the natural logarithms (base e) of the concentrations of bilirubin and creatinine (in milligrams per deciliter) and the international normalized ratio (INR):

$$MELD = [3.8 \times ln\,(Bilirubin)] + [11.2 \times ln\,(INR)] + [9.6\,ln\,(Creatinine)]$$

TIPS should be avoided in patients with a MELD score greater than 18 or Child-Pugh grade C disease (Table 3). These patients have a poor outcome because of deterioration in hepatocellular function following therapeutic portosystemic shunting. Not surprisingly, there is a high frequency (up to 40%) of portosystemic hepatic encephalopathy (PSE) after TIPS, which can be disabling and can even necessitate reduction in the shunt diameter to alleviate symptoms. TIPS occlusion was common in the past, but with newer covered stents patency is maintained.

As part of evaluation for TIPS placement, patients should undergo echocardiography to confirm that the cardiac ejection fraction is greater than 60%. This is done to prevent heart failure precipitated by an increased venous return after shunt placement. Because of the availability of TIPS, peritoneovenous shunting has fallen out of favor. Given the invasive nature of the procedure, along with its potential complications (disseminated intravascular coagulation, infection of the shunt, bleeding), this intervention is

TABLE 2	Diagnostic Tests on Ascites
TEST	**COMMENTS**
Cell count	If PMN >250 cells/mm³, infection is presumed
Culture	High sensitivity if infected
Albumin	Necessary to calculate SAAG
Total protein	Assists in determining cause of ascites
Gram stain	Assists in infectious/inflammatory work-up
LDH	High in malignant ascites
Amylase	Elevated in ascites secondary to pancreatitis
TB smear, culture, PCR	If TB is suspected
Cytology	Assists in diagnosis of malignant ascites
Triglycerides	Chylous ascites if >110 mg/dL
Bilirubin	To confirm leakage of bile in peritoneum

Abbreviations: LDH = lactate dehydrogenase; PCR = polymerase chain reaction; PMN = polymorphonuclear neutrophils; SAAG = serum-ascites albumin gradient; TB = tuberculosis.

TABLE 3 Child-Pugh Classification*

FACTOR	POINTS ASSIGNED		
	1	2	3
Ascites	Absent	Slight	Moderate
Bilirubin	<2 mg/dL	2–3 mg/dL	>3 mg/dL
Albumin	>3.5 g/dL (35 g/L)	2.8–3.5 g/dL	<2.8 g/dL
Prothrombin time seconds over control	<4	4–6	6
International normalized ratio	<1.7	1.7–2.3	>2.3
Encephalopathy	None	Grade 1–2	Grade 3–4

*A total score of 5–6 is considered grade A (well-compensated disease); 7–9 is grade B (significant functional compromise); and 10–15 is grade C (decompensated disease).

no longer considered in most centers. Management of ascites is typically only a temporizing measure because its development indicates that liver transplantation needs to be considered.

Spontaneous Bacterial Peritonitis

Bacterial infections are a major cause of mortality in cirrhotic patients. Translocation of enteric bacteria and bacterial products such as endotoxin alter hemodynamics even in the absence of infection. SBP is infection of the ascitic fluid with enteric aerobic organisms in the absence of a discrete source of infection such as a perforated viscus. Cirrhotic patients with ascites have a 10% annual incidence of SBP. It is the most common bacterial infection in cirrhotics with ascites, with a mortality rate of 49% in older series at 30 days, which has declined to 30% more recently, reflecting earlier recognition and the use of prophylactic antibiotics. The mortality rises when SBP is complicated by renal failure.

Diagnosis

Patients may be asymptomatic (Table 4), and on admission or readmission of a cirrhotic patient with ascites, diagnostic paracentesis is essential to exclude unrecognized SBP. A high index of suspicion is also necessary in cirrhotic patients with unexplained fever, impaired renal function, worsening hepatocellular function, nonspecific abdominal pain, or unexplained PSE. SBP is defined as positive ascitic fluid culture (one organism) and a polymorphonuclear neutrophil (PMN) count of 250 cells/mm³ or higher. Treatment with antibiotics is also indicated if the culture is negative but the PMN count is 250 cells/mm³ or greater, or if the culture is positive with one organism and the PMN count is 250 cells/mm³ or greater in a symptomatic patient. Diagnostic paracentesis revealing PMNs greater than 250 cells/mm³ and multiple enteric organisms suggests secondary bacterial peritonitis, and treatment should include antibiotics with prompt evaluation to exclude bowel perforation or an intraabdominal abscess.

TABLE 4 Incidence of Signs and Symptoms in Patients with Spontaneous Bacterial Peritonitis

SIGN OR SYMPTOM	INCIDENCE (%)
Fever	68
Abdominal pain	49
Abdominal tenderness	39
Rebound	10
Altered mental status	54

Adapted from Feldman M, Friedman LS, Brandt LJ (eds): Sleisenger & Fordtran's Gastrointestinal and Liver Disease, 8th ed. Philadelphia: Saunders Elsevier, 2006.

Treatment

Treatment of SBP involves the empiric administration of third-generation cephalosporins (e.g., cefotaxime [Claforan]) before bacterial culture results become available. The organisms most commonly involved are *Escherichia coli*, *Streptococcus* species, and *Klebsiella pneumoniae*. Ascitic fluid cultures are positive in only 50% to 60% of cases. Culture sensitivity is improved by bedside inoculation of aerobic and anaerobic blood culture bottles. For patients allergic to cephalosporins, alternatives include amoxicillin–clavulanate (Augmentin) and ciprofloxacin (Cipro). A 5-day antibiotic regimen is usually adequate, with resolution in 90% of cases. Repeat paracentesis 48 hours after starting antibiotics is useful to confirm clinical response, especially if the initial ascitic white blood cell count was in the thousands or there is concern about secondary peritonitis. Paracentesis should also be repeated after 5 days of antibiotics to confirm the response before withdrawing antibiotic therapy.

If the typical clinical response to antibiotics does not occur, important considerations include secondary bacterial peritonitis, intraabdominal abscess or bacterial resistance. Plasma volume expansion with albumin in addition to antibiotics decreases the incidence of renal dysfunction and improves survival. Albumin, unlike other volume expanders, improves cardiac function by decreasing arterial vasodilation. The recommended dosage of albumin is 1.5 g/kg at the time of diagnosis of SBP and 1.0 g/kg after 72 hours of antibiotic treatment if serum creatinine is greater than 1 mg/dL, blood urea nitrogen (BUN) is greater than 30 mgs/dL, or total bilirubin is greater than 4 mgs/dL.

After SBP, there is a 70% 1 year cumulative probability of a further episode; therefore, prophylaxis with antibiotics is appropriate. Other risk factors for SBP include an ascitic fluid protein content of less than 1 g/dL or variceal hemorrhage. Oral norfloxacin (Noroxin)[1] 400 mg daily or ciprofloxacin[1] 750 mg weekly can reduce the risk of SBP to 20% over 1 year. For patients with a fluoroquinolone allergy, trimethoprim–sulfamethoxazole (Bactrim)[1] one double-strength tablet daily may be administered. Primary prophylaxis for SBP is beneficial in patients with a low ascitic protein concentration (less than 1.0 g/dL). Antibiotics are helpful in cirrhotic patients admitted with gastrointestinal bleeding. Antibiotic therapy lowers infection rates, decreases the rate of further variceal bleeding, and improves survival. Improvements in earlier detection and treatment of this infection have had a major impact on reducing mortality. In addition, prophylaxis against SBP has lowered its incidence in cirrhotics at risk. Use of prophylactic antibiotics can encourage the emergence of resistant organisms, although fortunately response to cefotaxime is preserved. Rifaximin (Xifaxan),[1] a nonabsorbable antibiotic increasingly used in the management of hepatic encephalopathy, can also have a role in the prophylaxis of SBP.

Portosystemic (Hepatic) Encephalopathy

PSE is a syndrome of reversible neuropsychiatric dysfunction of varying severity that occurs on a background of portal hypertension with shunting of blood from the portal system into the systemic circulation. Despite its high incidence in cirrhotic patients, there is continuing controversy about its exact pathogenesis. Nitrogenous products from the gut are clearly implicated. Pathologically, there may be evidence of swelling of astrocytes in the brain. Ammonia and other toxins accumulate in the blood to impair cognitive and motor function.

Diagnosis

PSE is classified into three types (Table 5). The most common type has a gradual onset in cirrhotic patients and is referred to as type C. Type A is associated with acute liver failure, and type B is associated with portosystemic bypass (portocaval shunt) in the absence of cirrhosis. The clinical features of type C PSE include a wide range of neuropsychiatric symptoms. Stage 1 is characterized by alterations in consciousness and behavioral changes (inversion

[1]Not FDA approved for this indication.

TABLE 5 Types of Hepatic Encephalopathy

TYPE	DESCRIPTION
A	Acute liver failure
B	Portosystemic bypass without cirrhosis (portocaval shunt)
C	Chronic liver disease (cirrhosis)

of sleep/wake pattern, forgetfulness); stage 2 can include confusion and disorientation; stage 3 includes more profound symptoms, with lethargy and a stuporous state; and stage 4 is frank coma. Physical examination can elicit subtle findings such as mild tremor, as well as the more classic asterixis. Fetor hepaticus is a sweetish breath odor found in some patients with PSE.

The diagnosis of PSE remains clinical. Serum ammonia levels correlate poorly with the severity of encephalopathy. An increased level of serum ammonia per se is not an indication to treat a patient with liver disease in the absence of clinical evidence of PSE. Minimal encephalopathy is subclinical and is present in up to 70% of cirrhotic patients. It is diagnosed by psychomotor and neuropsychological tests only. Its progression to overt PSE seems to be related to deterioration of hepatocellular function.

Treatment

When a cirrhotic patient presents with overt PSE, management includes identification of a precipitating cause, which is present in more than 80% of cases and includes infection, noncompliance with medications, gastrointestinal bleeding, dehydration, electrolyte abnormalities, use of narcotics or sedatives, constipation, TIPS, and increased protein intake. Treatment of the precipitating cause, in addition to inducing a catharsis, is associated with improved cognitive and motor function. Upper gastrointestinal bleeding should be excluded by rectal examination and nasogastric lavage. An absence of improvement in mentation within 48 hours should lead to a further search for unrecognized precipitants (e.g., ongoing sepsis) or a separate neurologic diagnosis (e.g., subdural hematoma). Repeated admissions to hospital with easily reversible PSE suggests noncompliance with lactulose therapy, which remains the mainstay of treatment.

Available therapies for overt PSE counteract the effects of gut-derived bacterial neuroactive toxins. Therapy for overt PSE includes the induction of a catharsis with lactulose (Cephulac) or lactitol. Lactulose 15 to 30 mL should be given via nasogastric tube three times daily (in severe PSE) until loose bowel movements are observed, and thereafter to obtain two or three loose bowel movements daily. Lactulose enemas may be given in a less-alert patient. Cathartics used for PSE have frequent and troublesome common side effects, including abdominal cramping, diarrhea, and flatulence.

Outpatient therapy is initially with lactulose or lactitol titrated to obtain two or three soft bowel movements daily. These medications alter the pH in the colon and can promote ionization of ammonia, making it impossible for it to cross the mucosal barrier. A more acidic gut pH always reduces bacterial replication and production of nitrogenous products. The use of spironolactone along with furosemide decreases the incidence of hypokalemia, which promotes renal ammonia production. Traditionally, dietary protein restriction has been recommended in cirrhotics, often even in the absence of PSE, but rigorous evidence is lacking to support this strategy. It is more important for a patient with decompensated cirrhosis to maintain adequate nutrition. A nutritional evaluation is key in maintaining muscle mass in these patients.

If the cathartic effects of lactulose are poorly tolerated, nonabsorbable antibiotics can be used to inhibit production of bacterial toxins. Neomycin has been used longest, but its ototoxicity and nephrotoxicity preclude its use. Other antibiotics, such as metronidazole (Flagyl),[1] have also been used, but increasingly rifaximin (Xifaxan 550 mg twice daily) has become the antibiotic of choice,

[1]Not FDA approved for this indication.

despite its expense, to treat PSE. Rifaximin has been conclusively shown to reduce admissions to hospital for encephalopathy as well as maintaining remission from symptoms and improving quality of life in cirrhotic patients.

In patients with intractable and severe post-TIPS PSE, reduction or occlusion of the shunt may be necessary if pharmacologic treatment is not efficacious. Type A PSE associated with acute liver failure does not respond to standard medical therapy, which is futile in this circumstance, and urgent referral for liver transplantation is indicated. Cerebral edema, a common and often fatal complication of acute liver failure, can lead to cerebral herniation or intracranial hemorrhage, precluding liver transplantation.

Hepatorenal Syndrome

There are several potential explanations for renal dysfunction in patients with cirrhosis. Renal dysfunction can reflect glomerulonephropathy (hepatitis B, hepatitis C, immunoglobulin A nephropathy, diabetes mellitus), whereas the differential for acute renal dysfunction includes hypovolemia (diuretics, gastrointestinal bleeding, diarrhea), nephrotoxic drugs (aminoglycosides, NSAIDs, contrast dye), sepsis, and hepatorenal syndrome (HRS).

Diagnosis

The incidence of HRS in cirrhotic patients with ascites is up to 18% per annum. HRS in cirrhosis results from marked splanchnic and systemic vasodilation and decreased cardiac function, which lead to a decrease in effective arterial blood volume typical of more-advanced portal hypertension. Although the renal parenchyma is preserved, there is severe renal arterial vasoconstriction, low renal perfusion, and a decrease in the glomerular filtration rate. Clinically, the diagnosis of HRS is suspected when there is an increase in the creatinine level to greater than 1.5 mg/dL in the absence of shock, dehydration, infection, or nephrotoxic drugs.

Clinically, there are two types of HRS (Box 1). Type 1 HRS is defined as a severe, rapidly progressive increase in creatinine to greater than 1.5 mg/dL in less than 2 weeks. It is often precipitated by SBP, alcoholic hepatitis, or gastrointestinal hemorrhage. These patients tend to have floridly decompensated cirrhosis with tense ascites, PSE, and coagulopathy. The median survival time is 2 weeks. Type 2 HRS, with a median survival time of 6 months, is defined as a moderate and steady decline in renal function.

Evaluation of renal dysfunction in patients with liver disease should include an ultrasound study to determine the presence of ascites. If ascites is not present, the diagnosis of HRS is unlikely, and prerenal or intrinsic renal causes should be sought. If ascites is present, a work-up for sepsis (urinalysis, diagnostic paracenteses, and blood cultures) is indicated. Discontinuing all diuretics and nephrotoxic agents and introducing plasma volume expansion (intravenous fluids or albumin) is the initial intervention to correct renal dysfunction in cirrhotic patients. If renal function does not improve, HRS is likely. Additional clues that are helpful in the diagnosis of HRS are urine volume less than 500 mL/day, urine sodium concentration less than 10 mEq/L (despite plasma volume expansion), urine osmolality greater than that of plasma, protein secretion of less than 500 mg/day, and serum sodium concentration less than 130 mEq/L.

Box 1 Diagnostic Criteria for Hepatorenal Syndrome

Cirrhosis with ascites
Serum creatinine >1.5 mg/dL
No improvement of serum creatinine after at least 2 days with diuretic withdrawal and volume expansion
Absence of shock
No current or recent treatment with nephrotoxic drugs
Absence of parenchymal kidney disease

Adapted from Salerno F, Gerbes A, Ginès P, et al: Diagnosis, prevention and treatment of hepatorenal syndrome in cirrhosis. Gut 2007;56:1310–8.

Treatment

Treatment of HRS had been limited to establishing whether a reversible component in the renal dysfunction is present. Most data on the efficacy of therapeutic interventions are based on small retrospective and pilot comparative studies. Realistically, patients with severe HRS require either an improvement in liver function or liver transplantation for renal function to recover. Medical therapy can result in modest improvement in renal function. The combination of an α-agonist, midodrine (ProAmatine),[1] with octreotide (Sandostatin)[1] and albumin[1] can result in improvement of HRS. Vasoconstrictors such as terlipressin (Glypressin)[2] and norepinephrine (Levophed) improve renal function, with a decrease in serum creatinine in many treated subjects, although survival is not improved. Albumin administered with these medications can aid in vasoconstriction as well as plasma volume expansion and has antioxidant and anti-inflammatory properties. Terlipressin is expensive and is not yet available for use in the United States.

TIPS may improve renal function in patients with HRS. In a small prospective study of 14 patients, 10 patients who had initially responded to medical therapy (midodrine, octreotide, and albumin) and subsequently underwent TIPS had improvement in renal function. This study supported the possible use of this combination. In one study, TIPS was shown to improve survival to an average of 5 months, much better than the otherwise expected survival time of 2 weeks. TIPS can cause a precipitous deterioration in hepatocellular function in patients with more floridly decompensated liver disease, and its use should be entertained only in collaboration with a liver transplant center.

In patients with confirmed SBP, administration of albumin[1] on days 1 and 3 reduced the incidence of HRS from 33% to 10%. Also, the use of pentoxifylline (Trental)[1] 400 mg three times daily in patients with alcoholic hepatitis reduced the incidence of HRS from 35% to 8%.

Portopulmonary Hypertension

The prevalence of pulmonary hypertension as a complication of cirrhosis varies from 2% to 12.5% in candidates for liver transplantation. Before making a diagnosis of PPHTN, other causes of pulmonary arterial hypertension, such as recurrent pulmonary emboli, collagen vascular disease, intracardiac shunts, and medications, need to be excluded. The criteria for diagnosis of pulmonary arterial hypertension by right heart catheterization are mean pulmonary artery pressure greater than 25 mm Hg at rest or greater than 30 mm Hg with exercise; pulmonary capillary wedge pressure lower than 15 mm Hg; pulmonary vascular resistance greater than 120 dynes/sec/cm[5]; and transpulmonary gradient (pulmonary arterial diastolic pressure minus pulmonary capillary wedge pressure) greater than 10 mm Hg. The pathogenesis of PPHTN can reflect vasoconstrictive substances produced in the splanchnic circulation that bypass hepatic clearance. Candidate substances include serotonin, interleukin 1, glucagon, thromboxane B_2, endothelin 1, and vasoactive intestinal peptide. All have been detected in increased concentrations in patients with PPHTN.

Diagnosis

Symptoms of PPHTN include dyspnea on exertion, syncope, chest pain, fatigue, hemoptysis, and orthopnea. On physical examination, an accentuated pulmonic component of the second heart sound, right ventricular heave, and lower extremity edema are common. More than 60% of patients are asymptomatic at the time of diagnosis. Transthoracic echocardiography is used to estimate pressures. Patients who have right ventricular systolic pressures greater than 50 mm Hg or symptoms of right-sided heart failure should undergo right heart catheterization. In one third of these patients, the pulmonary vascular resistance is normal. Treatment should be initiated in patients who are symptomatic and have mean pulmonary arterial pressure greater than 35 mm Hg with increased pulmonary vascular resistance.

Treatment

Several drugs have been used to treat PPHTN with variable success. Epoprostenol (Flolan),[1] a prostacyclin (which directly dilates peripheral vessels), has often been used. Other agents have been used, including bosentan (Tracleer), an endothelin receptor antagonist; sildenafil (Revatio), a phosphodiesterase inhibitor; and iloprost (Ventavis),[1] a vasodilator. β-Blockers should be used cautiously in patients with PPHTN because of their cardiac depressant and pulmonary vasoconstrictive effects. Anticoagulation therapy should be considered, given the risk of venous stasis and pulmonary vascular thrombosis. Therapy should be attempted in concert with consideration for liver transplantation, which can arrest PPHTN. More-severe PPHTN is a contraindication to liver transplantation, especially if it does not improve with pharmacologic therapy. Liver transplantation can be delayed if patients have a good clinical response to medical therapy.

Hepatopulmonary Syndrome

In patients with liver disease, hypoxemia (increased alveolar-arterial gradient while breathing room air) and vascular dilations in the lung suggest the diagnosis of HPS. Its prevalence has been reported to be from 8% to 20% in transplantation candidates. The clinical features of HPS include the insidious onset of dyspnea, platypnea (shortness of breath exacerbated in upright position), orthodeoxia (hypoxemia in upright posture), clubbing, and cyanosis. Cutaneous spider nevi can reflect analogous vascular dilations in the lungs. A widened alveolar–arterial oxygen gradient on room air (>15 mm Hg, or >20 mm Hg in patients older than 64 years) should prompt evaluation for HPS in a patient with liver disease. A pulse oximetry reading of less than 97% on room air and an arterial partial pressure of oxygen (Pao_2) lower than 70 mm Hg on blood gas analysis indicate HPS in the absence of intrinsic cardiopulmonary diseases.

Diagnosis

The diagnosis of HPS can be confirmed with contrast echocardiography. Agitated saline to produce bubbles is injected intravenously. Bubbles resulting from vascular dilations in HPS appear three to six heartbeats after the appearance of contrast in the right side of the heart. If bubbles appear within three beats after injection, intracardiac shunting (e.g., atrial septal defect, patent foramen ovale) should be considered. If intrinsic cardiopulmonary disease is present, a technetium-labeled macroaggregated albumin scan can distinguish HPS. Normally, 20 mg of radiolabeled albumin gets trapped in the lung, but in a patient with pulmonary vascular dilations, the tracer escapes to elsewhere in the body. A shunt fraction of greater than 6% confirms the presence of HPS. Pulmonary angiography may be considered to rule out alternative causes of hypoxemia if noninvasive studies are not diagnostic.

Treatment

Patients with HPS have a median survival time of 10.6 months. Therapeutic approaches have included acetylsalicylic acid,[1] garlic powder,[7] indomethacin (Indocin),[1] methylene blue,[1] almitrine bismesylate (Duxil),[2] somatostatin analogues (Octreotide),[1] and plasma exchange, but currently none are recommended for use. Results of TIPS have been variable in HRS. Supplemental oxygen therapy has been shown to improve exercise tolerance and quality of life. Patients with HPS should be referred for liver transplantation evaluation, because transplantation increases survival, with impressive improvement in hypoxemia in about 85% of patients who undergo the procedure. However, resolution of symptoms can take up to 1 year. The 1-year survival after transplantation in HPS is 71%, compared with 90% in cirrhotic patients without HPS.

[1]Not FDA approved for this indication.
[2]Not available in the United States.

[1]Not FDA approved for this indication.
[2]Not available in the United States.
[7]Available as a dietary supplement.

Hepatic Hydrothorax

Hepatic hydrothorax is a pleural effusion greater than 500 mL in a cirrhotic patient without a cardiopulmonary explanation. Although patients can tolerate a large amount (more than 5 L) of ascites before becoming symptomatic, a hepatic hydrothorax greater than 1 L can cause shortness of breath and hypoxemia. It develops on the right side about 85% of the time, is left-sided in 13% of the cases, and is bilateral in 2%. Accumulation of a transudate in the pleural space is caused by portal hypertension with leakage of fluid from the peritoneal space through small defects in the diaphragm. With inspiration, there is an increase in negative intrathoracic pressure, facilitating fluid movement from the peritoneal space to the pleural space.

Diagnosis

Clinical features include dyspnea, nonproductive cough, chest discomfort, and even hypoxemia. Ascites is not always present, because it tends to be drawn into the pleural space. Less commonly, patients present dramatically, with severe dyspnea and hypotension in the presence of tension hydrothorax. In patients with fevers and pleuritic chest pain, infection of the pleural fluid needs to be excluded; its incidence in patients with hepatic hydrothorax is 13%.

Spontaneous bacterial empyema is defined as a PMN count greater than 500 cells/mm^3 or a positive bacterial culture in the absence of parapneumonic effusion. Like most bacterial infections in patients with cirrhosis, it is associated with a high mortality rate despite therapy. Spontaneous bacterial empyema should be promptly treated with antibiotics (Ceftriaxone 1–2 g daily) to cover organisms such as E. coli, Streptococcus, Enterococcus, Klebsiella, and Pseudomonas. After an effusion is recognized on chest radiography in a cirrhotic patient, especially when there has been a change in clinical status, diagnostic thoracentesis should be performed with analysis of fluid cell count, pH, Gram stain, culture, protein, and lactate dehydrogenase. Hepatic hydrothorax is typically transudative in nature. In the absence of infection, white cells should be scarce, fewer than 500 cells/mm^3 (PMNs <250 cells/mm^3); pH greater than 7.4; and total protein less than 2.5 g/dL. If atypical features of hepatic hydrothorax cause concern, such as an exclusively left-sided effusion, other nonhepatic causes of pleural effusion (e.g., pleural infection, congestive cardiac failure) need to be excluded. A confirmatory test for hepatic hydrothorax is a nuclear-tagged colloid albumin study. If hepatic hydrothorax is the source of pleural fluid, the nuclear-tagged albumin injected in the peritoneum should migrate and be identified in the thoracic cavity in the study. Alternative diagnoses should be sought if this tracer pattern is not observed.

Treatment

The management of hepatic hydrothorax is similar to management of ascites, as discussed earlier. For severely symptomatic patients and those whose disease is refractory to diuretics, frequent therapeutic thoracentesis is necessary. A need for frequent thoracentesis in a patient who is compliant with medical therapy should lead to consideration of TIPS, which is effective in up to 80% of patients with hepatic hydrothorax. The usual considerations regarding TIPS in a cirrhotic patient need to be addressed.

Indwelling chest tubes should be avoided, because they often lead to complications, including protein and electrolyte loss, infection, and fistula formation. Pleurodesis is usually ineffective in ablating the space between the parietal and the visceral pleura in patients with hepatic hydrothorax, and it can be associated with a variety of complications (e.g., fever, empyema, chest pain, pneumonia, incomplete expansion). Surgical repair of diaphragmatic defects has been reported in small case series, but clearly this is a major undertaking in a patient with decompensated cirrhosis.

Cirrhotic Cardiomyopathy

Cirrhotic cardiomyopathy is cardiac dysfunction in cirrhotic patients characterized by diminished contractility and impaired diastolic relaxation in the absence of intrinsic cardiac disease and can result in heart failure in decompensated cirrhotics. Q–T interval prolongation may be present and lead to ventricular tachyarrhythmias. Other consequences can include increased perioperative pulmonary edema, but improvement can occur in cardiac function with successful liver transplantation.

Hepatocellular Carcinoma

HCC is one of the most common fatal malignancies worldwide, with a rising incidence in the United States reflecting the consequences of chronic hepatitis C and hepatitis B infection as well as an increasing incidence of HCC related to nonalcoholic steatohepatitis. The incidence of HCC in patients with cirrhosis is 1% to 4% per year.

Diagnosis

The diagnosis is increasingly made radiologically. If two imaging techniques show that a mass in a cirrhotic liver has the characteristic features of HCC, with an arterial blood supply and rapid washout, a confident diagnosis can be made. In chronic hepatitis B infection, HCC can occur in the absence of cirrhosis. An α-fetoprotein level greater than 200 ng/mL is specific for HCC, although α-fetoprotein is not produced in up to 40% of HCCs, limiting the sensitivity of this test. A radiographically guided biopsy of the mass may be necessary if noninvasive testing is inconclusive.

Treatment

The prognosis and treatment options in HCC are related to tumor size and stage, underlying liver function, and the patient's performance status. Surgical resection or ablation is an initial option for those with Child-Pugh grade A cirrhosis, a single mass smaller than 5 cm, and a normal bilirubin level without portal hypertension. Liver transplantation is effective treatment, especially for patients who meet the Milan criteria (HCC with up to three tumors not more than 3 cm or one tumor not larger than 5 cm), provided that there is no vascular invasion and no metastasis. Transplantation within the Milan criteria results in long-term survival equivalent to that seen in cirrhotic patients without HCC. These patients are given priority for liver transplantation and often undergo radiofrequency ablation or transarterial chemoembolization if the waiting time will be protracted, in an effort to prevent tumor progression while awaiting transplantation. Patients with HCC outside the Milan criteria may be candidates for downsizing of the tumor prior to liver transplantation.

Transarterial chemoembolization can prolong survival in patients who are believed not to be candidates for resection or transplantation because it can lead to a modest increase in survival time. For symptomatic patients with inoperable tumors and marginal liver function, survival is poor, and systemic chemotherapy is of little value, although sorafenib (a tyrosine kinase inhibitor) has shown survival benefit compared with supportive care alone.

To detect and treat HCC at an early stage, screening and surveillance strategies are recommended. The following groups of patients are at high risk for HCC and should be in a surveillance program (Box 2 and Box 3): Asian men who are carriers of the hepatitis B virus (HBV) and are 40 years of age or older, Asian female HBV carriers who are 50 years of age or older, and all cirrhotic

---

Box 2	Surveillance for Hepatocellular Carcinoma in High-Risk Patients: Hepatitis B Carriers*

Asian men ≥40 years of age
Asian women ≥50 years of age
All cirrhotic hepatitis B carriers
Patients with family history of hepatocellular carcinoma
Africans >20 years of age

*For noncirrhotic hepatitis B carriers not listed here, surveillance is based on disease activity and clinical judgment.

Box 3   Surveillance for Hepatocellular Carcinoma in High-Risk Patients: Non-Hepatitis B Carriers

Cirrhosis of any etiology
Consider surveillance based on disease activity and clinical judgment:
- α1-Antitrypsin deficiency
- Nonalcoholic steatohepatitis
- Autoimmune hepatitis

Adapted from Bruix J, Sherman M; Practice Guidelines Committee, American Association for the Study of Liver Diseases: Management of hepatocellular carcinoma. Hepatology 2005;42:1208–36.

HBV carriers with a family history of HCC or cirrhosis of any etiology. Patients deemed to be at increased risk for HCC should be screened with twice-yearly ultrasound and measurement of AFP. If there is reason to suspect development of an HCC, such as rising AFP levels despite absence of a mass on ultrasound, additional abdominal imaging with magnetic resonance imaging or contrast computed tomography is necessary.

Special Considerations

Vaccination

Cirrhotic patients have increased morbidity and mortality if they contract viral or bacterial infections. All patients with chronic liver disease should be vaccinated against hepatitis A virus (HAV), HBV, pneumococcus, and influenza. At initial evaluation for chronic liver disease, total hepatitis A antibody and total hepatitis B core antibody should be ordered to determine preexisting immunity against HAV and HBV, and appropriate vaccines should be administered to nonimmune patients.

Osteopenia

The prevalence of osteopenia is high in patients with chronic liver disease, and there is a particularly high risk of osteoporosis in patients with primary biliary cirrhosis, primary sclerosing cholangitis, autoimmune disease, and alcoholic liver disease. Management of osteopenia can reduce morbidity before and after transplantation. All transplantation candidates should undergo screening for bone mineral density by dual-energy x-ray absorptiometry (DEXA), initially and repeated every 1 to 2 years. Hypothyroidism and disordered calcium and vitamin D metabolism should be excluded, and regular exercise should be encouraged. Concern about gastrointestinal irritation and bleeding from use of the oral bisphosphonates can be obviated by parenteral administration.

Liver Transplantation

With improvements in immunosuppression, surgical techniques, anesthesia, prophylaxis of common posttransplantation infections, and patient selection, liver transplantation has become the definitive intervention for decompensated cirrhosis, acute liver failure, and a subset of unresectable hepatic malignancies. Mean 1-year and 3-year survival rates after transplantation in the United States are about 90% and 80%, respectively. Liver transplantation should be considered once a cirrhotic patient has an index complication such as onset of ascites, and timely referral should be made before the patient becomes debilitated from recurrent complications of cirrhosis.

The most common indication for transplantation is decompensated cirrhosis (Box 4). Other important indications are HCC, acute liver failure, and metabolic liver disease. Most donor organs come from brain-dead but heart-beating donors and are allocated based on the severity of liver disease in the potential recipient. The organ allocation system is based on the MELD score (see earlier discussion), which ranges from 6 to 40 (Figure 1). The higher the MELD score, the lower the likelihood that the patient will be alive 3 months later, and the higher the patient's rank on the transplant list. Other determinants in allocation of organs are blood type, recipient's weight, and waiting time (for patients with

Box 4   Indications for Liver Transplantation

Chronic noncholestatic liver disorders (decompensated disease):
Chronic hepatitis C
Chronic hepatitis B
Autoimmune hepatitis
Alcoholic liver disease

Cholestatic liver disorders (decompensated disease):
Primary biliary cirrhosis
Primary sclerosing cholangitis
Biliary atresia
Alagille's syndrome
Nonsyndromic paucity of the intrahepatic bile ducts
Cystic fibrosis
Progressive familial intrahepatic cholestasis

Metabolic disorders causing cirrhosis:
α_1-Antitrypsin deficiency
Wilson's disease
Nonalcoholic steatohepatitis and cryptogenic cirrhosis
Hereditary hemochromatosis
Tyrosinemia
Glycogen storage disease type IV
Neonatal hemochromatosis

Metabolic disorders causing severe extrahepatic morbidity:
Amyloidosis
Hyperoxaluria
Urea cycle defects
Disorders of branched-chain amino acids

Primary malignancies of the liver:
Hepatocellular carcinoma
Hepatoblastoma
Fibrolamellar hepatocellular carcinoma
Hemangioendothelioma
Fulminant hepatic failure

Miscellaneous conditions:
Budd–Chiari syndrome
Metastatic neuroendocrine tumors
Polycystic disease
Retransplantation

Adapted from Murray KF, Carithers RL Jr: AASLD practice guidelines: Evaluation of the patient for liver transplantation. Hepatology 2005;41:1407–32.

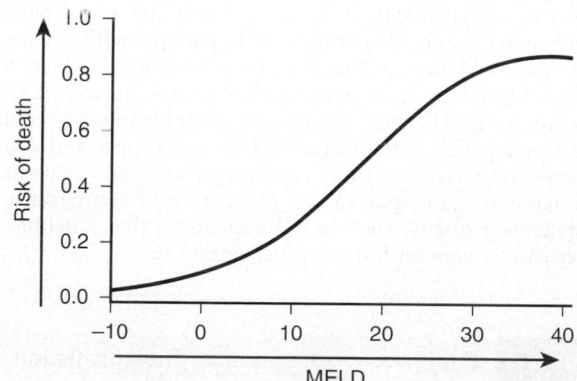

Figure 1. The Model for End-Stage Liver Disease (MELD) score predicts the risk of death over 3 months. See text for details.

identical MELD scores). Patients with fulminant hepatic failure, posttransplantation primary graft nonfunction, and hepatic artery thrombosis are given highest priority, independent of MELD.

A few indications (e.g., HCC, HPS) make patients eligible for a higher MELD score (priority), although this raises concern about reducing the organ supply for other potential recipients. The most common example of this situation is the cirrhotic patient with well-preserved hepatocellular function and a low MELD score whose indication for liver transplant is an HCC that meets Milan criteria. The organ allocation system under these circumstances awards extra MELD points to expedite transplantation, hopefully before metastatic spread has occurred. Specific etiologies of liver disease may be eligible for the highest priority for listing (status 1). An example is Wilson's disease with an acute presentation, because copper-chelating therapy is ineffective and can even lead to further deterioration. Any patient with acute liver failure with onset of hepatic encephalopathy within 26 weeks after recognition of liver disease of any etiology is also eligible for status 1.

Expansion of the organ donor pool to reduce deaths on the waiting list for transplantation has been possible with live donor transplantation, in which a healthy adult donates a major portion of his or her liver to another adult (right lobe) or to a child (left lobe). This remains a somewhat controversial approach because of the risk to the donor, especially with right lobe donation, because of the larger volume of hepatic tissue required for an adult patient. Another strategy is to split an adult graft, with the larger right lobe going to an adult recipient and the smaller left lobe to a pediatric recipient. In addition, organs from non–heart-beating donors harvested promptly after cardiac arrest are now used, albeit with concerns about inferior graft outcomes.

There are several important contraindications in liver transplantation (Box 5). Irreversible brain damage, as commonly occurs due to cerebral edema in acute liver failure, and advanced cardiopulmonary disease are absolute contraindications. PPHTN is not an absolute contraindication unless mean pulmonary pressures are greater than 35 mm Hg. In HPS, a PaO_2 of less than 50 mm Hg and a pulmonary artery shunt fraction greater than 30% are associated with a high mortality rate after transplantation. Extrahepatic malignancy or a history of malignancy with a disease-free period of less than 2 years, uncontrolled infection, and active alcohol intake or substance abuse are all contraindications. HIV infection is no longer a contraindication as long as it is well controlled on antiretroviral therapy. Advanced age is a relative contraindication, but biological rather than chronologic age is more pertinent, with particular attention to key comorbidities such as cardiovascular disease and diabetes mellitus.

The transplantation evaluation process typically involves a multidisciplinary team. Key components of the evaluation consist of separate medical and surgical evaluations; assessment of the severity of comorbid medical conditions, if any; identification of psychosocial aspects requiring intervention; and determination of financial and insurance status. Other important issues, such as the patient's willingness to undergo transplantation, a history of compliance with medical care, and the availability of a dependable support network, are also evaluated. In patients with a history of drug or alcohol abuse, a commitment to long-term sobriety and a drug-free lifestyle is an important prerequisite for acceptance for transplantation. The management of complications of cirrhosis is challenging. Given the disparity between supply and demand for donor organs, physicians care for increasingly tenuous cirrhotic patients. Anticipation and prevention of complications of end-stage liver disease such as SBP can ensure that potential candidates can survive until liver transplantation.

References

Angeli P, Gines P. Hepatorenal syndrome, MELD score and liver transplantation: An evolving issue with relevant implications for clinical practice. J Hepatol 2012;57:1135–40.

Arroyo V, Fernandez J, Ginès P. Pathogenesis and treatment of hepatorenal syndrome. Semin Liver Dis 2008;28:81–95.

Bajaj JS. The modern management of hepatic encephalopathy. Aliment Pharmacol Ther 2010;31:537–47.

Boyer TD, Haskal ZJ. The role of transjugular intrahepatic portosystemic shunt in the management of portal hypertension. Hepatology 2005;41:386–400.

Cárdenas A, Arroyo V. Management of ascites and hepatic hydrothorax. Best Pract Res Clin Gastroenterol 2007;21:55–75.

Forner A, Llovet JM, Bruix J. Hepatocellular carcinoma. Lancet 2012;31:1245–55.

Golbin JM, Krowka MJ. Portopulmonary hypertension. Clin Chest Med 2007;28:203–18.

Mandell MS. The diagnosis and treatment of hepatopulmonary syndrome. Clin Liver Dis 2006;10:387–405.

Runyon BA. Management of adult patients with ascites due to cirrhosis; an update. Hepatology 200;49:2087–107.

Tan HH, Martin P. Care of the liver transplant candidate. Clin Liver Dis 2011;15:779–806.

Tsochatzis EA, Bosch J, Burroughs AK. A new therapeutic paradigm for patients with cirrhosis. Hepatology 2012;56:1983–92.

DIVERTICULA OF THE ALIMENTARY TRACT

Method of
Aaron Sinclair, MD

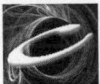

CURRENT DIAGNOSIS

- Endoscopy or barium swallow study may be used in the evaluation of most upper alimentary tract diverticula.
- Symptomatic small intestinal diverticula are difficult to diagnose and require a high index of suspicion and radiographic examination (nuclear medicine scans, capsule endoscopy, or computed tomography scans).
- Diverticulitis of the colon is most accurately identified and the treatment planned with computed tomography of the abdomen and pelvis.
- Diverticulitis of the colon that is slow to resolve may require additional imaging or direct visualization with endoscopy to identify an alternative diagnosis.

CURRENT THERAPY

- Most asymptomatic diverticula are identified incidentally and may only require monitoring.
- Surgical management of symptomatic diverticula may require surgical resection or endoscopic stenting.
- Early in the disease process, uncomplicated diverticulitis of the colon may be managed as an outpatient with a conservative no intervention approach or oral antibiotics.
- Complicated diverticulitis of the colon should be managed in conjunction with a surgeon and in the hospital with intravenous antibiotics.

A diverticulum is an abnormal saccular protrusion from the wall of the alimentary tract. Diverticula may be classified as either true or false. The wall of the alimentary tract is composed of submucosal, mucosal, and muscular layers. A false diverticulum is a protrusion of the submucosa and mucosa through a defect in the muscular wall of the alimentary tract. A true diverticulum is a protrusion of all layers of the alimentary tract wall. Many diverticula are asymptomatic and require no treatment. Some diverticula cause symptoms depending on their anatomic location or associated pathophysiologic complications (e.g., obstruction, infection, inflammation, or bleeding). This chapter categorizes alimentary canal diverticula by their location.

Box 5   Contraindications to Liver Transplantation

Absolute
Irreversible severe cardiopulmonary disease
Extrahepatic malignancy
Active substance abuse
Morbid obesity

Relative (varies by Transplant Center and Experience)
Age
HIV status

Esophagus

Zenker's Diverticulum

Zenker's diverticulum is a false diverticulum that develops in the upper posterior esophagus in an area known as Killian's triangle, located between the inferior pharyngeal constrictors and the cricopharyngeal muscles. Zenker's diverticulum typically presents after age 60 and has a male predominance for reasons that are unclear. It affects only 2 per 100,000 patients per year. Though it can be asymptomatic for years before the development of symptomatology, patients may experience dysphagia, aspiration, and regurgitation of undigested food. The exact cause is unclear but proposed mechanisms suggest a dysfunction in coordinated swallowing muscle movement and increased intraluminal pressure in the esophagus due to long-term upper esophageal sphincter irritation from acid reflux.

Diagnosis is primarily made through barium swallow, though small diverticula may be missed (Figure 1). Although endoscopic direct visualization is possible, caution should be exercised due to the risk of perforation. Small asymptomatic diverticula can be monitored. Zenker's diverticulum greater than 2 cm in size, regardless of symptomatology, should be surgically evaluated and repair considered. Methods for closure include endoscopic stapling or traditional surgical resection. Although most patients (>90%) demonstrate symptom improvement, recurrence rates can be as high as 35%.

Traction Diverticulum

Traction diverticula are the only true diverticula of the esophagus. Traction diverticula are rare. Their size tends to stay below 2 cm. Due to the mechanism of formation, traction diverticula are isolated to the middle third of the esophagus. The proposed mechanism is related to a precedent pulmonary infection, most commonly tuberculosis or histoplasmosis, with resultant mediastinal lymph node formation. After the active infection subsides, resultant fibrosis and scarring between the tissues surrounding the mediastinal lymph nodes and esophagus occurs. Initially, a small diverticulum develops from this fibrosis, which produces "traction" or a lack of mobility. Diverticular progression results when age-related changes from the dysfunction of coordinated swallowing muscle movement and increased intraluminal pressure in the esophagus develop. Surgical management is rarely needed unless these diverticula become symptomatic or complications, such as fistulas, occur.

Epiphrenic Diverticulum

Epiphrenic diverticula are false diverticula of the distal esophagus affecting only 0.015% of the general population. They are thought to arise secondary to mucosal injury from gastroesophageal reflux and muscle dysmotility. Occurring within 10 cm of the gastroesophageal junction, symptoms include dysphagia, spasmodic chest pain, and gastroesophageal reflux. With progression of diverticular size, obstruction can become a potential complication. Diagnostic measures start with barium swallow and may be followed with additional tests, including endoscopy, 24-hour pH probe, and esophageal manometry.

Management depends on patient symptoms and size of the diverticulum. If small (<5 cm) and asymptomatic, routine clinical and endoscopic surveillance is permissible. However, any symptomatology necessitates surgical evaluation and repair. Surgical options include open resection or laparoscopy. Partial fundoplication may be indicated depending on the severity of gastroesophageal reflux present as indicated by ancillary testing of the 24-hour pH probe.

Stomach

Gastric Diverticula

Gastric diverticula are rare with an endoscopic incidence of 0.01%. Most are asymptomatic and small (<3 cm). Symptoms may include epigastric pain, dyspepsia, and emesis. Rarely, ulcerations, perforations, or bleeding can occur. Diagnosis involves endoscopy, barium swallow, or contrast-aided computed tomography scan. Typical treatment includes a proton pump inhibitor and monitoring for symptom improvement. Persistent symptoms may necessitate gastrectomy of the diverticulum.

Small Intestine

Duodenal Diverticula

Diverticula located in the duodenum are relatively common, affecting up to 22% of the general population (Figure 2). Duodenal diverticula may be either true or false diverticula. The most common location is the second portion of the duodenum. The size and position of the diverticula may lead to complications such as obstruction of the sphincter of Oddi and/or impingement of the hepatobiliary tree drainage. This impingement may result in jaundice, right upper quadrant pain, or infection signs/symptoms

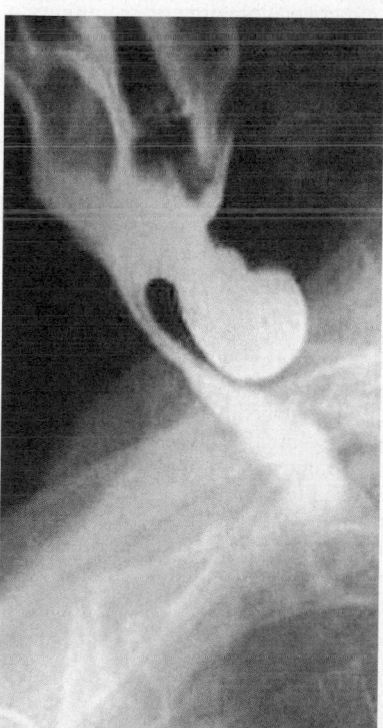

Figure 1. Zenker's diverticulum. (Image courtesy of Gastrolab—The Gastrointestinal Site. Available at http://www.gastrolab.net [accessed August 25, 2014].)

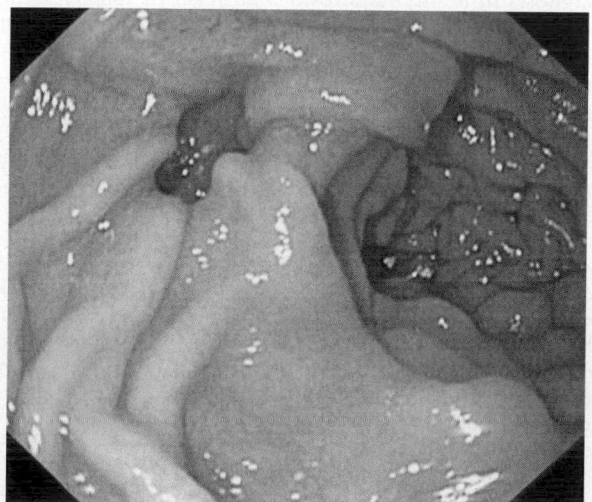

Figure 2. Duodenal diverticulum. (Image courtesy of Gastrolab—The Gastrointestinal Site. Available at http://www.gastrolab.net [accessed August 25, 2014].)

similar to cholecystitis. Although usually asymptomatic, on occasion ulcerative bleeding or perforation may occur.

Duodenal diverticula may be identified on barium swallow, contrast-enhanced computed tomography, or endoscopy. Duodenal diverticula found incidentally do not require treatment. If symptoms arise, endoscopic stenting/stapling, angiographic embolization, or surgical resection may be necessary.

Jejunal and Ileal Diverticula

Jejunal and ileal diverticula occur throughout the length of the small intestine. There does not appear to be any statistically significant relationship with morbidity or mortality of these types of diverticulum with respect to location, gender, size, number, etc. These false diverticula are located predominantly where the blood vessels penetrate the muscular wall of the mesenteric side of the bowel. Most are noted incidentally, but some manifest with symptoms secondary to bleeding, obstruction, or infection. These symptoms are believed to be due to bacterial overgrowth that may occur within the cavity of the diverticulum. Diagnosis can be made with capsule endoscopy or small bowel barium contrast follow-through study, although some may be noted on computed tomography with intravenous and oral contrast.

Asymptomatic jejunal and ileal diverticula should not be resected. Bacterial overgrowth symptoms may respond to antibiotic treatment and intestinal promotility drug therapy. Surgical intervention with small bowel resection is indicated if symptomatic diverticula persist.

Meckel's Diverticulum

A Meckel's diverticulum is a congenital anomaly that occurs due to incomplete closure of the vitelline duct. This duct typically obliterates during the ninth week of gestational age. Due to the embryological origin of the diverticulum, it is almost always located within 2 feet of the ileocecal valve. Meckel's diverticulum has a prevalence of approximately 1% to 2% of the population, with a 2:1 male predominance. Only 2% of all existing Meckel's diverticula will become symptomatic. The symptom most commonly associated with a Meckel's diverticulum is intussusception. This occurs due to residual fibrous attachments to the umbilicus causing a lead point for the proximal bowel to involute onto the distal bowel. It most commonly presents with bloody mucoid stools, abdominal pain, and vomiting in children under age 6. However, other symptoms may occur if ectopic tissue exists in the diverticulum. Gastric ectopic tissue may cause abdominal pain and bloody stools from ulceration of the underlying ileal tissue. Duodenal and pancreatic tissues have been identified in a Meckel's diverticulum but are very rare and do not typically cause symptoms.

Diagnosis in adults requires a high level of suspicion and is aided by the use of a technetium 99m (Tc^{99m}) scan to identify ectopic gastric mucosa in those patients with bleeding and symptoms of ulceration. For children with obstructive signs or symptoms, the diagnosis may be aided by ultrasound and/or computed tomographic scans. Plain film radiographs of the abdomen have low sensitivity and specificity for the diagnosis of intussusception. The choice of imaging procedure is dictated by the experience of the radiologic personnel performing the procedure.

Symptomatic Meckel's diverticulum should be surgically resected. Up to 90% of intussusception secondary to a Meckel's diverticulum may be reduced during diagnostic ultrasonography in children. Treatment of Meckel's diverticulum largely depends on age and symptomatology because operating on asymptomatic Meckel's diverticulum has been shown to have a fivefold increase in complications, such as postoperative bowel obstruction and infection. Many experts have advocated that incidental, asymptomatic Meckel's diverticulum should not be resected. Others advocate for resection for the following: healthy young children, healthy adults less than 50 years of age with palpable abnormalities suggestive of heterotrophic tissue, size longer than 2 cm, or a broad base wider than 2 cm.

Colon

Diverticulosis

The colon is where the majority of all diverticula occur in the alimentary tract. Due to this predominance, this condition is commonly termed *diverticulosis* or *diverticular disease*. Diverticulum of the colon is of the false type. The incidence increases with age. The incidence of diverticulosis approaches 20% at age 40 and increases to greater than 60% at age 80. Diverticulosis is most commonly located in the sigmoid colon.

The exact pathogenesis of diverticulosis is unclear. The proposed mechanism of colonic diverticular formation places an emphasis on intraluminal pressure buildup. The pressure across the colonic wall increases as the radius of the wall decreases. Accordingly, the radius is the smallest in the sigmoid colon and thus the most likely location of diverticulosis. Normally, pressure is constant throughout the colon. However, as diverticular disease develops, abnormal pressure segmentations occur resulting in pressure gradient changes in the colon. With increased pressure, the integrity of collagen and elastin in the wall muscle changes, the circular muscles thicken, colonic segments shorten, and the lumen narrows, leading to propagation of the disease. Several risk factors have been associated with the development of diverticular disease: smoking, lack of physical activity, and obesity. By increasing the amount of dietary fiber, it is theorized that the resultant bulking of the stools may decrease the pressure in the colon lumen and prevent diverticular disease progression. Yet, mixed results have been noted on studies with regard to fiber intake and diverticular development and progression of disease.

Colonic Diverticular Bleeding

Diverticula tend to develop where an arteriole penetrates the circular muscle layer of the colon. This results in vessels arching over the dome of the diverticulum. This leaves fragile vessels in a vulnerable position of a relatively thin mucosal layer prone to trauma and resultant diverticular bleeding. Bleeding typically manifests as hematochezia—a darkish to bright red bleeding that is typically characterized as brisk and acute in nature. Diverticulosis is attributed to 30% to 50% of all hematochezia. Fifteen percent of patients will experience at least one episode of bleeding in their lifetime, with a recurrent bleeding risk of up to 38%. Most patients presenting with diverticular bleeding are asymptomatic but some may experience bloating or cramping.

Selection of the diagnostic modality depends largely on the degree of bleeding and the cardiovascular stability of the patient. Although new technologies are emerging with enhanced computed tomography scanning, their availability is not widespread. Endoscopy is the preferred treatment modality for stable patients due to its potential for diagnosis and treatment options. Up to 80% of diverticular bleeding can be isolated with direct endoscopic visualization (Figure 3).

Endoscopic failure to identify or control diverticular bleeding may occur in the patient with massive or intermittent bleeding. Hemodynamically unstable patients may have a high complication risk from the bowel preparation, sedation, or the procedure. Radionuclide imaging can be considered in unstable patients, nondiagnostic endoscopy, or bleeding recurrence. Radionuclide imaging requires that bleeding be active (at least 0.05–0.1 mL/min) to accurately isolate the location of the diverticulum. Radionuclide imaging using technetium (99mTc) sulfur colloid (shorter half-life thus utilized for acute bleeding) or 99mTc pertechnetate (longer half-life more useful for intermittent bleeding)–labeled autologous red blood cells can be used to isolate the location of obscure gastrointestinal bleeding. However, numerous studies have produced highly variable sensitivities (26% to 91%). Many advocate for radionuclide imaging to be used as an ancillary test for directing more definitive treatments such as surgery or angiography-directed therapies. Angiography can be used if bleeding is active (at least 0.5 mL/min) and can isolate the bleeding location with a diagnostic yield of 40% to 78%. Angiography can be combined with embolization and/or vasopressin infusion to achieve hemostasis; however, complications may occur, including bowel infarction and contrast-induced nephrotoxicity.

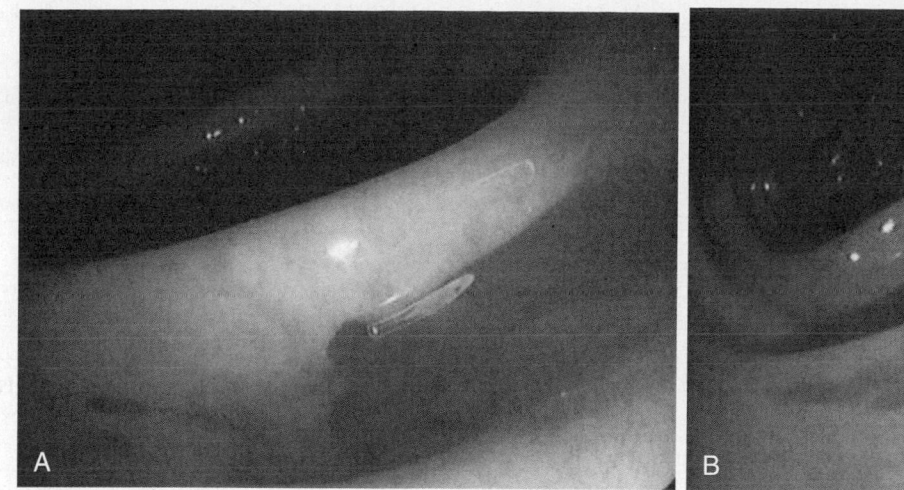
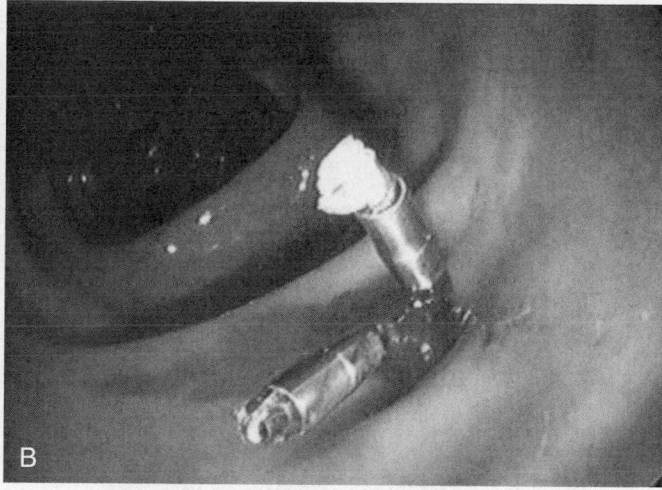

Figure 3. Colonoscopy in a patient with hematochezia from the source isolated to a diverticulum (**A**) and hemostasis noted after placement of two hemoclips (**B**). (Courtesy of Janak Shah.) (From Feldman M: Sleisenger and Fordtran's Gastrointestinal and Liver Disease, 9th ed. Philadelphia, Elsevier, Figure 117-8.)

Diverticulitis

Diverticulosis is largely asymptomatic. Only about 4% will develop inflammation and infection known as diverticulitis. The disease severity and complications occur along a spectrum. Colonic diverticula become filled with feces and obstruction may occur. With the resultant bacterial overgrowth, expansion of the diverticula occurs. Subsequent vascular compromise and microperforation may occur, leading to localized infection and inflammation. These microperforations are usually sequestered and may lead to small localized abscess formation. This process is generally referred to as uncomplicated diverticulitis. Complicated diverticulitis is classified when a localized abscess or infection infiltrates into adjacent organs or viscera causing macroperforations, fistulas, obstructions, or enlarged abscesses.

The clinical presentation may begin with mild left lower abdominal pain, fever, and leukocytosis. Patients who seek care later in the disease process may present with sepsis or diffuse peritonitis. Initial diagnosis should be accomplished with history, physical examination, radiographic imaging, and laboratory evaluation. Abdominal radiography may indicate severe complications of diverticulitis such as bowel perforation or bowel obstruction. With sensitivity and specificity approaching 100%, computed tomography with intravenous and oral contrast is the test of choice for diagnosis of diverticulitis and accompanying complications such as fistula, abscess, and/or colitis. Ultrasonography and magnetic resonance imaging can be used with high levels of sensitivity and specificity in centers with demonstrated expertise. Those patients with a past medical history of diverticulitis may be empirically treated. Imaging may be needed if no clinical improvement is noted within 48 hours.

Recent data indicates no added benefit with antimicrobial therapy; thus, uncomplicated diverticulitis may be treated without antibiotics. Traditional treatment includes supportive care and antibiotics for uncomplicated diverticulitis. Outpatient management is reasonable if the diagnosis is made early in the disease process. Uncomplicated diverticulitis responds to medical therapy in the majority of cases. Complicated diverticulitis occurs in 25% of all diverticulitis diagnoses, requiring a surgical evaluation and intervention. Optional antibiotic regimens for gram-negative coverage and anaerobic coverage are listed in Table 1. Inpatient management is recommended with any comorbid conditions, immunosuppression, high-grade fever, leukocytosis, and/or for elderly patients. Patient improvement should be seen within 48 hours. Those who do not improve should undergo additional evaluation such as repeat imaging or endoscopy. This is done to evaluate for underlying pathology such as cancer or inflammatory bowel disease, which would change the management strategy.

Follow-up scanning should also be considered for cases of slow-resolving diverticulitis. In up to 10% of computed tomography scans in which diverticulitis was the primary diagnosis, cancer could

TABLE 1	Antibiotic Therapy for Diverticulitis	
OPTIONAL REGIMENS		**DOSAGE (ADULT)**
Uncomplicated Diverticulitis		
Outpatient (10–14 Days)		
Ciprofloxacin (Cipro) and		500 mg PO bid
Metronidazole (Flagyl)		500 mg PO tid
Amoxicillin-Clavulanate (Augmentin)[1]		875 mg PO bid
Moxifloxacin (Avelox)		400 mg PO daily
Complicated Diverticulitis		
Inpatient Transitioning to Outpatient (10–14 Days Total)		
Piperacilin-tazobactam (Zosyn)[1]		3.375–4.5 g IV every 6 hours
Ticarcillin-clavulanate (Timentin)		3.1 g IV every 4 hours
Imipenem-cilastatin (Primaxin)		500 mg IV every 6 hours
Levofloxacin (Levaquin)[1] and		500 mg IV every 24 hours
Metronidazole		500 mg IV every 8 hours
Ceftriaxone (Rocephin) and		1 g IV every 24 hours
Metronidazole		500 mg IV every 8 hours

Abbreviations: bid = twice a day; IV = intravenously; tid = three times a day.
Adapted from Jacobs DO: Clinical practice. Diverticulitis. N Engl J Med 2007;357:2057–66.
[1]Not FDA approved for this indication.
Notes: Clindamycin (Cleocin) may be substituted in metronidazole intolerance/allergy. Antibiotics continued in complicated diverticulitis cases until negative cultures, clinical improvement, or sensitivities obtained on any surgical specimens.

not be fully excluded. A colonoscopy should be performed to evaluate the extent of diverticular disease and to rule out other comorbid pathology in all patients. Colonoscopy is typically recommended within 3 to 6 weeks after diverticulitis symptoms have resolved. Introduction of stool softeners and a high-fiber diet should begin immediately and continued indefinitely for all patients to help decrease the intraluminal pressure within the colon.

Diverticulitis that is complicated with abscess formation should be evaluated by a surgeon or radiologist for percutaneous drainage using computed tomography or ultrasonography (Figure 4). Depending on location, drainage tubes may be placed trans-anally for drainage. A general recommendation exists for radiologic evaluation and drainage if the abscess is greater than 2 cm.

New research to prevent recurrent diverticulitis with medical management is emerging. Mesalamine and rifaximin, in combination or

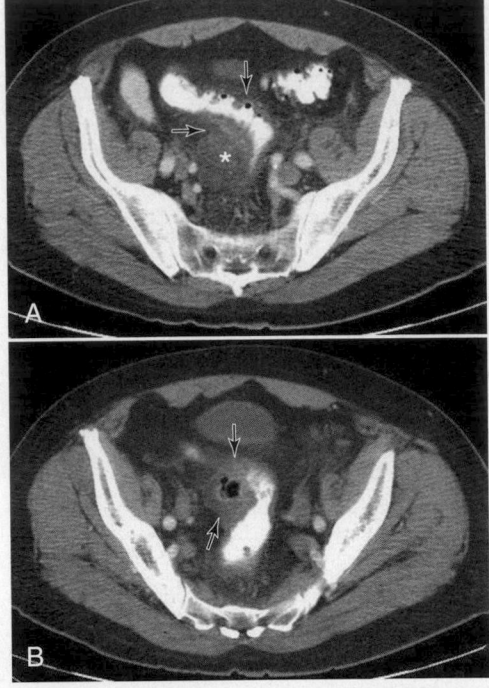

Figure 4. Diverticulitis. **A,** Computed tomography (CT) image demonstrates thickened wall of the sigmoid colon (arrows) with stranding in the adjacent fat (*) indicative of diverticulitis. Fat stranding refers to abnormally increased attenuation of fat from edema and engorgement of lymphatics. **B,** CT image slightly more caudal demonstrates an air-filled abscess cavity (arrows) with adjacent thickened sigmoid colon wall. (From McNally PR: GI/Liver Secrets Plus, 4th ed. Noninvasive Gastrointestinal Imaging: Ultrasound, Computed Tomography, Magnetic Resonance Imaging. Philadelphia, Mosby Elsevier, 2010, Figure 70-16.)

separately, may help prevent recurrent episodes of diverticulitis. Probiotics have not been shown to prevent recurrence. Fiber may be used as a beneficial supplement for the prevention of recurrent diverticulitis. Debate exists regarding elective segmental colectomy for patients who have experienced recurrent episodes of diverticulitis. Current recommendations suggest surgical consultation with discussion of the benefits and risks of surgery compared to the risks of recurrent diverticulitis. This discussion should take into account the diverticulitis frequency and severity, the impact on the patient's lifestyle, and the patient's other comorbid conditions. This consultation should at minimum occur after the fourth recurrence of diverticulitis in patients over age 50. Limited data are available as to whether a patient who has experienced less than four recurrent cases of diverticulitis or who is younger than age 50 would benefit from a segmental colectomy.

References

Aggerholm K, Illum P. Surgical treatment of Zenker's diverticulum. J Laryngol Otol 1990;104:312–4.
Choi JJ, Ogunjemilusi O, Divino CM. Diagnosis and management of diverticula in the jejunum and ileum. Am Surg 2013;79(1):108–10.
Fry RD, Mahmoud NN, Maron DJ, Bleier JIS. Colon and rectum. In: Townsend Jr CM, Beauchamp D, editors. Sabiston Textbook of Surgery. 19th ed. Philadelphia: Saunders; 2012. p. 1309–14.
Jacobs DO. Clinical practice. Diverticulitis. N Engl J Med 2007;357:2057–66.
Janes SE, Meagher A, Frizelle FA. Management of diverticulitis. BMJ 2006;332:271–5.
Kilic A, Schuchert MJ, Awais O, et al. Surgical management of epiphrenic diverticula in the minimally invasive era. JSLS 2009;13:160–4.
Maish MS. Esophagus. In: Townsend Jr CM, Beauchamp D, editors. Sabiston Textbook of Surgery. 19th ed. Philadelphia: Saunders; 2012. p. 1023–5.
Martinez-Cecilia D, Arjona-Sanchez A, Gomez-Alvarez M, et al. Conservative management of perforated duodenal diverticulum: a case report and review of the literature. World J Gastroenterol 2008;14:1949–51.
Mohan P, Ananthavadivelu M, Venkataraman J. Gastric diverticulum. CMAJ 2010;182:E226.
Morris AM, Rogenbogen SE, Hardiman KM, Hendren S. Sigmoid diverticulitis: a systematic review. JAMA 2014;311:287–97.
Mulder CJ, Costamagna G, Sakai P. Zenker's Diverticulum: treatment using a flexible endoscope. Endoscopy 2001;33:991–7.
Park JJ, Wolff BG, Tollefson MK, et al. Meckel diverticulum: the Mayo clinic experience with 1476 patients (1950–2002). Ann Surg 2005;241:529–33.
Shahedi K1, Fuller G, Bolus R, et al. Long-term risk of acute diverticulitis among patients with incidental diverticulosis found during colonoscopy. Clin Gastroenterol Hepatol 2013;11(12):1609–13.
Strate LL. Lower GI, bleeding: epidemiology and diagnosis. Gastroenterol Clin North Am 2005;34:643–64.
Verdonck J, Morton RP. Systematic review on treatment of Zenker's Diverticulum. Eur Arch Ororhinolargoi 2014; epub ahead of print.
Weizman AV, Nguyen GC. Diverticular disease: epidemiology and management. Can J Gastroenterol 2011;25:385–9.
Zani A, Eaton S, Rees CM, et al. Incidentally detected Meckel diverticulum: to resect or not to resect? Ann Surg 2008;247:276–81.

DYSPHAGIA AND ESOPHAGEAL OBSTRUCTION

Method of
Kumar Krishnan, MD; and John E. Pandolfino, MD

CURRENT DIAGNOSIS

- The evaluation of dysphagia begins with a careful history, though additional diagnostic testing is often required.
- Oropharyngeal dysphagia is best initially evaluated with a videoscopic fluoroscopy examination, whereas esophageal dysphagia is best evaluated with endoscopy.
- Esophageal dysphagia with negative endoscopy and biopsy should be evaluated next with esophageal manometry.

CURRENT THERAPY

- Underlying neuromuscular conditions such as amyotrophic lateral sclerosis, myasthenia gravis, or Guillain-Barré syndrome should be treated accordingly.
- Endoscopic therapy with dilation (often multiple) is the mainstay of treating fibrotic esophageal strictures regardless of etiology.
- Achalasia can be treated surgically or with dilation, which are equally effective. Minimally invasive endoscopic therapy for achalasia is promising and may provide a competing approach.

Dysphagia is a symptom generated by the perceived sensation of difficulty or inability to swallow. It ranges in severity from mild difficulty with no associated clinical sequelae, to a complete inability to swallow with aspiration and severe malnutrition. Dysphagia can coexist with and must be distinguished from odynophagia, which is pain when swallowing, with associated swallowing aversion. The etiology of dysphagia is protean and includes two main categories, mechanical obstruction and motor dysfunction.

Epidemiology

Dysphagia is a common condition. A recent investigation surveyed 790 ambulatory patients who were awaiting their annual primary care visit; 22.6% of patients reported dysphagia at least several times per month. Only half of these patients had discussed their symptoms with their physician. Elderly patients and women were more likely to note symptoms of dysphagia.

Pathophysiology

Effective swallowing and transfer of food bolus into the stomach requires multiple steps. These steps can be broadly placed into two phases: the oropharyngeal phase and the esophageal phase. The oropharyngeal phase of swallowing ultimately transforms the hypopharynx from a respiratory organ to a digestive organ. It requires five main coordinated steps to occur: (1) elevation of the soft palate and closure of the nasopharynx, (2) relaxation of the upper esophageal sphincter (UES), (3) traction opening of the UES, (4) closure of the laryngeal vestibule and hence airway protection, and

(5) propulsion of the food bolus by the tongue and pharyngeal constrictors. This process is a carefully coordinated neuromuscular phenomenon with both autonomic and volitional components.

The esophageal phase of swallowing begins when a food bolus passes through the UES. During swallowing, the rapidity of bolus transit into the stomach is accomplished primarily by gravity. Esophageal peristalsis is a secondary contributor that functions to strip the bolus and clear the esophagus. Primary peristalsis is associated with oropharyngeal swallowing and propagates down through the predominantly striated muscle esophagus via a sequential activation pattern originating from the brainstem. This continues into the smooth muscle esophagus where it also engages the intrinsic enteric nervous system to promote peristalsis through a similar but distinct mechanism. Secondary peristalsis is stimulated by distention of the proximal esophagus and will generate a propagating peristaltic contraction similar to primary peristalsis without a swallow-induced trigger. The strength, propagation velocity, and order of peristaltic contractions can be altered and this may lead to motor abnormalities associated with dysphagia.

Diagnosis

Dysphagia is never a normal symptom and always requires additional investigation. The first step in the diagnostic evaluation of dysphagia begins with a careful history to distinguish true dysphagia from other associated conditions such as odynophagia and globus sensation. Odynophagia can coexist with dysphagia; however, the predominant symptom is pain during swallowing. Globus is a sensation of a lump in the throat. It is likely a pharyngeal hypersensitivity that may coexist with other esophageal diseases or occur alone as a functional disorder. Unlike dysphagia, the symptoms in globus persist between swallows and may actually improve during the swallow.

After the above conditions have been ruled out, the next step focuses on distinguishing oropharyngeal dysphagia from esophageal dysphagia. Unfortunately, patients have a difficult time communicating their symptoms because localization of the point of perceived obstruction is hampered by poor discriminant capacity and may be masked by compensatory mechanisms. Localization of dysphagia to the throat or sternal notch is unreliable because the point of obstruction may be further down in the body. However, localization in the midchest or below is more reliable that the obstruction is esophageal in origin.

As a result, the most useful and underused test for distinguishing oropharyngeal and esophageal dysphagia focuses on observing the patient swallow sips of water in the office. Often this allows the distinction between oropharyngeal and esophageal dysphagia to become apparent. Patients with oropharyngeal dysphagia will have difficulty almost immediately after initiating a swallow, such as coughing, choking, and nasal regurgitation. Patients who can initiate a swallow without difficulty, but note symptoms soon after the swallow, are likely to have esophageal dysphagia. Furthermore, this exercise may be able to elicit associated odynophagia or regurgitation.

Physical examination plays a minor role in evaluating dysphagia outside of assessing the patient's baseline status to rule out malnutrition and dehydration because this will determine whether an expedited evaluation is required. A careful assessment of the oropharynx and a careful neck examination may unmask a mass lesion, and a neurologic examination should be performed if oropharyngeal dysphagia is suspected. Additionally, a skin examination and assessment of the oropharyngeal mucosa may be helpful in assessing for potential dermatologic diseases that are associated with esophageal dysphagia. Regardless of findings, most patients will ultimately be referred for diagnostic testing, and this is dependent on the anatomic zone of interest—oropharyngeal versus esophageal (Figure 1).

Diagnostic Testing
Oropharyngeal Dysphagia

Once a distinction is made that the patient is experiencing oropharyngeal dysphagia, the next step in the evaluation should be referral for a videoscopic swallowing examination. Standard upper endoscopy is of limited value given the general inability to evaluate lesions in the hypopharynx and the upper esophageal sphincter.

Videoscopic swallowing examinations have the added benefit of providing functional information in addition to anatomic information. They differ from a standard fluoroscopic examination (i.e., esophogram) by offering the patient various radiopaque food items of different consistency and are often performed by a speech pathologist. They can evaluate delay in initiation of pharyngeal swallowing, aspiration of solids and liquids, retrograde flow of ingested bolus, and residual pharyngeal contents.

If there is a suspicion for a malignancy or mechanical obstruction, a referral to otolaryngology is required. Direct laryngoscopy is used to evaluate for anatomic lesions in the nasopharynx and hypopharynx. In addition to anatomic abnormalities, function can be assessed by having the patient drink liquids with the nasal endoscope positioned in the hypopharynx. Oropharyngeal pooling of liquid indicates ineffective hypopharyngeal clearance and can suggest a high aspiration risk. Cross-sectional imaging is often an adjunct to the functional assessment of videoscopic imaging or direct laryngoscopy when an obstruction is noted without a clear lesion noted on direct examination.

Esophageal Dysphagia

If oropharyngeal dysphagia is excluded on history, the evaluation of dysphagia should proceed to upper endoscopy to rule out a mechanical obstruction. Although an esophogram can be used to assess for obstruction, most patients will eventually require endoscopy to obtain biopsies to rule out malignancy or eosinophilic esophagitis. Additionally, endoscopy has the added benefit of being therapeutic in some circumstances, and thus it is more cost-effective to begin the evaluation with endoscopy. If the endoscopy is negative, the next step is to perform esophageal manometry to rule out an esophageal motor disorder. If this is negative, a careful evaluation for the presence of gastroesophageal reflux disease (GERD) should be performed and if suspected, the patient may benefit from ambulatory reflux testing or an empiric trial of proton pump inhibitors. Patients with no evidence of obstruction, abnormal esophageal motor function, or evidence of GERD may be classified as having functional dysphagia if the symptoms fulfill the Rome III consensus (onset greater than 6 months before presentation with 3 months of symptoms).

Oropharyngeal Dysphagia
Differential Diagnosis

The etiology of oropharyngeal dysphagia can be broadly separated based on neuromuscular causes and anatomic causes (Table 1). The most common neurologic cause is cerebrovascular accident (CVA), with an incidence reported between 20% and 80%. CVAs involving the cerebrum, cerebellum, and brainstem can each lead to swallow dysfunction. Cerebral CVA can lead to impairment in mastication and the oral phase of swallowing and can interrupt normal pharyngeal peristalsis. CVA involving the brainstem can lead to disruption of the sensory afferents in the pharynx that help trigger pharyngeal swallow, and can also lead to motor dysfunction of laryngeal elevation, glottic closure, and cricopharyngeal relaxation/opening. Tumors in these areas can also produce similar effects.

A variety of neuromuscular disease can lead to bulbar symptoms, which manifest as dysphagia. This includes myasthenia gravis, amyotrophic lateral sclerosis (ALS), and Guillain-Barré syndrome (GBS). Clinicians need to be able to identify systemic manifestations of these conditions because dysphagia can often be the first manifestation of neuromuscular disorders.

The most common structural abnormalities of the hypopharynx associated with dysphagia are hypopharyngeal diverticula and cricopharyngeal bars. Acquired hypopharyngeal diverticula are most common in men after age 60 and typically present with symptoms of dysphagia, halitosis, post-swallow regurgitation, or even aspiration of material from the pharyngeal pouch. Hypopharyngeal diverticula are the result of a restrictive myopathy associated with diminished compliance of the cricopharyngeus muscle. The treatment of hypopharyngeal diverticula is cricopharyngeal myotomy with or without a diverticulectomy. Good or excellent results can be expected in 80% to 100% of Zenker's patients treated by transcervical myotomy combined with diverticulectomy or diverticulopexy. Small diverticula may spontaneously disappear following myotomy.

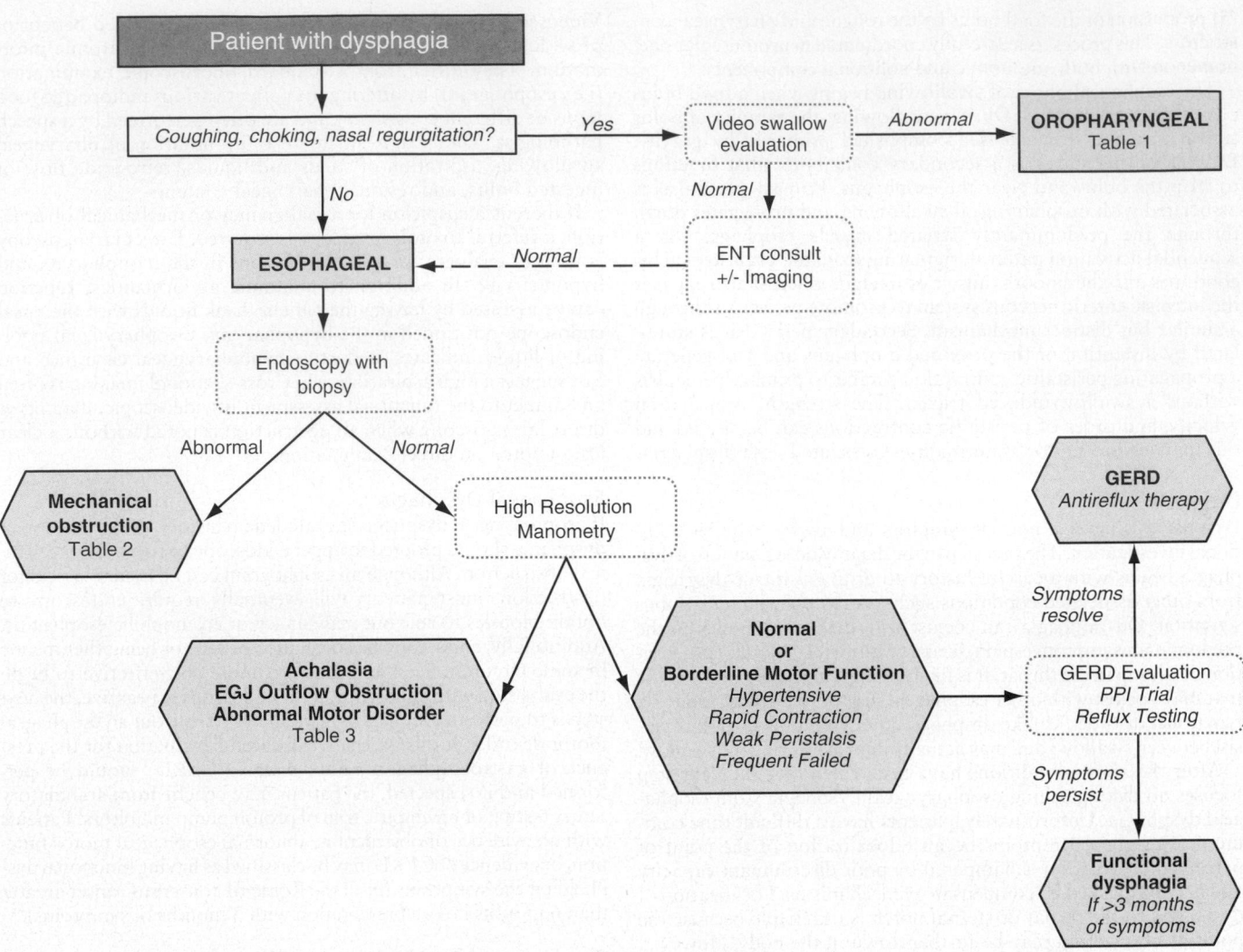

Figure 1. The workup of dysphagia and esophageal obstruction. The first step in the workup of dysphagia focuses on distinguishing oropharyngeal from esophageal dysphagia, which can be done with a history and careful assessment of swallowing during liquid swallows. The workup once this distinction is made is very different. Oropharyngeal dysphagia is typically evaluated by speech pathology and otolaryngology (ENT) based on the results of a videofluoroscopic swallow evaluation. Esophageal dysphagia is evaluated primarily with endoscopy because biopsies and interventions are often required. The primary indication for manometry is to rule out a major motor disorder in patients with a negative endoscopy. If manometry does not identify a major motor abnormality, a diagnosis of functional dysphagia should be considered; however, underlying GERD must also be addressed.

Other anatomic causes associated with oropharyngeal dysphagia that should be considered are cervical osteophytes and head and neck cancers. Cervical osteophytes are associated with cervical spine arthritis and may be confused with a cricopharyngeal bar because the dysphagia is structural and localized to the area of the upper esophageal sphincter. It is easily differentiated on contrast studies because the cervical osteophyte can be seen impinging on the upper sphincter. Additionally, head and neck lesions of the larynx, tonsil, tongue, oral cavity, vocal cord, and nasopharynx may also impair bolus transit into the esophagus. Rapid weight loss in a patient with oropharyngeal dysphagia warrants further evaluation for malignancy; however, it is often difficult to distinguish weight loss resulting from malignancy from weight loss secondary to dysphagia. Constitutional symptoms (night sweats, fever, etc.) associated with oropharyngeal dysphagia should raise the suspicion for lymphoma.

Management

The management of oropharyngeal dysphagia is dependent on the underlying cause. Neuromuscular conditions such as stroke may respond to speech therapy and rehabilitation. Systemic neuromuscular dysfunction from conditions such as myasthenia gravis, GBS, or ALS will require treatment of the underlying condition. Patients who cannot safely take oral nutrition may need a temporary enteral feeding tube until swallow function is intact.

Management of dysphagia in patients with head and neck cancers requires a multidisciplinary approach and treatment of the underlying malignancy. Some patients are able to take adequate nutrition with dietary modification (soft or full liquid diet) while undergoing therapy. Patients who are losing weight, are dehydrated, or are unable to meet nutritional requirement by dietary modification alone may require enteral nutrition in the form of a gastrostomy tube. Although endoscopic gastrostomy tube placement is typically safe, and routinely performed in patients with head and neck cancer, there are reports of seeding the gastrostomy tube tract with malignant cells from the pharynx. In such circumstances, a direct gastrostomy tube placed by a radiologist may be preferable.

Esophageal Dysphagia

Esophageal dysphagia can be easily separated into mechanical causes and motor abnormalities after upper endoscopy is performed. Mechanical causes can be further separated into malignant and benign causes of dysphagia, and motor disorders can be conceptualized as primary motor abnormalities versus borderline motor abnormalities. Patients who have symptoms in the context of a normal endoscopy (negative biopsies for eosinophilic esophagitis) and no evidence of a primary motor disorder may also have underlying GERD or functional dysphagia (see Figure 1).

TABLE 1 Oropharyngeal Dysphagia

Iatrogenic

- Medication side effects (chemotherapy, neuroleptics, etc.)
- Postsurgical muscular or neurogenic
- Radiation
- Corrosive (pill injury, intentional)

Infectious

- Diphtheria
- Botulism
- Lyme disease
- Syphilis
- Mucositis (herpes, cytomegalovirus, candida, etc.)

Metabolic

- Amyloidosis
- Cushing's syndrome
- Thyrotoxicosis
- Wilson's disease

Myopathic

- Connective tissue disease (overlap syndrome)
- Dermatomyositis
- Myasthenia gravis
- Myotonic dystrophy
- Oculopharyngeal dystrophy
- Polymyositis
- Sarcoidosis
- Paraneoplastic syndromes

Neurologic

- Brainstem tumors
- Head trauma
- Stroke
- Cerebral palsy
- Guillain-Barré syndrome
- Huntington's disease
- Multiple sclerosis
- Polio
- Postpolio syndrome
- Tardive dyskinesia
- Metabolic encephalopathies
- Amyotrophic lateral sclerosis
- Parkinson's disease
- Dementia

Structural

- Cricopharyngeal bar
- Zenker's diverticulum
- Cervical webs
- Oropharyngeal tumors
- Osteophytes and skeletal abnormalities
- Congenital abnormalities (cleft palate, diverticula, pouches, etc.)

TABLE 2 Esophageal Dysphagia (Mechanical)

Mucosal disease
  GERD (peptic stricture)
  Esophageal rings
  Esophageal cancer
  Caustic injury (e.g., lye ingestion, pill esophagitis, sclerotherapy)
  Radiation injury
  Infectious esophagitis
  Eosinophilic esophagitis
  Anastomotic stricture
  Submucosal disease
  Gastrointestinal stromal tumor
  Sarcoidosis
  Invasive carcinoma (primary or secondary)
Mediastinal disease
  Tumors (lymph nodes, lung cancer)
  Infection (histoplasmosis, tuberculosis)
  Vascular compression
  Dysphagia lusoria
  Dysphagia aortica

increasing. EoE is a condition characterized by marked eosinophilic infiltrate within the esophageal epithelium. This infiltrate results in characteristic endoscopic findings of esophageal rings, furrows, exudate, and eventually stricture formation. The most common symptom in patients with EoE is dysphagia, which often leads to food bolus impaction. Patients are typically young Caucasians and there is a clear male predominance. Atopic conditions are more prevalent in patients with EoE. Patients should initially be treated with proton pump inhibitor (PPI) therapy because there is an overlap between GERD and EoE. Patients with persistent eosinophilia on PPI therapy can be treated by swallowing inhaled formulations of steroids (fluticasone [Flovent],[1] budesonide [Pulmicort][1]) or a food elimination diet (avoid: soy, nuts, wheat, eggs, dairy, seafood) to reduce the inflammatory component of the disease. Additional therapy with dilation will be required in many patients because histologic improvement does not always result in regression of fibrotic strictures. The esophageal body is more prone to fracture in EoE, and deep mucosal tears are often associated with dilation therapy; thus these lesions may require a more gradual and careful dilation protocol.

Rings/Webs

Esophageal webs can exist along the length of the esophagus and lead to dysphagia. The classic triad of proximal esophageal web, iron deficiency anemia, and dysphagia is Plummer-Vinson syndrome. The etiology of this condition is not entirely known; however, it is thought that iron deficiency leads to a decrease in iron-dependent oxidative enzymes, which results in degradation of esophageal tissue, resulting in web formation. Interestingly, iron supplementation alone may result in resolution of symptoms. Whereas Plummer-Vinson syndrome is a rare condition, esophageal webs are relatively common and should prompt an evaluation for caustic pill injury if localized to the transition zone along the aortic impression or distal esophagus. Medications that can be associated with pill esophagitis include NSAIDs, tetracycline, iron, bisphosphonates, potassium, and quinidine.

Malignancy

Dysphagia is often the presenting symptom in a patient with esophageal cancer. There are two subtypes of mucosal cancer in the esophagus, squamous cell and adenocarcinoma. In general, esophageal cancer has a male predominance and is slightly more prevalent among African Americans. The racial disparity is largely due to squamous cell carcinoma, which has noted a sharp decline since the 1960s. Adenocarcinoma tends to be a disease of white men (SEER database). Squamous cell carcinoma typically occurs in the mid esophagus, whereas adenocarcinoma is localized to the distal esophagus where it is associated with intestinal metaplasia (Barrett's esophagus).

Differential Diagnosis: Mechanical Obstruction (Table 2)
Stricture

Fibrotic esophageal strictures are common and can be caused by erosive esophagitis (peptic stricture), radiation therapy, surgical anastomosis, eosinophilic esophagitis, and desquamating lesions (pemphigus, lichen planus, etc.). Peptic strictures are common and are the result of long-standing erosive esophagitis. They typically occur in the distal esophagus. Such patients often have underlying physiologic derangements that favor aggressive reflux (weak lower esophageal sphincter, hiatal hernia, poor esophageal clearance). Postsurgical anastomotic strictures are an unfortunate consequence of surgical therapy for esophageal disease, but these lesions are often amenable to endoscopic therapy.

Eosinophilic Esophagitis

Eosinophilic esophagitis (EoE) requires some focused discussion because its prevalence in patients presenting with dysphagia is

---

[1]Not FDA approved for this indication.

Management for Esophageal Obstruction

Endoscopic dilation therapy is the most common therapeutic intervention for patients with nonmalignant mechanical dysphagia. This can be done with a single, large-diameter dilating balloon or semirigid bougie over a guide wire. There has not been any convincing data to demonstrate superiority of balloon dilators over bougie dilators. In cases of membranous webs or Schatzki rings, the goal of endoscopic therapy is to tear the lesion with a single, large-diameter dilation. In the case of a Schatzki ring, postdilation PPI therapy is associated with decreased recurrence rates.

When treating fibrotic strictures (peptic, anastomotic, radiation, EoE), the goal should be gradual stretching of the stricture. The choice of initial dilation size is based on an estimate of the diameter of the stricture. The extent to which a stricture can be dilated is expressed by the endoscopic axiom of the "rule of threes." This refers to the approach whereby the diameter of the stricture is approximated, and no more than three subsequent dilations are performed at 1-mm intervals once resistance is noted. Though there is no controlled trial for support, this approach is used to minimize the most serious risks of dilation therapy, perforation and bleeding.

In patients with refractory strictures despite dilation therapy, several therapies have been attempted with variable efficacy. Temporary self-expanding stents have been placed to maintain lumen patency. When placed across a stricture, stents serve two purposes. First, they relieve symptoms of dysphagia by maintaining a patent lumen. In addition, the self-expanding nature of the stent provides ongoing radial force, which gradually stretches the lumen. The main disadvantage of stents is their tendency to migrate. Plastic and biodegradable stents are currently not available, but may be promising in the future.

An alternative endoscopic approach is incisional therapy with an electrocautery knife. This is used to make incisions in the mucosa and fibrotic submucosa. This approach has been best studied in the setting of refractory anastomotic strictures; however, no head-to-head comparisons have been made between incisional therapy and other modalities.

Treatment of malignant etiologies for dysphagia will ultimately depend on the tumor type and extent of disease. Benign tumors and early-stage lesions can be treated with endoscopic resection or surgery. Endoscopic therapy using stents is also an important component of the treatment of malignancy and may be used during the treatment phase of malignant disorders or as a palliative technique for later-stage disease.

Differential Diagnosis: Motility Disorders (Table 3)

Esophageal motor disorders are defined based on patterns of contractile vigor, propagation, and the presence of deglutitive relaxation. Multiple classifications have been proposed; however, a new technique using a more advanced high-resolution manometric system that provides greater detail and accuracy has become available. This classification scheme is based on previous conventional schemes with modifications based on refining disorders into clinically relevant phenotypes.

Achalasia

The diagnosis of achalasia is made by esophageal manometry and requires two main manometric criteria: (1) inability of the lower esophageal sphincter to relax and (2) absence of peristalsis. Recently achalasia has been subdivided into three different phenotypes using high-resolution manometry, which are associated with varying clinical outcomes. Patients typically describe both solid

TABLE 3 Esophageal Dysphagia (Abnormal Motor Function)

Achalasia
EGJ outflow obstruction
Absent peristalsis
Spasm
Jackhammer

and liquid dysphagia. Other common symptoms are regurgitation (especially nocturnal), chest pain, and aspiration. Weight loss and malnutrition may be dominant symptoms as the disease progresses. Given that there is no treatment to reverse absent peristalsis, the treatment is focused on improving esophagogastric junction (EGJ) opening by disrupting the poorly relaxing lower esophageal sphincter. This can be accomplished using pneumatic dilation with rigid balloons ranging in size from 3 to 4 cm or surgical myotomy. It appears that the two treatment approaches are associated with good outcomes with surgery having a more durable single intervention success rate and pneumatic dilation typically requiring multiple sessions. Botulinum toxin type A (Botox)[1] injected into the lower esophageal sphincter has been shown to reduce EGJ pressure and improve symptoms; however, this treatment only provides temporary relief and should only be reserved for poor surgical candidates or patients unwilling to undergo surgery or dilation. Occasionally, esophageal dilation may progress to a point where treatment with pneumatic dilation and myotomy are not adequate and esophagectomy must be performed to prevent severe complications, such as aspiration and severe malnutrition.

Esophagogastric Junction Outflow Obstruction

This pattern of motor disturbance is associated with preserved peristalsis and evidence of high pressures through the EGJ during swallowing. This may be an achalasia variant or could be associated with a subtle obstruction at the distal esophagus not evident on endoscopy. Thus, recognition of this pattern should prompt an evaluation for an infiltrating tumor or other potential etiology of obstruction. Treatment is focused on the underlying cause of the obstruction.

Absent Peristalsis

Absent peristalsis is defined as complete absence of contractile activity on all swallows in the context of a normal or low EGJ relaxation pressure. This pattern was previously categorized as scleroderma esophagus if it was found in the context of a hypotensive lower esophageal sphincter; however, this has been abandoned because this pattern may be found in patients with severe GERD without scleroderma. Treatment is focused on aggressive antireflux therapy and lifestyle modifications to reduce dysphagia and caustic injury to the esophagus.

Distal Esophageal Spasm

Distal esophageal spasm is a rare primary motor disorder that may present with dysphagia and chest pain. It is associated with impaired deglutitive inhibition of the esophageal body and results in unopposed activation of the cholinergic intrinsic neurons resulting in premature contractions associated with a rapid contractile velocity. The premature contraction is the most important aspect of this disorder and this has replaced an emphasis on peristaltic velocity because high-resolution manometry has shown that rapid contractions are usually associated with weak contractions. Treatment for this disorder is extremely difficult and focuses on medical management with smooth muscle relaxants, such as calcium channel blockers,[1] nitrates,[1] and 5-phosphodiesterase inhibitors.[1]

Jackhammer

Jackhammer esophagus is an extreme form of nutcracker esophagus associated with contractile vigor not encountered in asymptomatic controls or under normal conditions. Previous definitions for hypertensive esophagus had a significant overlap with data from cohorts of asymptomatic controls, and thus the clinical significance of these disorders was unclear. This pattern is associated with dysphagia and chest pain and is typically treated similar to distal esophageal spasm. This motor pattern can also be seen with distal esophageal obstruction, and this should be considered in the differential diagnosis because it would alter management to focus on the obstruction.

---

[1]Not FDA approved for this indication.

Borderline Motor Abnormalities

Borderline motor abnormalities are those associated with ineffective esophageal motility and mild abnormalities of peristaltic propagation (rapid contraction) or hypertensive contraction. These disorders are not considered to be primary motor disorders, and secondary cause for symptoms, such as GERD and visceral sensitivity, should be considered and treated.

Monitoring

Patients with dysphagia or esophageal obstruction should be monitored for three important complications:

- Evidence of aspiration and nocturnal regurgitation because these can be associated with severe complications, such as chemical pneumonitis and aspiration pneumonia.
- Malnutrition and dehydration because this may prompt more aggressive therapy or consideration of non-oral feeding methods.
- Progressive symptoms because this could lead to progression of the disease and early therapy may avoid the above complications.

Acknowledgment

This work was supported by R01 DK079902 (JEP) from the U.S. National Institutes of Health.

References

Bredenoord AJ, Fox M, Kahrilas PJ, et al. Chicago classification criteria of esophageal motility disorders defined in high resolution esophageal pressure topography. Neurogastroenterol Motil 2012;24(Suppl. 1):57–65.

Cook IJ, Kahrilas PJ. AGA technical review on management of oropharyngeal dysphagia. Gastroenterology 1999;116:455–78.

Drossman DA. The functional gastrointestinal disorders and the Rome III process. Gastroenterology 2006;130:1377–90.

Egan JV, Baron TH, Adler DG, et al. Esophageal dilation. Gastrointest Endosc 2006;63:755–60.

Francis DL, Katzka DA. Achalasia: update on the disease and its treatment. Gastroenterology 2010;139:369–74.

Liacouras CA, Furuta GT, Hirano I, et al. Eosinophilic esophagitis: updated consensus recommendations for children and adults. J Allergy Clin Immunol 2011;128:3–20e26; quiz 21–2.

Pandolfino JE, Kahrilas PJ. AGA technical review on the clinical use of esophageal manometry. Gastroenterology 2005;128:209–24.

Pandolfino JE, Kwiatek MA, Nealis T, et al. Achalasia: a new clinically relevant classification by high-resolution manometry. Gastroenterology 2008;135:1526–33.

Spechler SJ. AGA technical review on treatment of patients with dysphagia caused by benign disorders of the distal esophagus. Gastroenterology 1999;117:233–54.

Wilkins T, Gillies RA, Thomas AM, et al. The prevalence of dysphagia in primary care patients: a HamesNet Research Network study. J Am Board Fam Med 2007;20:144–50.

GASTRITIS AND PEPTIC ULCER DISEASE

Method of
Kyle Vincent, MD

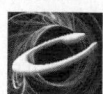

CURRENT DIAGNOSIS

- Diagnosis of gastritis and peptic ulcer disease is based on a history of dyspepsia and elimination of other conditions.
- *Helicobacter pylori* (*H. pylori*) and nonsteroidal antiinflammatory drugs (NSAIDs) are the most common cause of ulcer disease. Hypersecretory conditions such as Zollinger-Ellison syndrome are rare.
- If testing for *H. pylori* is indicated (test-and-treat strategy), serum IgG antibody, urea breath test, and fecal antigen test are available.
- Young patients with no "warning signs" can usually be managed on an outpatient basis without immediate endoscopy.
- Patients older than 55, with bleeding, anemia, loss of more than 10% of body weight, dysphagia, odynophagia, early satiety, history of previous malignancy, lymphadenopathy, abdominal mass, or a previously documented ulcer should undergo upper endoscopy promptly.

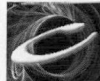

CURRENT THERAPY

- The two principal strategies are empiric treatment or test and treat.
- In areas with an *H. pylori* infection rate of less than 10%, a 4 to 8 week course of proton-pump inhibitors (PPIs) given empirically is appropriate.
- In patients who fail empiric PPI treatment or in areas with an *H. pylori* infection rate of greater than 10%, a test-and-treat strategy should be employed. A verified noninvasive *H. pylori* test should be used.
- First-line treatment of *H. pylori* consists of a PPI, clarithromycin (Biaxin), and amoxicillin (Amoxil), all taken twice a day for 14 days.
- NSAIDs should be discontinued or a standard dose PPI for ulcer prophylaxis used to treat any dyspepsia.

Epidemiology

An estimated 4 million Americans have active gastric ulcers, with 350,000 new cases diagnosed each year. The lifetime prevalence of this condition is about 10%. The incidence was previously higher in men but is currently equal in men and women. Familial clustering is now believed to result from transmission of *Helicobacter pylori* (*H. pylori*) from person to person or from a genetic predisposition to infection with *H. pylori* rather than a genetic predisposition to gastric ulcers.

Risk Factors

Most gastric and duodenal ulcers can be attributed to *H. pylori*, nonsteroidal antiinflammatory drugs (NSAIDs), severe physiologic stress, or hypersecretory conditions. In America, 10% of young adults harbor *H. pylori* infections; this incidence increases with age. Lower socioeconomic status and recent immigration from areas with high rates of infection also increase the incidence of *H. pylori* infection. Hypersecretory conditions such as Zollinger-Ellison syndrome are rare, estimated to be responsible for only 0.1% of all ulcers. These conditions should not be routinely considered except in refractory or recurrent cases or in patients who have multiple ulcers.

Pathophysiology

The low pH of gastric acid is required to kill ingested bacteria and to promote proteolysis and activation of pepsin. Postprandial gastric acid production is stimulated by expression of gastrin from G cells and is inhibited in a negative feedback loop by somatostatin from antral D cells. Contrary to previous beliefs, peptic ulcer disease is not simply due to excessive acid production. Almost all patients with gastric ulcer have normal acid production and only one-third of patients with duodenal ulcers have evidence of increased acid production. The protective mechanisms of the mucosa play an important role in maintaining mucosal integrity.

The gastric and duodenal mucosa forms a gelatinous layer that is impermeable to gastric acid and pepsin. Mucosal blood flow as well as the production of mucus and bicarbonate secretion is largely regulated by E type prostaglandins. Anything that can disrupt the balance between acid production and the protective barrier has the potential to cause loss of mucosal integrity and tissue exposure to gastric acid and pepsin with subsequent inflammation and potential ulceration.

Two major mechanisms contribute to gastritis and/or ulcer formation. *H. pylori* is a gram-negative curved rod that produces ammonia to control the surrounding pH. Ammonia is toxic to epithelial cells, causing gastritis or duodenitis and damaging mucosal integrity. Many patients with gastritis also have a marked decrease in the number of somatostatin-secreting antral D cells, leading to diminished feedback to control acid secretion during gastrin stimulation.

Prevention

The United States Preventative Task Force does not currently recommend routine screening for *H. pylori* in asymptomatic individuals. Prevention is based on avoidance or minimization of risk factors. Long-term NSAID use should be avoided. Prophylactic antisecretory medication should be considered when prolonged NSAID use is necessary. Proton-pump inhibitors (PPIs) have better protective efficacy than histamine receptor antagonists (H2RAs) when prolonged NSAID use is necessary. Patients with a previous history of ulcer disease who use steroids or are older than 65 years of age should strongly be considered for prophylaxis with an antisecretory medication. Because of the high risk of gastric ulceration, prophylaxis is recommended for patients experiencing severe physiologic stress, such as mechanical ventilation for longer than 48 hours, hypoperfusion, high-dose corticosteroids, and large surface-area burns (>35% total body surface). Histamine receptor antagonists such as famotidine (Pepcid),[1] cimetidine (Tagamet),[1] and ranitidine (Zantac)[1] or PPIs are recommended. Neither agent has shown clear superiority for prophylaxis in patients on steroids or undergoing physiologic stress.

No immunization against *H. pylori* is currently available but early stage animal trials are in progress.

Clinical Manifestations

Dyspepsia is defined by the American College of Gastroenterology as chronic or recurrent pain or discomfort centered in the upper abdomen. Discomfort is defined as a subjective negative feeling that is not painful. Discomfort can incorporate a variety of symptoms including early satiety or upper abdominal fullness. A thorough history is usually sufficient to establish the diagnosis and to differentiate gastritis and peptic ulcers from other common conditions. Gastritis and peptic ulcer disease are difficult to differentiate from each other based on history and physical examination alone, though patients with peptic ulcer disease tend to have symptoms more pronounced with food intake. A patient with a duodenal ulcer usually reports increased pain 2 to 3 hours after a meal; conversely, a patient with a gastric ulcer tends to have pain precipitated or exacerbated by food intake. However, these classical findings are not reliable diagnostic indicators. Physical examination is important to rule out serious complications from peptic ulcer disease. Patient with a rigid abdomen, rebound tenderness, or guarding should be evaluated with imaging and by a surgeon to rule out perforation. The most common physical finding in peptic ulcer disease is tenderness in the epigastrium.

Differential Diagnosis

The differential diagnosis for gastritis and peptic ulcer disease is broad given its nonspecific nature, but can be narrowed down fairly quickly by a good initial history. The differential diagnosis includes gastroesophageal reflux disease (GERD), cardiac disease, gastric cancer, pancreatitis, pancreatic neoplasm, biliary disease including cholelithiasis or cholecystitis, delayed gastric emptying, or bowel ischemia. Patients presenting with a predominant complaint of heartburn or abdominal pain with heartburn more than once per week, should be considered to have GERD until proven otherwise. Any symptoms associated with dyspnea or chest pressure should raise concern for a cardiac etiology. Biliary pain often radiates to the right shoulder and is associated with fatty or greasy foods. Patients with pancreatitis usually describe a severe boring type pain in the epigastrium. They may also get relief from leaning forward.

Diagnosis

While most dyspepsia symptoms can be treated on a nonurgent basis, specific "warning signs" should prompt referral or performance of upper endoscopy. These include age greater than age 55 years, bleeding, anemia, loss of more than 10% of body weight, dysphagia, odynophagia, early satiety, history of previous malignancy, lymphadenopathy, abdominal mass, or a previously documented ulcer.

H. pylori testing is the cornerstone of managing dyspepsia. However, most other laboratory studies are usually not helpful in establishing the diagnosis in uncomplicated peptic ulcer disease or gastritis but may be helpful in eliminating other conditions in the differential diagnosis.

Noninvasive Testing

Antibody test—Serum IgG antibodies are typically present at 21 days after the onset of *H. pylori* infection, but can persist long after active infection. Antibody testing has a sensitivity of 85% and specificity of 79%. The positive predictive value is greatly influenced by the prevalence of the organism in the community and is therefore less useful in areas with lower rates of *H. pylori* infection. The excellent negative predictive value makes IgG testing a good screening test. However, given that the IgG antibodies can persist for up to a year or longer after infection, it is not as helpful in the acute phase.

Urea breath test—This test identifies infection through urease activity. The patient ingests urea labeled with either ^{13}C or ^{14}C. In the presence of *H. pylori*, urease activity produces labeled CO_2 that is expired and can be collected and measured. The sensitivities and specificities of this test exceed 95%. It maintains a strong positive and negative predictive value despite the prevalence of *H. pylori*, but the test is not universally available.

Fecal antigen test—This assay uses either polyclonal or monoclonal antibodies to identify *H. pylori* antigens in the stool. The sensitivity and specificity exceed 90% in most studies. As with the breath test, it is unaffected by prevalence; however, both tests are affected by previous exposure to bismuth, antibiotics, and PPIs.

Treatment

The treatment of dyspepsia was revolutionized in the 1990s, following the discovery of the role of *H. pylori* in pathogenesis. For patients who present with dyspepsia but no "warning signs," two separate and approximately equivalent treatment strategies are recommended. The "test-and-treat" option recommends using a validated noninvasive test for *H. pylori* and treatment of positive tests. The "empiric" acid suppression option recommends treating with a PPI for 4 to 8 weeks without testing for *H. pylori*. The test-and-treat strategy is recommended for populations where the *H. pylori* infection rate is >10%. As the U.S. prevalence varies from 10% to 40% in different communities, either strategy may be appropriate. The test-and-treat strategy is more appropriate for most urban areas and in communities with a high immigrant population or known high rates of *H. pylori* infection. In populations with low *H. pylori* prevalence, such as high socioeconomic areas, empiric acid suppression is an appropriate first strategy, followed by *H. pylori* testing in those patients who have continued symptoms (Figure 1).

Several FDA-approved regimens are available to eradicate *H. pylori*. Additional well-studied regimens are recommended by the American College of Gastroenterology (Table 1). The current first-line treatment is with standard dose PPI, clarithromycin (Biaxin), and amoxicillin (Amoxil) for 10 to 14 days. This regimen has an eradication rate of 70% to 85%. Studies show no statistical difference between 7- and 10-day treatment regimens; however, there were trends toward higher eradication rates with the longer regime. In addition, these studies have not been duplicated in the U.S. population, where 7-day regimens have shown efficacy rates below 80%. Therefore regimens of less than 10 days are not recommended, and 14 days of treatment should be considered. In patients who are allergic to penicillin, metronidazole (Flagyl)[1] may be substituted for amoxicillin; however, resistance rates for metronidazole are more than double those for amoxicillin.

---

[1]Not FDA approved for this indication.

[1]Not FDA approved for this indication.

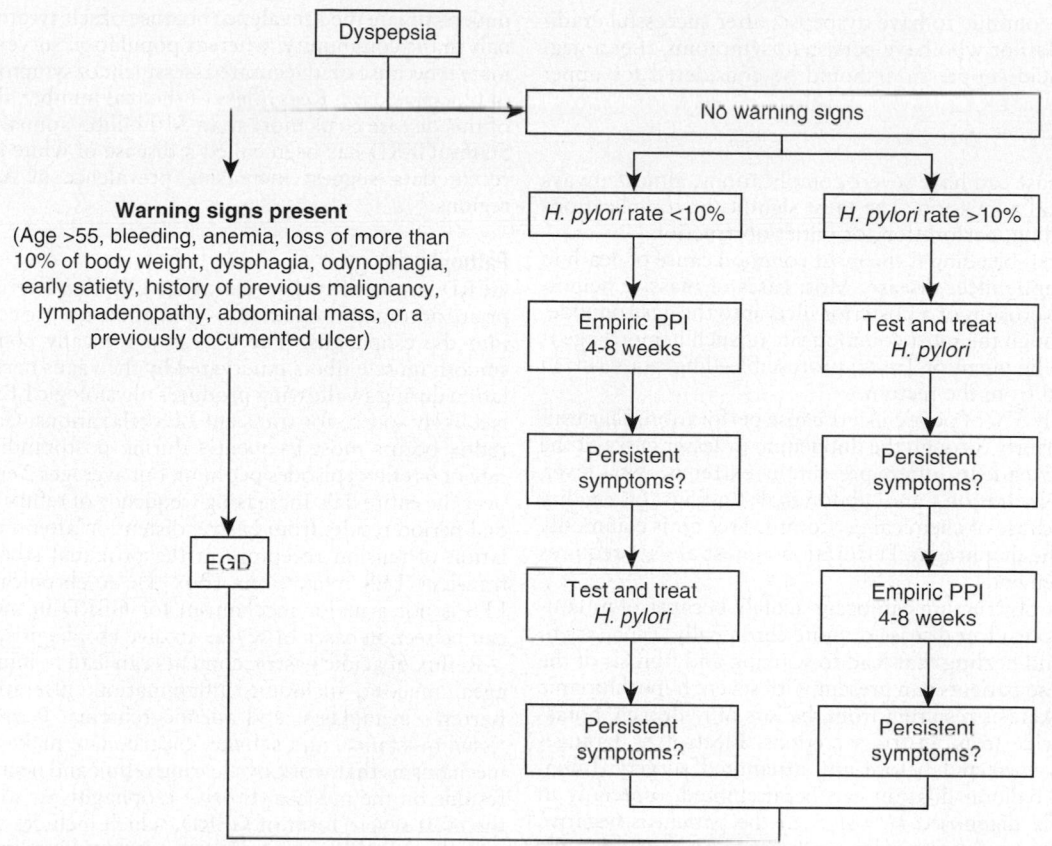

Figure 1. The treatment of dyspepsia.

TABLE 1	FDA-Approved *Helicobacter pylori* Regimens		
ANTACID*	**ANTIBIOTIC**		**DURATION**
Lansoprazole (Prevacid) 30 mg twice daily	Clarithromycin (Biaxin) 500 mg twice daily	Amoxicillin (Amoxil) 1 g twice daily[†]	10 d[‡]
Omeprazole (Prilosec) 20 mg twice daily	Clarithromycin 500 mg twice daily	Amoxicillin 1 g twice daily[†]	10 d[‡]
Esomeprazole (Nexium) 40 mg daily	Clarithromycin 500 mg twice daily	Amoxicillin 1 g twice daily[†]	10 d[‡]
Rabeprazole (Aciphex) 20 mg twice daily	Clarithromycin 500 mg twice daily	Amoxicillin 1 g twice daily[†]	7 d
H2RA as directed × 4 weeks + bismuth subsalicylate 525 mg four times a day	Metronidazole (Flagyl) 250 mg four times a day	Tetracycline 500 mg four times a day	14 d (except for H2RA which is × 4 weeks)

*H2RAs can replace the PPI in these regimens if the patient is unable to tolerate PPI, although this is not FDA approved.
[†]In patients with penicillin allergy, metronidazole (Flagyl) 500 mg twice daily can be substituted, although it is not FDA approved.
[‡]14-Day courses should be considered secondary to increased eradication rates.

H2RAs can be used at standard doses in patients who cannot tolerate PPI.

Monitoring

In most cases, routine testing for eradication of *H. pylori* is not required as it is neither practical nor cost-effective. Expert consensus supports testing for eradication in selected cases, including patients who have persistent symptoms despite the test-and-treat strategy, any patient with an *H. pylori*-associated ulcer, any patient who has had a resection of any early gastric cancer, or those with an *H. pylori*–associated mucosa-associated lymphoma tissue (MALT) lymphoma. In these patients, testing should be done no sooner than 4 weeks after the completion of eradication treatment. Patients requiring follow-up endoscopy, such as for an ulcer or MALT lymphoma, should undergo endoscopic testing for eradication. Patients who are not undergoing endoscopy can be tested for eradication with fecal antigen or urea breath testing. The serum antibody test is unreliable for follow-up, as it can remain positive for quite some time after successful treatment.

The most common causes of treatment failure are poor compliance with the medications and antibiotic resistance by the organism. Patient should be counseled on the side effects of his or her regimen and the importance of compliance. About 10% of patients report headaches and diarrhea with PPI use. Clarithromycin (Biaxin) can cause diarrhea, GI upset, and altered taste. Similar effects can be seen with amoxicillin and metronidazole. Metronidazole also has disulfiram-like effects if taken with alcohol. Bacterial resistance is relatively rare, with multicenter U.S. data showing resistance rates to be 37% for metronidazole, 10% for clarithromycin, 3.9% for both antibiotics, and 1.4% for amoxicillin. For patients with persistent *H. pylori* infections, a new regimen should be attempted that does not include previously used antibiotics.

Patients who continue to have dyspepsia after successful eradication of *H. pylori* or who have persistent symptoms after a negative test and acid suppression should be considered for upper endoscopy.

Complications

Peptic ulcer disease can have severe complications, almost always requiring hospital admission. The most significant complications are gastric bleeding, perforation, or outlet obstruction.

Gastrointestinal bleeding is the most common cause of death in patients with peptic ulcer disease. Most cases of massive hemorrhage are due to erosion of a posterior ulcer into the gastroduodenal artery. Although the most common site of such hemorrhage is proximal to the ligament of Treitz, profuse bleeding can result in bright red blood from the rectum.

Approximately 5% of peptic ulcers cause perforation. This usually occurs anteriorly through the duodenum or lesser curve of the stomach. These patients often present in extremis with fever, tachycardia, dehydration, and abdominal findings of rigidity and rebound because of chemical peritonitis. Free air is commonly present under the diaphragm. Perforation almost always requires surgical management.

Gastric outlet obstruction can occur acutely because of inflammation from peptic ulcer disease or more chronically secondary to inflammation and healing that lead to scarring and fibrosis of the duodenum. These patients can present with severe hypochloremic hypokalemic alkalosis resulting from the loss of hydrogen, potassium, and chloride from gastric secretions. Electrolyte derangements must be corrected before any attempted surgery. Initial treatment with balloon dilation can be attempted, especially in cases with newly diagnosed *H. pylori*. If the patient is negative for *H. pylori* or has successfully eradicated the organism, the long-term outcomes of dilation do not compare well to surgery.

References

Chey WD, Wong BC. The Practice Parameters Committee of the American College of Gastroenterology: American College of Gastroenterology guideline on the management of *Helicobacter pylori* infection. Am J Gastroenterol 2007;102:1808–25.

Helicobacter pylori and peptic ulcer disease: FDA approved drug regimens. Available at http://www.cdc.gov/ulcer/keytocure.htm (accessed December 30, 2013).

Mercer DW, Robinson EK. Stomach. In: Sabiston Textbook of Surgery. 18th ed. Philadelphia: Saunders; 2008. p. 1223–77.

Nordenstedt H, Graham DY, Kramer JR, et al. *Helicobacter pylori*—Negative gastritis prevalence and risk factors. Am J Gastroenterol 2013;108:65–71.

Surgical critical care evidence based-medicine guidelines: Stress ulcer prophylaxis. Available at http://www.surgicalcriticalcare.net/Guidelines/stress%20ulcer%20prophylaxis%202011.pdf (accessed December 15, 2013).

Talley NJ, Vakil NB. The Practice Parameters Committee of the American College of Gastroenterology: Guideline for the management of dyspepsia. Am J Gastroenterol 2005;100:2324–37.

GASTROESOPHAGEAL REFLUX DISEASE (GERD)

Method of
Jason R. Roberts, MD; and Donald O. Castell, MD

Gastroesophageal reflux disease (GERD) is a motility disorder of the lower esophageal sphincter (LES). The definition of this disease has evolved over time, reflecting better understanding of the roles that transient LES relaxations and acid/pepsin contact with esophageal mucosa play, as well as the ability to identify these events. The diagnosis of GERD has changed from identification of a hiatal hernia, to identification of erosive esophagitis, to the currently accepted patient-centered definition: any symptom or injury to esophageal mucosa resulting from reflux of gastric contents into the esophagus. GERD should not be confused with physiologic gastroesophageal reflux, which is not associated with symptoms or esophageal mucosal injury.

The prevalence of GERD is difficult to ascertain, although several studies have indicated it to be as high as 50% of adults in Western countries, with 10% to 18% experiencing heartburn on a daily basis. Studies using health care utilization data may underestimate the prevalence because of self-treatment by individuals in the community, whereas population surveys may overestimate it because of inaccurate assessment of symptoms and absence of objective data. Regardless of the real number, the management of this disease costs more than $10 billion annually in the United States. GERD has been called a disease of white males, although recent data suggest increasing prevalence in Asia and Pacific regions.

Pathophysiology

GERD is a motility disorder of the LES characterized by inappropriate or transient relaxations that allow gastric contents to reflux into the esophagus. The LES is a tonically contracted ring of smooth muscle fibers innervated by the vagus nerve. Vagal stimulation during swallowing produces physiologic LES relaxation and is a likely source for transient LES relaxations. Gastroesophageal reflux occurs most frequently during postprandial periods, at a rate of 6 reflux episodes per hour, but averages 2 episodes per hour over the entire day. Increasing frequency of reflux in the postprandial period results from gastric distention after a meal and stimulation of tension receptors in the proximal stomach leading to transient LES relaxations (Box 1). A chronically hypotensive LES is not a major mechanism for GERD in most patients but can be seen in cases of severe erosive esophagitis.

Reflux of acidic gastric contents can lead to injury of the esophageal mucosa, including inflammation, ulceration, stricturing, Barrett's metaplasia, and adenocarcinoma. Peristaltic clearance, tissue resistance, and salivary bicarbonate make up host defense mechanisms that work by clearing reflux and neutralizing the acid residue on the mucosa. Erosive esophagitis or strictures result in the most severe form of GERD, which includes nocturnal reflux with longer acid contact times, decreased salivary production, and lower frequency of swallowing during sleep.

Complications

Acid reflux can lead to significant morbidity if it is not recognized and treated appropriately. Habitual contact of acid and activated pepsin with the stratified squamous epithelium, along with impaired defense mechanisms, results in tissue injury (Box 2). The end result of this process can be ulceration, fibrosis with stricture formation, Barrett's esophagus, or adenocarcinoma. These complications can produce alarm symptoms (Box 3). Patients presenting with alarm symptoms should undergo immediate diagnostic evaluation with an esophagogastroduodenoscopy (EGD).

Erosive Esophagitis

The endoscopic finding of erosive esophagitis is seen in fewer than 50% of patients with heartburn. The severity is stratified according to the Los Angeles Classification of Esophagitis. Treatment with a proton pump inhibitor (PPI) for 4 to 12 weeks heals erosive esophagitis in 78% to 95% of cases. The healing effect of antisecretory therapy, and particularly PPIs, demonstrates the important role of acid reflux in causing tissue injury. The recurrence rates for

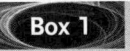

Box 1   Factors That Modulate Transient Lower Esophageal Sphincter Relaxation

Stimulants
- Gastric distention
- Pharyngeal intubation
- Upright orientation
- Foods (fatty foods, caffeine, alcohol)
- Tobacco

Inhibitors
- Recumbency
- Lateral decubitus (left side)
- Anesthesia
- Sleep

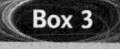

Box 2 — Esophageal Tissue Defense Mechanisms

Preepithelial
- Mucous layer
- Unstirred water layer
- Surface bicarbonate concentration

Epithelial Structures
- Cell membranes
- Intercellular junctional complexes (tight junctions, glycoconjugates/lipid)

Cellular
- Epithelial transport (Na^+/H^+ exchanger, Na^+-dependent Cl^-/HCO_3^- exchanger)
- Intracellular and extracellular buffers
- Cell restitution
- Cell replication

Postepithelial
- Blood flow
- Tissue acid-base status

Box 3 — Alarm Symptoms of Gastroesophageal Reflux Disease

Presence of any of the following symptoms requires immediate evaluation:
- Dysphagia
- Odynophagia
- Weight loss
- Spontaneous resolution of GERD symptoms
- Iron deficiency anemia
- Gastrointestinal bleeding

erosive esophagitis are high after discontinuation of PPI maintenance therapy (75%–92%), necessitating continuation of gastric acid suppression.

Strictures

Most strictures caused by GERD are peptic in origin and are located at the squamocolumnar junction. Patients with GERD and strictures, compared to those without strictures, are more likely to have a hypotensive LES, abnormal peristalsis, and prolonged acid clearance time. Stricture formation decreases the luminal diameter, resulting in solid food dysphagia. Dysphagia in these patients is often a combination of decreased luminal diameter and dysmotility of the distal esophageal body with low-amplitude peristalsis. Patients with GERD who develop dysphagia should have immediate barium radiography and an endoscopic evaluation.

Barrett's Esophagus

Barrett's esophagus (BE) is a premalignant condition that may evolve into esophageal adenocarcinoma. The histologic abnormality involves intestinal-like metaplasia of the stratified squamous epithelium. Epidemiologic studies show Barrett's to be more common among Caucasians, males, and the elderly (mean age, 60 years). The relative risk of esophageal adenocarcinoma (EAC) in BE patients was thought to be 30- to 125-fold with an incidence of 0.5% per patient year; however, recent population studies have shown a lower incidence of 0.12% to 0.13%. Despite the prevalent use of PPIs in the treatment of GERD, the incidence of adenocarcinoma has been increasing. Current guidelines encourage endoscopic surveillance for patients with Barrett's esophagus, yet there are sparse data showing the cost-effectiveness or mortality benefit of this strategy.

Adenocarcinoma

Approximately 50% of esophageal cancers are adenocarcinomas. Since the 1970s, the incidence has been rising for reasons that are still unknown. GERD is a risk factor for esophageal adenocarcinoma, and the risk increases with the duration and severity of GERD symptoms. There is a suggestion that cagA strains of *Helicobacter pylori* are protective against development of Barrett's esophagus and adenocarcinoma. The declining incidence of *H. pylori* may be a possible explanation for the rising incidence of adenocarcinoma.

Diagnosis

GERD is largely a clinical diagnosis under the current definition (i.e., any symptom or tissue injury resulting from reflux of gastric contents into the esophagus). Patients with the typical symptoms of heartburn and regurgitation most often associated with meals have a high pretest probability of having GERD. A well-obtained history and symptom questionnaire are usually sufficient to form a presumptive diagnosis and are more cost-effective than ambulatory reflux testing or EGD. An empiric trial of PPI therapy that leads to a significant reduction or resolution of symptoms likely confirms the diagnosis.

The pathophysiology of GERD is much more complex than previously thought. It involves more than acid reflux, because nonacid reflux with a pH greater than 4 can be a common source of symptoms. This entity is unmasked when PPI therapy is found to control gastric acid secretion and impedance-pH testing identifies a temporal relationship between symptoms and episodes of nonacid reflux.

Direct-to-consumer marketing and the availability of over-the-counter PPI medications (Prilosec OTC) have led to self-treatment of GERD-type symptoms and a consequent change in the type of patients seeking medical care for their symptoms. Patients with typical GERD symptoms that do not completely respond to therapy with PPIs, including over-the-counter and prescription PPIs, warrant a more detailed evaluation of their symptoms. A separate population requiring earlier diagnostic evaluation includes patients with exclusively atypical GERD symptoms such as cough, hoarseness, throat clearing, asthma attacks, and chest pain. Less commonly, patients presenting with signs or symptoms of tissue injury, such as solid food dysphagia, should also be more rigorously tested for GERD (Box 4).

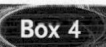

Box 4 — Clinical Spectrum of Gastroesophageal Reflux Disease–Related Symptoms and Tissue Injury

Esophageal

Symptomatic Syndromes
- Typical reflux syndrome
- Reflux chest pain syndrome

Syndromes with Tissue Injury
- Reflux esophagitis
- Reflux stricture
- Barrett's esophagus
- Adenocarcinoma

Extraesophageal

Established Association
- Reflux cough
- Reflux laryngitis
- Reflux dental erosions

Proposed Association
- Sinusitis
- Reflux asthma
- Pulmonary fibrosis
- Pharyngitis
- Recurrent otitis media

Patients who have symptoms associated with GERD, whether typical or atypical, are frequently treated empirically with PPI therapy. With a lack of discrimination regarding symptom types, this population is very heterogeneous and comprises patients with symptoms that are truly associated with GERD, not at all associated with GERD, and a combination of both. The pretest probability of GERD in this group is diluted, and nonresponders to empiric therapy are numerous. Partial responders and nonresponders to PPI therapy should undergo ambulatory reflux testing using combined multichannel intraluminal impedance (MII)-pH or standard pH. MII-pH catheters measure both esophageal pH changes and impedance changes that occur as an ion-rich refluxate passes a pair of ring electrodes, resulting in a drop in the resistance to a low-voltage current between the electrodes. The change in impedance can detect gastroesophageal reflux regardless of the acid content and can distinguish reflux types as liquid, gas, or mixed.

The goals of ambulatory reflux testing are to determine whether the esophageal acid contact time is abnormal, whether there are an abnormal number of reflux episodes, and whether a relationship between reflux and symptoms exists. The advantage of combined MII-pH is its ability to identify both acid and nonacid reflux, so that testing can be done while the patient is on acid-suppression therapy and the artifact of acidic food or beverage ingestion is eliminated; pH-only testing is affected by both of these conditions. The major disadvantage is that MII-pH testing is less available than conventional pH testing.

EGD is specific for detecting reflux-related tissue injury but is not sensitive, because fewer than 50% of patients with GERD-related heartburn have endoscopic findings of reflux. If erosive esophagitis or Barrett's esophagus is found on endoscopy, aggressive antisecretory therapy with a PPI is warranted.

A barium esophagram is unlikely to add useful diagnostic information in patients with GERD symptoms without dysphagia. It is a useful tool in distinguishing obstructive from nonobstructive dysphagia and may even be more sensitive than EGD in detecting causes of obstructive dysphagia. Achalasia is often mistaken for GERD during the onset of symptoms, and early use of esophagography may help make this diagnosis.

Management

GERD is predominantly a postprandial event involving transient LES relaxations. The primary focus in management of this disease is to eliminate or improve symptoms and prevent tissue injury. In most patients with recurrent GERD symptoms, this can be accomplished by controlling gastric acid secretion with antisecretory therapy. PPIs are the most effective pharmacologic therapy for improving symptoms and preventing tissue injury from acid reflux. Individuals with only occasional heartburn may successfully treat symptoms with a combination of lifestyle modifications and over-the-counter antacids, histamine 2 receptor antagonists, or a PPI.

Patients presenting with typical symptoms and a history consistent with GERD should be given a trial of PPI once daily for at least 4 weeks. A validated GERD symptom assessment questionnaire such as the Reflux Disease Questionnaire should be used as an initial screening tool, because symptom response is the primary outcome measure and subsequent questionnaire responses are useful in comparison with the initial responses for measuring treatment efficacy. If symptoms have not responded or have responded only partially after this trial, then the dosing or frequency of the PPI should be increased over another 4-week period. If the response is still unsatisfactory, diagnostic testing with ambulatory combined MII-pH or pH-only monitoring is indicated.

PPIs are an effective maintenance therapy for most patients with GERD and may be stepped down or used on demand, but GERD is a chronic condition with a high recurrence rate of symptoms without some form of maintenance therapy. This creates a large population of patients on antisecretory therapy for a disease with a low mortality rate, which raises the question of drug safety. There are insufficient data available that would warrant a recommendation against long-term PPI therapy. Clinical judgment in specific patient populations should be used to determine the optimal PPI regimen.

At present, pharmacologic reflux reduction therapy consists solely of the use of baclofen (Lioresal),[1] which has been shown to reduce transient LES relaxations and associated gastroesophageal reflux. The drawback of this medication is its unwanted side effects, which include somnolence and dizziness, limiting its tolerability and clinical utility as a stand-alone therapy.

Antireflux surgery is another alternative that is effective in limiting GERD symptoms in patients with a positive reflux-symptom relationship. Candidates for surgery include younger patients who do not want to continue chronic PPI therapy and patients with symptomatic nonacid reflux. Today, most antireflux surgery is performed laparoscopically with a 360-degree Nissen fundoplication. The associated mortality rate is small (0.5%–1%), and this approach is preferred to open laparotomy. Traditional predictors for surgical success have included the presence of typical symptoms (heartburn and regurgitation), symptom response to a trial of PPIs, and an abnormal ambulatory pH study. These criteria exclude the important group of patients with atypical symptoms or symptoms related to nonacid reflux. However, such patients should be considered candidates for antireflux surgery if a positive reflux-symptom relationship can be demonstrated.

Patients with alarm symptoms and those who are partial responders to PPI therapy should also undergo EGD to aid in determining the cause of the symptoms, such as obstructive dysphagia from peptic strictures, adenocarcinoma, and bleeding esophageal ulcers (which can cause anemia). EGD findings that suggest GERD are a result of acid reflux. However, the incidence of these findings has declined with the use of PPIs.

Nonerosive reflux disease is increasingly common as more patients are converted from acid refluxers to nonacid refluxers with PPI therapy. By definition, these patients have no findings on endoscopy to suggest ongoing GERD. Absence of endoscopic findings does not exclude GERD, however, because tissue injury can occur at the microscopic as well as the macroscopic level. Patients with either erosive esophagitis or nonerosive reflux disease have dilated intercellular spaces on electron microscopy.

As previously discussed, patients with GERD may develop Barrett's esophagus. The metaplastic transformation from normal stratified squamous epithelium to an intestinal-type, columnar-lined epithelium creates a premalignant lesion with a 0.5% per year risk of progression to adenocarcinoma. Screening for Barrett's esophagus remains controversial. There is no evidence that screening results in a mortality benefit due to early detection of esophageal adenocarcinoma. Screening of all patients with GERD for Barrett's esophagus is clearly not cost-effective, but it is reasonable to target the highest-risk populations, such as Caucasian men older than 50 years of age with chronic reflux symptoms. Current American College of Gastroenterology guidelines recommend surveillance endoscopy in patients with known Barrett's esophagus at intervals determined by the degree of dysplasia. Because there have been no long-term, controlled studies, it is a grade C recommendation.

---

[1]Not FDA approved for this indication.

References

Bonino J, Sharma P. Barrett's esophagus. Curr Opin Gastroenterol 2005;21:461–5.

Castell DO, Richter JE. The Esophagus. 4th ed. Philadelphia: Lippincott Williams & Wilkins; 2003.

Frye J, Vaezi M. Extraesophageal GERD. Gastroenterol Clin North Am 2008;37:845–58.

Hila A, Agrawal A, Castell D. Combined multichannel intraluminal impedance and pH esophageal testing compared to pH alone for diagnosing both acid and weakly acidic gastroesophageal reflux. Clin Gastroenterol and Hepatol 2007;5:172–7.

Hvid-Jensen F, Funch-Jensen P, et al. Incidence of adenocarcinoma among patients with Barrett's esophagus. NEJM 2011;365:1375–83.

Katz PO, Gerson LB, Vela MF. Guidelines for the Diagnosis and Management of Gastroesophageal Reflux Disease. Am J Gastroenterol 2013;108:308–28.

Mainie I, Tutuian R, Agrawal A, et al. Combined multichannel intraluminal impedance-pH monitoring to select patients with persistent gastro-oesophageal reflux for laparoscopic Nissen fundoplication. Br J Surg 2006;93:1483–7.

Mainie I, Tutuian R, Castell D. Comparison between the combined analysis and the DeMeester score to predict response to PPI therapy. J Clin Gastroenterol 2006;40:602–5.

Mainie I, Tutuian R, Shay S, et al. Acid and non-acid reflux in patients with persistent symptoms despite acid suppressive therapy: A multicentre study using combined ambulatory impedance-pH monitoring. Gut 2006;55:1398–402.

Savarino E, Zentilin P, Tutuian R, et al. The role of nonacid reflux in NERD: Lessons learned from impedance-pH monitoring in 150 patients off therapy. Am J Gastroenterol 2008;103:2685–93.

Vakil N, Van Zanten SV, Kahrilas P, et al. The Montreal definition and classification of gastroesophageal reflux disease: A global evidence-based consensus. Am J Gastroenterol 2006;101:1900–20.

Vakil N. Review article: Test and treat or treat and test in reflux disease. Aliment Pharmacol Ther 2003;17(Suppl. 2):57–9.

Verbeek RE, Siersema PD, et al. Surveillance and follow-up strategies in patients with high-grade dysplasia in Barrett's esophagus: a Dutch population-based study. Am J Gastroenterol 2012;107:534–42.

Wang KK, Sampliner RE. Updated guidelines 2008 for the diagnosis, surveillance and therapy of Barrett's esophagus. Am J Gastroenterol 2008;103:788–97.

HEMORRHOIDS, ANAL FISSURE, AND ANORECTAL ABSCESS AND FISTULA

Method of
Genevieve B. Melton-Meaux, MD; and Mary R. Kwaan, MD, MPH

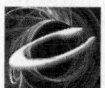

CURRENT DIAGNOSIS

- While most anorectal complaints are caused by a benign process, it is important to be mindful that the etiology can be a malignancy or other serious medical condition, such as anorectal Crohn's disease.
- A thorough, focused history is often the most helpful diagnostic tool for patients with anorectal complaints.
- In patients where no etiology for bleeding is found or where there has been a change in bowel movements, a further diagnostic work-up should be performed.
- Pain is the predominant symptom with anal fissure, thrombosed external hemorrhoids, and anorectal abscess but is not prominently featured with internal hemorrhoids.

CURRENT THERAPY

- External thrombosed hemorrhoids are treated with evacuation in their early development (<72 hours) but with expectant, supportive management only in their subacute phase.
- Most internal hemorrhoids can be treated with outpatient treatments, including measures to normalize bowel movements and hemorrhoidal banding or injection therapy.
- Anal fissures are treated conservatively with medical therapy but require operative therapy in a minority of cases.
- Anal fistula repair techniques have variable success rates; it may require multiple procedures to treat anal fistula effectively.

A number of conditions cause anorectal symptoms, but the majority of patients present with a complaint of "hemorrhoids." Most anorectal conditions can be diagnosed with a focused history and physical examination. Treatment is aimed at the relief of symptoms, education of the patient, and prevention of further symptoms. Although most anorectal complaints are caused by a benign process, it is important for clinicians to be mindful that in some cases the etiology can be a malignancy or other serious medical conditions, such as anorectal Crohn's disease.

History

A thorough, focused history is often the most helpful diagnostic tool for patients with anorectal complaints. Clinicians should inquire about pain, itching, discharge, extra tissue or a lump, and bleeding. It is particularly important to understand the patient's bowel habits with respect to constipation or diarrhea as well as any change in defecatory habits. Other relevant history items include previous anorectal procedures and related medical conditions such as Crohn's disease, malignancy, sexually transmitted diseases, or immunosuppression.

Pain is an important symptom to elicit from patients. In most cases, pain is the predominant symptom with anal fissure, thrombosed external hemorrhoids, and anorectal abscess. Although discomfort from internal hemorrhoids can cause aching, soreness, or itching in the setting of tissue prolapse, internal hemorrhoid disease is most often painless. In contrast, external hemorrhoids that are acutely thrombosed cause pain that is acute in onset, severe, and constant. Fissure pain is often described as a tearing sensation or the feeling of "razor blades" during bowel movements that can continue for more than an hour following defecation. Patients with anal fissures might also express a fear of having bowel movements because of pain. Anorectal abscess is often associated with pain, and patients can also present with an acute lump and sometimes fever.

Anal discharge and difficulty with anorectal hygiene are also common complaints. The discharge associated with prolapsing internal hemorrhoids might contain mucus or small amounts of stool. In contrast, an anorectal fistula or abscess can spontaneously drain with associated purulent and blood-tinged output.

When a patient has bleeding, specific details to inquire about include color (bright red versus dark blood), amount, frequency, and length of time. When no etiology for bleeding is found, further screening should be performed. Patients who are younger than 50 years and who have no other risk factors should undergo flexible sigmoidoscopy. A colonoscopy should be done when patients are 50 years of age or older who have abdominal pain, anemia, change in bowel habits, a family history of polyps or colon cancer, or a personal history of polyps or colon cancer.

Diagnosis

Although the prone jack-knife position allows the greatest exposure, the left lateral decubitus position with the knees up is preferred by patients and usually allows adequate exposure for the anorectal examination. It is critically important to have sufficient lighting with a self-lighted anoscope or a headlight as well as adequate instrumentation to perform the anoscopy. An adjunctive test that can also be helpful in patients where mucosal (hemorrhoidal) or full-thickness rectal prolapse is suspected is to have patients bear down on the commode and then to examine externally.

The perianal skin is the skin immediately surrounding the anal verge (Figure 1). Perianal inspection includes careful examination of the surrounding skin for excoriation, an external draining orifice in the case of an anorectal fistula, lichenified skin with chronic irritation, other dermatitis, and the presence of perianal lesions. The anal verge is the entrance to the anal canal and is defined by the intersphincteric groove. There is frequently a clear demarcation between hair-bearing and non–hair-bearing skin in this location. Careful retraction of the buttocks can help to visualize an anal fissure located at the anal verge and extending into the anal canal.

A digital rectal examination is helpful for assessing resting and squeeze anorectal tone, palpating the prostate in men, assessing for rectocele in women, detecting any palpable anorectal lesions, and evaluating for tenderness within the anal canal or at the level of the levator ani muscles at the anorectal ring. Anoscopy is used to visually examine the anal canal, which is between 4 and 5 cm in length starting at the anal verge and extending to the top of the anorectal ring (top of external sphincter and levator ani muscles). Within the anal canal is the dentate line, which acts as a landmark anatomically and is located approximately 2 cm from the anal verge. The dentate line represents the transition from squamous epithelial lining of the anus to the columnar epithelial lining of the rectum. Sensation above the dentate line is mediated by autonomic fibers

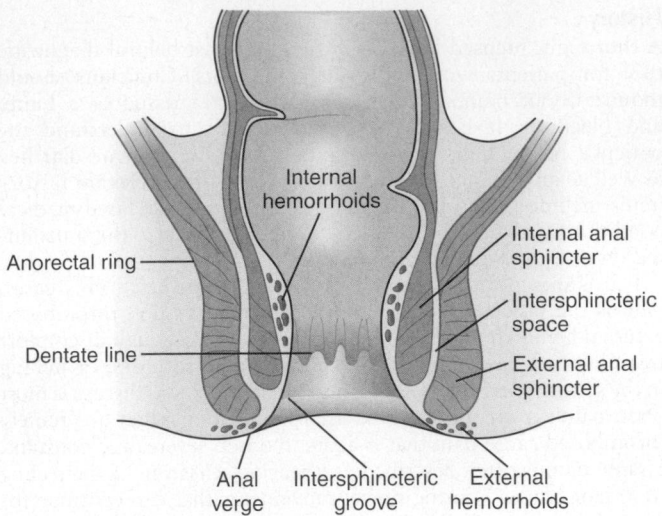

Figure 1. Anatomy of the anal canal.

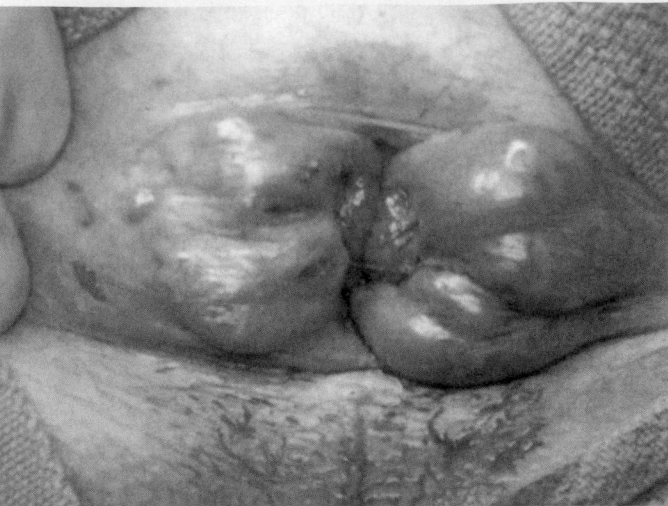

Figure 2. Prolapsing (grade III) hemorrhoids, with a prominent external component on the right and two sites of recent bleeding seen on the left.

and results in a relative lack of sensation in comparison to the highly sensitive, somatically innervated tissue below the dentate line. The dentate line is also the location of the crypt anal glands from which anorectal abscesses and fistulas originate.

Hemorrhoids

Hemorrhoids are the anal vascular cushions that are present as normal structures in everyone. In the case of internal hemorrhoids, these cushions are arteriovenous channels that have overlying mucosa, submucosal smooth muscle, and supportive fibroelastic connective tissue. It is believed that internal hemorrhoids function by aiding with fine control of fecal continence of liquids and gases. Internal hemorrhoids enlarge and become symptomatic as fixation by submucosal smooth muscle and connective tissue becomes disrupted and loosens. This results in a sliding or prolapsing of the anal canal lining and further engorgement of the internal hemorrhoid tissues. Common exacerbating factors include constipation, diarrhea, aging, and increased abdominal pressure that can occur with chronic straining, pregnancy, heavy lifting, and decreased venous return. Internal hemorrhoids are typically staged on a scale from I to IV based upon the extent of prolapse (Table 1).

Internal hemorrhoids, when symptomatic, most commonly present with painless bright red bleeding or prolapsing tissue (Figure 2). Patients describe bleeding with or after bowel movements. Other symptoms include itching and leakage of mucus in the setting of tissue prolapse. Pain is rarely a prominent symptom except in the case of mixed hemorrhoid disease, when there is a thrombosed external component, or in the case of stage IV incarcerated hemorrhoids.

The central principles for conservative treatment of internal hemorrhoids and for long-term prevention of worsening symptoms are the normalization of bowel habits and avoidance of straining. Ideal bowel habits include having regular, soft, and formed stool resulting in minimal straining with elimination. An ideal diet should have high fiber content along with sufficient fluid intake. A total of at least 30 g of fiber per day is generally

recommended. For the majority of patients, this is most easily achieved with the addition of a fiber supplement such as psyllium. Other medical treatment of hemorrhoids includes local anesthetic topical ointments, which relieve symptoms but do not improve the hemorrhoids, and steroid ointments, which symptomatically improve itching and irritation but also thin and atrophy the overlying tissue if used regularly.

Internal hemorrhoids might benefit from further treatment in the setting of persistent prolapse or bleeding. Injection sclerotherapy works through shrinking and scarring the internal hemorrhoid by injecting a sclerosing agent (most commonly phenol in olive oil). Alternatively, infrared coagulation may be administered at the apex of the hemorrhoid. Both procedures have moderate effectiveness but are considered to be less effective than rubberband ligation, which is widely used in the office setting, with good results.

Rubber-band ligation requires the use of a rubber-band ligator (either suction type or ligator with clamp) and is performed by placing a rubber band around excess hemorrhoidal tissue at the apex of the hemorrhoid. Rubber-band ligation works by strangulating and cutting off blood flow to the hemorrhoid and by creating a scar that helps to fix tissue into place. The band must be placed well above the dentate line to prevent pain. Most patients experience a sensation of pressure with the procedure. Rarely, this procedure can cause significant pain, bleeding, or a vasovagal reaction. In general, only one or two band applications are performed in the same setting to prevent excessive pain or a vasovagal reaction.

Surgical treatment for hemorrhoidal disease should be considered in patients with stage III or IV internal hemorrhoids. Surgery is also a consideration in cases where office procedures and conservative treatment have been ineffective or when internal hemorrhoids are circumferential. In the United States, most hemorrhoidectomies continue to be performed using a closed technique, where the hemorrhoid is excised and the defect sutured closed. More recently, stapled hemorrhoidectomy (sometimes called hemorrhoidopexy) has been introduced. The stapled technique appears to work best in cases where patients have more circumferential disease and is performed by excising the rectal mucosa and disrupting blood flow, thereby shrinking hemorrhoidal tissue and lifting the prolapsing tissue into the anal canal. Although stapled hemorrhoidectomy has been demonstrated to be effective and on average less painful, it does not address any external hemorrhoidal component, costs significantly more money, and has been associated with rare but severe complications, including pelvic sepsis.

External hemorrhoids are generally painless, except in the case of thrombosis, and normally appear as more prominent external perianal tissue or painless skin tags. Thrombosed external hemorrhoids, in contrast, are associated with severe pain and a

TABLE 1	Staging of Hemorrhoidal Disease
GRADE	**DESCRIPTION**
I	Protrude only inside the lumen; seen only with the anoscope
II	Protrude during defecation; reduce spontaneously
III	Protrude during defecation; require manual reduction
IV	Permanently prolapsed and irreducible

prominent external lump but not with bleeding or fever. On examination, an external thrombosed hemorrhoid appears as a prominent, blue, and firm perianal lump. It is also not uncommon for multiple hemorrhoids to thrombose. Patients who present within 72 hours of the onset of symptoms benefit from an evacuation of the thrombosed clot using local anesthetic (Figure 3). In contrast, patients who present after 72 hours should be treated expectantly with conservative supportive care, including sitz baths, normalization of bowel habits with fiber or stool softener, and pain management. The natural history in these cases is for the thrombosed clot to gradually be reabsorbed within several weeks.

Anal Fissure

An anal fissure is a tear in the anoderm extending proximally into the anal canal and initially resulting from a traumatic bowel movement. Fissures typically occur in the setting of constipation or frequent bowel movements. Although most superficial fissures resulting from trauma to the anorectal region will heal, some patients have prolonged symptoms, causing them to seek medical attention. The pathophysiology of anal fissures is still not completely understood but is related to local ischemia caused by hypertonia of the internal sphincter. The great majority of anal fissures are located at the posterior midline; some also occur at the anterior midline (Figure 4). Lateral fissures are rare and can be associated with anal malignancy, anorectal Crohn's disease, HIV, syphilis, or tuberculosis. In these cases, a biopsy should be strongly considered to confirm the diagnosis.

Patients who present with anal fissure most often have a tearing pain that is associated with bowel movements and that continues after defecation and bright red bleeding with bowel movements. Physical examination demonstrates a tear in the anoderm with exposed internal sphincter upon retraction of the buttocks. Chronic cases also demonstrate a sentinel tag overlying the distal aspect of the fissure.

Conservative treatment for acute anal fissures includes the normalization of bowel habits to minimize recurrent trauma to the anoderm and sitz baths for comfort. In cases in which the fissure is chronic or unresponsive to conservative treatment, topical therapy to relax the internal sphincter (i.e., a "chemical sphincterotomy") is prescribed. Classically, nitroglycerin ointment (0.2%–0.4%)[1,2] has been used but is associated with significant headaches and lightheadedness. Diltiazem ointment (2%)[1] is a commonly used alternative without associated side effects. Either ointment can be applied topically two to three times per day for approximately 8 weeks. Reported healing rates are similar and range from 40% to 100%. An alternative agent that can be used for chemical sphincterotomy is botulinum toxin A (Botox), which can be injected in the office or operating room with a single application into the internal sphincter. Although botulinum toxin A appears to be as effective as topical therapy, it is significantly more expensive.

---

[1]Not FDA approved for this indication.
[2]Not available in the United States.

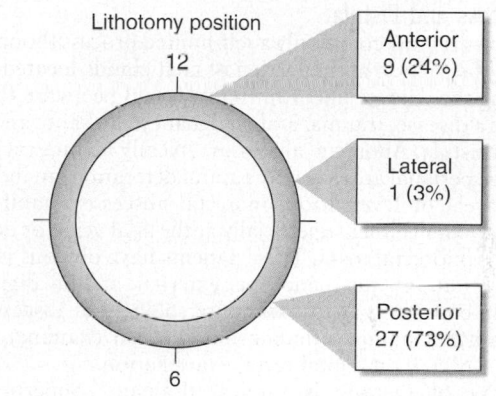

Figure 4. Distribution of the location of anal fissures.

Figure 3. Incision and evacuation of an external thrombosed hemorrhoid. **A,** A local anesthetic is injected into the subcutaneous surrounding tissue and at the base of the hemorrhoid. **B,** The skin over the hemorrhoid is lifted and a small elliptical excision of skin is made. **C,** The thrombotic clot is evacuated. Additional dissection is sometimes needed in the subcutaneous tissue to extract the clot. **D,** The appearance of the evacuated area. The incision is left open and the skin heals by secondary intention.

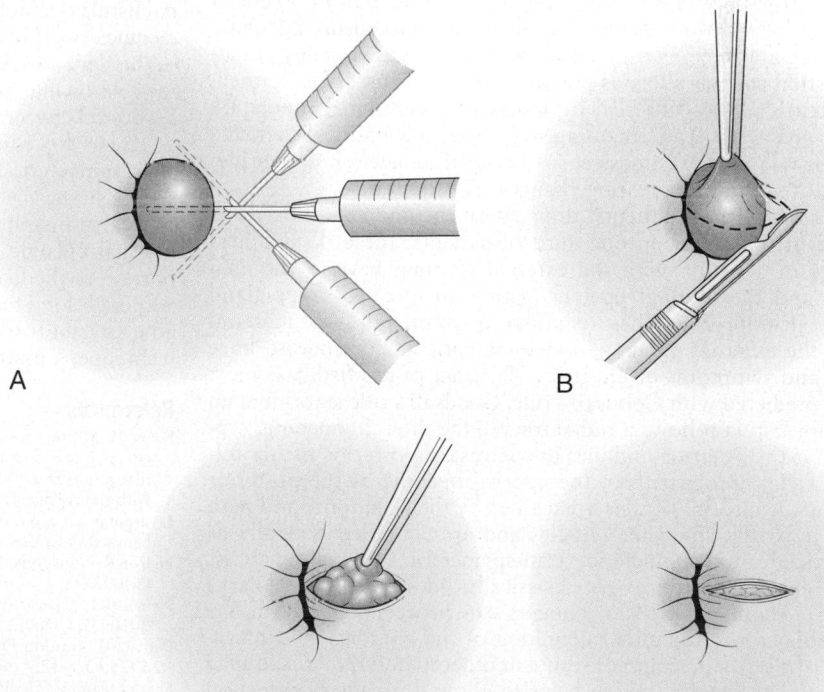

Surgical internal sphincterotomy is the most effective treatment for resolution of anal fissures but is associated with a risk of fecal incontinence, particularly in women, elderly patients, or others at risk for impaired continence. This procedure is performed in the outpatient setting and should be considered in cases where more-conservative dietary and medical treatments have failed. Internal sphincterotomy is performed by dividing the internal sphincter laterally, which prevents the formation of a keyhole defect with stool leakage, which can occur with the posterior division of the internal sphincter muscle. This procedure can be performed with an open approach (incising mucosa and exposing muscle) or a closed approach (using landmarks and then blindly dividing muscle) and can be full thickness (entire internal sphincter) or tailored (partial thickness and length). Most surgeons perform a tailored sphincterotomy from the level of the top of the fissure distally, with partial division of the internal sphincter muscle to decrease the risk of postoperative fecal incontinence.

Anorectal Abscess and Fistula

Anorectal abscess is most commonly a self-limited process thought to result from obstruction and infection of anal glands located in the crypts along the dentate line. Clinicians should be aware that perianal Crohn's disease, trauma, and malignancy can cause anorectal abscess or fistula. Anorectal abscesses typically manifest with acute pain in the perianal area, acutely painful defecation, an indurated painful area, or fever. Most anorectal abscesses manifest with pain and swelling either superficially at the anal verge or deeper within the ischiorectal fossa. These patients have obvious tenderness, induration, or fluctuance on external and/or digital examination. In contrast, patients with intersphincteric abscesses have severe pain but minimal findings on external examination and are only suspected on digital rectal examination.

The mainstay of therapy is surgical drainage. Superficial abscesses can be drained using local anesthesia, but more-extensive infections typically require general anesthesia. When the abscess is fluctuant and appears easily accessible, an incision and drainage with a local anesthetic can be considered in a motivated patient. Important principles in draining an anorectal abscess include keeping the patient comfortable, using aspiration with a large-bore (14- or 16-gauge) needle to help in the event of difficult localization, using a cruciate incision to ensure adequate drainage, and keeping the incision near the anus to keep any potential fistula tract as short as possible. After the abscess is drained, the area is allowed to heal by secondary intention. Patients are given analgesics and encouraged to take sitz baths. When the abscess is large and extensive, sometimes drainage tubes, débridement, or additional dressing changes are required.

In a majority of patients, drainage of the anorectal abscess is sufficient. However, in one-third of patients, these do not heal and form a fistula with the external opening beyond the anal verge and the internal opening within an infected crypt gland at the dentate line. These continue to drain purulent material from the external opening, and some patients continue to have signs and symptoms of infection. The tract of the fistula is most often predicted with Goodsall's rule. Goodsall's rule states that an anterior fistula follows a radial tract to the internal opening, typically at the anterior midline. In contrast, a posterior fistula follows a curvilinear path to the internal opening at the posterior midline. Anorectal fistulas are defined by their anatomy and path relative to the sphincter muscles and are classified typically as superficial, intersphincteric, transsphincteric, suprasphincteric, and extrasphincteric, as classically described by Parks (Figure 5). In most cases, patients can proceed directly to the operating room for initial definition of the anatomy and placement of a seton (a length of suture or other material that is looped through the fistula), which helps to allow drainage of infection within the tract, prevents recurrent infection, and allows the fistula to mature. Recurrent and complex fistulas may be better defined anatomically with the use of magnetic resonance imaging or endorectal ultrasound.

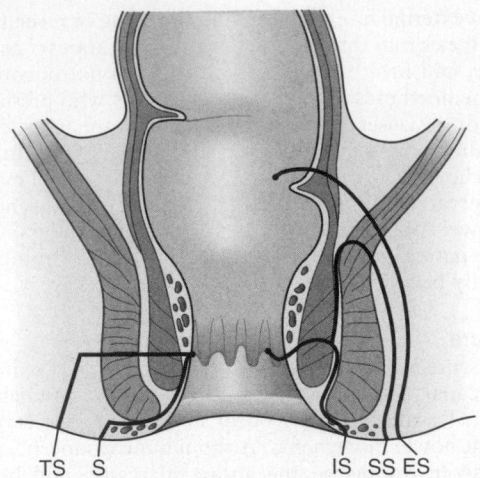

Figure 5. Classification of anal fistulas. *Abbreviations:* ES = extrasphincteric; IS = intersphincteric; S = superficial; SS = suprasphincteric; TS = transsphincteric.

Superficial, intersphincteric, or low transsphincteric fistulas can be treated with simple fistulotomy, which opens up the fistula tract and allows the tissue to heal by secondary intention. This, however, can result in impaired fecal continence, particularly if the fistula involves a significant amount of sphincter muscle.

Following this, a variety of methods can be used to repair the fistula. One classic technique is the use of a cutting seton, where a taut seton is progressively tightened over several weeks or months to form a scar in place of the fistula and muscle. A cutting seton may be painful, and the scar is associated with impaired continence in some cases. Fibrin glue has been proposed as a method to repair a fistula, but the long-term recurrence rate is high (>85%). Fistula plugs have also been proposed as a method to heal the fistula tract by repairing the internal opening and providing a scaffolding for fibrosis to occur. Although short- and medium-term success is reported to be approximately 30%, long-term results are not known.

Endorectal advancement flaps are the most well-established method to repair an anal fistula. With this technique, the internal orifice is closed and healthy tissue is brought down over the internal fistula opening to allow the area to heal. This procedure can be technically difficult: failure most commonly results from ischemia of the flap, and repeat flap procedures are often not anatomically feasible owing to scarring and fibrosis. Success rates have been reported between 50% and 80%.

A new procedure has been developed for transsphincteric and suprasphincteric fistulas called ligation of intersphincteric fistula tract. This has been reported in about a dozen centers as a method to treat transsphincteric fistulas and is performed by closing the internal opening and ligating and removing the intersphincteric portion of the fistula tract through an intersphincteric approach. Although long-term results are still unknown, reports are favorable (on the order of 80%) for the short-term success of this technique; a multicenter trial is ongoing.

References

Bleier JI, Moloo H, Goldberg SM. Ligation of the intersphincteric fistula tract: An effective new technique for complex fistulas. Dis Colon Rectum 2010;53:43–6.

Christoforidis D, Etzioni DA, Goldberg SM, et al. Treatment of complex anal fistulas with the collagen fistula plug. Dis Colon Rectum 2008;51:1482–7.

Jayaraman S, Colquhoun PH, Malthaner RA. Stapled versus conventional surgery for hemorrhoids. Cochrane Database Syst Rev 2006;(4), CD005393.

Nelson R. Nonsurgical therapy for anal fissure. Cochrane Database Syst Rev 2006;(4), CD003431.

Nelson RL. Operative procedures for fissure in ano. Cochrane Database Syst Rev 2010;(1), CD002199.

Parks AG, Gordon PH, Hardcastle JD. A classification of fistula-in-ano. Br J Surg 1976;63:1–12.

Shanmugam V, Thaha MA, Rabindranath KS, et al. Rubber band ligation versus excisional haemorrhoidectomy for haemorrhoids. Cochrane Database Syst Rev 2005;(3), CD005034.

Wang JY, Garcia-Aguilar J, Sternberg JA, et al. Treatment of transsphincteric anal fistulas: Are fistula plugs an acceptable alternative? Dis Colon Rectum 2009;52:692–7.

INFLAMMATORY BOWEL DISEASE: CROHN'S DISEASE AND ULCERATIVE COLITIS

Method of
Prabhakar P. Swaroop, MD; and Daniel K. Podolsky, MD

CURRENT DIAGNOSIS

- The most common clinical symptom of ulcerative colitis (UC) is bloody diarrhea, which is often associated with cramping abdominal pain.
- Clinical manifestations of Crohn's disease (CD) are highly variable, but the most common constellation is right lower quadrant abdominal pain and nonbloody diarrhea, often accompanied by weight loss and other constitutional symptoms.
- The hallmarks of CD are transmural inflammation, fistula formation, small-bowel fibrosis, and patchy inflammation; these may affect any segment of the gastrointestinal tract (with terminal ileal involvement in two thirds of patients). In contrast, inflammation in UC is limited to mucosa and submucosa and is diffuse, with the rectum most commonly involved. Inflammation extends proximally to varying degrees among patients.
- There is no single diagnostic test for inflammatory bowel disease; instead, the diagnosis is made based on several corroborative features.
- Potential infectious causes of symptoms should be ruled out.
- Endoscopic examination is valuable in establishing the extent of inflammation, obtaining mucosal biopsy specimens, and excluding certain infectious agents.
- Serology studies, such as anti–*Saccharomyces cerevisiae* antibodies (ASCA), perinuclear antineutrophilic cytoplasmic antibody (pANCA), anti-porin antibody (OmpC), and anti-flagellin antibody (CBir1), are occasionally useful to predict disease behavior.
- Lactoferrin and Calprotectin, which are inflammatory markers found in stool, can be used to assess for postoperative recurrence in patients with Crohn's disease. A few studies have demonstrated the utility of elevated inflammatory markers in predicting future clinical flares.
- Computed tomographic enterography can help distinguish inflammatory component from fibrosis.
- Rectal magnetic resonance imaging, endoscopic ultrasound, or examination under anesthesia can be used to fully delineate perianal fistulizing disease.
- In centers with available expertise, limited right lower quadrant ultrasound with doppler can be used for evaluation of ileal Crohn's disease.

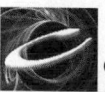

CURRENT THERAPY

- Mesalamine products in adequate dosage and appropriate formulation can be effective therapy for mild to moderately active ulcerative colitis (UC) and in maintaining remission.
- Mesalamine products may be effective in mild Crohn's disease (CD), and the formulation selected should be determined by disease location.
- Steroids are useful in patients with moderate to severe CD or UC, but their use should be limited as much as possible because of frequent side effects and complications.
- Immunomodulators such as Azathioprine (Imuran)[1] and 6-mercaptopurine (Purinethol)[1] may be used as an adjunct therapy to minimize steroid use in patients who are steroid dependent and to minimize formation of neutralizing antibodies in patients receiving antibody-based biologic agents.
- Anti–tumor necrosis factor (anti-TNF) biologic agents such as infliximab (Remicade) and adalimumab (Humira) are effective in patients with moderate to severe inflammatory CD or UC that is unresponsive to conventional treatments. Golimumab (Simponi), which is another anti-TNF agent, recently has been approved for induction and maintenance of remission in ulcerative colitis. It has been demonstrated to result in improvement of endoscopic appearance of colonic mucosa. Certolizumab pegol (Cimzia) may be used to maintain response. Immunomodulators and biologic agents may be used independently or in combination for treatment of inflammatory bowel disease and for maintaining surgically induced remission in CD.
- Risks of opportunistic infections, hematologic and cutaneous malignancies, and neurologic complications, in addition to other adverse effects of biologic therapy with or without immunomodulators, should be discussed with the patient.
- The proven role of antibiotics is limited to septic complications, perianal disease, small intestinal bacterial overgrowth, and pouchitis.
- Nataluzimab (Tysabri), an anti-α_4 agent, is effective in some patients with refractory CD, including those for whom anti-TNF therapy has failed.
- Another Integrin inhibitor, Vedolizumab (Entyvio) has been recently approved by FDA for induction and maintenance of remission and response in both Crohn's disease and ulcerative colitis.

[1]Not FDA approved for this indication.

Clinical Manifestations

The cardinal symptom of ulcerative colitis (UC) is bloody diarrhea. Symptoms of tenesmus and the sensation of incomplete evacuation may dominate in patients who have disease limited to the rectum. Although cramping abdominal pain is often present, it is a more prominent symptom in patients with Crohn's disease (CD).

Physical examination of patients with UC may detect left lower quadrant and left upper quadrant tenderness, and occasionally the extent of colonic involvement may be deduced by careful physical examination. Rebound tenderness, distention, or guarding suggests the development of the dreaded complication of toxic megacolon, which may supervene in patients with severe UC.

Patients with CD have more widely varying symptoms as a result of the highly variable sites of involvement and the range of phenotypic forms. Disease manifestations may be dominated by inflammatory activity per se, by fistula formation (fistulizing or perforating disease), or by stricture formation (stricturing disease). Perianal fistulas can be a distressing manifestation and may parallel clinical flares. The symptom complex of right lower quadrant pain, nonbloody diarrhea, and weight loss is most common because of the frequent involvement of the ileum. However, in CD with colonic involvement (with or without more proximal disease), symptoms may be indistinguishable from those of UC. Intestinal narrowing may be caused by edema due to inflammation, fibrosis from chronic inflammation, or a combination of these factors. The presence of a mass in the right lower quadrant suggests inflammatory ileal disease (and probably abscess formation), whereas right lower quadrant pain in conjunction with obstructive symptoms in the absence of a mass may be suggestive of stricture formation. Fistula disease can manifest with especially variable symptoms because of the many anatomic structures that can be involved (e.g., fecaluria and pneumaturia in those with fistulas to the bladder). Rectovaginal fistulas may lead to passage of air from the vagina. Patients with upper gastrointestinal CD may present with dysphagia, early satiety, and fear of food leading to weight loss.

Diarrhea is common but not universal in CD. Inflammation of the ileum or of the colon can cause diarrhea. Occasionally, diarrhea is caused by small intestinal bacterial overgrowth, especially in patients with fistulizing disease, or it may be induced by bile salts in those with ileal disease (or after ileal resection).

Diagnosis

Diagnosis of inflammatory bowel disease (IBD) is based on the combination of clinical features, laboratory abnormalities, imaging studies (e.g., upper gastrointestinal series with small bowel follow-through and abdominal computed tomography or magnetic resonance imaging or both), and endoscopic findings including examination of mucosal biopsies. None of these tests alone is diagnostic of IBD. In a patient with new symptoms and in those patients with flares if appropriate, infectious agents should be ruled out. Common pathogens that can mimic IBD are *Salmonella, Shigella, Aeromonas, Campylobacter, Yersinia, Clostridium difficile, Plesiomonas,* and parasites such as *Giardia lamblia* and *Entamoeba;* these should be ruled out. In an immunocompromised host (including patients with established IBD receiving immunosuppressive therapy), viral infections such as cytomegalovirus and herpes simplex virus may cause ulcers suggestive of IBD. Endoscopic imaging is often very useful. The constellation of findings in endoscopy and other studies, together with the histologic and clinical features, usually allows a reliable distinction between UC and CD. However, in as many as 10% of patients, it may not be possible to make the distinction with confidence, and such patients are said to have indeterminate colitis. The distinguishing features of UC and CD are presented in Table 1.

Hematologic abnormalities include evidence of microcytic anemia, elevated white blood cell count in peripheral blood, and thrombocytosis. Markers of inflammation such as erythrocyte sedimentation rate (ESR) and high-sensitivity C-reactive protein (hsCRP) may also be elevated, the latter more commonly in CD than in UC. Very high hsCRP may be associated with infections such as cytomegalovirus or *Clostridium difficile.*

Serologic measurements of perinuclear antineutrophilic cytoplasmic antibody (pANCA), anti–*Saccharomyces cerevisiae* antibodies (ASCA—immunoglobulin G and immunoglobulin A), anti-porin antibody (OmpC), and anti-flagellin antibody (CBir1) are occasionally helpful as corroborative evidence and to help identify patients who are at higher risk for complicating events. They may also be useful in differentiating between CD and UC in patients for whom colectomy is being considered when diagnostic ambiguity remains.

Hypoalbuminemia can be a sign of poor nutritional status, and these patients should be considered for total parenteral nutrition, particularly if surgery is being planned.

Among the imaging modalities commonly used in diagnosis and management of IBD, computed tomography of the abdomen and pelvis can alert physicians to perforation, bowel obstruction, and extent of inflammation. Computed tomographic enterography can be used to evaluate the degree and extent of inflammation in the small bowel (Figure 1). In cases of stenotic lesions of the small bowel, it can be especially helpful in identifying the inflammatory component, as evidenced by mural stranding. Lack of mural stranding in stenotic portions of small bowel suggests fibrosis, and if there is evidence of proximal dilation in a symptomatic patient, resection or strictureplasty should be considered. Ultrasound of the right lower quadrant can be an effective imaging

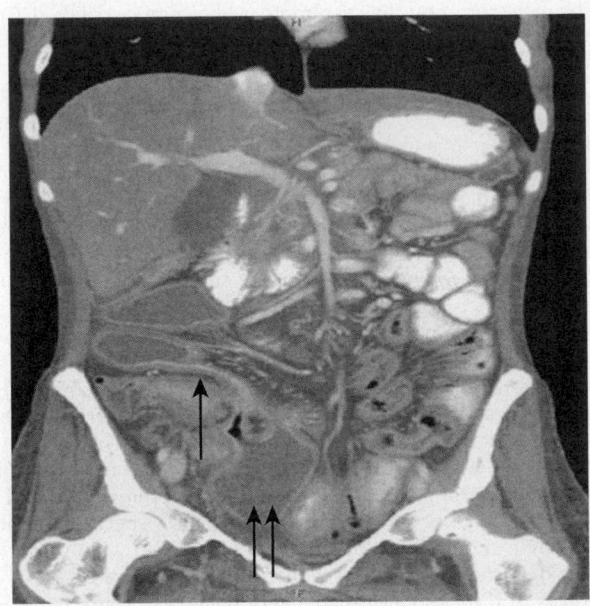

Figure 1. Computed tomographic enterography. Mural stratification; ileal wall thickening *(arrow)* suggestive of active inflammation; dilated loops of small bowel *(double arrow)* consistent with partial obstruction; and diffuse increased density of the subcutaneous and intraperitoneal fat compatible with anasarca are seen in this image. (Courtesy Dr. Cecelia Brewington, MD.)

TABLE 1   Distinguishing Features: Crohn's Disease and Ulcerative Colitis

FEATURES	CROHN'S DISEASE	ULCERATIVE COLITIS
Location	Any part of gastrointestinal tract	Colonic
Inflammation	Transmural	Mucosal/submucosal
Smoking	Smokers higher than expected	Appears to be protective
Risk of colorectal cancer	Elevated in colonic Crohn's	Elevated
Risk of intestinal cancer	Elevated in small-bowel Crohn's disease	NA
hsCRP	Elevation common	Elevation not common
Serology	ASCA, OmpC, CBir1	pANCA
Surgery	Recurrence common	Total proctocolectomy may be curative
Fistulas	Common	Very rare
FDA-approved biologic agents	Infliximab (Remicade), adalimumab (Humira), certolizumab pegol (Cimzia), natalizumab (Tysabri), vedolizumab (Entyvio)	Infliximab, adalimumab, golimumab, vedolizumab (Entyvio)
Immunomodulator therapy	Azathioprine (AZA, Imuran),[1] 6-mercaptopurine (6MP, Purinethol),[1] methotrexate (MTX, Trexall)[1]	AZA, 6MP, cyclosporine (Sandimmune, Neoral)[1]
Endoscopic features	Skip lesions	Contiguous involvement
Strictures	Common	Colorectal cancer unless proven otherwise
Genetic markers*	NOD2, ATG16L1, IRGM, IL23R, IL12B, STAT3, NKX2-3	IL12B, STAT3. NKX2-3

Abbreviations: ASCA = anti–*Saccharomyces cerevisiae* antibodies; CBir1 = anti-flagellin antibody; FDA = U.S. Food and Drug Administration; hsCRP = high-sensitivity C-reactive protein; NA = not applicable; OmpC = anti-porin antibody; pANCA = perinuclear antineutrophilic cytoplasmic antibody.
[1]Not FDA approved for this indication.
*Not approved for diagnosis. More than 50 genes have been associated with susceptibility to IBD.

modality in select patient populations to assess for postoperative recurrence, disease activity, and response to therapy.

Magnetic resonance imaging can be a helpful adjunct, along with examination under anesthesia and rectal endoscopic ultrasonography, in cases of perianal fistulizing disease.

Endoscopic examination is helpful to establish the extent of disease and obtain tissue for histologic examination. Esophagogastroduodenoscopy should be done if upper gastrointestinal CD is suspected. Single-balloon and double-balloon enteroscopy have allowed gastroenterologists to obtain tissue samples from jejunum and proximal ileum. Capsule endoscopy can be a useful alternative, although it does not allow tissue sampling and should not be used if even limited obstruction is suspected. Colonoscopy is helpful in diagnosis and during follow-up to assess response to various therapeutic modalities. It can also be used to obtain biopsy specimens from the colon and terminal ileum to be examined for findings of IBD or potentially confounding processes, including some infections. Stool Calprotectin can be a valuable tool to assess efficacy of therapies, monitor for postsurgical recurrence in patients with Crohn's disease, and differentiate between inflammatory and noninflammatory etiologies of diarrhea in patients with IBD.

Treatment

Once the diagnosis is confirmed, the treatment of IBD is based on manifestation, location, patient history, and severity of symptoms.

Treatment algorithms for IBD are usually divided into management of mild, moderate, and severe disease. The roles of various agents have evolved, and as more data are being accumulated, patients are treated earlier with agents that had been reserved for more severe disease in the past. Treatment goals for these patients are:

- Improving quality of life to as close to normal as possible
- Maintaining remission
- Avoiding surgery
- Minimizing the risk of steroid dependence
- Minimizing the risk of treatment-associated complications

Ulcerative Colitis

In the initial evaluation of UC patients, it is important to establish the extent and degree of inflammation and the concomitant presence of extraintestinal manifestations. Extent and severity of UC are judged on clinical symptoms, basic laboratory parameters (complete blood count and albumin level), and colonoscopic findings. Disease limited to the rectum and distal colon may be treated with local mesalamine therapy, in a suppository (Canasa), foam (Salofalk),[2] or enema (Rowasa) formulation. Newly diagnosed patients with mild to moderate disease activity should be given an appropriate oral formulation of mesalamine (Asacol). Mesalamine formulation as Asacol has been discontinued in the United States. Patients who are on Asacol can be switched to alternate mesalamine formulations, keeping in mind that the replacement agent should deliver an equivalent amount of mesalamine to the colon. One of the substitute mesalamine preparations is Delzicol, which delivers 400 mg of mesalamine per capsule. Antidiarrheal agents may provide symptomatic relief once infectious causes of colitis have been excluded. Colonic release budesonide (Uceris) recently has been approved for short-term (up to 16 weeks) therapy of mild to moderate ulcerative colitis.

If remission is achieved with a mesalamine formulation, the same dose of mesalamine is continued for maintenance of remission. For an occasional flareup suggested by symptoms of recurrence and documented by sigmoidoscopy or colonoscopy, steroids may be used. For patients who have frequent flareups (more than two per year), initiation of therapy with a conventional immunomodulator or biologic agent (infliximab, adalimumab, or golimumab) should be considered. Colonic release budesonide formulation utilizing MMX technology, marketed as Uceris, has been shown to be an effective but probably short-term (up to 16 weeks) therapy for active mild to moderate ulcerative colitis.

For patients with moderate disease unresponsiveness to mesalamine or severe disease, a topical, oral, or intravenous corticosteroid (depending on extent and severity) may be necessary, but it should be used for as short a period as possible, and, if it is not possible to taper and discontinue the steroid within 6 weeks, an immunomodulator should be added.

Surgical intervention should be considered for patients who have not responded to therapy with biologic agents, steroids, and/or cyclosporine (Neoral).[1] Patients who have high-grade dysplasia or colorectal cancer are also candidates for surgery.

Crohn's Disease

Optimal treatment of CD is based on many factors, including location, severity, specific clinical manifestation and complications, prior clinical course intervention, whether fistulas are present, potential fibrostenotic strictures, history of steroid dependence, history of failure with other agents, and contraindications (e.g., malignancy, opportunistic infections, tuberculosis, intolerance to medications). Before deciding on treatment options, it is important to delineate behavior (fistulizing, stricturing, or inflammatory), location (ileal, colonic, or ileocolonic), and severity and to assess for the presence of extraintestinal complications and nutritional deficiencies.

In patients with mildly active, localized ileocecal disease, treatment has historically begun with a suitable mesalamine product (although the effectiveness of this approach remains uncertain).[1] More recently, oral budesonide (Entocort EC, a steroid targeted to the ileum that undergoes extensive first-pass metabolism to minimize systemic steroid effects) has been used. For those with more extensive or severe disease, conventional systemic steroids (prednisone) may be used, but if it is not possible to wean the patient off steroids within 6 weeks, an immunodulatory agent should be started, typically 6-mercatopurine (Purinethol)[1]/azathioprine (Imuran)[1] or, in those unable to tolerate these agents, low-dose methotrexate (Trexall).[1] For patients with moderate to severe disease, treatment should include an anti-tumor necrosis factor (anti-TNF) agent with or without immunomodulator therapy. Natalizumab (Tysabri), an anti-α_4 integrin, is an alternative and may be used if anti-TNF therapy fails.

Before starting therapy with a biologic agent, patients should have a purified protein derivative (PPD) test and a hepatitis B surface antibody determination. Once biologic therapy begins, patients should continue to have an annual PPD test. QuantiFERON-TB Gold testing is a possible alternative to PPD for testing. This requires patients to come for testing once, as opposed to twice for PPD. We recommend checking for John Cunningham (JC) virus antibody before starting therapy with natalizumab. JC virus is a polyomavirus which is responsible for progressive multifocal leukoencephalopathy. Those testing positive should not be started on natalizumab. Patients who test negative should be tested for exposure at least twice a year.

Plans for alternative therapies should be made for patients who have not responded to a biologic agent within 12 weeks.

Perianal fistulizing disease, in the absence of abscess, can be treated with a combination of antibiotics, seton placement, immunomodulator therapy, and biologic agents. Complex perianal fistulizing disease may require a diverting ostomy.

Therapeutic Options
Mesalamine Preparations

Aminosalicylate preparations have been used for the treatment of UC and CD. Some data suggest that mesalamine has limited efficacy in patients with CD.

In patients with limited distal UC (e.g., proctitis), treatment may be begun with a mesalamine enema (Rowasa) or suppository

---

[2]Not available in the United States.

[1]Not FDA approved for this indication.

(Canasa). For more extensive disease, oral therapy (Asacol) or an appropriate substitute mesalamine product should be used.

Combination therapy (oral administration as well as enemas/suppositories) has been shown to be more effective in inducing remission than either modality alone. In general, the dosage that induces remission is used for maintenance of remission (Table 2).

Steroids

The National Co-operative Crohn's Disease Study and the European Co-operative Crohn's Disease Study demonstrated that steroids are efficacious in inducing remission but ineffective in maintaining remission. Among patients who have received steroids, about 26% will have a partial response, and 16% will have no response; among those who have had a complete or partial response, about 28% will become steroid dependent. The requirement for surgery is high in the latter group of patients; about 38% require surgery by the end of 1 year.

The adverse effects of steroids are many and varied and can be classified as early effects and delayed effects associated with prolonged use (>12 weeks). Acne, moon facies, mood changes, sleep disturbances, gastrointestinal intolerance, hyperglycemia, hypertension, weight gain, and ulcers of the gastrointestinal tract can be seen early. Formation of cataracts, aseptic necrosis, suppression of the hypothalamic-pituitary axis, and myopathy are associated with prolonged use. Loss of bone density, previously thought to occur only with chronic use, may be evident in bone density studies after as little as 2 weeks of therapy.

Budesonide (Entocort EC) is used for ileal inflammatory and right-sided colonic CD, with lower expected incidences of acne, moon facies, adrenal suppression, and loss of bone mineral density. Alternative therapies (immunomodulators, biologic agents) should be discussed with the patient if there has been no response to steroids in a few weeks.

Immunomodulatory Therapy

Azathioprine[1] and 6-mercaptopurine[1] are immunomodulators used as steroid-sparing agents for both CD and UC. Immunomodulators have been shown to modestly reduce the incidence of postsurgical recurrence in CD. The onset of action of these agents is slow, up to 3 to 4 months. Some toxicities are associated with genetic variants in the enzymes responsible for catabolism of azathioprine and 6-mercaptopurine, most notably thiopurine methyl transferase (TPMT). Most (89%) patients have wild-type

TPMT (full TPMT enzyme activity), 11% have intermediate enzyme activity, and 0.3% have none. In patients with full TPMT enzyme activity, therapy should be started with 1.5 mg/kg/day of 6-mercaptopurine or 2.5 mg/kg/day of azathioprine; those with intermediate activity should have the dosage reduced by half. Those who do not have any TPMT expression should not be started on these agents because of the high risk of bone marrow toxicity.

Some complications, including pancreatitis, hepatotoxicity, and serum sickness–like syndrome, cannot be predicted. It is recommended that patients starting these medications have a complete blood count and liver function tests performed every other week while their medications are being adjusted. Once they are on a stable dosage, these tests should be done every 2 to 3 months.

Parenteral methotrexate[1] 15 to 25 mg/week can be used to induce remission in patients with CD that has not responded to conventional agents. Once remission has been achieved, oral methotrexate[1] 15 mg can be used to maintain remission. Methotrexate is absolutely contraindicated in pregnancy. Leukopenia, hepatic fibrosis, nausea and vomiting, and hypersensitivity reactions are potential side effects. Risk of hepatic fibrosis is associated with a cumulative dose of more than 1.5 g, diabetes, and concomitant use of alcohol.

Cyclosporine

In patients with severe UC, intravenous cyclosporine (Sandimmune)[1] at a dose of 2 to 4 mg/kg/day has been shown to be effective in inducing remission. A significant proportion of these patients may still require colectomy within 1 year. Those patients who have achieved response and remission on intravenous cyclosporine should be started on oral cyclosporine (Neoral)[1] for a few months, together with prophylaxis against *Pneumocystis*. 6-Mercaptopurine or azathioprine can also be used as maintenance agents.

Side effects commonly seen with cyclosporine include renal dysfunction, seizures (particularly in patients with hypocholesterolemia), hypertension, gingival hyperplasia, electrolyte abnormalities, and hirsutism.

Biologic Agents

Infliximab is a chimeric (murine-human) monoclonal anti-TNF antibody that has been approved for induction and maintenance of remission in both CD and UC. It was initially approved for the treatment of fistulizing CD, and subsequent studies showed it to be effective in maintenance therapy as well. In several other studies, it was found to be efficacious in reducing steroid use, length of hospital stay, and surgical intervention and achieving mucosal healing. Infliximab is administered intravenously with or without premedication to avoid allergic reactions.

For induction, infliximab 5 mg/kg is administered at weeks 0, 2, and 6, and maintenance is begun at 5 mg/kg every 8 weeks. Some patients require dose escalation because of diminution of response or failure to maintain remission. In these patients, depending on the clinical scenario, the dose should be increased to 10 mg/kg or the interval reduced to every 6 weeks. In the past, infliximab was routinely used with concomitant immunomodulator therapy to reduce the possibility of infliximab antibodies, but this practice has been associated with a higher risk for a rare hepatosplenic T-cell lymphoma (predominantly in the pediatric population), leading to reconsideration of the need for concomitant immunomodulators in some patients. However, results from the recently released Study of Biologic and Immunomodulator Naive Patients in Crohn's Disease (SONIC) trial demonstrated the superiority of combination therapy over either immunomodulator or infliximab alone, especially in patients with elevated C-reactive protein and ulcers in their baseline colonoscopy. Because reactivation of latent tuberculosis has been reported, patients should undergo a PPD test or QuantiFERON-TB gold and chest radiography before beginning therapy. Available data, although limited, suggests that biologic agents (Infliximab, Adalimumab, Certolizumab and Tysabri) are safe for conception and pregnancy as well as breast feeding.

---

[1]Not FDA approved for this indication.

TABLE 2	Mesalamine Products Indicated for Ulcerative Colitis	
AMINOSALICYLATE PRODUCT	**DAILY DOSAGE**	**FREQUENCY**
Azulfidine (sulfasalazine tablet)	0.5 g–4 g	qid
Delzicol	2.4 g	tid
Pentasa (mesalamine controlled-release tablet)	2–4 g	qid
Colazal (balsalazide capsule)	6.75 g	tid
Dipentum (olsalazine capsule)	1 g	bid
Lialda (mesalamine delayed-release tablet)	2.4–4.8 g	qd
Canasa (mesalamine rectal suppository)*	1 g	qd
Rowasa (mesalamine rectal enema)†	4 g	qd
Apriso (mesalamine delayed and extended-release capsule)	1.5 g	qd

*Indicated for ulcerative proctitis.
†Indicated for distal ulcerative colitis.

---

[1]Not FDA approved for this indication.

Other Anti–Tumor Necrosis Factor Antibodies

Adalimumab

Recently, adalimumab (Humira), a recombinant fully human immunoglobulin targeting TNF, was approved for use in CD. In the CLASSIC and CHARM trials, adalimumab was demonstrated to be an effective agent in inducing and maintaining remission. It has also been shown to be effective in patients who have lost response to infliximab or are intolerant to it, but it has not yet been approved for treatment of UC. Serious reactions, reactivation of tuberculosis, allergic reactions, lupus-like reactions, and demyelinating diseases are some of the concerns.

For induction, adalimumab 160 mg is given subcutaneously at week 0, 80 mg at week 2, and then, for maintenance of remission, 40 mg every other week.

Certolizumab

Certolizumab (Cimzia) is a polyethylene glycolated Fab fragment of humanized anti-TNF monoclonal antibody approved for use in CD. In the PRECISE 1 and 2 studies, certolizumab was shown to result in modest improvement in response but no clinically significant improvement in remission.

Golimumab

Golimumab (Simponi) is another monoclonal TNF antibody that has been approved for the treatment of moderate to severe ulcerative colitis. It should be considered as one of the treatment options when patients have begun failing therapy with mesalamine products or are at risk for developing steroid dependence. After two starter doses it is a monthly self-injectable treatment.

Anti-α_4 Therapy

Natalizumab

Natalizumab (Tysabri) is a humanized monoclonal antibody against the α_4 integrin subunit, a molecule involved in cellular adhesion that is required for recruitment of key immune cells to sites affected by IBD. In several studies, it has been shown to be efficacious in inducing remission and maintaining response in CD patients. Enthusiasm has been tempered by the apparent risk for progressive multifocal leukoencephalopathy, a rare but fatal opportunistic infection. Before initiating therapy with this agent, patient will need to be enrolled in the TOUCH program (www.tysabri.com) and should be tested for evidence of prior exposure to JC virus. If the test is positive, alternative therapies should be considered. If the test is negative, JC virus antibody testing should be done at least twice a year while the patient is on natalizumab.

Vedolizumab (Entyvio) is another humanized α_4, β_7 integrin inhibitor that mediates its anti-inflammatory activity in the gastrointestinal tract via MAdCAM pathway. It does not affect CSF T lymphocyte immunophenotype and it activity seems to be localized in the gut.

The treatment regimens for UC and CD are summarized in Box 1.

Box 1 Summary of Treatment Regimen

Ulcerative Colitis

Proctitis
- Initial treatment choices
  - Mesalamine suppositories (Canasa) or enemas (Rowasa) to induce remission
  - Steroid foam enemas (Cortifoam) to induce remission
  - Mesalamine suppositories or enemas to maintain remission
- Second-line treatment choices
  - Oral mesalamine in combination with local therapy
  - Adjunctive treatment with antibiotics: ciprofloxacin (Cipro),[1] metronidazole (Flagyl),[1] or rifaximin (Xifaxan)[1]
  - Probiotics

Left-Sided Colitis
- Initial treatment choices
  - Oral mesalamine product with or without local therapy
- Second-line treatment choices
  - Oral or intravenous steroids budesonide (Uceris)
  - Immunomodulator therapy
  - Infliximab (IFX, Remicade), adalimumab (Humira), golimumab (Simponi)
  - Cyclosporine (Sandimmune)[1] on an inpatient basis (avoid cyclosporine after IFX therapy due to risk of severe immunosuppression)

Pancolitis
- Initial treatment choices
  - Oral mesalamine with a short course of oral or intravenous steroids including colonic-release budesonide
- Second-line treatment choices
  - Immunomodulator therapy
  - Infliximab, adalimumab, golimumab
  - Cyclosporine on an inpatient basis (avoid cyclosporine after IFX therapy due to risk of severe immunosuppression)

Crohn's Disease

Ileocecal Inflammatory Crohn's Disease
- First-line treatment
  - Oral mesalamine (ileo-colonic release mesalamine product for ileal disease; Pentasa for more proximal small-bowel disease)[1]
  - Budesonide (Entocort EC) 9 mg PO qd

- Immunomodulator therapy
- Biologic agents with or without concomitant immunomodulators

Ileal Stricturing Disease
- No proximal dilation
  - Trial with budesonide or biologic agents (patients with elevated hsCRP are more likely to respond)
- Proximal small-bowel dilation
  - Consider surgical approach

Internally Fistulizing Disease without Intraabdominal Abscess
- Stricture immediately distal to fistula
  - Surgical approach
- No stricture
  - Biologic agents with or without concomitant immunomodulators

Externally Fistulizing Disease without Intraabdominal Abscess
- Biologic agents with or without concomitant immunomodulators

Fistulizing Disease with Intraabdominal Abscess
- Intravenous antibiotics as appropriate
- Percutaneous drainage if appropriate
- Surgical drainage if indicated
- Biologic agents with or without concomitant immunomodulators once infectious process has been treated

Perianal Crohn's Disease without Abscess Formation
- Antibiotics: Ciprofloxacin (Cipro),[1] metronidazole (Flagyl),[1] rifaximin (Xifaxan)[1]
- Immunomodulators
- Biologic agents with or without concomitant immunomodulators
- Seton placement
- Diverting ostomy

Colonic Crohn's Disease
- Oral steroids to induce remission
- Immunomodulator therapy
- Biologic agents with or without concomitant immunomodulator therapy

[1]Not FDA approved for this indication.
Abbreviations: hsCRP = high-sensitivity C-reactive protein.

References

Booya F, Akram S, Fletcher JG, et al. CT enterography and fistulizing Crohn's disease: Clinical benefit and radiographic findings. Abdom Imaging 2009;34(4):467–75.

Feagan BG, Panaccione R, Sandborn WJ, et al. Effects of adalimumab therapy on incidence of hospitalization and surgery in Crohn's disease: Results from the CHARM study. Gastroenterology 2008;135(5):1493–9.

Ghosh S, Goldin E, Gordon FH, et al. Natalizumab for active Crohn's disease. N Engl J Med 2003;348(1):24–32.

Hanauer SB, Sandborn WJ, Kornbluth A. Delayed-release oral mesalamine at 4.8 g/day (800 mg tablet) for the treatment of moderately active ulcerative colitis: The ASCEND II trial. Am J Gastroenterol 2005;100(11):2478–85.

Lichtenstein GR, Yan S, Bala M. Infliximab maintenance treatment reduces hospitalizations, surgeries, and procedures in fistulizing Crohn's disease. Gastroenterology 2005;128(4):862–9.

Podolsky DK. Inflammatory bowel disease. N Engl J Med 2002;347(6):417–29.

Thomsen OO, Cortot A, Jewell D, et al. A comparison of budesonide and mesalamine for active Crohn's disease. International Budesonide-Mesalamine Study Group. N Engl J Med 1998;339(6):370–4.

Thukral C, Travassos WJ, Peppercorn MA. The role of antibiotics in inflammatory bowel disease. Curr Treat Options Gastroenterol 2005;8(3):223–8.

Xavier RJ, Podolsky DK. Unraveling the pathogenesis of inflammatory bowel disease. Nature 2007;448(7152):427–34.

INTESTINAL PARASITES

Method of
Nathan Thielman, MD, MPH; and Elizabeth Reddy, MD

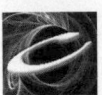

CURRENT DIAGNOSIS

Signs and Symptoms

- Watery diarrhea—Most protozoal infections: *Giardia, Blastocystis, Dientamoeba, Cryptosporidium, Cyclospora, Cystoisospora, Microsporidia*
- Dysentery—Most commonly *Entamoeba histolytica*; less commonly *Balantidium coli, Trichuris trichiura* (whipworm)
- Eosinophilia—Throughout chronic infection: *Strongyloides*, schistosomiasis, *Cystoisospora*; usually only in early infection: *Ascaris*, hookworm, whipworm
- Prolonged or severe diarrhea in HIV infection—Spore-forming protozoal infections: *Cryptosporidium, Cyclospora, Cystoisospora, Microsporidia*
- Visible worms passed in stool—*Ascaris, Taeniasis, Diphyllobothrium*

Diagnosis of Parasitic Infections

- Stool antigen assay—*Entamoeba histolytica, Giardia, Cryptosporidium*
- Serology*—Strongyloides, schistosomiasis
- Stool for ova and parasites—All intestinal parasites. Sensitivity increased with repeat examinations if necessary. Concentration, preservation, and staining improve diagnosis of certain pathogens.

Note: Key features of intestinal parasitic infection may overlap with other conditions, including nonparasitic infections, and extra-intestinal parasites.

*Optimal method of diagnosis in returned travelers and immigrants from endemic to nonendemic areas. Does not distinguish between active and resolved infections.

Intestinal parasites are a diverse group of pathogens with local and global significance. Immigration, international adoption, travel, and the frequency of HIV/AIDS and other immune-compromising conditions (e.g., malignancy, organ transplantation) have all contributed to a need for ongoing or increased awareness of parasitic infections in the United States. Persons who reside in chronic care facilities, children in daycare, and persons whose sexual practices increase the likelihood of fecal–oral contact are also at risk for acquiring intestinal parasitic infection.

Globally, intestinal parasites are responsible for an enormous burden of disease. Although these pathogens are rarely fatal, ongoing exposure to intestinal parasites among persons in endemic areas exacerbates malnutrition, carries multiple morbidities, and causes stunting of growth and development in children, all of which have far-reaching consequences.

Patients who present with diarrheal illness (especially prolonged or travel-associated), unexplained eosinophilia, or expulsion of worms should be evaluated for intestinal parasites. In such cases, a careful history should focus on the patient's country of origin, detailed travel and recreational activities, dietary habits and new or unusual food exposures, occupation, sexual history, sick contacts, and risks for or known immunodeficiency. Some specialists advocate obtaining a complete blood count with differential to assess eosinophil count in all international adoptees and immigrants from areas where parasitic infections are common. If eosinophilia is present, antibody testing for schistosomiasis and strongyloidiasis—two chronic parasitic infections with potentially serious consequences—should be performed, and appropriate therapy should be administered if infection is discovered. For key features of common intestinal parasitic infections, see the Current Diagnosis box.

Diagnosis of intestinal parasites has improved recently with the advent of quick, simple, and accurate stool antigen tests for some major pathogens, such as *Entamoeba, Giardia* and *Cryptosporidium* species. However, the fecal examination for ova and parasites is still the mainstay of diagnosis in many cases. Whenever possible, stool specimens should be sent to a laboratory with clinical expertise in parasitology, where wet preparation, concentration, or staining can identify most pathogens. Evaluation of fresh specimens and repeated examinations improve diagnostic sensitivity. Key diagnostic points are summarized in the Current Diagnosis box.

This review focuses on basic understanding, recognition, diagnosis and treatment of common intestinal parasites in the United States and throughout the world. Within each section, parasites are listed in order of relative clinical significance.

Protozoa: Amoebae, Flagellates, Ciliates

Entamoeba histolytica

Entamoeba histolytica, the cause of amoebic dysentery and amebic liver abscess, is a worldwide pathogen of major clinical significance. Approximately 10% of the world's population and up to 60% of children in highly endemic areas show serologic evidence of infection, and *E. histolytica* is estimated to cause 100,000 deaths per year globally. In the United States, infection is almost exclusively found among returned travelers, immigrants from endemic areas (especially Mexico and Central and South America), men who have sex with men (MSM), and institutionalized persons. *E. histolytica* exists in only two forms, the hardy cyst characterized by four nuclei, and the trophozoite, which has a single nucleus and survives poorly outside the human body. It is important to note that *Entamoeba dispar* and *Entamoeba moshkovskii*, which are morphologically identical to *E. histolytica* in stool microscopy, are now thought to be largely nonpathogenic species. Other *Entamoeba*, including *Entamoeba hartmanni, Entamoeba coli, Entamoeba polecki*, and others, can be individually identified on microscopy but are of uncertain pathogenicity and generally considered benign.

E. histolytica infection is acquired by ingestion of cysts in contaminated water or food or by fecal–oral contact, as can occur in chronic care facilities or with anal–oral sexual practices. Acquisition of the parasite can result in asymptomatic infection (most common), diarrheal illness, or extraintestinal infection, the latter most commonly manifest as amebic liver abscess. An appropriately robust layer of colonic mucin may be protective against symptomatic infection, whereas attachment to intestinal epithelium results in penetration of the organism into the submucosal layer, where extensive tissue destruction can take place in the form of apoptosis and lysis of cells, hence the name "histolytica."

Symptoms of classic amebic dysentery begin insidiously 1 to 2 weeks after infection. Diarrhea is almost universal and typically consists of numerous small-volume stools that can contain mucus or frank blood, or both. Stools are almost always heme positive if not grossly bloody. Abdominal pain and tenesmus are common; fever is present in approximately 30% of cases. Some persons have a chronic course characterized by weight loss, intermittent loose stools, and abdominal pain. Rare presentations of amebic dysentery include amebomas, which can mimic malignancy, and perianal ulcerations or fistulae. Severe disease can occur in the form of fulminant colitis or toxic megacolon; the latter almost universally requires colectomy. Young age, pregnancy, and corticosteroid use predispose to severe infection. Although persons with HIV infection or AIDS can develop invasive disease, *E. histolytica* does not appear to be a common opportunistic infection, and infection is curable in this population.

Amebic liver abscess is the most common extraintestinal complication of *E. histolytica*; cerebral and ocular amebiasis have also been reported. Amebic liver abscess affects children of both sexes equally, but it is up to nine times more common in men, indicating that hormonal milieu likely plays a role. Amebic liver abscess almost always manifests within 3 to 5 months of initial infection, but it can surface years later. Illness is characterized by fever and abdominal tenderness that worsen over several days to weeks. Weight loss, jaundice, and cough from diaphragmatic irritation can also occur. Symptoms of dysentery usually are not present, and diarrhea is reported in less than one third of cases. Laboratory abnormalities include leukocytosis, transaminitis, elevated alkaline phosphatase, and elevated sedimentation rate. Chest radiograph often demonstrates elevation of the right hemidiaphragm, and pleural effusion may be present. Rupture of the abscess can occur into the abdomen or pleuropulmonary space, manifesting as acute abdomen or empyema.

Diagnosis of intraintestinal *E. histolytica* infection has classically relied on stool microscopy, and this remains the only available method in much of the world. At least three stool specimens should be examined to improve sensitivity. Cysts visualized in stool might or might not indicate active infection and cannot be distinguished from *E. dispar* and *E. moshkovskii*. Presence of trophozoites with ingested red blood cells on stool preparation is diagnostic of dysentery secondary to *E. histolytica*, as are mobile amebae if seen within freshly examined biopsy material.

Diagnosis of *E. histolytica* infection has improved greatly with the advent of antigen tests, now available as enzyme-linked immunosorbent assays (ELISAs) and immunofluorescent probes. The Techlab ELISA antigen test is highly sensitive and specific and can be used on a freshly passed stool specimen, serum, or hepatic abscess material. It becomes positive with onset of symptomatic disease and resolves on treatment of infection. Other available antigen tests appear to function well but have not been as rigorously studied. Aspirate of liver abscess material may be necessary to distinguish from pyogenic liver abscess; a negative stool examination for *E. histolytica* does not preclude amebic liver abscess. In a patient at high risk for amebic liver abscess (e.g., young male immigrants), a trial of antimicrobial therapy can help in diagnosis because infection typically responds rapidly.

All patients who have confirmed *E. histolytica* infection and reside in nonendemic areas should be treated regardless of whether they are symptomatic, because invasive disease can develop in the future. Asymptomatic cyst passers may be treated with an intraluminal agent alone, such as paromomycin (Humatin) or iodoquinol (Yodoxin). In the United States, the most readily available effective treatment for patients with amebic colitis or liver abscess is metronidazole (Flagyl). It can be given intravenously for patients unable to tolerate oral medications. Experts recommend that a course of therapy with an intraluminal agent be given following the completed course of the systemic agent for all cases of invasive *E. histolytica*. See Table 1 for medications and doses.

Giardiasis

Giardia lamblia, also known as *Giardia intestinalis* or *Giardia duodenalis*, is the most commonly identified diarrheal parasitic infection in the United States, with an estimated 100,000 to 2.5 million cases per year. It is globally distributed and found in fresh water throughout mountainous regions of the United States and Canada. The organism is a flagellated aerotolerant anaerobe that exists in a cyst and trophozoite form. Cysts can survive for several weeks in cold water. Contaminated food and water are the most common sources of infection, but the organism can also be passed by person-to-person contact. In the United States, giardiasis is primarily diagnosed among international travelers, persons with recreational water exposure, institutionalized persons and children in day care, and persons with anal–oral sexual practices.

Illness can result from ingestion of as few as 10 to 25 cysts, which transform into trophozoites in the small intestine and attach to and damage the small bowel wall. Symptomatic disease begins insidiously over approximately 2 weeks in 25% to 50% of persons who ingest *Giardia* cysts. Others become asymptomatic cyst passers (5%–15%) or have no signs of infection (35%–50%). Hallmarks of infection are watery diarrhea, bloating, gas, abdominal pain, and weight loss; less commonly, patients have nausea, vomiting, or low-grade fever. Steatorrhea and malabsorption, particularly secondary to *Giardia*-induced lactase deficiency, can be observed. Chronic *Giardia* infection should be considered in the differential diagnosis for a long-standing diarrheal illness, especially if there is history of exposure to possibly contaminated water. Patients with common variable immune deficiency, X-linked agammglobulinemia, and IgA deficiency syndromes are at risk for fulminant and sometimes incurable disease, suggesting a significant role for humoral immunity in control of infection. Persons with HIV infection or AIDS have symptoms similar to those in patients without HIV and typically can be cured of infection with standard therapy.

Diagnosis of giardiasis is made by examination of fresh or preserved stool or by stool antigen assays. In the case of fecal examination, trophozoites may be directly visualized in fresh liquid stool; semiformed and preserved stool should be stained before examination. Currently, there are immunochromographic, direct fluorescence antibody, and ELISA tests for diagnosis of *Giardia*, including the ImmunoCard STAT! Cryptosporidium/Giardia Rapid Assay (Meridian Bioscience, Cincinnati, Ohio), which tests for both pathogens simultaneously. Although it is rarely necessary, the diagnosis can sometimes be made on duodenal biopsy.

For details of treatment options, see Table 1. Metronidazole[1] is the most commonly prescribed treatment in the United States and should be given for a 10-day course. Tinidazole (Tindamax), recently approved in the United States, appears to have excellent efficacy and improved tolerability over metronidazole. Nitazoxanide (Alinia) has also been shown to eradicate infection well and can be used as an alternative or in patients who fail a first course of treatment. Patients who fail first-line therapy might have a persistent source of infection (contaminated water source, close contact with an infected person), immune deficiency predisposing to difficult eradication, or persistence of cysts. Once possible sources of reinfection have been investigated and eliminated, relapsed infections should either be re-treated with a longer course of therapy (21–28 days) or treated with a different agent. Patients who fail more than one course of therapy should undergo immunologic work-up.

Prevention of *Giardia* infection, as with other parasitic infections, involves primarily close attention to personal hygiene, hand washing, and avoidance of ingestion of fresh unfiltered water. Boiling water or use of a 0.2- to 1-μm water filter offer optimal protection against *Giardia* and other parasitic pathogens, although such filters still might not protect against *Cryptosporidium*.

Blastocystis hominis

Blastocystis hominis, formerly considered a protozoan, has been reclassified as a fungus. It has a worldwide distribution found most commonly in tropical regions; it is present in humans and several other animals. In temperate regions, *B. hominis* is detected at a high rate among MSM. *B. hominis* was long thought to cause only asymptomatic colonization, but there is some evidence to suggest a

---

[1]Not FDA approved for this indication.

TABLE 1 Pharmacologic Treatment of Major Protozoan Infections

CLINICAL SITUATION	DRUG	ADULT DOSE	PEDIATRIC DOSE	COMMENTS
Amebiasis				
Entamoeba histolytica				
Asymptomatic	Recommended: Paromomycin* *or* Iodoquinol[†]	25–35 mg/kg/d in 3 doses × 7 d	25–35 mg/kg/d in 3 doses × 7 d	
		650 mg tid × 20 d	30–40 mg/kg/d (max 2 g) in 3 doses × 20 d	
	Alternative: Diloxanide furoate[‡]	500 mg tid × 10 d	20 mg/kg/d in 3 doses × 10 d	
Mild to moderate intestinal disease	Recommended: Metronidazole *or* Tinidazole[1,§]	500–750 mg tid × 7–10 d	35–50 mg/kg/d in 3 doses × 7–10 d	Treatment should be followed by a course of iodoquinol or paromomycin in the dosage used to treat asymptomatic amebiasis.
		2 g once daily × 3 d	≥3 y: 50 mg/kg once daily (max 2 g) × 3 d	
Severe intestinal or extraintestinal disease	Metronidazole *or*	500–750 mg tid × 7–10 d	35–50 mg/kg/d in 3 doses × 7–10 d	Treatment should be followed by a course of iodoquinol or paromomycin in the dosage used to treat asymptomatic amebiasis.
	Tinidazole[§]	2 g once daily × 5 d	≥3 y: 50 mg/kg once daily (max 2 g) × 5 d	
Balantidiasis				
Balantidium coli				
Symptomatic and asymptomatic disease	Recommended: Tetracycline[1,‖]	500 mg qid × 10 d	40 mg/kg/d (max 2 g) in 4 doses × 10 d	
	Alternatives: Metronidazole[1] *or* Iodoquinol[1,†]	500–750 mg PO tid × 5 d 650 mg tid × 20 d	35–50 mg/kg/d in 3 doses × 5 d 30–40 mg/kg/d (max 2 g) in 3 doses × 20 d	
Blastocystis hominis				
Symptomatic disease only				Organism's pathogenicity is uncertain.[¶]
Cryptosporidiosis				
Cryptosporidium				
Immune competent	Nitazoxanide	500 mg bid × 3 d	1–3 y: 100 mg bid × 3 d 4–11 y: 200 mg bid × 3 d ≥12 y: adult dose	FDA approved as a pediatric oral suspension for treating *Cryptosporidium* in immunocompetent children <12 y and for *Giardia*. It might also be effective for mild to moderate amebiasis. Nitazoxanide is available in 500-mg tabs and an oral suspension; it should be taken with food.
HIV-infected	No optimal therapy available			All HIV-infected patients with cryptosporidiosis should receive HAART whenever possible. Nitazoxanide, paramomycin, or paramomycin + azithromycin may have a role in decreasing diarrhea in chronic cases of HIV-infected persons.
Cyclosporiasis				
Cyclospora cayetanensis	Recommended: TMP-SMX (Bactrim, Septra)[1]	160 mg TMP, 800 mg SMX (1 DS tab) bid × 7–10 d	5 mg/kg TMP, 25 mg/kg SMX bid × 7–10 d	In immunocompetent patients, usually a self-limited illness. Immunosuppressed patients might need higher doses, longer duration (TMP-SMX qid × 10 d, followed by bid × 3 wk) and long-term maintenance.
	Alternative: Ciprofloxacin	500 mg PO bid × 7 d	(no recommended pediatric dose)[1]	
Dientamoebiasis				
Dientamoeba fragilis Symptomatic disease only	Iodoquinol[1,†] *or*	650 mg tid × 20 d	30–40 mg/kg/d (max 2 g) in 3 doses × 20 d	
	Paromomycin[1,*] *or*	25–35 mg/kg/d in 3 doses × 7 d	25–35 mg/kg/d in 3 doses × 7 d	
	Metronidazole[1]	500–750 mg tid × 10 d	35–50 mg/kg/d in 3 doses × 10 d	

TABLE 1 Pharmacologic Treatment of Major Protozoan Infections—cont'd

CLINICAL SITUATION	DRUG	ADULT DOSE	PEDIATRIC DOSE	COMMENTS
Giardiasis				
Giardia lamblia				
All symptomatic disease and asymptomatic carriage in nonendemic areas	Recommended: Metronidazole[1] *or*	250 mg tid × 5–7 d	15 mg/kg/d in 3 doses × 5 d	
	Nitazoxanide *or*	500 mg bid × 3 d	1–3 y: 100 mg bid × 3 d 4–11 y: 200 mg bid × 3 d	
	Tinidazole[§]	2 g once	50 mg/kg (max 2 g) once	Treatment should be followed by a course of iodoquinol or paromomycin in the dosage used to treat asymptomatic amebiasis. Albendazole, 400 mg daily × 5 d alone or in combination with metronidazole may also be effective.
	Alternatives:			
	Quinacrine[1,**] *or*	100 mg tid × 5 d	6 mg/kg/d (max 300 mg/d) tid × 5 d	Combination treatment with standard doses of metronidazole and quinacrine × 3 wk is effective for a small number of refractory infections. In one study, nitazoxanide was used successfully in high doses to treat a case of *Giardia* resistant to metronidazole and albendazole.
	Furazolidone *or*	100 mg qid × 7–10 d	6 mg/kg/d in 4 doses × 10 d	
	Paromomycin[1]	25–35 mg/kg/d in 3 doses × 7 d	25–35 mg/kg/d in 3 doses × 7 d	Nonabsorbed luminal agent; may be useful for treating giardiasis in pregnancy
Cystoisosporiasis				In immunocompetent patients, usually a self-limited illness. Immunosuppressed patients might need higher doses, longer duration (TMP-SMX qid × 10 d, followed by bid × 3 wk) and long-term maintenance. For isosporiasis in sulfonamide-sensitive patients, pyrimethamine 50–75 mg qd in divided doses (*plus* leucovorin 10–25 mg/d) is effective.
Cystoisospora belli	Recommended: TMP-SMX[1]	160 mg TMP, 800 mg SMX bid × 7–10 d	5 mg/kg TMP, 25 mg/kg SMX bid × 7–10 d	Ciprofloxacin is an alternative but may not be as effective.
Microsporidiosis				
Enterocytozoon bieneusi				
Intestinal disease	Fumagillin[+]	60 mg/d PO × 14 d		Oral fumagillin (Sanofi Recherche, Gentilly, France) is effective in treating *E. bieneusi* but is associated with thrombocytopenia and neutropenia. HAART can lead to microbiological and clinical response in HIV-infected patients with microsporidial diarrhea. Octreotide (Sandostatin) has provided symptomatic relief in some patients with large-volume diarrhea.
	Albendazole[1]	400 mg PO bid × 21 d	15 mg/kg/d in 2 doses (max 400 mg/dose)	
Encephalitozoon intestinalis				
Diarrheal or disseminated disease	Albendazole[1]	400 mg bid × 21 d	15 mg/kg/d in 2 doses (max 400 mg/dose)	

Abbreviations: DS = double strength; GI = gastrointestinal; HAART = highly active antiretroviral therapy; max = maximum; tab = tablet; TMP-SMX = trimethoprim-sulfamethoxazole.

Adapted from World Health Organization. Drugs for parasitic infections. Med Lett Drug Ther 2010: 8 (Suppl.).

[1]Not FDA approved for this indication.

*Should be taken with meals.

[†]Should be taken after meals.

[‡]The drug is not available commercially, but as a service it can be compounded by Panorama Compounding Pharmacy, 6744 Balboa Blvd., Van Nuys, CA 91406 (800-247-9767) or Medical Center Pharmacy, New Haven, CT (203-688-6816).

[§]A nitroimidazole similar to metronidazole, tinidazole is FDA approved and appears to be as effective and better tolerated than metronidazole. It should be taken with food to minimize GI adverse effects. For children and patients unable to take tablets, a pharmacist may crush the tablets and mix them with cherry syrup. The syrup suspension is good for 7 d at room temperature and must be shaken before use. Ornidazole, a similar drug, is also used outside the United States. Dosing recommendations are only available for children ≥3 years of age.

[||]Contraindicated in pregnant and breastfeeding women and children <8 y.

[¶]Clinical significance of these organisms is controversial; metronidazole 750 mg tid × 10 d, iodoquinol 650 mg tid × 20 d, or TMP-SMX11 double-strength tab bid × 7 d are effective. Metronidazole resistance may be common. Nitazoxanide is effective in children.

**Should be taken with liquids after a meal.

Intestinal Parasites

579

role in human disease, although this remains controversial. Ongoing molecular analysis might elucidate subtypes of *B. hominis* with varying degrees of pathogenicity in humans.

B. hominis has four forms: vacuolated, amoeba-like, granular, and cyst, the latter of which is likely to be the infectious form. It appears to be transmitted via the fecal–oral route, possibly from waterborne sources.

As suggested previously, the majority of infections appear to be entirely asymptomatic, and number of organisms does not appear to accurately predict severity of illness. Symptoms consist mainly of watery diarrhea, bloating, and abdominal cramps. There are typically no pathologic findings on colonoscopy and there are no reports of invasive disease. Infection is diagnosed by stool microscopy with use of a trichrome or hematoxylin-stained preserved specimen. The organism is susceptible in vitro to numerous antimicrobials. Bactrim[1] or metronidazole is the treatment of choice; details are listed in Table 1.

Dientamoeba fragilis

Dientamoeba fragilis was originally classified as an amoeba, but it is more closely related to the flagellates such as *Trichomonas vaginalis*. It is distributed worldwide, including in Western nations, and has only recently been recognized as a clinically significant pathogen, possibly because it is difficult to visualize without specific staining techniques. Illness has commonly been found in travelers and MSM, but it can affect anyone.

The parasite exists only in the trophozoite form. Despite its genetic relationship to the flagellates, *D. fragilis* does not have a flagellum and is immotile. Trophozoites range in size from 4 to 20 μm and are binucleate. Patients in the United States who have *D. fragilis* were found in some studies to harbor other intestinal parasites as well, such as *E. vermicularis* and *B. hominis*, and in general *D. fragilis* is more prevalent in areas of the world with limited public sanitation. These features support a fecal–oral mode of transmission for *D. fragilis*.

Most patients are asymptomatic; however, numerous case reports and small series describe patients with no other organisms identified to cause their symptoms who improve significantly after treatment and documented clearance of *D. fragilis* from their stool. Illness is typically subacute to chronic, characterized by abdominal pain, watery diarrhea, anorexia, fatigue, and malaise. Diagnosis can be difficult, because the parasite is fastidious. If *D. fragilis* is suspected, stool should be preserved with polyvinyl alcohol and quickly stained with iron–hematoxylin and trichrome. Polymerase chain reaction (PCR) has been used for diagnosis as well, but it is not readily available for use in most clinical settings.

For full treatment information, see Table 1. Iodoquinol (Yodoxin)[1] and metronidazole[1] have both been used successfully to treat *D. fragilis*.

Balantidium coli

Balantidium coli is the largest protozoan that infects humans, and the only ciliate. Balantidiasis is a relatively rare cause of illness and is found primarily in rural agrarian communities in Southeast Asia, Central and South America, and Papua New Guinea. *B. coli* is highly associated with animal farming, in particular, pigs; humans are incidental hosts. The parasite is transmitted by direct contact with animals or on ingestion of water or food contaminated by animal excrement. Persons with malnutrition or immune deficiency are particularly susceptible to infection.

B. coli invades the intestinal mucosa from the terminal ileum to the rectum. About one half of infections are asymptomatic; the other one half result in a subacute or chronic diarrheal illness with abdominal cramping, nausea, vomiting, weight loss, and occasional low-grade fever. Fewer than 5% of patients present with severe or even fulminant dysentery, and rare cases of colonic penetration with peritonitis, mesenteric lymphadenitis, or hepatic infection have been reported.

Diagnosis is made by visualization of trophozoites in fresh stool specimens or preserved and permanently stained samples. The trophozoite is large and ciliated; cysts are difficult to distinguish. It displays a distinct spiraling motility that can be seen under low power. On stained sample, visualization of *B. coli*'s characteristic macronucleus and spiral micronucleus can help confirm the diagnosis. All patients should be treated regardless of symptoms. Tetracycline[1] (Sumycin and others) is the therapy of choice; the infection also responds to metronidazole[1]; see Table 1 for dosing information.

Spore-Forming Protozoa and Microsporidia
Cryptosporidiosis

Cryptosporidium is a pathogen with worldwide distribution that is endemic to the United States. Humans are most commonly infected by the recently reclassified *Cryptosporidium hominis*, but *Cryptosporidium parvum*, primarily a bovine pathogen, also causes human disease. *Cryptosporidium* has caused multiple waterborne outbreaks in the United States and can be acquired secondary to recreational water exposure (e.g., swimming pools, water parks). The best-known outbreak occurred secondary to heavy rains that brought farm runoff into the drinking water supply in Wisconsin in 1984. It resulted in 430,000 documented cases of cryptosporidiosis and contributed to the deaths of dozens of persons with advanced HIV infection or malignancy.

Cryptosporidium is a coccidian, part of a group of spore-forming protozoa with a complex life cycle and a structure that allows mechanical penetration into host cells. *Cryptosporidium* can mature and reproduce entirely within human hosts, thereby enabling infection to occur both from environmental sources and by direct person-to-person contact. Its oocysts, the source of infection on ingestion, are markedly hardy; they can withstand heavy chlorination, survive for months in cold water, and are small enough to occasionally evade even the smallest available water filtration systems.

All persons are susceptible to infection, which usually is self-limited. Fulminant or chronic infection, or both, can be seen among patients with immune compromise secondary to HIV infection (especially those with CD4 <50), in patients with malignancy, and in malnourished children. As few as 100 oocysts can cause infection, which results when the parasite penetrates small bowel epithelium and replicates just beneath its surface. Villous flattening and small bowel wall edema are seen on pathologic examination from infected persons.

Asymptomatic infections occur but are relatively rare. Symptoms begin within several days to 1 week of ingestion of oocysts. The hallmark of infection is explosive watery diarrhea, which can be so voluminous as to resemble cholera and can cause significant dehydration and electrolyte imbalance. Abdominal discomfort, nausea, vomiting, fever, malaise, and myalgia can also be present, and weight loss is common. Illness lasts 1 to 2 weeks, but a substantial percentage of patients report a relapse of symptoms after initial improvement. The biliary tract can be involved, particularly in patients with HIV infection, and infection at other distant sites, such as the lungs, has rarely been reported.

Diagnosis of *Cryptosporidium* has improved dramatically in recent years with the advent of antigen tests, which are highly sensitive and specific and can be used on a single sample of fresh stool. The ImmunoCard STAT! Cryptosporidium/Giardia Rapid Assay is useful because it can detect both pathogens. When such tests are not available, stools submitted for examination should be fixed in formalin and stained for trophozoites or cysts; availability of multiple stool specimens improves the diagnostic sensitivity. Luminal fluid or biopsy specimens obtained during endoscopy can also reveal the organism.

Infection with *Cryptosporidium* is typically a self-limited illness in otherwise healthy persons, but symptoms can be improved and the course shortened with the antiparasitic nitazoxanide.

---

[1]Not FDA approved for this indication.

[1]Not FDA approved for this indication.

Cryptosporidium remains an extremely challenging and potentially devastating infection in immunocompromised patients, especially those with HIV and a low CD4 count (counts <200 increase risk of severe illness, and counts <50 markedly increase risk). Although anticryptosporidial therapies in this population have shown very limited efficacy, restoration of immune function with HAART often effects cure. Limited data suggest a trial of nitazoxanide may be reasonable in this circumstance as well. Appropriate supportive measures are also crucial in all patients with *Cryptosporidium*, including fluid and electrolyte replacement; avoiding lactose products is likely to be beneficial during the first 2 weeks after infection as the brush border regenerates. Appropriate treatment doses for nitazoxanide are listed in Table 1.

Prevention of *Cryptosporidium* infection requires a highly developed public water purification system including flocculation, sedimentation, and filtration. Use of 0.2- to 1-µm personal water filters for campers and hikers greatly reduces but does not eliminate risk of infection, whereas boiling water before drinking kills oocysts. Close attention to hygiene and avoidance of fecal–oral contact is the mainstay of prevention in the settings of institutional and community outbreaks.

Cyclospora Species

Cyclospora cayetanensis is a coccidian with structure similar to that of *Cryptosporidium*. Unlike *Cryptosporidium*, *C. cayetanensis* requires a period of development outside the human body, thereby eliminating the possibility of close person-to-person contact as a means of acquiring the infection. *C. cayetanensis* is distributed worldwide, most commonly in the tropics and subtropics where infection tends to exhibit seasonality. It has also been associated with food (e.g., raspberries) and waterborne outbreaks in temperate regions, including the United States, and in recent years it has become increasingly recognized as a cause of infectious diarrhea in returned travelers.

All persons are susceptible to infection, but those with HIV are at risk for more severe and prolonged disease, as seen with cryptosporidiosis and isosporiasis. Symptomatic disease appears to be most common in adults who do not have previous exposure to *Cyclospora*, such as travelers or persons who have relocated to endemic areas. Illness begins about a week after ingestion of sporulated oocysts and is characterized by watery diarrhea, abdominal cramping, bloating, anorexia, and weight loss. Low-grade fever can occur; marked fatigue is common and can last weeks or even months, and untreated infections can relapse after apparent resolution. Biliary involvement can occur in patients with HIV coinfection, as with cryptosporidiosis. Cyclosporiasis, similar to infection with other coccidians, causes damage to the small bowel epithelium, with resultant crypt flattening, edema, and inflammatory infiltrate. Lactose deficiency can remain for months following initial infection.

Diagnosis is made by stool examination. As with diagnosis of other parasitic infections, multiple stool specimens improve sensitivity. In the case of *Cyclospora*, concentration of the stool specimen also increases yield. If cyclosporiasis is suspected, specific testing should be requested, because the organism exhibits unique properties. Organisms are about two times the size of *Cryptosporidium* and can be seen with Kinyoun acid-fast stain. They also autofluoresce and can be visualized under ultraviolet microscopy. Currently there is no stool antigen assay, but PCR testing has been used in experimental and limited clinical settings to assist in diagnosis.

Cyclosporiasis is best treated with trimethoprim-sulfamethoxazole (Bactrim)[1]; ciprofloxacin[1] may be effective for patients who have a sulfa allergy. Patients with HIV infection can require longer courses of treatment or chronic suppressive therapy; appropriate antiretroviral therapy is also important in the treatment of severe or relapsing infections. See Table 1 for details.

Cystoisospora Species

Cystoisospora belli, formerly *Isospora belli*, is a large coccidian native to tropical areas. Similar to *Cyclospora*, it requires a period of maturation outside the human body and therefore cannot be spread directly from person to person. It appears to cause largely asymptomatic or mild infection in tropical areas to which it is endemic; the exception is among patients coinfected with HIV and particularly those with AIDS, in which it is a very common cause of chronic diarrhea in the Caribbean and Central America. Currently in wealthy countries it is found primarily in travelers returning from endemic areas.

Illness is typically mild and self-limited, consisting primarily of watery diarrhea. However, some immunocompetent persons can develop a chronic spruelike syndrome with malabsorption, and those with HIV infection or AIDS often have severe and prolonged diarrhea. *Cystoisospora* can invade to the lamina propria and can cause eosinophilia, which is different from other coccidian infections.

Diagnosis is made by observation of cysts in stool. As with *Cyclospora*, they can be visualized with acid-fast stains or ultraviolet microscopy. Stool may also contain Charcot–Leiden crystals. Infection in immunocompetent hosts responds well to antimicrobials; persons coinfected with HIV can require longer courses of therapy or chronic suppression, and appropriate antiretroviral therapy may be helpful as well. Trimethoprim-sulfamethoxazole (Bactrim)[1] is the treatment of choice. Ciprofloxacin (Cipro)[1] or pyrimethamine (Daraprim)[1] may be used in cases of sulfa allergy. Doses are listed Table 1.

Microsporidiosis

Microsporidia are eukaryotic organisms that have been recently reclassified as fungi based on molecular genotyping. They are distributed globally, and more than 100 genera have been identified, seven of which contain species known to be pathogenic in humans: *Encephalitozoon*, *Enterocytozoon*, *Trachipleistophora*, *Pleistophora*, *Nosema*, *Vittaforma*, and *Microsporidium*. These pathogens cause a wide variety of systemic and focal illness throughout the world.

Many immunocompetent patients in wealthy nations exhibit positive serology for certain types of microsporidial infections without a history of disease or travel. Microsporidia are most commonly associated with systemic infection in immunosuppressed persons, particularly those with HIV and a CD4 count of less than 100 or patients with organ transplants. Mode of transmission is not entirely clear, but the pathogen likely is spread both from water sources and possibly from close household contact.

Encephalitozoon intestinalis and *Enterocytozoon bieneusi* are responsible for intestinal microsporidial infections. *E. bieneusi* has been associated with self-limited diarrheal illness, *E. intestinalis* is commonly found in stool specimens throughout the developing world, but its pathogenicity is often not certain. Symptomatic infections, most often in patients coinfected with HIV, typically include a gradual onset of watery diarrhea, which may be worse in the morning and after oral intake. Significant volume and electrolyte depletion can occur, as well as fatigue, anorexia, weight loss, and malabsorption. *E. intestinalis* can disseminate and cause acute abdomen with peritonitis, cholangitis, nephritis, and keratoconjunctivitis, and *E. bieneusi* infection can result in cholangitis and nephritis as well as rhinitis, bronchitis, and wheezing. Other microsporidia are implicated in a wide variety of illness both in previously healthy and immunosuppressed hosts and include several ocular pathogens.

Diagnosis of microsporidiosis is attained by visualization of spores in stool or in tissue specimens. As suggested by their name, microsporidial spores are much smaller than those produced by spore-forming protozoal infections; most are approximately 1 µm in length and can easily be confused with bacteria or debris on slides. Special staining techniques have been described, but

Intestinal Parasites

---

[1]Not FDA approved for this indication.

[1]Not FDA approved for this indication.

electron microscopy is required for species identification. See Table 1 for details of treatment. Albendazole (Albenza)[1] is the treatment of choice for *Encephalitozoon intestinalis*.

Treatment of *Enterocytozoon bieneusi* is more challenging. Although some response to albendazole has been reported, oral fumagillin[2] may have more efficacy. Unfortunately, it is not currently commercially available in the United States. Use of appropriate antiretroviral therapy is perhaps the most important treatment for patients with HIV infection or AIDS and chronic microsporidial infections.

Helminths
Nematodes

Nematodes (roundworms) are cylindrical nonsegmented organisms that are found throughout the world both as free-living species and as human and animal pathogens. Nematodes are the most common type of human parasitic infestation, found in approximately one quarter of the world's population; often, susceptible hosts carry multiple different pathogenic nematodes. There are at least 60 species that have been shown to infect humans and 10 times that many that cause disease in other animals, but a few pathogens account for the bulk of human infections, in particular *Ascaris*, hookworm, and whipworm. These three organisms all require a period of maturation outside the human body—typically in warm, moist soil—underscoring the fact that repeated contact with fecally contaminated soil or food and water is necessary to sustain the cycle of infestation. *Strongyloides* and *Enterobius* are unique in that they can both complete their life cycle on or within human hosts and therefore can cause chronic infection and be transmitted directly by close person-to-person contact where there is the possibility of fecal–oral contamination.

Ascaris

Ascaris lumbricoides, the most common human helminthic infection, is estimated to affect 20% to 25% of the world's population. Up to 80% of community members are infected in heavily endemic areas, namely in Africa, Asia, and Central and South America. Cases of *Ascaris* infestation are also seen in rural areas in the southeastern United States. *A. lumbricoides* are white to pinkish worms that range from 10 to 40 cm in length; the infectious eggs are oval white bodies with an adherent mucopolysaccharide capsule that clings to multiple surfaces and aids in transmissibility of the parasite. Eggs are also remarkably durable, capable of surviving up to 6 years in moist soil and able to weather brief droughts and periods of freezing.

Fecal contamination of water, food, and environmental surfaces such as doorknobs and countertops provide the means of transmission for *Ascaris*, and recurrent infection occurs as long as living conditions that predispose people to infection remain unchanged. Lack of adequate public sanitation, use of human feces as fertilizer (night soil), and frequent contact with soil or shared contaminated surfaces among close household members are risk factors for infection. Persons who move to environments with improved sanitation typically lose their infection within 2 years as all the adult worms die. Eggs excreted by an infected person must mature outside the human body for approximately 2 weeks. On ingestion by a susceptible host, mature eggs hatch in the small intestine and release larvae, which penetrate the intestinal wall and travel through the venous circulation to the lungs, where they are coughed up and swallowed. They then undergo maturation into adult worms in the intestine and produce eggs by 2 to 3 months after initial infection. The eggs are excreted in the feces and mature outside the body to continue the cycle.

Most persons with *Ascaris* infection are asymptomatic. Approximately 15% of infected people have morbidity, which is associated with young age, large burden of worms, coinfection with other intestinal parasites, and genetic predisposition. In children, infection contributes to malabsorption of protein, fat, and vitamins A and C, and treatment of heavily infected children can improve their nutritional status. *Ascaris* infection can also cause intestinal, pancreatic, or biliary obstruction as a result of worm mass or worm migration. Despite the low incidence of obstructive complications per infected person, the *Ascaris*-related acute abdomen is a significant problem on a global level given the enormous number of people infected. Some patients with intestinal *Ascaris* infection report vague abdominal complaints, such as abdominal discomfort, nausea, vomiting or diarrhea, but these are relatively rare. Pulmonary migration of a large quantity of worms can produce Loeffler's syndrome, or eosinophilic pneumonitis.

Diagnosis is easily attained with standard saline stool preparation, and large numbers of eggs are typically seen. Larvae or worms can also sometimes be seen in sputum or stool samples. In cases of intestinal obstruction, worms may be visualized on upper gastrointestinal series, computed tomography, and even ultrasound. Eosinophilia with *Ascaris* infection is found only during the larval migratory phase, but not at all times. Chronic eosinophilia in an at-risk person suggests another parasitic infection, often *Strongyloides*.

All persons documented to carry *Ascaris* who have migrated to nonendemic areas should be treated to prevent complications in the future; in endemic areas, adults need only be treated if they are symptomatic. Children have been shown to benefit from intermittent anthelminthic therapy in heavily affected areas of the world.

For patients with intestinal obstruction, bowel rest and intravenous hydration are usually sufficient to relieve the obstruction, at which time anthelminthic therapy can be administered. In such cases, gastroenterology consultation should be obtained. In rare cases, surgical intervention is required. Treatment of pulmonary infection is controversial; however, most experts recommend steroid therapy for severe infections followed 2 to 3 weeks later (at the time full-grown worms will have migrated to the intestine) by administration of anthelminthic therapy.

The benzimidazoles (mebendazole [Vermox], albendazole [Albenza],[1] levamisole [Stromectol], and pyrantel pamoate [Pin-X]) all exhibit excellent activity against *Ascaris*. Doses and other options are listed in Table 2. Although albendazole and mebendazole carry a pregnancy class B label, they have been used in pregnant women, adolescent girls, and women of reproductive age without demonstrable effects on fetuses; most experts recommend holding treatment until the second trimester whenever possible.

Sanitary conditions that allow for proper management of human feces are crucial in control and prevention of *Ascaris* infection; boiling water kills the eggs.

Whipworm (Trichurasis)

Trichuris trichiura has become recognized in recent years as a worldwide pathogen with a scope similar to that of *Ascaris*. Sanitary conditions that predispose to ingestion of food and water contaminated with human feces place people at risk for infection; in many communities infection is hyperendemic, with almost universal carriage of the pathogen.

The adult organism is a small worm about 4 cm in length with a unique whip-like structure that allows its thin tail to become embedded in colonic crypts. Whipworm eggs have a characteristic barrel shape with mucous plugs at either end. Infection is acquired by ingesting *Trichuris* eggs that have undergone embryonation in the soil for 2 to 4 weeks after excretion from a previous host. Larvae emerge from eggs in the intestine and migrate into crypts, where they begin to mature. Egg production begins approximately 3 months later.

Most persons with whipworm carry few worms (approximately 20) and are asymptomatic. As with many other intestinal parasites, children are at greater risk for symptomatic infection, which can cause failure to thrive, anemia, clubbing, inflammatory colitis,

---

[1]Not FDA approved for this indication.
[2]Not available in the United States.

---

[1]Not FDA approved for this indication.

TABLE 2 Pharmacologic Treatment of Nematode, Trematode, and Cestode Infections

CLINICAL SITUATION	DRUG	ADULT DOSE	PEDIATRIC DOSE	COMMENTS
Anisakiasis				
Anisaka spp. or *Pseudoterranova decipiens*	No recommended medical therapy Surgical or endoscopic removal of worm	—	—	Successful treatment of a patient with *Anisakiasis* with albendazole has been reported.
Ascariasis				
Ascaris lumbricoides	Albendazole (Albenza)[1],* or	400 mg once	400 mg PO once	
	Mebendazole[†] (Vermox) or	100 mg bid × 3 d or 500 mg once	100 mg bid × 3 d or 500 mg once	
	Ivermectin[1],[†] (Stromectol)	150–200 µg/kg once	150–200 µg/kg once	In heavy infection, therapy may be given for 3 d.
Enterobiasis (Pinworm)				
Enterobius vermicularis	Mebendazole[†] or	100 mg once, repeat in 2 wk	100 mg once, repeat in 2 wk	Because all family members are usually infected, treatment of the entire household is recommended.
	Albendazole[1],* or	400 mg once, repeat in 2 wk	400 mg once, repeat in 2 wk	
	Pyrantel pamoate[‡]	11 mg/kg base (max 1 g) once; repeat in 2 wk	11 mg/kg base (max 1 g) once; repeat in 2 wk	
Hookworm				
Ancylostoma duodenale, Necator americanus	Albendazole[1],* or Mebendazole or	400 mg once 100 mg bid × 3 d or 500 mg once	400 mg once 100 mg bid × 3 d or 500 mg once	
	Pyrantel pamoate[‡]	11 mg/kg (max 1 g) × 3 d	11 mg/kg (max 1 g) × 3 d	
Schistosomiasis				
Schistosoma haematobium, Schistosoma mansoni	Praziquantel[§] or	40 mg/kg/d in 2 doses × 1 d	40 mg/kg/d in 2 doses × 1 d	
S. mansoni only	Oxamniquine[‖]	15 mg/kg once	20 mg/kg/d in 2 doses × 1 d	Praziquantel is first line, but oxamniquine may be effective in some patients in whom praziquantel is less effective. Contraindicated in pregnancy
Schistosoma japonicum, Schistosoma mekongi	Praziquantel[§]	60 mg/kg/d in 2 or 3 doses × 1 d	60 mg/kg/d in 3 doses × 1 d	
Strongyloidiasis				
Strongyloides stercoralis	Recommended: Ivermectin[†]	200 µg/kg/d × 2 d	200 µg/kg/d × 2 d	In immunocompromised patients or in patients with disseminated disease, it may be necessary to prolong or repeat therapy or use other agents. Veterinary parenteral and enema formulations of ivermectin are used in severely ill patients unable to take oral medications.
	Alternative: Albendazole[1],*	400 mg bid × 7 d	400 mg bid × 7 d	
Tapeworm				
Taenia solium (intestinal disease), *Taenia saginata, Diphyllobothrium latum*	Praziquantel[1] or Niclosamide[¶]	— 2 g once	— 50 mg/kg once	Available in the United States only from the manufacturer
Trichurasis (Whipworm)				
Trichuris trichiura	Recommended: Mebendazole	100 mg bid × 3 d or 500 mg once	100 mg bid × 3 d or 500 mg once	
	Alternatives: Albendazole[1],* or	400 mg daily × 3 d	400 mg daily × 3 d	
	Ivermectin[†]	200 µg/kg daily × 3 d	200 µg/kg daily × 3 d	

Adapted from World Health Organization. Drugs for parasitic infections. Med Lett Drug Ther 2010: 8 (Suppl.).
[1]Not FDA approved for this indication.
*Should be taken with a fatty meal.
[†]Safety of Ivermectin in young children (<15 kg) and pregnant women not yet established. Ivermectin should be taken on an empty stomach with water.
[‡]Limited availability; can be mixed with juice or water to improve palatability.
[§]Should be taken with liquids during a meal.
[‖]Limited or no availability in the United States.
[¶]Available in the U.S. only from the manufacturer. Must be chewed or crushed thoroughly and swallowed with a small amount of water. Limited or no availability in the United States.

and rectal prolapse. Adults with a high worm burden can also experience inflammatory colitis characterized by frequent—often bloody—diarrhea and tenesmus. Infection has been shown to result in production of tumor necrosis factor (TNF)-α by lamina propria cells in the colon, which can contribute to poor appetite and wasting that can be seen with significant infection.

Diagnosis is made by standard stool microscopy without a need to concentrate stool, because large numbers of eggs are excreted. Worms can also be seen on colonoscopy, or they can be visualized grossly in cases of rectal prolapse. Eosinophilia may be seen.

Treatment of symptomatic infections can be accomplished with mebendazole, albendazole,[1] or ivermectin (Stromectal)[1]; see Table 2 for details.

Hookworm (Necator americanus and Ancylostoma duodenale)

Like other helminthic infections, hookworm affects a substantial portion of the world's population, particularly in rural subtropical and tropical communities where human feces is used as a component of fertilizer. Infection results primarily from parasite penetration into the skin; therefore persons with an agrarian lifestyle and significant soil contact are at greatest risk.

Two species are responsible for the majority of human hookworm: *Necator americanus* and *Ancylostoma duodenale*. *Ancylostoma braziliense*, a canine intestinal pathogen, causes cutaneous larval migrans in humans because the pathogen cannot penetrate the human dermis. Of the two common forms of human hookworm, *N. americanus* is smaller and a less aggressive pathogen with a longer life span than *A. duodenale*. Both parasites are found in warm climates throughout the world; *A. duodenale* exists in smaller pockets, whereas *N. americanus* is widely distributed throughout impoverished rural areas of the tropics in the Americas, Asia, and Africa.

Hookworms are small helminths, between 0.5 and 1 cm in length. Infection results from larval penetration of the skin on contact with contaminated soil. An intensely pruritic, erythematous, papulovesicular rash called *ground itch* can develop at the site of entry. Parasites then enter the venous or lymphatic circulation and travel to the lungs, at which point an urticarial rash with cough can develop. The larvae are swallowed and migrate to the small intestine, where they attach to the bowel wall with teeth or biting plates and take a continuous blood meal by sucking with strong esophageal muscles. As the hookworms lodge in the small intestine, peripheral eosinophilia peaks, and gastrointestinal discomfort with or without diarrhea can result. Large oral ingestion of *A. duodenale* can cause Wakana syndrome, characterized by cough, shortness of breath, nausea, vomiting, and eosinophilia. The most important clinical manifestation of hookworm infection is iron-deficiency anemia, which can be mild or severe and may be accompanied by malabsorption of protein in hosts with heavy burden of disease. Infants and pregnant women can become extremely ill or even die as a result of the anemia.

Hookworm may be difficult to diagnose because light infections often do not produce enough eggs to be readily seen on stool examination; stool should therefore be concentrated if infection is suspected. Eggs do not appear in stool until approximately 2 months after infection, so patients with pulmonary complaints will not yet have a positive stool examination.

Hookworm infection can be eradicated with benzimidazole antihelminthics; see Table 2 for details. Prevention of hookworm infection, as with other parasites, lies in improved sanitary conditions; wearing shoes is especially important because the majority of infections are acquired through the skin. Mass anthelminthic treatment campaigns have shown some efficacy in reducing disease in children; however, reinfection and concern for development of resistance continue to present significant challenges. Candidate vaccines are currently under investigation.

Strongyloides

Strongyloides stercoralis is a global pathogen that is estimated to affect as many as 100 million people, mostly in tropical regions of the world. In recent years, it has become more commonly recognized in the United States among immigrants as a cause of chronic eosinophilia as well as symptomatic infection.

Strongyloides infection results when filariform larvae dwelling in fecally contaminated soil penetrate the skin or mucous membranes of a susceptible host. Larvae move to the lungs and subsequently to the trachea, where they are coughed up and swallowed. Females, about 2 cm in length, lodge in the lamina propria of the duodenum and proximal jejunum where they begin to oviposit. Rhabditiform larvae emerge from these eggs and either repenetrate the intestinal wall or are passed into the feces, at which point they can begin a free-living cycle and reproduce sexually, or can molt directly into an infectious form ready to enter a subsequent susceptible host.

Persons infected with *Strongyloides* are typically asymptomatic. Those who have symptoms might report abdominal discomfort, diarrhea alternating with constipation, or, rarely, blood-tinged stool. Severe intestinal infections can occur and are manifest by chronic watery or mucousy diarrhea. In such cases, colonoscopy reveals excessive bowel wall thickening and copious secretions, or edema (catarrhal enteritis or edematous enteritis). Parasite migration through the dermis can manifest as serpiginous, erythematous, and pruritic patches along the buttocks, perineum, and thighs, known as *larvae currens*.

Strongyloides appear to attain a balanced state in their host, with similar numbers of adult worms throughout the many years of infection. During periods of host immunocompromise, in particular in patients taking corticosteroids, *Strongyloides* can enter into a state of rapid autoinfection and rampant reproduction called *hyperinfection syndrome*, which results in devastating illness. Persons with HIV infection do not seem to be at particular risk for symptomatic disease or hyperinfection, but hyperinfection has been linked to HTLV-1 infection. *Strongyloides* has also caused hyperinfection in organ transplant patients whose donor had been infected asymptomatically with the parasite. Although it has long been thought that steroid-induced immune compromise was the major trigger for hyperinfection, growing evidence suggests that steroids themselves may be the culprit by directly inducing the accelerated life cycle in the parasite.

The hyperinfection syndrome is characterized by systemic illness with fever, cough, hypoxia, patchy or diffuse pulmonary infiltrates with alveolar microhemorrhages, and dermatitis; it can include myocarditis, hepatitis, splenic abscess, meningitis and cerebral abscess, and endocrine organ involvement. Larvae migrating out of the intestines can drag bacteria with them, resulting in gram-negative or polymicrobial sepsis. The prognosis of *Strongyloides* hyperinfection syndrome is grave even with highly effective anthelminthic treatment given the diffuse nature of this disease. However, earlier recognition and intensive supportive care result in cure.

Diagnosis of uncomplicated *Strongyloides* infection in endemic areas can be challenging because few larvae are passed in stool, and numerous examinations may be necessary to detect them. ELISA is available and is highly sensitive, but it does not distinguish between active and past infections. It is, however, the test of choice for persons who have migrated to nonendemic areas, and all persons in this setting should be treated. Ivermectin is the treatment of choice; see Table 2 for dosing. During the first days of treatment, patients can experience intense dermal pruritis as parasites die. Eosinophilia and positive ELISA can persist for months even after effective therapy.

Enterobius vermicularis

Human pinworm infection, caused by the thread-like nematode *Enterobius vermicularis*, is found throughout the world and continues to be diagnosed commonly in the United States, especially in children. Its persistence is likely related to the fact that pinworm does not require a period of maturation outside the human body,

---

[1]Not FDA approved for this indication.

and autoinfection or transmission by very close contact sustains the parasite within communities. *E. vermicularis* is at maximum 1 cm long with a tapered tail, and dwells in the cecum, appendix, and adjacent colon. At night, female worms travel to the anus and lay small (25–50 μm), double-walled oval eggs in the perianal skin. Within 6 hours, the eggs embryonate within their capsule and are infectious. In scratching the perianal area and subsequently bringing his or her hand to the mouth, the host ingests the embryos, which then hatch in the bowel about 2 months later and continue the cycle of infection. Embryonated eggs can also attach to bedclothes, thereby placing other household members with close contact at risk for infection. In family groups, infection is associated with close living quarters, poor hand washing, and infrequent washing of clothes and sheets. It can also be prevalent in among institutionalized persons.

Infection is often asymptomatic, but it can cause perianal itching, which helps to facilitate persistent infection by encouraging frequent touching of the perianal area. Rarely, worms migrate into ectopic foci and produce painful genitourinary tract disease with granulomatous inflammation; pinworm infection rarely results in pain that mimics acute appendicitis.

Pinworm infestation is best diagnosed by the classic Scotch tape test, which involves placing and immediately removing a piece of sticky tape firmly across the perianal area early in the morning when the eggs have been deposited. The tape can then be brought into a physician's office or laboratory, where it is placed sticky-side down for microscopic examination to detect the eggs. Three specimens should be examined if necessary to improve the sensitivity. It is also sometimes possible to see the worms directly on the perianal region, although they are so small that they may easily be mistaken for residual bits of toilet paper. *E. vermicularis* is susceptible to standard anthelminthic therapies as listed in Table 2. All household contacts should be empirically treated with the same regimen to avoid reintroducing infection from family members who may be asymptomatically carrying the parasite. Careful laundering of all bedclothes is recommended as well.

Anisakiasis

Anisakiasis is a descriptive term for human infection with parasites of two distinct genera: *Anisakis* and *Pseudoterranova*. Humans are incidental hosts for these roundworms that inhabit multiple species of fish and other marine animals (tuna, mackerel, hake, cod, sardines, and cephalopods) as intermediate hosts, and marine mammals such as whales, seals, sea lions, and walruses as final hosts. Humans acquire the parasite in its larval stage by eating raw fish (e.g., sushi, ceviche), and therefore the condition predominates in cultures where uncooked fish is consumed. Cases are most commonly reported from Japan but are seen throughout the world in other coastal nations and among restaurateurs.

On consumption of fish with anisakid larvae embedded in its musculature, humans can experience immediate symptoms in the form of itching or burning in the throat, which can provoke coughing that expels the parasite. If the parasite is swallowed, the larva attempts to embed in the gastric musculature at the pylorus. This can produce acute, short-lived epigastric abdominal pain and possibly immediate vomiting, at which point the parasite might again be ejected. If the larva does manage to penetrate gastric tissue, it dies because it is incapable of further tissue invasion in humans. An intense inflammatory response to the dead pathogen can then result, with gastric pain, nausea, and occasionally diarrhea with blood or mucus if a gastric ulcerative lesion has resulted.

Rare cases have been reported in which the larva penetrates the peritoneum, causing focal peritonitis and abscess formation. *Pseudoterranova* appears to cause milder symptoms and less tissue invasion, and the worm might simply be vomited several days after initial ingestion and presented to a physician, often by an alarmed patient. Because the vast majority of infections are caused by a single organism, vomiting of the parasite results in a definitive cure and patients can be reassured. Diagnosis in patients with ongoing symptoms related to an embedded parasite is ultimately endoscopic. Effective cure results on endoscopic or surgical removal of the worm.

Trematodes

Schistosomiasis

Schistosomes are freshwater pathogens with areas of endemicity in Africa, South America, Southeast Asia, and parts of the Middle East. These small trematodes cause varied, often chronic infections that can carry significant morbidity, although some species cannot invade beyond the dermis in humans and result strictly in cercarial dermatitis or swimmer's itch. There are five species of schistosomes known to cause disease in humans: *Schistosoma haematobium*, found through much of Africa and parts of the Middle East; *Schistosoma mansoni*, also native to Africa and the Middle East as well as Latin America; *Schistosoma japonicum*, present in China, Southeast Asia, and the Philippines; *Schistosoma mekongi*, found only in the Mekong River basin in Southeast Asia; and *Schistosoma intercalatum*, endemic only in West Africa.

All persons who come in contact with schistosomes are at risk for infection, even after only very brief exposure to fecally contaminated freshwater in which the intermediate hosts of the pathogen (snails) reside. Frequency and degree of infection tend to be highest in children in endemic areas and then level off in the early teenage years, likely secondary to level of environmental exposure and possibly to host immunity. *S. haematobium* causes disease in the genitourinary system; the others cause intestinal, hepatic, and sometimes pulmonary diseases.

Infection is acquired rapidly on contact with freshwater (including brief swims or by repeated splashing, as can occur during river rafting), when free-living fork-tailed schistosomal larvae penetrate human skin and lose their tail. These schistomorula can cause intense itching and a papulovesicular, pruritic rash at the site of penetration, swimmer's itch. Invasive schistomorula then enter the venous bloodstream and ultimately lodge in gut mesenteric and portal venules, where maturation occurs, and male and female forms join and mate for life. Females begin to oviposit, and the resultant inflammatory response to the eggs can cause either acute illness or chronic fibrosis and granulomatous inflammation of the tissues in which they reside.

Acute illness, called *Katayama fever*, is more common among hosts who have not been previously exposed to the organism and can be quite severe, even fatal. Katayama fever begins 4 to 8 weeks after exposure to the schistosomes, with fever, cough, abdominal pain, hepatomegaly, and lymphadenopathy. Eggs might not yet be present in the stool at the time of diagnosis. Chronic schistosomiasis is a slowly progressive illness. *S. haematobium* infection is manifest by gross or microscopic hematuria, urinary symptoms, and chronic bacterial urinary tract infections; ultimately ureteral fibrosis, hydronephrosis, and granulomatous genital lesions also can ensue. In infection with other invasive schistosomes, chronic illness can manifest as abdominal pain and diarrhea, which is often bloody, with associated iron-deficiency anemia. Hepatomegaly is often the first clinical finding in chronic intestinal schistosomiasis. Over many years, hepatic congestion and fibrosis can result in liver failure, and the pulmonary vasculature can be involved as well, which causes pulmonary hypertension and cor pulmonale.

Diagnosis of schistosomiasis is by observation of eggs in stool (intestinal disease), urine (urinary tract disease), or biopsy specimens, or by serum antibody testing. Concentration of stool may be necessary to detect the pathogen. The eggs of the three most common species of schistosomes can be readily identified microscopically: *S. haematobium* has an inferior spine, *S. mansoni* an inferolateral spine, and *S. japonicum* lacks a spine. Eosinophilia is a hallmark of chronic infection and is a common cause of asymptomatic eosinophilia among immigrants from schistoendemic regions of the world. Serology is highly sensitive and specific but cannot distinguish acute, chronic, or cleared infection; it is very useful when attempting to diagnose infection in returned travelers.

All patients with schistosomiasis should be treated, and those with chronic manifestations might experience significant regression of even late-stage organ-specific disease. Treatment of choice is with praziquantel; see Table 2 for details.

Prevention of schistosomiasis involves improving access to treated water and exploration of avenues to eliminate the intermediate snail hosts. Host immunity does appear to occur, and efforts are under way to better understand and induce such immunity in the form of a vaccine.

Cestodes

Taeniasis

Human tapeworm infection has long been implicated in North American oral folklore as a cause of insatiable appetite and excessive weight loss. In reality, despite their impressive size of up to 12 meters, tapeworm infection tends to be minimally symptomatic.

Taenia solium, pork tapeworm, and *Taenia saginata*, beef tapeworm, are the two most common flatworm infections of humans worldwide and occur in any setting in which raw or undercooked meat is served and cattle and pigs have access to feed contaminated with human feces. *T. saginata* is still found in areas of North America and Europe, as well as in Central and South America and Africa; *T. solium* is common throughout Mexico, Central and South America, Africa, China, and the Indian subcontinent. Although humans are the definitive hosts for both parasites, *T. solium* is best known for its pathogenicity in the form of cysticercosis. Cysticercosis is not an intestinal parasitic infection.

Domesticated animals acquire infection on ingestion of eggs excreted by humans; the eggs mature in their musculature and develop a scolex. When humans consume infected meat, the scolex attaches in the small intestine, and the adult tapeworm develops over approximately 2 months. Adult tapeworms are made up of hundreds to thousands of gravid proglottids and can live for up to 25 years. Symptoms tend to be mild or absent but can include nausea, abdominal pain, loose stools, anal pruritus, and occasionally weakness or increased appetite, especially in children. Serious illness rarely results when a tapeworm becomes lodged in the biliary or pancreatic ducts or is coughed up and aspirated. Some patients come to medical attention when the worm is noted emerging from the anus or on extrusion of proglottids in the stool.

Diagnosis of taeniasis can be made on visualizing the round eggs in stool; however, the species cannot be determined unless a segment of the worm is examined. Serum antibody and antigen tests, as well as stool PCR, have been developed for diagnosis but are not widely used in clinical practice. Eosinophilia and elevated IgE levels may be present. Single-dose praziquantel[1] (see Table 2) is curative in almost all cases, but infectious eggs can still be released in the feces for a time; ingestion of these could result in the subsequent development if cysticercosis, so patients should be counseled to avoid fecal–oral contact.

Proper cooking of meat is the mainstay of prevention; disposal of human waste away from animals would also be effective in interrupting the life cycle.

Diphyllobothriasis

Diphyllobothrium latum is the longest parasite known to infect humans (10–12 m). It is found in freshwater lakes in areas of the Americas, Northern Europe, Africa, China, and Japan and has a complex life cycle involving two intermediate hosts: crustaceans and small fish. Humans and other fish-eating mammals are the definitive hosts and acquire the infection on ingestion of raw fish or roe.

The organism attaches within the small intestine, and hosts are usually asymptomatic. Infected persons might complain of increased appetite, nausea, or abdominal discomfort. Many present after passage of portions of the tapeworm in stool, as with taeniasis; in others, diagnosis is on stool examination done for other purposes or during screening colonoscopy. As with other worms, the parasite occasionally migrates into biliary ducts or causes intestinal obstruction. Attachment of the parasite higher in the intestine can result in decreased levels of vitamin B_{12}. Rarely, pernicious anemia develops as a result (tapeworm anemia).

Diagnosis is made either by seeing eggs in unconcentrated stool or by encountering the adult worm. Eosinophilia is present in a

---

[1]Not FDA approved for this indication.

minority of cases. Treatment with praziquantel[1] is curative; see Table 2. Vitamin B_{12} supplementation is necessary in cases of severe or symptomatic deficiency, but it will not recur once the tapeworm is eliminated. Prevention involves not ingesting undercooked fish.

---

[1]Not FDA approved for this indication.

References

Abubakar I, Aliyu SH, Hunter PR, Usman NK. Prevention and treatment of cryptosporidiosis in immunocompromised patients. Cochrane Database Syst Rev 2007; (1): CD004932.

Bethony J, Brooker S, Albonico M, et al. Soil-transmitted helminth infections: Ascariasis, trichiurasis, and hookworm. Lancet 2006;367(9521):1521–32.

Boggild A, Yohanna S, Keystone J, Kain K. Prospective analysis of parasitic infections in Canadian travelers and immigrants. J Travel Med 2006;13:138–44.

Boulware DR, Stauffer WM, Hendel-Paterson RR, et al. Maltreatment of Strongyloides infection: Case series and worldwide physicians-in-training survey. Am J Med 2007;120:545.e1–545.e8.

Concha R, Hartington Jr W, Rogers AI. Intestinal strongyloidiasis: Recognition, management, and determinants of outcome. J Clin Gastroenterol 2005;39(3):203–11.

Drugs for Parasitic Infections. Treatment Guidelines from the Medical Letter, 2013. (11) p. e1–e31.

Goodgame RW. Understanding intestinal spore-forming protozoa: Cryptosporidia, microsporidia, isospora, and cyclospora. Ann Intern Med 1996;124(4):429–41.

Guerrant R, Walker D, Weller P, editors. Tropical Infectious Diseases: Principles, Pathogens, and Practice. Philadelphia: Churchill Livingstone; 1999.

Huang DB, White AC. An updated review on Cryptosporidium and Giardia. Gastroenterol Clin North Am 2006;35:291–314.

Mandell G, Bennett J, Dolin R, editors. Mandell, Douglas and Bennett's Principles and Practice of Infectious Diseases. 5th ed. Philadelphia: Churchill Livingstone; 2005.

Pardo J, Carranza C, Muro A, et al. Helminth-related eosinophilia in African immigrants, Gran Canaria. Emerg Infect Dis 2006;12(10):1587–9.

Stark D, Beebe N, Marriott D, et al. Dientamoebiasis: Clinical importance and recent advances. Trends Parasitol 2006;22(2):92–6.

IRRITABLE BOWEL SYNDROME

Method of
Brenda R. Velasco, MD; Robert S. Fisher, MD; and Nicholas Wilson, MD

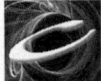

CURRENT DIAGNOSIS

- Detailed history and physical examination to elicit red flags and exclude secondary causes
- Appropriate laboratory and imaging studies based on symptoms
- Identification of the subcategory of irritable bowel syndrome that best describes the patient's symptoms

CURRENT THERAPY

- Establishment of a strong physician-patient relationship
- Dietary and behavioral modifications
- Pharmacotherapy based on the subcategory of irritable bowel syndrome

Epidemiology

Irritable bowel syndrome (IBS) is one of the most common functional gastrointestinal disorders, with a worldwide prevalence estimated to be between 10% and 20%. It is a syndrome characterized by chronic abdominal pain or discomfort and irregular bowel habits that has a significant impact on affected individuals and society. The diagnosis of IBS is based on the absence of detectable structural or biochemical causes and the presence of a constellation of symptoms as outlined by the so-called Rome III criteria (Box 1).

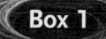

Box 1 — Rome III Criteria for the Diagnosis of Irritable Bowel Syndrome

Recurrent abdominal pain or discomfort (with onset at least 6 months before diagnosis) that

- Occurred on at least 3 days per month in the last 3 months, and
- Is associated with two or more of the following:
  - Improvement with defecation
  - Onset associated with a change in frequency of stool
  - Onset associated with a change in form (appearance) of stool

Adapted from Longstreth GF, Thompson WG, Chey WD, et al: Functional bowel disorders. In Drossman DA, Corazziari E, Delvaux M, et al. (eds): Rome III: The functional gastrointestinal disorders, 3rd ed. McLean, VA, Degnon, 2006, p 487–555.

Box 2 — Subgroups of Irritable Bowel Syndrome (IBS)

- IBS with diarrhea (more common in men)
- IBS with constipation (more common in women)
- IBS with mixed bowel habits (previously known as IBS with alternating bowel habits based on Rome II criteria)
- IBS unsubtyped (not enough stools are abnormal to meet criteria for any other subtype)

Adapted from Longstreth GF, Thompson WG, Chey WD, et al: Functional bowel disorders. In Drossman DA, Corazziari E, Delvaux M, et al. (eds): Rome III: The functional gastrointestinal disorders, 3rd ed. McLean, VA, Degnon, 2006, p 487–555.

Bloating or visible abdominal distention often is present in patients with IBS but is not considered essential for diagnosis. The Rome III diagnostic criteria divide IBS into subgroups based on stool form and not frequency. Each of the top three IBS subgroups constitutes approximately one third of all IBS patients (Box 2).

Gender differences have been documented in terms of both prominent symptoms and response to treatment. In the community, the ratio of women to men with IBS is estimated to be between 2:1 and 4:1; this difference is greater in the population of IBS patients who seek health care. Women with IBS report greater overall IBS symptom severity, greater intensity of abdominal pain and bloating, greater impact of symptoms on daily life, and lower health-related quality of life, compared to men with IBS. The estimated prevalence of IBS in children is similar to that in adults, and newly diagnosed adults frequently report symptoms of IBS (or other related functional gastrointestinal symptoms) dating back to childhood. The most common age group seen by physicians for treatment of IBS is 20- to 50-year-olds. Patients with a diagnosis of IBS are at increased risk for other, nongastrointestinal functional disorders, such as fibromyalgia, chronic pelvic pain, interstitial cystitis, and migraine headaches.

IBS is associated with substantial economic costs, including the direct costs of excess physician visits, diagnostic testing, medications, hospitalizations, and surgeries and indirect costs from absenteeism and decreased productivity at work (presenteeism). Patients with IBS have been reported to miss three times as many days of work compared to those without bowel symptoms. In 2006, there were at least 2.4 to 3.5 million U.S. physician visits for IBS. The annual direct and indirect costs of IBS were recently estimated to be at least $1.6 billion and $19 billion, respectively.

Pathophysiology

The pathophysiology of IBS is multifactorial and complex (Box 3). Altered bowel motility, visceral hypersensitivity, central nervous system effects, an imbalance in neurotransmitters, and alterations in epithelial barrier function with increased mucosal immune

Box 3 — Pathophysiologic Factors of Irritable Bowel Syndrome

- Altered bowel motility
- Visceral hypersensitivity
- Altered epithelial permeability
- Intramucosal immune activation
- Central nervous system effects
- Neurotransmitter imbalance (i.e., serotonin)
- Infection
- Psychosocial factors
- Genetics

activation have all been considered. In addition, roles for infection, small-bowel bacterial overgrowth, abnormal colonic bacterial flora, genetics, and environmental and psychosocial factors have been proposed.

In about 10% of patients the onset of IBS-like symptoms can be attributed to a preceding episode of acute viral or bacterial gastroenteritis. Furthermore, a longer duration of the acute illness confers a higher risk of eventually developing IBS. Altered contractility of the colon and small bowel has been described in patients with IBS and may be related to ingestion of food and psychological or physical stress. For example, there have been reports of an exaggerated contractile response of the colon (gastrocolic reflex) and small intestine to a high-fat meal.

Patients with IBS also perceive pain abnormally related to irregular small bowel motor activity. There are studies using balloon distention of the rectosigmoid and the ileum that suggest patients with IBS perceive pain and bloating at balloon volumes and pressures significantly lower than those required by normal subjects to elicit similar symptoms. Functional magnetic resonance imaging and positron emission tomography of the brain have revealed different levels of activity in the thalamus and the anterior cingulate cortex after balloon distention of the rectum in patients with IBS compared to normal subjects. This phenomenon is referred to as visceral hypersensitivity.

Both altered motility and visceral hypersensitivity could be mediated by imbalances of neurotransmitters, including serotonin, which has a significant presence in the gastrointestinal tract and known associations with symptoms including nausea, vomiting, abdominal pain, and bloating. Increased concordance of IBS in monozygotic versus dizygotic twins and familial aggregation in IBS may support a genetic component to IBS. Additionally, there are reports that IBS is more frequent and more severe in women with a history of physical and/or sexual abuse.

Finally, a growing body of evidence describes compromised epithelial barrier function in patients with IBS. This alteration in permeability may be related to altered expression of tight junction proteins. Expression of the epithelial tight-junction protein E-cadherin was significantly lower in cecal samples from patients with mixed-type or diarrhea-predominant IBS compared to controls, and levels of E-cadherin expression were also associated with symptom duration and severity of abdominal pain. IBS patients also have increased numbers of immune cells in the gut mucosa including mast cells, T lymphocytes, and enteroendocrine cells. The inflammatory mediators released by these cells and their presence in the mucosa could relate to the impaired epithelial barrier function in IBS and abnormal enteric nervous system signaling that leads to gut hypersensitivity.[1]

Evaluation

Current clinical guidelines recommend that IBS can generally be diagnosed without additional testing beyond careful history taking, a general physical examination, and routine laboratory studies to exclude other organic causes in patients who have symptoms that meet the Rome criteria and who do not have alarm warning signs (red flags).

[1] Not FDA approved for this indication.

The red flags include, but are not limited to, blood in the stool (gross or occult), anemia, anorexia, weight loss, fever, family history of colon cancer, inflammatory bowel disease or celiac disease, onset of the first symptom after 50 years of age, nocturnal symptoms that awaken the patient from sleep, and a major change in symptoms. Routine laboratory tests have been suggested to include a complete blood count (CBC), thyroid function studies, stool studies for ova and parasites, and a comprehensive metabolic panel. In addition, it has recently been proposed that patients being evaluated for IBS-like symptoms who have a predominance of diarrhea be screened with serologic tests for celiac disease.

If the patient meets the Rome III criteria and does not have any red flags, classification of the IBS into one of the subcategories is recommended to guide and facilitate empiric therapy. If a red flag is present, diagnostic tests should be performed as appropriate based on the presenting symptoms, signs, and laboratory findings. The differential diagnosis for IBS-like symptoms is significant and should always be considered when evaluating patients (Box 4).

Treatment

Treatment of IBS involves a multilevel approach. One of the most important components is the establishment of a strong physician-patient relationship; this is done by being nonjudgmental and allowing for a patient-centered interview. Be sure to acknowledge the patient's symptoms, identify whether any of them are stress-related, and determine whether comorbid psychological symptoms exist. Addressing psychosocial factors may improve health status and treatment response. Another component of treatment involves dietary modification. Although some patients may identify certain foods that precipitate or exacerbate their symptoms, reduction or exclusion or specific foods has not shown significant benefit in the literature. However, there is increasing evidence to support a diet low in fermentable oligo-, di-, and monosaccharides, and polyols (FODMAPs), including a recent randomized controlled trial that showed a diet low in FODMAPs in patients with IBS effectively reduced functional gastrointestinal symptoms.[2] Pharmacotherapy is guided by the predominant symptom; placement of each patient into an IBS subcategory is useful (Table 1). In addition, alternative therapies, including complementary medicines and psychotherapy, are often coupled with the available FDA-approved pharmacotherapy in an effort to treat IBS (Box 5).

Although almost all of these agents have been tested in randomized, controlled studies, only three – alosetron (Lotronex), lubiprostone (Amitiza), and linaclotide (Linzess) – are currently approved by the FDA for treatment of IBS. Alosetron is a serotonin 5-HT3 antagonist that received FDA approval for treatment of IBS with diarrhea in adult women at a dose of 1.0 mg twice daily. Because of reports of ischemic colitis and bowel perforations, it was removed from the market. It has now been reintroduced on a restricted basis for use in patients with refractory disease.

[2]Not available in the United States.

Box 4 — Differential Diagnosis for Irritable Bowel Syndrome

- Colon malignancy
- Lymphoma of the gastrointestinal tract
- Inflammatory bowel disease (Crohn's disease, ulcerative colitis)
- Diverticulitis
- Peptic ulcer disease
- Biliary or liver disease
- Chronic pancreatitis
- Celiac disease
- Small-bowel bacterial overgrowth
- Parasites
- Endometriosis
- Medication-induced symptoms

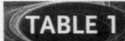

TABLE 1 Pharmacotherapy for Irritable Bowel Syndrome According to Symptom

SYMPTOM	INITIAL DOSE	TARGET DOSE
Diarrhea		
Loperamide (Imodium)	2 mg/d	2–8 mg/d
Diphenoxylate and atropine (Lomotil)[1]	5 mg	up to 20 mg/d
Alosetron (Lotronex)*	0.5 mg bid	up to 1 mg bid
Constipation		
Fiber (over-the-counter products)		
Laxatives and secretory stimulants		
Polyethylene glycol 3350 (MiraLAX)[1]	17 g/d	up to 34 g bid
Lactulose (Cephulac)[1]	10–20 g/d	up to 40 g/d
Lubiprostone (Amitiza)	8 µg bid	
Linaclotide (Linzess)		290 µg/d
Osmotic laxatives		
Stimulant laxatives		
Prokinetics		
Tegaserod (Zelnorm)[2]	6 mg bid	
Bloating		
Rifaximin (Xifaxan)[1]		400 mg tid[3]
Probiotics (*Bifidobacterium infantis* 35624; Bifantis)[7]		1 capsule per day
Pain		
Dicyclomine (Bentyl)	10 mg qid	40 mg qid
Hyoscyamine (Levsin)[1]	0.25 mg SL/PO q4h prn	maximum 1.5 mg/d
Tricyclic antidepressants[1]		
Amitriptyline (Elavil)	10 mg qhs	10–75 mg qhs
Desipramine (Norpramin)	10 mg qhs	10–75 mg qhs
Nortriptyline (Pamelor)	10 mg qhs	10–75 mg qhs
Selective serotonin-reuptake inhibitors[1]		
Paroxetine (Paxil)	10 mg qhs	10–60 mg qhs
Citalopram (Celexa)	5 mg qhs	5–20 mg qhs
Fluoxetine (Prozac)	20 mg qhs	20–40 mg qhs

[1]Not FDA approved for this indication.
[2]Not available in the United States.
[3]Exceeds dosage recommended by the manufacturer.
[7]Available as a dietary supplement.
*Available only to physicians enrolled in the Prescribing Program for Lotronex.

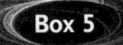

Box 5 — Alternative Management of Irritable Bowel Syndrome

Complementary Medicines
- Herbal medicines
- Megavitamins
- Folk remedies
- Microbial food supplements (prebiotics, probiotics, fungi)

Psychotherapy
- Cognitive behavioral therapy
- Relaxation therapy
- Contingency management
- Biofeedback
- Hypnosis

The recommended dosing is to begin with 0.5 mg once daily and slowly increase the dose to 1.0 mg twice daily if necessary. Lubiprostone, a prostaglandin-derived bicyclic fatty acid, is FDA approved for use in women with IBS with constipation at a dose of 8 mcg twice daily. Lubiprostone acts on epithelial surface chloride channels to increase intraluminal chloride and water in the small intestine and colon, and leads to decreased intestinal transit time and quicker passage of stool. There have been no serious adverse effects reported in placebo-controlled, randomized, controlled trials or long-term extension studies of lubiprostone, and there are currently no restrictions on the duration of use. The most common side effects are mild to moderate diarrhea and nausea, and it is recommended to take with food.[3] Linaclotide is another novel agent that is FDA approved for treatment of IBS with constipation at a dose of 290 mcg daily. Linaclotide binds and agonizes guanylate cyclase on the intraluminal surface of the intestinal epithelium and subsequently leads to chloride and bicarbonate secretion into the intestinal lumen. This results in increased intraluminal fluid and decreased intestinal transit time. Linaclotide may also decrease visceral pain sensation.[4] Another agent, Tegaserod, a 5-HT4 agonist, was previously approved by the FDA for treatment of IBS with constipation in women, however it was subsequently removed from the market because of increased serious cardiovascular side effects.

---

[3]Exceeds dosage recommended by the manufacturer.
[4]Not yet approved for use in the United States.

References

Gershon MD, Tack J. The serotonin signaling system: From basic understanding to drug development for functional GI disorders. Gastroenterology 2007;132:397–414.

Halmos FP, Power VA, Shepherd SJ, Gibson PR, Muir JG. A diet low in FODMAPs reduces symptoms of irritable bowel syndrome. Gastroenterology 2014;146: 67–75 e65.

Horwitz BJ, Fisher RS. The irritable bowel syndrome. N Engl J Med 2001;344:1846–50.

Longstreth GF, Thompson WG, Chey WD, et al. Functional bowel disorders. In: Drossman DA, Corazziari E, Delvaux M, et al, editors: Rome III: The functional gastrointestinal disorders. 3rd ed. McLean, VA: Degnon; 2006. p. 487–555.

Mayer EA. Irritable bowel syndrome. N Engl J Med 2008;358:1692–9.

Park M, Camilleri M. Genetics and genotypes in irritable bowel syndrome: Implications for diagnosis and treatment. Gastroenterol Clin North Am 2005;34:305–17.

Quigley EM, Flourie B. Probiotics and irritable bowel syndrome: A rationale for their use and an assessment of the evidence to date. Neurogastroenterol Motil 2007;19:166–72.

Rothstein RD, Friedenberg FK. Linaclotide: a novel compound for the treatment of irritable bowel syndrome with constipation. Expert Opin Pharmacother 2013;14: 2125–32.

Schey R, Rao SS. Lubiprostone for the treatment of adults with constipation and irritable bowel syndrome. Dig Dis Sci 2011;56:1619–25.

Videlock EJ, Chang L. Irritable bowel syndrome: Current approach to symptoms, evaluation, and treatment. Gastroenterol Clin North Am 2007;36:665–85.

Wilcz-Villega E, McClean S, O'Sullivan M. Reduced E-cadherin expression is associated with abdominal pain and symptom duration in a study of alternating diarrhea predominant IBS. Neurogastroenterol Motil 2014;26:316–25.

MALABSORPTION

Method of
Lawrence R. Schiller, MD

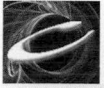

CURRENT DIAGNOSIS

- Recognize the presence of generalized malabsorption by the combination of typical symptoms: diarrhea, greasy stools, flatulence, weight loss, fatigue, edema.
- Recognize the presence of specific malabsorption by associated symptoms and those symptoms particular to deficiency states of the malabsorbed substance: flatus, diarrhea, anemia, dermatitis, glossitis, neuropathy, paresthesias, tetany, ecchymosis.
- Documentation of generalized malabsorption is best done by stool analysis demonstrating steatorrhea and acid stools (reflecting carbohydrate malabsorption). Diagnosis depends on visualization of the small bowel by endoscopy or radiography and small bowel biopsy. Additional tests may be needed.
- Documentation of specific malabsorption is best done by demonstrating low blood levels of the malabsorbed substance or by tests designed to measure absorption of that substance. Diagnosis depends on studies designed to identify the likely diagnosis for a given situation.

CURRENT THERAPY

- Once a diagnosis is reached, therapy can be directed toward that specific problem:
  - Gluten-free diet for celiac disease
  - Antibiotics for bacterial overgrowth
  - Lactose-free diet for lactase deficiency

Every day the average human being consumes 2000–3000 kcal of food, much of it in the form of polymers or other complex molecules that must be digested and absorbed by the gut. The processes of digestion and absorption are complex and are readily disturbed by pathologic processes. More than 200 conditions have been described that can adversely affect nutrient absorption.

Strictly speaking, *maldigestion* refers to impaired hydrolysis of nutrients, usually due to lack of luminal factors, such as bile acids and pancreatic enzymes, and *malabsorption* refers to impaired mucosal transport. For clinical purposes, "malabsorption" is used to describe both processes.

Malabsorption can be generalized (panmalabsorption) or limited to a specific category of nutrients. Generalized malabsorption is usually due to maldigestion or to extensive mucosal dysfunction. Specific malabsorption occurs when a single transporter is disabled.

The causes of malabsorption can be divided into three categories: impaired luminal hydrolysis, impaired mucosal function (mucosal hydrolysis, uptake, packaging, and excretion), and impaired removal of nutrients from the mucosa (Box 1).

Diagnosis
Symptoms and Signs
Most patients with panmalabsorption have changes in their stools (Box 2). Steatorrhea (excess fat in stools) is characterized by pale color, bulkiness, greasiness, and a tendency to float (probably because of incorporated gas). Occasionally patients with malabsorption present with watery stools due to the osmotic effects of unabsorbed carbohydrates and short-chain fatty acids.

Abdominal distention and excess flatus also commonly occur due to fermentation of unabsorbed carbohydrate by colonic bacteria. This can occur not only with panmalabsorption but also with specific malabsorption of carbohydrate (e.g., lactase deficiency).

Weight loss is typical with severe panmalabsorption, but it might not be very prominent with lesser degrees of malabsorption due to compensatory hyperphagia. Weight loss is most prominent early in the course of the illness, but body weight usually stabilizes as calorie absorption and body weight come into balance again. This is in contrast to illnesses like cancer or tuberculosis that produce continuing weight loss. If a patient with malabsorption has continuing weight loss, inflammatory bowel disease or lymphoma should be considered.

Abdominal pain is usually not present with malabsorption, although some cramping may be associated with diarrhea. Severe pain should bring chronic pancreatitis, Zollinger-Ellison syndrome, lymphoma, Crohn's disease, or mesenteric ischemia to mind.

Constitutional symptoms of fatigue and weakness commonly occur, even early in the course. In contrast, appetite is impaired only late in the course of most malabsorption states. Edema is uncommon until late in the course unless protein-losing enteropathy is present.

Vitamin and mineral deficiencies can lead to several symptoms or signs. Glossitis and cheilosis are common in patients with water-soluble vitamin deficiencies. Florid beriberi, pellagra, and

Box 1 — Causes of Malabsorption or Maldigestion

- Impaired luminal hydrolysis or solublization
  - Bile acid deficiency
  - Impaired mucosal hydrolysis, uptake, or packaging
  - Pancreatic exocrine insufficiency
  - Postgastrectomy syndrome
  - Rapid intestinal transit
  - Small bowel bacterial overgrowth
  - Zollinger-Ellison syndrome
- Brush border or metabolic disorders
  - Abetalipoproteinemia
  - Glucose-galactose malabsorption
  - Lactase deficiency
  - Sucrase-isomaltase deficiency
- Mucosal diseases
  - Amyloidosis
  - Chronic mesenteric ischemia
  - Crohn's disease
  - Celiac sprue
  - Collagenous sprue
  - Eosinophilic gastroenteritis
  - Immunoproliferative small intestinal disease (IPSID)
  - Lymphoma
  - Nongranulomatous ulcerative jejunoileitis
  - Olmesartan enteropathy
  - Radiation enteritis
  - Systemic mastocytosis
- Infectious diseases
  - AIDS enteropathy
  - *Mycobacterium avium-intracellulare*
  - Parasitic diseases
  - Small bowel bacterial overgrowth
  - Tropical sprue
  - Whipple's disease
- After intestinal resection
- Chronic mesenteric ischemia
- Impaired removal of nutrients
  - Lymphangiectasia

Box 2 — Symptoms and Signs of Malabsorption or Maldigestion

- Changes in stool characteristics
  - Floating stools
  - Pale, bulky, greasy stools
  - Watery diarrhea
- Increased colonic gas production
  - Abdominal distention
  - Borborygmi
- Vitamin and mineral deficiencies
  - Anemia
  - Cheilosis
  - Glossitis
  - Dermatitis
  - Neuropathy
  - Night blindness
  - Osteomalacia
  - Paresthesia
  - Tetany
- Ecchymosis
- Fatigue, weakness
- Edema
- Weight loss, muscle wasting

Box 3 — Systemic Diseases Associated with Malabsorption or Maldigestion

Endocrine Diseases
- Addison's disease
- Diabetes mellitus
- Hypoparathyroidism
- Hyperthyroidism, hypothyroidism

Collagen-Vascular and Miscellaneous Diseases
- AIDS
- Amyloidosis
- Scleroderma
- Vasculitis (systemic lupus erythematosus, polyarteritis nodosa)

scurvy are not commonly seen unless malabsorption has been particularly severe or long-lasting. Fat-soluble vitamin deficiencies also are unlikely to develop except when malabsorption has been long-standing because of substantial body stores.

Miscellaneous findings occasionally seen in patients with malabsorption can provide clues to the diagnosis. Aphthous ulcers in the mouth may be seen with celiac disease, Behçet's syndrome, or Crohn's disease. Hyperpigmentation is seen in Whipple's disease, and dermatitis herpetiformis (pruritic, blistering skin lesions) is seen in celiac disease. Scleroderma can manifest with tight skin, digital ulceration, nail changes, and Raynaud's phenomenon. Chronic sinusitis, bronchitis, and recurrent pneumonia suggest cystic fibrosis or IgA deficiency. Several systemic diseases can be associated with malabsorption syndrome (Box 3).

Tests

Routine Laboratory Tests

Routine laboratory tests (Box 4) commonly are abnormal in patients with established malabsorption syndrome. Anemia is common but not universal. Iron deficiency anemia may be the only finding in some patients with celiac disease. Microcytic anemia may be present in Whipple's disease (due to occult blood loss) and in lymphomas manifesting with malabsorption. Macrocytic anemia due to folate or vitamin B_{12} deficiency can occur in short bowel syndrome, small bowel bacterial overgrowth, or ileal disease. Lymphopenia may be present in patients with AIDS or lymphangiectasia.

Electrolyte abnormalities may be due to a combination of poor intake and excess loss in stool. Renal function usually is well maintained in malabsorption syndrome, but blood urea nitrogen may be low due to poor protein absorption, and serum creatinine concentration may be low due to depletion of muscle mass. Serum calcium levels may be low due to malabsorption, vitamin D deficiency, or intraluminal complexing of calcium by fatty acids. Hypomagnesemia can produce hypocalcemia or hypokalemia that is resistant to intravenous repletion. Serum phosphorus, cholesterol, and triglyceride levels may be reduced due to poor intake or malabsorption. Liver tests may be abnormal due to fatty liver. Serum protein and albumin levels are well preserved in patients with malabsorption unless protein-losing enteropathy or an acute illness is present.

Prothrombin time is normal unless vitamin K malabsorption (typically associated with steatorrhea), anticoagulant therapy, antibiotic therapy, or colectomy is present.

Assays are available for several potentially malabsorbed substances, including iron, vitamin B_{12}, folate, 25-hydroxyvitamin D, and β-carotene. Malabsorption tends to lower blood levels, but substantial body stores of many of these can mitigate the reduction in concentration that otherwise might occur. Thus, the sensitivity and specificity of these assays for malabsorption are poor.

Tests for Malabsorption

Fat Malabsorption. The simplest test for fat malabsorption is a qualitative microscopic examination of stool using a fat-soluble stain, such as Sudan III. The finding of more than 5 stained droplets per high power field is abnormal and correlates well with

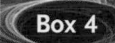

Box 4 Laboratory Tests for Evaluation of Malabsorption or Maldigestion

Routine Blood Tests
- Complete blood count
- Hemoglobin/hematocrit
- Platelet count
- WBC differential count

Biochemistry Tests
- Blood urea nitrogen
- Potassium
- Prothrombin time
- Serum albumin
- Serum calcium
- Serum creatinine

Blood Levels of Potentially Malabsorbed Substances
- Serum iron, vitamin B_{12}, folate, 25-OH vitamin D, carotene

Fat absorption
- Qualitative fecal fat
- Quantitative fecal fat

Protein Absorption and Protein-Losing Enteropathy
- α_1-Antitrypsin clearance
- Fecal nitrogen excretion

Carbohydrate Absorption
- Osmotic gap in stool water
- Quantitative excretion (anthrone)
- Stool pH <5.5
- Stool reducing substances
- D-Xylose absorption test
- Oral glucose, sucrose, and lactose tolerance tests
- Breath hydrogen tests

Vitamin B_{12} Absorption
- Schilling test with intrinsic factor

Bile Acid Malabsorption
- ^{14}C-glycocholic acid breath test
- Fecal bile acid excretion
- Radiolabeled bile acid excretion
- ^{75}SeHCAT retention

Small Bowel Bacterial Overgrowth
- ^{14}C-glycocholic acid breath test
- ^{14}C-xylose breath test
- Glucose breath hydrogen test
- Quantitative culture of jejunal aspirate

Exocrine Pancreatic Insufficiency
- Dual-labeled Schilling test
- Secretin/CCK test
- Stool chymotrypsin concentration

Serologic Testing for Celiac Disease
- Anti-tissue transglutaminase antibody (IgA)
- Anti-endomysial antibody (IgA)

Abbreviations: CCK = cholecystokinin; SLE = systemic lupus erythematosus; ^{75}SeHCAT = selenium-75-labeled taurohomocholic acid; WBC = white blood cell.

---

quantitative measurement of fecal fat excretion. The test is subject to false-positive results with some drugs and food additives, such as mineral oil, orlistat, and olestra.

A more precise estimate of fat absorption is obtained by a quantitative analysis of a timed stool collection (48 or 72 hours). During the collection, a diary of dietary intake should be maintained so that fat excretion can be assessed as a percentage of intake. Normal fat excretion is <7% of intake when stool weight is normal, but it can be twice as high due to voluminous diarrhea without indicating defective mucosal transport of fat. Thus, fat excretion must be judged against stool weight. Stool fat concentration (grams of fat per 100 grams of stool) also is of value. Pancreatic exocrine insufficiency is associated with high fecal fat concentration (>10 g/100 g stool) because unlike hydrolyzed fat, unhydrolyzed fat does not stimulate colonic water and electrolyte secretion that would dilute fecal fat concentration.

Protein Malabsorption. Fecal nitrogen excretion can be employed as a marker of protein malabsorption, but is not often used in clinical medicine because it adds little to the evaluation. If protein-losing enteropathy is suspected, an α_1-antitrypsin clearance study can be done. In this study, fecal excretion of α_1-antitrypsin, a serum protein that is relatively resistant to hydrolysis by luminal enzymes, is divided by serum concentration of α_1-antitrypsin, and the volume of serum leaked into the lumen can be calculated. Values of more than 180 mL/day are associated with hypoalbuminemia.

Carbohydrate Malabsorption. Carbohydrate malabsorption is difficult to measure directly because fermentation of malabsorbed carbohydrate by colonic bacteria reduces the amount of intact carbohydrate that can be recovered in stool. Indirect estimates of carbohydrate malabsorption can be made by examining fecal pH (<5.5 with carbohydrate malabsorption) or fecal osmotic gap (> 100 mOsm/kg with osmotic diarrhea). Oral carbohydrate tolerance tests may be used to evaluate absorption of sugars, such as lactose or fructose. Following an oral load of a given sugar, blood glucose levels are monitored; failure of blood glucose to increase suggests malabsorption.

Another test for carbohydrate malabsorption is the D-xylose absorption test. In this test, a 25-gram dose of D-xylose is given orally; blood xylose levels are measured 1 and 3 hours later, and urinary excretion of xylose is measured for 5 hours. Failure of blood xylose to rise above 20 mg/dL at 1 hour or above 22.5 mg/dL at 3 hours or failure of urinary excretion to exceed 5 g in 5 hours suggests malabsorption. In addition, because xylose does not require pancreatic enzymes or bile acids for absorption, an abnormal D-xylose test suggests a mucosal problem as the cause for malabsorption. The results of this test can be misleading if the patient is dehydrated or has ascites, if renal function is compromised, or if bacterial overgrowth is present in the upper small bowel.

Breath hydrogen testing is another method to assess carbohydrate absorption. If substrates such as lactose or sucrose are not absorbed in the small intestine, they pass into the colon, where bacterial fermentation produces hydrogen gas. The hydrogen is absorbed into the bloodstream and then is exhaled. The concentration of hydrogen in exhaled breath can be measured easily; a rise of more than 10 to 20 ppm after ingestion of a specific substrate is consistent with malabsorption. False-positive results can be seen in patients with small bowel bacterial overgrowth, and false-negative results can be seen in patients who lack hydrogen-producing flora or who have been on antibiotics recently.

Vitamin B_{12} Malabsorption. Although the Schilling test can be used to measure Vitamin B_{12} absorption, commercial testing kits are no longer available in the United States. For purposes of a malabsorption evaluation, Part II of the Schilling test could be used to measure radiolabeled B_{12} absorption with intrinsic factor. Recovery of less than 9% of the radiolabeled B_{12} in the urine is abnormal and suggests ileal dysfunction. The test may be falsely positive in patients with pancreatic exocrine insufficiency, small bowel bacterial overgrowth, or renal failure.

Bile Acid Malabsorption. Tests for bile acid malabsorption are not widely available in the United States. Direct measurement of bile acid excretion has been used mainly in research studies. Retention of a radioactive taurocholic acid analogue (SeHCAT, selenium-75-labeled taurohomocholic acid) is used in Europe to assess bile acid malabsorption. A breath test using ^{14}C-glycocholic acid has been used for evaluating small bowel bacterial overgrowth, but it may have application for assessing bile acid malabsorption as well.

Small Bowel Bacterial Overgrowth. The gold standard method used to test for small bowel bacterial overgrowth in the upper intestine is quantitative culture of jejunal fluid. The sample can be obtained during endoscopy and sent to the laboratory with instructions to quantitate the aerobic and anaerobic flora. Finding more than 10^5

bacteria per mL confirms bacterial overgrowth. Breath tests using glucose, ^{14}C-xylose, and lactulose also have been described for this purpose.

Pancreatic Exocrine Insufficiency. Tests for pancreatic exocrine insufficiency are not commonly used. The gold standard test is a secretin test. This study requires duodenal intubation, injection of secretin, and measurement of bicarbonate output. A tubeless test, the bentiromide test, had average clinical utility; it is no longer available in the United States. Measurement of fecal chymotrypsin or elastase activity is only moderately useful in predicting the presence of exocrine pancreatic insufficiency. For most situations, a therapeutic trial using a high dose of pancreatic enzymes with monitoring of the effect on steatorrhea is the best that can be done.

Evaluation of Suspected Malabsorption

When malabsorption is suspected because of the history, physical findings, and setting, the physician must decide if the malabsorption involves a specific nutrient or represents a generalized process (Figure 1). If the malabsorption seems to be specific, a diet and symptom diary, breath tests using the presumptively malabsorbed substrate, and stool pH to identify acid stools seen with carbohydrate malabsorption are reasonable diagnostic maneuvers.

Suspected generalized malabsorption requires a more intense evaluation. Steatorrhea should be confirmed with either a qualitative fecal fat test (e.g., Sudan stain) or a quantitative stool collection for measurement of fat excretion. If steatorrhea is confirmed, the small bowel should be visualized with either capsule endoscopy or radiography (small bowel follow-through examination or computed tomography) and biopsied from above by enteroscopy and from below by colonoscopy. During enteroscopy, an aspirate of small bowel contents can be obtained for quantitative culture to look for small bowel bacterial overgrowth. An alternative method to detect small bowel bacterial overgrowth is breath testing (see earlier). Stool samples also should be examined with microscopy or immunoassay for the presence of parasites that may be associated with malabsorption.

This sequence of evaluation often leads to a specific diagnosis. When it does not, empiric trials of pancreatic enzyme replacement or bile acid supplementation can lead to a presumptive diagnosis of pancreatic exocrine insufficiency or bile acid deficiency. Hard endpoints (e.g., quantitative fat excretion) should be used to assess the effectiveness of these empiric trials.

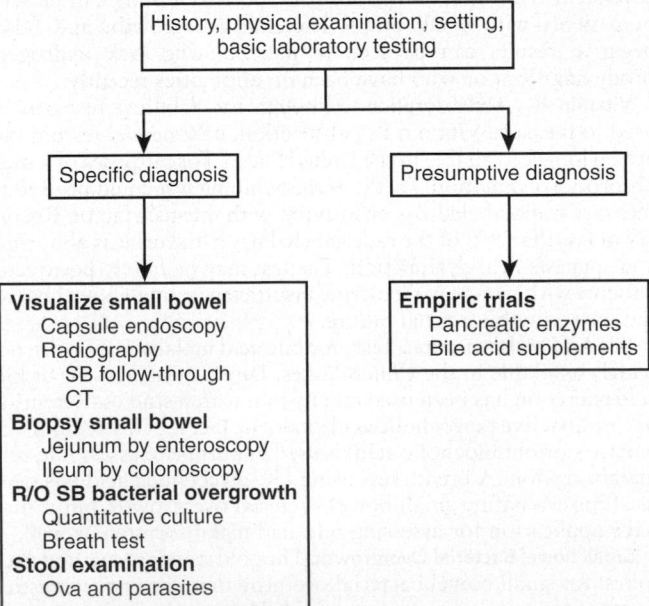

Figure 1. Flow chart for evaluation of malabsorption or maldigestion. *Abbreviations:* CT = computed tomography; R/O = rule out; SB = small bowel.

Specific Disorders Associated with Malabsorption
Malabsorption of Specific Nutrients
Disaccharidase Deficiency

Ingested disaccharides such as lactose and sucrose and starch-digestion products such as maltotriose and α-limit dextrins must be hydrolyzed by brush border enzymes into monosaccharides for absorption by the mucosa. If these brush border enzymes are not active or if the brush border is damaged, malabsorption of the specific carbohydrate substrate results. This can result in gaseousness or osmotic diarrhea when those substrates are ingested. This rarely occurs on a congenital basis, but it commonly occurs as an acquired disorder.

Lactase deficiency is the most common acquired disaccharidase deficiency. Infant mammals all rely on lactose as the carbohydrate source in milk, but lactase activity is shut off after weaning in most species. Most human populations lose lactase activity during adolescence as a normal part of maturation. Members of the northern European gene pool might maintain lactase activity into adult life, but lactase activity declines gradually in many. At some point the amount of lactose ingested might exceed the ability of the remaining enzyme to hydrolyze it, resulting in lactose malabsorption and symptoms. This also can occur with acute conditions such as gastroenteritis that can disturb the mucosa and temporarily reduce lactase activity. Patients might not recognize lactose ingestion as a cause of their problem because they have not had difficulty tolerating lactose in the past. Restriction of lactose in the diet (or use of products that have predigested lactose) mitigates symptoms. Use of exogenous lactase as a tablet may only be partially effective because of incomplete hydrolysis of ingested lactose.

Transport Defects at the Brush Border

Glucose-galactose malabsorption is a rare congenital disorder resulting from an inactive hexose transporter in the brush border. Hydrolysis of lactose is intact, but transport across the apical membrane of the enterocyte fails to occur. Fructose absorption, which is mediated by a different carrier, is unaffected.

In all human beings, the ability to absorb fructose is limited by the availability of carriers in the brush border and may be overwhelmed when excess fructose is ingested. This can occur relatively easily nowadays, because high-fructose corn syrup is used frequently as a sweetener in commercial products such as soda pop. Limiting the amount of fructose ingested will reduce symptoms.

Abetalipoproteinemia is a rare condition that prevents absorption of long-chain fatty acids due to failure to form chylomicrons. Use of medium-chain triglycerides that do not require transport in chylomicrons can bypass this defect.

Pernicious anemia develops when failure to secrete intrinsic factor in the stomach prevents vitamin B_{12} absorption by the ileal mucosa. Parenteral replacement with cyanocobalamin by injection (Cyanoject) or nasal spray (Nascobal) is necessary.

Generalized Malabsorption
Celiac Disease

Celiac disease (also known as celiac sprue) is a disorder in which the mucosa of the small bowel is damaged due to activation of the mucosal immune system by ingestion of gluten, a protein component found in wheat, barley, and rye. People who have HLA-DQ2 or DQ8 are susceptible to this condition because these specific antigen-presenting proteins produce particularly strong reactions by interacting with a unique peptide digestion product of gluten. Tissue transglutaminase, an enzyme produced in the mucosa, is an important cofactor in pathogenesis by amplifying the immunogenicity of gluten peptide fragments and is the target of autoantibodies that are characteristic of this disease. The condition produces generalized malabsorption by destroying the villi of the small intestine, reducing the surface area available for absorption.

In addition to malabsorption syndrome with diarrhea and weight loss, celiac disease can produce a host of nonspecific symptoms, including abdominal pain, fatigue, muscle and joint pains, and headaches and seemingly unrelated problems such as iron deficiency anemia, abnormal liver tests, and osteoporosis. These protean manifestations mean that celiac disease must be considered in the differential diagnosis of many conditions. The clinical course is quite variable, with symptoms coming and going. Symptoms can develop during childhood and produce growth retardation or first become manifest in adulthood.

Testing for celiac disease has been simplified by the development of an assay for anti–tissue transglutaminase antibodies. This test largely supplants measurement of antigluten antibodies, although these remain of some use in evaluating adherence to a gluten-free diet. IgA antibodies are the most useful for diagnosis, but IgA deficiency is common enough that an IgA level should be measured concomitantly.

Although serologic tests have high sensitivity and specificity, the implications of adhering to a gluten-free diet are so extreme that the diagnosis of celiac disease should be confirmed whenever possible by small bowel mucosal biopsy, now obtained routinely by endoscopy. An empiric trial of a gluten-free diet may be difficult to interpret because many persons with gastrointestinal symptoms improve with dietary carbohydrate restriction. Wheat starch is particularly hard to digest (due to gluten coating wheat starch granules), and ordinarily 20% of wheat starch is not absorbed by the small bowel and enters the colon.

Treatment of celiac disease at present involves strict lifetime exclusion of gluten from the diet. This is a difficult regimen that excludes most processed foods. Assistance of a dietitian is most helpful. The prognosis with effective treatment is very good. Symptoms should respond to the diet within weeks; failure to do so should prompt an examination of compliance with the diet or reconsideration of the diagnosis. Failure to respond may be seen when lymphoma or adenocarcinoma complicate the course of celiac disease or in cases of "refractory sprue" or "collagenous sprue," which can have a different autoimmune basis from classic celiac disease and which might respond to immunosuppressive drugs such as corticosteroids or azathioprine (Imuran).[1] Persistent diarrhea may be observed in patients with celiac disease who have concomitant microscopic colitis, another condition that is linked to HLA-DQ2 and HLA-DQ8.

Inflammatory Diseases

Diseases that produce extensive mucosal damage by inflammation cause generalized malabsorption by reduction of mucosal surface area, by promotion of small bowel bacterial overgrowth, by ileal dysfunction, or by development of enteroenteral or enterocolic fistulas. Examples include jejunoileitis due to Crohn's disease, nongranulomatous ulcerative jejunoileitis, radiation enteritis, and chronic mesenteric ischemia. With Crohn's disease, previous resection can add to the problem (see later). Therapy aimed at the underlying process can improve absorption; in some cases (e.g., radiation enteritis) no effective therapy is available for the underlying problem, and symptomatic management is all that is possible. This includes use of antidiarrheal drugs to prolong contact time between luminal contents and the small bowel mucosa, ingestion of a reduced fat diet to reduce steatorrhea, and use of vitamin and mineral supplements to prevent deficiency states.

Infiltrative Disorders

Several conditions involve infiltration of the intestinal mucosa with cells or extracellular matrix that impede absorption or modify mucosal function by secretion of cytokines and other regulatory substances. These include eosinophilic gastroenteritis, systemic mastocytosis, immunoproliferative small intestinal disease (IPSID), lymphoma, and amyloidosis. These conditions are diagnosed by mucosal biopsy, but special stains might have to be employed to identify the infiltrating cells or matrix accurately.

Treatment of the underlying processes can improve absorption, but it is not uniformly effective. For eosinophilic gastroenteritis, a hypoallergenic (elimination) diet and corticosteroids may be useful. Mild systemic mastocytosis is treated with the mast cell-stabilizer sodium chromoglycate, H_1- and H_2-receptor antagonists, and

low-dose aspirin. More advanced disease might respond to interferon or cytotoxic chemotherapy. IPSID initially is treated with antibiotics because small bowel bacterial overgrowth may be a causative factor. Once malignant change has occurred, it is treated like lymphoma with cytotoxic chemotherapy. Amyloidosis affecting the gut is not amenable to therapy and is usually fatal.

Infectious Diseases

Small Bowel Bacterial Overgrowth. Small bowel bacterial overgrowth in the jejunum can produce generalized malabsorption. It can occur whenever the mechanisms that reduce overgrowth are compromised. These situations include achlorhydria or hypochlorhydria, motility disorders of the small intestine (e.g., diabetes mellitus or scleroderma), and anatomic alterations (e.g., diverticulosis, gastrocolic fistula, or blind loops postoperatively). Fat malabsorption is attributed to bacterial deconjugation of bile acid. Bacterial toxins or free fatty acids can produce patchy mucosal damage, leading to less efficient carbohydrate and protein absorption. Bacteria also can compete with the mucosa for uptake of certain nutrients such as vitamin B_{12}.

Diagnosis of small bowel bacterial overgrowth can be difficult (see earlier). Treatment consists of antibiotic therapy unless a surgically correctable anatomic defect is discovered. Tetracycline is no longer uniformly effective; amoxicillin–clavulinic acid (Augmentin), cephalosporins, ciprofloxacin (Cipro), metronidazole (Flagyl), and rifaximin (Xifaxan) may be employed. Therapy should be given for 1 to 2 weeks initially and then discontinued. It should be restarted when symptoms recur. If this occurs quickly, longer treatment periods should be considered. Continuous antibiotic therapy is needed rarely.

Tropical Sprue. Tropical sprue is a progressive, chronic malabsorptive condition occurring in both the indigenous population and in visitors residing in certain tropical countries for extended periods. The prevalence of tropical sprue seems to be decreasing for uncertain reasons. The disease starts as an acute diarrheal disease that becomes a persistent diarrhea associated with substantial weight loss and typically megaloblastic anemia. Villi become shortened and thickened (partial villous atrophy), but the flat mucosa of celiac disease is not usually present. Enterocytes have disrupted brush borders and can have megaloblastic changes; the submucosa has a chronic inflammatory infiltrate. Intestinal biopsy is required for diagnosis.

Currently, tropical sprue is believed to represent a form of bacterial overgrowth with organisms that secrete enterotoxins. Most patients have evidence of excessive gram-negative bacterial colonization of the jejunum. The declining prevalence of tropical sprue may be due to improved nutrition, better sanitation, or prompt treatment of acute diarrhea with antibiotics. Treatment consists of pharmacologic doses of folic acid (folate) (5 mg daily[3]), injection of cyanocobalamin (if deficient), and antibiotic therapy for 1 to 6 months. Tetracycline 250 mg four times a day or sulfonamide is the treatment of choice. Newer antibiotics have not been tested extensively in this condition. Improvement should be noted after a few weeks. The prognosis with treatment is excellent; without treatment, tropical sprue can be fatal. Recurrence can occur.

Whipple's Disease. Whipple's disease is a rare chronic bacterial infection with multisystem involvement. The small bowel typically is heavily infiltrated with foamy macrophages containing periodic acid–Schiff (PAS)-positive material, distorting the villi. Small bowel biopsy with special stains or electron microscopy or a specific polymerase chain reaction (PCR) is diagnostic. Foamy macrophages and bacteria can be found outside the intestine in lymph nodes, spleen, liver, central nervous system, heart, and synovium. Accordingly, symptoms are protean. The bacterium has been identified as *Tropheryma whippelii*, a relative of *Acinetobacter*. It does not appear to be very contagious, and no direct person-to-person transmission has been demonstrated. Presumably, differences in host resistance allow proliferation within macrophages without clearance of the bacteria.

---

[1]Not FDA approved for this indication.

[3]Exceeds dosage recommended by the manufacturer.

Whipple's disease occurs mainly in older white men, but women and all ethnic groups are susceptible. Patients can present with malabsorption syndrome or with symptoms related to the extraintestinal disease (arthritis, fever, dementia, headache, or muscle weakness). Gross or occult gastrointestinal bleeding can occur. Protein-losing enteropathy may be present.

Treatment with any of several antibiotics (penicillin, erythromycin, ampicillin, tetracycline, chloramphenicol, or trimethoprim-sulfamethoxazole [TMP-SMX]) produces excellent symptomatic responses within days to weeks, but it should be continued for months to years. Even with protracted courses, relapses are common.

Other Infections. *Mycobacterium avium–intracellulare* is another chronic bacterial infection that can cause malabsorption, particularly in patients with AIDS. Mucosal biopsy with special stains to distinguish it from Whipple's disease is essential. Antibiotic therapy can reduce the intensity of infection; clearance depends on immunologic reconstitution with antiretroviral therapy. Clarithromycin (Biaxin) and ethambutol (Myambutol) are recommended as initial therapy.

Parasitic diseases can produce malabsorption by competing for nutrients and causing mechanical occlusion of the absorptive surface and epithelial damage. Protozoa that may be associated with malabsorption include *Giardia lamblia*, *Isospora belli*, *Cryptosporidium*, and *Enterocytozoon bieneusi*. Tapeworms associated with malabsorption include *Taenia saginata* (beef tapeworm), *Hymenolepis nana* (dwarf tapeworm), and *Diphyllobothrium latum* (fish tapeworm).

Giardia lamblia is a cosmopolitan parasite acquired from contaminated water or from another person by fecal-oral transmission. Cysts are relatively hardy, and ingestion of as few as 10 cysts is sufficient to establish infection. Patients with dysgammaglobulinemia (especially IgA deficiency) are likely to become infected. Diagnosis depends on finding the organism (cysts or trophozoites) in stool by microscopy (sensitivity ~50% for a single specimen), or detection of giardia antigens by immunologic testing of stool (sensitivity >90%), or discovery of the organism on small bowel biopsy.

Therapy consists of a single dose of tinidazole (Tindamax) (2 g), metronidazole (Flagyl)[1] (250 mg three times a day for a week), nitazoxanide (Alinia) (500 mg twice a day for three days), or quinacrine[2] (100 mg three times a day for a week).

Isospora belli and *Cryptosporidium* spp. are coccidia, protozoa that disrupt the epithelium by intracellular invasion *(Isospora)* or by attaching to the brush border, destroying microvilli *(Cryptosporidium)*. Stool examination or small bowel biopsy can identify the organism. *Cryptosporidium* antigen can be discovered by immunoassay on stool with excellent sensitivity. *Isospora* can be treated with TMP-SMX[1] or furazolidone.[2] *Cryptosporidium* can be treated by nitazoxanide.

Microsporidia are intracellular organisms now believed to be most closely related to fungi and are implicated in diarrhea and malabsorption in patients with AIDS and other immunodeficiency states. Small bowel biopsy can show partial villous atrophy, and electron microscopy displays characteristic changes. Stool examination occasionally is helpful. No treatment is of proven value.

Tapeworms compete with their hosts for nutrients in the lumen. *Diphyllobothrium latum* can produce vitamin B_{12} deficiency. The others can result in more extensive nutritional deficiencies. Diagnosis is based on stool examination, and treatment depends on the particular organism identified.

Luminal Problems Causing Malabsorption

Pancreatic Exocrine Insufficiency. Pancreatic exocrine insufficiency is the most common luminal problem that results in maldigestion. Patients develop symptoms of malabsorption when pancreatic enzyme secretion is reduced by >90%. There are several clinical features that distinguish pancreatic exocrine insufficiency from mucosal disorders, such as celiac disease. When fat is not

digested, it is transported through the gastrointestinal tract as intact triglyceride, which can appear as oil in the stool. In contrast, if fat is digested but not absorbed, it is in the form of fatty acids that can produce secretory diarrhea in the colon, resulting in more voluminous, even watery stools. This has two important ramifications: Fecal fat concentration is lower with mucosal disease (typically <9% by weight), and hypocalcemia due to formation of soaps (calcium plus 2 fatty acids) is seen with mucosal disease but not with pancreatic exocrine insufficiency. In addition, patients with mucosal disease tend to have more problems with water-soluble vitamin deficiencies than those with pancreatic exocrine insufficiency. In some patients with pancreatic exocrine insufficiency, carbohydrate malabsorption can produce substantial bloating, flatulence, and watery diarrhea.

Tests to document pancreatic exocrine insufficiency are not widely available or are nonspecific (see earlier), and so diagnosis usually hinges on a consistent history, demonstration of anatomic problems in the pancreas (calcification or abnormal ducts), and documentation of a response of steatorrhea to empiric treatment with a large dose of exogenous enzymes.

Bile Acid Deficiency. Bile acid deficiency is a less common cause of maldigestion, and malabsorption in this setting is limited to fat and fat-soluble vitamins. The usual setting is a patient with an extensive ileal resection (see later), but this also occurs in certain cholestatic conditions in which bile acid secretion by the liver is markedly compromised, such as advanced primary biliary cirrhosis, or complete extrahepatic biliary obstruction. As with pancreatic exocrine insufficiency, stools tend to have high fat concentrations (>9% by weight) when bile acid secretion is limited by hepatic or biliary disorders.

Zollinger-Ellison Syndrome. Zollinger-Ellison syndrome produces several abnormalities that can affect absorption. High rates of gastric acid secretion produce persistently low pH in the duodenum, which precipitates bile acid and inactivates pancreatic enzymes. In addition, excess acid can damage the absorptive cells directly.

Postoperative Malabsorption

Substantial malabsorption can result from gastric surgeries. Weight loss can result from inadequate intake due to early satiety or symptoms of dumping syndrome. Malabsorption can result from impaired mechanical disruption of food, mismatching of chyme delivery and enzyme secretion, rapid transit, or small bowel bacterial overgrowth due to loss of the gastric acid barrier. In addition, gastric surgery sometimes brings out latent celiac disease.

Short intestinal resections are well tolerated, but more extensive resections produce diarrhea and malabsorption of variable severity. When these symptoms are associated with weight loss or dehydrating diarrhea, short bowel syndrome is said to exist. In general, nutrient absorptive needs can be met if at least 100 cm of jejunum are preserved, but fluid absorption will be insufficient and diarrhea may be profuse. The process of intestinal adaptation permits improved absorption with time; it depends on exposure of the absorptive surface to nutrients. Absorption of specific substances, such as bile acids or vitamin B_{12}, is reduced permanently by resection of the terminal ileum.

Malabsorption in short bowel syndrome is not due solely to loss of absorptive surface area. Gastric acid hypersecretion, bile acid deficiency, rapid transit (due to loss of the ileal brake), and bacterial overgrowth may be present. These conditions are amenable to treatment and therapy with antisecretory drugs, exogenous bile acids, opiate antidiarrheals, or antibiotics can produce substantial improvement. Injection of teduglutide, a glucagon-like peptide-2 intestinal growth factor, or growth hormone in combination with glutamine and a special diet have been approved as treatments for short bowel syndrome; they can reduce the volume of parenteral fluid or nutrients required. Results with small bowel transplantation are improving with the use of better immunosuppressive regimens, and it remains the only cure for select patients with post-resection malabsorption.

---

[1]Not FDA approved for this indication.
[2]Not available in the United States.

Attention to nutrition is vital in any patient with malabsorption. If adequate nutrition cannot be maintained by oral intake, nutritional therapy is needed. Because of impaired bowel function, success with enteral nutrition may be impossible; parenteral nutrition may be needed. It is important to distinguish between the need for supplemental fluid and electrolytes and the need for nutrients; total parenteral nutrition is not a good choice for patients who only require fluids and electrolytes.

References

Barkun AN, Love J, Gould M, Pluta H, Steinhart H. Bile acid malabsorption in chronic diarrhea: pathophysiology and treatment. Can J Gastroenterol. 2013;27:653–9.

Bechtold ML, McClave SA, Palmer LB, et al. The pharmacologic treatment of short bowel syndrome: new tricks and novel agents. Curr Gastroenterol Rep. 2014;16:392.

Brelian D, Tenner S. Diarrhoea due to pancreatic diseases. Best Practice Res Clin Gastroenterol 2012;26:623–31.

DiMagno MJ, DiMagno EP. Chronic pancreatitis. Curr Opin Gastroenterol. 2013;29:531–6.

Gorospe EC, Oxentenko AS. Nutritional consequences of chronic diarrhoea. Best Pract Res Clin Gastroenterol. 2012;26:663–75.

Guandalini S, Assiri A. Celiac disease: a review. JAMA Pediatr. 2014;168:272–8.

Hammer HF, Hammer J. Diarrhea caused by carbohydrate malabsorption. Gastroenterol Clin North Am 2012;41:611–27.

Jeppesen PB. Spectrum of short bowel syndrome in adults: intestinal insufficiency to intestinal failure. JPEN J Parenter Enteral Nutr 2014;38(1 Suppl):8S–13S.

Rubio-Tapia A, Hill ID, Kelly CP, et al. ACG clinical guidelines: diagnosis and management of celiac disease. Am J Gastroenterol 2013;108:656–76.

Schiller LR, Pardi DS, Spiller R, et al. Gastro 2013 APDW/WCOG Shanghai Working Party Report: Chronic diarrhea: Definition, classification, diagnosis. J Gastroenterol Hepatol. 2014;29:6–25.

Schwartzman S, Schwartzman M. Whipple's disease. Rheum Dis Clin North Am. 2013;39:313–21.

Vipperla K, O'Keefe SJ. Study of teduglutide effectiveness in parenteral nutrition-dependent short-bowel syndrome subjects. Expert Rev Gastroenterol Hepatol. 2013;7:683–7.

Wales PW, Nasr A, de Silva N, Yamada J. Human growth hormone and glutamine for patients with short bowel syndrome. Cochrane Database Syst Rev 2010;6(6): CD006321.

TUMORS OF THE COLON AND RECTUM

Method of
Pinckney J. Maxwell, IV, MD; and Gerald A. Isenberg, MD

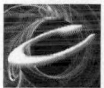

CURRENT DIAGNOSIS

- Screening of asymptomatic, average-risk patients should begin at 50 years of age.
- Colonoscopy should be performed if any screening test result is positive.
- Colonoscopy should be performed for any patient with signs or symptoms of colorectal cancer.
- Screening of high-risk patients—those with inflammatory bowel disease, familial adenomatous polyposis, or hereditary nonpolyposis colorectal cancer) and those with a significant positive family history—should begin at an earlier age and occur more frequently.

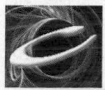

CURRENT THERAPY

- Patients with familial adenomatous polyposis or hereditary nonpolyposis colorectal cancer should undergo early, prophylactic colon resection.
- Colon tumors should be treated with segmental laparoscopic or open resection.
- Chemotherapy is offered for colon cancers with locally advanced, nodal (stage III), or metastatic (stage IV) disease.

- Rectal tumors that are small (<3 cm), involve <25% of the rectal circumference, are superficial (Tis or T1), lack nodal involvement, and have favorable pathologic characteristics should be removed by transanal techniques.
- Rectal tumors that are larger, are locally invasive, or have nodal involvement should be removed by formal open resection, with sphincter preservation if possible.
- Combination chemotherapy and radiation therapy is offered for advanced (stage II), nodal (stage III), or metastatic (stage IV) rectal cancer.
- Postoperative surveillance includes frequent office evaluations, measurements of carcinoembryonic antigen, endoscopy, and imaging.

Background, Epidemiology, and Etiology

Colorectal cancer is the third most common cancer in men and women, after prostate and lung/bronchus cancer in men and breast and lung/bronchus cancer in women. The American Cancer Society estimates that there will be 102,900 new diagnoses of colon cancer and 39,670 new diagnoses of rectal cancer in the United States in 2010. The incidence of colorectal cancer has been decreasing since the mid-1980s, with a more dramatic decrease occuring in the most recent decade. This decrease is likely related to an increase in screening with removal of precancerous polyps. The American Cancer Society expects an estimated 51,370 deaths from colorectal cancer in 2010, accounting for 9% of all cancer deaths. The mortality rate of colorectal cancer has similarly decreased since the mid-1980s, again with a sharper decline in the past decade most likely related to improved screening. Colorectal cancer is a highly treatable and frequently curable malignancy when it is detected early, highlighting the need for better screening.

The development of colorectal cancer is related to a number of factors, including age, diet, activity, environmental exposures, family history, and genetics. Ninety percent of colorectal cancers are diagnosed after the age of 50 years, and fewer than 5% of cases are diagnosed before the age of 40. The peak incidence of diagnosis is in the seventh decade of life. Dietary factors play a role in carcinogenesis. Western diets, containing high fat and low fiber, have been associated with increased rates of colorectal cancer, as has the intake of red or processed meats and alcohol. It is likely that the low-fiber Western diet slows transit time, leading to increased exposure to carcinogens. Activity level also can play a role in carcinogenesis: studies have shown an increase in cancer among those with sedentary jobs and a decreased incidence among those who exercise regularly. Exposure to cigarette smoke increases the risk of colorectal adenomas and cancers. The American Cancer Society Cancer Prevention Study II revealed that 12% of colorectal cancer deaths in the general U.S. population can be attributed to smoking. Family history and genetics also play a significant role in carcinogenesis, because approximately 10% of patients diagnosed have a first-degree relative with colorectal cancer.

Adenomatous Polyps

The progression from normal mucosa to an adenomatous polyp and then to an invasive colorectal cancer proceeds through a well-defined process over many years. Aberrant crypt foci develop into microadenomas and then into adenomatous polyps. Dysplastic cells develop within the polyp, continue to multiply, become a tumor and then break through the subepithelial barrier and invade the layers of the bowel wall, eventually spreading to pericolic tissues or to lymph nodes and distant sites. A number of genes have been implicated in carcinogenesis, including protooncogenes (*KRAS, SRC, MYC*), tumor-suppressor genes (*APC, DCC, TP53, MCC, DPC4*), and DNA-mismatch repair genes (*HMSH2, MLH1, PMS1, PMS2, GTBP*). Sporadic colorectal cancers develop as a result of several cumulative genetic insults involving these genes (Figure 1).

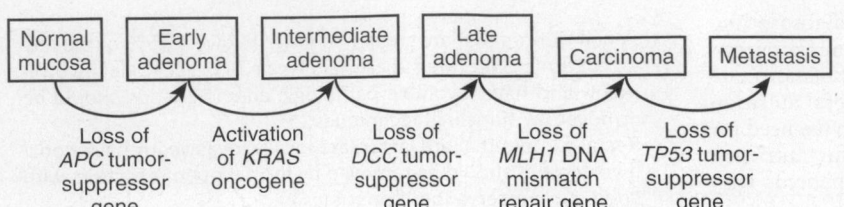

Figure 1. Sequence of progression from adenoma to carcinoma.

Familial Colorectal Cancer Syndromes

Familial adenomatous polyposis (FAP) is an inherited, non–sex-linked, mendelian dominant disease that accounts for approximately 1% of all colorectal cancers. The high penetrance of FAP means that there is a 50% chance of development of colorectal cancer among members of affected families. However, 20% of FAP patients have no family history, and their cases most likely represent new, spontaneous mutations. The disorder is caused by mutations in the tumor-suppressor *APC* gene, which is located on chromosome 5 (5q21–q22), or in the *MUTYH* gene, which is located on chromosome 1 (1p34.3–p32.1). FAP is characterized by the progressive development of hundreds or thousands of adenomatous polyps located throughout the entire colon. The clinical diagnosis is based on histologic confirmation of at least 100 adenomas. All patients eventually develop colorectal cancer. The adenomas typically appear by the mid-twenties, and cancers by the late thirties.

An attenuated form of FAP is recognized in which fewer adenomas (20–100) are identified. Adenomas and cancers develop somewhat later, at average ages of 44 and 56 years, respectively. FAP also exhibits extracolonic manifestations, including gastric, duodenal, and small-bowel polyps; osteomas and desmoid tumors (Gardner's syndrome); eye lesions (congenital hypertrophy of retinal pigment epithelium [CHRPE]); epidermoid cysts; and brain neoplasms (Turcot's syndrome).

Hereditary nonpolyposis colon cancer (HNPCC), also called Lynch syndrome, is an inherited, non–sex-linked, mendelian dominant disease with virtually complete penetrance. HNPCC is caused by a defect in any of a number of DNA-mismatch repair genes (*MLH1, MSH2, MSH6, PMS, PMS2*) that leads to high-level microsatellite instability (MSI-H). A number of criteria have been generated for the diagnosis of HNPCC, including the Amsterdam I and II criteria and the Bethesda guidelines (Box 1). According to the EPICOLON study, the revised Bethesda guidelines are the most discriminating set of clinical parameters for diagnosis of HNPCC.

HNPCC is subdivided into Lynch syndrome types I and II. Lynch type I refers to site-specific nonpolyposis colon cancer, and Lynch type II (formerly called familial cancer syndrome) refers to cancers that develop in the colon and related organs such as the endometrium, ovaries, stomach, pancreas, and proximal urinary tract, among others. Lynch syndrome differs from sporadic colorectal cancer in a number of important ways. It has an autosomal dominant inheritance, a predominance of proximal lesions (75% are found in the right colon), an excess of multiple primary colorectal cancers (18%), an early age at onset (average, 44 years), a significantly improved survival rate with right-sided lesions (53% at 5 years, compared with 35% for distal colorectal cancer in family members), and an increased risk for development of metachronous lesions (24%). Patients and family members of those diagnosed with HNPCC or FAP should undergo genetic testing to help improve future diagnosis and treatment options.

Inflammatory Bowel Disease

Both Crohn's disease and ulcerative colitis are associated with an increased risk of colorectal cancer; with the latter conferring approximately double the risk of the former. The duration and severity of Crohn's disease and the duration and extent (left-sided colitis versus pancolitis) of ulcerative colitis contribute to cancer risk in patients with inflammatory bowel disease. Cancer in Crohn's disease typically occurs in a stricture or bypassed segment.

Box 1 Diagnosis of Hereditary Nonpolyposis Colon Cancer (HNPCC)

Amsterdam I Criteria, 1990
- Three or more family members with histologically verified colorectal cancer, one of whom is a first-degree relative (parent, child, sibling) of the other two
- Two successive affected generations
- One or more colon cancers diagnosed before age 50 years
- Familial adenomatous polyposis has been excluded.

Amsterdam II Criteria, 1999
- Three or more family members with histologically verified HNPCC-related cancers (endometrium, ovary, stomach, small intestine, hepatobiliary, upper urinary tract, brain, or skin), one of whom is a first-degree relative (parent, child, sibling) of the other two
- Two successive affected generations
- One or more colon cancers diagnosed before age 50 years
- Familial adenomatous polyposis has been excluded.

Revised Bethesda Guidelines, 2002
- Colorectal cancer diagnosed in a patient who is younger than 50 years of age
- Presence of a synchronous, metachronous colorectal or other HNPCC-related malignancy, regardless of age
- Colorectal cancer with the high-level microsatellite instability (MSI-H) histology diagnosed in a patient who is younger than 60 years of age
  - Presence of carcinoma infiltrating lymphocytes, Crohn's-like lymphocytic reaction, mucinous/signet-ring differentiation, or medullary growth pattern
  - No general consensus based on this age
- Colorectal cancer diagnosed in one or more first-degree relatives with an HNPCC-related neoplasm
  - With one or more neoplasms being diagnosed before age 50 years
- Colorectal cancer diagnosed in two or more first- or second-degree relatives with HNPCC-related malignancies, regardless of age

---

Neoplasia in ulcerative colitis does not follow the adenoma-carcinoma development sequence seen in sporadic colorectal cancer, and this has important screening and treatment implications.

Evaluation

Screening Average-Risk Patients

Patients with no personal history of colorectal polyps or cancers, no personal history of inflammatory bowel disease, no symptoms suspicious for colorectal cancer, no family history of colorectal polyps or cancers, and no evidence of a familial or genetic syndrome may be screened as having average risk. The two main categories of screening tests are those that detect adenomatous polyps and cancers (flexible sigmoidoscopy, colonoscopy, double-contrast barium enema, and computed tomographic [CT] colonography) and those that primarily detect cancer (fecal occult blood testing, fecal immunohistochemical testing, and stool DNA testing). The goal of screening is to reduce mortality by reducing the incidence of advanced disease. It seems intuitive that tests that detect polyps, the premalignant phase of colorectal cancer, would be preferred to tests that detect only cancers. However, testing for polyps and cancers is usually procedure related, whereas testing for only cancers can be conducted on stool samples alone. Screening with simple stool samples has the potential to more easily increase overall screening.

Regardless of the method employed, testing in the average-risk, asymptomatic patient should begin at age 50 years. A total colonoscopy is required only every 10 years but involves oral bowel preparation and carries a small risk of perforation (approximately 1/1000). A flexible sigmoidoscopy is required every 5 years, in combination with annual fecal occult blood testing. Flexible sigmoidoscopy requires only enemas for preparation and carries a lower risk of perforation. Air-contrast barium enemas may be used for screening every 5 years, but they also require oral bowel preparation and are only diagnostic. CT colonography is an evolving method for screening every 5 years and offers the opportunity for more accessible screening; however, the procedure is limited in regard to identification of polyps smaller than 1 cm, also requires oral bowel prepation, and is only diagnostic. Fecal occult blood testing and fecal immunohistochemical testing are done annually. The interval for stool DNA testing is uncertain, and it tests only for a limited number of mutations. The most complete screening test, which allows removal of any precancerous lesions that are identified, remains the total colonoscopy.

Screening High-Risk Patients

High-risk patients include those with a personal history of colorectal polyps or cancers, a family history of colorectal cancer in a first-degree relative, Crohn's disease or ulcerative colitis, or a personal or family history of FAP or HNPCC. Screening in these patients has been adjusted for changes in incidence and age at onset of neoplasia (Table 1).

Symptoms and Diagnosis

Symptoms of colorectal cancer include bleeding (85%), a change in bowel habits, abdominal pain, malaise, and obstruction. Frequently, anemia is the only sign a patient exhibits. Patients with symptoms suspicious for colorectal cancer should undergo a colonoscopy. An anorectal source of bleeding should not preclude a complete colonic evaluation.

Management

Preoperative Management

Before operative intervention is undertaken, a complete evaluation should occur, including a careful history and physical examination, routine laboratory testing, and measurement of the level of carcinoembryonic antigen. A complete evaluation of the colon is essential, including colonoscopy with biopsy, or barium enema or CT colonography if colonoscopy is incomplete. Bowel preparation is no longer indicated as a routine preoperative measure for colonic surgery.

Preoperative staging should be undertaken for colorectal cancers. CT scanning of the abdomen and pelvis are indicated to aid in evaluating the extent of localized or metastatic disease and the presence of enlarged lymph nodes. Staging of rectal cancers includes determining the distance from the anal verge, frequently with the use of a rigid proctoscope; the depth of

TABLE 1	Screening High-Risk Patients for Colorectal Cancer		
RISK CATEGORY	**AGE TO BEGIN**	**RECOMMENDED TEST**	**COMMENT**
Personal history of <3 adenomas with low-grade dysplasia	5–10 y after the initial polypectomy	Colonoscopy	Examination interval should be based on other clinical factors, such as prior findings, family history, or endoscopist or patient preference.
Personal history of 3–10 adenomas, or 1 adenoma >1 cm, or any adenoma with villous features or high-grade dysplasia	3 y after the initial polypectomy	Colonoscopy	Adenomas require compete excision. If the follow-up is normal, the next examination should be in 5 y. Presence of >10 adenomas should raise suspicion of a familial syndrome.
Personal history of colorectal cancer	1 y after resection	Colonoscopy	Patients should undergo high-quality preoperative clearance. Follow up after normal examinations should be extended to 3 y and then to 5 y.
Family history of adenomas or cancer in a first-degree relative <60 y of age or in 2 first-degree relatives at any age	Age 40 y, or 10 y before the age at onset of youngest affected family member	Colonoscopy	Every 5 y
Family history of adenomas or cancer in a first-degree relative >60 y of age or in 2 second-degree relatives with cancer	Age 40 y	Colonoscopy	Screening should be initiated at an earlier age. Intervals are based on findings or on the average-risk patient.
FAP or suspected FAP	Age 10–12 y	Annual FS, counseling for genetic testing if showing polyps	Colectomy should be considered for positive genetic testing.
HNPCC or risk for HNPCC	Age 20–25 y, or 10 y before the age at onset of youngest affected family member	Colonoscopy, counseling for genetic testing	Every 1–2 y. Genetic testing should be offered to first-degree relatives of persons with a known DNA-mismatch repair gene defect or with 1 of the first 3 Bethesda criteria.
IBD, Crohn's disease, or chronic UC	8 y after the onset of pancolitis, or 12–15 y after the onset of left-sided colitis	Colonoscopies with random four-quadrant biopsies every 10 cm for dysplasia	Screening should be offered every 1–2 y, and patients are best referred to a center with experience in the surveillance and management of IBD.

Abbreviations: FAP = familial adenomatous polyposis; FS = flexible sigmoidoscopy; HNPCC = hereditary nonpolyposis colorectal cancer; IBD = inflammatory bowel disease.

invasion; and the presence of enlarged lymph nodes, using endorectal ultrasound or endoanal coil magnetic resonance imaging. Metastatic disease mandates neoadjuvant chemotherapy in the absence of acute symptoms of obstruction or exsanguination. Rectal cancers with evidence of local invasion into perirectal fat or adjacent structures or evidence of enlarged metastatic lymph nodes may benefit from neoadjuvant chemotherapy and irradiation. Preoperative staging allows for the application of neoadjuvant therapy in selected candidates, which can downstage and downsize tumors and can decrease rates of local recurrence in rectal cancer. Neoadjuvant therapy can also allow for sphincter-preserving procedures in patients with previously bulky or very low rectal tumors.

Surgery for Colonic Tumors

The primary therapy for tumors of the colon is operative. The basic principles of surgery for colon cancer are the following:

- Exploration: adequate visual, tactile, and potentially intraoperative hepatic ultrasound staging at the time of primary resection
- Removal of the entire cancer with enough proximal and distal bowel to encompass the possibility of submucosal lymphatic tumor spread
- Removal of the regional mesenteric pedicle, including draining lymphatics, based on the predictable lymphatic spread of the disease and the potential for regional mesenteric involvement without concurrent distant involvement
- En bloc resection of involved structures (T4 tumors)

Segmental colonic resections (right, transverse, left, or sigmoid colectomy) are undertaken based on the tumor location and blood supply with lymphatic drainage, specifically the ileocolic, middle colic, and left colic arteries. These arteries define a convenient anatomic boundary for standard colonic resection and also provide for adequate regional lymph node clearance, because the major draining lymphatics follow these blood vessels in the mesentery. Locally invasive tumors (T4) require en bloc resection of involved structures. Metastatic colonic tumors (M1) may require neoadjuvant chemotherapy before resection or palliation.

Numerous studies have verified that laparoscopic surgery is appropriate, and perhaps preferred, for colon cancer in experienced hands. The landmark Clinical Outcomes of Surgical Therapy (COST) trial in 2004 established that laparoscopic resection is equivalent to open resection for colon cancer.

Surgery for Rectal Tumors

Two approaches for rectal tumors are local excision and formal rectal resection. Local excision is the treatment of choice for a select, small group (3%–5% of all patients diagnosed with rectal cancer). Tumors amenable to transanal excision are small (<3 cm), involve less than 25% of the rectal circumference, are confined to the mucosa or submucosa (Tis or T1), lack nodal involvement by preoperative imaging, and have favorable pathologic characteristics (well or moderately differentiated with no lymphovascular invasion). Tumors in the lower or middle third of the rectum are accessible by simple transanal excision, but tumors of the upper rectum require the use of transanal endoscopic microsurgery (TEMS) techniques for resection. Local excision requires a 1-cm normal margin, but the defect usually does not require closure.

Tumors staged at T2 or greater require a formal resection, the type of which depends on the location of the tumor. Upper and middle rectal tumors can usually be managed with a low or very low anterior resection. Lower rectal tumors frequently require a proctectomy with coloanal anastomosis or an abdominoperineal resection. The goal of resection is to obtain a 5-cm distal margin, but lower tumors can be managed with a 2-cm distal margin. Very low tumors and those involving the sphincter mechanism require an abdominoperineal resection.

Rectal tumors with greater depth of rectal wall invasion (T3), evidence of fixation or local invasion (T4), or evidence of lymph nodal (N1–2) or metastatic (M1) disease mandates neoadjuvant chemoradiation therapy. Proctectomy requires a specimen-appropriate total mesorectal excision. This involves complete excision of all mesorectal tissue located behind the rectum with no carcinoma at the lateral or circumferential margins. The goal is to remove all malignant tissue, so as to reduce or eliminate the possibility of locally recurrent disease.

Locally advanced rectal tumors may preclude an effective or safe resection. Some indications for likely inoperability include extensive pelvic disease, invasion of ileofemoral vessels, extensive lymphatic involvement or significant lower extremity lymphedema, bony involvement, and life expectancy less than 3 to 6 months.

Laparoscopy is being performed for rectal malignancies in advanced centers, and studies are under way to verify the efficacy and safety of laparoscopic rectal resection in comparison with traditional open resection.

Complicated Disease

Colorectal tumors may manifest with complications such as obstruction, perforation, or significant bleeding. These presentations are generally related to more advanced disease and may preclude a complete staging work-up or potential neoadjuvant therapy. Unless patients are unstable or critically ill or the tumor is unresectable, the tumor should be appropriately resected. An ostomy is usually performed, whether as an end ostomy or as a proximal loop diversion for a primary anastomosis. Colonic stenting is an attractive option for obstructing lesions as palliation or as a bridge to resection after medical stabilization and staging for potential neoadjuvant therapy.

Surgery for High-Risk Conditions

High-risk conditions for the development of colorectal malignancies include FAP, HNPCC, and chronic ulcerative colitis. Surgical management may be prophylactic or possibly therapeutic after a malignancy has been diagnosed. The mainstay of operative management in FAP and chronic ulcerative colitis is a total proctocolectomy. Reconstructive options include an ileal pouch–anal anastomosis, a continent ileostomy (Kock pouch), or an end ileostomy. A total abdominal colectomy with ileorectal anastomosis may be performed for temporary preservation of rectal function in selected cases of chronic ulcerative colitis with rectal sparing and FAP with few rectal polyps, but this requires aggressive surveillance of the remaining rectal mucosa because of the risk of malignancy. Patients with HNPCC should also undergo subtotal colectomy with ileorectal anastomosis; because of the prevalence of associated gynecologic malignancies, a total hysterectomy with bilateral salpingo-oophorectomy should be offered to women as well.

Pathologic Staging and Adjuvant Therapy

Excellent pathologic sampling and review of the operative specimen provide important prognostic and therapeutic information. Current standards recommend that at least 12 lymph nodes be removed for adequate staging of colon cancer. The decision for adjuvant chemotherapy or radiation therapy or both is based on the pathologic staging. This information also provides prognostic information in terms of survival for the patient and family. A number of staging systems have been developed, but the tumor-node-metastasis (TNM) system is the one most commonly used in the United States (Table 2).

Chemotherapy is offered for patients who have colorectal cancers with locally advanced, nodal (stage III), or metastatic (stage IV) disease. The combination of chemotherapy and radiation therapy for advanced rectal cancer (stage II–IV) has decreased local recurrence and increased survival. Numerous protocols are available for treatment, with the standard of care being FOLFOX: oxaliplatin (Eloxatin), 5-fluorouracil (5-FU [Adrucil]), and leucovorin. Elderly patients and those with multiple comorbidities who may not be able to tolerate full-dose chemotherapy may be candidates for capecitabine (Xeloda) or 5-FU and leucovorin. Numerous study protocols are available at specialized centers evaluating other medications. Newer technologies continue to evolve, such as antiangiogenesis agents and immunomodulatory agents.

TABLE 2 Pathologic Staging Systems for Colorectal Cancer

PATHOLOGIC FEATURES	STAGE	TNM	DUKES	ASTLER-COLLER	5-YR SURVIVAL (%)
Depth of Invasion					
Lamina propria, muscularis mucosa	0	T0/Tis	A		>90
Submucosa	I	T1	A	B1	
Muscularis propria	I	T2	A	B1	
Subserosa, pericolic fat	II	T3	B	B1	70–85
Adjacent organs, perforation	II	T4	B	B2	55–65
Lymph Nodal Involvement					
None		N0			
1–3 nodes	III	N1	C	C1, C2	45–55
>3 nodes	III	N2	C	C1, C2	20–30
Distant Metastatic Disease					
Absent		M0			
Present	IV	M1	D		<5

Abbreviation: TNM = tumor-node-metastasis system.

Metastatic Disease

Surgical therapy is also available for metastatic disease in certain situations. Metastatic liver lesions amenable to resection can be addressed at the time of colon resection or after the patient has healed from colectomy. The lesions could be resected or treated with radiofrequency ablation, a newer technology that allows in situ destruction of liver lesions. Similarly, selected pulmonary metastases can be resected, possibly with the use of minimally invasive thoracoscopic techniques.

Surveillance

Surveillance for colon and rectal cancer is a lifelong process. Patients are seen and examined in the office every 3 months for 2 years, then every 6 months for 3 years, and then yearly for 5 years. Levels of carcinoembryonic antigen are measured at each office visit, but current literature recommends obtaining levels every 3 months for 3 years as a marker for tumor recurrence in stage II–III patients. Colonoscopy should be performed at 1 year postoperatively, assuming a high-quality preoperative study has cleared the rest of the colon. A normal colonoscopy at 1 year postoperatively would allow the next surveillance colonoscopy to be performed 3 years later. If that one is normal, subsequent examinations should be performed every 5 years. After the examination at 1 year postoperatively, the subsequent intervals should be shortened if there is evidence of HNPCC or if additional adenomas are found. As an addition to formal colonoscopies, flexible sigmoidoscopies are performed with each office visit for patients with rectal cancer. Routine imaging utilizing CT scans of the chest, abdomen, and pelvis is performed annually for 3 years in patients with colorectal cancer. Patients with increased or rising CEA levels, as noted by routine surveillance checks, or evidence of recurrent disease, as noted by history and physical examinations or routine surveillance imaging studies, can be evaluated with the use of positron emission tomography (PET), an emerging sensitive test for tumor recurrence.

References

American Cancer Society. Cancer Facts and Figures 2013, Atlanta, GA: American Cancer Society; 2013. Available at: http://www.cancer.org/Research/CancerFactsFigures/CancerFactsFigures/cancer-facts-figures-2013 [accessed August 25, 2014].

Beart RW, Steele Jr GD, Menck HR, et al. Management and survival of patients with adenocarcinoma of the colon and rectum: A national survey of the Commission on Cancer. J Am Coll Surg 1995;181:225–36.

Bentrem DJ, Okabe S, Wong WD, et al. T1 Adenocarcinoma of the rectum: Transanal excision or radical surgery? Ann Surg 2005;242:472–9.

Clinical Outcomes of Surgical Therapy Study Group. A comparison of laparoscopically assisted and open colectomy for colon cancer. N Engl J Med 2004;350:2050–9.

Desch CE, Benson 3rd. AB, Somerfield MR, et al. Colorectal cancer surveillance: 2005 update of an American Society of Clinical Oncology Practice Guideline. J Clin Oncol 2005;23(33):8512–9.

Floyd ND, Saclarides TJ. Transanal endoscopic microsurgical resection of pT1 rectal tumors. Dis Colon Rectum 2005;49:164–8.

Lan Y-T, Lin J-K, Li AF-Y, et al. Metachronous colorectal cancer: Necessity of postoperative colonoscopic surveillance. Int J Colorectal Dis 2005;20:121–5.

Levin B, Lieberman DA, McFarland B, et al. Screening and surveillance for the early detection of colorectal cancer and adenomatous polyps, 2008: A joint guideline from the American Cancer Society, the US Multi-Society Task Force on Colorectal Cancer, and the American College of Radiology. For the American Cancer Society Colorectal Cancer Advisory Group, the US Multi-Society Task Force, and the American College of Radiology Colon Cancer Committee. Gastroenterology 2008;134:1570–95.

Maetani I, Tada T, Ukita T, et al. Self-expandable metallic stent placement as palliative treatment of obstructed colorectal carcinoma. J Gastroenterol 2004;39:334–8.

Pinol V, Castells A, Andreu M, et al. Accuracy of Revised Bethesda Guidelines, microsatellite instability, and immunohistochemistry for the identification of patients with hereditary nonpolyposis colorectal cancer. JAMA 2005;293:1986–94.

Rex DK, Kahi CJ, Levin B, et al. Guidelines for colonoscopy surveillance after cancer resection: A consensus update by the American Cancer Society and the US Multi-Society Task Force on Colorectal Cancer. Gastroenterology 2006;130:1865–71.

Sauer R, Becker H, Hohenberger W, et al. for the German Rectal Cancer Study Group: Preoperative versus postoperative chemoradiotherapy for rectal cancer. N Engl J Med 2004;351:1731–40.

Stipa F, Chessin DB, Shia J, et al. A pathologic complete response of rectal cancer to preoperative combined-modality therapy results in improved oncological outcome compared with those who achieve no downstaging on the basis of preoperative endorectal ultrasonography. Ann Surg Oncol 2006;13(8):1047–53.

Winawer SJ, Zauber AG, Fletcher RH, et al. Guidelines for colonoscopy surveillance after polypectomy: A consensus update by the US Multi-Society Task Force on Colorectal Cancer and the American Cancer Society. CA Cancer J Clin 2006;56:143–59.

TUMORS OF THE STOMACH

Method of
Scott A. Hundahl, MD

CURRENT DIAGNOSIS

- Intestinal metaplasia, which predisposes to cancer, results from chronic *Helicobacter pylori* infection.
- In the United States, screening studies are reserved for those with definite risk factors.
- Pretreatment staging drives subsequent treatment and involves endoscopy, endoscopic ultrasound, helical computed tomography, and often laparoscopy or mini-laparotomy.

- Mucosal abnormalities can be largely absent in early gastrointestinal stromal tumors, small carcinoids, and even diffuse-type linitis plastica. Deep endoscopic biopsies are required.

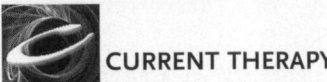 CURRENT THERAPY

Adenocarcinoma
- To ensure complete surgical resection, resection should be customized (e.g., gross margin, use of endoscopic mucosal resection for certain mucosal tumors).
- Survival is highest with low Maruyama Index surgery.
- Adjuvant therapy options include preoperative chemotherapy (± postoperative treatment), or postoperative chemoradiation

Gastrointestinal Stromal Tumors
- Node dissection is not indicated.

Gastric Lymphoma
- For aggressive diffuse-type lymphomas, chemotherapy with or without radiation therapy is now the mainstay of treatment. Surgery is reserved for complications such as acute perforation.
- Superficial mucosa-associated lymphoid tissue tumors can sometimes be treated by simply eliminating *Helicobacter pylori* infection. It comes back if reinfection occurs, however.

Gastric Adenocarcinoma
Thanks to happy accident rather than specific planning, over the past 80 years, gastric adenocarcinoma has changed from the most-common solid organ malignancy in the United States to a relatively uncommon disease. Worldwide, however, it remains a scourge second only to lung cancer.

Classification and Epidemiology
Several classification schemes exist. Two are commonly used. Bormann's morphologic classification relies on gross characteristics of the tumor. The histologic classification of Lauren, first described by Jarvi and Lauren in 1951, divides gastric adenocarcinomas into intestinal (gland-forming) and diffuse (discohesive) types, based on their microscopic appearance. Several other classification schemes have been proposed, including Broder's classification of differentiation, the World Health Organization (WHO) classification, the Nagayo–Komagome classification, the Ming classification, and the Goseki classification, but none eclipses the Lauren classification.

Epidemiologically, three patterns of disease can be discerned, with *Helicobacter pylori* infection playing an important role in the first two patterns: intestinal-type tumors arising from the lesser curve and distal stomach, related to *H. pylori*–associated atrophic gastritis and intestinal metaplasia; diffuse-type tumors involving the body of the stomach, often associated with intense *H. pylori*–associated inflammation but not associated with significant intestinal metaplasia; and intestinal-type tumors of the gastroesophageal junction.

In high-incidence regions of the world, such as Japan and Korea, up to two thirds of gastric adenocarcinomas are of the first type and are strongly associated with chronic multifocal atrophic gastritis and intestinal metaplasia from chronic *H. pylori* infection. The process usually begins at the antrum–corpus junction along the lesser curvature and predisposes to cancers of the intestinal type occurring in the sixth or seventh decades of life. The second type of gastric adenocarcinoma, also associated with *H. pylori*, afflicts younger persons in the fourth and fifth decades of life. The last type, seen in lower-incidence regions of the world such as the United States, is associated with chronic gastroesophageal reflux and Barrett's esophagitis.

Epidemiologists and public health experts estimate that more than 40% of gastric adenocarcinomas worldwide can be attributed to chronic *H. pylori* infection. Strains containing the *cagA* gene appear more dangerous. The infection usually starts by the second or third decade, and unless it is successfully treated, it gives rise to chronic inflammation, atrophic gastritis, and eventually intestinal metaplasia, which is a premalignant histologic condition. Dietary factors such as high salt and high nitrates can accentuate this progression as well as the march to cancer. As the condition progresses, acid-producing oxyntic mucosa is progressively wiped out, gastric pH increases, and bacterial overgrowth with non–*H. pylori* bacteria is facilitated. The original *H. pylori*, which requires an acid environment to thrive, often disappears at this point.

Once intestinal metaplasia is established, dietary factors become particularly important in mitigating the risk of cancer development. Protective factors include intake of vitamin C, fresh fruits and vegetables, and antioxidants. The association of *H. pylori* infection with the development of intestinal metaplasia suggests that early detection and elimination of this infection might prevent gastric cancer. Unfortunately, in high-incidence areas, reinfection from contaminated water supply and other sources is common, thus undermining the strategy. Also, in prevention trials to date, benefit appears restricted to the subgroups without preexisting intestinal metaplasia.

Risk Factors
Risk factors other than *H. pylori* infection include low socioeconomic status, smoking, a diet deficient in fresh fruits and vegetables or high in salt-preserved high-nitrate foods, previous gastric ulcer, ionizing radiation, family history, and previous gastric resection. Blood group A is associated with higher risk of developing a diffuse-type tumor. Predisposing genetic conditions include the Lynch's syndrome (hereditary nonpolyposis colorectal cancer [HNPCC], a condition with microsatellite instability due to deficient DNA repair enzymes), as well as dominantly inherited germline mutations in the E-cadherin gene.

Diagnosis
In Western populations, by the time gastric cancer causes symptoms, the disease is often relatively advanced. In a large National Cancer Data Base survey of U.S. patients, presenting ascribable symptoms included weight loss (62%), abdominal or epigastric pain (52%), nausea (34%), anorexia (32%), early satiety (32%), dysphagia (26%), and melena (18%).

Mass screening combining upper GI series, endoscopy, and serum pepsinogen I/II ratio have proved beneficial in high-incidence areas such as Japan, but they cannot be justified in the United States, where incidence is low. However, for defined risk groups, such as those with established atrophic gastritis and established intestinal metaplasia, strong family history, and those with HNPCC syndrome, surveillance screening should definitely be considered. For those with hereditary E-cadherin mutations associated with gastric cancer, prophylactic total gastrectomy is recommended.

In the United States, diagnosis is usually made by upper endoscopy. One should be aware that diffuse-type cancers manifesting as linitis plastica are often associated with minimal visible mucosal changes, and deep biopsies are often required for establishing the diagnosis. Furthermore, small, early gastric cancers (defined by the Japanese as in situ and T-1 cancers, with or without node involvement) can be associated with particularly subtle mucosal changes, presenting a challenge for even the most experienced endoscopist. Chromoendoscopy and other sophisticated mucosal imaging techniques have been used to identify such changes but are not yet standard.

Extent-of-disease studies for gastric adenocarcinoma include endoscopic ultrasound (good for estimating depth of tumor and visualizing immediately adjacent nodes), and helical CT scanning, which is good for evaluating extraluminal extent of disease, intraabdominal or mediastinal extension or spread, and liver or lung metastases. Because even high-resolution CT scanning can miss small peritoneal implants, extraregional nodal spread, and small liver metastases, staging laparoscopy or minilaparotomy are valuable adjuncts and should be considered mandatory if any preoperative chemotherapy is considered.

Staging

Seventh Edition American Joint Committee on Cancer/International Union Against Cancer (AJCC/UICC) staging, to be applied to cases diagnosed after Jan. 1, 2010, mandates a number of major changes. For example, any tumor arising in the upper 5 cm of the stomach and extending cephalad to involve the esophagogastric junction is now deemed an esophageal cancer. Also, to avoid confusion, 7th Edition staging now harmonizes the T-category designations among esophagus, small intestine, and colon sites. T1 tumors, which involve mucosa or submucosa, are now sub-categorized T1a or T1b accordingly. T2 tumors involve the muscularis propria. T3 tumors penetrate to subserosal connective tissue without breaching the visceral peritoneum. T4 tumors breach the serosa (T4a) or invade adjacent structures (T4b). Nodal categories have also changed, with N1 now reflecting 1 to 2 nodes involved, N2 designating 3 to 6 nodes involved, and N3 designating 7 or more nodes involved. In the overall TNM staging matrix, Stage IV is now restricted to patients with documented peritoneal (including positive peritoneal washing cytology), distant-organ, or extraregional nodal metastases. As a result of these changes, stage migration between 6th edition and 7th edition AJCC/UICC staging is high, more than 50% in most reports.

Treatment

Curative treatment of gastric cancer involves, as main therapy, complete negative-margin surgical resection of disease. For select tumors, such resection sometimes follows up-front chemotherapy. For localized in situ and select T1 tumors, endoscopic mucosal resection and minimally invasive techniques have been successfully employed. Unfortunately, most tumors in the United States are discovered at a stage where formal open surgery is required.

To secure a histologically negative mural margin of resection, a gross margin of 2 cm is usually adequate for exophytic, noninfiltrating tumors, and a margin of at least 5 to 6 cm of grossly normal tissue is recommended for ulcerated or infiltrating tumors or diffuse histology. Closest mural margins are generally checked by frozen section at the time of surgery to confirm adequacy of resection. Total gastrectomy is not indicated as a routine procedure, except in diffuse-type tumors involving most of the stomach (linitis plastica), but it is warranted whenever required for a negative-margin resection.

Routine splenectomy in the treatment of gastric cancer, as well as routine distal pancreatectomy (performed in the past to clear splenic nodes), should be avoided unless definitely required for complete resection of visible or palpable disease.

The optimal extent of lymph node dissection in this disease has generated—and continues to generate—international controversy. Although several prospective randomized trials to date in non-Asian populations—none perfect—fail to demonstrate that routine extensive lymphadenectomy increases survival, it has also been shown that insufficient lymphadenectomy definitely compromises survival. A prospective randomized single-institution trial in Taipei has documented survival benefit associated with radical lymph node dissection. The adequacy of lymphadenectomy for a given case can be quantified using the Maruyama Index of Unresected Disease. In both a large U.S. adjuvant chemoradiation trial and in a blinded reanalysis of a large Dutch surgical trial, low Maruyama Index score correlates with survival. Moreover, a dose–response effect is seen for the extent of surgical clearance of node groups at risk. Using the Maruyama computer program to predict the extent of nodal spread for a given cancer case before surgery is one way to facilitate a low Maruyama Index operation.

Sentinel node biopsy, an established technique in the treatment of other cancers, has largely failed to win support in cancer of the stomach owing to the organ's lymphatic complexity and relatively high reported false-negative rates.

A large North American prospective randomized trial of postoperative adjuvant 5-fluorouracil–based chemoradiation in completely resected gastric cancer revealed a significant increase in disease-free and overall survival with this treatment. The postoperative nature of this trial thwarted implementation of surgical guidelines, and the extent of node dissection for most patients in the trial was suboptimal. Practitioners in some countries, such as Japan, dismiss the necessity of adjuvant postoperative adjuvant chemoradiation with the (unproved but reasonable) argument that this is only a salvage technique for inadequate surgery. A separate Korean chemoradiation series has shown benefit even for radically treated cases, however. For patients with good postoperative performance status, good organ function, and adequate nutrition, postoperative adjuvant chemoradiation therapy remains the standard in North America.

A recent U.K. study of preoperative plus postoperative ECF (epirubicin [Ellence],[1] cis-platinum, and continuous-infusion 5-fluorouracil [Adrucil]) chemotherapy versus surgery alone has shown encouraging results for ECF, with a significant improvement in survival. Previous preoperative chemotherapy trials, using other regimens, have been negative, however. Preoperative ECF chemotherapy is now recommended by some, and this is especially the case for localized advanced tumors considered borderline resectable.

In Korea, a positive trial of adjuvant perioperative intraperitoneal chemotherapy has been reported. Considerable morbidity and mortality are associated with this adjuvant treatment, however, and it is unlikely it will be implemented without refinement and successful independent duplication of results.

For localized disease deemed not resectable to negative margins, both chemotherapy and chemoradiation have been used to convert such tumors to potentially resectable status. With successful negative-margin resection, some of these patients indeed survive free of disease long term. When localized unresected disease is documented to exist, administering chemoradiation with 5-fluorouracil as a radiation sensitizer can also result in some degree of 5-year survival (per reports, >10%).

Gastrointestinal Stromal Tumors

Gastrointestinal stromal tumors (GISTs) manifest as submucosal spindle cell tumors in the sarcoma family. In contrast to leiomyosarcomas and other spindle cell sarcomas, they express the antigen CD117 and most (>80%) tumors have activating mutations of c-KIT. Formerly considered rare, approximately 5000 of these tumors per year are now diagnosed in the United States. Owing to pattern of growth in the gastric wall, deep to the mucosa, early symptoms are unusual and these tumors often grow to massive size before mucosal ulceration and hemorrhage (or other major symptoms) finally develop. GISTs are classified as sarcomas. Even low-risk GISTs (<5 cm and <1 mitosis per 10 high-power fields) can metastasize, and no GIST can be considered truly benign.

Treatment of localized primary GISTs consists of complete surgical resection, and a 2-cm margin of grossly normal tissue usually accomplishes this. Specific lymph node dissection is not indicated for this histology. Surgical series indicate that approximately 50% of primary gastric tumors metastasize and recur within 5 years. For patients with widespread metastases, generally located in the peritoneal cavity or the liver, first-line therapy is now a well-tolerated oral agent, imatinib mesylate (Gleevec or STI-571) at an initial dose of 400 mg daily, which generates partial responses in more than 50% of cases and stable disease in an additional 25% of cases. Side effects are minimal, and 1-year survival in treated patients is approximately 85%. On the basis of a completed American College of Surgeons Oncology Group (ACOSOG) trial, patients who have all disease completely resected should receive postoperative adjuvant therapy for 1 year.

---

[1]Not FDA approved for this indication.

For tumors resistant to imatinib, SU11248, sunitinib malate (Sutent), is now used as effective second-line therapy. Additional targeted biological agents are under active investigation.

Carcinoid Tumors

Carcinoid tumors of the stomach are similar in behavior to small bowel carcinoids. When small (<1 cm), and unassociated with invasion of the muscularis propria, local excision to negative margins is generally deemed sufficient. For such tumors, endoscopic resection has an established role. However, even small tumors can metastasize to lymph nodes. Wider gastrectomy with lymph node dissection is generally recommended for gastric tumors larger than 1 cm. Many of these tumors are associated with serum hypergastrinemia; those without this finding tend to be more aggressive. When metastatic to the liver or other organs, surgical cytoreduction (or other means of tumor ablation) can offer considerable palliation to those with carcinoid syndrome, and this should always be considered. Octreotide therapy is now a palliative mainstay in all patients with carcinoid syndrome.

Gastric Lymphomas

Gastric lymphomas encompass most of the lymphoma subtypes, but low-grade, mucosa-associated B-cell lymphomas (B-cell MALT lymphomas) deserve special mention because they are strongly associated with *H. pylori* infection. Indeed, localized cases can be controlled simply by treating the *H. pylori* infection. In such cases, molecular studies indicate persistence of the offending lymphoid clone in about one half of cases. However, and, particularly if *H. pylori* infection recurs, the lymphoma in such cases returns.

Aggressive, high-grade, diffuse-type B-cell gastric lymphomas, stage IE and IIE, once treated with multimodal therapy, are now treated with chemotherapy alone as the primary treatment, with or without radiotherapy. Surgical intervention is now reserved for emergencies, such as perforation.

For further information on this and other gastrointestinal lymphomas, please see the chapter on lymphoma.

References

Cunningham D, Allum WH, Stenning SP, et al. Perioperative chemotherapy versus surgery alone for resectable gastroesophageal cancer. N Engl J Med 2006;355(1):11–20.

Ferrucci PF, Zucca E. Primary gastric lymphoma pathogenesis and treatment: What has changed over the past 10 years? Br J Haematol 2007;136(4):521–38.

Fritz AG, Greene FL, Trotti A, editors. AJCC Cancer Staging Manual. 7th ed. 2010.

Hundahl SA, Macdonald JS, Benedetti J, et al. Surgical treatment variation in a prospective, randomized trial of chemoradiotherapy in gastric cancer: The effect of undertreatment. Ann Surg Oncol 2002;9(3):278–86.

Hundahl SA, Peeters KC, Kranenbarg EK, et al. Improved regional control and survival with "low Maruyama Index" surgery in gastric cancer: Autopsy findings from the Dutch D1-D2 Trial. Gastric Cancer 2007;10(2):84–6.

Macdonald JS, Smalley SR, Benedetti J, et al. Chemoradiotherapy after surgery compared with surgery alone for adenocarcinoma of the stomach or gastroesophageal junction. N Engl J Med 2001;345(10):725–30.

Modlin IM, Kidd M, Latich I, et al. Current status of gastrointestinal carcinoids. Gastroenterology 2005;128(6):1717–51.

Siehl J, Thiel E. C-kit, GIST, and imatinib. Recent Results. Cancer Res 2007;176:145–51.

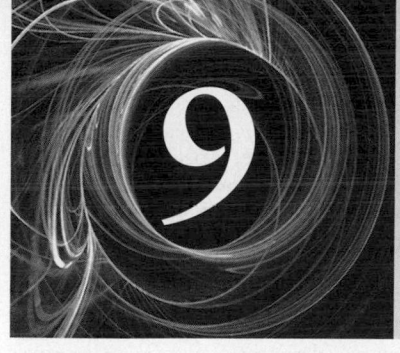

9 Rheumatology and the Musculoskeletal System

ANKYLOSING SPONDYLITIS

Method of
John D. Reveille, MD

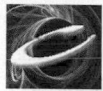

CURRENT DIAGNOSIS

- The diagnosis of ankylosing spondylitis rests on the presence of inflammatory back pain or restriction of spinal mobility in the presence of radiographic sacroiliitis.
- Generally, sacroiliitis as determined by standard radiographs does not appear until after 7 to 10 years of inflammatory back pain.
- When inflammatory back pain is present with other stigmata of spondyloarthritis (e.g., uveitis, enthesitis, inflammatory bowel disease) and standard radiographs are normal, MRI scanning of the sacroiliac joints or HLA-B27 testing, or both, can provide important diagnostic information.

CURRENT THERAPY

- Nearly half of patients with ankylosing spondylitis respond to high doses of nonsteroidal antiinflammatory drugs (NSAIDs) alone.
- Disease-modifying anti-rheumatic drugs (DMARDs), such as sulfasalazine (Azulfidine),[1] methotrexate (Trexall),[1] or leflunomide (Arava)[1], are effective for peripheral arthritis but not for axial disease.
- Anti–tumor necrosis factor treatment is very effective in controlling inflammatory symptoms in patients who do not respond adequately to NSAIDs and DMARDs.

[1]Not FDA approved for this indication.

The term *ankylosing spondylitis* (AS), part of the spectrum of disease known as axial spondyloarthritis, comprises a group of chronic inflammatory diseases characterized by spinal and peripheral joint oligoarthritis, inflammation of the attachments of ligaments and tendons to bones (enthesitis), and, at times ocular or cardiac manifestations.

Epidemiology
The prevalence of AS parallels the frequency of HLA-B27. AS occurs in approximately 0.5% of persons of European descent and eastern Asian descent, with B27 seen in 8% and 6%, respectively. Higher incidences of AS are reported in eastern Europe and Scandinavia, where HLA-B27 is more common, and in certain Native American groups. AS is rare in Africans and Japanese, where HLA-B27 is rare. Men are affected three times more commonly than women. Recent data from the National Health and Nutrition Examination Survey have estimated the prevalence of axial spondyloarthritis to occur in more than one percent of the U.S. population.

Pathophysiology
AS is caused primarily by genetic factors, with a sibling recurrence risk ratio as high as 82 and twin-based studies estimating disease heritability to exceed 90%. The major histocompatibility complex (MHC) gene HLA-B27 confers the greatest known risk for AS and is found in up to 90% of patients of European and East Asian ancestry (although AS patients from the Middle East and Africa have lower B27 frequencies).

How HLA-B27 contributes to the pathogenesis of AS is not known. One theory is the arthritogenic peptide hypothesis: that AS results from HLA-B27 binding a unique peptide or a set of antigenic peptides derived from either triggering microorganisms or from self proteins. To date, however, none have been identified. In fact, recent data have shown that another gene that has been associated with AS worldwide: endoplasmic reticulum aminopeptidase (ERAP1)-which is involved in trimming peptides to the optimal length for loading onto the peptide binding groove for MHC class I presentation interacts with HLA-B27, resulting in *aberrant peptide presentation*. Secondly, HLA-B27 heavy chains self-associate to form homodimers, which can with misfold in the endoplasmic reticulum, resulting in a proinflammatory unfolded protein response and be recognized at the cell surface by natural killer cells. A third hypothesis is that AS results from inability to effectively combat certain infections, such as from gut infection (i.e. alterations in the gut microbiome). HLA-B27–positive persons are more efficient at dealing with certain infections (hepatitis C and HIV) and less efficient at dealing with others (*Salmonella, Shigella, Chlamydia* species, and others). Older studies have implicated *Klebsiella pneumoniae*, although recent data have not borne this out. How these factors initiate disease onset is not known.

Less than 5% of HLA-B27–positive people in the general population develop AS or other spondyloarthritis, as opposed to 20% of HLA-B27–positive relatives of AS patients. Data from family studies and genomewide association studies have shown that most of the overall genetic risk for AS comes from HLA-B27. Other MHC genes, such as HLA-B60 (B*40:01) and MICA all contribute to susceptibility.

Over 42 non-MHC genes have been implicated in AS susceptibility, including those involved in IL-17 mediated immunity (*IL23R, TYK2, IL6R, IL7R?, IL7?, IL1R2/IL1R1, IL12B*), CD8 T cell function (*RUNX3, EOMES, IL7R*), peptide presentation (*ERAP1, ERAP2, LNPEPP, NPEPPS*), microbial sensing (*CARD9, NOS2*) as well as a number of others relevant to immune function (*ZMIZ1, FCGR2A, KIF21B, SH2B3, TNFRSF1A, GPR65, SULT1A1, GPR35, BACH2, ICOSLG, NKX2-3*).

Clinical Manifestations
The hallmark of AS is inflammatory back pain. This pain is classically characterized as a dull pain in the low back or in the buttocks and hips that begins before the age of 40 years, has an insidious onset, and lasts longer than 3 months. Inflammatory back pain is

associated with morning stiffness lasting 30 minutes or longer, which responds readily to nonsteroidal antiinflammatory drugs (NSAIDs), is relieved with activity and worsened with rest, and often awakens the patient during the second half of the night. As the disease progresses, patients can develop limitation of spinal mobility, loss of lumbar and cervical lordosis, and kyphotic deformities of the spine. This limitation of motion is initially the result of axial inflammation and muscle spasm but is contributed to over time by ossification of the ligamentous structures and ultimately bony fusion of the sacroiliac joints, apophyseal joints, and the outer fibers of the annulus fibrosis of the intervertebral disks.

Arthritis of the hips occurs in approximately 50% of patients with AS. About 10% of AS patients have arthritis of the joints of the hands, feet, wrists, and ankles. Enthesitis, inflammation of tendinous or ligamentous insertions onto bone, is one of the most characteristic findings of the AS and other spondyloarthritides, especially in the Achilles tendon and the plantar fascial insertions, although involvement of the ligamentous and tendinous insertions onto the pelvic bones is also encountered. Dactylitis or sausage digits—fusiform swelling of the entire digit due to inflammation and swelling of the flexor tenosynovium—also occasionally occurs.

AS also affects the gastrointestinal tract and eyes. About 6% of AS patients have inflammatory bowel disease (Crohn's disease or ulcerative colitis), and asymptomatic bowel inflammation is seen on ileocolonoscopy in up to 50% of patients with AS. Anterior uveitis occurs in about 40% of AS patients. It is usually unilateral with sudden onset, manifesting as a painful red eye with photophobia and blurred vision. It can recur periodically, although is rarely associated with permanent loss of vision. Similarly, about 10% of AS patients have psoriasis.

Diagnosis

The diagnosis of AS rests on the presence of inflammatory spinal pain or restriction of spinal and chest wall motion occurring in the setting of radiographic sacroiliitis (sclerosis, erosion, and even ankylosis of the sacroiliac joints). Plain radiographs of the spine show Romanus lesions (shiny corners) and squaring of the vertebral body owing to erosions at the attachments of the spinal ligaments early in disease, followed by formation of syndesmophytes owing to ossification of the outer layer of the annulus fibrosis and eventual ankylosis of the spine, producing a bamboo spine appearance.

Abnormalities on standard radiographs typically are not seen until up to 8 to 11 years after disease onset, leading to a significant delay in diagnosis and initiation of therapy. Radiographic changes can be detected with magnetic resonance imaging (MRI) years before the appearance of radiographic disease, with bone marrow edema adjacent to the inflamed sacroiliac joint and spinal joints. This preradiographic disease has resulted in the concept of axial spondyloarthritis, for which new criteria have been developed based on the presence of inflammatory back pain accompanied by the presence of a positive MRI or HLA-B27 typing and other spondyloarthritis features (e.g., uveitis, enthesitis).

Differential Diagnosis

Diffuse idiopathic skeletal hyperostosis (DISH) is a disease of older persons, predominantly men, characterized by low back pain and stiffness. Characteristic findings are flowing calcification and ossification along the anterolateral segment of at least four contiguous vertebral bodies with the relative preservation of intervertebral disk height and the absence of apophyseal joint ankylosis. The sacroiliac joints are characteristically spared or show degenerative changes but not erosion or fusion, and the back pain is usually mechanical in nature.

Osteitis condensans ilii is a condition primarily noted in young multiparous women. It consists of increased bone density generally confined to a triangular area along the inferior aspect of the ilium adjacent to the sacroiliac joint. It is usually asymptomatic, and erosions and intra-articular ankylosis are rare.

Ochronosis is a rare hereditary metabolic disease in which the enzyme homogentisic acid oxidase is absent. It is characterized by abnormal pigmentation of the sclerae and ears. Ochronotic arthropathy manifests in the fourth decade, especially in the hips, knees, and shoulders. Although the spine can appear fused as in AS, characteristic findings include loss of disk height and calcification of the disks, which are not seen in AS.

Treatment

A great deal of educational information is available for patients (www.spondylitis.org). Unsupervised recreational exercise improves pain and stiffness, and back exercise improves pain and function in patients with AS, but these effects differ with disease duration. Health status is improved when patients perform recreational exercise at least 30 minutes per day and back exercises at least 5 days per week.

NSAIDs, used in high (antiinflammatory) doses on a daily basis, remain the starting point of treatment of spondylitis, and up to half of AS patients attain satisfactory symptom control with these agents alone. There are no strong data to suggest the superiority of any specific NSAID in patients with AS.

Disease-modifying antiinflammatory drugs (DMARDs), especially sulfasalazine (Azulfidine)[1] in doses of 2 to 3 g/day, but also methotrexate (Trexall)[1] (up to 25 mg once a week) and leflunomide ([Arava][1] 20 mg per day) are effective in the treatment of peripheral joint involvement in AS, although not in axial disease.

Glucocorticoids such as prednisone (5–15 mg/day) are occasionally used by clinicians to augment the effect of NSAIDs, although owing to unproven efficacy and side effects, including osteoporosis, they are not recommended unless other treatments are not available. Intraarticular and peritendinous injections of depot steroids can provide relief of local flare-ups, although injecting around the Achilles tendon is not recommended because of the risk of tendon rupture.

TNF-α blockers have become a mainstay in AS treatment for those not responding to NSAIDs and DMARDs. Currently five are approved by the FDA for use in AS. Four are injected subcutaneously, including the soluble TNF-α receptor etanercept (Enbrel), given at 50 mg weekly, and the TNF-α monoclonal antibodies adalimumab (Humira) 40 mg every 2 weeks and golimumab (Simponi) 50 mg once a month and certolizumab pegol, 200 mg twice a month or 400 mg once per month. In addition, the TNF-α monoclonal antibody infliximab (Remicade) is infused at 5 mg/kg every 6 to 8 weeks intravenously. These medications have been shown to be beneficial in both the axial and peripheral manifestations of AS. Onset of action is rapid, and improvement is seen not only clinically but also on MRI, with clearing of bone marrow edema. Anti-TNF treatment is expensive, and complications can include infusion or injection site reactions, infections (especially from *Mycoplasma tuberculosis*), lymphoma (though not other malignancies), and the development of antinuclear antibodies following anti-TNF treatment, although reports of patients developing systemic lupus erythematosus or other connective tissue disease are rare.

Patients with AS also require surgical treatment on occasion. Total hip arthroplasty is the most common surgical procedure in patients with AS, and heterotopic new bone formation can be a potential problem. Patients with AS are at increased risk for vertebral fracture, often resulting in neurologic compromise due to osteoporosis. In general, halo vest immobilization is recommended. Surgical intervention may be necessary when neurologic impairment is seen. Also, osteotomies (open, polysegmental, and closing wedge) are occasionally employed to correct the fixed kyphotic deformities seen in patients with advanced AS.

Monitoring

The most widely used clinical measure of disease activity is the Bath Ankylosing Spondylitis Disease Activity (BASDAI) measure, a self-reported questionnaire consisting of six 10-cm horizontal visual analogue scales. This has been replaced recently by the Ankylosing Spondylitis Disease Activity Score (ASDAS), which includes elements of the BASDAI, a patient global assessment of

---

[1]Not FDA approved for this indication.

disease activity, and C-reactive protein (CRP) or erythrocyte sedimentation rate (ESR) assessments. It measures severity of fatigue, spinal and peripheral joint pain, localized tenderness, and morning stiffness. Functional impairment is measured by the Bath Ankylosing Spondylitis Functional Index (BASFI), another self-reported questionnaire with ten 10-cm visual analogue scales, including eight AS-specific questions and two on coping and daily life. Spinal mobility can be assessed by specific physical examination maneuvers, such as the Schober test, which measures lumbar flexion; chest wall expansion, which assesses costovertebral joint involvement; the occiput-to-wall measurement, which assesses cervical extension; and the lateral bending maneuver.

Laboratory markers of disease include C-reactive protein (CRP) and erythrocyte sedimentation rate (ESR). Radiographic severity is measured by the Modified Stoke Ankylosing Spondylitis Spinal Score (mSASSS), a detailed scoring system comparable to the modified Sharp Score in rheumatoid arthritis. However, standard radiographs are complicated by low sensitivity to change and are not useful in gauging disease activity. MRI scanning is more helpful, particularly in measuring early or "pre-radiographic" disease activity, and has its highest specificity in the sacroiliac joints.

Complications

Cardiac manifestations, including conduction abnormalities and aortic valvular insufficiency, occasionally are seen in AS patients. The spectrum of pulmonary involvement in AS ranges from restricted chest wall movement from costovertebral joint fusion to a rare upper lobe–predominant interstitial lung disease. Other complications of AS include osteoporosis; spinal fracture, often accompanied by neurologic compromise; atlantoaxial subluxation; cauda equina syndrome; secondary amyloidosis; sleep disturbance; and depression.

References

Braun J, Inman R. Clinical significance of inflammatory back pain for diagnosis and screening of patients with axial spondyloarthritis. Ann Rheum Dis 2010;69: 1264–8.
Cortes A, Hadler J, Pointon JP, et al. Identification of multiple risk variants for ankylosing spondylitis through high-density genotyping of immune-related loci. Nat Genet 2013;45:730–8.
Gensler L, Inman R, Deodhar A. The "knowns" and "unknowns" of biologic therapy in ankylosing spondylitis. Am J Med Sci 2012;343:360–3.
Lukas C, Landewé R, Sieper J, et al. Development of an ASAS-endorsed disease activity score (ASDAS) in patients with ankylosing spondylitis. Ann Rheum Dis 2009;68:18–24.
Reveille JD. The MHC, and ankylosing spondylitis. Clin Rheum 2014;33:749–57.
Reveille JD, Ximenes A, Ward MM. Economic considerations of the treatment of ankylosing spondylitis. Am J Med Sci 2012;343:371–4.
Rudwaleit M, van der Heijde D, et al. The development of Assessment of SpondyloArthritis International Society classification criteria for axial spondyloarthritis (part II): Validation and final selection. Ann Rheum Dis 2009;68:770–6.
Stolwijk C, Boonen A, van Tubergen A, Reveille JD. Epidemiology of spondyloarthritis. Rheum Dis Clin North Am 2012;38:441–76.

BURSITIS, TENDINITIS, MYOFASCIAL PAIN, AND FIBROMYALGIA

Method of
Keith K. Colburn, MD

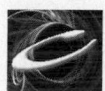

CURRENT DIAGNOSIS

Bursitis and Tendinitis
- Localized tenderness is usually palpated directly over an affected bursa or tendon.
- Most often, active range of motion in the affected tendon or bursa is painful, but unlike with arthritis, passive range of motion is often painless.
- With a few exceptions, blood tests and x-rays are usually normal.

Fibromyalgia
- Typical presentation includes a greater than 3 month history of chronic, widespread pain both above and below the waist and on both sides of the body in the absence of another condition to explain the pain.
- Though diagnosis no longer requires the presence of at least 11 of 18 tender points by digital paplation, assessment of bilaterally standardized tender points should remain part of the physical examination.
- Signs and symptoms include sleep disturbance, fatigue, paresthesias, stiffness, depression, dry eyes and mouth, Raynaud's syndrome, and headaches.

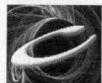

CURRENT THERAPY

Bursitis and Tendinitis
- Use conservative measures first: rest, modifying wear and tear activities, applying heat or ice or both, physical therapy, weight loss, splinting, topical analgesics, nonsteroidal antiinflammatory drugs (NSAIDs) and well-placed lidocaine injections with or without corticosteroids.
- Corticosteroid injections are best administered after 1-10 mL of lidocaine has been injected with a separate syringe, leaving the needle in place while changing the syringe. This prevents subcutaneous fat atrophy at the injection site from the corticosteroid. Inject around, not into a tendon to avoid tendon rupture.
- For the patient's comfort use a 25- or 27-gauge needle of appropriate length. Ethyl chloride spray on the skin obscures the pain of the needle stick. Adding sodium bicarbonate[1] to the syringe neutralizes the stinging sensation of lidocaine.
- Surgery for bursitis and tendinitis are reserved for cases unresponsive to conservative measures.

Fibromyalgia
- Daily aerobic exercise, starting with as little as 5 minutes at first, progressing to between 30 and 60 minutes, but even some exercise is beneficial.
- Psychological therapy to help with coping mechanisms and to aid in family support systems.
- Medication for pain includes starting one of the following drugs: gabapentin (Neurontin)[1] in graduating doses from 300 mg at bedtime up to 3600 mg per day in divided doses; pregabalin (Lyrica) from 25 to 50 mg increasing to 225 to 300 mg twice daily[3]; duloxetine (Cymbalta) 30 to 60 mg daily; milnacipran (Savella) 25 mg increased to 50 to 100 mg twice daily, or tramadol (Ultram) 50 mg increased to as high as 100 mg four times per day.
- Other potentially helpful medications include zolpidem (Ambien) 10 mg at bedtime for stage III-IV sleep; amitriptyline (Elavil)[1] 25 to 100 mg; or trazodone (Desyrel)[1] 50 to 150 mg 2 hours before bedtime. Muscle relaxants such as tizanidine (Zanaflex) 4 to 8 mg at bedtime or three times daily; baclofen (Lioresal) 10 to 20 mg at bedtime or three times daily, or cyclobenzaprine (Flexeril) 10 mg at bedtime or three times daily are often helpful for muscle tightness.
- Antidepressants such as sertraline (Zoloft)[1] 50 to 100 mg daily also can be helpful.
- Avoid narcotics, NSAIDs (rarely helpful), prolonged bed rest and inactivity, and expensive or dangerous alternative therapies.

[1]Not FDA approved for this indication.
[3]Exceeds dosage recommended by the manufacturer.

Soft tissue rheumatism is a term that describes musculoskeletal pain and other symptoms not caused by arthritis. Bursitis, tendinitis, myofascial pain syndrome, and fibromyalgia belong to this group of disorders. These maladies can occur in the absence of systemic disease. They are associated with persistent mild trauma and overuse of muscles, bursae, tendons, entheses, ligaments, and fascia. Localized tendinitis or bursitis are very specific and may be self-limiting, relieved by topical or oral antiinflammatory medications, or treated with a well-placed injection. Fibromyalgia is more diffuse and may be very difficult to treat. There are no abnormal laboratory tests consistently associated with soft tissue rheumatism. Radiologic tests and scans can show abnormalities of soft tissue; however, it is only occasionally necessary to do expensive tests to get an accurate diagnosis of these conditions. Diagnosis requires a good history and a careful physical examination of the musculoskeletal system.

Bursitis and Tendinitis

Bursitis and tendinitis can occur in any one of hundreds of locations throughout the body. A bursa is a synovial membrane–lined sac containing synovial fluid found in areas of potential friction, such as where tendons, ligaments, and bone rub against each other. Bursitis and tendinitis are considered together by regions of the body because diagnosis and treatment share some common principles.

General Principles
Diagnosis
Localized tenderness is usually palpated directly over an affected bursa or tendon. Most often, active range of motion in the affected tendon or bursa is painful, but unlike with arthritis, passive range of motion is often painless. Blood tests and x-rays are usually normal.

Treatment
Use conservative measures first in treating bursitis and tendinitis. These include rest, modifying wear-and-tear activities, heat or ice (or both), physical therapy, weight loss, splinting, topical analgesics, nonsteroidal antiinflammatory drugs (NSAIDs), and well placed lidocaine (Xylocaine) injections with or without corticosteroids. There are numerous NSAID preparations including naproxen (Naprosyn) 500 mg twice daily, ibuprofen (Motrin)[1] 400 to 800 mg every 6 to 8 hours, and the cyclooxygenase (COX)-2 selective agents including celecoxib (Celebrex)[1] 100 to 200 mg once or twice daily. If the patient is taking aspirin, even a baby aspirin, the COX-2 effect is eliminated. A proton pump inhibitor such as lansoprazole (Prevacid) 15 to 30 mg daily with a traditional NSAID gives the equivalent gastrointestinal protection of the COX-2 agents.

Corticosteroid injections using 0.5 to 1.0 mL of methylprednisolone acetate (Depo-Medrol) or triamcinolone acetonide (Kenalog-40) are best administered after 1 to 10 mL of lidocaine (Xylocaine) has been injected with a separate syringe, leaving the needle in place while changing the syringe. This prevents subcutaneous fat atrophy at the injection site from the corticosteroid. Inject around, not into, a tendon to avoid tendon rupture.

For the patient's comfort, a 25- or 27-gauge needle of appropriate length should be used. Ethyl chloride spray on the skin obscures the pain of the needle stick. Adding sodium bicarbonate[1] to the syringe neutralizes the stinging sensation of lidocaine.

Surgery for bursitis and tendinitis are reserved for cases unresponsive to conservative measures.

Specific Areas
Shoulder Region
Shoulder pain is a common problem that increases with age. Because the shoulder has an extensive range of motion, it is one of the most unstable joints in the body.

Rotator cuff tendinitis or the impingement syndrome is reported to be the most common cause of shoulder pain, but in our rheumatology clinics, bicipital tendinitis seems to be a more common cause of shoulder pain. Subacromial bursitis may be secondarily present with the impingement syndrome. Pain on active abduction and internal rotation of the glenohumeral joint and aching over the deltoid area are the main symptoms of this condition. The impingement syndrome may be acute from a recent injury or chronic with calcific tendinitis sometimes seen on x-rays.

Rotator cuff tears may be partial or complete, acute or chronic, extremely painful or hardly felt. Weakness and pain on abduction, night pain, and tenderness on palpation can indicate the presence of a torn rotator cuff. The diagnosis may be established by a shoulder arthrogram, ultrasonography, or magnetic resonance imaging (MRI). Incomplete tears often are best treated by conservative means; over time they often become complete tears. Complete tears can often be surgically repaired, especially if they are acute and occur in younger patients.

Bicipital tendinitis often manifests as anterior shoulder pain. Often the pain is diffuse or felt as referred pain to the posterior shoulder or subacromial area. Rolling the long head of the inflamed biceps tendon under the examiner's thumb elicits localized tenderness. Rupture of the long head of the biceps tendon manifests as an enlargement of the distal end of the biceps muscle. This complication is usually not repaired except in a young person because it results in only a minor loss of strength in the biceps muscle.

Adhesive capsulitis or frozen shoulder manifests as generalized pain and tenderness of the shoulder area with a marked loss of active and passive range of motion and muscle atrophy. Inflammatory arthritis, diabetes, immobility, low pain threshold, depression, or improper treatment of a painful shoulder can result in a frozen shoulder. Arthrography demonstrates a contracted joint capsule space. Less-common painful conditions associated with the shoulder region include the thoracic outlet syndrome, brachial plexopathy, and neuropathies.

Anterior Chest Wall
Pain in the anterior chest wall is common and often needs to be differentiated from cardiac, pulmonary, or gastrointestinal pain. Point tenderness helps delineate actual chest wall pain from internal organ generated pain. Costochondritis (Tietze's syndrome) is manifested by tenderness at the costochondral junction of the anterior ribs. Xiphodynia is characterized by tenderness and pain over the xiphoid area.

Elbow Region
Olecranon bursitis occurs with repetitive mild trauma and abrasion over the elbow or with an inflammatory condition including gout, pseudogout, rheumatoid arthritis, or an infection. Aspiration of an uninfected bursa alone or combined with an injection of a corticosteroid is the usual treatment. Crystal identification with a polarized microscope is helpful to differentiate gout or pseudogout from infection. Antibiotic treatment, after a Gram stain and culture of purulent fluid, is indicated in a suspected infected bursa.

Lateral epicondylitis or tennis elbow and medial epicondylitis or golfer's elbow are common findings in the repetitive use of one's arms. Tenderness is elicited by pressing the extensor or flexor tendons 1 to 2 cm distal to the epicondyle. Shaking hands or lifting a bag causes pain in the same location. A soft forearm brace may be helpful if patients would prefer not to have an injection of the tender spot.

Ulnar nerve entrapment and tendinitis of the musculotendinous insertion of the biceps are conditions also found in the elbow region.

Hand and Wrist Region
A ganglion is a cyst arising from a tendon sheath or a joint, commonly located on the dorsum of the wrist. It is lined with synovium and contains a thick, jelly-like liquid. De Quervain's tenosynovitis is inflammation and tenderness of the sheath of the abductor pollicis longus and extensor pollicis brevis tendons located over the radial styloid. Repetitive trauma, pregnancy, and systemic rheumatoid diseases are causes for this disorder.

Carpal tunnel syndrome caused by the compression of the median nerve by the surrounding structures in the wrist is the most common cause of numbness and tingling in the hands. A positive Tinel's or Phalen's sign with a confirming nerve conduction test makes the diagnosis fairly simple. Trauma, pregnancy, and a host of metabolic or inflammatory diseases are often responsible for this condition. Treatment starts with wrist splinting at night. The use of 200 mg of vitamin B_6 (pyridoxine)[1] daily until the

---

[1]Not FDA approved for this indication.

[1]Not FDA approved for this indication.

symptoms subside may be controversial, but in my opinion it often seems to be very helpful. If these measures are unsuccessful, a corticosteroid injection on the ulnar side of the carpal tunnel, a few millimeters away from the median nerve, usually relieves the numbness and tingling, often for months. In many patients, surgery is eventually required to release the median nerve.

Other, less-common hand and wrist soft-tissue problems include pronator teres syndrome, anterior interosseous nerve syndrome, radial nerve palsy, ulnar nerve entrapment at the wrist, volar flexor tenosynovitis, and Dupuytren's contractures.

Hip Region

The trochanteric bursa lies on the posterior portion of the greater trochanter. Pain from trochanteric bursitis is felt in the trochanteric area and lateral thigh, and it is often inaccurately thought to be hip joint pain. Hip joint pain is usually felt in the groin and high in the buttock. Excessive trauma to the bursal area, such as an unusual amount of exercise like an excessively long hike, can precipitate trochanteric bursitis. Osteoarthritis of the lumbar spine or hip, scoliosis or leg length discrepancies, and age can contribute to trochanteric bursitis.

Iliopsoas (iliopectineal) bursitis causes groin and anterior thigh pain and is made worse on passive hyperextension, and sometimes flexion, of the hip with resistance.

Ischial (ischiogluteal) bursitis or weaver's bottom is caused by trauma or sitting a long time on hard surfaces. Pain from ischial bursitis is felt down the back of the thigh, with point tenderness over the ischial tuberosity. Soft seating cushions and a corticosteroid injection of the bursa usually helps the pain.

Piriformis syndrome manifests as pain over the buttocks, sometimes radiating down the back of the thigh and leg. Trauma is usually involved in the etiology. The diagnosis is often made on rectal or vaginal examination.

Meralgia paresthetica is caused by the compression of the lateral femoral cutaneous nerve (L2-L3). It causes intermittent burning pain, hyperesthesia, and numbness of the anterolateral thigh. This syndrome is seen most often in patients with obesity, diabetes, or pregnancy.

Knee Region

Popliteal cysts or Baker's cysts are associated with knee joint effusions, causing a synovial herniation into the popliteal fossa. The cyst can rupture and dissect down the calf, often to the ankle, where it can leave a purpuric crescent sign beneath the malleolus. A ruptured Baker's cyst is acutely painful and must be differentiated from thrombophlebitis. An arthrogram or ultrasound examination of the knee may be used to diagnose a Baker's cyst with or without a rupture. An ultrasound for a DVT or venogram can exclude concomitant thrombophlebitis if necessary. Surgical removal of the cyst may be necessary if an injection of a corticosteroid is ineffective.

Anserine bursitis is diagnosed by tenderness over the medial aspect of the knee an inch or two below the joint line and predominantly occurs in obese, middle-aged to elderly women with osteoarthritis of the knee and in patients with fibromyalgia.

Prepatellar bursitis or housemaid's knee presents as a mildly tender swelling over the patella. It is usually caused by trauma from frequent kneeling. Aspiration of the bursa is important because septic prepatellar bursitis is occasionally present. Because this bursa does not communicate with the knee joint, treatment with oral antibiotics appropriate for the organism cultured is adequate. For sterile bursitis, an injection of a corticosteroid is helpful as protection of the knee from trauma.

Less-common painful soft-tissue conditions of the knee include patellar tendinitis, popliteal tendinitis, medial plica syndrome, rupture of the quadriceps tendon and infrapatellar tendon, and patellofemoral pain syndrome (chondromalacia patellae).

Ankle and Foot Region

Achilles tendinitis has two predominant causes. One is trauma; the other is a group of inflammatory conditions including rheumatoid arthritis, ankylosing spondylitis, reactive arthritis, and pseudogout. Tenderness,

pain, and swelling occur proximal to or at the Achilles tendon attachment to the calcaneus. Shoe corrections, heel lifts, a splint with plantar flexion, and careful stretching of the tendon constitute the safest treatments. The inflamed Achilles tendon is vulnerable to rupture, especially if a corticosteroid is injected around it (which is not recommended). The differential diagnosis of Achilles tendinitis includes retrocalcaneal bursitis and subcutaneous Achilles bursitis.

Plantar fasciitis is characterized by burning, lancing, or aching pain and tenderness over the plantar surface of the heel from a variety of kinds of trauma or overuse.

Tarsal tunnel syndrome is caused by compression of the posterior tibial nerve, posterior and inferior to the medial malleolus. A positive Tinel's sign may be elicited by percussion over the entrapment site. Numbness, paresthesias and burning pain are felt from the toes to the medial malleolus. Changing shoes and using conservative therapy, such as NSAIDs, topical analgesics or local steroid injections might help in the treatment of this condition, but surgery is often needed to decompress the nerve and provide relief.

Morton's neuroma is an entrapment neuropathy of the interdigital nerve most commonly found between the third and fourth toes. This condition is often detected in middle-aged women wearing high heels or tight shoes. Pain is often felt in the fourth toe as a burning, aching pain with paresthesias. Treatment consists of a metatarsal bar or a corticosteroid injection in the web space of the toe where the tenderness is palpated. If these are unsuccessful, surgery to remove the neuroma may be necessary.

Other causes of nonarthritic foot pain include posterior tibial tendinitis, hallux valgus, bunionette (tailor's bunion) of the fifth toe, hammer toes, metatarsalgia, pes planus (flat foot), pes cavus (claw foot), and a variety of tendon ruptures or displacements including the Achilles, posterior tibialis and the peroneal tendons.

Myofascial Pain Syndrome

Myofascial pain syndromes are often referred to as localized or regional fibromyalgia. They include regional pain disorders including chronic whiplash, repetitive strain syndrome, and temporomandibular joint syndrome. Myofascial pain is characterized by the presence of trigger points, defined as localized areas of deep muscle tenderness located in a taut band in the muscle. Unlike in the tender points of fibromyalgia, when these are palpated the pain is referred to distant zones of perceived pain. Treatment includes injecting the trigger points (see the treatments for bursitis and tendinitis) and often adding the treatment modalities outlined in the fibromyalgia section.

Complex Regional Pain Syndromes

Formerly referred to as reflex sympathetic dystrophy, Sudek's atrophy, causalgia, or shoulder–hand syndrome, among other terms, this condition was named complex regional pain syndrome in 1995. It is described as regional pain usually related to nerve injury, trauma, surgery, myocardial infarction, or stroke. The pain is usually worse than should be expected from the inciting injury. It is associated with pain, edema, and skin temperature and color changes. Treatment is complex and requires the help of physiatrists, physical therapists, and pain clinics.

Fibromyalgia Syndrome

Fibromyalgia is a chronic, diffuse pain syndrome of unknown etiology. It is characterized by widespread musculoskeletal pain of variable intensity and specific tender points to palpation (see later). Fibromyalgia is associated with a lack of deep sleep and a relative intolerance of physical activities due to pain.

Clinical Manifestations and Diagnosis

Signs and symptoms include sleep disturbance, fatigue, paresthesias, stiffness, depression, dry eyes and mouth, Raynaud's syndrome, bladder pain (interstitial cystitis) and headaches. Fibromyalgia is remarkable for the lack of abnormal laboratory and radiologic tests routinely done for rheumatologic diseases. Fibromyalgia may be associated with other diseases and can improve when the other disease is treated. On the other hand, concurrent fibromyalgia (Box 1),

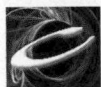

Box 1 · Conditions Associated or Concurrent with Fibromyalgia

Conditions Associated with Fibromyalgia
Hypothyroidism
Polymyalgia rheumatica
Tapering off corticosteroids
Drugs: lipid-lowering and antiviral agents
Cervical stenosis (?)
Malignancy
Viral infections: parvovirus, Lyme disease, hepatitis C, others

Conditions Concurrent with Fibromyalgia
Chronic fatigue syndrome
Autoimmune diseases such as systemic lupus erythematosus or
    rheumatoid arthritis
Myofascial pain syndrome
Irritable bowel syndrome
Gulf War syndrome
Migraine headaches
Interstitial cystitis

including that found in approximately 30% of patients with rheumatoid arthritis and systemic lupus erythematosus, might not respond to treatment of the other disease. Although the term "concurrent" fibromyalgia is out of favor, I find it still useful when fibromyalgia is associated with other conditions regularly.

Presentation includes a history of chronic, widespread pain both above and below the waist and on both sides of the body in the absence of another condition to explain the pain and that has lasted longer than 3 months. In the past, the diagnosis was based on the presence of at least 11 out of 18 tender points by digital palpation at previously published locations. The diagnosis based on tender points is being dropped from the criteria, but the tender points should still be assessed on physical examination. Tender point sites include bilateral locations on the occiput, anterior lower neck (C5-C7), trapezius, supraspinatus, second anterior costochondral junction, lateral epicondyle, buttocks in the upper outer quadrant, greater trochanters, and medial fat pad of the knees. Digital palpation of the tender points is done at about 4 kg of force, which is roughly enough pressure to blanch the thumbnail.

Treatment

It is extremely important that patients are made aware by the treating physician that they own this diagnosis and it requires effort on their part to get better. Treatment with narcotics should be avoided if at all possible because they seldom relieve pain caused by fibromyalgia for an adequate length of time. Self-motivated patients might find relief for a significant portion of their discomfort in combining aerobic exercise with a well-thought-out drug and psychological treatment program. Refer patients to support groups backed by organizations like the Arthritis Foundation.

Initial Treatment

Daily aerobic exercise, starting with as little as 5 minutes at first, progressing to between 30 and 60 minutes, is ideal. Emphasize to patients that without the progressive aerobic exercise part of treatment—walking, swimming in warm water, bicycling, jogging, or other exercise—they are unlikely to improve very much no matter what medications they take. It usually takes 6 to 12 months of exercise by unusually motivated patients to attain the level of fitness that is likely to diminish most or all the pain. Even some exercise is still beneficial.

Pregabalin (Lyrica) is the first medication approved by the FDA for the treatment of fibromyalgia. The dosage is 150 to 225 mg two times per day. The antidepressant duloxetine (Cymbalta) has been approved by the FDA for fibromyalgia at a dose of 60 mg once daily for pain.[3] Duloxetine may be used secondarily for depression.

[3]Exceeds dosage recommended by the manufacturer.

The newest FDA-approved drug for fibromyalgia is milnacipran (Savella) 50 mg twice daily (starting at 10 mg/day and titrated to arrive at the recommended dose in 1 week). Gabapentin (Neurontin)[1] 1800 to 3600 mg daily, in progressive, divided doses, may be used primarily for pain. Tramadol (Ultram) 50 mg, progressively titrated up to 8 tablets daily in divided doses, may be given for pain. Zolpidem (Ambien) 10 mg at bedtime can help with sleep disturbances. This drug is less habit forming and gives the deepest (i.e., state 3 or 4) sleep of any sleeping medications.

Psychological therapy should be considered to help with coping mechanisms and to aid in family support systems.

Second-line Treatment

Other medications may be added onto, or substituted for, one of the first-line medications, depending on drug interactions and efficacy. Amitriptyline (Elavil) 10 to 200[3] mg or trazodone (Desyrel) 25 to 250 mg at bedtime may help with sleep disturbance,[1] depression, and mild pain relief.[1] A selective serotonin reuptake inhibitor (SSRI), such as sertraline (Zoloft) 50 mg daily, may be useful for depression and mild pain relief.[1]

Other Tested and Possibly Helpful Treatments

Muscle relaxants including tizanidine (Zanaflex)[1] 4 to 8 mg three times a day, baclofen (Lioresal)[1] 10 to 20 mg three times a day, or cyclobenzaprine (Flexeril)[1] 10 mg at bedtime may be helpful for pain and rest. Magnesium[1] 500 mg combined with malic acid[7] 1200 to 2400 mg daily might be helpful for fatigue.

Treatments to Avoid

Narcotics should be avoided. NSAIDs are rarely helpful. Prolonged bed rest and inactivity are counterproductive. Expensive or dangerous alternative therapies should be avoided.

[1]Not FDA approved for this indication.
[3]Exceeds dosage recommended by the manufacturer.
[7]Available as a dietary supplement.

References

Biundo Jr JJ. Regional rheumatic pain syndromes. In: Klippel JH, Stone JH, Crofford LJ, White PH, editors. Primer on the Rheumatic Diseases. 13th ed. Atlanta: Arthritis Foundation; 2008. p. 68–86.

Dadabhoy D, Clauw DJ. The fibromyalgia syndrome. In: Klippel JH, Stone JH, Crofford LJ, White PH, editors. Primer on the Rheumatic Diseases. 13th ed. Atlanta: Arthritis Foundation; 2008. p. 87–93.

Fransen J, Russell IJ. Medical management of fibromyalgia. In: Fransen J, Russell IJ, editors. The Fibromyalgia Help Book. St. Paul: Smith House Press; 1996. p. 35–58.

Goldenberg DL. Fibromyalgia and related syndromes. In: Hochberg MC, Silman AL, Smolen JS, et al., editors. Rheumatology. 3rd ed. St Louis: Mosby; 2003. p. 701–12.

Sheon RP. Overview of soft tissue rheumatic disorders. 2009. UpToDate, online 17.3, www.uptodate.com.

COMMON SPORTS INJURIES

Method of
Andrew S.T. Porter, DO

CURRENT DIAGNOSIS

- Lateral Ankle Sprain—Pain over lateral ankle ligament(s) with localized swelling. Often associated with laxity and pain with anterior drawer and/or talar tilt test. Obtain x-rays based on the Ottawa ankle and foot rules.
- Medial Ankle Sprain—Less common than lateral ankle sprain. Pain in the deltoid ligament with localized swelling. Obtain x-rays based on Ottawa ankle and foot rules.
- High Ankle Sprain—Syndesmotic injury. Pain with squeeze test and/or dorsiflexion with external rotation.

- Osteochondral Ankle Injuries—Most commonly seen in the talar dome. Associated with an ankle inversion injury and ankle pain. Often have a joint effusion and soft tissue swelling and can have mechanical symptoms (catching, locking, crepitus, and a feeling of giving way). Obtain x-rays initially and then magnetic resonance imaging (MRI) to grade degree of injury.
- Anterior Cruciate Ligament (ACL) Injuries—Most common after noncontact injuries. Physical examination reveals a diffuse knee effusion, positive Lachman, and/or anterior drawer test. Obtain x-rays then MRI for further evaluation.
- Posterior Cruciate Ligament (PCL) Injuries—Occur with varus/valgus stress with the knee in full extension. Physical examination reveals a positive posterior drawer and sag sign. Obtain x-rays then MRI for further evaluation.
- Medial Collateral Ligament (MCL) Injuries—Occur with valgus stress or twisting with or without contact. Physical examination reveals localized effusion and a positive valgus stress testing and tenderness to palpation along the MCL. Graded 1 to 3.
- Osteochondral Knee Injuries—Most commonly seen in the femoral condyle. Associated with a knee injury. Knee pain and, often, mechanical symptoms of the knee. Palpation of the femoral condyles with the knee in flexion reproduces pain. Obtain x-rays initially and then MRI to grade degree of injury.
- Mallet Finger—Disruption of the extensor mechanism insertion into the distal phalanx.
- Jersey Finger—Occurs after avulsion of the flexor digitorum profundus tendon from its insertion on the distal phalanx.
- Proximal Interphalangeal (PIP) Joint Dorsal Dislocation—Injury to the volar plate with or without an avulsion fracture.
- Scaphoid Fracture—Pain over the scaphoid with or without a fall on an outstretched hand injury is a scaphoid fracture until proven otherwise. Obtain wrist x-rays with a scaphoid view.
- Tendinosis—Repetitive chronic tendon injuries result in scarring, disorganization of fibers, degeneration and are without an inflammatory component.
- Stress Fractures—Most often seen in active patients as a result of excessive stress on normal bone from overactivity or normal stress on a bone that is deficient (osteoporotic, poor nutrition, or in female athlete triad). History is positive for bone pain, and physical examination reveals tenderness to palpation in the affected bone and often a positive tuning fork test, hop test, and fulcrum test. Obtain x-rays first, then MRI or bone scan if needed.
- Spondylolysis/Spondylolisthesis—Most often seen in young athletes with insidious onset low back pain and history of repetitive extension. Positive stork test. X-rays initially, and if negative, may proceed with limited CT and SPECT scan or MRI.

- Osteochondral Knee Injuries—Degree of injury is graded via MRI, and this guides treatment and RTP.
- Mallet Finger—Treat with continuous full-extension stack splinting of the distal interphalangeal joint for 6 weeks and then nighttime splinting and activity splinting for 6 weeks.
- Jersey Finger—Treatment is referral to orthopedic surgeon for surgical intervention.
- PIP joint dorsal dislocation—Reduce dislocation and obtain x-rays. Treat with progressive extension blocking splint with 30° to 40° of flexion and decrease by 10° per week.
- Scaphoid Fracture—If x-rays with scaphoid view are negative, place in a short-arm thumb spica cast and follow up in 2 weeks. If x-rays remain negative but pain persists, obtain a CT or MRI. Treat nondisplaced scaphoid fractures with short-arm (4) thumb spica cast: proximal-third fractures 12 to 20 weeks, middle-third fractures 10 to 12 weeks, and distal-third fractures 4 to 6 weeks.
- Tendinosis—Treat by creating inflammation to facilitate healing.
- Stress Fractures—Treat with general treatment for stress fractures plus specific treatment based on stress fracture site.
- Spondylolysis/Spondylolisthesis—Treat with extension blocking brace, rest, rehabilitation with core strengthening and lower extremity flexibility, and gradual RTP.

Ankle Injuries

The ankle is the most common joint injured in athletes. Ankle sprains are common, as they represent 25% of all sports-related injuries. The Ottawa ankle and foot rules help in the decision to obtain x-rays (Box 1). In general, treatment will consist of RICE (rest, ice, compression, elevation), early mobilization, and rehab. Prevention of ankle injuries is important and consists of ankle braces, ankle taping, neuromuscular training program, and regular sport-specific warm-up exercises.

Lateral Ankle Sprain

The most common ankle sprain is a lateral inversion sprain that results from landing on an inverted foot with or without plantarflexion. The lateral ankle ligaments are the anterior talofibular ligament (ATFL), calcaneofibular ligament, and the posterior talofibular ligament. The ATFL is the most commonly sprained ligament. Lateral ankle sprains are most commonly treated with RICE initially, then early ambulation, range of motion, progression into strengthening, and then proprioception rehabilitation. Proprioception rehabilitation includes balancing on one leg and performing balancing exercises on a wobble board. For example, patients can balance on one leg when brushing their teeth. Athletes should return to play (RTP) with a lace-up/velcro ankle brace after injury with or without taping. This added stability will help prevent future ankle injuries and also decrease the severity of ankle

CURRENT THERAPY

- Lateral Ankle Sprain—Treat with RICE (rest, ice, compression, elevation) and early rehab. Return to play (RTP) is generally 1 to 4 weeks and is based on functional progression. RTP with ankle brace.
- Medial Ankle Sprain—Treat with RICE and early rehab. RTP with ankle brace.
- High Ankle Sprain—Treat with RICE and boot for 1 to 3 weeks and then rehab. RTP takes a longer time compared with lateral ankle sprain.
- Osteochondral Ankle Injuries—Degree of injury is graded via MRI, and this guides treatment and RTP.
- ACL Injuries—ACL tears often need reconstruction that is individualized in active patients who require knee stability.
- PCL Injuries—Isolated PCL injuries often heal conservatively with protected weight bearing in an extension brace and knee rehab.
- MCL Injuries—Often heal conservatively with bilateral hinged knee brace and knee rehab. Generally, RTP in 2 to 6 weeks.

Box 1   Ottawa Ankle and Foot Rules

- An ankle x-ray series is indicated if there is pain in the malleolar zone and any of these findings are made:
  - Tenderness over the lateral malleolus
  - Tenderness over the medial malleolus
  - Inability to bear weight four steps immediately after the injury or in the emergency department or physician's office
- A foot x-ray series is indicated if there is pain in the midfoot zone and any of these findings are made:
  - Tenderness over the base of fifth metatarsal
  - Tenderness over the navicular bone
  - Inability to bear weight four steps immediately after the injury and in the emergency department or physician's office

*X-rays are indicated if any of these criteria are met.
Data from Bachmann and colleagues (2003) and Tiemstra (2012).

injuries. Most athletes will RTP in a few days to 4 weeks; this return is based on pain, obtaining full active range of motion and full strength, and functional stability.

Medial Ankle Sprain

Medial ankle ligament sprains are rare, account for <10% of ankle injuries, and are often accompanied with a lateral malleolar fracture or syndesmotic injury. The medial ankle ligament is the deltoid ligament and is injured via external rotation or eversion. These ankle sprains are treated similarly to lateral ankle sprains.

High Ankle Sprain

High ankle sprains, also known as syndesmotic ankle sprains, occur through forced external rotation of a dorsiflexed foot most commonly but also occur by forced internal rotation of a fixed plantar flexed foot. The syndesmotic ligaments connect and stabilize the distal tibia to the distal fibula. The syndesmotic ligaments are the anterior tibiofibular ligament, posterior tibiofibular ligament, transverse tibiofibular ligament, interosseous ligament, and the interosseous membrane. Palpate the fibular head for pain. Pain on palpation of the fibular head might indicate a maisonneuve fracture, a fracture of the proximal third of the fibula associated with syndesmotic disruption. A high ankle sprain has a longer healing time compared to a lateral ankle sprain. Often these need immobilization with a boot or cast for 1 to 4 weeks to help with healing before beginning rehab. RTP after a high ankle sprain depends on pain, achieving a full active range of motion, full strength, and functional stability. Incomplete healing of a high ankle sprain can result in distal tibia and fibula instability.

Osteochondral Ankle Injuries

Osteochondral injuries are injuries to the articular surface of a joint. These injuries range from small undisplaced depressions and cracks in the osteochondral surface to small pieces of articular cartilage and bone that break off of the articular surface and float within the joint. Osteochondral injuries occur most commonly on weight bearing articular surfaces. In osteochondral injuries, osteonecrosis of subchondral bone occurs, resulting in separation of cartilage and subchondral bone from underlying, well-vascularized bone. The term "osteochondral lesion" (OCL) is favored over the previously used term "osteochondritis dessicans" because

there might not be an inflammatory component of the injury. OCLs are often associated with repeated trauma or overuse in athletes. OCLs typically present with pain in the affected joint and can develop with a specific injury or over several months in highly active athletes. OCLs are more common in younger patients with open physes (growth plates) and are referred to as juvenile OCLs. Adult OCLs describe this condition in skeletally mature patients.

Osteochondral injuries are a cause for pain in up to 25% of ankle injuries and need to be considered when a patient presents with ankle pain. Acute osteochondral injuries in the ankle most commonly affect the talar dome (Figures 1–3) but can also be found in the distal tibia (Figure 4). OCLs are first evaluated by x-rays (see Figures 1 and 2) and then graded by magnetic resonance imaging (MRI) (Table 1). CT scan (see Figure 3) is sometimes utilized as well. Grade 1 to 3 juvenile OCLs and grade 1 to 2 adult OCLs are treated conservatively. Conservative treatment consists of no weight bearing (NWB) in a cast or boot for 6 to 10 weeks followed by partial weight bearing (PWB) to full weight bearing (FWB) over 2 to 6 weeks, followed with an ankle brace for 3 months, and ensuring adequate calcium and vitamin D intake to facilitate healing. Nonsteroidal antiinflammatory drugs (NSAIDs) should be avoided because they can slow bone healing, and OCLs are probably not an inflammatory process. For grade 4 juvenile OCLs, grade 3 and 4 adult OCLs, and those that have not clinically healed with conservative care operative treatment is required. Operative treatment options depend on OCL size and type and include removal of the OCL followed by transchondral drilling and microfracture to stimulate fibrocartilage formation, fixation of the OCL with an osteochondral allograft, osteochondral autograft transfer, and autologous chondrocyte implantation.

Knee injuries—The knee joint lacks intrinsic bone stability, so most stability is from the major knee ligaments.

Anterior Cruciate Ligament Injuries

The anterior cruciate ligament (ACL) is the key stabilizer of the knee and is one of two major intraarticular knee ligaments, the other being the posterior cruciate ligament (PCL). Most ACL tears occur from noncontact injuries. Women experience ACL tears up to nine times more often than men. The main function of the ACL is to prevent excessive anterior tibial translation relative to the femur. Patients who sustain an injury to their ACL often describe hearing a pop, feeling instability in their knee, experiencing pain

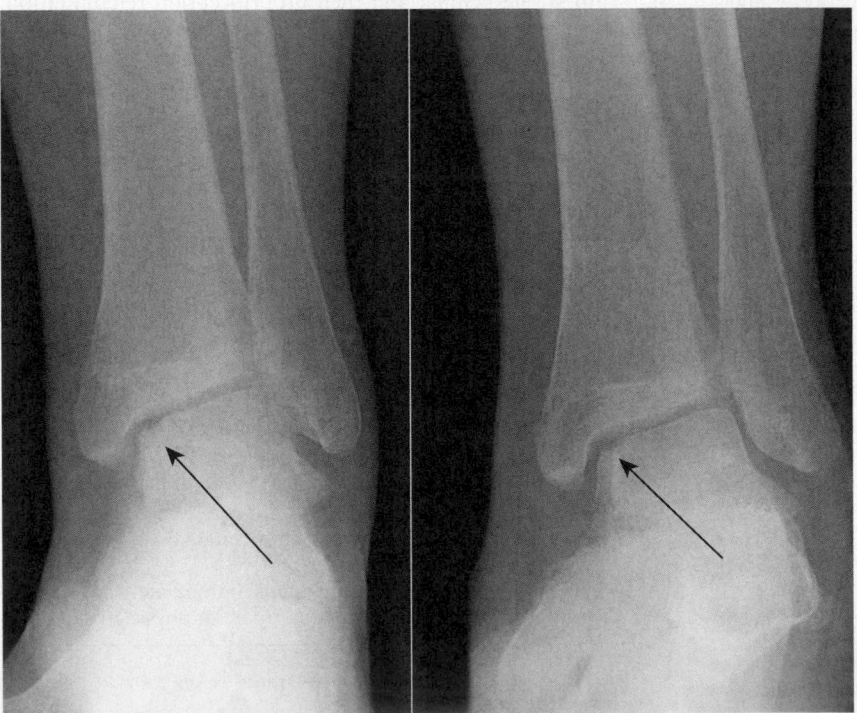

Figure 1. X-rays of the left ankle, AP and mortise views, which demonstrate a grade 2 osteochondral lesion (OCL) along the medial talar dome.

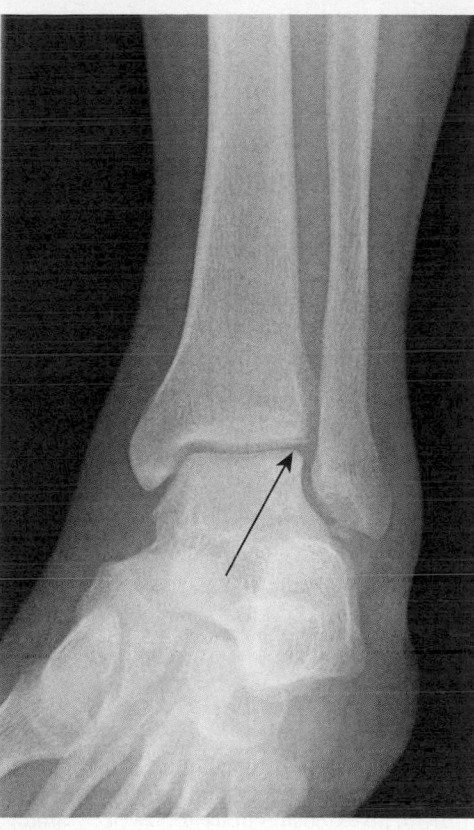

Figure 2. X-ray of the left ankle, mortise view, which demonstrates a grade 4 OCL along the lateral talar dome.

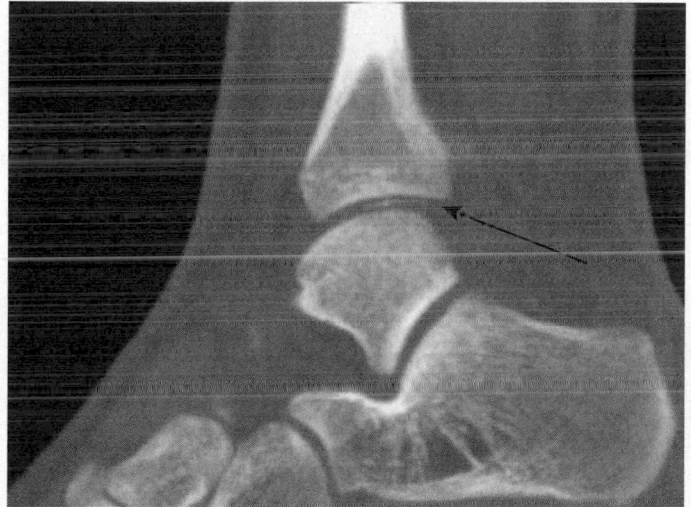

Figure 3. CT scan without contrast. Sagittal image of ankle, which demonstrates a grade 4 OCL of the talar dome.

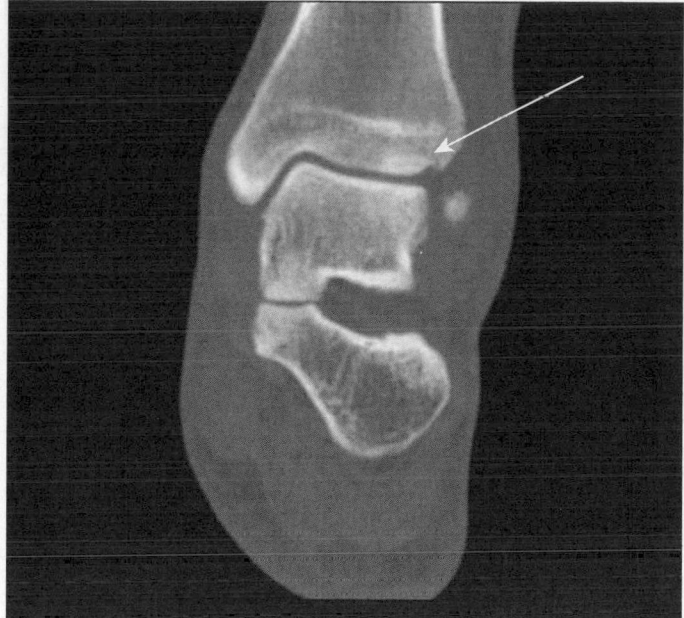

Figure 4. CT scan without contrast. Coronal image of ankle, which demonstrates a grade 1 OCL of the distal lateral tibia.

TABLE 1	Classification of Osteochondral Lesions	
STAGE	**PLAIN X-RAY FINDINGS**	**MRI FINDINGS**
1	Depressed osteochondral fragment	Articular cartilage thickening and low signal changes in subchondral bone
2	Osteochondral fragment attached by bone	Articular cartilage breached, no synovial fluid around fragment
3	Detached nondisplaced fragment	Articular cartilage breached, synovial fluid around fragment
4	Displaced fragment	Loose foreign body

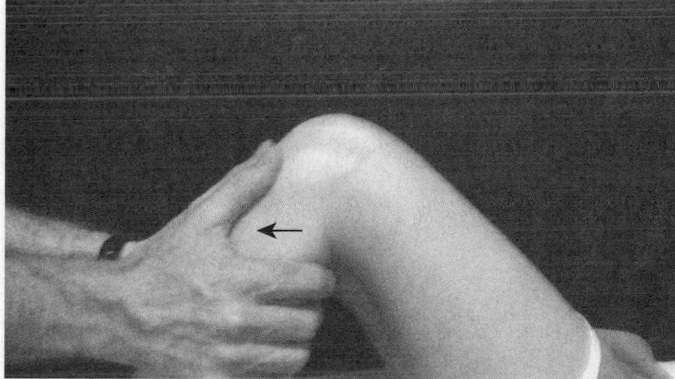

Figure 5. Anterior drawer test for ACL laxity. Patient's knee is flexed 90°. Examiner applies anterior force to the tibia in relation to the patient's femur to evaluate for laxity.

immediately after the injury, and develop an associated knee effusion. On-the-field evaluation is ideal in an ACL injury, as the hamstrings will often start to tighten up shortly after the injury, preventing anterior tibial translation. This will prevent an isolated test of the ACL and give the false impression that an ACL endpoint is present when in fact the ACL is completely torn. The anterior drawer (Figure 5) and Lachman test (Figure 6) are the main physical exam tests to evaluate the ACL. Obtain x-rays and then MRI if an ACL tear is suspected. The blood supply to the ACL is poor and is provided by the middle geniculate artery off of the popliteal artery. Because of the poor blood supply, ACL tears often need reconstruction if athletes want to return to a high level of activity, and knee stability is needed. ACL reconstruction timing is

important and often will occur 3 to 4 weeks after injury to allow for swelling to decrease, ROM and strength to improve, and inflammation to decrease. Also during this presurgical time, it is important to have patients perform pre-hab (presurgical rehabilitation), focusing on AROM and knee strengthening. A knee effusion will cause the quadriceps muscles to weaken and atrophy.

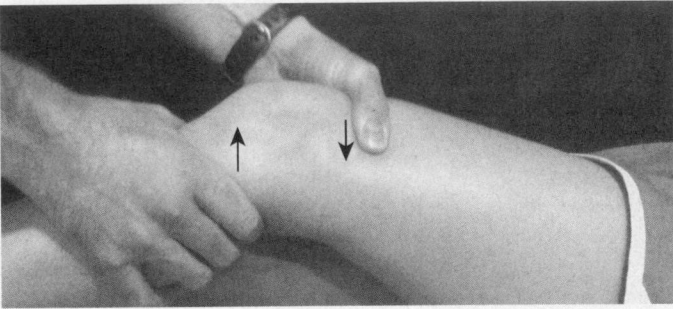

Figure 6. Lachman test for ACL laxity. Patient's knee is flexed 20°–30°. Examiner grasps the distal femur and proximal tibia and applies anterior force to the tibia and posterior force to the femur to evaluate for ACL laxity.

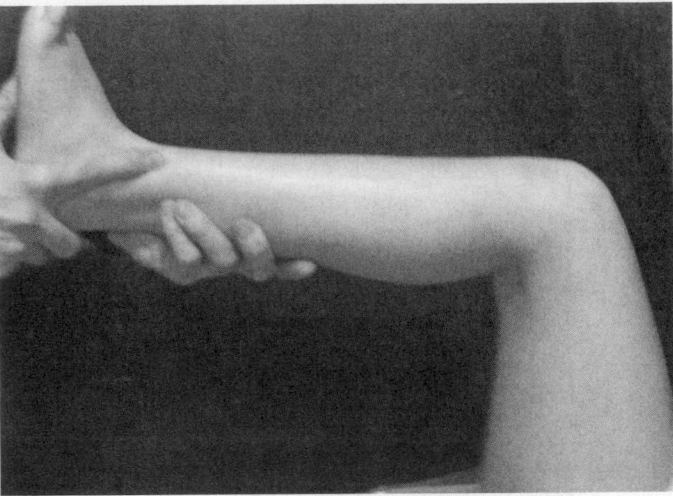

Figure 8. Sag sign test for PCL laxity. Examiner views the tibia condyles from the lateral side to evaluate for a posterior sag (displacement) in the appearance that would indicate a PCL injury.

Hamstring tendon autograft, patella tendon autograft, quadriceps tendon autograft, and allograft are all used for ACL reconstruction. Each graft has advantages and disadvantages and should be discussed with the orthopedic surgeon before reconstruction and individualized for each patient. Continuing to participate in high-level activity after an ACL tear if undiagnosed can lead to a knee dislocation and further intraarticular knee injury.

PCL Injuries

The PCL is the other major intraarticular knee ligament. Isolated PCL injuries are much less common than ACL injuries and make up only 3.5% of ligamentous knee injuries in sports, with the remaining 96.5% of PCL injuries associated with multiligamentous knee injuries. PCL injuries, unlike ACL injuries, are the result of external forces (e.g., a soccer player sliding into the goal post and tearing his or her PCL). The main function of the PCL is to resist posterior tibial translation. Posterior drawer testing (Figure 7) and a sag sign test (Figure 8) are the physical exam tests used to evaluate the PCL. Obtain x-rays then MRI if a PCL tear is suspected. The blood supply to the PCL is better than the blood supply to the ACL. Isolated PCL injuries (grades 1 and 2) are treated conservatively because surgical reconstruction has not been shown to be helpful. Conservative treatment consists of protected weight bearing in an extension brace followed by quadriceps rehabilitation and ROM exercises. RTP is generally 4 to 6 weeks after a PCL injury. Surgical intervention is recommended for associated injuries to the ACL, medial collateral ligament (MCL), and posterior lateral corner (grade 3 PCL injury).

MCL Injuries

The MCL is an extraarticular ligament that resists knee valgus forces. An MCL sprain results from a valgus stress to a partially flexed knee. Athletes will present with localized pain and swelling along the medial aspect of the knee. Most MCL injuries are isolated ligament injuries, but more severe MCL injuries can involve tears of the medial meniscus and ACL, commonly referred to as the "terrible triad." The MCL is examined by palpation and valgus stress testing at 0° and 30° of knee flexion. MCL injuries are graded 1, 2, or 3 depending on severity of injury. A patient with a grade 1 MCL sprain has pain in the MCL but no valgus stress testing laxity. A grade 2 MCL sprain has valgus stress testing laxity but a solid endpoint. A grade 3 MCL sprain has no endpoint with valgus stress testing. Thankfully, the MCL has a rich vascular supply and can often heal conservatively. Treatment consists of RICE for the first 1 to 2 weeks and a bilateral hinged knee brace to facilitate healing. Weight bearing and ROM and strengthening exercises are started when they are tolerable. RTP after an MCL injury depends on the grade and generally takes 2 to 6 weeks.

Osteochondral Knee Injuries

Osteochondral injuries occur in the knee as well as in the ankle. Osteochondral injuries of the knee most commonly affect the lateral aspect of the medial femoral condyle but can be found anywhere along the medial or lateral femoral condyle, patella, or trochlea. History is significant for knee pain, with or without swelling and mechanical symptoms (catching, locking, crepitus, and feeling of giving way). On palpation, patients can have pain in the affected area with knee flexion with or without crepitus. Obtain x-rays initially (Figure 9) and then grade the OCL severity by MRI (Figure 10). CT scans are also utilized sometimes. Grade 1 to 3 juvenile knee OCLs and grade 1 to 2 adult knee OCLs are treated conservatively. Grade 4 juvenile OCLs, grade 3 to 4 adult OCLs and all OCLs that have failed conservative care are treated operatively.

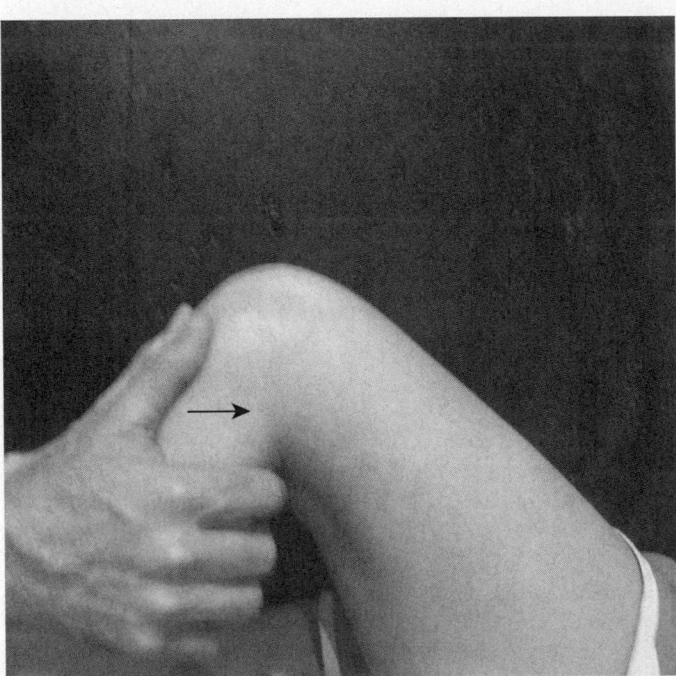

Figure 7. Posterior drawer test for PCL laxity. Patient's knee is flexed 90°. Examiner applies posterior force to the tibia in relation to the patient's femur to evaluate for laxity.

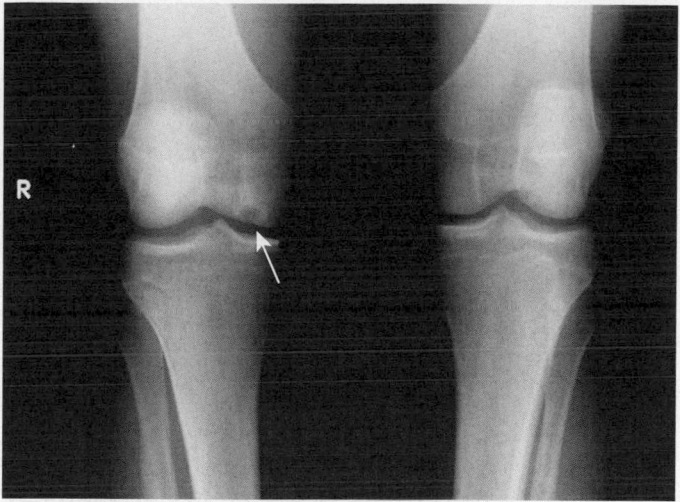

Figure 9. X-ray of the bilateral knees, AP view, which demonstrates a grade 1 OCL along the right knee medial femoral condyle.

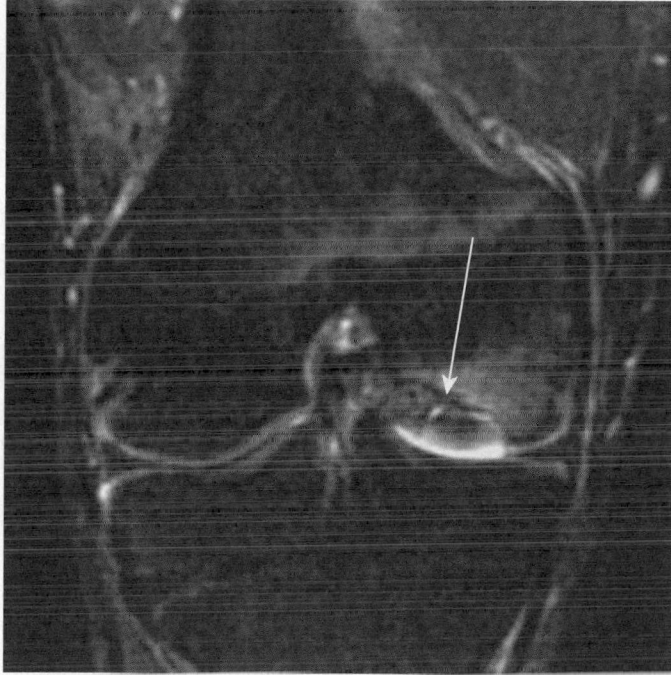

Figure 10. Magnetic resonance imaging (MRI) of the right knee, without contrast. Coronal T2 fat saturation image, which demonstrates a grade 4 OCL of the medial femoral condyle.

Hand Injuries

Mallet Finger

A mallet finger occurs after forced flexion of an actively extended distal interphalangeal (DIP) joint, resulting in disruption of the extensor mechanism insertion into the distal phalanx. Patients with a mallet finger are unable to actively extend the DIP joint. This injury can be associated with an avulsion fracture (Figure 11). For acute injuries, general treatment consists of continuous extension splinting of the DIP joint (0° to 10° of hyperextension) for at least 6 weeks. The 6-week clock starts over if the DIP joint is allowed to flex at all during the initial 6 weeks of treatment or if, at the end of the 6 weeks, the mallet finger is not completely healed. After the initial 6 weeks, it is recommended to continue with nighttime splinting and activity splinting for another 6 weeks to ensure adequate healing and avoidance of surgery. To perform this splinting, a stack splint is well tolerated and

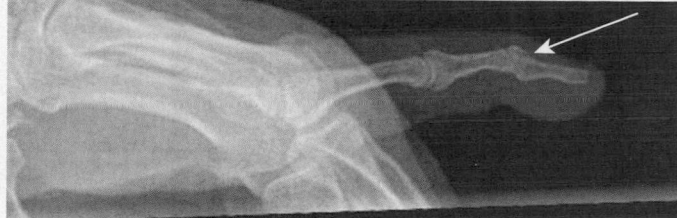

Figure 11. X-ray of the left hand, lateral view, which demonstrates a mallet finger of the fifth finger. Note the flexion of the DIP joint and avulsion fracture of the distal phalanx that involves about 30% of the joint space.

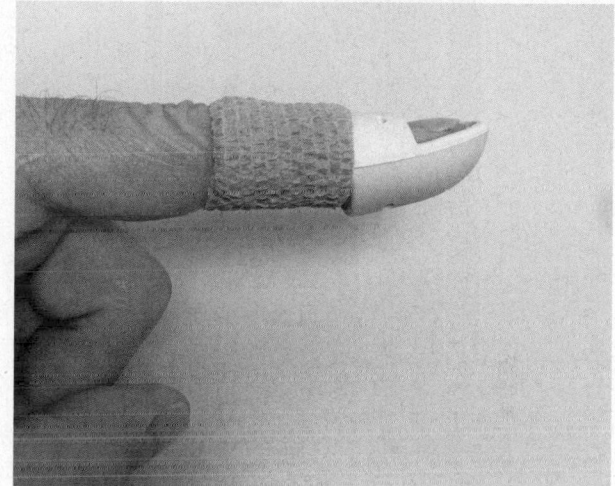

Figure 12. Stack splint with Coban wrap added for stability that immobilizes the DIP joint at neutral to 5° of hyperextension.

is protective (Figure 12). Orthopedic referral is indicated if the patient is unable to obtain full passive extension of the DIP joint or if the avulsion fracture involves over 30% of the joint space.

Jersey Finger

A jersey finger results from the avulsion of the flexor digitorum profundus tendon from its insertion on the distal phalanx. This commonly occurs in football and rugby players when the tip of their flexed finger is caught in a jersey and the DIP joint of the finger is then forcefully extended. After this injury occurs, the patient is unable to actively flex the DIP joint. Treatment is urgent referral to an orthopedic surgeon for surgical intervention.

Proximal Interphalangeal Joint Dorsal Dislocation

Proximal Interphalangeal (PIP) joint injuries are the most common joint injuries in sports. Most PIP dislocations are dorsal and result from hyperextension with an axial load. Dislocations are described by the position of the distal fragment in relation to the proximal fragment. PIP dorsal dislocations cause injury to the volar plate with or without avulsion fracture. Pre-reduction x-rays are preferred if they can be obtained promptly (Figure 13). X-rays of the finger with at least one view being a true lateral view should be obtained to rule out fracture. However, many PIP dorsal dislocations occur on the playing field and it is reasonable to reduce these dislocations, buddy tape the affected finger, and allow the patient to RTP with x-rays obtained after the athletic competition. Reduction is usually uncomplicated and is performed urgently via hyperextending the joint, applying traction in plane with the finger, then flexing the joint. Post-reduction films are a necessity (Figure 14). Stability testing of the collateral ligaments should be performed after the reduction. Full flexion and extension of the PIP joint will be possible if the joint

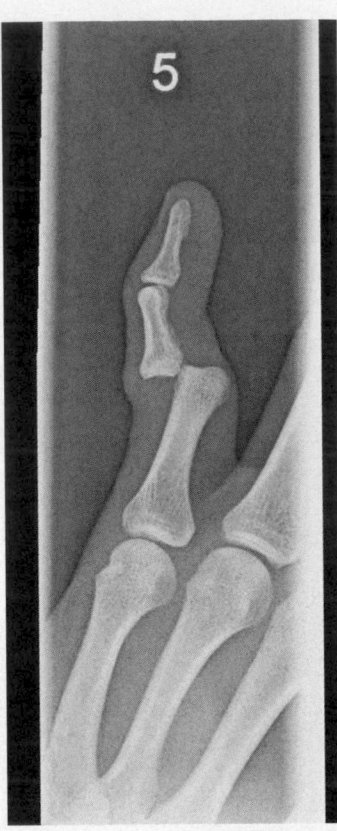

Figure 13. X-ray of the left hand, oblique view, which demonstrates a proximal interphalangeal (PIP) joint dorsal and lateral dislocation.

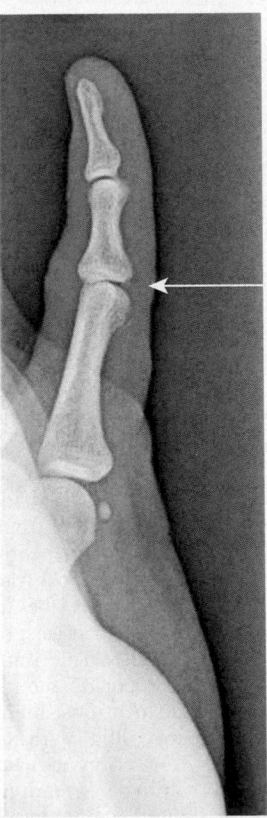

Figure 14. X-ray of the left hand, lateral status postreduction view, which demonstrates a relocated proximal interphalangeal (PIP) joint. Note the avulsion fracture of the middle phalanx.

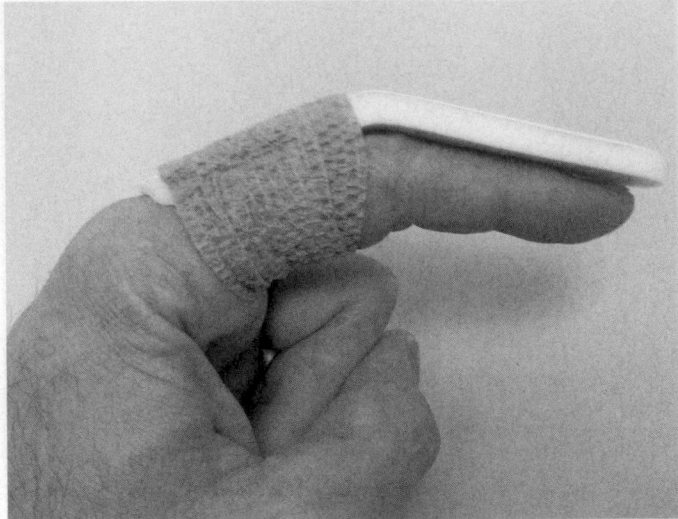

Figure 15. Dorsal extension blocking splint at 30°–40° of flexion at the PIP joint. Note that there is no pressure over the PIP joint volar plate and that flexion and extension at the DIP joint is possible.

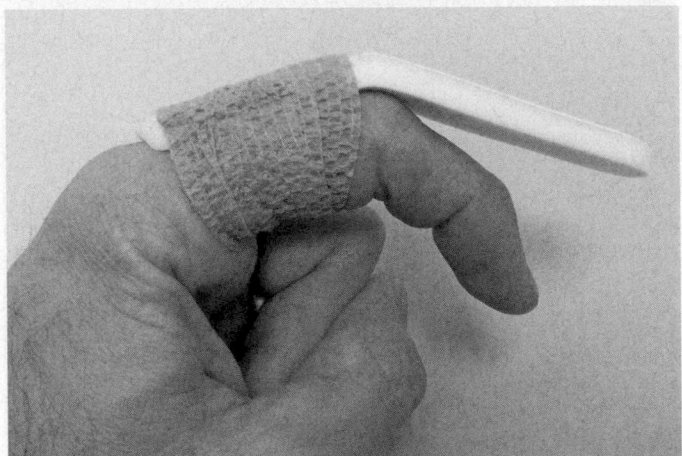

Figure 16. Dorsal extension blocking splint at 30°–40° of flexion at the PIP joint. This figure illustrates the freedom of motion that is possible at the PIP joint (full flexion and limited extension) and the DIP joint (full flexion and extension).

is stable. A stable joint without a large avulsion fragment should be treated with a progressive extension blocking splint (Figures 15 and 16). Start with 30° to 40° of flexion and decrease by 10° per week over 3 to 4 weeks, then buddy tape the injured finger with activity PRN (8). Some PIP dorsal dislocations have a lateral component to them and these are treated similar to pure dorsal dislocations (see Figure 13). Orthopedic surgeon referral is indicated if there is a large avulsion fracture or the joint is unstable.

Scaphoid Fracture

The scaphoid bone is the most common carpal bone that is fractured and is a common injury that is encountered in primary care. Interestingly, scaphoid fractures occur most commonly in young men. Scaphoid fractures occur less commonly in young children and the elderly because of the relative weakness of the distal radius compared with the scaphoid in these age groups. Often a scaphoid fracture is caused by a FOOSH (fall on an outstretched hand) injury. On physical examination, if the patient has pain over the scaphoid tubercle or in the anatomical snuffbox with or without a history of a FOOSH injury, the clinician needs to have a high index of suspicion for a scaphoid fracture when evaluating the wrist x-rays. Obtain the standard wrist x-rays (AP, lateral, and oblique views) plus a dedicated scaphoid view (AP with ulnar deviation) and be

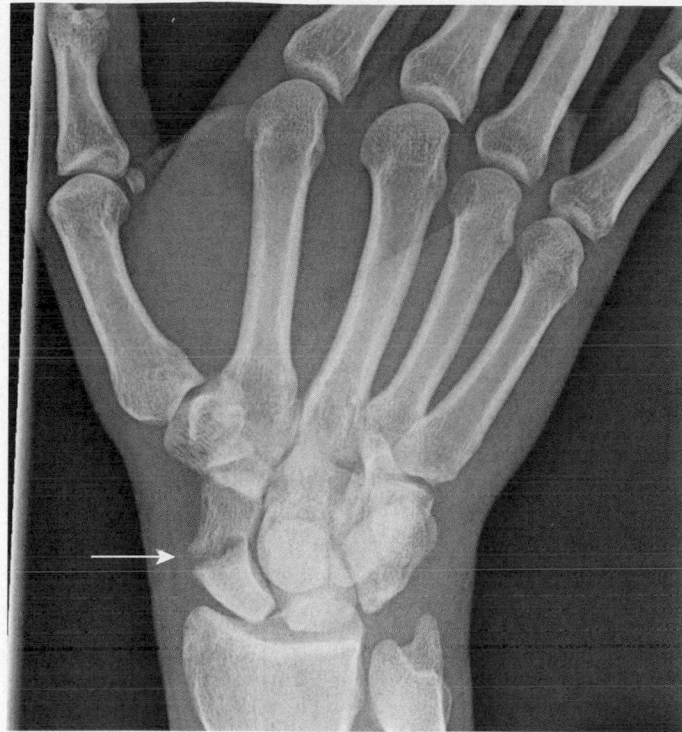

Figure 17. Scaphoid view x-ray (AP view with ulnar deviation) is important to obtain in addition to your standard wrist views (AP, lateral, and oblique) when scaphoid fracture is suspected. This scaphoid fracture was not seen on the x-rays on the day of the injury. Patient continued to have wrist pain and then presented 10 weeks later and x-rays were obtained demonstrating the scaphoid fracture.

aware that early imaging with x-rays is often unrevealing for a scaphoid fracture (Figure 17). If a fracture is not seen on x-rays, the clinician needs to have a high index of suspicion for a scaphoid fracture, place the patient in a short-arm thumb spica cast and have the patient follow up in 2 weeks. If repeat x-rays remain negative and the patient continues to have scaphoid pain, proceed with an MRI of the wrist with T2 fat saturation views or a CT scan. If a scaphoid fracture is noted on imaging, the location of the scaphoid fracture will guide treatment. Because the blood supply to the scaphoid is distal to proximal, scaphoid fractures are harder to heal than other carpal fractures. Nondisplaced middle-third or

proximal-third scaphoid fractures are treated with a long- or short-arm thumb spica cast with the wrist at 20° to 30° of extension and the thumb in slight extension and abduction for 10 to 20 weeks. Middle-third fractures should be immobilized for 10 to 12 weeks. Proximal-third fractures should be immobilized from 12 to 20 weeks. It is much easier to regain flexion in the wrist after casting than it is to regain extension. If the elbow is incorporated in the cast, it should be casted at 90° of flexion. A long-arm cast may decrease healing time, but it does not improve nonunion rates. A nondisplaced distal-third fracture should be treated in a short-arm thumb spica cast for 4 to 6 weeks. For displaced fractures or non-healing fractures, a referral to an orthopedic surgeon is recommended. Use acetaminophen for pain control and avoid nonsteroidal anti-inflammatory drugs (NSAIDs) because NSAIDs can impair bone healing. Ensure adequate energy availability via diet and adequate calcium and vitamin D intake (7), and avoid tobacco exposure to help heal the fracture. Bone health and bone nutrition are a part of the big picture in fracture healing.

Overuse Injuries

Tendinosis

The paradigm and management of tendon overuse injuries is changing. The term tendinitis is generally used to refer to painful overuse tendon conditions and implies that inflammation is present. However, the most common pathology in chronic painful tendons is tendinosis. Tendinosis occurs after repetitive injuries to a tendon results in intertendinous scarring, disorganization of tendon fibers and degeneration. Tendinosis does not have an inflammatory component. Early on in a tendon injury, there is inflammation resulting in tendinitis, but after about 6 weeks this generally evolves into tendinosis. Early activity modification and treatment of tendinitis with NSAIDs and rehabilitation may prevent the development of tendinosis. Tendinosis is a problematic condition that affects many active people, young and old. To address these more chronic tendon injuries, healing is facilitated by creating an inflammatory response. To create inflammation, treatments such as eccentric strengthening (Figure 18), deep soft tissue massage with tools (e.g., gua sha or Graston®, or ASTYM®) (Figure 19), nitroglycerin patches (Nitro-Dur),[1] and musculoskeletal ultrasound-guided percutaneous needle tenotomy (with or without injection of autologous blood, prolotherapy, or platelet-rich plasma) have all been utilized and have been shown to be effective (Table 2). It is important to avoid NSAIDs when

[1]Not FDA approved for this indication.

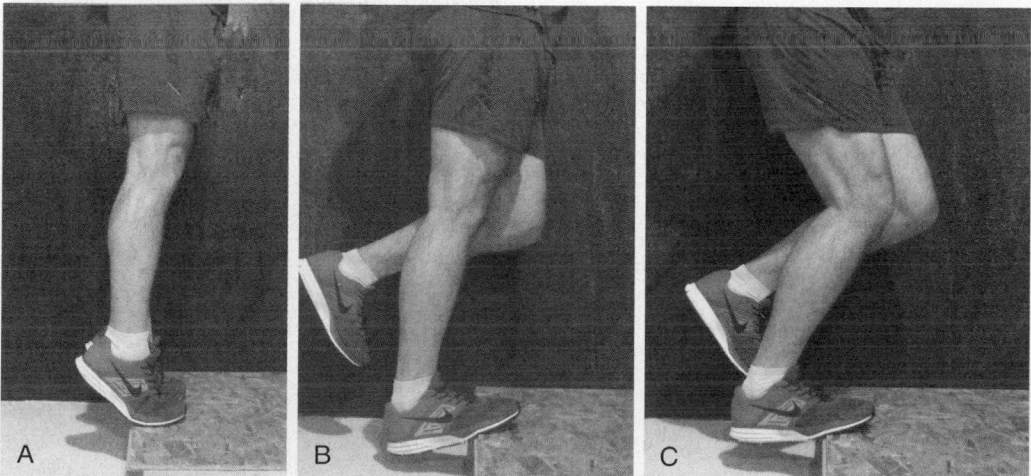

Figure 18. Eccentric exercises for Achilles tendinosis. (**A**) Patient begins with the injured leg straight and the ankle in flexion. The assistance of the uninjured leg was utilized to get in this starting position. (**B**) The ankle of the injured leg (right leg, in this case) is slowly lowered in a controlled fashion to full dorsiflexion to eccentrically strengthen (while lengthening the calf muscles) the right Achilles tendon. The left leg is then brought back down, and full plantarflexion in both ankles is performed, recruiting the uninjured leg to assist with getting back to position (**A**). (**C**) The eccentric exercise from (**B**) is repeated with the knee bent at 45°.

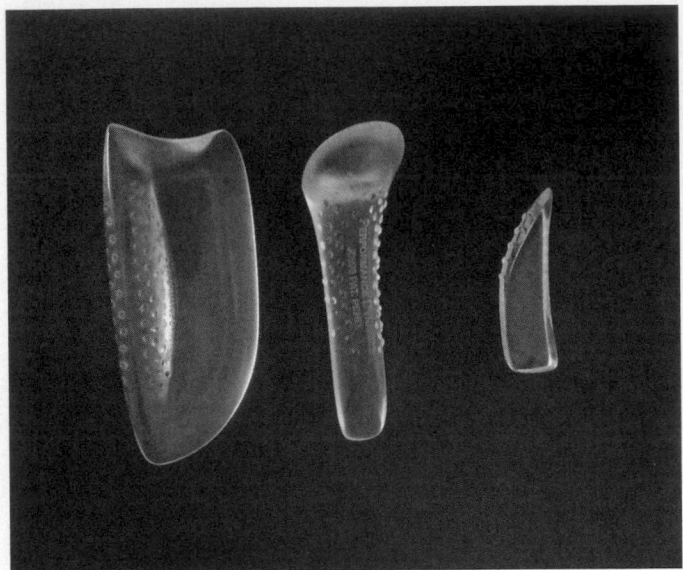

Figure 19. ASTYM® tools.

TABLE 2	Treatment of Tendinosis

TREATMENT MODALITY	DESCRIPTION
Deep soft tissue massage with tools (gua sha, Graston®, ASTYM®) (Figure 19)	One to three times per week for 4–6 wk; most common with athletic trainer certified or physical therapist
Nitroglycerin patches (Nitro-Dur)[1]	0.2 mg/h patch, cut in half and apply Q24 h to a different location on tendon for at least 6 wk
Eccentric strengthening (Figure 18)	3 sets of 15 exercises, twice daily, for 12 wk
Musculoskeletal ultrasound-guided percutaneous needle tenotomy with or without autologous blood injection, prolotherapy, or platelet-rich plasma	Referral to primary care sports medicine physician

[1]Not FDA approved for this indication.

trying to create inflammation because NSAIDs will prevent the inflammatory response. This concept of tendinosis diagnosis and treatment can be utilized for tendons throughout the body and is most commonly applied to the Achilles tendon, patella tendon, iliotibial (IT) band, piriformis, gluteus medius, hamstrings, biceps, common elbow flexor tendon, and common elbow extensor tendon.

Stress Fractures

Stress fractures occur when osteoclastic activity overwhelms osteoblastic activity. Bone injury unfolds over a continuum of time, starting with normal bone that progresses to stress reaction, then stress fracture, and finally fracture if the bone continues to be injured. This can occur as a result of excessive stress on normal bone from overactivity or normal stress on a bone that is deficient (osteoporotic, poor nutrition, or in female athlete triad). Stress fractures are common injuries in athletes and occur most often in the lower extremities. Running sports account for 69% of stress fractures. Stress fractures should be considered in someone who is active, presents with bone pain, and who performs repetitive activities with limited rest or with a recent increase in activity. Physical examination tests to perform in the area of interest are palpation, the tuning fork test, the fulcrum test, and the hop test (Table 3). If a stress fracture is suspected, x-rays should be obtained, keeping in

TABLE 3	Stress Fracture Physical Exam Tests

PHYSICAL EXAM TEST	POSITIVE TEST
Palpation	Pain over affected bone with palpation
Stork test (Figure 22)	Back extension with rotation while standing on one leg increases pain in the pars interarticularis region
Fulcrum test	Pain in fracture site while applying a bending force (e.g., over the exam table) to distal extremity while proximal extremity is kept relatively immobilized
Hop test	Hopping 10 times on affected leg reproduces pain at fracture site
Tuning fork test	Vibrating tuning fork over fracture site results in pain at site

mind that it takes 2 to 3 weeks for signs of stress fracture (i.e., periosteal reaction, callus formation, fracture line) to show up on an x-ray, and often stress fractures do not show up on x-rays. If x-rays are negative and a diagnosis is needed to help guide care and RTP, a bone scan or MRI with T2 fat saturation views (Figures 20 and 21) should be obtained. The bone scan and MRI are equally sensitive, but an MRI is more specific and avoids patient radiation exposure. An MRI is more expensive. Because a bone scan can stay positive for up to 18 months, clinical progress should not be monitored with a bone scan.

To prevent stress fractures, athletes should distribute loading forces on the bone with cross training and biomechanical adjustments (i.e., orthotics, proper shoes, stretches, strengthening, running mechanics), consume sufficient calories to maintain adequate energy availability, and ensure appropriate intake of calcium and vitamin D. A study by Lappe of female Navy recruits showed reductions in stress fractures in those consuming 2000 mg of

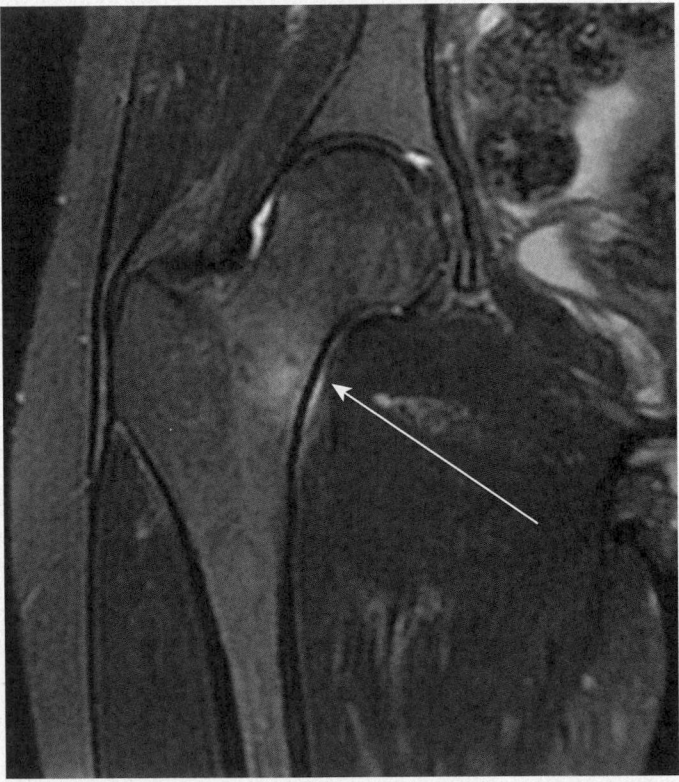

Figure 20. MRI of the right hip without contrast. Coronal T2 fat saturation image demonstrates a compression-sided femoral neck stress fracture (note surrounding bone edema in white).

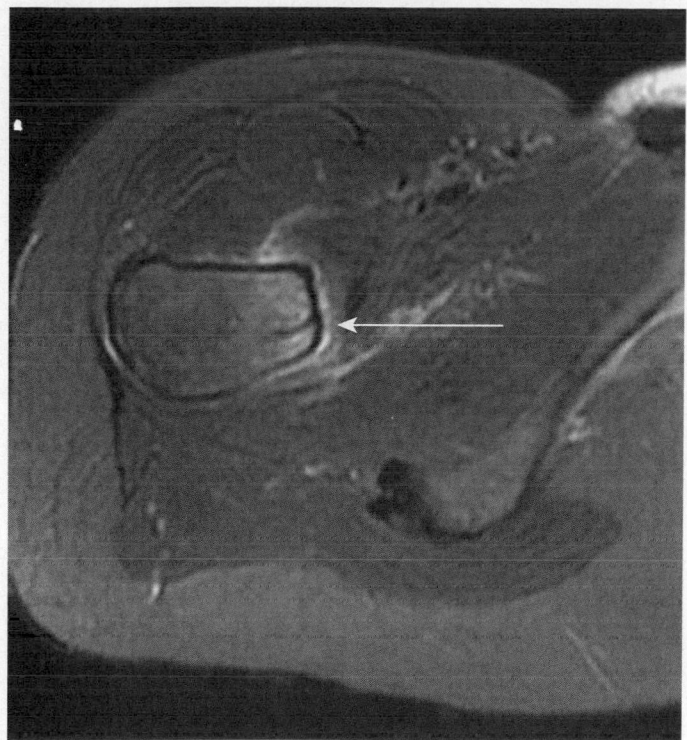

Figure 21. MRI of the right hip without contrast. Axial T2 fat saturation image that demonstrates a compression-sided femoral neck stress fracture (note fracture line in black and surrounding bone edema in white) that measures up to 11 mm.

calcium[1] and 800 IU vitamin D[1] daily, either as a supplement or through consumption of dairy products. Tobacco should be avoided. Additionally, women of child bearing age should try to maintain regular menses by consuming adequate calories and avoiding a negative energy balance.

General treatment for stress fractures can be grouped into nutrition, medication, and biomechanical recommendations. Nutrition recommendations include optimizing energy availability in the diet, ensuring adequate calcium and vitamin D intake, and avoidance of tobacco exposure. Medication recommendations include using acetaminophen as needed for pain control and avoidance of NSAIDs. Biomechanical recommendations are to offload the affected bone and reduce activity to pain-free functioning and pain-free cross-training. Crutches may be needed to offload the injured area even more than a walking boot/cast or steal shank. The patient may require complete non-weight bearing (NWB) with the overall goal being to obtain pain-free ambulation during the initial treatment. Tables 4 and 5 outline recommended guidelines for protected weight bearing for specific stress fracture sites. Additional recommendations are to begin a rehabilitation program when tolerated and to stretch and strengthen supporting structures. Start a gradual increase in activity when the patient is pain-free.

Because of their propensity for delayed healing and nonunion, certain stress fractures are considered high risk, necessitate prompt treatment, and may ultimately require surgical fixation. Low-risk stress fractures have a lower incidence of delayed healing and nonunion. High-risk stress fractures that appear stable and nondisplaced can be treated nonoperatively with close follow-up. Consider referral to an orthopedic surgeon for failed conservative treatment. Biomechanical forces along the bone with activity are used to classify tibia and femur stress fractures as either compression-sided or compression-sided. For example, when running, the tibia and femur have different forces exerted on different parts of the bone. The tibia compresses posteriorly, so there is

TABLE 4 High-Risk Stress Fracture Initial Treatment

HIGH-RISK STRESS FRACTURE	INITIAL TREATMENT (IF STABLE AND NONDISPLACED)
Femoral neck (compression side) (Figures 20 and 21)	NWB for 6–8 wk then PWB to FWB over next 6–8 wk
Anterior tibia (tension side)	NWB for 6–8 wk then PWB to FWB over next 6–12 wk
Medial malleolus	Pneumatic lower leg boot for 6–8 wk
Navicular	NWB cast/boot for 6 wk then 6-wk RTP progression
Base of fifth metatarsal (Jones)	NWB cast/boot 6–8 wk
May consider surgery for quicker RTP	
Sesamoids	NWB cast/boot 6 wk

Abbreviations: NWB—non-weight bearing; PWB=partial weight bearing; FWB=full weight bearing.

TABLE 5 Low-Risk Stress Fracture Initial Treatment

LOW-RISK STRESS FRACTURE	INITIAL TREATMENT
Sacrum/pelvis	WBAT 7–12 wk
Femoral shaft	WBAT 6–8 wk
Posterior medial tibia (compression side)	WBAT boot 2–12 wk (longer time with cortical break) then transition to pneumatic tibial brace
Fibula	WBAT 1–4 wk
Metatarsal (2nd–5th)	Steel shank/walking boot 3–6 wk

Abbreviations: WBAT=weight bearing as tolerated.

more compression along the posterior tibia and more tension along the anterior aspect of the tibia. The femoral neck compresses inferiorly and medially with running, so there is more compression along the inferior medial aspect of the femoral neck and more tension along the superior lateral aspect of the femoral neck. These variable forces on different parts of the bone affect the potential for delayed healing and nonunion.

Spondylolysis and Spondylolisthesis

Spondylolysis is a nondisplaced stress fracture of the pars interarticularis. Spondylolisthesis occurs when there is bilateral spondylolysis with listhesis (slippage) of the vertebral body. Spondylolisthesis is graded 1 to 4 depending on how much slippage is present with each grade, accounting for 25% (i.e., grade 1 = 0–25%).

When a young athlete presents with low back pain, spondylolysis needs to be considered: this can be the cause of their pain up to 47% of the time. Spondylolysis is an overuse injury caused by repetitive hyperextension and/or rotation and has increased incidence in ballet dancers, gymnasts, divers, soccer players, and football linemen. L4 is the most common level for a spondylolysis. The history is significant for insidious onset of deep pain in the low back exacerbated by extension. Physical examination shows a positive Stork test (see Table 3), often with reproduction of pain on the side of weight bearing (Figure 22). If history and physical exam are suggestive of a pars interarticularis injury, x-rays of the lumbar spine, including oblique views, should be obtained. Oblique view x-rays provide the best view to identify a spondylolysis even though they only demonstrate spondylolysis about 30% of the time when it is present (Figure 23). If x-rays are negative, proceed with MRI or with SPECT scan. If the SPECT scan is positive (Figure 24), then proceed with limited CT scan (Figures 25 and 26). If radiation exposure is a concern, thinly sliced stacked

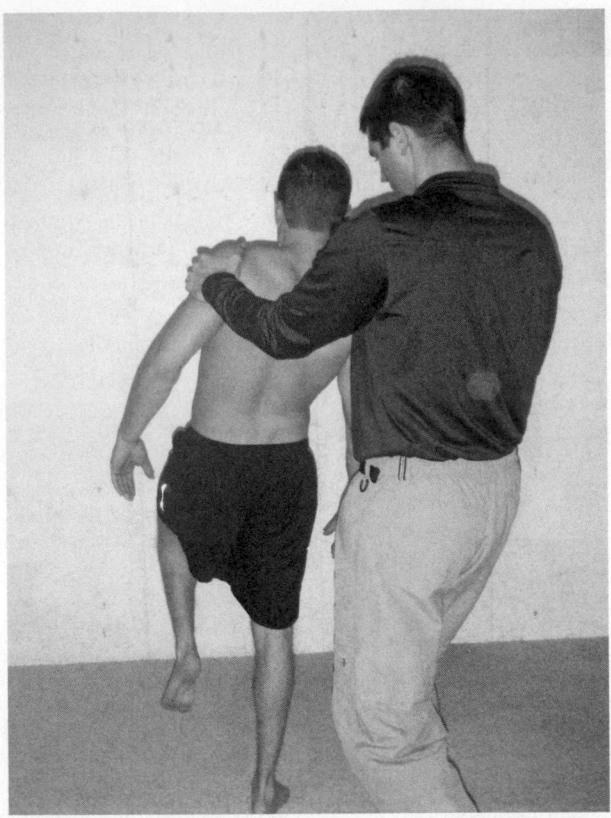

Figure 22. Stork test: To assess localized spondylolysis pain, a single leg hyperextension rotation test (stork test) is performed. The patient stands on one leg and hyperextends and rotates the spine. Reproduction of the patient's pain is suggestive of a spondylolysis.

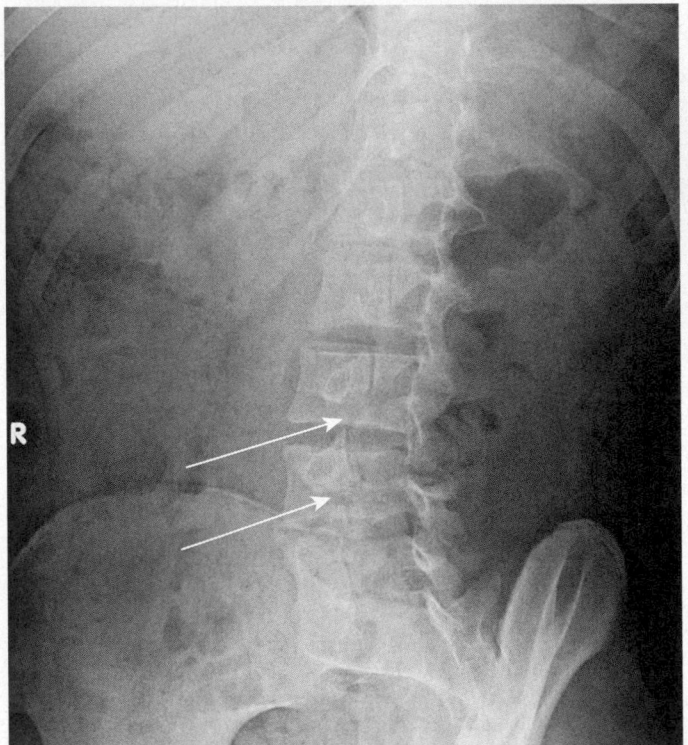

Figure 23. Oblique view x-ray of the lumbar spine, which demonstrates a L3 and L4 spondylolysis.

axial cuts with T2 fat saturation views in all planes using a high-definition MRI is the test of choice. Even with high-definition thinly sliced MRI images, the MRI can skip over the fracture line and the bone edema of a pars interarticularis injury. A spectrum of

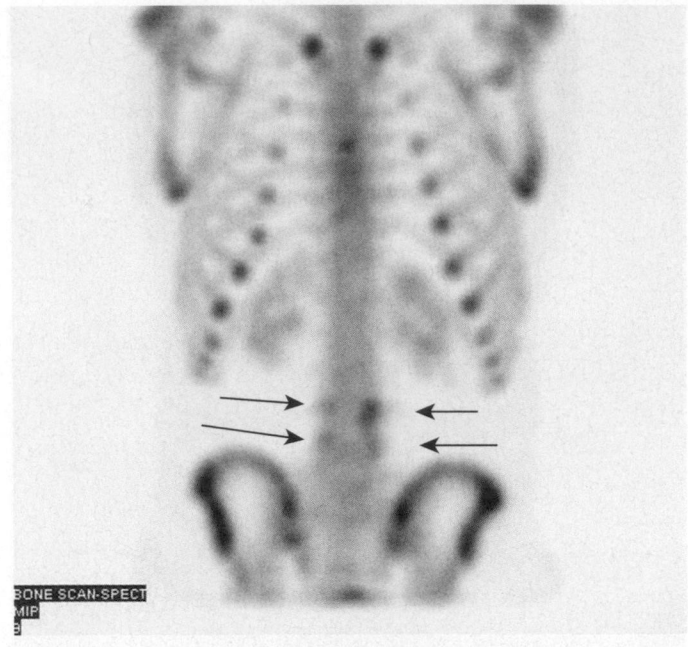

Figure 24. SPECT scan lumbar spine, PA view, which demonstrates an acute bilateral L3 and L4 spondylolysis.

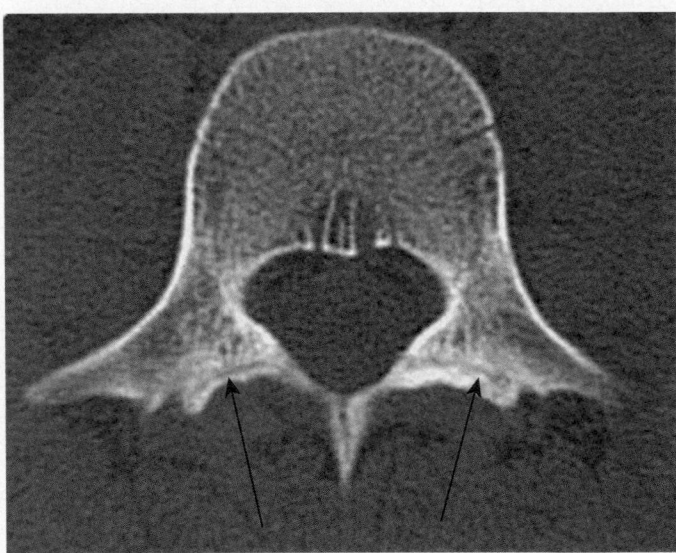

Figure 25. CT scan without contrast. Axial image at L3 shows bilateral pars interarticularis fractures that appear acute with jagged and nonsclerotic fracture edges.

recommended treatments and conservative approaches that allow for a prompt and safe RTP are reasonable. For acute spondylolysis, the recommended treatment consists of a warm and form-extension-blocking back brace worn all day except for showering and bathing (23–24 hours per day) for the first month of treatment in conjunction with rest from activity. During the second month, use of the brace during the day and with rehabilitation is suggested. Rehabilitation consists of core strengthening and lower extremity flexibility. The third month consists of a gradual return to activity, continuing core strengthening and flexibility, and wearing the brace with activity. When treating spondylolysis, a healed pars interarticularis injury is defined as pain-free activity that may include bony union of the pars interarticularis stress fracture or fibrous nonbony union. Generally, the patient should wear the brace for at least 1 year with activity and sometimes longer depending on the severity of injury. Utilize acetaminophen for pain, avoid NSAIDs, ensure adequate energy availability,

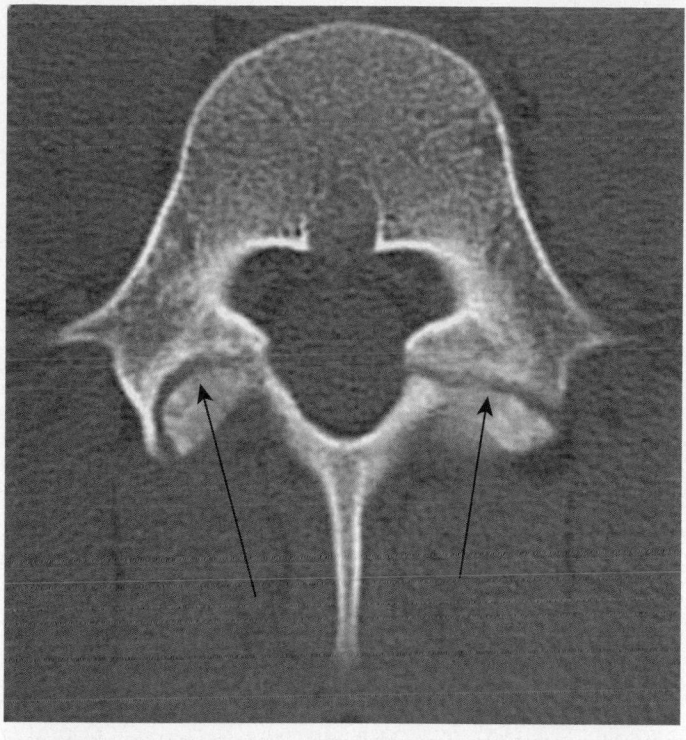

Figure 26. CT scan without contrast. Axial image at L4 shows bilateral pars interarticularis fractures. Right L4 pars fracture appears more chronic in appearance, with sclerotic fracture edges on the lateral aspect. Left L4 pars fracture appears more acute, with more jagged-appearing edges.

maximize calcium and vitamin D intake, and avoid tobacco exposure to facilitate bone healing.

The general goal for spondylolisthesis treatment is to prevent further slippage; treatment is similar to that for spondylolysis. Surgical referral is indicated for grade 2, 3, or 4 spondylolisthesis (Figure 27).

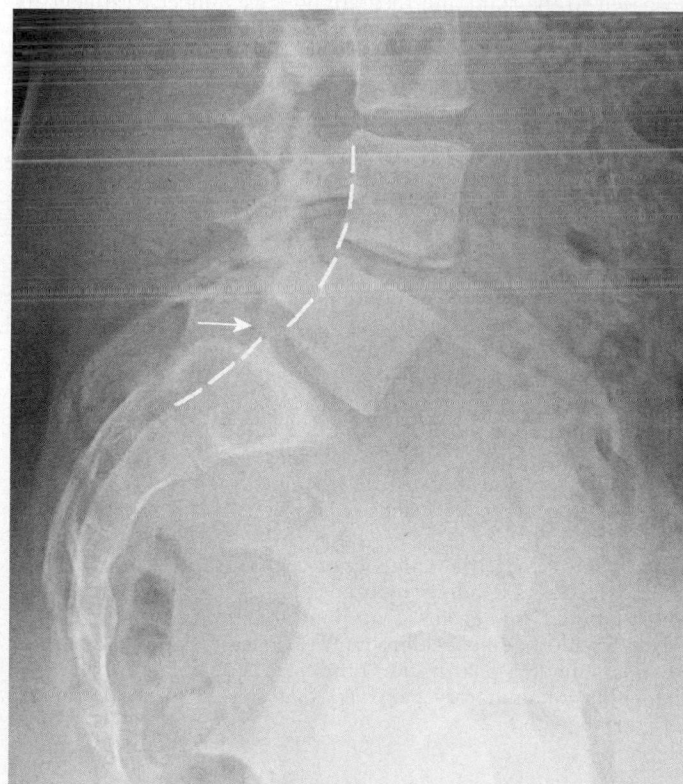
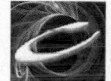

Figure 27. Lateral view x-ray of the lumbar spine, which demonstrates a grade 1 L4 spondylolisthesis.

References

Almekinders LC. Anti-inflammatory treatment of muscular injuries in sports. Sports Med 1993;15:139–45.

Bachmann LM, Kolb E, Koller M, et al. Accuracy of Ottawa ankle rules to exclude fractures of the ankle and mid-foot: Systematic review. Br Med J 2003;326:417–24.

Beynnon BD, Johnson RJ, Brown L. Knee. In: DeLee JC, Drez D, Miller MD, editors. DeLee & Drez's Orthopaedic Sports Medicine Principles & Practice. 3rd ed. Philadelphia: Elsevier; 2009. p. 1579–847.

Gellman H, Caputo RJ, Carter V, et al. Comparison of short and long thumb-spica casts for non-displaced fractures of the carpal scaphoid. J Bone Joint Surg Am 1989;71:354–7.

Haskell A, Mann RA. Foot and ankle. In: DeLee JC, Drez D, Miller MD, editors. DeLee & Drez's Orthopaedic Sports Medicine Principles & Practice. 3rd ed. Philadelphia: Elsevier; 2009. p. 1865–2205.

Kaeding C, Best TM. Tendinosis: Pathophysiology and nonoperative treatment. Sports Health 2009;1:284–92.

Lappe J, Cullen D, Haynatzki G, et al. Calcium and vitamin D supplementation decreases incidence of stress fractures in female navy recruits. J Bone Miner Res 2008;23:741–9.

Leggit JG, Meko CJ. Acute finger injuries: Part I. Tendons and ligaments. Am Fam Physician 2006;73:810–6.

Liem BC, Truswell HJ, Harrast MA. Rehabilitation and return to running after lower limb stress fractures. Curr Sports Med Rep 2013;12:200–7.

Purcell L, Micheli L. Low back pain in young athletes. Sports Health 2009;1:212–22.

Simon AM, Manigrasso MB, O'Connor JP. Cyclo-oxygenase 2 function is essential for bone fracture healing. J Bone Miner Res 2002;17:963.

Tiemstra JD. Update on acute ankle sprains. Am Fam Physician 2012;85:1170–6.

CONNECTIVE TISSUE DISORDERS

Method of
Molly Hinshaw, MD; and Susan Lawrence-Hylland, MD

CURRENT DIAGNOSIS

Lupus Erythematosus

- The erythematous-violaceous and variably pruritic, tender, or scaly eruption is photosensitive.
- Mild to moderate systemic involvement may include arthritis and pleurisy.
- Severe systemic involvement may include nephritis, cerebritis, vasculitis, and severe cytopenias.
- Associated findings include antiphospholipid antibodies associated with thromboembolism or stroke, Raynaud's phenomenon, and sicca symptoms.

Dermatomyositis and Polymyositis

- Photosensitive, violaceous-erythematous, poikilodermatous, and variably scaly patches occur around eyes, on extensor extremities (especially over joints), upper back, scalp, and dystrophic nail folds with prominent telangiectasias.
- Patients may have or develop myositis or pulmonary involvement.
- Age-appropriate cancer screening is required for adults.

Scleroderma

- Patients have firm, variably pruritic, and indurated plaques.
- Localized scleroderma (i.e., morphea or asymmetric sclerotic plaques) may be seen.
- Limited systemic sclerosis is characterized by symmetric sclerosis of distal extremities, and patients may have systemic disease.
- Diffuse systemic sclerosis is characterized by symmetric sclerosis of the trunk and proximal extremities, and patients may have systemic disease.
- Sclerodactyly (i.e., thickening of skin of digits) may occur in patients with systemic sclerosis.
- Pulmonary, cardiac, and gastrointestinal screening should be done for patients with systemic sclerosis.
- Patients with systemic sclerosis should be evaluated and monitored for renal crisis.
- Raynaud's phenomenon may develop in patients with systemic sclerosis.

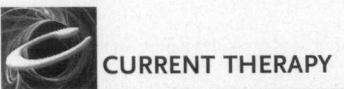

CURRENT THERAPY

Lupus Erythematosus
- Patients should be counseled on photoprotection measures.
- Localized cutaneous disease is treated with medium- to high-potency topical corticosteroids, and intralesional triamcinolone acetonide 10 mg/mL (Kenalog-10) is added if needed.
- Mild to moderate systemic involvement is treated with low- to medium-potency prednisone 5 to 20 mg/day and with antimalarials.
- Severe disease is treated with prednisone 1 mg/kg/day with a taper based on clinical response. Steroid-sparing agents include azathioprine (Imuran),[1] mycophenolate mofetil (CellCept),[1] methotrexate (Rheumatrex),[1] and cyclophosphamide (Cytoxan).[1]
- Thromboembolism or stroke is treated by anticoagulation with warfarin (Coumadin), aspirin, or heparin.
- Sicca syndrome is treated with frequent water intake, saliva replacement, artificial tears, routine dental care, and pilocarpine (Salagen).

Dermatomyositis and Polymyositis
- Patients should be counseled on photoprotection measures.
- Medium-potency topical corticosteroids and calcineurin inhibitors are used for cutaneous disease.
- Prednisone 1 mg/kg/day is first-line therapy for muscle or pulmonary disease.
- Methotrexate[1] 10 to 25 mg/week is a steroid-sparing agent used for muscle involvement.
- Hydroxychloroquine (Plaquenil)[1] 200 mg/day is used for persistent skin involvement.

Scleroderma
- For localized scleroderma, UVA[1] 20 to 60 J/cm^2 or psoralen plus UVA (PUVA) is used to resolve established lesions; high-potency corticosteroids and calcipotriene (Dovonex)[1] may help to reduce pruritus and inflammation in new lesions; and systemic prednisone[1] or methotrexate[1] may be used for rapidly progressive new lesions.
- Treatment of systemic sclerosis is primarily aimed at limiting complications.
- Physical therapy is used for contractures.
- Systemic sclerosis is treated with cyclophosphamide (Cytoxan),[1] mycophenolate mofetil (CellCept),[1] methotrexate[1] 10 to 25 mg/week, and photopheresis.
- Renal crisis is treated with captopril (Capoten)[1] 6.25 mg three to six times/day and titrated to effect.
- Raynaud's is treated with warming techniques, calcium channel blockers, antiadrenergic agents, antiplatelet drugs, and topical vasodilators.

[1]Not FDA approved for this indication.

Lupus Erythematosus

Lupus erythematosus is an autoimmune connective tissue disease that may localize to the skin or involve several organ systems. A complete review of systems with evaluation of positive findings is necessary to thoroughly assess patients for signs of systemic lupus as defined by the American Rheumatism Association. Cutaneous lupus erythematosus manifests in chronic, subacute, and acute forms. A punch biopsy from within an erythematous lupus lesion is useful for confirming the diagnosis.

Clinical Features

Discoid lupus and tumid lupus are the two forms of chronic cutaneous lupus erythematosus. Discoid lupus lesions are tender or pruritic, erythematous to violaceous, scaly plaques that typically occur on sun-exposed skin. The lesions resolve with scarring, and when the lesions affect the scalp, they cause scarring alopecia. Tumid lupus manifests as pruritic, erythematous to violaceous, nonscaly plaques that typically preferentially affect the face and trunk.

The lesions of subacute cutaneous lupus erythematosus occur as erythematous to violaceous, scaly macules and as annular or polycyclic patches. These lesions are commonly located on sun-exposed skin and heal without scarring.

Acute cutaneous lupus erythematosus is exemplified by malar erythema (i.e., butterfly rash) and by poikiloderma (i.e., hyperpigmentation, telangiectasias, and epidermal atrophy). It is a manifestation of systemic lupus erythematosus (SLE). Cutaneous lesions may be widespread. In addition to the American Rheumatism Association criteria, patients with SLE may also develop Raynaud's phenomenon, hypercoagulability, and overlap syndromes with Sjögren's disease, dermatomyositis, and other conditions.

Hydrochlorothiazide (HydroDIURIL), terbinafine (Lamisil), minocycline (Minocin), procainamide (Pronestyl), hydralazine (Apresoline), and isoniazid (Nydrazid) are a few of the pharmaceutical agents that cause drug-induced lupus. This disease manifests with synovitis, photosensitivity, and positive serology results, and it may have cutaneous lesions that do not necessarily abate with cessation of the medication.

Management
Prevention

All patients with lupus erythematosus should be counseled on photoprotection, including protecting skin from sunlight and avoiding sun exposure during peak hours (i.e., between 10 AM and 2 PM). Ultraviolet A and B wavelengths may cause lupus to flare. Broad-spectrum sunscreen with an SPF of 30 or higher and that contains titanium, zinc, Mexoryl (L'Oreal), or Helioplex (Neutrogena) should be used whenever patients are outdoors. Photoprotective clothing, available from multiple vendors, is useful for limiting sun exposure.

Patients with lupus are relatively immunosuppressed by their disease. Vaccinations should be kept up to date, although there is a debate about the necessity and safety of vaccination against meningococcal disease (*Neisseria meningitidis*) (Menactra, Menomune), varicella-zoster virus (Zostavax), and *Streptococcus* (Pneumovax).

Treatment of Cutaneous Lupus Erythematosus

Medium-potency topical corticosteroids should be used for lupus localized to the skin, and they are used as adjunct treatment for patients with systemic lupus. Use of triamcinolone 0.1% cream (Flutex) for lesions on the head and neck until symptoms subside or up to 2 weeks continuously is an appropriate starting strength. Ointment-based vehicles are useful for lesions on the trunk and extremities. They are also the vehicles of choice on the scalp of patients of African American descent. Foam or liquid- or lotion-based corticosteroids work well in the scalp of other ethnic groups and can be used on the trunk and extremities. If lesions persist, the corticosteroid can be occluded, or intralesional injections with triamcinolone can be repeated monthly as needed. Intralesional triamcinolone acetonide at concentrations of 5 mg/mL (Kenalog) can be injected into lesions on the face or neck and doses of 10 to 20 mg/mL (Kenalog-10, Kenalog) into lesions on the trunk or extremities. Intralesional corticosteroids may cause mild discomfort, atrophy of the skin or subcutis, or stretch marks. Topical calcineurin inhibitors such as pimecrolimus (Elidel)[1] or tacrolimus (Protopic)[1] may be used for maintenance treatment but are not recommended for new or active lesions because they do not work quickly. Recurrent or refractory cutaneous lesions require systemic treatment.

Treatment of Systemic Lupus Erythematosus

Antimalarials, including hydroxychloroquine (Plaquenil),[1] are disease-modifying agents that limit the progression of lupus. Hydroxychloroquine, chloroquine (Aralen),[1] and quinacrine[2] (at compounding pharmacies) raise the pH of inflammatory cells, inhibiting inflammatory pathways that cause end-organ damage in patients with SLE.

[1]Not FDA approved for this indication.
[2]Not available in the United States.

Hydroxychloroquine is typically used first at 200 mg daily for 2 weeks and then increased to 400 mg daily. Patients need laboratory monitoring and a baseline and then yearly eye examination because the medication may be deposited in the retina over time. Hydroxychloroquine exerts its effects within 2 to 3 months of beginning treatment. Its effects are diminished in smokers.

Depending on end-organ involvement in SLE, immunosuppression with systemic corticosteroids such as prednisone at doses of 1 mg/kg/day is appropriate. Steroid-sparing drugs such as methotrexate (Rheumatrex),[1] acitretin (Soriatane),[1] or mycophenolate mofetil (CellCept)[1] are added. After signs of inflammation subside, prednisone is tapered.

Treatment of Musculoskeletal Manifestations

Arthralgia is a common complaint that can usually be managed with acetaminophen or nonsteroidal antiinflammatory drugs (NSAIDs). For true arthritis unresponsive to the previously described measures, hydroxychloroquine[1] 200 mg twice daily can be added. After that, treatments similar to those used for rheumatoid arthritis can be added, although the antitumor necrosis factor agents usually are avoided in lupus. Methotrexate[1] 7.5 to 25 mg PO once weekly may be used along with folic acid[1] 1 mg daily to help limit side effects. Routine toxicity monitoring includes frequent complete blood cell counts and liver tests. Azathioprine (Imuran)[1] 0.5 to 2 mg/kg can be used with frequent monitoring of complete blood cell counts and liver tests. A sample for testing the thiopurine methyltransferase activity level should be drawn before initiating therapy because a genetic deficiency can lead to severe pancytopenia. Leflunomide (Arava)[1] 10 to 20 mg PO once daily can be used with frequent blood cell counts and liver tests. Low-dose glucocorticoids (prednisone 5–10 mg/day) may be used as a bridge to steroid-sparing therapy and to treat intermittent flares.

Treatment of Hematologic Manifestations

Autoimmune cytopenias are common and are often a defining feature of SLE. Lymphopenia (absolute lymphocyte count <1500 cells/microliter) does not require therapy. Hemolytic anemia in SLE is the result of antierythrocyte antibodies that activate complement, and it is treated with prednisone at a dose based on clinical severity. Typically, 1 mg/kg/day, or approximately 60 mg, is used for 4 to 6 weeks, with gradual tapering as long as the response is maintained. For severe hemolytic anemia, pulse methylprednisolone (Solu-Medrol) 1 g IV for 3 consecutive days can be tried, followed by the previously described standard dosing. For patients who do not respond to glucocorticoids or are unable to taper prednisone to low doses, other treatments can be used. They may include azathioprine[1] 1.5 to 2.5 mg/kg/day, mycophenolate mofetil[1] 1000 to 2000 mg/day in divided doses, danazol (Danocrine)[1] 300 to 600 mg/day in divided doses, intravenous immunoglobulin,[1] or rituximab (Rituxan)[1] 375 mg/m² weekly for four doses.

Immune thrombocytopenia results from antiplatelet antibodies that identify platelets for early destruction. Treatment is indicated when patients have signs or symptoms of spontaneous bleeding or when the platelet count drops below 50,000/mL. The initial treatment approach with glucocorticoids is similar to that used for hemolytic anemia. For patients with chronic thrombocytopenia or for those who cannot achieve an acceptable long-term dose of prednisone, steroid-sparing agents, including azathioprine,[1] mycophenolate mofetil,[1] danazol,[1] rituximab,[1] and intravenous immunoglobulin[1] can be used in doses similar to those used for hemolytic anemia. Dapsone,[1] cyclosporine (Sandimmune, Neoral),[1] and cyclophosphamide (Cytoxan)[1] have also been used.

Thrombotic thrombocytopenia purpura may occur in SLE, and it must be differentiated from immune thrombocytopenia because treatment requires emergent plasmapheresis. Manifestations of thrombotic thrombocytopenia purpura include fever, microangiopathic hemolysis, and central nervous system and renal abnormalities.

Antiphospholipid antibodies include the lupus anticoagulant, anticardiolipin antibodies, and β_2-glycoprotein. They are associated with coagulopathy, thrombocytopenia, late-trimester miscarriage, and heart valve abnormalities. Antiphospholipid antibodies that can be determined with blood testing but are not associated with thromboembolism do not require treatment. Low-dose aspirin[1] may be considered but has not been shown to prevent future thrombosis. Hydroxychloroquine[1] 200 mg twice daily has been shown to reduce the risk. Patients with antiphospholipid antibodies who develop thromboembolism need lifelong treatment with warfarin (Coumadin). A goal international normalized ratio (INR) remains controversial because different studies advocate for high-intensity warfarin (INR >3) or low-intensity therapy (INR >2). For women who have suffered a miscarriage determined to be related to antiphospholipid antibodies, low-dose aspirin and heparin 5000 units SQ twice daily may increase the likelihood of a successful pregnancy.

Treatment of Renal Manifestations

Many patients with SLE have mild to severe renal involvement. Diagnosis by renal biopsy is important to establish the type of kidney involvement. Lupus nephritis is considered one of the more severe manifestations of the disease, and treatment is aimed at preventing renal failure. Treatment should be coordinated with a rheumatologist or nephrologist.

Class I disease requires no specific therapy. The class IIb pattern with more than 1 g of proteinuria can be treated with moderate-dose prednisone (20 mg/day for 6 weeks to 3 months), followed by tapering. Class III and IV patterns of disease have the same prognosis and are treated similarly with high-dose prednisone (1 mg/kg/day) for at least 6 weeks before tapering, based on clinical response, by 10 mg a week to a maintenance of 10 to 15 mg/day. In addition to prednisone, cytotoxic therapy is initiated with cyclophosphamide[1] 0.5 to 1 g/m² of body surface area monthly for 6 months and tapered to every 3 months, based on clinical response, for a total of 2 to 3 years. Cyclophosphamide has serious toxicities, including hemorrhagic cystitis, bone marrow suppression, infertility, teratogenicity, and increased risk of malignancy. 2-Mercaptoethane sulfonate sodium (Mesna)[1] can be given with each infusion to minimize bladder toxicity. Class V disease can be treated with prednisone alone, similar to class IIb disease, unless there are coexisting features of class III or IV disease, for which treatments outlined previously should be implemented.

An acceptable alternative to cyclophosphamide for class III and IV disease is mycophenolate mofetil[1] 2 to 3 g/day in divided doses combined with corticosteroids (dosing outlined earlier). This appears to be an effective therapy with fewer side effects than traditional therapy.

Treatment of Nervous System Manifestations

Neuropsychiatric involvement is common in patients with lupus. Symptoms can range from mild to severe and include headache, aseptic meningitis, neuropathy, myelopathy, cognitive dysfunction, seizures, cerebritis, and stroke. A thorough evaluation is necessary to define the cause of nervous system dysfunction and differentiate it from a medication side effect. For seizures, antiepileptic therapy is used, preferably in coordination with a neurologist. Lupus cerebritis and transverse myelitis are two of the more serious manifestations that need to be treated emergently with aggressive immunosuppression in coordination with a rheumatologist or neurologist. Treatment includes high-dose corticosteroids and cyclophosphamide,[1] similar to treatment for lupus nephritis.

Dermatomyositis and Polymyositis

Clinical Features

Dermatomyositis may affect skin and muscle. Cutaneous dermatomyositis manifests with violaceous erythema of characteristic areas, including the periorbital skin (i.e., heliotrope rash), upper back (i.e., shawl sign), dorsal hands (i.e., Gottron's papules), scalp, lateral thighs (i.e., holster sign), and periungual skin, where dilated capillary loops and erythema are observed. Patients may report muscle weakness. As in lupus, a punch biopsy of an actively inflamed cutaneous lesion shows characteristic features.

Evaluation of patients with cutaneous dermatomyositis is not complete without assessment for systemic involvement. Serum aldolase is the most specific marker for myositis, and it can be used as a measure of response to treatment. Creatinine kinase and alanine aminotransferase levels may be elevated but are not specific indicators. An electromyogram shows dampening of signals, and a muscle biopsy shows a characteristic pattern of myositis. Inflammatory lung disease, diagnosed by the characteristic pattern on chest computed tomography, bronchoalveolar lavage, or biopsy, may be life limiting and therefore should be treated aggressively, similar to lung disease in scleroderma. Adult patients should have age-appropriate cancer screening because dermatomyositis is a paraneoplastic phenomenon in 10% to 50% of patients.

Some patients present with characteristic cutaneous dermatomyositis but no systemic involvement (i.e., dermatomyositis sine myositis). The risk of concurrent or subsequent cancer development is thought to be increased. These patients require monitoring for systemic involvement that may develop over time.

Treatment

Patients with dermatomyositis need photoprotection similar to patients with lupus. Periodic evaluation by clinical examination and review of systems allows for early intervention for developing visceral or muscle involvement.

Cutaneous dermatomyositis is treated the same as lupus (see earlier). Dermatomyositis with systemic involvement is initially treated with immunosuppression using prednisone at doses of 1 mg/kg/day. Steroid-sparing agents are incorporated early in the disease and include antimalarials (methotrexate,[1] azathioprine,[1] and mycophenolate mofetil[1]) at doses that are used in treating lupus.

Scleroderma
Clinical Features

Scleroderma is a sclerosing condition of skin or viscera, or both. The cause is unknown, but transforming growth factor-β plays a role. Type I and III collagens are excessively produced, as are other substances, including glycosaminoglycans, tenascin, and fibronectin.

Cutaneous scleroderma without Raynaud's phenomenon or clinically relevant systemic involvement is also known as *morphea*. Morphea has different distribution patterns, including guttate, linear, segmental, or diffuse distribution, but it is always characterized by indurated plaques that are inflammatory initially, have an advancing inflammatory ("lilac") border as they progress, and then become hyperpigmented. The cutaneous lesions may restrict movement of joints and can cause restricted growth of underlying structures, particularly when they develop in childhood.

Systemic sclerosis may affect the respiratory, renal, cardiovascular, genitourinary, and gastrointestinal systems and vascular structures. Raynaud's phenomenon may be the first presenting symptom of systemic sclerosis, and it can be severe, leading to digital ulcerations and autoamputation. The American College of Rheumatology has defined criteria for the diagnosis.

Tests for antinuclear antibodies are positive in approximately 95% of patients, who typically present with a homogeneous or speckled pattern. A nucleolar pattern is more specific for systemic sclerosis. Anticentromere antibodies are present in 60% to 90% of patients with limited disease but are rare in diffuse disease. Topoisomerase I (Scl-70) antibodies are positive in 30% of patients with diffuse disease and are associated with pulmonary fibrosis. Anti-PM-Scl antibodies are present in overlap syndromes and are associated with myositis and renal involvement.

Treatment
Treatment of Limited Scleroderma

For limited scleroderma, treatment with topical medium-potency corticosteroids such as triamcinolone 0.1% ointment (Kenalog) plus calcipotriene (Dovonex)[1] 0.005% cream or intralesional triamcinalone[1] 20 mg/mL may slow progression of active lesions or improve the pruritus and cutaneous stiffness that typify cutaneous scleroderma. For rapidly evolving disease, prednisone[1] 1 mg/kg/day and methotrexate[1] 15 to 20 mg/week may help slow progression of disease. UVA[1] given over 36 treatments at doses of 30 to 60 mJ/cm^2 or PUVA (oral methoxsalen [8-MOP] 10 mg taken 2 hours before treatment with UVA light) can soften the existing plaques of morphea.

Treatment of Systemic Sclerosis: Raynaud's Phenomenon

First-line treatment for Raynaud's phenomenon is preventive, with cold avoidance and the use of warming techniques. If pharmacotherapy is required, extended-release calcium channel blockers such as nifedipine (Procardia XL)[1] starting at 30 mg/day or amlodipine (Norvasc)[1] starting at 5 mg/day may be useful. If this is not helpful, the α-blocker prazosin (Minipress)[1] 1 mg three times daily or the angiotensin receptor blocker losartan (Cozaar)[1] 50 mg daily may be helpful. Antiplatelet therapy with low-dose aspirin[1] (81 mg/day) or dipyridamole (Persantine)[1] 50 to 100 mg three or four times daily may be useful. Topical vasodilators such as nitroglycerin ointment (Nitro-Bid)[1] applied to the base of the affected finger three times daily can be helpful in refractory disease. Digit-threatening ischemia may be treated with an intravenous prostaglandin such as alprostadil (Prostin VR)[1] or iloprost (Ilomedine),[5] which require peripheral or central access. Patients with severe recurrent digital ischemia may ultimately benefit from surgical sympathectomy.

Treatment of Gastrointestinal Manifestations

The most common gastrointestinal manifestation is esophageal reflux caused by esophageal dysmotility. Proton pump inhibitors such as omeprazole (Prilosec)[1] 20 mg twice daily should be used and may prevent the development of esophageal strictures. Prokinetic drugs such as metoclopramide (Reglan)[1] 10 mg four times daily can be helpful. Erythromycin[1] 500 mg three or four times daily can help esophageal and gastric hypomotility. Small bowel hypomotility can lead to bacterial overgrowth, resulting in malabsorption and diarrhea. Rotating antibiotics that include metronidazole (Flagyl),[1] ciprofloxacin (Cipro),[1] and amoxicillin/clavulanate (Augmentin)[1] can be used.

Treatment of Pulmonary Manifestations

Inflammatory lung disease occurs commonly in patients with scleroderma and can be life limiting. Cyclophosphamide[1] at doses of up to 2 mg/kg/day for up to 2 years may slow progression of pulmonary disease. Pulmonary hypertension occurs more commonly in limited systemic sclerosis than in diffuse disease. Symptomatic patients may receive treatment with prostacyclin analogues, which require continuous infusions. The endothelin receptor antagonist bosentan (Tracleer)[1] can be given orally starting at 62.5 mg twice daily. Liver tests should be monitored frequently. At this point, care is typically coordinated with a cardiologist to monitor disease progression and treatment response. Anticoagulation for pulmonary hypertension may improve survival because of the frequent occurrence of pulmonary arterial thrombosis.

Treatment of Renal Manifestations

Angiotensin-converting enzyme (ACE) inhibitors (e.g., captopril [Capoten[1]] beginning at 6.25 mg three to six times daily and titrated for blood pressure control) have dramatically reduced the incidence of renal failure and death due to renal crisis. Avoidance of prednisone at doses greater than 15 mg/day is also important in reducing the risk of renal crisis.

---

[1]Not FDA approved for this indication.

[1]Not FDA approved for this indication.
[5]Investigational drug in the United States.

References

Atzeni F, Bendtzen K, Bobbio-Pallavicini F, et al. Infections and treatment of patients with rheumatic diseases. Clin Exp Rheumatol 2008;26(Suppl. 48):S67–73.

Dziadzio M, Denton CP, Smith R. Losartan therapy for Raynaud's phenomenon and scleroderma. Arthritis Rheum 1999;42(12):2646–55.

Ginzler EM, Dooley MA, Aranow C, et al. Mycophenolate mofetil or intravenous cyclophosphamide for lupus nephritis. N Engl J Med 2005;353(21):2219–28.

Iorizzo LJ, Jorizzo JL. The treatment and prognosis of dermatomyositis: An updated review. J Am Acad Dermatol 2008;59:99–112.

Matucci-Cerinic M, Steen VD, Furst DE, et al. Clinical trials in systemic sclerosis: Lessons learned and outcomes. Arthritis Res Ther 2007;9(Suppl. 2):S7.

Nihtyanova SI, Denton CP. Current approaches to the management of early active diffuse scleroderma skin disease. Rheum Dis Clin North Am 2008;34:161–79.

Pisoni CN, Sanchez FJ, Karim Y, et al. Mycophenolate mofetil in systemic lupus erythematosus: Efficacy and tolerability in 86 patients. J Rheumatol 2005;32:1047–52.

Steen VD. The many faces of scleroderma. Rheum Dis Clin North Am 2008;34:1–15.

Subcommittee for Scleroderma Criteria of the American Rheumatism Association Diagnostic and Therapeutic Criteria Committee. Preliminary criteria for the classification of systemic sclerosis (scleroderma). Arthritis Rheum 1980;23:581–90.

Tan EM, Cohen AS, Fries JF, et al. The 1982 revised criteria for the classification of lupus erythematosus. Arthritis Rheum 1982;25:1271–2.

Wallace DD. Lupus Erythematosus. 7th ed. Philadelphia: Lippincott Williams & Wilkins; 2006.

JUVENILE IDIOPATHIC ARTHRITIS

Method of
James N. Jarvis, MD

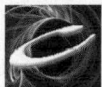

CURRENT DIAGNOSIS

- Isolated musculoskeletal pain is almost never the presenting complaint of children with chronic forms of arthritis. Relatively *painless* joint swelling, often associated with gait disturbance, is more common.
- The laboratory has very limited use in making the diagnosis of juvenile idiopathic arthritis (JIA). Anti-nuclear antibody (ANA) tests have limited utility because they are so commonly positive in perfectly healthy children (as many as 30%), and the titers that healthy children have directly overlap those seen in children with JIA. Thus, the test cannot discriminate a healthy child from one with JIA and should not be used for that purpose. Rheumatoid factor (RF) tests have the opposite problem: They are seldom positive in children with JIA, and only the minority of children with positive RF tests have JIA or any other rheumatic disease. The low positive and negative predictive values of the test make it virtually useless for diagnostic purposes. This test should never be ordered as a means of evaluating musculoskeletal pain in children.
- The hallmark for making the diagnosis of JIA is the presence of warm, thickened synovial membranes that can be palpated around the joints of affected children. The presence of hypertrophic synovial tissue around the joint(s) of a child with a typical history and clinical setting is virtually diagnostic of JIA.

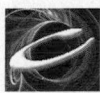

CURRENT THERAPY

- Nonsteroidal antiinflammatory drugs
- Systemic glucocorticoids in select instances
- Oral or subcutaneous methotrexate (particularly for polyarticular disease)
- Anti-TNF (tumor necrosis factor) therapies, particularly for polyarticular disease
- Anti-IL-1 (interleukin-1) therapies, particularly in systemic disease

The term *juvenile idiopathic arthritis* (JIA) is now the internationally accepted term to describe a family of illness characterized by chronic inflammation of synovial membranes. It replaces, but does not completely overlap, the diagnostic classification system that used the term *juvenile rheumatoid arthritis*. Three major phenotypes of JIA are recognized: oligoarticular, polyarticular, and systemic. In addition, the accepted international classification scheme recognizes other subtypes (e.g., enthesitis-associated arthritis, which overlaps the family of conditions previously designated *spondyloarthropathies*) that have distinct clinical phenotypes and that the clinician must recognize against the general background of children presenting with musculoskeletal complaints. Because each of these subtypes represents a distinct phenotype based on presentation, age of onset, differential diagnosis, and therapy, each of these illnesses is described as a distinct entity.

Oligoarticular Juvenile Idiopathic (Pauciarticular) Arthritis (Pauciarticular Juvenile Rheumatoid Arthritis)

Epidemiology
Oligoarticular JIA (*pauciarticular JRA* under the old American College of Rheumatology criteria) is typically a disease of preschoolers of European descent. This subtype of JIA is quite rare in African American children, children from the Indian subcontinent, and Native American children.

Risk Factors
Specific human leukocyte antigen (HLA) alleles, particularly in the class II locus, are known to confer risk for this JIA subtype. However, different alleles are seen in different ethnic subgroups, even in European populations. Thus, the presence of specific HLA alleles is not clinically useful for the diagnosis of most forms of monoarticular JIA. Older boys presenting with monoarthritis might, in fact, have what is now termed enthesitis-associated arthritis (EAA), for which the presence of class I HLA allele B27 can often be a diagnostic clue, because this allele is a major risk factor for developing EAA.

Young age (onset before the age of 3 years) and the presence of antinuclear antibodies (ANA) are specific risk factors for the development of uveitis in children with established disease. Slit-lamp examinations (see "Complications") are recommended every 4 months for children in this high-risk group.

Pathophysiology
The pathophysiology of this form of JIA is not well understood. Once generally accepted as an autoimmune disease, the high percentage of autoantibodies (especially ANA) in perfectly healthy children makes it more difficult to assess their pathologic significance in children with arthritis. Under any circumstances, what is generally accepted is that leukocyte invasion of the synovium transforms it into a growing, locally invasive tissue that secretes cytokines (thus sustaining the inflammatory process) and proteolytic enzymes that can injure surrounding joint structures.

Prevention
This illness is not known to be preventable.

Clinical Manifestations
Children with pauciarticular JIA typically present with a combination of relatively painless joint swelling, often in combination with gait disturbance. The gait disturbance, when present, is typically more prominent after periods of inactivity (e.g., first thing in the morning or after a nap). Verbalized musculoskeletal pain is almost never a prominent presenting complaint. Although children seldom verbalize pain, they might express some distress when the affected joint is moved.

Diagnosis
This illness typically occurs in preschool children, with a female-to-male ratio of about 3:1. In older children and teenagers with monoarticular disease, diagnoses other than JIA should be considered. Children typically present with relatively painless swelling of a lower extremity joint.

Gait disturbance, most prominent after periods of inactivity (e.g., first thing in the morning or after an afternoon nap), is often a prominent symptom. Careful palpation of lower extremity joints typically reveals warm, thickened synovial tissue. An effusion might or might not be present if the affected joint is a knee. Laboratory tests are not particularly helpful, except in excluding other diagnoses (e.g., Lyme disease, leukemia).

The diagnosis is typically established on the basis of the history and physical examination. Laboratory studies may be necessary to exclude other causes of monoarticular or oligoarticular joint swelling, particularly in children not in the typical demographic (e.g., older children or children of non-European ancestry). No single laboratory test or set of laboratory tests establishes the diagnosis. ANA and rheumatoid factor (RF) tests are particularly unhelpful, because of the low positive predictive value of the former and the low positive and negative predictive values of the latter.

Differential Diagnosis

In a typical clinical setting, the diagnosis is usually straightforward. In areas of North America and Europe where Lyme disease is endemic, Lyme disease is a more common cause of monoarticular joint swelling than oligoarticular JIA. Lyme arthritis can usually be established or excluded on the basis of a screening enzyme-linked immunosorbent assay (ELISA) and Western blot analysis. In preschoolers presenting with severe musculoskeletal pain in a lower extremity joint, acute lymphocytic leukemia should be considered and investigated with one or more complete blood counts (CBC, performed serially), a serum lactate dehydrogenase (LDH), and possibly plain films to examine for periosteal elevation around the affected joint. In children from ethnic groups not typically within the oligoarticular JIA risk group (e.g., Native American children), a more determined search for nonrheumatic causes of monoarticular arthritis (e.g., tuberculosis) may be advisable.

Treatment

The goals of treatment are to rapidly re-establish normal function, prevent further intrusiveness of the disease process into normal activities, and prevent damage to the affected joint(s) and atrophy of the surrounding muscles. Rapid restoration of normal function is increasingly being addressed by the use of intraarticular steroid injections. Daily administration of nonsteroidal antiinflammatory drugs (NSAIDs; e.g., naproxen [Naprosyn], 10–20[3] mg/kg/day) can often accomplish this same aim but take considerably longer to demonstrate efficacy. In a few cases, synovitis is intractable even with the combination of NSAIDs and joint injection, and in these cases, methotrexate, given either orally or subcutaneously at 10 to 20 mg/m^2/week, typically provides good disease control. Treatment of uveitis is discussed later.

Monitoring

The disease process itself is monitored by interim histories and physical examinations. Slit-lamp examinations are a critical component of the monitoring of all children with JIA, because uveitis is typically indolent and asymptomatic. Children on daily NSAIDs should have a CBC (to monitor for occult blood loss) as well as comprehensive metabolic panel and urinalysis (to monitor for renal toxicity) at least twice a year. The same laboratory studies should be performed in children on methotrexate, although pediatric rheumatologists typically monitor more frequently (every 3–4 months) in children on that drug.

Complications

Before effective therapies were available, muscle atrophy and joint contracture were common complications of this form of JIA. Such sequelae are rare with current approaches to treatment. Uveitis remains the single most common and serious complication of this form of JIA and, even with new and more aggressive therapies, uveitis often results in loss of some visual acuity in the affected eye(s). Diagnosis of this complication can only be made under slit-lamp examination, because signs and symptoms develop only later, when visual acuity is already severely compromised. Children in the highest risk group should have slit-lamp examinations at least three times per year. The high-risk group includes children with a new diagnosis, who are 3 years of age or younger, and who are ANA positive; note that the ANA in this setting is used for prognostic, not diagnostic, purposes. The risk of uveitis is lifelong, and slit-lamp examinations should continue on a yearly basis throughout adulthood.

First-line therapy for uveitis typically includes topical corticosteroids. However, methotrexate and anti–tumor necrosis factor (TNF) monoclonal antibodies (infliximab [Remicade],[1] adalimumab [Humira]) have been shown to be effective in children with disease that is refractory, persistent, or recurrent.

Oligoarticular (pauciarticular) juvenile idiopathic arthritis

Epidemiology

Polyarticular JIA occurs in all age groups (although cases diagnosed in children younger than 1 year of age are rare) and in all ethnic groups. Polyarticular disease is further subcategorized based on the presence or absence of immunoglobulin M (IgM) RFs detected by standard laboratory tests. RF-positive children tend to be older (school-aged children and adolescents) and have severe synovitis, morning stiffness, and other constitutional symptoms. This subtype is more strongly represented among African American and Native American patients, where it represents as many as 50% of all cases of polyarticular JIA. It is rare in European and European-descended children, representing only 10% of all cases of JIA in that population.

RF-negative JIA occurs at all ages in European and European-descended children, from preschool ages to adolescence. African American and Native American children tend to be school-aged or adolescents.

Risk Factors

Specific HLA class II alleles are known to confer risk for RF-negative polyarticular JIA, but, as with pauciarticular disease, these associations vary among different ethnic groups and are not sufficiently strong to be useful diagnostically. Alleles subsumed under the HLA-DR4 group are associated with RF-positive disease, particularly in Native Americans.

Pathophysiology

The pathophysiology of polyarticular JIA is poorly understood. It was once thought to be a typical autoimmune disease in which autoreactive T cells initiate an immune reaction against (unknown) joint or synovial antigens, but that concept has come under challenge. Disease biomarker studies have suggested an important role for innate immunity in this JIA subtype, particularly monocytes and neutrophils. Under any circumstances, leukocyte infiltration of the synovium transforms it into a proliferating, invasive, and immunologically active tissue. Secretion of both cytokines and proteolytic enzymes plays an important role in causing local tissue damage. Gene expression profiling studies of peripheral blood suggest important roles for interferon (IFN)-γ and TNF-α in either initiating or sustaining the chronic inflammatory response.

Prevention

This illness is not known to be preventable. Given the strong association between tobacco smoking and HLA-DR4–positive RA in adults, it is possible that measures used to prevent tobacco abuse could reduce the incidence of disease in high-risk populations, such as members of specific Native American tribes.

---

[3]Exceeds dosage recommended by the manufacturer.

[1]Not FDA approved for this indication.

Clinical Manifestations

Because of the wide age range affected, clinical manifestations vary significantly for this JIA subtype. Preschoolers typically present with joint swelling and gait disturbance. Failure to gain or loss of major motor milestones is a fairly rare but well-described presentation in this age group. Joint swelling is the most common presenting complaint in older children and adolescents. Less than 20% of children with JIA verbalize pain at all on initial presentation. Morning stiffness lasting for an hour or more is typically seen in all age groups. Older children with wrist or finger involvement (or both) commonly complain of difficulty with fine motor tasks, such as playing a musical instrument.

Diagnosis

As with oligoarticular JIA, musculoskeletal pain is not a common complaint at presentation in children with polyarticular JIA. Joint swelling, gait disturbance, or, in younger children, loss of (or failure to achieve) major motor milestones are more common presentations.

As with oligoarticular JIA, the laboratory is of limited utility. The diagnosis is made on the basis of the history and physical examination. The critical physical finding in polyarticular JIA is the presence of warm, thickened synovial membranes, typically including both large (knees, ankles) and small (fingers, toes) joints.

The diagnosis is established on the basis of a typical history (swelling in multiple joints, morning stiffness) and a physical examination demonstrating warm, thickened synovial membranes around multiple joints. Involvement of at least one wrist and small joints of the hands is typical. As with all other forms of childhood-onset arthritis, the laboratory is only of marginal use in making the diagnosis and is more useful in excluding other diagnoses. RF tests are singularly unhelpful and should not be ordered for diagnostic purposes. ANA tests are helpful only in excluding the diagnosis of systemic lupus erythematosus (SLE; see later under "Differential Diagnosis"). Thrombocytosis and mild anemia may be seen in severely affected children, but in such cases the history and physical examination have usually established the diagnosis without need of the laboratory.

Differential Diagnosis

Acute postinfectious arthritis can mimic polyarticular JIA. A distinguishing feature of postinfectious arthritis is the prominence of joint pain as a presenting complaint. Acute RF occasionally mimics polyarticular JIA, but the joint swelling of acute RF is typically exceptionally painfully and migratory (i.e., swelling moves from joint to joint and seldom lasts more than 24 hours in any given joint).

Acute leukemia occasionally manifests with painful swelling in multiple joints and should be considered in a child with swelling and severe musculoskeletal pain.

SLE is another entity that can present with swelling in multiple joints and constitutional symptoms. ANA tests may be helpful in establishing this diagnosis if the titer is 1:1080 or more. Titers between 1:320 and 1:640 are ambiguous, because these results can be seen in healthy children and in children with JIA. Serum C3 and C4 levels and a urinalysis should always be drawn when an ANA test is being requested for diagnostic purposes, because most children with SLE have low serum complement levels and an abnormal urinalysis. Thus, abnormal results from these tests can often clarify the ambiguity that emerges with ANA titers between 1:320 and 1:640.

Treatment

The goals of therapy for polyarticular JIA are identical to those for pauciarticular JIA: to rapidly reestablish normal function, prevent further intrusion of the disease process into normal activities, and prevent damage to the affected joint(s) and atrophy of the surrounding muscles. Very few children with polyarticular JIA have adequate clinical responses on NSAIDs alone, although these

drugs (most commonly naproxen, 10–20[3] mg/kg/day in two divided doses) are often used.

More aggressive treatment approaches are now typical in pediatric rheumatology, supported by recently published data that demonstrate that only 5% of children with this disease achieve remission within 5 years. Combinations of methotrexate (10–20 mg/m² given orally or subcutaneously), NSAIDs, and oral steroids are often used in children as first-line treatment. Joint injections with triamcinolone (Aristopan) are used to quickly restore function when activities of daily living or comfort are compromised by synovitis in one or a few joints. TNF inhibitors (etanercept [Enbrel], infliximab,[1] adalimumab) have all shown efficacy in children who have failed methotrexate, and there is a growing trend to use these drugs earlier in the disease course or even at presentation in severely affected children.

There is limited experience in pediatric rheumatology with the IL-1 inhibitor anakinra (Kineret),[1] particularly in JIA, and many children find the required daily injections burdensome. Inhibitors of T cell costimulation signals (e.g., abatacept [Orencia]) have shown some efficacy in children but are generally reserved for children who have failed other therapies. Autologous stem cell transplantation has been shown to be efficacious in children who have failed multiple therapies and have a poor quality of life because of severe, persistent synovitis.

Monitoring

Monitoring for NSAIDs and methotrexate is described under the section on oligoarticular arthritis. Potential hepatic, renal, and bone marrow toxicities of TNF inhibitors are monitored exactly as is done for methotrexate. Because the TNF inhibitors can unmask latent tuberculosis, a PPD is required before starting anti-TNF therapy. All children with polyarticular JIA should be monitored for uveitis through routine slit-lamp examinations (see below).

Children on methotrexate and etanercept (with or without concomitant corticosteroid therapy) should be considered immunosuppressed. Thus, fever, unexplained pulmonary infiltrates, or other signs of infection might need to be investigated more vigorously than in an otherwise healthy child. Fever is almost never a sign of the underlying arthritis.

Complications

Uveitis is a complication of all forms of JIA, including polyarticular JIA. As with oligoarticular JIA, younger children who are ANA positive are at highest risk for this complication, and routine slit-lamp examinations are recommended. Treatment of uveitis is described in the section on oligoarticular arthritis. Anemia of chronic inflammation is often seen in children with severe polyarticular JIA. The most efficient way of treating this complication is to resolve the inflammatory process as rapidly as possible, and providing oral iron can attenuate or resolve this problem.

A severe, albeit rare, complication of polyarticular JIA is an entity called *macrophage activation syndrome*. This severe, sometimes fatal, complication is described in detail in the section on systemic disease.

Severe joint destruction is becoming rare in children with polyarticular JIA, but it still occurs, particularly in children who are RF positive. Joint replacement surgery has sometimes been useful in this setting.

Systemic-Onset Juvenile Idiopathic Arthritis

Epidemiology

All age groups are affected by systemic-onset JIA. This is one of the few forms of JIA that affects boys and girls equally. After RF-positive polyarticular JIA, this is the rarest form of JIA. However, this form of JIA may be proportionally more common in some Asian countries, including Japan.

Risk Factors

There are no known risk factors for this illness. Unlike other types of JIA, there are no convincing HLA associations with this subtype.

---

[1]Not FDA approved for this indication.
[3]Exceeds dosage recommended by the manufacturer.

Pathophysiology

As with all the other forms of JIA, the pathophysiology of this illness is poorly understood. Mouse models that overexpress human IL-6 mimic many of the features of the human illness, including growth failure. The importance of IL-6 has been corroborated in gene-expression studies from Japan. Gene-expression profiling in affected children also demonstrates a prominent role for IL-1 and IL-1–regulated genes. These findings together suggest an important role for innate immunity in disease pathogenesis. How these findings fit together, or how they explain the chronic synovitis that eventually evolves during or after the febrile phase of the disease, remains to be elucidated.

Prevention

There are no known preventive measures for systemic-onset JIA.

Clinical Manifestations

Children typically present with fever and rash. The fever commonly occurs at regular intervals once, twice, or three times a day. When the fever is present, the child can appear to be quite ill. In contrast, between febrile episodes, the child can appear active, playful, and near normal. The patterned occurrence of the fever and the child's often-robust appearance between febrile episodes are important clues to the diagnosis. Once the febrile episodes begin, they invariably occur daily. Other diagnoses should be pursued in a child with intermittent fever who goes entire days without a febrile episode. The characteristic salmon-colored rash may be present all the time or appear only with the fever. In cases where the rash is continuously present, it can become more prominent during febrile periods. The rash is macular, often confluent in areas, and present on the trunk and extremities but not usually the palms and soles.

The synovitis might appear at the time of the fever and rash or only appear days, weeks, or months later. The presence of joint pain is not diagnostically useful, because many febrile children have this complaint. The presence of morning stiffness or gait disturbance should prompt a very careful examination of the lower extremities for proliferative synovium around the knees, ankles, or small joints of the feet.

An acute phase response is quite typical, and its absence should lead to the pursuit of other diagnoses. White blood cell counts of more than 20,000/mm^3 are common, and counts below 15,000 mm^3 relatively uncommon. Platelet counts are typically greater than 500,000/mm^3, and it is not unusual to see erythrocyte sedimentation rates of more than 80 mm/hour.

Diagnosis

Fever and rash are the typical presenting complaints in children with systemic-onset JIA. The fever typically occurs daily, not intermittently. Other diagnostic entities (e.g., Epstein-Barr virus [EBV] infection) should be considered in children with intermittent fever. The fever typically occurs regularly, in a once, twice, or (more rarely), thrice daily pattern. When the fever is present, the child usually appears quite ill; affected children appear surprisingly well in periods between febrile episodes. Querying parents and caretakers for this very typical feature of the disease can be useful diagnostically. The rash, when present, typically intensifies when the fever is present. A brisk acute phase response is typically seen. White blood cell counts of more than 20,000/mm^3 and platelet counts of more than 500,000/mm^3 are common.

The diagnosis is made based on the history and physical examination and the exclusion of other explanations for fever. The diagnosis can be challenging to make in children who have not yet developed synovitis. This is one form of JIA where the laboratory can be somewhat helpful, because the absence of leukocytosis and thrombocytosis makes systemic onset JIA less likely. Determined efforts to exclude infection, malignancy, and other inflammatory disorders (e.g., Kawasaki's disease) are often required before the diagnosis of systemic-onset JIA can be established.

Differential Diagnosis

The differential diagnosis for systemic JIA is broad and includes infectious (e.g., EBV and cytomegalovirus [CMV] infection), malignant (e.g., lymphoma, neuroblastoma, and leukemia), and other inflammatory (e.g., Kawasaki's disease) etiologies. The latter can be difficult to exclude in a toddler and, thus, the importance of the details of the history and physical; for example, toddlers with Kawasaki's disease are typically irritable even when they are afebrile, but children with systemic-onset JIA often appear quite comfortable between febrile episodes. Younger children (younger than 10 years) might not make the heterophile antibody that is detected in the monospot test for EBV, and antibody titers to specific EBV antigens (usually available in standard EBV antibody panels) should be requested to exclude this diagnosis. Bone marrow examination may be required to exclude malignancy, especially if corticosteroid therapy is anticipated.

Treatment

Corticosteroids, given either as daily oral prednisone (1–2 mg/kg/day) or as methylpredisolone (Medrol) pulses (500 mg/m^2/dose) are usually effective in controlling the systemic symptoms. In Japan, where systemic disease is quite common, anti–IL-6 monoclonal antibody therapy with tocilizumab (Actemra)[1] has been shown to be effective in controlling both systemic and articular disease. Clinical trials of tociluzimab are under way in North America. Recent work has also shown promising results for the IL-1 receptor antagonist anakinra,[1] based on measured clinical efficacy and responses measured by gene expression profiling. The longer acting agent, canakinumab, has shown efficacy in children with systemic JIA and is approved for that use. Canakinumab may be better tolerated by children because of its monthly dosing schedule. Methotrexate (10–20 mg/m^2/week) remains a standard treatment for persistent articular disease, which is typically treated using approaches much like those used for polyarticular disease. Cyclosporine (Neoral)[1] has demonstrated some efficacy for both systemic and articular disease in children who have failed other agents.

Monitoring

Monitoring is the same as for polyarticular JIA. Uveitis is not as common in systemic-onset JIA as in other forms of JIA.

Complications

The hematologic and articular complications of systemic-onset JIA are essentially the same as those seen in polyarticular disease. A serious, sometimes lethal, complication of systemic JIA is macrophage activation syndrome. Macrophage activation syndrome comprises endothelial cell activation and hepatic and cerebral dysfunction typically heralded by otherwise unexplained decreases in serum hemoglobin, white blood cell, and platelet counts. Elevations in serum ASL/ALT and serum ferritin are other diagnostic clues. Bone marrow aspiration might reveal erythrophagocytic macrophages; their presence is diagnostic, but their absence does not exclude macrophage activation syndrome and should not delay therapy. The development of macrophage activation syndrome should be considered a medical emergency, and affected children should be referred immediately to facilities with experience in caring for this complication.

Enthesitis-Associated Arthritis

Epidemiology

Enthesitis-associated arthritis describes a group of arthritides characterized by male predilection, involvement of the axial skeleton (e.g., hips, sacroiliac joints, cervical spine), extraarticular inflammation (bursae, tendon insertions or enthuses, plantar fascia), and acute uveitis. This is the most common form of childhood-onset arthritis on the Indian subcontinent and in some Native American tribes. It might also be more common among children from Mexico and Central America than it is among European and European-descended children.

---

[1]Not FDA approved for this indication.

Risk Factors

HLA-B27 represents an important risk factor in all populations. Between 80% and 90% of European Americans with enthesitis-associated arthritis are HLA-B27 positive. African American patients are less commonly HLA-B27 positive (60%–70%), so the absence of HLA-B27 should not exclude the diagnosis in this population.

Pathophysiology

Current evidence suggests a causative role for HLA-B27. Rats expressing the human HLA-B27 gene develop a clinical picture nearly identical to the human disease. HLA-B27 transgenic rats raised in germ-free environments do not develop the disease, suggesting that normal commensural flora, particularly intestinal flora, play an important role. The connection between gastrointestinal flora and human disease is corroborated by the development of postinfectious arthritic syndromes (e.g., Reiter's syndrome) in HLA-B27-positive adolescents and adults after salmonella, shigella, or chlamydia infection. Finally, the high prevalence of arthritis strongly resembling enthesitis-associated arthritis in patients with inflammatory bowel disease suggests a link between the arthritis and loss of integrity of the gastrointestinal mucosal barrier. Recent research interest has therefore focused on antigen processing by gut-associated lymphoid tissue, although no single pathogenic model has emerged.

Prevention

There are no known preventive measures.

Clinical Manifestations

Enthesitis-associated arthritis demonstrates a wide variety of clinical presentations. The practitioner may be confronted with a preschool or school-aged boy with monoarticular joint swelling virtually indistinguishable from oligoarticular JIA (male sex and the older age of the child may be important diagnostic clues). School-aged and adolescent patients often present with unilateral or bilateral hip pain. The pain is characteristically worse in the morning and better with activity, which helps distinguish it from other causes of hip pain in teens (e.g., slipped capital femoral epiphysis), which typically cause pain that is worse with activity and better with rest. Finally, some patients present with an acute polyarthritis very similar to polyarticular JIA. Selective involvement of the distal interphalangeal joints of the fingers with sparing of the proximal interphalangeal joints is a typical pattern. Low back pain is very seldom a presenting complaint, unlike in adults with HLA-B27–mediated forms of arthritis.

Diagnosis

The disease typically occurs as a monoarthritis, often involving the hip. This is the only form of JIA where pain is typically a prominent presenting complaint. Hip pain, made worse with rest and better with activity, is a common presenting complaint. Unlike in adults, back pain is only an infrequent presenting complaint in children. The diagnosis is supported (but not established) by the presence of HLA-B27 on peripheral blood leukocytes.

As with all the other forms of JIA, the diagnosis is established on the basis of the history and physical examination. Hip disease typically is associated with pain on internal and external rotation of the affected hip(s), with some loss of range of motion. The presence of extraarticular inflammation (e.g., pain or swelling around the Achilles tendons, plantar fasciitis, bursitis of the hips or shoulders) can be helpful diagnostic clues. Nail pitting, sometimes with frank onycholysis, is sometimes seen. Diffuse swelling of a single toe (sausage toe) is a characteristic finding, as is painful arthritis of the first metatarsophalangeal joint.

The laboratory can be helpful in making the diagnosis. HLA-B27 is present in 80% to 90% of patients of European descent. Elevations in erythrocyte sedimentation rate or anemia associated with chronic inflammation are sometimes seen. Imaging studies of the hips can show cartilage loss with or without periarticular demineralization. Changes in the sacroiliac joints are seldom seen at presentation but they can evolve over the course of the disease; their appearance strongly supports the diagnosis.

Differential Diagnosis

Because of the broad spectrum of clinical presentations, the differential diagnosis is likewise broad. Transient synovitis of the hip must be considered in younger children complaining of hip pain. In older children, this same complaint can raise the possibility of Legg-Calvé-Perthes disease, slipped capital femoral epiphysis, idiopathic avascular necrosis, or axial skeletal tumors (e.g., Ewing's sarcoma). Hip pain in children is almost always an indication for obtaining plain films.

Oligoarticular JIA and polyarticular JIA are almost always considered in patients presenting with peripheral arthritis. Acute, self-limited, postinfectious arthritis is sometimes in the differential diagnosis.

Treatment

Therapeutic goals and approaches are virtually identical to those for polyarticular JIA.

Monitoring

See the section on polyarticular JIA.

Complications

Acute, painful uveitis is a common complication of this form of arthritis and can even be the presenting complaint. Pain; red, inflamed sclerae; and photophobia almost invariably lead patients to seek medical attention quickly. Most patients with acute uveitis respond well to topical corticosteroids. Inflammation of the genital tract (sterile urethritis, balanitis) are less common complications.

Progressive joint destruction, particularly in affected hips, can occur even with aggressive management. Sacroiliitis can be seen in older patients or patients with long-standing disease. Frank ankylosis of the spine is rare before adulthood.

Acknowledgment

Special thanks to Ms. Lucy Chen for proofreading and editing and for helpful comments on this chapter.

References

Allantaz F, Chaussabel D, Stichweh D, et al. Blood leukocyte microarrays to diagnose systemic onset juvenile idiopathic arthritis and follow the response to IL-1 blockade. J Exp Med 2007;204:2131–44.

Foster CS. Diagnosis and treatment of juvenile idiopathic arthritis-associated uveitis. Curr Opin Ophthalmol 2003;14:395–8.

Hashkes PJ, Laxer RM. Update on the medical treatment of juvenile idiopathic arthritis. Curr Rheum Rep 2006;8:450–8.

Hayward K, Wallace CA. Recent developments in anti-rheumatic drugs in pediatrics: treatment of juvenile idiopathic arthritis. Arthritis Res Ther 2009;11:216.

Ilowite NT. Update on biologics in juvenile idiopathic arthritis. Curr Opin Rheumatol 2008;20:613–8.

Jarvis JN. Commentary: Ordering laboratory tests for suspected rheumatic disease. Pediatr Rheumatol 2008;6:19.

McGhee JL, Kickingbird L, Jarvis JN. Clinical utility of ANA tests in children. BMC Pediatr 2004;4:13.

McGhee JL, Burks F, Sheckels J, Jarvis JN. Identifying children with chronic arthritis based on chief complains: Absence of predictive value for musculoskeletal pain as an indicator of rheumatic disease in children. Pediatrics 2002;110:354–9.

Tse SM, Laxer RM. Juvenile spondyloarthropathy. Curr Opin Rheumatol 2003;15:374–9.

OSTEOARTHRITIS

Method of
David H. Neustadt, MD

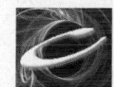

CURRENT DIAGNOSIS

- Improved understanding and knowledge of the pathogenesis of osteoarthritis have led to increasing optimism for the 20 to 30 million osteoarthritis sufferers in the United States.
- Osteoarthritis is now known to involve inflammatory mechanisms, not mechanical wear and tear, as believed in the past.

627

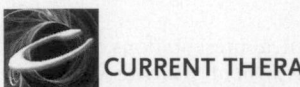

CURRENT THERAPY

- Although there is no cure for osteoarthritis, coping strategies including simple measures such as weight reduction and modification of activities to reduce stress and load on the joints should be emphasized.
- Pharmacotherapy includes acetaminophen (Tylenol), other simple analgesics, and judicious use of nonsteroidal antiinflammatory drugs. Opioids should be avoided, except during the first few days of post-operative surgery when joint replacement procedures have been carried out.
- When usual medical measures fail to control the pain of osteoarthritis, intraarticular injections of a corticosteroid is the next step.
- A painful effusion is the major indication for arthrocentesis, aspiration, and if fluid is not infectious, instillation of a corticosteroid preparation.
- After a corticosteroid injection for knee osteoarthritis, increased therapeutic response results if a postinjection rest regimen is imposed. The patient remains in bed or at rest for 3 days and then uses walking devices (cane or crutches) for 2 to 3 weeks.
- The main factors that influence the therapeutic response from a series of hyaluronan injections are the extent of loss of cartilage and severity of the osteoarthritis disease in the affected knee.
- Total knee and hip replacement procedures are considered when nonoperative management fails to adequately control symptoms and pain.

Osteoarthritis (OA) (degenerative joint disease) is the most commonly encountered rheumatic disorder and the major cause of disability and reduced activity after 50 years of age. Radiographic evidence of OA is found in up to 85% of people older than 65 years. Autopsies indicate evidence of OA in weight-bearing joints of almost all persons by the age of 45 years.

In spite of the evidence of pathologic changes of OA found in Java and Neanderthal human skeletons and dinosaur skeletons, OA was confused with rheumatoid arthritis (RA) until the turn of the 20th century. It is characterized pathologically by involvement of cartilage, varying from fissures and microfibrillations in early disease to erosive destruction in advanced disease. Weight-bearing or shearing forces are transmitted to the subchondral bone, leading to sclerosis, cyst formation, and bone remodeling. Osteophytes (spurs) develop at the margins of joints, and new cartilage proliferates over these bony spurs.

An inflammatory component is present in most patients with symptomatic OA. The traditional belief that OA is simply a wear-and-tear condition associated with the stress of advancing years is not tenable. This mistaken belief is considered the major reason for the relatively slow progress of cartilage and bone research and investigation into the etiology and pathogenesis of OA. During the past decade, much new knowledge on cartilage, including metabolic changes, genetic mutations, metalloproteinases, and possible diagnostic biomarkers and inflammatory mediators, has fostered considerable excitement and interest in new approaches for the prevention, monitoring, and treatment of OA.

Although the cause of OA is unknown, contributing factors include genetic history, trauma, overweight, overuse of joints, and aging. An additional risk factor recognized more recently is leg length disparity (inequality), which seems to be associated with greater hip or knee joint pain. OA may be classified into primary (idiopathic) and secondary forms. Secondary OA results from trauma or repetitive overuse of a specific joint; an inflammatory form of arthritis such as RA, repeated attacks of gout, or septic arthritis; developmental problems such as congenital dysplasia of a hip or slipped capital femoral epiphysis; or metabolic and miscellaneous causes including hemophiliac arthropathy, ochronosis (alkaptonuria), and osteonecrosis. Thus, OA may be considered a (final) common pathway resulting from a host of many different problems.

Joints commonly affected in OA include the large, weight-bearing, and frequently used joints, such as the hips and knees, spine, distal interphalangeal (DIP) joints (Heberden's nodes), and trapeziometacarpal (carpometacarpal thumb base) and first metatarsophalangeal joint (bunion). Joints often spared in OA include the metacarpals, the wrists, the shoulders, and the ankles (except in ballet dancers).

Clinical Features

The onset of OA is insidious, and the course is slowly progressive. Clinical features include variable pain and mild stiffness, with associated limited motion; bony enlargement with or without tenderness; synovitis of the knees; and functional impairment with malalignment (varus or valgus deformities) when advanced involvement of the knees or hips develops. There are no specific laboratory abnormalities or specific (disease) markers of the disease, except in ochronosis.

Radiographs and other imaging procedures demonstrate evidence of OA, manifested chiefly by a narrowed joint space (loss of cartilage), osteophyte formation, and secondary subchondral sclerosis. There may be a poor correlation between symptoms and underlying abnormal structural findings on x-ray images. Special subsets of OA and significant associated conditions include inflammatory (cystic erosive) OA, calcium pyrophosphate dihydrate disease (chondrocalcinosis), and diffuse idiopathic skeletal hyperostosis (DISH).

Treatment

The optimal management program for OA should be individualized to the specific problems and clinical syndromes presented by each patient (Box 1).

General Considerations

Realistic reassurance that the patient does not have a serious, potentially crippling disease such as RA and adequate understanding of what to expect are of paramount importance for successful management. Education of the patient is the basic foundation of the treatment program. The updated OA booklet provided by the National Arthritis Foundation is a useful supplement to education. Involving spouses and other family members in coping skills training may be helpful. Understanding the patient's problem permits reasonable delegation of responsibilities for chores and engaging in activities. Patients and spouses who are better informed about the disease and its outlook are generally better able to cope with the condition. Cognitive behavior techniques can help patients confront the variability of symptoms, the effects of rest and exercise, and emotional aspects.

Prophylactic Measures

Reducing the impact of the load and shearing force on an osteoarthritis joint not only can diminish symptoms but also can retard progression of the disease. Explaining the biomechanical factors enables the patient to understand the need for rest and protection of the affected joints. Weight reduction by dietetic means is

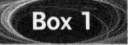

Box 1   Comprehensive Management Program for Osteoarthritis

Education of the patient and family
Coping measures: Rest and modification of activities of daily living
Measures to reduce joint loading
Physical therapy, occupational therapy, assistive devices
Pharmacotherapy
Intraarticular therapy (corticosteroid suspensions and hyaluronan)
Total joint replacement procedure

Box 2	Measures to Protect Knees

Avoid knee bending during weight bearing
Avoid steps when possible
Use high chair or high stool
Use elevated toilet seat
Use cane, crutches, or walker for prolonged walking
Do isometric quadriceps muscle-strengthening exercises

---

strongly encouraged for the obese patient. Protective and preventive measures for the knee include avoiding weight-bearing knee bending, stair climbing, jogging, and prolonged walking. Knee loading during weight bearing can be avoided by using a high chair or stool, elevated toilet seat, knee supports or braces, and walking devices (Box 2).

Nonpharmacologic Therapy

The most important aspect is specific instructions for balanced rest and exercise (preferably at home). Exercises should be mainly isometric (nonmovement), such as quadriceps muscle strengthening, stretching, and range-of-motion exercises.

Instructions should be given for joint protection with measures to conserve energy and on the use of any needed assistive aids, such as canes, crutches, walkers, splints, back supports and braces, cervical supporting collars, and proper shoes with any needed modifications and orthotics.

Heat modalities should be prescribed in the form of hot showers or tub soaks, hot packs such as a Bed Buddy (microwavable cervical collar or back wrap), and a warm pool for water aerobic exercises. These measures ameliorate discomfort and facilitate the exercise program. Diathermy, short wave, and ultrasound methods are relatively expensive and of questionable benefit. The use of a hot tub or whirlpool bath, especially after exercise or work, may be of palliative benefit.

Job and recreational activities must be assessed and modified if necessary to avoid overuse of affected joints. Sexual counseling may be needed, especially in some patients with severe knee, hip, or back involvement.

Pharmacotherapy

The basic program of education and reassurance of the patient, joint rest and protection, and physical measures can control symptoms in some patients with early mild OA. Many patients, however, require drug therapy. Although no available drugs predictably reverse or halt the inexorable progression of the disease, the drugs do reduce pain and inflammation, enhancing the patient's quality of life.

Analgesics

Some patients with OA have minimal inflammation and can be managed with analgesics alone. Analgesic agents (non-narcotic) currently available include acetaminophen (Tylenol) and tramadol (Ultram). Effective dosages of acetaminophen are 1.0 to 1.3 g administered every 8 hours or three or four times daily (do not exceed 4 g/day). Adverse effects are rare, but caution must be exercised in patients who have preexisting renal or liver conditions. Tramadol can be given in 50-, 100-, 200-, or 300-mg tablets up to two to three times daily for pain relief (do not exceed 400 mg of immediate-release tablets per day or 300 mg of extended-release tablets per day). These drugs are generally well tolerated, and nausea, vomiting, and dizziness are the most common adverse effects. A combination preparation, Ultram 37.5 plus acetaminophen (Ultracet), is available. Propoxyphene (Darvon and Darvon products), longstanding, useful, and safe analgesics, unfortunately have been removed from the approval list by the Food and Drug Administration (FDA). Duloxetine (Cymbalta) 60 mg daily was introduced as a compound for pain

caused by fibromyalgia syndrome. Recently, the drug received approval by the FDA for mild to moderate pain resulting from OA. Duloxetine has minor adverse effects, the most common of which is nausea that usually subsides when the medication is continued for a period of approximately 6 to 10 days. In large, controlled clinical trials, nausea occurred in up to 24% of patients taking duloxetine versus 8% of the placebo group. The drug has been reported as occasionally causing mild renal lab alterations. Discontinuing the drug brings about clearing of the renal dysfunction within 1 to 2 weeks. Duloxetine is considered relatively safe when the patient is seen for a checkup every 2 to 3 months and has laboratory tests to include routine urinalysis, serum creatinine, and BUN. Patients who have a history of elevated blood pressure should be cautioned to have their blood pressure checked every 2 to 3 months. Duloxetine is contraindicated in patients taking monoamine oxidase inhibitors (MAOIs). Rare interactions can cause a serious reaction. The drug is known to cause mydriasis occasionally. In view of this problem it should not be used in patients who have uncontrolled narrow-angle glaucoma. Duloxetine may increase the risk of bleeding; therefore patients should be cautioned about taking the medication with aspirin or other possible anticoagulants. In a double-blind, randomized, placebo-controlled study of patients with chronic pain due to OA of the knees, there was significant improvement with duloxetine versus the placebo. I advise avoiding regular use of opioids. Opioids may be needed occasionally for intense pain, but the benefits are limited owing to the common gastrointestinal adverse events and the potential for addiction.

Antiinflammatory Agents

A much-discussed report compared acetaminophen 4 g/day with ibuprofen (Advil, Motrin) 1200 to 2400 mg/day in OA of the knee. The clinical results demonstrated no significant difference in efficacy among the three treatment groups. Critical analysis of this comparative study, however, discloses a short duration of the treatment trial (4 weeks) and a relatively low antiinflammatory dosage (up to 2400 mg) of ibuprofen. In my experience and that of many others, pain in OA patients is often not adequately controlled with pure analgesics, whereas nonsteroidal antiinflammatory drugs (NSAIDs) in adequate dosage can provide significant clinical improvement.

Nonacetylated salicylates are widely used in OA. Compounds currently available include salsalate, choline magnesium trisalicylate, and magnesium salicylate. These agents are weak prostaglandin (cyclooxygenase) inhibitors, thus avoiding the anticlotting effect and potential adverse effect on the gastrointestinal tract and kidneys. Side effects are relatively uncommon and minor with nonacetylated salicylates when administered in a dosage of 1 to 1.5 g twice daily. Gastrointestinal and cardiovascular problems have not been reported. Salicylism with ototoxicity is a rare side effect.

If simple analgesics and salsalate fail to provide adequate relief, one of the many currently available NSAIDs may be selected for a therapeutic trial. Clinical trials with naproxen, diclofenac, and sulindac showed significantly greater improvement of the NSAID when compared with high-dose acetaminophen. The chief limiting factor in the use of NSAIDs is the possible induced gastric pathologic changes, disturbed renal function, and potential increased cardiac events.

Cost and compliance also must be given consideration. Many of the NSAIDs are now available in dosage forms that can be given once or twice daily, which helps overcome the compliance problem.

Currently available NSAIDs are all similar in their proposed mechanism of action but vary considerably in their pharmacokinetics, dosage, clinical response, and side effects. The variability of the effects of different NSAIDs in patients is significant and unpredictable. All NSAIDs are metabolized in the liver, except two available compounds, sulindac (Clinoril) and nabumetone

(Relafen), which are called prodrugs; they are not converted to active drugs until after absorption and hepatic biotransformation. The prodrug effect might partially spare the gastrointestinal tract and also produces less suppression of renal prostaglandins. Etodolac (Lodine) reportedly has fewer gastric complications, and endoscopy does not demonstrate the typical gastric erosions found in the gastric mucosa of the majority of patients taking older NSAIDs.

Concomitant prophylactic use of misoprostol (Cytotec) has been recommended to protect gastric mucosa in patients with a previous history of peptic ulcer or gastrointestinal bleeding. Unfortunately, misoprostol causes cramps and diarrhea in a relatively high percentage of patients. A gastroprotective agent, such as a proton pump inhibitor, will reduce the risk of gastrointestinal adverse effects.

The question of potential deleterious effect on cartilage versus chondroprotective properties by various NSAIDs remains controversial.

Cyclooxygenase 2 Inhibitors

Prostaglandin synthesis in humans is catalyzed by two enzyme forms of cyclooxygenase: cyclooxygenase 1 (COX-1) and cyclooxygenase 2 (COX-2).

COX-1 is constitutively expressed and is considered responsible for suppression of physiologic functions including gastric mucosal protection. In contrast, COX-2 is induced by inflammatory mediators and is responsible for inflammation without any significant effect on the gastric mucosa. The development of agents that selectively inhibit the COX-2 pathway without significant gastrointestinal adverse effects was considered an extremely important advance.

Currently only one COX-2–specific inhibiting NSAID is FDA approved and available. Celecoxib (Celebrex) is equivalent to the older nonselective NSAIDs with regard to therapeutic effectiveness, but the risk of gastrointestinal toxicity and adverse effects on platelet aggregation is lessened. The risk of renal side effects is probably comparable with that of the conventional NSAIDs. A trial assessing the effect of celecoxib on cardiovascular events found a slightly higher risk of cardiovascular events but chiefly only at higher doses (400 mg/day or greater). Celecoxib can be used with low-dose aspirin (81 mg) daily and anticoagulants including warfarin (Coumadin).

Intraarticular Injections

Corticosteroids

After many years of controversy concerning intraarticular corticosteroid therapy in OA, there is now consensus that this form of therapy is of considerable value when it is indicated and skillfully administered. Although early on it is still preferable to attempt to control symptoms by simple measures with oral therapy, rather than by local injection, when faced with relatively acute painful conditions such as synovitis of the knee or inflamed Heberden's nodes, quick and sometimes lasting relief can be obtained with intrasynovial steroid injection. This form of treatment is considered an adjunct to a conventional management program.

A painful knee effusion is the most common indication for arthrocentesis followed by a local corticosteroid injection. The remote potential deleterious effect of instability developing in the knee can be avoided by giving injections at infrequent intervals and prescribing a strict postinjection rest regimen. Specific instructions are given to the patient to refrain from weight-bearing activity for 3 days, except getting up for meals and going to the bathroom. The patient is advised to reduce loading of the injected knee by using a cane or crutches with a three-point gait during weight bearing for 2 to 3 weeks after the procedure. This rest regimen delays escape of the steroid suspension from the joint cavity

and promotes a longer duration of response to the injection. I have observed numerous patients with OA of the knee associated with large recurrent synovitis who had been given three to five or more local injections with only transient benefit. When a strict postinjection rest program was imposed, these patients obtained substantial improvement in the duration of the effect, and some achieved indefinite "cures." The remote risk of introducing infection from the procedure is minimized by adhering to a meticulous aseptic technique.

Another important indication for arthrocentesis and intraarticular steroid therapy is OA associated with crystal synovitis due to calcium pyrophosphate dihydrate disease (CPPD) pseudo-gout or pseudogout. Diagnosis is confirmed by radiographic findings of chondrocalcinosis and polarized microscopic identification of the specific crystals in the fluid. Treatment, including aspiration and administration of intraarticular steroids, is usually successful in controlling the acute synovitis.

Hyaluronans (Hyaluronic Acid, Hyaluronate)

Intraarticular hyaluronan, approved by the FDA in 1997 as a new procedure for clinical use in OA of the knee, represents a valuable addition to the therapeutic armamentarium for the treatment of OA. The clinical use of intraarticular hyaluronan in painful OA of the knee was introduced in Europe in the 1990s. The mechanism of action of hyaluronate is termed *viscosupplementation*, an effort to restore normal viscoelastic properties to the pathologically altered synovial fluid. Other possible beneficial effects include protection of the chondrocytes, antiinflammatory effects, and improvement of the mechanics of joint motion.

Numerous preparations of FDA approved hyaluronan preparations are in wide use in the United States. Initially, all hyaluronans were extracted from rooster combs. Table 1 lists the more common hyaluronans that are available for injecting knee osteoarthritis. The hyaluronan products are injected in a series of three, four, or five at weekly intervals in accordance with the patient's response. All the hyaluronans are highly purified natural preparations except Hylan G-F20, which is cross-linked with added formaldehyde and vinyl sulfone in an effort to increase retention in the joint cavity. Effectiveness and duration of improvement are similar with all the products. Undesirable complications and adverse effects are limited to rare local mild pain, with the exception of the cross-linked Hylan G-F20, which can cause a severe acute inflammatory reaction (SAIR, or pseudoseptic reaction) in approximately 2% to 8% of patients injected with the product.

Newer hyaluronan products are non–animal-derived preparations that are developed from biological fermentation of streptococcal origin. Until recently, these hyaluronans have been

---

TABLE 1 Some Common FDA-Approved Hyaluronans and Their Molecular Weights

PRODUCT	MW (kDa)	DOSE (WEEKLY)
Hylan G-F20 (Synvisc)*	5000–6000	3 × 16 mg
High-molecular-weight hyaluronan (Orthovisc)	1000–2900	3–4 × 30 mg
Sodium hyaluronate (Hyalgan)	500–720	3–5 × 20 mg
Sodium hyaluronate (Supartz)	620–1200	5 × 25 mg
1% Sodium hyaluronate (Euflexxa)†	2400–3600	3 × 20 mg

*Not pure; contains formaldehyde and vinyl sulfones. Human synovial fluid MW is 350–500 kDa.
†Derived from biologic fermentations.

available only in Europe. One of these products (Euflexxa) has been approved by the FDA for use in the United States. This preparation would be especially useful in the rare patient who is allergic to avian products. Hyaluronan therapy has been studied in other specific joints including the hip, shoulder, ankle, and first carpometacarpal joints. Approval from the FDA is expected. Drawbacks of intraarticular hyaluronan include difficulty injecting and limited response in patients with extreme obesity and severe advanced osteoarthritis of the knee (grade 4 Kellgren classification). Re-treatment with intraarticular hyaluronic acid 1 year after the first series is safe and effective in patients whose initial course of therapy was successful. A new hyaluronan preparation (Monovisc) has been developed, containing 4 or 5 times the amount of hyaluronan used in the usual knee injection, which is given in a series of 3 or 4 weekly injections. Monovisc is a cross-linked sodium hyaluronate. It is designed to treat the symptoms of osteoarthritis with only one injection. The response and results have not been compared directly in a clinical trial to date. The approach, if effective, would simplify the procedure, especially for "needle shy" patients.

Joint Lavage and Arthroscopy

Lavage of the arthritic knee may be performed with arthroscopic visualization. The authors of a recent double-blind, sham-controlled evaluation concluded that "most, if not all" of the effects of tidal irrigation seem to be attributable to a placebo effect. Arthroscopy permits inspection of the joint cavity. Associated abnormalities such as ligamentous and meniscal tears can be observed in conjunction with osteoarthritis. Calcified loose bodies can be removed, and débridement can be carried out.

Treatment of Cystic Erosive (Inflammatory) Osteoarthritis

Cystic erosive OA is the genetically determined clinical syndrome manifested by lumpy-bumpy fingers with involvement of the DIP joints (Heberden's nodes) and proximal interphalangeal joints (Bouchard's nodules). It rarely causes significant pain except during the early developing stage. It is important to strongly reassure the patient that this is not a serious crippling disease, emphasizing the distinction of the knobby nodes from the swelling of the synovitis of RA. However, if the thumb base joint (trapeziometacarpal, first carpometacarpal) is involved, abduction splinting or local injection may be necessary for relief of pain.

Occasionally, when OA of the fingers is symptomatic, warm soaks; application of an analgesic balm, such as triethanolamine, after the warm soaks; and the wearing of spandex gloves during sleep at night are useful. When a digital node is inflamed, local instillation of a few drops of a corticosteroid suspension often provides prompt relief.

If symptoms persist, a cautious trial with one of the topical analgesic pepper plant creams (capsaicin) such as Zostrix may be worthwhile. Capsaicin is an inhibitor of substance P, the neuropeptide pain mediator. The topical cream is safe, and a local burning or transient stinging sensation during application is the only troublesome adverse effect. The stinging diminishes with use after a few days.

New Approaches
Disease-Modifying Drugs

The purpose of the investigational disease-modifying drugs is to play a role in either enhancing the biosynthesis of cartilage matrix or preventing enzymatic degradation and inhibiting catabolic cytokine activity in an attempt to induce cartilage repair and restore joint homeostasis.

Tetracycline (Sumycin)[1] and its congeners [doxycycline (Vibramycin),[1] minocycline (Dynacin)[1]] have shown evidence of inhibiting enzymatic degradation of cartilage, including that by stromelysin, collagenase, and gelatinase, in dog, guinea pig, and rabbit models of OA. A proposed long-term clinical trial in human subjects is in progress.

Hydroxychloroquine (Plaquenil)[1] and chloroquine (Aralen)[1] have been administered successfully for many years in RA and systemic lupus erythematosus. Recently, anecdotal and retrospective uncontrolled studies have reported the efficacy of hydroxychloroquine in retarding the progression of inflammatory (cystic) erosive OA. It has been suggested that the beneficial action of hydroxychloroquine is due to its inhibitory effects on lysosomal enzymes and the secretion of interleukin-1. Experience thus far suggests that this agent may be promising in inflammatory OA.

Other novel therapeutic approaches that are under study but lack conclusive significant data at this time include insulin-like growth factors, transforming growth factor-β, and glucosamine, a proteoglycan component and a growth factor for cartilage. In ongoing studies, an antinerve growth factor antibody, fully humanized, effectively reduces pain and improves function in subjects with knee osteoarthritis. Undesirable effects so far are minor, including a rare, transient, mild peripheral neuritis.

Chondrocyte Transplantation

Chondrocyte transplantation was initially developed and carried out in Sweden for localized cartilage damage resulting from trauma in young subjects. A subsequent report described relatively successful treatment of 23 patients who had chondral defects of the knee and were given autologous chondrocyte transplantation combined with periosteal grafting. The expectation that the procedure will "cure" OA lesions remains an unmet possibility for the future. Regeneration of articular cartilage is a complex process and will require long-term evaluation of the function of the new cartilage and prospective controlled clinical studies to confirm the value of the procedure.

Gene Therapy

Gene therapy is an exciting new technology that holds promise for the future but requires considerable further investigation and refinement. Techniques to introduce gene transfer in conjunction with autologous cultured chondrocytes are being explored.

Glucosamine and Chondroitin Sulfate

Glucosamine[7] and chondroitin[7] sulfate are over-the-counter nutraceuticals (dietary supplements) that have considerable anecdotal data touting their symptom-modifying effects. Some reports have suggested that glucosamine can retard or modify structural changes of OA, but convincing evidence for this effect is lacking. The drugs are well tolerated and have no significant adverse effects. Recently published studies have no evidence or significant data demonstrating that either of these preparations used alone or in combination prevents or reduces pain in osteoarthritis of the knee. These so-called neutraceuticals cause no serious adverse effects, but any true clinical value remains to be shown.

Surgery

When appropriate medical (nonoperative) management fails to adequately control pain, and functional disability significantly interferes with lifestyle, surgical options should be considered.

---

[1]Not FDA approved for this indication.
[7]Available as a dietary supplement.

Available procedures include osteotomy for joint malalignment (varus knee deformities); arthroscopy, especially for specific lesions such as calcified loose bodies or meniscal tears; and arthrodesis (fusion) for unstable joints, when joint replacement is not indicated or declined. Arthrodesis may be the optimal procedure in young, overweight, active patients with severe OA involving a single knee.

Partial or total arthroplasty, especially total knee and hip replacement, may be carried out in patients in whom medical management fails to adequately control symptoms. An estimated 125,000 total hip replacements, most of which are for OA, are performed each year in the United States. Total knee replacement (total knee arthroplasty) is an increasingly gratifying operation for advanced knee OA. Innovative approaches and new techniques, including the development of minimally invasive procedures (MIS), bodes well for the future.

References

Chappell AS, Desaiah D, Liu-Seifert H, et al. A double-blind, randomized, placebo-controlled study of the efficacy and safety of duloxetine for the treatment of chronic pain due to osteoarthritis of the knee. Pain Practice 2011;11:33–41.

Hunter DJ. Clinical therapeutics: Viscosupplementation for osteoarthritis of the knee. N Engl J Med 2015;372:1040–7.

Mandell BF, Lipani J. Refractory osteoarthritis. Differential diagnosis and therapy. Rheum Dis Clin North Am 1995;21:163–78.

Neustadt DH. Intra-articular injections for osteoarthritis of the knee. Cleve Clin J Med 2006;73:897–910.

Neustadt DH. Current approach to therapy for osteoarthritis of the knee. Louisville Med 2004;51:341–3.

Neustadt DH, Altman RD. Intra-articular therapy. In: Moskowitz RW, Howell DS, Goldberg VM, et al., editors. Osteoarthritis, Diagnosis and Medical/Surgical Management. 4th ed. Philadelphia: Lippincott Williams & Wilkins; 2007. p. 287–301.

Poole AR, Howell DS. Etiopathogenesis of osteoarthritis. In: Moskowitz RW, Howell DS, Goldberg VM, et al., editors. Osteoarthritis, Diagnosis and Medical/Surgical Management. 4th ed. Philadelphia: Lippincott Williams & Wilkins; 2007. p. 27–49.

Sharma L, Kapoor D, Issa S. Epidemiology of osteoarthritis. In: Moskowitz RW, Howell DS, Goldberg VM, et al., editors. Osteoarthritis, Diagnosis and Medical/Surgical Management. 4th ed. Philadelphia: Lippincott Williams & Wilkins; 2007. p. 1–26.

Steinbrocker O, Neustadt DH. Aspiration and Injection Therapy. Arthritis and Musculoskeletal Disorders: A Handbook on Technique and Management. Hagerstown MD: Harper & Row; 1972.

OSTEOPOROSIS

Method of
Alexei DeCastro, MD; and Peter J. Carek, MD, MS

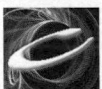

CURRENT DIAGNOSIS

- Evaluation of risk factors for osteoporosis and related fractures is always recommended.
- Routine bone mineral density to evaluate women ages 65 years and older is recommended.
- In postmenopausal women younger than 65 years, bone mineral density testing may be indicated depending on evaluation of fracture risk.
- Determination of bone mineral density is indicated for those with osteoporotic fractures to determine the severity of the disorder.
- Clinical and laboratory evidence of secondary causes of osteoporosis should be pursued in all patients with osteoporosis.
- Current evidence is insufficient to recommend screening for osteoporosis in men.

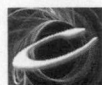

CURRENT THERAPY

- A comprehensive nutritional orientation targeting normal body weight is recommended. Additionally, healthy bone orientation requires adequate ingestion of calcium and vitamin D. Calcium intake should be at least 1200 mg/day, including supplements, when necessary. Vitamin D should be prescribed for persons at risk of insufficiency at doses of 800 to 1000 IU.
- Weight-bearing and muscle-strengthening exercises are important tools to reduce the risk of falls and fracture.
- Pharmacologic therapy is indicated for those with vertebral fracture or hip fracture.
- Pharmacologic therapy is indicated for those with bone mineral density T-scores of −2.5 standard deviations or less at the lumbar spine, at the femoral neck, or the total hip, after proper evaluation.
- Pharmacologic therapy is indicated for postmenopausal women and men ages 50 years and older who have lower bone mass (T-score −2.5 to −1.0) at the femoral neck, the total hip, or the lumbar spine if the 10-year hip fracture probability is 3% or more or if the 10-year probability of a major osteoporosis-related fracture is 20% or more based on the U.S.-adapted World Health Organization (WHO) absolute fracture risk model.
- The drugs currently approved by the FDA for preventing or treating osteoporosis include bisphosphonates (alendronate [Fosamax], ibandronate [Boniva], risedronate [Actonel], and zoledronate [Reclast]), calcitonin (Miacalcin), estrogens or hormone therapy, raloxifene (Evista), and parathyroid hormone (PTH) (1-34) (teriparatide [Forteo]).
- The assessment of therapeutic response can be monitored by bone mineral density. Normally, bone mineral density testing is repeated every 2 years after starting pharmacotherapy. However, in some conditions (e.g., glucocorticoid therapy) 1-year intervals may be warranted.

Osteoporosis is a skeletal disease characterized by low bone mass and structural deterioration of bone tissue that is associated with decreased bone strength and increased susceptibility to fractures. Its clinical relevance is increasing due to the associated morbidity and mortality associated with the disease. The signs and symptoms of osteoporosis, such as back pain, height loss, and thoracic kyphosis, not only are usually late manifestations of previously unrecognized vertebral fractures but can also be important risk indicators for future fractures. The overwhelming challenge to primary care clinicians is to find the best screening method to identify those patients with the highest risk for fracture who would benefit from a preventive or therapeutic intervention.

The WHO has defined osteoporosis as a condition in which bone mineral density (BMD) assessed by dual-energy x-ray absorptiometry (DEXA) at the spine, hip, or forearm is decreased. Osteoporosis is defined as a bone mineral density more than −2.5 standard deviations (SD) below the normal young adult mean (T-score ≤ -2.5), whereas osteopenia, a milder degree of bone loss, is defined as a T-score between −1.0 and −2.5 SD. Although the risk of fracture increases significantly with decreasing BMD, large observational studies have demonstrated that osteoporotic fractures can occur across a wide spectrum of BMDs. These events may be related not only to bone quantity but also to bone quality, a component not measured by DEXA scans. Qualitative determinants of bone strength include trabecular perforation, microcracks, mineralization defects, bone geometry, cell death, changes in bone size, and changes in bone turnover. Even though a low BMD defines osteoporosis, this diagnosis should not be excluded in at-risk patients, particularly those with a personal or family history of a fragility fracture (fractures that occur spontaneously). In other words, osteoporosis may be either a radiographic or a clinical diagnosis.

Although there is no universally accepted screening tool for patients at risk for osteoporotic fracture, the WHO and U.S. Preventive Services Task Force (USPSTF) recommend screening in women >65 and in younger women whose fracture risk is the same as or greater than that of a 65-year-old white woman who has no additional risk factors (Level B). They use a targeted approach to screen for osteoporosis based on the 10-year absolute risk of major osteoporotic fracture. The FRAX (Fracture Risk Assessment) tool, which considers several major independent fracture risk factors, including BMD of the hip, may be superior in demonstrating the long-term fracture risk of a given patient. Other independent risk factors such as previous fracture history, age older than 65 years, glucocorticoid use, alcohol abuse, and recent weight loss are also considered, but these factors are easily attainable clinical information. Nevertheless, many women with osteoporosis go unrecognized and untreated. In one study, it was reported that only 49% of women were evaluated and treated despite these screening guidelines.

Epidemiology

Osteoporosis is the most common metabolic disorder of the skeleton. Worldwide, 200 million women suffer from osteoporosis and have a lifetime risk of fracture between 30% and 40%. In men, the lifetime risk of osteoporotic fracture is currently about 13%, but it is projected to rise with an increased life expectancy. In the United States, approximately 8 million women and 2 million men have osteoporosis and 34 million men and women have osteopenia. After the fourth decade, fracture rates in women are twice those in men. In addition, hip fracture has a seasonal influence, with an increase during winter months in temperate countries. Hip fractures are reported to cause a mortality rate of 10% to 20% at 12 months, and up to 25% of those with hip fractures require long-term nursing home care. Ethnicity may also influence the incidence of skeletal failure: adult African Americans have fewer fractures than whites or Asians. Approximately one in two white women will have an osteoporotic fracture in their lifetime.

Risk Factors

Risk factors for osteoporosis should be considered at any routine visit. Nonmodifiable risk factors are genetic background, advancing age, female sex, Asian or white ethnicity, personal history of fracture, family history of fracture in a first-degree relative, and rheumatoid arthritis. Modifiable risk factors consist of low body weight, hormonal deficiencies, long-term use of medications that affect skeletal homeostasis (e.g., glucocorticoids, immunosuppressive medications, anticonvulsants), smoking, alcohol abuse, an inactive lifestyle, and a lifetime diet low in calcium and vitamin D.

Tools are available to help identify patients who are at high risk for osteoporosis. These tools use clinical risk factors to estimate a newly diagnosed patient's absolute fracture risk over a defined time interval. One such tool is a risk calculator called the Simple Calculated Osteoporosis Risk Estimation (SCORE) tool, which is a six-item instrument that may be used to predict women who may benefit from DEXA screening. However, the USPSTF uses the WHO's FRAX (Fracture Risk Assessment) tool, which incorporates other risk factors and then provides a 10-year absolute fracture risk. It uses easily attainable history such as age, body mass index (BMI), parental fracture history, and tobacco and alcohol use. The FRAX tool incorporates previous DEXA results but does not require this information in order to estimate fracture risk. Therefore, it can be used to predict which women may benefit

from DEXA screening. (The USPSTF recommends using a 9.3% 10-year fracture risk threshold to screen women 50–64 years of age).

Pathophysiology

Although osteoporosis is often thought of as synonymous with decreased BMD, this association is not always present. Several factors can lead to decreased bone strength: small bone size, unfavorable anatomy such as increased length of the femoral neck, cortical porosity, decreased viability of osteocytes, and others.

Peak bone mass is the maximum bone mass achieved in life, which typically occurs in the patient's third decade. Differences in the peak bone mass may be secondary to genetic, hormonal, and environmental variables. The contribution of genetic variants may be small. There are no clear studies that associate genetic variants with fracture risk or BMD loss. African Americans have higher BMDs than Caucasians, and Asian Americans have lower BMDs than Caucasians. However, it is reported that Hispanics and Asian Americans have lower hip fracture rates than whites. Increases in body size and skeletal load also play a role in peak bone mass. Physical activity during childhood also enhances bone mass, whereas chronic diseases during childhood may adversely affect BMD.

Age-related bone loss is a large factor in the development of osteoporosis. Bone resorption begins to overtake bone formation with advancing age, most commonly after age 65. Men, however, are less likely to develop bone loss because of greater bone gain during puberty and no sudden loss of estrogen. Also, there is evidence that aging itself seems to be an independent risk factor for bone loss. However, there are other contributing factors to age-related decline of bone mass such as loss of muscle strength, which may increase the risk for falls, and the severity of falls.

Hormonal deficiency causes bone loss by unbalancing the homeostasis normally present and the bone remodeling rate (i.e., osteoclasts vs. osteoblasts; bone formation and bone resorption). Estrogen loss initially affects trabecular bone after menopause. After a few years, bone loss continues to occur more slowly and primarily affects cortical sites. This slower phase is associated with a decreased number of osteoblasts and a slower bone formation rate. It is also theorized that androgen loss has detrimental effects on BMD, but it is uncertain how much. Still, both sex hormone deficiencies play a role in bone loss in both men and women.

Prevention

Prevention of osteoporosis is important because bone loss associated with the disease is mostly irreversible. Treatment may only stabilize the disease by increasing BMD, and reduce the fracture risk, but does not restore bone strength. Limitations in the development of peak bone mass during adolescence may determine bone strength decades later. Therefore, prevention starts with good nutrition, physical activity, and exercise that optimize bone mass during bone-forming years. Other lifestyle factors that can be modified are discouraging cigarette smoking and excessive alcohol intake. Medications that may be harmful to bone health, such as glucocorticoids and anticonvulsants, should be closely monitored and used for the minimum duration.

Calcium and vitamin D are both physiologically vital in bone formation. Some studies have shown increases in BMD and reduction of fracture risk in a geriatric population that was given both calcium and vitamin D. The Recommended Daily Allowance (RDA) of elemental calcium for postmenopausal women is 1200 mg, and the RDA for vitamin D is 600 IU. However, it is difficult to obtain proper levels of vitamin D through nutrition and natural sunlight. Previous recommendations varied on the proper daily dosing for both calcium and vitamin D. New evidence, however, does not support supplementation with daily vitamin D or calcium to reduce the risk of fractures in adults, according to the USPSTF.

Clinical Manifestations

There are typically no clinical manifestations of osteoporosis until the patient actually has a fracture. The signs and symptoms associated with osteoporosis correspond to direct or indirect manifestations of these fractures. For example, vertebral fractures may be asymptomatic and can be clinically inconspicuous. Patients may have height loss, back pain, and thoracic kyphosis, which can cause respiratory limitation and intestinal constipation. A fracture may be the first sign of a systemic disease associated with osteoporosis, as well as a complication from glucocorticoid therapy or solid organ transplantations. Many factors may contribute to the osteoporosis after organ transplantation such as immunosuppressive medications or derangements of the parathyroid-calcium-vitamin D and the pituitary-gonadal axes.

Diagnosis

Osteoporosis is diagnosed either clinically or radiographically. It can be established after the occurrence of a fragility fracture, such as a low-trauma fracture of appendicular or axial bones, excluding the skull. The initial evaluation includes a history to assess for clinical risk factors for fracture, evaluation for other conditions that contribute to bone loss, a physical examination, and basic laboratory tests. Secondary causes of osteoporosis should always be excluded. Most cases of osteoporosis are diagnosed by DEXA scan of the total hip, femoral neck, or lumbar spine, with a T-score of -2.5 or below. The USPSTF recommends screening for osteoporosis in women ages 65 years or older and in younger women whose fracture risk is equal to or greater than that of a 65-year-old white woman who has no additional risk factors (Grade B recommendation). Bone mass measurements by DEXA must be interpreted in relation to the patient's age, ethnicity, fracture history, family background, previous medications, timing of menopause, and other concomitant disorders.

Other techniques for measuring bone mass besides DEXA scans exist. These include ultrasound of the calcaneus, wrist, and finger and computed tomography (CT) of the spine and peripheral quantitative CT of the wrist and tibia. However, these modalities may be limited by factors such as radiation exposure and cost. DEXA scans give an accurate and precise estimate of BMD and has been a proven, cost-effective tool.

DEXA results are expressed as a T-score and a Z-score. The T-score was established by the WHO, and is the number of standard deviations (SD) difference between the patient's BMD and a young-adult reference population. The T-score should be used in the evaluation of men and women older than age 50 or postmenopausal women. The T-score provides an indication of the risk for developing fractures, and this risk increases exponentially with decreasing T-scores. A T-score that is 2.5 SD or more below the young-adult mean is diagnostic of osteoporosis; a T-score that is 1 to 2.5 SD below the mean is defined as low bone mass (osteopenia). A T-score below -2.5 SD plus a fragility fracture is termed *severe osteoporosis*. BMD measurements may be different across various bone sites in the same patient. These discrepancies may likely be related to differences in skeletal compartments (trabecular vs. cortical) at distinct sites. The lowest T-score of the lumbar spine, femoral neck, and total hip should be used to classify the degree of osteoporosis.

The Z-score is the number of standard deviations the patient's BMD differs from a reference population of the same age, sex, and ethnicity. A low Z-score of less than -2.0 is below the expected BMD range for age and may help identify patients who need further evaluation for secondary causes of osteoporosis such as long-term corticosteroid steroid use or the adolescent female athlete triad. Z-scores should be used in the evaluation of adult men and women less than age 50, premenopausal women,

and children because there is no comparison of the BMD of a child to an adult who has achieved peak bone mass.

Biochemical markers reflect the activity of the bone-remodeling unit. These markers, such as urinary pyridinoline and deoxypyridinoline, are called bone turnover markers. Their roles in the management of osteoporosis have not been well established. Future use of these biochemical markers may be helpful in determining risk and for monitoring patients treated with active drugs.

Differential Diagnosis

A comprehensive workup of osteoporosis should always include an evaluation of secondary causes of osteoporosis. If clinical evaluation does not support a secondary cause, there is currently little evidence for additional testing in postmenopausal women. However, in premenopausal and perimenopausal women, additional testing should be considered if there is no clear etiology found by history and physical examination.

More than 50% of men with vertebral collapse fractures are reported to have secondary causes of osteoporosis. Common causes of osteoporosis in men are long-term use of glucocorticoids, hypogonadism, alcohol abuse, myeloma, and gastrointestinal, thyroid, and parathyroid disorders. Most recommendations for the screening and diagnosis are based on expert opinion. The National Osteoporosis Foundation (NOF) and the International Society for Clinical Densitometry recommend screening all men 70 years and older and men 50 to 69 years of age with risk factors. However, the USPSTF guidelines state that there is insufficient evidence to support screening for osteoporosis in men.

Treatment

Nonpharmacologic Therapy

Nondrug therapy includes addressing risk of falls, diet, exercise, and smoking. Preventing the fall to avoid fragility fracture is the first step in treating osteoporosis. Vision deficits, gait abnormalities, cognitive impairment, dizziness, and balance problems need to be addressed in order to prevent falls. Performing a formal home safety evaluation and modifying the patient's living environment by improving lighting and removing loose rugs can enhance safety. Physical therapy evaluation and treatment can address both balance and gait issues. Medications need to be reviewed that pose a risk of falls due to their side-effect profile.

Ensuring adequate nutrition is an initial approach in treating osteoporosis, especially calcium and vitamin D. Studies showing the efficacy of calcium on fracture prevention and treatment are mixed, but there is some evidence from several meta-analyses that there are decreased fracture rates in women older than 65 years who take calcium and vitamin D supplementation as a preventive measure. Optimal dosing is not standardized, but a daily intake of at least 1200 mg of calcium is recommended for all women with osteoporosis. Supplementation to dietary intake of calcium is often needed. Both calcium carbonate and calcium citrate can be used, but caution should be used due to constipation and gastrointestinal upset. Concerns about renal adverse events, particularly nephrocalcinosis, exist when the calcium dose is greater than 2000 mg per day from dietary plus supplemental sources.

The NOF recommends 800 to 1000 IU of vitamin D daily for persons 50 years and older. Because it is difficult to consume this amount of dietary vitamin D, supplementation is important. Even with mild vitamin D insufficiency bone loss can often follow. Some studies suggest that a serum 25-hydroxyvitamin D level of at least 30 ng/mL is needed to reduce falls and improve physical function in the elderly. For most individuals 50 years and older, the NOF recommends 800 to 1000 IU of vitamin D daily. Supplementation is important because it is difficult to consume this amount of dietary vitamin D. In patients with vitamin D insufficiency, administration of 50,000 IU of oral ergocalciferol (vitamin D_2 [Drisdol])[1] given once weekly for 8 weeks is safe and effective. This is followed by

---

[1]Not FDA approved for this indication.

a maintenance dosage of 50,000 IU every 2 to 4 weeks of oral cholecalciferol (vitamin D$_3$)[1] at 1000 IU daily. Vitamin D deficiency is diagnosed with baseline serum levels in the workup for secondary osteoporosis, and measurement of levels following treatment is important because of the possible risk of vitamin D toxicity. However, the optimal interval for testing is not known. The goal of treatment is a 25-hydroxyvitamin D level greater than 30 ng/mL (74 nmol/L).

Regular physical activity and performing aerobic, weight-bearing, and resistance exercises are effective in increasing spine BMD. Patients should exercise at least 30 minutes three times per week. However, there is no evidence that high-intensity exercise provides greater benefit. Smoking cigarettes may accelerate bone loss and cessation unquestionably has positive health benefits while reducing risk for fracture.

Pharmacologic Treatment

All drugs approved by the FDA for osteoporosis therapy reduce fracture risk at least at the spine. Most of the antifracture effects of these medications are not due to an increase in BMD but rather to an improvement in qualitative measures of bone strength. Two main classes of medications are available for osteoporosis: antiresorptives, which decrease bone resorption, and anabolics, which promote bone formation. The antiresorptive drugs approved by FDA to treat or prevent osteoporosis are noted in Table 1: bisphosphonates, including alendronate (Fosamax), risedronate (Actonel), zoledronic acid (Reclast), and ibandronate (Boniva); estrogen therapy; the selective estrogen receptor modulators (SERM) raloxifene (Evista) or a conjugated estrogen combined with bazedoxifine (Duavee); and calcitonin (Miacalcin). The bisphosphonates impair osteoclastic resorption through the inhibition of farnesyl diphosphate synthase, a key enzyme that supports osteoclast activity. Estrogen and raloxifene (an SERM) inhibit osteoclastogenesis through the RANKL (receptor activator of nuclear factor kappa B ligand)/osteoprotegerin (OPG) (also known as osteoclastogenesis inhibitory factor) system. Estrogen and raloxifene stimulate the synthesis of OPG and inhibit RANKL expression in osteoblasts resulting in a signal to reduce the production of osteoclasts. Another medication with a different mechanism is calcitonin, which acts directly on osteoclasts by inhibiting their activity through the calcitonin receptor.

There are different approved indications for these drugs in osteoporosis. Alendronate and risedronate are indicated for the prevention and treatment of postmenopausal osteoporosis,

---

[1]Not FDA approved for this indication.

treatment of osteoporosis in men, and treatment of glucocorticoid-induced osteoporosis. Ibandronate and raloxifene are approved only for prevention and treatment of postmenopausal osteoporosis. It may be noted that daily and intermittent uses of ibandronate have demonstrated antifracture effectiveness at the spine only. Weekly and monthly dosing may increase compliance with taking bisphosphonates. Zoledronic acid 5 mg by intravenous (IV) administration is approved for once-yearly treatment of postmenopausal osteoporosis, and 5 mg IV administered once every other year is approved to prevent osteoporosis. Calcitonin is approved for treating postmenopausal osteoporosis. Estrogen is approved only for the prevention of osteoporosis.

The proper duration of therapy for oral bisphosphonate therapy is unknown. Low-risk patients may consider discontinuing therapy after risks and benefits are weighed. However, IV bisphosphonates may be used for high-risk patients who cannot tolerate or are noncompliant with oral therapy, or even those currently hospitalized for hip fracture.

Side effects of oral bisphosphonates include esophageal and gastric irritation and musculoskeletal pain. They must be taken with a full glass of water, and a 30- to 60-minute wait is required before reclining or any oral intake to lower the risk of upper gastrointestinal adverse effects. IV bisphosphonates are associated with hyperthermia, episcleritis, uveitis, and hypocalcemia. Alendronate and risedronate have been well studied and both have excellent long-term safety profiles. There have been reports of subtrochanteric fractures during prolonged treatment with bisphosphonates, particularly alendronate. Young women are particularly prone to these fractures, which often require surgical intervention. Prodromal symptoms that have been linked to this syndrome include proximal femur pain and evidence of previous stress fracture or cortical thickness on x-ray. Osteonecrosis of the jaw is a rare but serious complication observed in patients treated with bisphosphonates. Usually, these patients are on higher doses of IV infusions to treat bone metastases associated with cancer.

Raloxifene, an SERM given daily, improves BMD and reduces the risk of vertebral fractures, but not the hip. However, it can exacerbate the vasomotor symptoms of menopause. Although raloxifene increases serum levels of high-density lipoprotein (HDL) cholesterol, it increases the risk of thromboembolic events. Raloxifene may be considered in postmenopausal women with osteoporosis who cannot tolerate bisphosphonates, have no vasomotor symptoms, have a low risk of venous thromboembolism, and have a high breast cancer risk score. However, a new SERM, bazedoxifine as paired with conjugated estrogens (Duavee) has been approved for use in women with hot flashes associated with menopause and also for the prevention of osteoporosis.

TABLE 1 Efficacy of Approved Drugs for Osteoporosis Treatment on Fracture Risk

MEDICATION	ROUTE	DOSE	CLINICAL EVIDENCE OF EFFICACY		
			VERTEBRAL	HIP	NONVERTEBRAL
Alendronate (Fosamax)	Oral	Oral 10 mg qd or 70 mg weekly	+	+	+
Risedronate (Actonel)	Oral	5 mg qd or 35 mg weekly	+	+	+
Zoledronic acid (Reclast)	IV	5 mg yearly	+	+	+
Ibandronate (Boniva)	Oral IV	150 mg monthly 3 mg q3mo	+ +	− −	− −
Raloxifene (Evista)	Oral	60 mg qd	+	−	−
Calcitonin (Miacalcin)	Nasal SC	200 IU qd 100 IU	+ −	− −	− −
Conjugated equine estrogen (Premarin)	Oral	0.624 mg qd	+	+	NR
Medroxyprogesterone (Provera)	Depot	2.5 mg qd	+	+	NR
Teriparatide (Forteo)	SC	20 mg qd	+		+

Abbreviations: IU = international units; IV = intravenous; NR = not reported; SC = subcutaneous.

PTH (1-34) (teriparatide [Forteo]) has recognized antifracture effects on both vertebral and nonvertebral sites, and it is the only anabolic option available for treating postmenopausal osteoporosis. Currently, it is recommended that PTH (1-34) therapy (20 mg SC daily) should be limited to 2 years for the treatment of postmenopausal women and hypogonadal men with osteoporosis. Adverse effects may include orthostatic hypotension, hypercalcemia, nausea, arthralgia, risk of renal stones, and leg cramps. There are reports of increased risk of osteosarcoma, which has only been seen in rats exposed to high doses. Consequently, teriparatide is contraindicated in patients with risk of osteosarcoma, such as those with Paget disease of the bone, previous skeletal radiation, or unexplained elevations of alkaline phosphatase; therefore a baseline alkaline phosphatase level before initiation of therapy is recommended. It should be used in the treatment of postmenopausal women with severe bone loss, men with osteoporosis who have a high risk of fractures, and patients who have not improved on bisphosphonates. No evidence exists that indicates combining anticatabolic and anabolic classes of drug provides additive results. However, it is recommended that after a period of 2 years of intermittent PTH (1-34), bisphosphonates should be started to avoid posttreatment bone loss.

Strontium ranelate (Protelos)[2] is an orally administered medication that is capable of stimulating bone formation and inhibiting bone resorption. After 3 years of treatment, strontium ranelate preserves or enhances trabecular microarchitecture and increases cortical thickness. Strontium is not approved for the treatment of osteoporosis in the United States.

Denosumab (Prolia), 60 mg subcutaneously twice a year, is a human monoclonal antibody that works by inhibiting bone resorption and most recently has been approved for treatment of men and postmenopausal women with osteoporosis who are at high risk for fracture (history of fragility fracture, multiple risk factors, or intolerant to other therapy). In a large trial involving more than 7000 postmenopausal women, denosumab was administered for 3 years and showed significant efficacy in reducing the risk of vertebral, nonvertebral, and hip fractures compared to placebo. The safety profile of denosumab has been demonstrated in long-term trials, although there was a reported modest increase in skin infections with continued use.

New Agents

A new SERM, lasofoxifene (Fablyn),[5] is in clinical development. It has demonstrated antifracture effects but still awaits FDA approval. An inhibitor of cathepsin K,[5] which is an osteoclast enzyme required for resorption of bone matrix, is under clinical investigation and currently is in phase III trials. Duavee, a combination product pairing a new SERM, bazedoxifine, with conjugated estrogens has been approved for use in women with hot flashes associated with menopause and also for the prevention of osteoporosis.

---

[2]Not available in the United States.
[5]Investigational drug in the United States.

References

Bilezikian JP. Efficacy of bisphosphonates in reducing fracture risk in postmenopausal osteoporosis. Am J Med 2009;122(Suppl. 2):S14–21.

Bischoff-Ferrari HA, Dawson-Hughes B, Staehelin HB, et al. Fall prevention with supplemental and active forms of vitamin D: a meta-analysis of randomised controlled trials. BMJ 2009;339:b3692.

Committee to Review Dietary Reference Intakes for Vitamin D and Calcium. Dietary reference intakes for calcium and vitamin D. Washington, DC: Institute of Medicine; 2010.

eVitamin D and calcium supplementation to prevent fractures in adults: U.S. Preventive Services Task Force Recommendation Statement. Free Online First. Available at http://www.uspreventiveservicestaskforce.org/uspstf12/vitamind/finalrecvitd.htm.

Hippisley-Cox J, Coupland C. Predicting risk of osteoporotic fracture in men and women in England and Wales: prospective derivation and validation of QFracture scores. BMJ 2009;339:b4229.

Khosla S, Melton LJ. Clinical practice. Osteopenia. N Engl J Med 2007;356:2293–300.

Moyer V. To supplement or not to supplement: the U.S. Preventive Services Task Force recommendations on calcium and vitamin D. Ann Intern Med 2013;158:691–6.

Rosen CJ. Clinical practice. Postmenopausal osteoporosis. N Engl J Med 2005;353:595.

Rosen CJ. Bone remodeling, energy metabolism, and the molecular clock. Cell Metab 2008;7:7–10.

Sambrook P, Cooper C. Osteoporosis. Lancet 2006;367:2010–8.

Schousboe JT, Taylor BC, Fink HA, et al. Cost-effectiveness of bone densitometry followed by treatment of osteoporosis in older men. JAMA 2007;298:629–37.

Sweet MG, Sweet JM, Jeremiah MP, et al. Diagnosis and treatment of osteoporosis. Am Fam Physician 2009;79:193–200.

Uitterlinden AG, Ralston SH, Brandi ML, et al. The association between common vitamin D receptor gene variations and osteoporosis: a participant-level meta-analysis. Ann Intern Med 2006;145:255–64.

U.S. Department of Health and Human Services. Bone health and osteoporosis: a report of the surgeon general. Rockville, MD: U.S. Department of Health and Human Services, Office of the Surgeon General; 2004.

U.S. Preventive Services Task Force. Screening for osteoporosis in post-menopausal women: recommendations and rationale, Rockville, MD: Agency for Healthcare Research and Quality; September 2002. Available at http://www.uspreventiveservicestaskforce.org/uspstf/uspsoste.htm.

Wells GA, Cranney A, Peterson J, et al. Alendronate for the primary and secondary prevention of osteoporotic fractures in postmenopausal women. Cochrane Database Syst Rev 2008;1, CD001155.

PAGET'S DISEASE OF BONE

Method of
Ian R. Reid, MD

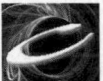

CURRENT DIAGNOSIS

- Suspect the presence of Paget's disease in those patients with bone pain, bone deformity, isolated elevation of alkaline phosphatase, or lytic/sclerotic lesions on radiographs.
- Paget's disease is diagnosed from plain radiographs.
- Bone scintigraphy identifies the affected bones and allows some assessment of disease activity.
- Biochemical markers of bone turnover allow more precise assessment of turnover and response to therapy.
- Serum total alkaline phosphatase activity is the most cost-effective marker, although bone-specific alkaline phosphatase and procollagen type I N-terminal propeptide (PINP) are marginally more sensitive.

CURRENT THERAPY

- Zoledronate (zoledronic acid, Reclast) 5 mg given as a single infusion over 15 minutes; retreatment is seldom required within 5 years.
- Alendronate (Fosamax) 40 mg/day for 6 months; retreatment may be required between 2 and 6 years.
- Risedronate (Actonel) 30 mg/day for 2 months; retreatment may be required between 1 and 5 years.

Paget's disease is a focal skeletal condition in which one or more bones has a clearly circumscribed area of increased turnover (Figure 1A). Either osteoblasts or osteoclasts may predominate at a given time, resulting in sclerosis or lysis, respectively. Areas that are initially lytic often become sclerotic later, and it is common to see both changes within the same bone (see Figure 1B). Unaffected areas of the skeleton are completely normal, in marked contrast to some rare congenital conditions which are sometimes (inappropriately) referred to as early-onset or juvenile Paget's disease. Such conditions (e.g., familial expansile osteolysis, idiopathic hyperphosphatasia) have different etiologies, clinical presentations, and responses to treatment when compared to Paget's disease.

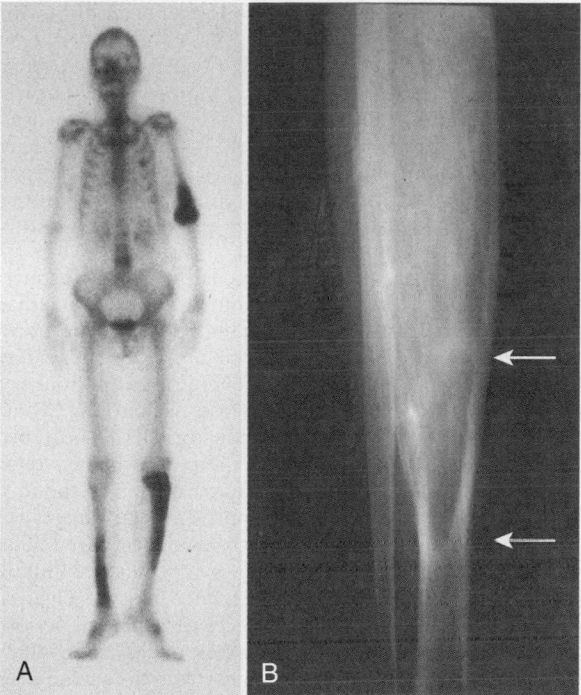

Figure 1. A, Bone scintigram in a patient with Paget's disease, demonstrating the multifocal nature of the condition and the presence of normal bone at other sites. **B,** Tibia affected by Paget's disease. The upper tibia is of increased density and width as a result of osteoblast overactivity, whereas the lower part of the affected bone shows a lytic region *(between arrows)* resulting from osteoclastic bone resorption. Below this, the bone is normal. (Copyright I. R. Reid, used with permission.)

Etiology

Within pagetic bone, there is a loss of the usual tight control of bone cell function, and the bone-resorbing cells (osteoclasts) and bone-forming cells (osteoblasts) both exhibit overactivity. In the case of osteoclasts, this leads to local areas of bone loss, which can result in deformity or fracture. Osteoblast overactivity leads to the random laying down of new bone, which is disorganized in its structure, mechanically inadequate, and prone to deformity. Osteoblast overactivity can also lead to bone expansion, resulting in bone pain, premature arthritis (if it affects articular surfaces), and nerve compression (e.g., in the spine or skull). Figure 1B shows the effects of osteoblast and osteoclast overactivity on the structure of an affected tibia. The disease progresses along a long bone at a rate of about 1 cm per year, so most patients have had active disease for 1 or more decades before presentation. Typically, the disease progresses until the entire bone is involved. However, Paget's disease does not spread from one bone to another, so the number of affected bones remains constant throughout the disease course.

Paget's disease sometimes runs in families, and about 10% of patients are reported to have an affected relative. This observation has led to much work seeking genetic associations of the condition. It is now apparent that mutations of the gene for sequestosome 1 are associated with Paget's disease in some families. Other research has focused on possible environmental causes, and a slow viral infection has been suggested. Evidence that the prevalence of Paget's disease has decreased in recent decades would be consistent with altered exposure to an environmental agent. However, both the genetic and environmental hypotheses fail to account for the focal nature of the condition, which in some ways resembles a benign neoplasm.

Altered gene expression in osteoblasts and bone marrow stromal cells from pagetic bone has been demonstrated recently, including increased levels of dickkopf-1, interleukin-1, and interleukin-6. These changes are likely to result in stimulation of osteoclast proliferation and inhibition of osteoblast growth, leading to development of the characteristic lytic bone lesions. This work suggests that the key abnormality may reside in the osteoblast, rather than the osteoclast, as was assumed in the past. Uncertainties remain regarding the primary abnormality giving rise to this condition.

Epidemiology

Paget's disease is classically a condition of older adults, most patients being older than 60 years of age at diagnosis. There is a male preponderance in some studies. It is overwhelmingly a condition of individuals with European forebears, particularly from the United Kingdom and Western Europe (excluding Scandinavia), where about 6% to 7% of the older population is affected. Among older white Americans, the prevalence is about 2%. There is some evidence that prevalence and disease severity are both declining, possibly reflecting change in an environmental etiologic factor. It is extremely uncommon in individuals with predominantly Asian or Polynesian ancestry, although it is observed in some black populations.

Clinical Presentation

The most common symptoms attributable to Paget's disease are bone and joint pain. The bone pain is typically worse at rest and may trouble patients particularly at night. With skull involvement, pounding headaches can result. If Paget's disease leads to deformity of joint surfaces, premature arthritis occurs. This is particularly common at the hips. Deformity in long bones can occur, and involvement of the radius or weight-bearing bones of the lower limb often manifests in this way. Microfractures, which can be very painful, sometimes occur over the convexity of a deformed, weight-bearing bone. These can progress to complete fractures. Fractures can also occur through an area of active lytic disease in a weight-bearing bone.

Deafness is a common manifestation of Paget's disease and is caused by involvement of the bones of the middle ear or compromise of the eighth cranial nerve. More rarely, other neurologic syndromes can arise from nerve entrapment, including paraplegia as a result of spinal cord involvement.

Some pagetic patients are asymptomatic and are diagnosed because of an incidental finding of elevated circulating levels of alkaline phosphatase. The diagnosis may also result from an incidental radiographic finding, such as in studies of the urinary tract. Commonly, only one or two bones are involved, although disease may be more widespread. The pelvis, vertebral bodies, long bones, and skull are the most common sites, but almost any bone can be involved.

Diagnosis

Serum alkaline phosphatase, the most widely available marker of osteoblast activity, is usually elevated; however, if only one bone is involved, this test can be normal. In any patient with an elevation of alkaline phosphatase, it is important to determine whether this is coming from liver or bone. This question is usually addressed by other liver function tests, although assays of bone-specific alkaline phosphatase and of other osteoblast-specific markers (e.g., procollagen type I N-terminal propeptide [PINP]) are available. If the elevation of alkaline phosphatase is bony in origin, it is important to rule out other bone conditions such as metastatic cancers (e.g., breast, prostate). This is usually done by identifying the sites of skeletal abnormality on a bone scintigram and then obtaining plain radiographs of the abnormal areas.

Paget's disease has a characteristic appearance on plain radiographs, showing either bony rarefaction or sclerosis (depending on whether the osteoclastic or osteoblastic phase is predominating), disorganization of trabecular architecture, and the other abnormalities already discussed (e.g., deformity). Bone biopsy is not usually necessary to confirm the diagnosis.

Other biochemical markers of osteoblast or osteoclast activity, such as breakdown products of bone collagen, have been used in Paget's disease. Total alkaline phosphatase, bone alkaline phosphatase, PINP or N-terminal telopeptide of type I collagen (NTX) identified more than 95% of pagetic subjects in one cohort of pagetic subjects, although the poorer precision of NTX reduced its utility in monitoring the effects of treatment. Osteocalcin, C-telopeptide of type I collagen, and urinary free deoxypyridinoline are less useful for assessment of baseline activity and monitoring response to therapy. Total alkaline phosphatase remains the most widely used test because of its low cost and wide availability.

Treatment

Treatment of Paget's disease almost always relies on the potent bisphosphonates. These compounds have a very high affinity for the bone surface, where they remain for years. They are ingested by osteoclasts when bone is resorbed and inhibit a key enzyme in the mevalonate pathway, farnesyl pyrophosphate synthase. This results in disruption of the osteoclast cytoskeleton and cell death. Bisphosphonates are preferentially taken up at sites of high bone turnover, which accounts for their utility as bone scintigraphy agents, and therefore target active pagetic bone.

The injectable bisphosphonate pamidronate (Aredia) has been used for many years in the treatment of Paget's disease. It is typically given as a series of infusions of 60 to 90 mg, each administered over a period of 1 to 2 hours. Pamidronate produces partial or complete remissions of disease activity that last for up to several years. The first administration of the drug may be accompanied by mild flu-like symptoms, which settle over 24 to 48 hours and usually do not recur. Their resolution can be hastened by the use of paracetamol (acetaminophen, Tylenol) or similar agents.

More recently, potent oral bisphosphonates such as alendronate (Fosamax) and risedronate (Actonel) have become widely used. These are administered daily over periods of 2 to 6 months and produce good disease control. The duration of treatment chosen in the pivotal clinical trials was arbitrary to some extent, and individual patients may require longer or shorter initial courses to achieve remission. Oral bisphosphonates have a very low bioavailability. Therefore, they must be taken in a fasting state, with a glass of water, and at least 30 minutes before consumption of food or other fluids. Positively charged ions (including calcium supplements, antacids, and mineral supplements) bind avidly to bisphosphonates and impair their absorption, so they must be taken at a different time of day. Potent bisphosphonates can cause irritation to the upper gastrointestinal tract and should not be prescribed to patients with inflammation or ulceration in that region. Patients should remain upright for 30 minutes after taking oral bisphosphonates to minimize the risk of reflux and associated esophagitis or ulceration.

The latest addition to the therapeutic armamentarium in managing Paget's disease is the more potent intravenous bisphosphonate zoledronate (Reclast), which is administered in a single dose of 5 mg over 15 minutes. It was recently compared with the standard 2-month course of risedronate in two randomized, controlled trials. At 6 months, 96% of patients receiving zoledronate had a therapeutic response, compared with 74% of those randomized to risedronate ($P < 0.001$). Alkaline phosphatase levels normalized in 89% of patients in the zoledronate group and in 58% of those in the risedronate group ($P < 0.001$). Zoledronate showed a more rapid onset of action and superior effects on quality-of-life measures. Perhaps the most impressive data with zoledronate have been those from the open follow-up of responders in these studies. Six years after drug administration, relapse had occurred in 0.7% of those receiving zoledronate but in 20% of risedronate-treated patients. Therefore, zoledronate produces much more sustained responses to therapy than have hitherto been possible.

Potent bisphosphonates can cause mild hypocalcemia, which is usually asymptomatic and not a cause for concern. However, in patients with vitamin D deficiency, hypocalcaemia can be more severe and sustained. Therefore, it is important to ensure that patients are vitamin D sufficient before receiving these drugs—a serum 25-hydroxyvitamin-D level greater than 50 nmol/L is more than adequate. Many physicians prescribe calcium to patients receiving bisphosphonate therapy (given in the evening if the oral bisphosphonate is given in the morning) as a further protection against hypocalcemia.

In the past, the weak bisphosphonate etidronate (Didronel) was used to treat Paget's disease. This is much less effective than the agents discussed previously. If used in high doses or for more than a few months, it carries the risk of producing osteomalacia, which can lead to bone pain and fractures. Therefore, it no longer has a place in the treatment of Paget's disease. Calcitonin (Miacalcin Injection) has also been relegated to an historical role only, because its efficacy is much less than that of the potent bisphosphonates and its effects are rapidly reversed after cessation of therapy.

There are several philosophical approaches to Paget's disease management, none of which is strictly evidence based. There is general agreement that patients with symptoms attributable to Paget's disease should receive treatment. This is clear-cut in patients who have bone pain at the site of a pagetic lesion, but it is a common observation that antipagetic drugs can produce variable degrees of improvement in pain from joints adjacent to pagetic bone. Patients with neurologic complications from spinal cord or other nerve entrapments also improve with antipagetic therapy.

Treatment aimed at preventing complications of Paget's disease is variably endorsed, because there is no clinical trial evidence that treatment prevents the progression of deformity, the development of pagetic symptoms, or fracture. However, it is clear that treatment leads to a restoration of normal bone histology (Figure 2) and radiographic healing of lytic lesions and that, in the absence of such intervention, both bone lysis and deformity progress. It seems unreasonable to withhold safe therapies that are able to halt histologic and radiologic disease progression. Therefore, many experienced physicians endorse the provision of antipagetic therapy for individuals with lytic lesions in long bones; lesions at sites that are likely to lead to neurologic complications, arthritis,

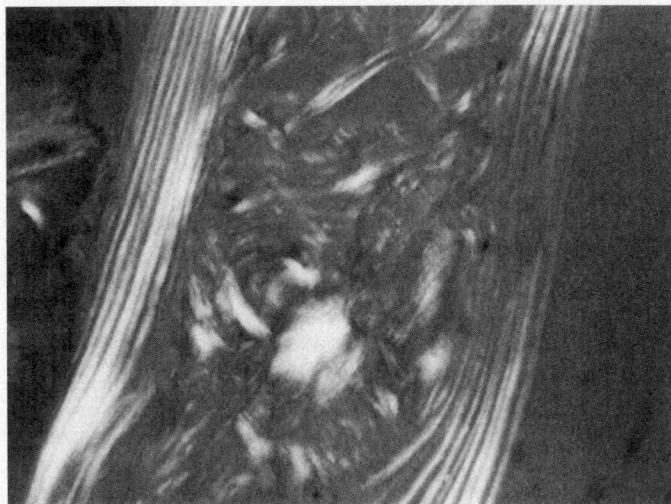

Figure 2. Section of a bone trabecula affected by Paget's disease, viewed under polarized light to show orientation of lamellae. In the center of the trabecula, the collagen fibers are chaotically laid down (woven bone), consistent with active Paget's disease. Over the outer surfaces, collagen is organized in parallel lamellae, indicating the restoration of normal bone microarchitecture after treatment with alendronate. (Reprinted with permission from: Reid IR, Nicholson GC, Weinstein RS, et al: Biochemical and radiologic improvement in Paget's disease of bone treated with alendronate: A randomized, placebo-controlled trial. Am J Med 1996;101:341–48.)

or deformity; or involvement of the skull that could compromise hearing. Expert opinion also supports the use of antipagetic therapy before elective surgery on pagetic bone, because this approach reduces the vascularity of pagetic bone and results in less perioperative blood loss. On the other hand, Paget's disease in asymptomatic patients whose future risk of complications is thought to be low (e.g., with involvement of the ilium) is commonly managed without specific pharmaceutical intervention, although the availability of a safe, single-dose treatment with zoledronate is increasing the inclination to treat.

When providing treatment targeted at these goals, it is important to consider how adequacy of therapy can be judged. In the case of patients with pain, maximal relief of pain is an important endpoint. Lytic lesions should be treated and monitored with sequential radiographs until healing is apparent. Activity at other sites can be assessed indirectly with biochemical markers of bone turnover, although these are much less sensitive in patients with monostotic disease. In this context, there can be considerable residual activity at a single affected site without the markers being abnormal. Bone scintigrams provide the most sensitive method of assessing local disease activity.

In the past, Paget's disease caused substantial morbidity in the elderly population. However, it is now possible to achieve adequate and sustained disease control with use of the potent bisphosphonates. Prompt use of these agents, when indicated, can be expected to halt disease progression and to effectively prevent the development of significant complications from this condition.

References

Kanis JA. Pathophysiology and Treatment of Paget's Disease of Bone. London: Martin Dunitz; 1991.

Lyles KW, Siris ES, Singer FR, et al. A clinical approach to diagnosis and management of Paget's disease of bone. J Bone Miner Res 2001;16:1379–87.

Miller PD, Brown JP, Siris ES, et al. A randomized, double-blind comparison of risedronate and etidronate in the treatment of Paget's disease of bone. Am J Med 1999;106:513–20.

Ralston SH, Langston AL, Reid IR. Pathogenesis and management of Paget's disease of bone. Lancet 2008;372:155–63.

Reid IR, Davidson JS, Wattie D, et al. Comparative responses of bone turnover markers to bisphosphonate therapy in Paget's disease of bone. Bone 2004;35:224–30.

Reid IR, Miller P, Lyles K, et al. Comparison of a single infusion of zoledronic acid with risedronate for Paget's disease. N Engl J Med 2005;353:898–908.

Reid IR, Nicholson GC, Weinstein RS, et al. Biochemical and radiologic improvement in Paget's disease of bone treated with alendronate: A randomized, placebo-controlled trial. Am J Med 1996;101:341–8.

Selby PL, Davie MWJ, Ralston SH, et al. Guidelines on the management of Paget's disease of bone. Bone 2002;31:366–73.

POLYMYALGIA RHEUMATICA AND GIANT CELL ARTERITIS

Method of
Barri J. Fessler, MD, MSPH

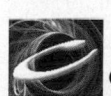

CURRENT DIAGNOSIS

Polymyalgia Rheumatica
- Age at onset is 50 years or older.
- Symptoms include pain and stiffness in neck, bilateral shoulders and upper arms, hips, and proximal thighs. Weakness is *not* a feature of polymyalgia rheumatica and should prompt a search for other diagnoses.
- Erythrocyte sedimentation rate is ≥40 mm/h.*
- Exclude other diagnoses that can cause similar symptoms.
- Up to 20% of patients with polymyalgia rheumatica also have giant cell arteritis.

Giant Cell Arteritis
- Age at onset is 50 years or older.

- Symptoms can include new-onset headache, jaw claudication, scalp tenderness, and vision loss or diplopia.
- Fevers, anorexia, weight loss, or hoarseness may also be present.
- Polymyalgia rheumatica is seen in 40% to 60% of patients with giant cell arteritis.
- The temporal artery may be tender to palpation or have decreased pulsations.
- Erythrocyte sedimentation rate is at least 40 mm/hour.*
- Temporal artery biopsy is the gold standard for diagnosis; however, the biopsy may be negative owing to patchy involvement of the arteries.
- Giant cell arteritis can present as a fever of unknown origin.

*A normal sedimentation rate may be seen in up to 20% of patients and should not exclude a diagnosis.

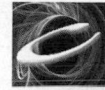

CURRENT THERAPY

Polymyalgia Rheumatica
- Corticosteroids (e.g., prednisone[1] 15–20 mg daily) are used with a gradual taper. If prednisone is tapered too rapidly, the symptoms will return. Patients are generally treated for at least 1 year.
- Rarely are higher doses of prednisone required. If symptoms do not respond to prednisone 30 mg daily, the diagnosis should be reevaluated.

Giant Cell Arteritis
- Corticosteroids (e.g., prednisone[1] at 1 mg/kg/day or 60 mg daily) are followed by a gradual taper.
- Patients are generally on treatment for at least 1 to 2 years. Some patients require low doses of prednisone indefinitely.
- One aspirin[1] daily, unless contraindicated (possibly with a proton pump inhibitor in high-risk patients), is used to decrease the risk of ischemic events.
- Prophylaxis for steroid-induced osteoporosis includes calcium, vitamin D, and a bisphosphonate unless contraindicated.

[1]Not FDA approved for this indication.

Polymyalgia rheumatica (PMR) and giant cell arteritis (GCA) are systemic inflammatory disorders of unknown etiology. Each condition can occur in isolation or in conjunction with the other; 15% to 20% of patients with PMR have GCA, and 40% to 60% of patients with GCA have PMR. For both conditions, onset is in people older than 50 years, women are more commonly affected than men, and significant elevations in acute phase reactants are typically seen in the majority of patients. The prevalence of GCA is highest in Scandinavian countries and regions with people of Northern European descent. It is rare in blacks and Hispanics.

Polymyalgia Rheumatica

Clinical Presentation

PMR is characterized by aching, pain, and stiffness in the muscles of the neck, shoulder, and hip girdle. Symptoms initially may be unilateral, but they eventually become bilateral. The pain typically radiates toward the elbows and knees. Weakness is not a feature of PMR. Fatigue, anorexia, weight loss, and low-grade fevers may be seen. Half of patients develop an asymmetric arthritis affecting the knees and wrists or diffuse pitting edema of the hands and feet. The erythrocyte sedimentation rate (ESR) is usually more than 40 mm/h; up to 20% of patients have a normal ESR.

Diagnosis

The diagnosis of PMR depends upon a combination of symptoms, elevated ESR, exclusion of other diseases, and response to corticosteroids. Diseases to be excluded include elderly-onset rheumatoid arthritis, spondyloarthropathy, crystal-induced arthritis, polymyositis, malignancy, and infection.

Treatment
Treatment of PMR is with moderate doses of corticosteroids (e.g., prednisone[1] 15–20 mg daily). The majority of patients experience rapid and dramatic relief of symptoms within 24 to 48 hours. If there is no clinical improvement, the prednisone dose can be increased to 30 mg daily. If there is still no response, the diagnosis of PMR needs to be questioned. Following relief of symptoms the prednisone is gradually tapered in small increments every 2 to 4 weeks; relapse is common if taper is too rapid. Successful tapering is based on suppression of symptomatology, not the level of the ESR. Treatment duration is typically 1 to 2 years.

Giant Cell Arteritis
Clinical Presentation
GCA, also known as temporal arteritis, is a vasculitis characterized by granulomatous inflammation in the wall of medium and large arteries, especially the proximal aorta and its branches. It typically manifests with new-onset severe headache, usually located over the temporal area, which is constant and interferes with sleep. The temporal artery may be thickened, nodular, and tender, with diminished or absent pulsation. The vertebral, ophthalmic, posterior ciliary, and central retinal arteries and the internal and external carotid arteries may be affected in addition to the temporal artery. Half of patients have jaw claudication or scalp tenderness (or both). Symptoms of PMR are common, occurring in 40% to 60% of patients with GCA.

Vision disturbances (e.g., diplopia, amaurosis fugax) due to optic nerve ischemia can occur as an early manifestation or during the tapering of corticosteroids. Vision loss may be irreversible if not treated expeditiously.

Fever, malaise, and weight loss may be present. Rarely GCA manifests as a fever of unknown origin (FUO) without the other more typical symptoms.

Aortic arch involvement occurs in 10% to 15% and can manifest with claudication of the arms or legs, with bruits present over affected arteries. Strokes are seen in 3% to 7% of patients owing to ischemia in the vertebrobasilar or carotid arteries. Thoracic aortic aneurysms can develop years after initial diagnosis of GCA and are an important late complication.

Diagnosis
Laboratory testing demonstrates an elevated ESR (≥50 mm/hour) in 80% of patients. A normal ESR does not rule out the diagnosis. Anemia of chronic disease is often present.

A temporal artery biopsy should be obtained, if possible, but should not delay onset of treatment. Because the arterial inflammation occurs in a patchy distribution, a temporal artery biopsy of 3 to 4 cm in length should be obtained to minimize the false-negative rate. Histopathologic evidence is the gold standard for diagnosis; however, the diagnosis of GCA may be established clinically based on characteristic signs and symptoms without a biopsy.

Treatment
Treatment with high-dose corticosteroids (e.g., prednisone[1] 60 mg daily or 1 mg/kg/day equivalent) is initiated once the diagnosis of GCA is entertained; treatment should not be postponed while awaiting temporal artery biopsy. If vision loss has occurred, some advocate treatment with intravenous methylprednisolone (Solu-Medrol)[1] (1000 mg daily for 3 days) followed by high-dose daily oral prednisone. Alternate-day treatment is not recommended owing to the higher rate of disease flare-up. Following clinical response, corticosteroids are tapered gradually every 2 to 4 weeks. Relapse of symptoms can occur at any time in up to 60% of patients. The decision to increase the dose of steroids is based on recurrence of clinical symptoms; an elevated ESR in the absence of symptoms is not a reason to increase the prednisone dose. Treatment duration

[1]Not FDA approved for this indication.

is usually 1 to 2 years; however, a subset of patients require chronic steroid treatment. Aspirin,[1] unless contraindicated, is an important adjunctive treatment because studies suggest a decreased risk of vision loss and central nervous systemic events.

[1]Not FDA approved for this indication.

References
Dasgupta B, Matteson EL. Maradit-Kremers: Management guidelines and outcome measures in polymyalgia rheumatica. Clin Exp Rheumatol 2007;25:S130–6.
Gonzalez-Gay MA, Vazquez-Rodriguez TR, Gomez-Acebo I, et al. Strokes at time of disease diagnosis in a series of 287 patients with biopsy-proven giant cell arteritis. Medicine (Baltimore) 2009;88:227–35.
Hernandez-Rodriguez J, Cid MC, Lopez-Soto A, et al. Treatment of polymyalgia rheumatica: A systematic review. Arch Intern Med 2009;169:1839–50.
Marie I, Proux A, Duhaut P, et al. Long-term follow-up of aortic involvement in giant cell arteritis. Medicine (Baltimore) 2009;88:182–92.
Michet CJ, Matteson EL. Polymyalgia rheumatica. BMJ 2008;336:765–9.
Salvarani C, Cantini F, Hunder G. Polymyalgia rheumatica and giant cell arteritis. Lancet 2008;372:234–45.
Warrington KJ, Matteson EL. Management guidelines and outcome measures in giant cell arteritis. Clin Exp Rheumatol 2007;25:S137–41.

RHEUMATOID ARTHRITIS

Method of
Arthur Kavanaugh, MD; and Sriharsha Cherukumilli Grevich, MD

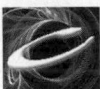

CURRENT DIAGNOSIS

Criteria for classifying patients as having RA:
- Presence of clinical synovitis (swelling) in at least one joint not explained by another disease (e.g., psoriatic arthritis, systemic lupus erythematosus, or other rheumatic diseases manifest with inflammatory arthritis)
- Having a cumulative score of at least 6 out of 10 from the following four categories (using highest score from each category):

	Points
1 large joint	0
2–10 large joints	1
1–3 small joints	2
4–10 small joints	3
>10 joints with inclusion of at least 1 small joint (may also include joints other than those listed above, except for the excluded joints)	5

I. Joint involvement (includes tender or swollen joints indicative of active synovitis; large joints include shoulders, elbows, hips, knees, and ankles. Small joints include metacarpophalangeal joints, proximal interphalangeal joints, second through fifth metatarsophalangeal joints, thumb interphalangeal joints, and wrists. Distal interphalangeal joints, first carpometacarpal joints, and first metatarsophalangeal joints are excluded.)

II. Serologic categories (RF = rheumatoid factor, ACPA = anti-citrullinated protein antibody. Negative value is ≤ULN (upper limit of normal for respective lab test); low-positive is >ULN but ≤3 × ULN; high-positive is >3 × ULN)

	Points
Negative RG and negative ACPA	0
Low-positive RF or low-positive ACPA	2
High-positive RF or high-positive ACPA	3

III. Acute-phase response

	Points
Normal CRP and normal ESR	0
Abnormal CRP or abnormal ESR	1

IV. Duration of symptoms (based on patient self-reported symptoms of synovitis)

	Points
< 6 weeks	0
≥ 6 weeks	1

Other patients classified as having RA:
- Patients with radiographic changes that are very characteristic of rheumatoid arthritis (e.g., periarticular bony erosions) who have fulfilled the above criteria in the past
- Patients with longstanding symptoms (either active or inactive and with or without treatment) who have fulfilled the above criteria in the past based on retrospective data

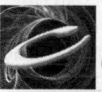

CURRENT THERAPY

Nonpharmacologic Treatment
- Patient and family education and longitudinal supportive care should be provided by physicians and their staff
- Physical therapy and occupational therapy assists patients with compromised activities of daily living
- Dynamic and aerobic conditioning exercises improve mobility, strength, and psychological well-being

Pharmacologic Treatment
NSAIDs and Selective Cyclooxygenase 2 (COX-2) Inhibitors
- Joint function is improved by reducing joint pain and swelling

Glucocorticoids
- Glucocorticoids can relieve signs and symptoms of disease and may slow its progression
- Low-dose glucocorticoids, such as < 10 mg of prednisone daily or the equivalent, should be administered
- Local injections of depot formulations of corticosteroids are given
- Bridge therapies should be given for flare-ups or when patients are starting treatment

Disease-Modifying Antirheumatic Drugs (DMARDs)
- DMARDs can preserve joint integrity and function by reducing joint damage
- Commonly used DMARDs:
  - Methotrexate (Rheumatrex) oral, 7.5–25 mg/week; SC injection (Otrexup) 7.5–25 mg/week
  - Hydroxychloroquine (Plaquenil) oral, 200 mg twice daily
  - Sulfasalazine (Azulfidine-EN Tabs) oral, 1000 mg twice or three times daily[3]
  - Leflunomide (Arava) oral, loading dose 100 mg/day for 3 days then 20 mg/day in a single dose, if tolerated; otherwise, 10 mg/day
  - Cyclosporine A (Neoral, Gengraf) oral, 2.5–4 mg/kg/day in divided doses (twice daily)
  - Combinations of DMARDs that have been effective in RA include methotrexate plus cyclosporine, methotrexate plus leflunomide, and methotrexate plus sulfasalazine plus hydroxychloroquine
  - Tofacitinib (Xeljanz): Oral 5 mg twice daily (monotherapy or in combination with nonbiologic disease-modifying antirheumatic drugs).

Biologic Response Modifiers (Biologics)
- Biologics are commonly used in combination with methotrexate, or less commonly with other DMARDs
- They slow or prevent disease progression (particularly TNF inhibitors) and can induce remission
- TNF-α inhibitors include the following:
  - Infliximab (Remicade) IV infusion, doses between 3–10 mg/kg (mean dose, ≈5 mg/kg) with additional similar doses at 2 and 6 weeks after the first infusion and then every 8 weeks thereafter
  - Etanercept (Enbrel) SC injection, 50 mg/week as a single dose or 25 mg biweekly[3]
  - Adalimumab (Humira) SC injection, 40 mg every other week (also approved for use weekly)
  - Certolizumab pegol (Cimzia) SC injection, 400 mg initial dose with additional similar doses at 2 and 4 weeks after initial dose and then every 4 weeks thereafter (or 200 mg every other week)
  - Golimumab (Simponi) SC injection 50 mg once a month. Also available as IV infusion (Simponi Aria), 2 mg/kg with additional similar doses at 4 weeks after the first infusion and then every 8 weeks thereafter
  - Anti-CD20 antibody: Rituximab (Rituxan) IV infusion, two 1000-mg infusions separated by 2 weeks; further treatments are typically given after 6 months when disease activity recurs
  - CTLA-4-immunoglobulin: abatacept (Orencia) IV infusion, dosage between 500 and 1000 mg based on weight (dose approximates 10 mg/kg). Initial dose is followed by doses 2 and 4 weeks later, with further doses every 4 weeks thereafter. Also available SC injection 125 mg/week given within a day following a single IV loading dose
- Interleukin-1 receptor antagonist: anakinra (Kineret) SC injection 100 mg/day
- Interleukin-6 receptor antibody: tocilizumab (Actemra) IV infusion, dosage between 4 and 8 mg/kg in adults (maximum dose 800 mg) every 4 weeks. Also available in SC injection: 162 mg every 2 weeks, with the option to move to weekly (patients ≥ 100 kg can start at 162 mg weekly)

Surgical Treatment
- Surgery is used for patients with intolerable pain, loss of range of motion, or structural joint damage that leads to limitation of function
- Procedures include joint fusion, synovectomy, total joint arthroplasty, and partial joint replacement or remodeling

---

[3] Exceeds dosage recommended by the manufacturer.

Epidemiology
Rheumatoid arthritis (RA) is a progressive, systemic inflammatory disease that affects about 0.5% to 1% of the population worldwide. RA is associated with substantial morbidity and accelerated mortality and exerts a tremendous economic toll on affected patients, their families, and society. Women are three to four times more likely to be affected than men. The peak age of onset is between 40 and 60 years, but it is possible to get RA at any age. RA also affects the elderly and young children.

Pathophysiology
Even though there has been progress in deciphering the cellular and molecular mechanism of RA, the cause is still not fully defined. RA is characterized by synovial and vascular proliferation with the formation of pannus tissue, which results in damage to articular cartilage and adjacent subchondral bone. Activation of specific CD4$^+$ T cells, potentially in response to unidentified antigens, in an immunogenetically susceptible individual is hypothesized to be an early event in this process. Activated T cells orchestrate a cell-mediated immune response, stimulating and interacting with monocytes or macrophages, synovial fibroblasts, osteoclasts, B cells, and many other cell types. The cascade of inflammatory mediators that is released contributes to the sustenance of the ongoing immune activation and directly causes signs, symptoms, and sequelae of the disease, such as destruction of joints. Joint destruction, which may be considered the sequela of untreated inflammation over time, correlates directly with functional disability. Impaired function correlates with many key outcomes, such as increased mortality and greater costs.

Diagnosis
RA diagnosis is mainly clinical based on physical findings, patient history and ongoing observation of symptoms, signs, and response to therapy. The 2010 American College of Rheumatology

(ACR)/EULAR classification criteria for the diagnosis of RA is presented above in the current diagnosis section.

Treatment

The main goals of treatment for RA are to alleviate pain, prevent or limit joint damage, optimize quality of life, avoid complications of therapy, and improve or preserve function. Novel therapies with specific targets are being designed based on the improved understanding of the pathophysiology of RA. Adoption of an aggressive approach early in the course of the disease is thought to be the best way to prevent irreversible joint damage and to spare patients years of pain and discomfort. Remission, once a purely hypothetical consideration, is now considered to be an appropriate and attainable goal, largely because of the introduction of new therapies, particularly biologic agents, and new treatment paradigms, particularly the frequent assessment of disease activity with resultant changes in treatment to achieve low disease activity.

Treatment response in clinical trials is typically measured using the ACR criteria for measuring improvement of arthritis. The ACR20 refers to 20% improvement in tender and swollen joint counts and 20% improvement in three of the five additional measures: patient and physician global assessments of arthritis, pain, disability, and an acute-phase reactant, such as the erythrocyte sedimentation rate (ESR) or C-reactive protein (CRP). Variations that define higher levels of response—the ACR50 and ACR70, which require improvements in individual measures exceeding 50% and 70%, respectively—are more stringent outcomes. The Health Assessment Questionnaire (HAQ) and Short Form 36 (SF-36) are used to calculate functional disability and health-related quality of life, respectively. Joint damage in patients with RA is assessed by quantifying radiographic changes characteristic of RA, including joint space narrowing and periarticular bony erosions.

Treatment of RA begins after the diagnosis is established, baseline activity is assessed, and prognosis is estimated. Therapy is initiated with patient education about the disease and the treatments available. Symptoms can be controlled to some extent with nonsteroidal antiinflammatory drugs (NSAIDs) and low-dose oral glucocorticoids or glucocorticoid joint injections. Ideally, disease-modifying antirheumatic drugs (DMARDs) should be started soon after diagnosis is established (e.g., within 3 months). Further care is determined by assessing disease activity and response to treatment. The Current Therapy box lists commonly used treatments for RA and includes trade names and usual maintenance doses for these drugs.

Analgesics and Nonsteroidal Antiinflammatory Drugs

Analgesics (e.g., acetaminophen, tramadol [Ultram], opioids) are used to relieve pain, but they do not reduce inflammation or prevent joint destruction. NSAIDs (e.g., aspirin, ibuprofen [Motrin], naproxen [Naprosyn], ketoprofen [Orudis], piroxicam [Feldene], diclofenac [Voltaren], celecoxib [Celebrex]) reduce pain and inflammation (at higher doses) but do not slow joint damage. These drugs are used as adjuncts but are not usually the sole treatment for RA because they do not prevent disease progression.

Although many over-the-counter analgesics and NSAIDs are available and are perceived by patients to be benign, they are not risk-free. Narcotic analgesics should be used with caution because of their potential for habituation and toxicity with chronic use. NSAIDs work by inhibiting cyclooxygenase enzyme isoforms COX-1 and COX-2. COX-1 is constitutively expressed by many cells, whereas COX-2 production is usually increased at sites of inflammation. Side effects with chronic use of NSAIDs include gastrointestinal irritation, rash, fluid retention, and the potential for renal toxicity. Acetaminophen (Tylenol), a non-NSAID COX inhibitor, does not cause gastrointestinal irritation, but it may cause severe hepatotoxicity, and it potentially interacts with warfarin (Coumadin). The frequency of NSAID-induced ulcers can be reduced with concomitant use of proton pump inhibitors or misoprostol (Cytotec). COX-2 inhibitors were developed because their more specific activity was expected to control signs and symptoms of arthritis with less risk of gastrointestinal complications. However, two of the three COX-2 inhibitors approved in the United

States were withdrawn because of concerns about thrombotic and atherosclerotic toxicities. The remaining available COX-2 inhibitor, celecoxib, seems to have a safety profile comparable to other NSAIDs in that regard.

Glucocorticoids

Oral glucocorticoids at lower doses (e.g., <10 mg prednisone equivalent per day) are often used to control pain, inflammation, and stiffness, and they can potentially slow the progression of joint damage. However, because of the possibility of significant side effects, especially with long-term use at a high dose, glucocorticoids are most commonly used for short-term treatment of very active or aggressive RA, usually in combination with NSAIDs and DMARDs. They are often tapered when the disease is under control.

Side effects of glucocorticoids include changes to appetite and weight, glucose intolerance or hyperglycemia, infection, osteoporosis, mood and sleep disturbances, hypertension, suppression of the hypothalamic-pituitary axis, and interference with wound healing, among others. Administering calcium and vitamin D supplementation, bisphosphonates, calcitonin (Miacalcin),[1] parathyroid hormone (teriparatide [Forteo]),[2] and estrogen[2] or testosterone[2] replacement can reduce the risk of bone loss in patients taking corticosteroids.

Intraarticular glucocorticoid injections can provide dramatic but usually temporary clinical improvement in patients who have a disease flareup in a single or a few joints. Most clinicians think that no more than one injection in any 3-month period should be made in a given joint. The need for more repeated injections suggests that the overall treatment plan requires reevaluation.

Disease-Modifying Antirheumatic Drugs

DMARDs are the mainstay of treatment for RA because they can modify various aspects of the immune and inflammatory responses, potentially controlling signs and symptoms of disease and slowing its progression. Extensive clinical studies of DMARDs have demonstrated reductions in joint damage, preservation of joint function, and higher rates of productivity. DMARDs are considered first-line therapy for all patients with newly diagnosed RA. The standard of care is to initiate DMARD therapy early, such as within the first 3 months of the disease for patients with established RA who, despite adequate treatment with NSAIDs, have ongoing joint pain, significant morning stiffness or fatigue, active synovitis, evidence of active inflammation (e.g., persistent elevation of the ESR or CRP level, actively inflamed joints), or radiographic joint damage. Because DMARDs may take 2 to 6 months to reach full effect, NSAIDs and sometimes glucocorticoids can be used in the interim to reduce pain and swelling. The duration of DMARD use may be limited by loss of efficacy or development of toxicity.

Methotrexate (Rheumatrex) is the most commonly used DMARD because of its oral, once-weekly administration, well-defined safety profile, demonstrated efficacy, and low cost. Sulfasalazine (Azulfidine EN-tabs) or hydroxychloroquine (Plaquenil) tend to be used in persons whose disease is considered milder or more slowly progressive. They are also used in combination with methotrexate for aggressive disease. Leflunomide (Arava) was shown in several phase III trials to offer comparable efficacy to methotrexate and sulfasalazine against active RA. Older drugs in this class (e.g., parenteral or oral gold [gold sodium thiomalate[2] or auranofin], azathioprine [Imuran], D-penicillamine [Cuprimine]) were shown to be effective in older clinical trials, but they are much less commonly used now largely because of lower efficacy and poor tolerability.

In RA, methotrexate's mechanism of action may be related to its inhibition of inflammation, presumably by increasing the local release of adenosine. Clinical response may take 6 to 8 weeks to be seen. The mean dose used among RA patients worldwide is approximately 17.5 mg/week, although many clinicians initiate

---

[1]Not FDA approved for this indication.
[2]Not available in the United States.

therapy at lower doses to help ensure tolerability. Most clinicians consider 25 mg/week to be a maximum dose. Higher doses are not clearly associated with better disease control but may be associated with more toxicity. Parenteral administration may be used at doses higher than 15 mg/week because of more predictable absorption. Many RA patients have taken methotrexate successfully for years, attesting to its efficacy and safety.

Leflunomide (Arava) is a prodrug that is actively metabolized after oral administration. This active metabolite inhibits dihydroorotate dehydrogenase, which interferes with pyrimidine synthesis and ultimately leads to inhibition of activated T cells and other cells. To minimize toxicity, the maintenance dose of 20 mg/day can be reduced to 10 mg/day.

Tofacitinib (Xeljanz) is an oral Janus kinase (JAK) inhibitor for treatment of moderate to severe RA. It can be used as a monotherapy or in combination with methotrexate or another nonbiologic DMARD. Tofacitinib has been shown to be a more effective monotherapy agent than methotrexate in reducing signs and symptoms of rheumatoid arthritis and the progression of structural joint damage. In patients with inadequate response to methotrexate or TNF inhibitor therapy, tofacitinib has been shown to be effective as a single agent or in combination with methotrexate.

Although DMARDs represent a major advance in the management of RA, they are not without risks or limitations. Methotrexate is associated with rare but serious side effects, including bone marrow suppression, hypersensitivity pneumonitis, and hepatotoxicity. It may also slightly increase the risk of infection. It must be used with caution in patients with preexisting liver disease, renal impairment, significant pulmonary disease, or alcohol abuse. Less serious but common side effects of methotrexate include stomatitis, gastrointestinal effects, headache, fatigue, and liver transaminase elevations. Folic acid supplementation can prevent many of the minor side effects. Leflunomide can lead to elevated liver enzyme levels, weight loss, hypertension, diarrhea, reversible alopecia, and myelosuppression. Leflunomide inhibits cytochrome P-450 (CYP) 2C9, so there is a theoretical potential for interactions with other drugs that are also CYP2C9 substrates. Methotrexate and leflunomide necessitate regular monitoring of liver enzymes and complete blood cell counts at regular intervals. Treatment should be stopped for any persistent or severe abnormalities. Common side effects of tofacitinib include a risk of infections, lymphopenia, neutropenia, hyperlipidemia, liver function test abnormalities and increased serum creatinine levels. To prevent serious adverse effects, especially infections, tofacitinib should not be used in combination with a biologic agent or azathioprine or cyclosporine.

Other side effects seen with various DMARDs include gastrointestinal intolerance and rash. Although antimalarial drugs (e.g., hydroxychloroquine) have been reported to cause ocular toxicity, with current dosages and preparations, this reaction is rare. Sulfasalazine may cause cutaneous adverse events (e.g., urticaria, maculopapular rash, photosensitivity) and hematologic side effects. Cyclosporine's use has been limited by its toxicity; side effects include headache, tremors, hypertension, and renal insufficiency. Patients taking cyclosporine (Neoral) require regular monitoring of blood pressure and serum creatinine levels. Some DMARDs (e.g., cyclophosphamide [Cytoxan],[1] chlorambucil [Leukeran],[1] azathioprine [Imuran]) may promote the development of secondary malignancies. Some DMARDs are teratogenic and abortifacient and therefore should not be used during pregnancy or breastfeeding and must be discontinued for an appropriate amount of time, typically 3 months or more, before any attempts to conceive.

Biologic Response Modifiers

The introduction of biologic agents was driven largely by three factors: recognition of the unmet clinical need for more effective treatments based on an appreciation of the significantly poor outcomes of uncontrolled RA; improved understanding of the immunopathogenesis of RA; and advances in biopharmaceutical science

---

[1]Not FDA approved for this indication.

allowing the development of specific inhibitors of relevant targets within the dysregulated immune system.

Traditional therapies such as NSAIDs, corticosteroids, and DMARDs may help ameliorate the symptoms of RA, but they rarely induce sustained remission, and they can have toxicities that prevent their long-term use. Newer therapies, many of which are large protein molecules such as monoclonal antibodies or soluble receptor constructs, are referred to as biologic agents. Biologic agents, particularly inhibitors of tumor necrosis factor (TNF), have changed the treatment paradigm for RA. They can inhibit various components of the immune system and inflammatory response that are central to the pathogenesis of RA. The goal is to adopt an early, proactive approach to treatment to prevent the damage from chronic synovial inflammation. Studies have shown that biologic agents can slow disease progression, control signs and symptoms of disease, improve function, and improve quality of life. They are typically used in combination with DMARDs, most commonly methotrexate, to potentiate treatment responses. This newer class of antirheumatic drugs can be further sub-classified according to their specific target or mechanism.

TNF-α Inhibitors
Use of TNF-α inhibitors in combination with methotrexate is considered by many to be the gold standard for treatment of RA. TNF-α is a soluble 17-kDa protein homotrimer that binds to two receptors: type 1 TNF receptor and type 2 TNF receptor. A versatile, multipotent cytokine, it induces production of other inflammatory cytokines such as interleukin 1 (IL-1), IL-6, and granulocyte-monocyte colony-stimulating factor (GM-CSF) and chemokines such as IL-8. TNF-α causes tissue destruction by promoting release of matrix metalloproteinases, upregulates cell trafficking through adhesion molecules and chemokines, increases the breakdown of proteoglycans in the cartilage, and potentiates osteoclast differentiation and activation. There is abundant evidence that TNF inhibition dramatically improves patient outcomes for RA and other autoimmune systemic inflammatory conditions, including psoriasis, psoriatic arthritis, ankylosing spondylitis, and inflammatory bowel disease.

Most RA patients respond to TNF-α inhibitors with a reduction in signs and symptoms, improved quality of life, and preservation of functional status; some even achieve clinical remission of disease. Radiographic evidence shows that TNF-α inhibitors inhibit radiographic disease progression to an extent not seen with any previous agents. From an immunologic standpoint, TNF-α inhibitors do not represent a cure, and maintenance of clinical efficacy almost always requires continued therapy, certainly for patients with long-standing RA. Five of the available biologic agents are inhibitors of TNF-α: infliximab (Remicade), etanercept (Enbrel), adalimumab (Humira), golimumab (Simponi), and certolizumab pegol (Cimzia).

Infliximab, a chimeric human/mouse monoclonal anti-TNF-α monoclonal antibody, was shown to be effective initially in open trials, followed soon by double-blind, placebo-controlled, randomized clinical trials. Inhibition in the progression of joint damage and improvement in health-related quality of life and functional status were observed in patients treated with infliximab. It is used mostly in combination with methotrexate, which decreases immunogenicity and produces synergy in clinical outcomes.

Etanercept is a recombinant form of the human receptor that is fused to the Fc fragment of the human immunoglobulin G1. Clinical trials have shown etanercept to be effective in improving the signs and symptoms of RA when used as monotherapy and in combination with methotrexate; it also inhibits disease progression and optimizes functional status and quality of life.

Adalimumab is a human anti-TNF-α monoclonal antibody. The efficacy of adalimumab on the signs and symptoms of RA has been proved in various studies, and it has demonstrated benefit in terms of improving quality of life and functional status and in attenuating the progression of joint damage.

Certolizumab pegol is a PEGylated Fab′ fragment of a humanized monoclonal anti-TNF antibody. Golimumab is a human anti-TNF-α monoclonal antibody. Both of these agents have been shown to improve signs and symptoms of disease and physical function and to prevent disease progression in patients with active RA.

TNF antagonists exhibit a rapid onset of action, provide significant clinical response, improve quality of life, and most importantly, substantially inhibit radiographic progression of disease. Most patients on TNF antagonists are still treated with methotrexate because studies have shown that TNF antagonists work better in this combination. There are some safety concerns because reports of opportunistic infections, tuberculosis, lymphoma, administration reactions, immune or autoimmune responses, and demyelinating syndromes have emerged with TNF antagonist treatment. Some patients do fail to respond or eventually lose the ability to respond. Other biologic agents can be effective for patients who fail anti-TNF therapy.

B-Cell Directed Therapy

Mounting evidence suggests that B cells play an active role in RA. B cells can accumulate in the synovium, form aggregates, produce autoantibodies such as rheumatoid factor (RF), and function as antigen-presenting cells that aid in the activation of $CD4^+$ T cells. These findings provide the rationale for targeting B cells in RA patients. Rituximab (Rituxan) is a monoclonal antibody directed against the CD20 antigen found on the surface of B cells. When bound to CD20, rituximab depletes B cells through various mechanisms, including complement-mediated lysis, antibody-dependent cytotoxicity, and apoptosis.

Rituximab treatment induced depletion of peripheral-blood B cells for 6 months or longer, but the levels of immunoglobulins in the serum (IgG, IgA, IgM) did not change substantially. RF levels decreased substantially. Despite the prolonged depletion of peripheral-blood B cells, the overall incidence of infection was similar in the control group and the rituximab groups. However, an increased rate of infusion-related reactions was identified for the rituximab group compared with the placebo group. In patients with active RA who failed one or more anti-TNF-α therapies, rituximab significantly reduced signs, symptoms, fatigue, and disability and improved health-related quality of life.

T-Cell Directed Therapy

T-cell activation plays a central role in the pathogenesis of RA. For example, the rheumatoid synovium contains a preponderance of $CD4^+$ T cells. It is thought that these cells are stimulated by arthritogenic antigens to initiate synovial inflammation. Cytotoxic T lymphocyte-associated antigen 4 (CTLA4) is expressed on the surface of T cells within days after they have become activated. CTLA4 binds to and prevents CD80 and CD86 from binding to CD28, thereby effectively blocking the costimulatory signal required for activation of T cells. Blocking CD28 costimulation has been shown to induce T-cell anergy.

Abatacept (Orencia), an inhibitor of T-cell costimulation, is a fusion protein construct consisting of the extracellular component of CTLA4 fused to the Fc region of human IgG, which increases its half-life. The high affinity of CTLA4-Ig for CD28 prevents B7-mediated costimulation. Abatacept has improved signs and symptoms of disease, helped to maintain physical function, and reduced progression of joint damage in patients with active disease despite concomitant methotrexate. Similarly, it improved signs and symptoms, physical function, and health-related quality of life in RA patients refractory to TNF-α inhibition.

Interleukin-1 Receptor Antagonist

Interleukin-1 (IL-1) appears to have a prominent role in synovial inflammation and displays many overlapping effects with TNF-α. RA patients have increased levels of IL-1 in the plasma and synovial fluid, and its concentration has been correlated with disease activity. Similar to TNF-α, IL-1 can activate a variety of inflammatory cells and mediators using some overlapping signal transduction pathways.

Anakinra (Kineret) is a subcutaneously administered IL-1 receptor antagonist. Anakinra has been shown in several studies to reduce the signs and symptoms of RA; however, the extent of improvement is less than that seen with TNF antagonists. Combination therapy with anti-IL-1 and anti-TNF is contraindicated because of an observed increase in the risk of adverse events in a study in which patients were treated with anakinra and etanercept. Anakinra usually is well tolerated, and the most common side effect is injection site reactions. The need for daily injectable administration and the modest efficacy compared with TNF inhibitors have limited the use of anakinra.

IL-6 Receptor Antibody

IL-6 is an inflammatory cytokine that may contribute to the immune-pathophysiology of several autoimmune systemic inflammatory disorders, including RA. To date, the greatest experience with IL-6 inhibition has been with tocilizumab (Actemra), a humanized monoclonal antibody with specificity toward the IL-6 receptor (IL-6R). Tocilizumab has been proven effective in various subsets of RA patients, including those previously exposed to TNF inhibitors, and it is approved in many countries worldwide for the treatment of RA. In addition, it has been approved for use in patients with systemic juvenile idiopathic arthritis (sJIA), a potentially devastating condition characterized by abundant systemic inflammation. It has been shown to reduce signs and symptoms and improve functional status and to inhibit radiographic progression in patients with active RA. Potential adverse effects that may be associated with IL-6 inhibition include risk for infection, alteration in serum lipid profiles, decreased neutrophil counts, and elevated liver function tests.

Biologic agents have different mechanisms, methods of delivery, and side effects. A patient who does not respond to or cannot tolerate one may still have a good outcome with another. Although they are commonly used in combination with methotrexate, biologic agents usually are not given in combination with each other, because this approach may increase risk without much increase in benefit. Because biologic agents modulate part of the immune response, there is concern about potential side effects related to impaired immune function, such as increased risk of minor and serious infections and secondary malignancies.

Biologic agents require parenteral administration: subcutaneous injections (e.g., etanercept, adalimumab, anakinra, certolizumab, golimumab) or intravenous infusions (e.g., infliximab, abatacept, rituximab, tocilizumab). These routes are less convenient than orally administered drugs and can be associated with administration reactions, such as injection-site or infusion reactions. Biologic agents are also more expensive than traditional DMARDs, which has affected their use. However, the increased clinical benefit seen with these agents needs to be considered in any comprehensive cost-efficacy analysis.

Conclusions

RA is a prevalent disease and a leading cause of physical disability. There is no cure for RA. However, with available agents applied appropriately, clinical remission is the goal of therapy and is a realistic expectation for some patients. When remission is not achieved, the rheumatologist must look for the most effective combination of therapies to alleviate pain, maintain function, and maximize quality of life. Methotrexate is still the mainstay of long-term care, but newer biologic DMARDs provide additional benefits. The role of biologic agents is still evolving. Their use is often reserved for patients who fail to respond to methotrexate, but the trend is toward earlier use of these agents. NSAIDs and glucocorticoids are useful for bridge therapy in patients with acute symptoms, especially while waiting for DMARDs to reach their maximal effect. Patients should be evaluated periodically for evidence of disease activity and progression and for drug toxicity. The management strategy should be changed if there is progressive joint damage or evidence of ongoing activity after 3 months of maximal treatment, or if treatment is poorly tolerated.

References

Aletaha D, Neogi T, Silman AJ, et al. 2010 Rheumatoid arthritis classification criteria: An American College of Rheumatology/European League Against Rheumatism collaborative initiative. Arthritis Rheum 2010;62:2569–81.

American College of Rheumatology Subcommittee on Rheumatoid Arthritis Guidelines. Guidelines for the management of rheumatoid arthritis 2002 update. Arthritis Rheum 2002;46:328–46.

Chang J, Kavanaugh A. Novel therapies for rheumatoid arthritis. Pathophysiology 2005;12:217–25.

Doan QV, Chiou CF, Dubois RW. Review of eight pharmacoeconomic studies of the value of biologic DMARDs (adalimumab, etanercept, and infliximab) in the management of rheumatoid arthritis. J Manag Care Pharm 2006;12:555–69.

Felson DT, Anderson JJ, Boers M, et al. American College of Rheumatology: Preliminary definition of improvement in rheumatoid arthritis. Arthritis Rheum 1995;38:727–35.

Lee E, Fleischmann R, Hall S, et al. Tofacitinib versus methotrexate in rheumatoid arthritis. N Engl J Med 2014;370(25):2377–86.

Mircic M, Kavanaugh A. The clinical efficacy of tocilizumab in rheumatoid arthritis. Drugs Today (Barc) 2009;45:189–97.

Olsen NJ, Stein M. New drugs for rheumatoid arthritis. N Engl J Med 2004;350:2167–79.

Scott D, Kingsley G. Biologics in Rheumatoid Arthritis. Inflammatory Arthritis in Clinical Practice. London: Springer; 2007 p. 86–96.

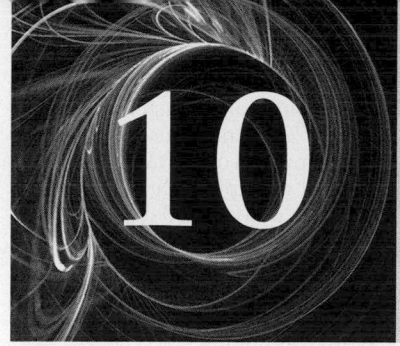

10 The Nervous System

ACUTE FACIAL PARALYSIS

Method of
Steven Meyers, MD

CURRENT DIAGNOSIS

- Typical cases of acute facial paralysis are diagnosed based on examination and do not require additional evaluation.
- All patients with acute facial paralysis should have a complete neurologic and head and neck examinations.
- The presence of atypical features such as a slowly progressive course, failure to improve, recurrent attacks, or other neurologic findings should prompt additional evaluation with computed tomography (CT) or magnetic resonance imaging (MRI) of the head and a specialist consultation.

CURRENT THERAPY

- Steroid therapy, such as prednisone[1] 60–80 mg daily for 7 days, initiated within 3 days of onset of the facial paralysis, increases the chances of recovery
- The use of antiviral therapy remains controversial without strong evidence of benefit, but valacyclovir (Valtrex)[1] 1000 mg three times daily for 7 days may be beneficial in patients with severe paralysis.
- Eye care with artificial tears, ophthalmic ointments at night, and eye protection should be used in patients with severe facial paralysis.

[1]Not FDA approved for this indication.

Acute facial nerve paralysis, or Bell's palsy, is a common disorder manifesting with the acute to subacute onset of unilateral paralysis of the muscles of facial expression. The Scottish physician Sir Charles Bell described cases of facial paralysis due to trauma in the 1800s, and the idiopathic condition carries his name today. However, there are many possible causes of facial paralysis, and each patient requires a careful history and complete neurologic examination to exclude these possibilities.

Epidemiology and Risk Factors

The annual incidence rate is between 13 and 34 cases per 100,000 population. All age ranges can be affected, but persons between the ages of 15 and 40 years are most commonly affected. Diabetics, pregnant women in the third trimester, and women in the immediate postpartum period are at increased risk. There is no gender, race, or geographic predilection.

Pathophysiology

The seventh cranial, or facial, nerve arises from the pontomedullary junction and runs in close proximity to the eighth cranial nerve to the internal auditory meatus. The nerve then runs through the bony fallopian canal before exiting the skull at the stylomastoid foramen. The labyrinthine portion of the fallopian canal is very narrow, and it is postulated that swelling of the nerve results in compression in this region.

Three branches arise from the facial nerve within the fallopian canal. The greater petrosal nerve arises from the geniculate ganglion, passes to the pterygopalatine ganglion, and eventually supplies innervation to the lacrimal and palatine glands. The second branch is the nerve to the stapedius muscle in the middle ear. The final branch is the chorda tympani, which supplies taste sensation from the anterior two thirds of the tongue.

The pathophysiology of Bell's palsy is uncertain, but a viral cause is the most commonly accepted hypothesis. Many different viruses have been associated with facial paralysis, with herpes simplex virus (HSV) having the strongest evidence. HSV-1 DNA has been detected by polymerase chain reaction assay in endoneural fluid in patients with Bell's palsy undergoing facial nerve decompression.

Herpes zoster is another virus associated with facial nerve paralysis. Herpes zoster oticus (Ramsey Hunt syndrome) is diagnosed when vesicles are seen in the external auditory canal or on the auricle. Other viruses implicated include cytomegalovirus, Epstein–Barr virus, adenovirus, rubella, mumps, influenza B, and coxsackievirus.

The histopathology of the facial nerve supports an inflammatory etiology with findings similar to those seen in herpes zoster infection. The perineurium is edematous, with diffuse infiltration of inflammatory cells between nerve bundles and surrounding the intraneural vessels.

Clinical Manifestations

The clinical presentation of Bell's palsy is typically dramatic and very stereotypical. Pain behind the ear in the region of the mastoid can precede the onset of weakness by hours to days. Weakness of the muscles of facial expression on one side progresses over a period up to 48 hours. Progression over more prolonged periods raises the possibility of a neoplasm affecting the nerve. The degree of weakness can range from quite subtle to complete paralysis of all muscles of facial expression. Typical features include inability to close the eye, sagging of the eyelid, loss of the nasolabial fold, and inability to wrinkle the forehead muscles. Sparing of the forehead muscles suggests a central or upper motor neuron lesion because these muscles receive bilateral innervation. Additional symptoms that may be reported include hyperacusis due to paralysis of the stapedius muscle, loss of taste in the anterior tongue due to involvement of the chorda tympani, and decreased tearing due to dysfunction of the parasympathetic innervation of the lacrimal gland. However, most patients actually report increased tearing from the affected eye owing to diminished blinking.

Diagnosis and Differential Diagnosis

There is no specific diagnostic test for Bell's palsy. The diagnosis is based on a typical history and examination. Atypical features mandate a search for other causes. A slowly progressive course, parotid gland mass, or involvement in selected branches of the facial nerve can suggest neoplastic compression. Vesicles over the ear or internal auditory canal suggests herpes zoster infection. Patients should be asked about preceding fevers, rashes, and arthralgias, which can prompt evaluation for Lyme disease. However, in the absence of these features, routine serologic testing is not recommended. Sarcoid is a rare cause of usually bilateral facial paralysis. The onset of facial paralysis in the setting of head injury, particularly in the presence of ipsilateral hearing loss, should prompt imaging of the skull base to rule out a temporal bone fracture (Box 1).

Treatment

Treatment of Bell's palsy can be divided into three categories: general medical therapy, specific medical therapy, and surgical therapy. General medical care includes proper eye care. Reduced blinking and inability to completely close the eye increases the risk of corneal abrasion and ulceration. Artificial tears and ophthalmic ointments can prevent these complications. Patients should be instructed to use proper eye protection to prevent injuries. Facial muscle massage and facial nerve stimulation have no evidence to support their use.

Medical Therapy

Specific medical therapy includes glucocorticoid and antiviral medications. Glucocorticoid therapy has been demonstrated to be effective in both meta-analyses and randomized trials. The two largest trials of glucocorticoid and antiviral therapy demonstrated benefit for steroids but no benefit for antiviral therapy when used either alone or in combination with steroids. Treatment in these trials was begun within 72 hours of onset of paralysis and consisted of relatively high dose prednisolone (Millipred)[1] 50 to 60 mg daily for 10 days. Antiviral therapy evaluated included acyclovir (Zovirax)[1] 400 mg five times daily for 10 days and valacyclovir (Valtrex)[1] 1000 mg three times daily for 7 days, neither of which showed benefit.

Smaller, lower-quality studies have suggested a benefit of combining antiviral therapy with glucocorticoids, particularly in patients with more severe baseline dysfunction.

Surgical Therapy

Surgical decompression of the facial nerve is not recommended. A 2011 Cochrane review and a 2001 review by the American Academy of Neurology both found no good evidence supporting this treatment modality. Only two small randomized studies showed no differences in outcome between surgical and medical therapy.

Monitoring and Complications

The overall prognosis of Bell's palsy is favorable. In one study of untreated patients, 85% showed signs of recovery within 3 weeks. Ultimately, 71% experienced complete recovery and an additional 13% were felt to have only slight residual weakness. The degree of weakness at onset is an important prognostic indicator: 94% of patients with incomplete paralysis experienced complete recovery. The absence of any improvement, no matter how small, at 3 to 4 months should raise concern regarding the diagnosis and lead to a search for alternative etiologies.

Motor nerve conduction studies, or electroneurography, can be used to help predict prognosis in selected patients. Patients with incomplete lesions that have an excellent prognosis do not require further evaluation. Motor nerve conduction studies involve stimulating the facial nerve electrically and recording muscle responses with surface electrodes over appropriate muscles. The amplitude of the evoked muscle response on the affected side at 10 days can be compared to the unaffected side, giving an estimate of the degree of axonal loss. A 90% drop in amplitude predicts less than complete recovery, and loss greater than 98% predicts significant residual weakness and synkinesis.

In severe cases of facial paralysis, attention to good eye care as previously discussed is important to prevent eye damage and vision loss.

During recovery from severe nerve injury, axonal regrowth may be misdirected, resulting in synkinesis. Voluntary activation of one muscle group can cause activation of other muscles. Attempts at blinking can result in twitching of the mouth, or smiling can cause involuntary blinking. Misdirection of autonomic fibers can result in the syndrome of "crocodile tears," involuntary lacrimation while eating.

Recurrent attacks of facial paralysis on the ipsilateral or contralateral side occur in up to 15% of patients even after many years. Additional recurrences are quite rare, being reported at a rate between 1% and 3%.

> ## Box 1   Differential Diagnosis of Acute Facial Nerve Paralysis
>
> **Idiopathic**
> Idiopathic cases account for 65%
>
> **Infectious**
> Common
> - Herpes zoster
> - Herpes simplex
> - Borreliosis
> Uncommon
> - Lyme disease
> - Epstein–Barr virus
> - Human immunodeficiency virus
> - Tuberculosis
> Rare
> - Acute otitis media
> - Chronic otitis media
>
> **Trauma**
> Temporal bone fractures
> Penetration wounds
>
> **Neoplasm**
> Parotid
> Metastases
> Schwannoma
> Cholesteatoma
>
> **Metabolic and Toxic**
> Diabetes
> Thyroid disease
> Alcoholism
> Carbon monoxide poisoning (rare)
>
> **Other**
> Sarcoidosis
> Multiple sclerosis
> Sjögren syndrome

---

[1]Not FDA approved for this indication.

References

Engstrom M, Berg T, Stjernquist-Desatnik A, et al. Prednisolone and valaciclovir in Bell's palsy: A randomised, double-blind, placebo-controlled, multicentre trial. Lancet Neurol 2008;7:993–1000.

Gilden DH. Bell's palsy. N Engl J Med 2004;351:1323–31.

Grogan PM, Gronseth GS. Practice parameter: Steroids, acyclovir, and surgery for Bell's palsy (an evidence based review): Report of the Quality Standards Subcommittee of the American Academy of Neurology. Neurology 2001;56:830–6.

Peitersen E. The natural history of Bell's palsy. Am J Otol 1982;4:107–11.

Ronthal M. Bell's palsy: Pathogenesis, clinical features, and diagnosis in adults, Up to Date December 22, 2011;Available at http://www.uptodate.com/contents/bells-palsy-pathogenesis-clinical-features-and-diagnosis-in-adults?source=search_result &search=bell%27s+palsy&selectedTitle=2~26 [accessed 27.08.14].

Ronthal M. Bell's palsy: Prognosis and treatment in adults, Up to Date May 10, 2012;Available at, http://www.uptodate.com/contents/bells-palsy-prognosis-and-treatment-in-adults?source=search_result&search=bell%27s+palsy&selectedTitle=1~26[accessed 27.08.14].

Sullivan FM, Swan IR, Donnan PT, et al. Early treatment with prednisolone or acyclovir in Bell's palsy. N Engl J Med 2007;357:1598–607.

Yeo SG, Lee YC, Park DC, Cha CI. Acyclovir plus steroid vs steroid alone in the treatment of Bell's palsy. Am J Otolaryngol 2008;29:163–6.

ALZHEIMER'S DISEASE

Method of
Philip D. Sloane, MD, MPH; and Daniel I. Kaufer, MD

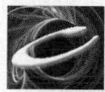

CURRENT DIAGNOSIS

- Routine screening for cognitive impairment is controversial but may be beneficial for early diagnosis and identifying treatable causes.
- Combining the Mini-Cog screening test with screening questions on the informant-based AD8 provides a rapid, sensitive, validated screening assessment.
- A comprehensive dementia evaluation includes a battery of cognitive tests, a laboratory panel for treatable causes, a neurologic examination, a brain MRI, and other testing (e.g., depression screen), as indicated.
- The diagnosis of Alzheimer's disease (AD) continues to rest on having a presentation and course of dementia that is consistent with the disease, and ruling out other identifiable etiologies.
- AD often coexists with cerebrovascular disease; atypical and non-AD dementias generally merit a consultation with a neurology or geriatric specialist.

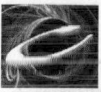

CURRENT THERAPY

- Patient and family education and support are the cornerstones of effective care.
- Preventive measures with the strongest supporting evidence include hypertension control; head injury prevention; physical, cognitive, and social activity; and a Mediterranean diet.
- Cholinesterase inhibitors and memantine (Namenda) alone or jointly have a modest effect on improving or slowing cognitive decline.
- The primary approach to managing behavioral symptoms is person-centered care using dementia-focused communication skills.
- First-line drug agents that may help control behavioral symptoms include cholinesterase inhibitors and mood stabilizers; antipsychotics may be helpful for moderate to severe agitation.

Alzheimer's disease (AD) and related disorders of cognitive function are a common and growing issue for all clinicians who provide care to older adults. In discussing this condition, several related but distinctly different terms are used:

- *Cognitive impairment* refers to the presence of one or more measurable deficits in cerebral function when compared with normal persons of the same age.
- *Dementia* refers to cognitive impairment that represents a decline from that person's baseline and is associated with demonstrative changes in the person's everyday function.
- *AD* is the most common cause of dementia; it has a characteristic pathophysiology and clinical presentation.

Lack of a simple, reliable diagnostic test makes it difficult to know with certainty how many persons in the United States currently have AD, but estimates place the number between 5 and 8 million. Onset can occur when people are in their 40's or 50's, but it is largely a disease of older persons, with the prevalence approximately doubling every 5 years after age 65. By age 85 to 90, up to 50% of individuals will meet criteria for dementia, often with mixed features of AD and cerebrovascular disease.

Risk Factors

Numerous risk factors have been associated with AD (Table 1); however, the strongest ones—age and a positive family history—cannot be modified. Of the modifiable risk factors, current emphasis is being placed on reduction of risk factors for atherosclerotic disease (especially hypertension) and traumatic brain injury, particularly sports-related concussions.

Pathophysiology

AD results from the gradual loss of connections between, and eventual death of, neurons in the cerebral cortex. The cause of this neuronal loss remains incompletely understood. For over a century, the accumulation of amyloid deposits outside neuronal cells, and of neurofibrillary tangles within neuronal cells, have been known to be pathological hallmarks of the disease. New brain imaging techniques have shown that amyloid deposits may begin decades before the onset of clinical signs, whereas the presence of neurofibrillary tangles composed of abnormal tau protein is much more strongly correlated with disease severity. Genetic mutations that cause AD and the strongest known AD genetic risk factor, the epsilon 4 allele of the apolipoprotein E locus, have led to a primary focus on abnormal amyloid protein processing, but amyloid-based therapeutics to date have been ineffective.

Despite intensive research efforts, the precise mechanisms and interrelationships between extracellular amyloid plaque and intracellular neurofibrillary tangle deposition remains elusive.

Prevention

With the disappointing lack of progress in developing safe, effective new medications to treat AD, increased emphasis is being placed on prevention through (a) modification of vascular risk factors, prevention of neural injury, and buildup of neuronal reserves (see Table 1). Among the preventive measures that can be recommended to persons with a family history of AD or other risk factors for the disease include:

- Control of hypertension, with the goal of a blood pressure of 130 to 140 or 80 to 90. Lower blood pressures are not generally advocated, especially in older persons, because of concern that more aggressive blood pressure reduction in persons with existing vascular disease may reduce cerebral perfusion, leading to ischemic damage.
- Reduction in other cardiovascular risk factors by not smoking and by treating hyperlipidemia and diabetes.
- Avoidance of and/or treatment of anything else that causes injury to brain cells, including head trauma, alcoholism, and obstructive sleep apnea.
- Maintenance of good general health by engaging in regular physical activity, being socially active, and adhering to healthy dietary principles, such as the Mediterranean diet.
- Promotion of brain use and activity through such activities as learning a language and doing puzzles.

Clinical Features

Diagnostic criteria for *dementia* include a chronic, progressive disease characterized by (a) memory impairment; (b) impairment of one or more other aspects of neurologic function, such as executive function, visuospatial function, aphasia, apraxia, and/or agnosia; and (c) significant reduction in social or occupational function from the person's previous level of performance, which is not explained by another psychiatric or neurologic disorder. Diagnostic criteria for *AD* include meeting all criteria for dementia and

TABLE 1 Major Risk Factors for Alzheimer's Disease and Evidence of Ability to Modify Risk

RISK FACTOR	DIRECTION OF EFFECT	MODIFIABLE?/ STRATEGY	EVIDENCE OF RISK REDUCTION*
Older age	↑	No	–
Family history of Alzheimer's	↑	No	–
Head injury history	↑	Yes/head protection in sports	B
Hypertension	↑	Yes/treat to ≤140/90	A
Other cardiovascular risk factors	↑	Yes/risk factor reduction	C
Apolipoprotein E4 allele	↑	No	–
Physical activity	↓	Yes/aerobic and strength training	B
Mediterranean diet	↓	Yes/diet modification	B
Diabetes	↑	Yes/treatment to reduce HbA1c	C
Moderate alcohol use	↓	Yes/encourage limited use	C
Heavy alcohol use	↑	Yes/successful alcoholism treatment	C
Cognitive and social activity	↓	Yes/brain health activities	B

*A = consistent, good-quality patient-oriented evidence; B = inconsistent or limited-quality patient-oriented evidence; C = consensus, disease-oriented evidence, usual practice, expert opinion. For information about the SORT evidence rating system, see http://www.aafp.org/afpsort.xml.

ruling out delirium and the other dementias (see next section). Over time, these criteria may change: In 2011 the Alzheimer's Association and the National Institute on Aging defined AD to include a preclinical stage and mild cognitive impairment (MCI); however, at present, these definitions are for research purposes only.

The cardinal feature of AD is short-term memory loss or difficulty learning new information, which is often accompanied by a lack of awareness or concern of the memory problem. Word-finding difficulties, loss of time orientation, getting lost or misplacing things, and impaired judgment and planning are other common features. On average, the person with AD lives 6 to 10 years after the diagnosis and progresses through several stages. Over time, progressive cognitive disturbances become more pervasive, leading to impairment in instrumental activities of daily living (IADLs) and later even basic activities of daily living (ADLs). Ultimately, if the person does not die from some other cause, they will progress to being unable to express themself verbally and will be relatively immobile, with contractures, swallowing problems, cachexia, weight loss, and eventually death.

Differential Diagnosis
The most important considerations in the differential diagnosis of AD are the following:
- Vascular dementia (VaD). There are two general types: (a) cortical—resulting from multiple infarcts in the cerebral cortex, and (b) subcortical—resulting from small-vessel disease with multiple lacunar infarcts. Presentation is highly variable; however, memory deficits are typically less prominent than in AD.
- Frontotemporal dementia (FTD). This diagnosis is relatively uncommon but accounts for about half of all cases before age 65. The clinical presentation is highly variable, depending on the lateral distribution of pathological changes. Language disturbances involving expression or comprehension, or prominent changes in behavior and personality (e.g., apathy, disinhibition, repetitive motor behaviors, loss of empathy) are the two main clinical subtypes (left and right side predominant, respectively). Clinical diagnosis can be aided by MRI brain imaging showing severe focal atrophy in the frontal and/or temporal lobes.
- Lewy body dementia (LBD) and Parkinson's disease dementia (PDD). Characteristics include parkinsonian motor signs (bradykinesia, rigidity, and tremor), prominent visual hallucinations, and sleep-wake disturbances (e.g., fluctuating arousal, daytime somnolence, acting out dreams). LBD is used to describe the syndrome when cognitive symptoms predominate; PDD refers to late-occurring dementia in a patient with Parkinson's disease.
- Rare but distinctive forms of dementia. These include progressive supranuclear palsy, normal pressure hydrocephalus, Creutzfeldt-Jakob disease, postanoxic dementia, posttraumatic brain injury, chronic subdural hematoma(s), and Huntington's disease.
- MCI. This is a condition in which the person is able to carry out his or her normal activities but has deficits in certain areas of higher function such as short-term memory, judgment, and planning. There are two kinds of MCI, amnestic, which is characterized by isolated short-term memory loss, and nonamnestic, in which one or more other cognitive domains are affected. Amnestic MCI is particularly likely to progress to AD and in such cases reflects a prodromal stage of the disease.
- Delirium. In contrast to the dementias, delirium tends to be subacute or acute in onset and to be completely or partially reversible. Key characteristics include fluctuating consciousness, confusion, and hallucinations or delusions. The cause is usually identifiable and is most often because of medication, stress (such as infection or surgery), or a metabolic disturbance. Delirium often coexists with dementia as one of its biggest risk factors is cognitive impairment.
- Depression. Decades ago, depression was at times mistaken for dementia and termed "pseudodementia," because people with depression often say "I don't know" in response to cognitive status questions. Improved interviewing techniques and routine use of depression screening tests as part of dementia evaluations have largely eliminated this confusion. However, depression remains an important consideration in the dementia evaluation because it frequently coexists with dementia, particularly in early stages of the illness.

Screening for Cognitive Impairment
Whether to screen for AD is highly controversial. Advantages of early diagnosis include offering earlier treatment and research participation, allowing the person an opportunity to make life-planning decisions at a point where his or her residual cognitive

function is at its best, helping family understand what is happening and learn how best to provide support, providing guidance to patient and family about managing finances wisely and avoiding scams, and providing time for decision making about such things as durable power of attorney and advance-care planning. Medicare currently requires cognitive screening as part of the welcome-to-Medicare visit; in addition, we recommend screening anyone age 75 and older and anyone for whom a memory lapse or vagueness noted in an interview or an error in judgment (e.g., causing an auto accident) raises suspicion of cognitive impairment.

Primary care physicians can conduct expedient, reliable screening for dementia by simultaneously administering the Mini-Cog and the AD8. Both can be administered by a nurse or medical assistant, and each takes less than 3 minutes.

- The *Mini-Cog* is administered directly to the person being screened. It consists of asking the person to remember three items; to draw a clock face, putting in the numbers and placing the hands at "10 after 11"; and then to recall the three items. A positive screen occurs if the person cannot recall any of the items (regardless of the clock drawing), or if they recall one to two items and the clock is drawn incorrectly.
- The *AD8* requires the person being screened to be accompanied by a spouse, child, or other person who knows him or her well. It inquires about whether the person has had a change over the past several years in eight areas: judgment, interest in hobbies/activities, repeating things, learning, orientation, financial management, remembering appointments, and other memory. A change in two or more items is a positive screen.

Downloadable, printable copies of both instruments with instructions are available at http://www.ncalzheimers.org/.

Diagnostic Evaluation

There are five general steps in a diagnostic evaluation for AD: (1) history; (2) cognitive assessment; (3) physical examination, with a focus on the neurologic evaluation; (4) laboratory testing; and (5) establishment of a working diagnosis (including consideration of and attempts to rule out other depression, delirium, and non-Alzheimer's dementias). Each of these is discussed below.

History

Patients suspected of having AD typically present either because a family member reports changes in their behavior and function, or because of a positive screening evaluation. Judgment and decision making can be impaired early in the disease, which may lead to an incident that draws attention to the problem. Examples include auto accidents, an uncharacteristic purchase, problems managing a household budget, or being victimized by a scam. With increasing publicity and openness regarding the disease, however, we are beginning to see more persons present with memory concerns, some of whom go on to have MCI or AD.

The person with the illness rarely gives a reliable history, so the primary source of historical information about functional change needs to be a family member close to the individual. Such a history typically includes gradual decrease in function in multiple domains including memory, plus unusual behaviors such as repeating oneself, getting lost while driving, having trouble managing a checkbook, saying things that the person normally wouldn't have said, and difficulty making decisions.

An important element of the history should be questions aimed at identifying other potential causes of cognitive impairment, such as alcoholism, illicit drug use, and prescription medications.

In addition, inquiry as to the person's psychiatric history should be undertaken as well as screening for anxiety and depression. A formal screening tool, such as the Geriatric Depression Scale or the Patient Health Questionnaire nine-item depression screen (PHQ-9) is recommended.

Cognitive Status Examination

The cognitive status examination should include a standardized cognitive status battery, both for comparison with other patients and to provide a numerical result that can be followed over time. We recommend either the St. Louis University Mental Status Examination (SLUMS) or the Montreal Cognitive Assessment examination (MOCA), both of which cover a wide range of cognitive domains, detect cognitive impairment earlier than older tests (such as the Mini-Mental State Examination), have been validated in many populations, and are freely available in the public domain (i.e., available for download from the Internet).

The standardized examination should be supplemented by several other components to help round out the evaluation, identify behavioral issues, and screen for non-Alzheimer's dementias. Supplementary examination components that are useful include

- Verbal fluency testing—naming as many objects, such as animals, as they can in 1 minute (category fluency) and as many words beginning with a single letter such as "F" as they can in 1 minute (letter fluency). These not only tap into early loss cognitive areas but also help differentiate between AD (where category fluency tends to be more impaired) and other dementias where impairment is similar (e.g., VaD) or letter fluency tends to be more impaired (e.g., FTD and LBD).
- Trails B test—this is a timed paper-and-pencil test; it is a particularly sensitive test for early cognitive changes in nonmemory domains (visuospatial and executive).
- Psychological and behavioral symptom evaluation—this is best obtained from a family member using a questionnaire tool such as the Neuropsychiatric Inventory (NPI).

Physical Examination

The physical examination should focus on neurologic function, looking for signs that suggest a diagnosis other than AD. In particular, the examination should look for asymmetry in strength and/or motor function (suggesting one or more prior strokes), tremor and bradykinesia (suggesting parkinsonism or LBD), abnormalities of eye movement—especially inability to gaze downward (suggesting primary supranuclear palsy), peripheral neuropathy (suggesting the possibility of vitamin B12 deficiency, hypothyroidism, alcoholism, or neurosyphilis [although diabetes is more often the cause]). In addition, a screening examination for cardiovascular and pulmonary function should be conducted.

Laboratory Testing and Neuroimaging

If the cognitive status examination confirms dysfunction, then a laboratory battery should be conducted largely to help identify remediable causes of cognitive impairment. Basic testing should include a complete blood count, blood glucose, electrolytes, renal function (BUN/creatinine), thyroid function, liver function tests, vitamin B12 level, and, if appropriate, a serologic test for syphilis.

Although research advances in brain imaging offer promise for more early and definitive diagnosis, a routine brain MRI remains the standard of practice. It can identify cerebrovascular disease as discrete old infarcts (usually cortical) or as greater-than-normal deep white-matter changes (leukoariosis; suggests subcortical vascular disease). The MRI is also useful in ruling out tumor or normal pressure hydrocephalus and in identifying focal cortical atrophy consistent with FTD.

Recently, positive emission tomography (PET) scanning for brain amyloid (florbetapir F 18 or Amyvid) has become commercially available, but is currently reimbursed by Medicare only if done as part of a research protocol. It is anticipated that amyloid PET imaging will have an emerging use in helping identify which persons with MCI have early AD. At present, however, the only clinical indication for routine metabolic brain PET reimbursed by Medicare is to distinguish FTD from AD.

TABLE 2   Differential Diagnosis of Alzheimer's Disease

DIAGNOSIS	TYPICAL PRESENTING HISTORY	KEY EXAMINATION FINDINGS	BRAIN IMAGING/LAB FINDINGS
Alzheimer's disease (AD)	Progressive, gradual onset; behavioral symptoms variable		
Mild	Short-term memory loss; IADL and judgment problems	Essentially normal	Normal CT or medial temporal atrophy; +amyloid brain PET scan
Moderate	ADL impairment; prominent memory deficits and confusion	May have frontal release signs	Medial temporal and parietal lobe atrophy; +amyloid PET scan
Mild cognitive impairment (MCI)	Impaired short-term memory without functional impairment	Isolated short-term memory loss and/or other minor cognitive deficits	Variable medial temporal atrophy (nonspecific)
Vascular dementia (VaD)	Stepwise progression; stroke history and/or vascular risk factors; gait problems early	Abnormal neurologic examination with lateralizing findings (may be subtle)	MRI shows cortical and/or subcortical infarcts, leukoariosis
Frontotemporal dementia (FTD)	Behavioral, personality, language changes; apathy	Variable, gait apraxia, frontal release signs	Marked atrophy in frontal and/or temporal lobes
Lewy body dementia (LBD)	Fluctuating attention, visual hallucinations, gait/motor/sleep disturbance (act out dreams)	Limb rigidity, bradykinesia, may see intention tremor and gait disturbance	MRI nondiagnostic
Parkinson's dementia	History of Parkinson's disease, later-onset cognitive dysfunction	Limb rigidity, bradykinesia, resting tremor, gait disturbance	MRI nondiagnostic
Delirium	Acute onset; identifiable pharmacologic, metabolic, toxic, or infectious cause	Fluctuating attention, fidgety, agitated, tremulous, or apathetic; may be obtunded	Diffuse EEG slowing, evidence of drug or metabolic toxicity, infection

Establishment of a Working Diagnosis

Because no gold-standard clinical test exists for diagnosing AD, the evaluation usually results in a working diagnosis. If the evaluation raises suspicions that a non-AD dementia may be involved (Table 2), then consultation with a specialist in neurology or geriatric medicine is advised. General principles of management apply to all dementias; however, different dementias respond differently to certain medications discussed later in this chapter, and so consultation may help direct appropriate therapeutic interventions in addition to clarifying diagnosis

Treatment

In managing AD, the physician needs to treat at least two individuals: the person with the disease and the person (or persons) who serve as the primary caregiver. A common thread in this dualistic approach is to promote safety and quality of life for all involved. While cognitive function is the key to diagnosis, behavioral symptoms are often the most important to address in management. Table 3 reviews the main therapeutic targets and interventions.

Counseling and Caregiver Support

The patient and caregiver should be counseled about the disease course, about increased safety risks from such things as operating machinery and driving a motor vehicle, about the desirability of establishing a durable power of attorney for health care decisions, and about the value of having conversations early on about desires for end-of-life care, including completion of advance directives. As the disease progresses, regular meetings with the patient and family are important, so as to anticipate and address key decision points.

AD leads to progressive dependency; maintaining the health and well-being of the caregiver(s) is a critical component of care. Make sure the caregiver has a physician and is under treatment for any medical problems he or she may have. In addition, the caregiver should be advised about community resources that can provide assistance, such as the local chapter of the Alzheimer's Association, programs for persons with early-stage dementia, support programs for caregivers, local adult day care centers, and respite programs. In addition, because the majority of persons with AD spend their final days in a nursing home or assisted living community, health care providers should be prepared to provide support for that decision when appropriate.

Management of Cognitive Symptoms

The lack of novel therapeutic approaches during the past 10 years, in spite of very active research, has been a major disappointment. The cholinesterase inhibitors and memantine (Namenda) remain mainstays of treatment. Key points in using these drugs include the following (see Table 4):

• There is no demonstrated value to withholding drugs for later, when the patient gets worse.

• The overall benefit of treatment may be difficult to assess clinically; "real-world" changes noted by caregivers may be more important than cognitive test scores.

• Side effects are largely gastrointestinal (pain, bloating, nausea). Treatment should involve reducing the dose or switching to another agent. Donepezil (Aricept), while generally given at bedtime, may cause leg cramps, insomnia, or vivid bizarre dreams that often abate by switching to morning dosing.

• Studies indicate that combining a cholinesterase inhibitor with memantine produces a modest additive benefit.

• Long-term treatment effects involve symptom reduction and are not cumulative; if the efficacy of one or more drug treatments is in question, it is reasonable to pursue a sequential trial taper and withdrawal (resuming the previous dose or medication if acute decline is noted by informants).

• Ensuring adequate sleep, activity, and nutrition is important for optimizing the patient's functional abilities.

| TABLE 3 | Alzheimer's Disease Management Strategies |

OUTCOME TO BE AFFECTED	INTERVENTION	COMMENTS	LEVEL OF EVIDENCE*
Cognitive symptoms (memory, judgment, etc.)	Cholinesterase inhibitors (donepezil [Aricept], rivastigmine [Exelon], galantamine [Razadyne], memantine [Namenda])	Effective for mild, moderate, and severe dementia. Effect equal to slowing decline by 6 months	A
	Medical food; Caprylidene (Axona)	Modest benefits in apo E4 negative subjects only	B/C
	Cognitive training	Improved ability specific to the abilities trained	B
	Physical activity and adequate rest	Improved alertness and physical function; reduced depression	B
Behavioral symptoms (agitation, resistance to care, physical violence)	Individualized, person-centered ADL care	Reduced agitation; improved quality of life	A
	Cognitive enhancers (e.g., donepezil, memantine)	Effects modest but fewer adverse effects than other medications	A
	Antipsychotic drugs	Only a minority of patients clearly benefit; high adverse effect profile; "black box" warning on atypical antipsychotics for increasing cardiovascular disease but typical antipsychotics also have adverse effects	A
	Anticonvulsants	Carbamazepine (Tegretol)[1] reduces agitation, anxiety, and restlessness; ataxia and hematologic toxicity occur	B
Caregiver stress, burden, and depression	Education, group programs, respite services	Early disease—education and group activities for caregiver and person with dementia; respite Moderate/advanced disease—caregiver support group; respite	A
Depression in persons with dementia	Selective seratonin reuptake inhibitors (SSRIs) (sertraline [Zoloft], citralopram [Celexa])	Mild to moderate effects on mood; no effect on agitation, aggression	A
	Physical activity/exercise	Formal program of caregiver education and exercise for the person with dementia; improved depression	B
Quality of life; well being	Pleasant sensory stimulation		A

*A = consistent, good-quality patient-oriented evidence; B = inconsistent or limited-quality patient-oriented evidence; C = consensus, disease-oriented evidence, usual practice, expert opinion. For information about the SORT evidence rating system, see http://www.aafp.org/afpsort.xml.
[1]Not FDA approved for this indication.

653

| TABLE 4 | Drug Therapy for Cognitive Symptoms in Alzheimer's Disease |

	DONEPEZIL (ARICEPT™)	RIVASTIGMINE (EXELON™ TRANSDERMAL PATCH)	GALANTAMINE (RAZADYNE™)	MEMANTINE (NAMENDA™)
Mechanism	Cholinesterase-inhibitor	Cholinesterase-inhibitor	Cholinesterase-inhibitor	NMDA antagonist
Doses	5, 10, 23 mg	4.6, 9.5, 13.3 mg	4, 8, 12 mg 8*, 16*, 24 mg*	5, 10 mg 7*, 14*, 21*, 28 mg*
Target dose	5–10 mg/d	4.6–13.3 mg/d	16–24 mg/d	10–20 mg/d 28 mg/d*
Half-life	70 h	>24 h	6–8 h	60–80 h
Dosing	qd	qd[†]	bid/qd*	bid/qd
Metabolism	Hepatic	Nonhepatic	Hepatic	Nonhepatic
Protein-binding	96%	40%	19%	45%
Most common adverse effects	Nausea (13%) Diarrhea (10%) Insomnia (8%)	Nausea (12%) Vomiting (10%) Diarrhea (6%)	Nausea (12%) Vomiting (9%) Anorexia (6%)	Headaches (3%) Dizziness (2%) Constipation (2%)

*Extended release formulations qd.
[†]Transdermal patch (oral dosing with high incidence of GI side effects not listed).

Management of Behavioral Symptoms

A wide variety of behavioral symptoms can develop. Among the more common are (a) early in the disease—repetitive questions, wandering, and refusing assistance; (b) in the mid-stage of the disease—resistance to care, agitation or pacing, verbal and physical agitation and aggression, and antisocial behaviors such as inappropriate sexual remarks; (c) late in the disease—resistance to care, and screaming.

The key to managing most behavioral symptoms rests on nonpharmacologic approaches involving good dementia communication skills. Key elements include making eye contact before speaking; using simple language; speaking slowly, clearly, and in a low-pitched voice; communicating caring through such actions as smiling and giving a hug; asking only one question at a time and allowing the patient adequate time to respond; breaking instructions into small steps and presenting one at a time; and backing off and trying later if the person becomes agitated or refuses. If the person doesn't seem to understand a statement, repeat the statement using the same wording; if this does not work, rephrase and allow time for processing. When a specific problem develops, such as resistance to care or unwanted exiting, caregivers should use a structured problem-solving approach that defines the symptom, tries to identify reasons (including emotions and delusions) behind the symptom, and develops a management strategy to try and evaluate, using a quality improvement approach.

At times, however, families or facility caregivers report aggressive, frightening, or socially unacceptable behaviors that do not remit even in spite of excellent psychosocial, personalized care. In these situations, medical providers are often asked for a prescription. Sometimes all that is needed is time, as aberrant behaviors tend to moderate over time. If a medication is needed, the first step should be a cholinesterase inhibitor, which has been shown to have potential benefits on apathy, delusions, and purposeless motor behaviors. If that is unsuccessful, then an antipsychotic or anticonvulsant should be considered, starting at a low dose and increasing until improvement is seen or intolerable side effects occur. Patients who demonstrate, or later develop, prominent behavioral features (e.g., visual hallucinations, disinhibition) should be referred to an appropriate specialist in neurology, geriatrics, or psychiatry.

Monitoring

Patients and caregivers should be reevaluated every 3 to 6 months. If the person with AD resists going to the doctor (a common feature early in the disease), then some of these check-in evaluations can be handled by telephone. Indeed, telephone consultation is highly valued by caregivers, for whom a trip to the doctor can be costly and disruptive. To help provide readily available consultation, primary care practices are encouraged to designate a nurse, nurse practitioner, or physician assistant to focus on dementia treatment and care. This focus would include coordinating dementia screening in the practice, knowing each of the patients and families with dementia, coordinating a support group (if the practice chooses to have one), and responding to questions from caregivers. Local caregiver support groups and websites such as www.alzheimers.gov and Alzheimer Disease Education and Referral (ADEAR) can provide useful information about research opportunities and broader aspects of dementia care.

References

Jack Jr CR, Albert MS, Knopman DS, et al. Introduction to the recommendations from the National Institute on Aging—Alzheimer's Association workgroups on diagnostic guidelines for Alzheimer's disease. Alzheimers Dement 2011;7:257–62.

Galvin JE, Sadowski CH. Practical guidelines for the recognition and diagnosis of dementia. J Am Board Fam Med 2012;25:367–82.

Odenheimer G, Borson S, Sanders AE, et al. Quality improvement in neurology: Dementia management quality measures. Neurology 2013;81:1545–9.

BRAIN TUMORS

Method of
Ryan Merrell, MD

CURRENT DIAGNOSIS

- Subacute to chronic onset of generalized and/or focal neurologic symptoms should alert the physician to order neuroimaging to investigate the possibility of a brain tumor.
- Magnetic resonance imaging (MRI) is preferable to computed tomography (CT) for imaging tumors.
- A biopsy or resection is necessary to diagnose a primary brain tumor or a metastatic tumor of unknown primary origin. The diagnostic yield is increased with a resection.
- Neuroimaging suggestive of meningioma does not require a tissue diagnosis and in many cases can be followed closely with serial neuroimaging.
- If a primary CNS lymphoma is suspected, corticosteroids should not be given unless absolutely necessary in order not to confound the biopsy diagnosis.

CURRENT THERAPY

- Surgical resection is preferred for patients with most types of brain tumors as long as the resection does not leave the patient with permanent neurologic deficits.
- Whole-brain radiotherapy and stereotactic radiosurgery are the primary treatment modalities for patients with metastatic brain tumors.
- Surgical resection is preferred for patients with large or symptomatic meningiomas that are surgical accessible and in patients who can tolerate surgery.
- Patients with gliomas are treated with fractionated radiotherapy or chemotherapy alone or in combination.
- Patients with primary CNS lymphoma are treated with high-dose methotrexate alone or in combination with other chemotherapy drugs.

Brain tumors are categorized as metastatic or primary. The incidence and prevalence of metastatic tumors outweigh those of primary tumors up to 10:1. Lung and breast carcinoma make up the majority of metastatic tumors, largely because of their increased prevalence in the population compared to other tumors. Melanoma is a less prevalent malignancy but has a high propensity to metastasize to the brain. Meningioma is usually a benign tumor that is found most often in the fourth through sixth decade, with a female-to-male ratio of 2:1. Gliomas are primary brain tumors that are categorized as high-grade gliomas or low-grade gliomas. High-grade gliomas usually affect patients in the fifth and sixth decades and older, whereas low-grade gliomas usually affect patients in the third and fourth decades. Primary central nervous system (CNS) lymphoma is a rare tumor that usually affects patients in the sixth decade and older.

There are very few identifiable risk factors for brain tumors. The histology of the primary neoplasm confers the risk of brain metastases because lung cancer, breast cancer, and melanoma are more likely to metastasize to the brain, whereas colorectal, ovarian, and prostate cancers are less likely to metastasize to the brain. Past exposure to ionizing radiation and a family history of a genetic cancer syndrome are the only known risk factors for primary tumors. Despite much press, cell phone use has not been irrefutably shown to be a risk factor for brain tumors. Immunocompromise such as HIV infection is a well-known risk factor for primary CNS lymphoma.

Brain tumors manifest with the subacute or chronic onset of generalized symptoms such as confusion, headaches, seizures, and nausea or focal symptoms and signs such as visual field deficit, loss of language, unilateral weakness, sensory neglect, or difficulty walking. There are no symptoms or signs specific to any brain tumor because the anatomic location of the tumor in the brain dictates the presentation. These symptoms and signs should prompt neuroimaging with MRI. MRI has largely replaced CT for evaluating brain tumors, although CT serves as a quick screening modality and must be used in patients who have contraindications to MRI. Radiographic features on MRI can predict the type of tumor but cannot accurately confirm the pathology. A tissue diagnosis through a biopsy or surgical resection is necessary to confirm the pathology, except in patients with metastatic tumors with a known primary tumor. The differential diagnosis of mass lesions in the brain includes abscess, demyelinating lesion, inflammatory disease, and other infections such as toxoplasmosis and cysticercosis.

A biopsy or surgical resection provides the definitive diagnosis of the tumor. For most tumors, a resection is preferred when safely possible, because the greater amount of tissue obtained avoids the sampling error that can occur with a biopsy. The goal of surgery for all brain tumors is to provide a maximal resection while leaving the patient free of permanent neurologic deficits. Metastatic brain tumors are classified according to the cell of origin. Primary brain tumors are classified according to the World Health Organization (WHO) classification system. Additional molecular classification that can provide prognostic and therapeutic information is often obtained on select primary brain tumors. Oligodendroglioma is a primary brain tumor that has well-characterized chromosomal deletions on the short arm of chromosome 1 and the long arm of chromosome 19 (1p/19q co-deletion) that have been shown to predict improved survival and increased sensitivity to treatment. Similarly, O-6-methylguanine-DNA-methyltransferase (MGMT) promoter methylation is a marker that predicts improved survival and may predict improved response to treatment in high-grade glioma.

A major challenge to treating brain tumor is to find drugs that cross the blood–brain barrier. Many chemotherapy drugs used to treat systemic tumors are too large or hydrophilic to cross the blood–brain barrier. Treatments designed to circumvent the blood–brain barrier have only been modestly successful to date.

Metastatic Tumors

Metastatic brain tumors are the most common brain tumors, with as many as 170,000 new cases diagnosed in the United States each year. Metastatic tumors can occur with or without evidence of a primary neoplasm. Findings on brain MRI suspicious for a metastatic tumor should prompt an investigation for a primary malignancy with body imaging (Figure 1). The discovery of a systemic mass that can be biopsied might avoid a brain biopsy or resection in select patients. Occasionally, after an extensive evaluation, no evidence of a primary tumor is found. About 50% of patients have a single metastasis, and the rest have multiple tumors. In general, prognosis is poor, but some patients with less-aggressive primary tumors (breast, non–small cell lung carcinoma) can achieve long-term survival.

Tumors can metastasize to the nervous system through infiltration of the cerebrospinal fluid (CSF), a process termed *leptomeningeal carcinomatosis* or *carcinomatous meningitis*. Symptoms suggesting leptomeningeal carcinomatosis include altered mental status, headaches, loss of vision, double vision, slurred speech, difficulty swallowing, and lower extremity pain and weakness. Brain MRI can show enhancement of the meninges, and CSF from lumbar puncture shows low glucose and elevated protein with malignant cells. A lumbar puncture is not necessary to confirm the diagnosis in a patient with a known primary malignancy and characteristic clinical presentation and MRI findings. The prognosis is poor, on the order of several months. Patients with lymphoma and breast cancer might realize longer survival.

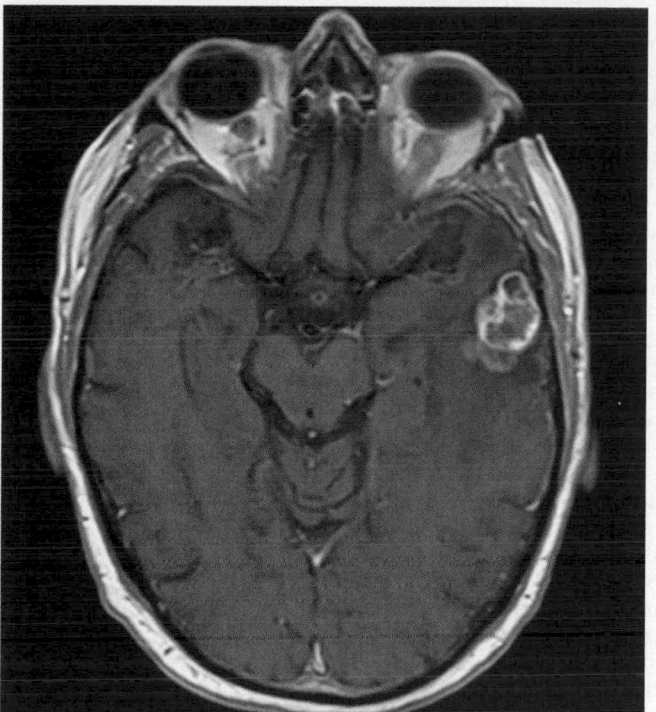

Figure 1. Contrast-enhanced magnetic resonance image shows a homogeneously enhancing mass with surrounding edema at the gray–white junction, suggesting a metastatic tumor.

Several factors determine the approach to treatment of metastatic tumors. The age, comorbidities, functional status, degree of neurologic impairment, and extent of the systemic disease determine whether surgery is indicated. Solitary metastases and large symptomatic tumors in patients with multiple tumors are generally resected in patients who are good surgical candidates. Whether a patient undergoes surgical resection or not, radiotherapy is the mainstay of treatment for metastatic tumors.

The two approaches to radiotherapy are whole-brain radiotherapy and stereotactic radiosurgery. In whole-brain radiotherapy, a dose of radiation is fractionated into several treatment sessions and given to the entire brain. In stereotactic radiosurgery, a high dose of radiation is given only to areas of brain involved with tumor and often in one treatment session. The effectiveness of whole-brain radiotherapy versus stereotactic radiosurgery has not been established in large randomized trials. Whole-brain radiotherapy is more suited for patients with multiple metastases or large tumors (more than 3 cm diameter). Stereotactic radiosurgery is indicated for patients with fewer than four metastases, for smaller-volume tumors (less than 3 cm diameter), and for radioresistant tumors such as melanoma. Whole-brain radiotherapy has the advantage of treating the visible and undetectable tumors, but it carries a risk of delayed neurotoxicity that often manifests as cognitive impairment. Stereotactic radiosurgery has the advantage of local control by treating the visible tumors and carries less risk of delayed neurotoxicity. Stereotactic radiosurgery can be repeated if new tumors develop in areas of brain not previously radiated. The disadvantage of stereotactic radiosurgery is the potential for new tumors to develop in areas of brain not treated.

There is no specific role for chemotherapy for metastatic solid tumors, although some chemotherapy drugs used to treat systemic disease can cross the blood–brain barrier.

Treatment of leptomeningeal carcinomatosis involves chemotherapy or radiotherapy. Chemotherapy is often administered directly into the spinal fluid (intrathecal), usually through a ventricular (Omaya) reservoir. Alternatively, chemotherapy can be given systemically. Common chemotherapeutic agents include methotrexate (Methotrexate PF), cytarabine (Cytarabine PF), and thiotepa.[1] Radiotherapy is usually only used as a salvage treatment after chemotherapy failure.

Meningiomas

Meningiomas are the most common primary brain tumor, accounting for more than 32% of all tumors. Meningiomas arise from the arachnoid cap cells. They are often discovered incidentally when a patient undergoes neuroimaging for symptoms that are unrelated to the meningioma. The radiographic appearance of meningiomas is one of the most specific of all brain tumors and allows a confident diagnosis without the need for a confirmatory biopsy (Figure 2). The most common radiographic mimicker is a metastatic tumor to the meninges, but usually a patient in this circumstance has a known history of malignancy. Small meningiomas may be followed with serial imaging. Meningiomas that correlate with neurologic deficits or tumors that have grown significantly over time should be treated.

Surgical resection is the preferred treatment if it can be safely accomplished, but it should be avoided in the elderly. Meningiomas are graded WHO I to III; 90% are grade I (benign), and grade III (anaplastic) are the most aggressive and likely to recur. Complete resection is curative in most cases, but some meningiomas recur. If recurrent tumors are large or symptomatic, surgery is the preferred treatment if possible. Radiotherapy, either fractionated or stereotactic radiosurgery, can be used postoperatively to treat residual tumor or to treat tumors that cannot be resected. Meningiomas have an intermediate response to radiotherapy, and grade III tumors often show minimal response.

There is no defined chemotherapy for meningiomas, although several drugs are being actively investigated.

Gliomas

Gliomas consist of astrocytomas, oligodendrogliomas, and ependymomas, in decreasing order of prevalence. It was once thought that these tumors derived from mutations of normal glial cells, but

---

[1]Not FDA approved for this indication.

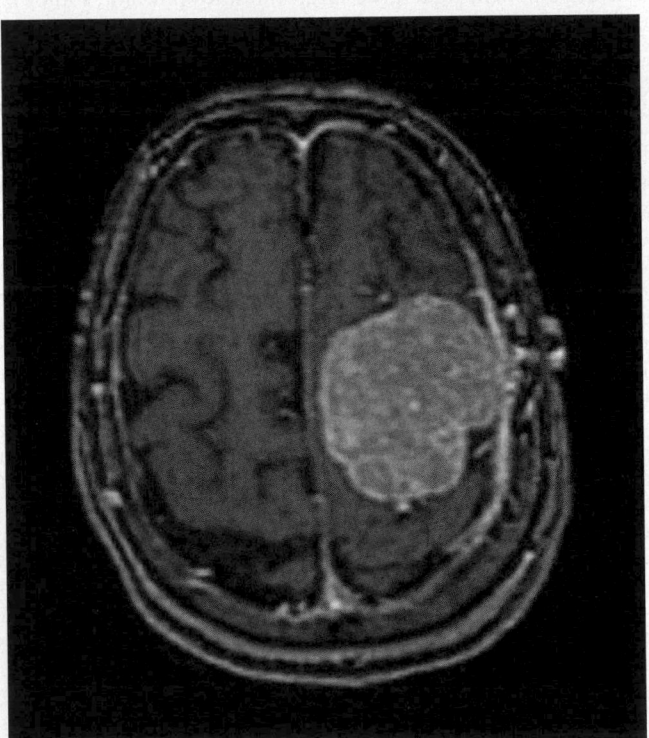

Figure 2. Contrast-enhanced magnetic resonance image shows a homogeneously enhancing mass arising from the dura, with the typical appearance of a meningioma.

TABLE 1 World Health Organization Classification of Common Gliomas in Adults

SUBTYPE	WORLD HEALTH ORGANIZATION GRADE
Low-Grade Gliomas	
Astrocytoma	II
Oligodendroglioma	II
Oligoastrocytoma	II
High-Grade Gliomas	
Anaplastic astrocytoma	III
Anaplastic oligodendroglioma	III
Anaplastic oligoastrocytoma	III
Anaplastic ependymoma	III
Glioblastoma	IV

it is increasingly recognized that gliomas derive from brain tumor progenitor cells. Glioblastoma is the most malignant glioma and accounts for 60% to 70% of all gliomas. Gliomas are classified by the glial cells from which they originate and the histologic features that give them a grade according to the WHO classification (Table 1). Grade III and IV tumors are high-grade gliomas, and grade II tumors are low-grade gliomas. Grade I glioma (pilocytic astrocytoma) is rarely seen in adults. A maximal surgical resection that leaves the patient with minimal neurologic deficits is the preferred initial treatment for all grades of gliomas.

High-Grade Gliomas

Most high-grade gliomas are glioblastoma or anaplastic astrocytoma (WHO grade III); anaplastic oligodendroglioma and anaplastic ependymoma are less common. The brain MRI often shows a ring-enhancing mass centered in the white matter surrounded by edema and causing mass effect (Figure 3). A maximal surgical resection that leaves the patient without permanent neurologic deficits is the goal in high-grade glioma. A maximal resection, younger age, and good performance status are favorable prognostic factors. Methylation of the MGMT promoter correlates with improved survival. High-grade gliomas are aggressive, incurable tumors; the median survival for glioblastoma is 14 to 18 months and for anaplastic astrocytoma is 2 to 2.5 years.

Treatment of high-grade glioma is based on the histology of the tumor. Glioblastoma is the only high-grade glioma with a standard treatment, but anaplastic astrocytoma are often treated like glioblastoma. The standard treatment consists of fractionated radiotherapy given over 6 weeks with temozolomide (Temodar), an oral chemotherapeutic drug. Temozolomide is given 1 month after the completion of radiotherapy until tumor progression, which occurs on average around 7 months after the original diagnosis for glioblastoma (Table 2). Patients with glioblastoma and anaplastic astrocytoma are usually treated with 6 to 12 months of temozolomide or until tumor recurrence. Careful consideration should be given to neuroimaging findings suggesting tumor progression within the first 6 months after radiotherapy because these changes can reflect radiation necrosis (pseudoprogression) rather than true tumor progression.

In the setting of tumor progression, salvage chemotherapy is the mainstay of treatment. Bevacizumab (Avastin), a drug that inhibits blood vessel formation around tumors, is the most common drug that is given at tumor recurrence. Bevacizumab is sometimes combined with other drugs such as irinotecan (CPT-11 [Camptosar]).[1] Temozolomide given in low dose daily is another standard approach for recurrent high-grade glioma. Experimental chemotherapy through a clinical trial is a common option used in

---

[1]Not FDA approved for this indication.

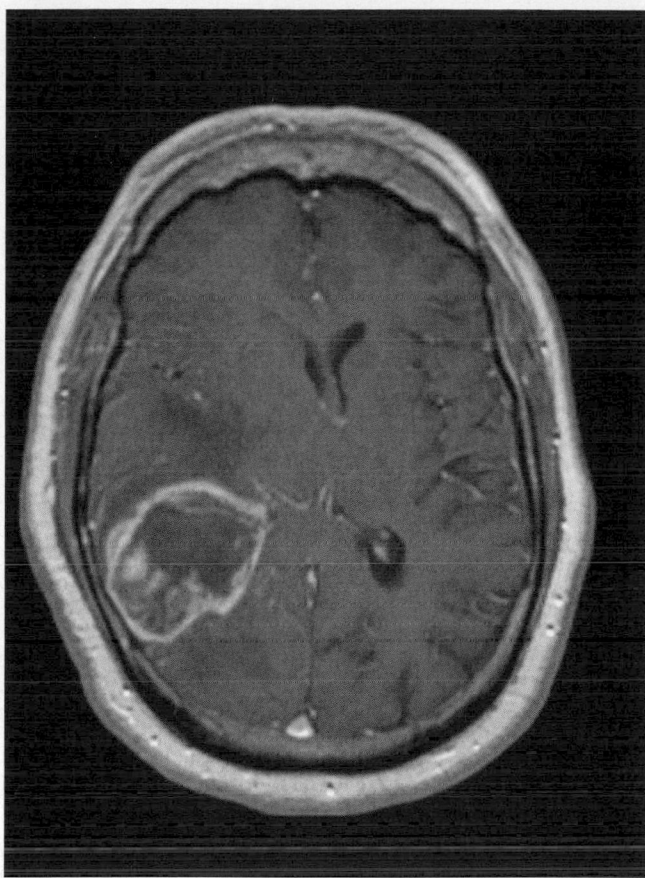

Figure 3. Contrast-enhanced magnetic resonance image shows a ring-enhancing mass with surrounding edema with the typical appearance of glioblastoma.

TABLE 2	Common Chemotherapy for Gliomas	
GENERIC NAME	**TRADE NAME**	**DOSE**
Temozolomide	Temodar	75 mg/m² daily during radiotherapy, 150–200 mg/m² after radiotherapy on 5 d per 28 d schedule 50 mg/m² daily or 75 mg/m² 3 wk on, 1 wk off, for recurrent high grade glioma
Bevacizumab	Avastin	10 mg/kg every 2 wk

recurrent high-grade glioma. Occasionally, surgical resection is indicated to improve symptoms, but it has not been shown to improve survival. Likewise, focused radiation such as stereotactic radiosurgery has not been shown to affect survival.

Anaplastic oligodendroglioma treated with radiation followed by chemotherapy, either PCV (procarbazine [Matulane[1]], CCNU [Lomustine], vincristine[1]) or temozolomide while anaplastic ependymoma is usually treated with radiotherapy alone.

Low-Grade Gliomas

Despite being lower-grade tumors, low-grade gliomas are not benign. The natural history is that patients with low-grade gliomas ultimately progress to high-grade glioma. Low-grade gliomas

---

[1]Not FDA approved for this indication.

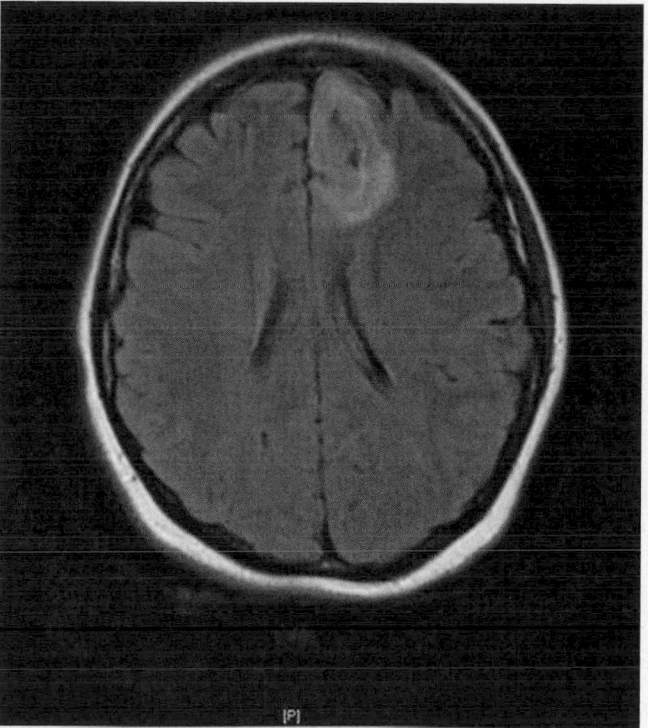

Figure 4. Fluid-attenuated inversion recovery (FLAIR) magnetic resonance image shows a nonenhancing tumor abutting the cerebral cortex with the typical appearance of a low-grade glioma. The tumor proved to be a grade II oligodendroglioma.

account for about 15% of all primary brain tumors. Low-grade gliomas are more likely to manifest with seizures than high-grade gliomas. The brain MRI often shows a nonenhancing mass with involvement of white matter and sometimes abutting the cerebral cortex (Figure 4). Prognosis varies considerably by tumor histology: Patients with astrocytoma live 5 to 10 years after diagnosis, whereas patients with oligodendroglioma live 10 to 15 years after diagnosis.

There is no accepted standard treatment for low-grade gliomas. Tumor histology and individual patient characteristics guide treatment decisions. Tumors with oligodendroglial features are more sensitive to chemotherapy than their astrocytic counterparts, especially those with chromosomal 1p/19q co-deletions. The results of a recent randomized clinical trial revealed superior progression free survival and overall survival in patients with low grade gliomas treated with radiation followed by adjuvant PCV.

In the absence of a head to head clinical trial of PCV with temozolomide, many clinicians would use temozolomide in place of PCV since temozolomide is better tolerated. It still common practice to take a watch and wait approach in select patients with newly diagnosed low grade glioma who have had a gross total resection. When patients with low-grade gliomas have findings on neuroimaging that suggest progressive tumor, a surgical resection or biopsy is often conducted to alleviate symptoms and to establish the grade of the tumor. Patients with low-grade gliomas that progress to high-grade glioma are treated similarly to patients with de novo high-grade glioma but with consideration to previous treatments.

Primary Central Nervous System Lymphoma

Primary CNS lymphoma is a rare non-Hodgkin lymphoma that affects the brain, eyes, meninges, and spinal cord and accounts for about 5% of all brain tumors. This tumor is associated with the immunocompromised state, but it has a significant incidence in the immunocompetent. The characteristic radiographic appearance suggests but does not confirm the diagnosis (Figure 5). If primary

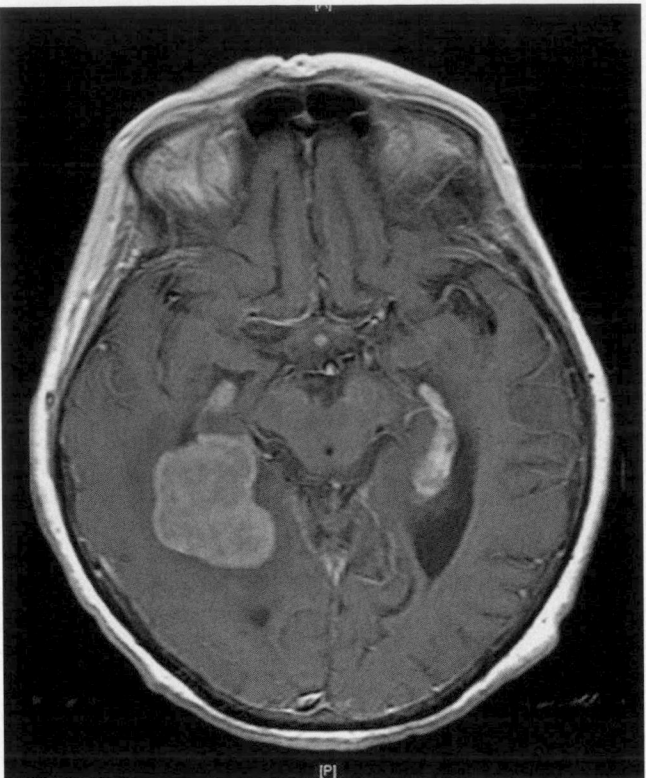

Figure 5. Contrast-enhanced magnetic resonance image shows a homogenously enhancing mass near the surface of the ventricle, suggesting primary central nervous system lymphoma.

CNS lymphoma is suspected, corticosteroids should not be given unless they are necessary to reduce increased intracranial pressure. This is because corticosteroids are directly cytotoxic to lymphoma cells, which can confound the tissue diagnosis. Occasionally, the diagnosis can be obtained through CSF testing, but a brain biopsy is often necessary.

Surgical resection has no role in treating this tumor because lymphoma is sensitive to chemotherapy and radiotherapy. Staging tests are necessary to rule out a systemic lymphoma that has metastasized to the CNS. Despite being incurable, primary CNS lymphoma is a more treatable tumor, and many patients live 5 years or longer after diagnosis.

Primary CNS lymphoma is treated with intravenous or intrathecal chemotherapy with or without radiotherapy. Methotrexate is the principal drug used either alone or in combination with other chemotherapy drugs. High doses of methotrexate ($3.5-8$ g/m^2)[3] must be used to overcome the blood–brain barrier. Owing to the potential for renal toxicity, high-dose methotrexate must be given in a setting where kidney function can be carefully monitored (usually the inpatient setting).

Radiotherapy was previously used as an initial treatment, but it is associated with profound cognitive impairment, especially in patients older than 60 years. However, more recent approaches have used lower doses of radiotherapy combined with chemotherapy with less neurotoxicity reported. Opinion is divided about the use of radiotherapy. Chemotherapy can also be used as a salvage treatment. Besides methotrexate, other commonly used chemotherapy drugs include cytarabine,[1] etoposide (Toposar),[1] rituximab (Rituxan),[1] and procarbazine (Matulane).[1] In younger patients, an increasingly used treatment at the time of relapse is high-dose chemotherapy with autologous stem cell transplantation. This approach is increasingly being investigated in the newly diagnosed setting.

[1]Not FDA approved for this indication.
[3]Exceeds dosage recommended by the manufacturer.

References

Ellis TL, Neal MT, Chan MD. The role of surgery, radiosurgery, and whole brain radiation therapy in the management of patients with metastatic brain tumors. Int J Surg Oncol 2012;2012:952345.

Gerstner ER, Batchelor TT. Primary central nervous system lymphoma. Arch Neurol 2010;67:291–7.

Norden AD, Drappatz J, Wen PY. Advances in meningioma therapy. Curr Neurol Neurosci Rep 2009;9:231–40.

Sanai N, Chang S, Berger MS. Low-grade gliomas in adults. J Neurosurg 2011;115:948–65.

Wen PY, Kesari S. Malignant gliomas in adults. N Engl J Med 2008;359:492–507.

GILLES DE LA TOURETTE SYNDROME

Method of
Steve W. Wu, MD; and Donald L. Gilbert, MD, MS

CURRENT DIAGNOSIS

- Multiple motor and one or more vocal tics have been present for some time during the illness, although not necessarily concurrently.
- The tics may wax and wane in frequency but have persisted for more than 1 year since first tic onset.
- Onset occurs before age 18 years.
- The disturbance is not caused by the direct physiologic effects of a substance or a general medical condition.

Gilles de la Tourette syndrome, or Tourette syndrome, was named after French neurologist Georges Gilles de la Tourette, who in 1885 described a series of nine patients with chronic tics. Tourette syndrome is a neuropsychiatric illness that begins in childhood. It is characterized by multiple motor and vocal tics that last for longer than 1 year (see Current Diagnosis box). The prevalence of Tourette syndrome varies greatly among epidemiologic studies, ranging from 0.1% to 3.8%. The prevalence of tic disorders is even higher, especially in children requiring special education.

Simple motor tics are sudden, brief, patterned movements such as eye blinking, facial grimace, head jerk, or shoulder shrug. Complex motor tics can involve a series of simple tics or a seemingly purposeful action, such as jumping, touching, or copropraxia (i.e., performing obscene gestures). Simple vocal tics consist of sounds such as throat clearing, sniffing, and coughing. Patients with complex vocal tics may exhibit echolalia (i.e., repeating others' words), palilalia (i.e., repeating their own words), or coprolalia (i.e., utterance of foul language).

Older children and adolescents often describe a premonitory urge before their tics. Tics can usually be transiently suppressed and are often diminished during focused mental or physical activities. Unlike myoclonus or chorea, tics usually do not affect activities of daily living or occupational or recreational activities. After the brief suppression, the release of the tic often brings relief to the patient. Tic severity commonly worsens during times of emotional stress. Fatigue or illness may also increase tics. Parents often notice more tics when the child is bored or unoccupied with an activity. Tics can occur during light sleep and rapid eye movement (REM) sleep.

Clinical Course

The onset of tics can occur after children are 3 years old, but they usually begin in children 6 to 7 years old. Children often present with motor tics first, followed by the development of vocal tics. Tics often wax and wane in the course of Tourette syndrome. During the early school years, tics often can go unnoticed or be mislabeled as a habit. If tics are noticed by fellow students, bullying is typically not an issue at this age. However, when parents notice the tics, they are often distressed and frequently tell their children to stop the movements.

Tic severity usually increases in the later elementary school years and into adolescence. This is the time when social interference such as bullying begins to occur. By late adolescence and early adulthood, most patients with Tourette syndrome have minimal tics, and some may "outgrow" tics. Because of this pattern, most individuals presenting for medical attention for tics are children.

Patients with Tourette syndrome frequently present with comorbid attention-deficit/hyperactivity disorder (ADHD) and obsessive-compulsive disorder (OCD). They also tend to have more sleep problems, anxiety, and mood disorders.

Diagnosis and Differential Diagnosis

Diagnosis of tic disorders depends on correctly recognizing that the abnormal movements are tics by means of a careful history and thorough physical examination. Laboratory and imaging studies are rarely needed.

Tics may resemble other abnormal movements, such as stereotypy, chorea, ballism, dystonia, and myoclonus. *Stereotypies* are repetitive, simple movements that are suppressible and that usually occur when a child is excited. Stereotypies usually start when the child is younger than 3 years. *Chorea* consists of a sequence of random, continual, involuntary, nonpurposeful, nonrhythmic movements. Choreic movements often flow from one body part to another. *Ballism* is a large-amplitude choreic movement affecting the proximal limb. *Myoclonus* is an involuntary, sudden, shocklike movement. Chorea, ballism, and myoclonus cannot be volitionally suppressed. *Dystonia* is produced by co-contraction of agonist and antagonist muscles, leading to abnormal postures, and its twisting movements typically are slower than tics.

Vocal tics may sometimes lead to the misdiagnosis of asthma, chronic cough, or allergic rhinitis. Other primary tic disorders include Provisional Tic Disorder, Persistent (Chronic) Motor or Vocal Tic Disorder, Other Specified Tic Disorder and Unspecified Tic Disorder (DSM-5).

Tics are nonspecific and may occur in drug-induced movement disorders, after head trauma, and in a variety of neurodevelopmental and neurodegenerative disorders. Complex or atypical cases with multiple comorbidities or multiple abnormalities identified on a general or neurologic examination should be referred for specialist consultation.

A controversial diagnosis in which tics or OCD may occur is called pediatric autoimmune neuropsychiatric disorders associated with streptococcal infections (PANDAS). Criteria for this diagnosis classically include abrupt appearance in prepubertal children of tics or OCD on two or more occasions after documented group A β-hemolytic streptococcal (GABHS) infections. The paradigm for this diagnosis is rheumatic (Sydenham's) chorea; however, PANDAS has no arthritis, carditis, or nephritis and is not thought to be a rheumatic disease. As a result of recent epidemiological studies, tics are no longer considered a primary symptom of PANDAS. The following interventions are not routinely recommended: diagnostic throat cultures and antistreptococcal antibody tests; therapeutic or preventive antibiotics; and immune-modulating therapies such as steroids, intravenous immunoglobulins, or plasmapheresis. Specialty consultation should be considered.

Treatment

There are many factors to consider when treating a patient with Tourette syndrome, including the presence of common symptoms such as inattentiveness, hyperactivity, obsessive or compulsive behaviors, depression, and anxiety (Box 1). When deciding to treat the patient, it is important to prioritize all the neuropsychiatric symptoms and provide accurate educational information. Tics may not always need to be treated medically, and if treatment is needed, tics may not be the first symptom to manage. Daily tic-suppressing medication is considered when there is functional

---

Box 1 Therapeutic Approach for Tourette Syndrome

- Educate the patient and family about tics and how tics often diminish spontaneously. Long-term reductions in tics may occur in the late teens, irrespective of pharmacologic therapy.
- Rank the tics, attention-deficit/hyperactivity disorder (ADHD), obsessive-compulsive disorder (OCD), anxiety, mood problems, learning problems, and behavior problems in order of the patient's or the family's perception of severity.
- Consider nonpharmacologic and pharmacologic treatment for each symptom in the order of perceived severity or impairment.
- Provide information to educate teachers and classmates to reduce social impairment.
- If the patient has learning problems, encourage formal assessment through the school or a psychologist. These children may qualify for modified educational methods.
- If ADHD is the most concerning problem, consider treating with clonidine[1] (Kapvay), guanfacine[1] (Intuniv), atomoxetine (Strattera), or methylphenidate (Ritalin). Stimulants are *not* absolutely contraindicated in patients with Tourette syndrome. However, if symptoms of OCD, anxiety, or pervasive developmental disorder are present, ticcing or compulsions may escalate on stimulants. If a patient has done well for months to years on stimulants for ADHD before an exacerbation of tics, it usually is not necessary to discontinue stimulants.
- If behavior problems are the most concerning problem or if a first-degree family member has a bipolar or psychotic disorder, refer the patient to a psychologist or psychiatrist.
- Anxious parents often worsen tic severity. If the family's anxiety is excessive, refer family members to a psychologist.
- If OCD or generalized anxiety disorder is the most severe problem, treatment with a selective serotonin reuptake inhibitor may be considered.
- Do not begin treatment with more than one central nervous system drug simultaneously. Start one, wait 2 to 4 weeks, and then reassess all symptoms before starting the next medication.
- Monitor the benefits and side effects at regular intervals.
- Maintain stable dosing during the school year; consider tapering medications in the summer.
- Consider weaning tic-suppressing medications in the middle to late teen years if tics wane.

[1]Not FDA approved for this indication.

---

interference, social interference, pain, or classroom or occupational disruption.

The first step in treating Tourette syndrome is educating the patient, parents, and other adult caregivers. Parents, teachers, and other adult caregivers are discouraged from telling the child to stop ticcing because this produces emotional anxiety that may worsen the tics. Educational materials for teachers often promote a conducive environment for the child at school. The patient is encouraged to openly talk about his or her disorder to classmates to promote understanding and minimize bullying. Newer cognitive-behavioral treatments for tic suppression appear to be helpful for children and adolescents, and they should be considered.

Clinical trials enrolling patients with Tourette syndrome are usually small and show small effect sizes. Most commonly used tic-suppressing medications belong to two classes: α_2-adrenergic agonists and dopamine receptor blocking agents (Table 1). Other agents may show modest benefit. Because Tourette syndrome is a chronic, nonfatal disorder, it is prudent to start treatment with medications that carry the least side effects. For this reason, α_2-adrenergic agonists are usually the first-line treatment. Although it is unclear what the second-line agents should be, it is reasonable in many cases to restrict dopamine receptor blocking agents to the most severe cases.

TABLE 1 Therapy for Tics in Tourette Syndrome

MEDICATION	STARTING DOSE	TITRATION	GOAL DOSE
Clonidine (Kapvay)	0.05 mg qhs	0.05 mg every 3–7 d	0.05–0.1 mg tid
Clonidine patch (Catapres-TTS)[1]	Catapres TTS-1 weekly*	Weekly as needed	Catapres TTS-1, TTS-2, or TTS-3 weekly*
Guanfacine (Intuniv)	0.5 mg qhs	0.5 mg every 3–7 d	1–4 mg divided bid
Baclofen (Lioresal)[1]	10 mg qhs	10 mg every 3–7 d	40–90 mg/d divided bid/tid
Clonazepam (Klonopin)[1]	0.5 mg qhs	0.5 mg every wk	1–2 mg bid
Topiramate (Topamax)[1]	25 mg qhs	25–50 mg weekly	50–100 mg bid
Pimozide (Orap)	1 mg qhs	1 mg every 3–5 d	1–4 mg/d divided daily or bid
Haloperidol (Haldol)	0.25–0.5 mg qhs	0.25–0.5 mg every 5–7 d	1–4 mg/d divided daily or bid
Fluphenazine (Prolixin)[1]	0.5 mg qhs	0.5 mg every 3–5 d	1–4 mg/d divided daily or bid
Risperidone (Risperdal)[1]	0.5 mg qhs	0.5 mg every 3–5 d	1–4 mg/d divided daily or bid
Ziprasidone (Geodon)[1]	20 mg qhs	20 mg every wk	20–80 mg/d divided daily or bid
Aripiprazole (Abilify)[1]	1 mg HS	1 mg every wk	1–20 mg daily or divided bid
Botulinum toxin type A (Botox)[1]	Not applicable	Not applicable	30–300 units in one or more focal sites, injected once every 3 mo

[1]Not FDA approved for this indication.

*The system areas are 3.5 cm^2 (Catapres TTS-1), 7.0 cm^2 (Catapres TTS-2), and 10.5 cm^2 (Catapres TTS-3), and the amount of drug released is directly proportional to the area.

α_2-Adrenergic Agonists

Clonidine (Catapres)[1] and guanfacine (Tenex)[1] are α_2-adrenergic agonists often used to treat tics. Several randomized trials have shown that these agents reduce tic and ADHD symptoms. The main side effects are sedation and lightheadedness due to mild hypotension. Sedation is more common with clonidine. The clonidine patch (Catapres-TTS)[1] may produce less peak sedation, but it commonly produces local skin irritation.

Dopamine Receptor Blocking Agents

Typical and atypical neuroleptics are dopamine receptor blocking agents that can be used to treat tics. Neuroleptics such as pimozide (Orap) and haloperidol (Haldol) can be very effective in tic suppression, but they can cause acute akathisia, dystonic reactions, cognitive blunting, acute anxiety with somatizations and school refusal, sedation, weight gain, metabolic syndrome, and QT prolongation. Monitoring for tardive dyskinesia is also important. Some experts recommend baseline electrocardiograms, particularly for individuals with personal or family history of cardiac arrhythmias. Weight gain and metabolic syndrome should be considered when starting neuroleptics, particularly risperidone (Risperdal) and aripiprazole (Abilify).[1] Some experts recommend obtaining baseline values for weight, blood pressure, fasting glucose, and lipid profile, with follow-up monitoring every 3 months to detect drug-induced metabolic syndrome. Diet modification, routine exercise, or medical therapy may be needed.

Other Tic-Suppressing Medications

Several small, controlled studies show benefit for topiramate (Topamax),[1] dopamine agonists,[1] baclofen (Lioresal),[1] benzodiazepines,[1] and botulinum toxin type A (Botox)[1] injections for focal, strong tics. Tetrabenazine (Xenazine)[1] has been reported to reduce tics.

Behavioral Therapy

Recent clinical trials show that Comprehensive Behavioral Intervention for Tics, in which the patient learns to increase self-awareness of tics and premonitory urges and to perform antagonistic movements, reduces tics.

[1]Not FDA approved for this indication.

Treatment of Comorbid Conditions

ADHD and OCD are common comorbid conditions in Tourette syndrome. These comorbid symptoms are often more debilitating than the tics. Concern about stimulant therapy worsening tics was addressed by the Tourette Syndrome Study Group in the landmark Treatment of ADHD in Children with Tics (TACT) study. In this study, children treated with methylphenidate (Ritalin) had, on average, reduced tic severity, contrary to the widely held belief that stimulants exacerbate tics.

Medical treatment options for ADHD include psychostimulants, α_2=adrenergic agonists guanfacine (Intuniv) and clonidine (Kapvay), and the selective norepinephrine reuptake inhibitor atomoxetine (Strattera). OCD management includes cognitive-behavioral therapy, clomipramine (Anafranil), and any of the selective serotonin reuptake inhibitors.

Summary

Tourette syndrome is a complex neuropsychiatric illness with many potential symptoms that may need medical and nonmedical therapies. Cooperation among the primary care physician, neurologist, psychiatrist, and psychologist is imperative for the comprehensive care of severely affected patients. If a patient has mild tics and few or no comorbid symptoms, medical therapy may not be needed. However, if the tics are severe in the presence of many neuropsychiatric symptoms, it is reasonable to refer patients to specialists.

References

Bloch MH, Panza KE, Landeros-Weisenberger A, Leckman JF. Meta-analysis: treatment of attention-deficit/hyperactivity disorder in children with comorbid tic disorders. J Am Acad Child Adolesc Psychiatry 2009;48:884–93.

Gilbert DL, Jankovic J. Pharmacological treatment of tourette syndorme. Journal of Obsessive-Compulsive and Related Disorders 2014;3:407–14.

Leckman JF, King RA, Gilbert DL, et al. Streptococcal upper respiratory tract infections and exacerbations of tic and obsessive-compulsive symptoms: a prospective longitudinal study. J Am Acad Child Adolesc Psychiatry 2011;50:108–118 e3.

Piacentini J, Woods DW, Scahill L, et al. Behavior therapy for children with Tourette disorder: a randomized controlled trial. JAMA 2010;303:1929–37.

Zinner SH, Mink JW. Movement disorders I: tics and stereotypies. Pediatr Rev 2010;31:223–33.

HEAD INJURIES

Method of
Todd W. Vitaz, MD

CURRENT DIAGNOSIS

Classification of Head Injuries
- Closed versus penetrating
- Isolated versus multisystem injuries
- Severity
  - Mild (GCS 13–15)
  - Moderate (GCS 9–12)
  - Severe (GCS 3–8)

Pathologic Findings with Closed Head Injuries
- Skull fractures
- Epidural hematomas
- Subdural hematomas
- Parenchymal contusions
- Intraparenchymal hematomas
- Diffuse axonal injury

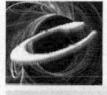

CURRENT THERAPY

Management of Elevated Intracranial Pressure
- Prevention of venous engorgement
- CO_2 control (mild hyperventilation)
- Sedation and pain control
- Cerebrospinal fluid drainage
- Mannitol
- Lasix
- Hypertonic saline
- Decompressive craniectomy
- Pentobarbital coma

Traumatic brain injury (TBI) most commonly results from motor vehicle crashes (MVC) and typically affects males in the 2nd through 4th decades of life. These sudden random acts can have long-lasting effects on the patient and family, but these events also impact society as a whole when a young, viable, working-age individual becomes suddenly disabled and dependent on the care of others. TBI has no regard for age or gender, however, and can be seen in infants as a result of nonaccidental trauma as well as in geriatric patients following falls. The management of these patients can become extremely complicated and often requires the close interaction of numerous health care providers ranging from trauma, orthopedic, and neurologic surgeons to nurses, social workers, and speech, occupational, and physical therapists. Unfortunately, current interventions are still limited to the avoidance or minimization of secondary injury and rehabilitative intervention. However, when these patients are managed with aggressive, comprehensive, multidisciplinary approaches, the outcomes at times can be rewarding.

TBI can be categorized based on numerous factors. Most commonly it is differentiated based on mechanism and injury type (closed versus penetrating), whether it has occurred with or without systemic injuries (isolated versus multisystem), and the severity (mild, moderate, severe). The Glasgow Coma Scale (GCS) (Table 1), which was initially developed as a prognostic indicator following closed head injury, has become the principal triage tool for evaluating these patients. Patients are scored based on their best response in each of the three categories (eye opening, verbal responses, and motor score) and then subdivided into mild

BEST MOTOR SCORE	BEST VERBAL RESPONSE	BEST EYE OPENING
6 Obeys commands	5 Normal speech	4 Spontaneous
5 Localizes to pain	4 Confused	3 To voice
4 Withdraws to pain	3 Inappropriate words	2 To pain
3 Flexor posturing	2 Incomprehensible sounds	1 No eye opening
2 Extensor posturing	1 No verbal response	
1 No motor response	Intubated patients receive a 1 with the suffix T added to score	

TABLE 1 Glasgow Coma Scale

(13–15), moderate (9–12), and severe (3–8). One caveat to this assessment tool is that it can be affected by numerous alterations, such as hypoxia, hypotension, hypothermia, intoxication, infection, and other metabolic derangements, which are commonly seen in the trauma population.

Pathology

Another common classification system following TBI is based on pathophysiologic findings. Concussion commonly occurs following mild or moderate TBI as the result of transient (typically seconds to minutes) neurologic dysfunction in the setting of a normal computed tomography (CT) scan. Brief loss of consciousness, commonly with amnesia regarding the event, is not uncommon and is often associated with nausea, vomiting, headache, dizziness, and transient visual obscuration. These symptoms may persist for several hours to weeks as part of the *postconcussive syndrome* and, in rare instances, especially following repetitive injury, these alterations may become long-lasting. As a result of these persistent problems, in addition to a better understanding of the neurocognitive effects following this type of injury, there has been an enormous emphasis placed on their prevention (see text following).

Skull fractures may occur in isolation or be associated with other types of brain injuries. They are commonly classified based on whether they are open (overlying laceration) or closed, linear or comminuted, and nondepressed or depressed. Skull fractures occur either as the result of a large force directed to a small area (i.e., depressed skull fracture following a blow to the head with a golf club) or when larger forces are dissipated throughout the skull resulting in fracture through the weakest area (linear fractures through frontal skull base petrous, or squamous temporal bone). Linear fractures are commonly associated with raccoon eyes (frontal skull base fractures), Battle's sign (posterior skull base fracture), cerebrospinal fluid leak (otorrhea or rhinorrhea), or olfactory, facial or acoustic nerve injury (amnesia, facial palsy, sensorineuronal deafness).

In addition, temporal bone fractures may also be associated with epidural hematomas (EDHs). These extra-axial blood clots are most commonly caused by laceration of the middle meningeal artery and result in accumulation of *high-pressure arterial bleeding* in the potential space between the dura and skull. EDHs are more commonly seen in younger individuals, probably because of the decreased skull thickness and lack of adhesions between the skull and dura mater in this population. Commonly, these lesions appear on CT scan as lens-shaped, extra-axial hematomas most often in the temporal region and can be rapidly expansive secondary to the high-pressure arterial bleeding. The clinical course in these patients is classically described by a brief loss of consciousness from the initial concussion, followed by a "lucid interval" in which the patient may be awake and alert, which then gives way to another episode of decreased mental status that may be rapidly progressive and associated with signs of brain stem compression (flexor or extensor posturing, dilated nonreactive pupil). EDHs are usually treated surgically unless they are extremely small and constitute one of the few true neurosurgical emergencies where mere minutes may make an enormous difference in the patient's outcome.

Unlike EDHs, subdural hematomas (SDHs) are often associated with other types of brain injury and thus typically involve an altered level of consciousness (LOC) from the onset. SDHs are typically caused by bleeding from bridging veins that get torn when the brain moves within its cerebrospinal fluid (CSF) buffer while the veins remain tethered at their dural insertions; however, other causes such as venous or arterial hemorrhage from a brain laceration also exist. CT scanning reveals that these lesions commonly appear more crescent-shaped but never cross the dural boundaries (falx or tentorium). Unlike the high-pressure EDHs, SDHs typically expand at a slower rate but still cause devastating neurologic dysfunction from compression of the underlying brain. In addition, mortality rates tend to be higher with worse outcome for SDH as a result of the common underlying brain injury. Once again, these extra-axial clots frequently require surgical evacuation unless they are small and fail to have substantial compression on the underlying brain, where they are managed with serial imaging and close neurologic observation. In patients for whom a small SDH is not treated surgically, the physician must remain cognizant of the fact that a small proportion of these will increase in size between 1 and 4 weeks following the trauma and can be a cause of delayed deterioration or increased headache and new neurologic findings.

Intraparenchymal hematomas occur quite commonly following TBI and can be either hemorrhagic or nonhemorrhagic. These lesions range in size from 1 to 2 mm up to several centimeters, and can cause a full range of symptoms and neurologic findings based on their location, size, and degree of compression on surrounding structures. Just like extra-axial hematomas, these lesions may increase in size and commonly coalesce or mature and *blossom* during the first 12 to 24 hours following the trauma. In addition, larger hematomas incite an inflammatory reaction in the surrounding brain, resulting in increased edema around the lesion, which may result in increases in the intracranial pressure (ICP) (commonly seen on postinjury days [PIDs] 3–7). Management of these lesions depends on their size, location, and associated findings and ranges from serial observation and repeat imaging, surgical evacuation of the hematoma, or decompressive craniectomy with or without lobectomy.

The final category of pathologic abnormalities following TBI occurs as the result of shear injury to the axons themselves, called diffuse axonal injury (DAI). This is caused by either acceleration and deceleration or rotational forces to the axons resulting in micro- or macroscopic areas of injury and axonal transection. Most commonly this is encountered in the setting where a patient clinically has signs of a severe TBI, often with a GCS score less than 6; however, the CT scan is either unimpressive or shows only small areas of petechial hemorrhage. In addition, ICP recording typically shows normal or only slightly elevated values. Magnetic resonance imaging (MRI) is commonly used in this subset of patients and can be used as a predictive indicator for determining the severity of injury, especially if CT is negative. MRI commonly shows areas of increased intensity on fluid attenuation inversion recovery (FLAIR) and T2-weighted sequences in the brainstem, diencephalon, deep white matter tracts, or corpus callosum. Recovery following this type of injury is variable and depends more on the injury location (reticular activating system of brainstem versus supratentorial white matter tracts) than on the injury volume.

In addition to these abnormalities, patients with TBI are also at risk for damage to the spinal cord and vertebral and carotid arteries. Thus, patients with altered LOC should be assumed to have spinal instability and possible spinal cord injury (SCI); they should remain immobilized until the absence of these can be confirmed. The incidence of carotid and vertebral artery injury associated with severe TBI is unknown, but patients with facial or cervical fractures and those with soft tissue neck or chest injury (seat belt sign) have been found to be at higher risk. The appropriate screening for and treatment of these injuries have become a topic of intense debate in recent years but should be suspected in a patient with focal neurologic findings without identifiable cause on other imaging.

Intracranial Pressure and the Monroe-Kellie Doctrine

Regardless of the pathophysiologic type of injury, the end result commonly is the generation of increases in the ICP, which can then lead to secondary brain injury. ICP dynamics are easily understood if one considers the principles of the volume pressure relationships outlined by the Monroe-Kellie doctrine. The basis of this principle resides on the fact that the skull is a fixed and rigid volume; because of this any changes to the volume of its contents will directly affect the pressure within this rigid space. In simplest terms the intracranial cavity contains blood, water, and tissue. Blood may be intravascular (IV) or extravascular (EV) in the case of extra-axial blood clots; water includes not only CSF, which may build up in cases of hydrocephalus, but also edema following traumatic injuries; brain parenchyma typically compromises the tissue component, but in select instances tumors or cysts may also fall into this category.

As increases in any or all three of these categories occur, the pressure inside the cranial cavity increases proportionally. At first, compensatory changes occur, which accommodate for these increases, resulting in only mild pressure changes; however, eventually a critical volume is reached where the compensatory mechanisms are saturated, resulting in rapid and dramatic pressure changes. The following scenario illustrates these principles. A patient is involved in a motor vehicle crash and suffers a head injury with a small epidural hematoma. Initially he is awake and alert without any focal neurologic findings. The epidural hematoma creates an increase in the EV blood component of the Monroe-Kellie doctrine; however, compensatory changes in intracranial CSF volume result in decreases in the water component, thus preventing significant changes in ICP. However, the hematoma continues to enlarge, causing increases in ICP exhibited clinically by slow deterioration in the patient's level of consciousness. The patient is now intubated and mildly hyperventilated, causing vasoconstriction, thereby decreasing the intravascular blood component and reducing ICP with an improvement in the patient's neurologic condition. Unfortunately, as the operating room (OR) is being prepared, the patient suffers a rapid decrease in his level of consciousness, becoming unresponsive with flexor posturing and a nonreactive pupil. Although the hematoma has expanded at a constant rate over time, the rapid change in the patient's condition is the result of him reaching the critical point where all compensatory mechanisms have been exhausted, thus causing profound, rapid changes in the patient's ICP.

Treatment of Elevated Intracranial Pressure

Acute changes in ICP result in altered LOC, and at times other localizing neurologic findings such as *blown* (dilated, nonreactive) pupils and flexor or extensor posturing, and such findings may be the sign of impending herniation and death without immediate intervention. In a patient without a ventricular drain already in place, hyperventilation is the most rapid mechanism for acutely lowering elevated ICP. Currently, aggressive hyperventilation (Pco_2 <30) is recommended only for short durations in cases of impending cerebral herniation while patients are being stabilized. As stated previously, hyperventilation causes vasoconstriction, which reduces intravascular blood within the cranial vault and almost instantaneously lowers ICP. However, several studies have now shown that the routine use of aggressive hyperventilation in the management of patients with severe closed head injury (CHI) results in decreased outcomes because of hypoxic injury and possible stroke caused by the sustained hyperventilation. Our current practice is to maintain Pco_2 values between 35 and 38 with controlled ventilation in all patients with severe CHI; because of this, we leave all these patients intubated and mechanically ventilated until their ICPs normalize and all other therapies are withdrawn.

Adequate sedation and pain control are also important elements of ICP control. Patients who are restless and agitated will have higher ICPs than similar patients who are resting quietly in bed. Another important point is the prevention of venous congestion. This occasionally is evident in cervical collars, which are fastened too tightly or with the use of trach ties that are wrapped too tightly around the neck to hold the endotracheal tube in place.

Several medications are available for the treatment of elevated ICP, with the most common one being mannitol. Although this agent acts as an osmotic diuretic and helps pull excess interstitial fluid into the vascular space and thus lower ICP, there are several other hypothetical mechanisms that probably also increase its efficacy such as increasing RBC flexibility, decreasing RBC and platelet clumping in small arterioles and capillaries, and increasing intravascular volume, thus improving cardiac function. Other diuretics such as furosemide (Lasix)[1] or urea (Ureaphil) may also be used but have less dramatic effects on ICP. Hypertonic saline (NaCl 3% to 5%)[1] has also been used more recently by some physicians and has been shown to have many of the same effects as mannitol.

CSF diversion is one of the simplest, quickest-acting methods for decreasing ICP, especially if a ventricular drain is already in place. The emergent surgical evacuation of mass lesions such as large epidural, subdural, or intraparenchymal hematomas is also extremely effective for controlling ICP, and in many instances it is also lifesaving. However, in some instances, underlying brain injury or stroke from prolonged brain compression may be exhibited as massive intraoperative brain swelling and in these instances may necessitate that the bone flap be left off (craniectomy).

Management of Severe Closed Head Injury

The current recommendations of the Brain Trauma Foundation Guidelines for the management of closed head injuries call for the placement of ICP monitors in all patients who fall into the severe category (GCS score <9). At our institution we routinely place combination intraventricular monitors and drains in all patients with a postresuscitation GCS score of less than 7. Monitors are inserted into patients with a GCS score of 7 to 9 on an individual basis depending on whether there are distracting reasons, such as intoxication, to cause the altered LOC. If patients are intubated and not following commands but are purposeful in their movements, we will sometimes elect not to place a ventriculostomy and follow the patient's clinical course over several hours. Other factors include CT findings and the need to go to the operating room during the acute period for the treatment of other life-threatening injuries, age, or for heavy sedation secondary to other injuries or pulmonary problems. At times patients in this GCS range will be given 6 to 12 hours and treated medically to see whether or not they improve prior to placement of an ICP monitor.

Once an ICP monitor and drain have been placed, elevations in ICP are treated in a systematic order. Target values include attempts to keep ICP less than 15 to 20 and cerebral perfusion pressure (CPP) greater than 60. Low CPP (CPP = mean arterial blood pressure [MAP] − ICP) is caused by either elevated ICP or low MAP. For patients with low MAP or uncontrolled ICP, vasopressors may be used to increase blood pressure (BP) and central venous pressure. At the University of Louisville, dopamine (Intropin) is used as a first-line agent, followed by phenylephrine (Neo-Synephrine) and norepinephrine (Levophed) in refractory cases. ICP elevations are initially treated with adequate sedation and pain control, such as midazolam (Versed),[1] propofol (Diprivan), and/or morphine (Lioresal),[1] to prevent agitation and elevated airway pressures, which can further increase ICP and intermittent CSF diversion. In cases where this fails to control ICP, mannitol is then added to the treatment protocol along with

more continuous CSF diversion and finally chemical paralysis. Mannitol is administered as a bolus infusion in doses ranging from 0.25 to 1.0 mg/kg body weight every 4 to 8 hours with the endpoints being either ICP control or measured serum osmolarity greater than 315 mOsmL.

Patients who continue to have sustained increases in their ICP despite these interventions are considered to have refractory ICP and at our facility are considered for one of two potential salvage treatments. Pentobarbital (Nembutal)[1] coma has been used successfully on occasion in young patients without mass lesions to decrease the metabolic demands of the brain during these periods of sustained ICP. Patients need to be chosen wisely for this therapy because it carries enormous risks in addition to the possibility of preserving the patient in a long-term, nonfunctional, persistent vegetative state. Initiation of pentobarbital coma causes severe hypotension, and patients almost always require the use of pressors in addition to volume expansion. At our facility we also place all of these patients on a Rotorest bed in an attempt to minimize the pulmonary complications that frequently occur with the use of this technique.

The second salvage therapy is decompressive craniectomy. This procedure involves the removal of a significant area of skull, typically almost an entire hemisphere or both frontal regions with opening of the dura. This permits the injured, swollen brain to herniate through the opening and is the only intervention that increases the volume of the intracranial compartment, thereby reducing pressure. In addition, this technique allows for the evacuation of large hemorrhagic contusions, or in cases of extreme ICP elevations it can be coupled with either frontal or temporal lobectomy. Once again, patients must be selected carefully for this intervention. Decompressive craniectomy is used much more frequently than pentobarbital coma at our institution. We use this strategy for patients with elevated ICP—more than 30 to 40 for more than 30 minutes—or a significant change in neurologic condition that is nonresponsive to all other interventions. In order for either of these two salvage approaches to be effective, they must be used at the first signs of refractory ICP prior to the occurrence of complications such as ischemic infarcts, brainstem compression, or hemorrhage.

Patients treated with decompressive craniectomies are at risk for significant alterations in CSF dynamics, which may result in delayed deterioration. Signs of hydrocephalus, either in the form of ventriculomegaly or extra-axial or interhemispheric CSF fluid collections, will be evident in 50% to 80% of these patients. When necessary these patients will be treated with external ventricular or subdural drains followed by early cranioplasty (replacement of the bone plate). In many instances these changes will resolve following cranioplasty and therefore avoid the need for ventriculoperitoneal shunting, with its associated risks and complications.

All patients with abnormal head CT scans (regardless of GCS score) are treated with close neurologic observation, most commonly in an intensive care unit (ICU) setting, and serial CT scans (4–6 hours later and on PID 1), and they are placed on 7 days of phenytoin (Dilantin). Temkin and colleagues showed that patients with post-traumatic intracranial hemorrhage were at increased risk of suffering seizures in the acute period; treatment with antiepileptics beyond 7 days did not decrease the risk of these patients developing epilepsy or delayed seizures, but there were increased risks associated with side effects from medication administration. Patients who experience a seizure following CHI (with the exception of acute post-traumatic seizures) should be maintained on antiepileptics for at least 3 to 6 months and possible indefinitely depending on their clinical condition and EEG results. Patients with acute post-traumatic seizures (within the first several minutes following the event) are not felt to be at increased risk for developing further seizures and receive the routine 7-day treatment. At the University of Louisville we have found that changing phenytoin dosing to a weight-based schedule (15 mg/kg load, 2 mg/kg every 8 hours unless elderly [≥70 years old], then 2 mg/kg every 12 hours)

---

[1]Not FDA approved for this indication.

[1]Not FDA approved for this indication.

increases the chance of achieving a therapeutic dose earlier in the treatment course and lowers the costs of monitoring these agents.

Finally, the treatment of these patients requires a tight-knit group of specialists and ancillary service providers with open communication channels. We have found that the use of a time-independent phased outcome clinical pathway helps maximize the level of patient care and maintain cost-effectiveness. By using such an approach all routine interactions are initiated at the time of admission and each care provider has a clear role and responsibility; one of the most important aspects of this system is the involvement of a clinical coordinator whose responsibility includes ensuring that all aspects of patient care and family education are completed at the appropriate intervals. We believe another key component is our philosophy toward early feeding (prior to PID 3) and early tracheotomy and percutaneous endoscopic gastrostomy (PEG) feeding tube placement in a majority of these individuals (PID 4). We have shown that such an aggressive approach to these issues helps reduce infectious complications and minimizes length of ICU stay.

Treatment of Mild and Moderate Traumatic Brain Injury

In many circumstances patients with moderate TBI are treated almost as though they had severe TBI, with the exception of invasive ICP monitoring. Many patients will be intubated at the time of admission and require sedation and adequate pain management. This can be difficult because it is of utmost importance to maintain the ability to perform serial neurologic examinations. Therefore, we commonly use a combination of propofol (Diprivan) infusions and intermittent morphine (Lioresal)[1] injections in these patients, thereby allowing hourly assessment of neurologic function. We have found that a subset of patients (older than age 45 years, multisystem trauma, presence of early pneumonia) with moderate TBI requires more aggressive treatment with early tracheostomy and PEG tube placement and, at times, ICP monitors.

The subset of patients with moderate TBI who are not intubated at the time of admission are also watched closely in the ICU. Once again, close monitoring of neurologic function and vigorous pulmonary toilet is of key importance because some patients may be lethargic and are at risk of pulmonary decompensation. We have found ipratropium (Atrovent)[1] and albuterol (Proventil)[1] nebulizers and early mobilization minimize pulmonary problems. Patients with progressive lethargy, worsening neurologic function, hypoxia, hypercapnia, or the inability to protect their airways are intubated and placed on mechanical ventilation. Once again, patients unable to tolerate a diet by PID 3 have a nasogastric feeding tube placed to allow for early enteral nutritional support; however, PEG tubes are not placed until later in the hospital course in the predischarge phase because many patients in this category will improve throughout their hospitalization and be able to tolerate an oral diet by the time of discharge.

Patients with mild TBI are treated over a much wider continuum, ranging from discharge from the emergency room (ER) with appropriate adult supervision to observation in the ICU to immediate surgical treatment of mass lesions. The two most important factors in determining treatment algorithms for these patients are presence or absence of abnormal CT findings and neurologic function, with associated symptoms such as nausea, vomiting, dizziness, or visual problems. Headache is a common complaint in all of these patients and must be taken in context with other complaints and imaging results. Patients with severe headaches, dizziness, and vomiting (postconcussive syndrome) may commonly require a brief hospital stay to allow for delayed imaging and at least partial resolution of some of the complaints.

Early and Delayed Neurologic Changes

Any patient suffering a significant neurologic injury requires close neurologic monitoring. Although most patients remain unchanged or show gradual improvement in the early phases, a small percentage will show signs of neurologic deterioration. At first these signs may be subtle (agitation, mild increase in lethargy, protracted vomiting); but eventually they may become more profound and can be precursors to impending neurologic demise and death. When these changes are the result of either expanding mass lesions or increases in ICP, treatment instituted in the early phases is more likely to be successful compared to instances when interventions are performed under conditions associated with cerebral herniation syndromes. Thus any patient showing persistent signs of neurologic decline should be promptly evaluated by a physician and many may also require repeat CT scanning.

However, not all neurologic changes are the result of changes in ICP or expansion of mass lesions, and such irregularities may be caused by a long list of other metabolic or neurologic conditions. Some of the more common causes are seizures, strokes (especially from carotid or vertebral dissections), electrolyte imbalances, hypoxia, hypercarbia, fever, excess sedation, or drug and/or alcohol withdrawal.

Concussions and Sports-Related Injuries: Return to Play Guidelines

Over the past 2 decades, knowledge regarding the detrimental effects of repetitive mild head injuries has led to intense public debate concerning whether athletes should be allowed to return to play following such injuries. Concussions are not uncommon among participants in competitive sports including football, hockey, baseball, and soccer. Concerns regarding the full negative impact of repetitive, almost innocuous injury have led many youth soccer leagues to ban or modify rules regarding *heading* of the ball. In addition, other concerns exist following more severe concussions, including development of other life-threatening neurologic injuries such as subdural or epidural hematomas, development of the double-impact syndrome (rapid, uncontrolled increases in ICP following sequential minor traumas), and the long-term neuropsychological impact of these injuries. As a result of these concerns, the guidelines concerning when and if an athlete should be allowed to return to play have undergone modification since development of the earlier criteria. Because of these frequent changes, readers are encouraged to check with their local medical agencies or recent publications and Internet sources if faced with these issues. In short, if a player loses consciousness or has persistent symptoms (>15–20 minutes), he or she should not be allowed to return to play on that day or even not for 1 to 2 weeks following the complete resolution of all symptoms. It should also be stressed that an individual may have a concussion without loss of consciousness and that concussion is defined as any transient change in mental status. To this end many organizations including the National Football League have developed a sideline neuropsychological screening test that can often help illustrate these deficits even when the athlete appears normal.

Restorative Therapies

Patients suffering any type of TBI can have long-lasting cognitive, psychological, and emotional dysfunction in addition to their functional and neurologic deficits. Although most people assume that the resolution of decreased alertness and consciousness symbolizes resolution of the overall neurologic injury, this is not the case in most patients. In our series of patients with moderate TBI, we found that almost 50% of patients at median follow-up of 27 months complained of persistent emotional or cognitive problems that interfered with their lifestyle despite the fact that they all were discharged from the hospital with a GCS score of 14 to 15. Long-term speech and cognitive therapies as well as individual, group, and family counseling will be helpful for many of these patients.

In the late hospital and early rehabilitative stages, numerous pharmacologic agents may be helpful to overcome some of the neurologic side effects following TBI. Patients with autonomic storms (intermittent episodes of diaphoresis, tachycardia, fever, agitation) may respond to adrenergic antagonists such as clonidine

---

[1]Not FDA approved for this indication.

(Catapres)[1] or propanolol (Inderal),[1] in addition to volume resuscitation, morphine (Lioresal),[1] baclofen,[1] and bromocriptine (Parlodel).[1] Patients with hypoarousal are treated with amantadine[1] (Symmetrel), 100 mg at 8 AM and 12 PM, and bromocriptine,[1] 5 to 15 mg every day. Trazodone (Desyrel), 50 to 100 mg at bedtime, may be helpful in restoring sleep-wake cycles, whereas risperidone (Risperdal),[1] olanzapine (Zyprexa),[1] and quetiapine (Seroquel)[1] may be helpful to control agitation and combativeness during the subacute recovery phases.

Future Considerations

The previously mentioned treatment strategies include what is considered common practice at the University of Louisville; however, newer, more aggressive treatments and monitoring capabilities are always being developed. Some of the newer monitoring systems under development include cerebral oximetry measurements (frequently through invasive indwelling catheters) and cerebral microdialysis systems, in which continuous assessments are performed to determine the concentrations of critical markers such as lactate in the brain or CSF. Both of these methods provide physiologic feedback for the metabolic environment of the brain, are sensitive enough to predict changes in regional oxygenation, and have been found to be correlated with outcomes in small nonrandomized studies.

---

[1]Not FDA approved for this indication.

References

Brain Trauma Foundation. Management and Prognosis of Severe Traumatic Brain Injury. New York: Brain Trauma Foundation; 2000.
McIlvoy L, Spain DA, Raque G, et al. Successful incorporation of the Severe Head Injury Guidelines into a phased-outcome clinical pathway. J Neurosci Nurs 2001;33(2):72–882.
Miller PR, Fabian TC, Bee TK, et al. Blunt cerebrovascular injuries: Diagnosis and treatment. J Trauma 2001;51(2):279–86.
Temkin NR, Dikmen SS, Wilensky AJ, et al. A randomized, double-blind study of phenytoin for the prevention of post-traumatic seizures. N Engl J Med 1990;323:497–502.
Vitaz TW, McIlvoy L, Raque GH, et al. Development and implementation of a clinical pathway for severe traumatic brain injury. J Trauma 2001;51(2):369–75.
Vitaz TW, McIlvoy L, Raque GH, et al. Development and implementation of a clinical pathway for spinal cord injuries. J Spinal Disord 2001;14(3):271–6.
Vitaz TW, Jenks J, Raque GH, Shields CB. Outcome following moderate traumatic brain injury. Surg Neurol 2003;60(4):285–91.

INTRACEREBRAL HEMORRHAGE

Method of
Jonathan Rosand, MD, MSc

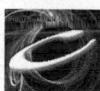

CURRENT DIAGNOSIS

- Obtain a thorough history, including time of symptom onset
- Imaging of the cerebral vessels should be performed in all patients younger than 55 years and should be strongly considered in all patients in whom underlying aneurysm or arteriovenous malformation is suspected.
- Obtain contrast-enhanced neuroimaging if underlying cerebral mass or tumor is suspected.

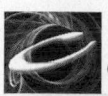

CURRENT THERAPY

- Maintain airway, breathing, and circulation; stabilize the neck if fracture is considered.
- Detect and emergently correct coagulopathy.

- Arrange an emergent neurosurgical consultation for cerebellar hemorrhage.
- Maintain systolic blood pressure ≤140 mm Hg using intravenous agents. Reduce systolic blood pressure to 180 mm Hg for patients whose systolic pressure is greater than 220 mm Hg.

Epidemiology

Intracerebral hemorrhage (ICH) is most often the acute manifestation of a chronic, progressive disorder of the blood vessels of the brain. With an estimated incidence rate of between 35 and 45 cases per 100,000 population in Europe and North America, ICH generally accounts for between 10% and 15% of acute strokes on those continents. The incidence is higher in East Asia, with estimates that ICH accounts for as many as 30% to 40% of acute stroke cases in those countries. Hospital-based series consistently reveal an acute mortality from ICH ranging between 35% and 65% and substantial permanent disability in at least 50% of survivors. Because mortality figures are all confounded by the fact that withdrawal of aggressive care by clinicians and families is a very common precipitant of death in these patients and often occurs in patients whose ICH is survivable, it is more useful to focus on rates of disability among survivors when discussing prognosis (see later).

Risk Factors

Risk factors for primary ICH include chronic conditions, chronic exposures, and acute physiologic derangements. Secondary ICH refers to hemorrhage that develops in the setting of vascular malformations, including saccular aneurysms, brain tumor, cerebral venous thrombosis, or hemorrhagic conversion of an ischemic infarct. Among patients older than 55 years, who account for the majority of cases, chronic hypertension, cerebral amyloid angiopathy, and chronic use of antithrombotic medication are the leading risk factors for primary ICH. History of a prior stroke, chronic alcohol use, and family history of ICH also contribute, and patients with severe coagulopathy, cocaine abuse, and liver disease are also at higher risk for ICH. Accumulating data suggest that aggressive lowering of serum cholesterol or chronic use of statin therapy can increase risk for ICH in the elderly. Although chronic hypertension has long been identified as contributing to the largest proportion of ICH cases, recent population-based studies demonstrate a substantial fall in hypertension-associated ICH. In parallel, however, the aging of the population has led to the broader use of antithrombotic medications as well as increases in the prevalence of amyloid angiopathy. The result is that ICH incidence rates have not fallen.

Pathophysiology

ICH arises when a blood vessel within the brain ruptures and blood leaks out to form a hematoma. Because the skull is fixed in volume and is completely filled by brain, blood, and CSF, any accumulation of blood within the brain must necessarily compress, distort, and disrupt surrounding brain structures. The result is that the damage caused by ICH is due the mass effect of the hematoma as well as the toxic effects of the blood itself. The volume of blood that leaks out is thus the most potent predictor of outcome from ICH. In addition, extravasated blood can enter the CSF drainage system, leading to hydrocephalus, another predictor of poor outcome.

Bleeding in ICH often occurs over hours, a phenomenon that can be documented with serial head computed tomography (CT) scans. The volume of ICH can be compared between a CT scan obtained at the time of presentation to the emergency department and one obtained several hours later. The shorter the time interval between symptom onset and presentation to the emergency department, the more likely the patient is to have ongoing bleeding and hematoma expansion after the initial CT scan.

Location of the ICH within the brain can be a clue to the underlying vessel abnormality responsible for the rupture. Among patients 55 years and older, hemorrhage in lobar locations, the junction of the cortical gray matter and underlying white matter, are most commonly a manifestation of underlying cerebral amyloid angiopathy, although other underlying conditions such as chronic hypertension and an underlying vascular malformation may instead be responsible. By contrast, hemorrhages centered in the deep gray structures of the basal ganglia, thalamus, and the brain stem arise most often as a complication of chronic hypertension, with amyloid angiopathy playing no role. Hemorrhages in the cerebellum can arise from any of these conditions.

ICH in the setting of chronic antithrombotic therapy is increasing in incidence as use of anticoagulants becomes increasingly widespread. Although it is likely that excessive doses of antithrombotic medication (e.g., supratherapeutic prothrombin times in patients receiving warfarin [Coumadin]) can cause ICH in the absence of an underlying chronic disorder of the blood vessels of the brain, the majority of ICH cases in patients receiving antithrombotic medication occur in the absence of an overdose. This suggests that the majority of cases of antithrombotic-associated ICH arise in patients with an underlying disorder of the cerebral vessels such as cerebral amyloid angiopathy or hypertensive vasculopathy.

Recurrent ICH is common among survivors of ICH. In particular, patients 55 years and older who survive a lobar hemorrhage have a risk of recurrent lobar ICH in the range of 10% per year. The explanation for this is likely the inexorable progression of the underlying blood vessel disease, amyloid angiopathy. On the other hand, whereas survivors of ICH in the nonlobar regions are also at high risk for recurrent ICH, adequate control of hypertension following the initial ICH appears to substantially reduce that risk, suggesting that hypertension-related disease of the cerebral blood vessels can be arrested.

Prevention

Adequate control of chronic hypertension reduces the incidence of ICH in addition to reducing the incidence of a broad range of cardiovascular and other conditions. Although no specific therapies are shown to be effective in preventing ICH in patients with cerebral amyloid angiopathy, recognition of this condition might become useful in selecting patients for long-term antithrombotic use. Chronic statin therapy can increase risk of ICH, but more studies are required to inform the decision to withhold statins from patients at high risk for ICH.

Clinical Manifestations

Symptomatic ICH manifests with an acute stroke syndrome such as the sudden development of impaired consciousness, language difficulty, disorientation, or weakness. Nausea and vomiting can be prominent, particularly in patients with cerebellar hemorrhages as well as those who rapidly develop substantial mass effect or hydrocephalus. Headache and seizure at the onset of symptoms are more common in ICH than in ischemic stroke.

Small asymptomatic ICH occurs in the setting of diseases like chronic hypertension and cerebral amyloid angiopathy. These hemorrhages, usually only detectable on magnetic resonance imaging (MRI) of the brain that includes susceptibility-weighted sequences sensitive to the permanent hemosiderin deposits left by all hemorrhages, are increasingly recognized as contributing to age-related deterioration in cognition and memory, as well as gait.

Diagnosis

ICH is a medical emergency. Rapid diagnosis and urgent critical care management (airway, breathing, circulation) are essential, particularly because ICH patients can deteriorate rapidly within hours of presentation. Noncontrast CT scan of the brain is the gold standard for confirming acute ICH, and all patients with suspected acute stroke or ICH should undergo an emergent noncontrast CT scan. In centers where emergent MRI is available, it can be substituted for noncontrast CT only if susceptibility-weighted

sequences are performed. Angiographic imaging in the form of traditional catheter-based angiography or CT angiography should be performed in any patient younger than 55 years or in patients in whom underlying vascular malformation or ruptured saccular aneurysm is suspected. The history and laboratory evaluation, summarized in Box 1, should be focused on identifying possible contributing causes as well as targets for treatment.

Differential Diagnosis

Emergent neuroimaging can confirm the presence of ICH (Box 2). For patients in whom the history is not obtainable, or who have

---

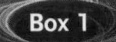 **Box 1** Focused Evaluation of Intracerebral Hemorrhage

Assess airway, breathing, circulation

History
Time of symptom onset (or when last seen well)
Recent trauma or surgery
Headache
Seizures
Alcohol or drug abuse
History of hypertension
Prior stroke
Liver disease
Cancer
Coagulopathy
Medications, including antithrombotics

Physical Examination
General physical examination
Glasgow Coma Scale
NIH stroke scale

Neuroimaging
Computed tomography, magnetic resonance imaging
Angiography for patients younger than 55 years or in whom an underlying vascular lesion is suspected
Venography if venous sinus thrombosis is suspected
Cervical spine imaging if trauma is suspected

Laboratory
Electrolytes
Complete blood count
Coagulation panel
Toxicology screen
Electrocardiogram

Abbreviation: NIH = National Institutes of Health.

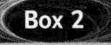 **Box 2** Differential Diagnosis of Intracerebral Hemorrhage

Primary Intracerebral Hemorrhage
Cerebral small-vessel disease
Cerebral amyloid angiopathy
Hypertensive vasculopathy

Secondary Intracerebral Hemorrhage
Vascular malformations
Cerebral venous thrombosis
Hemorrhagic conversion of an ischemic infarct
Moya moya disease
Cerebral vasculitis
Bacterial endocarditis
Brain tumor
Trauma

associated trauma, it is sometimes difficult to distinguish traumatic from nontraumatic ICH. It is therefore essential to examine head imaging for skull fractures and the presence of subdural or subarachnoid hemorrhage, which might be traumatic in origin.

Treatment

After the focused evaluation (see Box 1) is completed, emergency care is devoted to preventing neurologic deterioration (Box 3). Blood pressure elevation is common in ICH; clinical trials are under way to investigate the benefit of blood pressure reduction, and accumulating data suggest that reducing the blood pressure acutely to a systolic reading of 140 is safe and improves outcome.

Because ICH is a devastating condition that most commonly affects the elderly, physicians and families are often confronted with the question of whether their patient or loved one would choose to survive the event. Accurate prediction of prognosis is essential to guide such decision-making. In this context, tools that predict mortality are of limited utility, as they do not give any guidance on the likelihood of functional recovery among survivors. The FUNC score (Table 1) enables prediction of the likelihood of recovering functional independence for patients with primary ICH. Tools such as the FUNC score calculator (http://www.massgeneral.org/stopstroke/funcCalculator.aspx) can be useful in guiding decisions about aggressiveness of care, but their precision remains to be proved. Clinicians are therefore advised to provide care according to the principles outlined in this chapter for all patients at the outset, and to proceed to limitation of aggressive care no sooner than 48 hours after admission to an intensive care unit.

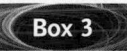

Box 3 Targeted Therapy to Prevent Deterioration in Acute Intracerebral Hemorrhage

Neck stabilization in any patient at risk for cervical spine injury
Anticoagulant-associated ICH: Correct prothrombin time as rapidly as possible using intravenous vitamin K and fresh frozen plasma or prothrombin complex concentrate; recommendations regarding reversal of newer agents such as dabigatran are currently in formulation.
Severe thrombocytopenia or coagulation factor deficiency: Platelet and/or factor replacement. There are no data to support the use of platelet transfusion in ICH patients taking oral antiplatelet agents.
Blood pressure: For patients whose systolic BP is 150 to 220 mm Hg, reduce systolic BP to 140 mm Hg using intravenous agents. Reduce systolic BP to 180 mm Hg for patients whose systolic BP is >220 mm Hg.
Avoid hypoglycemia.
Maintain euthermia.
Anticonvulsant medication: Only in patients who have had a seizure.
External ventricular drainage catheters: Consider for any patient with hydrocephalus or intraventricular hemorrhage.
Emergent surgical clot removal: Indicated for cerebellar hemorrhage with brain stem compression or neurologic deterioration.
Prevention of deep venous thrombosis: Intermittent pneumatic compression device and elastic stockings. Low-dose heparin should be started once serial CT scans confirm that bleeding has stopped and there is no longer any ICH expansion occurring.
Rehabilitation: Multidisciplinary rehabilitation should be offered to all ICH patients.

Abbreviations: BP = blood pressure; CT = computed tomography; ICH = intracerebral hemorrhage.

TABLE 1 FUNC Score

COMPONENT	FUNC SCORE POINTS
ICH Volume (cm³)	
<30	0
30–59	2
≥60	3
Age (y)	
<70	0
70–79	1
≥80	2
ICH Location	
Lobar	0
Deep	1
Infratentorial	2
Glasgow Coma Scale Score	
≥8	0
<8	2
Pre-ICH Cognitive Impairment	
No	0
Yes	1
Total FUNC score	0–10

Abbreviation: ICH = intracerebral hemorrhage.

Monitoring

Initial monitoring of the ICH patient is best provided by an intensive care unit with neurointensive care specialists available. Because subclinical seizures are common in ICH patients, EEG monitoring should be considered in any patient who has had a seizure or whose level of consciousness is altered. Invasive monitoring of intracranial pressure should be considered in patients with evidence of shift of the intracranial contents on neuroimaging.

Complications

Prevention of ICH, particularly recurrent ICH, is increasingly recognized as a priority in making decisions about whether or not to offer chronic anticoagulation to elderly patients with atrial fibrillation, prosthetic heart valves, and other conditions accompanied by high risk of thromboembolic ischemic stroke. Given the established benefit of antithrombotic therapy for preventing ischemic stroke, decision-analysis models suggest that only patients at very high risk for ICH might benefit from antiplatelet therapy rather than anticoagulation, or even neither therapy. Factors that must be considered include the patient's presumed risk for ICH, risk for thrombembolic stroke, expected outcomes from each should they occur, and the patient's preferences. At the present, patients who have survived a lobar ICH and are therefore at very high risk for recurrent ICH should be considered candidates for antiplatelet or no antithrombotic therapy at all.

References

Becker KJ, Baxter AB, Cohen WA, et al. Withdrawal of support in intracerebral hemorrhage may lead to self-fulfilling prophecies. Neurology 2001;56:766–72.
Eckman MH, Rosand J, Knudsen KA, et al. Can patients be anticoagulated after intracerebral hemorrhage? A decision analysis. Stroke 2003;34:1710–6.
Eckman MH, Wong LK, Soo YO, et al. Patient-specific decision-making for warfarin therapy in nonvalvular atrial fibrillation: How will screening with genetics and imaging help? Stroke 2008;39:3308–15.
Kothari RU, Brott T, Broderick JP, et al. The ABCs of measuring intracerebral hemorrhage volumes. Stroke 1996;27:1304–5.

Morgenstern LB, Hemphill JC, Anderson C, et al. Guidelines for the management of spontaneous intracerebral hemorrhage in adults: 2010 update. Stroke 2010;Epub ahead of print.

Rost NS, Smith EE, Chang Y, et al. Prediction of functional outcome in patients with primary intracerebral hemorrhage: The FUNC score. Stroke 2008;39:2304–9.

ISCHEMIC CEREBROVASCULAR DISEASE

Method of
Alvaro Cervera, MD; and Geoffrey A. Donnan, MD

Treatment of ischemic stroke has improved significantly in the past few years, and mortality and disability rates due to this condition have decreased. The demonstration of efficacy of thrombolysis in the management of patients in stroke units has been crucial in this achievement. Control of vascular risk factors has decreased the number and severity of events. Improved management has included high-quality rehabilitation, which is started as soon as possible to improve the recovery (i.e., functional independence) of stroke survivors.

The multidisciplinary management of stroke can be improved with specific educational programs aimed at increasing awareness of stroke in the general population and among professionals. The concept of *time is brain* has a great value in emphasizing that stroke is an emergency. Because the window for the available time-dependent treatments is very narrow, avoiding delay is the major goal in the prehospital phase of acute stroke care. All stroke patients must be transported as soon as possible to the closest hospital with a stroke unit. In rural or remote areas with no stroke unit facilities, telemedicine has proved to be a valid alternative.

Prevention

Lifestyle modification can be a major contributor to reducing the risk of ischemic stroke. Strategies to achieve this protection include avoiding smoking and excessive alcohol consumption; keeping a low–normal body mass index; practicing regular exercise; and having a diet low in salt and saturated fat, high in fruit and vegetables, and rich in fiber. There is no need to add vitamin supplements to the diet because they have not been found to affect stroke prevention.

Regular assessment of vascular risk factors (e.g., hypertension, diabetes, hypercholesterolemia) is important because their control can reduce significantly the incidence of vascular events. Blood pressure should be managed with diet and pharmacologic therapy, aiming at normal levels of 120/80 mm Hg. After an ischemic stroke, blood pressure should be lowered even in patients with normal blood pressure. Diabetes should be managed with lifestyle modification and pharmacologic therapy as required, and blood pressure needs to be more tightly controlled in these patients (<130/80 mm Hg). The best antihypertensive treatments for diabetics are angiotensin-converting enzyme (ACE) inhibitors or angiotensin receptor antagonists. Hypercholesterolemia should be managed with lifestyle modification and a statin. After a noncardioembolic ischemic stroke, statins are beneficial in all patients for secondary prevention.

Postmenopausal hormone replacement therapy should be avoided for the primary or secondary prevention of stroke because it can increase the risk of new vascular events. Other strategies to prevent stroke include the treatment of obstructive sleep apnea with continuous positive airway pressure (CPAP) breathing.

Antithrombotic Therapy

Low-dose aspirin can be used for the primary prevention of stroke in women or of myocardial infarction in men. Nevertheless, its effect is very small, and it cannot be recommended on a population-wide basis. Aspirin is beneficial for the prevention of stroke in patients with asymptomatic carotid stenosis.

In patients with atrial fibrillation, aspirin can prevent ischemic events in those younger than 65 years and free of vascular risk

TABLE 1	Prevention of Stroke in Patients with Atrial Fibrillation
PREVENTION	**THERAPY**
Primary prevention	
No risk factors	<65 years old: aspirin 65–75 years old: aspirin or warfarin >75 years old: warfarin
Risk factors*	All age groups: warfarin
Secondary prevention	All groups: warfarin

*Previous systemic embolism, high blood pressure, or poor left ventricular function.

factors. In patients older than 65 years, anticoagulation is the first option, although aspirin is an alternative for those younger than 75 years without other risk factors (Table 1). In all patients with atrial fibrillation who have suffered a stroke, anticoagulation should aim for an international normalized ratio (INR) of 2.0 to 3.0. Patients with prosthetic heart valves should also receive anticoagulation, and the target INR depends on the prosthesis type. Dabigatran, a direct thrombin inhibitor, has recently shown to be more effective than warfarin in non-valvular atrial fibrillation at high doses (150 mg twice daily) and is associated with a lower hemorrhagic risk at low doses (110 mg twice daily).

After ischemic stroke, all patients should receive antithrombotic therapy. Antiplatelet agents are the first choice unless anticoagulation is required. The most effective regimen is aspirin and extended-release dipyridamole combined (Aggrenox). However, after the PRoFESS trial failed to show the noninferiority criteria for aspirin plus dipyridamole compared with clopidogrel (Plavix), this superiority is not clear. Aspirin plus dipyridamole, clopidogrel, or aspirin alone are acceptable therapies for secondary stroke prevention. Triflusal[2] and cilostazol (in Asian populations) are other alternatives. The combination of aspirin and clopidogrel is not recommended after stroke, except if there is an association with unstable angina or non-Q-wave myocardial infarction or if there has been a recent stenting.

Anticoagulation is usually indicated for secondary prevention if the stroke cause is cardioembolic and in specific situations such as aortic arch atheroma, fusiform aneurysms of the basilar artery, cervical artery dissection, or patent foramen ovale in the presence of proven deep venous thrombosis. However, level one evidence is lacking for these approaches.

Management of Carotid Stenosis

In patients with asymptomatic carotid stenosis (≥60%), surgery is indicated only if the risk of stroke is high. Endarterectomy is the treatment of choice if the stenosis is symptomatic (i.e., has been associated with an ipsilateral stroke or transient ischemic attack) and severe (70%–99%). Surgery should be performed in centers with a perioperative complication rate of less than 6% and as soon as possible after the last ischemic event.

Endarterectomy may be indicated for certain patients with moderate stenosis (50%–69%), although it should be performed only in centers with a perioperative complication rate of less than 3% to be effective. In cases of symptomatic carotid lesions, angioplasty plus stenting is recommended only for selected patients, mainly younger than 70 years old. If stenting is performed, a combination of clopidogrel and aspirin is required immediately before the procedure and for at least 1 month to prevent stent thrombosis.

In patients with intracranial atheromatosis and stroke recurrences despite appropriate antiplatelet therapy, endovascular treatment may be a reasonable choice.

[2] Not available in the United States.

Management of Acute Ischemic Stroke

All stroke patients should be treated in a stroke unit, because this is associated with a reduction of death, dependency, and the need for institutional care. This effect is seen for all types of patients, irrespective of gender, age, stroke subtype, and stroke severity. Patients with stroke should have a careful clinical assessment, including a neurologic examination. The use of a stroke rating scale, such as the National Institutes of Health Stroke Scale (NIHSS), provides important information about the severity of stroke.

Urgent cranial computed tomography (CT) is mandatory after an ischemic stroke before starting any therapy. Alternatively, magnetic resonance imaging (MRI) can be performed and can provide additional information about the selection of patients for thrombolytic therapy beyond 3 hours. However, there is not enough evidence to recommend its routine use in the acute stroke setting.

For the detection and early management of the medical complications of stroke, neurologic status, pulse, blood pressure, temperature, and oxygen saturation should be monitored. Similarly, serum glucose levels need to be monitored and hyperglycemia treated with insulin accordingly. Normal saline is recommended for fluid replacement during the first 24 hours after stroke. If the patient has fever, treatment with paracetamol (acetaminophen) may be used while sources of infection are being sought. Reducing blood pressure is recommended only in patients with extremely high blood pressure or when indicated by other medical conditions. Blood pressure should be lowered gradually, avoiding abrupt changes.

Thrombolysis

All patients with an ischemic stroke within 3 hours of onset should receive thrombolytic treatment with intravenous tissue plasminogen activator (tPA [Activase]) unless contraindicated, because it is effective in improving stroke outcome (Box 1). The ECASS III clinical trial showed that this effect could also be obtained over a longer period (4.5 hours). Based on the available evidence, thrombolysis with tPA can be given in ischemic stroke within 4.5 hours of onset, provided that it is approved by the local regulatory authorities. There is also evidence from phase II trials (e.g., EPITHET) that selecting patients with MRI to assess the penumbra can be an appropriate tool to extend the time to more than 3 hours, because tPA was associated with increased reperfusion in these patients and a trend toward better outcomes. Nevertheless, increasing the time window does not mean that treatment can be delayed. As evidenced by pooled analysis, earlier treatment results in a better outcome. There is little evidence that thrombolysis is effective in patients older than 80 years, but the available information indicates that it is safe.

Intraarterial administration of a thrombolytic agent within a 6-hour time can be an alternative therapy. Another treatment, which has been approved by some regulatory authorities, is the MERCI device. It mechanically removes the thrombus, which can be associated with thrombolytic therapy. However, no evidence for the clinical efficacy of mechanical devices has been derived from randomized clinical trials.

Antithrombotic Drugs

All patients should receive a low dose of aspirin daily, and this should be started within 48 hours after stroke onset. The use of other antiplatelet agents during the acute phase of stroke cannot be recommended based on available evidence. Similarly, early administration of unfractionated heparin, low-molecular-weight heparin, or heparinoids is not indicated in acute ischemic stroke patients.

Treatment of Stroke Complications

Brain edema develops between the second and fifth day after stroke onset and is the cause of early deterioration and death. In the case of a malignant infarction of the middle cerebral artery, the mortality rate is 80%. In patients younger than 60 years with this pattern of cerebral infarction, hemicraniectomy has been effective in reducing mortality and severe disability, as shown in the pooled analysis of the DECIMAL, DESTINY, and HAMLET trials. Surgery needs to be performed within 48 hours after symptom onset. Surgical decompression is also indicated in the case of large cerebellar infarctions that compress the brainstem.

Stroke-associated infections require appropriate antibiotics, but prophylactic administration is discouraged. Venous thromboembolism is a frequent complication after stroke, but its incidence can be reduced with appropriate hydration and graded compression stockings. If the risk of deep venous thrombosis or pulmonary embolism is high, the use of subcutaneous heparin or low-molecular-weight heparin is beneficial. Early mobilization is an effective way of preventing complications such as aspiration pneumonia or pressure ulcers. Anticonvulsants are administered only to prevent recurrent seizure but are not used prophylactically.

In stroke patients at risk for falls, hip fracture can be prevented with bisphosphonates. In case of urinary incontinence, specialist assessment and management are recommended. Dysphagia is common after stroke and is associated with a higher incidence of medical complications and increased mortality. Malnutrition also predicts a poor functional outcome and increased mortality, and it is important to assess the swallowing capacity and the nutritional status of the patient.

Rehabilitation should be started after admission to the stroke unit. The optimal timing of first mobilization is unclear, but mobilization within the first few days appears to be well tolerated. The AVERT study demonstrated that very early mobilization (i.e., within 24 hours of symptom onset) is safe and feasible. An ongoing study is assessing its efficacy and cost-effectiveness. It is important to assess cognitive deficits and depression during the patient's hospital stay, because this may require specific intervention, although evidence about the type is lacking.

| **Box 1** | Treatment of Acute Ischemic Stroke: Intravenous Administration of Tissue Plasminogen Activator |

- Infuse 0.9 mg/kg (maximum dose 90 mg) of tissue plasminogen activator (tPA) over 60 minutes, with 10% of the dose given as a bolus over 1 minute.
- Admit the patient to a stroke unit for monitoring. Perform neurologic assessment and blood pressure measurement every 15 minutes during the infusion, every 30 minutes thereafter for the next 6 hours, and then hourly until 24 hours after treatment. Administer antihypertensive medications to maintain systolic blood pressure ≤180 and diastolic ≤105.
- If intracranial hemorrhage is suspected, discontinue the infusion and obtain an emergency CT scan.
- Obtain a follow-up CT scan at 24 hours before starting anticoagulants or antiplatelet agents.

References

Adams Jr HP, del Zoppo G, Alberts MJ, et al. Guidelines for the early management of adults with ischemic stroke: A guideline from the American Heart Association/American Stroke Association Stroke Council, Clinical Cardiology Council, Cardiovascular Radiology and Intervention Council, and the Atherosclerotic Peripheral Vascular Disease and Quality of Care Outcomes in Research Interdisciplinary Working Groups: The American Academy of Neurology affirms the value of this guideline as an educational tool for neurologists. Stroke 2007;38:1655–711.

Bernhardt J, Dewey H, Thrift A, et al. A very early rehabilitation trial for stroke (AVERT): Phase II safety and feasibility. Stroke 2008;39:390–6.

Davis SM, Donnan GA, Parsons MW, et al. Effects of alteplase beyond 3 h after stroke in the Echoplanar Imaging Thrombolytic Evaluation Trial (EPITHET): A placebo-controlled randomised trial. Lancet Neurol 2008;7:299–309.

European Stroke Organisation (ESO). Executive Committee; ESO Writing Committee: Guidelines for management of ischaemic stroke and transient ischaemic attack 2008. Cerebrovasc Dis 2008;25:457–507.

Hacke W, Kaste M, Bluhmki E, et al. Thrombolysis with alteplase 3 to 4.5 hours after acute ischemic stroke. N Engl J Med 2008;359:1317–29.

Kent DM, Thaler DE. Stroke prevention—Insights from incoherence. N Engl J Med 2008;359:1287–9.

Sacco RL, Diener HC, Yusuf S, et al. Aspirin and extended-release dipyridamole versus clopidogrel for recurrent stroke. N Engl J Med 2008;359:1238–51.

Vahedi K, Hofmeijer J, Juettler E, et al. Early decompressive surgery in malignant infarction of the middle cerebral artery: A pooled analysis of three randomised controlled trials. Lancet Neurol 2007;6:215–22.

MIGRAINE HEADACHE

Method of
Anne Walling, MB, ChB

CURRENT DIAGNOSIS

- Recurrent headaches occur along with nausea/vomiting and/or photophobia and phonophobia.
- Each episode lasts 4 to 72 hours and usually ends with sleep.
- The headache has at least two of the classic features: it is unilateral, pulsating, moderate-to-severe intensity, and/or aggravated by movement.
- Five similar episodes must occur for diagnosis.
- No other condition better accounts for symptoms.

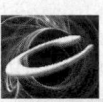

CURRENT THERAPY

Acute Migraine Episodes
- Nonsteroidal antiinflammatory drugs (NSAIDs)
- Triptans
- Ergots
- Antiemetics
- Isometheptene-containing products
- Combination medications

Prophylaxis
- β-Blockers
- Tricyclic antidepressants
- Anticonvulsants
- Petasites (butterbur)

Definition

Migraines are episodic headaches accompanied by nausea and/or photophobia plus phonophobia. The headache must last 4 to 72 hours and have at least two defining features (it is unilateral, pulsating, moderate-to-severe intensity, and/or aggravated by movement). Five attacks and the exclusion of other conditions are required for diagnosis. Patients with migraine may also suffer from other types of headaches (e.g., tension).

Epidemiology

About 23 million U.S. adults (18% of women, 6% of men) report migraine. Onset is usually between ages 12 and 30. Prevalence peaks in young adults. Migraine is diagnosed in about 30% of family medicine headache patients. A positive migraine diagnosis by a family physician is over 95% accurate, but cases may be misdiagnosed, especially as a tension or sinus headache.

Risk Factors

Besides age and female sex, the biggest risk factor is family history.

Pathophysiology

Migraine results from complex interactions among multiple genetic and environmental factors. The primary neuronal process may be a depolarizing wave (Leão's cortical spreading depression) activating the trigeminal nerve afferents and causing vasoactive neuropeptide release, local inflammation, vascular instability, and blood-brain barrier changes. The type and location of symptoms depend on which parts of the complex trigeminovascular system are activated. This system innervates pain-sensitive blood vessels and meninges and connects with various areas of the brain, including the thalamus and sensory cortex. Biochemically, serotonin, calcitonin gene-related peptide (CGRP), and other substances are implicated in migraine.

The suspected role of right–left cardiac shunts, especially patent foramen ovale, has not been validated.

Prevention

The vulnerability to migraine cannot be eliminated, but patients can be assisted to reduce the number of attacks and minimize the negative impact of migraine through a consideration of triggers and use of prophylaxis.

Triggers

Some migraineurs have specific precipitants for an attack. The strongest evidence is for stress, menstruation, missed meals, weather changes, and sleep disturbances. Migraines may be associated with stress or its relief (weekend migraine). Avoiding or minimizing triggers may reduce the likelihood of a migraine.

Prophylactic Medications

The U.S. Headache Consortium (USHC) recommends discussing prophylaxis with patients who meet the following criteria:
- They have severe and/or frequent symptoms that disrupt daily activities despite adequate treatment.
- They have a poor efficacy or inability to use standard treatments for acute attacks (e.g., because of adverse effects, contraindications, cost).
- They have specific rare migraine syndromes associated with dangerous neurologic complications (basilar migraine, prolonged aura, hemiplegic migraine).

Successful prophylaxis depends on balancing potential benefit against adverse effects and the demands of adherence to long-term medications. Selection of a prophylactic medication depends on patient factors (personal preferences, comorbidities such as hypertension and depression) and medication concerns (including efficacy, cost, pharmacokinetics, adverse effects, and medication interactions).

Prophylactic medication should be started at a low dose and gradually increased until benefit is demonstrated or adverse effects outweigh benefits. Individual patients show enormous variation in the effective dose of prophylactic medication. An adequate trial of prophylaxis requires several months. A patient may have poor outcomes from one agent but good response to an agent from a different class. A headache diary is useful to monitor symptoms and adverse effects. Therapy should be reevaluated every 3 to 6 months.

The USHC evidence-based recommendations for migraine prophylaxis based on efficacy and potential adverse effects have been updated by the American Academy of Neurology (AAN) (Table 1). The AAN (2012) and European (2009) guidelines confirm the use of certain beta-blockers and antiepileptic medications and also for the first time rate herbal and complementary treatments. Level A evidence was established for petasites (butterbur extract)[1] 50 to 75 mg twice daily. Magnesium (400–600 mg),[2] feverfew[1] (as MIG-99 extract, 6.25 mg three times daily), and riboflavin[2]

---

[1]Not FDA approved for this indication.
[2]Not available in the United States.

TABLE 1	Medications for Migraine Prophylaxis			
	β-BLOCKERS	ANTIEPILEPTICS	ANTIDEPRESSANTS	OTHERS
Level A: Established efficacy	Metoprolol (Lopressor)[1] 100–200 mg/d Propranolol (Inderal) 40–240[2] mg/d Timolol (Blocadren) 10–15 mg bid	Divalproex sodium (Depakote ER) 750–1500 mg/d[2] Sodium valproate (Depakene)[1] 800–1500 mg/d[2] Topiramate (Topamax) 25–100 mg/d		Frovatriptan (Frova)[1] 2.5 mg daily or bid*
Level B: Probably effective	Atenolol (Tenormin)[1] 50–200 mg/d Nadolol (Corgard)[1] 20–160 mg/d		Amitriptyline (Elavil)[1] 50–150 mg/d Venlafaxine (Effexor)[1] 75–150 mg/d	Fenoprofen (Nalfon)[1] 1800 mg/d Ibuprofen (Motrin)[1,†] Ketoprofen (Orudis)[1] 150 mg/d Naproxen (Naprosyn)[1,†] Naproxen sodium (Anaprox)[1] 1100 mg/d Naratriptan (Amerge)[1] 1 mg bid × 5 days premenses Zolmitriptan (Zomig)[1] 2.5 mg bid or tid*
Level C: Possibly effective	Nebivolol (Bystolic)[1] 5 mg/d Pindolol (Visken)[1,†]	Carbamazepine (Tegretol)[1] 600 mg/d		Mefenamic acid (Ponstel)[1] 1500 mg/d Flurbiprofen (Ansaid)[1] 200 mg/d Cyproheptadine (Periactin)[1,†] Lisinopril (Prinivil)[1,†] Candesartan (Atacand)[1,†] Clonidine (Catapres)[1] 0.075–0.15 mg/d Guanfacine (Intuniv)[1] 1 mg/d
Level U: Insufficient or conflicting data for efficacy	Bisoprolol (Zebeta)[1,†]	Gabapentin (Neurontin)[1] 900–2400 mg/d	Protriptyline (Vivactil)[1,†] Fluvoxamine (Luvox)[1,†] Fluoxetine (Prozac)[1] 20–40 mg/d	Aspirin[1] 1300 mg/d Indomethacin (Indocin)[1,†] Nicardipine (Cardene)[1,†] Nifedipine (Procardia)[1,†] Nimodipine (Nimotop)[1] 120 mg/d Verapamil (Calan)[1] 240–320 mg/d Acetazolamide (Diamox)[1] 250 mg bid Warfarin (Coumadin)[1,†] Cyclandelate (Cyclospasmol)[3,†]
Other: Possibly/ probably ineffective	Acebutolol (Sectral)[1]	Lamotrigine (Lamictal)[1] Clomipramine (Anafranil)[1] Clonazepam (Klonopin)[1] Oxcarbazepine (Trileptal)[1] Telmisartan (Micardis)[1]		

Sources: Silberstein SD, Holland S, Freitag F, et al. Evidence-based guideline update: Pharmacologic treatment for episodic migraine prevention in adults: Report of the Quality Standards Subcommittee of the American Academy of Neurology and the American Headache Society. Neurology 2012;78:1337–45; Silberstein SD, Holland S, Freitag F, et al. Evidence-based guideline update: NSAIDs and other complementary treatments for episodic migraine prevention in adults: Report of the Quality Standards Subcommittee of the American Academy of Neurology and the American Headache Society. Neurology 2012;78:1346–53. Dosages from Becker WJ, Gawel M, Mackie G, et al. Migraine treatment. Can J Neurol Sci 2007;34:S10–19 and Evers S, Afra J, Frese A, et al. EFNS guideline on the drug treatment of migraine: Revised report of an EFNS task force. Eur J Neuro 2009;16:968–81; Ramadan NM, Silberstein SD, Freitag F, Gilbert TT, Frishberg BM. Evidence-based guidelines for migraine headache in the primary care setting: Pharmacological management for prevention of migraine. U.S. Headache Consortium, 2000. Available at www.aan.com/professional/practice.

[1]Not FDA approved for this indication.
[2]Exceeds dosage recommended by the manufacturer.
[3]Not available in the United States.
*Short-term use only.
[†]Dosage not established.

(400 mg) were classified as level B. Coenzyme Q[1] (100 mg tid) was classified as level C and omega-3[1] (3 g twice daily) as level U.

Nonpharmacologic Therapies

Nondrug therapies to prevent attacks may be preferred by some patients, including those who have had limited success with medications. The four main types of nonpharmacologic therapies are relaxation training, biofeedback therapy, cognitive-behavioral training (stress-management training), and physical treatments (acupuncture, cervical manipulation, and mobilization therapy).

Each may be used alone or in combination with other therapies, including medications.

Research evidence is lacking or controversial for many of these therapies. The USHC concluded that relaxation training, thermal biofeedback combined with relaxation training, and cognitive-behavioral therapy are all modestly effective in preventing migraine (Grade A); behavioral therapy (relaxation, biofeedback) combined with preventive drug therapy (propranolol [Inderal], amitriptyline [Elavil][2]) may provide additional clinical improvement (Grade B); but no recommendations could be made for

[1]Not FDA approved for this indication.

[2]Not available in the United States.

hypnosis, acupuncture, transcutaneous electric neuromuscular stimulation, cervical manipulation, occlusal adjustment, and hyperbaric oxygen as preventive or acute therapy for migraine.

Clinical Manifestations

Prodrome: About 60% of migraineurs experience 1 to 2 days of symptoms such as yawning, intense hunger, mild euphoria, or depression/irritability before an attack.

Aura

About 25% of migraineurs report consistent, specific neurologic changes about 5 to 60 minutes before the onset of headache. Common aura symptoms include visual (flashing lights, zigzag lines, scotoma), sensory (paresthesia, numbness), or speech disturbances.

Symptoms

Migraine combines a specific type of headache (unilateral, throbbing, moderate-to-severe, worse with activity) with other diagnostic symptoms (nausea/vomiting and/or photophobia/ phonophobia). Many patients also experience vertigo, allodynia, and fatigue. Additional symptoms may be prominent in migraine subtypes such as basilar or ophthalmoplegic migraine. Patients vary enormously in the symptom pattern as well as in the frequency, intensity, and impact of attacks. Some have infrequent episodes with mild symptoms, whereas others are incapacitated by recurrent, severe attacks.

Duration and Complications

Classically, migraine patients lie still in a dark room until sleep resolves symptoms. Afterward, some patients feel refreshed, others are tired, and others experience localized skull tenderness or headache on movement.

Status migrainosus is debilitating migraine lasting more than 72 hours. The patient may be dehydrated, exhausted, and/or suffering adverse medication effects. Very rarely, migraine subtypes (basilar, ophthalmoplegic, hemiplegic) are complicated by seizure or cerebral infarction. Chronic migraine (defined as symptoms on more than 15 days per month) requires investigation, especially for medication-rebound headache. With inappropriate therapy, migraine can transform into chronic daily headache.

Diagnosis

Migraine diagnosis depends on history. Identifying classic symptoms has a high probability of accurate diagnosis (Table 2). The headache pattern should distinguish migraine from other primary headaches (e.g., tension, cluster). The clinical history and examination target identifying conditions that could cause secondary headache. Neurologic examination must be documented, because change over time is crucial in detecting the rare cases of intracranial pathology that present with migraine-type symptoms.

Diagnostic imaging is not indicated in migraine patients with normal neurologic examination. Guidelines recommended imaging only for atypical symptoms or "red flag" indications of serious pathology but recognize that some patients may require testing for excessive anxiety (Table 3). Other testing (e.g., complete blood count, sedimentation rate, analysis of cerebrospinal fluid) are

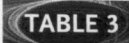

TABLE 2 Diagnostic Probability of Symptoms for Migraine (POUND Mnemonic)

Character of headache described as pulsing or throbbing
Duration average **O**ne day (4–72 h)
Location **U**nilateral
Associated symptoms include **N**ausea or Vomiting
Severity ranked as **D**isabling
Probability of migraine 92% with 4 POUND symptoms, 64% with 3, 17% with 0–2.

From Gilmore and Michael (2011).

TABLE 3 "Red Flag" Findings Associated with Increased Risk of Underlying Pathology in Headache

Acute onset
Occipitonuchal location
Age greater than 55 years
Associated symptoms (fever, neurologic symptoms, mental status changes)
Abnormal neurologic examination

Adapted from Silberstein (2000).
Notes: Headache type, severity, characteristics, or duration were not risk factors; increasing frequency and headache awakening from sleep were positively associated. In the ER setting, patients over 50 years of age with acute onset and neurologic signs had 98.6% specificity for serious intracranial pathology.

selected to identify specific potential causes of symptoms in individual patients. Guidelines stress that testing should be done only if results are likely to change management.

Differential Diagnosis

Other recurrent headaches, especially tension or cluster, can usually be distinguished by the combination of features (unilaterality, nausea, photo/phonophobia) and pattern (frequency of occurrence and duration).

Intracranial pathology (including acute or chronic bleeding, infection, or space-occupying lesions) can cause headache resembling migraine. This can also occur with head and neck conditions such as temporal arteritis, sinusitis, temporomandibular joint syndrome, and various neuralgias as well as systemic conditions including carbon monoxide poisoning, sudden rise in blood pressure, or medication adverse effect. Diagnosis depends on recognizing that the clinical picture is not completely congruent with migraine, and also on identifying risk factors, symptoms, and signs, along with positive targeted testing for the underlying condition.

Treatment

Treatment goals for acute migraine are rapid symptom control, minimizing adverse effects, preventing recurrence, and optimizing function. Self-management and efficient use of resources are priorities. The USHC guidelines (2000) and more recent European guidelines (2009) are based on research evidence. Individual patients vary enormously in response to specific medications and in the effective dose. Patients who do not respond to an appropriate dose of one medication may have good outcomes from another agent in the same class or one from a different class. Medications should be taken in adequate dosage as early as possible during a migraine attack. Nonoral formats or adjunct medications may be necessary because of vomiting or poor absorption resulting from gastric stasis.

Many medications have antimigraine activity (Table 4). Considerations in selecting an agent include patient comorbidities (e.g., hypertension) and the medication's adverse effects. Cost may be a significant concern.

Of first-line therapies, NSAIDs or combination analgesics with caffeine are recommended for mild-to-moderate attacks or more severe attacks that have previously responded to these agents. Evidence also supports intramuscular ketorolac (Toradol)[2] as a useful strategy for vomiting patients.

Triptans are recommended for moderate-to-severe migraine and for mild-to-severe attacks that have not responded adequately to other first-line therapies. Individual triptans have comparable efficacy and tolerability but differ in speed of onset and duration of action. This allows for the selection of an agent with pharmacokinetics that correspond to the patient's migraine symptom pattern. The most effective agent and dose for each patient can only be established by experience. Triptans may be combined

---

[2]Not available in the United States.

TABLE 4	Medications for Treatment of Acute Migraine	
	MEDICATION (INITIAL ORAL DOSE mg)	**LEVEL OF EVIDENCE**
First Line	Aspirin (250 mg), acetaminophen (250 mg), caffeine (65 mg) (Excedrin Migraine)	A
	NSAIDs:	
	Naproxen (Naprosyn) (250–500 mg)	A
	Ibuprofen (Motrin) (200–800 mg)	A[†]
	Aspirin*	A
	Triptans:	
	Almotriptan (Axert) (6.25–12.5 mg) tab	A
	Eletriptan (Relpax) (20–40 mg) tab	A
	Frovatriptan (Frova) (2.5 mg) tab	A
	Naratriptan (Amerge) (1–2.5 mg) tab	A
	Rizatriptan (Maxalt) (5–10 mg) tab (also oral disintegrating tab)	A
	Sumatriptan (Imitrex) (25–100 mg) tab (also nasal spray [5–20 mg], subcutaneous injection [6 mg])	A
	Zolmitriptan (Zomig) (2.5, 5 mg) tab (also oral disintegrating tab, nasal spray [2.5, 5 mg])	A
Other Agents	Ergots:	
	Dihydroergotamine nasal spray (Migranal [1 spray each nostril])	B
	Dihydroergotamine IV (D.H.E. 45) IV (0.5–1 mg), IM (0.5–1 mg), SC (1 mg)	B
	Ergotamine (Ergomar) (2 mg) tab	B
	Ergotamine (2 mg) plus caffeine (200 mg) tab (Cafergot)	
	Antiemetics:	
	Prochlorperazine (Compazine)[1] IV (10 mg), PR (25 mg)	B
	Metoclopramide (Reglan)[1] (10 mg) oral, IM, IV	B
	Isometheptene-containing product:	
	Acetaminophen 325 mg +dichloralphenazone 100 mg +isometheptene 65 mg (Midrin)	B

[1]Not FDA approved for this indication

*Doses <1000 mg in combination with antiemetics and other agents in studies.

[†]Not included in U.S. Headache Consortium Guidelines, 2000.

synergistically with NSAIDs. Potential triptan adverse effects include vasoconstriction and serotonin syndrome.

Ergotamines are effective in migraine but limited by adverse effects, especially vasoconstriction. They are less effective than triptans but may have good results in some patients. Nasal spray is useful if the patient cannot take oral medications. In emergency room studies, parenteral dihydroergotamine (D.H.E. 45) combined with antiemetics has been as effective as opiates. Opiates are rarely appropriate for migraine. Studies show that other agents are more effective with fewer adverse effects and no risk of addiction or exploitation.

Monitoring

Regular monitoring can allow for the adjustment of medication for maximum efficacy and minimal adverse effects, promote healthy lifestyles, and aid in screening for migraine comorbidities, especially depression. Conversion to chronic daily headache by overuse of medications is a major concern.

References

Gilmore B, Michael M. Treatment of acute migraine headache. Am Fam Physician 2011;83:271–80.

Headache Classification Committee of the International Headache Society. Classification and diagnostic criteria for headache disorders, cranial neuralgia, and facial pain. Cephalalgia 1988;8:1–96.

Lipton RB, Stewart WF, Diamond S, et al. Prevalence and burden of migraine in the United States: Data from the American Migraine Study II. Headache 2001;41:646–57.

Silberstein SD. Practice parameter: Evidence-based guidelines for migraine headache (an evidence-based review): Report of the Quality Standards Subcommittee of the American Academy of Neurology. Neurology 2000;55:754–62.

http://www.americanheadachesociety.org/professionalresources/USHeadache ConsortiumGuidelines.asp.

MULTIPLE SCLEROSIS

Method of

B. Mark Keegan, MD

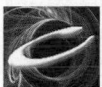

CURRENT DIAGNOSIS

- Multiple sclerosis (MS) is an autoimmune demyelinating disease of the central nervous system (CNS).
- Diagnosis is secured from having repeated CNS demyelinating attacks and/or new CNS demyelinating lesions on magnetic resonance imaging (MRI) or progressive neurologic dysfunction consistent with MS with no better alternative explanation.

CURRENT THERAPY

- Acute attacks of multiple sclerosis (MS) are treated with high-dose corticosteroids and, in severe cases, plasma exchange.
- Therapy is directed at relapsing–remitting disease with interferon β1, glatiramer acetate (Copaxone), fingolimod, teriflunomide, dimethyl fumarate, and natalizumab (Tysabri). Therapy for secondary progressive MS (typically with ongoing relapses) is mitoxantrone (Novantrone).
- Novel MS medications, including further oral medications, and infusion-based monoclonal antibodies, are currently under scientific evaluation.

Multiple sclerosis (MS) is an autoimmune inflammatory demyelinating disease of the central nervous system (CNS) that affects approximately 400,000 people in the United States alone.

Risk Factors

Women are at least twice as likely to develop MS as are men. Other known risk factors for developing MS include ethnicity, genetic background, and environmental exposures. Persons of European ethnicity, particularly those born and reared in extreme northern or southern latitudes, are particularly susceptible to MS. African Americans are less likely to be diagnosed with MS than European Americans, but they have a more severe clinical course. Genetic susceptibility is associated with the major histocompatibility (MHC) allele HLA-DRB1 as well as interleukin-2 and interleukin-7 receptors. Low serum vitamin D levels are associated with an increased risk of development of MS in whites but are of unclear significance in the severity of its clinical course. There are intriguing but as yet unproven associations with infection with Epstein-Barr virus (infectious mononucleosis), particularly if this is contracted later in adolescence. Exposure to Epstein-Barr virus may be necessary but insufficient for developing MS. Cigarette smoking is associated with an increased risk of development of MS and likely is associated with an increased severity and clinical course of MS, including that of cognitive impairment.

Pathophysiology

The etiology and pathophysiology of MS as a whole remains uncertain. However, most evidence supports an inflammatory demyelinating disease induced by uncertain environmental factors in a genetically susceptible host. Animal studies including experimental allergic encephalomyelitis and Theiler's murine encephalomyelitis virus also point to an autoimmune inflammatory demyelinating etiology, possibly associated with viral infection. Studies that suggest chronic cerebrospinal vascular insufficiency has an important association with MS remain unconfirmed.

Pathophysiology likely varies among individual patients with MS. Four distinct pathologies in active demyelinating MS lesions have been described. Pattern 1 displays marked macrophage infiltration without humoral abnormalities. Pattern 2 shows distinct humoral abnormalities with complement activation and immunoglobulin (Ig) deposition. Pattern 3 involves primary oligodendrocyte degeneration and early loss of myelin-associated glycoprotein. Pattern 4 reveals oligodendrocyte dystrophy in periplaque white matter. Early studies suggest there could be a therapeutic advantage with different therapies for different types of demyelinating disease.

Prevention

Currently, there is no known way to prevent the development of MS. Patients with a single clinical attack of demyelination and abnormal magnetic resonance imaging (MRI) ("high-risk" clinically isolated syndrome) have a delayed onset to MS diagnosis with immunomodulatory therapy; however, there is no evidence to support that this prevents the eventual development of MS.

Clinical Manifestations

The clinical course of MS is varied. Approximately 85% of patients present with a relapsing–remitting course. This entails an acute impairment within the CNS, depending on the area of inflammation. A demyelinating cause of a focal neurologic symptom is suggested by an onset over hours to days, with a plateau of impairment over a few weeks. Symptoms then improve either spontaneously or with the use of corticosteroids over a number of days to weeks or longer. Following this, however, symptoms might not completely resolve. Inflammation within the optic nerve (optic neuritis) is heralded by painful, unilateral, central monocular visual deficit (central scotoma). Symptoms of brain stem dysfunction include binocular diplopia, sensory deficits unilaterally on the face and contralaterally on the arm and leg, significant dysarthria, and vertigo. Cerebellar dysfunction is seen with pure ataxia that is typically unilateral. Spinal cord inflammation is indicated by a distinctive, usually gradually rising sensory level of deficit that commonly is accompanied by bowel and bladder impairment and paraparesis or quadriparesis, depending on a thoracic versus cervical level of the lesion.

Progressive forms of MS include secondary progressive MS and primary progressive MS. These are heralded by a slow (months to years) but steady and insidious, progressive neurologic deficit, usually a progressive myelopathy of upper motor neuron gait disorder with spasticity, neurogenic bladder and bowel impairment, and progressive weakness. Occasionally, patients with progressive MS have insidious cerebellar ataxia or dementia in isolation or in association with the myelopathy. Secondary progressive MS is diagnosed when a patient has had a history of at least one clinical attack (relapse) with improvement in the past. Primary progressive MS is diagnosed in the entire absence of any prior relapse but with progressive CNS disease consistent with MS and typical MRI brain or spinal lesions, often with cerebrospinal fluid (CSF) or visual evoked potential abnormalities that support the diagnosis.

Diagnosis

The diagnosis of MS is formalized by the revised McDonald criteria. This entails having two or more clinical attacks (relapses) in the accompaniment of two or more objective lesions seen on clinical examination or with evidence for dissemination in space and time diagnosed by further development of new MRI lesions. Additionally, patients with a single clinical attack who have both the presence of MRI gadolinium enhancing lesions (indicative of prior MS lesions) and nongadolinium enhancing lesions (indicative of acute MS lesions) may now be diagnosed with MS. Progressive MS is diagnosed when there is progressive disease for at least 1 year and abnormal MRI scan of the brain and abnormal MRI scan of the spinal cord, with or without abnormal CSF and visual evoked potentials (Figure 1). An abnormal CSF examination is defined as elevated oligoclonal IgG bands within CSF that are not present in serum with or without elevations in the IgG index. Occasionally, visual evoked potentials and somatosensory evoked potentials are used to further document dissemination of MS within the CNS. Serologic investigations are done primarily to rule out MS mimickers depending on and directed by any accompanying systemic symptoms and the clinical setting in individual patients. These may include antinuclear antibodies (ANA for lupus), erythrocyte sedimentation rate, anticardiolipin antibodies, vitamin B_{12}, Lyme serology, and chest imaging for CNS sarcoidosis.

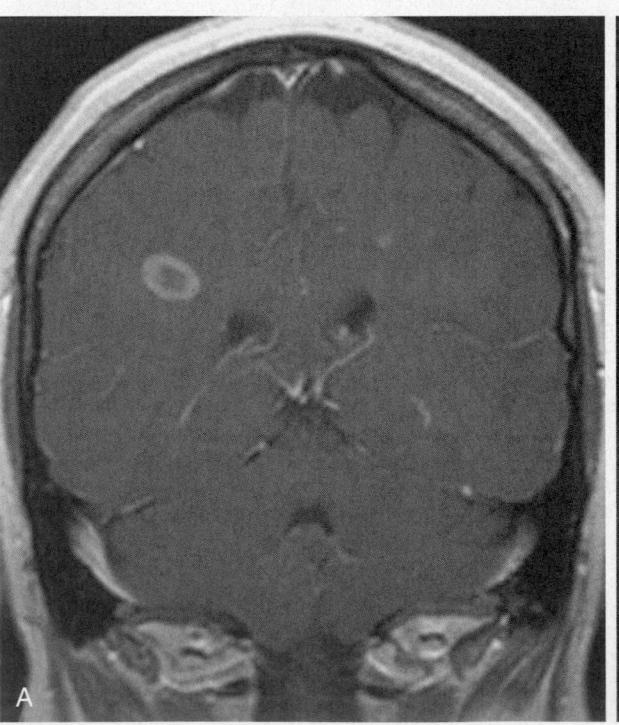
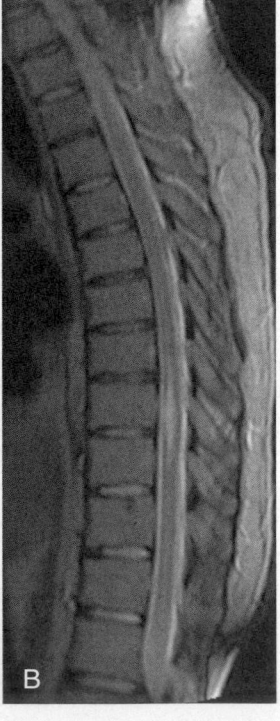

Figure 1. Magnetic resonance image showing brain T1 gadolinium-enhancing lesions (**A**) and T2 thoracic spine (**B**) typical of multiple sclerosis.

Differential Diagnosis

Other CNS demyelinating diseases can mimic relapsing or progressive MS. Acute disseminating encephalomyelitis is an acute, typically monophasic, and postinfectious CNS inflammatory demyelinating disease. It may be severe; however, if recurrent episodes occur separated by at least 3 months, a diagnosis of relapsing–remitting MS is by far more likely.

Neuromyelitis optica is an autoimmune disease with severe acute attacks but is relatively restricted to the optic nerves and spinal cord. Other brainstem and deep cerebral structures, such as the area postrema, cerebral white matter, and hypothalamus, can also be affected by neuromyelitis optica. Brain MRI scan is usually not consistent with MS, at least early on in the disease, and a specific autoantibody (neuromyelitis optica IgG) directed against the aquaporin 4 water channel is found in more than 70% of cases.

Progressive myelopathies that mimic primary progressive MS or secondary progressive MS include a compressive myelopathy from cervical spondylosis, disk disease, or neoplastic infiltration; nutritional deficiencies (such as vitamin B_{12} or copper deficiencies); paraneoplastic disease (usually associated with CRMP-5 auto-antibodies); or a vascular progressive cause due to dural arteriovenous fistula.

Optic neuritis may be mimicked by acute ischemic optic neuropathy. This condition is typically painless, occurs suddenly, and occurs in patients with advanced age and preexisting vascular risk factors.

Treatment

Acute demyelinating MS attacks (relapses) may be treated with high doses of corticosteroids. These may be given orally or intravenously; however, high doses of corticosteroids are necessary and are superior to low doses. For example, a typical regimen is intravenous methylprednisolone (Solu-Medrol) 1000 mg once daily for 3 to 5 days without oral corticosteroid tapering doses. The oral equivalent to this intravenous regimen is prednisone 1250 mg orally once daily for 5 days with no oral corticosteroid taper

following. Gastrointestinal intolerance occurs in some patients, and concomitant use of stomach-protecting agents such proton pump inhibitors may be recommended. Typical acute corticosteroid side effects include insomnia, irritability, and increased appetite as well as an extremely rare association with avascular hip necrosis. Chronic corticosteroid side effects such as diabetes mellitus, cataracts, and weight gain and cushingoid habitus are more associated with chronic corticosteroid use and not short courses of steroids.

Generally, only MS attacks that are associated with functional impairment (vision loss, diplopia, motor weakness, ataxia) are treated because clinical recovery is hastened but final clinical recovery is not found to be altered by this therapy. Rarely, patients have very severe acute attacks of MS or other demyelinating disease that does not improve with use of high-dose corticosteroids. In these rare patients, the use of plasma exchange (seven exchanges over approximately 14 days) is recommended. Approximately 45% of patients experience functional recovery within 1 month following plasma exchange. Side effects of plasma exchange therapy include paresthesias related to hypocalcemia, anemia, thrombocytopenia, or complications of central venous access that is required for many patients. Intravenous immunoglobulin (Gammagard)[1] has not yet been shown to improve severe clinical attacks of demyelinating disease.

Chronic therapy for relapsing–remitting MS includes the use of β1 interferon (IFN-β1), glatiramer acetate (Copaxone), natalizumab (Tysabri), alemtuzumab (Lemtrada), or, for secondary progressive MS (typically with ongoing attacks or new inflammatory lesions on MRI), mitoxantrone (Novantrone) (Table 1). First-line therapy for patients with relapsing–remitting MS is by injectable therapies with preparations of IFN-β1 or, alternatively, glatiramer acetate and with oral therapy with fingolimod (Gilenya),

---

[1]Not FDA approved for this indication.

TABLE 1 Approved Immunomodulatory Therapy for Relapsing–Remitting Multiple Sclerosis

MEDICATION	DOSING	SIDE EFFECTS	MONITORING	ADDITIONAL INFORMATION
Interferon β1a (Avonex)	30 µg IM injection 1×/wk	Flulike symptoms (fever, chills, arthralgias, myalgias, and headaches), elevated liver function tests, anemia, leukopenia, thrombocytopenia, depression. Localized injection-site rejections	CBC with differential, AST, ALT, ALP, and total bilirubin level every 3 mo while on therapy. Thyroid function cascade upon initiation of therapy	Premedication with acetaminophen can ameliorate any postinjection flulike symptoms. Ibuprofen and naproxen. Pregnancy category C medication
Interferon β1a (Rebif)	22 µg or 44 µg SC injection 3×/wk	Flulike symptoms (fever, chills, arthralgias, myalgias, and headaches), elevated liver function tests, anemia, leukopenia, thrombocytopenia, depression. Localized injection-site rejections	CBC with differential, AST, ALT, ALP, and total bilirubin level every 3 mo while on therapy. Thyroid function cascade upon initiation of therapy	Premedication with acetaminophen can ameliorate any postinjection flulike symptoms. Ibuprofen and naproxen. Pregnancy category C medication
Peginterferon β1a (Plegridy)	125 µg SC every 14 d	Flulike symptoms (fever, chills, arthralgias, myalgias, and headaches), elevated liver function tests, anemia, leukopenia, thrombocyto penia, and depression. Localized injection-site rejections	CBC with differential, AST, ALT, alkaline phosphatase, and total bilirubin level. Every three months while on therapy. Thyroid function cascade upon initiation of therapy	Premedication with acetaminophen may ameliorate any postinjection flulike symptoms. Ibuprofen and naproxen. Pregnancy category C medication

Continued

TABLE 1 Approved Immunomodulatory Therapy for Relapsing–Remitting Multiple Sclerosis—cont'd

MEDICATION	DOSING	SIDE EFFECTS	MONITORING	ADDITIONAL INFORMATION
Interferon β1b (Betaseron, Extavia)	250 μg SC injection every other day	Flulike symptoms (fever, chills, arthralgias, myalgias, and headaches), elevated liver function tests, anemia, leukopenia, thrombocytopenia, depression Localized injection-site rejections	CBC with differential, AST, ALT, ALP, and total bilirubin level every 3 mo while on therapy Thyroid function cascade upon initiation of therapy	Premedication with acetaminophen can ameliorate any postinjection flulike symptoms Ibuprofen and naproxen Pregnancy category C medication
Glatiramer acetate (Copaxone)	20 mg SC injection daily or 40 mg SC injection 3x/wk	Injection-site reactions (erythema, edema, pruritus, pain), transient chest pain, palpitations, facial flushing, anxiety, shortness of breath	None	Pregnancy category B medication
Fingolimod hydrochloride (Gilenya)	0.5 mg by mouth once daily	Headache, flu, diarrhea, back pain, liver enzyme elevations, and cough New FDA labeling required; investigating unexplained deaths occurring during treatment with fingolimod	Ophthalmologist review prior to therapy and in 3–4 mo for macular edema, repeated annually in those with diabetes mellitus or uveitis Serology for VZV-IgG to determine immunity CBC with differential, AST, ALT, alkaline phosphatase, and total bilirubin level, ECG ECG before first dose and following 6-hour monitoring; first dose must be monitored for 6 hours for heart-rate reduction and blood-pressure changes; 6-hour monitoring following oral dose must be repeated for patients who discontinue therapy for 14 or more consecutive days For VZV nonimmune patients, vaccination (two doses at least 1 month apart) before starting treatment is needed, and treatment may commence 1 month after the second VZV vaccination	Should not be used in patients with recent MI, unstable angina, stroke, TIA, 2nd- or 3rd-degree AV block, CHF, SSS without cardiac pacing, or QTc >500 ms, or with Class Ia or III antiarrhythmic drugs. Overnight continuous ECG monitoring recommended for those with: preexisting cardiac or cerebrovascular disease; recurrent syncope; severe, untreated obstructive sleep apnea; use of β-blockers; or prolonged QTc Pregnancy category C medication.
Teriflunomide (Aubagio)	7 mg or 14 mg PO once daily	Diarrhea, abnormal liver tests, nausea, influenza, alopecia, potential for hepatotoxicity, may cause significant birth defects if used during pregnancy (pregnancy category X), peripheral neuropathy, transient acute renal failure, and hyperkalemia	CBC monthly for the first 6 mo Liver enzymes Tuberculin skin test Pregnancy test (women of childbearing potential)	Prolonged half-life; recommend removal by activated charcoal or cholestyramine when required. Pregnancy category X medication
Dimethyl fumarate (Tecfidera)	120 mg PO twice daily for 7 days, then 240 mg PO twice daily	Flushing, abdominal pain, nausea, diarrhea	CBC Consider serum JCV Ab serology	CBC annually PML seen in individuals treated for psoriasis with related agent (fumaric acid)
Mitoxantrone hydrochloride (Novantrone)	12 mg/m² IV once every 3 mo	Nausea, skin extravasation reactions, neutropenia, alopecia, amenorrhea, cardiotoxicity, acute myelogenous leukemia	CBC, AST, ALT, bilirubin, creatinine, BUN, and urinalysis at baseline, chest x-ray, PPD skin test, transthoracic echocardiogram before every infusion and annually following therapy	Approved for SPMS Delivered commonly in oncology setting Dose reduction may be needed for prolonged neutropenia Cardiotoxicity may be delayed Pregnancy category D medication

MEDICATION	DOSING	SIDE EFFECTS	MONITORING	ADDITIONAL INFORMATION
Natalizumab (Tysabri)	300 mg IV once every 28 d	Urticaria and anaphylaxis, headache, arthralgias, nausea, fatigue, depression, infections (urinary tract, pneumonia, herpes simplex or reactivation)	Before treatment: JCV Ab serologic study, head MRI with or without gadolinium, CBC with differential, AST, ALT, alkaline phosphatase, and total bilirubin and pregnancy test if applicable; Every 6 months: JCV Ab serology if seronegative (no need to repeat if JCV Ab is seropositive; head MRI with and without gadolinium every 6 months while on therapy; if PML is suspected, discontinue therapy immediately, PLEX to remove drug, MRI head with and without gadolinium with diffusion-weighted imaging; CSF for JCV PCR	Monotherapy approved Risk of PML may be greater in patients with prolonged therapy and those previously treated with immunosuppressive medications Prescribing professional requires TOUCH enrollment Pregnancy category C medication
Alemtuzumab (Lemtrada)	IV infusion over 4 h × 2 treatment course First Course: 12 mg/day on 5 consecutive days. Second course: 12 mg/day on 3 consecutive days 12 months after the first treatment course	Infusion reactions with anaphylaxis. Autoimmune thyroid disorders, immune thrombocyto penia, antiglomerular basement membrane disease. Malignancies including thyroid cancer, melanoma and lymphoprolif erative disorders	CBC with differential, monthly for 48 months after last dose. Creatinine, urinalysis with urine cell counts periodically for 48 months after last dose. Baseline and yearly skin examinations	Premedicate with high dose corticosteroids, check VZV status and vaccinate those VZV antibody negative

Abbreviations: Ab = antibody; ALP = alkaline phosphatase; ALT = alanine aminotransferase; AST = aspartate aminotransferase; AV = atrioventricular; BUN = blood urea nitrogen; CBC = complete blood count; CHF = congestive heart failure; CSF = cerebrospinal fluid; ECG = electrocardiogram; FDA = U.S. Food and Drug Administration; JCV = JC virus; MI = myocardial infarction; MRI = magnetic resonance imaging; PCR = polymerase chain reaction; PLEX = plasma exchange; PML = progressive multifocal leukoencephalopathy; PPD = purified protein derivative; SPMS = secondary progressive multiple sclerosis; SSS = sick sinus syndrome; TIA = transient ischemic attack; TOUCH = Tysabri Outreach: Unified Commitment to Health; VZV-IgG = varicella zoster virus immunoglobulin G.

teriflunomide (Aubagio), and dimethyl fumarate (Tecfidera). The side-effect profile is well known for traditional injectable agents such as interferons and glatiramer acetate (see Table 1), and they have been safely used for many years. The short-term safety profile for oral therapies seemed satisfactory, but the long-term side-effect profile is still being assessed. For fingolimod, new federal FDA labeling was required in 2012 after the sudden death of a patient within 24 hours of first fingolimod dose and the occurrence of other unexplained deaths following initiation of fingolimod. Teriflunomide may be associated with liver disease and teratogenicity. Dimethyl fumarate is associated with flushing gastrointestinal discomfort, and rare patients treated for psoriasis with a related agent, fumaric acid, have developed PML as has one MS patient treated with dimethyl fumarate. Second-line therapy, if first-line medications are intolerable or if therapeutic response is suboptimal (continued MS attacks or marked ongoing and new inflammatory disease on MRI), includes agents such as natalizumab or mitoxantrone. The goal of chronic immunomodulatory therapy for MS is a reduction in clinical attacks of MS (somewhere between 30% and 60%, depending on the agent) and reduction in new inflammatory MRI lesions (somewhere between 40% and 90%, depending on the agent). Patients and health care professionals should realize that the medications are not a cure or for symptomatic benefit (making people feel better) but specifically for reduction in relapse-related disease.

Second-line immunomodulatory agents are effective in reducing MS attacks; however, they are rarely associated with serious side effects. Natalizumab, as monotherapy or in combination with other medications, is associated with the development of progressive multifocal leukoencephalopathy, a severely impairing, and often fatal, opportunistic brain infection caused by reactivation of dormant JC virus. In North America, natalizumab is only available through the TOUCH (Tysabri outreach: unified commitment to health) prescribing program. Risk factors for PML in natalizumab-treated patients include the presence of JC virus serum antibody (AB), duration of therapy of at least 2 years, and history of immunosuppressive medication therapy (e.g., methotrexate, azathioprine). Seropositivity of MS patients for JC virus antibody is approximately 56%. Seroconversion rate from JC virus Ab negativity to positivity is approximately 2% per year, and false-negative results are rare (less than 3%). Currently, no cases of PML have been found in patients persistently seronegative for JCV antibodies. Risk prevalence estimation after 2 years of treatment in JCV Ab positive patients range from 1:250 for those without history of immunosuppression to 1:90 in those with history of prior immunosuppressive therapy. Mitoxantrone is a chemotherapy agent that is the only approved medication for secondary progressive MS. It may be associated with pulmonary and urinary tract infections, alopecia, and cardiotoxicity. The lifetime cumulative dosing of mitoxantrone is restricted to no more than approximately 100 mg/m^2. Cases of acute myelogenous leukemia as well as acute or delayed cardiotoxicity are additional concerns associated with the use of mitoxantrone in MS patients, and close clinical and investigational (e.g., measuring ejection fraction by echocardiography) follow-up is needed.

Newly FDA approved for relapsing MS is alemtuzumab (Lemtrada) a monoclonal antibody (anti-CD52; T and B cells). Given the safety precautions that include autoimmune thyroid disease, immune thrombocytopenia and anti-glomerular basement membrane disease it is generally reserved for patients with inadequate response to other MS immunomodulatory medications.

Novel medications for MS are under therapeutic investigation. These include intravenous monoclonal antibodies that have a direct effect on inflammatory mediators such as daclizumab

---

[1]Not FDA approved for this indication.

[1]Not FDA approved for this indication.

(Zenapax)[1] (anti-CD25, IL2 receptor), and ocrelizumab[1] (anti-CD20 B cells; humanized form).

Monitoring

Most, if not all, MS patients should be followed by a neurologist at least occasionally. Recommendations for clinical assessment range from 6 to 18 months, depending on clinical activity of relapses and disability. The ideal scheduling of repeat brain MRI scans is controversial and varies depending on MS clinical activity, but general recommendations are every 1 to 2 years.

Complications

MS is one of the main causes for impairment at a young age and trails only acute trauma. Often patients need gait assistance when impairment becomes more severe. This includes the use of a single gait aid, such as a cane or walking stick, or an ankle-foot orthosis for symptomatic foot drop.

Patients often experience symptoms of neurogenic bladder dysfunction. This includes symptoms of urgency and urge-related incontinence. Bladder stimulants such as caffeine need to be avoided. Patients with this symptom should be investigated for completeness of bladder emptying. If there is severe impairment in bladder emptying, urinary catheterization often is recommended. If bladder emptying is complete or only mildly impaired (<100 mL postvoid residual), use of medications such as oxybutynin (Ditropan) or tolterodine (Detrol) may be recommended for urge-related symptoms; however, ongoing monitoring of bladder emptying is recommended. Some patients require formal urodynamic evaluation for complex bladder symptoms.

Fatigue is a common MS-related symptom. A complete sleep history to ensure appropriate sleep hygiene is imperative. This includes initiating sleep promptly, maintaining sleep throughout the night, and awakening feeling refreshed. Encouragement of a formal exercise program to facilitate restful sleep and daytime vigor is important. Obstructive sleep apnea, restless legs syndrome, and other parasomnias need to be ruled out as additional contributing factors to fatigue. If sleep hygiene is entirely normal and late afternoon fatigue remains a problem, pharmacologic therapy for MS-related fatigue can proceed. Pharmacologic recommendations are limited but include amantadine hydrochloride (Symmetrel)[1] 100 mg by mouth twice daily. Modafinil (Provigil)[1] has been shown in some studies to have an effect on MS-related fatigue at a dose of 200 mg by mouth once daily.

Spasticity associated with upper motor neuron weakness in the lower extremities may be treated with an active daily exercise program directed by physical therapists and physiatrists. Judicious use of baclofen (Lioresal) is helpful (starting at 10 mg once to three times by mouth daily no more than a maximum of 80 mg per day). Baclofen side effects include drowsiness and liver enzyme elevations. Some patients with significant lower extremity weakness are assisted in their gait by the leg support provided by spasticity, and if spasticity is reduced pharmacologically, this can in fact worsen their gait. Alternatives to baclofen include tizanidine (Zanaflex) and clonidine (Catapres).[1]

MS is a common CNS inflammatory demyelinating disease with heterogenous presentation and prognosis. Relapsing–remitting or attack-related MS is treated with corticosteroids to hasten resolution of acute relapses and chronic immunomodulatory medications such as IFN-β,[1] glatiramer acetate, fingolimod, teriflunomide, dimethyl fumarate, and natalizumab to reduce the number of future clinical attacks and new MRI lesions. Mitoxantrone is the only medication approved for secondary progressive MS, but is appears to improve primarily those with ongoing attacks or continued inflammatory lesions, and concerns regarding short- and long-term side effects have limited its use. Purely progressive forms of primary progressive MS and secondary progressive MS are not responsive to immunomodulatory or immunosuppressive medications. Symptomatic care is important in those patients, including the treatment of gait disorder, spasticity, neurogenic bladder dysfunction, and fatigue.

References

Cohen JA. Emerging therapies for relapsing multiple sclerosis. Arch Neurol 2009;66 (7):821–8.

Compston A, Coles A. Multiple sclerosis. Lancet 2008;372(9648):1502–17.

Hartung HP, Gonsette R, König N, et al. Mitoxantrone in progressive multiple sclerosis: A placebo-controlled, double-blind, randomised, multicentre trial. Lancet 2002;360(9350):2018–25.

Keegan BM. Therapeutic decision-making in a new drug era in multiple sclerosis. Semin Neurol 2013;33:5–12.

Keegan M, König F, McClelland R, et al. Relation between humoral pathological changes in multiple sclerosis and response to therapeutic plasma exchange. Lancet 2005;366(9485):579–82.

Lublin FD, Reingold SC. Defining the clinical course of multiple sclerosis: Results of an international survey. Neurology 1996;46:907–11.

Lucchinetti C, Parisi J, Lucchinetti CF. The pathology of multiple sclerosis. Neurol Clin 2006;23(1):77–105.

Polman CH, O'Connor PW, Havrdova E, et al. A randomized, placebo-controlled trial of natalizumab for relapsing multiple sclerosis. N Engl J Med 2006;354 (9):899–910.

Polman CH, Reingold SC, Edan G, et al. Diagnostic criteria for multiple sclerosis: 2005 revisions to the McDonald criteria. Ann Neurol 2005;58(6):840–6.

Wingerchuk DM, Lennon VA, Pittock SJ, et al. Revised diagnostic criteria for neuromyelitis optica. Neurology 2006;66(10):1485–9.

MYASTHENIA GRAVIS

Method of
Bryan Ho, MD

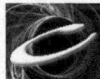

CURRENT DIAGNOSIS

- Myasthenia gravis is an autoimmune disease that affects the neuromuscular junction.
- Symptoms include fluctuating skeletal, ocular, or bulbar muscle weakness in any combination and of varying degrees of severity.
- Depending on the clinical severity, treatment can focus on controlling symptoms or can require chronic immunomodulating therapy. Thymectomy may also induce remission in many patients.
- Myasthenic crisis can be potentially life threatening due to rapid respiratory compromise and can be triggered by a wide variety of medications and acute illness.

CURRENT THERAPY

- Mild symptoms respond very well to anticholinesterase inhibitors, with pyridostigmine (Mestinon) being the most commonly used.
- Chronic control of symptoms can require oral immunosuppressive agents such as steroids, azathioprine (Imuran),[1] or mycophenolate mofetil (Cellcept).[1] If necessary, plasmapheresis or IV immunoglobulin (IVIg; Gammagard)[1] can be helpful to treat worsening symptoms or as maintenance therapy.
- A diverse range of medications can exacerbate myasthenic symptoms. Clinicians need to be mindful of this with their prescriptions for myasthenic patients.
- Myasthenic crisis is a medical emergency and requires aggressive supportive care. Such patients need to be hospitalized in an intensive care setting with close respiratory monitoring and intubation if necessary. Such patients require acute immunologic treatment with plasmapheresis or IVIg[1] to accelerate recovery followed by chronic immunomodulating therapy.

---

[1]Not FDA approved for this indication.

[1]Not FDA approved for this indication.

Epidemiology

Myasthenia gravis is often described as a disease of young women and old men. The disease most commonly occurs in women younger than 40 years and men between the ages of 50 and 70 years. However, it can certainly occur in men and women outside of these age ranges.

Risk Factors

Patients with immediate family members who have a history of autoimmune disease may be at higher risk for developing myasthenia gravis.

Pathophysiology

Myasthenia gravis may be the best understood of all the autoimmune disorders. Before discussing the pathophysiology, a brief overview of the neuromuscular junction may be useful.

The neuromuscular junction is the synapse between the motor unit axon and the motor end plate. An action potential arriving at the neuromuscular junction opens voltage-gated calcium channels, which trigger the release of acetylcholine into the synaptic cleft. The acetylcholine diffuses across the cleft and binds to receptors in the motor end plate, which leads to depolarization and ultimately to muscle activation. To prevent involuntary sustained muscle activation, the acetylcholine is rapidly broken down by acetylcholinesterase in the synaptic cleft.

In myasthenia gravis, autoantibodies bind to the acetylcholine receptors in the motor end plate but do not activate them. Thus, there is competitive inhibition with the endogenous acetylcholine released in the synaptic cleft, leading to reduced activation of the motor end plate.

The muscle tissue itself is healthy and a muscle biopsy is unremarkable.

Prevention

The primary disease itself is not preventable. However, myasthenic exacerbations can be triggered by many types of medications, particularly β-blockers, aminoglycosides, and neuromuscular junction–blocking agents, among many others (Box 1). These agents should be avoided if possible or used with extreme caution if they are medically necessary. Systemic medical illnesses can also trigger myasthenic crisis, particularly upper respiratory infections. These patients can deteriorate quickly, so close monitoring is essential.

Clinical Manifestations

The hallmark of myasthenia gravis is pure motor weakness involving ocular, bulbar, or skeletal muscles in any combination and that fluctuates over time. Ocular myasthenic symptoms generally include diplopia and ptosis. Patients can present with oculoparesis that can mimic isolated cranial nerve III, IV, or VI palsies in any combination and is a common feature in myasthenic patients. Bulbar symptoms include dysarthria and dysphagia. Skeletal muscle weakness is usually affected more in the proximal muscles than the distal muscles. A common complaint is difficulty walking up stairs owing to hip flexor weakness, but any muscle group can be affected. There also tends to be a diurnal variation of the symptoms, with the weakness tending to get worse toward the end of the day after exertion but improving with rest. About half of patients with only ocular symptoms on initial presentation develop more generalized symptoms later in life.

Diagnosis

The diagnosis of myasthenia can often be made based on a careful history and detailed neurologic examination demonstrating the pattern of weakness and its variable nature. Laboratory testing and electromyography help to confirm the diagnosis. If the patient is not presenting with any symptoms at the time of the examination, muscle fatigability can often be induced. Sustained upward gaze can induce ptosis and unmask oculoparesis leading to diplopia. Prolonged speech can induce slurring or a nasal quality to the voice. Repetitive muscle movements can lead to clinically detectable weakness.

Box 1 Common Drugs That Can Exacerbate Myasthenia Gravis

Anesthetics
Halothane (Fluothane)
Ketamine (Ketalar)
Lidocaine (Xylocaine)
All neuromuscular blocking agents
Procaine

Antibiotics
Aminoglycosides
Fluoroquinolones
Tetracyclines
Erythromycin
Clarithromycin (Biaxin)
Clindamycin (Cleocin)

Antiepileptics
Gabapentin (Neurontin)
Phenytoin (Dilantin)

Antipsychotics
Chloropromazine (Thorazine)
Lithium (Eskalith, Lithobid)
Phenothiazines

Cardiovascular Agents
β-Blockers
Calcium channel blockers
Procainamide (Pronestyl)
Quinidine

Others
Anticholinergic agents
Cholinesterase inhibitors
Glucocorticoids
Narcotics
Statins

Another helpful bedside examination finding is the ice pack test. In a patient presenting with ptosis, applying an ice pack over the affected eye can lead to demonstrable improvement, supporting the diagnosis of myasthenia gravis.

Another way to confirm the diagnosis clinically is a Tensilon (edrophonium) test. To do this, there needs to be a clear observable sign of weakness, preferably ptosis, because this is difficult for the patient to simulate factitiously. Because of the risk of bradycardia, this test needs to be done with telemetry monitoring, with atropine 1 mg on hand at the bedside. An initial test dose of edrophonium 2 mg is given intravenously and the patient is observed for any side effects. If the patient tolerates this dose, another 8 mg (10 mg total) is given. The patient is monitored for any clinical improvement in the weakness being observed; improvement supports the diagnosis of myasthenia. Some clinicians, if a skeletal muscle is observed, administer a placebo before the edrophonium. Improvement in symptoms with the placebo suggests a psychogenic component to the symptoms.

Serologic tests are available for confirming the clinical diagnosis of myasthenia gravis; the most useful are assays for detecting acetylcholine receptor antibodies (AChR-Ab). This test is very specific and has very low false-positive rates. It is fairly sensitive in generalized myasthenia (more than 80%) but less sensitive in detecting milder forms like ocular myasthenia (as low as 50%). In cases where clinical suspicion is high but the patient is AchR-Ab negative, another assay for antibodies to muscle-specific receptor tyrosine kinase (anti-MuSK) is available. Anti-MuSK is positive in up to 50% of AchR-Ab negative patients with myasthenia gravis. Up to 10% of patients with myasthenia gravis are seronegative for both assays.

Notably, patients who are AchR-Ab positive are more likely to have thymic abnormalities and thus can be predicted to benefit more from thymectomy. Conversely, patients who are seronegative or have anti-MuSK antibodies alone are less likely to have thymic pathology and may be expected to receive less benefit from thymectomy. Otherwise the medical approach to treatment is unchanged regardless of the presence or absence of serologic markers.

An autoimmune screen is also recommended in any patient being worked up for myasthenia gravis. Thus checking erythrocyte sedimentation rate, C-reactive protein, antinuclear antibodies, rheumatoid factor, and thyroid-stimulating hormone levels is advised.

Electromyography is very useful in confirming the diagnosis of myasthenia gravis as well as excluding other possible neuromuscular diagnoses. Electromyography should be viewed as an extension of the neurologic examination. If myasthenia gravis is suspected, the ordering physician should request that repetitive nerve stimulation and single-fiber electromyography (EMG) be done if the equipment is available. In repetitive nerve stimulation, a motor nerve to a clinically affected muscle is stimulated repeatedly at low frequencies. In myasthenia gravis, this test should demonstrate decrement in amplitude of the compound motor action potentials and has a sensitivity of roughly 75% for generalized myasthenia. Single-fiber EMG is a more time-consuming and technically difficult test that involves simultaneously measuring the motor action potentials of two muscle fibers innervated by the same motor nerve. The time between action potentials (referred to as "jitter") is measured, and increased jitter strongly suggests delayed neuromuscular transmission. Single-fiber EMG has a sensitivity up to 95%. Milder forms such as ocular myasthenia are more likely to have false negatives in either of these tests. However, even with single-fiber EMG, the sensitivity in these cases is greater than 90%.

In patients with a confirmed diagnosis of myasthenia gravis, a chest CT scan is recommended to evaluate for any gross thymic pathology. All myasthenic patients should be considered for thymectomy if there are no medical contraindications, even if there are no gross abnormalities on imaging.

Differential Diagnosis

Other neuromuscular junction disorders can manifest with features similar to myasthenia gravis, such as botulism, Lambert-Eaton syndrome, and cholinergic crisis. However, usually these conditions can be distinguished clinically, particularly by the presence of autonomic features that are not present in myasthenia gravis. Botulism is associated with ingestion of toxin from the bacteria *Clostridium botulinum,* usually from home-canned food, and generally occurs in infants rather than adults. In addition to oculobulbar and generalized weakness, these patients also present with dilated pupils, dry skin, and dry mucosal membranes. Lambert-Eaton myasthenic syndrome (LEMS) is due to autoantibodies to the presynaptic voltage-gated calcium channels and is often associated with underlying malignancy, usually small cell lung cancer. In contrast to myasthenia, weakness often spares the oculobulbar muscles and the weakness tends to improve rather than worsen with exercise. These patients are usually areflexic and also have other autonomic symptoms such as dry mouth and sexual dysfunction. Cholinergic crisis can occur with overdose of acetylcholine esterase inhibitors or exposure to pesticides with organophosphates, leading to excess cholinergic activity in the neuromuscular junction. In addition to bulbar, generalized, and respiratory weakness, these patients usually present with autonomic signs of cholinergic excess such as pupillary constriction, hypersalivation, and sweating.

Other neuromuscular conditions can lead to weakness that can mimic myasthenia gravis. Acute demyelinating polyneuropathy (Guillain-Barré syndrome), if severe, could appear similar to myasthenic crisis. However, the cerebrospinal fluid usually shows elevated protein, and EMG findings should show demyelination. Critical illness polyneuropathy and myopathy occur in patients with prolonged ICU courses, particularly if sepsis is part of the clinical picture, and EMG studies are helpful in clarifying the diagnosis. Inflammatory myopathies and motor neuron disease are also in the differential diagnosis, and EMG studies should be very helpful to elucidate the diagnosis in clinically uncertain cases.

In cases of pure ocular myasthenia, third, fourth, or sixth cranial neuropathies in any combination could be considered in the differential diagnosis. In the case of third nerve palsy, the pupil is usually involved as well, and the affected eye is deviated down and outward. There can also be ptosis. In fourth nerve palsy, the affected eye is usually elevated compared to the normal eye, leading to a vertical diplopia. In sixth nerve palsies, the eye is deviated inward and there is clear weakness in abducting the affected eye. Conversely, myasthenia gravis should be considered in any patients with isolated ocular weakness.

Treatment

Treatment for myasthenia gravis can be divided into symptomatic control, immunosuppression, and, in selected patients, thymectomy, depending on the severity of the disease.

Symptoms can be controlled in many patients with acetylcholinesterase inhibitors. Inhibition of acetylcholinesterase leads to prolonged action of acetylcholine in the synaptic cleft, partially overcoming the competitive inhibition with acetylcholine-receptor antibodies. This may be sufficient alone to address mild forms of the disease, such as in ocular myasthenia. The most commonly used agent in this class is pyridostigmine (Mestinon). Neostigmine (Prostigmin) is another alternative, though it is less often used.

Pyridostigmine

Pyridostigmine is effective for controlling mild symptoms. It should not be relied on as therapy for suspected myasthenic crisis or if respiratory compromise is a concern.

The dose is 30 to 90 mg, generally used every 3 to 6 hours as needed, and tailored to clinical response. Maximum dose should not exceed 120 mg per single dose. Patients typically get a response within 30 minutes. It is also available in a long-acting formulation (Mestinon TS 180 mg). The long-acting form is generally not recommended for daytime use owing to a less-predictable onset of action. It may be useful as a bedtime dose for patients who have severe morning weakness on awakening.

Side effects for acetylcholine esterase inhibitors are mostly gastrointestinal, with abdominal cramping, nausea and vomiting, and diarrhea being most common. Patients might find it helpful to take the medicine with some food. Other symptoms of cholinergic excess such as miosis, sweating, and hypersalivation can also occur. Overdose can lead to cholinergic crisis, with severe weakness, bradycardia, and hypotension being potentially life-threatening, but these effects generally do not occur if the medication is taken within recommended parameters.

If necessary, side effects can be alleviated with certain anticholinergic medications with little or no activation of nicotinic receptors. A commonly used agent for this purpose is glycopyrrolate (Robinul)[1] 1 mg taken with each pyridostigmine dose or as a stand-alone dose three times a day.

In patients with baseline weakness beyond mild bulbar or ocular symptoms or with progressively worsening symptoms, chronic immunosuppression may be necessary. The most commonly used agents are prednisone,[1] azathioprine (Imuran),[1] mycophenolate mofetil (Cellcept),[1] and cyclosporine (Sandimmune, Neoral), each with its own advantages and disadvantages.

Prednisone

Prednisone[1] is often the first agent used in long-term management of generalized myasthenia. Prednisone has the advantage of having relatively quick onset of action compared to other immunosuppressive agents used for chronic myasthenia. Some clinicians favor starting patients on high doses (1.5 mg/kg to a maximum dose of

---

[1]Not FDA approved for this indication.

100 mg) to achieve a quick clinical response initially, then tapering to the lowest dose possible to maintain control of symptoms. Other immunosuppressive treatments can be used in conjunction as steroid-sparing agents. The disadvantage with this strategy is that for unclear reasons, prednisone can exacerbate symptoms in the short term, and this risk increases with higher doses. Thus this strategy is generally initiated in the inpatient setting. Most clinicians, if possible, favor avoiding the risk of exacerbating symptoms and instead start at a lower dose (15–20 mg) and titrate the dose slowly based on the patient's clinical response. The drawback is that it generally takes longer to achieve significant symptomatic improvement.

Azathioprine

Azathioprine[1] can be used for chronic immunosuppression as a steroid-sparing agent. Patients are started on 50 mg/day and then titrated 50 mg/week to a target dose of 2 to 3 mg/kg/day. During the first few weeks, some patients have to discontinue the medication owing to a systemic reaction involving fever, abdominal pain, nausea, and vomiting. Patients also require weekly monitoring of complete blood counts and liver function during the titration phase. Upon reaching the target dose, monitoring can be extended to every 3 months. The medication can take up to 6 months to take effect.

Mycophenolate Mofetil

Mycophenolate mofetil[1] is less well studied than azathioprine, but from clinical experience, it appears to be efficacious in chronic treatment of myasthenia and has become preferred owing to better side-effect profile, faster onset of action (usually within 3 months), and no need for regular monitoring of liver function. Patients start on 1 g twice a day, titrated by 500 mg a month until a target dose of 1.5 g twice a day is reached. Side effects include diarrhea, abdominal pain, and nausea. Less commonly, leukopenia can occur.

Cyclosporine

Cyclosporine[1] is viewed by most clinicians as a second-line agent for patients who fail treatment with azathioprine and mycophenolate mofetil. Patients can start on 3 mg/kg daily divided in two doses, titrated up to 6 mg/kg daily. The dose should be adjusted to a trough cyclosporine level between 50 and 150 ng/mL. Kidney function also needs to be monitored. Cyclosporine tends to take effect within 2 to 3 months of drug initiation.

Plasmapheresis and Intravenous Immunoglobulin

Plasmapheresis and intravenous immunoglobulin (IVIg, Gammagard)[1] have been shown to be effective in the acute management of myasthenia and are mainstays of treatment in myasthenic crisis. These treatments are also useful as bridging therapies in patients transitioning to chronic immunosuppression or as prophylaxis for patients at risk for myasthenic crisis. Plasmapheresis directly removes circulating acetylcholine receptor antibodies, leading to alleviation of symptoms. The mechanism of action of intravenous immunoglobulin is less clear. It may be due to the pooled immunoglobulin binding to the autoantibodies, in turn preventing them from binding to the acetylcholine receptors.

Plasma exchange typically involves five sessions spread over 1 to 2 weeks. Clinical response correlates with the reduction in acetylcholine receptor antibody levels, though it is not necessary to check levels routinely during exchanges. Patients often have a clinical response within a few days after initiation of treatment. The most common significant complication of the procedure is hypotension and other cardiac issues. Because the procedure requires catheter placement, infection and thrombosis are also potential risks.

IVIg therapy is typically given at a dose of 2 g/kg divided over 5 days. An IgA level should be checked before starting the therapy in a treatment-naïve patient because patients with IgA deficiency are at risk for developing an anaphylactic reaction to the infusion. Patients generally respond within a week of initiation.

Complications of treatment are uncommon but include thrombotic events such as stroke and myocardial infarction. It should also be used with caution in patients with congestive heart failure owing to the fluid load. There is also a risk of acute renal failure. Aseptic meningitis can also occur.

Comparatively, plasmapheresis and IVIg have roughly equivalent efficacy, so the choice is based on the clinical scenario, preference of the treating physician, and available resources. If one treatment fails to confer any clinical improvement, it is perfectly reasonable to attempt the other.

Thymectomy

Thymectomy should be strongly considered in any patient who is younger than 60 years and has no medical contraindications for the surgery. It should also be considered in older patients with significant weakness beyond mild ocular or bulbar symptoms. A significant number of patients achieve significant improvement or full remission of symptoms after thymectomy, even if no thymic pathology is found at the time of surgery.

Myasthenic Crisis

Any myasthenic patient, regardless of how mild the baseline symptoms are, has a risk of developing myasthenic crisis at some point in his or her lifetime. Myasthenic crisis is often precipitated by systemic illness, particularly upper respiratory infections, and a wide variety of medications are also known to exacerbate myasthenia symptoms. Any myasthenic patient complaining of worsening symptoms, particularly dyspnea, should be evaluated urgently because the patient can quickly decompensate. Such patients also should not be managed by adjusting their cholinesterase inhibitor regimen alone because symptomatic control is insufficient to forestall further progression into crisis.

These patients require immunomodulating therapy with either plasmapheresis or IVIg.[1] They should also be monitored in an intensive care unit setting with frequent respiratory mechanics assessed at least two or three times a day. If forced vital capacity (FVC) is less than 20 mg/kg or the net inspiratory force (NIF) is less than −30 cm H_2O, elective intubation is strongly advised. Either plasmapheresis or IVIg therapy should be started. A thorough work-up should be done to search for the underlying trigger (e.g., infection, new medication), and any triggers that are found should be treated or removed. Once stabilized, the patient should also begin taking chronic immunomodulation, if this medication is not already used. Prednisone[1] is most commonly used initially because its onset of action is faster than the other options.

Monitoring

Patients should be monitored as outpatients on a regular basis to ensure stability of symptoms and adequate symptomatic response, as well as monitoring laboratory studies, depending on the chronic immunomodulating medication being used. Acute deterioration in symptoms needs to taken very seriously, with a low threshold for urgent evaluation and hospitalization.

Complications

The dreaded complication of myasthenia is myasthenic crisis leading to fulminant generalized weakness and respiratory failure, often precipitated by systemic illness or other medications. Because patients can deteriorate rapidly, patients in whom symptoms appear to be worsening acutely need to be evaluated urgently. See "Myasthenic Crisis" earlier for further discussion.

---

[1]Not FDA approved for this indication.

References

Drachman DB. Myasthenia gravis. N Engl J Med 1994;330:1797–810.

Hoch W, McConville J, Helms S, et al. Auto-antibodies to the receptor tyrosine kinase MuSK in patients with myasthenia gravis without acetylcholine receptor antibodies. Nat Med 2001;7:365–8.

Keesey JC. Clinical evaluation and management of myasthenia gravis. Muscle Nerve 2004;29(4):484–505.

---

[1]Not FDA approved for this indication.

McConville J, Farrugia ME, Beeson D, et al. Detection and characterization of MuSK antibodies in seronegative myasthenia gravis. Ann Neurol 2004;55:580–4.

Ropper AH, Brown RH. Adam and Victor's Principles of Neurology. 8th ed. New York: McGraw-Hill; 2005.

Saperstein DS, Barohn RJ. Management of myasthenia gravis. Semin Neurol 2004;24:41–8.

OPTIC NEURITIS

Method of
Heather E. Moss, MD, PhD

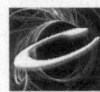

CURRENT DIAGNOSIS

- Vision is impaired, including visual acuity, visual field, and/or color perception.
- Patients have eye pain that is worse with eye movement.
- There is a relative afferent papillary defect if only one eye is affected.
- The anterior optic nerve has a normal appearance in two thirds of affected patients.

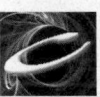

CURRENT THERAPY

- Consider IV methylprednisolone (Solu-Medrol) followed by oral steroids.
- Avoid oral steroid monotherapy.
- If brain MRI suggests a high-risk, clinically isolated syndrome, consider disease-modifying therapy to delay progression to MS.
- If the patient's history suggests MS or NMO, consider treatment for these conditions.

Epidemiology

The incidence of optic neuritis is approximately 1 to 5 in 100,000. Though it typically affects women in their fourth decade of life, 1 in 4 patients are male, and patients have been reported ranging from the first to seventh decades of life. Optic neuritis occurs worldwide in persons of various ethnicities.

Optic neuritis can be classified as a clinically isolated syndrome or in association with a disease such as multiple sclerosis (MS) or neuromyelitis optica (NMO). Approximately half of patients with optic neuritis as a clinically isolated syndrome develop MS. A small percentage develop NMO.

Risk Factors

A diagnosis of a disease associated with optic neuritis, such as MS or NMO, increases the risk of developing optic neuritis. In one study, more than 70% of patients with MS and 100% of patients with NMO had unilateral optic neuritis at some point.

Pathophysiology

Most optic neuritis occurs as a result of inflammation causing demyelination of the ganglion cell axons that compose the optic nerve. This is thought to be an immune-mediated process.

Prevention

Disease-modifying therapies have been shown to reduce risk of neurologic relapses in patients with MS or NMO. These therapies presumably also decrease the risk of MS- or NMO-associated optic neuritis because optic neuritis is a common relapse syndrome in these conditions.

Clinical Manifestations

A typical optic neuritis patient experiences acute or subacute loss of vision characterized by decreased visual acuity, visual field loss, and/or color vision loss, accompanied or preceded by pain in the affected eye that is worse with eye movements. However, 8% of patients do not have pain. Other symptoms include positive visual phenomena in 30% of patients. Other signs include a relative afferent papillary defect in cases where one eye is affected and a mildly swollen optic nerve head in approximately one third of patients.

The natural history of clinically isolated optic neuritis includes resolution of pain 3 to 5 days after onset and nadir of vision 7 to 14 days after onset. Spontaneous improvement in vision is typically evident within 3 weeks, and almost 70% of affected patients recover 20/20 visual acuity. Optic neuritis associated with MS shares similar features. Optic neuritis associated with NMO tends to have less recovery of vision.

Diagnosis

The diagnosis is based on the clinical presentation. Where there is uncertainty, magnetic resonance imaging (MRI) of the orbits, including fat-saturated sequences (T2 and T1 with and without gadolinium contrast) can help to visualize inflammation in the retrobulbar optic nerve.

Optic neuritis is often associated with other demyelinating syndromes, most commonly MS. Therefore it is important to screen for historical and current neurologic impairment through history and examination. MRI of the brain has been shown to be an important prognostic indicator for development of MS in patients who present with their first episode of clinically isolated optic neuritis. MRI of the brain showing 0, 1, or more than 3 lesions typical for MS is associated with a 25%, 60%, and 78%, respectively, risk of progression to clinically definite MS.

Less commonly, optic neuritis is associated with other demyelinating syndromes such as NMO. This should be considered in patients with severe vision loss, bilateral involvement, or history of prior optic neuritis or transverse myelitis. A serum antibody (anti-aquaporin 4 or NMO antibody) has been identified as a pathologic agent in this disorder. Testing for this is commercially available with a published sensitivity and specificity of 63% and 99%, respectively. Research is ongoing to define the role of this test in establishing prognosis following a first clinically isolated episode of optic neuritis.

Differential Diagnosis

Other diagnostic considerations in a patient with unilateral painful vision loss without explanatory pathology evident on ophthalmic examination include other optic neuropathies such as those due to sarcoidosis, lupus, vasculitis, neoplastic, vascular, and infectious causes. Atypical features for optic neuritis such as systemic symptoms, history of cancer, pain that persists beyond 2 weeks, progressive vision loss beyond 14 days, no spontaneous improvement in vision, retinal hemorrhages, cotton-wool spots, or macular exudates should prompt diagnostic evaluation for etiologies other than optic neuritis.

Treatment and Monitoring

The Optic Neuritis Treatment Trial (ONTT) was a randomized trial comparing placebo, oral prednisone, and IV methylprednisolone (1 g/day IV for 3 days) followed by oral prednisone (1 mg/kg per day for 11 days) for acute optic neuritis. IV steroids hastened recovery of vision without affecting final visual outcome compared with placebo treatment. Treatment with oral prednisone alone was associated with an increased risk of relapse compared with placebo treatment. The 15-year follow-up results, published in 2008, demonstrated persistence of visual recovery.

Based on the ONTT results, many clinicians offer IV steroid treatment to hasten visual recovery. Monotherapy with oral prednisone should be avoided. Regardless of the decision to treat or not with IV steroids, all patients should be monitored closely. Continued progression of vision loss, failure to spontaneously recover vision, or persistent pain should prompt additional diagnostic work-up as well as consideration for additional IV steroid therapy for atypical optic neuritis. If this is not effective, plasma exchange has been reported as an effective acute therapy for atypical optic neuritis.

In patients with a clinically isolated syndrome, consideration should be given to institution of disease-modifying therapy for MS based on the presence of lesions on brain MRI. Several clinical trials have shown an association between early treatment with MS therapies and decreased incidence of progression to clinically definite MS in patients with a recent clinically isolated syndrome and clinically silent lesions on brain MRI.

In patients who meet diagnostic criteria for either MS or NMO, consideration should be given to treating the underlying disease.

Complications

Though more than 70% of patients with optic neuritis recover objectively normal visual acuity, many have residual subjective visual disturbances. These often worsen or recur in heat, which is known as Uhtoff's phenomenon.

Complications of steroid therapy include insomnia, agitation, and stomach irritation. Long-term side effects of steroid treatment for this condition are rare owing to the brief period of treatment. Complications of disease-modifying therapies for MS and NMO are reviewed elsewhere.

References

Beck RQ, Cleary PA, Anderson MM, et al. A randomized, controlled trial of corticosteroids in the treatment of acute optic neuritis. The Neuritis Study Group. N Engl J Med 1992;326:581–8.

Hickman SJ, Ko M, Chaudhry F, et al. Optic neuritis: An update on typical and atypical optic neuritis. Neuro-ophthalmology 2008;32:237–48.

Kinkel RP, Dontchev M, Kollman C, et al. Association between immediate initiation of intramuscular interferon beta-1a at the time of a clinically isolated syndrome and long-term outcomes: A 10-year follow-up of the controlled high-risk Avonex multiple sclerosis prevention study in ongoing neurological surveillance. Arch Neurol 2012;69:183–90.

Merle H, Olindo S, Bonnan M, et al. Natural history of the visual impairment of relapsing neuromyelitis optica. Ophthalmology 2007;114:810–5.

Optic Neuritis Study Group. The clinical profile of optic neuritis: Experience of the optic neuritis treatment trial. Arch Ophthalmol 1991;109:1673–8.

Optic Neuritis Study Group. Multiple sclerosis risk after optic neuritis: Final optic neuritis treatment trial follow-up. Arch Neurol 2008;65:727–32.

Optic Neuritis Study Group. Visual function 15 years after optic neuritis. Ophthalmology 2008;115:1079–82.

Polman CH, Reingold SC, Edan G, et al. Diagnostic criteria for multiple sclerosis: 2005 revisions to the "McDonald Criteria." Ann Neurol 2005;58:840–6.

Roesner S, Appel R, Gbadamosi J, et al. Treatment of steroid-unresponsive optic neuritis with plasma exchange. Acta Neurol Scand, published online November, 2, 2011 http://dx.doi.org/10.1111/j.1600-040.2011.01612.x.

Sellner J, Boggild M, Clanet M, et al. EFNS guidelines on diagnosis and management of neuromyelitis optica. Eur J Neurol 2010;17:1019–32.

Smith CH. Optic neuritis. In: Miller NR, Neumann NJ, editors. Walsh & Hoyt's Clinical Neuro-Ophthalmology. 6th ed. Philadelphia: Lippincott Williams & Wilkins 2005. p. 294–338.

Wingerchuk DM, Lennon VA, Lucchinetti CF, et al. The spectrum of neuromyelitis optica. Lancet Neurol 2007;6:805–15.

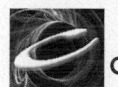

PARKINSON DISEASE

Method of
John D. Gazewood, MD, MSPH

CURRENT DIAGNOSIS

- Clinical diagnosis
  - Rigidity
  - Bradykinesia
  - Resting "pill-rolling" tremor
- Postural instability
- Sustained response to carbidopa/levodopa or dopamine agonist

- Frequent re-evaluation
- Imaging
  - Single photon emission computer tomography (SPECT) to differentiate essential tremor
  - Functional magnetic resonance imaging (fMRI) progressive supranuclear palsy

CURRENT THERAPY

- Early disease
  - Patients over age 70: levodopa/carbidopa
  - Patient under age 60: dopamine agonist or monoamineoxidase B (MAO-B) inhibitor
- Patients between 60 and 70: one of above agents
- On-off phenomenon
  - Levodopa/carbidopa with dopamine agonist or catechol-O-methyltransferase (COM-T) inhibitor
- Dyskinesias
  - Amantadine
- Advanced disease
  - Deep brain stimulation of subthalamic nucleus or globus pallidus interna

Parkinson disease (PD) is a common degenerative neurologic disorder characterized by bradykinesia and pathologically defined by the presence of Lewy bodies in the dopaminergic neurons of the substantia nigra.

Epidemiology

PD is rare in patients below 60 years of age. The prevalence is approximately 1% in people aged 60 and older. The prevalence among African Americans and Asian Americans is about half that of the white population. With a growing elderly population, the number of PD sufferers is expected to double by 2030. PD is not distributed equally across geographic areas. In the United States, higher rates of PD are found in the Midwest/Great Lakes region and in the Northeast Seaboard.

Risk Factors

Epidemiologic studies have consistently shown an association between exposure to pesticides and herbicides and risk of PD. Nicotine exposure, primarily through cigarette smoking, is associated with a lower risk of PD. Coffee drinkers also have lower rates of PD. First degree relatives of PD patients have a two-fold increased risk.

Pathophysiology

The etiology of PD is not understood. While there are several genetic mutations implicated in sporadic PD, including *LRRK2* and *Parkin*, their role is unclear. At this time, it seems likely that PD arises as a result of complex interactions between genes that promote or inhibit development of PD and environmental factors.

Post-mortem analysis of PD patients' brains show neuronal loss and Lewy bodies in the substantia nigra. Lewy bodies are intracytoplasmic inclusions containing α-synuclein and ubiquitin. While the striatum, which receives neuronal inputs from the substantia nigra, appears normal, the loss of dopaminergic input into the striatum from the substantia nigra leads to the motor symptoms of PD, which typically begin when 70% to 80% of the dopaminergic neurons in the substantia nigra are lost.

Prevention

Although there are no measures proven to prevent PD, given the observed epidemiology, it is reasonable to recommend that people minimize exposure to herbicides and pesticides.

Clinical Manifestations

PD first manifests with the hallmark symptoms of bradykinesia, tremor, rigidity, and postural instability. Symptoms begin on one side and gradually progress.

Bradykinesia refers to generalized slowness of movement. Bradykinesia makes it difficult for patients to perform fine motor tasks, such as key-boarding or writing, as well as initiating movement with large muscle groups. Patients may complain of trouble turning over in bed or standing up from a chair, as well as weakness or fatigue.

The "pill-rolling" tremor of PD is a resting tremor with a frequency of 3 to 7 Hz, and is most noticeable when the patient is sitting quietly or walking. Less commonly, the tremor can be present in the legs, lips, jaws or tongue. The tremor improves with action and with sleep.

Rigidity is increased resistance to passive range of motion about a joint. Rigidity can be focal or widespread, and may lead to complaints of pain and stiffness.

Diagnosis

The diagnosis of PD is made clinically, and is suggested by the presence of tremor, rigidity, bradykinesia, postural instability, gradual progression, and a sustained response to levodopa. The London brain bank criteria have been found to have good predictive value in advanced disease, but there are no good clinical prediction rules for diagnosis of early disease.

Historical features that increase the likelihood of PD include tremor of head or limbs; bradykinesia and rigidity; decreased facial expression; difficulty arising from a chair, loss of balance, feet freezing; shuffling gait, trouble turning in bed and opening jars, and micrographia. The absence of rigidity and bradykinesia make PD less likely, as do a history of falls.

On examination, the clinician should look for the typical tremor with the patient sitting and hands resting in the lap. Having the patient do mental calculations or move the contralateral limb may increase a tremor or bring out a latent tremor. The tremor will improve with use of the affected limb. Bradykinesia can be observed via several maneuvers. Perform a get-up and go test, and watch for difficulty arising from a chair, decreased arm swing, and decreased stride length, as well as difficulty turning. Provocative maneuvers—repeatedly circling the hands in front of the body; pinching the thumb and forefinger together repeatedly with the right hand and then with the left hand, circling one hand and then the other, and then pinching thumb and forefinger together with one hand while circling with the other can reveal bradykinesia, as will asking the patient to repeatedly tap their heel to the floor. The examiner can detect rigidity by passively rotating the wrist and/or flexing and extending the forearm, and noting resistance. Jerky resistance is typical of "cogwheel" rigidity, whereas smooth resistance is typical of lead-pipe rigidity: both can be present in PD. A positive glabellar tap test also increases the likelihood of PD.

A sustained response to levodopa/carbidopa (Sinemet) or a dopamine agonist helps confirm the diagnosis. The "acute challenge test," using either levodopa/carbidopa or apomorphine (Apokyn) is no longer recommended.

Imaging is not routinely needed. In rare instances, magnetic resonance imaging can help differentiate PD from multisystem atrophy, and single-photon emission computed tomography may distinguish PD from essential tremor.

PD shares features with a number of other conditions, making diagnosis, particularly in the early stages, challenging. Repeated evaluation over the course of the illness is important, as is careful attention to response to treatment. The absence of a sustained response to appropriate therapy early in the course of the illness should lead to re-evaluation. Uncertainty about the diagnosis warrants consulting a clinician experienced in diagnosis.

Differential Diagnosis

Diseases with a tremor, parkinsonian symptoms or gait impairment should be considered in the differential of a patient with suspected PD. Diseases that are most commonly mistaken for PD by primary care physicians include essential tremor, vascular parkinsonism, progressive supranuclear palsy and drug-induced parkinsonism. These conditions, as well as differentiating signs and symptoms, are listed in Table 1.

Findings that make a diagnosis of PD less likely include a history of traumatic, vascular or infectious brain injury and use of antidopaminergic drugs within the previous 6 months. The time course of disease progression is helpful in distinguishing PD from other neurologic diseases. Presentation of dementia, significant autonomic insufficiency, frequent falls, and apraxia early in the disease course make PD unlikely. Symmetric findings on examination, as well as cerebellar signs, spasticity and hyper-reflexia, and inability to name objects despite intact sensation all point away from PD. Individuals less than age 50 who present with PD may have an inherited form of the disorder, and should also be evaluated for Wilson disease. Younger adults and adolescents who present with parkinsonian features likely have dopa-responsive dystonia.

Treatment

Early Disease

Treatment begins when symptoms impair an individual's ability to carry out their usual daily routine. Three classes of medications are effective for early disease: levodopa/carbidopa (Sinemet), dopamine agonists, and monoamine oxidase inhibitors (Table 2). Levodopa/carbidopa is the most effective of these three classes of medications, but motor-related complications, such as dyskinesias, develop at a rate of 10% per year, and are more problematic in younger patients. Dopamine agonists, which directly stimulate dopamine receptors, are less likely to lead to dyskinesias in head to

TABLE 1	Characteristics of Conditions Considered in Differential Diagnosis of Parkinsonism
CONDITION	**FEATURES**
Essential tremor	Symmetric postural tremor; worsens with movement; affects distal extremities, head and speech; family history common
Vascular parkinsonism	May have focal neurologic finding; stepwise progression; poor response to carbidopa/levodopa; basal ganglia and/or thalamic infarcts present on CNS imaging
Drug-induced parkinsonism	Clinical features similar to PD; symptoms improve after withdrawal of medicine; anti-emetics and psychotropic drugs most common cause
Dementia with Lewy bodies	Onset of dementia and hallucinations at same time as motor symptoms; fluctuating mental status; poor response to carbidopa/levodopa
Progressive supranuclear palsy	Parkinsonism accompanied by falls and minimal response to dopaminergic treatment, with later development of supranuclear gaze palsy
Multiple system atrophy	Parkinsonism accompanied by early autonomic dysfunction and poor response to dopaminergic treatment and ataxia
Corticobasal degeneration	Cognitive impairment, asymmetrical limb dysfunction and minimal response to dopaminergic treatment, with absence of tremor

TABLE 2 Drugs for Parkinson disease	
DRUG	**DOSING**
Carbidopa/levodopa (Sinemet)	Initial: 25/100—½ to 1 tab tid Maximum: 1500 mg levodopa in divided dosages
Dopamine agonists	
Pramipexole (Mirapex)	Initial: 0.125 tid Maximum: 4.5 mg a day
Pramipexole ER (Mirapex ER)	Initial: 0.375 mg a day Maximum: 4.5 mg a day
Ropinorole (Requip)	Initial: 0.25 mg tid Maximum: 8 mg tid
Ropinorole ER (Requip ER)	Initial: 2 mg a day Maximum: 24 mg a day
Rotigotine (transdermal) (Neupro)	Initial: 2 mg/24 hours Maximum: 16 mg/24 hours[2]
MAOB inhibitors	
Rasagiline (Azilect)	Initial: 0.5 mg a day Maximum: 1 mg a day
Selegiline (Eldepryl)	Initial: 5 mg a day Maximum: 5 mg bid with breakfast and lunch
COMT inhibitors	
Entacapone (Comtan)	Initial: 200 mg with each dose of levodopa Maximum: 8 tablets (1600 mg) a day
Other	
Amantadine (Symmetrel)	Initial: 100 mg bid

[2]Exceeds dosage recommended by the manufacturer.

head comparisons with levodopa/carbidopa. However, these same trials demonstrated that they are less effective and resulted in a higher drop-out rate than levodopa/carbidopa. Monoamine oxidase inhibitors are the best tolerated but least effective. There are no drugs that slow progressive neuron loss in PD. The initial choice of medication should be made taking into account the severity of the patient's symptoms and age, after a discussion of benefits and burdens with patients. Most experts recommend initiating therapy with a dopamine agonist for patients younger than 60 years old, and levodopa/carbidopa for patients over the age of 70. For patients between these ages, the initial choice of medication is less clear. The evidence does not support the use of combination therapy in early disease to delay the development of dyskinesias.

Levodopa/carbidopa is started at a dose of ½ to 1 tablet of the 25/100 immediate release tablet three times a day. The dose can be titrated to 2 to 3 tablets of the 25/100 tablet, increasing the dose weekly by a half-tablet at all doses, until the patient's symptoms are controlled. In early disease, patients will develop a sustained response to dopamine, with good control of symptoms throughout the day. Patients should take levodopa/carbidopa on an empty stomach, as dietary protein competes with dopamine for receptors sites on trans-gut amino acid transporters. The main side effects of levodopa/carbidopa that patients will experience are nausea and orthostatic hypotension. For nausea, patients may try taking their medication with a small nonprotein snack, such as saltine crackers. Adding additional carbidopa to each dose of levodopa/carbidopa can also help. Trimethobenzamide (Tigan)[1] and ondansetron

(Zofran),[1] nondopamine blocking nausea agents may be effective. There is no benefit to use of sustained release levodopa/carbidopa.

The oral dopamine agonists, pramipexole (Mirapex) and ropinirole (Requip), and the transdermal agonist rotigotine (Neupro) are started at the lowest dose and titrated slowly to effect. In addition to nausea, these agents can cause sleepiness, edema, and hallucinations, as well as compulsive repetitive behaviors, pathologic gambling or shopping, and hypersexuality. Older dopamine agonists, such as bromocriptine (Parlodel), can cause pleural and retroperitoneal fibrosis and cardiac valvulopathies and should not be used. Rasagiline (Azilect) and selegiline (Eldepryl) are monoamine oxidase B (MAO-B) inhibitors that can delay use of levodopa/carbidopa in patients with mild disease, but also cause nausea and orthostatic hypotension.

Later Disease

As the disease progresses, bradykinesia, rigidity and tremor worsen. For patients taking dopamine agonists or MAO-B inhibitor increasing the dose may help, but these patients will eventually require the addition of levodopa/carbidopa. Patients taking levodopa/carbidopa will eventually develop motor fluctuations and will initially notice that the symptoms recur near the end of dosing intervals ("wearing off"). For these patients, increase the frequency of the effective dose, not the amount of the dose. Eventually, patients will notice more abrupt and sudden fluctuations in effect ("on-off" phenomenon). There are three classes of medications that can be added to increase "on time" to patients on levodopa/carbidopa: monoamine oxidase inhibitors, dopamine agonists, and catechol O-methyltransferase (COM-T) inhibitors, which decrease peripheral dopamine metabolism. The COM-T inhibitor entacapone (Comtan) is preferred to tolcapone (Tasmar), which can cause fatal hepatotoxicity. In addition to oral and transdermal dopamine agonists, an injectable agonist, apomorphine (Apokyn), is effective in reducing off-time; its use should be supervised by a specialist in movement disorders. Dopamine agonists are probably the most effective medications for reducing off-time. With addition of any of these agents, the dose of levodopa/carbidopa can often be reduced. All of these agents increase the occurrence of dyskinesias.

Dyskinesias eventually develop, often around the same time that wearing-off or on-off symptoms begin. Dyskinesias are choreaform movements affecting a limb, trunk, head, neck, or a combination of areas. Dyskinesias are due to excessive dopamine stimulation. If patients find them bothersome, treat them by reducing the dose of levodopa/carbidopa and decreasing the dosing interval. Unfortunately this will often lead to worsening of other parkinsonian motor symptoms. Amantadine (Symmetrel) can also reduce dyskinesias, although the effect is modest.

For patients whose symptoms cannot be adequately controlled by optimal medical therapy, consider referral for deep brain stimulation, which targets either the subthalamic nucleus or the globus pallidus interna. Patients who have had a good response to levodopa/carbidopa, few comorbidities, no cognitive impairment, and either no depression or who have well controlled depression are likely to have a good response. Patients who have surgery have gains in on-time and improvements in motor function and quality of life. Surgery does not slow disease progression, however, and patients will ultimately develop treatment resistant symptoms. Surgical risks include intracranial hemorrhage, stroke, infection, lead migration, misplacement or fracture, and death. Patients undergoing surgery area are at increased risk for depression.

Physical therapy is an important intervention in both early and later disease. For patients with mobility impairment, physical therapy improves balance, motor strength and walking speed. Speech therapy aimed at increasing speech volume is effective in patients with hypophonia. While lacking evidence of effectiveness, occupational therapy might help patients maintain work, family, or social roles.

[1]Not FDA approved for this indication.

[1]Not FDA approved for this indication.

Complications

In addition to functional impairment and disability from motor disease, PD also has cognitive, neuropsychiatric, and autonomic nervous system manifestations. Sleep disturbances occur in almost half of PD patients, including insomnia, nightmares, excessive daytime sleepiness, and rapid-eye movement sleep behavior disorder. Sleep disturbances are often due to sleep fragmentation, and may respond to usual treatments for insomnia. For patients who have difficulty with bed mobility or tremor that affects sleep, prescribe a night-time dose of levodopa/carbidopa. Restless leg syndrome is common in PD and responds to the usual treatments. Rapid eye movement sleep disorder occurs commonly and can occur prior to the onset of motor symptoms. It is characterized by dream-enactment behaviors such as kicking and screaming. Confirm the diagnosis with polysomnography and treat with benzodiazepines.

Fatigue is present in up to a third of patients with PD at the time of diagnosis and may respond to methylphenidate (Ritalin).[1] Daytime drowsiness in PD may be due to sleep disorders and the effect of PD medication. Modefinil (Provigil)[1] has improved scores on the Eppworth sleepiness scale, but has not actually improved sleep parameters in PD patients. There is no effective treatment for sleep attacks in patients with PD. Counsel these patients to avoid driving or operating machinery.

Depression has been reported in up to 80% of PD patients, and can be difficult to distinguish from apathy. The motor symptoms of PD can mimic signs of depression, such as psychomotor slowing. Use of a depression inventory can aid in diagnosis. Desipramine (Norpramin) and nortriptyline (Pamelor) have effectively treated depression in PD; however, their side effect profiles complicate their use. Select a medication for depression—a tricyclic antidepressant (TCA), serotonin-norepinephrine (SNRI) or selective serotonin reuptake inhibitors (SSRI)—based on the patient's co-morbidities and risk for drug interactions.

Psychosis manifests commonly as visual hallucinations. Evaluate the patient for potential causes of delirium, and treat if present. Reassure patients and families in regards to mild, nonfrightening hallucinations. Prescribe quetiapine (Seroquel) for psychosis that requires pharmacologic therapy. Clozapine (Clozaril) is more effective, but the risk of agranulocytosis and need for monitoring make it the second-line agent in the United States. Do not use other antipsychotics, which can worsen motor symptoms of PD. Pimavanserin is new antipsychotic agent that has been found, in one randomized controlled trial, to reduce psychotic symptoms (NNT = 7) and caregiver burden (NNT = 13). The drug is not yet available; the manufacturer is applying for a New Drug Approval in 2015.

Autonomic symptoms include drooling, dysphagia, constipation, voiding dysfunction, erectile dysfunction and orthostatic hypotension. Treat drooling with glycopyrrolate (Robinul) or botulinum toxin type A (Botox).[1] Dysphagia is worse during "off" times; adjusting PD medications to reduce "off" time may help, as may speech therapy. In a randomized trial, polyethylene glycol solution (Miralax) was effective in reducing constipation. No treatments are proven to affect urinary symptoms in PD. It is reasonable to try usual symptomatic treatments, such as antimuscarinic agents. Sildenafil (Viagra) has been shown to improve erectile dysfunction in PD. For patients with orthostatic hypotension, lower antihypertensive dosages if possible and encourage increased fluid and salt intake. Consider use of fludrocortisone[1] or midodrine (Proamatine), even though there is no data to support their use in PD, and monitor for supine hypertension.

Cognitive impairment occurs frequently in PD, and up to 80% of patients will develop dementia at 20 years after diagnosis. Rivastigmine (Exelon) is approved for use in PD. Donepezil (Aricept)[1] is also effective, and it is generally better tolerated than rivastigmine. It is unclear which drug is more effective. Memantine (Namenda)[1] is of uncertain benefit.

PD patients will experience progressive decline in motor and cognitive function, and have about a two-fold increased mortality risk. At age 70, men with PD have a median life expectancy of 8 years and women a median life expectancy of 11 years. Effective treatment can delay disability and improve quality of life.

References

Ahlskog JE. Cheaper, simpler, and better: Tips for treating seniors with Parkinson disease. Mayo Clin Proc 2011;86:1211–6.

Chou KL. In the clinic: Parkinson disease. Ann Int Med 2012;157:ITC5–1–16.

Connolly BS, Lang AE. Pharmacological treatment of Parkinson disease: A review. JAMA 2014;311:1670–83.

Cummings J, et al. Pimavanserin for patients with Parkinson's disease psychosis: a randomised, placebo-controlled phase 3 trial. Lancet 2014;383:533–40.

Drugs for Parkinson's Disease. Treat Guidel Med Lett 2013;11:101–6.

Fritsch T, Smyth KA, Wallendal MS, et al. Parkinson disease: research update and clinical management. South Med J 2012;105:650–6.

Gazewood JD, Richards RR, Clebak K. Parkinson disease: an update. Am Fam Physician 2013;87:267–73.

Okun MS. Deep-brain stimulation for Parkinson's disease. N Engl J Med 2012;367:1529–38.

Rao G, Fisch L, Srinivasan S, et al. Does this patient have Parkinson disease? JAMA 2003;289:347–53.

Scottish Intercollegiate Guidelines Network. Diagnosis and Pharmacological Management of Parkinson's disease: A National Clinical Guideline. Edinburgh: Scottish Intercollegiate Guidelines Network; January, 2010. Available at http://www.sign.ac.uk/pdf/sign113.pdf [accessed Feb 2, 2013].

Stowe R, Ives N, Clarke CE, et al. Evaluation of the efficacy and safety of adjuvant treatment to levodopa therapy in Parkinson's disease patients with motor complications. Cochrane Database Syst Rev 2010;7:CD007166.

PERIPHERAL NEUROPATHIES

Method of
Kerrie Schoffer, MD

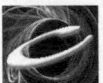

CURRENT DIAGNOSIS

- The five-step approach to classify neuropathies based on fiber type, pattern of distribution, temporal course, pathology, and key features allows a tailored diagnostic evaluation.
- Electrodiagnostic testing provides a useful adjunct to the clinical evaluation.
- The cause of neuropathy might not be found in 20% of patients, but there are treatments for several known etiologies, as well as specific medications to treat neuropathic pain.

Disorders of the peripheral nerve system (PNS) include pathology affecting the spinal cord roots (radiculopathies), the dorsal root ganglia (neuronopathies), the brachial, lumbar, and sacral plexuses (plexopathies), and the terminal nerve (mononeuropathies) or nerves (polyneuropathies). They are among the most common and challenging problems in medical practice, with literally hundreds of conceivable causes. An organized diagnostic approach consists of first categorizing the neuropathy based on clinical and electrophysiologic assessments and then performing a tailored diagnostic evaluation. However astute the diagnostician, the cause of a neuropathy might not found in up to 20% of patients.

Anatomy

Four types of fibers are found in the PNS: motor, large fiber sensory, small fiber sensory, and autonomic. Motor fibers extend peripherally to the neuromuscular junction of their respective muscles and have their cell bodies in motor neurons located in the spinal cord. Conversely, sensory fibers receive information from peripheral sensory receptors and transfer this to cell bodies in the dorsal root ganglia, located near, but outside, the spinal cord. Large, myelinated sensory fibers supply information regarding position and vibration. Small myelinated axons, composed of autonomic and sensory fibers, are responsible for light touch, pain, temperature, and parasympathetic and sympathetic information.

Damage can occur to the cell bodies (neuronopathy), nerve fibers (axonopathy), or to the surrounding myelin sheath (myelinopathy). Myelinopathies principally affect only the coating around the nerve, and an axonopathy results in degeneration of both the axon and

---

[1]Not FDA approved for this indication.

myelin. The most distal segments usually degenerate first, in a process termed *Wallerian degeneration*, resulting in a dying-back neuropathy and a stocking and glove clinical pattern. Neuronopathies affect either the motor neuron or dorsal root ganglion and result in degeneration of both peripheral and central processes.

Five-Step Approach to Neuropathies

When evaluating neuropathy, the differential diagnosis can be limited by asking five key questions:

- What is the *fiber type* involved (motor, large sensory, small sensory, autonomic, combination)?
- What is the *pattern of distribution* (distal or proximal, symmetric or asymmetric)?
- What is the *temporal course* (acute, chronic, progressive, stepwise, relapsing–remitting)?
- Are there any *key features* pointing to a specific etiology?
- What is the *pathology* (axonal, demyelinating)?

Fiber Type

The PNS produces symptomatology in only two ways: negative symptoms (weakness, numbness), which reflect loss of nerve signaling, or positive symptoms (tingling, burning) due to inappropriate spontaneous nerve activity. Box 1 lists symptoms and signs that suggest localization to the peripheral nerves and point specifically to motor, sensory, or autonomic involvement. When inquiring about symptoms, it is important to ask the patient to be as specific as possible. Many patients simply describe an area as numb when, in fact, they are experiencing tingling or even weakness.

A detailed motor examination should include inspection for atrophy, particularly in the distal extensor digitorum brevis and first dorsal interosseous muscles, and for fasciculations (visible twitches of muscle), which are best seen using tangential light. Strength should be tested against resistance, as well as with active maneuvers such as walking on the heels and toes to assess distal strength and rising from a squatting position to examine proximal muscles. Facial muscles should also be tested. When assessing deep tendon reflexes, ensure the reflex is truly absent by asking the patient to concurrently perform a Jendrassic maneuver (pulling against interlocking fingers) or clench the jaw. Note that the reflex arc consists of large-diameter afferent sensory input as well as motor nerve output, so that dysfunction of either can impair reflexes. Tone is sometimes reduced in peripheral nerve diseases.

On sensory examination, sensation should be tested with a pin and a 128-Hz vibratory tuning fork, beginning at the big toe level and moving progressively more proximal. Likewise, position testing should begin distally, with fingers placed on the lateral sides of the big toe and progressively smaller movements tested. Severe loss of position sense can result in athetoid movements of the fingers when the eyes are closed (pseudoathetosis) or a positive Romberg's sign. Temperature can be tested informally by placing a cold tuning fork on the skin. Foot injuries may be apparent with severe sensory loss.

Other important signs include high arches and hammertoe deformities, which suggest a long-standing neuropathy causing differences in muscular force. Demyelinating neuropathies, amyloidosis, and leprosy can cause nerve thickening, which is felt best in the dorsal cutaneous nerve of the foot or the great auricular nerve. Superficial nerves, such as the ulnar nerve at the elbow, can be palpated when appropriate. Postural blood pressure should be assessed for a blood pressure drop more than 20 mm Hg systolic or more than 10 mm Hg diastolic, following 5 minutes of supine rest at a minimum, to test autonomic functioning.

Several other levels of the nervous system can mimic symptoms of PNS disease. Myelopathy and motor neuron disease can manifest with weakness similar to motor neuropathies, although upper motor neuron features such as spasticity and increased reflexes are clues. Myopathies can also cause weakness, but usually more proximal than distal and without any sensory impairment. Isolated sensory involvement should be a red flag that the dorsal root ganglia may be the site of involvement rather than the peripheral nerve; this is particularly important because neuronopathies have a limited differential.

Pattern of Distribution

The pattern of distribution should be classified in two ways: symmetric or asymmetric and distal or proximal. Putting this together with the fiber type, six patterns of PNS disorders can be appreciated, with specific differentials (Table 1).

The symmetric distal sensorimotor neuropathy (pattern 1) manifests in a stocking-and-glove distribution and is the most common type of polyneuropathy. Once the level of the upper calves is reached, fibers of the same length in the fingertips begin to be affected. Sensorimotor polyneuropathies that affect both the distal and proximal nerves (pattern 2) should alert the physician to think of inflammatory neuropathies, such as Guillain-Barré syndrome (GBS) and chronic inflammatory demyelinating polyneuropathy (CIDP).

Asymmetric patterns (pattern 3) are often a result of trauma or compression, such as that seen in mononeuropathies, radiculopathies, and plexopathies. A pattern that affects multiple anatomically separated nerves is termed *mononeuritis multiplex* and is usually the result of a more diffuse process, such as diabetes or vasculitis.

Predominant motor neuropathies (pattern 4) are often proximal, such as diabetic amyotrophy. An exception is lead neuropathy, which affects motor fibers in a distal radial and peroneal distribution. Pure sensory neuropathies (pattern 5) are more likely to be distal, with the exception of a rare few such as Tangier disease, which manifests with a bathing-suit pattern. Neuropathies with autonomic impairment have a limited differential (pattern 6).

Additionally, involvement of the cranial nerves is only seen in a few causes of neuropathy. GBS, CIDP, Lyme disease, sarcoidosis, HIV-associated neuropathy, and Tangier disease are examples.

Temporal Course

Acute neuropathies are relatively rare and suggest an etiology such as GBS, acute intermittent porphyria, ischemia, toxins (thallium toxicity), drugs, or infections (diphtheric neuropathy). Subacute onset (>8 weeks) is seen in nutritional deficiencies, metabolic

---

Box 1 Signs and Symptoms of Peripheral Nervous System Disease by Fiber Type

Motor
- Cramps
- Fasciculations
- Hyporeflexia
- Hypotonia
- Muscle atrophy
- Myokymia
- Pes cavus
- Weakness

Large Fiber Sensory
- Decreased vibration and position
- Hyporeflexia
- Pins and needles
- Tingling
- Unsteady gait, especially at night or with eyes closed

Small Fiber Sensory
- Burning
- Decreased pain sensation
- Decreased temperature sensation
- Jabbing

Autonomic
- Decreased or increased sweating
- Heat intolerance
- Impotence
- Postural hypotension
- Urinary retention

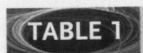

TABLE 1 Causes of Neuropathy by Pattern Type

CAUSES	POTENTIALLY USEFUL TESTS
Sensorimotor	
Symmetric and Distal	
Metabolic disorders	OGTT, LFT, creatinine, TSH, vitamin B₁₂
Hereditary disorders (CMT)	EMG/NCS
Infections (HIV, leprosy)	HIV test, review of medical and social history
Toxins (drugs, alcohol, arsenic, thallium)	
Symmetric, Proximal, and Distal	
Inflammatory neuropathies (GBS, CIDP)	EMG/NCS, CSF
Asymmetric	
Mononeuropathy, radiculopathy, plexopathy	EMG/NCS
Mononeuritis multiplex	ANA, RF, ESR, ANCA, nerve bx
Vasculitis	
Diabetes	OGTT
HIV	HIV test
Multifocal CIDP	CSF
Rare: porphyria, leprosy, HNPP	
Pure Motor	
Proximal	
Diabetic amyotrophy	OGTT
MMNCB	EMG/NCS
Motor variants of GBS, CIDP, MGUS	CSF, SPE, IF
Lymphoma	CBC
Distal	
Rare: Lead toxicity, porphyria	
Pure Sensory	
Neuropathies	
Nonsystemic vasculitis neuropathy	Nerve bx
Chronic gluten enteropathy	Antigliadin antibodies
Vitamin E deficiency	Vitamin E level
Distal, demyelinating, symmetric neuropathy	SPE, IF
Rare: primary biliary cirrhosis, Crohn's disease	
Neuronopathies	
Paraneoplastic neuronopathy	Anti-Hu/CV2, Imaging
Sjögren's syndrome	Lip biopsy
HIV-related sensory neuronopathy	HIV test
Miller Fisher variant	EMG/NCS
Drugs (see Box 4)	Medication review
Autonomic	
Diabetes	OGTT
GBS	EMG/NCS
Paraneoplastic sensory neuropathy	Anti-Hu, CV2, imaging
HIV-related neuropathy	HIV test
Vincristine (Oncovin)	Medication review
Thiamine deficiency	Alcohol history
Rare: porphyria, hereditary autonomic neuropathy, amyloidosis	

Abbreviations: ANA = antinuclear antibodies; ANCA = antineutrophilic cytoplasmic antibodies; bx = biopsy; CBC = complete blood count; CIDP = chronic inflammatory demyelinating polyneuropathy; CMT = Charcot-Marie-Tooth disease; CSF = cerebrospinal fluid; EMG/NCS = electromyography/nerve conduction studies; ESR = erythrocyte sedimentation rate; GBS = Guillain-Barré syndrome; HIV = human immunodeficiency virus; HNPP = hereditary neuropathy with liability to pressure palsies; IF = immunofixation; LFT = liver function tests; MGUS = monoclonal gammopathy of unknown significance; MMNCB = multifocal motor neuropathy with conduction blocks; OGTT = oral glucose tolerance test; RF = rheumatoid factor; SPE = serum protein electrophoresis; TSH = thyroid-stimulating hormone.

neuropathies, paraneoplastic syndromes, and CIDP. A chronic course is typical of hereditary neuropathies, a stepwise pattern can be seen in mononeuropathy multiplex, and a relapsing-remitting course occurs with intermittent exposure to a toxin or drug and in CIDP.

Key Signs
Sometimes, there is a key classic feature on history or examination that significantly narrows the differential immediately. Box 2 includes a checklist of items for inquiry and observation during assessment of neuropathy.

Pathology and the Role of Neurophysiology
Nerve conduction studies (NCSs) and electromyography (EMG) are highly specialized tests that are performed principally by neurologists. NCSs electrically activate peripheral nerves at particular sites and then assess for abnormal transmission from the stimulation point to the final muscle response. EMG involves placing a small needle into the muscle to observe both the sound and appearance of the muscle at rest and with motor units firing. Because NCSs can only be performed at points where the nerve is

Box 2 Key Diagnostic Features

Medical History
- Connective tissue disease
- Diabetes
- Renal disease
- Thyroid disease

Surgical History, Trauma
- Compression neuropathies

Medication History
- Drug-induced neuropathy

Family History, High Arches
- Inherited neuropathy

Nutrition, Alcohol Use
- Alcoholic neuropathy
- Vitamin deficiency

Occupational Exposures
- Toxic neuropathy

History of Weight Loss
- Amyloidosis
- HIV
- Malignancy

Recent Infection, Travel
- Diphtheria
- Guillain-Barré syndrome
- HIV
- Leprosy
- Lyme disease

Dry Eyes and Mouth
- Sarcoidosis

Severe Pain
- Amyloidosis
- Diabetes
- Guillain-Barré syndrome
- HIV
- Vasculitis

Skin Lesions
- Anesthetic patches (leprosy)
- Bullous lesions (porphyria)
- Hyperpigmentation (osteosclerotic myeloma)
- Mee's lines (arsenic or thallium poisoning)
- Orange tonsils (Tangier disease)
- Angiokeratomas (Fabry's disease)

superficial (most often distal), EMG is needed to assess for more proximal damage such as radiculopathy. EMG can also rule out other mimics of PNS disease, such as myopathy.

For the general physician, the most important thing is being able to interpret the results of these tests. Often, a report will be received back such as: "There is evidence of a symmetric distal axonal sensorimotor neuropathy." An NCS/EMG study should be able to specify the distribution and if motor or sensory fibers are involved. Autonomic and small sensory fibers are not tested well by EMG, so the diagnosis of these types of neuropathies is often clinical or requires more specialized testing. Thus, a normal NCS/EMG does not rule out neuropathy.

A further feature that electrophysiology can add is whether the pathology is demyelinating or axonal. Demyelination is characterized by slowed conduction velocity, temporal dispersion of the muscle action potential, and conduction block. Hereditary demyelinating neuropathies, such as Charcot-Marie-Tooth disease, do not show the latter two features, which are only seen in acquired neuropathies. Axonal disease is characterized by modest slowing of velocities and more marked reduction in the amplitudes of the muscle and sensory action potentials. On EMG, there are fibrillations within 3 weeks of the neuropathic injury, indicating spontaneous firing of denervated muscle. Enlarged and prolonged motor unit potentials indicate subsequent regeneration, which occurs after several weeks to months.

Demyelination has a limited differential (Box 3) and often a better prognosis, because myelin can start to regenerate within a few days. Axonal regeneration proceeds at a far slower rate of 1 to 3 μm/day, and nerves with proximal lesions must go a long distance to reinnervate their muscle and might never reach their goal.

Investigations

Once the neuropathy has been subclassified, investigations for the specific causes in that pattern class should be undertaken (see Table 1). Several recent papers suggest that 2-hour oral glucose tolerance testing (OGTT) is the best test for glucose intolerance due to the relatively low sensitivity of serum glucose levels and glycosylated hemoglobin (HbA1c). Likewise, vitamin B_{12} levels have a low sensitivity, and serum metabolites methylmalonic acid (MMA) and homocysteine (Hcy) should be measured in patients with a result less than 300 pg/mL to improve diagnostic accuracy. These metabolites can be falsely increased with hypovolemia, renal insufficiency, hypothyroidism, and increased age, but a return to normal levels 1 to 2 weeks after beginning replacement therapy indicates this is the cause. The combination of elevated gastrin and anti-parietal cell antibodies may be used to diagnose pernicious anemia. The yield of general testing for other vitamin deficiencies in polyneuropathy is relatively low.

Antinuclear antibodies (ANA) probably are usually only significant in the context of suggestive features (abrupt onset, mononeuropathy multiplex pattern, arthralgia or arthritis, fevers, rash, or renal abnormalities) because they are positive in about 3% of normal patients. However, referral to a rheumatologist should be considered with a very high titer (>1:1280).

The erythryocyte sedimentation rate (ESR) is often elevated, especially in older patients. Rates greater than 70 mm/hour tend to be more meaningful, particularly with a mononeuritis multiplex pattern.

Serum protein electrophoresis lacks sensitivity, and immunofixation should be ordered if there is high suspicion of a paraproteinemia. If an elevated monoclonal antibody is found, a 24-hour urine test for Bence Jones proteinuria, skeletal survey, CBC, renal function tests, and serum calcium should be ordered. If the M protein is greater than 2.5 g/dL or if abnormalities are detected on these tests, referral to a hematologist for bone marrow aspiration is required. Polyclonal antibodies are not associated with neuropathy.

If there is suspicion of amyloidosis, a rectal, abdominal fat, or sensory nerve biopsy can be undertaken. Sural nerve biopsy is reserved for difficult diagnostic situations because it causes a permanent area of numbness with possible dysesthesias over the biopsied area. Suspicion of vasculitis is the most common indication, but pathology can also be seen in leprosy and with tumor infiltrate.

In approximately 20% of patients, an underlying cause of neuropathy is not found. These patients are said to have a cryptogenic sensory or sensorimotor neuropathy. A distinct clinical picture has emerged, most commonly of a patient in the sixth or seventh decade manifesting with distal dysesthesias and possibly with mild weakness and sensory ataxia. These patients tend not to develop significant disability, and treatment is mainly for neuropathic pain.

Treatment
Mononeuropathies

The most common cause of mononeuropathy is nerve compression, and surgical treatment is often a consideration for these patients. The four most common locations are median neuropathy at the wrist (carpal tunnel syndrome), ulnar neuropathy at the elbow, peroneal neuropathy at the fibular head, and facial nerve palsy (Bell's palsy).

Carpal tunnel syndrome manifests with pain and numbness principally in the first three digits, although it is often poorly localized. Classic features include pain at night and shaking out the hand to relieve pain. For milder symptoms, a nighttime splint, which prevents wrist flexion and high pressure in the carpal tunnel, is often helpful. Local corticosteroid injections can provide relief, and surgical decompression has a very high success rate.

Ulnar neuropathy manifests with numbness of the fourth and fifth digits and wasting of the interosseous muscles, often with pain localized to the elbow. Peroneal neuropathies manifest with foot drop and numbness on the dorsum of the foot. In both cases, avoidance of pressure over the nerve often leads to improvement. Surgery might improve symptoms, but less reliably so than carpal tunnel surgery.

Bell's palsy is an inflammatory rather than compressive process, presumably due to a viral etiology. Treatment is controversial, but early (within 14 days) use of prednisone[1] 60 mg daily, decreasing by 10 mg steps every 2 days, along with acyclovir (Zovirax)[1] 800 mg five times daily for 7 days has been advocated. About 15% of patients have residual facial weakness.

Guillain-Barré Syndrome

GBS often begins following gastroenteritis with *Campylobacter jejuni*, or an upper respiratory tract infection, due to a presumed autoimmune response directed against myelin. The incidence is 1 or 2 per 100,000 persons per year. Characteristic features are ascending weakness, areflexia, and sensory and autonomic symptoms progressing over a few days up to 4 weeks. Facial diplegia and pain can occur. Electrophysiology shows acute demyelination with conduction blocks, and cerebrospinal fluid (CSF) reveals an

---

Box 3 Demyelinating Neuropathies

- Charcot-Marie-Tooth disease
- Hereditary neuropathy with liability to pressure palsies
- Inflammatory neuropathies
- Monoclonal gammopathies and paraproteinemias
- Multifocal motor neuropathy with conduction block
- Neuropathies caused by drugs such as amiodarone (Cordarone) and suramin[2]
- Neuropathies caused by infections (diphtheria) or toxins (arsenic)

[2]Not available in the United States.

[1]Not FDA approved for this indication.

increase in protein with a cell count of fewer than 5 white blood cells (cytoalbuminologic dissociation) in more than 80% of patients after 2 weeks. A CSF pleocytosis of more than 10 lymphocytes/mm³ should alert the physician to another cause such as sarcoidosis, Lyme disease, or early HIV.

The Miller-Fisher variant is characterized by specific clinical features of sensory ataxia, areflexia, and ophthalmolplegia. *C. jejuni* infection has been correlated with more severe variants, such as acute motor axonal neuropathy (AMAN) and acute motor and sensory axonal neuropathy (AMSAM), which damage axons in addition to myelin. *C. jejuni*–related GBS correlates with anti-GM1 antibodies, although they are not prognostic or specific. Recovery can take months to years. Only 20% of patients are left without residual deficit. About 5% to 10% have significant persistent disability, and the mortality rate is 5%.

During early treatment, patients might require admission to intensive care, with close monitoring of pulmonary function tests for respiratory compromise. Diaphragmatic weakness correlates with neck flexion and extension and shoulder abduction. The patient should be intubated when the forced vital capacity (FVC) declines to less than 15 mL/kg or when negative inspiratory flow (NIF) is less than −20 to −30. Monitoring of the cardiac rhythm is important due to dysautonomia.

The preferred treatment is intravenous immunoglobulin (IVIg)[1] at a dose of 0.4 g/kg/day for 5 days. This is generally well tolerated, and adverse side effects such as myalgia, headache, or flu-like symptoms often resolve with a reduced infusion rate. If IVIg is contraindicated (renal failure, IgA deficiency), plasmapheresis can be initiated with four alternate-day exchanges over 7 to 10 days for a total of 200 to 250 mL/kg. Both plasmapheresis and IVIg continue to work for several weeks after the treatment period, but if patients experience a secondary worsening after successful treatment, a second dose may be initiated. Steroids were reviewed recently by a Cochrane systematic review and were not found to be of benefit in GBS.

Chronic Inflammatory Demyelinating Polyneuropathy

This neuropathy is pathologically similar to GBS, but progression is longer than 8 weeks, often with a relapsing-remitting course. Symmetric distal and proximal weakness and sensory impairment, hyporeflexia, and cytoalbuminergic dissociation in the CSF is the classic presentation, although there are variants.

Treatment is either IVIg[1] or prednisone. IVIg is given initially at 0.4 g/kg/day for 5 days, and then the dose and frequency are reduced over time. Prednisone is given 1 mg/kg/day until improvement, followed by a slow tapering of 5 mg every 2 to 3 weeks over a period of months. Response is usually seen within 4 weeks. Refractory patients have been treated with repeated plasmapheresis treatments or immunosuppressive therapy with cyclosporine (Sandimmune).[1]

Multifocal Motor Neuropathy

Multifocal motor neuropathy (MMN) is not a common disorder but is important not to mistake for motor neuron disease because it has a very different prognosis and treatment. Patients present with progressive asymmetric distal weakness, often of the arm, without sensory loss and with less atrophy than would be expected for the degree of weakness. Unlike motor neuron disease, there are no upper motor neuron signs. It is different from multifocal acquired demyelinating sensory and motor neuropathy (MADSAM), an asymmetric variant of CIDP, in that loss of reflexes and weakness involves only the affected limb, there is a relatively normal CSF protein concentration, and sensory nerve conduction studies are normal. Diagnosis is supported by finding conduction blocks in sites not usually associated with compression. The GM1 antibody is elevated in 60% of cases. Repeated treatments with IVIg[1] or cyclophosphamide (Cytoxan)[1] are common choices. Rituximab (Rituxan),[1] a monoclonal antibody, has also been used. Prednisone classically worsens the condition.

Diabetic Neuropathy

Diabetes is one of the most common causes of neuropathy. Patients can present with a symmetric distal neuropathy, autonomic proximal diabetic neuropathy, mononeuritis multiplex, compressive and cranial neuropathies, and trunk polyradiculopathies.

The distal symmetric sensory polyneuropathy (DSPN) correlates with the duration of the diabetes, control of hyperglycemia, and presence of retinopathy and nephropathy. The exact etiology is unknown, but theories include a metabolic process involving aldose reductase, ischemic damage, or an immunologic disorder. Typical symptoms include lancinating pains or burning, worse at night, and possible dysautonomia. Atrophy may be noted in the foot muscles, but severe weakness is atypical. NCS may be normal because small fibers are primarily affected. Treatment includes blood sugar control to limit progression and symptom control for neuropathic pain. Gabapentin (Neurontin)[1] and tricyclic antidepressants are common choices (see later). Drugs such as QR-333, a topical compound that contains quercetin, a flavonoid with aldose reductase–inhibitor effects, are being investigated specifically for diabetic neuropathy.

Autonomic neuropathy is treated symptomatically, with fludrocortisone (Florinef)[1] 0.1 mg/day for orthostatic hypotension, meto-clopramide (Reglan) 10 mg before meals for gastroparesis, and sildenafil (Viagra) 25 mg 1 hour before sexual intercourse for impotence.

Proximal diabetic neuropathy (diabetic amyotrophy) manifests typically with unilateral pain in the anterior thigh followed by step-wise progression over weeks to months of quadriceps weakness, atrophy of the proximal leg muscles, and a reduced knee reflex, with occasional contralateral leg involvement. The ESR may be elevated and CSF protein mildly increased (120 mg/dL on average). NCS and EMG reflect multifocal active axonal damage (fibrillations) to the lumbar plexus and roots. Small retrospective studies have reported that IVIg[1] and other forms of immunosuppressive therapy are effective in treating patients with proximal diabetic neuropathy. A short course of corticosteroids (prednisone[1] 50 mg/day for 1 week, then tapering by 10 mg/week) can be used to ease pain in severe cases, with close monitoring of the glucose level, but overall prognosis is quite good, ranging from 1 to 18 months of recovery phase (mean of 6 months) and partial or complete restoration of strength in approximately 70% of patients.

Paraproteinemic Neuropathies

Multiple myeloma, Waldenström's macroglobulinemia, cryoglobulinemia, osteosclerotic myeloma (POEMS syndrome), and monoclonal gammopathy of unknown significance (MGUS) are associated with monoclonal antibodies directed at PNS components, such as myelin-associated glycoprotein (MAG). Neuropathies associated with an immunoglobulin (Ig)M monoclonal protein (approximately 60%) are typically distal, demyelinating, and symmetric, whereas IgG (30%) and IgA (10%) gammopathies can be axonal or demyelinating. In terms of treatment, the distal demyelinating neuropathy of IgM paraproteinemias tends to be treatment refractory. IgG and IgA gammopathies can mimic the demyelination pattern seen in CIDP, and patients with any antibody and this pattern should receive immunotherapy as recommended for CIDP (see earlier). Axonal neuropathies and IgM, IgG, or IgA gammopathies have a less clear relationship and are typically not responsive to treatment.

Hereditary Neuropathies

Charcot-Marie-Tooth (CMT) disease is among the most common of genetic neuromuscular disorders, and more than 30 genes have been identified. Clues are a history of difficulty running in childhood, high arches, hammertoes, ankle weakness, and nerve hypertrophy developing in teenage years. Depending on the subtype, the neuropathy may be axonal or demyelinating, but the most common type (CMT-1) is caused by an autosomal dominant gene

---

[1]Not FDA approved for this indication.

[1]Not FDA approved for this indication.

encoding peripheral myelin protein 22 and is easily diagnosed by the relatively uniform slowing on nerve conduction velocities (<25% of lower limits of normal). Patients have a mild course and remain ambulatory throughout life in most cases.

Hereditary neuropathy with liability to pressure palsies (HNPP) is another dominantly inherited neuropathy in which patients have recurrent episodes of isolated mononeuropathies, typically affecting, in order of decreasing frequency, the common peroneal, ulnar, radial, and median nerves. Most attacks are sudden onset, painless, and followed by complete recovery. There is no treatment other than preventive measures.

Toxic and Nutritional Neuropathies

Treatment of toxic and nutritional neuropathies involves detection and removal of the underlying cause. A thorough review of medications, occupational exposures, and nutritional risk factors is essential (Box 4). Drug toxicity is much more common than

---

Box 4　Causes of Toxic and Nutritional Neuropathies

Drug Toxins
Axonal
- Colchicine
- Dapsone
- Disulfiram
- Ethambutol
- Hyralazine
- Isoniazid
- Metronidazole
- Nitrofurantoin
- Nitrous oxide
- Nucleosides
- Paclitaxel
- Phenytoin
- Tacrolimus
- Vincristine

Demyelinating
- Amiodarone (Cordarone)
- Chloroquine (Aralen)
- Gold
- Suramin[2]

Neuronopathy
- Cisplatin (Platinol-AQ)
- Pyridoxine (vitamin B_6)
- Thalidomide (Thalomid)

Environmental Toxins
- Acrylamide (plastics)
- Allyl chloride (insecticides)
- Arsenic
- Carbon disulfide (cellophanes)
- Ethylene glycol (antifreeze)
- Ethylene oxide (sterilizer)
- Hexacarbons (glue)
- Lead
- Mercury
- Methyl bromide (fumigant)
- Organophosphates (insecticides)
- Thallium (pesticides)
- Trichloroethylene (drycleaning)
- Vacor (rodenticide)

Vitamin Deficiencies
- B_1 (alcoholism)
- B_3 (alcoholism)
- B_6 (isoniazid use)
- B_{12} (vegans, pernicious anemia)
- E (cholestasis and abetalipoproteinemia)

[2]Not available in the United States.

---

environmental toxicity. Incidence of neuropathy does not always correlate with the dosage and duration of exposure. For instance, amiodarone neuropathy has been reported with dosages as low as 200 mg/day and durations as short as 1 month. Symptoms might not improve, or might even worsen, for several weeks after the drug is stopped before improvement starts, a phenomenon known as *coasting*.

Cisplatin can cause a neuropathy that overlaps in symptomatology with paraneoplastic sensory neuronopathy, and dapsone is associated with a motor axonopathy. Gold neuropathy can have prominent myokymia and can mimic GBS.

Specific treatments for drug-induced neuropathies include cyanocobalamin (vitamin B_{12})[1] for nitrous oxide neuropathy and pyridoxine (vitamin B_6)[1] for hydralazine and isoniazid neuropathies. Excessive vitamin B_6 can also *cause* a neuropathy. Glutamine[7] and vitamin E[1] 300 mg twice a day has shown promise for paclitaxel neuropathy, and neuroprotective agents such as nerve growth factor are being investigated for cisplatin-induced neuropathy. Tacrolimus can cause a CIDP-like neuropathy that responds to IVIg[1] or plasmapheresis.

One of the most common nutritional neuropathies is caused by thiamine deficiency and is associated with alcohol consumption of at least 100 g per day. Patients present with burning feet, and early alcohol abstinence and treatment with thiamine denotes better chance of recovery. Vitamin B_{12} deficiency is vital not to miss and can manifest with a subacute combined degeneration, whereby patients have a superimposed myelopathy and neuropathy (spasticity but reduced reflexes). Sudden-onset symptoms, particularly in the feet and hands simultaneously, are also suggestive.

Metabolic and Infectious Neuropathies

Peripheral neuropathy can complicate renal failure, hypothyroidism, biliary cirrhosis, porphyria, Tangier disease, Fabry's disease, and mitochondrial diseases.

Early in the course, HIV can manifest as a GBS-like syndrome, although with CSF pleocytosis. This typically responds to IVIg[1] and plasmapheresis. In later stages, patients might develop a distal symmetric polyneuropathy, although it is important to determine if this might be due to nucleoside reverse transcriptase inhibitors, nutritional deficiency, or infection. Cranial neuropathies, sensory neuronopathy, lumbosacral polyradiculopathies, and mononeuritis multiplex also occur.

Leprosy is the most common treatable neuropathy worldwide. Tuberculoid leprosy leads to hypopigmented patches with loss of pain and temperature sensation. Lepromatous leprosy, a more severe form seen in immunosuppressed persons, can cause ulnar, common peroneal, and facial neuropathies. Treatment involves a long-term multidrug regimen of dapsone and rifampin (Rifadin).[1]

Herpes zoster can cause a postherpetic neuralgia, defined as pain persisting for more than 6 weeks after the rash appears. Early treatment with acyclovir (Zovirax) (800 mg five times daily for 7 days) can reduce the duration of the acute phase. Chronic discomfort is treated with medications for neuropathic pain (see later).

Lyme disease, caused by *Borrelia burgdorferi*, begins with erythema migrans, followed by multifocal peripheral and cranial neuropathies, particularly facial diplegia. CSF lymphocytic pleocytosis plus serologic demonstration of *B. burgdorferi* infection on serum or CSF are the diagnostic features. Early stages are treated with a 3-week course of doxycycline[1] 100 mg twice daily, and intravenous penicillin G[1] should be given in the late stages.

[1]Not FDA approved for this indication.
[7]Available as a dietary supplement.

Carcinomatous Neuropathy

Tumors can cause neuropathy by compression, metastatic spread, paraneoplastic antibodies, hemorrhage, and treatment with chemotherapy or radiation therapy. A distal sensorimotor neuropathy is associated with many different tumors and seldom precedes tumor diagnosis. Pathogenesis can include toxic, nutritional, and immunologic causes. A sensory neuronopathy is less common, but often precedes tumor diagnosis, thus warranting a careful work-up. Lung, breast, ovary, and gastrointestinal tract cancers are the most likely associated types. Imaging and paraneoplastic antibodies (particularly anti-Hu and anti-CV2, most commonly associated with lung cancer) may help in making the diagnosis. Treatment focuses on the underlying neoplasm.

Vasculitic Neuropathy

Vasculitis can be primary (polyarteritis nodosa, Wegener's granulomatosis, Churg-Strauss syndrome, microscopic polyangitis) or secondary (connective tissue diseases, systemic infections, drug reactions). It classically manifests with a painful mononeuritis multiplex with asymmetric patchy features, reflecting multifocal ischemic damage. If the patient's vasculitis is restricted to the PNS, serologic testing for these disorders is often negative. In this case, a sural nerve biopsy might reveal fibrinoid necrosis and perivascular inflammation.

Treatment needs to be carefully undertaken with intravenous methylprednisolone (Solu-Medrol)[1] for 3 days followed by oral prednisone. In many cases, other immunosuppressive drugs are eventually used.

Neuropathic Pain

Often pain is the most predominant and distressing feature of neuropathy. Several classes of medications can be tried (Table 2), although it is important to counsel the patient that complete abolition of pain is unlikely. A trial period should be undertaken for at least 6 to 8 weeks before concluding that the patient does not respond. A combination of agents with different mechanisms can have an advantage over monotherapy for the nonresponsive patient.

First-line treatment is generally with tricyclic antidepressants. Serotonin and noradrenaline reuptake inhibitors such as amitriptyline[1] (Elavil), imipramine[1] (Tofranil), and clomipramine[1] (Anafranil) may be marginally more effective than those with relatively selective noradrenergic effects such as desipramine and nortriptyline. However, nortriptyline and desipramine are less sedating. Selective serotonin reuptake inhibitors appear to be less effective. Second-line antidepressants include venlafaxine[1] (Effexor), bupropion[1] (Wellbutrin), and the recently approved duloxetine (Cymbalta), which have the advantage of better tolerability due to less muscarinic, histaminergic, and α-adrenergic affinity.

The typical next class of medications to try is the antiepileptics. Gabapentin[1] is a common choice and is generally well tolerated. Pregabalin (Lyrica) is a newer related agent that, unlike gabapentin, exhibits linear pharmacokinetics and can be initiated at a therapeutic dose without a long titration. Second-line choices include lamotrigine[1] (Lamictal), carbamazepine[1] (Tegretol), and topiramate[1] (Topamax). Valproate[1] (Depacon) and zonisamide[1] (Zonegran) have limited evidence, and phenytoin[1] (Dilantin) can cause neuropathy. Oxcarbazepine[1] (Trileptal), like carbamazepine, slows the recovery rate of voltage-activated sodium channels, but it also inhibits high-threshold N-type and P/Q-type calcium channels and reduces glutamatergic transmission. As a result, it can modulate both peripheral and central neuropathic pain pathways, and several studies into its efficacy are under way.

Topical creams, such as capsaicin (Zostrix), an extract of chili, can be tried. Capsaicin works by depleting substance P and can temporarily worsen pain by causing a burning sensation. Lidocaine[1] (Xylocaine) can be also used topically.

Other agents for severe neuropathies include opioid agents, such as tramadol (Ultram), which has low-affinity binding for μ-opioid receptors coupled with mild inhibition of norepinephrine and serotonin reuptake. Slow-release opioids, such as oxycodone (OxyContin) 30 to 60 mg/day, can help, and risk of addiction is low in this population. Glutamate antagonists, such as dextromethorphan[1] (Delsym), have shown benefit in some studies, as has mexiletine[1] (Mexitil), a class IB antiarrhythmic agent and oral analogue of lidocaine. Nonpharmacologic therapies, such as transcutaneous electrical nerve stimulation (TENS) and acupuncture, might also provide adjunctive relief.

[1]Not FDA approved for this indication.

[1]Not FDA approved for this indication.

TABLE 2	Select Neuropathic Pain Medications	
DRUG	**DOSAGE**	**SIDE EFFECTS**
Amitriptyline (Elavil)[1]	10 mg/d, increasing weekly by 10 mg, up to 150 mg/d	Dry mouth, sedation, urinary retention, cardiac arrhythmias, orthostatic hypotension, constipation, weight gain Contraindications: cardiac arrhythmias, CHF, recent MI, narrow angle glaucoma, urinary retention
Capsaicin (Zostrix)	0.075% cream applied tid to qid	Sneezing, coughing, rash, skin irritation
Carbamazepine (Tegretol)[1]	100 mg bid, increasing by 100 mg weekly Max: 1200 mg/d	Somnolence, dizziness, nausea, gait changes, urticaria, hyponatremia, pancytopenia, hepatic dysfunction Obtain baseline and 6-wk CBC and LFT
Gabapentin (Neurontin)[1]	300 mg on day 1, 600 mg on day 2, 900 mg on day 3 Max: 3600 mg/d	Sedation, fatigue, dizziness, confusion, tremor, weight gain, peripheral edema, headache Reduce dose in renal insufficiency
Lamotrigine (Lamictal)[1]	25 mg at night for 2 wk, increasing weekly by 25–50 mg Max: 400 mg/d	Severe rash (especially if increased too quickly), dizziness, unsteadiness, drowsiness, diplopia
Tramadol (Ultram)	50 mg bid Titrate 50 mg every 3–7 d, using a tid or qid schedule Max: 100 mg qid	Constipation, headache, nausea Risk of seizures with neuroleptics and antidepressants Reduce dose with hepatic or renal dysfunction

[1]Not FDA approved for this indication.
Abbreviations: CBC = complete blood count; CHF = congestive heart failure; LFT = liver function test; max = maximum; MI = myocardial infarction.

References

Donofrio PD, Albers JW. AAEM minimonograph 34. Polyneuropathy: Classification by nerve conduction studies and electromyography. Muscle Nerve 1990;13:889–903.

Dworkin RH, Backonja M, Rowbotham MC, et al. Advances in neuropathic pain: Diagnosis, mechanisms, and treatment recommendations. Arch Neurol 2003;60:1524–34.

Grant I, Benstead TJ. Differential diagnosis of peripheral neuropathy. In: Dyck PJ, Thomas PK, editors. Peripheral Neuropathy. Philadelphia: Saunders; 2005.

Poncelet AN. An algorithm for the evaluation of peripheral neuropathy. Am Fam Physician 1997;57(4):755–64.

Stewart JD. Focal peripheral neuropathies. New York: Raven Press; 1993.

REHABILITATION OF THE STROKE PATIENT

Method of
Marlís González-Fernández, MD, PhD; and Dorianne Feldman, MD

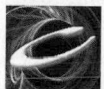

CURRENT THERAPY

- Stroke rehabilitation improves functional outcomes.
- A comprehensive rehabilitation team composed of physicians, nurses, therapists, and community reintegration professionals can achieve the best outcomes.
- Early evaluation of family support and the home environment is critical to prevent unnecessary institutionalization.
- Evaluation and management of modifiable stroke risk factors, such as smoking, hypertension, and diabetes, are imperative during stroke rehabilitation to prevent stroke recurrence.
- Rehabilitation of the stroke patient can be hindered by conditions such as pneumonia (usually caused by aspiration), deep venous thrombosis, urinary tract infections, shoulder pain, depression, and spasticity. Early identification and treatment of these conditions are necessary to maximize functional outcomes.

According to the National Center for Health Statistics, 5.6 million Americans live with the disability caused by a previous stroke.

Stroke is the leading cause of permanent disability in adults. Conservative estimates suggest that about 45% of stroke patients have moderate to severe disabilities requiring rehabilitation.

The goals of stroke rehabilitation are to maintain and optimize medical management, to maximize functional recovery, to minimize disability, and to improve quality of life and participation in society. The rehabilitative approach endeavors to provide patient-centered care that is organized, comprehensive, and specific to the needs of the stroke patient. The concerted efforts of the patient, family, and rehabilitation team are essential for achieving these goals. Recovery after stroke can be a long and challenging process for the patient and the family. Although functional gains occur most rapidly in the first year after a stroke, additional motor recovery is possible beyond 1 year when patients are involved in targeted rehabilitation programs.

The rehabilitation team is composed of rehabilitation physicians (physiatrists), other physicians such as neurologists and neurosurgeons, rehabilitation nurses, occupational therapists, physical therapists, speech and language pathologists, rehabilitation neuropsychologists, social workers, case managers, nutritionists, vocational counselors, and pharmacists. A goal of the acute inpatient rehabilitation team is discharging the patient to the least restrictive environment, ideally home. To accomplish this goal, it is critical to evaluate family support and the home environment.

Rehabilitation should start as part of the acute stroke inpatient stay. The decision-making process to determine the appropriate rehabilitation setting after discharge is described in Figure 1. Speech-language pathologists, physical therapists, and occupational therapists evaluate deficits in cognition, communication, deglutition, mobility, and activities of daily living. The severity of deficits in these major areas and the ability of the patient to tolerate therapy determine the appropriate rehabilitation setting.

Stroke patients with mild deficits are able to return home with home or outpatient therapy services. Patients with moderate to severe strokes benefit from more intensive therapy in an institutional setting. Comprehensive inpatient rehabilitation is suitable for patients with moderate to severe deficits who can tolerate intensive rehabilitation (3 h/day for 5 days each week or 15 hours of therapy over a 7 day period). If the severity of deficits or medical comorbidities limits the ability of the patient to participate in intensive therapy, alternate settings can be considered.

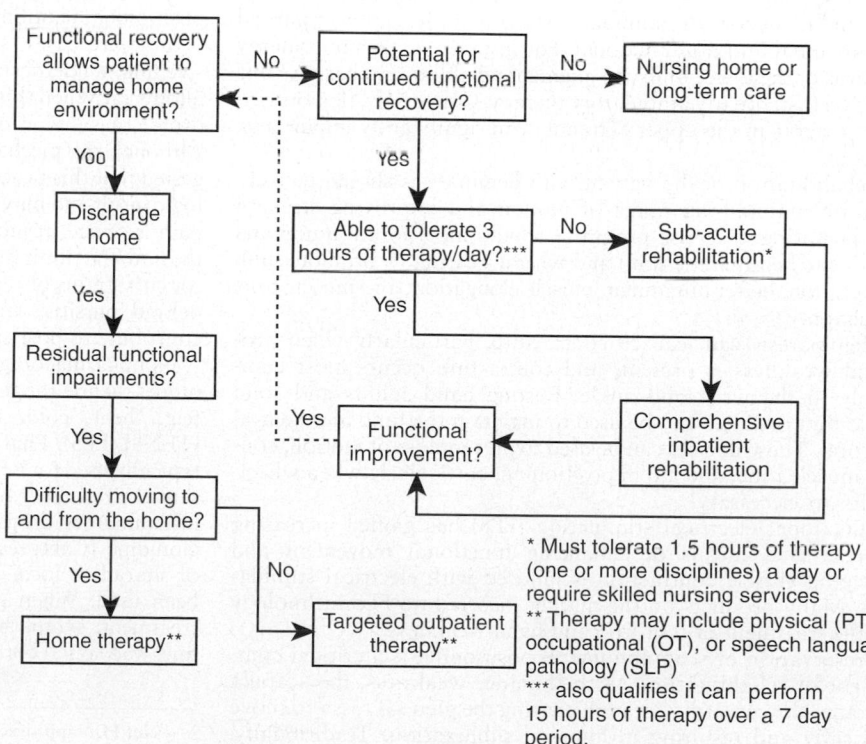

Figure 1. Determination of rehabilitation needs of patients being discharged after an acute stroke.

During the inpatient rehabilitation stage, medical management focuses on secondary stroke prevention: diet; exercise; smoking cessation; and reducing complications, including optimizing blood pressure control while maintaining cerebral perfusion, preventing and treating lipid disorders, and managing post-stroke pain, depression, and abnormal muscle tone. During this stage, much of the rehabilitation effort is directed toward educating stroke survivors about complications and the importance of adherence to medical recommendations.

Medical complications, such as deep venous thrombosis and related thromboembolism, pneumonia (usually related to aspiration), skin breakdown, and urinary infections, can hinder a patient's recovery. Early identification of these complications is necessary to maintain progress in the rehabilitation effort. Other complications, such as seizures and cardiac decompensation, are possible and should be monitored.

Stroke often causes significant impairment and activity limitations. Deficits in strength, swallowing, vision, balance, muscle tone, communication, comprehension, cognition, attention, sensory perception, and bladder function are common and can cause difficulty completing activities of daily living, walking, transferring to and from different surfaces, and getting in and out of the bed. Post-stroke depression, fatigue, and pain are common and should be addressed to maximize participation in rehabilitative efforts.

Transition to the chronic phase begins after the patient is medically stable and inpatient therapy goals are met. Outpatient therapy services are initiated in conjunction with physiatric, primary care, and neurologic follow-up.

Hemiparesis

Hemiparesis, or one-sided weakness, is one of the most frequent complications after stroke. Recovery of motor function varies. Often, it is limited by muscle atrophy, co-contraction of agonists and antagonists, and abnormal tone. Usually, motor recovery is preceded by the development of patterned muscle movements, or synergies. Synergies occur when select muscles contract in a predictable manner. In the paretic upper extremity, a flexion synergy pattern (i.e., humeral adduction, internal rotation, elbow flexion, forearm pronation, and wrist and finger flexion) is common. In the lower extremity, extension synergies (i.e., hip internal rotation, adduction, extension, knee extension, and ankle extension and inversion) predominate. These patterns can be regarded as functional and nonfunctional. For instance, extension synergy patterns of the lower limb can augment rehabilitation because this position fosters early ambulatory therapy. Conversely, flexion synergy patterns in the upper extremity can significantly impair arm function.

Rehabilitation of the patient with hemiparesis should concentrate on maintaining range of motion and improving strength and posturing. Exercise programs should incorporate functional use of the hemiparetic limb and weight bearing to promote limb recognition, better alignment, muscle elongation, and muscle tone reduction.

Hemiparesis can lead to contracture, particularly when profound weakness is present, and contracture occurs most commonly in the wrist and ankle. Resting hand splints and solid ankle-foot orthoses can be used to maintain the limb in a neutral position. These devices can be used to prevent loss of motion, control muscle tone, and aid in positioning, particularly when wheelchairs are necessary.

Functional electrical stimulation (FES) has gained increasing interest as a means of enhancing functional movement and strength. Muscle contraction is induced with electrical stimulation. Many products on the market incorporate FES technology for the treatment of footdrop and hand weakness.

Preservation of scapulohumeral positioning is a critical component of rehabilitation. With shoulder weakness, the scapula becomes downwardly rotated, causing the glenoid fossa to move vertically and resulting in humeral subluxation. Traditionally, shoulder slings have been prescribed for the hemiplegic shoulder, but their effectiveness in preventing subluxation is questionable.

FES has been used to augment motor return in the hemiplegic shoulder and prevent subluxation. Despite advances in the treatment of the hemiplegic shoulder, it is still unclear which therapeutic interventions should constitute the standard of care.

Constraint-induced therapy (CIT), a therapeutic approach in which the nonparetic limb is restrained, can improve functional movement of the paretic upper extremity in patients with residual hand and wrist movement, even in patients more than 1 year after a stroke. More recently, CIT concepts have been applied to the treatment of aphasia. By limiting the use of nonverbal communication and stimulating verbal output, participants were able to improve language performance and communication.

Weight-supported treadmill training has been proposed to enhance gait training after a stroke. Although a recent clinical trial showed no clear benefit from weight-supported treadmill training on improving gait speed, walking ability, or balance, some advocate for continued research on the effects of this training on overall health, including maintaining bone mass and decreasing insulin resistance.

Dysphagia

Dysphagia after stroke occurs acutely in approximately 50% of stroke patients. Identifying dysphagia in this population is essential for preventing associated morbidity and mortality. Stroke patients with dysphagia are at risk for dehydration, malnutrition, and aspiration pneumonia. As allowed by their overall clinical status and consciousness level, stroke patients should be evaluated as early as possible during their acute hospital stay. Trained clinicians (most commonly speech-language pathologists) should evaluate the patient to make recommendations regarding further dysphagia evaluation or testing and the need for diet modifications or dysphagia rehabilitation.

Hemiplegic Shoulder Pain

Stroke survivors with residual hemiparesis or weakness are at risk for pain syndromes (particularly in the upper extremity), which can significantly limit rehabilitation efforts. These pain syndromes are usually multifactorial. In the rehabilitation setting, prevention of shoulder pain is key, and interventions should focus on proper positioning, handling, and transfer techniques.

In severe cases, shoulder pain can be accompanied by hand swelling, tenderness, skin changes, erythema, hyperhidrosis, and allodynia. When this occurs, it is referred to as shoulder-hand syndrome, a subtype of complex regional pain syndrome (CRPS). Although the mechanism and cause are unclear, it has been suggested that this process is the result of an overreaction to a neurologic insult and may be inflammatory in nature. In some cases, the pain is severe, resulting in decreased and guarded movements of the limb that limit functional use. Shoulder pathology such as rotator cuff strains or tears, bicipital tendonitis, subacromial and subdeltoid bursitis, and glenohumeral subluxation or dislocation contribute to post-stroke shoulder pain and should be treated.

Nonpharmacologic treatment focuses on desensitization techniques, gentle range-of-motion exercises, and physical modalities (e.g., heat, cold, transcutaneous electrical nerve stimulation [TENS], FES). Pharmacologic management includes medications typically used for neuropathic pain syndromes, such as anticonvulsants, tricyclic antidepressants (TCAs), nonsteroidal anti-inflammatory drugs, topical agents (e.g., lidocaine [Xylocaine],[1] clonidine [Catapres-TTS],[1] capsaicin [Zostrix][1]), and injections of steroid or local anesthetics. Antispasmodic medications have been used. When pain relief is not achieved with conservative treatment, sympathetic blocks can be considered. Sympathectomies and spinal cord stimulators can be considered as last resorts.

---

[1]Not FDA approved for this indication.

TABLE 1 Neuropharmacologic Agents Commonly Used During Stroke Rehabilitation

DRUG CLASS	DRUG NAME	INDICATION	POTENTIAL PROBLEMS
Benzodiazepines	Diazepam (Valium)	Agitation,[1] spasticity	Sedation, confusion, sundowning
	Lorazepam (Ativan)	Agitation,[1] seizures	Sedation, paradoxical reactions, confusion, sundowning
Tricyclic antidepressants (TCAs)	Nortriptyline (Pamelor)	Depression, neuropathic pain,[1] central pain[1]	Anticholinergic effects, sedation
	Amitriptyline (Elavil)		
Selective serotonin reuptake inhibitors (SSRIs)	Sertraline (Zoloft)	Depression, stimulation[1]	Long titration period, suicidal ideations, serotonin syndrome, syndrome of inappropriate antidiuretic hormone (SIADH), somnolence, seizures
	Escitalopram (Lexapro)		
	Citalopram (Celexa)		
	Fluoxetine (Prozac)	Depression motor recovery[1]	As above for other SSRIs
Stimulants	Modafinil (Provigil)	Drowsiness,[1] decreased alertness,[1] impaired concentration,[1] diminished attention[1]	Arrhythmia, seizures, hepatotoxicity, blood pressure changes
	Methylphenidate (Ritalin)		

[1]Not FDA approved for this indication.

Spasticity

Spasticity after stroke can significantly impact rehabilitation. The classic upper extremity flexor synergy pattern (i.e., adducted shoulder with flexed elbow, wrist, and fingers) can markedly interfere with the function of the affected arm. Conversely, the classic lower extremity extensor synergy pattern (i.e., extended hip and knee and ankle plantar flexion) can be advantageous for ambulation if plantar flexion can be controlled by physical or pharmacologic agents. If untreated, these patterns can lead to abnormal positioning and contracture.

Treatment of spasticity after stroke should address positioning and exacerbating factors. Splinting or bracing, appropriate wheelchair sitting position, and physical therapy techniques are important to prevent contracture and promote motor recovery. Painful or noxious stimuli can exacerbate spasticity. Shoulder pain, pressure sores, deep venous thrombosis, bladder distention, and constipation are examples of stimuli that can exacerbate spasticity. Pharmacologic treatment should take into account the presence of these triggers because spasticity is likely to improve after the stimuli are resolved or relieved.

Pharmacologic treatment of post-stroke spasticity presents some challenges. Effective antispasticity agents such as baclofen (Lioresal) or tizanidine (Zanaflex) can cause somnolence or weaken unaffected muscles, which can significantly affect rehabilitation. Localized treatments such as botulinum toxins (Botox, Dysport, Myobloc, Xeomin)[1] injections or phenol blocks[1] can be useful, because treatment can be directed toward muscles that are affecting functional use of the limbs. Surgical interventions can be used for patients with severe spasticity limiting functional positioning or for those with the potential for functional grip if tendon lengthening or transfer can be considered.

Cognitive Dysfunction

Stroke patients can experience many cognitive deficits, including visuospatial neglect, cognitive-linguistic deficits, apraxia, memory loss, and attention deficits. Cognitive rehabilitation should concentrate on treatment of the specific deficits of the patient. Visuospatial rehabilitation (including scanning training) is recommended for deficits associated with visual neglect after right stroke. Cognitive-linguistic therapies are recommended for left hemispheric stroke patients with language deficits. Treatment of apraxia should include specific gestural and strategy training.

The use of medications that may impair cognitive function should be limited. Medications that are commonly considered during a stay in a rehabilitative facility that may have a significant impact on cognition and rehabilitation are highlighted in Table 1.

Depression and Neuropharmacology

Depression can be seen in up to one half of all stroke patients. It has been associated with poor functional outcomes and more severe impairments. Vegetative symptoms can have a significant impact on rehabilitative efforts because participation in therapy is critical.

Psychoactive drugs can be beneficial and should be considered. Selective serotonin reuptake inhibitors (SSRIs) are recommended in this population because of a better side effect profile and because of the undesirable anticholinergic side effects of TCAs. In cases unresponsive to treatment with SSRIs, nortriptyline (Pamelor) may be helpful. In the rehabilitation setting, when rapid short-term improvement in symptoms is necessary to increase participation in therapy, the use of psychostimulants (e.g., methylphenidate [Ritalin][1]) may be indicated. Table 1 shows the neuropharmacologic agents commonly used during stoke rehabilitation. Psychotherapy has been associated with modest improvement in post-stroke depression and is considered to be part of a multidisciplinary approach. Research has demonstrated the benefit of the antidepressant fluoxetine (Prozac)[1] on motor recovery; administration of the drug for 3 months as an adjunct to physical therapy improved motor functioning in post-stroke patients.

Bladder Dysfunction

Bladder dysfunction after stroke depends on the stroke's location. During the rehabilitation phase, the most common problem is urinary incontinence and urgency associated with uninhibited bladder contraction. Ultrasound bladder scans (usually every 4 h and after voiding) should be ordered to detect bladder distention and urinary retention. It is standard practice to intervene when bladder volumes are greater than 500 mL. If volumes exceed this cutoff point, intermittent catheterization should be started. Intermittent catheterization is preferable to indwelling catheters because the risk of urinary tract infection is higher with the latter. Bladder scans are usually discontinued when post-voiding residual volumes at 3- to 4-hour intervals are low (<150 mL) for a period of 24 to 48 hours.

[1]Not FDA approved for this indication.

[1]Not FDA approved for this indication.

Mobility and Use of Adaptive Equipment

Activity limitations vary among stroke survivors and can include difficulties with bed mobility, wheelchair propulsion, transfers, gait, stairs, and the basic activities of daily living. The goal of physical therapy and occupational therapy is to maximize functional independence. Addressing mobility limitations is fundamental in stroke rehabilitation because it is related to long-term care needs and independence.

Transfer training comprises learning how to maneuver from one surface or height to another. Ideally, patients should learn to roll and transfer toward the involved and uninvolved sides; however, early mobility efforts are directed to the uninvolved side to minimize the risk of injury.

Gait deviations are common after stroke and interfere with safety and efficiency of locomotion. If an assistive device is needed, the goal of physical therapy is to progress to the least restrictive device possible. Hemiwalkers and wide-based quad canes provide the most stability. An ankle-foot orthosis may be indicated for patients with decreased ankle control and footdrop. Instruction in ascending or descending stairs depends on assistive device requirements. With weakness, stairs are ascended by initiating movement with the uninvolved or stronger lower extremity. This process is reversed when descending.

For some stroke survivors, functional ambulation is not a realistic goal. In these cases, the wheelchair becomes the primary means of locomotion. Wheelchair prescription requires considerable skill and training and must take into account posturing, body habitus, cognition, physical fitness level, and the home environment. An appropriate wheelchair prescription is required to maximize mobility and prevent complications such as shoulder pain. Physical and occupational therapists should evaluate the patient before providing wheelchair recommendations to vendors. Hemi wheelchairs (i.e., wheelchairs situated closer to the ground) and one-arm drive wheelchairs allow hemiplegic patients to use the uninvolved side for wheelchair propulsion. Lap boards with arm supports can be added to improve hemiparetic arm posturing and sitting symmetry.

For some stroke survivors, the ability to return to driving is considered one of the most important long-term rehabilitation goals. Formal driving rehabilitation programs are available to evaluate and improve driver safety. Driver rehabilitation specialists perform vision, cognitive, and perceptual examinations. Perception tests assess reaction times to visual and auditory stimuli. Values for vision and reaction times are standardized and state-dependent. Specialists should also perform a behind-the-wheel assessment, beginning in a parking lot and progressing to the negotiation of more complex traffic situations. Many modifications can increase independence and assist with a return to driving, including a spinner knob, which can be attached to the steering wheel to allow one-arm control; hand controls for acceleration and braking; left foot pedals to compensate for right foot impairment; and wheelchair lifts.

Adaptive equipment, including bracing, shoe modification, and other tools, increases independence through completion of activities of daily living (e.g., long-handled sponge, reacher, shoe horn, mirror, sock aids) and is extremely beneficial for those with moderate to severe strokes, particularly if hemiparesis is dense (Figure 2). Silverware, pens, and other utensils can be modified for easier maneuverability. Multipodus boots can be used to prevent plantar flexion contracture development in the hemiparetic limb.

Falls

Falls are common after moderate to severe strokes. In rehabilitation settings, fall prevention usually requires a multimodal approach. Strategies include use of bed-chair alarms, placing those at risk close to the nursing station, wearing skid socks, limiting or refraining from polypharmacy, eliminating slick or irregular floors, and in some cases, providing a sitter for closer monitoring. Physical and occupational therapists must include general safety and fall recovery as part of the treatment plan.

Visual Impairment

Depending on the location of the stroke, the visual system may be involved. One of the most debilitating visual impairments is visuospatial neglect, a complication of right hemisphere strokes. Left-sided stimuli are not attended to or recognized, and affected individuals must learn to deal with this deficit. Other complications include gaze weakness or paralysis, diplopia, visual field loss, ptosis, tracking disorders, decreased visual acuity, and cortical blindness.

Screening for primary visual skills, including visual acuity, visual fields, and visual tracking, should be done by physiatrists, neurologists, and occupational therapists. If problems are identified, patients should be referred to neuro-ophthalmologists and low-vision rehabilitation programs. Visual acuity problems often can be addressed by incorporating the use of glasses into the therapy session or by changing the prescription. Eye movement disorders and visual field deficits usually lessen as time elapses and may respond to treatment with prisms, head positioning, and unilateral eye occlusion with tape or a patch technique. Prism therapy has also shown promise in treating hemispatial neglect. Those with continued visual field impairment should be taught eye movement techniques to expand the visual area.

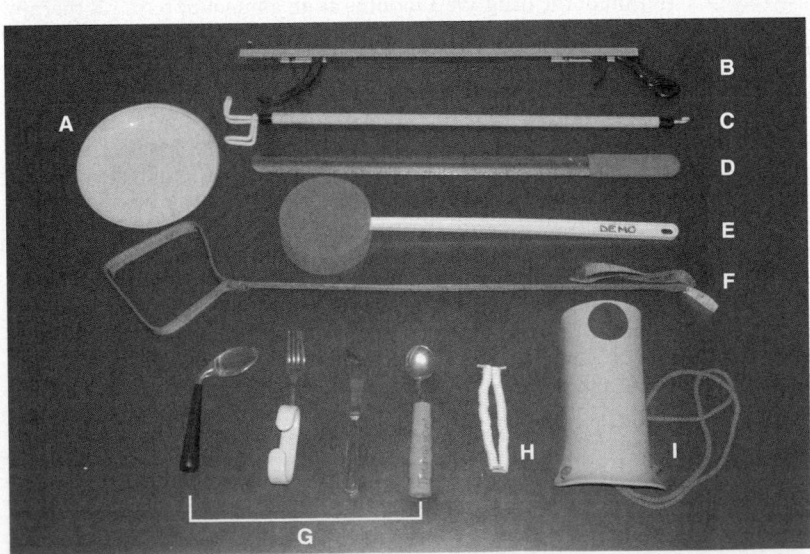

Figure 2. Adaptive equipment commonly used during stroke rehabilitation. The tapered front scoop dish (**A**) has nonskid feet to keep the plate from sliding. The curved edge simplifies scooping food. The dish is especially suited for individuals who have limited flexibility, have decreased motor coordination, or feed using one hand, such as a hemiparetic stroke patient. The reacher (**B**) is used to get items from the floor. The long-handled dressing aid (**C**) is used to reach clothes on the floor or to bring clothes up the paretic side. The long-handled shoe horn (**D**) aids with slipping into shoes. The long-handle sponge (**E**) is used for reaching the involved side while bathing or when the shoulder range of motion does not allow reaching. The leg lifter (**F**) and the sound upper limb can be used to assist in moving the paretic lower limb. Adapted feeding utensils (**G**) are used for patients with grip weakness or difficulties with upper limb range of motion; *left to right*: bent-handle spoon, no-grip fork, rocker bottom knife, and thick-handle spoon. No-tie laces (**H**) are elastic shoelaces that do not require tying. When using the sock-donning aid (**I**), the sock slides onto the plastic portion of the device, and the strap is used to pull the sock with the device on the foot.

Brain-Based Therapies: Noninvasive Brain Stimulation

Repetitive transcranial magnetic stimulation (rTMS) applies a brief magnetic field to the scalp with enough intensity to penetrate the skull and induce neuronal activation. Some promising results have been seen when rTMS is used after stroke. A second modality, transcranial direct current stimulation (tDCS), applies low-voltage electrical current to stimulate or modify neuronal activity in the brain cortex. The stimulation is applied to discrete areas of the head to target affected areas. Although the side-effect profile of these techniques is positive, more research is necessary to determine best candidates for treatment and optimal treatment protocols.

Robotics

The aim of robotic technology is to use an adjustable, programmable device to augment mobility in a task-specific manner. Robots can serve in an assistive (perform desired function) or therapeutic capacity (enhance gait or upper extremity function) and are suitable for this purpose as they not only enable more intensive therapy than conventional modes but also incorporate a greater degree of activity repetition. Present recommendations are for use as an adjunct to traditional rehabilitation interventions.

Conclusions

Stroke rehabilitation requires the concerted efforts of the patient, family, and medical professionals. A multidisciplinary team with training to address the particular impairments and functional limitations of the stroke patient is critical. The physician's efforts should focus on preventing complications and treating stroke sequelae with the primary goal of improving overall function and participation in society.

References

Barrett AM, Oh-Park M, Chen P, et al. Neurorehabilitation: Five new things. Neurol Clin Pract 2013;3:484.

Bhakta BB. Management of spasticity in stroke. Br Med Bull 2000;56:476.

Cicerone KD, Dahlberg C, Malec JF, et al. Evidence-based cognitive rehabilitation: Updated review of the literature from 1998 through 2002. Arch Phys Med Rehabil 2005;86:1681.

Chang WH, Kim YH. Robot-assisted therapy in stroke rehabilitation. J Stroke 2013a;15:174.

Chollet F, Tardy J, Albucher JF, et al. Fluoxetine for motor recovery after acute ischaemic stroke (FLAME): A randomised placebo controlled trial. Lancet Neurol 2011;10:123.

Hackett ML, Anderson CS, House A, et al. Interventions for treating depression after stroke. Cochrane Database Syst Rev 2008;CD003437.

Jones SA, Shinton RA. Improving outcome in stroke patients with visual problems. Age Ageing 2006;35:560.

Kelly-Hayes M, Beiser A, Kase CS, et al. The influence of gender and age on disability following ischemic stroke: The Framingham Study. J Stroke Cerebrovasc Dis 2003;12:119.

Lannin NA, Cusick A, McCluskey A, et al. Effects of splinting on wrist contracture after stroke: A randomized controlled trial. Stroke 2007;38:111.

Legg L, Drummond A, Leonardi-Bee J, et al. Occupational therapy for patients with problems in personal activities of daily living after stroke: Systematic review of randomised trials. BMJ 2007;335:922.

Pertoldi S, Di Benedetto P. Shoulder-hand syndrome after stroke. A complex regional pain syndrome. Eura Medicophys 2005;41:283.

Poole D, Chaudry F, Jay WM. Stroke and driving. Top Stroke Rehabil 2008;15:37.

Starkstein SE, Mizrahi R, Power BD. Antidepressant therapy in post-stroke depression. Expert Opin Pharmacother 2008;9:1291.

Stein J. Stroke. In: Frontera WR, Silver JK, editors. Essentials of Physical Medicine and Rehabilitation. Philadelphia: WB Saunders; 2002. p. 778–83.

Stein J, Harvey RL, Macko RF, et al. Stroke Recovery & Rehabilitation. New York: Demos Medical Publishing; 2009.

Umphred DA. Neurological Rehabilitation. St Louis: Mosby Elsevier Health Science; 1995.

van Wijk I, Algra A, van de Port IG, et al. Change in mobility activity in the second year after stroke in a rehabilitation population: Who is at risk for decline? Arch Phys Med Rehabil 2006;87:45.

Wolf SL, Winstein CJ, Miller JP, et al. Effect of constraint-induced movement therapy on upper extremity function 3 to 9 months after stroke: The EXCITE randomized clinical trial. JAMA 2006;296:2095.

Chang WH, Kim YH. Robot-assisted therapy in stroke rehabilitation. J Stroke 2013b;15:174.

SEIZURES AND EPILEPSY IN ADOLESCENTS AND ADULTS

Method of
Sofia Dobrin, MD

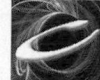

CURRENT DIAGNOSIS

- Obtain a thorough history, especially from witnesses of the paroxysmal event.
- Perform a thorough physical and neurologic examination.
- Laboratory testing includes blood glucose, complete blood cell count, electrolytes, liver function tests, and toxicology screening.
- Perform lumbar puncture if central nervous system (CNS) infection is suspected
- Neuroimaging should be performed, preferably magnetic resonance imaging (MRI). Computed tomography (CT) is acceptable in the acute setting to exclude hemorrhage; neoplasms may be missed by head CT.
- Routine electroencephalogram (EEG) with sleep deprivation and activation procedures should be performed when possible.

CURRENT THERAPY

- Select an antiepileptic drug (AED) based on seizure type and epilepsy syndrome.
- Consider side-effect profile and the patient's unique characteristics.
- Consider convenience (dosing schedule) and cost.
- Aim for monotherapy whenever possible.
- "Start low and go slow" when initiating AED therapy.
- Overlap drugs when switching AEDs and gradually withdraw the first drug when the second is effective.
- Refer to an epilepsy center for consideration of surgery if seizures are refractory to two AEDs.
- After a minimum 2-year seizure-free period, consider withdrawing AEDs for epilepsy of unknown etiology or syndromes known to resolve.

All patients with epilepsy experience seizures, but not all patients with a seizure have epilepsy. An epileptic seizure is a transient occurrence of signs and symptoms resulting from abnormal excessive or synchronous neuronal activity in the brain. Epilepsy is a disorder of the brain characterized by an enduring predisposition to generate epileptic seizures and by the neurobiologic, cognitive, and psychosocial consequences of this condition. The diagnosis of epilepsy requires the occurrence of at least one epileptic seizure. In practice, however, epilepsy is most commonly diagnosed after two or more unprovoked seizures.

Seizures can be acute symptomatic or unprovoked. Acute symptomatic seizures occur at the time of a systemic insult, such as during alcohol withdrawal or in the setting of severe hypoglycemia, or in close temporal association with a brain insult, such as in acute head trauma. The condition leading to the seizure is thought to disrupt normal brain neuronal physiology in a transient fashion. Unprovoked seizures occur in the absence of such precipitating factors. Recurrent provoked seizures do not constitute epilepsy and therefore do not require treatment with antiepileptic medication.

Epilepsy has many causes including structural (e.g., tumors, strokes, vascular abnormalities), metabolic, infectious, and genetic. Often, no clear cause can be determined. Several epilepsy syndromes have been recognized with clustering of symptoms and signs in epilepsies, which aids in accurate diagnosis and management of seizure disorders.

Epidemiology

Epilepsy is a common disease affecting about 50 million people worldwide. The lifetime risk for developing epilepsy is estimated at about 3% to age 80 years. The average annual incidence of epilepsy is about 55 per 100,000 population in the United States and in Europe. The highest incidence rates are in infants younger than 1 year and in those older than 60 years. Men tend to be affected slightly more than women. Studies in several countries have shown similar prevalence and incidence rates as in the United States. The lifetime risk of a single seizure from any cause is estimated at about 10%.

Classification

A standardized classification system for seizures and epilepsy was developed to create a common language and facilitate communication among clinicians and researchers as well as to aid in diagnosis and management. The International League against Epilepsy (ILAE) classifications were first published in 1960 and last updated officially in 1981 for seizures and in 1989 for epilepsies and are mostly based on concepts formulated prior to modern neuroimaging and genomic research. The ILAE Commission on Classification and Terminology has recently revised concepts, terminology, and approaches for classifying seizures and forms of epilepsy. The two major categories of seizures, generalized and partial, are redefined as generalized and focal. Generalized seizures originate within, and rapidly engage, bilaterally distributed networks. Focal seizures originate within networks limited to one hemisphere of the brain. The classification of generalized seizures has been simplified, specifically with the elimination of neonatal seizures as a subcategory and with a simplified subclassification of absence seizures (Box 1). The distinction between the different types of focal seizures based on level of consciousness (e.g., simple partial, complex partial, and partial seizures secondarily generalized) is eliminated in the revised classification scheme. Focal seizures are now described based on their manifestations, such as dyscognitive or focal motor (Box 2).

In the former classification scheme, epilepsies were subdivided into three categories based on etiology: idiopathic, symptomatic, or cryptogenic syndromes, indicating a presumed genetic cause, underlying brain lesion, or suspected but unidentified brain lesion, respectively. In the revised classification scheme, these are now referred to as genetic, structural–metabolic, and unknown (Box 3). Genetic epilepsy is the direct result of a known or presumed genetic defect. In structural–metabolic epilepsy there

---

Box 1   Classification of Seizures

Generalized Seizures
Tonic–clonic (in any combination)
Absence
- Typical
- Atypical
- Absence with special features
  - Myoclonic absence
  - Eyelid myoclonia
Myoclonic
- Myoclonic
- Myoclonic atonic
- Clonic
- Tonic
- Atonic

Focal seizures
Unknown
- Epileptic spasms

Box 2   Descriptors of Focal Seizures According to Degree of Impairment during Seizure

Without impairment of consciousness or awareness
- With observable motor ("focal motor") or autonomic ("autonomic") components (replaces the term "simple partial seizure")
With impairment of consciousness or awareness ("dyscognitive") (replaces the term "complex partial seizure")
Evolving to a bilateral, convulsive seizure (involving tonic, clonic, or tonic and clonic components) (replaces the term "secondarily generalized seizure")

Box 3   Terminology for Underlying Cause

Genetic
Childhood absence epilepsy
Autosomal dominant nocturnal frontal lobe epilepsy
Dravet syndrome

Structural–Metabolic
Cortical malformations
Cortical dysplasias
Metabolic abnormalities

Unknown
Epilepsy of infancy with migrating focal seizures
Myoclonic epilepsy in infancy
Benign rolandic epilepsy
Panayiotopoulos syndrome
Benign occipital epilepsy of the Gastaut type

---

is a distinct structural or metabolic condition that is associated with a significantly increased risk of developing epilepsy. Unknown epilepsy suggests that the underlying cause is not yet identified.

Another change in the revised classification is the recognition of the concept of "electroclinical syndrome" to mean a complex of clinical features, signs, and symptoms that together define a distinctive, recognizable clinical disorder. These are based on typical age of onset, EEG characteristics, seizure types, and other characteristics. The diagnosis of these syndromes helps determine treatment and prognosis.

Diagnosis

Making a diagnosis of epilepsy has important medical and psychosocial implications for patients. An incorrect diagnosis of epilepsy has many negative consequences, including unnecessary restrictions on driving, working, and recreational activities; exposure to potentially toxic antiepileptic drugs (AEDs); and dealing with societal stigma associated with a chronic disease. An accurate diagnosis of epilepsy is based on obtaining a thorough history, conducting a thorough physical and neurologic examination, and performing appropriate testing.

Detailed descriptions from the patient and a witness about the triggering factors, prodromal symptoms, ictal phase, and postictal phase are of paramount importance. Common triggering factors are sleep deprivation, stress, drug intake, and alcohol withdrawal. Witnesses should be questioned about altered consciousness, duration of each phase, automatism, or head turning as well as any abnormal movements such as tonic, tonic–clonic, or myoclonic activity and the spread of the abnormal movements if they start focally; falling; urinary or bowel incontinence; and tongue biting. Postictal confusion, fatigue, sleeping, focal neurologic signs, and muscle aches often follow a generalized tonic–clonic (GTC) seizure; it is extremely rare for someone to recover full consciousness immediately after a GTC seizure.

Additional important features of the history to obtain include age at onset of events, family history of seizures, birth trauma or injury, childhood febrile illnesses and associated seizures, and history of significant head injury. An important clue to the diagnosis and localization of epilepsy lies in the detailed description of events that take place during recurrent paroxysmal events (semiology) and consistent clinical features with little variation between events (stereotypy).

The presence of an aura, a subjective sensation or motor phenomenon that precedes a generalized or focal seizure, also favors the diagnosis of epilepsy. An aura is actually a focal seizure without impairment of consciousness. The characteristics of an aura may also provide clues to the localization or origin of a seizure. For example, sensations of déjà vu, epigastric rising, and exaggerated emotions of fear or fright are common auras of temporal lobe epilepsy. Muscle and motor activity, forced eye deviation, and speech arrest or disturbances are typically seen in frontal lobe epilepsy. Parietal lobe epilepsies can have auras of paresthesias or sensory phenomena, whereas occipital lobe epilepsy can have positive basic visual phenomena such as flashes or colors experienced as an aura.

Several features of the history and physical or neurologic examination, such as the presence of specific generalized or focal neurologic deficits, predict a higher risk of seizure recurrence and help classify the type of seizure or epilepsy. For instance, the finding of transient unilateral hemiparesis when examining a patient soon after a suspected seizure, or a clinical history to support such a finding, is consistent with a Todd paralysis and suggests a focal-onset seizure involving the motor cortex contralateral to the weakness.

The evaluation of a first seizure is aimed at determining whether it was provoked by a transient cause and thus is an acute symptomatic seizure, or if it was unprovoked, resulting from underlying epilepsy. In the initial evaluation it is crucial to exclude acute life-threatening etiologies such as infection, neoplasm, or hemorrhage. Basic laboratory tests are usually indicated including blood glucose, complete blood count, electrolytes (particularly sodium), liver function tests, and toxicology screening to exclude infections, electrolyte abnormalities, organ dysfunction, and drug intoxication/withdrawal. A lumbar puncture should be performed if a CNS infection is suspected, such as in a febrile patient.

A routine electroencephalogram (EEG) is an essential component of the initial work-up of a patient with suspected epilepsy. Although an EEG can show many different abnormalities, true epileptiform activity, spike and slow wave complexes and sharp waves, have a high correlation with clinical seizures.

In a nonemergent situation, performing an MRI is important in the initial work-up of a patient with suspected epilepsy, especially when focal seizures are suspected. MRI is more sensitive and more likely to show significant abnormalities than is CT. If MRI is not available or in an acute or emergent setting, a noncontrast head CT may be substituted. Finding a lesion with the potential for being the seizure focus would correlate with focal seizures. A common example of this is mesial temporal sclerosis characterized by atrophy and gliosis of the hippocampus in the temporal lobe. Histopathologically, this is represented by neuronal loss and gliosis of the hippocampus and several mesial temporal structures. Mesial temporal sclerosis correlates with temporal lobe epilepsy and has been associated with good surgical resection outcomes. High resolution cuts through the temporal lobes on MRI have been shown to detect mesial temporal sclerosis.

The evaluation of recurrent seizures is aimed at defining the underlying cause of epilepsy or the epilepsy syndrome. Evaluation is similar to that for a single unprovoked seizure; however, the therapeutic and prognostic implications for a patient with epilepsy are very different. A routine EEG is indicated because it can reveal interictal focal or generalized epileptiform discharges and aid in classifying the seizure type and epilepsy syndrome. However, a normal EEG does not exclude clinical epilepsy. The yield of recording epileptiform activity on routine EEG can be improved by performing the test with sleep deprivation and recording a period of sleep. Activation procedures of intermittent photic stimulation and hyperventilation should also be performed whenever possible to increase the yield of finding EEG abnormalities. Nevertheless, in patients ultimately shown to have epilepsy, the initial EEG shows epileptiform activity in about 50% of recordings. The yield increases with repeat studies, but only to a point, and doing more than four routine EEGs on a single patient is unlikely to be helpful in capturing epileptiform activity.

The diagnostic evaluation of intractable epilepsy is discussed in a later section.

Differential Diagnosis

In making a diagnosis of a seizure or epilepsy, it is important to consider other conditions that can mimic seizures. Psychogenic nonepileptic seizures are the most common condition misdiagnosed as epilepsy, followed by syncope. Other transient and often recurrent conditions that can be misdiagnosed as epilepsy include migraine, transient ischemic attack (TIA), transient global amnesia, dizziness or vertigo, delirium, sleep disorders, and movement disorders.

Psychogenic nonepileptic seizures, formerly called pseudoseizures or psychogenic seizures, present a particular challenge to health care providers when evaluating atypical seizure-like events. It can be especially difficult to distinguish between true epileptic seizures and psychogenic nonepileptic seizures because both can occur in the same patient. Some features that suggest psychogenic nonepileptic seizures include lack of response to AEDs, comorbid personality or psychological disorders, certain ictal movements such as pelvic thrusting and back arching, and ictal eye closure. Ictal stuttering, bringing a stuffed animal to the epilepsy monitoring unit, pseudosleep, a history of fibromyalgia or chronic pain, a history of physical, emotional, or sexual abuse, and having a seizure during an outpatient epilepsy clinic visit have all been associated with the diagnosis of psychogenic nonepileptic seizures.

Syncope is typically characterized by sudden atonic loss of consciousness. Convulsive syncope is a variant that can easily be confused with an epileptic seizure. Abnormal movements including tonic posturing and clonic or myoclonic activity occur during convulsive syncope in response to sudden and transient cerebral anoxia and ischemia. EEG during an attack shows diffuse slowing of the background rhythms but no epileptiform activity. Syncope is distinguished from an epileptic seizure by the presence of presyncopal symptoms (nausea, flushing, and lightheadedness), brief loss of consciousness, and the return of normal cognition within seconds after arousal. Motor symptoms such as clonic jerking or stiffening often accompany prolonged syncope, especially if the patient is maintained in an upright position, and can resemble an epileptic seizure; however, consciousness returns immediately after syncope despite the motor symptoms, whereas it does not return for at least minutes after a GTC seizure.

Migraine headaches can be accompanied by complex visual phenomena or sensorimotor symptoms, which could be confused with seizures. However, visual auras associated with seizures usually evolve and last seconds, whereas migraine auras tend to develop over minutes. Postictal headaches may be confused with migraine. Complicated migraine with hemiparesis may be mistaken for postictal Todd paralysis. A history of migraine headaches and preservation of normal consciousness help identify the spells as migraine. Rarely, basilar migraines and acute confusional migraine are accompanied by loss of consciousness.

TIAs should almost never be mistaken for seizures because TIAs usually cause focal negative phenomena, such as weakness, numbness, aphasia, or ataxia, whereas seizures usually cause positive phenomena such as jerking, tingling, automatisms, or movements. Rarely, TIA can have positive symptoms, as in limb-shaking TIA. These consist of brief myoclonic or rhythmic motor activity corresponding to transient cerebral ischemia due to focal arterial stenosis supplying the motor cortex. TIAs of vertebrobasilar artery territory origin occasionally cause loss of consciousness and falls that could be confused with seizures, but vertebrobasilar TIA is usually accompanied by neighborhood signs. Transient global amnesia, which is sudden-onset alteration of anterograde memory and confusion, can mimic seizures and nonconvulsive status epilepticus. Patients with transient global amnesia can perform complex tasks such as calculating, reading, and writing despite appearing confused, whereas patients with nonconvulsive status epilepticus cannot.

Some sleep disorders, movement disorders, and hypoglycemia can mimic seizures. Cataplexy attacks of narcolepsy precipitated by emotional stimuli manifest with sudden loss of muscle tone but preservation of consciousness. Other narcolepsy symptoms such as excessive daytime sleepiness, hypnagogic hallucinations, and sleep paralysis help to make the diagnosis. Parasomnias, arousal disorders, and periodic limb movements in sleep can rarely be confused with epileptic seizures. Hemifacial spasms could be mistaken for simple partial seizures, and myoclonus, which can be epileptic or nonepileptic, can also be difficult to distinguish from seizures. EEG can play a role in making the correct diagnosis.

Treatment

The decision whether or not to treat is just as important as what drug to use. In general, patients with an acute symptomatic seizure do not require treatment with AEDs, because they are thought to have a transient reversible etiology causing their seizure as opposed to having underlying epilepsy. They are best managed by treating the provoking factor (e.g., correcting an electrolyte

abnormality or discontinuing an offending drug or medication). If an acute symptomatic etiology cannot be found, then the patient's seizure most likely represents underlying epilepsy. Still, the rate of recurrence after a first such seizure ranges in the literature from about 30% to 55%.

Factors that have been shown to increase risk of recurrence include a remote symptomatic etiology, abnormal neurologic examination, and first seizure onset out of sleep. Family history of seizures or epilepsy and EEG abnormalities have been shown to increase risk in some, but not all, studies. If any of these factors are present, treatment may be warranted even after a single event. In addition, early treatment should be considered in any patient for whom the consequences of a recurrent seizure would be significant, such as related to driving, working, or general safety. Once two or more seizures have occurred, risk of recurrence is well over 50%, closer to about 70% in most studies, and treatment with AEDs is recommended.

The treatment of epilepsy involves choosing among the many AED options available (currently 14 first-line AEDs in the United States) by considering spectrum of efficacy, pharmacokinetic and pharmacodynamic properties, and the patient's comorbidities (Tables 1 and 2). The goal of therapy should be complete seizure freedom with no side effects. This goal can be achieved by following some basic principles.

10 The Nervous System

700

TABLE 1 Dosage and Side Effect Profile of Commonly Prescribed Antiepileptic Drugs

DRUG	HALF-LIFE	INITIAL DOSAGE	MAINTENANCE DOSAGE	INCREMENT	DOSING SCHEDULE	ADVERSE EFFECTS
Carbamazepine (Tegretol)	12–17 h	200 mg bid	600–1800[3] mg	200 mg q wk	tid–qid	Hyponatremia, leukopenia, rare aplastic anemia and hepatitis
Gabapentin (Neurontin)	5–7 h	300 mg qd	1200–3600 mg	300 mg q3–7d	tid	60% removed by hemodialysis, prolonged half-life to 51 h with hemodialysis. Dosed 300 mg after hemodialysis
Lacosamide (Vimpat)	13 h	50 mg qd	300–600 mg[3]	100 mg q wk	bid	Extra 50% of dose after each hemodialysis. Can prolong PR interval at high doses
Lamotrigine (Lamictal)	25 h alone; 60 h with VPA	6.25–12.5 mg qd to qod	400 mg alone 100 mg with VPA	12.5–25 mg	bid q2wk	Life-threatening rash, especially with rapid titration and VPA. Titration and maintenance doses vary based on other AEDs
Levetiracetam (Keppra)	7 h	500 mg qd	2000–4000[3] mg	500 mg q wk	bid	Decrease dose in chronic renal insufficiency, severe hepatic disease
Oxcarbazepine (Trileptal)	9–11 h	300 mg qd	900–2400 mg	300 mg q wk	bid	Hyponatremia. Fewer side effects than carbamazepine
Phenobarbital	80–100 h	30–60 mg qd	60–120 mg	30 mg q1–2wk	qd–bid	Sedation, Dupuytren's contractures, rebound seizures with rapid tapering
Phenytoin (Dilantin)	22 h	200 mg qd	200–300 mg	100 mg q wk	qd–bid	Gum hypertrophy, hirsutism, cerebellar ataxia or atrophy, peripheral neuropathy, rare hypersensitivity, hepatitis
Pregabalin (Lyrica)	6 h	50 mg qd	150–600 mg	50 mg q3–7d	bid–tid	Weight gain
Topiramate (Topamax)	21 h	25 mg qd	200–400 mg	25 mg q1–2wk	bid	Cognitive impairment at >400 mg/day, rare kidney stones, glaucoma, oligohidrosis
Valproic acid (Depakene)	9–16 h	250 mg qd	750–3000 mg	250 mg q3–7d	tid–qid	Tremor, weight gain, alopecia, thrombocytopenia. Rare hepatitis and pancreatitis. Risk of teratogenesis and neural tube defects
Zonisamide (Zonegran)	63 h	100 mg qd	200–400 mg	100 mg q2wk	bid	Kidney stones, oligohidrosis, rare blood dyscrasias

[3]Exceeds dosage recommended by the manufacturer.
Abbreviations: AED = antiepileptic drug; VPA = valproic acid.

TABLE 2 Choice of Antiepileptic Drug in Special Situations

SPECIAL SITUATION	DRUG OF CHOICE	COMMENTS
Partial seizures	Carbamazepine, lamotrigine, levetiracetam, oxcarbazepine, topiramate, gabapentin	
Refractory partial seizures	Lacosamide, pregabalin, zonisamide	Second-line treatment
Generalized epilepsies	Lamotrigine, topiramate, valproic acid,[1] zonisamide[1]	Avoid valproic acid in women
Absence seizures	Ethosuximide, lamotrigine,[1] valproic acid, topiramate[1]	Ethosuximide is the choice for only pure absence seizures and is insufficient in other associated generalized tonic–clonic or myoclonic seizures
Juvenile myoclonic epilepsy	Valproic acid,[1] topiramate,[1] lamotrigine,[1] zonisamide,[1] levetiracetam	Avoid valproic acid in women
Myoclonic seizures	Clonazepam, valproic acid,[1] levetiracetam	Lamotrigine occasionally exacerbates myoclonic seizures
Women of childbearing potential	Lamotrigine, topiramate, levetiracetam, oxcarbazepine	Avoid enzyme-inducing agents that alter steroid hormones and OCP levels; use OCPs with ≥50 µg of estrogen; OCPs increase the elimination of lamotrigine. Significant increased risk of teratogenicity with valproic acid
Elderly patients	Lamotrigine, gabapentin, levetiracetam, topiramate	Avoid polypharmacy and highly protein-bound AEDs and AEDs with high drug–drug interactions
Depression	Lamotrigine,[1] topiramate[1]	
Bipolar disorder	Valproic acid,[1] carbamazepine, lamotrigine, topiramate[1]	
Migraine	Valproic acid, topiramate	Consider the choice according to sex, side-effect profile, and seizure type
Chronic pain	Pregabalin,[1] gabapentin[1]	
Neuropathic pain	Carbamazepine,[1] gabapentin,[1] pregabalin	

[1]Not FDA approved for this indication.
Abbreviations: AED = antiepileptic drug; OCP = oral contraceptive pill.

First, choose a drug that is effective for the seizure type or epilepsy syndrome. All current AEDs, except ethosuximide (Zarontin), are effective against focal onset seizures. Five AEDs are broad spectrum and are effective against both focal onset and generalized seizures: valproate (Depakene), lamotrigine (Lamictal), topiramate (Topamax), zonisamide (Zonegran),[1] leviteracetam (Keppra). Choose a broad-spectrum drug when seizure type is unknown. Head-to-head studies can favor a single drug, but there is no consistent evidence for superiority of one drug over another. Some recommendations can be made based on common clinical experience and the SANAD (Standard and New Antiepileptic Drugs) open-label clinical trials that compared some AEDs in a large number of patients (see Table 1).

Next, consider the drug side-effect profile and the patient's unique characteristics. Comorbidities such as depression, migraine or other chronic pain, and obesity can guide AED choice based on side-effect profiles. Consider convenience (drug-dosing schedule) and cost when selecting an AED. Less-frequent dosing leads to better compliance. Aim for monotherapy whenever possible to decrease risk of side effects. It is best to "start low and go slow" when initiating therapy. Most side effects are experienced at the start of therapy and can be avoided by starting with a low enough dosage and increasing more slowly than recommended by the manufacturer. The maintenance dosages cover a wide range because there is no set final dosage for any of the AEDs.

Finally, push the dose until seizure freedom is achieved or side effects occur. This is the only way to determine that the drug is ineffective. If side effects do occur, reduce the dosage to the maximum tolerated.

Serum drug levels are available for conventional and essentially all new AEDs, but the levels of new AEDs are of very limited utility because they are effective over a wide range of serum levels. Most patients do not need routine monitoring of blood levels. Drug levels can provide a general guide and can help guide dosage increases by warning that toxicity can occur with further increases if levels are in the upper limit of the established therapeutic range. If seizure control is not improved or side effects occur at low dosages, then checking a serum level can help to uncover unexpectedly low levels due to fast metabolism or noncompliance, a problem especially common among adolescents. Ultimately, management decisions should be based on clinical history and not serum drug levels.

When switching from one AED to another, drugs should be overlapped, with the new drug increased to the target dosage to determine that it is effective before gradually withdrawing the first drug. This affords at least some protection from seizures at all times.

After a minimum 2-year seizure-free period, a trial of drug withdrawal may be considered in certain patients, especially in those with an unknown etiology. Patients who have a normal MRI and EEG and who do not have primary generalized epilepsy likely have a lower risk of seizure recurrence after drug withdrawal. Drug withdrawal is usually not logical in patients who have an epilepsy syndrome with a known lifelong tendency to seizures, such as juvenile myoclonic epilepsy.

It is important to note that AEDs as a class have been associated with a risk of suicidality, leading to an FDA warning issued in 2008; however, people with epilepsy have a greater risk of mood disorders, anxiety, and suicidality than in the general population, and the relationship among these factors is complex.

[1]Not FDA approved for this indication.

Characteristics of Specific Antiepileptic Drugs

Phenytoin

Phenytoin (Dilantin, Phenytek) is the most widely used and familiar AED despite having the most problematic side effects. Mechanism of action is thought to be through use-dependent sodium channel blockade. The metabolism of phenytoin is saturable, which means that it shows zero-order kinetics at high blood levels. Very steep elevations in the blood level can occur with even small dosage increases when the blood level is near 20 µg/mL, despite the occurrence of a linear increase in blood level with dosage increases when blood levels are below 20 µg/mL. For example, the blood level may be 10 µg/mL with 200 mg/day and then increase to 15 µg/mL with 300 mg/day and then increase to 20 µg/mL with 400 mg/day, but with an increase to 500 mg/day the level might skyrocket to more than 30 µg/mL if metabolism is saturated.

Phenytoin's idiosyncratic side effects of hepatitis and blood dyscrasias are rare. Cumulative side effects of phenytoin occur over many years and include gum hypertrophy, hirsutism, coarsening of features, ataxia due to cerebellar atrophy, peripheral neuropathy, and osteoporosis. All patients on phenytoin should receive calcium and vitamin D because phenytoin induces the metabolism of vitamin D, thus lowering its level and causing osteoporosis. Phenytoin is prone to drug–drug interactions, and it increases clearance of oral contraceptives and decreases their effectiveness.

Intravenous phenytoin solution is very basic (pH 11), which often causes venous irritation and can cause purple glove syndrome and severe acute necrosis leading to amputation. Intravenous phenytoin is mixed in polyethylene glycol, causing bradycardia and hypotension, which limits the rate of infusion to less than 50 mg/minute. This can be a significant problem in the treatment of status epilepticus or frequent seizures.

Fosphenytoin (Cerebyx) is a phenytoin prodrug in which the phosphate group is rapidly cleaved off upon entering the bloodstream, yielding phenytoin. It is mixed in an aqueous solution and has a more neutral pH; thus it is much better tolerated and can be given as fast as 150 mg/minute.

Carbamazepine

Carbamazepine (Carbatrol, Tegretol), like phenytoin, is metabolized by the liver and induces hepatic metabolism. It also undergoes autoinduction, inducing its own metabolism for up to 3 weeks after initiating it, so that steady-state blood levels are not achieved for several weeks. Carbamazepine has a relatively narrow therapeutic window, with usual therapeutic blood levels of between 4 µg/mL and 12 µg/mL. It has a similar mechanism of action to phenytoin's. It is indicated for simple partial, complex partial, and GTC seizures. It commonly causes acute toxicity (ataxia, diplopia, and lethargy) with only a small increase in the dosage.

Carbamazepine does not have cumulative side effects, but it rarely causes serious idiosyncratic side effects including blood dyscrasias, hepatitis, and hyponatremia. Mild leukopenia is common and does not require intervention unless the white blood cell count falls below 3000 per mm³. Very rarely it can cause bone marrow suppression with aplastic anemia. Extended-release preparations (Carbatrol, Tegretol XR), which can be dosed twice daily, are preferable to standard preparations, which must be dosed every 8 hours. Like phenytoin, it increases the clearance of oral contraceptives and decreases their effectiveness.

Valproic Acid

Valproic acid is available as valproic acid and sodium divalproex (Depakote) and in an extended-release form (Depakote ER). Valproic acid affects many systems and so has several potential mechanisms of action, including through sodium-channel blockade and augmenting γ-aminobutyric acid (GABA) inhibition. It is most commonly used for primary generalized seizures such as in juvenile myoclonic epilepsy[1] and syndromes with absence seizures, but it is also effective for focal seizures. It often causes dyspepsia and other gastrointestinal side effects. Sodium divalproex is immediately cleaved to valproate in the stomach, but this preparation has much better gastrointestinal tolerance. Valproate is usually dosed every 8 hours because of its relatively short half-life. Depakote ER was approved for once-daily dosing for migraine headaches, but it is actually released over fewer than 24 hours, so twice-daily dosing is more useful for the treatment of epilepsy. Valproate is available as an intravenous preparation (Depacon), dosed identically to the oral forms.

Valproate is usually well tolerated, but it occasionally causes weight gain, alopecia, tremor, and thrombocytopenia. It can cause potentially fatal hepatitis and pancreatitis. Hepatitis occurs in only 1 in 40,000 adult patient exposures, but it is much more common in children (as many as 1 in 500) who are taking multiple AEDs and have mental retardation, possibly because they have an undiagnosed metabolic abnormality. It has been suggested that L-carnitine (levocarnitine, Carnitor)[1] supplementation might reduce the risk of hepatitis. Although this has not been demonstrated, it is prudent for children who have unknown causes of mental retardation and who are taking valproate to take carnitine.

The overall risk of birth defects associated with valproate is approximately 10%, and the rate is only approximately 2% in the general population and seemingly not more than approximately 4% for any other AED. Of even greater concern is that valproate is more often associated with neural tube defects such as spina bifida. Folic acid supplementation at 4 mg/day is recommended because it reduces the risk of neural tube defects in all pregnant women. Valproate is a poor choice for women of childbearing potential, and if they are on valproate, they should use an effective method of birth control and take folic acid.

Phenobarbital

Phenobarbital has fallen out of favor as an AED because it occasionally induces lethargy, depression, and learning difficulties. However, it is usually well tolerated in adults, is effective for partial-onset and primary GTC seizures, is inexpensive, and can be given intravenously. It can be dosed once per day and has a very long half-life, which is an advantage in poorly compliant patients. Primidone (Mysoline) is an infrequently used prodrug of phenobarbital that also has its own antiseizure effects but less often causes lethargy.

Ethosuximide

Ethosuximide is unique because it is the only AED that is effective exclusively for absence seizures and is not effective for other types of seizures. It is usually well tolerated, but occasionally it causes nausea, anorexia, headache, and blood dyscrasias. It can be dosed once per day because of its very long half-life, but it is usually better tolerated dosed twice daily.

Felbamate

Felbamate (Felbatol) is highly effective for the most intractable epilepsies, such as the Lennox–Gastaut syndrome, as well as for partial-onset seizures despite frequent side effects of anorexia, insomnia, and agitation and the common occurrence of AED interactions. However, it can cause aplastic anemia and fulminant hepatitis, so it is only indicated for intractable epilepsy, in cases where the potential benefit outweighs the risk of potentially fatal side effects. Its use should probably be limited to epilepsy centers.

Gabapentin

Gabapentin (Neurontin) is very well tolerated and has no pharmacokinetic interactions because it is renally excreted unchanged. It is indicated for partial seizures with and without secondary generalization. It has engendered an unwarranted poor reputation as an AED because some have thought that it is ineffective. Clinical studies have examined doses that statistically reduced the frequency of seizures with minimal side effects but were not high

---

[1]Not FDA approved for this indication.

[1]Not FDA approved for this indication.

enough to determine the maximum tolerated dosage; thus it was approved and initially used at relatively low dosages of 900 to 1800 mg/day. However, clinical experience suggests that dosages of as much as 3600 mg/day may be required to be effective for most patients. On the other hand, very high dosages might not increase blood levels because drug absorption may be saturated at dosages above 4000 mg/day.

Lamotrigine

Lamotrigine (Lamictal) is particularly useful because it is effective for partial seizures, generalized seizures, and Lennox-Gastaut syndrome. It is severely affected by hepatic enzyme-inducing or enzyme-inhibiting AEDs so that its dosing is drastically different depending on concomitant AEDs. When taken alone (or with a combination of an enzyme inducer and inhibitor), the half-life of lamotrigine is about 25 hours, but this is reduced to 12 hours when it is taken with enzyme inducers (such as phenytoin, phenobarbital, carbamazepine) and prolonged to as much as 60 hours when taken with valproate, an enzyme inhibitor. Oral contraceptives decrease the half-life to 12 hours, necessitating dosage adjustment.

The only potentially serious side effect of lamotrigine is rash. Mild rash is common and was present in as many as 1 in 50 children and 1 in 1000 adults during initial clinical studies. The rash can be life threatening in the form of Stevens–Johnson syndrome or toxic epidermal necrolysis, but the incidence of serious rash, as lamotrigine is used today, is probably only about 1 in 40,000. The rash is most likely to occur after the first 3 weeks of therapy, but it can occur at any time, and it is most common with high initial doses and titration rates and when taken with valproic acid. A slow titration rate decreases the risk of rash. In fact, the rate is so slow that patients are unlikely to see an effect for many weeks or months and can require encouragement from the physician. When a rash is reported, the patient must be examined immediately, and serious consideration must be given to stopping the drug.

Levetiracetam

Levetiracetam Keppra is very well tolerated and has not been associated with serious side effects. It occasionally causes significant irritability and/or depression that necessitates stopping the drug. It can be titrated relatively rapidly so that its effectiveness in a patient can be determined in a short time. It is primarily excreted unchanged, so it does not have significant drug interactions. Levetiracetam is available in an intravenous preparation, dosed the same as the oral form.

Oxcarbazepine

Oxcarbazepine (Trileptal) is a derivative of carbamazepine, and its mechanism of action is similar to carbamazepine's. The primary CNS side effects of carbamazepine are due to epoxide-10,11-carbamazepine, a metabolite produced by oxidation. Oxcarbazepine cannot undergo this conversion and thus does not produce this metabolite. Therefore, it is better tolerated than carbamazepine and is less likely to cause diplopia and ataxia, although it is not clear whether it causes less sedation. The incidence of blood dyscrasias also appears lower than with carbamazepine, but hyponatremia seems more common than with carbamazepine. It does not induce AED-metabolizing liver enzymes (although it does affect other liver enzymes) or undergo autoinduction. The daily dose cannot be directly converted from the carbamazepine dose. It is effective as monotherapy, so it is likely that in the future oxcarbazepine will entirely replace carbamazepine.

Tiagabine

Tiagabine (Gabitril) is approved as add-on therapy for partial-onset seizures. It is the only AED that was designed for a specific mechanism of action; it inhibits the reuptake of GABA in the synaptic cleft. It has a very short serum half-life, but it affects the GABA transporter for at least 12 hours so it can be dosed twice a day. Some patients require more frequent dosing. It is not associated with any end-organ toxicity, but it can exacerbate myoclonic and absence seizures and precipitate nonconvulsive status epilepticus in those who are predisposed, usually patients with generalized epilepsy. Thus, it is uncommonly prescribed.

Topiramate

Topiramate (Topamax) is effective for partial seizures and some types of generalized seizures, especially the Lennox–Gastaut syndrome. It has acquired an unwarranted reputation for causing cognitive side effects. The source of this is probably the design of clinical studies, which appropriately determined the maximum tolerated dose by finding the dose at which an unacceptable incidence of side effects occurs. Considering all topiramate clinical studies together, the incidence of subject dropout in those treated with more than 400 mg/day was twice that of the group treated with less than 400 mg/day, which was approximately equal to dropout in the placebo group. This indicates that the average maximum tolerated dose is about 400 mg/day, so it should usually be used at a dose lower than this. Topiramate is a weak carbonic anhydrase inhibitor and can cause kidney stones and metabolic acidosis; the use of other carbonic anhydrase inhibitors is relatively contraindicated. Acute narrow-angle glaucoma has been reported in a few cases and requires immediate discontinuation.

Zonisamide

Zonisamide (Zonegran) appears to be effective for both focal and some generalized[1] epilepsies. It is approved as adjunctive treatment for partial seizures in adults. Its pharmacology is not well described, but it is metabolized by multiple mechanisms and has a very long half-life, which might allow it to be dosed once per day. It rarely causes kidney stones. It also can cause oligohydrosis (reduced sweating) and has rarely been associated with blood dyscrasias.

Pregabalin

Pregabalin (Lyrica) is approved as adjunctive treatment of partial seizures in adults. It is not metabolized significantly, so it is excreted unchanged in urine. It does not bind to plasma proteins. Common side effects are dizziness, weight gain, pedal edema, and somnolence.

Vigabatrin

Vigabatrin (Sabril) is approved for infantile spasms in children ages 1 month to 2 years and for adult use in combination with other medications to treat complex partial seizures that have not responded adequately to previous drug therapies. It reversibly inhibits the major degradative enzyme for GABA (GABA-transaminase). It does not bind to plasma proteins. It is eliminated primarily by the kidneys. The side effects can be serious. Peripheral visual field defects can be seen in about 25% to 50% of adults and about 15% of children. Psychotic disorders and hallucinations are rare but also can be seen. Therefore it is recommended to have cognitive and age-appropriate vision testing at baseline and repeated at intervals. If it is effective, then it will be effective within 12 weeks. If there is significant reduction in seizures or the patient becomes seizure free, then the continuation of therapy depends on the risk-to-benefit ratio, and the patient or the caregiver should be involved in decision making. If there is no benefit after 12 weeks of treatment, it should be discontinued. Its use should be limited primarily to epilepsy centers.

Rufinamide

Rufinamide (Banzel) is approved as adjunctive therapy for seizures associated with Lennox–Gastaut syndrome, a severe form of epilepsy. The proposed mechanism of action is the limitation of sodium-dependent action potential firing. There seem to be a good cognitive and psychiatric adverse effect profile and few drug interactions. Rufinamide use is most appropriate when Lennox–Gastaut patients have failed other therapies.

---

[1]Not FDA approved for this indication.

Lacosamide

Lacosamide (Vimpat) is approved as adjunctive therapy in the treatment of partial-onset seizures in adults. It has a unique mechanism of action with selective enhancement of voltage-gated sodium channel slow inactivation. Lacosamide has a favorable pharmacokinetic profile with near 100% bioavailability, minimal protein binding, and few drug–drug interactions. The most common adverse effects include diplopia, headache, dizziness, and nausea. At high doses, lacosamide can induce P-R interval prolongation. It is dosed twice a day and is available in an intravenous formulation.

Clobazam

Clobazam (Onfi) was recently approved in the United States for adjunctive treatment of seizures associated with Lennox–Gastaut syndrome. Clobazam is an antiepileptic of the benzodiazepine class. The most common adverse effects are sedation related (sedation, somnolence, drowsiness). Clobazam is dosed twice daily and should be dosed according to body weight. It is primarily metabolized in the liver, and thus dosing should be adjusted in those with hepatic impairment.

Ezogabine

Ezogabine (Potiga), a potassium-channel opener, is approved as an adjunctive treatment of partial-onset seizures in adults. Urinary retention was reported in approximately 2% of patients in clinical trials. In October 2013, the FDA added a boxed warning due to risks of retinal abnormalities, potential vision loss, and skin discoloration that may occur with use of ezogabine. This drug should therefore be limited only to patients who have failed several alternative treatments and for whom the benefits outweigh the potential risk of vision loss. All patients taking ezogabine should have baseline and periodic (every 6 months) visual monitoring by an ophthalmic professional.

Perampanel

Perampanel (Fycompa), an AMPA glutamate receptor antagonist, is approved as an adjunctive treatment of partial-onset seizure in patients aged 12 years and older. Perampanel is extensively metabolized by the liver. Dose adjustments are recommended in those with mild and moderate hepatic impairment, and the drug should not be used in patients with severe hepatic or renal impairment, including those on hemodialysis. Common side effects include dizziness, somnolence, headache, fatigue, irritability, gait disturbance and falls. There is a boxed warning of serious neuropsychiatric effects including alteration of mood and aggression. Perampanel is classified as a Schedule III drug by the U.S. Drug Enforcement Administration (DEA) due to its potential for abuse.

Eslicarbazepine

Eslicarbazepine (Aptiom) was approved by the United States FDA in 2013 as an adjunctive treatment of partial-onset seizures in adults. It is structurally similar to carbamazepine and oxcarbazepine. It is believed to act through preferential blockade of voltage-gated sodium channels in rapidly firing neurons, but there may be additional mechanisms of action. Common side effects include dizziness, drowsiness, headache, nausea, and diplopia. Eslicarbazepine has also been associated with an increase in the PR interval, abnormal liver function tests, and hyponatremia.

Special Patient Populations

Women

Women with epilepsy face unique challenges throughout their lifespan related to the interaction of hormones, epilepsy, and AEDs. Women with epilepsy have increased rates of infertility due to intrinsic hormone changes, anovulatory cycles, irregular menstrual cycles, and sexual dysfunction. This can be compounded by the effects of AEDs, especially valproate, which is associated with polycystic ovary disease, as well as the enzyme-inducing AEDs, which can alter endogenous steroids.

Enzyme-inducing AEDs can decrease the efficacy of oral contraceptives (OCs), leading to unwanted pregnancies. Valproate, gabapentin, lacosamide, levetiracetam, pregabalin, tiagabine, and zonisamide do not affect OCs. Oxcarbazepine has an inconsistent effect, and topiramate at higher doses (greater than 200 mg) decreases OCs' efficacy. The benefits of OCs with higher hormone concentration remain unproven, and therefore a back-up barrier method or changing to a non–enzyme-inducing AED is recommended to prevent unwanted pregnancy. OCs can significantly reduce the serum concentration of lamotrigine, leading to breakthrough seizures, but the effect is variable.

The risk of major congenital malformations related to AEDs is a major concern for women with epilepsy. In general, the risk to the fetus from seizures, especially convulsions, is thought to be greater than the risk to the fetus from AEDs. It is generally recommended to continue AEDs at the lowest effective dose and to avoid polypharmacy. Birth defects occur in 1.6% to 2.3% of all live births in the general population. With the exception of valproic acid, rates of major congenital malformations for women taking AEDs are about twice those of the general population. Patients should be reassured that more than 90% of women with epilepsy have normal, healthy children.

Valproic acid is the AED that clearly has the higher teratogenicity rate (6.2%–10.7%). It has also been shown to reduce cognitive outcomes. Therefore it should not be used as a first-line treatment in women of childbearing potential. All women of childbearing potential, with or without epilepsy, should take at least 0.4 mg of folic acid daily prior to conception and during pregnancy to decrease the risk of major congenital malformations.

Breast-feeding is a common postpartum concern for women with epilepsy. Primidone (Mysoline) and levetiracetam probably transfer into breast milk in amounts that may be clinically important, whereas valproate, phenobarbital, phenytoin, and carbamazepine likely do not. The effects on infant health and development are unknown, however, and most experts believe that taking AEDs does *not* generally contraindicate breast-feeding because the probable benefits outweigh the risks.

Enzyme-inducing AEDs induce the metabolism of vitamin D, increasing the risk of osteoporosis. Long-term AED use has been associated with an increased risk of fracture, particularly in women. Therefore, supplemental vitamin D and calcium should be recommended.

Elderly Patients

Elderly patients with epilepsy have several unique characteristics. Altered physiology during aging and possible polypharmacy for other medical conditions need to be considered when selecting an AED. The incidence of epilepsy is high among elderly people, increasing after the age of 75 years. The recognition of seizures may be difficult owing to atypical clinical presentations. The most common presumed cause is stroke. Alzheimer's disease and head injury are other common causes. Complex partial and simple partial seizures are the most common presentation, especially in the form of memory lapses, confusion, change in mental status, and staring.

When initiating an AED, lower dosages are required owing to decreased renal and hepatic clearance. An age-related decrease in serum albumin increases the free fraction of the protein-bound AEDs. Phenytoin is particularly poorly tolerated in the elderly and in addition can have a prolonged half-life so that levels are unexpectedly high. Some new AEDs are better tolerated and less likely to cause drug interactions. Gabapentin is particularly desirable because it has no drug interactions. Lamotrigine, oxcarbazepine, and levetiracetam are also usually well tolerated and often selected as first-line agents in this age group.

Refractory Epilepsy

An estimated one third of people with epilepsy do not respond adequately to AEDs. Patients with refractory epilepsy, defined by failure of two AEDs, should be referred to an epilepsy center for diagnosis and consideration of the many therapeutic options currently available. In addition to a careful history and physical examination directed at determining seizure type, neuroanatomic site of seizure origin, and the epilepsy syndrome or etiology, the most important diagnostic test for evaluating intractable seizures is prolonged simultaneous video and EEG monitoring. Video EEG may need to continue for days or weeks to capture enough spells to make a correct diagnosis. Tools such as MRI of the brain with special acquisition protocols, positron emission tomography (PET), and single photon-emission CT (SPECT) may be used to help reveal abnormalities that are not obvious on routine imaging.

Surgery to resect the epilepsy focus is the only currently available method of curing epilepsy. The seizure-free outcomes after epilepsy surgery have been reported at about 52% at 5 years and 47% at 10 years. Extratemporal resections have an unfavorable outcome compared with temporal resections. Devices such as vagal nerve stimulation have an increasingly important role in the treatment of refractory epilepsy and have been shown to significantly reduce seizure frequency. Continuous deep brain stimulation, which uses electricity to stimulate the anterior nucleus of the thalamus, is not yet approved by the FDA. Responsive cortical stimulation is a treatment option for patients with refractory focal epilepsy and a well defined seizure focus when surgery is not possible. The device monitors and interrupts abnormal electrical activity in the brain before a seizure occurs and was approved by the US FDA in 2013.

References

Berg AT, Berkovic SF, Brodie MJ, et al. Revised terminology and concepts for organization of seizures and epilepsies: Report of the ILAE Commission on Classification and Terminology, 2005–2009. Epilepsia 2010;51:676–85.

Britton JW. Antiepileptic drug therapy: When to start, when to stop. Continuum Lifelong Learning Neurol 2010;16:105–20.

Drazkowski JF, Chung SS. Differential diagnosis of epilepsy. Continuum Lifelong Learning Neurol 2010;16:36–56.

Fisher RS, Boas WVE, Blume W, et al. Epileptic seizures and epilepsy: Definitions proposed by the International League Against Epilepsy (ILAE) and the International Bureau for Epilepsy (IBE). Epilepsia 2005;46:470–2.

Harden CL, Meador KJ, Pennell PB, et al. Management issues for women with epilepsy—focus on pregnancy (an evidence-based review): II. Teratogenesis and perinatal outcomes: Report of the Quality Standards Subcommittee and Therapeutics and Technology Subcommittee of the American Academy of Neurology and the American Epilepsy Society. Epilepsia 2009;50:1237–46.

Harden CL, Pennell PB, Koppel BS, et al. Management issues for women with epilepsy—focus on pregnancy (an evidence-based review): III. Vitamin K, folic acid, blood levels, and breast-feeding: Report of the Quality Standards Subcommittee and Therapeutics and Technology Assessment Subcommittee of the American Academy of Neurology and the American Epilepsy Society. Epilepsia 2009;50:1247–55.

Hesdorffer DC, Logroscino G, Benn EKT, et al. Estimating risk for developing epilepsy: A population-based study in Rochester, Minnesota. Neurology 2011;76:23–7.

Krumholz A, Wiebe S, Gronseth G, et al. Practice parameter: Evaluating an apparent unprovoked first seizure in adults (an evidence-based review): Report of the Quality Standards Subcommittee of the American Academy of Neurology and the American Epilepsy Society. Neurology 2007;69:1996–2007.

Marson AG, Al-Kharusi AM, Alwaidh M, et al. The SANAD study of effectiveness of carbamazepine, gabapentin, lamotrigine, oxcarbazepine, or topiramate for treatment of partial epilepsy: An unblinded randomised controlled trial. Lancet 2007;369:1000–15.

Marson AG, Al-Kharusi AM, Alwaidh M, et al. The SANAD study of effectiveness of valproate, lamotrigine, or topiramate for generalised and unclassifiable epilepsy: An unblinded randomised controlled trial. Lancet 2007;369:1016–26.

Tisi J, Bell GS, Peacock JL, et al. The long-term outcome of adult epilepsy surgery, patterns of seizure remission, and relapse: A cohort study. Lancet 2011;378:1388–95.

SLEEP DISORDERS

Method of
Erik K. St. Louis, MD; and Timothy I. Morgenthaler, MD

Sleep is a universal biological imperative for all mammals. Sleep deprivation and sleep disorders are frequent and underappreciated determinants of health status. Sleep is essential for survival, and sleep loss and sleep disorders are associated with major health problems, including cardiovascular, metabolic, neuropsychiatric, and neoplastic disorders, as well as neurobehavioral-associated accidents and risks. Healthy sleep must be regarded along with nutrition and exercise as key pillars for good health.

Recent evidence has suggested that a chief purpose of sleep may be to maintain cerebral metabolic homeostasis, clearing waste products that accumulate during wakefulness such as beta-amyloid, a protein known to abnormally accumulate in Alzheimer's disease. Insufficient sleep quantity appears to be associated with a variety of health problems and may contribute to mortality and dementia risk. Total sleep deprivation, as well as selective deprivation of nonrapid eye movement (NREM) or rapid eye movement (REM) sleep, may be lethal in laboratory animals. Adequate sleep quality is similarly necessary to ensure optimal daytime functioning because basic vigilance, attention and cognitive performance, and overall quality of life are each substantially eroded by disordered sleep, and insufficient sleep and sleep-disordered breathing (SDB) pose significant health hazards. Unfortunately, insufficient sleep quantity and quality is a widespread public health crisis in children and adults worldwide in the developed world, and primary sleep disorders are a highly prevalent cause of morbidity, an important contributor to mortality, and a public health hazard that raises risk for motor vehicle collisions and catastrophic occupational injuries and accidents.

The clinical specialty of sleep medicine initially emerged during the 1970s and 1980s, surrounding growing clinical application of diagnostic polysomnography (PSG). While the main diagnostic use remains evaluation and initial treatment for SDB, PSG and related techniques have tremendous utility for the evaluation of selected patients with nocturnal events, periodic limb movement disorder (PLMD), narcolepsy and related primary central nervous system (CNS) hypersomnias.

In this chapter, we review the classification of common sleep disorders, a practical bedside approach toward interviewing and examining patients with sleep problems, advantages and limitations of diagnostic implements within the sleep laboratory, and summarize diagnostic and therapeutic approaches to common sleep disorders.

The International Classification of Sleep Disorders

The International Classification of Sleep Disorders (ICSD) provides a common nomenclature and taxonomy for disorders of sleep for clinicians and researchers alike. The most current ICSD, ICSD-2, divides sleep disorders into eight distinct categories. The ICSD-2 nomenclature is shown in Box 1, and the most common sleep complaints and disorders are presented and discussed in detail throughout this chapter. At the time of this writing, the ICSD-3 release is imminent but not yet available.

Clinical Approach to the Sleep Medicine Patient: The Interview and Examination

The three most common clinical presenting sleep-related complaints are hypersomnia, insomnia, and unusual behaviors or events at night (parasomnias). Hypersomnia, which is excessive sleepiness during waking hours, is often multifactorial and may be related to insufficient sleep quantity, quality, or timing; SDB; sedating medications; or certain medical, psychiatric, or neurologic conditions. Insomnia may be regarded as a problem in initiating or maintaining sleep under conditions that are normally conducive to sleep. Parasomnias are unusual behaviors that are often dangerous to the patient or bed partner during sleep.

Insomnia is a subjective complaint. To some patients it is not at all bothersome to require 20 to 30 minutes to fall asleep, while to others it seems very wrong. While insomnia is fundamentally a subjective symptom, the manifestations follow common patterns. Sleep latency, the time taken to fall asleep, varies significantly, but initial sleep latency longer than 30 minutes may be considered prolonged, once proper sleep-conductive conditions have been established (lights off, dark and quiet sleep environment without distracting stimuli). There is also significant variation in what degree of subjective sleep disruption reflects sleep-maintenance

Insomnia and Inadequate Sleep Hygiene
Primary insomnias
Idiopathic insomnia
Psychophysiologic insomnia
Paradoxical insomnia

Secondary insomnias
Insomnia due to mental disorder
Inadequate sleep hygiene
Behavioral insomnia of childhood
Adjustment insomnia
Insomnia due to drug or substance (alcohol)
Insomnia due to medical condition
Insomnia not due to substance of known physiologic condition, nonorganic
Physiologic (organic) insomnia, unspecified

Sleep-Related Breathing Disorders
The continuum of obstructive sleep-disordered breathing: snoring, Upper-airway resistance syndrome, and obstructive sleep apnea (OSA)
Central sleep apnea
• Primary central sleep apnea
• Due to Cheyne-Stokes breathing pattern
• Due to high-altitude periodic breathing
• Due to medical condition, not Cheyne-Stokes
• Due to drug or substance
Primary sleep apnea of infancy
Complex sleep apnea syndrome
Sleep-related hypoventilation
• Sleep-related nonobstructive alveolar hypoventilation, idiopathic
• Congenital central alveolar hypoventilation syndrome
• Due to lower airways obstruction, neuromuscular and chest wall Disorders, pulmonary parenchymal or vascular pathology
• Unspecified

Narcolepsy and Primary CNS Hypersomnias
Narcolepsy
• With cataplexy
• Without cataplexy
• Due to medical condition
• Unspecified
Recurrent hypersomnia
• Kleine-Levin syndrome
• Menstrual-related hypersomnia
Idiopathic hypersomnia
• With long sleep time
• Without long sleep time
Behaviorally induced insufficient sleep syndrome
Hypersomnia due to medical condition, drug, or substance (alcohol)
Hypersomnia not due to substance or known physiologic condition
Physiologic hypersomnia (unspecified)

Circadian Sleep Disorders
Delayed sleep-phase syndrome

Advanced sleep-phase syndrome
Irregular sleep-wake type
Nonentrained type (free running)
Jet lag type
Shift-work type
Due to medical condition
Other
Due to drug or substance (alcohol)

Parasomnias
Disorders of arousal from NREM sleep
Confusional arousals
Sleepwalking
Sleep terrors

Parasomnias usually associated with REM sleep
REM sleep behavior disorder
Recurrent isolated sleep paralysis
Nightmare disorder

Other parasomnias
Sleep-related dissociative disorders
Sleep enuresis
Sleep-related groaning (catathrenia)
Exploding head syndrome
Sleep-related hallucinations
Sleep-related eating disorder
Parasomnias due to drug or substance (alcohol)
Parasomnias due to medical condition

Sleep-Related Movement Disorders
Restless leg syndrome
Periodic limb movement disorder
Sleep-related leg cramps
Sleep-related bruxism
Sleep-related rhythmic movement disorde
Sleep-related movement disorder, unspecified, due to drug or substance, due to medical condition

Isolated Symptoms, Apparently Normal Variants, and Unresolved Issues
Long sleepers
Short sleeper
Snoring
Sleep talking
Sleep starts (hypnic jerks)
Benign sleep myoclonus of infancy
Hypnagogic foot tremor and alternating leg muscle activation during sleep
Propriospinal myoclonus at sleep onset
Excessive fragmentary myoclonus

Other Sleep Disorders
Physiologic sleep disorder, unspecified
Environmental sleep disorder
Fatal familial insomnia

Abbreviations: CNS = central nervous system; NREM = non–rapid eye movement [sleep]; REM = rapid eye movement [sleep].

insomnia, as normal individuals may briefly awaken as often as 10 to 15 times each hour, with most such arousals being below the threshold of conscious awareness. Multiple nocturnal awakenings that are disturbing to the patient, especially when there is difficulty reinitiating sleep and prolonged wake after sleep-onset time, may be regarded as sleep-maintenance insomnia. Patients admitting to insomnia should be asked to estimate what amount of their problem is ascribable to an active mind or worries, restless legs, or body pain. Disturbing influences in the sleep environment such as the ambient light, temperature, and noise conditions in the bedroom should be sought. A precise diagnosis is not possible without

detailed knowledge of sleep and wake behavior over the entire circadian cycle during a more protracted time, such as 1 to 2 weeks. A sleep diary can be very helpful in gaining needed insights for diagnosis. Increasingly, helpful information about timing and duration of sleep may be logged in applications for personal mobile computing devices.

The patient and physician may at times have difficulty differentiating between hypersomnia and complaints of fatigue (a sense of lacking enough energy to carry out usual daily activities, without the tendency toward dozing or nodding off inadvertently). A quick, incisive bedside test that helps distinguish between hypersomnia and fatigue is the Epworth Sleepiness Scale (ESS), a short questionnaire asking the patient his or her likelihood of dozing inadvertently during usual permissive daytime sedentary settings including reading, watching television, or traveling in a car. An online version is available at http://www.stanford.edu/~dement/epworth.html. Scores over 10 are considered abnormal and indicative of a possible underlying primary sleep disorder and suggest the need for further evaluation. Complaints of hypersomnia must be placed into the context of the sleep history with particular emphasis on the quantity, timing, and quality of sleep.

Patients may also present with complaints of disturbing or unusual activities during sleep (parasomnias). Key diagnostic points in determining the diagnosis for parasomnias include their onset, duration, frequency, time of night, stereotypy, injuries sustained, and whether there is any further behavioral change following the parasomnia episode.

Collateral history obtained from a bed partner may be particularly instructive. Patients should be asked whether they are reported to snore, whether the snoring is intermittent or constant, and if the snoring volume is related to sleeping in a supine position. Disruptive snoring loud enough to be heard outside a closed bedroom door, or witnessed stop-breathing episodes indicating apneas or self-awareness of arousals related to a snort or gasp, are particularly suggestive symptoms of obstructive sleep apnea (OSA). Symptoms such as morning dry mouth and sore throat, frequent morning headaches, or heartburn may indicate a higher likelihood of significant SDB. Patients should be asked about awareness of restless legs symptoms or movements during sleep, and whether they have been told of peculiar sleep-related behaviors or evidence of acting out their dreams, yelling or thrashing in sleep, or exhibiting sleep walking or other amnestic behaviors during sleep.

In addition to a detailed sleep history, taking a thorough general medical history is important because sleep disorders are frequently tightly linked to other diseases. OSA is closely associated with hypertension, coronary artery disease, cerebrovascular disease, atrial fibrillation, obesity, and the metabolic syndrome. Congestive heart failure, even when well compensated, is frequently associated with central sleep apnea syndrome. Restless legs syndrome and periodic limb movements in sleep (PLMS) are more common in patients with spinal cord or peripheral nerve pathologies. Hypoventilation is more prevalent in patients with neuromuscular disease; advanced obstructive lung disease; kyphosis; and in traumatic, vascular, neoplastic, or degenerative disorders that affect the medullary centers of the brain. Various genetic syndromes such as trisomy 21 produce craniofacial abnormalities predisposing to OSA due to anatomic narrowing of the upper airway.

Physical examination in sleep medicine focuses upon signs indicating predisposition or associated sequelae of SDB. Careful inspection of the oropharynx and nares is particularly important because significant oropharyngeal narrowing is the chief anatomic substrate for obstructive SDB, while nasal septal deviation or other nasal obstruction, in addition to a thickened neck and overweight body habitus, may also contribute toward sleep apnea. Careful inspection for signs of neuromuscular disease, such as fasciculations or thoracoabdominal paradox, may help detect the underlying cause for sleep-related hypoventilation. Elevated blood pressure, a cardiac gallop, wet rales, and peripheral edema may be present as signs of systemic hypertension, heart failure, or cor pulmonale associated with untreated SDB.

Diagnostic Tools in the Sleep Laboratory

Polysomnography

Laboratory PSG is the "gold standard" for formal assessment of suspected SDB, hypersomnia, or parasomnias. PSG is a diagnostic test most often performed in a sleep laboratory; attended by trained technicians; and combining evaluation of sleep, breathing, and movement. During PSG, several polygraphic physiologic variables are analyzed, including electroencephalography (EEG) as well as chin electromyography (EMG) to allow determination of sleep staging, limb EMG leads to analyze periodic leg or arm movements that may disrupt sleep, oronasal airflow measured by a thermistor and nasal pressure sensors, electrocardiography, and respiratory effort measured by inductance plethysmography or piezocrystal monitors. Body position is also analyzed to delineate effects of sleeping position on breathing.

Each 30-second epoch of the polysomnogram is subsequently scored by a PSG technologist as either wake, NREM sleep (N1 or N2 light NREM, or N3 slow wave sleep), or REM sleep according to well-defined guidelines. Sleep architecture, or the composition of sleep by different stages, varies greatly by age, but in middle-aged adults is approximately 60% to 75% N1-N2, 10% to 20% N3, and 15% to 25% REM sleep. Children usually have higher, and elderly individuals have lower, percentages of N3 and REM. Arousals from sleep and their mechanisms, whether due to breathing, movement, or spontaneous causes, are determined. Accordingly, a precise determination of the duration of a patient's total sleep time, sleep efficiency (total time spent asleep divided by time in bed), and disrupting influences on sleep, such as abnormal respiration or movement, may be determined. The effects of confounding medications and medical disorders on sleep architecture, such as selective-serotonin reuptake inhibitors (SSRI) that suppress and delay REM sleep, or benzodiazepines that reduce the N3 and REM amounts and increase sleep stage shifting leading to heightened light NREM N1 and N2, must also be considered.

Attended PSG is advantageous because it allows precise measurement of sleep and relevant cardiorespiratory and neurologic behaviors and allows intervention with therapeutic positive airway pressure (PAP) trials if indicated. Disadvantages of PSG include patient inconvenience, a foreign sleep environment, and expenses due to highly trained personnel and technology. For those patients whose disease severity is difficult to predict, or who may have other complicating medical illnesses that would render interpretation of an out-of-center cardiopulmonary sleep test inaccurate (such as those with significant cardiopulmonary or neurologic diseases), or those who may require noncontinuous PAP modalities, or for those with parasomnia symptoms, attended PSG and treatment design is needed. Split-night PSG remains a cost-effective strategy for many patients.

PSG is currently the only way to actually measure sleep; although the sleep state is currently defined by the variables measured in PSG (EEG, EMG, and EOG), the science of sleep medicine may develop other ways of characterizing the sleep state that are more convenient, precise, and correlate even better with health and disease.

Home Sleep Apnea Testing

PSG is comprehensive, but for patients with characteristic clinical presentations for OSA syndrome, it is often possible to arrive at a diagnosis using a significantly reduced number of recording channels that may be conducted in the home setting. A recent systematic review concluded that many commercially available home monitoring devices do not perform well in sensitivity or specificity. The best out-of-center testing devices use similar measures as PSG but exclude EEG, EMG, or EOG channels needed to score sleep. Thus, these devices typically measure at a minimum airflow using thermistors and nasal pressure transducers, breathing effort using respiratory impedance plethysmography, oxygen saturation using pulse oximetry, and snoring. Using these signals, the frequency of apneas and hypopneas per hour of recording, called the respiratory event index (REI), may be determined. Some testing devices add markers for sleep, such as actigraphy (see below), position sensors, or pattern recognition of pulse or autonomic variability to estimate sleep time (called peripheral arterial tonometry). Home sleep apnea testing (HSAT) devices are thus far only considered for evaluation of OSA syndrome and are not suitable for diagnostic evaluation of other sleep disorders. Because of limited sensitivity, they are best employed when there is a high pretest probability that the patient has at least moderately severe OSA syndrome. Patients appropriate for HSAT would be those who satisfy three criteria: have a high likelihood of having at least moderately severe OSA, will be good candidates for either autotitrating continuous PAP (CPAP) or an oral appliance, and do not have underlying diseases that either will obscure HSAT or who may have other disorders that require PSG for diagnosis. Because of the poor sensitivity of HSAT, a negative result should be cause for PSG: the patient should have had a high pretest probability for having at least moderately severe OSA.

For medically uncomplicated patients fitting the above criteria, using HSAT followed by APAP most often leads to similar results as attended PSG with CPAP therapy based upon in-lab titration of pressure. This strategy is increasingly being used, largely owing to reduced costs. These good results depend, however, upon expert PAP mask fitting and follow-up. It is best to remember that treatment is chronic and requires ongoing follow-up. More is written about this in the section on OSA below.

Multiple Sleep Latency and Maintenance of Wakefulness Testing

The multiple sleep-latency test (MSLT) provides an objective measure of sleepiness compared with normal individuals lacking primary sleep disorders. The chief clinical indication for MSLT is for evaluation of narcolepsy and related primary CNS hypersomnias such as idiopathic hypersomnia and Kleine-Levin syndrome. A MSLT is carried out during the daytime in a sleep laboratory following nocturnal PSG, with four or five nap opportunities at standard times and intervals, usually at 9:00 and 11:00 AM and 1:00, 3:00, and 5:00 PM. Careful inspection of each nap is subsequently performed to determine the timing of sleep onset relative to commencement of each nap, and whether REM sleep occurs during each nap. A mean sleep latency is then calculated from the average initial sleep latency from each nap. Mean sleep latencies shorter than 8 minutes are considered abnormal and indicative of pathologic excessive daytime sleepiness. Whether or not a sleep-onset REM period (a SOREM, i.e., reaching REM sleep within 15 minutes of sleep onset during a nap) is captured is also considered and tabulated. More than one SOREM is abnormal and is consistent with the diagnosis of narcolepsy.

There are several considerations prior to performing and interpreting a valid MSLT. Patients should be instructed to sleep well for at least 2 weeks preceding the study, to allow at least 6 to 7 hours per night (and when possible, extending time in bed to 8-9 hours), and many sleep specialists document the quantity of sleep before the test with actigraphy monitoring or a sleep diary to ensure adherence to this recommendation and exclude the contaminating influence of insufficient sleep quantity. If it is safe and practically possible to do so, patients should be instructed to taper or discontinue sedative, stimulant, or REM suppressant medications (i.e., opiate analgesics, antidepressants, or other psychotropic or CNS active drugs) with the oversight and permission of other relevant treating primary care, psychiatry, and pain physicians at least 2 weeks prior to MSLT, and certain psychotropic drugs such as fluoxetine (Prozac) with a long elimination half-life should be discontinued for at least a month prior to MSLT to avoid decrease in MSLT sensitivity for delay of REM latency. Patients should undergo a full-night diagnostic PSG the night before a MSLT study to ensure that there is not another primary sleep disorder, such as SDB or PLMD, that could provide an alternative reason for significant sleepiness and to ensure that sufficient sleep quantity of 6 hours or more is obtained.

While the MSLT is designed to assess sleepiness, the maintenance of wakefulness test (MWT) is used to assess the ability to remain awake. The MWT is most useful when an objective measure of the effectiveness of treatment for disorders causing hypersomnolence is needed. The patient is seated in a dim room in a comfortable, semi-reclined position and asked to remain alert but passive for four 40-minute periods that are 2 hours apart. EEG, EOG, and chin EMG are measured, and the signals are analyzed to detect any epochs of unequivocal sleep during each 40-minute period. Normal patients have a mean time to epochs of unequivocal sleep of 30.4 minutes; however, the data is not

normally distributed, and 42% of all patients remain awake for the entire 40 minutes on all four opportunities. Since simulated and actual driving performance is compromised with sleep times of 19 minutes or less on MWT, this is a reasonable threshold for the distinction of clinically significant daytime sleepiness, and driving or other safety sensitive tasks should be curtailed when sleep latencies are 19 minutes or shorter.

Actigraphy Monitoring

Wrist actigraphy monitoring is utilized to provide a rigorous estimation of sleep quantity and its circadian pattern. The actigraphy monitor may be worn like a wristwatch and contains an accelerometer that detects movements, which are recorded over time periods lasting up to weeks. The magnitude and pattern of movements may be analyzed and modeled to infer the sleep-wake pattern and provides a graphic representation of the patient's sleep schedule. The test is used in the evaluation of suspected circadian rhythm disorders, to assess response to treatment of insomnia, and for investigating patients with hypersomnia prior to PSG and MSLT to more accurately document the adequacy of sleep prior to the assessment for sleepiness. Recent applications utilizing the accelerometer in smartphones and wrist-worn fitness devices show promise, but most have not been validated as diagnostic tools.

Diagnostic and Therapeutic Approach to Common Sleep Disorders

Insomnia

The insomnia disorders all share three basic components: repeated complaints of insomnia, which may involve difficulties falling asleep, staying asleep, poor sleep quality, or waking undesirably early; an adequate time and opportunity for sleep; and a complaint of resultant daytime impairment. Insomnia is the most common of sleep complaints: nearly 45% of people were affected intermittently within the past year in some large studies, and up to 15% suffer chronic insomnia disorders. Risks for insomnia include female sex, older age, and a psychiatric or medical comorbidity. Chronic insomnia should be distinguished from acute insomnia, which may occur in anyone occasionally (e.g., the night before an important job interview, or during increased stress). Some suggest a 3-month duration of the above symptoms to define chronicity, but there is evidence to suggest that as few as 30 days of symptoms may be clinically significant.

Insomnia may be classified as primary or secondary, with secondary insomnia being far more common (see Box 1). Idiopathic insomnia begins in childhood, is lifelong, and appears as a manifestation of neurologic hyperarousal, with demonstrable increases in cerebral metabolism via functional MRI and increases in beta and theta EEG activity as well as generalized increased metabolism and stress hormone production compared with normals in either wake or sleep states. To a lesser extent, these same markers for hyperarousability are seen in other causes of primary insomnia (see Box 1).

In the past, secondary insomnia was thought to be a result or accompaniment of an underlying illness. This may be incorrect. For example, it has previously been thought that treatment of secondary insomnia ought to focus on treatment of the underlying disorder. Newer evidence indicates that this approach may be suboptimal for the following reasons: secondary insomnia does not reliably improve when the underlying disorder does; secondary insomnia in general responds to treatment directed at insomnia; and in some cases, the underlying disorder, such as depression, responds better to treatment when the insomnia is addressed directly and concurrently. Furthermore, in several illnesses, such as depression, insomnia may predate the depression by months, and insomnia is a risk factor for future development of many psychiatric illnesses. For these reasons, many now prefer the term "comorbid insomnia" to secondary insomnia.

Chronic insomnia may be preceded in predisposed individuals by precipitating factors such as illness or stress and may be propagated by behavioral or maladaptive cognitive factors. Some individuals, such as those with idiopathic insomnia, do not appear to require precipitating or propagating factors to develop chronic insomnia. They are prototypic for an underlying predisposition toward insomnia. These individuals manifest insomnia from infancy and persist despite optimization of sleep hygiene and habit. However, in most cases of insomnia, precipitating and/or propagating influences may be found through careful interview and help establish a secure diagnosis.

As a prototype of insomnia largely due to precipitating and propagating influences, adults with psychophysiologic insomnia not infrequently have identifiable precipitating causes that may be traumatic, stressful periods or struggles, medical illness, drugs, or toxins. However, even when the cause is removed, a conditioned response built upon associated and at times maladaptive sleep-related behaviors ensues. Instead of beginning to relax for sleep under permissive circumstances, the affected patient experiences paradoxical arousal as they approach their sleep conditions. The patient under the influence of the precipitating cause may have spent many hours worrying, uncomfortable, clock-watching, or otherwise raising their anxiety levels. Propagating factors include these same behaviors that help maintain sleeplessness once it has begun and may additionally include irregular sleep schedules and the use of drugs. Abuse of alcohol may contribute or be secondary to the sleep disturbance.

Effective treatment strategies for insomnia focus on removing any residual precipitating influences and mitigating or eliminating propagating influences. The main therapies for insomnia are sleep hygiene, behavioral therapies, cognitive therapies, and pharmacologic therapies. Patients often respond best to combined modalities. There is high-level evidence that combined cognitive/behavior therapies (CBT) are at least as effective as pharmacologic therapy for most patients with insomnia. CBT also appears to have enhanced rates of insomnia remission, so these approaches ought generally to be employed first. The addition of hypnotics to CBT has resulted in more rapid remission in some, but not all, studies. Growing recognition of the adverse effect profile of sedative-hypnotic drugs, particularly zolpidem (Ambien), which has been associated with heightened risks of falls and sleep walking, sleep

eating, and related amnestic behaviors, has also encouraged a shift toward an earlier application of behavioral approaches to coping with insomnia.

In childhood, the most common causes of insomnia include limit-setting sleep disorder and sleep-onset association disorder. Limit-setting sleep disorder may occur when parents fail to establish and enforce an appropriate nightly bedtime, so that their child may subsequently stall and refuse to go to bed in a timely fashion. Sleep-onset association disorder results when a child cannot fall asleep until a usual condition is present, such as being held, rocked, or fed. Appropriate advice and treatments include strict limit-setting for bedtime resistance; maintaining regular sleep schedules with avoidance of napping during the daytimes; and curtailing disrupting influences, such as television watching, gaming, and computer use. Suggesting a nightly cell phone or personal device (i.e., iPod, iPad, or Wii U) check-in procedure is especially helpful in teenage children, and caffeinated soda and excessively stimulating activities should be avoided during the evenings. Selected children benefit from incentives such as a patient-parent contract that offers privileges for slightly later bedtimes on weekends after the child adheres regularly to a specified sleep schedule during school nights.

Four considerations for restoring normal sleep hygiene to discuss with all insomnia patients in the office include these three central concepts:

- Maintain a regular sleep schedule. Go to bed and arise at the same time each day. Ideally, the schedule should match the patient's biologic clock, with nocturnal sleep and bedtime/rise time matching their tendency for sleepiness and alertness (sleep education/hygiene).
- Avoid lying sleepless in bed. After 20 to 30 sleepless minutes spent trying to fall asleep, the patient should be instructed to leave the bedroom to pursue a quietly distracting activity, such as reading mundane material or watching a boring television program, and waiting until he or she feels sleepy enough to return to bed. Patients should explicitly avoid reading in bed, listening to the radio in bed, or watching television in bed if they are having difficulty initiating or maintaining sleep. This is a practical form of stimulus control (Table 1).

TABLE 1	Therapeutic Tools for Treating Insomnia		
THERAPY TYPE	**SPECIFIC THERAPIES/COMPONENTS**		**GOALS**
Education/sleep hygiene	Improve knowledge about behaviors that foster or hinder healthy sleep		Improve opportunity and environment for sleep
Behavioral therapies	Stimulus control • Unmodified extinction • Graduated extinction • Positive routines/faded bedtime with response cost • Scheduled awakenings		Dissociate anxiety or conditioned autonomic response from the process or location of going to sleep
	Sleep restriction		Increase pressure for sleep by decreasing the time allotted for sleep, increasing the probability of successful sleep attempts
	Relaxation training • Progressive muscle relaxation • Passive relaxation • Autogenic training-biofeedback • Imagery training • Meditation • Hypnosis		Reduce physiologic and/or cognitive arousal that hinders or disrupts sleep
	Paradoxical intention		Reduce performance anxiety that confounds ability to successfully go to sleep
Cognitive therapies	Cognitive restructuring Decatastrophizing Reappraisal Attention shifting		Decrease unrealistic expectations about sleep, misconceptions, or misattributions regarding causes of insomnia, consequences of insomnia, ability to control sleep; produce a more appropriate and adaptive mind-set
Pharmacologic therapies	Hypnotics Sedating antidepressants Herbal supplements		Enhance sleepiness at appropriate times or to enhance convenience of sleep time and/or duration

- Avoidance of clock-watching behavior. Patients should be instructed to remove clocks from their bedrooms or hide the clock face so as to make the insomnia period timeless and of uncertain duration. Falling asleep should not be a race against time, and repetitive checking of the time only serves to reinforce anxiety and further activate the mind (see stimulus control, Table 1). For the same reason, when watching television, discourage patients from watching news shows with scrolling tickertape newsflashes with clock time shown.
- Schedule thinking time earlier in the evening, well in advance of the sleep period. Patients who worry, plan, or think out their problems in bed should be encouraged to schedule a time earlier in the evening, well in advance of their normal bedtime, to attempt to work out these concerns prior to carrying them into bed. This "constructive worry" or "worry time" represents a practical form of cognitive and stimulus control therapy.

There are numerous other associated issues and behaviors that may be useful for application in selected patients, such as cutting down overall time in bed (sleep restriction), establishing a regular and relaxing bedtime routine (such as by taking a relaxing bath, listening to soothing music, or having a light snack before bed), avoiding daytime naps, avoiding caffeinated beverages after noontime, and establishing a regular morning exercise routine and avoiding evening exercise. It is important for the physician to avoid overloading the patient with too many considerations and tasks at once, however, as the burden of implementing these suggestions then becomes tantamount to too many obtrusive "swing thoughts" during a golf swing. One or two concepts to start with are sufficient, and once mastered and implemented, the patient can gradually phase in other ideas over time. Relaxation training and cognitive behavioral therapy can be very helpful in selected receptive patients who have failed the above typical self-help measures,

and as a last resort, periodic or even scheduled chronic pharmacotherapy can also be implemented.

There are now several highly effective and tolerable hypnotic medications available for short-term, intermittent, and chronic use. The class of nonbenzodiazepine receptor agonists (the so-called "Z" drugs, or zolpidem, zaleplon [Sonata], and ezopiclone [Lunesta]) are preferred by most sleep specialists but remain costlier than the older generation choices, including the benzodiazepines—which have adverse effects on sleep architecture—as well as diphenhydramine (Benadryl) and trazodone (Desyrel),[1] which each have less specific sleep-promoting effects and more adverse effects and potential for drug-drug interactions, especially in elderly patients. The clinical pharmacology of the most commonly prescribed and most useful hypnotic medications are summarized in Table 2. A concern with each of these may be the potential for habituation of efficacy; fall risk; and the potential to cause sleepwalking, sleep eating, or other amnestic behaviors during sleep. If these adverse effects result, the hypnotic drug should be promptly discontinued with a shift toward the use of cognitive behavioral therapy strategies. In women, zolpidem should be used with particular caution given the slower metabolism of the drug, thereby promoting vulnerabilities to carryover sedation and unpleasant "hangover" type feelings the next morning. Pharmacologic therapy of insomnia may be bolstered in the future by the advent of suvorexant (MK-4305),[2] a novel hypocretin antagonist that has a wake-suppressing rather than sleep-promoting mechanism of action. However, the higher doses that were primarily studied were determined as overly sedating and unsafe by the FDA at

---

[1]Not FDA approved for this indication.
[2]Not available in the United States.

TABLE 2	Clinical Pharmacology of Hypnotic Medications				
	MECHANISM OF ACTION	**DOSAGE (mg)**	**DURATION OF ACTION (T½)**	**TYPICAL ADVERSE EFFECTS**	**INTERACTIONS**
Older Hypnotics					
Diphenhydramine (Benadryl)	H1	25–50	Intermediate (2.4–9.3 h)	Dry mouth, constipation, urinary retention	Nonsignificant
Trazadone (Desyrel)[1]	SRI	50–150	Short (3–6 h)	Dry mouth, dizziness, rash	CYP substrate; several others
Triazolam (Halcion)	BRA	0.125–0.5	Short (1.5–5.5 h)	Tolerance	CYP induction
Lorazepam (Ativan)[1]	BRA	0.5–2.0	Intermediate (10–20 h)	Tolerance	CYP induction
Melatonin[2]	MT1-MT2	1–3	Ultra-short (35–50 min)	Hangover type effect	None
Newer Hypnotics					
Zolpidem (Ambien)	NBRA	5, 10	Short (2–2.6 h)	Amnestic behavior	Numerous
Zaleplon (Sonata)	NBRA	5, 10	Short (1 h)	Headache, amnestic behavior	Several
Eszopiclone (Lunesta)	NBRA	1–3	Intermediate (6 h)	Headache, amnestic behavior, rash possible	Nonsignificant
Ramelteon (Rozerem)	MT1-MT2	8, 16	Short (1–2.6 h)	Hyperprolactinemia	Ketoconazole (Nizoral), rifampin

[1]Not FDA approved for this indication.
[2]Not available in the United States.
Abbreviations: t½ = half-life of drug; h = hours; H1 = antihistaminergic H1 receptor blocker; SRI = serotonin reuptake inhibitor; BRA = benzodiazepine receptor agonist; CYP substrate = metabolized by cytochrome metabolism, susceptible to enzyme inhibition and elevated serum levels by multiple drugs; CYP induction = cytochrome enzyme inducer, may cause multiple potential drug-drug interactions via this mechanism; NBRA = nonbenzodiazepine benzodiazepine receptor agonist; MT1/MT2 = melatonin type 1 and type 2 receptor agonist.

the current time, so that further clinical testing will most likely be necessary before approval and clinical use is possible.

Sleep-Disordered Breathing

Breathing during sleep is carefully regulated to maintain homeostasis of oxygen, carbon dioxide, and blood pH. The mechanisms and homeostatic set points for ventilation vary systematically between wake, non-REM sleep, and REM sleep. In wake, the resulting ventilatory pattern is governed by careful integration of classic feedback systems designed to keep blood pH at approximately 7.40, arterial $Paco_2$ at approximately 38 to 45 mm Hg, and Pao_2 greater than approximately 60 mm Hg with cortical influences that govern functions such as speaking, laughing, eating, singing, and other voluntary activities. During non-REM sleep, ventilation is considerably more rhythmic and is governed almost exclusively by the chemoresponsive feedback systems indicated above; during REM sleep, the chemoresponsive feedback system is further influenced by additional input from REM-influenced neurons, resulting in a less rhythmic and less-carefully regulated metabolic milieu.

Significant deviation from these norms is termed "sleep-disordered breathing" (SDB), and is marked by several distinct event types. Apneas are total or near-total cessations of airflow. Hypopneas are significant declines in tidal volume sufficient to result in significant reduction in oxygenation. Excess effort for breathing may result in arousals from and disturbance of sleep, and are termed respiratory effort-related arousals (RERAs). These types of events are often related as a rate, either as the apnea-hypopnea index (AHI; apneas + hypopneas per hour of sleep), the respiratory disturbance index (apneas + hypopneas + RERAs per hour of sleep), or the REI (apneas + hypopneas per hour of recording when sleep is not measured directly). In addition to these types of SDB, the general baseline minute ventilation may fall to the point where sustained hypoventilation takes place during sleep, termed sleep-related alveolar hypoventilation.

Obstructive SDB: Snoring and OSA

The dynamic upper-airway obstruction, which occurs as a result of sleep in some persons, leads to a continuum of SDB varying from mild snoring to hypopneas to obstructive apneas. The likelihood and extent of upper-airway collapse is determined by the neural input into the dilating upper-airway muscles, influence of sleep state, and upper-airway anatomy. Obstructive events are more likely to occur in REM sleep when muscle tone is lowest, during transitions from lighter non-REM sleep to deep non-REM sleep when sleep is unstable, or when muscle tone is decreased by substances such as alcohol or drugs. The single biggest risk factor for snoring or OSA is obesity, wherein fatty deposition reduces upper-airway dimension, humeral factors reduce net dilating forces of the muscles, and the mechanical effects of obesity reduce lung volumes and the stabilizing effect of tracheal traction on the upper airway. Beyond obesity, many but not all patients have a predisposing anatomy of a narrowed oropharynx, such as a low-lying palate or redundant soft palate tissue, a thickened tongue base, or a narrow hypopharynx, although nasal anatomy with septal deviation or chronic congestion may also aggravate the problem.

Snoring without other symptoms, signs, or polysomnographic evidence of upper-airway obstructions such as hypersomnia, frequent associated arousals, or significant airflow limitation is termed primary snoring. While snoring may be a socially objectionable symptom or disruptive to the patient's sleep partner, snoring in isolation is otherwise not considered to be abnormal and such patients may be reassured if their bed partners are not bothered by their snoring. If treatment is desired, options include relieving nasal obstruction if present, commercially available lubricant throat sprays, maxillary-mandibular advancement (MMA) devices, and nasal or upper-airway surgical approaches such as nasal septal repair or uvulopalatopharyngoplasty (UPPP, or UP3 procedure). An otorhinolaryngology consultation may be helpful in determining which surgical approaches may be most beneficial for the individual.

OSA is an extremely common public health problem present in 2% to 4% of the general population and has been linked to development of hypertension and is a risk factor for incidental development of stroke, coronary artery disease, congestive heart failure, and atrial fibrillation. OSA has been shown to be associated with a wide variety of endothelial and metabolic abnormalities that favor vascular disease, and when patients with moderate to severe OSA are compared to normals or treated OSA patients, they appear to have a higher mortality and cardiovascular event frequency. Thus, the two main reasons to detect and treat OSA are to improve symptoms and to decrease cardiovascular risks. There are good data to show that treatment of OSA improves symptoms and quality of life. Data regarding the reversal of cardiovascular risk are not as firm, mostly consisting of retrospective studies with methodological and biasing issues. Nonetheless, most experts agree that at least moderate and severe OSA ought to be treated, regardless of symptom severity.

OSA severity is rated by the polysomnographic AHI, the hourly rate of apneas and hypopneas averaged over the total sleep time, or, in the case of HSAT, by the REI. An AHI of 4 per hour or less is considered normal. Mild OSA is diagnosed with an AHI of 5 to 14 per hour, moderate OSA with AHI of 15 to 29 per hour, and severe OSA with AHI being 30 per hour or higher. In most laboratories, correlation of the AHI with specific sleep stages and body positions is usually performed to determine whether positional therapy may be offered, as many patients have OSA only during the supine sleep position (position-dependent OSA), and some manifest OSA only during REM sleep in the supine position.

A form of OSA called the upper-airway resistance syndrome is defined by a clinical complaint of hypersomnia, often accompanied by snoring but without an abnormally high frequency of overt apneas or hypopneas resulting in significant decline in oxygen saturation. PSG confirms repetitive arousals related to the increased respiratory effort (respiratory effort-related arousals, or RERAs, during PSG) required to overcome upper-airway obstruction. Because of the similar pathogenesis and treatment response to relieve upper-airway obstruction, this is considered a variant of OSA.

Therapeutic options for snoring and sleep apnea include reducing nasal congestion or obstruction, positional therapy, nasal continuous positive airway pressure, oral appliances, the nasal expiratory positive airway pressure device, oral pressure therapy (OPT), or surgical management (Table 3). Patients with OSA have higher morbidity from vascular events and higher motor vehicle accident rates. Assessment and appropriate counseling for weight loss, cardiovascular risk factors, and driving while untreated (or extreme caution) should be part of a treatment plan.

Weight loss. Weight loss may reduce soft tissue in the neck, making the oropharynx less compressible. The improvement in lung volumes accompanied by weight loss also favor enhancement of longitudinal traction on the upper airway, the so-called "tracheal tug." About 30% to 40% of patients who are able to achieve substantial weight loss may become cured of their OSA. Careful follow-up is needed because many remissions are not permanent. Alcohol and other substances that reduce upper-airway tone or cause sedation or reduced responsiveness worsen OSA and should be prudently avoided.

Positional therapy. Among the lifestyle or behavioral changes, positional therapy involves employing one or more simple strategies to enforce sleep only in nonsupine body positions, usually on the side. One method is the "tennis ball in T-shirt" approach. The patient wears a snug-fitting T-shirt with a pocket sewn onto the back between the shoulder blades with two or three tennis or whiffle balls inserted into it to discourage the patient from turning onto the back during sleep. Other options include similar commercially marketed shirts or vests (the FDA-approved ZZoma sleep apnea pillow, the "snoring backpack," and similar strategies) and body pillows propped or wedged behind the patient or hugged by the patient. Unfortunately, shoulder or hip pain often limits the application of positional therapy, especially in elderly persons, and long-term adherence or compliance remains poor, with only about

TABLE 3	Treatment of Sleep-Related Breathing Disorders		
SLEEP-RELATED BREATHING DISORDER	**TREATMENT MODALITY**		**GOAL**
OSA syndrome	Lifestyle/behavior modification	• Weight loss	Reduced weight may result in improvement airway patency
		• Alcohol avoidance	Alcohol worsens OSA; avoidance of exacerbating factor is encouraged
		• Positional therapy	Enhance airway patency by nonsupine sleeping
	Positive airway pressure	• Continuous positive airway pressure (CPAP)	Counteract collapsing forces in upper airway; "stent" open the upper airway
		• Bilevel positive airway pressure (BPAP)	End expiratory pressure stents open airway; inspiratory pressure enhances minute ventilation or decreases hypopneas
		• Autotitrating positive airway pressure (APAP)	Uses feedback algorithms to adjust pressure in response to airway conditions in order to provide airway patency with minimal mean pressure
	Oral appliances	• Mandibular positioning devices • Tongue retention devices	Enhance airway patency by stabilizing lateral pharyngeal walls and enhancing AP airway dimensions at the velopharyngeal level
	Surgical modification of the upper airway	• Palatal surgeries (uvulopalatopharyngoplasty, others) • Maxillo-mandibular advancement	Enhance airway patency by reconfiguring soft tissues and/or skeletal structures
Central sleep apnea syndromes	Correct underlying disorders (treat heart failure, etc.)	• Various	Reduce stimuli to ventilatory hyperresponsiveness
	Gases	• Oxygen	Reduce responsiveness to variation in CO_2
	Positive airway pressure	• CPAP	Reduce stimulation to ventilate by decreasing lung water, improving V/Q matching, reducing airway resistance
		• Noninvasive positive pressure ventilation (NIPPV), also referred to as BPAP-ST	Provide ventilatory assistance in order to avoid hypercapnia/hypoxemia associated with central apneas or hypopneas, thus reducing hyperventilatory feedback
		• Adaptive servoventilation	Provide ventilatory assistance in proportion to needs, reducing or eliminating variability in ventilation and ventilatory drive; avoid hypercapnia/hypoxemia associated with central apneas or hypopneas, thus reducing hyperventilatory feedback.
Hypoventilation syndromes	Positive airway pressure	• Noninvasive positive pressure ventilation (NIPPV), also referred to as BPAP-ST	Provide ventilatory assistance in order to avoid hypercapnia/hypoxemia associated with central apneas or hypopneas
		• Tracheostomy with mechanical ventilation	Provide ventilatory assistance in order to avoid hypercapnia/hypoxemia associated with central apneas or hypopneas, protect or control airway

one-third of patients able to perpetuate positional therapy strategies in long-term follow-up. Patients with position-dependent OSA should be counseled to be cautious for development of severe OSA problems during any future anticipated prolonged periods of supine sleep, such as postoperative recovery periods following surgery or following a major injury.

Positive airway pressure. The mainstay of treatment for OSA for the majority of patients remains positive airway therapy (PAP). The main components of PAP appliances are the blower unit, which delivers calibrated pressures to hold open the airway; tubing to conduct the pressurized air to the patient; an interface such as a nasal or oronasal mask; and a harness to hold the mask firmly to the patient's face during use. Of the PAP therapies, CPAP, which delivers a continuous set pressure between 5 and 20 cm H_2O, is usually first tried in the setting of PSG; in many sleep centers, the practice of performing split-night PSG (an initial diagnostic phase followed by a treatment phase of CPAP titration toward an optimal pressure for the individual patient) allows diagnosis and treatment prescription to occur in an efficient manner. If an optimal pressure cannot be determined by laboratory titration or data is not available to guide prescription of a specific pressure for a patient, application of an autotitrating PAP device may be considered, offering flexibility for delivering a relatively wide range of self-adjusting treatment pressures as the patient changes sleep position and enters different sleep stages through the night with accordingly varying apnea severity. Autotitrating PAP has been found to be efficacious in most patients diagnosed with OSA by HSAT. However, close clinical follow-up is needed in all patients who have recently started PAP.

PAP is typically delivered through an interface chosen as most comfortable by the patient, either a nasal mask, nasal pillows, or an oronasal. Nasal pillows, a type of cannula that provides a tight seal within the nares, are most effective at lower treatment pressures; they may be favored by many patients with claustrophobia but tend to dislodge at higher pressures or with frequent nocturnal movement. Nasal masks of various types are used in many patients, but if mouth breathing and consequent leak are a problem, a chin strap may be added, or an oronasal face mask may be substituted. Many newer PAP machines offer the feature of pressure relief during exhalation, which may enhance patient tolerability at higher level PAP pressures by "giving way" as the patient expires. Bilevel positive airway pressure (BPAP) may also be employed at higher treatment pressures if CPAP is not well tolerated. Setting a pressure delta ≥4 cm between the inspired and expired pressure may also add a degree of positive pressure ventilation for patients with concurrent sleep-related hypoventilation from an intrinsic pulmonary disease or neuromuscular respiratory muscle weakness.

Oral appliances. Oral appliances may be fitted by a dental sleep specialist. They provide a means of advancing the mandible that pull the tongue base forward slightly, opening the oropharyngeal airway to some degree and obviating some apnea and hypopnea events. The device is most effective for mild to moderate severity and supine position-dependent OSA and generally less predictably effective for most cases of severe OSA. However, the use of oral appliances is increasing due to greater availability of competent dental professionals working with the devices, awareness that for some patients adherence is better with OAs than PAP, and improvements in appliance design that allow enhanced efficacy in some instances. Because oral appliances are less reliably effective in controlling SDB, repeat testing—either with out-of-center sleep testing or PSG after maximal adjustment—is needed to confirm efficacy.

Nasal valve appliances. An expiratory nasal resistance valve appliance has been approved recently for treatment of OSA. The device may be an alternative for some patients with OSA who fail to tolerate CPAP therapy. The device is a small, disposable oval appliance that is affixed over each of the patient's nares by self-adhesive with an airflow port that offers resistance to expiratory airflow, thereby producing expiratory positive airway pressure and preserving nasal and oropharyngeal airway patency with minimal impedance to inspiratory airflow. The device was proven to significantly reduce polysomnographic AHI and subjective sleepiness on the ESS in a recently published sham-controlled randomized trial. Because they are disposable, a new device must be affixed each night. Appropriate patient characteristics and long-term results are not yet clear, but these may be considered in patients who do not prefer CPAP or oral appliances and are agreeable to follow-up to ensure efficacy.

Oral pressure therapy. A newer option for treatment of mild to moderate OSA is OPT (Winx™), which combines an oral appliance with negative intraoral pressure to help keep the tongue and soft palate in a more anterior position, enlarging the retrolingual and retropalatal space. There is as yet limited experience with the device; however, this may be an option for some patients who are averse to or intolerant of other therapies.

Surgery. Surgical options are principally of two basic approaches, palatal approaches, tongue-based procedures (genioglossus advancement, hyoid myotomy and suspension, lingualplasty), or MMA. Palatal approaches such as UPPP, or "UP3" performed by otorhinolaryngologists are effective for relief of snoring but mostly ineffective for treatment of OSA, especially if severity is moderate or greater in degree. MMA appears to be quite effective in mild to moderate OSA and can even be applied with good effect even in selected severe OSA cases; however, morbidity from perioperative pain is considerable and long-term outcomes remain unclear. Hypoglossal nerve stimulation implantation is one promising experimental surgical approach for PAP-intolerant patients that remains in development, with a recently published randomized controlled trial demonstrating efficacy and reasonable tolerability; however, this device was only very recently FDA approved and remains unavailable for clinical use at the time of this writing, and its future role and scope of use in OSA management remains to be determined.

Central Sleep Apnea Syndrome

Central sleep apnea syndrome results from an unstable ventilatory drive during sleep, resulting in periods of insufficient ventilation and compromise of gas exchange despite a patent oropharyngeal airway. Clinically, patients may share similar symptoms with those with OSA, including snoring, except patients with central sleep apnea more frequently complain of insomnia than hypersomnia.

Central sleep apnea has a heterogeneous pathophysiology and may be idiopathic or due to high-altitude-induced periodic breathing, due to Cheyne-Stokes breathing, or narcotic-induced. Neurologic causes—such as brainstem infarction or neurodegenerative disorders, including multiple system atrophy—may also cause central apnea. In heart failure, the presence of central sleep apnea syndrome or Cheyne-Stokes breathing imparts a poor prognosis. A high-quality clinical trial showed that on average, CPAP did not reduce mortality. However, central sleep apnea is often at least partially resistant to treatment with conventional nasal CPAP therapy, and while CPAP may effect improved mean oxygenation, frequent arousals that fragment sleep often continue. There is emerging evidence that noninvasive positive airway pressure ventilation (NIPPV) therapy, particularly adaptive servoventilation (ASV), may be superior to conventional CPAP for treatment of central sleep apnea syndrome. Trials to determine if these more effective PAP therapies might reduce mortality in CSA patients with heart failure are underway. In the meanwhile, at least symptomatic patients with CSA ought to be treated.

Complex Sleep Apnea Syndrome

Complex sleep apnea syndrome is a subtype of central sleep apnea wherein patients have significant obstructive/anatomical problems with ventilation, but also have unstable ventilatory patterns noted in patients with central sleep apnea syndromes. These patients have a clinical and PSG presentation of OSA, but once the upper airway is opened with CPAP, they experience frequent central apneic events that may or may not later resolve with continued exposure to PAP in the home setting. Some patients clearly continue to manifest frequent central sleep apneic events more than five times per hour, leading to the suboptimal outcomes of persisting clinical complaints of hypersomnia and medical risk. Complex sleep apnea syndrome may occur in as many as 4% to 15% of those with OSA. There is emerging evidence that alternative modes of PAP—such as BPAP therapy, particularly ASV—may be superior to conventional CPAP for treatment of the complex sleep apnea syndrome. A randomized controlled trial recently showed that ASV more reliably relieves SDB, while CPAP fails to control SDB in up to one-third of cases.

Sleep-Related Hypoventilation

The causes of hypoventilation during sleep include primary pulmonary parenchymal disorders, neuromuscular conditions affecting bellows musculature, or restrictive physiology of the chest wall accompanying kyphoscoliotic disorders or morbid obesity. While each of these disorders may also ultimately cause daytime hypoventilation, sleep recumbency, especially supine sleep positioning, and REM sleep stage (which leads to relative paralysis of the chest wall and sole dependency on diaphragmatic excursion to drive respiratory effort) often lead to exclusive or initial sleep-related hypoventilation with subsequent medical risk consequent to suboptimal nocturnal oxygenation. Failure to treat significant nocturnal hypoventilation may result in the development of sequelae of hypoxemia such as polycythemia, pulmonary hypertension, and right heart failure, or of hypercapnic respiratory failure. Treatment most often involves use of NIPPV (see Table 4). A newer modality of positive pressure ventilation, average volume-assured pressure support ventilation (AVAPS™), consists of a short delivery of a provider-set tidal volume, which, when coupled with a set backup respiratory rate, assures delivery of a minimum minute ventilation, even when changes in the patient's muscular strength or ventilatory load change. These therapies are best titrated in the context of a supervised overnight laboratory polysomnogram under the direction of a sleep or pulmonary medicine specialist. One must be careful not to resort to the potentially dangerous solution of added oxygen therapy alone in severe COPD or neuromuscular etiologies of sleep-related hypoventilation, because as ventilation fails and hypercapnea results, the hypoxic drive to breathe may become the chief factor leading to continued ventilatory effort and oxygen in this context may precipitate acute respiratory failure in some individuals. A morning arterial blood gas on room air following PSG is indicated to assess for potential hypercapnea and assess the impact of ventilatory support. In the context of severe hypercapnea (i.e., P_{CO_2} of 55 or greater), serial arterial blood gases to monitor the effects of ventilatory support, oxygenation, and accumulating hypercapnea may help determine whether nocturnal mechanical ventilatory support is indicated.

Narcolepsy and Primary CNS Hypersomnias

Narcolepsy is the prototypical primary CNS hypersomnia. Narcolepsy is categorized further as narcolepsy with or without cataplexy, a distinctive and highly specific symptom characterized by emotionally provoked muscle atonia intruding into wakefulness that is seen in a minority of patients overall and may precede but more often follows onset of the main symptom of hypersomnia. The full clinical pentad of narcolepsy also includes symptoms of sleep paralysis, the inability to move the body upon awakening, hypnogogic hallucinations, the intrusion of dream imagery and mentation into conscious awareness following awakening, and sleep-maintenance insomnia, with frequent nocturnal arousals and difficulty maintaining sleep. However, narcolepsy is most frequently monosymptomatic, with the sole symptom being pervasive, enduring sleepiness and decreased vigilance with a tendency toward dozing off inadvertently in permissive settings and the overwhelming desire to nap during the daytime, especially in the afternoons. Naps are most often highly refreshing; scheduled naps can be utilized to therapeutic advantage or indeed, in rare patients, as the sole treatment for those bent on avoiding stimulant pharmacotherapy. Narcolepsy is relatively uncommon, affecting approximately 1:2000 of the general population. While the etiology of narcolepsy remains unknown, most experts continue to favor a long hypothesized autoimmune cause. Major advances in the understanding of the neurobiology of narcolepsy over the past two decades have included the clear linkage of the HLA DQB1*0602 haplotype in up to 90% patients having narcolepsy with cataplexy, discovery of wake-promoting hypocretin/orexin peptides produced by the perifornical posterolateral hypothalamus, and low to unmeasurable CSF hypocretin in nearly 90% of narcolepsy with cataplexy patients. Within the last few years, epidemic narcolepsy-cataplexy following H1N1 vaccination in Europe and Asia also provided further support for the autoimmune hypothesis of narcolepsy. Unfortunately, these tantalizing discoveries have not yet yielded clear insight into pathogenic mechanisms nor more specific therapies for patients, and the mainstay of treatment for the condition remains the use of older stimulant and wake-promoting medications, or prescribed therapeutic napping, as naps are most often highly refreshing and restorative in narcolepsy patients. Supportive laboratory evidence for narcolepsy includes a relatively normal polysomnogram to exclude other causes of hypersomnia such as OSA or PLMD, followed by a confirmatory MSLT, which demonstrates mean sleep latency shorter than 8 minutes and two or more sleep-onset REM periods during four or five nap opportunities.

Idiopathic hypersomnia is a closely related condition often difficult to distinguish from narcolepsy without cataplexy, although a few nuanced clinical features tend to distinguish it from narcolepsy, chiefly a characteristically reported unrefreshing nocturnal sleep and nap quality. Idiopathic hypersomnia has previously been further subclassified as variants with or without prolonged sleep period, although these phenotypes are overlapping and current diagnostic standards have eliminated this distinction. Other similar enigmatic and poorly understood primary CNS hypersomnias include posttraumatic hypersomnia when there is a history of temporally related antecedent substantial head injury, and recurrent hypersomnia, also known as the Kleine-Levin syndrome, which in addition to hypersomnia includes other neuropsychiatric sequelae such as cognitive and behavioral changes like hypersexuality and hyperphagia. Hypersomnia is also commonly associated with as many as 50% of those with myotonic dystrophy type 1.

The mainstay of treatment for each of these conditions is stimulant and wake-promoting agent therapy, with the goal of improved vigilance and psychomotor functioning. Stimulants and wake-promoting agents range in intensity from lower to higher intensity and efficacy/tolerability options, from modafinil (Provigil) and armodafinil (Nuvigil) on the milder end of the spectrum—although selected narcolepsy patients respond quite selectively to these drugs—to methylphenidate (Ritalin), and to the amphetamines (Adderall). Relevant clinical pharmacology of the stimulant medications commonly used in clinical practice are summarized in Table 4. Patients with uncontrolled hypersomnias should be cautioned against driving, operating dangerous machinery, or engaging in other similarly dangerous activities or hobbies while they are drowsy, as they may be prone to sudden and unpredictable sleep attacks.

Circadian Rhythm Sleep Disorders

Circadian rhythm sleep disorders result in misalignment of the timing of the sleep period relative to the desired bed and rise times, resulting in concurrent insomnia and hypersomnia symptoms despite normal total sleep time. The most common circadian rhythm disturbances are actually exogenous influences on the patient and his/her circadian axis, which in these cases is functioning normally but is unable to adjust rapidly enough to the required new temporal milieu. These exogenous disorders include jet lag syndrome and shift-work sleep disorder, resulting either from imposed transmeridian travel or alternating work shifts, respectively, that disturb the patient's environmental entraining cues and homeostatic drives for sleep and wakefulness, thereby resulting in misalignment of the patient's endogenous biological sleep drive and typical sleep schedule to the clock time and environment to which they must rapidly adapt.

Jet lag syndrome results when an individual crosses across several transmeridian time zones in a single day. Crossing one or two time zones is usually not too difficult for the traveler to accommodate, but crossing three time zones typically causes symptoms of jet lag. Flying eastward is generally much more difficult than flying westward, as patients more easily accommodate phase delay then phase advancing, or "loss" of time. Treatments for jet lag syndrome usually involve efforts to rapidly reentrain the patient to the new environment, and protocols for advance prepartion including setting back (for eastward travel) or setting ahead (for planned westward travel) one's daily routine 2 to 3 weeks prior to the trip so that the traveler is already partially reset in his or her circadian routine before departing. Also critical is attempting to rapidly adapt to the new time zone, such as by seeking regular sunlight exposure during the daytime and avoiding light exposure in the evening. Brief use of a hypnotic medication and regular daily doses of melatonin[3] 0.5 to 5.0 mg at bedtime for the first few nights after arrival can help reset the sleep schedule in the new time zone.

Shift-work sleep disorder results from workers who must constantly and regularly alter or rotate their work schedules between different shifts (so-called "swing shifts") or workers who must accommodate a regularly scheduled second or third shift (i.e., shifts other than a day shift). Shift workers often have difficulty adapting and shifting their sleep-wake schedules and develop symptoms of insomnia or hypersomnia. Shift workers must be educated to prioritize regularly obtaining a sufficient quantity of sleep, regardless of their work circumstances. Swing shift workers should also be counseled to avoid working more than five night shifts in a row, as night shift work frequently leads to a greater degree of sleep deprivation over time. Shift workers should also be counseled to avoid rotating swing shifts whenever possible, to strictly avoid scheduling overtime duty, and to avoid long commutes (and to exercise special caution to avoid drowsy driving). Judicious use of caffeinated beverages, or prescribed stimulant therapy with modafinil may be helpful for enhancing vigilance in some patients, but should be used with caution.

The two most common endogenous circadian disorders are delayed sleep-phase syndrome (DSPS) and advanced sleep-phase syndrome (ASPS), disorders that are most prevalent in opposite extremes of life. DSPS is seen most often in adolescents and young

TABLE 4 Clinical Pharmacology of Stimulant and Wake-Promoting Medications

	MECHANISM OF ACTION	DOSAGE (mg)	DURATION OF ACTION (T½)	TYPICAL ADVERSE EFFECTS	INTERACTIONS
Modafinil (Provigil)	Unknown	100–600	Intermediate (15 h)	Tremor, jitteriness, palpitations, hypertension	Oral contraceptives
Armodafinil (Nuvigil)	Unknown	150–450	Intermediate (15 h)	Tremor, jitteriness, palpitations, hypertension	Oral contraceptives
Methylphenidate (Ritalin)	DNRI	15–100[1]	Short (2–4 h)	Tremor, jitteriness, palpitations, hypertension	Nonsignificant
Methylphenidate SR (Concerta)[2]	DNRI	18–72	Intermediate (3.5 h)	Tremor, jitteriness, palpitations, hypertension	Nonsignificant
Amphetamine/ dextroamphetamine (Adderall)	DNRI	15–100[1]	Intermediate (10–13 h)	Tremor, jitteriness, palpitations, hypertension, QTc prolongation	Beware MAOIs, SSRIs, SNRIs, TCAs, bupropion (Wellbutrin)
Dextroamphetamine (Dexedrine)	DNRI	15–100[1]	Long (10–28 h)	Tremor, jitteriness, palpitations, hypertension, QTc prolongation	Beware MAOIs, SSRIs, SNRIs, TCAs, bupropion
Lisdexamfetamine (Vyvanse)[2]	DNRI	20–100[1]	Short (<1 h as prodrug) (10–28 h as dextroamphetamine)	Tremor, jitteriness, palpitations, hypertension, QTc prolongation	Beware MAOIs, SSRIs, SNRIs, TCAs, bupropion
Methamphetamine (Desoxyn)[2]	DNRI	15–100[1]	Intermediate (9–15 h)	Tremor, jitteriness, palpitations, hypertension, QTc prolongation	Beware MAOIs, SSRIs, SNRIs, TCAs, bupropion

[1]Not FDA approved for this indication.
[2]Not available in the United States.
Abbreviations: *t½* = half-life of drug; h = hours; DNRI = dopamine and norepinephrine monoamine reuptake inhibitor; QTc = corrected QT interval; MAOI = monoamine oxidase inhibitor; SSRI = serotonin selective reuptake inhibitor; SNRI = selective norepinephrine reuptake inhibitor; TCA = tricyclic antidepressant (the potential interaction with all these agents is largely theoretical concern for potentiation of serotonin syndrome).

adults who are biological night owls in their circadian preference, preferring a delayed bedtime and rise time (i.e., bedtimes well past midnight and subsequent arising times in the late morning or early afternoon). DSPS patients have an extreme and enduring form of this tendency, however, resulting in persisting misalignment of the patient to societal norms. Adolescent and young adult patients present with profound intractable initial insomnia due to their inability to fall asleep at a conventional bedtime as required for school or most daytime occupations, and profound daytime hypersomnia due to their inability to arise and function in the morning hours. Diagnosis is easily recognized by clinical history and sleep diaries, with or without adjunctive actigraphy to objectively verify the pattern of consistent delayed sleep-phase periods. Contrarily, ASPS is more common in elderly individuals who are biological larks (i.e., preferring an early bedtime and early rise time by nature). However, the ASPS elderly are unable to stay awake for desired evening activities (often even unable to go out to dinner with friends), and awaken undesirably early in the morning with a consequent inability to fall back asleep in early morning hours. The presentation can mimic depression, whose hallmark biological sign is often noted to be an early morning awakening; care should be taken to carefully distinguish between these two diagnoses. Treatment of each is difficult; options include specifically

timed bright light therapy, with or without light restriction, and timed administration of low dose melatonin.[3] The time of administration differs for the two disorders, and is determined by the patient's own endogenous dim light melatonin onset and arise time, and the phase response curve for light and melatonin administration. Bright light therapy is administered at approximately 2500 lx intensity for at least 30 minutes. The timing of bright light administration is first thing in the morning after arising in DSPS, where a phase-advancing influence is desired; for ASPS patients, bright light is prescribed in the late afternoon and early evening hours where it will have a phase-delaying effect. Weeks to a few months of regular therapy are necessary to achieve effect. Adherence is difficult and compliance unable to be verified. Specifically timed melatonin given at very low doses for this indication (contrary to its use in higher supraphysiologic doses as a hypnotic agent by many patients in other contexts of insomnia, or its high-dose use in REM sleep behavior disorder [RBD]) may also be administered, but its dose and timing are complicated; it must be given in accordance with the circadian phase response curve to have optimal effects and to avoid complicating the problem. For most patients with DSPS, melatonin 0.5 mg should be administered at approximately 6 PM (i.e., after the time point of 8 hours following the usual rise time, when the phase response curve shifts so that

[3]Exceeds dosage recommended by the manufacturer.

[3]Exceeds dosage recommended by the manufacturer.

melatonin administration will have a phase-advancing effect); in ASPS, melatonin would instead be given prior to the time point of 8 hours following the patient's usual rise time (so as to have a phase-delaying effect). Adjunctive light restriction is recommended in the late afternoon and evenings for DSPS to avoid precipitating additional phase delays—such as the avoidance of working with luminescent computer screens or viewing video media from close distance in the late evenings—and some experts advocate the use of commercially available blue light restricting glasses as biologically reasonable, as blue light stimuli in evening hours may exacerbate phase delay and confound other recommended treatment effects. However, the efficacy of blue light restriction currently lacks explicit evidence from large clinical trials. As a last resort, the measure of chronotherapy, a progressive delay of bedtime every few days, is prescribed, with the bed and rise times being progressively and successively delayed until the desired bed and rise times are achieved. Attempts to then entrain the patient on this schedule with the aforementioned measures are again attempted with scheduled bright light and prescribed timed melatonin dosing. This is a lengthier process for DSPS patients and necessitates work restriction during the approximate 2-week time frame necessary to achieve a turnaround of the desired patient's sleep/wake schedule.

Parasomnias and Other Nocturnal Events

Parasomnias are nocturnal events that disrupt sleep but usually do not appreciably disturb sleep quality. As such, nocturnal events do not typically present with symptoms of insomnia or hypersomnia unless there are other comorbid primary sleep disorders such as OSA, which is a frequent comorbidity presenting along with the parasomnias, especially in adult patients.

Parasomnias may arise from either NREM or REM sleep. The NREM parasomnias are essentially all variations on the theme of disorders of arousal, where the behavioral sleep state lingers into awakening, leaving arousal from sleep incomplete. Consequent clinical manifestations are surprisingly heterogeneous and often age related, with specific syndromes such as night terrors in children, sleep walking and confusional arousals seen in children and adults, and sleep eating behavior seen almost exclusively in adults, especially those receiving zolpidem or other newer prescribed hypnotics. NREM disorders of arousal are especially common in children in the first decade of life and are regarded as a relatively normal variant (and perhaps in some cases simply representing an exaggerated manifestation of the physiological difficulty in arousing from the characteristically deeper N3 NREM sleep inherent in the developing brain). As such, pediatric parasomnias are frequently outgrown; however, in some patients, they do endure throughout life. In adult patients who present with newly evolved nocturnal events proven to be NREM disorders of arousal, one should be highly suspicious of comorbid primary sleep disorders that provoke arousing events, such as SDB or PLMD.

REM parasomnias include nightmares and RBD. Nightmares are undesirable, disturbing dreams that lead to sudden arousal from sleep with heightened autonomic sequelae of sweating, hypervigilance, tachycardia, and tachypnea. Nightmares and vivid dreaming are present in between 10% and 50% of normal young children and in about 50% of adults, but become abnormally disturbing in content or frequency much less frequently, and the true prevalence of nightmare disorder remains unknown. Patients who present with a chief complaint of frequent nightmares should be reassured as to their biological nature and receive a detailed physical and neurologic history and examination to exclude potential provoking comorbid causes such as a recent medication change in type or dosage, mood or anxiety disorder, or primary sleep disorder such as SDB. If no certain readily reversible triggering cause may be identified, referral for consideration of hypnosis or pharmacotherapy with clonazepam may be helpful in some cases.

Nightmares that involve flashbacks of previous traumatic events, most often also with similar daytime flashbacks, suggest the alternative diagnosis of posttraumatic stress disorder (PTSD) and the need for psychiatric evaluation. Recent evidence has suggested that alpha-blocking medications such as terazosin (Hytrin)[1] may be helpful in suppressing nightmares associated with PTSD.

RBD is characterized by potentially injurious dream enactment behaviors that mirror frightening dream content (characteristically involving fighting off attackers or defending oneself against assailants). In RBD, bed partners will describe objective witnessed dream enactment manifested by violent limb thrashing movements and screaming or shouting vocalization during sleep. While RBD patients rarely leave the bed and sleepwalk, falls or other injurious behavior to self or the bed partner are frequent. Importantly, RBD is strongly associated with future development of neurodegenerative disorders. Elderly patients newly diagnosed with RBD harbor up to an 81% risk of developing Parkinsonism within 15 years of symptom onset, with a shorter-term risk of 30% to 50%, so that all patients with RBD require serial neurologic examinations and follow-up. RBD in young adults may, however, be caused by antidepressant medications, especially the SSRIs, and removal of the offending drug may lead to resolution of dream enactment in some cases. Diagnosis of RBD is by clinical history as well as confirmatory evidence for increased REM sleep muscle tone evident on polysomnographic electromyogram (EMG) leads in the chin and limbs (so-called REM sleep without atonia). Treatment options include melatonin,[3] initially at doses of 3 to 6 mg and gradually titrating toward 12 mg nightly as needed to suppress witnessed injurious behaviors, or clonazepam (Klonopin)[1] 0.5 to 1.0 mg increased to 2 to 3 mg nightly. Great care should be taken to first exclude comorbid OSA prior to use of clonazepam, a potential respiratory and upper-airway suppressant.

Nocturnal epilepsies or psychogenic nonepileptic spells may also arise from sleep or apparent sleep and are additional diagnostic considerations in the differential diagnosis of parasomnias. A high degree of stereotypy (one attack being essentially identical to the next) with multiple attacks within a single night are features suggestive of organic partial extratemporal (frontal lobe) epilepsy, even in the absence of EEG changes between or during an episode. In children, benign rolandic epilepsy may lead to stereotyped episodes of facial twitching and drooling, with or without secondary generalized tonic clonic seizures. Children or adults with autosomal dominant nocturnal frontal lobe epilepsy (ADNFLE) may present with bizarre brief motor behavior (typically of 10- to 60-second duration) without postictal sleepiness. ADNFLE has recently been mapped in several kindreds as a channelopathy, producing a defect of the neuronal nicotinic acetylcholine receptor. Psychogenic nonepileptic spells are instead characterized by non-stereotypic and often prolonged attacks that arise from a behavior state of apparent sleep that is instead confirmed during video-EEG PSG to represent normal waking EEG background. Distinguishing features for the differential diagnosis of nocturnal events are shown in Table 5.

Sleep-Related Movement Disorders

Sleep-related movement disorders include restless leg syndrome (RLS), periodic limb movement disorder (PLMD), leg cramps, bruxism, rhythmic movement disorder, and others.

RLS and PLMS

Diagnosis of RLS is based completely on a clinical history and typically requires four central elements of the described symptoms: an uncomfortable urge to move the legs, with or without uncomfortable leg sensations; temporary relief by movement; symptoms occurring solely or predominantly at rest; and nocturnal worsening of symptoms. About 50% of patients with RLS will carry a positive family history of the disorder, but positive family history is not necessary for the diagnosis. The nature of the symptoms as described

---

[1]Not FDA approved for this indication.
[3]Exceeds dosage recommended by the manufacturer.

---

[1]Not FDA approved for this indication.

TABLE 5 Distinguishing Features of Nocturnal Events

	PREMONITORY SYMPTOMS	BEHAVIORAL CHARACTERISTICS	DURATION	FREQUENCY	EEG/PSG FINDINGS
NREM Parasomnias					
Night terrors	None	Inconsolable screaming	Minutes	1 or less nightly	Arousal from N2-N3
Confusional arousals	None	Confused, amnestic	Seconds to minutes	1 or less nightly	Arousal from N3 > N2
Sleepwalking	None	Ambulation, amnesia	Minutes	1 or less nightly	Arousal from N3 ≫ N2
REM Parasomnias					
Nightmares	Dream recall	Arousal, frightened, palpitations	Seconds	Generally 1/nightly	Arousal from REM
RBD	Variable dream recall	Thrashing, complex motor behavior	Seconds to minutes	>1/night, second > first half	REM sleep without atonia
Epilepsies					
BECTS	Facial twitching, hypersalivation	Focal motor or GTC, postictal	Seconds to minutes	>1/night	Arousal from NREM, IEDs, EEG pattern
ADNFLE	Bizarre stereotyped motor behavior	Focal motor, bizarre motor	Seconds, <1 min	1 or multiple attacks/night	Arousal from N2
TLE	Aura variable	CPS, postictal	1–2 min	1 or multiple attacks/night	Arousal from N2
Psychogenic spells	Variable	Variable	often >5 min	1 or multiple attacks/night	Normal awake EEG

Abbreviations: NREM = nonrapid eye movement sleep; N2 = stage 2 NREM sleep; N3 = stage 3 NREM sleep; REM = rapid eye movement sleep; IEDs = interictal epileptiform discharges; EEG = electroencephalogram; PSG = polysomnogram; BECTs = benign epilepsy of childhood with centro-temporal spikes; ADNFLE = autosomal dominant nocturnal frontal lobe epilepsy; TLE = temporal lobe epilepsy; RBD = REM sleep behavior disorder.

by the patient may be quite variable with regard to the symptom quality, location or distribution, temporal occurrence, frequency, and severity. RLS symptoms are usually described as uncomfortable, although not really painful, with a sense of a creepy-crawly or prickling discomfort, often below the knees and centered about the shins or calves, but sometimes more proximally in the thighs, or even isolated to the feet and ankles. Symptoms may occur in the arms as well, especially proximally near the shoulders. Augmentation is common, occurring in about 50% of patients treated with dopaminergic drugs and involves a worsening of the symptoms: symptom onset occurs earlier during the day, becomes more intense, and spreads up to the arms. RLS has been linked to deficient iron stores and dopaminergic neurotransmission in the brain and is more common in patients with parkinsonism, multiple sclerosis, epilepsy, and in those with chronic renal insufficiency.

While PLMs are seen in 80% to 90% of RLS patients, PLMS is not necessary for the diagnosis of RLS. Furthermore, PLMs are also extremely frequent in the general population, seen in 5% to 15% of younger adults and as many as 45% of elderly individuals. PLMD is diagnosed when PLMS is thought to cause daytime hypersomnia.

Nonpharmacologic treatments including warm or cool baths, massage, stretching, or even the application of spontaneous compression devices have been reported to be effective anecdotally and in small case series, but an evidence basis for these measures remains poor, and most patients seeking medical care for the symptom have severe enough symptoms to merit pharmacologic treatment.

Iron and pharmacologic treatments for RLS are outlined in Table 6. Iron deficiency, or even low normal body iron stores, may worsen or precipitate symptoms. Measuring a serum ferritin should be considered early in all RLS patients, with iron replacement therapy begun if serum ferritin values are less than 50 mcg/L. Iron therapy can be constipating or cause GI distress, and the formulation of ferrous gluconate with added vitamin C (Ferrex 150

Plus, Vitelle Irospan)[1] is often well tolerated by those who cannot stomach ferrous sulfate.

Carbidopa-levodopa (Sinemet)[1] may be used for patients with only intermittently disturbing symptoms, but chronic nightly use of carbidopa-levodopa, especially above a dosage of 200 mg daily, may raise the risk of augmentation. For nightly use, the newer dopaminergic agonist medications pramipexole (Mirapex) or ropinirole (Requip) remain a mainstay of treatment. Pramipexole may be initiated at 0.125 to 0.25 mg nightly and titrated every few days to the 0.375 to 0.50 mg range or beyond if needed for symptom control. Doses beyond 1.0 mg[1] are typically not additionally effective. Ropinirole may be initiated at 0.5 to 1.0 mg with gradual upward titration to the 4 to 6 mg[4] range as needed and tolerated. Generally, dosing 1 hour prior to bedtime is sufficient, but if earlier evening or late afternoon symptoms emerge, cautious application of divided doses may be utilized, and some experts advice at least a low morning dosage administered daily to achieve a more chronic steady state of dopamine administration since this may be a sensible strategy to minimize augmentation risk. For either initial first-line therapy, or particularly when patients are beginning to experience earlier symptom onset during the day and may have failed the other short-acting dopaminergic drugs pramipexole and ropinirole, a rotigotine (Neupro) patch has been an advent in RLS management and often may be substituted for those other agents to provide more day-long symptom relief and reduce a growing augmentation tendency. Rotigotine offers several other advantages, as its transdermal delivery system provides continuous day-long release of medication that may minimize peak/trough serum concentration variation and minimize the occurrence of other potential adverse effects. Rotigotine also appears to result

---

[1]Not FDA approved for this indication.
[4]Not yet approved for use in the United States.

TABLE 6 Clinical Pharmacology of Treatments for Restless Leg Syndrome

	MECHANISM OF ACTION	DOSAGE	TYPICAL ADVERSE EFFECTS	INTERACTIONS
Iron Replacement				
Ferrous sulfate[1]	Fe	324 mg tid	Nausea, constipation	None
Ferrous fumarate + vit C	Fe	200/125 mg tid	Nausea, constipation	None
Carbidopa-Levodopa (Sinemet)[1]	DA	25/100 1–2 prn	Nausea, dizziness, ICD	None
Pramipexole (Mirapex)	DA	0.125–1.0 mg[2] qhs	Nausea, dizziness, ICD	None
Ropinirole (Requip)	DA	1–6 mg[2] qhs	Nausea, dizziness, ICD	None
Rotigotine (Neupro)	DA	1–3 mg qAM	Nausea, dizziness, ICD	None
Gabapentin (Neurontin)[1]	Unknown	300–1200 mg qhs	Nausea, dizziness, pedal edema, weight gain	None
Gabapentin Enacarbil (Horizant)	Unknown	600 mg 1200 mg + q6pm	Nausea, dizziness, pedal edema, weight gain	None
Pregabalin (Lyrica)[1]	Unknown	100–600 mg qhs	Nausea, dizziness, pedal edema, weight gain	None
Tramadol (Ultram)[1]	MRA	50 mg 400 mg qhs	Nausea, dizziness	None
Oxycodone[1]	MRA	5–15 mg	Nausea, dizziness	None

[1]Not FDA approved for this indication.
[2]Exceeds dosage recommended by the manufacturer.
Abbreviations: mg = milligrams; Fe = iron replacement; DA = dopamine agonist; MOR = mu opiate receptor agonist.

in augmentation less frequently than other dopaminergic drugs. All patients receiving dopaminergic agents should be counseled upfront about the approximate 15% idiosyncratic risk of impulse control disorder symptoms (such as pathologic gambling, shopping, or hoarding/punding behaviors), and be forewarned that should such problems result, the medication must be withdrawn and another nondopaminergic drug substituted for symptom control. Typical dose-related adverse effects are also described further in Table 6.

For patients who are intolerant or resistant to the dopaminergic drugs, gabapentin (Neurontin)[1] has become the preferred second-line medication, dosed 300 to 1200 mg every night at bedtime as needed and tolerated. Gabapentin enacarbil (Horizant) is a prodrug of gabapentin that is better absorbed and carries an indication for RLS, but generic gabapentin is also frequently effective and well tolerated, and there has been no head-to-head trial showing superiority of the more expensive prodrug gabapentin enacarbil over that of gabapentin. Other alternatives include clonazepam[1] and tramadol (Ultram).[1] For patients unresponsive to these measures, opiate treatment with oxycodone (Roxicodone)[1] 5 to 15 mg at bedtime, hydromorphone (Dilaudid),[1] or methadone (Dolophine)[1] are often effective; small case series suggest other alternatives for refractory RLS such as carbamazepine (Tegretol),[1] oxcarbazepine (Trileptal),[1] and lamotrigine (Lamictal).[1] The impact of comorbid OSA should also be considered, as optimization of treatment for SDB may improve both subjective RLS symptoms as well as PLMD frequency in many patients.

Sleep-Related Leg Cramps
Sleep-related leg cramps are a common and enigmatic problem affecting 7% to 10% of children and up to 70% of elderly adults. Unfortunately, despite their extremely common occurrence and impact on the quality of life of cramp sufferers, little is known about the pathophysiology or treatment of this condition. Cramps are painful, involuntary sustained muscle contractions, lasting 2 to 10 minutes and affecting the unilateral or bilateral calves, thighs, or feet, with residual tenderness of the affected muscle lasting up to an hour or longer. The clinical approach to sleep-related leg

cramps is to first determine whether they are also present during daytime in addition to sleep. If daytime cramping is prominent, exclusion of a precipitating neuromuscular disorder is paramount, including amyotrophic lateral sclerosis, peripheral neuropathy, myositis, or cramp-fasciculation syndrome. In elderly men, peripheral vascular disease and other systemic medical comorbidities are also common. (The reader is referred to the chapter on neuromuscular disorders for further advice on the diagnosis of these conditions.) A neurologic examination should be conducted on all cramp sufferers, and those having sensorimotor findings, fasciculations, or pathologic reflex findings should be referred for EMG, serum creatinine kinase, or additional blood and urine tests for exclusion of symptomatic causes of neuropathy as appropriate. While additional testing for electrolyte abnormalities such as hypomagnesemia, hypocalcemia, hyponatremia, and hypokalemia can be considered, they are of extremely low yield. When examination findings are normal and cramps are isolated to the sleep state, further diagnostic work-up can usually be avoided. Symptomatic treatment measures for sleep-related leg cramps include tonic water with lemon and advising adequate hydration and nightly stretching of the calves and thighs. For refractory frequent cramp sufferers, prescription quinine sulfate (Qualaquin)[1] or a sodium-channel blocking anticonvulsant such as carbamazepine[1] or oxcarbazepine[1] may also be considered.

Sleep-Related Bruxism
Sleep-related bruxism, rhythmic grinding of the teeth during sleep, may lead to significant tooth wear and dental or jaw pain. The condition is usually idiopathic, although it may be associated with psychiatric conditions such as mood or anxiety disorders, especially if it is also present during daytime. Treatment usually involves dental referral for consideration of a fitted mouth guard, although in extreme cases pharmacotherapy with clonazepam[1] or consideration of botulinum toxin (Botox)[1] may be necessary.

Movement Disorders
Sleep-related rhythmic movement disorder usually occurs in patients with psychomotor maldevelopment and involves repetitive head and neck or axial body movements. This behavior is not strictly voluntary and often persists during PSG into deep drowsiness or light NREM sleep, so behavioral treatments alone are often ineffective. Head banging behavior, sometimes into the

[1]Not FDA approved for this indication.

headboard of the bed, can be injurious at times: a protective helmet or treatment with clonazepam is advisable in some cases. Most other movement disorders, such as organic tremors, myoclonus, or dyskinesias generated by the basal ganglia, are suppressed during sleep but may reemerge during drowsiness or nocturnal awakenings.

Isolated Symptoms, Apparently Normal Variants, and Unresolved Issues

These conditions are felt largely to represent either normal variants or otherwise largely benign disorders. The definition of long and short sleepers are somewhat arbitrary, but may be considered as greater than 10 hours or shorter than 5 hours of habitual sleep. Short or long sleep time are each assumed to be variants of normal behavior in the absence of hypersomnia or nighttime symptoms of insomnia.

Sleep talking, or somniloquy, in isolation is rarely of concern. History is often lifelong in such patients. When sleep talking is newly evolved in an elderly individual or a younger patient receiving antidepressant therapy, RBD should be considered in the differential diagnosis, and the patient should be questioned about other potential evidence for dream enactment behavior. A careful medication history and neurologic examination alone will usually dictate whether further evaluation with PSG may be indicated, but in most cases isolated sleep talking is not a cause for concern.

Sleep starts, hypnic jerks or physiologic myoclonus are near universal in their occurrence and often associated with recent excessive caffeine intake or emotional or physical stress. A history of occurrence of jerks limited to the arms, legs, or axial musculature causing arousal within the first 5 to 10 minutes of sleep, and lacking later recurrence during the night, is typical. Reassurance and avoidance of precipitating factors is advised; however, if hypnic jerks are excessive or recur later in the night, PSG is occasionally necessary to distinguish this benign diagnosis from PLMD or propriospinal myoclonus. Propriospinal myoclonus at sleep onset is characterized by myoclonic jerks having their primary and earliest onset in abdominal and axial muscles prior to spreading to the limbs and may be associated with thoracic spinal cord pathology. Spinal imaging with MRI is advised. Treatment with clonazepam[1] is usual for this uncommon diagnosis.

Other Sleep Disorders

Environmental sleep disorder results from undesirable influences in the patient's sleep environment that serve to regularly distract or disturb him or her from initiating or maintaining sleep. Typical influences include a bed partner who snores loudly or who causes bed motion due to restless or disturbed sleep; pets who sleep in bed with the patient and cause awakening; environmental noise from neighborhood dogs, car alarms, or neighboring freeway or train way; too much outdoor ambient light; or undesirable household ambient temperature. There is considerable overlap in this category of problems with inadequate sleep hygiene, as activating stimuli in the environment may lead the patient toward chronic insomnia and adapting undesirable sleep-related behaviors that serve to further disrupt restful sleep.

Fatal familial insomnia is a tremendously rare, autosomal dominant variant form of familial Creutzfeldt-Jakob disease, a prion disorder that leads to progressive insomnia and progressive cognitive impairment, with death inevitably occurring within 3 years of onset. Aggregate prion protein accumulates in the thalamus and other brain regions, and relentlessly progressive insomnia, panic disorder, hallucinosis, and dementia ensue. Unfortunately, no treatments are currently known for this rare disorder.

Conclusions

Sleep disorders are common and result in significant patient morbidity, daytime dysfunction, and impaired quality of life. Untreated SDB may also raise the risk for hypertension, vascular events, and mortality. The most common presenting symptoms of sleep disorders include insomnia, characterized by difficulty initiating and maintaining sleep with poor sleep quality, and hypersomnia, the symptom of excessive daytime sleepiness. Evaluation begins with a detailed history and physical examination, which in select cases may require support and clarification by PSG and multiple sleep-latency testing. Fortunately, effective therapies are available for the majority of sleep disorders. Insomnia typically requires behavioral or pharmacologic interventions, while SDB may be effectively treated in most cases with PAP therapy. Primary CNS hypersomnias including narcolepsy require stimulant management in most cases, while most parasomnias benefit from clonazepam. Circadian sleep disorders may require timed light and melatonin therapies. Patients having RLS and PLMD should be evaluated for iron deficiency and may enjoy symptom control through dopaminergic or other alternative symptomatic treatments. The majority of patients with sleep disorders benefit from a careful clinical evaluation and appropriately selected therapies.

---

[1]Not FDA approved for this indication.

References

American Academy of Sleep Medicine. International Classification of Sleep Disorders: Diagnostic and Coding Manual. 2nd ed. Westchester, IL: American Academy of Sleep Medicine; 2005.

Chesson AL, Anderson WL, Pancer JP, Wise M. Practice parameters for the indications for polysomnography and related procedures: An update for 2005. Sleep 2005;28:499–521.

Collop NA, Tracy SL, Kapur V, et al. Obstructive sleep apnea devices for out-of-center (OOC) testing: Technology evaluation. J Clin Sleep Med 2011;7:531–48.

Johns MW. A new method for measuring daytime sleepiness: The Epworth sleepiness scale. Sleep 1991;14:540–5. Also available online in a patient fillable version at, http://www.stanford.edu/~dement/epworth.html.

Kushida CA, Littner MR, Morgenthaler T, et al. Indications for positive airway pressure treatment of adult obstructive sleep apnea patients: A consensus statement. Chest 1999;115:863–6.

Luyster FS, Strollo Jr PJ, Zee PC, et al. Sleep: A health imperative. Sleep 2012;35:727–34.

Morgenthaler TI, Lee-Chiong T, Alessi C, et al. Standards of Practice Committee of the American Academy of Sleep Medicine. Practice parameters for the clinical evaluation and treatment of circadian rhythm sleep disorders. Sleep 2007;30:1445–59.

Schutte-Rodin S, Broch L, Buysse D, et al. Clinical guideline for the evaluation and management of chronic insomnia in adults. J Clin Sleep Med 2008;4:487–504.

Silber MH, Becker PM, Earley C, et al. Willis-Ekbom Disease Foundation revised consensus statement on the management of restless legs syndrome. Mayo Clin Proc 2013;88:977–86.

St. Louis EK. Key sleep neurologic disorders: Narcolepsy, restless legs syndrome/Willis-Ekbom disease, and REM sleep behavior disorder. Neurol Clin Pract 2014;4:16–25.

Wise MS, Arand DL, Auger RR, et al. American Academy of Sleep Medicine. Treatment of narcolepsy and other hypersomnias of central origin. Sleep 2007;30:1712–27.

TRIGEMINAL NEURALGIA

Method of
B. Wayne Blount, MD, MPH; and Jennifer Burkmar, MD, MBA

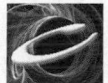

CURRENT DIAGNOSIS

IHS Diagnostic Criteria for Trigeminal Neuralgia (TN)
Classical

A. Paroxysmal attacks of pain last from a fraction of a second to 2 minutes, affecting one or more divisions of the trigeminal nerve and fulfilling criteria B and C.
B. Pain has at least one of the following characteristics:
   a. Intense, sharp, superficial, or stabbing.
   b. Precipitates from trigger zones or by trigger factors.

C. Attacks are stereotyped in the individual patient.
D. There is no clinically evident neurological deficit.
E. The pain is not attributed to another disorder.

Symptomatic: A, B, and C are the same as above
D. A causative lesion, other than vascular compression, has been found.

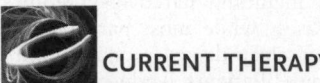

CURRENT THERAPY

For classical TN (CTN):
Carbamazepine (Tegretol) is first line at 100–2400[1] mg per day (NNT = 2.5). If it is not effective, alternative therapies can be added or substituted.
For symptomatic TN (STN), address the underlying cause.

---

[1]Not FDA approved for this indication.

Epidemiology and Risk Factors

The annual incidence of TN is 4.3 per 100,000 with a slight predominance in females (1.74:1) and no racial predilection. The typical age of onset is 60 to 70 years. CTN is rarely seen before age 40, but there is a high rate of misdiagnosis of TN.

Risk factors include multiple sclerosis with an incidence of 1% to 2% and hypertension with a slightly higher rate than the general population. Most cases are sporadic although there are some familial patterns.

Pathophysiology

The pathophysiology has not been determined. It is postulated that demyelination occurs secondary to neurovascular compromise of aberrant or tortuous vessels near or at the dorsal root. Demyelinated axons are prone to ephaptic conduction: ectopic impulses are transferred from nonpain fibers to pain fibers. Patients with CTN have also been found to have compression from a sharper-than-normal trigeminal-pontine angle and subsequent nerve atrophy. Other etiologies include tumors at the nerve root, amyloidosis, arteriovenous (A-V) malformation, bony compression, and small infarcts in the pons and medulla.

With the pathophysiology unknown, prevention is not realistic.

Clinical Manifestations

TN is characterized by severe episodes of unilateral, lancinating pain lasting from 1 second to 2 minutes in the distribution of the trigeminal nerve. This might recur from a few times daily to hundreds of times daily. It is also referred to as *tic douloureux* because of characteristic facial spasms that are often present. Episodes may be random and unprovoked or triggered by otherwise benign stimuli. Typical triggers include talking, smiling, chewing, teeth brushing, shaving, wind, and applying make-up. The right side of the face is affected more often than the left (1.5:1). The most commonly affected branch is the maxillary branch. The ophthalmic branch is the least affected. Some individuals experience spontaneous remission, but most cases persist. The typical course is multiple episodic attacks over many years.

TN can be classified as either classical or symptomatic. CTN accounts for >85% of cases and is attributed to neurovascular compromise. STN is less common and attributed to a variety of underlying conditions, including previous trauma, secondary systemic disease, or other pathologies such as tumors, cysts, demyelination, or A-V malformations.

Differential Diagnosis

The diagnosis of TN is clinical. Painful attacks that can be induced by minimal stimulation of trigger zones are nearly pathognomonic for TN. Consider alternate diagnoses if red flags or other atypical features are present (Table 1). It is imperative to differentiate STN, as it is secondary to an underlying disorder that is the target of treatment.

The approach to diagnosis is to consider TN in all patients who present with unilateral facial pain, to distinguish classical from symptomatic, to look for red flags (Table 2), and to do a focused physical. Laboratory testing is not helpful for typical symptoms associated with TN. Plain or dental radiographs can be useful when TMJ or dental pain is considered as a differential diagnosis. Magnetic resonance imaging of the brain is the test of choice to identify tumors, multiple sclerosis, or other etiologies. Trigeminal reflex testing is not routinely recommended. See Table 2 for the differential diagnoses of TN.

Treatment

Medical treatment should be initiated for all newly diagnosed TN. Surgery can be considered for those who fail to respond to, or are unable to tolerate, medical treatment.

Medical Treatment

Carbamazepine (Tegretol) is considered a first-line treatment for CTN in a dose of 100 to 2400[1] mg/day. If relief is not achieved, alternative therapies can be added or substituted. Baclofen (Lioresal)[2] 10 to 80 mg daily has shown efficacy in some studies. Other alternatives include phenytoin (Dilantin),[2] gabapentin (Neurontin),[2] lamotrigine (Lamictal),[2] topiramate (Topamax),[2] clonazepam (Klonopin),[2] valproic acid (Depakene),[2] pimozide (Orap),[2] and topical capsaicin (Zostrix). In a recent Cochrane review, there was insufficient evidence for nonepileptic agents in TN.

---

[1]Not FDA approved for this indication.
[2]Not available in the United States.

TABLE 1	Atypical Features Suggesting Symptomatic TN or Alternative Diagnosis
Abnormal neurologic examination	Hearing loss or abnormality
Abnormal oral, dental, or ear exam	Numbness
Age <40 years	Pain episodes lasting >2 min
Bilateral symptoms	Pain outside of trigeminal distribution
Dizziness or vertigo	Visual changes

TABLE 2	Differential Diagnosis of TN
Dental pain	Intracranial tumor
Sinusitis	Giant cell arteritis
Multiple sclerosis	Otitis media
Paroxysmal hemicranias	Postherpetic neuralgia
Temporomandibular joint syndrome	Trigeminal neuropathy
Migraine	
Short-lasting unilateral neuralgiform headaches with conjunctival injection and tearing (SUNCT)	
Short-lasting unilateral neuralgiform headaches with autonomic features (SUNA)	
Atypical (shorter) cluster-syndrome	

Surgical Treatment

Surgery for TN is unusual. Both percutaneous and open surgeries can provide short-term relief, but recurrence is common. Percutaneous procedures include radiofrequency rhizotomy, balloon compression, glycerol injection, and gamma knife stereotactic radiosurgery. These procedures typically have shorter-term results than open surgery and have a higher risk of sensory loss.

Open procedures have less symptom recurrence and sensory loss. Given the invasive nature of exploration of the posterior fossa, they may be better for younger, healthy patients. Techniques include partial trigeminal rhizotomy and microvascular decompression. Patients who had microvascular decompression had the best outcomes with >70% with relief at 10 years. Behavioral treatments are not usually helpful, unless TN results in chronic pain.

Monitoring

Typically, follow-up starts at least weekly and extends as pain relief is achieved. The goal in follow-up for most patients is complete remission, but with a secondary goal of achieving a balance between pain relief and medication side effects. Most patients can try a medication-free trial after 4 to 6 symptom-free months. Complications are chronic pain if the acute pain is not controlled, problems with underlying etiologies, and medication side effects.

References

Abhinav K, Love S, Kalantzis G, et al. Clinicopathological review of patients with and without multiple sclerosis treated by partial sensory rhizotomy for medically refractory trigeminal neuralgia: A 12-year retrospective study. Clin Neurol Neurosurg 2012;114:361–5.

Balasundram S, Cotrufo S, Liew C. Case series: Non vascular considerations in trigeminal neuralgia. Clin Oral Invest 2012;16:63–8.

Ha SM, Kim SH, Yoo EH, et al. Patients with idiopathic trigeminal neuralgia have a sharper-than-normal trigeminal-pontine angle and trigeminal nerve atrophy. Acta Neurochir 2012;154:1627–33.

Krafft RM. Trigeminal neuralgia. Amer Acad Fam Phys 2008;77:1291–6.

Leone C, Biaslotta A, La Cesa S, et al. Pathophysiological mechanisms of neuropathic pain. Future Neurol 2011;6:497–509.

Napenas JJ, Zakrzewska JM. Diagnosis and management of trigeminal neuropathic pains. Pain Manag 2011;1:353–65.

Obermann M, Holle D, Katsarava Z. Trigeminal neuralgia and persistent idiopathic facial pain. Expert Rev Neurother 2011;11:1619–29.

VIRAL MENINGITIS

Method of
Joanna Thomson, MD, and Samir S. Shah, MD

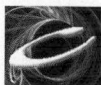

CURRENT DIAGNOSIS

- Typical presentation includes fever, headache, and neck stiffness or pain. Constitutional symptoms include mild lethargy, myalgias, nausea, and vomiting.
- Neonates often present with nonspecific signs and symptoms including lethargy, irritability, and poor feeding.
- Cerebrospinal fluid (CSF) profile should be performed. Results show elevated white blood cell count (often but not always with mononuclear cell predominance), normal to slightly elevated protein, normal glucose, normal to slightly elevated opening pressure, and negative bacterial Gram stain and culture.
- Diagnostic polymerase chain reaction (PCR) and serologic studies can identify the etiologic agent.
- Consider neuroimaging before lumbar puncture if there is concern for increased intracranial pressure or if encephalitis is possible.

CURRENT THERAPY

- Symptomatic and supportive management includes analgesia, antipyretics, antiemetics, and intravenous fluids.
- Hospitalization is recommended for infants (younger than 1 year), elderly patients (older than 65 years), and immunocompromised patients, as well as for patients presenting with altered mental status, seizures, focal neurologic signs, or the absence of classic viral CSF findings.
- Few medications, with the exception of acyclovir (Zovirax) for HSV, effectively treat viral meningitis.

Epidemiology

The true epidemiology of viral meningitis is unknown because it is not a reportable disease. However, the Centers for Disease Control and Prevention (CDC) estimate 25,000 to 50,000 hospitalizations per year. There is also yearly variation in disease burden. Causes of viral meningitis vary by age group, immune status, season, and geography. There is increased incidence in summer and early fall owing to the high prevalence of enteroviruses and arthropod-borne viruses (arboviruses). Common etiologic agents include enteroviruses, herpes simplex virus (HSV), arboviruses, lymphocytic choriomeningitis virus (LCMV), cytomegalovirus (CMV), varicella zoster virus (VZV), and Epstein–Barr virus (EBV). See Table 1 for features of the common and some less-common viral agents that cause meningitis.

Pathophysiology

Viral infection begins at the mucosal surface of the respiratory tract or gastrointestinal tract, with viral replication occurring in regional lymph nodes. A secondary viremia then occurs that provides access to the central nervous system (CNS). Symptoms of viral meningitis are due to either an immune response to the virus within the CNS (e.g., enterovirus) or direct viral invasion of neural tissue (e.g., HSV1/2).

Prevention

To prevent spread of viral agents responsible for meningitis, handwashing and other infection-control measures are most important. The infection-control precautions necessary during patient contact depend on mode of transmission of the virus (see Table 1). Vaccines are available for some of the viruses that are known to cause meningitis, including polio (an enterovirus), mumps, measles, and varicella.

Clinical Manifestations

Viral meningitis can be difficult to distinguish from bacterial meningitis. Fever, headache, and neck stiffness and pain are the usual presenting complaints. Headache can be localized to the frontal or retro-orbital areas and may be associated with photophobia. Although neck stiffness and pain are usually present, neck rigidity (positive Kerning's sign or positive Brudzinski's sign) is not always present on examination. Constitutional symptoms can include lethargy, myalgias, and nausea or vomiting. There is often a history of concomitant viral respiratory or gastrointestinal illness at the time of presentation. Seizures can occur with viral causes of meningitis, especially HSV, but should prompt consideration of other diagnostic possibilities.

In contrast to children and adults, neonates often present with nonspecific findings such as lethargy, irritability, and poor feeding. See Table 1 for clinical manifestations associated with specific etiologic agents.

Viral meningitis can also manifest with signs of encephalitis, in which case the encompassing diagnosis is meningoencephalitis. Encephalitis or meningoencephalitis are likely if any of the following are present: altered mental status, seizures, focal neurologic deficits (including aphasia, anosmia, ataxia, cranial nerve deficits, motor weakness, or involuntary movements), or behavioral changes.

TABLE 1 Clinical and Laboratory Characteristics of Viral Meningitis

VIRUS	TRANSMISSION	KEY CLINICAL FEATURES	DIAGNOSIS	COMMENTS
Enterovirus	Fecal-oral	May have rash on exam (e.g. Coxsackie, hand–foot–mouth) Patients with impaired humoral immunity or those <2 wk old can present with a sepsis-like syndrome with multiorgan dysfunction, DIC, cardiovascular collapse	CSF enterovirus PCR	More prevalent in summer and fall
Herpes simplex viruses 1 and 2	Vertical transmission during birth (HSV2), horizontal transmission via contact (HSV1 or HSV2)	10%–30% of adults have symptoms of meningitis with primary HSV2 infection; look for genital vesicular lesions on exam Mollarets meningitis: >3 episodes of fever and meningismus lasting 2–5 d, with spontaneous resolution; often due to chronic HSV2 CNS infection	CSF HSV1/HSV2 PCR	Meningitis is uncommon with nonprimary HSV2 infection
Arboviruses	Subcutaneous inoculation via mosquito or tick Prevention: Minimize tick and mosquito exposure with personal protection measures including insect repellents and covering exposed skin		CSF arboviral PCR	More prevalent in summer and fall Geographic distribution within the United States: Eastern equine encephalitis: Eastern U.S. Western equine encephalitis: Western U.S. St. Louis encephalitis: Across the U.S. (majority of cases in Central and Eastern U.S.) West Nile virus: Across the U.S. California encephalitis (LaCrosse): Midwestern, mid-Atlantic, and Southeastern U.S.
Lymphocytic choriomeningitis virus	Virus is present in rodent secretions, feces, and urine Ingestion of contaminated food, exposure of open wounds, or inhalation of aerosolized virus Lab workers, pet owners, and those living in impoverished conditions are highest risk for illness	Accompanied by a flulike illness	Serum LCMV titers (acute and convalescent) CSF findings: May have decreased glucose and WBC count >1000/mL	More prevalent in winter and spring
Cytomegalovirus	Exposure to infected body fluids (e.g., saliva, blood)		CSF CMV PCR	Reactivation of prior infection typically only occurs in the immunosuppressed
Epstein–Barr virus	Exposure to infected body fluids (e.g. saliva, blood)	Alice in Wonderland syndrome: altered body image and distortion of visual perception	CSF EBV PCR	Most common neurologic complication with primary infection
HIV	Exposure to contaminated blood or other body fluids (e.g., transfusion, sexual contact, percutaneous blood exposure)	During primary infection, a subset have meningitis or meningoencephalitis May expect thrush and cervical lymphadenopathy	HIV studies	Treatment with HAART
Human herpesvirus 6	Respiratory	Roseola: febrile illness followed by viral exanthem	CSF HHV6 PCR	HHV6 has been demonstrated in the CSF of asymptomatic persons Immunosuppressed persons at risk for symptomatic infection and reactivation

VIRUS	TRANSMISSION	KEY CLINICAL FEATURES	DIAGNOSIS	COMMENTS
Varicella	Respiratory	Typical vesicular skin lesions of chickenpox on exam CSF pleocytosis has also been demonstrated with reactivation; can also occur in the absence of cutaneous findings of herpes zoster ("zoster sine herpete")	CSF VZV PCR	Rarely diagnosed during acute chickenpox infection; usually a postinfectious complication Other neurologic sequelae of varicella infection are more common than aseptic meningitis; most common is cerebellar ataxia
Mumps	Respiratory	Parotitis on exam is the most prominent sign of infection Aseptic meningitis can precede or follow clinical exam findings CSF profile can demonstrate an unusually high protein with a mild pleocytosis and normal glucose	Serum titers	More common in winter and spring
Measles	Respiratory	CSF pleocytosis in ≤30% of patients with measles; patients are usually without clinical meningitis	Serum titers	In the United States, most cases are imported (e.g., occur in returning travelers)
Influenza	Respiratory	Aseptic meningitis is a less common neurologic complication of influenza infection (encephalopathy is more common)	CSF influenza PCR	More prevalent in winter Increased risk of neurologic complication in young patients and in those with pre-existing medical disease

Abbreviations: CMV = cytomegalovirus; CNS = central nervous system; CSF = cerebrospinal fluid; DIC = disseminated intravascular coagulopathy; HHV = human herpesvirus; HSV = herpes simplex virus; LCMV = lymphocytic choriomeningitis virus; PCR = polymerase chain reaction; VZV = varicella zoster virus; WBC = white blood cell.

Diagnosis

Diagnosis of viral meningitis requires lumbar puncture for CSF studies including cell count, protein, glucose, Gram stain and culture, and specific viral studies. Although a lymphocytic pleocytosis is associated with viral infections, most viral CNS infections initially have a neutrophilic pleocytosis. However, neutrophilic pleocytosis is also associated with bacterial meningitis. In viral meningitis, though CSF protein is normal to slightly elevated, CSF glucose is normal, and no organisms are identified on CSF bacterial Gram stain or culture compared with elevated CSF protein, low CSF glucose, and positive CSF bacterial culture in bacterial meningitis.

Studies to identify a specific virus as the etiologic agent are recommended for patients with severe illness or a complicated course. Viral cultures of CSF are not generally useful given their poor sensitivity, and serologic viral studies require both acute and convalescent titers to demonstrate antibody response to the suspected viral antigen. CSF PCR studies that detect viral DNA or RNA are more sensitive than viral culture and provide more rapid results than serologic viral studies (see Table 1). In some cases, it is useful to perform viral PCR studies on blood (HSV, EBV, CMV, and human herpesvirus [HHV]6), urine (CMV), stool (enterovirus), and skin vesicles (HSV) to further support the diagnosis. However, a positive PCR study from blood, urine, stool, or skin does not provide direct evidence of CNS infection by the same virus. For example, enterovirus isolated from the stool can represent asymptomatic infection or prior infection but may also be isolated from the stool at the same time as concomitant enteroviral meningitis.

Most other testing is not helpful, but further testing (including complete blood count, renal profile, liver function, pancreatic enzymes, and HIV studies) should be guided by the patient's presentation and clinical status.

Neuroimaging (computed tomography [CT] or magnetic resonance imaging [MRI]) should be obtained before lumbar puncture if there is concern for increased intracranial pressure. It is also recommended if symptoms of encephalitis are present (including altered consciousness, seizures, focal neurologic deficits, behavioral changes) to exclude other CNS disease.

Differential Diagnosis

The major item on the differential diagnosis for viral meningitis is bacterial meningitis. The bacterial meningitis score, validated in children 29 days to 19 years, is a clinical prediction rule that identifies patients as at very low risk (0.1%) for bacterial meningitis if they lack all of the following: positive CSF Gram stain, CSF absolute neutrophil count (ANC) of at least 1000 cells/μL, CSF protein of at least 80 mg/dL, peripheral blood ANC of at least 10,000 cells/μL, and a history of seizure before or at the time of presentation. C-reactive protein (CRP) is not generally useful in differentiating between bacterial and viral infections, because CRP can be high in viral meningitis and low in the initial stages of bacterial disease. Although it is not yet routinely used, elevated serum procalcitonin levels (>0.5 μg/mL in children and >0.2 μg/mL in adults) and elevated CSF lactate (>35 mg/dL) are more sensitive and specific than CRP for distinguishing viral from bacterial meningitis; elevated values are more typical of bacterial infection.

Other diagnoses to consider include parameningeal infections (i.e., subdural or epidural empyema, brain abscess), meningitis due to fungi, mycobacteria, rickettsia, mycoplasma, parasites, and other CNS infectious or inflammatory processes including malignancy, drug exposure, or rheumatologic disease (e.g. systemic lupus erythematosus).

Treatment

Symptomatic care remains the mainstay of therapy for viral meningitis. Therapy should be directed at pain and fever control (e.g., ibuprofen [Motrin], acetaminophen [Tylenol], ketorolac [Toradol]), management of nausea and vomiting (e.g., ondansetron [Zofran]), and intravenous fluids. Hospitalization is recommended for patients younger than 1 year, the elderly, and the immunocompromised. Patients who present with altered mental status, seizures, focal neurologic signs, or a CSF profile that does not have the classic viral profile should also be hospitalized for clinical management and for antibiotic treatment until bacterial meningitis can be excluded. Advanced care including management of respiratory failure, cardiovascular instability, seizures, disturbed fluid and electrolyte balance, and cerebral edema may be necessary.

Empiric antibiotic coverage may be considered while awaiting CSF culture results in the young, elderly, and immunocompromised, especially if there is suspicion of bacterial meningitis or partially treated bacterial meningitis.

Acyclovir should be initiated in cases of suspected HSV while waiting PCR confirmation. Dosing of acyclovir is age and weight dependent: 20 mg/kg per dose IV every 8 hours for patients younger than 12 years; 10 mg/kg per dose IV every 8 hours for patients older than 12 years.

In the immunocompromised patient, HHV6 may be treated with foscarnet (Foscavir)[1] or ganciclovir (Cytovene),[1] and CMV may be treated with ganciclovir, valganciclovir (Valcyte), foscarnet, or cidofovir (Vistide). Case reports suggest benefit of such antiviral therapies in the immunocompromised, but no controlled trials have been performed.

Complications

The prognosis of viral meningitis depends on cause and severity of illness as well as age. Non-HSV viral meningitis has low mortality rates in adults and children alike. Mortality and morbidity are associated with other organ system involvement, including meningoencephalitis. Although up to 10% of infants hospitalized with non-HSV viral meningitis experience seizures, altered mental status, or increased intracranial pressure during the acute illness, studies have shown no evidence of long-term neurodevelopmental delay. Most adults recover fully within a week without long-term sequelae. Persistent neurologic sequelae (including headaches, incoordination, concentration difficulties, muscle weakness, and focal neurologic deficits) occur more often in patients with meningoencephalitis.

---

[1]Not FDA approved for this indication.

HSV is associated with high rates of morbidity and mortality. Neonatal isolated CNS HSV has a 4% mortality rate even with acyclovir treatment; mortality is 50% without acyclovir treatment. Unfortunately, acute treatment does not affect morbidity, as 70% of infants with neonatal CNS HSV infection will suffer from neurodevelopmental impairments. Recent studies have demonstrated improved outcomes in these infants with long-term oral acyclovir suppression therapy. Outside of the neonatal period, CNS HSV infection has a 28% mortality rate with antiviral treatment (70% mortality rate without treatment). Long-term neurologic sequelae occur in two thirds of survivors who received antiviral therapy, compared with virtually all of those who did not receive treatment.

References

Dubos F, Korczowski B, Aygun DA, et al. Serum procalcitonin level and other biological markers to distinguish between bacterial and aseptic meningitis in children: A European multicenter case cohort study. Arch Pediatr Adolesc Med 2008;162:1157–63.

Hawkes MT, Vaudry W. Nonpolio enterovirus infection in the neonate and young infant. Paediatr Child Health 2005;10:383–8.

James SH, Kimberlin DW, Whitley RJ. Antiviral therapy for herpesvirus central nervous system infections: Neonatal herpes simplex virus infection, herpes simplex encephalitis, and congenital cytomegalovirus infection. Antiviral Res 2009;83:207–13.

Khetsuriani N, Quiroz ES, Holman RC, Anderson LJ. Viral meningitis associated hospitalizations in the United States, 1988–1999. Neuroepidemiology 2003;22:345–52.

Kimberlin DW, Lin CY, Jacobs RF, et al. Safety and efficacy of high-dose intravenous acyclovir in the management of neonatal herpes simplex virus infections. Pediatrics 2001;108:230–8.

Kimberlin DW, Whitley RJ, Wan W, et al. Oral acyclovir suppression and neurodevelopment after neonatal herpes. N Engl J Med 2011;365:1284–92.

Nigrovic LE, Fine AM, Monuteaux MC, et al. Trends in the management of viral meningitis at United States children's hospitals. Pediatrics 2013;131:670–6. [PMID: 23530164].

Nigrovic LE, Kuppermann N, Macias CG, et al. Clinical prediction rule for identifying children with cerebrospinal fluid pleocytosis at very low risk of bacterial meningitis. JAMA 2007;297:52–60.

Rorabaugh ML, Berlin LE, Heldrich F, et al. Aseptic meningitis in infants younger than 2 years of age: Acute illness and neurologic complications. Pediatrics 1993;92:206–11.

Rotbart HA. Viral meningitis. Semin Neurol 2000;20:277–92.

Sakushima K, Hayashino Y, Kawaguchi T, et al. Diagnostic accuracy of cerebrospinal fluid lactate for differentiating bacterial meningitis from aseptic meningitis: A meta-analysis. J Infect 2011;62:255–62.

Viallon A, Zeni F, Lambert C, et al. High sensitivity and specificity of serum procalcitonin levels in adults with bacterial meningitis. Clin Infect Dis 1999;28:1313–6.

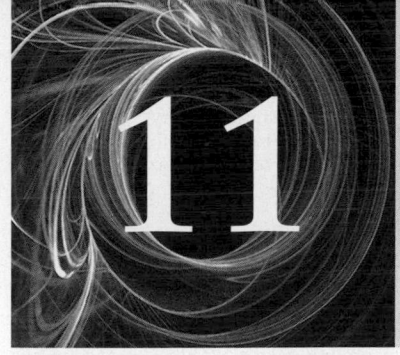

11 Endocrine and Metabolic Disorders

ACROMEGALY

Method of
Moises Mercado, MD

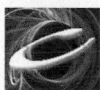

CURRENT DIAGNOSIS

Clinical
- Headaches, visual field defects
- Coarse features, increased size of hands (rings) and feet (shoes)
- Thick, oily skin, skin tags, acanthosis nigricans
- Arthralgias, osteoarthritis
- Paresthesias, carpal tunnel syndrome
- Hypertension, arrhythmia, heart failure
- Glucose intolerance, diabetes, hypertrygliceridemia
- Snoring, sleep apnea
- Risk of colon polyps or colon cancer
- Risk of thyroid cancer

Biochemical
- Glucose-suppressed growth hormone >0.4 ng/mL by ultrasensitive assays or >1 ng/mL by old radioimmunoassays
- Elevated age-adjusted insulin-like growth factor 1

Imaging
- Magnetic resonance imaging

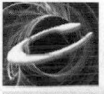

CURRENT THERAPY

- If a pituitary surgeon is available: Transsphenoidal surgery for microadenomas, intrasellar macroadenomas, and debulking or decompressing surgery in invasive macroadenomas
- Depot Somatostatin analogues (lanreotide autogel or octreotide LAR) as secondary treatment for patients failing surgery or waiting for radiotherapy effect to occur and as a primary treatment for patients with inaccessible lesions, contraindications for surgery, or preference
- Dopamine agonists: Cabergoline (DOSTINEX) is effective alone or in combination with somatostatin analogues in 15% to 30% of patients
- Growth hormone receptor antagonists: Pegvisomant (Somavert) for patients resistant or intolerant to somatostatin analogues and who have tumors >5 mm from the optic chiasm
- Radiotherapy for patients resistant or intolerant to pharmacologic therapy, with clinically and biochemically active disease and a tumor remnant on MRI

Acromegaly is a disorder resulting from an excessive secretion of growth hormone (GH), with a prevalence of 40 to 60 cases per million and an annual incidence of 3 to 4 per million.

Physiology, Biochemistry, and Regulation of the GH/IGF-1 Axis

GH secretion is regulated at the hypothalamus (Figure 1). The pulsatile secretion of GH-releasing hormone (GHRH) stimulates somatotroph proliferation and GH gene transcription, whereas somatostatin, which is secreted tonically, inhibits GH synthesis. These two hypothalamic signals result in the pulsatile secretion of pituitary GH, with most pulses occurring during the night. GH is also stimulated by ghrelin, a hypothalamic and gastrointestinal orexigenic hormone that binds specific receptors in the somatotroph known as GH-secretagogue receptors. GH exerts its actions through a specific membrane receptor located predominantly in the liver and cartilage, but ubiquitously present in all tissues. One molecule of GH interacts with two molecules of GH receptor, resulting in functional dimerization and conformational changes that lead to the phosphorylation of several kinases and eventually the interaction with target genes such as the insulin-like growth factor (IGF)-1 gene.

IGF-1 is closely related to proinsulin and circulates in plasma bound to six binding proteins (IGFBPs) that are synthesized and released by the liver. IGFBP3 is the most important of these binding proteins and is also GH dependent; it forms a heterotrimeric complex composed of BP3, IGF-1, and the acid-labile subunit (ALS). IGF-1 is responsible for most of the trophic and growth-promoting effects of GH. Blood levels of IGF-1 are increased during puberty, coinciding with the acceleration of somatic growth, and decline with aging. Malnutrition, poorly controlled type 1 diabetes, hypothyroidism, and liver failure all result in diminished IGF-1 concentrations. IGF-1 is the main player in GH negative feedback regulation and it acts at both the pituitary and the hypothalamic levels. Glucose regulates GH release by increasing (hyperglycemia) or decreasing (hypoglycemia) somatostatin synthesis in the hypothalamus. Exercise and amino acids such as arginine also stimulate GH secretion.

Etiopathogenesis of Growth Hormone–Secreting Tumors

The molecular pathogenesis of pituitary tumors includes the inactivation of tumor suppressor genes, the activation of oncogenes, and the trophic effect of factors such as the hypothalamic releasing hormones. Approximately 40% of GH-producing tumors in whites harbor somatic point mutations of the α subunit stimulatory G protein coupled to the GHRH receptor (GSPα mutations). This molecular alteration causes constitutive activation of the GHRH receptor, resulting in an increased transcription of the GH gene and the promotion of somatotroph proliferation. Acromegalic patients whose tumors harbor GSPα mutations usually have a more benign clinical course and appear to be more susceptible to management with somatostatin analogues. Nonwhite acromegalic populations, including persons of Japanese, Korean, and Mexican heritage, have a much lower prevalence of GSPα mutations.

Other molecular events should be present in GSPα-negative somatotrophinomas. Menin is a protein encoded by a tumor suppressor gene located on the short arm of chromosome 11. Inactivating mutations of menin are the molecular basis of type 1

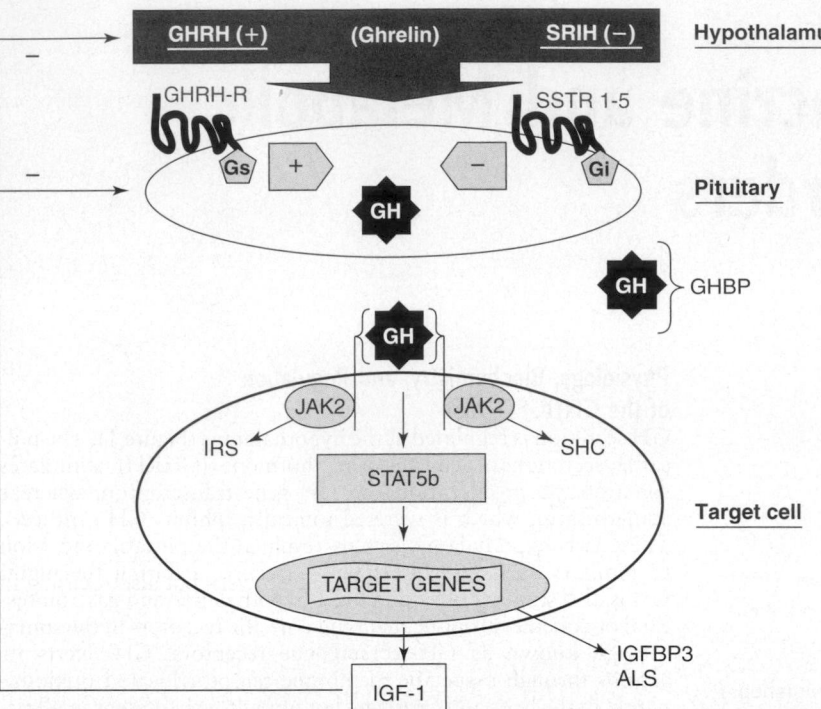

Figure 1. GH is regulated positively by GHRH and negatively by somatostatin. Fifty percent of circulating GH is bound to the GH binding protein, which represents the extracellular portion of the GH receptor. One molecule of GH dimerizes two molecules of GH receptor, and the ensuing signal transduction results in IGF-1 synthesis and secretion, which exerts negative feedback on GH secretion at the hypothalamic and pituitary levels. *Abbreviations:* ALS = acid-labile subunit; GH = growth hormone; GHRH = growth hormone–releasing hormone; IGF = insulin-like growth factor; IGFBP3 = insulin-like growth factor binding protein 3; IRS = insulin receptor S; JAK2 = Janus kinase 2; SRIH = somatostatin; SSTR = somatostatin receptor.

multiple endocrine neoplasia (MEN1); however, GH-secreting tumors occurring out of this context do not have such genetic abnormalities. Inactivating mutations of other putative tumor-suppressor genes located relatively close to the menin locus have been described in several kindreds with familial acromegaly; however, they do not seem to play an important oncogenic role in the sporadic form of the disease. Other genetic alterations such as underexpression of GADD 45γ (growth arrest and DNA damage-inducible protein) and overexpression of the securing molecule PTTG (pituitary tumor transforming gene) have also been shown to be involved in the molecular pathogenesis of acromegaly. Although hereditary acromegaly is rare (less than 2% of the cases), familial somatotrophinomas account for 30% of the tumors seen in the syndrome of familial isolated pituitary adenomas. Patients with isolated familial somatotrophinomas are younger and usually have more aggressive tumors than subjects with sporadic acromegaly. Affected members do not show any molecular alterations in the MEN1 gene. However, 15% of 73 tested families harbor inactivating, germline mutations of the AIP (aryl hydrocarbon interacting protein) gene located on chromosome 11q13.3.

In more than 90% of cases, acromegaly is caused by a sporadic pituitary adenoma. In approximately 70% of these patients, these benign epithelial neoplasms are larger than 1 cm in diameter and are known as *macroadenomas*, whereas one third of the patients harbor lesions smaller than 1 cm or *microadenomas*. One third of the patients have tumors that cosecrete GH and prolactin (PRL) (mammosomatoroph cell adenomas). Real pituitary GH-secreting carcinomas, with documented metastasis as the irrefutable malignancy criterion, are exceedingly rare. On rare occasions, acromegaly results from GHRH-secreting neuroendocrine tumors, usually located in the lungs, thymus, or endocrine pancreas. In this scenario, the ectopically produced GHRH leads to hyperplasia of the somatotroph, with the consequent excessive production of GH. Even less common are GH-secreting tumors arising in ectopic pituitary tissue, usually located in the sphenoid sinus. A case of GH-secreting lymphoma has been reported.

Clinical Manifestations

Acromegaly develops insidiously over many years. An 8- to 10-year delay in diagnosis has been estimated from the beginning of the first symptom. Clinical characteristics are often attributed to aging. Symptoms and signs can be divided into those resulting from the compressive effects of the pituitary tumor and those that are a consequence of the GH and IGF-1 excess.

Local Tumor Effects

Headache results from an increase in intracranial pressure and from the effects of GH itself; it is usually described as a dull pain that persists throughout the day. Occasionally, large tumors invading laterally into the cavernous sinuses give rise to cranial nerve syndromes, usually third and sixth. Visual field defects are relatively common with macroadenomas extending superiorly and compressing the optic chiasm. This usually results in different combinations of bitemporal homonymous hemianopia or quadrontopia.

Consequences of the GH/IGF-1 Excess
Skeletal Growth and Skin Changes
A GH excess developing before the pubertal closure of epiphyseal bone leads to an acceleration of linear growth, and this results in gigantism. Once the patient is in adulthood, the GH/IGF-1 excess results in acral enlargement, which is manifested by increases in ring and shoe sizes as well as enlargement of the nose, supracilliary arches, frontal bones and mandible. There is thickening of soft tissues of the hands and feet; hands are fleshy and bulky and the heel pad is increased. The skin is thickened due to the deposition of glycosaminoglycans and excessive collagen production. Hyperhidrosis and seborrhea occur in 60% of patients; skin tags (previously associated with colon cancer) and acanthosis nigricans are common.

Musculoskeletal System
Generalized arthralgias are present in the majority (80%) of patients. Degenerative osteoarthritis is more common than in the general population. Paresthesias of the hands and feet and a proximal painful myopathy are often reported. Nerve entrapment syndromes such as the carpal tunnel syndrome occur in nearly half of patients.

Cardiovascular System
Arterial hypertension is found in 30% of patients, and when associated with diabetes it contributes to the increased mortality rate of the disease. Hyperaldosteronism with low renin levels and the resulting sodium retention play an important role in the

pathogenesis of hypertension, but other contributors such as an increased sympathetic tone are also present. Echocardiographic findings include left ventricular and septal hypertrophy with varying degrees of diastolic dysfunction. Symptomatic cardiac disease develops in 15% of patients and is usually due to coronary artery disease, heart failure, and arrhythmias. Although the existence of an acromegalic cardiomyopathy is still controversial, there are patients without hypertension and with angiographically normal coronaries, who develop severe congestive heart failure, in whom histologic evidence of subendocardial, subepicardial, and myocardial fibrosis and necrosis has been documented.

Respiratory Abnormalities
The majority of patients with acromegaly are affected by loud snoring. A significant fraction of these have sleep apnea (with both central and obstructive components) with significant drops in oxygen saturation, which can be complicated by arrhythmias, daytime somnolence, and chronic fatigue.

Abnormalities in Glucose Metabolism
Chronic GH hypersecretion creates a state of insulin resistance, and glucose intolerance has been reported in 30% to 50% of patients with acromegaly; the percentage with fasting hyperglycemia can be close to 30%, depending on the population. Hyperglycemia has correlated with GH concentrations in some studies and with IGF-1 levels in others.

Abnormalities in Lipid Metabolism
The classic lipid profile consists of diminished total cholesterol, along with elevated triglyceride concentrations. Intermediate-density lipoprotein (IDL) particles and lipoprotein(a) might also be elevated, and there is a higher percentage of the more atherogenic type II low-density lipoprotein (LDL).

Bone and Calcium Metabolism
Acromegaly is associated with hypercalciuria and hyperphosphatemia. High serum 25 hydroxyvitamin D_3 and urinary levels of hydroxyproline can be found, reflecting a state of increased bone turnover. Cortical bone mineral density is elevated, whereas trabecular bone mass is diminished.

Neoplasia
Retrospective studies suggested that colonic adenomatous polyps and adenocarcinoma were more frequent in acromegalic patients than in the general population. Prospective studies have demonstrated that the risk, albeit smaller than previously thought, is real and probably justifies screening colonoscopy in these patients. Patients with uncontrolled acromegaly have a higher risk of recurrence of premalignant polyps and a higher mortality rate from colon cancer compared with subjects with biochemically controlled disease and the general population. Recently, an increased incidence of well-differentiated thyroid carcinoma has been documented.

Associated Endocrine Abnormalities
A euthyroid goiter is often found but seldom requires specific treatment. Hypopituitarism occurs variably, depending on the size and extension of the tumor and whether the patient has undergone surgery or radiation therapy. Hypogonadotropic hypogonadism is the most common pituitary deficiency, occurring in 20% of patients. A decreased libido is a common presenting complaint in both male and female patients with acromegaly; women often have menstrual and ovulatory disturbances and men complain of impotence.

Although an elevated PRL is common, it does not always reflect cosecretion of this hormone by the somatotrophinoma, but rather an interruption of the descending dopaminergic tone by the tumor compressing the pituitary stalk. Central hypocortisolism and hypothyroidism are less common.

GH-secreting pituitary adenomas are the second, after prolactinomas, pituitary tumor occurring in the context of MEN1 (multiple parathyroid adenomas, pituitary adenoma, and pancreatic islet cell tumors). Acromegaly can also develop in patients with the McCune-Albright syndrome (polyostotic fibrous dysplasia, café au lait spots, and endocrinopathies such as sexual precocity and autonomous thyroid nodules), and occurs in the context of the Carney complex.

Mortality
Life expectancy in patients with acromegaly is decreased by about 10 to 15 years, and the standardized mortality ratio is 1.5 to 2. Most patients die of cardiovascular causes, followed by cerebrovascular events, respiratory abnormalities, and neoplastic diseases. Hormonal control has a definite impact on survival. Lowering serum GH to less than 2.5 ng/mL results in reduction of the mortality rate to levels comparable with the general population. These safe GH levels were obtained using old radioimmunoassays, and there are no equivalent studies using ultrasensitive GH assays. IGF-1 levels have not been as good as GH as independent predictors of mortality. Other factors associated with an increased mortality include advanced age and the presence of hypertension and diabetes. Mortality rate in acromegaly can be reduced to that seen on the general population when patients are treated using a multidisciplinary approach aiming at controlling not only the GH and IGF-1 levels, but also focusing in the management of comorbidities.

Biochemical Diagnosis
Due to the pulsatile nature of GH secretion, random determinations of this hormone are not useful in the diagnosis of acromegaly. The gold standard for the diagnosis is the measurement of GH after an oral glucose load of 75 g; current guidelines state that suppression to less than 0.4 ng/mL (using ultrasensitive assays), reliably excludes the diagnosis. Situations associated with decreased suppression of GH by glucose include puberty, pregnancy, use of oral contraceptives, uncontrolled diabetes, and renal and hepatic insufficiency.

IGF-1 levels reflect the integrated concentrations over 24 hours of GH and correlate well with clinical activity. Blood IGF-1 concentrations decrease with age, reflecting the parallel decline of the somatotropic axis. There is a gender difference in IGF-1 (premenopausal women have lower levels than age-matched male subjects). Other conditions that lower IGF-1 levels include malnutrition, uncontrolled diabetes, and hepatic and renal failure. Normal ranges for IGF-1 should be established in each particular center based on age. The determination of other GH-dependent peptides such as IGFBP3 and ALS has not proved to be superior to IGF-1.

Imaging
Pituitary magnetic resonance imaging (MRI) with gadolinium enhancement allows visualization of lesions as small as 2 or 3 mm in diameter. High-resolution computed tomography (CT) is a reasonable alternative, although it is much less sensitive. An ectopic source of GHRH should be suspected when the MRI is completely normal. In these rare cases, serum GHRH should be measured and the ectopic tumor should be sought, usually with high-resolution CT of the chest and abdomen.

Treatment
The decision as to what therapeutic modality should be used has to take into account medical issues (cardiopulmonary comorbidities, size, and extension of the tumor) as well as the local characteristics of the treating center. The latter refers to the availability of pituitary surgeons and radiotherapeutic technologies as well as the economic feasibility of pharmacologic therapy.

Surgery
Transsphenoidal surgery has been the traditional treatment for acromegaly and achieves biochemical cure (achievement of a post-glucose GH <1 ng/mL and normalization of IGF-1) in 80% to 90% of microadenomas. According to the latest published acromegaly consensus, biochemical cure is defined as a glucose-suppressed GH of 0.4 ng/mL as well as a normal age-adjusted IGF-1. Cure rates for macroadenomas are much lower (40%–50%),

and invasive lesions have a very slight chance (<10%) of being cured by surgery. Even though surgery often fails to achieve a full biochemical cure, debulking the pituitary adenoma relieves optic chiasm compression and can result in a sufficient decrement of tumor mass (and therefore of GH production) to allow better results with either pharmacologic or radiotherapeutic regimens.

Pharmacologic Therapy

Somatostatin analogues are the most commonly used medical treatment for acromegaly. Somatostatin inhibits GH secretion and somatotroph cell growth via its interaction with five different somatostatin receptor (SSTR) subtypes. The development of long-acting somatostatin analogues such as octreotide (Sandostatin) and lanreotide (Somatuline) overcame the pharmacologic difficulties of native somatostatin (short half-life, rebound GH secretion, and need for IV administration) and resulted in a more potent inhibition of GH secretion. The most commonly used preparations are intramuscular octreotide LAR (long-acting repeatable) and subcutaneous lanreotide autogel, which are administered every 4 weeks. Doses of octreotide-LAR range from 10 to 40 mg and those of lanreotide autogel from 60 to 120 mg, both administered every 4 weeks; although in specific patients the interval of injection can be increased to every 6 or even 8 weeks, thus diminishing the cost of therapy. Octreotide and lanreotide have very high affinities for SSTR-2 and to a lesser extent SSTR-5, which are precisely the most commonly expressed somatostatin receptors in GH-secreting adenomas.

When used after surgery has failed, somatostatin analogues can achieve a safe and a normal IGF-1 in 25% to 35% of patients. Primary treatment with somatostatin analogues is increasingly being used in patients with invasive tumors, when cardiopulmonary contraindications are present, and more recently as a result of the patient's or treating physician's preference. In these settings, biochemical success rates (achievement of a GH <2.5 ng/mL and normalization of IGF-1) have ranged between 30% and 80%, and more than 80% report significant relief of symptoms. More recent trials performed in unselected populations reveal that the real success rate lies between 25% and 35%. Tumor shrinkage occurs in 70% of primarily treated patients. Overall, treatment success is directly related to the abundance of SSTR-2 and SSTR-5 in the tumor. Lower pretreatment GH levels are also associated with a better response to somatostatin analogues. Side effects of somatostatin analogues, including nausea, abdominal pain, alopecia, and biliary sludge, occur in 20% of subjects. The currently recommended biochemical targets when treating patients with somatostatin analogues are the achievement of a GH of 1 ng/mL and an IGF-1 level within the normal age-adjusted range patients with somatostatin analogues is 1 ng/mL.

Pegvisomant is a GH mutant that prevents functional dimerization of the GH receptor, thus acting as an antagonist. Its use results in normalization of IGF-1 in more than 70% of patients, while increasing GH levels. Concern about adenoma growth due to the abolition of IGF-1 negative feedback on the tumoral somatotroph prevents its use in patients with very large lesions in close proximity to the optic chiasm. Transient elevations of liver aminotransferases can occur, although this seldom requires drug discontinuation. Pegvisomant does not compromise insulin secretion, as somatostatin analogues do. GH-receptor antagonists are expensive and should not be used as primary treatment; they are currently indicated in patients who are intolerant or have failed somatostatin analogue therapy.

Few patients respond marginally to difficult-to-tolerate large doses of bromocriptine. Newer dopamine agonists, such as cabergoline, are better tolerated and achieve biochemical control in 20% to 30% of patients. Combination treatment with cabergoline and octreotide appears to be promising in cases resistant to somatostatin analogues.

Radiation Therapy

Both external-beam radiotherapy and radiosurgery are indicated in patients with persistent disease and a demonstrable tumor remnant who are either intolerant or resistant to pharmacologic treatment. Biochemical success occurs in 20% to 60% and requires many years to become apparent. Hypopituitarism, involving at least two axes, develops in more than 50% of patients within 10 years. Serious adverse effects such as brain necrosis and optic nerve damage seldom occur with the currently used techniques that minimize radiation to the normal surrounding tissues.

Novel pharmacologic therapies are being developed, some of which will likely become useful particularly in patients who do not respond to current somatostatin analogues. These include the so-called "universal" somatostatin analogue pasireotide, which is capable of interacting not only with the SSTRs 2 and 5, but also with subtypes 1 and 3. Pasireotide seems to be slightly more effective than octreotide in achieving GH and IGF-1 targets; however, its major drawback is the worsening of hyperglycemia. Dopastatin is a recently developed chimeric compound which behaves both as an analog and as a dopamine agonist; clinical trials had to be discontinued at its early stages due to lack of efficacy.

References

Beckers A, Daly AF. The clinical, pathological and genetic features of familial isolated pituitary adenomas. Eur J Endocrinol 2007;157:371–82.

Bevan JS. Clinical review: The antitumoral effects of somatostatin analog therapy in acromegaly. J Clin Endocrinol Metab 2005;90:1856–63.

Colao A, Ferone D, Marzullo P, Lombardi G. Systemic complications of acromegaly: Epidemiology, pathogenesis and management. Endocr Rev 2004;25:102–52.

Dekkers OM, Biermasz NR, Pereira AM, et al. Mortality in acromegaly: A metaanalysis. J Clin Endocrinol Metab 2008;93:61–7.

Espinosa E, Ramirez C, Mercado M. The multimodal treatment of acromegaly: Current status and future perspectives. Endocr Metab Immune Disord Drug Targets 2014;14:169–81.

Espinosa-de-Los-Monteros AL, González B, Vargas G, et al. Clinical and biochemical characteristics of acromegalic patients with different abnormalities of glucose metabolism. Pituitary 2011;14:231–5.

Espinosa-de-Los-Monteros AL, Sosa E, Cheng S, et al. Biochemical evaluation of disease activity after pituitary surgery in acromegaly: A critical analysis of patients who spontaneously change disease status. Clin Endocrinol 2006;64:245–9.

Espinosa de los Monteros AL, Gonzalez B, Vargas G, et al. Octreotide LAR treatment of acromegaly in "real life": long term outcome at a tertiary care center. Pituitary, 2015;18:290–6.

Freda P. Current concepts in the biochemical assessment of the patient with acromegaly. Growth Horm IGF Res 2003;13:171–84.

Freda P, Katznelson L, van der Lely AJ, et al. Long-acting somatostatin analog therapy of acromegaly: A meta-analysis. J Clin Endocrinol Metab 2005;90:4465–73.

Giustina A, Chanson P, Bronstein MD. A consensus on criteria for cure of acromegaly. J Clin Endocrinol Metab 2010;95:3141–8.

Giustina A, Chanson P, Kleinberg D, et al. Expert consensus document: A consensus on the medical treatment of acromegaly. Nat Rev Endocrinol 2014;10:243–8.

Holdaway IM, Rajasoorya RC, Gamble GD. Factors influencing mortality in acromegaly. J Clin Endocrinol Metab 2004;89:667–74.

Kopchick JJ, Parkinson C, Stevens EC, Trainer PJ. Growth hormone receptor antagonists: Discovery, development, and use in patients with acromegaly. Endocr Rev 2002;23:623–46.

Melmed S. Acromegaly: Pathogenesis and treatment. J Clin Invest 2009;119:3189–202.

Mercado M, Gonzalez B, Vargas G, et al. Successful mortality reduction and contra of comorbidities in patients with acromegaly followed at a highly specialized multidisciplinary clinic. J Clin Endocrinol Metab 2014;99:4438–46.

Vance ML, Laws ER. Role of medical therapy in the management of acromegaly. Neurosurgery 2005;56:877–85.

ADRENOCORTICAL INSUFFICIENCY

Method of
Justin Moore, MD

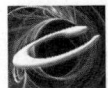 **CURRENT DIAGNOSIS**

- A first-waking or random cortisol level greater than 13 µg/dL effectively rules out adrenocortical insufficiency.
- If the first-waking cortisol level is less than 13 µg/dL, further testing with the high-dose (250 µg) cosyntropin (Cortrosyn) stimulation test is appropriate.
- A peak cortisol level less than 18 µg/dL after administration of cosyntropin is diagnostic of adrenocortical insufficiency.
- If adrenocortical insufficiency is present, an elevated endogenous ACTH level (typically >100 pg/mL) is generally indicative of primary adrenocortical insufficiency, and a normal or low endogenous ACTH level is generally indicative of secondary adrenal insufficiency.

- If primary adrenocortical insufficiency is present, serum testing for anti-adrenal antibodies may be useful.
- If secondary adrenocortical insufficiency is present and not thought to be secondary to exogenous glucocorticoid use, magnetic resonance imaging (MRI) of the pituitary sella is appropriate.

 CURRENT THERAPY

- For adrenal crisis in patients with known adrenocortical insufficiency, administer hydrocortisone injection (Solu-Cortef) 50 to 100 mg IV every 6 to 8 hours along with generous volumes of saline.
- For chronic steroid replacement, oral hydrocortisone (Cortef) can be dosed at roughly 10 to 12 mg/m^2 body surface area per day divided into two or three doses, with one half to two thirds of the daily dose given upon waking.
- In case of nausea or vomiting, patients should be dispensed hydrocortisone injection with instructions for home use of 50 to 100 mg IM every 6 to 8 hours.
- In patients with primary adrenocortical insufficiency, fludrocortisone (Florinef) should be added to the treatment regimen, with the typical dose falling between 50 and 100 µg once or twice daily.
- In women with primary adrenocortical insufficiency, consideration should be given to 25 to 50 mg dehydroepiandrostenedione (DHEA)[7] daily.
- Patients should wear a medical alert bracelet or necklace.

[7]Available as dietary supplement.

Epidemiology

Primary adrenocortical insufficiency, also known as Addison's disease, has a prevalence of 93 to 140 cases per million persons. More than 90% of Addison's disease in the developed world is secondary to autoimmune adrenalitis. Secondary adrenocortical insufficiency has a prevalence of 150 to 280 cases per million persons. Therapeutic glucocorticoid administration is thought to be the most common etiology of secondary adrenocortical insufficiency. Both primary and secondary adrenocortical insufficiencies are more common in women than in men.

Risk Factors

Primary Adrenocortical Insufficiency
A personal or family history of autoimmune disease, particularly autoimmune polyglandular syndrome types 1 or 2, type 1 diabetes, Hashimoto's disease, or vitiligo, is a risk factor for autoimmune adrenalitis. Multiple medications are a risk factor for adrenocortical dysfunction. Antifungals, particularly ketoconazole (Nizoral), inhibit adrenocortical function. The anesthetic etomidate (Amidate) is a powerful inhibitor of adrenal function, and adrenal crisis has been associated with as little as a single dose. The presence of an infiltrative or infectious disease associated with adrenal destruction (Box 1) is associated with risk for primary adrenocortical insufficiency. Use of anticoagulant medications or the presence of a coagulopathy, particularly antiphospholipid antibody syndrome, is a risk factor for adrenal hemorrhage. Other less-common risk factors for primary adrenocortical insufficiency include a family or personal history of congenital adrenal hyperplasia or adrenoleukodystrophy.

Secondary Adrenocortical Insufficiency
The most powerful risk factor for secondary adrenocortical insufficiency is prolonged use of exogenous glucocorticoids.

The presence of a tumor of the hypothalamic–pituitary region or a history of treatment of such tumors with surgery or radiation is a risk factor. Pregnancy is a risk factor for secondary adrenocortical

Box 1   Causes of Primary Adrenocortical Insufficiency

Autoimmune
Autoimmune polyglandular syndromes 1 and 2

Infectious
Tuberculosis
Histoplasmosis
Blastomycosis
Coccidiomycosis
Cryptococcosis
Human immunodeficiency virus
Cytomegalovirus

Hemorrhagic
Sepsis
Anticoagulation
Anti-phospholipid antibody syndrome

Neoplastic
Metastatic breast cancer
Non-small cell lung cancer
Colon cancer
Renal cell cancer

Drugs
Ketoconazole (Nizoral)
Aminoglutethimide (Cytadren)
Mitotane (Lysodren)
Etomidate (Amidate)

Infiltrative Diseases
Sarcoidosis
Hemochromatosis
Amyloidosis

Familial or Genetic
Adrenoleukodystrophy
Adrenomyeloneuropathy
Familial glucocorticoid deficiency
Congenital adrenal hyperplasia
Adrenocorticotropic hormone (ACTH) resistance syndromes

insufficiency by two mechanisms: autoimmune lymphocytic hypophysitis, which most commonly affects women during or shortly following pregnancy, and Sheehan's syndrome, characterized by pituitary apoplexy secondary to hypotension or blood loss in the postpartum period.

Pathophysiology

Primary adrenocortical insufficiency, or Addison's disease, is characterized by a defect in the adrenal cortex, resulting in insensitivity to adrenocorticotropic hormone (ACTH). Secondary adrenocortical insufficiency is the result of insufficient secretion of endogenous ACTH, owing to a synthetic defect in the pituitary or hypothalamus.

Prevention

No clinically practical strategy for preventing primary adrenocortical insufficiency exists. Glucocorticoid-associated secondary adrenocortical insufficiency may be prevented through judicious use of systemic glucocorticoids, with efforts made to limit administration of the glucocorticoid to the lowest effective dose for the shortest possible time. For patients on oral glucocorticoids, effort should be made to reduce the dose as aggressively as the treated condition allows. This can require a prolonged taper, with dose increments as small as 2.5 to 5 mg every 2 to 4 weeks. Once a dose of 1 to 2 mg prednisone or prednisone equivalent per day is reached, a first morning cortisol level of greater than 10 ng/dL after 24 hours of abstinence from the glucocorticoid usually predicts normal adrenal function. If glucocorticoids are discontinued, stress-dose glucocorticoids should be continued for 1 year in case of fever, severe emotional distress, or elective surgery.

Clinical Manifestations

Primary Adrenocortical Insufficiency

The presentation of Addison's disease is sometimes dramatic, and Addison's 1855 description of weakness, fatigue, anorexia, salt craving, and orthostatic hypotension is still largely accurate. Symptoms are often subtle and nonspecific, consisting of weight loss, nausea, and abdominal pain. The skin and buccal mucosa are often hyperpigmented, owing to the effect of excess ACTH on cutaneous melanocortin receptors. Vitiligo may be present. Hyponatremia and hyperkalemia (as a result of mineralocorticoid deficiency) are often present along with azotemia and occasionally hypercalcemia. Eosinophilia has been reported.

Secondary Adrenocortical Insufficiency

The presentation of secondary adrenocortical insufficiency is usually insidious, with weight loss, fatigue, and malaise as presenting features. This often leads to a delay in diagnosis. Because production of mineralocorticoid is relatively intact in secondary adrenocortical insufficiency, electrolyte abnormalities are less common. Hyperpigmentation is not present, reflecting normal or low ACTH levels. Laboratory abnormalities are less common, but hypoglycemia is occasionally seen. Because isolated ACTH deficiency is rare, physical examination findings consistent with other pituitary hormone abnormalities, such as hyperprolactinemia, hypogonadism, growth hormone deficiency, or hypothyroidism, may be present.

Diagnosis

A first-morning cortisol (within 2 hours of waking) of 3 µg/dL or less has a relatively high predictive value for adrenocortical insufficiency, but it should be confirmed with further testing. A first-morning cortisol level greater than 13 µg/dL effectively rules out adrenocortical insufficiency, but further testing should be performed if clinical suspicion is high. Given its technical nature and potential hazards to patients, insulin tolerance testing has largely been replaced by stimulation testing with synthetic cosyntropin (Cortrosyn, tetracosactrin [Synacthen][2]) containing the first 24 amino acids of human ACTH.

In high-dose testing, a cortisol level is checked before and 30 minutes and/or 1 hour after 250 µg of cosyntropin is administered (IM or IV), whereas low-dose testing substitutes a 1 µg dose of cosyntropin. A peak cortisol level greater than 18 µg/dL defines a normal response. Cosyntropin testing should not be used in cases in which sufficient time has not elapsed to allow adrenal atrophy, such as after recent pituitary surgery, because adrenal atrophy must have occurred for the adrenal response to cosyntropin to be blunted. The high-dose (250 µg) test remains the standard, because a significant portion of normal patients fail the 1 µg test if a cortisol cutoff of 18 µg/dL is used. A low or normal waking plasma ACTH level indicates secondary adrenocortical insufficiency. An elevated ACTH level (>100 pg/mL) typically indicates primary adrenocortical insufficiency, although care must be taken not to mistakenly draw an ACTH level after administering exogenous cosyntropin.

Once the diagnosis of adrenocortical insufficiency has been established, an etiology should be sought (Box 2, and see Box 1). Serology for anti-adrenal antibodies is useful in primary adrenocortical insufficiency, given the huge fraction of these patients with autoimmune adrenalitis. The presence of other autoimmune diseases is even more suggestive. Enlarged adrenal glands with high-density areas or calcification on computed tomography can suggest granulomatous disease or neoplasm. Fluid collections around the adrenals during an acute adrenal crisis sometimes indicate adrenal hemorrhage. Secondary adrenocortical insufficiency is most often associated with chronic glucocorticoid therapy but may be caused by a number of other diseases (see Box 2). MRI in patients with secondary adrenocortical insufficiency is helpful if exogenous steroids have been excluded as the cause of adrenocortical insufficiency. Testing of the other hypothalamic–pituitary axes is also helpful in this clinical scenario, because isolated ACTH deficiency is relatively rare.

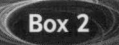

Box 2 · Etiologies of Secondary Adrenocortical Insufficiency

Chronic steroid therapy, either oral or parenteral

Pituitary Injury
Transsphenoidal or transcranial surgery
Radiation to the sella
Infarction (Sheehan's)
Closed head injury

Tumors of the Sella
Pituitary adenoma
Craniopharyngioma
Meningioma
Rathke's cleft cyst
Metastatic cancer

Infiltrative Diseases
Sarcoidosis, tuberculosis, or other granulomatous diseases
Lymphocytic hypophysitis
Idiopathic ACTH deficiency

Differential Diagnosis

The differential diagnosis of primary adrenocortical insufficiency includes other systemic illnesses associated with orthostatic hypotension and electrolyte abnormalities, including dehydration and distributive shock. The hyperpigmentation seen in Addison's disease can mimic the hyperpigmentation sometimes present in ACTH-dependent Cushing's syndrome or in hemochromatosis. Because the presentation of secondary adrenocortical insufficiency is often subtle, the differential diagnosis is broad and includes a number of illnesses associated with fatigue, weight loss, and malaise, including occult malignancies, renal or hepatic dysfunction, and electrolyte disturbances.

Treatment

In critical illness, if the diagnosis is not established and diagnostic testing is required, the initial steroid of choice is dexamethasone (Decadron) 1 to 4 mg IV every 12 hours until testing is complete. Because dexamethasone does not compete with the cortisol assay, cosyntropin stimulation testing may be performed while the patient is on treatment. Baseline cortisol and ACTH levels should preferably be drawn prior to initiation of dexamethasone, but treatment should not be delayed if testing cannot be obtained promptly.

If a patient with known adrenocortical insufficiency presents in adrenal crisis, hydrocortisone 50 to 100 mg IV every 6 to 8 hours is an appropriate initial therapy, with the dose tapered to an appropriate oral dose as the patient's condition improves. Mineralocorticoids are not required for treatment of acute adrenal crisis, but they should be re-initiated in primary adrenocortical insufficiency when the crisis abates. Fludrocortisone is the available drug, and the typical dose is 50 to 100 µg (0.05 to 0.1 mg) once or twice daily. Development of hypertension or hypokalemia should prompt a reduction in the fludrocortisone dose.

Glucocorticoid replacement may be accomplished with oral hydrocortisone two or three times daily. One half to two thirds of the daily dose is given upon waking, and the dosage is roughly 10 to 12 mg/m[2] body surface area per day. This dosage should be doubled or tripled for 3 or more days in case of fever, severe emotional distress, or elective surgery.

In case of nausea or vomiting, patients should be dispensed hydrocortisone injection with instructions for home self-administration of 50 to 100 mg IM every 6 to 8 hours until vomiting ceases.

Patients should wear a medical alert bracelet or necklace.

Dehydroepiandrostenedione (DHEA)[7] 25 to 50 mg PO daily should be considered in women with primary adrenocortical insufficiency, particularly if they have low energy or low libido.

---

[2]Not available in the United States.

[7]Available as dietary supplement.

Monitoring

Should hypokalemia or hypertension develop after initiation of therapy, the fludrocortisone dosage should be reduced. Patients should be interviewed and examined for indicators of excess glucocorticoid replacement, such as weight gain, striae, facial plethora, osteoporosis, or glucose intolerance.

Complications

Adrenal crisis in patients with known adrenal insufficiency occurs at a rate of approximately six cases per 100 patient-years. Precipitating causes of adrenal crisis are mainly gastrointestinal infection and other causes of fever, with other stressful events (pain, surgery, emotional distress, heat, and pregnancy) occurring less commonly. Iatrogenic Cushing's syndrome can develop if the dose of glucocorticoid replacement is not carefully monitored.

References

Arlt W, Allolio B. Adrenal insufficiency. Lancet 2003;361:1881–93.

Dorin RI, Qualls CR, Crapo LM. Diagnosis of adrenal insufficiency. Ann Intern Med 2003;139:194–204.

Hahner S, Loeffler M, Bleicken B, et al. Epidemiology of adrenal crisis in chronic adrenal insufficiency: The need for new prevention strategies. Eur J Endocrinol 2010;162:597–602.

Husebye ES, Allolio B, Arlt W, Badenhoop K, Bensing S, Betterle C, et al. Consensus statement on the diagnosis, treatment and follow-up of patients with primary adrenal insufficiency. J Intern Med 2014;275(2):104–15. http://dx.doi.org/10.1111/joim.12162. Epub 2013 Dec 16. Review. PubMed PMID: 24330030.

Kazlauskaite R, Evans A, Villabona C, et al. Corticotropin tests for hypothalamic-pituitary adrenal insufficiency: A meta-analysis. J Clin Endocrinol Metab 2008;93(11):4245–53.

CUSHING'S SYNDROME

Method of
Madson Q. Almeida, MD; Maya Lodish, MD; and Constantine A. Stratakis, MD, PhD

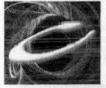

CURRENT DIAGNOSIS

- Cushing's syndrome remains one of the most challenging diagnoses in endocrine medicine.
- Cushing's disease is caused by corticotropin (ACTH)-producing pituitary adenomas (corticotropinomas) and constitutes the most common cause of endogenous Cushing's syndrome, although its prevalence varies across different age groups.
- Growth failure in children, facial plethora and rounded face, central fat deposition, supraclavicular fat accumulation, buffalo hump, purple striae, thin skin, and proximal myopathy are relatively sensitive clinical features of Cushing's syndrome.
- Ectopic ACTH syndrome occasionally has an unusual presentation of rapid onset, severe weakness, and hypokalemia without classic symptoms of Cushing's syndrome.
- A urinary free cortisol test is the most cost-effective and reliable outpatient screening test.
- A 1-mg overnight dexamethasone screening test is less useful and more expensive than the urinary free cortisol test, but it provides a good alternative for patients in whom urinary collection is impossible or unreliable.
- Midnight salivary cortisol levels greater than 3.6 nmol/L (0.13 μg/dL) have a sensitivity and specificity of approximately 95% for the diagnosis of Cushing's syndrome.
- Undetectable ACTH levels (<1 pmol/L or <5 pg/mL) indicate a primary autonomous adrenocortical disease.
- Postcontrast spoiled gradient-recalled acquisition (SPGR) magnetic resonance imaging (MRI) is superior to conventional MRI for the localization of corticotropinomas in children and adults.
- Computed tomography (CT) is used to investigate adrenal disease in patients with ACTH-independent Cushing's syndrome. Usually, conventional MRI is less useful owing to motion artifacts.

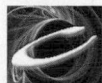

CURRENT THERAPY

- The initial therapy of choice for patients with Cushing's disease is transsphenoidal surgery of the pituitary gland to remove the responsible adenoma.
- Transsphenoidal surgery has a success rate greater than 80% in most experienced centers. Lower success rates and higher incidence of relapse are recorded in less-experienced centers.
- Laparoscopic adrenalectomy has become the treatment of choice for benign adrenal lesions with a diameter of less than 6 cm.
- In stages I to III adrenocortical carcinoma, complete tumor resection offers the best chance for cure.
- Mitotane, an adrenolytic agent, is used in the treatment of metastatic adrenocortical carcinoma and also as an adjuvant for tumors with a high risk of recurrence.
- Medical treatment with ketoconazole,[2] metyrapone,[1] aminoglutethimide, and mitotane[1] may be used to control hypercortisolism in preparation for surgery; medical adrenalectomy may also be used in cases of cyclic Cushing's syndrome.
- Pasireotide (Signifor) and mifepristone (Korlym) may be used for the treatment of Cushing's disease that cannot be cured by surgery and/or irradiation.
- The most effective treatment option for ectopic ACTH syndrome is resection of the tumor. Somatostatin analogues and various chemotherapeutic regimens have been used in the treatment of metastatic tumors.

[1]Not FDA approved for this indication.
[2]Not available in the United States.

Definition and Epidemiology

Cushing's syndrome remains one of the most difficult diagnoses in endocrinology. By definition, Cushing's syndrome is a multisystem disorder that develops in response to glucocorticoid excess. Iatrogenic Cushing's syndrome is common, but endogenous Cushing's syndrome is a rare condition, with an estimated incidence of 0.7 to 2.4 per million population per year. The etiology of Cushing's syndrome may be excessive adrenocorticotropic hormone (ACTH) production from the pituitary gland, ectopic ACTH secretion by nonpituitary tumors, or autonomous cortisol hypersecretion from adrenal hyperplasia or tumors (Table 1). Cushing's disease refers to the subset of Cushing's syndrome cases caused by an ACTH-producing pituitary adenoma. Cushing's disease is the most common cause of spontaneous Cushing's syndrome in almost all ages, including older children and adolescents. Approximately 20% to 30% (with the exception of very young children) of endogenous Cushing's syndrome is caused by primary adrenocortical diseases that are not ACTH-dependent. Cushing's disease and

TABLE 1	Etiology of Cushing's Syndrome in Older Children, Adolescents, and Young Adults*
SYNDROME	**% OF TOTAL**
ACTH-dependent	
Cushing's disease	60–70
Ectopic ACTH syndrome	5–10
Ectopic CRH syndrome	<1
ACTH-independent	
Adrenocortical adenoma	10–15
Adrenocortical carcinoma	5
Bilateral adrenocortical disease	5–10

*In infants and younger children, the distribution is different.
Abbreviations: ACTH = adrenocorticotropic hormone; CRH = corticotropin-releasing hormone.

adrenocortical adenomas occur more commonly in women, with a female-to-male ratio of 3–5:1.

Pathophysiology

Cortisol inhibits the biosynthesis and secretion of corticotropin-releasing hormone (CRH) and ACTH in a negative-feedback loop that is tightly controlled. The hallmark of Cushing's syndrome is the absence of suppression of cortisol levels after low-dose dexamethasone (Decadron) administration owing to autonomous ACTH secretion by a tumor or autonomous glucocorticoid production by a primary adrenocortical disease. It is essential to understand that all diagnostic testing in Cushing's syndrome relies on the disturbance of this feedback mechanism, as revealed by dexamethasone, CRH (corticorelin ovine triflutate [Acthrel]), and all related testing.

ACTH-producing pituitary adenomas are microadenomas (<1 cm in diameter) in 80% to 90% of cases. Macroadenomas are rare and often invasive, with extension outside of the sella turcica. Chronic ACTH hypersecretion commonly leads to secondary adrenocortical hyperplasia.

Ectopic ACTH secretion is most often associated with small cell lung carcinoma, which accounts for half of the cases in adult patients with Cushing's syndrome. The ectopic ACTH syndrome causes severe hypokalemia and is usually underdiagnosed in patients during advanced stages of neoplasia. Other tumors causing the syndrome are bronchial, thymic, and pancreatic carcinoids; medullary thyroid carcinoma; pheochromocytoma; or other rare neuroendocrine tumors, especially in pediatric patients.

Adrenocortical tumors are more often adenomas that are usually smaller than 5 cm. Adrenocortical carcinomas are rare but very aggressive neoplasms; they most commonly occur as large nonsecreting abdominal masses at diagnosis, and only rarely does Cushing's syndrome develop.

Up to recently, only two types of primary adrenal hyperplasias that are ACTH-independent and cause Cushing's syndrome were known: primary pigmented nodular adrenocortical disease (PPNAD) and ACTH-independent macronodular adrenocortical hyperplasia, also known as massive macronodular adrenocortical disease.

Table 2 lists no fewer than six types of bilateral adrenocortical hyperplasias. They are divided into two groups of disorders, macronodular and micronodular hyperplasias, on the basis of the size of the associated nodules. In macronodular disorders, the greatest diameter of each nodule exceeds 1 cm; in the micronodular group nodules are less than 1 cm. Although nodules less than 1 cm can occur in macronodular disease (especially the form associated with McCune-Albright syndrome), and single large tumors may be encountered in PPNAD (especially in older patients), the size criterion has biological relevance, because we rarely see a continuum in the same subject: most patients have either macronodular or micronodular hyperplasia. We use two additional basic characteristics in this classification of bilateral adrenocortical hyperplasias: presence of tumor pigment and status (hyperplasia or atrophy) of the surrounding cortex.

Pigment in adrenocortical lesions is rarely melanin; most of the pigmentation in adrenocortical adenomas and bilateral adrenocortical hyperplasias that produce cortisol is lipofuscin. The accumulation of lipofuscin-like material results from the progressive oxidation of unsaturated fatty acids by oxygen-derived free radicals in lysosomes. Lipofuscin pigmentation appears macroscopically as light brown to occasionally dark brown or even black discoloration of the tumor or hyperplastic tissue. Lipofuscin can be seen with a light microscope, but it is better detected by electron microscopy. Massive macronodular adrenocortical disease is a bilateral disease and may be caused by abnormal hormone receptor expression or activating mutations of $G_S\alpha$, which lead to stimulation of steroidogenesis. About 30% to 50% of the cases may be caused by ARMC5 mutations. Another cause of ACTH-independent Cushing's syndrome is primary pigmented nodular adrenocortical disease, usually associated with a syndrome of cardiac myxomas, lentigines, and schwannomas (Carney's complex).

TABLE 2 Bilateral Adrenal Hyperplasias Causing Cushing's Syndrome

LESION	AGE GROUP	HISTOPATHOLOGY	GENETICS	GENE, LOCUS
Macronodular Hyperplasias (Multiple Nodules >1 cm Each)				
Bilateral macroadenomatous hyperplasia	Middle age	Distinct adenomas (usually 2 or 3) with internodular atrophy	MEN1, FAP, MAS, HLRCS; isolated (AD); other	Menin, *APC,GNAS*, FH, ectopic GPCRs, ARMC5, PRKACA 5
Bilateral macroadenomatous hyperplasia of childhood	Infants, very young children	Distinct adenomas (usually 2 or 3) with internodular atrophy; occasional microadenomas	MAS	*GNAS*
ACTH-independent macronodular adrenocortical hyperplasia, also known as massive macronodular adrenocortical disease	Middle age	Adenomatous hyperplasia (multiple) with internodular hyperplasia of the zona fasciculata	Isolated, AD	Ectopic GPCRs; WISP2 and Wnt-signaling; 17q22-24, other; ARMC5, PRKACA 5
Micronodular Hyperplasias (Multiple Nodules <1 cm Each)				
Isolated primary pigmented nodular adrenocortical disease	Children; young adults	Microadenomatous hyperplasia with (mostly) internodular atrophy and nodular pigment (lipofuscin)	Isolated, AD	*PRKAR1A, PDE11A; PDE8B;* 2p16; PRKACA 5 other
Carney complex–associated primary pigmented nodular adrenocortical disease	Children; young and middle aged adults	Microadenomatous hyperplasia with (mostly) internodular atrophy and (mainly nodular) pigment (lipofuscin)	CNC (AD)	*PRKAR1A,* 2p16; other
Isolated micronodular adrenocortical disease	Mostly children; young adults	Microadenomatous, with hyperplasia of the surrounding zona fasciculata and limited or absent pigment	Isolated, AD; other	*PDE11A, PDE8B;* other; 2p12-p16, other

Abbreviations: ACTH = adrenocorticotropic hormone; AD = autosomal dominant; *APC* = adenomatous polyposis coli gene; cAMP = cyclic adenosine monophosphate; CNC = Carney complex; FAP = familial adenomatous polyposis; FH = fumarate hydratase; *GNAS* = gene coding for the stimulatory subunit alpha of the G-protein (Gsα); GPCR = G-protein-coupled receptor; HLRCS = hereditary leiomyomatosis and renal cancer syndrome; MAS = McCune–Albright syndrome; MEN1 = multiple endocrine neoplasia type 1; *PDE8B* = phosphodiesterase 8B gene; *PDE11A* = phosphodiesterase 11A gene; *PRKAR1A* = protein kinase, cAMP-dependent, regulatory, type I, alpha gene; WISP2 = Wnt1-inducible signaling pathway protein 1; Wnt = wingless-type MMTV integration site family.

TABLE 3 Clinical Manifestations of Cushing's Syndrome

SIGNS AND SYMPTOMS	INCIDENCE (%)
Central obesity	97
Plethora	89
Moon facies	89
Decreased libido	86
Atrophic skin and easy bruising	75
Decreased linear growth	70–80
Menstrual irregularities	80
Hypertension	76
Hirsutism	56
Depression or emotional lability	67
Glucose intolerance/diabetes mellitus	70
Purple striae	60
Buffalo hump	54
Osteoporosis	50
Headache	10

Clinical Manifestations

The clinical presentation of Cushing's syndrome is variable and differs in severity (Table 3). Truncal obesity is the most common clinical sign and is usually the initial manifestation in most patients. Growth failure in children is the most reliable sign of Cushing's syndrome, especially when combined with continuing weight gain. Other symptoms include central fat deposition, supraclavicular fat accumulation, buffalo hump, plethora, rounded face, purple striae, thin skin, proximal muscle weakness, hypertension, impaired glucose metabolism, gonadal dysfunction, and hirsutism (see Table 3). Diabetes mellitus and hypertension also develop. Osteoporosis, mood disorders, emotional lability and cognitive deficits are commonly observed. Proximal myopathy is common, especially in older patients. Ectopic ACTH syndrome caused by small cell lung cancer can have an unusual presentation characterized by rapid onset, severe weakness, and associated hypokalemia without classic symptoms of Cushing's syndrome. In contrast, ACTH-secreting carcinoids manifest with typical clinical manifestations.

Diagnosis

Confirmation of the Diagnosis

The initial evaluation should always include a careful clinical history and physical examination. Reliable symptoms and signs of Cushing's syndrome (see Table 3) should be present in any patient who undergoes evaluation for Cushing's syndrome; patients with no reliable symptoms and signs of Cushing's syndrome should not be investigated, as this often leads to unnecessary, extensive, and expensive testing. It is essential to investigate the use of exogenous glucocorticoids and other conditions that may be associated with mild hypercortisolism, such as alcoholism, anorexia nervosa, severe depression, and morbid obesity; these are pseudo-Cushing's states and are often difficult to exclude, especially in older or chronically ill patients.

The first task in the work-up of any patient is documentation of hypercortisolism. On an outpatient basis, this is typically done through the urinary free cortisol test. This is the most cost-effective and reliable outpatient screening test. We typically recommend collections over two or three consecutive days so that we avoid errors due to over- or undercollection that are not uncommon with single 24-hour studies. The results of the test need to be corrected for body surface area, as long as total creatinine excretion is normal. A 1-mg overnight dexamethasone test is less useful and more expensive, but it provides a good alternative for patients in whom urinary collection is impossible or unreliable. During these screening tests for hypercortisolism, patients should avoid any activation of the hypothalamic-pituitary-adrenal axis by stress, especially physical. The baseline measurements may be repeated as needed, because cyclic hypercortisolism often precedes overt Cushing's syndrome (Figure 1).

A 24-hour urinary free cortisol excretion of greater than 250 nmol per 24 hours (90 µg/24 hours measured by radioimmunoassay) is highly specific for the diagnosis of hypercortisolism. However, pseudo-Cushing's states are often associated with abnormal levels of 24-hour urinary free cortisol. Administration of 1 mg dexamethasone (15 µg/kg for children) at 11 PM results in suppression of the hypothalamic-pituitary-adrenal axis in normal persons and a fall in plasma and urinary cortisol levels. At 8 AM, serum cortisol should be less than 50 nmol/L (1.8 µg/dL). Unfortunately, dexamethasone is primarily metabolized by the cytochrome P-450 (CYP) system; several drugs, such as phenobarbital, carbamazepine (Tegretol), and rifampicin (Rifadin), that induce the activity of CYP3A4 can lead to false-positive tests. Oral contraceptives also interfere with serum cortisol levels owing to an increase in corticosteroid-binding globulin and by increasing dexamethasone metabolism. The test can only be interpreted if the serum dexamethasone levels reach the expected range; however, this additional requirement can make the test significantly more cumbersome and expensive.

Once hypercortisolism is suspected by the urinary free cortisol or the overnight dexamethasone test, the patient may undergo testing of the cortisol diurnal rhythm. The lack of circadian rhythm of cortisol is the earliest consistent biochemical abnormality of Cushing's syndrome, even in situations of cyclic or other atypical forms of Cushing's syndrome. Serum or salivary cortisol levels at midnight may be used for this test. Normally, the level of serum cortisol begins to rise at 3 to 4 AM and reaches a peak at 7 to 8 AM, falling during the day. A sleeping midnight serum cortisol level lower than 50 nmol/L (1.8 µg/dL) excludes the diagnosis of Cushing's syndrome, whereas a midnight serum cortisol higher than 207 nmol/L (7.5 µg/dL) is highly suggestive of Cushing's syndrome. This test does require inpatient admission. Salivary cortisol levels have an excellent correlation with serum cortisol levels and offer an easy and convenient outpatient way of evaluating circadian rhythm; saliva is also stable at room temperature (for up to 7 days). Midnight salivary cortisol levels greater than 3.6 nmol/L (0.13 µg/dL) have a sensitivity and specificity of approximately 95% for the diagnosis of Cushing's syndrome (see Figure 1).

After the biochemical confirmation of hypercortisolism, the next step is to investigate the source (see Figure 1). Baseline ACTH plasma levels greater than 2 to 5 pmol/L (>20–25 pg/mL) are diagnostic of ACTH-dependent Cushing's syndrome. On the other hand, undetectable ACTH levels (<1 pmol/L or 5 pg/mL) indicate a primary autonomous adrenocortical disease. Values in between should be further investigated with dynamic testing.

High-Dose Dexamethasone Testing

Oral dexamethasone is administered as 2 mg every 6 hours for 48 hours or as a single 8 mg (120 µg/kg for children) overnight dose. Urinary and serum cortisol levels are suppressed by more than 50% in most patients with Cushing's disease.

Corticotropin-Releasing Hormone Testing

Synthetic ovine CRH (corticorelin ovine triflutate [Acthrel]) or human[1] CRH is administered intravenously (100 µg), and plasma ACTH and cortisol levels are measured at 15-minute intervals during the next 60 minutes. Patients with Cushing's disease typically have an increase in ACTH or cortisol level of 35% and 22%, respectively. This test has a sensitivity of approximately 85% for the diagnosis of Cushing's disease, but it is often falsely positive in patients

[1]Not FDA approved for this indication.

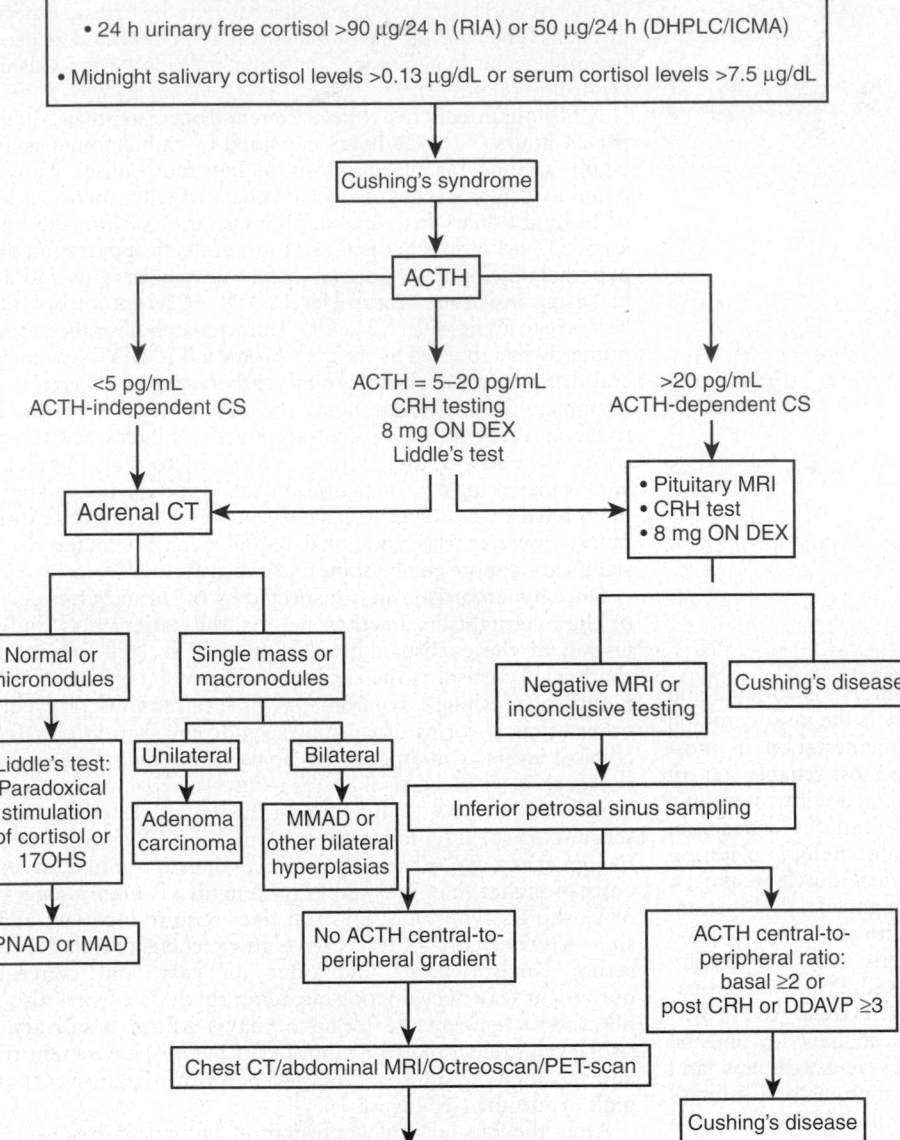

Screening

- Post-1 mg ON DEX 8 AM serum cortisol >1.8 µg/dL
- 24 h urinary free cortisol >90 µg/24 h (RIA) or 50 µg/24 h (DHPLC/ICMA)
- Midnight salivary cortisol levels >0.13 µg/dL or serum cortisol levels >7.5 µg/dL

Cushing's syndrome

ACTH

<5 pg/mL
ACTH-independent CS

ACTH = 5–20 pg/mL
CRH testing
8 mg ON DEX
Liddle's test

>20 pg/mL
ACTH-dependent CS

Adrenal CT

- Pituitary MRI
- CRH test
- 8 mg ON DEX

Normal or micronodules

Single mass or macronodules

Negative MRI or inconclusive testing

Cushing's disease

Liddle's test: Paradoxical stimulation of cortisol or 17OHS

Unilateral

Bilateral

Adenoma carcinoma

MMAD or other bilateral hyperplasias

Inferior petrosal sinus sampling

PPNAD or MAD

No ACTH central-to-peripheral gradient

ACTH central-to-peripheral ratio: basal ≥2 or post CRH or DDAVP ≥3

Chest CT/abdominal MRI/Octreoscan/PET-scan

Cushing's disease

Ectopic ACTH-secreting tumor

Figure 1. Algorithm for evaluating patients with Cushing's syndrome. *Abbreviations:* ACTH = adrenocorticotropic hormone; CRH = corticotropin-releasing hormone; CS = Cushing's syndrome; CT = computed tomography; DDAVP = desmopressin; DHPLC = denaturing high-performance liquid chromatography; ICMA = immunochemiluminometric assay; MAD = micronodular disease; MMAD = massive macronodular adrenocortical disease; MRI = magnetic resonance imaging; 17OHS = 17-hydroxysteroids; ON DEX = overnight dexamethasone; PET = positron emission tomography; PPNAD = primary pigmented nodular adrenocortical disease; RIA = radioimmunoassay.

with adrenal, ACTH-independent Cushing's syndrome, who do not have a fully suppressed hypothalamic-pituitary-adrenal axis.

Inferior Petrosal Sinus Sampling

None of the noninvasive tests are 100% accurate in distinguishing pituitary (Cushing's disease) from ectopic sources of ACTH. Inferior petrosal sinus sampling (IPSS) is indicated in all cases where an ACTH-dependent source of hypercortisolism is expected but the diagnosis of Cushing's disease versus an ectopic source remains uncertain. Typically, IPSS is done when the ovine CRH and dexamethasone tests are in disagreement or when the pituitary imaging by magnetic resonance imaging (MRI) is negative. An ACTH gradient of central-to-peripheral ACTH levels of 2 or more suggests Cushing's disease. When ovine CRH, human CRH, or desmopressin (DDAVP) testing is performed during IPSS, the diagnostic accuracy of IPSS increases. After ovine CRH stimulation, a central-to-peripheral ratio of ACTH levels of 3 or more suggest the diagnosis of Cushing's disease with specificity and sensitivity greater than 95%. The test is less useful for suggesting the tumor location (right versus left side of the pituitary gland).

Imaging Studies
Pituitary Magnetic Resonance Imaging
Unfortunately, less than 50% of ACTH-producing pituitary adenomas are detectable with MRI, even with the use of contrast enhancement. Typically, we recommend against obtaining an MRI until ACTH dependency is established, because as many as 20% of the patients have an incidental pituitary microadenoma. To avoid false-negative and false-positive imaging, several centers have sought improved methods for MRI detection of ACTH-producing tumors. Our studies demonstrated that postcontrast spoiled gradient-recalled acquisition (SPGR) MRI in addition to the conventional T1-weighted spin echo was superior to conventional MRI for the diagnostic evaluation of corticotropinomas in both children and adults.

Adrenal Imaging
Computed tomography (CT) and MRI are used to investigate adrenal disease in patients with ACTH-independent Cushing's syndrome. Adrenal tumors larger than 6 cm are highly suspicious for adrenocortical carcinomas. The fat content contributes to the

differentiation between benign and malignant adrenal tumors. Measurement of Hounsfield units (HU) in unenhanced CT is of great value in differentiating malignant from benign adrenal lesions. Adrenal lesions with an attenuation value of more than 10 HU in unenhanced CT or an enhancement washout of less than 50% and a delayed attenuation of more than 35 HU (on 10- to 15-min delayed enhanced CT) are suspicious for malignancy. MRI with dynamic gadolinium-enhanced and chemical shift technique is as effective as CT in distinguishing malignant from benign lesions. However, MRI is much less useful for detecting adrenal nodularity owing to motion artifacts. Thus, especially for detecting small unilateral adrenocortical adenomas or bilateral micronodular hyperplasia, we recommend a dedicated (thin-sliced) adrenal CT rather than MRI.

Ectopic Adrenocorticotropic Hormone Syndrome

High Resolution Chest-CT 7 and abdominal MRI are the recommended imaging procedures in patients with an IPSS that indicates a nonpituitary ACTH-producing source. Additionally, somatostatin receptor scintigraphy is a useful and complementary tool in the evaluation of patients with ectopic ACTH-dependent Cushing's syndrome. Recent studies have demonstrated a higher sensitivity of somatostatin receptor scintigraphy in comparison to CT or MRI for diagnosing occult ectopic tumors. Additional methods include PET-CT and FDG scans.

Treatment

Untreated chronic hypercortisolism is associated with high morbidity and mortality owing to diabetes mellitus, hypertension, cardiovascular disease, thromboembolism, and suppression of the immune system. Cushing's syndrome should be treated effectively; patients should be closely monitored to rapidly detect recurrent disease.

Treatment of Pituitary Corticotropinomas
Transsphenoidal Pituitary Surgery

The initial therapy of choice for patients with Cushing's disease is transsphenoidal surgery. This procedure is associated with low mortality and morbidity, but complications can include cerebrospinal fluid leaks, meningitis, hypopituitarism, and venous thromboembolism. The success rate for transsphenoidal surgery varies between 60% and 80%, but in experienced centers can be as high as 90% to 95%. Relapses are rare when surgery is performed in an experienced tertiary care center; it can be as high as 30% in less-experienced centers. Postoperative morning serum cortisol levels of less than 50 nmol/L (2 μg/dL) are highly predictive of remission and a low recurrence rate of less than 10% at 10 years.

After successful transsphenoidal surgery, glucocorticoid replacement therapy (hydrocortisone at 12–15 mg/m²/day; 20–30 mg daily in adults) is mandatory until the hypothalamic-pituitary-adrenal axis recovers from the chronic exposure to glucocorticoid excess; this usually takes place within a year after surgery. For recurrent disease, the choice of second-line therapy remains controversial. Repeat surgery can be successful when residual tumor is detectable on MRI imaging, but it carries a high risk of hypopituitarism. Irradiation is recommended in most cases where a tumor is not seen on MRI.

Radiotherapy

Radiotherapy has been used to suppress pituitary secretion of ACTH, but its success rate is variable (50% in some series). It can take as long as 5 years for a full effect; hypopituitarism develops in more than 70% of the patients over a period of 10 to 20 years after the therapy is completed. Stereotactic radiosurgery with gamma knife is associated with a more-rapid effect and a lower risk of hypopituitarism, but it has not been extensively studied.

Medical Treatment to Control Secretion of Adrenocorticotropic Hormone

Cushing's disease responds to the dopamine agonist cabergoline (Dostinex)[1] with a normalization of cortisol production in as many as 40% of the cases. The peroxisome proliferator-activated receptor γ (PPAR-γ) agonist rosiglitazone (Avandia) was demonstrated to be effective in animal models, but it was unsuccessful in controlling ACTH oversecretion in patients with Cushing's disease. A new agent, SOM-230 (pasireotide),[2] blocks both type 2 and type 5 somatostatin receptors and reduces ACTH secretion in vitro. Mifepristone, a glucocorticoid receptor antagonist, recently became available for patients who failed surgical or irradiation therapies (see also below).

Bilateral Adrenalectomy

Bilateral adrenalectomy offers a definitive treatment that provides immediate control of hypercortisolism, but this surgery should be reserved for patients with Cushing's disease who have failed all other treatments. Bilateral adrenalectomy in active Cushing's disease often leads to Nelson's syndrome, a condition characterized by unabated progression of a corticotropinoma (owing to the lack of negative feedback by cortisol), very high ACTH levels, and high morbidity.

Treatment of Adrenal Disease
Adrenocortical Tumors

For adrenocortical tumors, the recommended treatment is surgical. Laparoscopic adrenalectomy has become the treatment of choice for benign adrenal lesions with a diameter of less than 6 cm. In stages I to III adrenocortical carcinoma, complete tumor removal by a well-trained surgeon offers by far the best chance for cure. Surgery often needs to be extensive, with en bloc resection of invaded organs, and regularly includes lymphadenectomy. Surgery for local recurrences or metastatic disease is accepted as a valuable therapeutic option and was associated with improved survival in retrospective studies. The overall 5-year survival in different series ranged between 16% and 38%. Median survival for metastatic disease (stage IV) at the time of diagnosis is still consistently less than 12 months.

Radiotherapy has been considered ineffective for treatment of adrenocortical cancer, but it can be indicated to control localized disease not amenable to surgery.

Mitotane (o,p'-DDD [Lysodren]) is the only adrenal-specific agent available for treating adrenocortical cancer. Mitotane is indicated in metastatic adrenocortical carcinoma and can also be used as an adjuvant for tumors with a high risk of recurrence. Mitotane exerts a specific cytotoxic effect on adrenocortical cells, leading to focal degeneration of the fascicular and particularly the reticular zone. In most patients, treatment should be initiated with a dose that does not exceed 1.5 g/day; this is then rapidly increased, depending on gastrointestinal symptoms, to 5 to 6 g/day. This high-dose regimen requires measurement of mitotane blood levels 14 days after initiation of therapy. The dose is then adjusted according to the medicine's plasma concentrations (which should be greater than 14 mg/L) and tolerance of the side effects. Because mitotane treatment induces adrenal insufficiency and increases the metabolic clearance of glucocorticoids, glucocorticoid replacement is indicated, often at higher than normal doses owing to increased clearance.

Cytotoxic Chemotherapy

Cytotoxic chemotherapy includes etoposide (VePesid),[1] doxorubicin (Adriamycin),[1] and cisplatin (Platinol),[1] or streptozocin (Zanosar)[1] plus mitotane. Chemotherapy has limited efficacy for advanced adrenocortical cancer and is associated mainly with partial responses.

Bilateral Adrenal Hyperplasias

The treatment of choice for bilateral adrenal hyperplasias associated with ACTH-independent Cushing's syndrome is bilateral adrenalectomy. Patients require lifelong replacement therapy with

---

[1]Not FDA approved for this indication.
[2]Not available in the United States.

TABLE 4	Medical Treatment for Hypercortisolism		
MEDICATION	**INITIAL DOSE**	**MAXIMUM DOSE**	**ADVERSE EFFECTS**
Ketoconazole (Nizoral)[1]	100–200 mg bid/tid	1200 mg	Nausea, vomiting, abdominal pain, weakness, hypothyroidism, gynecomastia, hepatotoxicity, hypertriglyceridemia
Metyrapone (Metopirone)[1]	250 mg qid	6000 mg	Headache, alopecia, hirsutism, acne, nausea, abdominal discomfort, hypertension, weakness, leucopenia
Mitotane (Lysodren)[1]	500 mg tid	9000 mg	Nausea, vomiting, anorexia, diarrhea, ataxia, confusion, skin rash, hepatotoxicity
Aminoglutethimide (Cytadren)	250 mg qid	2000 mg/d	Lethargy, nausea, anorexia, hypothyroidism, somnolence

[1]Not FDA approved for this indication.

glucocorticoids and mineralocorticoids, and they should be adequately educated about the risk of acute adrenal insufficiency.

Treatment of Ectopic Corticotropin Syndrome

The choice of treatment for ectopic ACTH syndrome depends on tumor identification, localization, and classification. The most effective treatment option is surgical resection, although this is not always possible in metastatic disease or in the case of occult tumors. Because the ectopic ACTH syndrome is usually severe and occult tumors can become evident at imaging studies only during the follow-up, medical treatment to control hypercortisolism is often necessary. Bilateral adrenalectomy may be an option to be considered when the hypercortisolism cannot be controlled by other treatment options.

Medical Adrenalectomy

Several drugs that inhibit steroid synthesis are often effective for rapidly controlling hypercortisolism in preparation for surgery, after unsuccessful transsphenoidal surgery or removal of an adrenal tumor such as extensive cancer, or while awaiting the full effect of radiotherapy in recurrent Cushing's disease (Table 4).

Most experience with inhibitors of steroidogenesis has been with metyrapone (Metopirone)[1] and ketoconazole (Nizoral),[1] two medications that appear to be more effective and better tolerated than aminoglutethimide (Cytadren). Metyrapone reduces cortisol and aldosterone production by inhibiting 11β-hydroxylation in the adrenal cortex. Ketoconazole is a broad-spectrum antifungal drug, which inhibits c17-20 desmolase, cholesterol side-chain cleavage, and 11β-hydroxylation. Ketoconazole is also associated with inhibition of testosterone biosynthesis and gynecomastia.

RU-486, or mifepristone (Korlym), is an antagonist of the progesterone and glucocorticoid receptors. Unexpectedly, the treatment of Cushing's disease with this glucocorticoid antagonist has been associated with increased ACTH secretion and consequent stimulation of cortisol production. RU-486 may be more useful in ectopic ACTH-producing tumors and in adrenal Cushing's syndrome, but its efficacy and potential side effects when administered chronically are currently unknown.

---

[1]Not FDA approved for this indication.

References

Allolio B, Fassnacht M. Clinical review: Adrenocortical carcinoma: Clinical update. J Clin Endocrinol Metab 2006;91:2027–37.

Assié G, Libé R, Espiard S, et al. ARMC5 mutations in macronodular adrenal hyperplasia with Cushing's syndrome. N Engl J Med 2013;369(22):2105–14.

Batista D, Courkoutsakis NA, Oldfield EH, et al. Detection of adrenocorticotropin-secreting pituitary adenomas by magnetic resonance imaging in children and adolescents with Cushing disease. J Clin Endocrinol Metab 2005;90:5134–40.

Batista DL, Riar J, Keil M, Stratakis CA. Diagnostic tests for children who are referred for the investigation of Cushing syndrome. Pediatrics 2007;120:e575–e586.

Bertagna X, Guignat L, Groussin L, Bertherat J. Cushing's disease. Best Pract Res Clin Endocrinol Metab 2009;23:607–23.

Biller BM, Grossman AB, Stewart PM, et al. Treatment of adrenocorticotropin-dependent Cushing's syndrome: A consensus statement. J Clin Endocrinol Metab 2008;93:2454–62.

Boscaro M, Arnaldi G. Approach to the patient with possible Cushing's syndrome. J Clin Endocrinol Metab 2009;94:3121–31.

Feelders RA, Hofland LJ. Medical treatment of Cushing's disease. J Clin Endocrinol Metab 2013;98(2):425–38.

Newell-Price J, Trainer P, Besser M, Grossman A. The diagnosis and differential diagnosis of Cushing's syndrome and pseudo-Cushing's states. Endocr Rev 1998;19:647–72.

Terzolo M, Angeli A, Fassnacht M, et al. Adjuvant mitotane treatment for adrenocortical carcinoma. N Engl J Med 2007;356:2372–80.

DIABETES INSIPIDUS

Method of
Rami Mortada, MD

CURRENT DIAGNOSIS

- Diabetes insipidus (DI) is a disorder of excess urine production (i.e., "diabetes") that is dilute and tasteless (i.e., "insipidus"). DI contrasts with the concentrated and sweet urine in diabetes mellitus.
- Patients with DI present with polyuria and polydipsia; urine output is usually more than 40 mL/kg/day or more than 3 L/day.
- There are three subtypes of DI:
  - Central DI: due to relative or absolute lack of vasopressin
  - Nephrogenic DI: due to partial or total resistance to the renal antidiuretic effects of vasopressin
  - Dipsogenic DI (also called primary polydipsia): where polyuria is secondary to excessive, inappropriate fluid intake
- Initial labs should include plasma sodium and urine osmolality. Under normal physiologic conditions, the urine osmolality is less than 300 mOsm/L, but if the patient does not have sufficient fluid intake, the urine osmolality can be higher.
- The diagnosis is confirmed by examining urine output and osmolality. It can be followed by an assessment of renal response to the synthetic arginine vasopressin (AVP) analogue desmopressin (DDAVP).
- In primary polydipsia, urine concentration is normal in response to dehydration.
- In central DI, urine concentration does not increase appropriately with dehydration, but does respond to desmopressin (DDAVP). After dehydration in central DI, urine osmolality remains <300 mOsm/kg, and plasma osmolality is >290 mOsm/kg. Urine osmolality rises to >750 mOsm/kg after desmopressin.
- In nephrogenic DI, urine concentration does not increase appropriately with either dehydration or exogenous desmopressin.

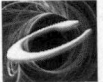

CURRENT THERAPY

- The treatment goal is to control polyuria and ensure electrolyte stability.
- In Central DI:
  - The mild form might not require treatment.

- Significant polyuria can be treated with desmopressin in divided doses: nasal spray 5 to 100 mcg/day; tablets 100 to 1000 mcg/day; or parenterally 0.1 to 2.0 mcg/day.
  - Overtreatment can cause hyponatremia.
- In Nephrogenic DI:
  - Urine output should not be expected to normalize after DDAVP administration.
  - Correct the culprit cause (hypercalcemia or lithium [Eskalith, Lithobid] cessation).
  - Follow a low-sodium, low-protein diet, as tolerated.
  - Hydrochlorothiazide[1] 25 to 50 mg/day may be taken either alone or in combination with indomethacin (Indocin) 25 to 50 mg twice daily.
  - Symptoms may respond partly to high-dose desmopressin (e.g., 4 mcg IM twice daily).
- Primary polydipsia is treated by limiting an excessive fluid intake.

[1]Not FDA approved for this indication.

Physiology of Antidiuretic Hormone

Arginine vasopressin (AVP), also known as antidiuretic hormone (ADH), is a neurohypophysial hormone. It is a peptide hormone that promotes water retention by increasing the permeability of the kidney's collecting duct and distal convoluted tubule to water. It also increases peripheral vascular resistance, which in turn increases arterial blood pressure. In the clinical setting, the terms AVP, ADH, and vasopressin are used interchangeably.

Vasopressin is considered the main hormone involved in the regulation of water homeostasis and osmolality. The regulation and synthesis of vasopressin is under the influence of two systems: osmotic and pressure/volume status. In the case of osmoregulation, a small increase in plasma osmolality produces a parallel increase in vasopressin secretion; a small decrease in plasma osmolality causes a parallel drop in vasopressin.

Vasopressin is one among other hormones and systems that are involved in the regulation of volume and blood pressure. Other factors influence vasopressin production. For example, glucocorticoids inhibit secretion, whereas nausea and vomiting have a stimulatory effect.

Pathophysiology of Diabetes Insipidus

The kidneys exercise one of their urine-concentrating abilities by promoting water retention. If the concentration of vasopressin is decreased, polyuria occurs and diluted urine is excreted. A decrease in total body water results in an increase in the plasma osmolality. If the physiologic response is intact, thirst is stimulated, which leads to an increase in water consumption and the correction of plasma osmolarity. Therefore, unless there is a dysregulation in the thirst mechanisms or water consumption is limited due to a lack of availability (e.g., decreased level of consciousness, immobility, or physical restraints) severe dehydration does not develop.

Clinical Causes

There are three subtypes of diabetes insipidus (DI).
- DI secondary to excess water intake (primary polydipsia)

  Primary polydipsia is a disorder characterized by inappropriate excess fluid intake due to a disordered thirst sensation seen mostly in patients with psychiatric illnesses. A central defect in thirst regulation plays an important role in the pathogenesis of primary polydipsia. Such patients continue drinking even if the plasma osmolality falls below normal. It is not easy to achieve or maintain a low plasma osmolality because vasopressin secretion will normally be suppressed by the fall in plasma osmolality, resulting in rapid excretion of the excess water. If vasopressin regulation is intact, primary polydipsia should not lead to clinically important disturbances in the plasma sodium concentration unless hyposmolar fluid intake overwhelms the kidneys' ability to excrete excess water. Thus, the serum sodium concentration is usually normal or slightly reduced in primary polydipsia. These patients may be asymptomatic or present with complaints of polydipsia and polyuria. In rare circumstances where water intake exceeds the kidneys' ability to excrete the water load of about 500 mL/hour, symptomatic severe hyponatremia might result in severe psychosis. Psychosis from hyponatremia in primary polydipsia is most commonly seen in institutionalized patients or in individuals attempting to dilute their urine to avoid a positive urine drug test.
- DI secondary to a decrease in or absence of vasopressin secretion (central DI)

  Central DI may be caused by genetic anomalies of the vasopressin gene (Table 1). Familial neurohypophyseal DI is characterized by the onset of DI with polyuria and polydipsia in childhood or early adulthood. The most common MRI finding in familial neurohypophyseal DI is the progressive disappearance of the posterior pituitary bright spot in children. The normal pituitary bright spot seen on unenhanced T1-weighted MRI is thought to result from the T1-shortening effect of the vasopressin stored in the posterior pituitary. The disappearance of the bright spot corresponds to the disappearance of vasopressin stores in the posterior pituitary. Wolfram's syndrome is a rare autosomal recessive syndrome manifested by DI, diabetes mellitus, optic atrophy, and deafness.

  Central DI may be caused by mass lesions of the neurohypophysis, such as craniopharyngiomas, and primary germ cell tumors in childhood. DI can be the initial presentation. MRI often shows a thickened pituitary stalk and may show a hypothalamic mass. Metastasis to the pituitary usually is found with widespread metastatic disease and is twice as likely to involve the posterior pituitary than the anterior pituitary. DI can be associated with pituitary infiltration associated with lymphomas and leukemias.

  In granulomatous disease that affects the hypothalamic-pituitary axis, there is usually clear evidence of disease elsewhere in the body. MRI shows an absence of the pituitary bright spot and widening of the hypothalamic-pituitary stalk. Lymphocytic infundibuloneurohypophysitis is a new, well-recognized cause of autoimmune DI, characterized by MRI appearance of a thickened hypothalamic-pituitary stalk and large posterior pituitary gland mimicking a pituitary tumor. Pituitary abscess is a rare cause of pituitary mass and DI. In situations where the cause is not easily diagnosed, an autoimmune process should be suspected. In some patients, the cause is idiopathic.

  Central DI may be caused by surgery or trauma to the pituitary region. Vasopressin is normally secreted after any kind of surgical stress, and secretion is more pronounced after surgery to the pituitary region. Only a small percentage of patients undergoing pituitary surgery have permanent DI. A triphasic DI can occur after complete hypothalamic-pituitary stalk transection. The first phase is polyuric and appears within the first 24 hours after surgery. It is thought to be secondary to axonal shock with a resultant inability to release prefabricated vasopressin. The second phase is antidiuretic and starts on about

TABLE 1	Central Diabetes Insipidus (DI) Etiologies
Idiopathic	Unknown etiology
Genetic	Familial neurohypophyseal DI, Wolfram's syndrome (autosomal recessive)
Mass effect	Craniopharyngiomas, primary germ cell tumors, metastatic tumors
Infiltrative diseases	Lymphoma, leukemia, sarcoidosis, amyloidosis
Autoimmune	Lymphocytic infundibuloneurohypophysitis
Trauma	Motor vehicle accident, closed head trauma
Surgical	Surgical intervention at the pituitary region

day 6, after stalk injury. It is thought to be secondary to the unregulated release of vasopressin stores. The third phase, also polyuric, starts about day 12, after vasopressin stores have been depleted. It may result in permanent or partial DI or resolve to clinically asymptomatic disease.

The same patterns of DI that occur after pituitary surgery can be seen in patients who experience a closed head trauma. Three-quarters of traumatic induced DI are secondary to motor vehicle accidents. Trauma is usually severe and causes unconsciousness. There is a high association of anterior pituitary deficiency in association with DI induced by head trauma, so the possibility of central hypocortisolism should be considered and treated immediately. DI is reported in 50% to 90% of patients with brain death.

- DI secondary to the lack of renal response to vasopressin (nephrogenic DI)

Genetic anomalies resulting in a lack of renal response to vasopressin are caused by either a mutation in the V2 receptors or a mutation of the aquaporin 2 water channels gene. The majority of the cases are X-linked recessive disorders in males. Newborns present with polyuria, vomiting, constipation, and failure to thrive. Symptoms usually occur within the first week of life.

Acquired nephrogenic DI can be caused by a kidney disease that distorts the architecture of the kidney and impairs its urine-concentrating ability (e.g., polycystic kidney disease, sickle cell disease). Decreased function of vasopressin or downregulation of aquaporin 2 channels can be caused by hypokalemia, hypercalcemia, and relief of bilateral urinary tract obstruction. Drugs such as lithium (the most common cause of drug-induced nephrogenic DI) and demeclocycline (used clinically to treat a syndrome of inappropriate ADH secretion) may cause nephrogenic DI.

Clinical Manifestations

Patients with central DI typically present with polyuria, nocturia, and polydipsia. The serum sodium concentration in untreated central DI is often in the high normal range, which provides the ongoing stimulation of thirst that replaces urinary water losses. Moderate to severe hypernatremia can develop when thirst is impaired or if there is a lack of access to free water, such as the postoperative period in patients with unrecognized DI or infants with DI. For uncertain pathophysiologic reasons, patients with central DI may develop decreased bone mineral density at the lumbar spine and femoral neck, even if treated with desmopressin.

Nephrogenic DI in its mild form can be asymptomatic. Patients with moderate to severe nephrogenic DI, as with central DI, typically present with polyuria, nocturia, and polydipsia.

Primary polydipsia is the result of an abnormal compulsion to drink water. This disorder is most often seen in middle-aged women and in patients with psychiatric illnesses. The excessive water intake initially drives the excessive urination.

Diagnosis

Polyuria must be distinguished from simple urinary frequency in the absence of excess urine volume. The initial diagnostic approach should be to confirm polyuria, defined as greater than 30 mL/kg or 3 L/day, with a urine osmolality measuring less than 300 mOsm/L. Simple metabolic causes such as hyperglycemia,

uremia, and hypercalcemia should be excluded. A definitive diagnosis of DI requires testing of vasopressin production and action in response to osmolar stress. All forms of DI may be partial or complete. In primary polydipsia, the plasma sodium, blood urea nitrogen (BUN), and uric acid are relatively low. In other forms of DI, the plasma sodium and uric acid are relatively high and the BUN is relatively low.

Central DI usually has an abrupt onset resulting from destruction of more than 80% of vasopressin-secreting hypothalamic neurons. The etiology of polyuria is not always evident after history and lab tests are completed. In that case, a water restriction test (e.g., dehydration test or water deprivation test) is completed. The water deprivation test is an indirect assessment of the AVP axis, measuring renal concentrating capacity in response to dehydration. It can be followed by assessment of the renal response to the synthetic AVP analogue desmopressin to determine whether any defect identified in urine-concentrating ability can be corrected with AVP-replacement. Office testing is acceptable unless the patient cannot be watched closely. No food or water is allowed. The patient is watched for signs of dehydration and surreptitious water drinking. Baseline measurements include weight, plasma osmolality, sodium, BUN, glucose, and urine volume and osmolality. Weight, plasma osmolality, and urine osmolality are measured hourly. The test is ended if urine osmolality has not increased to more than 300 mOsm/kg for 3 consecutive hours, plasma osmolality has reached 295 to 300 mOsm/kg, or the patient has lost 3% to 5% of body weight. All initial measurements are repeated at the end of the water restriction test. Then, 5 units of aqueous AVP (Pitressin) is administered or 2 mcg of desmopressin is given subcutaneously and the plasma osmolality, sodium, BUN, glucose, and urine volume and osmolality are measured at 30, 60, and 120 minutes.

In primary polydipsia, urine concentration is normal in response to dehydration (Table 2).

In central DI, urine concentration does not increase appropriately with dehydration, but responds to desmopressin. Urine osmolality remains <300 mOsm/kg, accompanied by plasma osmolality >290 mOsm/kg after dehydration, and urine osmolality rising to >750 mOsm/kg after desmopressin administration.

In nephrogenic DI, urine concentration does not increase appropriately with either dehydration or exogenous desmopressin.

In practice, many results are indeterminate. If central DI is suspected, but the water deprivation test data are inconclusive, a reasonable approach is a therapeutic trial of 10 to 20 mcg intranasal desmopressin per day with close monitoring of plasma sodium. If the diagnosis is confirmed, pituitary function testing and cranial MRI should follow.

Treatment

The treatment goal is to improve polyuria and polydipsia symptoms while attempting to treat the etiologic factors (Table 3). This is achieved by appropriate correction of dehydration, if present, and replacing vasopressin or augmenting its effect on the target tissue.

Mild forms of central DI may not require pharmacological treatment. Desmopressin effectively treats polyuria and polydipsia. Desmopressin comes in different forms and dosages usually need to be divided.

TABLE 2 Values Before and After Water Restriction

	INITIAL PLASMA OSMOLALITY	INITIAL PLASMA SODIUM	POSTTEST URINE/ PLASMA OSMOLALITY	POSTTEST URINE/PLASMA OSMOLALITY + ADH
Normal	NL	NL	>1	>1
Central DI	High (high NL)	High (high NL)	<1	>1
Nephrogenic DI	High (high NL)	High (high NL)	<1	<1
Primary polydipsia	Low (low NL)	Low (low NL)	>1	>1

TABLE 3	Treatment Options for Diabetes Insipidus
Central DI	Divide doses of two to three times per day: Desmopressin nasal spray 5–100 mcg/d Desmopressin tablets 0.1–1 mg/d Desmopressin injection 0.1–2 mcg/d
Nephrogenic DI	Low-salt, low-protein diet HCTZ[1] 25 mg one to two times per day Indomethacin[1] 25–50 mg bid Amiloride[1] 5–10 mg bid
Primary polydipsia	Water restriction to less than 1.5 L/d

[1]Not FDA approved for this indication.

Hyponatremia from plasma dilution can be avoided by skipping treatment for a short period on a regular basis (e.g., on Sunday). No second dose of desmopressin should be given unless the patient has urine output after the first dose.

Nephrogenic DI may respond to the removal of the offending agent (e.g., lithium) or correction of the underlying electrolyte disturbance (e.g., hypercalcemia or hypokalemia). Drug-induced nephrogenic DI, however, may persist after discontinuation of the drug.

Patients should be instructed to eat a low-sodium, low-protein diet, resulting in a decrease in urine output secondary to the drop in solute excretion. If symptomatic polyuria persists, hydrochlorothiazide[1] can be started. Hydrochlorothiazide presumably acts by inducing mild hypovolemia that induces an increase in proximal sodium and water reabsorption, thereby diminishing water delivery to the vasopressin-sensitive sites in the collecting tubules and reducing the urine output. Indomethacin (Indocin[1]) is an add-on medication if there is not enough response. Given that prostaglandins antagonize the action of vasopressin, indomethacin inhibits renal prostaglandin synthesis and subsequently decreases urine output.

Amiloride (Midamor)[1] might be more effective for lithium-induced nephrogenic DI. This drug closes the sodium channels in the luminal membrane of the collecting tubule cells. These channels constitute the mechanism by which filtered lithium normally enters the collecting tubule cells and interferes with the collecting tubule response to ADH.

The approach to primary polydipsia treatment is reduction in fluid intake. Desmopressin treatment should be avoided due to the risk of hyponatremia.

Monitoring

Primary polydipsia is the most challenging of all types of DI to treat. It requires a multidisciplinary approach that frequently demands medical and psychiatric involvement.

In central DI, patients will require frequent follow-up to adjust desmopressin dosing. Once stable, patients can be seen less frequently to assess symptom control and to check plasma sodium levels to avoid overtreatment resulting in hyponatremia.

In nephrogenic DI, after the precipitating agent has been withdrawn, follow-up is needed to assess the reversibility of polyuria. If acquired nephrogenic DI becomes irreversible, patients might require prolonged pharmacological treatment. In both central and nephrogenic DI, the patient is advised to wear a medical alert bracelet stating the disease and the potential complications.

Acknowledgment

I would like to thank K. James Kallail, PhD, for his contribution to the final editing of this chapter.

References

Bockenhauer D, Bichet DG. Inherited secondary nephrogenic diabetes insipidus: Concentrating on humans. Am J Physiol Renal Physiol 2013;304:F1037–42.
Crowley RK, Sherlock M, Agha A, et al. Clinical insights into adipsic diabetes insipidus: A large case series. Clin Endocrinol (Oxf) 2007;66:475–82.

[1]Not FDA approved for this indication.

Fujiwara TM, Bichet DG. Molecular biology of hereditary diabetes insipidus. J Am Soc Nephrol 2005;16:2836–46.
Hannon MJ, Sherlock M, Thompson CJ. Pituitary dysfunction following traumatic brain injury or subarachnoid haemorrhage. Best Pract Res Clin Endocrinol Metab 2011;25:783–98.
Monnens L, Jonkman A, Thomas C. Response to indomethacin and hydrochlorothiazide in nephrogenic diabetes insipidus. Clin Sci (Lond) 1984;66:709–15.
Oiso Y, Robertson GL, Nørgaard JP, Juul KV. Clinical review: Treatment of neurohypophyseal diabetes insipidus. J Clin Endocrinol Metab 2013;98:3958–67.
Vande Walle J, Stockner M, Raes A, Nørgaard JP. Desmopressin 30 years in clinical use: A safety review. Curr Drug Saf 2007;2:232–8.

DIABETIC KETOACIDOSIS

Method of
Aidar R. Gosmanov, MD, PhD, DMSc; and Barry M. Wall, MD

CURRENT DIAGNOSIS

- Initial evaluation includes physical examination and comprehensive metabolic panel, serum osmolality, serum ketones and β-hydroxybutyrate, complete blood count, urinalysis, urine ketones, and arterial blood gases.
- Search for precipitating cases. Omission of insulin, underlying medical illness, cardiovascular events, gastrointestinal disorders, recent surgery, stress, medications, eating disorders, psychological stress, insulin pump malfunction, and infection are potential causes; white blood cell count greater than 25,000 suggests presence of infection.
- β-Hydroxybutyrate of 3.8 mmol/L or greater in adults indicates presence of diabetic ketoacidosis (DKA) even if serum ketones are negative.
- Patients with severe chronic kidney disease (CKD) require careful evaluation of acid–base status.

CURRENT THERAPY

- Start intravenous fluids early before insulin therapy.
- Potassium level should be more than 3.3 mEq/L before insulin therapy is initiated. Supplement potassium intravenously if needed.
- Initiate continuous insulin infusion at 0.14 U/kg per hour and measure bedside glucose every 1 hour to adjust the insulin-infusion rate.
- Avoid hypoglycemia during the insulin infusion by initiating dextrose-containing fluids and/or reducing the insulin infusion rate until DKA is resolved.
- Transition to subcutaneous insulin only when DKA resolution is established.

Epidemiology

In 2005, there were 120,000 hospitalizations for diabetic ketoacidosis (DKA), with an average length of stay of 3.6 days. The direct and indirect annual cost of DKA hospitalization is $2.4 billion. Overall, diabetic population–adjusted rates of DKA admissions fell by about 50% between 1996 and 2005.

Risk Factors

Omission of insulin is the most common precipitant of DKA. Infections, acute medical illnesses involving the cardiovascular system (myocardial infarction, stroke) and gastrointestinal tract (bleeding, pancreatitis), diseases of the endocrine axis (acromegaly, Cushing's syndrome), and stress of recent surgical procedures can contribute to the development of DKA by causing dehydration, increase in insulin counterregulatory hormones, and worsening of peripheral insulin resistance. Medications such as diuretics, β-blockers, corticosteroids, second-generation antipsychotics, and anticonvulsants can affect carbohydrate metabolism and volume status and therefore can precipitate DKA. Other factors that can contribute to DKA include psychological problems, eating disorders, insulin pump malfunction, and drug abuse. It is now recognized that new-onset type 2 diabetes mellitus can manifest with DKA. These patients are obese, mostly African American or Hispanic, and extremely insulin resistant on presentation.

Pathophysiology

Insulin deficiency, increased insulin counterregulatory hormones (cortisol, glucagon, growth hormone, and catecholamines), and peripheral insulin resistance lead to hyperglycemia, dehydration, ketosis, and electrolyte imbalance, which underlie the pathophysiology of DKA. The hyperglycemia of DKA evolves through accelerated gluconeogenesis, glycogenolysis, and decreased glucose utilization, all due to absolute insulin deficiency. Owing to increased lipolysis and decreased lipogenesis, abundant free fatty acids are converted to ketone bodies: acetoacetate and β-hydroxybutyrate (β-OHB). Hyperglycemia-induced osmotic diuresis, if not accompanied by sufficient oral fluid intake, leads to dehydration, hyperosmolarity, electrolyte loss, and subsequent decrease in glomerular filtration.

With decline in a renal function, glycosuria diminishes and hyperglycemia worsens. With impaired insulin action and hyperosmolar hyperglycemia, potassium uptake by skeletal muscle is markedly diminished, which, along with hyperosmolarity-mediated efflux of potassium from cells, results in intracellular potassium depletion. Potassium is lost via osmotic diuresis, causing profound total body potassium deficiency. Therefore, DKA patients can present with a broad range of serum potassium concentrations. A "normal" plasma potassium concentration still indicates that potassium stores in the body are severely diminished and the institution of insulin therapy and correction of hyperglycemia will result in hypokalemia.

On average, patients with DKA have the following deficit of water and key electrolytes: water 100 mL/kg, sodium 7 to 10 mEq/kg, potassium 3 to 5 mEq/kg, and phosphorus 1 mmol/kg.

Clinical Manifestations

Polyuria, polydipsia, weight loss, vomiting, and abdominal pain usually are present in patients with DKA. Abdominal pain can be closely associated with acidosis and resolves with treatment. Physical examination findings such as hypotension, tachycardia, poor skin turgor, and weakness support the clinical diagnosis of dehydration in DKA. Mental status changes can occur in DKA and likely are related to degree of acidosis and hyperosmolarity. A search for symptoms of precipitating causes such as infection, vascular events, or existing drug abuse should be initiated in the emergency department. Patients with hyperglycemic crises can be hypothermic because of peripheral vasodilation and decreased utilization of metabolic substrates.

Diagnosis

Diagnostic criteria for DKA include blood glucose higher than 250 mg/dL, arterial pH 7.30 or less, bicarbonate level 18 mEq/L or less, and adjusted for albumin anion gap greater than 10 to 12. Therefore, initial laboratory evaluation should include a comprehensive metabolic panel and arterial blood gases. Positive serum and urine ketones can further support the diagnosis of DKA but are not required. In early DKA, acetoacetate concentration is low, but it is a major substrate for ketone measurement by many laboratories; therefore, ketone measurement in serum by usual laboratory techniques has a high specificity but low sensitivity for the diagnosis of DKA. Conversely, β-OHB is an early and abundant ketoacid that can first signal development of DKA, but its measurement requires use of specific assay that is different from ketone measurement. β-OHB of 3.8 mmol/L or higher was shown to be highly sensitive and specific for DKA diagnosis.

In patients with chronic kidney disease stage 4 or 5, the diagnosis of DKA is challenging because of presence of chronic metabolic acidosis and possibility of mixed acid–base disorders on presentation with DKA. Anion gap greater than 20 supports the diagnosis of DKA in such patients.

Differential Diagnosis

Hyperglycemic hyperosmolar state is usually not associated with ketosis, but mixed hyperglycemic hyperosmolar state and DKA can occur. Clinical scenarios that may be accompanied by acidosis are described in Table 1. Starvation and alcoholic ketoacidosis are not characterized by hyperglycemia greater than 250 mg/dL. With hypotension or history of metformin (Glucophage) use, lactic acidosis should be suspected. Ingestion of methanol, isopropyl alcohol, and paraldehyde[2] can also alter anion gap and/or osmolality but are not associated with hyperglycemia.

Treatment

The therapeutic goals of management include optimization of volume status, hyperglycemia and ketoacidosis, electrolyte abnormalities, and potential precipitating factors. DKA management protocol is presented in Figure 1. Special considerations should be given to patients with congestive heart failure and CKD. These patients tend to retain fluids; therefore, caution should be exercised during volume resuscitation in these patient groups.

Bicarbonate therapy is not indicated in mild and moderate forms of DKA because metabolic acidosis should correct with insulin therapy. The use of bicarbonate in severe DKA is controversial owing to lack of prospective randomized studies. It is thought that the administration of bicarbonate actually results in peripheral hypoxemia, worsened hypokalemia, paradoxical central nervous system acidosis, cerebral edema in children and young adults,

---

[2]Not available in the United States.

TABLE 1 Laboratory Evaluation of Metabolic Causes of Acidosis

LAB VALUE	DKA	STARVATION KETOSIS	LACTIC ACIDOSIS	UREMIC ACIDOSIS	ALCOHOL KETOSIS	SALICYLATE POISONING	METHANOL OR ETHYLENE GLYCOL POISONING
pH	↓	Normal	↓	Mild ↓	↑↓	↑↓*	↓
Plasma glucose	↑	Normal	Normal	Normal	↓ or normal	Normal or ↓	Normal
Plasma ketones†	↑↑	Slight ↑	Normal	Normal	↑	Normal	Normal
Anion gap	↑	Slight ↑	↑	Slight ↑	↑	↑	↑
Osmolality	↑	Normal	Normal	↑ or normal	Normal	Normal	↑↑
Other	—	—	Lactate ↑	BUN ↑	—	Serum level +	Serum level +

*Respiratory alkalosis or metabolic acidosis.
†Acetest and Ketostix (Bayer, Leverkusen, Germany) measure acetoacetic acid only; thus, misleadingly low values may be obtained because the majority of "ketone bodies" are β-hydroxybutyrate.
Abbreviations: BUN = blood urea nitrogen; DKA = diabetic ketoacidosis.

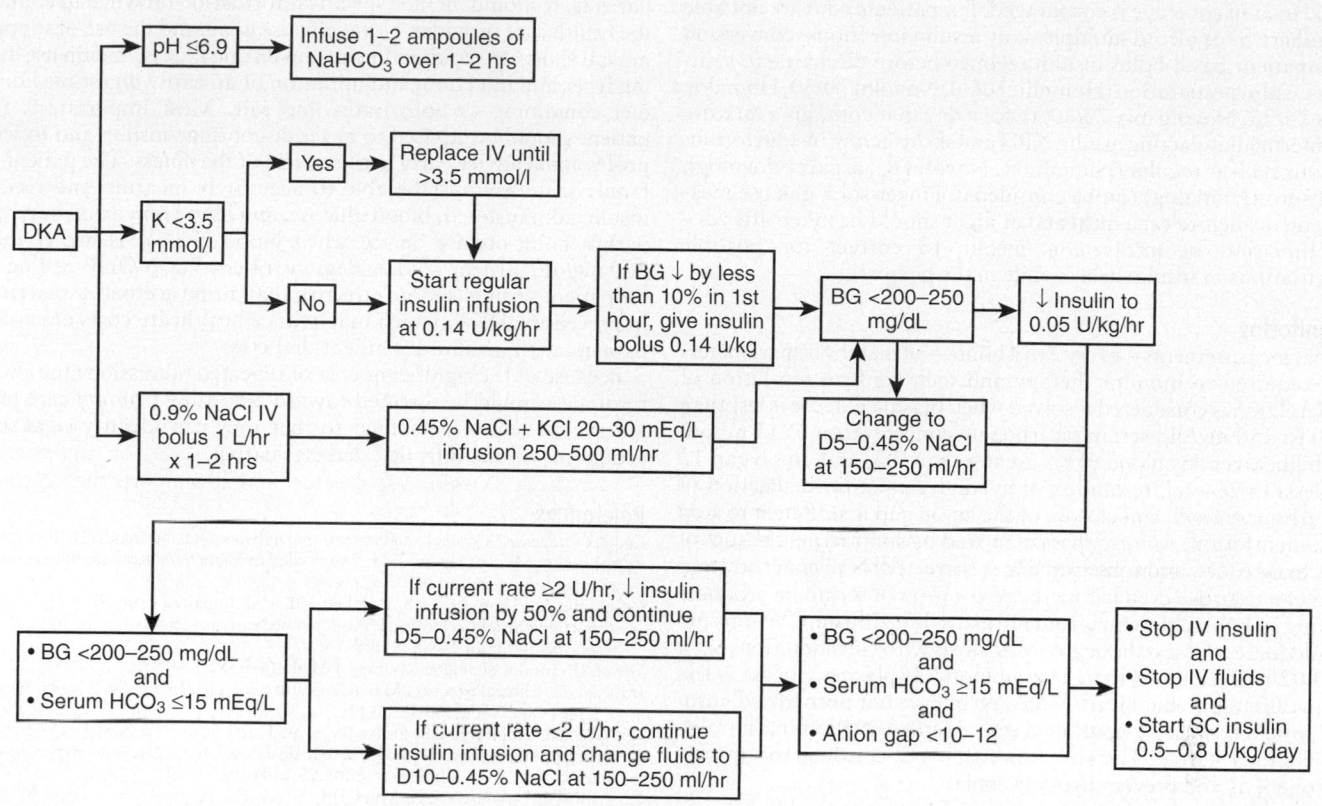

Figure 1. Workflow of management of adult DKA. *Abbreviation:* BG = blood glucose.

and an increase in intracellular acidosis. Because severe acidosis is associated with worse clinical outcomes and can lead to impairment in sensorium and deterioration of myocardial contractility, bicarbonate therapy may be indicated if the pH is 6.9 or less. Therefore, the infusion of 100 mmol (2 ampoules) of bicarbonate in 400 mL of sterile water mixed with 20 mEq potassium chloride over 2 hours and repeating the infusion until the pH is greater than 7.0 can be recommended pending the results of prospective trials.

A whole-body phosphate deficit in DKA can average 1 mmol/kg. Insulin therapy during DKA will further lower serum phosphate concentration. Prospective randomized studies have failed to show any beneficial effect of phosphate replacement on the clinical outcome in DKA. However, a careful phosphate replacement sometimes is indicated in patients with serum phosphate concentration less than 1.0 mg/dL and in those with cardiac dysfunction, anemia, or respiratory depression who have serum phosphate level between 1.0 and 2.0 mg/dL. Initial replacement strategy may include infusion of potassium phosphate at the rate of 0.1 to 0.2 mmol/kg over 6 hours depending on the degree of phosphate deficit (1 mL potassium phosphate solution for intravenous use contains 3 mmol phosphorous and 4.4 mEq potassium). Overzealous phosphate replacement can result in hypocalcemia; therefore, close monitoring of phosphorous and calcium levels is recommended. Patients who have renal insufficiency or hypocalcemia might need less-aggressive phosphate replacement.

When DKA is resolved, and independent of the patient's ability to tolerate oral intake, transition to subcutaneous insulin must be initiated. Patients are given intermediate (NPH) or long-acting insulin (detemir [Levemir], glargine [Lantus]) 2 hours before termination of intravenous insulin to allow sufficient time for injected insulin to start working (Table 2). When patient can eat, we recommend addition of short- or rapid-acting insulin for prandial glycemic coverage (see Table 2). This is the basal-bolus insulin regimen and provides physiologic replacement of insulin. It is common to see transition from intravenous to subcutaneous insulin using sliding-scale insulin only. This strategy as a sole approach should be discouraged because it cannot provide the necessary insulin requirement in patients recovering from hyperglycemic crisis and beta-cell failure.

If the patient used insulin prior to admission, the same dosage can be restarted in the hospital. Insulin-naïve patients require insulin at a total dose of 0.5 to 0.8 U/kg/day divided as 50% basal insulin and 50% as prandial insulin before each meal. Initially, after DKA resolution, given the possibility of fluctuating oral intake, use of

TABLE 2	Pharmacokinetics and Pharmacodynamics of Subcutaneous Insulin Preparations			
INSULIN	**ONSET OF ACTION**	**TIME TO PEAK**	**DURATION**	**TIMING OF DOSE**
Regular (Humulin R, Novolin R)	30–60 min	2–3 h	8–10 h	30–45 min before meal
Aspart (Novolog)	5–15 min	30–90 min	4–6 h	15 min before meal
Glulisine (Apidra)	15 min	30–90 min	5.3 h	15 min before meal
Lispro (Humalog)	5–15 min	30–90 min	4–6 h	15 min before meal
NPH (Humulin N, Novolin N)	2–4 h	4–10 h	12–18 h	Twice a day
Detemir (Levemir)	2 h	No peak	12–24 h	Once or twice a day
Glargine (Lantus)	2 h	No peak	20–24 h	Once a day

once-daily long-acting insulin such as glargine or detemir to provide basal insulin coverage is encouraged. For patients who are not able to adhere to or afford multiple daily insulin injections, conversion of inpatient basal-bolus insulin regimen before discharge to split-mix insulin preparation (Humulin 70/30, Novolin 70/30, Humalog mix 75/25, Novolg mix 70/30) twice a day that contains a mixture of intermediate-acting insulin NPH and short-acting insulin formulations such as regular (Humulin R, Novolin R), aspart (Novolog), or lispro (Humalog) can be considered. Finger-stick glucose measurements before each meal and at night should be taken after discontinuation of intravenous insulin to correct for possible fluctuations in insulin needs while in the hospital.

Monitoring

Serial measurements—every 2 to 4 hours—of metabolic parameters are required to monitor therapy and then confirm resolution of DKA. DKA is considered resolved when plasma glucose is less than 200 to 250 mg/dL, serum bicarbonate concentration is 15 mEq/L or higher, venous blood pH is greater than 7.3, and anion gap 12 or less. In general, resolution of hyperglycemia, normalization of bicarbonate level, and closure of the anion gap is sufficient to stop insulin infusion. Anion gap is calculated by subtracting the sum of Cl^- and HCO_3^+ from measured (not corrected) Na^+ concentration and can improve even before the restoration of serum bicarbonate owing to hyperchloremia from normal saline infusion. Venous pH is adequate to assess the degree of acidosis with consideration that it is 0.02 to 0.03 lower than arterial blood. If plasma glucose is less than 200 mg/dL but bicarbonate and pH are not normalized, insulin infusion must be continued and dextrose-containing intravenous fluids started. The latter approach will continue to suppress ketogenesis and prevent hypoglycemia.

Complications

Hypoglycemia is the most common complication and can be prevented by timely adjustment of insulin dosage and frequent monitoring of blood glucose levels. Hypoglycemia is defined as any blood glucose level below 70 mg/dL. If DKA is not resolved and blood glucose level is below 200 to 250 mg/dL, decrease in insulin infusion rate and/or addition of 5% or 10% dextrose to current intravenous fluids may be implemented (see Figure 1). For patients in whom DKA is resolved, strategies to manage hypoglycemia depend on whether patient is able to eat or not. For patients who are able to drink or eat, ingestion of 15 to 20 grams of carbohydrates—for example, four glucose tablets or 6 oz orange or apple juice or "regular" soft drink—is advised. In patients who are allowed nothing by mouth, are unable to swallow, or have altered level of consciousness, administer 25 mL 50% dextrose IV or give 1 mg glucagon (Glucagen) IM if no IV access present. Blood glucose should be rechecked in 15 minutes; only if the glucose level is less than 80 mg/dL should these steps be repeated.

Non–anion-gap hyperchloremic acidosis occurs from urinary loss of ketoanions, which are needed for bicarbonate regeneration and preferential reabsorption of chloride in proximal renal tubules secondary to intensive administration of chloride-containing fluids and low plasma bicarbonate. The acidosis usually resolves and should not affect treatment course. Cerebral edema has been reported in young adult patients. This condition is manifested by appearance of headache, lethargy, papillary changes, or seizures. Mortality is up to 70%. Mannitol (Osmitrol) infusion and mechanical ventilation should be used to treat this condition. Rhabdomyolysis is another possible complication resulting from hyperosmolality and hypoperfusion. Pulmonary edema can develop from excessive fluid replacement in patients with CKD or congestive heart failure.

Prevention

Discharge planning should include diabetes education, selection of an appropriate insulin regimen that the patient can understand and afford, and preparation of set of supplies for the initial insulin administration at home. Many cases of DKA can be prevented by better access to medical care, proper education, and effective communication with a health care provider during an intercurrent illness.

Sick-day management should be reviewed periodically with all patients. It should include specific information on when to contact the health care provider, blood glucose goals and the use of supplemental short- or rapid-acting insulin during illness, insulin use during fever and infection, and initiation of an easily digestible liquid diet containing carbohydrates and salt. Most importantly, the patient should be advised to never discontinue insulin and to seek professional advice early in the course of the illness. The patient or family member must be able to accurately measure and record insulin administered, blood glucose, and blood β-hydroxybutyrate with a point-of-care device when blood glucose is higher than 300 mg/dL. Recent studies demonstrated that b-OHB testing in outpatient setting is more effective than urine acetoacetate testing in preventing DKA, which may reduce healthcare costs of care of patients with insulin-dependent diabetes.

Because of the significant cost of repeated admissions for DKA, resources should be directed toward educating primary care providers and school personnel so that they can identify signs and symptoms of uncontrolled diabetes earlier.

References

Centers for Disease Control and Prevention: Diabetes data and trends: Diabetes complications. Available at http://www.cdc.gov/diabetes/statistics/complications_national.htm (accessed 08.07.12).

Gosmanov AR, Umpierrez GE, Karabell AH, et al. Impaired expression and insulin-stimulated phosphorylation of Akt-2 in muscle of obese patients with atypical diabetes. Am J Physiol 2004;287:E8–15.

Hirsch IB. Insulin analogues. N Engl J Med 2005;352:174–83.

Inzucchi SE. Clinical practice. Management of hyperglycemia in the hospital setting. N Engl J Med 2006;355:1903–11.

Kitabchi AE, Umpierrez GE, Fisher JN, et al. Thirty years of personal experience in hyperglycemic crises: Diabetic ketoacidosis and hyperglycemic hyperosmolar state. J Clin Endocrinol Metab 2008;93:1541–52.

Kitabchi AE, Umpierrez GE, Miles JM, Fisher JN. Hyperglycemic crises in adult patients with diabetes. Diabetes Care 2009;32:1335–43.

Kitabchi AE, Umpierrez GE, Murphy MB, Kreisberg RA. Hyperglycemic crises in adult patients with diabetes: A consensus statement from the American Diabetes Association. Diabetes Care 2006;29:2739–48.

Klocker AA, Phelan H, Twigg SM, Craig ME. Blood β-hydroxybutyrate vs. urine acetoacetate testing for the prevention and management of ketoacidosis in Type 1 diabetes: a systematic review. Diabet Med 2013;30(7):818–24.

Sheikh-Ali M, Karon BS, Basu A, et al. Can serum beta-hydroxybutyrate be used to diagnose diabetic ketoacidosis? Diabetes Care 2008;31:643–7.

Tzamaloukas AH, Ing TS, Siamopoulos KC, et al. Pathophysiology and management of fluid and electrolyte disturbances in patients on chronic dialysis with severe hyperglycemia. Semin Dial 2008;21:431–9.

Umpierrez GE, Smiley D, Kitabchi AE. Narrative review: Ketosis-prone type 2 diabetes mellitus. Ann Intern Med 2006;144:350–7.

DIABETES MELLITUS IN ADULTS

Method of
Anthony L. McCall, MD, PhD; and J. Terry Saunders, PhD

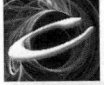

CURRENT DIAGNOSIS

- Screening for diabetes should be done in high-risk populations, especially:
  - Those with prediabetes or the metabolic syndrome.
  - High-risk ethnic groups (e.g., Native American, Latino American, African American).
  - History of gestational diabetes.
- Patients might present with atypical symptoms.
- Most diabetes is type 2 in adults, but type 1 does occur in adults, and delayed diagnosis is common.
- Cardiovascular risk should be aggressively screened for and treated.
- Complications should be documented and tracked.
  - Check fasting lipids or, if inconvenient, get non-fasting lipids focused on CV risk using a calculator.
  - Check renal function and albuminuria yearly.

- Have a low threshold for stress testing, with imaging for all patients who have symptoms.
- Refer for yearly eye examinations by an eye professional.
- Check feet for sensation, deformity, and circulation at regular visits.
- All patients should receive an educational assessment and training in self-management and self-monitoring of blood glucose.
- Take a diet history; this is especially important for patients on insulin.
- Get a baseline HbA1c and repeat 2 to 4 times per year (twice yearly if at glycemic goal).

CURRENT THERAPY

- Diabetes requires nutrition and behavioral self-management counseling as well as drug therapy.
- Individualize goals for every patient (for glycemia, lipids, BP)
- Base individualization on age, motivation, complications, diabetes duration, hypoglycemia risk
- Repeatedly encourage healthy eating and an active lifestyle.
- Prediabetes diagnosis represents an opportunity for behavioral and drug interventions.
- Metformin (Glucophage) is usually the first drug therapy.
- Don't expect one drug to do the job for very poorly controlled glycemia, especially if HgbA1c >9%.
- Dual defects (insulin resistance and secretion) should be addressed in most patients.
- Very insulin-resistant patients might need a dual insulin-resistance strategy.
- Therapy goals for both HbA1c and self-monitored blood glucose can be achieved in most patients.
- Cardiovascular risk reduction therapy is a very high priority—statins and BP control best.
- Consider use of new Omnibus calculator for when to start statin therapy.
- When patients have not met goals on two or three oral agents as therapy, basal insulin is often the most appropriate choice, particularly when patients are not near glycemic goals.
- For oral agent therapy, add—don't switch—unless side effects require it.
- When adding basal insulin, initially continue oral agent therapies.
- Threatening patients with insulin therapy is counterproductive.
- Follow the 3F rule: Fix the fasting glucose first, especially in patients with poor glycemic control. As control improves, pay attention to postmeal sugars.
- Prompt recognition of the need for meal insulin is critical to achieve glycemic goals.
- Usually start with a single-meal insulin dose for the largest meal.
- Balance meal and basal insulin; check post-meal BG.

Epidemiology

The Centers for Disease Control and Prevention (CDC) estimated that in 2012 the prevalence of diabetes in the United States was 29.1 million. Diabetes is diagnosed in 21 million persons and undiagnosed in 8.0 million. Type 2 diabetes mellitus (T2DM) is 90% to 95% of prevalent diabetes, and type 1 diabetes (T1DM) is about 5% to 10%. There are fewer persons with secondary or monogenic forms of diabetes, such as *maturity-onset diabetes of the young* (MODY). About 86 million people above the age of 20 in the United States are thought to have prediabetes.

The focus of this article is T2DM because it is the most prevalent form and is increasing rapidly in the United States and worldwide. A few comments are made on adult T1DM. This chapter emphasizes both lifestyle and pharmacologic treatments. Although prediabetes may not require drug therapy, it represents an important opportunity to prevent diabetes and initiate critical lifestyle changes.

Diagnosis and Classification of Diabetes and Prediabetes
Diagnosis

Most diabetes is diagnosed by random or fasting glucose (Table 1). Symptoms should be present (e.g., thirst, frequent urination) if random glucose criteria are used, but surprisingly, many people with diabetes are relatively asymptomatic. In the elderly, cognitive changes can occur and atypical symptoms such as prostatism or genital yeast infections can suggest the diagnosis. The American Diabetes Association (ADA) screening recommendations suggest screening every 3 years starting at age 45 for the general population, but they suggest earlier and more frequent screening in those with high risk. Elevated HbA1c when 6.5% or higher can be used for screening and diagnosis of diabetes.

Patients from diabetes-prone ethnic groups (e.g., Latin Americans, African Americans, Native Americans, Asian Americans of several types) or with a strong family history, polycystic ovary syndrome (PCOS), or gestational diabetes should have early and frequent screenings. High-risk persons include those with prediabetes (impaired glucose tolerance, impaired fasting glucose) or who meet the National Cholesterol Education Program (NCEP) criteria for the metabolic syndrome or its individual components (dyslipidemia, hypertension, central obesity, prediabetes). The metabolic syndrome is flawed, but this does not reduce the importance of fully documenting and treating cardiometabolic risk components in those with or at risk for T2DM in a targeted manner (see Box 1). Teach patients and clinicians about these risks and can encourage the overweight and sedentary to adopt a healthier lifestyle.

Classification

The classification of diabetes into its two most prominent types (T1DM and T2DM) seems straightforward in theory but in practice is increasingly confusing as more Americans become overweight. Although T1DM patients are traditionally lean, many now are overweight and some have metabolic syndrome characteristics. About 80% to 90% of persons with T2DM are overweight or have

DIAGNOSIS	GLUCOSE TEST	DIAGNOSTIC LEVEL	COMMENTS
Diabetes	Random	≥200 mg/dL	Plus classic symptoms*
Diabetes	Fasting	≥126 mg/dL	8-hour fast; need confirmation
Diabetes	Postglucose load (75 g in nonpregnant adults)	≥200 mg/dL at 2 h	Need confirmation
Diabetes	HbA1c†	6.5%	NGS standardized lab
Prediabetes	IFG Fasting	≥100 mg/dL	Decreased insulin secretion
Prediabetes	IGT Postglucose load (75 g)	140–199 mg/dL at 2 h	Increased insulin resistance
Prediabetes	HbA1c	5.7%–6.4%	NGS standardized lab

TABLE 1 Diagnosis and Classification of Diabetes and Prediabetes

*Polyuria, polydipsia, unexplained weight loss.
†NGS nationally standardized lab method.
Abbreviations: IFG = impaired fasting glucose; IGT = impaired glucose tolerance.

| Box 1 | Summary of Goals for Treatment |

Lifestyle

Medical Nutrition Therapy (individualized)
- Appropriate calories for weight, 5%–10% weight loss for obese patients
- Low saturated and trans fats, substitute with healthy fats
- Moderate, consistent carbohydrates (whole grains, vegetables, fruits with low glycemic effects)
- Foods that can reduce postmeal sugars (low glycemic load)
- Healthy fats and proteins (decreased saturated and trans fats, increased monosaturated fat; reduced consumption of animal protein)

Activity
- Consistent, regular activity tailored to complications and safety (ECG or stress test may be needed before starting an exercise program)

Glycemia: it is critical that these goals are individualized*
- Best possible without frequent or severe hypoglycemia
- HbA1c <7% generally; 6% or less if possible in selected patients early in disease course; 7%–8% may be appropriate in those with shortened lifespan

Self-Monitored Blood Glucose
- Preprandial 80–130[†] mg/dL; <110 ideally; 20–30 mg/dL higher is acceptable for high-risk patients
- Postprandial (1–2 h) <180 minimal; <140 ideal

Lipids
- All DM patients with overt ASCVD should be on high intensity statins
- DM patients <40 or >75 years old with CVD risk** consider medium intensity to high intensity statins
- DM patients 40-70 years old with CVD risk consider high intensity statins
- DM patients <40 without CVD risk statins are not recommended
- Blood Pressure[‡]
- Systolic <140 mm Hg
- Diastolic <90 mm Hg

---

*See ADA guidelines for factors.
**CVD risk factors include LDL cholesterol ≤100 mg/dL (2.6 mmol/L), high blood pressure, smoking, and overweight and obesity.
[†]80 mg/dL is too low for patients with high risk of hypoglycemia.
[‡]More aggressive BP goals may be appropriate for individual patients if there are no increase in risk of side effects. Relaxed criteria based on age, comorbidities, long duration of diabetes, behavioral, motivational criteria and others.
Abbreviations: ACS = acute coronary syndrome, ASCVD = atherosclerotic cardiovascular disease.

Pathophysiology

The primary causes of most adult diabetes are insulin resistance and lack of compensatory insulin secretion. Abnormalities in incretin hormone physiology may also underlie early pathophysiology although deficiency of GLP-1 is probably not the simple explanation. Insulin resistance is typically longstanding and begins at a young age because of heredity combined with environmental causes (sedentary lifestyle and calorie overconsumption with resultant overweight). Insulin secretory defects usually start about 10 years before diagnosis, and no therapy is proven so far to prevent progressive loss of insulin secretion. A few patients develop diabetes associated with malnutrition, but this is much less common. Longstanding insulin resistance is associated with dyslipidemia, central obesity, hypertension, and hyperglycemia. This long prodrome accounts for the common coexistence of cardiovascular disease and diabetes.

Cardiovascular Risk Management

Cardiovascular risk management in diabetes starts with lifestyle counseling and education. It is paramount that patients understand the intimate and direct links among diabetes, glycemic control, and cardiovascular disease. Drug interventions are ultimately needed for glycemia, lipid risks, and blood pressure in most patients. Women have higher relative risk and similar overall risk as men and are often undertreated. Specific recommended targets of therapy for diabetes in glycemia, blood pressure, dyslipidemia, and lifestyle are shown in Box 1.

Documenting and Following Complications

Patients should have a thorough examination and evaluation for complications at the time of diabetes diagnosis. About half of patients with newly diagnosed T2DM have established chronic complications, indicating delayed recognition of this disorder.

Neuropathy and circulatory signs and symptoms on foot examination should be assessed. Risk of ulcer and amputation can be gauged by 10-g Semmes-Weinstein monofilaments that test for severe neuropathy and attendant risk of ulceration. Retina examinations should be done by skilled eye professionals likely to pick up significant eye disease. High-risk patients (poor glycemic control, established retinopathy, especially if preproliferative or worse) should be referred promptly to an eye specialist. Pregnancy counseling should be given to all women of childbearing age with diabetes. Albumin-to-creatinine ratio in the urine should be assessed and kidney function (serum creatinine, estimated glomerular filtration rate [eGFR], and blood urea nitrogen [BUN]) should be tracked yearly. Many drugs for diabetes are dosed based on kidney function so it may be appropriate to track eGFR closely (e.g., every 3–6 months) when it is abnormal.

Home glucose monitoring should be taught to patients so they understand the effects of food, stress, and exercise on glycemic patterns. Diabetes education should be arranged for all patients, preferably by a diabetes educator. Diabetes is unique in being a self-managed condition where patient knowledge and skills are critical to avoiding complications. Moreover, behavioral management is critical to success in diabetes care.

Treatment

Behavioral Self-Management

Self-management of behavioral factors, including eating, physical activity, and psychological stress, is essential to good diabetes self-care. Ideally, professional support for behavioral self-management should be a coordinated, multidisciplinary effort involving expertise appropriate to a given patient from the areas of nutrition, nursing, physical activity, and behavioral counseling. The provider should develop basic behavior change skills and refer to appropriate multidisciplinary and community-based resources.

Quick, one-shot interventions seldom change longstanding patterns of behavior. Initial sessions should be scheduled close together (1–2 weeks), then further apart as the patient gains momentum and confidence. If multiple one-on-one sessions are

metabolic syndrome characteristics, but some are leaner and more active and do not have the metabolic syndrome. C-peptide measurements are not very helpful for those who are difficult to classify, but measuring three antibodies—including IA-2 (islet cell antigen 512), anti-GAD$_{65}$ (glutamic acid decarboxylase), and anti-insulin antibodies in high titers—can clarify a diagnosis of latent autoimmune diabetes. Younger age at onset, lean body habitus, severe loss of glycemic control with or without ketonemia, and weight loss all suggest insulin deficiency but might not be definitive.

Optimal glycemia goals must be individualized, but may be generally defined as hemoglobin A1c (HgbA1c) of less than 7% (see Table 1) as recommended by the ADA. Pre-prandial capillary blood glucose should be 80–130 mg/dL and postprandially at the peak (typically about 2 hours after meals) they should be generally less than 180 mg/dl. Individualizing glycemic goals should be based on several factors including: duration of diabetes, the age and life expectancy, comorbid conditions such as known cardiovascular disease, advanced microvascular complications, hypoglycemia unawareness and other individual patient considerations. Both HgbA1c and capillary blood glucose concentrations should be individualized to reduced hypoglycemic risk. A summary of other goals is given in Box 1.

impossible, other options such as group meetings, telephone support, or e-mail messaging should be considered.

Behavior change interventions should be highly individualized and specific. General advice about diet and exercise does not address the life experience or problems of a given patient and is often perceived as insensitive or unhelpful. Arriving at individualized objectives for behavior change can be accomplished using a simple three-step process composed of initial assessment, setting behavioral objectives, and follow-up and reassessment.

Initial Assessment

Initial assessment includes identifying salient features of social and family history that can affect efforts to change behavior. A nutrition assessment should be performed, including an appraisal of usual food intake, the patient's perception of problem eating behavior, and weight history. A physical activity assessment should also be conducted, focusing on past and current physical activity, preferences, perceived barriers, and general attitudes. Readiness to make changes in behavior should be assessed by asking how important a patient thinks it is to change a given area of behavior and how confident she or he is that she or he can succeed in making changes (on a 1 to 10 scale). Discussion of specific objectives for behavioral change should occur in areas where the patient indicates a definite readiness to begin. Finally, ask patients about current levels and sources of stress. Because depression is common with diabetes, patients should be screened for possible depression.

Behavioral Objectives

Setting behavioral objectives is initiated and facilitated by the provider, but the patient is responsible for selecting his or her own behavioral objectives. Objectives should be FIRM: *f*ew (1–3 at a time is plenty), *i*ndividualized to the patient's specific behavioral challenges, *r*ealistic (beware of trying to make big strides quickly), and *m*easurable. The patient should be encouraged to keep a daily record of progress on each objective. For those with access, phone and computer-based applications enhance the ease and accuracy of tracking. The primary focus of provider-patient discussions of progress should be on behavioral objectives, not outcomes.

Accurate knowledge of current behavior is key to setting behavioral objectives for nutrition and exercise. Obtaining a 3-day food record (2 work days and one non-work day) and a baseline for activity (we generally use a week of daily steps measured with a pedometer) provide a solid baseline for setting objectives.

A modest reduction in caloric consumption of around 250 to 500 kcal/day and moderate physical activity on the order of at least 150 minutes a week are the recommended approaches to weight loss. Reducing calories through decreased food consumption is more effective for weight loss than increasing energy expenditure through physical activity. Box 2 contains a checklist of healthy eating behaviors that can be used to stimulate patients' thinking about areas in which they might like to make changes. Note that an irregular pattern of eating often underlies unhealthy food choices. For example, staying up late encourages late-night snacking, which in turn can suppress interest in eating breakfast. Eating tends to be deferred to the afternoon or evening, perpetuating the cycle.

Physical activity plays an important role in weight maintenance. Higher levels of activity (200 min/week) may be required to prevent long-term weight regain. Box 3 lists ways that patients can become more active. It is worth repeating that the point of these and other suggestions is not to direct patients but to expand their thinking about what might work for them.

Follow-up and Reassessment

Follow-up and reassessment occur during each return visit, following a period of patient efforts to carry out mutually agreed on behavioral objectives. Reassessment focuses on the behavioral records kept by patients as well as on their verbal reports of difficulties and successes. Praise and encouragement are the order of the day. Efforts to initiate behavior change are highly responsive to external positive reinforcement, and the patient will need maximum external reinforcement until new behavior becomes self-sustaining. After review and discussion of patient records, new behavioral objectives or incremental changes in existing objectives are selected by mutual agreement, with the patient taking the lead.

A modest weight loss of 5% to 10% has a positive impact on cardiovascular risk factors and progression of diabetes. Reassure patients that medical goals for weight loss are achievable and worth the effort.

Box 2 Checklist of Healthy Eating Behaviors

☑ **Eat meals and snacks at set times to promote health.**
Examples:
- I will eat breakfast within 1 hour of getting up.
- I will not skip meals
- Other:..
....

☑ **Eat healthy carbohydrates.**
Examples:
- I will avoid regular soft drinks and choose water or diet soft drinks instead.
- I will eat 5–7 servings of fruits and vegetables every day.
- I will choose whole-grain breads and cereals.
- Other:..
....

☑ **Decrease serving sizes.**
Examples:
- I will keep a record of the food I eat and drink.
- I will know what counts as a serving size.
- When I am eating out, I will share or split an entrée and eat a salad.
- Other:..
....

☑ **Eat less fat and choose healthy fats.**
Examples:
- I will bake, broil, roast, grill, or boil instead of fry food.
- I will have a meatless meal at least once a week.
- I will choose fried or high-fat foods no more than once a week.
- I will drink fat-free or low-fat milk.
- I will use healthy oils (olive oil, canola oil) and buy tub margarine.
- Other:..
....

☑ **Make other healthy choices.**
Examples:
- I will drink plenty of fluids (at least 8 glasses of water or low-calorie fluid per day).
- I will limit how much alcohol I drink. (Women should drink no more than 1 alcoholic drink per day. Men should drink no more than 2 alcoholic drinks per day.)
- Other:..
....

Unpublished source: Virginia Center for Diabetes Professional Education, University of Virginia; Virginia Diabetes Council.

Box 3   Checklist for Physical Activity

☑ **Do something that you enjoy.**
Examples:
- I will take the stairs.
- I will park my car farther away and walk.
- I will walk.
- I will swim or do water exercises.
- I will ride a bike.
- I will use an exercise video.
- I will do yoga.
- Other:..
  ....

☑ **How often?**
Examples:
- ❑ Every day
- ❑ 3x/week
- ❑ 5x/week
- ❑ ....

☑ **How long?**
Examples:
- ❑ 10 minutes
- ❑ 15 minutes
- ❑ 20 minutes
- ❑ 30 minutes
- ❑ 60 minutes
- ❑ ___ minutes

☑ **Limit inactivity.**
Examples:
- I will watch no more than 1 hour of television per day.
- I will spend no more than 2 hours per day on the computer.
- Other:..
  ....

Unpublished source: Virginia Center for Diabetes Professional Education, University of Virginia; Virginia Diabetes Council.

When discussing changes in eating with patients, distinguish dieting from gradual behavioral changes that result in a lasting pattern of healthy eating. Diets are impermanent and run the risk of large weight losses followed by even larger weight gains. Gradual behavioral changes offer the possibility of permanent lifestyle changes.

Prohibiting or demonizing foods is counterproductive. It leads patients to think of food in moral extremes (e.g., "sugar is bad for my diabetes") rather than along a continuum of nutritional benefit and blood glucose control. Food prohibition also casts the provider as withholding and overly controlling. These traps can be avoided by exploring very small changes that are not perceived as significant losses.

Current nutrition therapy recommendations emphasize a flexible, individualized approach to macronutrient distribution and a carbohydrate-counting meal planning approach for individuals with type 1 diabetes. Patients should be encouraged to emphasize vegetables, fruits, whole grains, legumes, and dairy products as preferred sources of carbohydrate. Recommendations for achieving consistent, appropriate carbohydrate intake at meals are based on controlling postprandial blood glucose (<180 mg/dL 1–2 hours after beginning a meal). Carbohydrate counting and blood glucose pattern management are complicated and time-consuming to teach. Referral to a dietitian for medical nutrition therapy (MNT) or nutrition education through an ADA-recognized diabetes patient education program is recommended.

Stress reduction is important in controlling blood glucose and can also play a role by helping patients achieve a mental focus on their behavior-management efforts. We encourage patients to sit calmly for a period of 5 to 10 minutes each day, focusing on slow deep breathing and muscle relaxation. Activities such as yoga or tai chi also reduce stress and support awareness of body and mind. Box 4 contains suggestions for coping behaviors that may be useful to patients in dealing with stress.

Pharmacologic Therapy
Overview
Eventually, most patients with T2DM require drug treatment, often with multiple agents (combination therapy). Progressive insulin secretory loss probably is the primary explanation for the need to advance treatment. A resultant general rule with all therapies is *add, don't switch*, but it is important to remember that lifestyle modification should always be part of the therapy if possible. Table 2 lists major types of pharmacotherapeutic interventions with their usual hemoglobin (Hb) A1c lowering, balance of preprandial versus postprandial effects, and some comments

Box 4   Checklist of Coping Behaviors

Examples:
- Talk about how you feel to people you trust.
- Decide one small way to change your mood or old habit, and do it.
- Write down 10 good things about your life and think about and appreciate them.
- Organize your day with a "To Do" list.
- Learn how to relax through yoga, meditation, biofeedback, tai chi, deep breathing, or visual imagery.
- Take 30 minutes each day to relax through music, yoga, bath, writing, etc.
- Take time to have fun every day by exploring a new interest, watching a funny movie, going shopping, playing with a pet, etc.
- Get in touch with your spiritual side to help you feel better about yourself.
- Keep a stress diary to see what triggers your stress and discover better ways to react.
- Exercise every day to help you focus your energy on a more positive path.
- Keep your sleep cycle as regular as possible.
- Develop a favorite hobby.
- Other:.. ....

Unpublished source: Virginia Center for Diabetes Professional Education, University of Virginia; Virginia Diabetes Council.

---

on their actions and side effects. Table 3 lists classes of drugs, commonly used agents, and typical doses.

Recently the ADA and European Association for the Study of Diabetes (EASD) updated a joint consensus algorithm on controlling hyperglycemia in T2DM. In our practice, we similarly initiate behavioral self-management with and sometimes without medication. Metformin is the first medication usually started unless there are contraindications or intolerance. Commonly, ineffective early attempts by physicians to change behavior (e.g., giving general advice) lead to abandonment of this therapy. Referral to an ADA Recognized diabetes education program is a more efficacious alternative. A second oral medication may be initiated if patients cannot achieve glycemic goals. Commonly, we favor insulin secretagogues, especially glimepiride (Amaryl) or extended-release glipizide (Glucotrol XL), for their relatively low risk of hypoglycemia, convenient once-daily dosing, and low expense, or an oral incretin

DRUG TYPE	HBA1C LOWERING (%)	EFFECT ON GLYCEMIA		ACTIONS	SIDE EFFECTS/ COMMENTS
		PREPRANDIAL	POSTPRANDIAL		
SU and non-SU secretagogues	1.5–2.0*	++	+†	Direct and indirect secretagogue	Hypoglycemia, weight gain, rash
Biguanides	1.5–2.0*	+++	0	↓ hepatic glucose release, weight neutral	‡Adjust dose for CKD, lactic acidosis (rare)
Thiazolidinediones	0.5–1.5	+++	0	↑ insulin sensitivity in muscle, fat	Edema, CHF, fractures
Incretin agonists	0.8–1.5	+	++	Strong GLP-1 effects, ↑ insulin, ↓ glucogon, ↓ stomach emptying	Nausea, vomiting, weight loss§
DPP-4 inhibitors	0.6–0.8	+	++	Moderate GLP-1 effects, ↑ insulin, ↓ glucogon	Weight neutral
Colesevelam (bile acid sequestrant)	0.4–0.8	+	+	Mechanisms of action uncertain	Constipation, hypertriglyceridemia
Canagliflozin (SGLT inhibitor), Dapagliflozin, Empagliflozin	0.5–1.0	+	+	↓ renal tubule reabsorption of glucose	Altered kidney function, hypotension, UTI, Candida in groin
Pramlintide (amylin agonist)	0.5–0.7	0–+	++	↓ glucagon, slow stomach emptying	Hypoglycemia, GI upset, weight loss
Basal insulin	1.5–2.5	+++	0*	↓ hepatic glucose output, ↑ muscle glucose disposal	Hypoglycemia, weight gain
Meal insulin	1.0–2.0	0–+	++	↓ hepatic glucose output, ↑ muscle glucose disposal	Hypoglycemia, weight gain

*Older drugs may be less effective in well-controlled patients.
†Rapid acting secretagogues may have less fasting and more early postprandial effects.
‡Metformin dosing: Adjust for CKD stage 3a (45–60 eGFR); watch closely but continue, and in 3b (30–44 eGFR), reduce dose to ½ usual or less and check eGFR every 3 months.
§Although risk of pancreatitis exists, unclear if increased. Risk of pancreatic cancer not proven and based on controversial data.

drug. An alternative treatment strategy for heavier, more insulin-resistant patients is use of a thiazolidinedione, pioglitazone, effectively a dual insulin-resistance strategy (see Thiazolidinediones).

More reliably effective is the use of basal insulin treatment as a second agent to achieve control, although it is less accepted by many patients. Insulin initiation should be preceded by an open discussion of the patient's attitudes, beliefs, and possible fears regarding insulin. Insulin therapy should never be used as a threat or possible negative consequence for failure to carry out behavioral management. Many patients associate insulin with serious diabetes complications and mortality. A positive attitude about the value of insulin therapy and its natural presence and essential role in the body, along with reassurance that insulin can prolong life and improve its quality, can help to reduce initial fears enough to begin. Availability of many non-insulin medications has often moved insulin to later in the sequence but it can be used at any time.

Self-demonstration of injection technique using saline is also useful in overcoming fear of injections. Improvement in blood glucose control with insulin generally makes patients feel better, which further reinforces its perceived value. Use of insulin pens may increase acceptance of insulin treatment, patient convenience, and dosing accuracy.

It should be noted that an alternative algorithm for glycemic control therapy is proposed by the American College of Endocrinology. A patient-centered approach with emphasis on safely achieving goals and including patient choices and preferences is increasingly emphasized in both ADA and AACE guidelines.

Oral Agents

Secretagogues. These drugs enhance insulin secretion. There are first- and second-generation oral sulfonylureas; the latter are most commonly used. They are inexpensive, are moderately effective, and often can be dosed once daily. First-generation agents such as tolbutamide, chlorpropamide (Diabenese), and tolazamide (Tolinase) are less often used than the second-generation agents glyburide (Diabeta, Glynase), glipizide (Glucotrol), and glimepiride (Amaryl). Glyburide should not generally be used in elderly patients or those with renal disease due to hypoglycemia risk.

The dose-response characteristics of sulfonylureas suggest that one half the approved maximum dose achieves maximum HbA1c lowering, typically 1 to 1.5 percentage points (the latter with poorer baseline control). If the patient is not at goal with half-maximum doses, it is more effective to add a second agent than raise the dose. Common side effects include hypoglycemia, weight gain of about 2 kg, and, more rarely, hematologic or skin reactions.

Rapid secretagogues. The glinides (repaglinide [Prandin] and nateglinide [Starlix]), are more expensive and should be considered for patients who are sulfonylurea allergic, extremely erratic in eating, or at high risk for hypoglycemia.

Biguanides. Metformin is the only available agent in this class. It is useful in both obese and normal-weight T2DM patients. HbA1c lowering is typically about 1.5 percentage points in monotherapy or in combination therapy. Maximum efficacy is achieved with 2000 mg daily. The sustained-release preparation will last 24 hours if given with the evening meal.

Metformin's hypoglycemic mechanism is primarily by reduction of liver glucose production. It is cleared by the kidney, and the risk of lactic acidosis, a rare side effect with 50% mortality, may be increased in renal dysfunction. The original FDA guidelines suggesting serum creatinine should be less than 1.4 mg/dL in women and less than 1.5 mg/dL in men have largely been supplanted in practice with estimated glomerular filtration rate (eGFR), which should be assessed in all patients. Full doses of metformin appear safe down to eGFR of 45, but checking eGFR every 3 to 6 months is suggested. Between 30 and 44 eGFR, dose should be 1000 mg or less, and eGFR should be checked every 3 months. There may be

TABLE 3 Dosing Used for Noninsulin Agents

AGENT	DOSE
Thiazolidinediones	
Pioglitazone (Actos)	15, 30, 45 mg
α-Glucosidase Inhibitors	
Acarbose (Preset)	25, 50, 100 mg ac
Miglitol (Glyset)	25, 50 mg ac
Rosiglitazone~ (Avandia)	2, 4, 8 mg
Biguanides	
Metformin IR (Glucophage)	500, 850, 1000 mg*
Metformin ER	500, 750, 1000 mg
Glinides	
Nateglinide (Starlix)	60–120 mg ac
Repaglinide (Prandin)	0.5–4 mg ac
Sulfonylureas (Second Generation)	
Glipizide IR (Glucotrol)	2.5–20 mg
Glipizide ER (Glucotrol XL)	2.5–10 mg
Glimepiride (Amaryl)	1-4 mg
Glyburide (Glynase)	1.25-10, 1.5–6 mg
Incretins	
Exenatide (Byetta)	5, 10 µg
Exenatide QW Bydureon	2.0 mg
Liraglutide (Victoza)	0.6. 1.2, 1.8 mg
Albiglutide** (Tanzeum)	30, 50 mg
Dulaglutide (Trulicity)	0.75, 1.5 mg
DPP-4	
Sitagliptin (Januvia)	100, 50, 25 mg[†]
Saxagliptin (Onglyza)	5, 2.5 mg
Linagliptin (Tradjenta)	5 mg
Alogliptin (Nesina)	25, 12.5, 6.25 mg
Amylin Agonist	
Pramlintide (Symlin)	15, 30, 45, 60, 90, 120 µg[‡]
Bile Acid Sequestrant	
Colesevelam (Welchol)	1875–3750 mg
Dopamine Agonist	
Bromocriptine (Cycloset)	0.8–4.8 mg[§]
SGLT-2 Inhibitor	
Canagliflozin (Invokana)[$]	100, 300 mg
Dapagliflozin[$] (Farixga)	5, 10 mg
Empagliflozin[$] (Jardiance)	10, 25 mg

*Also available as a liquid preparation 500 mg/5 ml.
[†]Dose adjusted for renal function.
[‡]Pens come in range for type 1 (15–60 µg) and type 2 (60–120 µg).
~Restriction on use lifted as CVD risk not clearly increased.
[§]Take with food within 2 h of awakening.
[$]All of SGLT2 drugs use lower doses with moderate renal dysfunction and are contra-indicated in severe renal dysfunction.
**Powder reconstitutes in the pen before use with twist.

an increased lactic acidosis risk in patients with congestive heart failure (CHF) or respiratory insufficiency. Intravascular contrast administration should prompt holding the drug for 24 to 48 hours until renal function is confirmed to be adequate. GI side effects are common initially and are dose dependent but wane; they can require gradual titration. Sustained-release preparations have fewer GI side effects. Weight gain is less with this drug than with many others for diabetes. The United Kingdom Prospective Diabetes Study (UKPDS) found that risk of MI and death was reduced, making it a first choice for pharmacotherapy in most patients.

Thiazolidinediones. One thiazolidinedione (TZD) is used, and that is pioglitazone. Pioglitazone increases the sensitivity of muscle tissue

and fat to insulin action, probably through adipokines like adiponectin and muscle effects on adenosine monophosphate–activated protein kinase (AMPK), a fuel sensor enzyme, and through effects on glucagon. HbA1c lowering varies, dependent on whether patients are very insulin resistant (central adiposity, often hypertriglyceridemia) and whether there is adequate endogenous insulin secretion (short diabetes duration or secretagogues) or insulin is given.

Conversion to diabetes from prediabetes can be prevented by pioglitazone, but it is not commonly recommended. TZDs can precipitate edema, weight gain due to obesity, and occasionally congestive heart failure even absent a prior heart failure history. It is thus wise to track weight in all patients and limit gains to 5 or 6 pounds. The risk of heart failure is increased when TZDs are combined with insulin. TZDs have beneficial effects on lipids, and pioglitazone appears effective in reducing hypertriglyceridemia. Pioglitazone studies suggest reduced ischemic risk (stroke or myocardial infarction). Pioglitazone may increase heart failure, and new studies report more self-reported fractures in women, which suggests avoiding this medication with high risk of osteoporosis or fragility fractures. Some concerns exist about increased risk of bladder cancer, but risk specificity is unclear.

Incretins. Incretins are gut hormones that enhance food-induced insulin secretion. Incretin drugs either are receptor agonists (e.g., exenatide) for glucagon-like peptide-1 (GLP-1), perhaps the most important incretin, or they enhance endogenous levels for both GLP-1 and gastrointestinal insulinotropic polypeptide (GIP).

Exenatide is available as immediate release (Byetta) given twice daily and in once weekly slow release (Bydureon). There is a second available GLP-1 receptor agonist, liraglutide (Victoza), with once daily dosing. Two other agonists, albiglutide and dulaglutide, are approved by the FDA; they are given once weekly. The five incretin agonists increase meal insulin, decrease meal hyperglucagonemia, decrease rate of stomach emptying, and suppress appetite, which may cause a moderate weight loss. They work rapidly on injection. They have substantial GI side effects including nausea, vomiting, and diarrhea in a large minority of patients. Despite this, many patients favor them, probably because the side effects generally wane within weeks and there can be substantial weight loss in some very overweight patients. Typically, exenatide is given in doses of 5 µg twice daily at meals, advancing after a month to 10 µg twice daily. Liraglutide is usually started at 0.6 mg once daily and advanced to 1.2 and then 1.8 mg as needed and tolerated. Patients might report that nausea is more tolerable if they have a little food in their stomach at the time of dosing. Pancreatitis may rarely occur (case reports). Exenatide in a sustained-release once-weekly preparation is embedded into microspheres that permit slow release. The injections require a somewhat larger needle (23 gauge) that is short and well tolerated although somewhat more frequent site reactions and immunogenicity occur with this formulation. Adaptation to nausea seems quicker in longer-acting preparations (once daily or weekly) than in immediate-release exenatide).

Because incretin drugs all have a glucose-dependent insulin secretion and glucagon suppression, there is little risk for hypoglycemia used alone or when they are combined with metformin and TZDs; in contrast hypoglycemia is increased when combined with sulfonylureas or with insulin therapy. HbA1c lowering with exenatide has been 0.9 to 1.1 percentage points, and while albiglutide is similar to exenatide, liraglutide, dulaglutide, or sustained-release exenatide have similar to slightly more efficacy in lowering HbA1c but equal weight effects. Concerns are raised about pancreatitis risk and pancreatic dysplasia, but these remain inconclusive and controversial. Risk of medullary thyroid cancer prevents these drugs from use in patients with that disorder.

Dipeptidyl Peptidase-4 Inhibitors. Dipeptidyl peptidase-4 (DPP-4) is the enzyme that normally rapidly degrades the incretins GLP-1 and GIP to inactive proteolytic products. Inhibitors of DPP-4 have been shown to enhance GLP-1 and GIP levels to high physiologic levels and thereby reduce HbA1c concentrations, typically about 0.6 to 0.8 percentage points. At this writing, four drugs, sitagliptin (Januvia), saxagliptin (Onglyza), linagliptin (Tradjenta), and alogliptin (Nesina) are approved and appear to be similarly effective in recommended doses (see Table 3). Sitagliptin (standard dose 100 mg/d) and alogliptin (standard dose 25 mg/d) are excreted by the kidneys and thus should be given in lower doses (50 mg/d for sitagliptin and 12.5 mg/d for alogliptin) for those with moderate renal insufficiency (eGFR 30–50 for sitagliptin and 30–59 for alogliptin) and further reduced (25 mg/day and 6.25 mg/d, respectively) for those with severe renal dysfunction (GFR <30 mL/min). Saxagliptin is reduced from 5 mg per day to 2.5 mg per day in moderate renal insufficiency (eGFR <50), whereas linagliptin does not need dose adjustment with kidney disease. All have similar actions and probably potential side effects, including pancreatitis. These drugs are available in combination pills with metformin.

Because DPP-4 inhibitors are oral, they may be preferred to the injectable incretins. The side effects for these drugs are relatively minor, and these drugs cause little nausea, vomiting, or diarrhea. They also do not cause significant weight loss but, like metformin, appear to be weight neutral. Rare but serious allergic reactions such as angioedema and Stevens-Johnson syndrome have been reported in a few patients. Pancreatitis has been observed with this class of drugs rarely. Joint pain is a new uncommon side effect.

Amylin Agonists. Insulin is cosecreted with another beta cell hormone called amylin. The effects of amylin appear to be to help lower glycemia, reduce excess glucagon levels, curb appetite, and possibly reduce the rate of gastric emptying. A synthetic analogue of amylin, pramlintide (Symlin), is available as an injectable agent for treating both T1DM and T2DM as an adjunct to insulin. It lowers HbA1c about 0.5 to 0.7 percentage point. It also appears to have some weight loss effect, typically around 1 to 2 kg. Its action primarily controls glucose postprandially. Nausea and vomiting can occur in patients with either T2DM or T1DM but are worse in T1DM patients who require low doses at first (15 µg or less with meals) and slower titration. Those with T2DM usually start with 60 µg and can usually advance to 90 to 120 µg at meals.

Bile Acid Sequestrants. Colesevelam hydrochloride (Welchol), in either single or divided doses of 3.8 g daily, reduces hyperglycemia compared with placebo in patients with T2DM. A1c reductions range from 0.4% to 0.8% when used alone, with metformin, with sulfonylureas, and when used with insulin and other oral agents. Although this drug has already been approved for treatment of hyperlipidemia, it is now FDA approved also for T2DM. It has the potential, however, to increase triglycerides, and thus baseline fasting lipid values should be obtained and tracked, especially in hypertriglyceridemic patients-use is not recommended when baseline triglycerides exceed 250 mg/dL. There is little justification for its use alone or with thiazolidinediones, but it may be appropriate for some patients with T2DM not at goal on other therapies.

Dopamine Receptor Agonists. Bromocriptine, a dopamine receptor agonist in a rapid release formulation, is a relatively new addition to antidiabetes medications. Although its mechanism of action is not precisely clear, the drug will reduce premeal and postmeal blood sugars without changing insulin levels, which suggests a benefit to insulin action, perhaps through mediation of central nervous system mechanisms. Its side effects are somewhat similar to those of the bromocriptine used for pituitary disease. Nausea is a common initial side effect. Its efficacy is moderate, with HbA1c reductions of 0.5% or slightly more. Its preliminary data suggest a favorable cardiovascular safety profile associated with its use, which is reassuring. Usual starting doses are 0.8 mg once daily with gradual increase based on tolerance of nausea to bromocriptine in higher doses (up to 4.8 mg daily).

SGLT-2 Inhibitors. Three approved drugs are available; they are canagliflozin, dapagliflozin and empagliflozin. They act as inhibitors of sodium glucose transporters, which lead to a glucose diuresis from the kidney, a unique mechanism of action. This drug is effective in lowering HbA1c up to 1% or more with a relatively low risk of hypoglycemia when used alone or with other drugs such as metformin, but they may cause hypoglycemia when combined with insulin or insulin secretagogues such as sulfonylureas. These drugs may have favorable effects on blood pressure, partly from diuretic effects, and may cause postural hypotension. In monotherapy with these drugs, up to HbA1c reductions of 1%

may be seen. Added to metformin, the reduction is 0.5% to 0.75%. Additional benefits may include weight loss of 1.2 to 3.3 kg and a slight reduction in systolic blood pressure of up to 4 to 9 mm Hg, but postural hypotension symptoms or acute kidney injury may occur. Urinary infections are more common, but are treatable. *Candida* vulvovaginitis and balanitis are more common with SGLT-2 inhibitors. The usual starting dose is the lowest dose shown in table 3 once daily before the first meal. The dose may be advanced if needed for improving glucose control but only if the eGFR is equal to or greater than 60 mL/min/1.73 m^2 for canagliflozin, while for empagliflozin it should not be started if eGFR is <45 but for values above 45 no dose adjustment is needed, and for dapagliflozin it should not be started if eGFR is <60 and if >60 no dose adjustment is needed. For canagliflozin if the eGFR is between 45 and 60, the dose of should not be advanced beyond 100 mg, and if the eGFR is less than 45, the drug should not be used. Frequent monitoring of eGFR is recommended with values less than 60. These drugs should be used with caution in the event of significant renal dysfunction and should not be used in advanced liver or kidney dysfunction. Rarely, ketoacidosis can occur when used with insulin.

Insulin

Barriers to Insulin Use. Insulin deficiency underlies the genesis of both T1DM and T2DM. Progression of therapy to use of insulin, typically with oral agents in T2DM, also seems predicated on progressive loss of insulin secretion. Nonetheless, it is often started too late, and patients often are in very poor control when this is done. Reluctance by patients and physicians alike might underlie this. Physicians should understand that exogenous insulin in T2DM is needed, does not negatively alter life quality, and is more likely to achieve therapeutic targets. Moreover, exogenous insulin does not worsen insulin resistance, does not cause excess cardiovascular disease, and has a low frequency of severe hypoglycemia, especially when used relatively early in the disease. Table 4 lists common insulin preparations and some notes about kinetics and timing.

Starting Insulin: Use of Basal Insulin in Type 2 Diabetes. How should insulin be started? Practitioners should use temporary insulin for patients whose glycemia is initially poorly controlled or when patients temporarily have worse control due to illness or medications, such as glucocorticoids. It is unwise to use insulin as a threat because it creates a sense of personal failure and dread of insulin use. When therapy progresses but there is failure to achieve glycemic goals after one or two oral medications, use of basal insulin is often the best way to achieve euglycemia, especially if patients are much more than 1 percentage point from HbA1c goal (< 7%).

The Treat-to-Target Trial offers a good example of how to initiate insulin therapy. In this study, as often in our practice, patients start with a basal insulin either with NPH insulin or insulin glargine (Lantus). Insulin detemir (Levemir) represents another long-acting insulin analog option to be used similarly. Insulin is instituted as 10 U once daily, commonly in the evening near bedtime, followed by weekly increases of between 2 and 8 units depending on proximity to glucose goals, focusing on the fasting glucose.

This strategy is sometimes called the *fix the fasting first* rule. Average doses in that study were around 45 to 50 units for patients whose BMI was about 31 kg/m^2. An alternative initial dosing might be 0.2 U/kg body weight, but whatever the starting dose, a forced titration guided by patient self-monitoring with clear communication of target fasting glucose (90–130 mg/dL), size of increment (or decrement in case of hypoglycemia; usually 10%–20% of dose), and frequency of change (every 3–7 days) is necessary to get most patients to overall glycemic (HbA1c) goal. This strategy is referred to as *pattern management*. The intent is to use monitoring to adjust the insulin dose likely to affect the fasting glucose for basal insulin therapy. NPH and detemir usually can be used once daily, typically at bedtime. Patients using glargine may choose any time of the day as long as it is reasonably consistent, usually within an hour. Occasionally, twice-daily NPH or detemir is used. The new U-300 insulin glargine may be helpful in reduction of overnight hypoglycemia, as it has a flatter kinetic profile and longer duration of action.

TABLE 4	Insulin Preparations			
	PHARMACOKINETICS			
INSULIN TYPE	**ONSET (h)**	**PEAK (h)**	**DURATION (h)**	**COMMENTS**
Basal Insulins				
NPH (Humulin N, Novolin N)	0.5	4–10	18	Kinetics are dose dependent Peak effects exert meal action Dose at breakfast, bedtime, supper*
Glargine† (Lantus)	2–4	Little peak	24*	Dose can be given at any time of day if consistent
Glargine U-300 (Toujeo)#	3–4	No peak	30+	Dose at any time but consistently
Detemir† (Levemir)	2–3	Little peak		Kinetics are dose dependent Dose at breakfast, bedtime, supper*
Meal Insulins				
Regular (Humulin R, Novolin R)	0.25–0.5	2–3	5–8	Give 1/2 hour before meals Do not use at bedtime
Lispro (Humalog)	0.1–0.2	1.5–2.0	4	Dose up to 20 min before mealtime or immediately after
Aspart (Novolog)	0.1–0.2	1.5–2.0	4	Dose up to 20 min before mealtime or immediately after
Glulisine (Apidra)	0.1–0.2	1.5–2.0	4	Dose up to 20 min before mealtime or immediately after
Mixed Preparations				
NPH/regular (Humulin, Novolin)	70/30 dual kinetics based on components			Dosing 1/2 hour before meals Should not be dosed at bedtime
Lispro/NPLispro (Humalog 75/25)	75/25 dual kinetics based on components			Dosing at mealtime; should not be dosed at bedtime
Lispro/NPLispro Humalog 50/50	50/50 dual kinetics based on components			Dosing at mealtime, should not be dosed at bedtime
Aspart/NPAspart (NovoLog 70/30)	70/30 dual kinetics based on components			Dosing at mealtime; should not be dosed at bedtime

*Bedtime dosing may be preferred for some patients, especially those on low doses.
†Should not be mixed with other insulins or used in the same syringe that other insulin has been in.
#Advance dose no faster than every 3–4 days, slightly higher doses may be needed compared to U-100 insulin glargine.
Abbreviation: NPH = neutral protamine Hagedorn.

When and How to Add Meal Insulin. At some point, basal insulin therapy alone may be insufficient for glycemic control for T2DM patients. Usually this is a consideration in patients whose HbA1c values are over 9% to 9.5% or where the fasting goal is met but HbA1c or daytime glycemia remains elevated. The need for meal insulin is particularly likely to occur with larger meals, such as supper. Diagnostically, what is important is to have patients check either both before and after large meals or, if they are unwilling to check frequently, simply check about 2 to 3 hours after meals. Self-monitored glucose values that exceed even minimum postprandial glycemic guidelines (<180 mg/dL) indicate the need for meal insulin. A common mistake made in practice is to treat fasting hyperglycemia only with increases in basal insulin, when in some patients, the cause is overeating or lack of meal insulin the previous evening. This can be discerned by observing the pattern of glycemia, with lows often between meals or overnight and highs occurring after meals or at bedtime.

Fixed-Ratio Combined Insulins

A commonly employed strategy is to use fixed-ratio combination short-acting (either regular or rapid analog) insulin combined with intermediate insulin (NPH or neutral protamine modified rapid analog that mimics NPH timing). Examples of these preparations include 70/30 NPH and regular insulin, 75/25 neutral protamine lispro and lispro insulin (Humalog), and 70/30 neutral protamine aspart and aspart insulin (Novolog). These have the advantage of being able to achieve control very conveniently in T2DM patients who have quite poor control (HbA1c of 9.5% or more) with a simple twice-daily injection regimen. They also offer the advantage of greater dosing accuracy, especially when used with insulin pens. Important to the success of these formulations is consistent eating and carbohydrate intake with meals.

Unfortunately, when such consistency is not advised or followed, patterns of glycemia can be erratic and hypoglycemia can be significantly increased due to both components of the combination. Patients who skip meals are poor candidates for such treatments and should either switch to individual dosing of an insulin mixture or, even safer, use a basal bolus insulin regimen.

Adults with Type 1 DM

A significant minority of patients with a diagnosis of T2DM actually have a late onset of T1DM and typical autoimmunity (IA-2 antibodies, GAD-65 antibodies, and insulin antibodies). The diagnosis should certainly be suspected in patients who rapidly fail combination oral agent therapy. Nonobese body habitus, marked weight loss, extremely elevated glucose values, or a family or personal history of autoimmune disease (e.g., Hashimoto's or Graves' thyroid problems) should lead to diagnostic evaluation for such signs of autoimmunity.

T1DM patients need combined mealtime and basal insulin therapy. Although it is tempting to do so in a convenient fashion with combined preparations such as those with analogue fixed ratios, it usually is far preferable to use a better basal insulin, such as glargine or detemir combined with a rapid-acting analogue (separately injected) before meals. Sometimes an insulin pump is the best way for patients who have frequent hypoglycemia or marked variability to achieve good glycemic control safely. T1DM patients should preferably be seen by an endocrine specialist or other practitioner with extensive experience in T1DM management. Ready access to diabetes educators is an important key to success with both T1DM and T2DM.

Adults with Type 2 DM

Many T2DM patients eventually need mealtime insulin. For those on basal insulin alone, incretin mimetics[1] can be successfully used for meal-time control, because they effectively lower prandial hyperglycemia. If exenatide is used, then additional injections will be required at the two major meals of the day. If using an incretin-enhancer drug such as sitagliptin, injections are not required. This approach is useful with incretin agonists exenatide or liraglutide in patients who need to lose weight, who gain considerable weight with meal insulin, or who experience poor control despite attempts to regulate meal glycemia with short-acting insulins. Recent studies suggest possible benefit of combining long acting basal insulins with incretin receptor agonists.

---

[1]Not FDA approved for this indication.

References

Accord Study Group. Effects of intensive blood-pressure control in type 2 diabetes mellitus. N Engl J Med 2010;362:1575–85.

American Diabetes Association, Standards of Medical Care in Diabetes. Diabetes Care. 2015 January 2015 Volume 38, Supplement 1, S1-S93.

American Diabetes Association. Facilitating Behavior Change: Key Strategies for Empowering Your Patients, http://www.facilitatingbehaviorchange.org/2009.

Diabetes Prevention Program Research Group. The Diabetes Prevention Program (DPP): Description of lifestyle intervention. Diabetes Care 2002;25:2165–71.

Fox CS et al. Update on Prevention of Cardiovascular Disease in Adults With Type 2 Diabetes Mellitus in Light of Recent Evidence: A Scientific Statement From the American Heart Association and the American Diabetes Association Diabetes Care. 2015 Sep;38(9):1777–803.

Garber AJ, Abrahamson MJ, Barzilay JI, et al. American association of clinical endocrinologists' comprehensive diabetes management algorithm 2013 consensus statement-executive summary. Endocr Pract 2013;19:536–57.

Grundy SM, Cleeman JI, Daniels SR, et al. Diagnosis and management of the metabolic syndrome. An American Heart Association/National Heart, Lung, and Blood Institute Scientific Statement. Executive summary. Circulation 2005;112:2735–52.

Harja E, Lord J, Skyler JS. An analysis of characteristics of subjects examined for incretin effects on pancreatic pathology. Diabetes Technol Ther 2013;15:609–18.

Inzucchi SE et al. Management of hyperglycaemia in type 2 diabetes, 2015: a patient-centred approach. Update to a Position Statement of the American Diabetes Association and the European Association for the Study of Diabetes Diabetologia 2015;58: 429–42.

Kahn R, Buse J, Ferrannini E, Stern M. The metabolic syndrome: Time for a critical appraisal. Joint statement from the American Diabetes Association and the European Association for the Study of Diabetes. Diabetes Care 2005;8:2289–304.

Knowler WC, Barrett-Connor E, Fowler SE, et al. Reduction in the incidence of type 2 diabetes with lifestyle intervention or metformin. N Engl J Med 2002;346:393–403.

Lipska KJ, Bailey CJ, Inzucchi SE, Use of metformin in the setting of mild to moderate renal insufficiency. Diabetes Care 2011;34:1431–7.

Monnier L, Lapinski H, Colette C. Contributions of fasting and postprandial plasma glucose increments to the overall diurnal hyperglycemia of type 2 diabetic patients. Variations with increasing levels of HbA1c. Diabetes Care 2003;26:881–5.

Nesto RW, Bell D, Bonow RO, et al. Thiazolidinedione use, fluid retention, and congestive heart failure. A consensus statement from the American Heart Association and American Diabetes Association. Diabetes Care 2004;27:256–63.

Stone NJ, et al. 2013 ACC/AHA guideline on the treatment of blood cholesterol to reduce atherosclerotic cardiovascular risk in adults: a report of the American College of Cardiology/American Heart Association Task Force on Practice Guidelines. 2014;129(25 Suppl. 2):S1–45.

Riddle MC, Rosenstock J, Gerich J. The treat-to-target trial: Randomized addition of glargine or human NPH insulin to oral therapy of type 2 diabetic patients. Diabetes Care 2003;26:3080–6.

GOUT AND HYPERURICEMIA

Method of
Saima Chohan, MD

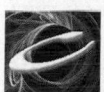

CURRENT DIAGNOSIS

- Gout is the most common inflammatory arthritis in men and is increasing in prevalence.
- A definitive diagnosis of gout requires demonstration of monosodium urate crystals in synovial fluid or tophi.
- Gouty arthritis often begins in the lower extremity joints.
- Septic arthritis, rheumatoid arthritis, and calcium pyrophosphate disease (pseudogout) can mimic gout and should be ruled out.

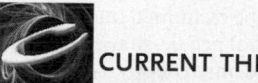

CURRENT THERAPY

- The goals of successful gout treatment include terminating the acute attack, preventing intermittent attacks, and undertaking long-term therapy to avoid chronic arthritis.
- Indications for chronic treatment of gout include frequent attacks, recurrent arthritis, and kidney disease.
- A serum urate level of less than 6.0 mg/dL is the goal when using urate-lowering therapy.
- Nonpharmacologic treatment includes lifestyle modification and dietary changes.
- The mainstay of urate-lowering therapies remains xanthine oxidase inhibition.

Epidemiology

Gout, or monosodium urate crystal deposition disease, is the most common inflammatory arthritis of men and is an increasingly common problem among postmenopausal women. It is a chronic disorder, affecting over 5 million people in the United States and increasing in both prevalence and incidence, especially in persons older than 65 years. Gout is often accompanied by serious comorbid disorders (hypertension, cardiovascular disease, chronic kidney disease, and all of the component features of the metabolic syndrome) and is managed in primary care practice in about 90% of affected persons. Therefore identifying risk factors, optimizing diagnosis, and choosing the appropriate treatment for gout are important skills for a wide array of caregivers.

Pathophysiology and Risk Factors

Uric acid is the end product of purine metabolism in humans. Hyperuricemia, a serum urate concentration exceeding urate solubility (6.8 mg/dL), is an invariable accompaniment of gout, though serum uric acid levels might not be elevated during an acute attack. Hyperuricemia predisposes affected persons to urate crystal formation and deposition, which lead to the inflammatory responses underlying the symptoms of gout. Thus, treatment of gout is aimed at reducing and maintaining serum urate concentration at subsaturating levels, usually set at less than 6.0 mg/dL.

Hyperuricemia

Risk factors for hyperuricemia include obesity, hypertension, hyperlipidemia, insulin resistance, renal insufficiency, and use of diuretics. Diets rich in certain foods are also associated with increased risk for gout. Many studies with large patient cohorts have demonstrated a relationship between hyperuricemia and hypertension, cardiovascular and peripheral vascular disease, chronic kidney disease, and diabetes mellitus. The association of hyperuricemia and metabolic syndrome has also been shown in children and adolescents. Interventional trials of asymptomatic patients with hyperuricemia and high cardiovascular risk must be performed before such treatment can be advocated.

Diagnosis

Acute gout is characterized by an abrupt onset of joint pain, erythema, and swelling, usually of one joint, but less commonly of more than one. The arthritis most often occurs first in a lower extremity joint, especially the first metatarsophalangeal (MTP) joint at the base of the great toe. The predilection for this site is thought to be secondary to cooler acral temperature or repeated trauma and pressure on this joint.

The gold standard for diagnosis of gout is the demonstration of monosodium urate crystals by polarized light microscopy, either in joint fluid aspirated during an acute attack or between attacks, or from material aspirated from suspected tophi. To aspirate the first MTP joint, the joint is first identified by palpating the space at the base of the metacarpal on the dorsal aspect while flexing and extending the toe. The needle is then inserted perpendicularly into the joint space to avoid the extensor hallucis tendon. Synovial fluid from affected joints should immediately be examined under polarized microscopy to confirm the diagnosis of needle-shaped crystals with negative birefringence. If polarized microscopy is unavailable, then fluid should be promptly sent in a sterile tube for crystal confirmation to an appropriate laboratory.

Unfortunately, the equipment and analytical expertise necessary to make this diagnosis are not widely available to primary care physicians. As a result, the diagnosis of acute gout is commonly made on clinical grounds, often using clinical and laboratory criteria established by organizations such as the American College of Rheumatology and the European League Against Rheumatism. These diagnostic guidelines emphasize the presence of signs of inflammation (swelling, warmth, redness, tenderness, and loss of joint function), abrupt onset, monoarticular involvement, occurrence in the first MTP joint, and presence of tophi.

The initial symptoms and signs of gout often occur after many years of asymptomatic hyperuricemia. In untreated or inadequately treated patients, the course of the disease often involves acute attacks at increasing frequency, with shortening of asymptomatic periods (called intercritical gout) and, ultimately, development of chronic joint disease (gouty arthropathy) and tophi (masses of urate crystals in a chronic inflammatory matrix) in bone, joints, skin, and even solid organs (Figure 1).

Indications for Treatment

Early in gout, patients might have attacks that are separated by years and manageable over the course of a few days with anti-inflammatory medications and adjuncts such as joint rest and application of ice. Over time, the attacks usually become more frequent, prolonged, and disabling, eventually requiring long-term urate-lowering treatment aimed at preventing urate crystal deposition and eventually abolishing acute flares and resolving tophi. Indications for urate-lowering (antihyperuricemic) therapy are listed in Box 1.

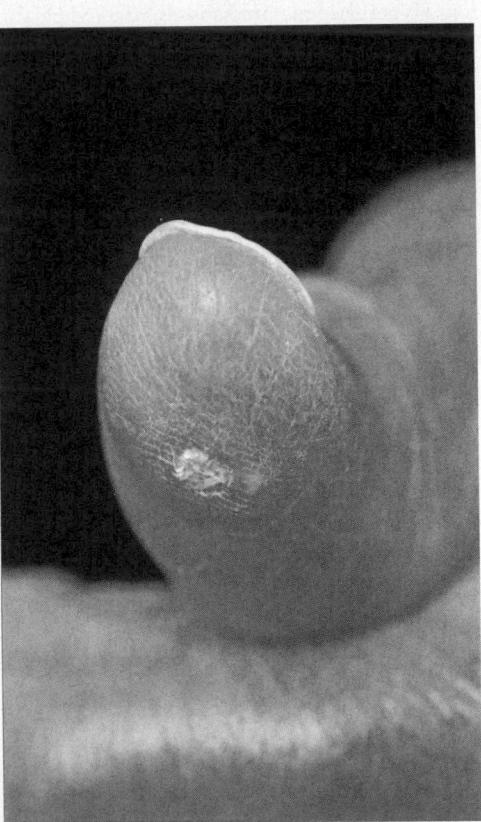

Figure 1. Intradermal urate deposit (tophus). (Reprinted with permission from Mandell BF: Gout and crystal deposition disease. In Weisman MH, Weinblatt ME, Louie JS, Van Vollenhoven R (eds): Targeted Treatment of the Rheumatic Diseases. Philadelphia, Saunders, 2010, 293–302).

Box 1	Indications for Urate-Lowering Therapy

- Frequent and disabling gouty attacks, often defined as two or three flares annually, though this is not evidence based; the decision to treat is based on both number of flares and the consequent disability resulting from flares
- Chronic gouty disease: clinically or radiographically evident joint erosions
- Tophaceous deposits: subcutaneous or intraosseous
- Gout with renal insufficiency
- Recurrent kidney stones
- Urate nephropathy
- Urinary uric acid excretion exceeding 1100 mg/d (6.5 mmol), when determined in men younger than 25 years or in premenopausal women

Treatment

Acute Gout

Gouty arthritis occurs suddenly, and attacks are often very painful and disabling. Patients describe acute onset of exquisite pain, swelling, erythema, and inability to bear weight on the afflicted joint. Occasionally, patients have constitutional symptoms including fever and chills, with an elevation of sedimentation rate and white blood cell count. To terminate an attack, nonsteroidal anti-inflammatory drugs (NSAIDs), colchicine (Colcrys), or corticosteroids can be offered. If given at full anti-inflammatory dosage, NSAIDs have a rapid onset and are quite efficacious in relieving pain and shortening the duration of an attack. The utility of this class of drugs may be limited by renal insufficiency, cardiovascular risk factors, and gastrointestinal bleeding. While indomethacin (Indocin), sulindac (Clinoril), and naproxen (Naprosyn) are all FDA approved for treating acute attacks of gout, nearly every drug in this class and the selective cyclooxygenase (COX) 2 inhibitors also have considerable efficacy. High-dose salicylate therapy lowers serum uric acid by interfering in renal urate transport; low-dose aspirin[1] has the opposite effect, but it is often continued in gout patients because of its overriding importance in managing coronary artery disease.

Oral colchicine has been used to treat gout for many years as an unproven drug with no FDA dosage recommendations or prescribing information. In July 2009, however, the FDA-approved Colcrys, a single-ingredient colchicine product, for the first day of treatment of acute gout attacks at a low-dose regimen of 1.2 mg followed by 0.6 mg in 1 hour (total 1.8 mg). With this regimen, colchicine can be used to abort an attack if taken immediately after the development of the first symptom of gout flare. Higher colchicine doses (0.6 mg every hour, until symptoms improve or until gastrointestinal symptoms of diarrhea, nausea, or vomiting develop, for a total of 4.8 mg over 6 h)[2] have traditionally been recommended. A randomized, placebo-controlled trial comparing the low-dose and high-dose regimens showed both approaches had equivalent efficacy in pain relief at 24 hours (compared with placebo). However, adverse gastrointestinal events were significantly less common with the low-dose regimen. In subjects warranting additional flare treatment, continued use of colchicine 0.6 mg twice daily (reducing to once daily as the flare subsides) is appropriate in persons with normal renal and hepatic function.

Gastrointestinal symptoms are generally the first clinical signs of colchicine toxicity in patients with normal renal and hepatic function. More serious toxicities do occur and include neuromyopathy, aplastic anemia, and worsening renal and hepatic function. Care should be used in patients with renal or hepatic impairment, and because of potentially serious drug-drug interactions, colchicine should be avoided in patients receiving cyclosporine (Neoral), clarithromycin (Biaxin), verapamil (Calan),

---

[1]Not FDA approved for this indication.
[2]Not available in the United States.

and amlodipine (Norvasc). Intravenous colchicine[3] is not available in Europe. The FDA has stopped the marketing of unapproved injectable colchicine products in the United States and discourages the compounding of IV colchicines because of reports of preparation errors causing deaths.

Corticosteroids provide a safe alternative for patients with contraindications to NSAIDs or colchicine. For isolated monoarticular attacks, especially of medium or large joints, aspiration of joint fluid and intraarticular injection with triamcinolone acetonide (Kenalog) 20 to 40 mg can quickly terminate an attack. For polyarticular attacks or attacks in smaller joints, systemic corticosteroids (oral or intramuscular) may be employed. Oral prednisone starting at 20 mg twice daily with a taper over 10 to 14 days is very effective. Patients can have rebound attacks if oral steroids are terminated too quickly, and thus methylprednisolone (Medrol) dose packs should be avoided. If intramuscular injection is used, a single dose of triamcinolone 40 mg may be employed.

There is interest in agents blocking the action of interleukin 1 (IL-1), a cytokine thought to play a major role in initiating and sustaining acute gouty inflammation. Anakinra (Kineret)[1] and canakinumab (Ilaris)[1] are potent injectable IL-1 inhibitors, and studies are ongoing to assess the utility of these agents to mitigate acute attacks. In 2013 canakinumab became the first biologic agent approved for acute gout in Europe. It was approved by the European Medicines Agency for symptomatic treatment of adult patients with frequent gouty arthritis attacks in whom NSAIDs and colchicine are contraindicated, are not tolerated, or do not provide an adequate response, and in whom repeated courses of corticosteroids are not appropriate. Rilonacept (Arcalyst)[1], which is also in this class, was declined approval for gout by the FDA in 2012 because of concerns about long-term safety.

Intercritical Gout
After an attack subsides, management is directed at preventing recurrent attacks. During acute attacks of gout, normal serum urate concentration is reported in up to 40% of affected patients, and thus it is not an accurate reflection of the true urate pool. Confirmation of hyperuricemia is best achieved either before the resolution of an attack or 2 to 4 weeks after it, in order to achieve an accurate serum urate concentration. There is a generalizable correlation between the serum urate level and risk for recurrent attack.

Prophylaxis of future attacks during early urate-lowering therapy can consist of colchicine (Colcrys) at doses of 0.6 mg once or twice a day (based on renal function) or NSAIDs. If chronic NSAIDs are used, acid-reducing medications such as proton pump inhibitors or histamine-2 blockers may be employed for patients at risk for gastrointestinal bleeding.

Long-Term Urate-Lowering (Antihyperuricemic) Therapy
The aim of urate-lowering therapy is to reduce and maintain serum urate at concentrations below those at which extracellular fluids are saturated with monosodium urate. In general, an ultimate serum urate concentration of less than 6.0 mg/dL is advised. Urate lowering can be achieved either by increasing urinary excretion or by decreasing production of urate.

Nonpharmacologic urate-lowering treatment begins with lifestyle changes. Diet and weight loss must be addressed. Obesity and weight gain are risk factors for gout, and weight loss has been shown to decrease the risk of gout. A purine-restricted diet has often been recommended to patients but is often unpalatable and impractical. Reduction in alcohol intake, namely beer and liquor, can effectively reduce urate levels. Similarly, reduced intake of red meat and shellfish also lowers the risk of recurrent gouty attacks. Studies have shown an increased frequency of attacks in patients who consume fruit juices and soft drinks containing high-fructose corn syrup, an ingredient not found in diet drinks.

Once the decision is made to institute serum urate-lowering therapy, the duration of treatment is indefinite and must be long-term to be effective. The majority of patients with gout and tophaceous disease will continue to have attacks if therapy is discontinued, and thus education is a key part of the treatment plan. Patients should be instructed that, with initiation of any urate-lowering therapy, they will be at increased risk for a flareup and thus must continue regular use of prophylactic agents as outlined above. At least 80% to 95% of cases of hyperuricemia and gout are attributable to impaired urate excretion, which is reflected in diminished urate clearance or fractional excretion of uric acid but not usually in low daily urine uric acid excretion. In practice, 24-hour urine collections are rarely performed. Patients are preferentially treated with xanthine oxidase inhibitors because of the easier dosing schedule and because many patients have contraindications to uricosurics such as renal insufficiency and kidney stones.

Uricosurics
Relative to medications aimed at urate synthesis, uricosurics are relegated to second-line treatment of patients with elevated urate burden or tophaceous disease. The most commonly used uricosuric agent in the United States is probenecid. This is a very effective drug that concentrates and promotes urinary excretion of urate. Its utility is limited in patients with renal insufficiency, and probenecid is not recommended as first-line therapy in patients with nephrolithiasis or uric acid overexcretion. The maintenance dose of probenecid required to achieve and maintain serum urate concentration at less than 6.0 mg/dL is 0.5 to 3 g/day,[4] administered in 2 or 3 daily doses. Once goal serum urate concentration is achieved with a uricosuric agent, the risk of uric acid calculi is diminished, because urinary uric acid excretion becomes normal.

Other drugs found to have uricosuric effects include fenofibrate (Tricor)[1], a fibric acid derivative used to treat hyperlipidemia, and the antihypertensives losartan (Cozaar)[1] and amlodipine (Norvasc).[1] These agents have mild uricosuric properties and may be useful adjuncts to urate lowering therapy. Skim milk ingestion has been shown to lower serum urate levels through uricosuric effects. Lower urate levels have also been seen in patients who consume coffee, but the mechanism of action is unknown.

Xanthine Oxidase Inhibitors
Allopurinol (Zyloprim) and febuxostat (Uloric) are the only FDA-approved xanthine oxidase inhibitors for the treatment of gout. Allopurinol, introduced in 1966, is approved in doses of 100 to 800 mg/day. More than 90% of patients with gout treated with urate-lowering medication in the United States are given allopurinol, but dosages of more than 300 mg/day are infrequently employed, and often patients do not achieve serum urate concentrations of 6.0 mg/dL or less. Appropriate use of allopurinol is limited for several reasons. There are genuine concerns about allopurinol drug interactions, gastrointestinal intolerance, rashes (ranging from mild to life-threatening), and the rare but sometimes fatal hypersensitivity syndrome. Allopurinol should be avoided with the immunosuppressives azathioprine (Imuran) and 6-mercaptopurine (Purinethol) because it can increase the risk of bone marrow toxicity, as these medications are partially metabolized by xanthine oxidase. Allopurinol should not be taken with ampicillin owing to increased risk of rash.

Effective dosing of allopurinol is often not achieved because of compliance with published but recently disputed recommendations for allopurinol dose reduction in states of renal impairment. Allopurinol should be initiated at 100 mg daily in patients with creatinine clearance of 40 mL/min or greater, and it should be titrated in 100-mg increments every 2 to 4 weeks, with the endpoint of dosing determined by achievement of serum urate concentration of 6.0 mg/dL or less.

---

[1]Not FDA approved for this indication
[3]Exceeds dosage recommended by the manufacturer.

[1]Not FDA approved for this indication.
[4]Not yet approved for use in the United States.

The FDA approved febuxostat (Uloric) in 2009. Unlike allopurinol, this is a nonpurine analogue and selective xanthine oxidase inhibitor that is not incorporated into purine nucleotides and does not appear to affect pyrimidine metabolism. Febuxostat is primarily metabolized by oxidation and glucuronidation in the liver, with little renal excretion of drug; this contrasts with the renal elimination of oxypurinol, the main allopurinol metabolite. The recommended starting dose of febuxostat is 40 mg daily, with an increase to 80 mg daily if serum urate concentrations do not reach goal urate levels in 2 weeks in patients with normal renal function. In Europe, higher dosages (80–120 mg daily)[5] have received approval, and studies have affirmed the efficacy and safety of dosing in this range. In the FOCUS trial, a 5-year study of efficacy and safety, febuxostat was shown to have durable maintenance of serum urate concentration at 6.0 mg/dL or less, nearly complete elimination of gouty flares, and resolution of baseline tophi in subjects. An advantage of febuxostat over allopurinol is that it can safely be taken by patients with creatinine clearance greater than 30 mL/min.

Pegloticase

Pegloticase (pegylated porcine recombinant uricase, Krystexxa) was granted FDA approval in 2010 for treatment of refractory gout. Humans lack the enzyme uricase, which converts uric acid to allantoin, a more soluble purine degradation product. Replacement of this missing enzyme allows direct conversion of urate to allantoin, with eventual depletion of increased body urate pools and control of disease, including resolution of tophi. Recombinant uricase therapy profoundly lowers serum urate concentration, as was demonstrated in two large trials. Pegloticase is approved at a dosage of 8 mg intravenously every 2 weeks.

Potential New Therapies

A number of other novel agents with new therapeutic targets for the treatment of acute and chronic gout are under investigation.

---

[5]Investigational drug in the United States.

References

Becker MA, Chohan S. We can make gout management more successful now. Curr Opin Rheumatol 2008;20:167–72.

Dalbeth N, Stamp L. Allopurinol dosing in renal impairment: Walking the tightrope between adequate urate lowering and adverse events. Semin Dial 2007;20:391–5.

Schumacher HR, Becker MA, Lloyd E, et al. Febuxostat in the treatment of gout: 5-year findings of the FOCUS efficacy and safety study. Rheumatology 2009;48:188–94.

Stamp L, O'Donnell JL, Zhang M, et al. Using allopurinol above the dose based on creatinine clearance is effective and safe in patients with chronic gout, including those with renal impairment. Arthritis Rheum 2011;63:412–21.

Sundy JS, Becker MA, Baraf HS, et al. Reduction of plasma urate levels following treatment with multiple doses of pegloticase (polyethylene glycol–conjugated uricase) in patients with treatment-failure gout. Results of a phase II randomized study. Arthritis Rheum 2008;58:2882–91.

Terkeltaub R, Furst DE, Bennett K, et al. High versus low dosing of oral colchicine for early acute gout flare. Arthritis Rheum 2010;62:1060–8.

Zhang W, Doherty M, Pascual E, et al. EULAR evidence based recommendations for gout. Part I: Diagnosis. Report of a task force of the standing committee for international clinical studies including therapeutics (ESCIT). Ann Rheum Dis 2006;65:1301–11.

Zhu Y, Pandya BJ, Choi HK. Comorbidities of gout and hyperuricemia in the US general population: NHANES 2007-2008. Am J Med 2012;125:679–87.

HYPERALDOSTERONISM

Method of
Jongoh Kim, MD; and Lawrence Chan, MD

CURRENT DIAGNOSIS

- Hyperaldosteronism may be suspected in patients with severe, resistant, or early-onset hypertension and hypertensive patients with family history, hypokalemia, metabolic alkalosis, and adrenal mass. Evaluation begins with measurement of morning plasma aldosterone concentration (PAC in ng/dL) and plasma renin activity (PRA in ng/mL/hr) in a sodium- and potassium-repleted state and off of significantly interfering medications (spironolactone [Aldactone], eplerenone [Inspra], amiloride [Midamor], triamterene [Dyrenium], potassium-wasting diuretics, and licorice-derived products[7]) for at least 4 weeks.

- Elevated PRA and PAC suggest secondary hyperaldosteronism; suppressed PRA and PAC suggest conditions mimicking hyperaldosteronism; suppressed PRA but elevated PAC suggests primary hyperaldosteronism (screening positive if PAC/PRA ratio >20–40 and PAC >15 ng/dL).

- Positive screening of primary hyperaldosteronism should be confirmed with one of the following tests: IV saline suppression, oral salt loading, fludrocortisone (Florinef)[1] suppression, or captopril (Capoten)[1] challenge test.

- Once primary hyperaldosteronism is biochemically confirmed, computed tomography (CT) of the adrenal glands is recommended to exclude adrenocortical carcinoma and help subtype primary hyperaldosteronism.

- If surgical treatment is considered, adrenal vein sampling is indicated to differentiate unilateral vs. bilateral lesions (may skip if the patient is <40 years of age and has a CT-confirmed unilateral adrenal nodule >1 cm). A cortisol-corrected aldosterone ratio from the high to the low side > 4:1 with cosyntropin (Cortrosyn) stimulation confirms unilateral aldosterone excess.

---

[1]Not FDA approved for this indication.
[7]Available as dietary supplement.

CURRENT THERAPY

- Laparoscopic adrenalectomy is recommended for unilateral disease. Otherwise, medical treatment with a mineralocorticoid receptor antagonist (MRA; spironolactone [Aldactone] or eplerenone [Inspra][1]) is recommended.

- Spironolactone: 12.5 to 25 mg/day titrated to a maximum dose of 400 mg/day to achieve normal blood pressure and normokalemia. Side effects include increased serum creatinine, hyperkalemia, gynecomastia, and menstrual irregularities.

- Eplerenone: 25 mg once or twice daily titrated to a maximum dose of 100 mg/day to achieve normal blood pressure and normokalemia. Side effects include increased creatinine, hyperkalemia, hypertriglyceridemia, increased liver enzymes, headache, and fatigue.

- Amiloride (Midamor)[1] or triamterene (Dyrenium)[1] (epithelial sodium channel antagonists) can be used in those who cannot tolerate MRAs or are still hypertensive/hypokalemic while on MRAs. Other antihypertensive agents are also added if necessary to control hypertension.

---

[1]Not FDA approved for this indication.

Introduction

Hyperaldosteronism is a state of excessive aldosterone secretion. Primary hyperaldosteronism occurs due to autonomous hypersecretion of aldosterone, whereas secondary hyperaldosteronism occurs due to activation of the renin angiotensin aldosterone system (RAAS). Primary hyperaldosteronism is the most common cause of secondary hypertension, and recent reports suggest that 5% to 20% of hypertensive patients have primary hyperaldosteronism (as opposed to less than 1%, as previously reported). Secondary hyperaldosteronism includes two different categories; one is compensatory activation of the RAAS due to decreased effective circulating volume, as in congestive heart failure and liver cirrhosis; the other is overactivity of the RAAS accompanied by hypertension, as in renovascular hypertension. There are also several conditions that mimic aldosterone excess through various mechanisms that present with hypertension and other metabolic perturbations. Except for the compensatory activation of the RAAS, these conditions cause secondary hypertension with or without other metabolic consequences, such as hypokalemia and metabolic alkalosis, which bring them to medical attention. This chapter covers the current approaches to hyperaldosteronism for patients suspected of having hypertension secondary to excess aldosterone production.

Pathophysiology

Aldosterone is a steroid hormone produced by the zona glomerulosa in the adrenal gland and contributes to volume and potassium homeostasis via its action primarily on the principal cells in the collecting tubule of the kidney. The main stimuli of aldosterone secretion are angiotensin II and hyperkalemia, which increase synthesis and activity of aldosterone synthase. Aldosterone and angiotensin II are part of the RAAS; plasma renin from the juxtaglomerular apparatus converts angiotensinogen to angiotensin I, and angiotensin-converting enzyme (ACE) converts angiotensin I to angiotensin II. Subsequently, angiotensin II stimulates secretion of aldosterone. Renin secretion is controlled by renal artery pressure, sodium delivery to the distal nephron, and sympathetic activation (via $\beta 1$). Increased effective arterial circulating volume from the action of aldosterone decreases renin secretion by negative feedback (Figure 1). Other minor factors involved in aldosterone secretion are adrenocorticotropic hormone and hyponatremia (which increase aldosterone secretion), and atrial natriuretic peptide (which decreases aldosterone secretion).

Aldosterone binds to the nuclear mineralocorticoid receptors. Activation of the mineralocorticoid receptors up-regulates the basolateral Na^+/K^+ pumps and the epithelial sodium channels (ENaC), leading to increased reabsorption of Na^+ and Cl^- and secretion of K^+ and H^+. The mineralocorticoid receptors can also be activated by other hormones with mineralocorticoid activity. Cortisol is able to bind to the mineralocorticoid receptors with similar affinity as aldosterone but normally is converted to inactive cortisone by 11β hydroxysteroid dehydrogenase 2 (11β HSD2). Mutations/inhibition of 11β HSD2 or very high cortisol levels above the capacity of 11β HSD2, as in Cushing's syndrome (particularly ectopic Cushing's syndrome), and glucocorticoid resistance can cause activation of the mineralocorticoid receptors.

Aldosterone precursors such as deoxycorticosterone have a weak mineralocorticoid effect but can cause features of hyperaldosteronism when they are present at very high levels as in some forms of congenital adrenal hyperplasias (11β hydroxylase deficiency or 17α hydroxylase deficiency) or deoxycorticosteroid-secreting tumors. Additionally, activating mutations of the ENaCs also cause increased sodium absorption and hypertension mimicking hyperaldosteronism (Liddle's syndrome).

Clinical Manifestations

Primary hyperaldosteronism usually presents with normokalemic hypertension. Hypokalemia is present only in 9% to 37% of cases and may indicate more severe cases. Patients with primary hyperaldosteronism usually do not develop severe volume overload or edema because of aldosterone escape possibly related to atrial natriuretic peptide, pressure natriuresis, or decreased sodium absorption at other nephron segments. Metabolic alkalosis, mild hypernatremia (due to reset osmostat from volume expansion), and hypomagnesemia may be observed. Glomerular filtration rate and urinary albumin excretion can be elevated independent of systemic hypertension. Cardiovascular morbidity and mortality are higher in primary hyperaldosteronism than in essential hypertension. Secondary hyperaldosteronism (when it is not from hypovolemia) and other conditions mimicking hyperaldosteronism can present with similar features as primary hyperaldosteronism plus specific manifestations for each disease entity. Depending on the mechanism of disease, more severe volume overload and pulmonary edema may be found (e.g., renovascular hypertension) because aldosterone escape may not work.

Evaluation
Screening

Hyperaldosteronism may be suspected based on severe or resistant hypertension, early onset hypertension without known risk factors, and hypertension with other features such as family history of hyperaldosteronism, early-onset hypertension, cerebrovascular accident at a young age, hypokalemia, metabolic alkalosis, and adrenal mass. Currently, there is no evidence-guided screening strategy. Some experts believe that routine screening for primary hyperaldosteronism is warranted in newly diagnosed hypertension considering its high prevalence, whereas others recommend that

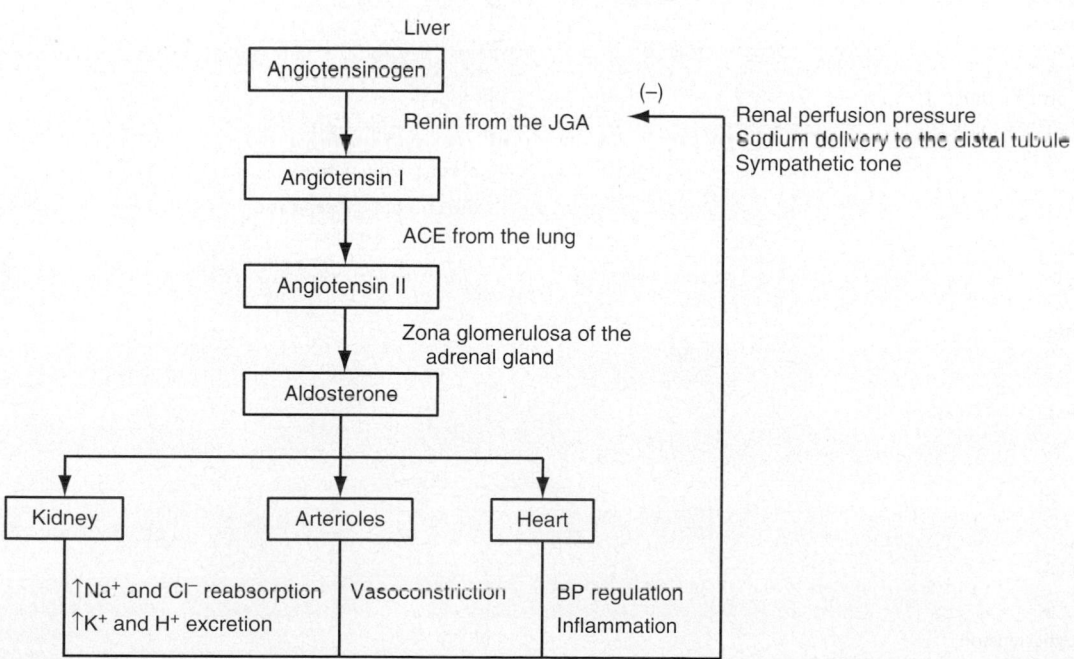

Figure 1. The renin-angiotensin-aldosterone system (RAAS). *Abbreviations:* ACE=angiotensin-converting enzyme; BP=blood pressure; JGA=juxtaglomerular apparatus.

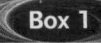

Groups with Relatively High Prevalence of Primary Hyperaldosteronism (Reported Prevalence of Primary Hyperaldosteronism is Provided if Available)

- Joint National Commission (JNC) 7 stage 2 hypertension (≥ 160–179/100–109 mmHg), prevalence 8%
- JNC 7 stage 3 hypertension (≥ 180/110 mm Hg), prevalence 13%
- Drug-resistant hypertension (>140/90 mm Hg despite 3 medications), prevalence 17%–23%
- Hypertension and hypokalemia (spontaneous or diuretic-induced)
- Hypertension and family history of early-onset hypertension or cerebrovascular accident at a young age (<40 years)
- Hypertension with adrenal incidentaloma, prevalence 1.1%–10%
- Hypertensive first-degree relatives of primary hyperaldosteronism patients

targeted screening is more appropriate. The recommendations of the Endocrine Society guidelines for primary hyperaldosteronism in 2008 provide helpful background information in selecting patients for screening (Box 1).

When a decision is made to screen for excessive mineralocorticoid effect, one should first examine the plasma renin and aldosterone levels; that is, plasma renin activity (PRA, ng/mL/hr) and plasma aldosterone concentration (PAC, ng/dL). It is important to note that several factors can affect PRA and PAC, such as age, medications, time of day, diet (salt intake), posture, method of blood collection, level of potassium, and level of creatinine (Table 1). Diuretics (both potassium sparing and wasting) and mineralocorticoid antagonists can have a significant effect on PRA and PAC. Angiotensin converting enzyme inhibitors/angiotensin receptor blockers (ACEI/ARB) and dihydropyridine calcium channel blockers can affect PRA and PAC modestly. Ideally, all medications and other factors that may affect PRA and PAC should be removed; unfortunately, it is not always practical and safe to do this because of the possibility of uncontrolled hypertension. If necessary, antihypertensive agents that affect PRA and PAC only minimally such as slow-release verapamil (Calan SR), hydralazine (Apresoline), prazosin (Minipress), doxazosin (Cardura), or terazosin (Hytrin) can be used. The Endocrine Society 2008 guidelines recommend certain caveats that optimize the chance for obtaining more easily interpretable PRA and PAC results (Box 2).

Patterns of PRA and PAC help differentiate among primary hyperaldosteronism, secondary hyperaldosteronism, and conditions mimicking hyperaldosteronism. Differential diagnoses according to different patterns of PRA and PAC are listed in Box 3. If both PRA and PAC are high, further investigation for causes of secondary hyperaldosteronism should follow. If both PRA and PAC are suppressed, further investigation for conditions that mimic hyperaldosteronism is indicated. Suppressed PRA and elevated PAC suggest primary hyperaldosteronism, and aldosterone renin ratio (ARR) should be calculated; ARR above 20–40 while PAC is greater than 15 ng/dL (to avoid false positive from very

TABLE 1 Medical Factors That May Affect Aldosterone and Renin Measurement

	EFFECT ON ALDOSTERONE	EFFECT ON RENIN	EFFECT ON ALDOSTERONE–RENIN RATIO
Medications			
β-Blocker	↓	↓↓	↑
Central α₂ agonists (clonidine [Catapres], α-methyldopa [Aldomet])	↓	↓↓	↑
NSAIDs	↓	↓↓	↑
K⁺ wasting diuretics	→↑	↑↑	↓
K⁺ sparing diuretics	↑	↑↑	↓
ACE inhibitors	↓	↑↑	↓
Adrenergic receptor binders	↓	↑↑	↓
Dihydropyridine Ca²⁺ blockers	→↓	↑	↓
Renin inhibitors	↓	↓ plasma renin activity	↑
		↑ direct renin concentration	↓
Potassium Status			
Hypokalemia	↓	→↑	↓
Potassium loading	↑	→↓	↑
Dietary Sodium			
Sodium restricted	↑	↑↑	↓
Sodium loaded	↓	↓↓	↑
Others			
Advanced age	↓	↓↓	↑
Renal impairment	→	↓	↑
Pregnancy	↑	↑↑	↓
Renovascular hypertension	↑	↑↑	↓
Malignant hypertension	↑	↑↑	↓

Abbreviation: NSAIDS = Nonsteroidal antiinflammatory drugs.

Box 2　Approach to Measure PRA and PAC

- Correct hypokalemia.
- Liberalize sodium intake.
- Withdraw the following agents that markedly affect PRA and PAC for at least 4 weeks: spironolactone (Aldactone), eplerenone (Inspra), amiloride (Midamor), triamterene (Dyrenium), potassium-wasting diuretic, and products from licorice.[7]
- If not diagnostic and hypertension can be controlled with relatively non-interfering medications, withdraw the following agents for at least 2 weeks: β-blockers, central α_2 agonists (clonidine [Catapres], methyldopa [Aldomet]), NSAIDs, ACEIs/ARBs, renin inhibitors, and dihydropyridine calcium channel antagonists.
- If necessary, start other antihypertensive agents that have fewer effects on ARR: slow-release verapamil (Calan-SR), hydralazine (Apresoline) (with verapamil to prevent reflex tachycardia), prazosin (Minipress), doxazosin (Cardura), and terazosin (Hytrin).
- Obtain blood for PRA and PAC mid-morning after the patient has been up for at least 2 hours and seated for 5–15 minutes.

[7]Available as dietary supplement.

Box 3　Differential Diagnoses According to PRA and PAC

Causes of Primary Hyperaldosteronism: ↓PRA and ↑PAC (>15 ng/dL); ARR > 20–40
- Most Common
  - Aldosterone-producing adenoma
  - Bilateral adrenal hyperplasia or idiopathic hyperaldosteronism
- Less Common
  - Unilateral hyperplasia or primary adrenal hyperplasia
  - Familial hyperaldosteronism type 1 or glucocorticoid remediable aldosteronism
  - Familial hyperaldosteronism type 2
  - Aldosterone-producing adrenocortical carcinoma
  - Ectopic aldosterone-secreting tumor (ovary, kidney)
  - Multiple endocrine neoplasia type 1

Causes of Secondary Hyperaldosteronism: ↑PRA and ↑PAC; ARR ≈ 10
- Renovascular hypertension
- Diuretic use
- Renin-secreting tumor
- Malignant hypertension
- Coarctation of the aorta

Causes of Conditions Which Mimic Mineralocorticoid Excess: ↓PRA and ↓PAC
- Congenital adrenal hyperplasia
- Exogenous mineralocorticoid
- Deoxycorticosterone producing tumor
- Cushing's syndrome
- 11β HSD2 deficiency
- Altered aldosterone metabolism
- Liddle's syndrome
- Glucocorticoid resistance

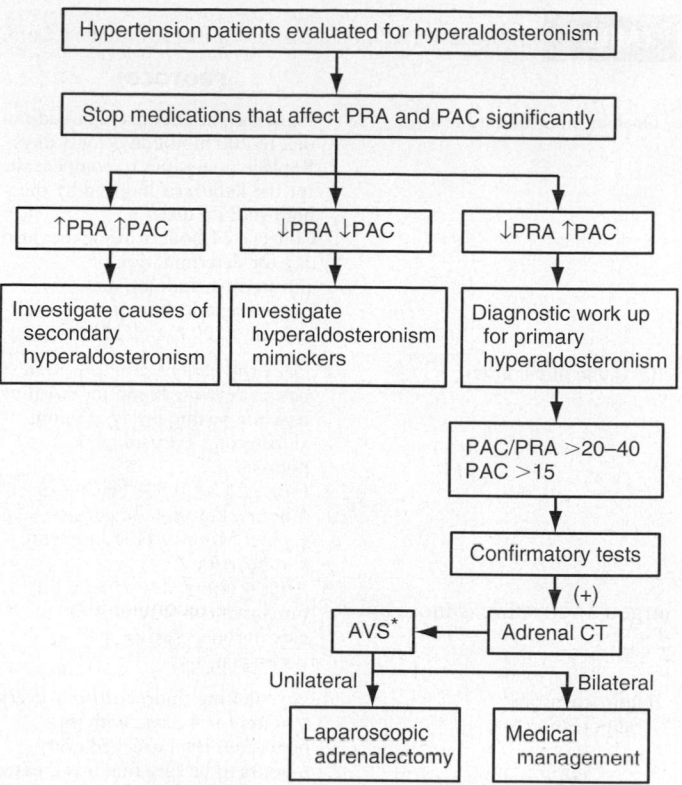

Figure 2. Evaluation of hyperaldosteronism. *Abbreviations*: AVS = adrenal vein sampling; CT = computed tomography; PAC = plasma aldosterone concentration in ng/dL; PRA = plasma renin activity in ng/ml/hr. *If surgical treatment is pursued. May skip if <40 years old with unilateral adrenal mass >1 cm.

Box 4　Adrenal Vein Sampling

- After both adrenal veins have been cannulated, draw baseline samples for PRA, PAC, ACTH, and cortisol from the IVC, right adrenal vein, and left adrenal vein.
- Inject 250 mcg of cosyntropin (Cortrosyn) after cannulation, or infuse 50 mcg cosyntropin per hour beginning 30 minutes before adrenal vein cannulation. This reduces stress-related fluctuations in aldosterone and cortisol values and augments the biochemical gradients (this step is controversial).
- Draw blood for aldosterone and cortisol levels at 5, 15, and 30 minutes from the peripheral site and from each adrenal vein.

low PRA raising ARR) is considered screening positive for primary hyperaldosteronism. Confirmatory tests should follow to avoid false positives. Diagnostic flow and subsequent management of hyperaldosteronism are summarized in Figure 2. Of note, there is no consensus on cut-off values for PRA, PAC, or ARR. In addition, PRA and PAC are often obtained in a less-than-optimal condition. Therefore, it is important to understand how PRA and PAC can be affected by various factors. For example, if ARR is positive while on medications that decrease PAC or increase PRA (thus decreasing ARR), ARR off this medication will be clearly positive. Screening tests should be repeated if results are inconclusive.

Confirmatory Tests of Primary Hyperaldosteronism

The positive screening test should be followed by confirmatory tests to avoid false positives. The confirmatory tests are designed to physiologically suppress aldosterone levels that would normally occur in the absence of primary hyperaldosteronism. However, some experts believe that some aldosterone-producing lesions are not completely independent of the RAAS, and confirmatory suppression tests can give false-negative results. Other experts think that confirmatory tests are not necessary for those with obvious clinical/biochemical features. Furthermore, there is no gold-standard confirmatory test. Therefore, factors such as cost, accessibility, feasibility, patient compliance, local expertise, and accuracy of assay should be taken into consideration in selecting confirmatory tests. The Endocrine Society guidelines in 2008 state that any of the following four confirmatory tests can be used: oral salt loading test, saline suppression test, fludrocortisone

TABLE 2 Protocols and Interpretation of Recommended Confirmatory Tests

	PROTOCOL	INTERPRETATION	REMARKS
Oral sodium loading test	1. Place the patient on a high-sodium diet (>200 mmol/day) for 3 days. 2. Replace potassium to compensate for the kaliuresis induced by the high-sodium diet. 3. Collect a 24-hour urine on the third day for determination of aldosterone, sodium, and creatinine; adequate if the urine sodium >200 mmol/24 hr	Confirmed if the 24-hour urine aldosterone is >12 mcg (33.3 nmol) to 14 mcg (38.8 nmol). Ruled out if the 24-hour urine aldosterone is <10 mcg (27.7 nmol). The test is equivocal if the value falls in between.	Do not perform this test in patients with severe uncontrolled hypertension, renal failure, cardiac failure/arrhythmias, or severe hypokalemia.
IV saline infusion test	1. Place the patient supine 1 hour before drawing blood for morning baseline fasting levels of renin, aldosterone, cortisol, and potassium. 2. Infuse 2 L of 0.9% NaCl over 4 hours, keeping the patient supine. Monitor blood pressure and heart rate. 3. After 4 hours, draw blood for measurement of renin, aldosterone, cortisol, and potassium.	Confirmed if the PAC is >10 ng/dL (277 pmol/L). Ruled out if the PAC is <5 ng/dL (139 pmol/L). If the PAC falls between these values, the test is equivocal.	Do not perform this test in patients with severe uncontrolled hypertension, renal failure, cardiac failure/arrhythmias, or severe hypokalemia.
Fludrocortisone[1] suppression test	1. Give 0.1 mg fludrocortisone every 6 hours for 4 days, with the potassium level checked every 6 hours to be sure that it is greater than 4 mmol/L. 2. Encourage a liberal sodium diet to keep urinary sodium excretion greater than 3 mmol/kg/day. 3. On day 4, draw blood for an upright 7 AM plasma cortisol level and 10 AM plasma aldosterone, renin, and cortisol levels.	Confirmed if the 10 AM PAC is >6 ng/dL, as long as PRA is <1 ng/ml/hr and the plasma cortisol at 10 AM is less than at 7 AM (to exclude the ACTH effect).	The test may require hospitalization. Risks include severe hypokalemia, QT changes, worsening of left ventricular function, hypertension, and frequent phlebotomy
Captopril[1] challenge test	1. Give 25–50 mg captopril after the patient has been upright for 1 hour. The patient remains upright throughout the test. 2. Draw blood for measurement of plasma renin, aldosterone, and cortisol at time 0, at 1 hour, and at 2 hours.	Normally, captopril suppresses PAC by more than 30% from baseline. Confirmed if there is no suppression of PAC and PRA remains suppressed. The false-negative rate for this test is high because suppression occurs in more than 30% of cases. A slight decrease in aldosterone can suggest bilateral adrenal hyperplasia.	

Abbreviations: ACTH = adrenocorticotropic hormone; PAC = plasma aldosterone concentration; PRA = plasma renin activity.
[1]Not FDA approved for this indication.

(Florinef)[1] suppression test, and captopril (Capoten)[1] challenge test (Table 2).

Subtype Classification of Primary Hyperaldosteronism
Once primary hyperaldosteronism is biochemically confirmed, subtype classification follows to guide treatment. Unilateral lesions such as aldosterone producing adenomas (APAs) can be treated surgically, whereas bilateral lesions such as bilateral adrenal hyperplasias (BAHs) are treated medically. Aldosterone-producing carcinoma is rare but should be ruled out. In this regard, CT of the adrenal glands should be done first to rule out aldosterone-producing carcinoma and obtain anatomic information. However, imaging studies are usually not reliable enough to lateralize lesions. If surgical treatment is considered, adrenal vein sampling should be performed. Young patients (<20 years of age) and those with family history of primary hyperaldosteronism should have genetic testing for glucocorticoid remediable aldosteronism (GRA) or familial hyperaldosteronism type 1 (FH-1), which is caused by the hybrid gene of 11β hydroxylase and aldosterone synthase (increased aldosterone synthesis by adrenocorticotropic hormone).

Imaging
CT/MRI scans of the adrenal glands provide one of five conclusions: normal adrenal glands, unilateral macroadenomas (>1 cm), minimal unilateral adrenal limb thickening, unilateral microadenomas (≤1 cm), and bilateral macroadenomas and/or microadenomas. APAs are typically smaller than 2 cm, and BAHs exhibit either normal or nodular changes. Aldosterone-producing adrenal carcinomas are almost always larger than 4 cm in diameter and have imaging characteristics suspicious for malignancy. However, there are limitations; small APAs may be missed, hyperplasia may be misread as adenomas, and nonfunctional tumors are radiologically indistinguishable from APAs. Although several studies suggested imaging criteria for different subtypes, no study has conclusively established specific criteria that differentiate among different subtypes of primary hyperaldosteronism. In fact, CT accurately lateralizes in only

[1]Not FDA approved for this indication.

about 50% to 70% of cases. Therefore, adrenal vein sampling is required to differentiate unilateral from bilateral lesions if surgical resection is being pursued. Some experts believe that individuals 40 years or younger with a unilateral adenoma larger than 1 cm do not need adrenal vein sampling because nonfunctioning tumors are uncommon in this young age group.

Adrenal Vein Sampling

Aldosterone levels are measured from adrenal venous blood samples obtained through adrenal vein cannulation to distinguish between unilateral and bilateral lesions. Unilateral lesions are associated with a marked increase in PAC on the side of the tumor (and suppressed PAC on the other side), whereas bilateral lesions have little difference between the two sides. Adrenal vein sampling (AVS) should be performed only by experienced physicians in part because recognition and successful cannulation of the right adrenal vein especially can be challenging. Complications of AVS include adrenal hemorrhage, adrenal infarction, adrenal vein perforation, and adrenal vein thrombosis, which occur only rarely (<2.5%) in the hands of a physician skilled in the procedure.

The use of cosyntropin (Cortrosyn) stimulation to minimize stress-induced fluctuation in aldosterone level is controversial, and some believe that it has no effect on AVS accuracy. If cosyntropin is not used, then AVS should be done in the morning after overnight recumbency to avoid postural aldosterone changes and reflect circadian aldosterone secretion.

In reality, different centers use different techniques, protocols, and interpretation criteria. The Endocrine Society guidelines in 2008 provide interpretation criteria with and without cosyntropin use. The first step for interpretation is to determine whether the procedure was done correctly. The adrenal vein-to-IVC cortisol ratio should be greater than 10:1 with cosyntropin given and greater than 3:1 without cosyntropin. If the ratio is significantly lower than these values, improper cannulation is implied. Next, divide the PAC values for the right and left adrenal veins by their respective cortisol values to correct the dilutional effect of the inferior phrenic vein flow into the left adrenal vein; this is termed the cortisol-corrected aldosterone (A/C). If cosyntropin is used, an A/C ratio of the high to the low side of greater than 4:1 indicates unilateral aldosterone hypersecretion, whereas an A/C ratio of less than 3:1 suggests bilateral aldosterone hypersecretion. These cutoffs were reported to have sensitivity of 95% and specificity of 100% for unilateral lesions. If the A/C ratio is between 3:1 and 4:1, the results of AVS should be interpreted in the context of CT, clinical findings, and other tests. Without cosyntropin, an A/C ratio of the high to low side of greater than 2 or an A/C ratio of the high side to the periphery greater than 2.5 plus an A/C ratio of the low side to the periphery of less than 1 (suppressed contralateral aldosterone secretion) is consistent with unilateral aldosterone excess.

Ancillary Tests

Clinical findings and other ancillary tests may help differentiate unilateral APAs from BAHs. BAHs will respond with increase in plasma aldosterone to postural stimulation, whereas APAs will not. Plasma 18-hydroxycorticosterone level tends to be higher in APAs as compared with BAHs. Iodocholesterol scintigraphy may be able to show functional correlation of anatomical abnormalities (but is not available at most centers). Interpretation criteria of these tests are listed in Table 3. Patients with APAs tend to be younger (<40 years), predominantly female, very hypertensive with marked hypokalemia (<3 mmol/L), and they tend to have a very high PAC (>25 mg/dL) as compared with those with BAHs.

Treatment

Treatment of secondary hyperaldosteronism and conditions mimicking hyperaldosteronism depends on their etiology. Treatment of primary hyperaldosteronism is discussed here. The goals of treatment of primary hyperaldosteronism are (1) normalization of the serum potassium in hypokalemic patients, (2) normalization of the blood pressure, and (3) reversal of the effects of hyperaldosteronism on the cardiovascular system. When a small group of patients

TABLE 3	Interpretation of Dynamic Testing	
TEST	**FINDINGS**
Screening Test	
PAC/PRA ratio	Positive if >20–40 with PAC >15 ng/dL
Confirmatory Tests	
Oral sodium loading test	Positive if 24-hr urine aldosterone excretion is >12–14 mcg
Saline infusion test	Positive if PAC after infusion is >10 ng/dL
Fludrocortisone[1] suppression test	Positive if upright PAC is >6 ng/dL on day 4 at 10 am
Captopril[1] challenge test	Positive if PAC does not decrease by 30% and PRA remains suppressed
AVS	
With cosyntropin stimulation	A/C ratio (the high to the low side) >4:1 → unilateral aldosterone excess A/C ratio 3:1 to 4:1 → unclear A/C ratio <3:1 → bilateral aldosterone excess
Without cosyntropin stimulation	A/C ratio from the high to the low side >2:1 → unilateral aldosterone excess A/C ratio from the high side to the periphery >2.5 and A/C ratio from the contralateral side to the periphery <1 → unilateral aldosterone excess
If Equivocal AVS	
Postural stimulation test	PAC falls or fails to rise by 30%: consistent with APAs PAC increases by at least 33%: consistent with BAHs
Recumbent 18-hydroxycorticosterone	>100 ng/dL is consistent with APAs
NP-59 iodocholesterol scintigraphy	Unilateral early uptake (<5 d): consistent with unilateral aldosterone excess Bilateral early uptake (<5 d): consistent with bilateral aldosterone excess Negative scan does not rule out either etiology

[1]Not FDA approved for this indication.
Abbreviations: A/C ratio = cortisol-corrected aldosterone ratio; APA = aldosterone producing adenomas; AVS = adrenal vein sampling; BAH = bilateral adrenal hyperplasia; PAC = plasma aldosterone concentration; PRA = plasma renin activity.

were followed after treatment with adrenalectomy or mineralocorticoid receptor antagonists (MRA), left ventricular mass was reduced (faster with adrenalectomy than MRA), glomerular filtration rate and urinary albumin secretion decreased and became similar to that in essential hypertension, and excessive cardiovascular risk compared to essential hypertension disappeared. Cardiovascular complications were rather related to age, duration of hypertension, and smoking. Therefore, timely diagnosis and treatment is essential. For unilateral lesions, surgical resection of the affected adrenal gland is recommended mainly to obviate the need for prolonged medical treatment and side effects. For bilateral lesions, medical treatment is recommended because surgical risk outweighs benefits. MRAs are a key component of medical treatment and used as a preoperative measure or maintenance treatment (GRA should be treated with the lowest dose of glucocorticoid that can normalize blood pressure and potassium levels rather than MRAs). A low-sodium diet (sodium <100 mEq/day = 2.3 g/day or salt 6 g/day) is also important, because left ventricular hypertrophy is associated with urine sodium excretion in primary hyperaldosteronism but not in essential hypertension. Other lifestyle changes include aerobic exercise, smoking cessation, and weight loss.

Unilateral Hypersecretion

Adrenalectomy, usually laparoscopic, is recommended. After adrenalectomy, blood pressure improves in all patients (maximal improvement in 1–6 months, sometime continues to fall up to 1 year), but 30% to 60% of patients have persistent hypertension. Blood pressure and potassium level should be controlled before surgery. MRAs such as spironolactone (Aldactone) and eplerenone (Inspra)[1] can be used to control blood pressure in patients awaiting adrenalectomy and also to prevent postoperative hypoaldosteronism. Postoperatively, normal saline is given to maintain volume status, MRAs and potassium supplements are discontinued, and antihypertensive medications may be reduced. To confirm biochemical cure, PAC and PRA should be checked shortly after the operation. Risk factors for persistent hypertension after adrenalectomy include older age, duration of hypertension (>5 years), use of two or more antihypertensive agents preoperatively, blood pressure higher than 165/100 mm Hg, low ARR preoperatively, low urine aldosterone, poor response to spironolactone preoperatively, family history of more than one first-degree relative with hypertension, and elevated serum creatinine level.

Bilateral Hypersecretion

MRAs and/or ENaC antagonists combined with other antihypertensives are used. One study showed that spironolactone had stronger antihypertensive effect than eplerenone, but there is insufficient evidence to choose one medication over another. Subtotal adrenalectomy has been tried, but only a minority of patients have responded with significant blood pressure improvement. Unilateral adrenalectomy, however, may help selected patients by debulking aldosterone-producing tissues.

Spironolactone is the most widely used MRA. It is very effective in decreasing blood pressure. The medication is initiated at 12.5 to 25 mg/day and can be titrated to 400 mg/day, with most patients requiring at least 200 mg/day. Potassium should be maintained at normal levels without use of potassium supplements. Use of spironolactone can be limited by side effects; antiandrogenic effects can cause gynecomastia in men and progesterone effect can cause menstrual irregularities in women. There are drug interactions to consider; spironolactone increases the half-life of digoxin (Lanoxin) and salicylates, and other NSAIDs may decrease the effectiveness of spironolactone. Serum potassium and creatinine should be closely monitored for the first 4 to 6 weeks, in particular for those with renal insufficiency or diabetes. Spironolactone is not recommended if creatinine clearance is less than 30 mL/minute.

Eplerenone[1] is a competitive and selective antagonist of the aldosterone receptors. It has a lower binding affinity to androgen and progesterone receptors than spironolactone. This leads to fewer side effects. Eplerenone is 25% to 50% less potent in antagonizing the aldosterone receptors than spironolactone. Eplerenone has a short half-life and may be more effective if given twice daily. Dosing is started at 25 mg once or twice daily, with a maximum dose of 100 mg/day. Again, serum potassium and creatinine should be closely monitored for the first 4 to 6 weeks in particular for those with renal insufficiency or diabetes. Other adverse effects include hypertriglyceridemia, increased liver enzymes, headache, and fatigue. Eplerenone is contraindicated if serum potassium is greater than 5.5 mEq/L at initiation, if creatinine clearance is less than 30 mL/minute, or if there is concomitant use of strong CYP3A4 inhibitors such as ketoconazole (Nizoral) and itraconzole (Sporanox).

ENaC antagonists, amiloride (Midamor)[1] and triamterene (Dyrenium),[1] can be used in patients who cannot tolerate MRAs or are still hypertensive/hypokalemic while on MRAs. Amiloride is prescribed at 10 to 20 mg/day in divided doses. Side effects include dizziness, fatigue, and impotence. Triamterene is dosed at 100 to 300 mg/day in divided doses, and its side effects are mainly dizziness and nausea. Addition of thiazide diuretics can help control blood pressure by relieving volume overload. If blood pressure remains uncontrolled, other antihypertensive agents such as ACEIs/ARBs or calcium channel blockers may be used.

---

[1]Not FDA approved for this indication.

References

Born-Frontsberg E, Reincke M, Rump LC, et al. Cardiovascular and cerebrovascular comorbidities of hypokalemic and normokalemic primary aldosteronism: results of the German conn's registry. J Clin Endocrinol Metab 2009;94:1125–30.

Catena C, Colussi G, Lapenna R, et al. Long-term cardiac effects of adrenalectomy or mineralocorticoid antagonists in patients with primary aldosteronism. Hypertension 2007;50:911–8.

Catena C, Colussi GL, Nadalini E, et al. Cardiovascular outcomes in patients with primary aldosteronism after treatment. Arch Intern Med 2008;168:80–5.

Funder JW, Carey RM, Fardella C, et al. Case detection, diagnosis, and treatment of patients with primary aldosteronism: an endocrine society clinical practice guideline. J Clin Endocrinol Metab 2008;93:3266–81.

Gordon RD, Gomez-Sanchez CE, Hamlet SM, et al. Angiotensin-responsive aldosterone-producing adenoma masquerades as idiopathic hyperaldosteronism (IHA: adrenal hyperplasia) or low-renin essential hypertension. J Hypertens 1987;5:S103–6.

Kempers MJ, Lenders JW, van Outheusden L, et al. Systematic review: diagnostic procedures to differentiate unilateral from bilateral adrenal abnormality in primary aldosteronism. Ann Intern Med 2009;151:329–37.

Mulatero P, Bertello C, Rossato D, et al. Roles of clinical criteria, computed tomography scan, and adrenal vein sampling in differential diagnosis of primary aldosteronism subtypes. J Clin Endocrinol Metab 2008;93:1366–71.

Parthasarathy HK, Ménard J, White WB, et al. A double-blind, randomized study comparing the antihypertensive effect of eplerenone and spironolactone in patients with hypertension and evidence of primary aldosteronism. J Hypertens 2011;29:980.

Pimenta E, Gordon RD, Ahmed AH, et al. Cardiac dimensions are largely determined by dietary salt in patients with primary aldosteronism: results of a case-control study. J Clin Endocrinol Metab 2011;96:2813–20.

Reincke M, Fischer E, Gerum S, et al. Observational study mortality in treated primary aldosteronism: the German conn's registry. Hyptertension 2012;60:618–24.

Rossi GP, Barisa M, Allolio B, et al. The adrenal vein sampling international study (avis) for identifying the major subtypes of primary aldosteronism. J Clin Endocrinol Metab 2012;97:1606–14.

Rossi GP, Bernini G, Caliumi C, et al. A prospective study of the prevalence of primary aldosteronism in 1,125 hypertensive patients. J Am Coll Cardiol 2006;48:2293–300.

Rossi GP, Seccia TM, Pessina AC. Adrenal gland: a diagnostic algorithm - the holy grail of primary aldosteronism. Nat Rev Endocrinol 2011;7:697–9.

Rossi GP. A comprehensive review of the clinical aspects of primary aldosteronism. Nat Rev Endocrinol 2011;7:485–95.

Sechi LA, Novello M, Lapenna R, et al. Long-term renal outcomes in patients with primary aldosteronism. JAMA 2006;295:2638–45.

Stowasser M. Update in primary aldosteronism. J Clin Endocrinol Metab 2009;94:3623–30.

Sukor N, Gordon RD, Ku YK, et al. Role of unilateral adrenalectomy in bilateral primary aldosteronism: a 22-year single center experience. J Clin Endocrinol Metab 2009;94:2437–45.

HYPERLIPIDEMIA

Method of
Jongoh Kim, MD; and Lawrence Chan, MD

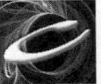

CURRENT DIAGNOSIS

- Hyperlipidemia is diagnosed based on the fasting lipid profile in the context of global cardiovascular risk. The exception is when the triglyceride level is greater than 500 mg/dL because of substantial risk of pancreatitis.
- Secondary causes of hyperlipidemia, such as hypothyroidism, alcoholism, uncontrolled diabetes mellitus, kidney disorders, pregnancy, and medications, should be thoroughly investigated and treated if found.
- Possibility of familial hyperlipidemia based on family history and physical findings should be considered because cardiovascular risk can be underestimated and treatment can be challenging.

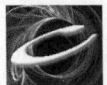

CURRENT THERAPY

- Therapy should be guided by goals of treatment based on estimated cardiovascular risk unless triglyceride level >500 mg/L, in which case lowering triglycerides to prevent pancreatitis is a priority.

- Low-density lipoprotein (LDL) cholesterol is a primary goal followed by non–high-density lipoprotein (HDL) cholesterol as a secondary goal.
- Therapeutic lifestyle changes should be initiated in everyone with LDL cholesterol above their target. Therapeutic lifestyle changes are also recommended for those with very high, high, or moderately high cardiovascular risk.
- Pharmacologic agents should be added if therapeutic lifestyle changes are not successful. Pharmacologic agents can be considered from the beginning for those with very high, high, or moderately high cardiovascular risk.
- Statin therapy is preferred if tolerated, and the intensity of therapy should be strong enough to lower LDL cholesterol at least by 30% to 40%
- Statins are the treatment of choice for their proven effects on cardiovascular outcomes. Other agents can be added based on response to statins and other targets such as high triglycerides or low-HDL cholesterol.
- All other cardiovascular risk factors should be treated aggressively at the same time.

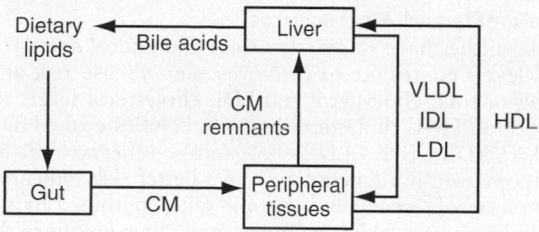

Figure 1. Overview of exogenous and endogenous pathways of lipid metabolism. *Abbreviations:* CM = chylomicrons; HDL = high-density lipoproteins; IDL = intermediate-density lipoproteins; LDL = low-density lipoproteins; VLDL = very–low-density lipoproteins.

Hyperlipidemia is a condition of elevated serum lipids and lipoproteins. Hyperlipidemia is associated with an increased risk of cardiovascular disease and, if the triglyceride level is greater than 500 mg/dL, pancreatitis. Unless the triglyceride level is greater than 500 mg/dL, the primary goal of management of hyperlipidemia is to decrease the risk of cardiovascular disease. In this regard, appropriate treatment of hyperlipidemia is essential in patients with established cardiovascular disease (secondary prevention), whereas detection and treatment of hyperlipidemia are guided by the risk of cardiovascular disease in asymptomatic patients (primary prevention).

The prevalence of hyperlipidemia varies with the definition of hyperlipidemia and the population studied. The percentage of U.S. adults with a total cholesterol level of 240 mg/dL or higher declined from 19% to 14% in men and from 21% to 15% in women from 1988 to 2008. This may be in part due to increased use of lipid-lowering medications, from 3.4% to 15.5%. However, major risk factors for cardiovascular disease actually have become more common: the prevalence of obesity (BMI $\geq$ 30 kg/m^2) increased from 19.9% to 31.6% in men and from 25.2% to 34.1% in women, and the prevalence of diabetes increased from 5.5% to 11.1% in men and from 4.6% to 6.3% in women over this period. Therefore, optimal treatment of hyperlipidemia to reduce cardiovascular risk is of paramount importance.

Various societies and professional organizations have published clinical guidelines for hyperlipidemia. The approach used in this chapter is mostly based on *The Third Report of the Expert Panel on Detection, Evaluation, and Treatment of High Blood Cholesterol in Adults (Adult Treatment Panel III)* published in 2002 and updated in 2004 by National Heart Blood Lung Institute (NHBLI). Recommendations from other recent guidelines are also integrated in this chapter. These guidelines include *The Lipoprotein Management in Patients with Cardiometabolic Risk, Consensus Statement from the American College of Cardiology Foundation and the American Diabetes Association (ACC/ADA) (2008), The European Society of Cardiology and European Atherosclerosis Society (ESC/EAS) Guidelines for the Management of Dyslipidaemias (2011)*, and the *American Association of Clinical Endocrinologists' (AACE) Guidelines for Management of Dyslipidemia and Prevention of Atherosclerosis (2012)*.

In November, 2013, the American College of Cardiology (ACC) and American Heart Association (AHA) released a new guideline in collaboration with National Heart Blood Lung Institute (NHBLI): *2013 ACC/AHA Guideline on the Treatment of Blood Cholesterol to Reduce Atherosclerotic Cardiovascular Risk in Adults: A Report of the American College of Cardiology/American Heart Association Task Force on Practice Guidelines*. This new guideline represents a substantial departure from previous guidelines in that it emphasizes the use of statins of appropriate strength according to the estimated cardiovascular risk without specific low-density lipoprotein (LDL) cholesterol targets. Similarities and differences of this new guideline compared with the others will be discussed later in the chapter.

Pathophysiology

Lipids have two main points of entry into the circulation: the gut (exogenous pathway) and the liver (endogenous pathway). The exogenous and endogenous pathways are interconnected by intermediate pathways (reverse cholesterol transport pathway and others). These pathways are outlined in Figure 1.

Exogenous Pathway

Lipids in food are emulsified by bile acids and then hydrolyzed into fatty acids and cholesterol by pancreatic lipases in the intestinal lumen. Inside the intestinal cells, fatty acids and cholesterol are reesterified and then packaged with apolipoprotein (Apo) B48 into chylomicrons. Chylomicrons are secreted into the intestinal lymph and delivered to the systemic circulation. At peripheral tissues, triglycerides are hydrolyzed by lipoprotein lipase with Apo CII acting as a cofactor. Released free fatty acids are then taken up for further metabolism or storage. Chylomicron remnants are taken up by the liver via the chylomicron remnant receptors.

Endogenous Pathway

The endogenous pathway begins in the liver with the synthesis of triglyceride-rich very–low-density lipoproteins (VLDLs). Microsomal triglyceride transfer protein facilitates the transfer of lipids onto Apo B100 and stabilizes the protein for secretion as VLDLs. VLDLs, as chylomicrons, undergo lipolysis by lipoprotein lipase, releasing free fatty acids, generating smaller particles called intermediate-density lipoproteins (IDLs, also known as VLDL remnants). IDLs are either removed by the liver or further processed into cholesterol-rich LDLs. LDLs are taken up into the liver or other cells via LDL receptors, a process regulated by cellular cholesterol requirement. Macrophages can also take up LDLs via the scavenger receptors and become foam cells. Foam cells play a key role in the development of atherosclerosis.

Reverse Cholesterol Transport

High-density lipoproteins (HDLs) are the major lipoproteins involved in the transport of cholesterol from peripheral tissues back to the liver. HDLs are synthesized by both the hepatocytes and the enterocytes in the form of small discoidal particles containing Apo AI and phospholipids. HDLs acquire additional lipids and apolipoproteins from triglyceride-depleted chylomicrons and VLDL remnants. HDLs remove free cholesterol from tissues with the help of Apo AI and esterify it with lecithin cholesterol acyltransferase. Cholesteryl esters are then transferred to Apo B 100-containing lipoproteins (VLDLs, IDLs, and LDLs) by cholesteryl ester transfer protein (CETP). HDLs can also be taken up directly by the liver class B type I scavenger receptors (SR-BI).

Plasma Lipids and Atherosclerosis

Multiple studies have shown that total cholesterol and LDL cholesterol levels contribute to cardiovascular disease risk and that lowering of total cholesterol and LDL cholesterol levels reduces the risk. Non-HDL cholesterol (i.e., total cholesterol − HDL cholesterol = VLDL + IDL + LDL cholesterol), reflects total atherogenic lipoprotein burden and may be a better risk indicator than LDL cholesterol, especially in people with combined hyperlipidemia, diabetes, metabolic syndrome, and chronic kidney disease. Elevated triglycerides, in particular nonfasting levels, also may be an independent cardiovascular risk factor. Even mildly elevated triglycerides (>150 mg/dL) can indicate metabolic syndrome, which is a strong risk factor for cardiovascular disease. Elevated triglycerides are often associated with low-HDL cholesterol and high levels of small, dense LDL particles (hyperlipidemia triad). HDL particles are considered protective against the formation of atherosclerotic plaque through reverse cholesterol transport and also possibly antiinflammatory and antioxidative activities. HDL cholesterol levels have been shown to be inversely associated with cardiovascular risk. However, the benefits of using drugs to lower triglycerides only and/or raising HDL cholesterol in reducing cardiovascular risk have not been proved. Table 1 shows the ATP III classification of lipid profile.

Evaluation

Global Cardiovascular Risk Assessment

The first step in assessing risk is to stratify global cardiovascular risk scores. Global risk scores estimate 10-year cardiovascular risk, which combines the effects of well-known risk factors, using one of several risk-calculation tools. Individual tools have developed based on large epidemiology studies examining a limited number of available risk factors. Traditional risk factors such as age, sex, cigarette smoking, cholesterol, diabetes, and blood pressure are able to predict 80% to 90% of the cardiovascular events in people 40 years or older. However, these tools may not accurately estimate cardiovascular risk in individuals with different demographics or unaccounted risk factors. The Framingham risk score, one of the most commonly used tools, provides several different risk assessment tools for different outcome measures (http://framinghamriskscore.com). The hard coronary heart disease (CHD) tool, used in the ATP III, incorporates age, sex, total cholesterol, HDL cholesterol, smoking, systolic blood pressure, and antihypertensive medications, and it predicts coronary death or myocardial infarction (http://hp2010.nhlbihin.net/atpiii/calculator.asp?usertype=prof). The SCORE, used in the ESC/EAS guidelines for the management of dyslipidemias, incorporates similar risk factors and predicts fatal cardiovascular events (www.heartscore.org). The Reynolds risk score incorporates high-sensitivity CRP and parental premature myocardial infarction, in addition to the risk factors mentioned above, and predicts major cardiovascular events (www.reynoldsriskscore.org).

In the ATP III, risk assessment begins with identifying the following cardiovascular risk factors: cigarette smoking, hypertension (BP ≥ 140/90 mm Hg) or use of antihypertensive agents, HDL cholesterol less than 40 mg/dL (≥60 mg/dL is a negative risk factor), age >45 years in men and >55 years in women, family history of premature CHD (male first-degree relatives <55 years, female first-degree relatives <65 years). The presence of zero or only one risk factor is considered as low risk (almost always, the risk for hard CHD over 10 years is <10%). If two or more risk factors are present without CHD or CHD equivalents, the Framingham risk score for the hard CHD over 10 years needs to be calculated. A risk of less than 10% is considered as moderate risk. If the risk is between 10% and 20%, it is considered as moderately high risk. If the risk is higher than 20%, it is considered as a CHD risk equivalent. Diabetes and clinical forms of atherosclerotic disease (abdominal aortic aneurysm, carotid artery disease—transient ischemic attack, stroke of carotid origin, greater than 50% obstruction of carotid artery, and peripheral vascular disease) are also considered as CHD equivalents. CHD and CHD equivalents belong to the high-risk group. Recently, chronic kidney disease with glomerular filtration rate less than 60 mL/minute/1.73 m^2 is also recognized as a CHD equivalent by some societies. The very–high-risk group was introduced in the ATP III update and more recent guidelines. The ATP III update defined the very–high-risk group as established cardiovascular disease plus multiple major risk factors (especially diabetes), severe and poorly controlled risk factors (especially continued smoking), multiple risk factors of the metabolic syndrome, and acute coronary syndrome. The therapeutic approach is determined by this risk stratification. Established cardiovascular disease itself and diabetes with other cardiovascular risk factor(s) are also considered as very high risk by some authorities (see the Treatment section and Tables 2 and 3).

The new 2013 ACC/AHA guideline focuses on identifying four subgroups of patients for whom the benefits of statin therapy outweigh the risk (Table 4). The new Pooled Cohort Equation is used to estimate a 10-year risk of atherosclerotic cardiovascular disease (nonfatal myocardial infarction, CHD death, and nonfatal and fatal stroke) for those aged 40 to 79 years, incorporating age, sex, race, HDL and total cholesterol, diabetes, hypertension, and smoking status (http://tools.cardiosource.org/ASCVD-Risk-Estimator). Statin therapy is recommended regardless of the baseline LDL cholesterol level in these four subgroups (see Table 4). The new guideline provides no recommendations for individuals requiring maintenance hemodialysis or with class II to IV ischemic systolic heart failure.

Measurement of Lipid Profiles

Lipid profiles should be measured as a part of global risk assessment, and the frequency of checkup is determined by age, sex, and risk factors for cardiovascular disease. A fasting lipid profile (fasting for 9–12 hours) is recommended to ensure the most precise lipid assessment, specifically triglycerides (subsequently LDL cholesterol if calculated using the Friedewald equation). Nonfasting lipid profile provides an accurate measurement of other lipids, including total cholesterol, HDL cholesterol, Apo B, and Apo AI. Recent studies showed that differences in triglyceride levels according to fasting time were small. Therefore, lipid values from nonfasting samples should not be ignored.

TABLE 1 The NCEP ATP III Classification of LDL, Total, and HDL Cholesterol and Triglycerides (mg/dL)

LDL Cholesterol (mg/dL)

<100	Optimal
100–129	Near optimal/above optimal
130–159	Borderline high
160–189	High
≥190	Very high

Total Cholesterol (mg/dL)

<200	Desirable
200–239	Borderline high
≥240	High

HDL Cholesterol (mg/dL)

<40	Low
≥60	High

Triglycerides (mg/dL)

<150	Normal
150–199	Borderline high
200–499	High
≥500	Very high

Abbreviations: ATP III = National Cholesterol Education Program Adult Treatment Panel III guidelines; HDL = high-density lipoprotein; LDL = low-density lipoprotein.

TABLE 2 — LDL Cholesterol Goals (mg/dL) and Levels for Initiating Lifestyle and Pharmacologic Interventions (The ATP III Update)

	RISK CATEGORY	GOAL (mg/dL)	LDL CHOLESTEROL LEVEL AT WHICH TO INITIATE TLC (mg/dL)	LDL CHOLESTEROL LEVEL AT WHICH TO INITIATE DRUG THERAPY (mg/dL)
High	CHD or CHD risk equivalents or 10-year risk of heart attack >20%	<100 (<70 if very high risk*)	>100	>100 (<100 optional)
Moderately high	2 or more risk factors and 10-year risk 10%–20%	<130 (<100 optional)	>130	>130 (100–129 optional)
Moderate	2 or more risk factors and 10-year risk <10%	<130	>130	>160
Lower	0–1 risk factor	<160	>160	>190

*Very high risk: acute coronary syndrome or established cardiovascular disease plus multiple major risk factors (especially diabetes), severe and poorly controlled risk factors (especially continued smoking), or multiple risk factors of the metabolic syndrome.

Abbreviations: ATP III = National Cholesterol Education Program Adult Treatment Panel III guidelines; CHD = coronary heart disease; LDL = low-density lipoprotein; TLC = therapeutic lifestyle changes.

TABLE 3 — LDL Cholesterol and Apo B Goals in More Recent Guidelines

	GOAL	
	LDL CHOLESTEROL (mg/dL)	APO B (mg/dL)
Very high risk: established cardiovascular disease or diabetes plus major cardiovascular risk factor(s)	70	80
High risk: 2 or more risk factors and/or 10-year risk >20%* or CHD equivalent (diabetes without any major cardiovascular risk factor)	100	90

Adapted from the lipoprotein management in patients with cardiometabolic risk, consensus statement from the American College of Cardiology Foundation and the American Diabetes Association (ACC/ADA) (2008), and the American Association of Clinical Endocrinologists' (AACE) guidelines for management of dyslipidemia and prevention of atherosclerosis (2012).

*10-year risk calculation is recommended in the ATP III and AACE guidelines; the presence of two or more major cardiovascular risk factors is considered as high risk in the ACC/ADA statement.

TABLE 4 — The Four Target Groups and Two Exceptions for Statin Therapy in the 2013 ACC/AHA Guideline

CHARACTERISTICS	TREATMENT
Clinical atherosclerotic cardiovascular disease*	<75 years: high-intensity statin >75 years or not candidate for high-intensity statin: moderate-intensity statin
LDL cholesterol >190 mg/dL	High-intensity statin
40–75 years with diabetes, LDL cholesterol 70–189 mg/dL	Moderate-intensity statin (may use high-intensity statin if 10 year risk ≥7.5%)
40–75 years without diabetes, LDL cholesterol 70–189 mg/dL, 10-year atherosclerotic cardiovascular risk[†] ≥7.5%	Moderate- to high-intensity statin
Maintenance hemodialysis	No recommendation
Ischemic systolic heart failure, NYHA class II–IV	No recommendation

*Coronary heart disease, stroke, and peripheral arterial disease of presumed atherosclerotic origin.

[†]10-year risk of nonfatal myocardial infarction, coronary heart disease death, and nonfatal and fatal stroke using the Pooled Cohort Equation (http://tools.cardiosource.org/ASCVD-Risk-Estimator).

LDL cholesterol is calculated either using the Friedewald equation (LDL cholesterol = total cholesterol − HDL cholesterol − triglycerides/5) or directly measured. The Friedewald equation should be used with appropriate caution: fasting state samples should be used, it becomes less accurate if triglycerides >200 mg/dL, not valid if triglycerides >400 mg/dL and LDL cholesterol can be underestimated at levels <70 mg/dL.

Apolipoproteins, including Apo B and Apo AI, may also be measured. The Apo B level (Apo B100) reflects the number of atherogenic lipoprotein particles and appears to be a better measure of cardiovascular disease than the LDL cholesterol level or the LDL particle size. Apo B level and Apo B/Apo AI ratio are as good as traditional lipid profiles and are especially useful in certain situations such as combined hyperlipidemia, metabolic syndrome, diabetes, and chronic kidney disease.

Other medical conditions may also affect lipid profiles. Secondary causes include hypothyroidism, nephrotic syndrome, dysgammaglobulinemia, use of progestin (especially those with androgenic activity), cholestasis, use of protease inhibitors, chronic kidney disease, uncontrolled diabetes, obesity, excessive alcohol intake, use of thiazide or β-blockers, use of corticosteroids, use of oral estrogen (not transdermal), and pregnancy. These conditions should be detected and treated, if appropriate, to improve control of hyperlipidemia.

Family history of premature cardiovascular disease and hyperlipidemia and physical findings such as xanthomas, xanthelasmas, and premature arcus cornealis may suggest familial hyperlipidemia. Familial hyperlipidemia can be associated with significantly high risk of cardiovascular disease, which could be underestimated by the global risk scores.

Treatment

Overview

Treatment is primarily aimed at lowering LDL cholesterol level, which has been shown to decrease the risk of cardiovascular disease in numerous studies unless the triglyceride level is higher than 500 mg/dL, in which case triglycerides should be lowered immediately to prevent pancreatitis. Every reduction of LDL cholesterol by 40 mg/dL is associated with about 20% reduction in cardiovascular risk. The absolute risk reduction by lowering LDL cholesterol is proportional to the global cardiovascular risk. Therefore, the targeted goal of LDL cholesterol is determined by the global cardiovascular risk.

The treatment goals and approaches according to the ATP III are summarized in Table 2. The optional goal of LDL cholesterol less than 70 mg/dL was added in the 2004 update for the very–high-risk group. Established cardiovascular disease itself and diabetes with other cardiovascular risk factor(s) are also considered as very high risk by some authorities. The goals for LDL cholesterol and Apo B in the very–high-risk and high-risk groups according to more recent guidelines are listed in Table 3. As a first line, therapeutic lifestyle changes should be initiated when LDL cholesterol is above the target range. People with very high, high, or moderately high risk should also start making therapeutic lifestyle changes regardless of their LDL cholesterol level. Medications may be added at the same time as therapeutic lifestyle changes for those with very high, high, or moderately high risk. If medications are indicated, statin is preferred because of proven efficacy that has been consistently shown in multiple clinical trials. The intensity of treatment should be strong enough to reduce LDL cholesterol level by at least 30% to 40%. Once the LDL cholesterol goal is achieved, then non-HDL cholesterol level should be controlled. The treatment goal for the non-HDL cholesterol is 30 mg/dL above the LDL cholesterol goal. Specific treatment of low-HDL cholesterol is controversial. CETP inhibitors, which specifically increase HDL cholesterol by blocking transfer of cholesterol to Apo B-containing lipoproteins, were not effective in reducing cardiovascular risk. The effect of increasing HDL cholesterol with niacin in people taking statins has not been encouraging. Generally, response to treatment can be evaluated in 6 weeks. Once under control, lipid profiles can be monitored every 4 to 6 months.

The ACC/AHA Task Force on Practice Guidelines issued a new guideline in 2013. The new approach recommends treating at-risk patients with statins of appropriate strength (reflecting the design of most published clinical trials), rather than titrating combinations of lipid-lowering medications to a preset target based on baseline cholesterol levels. Strength of the statin (high intensity: LDL cholesterol reduction >50%, moderate intensity: LDL cholesterol reduction 30%–50%) is determined by the global risk. The Pooled Cohort Equation, a new algorithm for risk calculation, is used to estimate the global risk in those with LDL cholesterol 70 to 189 mg/dL but without clinical atherosclerotic or diabetes (see Table 4). This new approach initially faced considerable skepticism because of the absence of LDL cholesterol targets, neglect of nonstatin therapy, and questionable validity of the new algorithm for risk calculation (the Pooled Cohort Equation). It is predicted that patients eligible for statin therapy may double according to the new guideline.

Part of the controversy over the new ACC/AHA guideline pertains to the risk-calculation tools, which have limitations: most of the risk calculators do not consider family history of premature cardiovascular events, which can lead to a serious underestimation of the risk in some patients (the Reynolds Risk Score includes family history of premature myocardial infarction); some of the risk calculators do not predict risk of stroke, which is another major cardiovascular event (the hard CHD tool in the ATP III predicts only fatal and nonfatal myocardial infarction whereas the new Pooled Cohort Equation predicts both nonfatal/fatal myocardial infarction and stroke); these risk calculators are not always validated beyond the original cohorts from which they were developed. The new risk prediction algorithm (the Pooled Cohort Equation) was also criticized for overestimating cardiovascular risk when applied to different cohorts. The panel who developed the algorithm countered that the criticism was largely based on data obtained from cohorts that include volunteers who tend to be healthier than the general population. On the other hand, validity of the algorithm has not been established by prospective clinical trials.

The 2013 ACC/AHA guideline focuses on the proven effects of statins on cardiovascular disease. It is predicted that patients eligible for statin therapy may double according to the new guideline and patients who are at high risk for cardiovascular disease will benefit from wider use of statins. Efficacy of adding other cholesterol lowering medications such as fibrates or niacin to achieve previously recommended target is limited (discussed below), but management of those who are not tolerant or contraindicated to moderate-high intensity statins is not well addressed. However, recent studies suggest that the high efficacy of the newly developed PCSK9 inhibitors may significantly change the landscape of effective cholesterol management in such individuals.

Therapeutic Lifestyle Changes

All patients with hyperlipidemia should be counseled on lifestyle modifications. Dietary modification to limit intake of lipids is an essential component, given that the main source of lipids is exogenous dietary fat. Saturated fatty acids and trans-unsaturated fatty acids increase LDL cholesterol while dietary fibers decrease LDL cholesterol. Carbohydrates do not affect LDL cholesterol but increase triglycerides and decrease HDL cholesterol, particularly if they have a high glycemic index. Intake of fructose, a component of sucrose, increases triglycerides and decreases HDL cholesterol. Body weight reduction and physical activity have a small effect on LDL cholesterol but reduce triglycerides and increase HDL cholesterol significantly. Alcohol intake has an adverse effect on triglycerides.

Individual patients will need different approaches based on their cardiovascular risk and lipid profiles. Generally, total dietary fat is recommended to constitute 25–35% of the total calorie intake mainly as mono- or poly-unsaturated fat, limiting saturated fat <7% and trans fat <1% of the total calorie intake. Therapeutic lifestyle changes include diets with emphasis on vegetables, fruits, whole grains, low-fat dairy products, poultry, fish, legumes, nontropical vegetable oils, and nuts as well as limited intake of sweets, sugar sweetened beverages, and red meats; further reduction of saturated fat (<5–6% of the total caloric intake) and trans fat; weight reduction; and increased regular physical activity. The amount of cholesterol intake is not well correlated with LDL cholesterol level and there is no recommended limit for intake. Management of other risk factors such as smoking cessation and controlling blood pressure in hypertensive patients and blood glucose in diabetics is also very important.

Pharmacologic Agents

The currently available lipid-lowering agents can be classified based on their mechanism of action into statins (3-hydroxy-3-methylglutaryl coenzyme A [HMG-CoA] reductase inhibitors), fibrates, niacin, bile acid sequestrants, and cholesterol absorption inhibitors such as ezetimibe (Zetia). These classes of agents differ with regard to degree and type of lipid lowering, and agents within the same group may differ in efficacy and side effects. Conventional dosing regimens and common adverse effects are summarized in Table 5. Expected changes in lipid profiles are shown in Table 6. The choice of drug depends on the specific lipid abnormalities and concurrent medical conditions. In general, statins are the most effective drugs to lower cardiovascular risk and are the treatment of choice when medications are indicated based on the global cardiovascular risk. If the primary goal is to lower triglycerides, fibrates or niacin may be more effective. If the treatment goal is not achieved by statins or statins are not tolerated, another agent should be used.

Statins

Statins are usually the first drug of choice in patients with high cholesterol levels to reduce cardiovascular risk. Statins are the only class of lipid-lowering agents that has been shown in multiple randomized clinical trials to improve cardiovascular outcomes in primary and secondary prevention. Furthermore, risk reduction was apparent in a wide range of patients, including men, women, smokers, those with diabetes, and those with hypertension as well as in older populations. Also, statins lead to the highest degree of LDL cholesterol reduction among all of the lipid-lowering agents. The approximate equipotent dosages of various statins and their cholesterol-lowering effects are listed in Table 7. The 2013 ACC/AHA guideline recommends moderate or high-intensity statins (see Table 7) based on the global risk (see Table 4). Statins inhibit HMG-CoA reductase, the rate-limiting enzyme in cholesterol biosynthesis. By blocking cholesterol biosynthesis, statins upregulate the LDL receptor on the hepatocytes and increase clearance of IDL and LDL. In addition to their direct effects on lipid metabolism, statins have been reported to have pleiotropic effects (e.g., reduced formation of reactive oxygen species, inhibition of platelet reactivity, and decreased vasoconstriction).

Statins are usually well tolerated. Potential common side effects include nonspecific gastrointestinal symptoms such as dyspepsia, headaches, fatigue, and myopathy. Hepatitis occurs in less than 1%. There is a small increase in risk of developing diabetes. It is recommended that the physician monitor for development of

TABLE 5   Major Drugs for Management of Hyperlipidemia

AGENT	STARTING DAILY DOSAGE	DOSAGE RANGE	MECHANISM	SIDE EFFECTS
Statins				
Lovastatin (Mevacor)	20 mg	10–80 mg	Decreased cholesterol synthesis, increased hepatic LDL receptors, decreased VLDL release	Myalgias, arthralgias, high liver enzymes, dyspepsia
Pravastatin (Pravachol)	40 mg	10–80 mg		
Simvastatin (Zocor)*	20–40 mg	5–80 mg		
Fluvastatin (Lescol)	40 mg	20–80 mg		
Atorvastatin (Lipitor)	10–20 mg	10–80 mg		
Rosuvastatin Crestor)	10 mg	5–40 mg		
Pitavastatin (Livalo)	2 mg	2–4 mg		
Fibrates				
Fenofibrate (Tricor)	48–145 mg	48–145 mg	Increased LPL activity, decreased VLDL synthesis	Dyspepsia, myalgia, gallstones, high liver enzymes
Gemfibrozil (Lopid)	1200 mg	1200 mg		
Fenofibric acid (Trilipix)	45–135 mg	45–135 mg		
Niacin				
Immediate release	250 mg	250–3000 mg	Decreased VLDL synthesis	Flushing, high glucose, uric acid, high liver enzymes
Extended release (Niaspan)	500 mg	500–2000 mg		
Bile Acid Sequestrants				
Cholestyramine (Questran)	8–16 g	4–24 g	Increased bile acid excretion, increased LDL receptors	Bloating, constipation, elevated triglycerides
Colestipol (Colestid)	2 g	2–16 g		
Colesevelam (Welchol)	3.75 g	3.75–4.375 g		
Cholesterol Absorption Inhibitors				
Ezetimibe (Zetia)	10 mg	10 mg	Deceased intestinal cholesterol absorption	High liver enzymes
Combination Therapies (single pill)				
Ezetimibe/simvastatin (Vytorin)	10/20 mg	10/10–10/80 mg		
Extended-release niacin/ simvastatin (Simcor)	500/20 mg	500/20 1000/20 mg		

*See the text for the FDA warning.

Abbreviations: LDL = low-density lipoprotein; LPL = lipoprotein lipase; TG = triglycerides; VLDL = very–low-density lipoprotein.

TABLE 6   Metabolic Effects of Each Lipid-Lowering Drug Class

	LDL CHOLESTEROL	HDL CHOLESTEROL	TRIGLYCERIDES
Statins	↓21%–55%	↑2%–10%	↓6%–30%
Fibric acids	↓20%–25%	↑6%–18%	↓20%–35%
Niacin	↓10%–25%	↑10%–35%	↓20%–30%
Bile acid sequestrants	↓15%–25%		May ↑
Cholesterol absorption inhibitors	↓10%–18%		

Adapted from lipoprotein management in patients with cardiometabolic risk, consensus statement from the American College of Cardiology Foundation and the American Diabetes Association (ACC/ADA) (2008), and American Association of Clinical Endocrinologists' (AACE) guidelines for management of dyslipidemia and prevention of atherosclerosis (2012).

myopathy clinically and hepatotoxicity with liver function tests (baseline and within 3 months and then periodically). Myopathy is one of the most common causes for cessation of statins. Myalgias can occur in about 10% to 20% of patients, which is much more often than reported in the clinical trials. The risk of rhabdomyolysis, however, is very low (0.1–0.2 per 1000 person-years). Risk for myopathy is increased in patients with advanced age, female sex, small body habitus, hypothyroidism, alcoholism, medical conditions (particularly liver or kidney disease), major surgery, excessive physical activity, history of myopathy, family history of myopathy, high-dose statins, and interacting medications or food such as grapefruit juice (>1 L/day). Simvastatin (Zocor), lovastatin (Mevacor), and atorvastatin (Lipitor) are primarily metabolized through CYP3A4, which is inhibited by protease inhibitors, cyclosporine (Neoral, Sandimmune), amiodarone (Cordarone, Pacerone), nondihydropyridine calcium channel blockers, fibrates, and other agents. Pravastatin (Pravachol) is metabolized by the kidney, not by the P450 system. Fluvastatin (Lescol) and rosuvastatin (Crestor) are primarily metabolized through CYP2C9. Simvastatin and lovastatin should be avoided in patients receiving protease inhibitors. Statin dosage should be reduced in patients taking cyclosporine. Because of significant risk of myopathy related to simvastatin, the FDA recommends that 80 mg/day should not be used unless the patient has been taking 80 mg safely for longer than 12 months. The FDA further recommends that the dose be limited to 20 mg if the patient is also taking amiodarone, amlodipine (Norvasc), or ranolazine (Ranexa), and to 10 mg/day if taking diltiazem (Cardizem), dronedarone (Multaq), or verapamil (Calan). Addition of fibrates increases the risk of myopathy; in patients on a statin, fenofibrate (Tricor) is preferred over gemfibrozil (Lopid), which has a much higher risk of rhabdomyolysis. Symptoms of statin myopathy are heaviness,

TABLE 7 Equipotency and Percentage Reduction in Total Cholesterol According to the Different Types and Doses of Statins					
REDUCTION IN TOTAL CHOLESTEROL (%)	**PRAVASTATIN (PRAVACHOL), mg**	**FLUVASTATIN (LESCOL), mg**	**SIMVASTATIN (ZOCOR),* mg**	**ATORVASTATIN (LIPITOR), mg**	**ROSUVASTATIN (CRESTOR), mg**
6–15	5	10	-	-	-
15–17	10	20	5	2.5	-
22	20	40	10	5	-
27	40†	80†	20†	10†	5†
32	80†		40†	20†	10†
37	-	-	(80)	40‡	20‡
42	-	-	-	80‡	40‡

Modified from Penning-van Beest and colleagues (2007).
*See the text for the FDA warning.
†Moderate-intensity statins (reduction of LDL cholesterol 30%–50%).
‡High-intensity statins (reduction of LDL cholesterol >50%).

stiffness, cramping associated with weakness during exertion, and tendon-associated pain. Location of symptoms can be at the thighs, at the calves, or generalized. Symptoms can be very nonspecific, and differentiating statin-related myopathy from other causes is not easy. Therefore, baseline symptoms, physical examination, and assessment of creatinine kinase level before the initiation of statins can be very helpful. Further decisions regarding stopping or switching medications can be made based on the severity of symptoms, level of creatinine kinase elevation, and presence of rhabdomyolysis. In patients who develop myopathy while on simvastatin or atorvastatin, if the decision is to continue treatment with a statin, one option is to cautiously switch them to pravastatin, fluvastatin, or rosuvastatin, which are less prone to cause myopathy. Furthermore, rosuvastatin has a long duration of action and can be taken once every other day, or weekly, if necessary. Theoretically, coenzyme Q10 may help statin-induced myopathy, but there is insufficient data to support its use. For patients who cannot tolerate statins, other agents should be used.

Fibrates
The effect of fibrates on cardiovascular outcomes is not as favorable as with statins or niacin. However, fibrates can be useful in subsets of patients with high triglycerides and low-HDL cholesterol. Recently, the ACCORD lipid trial showed that addition of fenofibrate to simvastatin in type 2 diabetic patients with cardiovascular risk factors did not improve cardiovascular outcomes, though there was a trend for better outcomes in a subgroup with triglycerides greater than 204 mg/dL and HDL cholesterol less than 34 mg/dL. Fibrates have multiple favorable metabolic effects including activation of peroxisome proliferator-activated receptor-α (contributing to the regulation of both lipid and carbohydrate metabolism), stimulation of lipoprotein lipase (increasing triglyceride hydrolysis), and downregulation of Apo CIII (improving lipoprotein remnant clearance as Apo CIII inhibits lipoprotein lipase). An enhanced VLDL-to-LDL conversion may lead to mild LDL cholesterol elevation in some patients. This effect may decrease over weeks as the LDL receptors are upregulated. Fibrates are generally well tolerated. The most common side effect is dyspepsia. Other side effects include myopathy and hepatic enzyme elevation, particularly when fibrates are added to statins. As mentioned above, fenofibrate is recommended when added to statins because of the high risk of rhabdomyolysis associated with gemfibrozil plus statins. Fibrates increase the risk of gallstones, and patients on warfarin (Coumadin) may need dose adjustment. Monitoring of liver enzymes is recommended, at baseline and within 3 months and then periodically. Creatinine level can be increased through unclear mechanisms.

Niacin
Niacin or nicotinic acid effectively decreases the hepatic production of VLDL and thus LDL cholesterol levels, and raises HDL cholesterol levels by reducing cholesterol transfer from HDL to Apo B-containing lipoproteins and HDL clearance by the liver. Niacin is the most potent agent available to increase HDL cholesterol. Several trials showed the effect of niacin in preventing cardiovascular disease. But the benefit of adding niacin to statins has not been proved. Niacin did not improve cardiovascular risk when added to simvastatin in patients with high risk for cardiovascular disease in the AIM HIGH study and the HPS2-Thrive study. There were excess adverse events and trends towards signs of harm among the niacin groups. The most common side effect of niacin is flushing. This can be avoided or minimized by initiating therapy with a low dose of niacin, taking an aspirin 1 hour before niacin, avoiding hot foods or beverages at the time the niacin is taken, or switching to extended-release forms (Niaspan). Hepatotoxicity can occur at any time. Immediate-release forms are less likely to cause hepatotoxicity than sustained-release forms (Slo-Niacin). Extended-release forms can minimally elevate transaminases but significant hepatotoxicity is rare. When switching to different forms, it is recommended that one should start with low doses and titrate up to achieve desired response. Liver function tests should be monitored regularly, at baseline and every 3 months for the first year and then periodically. Other side effects include pruritus, increased uric acid levels, and hyperglycemia.

Bile Acid Sequestrants
Bile acid sequestrants have been in clinical use for many decades. These agents promote fecal excretion of bile acids. The liver responds with increased integration of cholesterol into bile acid synthesis to maintain a stable bile acid pool. The consequent decrease in cholesterol in the liver leads to upregulation of the LDL receptor and enhanced LDL clearance from the plasma. HMG-CoA synthase activity can increase, so combination therapy with statins would be synergistic, especially in patients with a suboptimal response. Available agents are cholestyramine (Questran), colestipol (Colestid), and colesevelam (Welchol). Most side effects involve the gastrointestinal tract, with constipation and bloating being the most common. These agents may interfere with the absorption of warfarin, phenobarbital, levothyroxine (Synthroid), and digoxin (Lanoxin), among other medications. Patients on multiple medications should be advised to take bile acid sequestrants 1 hour before or 4 hours after taking the other medications. These agents can also cause elevation of triglyceride level. As they are not systemically absorbed, the bile acid sequestrants may be the preferred agents when systemic absorption is to be avoided, such as during pregnancy or lactation.

Cholesterol Absorption Inhibitors
Ezetimibe is the first in a new class of pharmaceutical agents that inhibit the sterol transporters in the intestine. Ezetimibe is a good add-on agent in people taking a statin if the LDL cholesterol goal is not achieved or high doses of statin cannot be tolerated. Ezetimibe was shown to modestly decrease cardiovascular events when added to simvastatin in high risk patients. Elevated liver enzymes have been reported but the risk of hepatotoxicity seems to be not different from that of placebo.

Several new lipid-lowering agents are under development. Among these, PCSK9 (proprotein convertase subtilisin/kexin type 9) inhibitors have shown promise in several phase 2–3 trials. The PCSK9 protein appears to control the number of LDL receptors. When it binds to the LDL receptor, the latter is destroyed with the LDL particle. Interference with PCSK9's LDL receptor-binding capacity or silencing the gene for PCSK9 allows the LDL receptor to recycle to the cell surface to remove more circulating plasma cholesterol. Individuals with loss-of-function mutations of PCSK9 have very low LDL cholesterol levels and are protected from CHD. Various PCSK9 inhibitors (mostly monoclonal antibodies) have been shown to decrease LDL cholesterol levels by >40–70% with no significant side effects when used as a single agent or added to maximal dose statin. Post-hoc analyses showed that addition of PCSK9 inhibitors for 12–18 months decreased cardiovascular events by 50%. Larger studies with longer follow up for cardiovascular outcome are underway. The Endocrinologic and Metabolic Drugs Advisory Committee of the US FDA recommended approval of two human monoclonal antibodies (alirocumab [Praluent], evolocumab [Repatha]) based on expected benefit especially for those with familial hypercholesterolemia. PCSK9 inhibitors enable reduction of LDL cholesterol to levels previously not achievable. In this regard, it is important to note that LDL cholesterol at levels <70 mg/dL can be underestimated by the Friedewald equation. The initial clinical trials appear quite exciting, though the long term safety of PCSK9 inhibition by the different treatment strategies remains to be established.

References

Brunzell JD, Davidson M, Furberg CD. Lipoprotein management in patients with cardiometabolic risk: Consensus conference report from the ADA and the ACC foundation. J Am Coll Cardiol 2008;51:1512–24.

Carroll MD, Kit BK, Lacher DA, et al. Trends in lipids and lipoproteins in U.S. adults, 1988–2010. JAMA 2012;308:1545–54.

Eckel RH, Jakicic JM, Ard JD, et al. 2013 ACC/AHA guideline on lifestyle management to reduce cardiovascular risk: A report of the American College of Cardiology/American Heart Association task force on practice guidelines. J Am Coll Cardiol 2014;63:2960–84.

Ginsberg HN, Elam MB, Lovato LC, et al. Effects of combination lipid therapy in type 2 diabetes mellitus. N Engl J Med 2010;362:1563–74.

Greenland P, Alpert JS, Beller GA, et al. 2010 ACCF/AHA guideline for assessment of cardiovascular risk in asymptomatic adults: A report of the American College of Cardiology Foundation/American Heart Association Task Force on Practice Guidelines developed in collaboration with the American Society of Echocardiography, American Society of Nuclear Cardiology, Society of Atherosclerosis Imaging and Prevention, Society for Cardiovascular Angiography and Interventions, Society of Cardiovascular Computed Tomography, and Society for Cardiovascular Magnetic Resonance. J Am Coll Cardiol 2010;56:e50–e103.

Grundy SM, Cleeman JI, Merz CNB, et al. Implications of recent clinical trials for the national cholesterol education program adult treatment panel III guidelines. Circulation 2004;110:227–39.

Huffman MD, Capewell S, Ning H, et al. Cardiovascular health behavior and health factor changes (1988–2008) and projections to 2020: Results from the National Health and Nutrition Examination Surveys (NHANES). Circulation 2012;125:2595–602.

Jellinger PS, Smith DA, Mehta AE, et al. American Association of Clinical Endocrinologists' guidelines for management of hyperlipidemia and prevention of atherosclerosis. Endocr Pract 2012;18:1–78.

Joy TR, Hegele RA. Narrative review: Statin-related myopathy. Ann Intern Med 2009;150:858–68.

Keaney JF, Curfman GD, Jarcho JA. A pragmatic view of the new cholesterol treatment guidelines. N Engl J Med 2014;370:275–8.

Otvos JD, Collins D, Freedman DS, et al. Low-density lipoprotein and high-density lipoprotein particle subclasses predict coronary events and are favorably changed by gemfibrozil therapy in the Veterans Affairs High-Density Lipoprotein Intervention Trial. Circulation 2006;113:1556–63.

Penning-van Beest FJA, Termorshuizen F, Goettsch WG, et al. Adherence to evidence-based statin guidelines reduces the risk of hospitalizations for acute myocardial infarction by 40%: A cohort study. Eur Heart J 2007;28:154–9.

Phan BAP, Dayspring TD, Toth PP. Ezetimibe therapy: Mechanism of action and clinical update. Vasc Health Risk Manag 2012;8:415–27.

Reiner Z, Catapano AL, De Backer G, et al. ESC/EAS guidelines for the management of dyslipidaemias: The task force for the management of dyslipidaemias of the European Society of Cardiology (ESC) and the European Atherosclerosis Society (EAS). Eur Heart J 2011;32:1769–818.

Ridker PM, Cook NR. Statins: New American guidelines for prevention of cardiovascular disease. Lancet 2013;382:1762–5.

Robinson JG, Farnier M, Krempf M, et al. Efficacy and safety of alirocumab in reducing lipids and cardiovascular events. N Eng J Med 2015;372:1489–99.

Sabatine MS, Giugliano RP, Wiviott SD, et al. Efficacy and safety of evolocumab in reducing lipids and cardiovascular events. N Eng J Med 2015;372:1500–9.

Stone NJ, Robinson J, Lichtenstein AH, et al. ACC/AHA guideline on the treatment of blood cholesterol to reduce atherosclerotic cardiovascular risk in adults: A report of the American College of Cardiology/American Heart Association task force on practice guidelines. J Am Coll Cardiol 2014;63:2889–934.

The HPS2-THRIVE Collaborative Group. Effects of extended-release niacin with laropiprant in high-risk patients. N Eng J Med 2014;371:203–12.

The AIM-HIGH Investigators. Niacin in patients with low HDL cholesterol levels receiving intensive statin therapy. N Engl J Med 2011;365:2255–67.

Third report of the National Cholesterol Education Program (NCEP) expert panel on detection, evaluation, and treatment of high blood cholesterol in adults (Adult treatment panel III) final report. Circulation 2002;106:3143–421.

HYPERPARATHYROIDISM AND HYPOPARATHYROIDISM

Method of
John P. Bilezikian, MD

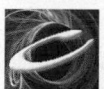

CURRENT DIAGNOSIS

Primary Hyperparathyroidism
- Most common cause of hypercalcemia.
- Diagnosis established by elevated serum calcium concentration and parathyroid hormone level that is frankly elevated or is in the upper range of normal.
- In some patients, the parathyroid hormone level is elevated but the serum calcium concentration is normal.

Hypoparathyroidism
- Much less common than primary hyperparathyroidism.
- Most often due to surgical removal of all parathyroid tissue or autoimmune destruction.
- Diagnosis is established by hypocalcemia and low parathyroid hormone levels.

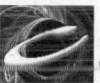

CURRENT THERAPY

Primary Hyperparathyroidism
- When symptoms are present, parathyroid surgery is indicated.
- In the absence of symptoms, surgery is recommended if any one of four criteria is met (see Table 2).
- Preoperative localization testing prior to surgery has become routine.
- Conservative management is reserved generally for those who do not meet surgical criteria.
- Prudent use of calcium and vitamin D is recommended, and ambulation is encouraged.
- Pharmacologic agents such as bisphosphonates show promise to increase bone density while calcimimetic therapy may be indicated to reduce the serum calcium level.

Hypoparathyroidism
- Acute management of hypocalcemia is a medical emergency and requires intravenous administration of calcium.
- Chronic treatment is based upon adequate calcium, vitamin D, and, often, the active vitamin D metabolite 1,25-dihydroxyvitamin D.
- Management with parathyroid hormone is under investigation.

Primary Hyperparathyroidism

Incidence and General Characteristics

Primary hyperparathyroidism (PHPT) is a relatively common endocrine disease with an incidence as high as 1 in 500 to 1 in 1000. The incidence of PHPT increased with the advent of the multichannel autoanalyzer in the 1970s. PHPT occurs in individuals of all ages but occurs most frequently in the sixth decade of life. Women are affected more often than men by a ratio of 3:1. PHPT in children is an unusual event. It might be a component of one of

TABLE 1	Differential Diagnosis of Hypercalcemia

Primary hyperparathyroidism
Malignancy
Other endocrinopathies
   Hyperthyroidism
   Pheochromocytoma
   Adrenal insufficiency
   VIPoma
Medications
   Lithium
   Thiazides
   Thyroid hormone
   Vitamin D
   Vitamin A
Granulomatous diseases
Familial hypocalciuric hypercalcemia
Immobilization

several endocrinopathies with a genetic basis, such as multiple endocrine neoplasia (MEN), type I or II. PHPT is caused by excessive secretion of parathyroid hormone (PTH) from one or more parathyroid glands. A benign, solitary adenoma is found in 80% of patients. Less commonly, in 15% to 20% of subjects, all four glands are hyperplastic. Four-gland parathyroid disease may occur sporadically or in association with the MEN syndromes. The most uncommon presentation of PHPT is parathyroid cancer, occurring in less than 0.5% of patients with PHPT.

Differential Diagnosis

The major diagnostic distinction to be made is between PHPT and malignancy, the other most common cause of hypercalcemia. These two etiologies account for more than 90% of all patients with hypercalcemia (Table 1). A much longer, complete list of potential causes of hypercalcemia is considered after these two etiologies are ruled out or if there is reason to believe that a different cause is likely. Today, PHPT presents most often as an asymptomatic disorder. In contrast, malignancy-associated hypercalcemia is usually found at a later stage of the malignant process and is associated with symptoms. Besides a major difference in clinical presentation between these two most common causes of hypercalcemia, the PTH immunoassay is a helpful distinguishing point. In patients with PHPT, the PTH level will be elevated or in the upper range of normal, whereas in malignancy, the PTH level is invariably suppressed.

Pathophysiology, Molecular Genetics, and Pathology

The pathophysiology of PHPT relates to the loss of normal feedback control of PTH by extracellular calcium. Why the parathyroid cell loses its normal sensitivity to calcium is not known. Genetic abnormalities that could be linked to sporadic parathyroid tumors have been described. A rearrangement of the cyclin D1/(PRAD1) protooncogene has been seen in some patients with PHPT. The rearrangement associates the PTH gene with the growth promoter cyclin D1. Tumor suppressors, such as the gene associated with MEN-I, have generated interest, as have potential abnormalities in the gene for the calcium-sensing receptor. Although the gene for the calcium receptor has been implicated in familial hypocalciuric hypercalcemia and neonatal severe hyperparathyroidism, there is little evidence for this genetic abnormality in the sporadic form of PHPT.

The typical parathyroid adenoma is an enlarged, oval-shaped, smooth, red-brown gland. A visible rim of normal yellow-brown parathyroid tissue is sometimes seen. The typical size of the parathyroid adenoma is smaller than it used to be, but still is much larger than a normal gland, which generally weighs 35 to 50 mg. Parathyroid adenomas are generally over 150 mg and can be much larger. Microscopically, the parathyroid adenoma consists of a network of cells arranged alongside a capillary network, resembling classic endocrine microanatomy. Fat cells are reduced or absent. The form of PHPT characterized by four-gland hyperplasia is seen grossly as uniformly enlarged glands. Microscopically, solid masses of chief cells are seen in the absence of fat cells. In contrast to the adenoma, in which a rim of normal tissue can sometimes be seen, normal tissue is absent in hyperplastic disease. The histological distinctions between adenomatous and hyperplastic disease are not always so clear.

Signs and Symptoms

PHPT is associated classically with skeletal and renal complications. In severe cases, the skeleton can be involved in a process called *osteitis fibrosa cystica*. Subperiosteal resorption of the distal phalanges, tapering of the distal clavicles, a "salt and pepper" appearance of the skull, bone cysts, and brown tumors of the long bones are all overt manifestations of hyperparathyroid bone disease. This form of hyperparathyroid bone disease is now most unusual in countries where multichannel screening is routine. Skeletal involvement in PHPT is detected much more often by dual energy x-ray absorptiometry (see later). Similar to the reduced incidence of gross skeletal disease, the kidney is also involved in PHPT much less commonly than before. Most series place the incidence of nephrolithiasis now to be no more than 15% to 20%. Nephrolithiasis, nevertheless, is still the most common complication of PHPT. Other renal features of PHPT include diffuse deposition of calcium–phosphate complexes in the parenchyma (nephrocalcinosis). The frequency of this complication is unknown. Hypercalciuria (daily calcium excretion of >250 mg in women or >300 mg in men) is seen in 30% to 40% of patients. PHPT may be associated with a reduction in creatinine clearance, in the absence of any other cause. Classic associations exist between PHPT and other organs, such as the neuromuscular system, the gastrointestinal tract, and the cardiovascular and articular systems, but such panopleistic features of PHPT are rarely seen today. More vexing are nonspecific elements associated with PHPT, such as easy fatigability, a sense of weakness, and a feeling that the aging process is advancing faster than it should be. This is sometimes accompanied by an intellectual weariness and a sense that cognitive faculties are less sharp. Whether these nonspecific features of PHPT are truly part of the disease process, reversible upon successful parathyroid surgery, remains under active investigation.

Clinical Forms of Primary Hyperparathyroidism

Asymptomatic PHPT with serum calcium levels within 1 mg/dL above the upper limits of normal is the most common clinical presentation. Most patients do not have specific complaints and do not show evidence of any target organ complications. In parts of the world where severe vitamin D deficiency is common, more symptomatic PHPT is seen. Unusual clinical presentations of PHPT include MEN-I and MEN-II, familial PHPT not associated with any other endocrine disorder, familial cystic parathyroid adenomatosis, jaw tumor syndrome, and neonatal PHPT. Over the past decade, yet another presentation of PHPT can be seen in individuals with normal serum calcium concentrations but elevated PTH levels. Potential secondary causes of elevated PTH levels have to be ruled out such as vitamin D deficiency, renal insufficiency, medications such as thiazide diuretics or lithium. Normocalcemic primary hyperparathyroidism, this newer phenotype of primary hyperparathyroidism, may represent in some patients the earliest stage of PHPT, when there is glandular overproduction of hormone, before hypercalcemia becomes evident.

Diagnosis and Evaluation

Hypercalcemia and elevated levels of PTH, or levels inappropriately in the upper range of normal with hypercalcemia, establish the diagnosis. The serum phosphorus concentration tends to be in the lower range of normal. Serum alkaline phosphatase activity may be elevated. More specific markers of bone formation (bone-specific alkaline phosphatase, osteocalcin) and bone resorption (urinary deoxypyridinoline, N- or C-telopeptide of collagen) tend to be in the upper range of normal. In some patients, the actions of PTH in altering renal acid-base handling leads to a small increase in the serum chloride concentration and a concomitant small decrease in the serum bicarbonate concentration. Urinary calcium excretion, when elevated, is not generally excessively high. The circulating 25-hydroxyvitamin D concentration is low, and the 1,25-dihydroxyvitamin D concentration tends to be in the upper range of normal, reflecting the disposition of parathyroid hormone to facilitate the conversion of 25-hydroxyvitamin D to 1,25-dihydroxyvitamin D.

Role of Bone Mass Measurement

Dual-energy x-ray absorptiometry shows a pattern of skeletal involvement that is consistent with the physiologic actions of PTH, namely a proclivity to be catabolic at cortical bone. Thus, the typical patient with PHPT shows reductions in bone density that are most marked in the distal third of the forearm, a cortical site, with much less involvement of the lumbar spine, a cancellous site. The hip region, a mixture of cortical and cancellous bone, shows changes that are intermediate between changes in the forearm and the lumbar spine. This classic densitometric presentation is not consistent with epidemiologic data that has suggested a more general increase in fracture risk, including vertebral fractures. More recently, application of non-invasive high resolution peripheral imaging by CT has shown reduced trabecular microstructure as well as cortical involvement in primary hyperparathyroidism.

Treatment
Localization Tests Prior to Surgery
Imaging of abnormal parathyroid tissue is accomplished accurately with technetium-99m sestamibi. Sestamibi is taken up by both thyroid and parathyroid tissue, but it persists in the parathyroid glands. Various approaches to the use of technetium-99m sestamibi include using the imaging agent alone, and thereby depending upon a difference in uptake kinetics between thyroid and parathyroid tissue, or in combination with iodine 123 (^{123}I). Combining sestamibi with single-photon emission computed tomography can be helpful. Ultrasound, computed tomography, and magnetic resonance imaging are also used to localize abnormal parathyroid tissue. In the hands of some experts, ultrasound and computed tomography can be very successful localization approaches. Invasive localization tests with arteriography and selective venous sampling for PTH are rarely used anymore. Non-invasive preoperative imaging has become routine in all patients who are to undergo parathyroid surgery. If there are no plans for parathyroid surgery, parathyroid imaging is not necessary or recommended.

Guidelines for Surgical Management of Primary Hyperparathyroidism
The Fourth International Workshop on the Management of Asymptomatic Primary Hyperparathyroidism was held in 2013, and the proceedings were published in 2014. The Workshop reviewed new data since the previous workshop in 2008 and suggested revised guidelines for surgical management (Table 2). The major changes are summarized here. Since dual energy absorptiometry alone may not be the best predictor of vertebral fracture risk in primary hyperparathyroidism, measures such as vertebral x-rays, vertebral fracture analysis (VFA), or newer imaging approaches such as High Resolution peripheral Computed Tomography are recommended. The 24-hour urinary calcium excretion is recommended and when elevated, further measurements of urinary risk factors for stones, such as a urinary biochemical stone risk factor analyses are recommended. Renal imaging by x-ray, ultrasound, or CT is recommended because of the appreciable incidence of silent renal stones or nephrocalcinosis.

Surgery
PHPT is cured when abnormal parathyroid tissue is removed. Asymptomatic patients are advised to have surgery if they meet current guidelines (see Table 2). Symptomatic patients are always advised to undergo parathyroid surgery if there are no medical contraindications. At the present time, a number of different surgical procedures can be performed. While the standard four-gland parathyroid gland operation under general or local anesthesia is still

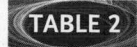

TABLE 2 2013 Guidelines for Parathyroid Surgery in Asymptomatic PHPT

MEASUREMENT	SURGERY RECOMMENDED IF
Serum calcium (>upper limit of normal)	>1.0 mg/dL (0.25 mmol/L)
Skeletal	a. BMD by DXA: T-score <−2.5 at lumbar spine, total hip, femoral neck or distal 1/3 radius* b. Vertebral fracture by x-ray, CT, MRI or VFA
Renal	a. Creatinine clearance <60 cc/min b. 24-hour urine for calcium >400 mg/day (>10 mmol/day) *and* increased stone risk by biochemical stone risk analysis c. presence of nephrolithiasis or nephrocalcinosis by x-ray, ultrasound, or CT
Age	<50

Adapted from Bilezikian et al: Guidelines for the Management of Asymptomatic Primary Hyperparathyroidism: Summary Statement from the Fourth International Workshop. J Clin Endocrinol Metab, 2014;99:3561.

performed, minimally invasive parathyroid surgery has gained in popularity. This procedure depends upon preoperative localization of the parathyroid adenoma by an imaging technology and confirmation of the success of abnormal gland removal with intraoperative PTH measurements before and minutes after parathyroidectomy. The circulating PTH level should fall to less than 50% of the preoperative value within minutes after removal of the parathyroid adenoma and be within the normal range. Minimally invasive parathyroid surgery, this latter approach, has become a standard for many parathyroid surgeons now.

Medical Management
In patients who do not meet surgical guidelines or who, for other reasons, will not undergo parathyroid surgery, the following medical principles apply. Adequate hydration and ambulation are always encouraged. Thiazide diuretics are to be avoided because they may lead to worsening hypercalcemia. Dietary intake of calcium should be moderate, avoiding both high- and low-calcium diets. Low-calcium diets theoretically could fuel abnormal parathyroid tissue to secrete more PTH. High-calcium diets could be detrimental by worsening hypercalcemia, especially if the 1,25-dihydroxy vitamin D level is elevated. Monitoring with annual measurements of the serum calcium and annual or every-other-year measurements of bone mass by dual-energy x-ray absorptiometry are recommended. In patients whose 25-hydroxyvitamin D level is low, careful replacement seems reasonable. The serum calcium concentration must be monitored to guard against the potential for worsening hypercalcemia in some patients.

Pharmacological management of primary hyperparathyroidism depends on the goal. If the goal is to increase bone mineral density, a bisphosphonate such as alendronate is reasonable and has been shown to be effective in this regard. One would not use bisphosphonate therapy instead of surgery, if the surgical guideline of low bone mineral density is met, unless the patient is not a candidate for parathyroid surgery. Bisphosphonate therapy in primary hyperparathyroidism has not been shown to reduce serum calcium or PTH concentrations.

If the goal of pharmacological therapy is to reduce the serum calcium, calcimimetic therapy with cinacalcet can be effective. Cinacalcet is approved by the FDA for the management of primary hyperparathyroidism. The serum calcium concentration typically becomes normal and remains within normal limits for as long as the drug is used. Interestingly, the serum PTH level falls only modestly and continues to be elevated despite correction of the hypercalcemia by the drug. Bone mineral density does not change. One would not use cinacalcet instead of surgery, if the guideline of hypercalcemia is met (>1mg/dL above normal) unless the patient is not a candidate for parathyroid surgery.

TABLE 3	Causes of Hypoparathyroidism
Parathyroid gland destruction	
Postsurgical	
Autoimmune	
Sporadic	
Polyglandular syndromes	
Activating antibodies against the calcium-sensing receptor	
Infiltration	
Iron, copper	
Malignancy	
Granulomatous	
Genetic	
Activating mutations of the calcium-sensing receptor	
Inactivating mutations in the PTH gene	
DiGeorge syndrome	
Impaired secretion and/or action of PTH	
Hypomagnesemia	
Pseudohypoparathyroidism	

Abbreviation: PTH = parathyroid hormone.

Hypoparathyroidism

Hypoparathyroidism is much more uncommon than is PHPT and, in fact, is defined in the United States as an orphan disease. Recent estimate place the prevalence at less than 100,000. Hypoparathyroidism results from the destruction, removal, or dysfunction of all parathyroid tissue.

Etiology

The most common causes of hypoparathyroidism are neck surgery and an autoimmune process (Table 3). Surgical hypoparathyroidism can follow the operation by many years and can occur after any neck surgery. Autoimmune destruction of the parathyroid glands can occur in an isolated fashion or in connection with a variety of polyglandular syndromes. Activating mutations of the calcium-sensing receptor or of the parathyroid gene itself can be associated with hypoparathyroidism. Parathyroid gland destruction is rarely due to infiltration of the glands by iron, copper, granulomas, or malignancy. In severe magnesium deficiency, parathyroid secretion is impaired along with a peripheral resistance to the actions of PTH. Mild hypoparathyroidism can become symptomatic in the presence of a potent bisphosphonate such as alendronate.

Clinical Features

Increased neuromuscular irritability is the clinical hallmark of hypoparathyroidism. Features of hypoparathyroidism can range from mild paresthesias around the mouth, fingers, and toes to muscle cramping, and, at their worst, carpal, pedal, or laryngospasm. Central nervous system seizure activity is also seen as a severe manifestation of hypocalcemia. These symptoms are due, in part, to the actual serum calcium level but also to the rate at which the serum calcium level falls. Rapid declines in the serum calcium concentrations are more likely to be associated with symptoms than are situations in which the serum calcium concentration has fallen gradually. If respiratory or metabolic alkalosis is present, symptoms can worsen because the partition between bound and free calcium is shifted to the bound state when the blood pH rises. Signs of hypocalcemia include the Chvostek sign (evoked facial nerve irritability), the Trousseau sign (carpal spasm when the blood pressure cuff is inflated to pressures above systolic), and a prolonged QT interval on the electrocardiogram. When severe hypocalcemia is present, impaired cardiac contractility, unresponsive to inotropic agents until the hypocalcemia is corrected, has been reported. Pseudopapilledema and subcapsular cataracts can be seen. In some individuals, hypoparathyroidism is detected only by an asymptomatic reduction in the serum calcium concentration. Pseudohypoparathyroidism is a group of genetic disorders of the PTH receptor/G-protein transduction system responsible for PTH action. In the type I variant, subjects have a classic phenotype (Albright's hereditary osteodystrophy) with short stature, brachydactyly, subcutaneous and basal ganglia calcifications, rounded facies, shortened neck, seizures, and below-average intelligence. The endocrine glands, such as the thyroid and gonads, can also be dysfunctional. In the type II form of pseudohypoparathyroidism, PHT resistance is present in the absence of the clinical phenotype.

Diagnosis

Hypocalcemia and an elevated serum phosphorus concentration in association with absent PTH levels confirm the diagnosis of hypoparathyroidism. In pseudohypoparathyroidism, PTH levels are elevated, reflecting the PTH-resistant state, but otherwise the biochemical findings of hypocalcemia and hyperphosphatemia are similar to those of hypoparathyroidism. The urinary calcium concentration is usually not elevated because the filtered load of calcium is low, but actually renal handling of calcium is impaired in this setting because of the lack of PTH. Such individuals have an increase in urinary calcium for the given filtered calcium load, even though the actual amount of urinary calcium excretion might not be excessive.

Treatment

The goals of treatment are to establish a serum calcium concentration that is not associated with symptoms or signs and to prevent long-term complications of hypocalcemia. Acute, symptomatic hypocalcemia is a medical emergency and must be treated urgently. The management of chronic hypocalcemia follows a different set of guidelines.

Acute Management

The initial approach is to infuse intravenously 1 to 2 ampules of calcium gluconate (90–180 mg of elemental calcium) diluted in 50 to 100 mL of 5% dextrose over a 10- to 15-minute period. If the acute symptoms are not quickly ameliorated, another 1 to 2 ampules can be administered. To raise the serum calcium concentration further, but more gradually, an infusion of 15 mg/kg of calcium gluconate in 1 L of 5% dextrose over 8 to 10 hours will raise the serum calcium concentration by 2 to 3 mg/dL. Because 1 ampule of calcium gluconate contains 90 mg of elemental calcium, 9 to 11 ampules of calcium gluconate are required for an average-size adult (60–70 kg). The serum calcium concentration should be monitored frequently. If the hypocalcemia is due to magnesium deficiency, these measures are also appropriate while magnesium is being replaced. Acute administration of magnesium without calcium will not immediately correct hypocalcemia because peripheral resistance to PTH, one component of hypocalcemia induced by magnesium deficiency, is not corrected for several days. Intravenous replacement of magnesium is 2.4 mg/kg, up to 180 mg, over a 10-minute period or a continuous infusion of 576 mg of magnesium over 24 hours.

Chronic Management

Oral calcium supplementation is required in virtually all patients. The amount varies but is generally in the range of 1 to 3 g in divided doses. The carbonate or citrated form of calcium is most commonly used. Calcium carbonate is generally preferred because it contains the highest amount of elemental calcium. When calcium preparations are given with meals, both the carbonate and the citrated form of calcium are equally bioavailable. The presence of food obviates the need for gastric acid when calcium carbonate is used.

Most patients also require vitamin D. The amount of ergocalciferol (vitamin D_2) or cholecalciferol (vitamin D_3) can be modest or as high as 200,000 IU daily (1.25–10 mg). These large amounts are required because the absence of PTH and hyperphosphatemia both sometimes limit the amount of vitamin D that ultimately is converted to 1,25-dihydroxy-vitamin D, the active metabolite in the kidney. Because activation of vitamin D is impaired, much more vitamin D is required. There is no impairment of the first activation step in the liver, namely, from vitamin D to 25-hydroxyvitamin D, the storage form. Because there is no impairment in this step, large amounts of 25-hydroxyvitamin D can accumulate in fat tissues. At times and unpredictably, these stores can be mobilized and lead to hypercalcemia. Sometimes, the hypercalcemia is severe, requiring emergent treatment. Other times, a simple adjustment in the amount of calcium and/or vitamin D is sufficient. In any event, patients receiving large doses of vitamin D should always be regularly monitored for serum calcium concentrations approximately every 3 to 6 months.

Although many patients with hypoparathyroidism can be adequately managed with oral calcium and vitamin D, many patients also require therapy with 1,25-dihydroxyvitamin D, the active metabolite of vitamin D. 1,25-Dihydroxyvitamin D is used in addition to, but not in place of, vitamin D because 1,25-dihydroxyvitamin D alone does not provide for smooth control. Perhaps this is because 1,25-dihydroxyvitamin D is not stored to any appreciable extent in fat tissue. The half-life of 1,25-dihydroxyvitamin D is as short as 6 hours. Therefore, patients managed without parent vitamin D but with 1,25-dihydroxyvitamin D as the only source of vitamin D are more likely to have unpredictable fluctuations in serum calcium concentration. The amount of 1,25-dihydroxyvitamin D ranges from 0.5 to 1.0 μg/day. Some patients require more. Enhanced gastrointestinal absorption of calcium with 1,25-dihydroxyvitamin D can lead to hypercalciuria because in hypoparathyroidism there is no PTH to facilitate calcium reabsorption in the renal tubule. Urinary calcium should be checked on a regular basis. If hypercalciuria occurs, the doses of 1,25-dihydroxyvitamin D, vitamin D and/or calcium should be adjusted downward. In this situation, a thiazide diuretic such as hydrochlorothiazide[1] can be used to reduce urinary calcium excretion.

Another reason for variability in the control of serum calcium concentration in hypoparathyroidism is a change in medications. For example, if a thiazide or loop diuretic is started for hypertension, the serum calcium concentration may increase or decrease, respectively. Glucocorticoids can lead to a reduction in the serum calcium concentration because glucocorticoids interfere with vitamin D action in the gastrointestinal tract. Bile-sequestering resins can interfere with vitamin D absorption. Midcycle changes in estrogen levels in premenopausal women can lead to altered control.

Hypoparathyroidism is one of the few endocrine disorders for which the replacement hormone, namely, PTH, is not yet available. A recent double-blind, placebo-controlled clinical trial of PTH(1-84) showed significant reductions in the need for oral calcium and 1,25-dihydroxyvitamin D while maintaining serum calcium levels. The protocol called for titration of PTH(1-84), injected subcutaneously, from 50 to 100 μg per day.

---

[1]Not FDA approved for this indication.

References

Arnold A, Shattuck TM, Mallya SM, et al. Molecular pathogenesis of primary hyperparathyroidism. J Bone Miner Res 2002;17(Suppl. 2):N30–N36.

Bilezikian JP, Khan A, Potts Jr JT, et al. Hypoparathyroidism in the adult: epidemiology, diagnosis, pathophysiology, target organ involvement, treatment, and challenges for future research. J Bone Miner Res 2011;26:2317–37.

Bilezikian JP, Khan AA, Potts Jr JT. 2009 Guidelines for the Management of Asymptomatic Primary Hyperparathyroidism: Summary Statement from the Fourth International Workshop. J Clin Endocrinol Metab, 2014;99:3561.

Bilezikian JP, Silverberg SJ. Primary hyperparathyroidism. In: Rosen C, editor. Primer on the Metabolic Bone Diseases and Disorders of Calcium Metabolism. 7th ed. Am Soc Bone Min Research, 2008. p. 302–6.

Cusano NE, Silverberg SJ, Bilezikian JP. Normocalcemic primary hyperparathyroidism. J Clin Densitometry 2013;16:33–9.

Eastell R, Brandi ML, Costa A, D'Amour P, Shoback DM, Thakker RV. Diagnosis of primary hyperparathyroidism. J Clin Endocrinol Metabol 2014 (in press).

Eastell R, Arnold A, Brandi ML, et al. 2009 Diagnosis of Asymptomatic Primary Hyperparathyroidism: Proceedings of the Third International Workshop. J Clin Endocrinol Metabol 2009;94:340–50.

Grey A, Lucas J, Horne A, et al. Vitamin D repletion in patients with primary hyperparathyroidism and coexistent vitamin D insufficiency. J Clin Endocrinol Metab 2005;90:2122–6.

Mannstadt M, Clarke BL, Vokes T, et al. Efficacy and safety of recombinant human parathyroid hormone (1-84) in hypoparathyroidism (REPLACE): a double-blind, placebo-controlled, randomised, phase 3 study. Lancet Diabetes Endocrinol 2013;1(4):275–83.

Marcocci C, Bollerslev J, Khan AA, Shoback D. Medical management of primary hyperparathyroidism: proceedings of the fourth International Workshop on the Management of Asymptomatic Primary Hyperparathyroidism. J Clin Endocrinol Metabol 2014;99(10):3607–18.

Peacock M, Bilezikian JP, Bolognese MA, Borofsky M, Scumpia S, Sterling LR, et al. Cinacalcet HCl reduces hypercalcemia in primary hyperparathyroidism across a wide spectrum of disease severity. J Clin Endocrinol Metabol 2011;96(1):E9–18.

Peacock M, Bilezikian JP, Klassen PS, et al. Cinacalcet hydrochloride maintains long-term normocalcemia in patients with primary hyperparathyroidism. J Clin Endocrinol Metab 2005;90:135–41.

Rubin MR, Bilezikian JP, McMahon DJ, et al. The natural history of primary hyperparathyroidism with or without parathyroid surgery after 15 years. J Clin Endocrinol Metab 2008;93:3462–70.

Shoback D. Clinical practice. Hypoparathyroidism. N Engl J Med 2008 Jul 24;359(4):391–403.

Silverberg SJ, Bilezikian JP. Primary hyperparathyroidism. In: DeGroot LJ, Jameson JL, editors. Endocrinology. Sixth Edition Philadelphia: Saunders Elsevier; 2010. p. 1176–97.

Silverberg S, Bilezikian JP. The diagnosis and management of asymptomatic primary hyperparathyroidism. Nat Clin Practice Endocrinol Metab 2006;2:494–503.

Silverberg SJ, Lewiecki EM, Mosekilde L, et al. 2009 Presentation of Asymptomatic Primary Hyperparathyroidism: Proceedings of the Third International Workshop. J Clin Endocrinol Metab 2009;94:351–65.

Stein EM, Silva BC, Boutroy S, Zhou B, et al. Primary hyperparathyroidism is associated with abnormal cortical and trabecular microstructure and reduced bone stiffness in postmenopausal women. J Bone Miner 2013;28(5):1029–40.

Udelsman R, Akerström G, Biagini C. The Surgical Management of Asymptomatic Primary Hyperparathyroidism. J Clin Endocrinol Metabol 2014 (in press).

Van Udelsman B, Udelsman R. Surgery in primary hyperparathyroidism: extensive personal experience. J Clin Densitom 2013;16:54–9.

Vignali E, Viccica G, Diacinti D, et al. Morphometric vertebral fractures in postmenopausal women with primary hyperparathyroidism. J Clin Endocrinol Metabol 2009;94(7):2306–12.

Walker MD, McMahon DJ, Inabnet WB, et al. Neuropsychological features in PHPT: a prospective study. J Clin Endocrinol Metab 2009;94(6):1951–8.

HYPERPROLACTINEMIA

Method of
Janet A. Schlechte, MD

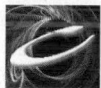

CURRENT DIAGNOSIS

- A history and physical examination; assessment of thyroid, liver, and kidney function; and a pregnancy test will exclude many causes of hyperprolactinemia.
- A single prolactin measurement is usually adequate for diagnosis.
- In patients with prolactinomas, prolactin levels generally parallel tumor size.

CURRENT THERAPY

- Medication-induced hyperprolactinemia is reversible upon discontinuation of the drug.
- A dopamine agonist is the treatment of choice for a prolactinoma.
- Discontinuation of therapy is usually associated with recurrence of hyperprolactinemia.

Epidemiology

Prolactin-secreting adenomas are the most common functioning pituitary tumors and are more common in women. Hyperprolactinemia occurs in about one third of patients with chronic kidney disease and resolves after successful transplantation. About 10% of patients with primary hypothyroidism have a small increase in serum prolactin, and hyperprolactinemia is reported in about 30% of women with polycystic ovarian syndrome. About 5% to 20% of patients with cirrhosis have elevated prolactin levels. Occasionally no cause of hyperprolactinemia can be identified (idiopathic hyperprolactinemia), and these patients might have pituitary adenomas too small to detect on magnetic resonance imaging (MRI).

Risk Factors

Estrogen can increase serum prolactin, and hyperprolactinemia is often detected after discontinuation of an oral contraceptive, but case control studies have shown no relation between the use of estrogen and the formation of prolactinomas.

Pathophysiology

The secretion of prolactin from pituitary lactotrophs is regulated by hypothalamic dopamine. Prolactin secretion is episodic, and serum levels are usually less than 25 ng/mL in women and less than 20 ng/mL in men. During pregnancy, estrogen induces hyperplasia of pituitary lactotrophs, which leads to a progressive increase in prolactin and a 10-fold elevation at term. In lactating women, prolactin levels remain elevated until about 6 weeks after delivery. The primary action of prolactin is to stimulate mammary tissue, but it is the prolactin-induced suppression of gonadotropins and sex steroids that brings patients to clinical attention.

Clinical Manifestations

In both sexes, hyperprolactinemia is associated with hypogonadism, infertility, and bone loss. In women galactorrhea is also commonly observed. Prolactin-secreting tumors in women are usually small and are rarely associated with pituitary hypofunction. Men with prolactinomas usually have large tumors and present with headaches, neurologic deficits, visual loss, and hypopituitarism in additional to gonadal dysfunction.

Diagnosis

A single measurement of serum prolactin obtained at any time of day is usually adequate to make the diagnosis of hyperprolactinemia. Stress can increase prolactin, and minimally elevated levels should be repeated before the diagnosis of hyperprolactinemia is confirmed. A history and physical examination; assessment of thyroid, liver, and kidney function; and a pregnancy test will exclude most causes of hyperprolactinemia. Provocative tests using thyrotropin-releasing hormone, levodopa (L-dopa), domperidone (Motillium),[5] nomifensine (Merital),[2] and insulin-induced hypoglycemia are not useful or necessary. When other causes of hyperprolactinemia have been excluded, gadolinium-enhanced MRI should be used to visualize the pituitary. In general, serum prolactin levels parallel tumor size. Prolactinomas larger than 1 cm are typically associated with prolactin levels greater than 250 ng/mL, and levels can exceed 1000 ng/mL.

Differential Diagnosis

Medications are the most common cause of hyperprolactinemia other than tumor (Box 1). By blocking dopamine receptors, metoclopramide (Reglan), phenothiazines, and risperidone (Risperdal) lead to prolactin levels greater than 200 ng/mL, but tricyclic antidepressants, verapamil (Calan), and estrogen cause only mild

---

[2]Not available in the United States.
[5]Investigational drug in the United States.

> ### Box 1 Causes of Hyperprolactinemia
>
> Prolactinomas
> Pregnancy
> Medications
> - Phenothiazines
> - Metoclopramide (Reglan)
> - Estrogen
> - Verapamil (Calan)
> - Butyrophenones
> - Risperidone (Risperdal)
> - Tricyclic antidepressants
> Primary hypothyroidism
> Renal failure
> Nonfunctioning pituitary tumors
> Hypothalamic disease
> Nipple stimulation
> Idiopathic

elevation. In general, medication-induced hyperprolactinemia is associated with prolactin levels between 25 and 100 ng/mL. Other causes of hyperprolactinemia include pregnancy, chest trauma, nipple stimulation, and hypothalamic disease.

Treatment

Medication-induced hyperprolactinemia is reversible, and it usually takes 3 to 4 days for prolactin to normalize after drug withdrawal. It is not always possible to discontinue a drug causing elevated prolactin. For example, in a patient with hyperprolactinemia, an antipsychotic agent should not be changed or discontinued without consulting the patient's psychiatrist. If a medication cannot be safety discontinued in a patient with medication-induced hyperprolactinemia, radiographic evaluation of the pituitary may be necessary to exclude a pituitary tumor.

The goals in treating a prolactinoma are to normalize prolactin, restore gonadal function and fertility, and reduce tumor size. The preferred treatment is a dopamine agonist, and the drugs approved for use in the United States are bromocriptine (Parlodel) and cabergoline (Dostinex). Both bind to pituitary dopamine receptors, thereby decreasing prolactin and reducing tumor size. Prolactin levels normalize within days of drug administration, and tumor shrinkage or disappearance is usually apparent 3 to 6 months after instituting therapy. Bromocriptine is less expensive, has a half-life of 8 hours, and must be given twice daily. Cabergoline has a half-life of about 24 hours and can be administered once or twice weekly. Both drugs are available in generic form.

Bromocriptine should be initiated at bedtime with a dose of 0.625 mg and a snack. After 1 week, twice-daily dosing should be initiated by adding a morning dose of 1.25 mg. At weekly intervals the dosage should be increased to a total of 5 mg daily, and after 6 to 8 weeks of therapy a prolactin level should be repeated. Most patients require 5 mg of bromocriptine daily. The starting dose of cabergoline is 0.25 mg weekly. After 1 week, twice-weekly dosing should be initiated by adding 0.25 mg. At weekly intervals the dose should be increased to a total of 0.5 mg twice weekly. After 6 to 8 weeks of therapy a prolactin level should be repeated. Most patients will require 1 mg of cabergoline *weekly*. Treatment with either drug can restore gonadal function without normalizing prolactin. If this occurs, it is not necessary to increase the dosage just to normalize the prolactin. The lowest dosage possible should always be used.

The major disadvantage of both dopamine agonists is that discontinuation usually leads to tumor regrowth and recurrence of hyperprolactinemia. Recent reports suggest that discontinuing therapy may be feasible in selected patients, but the optimal length of therapy has not been established and there are no precise criteria to predict which patients will benefit from drug withdrawal. I recommend a minimum of 2 years of therapy before considering withdrawal of therapy. Drug withdrawal is more likely to be successful if the prolactin has normalized and no tumor is visible on MRI before the drug is discontinued.

When fertility is the goal, bromocriptine is the treatment of choice. After starting bromocriptine a woman should use mechanical contraception until at least two regular menstrual cycles have occurred, and the drug should be discontinued as soon as pregnancy is confirmed. When administered in this fashion, bromocriptine has not been associated with an increased incidence of congenital malformations. Although cabergoline has *not* been associated with an increased risk of congenital malformations, it is not currently recommended because less information about its safety is available. It is not necessary to measure prolactin levels during pregnancy because rising levels do not reliably correlate with tumor enlargement. The risk of clinically significant tumor growth during pregnancy is less than 2%, so it is not necessary to perform serial MRI scans or visual field examinations during pregnancy in women who have small tumors. In contrast, there is a 15% to 30% risk of tumor enlargement during pregnancy in women with macroadenomas (>1 cm). With large or invasive tumors there is no single therapeutic option, and treatment must be individualized.

Monitoring

Small prolactinomas rarely progressively increase in size, so prevention of tumor growth is not an indication for treatment. It is crucial, however, to treat prolactin-induced gonadal dysfunction. When fertility is not desired, one option is to administer a dopamine agonist. Another option when fertility is not an issue is to use estrogen or testosterone *instead* of a dopamine agonist. Sex steroids are better tolerated and less expensive than either dopamine agonist and effectively treat hypogonadism and protect the skeleton. Short-term use of estrogen in women with prolactinomas has not been associated with tumor growth, but it should be used with caution in women with very large tumors. With either option, prolactin levels should be monitored yearly. Tumor growth is usually preceded by an elevation of serum prolactin, so it is not necessary to perform yearly MRI examinations. An MRI is indicated if clinical symptoms of tumor expansion occur or if the prolactin increases substantially.

Complications

Both dopamine agonists can cause nasal stuffiness, nausea, and orthostatic hypotension, but fewer women taking cabergoline demonstrate drug intolerance. Pleural thickening, retroperitoneal fibrosis, and cardiac valve regurgitation have been noted in patients who have Parkinson's disease and are taking high doses (3 mg daily) of cabergoline.[1] Long-term therapy of hyperprolactinemia with bromocriptine has not been associated with pulmonary complications, and clinically relevant valvular regurgitation has not been seen in patients who have prolactinomas and are taking 1 to 2 mg of cabergoline weekly.

Pituitary surgery may be necessary for occasional patients who cannot tolerate either of the dopamine agonists. When performed by an experienced neurosurgeon, transsphenoidal surgery normalizes prolactin in about 70% of patients with microadenomas and about 30% with macroadenomas, but recurrence of hyperprolactinemia is common.

[1]Not FDA approved for this indication.

References

Gillam MP, Molitch ME, Lombardi G, Colao A. Advances in the treatment of prolactinomas. Endocr Rev 2006;27:485–534.
Kilbanski A. Prolactinoma. N Engl J Med 2010;362:1219–26.
Molitch ME. Medication-induced hyperprolactinemia. Mayo Clin Proc 2005;80:1050–7.
Molitch ME. Prolactinomas and pregnancy. Pituitary 2005;8:31–8.

HYPERTHYROIDISM

Method of
William J. Hueston, MD

CURRENT DIAGNOSIS

- Hyperthyroidism or thyrotoxicosis is most often caused by Graves' disease, toxic nodular goiter (Plummer's disease), or acute thyroiditis.
- Common symptoms in hyperthyroidism are tachycardia, elevated systolic blood pressure, tremor, and anxiety. Patients with Graves' disease also might exhibit exophthalmos. In contrast, elderly patients can present with apathetic hyperthyroidism, which can be confused with hypothyroidism.
- Hyperthyroidism should be suspected in all patients who present with atrial fibrillation, palpitations, panic disorder, or unexplained tremors.
- Thyroid storm is an acute, life-threatening condition usually occurring in patients with undiagnosed or untreated hyperthyroidism placed under physiologic stress.
- An elevated free T_4, usually with a low thyroid-stimulating hormone is the hallmark of hyperthyroidism, and anti–thyroid-stimulating hormone antibodies can help identify Graves' disease.
- Ultimately, a thyroid scan and uptake are usually necessary to differentiate the cause of hyperthyroidism.

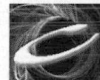

CURRENT THERAPY

- In patients with Graves' disease or autonomous thyroid nodules (toxic nodular goiter), short-term treatment includes thyroid suppression medications (such as methimazole [Tapazole]) and β-blockers (such as propranolol [Inderal][1]). Long-term management with radioiodine thyroid gland ablation is often pursued once symptoms are controlled.
- Patients with acute thyroiditis might need transient β-blockade but can often be managed expectantly until symptoms abate and thyroid hormone levels normalize. A small number of patients (~10%) have persistent hypothyroidism following an episode of illness.
- Thyroid storm is a medical emergency that requires close monitoring along with an antithyroid drug, β blockers, corticosteroids, and iodine-potassium solution (Lugol's solution).

[1]Not FDA approved for this indication.

Epidemiology

Hyperthyroidism is relatively uncommon and usually caused by three conditions: Graves' disease, toxic nodular goiter, or acute thyroiditis. Graves' disease is the most common cause of hyperthyroidism in the United States and usually affects younger patients from the teens to the 40s. Like other autoimmune diseases, women are at higher risk (seven to eight times) than men. Toxic nodular goiter accounts for 15% to 30% of hyperthyroid diagnoses. It usually occurs after age 50 years, is more common in women, and follows several decades of multinodular thyroid disease. A less-common cause is administration of amiodarone. Amiodarone is about one third iodine and can cause hyperthyroidism either through iodine-induced thyroid damage or from increased thyroxine synthesis owing to excessive iodine.

Box 1 Conditions Causing Hyperthyroidism

Graves' disease
Autonomous thyroid nodule (toxic nodular goiter)
Acute thyroiditis
- Hashimoto's thyroiditis
- Subacute granulomatous thyroiditis (de Quervain's thyroiditis)
- Subacute lymphocytic thyroiditis (silent or painless thyroiditis)
- Suppurative thyroiditis (bacterial infection of thyroid)
Excessive exogenous thyroid use
- Over-replacement after thyroid ablation or for hypothyroidism
- Thyroxine (Synthroid) abuse for weight loss
Iodine overconsumption
Amiodarone administration

Risk Factors

There are no known environmental or reversible risk factors for any of the causes of hyperthyroidism. Graves' disease is associated with a specific human leukocyte antigen (HLA) region on chromosome 6 (CTLA 4).

Pathophysiology

The most common causes of hyperthyroidism are shown in Box 1.

Graves' disease is an autoimmune disorder caused by antibodies against thyroid-stimulating hormone (TSH) receptors on the thyroid gland. Graves' disease is associated with many other autoimmune diseases, including pernicious anemia, vitiligo, type 1 diabetes mellitus, autoimmune adrenal disease, Sjögren's syndrome, rheumatoid arthritis, and lupus. As with these other disorders, the etiology is unknown.

Toxic nodular goiter, also known as Plummer's disease, results from the development of autonomous thyroid adenoma. Patients who develop a toxic nodular goiter usually have a long history of many other nodules that spontaneously burn out over time, but then develop a single large nodule (usually 2.5 cm or greater) that continues to produce thyroid hormone in such large quantities that patients become hyperthyroid. No clear cause is known for the development of the nodules.

Acute thyroiditis can also produce hyperthyroidism. Several different conditions can cause thyroiditis (see Box 1). The inflammation resulting in thyroiditis is thought to be related to subacute viral infections or autoimmune reactions; suppurative thyroiditis is a rare bacterial thyroid infection, usually caused by *Staphylococcus aureus*. During the acute period of thyroid inflammation, damage to the gland leads to the release of stored thyroxine from thyroid lakes, producing hyperthyroidism. However, after the initial release of thyroid hormone from the stored lakes, damage to the gland inhibits production of new thyroxine. After the initial surge in thyroid hormone levels, thyroxine levels drop, often to levels that can result in transient hypothyroidism. Most patients return to the euthyroid state after the thyroid gland heals, but about 10% of patients with acute thyroiditis remain chronically hypothyroid.

Other, less common causes of hyperthyroidism include excessive exogenous administration of thyroid medications. This is most commonly the result of over-replacement of thyroxine (Levoxyl, Synthroid) in patients with hypothyroidism, but it may be intentional for weight loss. Because thyroxine and triiodothyronine (T_3) are highly protein bound, over-replacement is most common if patients experience hypoproteinemia, such as in nephrotic syndrome, cirrhosis, or malnutrition.

Excessive iodine consumption can also lead to thyrotoxicosis.

Prevention

There are no known strategies to prevent hyperthyroidism. For patients with hypothyroidism, annual monitoring of TSH levels is recommended to ensure that patients receive the appropriate replacement dose and not over-replacement.

Clinical Manifestations

Patients with hyperthyroidism complain of a variety of symptoms that can include anxiety, tachycardia, wide-pulse pressure hypertension, palpitations, fine tremor, weight loss, heat intolerance, and, particularly in the elderly, confusion or delirium. Patients with Graves' disease also have ophthalmopathy characterized by lid retraction and exophthalmoses that can lead to optic nerve damage. In contrast, older patients can have few of the classic signs of hyperthyroidism and instead might complain of fatigue or weakness (apathetic hyperthyroidism), unexplained delirium, weight loss, heart failure, or isolated atrial fibrillation.

Some patients have a rapid escalation of symptom severity (thyroid storm) that is life-threatening if not identified and treated promptly. These patients usually have underlying thyrotoxicosis from Graves' disease complicated by a secondary physiologic stressor such as infection, surgery, or trauma. This is a medical emergency and needs immediate attention, including hospitalization with close observation.

On physical examination, patients with hyperthyroidism due to Graves' disease or thyroiditis might have a diffusely enlarged and mildly tender thyroid gland. In suppurative thyroiditis, the thyroid gland is red, hot, and very tender and accompanied by a fever and other systemic signs of severe infection. Patients with toxic nodular goiter can have palpable nodules in their thyroid gland and often have a single palpable nodule.

Diagnosis

Hyperthyroidism is diagnosed by finding an elevation in the free thyroxine (T_4) level accompanied by a low TSH level. Patients with Graves' disease often have positive anti–thyroid receptor antibody titers. Only anti-thyroglobulin receptor antibody testing is helpful because it can help differentiate Graves' disease from other causes. No other anti-thyroid tests are clinically indicated. Once the thyroid level abnormalities are found, a definitive diagnosis of the cause for the hyperthyroidism is needed to select the appropriate treatment strategy.

Other conditions can produce a depressed TSH but normal free T_4 levels. These include T_3 toxicosis and subclinical hyperthyroidism. T_3 toxicosis refers to situations where triiodothyronine (T_3) is produced in excess rather than thyroxine (T_4); this can occur in any of the conditions that can cause hyperthyroidism as well as in surreptitious triiodothyronine (Cytomel) ingestion.

Thyroid scanning and radiolabel uptake are usually necessary to differentiate the causes of hyperthyroidism. Thyroid scanning and uptake rely on the thyroid gland to concentrate radioactive molecules, such as iodine-131 (^{131}I) or technetium. Because of the risk of thyroid storm with iodine administration, patients should be treated with antithyroid drugs for 2 to 8 weeks before a scan and the drugs should be stopped at least 4 days before the test. Patients with Graves' disease show increases in uptake and diffuse distribution of the tracer throughout the thyroid gland. Patients with toxic nodular goiter also have increased uptake, but the isotope is concentrated in a one or a few focal areas, with the remainder of the thyroid gland suppressed. In contrast, patients with thyroiditis have decreased uptake of the radiolabel and a washed-out or mottled distribution on scanning.

Differential Diagnosis

Symptoms of hyperthyroidism also occur in patients with panic disorder and other anxiety conditions. These patients can have sinus tachycardia, tremor, and nervousness that mimic hyperthyroidism.

Treatment

Treatment depends on the cause of the hyperthyroidism (Table 1). In Graves' disease, immediate goals of treatment include reducing thyroid hormone production and blocking the peripheral effects of the excessive thyroid hormone. About 30% to 60% of patients, mostly adolescents, enter remission spontaneously, and the remission may be permanent. Remission rates are highest for those with a small goiter, no ophthalmopathy, thyroglobulin levels less than

TABLE 1	Treatment Strategies for Hyperthyroidism	
TREATMENT	**DRUG**	**DOSAGE**
Graves' Disease and Toxic Nodular Goiter		
Thyroid hormone suppression	Methimazole	Initial: 30–40 mg/d Maintenance: 5–15 mg/d
	Propylthiouracil	Initial: 300–400 mg/d Maintenance: 100–300 mg/d
β-Blockade	Propranolol[1]	10 mg qid
	Metoprolol (Lopressor)[1]	50–100 mg bid
Thyroid gland removal	Radioactive iodine ablation Thyroidectomy	
Acute Thyroiditis		
β-Blockade transiently May need thyroid replacement long term		
Thyroid Storm		
Thyroid hormone suppression	Propylthiouracil	300–400 mg/d
β Blockade	Propranolol[1]	1 mg/min IV to max 10 mg[3]
Iodine	Lugol's solution	1–2 gtt mixed in water tid
Cardiac and fluid monitoring	Dexamethasone (Decadron)[1]	2 mg q6h

[1]Not FDA approved for this indication.
[3]Exceeds dosage recommended by the manufacturer.

50 µg/mL, and thyroxine levels less than 20 µg/dL. Signs of remission include a decreased ratio of T_3 to T_4, lower thyroid-stimulating thyroglobulin levels, and decreased radioactive iodine uptake on rescanning. When remissions do occur, it is usually within a year of starting antithyroid medications.

For those who do not undergo spontaneous remission, which includes most adults, consideration should be given to thyroid gland ablation to permanently treat this condition. Although the dosage can be calculated to attempt to leave patients euthyroid, permanent hypothyroidism occurs in about half of all patients treated with radioactive iodine ablation.

The initial approach to toxic nodular goiter is similar to that for symptom control, but thyroid ablation should be recommended routinely because remissions are very rare.

Thyroid gland production of hormone can be reduced rapidly with either methimazole (Tapazole) or propylthiouracil. For treatment of Graves' disease, methimazole is the preferred treatment and has the advantage of less frequent dosing, which improves compliance. Propylthiouracil is an alternative that is recommended for women in the first trimester of pregnancy and patients who cannot tolerate methimazole. However, the FDA issued a black box warning about the use of propylthiouracil in 2010 because of liver toxicity; physicians should be aware of this and use propylthiouracil only when methimazole is not suitable. With both drugs, clinicians need to be aware of drug-associated agranulocytosis, which can result in life-threatening bacterial infections. In patients on either of these medications who develop a sore throat, fever, or other signs of infection, a white blood count should be done immediately to ensure that they are not neuropenic. Additionally, antithyroid drugs are associated with drug-induced lupus syndromes and other forms of vasculitis.

In addition to reducing production of thyroid hormone, initial therapy for patients with Graves' disease and toxic nodular goiter should include a β-blocker to reduce the tachycardia, tremor, hypertension, and anxiety. A β-blocker that crosses the blood-brain barrier, such as propranalol (Inderal)[1] or metoprolol (Lopressor),[1] is the best choice in this situation because these also reduce the central nervous system effects such as anxiety as well as the vascular problems caused by thyroid hormones.

Thyroid storm requires immediate attention and should be managed in the hospital setting, especially in older patients where tachycardia and hypertension can lead to cardiac instability. Prompt administration of β-blockers and propylthiouracil along with cardiac monitoring for dysrhythmias and appropriate fluid management are essential for managing this life-threatening condition. Once antithyroid drugs have been administered, iodine-potassium solution (Lugol's solution) at a dose of 1 or 2 drops three times a day should be administered, which will further reduce thyroid hormone production and reduce peripheral conversion of T_4 to T_3. Finally, corticosteroids also have been shown to rapidly reduce thyroid hormone levels in thyroid storm.

For long-term management, thyroid ablation with radioactive iodine (sodium iodide, ^{131}I) can restore patients to a permanent euthyroid state. However, radioactive iodine thyroid ablation often results in destruction of more thyroid than optimal, causing hypothyroidism. Radioactive iodine thyroid ablation is contraindicated in pregnancy. For patients in whom radioactive iodine is either contraindicated or not acceptable, thyroidectomy is an option. Thyroidectomy almost always results in permanent hypothyroidism as well as having other risks inherent in surgery including hypoparathyroidism and recurrent laryngeal nerve damage.

In patients with hyperthyroidism associated with acute thyroiditis, symptoms often resolve by the time the evaluation is complete. In the interim, symptoms can be managed with β-blockers. β-Blocker therapy can be discontinued fairly rapidly (2 to 3 weeks) after the initial onset of symptoms.

Monitoring

In patients on antithyroid drugs, thyroid hormone levels should be monitored frequently until they reach a stable euthyroid state. Any change in the patient's underlying health, especially changes that could alter protein levels, should prompt reevaluation. In addition, patients who have thyroid ablation need follow-up testing of TSH and free T_4 levels to ensure that sufficient thyroid tissue has been destroyed to reverse their hyperthyroidism but not make them hypothyroid. This should be done 6 to 8 weeks following ablation therapy.

Complications

Complications of hyperthyroidism include acute and chronic conditions. Acutely, the most concerning complications are cardiac dysrhythmias, especially atrial fibrillation. Chronically, excessive thyroxine is associated with cardiomyopathy and osteoporosis. In patients with ophthalmopathy, untreated Graves' disease can lead to progressive vision loss and blindness.

[1]Not FDA approved for this indication.

References

Cooper DS. Antithyroid drugs for the treatment of hyperthyroidism caused by Graves' disease. Endocrinol Metab Clin North Am 1998;27:225–47.

Kharlip J, Cooper DS. Recent developments in hyperthyroidism. Lancet 2009;373:1930–2.

Lazarus JH. Hyperthyroidism. Lancet 1997;349:339–43.

Nayak B, Hodak SP. Hyperthyroidism. Endocrinol Metab Clin North Am 2007;36 (3):617–56.

Zimmerman D, Lteif AN. Thyroxicosis in children. Endocrinol Metab Clin North Am 1998;27:109–26.

HYPOKALEMIA AND HYPERKALEMIA

Method of
Jie Tang, MD

CURRENT DIAGNOSIS

- The "initial approach" to the evaluation of dyskalemia is to determine if it is secondary to transcellular shifts (in vitro or in vivo) of potassium (K), or a result of a true change in total body K.
- A thorough history and physical will provide useful information regarding the causes of hypokalemia and hyperkalemia, especially in cases of low or high intake of K, and transcellular shifts.
- Key steps in the diagnostic approach to hypokalemia include assessments of urinary K excretion and acid-base status.
- Key steps in the diagnostic approach to hyperkalemia include assessments of renal function and aldosterone activity.

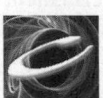

CURRENT THERAPY

- For both hypokalemia and hyperkalemia, it is critical to assess the underlying transcellular K shift, given the risk of rebound hyperkalemia after K repletion or hypokalemia after K restriction and removal.
- In cases of severe dyskalemia, close cardiac monitoring is needed.
- The aggressiveness of therapy for dyskalemia is directly related to the rapidity with which the condition has developed, the absolute level of serum K, and the clinical evidence of toxicity.
- In severe or symptomatic cases of hypokalemia, both intravenous and oral K repletion are often needed.
- In severe or symptomatic cases of hyperkalemia, supported by ECG abnormalities, both immediate temporizing measures and definitive therapy for K removal are necessary.

Epidemiology

Hypokalemia is defined as a serum K level of 3.5 mmol/L or lower. It is a common electrolyte disorder encountered in clinical practice. According to one study, serum K <3.6 mmol/L was found in up to 20% of hospitalized patients. The majority of these patients had serum K concentrations between 3.0 and 3.5 mmol/L, but as many as 25% had values <3.0 mmol/L. Even mild or moderate hypokalemia increases the risks of morbidity and mortality in patients with cardiovascular disease.

Hyperkalemia is defined as a serum K of 5.5 mmol/L or higher. The prevalence among hospitalized patients not yet on dialysis was reported to be about 3.3%, and among them, up to 10% had significant hyperkalemia (≥6.0 mmol/L). Hyperkalemia also carries a significantly increased risk of mortality.

Risk Factors

People most at risk for hypokalemia are those who are malnourished, with poor oral intake; those who use certain medications, such as diuretics; and those who have uncontrolled vomiting or diarrhea. People most at risk for hyperkalemia are those with reduced kidney function, those who have a history of diabetes mellitus, or those who take certain medications, such as angiotensin-converting enzyme inhibitors.

Pathophysiology

K is the most abundant cation in the human body. It regulates intracellular enzyme function and helps determine neuromuscular and cardiovascular tissue excitability. The total body store is approximately 55 mmol/kg of body weight. Over 98% of total body K is located in the intracellular fluid (primarily in muscle), and less than 2% in the extracellular fluid. A typical western diet provides 40 to 120 mmol of K per day. Tight control of the serum K is primarily accomplished by the kidney, where ~95% of body K is excreted. Under normal circumstances, K losses in stool and sweat are small. In addition, the interplay of several hormonal systems (insulin, catecholamine), serum tonicity, and the internal acid-base environment contribute to the exchange of K between the extracellular fluid and intracellular fluid, which helps keep the serum K concentration tightly controlled.

Hypokalemia occurs when there is a significant intracellular K shift or a reduced total body K store from poor intake, or excessive renal or extrarenal loss, whereas hyperkalemia develops when there is a significant extracellular shift, high body K load, and/or ineffective K elimination (aldosterone resistance/deficiency or reduced renal function).

Prevention

For patients at risk for hypokalemia, adequate dietary K intake is essential. Additional K supplements may be needed for patients taking high doses of diuretics (especially thiazide diuretics) or experiencing prolonged vomiting or diarrhea. For patients with hyperkalemia and severe kidney dysfunction, dietary K restriction is critical in maintaining body K balance. Sometimes, the empirical use of K exchange resin is needed to prevent hyperkalemia. Lastly, medications that contribute to hypokalemia or hyperkalemia should be avoided if possible.

Clinical Manifestations

Mild hypokalemia (serum K 3.0–3.5 mmol/L) is usually well tolerated. Moderate hypokalemia (serum K 2.5–3.0 mmol/L) may cause nonspecific symptoms, such as fatigue, weakness, muscle cramps, and constipation. When the serum K drops to <2.5 mmol/L, muscle necrosis and flaccid paralysis with eventual respiratory failure may occur. K depletion also causes supraventricular and ventricular arrhythmias, especially in patients on digitalis therapy. Although severe hypokalemia is more likely to cause complications, even minimal decreases in serum or total body K can be arrhythmogenic in patients with underlying heart disease or who are receiving digitalis therapy. Lastly, increases in systolic and diastolic blood pressures can occur in patients with hypokalemia while they are on a liberal salt diet. Overall, the likelihood of symptoms tends to correlate with the rapidity of the decrease in serum K.

As with hypokalemia, patients with hyperkalemia may present with nonspecific complaints such as fatigue and malaise. But the predominant manifestations in more severe hyperkalemia are neuromuscular and cardiac. Neuromuscular symptoms range from muscle weakness to paralysis. Cardiac arrhythmias, including asystole, ventricular tachycardia or fibrillation, and pulseless electrical activity, can also occur in severe hyperkalemia.

Diagnosis

Figures 1 and 2 illustrate the diagnostic approaches to hypokalemia and hyperkalemia. It is important to assess for pseudodyskalemia (in vitro shift of K) and dyskalemia from in vivo transcellular shift of K, because neither is associated with disturbances in total body K balance. Despite some limitations, Transtubular K gradient (TTKG) [(urine K/serum K)/(urine osmolarity/serum osmolarity)] remains a useful test in both conditions. It measures the amount of K secreted by the distal tubule corrected by water absorption in the medullary collecting tubules. Under a normal diet, the TTKG should be about 8. During hypokalemia or low dietary K intake, less K should be lost in the urine, and the TTKG will fall below 3. Levels >5 during hypokalemia indicate inappropriate urinary excretion of K. Of note, the TTKG can fall below 3 in hypokalemic patients who experience osmotic diuresis.

During hyperkalemia or high dietary K intake, more K should be excreted in the urine and the TTKG will be >10. Levels <5 during hyperkalemia indicate mineralocorticoid deficiency or resistance. Although cell shift of K and changes in total body K occur as isolated problems, they frequently occur simultaneously.

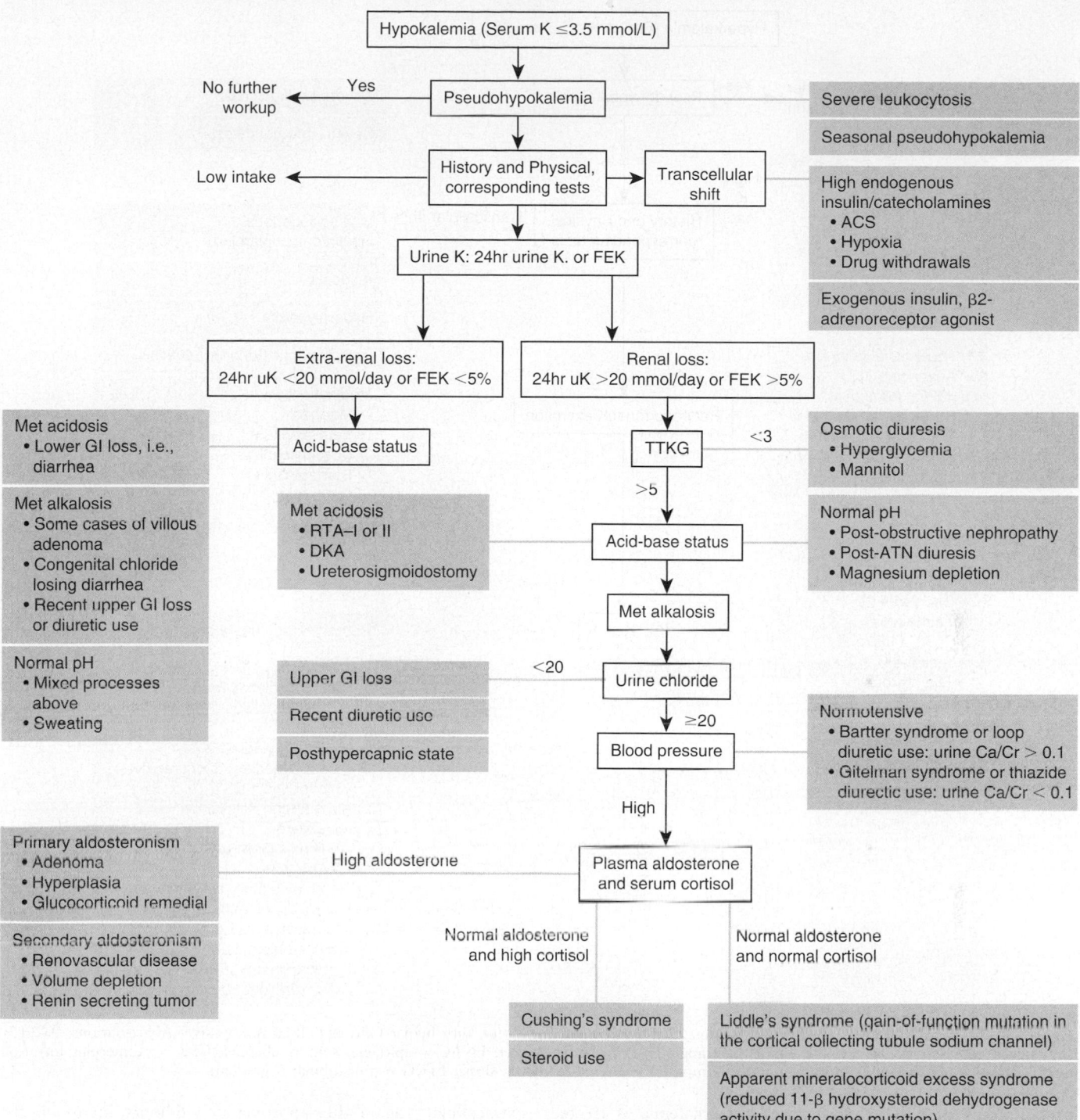

Figure 1. The diagnostic approach to hypokalemia. Abbreviations: ACS = acute coronary syndrome; ATN = acute tubular necrosis; DKA = diabetic ketoacidosis; FEK = fractional excretion of K; GI = gastrointestinal; Met = metabolic; RTA = renal tubular acidosis; TTKG = trans-tubular K gradient.

Differential Diagnosis

Figures 1 and 2 outline a diagnostic approach, including differential diagnosis, for hyperkalemia and hypokalemia.

Therapy

The treatment of hypokalemia depends on the underlying cause, the degree of K depletion, and the risk of K depletion to the patient. In general, hypokalemia secondary to cell shift is managed by treating underlying conditions. For example, hypokalemia in the setting of catecholamine increases, as in chest pain syndromes, is managed with appropriate treatments for the pain. However, when cell-shift hypokalemia is associated with life-threatening conditions such as paresis, paralysis, or hypokalemia in the setting of myocardial infarction, the administration of K is indicated. With K depletion, replacement therapy depends on the estimated degree of decreases in total body K. For example, decreases in total body K accompanied by a fall in serum K from 3.5 to 3.0 mmol/L are associated with a K deficit of 150 to 200 mmol. Decreases in serum K from 3 to 2 mmol/L are associated with 200- to 400-mmol additional decreases in total body K. K can be administered intravenously, but in limited quantities (10 mEq/h into a peripheral vein; 15–20 mEq/h into a central vein). Larger K requirements can only be accomplished by oral therapy or with dialysis.

The treatment of hyperkalemia depends on the presence or absence of ECG and neuromuscular abnormalities. In the absence

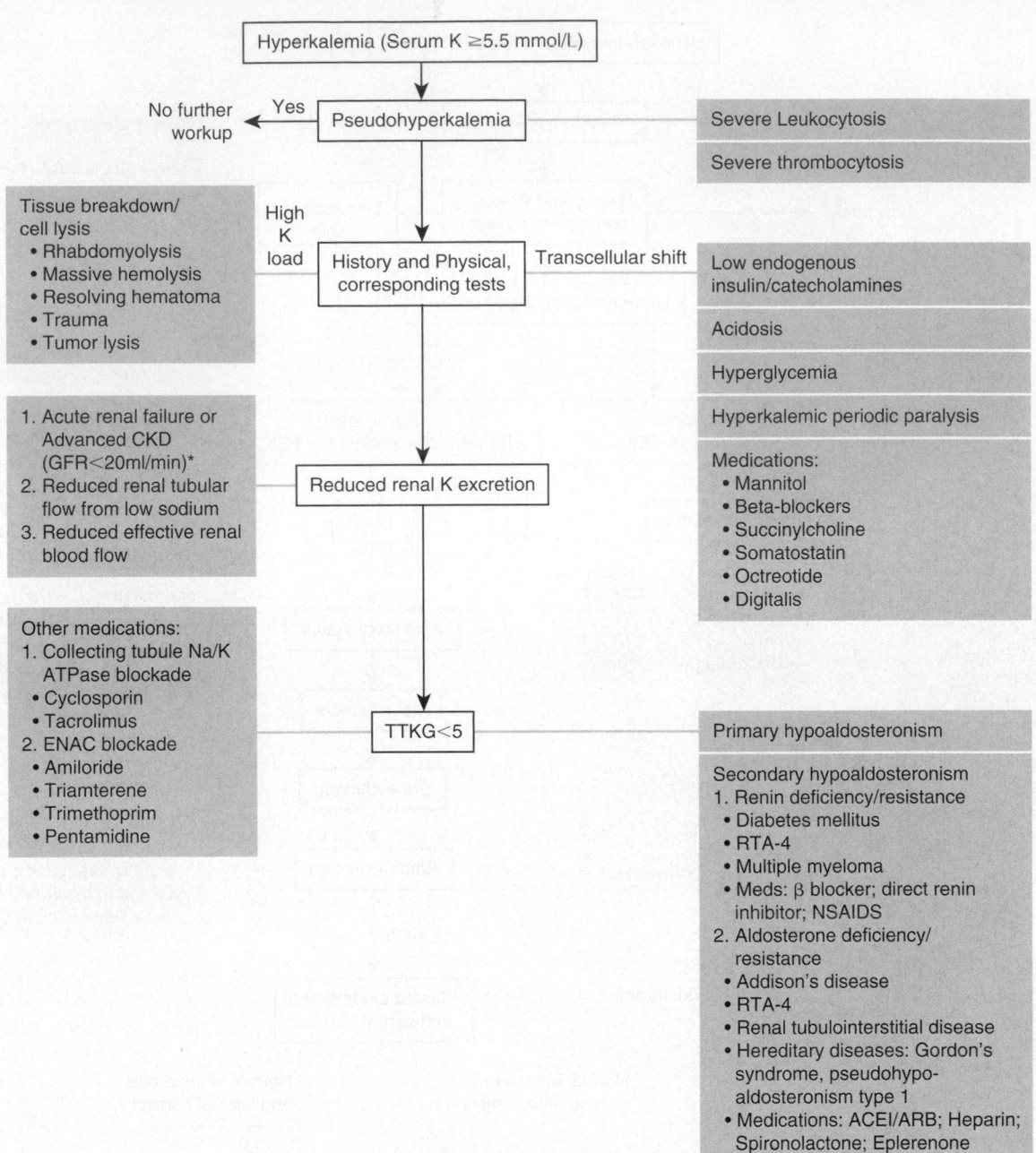

Figure 2. The diagnostic approach to hyperkalemia. *Hyperkalemia may occur with higher GFR if K load is excessive. Abbreviations: ACEI = angiotensin converting enzyme inhibitor; ARB = angiotensin receptor blocker; ENAC = epithelial sodium channel; GFR = glomerular filtration rate; NSAIDS = non-steroidal anti-inflammatory drugs; RTA = renal tubular acidosis; TTKG = transtubular K gradient.

of symptoms or ECG abnormalities, hyperkalemia is treated conservatively—for example, by decreasing dietary K or withdrawing offending drugs. In the presence of ECG abnormalities or symptoms, the goal of therapy is to stabilize cell membranes. First-line therapy includes calcium gluconate, 10 to 30 mL IV as a 10% solution (onset of action 1 or 2 min). Although the mechanism remains undefined, calcium "stabilizes" the cardiac membranes. Other therapies include 8.4% IV sodium bicarbonate,[1] 50 to 150 mEq (onset 15–30 min), and rapid-acting insulin[1] 5 to 10 units intravenously (onset 5–10 min). Insulin increases the activity of the Na-K-ATPase pump in skeletal muscle and drives K into cells. Glucose 50%, 25 g intravenously, is given simultaneously with insulin to prevent hypoglycemia. Albuterol inhalation solution 0.5%,[1] 20 mg in 4 mL normal saline by nebulizer (onset 15–30 min), also activates the Na-K-ATPase and drives K into cells. K driven intracellularly generally begins to move

extracellularly again after approximately 6 hours, increasing the serum K concentration. Therefore, therapy to remove K from the body should be started simultaneously. Reductions in total body K may be achieved through a K exchange resin. The primary K resin used is sodium polystyrene sulfonate (Kayexalate). One gram of this medication binds approximately 1 mEq of K and releases 1 to 2 mEq of sodium back into the circulation. This medication may be given orally (onset 2 h) or by enema with sorbitol to induce diarrhea (onset 30–60 min). If renal function is adequate, volume expansion with simultaneous diuresis can be attempted. Finally, hemodialysis is very effective in removing excess K.

Monitoring

Treatment for severe or symptomatic dyskalemia requires close cardiac monitoring and frequent laboratory testing to prevent overcorrection. If insulin and glucose are used in patients with hyperkalemia, blood sugars should be monitored for approximately 6 hours to identify and treat hypoglycemia from the insulin.

---

[1]Not FDA approved for this indication.

Complications

Complications from dyskalemia include cardiac arrhythmias, neuromuscular events, and, rarely, death. There are potential treatment-related complications if pseudodyskalemia or dyskalemia from in vivo transcellular shift are not recognized.

References

Paice BJ, Paterson KR, Onyanga-Omara F, et al. Record linkage study of hypokalaemia in hospitalized patients. Postgrad Med J 1986;62:187–91.
Gennari FJ. Hypokalemia. N Engl J Med 1998;339:451–8.
Stevens MS, Dunlay RW. Hyperkalemia in hospitalized patients. Int Urol Nephrol 2000;32:177–80.
Krishna GG, Kapoor SC. Potassium depletion exacerbates essential hypertension. Ann Intern Med 1991;115:77–83.

HYPONATREMIA

Method of
Beejal Shah, MD; and Susan L. Samson, MD, PhD

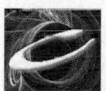

CURRENT DIAGNOSIS

- Perform a thorough history and physical examination with focus on the accurate assessment of volume status, neurologic symptoms and signs, current medications, and concurrent illnesses.
- Classify the hyponatremia as hypovolemic, euvolemic, or hypervolemic.
- Determine whether the hyponatremia is acute or chronic, based on the history and the clinical manifestations.
- Order the key laboratory tests, including a basic metabolic panel (serum sodium, glucose, blood urea nitrogen, and creatinine), plasma osmolality, urine osmolality, and urine sodium.

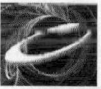

CURRENT THERAPY

- Severe and symptomatic hyponatremia should be treated with hypertonic saline (3%) at 1 to 2 mL/kg per hour. Neurologic status and serum sodium should be monitored every 2 to 4 hours. The objective is to raise sodium by 2 mEq/L per hour (or to >125 mEq/L) until deleterious neurologic symptoms improve. After this, the rate of infusion should be titrated to increase the serum sodium by 0.5 to 1.0 mEq/L per hour, with a maximum increase of 10 to 12 mEq/L over 24 hours and no more than 18 mEq/L over 48 hours, to avoid precipitating osmotic demyelination.
- As a general rule, the treatment of hyponatremia should be adjusted so that the serum sodium increases by 0.5 to 1.0 mEq/L per hour with a maximum increase of 10 to 12 mEq/L over 24 hours and no more than 18 mEq/L over 48 hours. Acute hyponatremia (<48 hours) may be treated more rapidly than chronic hyponatremia if dictated by neurologic findings. Treat SIADH with fluid restriction, medications, or observation; rule out adrenal insufficiency and hypothyroidism.
- Most cases of euvolemic hyponatremia are caused by the syndrome of inappropriate antidiuretic hormone (SIADH), which usually can be managed with fluid restriction, salt tablets, and demeclocycline (Declomycin)[1] in refractory cases.
- Discontinue thiazide diuretics in all cases of hypoosmolar hyponatremia.
- Hypovolemic and hypervolemic hyponatremia require therapy to correct the underlying cause (e.g., heart failure) and restore status to euvolemia.

- Conivaptan (Vaprisol) is a vasopressin receptor antagonist that is approved for inpatient management of euvolemic and hypovolemic hyponatremia. The same parameters apply for rate of sodium correction and monitoring as in conventional therapy.

[1]Not FDA approved for this indication.

Homeostasis maintains the concentration of sodium in the serum between 138 and 142 mEq/L (normal, 135–145 mEq/L) despite variations in water intake. Hyponatremia is defined as a serum sodium concentration of less than 135 mEq/L. It is one of the most common electrolyte abnormalities found in the inpatient setting, occurring in up to 2.5% of patients, and it is a significant marker for mortality, associated with a 60-fold higher risk of death. It is not clear whether hyponatremia itself is the cause of a more adverse prognosis or whether it echoes the degree of stress caused by illness. In the outpatient setting, chronic hyponatremia is most prevalent among the elderly and nursing home residents. The approach to management of hyponatremia is highly dependent on the underlying process. Establishing the correct etiology is critical, because inappropriate treatment can worsen hyponatremia. Therapy must be administered judiciously because of the risk of severe neurologic sequelae, including central nervous system demyelination. However, with a systematic approach to the differential diagnosis of hyponatremia, the correct diagnosis can be made and therapy initiated.

Clinical Presentation

Acute hyponatremia is defined as hyponatremia of less than 48 hours in duration. Mild symptoms include headache, nausea, vomiting, confusion, and weakness, which usually occur with a sodium level of less than 129 mEq/L. More severe neurologic manifestations—seizure and coma—are seen usually below a threshold of 120 mEq/L, although there currently is no evidence-based critical sodium level above which neurologic sequelae do not occur. The neurologic manifestations of acute or recurrent symptomatic hyponatremia can be delayed, so continued monitoring is important.

In contrast, patients with chronic hyponatremia more often are asymptomatic or have blunted symptoms. In elderly patients with mild chronic hyponatremia, subtle neurocognitive manifestations can occur, with decreased balance, lowered reaction speed, memory loss, and directed gait. Mild hypoosmolar hyponatremia is not independently associated with increased morbidity and mortality. Even so, the underlying etiology needs to be determined because of the potential for other factors (e.g., new medications, dehydration, occult illness) to contribute to the development of more severe hyponatremia with its potential for neurologic injury.

Regulation of Water Balance

Approximately two thirds of total body water is contained in the intracellular fluid (ICF) and one third as extracellular fluid (ECF). Plasma osmolality is tightly regulated between 280 and 290 mOsm/kg and reflects the osmolality of the ECF. A change in plasma osmolality results in a shift of total body water between the ECF and the ICF to maintain their osmolar equivalence. Because sodium is the major osmole in the ECF, hyponatremia most often is a manifestation of decreased osmolality, so-called hypoosmolar or hypotonic hyponatremia.

Renal Handling of Water

The major osmoregulatory hormone is arginine vasopressin, also called antidiuretic hormone, which is synthesized in the paraventricular and supraoptic nuclei of the hypothalamus. It is transported along axons to the posterior pituitary, where it is processed and stored in vesicles. Vasopressin secretion is regulated by osmotic and nonosmotic stimuli. Secretion occurs with a 1% to 2% rise in osmolality (>288 mOsm/kg), as detected by receptors in the anterolateral walls of the hypothalamus adjacent to the third

TABLE 1	Molecules That Regulate Vasopressin Secretion
STIMULATE VASOPRESSIN RELEASE	**INHIBIT VASOPRESSIN RELEASE**
Hormones and Neurotransmitters	
Acetylcholine (nicotinic)	Atrial natriuretic peptide
Histamine (H_1)	γ-Aminobutyric acid
Dopamine (D_1 and D_2)	Opioids (κ receptors)
Glutamine	
Aspartate	
Cholecystokinin	
Neuropeptide Y	
Substance P	
Vasoactive inhibitory peptide	
Prostaglandin	
Angiotensin II	
Pharmacologic Agents	
Vincristine (Oncovin)	Ethanol
Cyclophosphamide (Cytoxan)	Phenytoin (Dilantin)
Tricyclic antidepressants	Low-dose morphine
Selective serotonin reuptake inhibitors	Glucocorticoids Fluphenazine (Prolixin)
Nicotine	Haloperidol (Haldol)
Adrenaline (epinephrine)	Promethazine (Phenergan)
High-dose morphine	Butorphanol (Stadol)

ventricle. Vasopressin secretion is inhibited when the plasma osmolality is lower than 280 mOsm/kg. The major nonosmotic stimulus is a decrease in effective circulating volume, which is detected by baroreceptors in the aortic arch and carotid sinuses. Although this mechanism requires a large drop (10%–15%) in blood pressure, the secretory response is more robust than for increases in osmolality. As such, acutely lowered blood pressure can override the inhibitory signal of low osmolality because of the need to maintain perfusion. Other physiologic nonosmotic stimuli include catecholamines and angiotensin II, but there is a long list of hormones and pharmacologic agents that induce or repress vasopressin secretion (Table 1).

The renal site of action of vasopressin is the V_2 receptors on the basolateral membrane of collecting duct cells in the distal nephron. The hormone-receptor interaction initiates intracellular signaling via cyclic adenosine monophosphate–dependent pathways, resulting in translocation of cytoplasmic aquaporon-2 channels to the surface of the collecting duct luminal membrane. These channels allow movement of water back into the cell for later reabsorption into the circulation. This results in a net concentration of urine and decreased plasma osmolality.

Renal Handling of Sodium

In addition to renal water handling, sodium reabsorption and excretion are important for maintenance of water homeostasis. The renin-angiotensin-aldosterone system is activated by reduced arterial perfusion pressure sensed by the juxtaglomerular apparatus of the afferent renal arteriole. Reduced arteriole effective volume (low or perceived) is sensed by the juxtaglomerular apparatus, which secretes renin, activating the renin-angiotensin system. This cascade of events ultimately stimulates aldosterone secretion, which acts at the distal nephron to cause reabsorption of filtered sodium via Na^+,K^+-adenosine triphosphatase (ATPase)–dependent sodium channels.

Central Nervous System Response to Hyponatremia/Hypoosmolality

Osmolar equivalence between the ECF and ICF is closely maintained by shifts in water between the two compartments. The major symptoms and signs of hyponatremia are neurologic in nature and are a clinical manifestation of swelling of the cells in the central nervous system, which results in cerebral edema. The most devastating consequence is herniation due to anatomic limitations on brain volume within the confines of the skull. Premenopausal women are at the highest risk for brain injury from hyponatremia.

A major compensatory mechanism in the central nervous system is the extrusion from the cells of intracellular solutes, which prevents further water influx. In the first few hours, inorganic ions (potassium, sodium, chloride) move out of the cell. After a few days of persistent hypoosmolality, the cells further compensate by extruding organic osmoles (glutamate, taurine, inositol). The clinician must be aware of this protective adaptation, because it necessitates a slower time course of correction during treatment. A rapid rise in plasma osmolality from aggressive treatment causes water to rapidly shift out of the cells, resulting in demyelination of neurons. In the past, this was termed pontine demyelinosis, but it has also been reported for extrapontine neurons and is now referred to as osmotic demyelination. The sequelae are permanent and devastating. There is clinical progression from lethargy to a change in affect, to mutism and dysarthria, and finally to spastic quadriparesis and pseudobulbar palsy.

Classification and Differential Diagnosis of Hyponatremia

Initial evaluation of hyponatremia requires a systematic and sequential approach. First, a thorough history and physical examination are required. It is important to identify any history of brain injury, stroke, mental illness, or chronic illness and the patient's current medication usage. On examination, special attention should be paid to mental status and neurologic abnormalities; manifestations of cardiac, hepatic, or renal disease; and signs of adrenal insufficiency or hypothyroidism. From the assessment of volume status, the hyponatremia should be classified as hypervolemic, euvolemic, or hypovolemic; each of these conditions leads in a different direction for diagnosis and treatment of the underlying cause (Figures 1 and 2). Finally, it should be determined

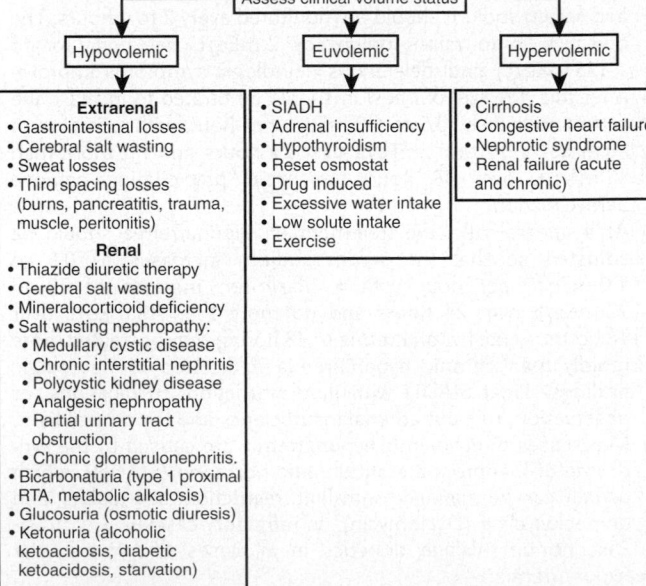

Figure 1. The differential diagnosis of hypoosmolar hyponatremia. *Abbreviations:* RTA = renal tubular acidosis; SIADH = syndrome of inappropriate antidiuretic hormone.

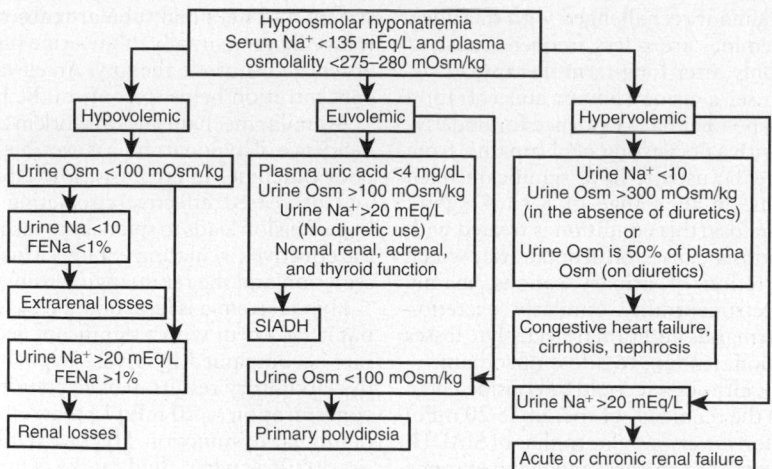

Figure 2. Laboratory findings in hypoosmolar hyponatremia. *Abbreviations:* FENa = fractional excretion of sodium; Osm = osmoles; SIADH = syndrome of inappropriate antidiuretic hormone.

whether the hyponatremia is acute (<48 hours) or chronic, because this can determine the time course of treatment.

For the laboratory work-up, essential basic tests are the serum sodium and potassium levels, renal function tests with blood urea nitrogen (BUN) and creatinine, and liver function tests. It is likely that these tests have already been performed, motivating the assessment of hyponatremia. After this, the plasma osmolality (P_{Osm}), urine osmolality (U_{Osm}), and urine sodium concentration are key diagnostic tests. P_{Osm} is directly measured in the laboratory and also can be calculated. Calculated osmolality is the sum of the concentrations of the known major osmoles—sodium and glucose—in the ECF and the BUN:

$$P_{Osm} = (2 \times Na) + (glucose) + (BUN)$$

The calculation is done in SI units. For sodium, mEq/L is the same as the SI unit, mmol/L; if glucose and BUN values were reported in mg/dL, they must be divided by 18 and 2.8, respectively, to convert to SI units (mmol/L). The directly measured osmolality should be within 10 to 12 mOsm/kg of the calculated value; an increased osmolar gap compared with the calculated value points toward the presence of additional osmoles in the plasma that are causing hypertonicity.

Because hyponatremia usually is a reflection of plasma osmolality, most patients also have a low P_{Osm}, and the clinician often can proceed to the differential diagnosis of hypoosmolar (or hypotonic) hyponatremia after excluding pseudohyponatremia (which usually has normal osmolality) and hyperosmolar hyponatremia. Pseudohyponatremia can occur if the plasma lipid or protein content is greatly increased in the plasma (usually to >6%–8% of volume), as in extreme hypertriglyceridemia and paraprotein disorders. These extra components decrease the aqueous portion of the plasma volume and thereby interfere with the laboratory measurement of sodium by dilutional, indirect methods such as flame photometry. Most laboratories now use direct measurement of sodium to avoid this problem.

Hyperosmolar hyponatremia can occur if there are additional osmoles present that cause water movement from the ICF into the ECF, resulting in ECF expansion and dilutional hyponatremia. Overall, the total body water and total body sodium are unchanged in this situation. An important clinical example occurs with hyperglycemia, and the reported sodium value should be corrected for high glucose by the clinician by adding 1.6 mEq/L to the measured Na for every 100 mg/dL rise in glucose above 200 mg/dL. Because glucose is included in the calculation of osmolality, there will be no significant osmolar gap.

Other osmotically active solutes encountered clinically are mannitol, which is used to manage increased intracranial pressure, and glycine, which is used for irrigation in urologic procedures. Mannitol and glycine are retained in the ECF and are not part of the calculated osmolality, so their presence results in an osmolar gap. High levels of alcohol or ethylene glycol also increase the osmolality, but these substances are so quickly metabolized that an osmolar gap may not be apparent by the time testing is performed.

Once pseudohyponatremia and hypertonicity have been ruled out, the diagnosis is narrowed to hypoosmolar hyponatremia. The combined physical examination and laboratory results allow classification of the patient as having hypervolemic hyponatremia with excess total body sodium, hypovolemic hyponatremia with a deficit of total body sodium, or euvolemic hyponatremia with near-normal total body sodium.

Hypovolemic Hyponatremia
The causes of hypovolemic hyponatremia can be classified as extrarenal or renal (see Figure 1). Signs of volume contraction are apparent on examination, including poor skin turgor, skin tenting (forehead), decreased or undetectable jugular venous pressure, dry mucous membranes, and orthostatic changes in blood pressure and pulse rate. If the volume status is not completely clear from the examination, laboratory values can be helpful (see Figure 2), but they need to be interpreted in the context of renal function tests. If the urine osmolality is less than maximally concentrated (<500 mOsm/kg), an infusion of 0.5 to 1 L of isotonic saline over 24 to 48 hours may help with differentiation. With hypovolemia, the sodium will begin to correct and the patient should improve clinically. Conversely, if the patient is actually euvolemic, such as with syndrome of inappropriate antidiuretic hormone (SIADH), discussed later, the serum sodium level will remain constant or decrease due to retention of free water with a concomitant increase in urinary sodium.

Extrarenal causes of hyponatremia include gastrointestinal losses and third-space losses such as in severe burns and pancreatitis. In the volume-depleted state, with intact renal function, the urine sodium is low (<10 mEq/L), reflecting a normal response by the kidney to maximally reabsorb sodium in response to volume depletion.

The renal causes of hypovolemic hyponatremia involve the inappropriate loss of sodium into the urine, and this is reflected by a urine sodium concentration of greater than 20 mEq/L.

Thiazide diuretics cause renal sodium loss, so the urine sodium is high. However, they also impair the kidney's diluting capacity, decreasing free water excretion and concentrating the urine. Only certain patients may be susceptible to hyponatremia while on thiazides. These patients may have an abnormally sensitive thirst response to the mild hypovolemia induced by the diuretics, causing increased water intake. Elderly women are the most susceptible, and hyponatremia can occur within days after initiation of thiazide therapy. Additional laboratory results reveal hypokalemia and a metabolic alkalosis. It is appropriate to stop the diuretic and restore potassium levels and volume status. Patients often have a recurrence of hyponatremia if rechallenged with thiazides. Loop diuretics, such as furosemide, are a less frequent cause of hyponatremia, which occurs only after long-term therapy.

In the absence of diuretic use, a urine sodium concentration greater than 20 mEq/L with hypovolemia is evidence for underlying renal pathology. Patients with salt-wasting nephropathy, from a number of causes (see Figure 1), usually have significant renal failure, with a creatinine value in the range of 3 to 4 mg/dL. Because of the large net sodium loss, this condition is treated with salt tablets. Renal tubular acidosis causes bicarbonaturia, which requires a compensatory excretion of urinary cations, mainly Na^+ and K^+, to maintain electroneutrality. Similarly, excretion of ketones into the urine also demands additional electrolyte losses in spite of ECF volume depletion, leading to a loss of sodium.

Cerebral salt wasting (CSW), although it could be considered an extrarenal cause, also involves the renal loss of sodium (>20 mEq/L). The biochemical presentation is very similar to that of SIADH, but the diagnosis of CSW is restricted to cases involving extreme central nervous system pathology. CSW is most commonly associated with subarachnoid hemorrhage but also has been reported with stroke, brain trauma, infection, metastases and after neurosurgery. Onset of CSW is usually within the first 10 days after the neurologic event.

CSW may be a protective mechanism against increased intracranial pressure. The proposed pathophysiologic mechanism of CSW is controversial, but one hypothesis is that the initiating event is a primary natriuresis, with renal loss of sodium, caused by the secretion of natriuretic peptides. Clinical studies have found both increased brain natriuretic peptide and increased atrial natriuretic peptide in neurosurgical patients with hyponatremia. Both hormones are vasodilators that increase the glomerular filtration rate while suppressing the renin-angiotensin system. This increases renal sodium losses as well as water excretion, resulting in volume depletion. Vasopressin levels rise in response to low volume, so that it becomes biochemically difficult to differentiate CSW from SIADH, with a urine sodium level greater than 20 mEq/L, low uric acid, and high urine osmolality. It is helpful if CSW patients have signs of volume depletion in combination with the laboratory results. Also, the hyponatremia of CSW responds to normal saline, whereas SIADH worsens with normal saline. CSW is relatively rare in most case series, and it is important to rule out other causes for natriuresis.

Hypervolemic Hyponatremia

There are a variety of causes of hypervolemic hyponatremia (see Figure 1), all of which are a result of decreased effective circulating volume. To correct this imbalance, the ECF expands, leading to fluid retention and hyponatremia. In spite of the increased total body water and low serum sodium on testing, all of these patients have some degree of total body sodium excess. In many cases, volume overload is clinically evident from the presence of subcutaneous edema, ascites, elevated jugular venous pressure, or pulmonary edema.

In congestive heart failure (CHF), patients can develop hyponatremia with only 2 to 3 L of fluid intake per day despite normal renal function. The decreased filling pressures and cardiac output of CHF are perceived as volume depletion, detected by the baroreceptors. This stimulates vasopressin secretion, overriding the signal of low osmolality detected by the hypothalamic osmoreceptors. This lack of inhibition of vasopressin secretion is believed to be the most important contributing factor to the development of hyponatremia. In addition, decreased right atrial pressures result in inhibition of secretion of atrial natriuretic peptide, contributing to the water and sodium gain. With the low perfusion pressure, there is a decrease in the glomerular filtration rate, which is sensed by the juxtaglomerular apparatus, causing neurohumoral activation of the renin-angiotensin system and sympathetic nervous system. This leads to increased circulating levels of catecholamines, angiotensin II, and aldosterone, further stimulating tubular sodium and water reabsorption. In the absence of diuretics, the urine sodium level is very low (<10 mEq/L) in patients with CHF because of activation of the renin-angiotensin-aldosterone

system and maximal tubular reabsorption of sodium. Also, there is less than maximally dilute urine (usually >300 mOsm/kg) in the absence of diuretic therapy. An elevated brain natriuretic peptide concentration helps to confirm the hypervolemia.

A similar mechanism is at work in cirrhotic patients, in whom the incidence of hyponatremia is even higher and is a strong predictor of poor outcome. In cirrhosis, low albumin results in third-spacing and decreased effective circulating volume. In addition, portal hypertension leads to splanchnic vasodilation, which also decreases the effective circulating volume. This serves to activate vasopressin secretion and the renin-angiotensin-aldosterone system.

Hyponatremia is less common in acute and chronic renal failure, but it can occur with a significant decrease in glomerular filtration rate accompanied by severe hypoalbuminemia. Interpretation of the laboratory results may be confounded by a high urine sodium concentration (>20 mEq/L) that reflects the concomitant presence of tubular dysfunction. Hyponatremia can develop in stage IV or V renal failure when fluid intake is in excess of 3 L/day.

Euvolemic Hyponatremia

Euvolemic hyponatremia is caused by impaired excretion of free water by the kidney. The differential diagnosis is more limited (see Figure 1) and the majority of cases are due to SIADH (Table 2). However, this often is a diagnosis of exclusion, and hypothyroidism and adrenal insufficiency must be ruled out clinically or biochemically in patients with euvolemic hyponatremia.

Hypothyroidism leads to reduced glomerular filtration rate and decreased flow to the distal nephron, causing maximal reabsorption of water to maintain arterial volume. Hypothyroidism has to be severe to cause hyponatremia and usually is obvious on examination. However, in the elderly population, apathetic hypothyroidism may be difficult to diagnose. Hypothyroidism can be confirmed by the presence of a high level of thyroid-stimulating hormone and a low level of free T_4 (thyroxine). Treatment involves thyroid hormone replacement and supportive care.

In primary adrenal insufficiency (Addison's disease), the concomitant aldosterone deficiency results in hyponatremia combined with hyperkalemia, prerenal azotemia, a urine sodium concentration greater than 20 mEq/L, and a urine potassium level lower than 20 mEq/L. In secondary or central adrenal insufficiency, the adrenal zona glomerulosa remains intact for the secretion of aldosterone. However, glucocorticoid deficiency still causes impaired water excretion, which can lead to dilutional hyponatremia. Vasopressin release may be stimulated by the nausea, vomiting, and orthostatic hypotension that occurs with adrenal insufficiency. Finally, corticosteroids normally inhibit vasopressin release, so their deficiency leads to enhanced vasopressin release, causing retention of free water that further contributes to the hyponatremia. The appropriate diagnostic test is a 250-μg ACTH (cosyntropin, Cortrosyn) stimulation test, although an extremely low 8 AM cortisol level (<3 μg/dL) can be diagnostic. Treatment consists of glucocorticoid replacement.

Syndrome of Inappropriate Antidiuretic Hormone

SIADH is the most common cause of euvolemic hypoosmolar hyponatremia. Edema, ascites, and orthostasis are absent, and thyroid, adrenal, and renal functions are normal. Recent diuretic use should be ruled out. The primary event is the release of vasopressin, which results in water retention. The increased intravascular volume stimulates a natriuresis, which actually is appropriate, but the resulting loss of sodium compounds the hyponatremia. There is an extensive list of causes of SIADH, usually involving pulmonary or central nervous system pathology (see Table 2). A number of medications also are known to stimulate vasopressin release or to potentiate its antidiuretic properties at the level of the kidney (see Tables 1 and 2).

The diagnosis of SIADH is suggested by a low P_{Osm} (<280 mOsm/kg) with a high U_{Osm} (>100 mOsm/kg), confirming water retention and an inappropriately concentrated urine. A spot urine sodium level will be greater than 20 mEq/L, and usually greater than 30 mEq/L. Other helpful laboratory findings include low plasma uric acid (<4 mg/dL), which has a positive predictive value of 73% to 100% for SIADH in this setting. In complicated

TABLE 2	Causes of SIADH		
CNS DISORDERS	**PULMONARY DISORDERS**	**MEDICATIONS**	**OTHER**
Mass lesions	Viral/bacterial pneumonia	Vasopressin analogues	Pain
Tumors	Positive-pressure ventilation	(Desmopressin [DDAVP])	Nausea
CNS abscess	Bronchogenic carcinoma (small cell)	NSAIDs	AIDS
Intracranial hemorrhage or hematoma	Acute respiratory failure	Tricyclic antidepressants	Prolonged exercise
Stroke	COPD	Phenothiazines	Idiopathic
CNS infections or inflammatory diseases	Tuberculosis	Butyrophenones	
Spinal cord lesions	Aspergillosis	SSRIs	
Acute psychosis	Pulmonary abscess	Morphine	
Pituitary stalk lesions		Opiates	
Hydrocephalus		Chlorpropamide (Diabinese)	
Dementia		Clofibrate (Atromid-S)[2]	
Guillain-Barré syndrome		Cyclophosphamide (Cytoxan)	
Head trauma		Vincristine (Oncovin)	
		Nicotine	
		Tolbutamide (Orinase)	
		Barbiturates	
		Acetaminophen (Tylenol)	
		ACE inhibitors	
		Carbamazepine (Tegretol)	
		Omeprazole (Prilosec)	

[2]Not available in the United States.

Abbreviations: ACE = angiotensin-converting enzyme; AIDS = acquired immunodeficiency syndrome; CNS = central nervous system; COPD = chronic obstructive pulmonary disease; NSAIDs = nonsteroidal antiinflammatory drugs; SSRIs = selective serotonin reuptake inhibitors.

cases confounded by use of diuretics, the fractional excretion of uric acid has a positive predictive value of 100% for SIADH when the calculated excretion is greater than 12%.

Reset osmostat can be considered a form of SIADH, but the hyponatremia is usually chronic, mild, and asymptomatic. Vasopressin release continues to be regulated, but at a lower threshold of plasma osmolality. The thirst threshold may be altered as well. Interventions to raise the sodium usually have short-lived effects, and the sodium resets at its previous value over time. Therefore, treatment is not recommended if the sodium level is stable and the patient is asymptomatic. A physiologic example of reset osmostat is seen in pregnancy, when the normal sodium range is lowered by 5 mEq/L.

Other Causes of Euvolemic Hypoosmolar Hyponatremia

Primary or psychogenic polydipsia should be considered in patients presenting with hyponatremia and a history of psychiatric illness and treatment. Almost 6% to 7% of psychiatric inpatients are at risk for hyponatremia from increased water intake. The polydipsia may be related to a lowered osmolar threshold for thirst, below the threshold of suppression of vasopressin secretion. This can be further complicated by the side effect of dry mouth caused by many psychiatric medications, which compounds the increased thirst and water intake. Because the kidney is capable of excreting up to 15 to 20 L/day of dilute urine, the fact that hyponatremia develops in these patients may point toward an additional and inappropriate increase in vasopressin release or sensitivity. These patients are clinically euvolemic because of renal excretion of the excess water and have otherwise normal laboratory results except for a dilute urine (<100 mOsm/kg), which is caused by vasopressin suppression and helps differentiate primary polydipsia from SIADH. However, some patients have mildly concentrated urine (>100 mOsm/kg), in which case the psychiatric history helps with the diagnosis.

Exercise-induced hyponatremia (e.g., from marathon running) is a form of euvolemic hypoosmolar hyponatremia primarily caused by excessive fluid intake during exercise. Vasopressin levels also may be inappropriately high, secondary to pain or the use of NSAIDs, which remove prostaglandin inhibition of vasopressin release. Low solute intake combined with high fluid intake also can cause hyponatremia, as with beer potomania or a low-protein "tea and toast" diet in elderly patients. In both cases, the lack of solute in the urine does not allow retention of water in the filtrate, so the excess water is not excreted.

Hyponatremia also is common after pituitary surgery (transsphenoidal or by craniotomy) and may be a result of damage to the hypothalamic-pituitary tract that causes release of preformed vasopressin from damaged neurons. Often, hyponatremia occurs as the second phase of the classic triphasic response: transient diabetes insipidus, transient SIADH, followed by permanent diabetes insipidus. Hyponatremia can be delayed up to 1 week postoperatively, and sodium should be monitored during the second week as well. Contributions by central adrenal insufficiency and hypothyroidism also are considerations after pituitary surgery, although with these conditions there will be obvious clinical manifestations in addition to the hyponatremia.

Management

The major considerations for choosing the type and time course of treatment for hyponatremia are the duration of hyponatremia (acute or chronic) and the presence of neurologic signs and symptoms, especially severe manifestations such as altered mental status or seizure (see Table 2). Treatment options for hyponatremia include fluid restriction, saline infusion (hypertonic or isotonic), vasopressin receptor antagonists (Conivaptan, [Vaprisol]), and demeclocycline (Declomycin).[1] Also, treatment of the underlying abnormality, such as CHF or salt wasting, and correction of volume status are important for hypovolemic or hypervolemic patients. Autocorrection may occur after initiation of therapy, especially in cases of hypovolemia, adrenal insufficiency, or thiazide use. Once treatment is started, the contribution of the nonosmotic stimulation of vasopressin secretion is removed, and the patient is able to raise the sodium level by 2 mEq/L per hour over 12 hours.

Acute Severe Symptomatic Hyponatremia

Acute severe hyponatremia is defined as a rapid fall in sodium in less than 48 hours to less than 120 mEq/L. Under these circumstances, most patients develop neurologic symptoms because of the rapid fluid shifts between the ECF and the ICF in the brain. If left untreated, it can result in irreversible neurologic damage and death. Because of the acute drop in sodium, initial rapid correction is acceptable and should not lead to osmotic demyelination. Treatment is aimed at raising the sodium enough to resolve the neurologic signs and symptoms. The goal is to raise the serum sodium by 1 to 2 mEq/L per hour or to greater than 125 mEq/L until symptoms resolve. Hypovolemic patients will respond to infusion of isotonic saline (normal saline 0.9%), especially if the urine sodium concentration is less than 30 mEq/L. If the neurologic findings are severe, hypertonic saline (3%) may

---

[1]Not FDA approved for this indication.

be infused at rate of 1 to 2 mL/kg per hour, or even up to 4 to 6 mL/kg per hour if the imbalance is life-threatening. A loop diuretic can be combined with the saline to enhance solute-free water excretion. Sodium levels should be monitored every 2 to 4 hours in patients undergoing hypertonic infusion. Once symptoms resolve, the rate of correction should be reduced to 0.5 to 1 mEq/hour, and the total rise in sodium should not exceed 8 to 12 mEq in 24 hours and no more than 18 mEq in 48 hours. No benefit has been observed for faster rates of correction of hyponatremia, whether acute or chronic. Useful formulas to determine the rate of infusion for fluids are provided in Figure 3. The formulas can only estimate the rate of correction, and sodium should be measured frequently.

Chronic Hyponatremia

Chronic hyponatremia is defined as a gradual fall in sodium over more than 48 hours. By this time, the brain has begun to compensate for hypoosmolality by extrusion of solutes. However, the patient is at risk of osmotic demyelination if hyponatremia is treated too aggressively. If the duration of hyponatremia is unknown, the recommendation is to assume that it is chronic. However, as with acute hyponatremia, severe neurologic symptoms and signs need to be treated with hypertonic saline until they resolve, after which the rate of correction can be slowed to 0.5 to 1 mEq/L per hour. Most cases of osmotic demyelination occur with correction rates of greater than 12 mEq/L in 24 hours, but there are cases reported with increases of 9 or 10 mEq/day. Asymptomatic hyponatremia can be treated with an infusion of isotonic saline calculated to raise the sodium by 0.5 to 1 mEq/hour. If the patient has a dilute urine (<200 mOsm/kg), water restriction may be sufficient.

Syndrome of Inappropriate Antidiuretic Hormone

The mainstays of treatment of SIADH are fluid restriction and treatment of the underlying cause. Mild SIADH usually can be controlled with fluid restriction alone.

In most cases of SIADH, the degree of fluid restriction required can be calculated. It is dependent on three factors: the daily osmolar load, the minimum U_{Osm}, and the patient's maximum urine volume. A typical diet has a daily osmolar load of 10 mOsm/kg of body weight. For a 70 kg person, this would be 700 mOsm/day. With SIADH, the urine osmolality is held constant for that particular patient, as revealed by a spot U_{Osm}. If the U_{Osm} is 500 mOsm/kg

and the solute load is 700 mOsm, the fluid load has to be less than 700/500 or 1.4 L/day just to maintain the serum sodium level. Fluid intake above this amount will cause the sodium to decrease.

When needed, salt tablets (sodium chloride tablet 1 g taken once to three times daily) can help to make up for renal loss of sodium in SIADH. With symptoms and severe hyponatremia, short-term use of hypertonic saline may also be instituted to restore sodium to the ECF compartment. Loop diuretics (e.g., furosemide [Lasix]) can increase free water clearance when given with solute (e.g., hypertonic saline or salt tablets). In refractory cases, demeclocycline (300–600 mg PO twice daily)[1] can be used. Demeclocycline (Declomycin) antagonizes the actions of vasopressin by inhibiting formation of cyclic adenosine monophosphate in the collecting duct. Long-term use is limited by the side effect of photosensitivity and by nephrotoxicity in patients with underlying liver disease. Vasopressin receptor antagonists also are important adjunct treatments (see later discussion). A less favored treatment is urea (powder or capsules),[1,6] which causes an osmotic diuresis and increased free water excretion.

Cerebral Salt Wasting

Management of CSW involves treatment of the underlying neurologic problem as well as volume replacement. CSW often is difficult to differentiate biochemically from SIADH, but the rise in vasopressin in CSW is secondary to volume depletion. As a result, CSW responds to volume replacement with isotonic saline, suppressing release of vasopressin, whereas SIADH worsens with this therapy. The recommended correction rate is 0.7 to 1.0 mEq/L per hour, with a maximum of 8 to 10 mEq per 24 hours. Salt tablets may also be given to replete total body sodium. Fludrocortisone (Florinef[1] 0.05 to 0.1 mg every 12 hours), an aldosterone receptor agonist, is a third-line treatment to encourage volume expansion and sodium retention, but the potassium concentration and blood pressure should be monitored. Fluid restriction is inappropriate for CSW and should be avoided, especially in patients with subarachnoid hemorrhage, because volume depletion can exacerbate cerebral vasospasm and cause infarction. The duration of CSW is usually 3 to 5 weeks.

---

[1]Not FDA approved for this indication.
[6]May be compounded by pharmacists.

Parameters for acute or chronic hyponatremia:
Do not increase serum Na by more than 10 to 12 mEq/l in 24 hrs and 18 mEq/l in 48 hrs

Symptomatic hyponatremia with severe neurologic symptoms (acute <48 hrs or chronic >48hrs)
1. Correct serum Na at a rate of 1–2 mEq/l per hour (for 2 to 4 hours) until symptoms have resolved
2. Correct Na at a rate of 0.5 to 1 mEq/l per hour, maximum 10–12 mEq/24h

Acute hyponatremia with mild symptoms
1. Correct at rate of 0.5 to 1 mEq/l per hour

Chronic hyponatremia with mild symptoms or asymptomatic
1. Correct at a rate of 0.5 mEq/l per hour with fluid restriction
2. Treat underlying etiology

Calculation of the rate of infusion of saline to correct hyponatremia
1. Change in serum sodium per liter infusate
$$(\Delta Na/L) = \frac{Infusate\ [sodium] - Serum\ [sodium]}{TBW + 1}$$
2. Amount of infusate (in L) required in 24hours
$$L = \frac{desired\ change\ in\ sodium\ (\Delta Na)\ over\ 24\ hrs}{\Delta Na/L\ (from\ 1.)}$$
3. Rate of infusate to raise serum Na by desired amount
$$ml/hr = \frac{L\ (from\ 2.) \times 1000\ mL/L}{24\ hr}$$
4. (Simplified) Hypertonic saline infused at 1–2 ml/kg per hour

Monitoring:
1. Monitor frequently for clinical improvement or worsening of symptoms
2. If on hypertonic saline or severely symptomatic check sodium q2–4hrs.
3. If undergoing treatment but asymptomatic, check sodium q6–12 h.

Infusate	Infusate [Na] (mmol/L)
5% sodium chloride in water	855
3% sodium chloride in water	513
Isotonic saline (0.9 %)	154
Ringer's lactate solution	130
0.45% sodium chloride in water	77
0.2% sodium chloride in water	34
5% dextrose in water	0

Total Body Water (TBW) is equal to 60% of body weight in young adult men and 50% in young adult women. Older patients have less TBW. In elderly males, TBW is equal to 50% of body weight and in elderly females it is 45%.

Figure 3. Treatment of hyponatremia. *Abbreviation:* TBW = total body water.

Vasopressin Receptor Antagonists

Vasopressin receptor antagonists, or vaptans, are a new class of nonpeptide drugs that have great potential for the treatment of dilutional hyponatremia. They block the binding of vasopressin to its receptors in the distal nephron, thereby inhibiting the insertion of aquaporin-2 channels into the membrane, increasing excretion of solute-free water by the kidneys, and resulting in a rise in serum sodium content. Currently, conivaptan (Vaprisol) is FDA approved for clinical use in euvolemic and hypervolemic hyponatremia in hospitalized patients, with the exception of patients with CHF or cirrhosis. Obviously, it is contraindicated in hypovolemic hyponatremia because of the water excretion that is induced. Conivaptan is given intravenously with a bolus of 20 mg over 30 minutes in 100 mL of 5% dextrose in water (D5W). After this, the drug (20 mg in 100 mL of D5W) is infused over 24 hours. Sodium is monitored every 2 to 4 hours, and the dose may be titrated to 40 mg per 24 hours to obtain an increase in sodium of 0.5 to 1.0 mEq/L per hour. During Vaprisol treatment, fluid restriction is liberal at 1.5 to 2.0 L/day. An oral formulation tolvaptan (Samsca) also is approved for outpatient treatment of hyponatremia associated with SIADH and CHF if it is clinically significant and Na is less than 125 mEq/L or it is resistant to other treatments. Tolvaptan is first initiated in the hospital setting, for careful monitoring of potassium and the rate of rise of sodium, at a dose of 15 mg once daily. It is titrated up with more than 24 hours between increased doses to a maximum of 60 mg once daily for a maximum of thirty days of therapy due to risks of hepatotoxicity. Tolvaptan is contraindicated in patients with liver disease, including cirrhosis, and liver tests should be performed promptly in patients with symptoms of hepatotoxicity. Inhibitors of the cytochrome P-450 3A4 isoenzyme (CYP3A4) are contraindicated, including ketoconazole (Nizoral), itraconazole (Sporanox), clarithromycin (Biaxin), ritonavir (Norvir), and indinavir (Crixivan). Additionally, the "vaptans" will alter the hepatic metabolism of other drugs that interact with Cyp 3A4, so all concurrent medications should be checked carefully for potential interactions.

Summary

Hyponatremia is a common electrolyte abnormality and is usually caused by decreased plasma osmolality. Accurate assessment of volume status is a key to determining the underlying cause and choosing the correct treatment approach. The biggest risk of hyponatremia and its treatment is the possibility of severe neurologic sequelae, including fatal cerebral edema and osmotic demyelination. Therefore, more aggressive initial treatment is needed in patients with neurologic manifestations (hypertonic saline), but a more conservative approach (e.g., fluid restriction) is needed for less symptomatic patients. Vasopressin antagonists are additional tools for the treatment of euvolemic or hypervolemic hyponatremia refractory to more conservative measures.

References

Andrøgué HJ. Consequences of inadequate management of hyponatremia. Am J Nephrol 2005;25:240–9.

Andrøgué HJ, Madias NE. Hyponatremia. N Engl J Med 2000;342(21):1581–9.

Cerdà-Esteve M, Cuadrado-Godia E, Chillaron JJ, et al. Cerebral salt wasting syndrome: Review. Eur J Intern Med 2008;19:249–54.

Ellison DH, Berl T. Clinical practice: The syndrome of inappropriate antidiuresis. N Engl J Med 2007;356:2064–72.

Fenske W, Störk S, Koschker A. Value of fractional uric acid excretion in differential diagnosis of hyponatremia patients on diuretics. J Clin Endocrinol Metab 2008;93:2991–7.

Hew-Butler T, Jordaan E, Stuempfle KJ. Osmotic and nonosmotic regulation of arginine vasopressin during prolonged exercise. J Clin Endocrinol Metab 2008;93:2072–8.

Palm C, Pistrosch F, Herbrig K, Gross P. Vasopressin antagonists as aquaretic agents for the treatment of hyponatremia. Am J Med 2006;119(Suppl. 1):S87–93.

Vaprisol conivaptan hydrochloride injection: Prescribing information. Deerfield, Ill: Astellas Pharma US, Inc; 2007.

Verbalis JG, Goldsmith SR, Greenberg A, et al. Hyponatremia treatment guidelines 2007: Expert panel recommendations. Am J Med 2007;120(11 Suppl. 1):S1–21.

Zada G, Liu CY, Fishback D, et al. Recognition and management of delayed hyponatremia following transsphenoidal pituitary surgery. J Neurosurg 2007;106:66–71.

HYPOPITUITARISM

Method of
Vanessa Ho, MD

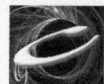

CURRENT DIAGNOSIS

- Symptoms can be vague. Having heightened awareness is key to making an early diagnosis with resultant proper treatment.
- The diagnosis of hypopituitarism is based on a combination of brain imaging studies and demonstration of insufficiency of one or more pituitary hormones.
- Always confirm the diagnosis before initiating treatment.

CURRENT THERAPY

- Primary treatment of hypopituitarism is cortisol replacement.
- Treatment for hypopituitarism can be an emergency in severe cases because cortisol is responsible for supporting peripheral vascular function.
- Use higher doses of cortisol in cases of stress such as illnesses or high-risk surgeries to aid in proper recovery.

Epidemiology

In one study published in 2001 comprising a population of 146,000 in northwestern Spain, the prevalence of hypopituitarism is as high as 45.5 cases per 100,000 individuals. The incidence is estimated to be 4.2 per 100,000 per year. About 50% of patients had 3 to 5 pituitary hormonal deficiencies, with luteinizing hormone/follicle-stimulating hormone (LH/FSH) being the most prevalent. Patients with tumor-induced hypopituitarism showed a tendency to suffer growth hormone (GH) deficiency more frequently than those resulting from nontumor causes.

Risk Factors

The most common cause of hypopituitarism is pituitary tumors (61%), followed by nonpituitary tumors (9%) (Table 1). Thirty percentage of cases are caused by nontumors. Nontumor causes include inflammatory diseases such as lymphocytic hypophysitis, sarcoidosis, hemochromatosis, and histiocytosis X. Infectious causes include tuberculosis and syphilis. Over the last few years, awareness and detection rates of hypopituitarism following traumatic brain injury (TBI) and subarachnoid hemorrhage (SAH) have steadily increased. Various studies have shown that cases of hypopituitarism resulting from postradiotherapy radiation damage are also on the rise. With radiation doses of 30 to 50 Gy, the incidence of GH deficiency can reach 50% to 100%; long-term gonadotropin, TSH, and ACTH deficiencies occur in 20% to 30%, 3% to 9%, and 3% to 6% of patients, respectively. With higher dose cranial irradiation (>60 Gy), or following conventional irradiation for pituitary tumors (30–50 Gy), multiple hormonal deficiencies occur in 30% to 60% after 10 years of follow-up.

Some degree of hypopituitarism is found in 35% to 40% of patients who have suffered TBI. A rule of three-quarters can be applied clinically for hypopituitarism after TBI: three-quarters of cases are male <40 years of age, three-quarters of cases occur after road traffic accidents, and three-quarters of cases manifest within 1 year.

Hypopituitarism has been observed in 19% of patients with ischemic stroke and 47% of patients with SAH, presenting as an isolated deficiency in most cases. Major risk factors for developing hypopituitarism after ischemic stroke include certain clinical conditions, such as preexisting diabetes mellitus and medical complications during hospitalization. Patients with Alberta Stroke Programme Early CT scores of 7 or less have a poorer prognosis

TABLE 1	Causes of Hypopituitarism

Pituitary and nonpituitary tumors

Pituitary surgery

Pituitary radiation

Inflammatory disease—lymphocytic hypophysitis, sarcoidosis, hemochromatosis, histiocytosis X

Infectious disease—tuberculosis, syphilis

Infarction—Sheehan's syndrome, also referred to as postpartum hypopituitarism, is attributed to infarction of the pituitary gland caused by hypovolemia from obstetric hemorrhage

Pituitary apoplexy—a potentially life-threatening syndrome that occurs as a result of hemorrhage, infarction, or hemorrhagic infarction within a pituitary tumor

Genetic diseases—multiple endocrine neoplasia-1 (MEN-1) is the most common; additional genetic problems are caused by pit-1 mutation

Traumatic brain injury

Stroke—both ischemic stroke and subarachnoid hemorrhage

Suppression of hypothalamic-pituitary axis by chronic exogenous steroid use

and a higher risk of developing hypopituitarism after an ischemic stroke compared with those with a score greater than 7.

Chronic exogenous steroid use is also a known cause of hypopituitarism. In one study published in 2009, Dr. Lansang and colleagues presented cases of hypopituitarism followed multiple intraarticular and epidural injections of steroids.

Pathophysiology

The pituitary gland is a pea-sized endocrine gland that sits at the base of the brain. Often referred to as the "master gland," the pituitary gland synthesizes and releases various hormones that affect several organs throughout the body (Figure 1). It is composed of two functionally distinct structures that differ in embryologic development and anatomy: the adenohypophysis (anterior pituitary) and the neurohypophysis (posterior pituitary). The anterior pituitary is responsible for GH, prolatin, adrenocorticotropic hormone (ACTH), thyroid-stimulating hormone (TSH), lutein (LH), and follicular-stimulating hormone (FSH). The posterior pituitary is responsible for vasopressin and oxytocin.

Therefore, any damage to the pituitary gland can cause an array of symptoms ranging from generalized weakness, generalized fatigue, low blood pressure, electrolyte abnormalities, mental confusion, and even disorientation.

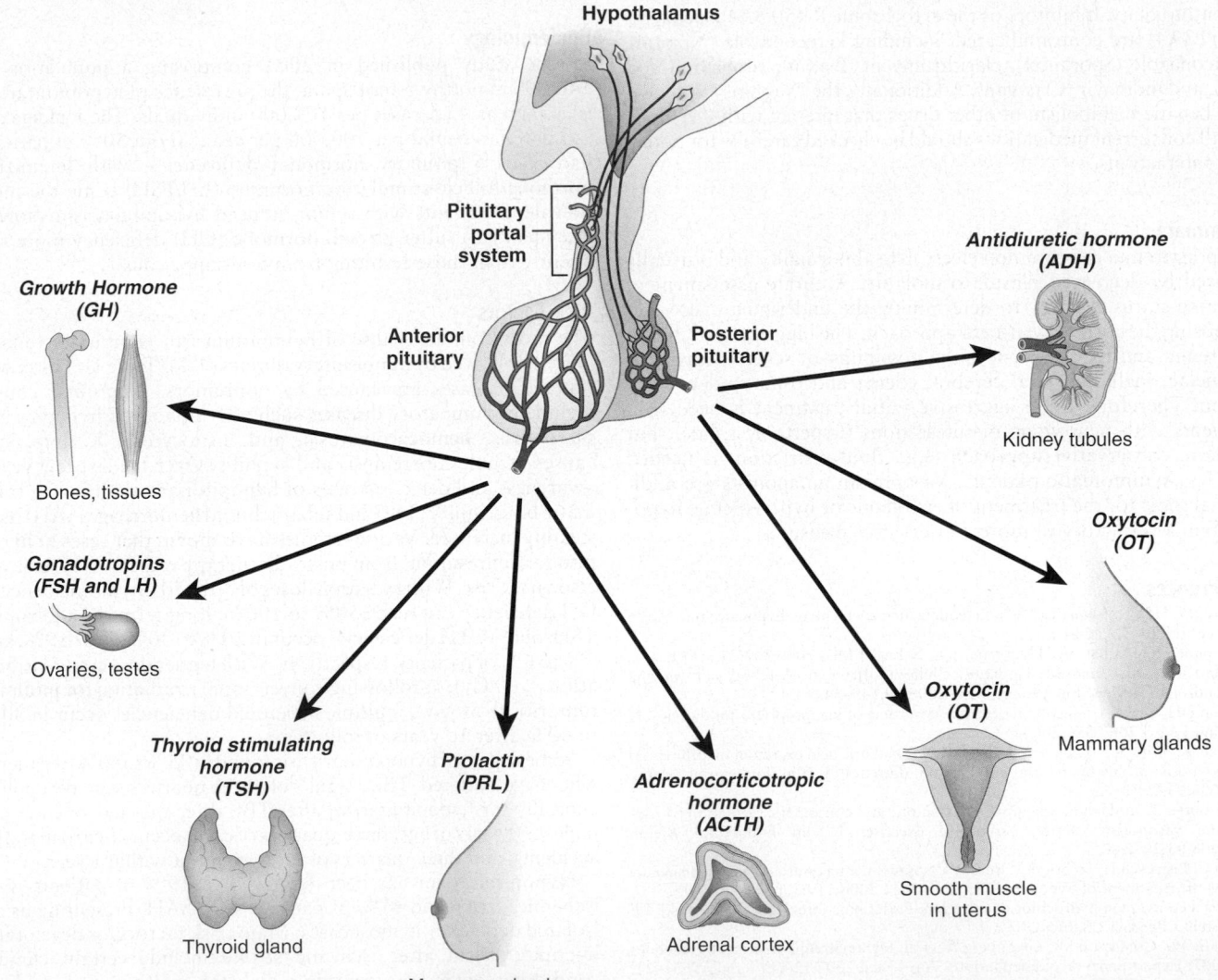

Figure 1. The pituitary gland.

Prevention

In most cases, the condition is not preventable. Awareness can lead to early detection and proper treatment. As little as 7.5 mg of prednisone/prednisolone (Millipred) or 0.75 mg of dexamethasone (Decadron) daily for more than 3 weeks can suppress the HPA axis. This suppression may last for months after the exogenous steroid is stopped. Therefore, to reduce the risk of developing suppression of the HPA axis, we recommend the use of steroids for the shortest time possible and in the smallest dose possible, and to taper down the steroids slowly if used for longer than 2 weeks.

Clinical Manifestation

Signs and symptoms of hypopituitarism vary, depending on which pituitary hormones are deficient and how severe the deficiency is. They may include

- ACTH deficiency—generalized fatigue, generalized weakness, failure to thrive, tachycardia, hypotension, electrolyte abnormalities, confusion and even disorientation
- TSH deficiency—fatigue, weight gain, cold intolerance
- Gonadotropin deficiency—decreased sex drive, infertility, hot flashes, irregular or no periods, inability to produce milk
- GH deficiency—failure to thrive and short stature in children; most adults are asymptomatic, but some may experience fatigue and weakness
- Anti-diuretic hormone (ADH) deficiency—polyuria, polydipsia, electrolyte abnormalities

Diagnosis

The diagnosis of hypopituitarism is based on a combination of high clinical suspicion, brain imaging studies, and demonstration of insufficiency of one or more pituitary hormones (Figure 2).

A. Corticotropin

1. Total cortisol level:

Normally, cortisol levels rise during the early morning hours and are highest at about 7 AM. They drop very low in the evening and during the early phase of sleep. Therefore, cortisol level should be measured early morning and no later than 9 AM. The normal level is between 4.0 and 22.0 mcg/dL. An early-morning serum cortisol level equal or less than 3 mcg/dL is abnormal. The next step is to repeat the test for confirmation and at the same time check a serum ACTH level to establish the diagnosis. A low or normal ACTH level is sufficient to make a diagnosis of

hypopituitarism versus a high ACTH level that suggests a diagnosis of primary adrenal insufficiency. If the cortisol level is borderline between 4.0 and 10.0 mcg/dL, an ACTH stimulation test should be performed to confirm the diagnosis.

2. ACTH stimulation tests:
- Metyrapone response test—or 11-Deoxycortisol (Compound S) test. The metyrapone test is used to evaluate inhibition of cortisol production with metyrapone (Metopirone) and a resultant increase of ACTH in response to the drop of cortisol. Metyrapone blocks cortisol production by inhibiting 11β-hydroxylase. The drop in cortisol stimulates ACTH secretion, which in turn increases plasma 11-deoxycortisol levels. The long version involves 24-hour inpatient admission because of the risk of hypotension. The short version involves the administration of a single dose of metyrapone at midnight and the measurement of serum cortisol in the morning. However, the inhibition of cortisol production may be partial, leading to a partial ACTH response and an inconclusive test result.

To conduct the metapyrone response test, metyrapone (30 mg/kg, maximum dose 3000 mg) is administered at midnight usually with a snack. The plasma cortisol and 11-deoxycortisol are measured the next morning between 8:00 and 9:00 AM. A plasma cortisol less than 220 nmol/L indicates adequate inhibition of 11β-hydroxylase. In patients with an intact hypothalamo-pituitary-adrenal (HPA) axis, CRH and ACTH levels rise as a response to the falling cortisol levels. This results in an increase of the steroid precursors in the pathway, including 11-deoxycortisol. Therefore, if the ACTH level rises and 11-deoxycortisol levels do not rise and remain less than 7 μg/dL, it is highly suggestive of impaired adrenal insufficiency. If neither ACTH or 11-deoxycortisol rise, it is highly suggestive of an impaired HPA axis at either the pituitary or hypothalamus.

- Cosyntropin (Cortrosyn) stimulation test—or ACTH stimulation test, is more appropriate than the metapyrone test to perform in an outpatient setting. It involves administering 0.25 mg of cosyntropin (Cortrosyn) to patients and measuring the serum cortisol level 60 minutes later. A 60-minute cortisol level of less than 18 mcg/dL is suggestive of abnormal pituitary response or hypopituitarism.

Figure 2. The diagnosis of hypopituitarism.

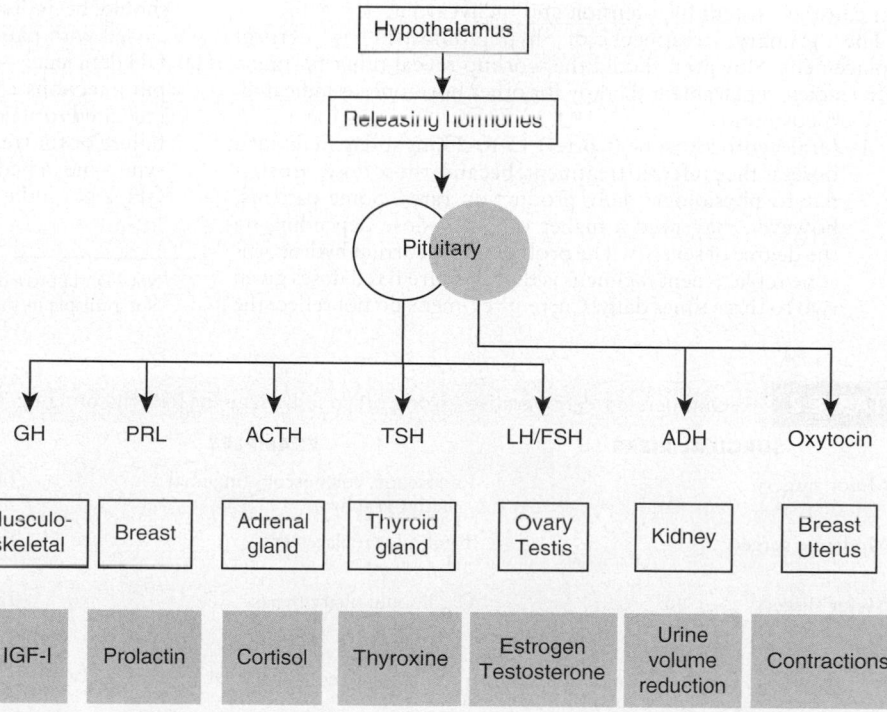

B. Thyrotropin—Patients who have pituitary or hypothalamic diseases may have secondary hypothyroidism. In primary hypothyroidism caused by thyroid gland disorders, the TSH level will be high. In pituitary or hypothalamic disease, the TSH level will be low. Thus, it is important to measure not only TSH but also "total T4" and "T3 uptake" or "free T4" levels to make the diagnosis.

C. Gonadotropins—Patients who have pituitary or hypothalamic diseases may have secondary hypogonadism. The characteristics of secondary hypogonadism are a low estrogen level in women or a low testosterone level in men and low or normal FSH and LH. On the contrary, primary hypogonadism caused by ovarian or testicular failure would result in low estrogen or testosterone levels and likely elevated FSH and LH.

D. GH—A measurement of basal serum GH concentration is not reliable. A diagnosis of GH deficiency is based on "serum IGF-1 concentration." A concentration lower than the age-specific normal level confirms the diagnosis of GH deficiency. Alternatively, a provocative test of GH secretion such as the arginine-GHRH test can be performed. Suboptimal increases in the serum GH concentration (less than 4.1 ng/mL) confirm the diagnosis of GH deficiency.

Differential Diagnosis

The differential diagnoses of hypopituitarism consist of isolated primary organ failure and deficiencies such as adrenal insufficiency, thyroid gland disorders, and primary ovarian or testicular failure.

Hypopituitarism may manifest several years after radiation exposure and in chronic Sheehan's syndrome. In acute pituitary failure, as in Sheehan's syndrome, the ACTH stimulation test may be normal because the adrenal glands are not atrophied in the acute setting; adrenal atrophy may require at least 3 months to develop. For many women, the symptoms of Sheehan's syndrome, such as fatigue, are nonspecific and often attributed to other things. It is possible for a woman to be symptom-free with Sheehan's syndrome. A woman might not realize that she has Sheehan's syndrome until she requires treatment for thyroid or adrenal insufficiency. Some women unknowingly live for years with pituitary insufficiency, then go into adrenal crisis triggered by extreme physical stressors, such as severe infection or surgery.

Treatment

Hypopituitarism can be an emergency in severe cases because of the risk of vascular collapse because cortisol is necessary for the maintenance of peripheral vascular function. Less severe cases can cause persistent hypotension and tachycardia.

The primary treatment of hypopituitarism is cortisol replacement. However, should the workup reveal other hormone deficiencies, replacement therapy for other hormones is indicated.

A. Corticosteroids
1. Oral hydrocortisone (Cortef) 15 to 25 mg a day in divided doses is the preferred treatment, because those doses are similar to physiologic daily production rates. Some patients, however, may need a higher or lower dose depending on the degree of severity. The problem with current hydrocortisone replacement regimens is that they are fixed doses given two to three times daily. Current regimens do not reflect the normal circadian pattern of physiologic cortisol concentrations, which rise highest in the morning, to an intermediate level in the afternoon, and to low levels in the evening, with a cortisol-free interval at night. The current replacement regimens inevitably result in temporary over- or underreplacement and, therefore, result in a poor quality of life and increased mortality. Recent effort has studied sustained-release once-a-day hydrocortisone therapy versus a thrice daily, weight-related, dosing regimen. Plenadren®[1] is a recently licensed modified-release formulation of hydrocortisone that provides the potential for once-daily dosing. Plenadren® provides cortisol concentrations in the afternoon but not in the evening; it does not provide an overnight rise in cortisol concentrations, such that patients have a long period of low cortisol concentrations from late afternoon to when they take their next morning dose. A pilot Chronocort®[2] formulation demonstrated delayed release and an overnight rise in cortisol after about 4 hours of administering 30 mg at 10 PM. Pharmacokinetic modeling of Chronocort® suggested that giving a 20-mg dose at 10 PM and a 10-mg dose at 7 PM could replicate the normal physiologic cortisol rhythm. Both are currently approved to be used in Europe and are in Phase 2 clinical trials in the United States.
2. Some authorities suggest prednisone or dexamethasone because of their longer duration of action. They can be given once a day, versus hydrocortisone, which is administered two to three times a day.
3. Patients may need a higher dose of hydrocortisone in times of illnesses or other stresses. Before planned surgeries, high-dose hydrocortisone (Solu Cortef) as stress doses for 1 to 3 days allows faster recovery (Table 2).

B. Thyroid deficiency—Thyroid deficiency from hypopituitarism is treated with T3 and T4 in a fashion similar to the treatment of primary hypothyroidism. However, treatment of secondary hypothyroidism should not be administered until adrenal function is restored and found to be normal. Treatment of the hypothyroidism alone may suppress other hormones produced by the pituitary gland and worsen the severity of other deficiencies. Similarly, TSH cannot be used as a guide for thyroid replacement in hypopituitarism; dose adjustment should be based on free T3 and free T4 levels instead.

C. Sex hormone deficiency—This includes testosterone, estrogen, and progesterone. The decision to initiate hormone therapy should be individualized. Risks and benefits should be discussed with patients extensively.

D. GH deficiency—GH replacement is now available as somatropin injections (Accretropin, Genotropin, Humatrope). GH is indicated for treatment of pediatric patients who have growth failure or for treatment of short stature associated with Turner syndrome in pediatric patients whose epiphyses are not closed. GH is not indicated for treatment of adult onset deficiency.

---

[1]Not FDA approved for this indication.
[2]Not available in the United States.

TABLE 2 Recommended Perioperative Hydrocortisone Dosage for Patients on Long-Term Steroid Therapy*

SURGICAL RISKS	EXAMPLES	RECOMMENDATIONS
Minor surgery	Endoscopy, colonoscopy, inguinal herniography	Take the usual morning dose. Then take 25 mg/day for 1 day starting before surgery
Moderate surgery	Total joint replacement	Take the usual morning dose. Then take 50–75 mg/day for 1–2 days
Major surgery	Cardiopulmonary bypass	Take the usual morning dose. Then 100–150 mg/day for 2–3 days

From Shawn (2012).
*Based on the recommendations of Salem M, Tainsh RE Jr, Bromberg J, Loriaux DL, Chernow B. Perioperative glucocorticoid coverage: A reassessment 42 years after emergence of a problem. Ann Surg 1994; 219:416-25.

Monitoring

Periodic serum cortisol levels are used to assess treatment adequacy and make adjustments as needed. Most studies use cortisol levels taken approximately 4 hours after the morning cortisol dose. The challenge of measuring serum cortisol levels is that cortisol sensitivity and concentrations vary between individuals. The total daily hydrocortisone dose should be based on the patient's clinical symptoms, not just cortisol level alone.

Complications

Most of the complications of hypopituitarism are caused by a failure to diagnose the condition. Having a high clinical suspicion is the key, especially after significant traumatic events such as cardiac arrests, acute emergency surgeries, or severe motor vehicle accidents. Inadequate replacement of hormone therapy can lead to persistent symptoms, whereas excessive replacement of hormones can lead to other conditions, such as Cushing's syndrome.

References

Regal M, Páramo C, Sierra SM, et al. Prevalence and incidence of hypopituitarism in an adult Caucasian population in northwestern Spain. Clin Endocrinol (Oxf) 2001;55:735–40.

Darzy KH, Shalet SM. Hypopituitarism following radiotherapy revisited. Endocr Dev 2009;15:1–24.

Garg MK. Hypopituitarism following external cranial irradiation for extrasellar tumors. Indian J Endocrinol Metab 2007;11:3–9.

Popovic V, Aimaretti G, Casanueva FF, et al. Hypopituitarism following traumatic brain injury. Growth Horm IGF Res 2005;15:177–84.

Benvenga S, Campenní A, Ruggeri RM, et al. Clinical review 113: Hypopituitarism secondary to head trauma. J Clin Endocrinol Metab 2000;85:1353–61.

Bondanelli M, Ambrosio MR, Zatelli MC, et al. Prevalence of hypopituitarism in patients with cerebrovascular diseases. J Endocrinol Invest 2008;31:16–20.

Lansang MC, Farmer T, Kennedy L. Diagnosing the unrecognized systemic absorption of intra-articular and epidural steroid injections. Endocr Pract 2009;15:225–8.

Zepf B. Adrenal insufficiency in acute severe illness. Am Fam Physician 2003;68:1416–20.

Lennernäs H, Skrtic S, Johannsson G. Replacement therapy of oral hydrocortisone in adrenal insufficiency: The influence of gastrointestinal factors. Expert Opin Drug Metab Toxicol 2008;4:749–58. http://dx.doi.org/10.1517/17425255.4.6.749.

Shaw M. When is perioperative 'steroid coverage' necessary? Cleve Clin J Med 2002;69:9–11.

HYPOTHYROIDISM

Method of
William J. Hueston, MD

CURRENT DIAGNOSIS

- Hypothyroidism is more common in women as they age.
- The signs and symptoms of hypothyroidism are nonspecific and can mimic other diseases found in the elderly, so clinicians need to have a high index of suspicion.
- The key diagnostic test is to find a low free T_4. The presence of an elevated TSH indicates primary hypothyroidism, and a low TSH indicates secondary hypothyroidism.
- There is insufficient evidence for screening for hypothyroidism in asymptomatic adults.

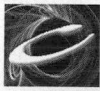

CURRENT THERAPY

- Thyroxine replacement with L-thyroxine (Synthroid, Levoxyl) is the treatment for hypothyroidism. Medication should be titrated to normalize the thyroid-stimulating hormone (TSH) level, which is usually achieved at an overall dose of 100 to 150 µg.
- Initial dosing for those with potential cardiac disease should be started low (25–50 µg/day) and advanced slowly every 6 to 8 weeks.
- Partial substitution of triiodothyronine (Cytomel) for thyroxine should be reserved for elderly patients with persistent neurocognitive dysfunction despite normalization of their TSH.

- Patients who have subclinical hypothyroidism with a TSH greater than 10.0 should be considered for treatment. Patients with a TSH lower than this do not require therapy.

Epidemiology

Hypothyroidism is second only to diabetes in the prevalence of endocrine disorders in adults in the United States. Hypothyroidism occurs in up to 18/1000 population, with women outnumbering men by approximately 10:1. Rates of hypothyroidism increase dramatically with age, so that about 2% to 3% of all older women have hypothyroidism, and the prevalence is up to 5% in nursing home populations.

Risk Factors

Thyroid conditions are more common in patients who have a family history of thyroid disorders. In addition, hypothyroidism as well as thyroid cancers are more common in patients who had neck irradiation in childhood. However, most cases of hypothyroidism occur in people who have no risk factors.

Pathophysiology

Several conditions can lead to hypothyroidism (Box 1). Two categories, hypothyroidism following thyroiditis and iatrogenic hypothyroidism secondary to treatment of Graves' disease, account for the overwhelming majority of cases of hypothyroidism in the United States.

The most common non-iatrogenic condition causing hypothyroidism in the United States is Hashimoto's thyroiditis. Most idiopathic hypothyroidism also represents Hashimoto's thyroiditis that has followed an indolent course. Hashimoto's thyroiditis, also called chronic lymphocytic thyroiditis, is the most common of the inflammatory thyroid disorders and the most common cause of goiter in the United States. The prevalence of Hashimoto's thyroiditis has been increasing dramatically since the 1960s in the United States, but the cause for this rise is unknown. In patients with acute thyroiditis, either subacute granulomatous (also known as de Quervain's) and subacute lymphocytic (also known as silent or painless), transient hypothyroidism is common following an acute attack, and 10% of these patients also develop long-term hypothyroidism.

Another common cause of hypothyroidism is a medical intervention to treat Graves' disease or thyroidectomy for chronic fibrocytic thyroiditis (Riedel's struma). Radioactive iodine ablation of the thyroid for Graves' disease often results in underproduction of thyroxine in the remaining tissue, necessitating thyroid replacement.

Box 1   Conditions Causing Hypothyroidism

Thyroiditis
Hashimoto's thyroiditis
Subacute granulomatous thyroiditis (de Quervain's thyroiditis)
Subacute lymphocytic thyroiditis (silent or painless thyroiditis)

Iatrogenic Hypothyroidism
Radioactive iodine treatment of Graves' disease
Thyroidectomy

Secondary Hypothyroidism (Pituitary Dysfunction)
Pituitary surgery
Intercranial radiation
Congenital panhypopituitarism

Other Causes
Infiltratative diseases (sarcoidosis, amyloidosis, hemochromatosis)
Drugs (lithium, interferon, amiodarone [Cordarone])
Iodine deficiency

A third uncommon cause of hypothyroidism that should not be overlooked is secondary hypothyroidism due to hypothalamic or pituitary dysfunction. These conditions are seen primarily in patients who have received intracranial irradiation or surgical removal of a pituitary adenoma.

Finally, a variety of other conditions including infiltration of the thyroid (amyloidosis, sarcoidosis), iodine deficiency, or medications (such as amiodarone [Cordarone] or interferon) can cause hypothyroidism.

Prevention

There are no known interventions to prevent hypothyroidism. According to their 2004 analysis, the U.S. Preventive Services Task Force found insufficient evidence to support early detection through routine screening of asymptomatic persons.

Clinical Manifestations

Individual who have hypothyroidism can present with a variety of symptoms, many of which are not specific. Consequently, clinicians must have a high index of suspicion for hypothyroidism when patients come in with any one or combination of the symptoms that could signal hypothyroidism.

Symptoms of hypothyroidism include lethargy, weight gain, hair loss, dry skin, constipation, poor concentration, trouble thinking or forgetfulness, and depression (Box 2). In older patients, hypothyroidism easily can be confused with Alzheimer's disease or other conditions that cause dementia. Patients who present with depression also should have their thyroid function assessed.

The thyroid examination in most patients with hypothyroidism is completely normal. Patients might have a painless goiter; tenderness in the thyroid is generally a sign of active inflammation consistent with acute thyroiditis. Once the thyroid inflammation has subsided, thyroid function might return to normal. Other physical findings that can occur with hypothyroidism include low blood pressure, bradycardia, nonpitting edema, generalized hair loss especially along the outer third of the eyebrows, dry skin, and a lag in the relaxation phase of reflexes that can be assessed most easily in the ankle jerk reflexes.

Diagnosis

The diagnosis of hypothyroidism is based on finding a low free thyroxine (T_4) level, usually with an elevation in the thyroid stimulating hormone (TSH) levels. For patients with hypothyroidism due to pituitary dysfunction, also called secondary hypothyroidism, both the free T_4 and the TSH levels are low.

One situation where clinicians need to be wary is evaluating thyroid status in patients who are severely ill. During times of acute physiologic stress, patients may have mildly elevated TSH levels that suggest hypothyroidism but are, in fact, euthyroid. This condition, called euthyroid sick syndrome, does not require treatment

with thyroid replacement and resolves within a few weeks of recovery, but it may be difficult to distinguish from preexisting or new-onset hypothyroidism. Clinicians need to use other clinical symptoms to try to differentiate euthyroid sick syndrome from hypothyroidism. Even though it does not require treatment, the presence of euthyroid sick syndrome in a critically ill patient is a poor prognostic sign.

In contrast to hyperthyroidism, there is no role for thyroid scans or iodine uptake testing in patients with hypothyroidism. The only exception to this is when the clinician identifies a mass on physical examination. In that situation, scanning or other imaging is essential to determine the malignancy potential of the mass.

Differential Diagnosis

The differential diagnosis for hypothyroidism is broad and depends on the primary complaints given by patients. For patients with slowed mentation, depressed affect, or confusion, clinicians should suspect depression. Patients with lethargy and a slow pulse and low blood pressure might have adrenal insufficiency. Patients with constipation need to have colonic obstruction from a mass considered as well. In the elderly, common drugs that can cause depression (such as centrally acting antihypertensive agents), bradycardia (such as β-blockers or calcium channel blockers), constipation (calcium channel blockers), hair loss, or confusion also should be considered.

In patients with pituitary failure, other pituitary hormones are likely to be deficient as well, so clinicians should look for evidence of adrenal and gonadotropic failure.

Treatment

The treatment for hypothyroidism is thyroxine replacement (Synthroid, Levoxyl). The usual dose required to achieve full replacement is between 100 μg and 150 μg, although patients who are treated with radioactive iodine and have some remaining thyroid activity might require lower doses. For patients with known heart disease or at risk for heart problems, doses should be initiated at 25 to 50 μg with increases of 25 μg every 4 to 6 weeks guided by TSH levels. Young patients who are at low risk for cardiac problems can be started at doses of 100 μg.

In choosing an agent to use for thyroid replacement, there is good evidence that generic substitutes are just as effective as brand-name drugs. A detailed study examining the metabolic effectiveness of a variety of generic drugs compared to a brand-name medication demonstrated no clinical or subclinical differences among preparations. So even though clinicians often hear that they should use a brand-name drug to maintain the stability of the replacement dose, this is not supported by the evidence.

One area of uncertainty is whether the addition of triiodothyronine (T_3, Cytomel) adds additional benefit to thyroid replacement with thyroxine. In some studies with elderly patients, subjects with continued neurocognitive dysfunction benefited from the addition of T_3 at a dose of 125 μg, with a concomitant decrease in the T_4 dose of 50 μg. However, subsequent studies of younger patients (aged 29–44 years) failed to find any benefits of partial T_3 substitution. Furthermore, studies of patients on doses of T_4 adequate to restore TSH levels to normal have been found to have normal T_3 levels. At this time, routine use of T_3 cannot be recommended; however, for selected elderly patients who have lingering confusion, depression, or slow mentation on adequate doses of T_4, a trial of T_3 partial substitution might be tried.

Another situation where there is controversy is the use of thyroid replacement in patients with a mildly elevated TSH and a normal free T_4. This condition, called subacute hypothyroidism or mild hypothyroidism, is more common in white elderly women. Some studies have shown clinical improvement in symptoms when low doses of T_4 are given to these patients, although the patient populations tend to be those with preexisting thyroid disease (such as Graves' disease), and studies have had only a small number of patients. An expert panel has suggested using the TSH level as an indication for therapy. Patients with a TSH less than 10 do not require any therapy. Treatment is reasonable in those with a TSH level of 10.0 because these

---

Box 2	Symptoms and Signs of Hypothyroidism

Common Symptoms
Lethargy
Weight gain
Constipation
Slowed mentation, forgetfulness
Depression
Hair loss
Dry skin
Neck enlargement or goiter

Physical Examination Findings
Goiter
Low blood pressure and slow pulse
Hair thinning or loss
Dry skin
Confusion
Depressed affect
Non-pitting edema

patients may be most symptomatic and have a progression to overt hypothyroidism of 5%.

Monitoring

In general, once a patient receives a full replacement dose of T_4 (usually between 100 and 150 μg) and has a TSH consistently in the normal range, there is little likelihood that their thyroid requirement will change over time. Although many advocate annual retesting of TSH to ensure patients are euthyroid, there is no evidence to show this is necessary.

Some conditions do warrant closer monitoring of the TSH level. Because T_4 and T_3 are highly protein bound, any conditions where a patient's serum protein status changes should prompt additional testing. This includes conditions that lower serum protein levels, such as liver disease, nephrotic syndrome, or malnutrition, as well as those where serum proteins are increased, such as pregnancy or initiation of estrogen therapy. Because patients' dietary protein usually decreases with advancing age, older patients whose diet declines can also require monitoring and a lowering of their T_4 dose over time.

Patients with subclinical hypothyroidism also might benefit from annual retesting of their free T_4 levels. Approximately 10% of patients with subacute hypothyroidism progress to hypothyroidism within 3 years of diagnosis. Because of this, yearly testing is recommended. Also, 50% of patients with subacute hypothyroidism have positive anti-thyroid antibodies; however, routine testing for these is not recommended.

Complications

Most of the complications of hypothyroidism are associated with undertreatment or overtreatment. Patients with inadequately treated hypothyroidism are at higher risk for cardiac disease. On the other hand, over-replacement of thyroxine increases the risk of both atrial fibrillation and osteoporosis.

In addition, Hashimoto's thyroiditis is associated with other endocrine autoimmune diseases such as Addison's disease and pernicious anemia. Clinicians should be aware of these associations and not overlook new endocrine disorders that might have clinical features similar to hypothyroidism.

Finally, patients with Hashimoto's hypothyroidism also are at higher risk for the future development of lymphoma. Clinicians should educate patients about the need to have newly enlarged lymph nodes evaluated and be aggressive about evaluating symptoms or signs consistent with the development of a lymphoma.

References

Bunevicius R, Kazanavicius G, Zalinkevicius R, Prange AJ. Effects of thyroxine as compared with thyroxine plus triiodothyronine in patients with hypothyroidism. N Engl J Med 1999;340:424–9.

Dong BJ, Hauck WW, Gambertoglio JG, et al. Bioequivalence of generic and brand-name levothyroxine products in the treatment of hypothyroidism. JAMA 1997;277:1205–13.

Helfand M, Crapo LM. Screening for thyroid disease. Ann Intern Med 1990;112:840–9.

Sawin CT, Chopra D, Azizi F, et al. The aging thyroid. Increased prevalence of elevated serum thyrotropin levels in the elderly. JAMA 1979;242:1386–8.

Surks MI, Ortiz E, Daniels GH, et al. Subclinical thyroid disease: Scientific review and guidelines for diagnosis and management. JAMA 2004;291(2):228–38.

U.S. Preventive Services Task Force: Screening for thyroid disease. Available at http://www.ahrq.gov/clinic/uspstf/uspsthyr.htm [accessed July 11, 2014].

OBESITY

Method of
Heather Wadams, MD, MHA; and Seema Kumar, MD

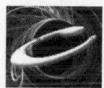

CURRENT DIAGNOSIS

- Body mass index (BMI) is calculated as weight in kilograms divided by height in meters squared (kg/m²). BMI is currently the preferred method for determining whether a patient is obese.

- Patients with a BMI of 30 or greater are considered obese; those with a BMI between 25 and 29.9 are considered overweight. For Asians, overweight is a BMI between 23 and 24.9 kg/m² and obesity a BMI >25 kg/m².
- Abdominal circumference should also be measured to assess for abdominal obesity.
- A waist circumference of >102 cm (40 in) in men or >88 cm (35 in) in women is considered indicative of abdominal obesity. A waist circumference of >80 cm in Asian females and >90 cm in Asian males is considered abnormal.

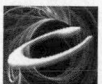

CURRENT THERAPY

- Treatment of patients with obesity requires a multidisciplinary team approach.
- Lifestyle modifications, including dietary changes and increased physical activity, remain first-line treatment for patients with obesity.
- Adjuvant pharmacotherapy may be considered for patients with a BMI greater than 30 kg/m² or a BMI of 27 to 30 kg/m² with concomitant weight-related complications.
- Bariatric surgery should be considered for patients with a BMI of 40 kg/m² or greater and for those with a BMI of 35 kg/m² or greater who have significant comorbidities such as severe diabetes, sleep apnea, or joint disease after nonsurgical weight loss attempts have failed.

Epidemiology

Obesity is a complex disease that represents a growing epidemic in the United States and worldwide. In the 2009 to 2010 National Health and Nutrition Examination Survey (NHANES), 35.5% of adult men and 35.8% of adult women were noted to be obese and there was no significant change noted compared with 2003 to 2008. In the United States, the lifetime risk of becoming overweight or obese is approximately 50% and 25%, respectively. There are disparities in the prevalence of obesity between ethnic groups, especially among women. In the United States, the prevalence of obesity is highest in non-Hispanic black women. The American Medical Association recently officially classified obesity as a disease due to its association with several comorbidities and increased mortality.

Diagnosis

Obesity is a condition marked by the accumulation of excess body fat. The body mass index (BMI) is the most practical way to evaluate the degree of excess weight. It is calculated from the weight (in kilograms) and the square of the height (in meters), as follows:

$$BMI = \frac{Weight}{Height^2}$$

The World Health Organization (WHO) and National Institutes of Health (NIH) define overweight as a BMI between 25 and 29.9 kg/m² and obesity as a BMI equal to greater than 30 kg/m² (Table 1). These guidelines apply to whites, Hispanics, and blacks. Because Asians can have higher percentage of body fat at a lower BMI, overweight for this particular ethnic group is a BMI between 23 and 24.9 kg/m², and obesity is a BMI equal to or greater than 25 kg/m². The BMI correlates with percentage of body fat and body fat mass as well as with mortality. The BMI may however overestimate the degree of body fat in athletes. However, for a given BMI, the degree of body fatness tends to be higher in women compared with men, and it is higher in older compared with younger people. The relationship between BMI and mortality appears to form a J- or U-shaped curve, with the lowest mortality rate seen in those with a BMI of about 25 kg/m² (Figure 1).

TABLE 1 Classification of Overweight and Obesity by BMI, Waist Circumference, and Associated Health Risk

		DISEASE RISK*	
CLASSIFICATION	BMI (kg/m²)	WAIST ≤102 cm (≤40 in) IN MEN OR ≤88 cm (≤35 in) IN WOMEN	WAIST >102 cm (>40 in) IN MEN OR >88 cm (>35 in) IN WOMEN
Underweight	<18.5	—	—
Normal†	18.5–24.9	—	—
Overweight	25.0–29.9	Increased	High
Obesity—class I	30.0–34.9	High	Very high
Obesity—class II	35.0–39.9	Very high	Very high
Extreme obesity—class III	>40	Extremely high	Extremely high

Reproduced from Clinical guidelines on the identification, evaluation, and treatment of overweight and obesity in adults: The evidence report. National Institutes of Health. Obes Res 1998;6(Suppl 2):51S–209S.

*Disease risk for type 2 diabetes, hypertension, and cardiovascular disease relative to normal weight and waist circumference.

†Increased waist circumference can also be a marker for increased risk even in persons of normal weight.

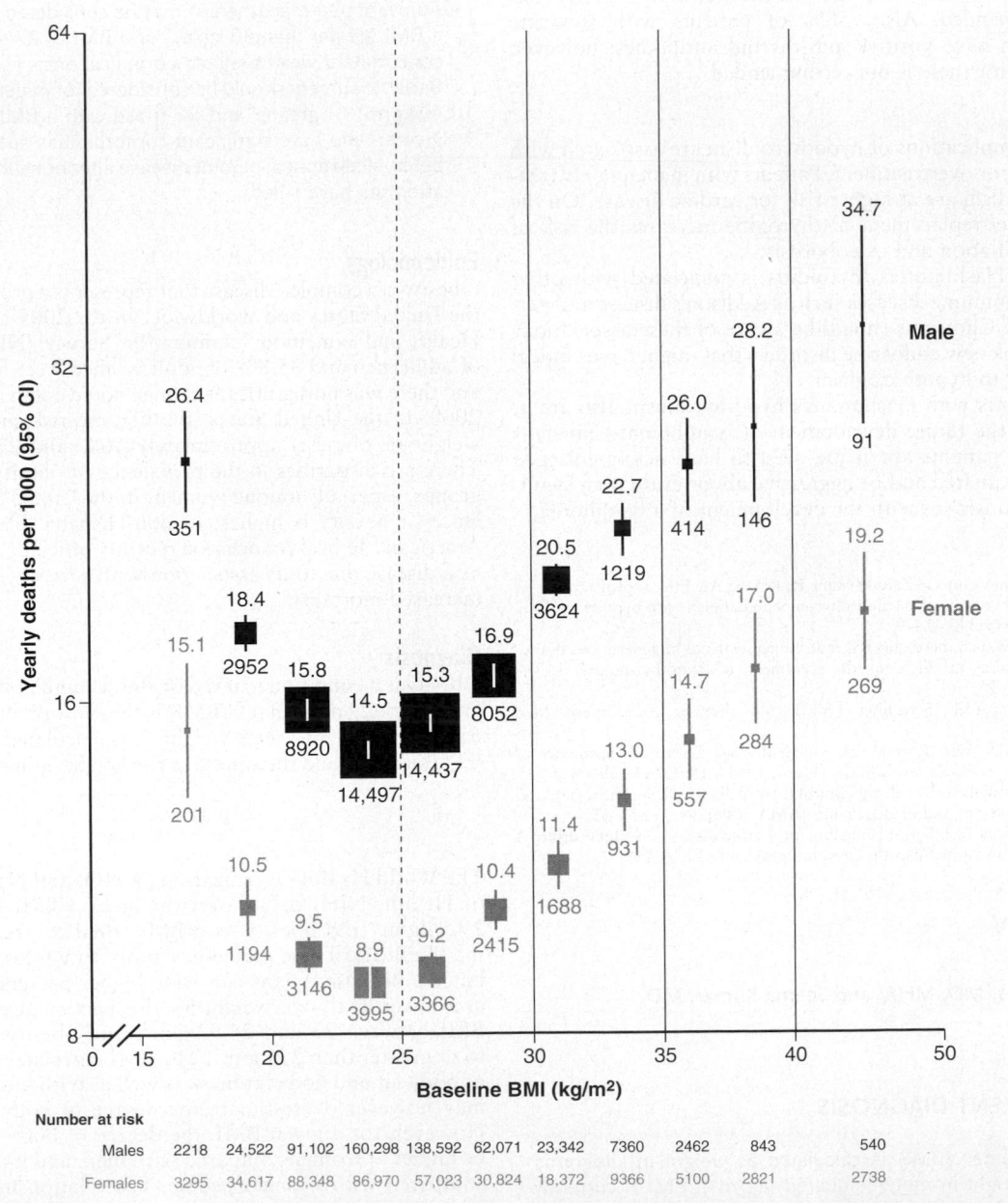

Figure 1. All-cause mortality versus body mass index (BMI) for each sex in the range of 15–50 kg/m² (excluding the first 5 years of follow-up). (From Whitlock G, Lewington S, Sherliker P, et al: Body-mass index and cause-specific mortality in 900,000 adults: Collaborative analyses of 57 prospective studies. Lancet 2009;373:1083).

Because people with abdominal (central) adiposity are more likely to develop many of the health conditions associated with obesity, waist circumference is an important adjuvant measurement to obtain when screening for obesity. Waist circumference is measured at the level of the top of the iliac crest with the measuring tape snug against the skin. In adults with a BMI of 25 to 34.9 kg/m², a waist circumference greater than 102 cm (40 in) for men and 88 cm (35 in) for women is associated with a greater risk of hypertension, type 2 diabetes, dyslipidemia, and coronary heart disease (CHD) (see Table 1). In patients with a BMI ≥ 35 kg/m², measurement of waist circumference is less helpful because it adds little to the predictive power of the disease risk classification of BMI; almost all individuals with this BMI also have an abnormal waist circumference. More precise measurement of abdominal fat can be made with abdominal computed tomography or magnetic resonance imaging. Alternative methods to assess body composition and degree of fatness include measurements of skin fold thickness, hydrostatic weighing, bioelectric impedance, and scanning by dual-energy x-ray absorptiometry. These methods require specialized equipment and trained personnel and are not used routinely in clinical practice.

Etiology and Pathophysiology

Obesity is a complex, multifactorial disease characterized by excessive caloric consumption and inadequate caloric expenditure. Many factors, including genetic and environmental influences, can contribute to the development of obesity. However, personal decisions regarding food choices, portion sizes, and level of activity also contribute to body size.

When evaluating a patient with obesity, it is important to rule out disorders such as Cushing's syndrome and hypothyroidism. Because many medications promote weight gain, including several antipsychotics, antidepressants, antiepileptics, sulfonylureas, and steroids (Table 2), it is prudent to obtain a complete medication history from any patient who is being evaluated for obesity. Single-gene mutations (e.g., in the melanocortin 4 receptor gene and leptin gene) and congenital syndromes (e.g., Prader-Willi, Bardet-Biedel, Cohen) typically cause early-onset obesity before 5 years of age.

Associated Comorbidities

Obesity is associated with a variety of other medical conditions that can increase morbidity and mortality. Comorbidities associated with obesity include metabolic syndrome and insulin resistance, type 2 diabetes, dyslipidemia, hypertension, coronary artery disease, degenerative joint disease, nonalcoholic fatty liver disease (NAFLD), and obstructive sleep apnea.

Insulin Resistance and Metabolic Syndrome

Insulin resistance is defined as a subnormal response to endogenous insulin. This results in pancreatic B-cell compensation with hypersecretion of insulin. Insulin resistance leads to various components of the metabolic syndrome, including low HDL cholesterol, high triglycerides, elevated blood pressure, and hyperglycemia. Patients may also manifest acanthosis nigricans and skin tags.

Type 2 Diabetes

The increasing prevalence of obesity has also resulted in an increasing prevalence of type 2 diabetes. More than 80% of type 2 diabetes can be attributed to obesity, but other factors, such as family history, are also involved. Criteria for the diagnosis of type 2 diabetes include a fasting glucose level greater than 125 mg/dL or glucose levels greater than 200 mg/dL during a 2-hour oral glucose tolerance test.

Hypertension

Hypertension is a common chronic disease, and it has been estimated that obesity is a major risk factor for hypertension. Hypertension is associated with an increased risk for stroke, myocardial infarction, heart failure, and kidney disease. Even a modest weight loss (5%–10% of initial weight) can lead to a significant fall in blood pressure and, often, decreased need for antihypertensive medications.

Dyslipidemia

A variety of blood lipid abnormalities are seen frequently in obese patients. These include elevated levels of total cholesterol, LDL cholesterol, and triglycerides and decreased levels of HDL cholesterol. Patients with central adiposity are at particularly high risk for the development of hypertriglyceridemia and low HDL. Screening for dyslipidemia should be done with a fasting lipid

TABLE 2 Drugs that Cause Weight Gain and Some Alternatives

CATEGORY	DRUGS THAT CAUSE WEIGHT GAIN	POSSIBLE ALTERNATIVES
Antipsychotics		
Conventional	Thioridazine (Mellaril)	Haloperidol (Haldol)
Atypical	Olanzapine (Zyprexa), clozapine (Clozaril), quetiapine (Seroquel), risperidone (Risperdal)	Ziprasidone (Geodon), aripiprazole (Abilify)
Lithium	Lithium carbonate (Eskalith)	
Antidepressants		
Tricyclics	Amitriptyline (Elavil), clomipramine (Anafranil), doxepin (Sinequan), imipramine (Tofranil), nortriptyline (Pamelor)	Protriptyline (Vivactil)
Selective serotonin reuptake inhibitors	Paroxetine (Paxil)	Other SSRIs
Other	Mirtazapine (Remeron)	Bupropion (Wellbutrin), nefazodone (Serzone)
Anticonvulsant drugs	Valproate (Depakene), carbamazepine (Tegretol), gabapentin (Neurontin)	Topiramate (Topamax), lamotrigine (Lamictal), zonisamide (Zonegran)
Antidiabetic drugs	Insulin, sulfonylureas, metiglinide, thiazolidinediones	Metformin (Glucophage), alpha-glucosidase inhibitors
Serotonin and histamine antagonist	Pizotifen[1]	
Antihistamines	Cyproheptidine (Periactin)	
Beta-adrenergic blockers	Propranolol (Inderal), atenolol (Tenormin), metoprolol (Lopressor)	
Steroid hormones	Glucocorticoids Progestins: megestrol acetate (Megace), medroxyprogesterone acetate (Provera)	

[1]Not available in the United States.
Copyright ©2001 George A Bray, MD. Reproduced with permission.

profile. However, if the testing opportunity is nonfasting, the total cholesterol and HDL values can still be measured.

Coronary Heart Disease

Comorbidities associated with obesity such as hypertension, insulin resistance, type 2 diabetes, and dyslipidemia lead to increased risk of cardiovascular disease in obese adults. Obesity is also associated with increased risk of CHD, heart failure, cardiovascular mortality, and all-cause mortality.

Respiratory Abnormalities

Obstructive sleep apnea is the most important respiratory problem associated with obesity. It is often underrecognized and inadequately treated. Patients may present with snoring, apneic episodes, excessive daytime somnolence, fatigue, irritability, and erectile dysfunction. Consequent nocturnal hypoxemia may result in arrhythmias, pulmonary hypertension, and right-sided heart failure. Treatment includes weight loss and use of continuous positive airway pressure at night. Other alterations in pulmonary function that may occur, include higher residual lung volume associated with increased abdominal pressure on the diaphragm, decreased lung compliance and increased chest wall impedance, ventilation-perfusion abnormalities, reduced strength and endurance of respiratory muscles, depressed ventilatory drive, and bronchospasm.

Gastroesophageal Disease

Obesity is associated with an increased risk of gastroesophageal reflux disease symptoms as well as erosive esophagitis, esophageal adenocarcinoma, and gastric carcinoma. It has been suggested that increased intragastric pressure and relaxation of the lower esophageal sphincter from gastric compression from surrounding adiposity contributes to the reflux rather than the type of diet consumed.

Hepatobiliary Disease

Obesity increases the risk of cholelithiasis and of NAFLD. The spectrum of NAFLD ranges from steatosis with mild disruption of the liver architecture by fat to steatohepatitis with varying degrees of fibrosis and cirrhosis. Increased liver transaminase levels and findings of steatosis on ultrasonography are both suggestive of NAFLD in obese patients. However, the definitive diagnosis remains histologic.

Osteoarthritis

The incidence of osteoarthritis is increased in obese subjects. Osteoarthritis commonly develops in the knees and ankles but can also affect non–weight-bearing joints. Weight loss results in decreased risk of osteoarthritis.

Cancer

For both men and women, increased BMI is associated with increased mortality from several cancers, such as those of the esophagus, colon and rectum, liver, gallbladder, pancreas, and kidney, as well as non-Hodgkin lymphoma and multiple myeloma. Additionally, obese men are at increased risk of death from stomach and prostate cancer, and obese women are at increased risk of death from cancers of the breast, uterus, cervix, and ovary.

Psychosocial Function

Obese subjects often are subjected to discrimination in education, employment, and health care. Overweight women have been noted to have lower household incomes and higher rates of household poverty than women who were not overweight, independent of their baseline socioeconomic status and aptitude test scores. Depression has also been seen in association with severe obesity, particularly in younger patients and in women.

Economic Consequences of Obesity

Overweight and obesity and their associated health problems have a significant economic impact on the health care system. Health care costs are higher in obese subjects compared to their normal weight counterparts. The higher costs are predominantly explained by the presence of CHD, hypertension, and diabetes.

Treatment

Patients must undergo a detailed history and physical examination before a treatment plan is initiated. Secondary causes of obesity, such as Cushing's syndrome and hypothyroidism, should be considered in the evaluation. A complete medication history is crucial to determining whether any medications may have promoted weight gain.

Laboratory studies should be directed at ruling out secondary causes in selected patients and ruling out comorbidities (fasting glucose, lipid profile, liver function tests). It is important that practitioners assess each patient's willingness to change and expectations for weight loss. Treatment should be based on the patient's BMI, risk factors, and willingness to lose weight. Patients who are in the precontemplative phase (i.e., in the early stages of thinking about it) are not likely to be successful despite appropriate counseling. Health care providers must enforce the idea that even a modest weight loss improves complications associated with obesity.

Treatment of obesity requires a multidisciplinary team approach. Lifestyle modifications, including dietary change and increased physical activity, represent first-line treatment for patients with obesity. Pharmacotherapy and bariatric surgery may be used as adjuvant therapies in certain patients.

The goal of treatment is to prevent the complications of obesity. The initial target goal of weight loss therapy is to decrease body weight by 5% to 10%. Once this target is achieved, further weight loss can be attempted if indicated. The rationales for this initial goal of moderate weight loss are that:

- It can decrease the severity of obesity-associated risk factors.
- It can set the stage for further weight loss, if indicated.
- It is realistic and can be achieved and maintained over time.

A reasonable timeline for a 5% to 10% reduction in body weight is 6 months of therapy. A period of weight maintenance should then occur. Further weight loss may be considered if the initial goal is achieved and then maintained for at least 6 months. It is important to inform patients that it is preferable to maintain a moderate amount of weight loss over time than to lose more weight but later regain it.

Behavior Modification

Behavior modification is an integral part of any weight loss program. Motivational interviewing (MI) is a client-centered, collaborative decision-making approach that is helpful in facilitating lifestyle modifications. MI helps the health care provider provide nonjudgmental feedback to patients, allowing for patients' resistance to change and encouraging patients to develop their own arguments for engaging in health behavior change.

The goal of behavioral therapy is to help patients make long-term changes in their eating behavior by modifying and monitoring their food intake, increasing their physical activity, and controlling cues and stimuli in the environment that trigger eating. Maintaining food diaries and activity records for self-monitoring are key elements in any successful behavioral weight loss program. Stimulus control is considered a key element in a behavioral program. It focuses on gaining control over the environmental factors that activate eating and eliminating or modifying the environmental factors that facilitate overeating.

This requires the availability of trained personnel such as psychologists and therapists. The behavioral strategies taught are aimed at decreasing caloric intake and increasing physical activity in the long term.

Dietary Therapy

The goal of dietary therapy, therefore, is to reduce the total number of calories consumed. A principal determinant of weight loss appears to be the degree of adherence to the diet, irrespective of the particular macronutrient composition. Recent data suggest that the so-called Mediterranean diet and low-carbohydrate diets may represent effective alternatives to the low-fat diet for weight loss. Thus, the macronutrient mix of the diet should be based upon patient preferences in order to improve long-term adherence. Often patients revert to their previous habit of eating and can regain the weight that was lost. Diets that incorporate the patient's preference and culture to find the optimal mix of macronutrients will have the best chance of success.

Approximately 22 kcal/kg is required to maintain a kilogram of body weight in a normal adult. Thus, the expected or calculated energy expenditure for a woman weighing 100 kg is approximately 2200 kcal/day. The variability of ±20% could give energy needs as high as 2620 kcal/day or as low as 1860 kcal/day. An average deficit of 500 kcal/day should result in an initial weight loss of approximately 0.5 kg/week (1 lb/week). However, after 3 to 6 months of weight loss, energy expenditure adaptations occur, which slow the body weight response to a given change in energy intake, thereby diminishing ongoing weight loss.

Patients should be counseled to avoid unnecessary calories from alcohol and sugary beverages such as soda and juice.

Very–low-calorie diets contain less than 800 kcal/day and are usually administered in the form of liquid supplements. Although these diets do produce significant and rapid weight loss, results are difficult to maintain in the long term. These diets require close monitoring by a health care professional. Side effects associated with very–low-calorie diets include fatigue, constipation, hair loss, and gallstones. These diets are strictly contraindicated in children and in pregnant and lactating women and are generally reserved for patients who require rapid weight loss for a specific purpose such as surgery.

Physical Activity

Physical activity is an integral component of therapy for obese patients and is most important in the prevention of weight regain. Physical activity also decreases the risks for cardiovascular disease and type 2 diabetes. Sedentary obese patients need to start their exercise program slowly and may require supervision from a health care professional. Initially, patients may be encouraged to increase their activities of daily living. For example, it may be suggested that they take the stairs instead of the elevator or that they park farther away from work or shopping. The intensity and duration of exercise should be increased gradually over time, with a goal of achieving 30 minutes of moderate-intensity activity on most days of the week to improve health (150 minutes/week) and 60 minutes of exercise of most days of the week to control body weight.

Ideally, adults should also perform muscle-strengthening exercises on 2 or more days per week. Patients should be encouraged to choose activities that they enjoy and to build these activities into their daily schedule. Sedentary activities, such as watching television, sitting in front of a computer screen, and playing video games, should be discouraged.

Pharmacotherapy

Pharmacotherapy (Table 3) is usually reserved for patients with a BMI greater than 30 kg/m^2 without complications or a BMI greater than 27 to 30 kg/m^2 with concomitant weight-related complications. These patients should have failed to achieve weight loss goals through diet and exercise alone. Pharmacotherapy must be used in conjunction with a program that includes dietary changes and physical activity.

The success may be measured by the degree of weight loss and improvement in associated risk factors. Weight loss should be more than 5% below baseline to be considered effective. A weight loss of 5% to 10% can significantly reduce the baseline risk factors for diabetes and cardiovascular disease and improvement in baseline risk factors after weight loss is an important criterion in the determination of whether to continue therapy.

Orlistat (Xenical) is recommended as the first-line drug for patients with dyslipidemia and/or diabetes. Orlistat is an inhibitor of pancreatic lipases that causes weight loss by limiting fat absorption. The recommended dose for adults is 120 mg PO three times daily with meals. A lower dose of 60 mg preparation (Alli) is available over the counter in the United States and several other countries. Orlistat has been shown to be effective for weight loss and prevention of weight regain. In a meta-analysis of 12 trials that included patients with and without diabetes and reported data with 12-month outcomes, patients randomly assigned to orlistat plus a behavioral intervention lost 5 to 10 kg (8% of baseline weight) compared with 3 to 6 kg in the control group (placebo plus behavioral intervention), for a mean placebo-subtracted difference of 3 kg. Weight loss was maintained with up to 24 to 36 months of orlistat treatment. Orlistat has also been shown to result in improved metabolic outcomes such as delay in development of type 2 diabetes in those that have impaired fasting glucose and improvement in blood pressure in hypertensive patients and in serum total and LDL cholesterol levels. Side effects associated with orlistat are mostly gastrointestinal and include cramping, flatus, fecal incontinence, oily spotting, and flatus with discharge. These side effects tend to decrease over time as patients learn to restrict their dietary intake to less than 30% fat. Severe cases of liver damage have been reported in patients taking orlistat. Orlistat may also interfere with the absorption of fat-soluble vitamins, so the use of a daily multivitamin supplement at bedtime is recommended.

Lorcaserin hydrochloride (Belviq) is a serotonin 2C receptor agonist that causes weight loss by causing appetite suppression. It

TABLE 3 Drugs Approved by the FDA for Treatment of Obesity		
DRUG	**DOSAGE**	**ADVERSE SIDE EFFECTS**
Pancreatic Lipase Inhibitor Approved for Long-Term Use		
Orlistat (Xenical)	120 mg tid before meals	Cramps, flatulence, diarrhea, oily spotting
Appetite Suppressants Approved for Long-Term Use		
Lorcaserin hydrochloride (Belviq)	10 mg bid	Headache, dizziness, nausea, nasopharyngitis
Phentermine/topiramate (Qsymia)	7.5 mg/46 mg/d*	Dry mouth, tachycardia, depression, anxiety
Noradrenergic Drugs Approved for Short-Term Use		
Phentermine (Adipex-P)	Immediate release: 15–37.5 mg/d	Increase in blood pressure or in heart rate, insomnia, nervousness Dry mouth, constipation Abuse potential due to amphetamine-like effects
Ionamin[1]	Slow-release resin 15–30 mg/d	
Diethylpropion (Tenuate)	Immediate release: 25 mg tid Controlled release: 75 mg every morning	Same
Benzphetamine (Didrex)	25–50 mg tid	Same
Phendimetrazine (Bontril PDM)	17.5–70 mg tid Extended release: 105 mg/d	Same

[1]Not available in the United States.
*Maintenance dose.

appears to have fewer adverse effects than orlistat, although long-term safety data are limited. The recommended dosage is 10 mg twice daily. Lorcaserin should be discontinued if patients do not lose 5% of their body weight in 12 weeks. The efficacy of lorcaserin appears similar to that of orlistat (mean difference in weight loss between active and placebo-treated groups approximately 3–4 kg). Common side effects include nausea, headache, dizziness, nasopharyngitis, and fatigue. Lorcaserin may increase the risk of symptomatic hypoglycemia in patients with type 2 diabetes on oral agents, necessitating a reduction in the dose of diabetes medications. Lorcaserin should not be used in individuals with creatinine clearance <30 mL/minute. It is contraindicated during pregnancy. In addition, lorcaserin should not be used with other serotonergic drugs (e.g., selective serotonin reuptake inhibitors, selective serotonin-norepinephrine reuptake inhibitors, bupropion [Wellbutrin], tricyclic antidepressants, and monamine oxidase inhibitors) because of the theoretical potential for serotonin syndrome.

Qsymia is a combination of phentermine (Adipex-P), an appetite suppressant, and topiramate, a medication used to treat epilepsy and migraine. The initial dose of phentermine/topiramate is 3.75/23 mg for 14 days, followed by 7.5/46 mg thereafter. If after 12 weeks, a 3% loss in bodyweight is not achieved, the dose can be increased to 11.25/69 mg for 14 days, and then to 15/92 mg daily. If an individual does not lose 5% of body weight after 12 weeks on the highest dose, phentermine/topiramate should be discontinued gradually, as abrupt withdrawal of topiramate can cause seizures. Qsymia is contraindicated during pregnancy due to an increased risk of orofacial clefts in infants exposed to the combination drug during the first trimester of pregnancy. Women of child-bearing age should have a pregnancy test before starting this drug and monthly thereafter. It is also contraindicated in patients with glaucoma, hyperthyroidism, and individuals who have taken monoamine oxidase inhibitors within 14 days. Clinicians who prescribe phentermine/topiramate are encouraged to enroll in a risk evaluation and mitigation strategy, which includes an online or print formal training module detailing safety information. Pharmacies that dispense Qsymia also require a specific certification and have to provide patients with a medication guide and brochure each time the drug is dispensed, detailing the risks of birth defects.

Side effects for Qsymia include tachycardia, paresthesias, dizziness, altered taste sensation, insomnia, and constipation. Qsymia is not recommended in patients with cardiovascular disease (hypertension or CHD) and may be considered for obese postmenopausal women and men without cardiovascular disease, particularly those who do not tolerate orlistat or lorcaserin.

Contrave, a combination of bupropion, an antidepressant/anorexiant with naltrexone, an opioid-receptor antagonist was approved by the Food and Drug Administration in September 2014 as an adjunct to diet and exercise in patients with BMI ≥30 kg/m² (or ≥27 kg/m² with comorbidities). The initial dose is one tablet (8 mg of naltrexone and 90 mg of bupropion) daily. After one week, the dose is increased to one tablet twice daily, and by week four to two tablets twice daily. If after 12 weeks the patient has not lost at least 5 percent of baseline body weight, the drug should be discontinued because benefit is unlikely. Contraindications include concomitant use of other bupropion-containing products, chronic opioid use, uncontrolled hypertension, eating disorder, seizure disorders, and use within 14 days of taking monoamine oxidase inhibitors. Side effects for bupropion-naltrexone include nausea, headache, constipation, insomnia vomiting, constipation, dizziness, and dry mouth.

Liraglutide (Saxenda) is a long acting glucagon-like polypeptide-1 (GLP-1) receptor agonist that is recommended for chronic weight management in conjunction with reduced-calorie diet and physical activity. It is recommended for patients with BMI ≥30 kg/m² or ≥27 kg/m² if one weight-related comorbidity is present. Liraglutide is administered subcutaneously in the abdomen, thigh, or upper arm once daily. The initial dose is 0.6 mg daily for one week. The dose can be increased at weekly intervals (1.2, 1.8, 2.4 mg) to the recommended dose of 3 mg. If after 16 weeks a patient has not lost at least 4 percent of baseline body weight, liraglutide should be discontinued, as it is unlikely the patient will achieve clinically meaningful weight loss with continued treatment. Liraglutide is contraindicated in those with a personal history or family history of medullary thyroid cancer or multiple endocrine neoplasia type 2 or 2B. Side effects for liraglutide include headache, nausea, vomiting, diarrhea, and constipation which tend to be dose-related. Hypoglycemia can occur in non-diabetics but at a lower frequency than type 2 diabetics.

Several sympathomimetic drugs (phentermine, benzphetamine [Didrex], diethylpropion [Tenuate], and phendimetrazine [Bontril PDM]) are approved for the short-term (up to 12 weeks) treatment of obesity. These drugs can increase blood pressure and have a potential for abuse and therefore are contraindicated in patients with CHD, hypertension, or hyperthyroidism or in patients with a history of drug abuse.

Vagal blockade device is available in the United States for the treatment of adults with a BMI of 40 to 45 kg/m² or of 35 to 39.9 kg/m² with at least one obesity-related comorbidity (eg, type 2 diabetes) who have failed a supervised weight management program within the past five years. The abdominal vagal nerve controls gastric emptying and signals the satiety center in the brain. Electric stimulation of the abdominal vagal nerve from the subcutaneously implanted device blocks vagal nerve conduction between the brain and the stomach, thereby reducing hunger. However, the specific mechanism for weight loss is unknown. Implantation of the device involves laparoscopically placing one lead on the anterior vagal trunk and the other on the posterior intra-abdominal vagal trunk. Adverse events include pain at the neuroregulator site, vomiting, surgical complications, nausea, heartburn, belching and dysphagia. Implantation of the device is contraindicated in patients at high risk for surgical complications, patients with other permanent implanted devices (eg, heart pacemaker, implanted defibrillator, neurostimulator), or patients likely to need magnetic resonance imaging (MRI) procedures.

Bariatric Surgery

Bariatric surgery should be considered for patients with a BMI greater than 40 kg/m² or a BMI greater than 35 kg/m² with significant comorbid conditions. Patients should be well informed and motivated and have failed a trial of nonsurgical weight loss. They should also be of acceptable risk for surgery. Contraindications to bariatric surgery include untreated major depression or psychosis, binge eating disorders, active drug or alcohol abuse, and the inability to comply with nutritional requirements including lifelong vitamin supplementation. A comprehensive preoperative evaluation and close extended follow-up after surgery are required. Bariatric surgery has been shown to result in a significant and sustained weight loss as well as resolution of many obesity-related complications, in most patients. Patients may lose more than 60% of their excess weight after bariatric surgery. There is increasing interest in the role of bariatric surgery as a treatment for type 2 diabetes in obese patients who have a BMI less than 35 kg/m². Several unblinded trials comparing bariatric surgery with medical therapy for type 2 diabetes have demonstrated significantly greater improvements in blood glucose control in patients who underwent bariatric surgery. However, long-term data are required before bariatric surgery procedures can be routinely recommended for the treatment of persistent hyperglycemia, resistant to multiple medications, in patients with mild obesity.

Bariatric procedures can be divided into three types: restrictive procedures, which decrease gastric volume and limit food intake; malabsorptive procedures, which alter digestion of food and decrease the effectiveness of nutrient absorption; and mixed procedures, which have components of both restriction and malabsorption. Currently, the most common procedures performed in the United States are the laparoscopic Roux-en-Y gastric bypass (RYGB), sleeve gastrectomy, and the laparoscopic adjustable band (a restrictive procedure) (Figure 2).

Roux-en-Y Gastric Bypass

The RYGB is characterized by a small (less than 30 mL) proximal gastric pouch that is divided and separated from the distal stomach and anastomosed to a Roux limb of small bowel, 75 to 150 cm in

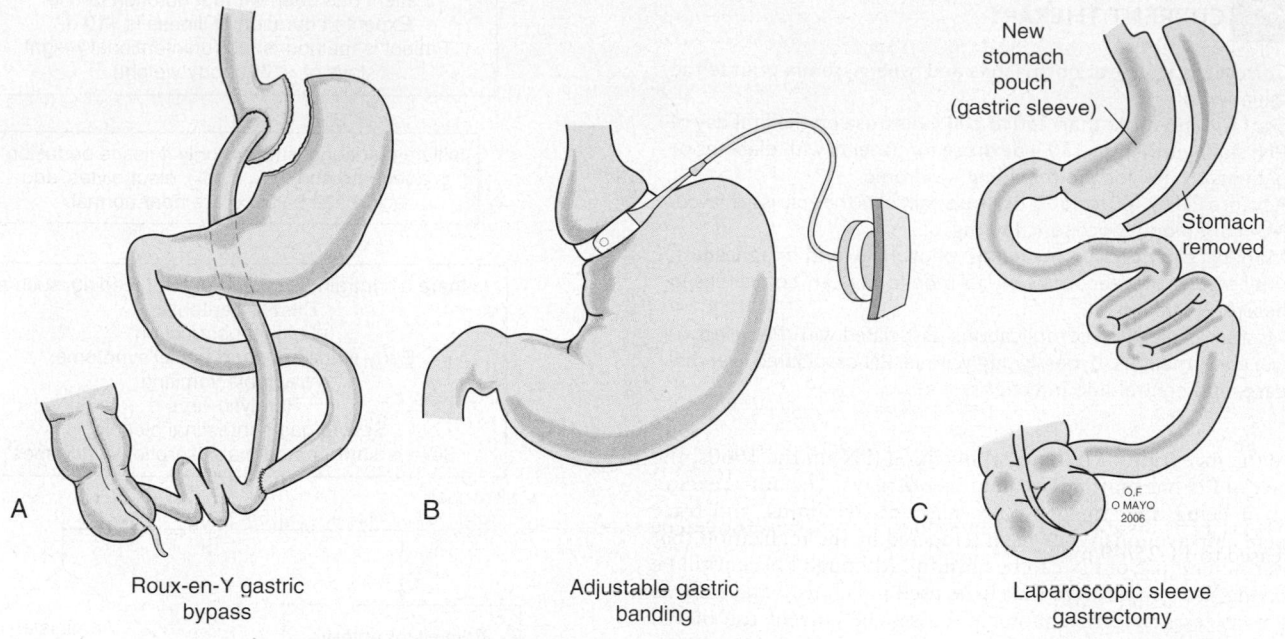

Common bariatric procedures

A — Roux-en-Y gastric bypass

B — Adjustable gastric banding

C — Laparoscopic sleeve gastrectomy

New stomach pouch (gastric sleeve)

Stomach removed

O.F O MAYO 2006

Figure 2. Techniques commonly used for the surgical treatment of obesity: Roux-en-Y gastric bypass (A), adjustable laparoscopic band (B), laparoscopic sleeve gastrectomy (C).

length. It is the most commonly performed bariatric procedure and involves the creation of a small pouch at the superior portion of the stomach. The pouch is then connected to the jejunum, bypassing the duodenum, where the majority of calories are absorbed. The mortality rate associated with gastric bypass is low (<1%), but patients can have significant postoperative complications, including pulmonary emboli, deep vein thromboses, leaks from the gastrointestinal tract, gastric remnant distention, stomal stenosis, ulcers, gallstones, and hernias. Patients are required to take lifelong vitamin and mineral supplementation because absorption of iron, vitamin B_{12}/folate, and others are affected.

Laparoscopic Sleeve Gastrectomy

Laparoscopic sleeve gastrectomy (LSG), the second-most commonly performed bariatric procedure, is emerging as a single-stage bariatric procedure. It is a restrictive, nonreversible procedure involving removal of about 85% of the stomach so that the remainder takes the shape of a tube or sleeve. Recent studies have shown that LSG has equivalent results to other procedures. There is durability of results 5 to 9 years following the procedure, but there is no long term data beyond this. Gastric-sleeve dilatations and staple-line leaks are the most common complications. LSG involves no foreign body, needs no invasive adjustments, and most likely avoids malabsorption of many micronutrients.

Laparoscopic Adjustable Gastric Band

Adjustable gastric banding is a purely restrictive procedure that compartmentalizes the upper stomach by placing a tight, adjustable prosthetic band around the entrance to the stomach. The gastric band consists of a soft, locking silicone ring that is connected to an infusion port placed in the subcutaneous tissue. The port can be accessed with a needle and syringe, and injection or removal of saline into the port may be used to manipulate the size of the band diameter, leading to greater or lesser degrees of restriction. Although weight loss with banding tends to be slower than with other weight loss procedures, the procedure is popular because it is performed laparoscopically and is reversible. Laparoscopic banding can also be associated with side effects such as stomal obstruction; band erosion, slippage, or prolapse; port malfunction; pouch or esophageal dilation; and infection.

Investigational procedures for weight loss include an intragastric balloon, endoluminal vertical gastroplasty, implantable gastric pacing, and endoscopic gastric intestinal bypass devices.

In conclusion, obesity is a growing public health problem that has significant short- and long-term consequences. Lifestyle modification with or without adjuvant therapies should be used to achieve a goal of modest weight loss. With modest weight loss, patients experience a decreased risk of mortality and improvement of obesity-related complications.

References

Bray GA, Ryan DH. Medical therapy for the patient with obesity. Circulation 2012;125:1695–703.

Jensen MD, Ryan DH, Donato KA, et al. 2013 AHA/ACC/TOS guideline for the management of overweight and obesity in adults: A report of the American College of Cardiology/ American Heart Association Task Force on Practice Guidelines and The Obesity Society. Obesity 2013;21.

Mechanick JI, Youdim A, Jones DB, et al. Clinical practice guidelines for the perioperative nutritional, metabolic, and nonsurgical support of the bariatric surgery patient—2013 update: Cosponsored by American Association of Clinical Endocrinologists, The Obesity Society, and American Society for Metabolic & Bariatric Surgery. Endocr Pract 2013;19:337–72.

Sacks FM, Bray GA, Carey VJ, et al. Comparison of weight-loss diets with different compositions of fat, protein, and carbohydrates. N Engl J Med 2009;360:859.

The Practical Guide: Identification, Evaluation, and Treatment of Overweight and Obesity in Adults. http://www.nhlbi.nih.gov/guidelines/obesity/prctgd_c.pdf.

PARENTERAL NUTRITION IN ADULTS

Method of
**Kris M. Mogensen, MS, RD, LDN, CNSC;
and Malcolm K. Robinson, MD**

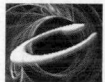

CURRENT DIAGNOSIS

- Reserve parenteral nutrition (PN) for patients with intestinal dysfunction or failure.
- Reserve PN for conditions such as short-bowel syndrome, severe malabsorption, ileus or intestinal dysmotility, intractable vomiting, and severe diarrhea.
- Always reevaluate the need for PN and work toward a transition to enteral nutrition, or an oral diet, if possible, to limit complications associated with PN.

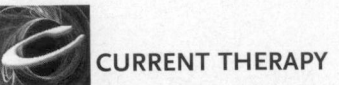

- Correct electrolyte abnormalities and hyperglycemia prior to the initiation of PN.
- Start with no more than 150 to 200 g dextrose on the first day of PN; start with 100 to 150 g dextrose for patients with diabetes or patients at risk for the refeeding syndrome.
- Advance PN by 100 to 150 g dextrose daily until the goal is achieved.
- Maintain blood glucose <180 mg/dL.
- Monitor electrolytes, including phosphate and magnesium, until stable; the frequency of lab monitoring can be decreased based on stability.
- Monitor closely for complications associated with PN: electrolyte abnormalities, hyper/hypoglycemia, PN-associated liver disease, and central line infections.

Since the inception of parenteral nutrition (PN) in the 1960s, the science of PN has matured in a number of ways. The initial excitement of being able to feed basic nutrients, vitamins, and trace elements intravenously has been tempered by the realization that indiscriminant use of PN can be harmful. Although PN can still be lifesaving, it is imperative that it be used judiciously and only as long as necessary. This chapter discusses the current use of PN in adult patients.

Indications and Contraindications

Enteral nutrition (EN) is the preferred method of nutrition support, primarily because it is associated with fewer infectious and metabolic complications. However, total PN (TPN), which is the provision of all nutrient requirements intravenously, may be indicated when feeding through the gastrointestinal (GI) tract is not possible. PN may be appropriately initiated in those who cannot receive enteral nourishment and are malnourished or at risk for developing malnourishment. Malnourishment can be defined as unintentional loss of more than 10% of usual body weight or greater than 7 to 10 days of inadequate nutrient intake. The body stores of well-nourished persons are generally sufficient to provide the essential nutrients, resist infection, promote wound healing, and support other necessary physiologic functions for this time period. In patients who are anticipated not to be able to receive adequate EN for longer than 10 days, it is not necessary to wait 10 days before initiating PN. This may include patients with short-bowel syndrome and others who are expected to have prolonged GI dysfunction.

According to the American Society for Parenteral and Enteral Nutrition (A.S.P.E.N.) guidelines, EN is contraindicated in conditions such as diffuse peritonitis, intestinal obstruction, early stages of short-bowel syndrome, intractable vomiting, paralytic ileus, severe GI bleeding, and severe diarrhea and malabsorption syndromes. Other relative contraindications to EN include severe pancreatitis and enterocutaneous fistulae, although depending on the clinical circumstances, EN may be indicated. PN and EN may be provided concomitantly, although in patients who are critically ill, PN should not be started until all strategies to maximize enteral feeding (such as the use of postpyloric feeding tubes and motility agents) have been attempted. PN support is unlikely to benefit a patient who will be able to take EN within 4 or 5 days after the onset of illness or who has a relatively minor injury (Figure 1).

There are four key steps to consider before initiating PN, including assessing nutritional status, determining energy needs, evaluating GI function, and estimating the length of time a patient will require PN (Box 1).

Assessment of Nutritional Status

Nutrient depletion is associated with increased morbidity and mortality, and the prevalence of malnutrition in hospitalized patients is approximately 50%. Therefore, it is imperative to identify patients who have or are at risk for developing protein-energy malnutrition or specific nutrient deficiencies. A patient's risk of developing malnutrition-related medical complications needs

Consider nutritional support if any are present:
Patient has been without nutrition for 7 d.
Expected duration of illness is >10 d.
Patient is malnourished (unintentional weight loss of >10% body weight).

Initiate nutritional support only if tissue perfusion is adequate and PO_2, PCO_2, electrolytes, and acid-base balance are near normal.

Is there a contraindication to enteral feeding, such as:
Diffuse peritonitis
Intestinal obstruction
Early stages of short bowel syndrome
Intractable vomiting
Paralytic ileus
Severe gastrointestinal bleeding
Severe diarrhea and malabsorption syndromes

No — Administer enteral nutrition

Yes — Administer parenteral nutrition

Enteral nutrition tolerated

Enteral nutrition not tolerated or partially tolerated

Figure 1. Determining route of feeding.

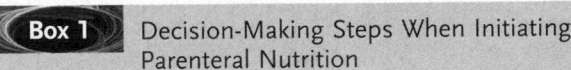

Box 1 Decision-Making Steps When Initiating Parenteral Nutrition

Assess the patient's nutritional status. Nutrition support (PN and/or EN) should not be initiated in well-nourished patients unless they have received a suboptimal diet for more than 7 d.

Determine if the patient has extreme energy needs (hypermetabolism) that warrant the early use of nutrition support (PN and/or EN) within 7 d of injury or illness. These are typically critically ill patients who have suffered severe burns or trauma.

Evaluate the function of the GI tract; if it is intact and can be used safely, PN should be avoided. PN support is indicated until enteral access is established and the patient can meet nutrient needs via tube feedings.

Estimate how long the patient will require PN support. If GI function is expected to return within 5 d, there is no known benefit of initiating PN.

Abbreviations: EN = enteral nutrition; GI = gastrointestinal; PN = parenteral nutrition.

to be quantified, and it is necessary to monitor the adequacy of nutritional therapy.

Nutrition assessment begins with a thorough history and physical examination in conjunction with select laboratory tests aimed at detecting specific nutrient deficiencies in patients who are at high risk for future abnormalities. The nutrition assessment should establish whether the patient will need maintenance therapy or nutrition repletion and should assess the status of the patient's GI tract, especially if nutrition support will be required.

A thorough history includes an assessment of recent weight changes, dietary habits, GI symptoms, and changes in exercise tolerance or physical abilities that would indicate functional capacity deficiencies. The physical examination includes inspecting for a loss of subcutaneous fat and muscle wasting, which indicate a loss of body energy and protein stores; edema and ascites, which can also indicate altered energy demands or decreased energy intake; and signs of vitamin and mineral deficits such as dermatitis, glossitis, cheilosis, neuromuscular irritability, and coarse, easily pluckable hair.

Several laboratory measurements have been used as nutritional biomarkers to aid the nutritional assessment. The serum proteins prealbumin, transferrin, and retinol-binding protein have a rapid turnover rate and short half-lives and therefore may be used as indicators of recent nutritional intake. However, these proteins are affected by the metabolic responses to stress and illness as well as other conditions, including iron status (transferrin) and renal status (retinol-binding protein, prealbumin). This can limit their usefulness during acute illness states.

Prealbumin is least affected by fluctuations in hydration status and by liver and renal function compared with other plasma proteins. However, prealbumin levels drop in acute inflammatory conditions during which the liver switches to acute-phase protein production and decreases prealbumin synthesis. A rise in C-reactive protein, a protein synthesized by the liver as part of the acute-phase response, indicates inflammatory states. Thus, C-reactive protein, when measured along with prealbumin, can help differentiate a low prealbumin due to nutritional inadequacy versus low prealbumin due to an acute-phase response.

The serum albumin concentration has traditionally been used as an indicator of nutritional status. Although it is a good preoperative predictor of outcome for patients undergoing surgery, it is affected by too many variables in the acute care setting to make it a reliable marker of nutritional status under such conditions or in the immediate postoperative period.

A simple and practical index of malnutrition is the degree of weight loss. Unintentional weight loss of greater than 10% within the previous 6 months indicates protein-energy malnutrition and is a good prognosticator of clinical outcome. Weight can also be compared with an ideal or desirable weight, or an index of body weight relative to height. The body mass index (BMI), reported as weight in kilograms divided by height in meters squared, is the best known such index and can be used to detect both undernutrition and overnutrition. This index is independent of height, and the same standards apply to both men and women. A BMI of 18.5 to 25 kg/m^2 is considered normal, 25 to 29.9 kg/m^2 is considered overweight, and greater than 30 kg/m^2 is considered obese. Patients with a normal or high BMI can still have nutrient deficiencies and therefore can be malnourished if they have recently lost a significant amount of weight. In addition, a BMI of 18 kg/m^2 or less in an adult indicates moderate malnutrition and a BMI less than 15 kg/m^2 is associated with increased morbidity.

Another practical tool for evaluating nutritional status is the subjective global assessment (SGA) that encompasses historical, symptomatic, and physical parameters. The SGA technique determines if nutrient assimilation has been restricted because of decreased food intake, maldigestion, or malabsorption; if any effects of malnutrition on organ function and body composition have occurred; and if the patient's disease process influences nutrient requirements. The findings of the history and physical examination are subjectively weighted to rank patients as being well nourished, moderately malnourished, or severely malnourished and are used to predict their risk for medical complications (Box 2).

Estimating Nutritional Requirements

Historically, TPN often provided nutrients in excess of actual requirements. This was based on the assumption that patients requiring nutritional intervention were severely depleted and required aggressive repletion, hence the misnomer "hyperalimentation." Overfeeding is associated with increased carbon dioxide production and difficulty weaning from a ventilator as well as metabolic complications, such as hyperglycemia, which can lead to increased infection, morbidity, and mortality. Thus,

Box 2   Subjective Global Assessment

Select the appropriate category with a checkmark, or enter a numeric value where indicated by #.

History
- Weight change
  Overall loss in past 6 mo: amount = # _____ kg; % loss = # _____.
  Change in past 2 wk: _____ increase, _____ no change, _____ decrease.
- Dietary intake change (relative to normal)
  _____ No change.
  _____ Change duration = # _____ wk.
  _____ Type: _____ suboptimal solid diet, _____ full liquid diet, _____ hypocaloric liquids, _____ starvation.
- Gastrointestinal symptoms (that persisted for >2 wk)
  _____ None, _____ nausea, _____ vomiting, _____ diarrhea, _____ anorexia.
- Functional capacity
  _____ No dysfunction (e.g., full capacity).
  _____ Dysfunction duration = # _____ wk.
  _____ Type: _____ working suboptimally, _____ ambulatory, _____ bedridden.
- Disease and its relation to nutritional requirements
  Primary diagnosis (specify): _____.
  Metabolic demand (stress): _____ no stress, _____ low stress, _____ moderate stress, _____ high stress

Physical (for each trait specify: 0 = normal, 1+ = mild, 2+ = moderate, 3+ = severe)
_____ Loss of subcutaneous fat (triceps, chest)
_____ Muscle wasting (quadriceps, deltoids)
_____ Ankle edema
_____ Sacral edema
_____ Ascites

SGA Rating (select one)
_____ A – Well nourished
_____ B = Moderately (or suspected of being) malnourished
_____ C = Severely malnourished

Reprinted with permission from Detsky AS; McLauglin JR, Baker JP, et al: What is subjective global assessment of nutritional status? JPEN 1987;11·8–13.

nutritional support should be titrated to match actual metabolic requirements.

In addition, there are times when *underfeeding* calories may be necessary and beneficial. In such cases, this is referred to as "permissive" underfeeding to distinguish it from underfeeding that occurs due to the unintentional inadequate delivery of nutrients. For example, permissive underfeeding may be appropriate for some critically ill obese patients who are receiving adequate protein. Such permissive underfeeding for critically ill individuals is now the recommendation of A.S.P.E.N. and the Society of Critical Care Medicine (SCCM).

Energy Requirements

There are four components of daily energy requirement. The first is the basal metabolic rate (BMR), which is the amount of energy expended under complete rest shortly after awakening and in a fasting state (12–14 hours). BMR varies with age, sex, and body size; correlates roughly with body surface area; and is proportional to lean tissue mass. This relationship holds true even among persons of different ages and sexes. Resting metabolic rate or resting energy expenditure (REE) represents the amount of energy expended 2 hours after a meal under conditions of rest and thermal neutrality. However, although it is often used synonymously with BMR, the REE is typically 10% higher.

The second component of daily energy expenditure is the thermic effect of exercise or the energy used in physical activity. The contribution of this component increases markedly during intense muscular work, and admission to a hospital generally results in a marked decrease in physical activity. Hospital activity in ambulatory patients accounts for a 20% to 30% increase in BMR. Critically ill patients who are on a ventilator generally have low activity levels (BMR increases by only 5%–10%) because the ventilator performs the work of breathing, and they are not ambulatory.

The third component of energy expenditure is diet-induced thermogenesis, the increase in BMR that follows food intake. The digestion and metabolism of exogenous nutrients, whether delivered to the gut or vein, result in an increase in metabolic rate. The magnitude of the thermic effect of food varies depending on the amount and composition of the diet and accounts for approximately 10% of daily energy expenditure.

Finally, acute illness adds an additional stress factor to the daily energy expenditure and correlates with disease severity. For example, a patient's metabolic rate increases by 10% to 30% after a major fracture, from 20% to 60% with severe infection, and from 40% to 110% with a severe third-degree burn. In addition, fever accelerates chemical reactions, and the BMR rises approximately 10% for each degree Celsius increase in temperature. Alternatively, cooling of febrile patients produces a reduction in BMR of approximately 10% per degree Celsius.

The first step of estimating energy requirements is to estimate the BMR. This is usually accomplished using one of several predictive equations. The most commonly used method is based on the predictive equations reported by Harris and Benedict in 1909. The Harris-Benedict equations are as follows:

$$BMR\ (men) = 66.47 + 13.75(W) + 5.0(H) - 6.76(A)$$

$$BMR\ (women) = 655.1 + 9.56(W) + 1.85(H) - 4.68(A)$$

where W is weight in kg, H is height in cm, and A is age in years. After the BMR is calculated, it is adjusted for the level of stress induced by injury or the disease process (Figure 2) and activity level. Activity factors for hospitalized patients are 1.0 to 1.1 for intubated patients, 1.2 for patients confined to bed, and 1.3 for patients out of bed. Therefore, the patient's energy requirements (total energy expenditure [TEE]) are finally calculated:

$$TEE = BMR \times Activity\ factor \times Stress\ factor$$

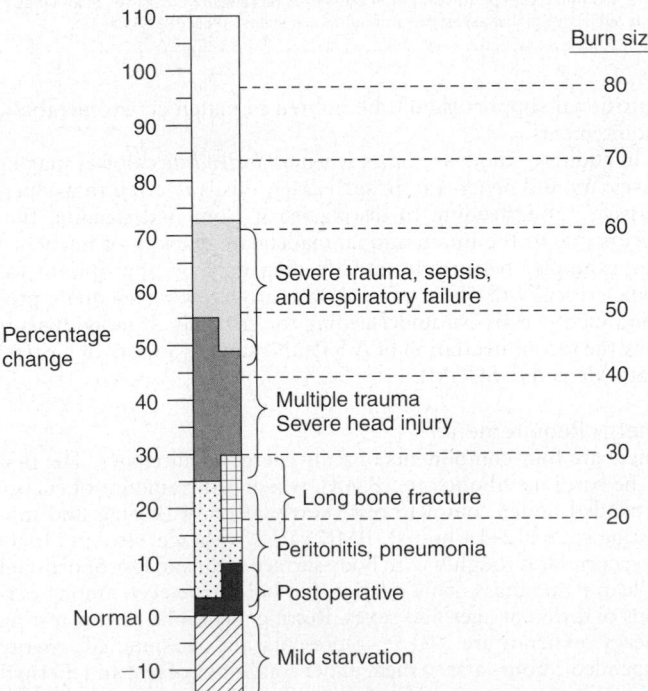

Figure 2. Percentage change in metabolic rate due to injury. (Adapted from Wilmore DW: The Metabolic Management of the Critically Ill, New York, Plenum Medical Books, 1977.)

The thermic effect of feeding is generally not included in the calculation of energy requirements for hospitalized patients.

Alternatively, some clinicians estimate energy requirements based on actual body weight. Thus, 20 to 25 kilocalories (kcal)/kg is administered to the critically ill intubated patient, and 30 kcal/kg is given to nonventilated patients in whom excessive energy intake is not a major concern.

Predicting energy expenditure in obese patients can be difficult because using predictive formulas with actual body weight can lead to high TEE and potentially to overfeeding. A factor of 18 to 21 kcal/kg has been validated in obese patients, and the Harris-Benedict equation using the average of actual and ideal weight and a stress factor of 1.3 predicts REE in acutely ill obese patients with a BMI of 30 to 50 kg/m².

Indirect calorimetry is a more precise, clinically practical, and individualized method to determine energy expenditure, particularly in patients in whom estimating requirements through predictive equations are difficult, such as those who continue to lose weight despite what appears to be an adequate caloric intake, who are critically ill, or who have rapidly changing energy needs.

Indirect calorimetry measures changes in oxygen consumption and carbon dioxide production to calculate the REE. Including a stress factor to account for injury is not necessary with indirect calorimetry because the measured energy expenditure accounts for the effects of disease state, stress, and trauma. However, the measurement occurs at rest, and therefore an activity factor of 1.0 to 1.3, depending on whether the patient is intubated, bedridden, or ambulatory, must be applied.

Nutrient Requirements

The recommended daily protein allowance for most healthy persons who are not hospitalized is 0.8 g/kg, or about 60 to 70 g of protein each day. The stressed, critically ill patient generally needs a higher dose of protein in the range of 1.0 to 1.5 g/kg/day. For most patients, providing protein beyond 1.5 g/kg/day is not beneficial. In fact, providing excess protein does not enhance uptake and can lead to increased ureagenesis, which can cause renal injury in some patients.

The calorie-to-nitrogen ratio for most PN solutions is typically about 150:1, with an acceptable range of 100:1 to 180:1. Nitrogen content is used as a marker for protein, and hence the two terms are used interchangeably. Usually, 6.25 g of protein is equal to 1.0 g of nitrogen. The conversion factor is slightly higher (6.4) for PN solutions, such as those with higher concentrations of crystalline amino acids.

Vitamin and mineral requirements are altered in certain disease states due to increased losses, greater use, or both. Guidelines for parenteral vitamin and trace elements, developed by the Nutrition Advisory Group of the American Medical Association, were approved by the U.S. Food and Drug Administration (FDA) in 1979 and amended in 2000 (Table 1).

Composition of Central and Peripheral Venous Solutions

Central venous access is required for providing TPN because of the hypertonicity of the formulas infused (1900 mOsm/kg). The infusion of a hypertonic solution into a peripheral vein, known as *peripheral parenteral nutrition* (PPN), can result in thrombophlebitis and venous sclerosis unless the PN is drastically diluted to lower the tonicity. To minimize the hypertonicity of PPN solutions, dextrose is limited to 5% to 10% and amino acids are limited to 2.5% to 3.5%. Lipids are isotonic and therefore provide a significant portion of the caloric substrate of PPN formulas.

Central venous solutions, which are prepared by the hospital's pharmacy, typically combine carbohydrate in the form of dextrose, protein as crystalline amino acids, and lipids from polyunsaturated long-chain triglycerides such as soybean oil or a safflower/soybean oil emulsion. Vitamins, electrolytes, and trace elements are added to the formulation as needed. Typical substrate profiles of carbohydrate, protein, and lipids in central PN are shown in Table 2. A usual PN prescription administers 1 to 2 L of a solution each day. Administration of 500 mL of a 20% fat

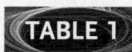

TABLE 1 Recommended Daily Doses of Parenteral Vitamins and Trace Elements

MICRONUTRIENT	PARENTERAL DOSE
Vitamins	
Vitamin A	3300 IU
Vitamin D	200 IU
Vitamin E	10 IU
Vitamin K	150 mcg
Ascorbic acid (vitamin C)	200 mcg
Folic acid	600 mcg
Niacin	40 mg
Riboflavin (vitamin B_2)	3.6 mg
Thiamine (vitamin B_1)	6 mg
Pyridoxine (vitamin B_6)	6 mg
Cyanocobalamin (vitamin B_{12})	5 mcg
Pantothenic acid	15 mg
Biotin	60 mcg
Trace Elements	
Zinc	2.5–5 mg
Copper	0.3–0.5 mg
Chromium	10–15 mcg
Manganese	60–100 mcg
Selenium	20–60 mcg

Data from American Medical Association, Department of Foods and Nutrition: Multivitamin preparations for parenteral use. A statement by the Nutrition Advisory Group, JPEN J Parenter Enteral Nutr 1979;3:258–62; Food and Drug Administration: Parenteral multivitamin products: Drugs for human use: Drug efficacy study implementation: Amendment, Federal Register 2000;65 (77):21200–1.

TABLE 2 Central Vs. Peripheral Parenteral Nutrition

PROPERTY	CENTRAL NUTRITION	PERIPHERAL NUTRITION
Daily calories	2000–3000	1000–1500
Protein	Variable	56–87 g
Volume of fluid required (mL)	1000–3000	2000–3500
Duration of therapy (d)	>7	5–7
Route of administration	Dedicated central venous catheter	Peripheral vein or multiuse central catheter
Substrate profile	55%–60% carbohydrate	30% carbohydrate
	15%–20% protein	20% protein
	25% fat	50% fat
Osmolarity (mOsm/L)	~2000	~600–900

emulsion one day each week is sufficient to prevent essential fatty acid deficiency. Alternatively, if additional calories from lipids are needed on a daily basis, they can be administered as a separate infusion or most commonly as part of the mixture of dextrose and amino acids, a technique known as *triple mix* or *three-in-one*.

Including intravenous (IV) fat emulsion into a parenteral admixture changes the conventional nutritional solution into an emulsion. Various electrolytes and micronutrients can adversely influence emulsion stability, and therefore their concentration in three-in-one solutions is limited to prevent "cracking" of the PN solution, in which microscopic or macroscopic precipitates are formed. The higher the cation valence, the greater the destabilizing influence to the emulsifier. Therefore, trivalent cations such as ferric ion (iron dextran) are more disruptive than divalent cations such as calcium or magnesium ions, which are more disruptive than monovalent cations such as sodium or potassium. No concentration of iron dextran is safe in triple-mix formulations. In-line filtration is necessary for all PN solutions, including triple-mix solutions, because it is impossible to visually detect precipitates until they are grossly incompatible and unsafe for infusion.

Once the basic solution is created, electrolytes are added as needed (Table 3). Sodium or potassium salts are given as chloride or acetate depending on the patient's requirements. Normally, equal amounts of chloride and acetate are provided. However, if chloride losses from the body are increased, which can occur in patients who have nasogastric tubes, then most of the salts should be given as chloride. Similarly, more acetate should be given to patients when additional base is required because acetate generates bicarbonate when it is metabolized. Sodium bicarbonate is incompatible with PN solutions and cannot be added to the mixture. Phosphate may be given as the sodium or potassium salt. Intravenous fat emulsions contain an additional 15 mmol/L of phosphate.

Commercially available preparations of fat-soluble and water-soluble vitamins, minerals, and trace elements are added to the nutrient mix unless they are contraindicated. Adequate thiamine is essential for patients receiving PN and can be provided separately. Vitamin K is now a component of standard IV multivitamin preparations; vitamin preparations without vitamin K are also available for those patients who may need a vitamin K restriction (e.g., patients on warfarin). Trace element preparations that include zinc, copper, manganese, and chromium are added to the PN solution in amounts consistent with the American Medical Association guidelines (see Table 1). Manganese accumulation can be toxic, and overexposure can lead to progressive neurodegenerative damage. Manganese is usually supplied in the PN solution at a daily dose of 0.5 mg as part of a multiple trace element additive. Because manganese is primarily eliminated via biliary excretion, patients with biliary obstruction or cholestasis can accumulate potentially toxic levels of manganese. Hence, manganese should be removed from the PN of patients with hyperbilirubinemia. Higher doses, 10 to 15 mg/day, of zinc are provided to patients with excessive GI losses.

Iron is not a part of commercial additive preparations because it is incompatible with triple-mix solutions and can cause anaphylactic reactions when it is given intravenously. Patients who need this trace element should receive it orally or by injection. Iron is not given to patients who are critically ill because hyperferremia can increase bacterial virulence, alter polymorphonuclear cell function, and increase host susceptibility to infection.

PPN is less commonly used than central PN and can be disadvantageous. Because of the low concentration of dextrose, greater volumes (typically >2 L/day) are required to provide sufficient calories, which might not be feasible in fluid-restricted patients. PPN generally does not approximate a patient's energy needs because PPN provides only 1000 to 1500 kcal/day, and a large percentage of the calories (60%) are derived from fat. High-fat infusions are undesirable because they are associated with impaired reticuloendothelial system function and are potentially immunosuppressive. There is no evidence that IV fat emulsions improve outcomes or significantly decrease nitrogen losses. Generally, PPN should be avoided unless it is combined with enteral feeding in patients who cannot tolerate full enteral feeding, patients who cannot get a central venous catheter, or patients with low body weights in whom PPN can meet at least two-thirds of estimated needs.

Administration and Venous Access

Typically, central PN solutions are administered into the superior vena cava. Access to this vein can be achieved by cannulation of the subclavian or internal jugular veins. Peripherally inserted

TABLE 3   Electrolyte Concentrations in Parenteral Nutrition

ELECTROLYTE	RECOMMENDED CENTRAL PN DOSES	RECOMMENDED PERIPHERAL PN DOSES	USUAL RANGE OF DOSES
Potassium (mEq/L)	30	30	0–120 (CVC)
			0–80 (PV)
Sodium (mEq/L)	30	30	0–150
Phosphate (mmol/L)	15	5	0–20
Magnesium (mEq/L)	5	5	0–16
Calcium (mEq/L) (as gluconate)	4.7	4.7	0–10
Chloride (mEq/L)	50	50	0–150
Acetate (mEq/L)	40	40	0–100

Abbreviations: CVC = central venous catheter; PN = parenteral nutrition; PV = peripheral vein.

central venous catheters (PICCs), typically inserted via an antecubital vein and advanced into the superior vena cava, are the most commonly used central venous access devices for providing PN. PICC placement offers the advantage of central venous access, while avoiding the risks associated with accessing the subclavian or jugular veins, such as hemothorax, pneomothorax, and arterial injury.

Tunneled catheters or catheters with indwelling ports should be considered for patients who will need prolonged central venous nutrition (e.g., >6 weeks). Patients who will be using their catheters solely for daily central PN and who require home IV feeding may be best served by a tunneled catheter rather than an indwelling port. Tunneled catheters may be more easily manipulated and cared for, which can minimize the risk of infection.

Inserting a dedicated line for infusing hypertonic solutions requires strict aseptic technique and maximal barrier protection: hat, mask, gown, and gloves must be worn. The position of the catheter tip in the superior vena cava is confirmed by chest x-ray before any concentrated solutions are administered. Once the position of the tip has been confirmed, the line should be used exclusively for administering the hypertonic nutrient solution.

Multiple-lumen central venous catheters are most commonly used. Although at least one lumen is dedicated to the infusion of the PN solutions, the other(s) may be used for monitoring, blood drawing, or medication. The rate of catheter sepsis associated with multiple-port catheters may be the same as or slightly greater than the rate associated with the use of single-port catheters. However, multiple-port PICCs are used to infuse PN solutions for a shorter time, which can minimize their inherent risk. Multiple-port catheters should be carefully maintained, including dressing changes, maintaining the dedicated lumen, careful handling of the other lumens, and removing the catheter as soon as it is no longer needed.

Infusion and Patient Monitoring

It is advisable to start with 1 L of central PN and increase the volume as needed, depending on the patient's metabolic stability. Blood glucose levels should be closely monitored and maintained at <180 mg/dL, tissue perfusion should be adequate, and P_{O_2}, P_{CO_2}, electrolytes (especially potassium, phosphate, and magnesium) and acid-base balance should be near normal before starting or advancing to the goal solution. The solutions should be administered using a volumetric pump set at a constant rate. It is important not to modify the infusion rate during any given day to try to compensate for excess or inadequate administration of the PN solution, such as when the PN solution arrives later than expected. A cyclic schedule (10–16 hour/day) for patients requiring long-term PN can be initiated once the patient is metabolically stable. In situations when the central PN solution must be suddenly discontinued, a 10% dextrose solution may be given at the same infusion rate as was used for the PN unless the patient is severely hyperglycemic. PN solutions may be administered at one half

the infusion rate to patients who are undergoing surgical procedures because circulating glucose and electrolyte levels are easier to control.

In addition to hyperglycemia, metabolic complications include hyper- and hypophosphatemia, hyper- and hypokalemia, hyper- and hypomagnesemia, and hyper- and hypocalcemia. Thus, it is important to monitor the patient's serum electrolytes closely, especially when initiating TPN. Once the patient has stabilized on the individual nutritional prescription, serum chemistries should be obtained at least twice weekly to measure chloride, CO_2, potassium, sodium, blood urea nitrogen, creatinine, calcium, and phosphate levels and once weekly for a full profile that includes liver function, magnesium, and triglyceride levels. Stable home PN patients may have less frequent chemistry monitoring, typically starting with once per week monitoring, then decreasing to twice per month and then monthly, depending on overall stability and clinical status.

Patients with Special Needs
Glucose Intolerance

Hyperglycemia is the most common metabolic complication related to PN, and glucose regulation may be especially difficult in patients who have diabetes mellitus or who develop insulin resistance in response to severe stress or infection. Control of blood glucose levels is important for all patients who receive PN because uncontrolled hyperglycemia may be associated with complications such as fluid and electrolyte disturbances and increased infection risk due to impairment of host defenses, including decreased polymorphonuclear leukocyte mobilization, chemotaxis, and phagocytic activity. Intensive insulin therapy, maintaining blood glucose concentrations between 80 and 110 mg/dL, was once considered standard practice for critically ill patients. However, other studies have demonstrated significant morbidity and mortality with this approach. For critically ill patients, a target blood glucose of 110 to 150 mg/dL is preferred, and for ambulatory patients, a target blood glucose of 140 to 180 mg/dL is recommended.

Patients with difficult glycemic control may best be managed by continuous insulin infusion, which is safe, effective, and more timely than subcutaneous insulin therapy. Hypoglycemia that occurs during this type of infusion generally is short lived and more easily corrected than hypoglycemia resulting from subcutaneous insulin administration. A separate IV insulin infusion can be used rather than adding incremental doses of insulin to the PN bag every 24 hours in patients for whom glycemic control is difficult. Many intensive care units (ICUs) have an insulin drip infusion protocol in which there are frequent checks of serum glucose and adjustments of the insulin infusion drip (e.g., every 1–2 hours) to maintain target glucose levels. The conventional approach of using sliding scale insulin to cover high blood glucose levels may be unsafe and ineffective, and repetitive doses of subcutaneous insulin in the edematous patient can have a cumulative effect leading to prolonged hypoglycemia. In addition, adjusting insulin in the PN bag every 24 hours might not achieve the desired rapid correction of hyperglycemia deemed appropriate based on the literature, which indicates worse outcomes for those with poor glucose control.

Abrupt discontinuation of PN can lead to hypoglycemia and should be avoided. Instead, it is recommended to decrease the PN infusion rate by one-half for the last hour of infusion prior to discontinuation to prevent rebound hypoglycemia.

Pancreatitis

Most cases of pancreatitis are mild, and nutritional support is not needed. However, 10% to 20% of patients with pancreatitis develop severe disease that results in a hypermetabolic, hyperdynamic, systemic inflammatory response syndrome that creates a highly catabolic stress state. In an evidence-based report evaluating nutrition support in acute pancreatitis patients, EN delivered to the small intestine (distal to the ligament of Treitz) is preferred over PN; EN patients are less likely to suffer from multiorgan failure, systemic infections, and death.

Initiation of PN should be delayed in patients with acute pancreatitis who cannot tolerate EN even though they might eventually require PN. Providing PN within 24 hours of admission has been shown to worsen outcome, and providing PN after resuscitation and abatement of the acute inflammatory process appears to improve outcome compared with standard therapy. Consequently, if EN is not feasible, the initiation of PN should be delayed for at least 5 days after admission to the hospital, when the peak period of inflammation has abated.

Acute Kidney Injury and Chronic Kidney Disease

Acute kidney injury (AKI) is associated with severe nutritional deficits. Most patients with AKI are catabolic and have energy requirements 50% to 100% greater than resting requirements, likely the result of other coexisting conditions such as sepsis, trauma, and burns. Energy is provided to patients with AKI in sufficient quantities to minimize protein degradation, generally in the range of 25 to 35 kcal/kg/day. Intravenous fat emulsions can be used as a source of concentrated energy in patients who require a fluid restriction.

Protein loss is accelerated and protein synthesis is impaired in patients with AKI. Loss of amino acids in the dialysate and renal replacement therapies add to the protein deficit and increase individual protein needs. Approximately 10 to 12 g of amino acids are lost with each dialysis therapy, depending on the type of dialyzer membrane, blood flow rate, and dialyzer reuse procedure, and approximately 10 to 16 g/day of amino acids are lost through continuous renal replacement therapies (CRRT). The provision of protein at 1.0 to 1.4 g/kg/day and 1.5 to 2.5 g/kg/day is recommended for AKI patients receiving hemodialysis and CRRT, respectively.

Protein is provided with a standard solution containing both essential and nonessential amino acids. Although some data suggest essential amino acids alone may be beneficial compared to a mixture of both essential and nonessential amino acids, the efficacy of using essential amino acid solutions remains uncertain. The goal is to provide adequate protein while treating the patient aggressively with dialysis to prevent the accumulation of nitrogenous waste products.

Fluid and electrolyte balance are often impaired in patients with AKI. The amount of fluid from the PN might need to be adjusted daily, depending on the phase of AKI, whether the patient is receiving dialysis, and whether dialysis is continuous or intermittent. Serum potassium and phosphate levels typically rise in patients with AKI until dialysis is initiated, at which time levels might drop, especially with the provision of PN. Potassium, phosphate, and magnesium levels need close monitoring and adjusting to correct imbalances. Acetate salts of potassium or sodium can be administered to help correct a metabolic acidosis.

Standard doses of the water-soluble vitamins and additional folic acid (1 mg/day total) and pyridoxine (vitamin B_6) (10 mg/day) might need to be added to the solution for patients who are being dialyzed because these vitamins are lost from the body in the dialysate bath. Thiamine losses are increased with CRRT and repletion (100 mg/day) must be provided for patients receiving this therapy. The dose of vitamin C might need to be restricted to 100 mg/day to prevent oxalate deposits. However, additional vitamin C (250 mg/day) should be provided to patients receiving CRRT. The supplementation of fat-soluble vitamins is usually not required, especially in patients who also are eating, because excretion of fat-soluble vitamins is reduced in renal failure. For example, serum vitamin A levels may be elevated in ARF due to enhanced hepatic release of retinol and retinol-binding protein, decreased renal catabolism, and decreased degradation of vitamin A transport protein by the kidneys. Vitamin D levels may be decreased because of impaired activation of 1,25-dihydroxycholecalciferol in the kidneys. In anuric patients, trace elements may be withheld from the PN solution; however, for prolonged PN, trace elements and fat-soluble vitamins should be monitored and replaced accordingly.

Patients with chronic kidney disease (CKD) also have nutritional deficits due to anorexia, amino acid losses into the dialysate, concurrent illness, metabolic acidosis, and endocrine disorders. However, unlike those suffering from AKI, patients with CKD have normal energy requirements. Protein intake generally is restricted in predialysis patients to 0.6 g/kg/day or 0.75 g/kg/day if the patient is malnourished. Protein is required in higher amounts in patients on dialysis, depending on the type of dialysis: 1.2 g/kg/day for hemodialysis; 1.2 to 1.5 g/kg/day for peritoneal dialysis. Predialysis patients who become acutely ill should be given protein 1.2 to 1.5 g/kg/day even if this precipitates the need for dialysis. Starvation from insufficient calories or protein in the patient with renal dysfunction increases the risk of nutritionally related complications and should be avoided in the severely ill patient regardless of the potential need for dialysis.

Intradialytic PN is the provision of IV amino acids, carbohydrates, and fat directly into the venous drip chamber of the hemodialysis unit during treatment. It is a method of providing additional calories and protein in malnourished chronic hemodialysis patients. It is associated with significant increases in body weight and serum albumin in patients with CRF. However, intradialytic PN is expensive and the benefits have not been fully elucidated. A typical solution contains about 1100 kcal and 50 g of protein, which is provided three times per week with hemodialysis. For example, intradialytic PN provides a patient with energy and protein requirements of 2500 kcal and 70 g of protein/day, respectively, only 20% of the weekly calorie and 30% of the weekly protein needs. Thus, intradialytic PN is reserved for patients with CRF who cannot ingest sufficient nutrients by mouth and who are not candidates for nutritional support via EN or PN due to GI intolerance or venous access problems or for other reasons. Appropriate use of intradialytic PN should be limited to a very small fraction of people who are on hemodialysis.

Hepatic Dysfunction and Liver Failure

Hepatic dysfunction is associated with a variety of abnormalities including metabolic abnormalities, malabsorption, maldigestion, anorexia, and early satiety due to ascites. Dietary restrictions also can contribute to malnutrition.

Protein intake in patients with stable chronic liver disease depends on the patient's nutritional status and protein tolerance. Nutritionally depleted patients can require as much protein as 1.5 g/kg estimated dry weight. In a minority of patients who have protein-sensitive hepatic encephalopathy, protein intake might need to be decreased to 0.5 to 0.7 g/kg/day and gradually increased to 1.0 to 1.5 g/kg/day, as tolerated. These patients have deranged plasma amino acid profiles, with increased concentrations of aromatic amino acids (phenylalanine, tyrosine, and tryptophan) and methionine and decreased branched-chain amino acids (leucine, isoleucine, and valine). Randomized, controlled trials that provided parenteral or enteral formulas enriched with branched-chain amino acids have been inconsistent and have had results including no benefit, improved morbidity, no change in mortality, and improvement in encephalopathy. These specialty products should be reserved for patients with disabling encephalopathy who do not tolerate standard proteins and have not responded to other therapies, such as lactulose or neomycin administration.

Energy requirements are difficult to predict in patients with liver failure. Whereas most patients have a normal metabolic rate, up to one-third may be hypermetabolic. Although providing 25 to 30 kcal/kg/day is a guideline for providing energy needs, basing requirements on indirect calorimetry is often recommended.

Fluid restriction due to ascites and edema often necessitates increasing the dextrose concentration in the PN so as to maintain sufficient calories in a restricted volume. Sodium is reduced in the formula because liver-failure patients excrete nearly sodium-free urine. Vitamin and mineral deficiencies often occur as a result of suboptimal nutrient intake, decreased absorption, decreased storage, and in some cases alcohol use, which decreases thiamine (vitamin B_1) and folate absorption. Copper and manganese may be contraindicated because a major route of excretion for these substances is the biliary system. Zinc deficiency is common in cirrhotic patients, and supplementation of this mineral may be necessary, especially if there are excessive GI losses.

Acute Respiratory Distress Syndrome
Patients with protein-calorie malnutrition have an increased incidence of pneumonia, respiratory failure, and acute respiratory distress syndrome (ARDS). Nutritional support is indicated in patients with ARDS, and underfeeding and overfeeding can be detrimental to pulmonary function.

Overfeeding calories, and particularly glucose, can lead to increased minute ventilation, increased dead space, and increased carbon dioxide production and ultimately to difficulty weaning from a ventilator. Hypercapnia from increased carbon dioxide production is the result of glucose combustion causing more carbon dioxide production and excess calories triggering lipogenesis. A healthy person increases ventilation in response to increased calories and thus avoids hypercapnia. However, patients with compromised ventilatory status might not be able to compensate with increased ventilation and can develop respiratory distress, acute respiratory failure, and difficulty weaning from mechanical ventilation. Thus, the use of indirect calorimetry measurements to determine energy expenditure is imperative in patients with ARDS.

Critically Ill Obese Patients
Obesity is a growing problem worldwide, and management of critically ill obese patients poses many challenges. These patients are at risk for hyperglycemia, hyperlipidemia, and hypercapnea, all of which can be exacerbated by metabolic changes associated with critical illness. As with any critically ill patient, obese patients will preferentially use protein and carbohydrate for energy and cannot effectively draw upon adipose tissue for energy. These patients require nutrition support to minimize loss of lean body mass.

The concept of "permissive underfeeding" has emerged as the preferred way to feed critically ill obese patients. Energy delivery is restricted to approximately 60% to 70% of estimated energy requirements and protein delivery is high (typically >2 g/kg ideal body weight [IBW]). This is to avoid hyperglycemia, hyperlipidemia, and hypercapnea while providing the protein required to spare lean body mass and support recovery. Small-scale studies employing this feeding method have demonstrated that patients can achieve positive nitrogen balance; one study found decreased ICU length of stay, decreased antibiotic days, and a trend toward decreased mechanical ventilation days.

Energy and protein delivery for critically ill obese patients is guided by BMI. The A.S.P.E.N.-SCCM guidelines recommend providing 11 to 14 kcal/kg actual weight or 22 to 25 kcal/kg IBW for patients with a BMI >30 kg/m². In comparing these recommendations to our experience with measuring REE in this population, we have found that this should be refined further by BMI. For patients with a BMI of 30 to 50 kg/m², 11 to 14 kcal/kg closely represented 60% to 70% of measured REE. For patients with a BMI >50 kg/m², 22 to 25 kcal/kg IBW represents 60% to 70% of measured REE. For protein delivery, A.S.P.E.N. and SCCM recommend protein provision of ≥2 g/kg IBW for patients with class I and class II obesity (BMI of 30 to 35 kg/m² and 35 to 40 kg/m², respectively) and for patients with class III obesity (BMI >40 kg/m²) protein provision should be ≥2.5 g/kg IBW.

Other Conditions and Nutritional Treatments
The catabolic response to major surgery, trauma, burn, and sepsis is characterized by a net breakdown of body protein stores to provide substrates for gluconeogenesis and acute-phase protein synthesis. Adequate nutrition can attenuate whole-body catabolism but rarely, if ever, prevents or reverses the loss of lean body mass during the acute phase of injury. Several strategies to prevent the loss of lean body mass have been investigated, including growth hormone, growth factors, and conditionally essential amino acids, such as glutamine.

Growth hormone is a potent anabolic agent, and administration to humans increases the rate of wound healing, decreases rates of wound infection, and decreases the catabolism and muscle wasting of critical illness. However, a large European trial found increased morbidity and mortality in patients with prolonged critical illness who received high doses of growth hormone. Thus, the use of growth hormone in patients who are in the acute phase of critical illness is not recommended.

Alternative anabolic agents such as oxandrolone (Oxandrin)[1] and testosterone[1] are being pursued to induce positive nitrogen balance and enhance wound healing in critically ill patients. These anabolic steroid hormones increase protein synthesis and can reduce the rate of protein breakdown. In a study of patients with alcoholic hepatitis, administration of oxandrolone was associated with lower mortality compared with patients receiving placebo. The patients receiving oxandrolone had improvements in the severity of their liver injury and the degree of malnutrition. Several studies have demonstrated a benefit of oxandrolone use in the burn patient population. Other anabolic steroid hormones, such as methandienone[2] and nandrolone decanoate (Deca Durabolin),[2] have been shown to increase protein anabolism and nitrogen balance in hospitalized patients.

Growth factors should be reserved for patients with major burns and documented impaired healing; patients who have large wounds or enterocutaneous fistulae and who have impaired healing; and patients with muscle wasting and weakness associated with AIDS; other failure to thrive conditions; and, in general, patients who have not responded to aggressive nutritional support but whose underlying disease processes are controlled. Growth factors have not been shown to decrease length of time on a respiratory in ICU patients. In fact, such factors can increase ventilator time and worsen outcome.

Glutamine-supplemented PN solutions administered to trauma or stressed patients can improve overall nitrogen balance, enhance muscle protein synthesis, improve intestinal nutrient absorption, decrease gut permeability, improve immune function, and decrease hospital stays and costs in some patient populations. A review of 14 randomized trials in surgical and critically ill patients found that glutamine supplementation was associated with reduced mortality, lower rates of infectious complications, and a decreased hospital stay. The greatest benefit was in patients receiving high-dose (>0.29 g/kg/day) parenteral glutamine.

However, a recent randomized trial of glutamine and antioxidant micronutrient supplementation in critically ill patients showed a trend toward increased 28-day mortality and significant in-hospital and 6-month mortality in patients receiving glutamine supplementation. There were limitations in this study in that baseline glutamine levels were not checked for all patients; in a subset of 66 patients with plasma glutamine levels evaluated, all had normal levels at baseline. This suggests that glutamine supplementation may not be appropriate for all critically ill patients. In addition, patients received approximately 50% of goal energy

---

[1]Not FDA approved for this indication.
[2]Not available in the United States.

requirements and approximately 45% of goal protein delivery from glutamine. The total amount of glutamine given in this study was significantly higher than the dose of glutamine usually recommended. This raises the possibility that there is an optimal "therapeutic window" for glutamine administration: giving too little glutamine may not be efficacious and giving too much may be toxic. Further study is required before a definitive recommendation can be given based on this study alone.

Patients with intestinal dysfunction requiring PN, such as those with short-bowel syndrome or mucosal damage following chemotherapy and/or irradiation, might benefit from glutamine-containing PN. Glutamine-containing PN might also be beneficial in patients with immunodeficiency syndromes, including AIDS, immune-system dysfunction associated with critical illness, and bone marrow transplantation; patients with severe catabolic illness, such as major burns; patients with multiple trauma; and patients with other diseases associated with a prolonged ICU stay.

Glutamine-supplemented solutions should not yet be considered routine care and should not be used in patients with significant renal insufficiency or in patients with significant hepatic failure. A recent A.S.P.E.N. position paper summarizes recommendations for use of both enteral and IV glutamine.

Common Complications and Management

Catheter Sepsis

Central venous catheter-related bloodstream infection ranges from 3% to 20% in hospitalized patients and is the most common complication of central venous catheters. The migration of microorganisms along the external surface of the catheter is likely the most common cause, followed by intraluminal contamination from manipulation of the catheter hub or IV connectors. The most common organisms associated with catheter-related bloodstream infections include *Staphylococcus epidermidis*, *Staphylococcus aureus*, *Enterococcus* spp., *Candida albicans*, and *Enterobacter* spp. as well

TABLE 4	Possible Etiologies and Treatment of Common Complications of Central Parenteral Nutrition	
PROBLEM	**POSSIBLE ETIOLOGY**	**TREATMENT**
Glucose		
Hyperglycemia, glycosuria, hyperosmolar nonketotic dehydration, or coma	Excessive dose or rate of infusion, inadequate insulin production, steroid administration, infection	Decrease the amount of glucose given, increase insulin, administer a portion of calories as fat
Diabetic ketoacidosis	Inadequate endogenous insulin production and/or inadequate insulin therapy	Give insulin Decrease glucose intake
Rebound hypoglycemia	Persistent endogenous insulin production by islet cells after long-term high-carbohydrate infusion	Give 5%–10% glucose before parenteral infusion is discontinued
Hypercarbia	Carbohydrate load exceeds the ability to increase minute ventilation and excrete excess CO_2	Limit glucose dose to 5 mg/kg/min Give greater percentage of total caloric needs as fat (up to 30%–40%)
Fat		
Hypertriglyceridemia	Rapid infusion Decreased clearance	Decrease rate of PN infusion Allow clearance (~12 h) before testing blood
Essential fatty acid deficiency	Inadequate essential fatty acid administration	Administer essential fatty acids in doses of 4%–7% of total calories
Amino Acids		
Hyperchloremia metabolic acidosis	Excessive chloride content of amino acid solutions	Administer Na^+ and K^+ as acetate salts
Prerenal azotemia	Excessive amino acids with inadequate caloric supplementation	Reduce amino acids Increase the amount of glucose calories
Miscellaneous		
Hypophosphatemia	Inadequate phosphorus administration with redistribution into tissues	Give 15 mmol phosphate/1000 IV kcal Evaluate antacid and Ca^{2+} administration
Hypomagnesemia	Inadequate administration relative to increased losses (diarrhea, diuresis, medications)	Administer Mg^{2+} (15–20 mEq/1000 kcal)
Hypermagnesemia	Excessive administration; renal failure	Decrease Mg^{2+} supplementation
Hypokalemia	Inadequate K^+ intake relative to increased needs for anabolism; diuresis	Increase K^+ supplementation
Hyperkalemia	Excessive K^+ administration, especially in metabolic acidosis; renal decompensation	Reduce or stop exogenous K^+ If ECG changes are present, treat with calcium gluconate, insulin, diuretics, and/or Kayexalate
Hypocalcemia	Inadequate Ca^{2+} administration; reciprocal response to phosphorus repletion without simultaneous calcium infusion	Increase Ca^{2+} dose
Hypercalcemia	Excessive Ca^{2+} administration; excessive vitamin D administration	Decrease Ca^{2+} and/or vitamin D administration
Elevated liver transaminases or serum alkaline phosphatase and bilirubin	Enzyme induction secondary to amino acid imbalances or overfeeding	Reevaluate nutritional prescription Cycle TPN Avoid overfeeding calories Consider administering carnitine

Abbreviations: ECG = electrocardiogram; PN = parenteral nutrition; TPN = total parenteral nutrition.

as resistant strains such as methicillin-resistant *S. aureus* and vancomycin-resistant enterococci. Primary catheter sepsis occurs when there are signs and symptoms of infection and the indwelling catheter is the only anatomic focus of infection. Secondary catheter infections are associated with another focus or multiple infectious foci that cause bacteremia and seed the catheter.

Management of patients with catheter infection depends on their clinical condition. With extremely ill patients with high fevers who are hypotensive or who have local signs of infection around the catheter site, the catheter should be removed, its tip cultured, and peripheral and central venous blood cultures obtained. In catheter-related bloodstream infection, the organisms that grow from the catheter tip are the same those identified in the peripheral blood culture, and typically more than 10^3 organisms are grown from cultures of the catheter tip.

Specific therapy should be initiated against the primary source in patients in whom a source of infection, other than the catheter tip, is present. Peripheral blood cultures should be obtained and blood cultures should not be taken from the central venous catheter port dedicated for PN because this increases the risk of contaminating the line. If the infection resolves, central venous feedings can be continued. If a secondary source is not identified and the symptoms persist, the catheter should be removed and its tip should be cultured. If the culture of the catheter tip returns positive or if the index of suspicion is high, appropriate antibiotic therapy is initiated. Central venous feeding can be resumed, maintaining euglyemia.

Occasionally, the situation arises in which a site of infection, other than the catheter, is identified, but signs and symptoms persist despite what is assumed to be adequate therapy. Again, if blood cultures are positive, the safest course of action may be to remove the catheter. If peripheral blood cultures are negative, the catheter may be changed over a guidewire and the catheter tip cultured to determine if it was contaminated. Central venous feedings may be continued during this interval if the patient is stable. If the catheter tip returns positive, a new catheter should be inserted at a different site. Changing the central venous catheter over a guidewire can also facilitate the diagnosis of primary catheter infections. Changing the site of catheter location, rather than guidewire exchange, is recommended in patients in whom infection is suspected.

Other Complications

Common complications, their etiologies, and treatments are outlined in Table 4. Prolonged administration of PN can result in altered hepatic function and changes in liver pathologic conditions that can lead to liver failure. One to 2 weeks after initiating PN, transaminases may be elevated, but this often resolves without any change in the composition of PN or rate of administration. However, in patients receiving long-term PN (>20 days), prolonged elevations of alkaline phosphatase followed by elevated levels of serum transaminases can occur, even after therapy is discontinued.

Serum levels of alkaline phosphatase and bilirubin initially remain normal, but they rise in many patients who receive long-term PN. Patients who do not receive lipids in the PN solution have more frequent and severe hepatic abnormalities, most likely due to higher carbohydrate loads. Excess glucose increases insulin secretion, which stimulates hepatic lipogenesis and results in hepatic fat accumulation. Fatty infiltration is the initial histopathologic change; it is readily reversible and might not be accompanied by altered liver function tests.

Longer PN therapy may be associated with cholestasis, cholelithiasis, steatosis, and steatohepatitis and can progress to active chronic hepatitis, fibrosis, and eventual cirrhosis. The management of PN-related liver dysfunction is summarized in Box 3.

Complications are minimized and nutritional therapy maximized when the care of patients who require specialized nutritional support is supervised by a nutrition support team. Ideally, the nutrition support team consists of a pharmacist, dietitian, nurse, and physician.

Box 3 Management of Parenteral Nutrition-Related Liver Dysfunction

Have the patient eat, if possible.
Avoid administering large amounts of glucose or protein calories.
Supply IV fat emulsions (up to 30% of total calories).
Cycle the parenteral nutrition, infusing for 10–12 h/d.
Reevaluate energy needs; reduce energy delivery if liver dysfunction persists.

References

Al-Omran M, Albalawi ZH, Tashkandi MF, Al-Ansary LA. Enteral versus parenteral nutrition in acute pancreatitis. Cochrane Database Syst Rev 2010; http://dx.doi.org/10.1002/14651858.CD002837.pub2, CD002837.

A.S.P.E.N. Board of Directors. Guidelines for the use of parenteral and enteral nutrition in adult and pediatric patients. JPEN J Parenter Enteral Nutr 2002;26:1SA–138SA.

Ayers P, Adams S, Boullata J, et al. A.S.P.E.N. parenteral nutrition safety consensus recommendations. JPEN J Parenter Enteral Nutr 2014;38:296–333.

Bistrian BR, McCowen KC. Nutritional and metabolic support in the adult intensive care unit: Key controversies. Crit Care Med 2006;34:1525–31.

Boullata JI, Gilbert K, Sacks G, et al. A.S.P.E.N. Clinical guidelines: Parenteral nutrition ordering, order review, compounding, labeling, and dispensing. JPEN J Parenter Enteral Nutr 2014;38(3):334–77.

Butler SO, Btaiche IF, Alaniz C. Relationship between hyperglycemia and infection in critically ill patients. Pharmacotherapy 2005;25:963–76.

Heyland DK, Dhaliwal R, Suchner U, Berger MM. Antioxidant nutrients: A systematic review of trace elements and vitamins in the critically ill patient. Intensive Care Med 2005;31:327–37.

Heyland D, Muscedere J, Wischmeyer PE, et al. A randomized trial of glutamine and antioxidants in critically ill patients. N Engl J Med 2013;368:1489–97.

Li Y, Tang X, Zhang J, Wu T. Nutritional support for acute kidney injury. Cochrane Database Syst Rev 2010; http://dx.doi.org/10.002/14651858.CD005426.pub2, CD005426.

McClave SA, Chang W-K, Dhaliwal R, Heyland DK. Nutrition support in acute pancreatitis: A systematic review of the literature. JPEN J Parenter Enteral Nutr 2006;30:143–56.

McClave SA, Martindale RG, Vanek VW, et al. Guidelines for the provision and assessment of nutrition support therapy in the adult critically ill patient: Society of Critical Care Medicine (SCCM) and American Society for Parenteral and Enteral Nutrition (A.S.P.E.N.). JPEN J Parenter Enteral Nutr 2009;33:277–316.

McMahon MM, Nystrom E, Braunschweig C, et al. A.S.P.E.N. Clinical guidelines: Nutrition support of adult patients with hyperglycemia. JPEN J Parenter Enteral Nutr 2013;37:26–36.

O'Grady NP, Alexander M, Burns LA, et al. Guidelines for the prevention of intravascular catheter-related infections, Clin Infect Dis 2011;52:e162–e193. Also available at http://www.cdc.gov/hicpac/BSI/BSI-guidelines-2011.html, accessed December 5, 2013.

Vanek VW, Matarese LE, Robinson M, et al. A.S.P.E.N. Position paper: Parenteral nutrition glutamine supplementation. JPEN J Parenter Enteral Nutr 2011;26:479–94.

PHEOCHROMOCYTOMA

Method of
Jan Schovanek, MD; and Karel Pacak, MD, PhD, DSc

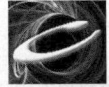

CURRENT DIAGNOSIS

- Hypertension is the most common clinical sign.
- A triad of headaches, palpitations, and sweating, with or without hypertension, indicates the possibility of a pheochromocytoma.
- Biochemical diagnosis of pheochromocytoma should be based on the determination of plasma free or urine fractionated metanephrines.
- Localization of pheochromocytomas should consist of anatomic imaging, preferably computed tomography (CT) or magnetic resonance imaging (MRI), and specific functional imaging by positron emission tomography (PET) and meta-iodobenzylguanidine (^{131}I-MIBG) scintigraphy.

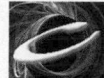

- Cost-effective genetic screening guided by family history, clinical features, and a gene-specific biochemical phenotype should be performed on most patients. The identification of a causative mutation should lead to presymptomatic genetic testing in a patient's relatives.

CURRENT THERAPY

- The optimal therapy for a pheochromocytoma is prompt surgical removal of the tumor.
- At least 1 to 2 weeks before the operation there should be adequate maintenance of blood pressure using mainly α-adrenoceptor blockers and possibly β-adrenoceptor blockers; less commonly, calcium channel blockers and metyrosine (Demser) may be used if indicated.
- For most pheochromocytomas, laparoscopy is the procedure of choice.
- Adrenal cortex–sparing surgery should be advocated in all patients with bilateral adrenal pheochromocytomas, if feasible.
- Clinical follow-up should be lifelong, especially in cases of an underlying germline mutation or with a large primary tumor greater than 5 cm.
- Management of malignant tumors requires a multidisciplinary approach, in which pharmacologic treatment, targeted radiotherapy, chemotherapy, and surgery play an important role.

The current (2004) WHO classification of endocrine tumors defines pheochromocytoma* as a tumor arising from catecholamine-producing chromaffin cells in the adrenal medulla. Closely related paragangliomas are divided into two groups: those arising from parasympathetic-associated tissues and those that arise from sympathetic-associated chromaffin tissue. Sympathetic paragangliomas were formerly designated as extra-adrenal pheochromocytomas. Pheochromocytomas and paragangliomas are characterized by the synthesis, metabolism, storage, and usually, but not always, secretion of catecholamines.

Parasympathetic paragangliomas are mainly located along the cranial and vagus nerves. Glomus or carotid body tumors, for example—head and neck paragangliomas—can be locally invasive but rarely develop metastases and are usually nonsecretory.

Sympathetic paragangliomas mainly arise in the abdomen from chromaffin tissue neighboring sympathetic ganglia. Less often, they originate from the pelvis and infrequently from the mediastinum (2%) and neck (1%). In the abdomen, they often derive from the organ of Zuckerkandl, a collection of chromaffin tissue around the origin of the inferior mesenteric artery (Figure 1).

Epidemiology

Pheochromocytomas can occur at any age, including in childhood, but most often they are detected in the fourth and fifth decades. There is no gender preference. In Western countries the prevalence of pheochromocytoma is estimated between 1:6500 and 1:2500, with an annual incidence of 3 to 8 cases per 1 million per year in the general population, although autopsies show a higher incidence. The pheochromocytoma-to-paraganglioma ratio is about 0.80 to 0.20. About 35% are familial, and 3% to 50% are malignant, depending on their genetic background.

Genetics

There are no lifestyle-related risk factors that increase the risk of pheochromocytoma. However, the understanding of the role of genetics has dramatically increased over the last years. Up to 35% of pheochromocytomas are hereditary, and a significant number of

---

*For the purpose of this chapter, the term *pheochromocytoma* also refers to paraganglioma unless otherwise specified.

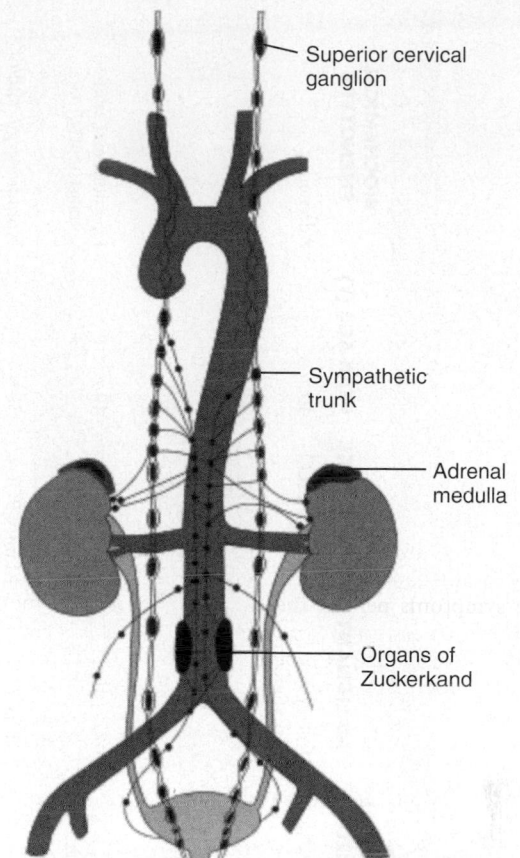

Figure 1. Anatomic distribution of chromaffin tissue. (Adapted from Lack E: Tumors of the adrenal gland and extra-adrenal paraganglia. In Armed Forces Institute of Pathology: Atlas of Tumor Pathology. Washington, DC, Armed Forces Institute of Pathology, 1997, pp 261–267.)

patients (up to 25% to 30%) with apparently sporadic tumors carry a germline mutation. Thus, gene mutations are the largest risk factor involved in the development of pheochromocytoma.

At present, at least 14 well-known susceptibility genes have been discovered that fall into two categories: major susceptibility genes and minor susceptibility genes. Major susceptibility genes represent about 85% to 90% of all hereditary tumors: the *VHL* gene, which causes von Hippel–Lindau syndrome; the *RET* gene, for multiple endocrine neoplasia (MEN) types 2A and 2B; the *NF1* gene in neurofibromatosis type 1; and the *SDHB* and *SDHD* genes in familial paraganglioma syndromes. Minor susceptibility genes include SDHA, SDHC, SDH5/SDHAF2, MAX, TMEM127, EGLN1/PHD2, IDH1, KIF1Bβ and HIF2α, which represent 10% to 15% of hereditary tumors. The list of susceptibility genes is constantly growing, with recently reported genes having a very low incidence; therefore, some of their characteristics have not yet been fully elucidated. We expect more genes to be reported in connection with familial pheochromocytoma but their relevance must be confirmed. The characteristics of hereditary tumors are described in Table 1.

Pheochromocytomas can occur as part of several syndromes, which are associated with additional clinical conditions (Box 1). A recently described Pacak-Zhuang syndrome connects novel mutations in the gene-encoding hypoxia-inducible factor 2α (HIF-2α) with paraganglioma, polycythemia, and somatostatinoma. Other rare syndromes that include pheochromocytomas are Carney triad and Carney–Stratakis syndrome, which are characterized by gastrointestinal stromal tumors and paragangliomas in *SDHB* and *SDHD* carriers. It is well established that renal cell carcinomas are also related to *SDHB*, *SDHC*, and *SDHD* gene mutations.

Genetic counseling is recommended for all patients with pheochromocytoma, but it would be neither appropriate nor

TABLE 1 Characteristics of Known Hereditary Pheochromocytomas

SYNDROME	MUTATION	GENE	PROTEIN FUNCTION	PENETRANCE	BILATERAL PHEO	MALIGNANT	PHEO OR PGL	PEAK AGE (Y)	BIOCHEMICAL PHENOTYPE
MEN2	10q11.2	RET	Receptor tyrosine kinase	~50%	50%–80%	Rarely malignant	Mainly PHEO	40	Adrenergic
VHL	3p25-26	VHL	von Hippel–Lindau protein/E3 ubiquitin protein ligase	10%–30%	50%	<5%	Mainly PHEO	30	Noradrenergic
NF-1	17q11	NF-1	Neurofibromatosis-related protein	1%–2%	16%	~10%	Mainly PHEO	50*	Adrenergic
	5p15	SDHA	Catalytic flavoprotein; A subunit of SDH	Has not been studied consistently	Has not been studied consistently	0%–14%	Mainly PGL	40	Has not been studied consistently
PGL4	1p36	SDHB	Catalytic iron-sulfur protein; B subunit of SDH	80%–100%† (by age 70 y)	Rarely	31%–71%	Mainly PGL	30	Noradrenergic and/or dopaminergic; sometimes silent
PGL3	1q21	SDHC	Membrane-spanning protein; C subunit of SDH	Has not been studied consistently	Has not been studied consistently	Rarely malignant	Mainly PGL	38	Noradrenergic and/or dopaminergic; often silent as HNPGL
PGL1	11q23	SDHD	Membrane-spanning subunit; D subunit of SDH	90%† if paternally transmitted (by age 70 y)	Has not been studied consistently	<5%	Mainly PGL	35–40	Noradrenergic and/or dopaminergic; often silent as HNPGL
PGL2	11q12.2	SDHAF2/SDHD5	Assembly factor for SDHA	~100% if paternally transmitted		Malignancy was not reported	Only PGL reported	30–40	Has not been studied consistently
	2q11.2	TMEM127	Transmembrane protein	Has not been studied consistently	33%	<5%	Mainly PHEO	43	Mixed adrenergic and noradrenergic
	14q23	MAX	bHLHLZ transcription factor	Has not been studied consistently (probably paternal transmission only)	67%	~25%	Mainly PHEO	32	Mixed adrenergic and noradrenergic

*Seldom seen in children.
†Our unpublished observations show lower penetrance.
Note: An adrenergic phenotype represents either an increase only in metanephrine or both metanephrine and normetanephrine; a noradrenergic phenotype represents an increase in both metanephrine and normetanephrine.
Abbreviations: bHLHLZ = basic helix-loop-helix leucine zipper; HNPGL = head and neck paraganglioma; MEN = multiple endocrine neoplasia; NF = neurofibromatosis; PGL = paraganglioma; SDH = succinate dehydrogenase; VHL = von Hippel–Lindau.

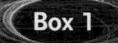

Box 1 — Main Clinical Features of Syndromes Associated with Pheochromocytoma

von Hippel–Lindau Syndrome

Type 1 (No Pheochromocytoma)
Renal cell cysts and carcinomas
Retinal and CNS hemangioblastomas
Pancreatic neoplasms and cysts
Endolymphatic sac tumors
Epididymal cystadenomas

Type 2 (with Pheochromocytoma)
Type 2A: Retinal and CNS hemangioblastomas
- Pheochromocytomas
- Endolymphatic sac tumors
- Epididymal cystadenomas
Type 2B: Renal cell cysts and carcinomas
- Retinal and CNS hemangioblastomas
- Pancreatic neoplasms and cysts
- Pheochromocytomas
- Endolymphatic sac tumors
- Epididymal cystadenomas
Type 2 C: Pheochromocytomas only

Multiple Endocrine Neoplasia Type 2

Type 2A (medullary thyroid carcinoma)
- Pheochromocytomas
- Hyperparathyroidism
- Cutaneous lichen amyloidosis
Type 2B (medullary thyroid carcinoma)
- Pheochromocytomas
- Multiple neuromas
- Marfanoid habitus
FMTC: familial medullary thyroid carcinoma only

Neurofibromatosis Type 1

Multiple benign neurofibromas on skin and mucosa
Café au lait skin spots
Iris Lisch nodules
Learning disabilities
Skeletal abnormalities
Vascular disease
CNS tumors
Malignant peripheral nerve sheath tumors
Pheochromocytomas

Paraganglioma Syndromes

Head and neck tumors
- Carotid-body tumors
- Vagal, jugular, and tympanic paragangliomas
Abdominal and/or thoracic paragangliomas
Pheochromocytomas
Renal cell carcinoma (SDHB)
Gastrointestinal stromal tumor (SDHB and SDHD)
Gastrointestinal stromal tumor (SDHB and SDHD)
Pacak-Zhuang Syndrome
Multiple paragangliomas
Multiple somatostinomas
Polythemia

Abbreviations: CNS = central nervous system; SDH = succinate dehydrogenase.
Adapted from Lenders JW, Eisenhofer G, Mannelli M, Pacak K: Phaeochromocytoma. Lancet 2005;366:665–75.

associated with other types of tumors and early diagnosis improves the prognosis of these patients.

Presymptomatic genetic testing in minors can raise ethical and legal issues, partly owing to the potential emotional impact of the results and the difficulty of obtaining individual informed consent for the testing of minors. To address these issues, the criteria for proper genetic testing should include several steps (Box 2).

Clinical Manifestations

The signs and symptoms of pheochromocytoma are mostly the result of the hemodynamic and metabolic actions of the often inconsistent and disorderly secreted catecholamines on α- and β-adrenoceptors. Most symptoms are nonspecific, including dyspnea, nausea, weakness, weight loss, visual disturbances, arrhythmias, and mental problems, but when a triad of headaches, palpitations, and sweating is accompanied by hypertension, pheochromocytoma should immediately be suspected. The typical episodic symptoms of catecholamine secretion seen in patients (e.g., palpitations, sweating, headache) may be caused by manipulation of the tumor, endoscopy, anesthesia, ingestion of food or beverages that contain tyramine, and certain medications. However, very often these symptoms occur spontaneously. Psychological stress does not seem to provoke a hypertensive crisis. Many patients have no symptoms or only minor ones. The diagnosis can therefore be easily missed. This is especially true in elderly patients.

Pheochromocytoma can also be discovered during preventive screening, as a result of signs and symptoms related to a mass effect of the tumor, and as incidental findings during imaging studies.

The primary clinical indicators for the diagnosis of pheochromocytoma are summarized in Box 3.

Differential Diagnosis

Pheochromocytoma is often referred to as "the great mimic," because it has signs and symptoms that are common in numerous other clinical conditions. As a result, this often leads to the misdiagnosis of pheochromocytoma. Consideration should be given to other conditions that are associated with sympathomedullary activation (e.g., hyperadrenergic hypertension, renovascular hypertension, panic disorders), because they mimic pheochromocytoma most closely. This overlap can be excluded by a normal response to the clonidine suppression test.

Biochemical Diagnosis

Missing a pheochromocytoma can have a fatal outcome. Therefore, tests with high sensitivity are needed to safely exclude a pheochromocytoma without using expensive and unnecessary biochemical follow-up or imaging studies.

Pheochromocytomas can secrete all, none, or any combination of catecholamines (epinephrine, norepinephrine, dopamine). After multiple studies at the National Institutes of Health (NIH), measurement of plasma free metanephrines (the O-methylated metabolites of parent catecholamines), which represent metabolism of catecholamines, but not their secretion, showed superior combined diagnostic sensitivity (98%) and specificity (92%) over all other tests examined, including urinary and plasma catecholamines, urinary total and fractionated metanephrines, and urinary vanillylmandelic acid (VMA). However, the relative advantage of measuring plasma free metanephrines compared to fractionated urinary metanephrines is small. Therefore, expert recommendations for initial biochemical testing include measurement of urine fractionated or plasma free metanephrines, or both if possible. The decision to rule out pheochromocytoma should be based on normal values of these tests, respecting for age-adjusted reference ranges.

The conditions under which blood samples are collected can be crucial to the reliability and interpretations of test results. The optimal circumstances are noted in Box 4. Besides these conditions, numerous foods and medications can cause direct or indirect interference in the measurement of catecholamines and metanephrines. This should be kept in mind when interpreting a positive

cost-effective to test for each disease-causing gene in every patient with a pheochromocytoma. An algorithm that takes family history, clinical characteristics, and biochemical phenotype into consideration is shown in Figure 2. In cases of confirmation of a hereditary disorder, one should offer specific genetic tests and genetic counseling to the patient's family members. Disease screening should be offered to presymptomatic relatives who have a diagnosed mutation, especially because familial syndromes are also

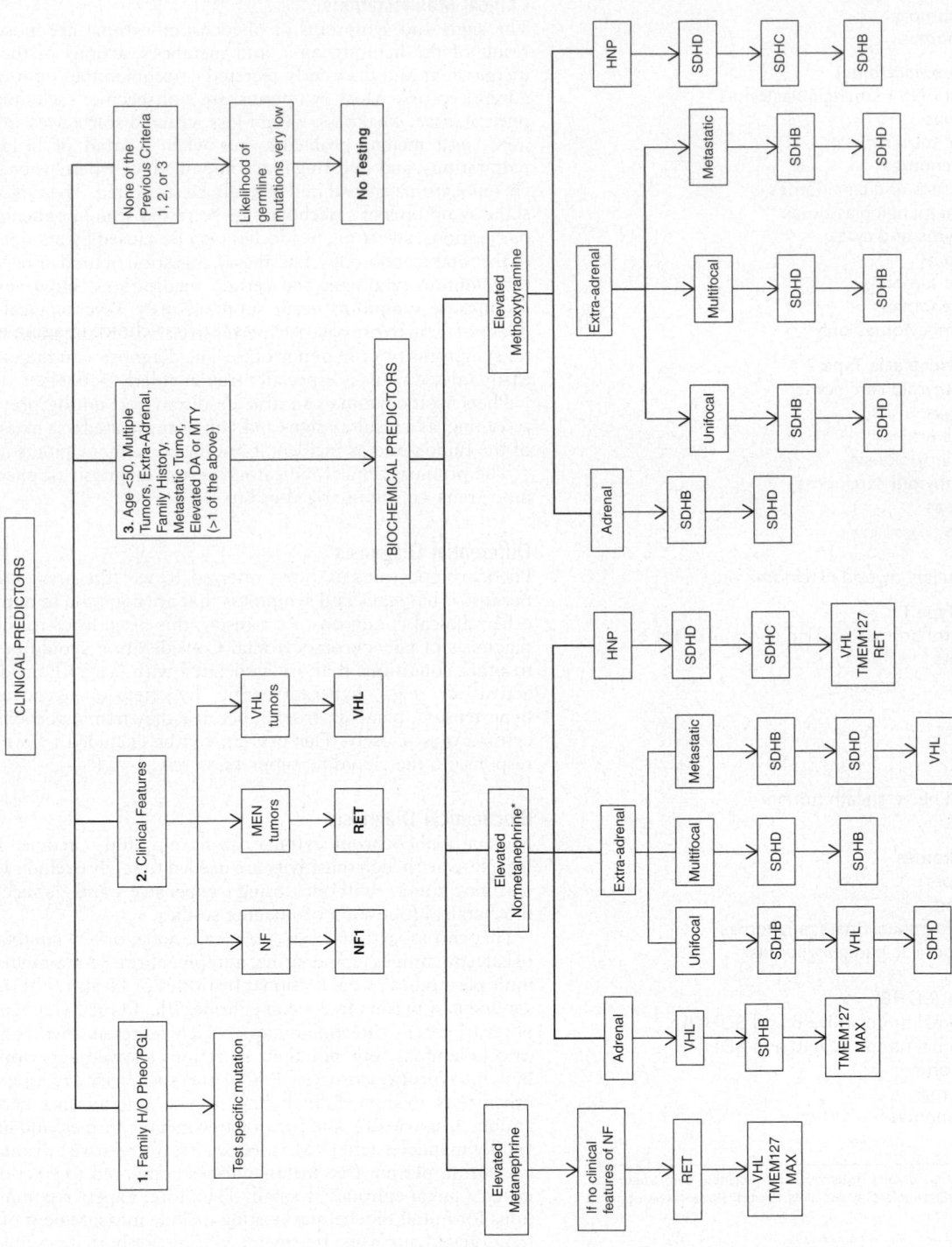

Figure 2. Suggested algorithm for genetic analysis in patients affected by pheochromocytoma or paraganglioma. If both normetanephrine and metanephrine are elevated, follow the algorithm for metanephrine. If both normetanephrine and methoxytyramine are elevated, follow the algorithm for methoxytyramine. *SDHAF2* mutation screening should be considered in patients who suffer exclusively from head and neck paragangliomas and who have familial antecedents, multiple tumors, or a very young age of onset and in whom the *SDHB/C/D* genes have been shown to be negative for mutations. In patients older than 50 years with benign adrenal tumors and no family history, consider *TMEM127* testing. *In a patient with elevated normetanephrine in whom clinical features and investigations do not clearly indicate which gene to test, perform immunohistochemistry before proceeding with testing. *Abbreviations:* DA = dopamine; H/O = history of; MTY = methoxytyramine. (From Karasek D, Shah U, Frysak Z, et al. An update on the genetics of pheochromocytoma. J Hum Hypertens. 2012 May 31. doi: http://dx.doi.org/10.1038/jhh.2012.20.)

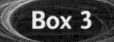

Box 2   Criteria for Proper Genetic Testing in Minors

Decision should be made by both parents after appropriate consultation with a geneticist.

Parents should be advised about how to inform their child about the hereditary disease and the reason for genetic testing.

The discussion of the most appropriate time for testing for each child should take into account the potential medical benefits and the minor's schedule (school schedule, birthdays, etc.).

Periods of medical examinations or hospitalization for the carrier parent should be avoided where possible.

Adapted from Lahlou-Laforet K, Consoli SM, Jeunemaitre X, Gimenez-Roqueplo AP. Presymptomatic genetic testing in minors at risk of paraganglioma and pheochromocytoma: Our experience of oncogenetic multidisciplinary consultation. Horm Metab Res 2012;44:354–8.

Box 3   Patients Who Should Be Evaluated for Pheochromocytoma or Paraganglioma

Anyone with a triad of headaches, sweating, and tachycardia, whether or not the subject has hypertension

Anyone with a known mutation of one of the susceptibility genes or a family history of pheochromocytoma

Anyone with an incidental adrenal mass

Anyone whose blood pressure is poorly responsive to standard therapy

Anyone who has had hypertension, tachycardia, or arrhythmia in response to anesthesia, surgery, or medications known to precipitate symptoms in patients with pheochromocytoma

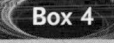

Box 4   Optimal Conditions for Blood Collection of Plasma-Free Metanephrines or Catecholamines

Patient is supine for at least 15 minutes before sampling.

Samples are collected through a previously inserted IV to avoid stress associated with the needle stick.

Patient has abstained from nicotine and alcohol for at least 12 hours.

Patient has fasted overnight before blood sampling.

test result. Tricyclic antidepressants, phenoxybenzamine (Dibenzyline), acetaminophen, monoamine oxidase inhibitors, and other drugs interfere with test results. Tricyclic antidepressants and phenoxybenzamine lead to elevated norepinephrine and normetanephrine levels. Patients with chronic kidney disease, particularly those on dialysis, commonly have elevated plasma metanephrines, even in the absence of pheochromocytoma. Use of liquid chromatography tandem mass spectrometry (LCMS/MS) is the recommended detection method, because it can remove potentially interfering substances. It is also faster, cheaper, and more specific than other techniques.

Besides the initial biochemical tests, which can exclude the disease, follow-up tests are required to establish the diagnosis. This is necessary because although the initial tests are specific, the diagnosis of pheochromocytoma is so rare that there are many false-positive results. Options for biochemical follow-up testing are repeated plasma or urinary metanephrine tests, additional sampling for plasma free or urinary fractionated catecholamines, and the clonidine (Catapres) suppression test. Biochemical follow-up testing is not necessary for patients with increases above four times the upper reference limit (URL) of plasma free metanephrines, which are almost always diagnostic for the presence of pheochromocytoma. The previously used glucagon stimulation test should be abandoned, because this test is insufficiently sensitive and can lead to hypertensive complications.

With the increasing proportion of familial tumors, it is important to highlight their different catecholamine profiles. The biochemical profile of a tumor can help guide genetic testing, as reflected in the genetic testing algorithm depicted in Figure 2. Biochemical measurements can also help identify metastatic tumors; a recent study introduced the O-methylated metabolite of dopamine, plasma methoxytyramine, as the most accurate biomarker for discriminating between patients with and without metastases. Several previous studies suggested that increased dopamine could have prognostic significance for metastatic pheochromocytomas, but later methoxytyramine was shown to be a more sensitive biomarker of a tumor's dopamine production than either plasma or urinary dopamine.

Based on these findings, an algorithm for biochemical diagnosis was designed and is shown in Figure 3.

Localization of pheochromocytoma

Imaging studies to locate pheochromocytoma should be initiated once there is clear biochemical evidence. For optimal results, anatomic imaging studies such as CT or MRI should be combined with high-specificity functional imaging studies. Computed tomography (CT) rather than magnetic resonance imaging (MRI) was suggested as the first-choice imaging modality because of its excellent spatial resolution of the thorax, abdomen, and pelvis. Use of MRI (T2-weighted) is recommended in patients with metastatic pheochromocytoma, for detection of skull base and neck paragangliomas in patients with surgical clips, in patients with an allergy to CT contrast and for patients in whom radiation exposure should be limited (children, pregnant women, patients with known germline mutations, and those with recent excessive radiation exposure).

Initial imaging should be focused on the adrenals. Negative imaging of the adrenals should be followed by CT or MRI scans of the abdomen and pelvis, where paragangliomas are most commonly located. If these scans are negative, chest and neck images should be obtained. Ultrasound is not recommended to localize pheochromocytoma. Exceptions include children and pregnant women when MRI is not available.

After anatomic imaging, which lacks the specificity to indisputably identify a mass as a pheochromocytoma, functional imaging methods can confirm a tumor as a pheochromocytoma. Functional imaging also detects most cases of metastatic and multifocal disease. They include ^{123}I MIBG scintigraphy, PET, and somatostatin receptor scintigraphy (Octreoscan), which is not recommended for hereditary tumors. PET scanning is preferred for comprehensive localization of metastatic disease. The most commonly used radiopharmaceuticals in PET scanning are ^{18}F-fluorodopamine (^{18}F-FDA), ^{18}F-3,4-dihydroxyphenylalanine (^{18}F-FDOPA), and ^{18}F-fluorodeoxyglucose (^{18}F-FDG). Different circumstances require different radiopharmaceuticals (Figure 4). The ^{18}F-FDOPA PET scan is recommended as the initial imaging modality for head and neck paragangliomas, and the ^{18}F-FDG PET scan is recommended for metastatic *SDHB*-related pheochromocytomas. The use of ^{123}I-MIBG scintigraphy in patients with known metastatic pheochromocytoma should be limited to the evaluation of whether a patient qualifies for ^{131}I-MIBG treatment. A combined PET–MRI scan has been introduced and might represent a novel advantageous imaging modality.

The algorithm described in Figure 4 provides the basis for diagnostic localization of pheochromocytoma.

If all tests return negative, it is advised to repeat noninvasive localization after 2 to 6 months.

Treatment

The optimal therapy for a pheochromocytoma is prompt surgical removal of the tumor, because an unresected tumor represents a time bomb waiting to explode with a lethal hypertensive crisis. In patients with extensive or metastatic disease, surgery can reduce the hormone secretion and prevent critical anatomic complications, such as urinary tract or cord compression or cardiac obstruction. Safe surgical removal requires the efforts of a team

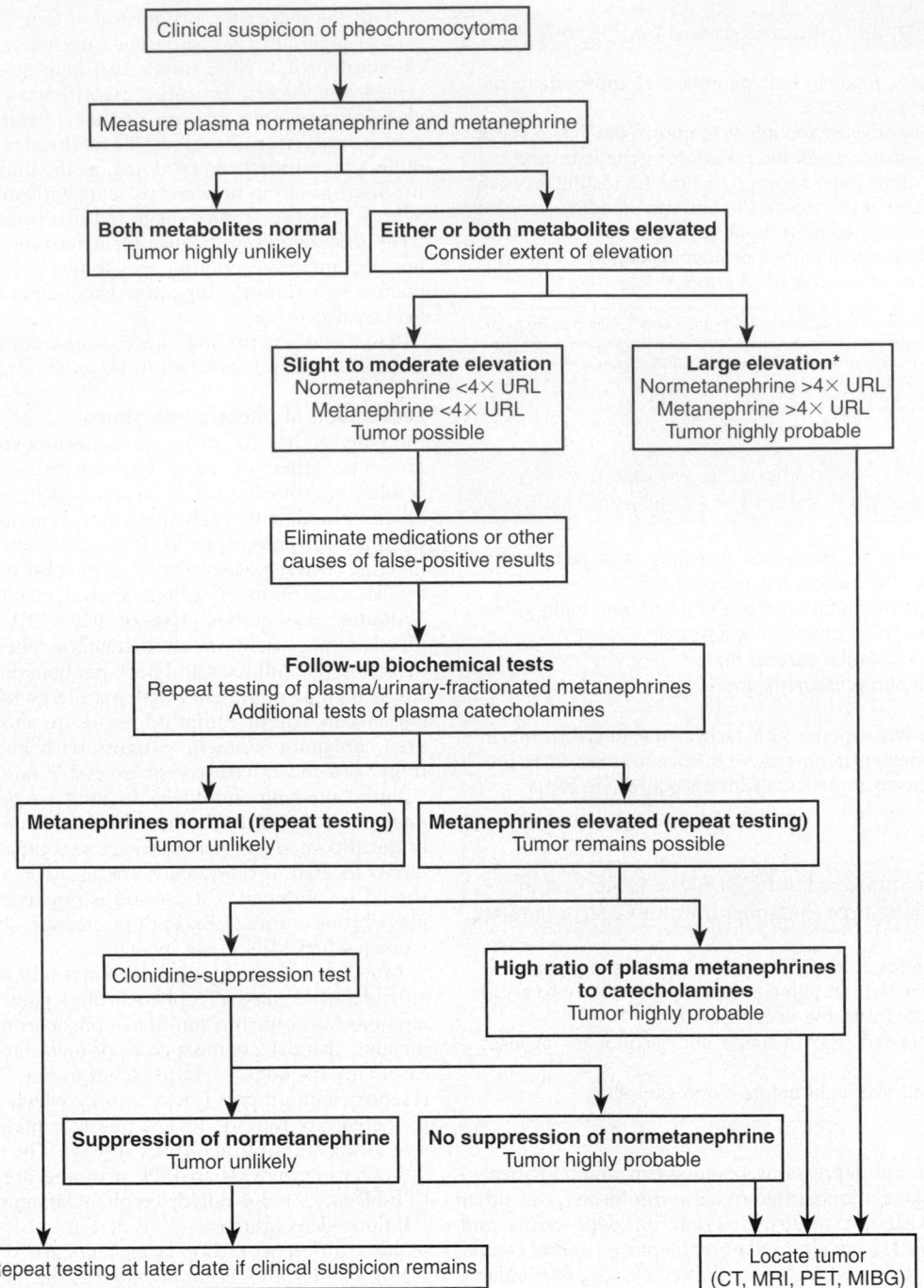

Figure 3. Algorithm for biochemical diagnosis. *It has been reported that venlafaxine (a serotonin–norepinephrine reuptake inhibitor) can cause an increase of more than four times the URL of normetanephrine. *Abbreviations:* MIBG = meta-iodobenzylguanidine; MRI = magnetic resonance imaging; PET = positron emission tomography; URL = upper reference limit.

made up of an internist, an anesthesiologist, and a surgeon, preferably in a center experienced with this demanding surgery.

Medical Therapy and Preparation for Surgery
The goal of preoperative medical treatment is to control hypertension, maintain stable blood pressure during surgery, minimize adverse effects during anesthesia, and reduce other clinical signs and symptoms caused by high plasma levels of catecholamines.

As soon as the diagnosis is made, blood pressure should be adequately treated for at least 2 weeks before the operation. With satisfactory pretreatment, perioperative mortality has fallen to less than 3%. α-Adrenergic blockade is the basis of medical management and preoperative preparation. The most commonly used nonselective α-adrenoceptor blocker is phenoxybenzamine, which

is also used for nonhypertensive patients. Other possibilities include α-blocking agents such as prazosin (Minipress), terazosin (Hytrin), and doxazosin (Cardura). Though these have a shorter duration of action and more often cause hypotension when initially administered for preoperative blood-pressure control, postoperative hypotension is more often seen with phenoxybenzamine. In addition to α-blockers, one can use β-blockers (especially when cardiac tachy- and other arrhythmias occur) and calcium-channel blockers such as nicardipine (Cardene). α-Methyl-L-tyrosine and metyrosine has limited use as a premedication. Diuretics should be avoided.

β-Blockers should never be used until α-adrenoceptor blockers have been administered for at least 2 to 3 days, because this can result in severe hypertensive crisis in patients with

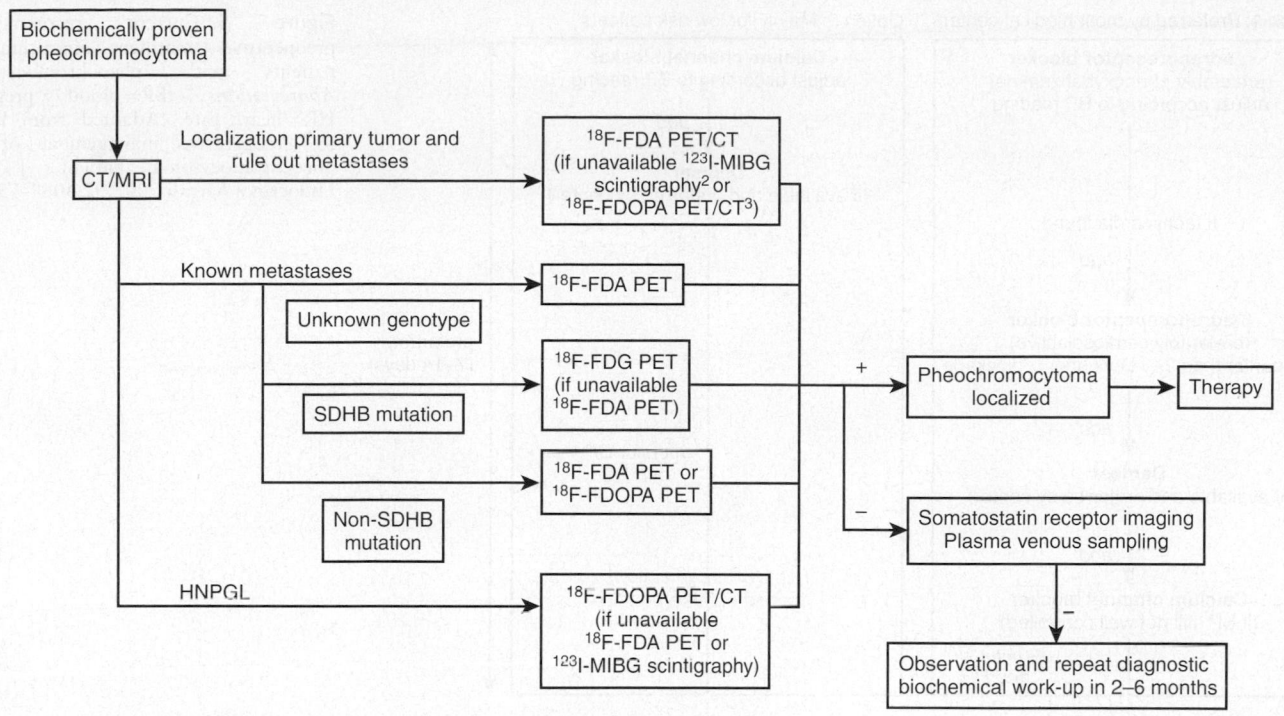

Figure 4. Recommended imaging studies for the localization of pheochromocytoma. [2], second choice; [3], third choice. *Abbreviations:* CT = computed tomography; [18] F-FDA = [18] F-fluorodopamine; [18] F-FDOPA = [18] F-3,4-dihydroxyphenylalanine; [18] F FDG = [18] F-fluorodeoxyglucose; HNPGL = head and neck paraganglioma; MIBG = meta-iodobenzylguanidine; MRI = magnetic resonance imaging; PET = positron emission tomography.

pheochromocytoma, which is believed to result from inhibition of β_2-adrenoceptor–mediated vasodilation (in the presence of catecholamine stimulation of incomplete α-adrenoceptor blockage). It might be presumed that cardioselective β_1-adrenoceptor–blocking drugs might be administered without adverse effect. Indeed, almost all adverse reactions to β-blockers in pheochromocytoma patients have involved nonselective β-blockers. Therefore, cardioselective β-blockers (such as atenolol, esmolol, and metoprolol) are favored over nonselective blockers for the management of patients with pheochromocytoma. Nevertheless, because of incomplete specificity and likelihood of some actions on β_2-adrenoceptors, even β-blockers deemed to be cardioselective should only be administered to patients with pheochromocytoma once there is adequate control of blood pressure by α-adrenoceptor blockade or other means.

Patients can be recommended a salt- and fluid-rich diet. A proposed algorithm for preoperative treatment is given in Figure 5.

Operative and Postoperative Management

After extensive preoperative preparation, surgery should be performed by an experienced surgical and anesthesiology team.

To ensure adequate preoperative preparation, several criteria have been proposed. First, targeted blood pressure should be below 140/90 mm Hg for at least 24 hours. Orthostatic hypotension should be present, but not below 80/45 mm Hg. In some cases, Doppler or conventional echocardiography are indicated in addition to ECG to detect the presence of cardiomyopathy or coronary artery disease. In patients with a large left adrenal pheochromocytoma, splenectomy is likely; therefore, vaccinations against *Streptococcus pneumoniae*, *Haemophilus influenzae*, and *Neisseria meningitidis* should be given preoperatively.

An experienced anesthesiologist should be aware of potential catecholamine release either as a side effect of the drugs used or as a result of tumor manipulation during the surgery.

A minimally invasive approach is the accepted standard for small, noninvasive, nonmetastatic pheochromocytomas and retroperitoneal paragangliomas, because of its significant postoperative

benefits. Locoregional invasion is difficult to establish preoperatively; therefore it has been recommended that potentially invasive tumors should be initially explored by laparoscopy or retroperitoneoscopy followed by conversion to open surgery in cases of critical adhesion. To prevent permanent glucocorticoid deficiency in patients with bilateral pheochromocytomas, adrenal cortex–sparing surgery is advocated. There are multiple potential hazardous events and situations during surgery, including anesthesia induction, tumor manipulation, hypotension, and hypoglycemia. The treatment of hypotension with pressor agents is not recommended, especially when long-acting β-blockers or metyrosine have been used; these paralyze the vascular bed in a dilated state. Instead, volume replacement is the treatment of choice.

Postoperative hypertension can indicate incomplete tumor resection. However, during the first 24 hours after surgery, hypertension is most likely attributed to pain, volume overload, or autonomic instability, all of which are treated symptomatically. If hypertension persists, any attempts to collect specimens for biochemical evidence of an incompletely resected tumor should be delayed for at least 5 to 7 days after surgery to ensure that the large increases in both plasma and urinary catecholamines produced by surgery have dissipated.

Close monitoring of blood glucose in the postoperative period is recommended, because its level can be decreased due to decreased glucose production and increased glucose utilization in the absence of the previous catecholamine excess and persistence of α-adrenoceptor blockers.

If the patient is hypotensive, hemorrhage should be excluded first; however, the most likely cause of hypotension is the prolonged effect of the α-adrenoceptor blockers in the presence of reduced plasma catecholamine levels.

Hypertensive Crisis

The most dangerous complication of pheochromocytoma is the occurrence of a hypertensive crisis. Hypertensive crisis can manifest as a severe headache, visual disturbances, acute myocardial infarction, congestive heart failure, or a cerebrovascular accident.

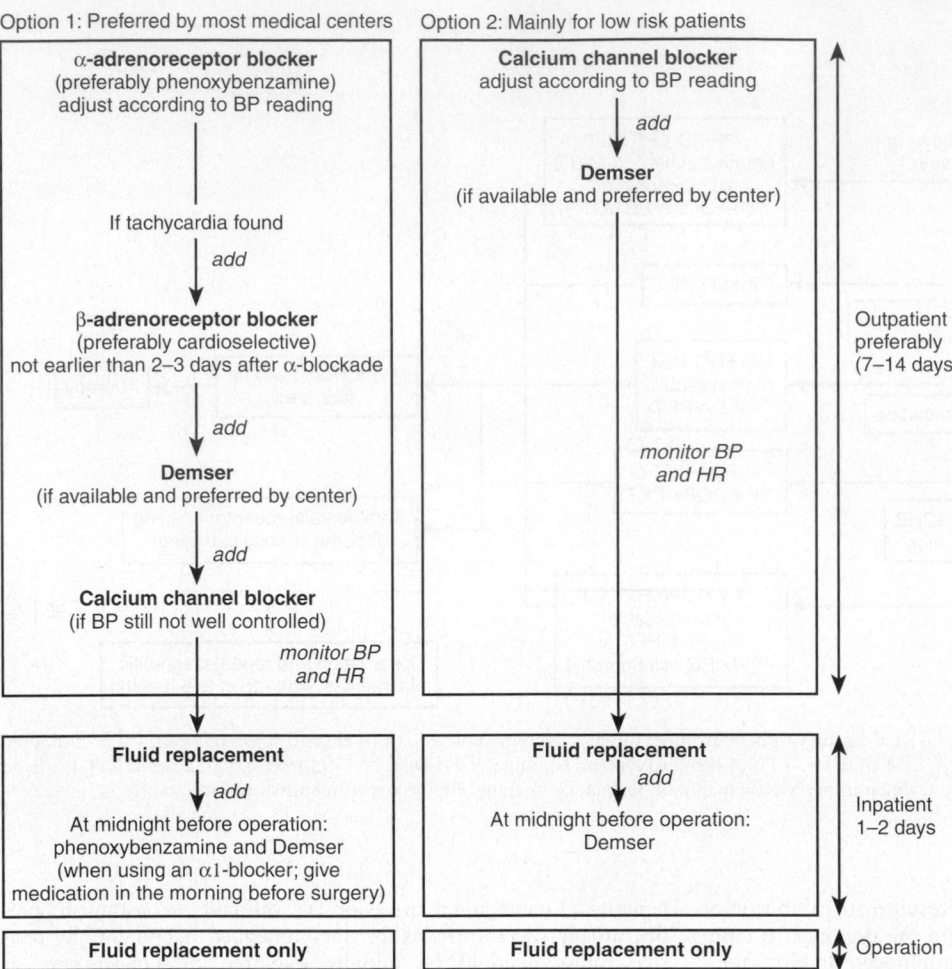

Option 1: Preferred by most medical centers | Option 2: Mainly for low risk patients

α-adrenoreceptor blocker
(preferably phenoxybenzamine)
adjust according to BP reading

If tachycardia found
add

β-adrenoreceptor blocker
(preferably cardioselective)
not earlier than 2–3 days after α-blockade

add

Demser
(if available and preferred by center)

add

Calcium channel blocker
(if BP still not well controlled)

monitor BP and HR

Fluid replacement
add
At midnight before operation:
phenoxybenzamine and Demser
(when using an α1-blocker; give
medication in the morning before surgery)

Fluid replacement only

Calcium channel blocker
adjust according to BP reading

add

Demser
(if available and preferred by center)

monitor BP and HR

Fluid replacement
add
At midnight before operation:
Demser

Fluid replacement only

Outpatient preferably (7–14 days)

Inpatient 1–2 days

Operation

Figure 5. Current recommended preoperative treatment algorithms in patients with pheochromocytoma. *Abbreviations:* BP = blood pressure; HR = heart rate. (Adapted from Pacak K: Preoperative management of the pheochromocytoma patient. J Clin Endocrinol Metab 2007;92:4069–79.)

814

It is treated with an intravenous bolus of 5 mg phentolamine (Regitine), a reversible nonselective α-adrenergic antagonist. Phentolamine has a very short half-life, and therefore the same dose can be repeated every 2 minutes until hypertension is adequately controlled. Phentolamine can also be given as a continuous infusion. Continuous intravenous infusion of sodium nitroprusside (Nitropress) or, in some cases, oral or sublingual nifedipine (Procardia),[1] can also be given to control hypertension.

Malignant Pheochromocytoma

Malignant pheochromocytoma is established only by the presence of metastases at sites where chromaffin cells are normally absent. Paragangliomas are malignant more commonly than pheochromocytomas (25% vs. 7%).

Pheochromocytoma metastasizes via hematogenous or lymphatic routes, and the most common metastatic sites are lymph nodes, bones, lung, and liver. About one half of malignant tumors are found at original presentation, and the other half develop at a median interval of 5.6 years, but they can be delayed up to 24 years. Based on the localization of the metastatic lesions, there are short-term and long-term survivors.

Up to 50% of malignant pheochromocytomas develop because of a germline mutation. *SDHB* mutations with the presence of pheochromocytoma represent about 70% or even more of the risk of malignancy (both in children and adults). Currently, there are several other independent factors of malignancy, including extra-adrenal localization (paragangliomas), the size of the primary tumor (larger than 5 cm), and high methoxytyramine level. Owing to the substantial amounts of methoxytyramine produced by a significant portion of metastatic pheochromocytomas, this measurement should also offer utility in patient management as a surrogate biomarker to assess tumor burden, disease progression, and response to treatment.

Malignant disease is often complicated by clinical manifestations of catecholamine excess and is invariably fatal. The 5-year survival probability after the diagnosis of the first metastasis is reported to be 36% in *SDHB* carriers and 67% in the absence of this mutation.

Successful management of malignant pheochromocytoma requires a multidisciplinary approach, where pharmacologic treatment, targeted radiotherapy, chemotherapy, and surgery can all play a part. While external-beam radiation has been used for inoperable tumors or for symptom palliation, especially in the treatment of bone lesions, surgical debulking is considered the mainstay of palliative treatment. About 30% of patients receiving CVD (cyclophosphamide, vincristine, and dacarbazine) exhibit clinical benefits; this number is much higher in patients with *SDHB*-related malignant tumors (about 70%–80%). Limited documented experience with other chemotherapeutic regimes is available. Somatostatin analogues can be used as an alternative option (for example, DOTATATE). Nowadays, a lot is expected from the novel molecular targeted therapies. In fact, some therapies have already been tested in clinical settings with new possible targets emerging, especially in HIF genes, the mTOR pathway and

[1]Not FDA approved for this indication.

Figure 6. Treatment algorithm for metastatic pheochromocytoma. Asterisk indicates that the risk of side effects from therapy exceeds the chance of benefit. *Abbreviations:* CVD = cyclophosphamide, vincristine, and dacarbazine [chemotherapy]; MIBG = meta-iodobenzylguanidine. (Adapted from Adjallé R, Plouin PF, Pacak K, Lehnert H: Treatment of malignant pheochromocytoma. Horm Metab Res 2009;41:687-896.)

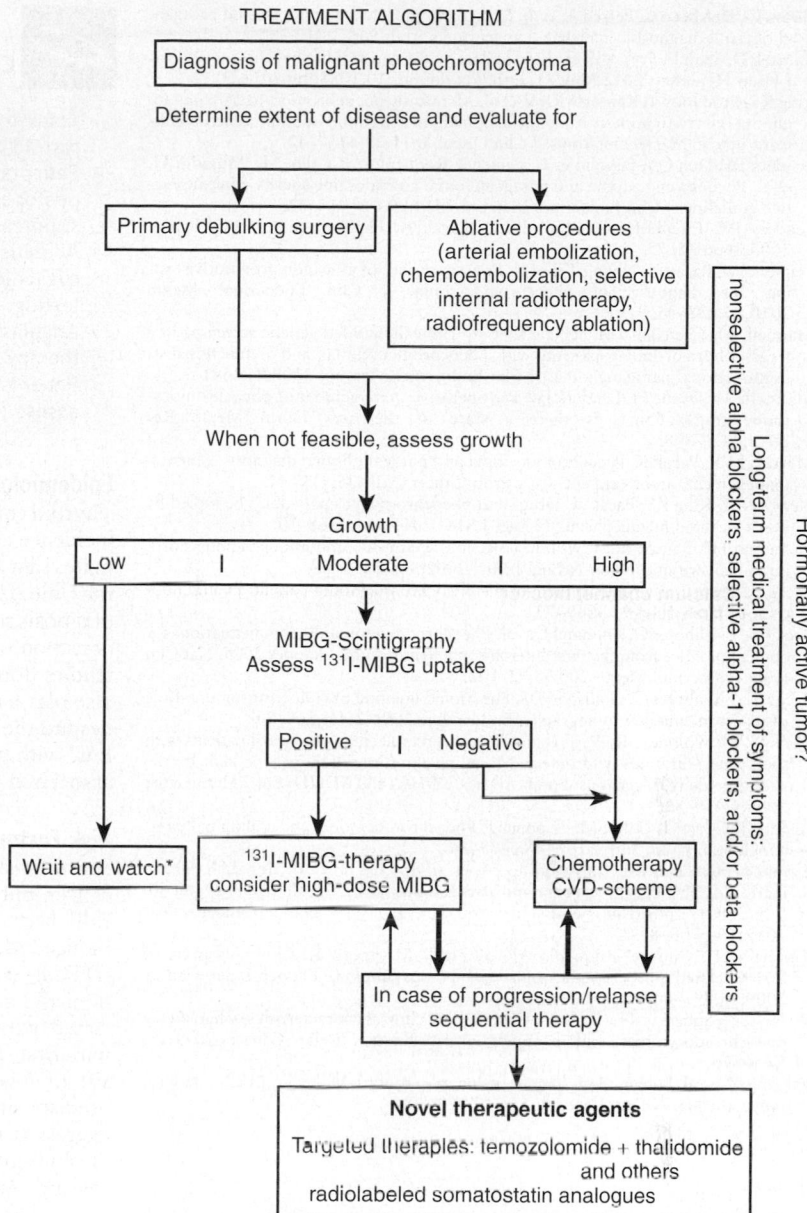

TREATMENT ALGORITHM

Hsp90. Individualized treatment should be performed with the intention to cure limited disease and achieve palliation for advanced disease. Figure 6 shows a proposed algorithm for the treatment of metastatic pheochromocytoma.

Prognosis and Monitoring

The long-term survival of patients after successful removal of a benign pheochromocytoma is essentially the same as that of age-adjusted normal subjects. Findings from a large study with a long-term follow-up showed a recurrence rate of 17%, with half the patients showing signs of malignant disease. Recurrences occur more often in patients with extra-adrenal disease and in patients with a hereditary disorder. At least 25% of patients remain hypertensive after treatment, but this is usually easily controlled with medication.

Clinical follow-up should be lifelong for all patients, but especially in those with an underlying hereditary disorder. The frequency of checkups, once a year or more often, and the kind of diagnostic measurements, only biochemical tests or also imaging studies, should depend on the characteristics of the pheochromocytoma. Follow-up must be more intensive in patients with hereditary and malignant pheochromocytoma.

References

Adjalle R, Plouin PF, Pacak K, Lehnert H. Treatment of malignant pheochromocytoma. Horm Metab Res 2009;41:687–96.

Amar L, Baudin E, Burnichon N, et al. Succinate dehydrogenase B gene mutations predict survival in patients with malignant pheochromocytomas or paragangliomas. J Clin Endocrinol Metab 2007;92:3822–8.

Ayala-Ramirez M, Feng L, Habra MA, et al. Clinical benefits of systemic chemotherapy for patients with metastatic pheochromocytomas or sympathetic extra-adrenal paragangliomas: Insights from the largest single-institutional experience. Cancer 2012;118:2804–12.

Bayley JP, Kunst HP, Cascon A, et al. SDHAF2 mutations in familial and sporadic paraganglioma and phaeochromocytoma. Lancet Oncol 2010;11:366–72.

Baysal BE. Screening: Correlation of genotype and phenotype in paraganglioma. Nat Rev Endocrinol 2009;5:594–5.

Eisenhofer G, Lenders JW, Siegert G, et al. Plasma methoxytyramine: A novel biomarker of metastatic pheochromocytoma and paraganglioma in relation to established risk factors of tumour size, location and SDHB mutation status. Eur J Cancer 2012;48:1739–49.

Eisenhofer G, Rivers G, Rosas AL, et al. Adverse drug reactions in patients with phaeochromocytoma: Incidence, prevention and management. Drug Saf 2007;30:1031–62.

Fishbein L, Nathanson KL. Pheochromocytoma and paraganglioma: Understanding the complexities of the genetic background. Cancer Genet 2012;205:1–11.

Gimenez-Roqueplo AP, Dahia PL, Robledo M. An update on the genetics of paraganglioma, pheochromocytoma, and associated hereditary syndromes. Horm Metab Res 2012;44:328–33.

Gimm O, DeMicco C, Perren A, et al. Malignant pheochromocytomas and paragangliomas: a diagnostic challenge. Langenbecks Arch Surg 2012;397:155–77.

Karasek D, Shah U, Frysak Z, et al. An update on the genetics of pheochromocytoma. J Hum Hypertens 2012 May 31. http://dx.doi.org/10.1038/jhh.2012.20.

King KS, Prodanov T, Kantorovich V, et al. Metastatic pheochromocytoma/paraganglioma related to primary tumor development in childhood or adolescence: Significant link to SDHB mutations. J Clin Oncol 2011;29:4137–42.

Lenders JW, Duh QY, Eisenhofer G, Gimenez-Roqueplo AP, Grebe SK, Murad MH, et al. Pheochromocytoma and paraganglioma: an endocrine society clinical practice guideline. J Clin Endocrinol Metabol 2014;99(6):1915–42.

Lenders JW, Eisenhofer G, Mannelli M, Pacak K. Phaeochromocytoma. Lancet 2005;366:665–75.

Lenders JW, Pacak K, Huynh TT, et al. Low sensitivity of glucagon provocative testing for diagnosis of pheochromocytoma. J Clin Endocrinol Metab 2010;95:238–45.

Mannelli M, Castellano M, Schiavi F, et al. Clinically guided genetic screening in a large cohort of Italian patients with pheochromocytomas and/or functional or nonfunctional paragangliomas. J Clin Endocrinol Metabol 2009;94:1541–7.

Mannelli M, Dralle H, Lenders JW. Perioperative management of pheochromocytoma/paraganglioma: Is there a state of the art? Horm Metab Res 2012;44:373–8.

Martucci VL, Pacak K. Pheochromocytoma and paraganglioma: diagnosis, genetics, management, and treatment. Curr Prob Cancer 2014;38(1):7–41.

Neary NM, King KS, Pacak K. Drugs and pheochromocytoma—don't be fooled by every elevated metanephrine. N Engl J Med 2011;364:2268–70.

Neumann HP, Bausch B, McWhinney SR, et al. Germ-line mutations in nonsyndromic pheochromocytoma. N Engl J Med 2002;346:1459–66.

Pacak K. Preoperative management of the pheochromocytoma patient. J Clin Endocrinol Metab 2007;92:4069–79.

Pacak K, Eisenhofer G, Ahlman H, et al. Pheochromocytoma: Recommendations for clinical practice from the First International Symposium, October 2005. Nat Clin Pract Endocrinol Metab 2007;3:92–102.

Pacak K, Eisenhofer G, Goldstein DS. Functional imaging of endocrine tumors: Role of positron emission tomography. Endocr Rev 2004;25(4):568–80.

Pasini B, McWhinney SR, Bei T, et al. Clinical and molecular genetics of patients with the Carney–Stratakis syndrome and germline mutations of the genes coding for the succinate dehydrogenase subunits SDHB, SDHC, and SDHD. Eur J Hum Genet 2008;16:79–88.

Renard J, Clerici T, Licker M, Triponez F. Pheochromocytoma and abdominal paraganglioma. J Visc Surg 2011;148:e409–16.

Timmers HJ, Chen CC, Carrasquillo JA, et al. Staging and functional characterization of pheochromocytoma and paraganglioma by ^{18}F-fluorodeoxyglucose (^{18}F-FDG) positron emission tomography. J Natl Cancer Inst 2012;104:700–8.

Timmers HJ, Gimenez-Roqueplo AP, Mannelli M, Pacak K. Clinical aspects of SDHx-related pheochromocytoma and paraganglioma. Endocr Relat Cancer 2009;16:391–400.

Welander J, Soderkvist P, Gimm O. Genetics and clinical characteristics of hereditary pheochromocytomas and paragangliomas. Endocr Relat Cancer 2011;18:R253–76.

Zhuang Z, et al. Somatic Hif-2α gain-of-function mutations in paraganglioma with polycythemia. N Engl J Med 2012;367:922–30.

THYROID CANCER

Method of
Rebecca B. Schechter, MD

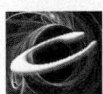

CURRENT DIAGNOSIS

- Thyroid nodules are typically diagnosed following recognition of a neck mass or found incidentally on radiology examinations performed for other reasons.
- History of thyroid irradiation and family history of thyroid cancer increase a patient's risk of developing thyroid cancer.
- Thyroid-stimulating hormone (TSH) should be measured to assess thyroid function.
- Patients with suppressed TSH levels should be evaluated for hyperfunctioning nodules.
- Hyperfunctioning nodules do not require fine-needle aspiration (FNA) biopsy.
- Most thyroid nodules are benign; ultrasonography-guided FNA biopsy of thyroid nodules is key to detecting thyroid cancer.
- About 25% of medullary thyroid cancer is inherited as an autosomal dominant mutation in the RET proto-oncogene.

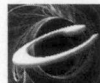

CURRENT THERAPY

- Total thyroidectomy is the preferred surgery for suspected thyroid cancer.
- Patients with differentiated thyroid cancer may also be treated postoperatively with radioactive iodine and thyroid hormone suppression therapy.
- All patients with medullary thyroid cancer require preoperative evaluation for pheochromocytoma and should undergo genetic testing.
- Anaplastic thyroid cancer can be treated with surgery, chemotherapy, and radiation, but the overall prognosis is poor.
- Patients with thyroid cancer require long-term follow-up to assess for recurrent disease.

Epidemiology

Thyroid cancer is the most common endocrine malignancy, and its incidence continues to rise. The National Institutes of Health estimates that 60,220 new cases of thyroid cancer will be diagnosed in the United States in 2013, representing more than a doubling in the diagnosis rate compared to 1990. This increase is in part due to the detection of small, incidental thyroid nodules found on radiology studies done for other reasons, but other unknown factors might also play a role. Luckily, most thyroid cancer has a good prognosis; despite the increase in diagnosis, the mortality rate has remained low, with about 1850 deaths per year. Death is most commonly associated with metastatic disease and high tumor burden.

Risk Factors

Several risk factors are associated with development of thyroid cancer, but radiation exposure is the only one that has unequivocally been shown to increase thyroid cancer risk. Most radiation-induced thyroid carcinomas are differentiated thyroid cancers (DTCs), with recurrence and mortality rates similar to those for nonirradiated DTCs. Family history of thyroid cancer is also associated with increased risk of thyroid cancer diagnosis. Persons with first-degree relatives with DTC have a 4- to 10-fold increased risk of developing thyroid cancer, although the inheritable genetic predisposition is usually unknown. Whether familial DTC is more aggressive than sporadic DTC is unclear. Increasing age, history of Hashimoto's thyroiditis, and female sex may be associated with thyroid cancer.

Pathophysiology

Thyroid carcinoma can be divided into those that originate from thyroid follicular cells and nonfollicular cells (Table 1). Follicular cell–derived cancers include DTC and undifferentiated thyroid cancer. DTC includes papillary, follicular, and Hürthle cell subtypes. Papillary cell cancer accounts for the large increase in thyroid cancer diagnosis. Undifferentiated thyroid cancer, or anaplastic thyroid cancer, accounts for only 2% of thyroid cancers

TABLE 1 Classification of Thyroid Cancers

TUMOR	ESTIMATED % OF CASES
Derived from Follicular Cells	
Anaplastic	2%
Differentiated	
Papillary	80%
Follicular	11%
Hürthle cell	3%
Derived from Calcitonin-Producing Cells	
Medullary	4%

but carries a uniformly poor prognosis. Non–follicular cell thyroid cancer, called medullary thyroid cancer, develops from calcitonin-producing cells and accounts for 4% of thyroid cancers. About 25% of medullary thyroid cancers are hereditary and are caused by autosomal dominant mutations in the *RET* proto-oncogene. Familial medullary thyroid cancer is collectively referred to as multiple endocrine neoplasia type 2 (MEN2).

Differentiated Thyroid Cancer

Constitutive activation of the MAP kinase (MAPK) pathway (Figure 1), leading to thyroid cell growth and proliferation, has been implicated in DTC initiation. Activating mutations in *BRAF* and *RET/PTC* rearrangements are commonly reported in papillary thyroid cancer. *RAS* mutations have been reported in follicular thyroid cancer. In addition, overexpression of vascular endothelial growth factor receptor (VEGF-R) likely plays an important role in DTC growth by stimulating angiogenesis. Increased VEGF expression has been associated with increased tumor size, lymph node metastases, and the development of distant metastatic spread.

Medullary Thyroid Cancer

Germline mutations in the *RET* proto-oncogene result in MEN2. Medullary thyroid cancer can be the only abnormality (familial type) or it can be associated with other findings (MEN2A and 2B), in which, importantly, there is a 50% risk of pheochromocytoma. Some cases are also associated with hyperparathyroidism. The location of the mutation strongly correlates with the phenotype and the age of onset. Approximately 30% to 50% of patients with sporadic medullary thyroid cancer have a somatic mutation in *RET*.

Anaplastic Thyroid Cancer

The pathogenesis of anaplastic thyroid cancer is not well understood. *BRAF* mutations have been reported in some anaplastic thyroid cancers, suggesting that it might develop from DTC. Mutations in the *p53* tumor suppressor gene may be important in the progression of DTC to anaplastic thyroid cancer.

Clinical Manifestations

The diagnosis of thyroid cancer is typically made after the recognition of a neck mass. Some patients present with hoarse voice or neck pain, but most are asymptomatic. For patients with palpable lesions, thyroid ultrasonography (US) is indicated to confirm presence, size, and quality of neck lesions. Commonly, nonpalpable thyroid nodules are found incidentally on radiology scans done for other unrelated reasons.

Diagnosis

The incidence of thyroid nodules increases with age, and more than 95% are benign. TSH should be measured; patients with suppressed TSH values could have one or more hyperfunctioning (toxic) nodules, and ^{123}I uptake and scanning should be performed. Nodules that are hot on scintigraphy are unlikely to be cancerous, and FNA biopsy is not necessary. For patients who are euthyroid or hypothyroid, the size and sonographic appearance of nodules are important to determine whether US-guided FNA biopsy is indicated. In general, solid hypoechoic nodules greater than 1.0 cm and mixed cystic–solid nodules greater than 1.5 to 2.0 cm in diameter should be biopsied. Lesions of any size with findings suggesting extracapsular growth or metastasis to cervical lymph nodes should be biopsied. In addition, smaller lesions in patients at greater risk for thyroid cancer (history of radiation, family history) should be evaluated.

Thyroid cytology can be classified into nondiagnostic (insufficient cells), benign, follicular lesion, suspicious, or malignant (Box 1). Nodules with nondiagnostic cytology should undergo repeat US-guided FNA biopsy; surgery can be considered for persistently nondiagnostic solid nodules. Lesions with benign cytology can be monitored for growth with repeat US in 6 to 18 months. Repeat biopsy can be considered if there is a greater than 50% increase in nodule volume or worrisome features. Follicular lesions are particularly challenging because their malignant potential cannot be determined via FNA biopsy. These lesions carry up to a 20% risk of malignancy, and surgery is generally recommended. Newly available genetic analysis of cytologic material may help to better determine the malignant risk of these indeterminate lesions. Suspicious or malignant nodules should be treated surgically.

Box 1   Fine Needle Aspiration Cytology and Associated Management

Nondiagnostic
Repeat USGFNA biopsy
Consider lobectomy if repeat biopsy is nondiagnostic

Benign
Repeat US in 6–18 months
Consider repeat USGFNA biopsy if >50% increase in nodule volume or suspicious features

Follicular Lesion
Surgery (lobectomy or total thyroidectomy)
If final pathology shows malignancy, return for completion thyroidectomy if lobectomy initially performed
Consider RAI and TSH suppression

Suspicious or Malignant
Papillary Thyroid Cancer
Total thyroidectomy with or without central lymph node dissection
Consider RAI and TSH suppression

Medullary Thyroid Cancer
Measure calcitonin and CEA
Evaluate for pheochromocytoma, hypercalcemia, *RET* proto-oncogene mutation
Total thyroidectomy plus central lymph node dissection with or without lateral lymph node dissection

Anaplastic Thyroid Cancer
Consider surgical resection and chemoradiation

Abbreviations: CEA = carcinoembryonic antigen; RAI = radioactive iodine; TSH = thyroid-stimulating hormone; US = ultrasound; USGFNA = ultrasound-guided fine needle aspiration.

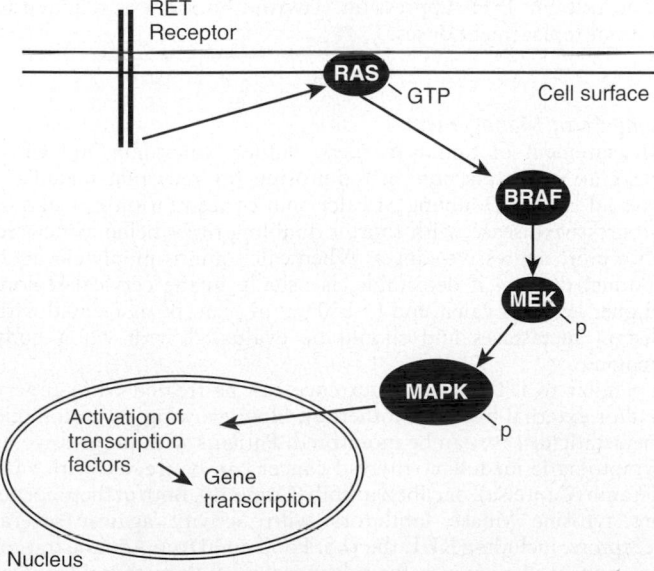

Figure 1. Schematic of the MAP kinase pathway.

Measurement of serum calcitonin may be useful to detect medullary thyroid cancer. However, in patients with no family history, calcitonin screening has not been shown to be cost-effective. If thyroid cytology is suspicious for medullary thyroid cancer, measurement of serum calcitonin and carcinoembryonic antigen (CEA) is indicated. Because up to 6% of patients with negative family histories have germline mutations in RET, patients with apparently sporadic medullary thyroid cancer should undergo preoperative evaluation for pheochromocytoma, hypercalcemia, and genetic testing.

The presentation of anaplastic thyroid cancer is more dramatic than in other thyroid malignancies. In 75% of cases, patients present with rapidly enlarging neck masses. In addition, compressive and invasive symptoms such as dyspnea, hoarseness, cough, and neck pain are observed. On examination, anaplastic thyroid cancer is a hard, fixed mass; it is often greater than 5 cm at presentation. Immediate tissue evaluation with biopsy is indicated.

Treatment
Differentiated Thyroid Cancer
Initial Therapy
Total (or near-total) thyroidectomy is the procedure of choice for suspected DTC. Small, isolated tumors (<1 cm) can be treated with lobectomy in selected cases. Abnormal lymph nodes seen on preoperative imaging should also be surgically removed. However, the role for prophylactic central-compartment lymph node dissection in DTC remains controversial. Potential complications from total thyroidectomy include transient or permanent hypoparathyroidism and damage to the recurrent laryngeal nerve.

Retrospective studies suggest that total thyroidectomy improves disease-free survival and reduces recurrence rates. Importantly, total thyroidectomy prepares patients for possible radioactive iodine (RAI, ^{131}I) therapy, the next step in DTC management.

RAI therapy allows easier surveillance for recurrent disease through imaging and improves the sensitivity of serum thyroglobulin (Tg), a protein made by thyroid follicular cells, as a tumor marker. Thyroid follicular cells take up serum iodine via the sodium–iodine symporter (NIS). Orally administered RAI can destroy normal cells remaining in the thyroid bed (thyroid remnant) as well as occult cancer cells. Because TSH stimulation increases the number and activity of NIS, patients are withdrawn from L-thyroxine therapy or treated with recombinant human TSH (rhTSH [thyrotropin alfa, Thyrogen]) to maximize RAI uptake. RAI therapy is commonly dosed empirically depending on the tumor stage. Low doses are appropriate for cancers confined to the thyroid, and higher doses are administered for more advanced tumors.

Benefits of RAI in high-risk patients include decreased disease progression and mortality. However, the advantages of RAI in low-risk patients (those with small tumors that are confined to the thyroid gland) are controversial. Although retrospective data suggest that in patients with isolated tumors greater than 1.5 cm, RAI can decrease their risk of recurrence, recent studies have called for a more judicious use of RAI in low-risk patients. In fact, low-risk patients treated with RAI may be at excess risk for developing a secondary cancer.

Patients who undergo thyroidectomy with or without RAI require thyroid hormone therapy. Because TSH stimulates thyroid growth, TSH suppression may be indicated in high-risk patients. In these patients, TSH suppression has been shown to decrease recurrence rates and cancer-related mortality. In low-risk patients, TSH suppression has not been shown to be beneficial, and L-thyroxine dosage can be adjusted for a normal TSH.

Long-Term Management
Surveillance testing is important to detect residual and recurrent DTC; timing and frequency of testing depend on a patient's risk for recurrence. Three main modalities are used

for monitoring patients: high-resolution US, serum thyroglobulin (Tg) measurements, and ^{131}I diagnostic total body scans. Neck US can detect disease in the thyroid bed and/or cervical lymph nodes. US-guided FNA biopsy of suspicious lesions can then be performed to confirm recurrence. Tg can be measured while a patient is on thyroid hormone or under conditions of stimulation (L-thyroxine withdrawal or following rhTSH). Stimulated Tg improves sensitivity for detecting disease. Total body scans are less sensitive than US and Tg measurements to detect recurrent disease. Nonetheless, total body scans can be useful for localizing disease, especially when Tg is detectable but neck US shows no disease and in patients whose Tg measurements are unreliable owing to the presence of anti-Tg antibodies.

Recurrent thyroid cancer can either grow locally in the neck or metastasize distantly. For localized measurable DTC, repeat surgery should be considered. Repeat RAI can be given for iodine-avid disease following surgery. For cervical disease not amenable to surgery and/or RAI, external beam radiotherapy may be considered. Metastatic cancer that is slow-growing may be monitored conservatively; some patients remain symptom-free with minimal cancer growth for years. For those with progressive disease, systemic therapy is indicated. Because cytotoxic chemotherapy is generally ineffective in DTC, newer targeted therapies should be considered.

Medullary Thyroid Cancer
Initial Therapy
Surgery is the primary treatment. Because medullary thyroid cancer often metastasizes to lymph nodes early, a preoperative neck US is important to guide surgery. At minimum, total thyroidectomy with bilateral central neck dissection is generally recommended. Many surgeons also perform ipsilateral and contralateral modified neck dissections if preoperative imaging suggests tumor.

Patients with positive tests for familial medullary thyroid cancer sometimes present without clear evidence of medullary thyroid cancer. These patients have a 90% lifetime risk of developing medullary thyroid cancer, and total thyroidectomy should be performed. Timing of prophylactic surgery depends on the specific mutation because some mutations result in aggressive, early-onset medullary thyroid cancer, even before 1 year of age.

Because calcitonin-producing cells do not take up iodine, there is no role for RAI in medullary thyroid cancer. In addition, because TSH does not stimulate growth of medullary thyroid cancer, there is no role for TSH suppression. Thyroid hormone is required in normal replacement doses.

Long-Term Management
Measurement of tumor markers, namely calcitonin and CEA, plays an important role in monitoring for recurrent medullary thyroid cancer. Doubling of calcitonin concentration is a sign of progressive disease, with shorter doubling times being associated with more aggressive cancer. When calcitonin is mildly elevated, residual disease, if detectable, is usually in the cervical region. Higher levels of calcitonin (>150 pg/mL) can be associated with distant metastases and should be evaluated with whole-body imaging.

Similar to DTC, local recurrence can be treated with surgery and/or external beam radiotherapy. Slow-growing asymptomatic metastatic disease can be monitored. Patients with progressive or symptomatic medullary thyroid cancer can be treated with vandetanib (Caprelsa), or cabozantinib (Cometiq). Both of these agents are tyrosine kinase inhibitors with activity against several receptors, including RET; the U.S. Food and Drug Administration has approved their use for advanced medullary thyroid cancer in 2011.

Anaplastic Thyroid Cancer

Standard treatment for anaplastic thyroid cancer is not well described because there is no clear evidence that any particular regimen is effective. Total thyroidectomy can be attempted, but it has not been shown to prolong survival except when tumors are small and confined to the thyroid. Hyperfractionated radiation therapy combined with radiosensitizing doses of doxorubicin (Adriamycin) with or without subsequent debulking surgery modestly improves survival in some patients.

Conclusion

US-guided FNA biopsy of thyroid nodules remains the gold standard method to detect thyroid malignancy. Most thyroid cancer responds well to standard therapy, but recurrence is common and long-term monitoring is essential. Treatment for patients with aggressive thyroid cancer remains suboptimal; external beam radiotherapy and/or targeted therapy should be considered in progressive cases.

References

Cooper DS, Doherty GM, Haugen BR, et al. Revised American Thyroid Association management guidelines for patients with thyroid nodules and differentiated thyroid cancer. Thyroid 2009;19:1167–214.

Gharib H, Papini E, Paschke R, et al. American Association of Clinical Endocrinologists, Associazione Medici Endocrinologi, and European Thyroid Association Medical guidelines for clinical practice for the diagnosis and management of thyroid nodules: Executive summary of recommendations. Endocr Pract 2010;16:468–75.

Iyer NG, Morris LG, Tuttle RM, et al. Rising incidence of second cancers in patients with low-risk (T1N0) thyroid cancer who receive radioactive iodine therapy. Cancer 2011;117:4439–46.

Jonklaas J, Sarlis NJ, Litofsky D, et al. Outcomes of patients with differentiated thyroid carcinoma following initial therapy. Thyroid 2006;16:1229–42.

Kloos RT, Eng C, Evans DB, et al. Medullary thyroid cancer: Management guidelines of the American Thyroid Association. Thyroid 2009;19:565–612.

National Cancer Institute. Thyroid Cancer. Available at http://www.cancer.gov/cancertopics/types/thyroid/ [accessed 08.07.12].

National Comprehensive Cancer Network. NCCN clinical practice guidelines in oncology: Thyroid carcinoma. Version 2.2012. PDF available at http://www.nccn.org/professionals/physician_gls/PDF/thyroid.pdf [accessed 08.07.12].

THYROIDITIS

Method of
Leigh M. Eck, MD

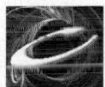

CURRENT DIAGNOSIS

- Thyroiditis is a term used to describe a diverse group of disorders associated with thyroid inflammation.
- Thyroiditis can be associated with a euthyroid state, thyrotoxicosis, or hypothyroidism.
- The clinical presentation of thyroiditis will direct the evaluation with useful testing to include measurement of thyroid hormone levels, thyroid antibody testing, white blood cell count, erythrocyte sedimentation rate, thyroid scintigraphy, and thyroid ultrasound.

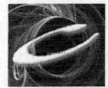

CURRENT THERAPY

- Abnormalities of thyroid hormone levels resulting from thyroiditis may be transient and require no or only short-term therapy.
- If symptomatic thyrotoxicosis is present, beta-blocker therapy should be initiated.
- Thyroiditis associated with persistent hypothyroidism is managed with synthetic thyroxine (T4, Levoxyl, Synthroid).
- Thyroid pain associated with subacute thyroiditis therapy is managed with a nonsteroidal antiinflammatory drug or, if ineffective, glucocorticoid therapy.

- Acute suppurative thyroiditis requires immediate parenteral antibiotic therapy as well as surgical drainage, if indicated.

Thyroiditis is a term used to describe a diverse group of disorders characterized by inflammation of the thyroid gland (Table 1). Presentation of thyroiditis is variable depending on the etiology. The most common thyroid disorder in the United States, Hashimoto's thyroiditis, most often presents with hypothyroidism. Other forms of thyroiditis may present with thyrotoxicosis because of inflammation in the thyroid gland resulting in the release of stored hormone. Painful thyroiditis is seen with subacute, suppurative and radiation-induced thyroiditis, while other variants are most often painless.

Epidemiology

The most common cause of hypothyroidism in iodine-sufficient areas of the world is *Hashimoto's thyroiditis*, also known as *chronic autoimmune thyroiditis*. Elevated serum antithyroid peroxidase antibody concentrations are found in ~5% of adults and ~15% of older women; overt hypothyroidism is seen in up to 2% of the population. A variant of chronic autoimmune thyroiditis, *postpartum thyroiditis*, is a destructive thyroiditis induced by an autoimmune mechanism that occurs within 1 year of parturition. Postpartum thyroiditis occurs in up to 10% of women in the United States. *Silent thyroiditis*, is indistinguishable from postpartum thyroiditis, with the exception of lack of temporal relationship to pregnancy. Silent thyroiditis may account for about 1% of all cases of thyrotoxicosis. Many medications are associated with an alteration in thyroid function testing; however, only a few are known to provoke an autoimmune or destructive inflammatory thyroiditis, including amiodarone (Cordarone), lithium, interferon alfa, interleukin-2, and tyrosine kinase inhibitors. *Riedel's thyroiditis* is a progressive fibrosis of the thyroid gland with a prevalence of only 0.05% among patients with thyroid disease requiring surgery. *Subacute thyroiditis* is the most common cause of thyroid pain. It occurs in up to 5% of patients with clinical thyroid disease. *Suppurative thyroiditis*, most commonly caused by bacterial infection, is rare because of the thyroid gland's encapsulation, high iodine content, rich blood supply, and extensive lymphatic drainage. *Radiation-induced thyroiditis* occurs in approximately 1% of patients who receive radioactive iodine therapy for hyperthyroidism.

Risk Factors

Hashimoto's thyroiditis is more common in women, particularly older women. Hashimoto's thyroiditis is associated with several gene polymorphisms, suggesting a role for genetic susceptibility. Subacute thyroiditis frequently follows an upper respiratory tract infection, with its incidence highest in summer. Suppurative thyroiditis is most likely to occur in patients with preexisting thyroid disease, those with congenital anomalies such as pyriform sinus fistula, and those who are immunosuppressed.

TABLE 1	Causes of Thyroiditis
Autoimmune thyroiditis: Hashimoto's thyroiditis, postpartum thyroiditis, silent thyroiditis	
Subacute thyroiditis, also known as de Quatrain's thyroiditis or subacute granulomatous thyroiditis	
Suppurative thyroiditis, also known as infectious thyroiditis or pyrogenic thyroiditis	
Riedel's thyroiditis, also known as fibrous thyroiditis	
Therapy induced thyroiditis: amiodarone (Cordarone), interferon-alpha, interleukin-2, lithium, tyrosine kinase inhibitors, radioactive iodine	

Pathophysiology

Hashimoto's thyroiditis, postpartum thyroiditis, and silent thyroiditis all have an autoimmune basis. The antithyroid immune response begins with activation of thyroid antigen-specific helper T cells. Once helper T cells are activated, they induce B cells to secrete thyroid antibodies; thyroid antibodies most frequently measured are those directed against thyroid peroxidase and against thyroglobulin. The mechanism for autoimmune destruction of the thyroid likely involves both cellular immunity and humoral immunity. Riedel's thyroiditis is the local involvement of the thyroid in a systemic disease, multifocal fibrosclerosis; the etiology of Riedel's thyroiditis is not known. Although a viral cause of subacute thyroiditis has been proposed, clear evidence for this proposed etiology is lacking. Suppurative thyroiditis is most often associated with a bacterial pathogen; however, fungal, mycobacterial, or parasitic infections may also be the cause. Although rare, radiation-induced thyroiditis may occur following the treatment of hyperthyroidism with radioactive iodine because of radiation-induced injury and necrosis of thyroid follicular cells and associated inflammation.

Clinical Manifestations

A symmetrical, painless goiter is frequently the initial finding in Hashimoto's thyroiditis. The usual course of Hashimoto's thyroiditis is gradual loss of thyroid function. Among patients with this disorder who have subclinical hypothyroidism, overt hypothyroidism occurs at a rate of about 5% per year. The classic presentation of postpartum thyroiditis occurs in only approximately 30% of afflicted women, with the characteristic sequence of hyperthyroidism, followed by hypothyroidism, and then recovery. Persistent hypothyroidism is seen in up to 30% of women following an episode of postpartum thyroiditis. Silent thyroiditis is marked by a similar characteristic sequence of thyroid hormone dysfunction. However, it is not temporally associated with pregnancy; 20% will have residual hypothyroidism. *Medication-induced thyroiditis* is variable in its presentation. Amiodarone (Cordarone), rich in iodine, is associated with hypothyroidism and hyperthyroidism; type 2 amiodarone-induced thyrotoxicosis is due to a destructive thyroiditis process. Lithium is more commonly associated with hypothyroidism. Interferon-alfa and interleukin-2 can cause both permanent and transient hypothyroidism likely related to the ability of these substances to induce or exacerbate thyroid autoimmune disease. Riedel's thyroiditis presents with neck discomfort or tightness, dysphagia, hoarseness, and a diffuse goiter that is hard, fixed, and often not clearly separable from the adjacent tissues. Generally, patients are euthyroid, and their antithyroid antibody concentrations are often high. Subacute thyroiditis manifests with a prodrome of myalgias, pharyngitis, low-grade fever, and fatigue with subsequent fever and neck pain, and up to 50% of patients have symptoms of thyrotoxicosis. Patients with suppurative thyroiditis are usually acutely ill with fever, dysphagia, dysphonia, anterior neck pain with erythema, and a tender thyroid mass. Radiation-induced thyroiditis presents 5 to 10 days following radioactive iodine treatment with neck pain and tenderness. In addition, there can be a transient exacerbation of hyperthyroidism.

Diagnosis and Differential Diagnosis

The diagnostic approach to suspected thyroiditis can be focused based on an association with thyroid pain and circulating thyroid hormone status (Figure 1). Hashimoto's thyroiditis is diagnosed when a goiter is found on examination with a subsequently noted elevation of thyroid antibodies or when subclinical or overt hypothyroidism is detected with associated elevated thyroid antibodies. Screening for postpartum thyroiditis with a measurement of TSH and free thyroxine should be undertaken in women presenting with symptoms of thyroid dysfunction in the postpartum period. If hyperthyroidism is present, thyroid scintigraphy (if not contraindicated, e.g., breastfeeding) or measurement of thyroid-stimulating immunoglobulins is helpful in the differentiation of postpartum thyroiditis from Graves' disease. The diagnostic approach to silent thyroiditis is similar. The laboratory hallmark of subacute thyroiditis is a markedly elevated erythrocyte sedimentation rate; the leukocyte count is normal or slightly elevated. Thyrotoxicosis may be present; if so, thyroid scintigraphy will reveal a low iodine uptake state. Thyroid antibody testing is typically normal. Thyroid ultrasound reveals a hypoechogenic gland with low to normal vascularity. Suppurative thyroiditis is typically associated with normal thyroid function. Leukocyte counts and erythrocyte sedimentation rates are elevated. Fine-needle aspiration with Gram stain and culture is the diagnostic test of choice. Radiation-induced thyroiditis should be considered if a temporal relationship to radioactive iodine treatment is present. If there is an exacerbation of hyperthyroidism immediately following radiation treatment for the same, consideration of radiation-induced thyroiditis due to the release of preformed thyroid hormone associated with destruction of follicular cells should be considered as an etiology of thyrotoxicosis in addition to the underlying disease process.

Treatment

Once overt hypothyroidism is present in the patient with Hashimoto's thyroiditis, treatment with synthetic L-thyroxine (Levoxyl, Synthroid) therapy is indicated. The average replacement dose of thyroxine in adults is approximately 1.6 mcg/kg body weight per day. Adjustment of dosage is undertaken every 6 weeks until a euthyroid status is achieved. The majority of women with postpartum thyroiditis will not need treatment during either the hyperthyroid nor hypothyroid phase. If symptomatic hyperthyroidism is present, beta-blocker therapy can be used; antithyroid medications have no utility in the management of postpartum thyroiditis. Women with symptomatic hypothyroidism should be treated with synthetic thyroxine therapy; in asymptomatic women, initiation of thyroxine therapy should be considered if TSH is >10 mU/L. Management of silent thyroiditis is the same as that for postpartum thyroiditis. Symptoms associated with Riedel's thyroiditis may be relieved with prednisone; a small case series associated improvement and even resolution of the process with Tamoxifen therapy. Surgery is indicated in Riedel's thyroiditis if compressive symptoms are present. The goal of therapy in subacute thyroiditis is to provide symptom relief. Nonsteroidal antiinflammatory medications are often adequate to control pain; if insufficient, glucocorticoid therapy should be initiated. Beta-blockade therapy can ameliorate symptoms of thyrotoxicosis if indicated. Suppurative thyroiditis is managed with appropriate antibiotics and drainage of any abscess; the disease may prove fatal if diagnosis and treatment are delayed. Pain associated with radiation-induced thyroiditis can be managed with nonsteroidal antiinflammatory therapy, or, if ineffective, a short course of glucocorticoid therapy. Radiation-induced thyroiditis is a self-limited process and will resolve spontaneously within days to weeks.

Monitoring

In the patient with Hashimoto's thyroiditis with a euthyroid state, routine TSH testing should be undertaken give the risk of development of overt hypothyroidism at 5% per year. Any woman who has had postpartum thyroiditis should be monitored very closely for thyroid dysfunction with future pregnancies, as reoccurrence is likely. For women who have fully recovered from postpartum thyroiditis, yearly TSH measurements should be considered because of underlying chronic autoimmune thyroiditis and risk for overt hypothyroidism. Although overall recurrence rates for silent thyroiditis have not been well established, a similar monitoring plan is warranted for this variant of chronic autoimmune thyroiditis. Subacute thyroiditis recurs in only about 2% of patients. Routine monitoring following resolution of process has not been defined.

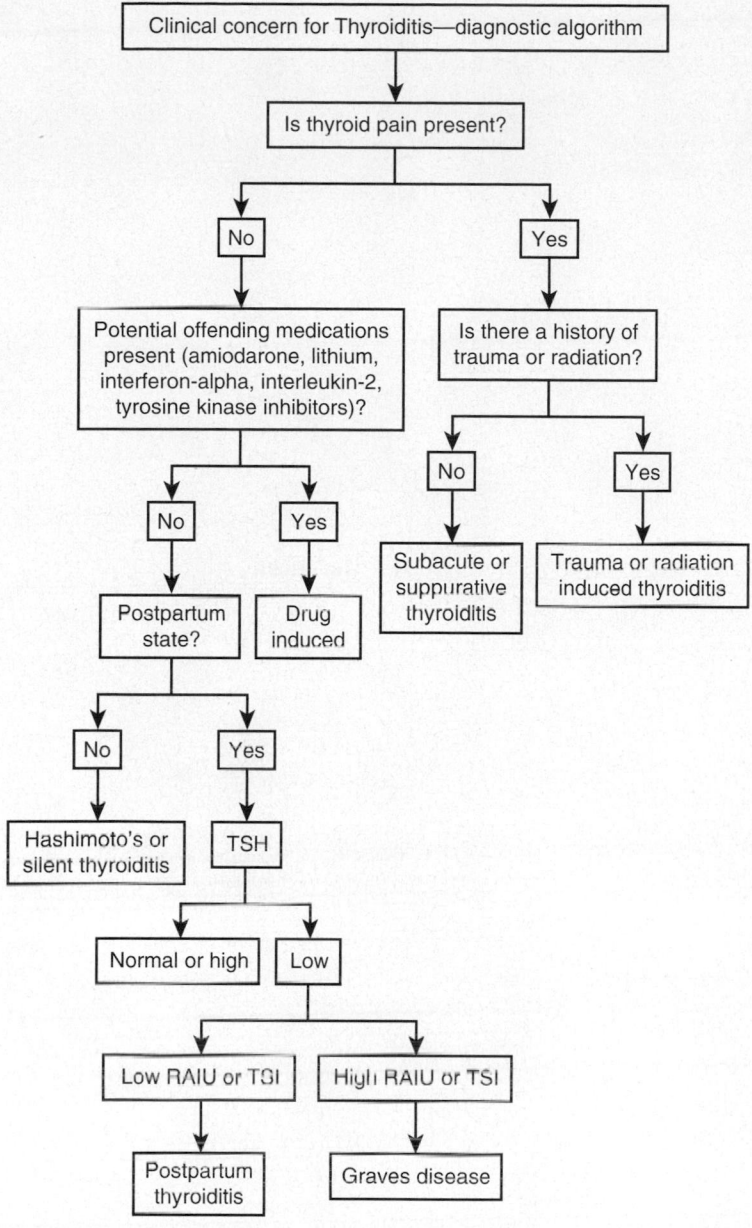

Figure 1. Clinical concern for thyroiditis—diagnostic algorithm. Abbreviations: RAIU = radioactive iodine uptake; TSI = thyroid-stimulating immunoglobulins.

References

Bogazzi F, Bartalena L, Martino E. Approach to the patient with amiodarone-induced thyrotoxicosis. J Clin Endocrinol Metab 2010;95:2529–35.

Cooper DS, Ladenson PW. The thyroid gland, In: Gardner DG, Shoback D, editors. Greenspan's Basic & Clinical Endocrinology. 9th ed. New York: McGraw-Hill; 2011. Available at http://accessmedicine.mhmedical.com/content.aspx?bookid=380&Sectionid=39744047 [accessed January 23, 2014].

De Groot L, Abalovich M, Alexander ED, et al. Management of thyroid dysfunction during pregnancy and postpartum: An Endocrine Society clinical practice guideline. J Clin Endocrinol Metab 2012;97:2543–65.

Pearce EN, Farwell AP, Braverman LE. Thyroiditis. N Engl J Med 2003;348:2646–55.

Samuels MH. Subacute, silent and postpartum thyroiditis. Med Clin North Am 2012;96:223–33.

12 Hematology

ACUTE LEUKEMIA IN ADULTS

Method of
Meir Wetzler, MD

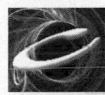

CURRENT DIAGNOSIS

Acute Myeloid Leukemia
- Diagnosis is made on 20% blasts or more; in patients with t(8;21) (q22;q22), inv(16)(p13q22) or t(16;16)(p13;q22), or t(15;17)(q22; q12) AML diagnosis is made even with less than 20% blasts.
- Separate entities are recognized based on specific chromosomal/molecular abnormalities.
- Presence of increased promyeloblasts facilitates diagnosis of acute promyelocytic leukemia.
- Presence of dysplastic eosinophils assists in the diagnosis of acute myeloid leukemia with inv(16)/t(16;16).
- Acute myeloid leukemia presentation is grouped based on presence of myelodysplastic changes, prior exposure to chemotherapy or radiotherapy, the presence of myeloid sarcoma, or Down syndrome.
- Acute myeloid leukemia with multilineage dysplasia is divided into subgroups based on prior history of myelodysplastic syndrome.

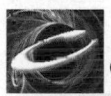

CURRENT THERAPY

Acute Myeloid Leukemia
- Treatment is divided into induction and post-remission therapy.
- Standard induction therapy for patients who have de novo acute myeloid leukemia and are younger than 60 years include combination therapy with cytarabine (cytosine arabinoside, ara-C [Cytosar]) and an anthracycline.
- All-*trans*-retinoic acid (tretinoin [Vesanoid]) and arsenic trioxide (Trisenox) are the new standard induction treatment for acute promyelocytic leukemia.

CURRENT DIAGNOSIS

Acute Lymphoblastic Leukemia
- There is no agreed-upon lower limit of blast percentage required for diagnosing acute lymphoblastic leukemia. Many treatment protocols use 25% blasts as the cut-off for diagnosis and in general, a diagnosis of acute lymphoblastic leukemia should be avoided if there are less than 20% blasts.
- The diagnosis includes B-lineage, T-lineage, and unspecified acute lymphoblastic leukemia.
- B-lineage, but not T-lineage categories are recognized as separate entities based on the presence of specific chromosomal or molecular abnormalities.

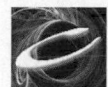

CURRENT THERAPY

Acute Lymphoblastic Leukemia
- The two most commonly used approaches include the Berlin-Frankfurt-Munster (BFM)-like and the hyper-cyclophosphamide (Cytoxan), vincristine (Oncovin), doxorubicin (Adriamycin), and dexamethasone (Decadron)[1] (CVAD) regimens.
- Imatinib mesylate (Gleevec) has significantly improved the outcome of t(9;22) acute lymphoblastic leukemia.
- Relapsed T-cell acute lymphoblastic leukemia benefits from the addition of nelarabine (Arranon).
- The use of pediatric regimens to treat adolescents and young adults has improved the outcome of these patients.
- Including anti-CD20 antibody in CD20-positive ALL leukemia has improved this disease's outcome.

[1]Not FDA approved for this indication.

Acute Myeloid Leukemia

Epidemiology
The age-adjusted incidence rate for acute myeloid leukemia (AML) is 4.05 per 100,000 men and women per year. The incidence increases with age and the median age at diagnosis is 67 years.

Risk Factors
Exposure to chemicals including benzene, petroleum products, herbicides, pesticides, and tobacco are associated with increased risk of AML. About 10% of patients exposed to chemotherapy or radiotherapy eventually develop therapy-related AML. Warfare and occupational exposure to ionizing radiation predispose to AML.

Pathophysiology
The pathophysiology of AML consists of maturation arrest at the blast level and activation of genes through several mechanisms (e.g., epigenetic silencing). One of the reasons for treatment failure in AML is the inability of current chemotherapy to kill the leukemia stem cells. These cells are quiescent, can self-renew, and have extensive proliferative capacity and the ability to give rise to differentiated progeny in a hierarchical pattern. Most of the chemotherapeutic agents traditionally used to treat AML are cell-cycle–active agents that primarily target dividing cells. These agents are highly unlikely to be effective against the quiescent leukemia stem cells. Therefore, new agents are being studied that target the leukemia stem cell.

Secondary AML, defined as AML following antecedent hematologic disorder or therapy for another disease, is associated with very poor outcome.

Prevention
Smoking cessation and avoiding exposure to offending agents, such as benzene, can prevent AML.

Clinical Manifestations
Patients might complain of fatigue or weakness, anorexia, or weight loss. Patients can also present with fever with or without source of infection, bleeding tendency, and sometimes bone pain, cough, or diaphoresis. Seldom patients present with soft tissue masses, called myeloid sarcoma, with or without bone marrow involvement.

On physical examination, fever, hepatosplenomegaly, lymphadenopathy, and evidence of infection and hemorrhage can be detected. Bleeding because of disseminated intravascular coagulopathy is more characteristic of **acute promyelocytic leukemia**. Infiltration of the gingiva, soft tissues, skin or meninges is more characteristic of monocytic leukemia. Patients with very high numbers of circulating blasts can develop signs of leukostasis such as headache, confusion, and dyspnea.

Diagnosis
AML is diagnosed if at least 20% blasts are present in the blood or bone marrow; except in patients with t(8;21)(q22;q22), inv(16) (p13q22), t(16;16)(p13;q22), or t(15;17)(q22;q12), where the diagnosis is made even with less than 20% blasts. Increased promyeloblasts are associated with t(15;17) and dysplastic eosinophils are characteristics of inv(16)/t(16;16). Auer rods, representing abnormal condensation of cytoplasmic granules, may be observed in myeloblasts.

AML presentation is grouped based on presence of myelodysplastic changes, prior exposure to chemotherapy or radiotherapy, the presence of myeloid sarcoma, or Down syndrome. AML with multilineage dysplasia is grouped into specific subtypes with or without the presence of prior multilineage dysplasia.

The AML blasts are characteristically myeloperoxidase-positive. If they are negative, expression of myeloid markers on their surface such as CD13 and CD33 is diagnostic. Blasts carrying t(8;21) often express lymphoid markers (e.g., CD19, PAX5, and cytoplasmic CD79a) and promyeloblasts with t(15;17) commonly express CD2.

Differential Diagnosis
The main alternative diagnosis is acute lymphoblastic leukemia (ALL).

Prognosis
Factors associated with worse outcome include older age (inability to survive induction either due to comorbidities or because of chemoresistance due to multidrug-resistance proteins), secondary presentation (prior chemotherapy for an unrelated disease or history of antecedent hematologic disorder), elevated white blood cell count (WBC >100 $\times$ 10^9/L), and poor performance status.

Karyotype aberrations (structural and numerical) assign patients into favorable, intermediate, and unfavorable subgroups (Table 1). In patients with normal karyotype, submicroscopic genetic aberrations further assign subgroups. *NPM1* mutations are found in 46% to 62% of AML patients, and they are associated with improved outcome if they are solely present. Detection of internal tandem duplications within the juxtamembrane domain of the *FLT3* gene, reported in about a third of the normal karyotype AML patients, predicts poor outcome, especially if the *FLT3*-ITD/*FLT3*-wild type allelic ratio is high. The deleterious prognostic significance of *FLT3* point mutations was demonstrated in younger patients; *FLT3*-ITD loses its prognostic effect in patients older than 70 years of age. Additional, less frequent, aberrations such as biallelic mutations of *CEBPA*, are associated with improved outcome, and partial tandem duplication of the *MLL* gene, *WT1* mutations, and overexpression of *BAALC*, *ERG* and *MN1* genes are associated with worse outcome in

GENETIC GROUP	**SUBSET[1]**
Favorable	t(8;21), inv(16) *NPM1*+/*FLT3*-WT (NK) Biallelic *CEPBA* (NK)
Intermediate-I	*NPM1*+/*FLT3*-ITD *NPM1*-/*FLT3*-ITD *NPM1*-/*FLT3*-WT
Intermediate-II	t(9;11) Others not favorable or adverse
Adverse	3q21-26, t(6;9), 11q23, -5, -7, abn(17p) complex

TABLE 1 New AML Standardized Reporting

normal karyotype AML. Submicroscopic genetic aberrations in the *KIT* gene adversely affect the outcome of t(8;21) and inv (16)/t(16;16).

Complete remission is defined as less than 5% blasts in the marrow, blood neutrophil count of at least 1×10^9/L, and platelet count at least 100×10^9/L without circulating blasts and disappearance of extramedullary disease, if such was present. Complete remission is necessary to achieve long-term survival or cure.

Treatment
Induction therapy for patients with newly diagnosed AML, in the absence of a clinical trial, consists of the combination of ara-C (Cytosar) at 100 to 200 mg/m²/day for 7 days as continuous infusion along with an anthracycline (e.g., daunorubicin [Cerubidine] or idarubicin [Idamycin]) administered intravenously over the first 3 days. Attempts to escalate ara-C during induction results in longer disease-free survival in some studies, and escalating anthracyclines improves complete remission rate and overall survival in patients younger than 65 years. Adding etoposide (Toposar)[1] can improve remission duration.

Multilumen right atrial catheters should be used to administer medications, fluid, and transfusions and to draw blood. Induction treatment can result in tumor lysis syndrome, characterized mainly by elevated uric acid. Therefore, allopurinol (Zyloprim) and hydration should be initiated early.

Patients who are allergic to allopurinol, who are unable to take oral medications, or who have uric acid nephropathy may be treated with rasburicase (recombinant uric acid oxidase, Elitek) or hemodialysis. Aggressive supportive care during the period of granulocytopenia and thrombocytopenia are necessary for the success of this treatment. Using recombinant growth factors has been reported to shorten median time to neutrophil recovery, but it has not resulted in improved outcome. Therefore, their use is controversial and should be restricted to clinical trials or according to published guidelines.

Platelet transfusions should maintain a platelet count greater than 10×10^9/L unless the patient has active bleeding or disseminated intravascular coagulation, when it may be necessary to maintain higher platelet counts. Similarly, red blood cell transfusions should maintain hemoglobin of greater than 8 g/dL unless patients have active bleeding, disseminated intravascular coagulopathy, or history of cardiovascular or pulmonary disease. All blood products should be leukodepleted by filtration and irradiated to prevent alloimmunization, fever, and transfusion-associated graft-versus-host disease.

Infections remain the most important cause of morbidity and mortality. Prophylactic antibiotics should be based on institutional antibiograms, and prophylactic antifungal and antiviral medications are highly recommended. Fever should be treated as resulting from bacterial and fungal infections.

After achieving complete remission, further treatment depends on the patient's age and prognostic factors. For example, high-dose

[1]Not FDA approved for this indication.

ara-C is more effective than standard-dose ara-C in younger AML patients, especially for those with t(8;21) and inv(16)/t(16;16) and those with normal karyotype AML.

Acute Promyelocytic Leukemia

Acute promyelocytic leukemia (APL), characterized by t(15;17) and its product *PML/RARα*, should be treated with all-*trans* retinoic acid (tretinoin [Vesanoid]), which induces differentiation of the leukemic blasts. During this differentiation process, the promyeloblasts lose their characteristic granules that can release enzymes causing disseminated intravascular coagulopathy. The most important side effect of tretinoin is the differentiation syndrome, characterized by increasing leukocyte counts, fever, shortness of breath, chest pain, pulmonary infiltrates, pleural and pericardial effusions, and hypoxia. Treatment for this complication includes steroids, chemotherapy, and supportive care.

Tretinoin and arsenic trioxide (Trisenox) represent the new treatment for APL. Because arsenic trioxide also exerts its effect through induction of differentiation, steroids are recommended for all patients preemptively. Approximately 90% of APL patients achieve complete remission, and this regimen results in prolonged disease-free survival.

Relapse

Once relapse occurs, patients are rarely cured with standard chemotherapy. Patients should be offered allogeneic stem cell transplantation in either first relapse or second remission; the outcome following second remission seems better. Second complete remission is more likely if the first remission lasted longer than 12 months and patients achieved complete remission following one induction course. The long-term disease-free survival following an allogeneic stem cell transplant in relapsed patients is about 40%.

Relapse in APL, in the absence of clinical trials, can respond to the combinations of tretinoin, arsenic trioxide, and an anthracycline.[1]

Novel Approaches and Future Directions

Novel approaches and future directions include targeted therapies for patients with *FLT3* and *KIT* mutations with specific tyrosine kinase inhibitors and targeting aberrant DNA methylation or histone deacetylation (or both) resulting in epigenetic silencing of structurally normal genes. Current hypomethylating agents approved for myelodysplastic syndromes (5-azacitidine [Vidaza][1] and decitabine [Dacogen][1]) are being studied in AML. The proteasome inhibitor bortezomib (Velcade)[1] is also being explored in AML.

Allogeneic stem cell transplantation reduces the relapse risk, but this beneficial effect is offset by its treatment-related mortality. Therefore, this approach should be reserved for patients with high-risk features such as intermediate and adverse karyotypes; those with high white blood cell counts at diagnosis; secondary AML; patients who do not achieve remission after standard induction treatment; and those in second remission and beyond.

Monitoring

Detection of minimal residual disease following complete remission by reverse-transcriptase polymerase chain reaction (PCR) of *PML/RARα* transcript predicts relapse. Therefore, sequential monitoring of *PML/RARα* is standard in APL. Detection of minimal residual disease in other types of AML is lagging behind, even though other fusion genes, such as t(8;21) and inv(16)/t(16;16), are available. Flow cytometry is being studied as a means to monitor minimal residual disease in AML.

---

[1]Not FDA approved for this indication.

Complications

The main risk following successful AML treatment is late development of secondary myelodysplastic syndromes and AML.

Acute Lymphoblastic Leukemia

Epidemiology

The age-adjusted incidence rate is 1.77 per 100,000 population per year. The median age at diagnosis is 14 years of age; about 60% of cases are diagnosed in patients younger than 20 years.

Risk Factors

Genetic predisposition to ALL is associated with Down syndrome, Fanconi's anemia, Bloom syndrome, neurofibromatosis type 1, and ataxia telangiectasia.

Pathophysiology

The theories about the origin of the leukemia-initiating cell in ALL vary. Some relate it to an already committed B- or T-lineage cell, and others propose that—at least in some ALL subtypes—the leukemia blasts might arise from a more phenotypically primitive hematopoietic stem cell. The most recent challenge to the leukemia-initiating cell theory is the report that B precursor blasts in various stages of differentiation displayed self-renewal capability, suggesting that leukemic lymphoid progenitors might not lose their self-renewal capability with maturation or are able to "move backward" in differentiation.

Secondary ALL, defined as ALL following another malignancy, irrespective whether patients received prior therapy, is rare. As in secondary AML, the outcome is extremely poor.

Prevention

Data suggest that early aspects of lifestyle and environment are associated with a decreased risk for ALL in children. For example, prolonged breast-feeding, daycare attendance, and early community-acquired infections are associated with a reduced incidence of childhood ALL. In the United States, ALL incidence rates are lower in rural communities compared with metropolitan areas. Finally, some data suggest that *Haemophilus influenzae* type b vaccine might reduce ALL risk.

Clinical Manifestations

The symptoms are not significantly different from those of patients with AML. Central nervous system (CNS) involvement is detected in approximately 10% of the cases and is more prevalent in T-cell ALL.

Diagnosis

The blasts range in size from homogeneous small cells with a high nuclear-to-cytoplasmic ratio and inconspicuous nucleoli to more-pleomorphic cells. Burkitt leukemia is characterized by medium-sized homogeneous cells with dispersed chromatin, multiple nucleoli, and a moderate amount of deep blue cytoplasm with clearly defined vacuoles. The "starry sky" appearance is composed of the tinted body macrophages (the stars) scattered among sheets of dark blue blasts (the sky).

ALL is characterized by blasts that are myeloperoxidase-negative and terminal deoxynucleotide transferase (TdT)-positive. CD10, CD19, cytoplasmic CD22, cytoplasmic CD79a, and PAX5 with variable expression of CD20 characterize B-lineage ALL, whereas CD1a, cytoplasmic CD3, CD7, CD4, and CD8 characterize T-lineage ALL. The presence of myeloid markers does not exclude the diagnosis of ALL.

Burkitt leukemia is characterized by B-cell–associated antigens and moderate to strong levels of membrane immunoglobulin M (IgM) with light chain restriction; the cells are TdT-negative and more than 99% Ki-67 positive. Burkitt's leukemia is a subtype of ALL whose hallmark is the t(8;14)(q24;q32) and its variants, t(2;8)(p12;q24) and t(8;22)(q24;q11). In these cases, *MYC*, located on 8q24, is activated and expressed at high levels, leading to uncontrolled cell proliferation. However, *MYC* translocations are not specific for Burkitt leukemia.

Differential Diagnosis

The main diagnosis in the differential is AML. The leukemia blasts can resemble hematogones, the normal lymphoid progenitors. Morphologic distinction between hematogones and residual ALL can be difficult. However, hematogones display the continuum of B-cell markers whereas the leukemic blasts overexpress or underexpress specific markers. For example, ALL with myeloid markers can be relatively easily distinguished from hematogones because the latter lack myeloid markers. Leukemia of ambiguous lineage includes biphenotypic leukemia, describing a single blast population expressing antigens from more than one lineage, and bilineage leukemia describing separate populations of blasts from more than one lineage. The two most common examples are those with t(9;22) and 11q23/*MLL* translocations.

Prognosis

Several factors are associated with worse outcome such as older age (inability to survive induction either owing to comorbidities or because of chemoresistance due to multidrug resistance proteins), secondary presentation (prior chemotherapy for an unrelated disease), elevated WBC count (>30 × 10^9/L in B-cell ALL; >100 × 10^9/L in T-cell ALL), immunophenotype (B-cell) CD20 expression and elevated lactate dehydrogenase, associated with CNS disease. Interestingly, persistence of normal residual hematopoiesis and intense leukemia cell mitotic index are associated with favorable outcome.

Recurring chromosomal abnormalities divide ALL into favorable, intermediate, and unfavorable subgroups (Table 2). Submicroscopic genetic aberrations further characterize the disease. For example, in T-cell ALL, activating somatic mutations in *NOTCH1* are described in about 50% of cases. NOTCH1 protein, either normal or aberrant, is cleaved by the γ-secretase complex, leading to its translocation to the nucleus where it induces *NOTCH1*-target gene transcription. This pathway is currently being targeted in clinical trials with γ-secretase inhibitors. Lack of *HOX11* expression and high *ERG* and *BAALC* expression predict adverse outcome in T-lineage ALL.

As in AML, achievement of complete remission is necessary to achieve long-term survival or cure. In addition, lack of cytoreduction on day 7 or 14 correlates with adverse prognosis in ALL.

Treatment

The two most commonly used approaches in ALL include the BFM (Berlin-Frankfurt-Munster) and the hyper-CVAD (cyclophosphamide, vincristine, doxorubicin [Adriamycin], and dexamethasone) regimens.

BFM-like regimens include induction with vincristine, prednisone,[1] daunorubicin, and pegylated asparaginase (Oncaspar); early intensification with cyclophosphamide (Cytoxan), ara-C (Cytosar), 6-mercaptopurine (Purinethol), and vincristine; CNS prophylaxis with either cranial radiation or high-dose methotrexate and ara-C; late intensification with doxorubicin, vincristine, dexamethasone,[1] cyclophosphamide, 6-thioguanine (Tabloid),[1] and ara-C; and maintenance with prednisone, vincristine, 6-mercaptopurine, and methotrexate (POMP) for a total of 24 months.

---

[1]Not FDA approved for this indication.

TABLE 2 Karyotype Risk Groups in Acute Lymphoblastic Leukemia

RISK GROUP	ABERRATION
Favorable	del(12p) or t(12p), t(14)(q11-q13), hyperdiploid
Intermediate	Normal karyotype, +21, del(9p) or t(9p)
Unfavorable	t(9;22), -7, +8, t(4;11), hypodiploid, t(1;19)

The hyper-CVAD regimen consists of eight alternating courses of CVAD with methotrexate and high-dose ara-C. CNS prophylaxis includes, in addition to the high-dose cytarabine and methotrexate, intrathecal methotrexate. Maintenance is conducted with POMP to complete 24 months.

The outcome following these different approaches results in approximately 30% to 40% 5-year survival. Supportive care guidelines are similar to those described in the AML section.

A major breakthrough occurred with the introduction of imatinib mesylate (Gleevec) for the treatment of t(9;22) ALL and its product *BCR/ABL*. Imatinib functions though competitive inhibition at the adenosine triphosphate (ATP) binding site of the ABL kinase in the inactive conformation, which leads to inhibition of tyrosine phosphorylation of proteins involved in BCR/ABL signaling. It shows a high degree of specificity for BCR/ABL, the receptor for platelet-derived growth factor and KIT tyrosine kinases. Imatinib does not affect the normal hematopoietic progenitor cells. Combining imatinib with chemotherapy, either sequentially (aiming to reduce toxicity) or concurrently, resulted in a significant improvement in disease-free survival over chemotherapy-alone approaches.

Four mechanisms of resistance to imatinib have been described to date: gene amplification, mutations at the kinase site, decreased intracellular imatinib levels, and alternative signaling pathways functionally compensating for the imatinib-sensitive mechanisms. Unique to ALL, kinase domain mutations can precede imatinib-based therapy and give rise to relapse in patients with de novo t(9;22) ALL. Alternating signaling pathways such as Src family kinase members—Lyn, Hck, and Fgr—have been shown to be elevated in hematopoietic cells of mice with t(9;22) ALL. Even in the presence of suppressed BCR/ABL, t(9;22) ALL cells can proliferate in the presence of stromal support.

Approaches to overcome these mechanisms of resistance include introduction of dasatinib (Sprycel), which is almost 300-fold more potent than imatinib, binds to the kinase domain in the open conformation, is resistant to most mutations, and is active against Src kinases. Dasatinib, as a single agent and in combination with chemotherapy, was tested in imatinib-resistant and imatinib-naïve t(9;22) ALL with encouraging results. Dasatinib and prednisone alone have been studied as front-line therapy in newly diagnosed t(9;22)[1] ALL with encouraging results. Similarly, nilotinib (Tasigna)[1] is about 30-fold more potent than imatinib, binds to the kinase domain in the inactive formation, and is resistant to most mutations. Nilotinib has promising activity in imatinib-resistant ALL as monotherapy. Recently, ponatinib (Iclusig) was approved for t(9;22) that failed prior treatment. Its unique role is in overcoming resistance generated by the presence of the T315I mutation, for which none of the other TKIs, have activity.

Nelarabine (Arranon) is a purine analogue shown to have significant activity in T-lineage ALL patients whose disease has not responded to or has relapsed following treatment with at least two chemotherapy regimens. In the adult clinical trial, the rate of complete remission was 31% and the overall response rate was 41%. The main toxicity was grade 3 to 4 neutropenia and thrombocytopenia. It is now going to be studied in newly diagnosed T-lineage ALL.[1]

Pediatric Regimens for Adolescents and Adults

Adolescents and young adults represent a challenging group for both pediatric and adult oncologists. Several groups have evaluated the outcome of patients aged 16 to 21 years based on their treatment on adult or pediatric protocols. Despite an assortment of treatment approaches among the different groups, the results of these retrospective analyses consistently demonstrated that adolescents and young adults treated on pediatric protocols had significantly better 5-year survival than those treated on adult protocols. Several reasons were suggested for these differences, including more-intensive use of non-myelosuppressive agents (e.g., steroids, L-asparaginase,

---

[1]Not FDA approved for this indication.

vincristine), earlier CNS prophylaxis, and longer maintenance in the pediatric protocols. Moreover, protocol adherence and compliance, by both treating physicians and patients, was raised as a contributing factor to outcome differences. Therefore, most groups offer pediatric regimens to adolescents and young adults (up to age 30 years and beyond) with encouraging results.

The treatment of adult Burkitt leukemia underwent significant improvement when pediatric regimens, including repetitive cycles of fractional alkylating agents and aggressive CNS therapy, were employed. Because Burkitt leukemia is characterized by strong CD20 expression, two groups successfully included anti-CD20 antibody, rituximab (Rituxan),[1] in their treatment regimens. In addition to the favorable outcome in these patients, concerns about increased infectious complications, due to the use of rituximab, were dismissed by these studies. This led to the addition of rituximab to CD20-positive ALL treatment protocol.

Allogeneic stem cell transplantation continues to represent an effective treatment approach for adult ALL. It is usually recommended to high-risk ALL patients in first remission and those in second remission and beyond. Offering allogeneic stem cell transplantation for standard-risk ALL is controversial.

Novel Approaches and Future Directions
The use of a bi-specific T cell–engaging antibody that directs cytotoxic T cells to CD19 expressing target cells resulted in a complete remission rate of 68% among relapsed or refractory ALL patients. In addition, a CD22 monoclonal antibody conjugated to calicheamicin has demonstrated a 50% overall response rate in relapsed or refractory ALL patients. Both studies are still ongoing, and plans to incorporate these novel approaches into the treatment armamentarium of newly diagnosed ALL are underway.

Monitoring
Minimal residual disease in ALL is one of the most powerful and informative parameters to guide clinical management. Two methods have been established to detect minimal residual disease: Flow cytometry relies on immunologic markers to identify residual leukemic cells, and PCR amplifies fusion transcript or uses antigen-receptor genes as targets to detect minimal residual disease.

Complications
The main risk following successful treatment of ALL is late development of secondary myelodysplastic syndromes and AML. Another complication is avascular necrosis due to steroid use.

---

[1]Not FDA approved for this indication.

References
Burnett A, Wetzler M, Lowenberg B. Therapeutic advances in acute myeloid leukemia. J Clin Oncol 2011;29:487–94.
Campana D. Role of minimal residual disease monitoring in adult and pediatric acute lymphoblastic leukemia. Hematol Oncol Clin North Am 2009;23:1083–98 vii.
DeAngelo DJ. Nelarabine for the treatment of patients with relapsed or refractory T-cell acute lymphoblastic leukemia or lymphoblastic lymphoma. Hematol Oncol Clin North Am 2009;23:1121–35 vii–viii.
Dohner H, Estey EH, Amadori S, et al. Diagnosis and management of acute myeloid leukemia in adults: Recommendations from an international expert panel, on behalf of the European LeukemiaNet. Blood 2010;115:453–74.
Forman SJ. Allogeneic hematopoietic cell transplantation for acute lymphoblastic leukemia in adults. Hematol Oncol Clin North Am 2009;23:1011–31 vi.
Jeha S, Pui CH. Risk-adapted treatment of pediatric acute lymphoblastic leukemia. Hematol Oncol Clin North Am 2003;23:973–90 v.
Kantarjian HM, Erba HP, Claxton D, et al. Phase II study of clofarabine monotherapy in previously untreated older adults with acute myeloid leukemia and unfavorable prognostic factors. J Clin Oncol 2010;28:549–55.
Lee HJ, Thompson JE, Wang ES, Wetzler M. Philadelphia chromosome-positive acute lymphoblastic leukemia: current treatment and future perspectives. Cancer 2010;117:1583–94.
Mrozek K, Harper DP, Aplan PD. Cytogenetics and molecular genetics of acute lymphoblastic leukemia. Hematol Oncol Clin North Am 2009;23:991–1010 v.
Nathan PC, Wasilewski-Masker K, Janzen LA. Long-term outcomes in survivors of childhood acute lymphoblastic leukemia. Hematol Oncol Clin North Am 2009;23:1065–82 vi–vii.
NCCN. Acute myeloid leukemia. Clinical Practice Guidelines in Oncology: National Comprehensive Cancer Network; 2010.
Ribera JM, Oriol A. Acute lymphoblastic leukemia in adolescents and young adults. Hematol Oncol Clin North Am 2009;23:1033–42 vi.
Sanz MA, Grimwade D, Tallman MS, et al. Management of acute promyelocytic leukemia: recommendations from an expert panel on behalf of the European LeukemiaNet. Blood 2009;113:1875–91.
Swerdlow SH, Campo E, Harris NL, et al. WHO Classification of Tumours of Haematopoietic and Lymphoid Tissues. In: Swerdlow SH, Campo E, Harris NL, et al., editors. WHO Classification of Tumours of Haematopoietic and Lymphoid Tissues. Lyon: IARC Press; 2008.
Thomas DA, O'Brien S, Kantarjian HM. Monoclonal antibody therapy with rituximab for acute lymphoblastic leukemia. Hematol Oncol Clin North Am 2009;23:949–71 v.

APLASTIC ANEMIA

Method of
Eva C. Guinan, MD

CURRENT DIAGNOSIS

- Patient must all meet hematologic criteria.
- Assess severity.
- Adequate cytogenetic analysis is essential.
- Consider diagnoses with treatment implications:
  - Causes of transient pancytopenia.
  - Evaluate for inherited bone marrow failure syndromes, paroxysmal nocturnal hemoglobinuria, myelodysplastic syndromes.
  - Evaluate for malignancy (leukemia, lymphoma), HIV.

CURRENT THERAPY

- Minimize interval between diagnosis and initiation of treatment.
- Determine if an MSD is available.
- If the patient is young and has an MSD, proceed to HCT with non-TBI regimen.
- If the patient has no MSD or is older, proceed to IST with CSA/ATG/steroid.
- For treatment failure, reconsider IST versus HCT options.

Abbreviations: ATG = antithymocyte globulin; CSA = cyclosporine; HCT = hematopoietic cell transplantation; IST = immunosuppressive therapy; MSD = matched sibling donor; TBI = total body irradiation.

The survival of patients with aplastic anemia has improved dramatically in the past several decades. Improved testing for underlying acquired and congenital genetic defects has served to better segregate patients with idiopathic aplastic anemia from those with the very different prognoses associated with inherited bone marrow failure syndrome (IBMFS) and myelodysplasia (MDS). For patients in the idiopathic (or acquired) aplastic anemia group, advances in transfusion medicine and other supportive care have also certainly contributed. Refinements in both major arms of treatment, immunosuppressive therapy (IST), and allogeneic hematopoietic cell transplantation (HCT), have also contributed to current outcomes (Figure 1). Although IST survival curves have been stable in the last decade, survival after HCT regardless of donor source has continued to improve. Greater understanding of pathophysiology and long-term treatment outcomes are having the largest impact on triage of therapy and standards of practice.

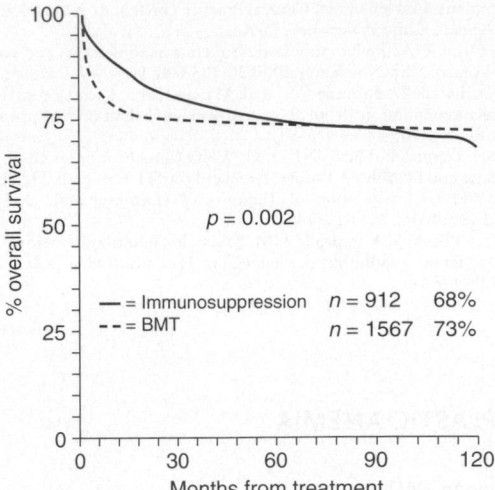

Figure 1. The actuarial survival of 2479 patients with acquired severe aplastic anemia. Group A received immunosuppressive therapy (IST) *(solid line)* as first-line therapy and Group B underwent hematopoietic stem cell transplant (BMT) *(dashed line)*. Ten-year survival was 73% with BMT and 68% with IST (*p* < 0.002). (Data from Locasciulli A, Oneto R, Bacigalupo A, et al: Outcome of patients with acquired aplastic anemia given first-line bone marrow transplantation or immunosuppressive treatment in the last decade: A report from the European Group for Blood and Marrow Transplantation [EBMT]. Haematologica 2007;92:11–18.)

Definition

There is no pathognomonic diagnostic test for aplastic anemia. Accordingly, aplastic anemia continues to be diagnosed by a combination of inclusion and exclusion criteria. The definition established by the International Agranulocytosis and Aplastic Anaemia Study states that patients must have bone marrow hypocellularity with two or more of the following: hemoglobin of less than 10 g/dL, platelet count of less than 50×10^9/L, and neutrophil count of less than 1.5×10^9/L. Most commonly, patients said to have aplastic anemia in fact have severe aplastic anemia, which is defined by the absolute neutrophil count (ANC) as shown in Box 1. Severity grading has become part of the diagnostic algorithm and is increasingly used as one predictor of outcome.

Differential Diagnosis

Because many conditions can fulfill these inclusion criteria, care must be taken to consider infectious, metabolic, and toxic exposures that could result in transient pancytopenia. Specific considerations are listed in many current reviews. These diagnoses are wide ranging and include hypoplastic presentations of lymphoma,

---

Box 1 — Severity Classification of Aplastic Anemia

Severe
Bone marrow cellularity <25%
and
Two peripheral blood findings:
- Absolute neutrophil count <0.5 × 10^9/L
- Platelet count <20 × 10^9/L
- Reticulocyte count <20 × 10^9/L

Very Severe
Same criteria as for severe
and
Peripheral blood absolute neutrophil count <0.2 × 10^9/L

Nonsevere (Moderate)
Hypocellullar bone marrow
and
Peripheral blood cytopenias not meeting criteria for severe aplastic anemia

---

leukemia, and MDS (including the subtype refractory cytopenia of childhood); anorexia; and transient severe bone marrow suppression due to drug exposure or, albeit rarely, a spectrum of acute viral illnesses.

Patients should be carefully evaluated for other conditions that can require an alternative management approach. A fraction of pancytopenic and hypocellular patients have clonal cytogenetic abnormalities despite well-reviewed histology that appears to be free of any evidence of dysplasia or infiltrative disease. Accordingly, best practice should include both fluorescent in situ hybridization (FISH) and routine cytogenetics, because the yield for the latter analysis may be inadequate given the hypocellularity of the bone marrow compartment.

Although the prognostic relevance of clonal cytogenetics remains somewhat debatable, evidence of clonality at diagnosis should certainly provoke consideration of MDS as an alternative diagnosis and mandate an aggressive plan of follow-up and determination of HCT donor status. Clonality also potentially alters immediate treatment depending on the clinical setting and most current literature. Among infectious problems, perhaps the most important consideration from a diagnostic and management perspective is HIV. However, viruses rarely cause a true aplastic picture, and their diagnosis, at present, does not have much therapeutic importance. Aplastic anemia can occur or recur during pregnancy and can resolve with either delivery or termination.

The most important alternative diagnosis is an inherited bone marrow failure syndrome (IBMFS) (Table 1), which should be considered in virtually all patients and certainly in all pediatric patients. Such a diagnosis has important implications for medical management of the extended family, for genetic counseling, for the choice of therapy, for prognosis of the patient, and, in the setting of HCT, for donor evaluation. A meticulous patient and family history and physical examination should be performed, although uninformative results do not eliminate the possibility of an IBMFS. IBMFS diagnosis by functional testing for cell surface molecules, telomere length, and chromosomal breakage has markedly improved. Genetic testing is available for some IBMFSs; however, it is clear that these syndromes are polygenic, and not all relevant genetic defects have been defined. Therefore, testing might not be diagnostic. Moreover, new genetic defects associated with aplastic anemia are still being discovered. As additional mutations are described and their epidemiology becomes better elucidated, this information should be of increasing value.

In addition to IBMFS, an evaluation for paroxysmal nocturnal hemoglobinuria (PNH) should be undertaken. A small clonal population of cells deficient in glycosylphosphatidylinositol (GPI)-linked proteins that characterize PNH can be found in 20% to 50% of both children and adults with aplastic anemia without a concurrent history of clotting or hemolysis. The presence of such cells does not imply a diagnosis of classic PNH, although some patients with apparent aplastic anemia do develop classic PNH. Ongoing clinical investigation into the relation of aplastic anemia and PNH might yield further information that will assist in therapeutic decision making.

Supportive Care

The goals of supportive care in aplastic anemia are alleviating symptoms of anemia and addressing the risks of hemorrhage and infection that result from pancytopenia. Appropriate precautions for minimizing alloimmunization should be taken, such as use of leukodepletion techniques and conservative transfusion goals.

Preemptive counseling can play as important a role as symptom management. There are few evidence-based guidelines for activities of daily living, such as the quality of diet, extent of exercise, and travel restrictions. The best standard is frequent, open communication between physician and patient. Some practical issues, however, are common. For example, the menstrual status of female patients should be ascertained immediately on diagnosis. Because severe menorrhagia can occur in the setting of protracted thrombocytopenia, use of hormonal therapy to suppress menstruation should be addressed with patients and with families of younger patients. Particular regard should be paid to anticipation of menarche in pubertal girls.

TABLE 1 Inherited Bone Marrow Failure Syndromes Commonly Associated with Pancytopenia*

SYNDROME	COMMON HEMATOLOGIC FINDINGS	DIAGNOSTIC TESTS AVAILABLE†
Amegakaryocytic thrombocytopenia	Thrombocytopenia with absent or hypolobulated megakaryocytes Macrocytosis Progressive pancytopenia with marrow hypoplasia	Gene mutation analysis
Dyskeratosis congenita	Macrocytosis Thrombocytopenia Progressive pancytopenia with marrow hypoplasia	Gene mutation analysis Telomere length (markedly shortened)
Fanconi anemia	Macrocytosis Single, bilineage, or trilineage cytopenia Progressive pancytopenia with marrow hypoplasia	Abnormal chromosomal breakage or sister-chromatid exchange in the presence of DNA cross-linkers Abnormal cell cycle progression Gene mutation analysis
Shwachman-Diamond syndrome	Neutropenia Progressive pancytopenia with marrow hypoplasia	Radiologic bony abnormalities Serum trypsinogen and isoamylase levels (may be decreased) Gene mutation analysis

*Diamond-Blackfan anemia, as well as less common disorders such as Pearson's, Seckel's, and Noonan's syndromes; cartilage–hair hypoplasia; and reticular dysgenesis, can progress to marrow failure meeting the definition of aplastic anemia.
†Clinically approved mutation testing is becoming increasingly available, but not all genetic defects have been defined for any of these disorders.

With regard to infectious risks, standards widely vary by practitioner and institution. Although the largest single cause of death in patients undergoing either HCT or IST is infection, there is no current standard for infection prophylaxis in aplastic anemia. Clinical trials to define the best possible approaches to this issue, including the role of novel broad-spectrum anti-infectives and their schedule of use, would be very important. At the least, a detailed history taken in the context of exposure and lifestyle issues should be used to develop a plan for fever and infection prophylaxis with which the patient can be compliant.

Benefit from the use of hematopoietic growth factors to support the ANC, or indeed any lineage, has been unclear in patients with idiopathic aplastic anemia. Prior concerns about the association of long-term use of granulocyte colony-stimulating factor (G-CSF) (Neupogen)[1] by pediatric aplastic anemia patients, in particular,

[1]Not FDA approved for this indication.

and subsequent development of MDS and acute myelogenous leukemia (AML), have not been confirmed in recent multicenter data.

Monitoring of iron status should be routine for patients with ongoing red cell transfusion needs. Chelation should be initiated according to accepted guidelines to minimize complications of iron overload.

Treatment

Observation is not a successful treatment option for patients with severe aplastic anemia; older, retrospective data demonstrate a 1-year mortality with supportive care alone of more than 80%, although current transfusion and support strategies should improve on this outcome. Nonetheless, a recent large report from the European Group for Blood and Marrow Transplantation demonstrates that decreased time from diagnosis to treatment, whether IST or HCT, is a highly significant predictor of survival. A triage of therapy is shown in Figure 2.

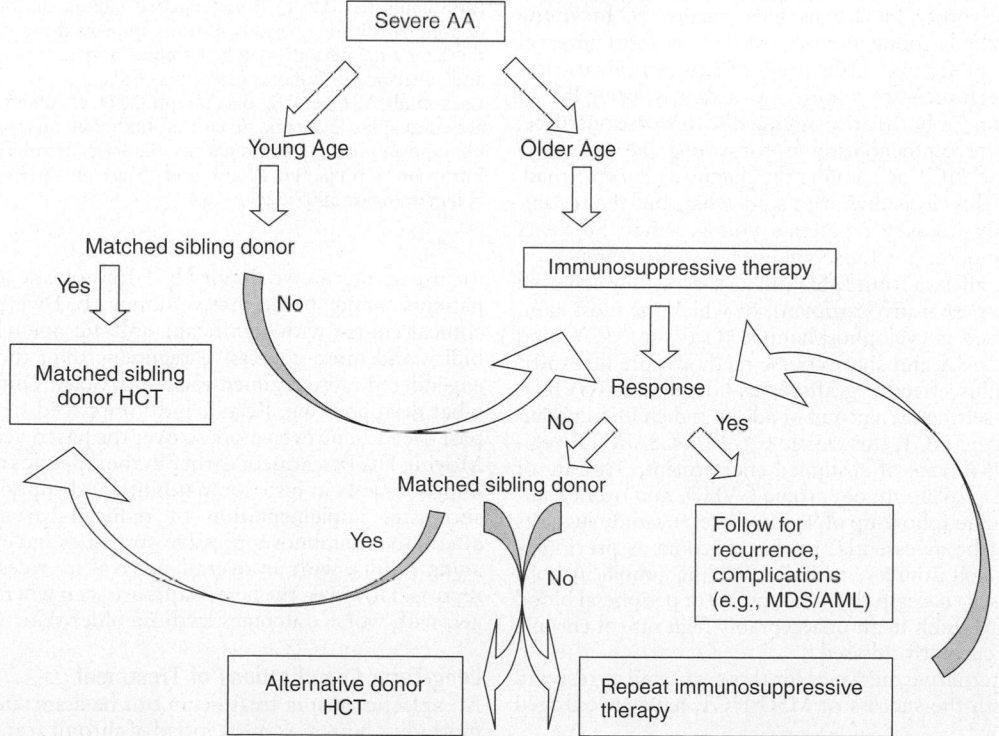

Figure 2. Triage of aplastic anemia (AA) therapies. The age limit suggested by young/old is variable from report to report, but generally sits in the 30- to 40-year-old range. *Abbreviations:* AML = acute myelogenous leukemia; HCT = hematopoietic cell transplant; MDS = myelodysplasia.

Immunosuppressive Therapy

It is generally held that a significant percentage of aplastic anemia has an immune pathogenesis. A variety of data on immune effector cell function and repertoire, cell surface phenotype, and cytokine production support this belief. In practice, this hypothesis is also supported by the observation that IST with cyclosporine (Neoral)[1] (CSA), antithymocyte globulin (ATG), and corticosteroids results in response in roughly 75% of patients. Horse ATG was shown to be superior to rabbit ATG in a recent randomized trial.

Younger patients generally have a higher likelihood of response. Children (<16 years) on IST with very severe aplastic anemia have better survival rates than similarly affected adults. Age does not affect the relative survival rate of patients with less severe aplastic anemia.

Randomized studies have demonstrated better response when IST agents are used in combination. Meta-analysis has also shown decreased all-cause mortality. In addition to their general immunomodulatory capacity, the immunologic effects of IST may be specific, because direct lympholytic and bone marrow stimulatory activities have been described. The addition of further immunosuppressive medications, such as mycophenolate or sirolimus, to this regimen has thus far not improved outcomes.

IST responses can be of varying degree and duration and can take 3 to 6 months to become evident. Often, responding patients continue to manifest some evidence of bone marrow failure, with mild degrees of cytopenia or residual macrocytosis commonly observed. Slow taper of CSA in IST responders is advisable, generally over longer than 6 months, and a significant fraction of patients demonstrate prolonged dependence on CSA for persistent hematologic improvement. A second course of IST in patients who failed a first course can produce response in 12% to 50% of patients. Complete or partial loss of response occurs in an appreciable number of patients, approximately one third, and can become manifest years after cessation of IST or immediately on CSA taper. Re-treatment with the same or a similar regimen is often successful.

Recent studies demonstrate that eltrombopag (Promacta), a thrombopoietin mimetic, has potential for multilineage efficacy in patients with severe aplastic anemia refractory to IST, and it has been FDA-approved for this indication.

Hematopoietic Cell Transplantation

HCT is the only truly curative therapy for aplastic anemia and produces stable survival rates in the range of 65% to 90%, depending on donor type and other HCT variables (Figure 3). In young patients with matched sibling donors (MSDs), a short interval from diagnosis to HCT, and little prior therapy, survival rates up to 97% have been recently reported. Conversely, prior IST or excessive transfusion (or both) are associated with worse outcome. Thus, the general recommendation is for young patients with MSDs to proceed to HCT as soon as the diagnosis is confirmed. The age cutoff for this decision varies somewhat, but the recommendation certainly holds for patients younger than 30 years and is often implemented for those younger than 40 years.

HCT for aplastic anemia from MSD can be successfully achieved with radiation-free preparative regimens, of which the most standard and widely used is cyclophosphamide (Cytoxan)[1] (CY) and ATG conditioning. CSA and short-course methotrexate (Trexall)[1] (MTX) provide highly effective graft-versus-host disease (GVHD) prophylaxis in this setting. In a group of adults and children undergoing MSD allogeneic HCT, this classic CY/ATG/CSA/MTX regimen produced a 96% rate of sustained engraftment, 3% rate of severe acute GVHD, 26% rate of chronic GVHD, and overall survival of 88% at median follow-up of 9 years. A recent study suggests that ATG may not be as essential to this outcome as previously thought. All stem cell sources, including sibling umbilical cord blood, have been used successfully, although use of peripheral blood stem cells appears to result in an unacceptably high rate of chronic GHVD and is not currently advised.

The dearth of alternative therapies for those who fail to respond to IST, coupled with the success of MSD HCT, have encouraged

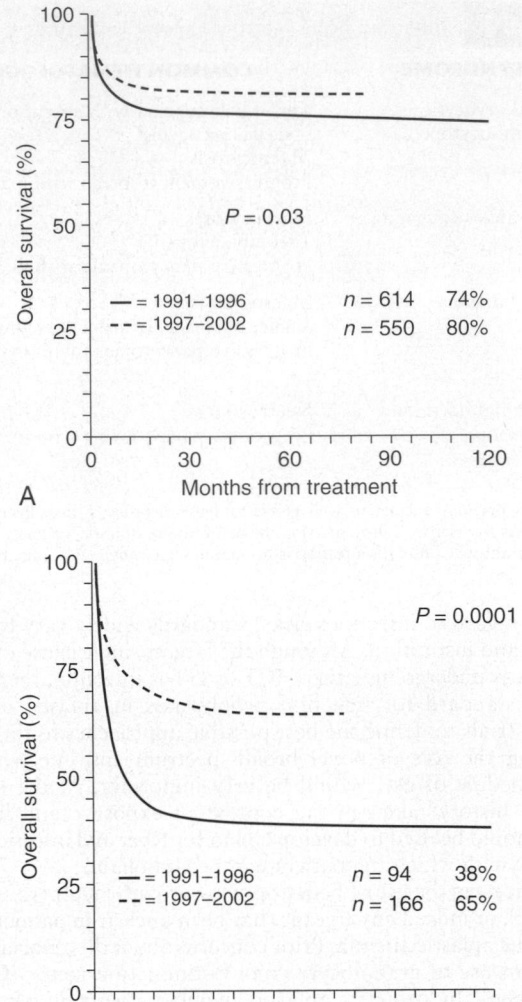

Figure 3. The actuarial survival of patients undergoing hematopoietic cell transplantation (HCT) from matched sibling donors (**A**) or alternative donors (**B**) by time periods. Results improved for both donor groups in the later time period (matched sibling donors 74% vs 80%, *P* = 0.03) and alternative donors (38% vs 65%, *P* = 0.0001). (Data from Locasciulli A, Oneto R, Bacigalupo A, et al. Outcome of patients with acquired aplastic anemia given first line bone marrow transplantation or immunosuppressive treatment in the last decade: A report from the European Group for Blood and Marrow Transplantation [EBMT]. Haematologica 2007;92:11–18.)

the use of alternative-donor HCT for aplastic anemia. Originally, patients coming to alternative-donor HCT were often late in their clinical course with significant aplastic anemia–associated morbidity and more aggressive regimens than those used for MSD engendered more regimen-related toxicity. Outcomes were somewhat disappointing. Results have improved significantly over the past decade, and even more so over the past 5 years (see Figure 3B). Moving HCT treatment earlier in therapeutic triage, coupled with improvements in histocompatibility and supportive care, and the successful implementation of reduced-intensity regimens and alternative immunosuppressive strategies have produced encouraging results, with an overall survival in excess of 70% in some reports. However, the best results are seen when patients are younger, with worse outcomes in those older than 40 years.

Long-Term Complications of Treatment

All aplastic anemia treatments can be associated with significant morbidity, be it the iron-overload of chronic transfusion or the more protean problems of IST or HCT. These include, in both cases,

---

[1]Not FDA approved for this indication.

significant regimen-related end-organ toxicity. The development of clonal cytogenetic abnormalities after IST is well described and occurs in patients of all ages, regardless of treatment response, and over a broad time frame. The rate of progression to frank AML is not predictable, although progression is most common in those with monosomy 7 or complex cytogenetic abnormalities. Patients with aplastic anemia who undergo HCT generally experience fewer toxicities than does the overall HCT population, in part due to the reduced intensity of aplastic anemia regimens. Growth and fertility may be well preserved, but persistent infectious complications, pulmonary insufficiency, dermatologic pathology, avascular necrosis, other bone and joint issues, hypothyroidism or other endocrine disturbances, and secondary malignancies can occur. Some of these conditions reflect the sequelae of chronic GVHD itself, and others reflect the toxicity of drugs used to manage GVHD. The toll of GVHD is real; decreased quality of life and overall survival are observed in the nearly one half of aplastic anemia patients experiencing chronic GVHD.

Conclusions

Improvements in diagnosis, supportive care, IST, and HCT have led to significant improvements in survival for patients with severe aplastic anemia. However, there are still controversies over the optimal choice of therapy for individual patients, and any given choice can lead to a number of serious regimen-related toxicities. Further insights into the pathophysiology of bone marrow failure, increased diagnostic accuracy for IBMFS, greater appreciation of the risk and epidemiology of late complications, and steady progress in therapeutics will hopefully combine to yield increasingly well-targeted and more-successful treatment.

Acknowledgments

Eva C. Guinan is a prior recipient of a Specified Established Researcher Award from the Aplastic Anemia & MDS International Foundation and the Distinguished Service Award of the Fanconi Anemia Research Foundation.

References

Ades L, Mary JY, Robin M, et al. Long-term outcome after bone marrow transplantation for severe aplastic anemia. Blood 2004;103:2490–7.
Desmond R, et al. Eltrombopag in aplastic anemia. Semin Hematol 2015;52(1):31–7.
Dokal I, Vulliamy T. Inherited bone marrow failure syndromes. Haematologica 2010;95:1236–40.
Frickhofen N, Heimpel H, Kaltwasser JP, Schrezenmeier H. Antithymocyte globulin with or without cyclosporin A: 11 year follow up of a randomized trial comparing treatments of aplastic anemia. Blood 2003;101:1236–42.
Fuhrer M, Burdach S, Ebell W, et al. Relapse and clonal disease in children with aplastic anemia (AA) after immunosuppressive therapy (IST): The SAA 94 experience. German/Austrian Pediatric Aplastic Anemia Working Group. Klin Padiatr 1998;210:173–9.
Gafter-Gvilli A, Ram R, Gurion R, et al. ATG plus cyclosporine reduces all-cause mortality in patients with severe aplastic anemia—systematic review and meta-analysis. Acta Haematol 2008;120:237–40.
Gurion R, Gafter-Gvili A, Paul M, et al. Hematopoietic growth factors in aplastic anemia patients treated with immunosuppressive therapy-systematic review and meta-analysis. Haematologica 2009;94:712–9.
Kurre P, Johnson FL, Deeg HJ. Diagnosis and treatment of children with aplastic anemia. Pediatr Blood Cancer 2005;45:770–80.
Locasciulli A, Oneto R, Bacigalupo A, et al. Outcome of patients with acquired aplastic anemia given first line bone marrow transplantation or immuno-suppressive treatment in the last decade: A report from the European Group for Blood and Marrow Transplantation (EBMT). Haematologica 2007;92:11–8.
Maciejewski JP, Risitano A, Sloand EM, et al. Distinct clinical outcomes for cytogenetic abnormalities evolving from aplastic anemia. Blood 2002;99:3129–35.
Marsh JCW, Ball SE, Cavenaugh J, et al. Guidelines for the diagnosis and management of acquired aplastic anaemia. Br J Haematol 2009;147:43–70.
Niemeyer CM, Baumann I. Classification of childhood aplastic anemia and myelodysplastic syndrome. Hematology Am Soc Hematol Educ Program 2011;2011:84–9.
Parker C, Omine M, Richards S, et al. Diagnosis and management of paroxysmal nocturnal hemoglobinuria. Blood 2005;106:3699–709.
Peinemann F, Grouven U, Kroger N, et al. First-line matched related donor hematopoietic stem cell transplantation compared to immunosuppressive therapy in acquired severe aplastic anemia. PlosOne 2011;6:e18572.
Scheinberg P. Nunez Olga, Weinstein B, et al. Horse versus Rabbit Antithymocyte Globulin in Acquired Aplastic Anemia N Engl J Med 2011;365:430–8.
Schrezenmeier H, Passweg JR, Marsh JC, et al. Worse outcome and more chronic GVHD with peripheral blood progenitor cells than bone marrow in HLA-matched sibling donor transplants for young patients with severe acquired aplastic anemia:
A report from the European Group for Blood and Marrow Transplantation and the Center for International Blood and Marrow Transplant Research. Blood 2007;110(4):1397–400.
Socie G, Gluckman E. Cure from severe aplastic anemia in vivo and late effects. Acta Haematol 2000;103:49–54.
Young NS, Calado RT, Scheinberg P. Current concepts in the pathophysiology and treatment of aplastic anemia. Blood 2006;108:2509–19.

BLOOD COMPONENT THERAPY

Method of
Theresa Nester, MD

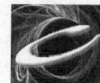

CURRENT DIAGNOSIS

- Fever greater than 1°C rise during or within 4 hours following transfusion should prompt evaluation of the patient and consideration of a transfusion reaction.
- Fever and pain are the most common manifestations of an acute hemolytic transfusion reaction.
- The point of the transfusion reaction laboratory investigation is to evaluate for hemolysis, either intravascular or extravascular. The majority of reactions are negative for hemolysis.
- The differential diagnosis of a transfusion reaction with respiratory symptoms includes febrile nonhemolytic and circulatory overload (common), allergic or anaphylactic reaction, transfusion-related acute lung injury, acute hemolytic reaction, and bacterial contamination (rare).

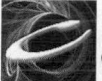

CURRENT THERAPY

- The decision to transfuse red cells to a patient should depend more on the clinical state of the patient than on an absolute trigger for hemoglobin or hematocrit.
- In an adult patient who has not had time to compensate for anemia, a transfusion trigger of less than 7 g/dL is reasonable.
- For severe autoimmune hemolytic anemia, maintenance of hemoglobin at greater than 4 g/dL in younger patients and greater than 6 g/dL in older patients or patients with cardiovascular disease is appropriate.
- Platelets are not typically indicated in thrombotic thrombocytopenic purpura, autoimmune thrombocytopenic purpura, and heparin-induced thrombocytopenia (HIT) unless the patient has significant bleeding.
- Currently available coagulation tests are not very useful for predicting bleeding in patients with end-stage liver disease. These patients establish a new equilibrium between coagulation, anticoagulation, and fibrinolysis that results in relatively less bleeding than predicted by the international normalized ratio.
- The goal during massive transfusion scenarios should be to prevent marked acidosis, hypothermia, and coagulopathy. The latter is often achieved with replacement of coagulation factors using plasma and/or cryoprecipitate within the first hour of the resuscitation.
- Cryoprecipitate is useful as a source of concentrated fibrinogen. In a patient who is actively bleeding and has a fibrinogen less than 100 mg/dL, cryoprecipitate is indicated.
- Fibrinogen concentrates are available for select patient populations.

Therapeutic Use of Blood Components

The community blood supply depends on two types of donors: whole blood donors and apheresis donors. Units of whole blood are centrifuged and then separated into components within a closed system. Using apheresis techniques, individual components of whole blood can be collected. Citrate is used to keep blood components from clotting.

The decision to transfuse blood to a patient should always include a consideration of the risks versus the benefits. Risks of transfusion-transmitted diseases are small with current testing standards. Transfusion reactions do occur; the most common ones are not life-threatening unless the patient cannot tolerate tachycardia or hypertension. Rarely, a patient experiences a life-threatening reaction. Thus it is important to ensure that the need for the blood component outweighs the risks. Additionally, in a bleeding patient, it is important to check coagulation parameters (platelet count, prothrombin time [PT], international normalized ratio [INR], activated partial thromboplastin time [aPTT], fibrinogen) in addition to hematocrit (Hct) to ensure that the component that will best address the bleeding is being used.

Red Cells
Indications
Red cells should be given to increase oxygen-carrying capacity. The hemoglobin (Hb) and Hct levels alone should not be used to determine the need for transfusion; rather, the patient's clinical picture should drive the decision to transfuse. The patient's intravascular volume status, cardiopulmonary function, and baseline vital signs in the presence of anemia should all be considered. When anemia has persisted over weeks and months, transfusion is often not indicated because compensatory mechanisms have had time to work.

Transfusion Triggers
In an adult patient who is not bleeding, transfusion of red cells is reasonable in almost all patients if Hb is less than 7 g/dL and Hct is less than 21%. Adult patients with evidence of organ dysfunction and inability to tolerate inadequate oxygenation may receive transfusion if the Hb is between 7 and 10 g/dL and the Hct is between 21% and 30%. Adult patients with rapid blood loss and hemodynamic instability may receive red cells to maintain the Hb at greater than 6 to 7 g/dL and the Hct at greater than 18% to 21%.

Dosage
One unit of packed red cells will increase the hemoglobin by 1 g/dL and hematocrit by 3% in the patient who is not bleeding or experiencing hemolysis (Table 1).

Autoimmune Hemolytic Anemia
Special Situation
When the autoantibody responsible for autoimmune hemolytic anemia reacts at body temperature, all red cell units can appear incompatible. This is because the antibody binds to an epitope common to all red cells, such as the band 3 protein. The clinician needs to decide when to transfuse the (apparently) incompatible units. In a patient who has never received a transfusion or been pregnant, there is little possibility of red cell alloantibodies in circulation, and the chance of hemolysis (beyond that being caused by the autoantibody) is low. For the patient who has received a transfusion or who has been pregnant in the past, the risk that a circulating red cell alloantibody is present and is being masked by the autoantibody is higher; special studies are available to reduce the risk of an alloantibody being overlooked. The transfusion trigger depends on whether the anemia is acute or chronic. For acute anemia, maintenance of hemoglobin at greater than 4 g/dL in younger patients and greater than 6 g/dL in older patients or patients with cardiovascular disease is appropriate.

Platelets
Platelets are required as part of normal clotting. The first stage of clot formation is development of a platelet plug over the site of endothelial injury.

Indications
The indications for platelet transfusion may be divided into prevention of bleeding and treatment of bleeding in the setting of thrombocytopenia or platelet dysfunction.

Transfusion Triggers
Prevention of Bleeding. In a stable patient with normal platelet function, transfusion is appropriate if the platelet count is less than 10,000/μL. One randomized, controlled trial has shown that transfusion at platelet counts of 5000/μL to 10,000/μL prevents bleeding in the stable patient. In a stable patient with other hemostatic abnormalities (e.g., on anticoagulation), transfusion is appropriate with a platelet count less than 50,000/μL.

Before a planned invasive procedure such as lumbar puncture, transfusion is appropriate with a platelet count of 50,000/μL. A patient undergoing major surgery should receive platelets if the count is less than 50,000 to 100,000/μL. The transfusion should take place as close to the procedure as possible so the platelets remain in circulation while the procedure is occurring.

Treatment of Bleeding. Platelets may be transfused with a major hemorrhage (e.g., gastrointestinal or genitourinary) and a platelet count less than 30,000 to 50,000/μL. For bleeding with major surgery or trauma, transfusion is appropriate for counts less than 80,000/μL. For bleeding into critical areas (e.g., central nervous system bleeding or diffuse alveolar hemorrhage), platelets may be given for counts less than 100,000/μL.

Dosage
Dosage is determined on the basis of the baseline platelet count, desired platelet count, and estimated blood volume. For a 70-kg patient, 3×10^{11} platelets (four to six units of pooled whole blood platelets or one unit of apheresis platelets) increases platelet count by approximately 30,000 to 50,000/μL in the absence of alloimmunization or excessive consumption. For prophylactic therapy, lower dosages have been shown to be as effective as higher dosages in the prevention of bleeding.

Out of ABO Group Platelet Transfusion
Because platelets can only be stored for a maximum of 5 days following collection, and the community platelet supply is collected from volunteer donors, a platelet product that is identical to the

TABLE 1	Component Therapy: Dosage and Expected Increment		
COMPONENT	**DOSE**	**EXPECTED INCREMENT**	**AVERAGE VOLUME**
Red cells	1 unit	Hct 3%, Hb 1 g/dL	250 mL
Whole blood platelets	1 unit	Platelet count increased by 5000–10,000/μL	50 mL/unit (1 pool of 6 = 300 mL)
Apheresis platelet	1 unit	Platelet count increased by 20,000–60,000/μL	300 mL/unit
Plasma	10 mL/kg	Factor levels increased by 20%	300 mL/unit
Cryoprecipitate	1 unit	Fibrinogen increased by 5 mg/dL	15 mL/unit
Prepooled cryoprecipitate	1 6-unit pool	Fibrinogen increased by 45 mg/dL	120 mL/pool

Abbreviations: Hb = hemoglobin; Hct = hematocrit.

patient's ABO type might not be available (Table 2 and Box 1). Thus it may be necessary to infuse a small volume of incompatible plasma (suspending the platelets) to the patient. There is, therefore, a small risk of hemolysis of the patient's red cells if the iso-agglutinin (anti-A or anti-B) titer in the donated plasma is high. Studies of healthy blood donors indicate that these antibody titers are typically low and do not precipitate hemolysis. Transfusion services often have policies that limit the amount of incompatible plasma a patient has received with platelet transfusion. Alternatively, some centers measure the antibody titer in the donated product and give high-titer products only to patients whose red cells lack the corresponding ABO antigen.

Unresponsiveness to Platelet Transfusion

A number of clinical factors can result in a patient's less-than-optimal response to platelet transfusion. In addition to consumption, some of these factors include splenomegaly, fever, and antifungal therapy. Patients who have been sensitized to foreign human leukocyte antigens through prior pregnancy or transfusion can also have a poor response to platelet transfusion. Transfusion medicine consultation regarding the evaluation of refractoriness to platelet transfusion may be indicated.

Special Situations

Uremia. Patients who are dialysis dependent might have an acquired platelet defect as a result of the uremic environment. Transfusion of platelets into this environment will render the transfused platelets dysfunctional. Thus if optimal platelet function is desired, dialysis should be performed frequently. Consider performing dialysis without heparin if the patient is actively bleeding.

Purpura and Thrombocytopenia. In patients with autoimmune thrombocytopenic purpura (ITP), thrombotic thrombocytopenic purpura (TTP), or heparin-induced thrombocytopenia (HIT), platelet transfusion is not indicated unless the patient has significant bleeding. Other therapies, such as steroid administration for ITP and plasma exchange for TTP, should be initiated to address the condition.

TABLE 2	ABO Compatibility*			
PATIENT'S ABO	**ANTIBODIES IN CIRCULATION**	**COMPATIBLE PACKED RED BLOOD CELLS**	**COMPATIBLE PLASMA**
O	anti-A, anti-B	O	O, A, B, AB
A	anti-B	O or A	A or AB
B	anti-A	O or B	B or AB
AB	None	O, A, B, AB	AB

*For platelet compatibility, see text.

Box 1	Rh(D) compatibility

Rh(D) negative patients should receive Rh negative red cell and platelet units.*†

Rh(D) positive patients can receive Rh positive or Rh negative red cells and platelet units.

Rh compatibility does not apply to acellular components (plasma and cryoprecipitate).

Only 15% of blood donors are Rh negative.

---

*In times of shortage, it becomes necessary to preserve the Rh(D) negative red cell inventory for females of childbearing potential (<50 years old).

†Platelet components contain very few red cells; Rho(D) immune globulin (RhoGAM) may be administered if prevention of anti-D formation is deemed appropriate. Consult with a transfusion medicine physician if further discussion is needed.

Plasma

Plasma contains all of the coagulation proteins needed for clot formation, as well as all of the fibrinolytic proteins that prevent systemic thrombosis. There are currently several kinds of plasma, such as fresh frozen, FP24, thawed, and liquid. All contain hemostatic levels of coagulation factors as long as they are stored appropriately. The effect of plasma transfusion on the PT and INR is 4 to 6 hours owing to the short half-life of coagulation factor VII. Thus other, longer-lasting means of restoring coagulation factors, such as vitamin K administration, should be undertaken.

When replacing coagulation factors with plasma, it is not necessary to have 100% factor replacement as the goal. Hemostasis is typically able to occur if circulating coagulation factor levels are between 40% and 50%. It is important to understand that the relationship between the INR and the percentage factor level is a logarithmic, rather than a linear, relationship (Figure 1). Thus whether the INR is 9 or 1.8, the initial dosage of plasma should be 10 to 20 mL/kg, with recheck of the laboratory values a few minutes after infusion. The more prolonged the INR, the more significant the impact of the dose on the INR.

Transfusion Triggers

For bleeding or imminent surgery that cannot be corrected in a timely manner by vitamin K administration, use plasma to correct an INR greater than 1.5 to 2.0. The exception is patients with end-stage liver disease (see later).

Dosage

At a dosage of 10 mL/kg, each unit has an average of 300 mL (3–5 units in a 70-kg adult). This dosage should increase circulating coagulation factors by 20% immediately after infusion.

Special Situations

Liver Disease. The INR is a less useful test in patients with end-stage liver disease. The destruction of liver tissue leads to decreased production of coagulation and fibrinolytic proteins such that a new balance is established. Patients with end-stage liver disease have been shown to have normal levels of circulating thrombin and reduced levels of certain anticoagulant proteins (e.g., protein C), which could explain why they do not bleed as often as predicted with the elevation in INR. Thus the prophylactic use of plasma to correct a mildly prolonged laboratory value in the absence of bleeding is not indicated. It will lead to unnecessary plasma infusion, and the risk of volume overload and transfusion reactions outweighs the benefit in these patients.

Massive Transfusion. In trauma patients, patients with ruptured aortic aneurysms, and patients with other arterial bleeding, massive transfusion may be necessary. The basic principles of such a scenario include taking steps early into the resuscitation to prevent the patient from becoming too cold, acidotic, or coagulopathic to reverse the situation. Some plasma (and cryoprecipitate,

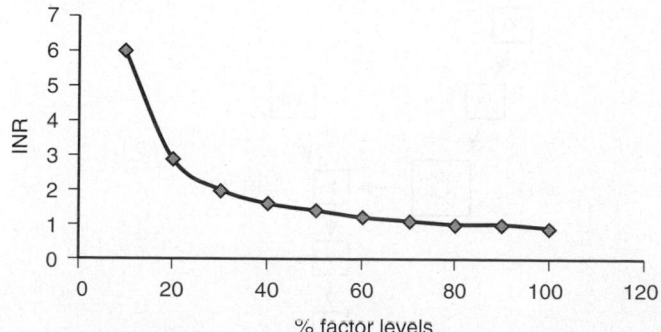

Figure 1. American Association of Blood Banks international normalized ratio (INR) compared with percentage factor levels. (Reprinted with permission from Nester T, AuBuchon J: Hemotherapy decisions and their outcomes. In Roback JD (ed): AAB Technical Manual, 17th ed. Bethesda, MD, American Association of Blood Banks, 2011, p 592.)

if the fibrinogen is very low) should be infused early into the resuscitation in order to help prevent coagulopathy. Red cells and plasma should be infused through a blood warmer, if possible.

Isolated Prolonged aPTT. Other than a deficiency in coagulation factor XI, bear in mind that the differential of an isolated prolonged aPTT includes entities that do not typically require plasma (refer to Figure 2). Hemophilia A, hemophilia B, and von Willebrand disease are no longer treated by plasma but can require factor concentrates to prevent bleeding. Systemic administration of heparin must be reversed by protamine, if fast reversal is desired. Note that plasma transfusion will not reverse the effect of heparin. One of the most common causes of a prolonged aPTT is a lupus anticoagulant; this is an antibody directed against phospholipids that typically leads to thrombosis rather than hemorrhage.

Intracranial Hemorrhage or Life-Threatening Bleeding. Reversal of anticoagulation in the setting of intracranial hemorrhage or life threatening bleeding depends on the anticoagulant. For patients taking warfarin (Coumadin), refer to Box 2.

Prothrombin complex concentrates (PCCs) may be used to replenish factors II, IX, and X rapidly. Two types of PCCs are available in the United States. A 4-factor PCC will replenish factors II, VII, IX, and X, and has been FDA approved for this indication. A 3-factor PCC lacks factor VII, thus a small dose of plasma will also be required. Inquire with a transfusion medicine physician or hematologist to determine if such a protocol exists in your facility. For other agents such as dabigatran (Pradaxa) and rivaroxiban (Xarelto), reversal may be significantly more difficult. See the guidelines by Cushman and colleagues (2011).

Cryoprecipitate

Cryoprecipitate contains fibrinogen, coagulation factors VIII and XIII, and von Willebrand factor. The most common current use is as a source of concentrated fibrinogen. It may also be used to treat hemorrhage in the rare patient with factor XIII deficiency.

Indications

Clinical scenarios that increase probability for low fibrinogen include any clinical situation where disseminated intravascular coagulation (DIC) may be present. These include obstetric bleeding, trauma involving head injury or crush injury, and sepsis. Clinical events that can lead to an isolated decrease in serum fibrinogen concentration include administration of L-asparaginase (Elspar) and surgeries that disrupt bladder or salivary gland endothelium. Fibrinogen concentrates are available for patients who will not accept cryoprecipitate.

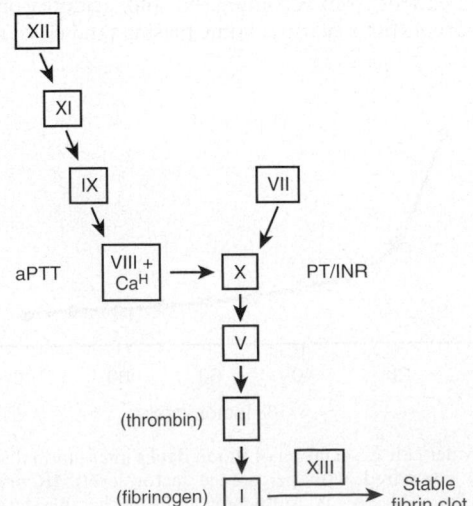

Figure 2. Coagulation cascade.

In vitro coagulation cascade (simplified)

XII → XI → IX → VIII + Ca^H → X ← VII

aPTT   VIII + Ca^H → X   PT/INR

X → V → II (thrombin) → I (fibrinogen) → XIII → Stable fibrin clot

---

INR Higher than Therapeutic but <5, No Significant Bleeding
Lower anticoagulant dosage.
Temporarily discontinue drug, if necessary.

INR >5 but <9, No Significant Bleeding
Omit 1 or 2 doses, monitor INR, resume when INR is in therapeutic range.
Alternative if patient is at increased risk of hemorrhage:
- Omit 1 dose
- Give 1–2.5 mg vitamin K orally.
For rapid reversal before urgent surgery:
- Give 2–4 mg vitamin K orally.
- Give 1–2 mg at 24 hours if INR remains elevated.

INR >9, No Significant Bleeding
Omit warfarin; give 2.5–5.0 mg vitamin K orally.
Closely monitor INR; give additional vitamin K, if necessary.
Resume warfarin at lower dose when INR is within therapeutic range.

Serious Bleeding at Any Elevation of INR
Omit warfarin.
Give 10 mg vitamin K by slow IV infusion.
Supplement with plasma or prothrombin complex concentrate depending on urgency of correction.
Vitamin K infusions may be repeated every 12 hours.

Life-Threatening Hemorrhage
Omit warfarin.
Give prothrombin complex concentrate with 10 mg vitamin K by slow IV infusion.
Repeat as necessary, depending on INR.

Abbreviation: INR = international normalized ratio.
From Nester T, AuBuchon J: Hemotherapy decisions and their outcomes. In Roback JD (ed): AAB Technical Manual, 17th ed. Bethesda, MD, American Association of Blood Banks, 2011, p 571–616.

Transfusion Triggers

Transfusion is appropriate in patients with low serum fibrinogen, typically less than 100 mg/dL.

Dosage

Dosage depends on the type of cryoprecipitate available. If the product requires resuspension in saline prior to pooling, then one unit (average 15 mL volume) will increase fibrinogen by 5 mg/dL. If the product has been pooled in plasma before freezing, then one unit will increase fibrinogen by 7 to 8 mg/dL; a six-unit pool will increase fibrinogen by 45 mg/dL. Check with the transfusion service laboratory regarding which product is available and the expected increment.

Special Situation

DIC is a state where fibrinogen is consumed at a faster rate than other circulating coagulation factors. This is because DIC is typically a thrombin-generating process (thrombin cleaves fibrinogen into fibrin for clot formation). Thus, although all coagulation factors are being consumed in DIC, timely repletion of fibrinogen by use of cryoprecipitate can result in more-timely cessation of bleeding in a patient with active DIC. The target value is fibrinogen at least 100 mg/dL. If the PT and INR are still prolonged with fibrinogen greater than 100 mg/dL, administration of plasma will replete other coagulation factors being consumed.

Transfusion Reactions

Reactions to transfusion are relatively common; life-threatening reactions are rare (Tables 3 and 4).

Because fever is a feature of both common and dangerous reactions, a transfusion reaction evaluation should be initiated with fever greater than 1°C above patient's baseline temperature at the start of the transfusion. The infusion of product should cease at least until the laboratory results are known and the patient has responded to treatment. The main point of the laboratory investigation is to evaluate the plasma for abnormal (usually red) color in an effort to detect intravascular hemolysis as quickly as possible. If the hemolysis, clerical, and direct antiglobulin test checks are negative, one might consider restarting the transfusion with careful surveillance of the patient. A direct antiglobulin test is also performed to detect the presence of antibody coating red cells in circulation; a positive result could indicate extravascular hemolysis, which is not as dangerous as intravascular hemolysis.

Most-Common Reactions

Febrile Nonhemolytic Reaction

Presentation. A febrile nonhemolytic transfusion reaction manifests as fever greater than 1°C rise above the patient's baseline, often accompanied by rigors. Hypertension, tachypnea, and transient decrease in oxygen saturation can also occur until the symptoms are treated. Evidence of hemolysis will be absent on laboratory evaluation. These reactions can manifest during or 2 to 3 hours following the transfusion.

Pathophysiology. Cytokines produced by white cells present in cellular blood components (red cell and platelet units) are responsible for the clinical presentation. Platelets also secrete cytokines; thus, leukoreduction of platelet units might not be successful in preventing the reaction.

Acute Management. Administration of an antipyretic is the routine treatment; meperidine (Demerol)[1] may be required to address severe rigors. Slow IV push of 25 mg as a first dose is recommended; an additional 25-mg dose can be given 10 to 15 minutes later if rigors persist.

Prevention with Future Transfusion. Antipyretic may be administered prior to transfusion. Ordering leukoreduced red cells and platelets (if the hospital inventory is not entirely composed of leukoreduced components) is also a preventive measure. For recurring reactions with platelets, volume reduction of the component can reduce the incidence.

Allergic Reaction of Mild Severity

Presentation. Urticaria or flushing occurs during a transfusion. Evidence of hemolysis is absent on laboratory evaluation.

Pathophysiology. Allergic reactions are immunoglobulin (Ig)E-mediated reactions against some allergen in the donor plasma. Because all blood components have some amount of plasma, it is possible to experience an allergic reaction with any blood product.

---

[1] Not FDA approved for this indication.

TABLE 3 Transfusion Reactions

MOST COMMON REACTIONS	INCIDENCE
Allergic reaction of mild severity	1:33 to 1:100
Febrile nonhemolytic reaction	1:100 to 1:1000 with leukocyte reduction
Transfusion-related circulatory overload	<1:100

MOST DANGEROUS REACTIONS	INCIDENCE
Acute hemolytic reaction	1:38,000 to 1:70,000
Anaphylactic reaction	1:20,000 to 1:50,000
Transfusion-related acute lung injury	1:1200 to 1:190,000
Bacterial contamination of red cell unit with Gram-negative organisms	1:1,000,000

TABLE 4 Transfusion Reactions with Respiratory Symptoms

REACTION	CLASSIC SIGNS	RELATIVE FREQUENCY	ACUTE MANAGEMENT (TRANSFUSION STOPPED IN ALL CASES)
Febrile nonhemolytic reaction	Transient tachypnea in the presence of rigors and fever	Common	Antipyretic ± meperidine (Demerol)[1]
Circulatory overload	Hypoxia Crackles in lower lung fields Increased BP Chest radiograph consistent with volume overload	Common	Diuresis
Allergic reaction of moderate severity	Wheezes Possible perioral or periorbital edema Possible hives	Uncommon	IV antihistamines and possibly epinephrine (Adrenalin)
Allergic reaction of marked severity	Wheezes, swollen lips, tongue, uvula Stridor or other signs of airway compromise Very decreased BP	Rare	Epinephrine IV fluids and airway management Bronchodilators and glucagon (GlucaGen)[1] for patient on β-blockers
Transfusion-related acute lung injury	Tachypnea and hypoxia during or within 6 h of transfusion Persisting for several hours Chest radiograph consistent with bilateral white out	Rare	Respiratory support of noncardiogenic pulmonary edema
Acute hemolytic reaction	Red urine and red serum Hypotension and diffuse oozing may be present Tachypnea (10% of patients)	Rare	Supportive (possibly ICU) care Administration of crystalloid solution Blood component therapy if DIC is present
Bacterial contamination with Gram-negative organism	Very decreased BP Fever Nausea, vomiting Possible tachypnea	Rare	Intensive care for support of Gram-negative sepsis

Abbreviations: BP = blood pressure; DIC = disseminated intravascular coagulation; ICU = intensive care unit.
[1] Not FDA approved for this indication.

Acute Management. Slowing the infusion rate may be all that is required to alleviate the reaction. Antihistamine administration also addresses the symptoms.

Prevention with Future Transfusion. A reaction of this type may be a one-time event. For patients with recurrent reactions, transfusing the blood product more slowly (maximum of transfusion over 4 hours) and/or premedication with antihistamines will reduce the incidence.

Transfusion Associated Circulatory Overload (TACO)

Presentation. The patient has respiratory distress, typically during the transfusion, and increase in blood pressure unless cardiac decompensation occurs. Tachycardia, tachypnea, and decrease in oxygen saturation are often present. Jugular venous distension may be seen. Radiographic findings include pleural effusions, perihilar edema, and increased vascular pedicle width.

Pathophysiology. The reaction results in cardiogenic pulmonary edema.

Acute Management. Diuretic should be administered. Supplemental oxygen may be required temporarily to improve oxygen saturation.

Prevention with Future Transfusion. Slowing the infusion rate with a maximum time of transfusion over 4 hours can prevent the reaction. Diuretic administration may be necessary in patients with poor heart function.

Most-Dangerous Reactions

Acute Hemolytic Transfusion Reaction (AHTR)

Presentation. The most common signs include fever with or without rigors and pain. The more commonly reported sites of pain include flank, back, chest, or abdomen. Nausea and vomiting and dyspnea can also occur. In more-severe presentations, hemodynamic instability is present, accompanied by oozing from line sites or petechial hemorrhage if DIC is occurring. Red or cola-colored urine is another manifestation of an acute hemolytic transfusion reaction and represents overwhelming of the kidneys' ability to recirculate free heme.

Pathophysiology. Red blood cells have proteins and carbohydrates on the cell surface that are antigenic. These epitopes are categorized into blood groups based on structure and sharing of a parent protein. A patient who lacks particular epitopes can develop antibodies through pregnancy or transfusion. Such red cell alloantibodies can then lyse transfused red cells that possess the cognate antigen. When time allows for pretransfusion testing, the antibodies are identified and antigen-negative units are provided. The ABO blood group system is unusual in that almost all patients older than 4 months have naturally occurring antibodies to the A and B antigens that they did not inherit. These antibodies are capable of activating complement and causing intravascular lysis when bound to their cognate antigen. Thus it is of utmost importance to avoid transfusing red cells against the ABO antibody in circulation. Refer to the ABO compatibility table (see Table 1).

Acute Management. Management is largely supportive. The end result of intravascular hemolysis and activation of the complement cascade can be shock, uncontrolled bleeding secondary to DIC, and renal failure. Therefore, prompt infusion of intravenous crystalloid solutions are indicated to maintain blood pressure and renal perfusion. The goal for urine flow rate should be more than 1 mL/kg per hour. Coagulation laboratory values should be obtained to determine if DIC is present; if so, component therapy to reverse the DIC is indicated. If the reaction is severe, intensive care is appropriate, because cardiac monitoring and mechanical ventilation may be necessary to support the patient.

Prevention with Future Transfusion. An acute hemolytic reaction is one of the most feared complications of transfusion. It is also often one of the most preventable. Great care should be given to the pretransfusion blood sample draw, comparing the label to the patient's unique identifiers, and labeling the tube at the patient's bedside as soon as the blood is in the tube. Just before transfusion, the unit label attached to the blood product should be compared with the patient's armband to ensure that the product is intended for this particular patient. To prevent intravascular hemolysis from antibodies directed against non-ABO antigens, pretransfusion testing (antibody screen or crossmatch) should be done in advance of the need for red cell transfusion for any patient whose clinical situation indicates a likelihood of needing blood. The exception is a patient who is hemodynamically unstable because of acute red cell loss, where uncrossmatched red cells are indicated. If the patient's identity is known, a call to the hospital transfusion service in this situation is warranted; explain that the patient needs uncrossmatched red cells and ask if there are transfusion records that indicate a need for antigen-negative units.

Allergic Reaction of Marked Severity (Anaphylaxis)

Presentation. Significant drop in blood pressure occurs, typically early into the transfusion. Wheezes, difficulty breathing, and stridor may be present. Tongue and/or facial edema as well as hives may be observed.

Pathophysiology. Anaphylaxis is an IgE-mediated reaction against an allergen in the donor plasma. In a patient with absolute IgA deficiency, naturally occurring anti-IgA can precipitate this reaction upon binding IgA in the plasma. Anti-haptoglobin antibodies can also induce a severe reaction.

Acute Management. Airway and blood pressure support should be provided with the patient recumbent and the lower extremities elevated. The treatment of choice is epinephrine (Adrenalin) 1 mg/mL, also labeled as 1:1000 or 0.1%, using an adult dosage of 0.3 to 0.5 mg per single dose, typically administered intramuscularly to the mid-quadriceps area. If symptoms persist, the dose may be repeated every 5 to 15 minutes for a maximum of three times, unless palpitations, tremors, or extreme anxiousness occurs. Supplemental oxygen should be administered and the airway maintained. Intravenous fluid administration is also recommended. Bronchodilators such as albuterol can be given as adjunctive treatment for bronchospasm that does not appear to respond to epinephrine. For patients on β-blockers, the addition of intravenous glucagon[1] (GlucaGen) 1 to 5 mg administered over 5 minutes, followed by infusion of 5 to 15 µg/minute, may be required. The addition of glucocorticoids can help prevent the biphasic reaction that occurs in some patients.

Prevention with Future Transfusion. Slow administration with careful observation of any transfusion is required. Premedication with intravenous antihistamines is appropriate. Steroids may be administered, although their effectiveness has not been confirmed through controlled trials. Epinephrine should be available at the bedside. For severe allergic reactions, a discussion with the transfusion service physician regarding washed components is appropriate.

Transfusion-Related Acute Lung Injury

Presentation. The signs of transfusion-related acute lung injury (TRALI) are difficulty breathing, tachypnea, and hypoxia during or within 6 hours of a transfusion of any blood component. Ideally, signs of underlying lung disease or circulatory overload are absent. Chest radiograph may show diffuse bilateral opacities (white-out). Diuretic administration does not result in improvement. The hypoxemia can progress to the point that the patient requires mechanical ventilation, and thus the patient should be closely monitored while the reaction is occurring.

Pathophysiology. The factors that result in TRALI are not entirely known. In a portion of cases, antibodies against white cell antigens are present in donor plasma. These antibodies are believed to bind the cognate antigens on the patient's white cells, leading to degranulation and a capillary leak syndrome involving the lungs. Other theories regarding the pathophysiology of TRALI exist. One such theory implicates biologically active substances such as lipids and cytokines in the stored blood products. These substances are believed to prime the patient's granulocytes and activate pulmonary endothelium, setting the stage for an additional trigger to cause

---

[1]Not FDA approved for this indication.

acute lung injury. Regardless of the cause of TRALI, the end result is an increase in pulmonary vascular permeability and noncardiogenic pulmonary edema. The estimated mortality rate from TRALI is 5% to 8%.

Acute Management. Management consists of supportive care, with particular regard to respiratory support. With adequate supportive care, the process most often reverses over 48 to 96 hours.

Prevention with Future Transfusion. Marked respiratory compromise is occasionally due to white cell antibodies in the patient, which bind cognate antigens in the donated red cell or platelet unit ("reverse TRALI"). In these cases, leukoreduction of cellular blood products may reduce the severity of subsequent transfusions, although solid evidence to support this is lacking. For TRALI caused by white cell antibodies in the donated product, there are no preventive measures for the clinician to take. The majority of U.S. blood suppliers provide plasma from only male donors, in an effort to reduce the incidence of TRALI caused by multiparous women with white cell antibodies.

Bacterial Contamination of a Blood Component

Presentation. The most-common presentation includes fever and rigors, nausea and/or vomiting, and possible onset of moderate hypotension during or after a platelet transfusion. Rarely, presentation includes signs of overt septic shock, including marked hypotension, typically early into the transfusion of a red cell or platelet component. Bacterial contamination of plasma or cryoprecipitate is extremely rare.

Pathophysiology. The most-common organisms to contaminate a platelet product are gram-positive organisms such as *Staphylococcus epidermidis*. These organisms are thought to be introduced into the collection bag via a skin plug that results from phlebotomy using a large-gauge needle when sterilization of the phlebotomy site has been ineffective.

The most common organisms to contaminate a red cell unit are gram-negative, endotoxin-producing organisms such as *Yersinia enterocolitica*. This organism is introduced into the blood product as a result of asymptomatic bacteremia in the donor, from sources such as the gastrointestinal tract. The donor-screening questionnaire and vital sign assessment at the time of donation help to make collection from such a donor a very rare event. Transfusion of a bacterially contaminated red cell unit is most often a fatal event. It is important to remember that platelets can also be contaminated by the same gram-negative, endotoxin-producing organisms; in this case, signs of septic shock may be manifest.

Acute Management. Blood cultures from the patient should be drawn and then prompt intravenous antibiotic administration should begin. Supportive care including inotropic agents and close nursing attention may be required.

Prevention with Future Transfusion. Bacterial contamination is associated with a donor product, and thus preventive measures for the patient do not apply. Blood suppliers perform bacterial detection tests on platelet components, and transfusion services have strict policies related to visual inspection of all blood products before they are issued to a patient-care area. However, these measures are not completely effective. The FDA recently approved pathogen inactivation technology for platelets which may further lower the risk.

Other Reactions
Delayed Hemolytic Transfusion Reaction

Presentation. The main finding with a delayed hemolytic transfusion reaction is usually an unexplained decrease in hematocrit within 2 to 7 days following transfusion. The patient often remains asymptomatic unless the decline in hemoglobin is poorly tolerated. Jaundice can occur, and laboratory values consistent with hemolysis may be positive (elevated indirect bilirubin, elevated lactate dehydrogenase, decreased haptoglobin). Rarely, signs of intravascular hemolysis can occur.

Pathophysiology. The most common source of this reaction is a red cell alloantibody that the patient developed with prior transfusion or pregnancy; the antibody titer wanes over time such that pretransfusion testing does not detect the antibody. A unit of red cells positive for the cognate antigen is then transfused, and within a few days the patient's memory B cell response produces the antibody again. Transfused cells are then cleared, most often by an extravascular mechanism.

Acute Management. Most transfusion services have a policy to notify the clinician that a serologic delayed hemolytic transfusion reaction is present on testing a new plasma sample from the patient. If the patient's hematocrit has declined, it may be useful to determine a clinical correlation by obtaining the laboratory values just described. This is of particular importance when the distinction between hemolysis and bleeding will lead to different management strategies for the patient. Although extravascular clearance of hemoglobin is fairly well tolerated by the kidneys, the conservative approach is to increase renal perfusion with intravenous crystalloid solutions if possible.

Prevention with Future Transfusion. For a patient who routinely receives care through one hospital system, the transfusion service will keep a record of the red cell alloantibody and provide antigen-negative cells for transfusion. The prevention, then, is to plan ahead for transfusion when possible, so that fully compatible units can be provided. Uncrossmatched red cells may be positive for the cognate antigen.

Allergic Reaction of Moderate Severity

Presentation. The patient has labile blood pressure, either hyper- or hypotension, accompanied by at least one of the following: throat scratchiness, respiratory wheezes, or perioral or periorbital edema. Hives may be present. Gastrointestinal symptoms such as crampy abdominal pain may also be present.

Pathophysiology. This is an IgE mediated reaction against an allergen in the plasma of the donated product.

Acute Management. Treatment is administration of intravenous antihistamines. If the respiratory component does not resolve, consider epinephrine administration and treat similarly to anaphylaxis (see previous section).

Prevention with Future Transfusion. Slower infusion of blood products can reduce further episodes of this type of reaction. If the patient is atopic, intravenous antihistamines may be administered as a premedication. If the patient requires chronic transfusion and experiences this type of reaction on a repeated basis, discussion with the transfusion service regarding washed components may be warranted.

Hypotensive Transfusion Reaction

Presentation. The patient has isolated hypotension (drop in systolic BP greater than 30 but less than 80 mm Hg) that responds quickly to cessation of the transfusion. The reaction classically occurs within the first 15 minutes of infusion of the blood product.

Pathophysiology. Pathophysiology is unclear. Some research indicates that the patient may have slower ability to metabolize bradykinin compared to other individuals.

Acute Management. Stop the transfusion.

Prevention with Future Transfusion. Prevention is unclear. In the author's experience, rate of infusion has a role. Slower infusion may help to prevent this type of reaction.

References

Abdel-Wahab OI, Healy B, Dzik WH. Effect of fresh-frozen plasma transfusion on prothrombin time and bleeding in patients with mild coagulation abnormalities. Transfusion 2006;46:1279–85.

Carson JL, Terrin ML, Noveck H, et al. Liberal or restrictive transfusion in high-risk patients after hip surgery. N Engl J Med 2011;365:2453–62.

Cushman M, Lim W, Zakai NA. 2011 Clinical Practice Guide on Anticoagulant Dosing and Management of Anticoagulant-Associated Bleeding Complications in Adults. Washington, DC: American Society of Hematology; 2011.

Kaatz S, Crowther M. Reversal of target-specific oral anticoagulants. J Thromb Thrombolysis 2013;36(2):195–202.

Lisman T, Porte RJ. Rebalanced hemostasis in patients with liver disease: Evidence and clinical consequences. Blood 2010;116:878–85.

Mazzei C, Popovsky M, Kopko P. Noninfectious complications of blood transfusion. In: Roback JD, editor. AABB Technical Manual. 17th ed. Bethesda, MD: American Association of Blood Banks; 2011. p 727–62.

Nester T, Jain S, Poisson J. Hemotherapy decisions and their outcomes. AABB Technical Manual. 18th ed. Bethsda, MD: AABB Press; 2014.

Kaufman RM, et al. Platelet transfusion: a clinical practice guideline from the AABB. Ann Internal Med 2015;162(3):205–13.

Holcomb JB, et al. Transfusion of plasma, platelets, and red blood cells in a 1:1:1 vs. a 1:1:2 ratio and mortality in patients with severe trauma: the PROPPR randomized clinical trial. JAMA 2015;313(5):471–82.

Slichter SJ, Kaufman RM, Assmann SF, et al. Dose of prophylactic platelet transfusions and prevention of hemorrhage. N Engl J Med 2010;362:600–13.

CHRONIC LEUKEMIAS

Method of
Katarzyna Jamieson, MD

CURRENT DIAGNOSIS

Chronic Myelogenous Leukemia
- Clinical symptoms
  - Constitutional symptoms
  - Splenomegaly (abdominal discomfort, early satiety)
- Laboratory parameters
  - Increased white blood cell count, commonly >100,000/µL, with differential counts showing granulocytes in all stages of differentiation, and two peaks involving neutrophils and myelocytes
  - Absolute basophilia
- Genetic parameters
  - Demonstration of *bcr-abl* by standard cytogenetic analysis, fluorescent in situ hybridization, or polymerase chain reaction

Chronic Lymphocytic Leukemia
- Clinical symptoms
  - B symptoms (fever, night sweats, and weight loss)
  - Lymphadenopathy and organomegaly
  - Recurrent infections
- Laboratory parameters
  - Increased white blood cell count with absolute lymphocytosis
  - Anemia, thrombocytopenia
- Immunophenotypic analysis (flow cytometry)
  - Demonstration of monoclonal population of light chain–restricted mature B lymphocytes expressing CD19, CD20 (dim), and CD23 and coexpressing pan-T cell antigen CD5

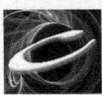

CURRENT THERAPY

Chronic Myelogenous Leukemia: Chronic Phase
- Initial therapy
  - Imatinib mesylate (Gleevec) 400–600 mg daily
  - Dasatinib (Sprycel)
  - Nilotinib (Tasigna)
- Second-line therapy:
  - Imatinib mesylate 800 mg daily
  - Dasatinib (Sprycel)
  - Nilotinib (Tasigna)
  - Bosutinib (Bosulif)
  - Ponatinib (Iclusig)
  - Omacetaxine (Synribo)
- High risk for failure:
  - Allogeneic stem cell transplantation

Chronic Lymphocytic Leukemia
- Chemotherapy drugs
  - Fludarabine (Fludara)
  - Deoxycoformycin (Pentostatin [Nipent])
  - Cyclophosphamide (Cytoxan)
  - Chlorambucil (Leukeran)
  - Bendamustine (Treanda)

- Targeted therapy drugs
  - Idelalisib (Zydelig)
  - Ibrutinib (Imbruvica)
- Immunotherapy (monoclonal antibodies):
  - Rituximab (Rituxan)
  - Alemtuzumab (Campath)
  - Ofatumumab (Arzerra)
  - Obinutuzumab (Gazyva)

Chronic Myelogenous Leukemia

Chronic myelogenous leukemia (CML) is a chronic myeloproliferative disorder defined by the presence of a chimeric gene, *bcr-abl*, encoded by translocation between chromosomes 9 and 22, the Philadelphia chromosome. Discovered in 1960, the Philadelphia chromosome was the first chromosomal abnormality implicated in carcinogenesis. This was followed by decades of unraveling of leukemogenic process, which culminated in a development of the *bcr-abl* inhibitor imatinib mesylate (Gleevec). As a result, in 2001 CML became the first human neoplasm in which the rationally designed therapeutic agent to target a carcinogenic pathway demonstrated great clinical efficacy.

Epidemiology and Risk Factors

CML accounts for 7% to 15% of all cases of leukemia in adults. The median age at diagnosis is 45 to 55 years. The disease is extremely rare in children and the overall incidence increases with age. There is slight male predominance, with a male-to-female ratio of 1.4 to 1.0. There is no association with geographic distribution or race. The etiology of CML is unknown. High-dose radiation exposure is the only well-established environmental risk factor. No genetic predisposition is thought to play any role in pathogenesis of CML.

Pathogenesis

bcr-abl is created by a reciprocal translocation of genetic material between the long arm of chromosome 9 (containing the protooncogene *c-abl*) and the long arm of chromosome 22 (containing the *bcr* gene). This is the Philadelphia chromosome, and it is correctly annotated t(9;22)(q34.1;q11.21). The translocation results in constitutive upregulation of tyrosine kinase activity of *abl*, which triggers downstream transduction pathways of a signaling cascade of oncogenic events.

The natural course of CML is one of inevitable progression from an initial chronic phase to a more-aggressive accelerated phase and eventually to a rapidly fatal myeloid or lymphoid blast phase. It is thought that the transformation proceeds as a consequence of the accumulation of additional molecular changes in genetically unstable *bcr-abl*–containing cells. Supportive of this hypothesis, up to 80% of patients with advanced CML have secondary cytogenetic abnormalities.

Clinical and Laboratory Characteristics

CML is a clonal myeloproliferative disorder that develops through accumulation of maturing cells of myeloid, erythroid, and megakaryocytic origin. CML has a biphasic or triphasic clinical course. Patients usually present in the initial chronic phase, exhibiting a cluster of specific clinical and laboratory features (listed in the Current Diagnosis box). More than half of patients with CML diagnosed in the chronic phase are asymptomatic, and the diagnosis is established following the incidental discovery of elevated white blood cell (WBC) count on a routine screening test.

The median time to the development of terminal blast phase is 3 to 6 years. The disease typically progresses through slow evolution into an accelerated phase and then blast phase, but it can transform rapidly directly into the blast phase. The detection of a change in the pace of the disease may be difficult and therefore definitions of accelerated phase vary and are imprecise. The blast phase is defined by the presence of extramedullary disease or at least 30% blasts or blasts and promyelocytes in the bone marrow or peripheral blood. Leukemic cells in blast phase are characterized by arrested maturation, and they proliferate rapidly, similar to acute leukemia cells. The symptoms of blast phase are also those typically seen in acute leukemia.

Diagnosis

The diagnosis of CML can be usually made with reasonable certainty based on the results of peripheral blood cell counts and examination of the peripheral blood smear (see the Current Diagnosis box). The detection of the Philadelphia chromosome or *bcr-abl* by cytogenetic analysis, fluorescent in situ hybridization (FISH), or polymerase chain reaction (PCR) confirms the diagnosis: all patients positive for the Philadelphia chromosome by standard cytogenetic analysis will have a *bcr-abl* fusion gene detectable by FISH or PCR; however, in approximately 5% of patients with *bcr-abl* detectable by FISH or PCR, the Philadelphia chromosome could not be appreciated by standard cytogenetics. The bone marrow biopsy is usually not necessary for diagnosis but should be performed for staging purposes in all patients with newly diagnosed CML.

Differential Diagnosis

At presentation, the differential diagnosis of CML usually involves distinction from leukemoid reaction. Among hematologic malignancies, CML may be difficult to differentiate from other myeloproliferative disorders (essential thrombocytosis, polycythemia vera, and mutagenic myeloid metaplasia), chronic neutrophilic leukemia, chronic myelomonocytic leukemia, juvenile chronic myeloid leukemia, and eosinophilic leukemia. In most cases, the detection of *bcr-abl* is sufficient to make the distinction. However, the differentiation between CML presenting in lymphoid-blast phase and Philadelphia chromosome–positive acute lymphoblastic leukemia might not be possible.

Prognosis

Before the effective therapies became available, the expected median survival of patients with CML was 39 to 47 months, with less than 20% surviving longer than 8 years. Allogeneic stem cell transplantation (SCT) and interferon (IFN) alfa-2b (Intron-A)[1] or INF alfa 2a (Roferon-A) in the 1990s improved median survival to 60 to 65 months. However, the availability of tyrosine kinase inhibitors (TKIs) in 2000s transformed CML into a chronic disease associated with near-normal life expectancy: The 8-year update of the IRIS trial (International Randomized Study of Interferon and STI- 571) reported 85% overall survival and 93% survival in patients with only CML-related deaths. At this time, it is still unclear if TKIs are capable of curing CML; and continuation of therapy to maintain the remission is generally considered the standard of care. However, the increasing body of evidence suggests that as many as 30% of imatinib-treated patients who stopped the treatment after ≥2 years of undetectable minimal residual disease by conventional PCR may be able to sustain their remission off treatment. Patients who are suboptimal responders, who are poor responders, or whose disease is refractory to imatinib have poorer prognosis than patients who met expected response criteria (Table 1). The Sokal prognostic score, originally derived from 800 patients treated in the early 1960s and 1970s, still helps to identify patients who are at high risk for failure in era of TKI.

Definitions of Response and Monitoring of Therapeutic Efficacy

The goal of CML therapy is the maximum possible reduction of leukemia burden. The status of the response is routinely evaluated by peripheral blood counts, cytogenetic analysis and FISH, and real-time quantitative PCR (RQ-PCR). The uniform criteria for hematologic, cytogenetic, and molecular responses have been developed to guide therapy and facilitate meaningful analysis of efficacy data across clinical trials (Tables 1 and 2). Close follow-up of response is critically important to predict when other therapies, such as alternative TKIs or transplantation, should be considered. Selective testing for bcr-abl kinase domain mutations is recommended for all patients who fail to respond to the first-line agent.

Treatment

Chronic Phase

Throughout most of the 20th century CML was considered incurable. The principal options for treating CML included busulfan (Myleran, Busulfex) or hydroxyurea (Hydrea). Such therapy, although successful in alleviating symptoms, did not alter the natural course of the disease. Introduction of allogeneic SCT in 1980s for the first time offered CML patients a prospect of cure. However, the high treatment-related morbidity and mortality associated with this procedure greatly limited its use to patients who were young and fit and for whom an HLA-identical donor could be identified. The alternative was treatment with IFN alfa 2b (Intron-A)[1] or IFN alfa 2a (Roferon-A), which offered prolongation of survival but generally only to a minority of patients who could tolerate it.

First-Line Therapy. In 2001, imatinib mesylate (Gleevec), the first selective bcr-abl tyrosine kinase inhibitor, was introduced into clinical practice. The trial that established imatinib as the treatment of choice for newly diagnosed CML in the chronic phase was the International Randomized Study of Interferon Alpha Versus STI571 (IRIS). Between June 2000 and January 2001 IRIS accrued and randomized 1106 patients to imatinib 400 mg daily versus what was then the standard of care, interferon alfa plus

[1]Not FDA approved for this indication.

[1]Not FDA approved for this indication.

TABLE 1 European LeukemiaNet Response Definitions for any TKI first line, and second line in case of intolerance, all patients (CP, AP, BP)

TIME AFTER DIAGNOSIS	FAILURE	WARNING/SUBOPTIMAL
Baseline		High risk Major route CCA/Ph+
3 mo	No CHR Ph+ >95%	BCR-ABL*>10% Ph+ 36–95%
6 mo	BCR-ABL >10% Ph+ >35%	BCR-ABL* 1–10% Ph+ 1–35%
12 mo	BCR-ABL*>1% Ph+ >0%	BCR-ABL* 0.1–1%
Then and at any time	Loss of CHR, CCyR or MMR Mutations** CCA/Ph+	CCA/Ph– (–7, or 7q–)

Abbreviations: CCgR = complete cytogenetic response; MMR = major molecular response; PCgR = partial cytogenetic response; Ph = Philadelphia chromosome. Major route CCA/Ph+ are clonal cytogenetic abnormalities in Ph+ cells: +8, 2nd Ph+ CCA/Ph+ are trisomy 8, [+der(22)t(9;22)(q34;q11)], isochromosome 17\[i(17)(q10)], trisomy 19, and ider(22)(q10)t(9;22)(q34;q11)

Reprinted with permission from Baccarani M, Deininger MW, Rosti G, et al: European LeukemiaNet recommendations for the management of chronic myeloid leukemia. Blood 2013;122(6):872–884. http://www.leukemia-net.org/content/leukemias/cml/recommendations/e8078/infoboxContent10260/PocketCard_UPDATE2013_105x165_final.pdf (accessed 20.8.2014).

*IS International Scale

**Confirmed by two consecutive tests, of which one is ≥1%

TABLE 2 European LeukemiaNet Definitions and Monitoring Recommendations

HEMATOLOGIC RESPONSE	CYTOGENIC RESPONSE	MOLECULAR RESPONSE
Definitions		
Complete: Platelet count <450 × 10⁹/L WBC count <10 × 10⁹/L Differential without immature granulocytes and with <5% basophils Nonpalpable spleen	Complete: Ph+ 0% Partial: Ph+ <35% Minor: Ph+ 36–65% None: Ph+ >95%	Complete: transcript nonquantifiable and nondetectable Major: ≤0.10
Monitoring		
Check every 2 wk until complete response achieved and confirmed, then every 3 mo unless otherwise required	Check at 3 and 6 mo, then every 6 mo until complete response achieved and confirmed; thereafter every 12 mo if molecular monitoring cannot be assured; check always for occurrence of treatment failure or unexplained cytopenia	Check every 3 mo until major response is achieved; conduct mutational analysis in case of failure, suboptimal response, or increase in transcript level

Abbreviations: Ph = Philadelphia chromosome; WBC = white blood cell.
Reprinted with permission from Baccarani M, Saglio G, Goldman J, et al: Evolving concepts in the management of chronic myeloid leukemia: Recommendations from an expert panel on behalf of the European LeukemiaNet. Blood 2006;108:1809–20; Baccarani M, Cortes J, Pane F, et al: Chronic myeloid leukemia: an update of concepts and management recommendations of European LeukemiaNet. J Clin Oncol 2009; 27:6041–51. Epub 2009 Nov 2.

subcutaneous cytarabine (Cytosar). After a median of 5 years, 382 of the 553 patients (69%) randomized to imatinib were still receiving it. The estimated progression-free survival was 83% and overall survival was 89%. The responding patients whose disease did not progress in any way in their first 3 years were unlikely to relapse and unlikely to suffer from late-onset side effects.

The recommended dose of imatinib for patients with CML in the chronic phase is 400 mg orally once daily. The drug is well tolerated by the majority of patients; the most common side effects are nausea, vomiting, edema (fluid retention), muscle cramps, skin rash, diarrhea, heartburn, and headache. Hematologic toxicity is quite common, particularly in patients with advanced CML, and the package insert contains exact guidelines for its management. Occasional severe hepatotoxicity has been reported.

Most patients with CML in the chronic phase today achieve and maintain excellent disease control with imatinib and seem to enjoy near-normal survival and quality of life. Given that continuation of TKI in a majority of patients seems necessary to maintain the remission, adherence to therapy is crucial and has recently become an avid focus of clinical investigations.

Since introduction of imatinib, three more second-generation TKIs have been developed and approved for treatment of CML: dasatinib (Sprycel), nilotinib (Tasigna) and bosutinib (Bosulif). All three have been studied extensively and demonstrated efficacy in the setting of imatinib failure. Dasatinib and nilotinib have subsequently been studied and received FDA approval for use as first-line agents. Phase III studies comparing dasatinib (DASISION) or nilotinib (ENESTnd) to imatinib as initial therapy for CML in the chronic phase demonstrated faster and deeper responses; however, a longer follow-up will be required to determine if this is going to translate into clinically significant long-term benefits such as improved survival. At this time the choice of a front line TKI is often determined by the patient's tolerance of the drug, as each of the TKIs has some unique and non-overlapping toxicities. Bosutinib has not yet been approved in the first-line setting. A randomized study comparing bosutinib to imatinib (BELA) in newly diagnosed patients indicated comparable response rates but higher rate of GI toxicity associated with bosutinib. Neutropenia, musculoskeletal events, and edema were less frequent.

A fourth generation TKI, ponatinib (Iclusig), is the newest agent of this class granted accelerated FDA approval after demonstrating high levels of response rates on PACE trial in heavily pretreated patients, including those carrying the T315I mutation. Soon after it's approval ponatinib received a black box warning in highlighting the increased risk of serious vascular events and hepatic toxicity. More recently an increased risk of serious complications associated with the long term use of the other second generation TKI have also been reported, emphasizing the relative safety of the first drug in this class, namely imatinib.

The long-term follow up of patients in the IRIS trial indicates that despite the favorable toxicity profile and efficacy, as many as 30% of patients will eventually fail imatinib therapy. Patients who are intolerant to first-line TKIs should be offered, and may be able to tolerate and respond to, other TKIs. Consensus recommends that patients who fail imatinib by progression or relapse should be screened for other medications that could affect metabolism and thus compromise the clinical efficacy of TKIs, for compliance and for *abl* mutations. More than 50 mutations in *bcr-abl* have been described, detection of which may help guide selection of second-line TKI therapy. Younger and otherwise fit patients should be evaluated for an allogeneic SCT.

Other Therapeutic Options. Patients who fail imatinib and/or second-generation TKI have particularly poor prognoses. Those who are not transplant candidates may be treated with omacetaxine (Synribo), which has recently been approved for patients resistant and/or intolerant to two or more tyrosine kinase inhibitors.

Advanced Phase

Imatinib mesylate is indicated for advanced CML in accelerated phase and blast phase. The recommended dosages are higher: 600 mg daily for CML accelerated phase and 800 mg daily for CML in the blast phase. Patients who satisfy criteria for acceleration are a heterogeneous group, because the disease biologically varies from slightly more advanced than late chronic phase to verging on blast phase. Up to 80% of patients achieve a hematologic remission, and approximately 40% achieve a complete cytogenetic response, which is considered a prerequisite to long-term survival. All second and third generation TKIs are approved for treatment of advanced CML: dasatinib at 140 mg once daily (or 70 mg twice daily), nilotinib at 400 mg twice daily, bosutinib 500 to 600 mg once daily, and ponatinib 45 mg once daily. Patients who progress to accelerated phase on the first-line TKI should be screened for *bcr-abl* mutations. In general the likelihood of response to a second-line TKI is 30 to 40 percent, and the identification of a mutation and selection of the second-line agent accordingly may improve those odds. Ponatinib is the only TKI with significant activity in CML associated with *T315I* mutation. Once the maximum response has been realized, patients who are suitable transplant candidates are offered an allogeneic stem cell transplantation.

Patients presenting in blast phase require a more-aggressive approach and are generally treated with a combination of TKI and chemotherapy or with a second-generation tyrosine kinase inhibitor with or without chemotherapy. Patients who achieve responses are immediately evaluated for an allogeneic SCT. The outcome of allogeneic SCT in advanced CML is much worse than in chronic phase, but a minority of patients can definitely be cured.

Allogeneic Stem Cell Transplantation

The curative potential of allogeneic SCT is well established, and transplantation remains the widely accepted regimen for patients who failed imatinib. Historically, in the pre-imatinib era the allogeneic SCT has been reported to produce long-term survival between 50% and 60%—and even as high as 80% for larger, more experienced centers—in patients who underwent transplantation in the chronic phase.

Chronic Lymphocytic Leukemia

CLL has historically been considered an indolent disease of older patients. The general approach to treatment was conservative and the few therapies available were only marginally effective; since the 1990s, new treatments namely purine analongs and monoclonal antibodies started to change the face of this disease. Intensive research over the past several years provided a greatly improved insight into the pathogenesis of CLL and lead to development of several targeted treatment approaches that will likely dramatically change the way we treat CLL. The availability of novel agents that are less toxic and more effective has rekindled hope that treatments with higher curative potential can be developed.

Epidemiology and Risk Factors:

The median age at diagnosis is 70 years. The incidence is higher in men, and the male-to-female ratio is 1.7:1. It is the most common leukemia in the Western world; it is rare is Asian people and remains rare in people of Japanese origin who live in Hawaii, suggesting a genetic rather than environmental predisposition. An increased risk of developing the disease has been described in first-degree relatives of patients with CLL.

Pathogenesis

CLL develops by progressive accumulation of genetically altered mature lymphocytes in the blood, bone marrow, and lymphoid tissue. The CLL cell of origin is a B cell arrested in its pathway of differentiation, intermediate between a pre-B cell and mature B cell. One of the most important genetic parameters defining clinical behavior and prognosis is the mutation status of the variable segments of immunoglobulin heavy chain *VH* gene: CLL with unmutated *VH* shows an unfavorable course with rapid progression, whereas CLL with mutated *VH* typically shows slow progression and long survival.

FISH detects genetic aberrations in more than 80% of patients with CLL. The FISH CLL panel typically includes probes for 13q, 11q, 17p, and 6q deletions and for 12q duplication. The most common abnormality is deletion of 13q, which occurs in more than 50% of patients. Persons showing 13q14 abnormalities have a relatively benign disease that usually manifests as stable or slowly progressive isolated lymphocytosis. Trisomy 12 is associated with atypical morphology and progressive disease. Deletions of bands 11q22-q23 are associated with extensive lymph node involvement, aggressive disease, and shorter survival. Deletion of 17p results in loss of function of *p53* and is associated with a particularly poor prognosis.

Clinical Manifestations

The clinical features of CLL are variable and depend on the stage of the disease. Up to 30% of patients with CLL are asymptomatic, and the diagnosis is established following the incidental discovery of leukocytosis and/or absolute lymphocytosis on routine screening tests. The remaining patients present with lymphadenopathy, splenomegaly, or B symptoms (fever, night sweats, and weight loss), alone or in combination. Anemia and thrombocytopenia are considered late signs of the disease but can be present at the time of diagnosis. Due to their immunocompromised state, patients can present with recurrent or persistent infections.

Diagnosis

The diagnosis of CLL requires demonstration of absolute lymphocytosis of greater than 5000/mL and an immunophenotypic evidence of monoclonal population of mature B cells expressing CD19, CD20 (dim), and CD23 and coexpressing pan–T-cell antigen CD5. The malignant cells express low density of monoclonal surface immunoglobulin (IgM or IgD) with either κ or λ light chain. Patients are evaluated and grouped prognostically based on physical examination and complete blood count. The bone marrow biopsy and CT scans are not required for diagnosis but may be indicated based on symptoms.

Differential Diagnosis

The immunophenotypic profile of CLL is quite characteristic, but at times it has to be differentiated from other low-grade lymphoproliferative disorders: hairy cell leukemia, prolymphocytic leukemia, (splenic) marginal zone lymphoma, and lymphoplasmacytic lymphoma. Most importantly, CLL needs to be differentiated from mantle cell lymphoma, which also coexpresses CD5 but is characteristically CD23 negative and cycline D1 positive by immunohistochemical staining.

Prognosis

The natural history of CLL is extremely variable, with survival times ranging from 2 to 20 (or more) years. Clinical staging using the Rai or Binet system provides a good estimate of prognosis but is not very reliable in an individual patient; for example, among patients presenting with early clinical stage disease, up to 30% never progress and eventually die of causes unrelated to CLL, and another 30% progress much more rapidly than expected. A number of additional prognostic factors are considered in estimating prognosis in an individual case: clinical characteristics such as age, sex, and performance status; laboratory parameters reflecting the tumor burden or disease activity such as lymphocyte count, lactate dehydrogenase (LDH), bone marrow infiltration pattern, or lymphocyte doubling time; serum markers such as soluble CD23 and β_2-microglobulin; and genetic markers such as genetic aberrations (see earlier), the *VH* mutation status, or its surrogate markers (CD38, ZAP-70).

Treatment

Early alkylating drug based treatment strategies in CLL offered control of symptoms but little impact on the natural course of the disease. The introduction of purine analogs in the 1980s represented a definite progress but it was not until they were combined with monoclonal antibodies that deeper and more meaningful remissions were experienced. The analyses of historical series suggests that immunotherapeutic regimens offer a modest prolongation of survival. The BCR pathway kinase inhibitors approved in the past few years are certainly very promising in this regard. However at present, short of allogeneic stem cell transplant, CLL is still considered incurable. Asymptomatic patients with CLL are followed expectantly. The treatment is initiated upon progression of the disease or appearance of symptoms such as rapid lymphocyte doubling time, bulky lymphadenopathy or organomegaly, disease-related B symptoms, and autoimmune or nonautoimmune cytopenias. CLL is quite sensitive to many chemo- and immunotherapeutic agents. However, remissions are rarely durable. The disease follows a remitting and relapsing pattern, and most patients receive at least a few different regimens throughout the course of their disease.

First-Line Therapy

The first-line treatment usually consists of purine analogue fludarabine (Fludara)-based chemotherapy in combination with the anti-CD20 monoclonal antibody rituximab (Rituxan). FR (fludarabine and rituximab) and FCR (fludarabine, cyclophosphamide [Cytoxan], and rituximab) are the chemoimmunotherapy combinations used most commonly. The overall response rates for these regimens are respectively 90% and 95%. FCR offers a higher complete remission rate of 70% vs 47% for FR; however, FR offers a more acceptable toxicity profile. Median overall survival with each of these regimens seems comparable: approximately 5 years. FCR may be particularly effective in CLL associated with del(11q). However, in general choice between the regimens is made based upon the patient's characteristics and the goals of therapy. The treatment cycles are administered every 28 days for up to 6 cycles.

Other treatment options used in the newly diagnosed progressive disease setting include PCR (deoxycoformycin (Pentostatin [Nipent]),[1] cyclophosphamide, and rituximab); bendamustine (Treanda); the anti-CD25 antibody alemtuzumab (Campath); or chlorambucil (Leukeran). Deoxycoformycin is another purine analogue, and the PCR regimen offers an alternative to FCR. The fludarabine-based regimens are only marginally effective in high-risk disease defined by the presence of del(17p). Patients with del(17p) either do not respond to initial treatment or relapse soon after achieving remission. Therefore, other therapies, including investigational therapies, are often offered in this setting. Alemtuzumab is the only FDA-approved agent that has demonstrated activity in cells lacking *p53* function, as seen in patients with deletion of chromosome 17p.

Bendamustine (Treanda) is a new alkylating agent approved for treatment of CLL in March 2008. Based on the results of a randomized trial, like fludarabine, it offers a higher response rate and progression-free survival in comparison to single agent chlorambucil. The toxicity of bendamustine seems intermediate between that of fludarabine and chlorambucil. In the past few years the combination of bendamustine and rituximab (BR) has become an acceptable alternative for patients who are unable to tolerate fludarabine due to co-morbid conditions or due to age. Many older patients too frail to tolerate either fludarabine or bendamustine could still be treated with chlorambucil combined with a novel anti-CD20 antibody either obinutuzumab (Gazyva) or ofatumumab (Arzerra). Both antibodies have been approved for this indication based on greater improvement in response rates and progression-free survival demonstrated in randomized trials. The initial results of those trials also suggest a benefit in overall survival.

Other Therapeutic Options

Relapsed disease occurs in a patient who achieved at least a partial remission that lasted more than 6 months after completion of treatment. Many of those patients can be re-treated successfully with the same medications or can be switched to an alternative strategy. Specifically, it has been demonstrated that patients initially treated with fludarabine often achieve another durable response upon re-treatment. Whether patients treated with fludarabine-containing combination regimens or other newer therapies such as alemtuzumab or bendamustine will respond to re-treatment equally well is not yet known.

Patients who fail to achieve at least a partial remission or whose disease progresses within 6 months from completion of treatment have refractory disease, which is associated with a poor prognosis. Patients refractory to fludarabine historically had expected median survival of 48 weeks and only an 11% likelihood of responding to other therapies, which included alkylating drugs, other purine analogs, high dose steroids, monoclonal antibodies (rituximab, alemtuzumab, ofatumumab). The year 2014 was remarkable for FDA approval of two novel agents for treatment of relapsed/refractory CLL. Ibrutinib (Imbruvica) is an oral BTK inhibitor. A randomized trial in relapsed/refractory CLL confirmed a superior response rate and survival when compared with ofatumumab. The drug produces rapid and sustained decrease in lymphadenopathy coupled by lymphocytosis. Idelalisib (Zydelig) is an oral inhibitor of PI3K kinase, which in combination with rituximab was shown to have a superior therapeutic activity over rituximab. A Phase III randomized trial was stopped prematurely after it demonstrated improved response rate and improved survival over rituximab alone.

Both drugs can be taken by mouth and are well tolerated. Interestingly both drugs generally induce only partial remission, yet, they translate to prolongation of survival. Furthermore it appears that continuation of the drugs is necessary to maintain remissions.

At this time it is still unclear what role these new drugs will play in treatment of CLL.

Patients are encouraged to participate in clinical trials. Those who are potential transplant candidates are considered for an allogeneic stem cell transplant.

---

[1]Not FDA approved for this indication.

Allogeneic stem cell transplantation remains the only potentially curative treatment modality. Unfortunately, data on the use of allogeneic stem cell transplantation is limited to small case series. Allogeneic stem cell transplantation is associated with considerable treatment-related morbidity and mortality and is usually not considered until definitive evidence of poor prognosis.

Complications

Major complications of CLL include cytopenias and immune dysfunction. Anemia and thrombocytopenia can result from direct infiltration of the bone marrow and hypersplenism, in which case response to treatment usually results in improvement. Splenectomy obtained either surgically or via splenic irradiation is clinically useful in patients with splenomegaly and profound cytopenias unresponsive to chemotherapy. Autoimmune hemolytic anemia and thrombocytopenia seen in a significant percentage of patients often respond to steroids. Danazol,[1] high-dose intravenous immunoglobulin (IVIg) (Gammagard),[1] cyclosporine (Neoral),[1] and rituximab[1] have all also been used in this setting.

Infections are the major cause of mortality in CLL. They result from hypogammaglobulinemia, impaired T-cell function, and neutropenia. Patients with repeat major bacterial infections are candidates for treatment with high-dose IVIg.[1] Patients treated with purine analogues and alemtuzumab are at high risk for opportunistic infections by herpes simplex virus and herpes zoster virus, *Listeria monocytogenes, Pneumocystis jirovecii,* and cytomegalovirus and should be offered prophylaxis with acyclovir (Zovirax),[1] trimethoprim-sulfamethoxazole (Bactrim), or aerosolized pentamidine (NebuPent) and antifungal agents. Patients receiving alemtuzumab should be monitored for cytomegalovirus reactivation or disease.

Patients with CLL have been reported to have a higher risk of developing other hematologic and solid malignancies. It is unknown how much of this increased risk is due to the underlying disease and accompanying chronic immunosuppression and how much is due to the treatments given. In 5% to 10% of patients with CLL, the disease transforms into an aggressive large-cell lymphoma (Richter's transformation) or prolymphocytic leukemia.

---

[1]Not FDA approved for this indication.

References

Baccarani M, Deininger MW, Rosti G, et al. European LeukemiaNet recommendations for the management of chronic myeloid leukemia: 2013. Blood 2013;122 (6):872–84.

Byrd JC, Rai K, Peterson BL, et al. Addition of rituximab to fludarabine may prolong progression-free survival and overall survival in patients with previously untreated chronic lymphocytic leukemia: an updated retrospective comparative analysis of CALGB 9712 and CALGB 9011. Blood 2005;105:49–53.

Deininger MW, O'Brien SG, Ford JM, Druker BJ. Practical management of patients with chronic myeloid leukemia receiving imatinib. J Clin Oncol 2003;21:1637–47.

Druker BJ, Guilhot F, O'Brien SG, et al. Five-year follow-up of patients receiving imatinib for chronic myeloid leukemia. N Engl J Med 2006;355:2408–17.

Goldman JM. Initial treatment for patients with CML. Am Soc Hematol Educ Program 2009;453–60.

Hallek M. Chronic lymphocytic leukemia: 2013 update on diagnosis, risk stratification and treatment. Am J Hematol 2013;88(9):803–16.

Hallek M. Signaling the end of chronic lymphocytic leukemia: new frontline treatment strategies. Blood 2013;122(23):3723–34.

Kantarjian H. Shah NP, Hochhaus A, et al. Dasatinib versus imatinib in newly diagnosed chronic-phase chronic myeloid leukemia N Engl J Med 2010;363:2260–70.

Keating MJ, Chiorazzi N, Messmer B, et al. Biology and treatment of chronic lymphocytic leukemia. Hematology Am Soc Hematol Educ Program 2003;153–75.

Lee SJ. Chronic myelogenous leukaemia. Br J Haematol 2000;111:993–1009.

Lozanski G, Heerema NA, Flinn IW, et al. Alemtuzumab is an effective therapy for chronic lymphocytic leukemia with *p53* mutations and deletions. Blood 2004;103:3278–81.

Saglio G, Kim DW, Issaragrisil S, et al. Nilotinib versus imatinib for newly diagnosed chronic myeloid leukemia. N Engl J Med 2010;362:2251–9.

Sokal risk score calculator. Available at: http://www.roc.se/sokal.asp (accessed 10.07.10).

Tam CS, O'Brien S, Wierda W, et al. Long-term results of the fludarabine, cyclophosphamide, and rituximab regimen as initial therapy of chronic lymphocytic leukemia. Blood 2008;112:975–80.

DISSEMINATED INTRAVASCULAR COAGULATION

Method of
Jaime Morales-Arias, MD

CURRENT DIAGNOSIS

- Disseminated intravascular coagulation (DIC) occurs in the presence of a life-threatening underlying illness and is characterized by systemic pathologic activation of the coagulation system.
- Symptoms may be secondary to either the underlying disease or to DIC, the most common manifestation being a bleeding diathesis.
- A combination of clinical and laboratory findings aid in making an accurate diagnosis.
- Depending on the underlying condition, laboratory abnormalities can vary. The most common laboratory findings are thrombocytopenia, elevated fibrin degradation products, elevated D-dimer assay, prolonged prothrombin time, prolonged activated partial thromboplastin time, low fibrinogen, and microangiopathic hemolytic anemia.
- A validated objective scoring system for the diagnosis of overt DIC based solely on laboratory data is available.

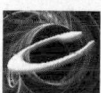

CURRENT THERAPY

- Prompt and efficacious treatment of the underlying condition is crucial.
- Aggressive supportive care measures are required.
- Platelet and factor replacement with fresh frozen plasma and cryoprecipitate may be indicated.
- Anticoagulation with heparin is used for selected cases.
- Activated protein C concentrates (drotrecogin alfa [Xigris]) are useful in disseminated intravascular coagulation secondary to severe sepsis.

Disseminated intravascular coagulation (DIC) is an acquired clinicopathologic syndrome that typically occurs as a consequence of a serious underlying condition. It is characterized by systemic activation of the coagulation system. This process initiates a cascade of events that includes the formation of fibrin clots and microthrombi with secondary end-organ ischemia and failure and concomitant consumption of coagulation factors and platelets that can result in hemorrhagic manifestations.

Epidemiology

DIC is a secondary thrombohemorrhagic phenomenon that occurs as a consequence of a multitude of disorders that pathologically activate and dysregulate the intravascular coagulation system. The most common causes are sepsis, cancer, and trauma. DIC is estimated to occur in approximately 1% of hospitalized patients, but it may be present in up to 30% to 50% of those with severe sepsis. DIC carries a high morbidity and mortality risk, usually depending on the severity of the underlying disease and the degree of the hematologic and thrombotic manifestations. Mortality rates have been reported to range from 31% to as high as 86% in some series. Advanced age is associated with a worse outcome.

Risk Factors

The main factor for the occurrence of DIC is the presence of a life-threatening underlying condition that abnormally activates the coagulation process. Severe sepsis (bacterial, viral, fungal) is the

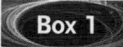

Box 1 — Underlying Conditions in Disseminated Intravascular Coagulation

Sepsis
- Meningococcemia
- Other organisms

Trauma and tissue damage
- Crush injury
- Burns
- Heat stroke

Malignancy
- Acute promyelocytic leukemia
- Solid tumors

Liver disease

Obstetric accidents
- Abruptio placentae
- Amniotic fluid embolism
- Eclampsia

Protein C and S deficiencies (purpura fulminans)
Kasabach-Merritt syndrome
Severe hemolytic transfusion reactions
Toxin exposures (snake and spider bites)
Severe pancreatitis

major cause. Additionally, serious trauma, especially head trauma, has a high correlation with DIC. Several pregnancy complications have also been implicated in the pathogenesis of DIC. Box 1 summarizes the most common causes.

Pathophysiology

The most common initiating event in DIC is the exposure of blood to tissue factor, which can be secondary to vascular endothelial damage or to activation of tissue factor by circulating monocytes in response to inflammatory cytokines. As a result, this aberrant exposure to tissue factor produces increased amounts of thrombin. In DIC, thrombin generation becomes so excessive that it cannot be counterregulated by the natural antithrombotic pathways, such as tissue factor pathway inhibitor and antithrombin III. Because thrombin activates fibrin, these events create a widespread systemic deposition of fibrin, thus stimulating the formation of microthrombi and end-organ ischemia and damage.

Thrombin promotes the release of tissue plasminogen activator from damaged endothelium. This phenomenon causes a secondary activation of the fibrinolytic pathway, generating fibrin degradation products that in turn interfere with fibrin polymerization and have a deleterious effect on platelet aggregation.

There is generalized consumption of fibrinogen, platelets, and coagulation factors (II, V, VIII), thus promoting bleeding. Coagulation inhibitors such as protein C also get depleted, further impairing the capacity to control the thrombotic manifestations. DIC can also induce a secondary microangiopathic hemolytic anemia, mostly due to intravascular fibrin causing mechanical damage and fragmentation of red blood cells.

Clinical Manifestations

Symptoms may be secondary to either the underlying disease or to DIC. The most common manifestation is that of a bleeding diathesis. A patient might initially have excessive oozing from venipuncture sites or mucosal surfaces, but more severe hemorrhages can also occur. Both venous and arterial thrombosis are seen in DIC and can manifest with secondary organ damage. Other signs include renal, hepatic, and neurologic impairment. Pulmonary hemorrhage and acute respiratory distress syndrome have been reported in severe cases. Table 1 summarizes the most common symptomatology in DIC.

TABLE 1	Clinical Symptoms in DIC
SIGN OR SYMPTOM	**INCIDENCE (%)**
Bleeding	64
Renal impairment	25
Hepatic impairment	19
Pulmonary manifestations	16
Shock	14
Thrombosis	7
Neurologic dysfunction	2

Diagnosis

No single test is diagnostic for DIC, but rather a combination of clinical and laboratory findings can aid in making an accurate diagnosis. Depending on the underlying condition, laboratory abnormalities can vary. However, the most common findings, in decreasing order of frequency, are thrombocytopenia, elevated fibrin degradation products or D-dimers, prolonged prothrombin time (PT), prolonged activated partial thromboplastin time (aPTT), and low fibrinogen. Thrombocytopenia occurs in 98% of patients with DIC, and the platelet count is less than 50,000 per microliter in 50% of them, making this an extremely sensitive, though nonspecific, marker. The PT and aPTT are prolonged in 75% and 60% of patients, respectively, reflecting the degree of consumption of coagulation factors.

Low fibrinogen is another marker for DIC, but its sensitivity has been reported to be as low as 28%. This may be due in part to the fact that fibrinogen is an inflammatory marker and may be falsely elevated in some conditions that cause DIC. Fibrin degradation products and D-dimers are elevated owing to the increased activation of the fibrinolytic pathway. The D-dimer assay has been shown to be more specific for DIC than the measurement of fibrin degradation products. In addition, the thrombin time may be elevated secondary to the increase in fibrin degradation products as well as to the hypofibrinogenemia. Measurement of anticoagulant proteins such as antithrombin III and protein C can demonstrate decreased levels in DIC, but there are limitations owing to the lack of availability of these assays in most centers. In addition, a review of the blood smear can reveal fragmented red blood cells in cases where DIC has caused a microangiopathic hemolytic anemia.

An objective scoring system for the diagnosis of overt DIC based solely on laboratory data has been established by the Scientific and Standardization Committee of the International Society of Thrombosis and Haemostasis (Box 2). It has been demonstrated to have a sensitivity of 91% and a specificity of 97% and to be an independent prognostic factor for mortality. Following the guidelines of the scoring system, patients with sepsis and DIC have been shown to have a mortality of 43%, as compared to only 27% for those without DIC.

Treatment

To control DIC, the precipitating disease needs to be treated vigorously and promptly. Additionally, aggressive supportive care measures, usually in an intensive care setting, are of utmost importance. In some cases this can indeed be enough. In other instances, a more specific treatment approach, such as replacing platelets or coagulation factor, may be necessary. This should not be based on laboratory parameters alone but rather on the clinical scenario and whether there is active bleeding, thrombosis, or organ dysfunction.

Platelet transfusions in nonbleeding patients are not usually indicated. They should be reserved for patients with a count of <50,000/μL and active bleeding or those who are perceived to be at an increased risk for bleeding, for example, in a preoperative or postoperative setting. A higher platelet count may be desired in specific situations, such as neurotrauma. Platelet support may also

Box 2	Scoring System for Overt Disseminated Intravascular Coagulation

1. Risk assessment: Does the patient have an underlying disorder known to be associated with overt DIC?
   - Yes: Proceed
   - No: Do not use this algorithm
2. Order global coagulation tests (platelet count, fibrin markers, PT, fibrinogen).
3. Score results.
   - Platelet count: >100 = 0, <100 =1, <50 = 2
   - Elevated fibrin markers such as D-dimers or FDP: No increase = 0, moderate increase = 2, strong increase = 3
   - Prolonged PT: <3 sec = 0, >3 sec but <6 sec = 1, >6 sec = 2
   - Fibrinogen level: >1 g/L = 0, <1 g/L = 1
4. Calculate score:
   - ≥5: compatible with overt DIC. Repeat score daily.
   - <5: Suggestive (not conclusive) for nonovert DIC. Repeat score in next 1 or 2 days.

Abbreviations: DIC = disseminated intravascular coagulation; FDP = fibrin degradation product; PT = prothrombin time.

be considered in nonbleeding patients if the count is significantly low (<20,000–30,000/mL).

The same rule applies to factor replacement with fresh frozen plasma. For patients without active bleeding, fresh frozen plasma is rarely indicated. However, in patients with a prolongation of the PT and aPTT and bleeding, or those perceived to be at an increased risk for bleeding or who are undergoing an invasive procedure, fresh frozen plasma should be considered. If the fibrinogen level is significantly low (<1 g/L), cryoprecipitate may be administered.

The use of anticoagulant therapy with heparin in patients with DIC has been controversial. Its use can potentiate the bleeding risks. However, heparin should be considered in cases where thrombosis predominates and is likely to lead to severe tissue injury. For example, heparin or other anticoagulant therapy should be given in the presence of dermal or acral ischemia that might rapidly progress to gangrene, as occurs in purpura fulminans and in some types of bacteremia. Indeed, anticoagulation has been demonstrated to reduce mortality from 90% to 18% in patients with purpura fulminans. Other instances in which heparin may be of benefit include DIC related to metastatic cancers, aortic aneurysms, retained dead fetus syndrome, and acute promyelocytic leukemias that are unresponsive to initial standard therapy. In addition, heparin therapy may be indicated in the presence of large vessel clots or in cases where intensive replacement of blood products alone has not been effective.

Replacement of anticoagulant factors, including administration of activated protein C (drotrecogin alfa [Xigris] and antithrombin concentrates (Thrombate III, ATryn),[1] is another strategy that has been evaluated. Clinical studies have shown a survival advantage for patients with severe sepsis and DIC using activated protein C, but there was a minor increased risk of bleeding (3.5% versus 2% in placebo), and caution should be exercised in this regard. After several clinical trials studying its potential efficacy in DIC, antithrombin administration has not been demonstrated to decrease mortality.

Antifibrinolytic therapy is usually contraindicated in DIC because of its risk of promoting thrombosis, but it may be considered in patients with severe bleeding whose primary process is a hyperfibrinolytic state. Agents include aminocaproic acid (Amicar) and tranexamic acid (Cyklokapron).[1]

Potential treatment agents undergoing trials include recombinant thrombomodulin, recombinant tissue factor pathway inhibitor, activated factor VII (Novoseven), and recombinant nematode anticoagulant protein c2.

---

[1]Not FDA approved for this indication.

References

Bernard GR, Vincent JL, Laterre PF, et al. Efficacy and safety of recombinant human activated protein C for severe sepsis. N Engl J Med 2001;344:699–709.

Bick RL. Disseminated intravascular coagulation current concepts of etiology, pathophysiology, diagnosis, and treatment. Hematol Oncol Clin North Am 2003;17:149–76.

Levi M, de Jonge E, van der Poll T. New treatment strategies for disseminated intravascular coagulation based on current understanding of the pathophysiology. Ann Med 2004;36:41–9.

Marder VJ, Feinstein DI, Colman RW, et al. Consumptive thrombohemorrhagic disorders. In: Colman RW, editor. Hemostasis and Thrombosis. 5th ed. Philadelphia: Lippincott Williams and Wilkins; 2006. p. 1571–600.

Seligsohn U, Hoots WK. Disseminated intravascular coagulation. In: Lichtman MA, editor. Williams Hematology. 7th ed. New York: McGraw Hill; 2006. p. 1959–79.

Siegal T, Seligsohn U, Aghai E, et al. Clinical and laboratory aspects of disseminated intravascular coagulation (DIC): A study of 118 cases. Thromb Haemost 1978;39:122–34.

Taylor FB, Toh CH, Hoots WK, et al. Towards definition, clinical and laboratory criteria, and a scoring system for disseminated intravascular coagulation. Thromb Haemost 2001;86:1327–30.

Toh CH, Hoots WK. The scoring system of the Scientific and Standardization Committee on Disseminated Intravascular Coagulation of the International Society on Thrombosis and Haemostasis: A 5-year overview. J Thromb Haemost 2007;5:604–6.

Warren BL, Eid A, Singer P, et al. Caring for the critically ill patient. High-dose antithrombin III in severe sepsis: A randomized controlled trial. JAMA 2001;286:1869–78.

HEMOCHROMATOSIS

Method of
Paul C. Adams, MD

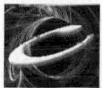

CURRENT DIAGNOSIS

- Consider the diagnosis in patients with Northern European ancestry.
- Initial testing is transferrin saturation or unsaturated iron binding capacity and serum ferritin.
- Secondary testing is the C282Y genetic test.
- More than 90% of typical hemochromatosis patients are homozygotes for the C282Y mutation.
- If genetic testing is not typical, reassess the diagnosis and consider secondary iron overload related to cirrhosis, alcoholism, viral hepatitis, or an iron-loading anemia.
- A number of other hemochromatosis genetic mutations are relevant to only a minority of patients.
- Not all patients need a liver biopsy.
- Siblings are at highest risk in a family study.

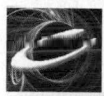

CURRENT THERAPY

- Iron overload from hemochromatosis is treated by the weekly removal of 500 mL of blood until the serum ferritin is in the low-normal range of approximately 50 µg/L.
- Some but not all patients require maintenance therapy with three to four phlebotomies per year. In some countries, this can be a voluntary blood donation.
- Excess alcohol, high doses of vitamin C, and iron supplementation should be avoided, but strict dietary restrictions are not recommended.
- Siblings and children of patients should be tested for hemochromatosis with transferrin saturation, ferritin, and genetic testing.

Hemochromatosis is the most common genetic disease in populations of European ancestry. The diagnosis can be elusive because of the nonspecific nature of the symptoms. With the discovery of the hemochromatosis gene (*HFE*) in 1996 came new insights into the pathogenesis of the disease and new diagnostic strategies.

A fundamental issue that arose after the discovery of the *HFE* gene is whether the disease hemochromatosis should be defined strictly on phenotypic criteria such as the degree of iron overload (i.e., transferrin saturation, ferritin, liver biopsy, hepatic iron concentration, iron removed by venesection therapy), or whether the condition should be defined as a familial disease in Europeans most commonly associated with the C282Y mutation of the *HFE* gene and varying degrees of iron overload. Because the genetic test has been increasingly used as a diagnostic tool, most studies now use a combination of phenotypic and genotypic criteria for the diagnosis of hemochromatosis.

Clinical Features

Although hemochromatosis is often classified as a liver disease, it should be emphasized that it is a systemic genetic disease with multisystem involvement. The liver is central in both diagnosis and prognosis. Hepatomegaly remains one of the more common physical signs in hemochromatosis, but it is not always present in the young, asymptomatic homozygote. In a study of 717 homozygotes from Australia, 8% of men and 1.7% of women had cirrhosis of the liver at the time of diagnosis. The prevalence of cirrhosis in asymptomatic or screened patients is much lower. It is likely that there are factors other than iron overload that contribute to cirrhosis in hemochromatosis. These can include the effects of alcohol or comodifying genes. The effect of iron depletion therapy is usually stabilization of the liver disease, and fibrosis improves with repeat liver biopsy after iron depletion. This accounts for the relatively small number of C282Y homozygotes that require liver transplantation. The other common clinical manifestations are arthralgias, pigmentation, congestive heart failure, impotence, and fatigue. Several large population studies failed to demonstrate an increase in diabetes compared with a control population. A population-based study estimated that only 28% of male and 1% of female C282Y homozygotes will develop symptoms of iron overload.

Diagnosis

A paradox of genetic hemochromatosis is that the disease is underdiagnosed in the general population and overdiagnosed in patients with secondary iron overload.

Preliminary population studies using genetic testing demonstrate a prevalence of homozygotes of approximately 1:227 among whites. The fact that many physicians consider hemochromatosis to be rare implies either a lack of penetrance of the gene (nonexpressing homozygote) or a large number of patients who remain undiagnosed in the community.

Diagnosis

Transferrin Saturation

Previous studies had suggested that transferrin saturation would be a good screening test and diagnostic test for hemochromatosis.

The sensitivity of transferrin saturation in population-screening studies designed to detect C282Y homozygotes (genotypic case definition) was only approximately 75%, and transferrin saturation can be in the normal range in young female homozygotes. A large biologic variation in transferrin saturation within an individual patient has also been reported.

Serum Ferritin

The relationship between serum ferritin and total body iron stores was clearly established by strong correlations with hepatic iron concentration and the amount of iron removed by venesection. However, ferritin can be elevated secondary to chronic inflammation and histiocytic neoplasms. A major diagnostic dilemma in the past was whether the serum ferritin concentration was related to hemochromatosis or to another underlying liver disease, such as alcoholic liver disease, chronic viral hepatitis, or nonalcoholic steatohepatitis. It is likely that most of these difficult cases can now be resolved by genetic testing.

Liver Biopsy

Liver biopsy was previously the gold-standard diagnostic test for hemochromatosis; however, it has shifted from a major diagnostic tool to a method of estimating prognosis and concomitant disease.

The need for liver biopsy seems less clear now in the young, asymptomatic C282Y homozygote in whom there is a low clinical suspicion of cirrhosis based on history, physical examination, and liver biochemistry. A large study conducted in France and Canada suggested that C282Y homozygotes with a serum ferritin concentration of less than 1000 μg/L, a normal aspartate transaminase (AST) concentration, and no hepatomegaly have a very low risk of cirrhosis. C282Y homozygotes with a ferritin level greater than 1000 μg/L, an elevated AST, and a platelet count of less than 200,000/mm^3 have an 80% chance of having cirrhosis. Hepatic elastography is another noninvasive tool to assess liver fibrosis in hemochromatosis.

Patients with cirrhosis have a 5.5-fold relative risk of death compared with noncirrhotic hemochromatosis patients. Cirrhotic patients are also at increased risk of hepatocellular carcinoma. Liver biopsy is considered in typical C282Y homozygotes with liver dysfunction and in potentially iron-overloaded patients without the typical C282Y mutation. Simple C282Y heterozygotes, compound heterozygotes (C282Y/H63D), H63D homozygotes, and patients with other risk factors (e.g., alcohol abuse, chronic viral hepatitis) who have moderate to severe iron overload (ferritin >1000 μg/L) may be considered for liver biopsy.

Since the introduction of genetic testing, hepatic iron concentration and hepatic iron index have become less useful in the diagnosis of hemochromatosis.

Genetic Testing

A major advance stemming from the discovery of the hemochromatosis gene is the use of a diagnostic genetic test. Most studies report that more than 90% of typical hemochromatosis patients were homozygotes for the C282Y mutation. A second minor mutation, H63D, was also described in the original report. Compound heterozygotes (C282Y/H63D) and, less commonly, H63D homozygotes, resemble C282Y homozygotes with mild to moderate iron overload. Genetic mutations involving ferroportin, hemojuvelin, transferrin receptor 2, ceruloplasmin, and hepcidin are associated with iron overload. It is likely that, as more mutations are found, they will be relevant to only a minority of patients. Commercial tests are rarely available for these rare genetic mutations.

Some patients with clinical pictures indistinguishable from genetic hemochromatosis are negative for the C282Y mutation. Most of these cases appear to be isolated, although a few cases of familial iron overload with negative C282Y testing have been reported. A negative C282Y test should alert the physician to question the diagnosis of genetic hemochromatosis and to reconsider secondary iron overload related to cirrhosis, alcoholism, viral hepatitis, or an iron-loading anemia. If no other risk factors are found, the patient should begin phlebotomy treatment, similar to any other hemochromatosis patient.

The interpretation of the genetic test in several settings is shown in Box 1. Genetic discrimination is a concern, given the widespread use of genetic testing, but discrimination has been rarely reported in screening studies. In the case of hemochromatosis, the advantages of early diagnosis of a treatable disease outweigh the disadvantages of genetic discrimination.

Family Studies

Once the proband case is identified and confirmed with the genetic test for the C282Y mutation, family testing is imperative. Siblings have approximately one in four chance of carrying the gene and should be screened with the genetic test (C282Y and H63D mutation), transferrin saturation, and serum ferritin. A cost-effective strategy now possible with genetic testing is to test the spouse for the C282Y mutation to assess the risk in the children. If the spouse is not a C282Y heterozygote or homozygote, the children will be obligate heterozygotes, assuming paternity and excluding another gene or mutation causing hemochromatosis. This strategy is particularly advantageous if the children are geographically separated or in different health care systems.

Treatment

The treatment of hemochromatosis continues to employ the medieval therapy of periodic bleeding. Blood is removed, with the patient in the reclining position over 15 to 30 minutes. Initial treatment consists of the weekly removal of 500 mL of blood. A hemoglobin test is done before each phlebotomy. If the hemoglobin concentration has decreased to less than 10 g/dL, the phlebotomy schedule is modified to 500 mL every 2 weeks. Phlebotomies are continued until the serum ferritin concentration is approximately 50 mcg/L. Serum ferritin levels are drawn monthly in patients with significant iron overload and increased to weekly as the ferritin decreases to <200 mcg/L. The concomitant administration of a salt-containing sport beverage (e.g., Gatorade) is a simple method of maintaining plasma volume during the phlebotomy.

Box 1 Interpretation of Genetic Testing for Hemochromatosis

"C282Y Homozygote"

This is the classic genetic pattern seen in more than 90% of typical cases. Expression of disease ranges from no evidence of iron overload to massive iron overload with organ dysfunction. Siblings have a one in four chance of being affected and should have genetic testing. For children to be affected, the other parent must be at least a heterozygote. If iron studies are normal, false-positive genetic testing or a nonexpressing homozygotic state should be considered

"C282Y/H63D Compound Heterozygote"

This patient carries two copies of the minor mutation. Most patients with this genetic pattern have normal iron studies. A small percentage have mild to moderate iron overload. Severe iron overload is usually seen in the setting of another concomitant risk factor (e.g., alcoholism, viral hepatitis)

"C282Y Heterozygote"

This patient carries one copy of the major mutation. This pattern is seen in approximately 10% of the white population and is usually associated with normal iron studies. In rare cases, the results of iron studies are high, in the range expected in a homozygote rather than a heterozygote. These patients may carry an unknown hemochromatosis mutation, and liver biopsy is helpful to determine the need for phlebotomy therapy

"H63D Homozygote"

Most patients with this genotype will have normal iron studies. A small percentage have mild to moderate iron overload. Severe iron overload is usually seen in the setting of another concomitant risk factor (e.g., alcoholism, viral hepatitis)

"H63D Heterozygote"

This patient carries one copy of the minor mutation. This pattern is seen in approximately 20% of the white population and is usually associated with normal iron studies. This pattern is so common in the general population that the presence of iron overload can be related to another risk factor. Liver biopsy is required to determine the cause of the iron overload and the need for treatment in these cases

"No HFE Mutations"

If iron overload is present without any mutations in the hemochromatosis gene (HFE), a careful history for other risk factors must be reviewed, and liver biopsy can be useful to determine the cause of the iron overload and the need for treatment. Most of these are isolated, nonfamilial cases. There are cases described involving genetic mutations in ferroportin, hemojuvelin, transferrin receptor 2, ceruloplasmin, and hepcidin genes. Genetic tests for these mutations are not widely available

Maintenance phlebotomies after iron depletion, consisting of three to four phlebotomies per year, are performed in most patients, although the rate of iron reaccumulation is highly variable. Maintenance therapy is initiated when the serum ferritin rises from 50 mcg/L to >300 mcg/L. The transferrin saturation remains elevated in many treated patients and does not normalize unless the patient becomes iron deficient. In some countries, patients with mild iron abnormalities are encouraged to become voluntary blood donors.

Chelation therapy[1] is not recommended for hemochromatosis. Patients are advised to avoid oral iron therapy and alcohol abuse, but there are no dietary restrictions. Patient support groups have been concerned by the practice of iron fortification of foods, but much of this iron is in an inexpensive form with poor bioavailability.

Hemochromatosis is a common and often underdiagnosed disease. Early diagnosis and treatment result in an excellent long-term prognosis. The development of a diagnostic genetic test has improved the feasibility of the goal of prevention of morbidity and mortality from hemochromatosis.

---

[1]Not FDA approved for this indication.

References

Adams PC, Reboussin DM, Barton JC, et al. Hemochromatosis and iron overload screening (HEIRS) study: Screening in a racially diverse of primary care population. N Engl J Med 2005a;352:1769–78.

Adams PC. Hemochromatosis case definition: Out of focus. Nat Clin Pract Gastroenterol Hepatol 2006;3:178–9.

Adams PC, Barton JC. How I treat hemochromatosis. Blood 2010;116:317–25.

Adams PC, Reboussin DM, Eckfeldt J, et al. A comparison of the unsaturated iron binding capacity to transferrin saturation as a screening test to detect C282Y homozygotes for hemochromatosis in 101,168 participants in the HEIRS study. Clin Chem 2005b;51:1048–52.

Allen KJ, Gurrin LC, Constantine CC, et al. Iron-overload-related disease in HFE hereditary hemochromatosis. N Engl J Med 2008;358:221–30.

Andersen R, Tybjaerg-Hansen A, Appleyard M, et al. Hemochromatosis mutations in the general population: Iron overload progression rate. Blood 2004;103:2914–9.

Bacon BR, Adams PC, Kowdley K, et al. Diagnosis and management of hemochromatosis: AASLD practice guidelines. Hepatology 2011;54:328–43.

Beaton M, Guyader D, Deugnier Y, et al. Non-invasive prediction of cirrhosis in C282Y-linked hemochromatosis. Hepatology 2002;36:673–8.

Cherfane CE, Hollenbeck RD, Go J, et al. Hereditary hemochromatosis: Missed diagnosis or misdiagnosis. Am J Med 2013;126:1010–5.

Falize L, Guillygomarch A, Perrin M, et al. Reversibility of hepatic fibrosis in treated hemochromatosis; A study of 36 cases. Hepatology 2006;44:472–7.

Gordeuk V, Lovato L, Vitolins M, et al. Relationship between dietary iron intake and serum ferritin concentration in HFE homozygotes. Can J Gastroenterol 2012;26:345–9.

Guyader D, Jacquelinet C, Moirand R, et al. Non-invasive prediction of fibrosis in C282Y homozygous hemochromatosis. Gastroenterology 1998;115:929–36.

HEMOLYTIC ANEMIA

Method of
Patricia A. Cornett, MD

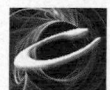

CURRENT DIAGNOSIS

- Anemia accompanied by reticulocytosis without evidence of bleeding or recovery from a nutritional anemia should prompt an evaluation for immune and nonimmune causes of hemolytic anemia.
- Key test results that help confirm the presence of hemolysis include elevated indirect bilirubin and lactate dehydrogenase (LDH) levels, often accompanied by a low haptoglobin level. Examination of the peripheral smear may reveal findings that guide further diagnostic testing.

- The direct antiglobulin test (DAT) can be an important initial test and if positive, would establish the diagnosis of immune-mediated hemolysis. Further testing will distinguish warm-antibody autoimmune hemolytic anemia (AIHA) from cold-antibody AIHA.
- A negative DAT should prompt evaluation for causes of nonimmune hemolysis. Both congenital and acquired red blood cell (RBC) disorders will require further diagnostic testing.

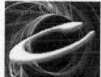

CURRENT THERAPY

- Patients with ongoing moderate to severe hemolysis should be treated with folate (folic acid),[1] 1 mg orally daily.
- RBC transfusion may be used for life-threatening situations. When the DAT is positive, least incompatible units should be used.
- Patients with warm AIHA are best treated with corticosteroids. Patients refractory to steroids or who cannot have their steroids tapered, will require second-line therapy such as splenectomy or rituximab (Rituxan).[1]
- Those patients with cold-antibody AIHA or paroxysmal cold hemoglobinuria (PCH) should avoid cold exposure; therapies used for warm AIHA are often not successful.
- Splenectomy can benefit selected patients with congenital hemolytic anemia. Vaccinations for Streptococcus pneumoniae, Haemophilus influenzae type B, and Neisseria meningitidis should be administered before surgery.
- Acquired causes of nonimmune hemolytic anemia are generally managed by treating the underlying cause or removing the offending agent.

---

[1]Not FDA approved for this indication.

Hemolysis, the premature destruction of red blood cells (RBC), leads to hemolytic anemia when the bone marrow cannot compensate for RBC loss. A useful classification divides the hemolytic anemias mechanistically into immune or nonimmune causes. Immune-mediated causes include autoimmune hemolytic anemia (AIHA) and alloantibody-induced hemolytic anemia (Box 1). AIHA occurs as a result of antibody production against self-RBC antigens. AIHA can be idiopathic or can occur secondary to drugs, infections, malignancies, or autoimmune disorders. Types of AIHA include warm-antibody AIHA, cold-antibody AIHA, paroxysmal cold hemoglobinuria (PCH), and medication-induced AIHA (see Box 1). Alloantibody-induced hemolytic anemia includes hemolytic transfusion reactions and hemolytic disease of the fetus and newborn. Nonimmune causes of hemolysis can be further classified into congenital disorders with defects in the RBC membrane, enzymes, or hemoglobin, and acquired disorders when, usually, the cause of hemolysis is by extrinsic influences on the RBC. Extrinsic factors causing direct injury to the RBCs include the microangiopathic hemolytic anemias, infections, toxins, and certain systemic illnesses. The one acquired cause of hemolytic anemia where the defect is due to an intrinsic RBC abnormality is paroxysmal nocturnal hemoglobinuria.

Pathophysiology

RBCs have a lifespan in the circulation of approximately 120 days. Senescent RBCs are removed from the circulation in the spleen. Hemolysis takes place either in the spleen or liver (extravascular hemolysis) or within the vasculature (intravascular hemolysis).

Immune Hemolytic Anemias

Immune hemolysis occurs due to antibodies directed against self-RBC antigens (AIHA) or antibodies directed against transfused RBCs.

Box 1 — Classification of Hemolytic Anemia

- Immune Hemolytic Anemia
  - Warm-antibody autoimmune hemolytic anemia
    - Primary or idiopathic warm-antibody AIHA
    - Secondary warm-antibody AIHA associated with
      - Lymphoproliferative disorders (e.g., Hodgkins Disease, non-Hodgkins lymphoma, chronic lymphocytic leukemia)
      - Rheumatologic or autoimmune diseases (e.g., systemic lupus erythematosus, rheumatoid arthritis, ulcerative colitis)
  - Cold-antibody autoimmune hemolytic anemia
    - Mediated by cold agglutinins
    - Idiopathic (primary) cold agglutinin disease
    - Secondary cold agglutinin hemolytic anemia associated with
      - Infections (e.g., *Mycoplasma pneumonia*, infectious mononucleosis)
      - Lymphoproliferative disorders
    - Mediated by cold hemolysins
      - Idiopathic (primary) paroxysmal cold hemoglobinuria (PCH)
      - Secondary PCH associated with
        - Infections (e.g., syphilis, viral infections)
        - Lymphoproliferative disorders
  - Mixed cold and warm autoantibodies
    - Primary or idiopathic mixed AIHA
    - Secondary mixed AIHA
      - Associated with rheumatologic diseases, especially SLE
  - Drug-immune hemolytic anemia
    - Hapten or drug-adsorption mechanism
    - Immune complex mechanism
    - Autoantibody mechanism
  - Allo antibody hemolysis
    - Acute transfusion reaction
    - Delayed transfusion reaction
    - Hemolytic disease of the fetus and newborn
- Nonimmune Hemolytic Anemia
  - Congenital hemolytic anemia
    - Membrane disorders (e.g., hereditary spherocytosis, hereditary elliptocytosis, hereditary pyropoikilocytosis, hereditary stomatocytosis)
    - Hemoglobinopathies (e.g., sickle cell disease, hemoglobin CC disease, unstable hemoglobins)
    - Enzyme disorders (e.g. G6PD deficiency)
  - Acquired hemolytic anemia
    - Microangiopathic (e.g., TTP, HUS, DIC, malignancy, vasculitis)
    - Infections (e.g., malaria, babesiosis)
    - Toxins (e.g., arsenic, lead, copper, insect or spider or snake bites)
    - Paroxysmal nocturnal hemoglobinuria
    - Other (liver failure, extensive burns)

Autoimmune Hemolytic Anemia

Warm AIHA. The antibodies most commonly involved in warm-antibody AIHA are of the IgG type. These IgG antibodies are typically directed against RBC Rh proteins. The antibodies bind RBCs at 37°C, allowing their Fc region to remain exposed. This region is recognized by Fc receptors on the macrophages of the spleen, resulting in fragmentation and ingestion of the antibody-coated RBCs. Partial or complete phagocytosis of the RBC ensures; if partial phagocytosis occurs, spherocytes are formed. Splenomegaly results from entrapment of RBCs in the spleen.

Cold-Antibody AIHA. Cold agglutinins are typically IgM autoantibodies that cause RBC agglutination at temperatures lower than 37°C, with maximal RBC agglutination at temperatures lower than 4°C. Cold agglutinins may occur in response to infection, as is commonly seen with *Mycoplasma* pneumonia and infectious mononucleosis. The IgM antibody usually reacts with I/i RBC antigen, resulting in complement activation by fixation of antibody to the antigen at low temperatures. Anti-I is characteristic of *Mycoplasma* pneumonia-induced hemolysis, whereas anti-i is characteristic of infectious mononucleosis

Paroxysmal Cold Hemoglobinuria. The Donath-Landsteiner autoantibody is a biphasic, polyclonal IgG that binds RBCs at cooler temperatures (4°C), activates complement, and results in intravascular hemolysis at warmer temperatures (37°C) due to complement fixation. This autoantibody is able to bind several RBC antigens, although its main target is the P antigen.

Medication AIHA. Medication-induced AIHA results from three proposed mechanisms based on the interactions among medications, RBC membrane antigens, and antibodies. These mechanisms are induced by drug or hapten adsorption, neoantigen formation, and autoantibody binding.

Alloantibody Hemolysis

Alloantibodies can occur in recipients of blood transfusions due to exposure to non–self-RBCs. Acute transfusion reactions are due to preformed antibodies in the recipient which attack donor RBCs leading to complement activation. Intravascular hemolysis occurs, often leading to disseminated intravascular coagulation (DIC) and acute renal failure. Delayed transfusion reactions occur 3 to 21 days after a transfusion due to an anamnestic antibody response from the recipient because of prior exposure to RBCs either through transfusions or pregnancy. The most common antibodies formed are anti-Kidd or directed against RH antigens. Typically, these antibodies are noncomplement binding and cause extravascular hemolysis.

Nonimmune Hemolytic Anemia

Congenital Hemolytic Anemia

The congenital nonimmune hemolytic anemias are caused by mutations affecting the RBC membrane, hemoglobin, or enzymes.

- Membrane Disorders

  The most common RBC membrane disorders are hereditary spherocytosis, hereditary elliptocytosis, and hereditary pyropoikilocytosis. Each disorder is caused by a defect in one of the cell wall proteins. The nature of the deformity depends upon the exact structural protein defect. Spherocytes (Figure 1), and to a lesser extent, elliptocytes (Figure 2), are not as deformable as the normal biconcave RBCs and are removed from the circulation by

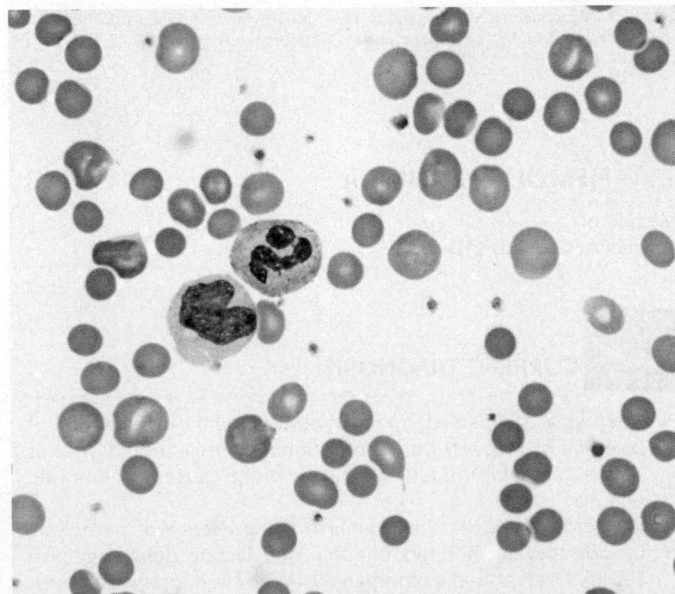

Figure 1. Hereditary spherocytosis. Peripheral blood film showing spherocytes.

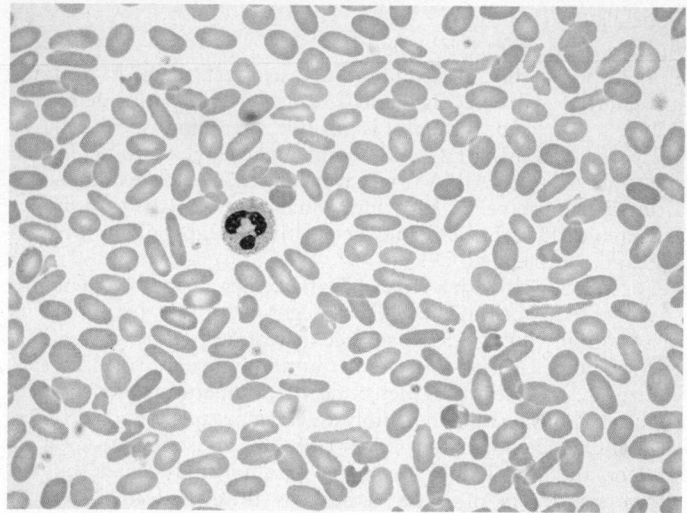

Figure 2. Hereditary elliptocytosis. Peripheral blood film showing elliptocytes.

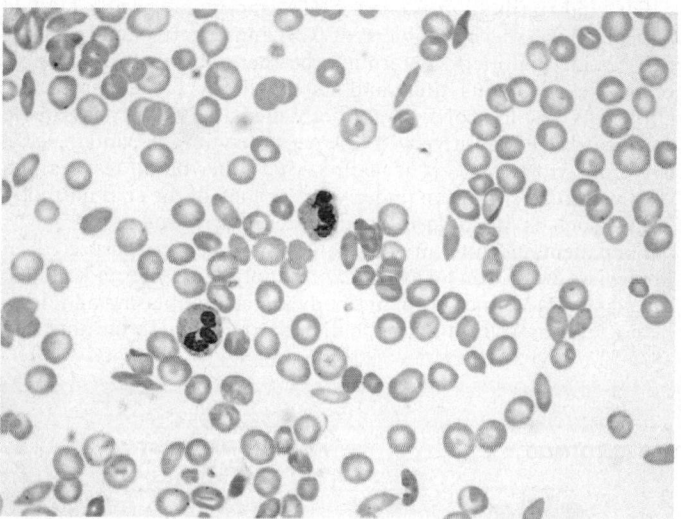

Figure 3. Sickle cell anemia. Peripheral blood smear showing sickle cells.

macrophages. This extravascular hemolysis typically occurs predominantly within the spleen. Patients with hereditary pyropoikilocytosis are double heterozygotes, usually inheriting two hereditary elliptocytosis mutations, resulting in the production of tiny, fragmented RBCs and severe hemolytic anemia.

- Hemoglobinopathies

   Hemoglobin is composed of four subunits held together by noncovalent forces. A number of mutations affect the forces maintaining this structural integrity and can result in degradation and precipitation of the hemoglobin within the cell. These unstable hemoglobins form precipitates, or Heinz bodies, attach to the membrane, and impair the deformability of the RBC, ultimately leading to removal of the cells within the spleen. Another hemoglobinopathy, and the most common, sickle cell disease, results from the replacement of valine for glutamic acid in the sixth position of the β-globin subunit. Sickle cell disease has a myriad of downstream physiologic effects that ultimately leads to hemolysis of the sickled RBCs (Figure 3).

- Enzyme Disorders

   The RBC relies on enzymes functioning in two glycolysis pathways to generate energy. Energy is required to maintain the RBC's biconcave shape as well as the integrity of the enzymes, hemoglobin, and membrane through its 120-day life span. The two metabolic pathways are the anaerobic glycolysis (Embden-Meyerhof) pathway and the aerobic glycolysis (hexose monophosphate) pathway. Enzyme defects in the Embden-Meyerhof pathway are generally associated with chronic hemolysis; enzyme defects in the hexose monophosphate pathway are often associated with episodic hemolysis. The most common defect affects the glucose-6-phosphate dehydrogenase (G6PD) enzyme. This enzyme is responsible for diverting glucose from the Embden-Meyerhof pathway to the hexose monophosphate pathway and for restoring intracellular reduced nicotinamide adenine dinucleotide phosphate, which functions as an antioxidant. Low levels of G6PD activity result in the inability of the cell to defend itself against oxidant stresses; absent levels result in chronic hemolysis.

Acquired Hemolytic Anemia

For the acquired nonimmune hemolytic anemias, hemolysis results from extrinsic forces affecting the RBC. In the microangiopathic hemolytic anemias, RBCs undergo fragmentation due to high sheer forces generated from abnormal vascular surfaces.

Infections can cause hemolysis due to direct invasion of the organism into the RBC (malaria, babesiosis) by release of products that can destabilize the red cell membrane (*Clostridia perfringens*), or by initiating DIC, resulting in microangiopathic hemolysis.

Certain toxic chemicals and physical agents can cause hemolysis through a variety of mechanisms affecting the RBC membrane or metabolism. These substances include arsenic; lead; copper; and insect, spider, and snake venoms.

Other systemic disease states causing hemolysis include liver failure and extensive burns. In liver failure, the ratio of cholesterol to phospholipid in the red cell membrane is altered, resulting in membrane instability and hemolysis. Patients with extensive burns can present acutely with a brisk hemolytic anemia; the heat from the burns likely causes mechanical and osmotic damage to RBCs.

The underlying defect in paroxysmal nocturnal hemoglobinuria is impaired production of a key anchoring cellular membrane protein. Loss of the anchoring protein, glycosylphosphatidylinositol, disrupts a number of cellular proteins including CD59, a protein inhibitor of complement-mediated lysis. Deficiency of CD59 leads to greater sensitivity of RBCs to hemolysis.

Clinical Manifestations

The clinical manifestations of all hemolytic anemias, in large part, depend upon the severity of the anemia and the rapidity of the hemoglobin decline as well as any associated manifestations related to the underlying cause. General symptoms of anemia include weakness, fatigue, lethargy, and palpitations. Physical examination not only includes the typical findings of anemia (pale sclerae and nail beds) but may also reveal icteric sclera and jaundice if the indirect bilirubin is sufficiently increased. Other clinical manifestations of the hemolytic anemias, particularly the congenital nonimmune causes but also seen in AIHA, include splenomegaly, formation of pigmented gallstones with the possibility of cholecystitis, and aplastic crisis due to viral infections. Aplastic crisis results from viral suppression of hematopoiesis. Because RBC survival at baseline is shortened, abrupt cessation of erythropoiesis results in a rapid fall in the hemoglobin level and relatively acute onset of symptomatic anemia.

As noted previously, hemolysis can occur in the intravascular or extravascular space, depending upon the etiology. Clinical manifestations of intravascular hemolysis versus extravascular hemolysis differ. Intravascular hemolysis, as might occur with PCH or an acute transfusion reaction can result in dark or cola-colored urine due to hemoglobinuria. Patients with acute transfusion reactions may also experience fevers and chills as well as flank pain. DIC, hypotension, and renal failure may ensue.

Specific manifestations of certain disorders can occur and may be helpful in establishing the diagnosis. For instance, patients with cold–antibody-mediated AIHA may experience acrocyanosis of their fingers, toes, nose, and ears, especially when exposed to the cold. Patients with PNH may present with abdominal pain, venous thrombosis, and may have, in addition to the hemolytic anemia, granulocytopenia and thrombocytopenia.

The AIHAs may be associated with other medical conditions. For instance, AIHA may also be associated with other viral or bacterial illnesses, as well as lymphoproliferative or rheumatologic disorders.

Diagnosis

Anemia that is accompanied by reticulocytosis is suggestive of a hemolytic process. Tests that support the presence of hemolysis include an elevated lactate dehydrogenase (LDH) and indirect bilirubin. In general, when hemolytic anemia is suspected due to these findings (reticulocytosis, elevated LDH, and indirect bilirubin), the first test to be performed is the peripheral smear examination. Abnormalities seen on the peripheral smear examination commonly suggest the cause of the hemolysis and direct further, specialized testing (Table 1).

Other tests that may be helpful to confirm the presence of hemolysis include serum haptoglobin, plasma and urinary free hemoglobin, and urinary hemosiderin. Haptoglobin, synthesized by the liver, binds any free hemoglobin in the plasma; the complex is then removed in hepatic parenchymal cells. If the rate of hemolysis exceeds the clearance rate of this complex, the haptoglobin level will be decreased. Haptoglobin is also an acute phase reactant; it can be elevated if there is acute inflammation present. Intravascular hemolysis can result in detection of free hemoglobin in the plasma if the plasma hemoglobin-binding proteins are saturated; urine hemoglobin will be detected if the capacity of renal tubular cells to absorb free hemoglobin is exceeded.

Hemoglobin that is filtered in the kidney is stored in the renal tubular cells and excreted in the form of hemosiderin. As these cells slough into the urine, the hemosiderin can be detected by a Prussian blue stain approximately 5 to 7 days following a hemolytic episode. This test is therefore helpful to detect intravascular hemolysis days after the hemolytic event.

For the hemolytic anemias, examination of the bone marrow is seldom helpful and generally not necessary in the diagnostic process.

Specialized Testing

Autoimmune Hemolytic Anemia

A polyspecific direct antiglobulin test (DAT), which contains reagents that will detect IgG and C3 antibodies, is performed when AIHA is suspected. If the test is positive, then monospecific DATs are performed using IgG and complement reagents to determine the subtype of AIHA (warm-mediated, cold-mediated, or Donath-Landsteiner). For individuals with warm–antibody-mediated AIHA, the DAT may be positive for IgG only or for both IgG and complement C3.

For individuals with a Donath-Landsteiner antibody, the monospecific DAT is positive for C3 but negative for IgG, because of its dissociation from the RBC surface at warmer temperatures. The presence of a Donath-Landsteiner antibody is confirmed by specialized testing aimed at detecting the temperature dependency of the antibody-mediated hemolysis. Plasma is incubated with normal RBCs and cooled to 4°C. If a Donath-Landsteiner antibody is present, the cold hemolysin in the plasma binds RBCs, but no hemolysis occurs until the sample is rewarmed to 37°C. At 37°C, the sensitized RBCs are hemolyzed by the complement present in plasma. The presence of hemolysis at 37°C following incubation at 4°C, but not at incubation at only 4°C or 37°C, constitutes a positive antibody test result.

For cold–antibody-mediated AIHA, the monospecific DAT is typically positive for complement (C3) and negative for IgG. Further testing is done to determine the thermal range of the antibody's reactivity, its titer, and its specificity for either the I/i antigen. A diagnosis of cold–antibody-mediated hemolysis is made when the DAT is positive with C3, negative with IgG, and the cold agglutinin titer at 4°C is at least >256. Other blood tests can be obtained to determine an underlying etiology of the cold-antibody AIHA, such as *Mycoplasma* and Epstein-Barr virus titers.

For patients in whom an acute transfusion reaction is suspected, an immediate evaluation for evidence of hemolysis must be undertaken, including a DAT and serum antibody screen and plasma and urine hemoglobin as well as haptoglobin. Both a DAT and serum antibody

---

TABLE 1   Classification of Nonimmune Hemolytic Anemias

DIAGNOSIS	PERIPHERAL SMEAR FINDINGS	ADDITIONAL TESTS
Congenital Disorders		
Membrane disorders		
Hereditary spherocytosis	Spherocytes	Ektacytometry
Hereditary elliptocytosis	Elliptocytes	Ektacytometry
Hereditary pyropoikilocytosis	Microcytes, fragments	Ektacytometry
Hemoglobin Disorders		
Sickle cell disease	Sickle cells, targets	Hemoglobin electrophoresis
Unstable hemoglobins	Bite cells	Supravital stain, hemoglobin electrophoresis, heat stability test
Enzyme Disorders		
G6PD deficiency	Bite cells, blister cells	Supravital stain, G6PD level
Others	Variable	Individual enzyme levels
Acquired Disorders		
Microangiopathic hemolytic anemias		
TTP, HUS, DIC, cancer, heart valves	Schistocytes, red blood cell fragments	Targeted to diagnosis
Infections		
Malaria, babesiosis, *Clostridium perfringens*	Parasite (malaria, babesiosis)	Giemsa stain (babesiosis)
Toxins, physical agents		
Arsenic, lead, copper	Basophilic stippling (lead)	Element levels
Insect, spider, snake venoms	Schistocytes, fragments	Targeted to diagnosis
Systemic diseases		
Liver disease	Acanthocytes, target cells	Liver function tests
Burns	Spherocytes, blister cells, fragments	Targeted to diagnosis
Paroxysmal nocturnal hemoglobinuria	Variable	Flow cytometry

Abbreviations: DIC = disseminated intravascular coagulation; G6PD = glucose-6-phosphate dehydrogenase; HUS = hemolytic-uremic syndrome; TTP = thrombotic thrombocytopenic purpura.

screen will be positive, and free hemoglobin should be detected in the plasma and urine. The haptoglobin will be low or undetectable. A delayed transfusion reaction is often not appreciated but should be suspected when the hemoglobin level falls more quickly than expected following a transfusion. The diagnosis can be made by demonstrating a new serum alloantibody in the recipient of the transfused blood. A urine hemosiderin can also be positive, reflecting hemolysis that occurred several days previously.

Congenital Hemolytic Anemias

The diagnosis of congenital nonimmune hemolytic anemias is often suspected when the anemia is long-standing. A family history of anemia, splenectomy, or gallstones can also be a clue to a congenital process. Peripheral smear examination is often helpful.

The membrane disorders all have findings on the peripheral smear (see Table 1), though these findings are not necessarily specific to the disorder. A specialized test, osmotic gradient ektacytometry, can be used to help in diagnosing these disorders.

For patients with certain enzymopathies, most notably G6PD deficiency, bite cells and blister cells may be seen in the peripheral smear during an acute hemolytic event (Figure 4). A supravital stain, such as crystal violet, brilliant cresyl blue, or methylene blue, can demonstrate Heinz bodies. G6PD deficiency is definitely diagnosed by the finding of low G6PD levels in the red cell; however, levels can be normal during the acute hemolytic event because RBCs with low levels have been removed from the circulation. If the diagnosis is still suspected after obtaining a normal result, a repeat test 2 to 3 months after the acute hemolytic episode should be performed. Most other RBC enzymopathies need to be diagnosed by specialized reference laboratories.

Hemoglobin electrophoresis should be performed to diagnose a suspected hemoglobinopathy. The most common hemoglobinopathy causing hemolysis, sickle cell anemia, is readily diagnosed by this test. However, other hemoglobinopathies causing hemolysis, specifically the unstable hemoglobins, may be electrophoretically silent. If the diagnosis of an unstable hemoglobinopathy is suspected, a supravital stain can demonstrate Heinz bodies and a heat stability test should be obtained for definitive diagnosis.

Acquired Nonimmune Hemolytic Anemias

The diagnosis of acquired causes of nonimmune hemolytic anemias is suspected when a hemolytic anemia is new in onset and previous hemoglobin levels have been normal. A notable exception to this general premise is in G6PD-deficient patients presenting with new anemia due to oxidant stresses. Even though the anemia

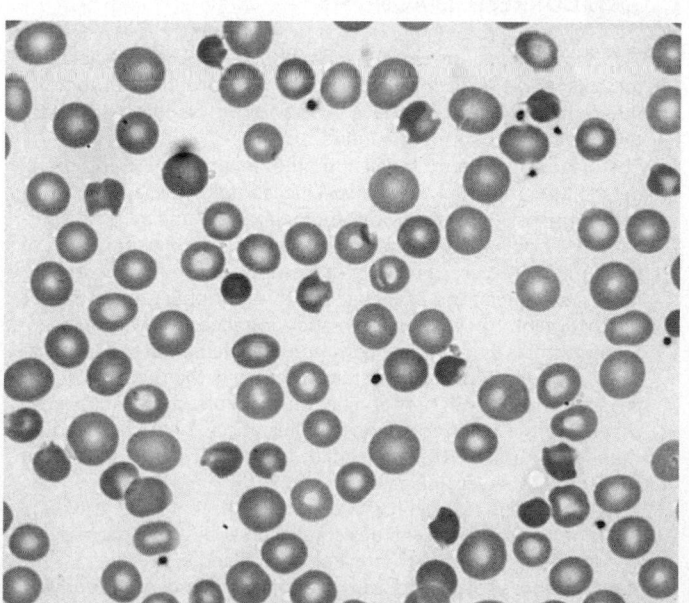

Figure 4. Glucose-6-phosphate dehydrogenase deficiency. Peripheral blood film showing bite cells and blister cells.

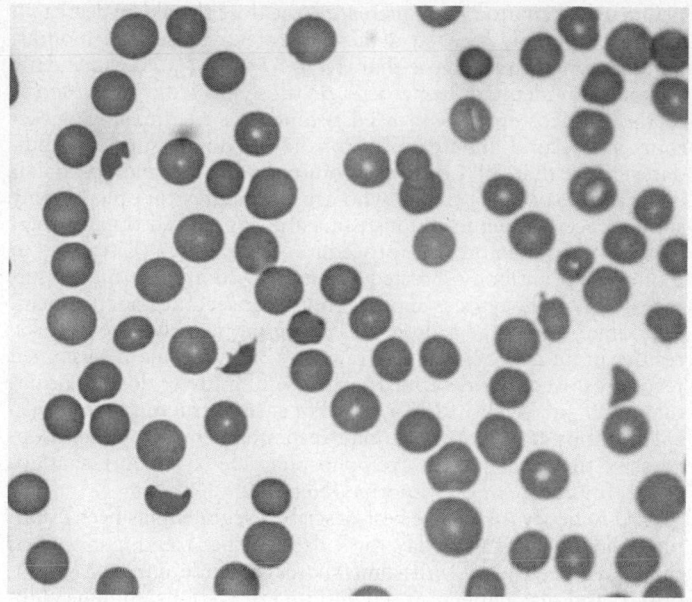

Figure 5. Microangiopathic hemolytic anemia. Peripheral blood film showing schistocytes and red blood cell fragments.

appears to be acquired, the key feature to recognize is the clinical context, which usually includes an infection or a precipitating event of a new drug.

The peripheral smear is usually very helpful in diagnosing the acquired causes of nonimmune hemolytic anemias. Microangiopathic changes found in thrombotic thrombocytopenia purpura (TTP), hemolytic-uremic syndrome (HUS), DIC, disseminated cancer, and heart valve hemolysis include schistocytes and RBC fragments. The ability to recognize these microangiopathic changes can be crucial, particularly in the diagnosis of conditions such as TTP and HUS, both of which require urgent management (Figure 5). The peripheral smear can also be diagnostic of certain infections (malaria, babesiosis). Other acquired causes are generally diagnosed by the clinical setting.

The diagnosis of paroxysmal nocturnal hemoglobinuria is made by flow cytometry using peripheral blood cells or bone marrow aspirate and the demonstration of deficiency of hematopoietic cell proteins normally linked to the anchoring glycosylphosphatidylinositol protein.

Differential Diagnosis

The differential diagnosis of the hemolytic anemias includes the reticulocytosis that can be seen with correction of anemia due to replacement of a deficiency (iron, folate, vitamin B_{12}) or recovery from bleeding.

Treatment

Immune Hemolytic Anemias
Autoimmune Hemolytic Anemias

The goal of AIHA treatment is to minimize or eliminate hemolysis. Some mild cases may not require medical intervention.

Warm-Antibody Hemolytic Anemia. For those patients with moderate to severe warm-antibody AIHA, corticosteroids are the treatment of choice. Approximately 80% of patients have a rapid response to corticosteroids, typically within 1 week after starting therapy. However, most responses are not sustained. The majority of adult patients receive high-dose oral prednisone 1 mg/kg/day during the initial phase of treatment. Intravenous methylprednisolone (Solu-Medrol) may also be used at daily doses of 100 to 200 mg.[2] In the pediatric population, prednisone is given at doses ranging from 2 to 6 mg/kg/day.[2] These high doses in adults and children are commonly maintained for approximately 2 weeks.

---

[2]Not available in the United States.

Once the hematocrit has increased, the dose should be decreased and subsequently tapered at a slow rate over several months. Patients who require more than 10 to 15 mg of prednisone daily to keep an adequate hematocrit or those who did not respond to the corticosteroids will need second-line treatment. Splenectomy is a second-line treatment for those who are surgical candidates. More than 50% of splenectomized patients have a partial or complete response. Patients who are candidates for splenectomy should receive immunizations against encapsulated organisms at least 2 weeks before the procedure. Rituximab (Rituxan),[1] a monoclonal antibody directed against CD20 antigen on the surface of B lymphocytes, is another choice for second-line treatment. Rituximab, given at a dose of 375 mg/m^2 weekly for 4 weeks, results in an overall response rate of 82% with many sustained responses. Recently described is the use of a lower dose of rituximab, 100 mg, weekly for 4 weeks. For cases refractory to steroids, splenectomy and rituximab may respond to other immunosuppressive therapies such as cyclophosphamide (Cytoxan), azathioprine (Imuran),[1] or cyclosporine (Neoral).[1]

Cold-Antibody AIHA. The best-described regimen has been cyclophosphamide 50 mg/kg/day for 4 days. Other treatment options that have been used with some success include danazol (Danocrine)[1] and plasmapheresis. High-dose intravenous immune globulin (Gammagard)[1] may be effective in some cases, but the response is short-lived (1–4 weeks).

In children, symptoms are usually mild and self-limited. A general approach is to avoid cold exposure. Supportive care to control the underlying disorder is recommended. RBC transfusions warmed to 37°C may be given for life-threatening situations, and the least incompatible unit should be used. For severe anemia, a trial of cytotoxic drugs such as cyclophosphamide[1] or chlorambucil (Leukeran)[1] may be used to decrease the cold agglutinin titer and the rate of hemolysis. Other alternatives that have been used with some success include rituximab[1] and interferon alfa-2b (Intron-A).[1] Plasmapheresis may be used to reduce or eliminate IgM antibodies. However, because its effect is not long-standing, it is used only in the acute setting. Eculizumab (Soliris),[1] an antibody to complement component 5 approved for use in paroxysmal nocturnal hemoglobinuria, has been reported to be successful in eliminating hemolysis in a patient with refractory cold agglutinin disease. Treatment with corticosteroids alone or in combination is generally not effective. In addition, splenectomy is not effective, because the liver is the predominant site of hemolysis.

Paroxysmal Cold Hemoglobinuria. For PCH, the mainstay of treatment is supportive care and avoidance of cold exposure. Warmed RBCs may be administered in cases of life-threatening hemolysis or symptomatic anemia. Most cases are self-limited; in the event PCH persists, measures used to treat AIHA can be employed.

Alloantibody Hemolysis

A suspected acute transfusion represents a true medical emergency. The transfusion must be stopped; intravenous access is maintained to provide fluids. All efforts to support the patient's blood pressure and urine output must be employed. For individuals with a delayed transfusion reaction, treatment is generally not necessary, although a transfusion may be needed to correct the anemia if symptoms due to the anemia develop.

Nonimmune Hemolytic Anemia

Congenital Hemolytic Anemias

For patients who have congenital hemolytic anemias and moderate to severe hemolysis, folate (folic acid)[1] replacement is recommended. Other treatments are more directed at the specific issues that can arise during the patient's lifetime. Because pigmented gallstone formation is common, cholecystectomy may be necessary. Splenectomy, to decrease the rate of hemolysis and improve the lifespan of circulating RBCs, may be recommended for patients who have moderate to severe ongoing hemolysis resulting in symptomatic anemia. Vaccinations for *Streptococcus pneumoniae*, *Haemophilus influenzae* type B, and *Neisseria meningitidis* should be administered before the splenectomy is performed. Patients with G6PD deficiency need to avoid oxidant drugs such as dapsone, primaquine, sulfamethoxazole (Gantanol), and other sulfa-based drugs. Parvovirus B19 infection in patients with congenital hemolytic anemias resulting in suppression of bone marrow erythropoiesis can manifest as aplastic crisis characterized by an abrupt fall in the hemoglobin. RBC transfusions may be necessary until bone marrow production recovers and erythropoiesis resumes.

Acquired Hemolytic Anemias

For patients with acquired causes of nonimmune hemolytic anemias, therapy is generally supportive, with RBC transfusions as clinically indicated, in addition to therapy directed at the underlying cause of the anemia. For example, infections should be treated appropriately; the underlying cause of DIC or HUS needs to be managed. For TTP and HUS, the initial management consists of emergent plasmapheresis. Exposure to any offending toxins needs to be eliminated; potentially, directed therapy to reduce toxin levels will be required. Specific therapy for paroxysmal nocturnal hemoglobinuria is now available; eculizumab, a humanized monoclonal antibody that inhibits the complement cascade, is used to reduce hemolysis and the need for RBC transfusions.

Monitoring

Patients with hemolytic anemia require frequent monitoring with periodic hemoglobin checks. Patients presenting with worsening anemia should have a reticulocyte count check; a decreased reticulocyte count should prompt an evaluation for reversible causes of anemia (e.g., folate, vitamin B$_{12}$, or iron deficiency) as well as monitoring for further decline in the hemoglobin. Patients with longstanding hemolysis should have periodic monitoring for cholelithiasis with abdominal ultrasounds.

HEMOPHILIA AND RELATED CONDITIONS

Method of
Meera Chitlur, MD; and Roshni Kulkarni, MD

CURRENT DIAGNOSIS

- The hemophilias and von Willebrand's disease (vWD) account for 80% to 85% of inherited bleeding disorders. Hemophilia A and B are X-linked, whereas vWD and rare bleeding disorders (RBDs) are autosomal disorders.
- The diagnosis of hemophilia and other inherited bleeding disorders should be confirmed by specific laboratory assays, because screening tests such as prothrombin time (PT) and activated partial thromboplastin time (aPTT) may be normal. Plasma levels of deficient factor determine clinical severity and management.
- Major complications associated with hemophilia are inhibitor development, hemarthrosis, and intracranial hemorrhage. Hemarthrosis is the most common and debilitating complication, and central nervous system bleeding is the most common cause of mortality in hemophilia. Mucosal bleeding and menorrhagia are the most common manifestations of vWD. Bleeding manifestations of RBDs are mild, although homozygotes can present with severe disease.
- Newborns have normal levels of factor VIII; therefore, the diagnosis of hemophilia A can be established at birth. Vacuum delivery should be avoided to prevent head bleeds.
- Women and adolescents with menorrhagia and no underlying pathology should be investigated for a bleeding disorder.

---

[1]Not FDA approved for this indication.

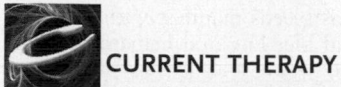

CURRENT THERAPY

- Early and effective treatment and prophylaxis can prevent repeated hemarthrosis and joint destruction in persons with hemophilia. Patients should be tested annually for the presence of inhibitors.
- Wherever available and indicated, recombinant factor concentrates are preferred over plasma-derived products due to potential risk of pathogen transmission. Cryoprecipitate is not recommended. For mild and moderate hemophilia A and von Willebrand's disease, the use of desmopressin coupled with antifibrinolytics can obviate the use of concentrates. Continued vigilance should be implemented for new and emerging blood-borne pathogens.
- All patients with inherited bleeding disorders should be immunized against hepatitis A and B and followed in close collaboration with the local hemophilia treatment center (http://www2a. cdc.gov/ncbddd/htcweb/index.asp). The National Hemophilia Foundation's (www.hemophilia.org) Medical and Scientific Advisory Committee (MASAC) guidelines for updated recommendations and product choice should be followed.

Hemophilia A and Hemophilia B

Hemophilia is an X-linked congenital bleeding disorder caused by a deficiency of factor VIII (hemophilia A) or factor IX (hemophilia B). Hemophilia A is the most common severe bleeding disorder and affects 1 in 5000 males in the United States; hemophilia B occurs in 1 in 30,000 males.

Pathophysiology

The factor VIII gene is one of the largest genes and spans 186 kb of genomic DNA at Xq28. Inversion mutations account for 40% of severe hemophilia A, and deletions, point mutations, and insertions account for the remainder.

Hepatic and reticuloendothelial cells are presumed sites of factor VIII synthesis. Factor VIII is synthesized as a single chain polypeptide with three A domains (A1, A2, and A3), a large central B domain, and two C domains (Figure 1). The binding sites for von Willebrand's factor (vWF), thrombin, and factor Xa are on the C2 domain, and factor IXa binding sites are on the A2 and A3 domains. The B domain can be deleted without any consequences. vWF protects factor VIII from proteolytic degradation in the plasma and concentrates it at the site of injury.

The factor IX gene is 34kb long and located at Xq26. It is a vitamin K–dependent serine protease composed of 415 amino acids. It is synthesized in the liver and its plasma concentration is about 50 times that of factor VIII. Gene deletions and point mutations result in hemophilia B.

Role of Factors VIII and IX in Coagulation

Factor VIII circulates bound to vWF. It is a cofactor for factor IX and is essential for factor X activation. In the classic coagulation cascade, activation of the intrinsic or extrinsic pathway of coagulation results in sufficient thrombin generation. However, this does not explain bleeding in hemophilia, because the extrinsic pathway is intact. This led to the revised cell-based model of coagulation.

The revised pathway incorporates all coagulation factors into a single pathway initiated by FVII and tissue factor. The contact factors (XI, XII, kallikrein, and high-molecular-weight kininogen) are not essential but serve as a backup. Following injury, encrypted tissue factor is exposed and forms a complex with factor VIIa. The tissue factor–factor VIIa complex activates factor IX to IXa (which moves to the platelet surface) and factor X to Xa. This generates small amounts of thrombin that activates platelets, converts platelet factor V to Va and factor XI to XIa, and releases factor VIII from vWF and activates it. The factor XIa activates plasma factor IX to IXa on the platelet surface, which together with factor VIIIa forms the tenase complex (factor VIIIa/IXa) that converts large amounts of factor X to Xa. Factor Xa forms a prothrombinase complex with FVa and converts large amounts of prothrombin to thrombin, called *thrombin burst*. This results in the conversion of sufficient fibrinogen to fibrin to form a stable clot. (Animations are available at the Foundation of Women and Girls with Blood Disorders (www.fwgbd.org and www.reddymed.com).

In hemophilia, lack of factor VIII or IX produces a profound abnormality. Factor Xa generated by FVIIa and tissue factor is insufficient because it is soon inhibited by tissue factor pathway inhibitor (negative feedback), and factors VIII and IX, which are required for amplifying the production of Xa, are absent. The primary platelet plug formation and initiation phases of coagulation are normal. Any clot that is formed (from the initiation phase) is friable and porous.

Clinical Features

The diagnosis of hemophilia is often made following a bleeding episode or because of a family history; 30% of cases, however, have no family history. Based on the plasma levels of factor VIII or IX (normal levels are 50%–150%) that correlate with severity and predict bleeding risk, hemophilia is classified as mild (>5%), moderate (1%–5%) and severe (<1%) (Table 1). Approximately 65% of persons with hemophilia have severe disease, 15% have moderate disease, and 20% have mild disease. Most severe disease

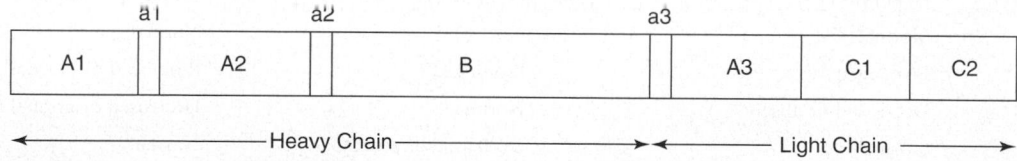

Figure 1. Factor VIII protein structure.

TABLE 1	Hemophilia Severity and Clinical Manifestations		
CHARACTERISTICS	**SEVERE (50%–70%)**	**MODERATE (10%)**	**MILD (30%–40%)**
Factor VIII or IX activity (normal 50%–150%)	<1%	1%–5%	>5%
Age of diagnosis	At birth to 2 y	Childhood or adolescence	Adolescence or adult
Bleeding patterns	2–4/mo	4–6/y	Rare
Clinical manifestations	Hemarthroses, muscle, central nervous system, gastrointestinal bleeding, hematuria	Bleeding into joints or muscle following minor trauma, surgical procedure, dental bleeding Rarely spontaneous	Surgical procedures (including dental) and major trauma

manifests by 4 years of age; moderate or mild disease is diagnosed later and often following bleeding secondary to trauma or surgery.

Hemophilia can be diagnosed in the first trimester, using chorionic villus sampling and gene analysis. In the second trimester, fetal blood sampling can be performed. Prenatal diagnosis to determine fetal gender can aid in the management of pregnancy and delivery.

The hallmark of severe hemophilia is hemarthrosis, or bleeding into the joint, that can occur spontaneously or with minimal trauma. Although the immediate effects of a joint bleed are excruciating pain, swelling, warmth, and muscle spasm, the long-term effects of recurrent hemarthrosis include hemophilic arthropathy, which is characterized by synovial thickening, chronic inflammation, and repeated hemorrhages resulting in a target joint. Knees, elbows, ankles, hips, and shoulders are commonly affected. Disuse atrophy of surrounding muscles leads to further joint instability. Limitation of joint range of motion due to hemarthrosis often correlates positively with older age, nonwhite race, and increased body mass index, and it affects quality of life.

Muscle hematomas, another characteristic site of bleeding, can lead to compartment syndrome, with eventual fibrosis and peripheral nerve damage. Iliopsoas bleeds manifest with pain and flexion deformity. Gastrointestinal bleeding and hematuria occur less often.

Central nervous system (CNS) hemorrhage is a rare but serious complication with a 10% recurrence rate and is the leading cause of mortality in hemophiliacs. Although most newborns with severe hemophilia experience an uneventful course following vaginal delivery, vacuum extraction is associated with an increased CNS bleeding risk. The incidence of intracranial hemorrhage in newborns with hemophilia is 1% to 4%.

Diagnosis

Hemophilia A and B are clinically indistinguishable, and specific factor assays are the only way to differentiate and confirm the diagnosis. Both should be differentiated from von Willebrand's disease (vWD). The prothrombin time (PT), platelet function analyzer (PFA-100), and fibrinogen are normal. (PFA, a platelet-function screening test, is replacing bleeding time, because the bleeding time has low sensitivity and specificity and is operator dependent.) The activated partial thromboplastin time (aPTT) is prolonged when the factor levels are below 30%. Table 2 shows the characteristics and

TABLE 2	Hemophilias and von Willebrand's Disease: Key Characteristics and Differences		
CHARACTERISTIC	**HEMOPHILIA A**	**HEMOPHILIA B**	**VON WILLEBRAND'S DISEASE**
Incidence	1:5000	1:30,000	1%–3% of U.S. population
Abnormality	Factor VIII deficiency	Factor IX deficiency	vWF (qualitative and quantitative defect)
Inheritance	X-linked, affects males Gene at the tip of X-chromosome	X-linked, affects males Gene at the tip of X-chromosome	Autosomal dominant (gene: chromosome 12) Some are recessive or compound heterozygotes
Production site	Unknown, liver endothelium	Liver (vitamin K dependent)	Megakaryocytes and endothelial cells
Function	Cofactor; forms tenase complex with factor IX and activates factor X, leading to thrombin burst that results in conversion of large amounts of fibrinogen to fibrin	Serine protease (inactive form: zymogen) activated by factor XI or VIIa; forms a tenase complex with factor VIII and activates factor X	Platelet adhesion to site of injury or damaged endothelium Protects factor VIII from proteolysis
Classification (normal levels 50%–150%)	Mild (>5%) Moderate (1–5%) Severe (<1%)	Mild (>5%) Moderate (1–5%) Severe (<1%)	Type 1 Type 2 (2A, 2B, 2M, 2N) Type 3
Clinical presentation	Positive family history (30% new mutation) Hemarthroses, hematomas, hematuria, intracranial hemorrhage, gastrointestinal hemorrhage, etc.	Positive family history (30% new mutation) Milder disease, although identical hemorrhage sites as hemophilia A	Positive family history Mucocutaneous bleeding (epistaxis, menorrhagia, postdental bleeding) Type 3 can manifest as hemophilia A
PFA, bleeding time	Normal	Normal	May be prolonged
PT	Normal	Normal	Normal
aPTT	Prolonged	Prolonged	Prolonged or normal
Factor VIII assay	Decreased or absent	Normal	Decreased or normal (absent type 3)
Factor IX assay	Normal	Decreased or absent	Normal
VWF:Ag	Normal	Normal	Decreased or absent (type 3)
VWF:RCo	Normal	Normal	Decreased or abnormal
VWF multimeres	Normal	Normal	Abnormal in types 1, 2A, 2B; absent in type 3
Specific treatment	Recombinant factor VIII (preferred) Pathogen-safe plasma-derived concentrates DDAVP for mild cases	Recombinant factor IX Pathogen-safe plasma-derived concentrates DDAVP ineffective	DDAVP (intranasal or intravenous) vWF concentrates (pathogen-safe plasma derived)
Inhibitor patients	Immune tolerance, recombinant factor VIIa, APCC	Immune tolerance, recombinant factor VIIa	Inhibitors are rare
Adjunct therapy	Antifibrinolytics	Antifibrinolytics	Oral contraceptives, antifibrinolytics

Abbreviations: APCC = activated prothrombin complex concentrates; aPTT = activated partial thromboplastin time; DDAVP = desmopressin; PFA = platelet function analyzer; PT = prothrombin time; RCo = ristocetin cofactor; VWF = von Willebrand factor; VWF:Ag = von Willebrand factor antigen.

differences between the hemophilias and vWD. Female carriers may be asymptomatic except for those with extreme lyonization resulting in low factor VIII or IX levels. However some carriers may experience bleeding episodes even with levels of FVIII or IX in the 40% range. Factor VIII levels increase throughout pregnancy and drop to prepregnancy levels following delivery, but factor IX levels remain constant throughout pregnancy.

Treatment

The treatment for hemophilia consists of replacement therapy with intravenous factor VIII or factor IX concentrates produced by purification of donor plasma (plasma derived) or in cell culture bioreactors (recombinant). Careful screening of donors combined with heat treatment and viral inactivation methods have made plasma-derived products safer. Plasma-derived and recombinant products appear to have equivalent clinical efficacy. Recombinant factor concentrates are recommended, but if they are not available, plasma-derived concentrates can be used. Cryoprecipitate is no longer recommended because of concerns regarding pathogen safety.

Treatment administered only during bleeding symptoms is known as *episodic therapy*, and periodic administration of factor concentrates to prevent bleeding is known as *prophylactic therapy*. Response to treatment is more effective when it is administered early. Although prophylaxis prevents the development of joint disease, the high cost of factor replacement coupled with the need for venous access makes it expensive and difficult and out of reach for patients in the developing world.

The goal of treatment is to raise factor levels to approximately 30% or more for minor bleeds (hematomas or joint bleeds) and 100% for major bleeds (CNS or surgery). Giving 1 U/kg of factor concentrate raises plasma factor VIII levels by 2% and factor IX levels by 1.5% (except with the recombinant factor IX product, where it increases by 0.8%). The half-life of factor VIII is approximately 8 to 12 hours and that of factor IX is up to 24 hours. Factor concentrates can also be given by continuous infusion (3–4 U/kg/hour). The bolus dose varies from 25 to 50 U/kg depending on the severity, site, and type of bleeding and is dosed to the available vial size because of the cost of the products. Table 3 lists the dosing schedule for various types of bleeds.

For short term therapy (before dental procedures and minor bleeding episodes) in mild hemophilia A and vWD, the synthetic vasopressin analogue desmopressin acetate (DDAVP [Stimate]) is useful. It increases plasma concentrations of coagulation factor VIII and vWF three- to fivefold by releasing the endothelial stores. A DDAVP trial to determine response is helpful in selecting patients who might benefit from such therapy. For hemostatic purposes, intravenous (0.3 µg/kg in 50 mL of normal saline infused over 15–30 min) or intranasal dose (150 µg) can be used. The intranasal dose is 15 times larger than that recommended for diabetes insipidus. A multidose intranasal spray formulation (Stimate nasal spray) delivers 150 µg per spray. The recommended dosage is one spray for patients who weigh less than 50 kg and two sprays (one in each nostril) for those who weigh more than 50 kg. Desmopressin is ineffective in hemophilia B. Aspirin and aspirin-containing compounds should be avoided in persons with bleeding disorders because they interfere with platelet function and can exacerbate bleeding.

Antifibrinolytics such as ε-aminocaproic acid (Amicar) and tranexamic acid (Cyklokapron or Lysteda) are used as adjunct therapies and in mild hemophilia and can decrease the need for factor concentrates. The recommended dosage for ε-aminocaproic acid is 75 to 100 mg/kg/dose IV or orally every 4 to 6 hours (maximum 30 g/24 hours). The recommended dosage for tranexamic acid is 10 mg/kg/dose IV or 25 mg/kg body weight orally, three times daily.

For prophylaxis, factor VIII 25 to 40 U/kg administered every other day or factor IX 25 to 40 U/kg twice weekly (because of the longer half-life of factor IX) is aimed at preventing joint disease. Prophylaxis may begin at 1 to 2 years of age and is continued lifelong. Self-infusion before any planned strenuous activity is recommended. Because of the complications of central venous catheters (infections, thrombosis, and mechanical), use of a peripheral vein is encouraged. Over the last 2 years various modified factor products with prolonged half lives have been developed with an aim to decrease the frequency of infusions and improve quality of life for patients with hemophilia. These include PEGylation, fusion proteins with fusion of the factor protein to the Fc fragment of an immunoglobulin or albumin. In March 2014, the US FDA approved the first long acting Factor IX Fc fusion protein (Alprolix) for use in patients with hemophilia B after safety and efficacy was established in initial clinical trials in adult patients with Hemophilia B. More recently in June 2014, rFVIII Fc fusion (Eloctate) was approved by the FDA for the treatment and prophylaxis of bleeding episodes in hemophilia A. Clinical trials are still ongoing with other prolonged half life factor concentrates.

TABLE 3 Treatment of Bleeding Episodes and Desired Plasma Levels in Hemophilias A and B

TYPE OF BLEEDING	DESIRED FACTOR LEVEL (%)	FACTOR VIII DOSE (U/kg)	FACTOR IX DOSE (U/kg)	DURATION OF TREATMENT (DAYS)	COMMENTS (DOSE FACTOR TO THE CLOSEST VIAL)
Persistent or profuse epistaxis Oral mucosal bleeding (including tongue and mouth lacerations)	20–30	10–15	20–30	1–2	Local pressure, antifibrinolytics, fibrin glue for local control, nosebleed QR for epistaxis Sedation in small children with tongue laceration
Dental procedures	30–50	15–25	30–50	1 h before procedure	Antifibrinolytics for 7–10 d
Acute hemarthrosis, intramuscular hematomas	30–60	15–50	30–60	1–3	Use lower doses if treated early. Non–weight bearing on affected joint.
Physical therapy	30–50	15–25	30–50	Treat before PT	Consider synovectomy (surgical, radioisotope or chemical) for target joints.
Life-threatening bleeding such as intracranial hemorrhage, major surgery, and trauma	80–100	40–50	80–100	10–14 d	Bolus dose followed by continuous infusion (3–4 U/kg/h); may switch to bolus before discharge
Gastrointestinal bleeding	30–50	15–25	30–50	2–3	May use oral antifibrinolytics
Persistent painless gross hematuria	30–50	15–25	30–50	1–2	Increase PO or IV fluids with low-dose antifibrinolytics; Risk of clotting in the urinary tract with factor replacement

Abbreviation: PT = physical therapy.

Complications of Treatment

One of the most serious complications of hemophilia treatment is the development of inhibitors or neutralizing antibodies (immunoglobulin [Ig]G) that inhibit the function of substituted factor VIII and factor IX. Approximately 5% to 10% of all hemophiliacs and up to 30% of patients with severe hemophilia A develop inhibitors. The incidence of inhibitors in hemophilia B is lower (1%–3%). Most factor VIII inhibitors arise after a median exposure of 9 to 12 days in patients with severe hemophilia A. They can be transient or permanent and should be suspected if a patient fails to respond to an appropriate dose of clotting factor concentrate. Inhibitors can exacerbate bleeding episodes and hemophilic arthropathy.

Inhibitor levels, measured using Bethesda units (BU), are classified as high titer (>5 BU) or low titer (<5 BU). In patients with low titer inhibitors, higher than normal doses of factor VIII or IX may be used to treat bleeding. For those with high-titer inhibitors, agents that bypass factor VIII or factor IX are used. These include recombinant activated factor VII and, in the case of hemophilia A, activated prothrombin complex concentrates (APCC) or recombinant porcine factor VIII (currently in prelicensure clinical trials). Immune tolerance induction, a long-term approach designed to eradicate inhibitors, is effective in 70% to 85% of patients with severe hemophilia A; the most important predictor of success of immune tolerance induction is an inhibitor titer of less than 10 BU at the start of immune tolerance induction.

Although inhibitors are rare in hemophilia B, they can result in anaphylaxis with exposure to factor IX–containing products. Immune tolerance regimens are associated with nephrotic syndrome and are successful in eradicating the inhibitor only in 40% of cases.

Another important complication of treatment is the transmission of bloodborne pathogens such as hepatitis B and C viruses and HIV. In the 1970s, lyophilized plasma factor concentrates of low purity resulted in the transmission of HIV, causing the deaths of many hemophiliacs. Currently, donor screening for pathogens coupled with viral attenuation by heat or solvent detergent technology make these products pathogen safe. However, nonenveloped virus (parvovirus and hepatitis A) and prions can resist inactivation and can be potentially transmitted.

Patients with bleeding disorders should be encouraged to attend the comprehensive hemophilia treatment centers, where they are educated, trained to self-infuse and calculate dosage, maintain treatment logs, and call for serious bleeding episodes. The mortality rate among patients who receive care at hemophilia treatment centers (HTCs) is lower than among those who do not: 28.1% versus 38.3%, respectively. At the HTCs, Hemovigilance for blood borne and emerging pathogens was maintained through participation in the Centers for Disease Control and Prevention's (CDC) Universal Data Collection (UDC) project. The grant cycle of the UDC was completed in 2012, and a new surveillance instrument is currently in use that incorporates collecting information on co-morbidities and complications of bleeding disorders in this population.

Routine vaccination against hepatitis A and B is recommended. Gene therapy offers promise of a cure but has not yet become reality. Two gene-therapy trials for hemophilia B had shown subtherapeutic or transient expression of factor IX. In December 2011, Nathwani and colleagues reported that a single injection of FIX expressing adenovirus-associated virus (AAV) vector was effective in treating patients with Hemophilia B for more than a year. This has been a significant breakthrough in the treatment of hemophilia.

von Willebrand's Disease

von Willebrand's disease (vWD) is an inherited (autosomal dominant) bleeding disorder caused by deficiency or dysfunction of von Willebrand factor (vWF), a plasma protein that mediates platelet adhesion at the site of vascular injury and prevents degradation of factor VIII. A defect in vWF results in bleeding by impairing platelet adhesion or by decreasing factor VIII.

vWF is synthesized in endothelial cells and undergoes dimerization and multimerization, forming low-, intermediate-, and high-molecular-weight (HMW) multimers. The HMW multimers are most effective in promoting platelet aggregation and adhesion. Circulating HMW multimers are cleaved by the protease ADAMTS13, which is deficient in patients with thrombotic thrombocytopenic purpura.

vWD is the most common bleeding disorder, affecting 1% or more of the population. It occurs worldwide and affects all races. vWD is classified into three major categories: partial quantitative deficiency (type 1), qualitative deficiency (type 2), and total deficiency (type 3). There are several different variants of type 2 vWD: 2A, 2B, 2N, and 2M based on the phenotype. About 75% of patients have type 1 vWD.

Clinical Presentation

Mucous membrane–type bleeding (e.g., menorrhagia, epistaxis) and excessive bruising are characteristic clinical features in vWD. Bleeding manifestations vary considerably, and in some cases, the diagnosis is not suspected until excessive bleeding occurs with a surgical procedure or trauma. Although excessive menstrual bleeding may be the initial manifestation, it takes 16 years for a diagnosis of bleeding disorder. It is for this reason that the American College of Obstetrics and Gynecology recommended screening for hemostatic disorders in all adolescents and women presenting with menorrhagia and no pathology and before hysterectomy for menorrhagia. In infants or small children with type 3 (severe) vWD, excessive bruising and even joint bleeding (due to very low levels of factor VIII) can mimic hemophilia A.

Diagnosis

Laboratory evaluation for vWD requires several assays to quantitate vWF and characterize its structure and function. Many variables affect vWF assay results, including the patient's ABO blood type. Persons of blood group AB have 60% to 70% higher vWF levels than those of blood group O. Thus, some laboratories interpret vWF levels referenced to specific normal ranges for blood types.

Clinical conditions and disorders with elevated vWF levels include pregnancy (third trimester), collagen vascular disorders, following surgery, in liver disease, and in disseminated intravascular coagulation. Low levels are seen in hypothyroidism and days 1 to 4 of the menstrual cycle.

Symptoms are modified by medications like aspirin or nonsteroidal antiinflammatory drugs (NSAIDs), which can exacerbate the bleeding; oral contraceptives can decrease the bleeding in women with vWD by increasing vWF levels. vWF levels in African American women are 15% higher than in white women. Clinical symptoms and family history are important for establishing the diagnosis of vWD, and a single test is sometimes not sufficient to rule out the diagnosis.

Initial work-up should include a complete blood count, aPTT, PT, fibrinogen level, or thrombin time. These tests do not rule out vWD but help to rule out thrombocytopenia or factor deficiency as the cause for bleeding. The closure times on the PFA-100, which has replaced the bleeding time as a screening test in some centers, may be prolonged. The aPTT in vWD is only abnormal when factor VIII is sufficiently reduced.

Specific tests for vWD include ristocetin cofactor assay, a factor VIII activity, and vWF antigen (vWF Ag) assay. The Ristocetin cofactor activity measures induced binding of vWF to platelet glycoprotein Ib and is the best functional assay of vWF activity. Multimer analysis is done by agarose gel electrophoresis using anti-vWF polyclonal antibody and is available at reference laboratories.

In type I vWD, the vWF is subnormal in amount, with normal multimer structure. Those with types 2A and 2B vWD lack the HMW multimers. In type 2B, the vWF has a heightened affinity for platelets, often resulting in some degree of thrombocytopenia from platelet aggregation. A useful laboratory test for type 2B is the low-dose ristocetin-induced platelet aggregation (RIPA) assay.

In type 3 (severe) vWD, the affected person has inherited a gene for type I vWD from each parent, resulting in very low levels (3%) of vWF (and low factor VIII, because there is no vWF to protect factor VIII from proteolytic degradation). Less commonly, a person with type 3 is doubly heterozygous. Table 4 provides a quick overview of the laboratory findings in the different variants of vWD.

Treatment

In type 1 vWD (with subnormal levels of normally functioning vWF), the treatment of choice is DDAVP, which causes a rapid release of vWF from storage sites. It can be given intravenously or by the intranasal route. The recommended dose for IV use is 0.3 µg/kg, given in saline over 10 minutes. Most persons with type 1 vWD have a two- to four-fold increase in plasma levels of vWF within 15 to 30 minutes following infusion. The IV route is often used for surgical coverage or for a severe bleeding episode requiring hospitalization. When necessary, repeat doses may be given at 12- to 24-hour intervals. Tachyphylaxis is less commonly seen in vWD patients than in hemophilia patients. It is important to monitor free water intake following DDAVP administration because it can cause hyponatremia and seizures.

The concentrated form of desmopressin for intranasal use (Stimate nasal spray) may be used. The recommended dosage is one 150-µg spray for patients who weigh less than 50 kg and two sprays (one in each nostril) for those who weigh more than 50 kg. Some young women with menorrhagia have benefited from its use at the onset of menses, with a second dose after 24 hours. Others have used it approximately 45 minutes before invasive dentistry, with good results.

In the type 2 variants (vWF produced is abnormal), desmopressin can cause an increase in abnormal vWF. Although some persons with type 2A might respond, desmopressin is seldom useful in type 2 and might even be contraindicated (as in type 2B, where it can exacerbate the thrombocytopenia).

In type 3 vWD, desmopressin is ineffective because there is no vWF to be released from storage sites. For type 3 patients and in persons with type 1 vWD who do not respond adequately to desmopressin, an intermediate-purity plasma-derived concentrate rich in the hemostatically effective HMW multimers of vWF (such as Humate P) should be used to treat moderately severe or severe bleeding episodes and for before surgery.

As in hemophilia, antifibrinolytics are an effective adjunctive treatment for invasive dental procedures or other bleeding in the oropharyngeal cavity. These may be effective even when used alone in some vWD women with menorrhagia. For epistaxis, Nosebleed QR, a hydrophilic powder, can help.

Special Situations

Pregnancy

vWF (and factor VIII) levels increase during the third trimester of pregnancy, and women with type 1 vWD have a decrease in bruising or other bleeding symptoms. However, those with type 2 vWD (abnormal vWF) and type 3 (no vWF) have no change in the bleeding tendency. Even in type 1 vWD, vWF levels fall following delivery, so treatment (with IV desmopressin or Humate P) may be needed.

Acquired von Willebrand's Disease

Acquired vWD occurs in persons who do not have a lifelong bleeding disorder. Conditions associated with acquired vWD include underlying autoimmune disease (lymphoproliferative disorders, myeloproliferative disorders, or plasma cell dyscrasias), valvular and congenital heart disease, Wilms' tumor, chronic renal failure, and hypothyroidism. The mechanism of acquired vWD is unknown. Medications such as valproic acid can also cause vWD. Removal of the underlying condition often corrects the vWF. Desmopressin, Humate P, recombinant factor VIIa, or plasma exchange may be tried, if necessary, to treat bleeding.

Rare Bleeding Disorders

The rare bleeding disorders account for 3% to 5% of inherited coagulation deficiencies, other than factor VIII, factor IX, or vWF deficiencies. They are autosomal recessive and affect both sexes. The prevalence of rare bleeding disorders ranges from 1:500,000 to 1:2,000,000. Bleeding manifestations are restricted to persons who are homozygotes or compound heterozygotes. Rare bleeding disorders are common in countries such as Iran, where consanguineous marriages are customary. Ashkenazi Jews are particularly affected by factor XI deficiency. Deficiency of factor XII is a risk factor for thrombosis, but not for bleeding. Most cases of rare bleeding disorders are identified by abnormal screening tests coupled with specific factor assays.

Factor concentrates (recombinant or plasma derived) are available for some of the deficiencies (mostly in Europe, but not in the United States). Fibrogammin P, a plasma-derived virally purified FXIII concentrate, is now licensed and commercially available in the United States under the trade name of Corifact. In addition, a Phase III clinical trial for Recombinant FXIII is now ongoing to evaluate its safety and efficacy in the treatment of congential FXIII subunit A deficiency. The advantages of concentrates are pathogen safety and small volume. The use of antifibrinolytics and fibrin glue as adjunct therapy for bleeding manifestations is encouraged. Table 5 lists the inheritance, frequency, manifestations, and treatments of the rare bleeding disorders.

| TABLE 4 | Clinical Variants of von Willebrand's Disease |

TYPE	FACTOR VIII	vWF AG	RISTOCETIN COFACTOR	RIPA	MULTIMER
1	↓	↓	↓	↓ or normal	Normal
2A	↓ or normal	↓↓	↓	↓↓	Large and intermediate multimers absent
2B	↓ or normal	↓↓	↓ or normal	↓ to low dose	Large multimers absent
2M	Variably ↓	Variably ↓	↓	Variably ↓	Normal
2N	↓↓	Normal	Normal	Normal	Normal
3	↓↓↓↓	↓↓↓↓	↓↓↓↓	None	Absent
Platelet type	↓ or normal	↓ or normal	↓	↓ to low dose	Large multimers absent

Abbreviations: Ag = antigen; RIPA = ristocetin-induced platelet aggregation; vWF = von Willebrand factor.

TABLE 5		Rare Bleeding Disorders: Inheritance, Clinical Features, and Treatment					
FACTOR	**PREVALENCE**	**TYPE**	**INHERITANCE**	**MANIFESTATION AND DIAGNOSIS**	**TREATMENT**	**HEMOSTATIC LEVELS**	**HALF-LIFE**
Factor I	1:1,000,000	Afibrinogenemia Dysfibrinogenemia Hypofibrinogenemia	AR AD AD	Mild bleeding CNS, umbilical, joint bleeding Recurrent miscarriage PT, aPTT, TT prolonged Low FI levels Paradoxical thrombosis	FFP 15–20 mL/kg Cryoprecipitate 1 bag/5–10 kg Fibrinogen concentrate (RiaSTAP) Treatment q3–5d	50 mg–1 g/dL	2–5 d
Factor II	1:2,000,000	Type I: hypoprothrombinemia Type II: dysprothrombinemia	AR AR	Hematomas, hemarthroses, menorrhagia CNS, umbilical, postpartum hemorrhage PT abnormal	FFP, PCC 20–30 U/kg for prophylaxis or treatment	20%–30%	3–4 d
Factor V	1:1,000,000	Parahemophilia, labile factor, proaccelerin, Owren's disease	AR	Mucosal bleeding, postpartum hemorrhage, CNS bleeding Platelet factor V deficiency more reflective of bleeding potential Prolonged PT, aPTT Normal TT	FFP Platelet transfusions Antiplatelet antibodies can develop with repeated platelet transfusions	15%–20%	36 h
Factor VII	1:500,000	Proconvertin or stable factor	AR	Menorrhagia; mucosal, muscle, intracranial bleeds (15%–60%); hemarthrosis Prolonged PT Normal aPTT, TT, FI, liver functions	Recombinant factor VIIa, 15–30 µg/kg q2h for major bleeds FFP, PCC 20–30 U/kg for prophylaxis or treatment Plasma-derived factor VII concentrates[2]*	15%–20%	4–6 h
Factor X	1:1,000,000		AR	Menorrhagia; umbilical, joint, mucosal, muscle, intracranial bleeding Prolonged PT, aPTT	FFP, PCCs 20–30 U/kg	15%–20%	24–48 h
Factor XI (common in Ashkenazi Jews)	1:1,000,000		AR	Post-traumatic bleeding, menorrhagia Prolonged aPTT Normal PT	Hemoleven,* FFP 15–20 mL/kg Inhibitors can occur	15%–20%	
Factor XIII	1:2,000,000		AR	Intracranial, joint, umbilical bleeding Delayed wound healing Recurrent miscarriages PT, aPTT normal ↓FXIII assay	Factor XIII concentrate (Cortifact) 40 IU/kg q28d to maintain trough level of 5%–20% FFP 15–20 mL/kg Tretten, a recombinant FXIII-A subunit concentrate 35 units/kg /month for prophylaxis. Use in patients with FXIII A subunit deficiency Cryoprecipitate 1 bag/5–10 kg q3–4wk	2%–5%	11–14 d

FACTOR	PREVALENCE	TYPE	INHERITANCE	MANIFESTATION AND DIAGNOSIS	TREATMENT	HEMOSTATIC LEVELS	HALF-LIFE
Combined factor V and VIII	1:2,000,000			Mucosal bleeding Prolonged PT, aPTT (dispropor-tionately)	Factor VIII concentrates and FFP	15%–20%	
Vitamin K–dependent multiple deficiencies	1:2,000,000			Umbilical stump, intracranial, postsurgical bleeding Skeletal abnormalities Hearing loss	Oral vitamin K, FFP, PCC	15%–20%	

TABLE 5 Rare Bleeding Disorders: Inheritance, Clinical Features, and Treatment—cont'd

Abbreviations: AD = autosomal dominant; aPTT = activated partial thromboplastin time; AR = autosomal recessive; CNS = central nervous system; FFP = fresh frozen plasma; FI = fibrinogen; PCC = prothrombin complex concentrate; PT = prothrombin time; TT = thrombin time.
[2]Not available in the United States.
*Available in Europe.

References

Arnold WD, Hilgartner MW. Hemophilic arthropathy. Current concepts of pathogenesis and management. J Bone Joint Surg Am 1977;59(3):287–305.

Bolton-Maggs PH, Pasi KJ. Haemophilias A and B. Lancet 2003;361(9371):1801–9.

Gill JC, Wilson AD, Endres-Brooks J, Montgomery RR. Loss of the largest von Willebrand factor multimers from the plasma of patients with congenital cardiac defects. Blood 1986;67(3):758–61.

Hoffman M, Monroe 3rd. DM. A cell-based model of hemostasis. Thromb Haemost 2001;85(6):958–65.

Miller CH, Dilley AB, Drews C, et al. Changes in von Willebrand factor and factor VIII levels during the menstrual cycle. Thromb Haemost 2002;87(6):1082–3.

Miller CH, Dilley A, Richardson L, et al. Population differences in von Willebrand factor levels affect the diagnosis of von Willebrand disease in African-American women. Am J Hematol 2001;67(2):125–9.

Mulder K, Llinas A. The target joint. Haemophilia 2004;10(Suppl. 4):152–6.

National Hemophilia Foundation Medical and Scientific Advisory Council (MASAC). MASAC recommendations concerning the treatment of hemophilia and other bleeding disorders, Available at http://www.hemophilia.org/Researchers-Healthcare-Providers/Medical-and-Scientific-Advisory-Council-MASAC/MASAC-Recommendations (accessed August 5, 2015).

Pabinger-Fasching I, Pipe S. Innovations in coagulation: improved options for treatment of hemophilia A and B. Thromb Res 2013;131(2):S1.

Pierce GF, Lillicrap D, Pipe SW, Vandendriessche T. Gene therapy, bioengineered clotting factors and novel technologies for hemophilia treatment. J Thromb Haemost 2007;5(5):901–6.

Shapiro A. Development of long-acting recombinant FVIII and FIX Fc fusion proteins for the management of hemophilia. Expert Opin Biol Ther 2013;13(9):1287–97.

Soucie JM, Nuss R, Evatt B, et al. Mortality among males with hemophilia; Relations with source of medical care. The Hemophilia Surveillance System Project Investigators. Blood 2000;96(2):437–42.

Veldman A, Hoffman M, Ehrenforth S. New insights into the coagulation system and implications for new therapeutic options with recombinant factor VIIa. Curr Med Chem 2003;10(10):797–811.

Warrier I, Ewenstein BM, Koerper MA, et al. Factor IX inhibitors and anaphylaxis in hemophilia B. J Pediatr Hematol Oncol 1997;19(1):23–7.

HODGKIN LYMPHOMA

Method of
Jeremy S. Abramson, MD

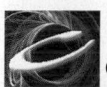

CURRENT DIAGNOSIS

- Hodgkin lymphoma typically presents as painless lymphadenopathy in young people.
- Systemic symptoms are often absent, but may include "B" symptoms (fevers, drenching night sweats, or weight loss) or diffuse pruritus.
- Definitive diagnosis is by tissue biopsy, ideally by excisional lymph node biopsy. Fine-needle aspiration (FNA) is insensitive for the diagnosis of Hodgkin lymphoma and should be avoided.

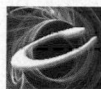

CURRENT THERAPY

- Treatment is guided by clinical stage using the Ann Arbor staging system.
- Limited-stage disease (stages I–IIA) without adverse risk factors (also called "early favorable") may be treated with combined-modality therapy (ABVD × 2 cycles followed by 20 Gy involved-field radiation), or 4 to 6 cycles of ABVD alone. Stanford V is an alternative option.
- Limited-stage disease (I–IIA) with adverse risk factors (also called "early unfavorable") may be treated with combined-modality therapy (4 cycles of ABVD followed by 30 Gy involved-field radiotherapy), or with 6 cycles of ABVD alone. Patients with bulky disease at presentation should receive combined-modality therapy.
- Advanced-stage disease (Ann Arbor stage IIB-IV) should be treated with ABVD for 6 cycles. Radiation should be included for bulky stage II disease, and may be considered for consolidation of bulky presenting sites in stage III–IV disease. Escalated BEACOPP is an alternative treatment option.
- Selection of treatment should be informed by the toxicity profiles of available therapies as well as the location of disease and the age and comorbidities of the patient.

Epidemiology

Hodgkin lymphoma is cancer of lymphoid tissue accounting for approximately 9000 new cases every year in the United States, and 1200 deaths. The median age of diagnosis is 35 years, but there is a bimodal distribution with the highest peak in the early 20s and then a rising incidence after the age of 60.

Pathology

Pathologically, Hodgkin lymphoma is broadly categorized as either classical Hodgkin lymphoma (CHL) or nodular lymphocyte predominant Hodgkin lymphoma (NLPHL) (Table 1). CHL includes four histologic subtypes, which are grouped together because of a common malignant cell—the Hodgkin Reed-Sternberg (HRS) cell—and shared natural history, prognosis, and approach to therapy. These subtypes, in order of frequency, are Nodular Sclerosis (NSHL), Mixed Cellularity (MCHL), Lymphocyte Rich (LRHL), and Lymphocyte depleted (LD).

NSHL accounts for approximately 70% of new cases of HL in the United States, and occurs with a female predominance. All other subtypes of CHL occur more frequently in men. NLPHL accounts for only about 5% of new cases of HL each year, and occurs more commonly in men than in women.

TABLE 1	Classification of Hodgkin Lymphoma	
Classic Hodgkin lymphoma		95%
Nodular sclerosis		75%
Mixed cellularity		15%
Lymphocyte rich		5%
Lymphocyte depleted		5%
Nodular lymphocyte-predominant Hodgkin lymphoma		5%

Risk Factors

Most cases of Hodgkin lymphoma are sporadic, though a few risk factors have been identified. An increased risk of CHL among first-degree family members points to a heritable genetic susceptibility. Identical twins of CHL patients have a markedly increased risk of developing CHL, while other first-degree relatives are four times likelier to develop CHL than the general population. Given the low overall incidence in the population, the absolute risk of CHL among first-degree relatives remains quite low.

NSHL occurs more frequently in the Western world and is associated with a favorable socioeconomic status. MCHL, on the other hand, is the most common subtype in developing countries, and is often associated with underlying Epstein-Barr virus (EBV) infection, but the absolute risk of developing CHL after infectious mononucleosis remains low at approximately 1 in 1000. The median time to CHL diagnosis after infectious mononucleosis is 4 years. HIV infection is associated with a tenfold increased risk of developing CHL, related to the immune suppression and increased rate EBV transformation. Risk is similarly increased in other immunosuppressive states such as congenital immunodeficiency and following solid organ or hematopoietic stem cell transplantation.

Clinical Manifestations

CHL most commonly presents with painless lymphadenopathy. The most common locations are in the neck (75%) and mediastinum (60%), followed by the axillae, retroperitoneal, and inguinal lymph nodes. Nodes are generally mobile and firm or rubbery on examination. The spleen is involved in approximately 20% of cases. Extranodal sites are uncommonly involved, including bone marrow, lungs, liver, bone, and other sites. Patients with bulky mediastinal disease may present with dyspnea, chest pressure, or cough, though even large mediastinal masses may be asymptomatic. Superior vena cava syndrome is uncommon. Systemic "B" symptoms (fever >38°C, unintentional weight loss of >10% of body weight over 6 months, and drenching night sweats) occur in approximately one third of patients at diagnosis. Generalized pruritus is not considered a "B" symptom but is present in a minority of patients, in whom it may presage the diagnosis by many months. Pain at involved nodal or bony sites with alcohol ingestion is rarely present, but is unique and the mechanism is not understood. Notable laboratory findings at diagnosis are typically mediated by cytokine production associated with the lymphoma, and may include anemia, thrombocytosis, leukocytosis, eosinophilia, lymphopenia, and hypoalbuminemia. The degree of these laboratory abnormalities typically tracks with increased disease burden. Hypercalcemia is an uncommon presenting feature, and is most commonly caused by increased production of calcitriol. Rarely, CHL can present with paraneoplastic cholestatic liver disease characterized by fevers and high conjugated bilirubin levels, but usually without frank infiltration by Hodgkin lymphoma on liver biopsy.

NLPHL presents in the majority of cases with localized painless peripheral adenopathy. Most patients are men between the ages of 30 and 50. The systemic "B" symptoms and laboratory abnormalities occasionally seen at presentation in CHL are rare in NLPHL.

Diagnosis

Diagnosis of HL requires pathologic examination, ideally performed by excisional biopsy, which obtains the largest amount of tissue for analysis and preserves tissue architecture. Hodgkin lymphoma may be difficult to diagnose on small biopsies because the malignant cells represent only about 1% of the overall tumor cellularity, while the majority is comprised of polyclonal reactive lymphocytes, neutrophils, and eosinophils. Inadequate tissue sampling may therefore falsely suggest a reactive inflammatory process as opposed to the underlying malignancy. Core needle or mediastinoscopic biopsies may be used for deep nonpalpable lesions where excisional surgical biopsies are not possible. Fine-needle aspiration (FNA) should not be used for diagnosis when lymphoma is suspected in the differential diagnosis because of the high rate of false-negative results. On histologic examination of CHL, the involved tissue is effaced by an infiltration of malignant Hodgkin Reed-Sternberg (HRS) cells amidst a rich inflammatory background. The classic HRS cell is typically large with abundant cytoplasm and a bilobed nucleolus, each with a single large eosinophilic nucleolus giving it the classic "owl's eye" appearance (Figure 1). Mononuclear variants also occur. By immunohistochemistry, the HRS cells usually stain positively for surface markers CD30 and CD15, and are usually negative for the pan-lymphoid marker CD45 and the B-cell marker CD20. The inflammatory microenvironment in NSHL is further characterized by dense bands of fibrosis from which its name is derived.

NLPHL is similarly characterized pathologically by infrequent atypical malignant cells amidst a polyclonal inflammatory microenvironment composed primarily of small lymphocytes in large nodular meshworks of follicular dendritic cells. The malignant lymphocyte-predominant (LP) cell is quite different from the HRS cells of CHL, in that it expresses CD45 and CD20, and does not express CD30 or CD15.

Differential Diagnosis

The differential diagnosis of lymphadenopathy is quite broad, and includes a wide range of malignancies, including lymphomas and solid tumors, infections, autoimmune diseases, hypersensitivity syndromes, and others. Diagnostic evaluation is guided by the clinical presentation as well as the size, location, and examination characteristics of the adenopathy.

Staging and Risk Stratification

Following confirmation of a pathologic diagnosis, patients with Hodgkin lymphoma undergo staging studies to determine the extent of disease involvement. Unlike many other cancers, Hodgkin lymphoma is highly curable regardless of stage, but the staging does assist in treatment selection and risk stratification. Staging is based on the Cotswold modification of the Ann Arbor Staging system (Table 2). This system was developed for Hodgkin lymphoma based on the tendency for HL to spread predictably via lymphatic

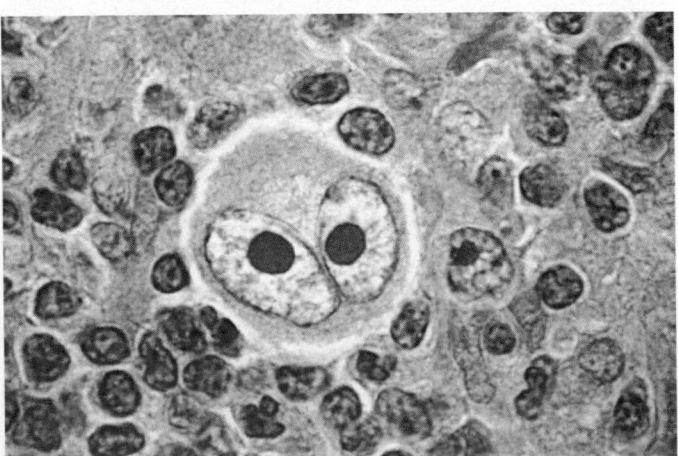

Figure 1. Classic Reed–Sternberg cell demonstrating large size, multinucleated nucleus, and prominent eosinophilic nucleolus.

TABLE 2	Ann Arbor Staging Sytem (Cotswold Modification)
STAGE	**DEFINITION**
I	Confined to single lymph node region or limited involvement of a single extranodal site (IE)
II	Confined to two or more lymph node regions on the same side of the diaphragm
III	Lymph node regions involved on both sides of the diaphragm
IV	Extensive involvement of one or more extranodal sites
MODIFIERS	
E	Localized focus of extranodal disease or localized extension of nodal disease into an extranodal site (e.g., hilar lymph node invading the lung)
A	Absence of "B" symptoms: fever (>38 °C), drenching night sweats, or unintentional loss of greater than 10% body weight over the previous 6 months.
B	Presence of "B" symptoms
S	Splenic involvement (the spleen is considered a nodal site)
X	Bulky disease (greater than 10 cm or greater than 1/3 the width of the maximal intrathoracic diameter)

spread to adjacent nodal regions. Limited-stage disease is therefore confined to either a single lymph-node region (stage I) or multiple lymph-node regions on a single side of the body (stages II), whereas advanced-stage disease involves nodal regions on both sides of the diaphragm (stage III) or with extensive involvement of an extranodal site (stage IV) such as the lungs, liver, bone, or bone marrow. Additional letters may be added to the numeric stage to denote the absence or presence of "B" symptoms ("A" or "B"), bulky disease measuring greater than 10 cm ("X") or splenic involvement ("S"). Stage IIB disease is typically categorized as advanced stage.

Staging begins with a physical examination with careful attention paid to all palpable lymph node regions, the spleen, and Waldeyer's ring. Radiographic staging is performed with whole-body computed tomographic (CT) scans, ideally in conjunction with a Positron Emission Tomography (PET) scan as a combined PET/CT scan, which enhances the sensitivity over CT scans alone. Bone-marrow biopsy is often not performed in modern staging because of the enhanced sensitivity of PET scans in detecting bone marrow involvement in HL, which is often patchy in nature, and because of the incorporation of systemic therapy into the treatment plans of virtually all patients with either limited-stage or advanced-stage disease, ensuring that any sites of subclinical disease are still exposed to lymphoma-directed therapy. Similarly, staging laparotomy is never performed for modern staging given the sensitivity of modern radiographic techniques.

Additional pretreatment studies include routine laboratory testing with a complete blood count and differential; erythrocyte sedimentation rate; and complete metabolic panel including liver function, renal function, calcium and albumin. Given the association of HIV infection in a minority of cases, HIV antibody testing at baseline is recommended. Assessment of left ventricular function with an echocardiogram or MUGA scan as well as pulmonary evaluation with pulmonary function testing should be checked in anticipation of doxorubicin and bleomycin containing therapy, respectively. Though most chemotherapy for Hodgkin lymphoma carries only minimal risk of sterility, fertility counseling for patients in their childbearing years is recommended prior to initiation of therapy.

Risk Stratification

Though Hodgkin lymphoma is a highly curable disease, clinical and laboratory variables can stratify patients into lower and higher risk groups. The cure rate for limited-stage CHL with modern therapy is greater than 85%. Identified risk factors can place patients into an "early favorable" or "early unfavorable" category, though, importantly, the vast majority of patients in both groups will be cured of their disease with initial therapy. Adverse risk factors denoting early unfavorable disease include age greater than 50 years, bulky mediastinal mass, involvement of more than three nodal areas, extranodal disease, presence of systemic "B" symptoms, and an elevated erythrocyte sedimentation rate.

Within advanced-stage CHL, multivariable analysis identified seven adverse risk factors that are summed to generate the International Prognostic Score (IPS). These adverse risk factors at the time of diagnosis are male gender, age greater than 45 years, stage IV disease, serum albumin less than 4.0 g/dL, hemoglobin concentration less than 10.5 g/dL, white cell count greater than 15,000/mm^3, and lymphopenia (<600 cells/mL or <8% of white cells). Data in the modern era with ABVD (doxorubicin [Adriamycin], bleomycin [Bleoxane], vinblastine [Velban] and dacarbazine [DTIC-Dome]) show 5-year freedom from progression ranging from 62% in the highest risk patients to 88% in the lowest risk patients, and 5-year overall survival ranging from 67% to 98%.

Prognosis in NLPHL is generally more favorable than that in classical HL, owing to a significantly more indolent natural history and higher likelihood of presenting as localized disease. Although late relapses may occur, very few patients die from NLPHL.

Treatment

Limited-Stage Classical Hodgkin Lymphoma

Standard therapy for limited-stage (stage I-IIA) CHL has most commonly included combined-modality therapy with systemic chemotherapy followed by involved-field radiation. This standard evolved over many years, during which time randomized clinical trials demonstrated improved overall survival favoring combined modality therapy compared to radiation alone, and showed no benefit to extended-field radiation over narrower radiation fields.

Patients with nonbulky limited-stage disease and absence of adverse risk factors ("early favorable") may receive only 2 cycles of chemotherapy with ABVD followed by 20 Gy of radiation therapy to all involved fields. Bulk is defined as greater than one third of the maximum thoracic diameter greater than or equal to 10 cm in maximal diameter. Among patients with limited-stage disease with presenting bulk or presence of adverse risk factors ("early unfavorable"), combined-modality therapy is intensified to consist of 4 cycles of ABVD followed by 30 Gy of involved-field radiotherapy. Similar excellent results have been obtained with the Stanford V regimen, which is an 8- to 12-week chemotherapy program including mechlorethamine (Mustargen), doxorubicin, vinblastine, prednisone, vincristine (Oncovin, Vincasar PFS), bleomycin, and etoposide (Toposar),[1] along with involved-field radiation therapy. Treatment intensification with the escalated BEACOPP regimen (bleomycin, etoposide,[1] doxorubicin [Adriamycin], cyclophosphamide (Cytoxan), vincristine [Oncovin], procarbazine [Matulane] and prednisone) has been compared to ABVD in early unfavorable disease, each followed by involved-field radiation therapy, and found no difference in overall survival to favor the intensified approach. ABVD remains the most commonly employed chemotherapy backbone for limited-stage Hodgkin lymphoma given the tolerability of the regimen and reduced reliance on alkylating agents.

Radiation therapy in young patients with Hodgkin lymphoma has prompted safety concerns given the increased incidence of late toxicities from mediastinal radiotherapy, including increased risk of secondary malignancies such as breast cancer, thyroid cancer, and lung cancer, as well as heart disease and lung disease. A large randomized trial comparing chemotherapy alone to combined-modality therapy showed a small increased risk of recurrence in patients who receive chemotherapy alone, but an improved overall

---

[1]Not FDA approved for this indication.

survival 10 years after completion of therapy favoring chemotherapy alone, due to an excess of nonlymphoma deaths in the irradiated patients. Notably, the radiation employed in this trial was more extensive than modern involved-field radiotherapy, which may have overestimated the rate of late radiation events, but 94% of patients receiving ABVD alone remained alive and well 12 years later, demonstrating outstanding results from the radiation-sparing approach. These data support consideration of ABVD chemotherapy alone for 4 to 6 cycles in patients with nonbulky limited-stage Hodgkin lymphoma. Patients with bulky disease have not been included in a randomized trial sparing radiation, and so combined-modality therapy remains the standard of care for such patients. Ongoing clinical trials in limited-stage disease are evaluating the role of early interim PET scanning in guiding intensity of chemotherapy and inclusion of radiation therapy.

Advanced-Stage Classical Hodgkin Lymphoma

Advanced-stage CHL (Ann Arbor stages IIB-IV) had been a nearly uniformly fatal disease prior to the development of effective combination chemotherapy with the introduction of MOPP (mechlorethamine, vincristine [Oncovin], procarbazine, and prednisone) at the National Cancer Institute in 1964. ABVD subsequently emerged as an alternative to MOPP, and was confirmed to have improved efficacy and reduced toxicity in a randomized trial that defined it as the standard of care. Modern outcomes with ABVD for advanced-stage disease produce 5-year freedom from progression and overall survival of 78% and 90%, respectively. ABVD is administered on days 1 and 15 of a 28-day cycle for 6 total cycles. Consolidative radiation therapy is not routinely administered in advanced-stage disease, except in the setting of an incomplete response to chemotherapy alone, or to bulky sites of disease at presentation.

The escalated BEACOPP regimen has been extensively explored as an alternative to ABVD, and does modestly decrease the rate of recurrence, but without a clear impact on overall survival. Stanford V has also been evaluated in several randomized trials of advanced-stage disease without evidence of superiority over ABVD. In the absence of an overall survival benefit favoring escalated BEACOPP or Stanford V, and the increased treatment-associated toxicity associated with intensified therapy, most practitioners in North America continue to favor ABVD as the standard of care for advanced-stage disease, though this remains a subject of worldwide debate.

Treatment of Relapsed Hodgkin Lymphoma

Though the majority of patients with CHL will be cured with initial treatment, approximately 15% of patients will relapse and require additional therapy. Patients who relapse with localized disease greater than 1 year after completion of initial therapy and without systemic "B" symptoms may be treated with conventional-dose second-line chemotherapy followed by involved-field radiation. The majority of patients, however, will relapse in less than 12 months or with more advanced disease, for which conventional-dose chemotherapy offers a disappointingly low chance of cure. In such patients, second-line chemotherapy followed by high-dose chemotherapy with autologous stem cell support offers a cure rate approaching 50% and is the modern treatment of choice. Patients who relapse after high-dose chemotherapy may be candidates for allogeneic stem cell transplantation with curative intent, but success rates are low, and risks of treatment-associated morbidity and mortality are significant.

For patients who are not candidates for intensive therapy, or who relapse after stem cell transplantation, multiple chemotherapy options are available that may offer palliative disease control. An appealing option at relapse is the antibody drug conjugate brentuximab vedotin (Adcetris), which is a monoclonal antibody against CD30 bound to the microtubule toxin monomethyl auristatin E (MMAE). This targeted therapy is FDA approved for relapsed Hodgkin lymphoma based on an overall response rate

of 75% and complete response rate of 34% in patients relapsing after high-dose chemotherapy and autologous stem cell transplantation. Clinical trials incorporating brentuximab vedotin into upfront therapy in both limited- and advanced-stage Hodgkin lymphoma are ongoing.

Treatment of Nodular Lymphocyte-Predominant Hodgkin Lymphoma

Nodular lymphocyte-predominant Hodgkin lymphoma (NLPHL) follows a unique natural history from CHL, and is typically treated with less-intensive therapy. Limited-stage NLPHL usually presents at peripheral locations rather than the mediastinum, and may be treated with involved-field radiation alone (without chemotherapy), which produces a 10-year overall survival in excess of 95%. Advanced-stage NLPHL is uncommon, but may be treated with rituximab (Rituxan)[1] because of the CD20 positivity of the malignant LP cells, with encouraging single-agent activity. Combination chemotherapy with either ABVD or with alkylator-based regimens is also effective.

Monitoring

Patients on therapy for Hodgkin lymphoma are evaluated for response using PET and CT scans, ideally as a combined-modality PET/CT scan. A complete response on PET/CT following 2 cycles of chemotherapy predicts for an extremely favorable prognosis, while a persistent positive PET scan is associated with a high rate of treatment failure. Clinical trials evaluating treatment intensification for patients with positive PET scans after 2 cycles of chemotherapy are ongoing, but presently there is no evidence that intensified therapy overcomes the negative prognostic effect of interim PET positivity, and so treatment modification based on interim PET results is not recommended outside of a clinical trial. Patients undergoing therapy for Hodgkin lymphoma are also evaluated with routine blood counts and chemistries to assess for treatment-associated marrow and organ toxicity. Patients receiving bleomycin are typically evaluated every 2 cycles with repeat pulmonary function tests in order to detect early evidence of bleomycin lung injury, though the predictive value of pulmonary function testing is controversial. Following completion of therapy, PET/CT scans should also be employed for end-of-treatment restaging, where it increases sensitivity over CT scans alone, particularly in the assessment of residual masses, which often represent residual scar tissue and debris of successfully treated disease.

Once patients achieve remission, they are followed by their oncologist in cooperation with their primary care physician to assess for relapse as well as late treatment-associated toxicities. Patients are monitored with periodic history and physical examination. CT scans are typically performed every 6 months for 2 to 3 years after completion of therapy, and thereafter only if prompted by concerning signs, symptoms, or physical findings. There is no role for PET scans in the routine follow-up of Hodgkin lymphoma after remission has been achieved. Following completion of radiographic surveillance, periodic history and physical examination continue, as does laboratory evaluation, to monitor for the development of uncommon late toxicities, including secondary malignancies, heart disease, and lung disease. Specific monitoring is dependent in part on the precise treatment the patient received.

Complications

Combination chemotherapy may be associated with fatigue, bone marrow suppression, increased susceptibility to infection, gastrointestinal upset, constipation, peripheral neuropathy, and mouth sores, among other complications. Doxorubicin carries a low risk of myocardial injury and congestive heart failure, and bleomycin carries a risk of lung injury, which may be life threatening. The risk of bleomycin lung injury persists lifelong, and may be precipitated

[1]Not FDA approved for this indication.

by exposure to high inspired fractions of oxygen or other pulmonary insults. Risks of myelodysplasia and secondary leukemia as well as impaired fertility are rare after ABVD, but occur with increased frequency following MOPP, escalated BEACOPP, and high-dose chemotherapy.

Radiation-associated toxicities may occur decades following completion of therapy, and are a function of dose and volume of tissue exposure. Secondary malignancies steadily increase beginning approximately a decade after completion of therapy, and include breast cancer, lung cancer, thyroid cancer, gastrointestinal cancers, urogenital cancers, melanoma, and non-Hodgkin lymphomas, among others. Age-appropriate cancer screening is recommended as well as consideration of breast MRI for women who received mediastinal radiation as children or young adults.

Mediastinal radiation, particularly in combination with doxorubicin-containing chemotherapy, confers multiple cardiac risks to be aware of in long-term follow-up, including premature coronary artery disease, cardiomyopathy, valvular heart disease, and restrictive pericarditis. Lung exposure to radiation, particularly in concert with bleomycin, also confers a risk of radiation pneumonitis or late radiation fibrosis. Radiation to the neck may be associated with dental caries, dry mouth, thyroid dysfunction, and cerebrovascular disease. Long-term care of the Hodgkin lymphoma patient requires attention to risk not only of relapse, but of the many late complications of therapy that may have substantial impact on long-term morbidity and mortality in Hodgkin lymphoma survivors.

References

Advani RH, Hoppe RT, Baer D, et al. Efficacy of abbreviated Stanford V chemotherapy and involved-field radiotherapy in early-stage Hodgkin lymphoma: mature results of the G4 trial. Ann Oncol 2013;34:1044–8.

Canellos GP, Anderson JR, Cella DF, et al. Chemotherapy of advanced Hodgkin's disease with MOPP, ABVD, or MOPP alternating with ABVD. N Engl J Med 1992;327:1478–84.

Chen RC, Chin MS, Ng AK, et al. Early-stage, lymphocyte-predominant Hodgkin's lymphoma: patient outcomes from a large, single-institution series with long follow-up. J Clin Oncol 2010;28:136–41.

Diehl V, Sextro M, Franklin J, et al. Clinical presentation, course, and prognostic factors in lymphocyte-predominant Hodgkin's disease and lymphocyte-rich classical Hodgkin's disease: report from the European Task Force on Lymphoma Project on Lymphocyte-Predominant Hodgkin's Disease. J Clin Oncol 1999;17:776–83.

Eichenauer DA, Fuchs M, Pluetschow A, et al. Phase 2 study of rituximab in newly diagnosed stage IA nodular lymphocyte-predominant Hodgkin lymphoma: a report from the German Hodgkin Study Group. Blood 2011;118:4363–5.

Engert A, Plütschow A, Eich HT, et al. Reduced treatment intensity in patients with early-stage Hodgkin's lymphoma. N Engl J Med 2010;363:640–52.

Ferme C, Eghbali H, Meerwaldt JH, et al. Chemotherapy plus involved-field radiation in early-stage Hodgkin's disease. N Engl J Med 2007;357:1916–27.

Gallamini A, Hutchings M, Rigacci L, et al. Early interim 2-[18 F]fluoro-2-deoxy-D-glucose positron emission tomography is prognostically superior to international prognostic score in advanced-stage Hodgkin's lymphoma: a report from a joint Italian-Danish study. J Clin Oncol 2007;25:3746–52.

Goldin LR, Bjorkholm M, Kristinsson SY, et al. Highly increased familial risks for specific lymphoma subtypes. Br J Haematol 2009;146:91–4.

Hjalgrim H, Askling J, Rostgaard K, et al. Characteristics of Hodgkin's lymphoma after infectious mononucleosis. N Engl J Med 2003;349:1324–32.

Meyer RM, Gospodarowicz MK, Connors JM, et al. ABVD alone versus radiation-based therapy in limited-stage Hodgkin's lymphoma. N Engl J Med 2012;366:399–408.

Moccia AA, Donaldson J, Chhanabhai M, et al. International Prognostic Score in advanced-stage Hodgkin's lymphoma: altered utility in the modern era. J Clin Oncol 2012;30:3383–8.

Moskowitz CH, Nimer SD, Zelenetz AD, et al. A 2-step comprehensive high-dose chemoradiotherapy second-line program for relapsed and refractory Hodgkin disease: analysis by intent to treat and development of a prognostic model. Blood 2001;97:616–23.

Schmitz N, Pfistner B, Sextro M, et al. Aggressive conventional chemotherapy compared with high-dose chemotherapy with autologous haemopoietic stem-cell transplantation for relapsed chemosensitive Hodgkin's disease: a randomised trial. Lancet 2002;359:2065–71.

Swerdlow SH, Campo E, Harris NL, et al. WHO classification of tumours of hematopoietic and lymphoid tissues. Lyon: WHO; 2008.

Viviani S, Zinzani PL, Rambaldi A, et al. ABVD versus BEACOPP for Hodgkin's lymphoma when high-dose salvage is planned. N Engl J Med 2011;365:203–12.

Younes A, Gopal AK, Smith SE, et al. Results of a pivotal phase II study of brentuximab vedotin for patients with relapsed or refractory Hodgkin's lymphoma. J Clin Oncol 2012;30:2183–9.

IRON DEFICIENCY ANEMIA

Method of
Paul Paulman, MD

CURRENT DIAGNOSIS

Symptoms
- Fatigue
- Poor exercise tolerance
- Weakness
- Irritability
- Poor concentration
- Dry mouth
- Headache
- Pica

Signs
- Pallor
- Systolic heart murmur if anemia is present
- Atrophy of lingual papillae
- Koilonychia
- Chlorosis

Laboratory Findings
- Decreased iron seen on bone marrow aspirate (gold standard)
- Low serum ferritin (diagnostic)
- Low serum iron level
- High serum iron-binding capacity
- Low serum hemoglobin
- Low mean corpuscular hemoglobin
- Low mean corpuscular volume
- Variations in size and shape of red blood cells

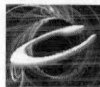

CURRENT THERAPY

Oral Replacement
- Ferrous sulfate (or other equivalent iron preparation) 325 mg three times daily.
- Add ascorbic acid tablet 500 mg with each iron tablet to increase iron absorption.
- Consider enteric-coated tablets to decrease gastrointestinal problems associated with oral iron therapy.

Parenteral Replacement
- If oral therapy is not tolerated, parental preparations including iron dextran, iron sucrose, or ferric gluconate may be used.

Unstable Patient
- If the patient is hemodynamically unstable due to anemia, consider blood transfusion.

Treatment Endpoint
- Iron deficiency has been corrected if the serum ferritin is 50 ng/mL or more.

Epidemiology

Iron is necessary for production of erythrocytes and the normal functioning of several iron-containing cellular enzymes. Iron deficiency is defined as the decrease of total iron stores in the body. Iron deficiency anemia results when iron deficiency is severe enough to decrease erythropoiesis. The most common cause of iron deficiency in the U.S. adult population is blood loss. The most common sources of blood loss are menstrual and gastrointestinal. Other causes of iron deficiency include inadequate intake during high-demand states such as pregnancy, early childhood, or erythropoietin therapy. A diet low in iron-rich foods (vegetarian or vegan) can lead to iron deficiency.

Gastrointestinal diseases including Crohn's disease, sprue, and postgastrectomy states can decrease iron absorption from the gastrointestinal tract, resulting in iron deficiency. Chronic inflammatory states can lead to decreased use of available iron stores, leading to symptoms of iron deficiency.

Iron deficiency is the most common micronutrient deficiency in the world. Iron deficiency affects approximately 2% to 5% of children and adolescents in the United States and 4% of the U.S. adult population, including 20% of women of childbearing age, 50% of pregnant women, and 2% of men.

Risk Factors

Risk factors for iron deficiency include age, socioeconomic status, sex, diet, disease, and medical treatment. Infants, children, and adolescents are at risk, especially during periods of rapid growth. Low socioeconomic status, including minority population group and low income, increase the risk for iron deficiency. Risk is increased in women during the childbearing years and during pregnancy and breastfeeding. Diets low in iron-rich foods, including vegan and vegetarian diets, increase the risk.

Any illness or therapy that leads to decreased absorption of iron or loss of blood also increases the risk. Gastrointestinal diseases causing blood loss or decreased iron absorption can lead to iron deficiency. Antacids cause decreased iron absorption and nonsteroidal antiinflammatory drugs (NSAIDs) cause gastrointestinal blood loss. Erythropoietin therapy depletes iron stores because of increased hematopoiesis. Frequent phlebotomy, including repetitive blood donation or treatment for polycythemia or hemochromatosis, decreases iron stores.

Pathophysiology

Total body iron stores for men are approximately 3.5 g and for women are about 2.5 g. More than 70% of body iron is found in hemoglobin, and the remainder is contained in myoglobin, tissue enzymes, and storage or transport proteins. Iron absorption takes place almost exclusively in the duodenum and upper jejunum. In a non–iron-deficient state, only about 6% to 10% of iron from food is absorbed (1 mg of 15 mg/day of dietary iron). Factors that increase iron absorption from the gut include ingestion of heme (meat) iron, iron-deficient states, and coadministration of vitamin C (ascorbic acid). Factors that decrease iron absorption include ingestion of certain foods including vegetable fiber phytates, tea tannates, bran, and medications including tetracyclines and antacids.

Iron deficiency develops in stages. During the early stage, iron needs exceed iron intake and body iron stores are depleted, causing an increase in absorption of dietary iron. As this process continues, erythropoiesis is impaired, leading to iron deficiency anemia, and dysfunction of iron-containing cellular enzymes can occur. This enzyme dysfunction can contribute to the fatigue and loss of stamina seen in patients with iron deficiency anemia. Iron deficiency during childhood can result in deficiencies in growth and cognitive function.

Prevention

Prevention of iron deficiency is focused on providing supplemental dietary iron to populations at risk for iron deficiency. Current recommendations include elemental iron supplementation (1 mg/kg/d) for breast-fed infants after 6 months of age and iron supplementation of infant formula (12 mg/L elemental iron) for formula-fed infants. Iron-enriched cereals should be among the first solid foods offered to infants. Whole cow's milk should be avoided during the first year of life to decrease the possibility of occult gastrointestinal bleeding. Supplemental iron should be taken during pregnancy and breast-feeding.

Clinical Manifestations

Patients with iron deficiency may be asymptomatic. The presence of symptoms and signs of iron deficiency depend on the degree of deficiency, the time course of the development of iron deficiency, and the overall physiologic state of the patient. Common symptoms of iron deficiency include fatigue, weakness, irritability, poor concentration, exercise intolerance, dry mouth, and headache. Severe iron deficiency can cause pica, a craving to eat substances such as ice, dirt, clay, or paint. Signs of iron deficiency include pallor and a systolic heart murmur if anemia is present, alopecia, atrophy of lingual papillae, koilonychias, and chlorosis.

Diagnosis

The gold standard for diagnosis of iron deficiency is the demonstration of decreased iron available for erythropoiesis on a bone marrow aspiration sample. The wide availability of reliable serum iron markers makes bone marrow sampling for diagnosis of iron deficiency unnecessary in most cases. A low serum iron is characteristic of both iron deficiency and anemia of chronic disease. Serum total iron binding capacity is decreased in iron deficiency and elevated in anemia of chronic disease. Serum iron and total iron binding capacity are often ordered together. Many authorities think serum ferritin determination is the most useful laboratory test for iron deficiency. Ferritin levels reflect the quantity of iron stored in the reticuloendothelial system. A low serum ferritin level is diagnostic of iron deficiency. Serum ferritin levels can be falsely elevated in the presence of inflammation.

The diagnosis of iron deficiency anemia requires a decline in serum hemoglobin to less than 13 g/dL in men or 12 g/dL in women along with a decreased mean corpuscular volume and mean corpuscular hemoglobin and the presence of iron deficiency. Other findings in iron deficiency anemia include variation in erythrocyte shape and size (poikilocytosis and anisocytosis) and elevation in the coefficient of red blood cell distribution width (RDW).

Because gastrointestinal blood loss is a common cause of iron deficiency anemia, patients who present with iron deficiency anemia should be considered for appropriate screening for gastrointestinal conditions, including malignancies.

Differential Diagnosis

The differential diagnosis of iron deficiency includes causes of fatigue and exercise intolerance such as hypothyroidism, electrolyte disturbances due to diuretic therapy, left ventricular dysfunction, chronic lung disease, malignancies, or liver disease.

Anemia of chronic disease can mimic iron deficiency anemia. Differentiating characteristics of the two types of anemia can be found in Table 1.

Treatment

Iron may be replaced via oral or intravenous routes. The most cost-effective oral iron preparation is a non–enteric-coated ferrous sulfate tablet. The most common oral iron replacement regimen consists of one 325 mg ferrous sulfate tablet (Feosol) by mouth three times daily. Each 325 mg ferrous sulfate tablet contains 65 mg of elemental iron.

Other iron salts, ferrous gluconate (Fergon) and ferrous fumarate (Ferro-Sequels) are available for oral replacement. The

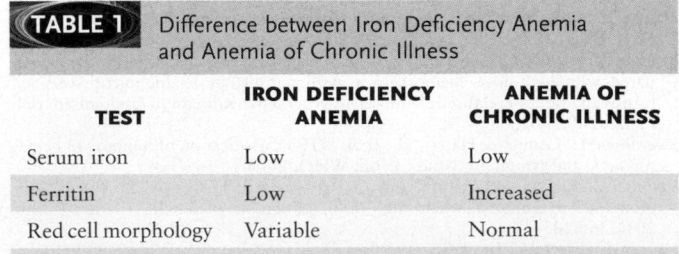

TABLE 1	Difference between Iron Deficiency Anemia and Anemia of Chronic Illness	
TEST	**IRON DEFICIENCY ANEMIA**	**ANEMIA OF CHRONIC ILLNESS**
Serum iron	Low	Low
Ferritin	Low	Increased
Red cell morphology	Variable	Normal
C-reactive protein	Normal	Increased

absorption of oral iron is enhanced by taking the pills on an empty stomach or with an ascorbic acid tablet (500 mg). Because of the gastric distress often caused by oral iron replacement, most practitioners prescribe enteric-coated iron tablets.

Patients who cannot take or cannot tolerate oral iron can be treated with intravenous iron preparations, iron dextran (InFeD), iron sucrose (Venofer),[1] ferric gluconate (Ferrlecit)[1], or ferumoxytol (Feraheme). Because of the pain associated with the injection and other problems, intramuscular iron is seldom used.

Patients who are severely anemic and hemodynamically unstable may be candidates for blood transfusion. To determine the total dose of iron needed to correct the deficiency, the total iron deficit (depleted stores plus the deficit in red cell hemoglobin iron) should be calculated before beginning therapy. Because the most common cause of iron deficiency is blood loss, the management of iron deficiency should include identification of the source and cause of blood loss.

Monitoring

The earliest marker for successful iron replacement is an increase in the reticulocyte count, which occurs within 5 to 10 days of initiation of iron replacement. A hemoglobin increase of 2 g/dL is considered an appropriate response to oral iron replacement. Complete blood counts should be obtained at 1 month and 2 months after beginning replacement therapy. Iron deficiency should be corrected after 2 months of replacement therapy. Treatment of iron deficiency should continue until the serum ferritin reaches a level of 50 ng/mL. Darkening of stools after 2 or 3 days of starting oral iron replacement is a reliable marker of compliance.

Complications

If properly treated, iron deficiency has few complications in adults. Untreated iron deficiency in infants and small children can lead to cognitive development and growth deficits. Treating iron deficiency without identifying the source and cause of blood loss could result in delay or failure to diagnose gastrointestinal malignancies or other serious clinical problems.

---

[1]Not FDA approved for this indication.

References

Anderson GJ, Frazer DM, Mclaren GD. Iron absorption and metabolism. Curr Opin Gastroenterol 2009;25:129–35.

Anemias caused by deficient erythropoiesis. Beers MH, Porter RS, Jones TV, et al., Merck Manual of Diagnosis and Therapy. 18th ed. Whitehouse Station, NJ: Merck Research Laboratories; 2006.

Clark SF. Iron deficiency anemia: Diagnosis and management. Curr Opin Gastroenterol 2009;26:122–8.

Clark SF. Iron deficiency anemia. Nutr Clin Pract 2008;23:128–41.

Cook JD. Diagnosis and management of iron deficiency anaemia. Best Pract Res Clin Haematol 2005;18:319–32.

Oski FA. The nonhematologic manifestations of iron deficiency. A J Di Child 1979;133:315–22.

MULTIPLE MYELOMA

Method of
Robert A. Kyle, MD; and S. Vincent Rajkumar, MD

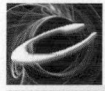

CURRENT DIAGNOSIS

- Malignant clonal plasma cell disorder
- Characterized by presence of a monoclonal immunoglobulin in the serum or urine in most patients
- Typical manifestations include anemia, osteolytic bone lesions, and renal failure

- Initial workup should include a bone marrow aspiration and biopsy with fluorescent in situ hybridization studies to determine molecular cytogenetic type
  - Standard risk: trisomies (hyperdiploidy), t(11;14), and t(6;14)
  - Intermediate risk: t(4;14)
  - High risk: 17p-, (t14;16) or t(14;20)

CURRENT THERAPY

- Do not begin treatment until symptomatic multiple myeloma develops (CRAB: *c*alcium elevated, *r*enal failure, *a*nemia, *b*one lesions) or other myeloma defining events are present.
- Decide whether an autologous stem cell transplant is feasible. If it is, one must avoid melphalan (Alkeran) therapy as initial treatment.
- Initial therapy is typically lenalidomide (Revlimid) plus low-dose dexamethasone (Decadron) (Rd),* or bortezomib (Velcade) combined with cyclophosphamide (Cytoxan) and low-dose dexamethasone (VCD).[1] High-risk patients are candidates for lenalidomide, bortezomib, and dexamethasone (VRd)[1]
- Patients who are candidates for autologous stem cell transplantation should collect stem cells after 3-4 cycles of induction. After collection, patients proceed to either early transplantation, or resume initial therapy and postpone transplant until relapse.
- Patients who are not stem cell transplant candidates receive initial therapy for a duration of approximately 12 months. However, in the case of Rd, therapy is continued until progression if tolerated.
- Relapsed or refractory myeloma should be treated with one of the active drugs given alone or in combination. Active agents include thalidomide, lenalidomide, bortezomib, carfilzomib (Kyprolis), pomalidomide (Pomalyst), corticosteroids, anthracyclines, and alkylators.

---

[1]Not FDA approved for this indication.
*Not FDA approved unless patient has had at least one prior treatment; induction therapy is considered off label use.

Multiple myeloma is characterized by the neoplastic proliferation of clonal plasma cells. It is typically associated with a monoclonal (M) protein in the serum and/or urine.

Epidemiology

In the United States, multiple myeloma constitutes 1% of all malignant diseases and slightly more than 10% of hematologic malignancies. The annual incidence is 4 to 5 per 100,000; the incidence in African Americans is twice that in whites. The apparent recent increase in rates is probably caused by increased availability and use of medical facilities and improved diagnostic techniques, particularly in the older population. The median age at diagnosis is approximately 70 years.

Risk Factors

The cause of multiple myeloma is unclear. Exposure to radiation might play a role. Persons in agricultural occupations who are exposed to pesticides, herbicides, or fungicides have an increased risk of multiple myeloma. Benzene and petroleum products, hair dyes, engine exhaust, furniture worker products, obesity, and chronic immune stimulation have also been reported as risk factors. The risk of developing multiple myeloma is higher for patients with a first-degree relative with the disease. Clusters of two or more first-degree relatives or identical twins have been recognized.

Clinical Manifestations

Weakness, fatigue, bone pain, recurrent infections, and symptoms of hypercalcemia or renal insufficiency should alert the physician to the possibility of multiple myeloma. Anemia is present in 70% of patients at the time of diagnosis. An M protein is found in the serum or urine in more than 97% of patients with multiple myeloma by immunofixation studies and the serum-free light chain assay. Lytic lesions, osteoporosis, or fractures are present at diagnosis in 80% of patients and can be detected by conventional radiography. Magnetic resonance imaging (MRI) and positron emission tomography/computed tomography (PET/CT) are helpful in patients who have skeletal pain but no abnormality on radiographs or when spinal cord compression is suspected. Hypercalcemia is present in 15% of patients, and the serum creatinine value is 2 mg/dL or greater in almost 20% of patients at diagnosis.

Diagnosis

If multiple myeloma is suspected, the patient should have, in addition to a complete history and physical examination:

- Determination of values for hemoglobin, leukocytes with differential count, platelets, serum creatinine, calcium, and uric acid
- A radiographic survey of bones, including humeri and femurs
- Serum protein electrophoresis with immunofixation
- Quantitation of immunoglobulins, serum free light chain (FLC) assay
- Bone marrow aspirate and biopsy
- Routine urinalysis
- Electrophoresis and immunofixation of an adequately concentrated aliquot from a 24-hour urine specimen
- Fluorescence in situ hybridization (FISH) and conventional cytogenetics
- Measurement of β_2-microglobulin, C-reactive protein, and lactate dehydrogenase

Box 1 lists the International Myeloma Working Group updated criteria for diagnosis of myeloma and related disorders. Metastatic carcinoma, lymphoma, leukemia, and connective tissue disorders can resemble multiple myeloma and must be considered in the differential diagnosis. Patients with multiple myeloma must be differentiated from those with monoclonal gammopathy of undetermined significance (MGUS) and smoldering (asymptomatic) multiple myeloma (SMM). Patients with MGUS and SMM may remain stable for long periods and not require treatment (see Box 1). The patient's symptoms, physical findings, and all laboratory and radiographic data must be considered in the decision to begin therapy. If there are doubts about whether to begin treatment, therapy should be withheld and the patient should be reevaluated in 2 to 3 months. No evidence indicates that early treatment of multiple myeloma is advantageous.

| **Box 1** | International Myeloma Working Group Diagnostic Criteria |

Monoclonal Gammopathy of Undetermined Significance
- Serum M protein <3 g/dL
- Clonal bone marrow–plasma cells <10%
- Absence of end-organ damage (CRAB) attributable to a plasma cell proliferative disorder

Smoldering Multiple Myeloma
- Serum M protein ≥3 g/dL and/or clonal bone marrow–plasma cells 10–60%
- Absence of myeloma defining events or amyloidosis

Multiple Myeloma
- Presence of clonal bone marrow plasma cells 10% or greater or biopsy proven plasmacytoma
- Presence of end-organ damage (CRAB) thought to be related to a plasma cell proliferative disorder or other myeloma defining event (clonal bone marrow plasma cells 60% or higher, serum free light chain ratio 100 or more provided involved free light chain level is 100 mg/L or more, more than one focal lesion on magnetic resonance imaging)

Abbreviations: CRAB = calcium elevated, renal failure, anemia, bone lesions; M = monoclonal.
Derived from Rajkumar SV, Dimopoulos MA, Palumbo A, et al. International Myeloma Working Group updated criteria for the diagnosis of multiple myeloma. Lancet Oncol 2014;15:e538-e548.

Treatment

Patients with symptomatic multiple myeloma may be classified as having high-risk, intermediate-risk, or standard-risk disease. High-risk disease is defined as the presence of del(17p), t (14;16), or t(14;20) with FISH. The presence of t(4;14) is considered intermediate-risk disease. Lactate dehydrogenase, circulating plasma cells, and β_2-microglobulin levels are additional important risk factors. Approximately 15% to 20% of patients with symptomatic multiple myeloma have high-risk disease.

If clinical trials are not available, one may separate patients into those eligible for an autologous stem cell transplant (SCT) versus those not eligible. An autologous SCT adds about 1 year of survival on average when compared with patients treated with conventional-dose chemotherapy alone.

Eligibility for autologous SCT in multiple myeloma varies from country to country. In the United States, decisions are made on a patient-by-patient basis depending on the physiologic age rather than the chronologic age. In most institutions, patients older than 70 years or with serum creatinine greater than 2.5 mg/dL, Eastern Cooperative Oncology Group (ECOG) performance status of 3 or 4, or New York Heart Association (NYHA) functional status class III or IV are considered ineligible for autologous SCT. Although patients with kidney failure may have an autologous SCT, the morbidity and mortality are higher.

Initial Therapy for Transplant-Eligible Patients

Lenalidomide (Revlimid) is an analogue of thalidomide and is an immunomodulatory agent. Lenalidomide 25 mg daily on days 1 to 21 plus dexamethasone (Decadron) 40 mg weekly for each 28-day cycle is an effective regimen.[1] Bortezomib (Velcade) once weekly (preferably administered subcutaneously) plus cyclophosphamide (Cytoxan) 300 mg/m² orally once weekly plus dexamethasone 40 mg once weekly (VCD)[1] produces a high response rate and is another effective regimen for initial therapy, particularly for intermediate-risk patients and in patients presenting with acute renal failure. Bortezomib should be given at weekly intervals because it is equally efficacious and is associated with less peripheral neuropathy. It is also preferable to administer bortezomib subcutaneously to diminish the risk of neuropathy. Other useful regimens include bortezomib, thalidomide (Thalomid), and dexamethasone (VTD)[1] and bortezomib, lenalidomide, dexamethasone (VRd).[1] There have been no phase III trials comparing any of these regimens. We prefer lenalidomide plus low-dose dexamethasone in standard-risk patients; bortezomib plus cyclophosphamide plus dexamethasone in intermediate-risk patients; and bortezomib, lenalidomide, and dexamethasone in high-risk patients.

Autologous Stem Cell Transplantation

Following 3 to 4 months of induction therapy with one of the initial regimens, one must collect the stem cells in patients eligible for transplantation. The stem cells must be collected before the patient is exposed to prolonged therapy, especially melphalan (Alkeran). Granulocyte colony-stimulating factor (G-CSF, Neupogen) with or without cyclophosphamide (Cytoxan)[1] is used for mobilizing stem cells. G-CSF plus cyclophosphamide is preferred in patients who are treated with lenalidomide plus dexamethasone induction, who are older than 65 years, or who have received such therapy for over 4 months. Plerixafor (Mozobil) may also be used for mobilization of hematopoietic stem cells. It is advisable to collect 6×10^6 CD34+ cells/kg, which is sufficient for two transplants in patients less than 65 years of age.

The timing of autologous SCT takes into account the patient's wishes, and it may be done early (when the patient recovers from stem cell collection) or delayed until relapse. There is no difference in overall survival among patients who receive an autologous SCT immediately following collection of stem cells and those who receive it at first relapse. In general, we prefer an early transplant because this provides a better quality of life and time without therapy.

Melphalan[3] 200 mg/m² is the preferred conditioning regimen for autologous SCT. This regimen has fewer adverse side effects than melphalan[3] 140 mg/m² plus total body irradiation. If a

---

[1]Not FDA approved for this indication.

patient obtains a VGPR or CR with the first transplant, little benefit results from a second (tandem) transplant.

The mortality rate with autologous SCT is approximately 1%. Unfortunately, multiple myeloma is not eradicated, and the autologous peripheral stem cells are contaminated by myeloma cells or their precursors.

Bone marrow transplantation from an identical twin donor (syngeneic) is the treatment of choice if such a donor is available. Results are superior to allogeneic transplantation.

Maintenance Therapy Following Autologous Stem Cell Transplantation

In a large prospective study, multiple myeloma patients were given a tandem transplant and then randomized to no maintenance, pamidronate (Aredia)[1] maintenance, or pamidronate plus thalidomide maintenance. Although thalidomide improved the response rate and overall survival, it often resulted in peripheral neuropathy. Moreover, the overall survival benefit was lost with longer follow-up.

Two randomized trials have tested the value of lenalidomide as maintenance therapy following stem cell transplantation. An overall survival benefit has been seen in one. An increased risk of second cancers was noted in both trials. Further follow-up is needed. In another randomized trial improved overall survival with bortezomib maintenance has been reported, but it is not clear whether the benefit is due to the maintenance therapy or differences in induction therapy between the two groups. We recommend that low-risk patients who have obtained a VGPR from autologous SCT be followed without maintenance therapy unless they are part of a clinical trial. Maintenance, usually for a fixed duration, is considered in intermediate and high-risk patients and in patients who fail to achieve a VGPR following autologous SCT. In intermediate and high-risk patients bortezomib-based maintenance is preferred. In standard risk patients who fail to achieve a VGPR following stem cell transplantation lenalidomide maintenance is preferred.

Allogeneic Transplantation

Allogeneic bone marrow transplantation has been tested in myeloma but treatment-related mortality is high and graft-versus-host disease is a troublesome problem. Further, only 5% to 10% of patients with multiple myeloma are eligible. Allogeneic transplantation is currently not recommended for routine use outside of a clinical trial. An exception to this are young patients with high-risk disease in first relapsed after autologous transplantation who are willing to assume the high treatment-related mortality associated with allogeneic SCT.

Nonmyeloablative allogeneic (mini-allo) transplant following autologous SCT has been tested but has not been consistently shown to be superior to autologous SCT. The mortality is 10% to 15%, and there is a substantial risk of graft-versus-host disease. Efforts are being made to reduce the toxicity of this approach. Currently, we believe that nonmyeloablative approaches should be limited to clinical trials.

Initial Therapy for Patients Who Are Ineligible for Autologous Stem Cell Transplantation

Since the 1960s, alkylating agent–based chemotherapy with oral administration of melphalan and prednisone[1] (MP) has been the standard of therapy, producing an objective response in 50% to 60% of patients and a median survival of 2 to 3 years. Various combinations of alkylating agents have been developed, but a large meta-analysis, based on data from 6633 patients in 30 trials comparing MP with various combinations of alkylating agents, was performed by the Myeloma Trialists' Collaborative Group. Although the response rate was higher with combination chemotherapy, there was no survival benefit over melphalan.

The addition of thalidomide to MP (MPT regimen)[1] has been found to produce overall survival improvement in 3 of the 6 randomized trials conducted so far. In contrast, a regimen of melphalan, prednisone, and lenalidomide has not demonstrated a survival benefit compared with MP.

Another option for patients who are not candidates for transplantation is bortezomib (Velcade) plus MP (the VMP regimen). VMP is superior to MP in terms of overall survival. Peripheral neuropathy is lower with once-weekly bortezomib.

However, melphalan-based regimens have several adverse effects, and are falling out of favor. Further in a recent randomized trial, Rd was found to be superior to MPT. Thus, the initial therapy for patients not eligible foe transplantation now resembles that of transplant eligible patients. Currently, we prefer MPT, VCD[1] or Rd for standard-risk myeloma patients, VCD or VMP for intermediate-risk patients, and VMP or VRd[1] for high-risk patients.

We continue the initial chemotherapy regimen for approximately 12 months; however, if Rd is used, treatment is continued till progression if treatment is well-tolerated. There is risk of myelodysplasia from continued treatment with alkylating agents. The role of thalidomide, bortezomib, and lenalidomide for maintenance therapy in transplant-ineligible patients has not been proved.

In general, lenalidomide or thalidomide therapy requires prophylaxis with aspirin[1] (81 mg or 325 mg daily) against deep venous thrombosis. If lenalidomide or thalidomide is given with high-dose dexamethasone,[1] doxorubicin (Adriamycin),[1] liposomal doxorubicin (Doxil), or erythropoietin (Epogen, Procrit), then full-dose warfarin (Coumadin)[1] or a low-molecular-weight heparin[1] should be given. Anticoagulation is also recommended for patients who have a history of previous thromboembolic events, are on bedrest, are obese, or have any other risk factors for thrombosis. Bortezomib does not produce a higher risk of thromboembolic events.

Relapsed or Refractory Multiple Myeloma

Almost all patients with multiple myeloma who survive eventually relapse. If relapse occurs more than 6 months after treatment is discontinued, the initial chemotherapy regimen should be reinstituted. Most patients respond again, but the duration and quality of response are usually inferior to the initial response. Since the turn of the century, thalidomide, bortezomib, and lenalidomide have been introduced and have revolutionized the treatment of patients with relapsed or refractory disease. Objective responses occur in approximately one third of patients and have a median duration of approximately 12 months. The addition of dexamethasone increases the response rate.

Thalidomide

Thalidomide (Thalomid) is usually instituted in a dose of 50 to 100 mg daily and, if necessary, escalated to 200 mg daily if tolerated. The duration of response is approximately 1 year. Side effects include sedation, fatigue, constipation, rash, deep venous thrombosis, edema, bradycardia, and hypothyroidism. Virtually all patients develop a sensorimotor peripheral neuropathy. The use of thalidomide in pregnancy is contraindicated, and the STEPS program (System for Thalidomide Education and Prescribing Safety) must be followed to prevent teratogenic effects.

Bortezomib

Bortezomib (Velcade) is a proteasome inhibitor that produces a response rate of approximately 35% in patients with relapsed or refractory myeloma. The median duration of response is 12 months. The response to bortezomib is rapid and usually occurs within 1 to 2 months.

Adverse effects include fatigue, anorexia, nausea, vomiting, fever, diarrhea, constipation, anemia, asthenia, neutropenia, and thrombocytopenia. The most troublesome side effect is peripheral neuropathy, which occurs in 35% to 40% of patients. The neuropathy is often painful, but does improve in most patients after discontinuing bortezomib. The risk of neuropathy can be greatly reduced by using bortezomib in a once weekly subcutanoeus schedule.

Lenalidomide

Lenalidomide (Revlimid) produces an objective response in approximately 30% of patients with relapsed or refractory multiple myeloma. The major side effects are cytopenias, and the dose needs to be modified accordingly.

Multiple Myeloma

---

[1]Not FDA approved for this indication.
[3]Exceeds dosage recommended by the manufacturer.

---

[1]Not FDA approved for this indication.

Carfilzomib

Carfilzomib (Kyprolis) is a new proteasome inhibitor approved for the therapy of patients with multiple myeloma who have received at least 2 prior therapies, including both an immunomodulatory agent and bortezomib, and have disease progression on or within 60 days of the completion of the last therapy. Carfilzomib needs to be administered intravenously twice weekly. In a recent randomized trial, the combination of carfilzomib, lenalidomide, and dexamethasone (KRd) was found to have superior response rate, progression free survival, and overall survival compared with Rd.

Pomalidomide

Pomalidomide (Pomalyst) is an analog of lenalidomide and thalidomide. It has shown significant clinical activity in patients who are refractory to both bortezomib and lenalidomide (dual refractory). It is approved for patients with multiple myeloma who received at least 2 prior therapies, including both lenalidomide and bortezomib, and have disease progression on or within 60 days of the completion of the last therapy. It is administered orally at a dose of 2–4 mg daily for 21 days every 28 days. The major side effects are cytopenias and fatigue.

Panobinostat

Panobinostat (Farydak) is a pan-deacetylase inhibitor that is approved for the treatment of multiple myeloma in patients who have received at least 2 prior therapies, including both an immunomodulatory agent and bortezomib. It is administered orally at a starting dose of 20 mg three times a week for 2 weeks every 3 weeks. It is given in combination with bortezomib and dexamethasone. It is associated with severe diarrhea in approximately 25% of patients, so use must be restricted to younger patients in good performance status who have failed other treatments but are not yet refractory to bortezomib. If the drug is used, the dose must preferably be lower than the approved label dose, and the dose of bortezomib and dexamethasone must also be reduced to a once weekly schedule. The drug approval carries a black-box warning concerning cardiac arrhythmias and severe diarrhea.

Other New Drugs

New drugs that are in clinical trials include new proteasome inhibitors (NPI-0052 [marizomib][5] and MLN9708 [ixazomib][5]), and anti-CD38 monoclonal antibodies (e.g., daratumumab)[5]. Bendamustine (Treanda)[1] and Elotuzumab (HuLuc63)[5] are also being studied.

Supportive Therapy
Radiotherapy

Palliative radiation in a dose of 20 to 30 Gy should be limited to patients who have disabling pain and a well-defined focal process that has not responded to chemotherapy. Analgesics in combination with chemotherapy usually can control the pain. This approach is preferred to local radiation because pain often occurs at another site, and local radiation does not benefit the patient with systemic disease. In addition, the myelosuppressive effects of radiotherapy and chemotherapy are cumulative and can restrict future therapy. Radiation is required for spinal cord compression from plasmacytoma. Postsurgical radiation after stabilization of fractures or impending fractures is rarely needed.

Hypercalcemia

Hypercalcemia must be suspected if the patient has anorexia, nausea, vomiting, polyuria, increased constipation, weakness, confusion, stupor, or coma. If it is untreated, renal insufficiency usually develops. Hydration, preferably with isotonic saline and prednisone (25 mg orally four times daily), is effective in many patients with mild to moderate hypercalcemia (calcium <13 mg/dL). If more-severe hypercalcemia occurs, zoledronic acid (Zometa) at a dose of 4 mg intravenously over 15 minutes or pamidronate (Aredia) 90 mg given intravenously over at least 2 hours is indicated. Calcitonin (Miacalcin) may be used if rapid reduction of calcium levels is needed. Hemodialysis may be necessary for extremely severe hypercalcemia. The dosage of prednisone must be reduced and discontinued as soon as possible.

Renal Insufficiency

Approximately 20% of patients with multiple myeloma have a serum creatinine level of 2.0 mg/dL or more at diagnosis. Myeloma kidney (cast nephropathy) and hypercalcemia are the two major causes. Myeloma kidney is characterized by the presence of large, waxy, laminated casts in the distal and collecting tubules. Some light chains are very nephrotoxic, but no specific amino acid sequence of the nephrotoxic light chain has been identified.

Dehydration, infection, nonsteroidal antiinflammatory agents, and radiographic contrast media can contribute to acute kidney failure. Hyperuricemia or amyloid deposition can produce renal insufficiency. Nephrotic syndrome rarely occurs in multiple myeloma unless amyloidosis is present.

Maintenance of a high fluid intake producing 3 L of urine per 24 hours is important for preventing kidney failure in patients with Bence Jones proteinuria. If hyperuricemia occurs, allopurinol (Zyloprim) in doses of 300 mg daily provides effective therapy.

Acute kidney failure should be treated promptly with appropriate fluid and electrolyte replacement. Patients with kidney failure should be treated with either VCD or VTD to reduce the tumor mass as quickly as possible. A trial of plasmapheresis is reasonable in an attempt to prevent chronic dialysis. Hemodialysis and peritoneal dialysis are equally effective and are necessary for patients with symptomatic azotemia.

Anemia

Almost every patient with multiple myeloma eventually becomes anemic. Increased plasma volume from the osmotic effect of the M protein can produce hypervolemia and can spuriously lower the hemoglobin and hematocrit values. Patients with significant symptoms should be considered for red blood cell transfusion. If a transfusion is indicated, irradiated leukocyte-reduced red cells are preferred.

In patients with newly diagnosed myeloma, induction chemotherapy is often associated with a prompt improvement in hemoglobin levels, so it is better to avoid the use of erythropoietin. Erythropoietin (Epogen) should be seriously considered in relapsed patients receiving chemotherapy who have a persistent, symptomatic hemoglobin level of 10 g/dL or less.

Erythropoietin reduces the transfusion requirement and increases hemoglobin concentration in more than half of patients. Those with low serum erythropoietin values are more likely to respond. Most physicians proceed with a trial of erythropoietin 150 U/kg three times weekly, or 40,000 U once a week. Darbepoetin, a long-lasting erythropoietin (Aranesp), may be given weekly or biweekly. Erythropoietin should be discontinued when the hemoglobin reaches 11 g/dL.

Skeletal Lesions

Bone lesions manifested by pain and fractures are a major problem. A skeletal radiographic survey should be repeated at 6-month intervals, or sooner if pain develops. Patients should be encouraged to be as active as possible because confinement to bed increases demineralization of the skeleton. Trauma must be avoided because even mild stress can result in a fracture. Fixation of long bone fractures or impending fractures with an intramedullary rod and methyl methacrylate gives excellent results.

All patients with multiple myeloma who have lytic lesions, pathologic fractures, or severe osteopenia should receive an IV bisphosphonate. Pamidronate (Aredia) 90 mg intravenously over 2 hours every 4 weeks or zoledronic acid (Zometa) 4 mg intravenously over 15 minutes every 4 weeks are equally efficacious. The dosage of bisphosphonates should be reduced with renal insufficiency. Because renal insufficiency or nephrotic-range proteinuria can occur, serum creatinine and 24-hour urine protein monitoring is necessary. One should seriously consider stopping the IV bisphosphonate in patients who have responsive or stable disease after 2 years of therapy. In other patients we recommend reducing the dose to once every 3 months.

Bisphosphonates should be resumed upon relapse with new-onset skeletal-related events. Osteonecrosis of the jaw can occur

---

[1]Not FDA approved for this indication.
[5]Investigational drug in the United States.

in patients receiving bisphosphonates. Although the relationship is unclear, it is essential to obtain a complete dental evaluation and perform preventive dental treatment before beginning bisphosphonates. The patient should practice good oral hygiene during therapy. Invasive procedures (especially dental extractions) should be avoided during bisphosphonate therapy. Osteonecrosis of the jaw should be managed conservatively.

Vertebroplasty or kyphoplasty may be helpful for patients with an acute compression fracture of the spine. Both have been associated with pain relief. Results appear to be better when the procedure is performed shortly after the compression fracture. Leakage of the methyl methacrylate is a potential adverse event. A choice between vertebroplasty and kyphoplasty depends upon the expertise of the physician performing the procedure.

Infections
Bacterial infections are more common in patients with myeloma than in the general population. All patients should receive pneumococcal and influenza immunizations despite their suboptimal antibody response. Substantial fever is an indication for appropriate cultures, chest radiography, and consideration of antibiotic therapy. The greatest risk for infection is during the first 2 months after chemotherapy is initiated. The use of prophylactic antibiotics is controversial. Antiviral prophylaxis (acyclovir [Zovirax] 400 mg twice daily or valacyclovir [Valtrex] 500 mg once daily) should be given to all patients receiving bortezomib because of the increased risk of herpes zoster. Intravenous immunoglobulin (IVIg, Gammagard)[1] may be helpful in selected patients who have recurrent serious infections despite the use of prophylactic antibiotics. It is inconvenient, associated with side effects, and very expensive. Consequently, few of our patients receive IVIg.

Hyperviscosity Syndrome
Symptoms of hyperviscosity can include oronasal bleeding, gastrointestinal bleeding, blurred vision, neurologic symptoms, or congestive heart failure. Most patients have symptoms when the serum viscosity measurement is more than 4 cP, but the relationship between serum viscosity and clinical manifestations is not precise. The decision to perform plasmapheresis, which promptly relieves the symptoms of hyperviscosity, should be made on clinical grounds rather than serum viscosity levels. Hyperviscosity is more common in immunoglobulin (IgA) myeloma than in IgG myeloma.

Extradural Myeloma (Cord Compression)
The possibility of cord compression must be considered if weakness of the legs or difficulty in voiding or defecating occurs. The sudden onset of severe radicular pain or severe back pain with neurologic symptoms suggests compression of the spinal cord. MRI or CT of the entire spine must be performed immediately. Radiation therapy in a dose of approximately 30 Gy is beneficial in about one half of patients. Dexamethasone (Decadron)[1] should be administered in addition to radiation therapy. Surgical decompression is necessary only if the neurologic deficit does not improve.

Venous Thromboembolism
Patients with multiple myeloma have an increased risk of venous thromboembolism. This is due to the malignancy itself as well as therapy with lenalidomide or thalidomide with corticosteroids. Aspirin[1] given prophylactically is beneficial. If there is a history of previous thromboembolic events or if other risk factors are present, anticoagulation with full-dose warfarin or low-molecular-weight heparin is indicated.

Emotional Support
All patients with multiple myeloma need substantial and continuing emotional support. The physician's approach must be positive in emphasizing the potential benefits of therapy. It is reassuring for patients to know that some survive for 10 years or more. It is vital that the physician caring for patients with multiple myeloma has the interest and capacity for dealing with incurable disease over the span of years with assurance, sympathy, and resourcefulness.

[1]Not FDA approved for this indication.

References
Attal M, Lauwers-Cances V, Marit G, et al. Lenalidomide maintenance after stem-cell transplantation for multiple myeloma. N Engl J Med 2012;366:1782–91. http://dx.doi.org/10.1056/NEJMoa1114138, Prepublished on 2012/05/11 as.

Krishnan A, Pasquini MC, Logan B, et al. Autologous haemopoietic stem-cell transplantation followed by allogeneic or autologous haemopoietic stem-cell transplantation in patients with multiple myeloma (BMT CTN 0102): a phase 3 biological assignment trial. Lancet Oncol 2011;12:1195–203. http://dx.doi.org/10.1016/S1470-2045(11)70243-1, Prepublished on 2011/10/04 as.

Kumar SK, Rajkumar SV, Dispenzieri A, et al. Improved survival in multiple myeloma and the impact of novel therapies. Blood 2008;111:2516–20.

Kyle RA, Rajkumar SV. Epidemiology of the plasma-cell disorders. Best Pract Res Clin Haematol 2007;20:637–64.

Kyle RA, Yee GC, Somerfield MR, et al. American Society of Clinical Oncology 2007 clinical practice guideline update on the role of bisphosphonates in multiple myeloma. J Clin Oncol 2007;25:2464–72.

Lacy MQ, Hayman SR, Gertz MA, et al. Pomalidomide (CC4047) plus low-dose dexamethasone as therapy for relapsed multiple myeloma. J Clin Oncol 2009;27:5008–14.

McCarthy PL, Owzar K, Hofmeister CC, et al. Lenalidomide after stem-cell transplantation for multiple myeloma. N Engl J Med 2012;366:1770–81.

Mikhael JR, Dingli D, Roy V, et al. Management of newly diagnosed symptomatic multiple myeloma: updated mayo stratification of myeloma and risk-adapted therapy (mSMART) consensus guidelines 2013. Mayo Clin Proc 2013;88: 360–76.

Moreau P, Pylypenko H, Grosicki S, et al. Subcutaneous versus intravenous administration of bortezomib in patients with relapsed multiple myeloma: a randomised, phase 3, non-inferiority study. Lancet Oncol 2011;12:431–40. http://dx.doi.org/10.1016/S1470-2045(11)70081-X, Prepublished on 2011/04/22 as.

Palumbo A, Hajek R, Delforge M, et al. Continuous lenalidomide treatment for newly diagnosed multiple myeloma. N Engl J Med 2012;366:1759–69.

Rajkumar SV, Jacobus S, Callander NS, et al. Lenalidomide plus high-dose dexamethasone versus lenalidomide plus low- dose dexamethasone as initial therapy for newly diagnosed multiple myeloma: an open-label randomised controlled trial. Lancet Oncol 2010;11:29–37.

Rajkumar SV, et al. International Myeloma Working Group updated criteria for the diagnosis of multiple myeloma. Lancet Oncol 2014;15:e538–48.

Siegel DS, Martin T, Wang M, et al. A phase 2 study of single-agent carfilzomib (PX-171–003-A1) in patients with relapsed and refractory multiple myeloma. Blood 2012;120:2817–25.

Sonneveld P, Schmidt-Wolf IGH, van der Holt B, et al. Bortezomib induction and maintenance treatment in patients with newly diagnosed multiple myeloma: results of the randomized phase III HOVON-65/ GMMG HD4 trial. J Clin Oncol 2012;30:2946–55.

Stewart AK, et al. Carfilzomib, lenalidomide, and dexamethasone for relapsed multiple myeloma. N Engl J Med 2015;372(2):142–52.

MYELODYSPLASTIC SYNDROMES

Method of
Jamile M. Shammo, MD

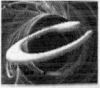

CURRENT DIAGNOSIS

- Myelodysplastic syndromes are diseases of the elderly.
- Chronic unexplained cytopenias should be evaluated to rule out myelodysplastic syndromes.
- Bone marrow biopsy with cytogenetic testing is necessary to make the diagnosis.
- The international prognostic scoring system (IPSS) is an important tool for risk stratification and choice of therapy.

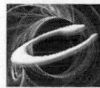

CURRENT THERAPY

- Myelodysplastic syndromes are divided into two broad categories per the IPSS: low-risk and high-risk disease.
- Patients with low-risk disease should receive supportive care and hematopoietic growth factors; those with del 5q abnormality should be treated with lenalidomide (Revlimid).
- Patients with high-risk disease should be treated with a hypomethylating agent and should be considered for allogeneic stem cell transplantation.

Epidemiology
The myelodysplastic syndromes (MDS) represent a group of heterogeneous clonal stem cell disorders that affect the elderly.

The reported annual incidence of approximately 3.3 per 100,000 of the general U.S. population is highest among whites and non-Hispanics. The onset of MDS before the age of 50 years is rare; the incidence rises with age such that in patients older than 70 years, the incidence exceeds 20 per 100,000 persons. Men are nearly twice as likely to be affected as women (4.5 vs. 2.7 per 100,000 per year).

Risk Factors

De novo or primary MDS refers to cases in which no prior toxic exposure can be documented. Therapy-related MDS, on the other hand, occurs in patients who have been treated with chemotherapy or radiotherapy or both. Median onset of therapy-related MDS varies with the agents used and is usually 2 to 5 years after initial exposure to chemotherapy.

Tobacco use and occupational exposure to solvents and agricultural chemicals have also been associated with the development of MDS. A minority of MDS cases might have evolved from an antecedent hematologic disorder such as aplastic anemia or paroxysmal nocturnal hemoglobinuria. Several rare and inherited genetic disorders have been associated with a higher risk of developing MDS, such as Fanconi's anemia, dyskeratosis congenita, Diamond-Blackfan syndrome, and Shwachman-Diamond syndrome.

Pathophysiology

A variety of pathophysiologic processes have been described in association with MDS, resulting in ineffective hematopoiesis and peripheral cytopenias. These processes include excessive apoptosis of myeloid progenitors, abnormal responses to cytokines and growth factors, epigenetic aberrations resulting in gene silencing, chromosomal abnormalities, and a defective bone marrow microenvironment. Recently, several somatic point mutations affecting multiple genes have been identified in up to 50% of MDS patients. However, the initiating event or molecular pathway is unknown.

Clinical Manifestations

Some patients with MDS are asymptomatic, but the majority present with peripheral blood cytopenias of which anemia is the most common. Patients might complain of fatigue, weakness, and exercise intolerance. Those with significant neutropenia and thrombocytopenia can present with infections or bleeding. Systemic symptoms are less common, but when present they can herald disease progression to more-advanced forms. Similarly, the presence of Sweet's syndrome (acute febrile neutrophilic dermatosis) can herald transformation to acute leukemia. Organomegaly and lymphadenopathy are uncommon. Infection is the cause of death in approximately 20% to 35% of cases. Transformation to acute leukemia occurs in about 30% of all patients.

Diagnosis

The diagnosis of MDS can be challenging, because its clinical and pathologic characteristics can overlap with other disorders such as aplastic anemia, myeloproliferative neoplasms, and acute leukemia.

A thorough history and physical examination should be performed on every patient with one or more peripheral blood cytopenias, along with basic laboratory tests such as iron studies, vitamin B$_{12}$, and folic acid levels. However, many disorders can cause pancytopenia; therefore, consideration for a hematology referral should be entertained for the evaluation of pancytopenia or persistent otherwise-unexplained cytopenias, in which case a bone marrow biopsy may be necessary.

The diagnosis of MDS requires an evaluation of the peripheral blood smear, a bone marrow biopsy and aspirate to ascertain the presence of myeloid dysplasia; iron stains, which are necessary for the detection of ring sideroblasts; and cytogenetic studies to detect abnormal clones. Bone marrow dysplasia involving at least 10% of the cells of a specific myeloid lineage is the hallmark of MDS. Cytogenetic abnormalities can be found in up to 70% of patients with de novo MDS and 95% of of patients with therapy-related MDS, and their presence can aid in making the diagnosis, particularly when dysplastic features are not prominent.

Differential Diagnosis

MDS should be distinguished from a broad number of disorders including megaloblastic anemia, aplastic anemia, large granular lymphocyte leukemia, myelofibrosis, copper deficiency, and HIV infection, which can cause anemia and dysplastic features in the bone marrow. Exposure to certain drugs and toxins can result in marrow dysplasia. These include mycophenolate mofetil (Cellcept), ganciclovir (Cytovene), lead, and excess zinc. Such changes are reversible once the offending agent is discontinued. The diagnosis of MDS can be made by performing a bone marrow biopsy to detect dysplasia and rule out other disorders that can also cause pancytopenia.

Classification and Risk Stratification

Since 1982, there have been various proposals for the classification and risk stratification of MDS. The French-American-British (FAB) classification scheme was the first attempt developed to address the broad range of morphologic features and clinical outcomes in MDS. It identified five subtypes based on morphology and percentage of marrow blasts: refractory anemia (RA), refractory anemia with ringed sideroblasts (RARS), refractory anemia with excess blasts (RAEB), refractory anemia with excess blasts in transformation (RAEB-t), and chronic myelomonocytic leukemia (CMML). This classification allowed MDS to be separated into distinct subsets relative to survival and acute leukemia evolution.

The World Health Organization (WHO) revised the FAB system to further refine MDS subsets by adding a category of refractory cytopenia with multilineage dysplasia, recognizing 5q-deletion syndrome as a separate clinical and pathologic entity, and lowering the blast percentage from 30% to 20% to diagnose acute myelogenous leukemia (AML). The WHO system was revised in 2008 to recognize the entity of refractory cytopenia with unilineage dysplasia, among other changes (Table 1).

The International Prognostic Scoring System (IPSS) was introduced to address the variability in prognosis within FAB subtypes. It predicts survival and risk of evolution to acute leukemia. The IPSS is calculated by adding scores assigned to three variables: blast cell count, cytogenetics, and number of cytopenias, thereby identifying four distinct groups (Table 2). The IPSS is the most widely used clinical tool to predict the prognosis and clinical behavior of patients with various forms of MDS and to guide choice of therapy (Table 3). A revised version of the IPSS (IPSS-R) is available.

Treatment

A variety of therapeutic options exist for the treatment of MDS patients spanning the spectrum from supportive care to allogeneic stem cell transplantation. Choice of therapy should take into account the patient's age, comorbidities, and the IPSS score.

The treating physician should consider the ultimate goal of therapy and whether it is intended to cure, extend survival, or merely palliate symptoms. In the first decade of the 21st century, several novel therapeutic options for MDS have emerged.

Supportive Care

Supportive care has been the cornerstone of MDS therapy for decades; it includes red blood cell transfusion for symptomatic anemia, platelet transfusion to reduce the risk of or to treat bleeding, and use of hematopoietic growth factors such as erythropoiesis stimulating agents (ESA) and colony-stimulating factors such as granulocyte colony-stimulating factor (G-CSF) (Filgrastim [Neupogen])[1] and granulocyte-macrophage colony-stimulating factor (GM-CSF) (Sargramostim [Leukine]).[1]

There are two currently available ESAs: a recombinant human erythropoietin (rhu-EPO; epoetin alfa [Epogen, Procrit])[1] and a super-sialylated form of EPO (darbepoetin alfa [Aranesp]).[1] These are considered the standard of care for the treatment of anemia in

---

[1]Not FDA approved for this indication.

TABLE 1 WHO 2008 Classification of Myelodysplastic Syndromes

DISEASE	BLOOD FINDINGS	BONE MARROW FINDINGS
Refractory cytopenias with unilineage dysplasia (RCUD) Refractory anemia (RA) Refractory neutropenia (RN) Refractory thrombocytopenia (RT)	Unicytopenia or bicytopenia* No or rare blasts (<1%)†	Unilineage dysplasia: ≥10% of the cells in one myeloid lineage <5% blasts <15% of erythroid precursors are ring sideroblasts
Refractory anemia with ring sideroblasts (RARS)	Anemia No blasts	>15% of erythroid precursors are ring sideroblasts Erythroid dysplasia only <5% blasts
Refractory cytopenia with multilineage dysplasia (RCMD)	Cytopenia(s) No or rare blasts (<1%)† No Auer rods <10^9/L monocytes	Dysplasia in ≥10% of the cells in ≥2 myeloid lineages (neutrophils, erythroid precursors, megakaryocytes) <5% blasts in marrow No Auer rods ±15% ring sideroblasts
Refractory anemia with excess blasts-1 (RAEB-1)	Cytopenia(s) <5% blasts† No Auer rods <10^9/L monocytes	Unilineage or multilineage dysplasia 5 5%–9% blasts No Auer rods
Refractory anemia with excess blasts-2 (RAEB-2)	Cytopenia(s) 5%–19% blasts ±Auer rods‡ <10^9/L monocytes	Unilineage or multilineage dysplasia 10%–19% blasts ±Auer rods‡
Myelodysplastic syndrome, unclassified (MDS-U)	Cytopenias ≤1% blasts†	Unequivocal dysplasia in <10% of cells in one or more myeloid cell lines when accompanied by a cytogenetic abnormally considered as presumptive evidence for a diagnosis of MDS <5% blasts
MDS associated with isolated del(5q)	Anemia Usually normal or increased platelet count No or rare blasts (<1%)	Normal to increased megakaryocytes with hypolobated nuclei <5% blasts Isolated del(5q) cytogenetic abnormality No Auer rods

*Bicytopenia is occasionally observed. Cases with pancytopenia should be classified as MDS-U.
†If the marrow myeloblast percentage is <5% but there are 2%–4% myeloblasts in the blood, the diagnostic classification is RAEB-1. Cases of RCUD and RCMD with 1% myeloblasts in the blood should be classified as MDS-U.
‡Cases with Auer rods and <5% myeloblasts in the blood and <10% in the marrow should be classified as RAEB-2.

TABLE 2 International Prognostic Scoring System for MDS (IPSS)

	SCORE VALUE				
PROGNOSTIC VARIABLE	0	0.5	1.0	1.5	2.0
Marrow blasts (%)	<5	5–10	11–20	—	21–30
Karyotype*	Good	Intermediate		Poor	
Cytopenia†	0/1	2/3			

*Cytogenetics: Good = normal, -Y alone, del(5q) alone, del(20q) alone; Poor = complex (≥3 abnormalities) or chromosome 7 anomalies; Intermediate = other abnormalities. This excludes karyotypes t(8;21), inv16 and t(15;17), which are considered to be AML, not MDS.
†Cytopenias: neutrophil count <1800/μL, platelets <100,000/μL, Hb <10 g/dL.

TABLE 3 Survival and Progression by IPSS Risk Category

RISK CATEGORY	% IPSS POP.	OVERALL SCORE	MEDIAN SURVIVAL (Y) IN THE ABSENCE OF THERAPY	25% AML PROGRESSION (Y) IN THE ABSENCE OF THERAPY
Low	33	0	5.7	9.4
Intermediate 1	38	0.5–1.0	3.5	3.3
Intermediate 2	22	1.5–2.0	1.2	1.1
High	7	≥2.5	0.4	0.2

Abbreviation: IPSS = International Prognostic Scoring System.

patients with low-risk MDS. A predictive model for response to such treatment has been developed by the Nordic MDS study group to guide patient selection. In general, patients with a serum EPO level less than 500 mU/mL and low transfusion burden are likely to respond by improving their hemoglobin level and reducing their need for transfusions.

Immunomodulatory Drugs

The novel class of immunomodulatory drugs includes thalidomide (Thalomid)[1] and lenalidomide (Revlimid). Thalidomide was investigated initially with some success in patients with low-risk disease. However, its use was compromised because of poor tolerability. Lenalidomide has been approved for the treatment of patients with low-risk MDS who harbor deletion 5q abnormality, because it was shown in clinical trials to result in transfusion independence in about two thirds of such patients.

Hypomethylating Agents

Currently, two hypomethylating agents are approved for the treatment of MDS: 5-azacitidine (Vidaza) and decitabine (Dacogen). These agents are cytosine analogues known to inhibit and deplete DNA methyltransferase, which adds a methyl group to cytosine residues in newly formed DNA, resulting in the formation of a hypomethylated DNA in vitro. The exact mechanism of action in vivo has not yet been identified.

Results of randomized clinical trials comparing these agents to best supportive care in patients with MDS have demonstrated a statistically significant improvement in response rate and hematologic improvement. It has been shown for the first time that treatment with 5-azacitidine, when compared to other conventional therapies in MDS, resulted in prolonged survival in patients with high-risk disease by the IPSS. Both drugs have myelosuppressive properties and comparable response rates.

Immunosuppressive Therapy

Immunosuppressive therapy with antithymocyte globulin (Thymoglobulin)[1] or cyclosporine (Neoral)[1] (or both) was evaluated in several clinical trials and was shown to result in durable hematological responses in a subset of MDS patients, specifically, younger patients with low-risk disease, hypocellular marrows, human leukocyte antigen (HLA)-DR 15 phenotype, and low transfusion need.

Hematopoietic Stem Cell Transplantation

Allogeneic stem cell transplantation is the only curative therapy for MDS patients; this option is feasible for a small subset: typically, younger patients with good performance status and an available HLA-matched donor. Approximately 40% of patients can be cured with this modality. The recent introduction of reduced-intensity conditioning regimens and nonmyeloablative transplants has resulted in expanding the age limit for performing the procedure, reducing transplant-related complications and mortality. However it has been associated with a higher risk of relapse. Because stem cell transplantation is associated with a high rate of treatment-related death—estimated at 39% at 1 year—and the development of acute and chronic graft versus host disease, such treatment is recommended to patients with high-risk disease. Patients with low-risk MDS may be considered for transplant at disease progression.

Conclusion and Future Direction

MDS is a chronic disease characterized by features reminiscent of bone marrow failure states with a variable propensity for leukemic evolution. It is curable only by allogeneic stem cell transplantation, which is feasible in only a small subset of patients. For all others, the treatment goal is aimed at improving quality of life and prolonging survival. A variety of ongoing clinical trials are evaluating novel agents and combinations of drugs to further optimize the outcome of patients with this disease. Meanwhile, a great deal of research is focused on understanding the molecular underpinning of this disease to enhance our understanding of the biology of this heterogenous disorder.

[1]Not FDA approved for this indication.

References

Bejar R, Stevenson K, Abdel-Wahab O, et al. Clinical effect of point mutations in myelodysplastic syndromes. NEJM 2011;364:2496–506.

Bennett JM, Catovsky D, Daniel MT, et al. Proposals for the classification of the myelodysplastic syndromes. Br J Haematol 1982;51:189–99.

Brunning RD, Porwit A, Orazi A, et al. Myelodysplastic syndromes/neoplasms. In: Swerdlow S, Campo E, Lee Harris N, et al., WHO Classification of Tumors of Hematopoietic and Lymphoid Tissues. 4th ed. Lyon, France: IARC; 2008. p. 88–103.

Cutler CS, Lee SJ, Greenberg P, et al. A decision analysis of allogeneic bone marrow transplantation for the myelodysplastic syndromes: Delayed transplantation for low-risk myelodysplasia is associated with improved outcome. Blood 2004;104(2):579–85.

Fenaux P, Mufti GJ, Hellstrom-Lindberg E, et al. Efficacy of azacitidine compared with that of conventional care regimens in the treatment of higher-risk myelodysplastic syndromes: A randomized, open-label, phase III study. Lancet Oncol 2009;10:223–32.

Godley LA, Larson RA. Therapy-related myeloid leukemia. Semin Oncol 2008;35:418–29.

Greenberg PL. The smoldering myeloid leukemic states: Clinical and biologic features. Blood 1983;61:1035–44.

Greenberg P, Cox C, LeBeau MM, et al. International scoring system for evaluating prognosis in myelodysplastic syndromes. Blood 1997;89:2079–88.

Greenberg PL, Tuechler H, Schanz J, et al. Revised International Prognostic Scoring System (IPSS-R) for myelodysplastic syndromes. Blood 2012;120:2454–65.

Hellstrom-Lindberg E, Negrin R, Stein R, et al. Erythroid response to treatment with G-CSF plus erythropoietin for the anaemia of patients with myelodysplastic syndromes: Proposal for a predictive model. Br J Haematol 1997;99(2):344–51.

Kantarjian H, Issa JP, Rosenfeld CS, et al. Decitabine improves patient outcomes in myelodysplastic syndromes: Results of a phase III randomized study. Cancer 2006;106(8):1794–803.

List A, Dewald G, Bennett J, et al. Lenalidomide in the myelodysplastic syndrome with chromosome 5q deletion. N Engl J Med 2006;355(14):1456–65.

Ma X, Does M, Raza A, Mayne ST. Myelodysplastic syndromes: Incidence and survival in the United States. Cancer 2007;109(8):1536–42.

Martino R, Iacobelli S, Brand R, et al. Retrospective comparison of reduced-intensity conditioning and conventional high-dose conditioning for allogeneic hematopoietic stem cell transplantation using HLA-identical sibling donors in myelodysplastic syndromes. Blood 2006;108:836–46.

Molldrem J, Leifer E, Bahceci E, et al. Antithymocyte globulin for treatment of the bone marrow failure associated with myelodysplastic syndromes. Ann Intern Med 2002;137(3):156–63.

Nisse C, Lorthois C, Dorp V, et al. Exposure to occupational and environmental factors in myelodysplastic syndromes: Preliminary results of a case-control study. Leukemia 1995;9:693–9.

Owen C, Barnett M, Fitzgibbon J. Familial myelodysplasia and acute myeloid leukaemia—a review. Br J Haematol 2008;140:123–32.

Rollison DE, Howlader N, Smith MT, et al. Epidemiology of myelodysplastic syndromes and chronic myeloproliferative disorders in the United States, 2001–2004 using data from the NAACCR and SEER programs. Blood 2008;112:45–52.

Silverman LR, Demakos EP, Peterson BL, et al. Randomized controlled trial of azacitidine in patients with the myelodysplastic syndrome: A study of the Cancer and Leukemia Group B. J Clin Oncol 2002;20(10):2429–40.

Soppi E, Nousiainen T, Seppa A, Lahtinen R. Acute febrile neutrophilic dermatosis (Sweet's syndrome) in association with myelodysplastic syndromes: A report of three cases and a review of the literature. Br J Haematol 1989;73(1):43–7.

Tefferi A, Vardiman JW. Myelodysplastic syndromes. N Engl J Med 2009;361(19):1872–85.

Vardiman JW, Harris NL, Brunning RD. The World Health Organization (WHO) classification of myeloid neoplasms. Blood 2002;100:2292–302.

NEUTROPENIA

Method of
Laurence A. Boxer, MD

CURRENT DIAGNOSIS

- Neutropenia is defined as a blood absolute neutrophil count that is less than two standard deviations below the normal population mean.
- Neutropenia can be inherited or acquired.
- Neutropenia usually arises from decreased production of neutrophil precursor cells in the marrow.
- Neutropenia can result from accelerated destruction of neutrophils.
- Neutropenia can occur with pancytopenia.

- Isolated neutropenia can occur with chronic idiopathic neutropenia or drug-induced neutropenia.
- Neutropenia can indicate an underlying systemic disease.
- Severe chronic neutropenia (ANC counts less than 500/µL) increases susceptibility to bacterial or fungal infections.

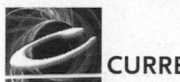

CURRENT THERAPY

- Therapy with granulocyte colony-stimulating factor (G-CSF) increases blood neutrophil counts for many types of neutropenia.
- Hematopoietic stem cell transplantation is indicated in patients who develop myelodysplasia or acute myelogenous leukemia in disorders such as severe congenital neutropenia or Shwachman–Diamond syndrome.
- Hematopoietic stem cell transplantation is useful for aplastic anemia or hemophagocytic lymphohistiocytosis complicating congenital syndromes of neutropenia.

Neutropenia is an absolute neutrophil count (ANC), calculated as the white blood cell (WBC) count times percentage of neutrophils and bands, more than two standard deviations below the normal mean. Normal neutrophil counts must be stratified for age and race. Neutropenia may be characterized as mild, moderate, or severe. Mild neutropenia has an ANC of 1000 to 1500/µL; moderate neutropenia has an ANC 500 to 1000/µL, and severe neutropenia has an ANC of less than 500/µL. The stratification aids in predicting the risk of pyogenic infections; only patients with severe neutropenia are at risk for pyogenic infection and susceptible to life-threatening infections.

Normal values for the total WBC change during childhood and into adolescence. The mean WBC and neutrophil count at birth are high, followed by a rapid fall beginning at 12 hours after birth until of the end of the first week. Thereafter, values are stable until 1 year of age. A slow, steady decline in the WBC count occurs throughout childhood until it reaches the adult value during adolescence.

For persons older than 12 months, the lower limit of normal for the neutrophil count is 1500/µL in whites and 1200/µL for blacks. The relatively lower limit in blacks is linked to the absence of the Duffy blood group antigen on red cells, also known as the Duffy antigen receptor for chemokines (DARC). Although the mechanism for the association of neutropenia with the lack of the DARC on red blood cells is unknown, it is possible that antigen expression regulates neutrophil storage within the bone marrow and mediates neutrophil release from the bone marrow.

Epidemiology

Neutropenia is a relatively common finding. Acute neutropenia is often well tolerated and normalizes rapidly. Neutropenia is sometimes a secondary finding in a patient who has far more significant disorders and who may be at risk for infectious complications and might require a thorough investigation. Congenital and cyclic neutropenia are quite rare; they occur in one case per million population. Both congenital and cyclic neutropenia occur much more commonly in whites compared to blacks.

Pathophysiology

Acute neutropenia evolves over a few days and occurs when neutrophil use is rapid and production is impaired. Chronic neutropenia can last months or years and can arise from reduced production, increased destruction, or excessive splenic sequestration of neutrophils. Neutropenia may be classified by whether it arises secondarily to causes extrinsic to marrow myeloid cells (Table 1), which is common; as an acquired disorder of myeloid progenitor cells (Table 2), which is less common; or as an intrinsic defect affecting proliferation and maturation of myeloid progenitor cells, which is rare (Table 3).

Transient neutropenia often follows viral infections. Neutropenia accompanying common childhood viral diseases occurs during the first or second day of illness and can persist for 3 days. Often it corresponds to a period of acute viremia. Bacterial sepsis can be a serious cause of neutropenia. In contrast, chronic neutropenia can accompany infection with Epstein–Barr virus, cytomegalovirus, or HIV.

Etiology
Drug-Induced Neutropenia

Drug-induced neutropenia constitutes one of the most common causes of neutropenia in adults. The majority of patients are older than 65 years. Drug-induced neutropenia has several underlying mechanisms, including immune mediation, hypersensitivity reactions, direct toxic effects, and idiosyncratic causes that are distinct from the severe neutropenia that predictably occurs after administration of cytoreductive cancer drugs or radiotherapy.

Drug-induced neutropenia secondary to immune mechanisms often develops quickly and is accompanied by fever. Drugs such as propylthiouracil or penicillin that act as haptens can stimulate antibody formation, whereas drugs such as quinine induce immune-complex formations. The antidepressant drugs and antipsychotic drugs are major causes of neutropenia. Patients

TABLE 1 Causes of Neutropenia Extrinsic to Marrow Myeloid Cells

CAUSE	ETIOLOGIC FACTORS AND AGENTS	ASSOCIATED FINDINGS
Infection	Viruses, bacteria, protozoa, rickettsia, fungi	Redistribution from circulating to marginating pools, impaired production, accelerated destruction
Drug induced	Phenothiazines sulfonamides, anticonvulsants, penicillins, aminopyrine	Hypersensitivity reaction (fever, lymphadenopathy, rash, hepatitis, nephritis, pneumonitis, aplastic anemia), antineutrophil antibodies
Immune neutropenia	Alloimmune, autoimmune	Variable arrest from metamyelocyte to segmented neutrophils in bone marrow
Reticuloendothelial sequestration	Hypersplenism	Anemia, thrombocytopenia, neutropenia
Bone marrow replacement	Malignancy (lymphoma, metastatic solid tumor, etc.)	Presence of immature myeloid and erythroid precursors in peripheral blood
Cancer chemotherapy or radiation therapy to bone marrow	Suppression of myeloid cell production	Bone marrow hypoplasia, anemia, thrombocytosis

Reprinted with permission from Newburger PE, Boxer LA. Leukopenia. In Kliegman RM, Stanton BF, St. Gene III JW, et al (eds). Nelson Textbook of Pediatrics, 19th ed. Philadelphia: Saunders, 2011, p. 747.

TABLE 2   Acquired Disorders of Myeloid Cells

CAUSE	ETIOLOGIC FACTORS AND AGENTS	ASSOCIATED FINDINGS
Aplastic anemia	Stem cell destruction and depletion	Pancytopenia
Vitamin B_{12} or folate deficiency	Malnutrition; congenital deficiency of B_{12} absorption, transport, and storage; vitamin avoidance	Megaloblastic anemia, hypersegmented neutrophils
Acute leukemia, chronic myelogenous leukemia	Bone marrow replacement with malignant cells	Pancytopenia, leukocytosis
Myelodysplasia	Dysplastic maturation of stem cells	Bone marrow hypoplasia with megaloblastoid red cell precursors, thrombocytopenia
Prematurity with birth weight <2 kg	Impaired regulation of myeloid proliferation and reduced size of postmitotic pool	Maternal preeclampsia
Chronic idiopathic neutropenia	Impaired myeloid proliferation and/or maturation	None
Paroxysmal nocturnal hemoglobinuria	Acquired stem cell defect secondary to mutation of *PIG-A* gene	Pancytopenia, thrombosis

From Newburger PE, Boxer LA. Leukopenia. In Kliegman RM, Stanton BF, St. Gene III JW, et al (eds). Nelson Textbook of Pediatrics, 19th ed. Philadelphia: Saunders, 2011, p. 748.

TABLE 3   Intrinsic Disorders of Myeloid Precursor Cells

SYNDROME	INHERITANCE	GENE	CLINICAL FEATURES (INCLUDING STATIC NEUTROPENIA UNLESS OTHERWISE NOTED)
Primary Disorder of Myelpoiesis			
Cyclic neutropenia	AD	*ELA2*	Periodic oscillation (21-day cycles) in ANC
Severe congenital neutropenia	AD XL	*ELA2, GFL1,* others *WAS*	Risk of MDS and AML Neutropenic variant of Wiskott–Aldrich syndrome
Kostmann's syndrome	AR	*HAX1*	Neurologic abnormalities, risk of MDS and AML
Disorders of Ribosomal Function			
Shwachman–Diamond syndrome	AR	*SBDS*	Pancreatic insufficiency, variable neutropenia, other cytopenias, metaphyseal dysostosis
Dyskeratosis congenital	Telomerase defects XL AD AR	 *DKC1* *TER* *TERT*	Nail dystrophy, leukoplakia, reticulated hyperpigmentation of the skin 30%–60% develop bone marrow failure
Disorders of Granule Sorting			
Chédiak–Higashi syndrome	AR	*LYST*	Partial albinism, giant granules in myeloid cells, platelet storage-pool defect, impaired NK cell function, hemophagocytic lymphohistiocytosis
Griscelli's syndrome type II	AR	*RAB27a*	Partial albinism, impaired NK cell function, hemophagocytic lymphohistiocytosis
Cohen's syndrome	AR	*COH1*	Developmental delay, facial dysmorphism, retinopathy
Hermansky–Pudlak syndrome type II	AR	*AP3P1*	Cyclic neutropenia, partial albinism
p14 deficiency	Probable AR	*MAPBPIP*	Partial albinism, decreased B and T cells
Disorders of Metabolism			
Glycogen storage disease, type 1b	AR	*G6PT1*	Hepatic enlargement, growth retardation, impaired neutrophil motility
G6Pase, catalytic subunit 3, deficiency	AR	*G6PC3*	Structural heart defects, urogenital abnormalities, venous angiectasia
Barth's syndrome	XL	*TAZ1*	Episodic neutropenia, dilated cardiomyopathy, methylglutaconic aciduria, pancytopenia
Pearson's syndrome	Mitochondrial (DNA deletions)		Vacuolization of erythroid and myeloid precursors, ringed sideroblasts, pancytopenia
Neutropenia in Disorders of Immune Function			
Common variable immunodeficiency	Familial sporadic	*TNFRSF13B*	Hypogammaglobulinemia, other immune system defects

TABLE 3   Intrinsic Disorders of Myeloid Precursor Cells—cont'd

SYNDROME	INHERITANCE	GENE	CLINICAL FEATURES (INCLUDING STATIC NEUTROPENIA UNLESS OTHERWISE NOTED)
IgA deficiency	Unknown	Unknown or *TNFRSF13B*	Decreased IgA
Severe combined immunodeficiency	AR, XL	Multiple loci	Absent humoral and cellular immune function
Hyper-IgM syndrome	XL	*HIGM1*	Absent IgG, elevated IgM, autoimmune cytopenia
WHIM syndrome	AD	*CXCR4*	Warts, hypogammaglobulinemia, infections, myelokathexis
Cartilage–hair hyperplasia	AR	*RMKP*	Lymphopenia, short-limbed dwarfism, metaphysical chondrodysplasia, fine sparse hair
Schimke immune–osseous dysplasia	Probable AR	*SMARCAL1*	Lymphopenia, pancytopenia, spondyleopiphyseal dysplasia, growth retardation, renal failure

Abbreviations: AD=autosomal dominant; AML=acute myelogenous leukemia; ANC=absolute neutrophil count; AR=autosomal recessive; Ig=immunoglobulin; MDS=myelodysplasia; NK=natural killer; WHIM=warts, hypogammaglobulinemia, infections, and myelokathexis; XL=X-linked.
Modified with permission from Newburger PE, Boxer LA. Leukopenia. In Kliegman RM, Stanton BF, St. Gene III JW, et al (eds). Nelson Textbook of Pediatrics, 19th ed. Philadelphia Saunders, 2011, p. 748.

receiving these drugs need to be monitored to assure that they are not developing neutropenia. Late-onset neutropenia can occur after rituximab (Rituxan) therapy, but the mechanism of neutropenia remains unknown. Neutropenia associated with anticonvulsants is rare and arises from a hypersensitivity reaction to the arene oxide metabolites.

Drug-induced neutropenia often is accompanied by fever, rash, lymphadenopathy, hepatitis, nephritis, pneumonitis and sometimes aplastic anemia. In all instances, the offending drugs causing neutropenia should be discontinued.

Bone Marrow Disorders

Various acquired bone marrow disorders lead to neutropenia and are accompanied by anemia and thrombocytopenia. Hematologic malignancies and metastatic solid tumors suppress myelopoiesis by infiltrating the bone marrow. Neutropenia often accompanies myelodsysplastic disorders or pre-leukemia syndromes, which are characterized by peripheral cytopenias and macrocytic blood cells. Aplastic anemia can arise from immune-mediated damage to stem cells, leading to neutropenia and other cytopenias.

Splenic Enlargement

Splenic enlargement resulting from intrinsic splenic disease such as storage diseases or systemic causes of splenic hyperplasia arising from inflammation, neoplasia, or hemolytic anemias can lead to neutropenia. Most often the neutropenia is mild to moderate and is accompanied by corresponding degrees of thrombocytopenia and anemia. Cytopenias are often improved by successfully treating the underlying disease. In selected cases, splenectomy is a necessary option to restore the neutrophil count, but this maneuver results in increased risk of infections by encapsulated bacterial infections.

Immune Neutropenia

Immune neutropenia is associated with circulating anti-neutrophil antibodies. The antibodies lead to neutrophil destruction by complement-mediated lysis or splenic phagocytosis of antibody-coated neutrophils. The causes of immune neutropenia include alloimmune neonatal neutropenia. This form of neonatal neutropenia occurs after transplacental passive transfer of maternal alloantibodies directed against specific antigens on the infant's neutrophils. This disorder occurs in 0.3% of pregnancies and is accompanied with delayed separation of the umbilical cord. The infant can suffer mild skin infections, fever, and pneumonia within the first or second week of life. Neutropenia resolves by 7 weeks of age, reflecting the decay of maternal antibodies in the infant's circulation. Supportive care and appropriate antibiotics for clinical infection often is the only treatment required. In selected cases,

the neutropenia does respond to granulocyte–colony stimulating factor (G-CSF). The use of G-CSF may be required in infants with pneumonia or sepsis.

Neutropenia in the newborn can also arise from the passive transfer of antibodies from the mother, who may herself have neutropenia arising from disorders such as systemic lupus erythematosus. Management is the same as in patients with alloimmune neonatal neutropenia.

Autoimmune Neutropenia

Autoimmune neutropenia in older children or adults is analogous to autoimmune hemolytic anemia and immune thrombocytopenia. The disorder is distinguished from other forms of neutropenia by the demonstration of anti-neutrophil antibodies and the appearance of myeloid hyperplasia on bone marrow examination. Autoimmune neutropenia can accompany a variety of autoimmune disorders and can occur in children with congenital or acquired immune deficiencies, including common variable immune deficiency or autoimmune lymphoproliferative syndrome. Treatment with G-CSF (filgrastim [Neupogen]) is usually effective in raising the ANC and preventing infection.

Autoimmune neutropenia of infancy is often a benign condition. In one study, it occurred with an annual incidence of approximately one per 100,000 among children between infancy and ten years. The age of diagnosis usually is between 5 and 15 months and it is not associated with other autoimmune diseases. Children with autoimmune neutropenia of infancy can present with minor infections such as otitis media, gingivitis, respiratory tract infections, and cellulitis. Diagnosis often is considered following a blood count revealing neutropenia. In the 20% of children with more-severe infections, G-CSF therapy is recommended. The median duration of disease is approximately 17 months.

Ineffective Myelopoiesis

Ineffective myelopoiesis can result from congenital or acquired vitamin B_{12} or folic acid deficiency. Though vitamin deficiencies are rare in pediatrics, neutropenia can accompany starvation or marasmus in infants and can be seen in adolescents with anorexia nervosa or the extended use of antibiotics, such as trimethoprim–sulfamethoxazole (Bactrim), which can inhibit folic acid metabolism.

The intrinsic disorders of myeloid precursors affect proliferation and maturation of myeloid precursor cells and are rare. Table 3 presents a classification based on genetics and molecular mechanisms; selected disorders are discussed later.

Severe congenital neutropenia is a rare heterogeneous disorder characterized by chronic severe neutropenia (ANC less than 200/µL) and arrest of neutrophil maturation at the promyelocyte/myelocyte stage owing to a constitutional genetic defect. Severe congenital neutropenia is usually diagnosed in the first year of life; patients present with frequent and/or life-threatening infections. Autosomal recessive, autosomal dominant, and sporadic forms exist. The autosomal recessive form is known specifically as Kostmann's syndrome and is due to *HAX1* mutations. The majority of the autosomal dominant forms of severe congenital neutropenia are attributed to *ELANE* mutations (formerly known as *ELA2*). Patients typically show monocytosis and eosinophilia and suffer from recurrent, severe pyogenic infections, especially of the skin, mouth, and rectum. The anemia of chronic inflammation is often present. Approximately 20% of patients develop acute myelogenous leukemia or myelodysplasia associated with monosomy 7.

Cyclic Neutropenia
Cyclic neutropenia is characterized by regular oscillations in neutrophil number, with a mean of 21-day cycles and a nadir period of 3 to 6 days associated with reciprocal monocytosis due to mutations in the *ELANE* gene. Patients present with recurrent fevers, mouth ulcers, and other infections. Serious infections can occur during the ANC nadirs including pneumonia, periodontitis, and recurrent ulcerations of the oral, vaginal, intestinal, and rectal mucosa leading to life-threatening gram-negative infections or clostridial sepsis. Many adult patients experience abatement of symptoms, and the cycles tend to be less noticeable.

Disorders of Ribosomal Function
Shwachman–Diamond syndrome is an autosomal recessive disorder characterized by pancreatic insufficiency and neutropenia. Shwachman–Diamond syndrome is caused by proapoptotic mutations of the *SBDS* gene, which encodes a protein that is involved in ribosome biogenesis or RNA processing. In most patients, the initial symptoms are usually diarrhea or failure to thrive because of malabsorption. In infancy the disorder is often accompanied by neutropenia with ANC less than 1000/µL and is associated with hypoplastic myelopoiesis. Myelosplasia and acute myeloid leukemia have been associated with this syndrome.

Dyskeratosis congenita consists of a classical triad of abnormal skin pigmentation, nail dystrophy, and oral leukoplakia. Other common abnormalities include epiphora, developmental delay, pulmonary disease, and hair loss. Often the classical triad is not present. The mean age of onset is 10 years. Pancytopenia is the hematologic form of dyskeratosis congenita. Approximately 50% of patients develop aplastic anemia. Genetic defects have been identified in about 60% of patients, of whom the large majority have the X-linked form caused by mutations in the *DKC1* gene encoding the nucleolar protein dyskerin, resulting in defective ribosomal function. Ten percent of patients with autosomal dominant disease have associated mutations in the telomerase components. Screening can be accomplished by identifying short telomeres.

Disorders of Metabolism
Barth's syndrome is an X-linked recessive disorder caused by mutations in the tafazzin gene. It is characterized by cardiomyopathy, skeletal muscle weakness, neutropenia, and growth retardation. The ANC in Barth's syndrome ranges from 500/µL to 1500/µL. There is a wide variation in clinical presentation. Patients can have severe debilitating disease to nearly asymptomatic forms. Patients have reduced concentrations and altered composition of cardiolipin in the inner mitochondrial membrane, which leads to changes in mitochondrial architecture and function. The mechanism of neutropenia remains unknown.

Glycogen storage disease type 1b (GSD1b) represents an inborn error of metabolism and is caused by inherited defects of the glucose-6-phosphatase complex, which has roles in both glycogenolysis and gluconeogenesis. Clinical features include hypoglycemia, hyperlipidemia, and hyperuricemia with hepatomegaly, growth retardation, osteopenia, and kidney enlargement. Neutropenia and neutrophil dysfunction are hallmarks

of GSD1b. The ANC often falls below 500/µL. Both myeloid hypercellularity and hypocellularity have been reported in bone marrows.

Severe congenital neutropenia has been associated with mutations of glucose-6-phosphatase catalytic subunit 3 (GSPC3) gene. The metabolic disorder is associated with severe permanent neutropenia with granulocyte maturation arrest and several other clinic manifestations, including highly superficial visible veins, urogenital malformation, and cardiac disorders.

Genetic Disorders
The constellation of autosomal recessive disorders combining neutropenia with partial albinism features and defective vesicular transport is derived from abnormalities in formation or trafficking of lysosome-related organelles.

Chédiak–Higashi syndrome is an autosomal recessive disorder characterized by increased susceptibility to infections arising from defective intercellular granule movement. The syndrome includes partial oculocutaneous albinism, a mild bleeding diathesis, progressive peripheral neuropathy, and a predisposition to the hemophagocytic syndrome following viral infections. Chédiak–Higashi syndrome is characterized by the presence of giant cytoplasmic granules in neutrophils, monocytes, and lymphocytes and arises as a disorder of subcellular vesicular dysfunction with increased fusion of cytoplasmic granules in all granule-bearing cells. Chédiak–Higashi syndrome derives from mutations in the lysosomal-trafficking regulator gene *LYST*. The only treatment to cure is hematopoietic stem cell transplantation.

Griscelli syndrome type II is a rare autosomal disorder characterized by hypopigmentation of the skin, presence of large clumps of pigment in the hair shafts, and abnormal accumulation of end-stage melanosomes in melanocytes. Unlike Chédiak–Higashi syndrome, peripheral granulocytes do not exhibit giant granules. Patients have mild neutropenia, which is caused by a mutation in *RAB27a*; the mutation leads to a predisposition to the hemophagocytic syndrome. The only curative to treatment is hematopoietic stem cell transplantation.

Disorders of Immune Function
Congenital immunologic disorders that have severe neutropenia as a clinical feature include common variable immune deficiency, X-linked hyper-IgM syndrome, and WHIM (warts, hypogammaglobulinemia, infections, myelokathexis) syndrome. WHIM syndrome arises from a mutation of receptors mediating adhesion to the extracellular matrix in myeloid cells (see Table 3).

Idiopathic Neutropenia
Acquired idiopathic chronic neutropenia affects children and adults. Patients have an ANC persistently less than 500 µL and are afflicted with recurrent pyogenic infections involving the skin, mucous membranes lungs, and lymph nodes. Bone marrow examination reveals variable patterns of myeloid formation.

Clinical Manifestations
Patients with neutrophil counts less than 500/µL chronically are at substantial risk for developing infections, primarily from the endogenous flora or from nosocomial organisms. Often patients with isolated chronic neutropenia with ANC less than 200/µL do not experience serious infection because the remainder of the immune system remains intact. In contrast, patients whose neutropenia is secondary to acquired disorders of production such as with cytotoxic therapy, immunosuppressive drugs, or radiation therapy are likely to develop serious bacterial infection because the neutropenia is also accompanied by compromised immune function.

Among the most common clinical presentations of profound neutropenia are fever greater than 38 °C, aphthous stomatitis, gingivitis, cellulitis, furunculosis, perirectal inflammation, colitis, sinusitis, and otitis media. In patients whose ANC is less than

200/μL, hepatic abscesses, recurrent pneumonias, and septicemia can occur. Isolated neutropenia does not heighten the patient's susceptibility to parasitic or viral infections or to bacterial meningitis. Among the most common pathogens causing infections in neutropenic patients are *Staphylococcus aureus* and Gram-negative bacteria. The common signs and symptoms of infection and inflammation such as exudate, fluctuant abscesses, and regional lymphadenopathy are generally reduced in the absence of neutrophils because of the inability to form pus.

Diagnosis

Evaluation of patients with neutropenia begins with a thorough history, physical examination, family history, and screening laboratory tests (Table 4). Isolated absolute neutropenia has a limited number of causes (see Tables 1 to 4). Attention to the duration and severity of the neutropenia influences the extent of laboratory examination. Patients with chronic neutropenia beginning in infancy and a history of recurrent fevers and chronic gingivitis should have WBC counts and differential determined three times weekly for 6 weeks to evaluate the periodicity of cyclic neutropenia. Bone marrow aspiration and biopsy should be performed on selective patients to assess cellularity. Cytogenetic analysis with special stains for detecting leukemia and other malignant disorders should be attained. In patients with suspected intrinsic defects in myeloid progenitors, the selection of further laboratory tests is determined by the duration and severity of the neutropenia and associated physical findings (see Table 4).

Patients with severe chronic neutropenia, cyclic neutropenia, or idiopathic neutropenia should have blood counts attained at least twice yearly. Patients with severe congenital neutropenia should have complete blood counts obtained quarterly and annual bone

TABLE 4	Diagnostic Approach to Patients with Leukopenia

EVALUATION	ASSOCIATED CLINICAL DIAGNOSES
Initial Evaluation	
History of acute or chronic neutropenia	
General medical history	
Physical examination: stomatitis, gingivitis, dental defects, congenital anomalies	Congenital syndromes (Shwachman–Diamond, Wiskott–Aldrich, Fanconi anemia, dyskeratosis congenital, glycogen storage disease type Ib, disorders of vesicular transport, glucose-6-phosphate, catalytic subunit 3, immune deficiencies)
Spleen size	Hypersplenism
History of drug exposure	Drug-associated neutropenia
Complete blood count with differential and reticulocyte counts	Neutropenia, aplastic anemia, autoimmune cytopenias
Absolute Neutrophil Count <1000/μL, Evaluation of Acute-Onset Neutropenia	
Repeat blood counts in 3–4 wk	Transient myelosuppression (e.g., viral)
Serology and cultures for infectious agents	Active chronic infection with viruses (e.g., EBV, CMV), bacteria, mycobacteria, rickettsia
Discontinue drug(s) associated with neutropenia	Drug-associated neutropenia
Test for the presence of anti-neutrophil antibodies	Autoimmune neutropenia
Measure quantitative immunoglobulins (IgG, IgA, and IgM), lymphocyte subsets	Neutropenia associated with disorders of immune function
Absolute Neutrophil Count <500/μL on Three Separate Tests	
Bone marrow aspiration and biopsy, with cytogenetics	Severe congenital neutropenia, cyclic neutropenia, Shwachman–Diamond syndrome, myelokathexis; chronic or benign or idiopathic neutropenia
Serial CBCs (3/wk × 6 wk)	Cyclic neutropenia
Exocrine pancreatic function	Shwachman–Diamond syndrome
Skeletal radiographs	Shwachman–Diamond syndrome, cartilage–hair hypoplasia, Fanconi anemia
Absolute Lymphocyte Count <1000/μL	
Repeat blood counts in 3–4 wk	Transient leukopenia (e.g., viral)
Absolute Lymphocyte Count <1000/μL on Three Separate Tests	
HIV-1 antibody test	HIV-1 infection, AIDS
Quantitative IgG, IgA, IgM, lymphocyte subsets	Congenital or acquired disorders of immune function
Pancytopenia	
Bone marrow aspiration and biopsy	Bone marrow replacement by malignancy, fibrosis, granuloma, storage cells
Bone marrow cytogenetics	Myelodysplasia, leukemia
Vitamin B$_{12}$ and folate levels	Vitamin deficiencies

Abbreviations: ANC = absolute neutrophil count; CBC = complete blood count; CMV = cytomegalovirus; EBV = Epstein–Barr virus; Ig = immunoglobulin.
Modified with permission from Newburger PE, Boxer LA. Leukopenia. In Kliegman RM, Stanton BF, St. Gene III JW, et al (eds). Nelson Textbook of Pediatrics, 19th ed. Philadelphia Saunders, 2011, p. 747.

marrow aspirates with cytogenetics to determine if there is progression in those patients to myelodysplasia and/or acute myelogenous leukemia.

Treatment

Management of acquired transient neutropenia associated with malignancies, chemotherapy, or immunosuppressive chemotherapy requires prompt attention to the treatment of infections with broad-spectrum antibiotics. Often the infections are heralded only by fever, and sepsis is a cause of early death. It is imperative to treat infections early even before the results of blood cultures are known.

Therapy for severe chronic neutropenia is dictated by the clinical manifestation. Patients with severe chronic neutropenia with no evidence of repeated bacterial infections or chronic gingivitis require no specific therapy. Superficial infections in children with mild to moderate neutropenia may be treated with appropriate oral antibiotics. For patients who have invasive or life-threatening infections, broad-spectrum intravenous antibiotics should be started promptly.

Administration of G-CSF (filgrastim) can provide effective treatment of severe chronic neutropenia including severe congenital neutropenia, cyclic neutropenia, and chronic symptomatic idiopathic neutropenia. The routine use of G-CSF for the primary prophylaxis of neutropenia following chemotherapy for solid tumors of lymphoma may be indicated when therapeutic regimens are associated with an expected rate of febrile neutropenia of at least 20%. When neutropenia arises from sepsis, G-CSF can prove useful in patients with documented infections that do not respond to appropriate antimicrobial therapy, or when a prolonged delay in marrow recovery is anticipated, such as is found in the bone marrow transplant setting. Doses ranging from 2 to 50 µg/kg per day lead to dramatic increases in neutrophil counts, resulting in marked attenuation of infection and inflammation. Use of G-CSF is often helpful in patients who have immune or drug-induced neutropenias. Long-term use of G-CSF is often accompanied by moderate splenomegaly and mild thrombocytopenia.

Autoimmune neutropenia may be responsive to intermittent corticosteroids, especially if it is part of an underlying disease process such as systemic lupus erythematosus. Hematopoietic stem cell transplantation is indicated in patients who develop myelodysplasia or acute myelogenous leukemia as seen in disorders such as severe congenital neutropenia or Shwachman–Diamond syndrome. In those two disorders, chemotherapy is ineffective. Hematopoietic stem cell transplantation is also useful for aplastic anemia or hemophagocytic lymphohistiocytosis complicating syndromes mentioned earlier.

References

Boxer LA, Newburger PE. A molecular classification of congenital neutropenia syndromes. Pediatr Blood Cancer 2007;49:609–14.

Boxer LA, Blackwood RA. Leukocyte disorders: Quantitative and qualitative disorders of the neutrophil, Part 1. Pediatr Rev 1996;17:19–28.

Boztug K, Rosenberg PS, Dorda M, et al. Extended spectrum of human glucose-6-phosphatase catalytic subunit 3 deficiency: Novel genotypes and phenotypic variability in severe congenital neutropenia. J Pediatr 2012;160:679–83.

Bruin LA, Dassen A, Pajkrt D, et al. Primary autoimmune neutropenia in children: A study of neutrophil antibodies and clinical course. Vox Sang 2005;88:52–9.

Dale DC. Neutropenia and neutrophilia. In: Litchman MA, Buetler E, Kipps TJ, et al., editors: Williams Hematology. 8th ed. New York: McGraw Hill; 2010. p. 939–50.

Fioredda F, Calvillo M, Bonanomi S, et al. Congenital and acquired neutropenias consensus guidelines on therapy and follow-up in childhood from the Neutropenia Committee of the Marrow Failure Syndrome Group of the AIEOP (Associazione Italiana Emato-Oncologia Pediatrica). Am J Hematol 2012;87(2):238–43.

Grann VR, Ziv E, Joseph CK, et al. Duffy (Fy), DARC, and neutropenia among women from the United States, Europe and the Caribbean. Br J Haematol 2008;143:288–93.

Klein C, Grudzien M, Appaswamy G, et al. HAX1 deficiency causes autosomal recessive severe congenital neutropenia (Kostmann disease). Nat Genet 2007;39:86–92.

Melis D, Fulceri R, Parenti G, et al. Genotype/phenotype correlation in glycogen storage disease type 1b: A mutlicentre study and review of the literature. Eur J Pediatr 2005;164:501–8.

Welte K, Boxer LA. Severe chronic neutropenia: Pathophysiology and therapy. Semin Hematol 1997;34:267–78.

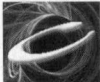

NON-HODGKIN LYMPHOMA

Method of
Andrew M. Evens, DO, MSc

CURRENT DIAGNOSIS

- The etiology of non-Hodgkin lymphoma (NHL) is not known, although several risk factors and conditions are associated with an increased risk of developing lymphoma, including congenital immunosuppression conditions (ataxia-telangiectasia, Wiskott-Aldrich syndrome, and X-linked lymphoproliferative syndrome), acquired immunodeficiency states (e.g., HIV and following any solid organ transplantation), viruses (e.g., human T-lymphotrophic virus (HTLV)-1 and hepatitis C virus), and autoimmune disorders (e.g., Sjögren's syndrome, celiac sprue, and systemic lupus erythematosus).
- Patients most commonly present clinically with enlarged lymph nodes, splenomegaly, and bone marrow involvement, but they may also present with other extranodal disease sites (e.g., stomach, skin, liver, bone, brain).
- NHL has many different clinicopathologic subtypes—more than 60 types are included in the WHO classification of lymphoid neoplasms. The natural history and prognosis of these vary greatly from indolent and slow-growing types (over many years) to highly aggressive (within weeks) types.
- Excisional lymph node resection is the gold standard procedure in establishing the precise NHL histology. Expert hematopathology review incorporating morphologic, immunophenotypic, and genetic features is essential for an accurate diagnosis.

CURRENT THERAPY

- Indolent lymphomas are low-grade and represent slow-growing non-Hodgkin lymphoma (NHL) that may remain stable with low tumor burden not warranting therapy for several years. The disease is highly responsive to treatment with a variety of treatment options (remission rates exceeding 90% with combined rituximab/chemotherapy), although the clinical course is characterized by repetitive relapses. Outside of early-stage disease and therapy with allogeneic stem cell transplantation, low-grade NHLs are not curable.
- Transformation of follicular lymphoma to a high-grade NHL occurs in 30% to 50%, or 3% to 4% of patients each year; it is less common in other indolent subtypes. Transformation is typically heralded by an aggressive change in the patient's clinical condition.
- Diffuse large B-cell lymphoma (DLBCL), the most common aggressive NHL, is curable in all stages in the majority of patients with rituximab (Rituxan)-based chemotherapy. A variety of primary extranodal DLBCL clinical subtypes warrant specialized therapy, such as primary central nervous system lymphoma.
- Long-term survivors are at increased risk for second cancers. The highest relative risk of developing a secondary malignancy occurs more than 21 to 30 years after original diagnosis. Patients who received an anthracycline (e.g., doxorubicin [Adriamycin]) as part of therapy are at a long-term increased risk for cardiovascular disease.

The term *malignant lymphoma* was originally introduced by Billroth in 1871 to describe neoplasms of lymphoid tissue. Generally speaking, lymphomas are neoplasms of the immune system. Traditionally, lymphomas are divided into Hodgkin lymphoma (HL) and non-Hodgkin lymphoma (NHL).

There are many different clinicopathologic subtypes of NHL (>60). By cell of origin, the majority of NHLs are of B-cell origin (85%–90%); T-cell NHLs account for 10% to 15% of lymphomas in the United States, whereas natural killer cell or histiocytic lymphomas are rare (<1%).

NHLs manifest most commonly clinically with involvement of lymph nodes, spleen, and bone marrow, but they can involve other extranodal sites (stomach, skin, liver, bone, brain, etc.). Peripheral blood involvement uncommonly occurs (leukemic phase of lymphoma). The natural history and prognosis vary greatly among the different subtypes of NHL from indolent subtypes that are often slow growing (i.e., therapy not warranted for years) to very aggressive and rapidly fatal types (within weeks) if not treated. Most NHL subtypes are highly treatable with initial remission rates over 90% to 95% using combined rituximab/chemotherapy; however, indolent NHLs are generally incurable, whereas the goal of treating most aggressive NHLs is cure.

Epidemiology

Currently, NHL represents approximately 5% of all cancer diagnoses, being the sixth most common cancer in women and the seventh in men. Estimates from the American Cancer Society indicate that in 2015 approximately 71,850 new cases of NHL will be diagnosed in the United States and approximately 19,790 people will die of the disease.

Geographic Distribution

The incidence of NHL varies throughout the world, in general being more common in developed countries, with rates in the United States of more than 15 per 100,000 compared with 1.2 per 100,000 in China. In the United States, the incidence rates of NHL more than doubled between 1975 and 1995 (Figure 1), representing one of the largest increases of any cancer. The increases have been more pronounced in whites, males, the elderly, and those with NHL diagnosed at extranodal sites. Similar findings have been reported in other developed countries. The incidence rates of NHL began to stabilize in the late 1990s, although the temporal trends vary by histologic subtype. Some of the increase may be related to improved diagnostic techniques and access to medical care and the increased risk of NHL attributable to HIV infection. However, additional factors are likely responsible for this unexpected increase in incidence.

Age

Overall, NHL incidence rises exponentially with increasing age. In persons older than 65 years, the incidence is 92.1 per 100,000 population compared with 7.1 per 100,000 population for persons aged 20 to 49 years (Figure 2). Except for high-grade lymphoblastic and Burkitt's lymphomas (the most common types of NHL seen in children and young adults), the median age at presentation for most subtypes of NHL exceeds 55 years.

Race and Ethnicity

Incidence varies by race and ethnicity, with whites overall having a higher risk than African Americans and Asian Americans (incidence rates increased 50% to 60% in whites compared with blacks). Most NHL subtypes are more common in whites than in blacks; however, peripheral T-cell lymphoma, mycosis fungoides, and Sézary syndrome occur more often in blacks than in whites.

Etiology and Risk Factors

Chromosomal Translocations and Molecular Rearrangements

Nonrandom chromosomal and molecular rearrangements play an important role in the pathogenesis of many lymphomas and often correlate with histology and immunophenotype. These chromosomal changes often result in oncogenic gene products; for example, t(11;14)(q13;q32) translocation results in overexpression of *bcl-1* (cyclin D1) in mantle-cell lymphoma, while translocation with 8q24 leads to c-*myc* overexpression in nearly all Burkitt's lymphomas and in 10-15% of patients with diffuse large B-cell lymphoma. Research to discover more information regarding the prognostic and pathogenic importance of these oncogenes continues, although they are currently used primarily in clinical practice for diagnostic purposes. Additionally, these genes serve as potential targets for novel therapeutics.

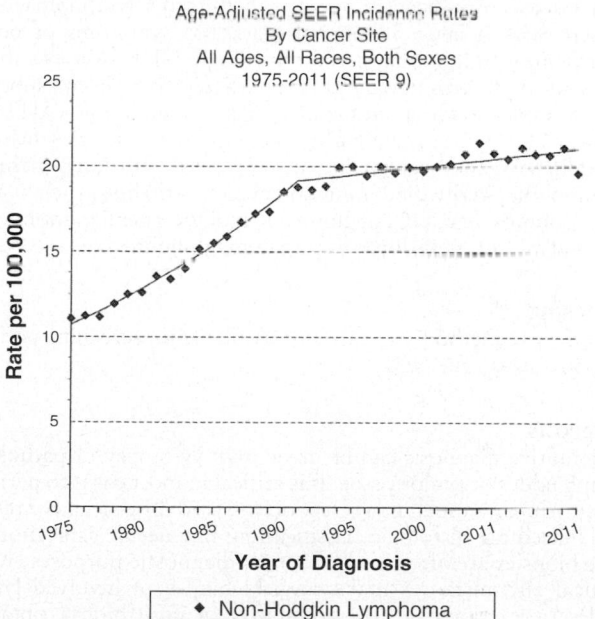

Figure 1. Surveillance Epidemiology and End Results (SEER) incidence rates for non-Hodgkin lymphoma since 1975. Rates are per 100,000 and are age-adjusted to the 2000 US Std Population (19 age groups - Census P25-1130). The modeled rates are the point estimates for the regression lines calculated by the Joinpoint Regression Program (Version 4.1.0, April 2014, National Cancer Institute). Incidence source: SEER 9 areas (San Francisco, Connecticut, Detroit, Hawaii, Iowa, New Mexico, Seattle, Utah, and Atlanta).

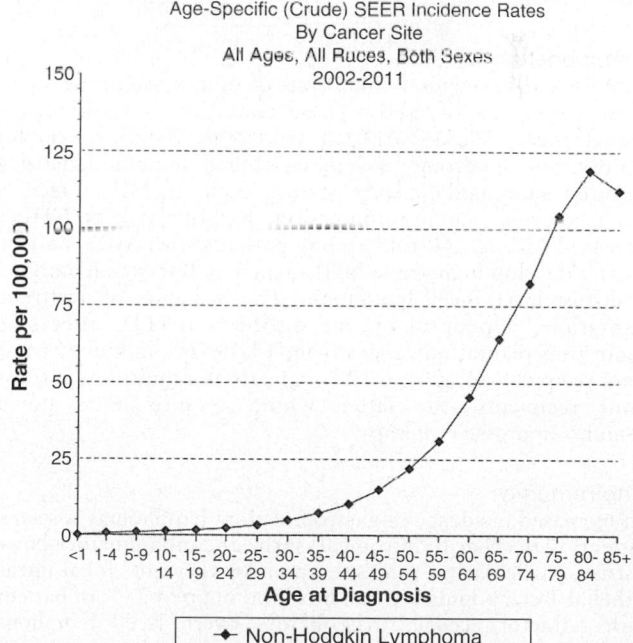

Figure 2. Surveillance Epidemiology and End Results (SEER) age-specific incidence rates for non-Hodgkin lymphoma. Incidence source: SEER 18 areas (San Francisco, Connecticut, Detroit, Hawaii, Iowa, New Mexico, Seattle, Utah, Atlanta, San Jose-Monterey, Los Angeles, Alaska Native Registry, Rural Georgia, California excluding SF/SJM/LA, Kentucky, Louisiana, New Jersey and Georgia excluding ATL/RG).

Environmental Factors

Environmental factors may also play a role in the development of NHL, including particular occupations (e.g., chemists, painters, mechanics, machinists) and chemicals (solvents and pesticides). Patients who receive chemotherapy or radiation therapy for any indication are also at increased risk for developing NHL as a secondary cancer as discussed later.

Viruses

Several viruses have been implicated in the pathogenesis of NHL, including Epstein-Barr virus, human T-cell lymphotropic virus 1 (HTLV-1), Kaposi's sarcoma–associated herpesvirus (KSHV, also known as human herpesvirus 8 [HHV-8]), and hepatitis C virus (HCV). Meta-analyses have shown 13% to 15% seroprevalence of HCV in certain geographic regions among persons with B-cell NHL. Further, HCV infection is associated with the development of clonal B-cell expansions and certain subtypes of NHL, particularly in the setting of essential (type II) mixed cryoglobulinemia. HTLV-1 is a human retrovirus that establishes a latent infection through reverse transcription in activated T-helper cells. A minority (5%) of carriers will develop adult T-cell leukemia lymphoma. KSHV-like DNA sequences are often detected in primary effusion lymphomas in patients with HIV infection and in those with multicentric (plasma cell variant) Castleman's disease.

Bacterial Infections

Gastric mucosa-associated lymphoid tissue (MALT) lymphoma is seen most often, but not exclusively, in association with *Helicobacter pylori* infection. Infection with *Borrelia burgdorferi* has been detected in about 35% of patients with primary cutaneous B-cell lymphoma in Scotland. Studies indicate that *Campylobacter jejuni* and immunoproliferative small intestinal disease are related. European reports have noted an association between infection with *Chlamydia psittaci* and ocular adnexal lymphoma. The infection was found to be highly specific and does not reflect a subclinical infection among the general population. Furthermore, remission of NHL to antibiotics have been reported. Attempts to confirm this association in the Western hemisphere have been unsuccessful.

Immunodeficiency

Patients with congenital conditions of immunosuppression are at increased risk of NHL. These conditions include ataxia-telangiectasia; Wiskott-Aldrich syndrome; X-linked lymphoproliferative syndrome; severe combined immunodeficiency; acquired immunodeficiency states, such as HIV infection; and iatrogenic immunosuppression. Relative risk of NHL is increased 150- to 250-fold among patients with AIDS; patients usually develop high grade NHLs, such as Burkitt's lymphoma or diffuse large B-cell lymphoma. The incidence of posttransplantation lymphoproliferative disorders (PTLD) after solid organ transplantation ranges from 1% to 2% in kidney transplant recipients to 10% to 12% in heart and multi-organ transplant recipients, the latter whom require more potent immunosuppressive therapy.

Autoimmunity

An increased incidence of gastrointestinal lymphomas is seen in patients with celiac (nontropical) sprue and inflammatory bowel disease, particularly Crohn's disease. An aberrant clonal intraepithelial T-cell population can be found in up to 75% of patients with refractory celiac sprue before overt T-cell lymphoma develops. Sjögren's disease is associated with a 6-fold increased risk of NHL overall with risk varying in part on severity of disease (5 to 200 times); moreover, the risk specifically of parotid marginal zone lymphoma is increased 1000-fold. Additionally, systemic lupus erythematosus and rheumatoid arthritis have been associated with a slightly increased risk of B-cell lymphoma.

Genetic Susceptibility

Several studies have implicated a role for genetic variants in the risk of NHL, including genes that influence DNA integrity and methylation, genes that alter B-cell survival and growth, and genes that involve innate immunity, oxidative stress, and xenobiotic metabolism.

Signs and Symptoms

Fever, weight loss, and night sweats, referred to as B symptoms, are more common in advanced and aggressive subtype NHLs, but they may be present at all stages and in any histologic subtype.

Low-Grade or Indolent Lymphomas

Painless, slowly progressive peripheral adenopathy is the most common clinical presentation in patients with low-grade lymphomas. Patients sometimes report a history of waxing and waning adenopathy before seeking medical attention. Spontaneous regression of enlarged lymph nodes can occur, which may cause a low-grade lymphoma to be confused with an infectious condition. Primary extranodal involvement and B symptoms are uncommon at presentation; however, both are more common in advanced or end-stage disease and in particular indolent NHL subtypes (e.g., gastric MALT and nongastric extranodal MALT). Bone marrow is frequently involved, sometimes in association with cytopenias. Splenomegaly is seen in about 40% of patients, but the spleen is rarely the only involved site besides the specific subtype of splenic marginal zone lymphoma.

High-Grade or Aggressive Lymphomas

The clinical presentation of high-grade lymphomas is more varied. Although the majority of patients present with adenopathy, more than one third present with extranodal involvement alone or with adenopathy, the most common sites being the gastrointestinal tract (including Waldeyer's ring), skin, bone marrow, sinuses, genitourinary tract, bone, and central nervous system. B symptoms are more common, occurring in about 30% to 40% of patients. Lymphoblastic lymphoma often manifests with an anterior superior mediastinal mass, superior vena cava syndrome, and leptomeningeal disease. American patients with Burkitt's lymphoma often present with a large abdominal mass and symptoms of bowel obstruction. In addition, certain histologic NHL subtypes manifest with symptoms unique to that particular lymphoma subtype; for example, angioimmunoblastic T-cell lymphoma (AITL) in addition to lymphadenopathy presents with disease features including organomegaly, skin rash, pleural effusions, arthritis, eosinophilia, and varied immunologic abnormalities such as positive Coombs' test, cold agglutins, hemolytic anemia, antinuclear antibodies, and polyclonal hypergammaglobulinemia.

Screening

No effective methods are currently available for screening patients or populations for NHL.

Diagnosis

A definitive diagnosis can be made only by biopsy of pathologic lymph nodes or tumor tissue. It is critical in most cases to perform an *excisional* lymph node resection to avoid false-negative results and inaccurate histologic classification; fine-needle aspirations or core biopsies are often insufficient for diagnostic purposes. When clinical circumstances make surgical biopsy of involved lymph nodes or extranodal sites prohibitive, a core biopsy obtained under CT or ultrasonographic guidance may suffice, but it often requires the integration of histologic examination and immunophenotypic and molecular studies for accurate diagnosis. A formal review by an expert hematopathologist is mandatory. In addition to morphologic review and immunostaining of tissue, other studies such as detailed cellular immunophenotyping and genotyping for relevant oncogenes are often needed to complete the diagnosis.

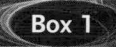

In addition to a detailed history and physical examination, baseline staging studies are warranted. These consist of blood tests (complete blood count with differential, complete metabolic panel including liver function tests, and lactate dehydrogenase), CT of chest, abdomen, and pelvis, and bilateral bone marrow biopsy and aspirate (Box 1). For aggressive NHL histologies, functional imaging is advocated (i.e., FDG-PET [fluorodeoxyglucose (^{18}F) positron emission tomography]), as is assessment of ejection fraction in anticipation of anthracycline-based chemotherapy. Testing for history of hepatitis B virus (HBV) is recommended, especially before starting anti-CD20 antibody therapy; evidence suggests that anti-CD20 antibody therapy (e.g., rituximab) increases the risk of HBV reactivation above the known rate of chemotherapy-associated reactivation. HIV serology should be obtained in patients with relevant risk factors, especially for diffuse large B-cell lymphoma (DLBCL) and Burkitt's lymphoma. HTLV-1 serology is recommended in patients who present with cutaneous T-cell lymphoma lesions, especially if they have hypercalcemia.

Examination of cerebrospinal fluid and consideration of intrathecal chemotherapy prophylaxis is applicable for patients with DLBCL with bone marrow, epidural, testicular, paranasal sinus, breast, or multiple extranodal sites (especially when in conjunction with elevated lactate dehydrogenase). Testing is mandatory for high-grade lymphoblastic lymphoma and Burkitt's lymphoma and its variants and primary central nervous system lymphoma if there is no evidence of increased intracranial pressure. Upper gastrointestinal endoscopy or gastrointestinal series with small bowel follow-through is recommended in patients with head and neck involvement (tonsil, base of tongue, nasopharynx) and those with primary gastrointestinal disease. Mantle cell lymphoma is associated with a high incidence of occult gastrointestinal involvement. In addition, MRI of the complete craniospinal axis and ocular examination is advocated with any brain or leptomeningeal disease involvement to rule out multifocal disease.

Classification

The 1965 Rappaport's Classification of malignant lymphomas was based solely on architecture and cytology. Since then, with the help of advanced cellular and genetic technologies, numerous new unique NHL entities have emerged. The latest classification is that of the World Health Organization (WHO) of 2008, which emphasizes immunophenotyping, genotyping, and clinical features (Box 2). Another way to group the many different lymphoma histologies is by clinical presentation and prognosis (Table 1).

Prognosis

International Prognostic Index

The International Prognostic Index was developed as a prognostic factor model for aggressive NHLs treated with doxorubicin-containing regimens (Box 3). In the pre-rituximab era, persons with no risk factors or one risk factor had a predicted 5-year overall survival of 73%, compared with 26% for high-risk patients with four or five risk factors. In the post-rituximab era, the survival rates have improved (see Box 3). A variant of the International Prognostic Index (IPI) is also useful in predicting outcome in patients with follicular low-grade lymphoma (FLIPI) or mantle cell lymphoma (MIPI) and in patients who have relapsed or refractory large B-cell lymphoma.

Molecular Profiling

DNA microarray technology for gene expression profiling has identified distinct prognostic subgroups in many NHL subtypes including DLBCL and follicular NHL. Patients with germinal center B-like DLBCL have an improved overall survival compared with other molecular profiles. Recent studies in follicular NHL have identified gene expression signatures that also predicted survival. Interestingly, the genes that defined the prognostic signatures were not expressed in the tumor cells, but were expressed by the nonmalignant tumor-infiltrating cells—primarily T cells, macrophages, and dendritic cells.

Treatment

The therapeutic approach for NHL differs for each clinicopathologic subtype. Chemotherapy remains the most important modality. However, in some instances, radiation therapy or, rarely, surgical resection plays a role. Biological approaches, including monoclonal antibodies and antibody-drug conjugates have shown significant activity and are now incorporated into most treatment paradigms. Autologous and allogeneic stem-cell transplantation are mostly reserved for patients with recurrent or refractory disease.

Indolent B-Cell Non-Hodgkin's Lymphomas

Indolent lymphomas are low-grade and represent slow-growing NHLs that may be stable with low tumor burden that may not warrant therapy for several years. The disease is responsive to treatment (remission rates above 90% with combined rituximab/chemotherapy), although the clinical course is characterized by repetitive relapses. Outside of early-stage disease and therapy with an allogeneic stem cell transplant, low-grade NHLs are not curable. The median survival of patients with advanced-stage follicular lymphoma in the pre-rituximab era was 9 to 10 years, although that is longer now (approximately 12–14 years). Transformation to a high-grade NHL occurs in 30% to 50% (3%–4% of patients each year) of follicular lymphoma patients (less common in other indolent subtypes) and is typically heralded by an aggressive change in the patient's clinical condition (e.g., B symptoms, rapidly rising LDH).

General Principles

Only a minority of patients present with early-stage disease (i.e., stage I or II). Radiotherapy is a valid treatment option for these patients (especially stage I), and associated 15- to 20-year disease-free survival rates are greater than 50%. Treatment for patients with advanced-stage disease ranges from observation (i.e., watchful waiting) to anti-CD20 monoclonal antibody therapy (rituximab [Rituxan]) with or without chemotherapy. Treatment choice depends in part on tumor burden and the patient's individual disease characteristics and baseline functional status. Treatment with frontline rituximab chemotherapy (outpatient

---

Box 2 WHO Classification of the Mature B-Cell, T-Cell, and Natural Killer–Cell Neoplasms (2008)

Mature B-Cell Neoplasms
Chronic lymphocytic leukemia, small lymphocytic lymphoma
B-cell prolymphocytic leukemia
Splenic marginal zone lymphoma
Hairy cell leukemia
Splenic lymphoma/leukemia, unclassifiable*
• Splenic diffuse red pulp small B-cell lymphoma*
• Hairy cell leukemia-variant*
Lymphoplasmacytic lymphoma
Waldenström macroglobulinemia
Heavy chain diseases
• Alpha heavy chain disease
• Gamma heavy chain disease
• Mu heavy chain disease
Plasma cell myeloma
Solitary plasmacytoma of bone
Extraosseous plasmacytoma
Extranodal marginal zone lymphoma of mucosa-associated lymphoid tissue (MALT lymphoma)
Nodal marginal zone lymphoma
Pediatric nodal marginal zone lymphoma*
Follicular lymphoma
Pediatric follicular lymphoma*
Primary cutaneous follicle center lymphoma
Mantle cell lymphoma
Diffuse large B-cell lymphoma (DLBCL), NOS
• T-cell histiocyte rich large B-cell lymphoma
• Primary DLBCL of the central nervous system
• Primary cutaneous DLBCL, leg type
• EBV⁺ DLBCL of the elderly*
• DLBCL associated with chronic inflammation
Lymphomatoid granulomatosis
Primary mediastinal (thymic) large B-cell lymphoma
Intravascular large B-cell lymphoma
ALK⁺ large B-cell lymphoma
Plasmablastic lymphoma
Large B-cell lymphoma arising in HHV-8–associated multicentric Castleman disease
Primary effusion lymphoma
Burkitt's lymphoma
B-cell lymphoma, unclassifiable, with features intermediate between diffuse large B-cell lymphoma and Burkitt lymphoma

B-cell lymphoma, unclassifiable, with features intermediate between diffuse large B-cell lymphoma and classic Hodgkin lymphoma

Mature T-Cell and Natural Killer–Cell Neoplasms
T-cell prolymphocytic leukemia
T-cell large granular lymphocytic leukemia
Chronic lymphoproliferative disorder of NK cells*
Aggressive NK cell leukemia
Systemic EBV⁺ T-cell lymphoproliferative disease of childhood
Hydroa vacciniforme-like lymphoma
Adult T-cell leukemia/lymphoma
Extranodal NK/T-cell lymphoma, nasal type
Enteropathy-associated T-cell lymphoma
Hepatosplenic T-cell lymphoma
Subcutaneous panniculitis-like T-cell lymphoma
Mycosis fungoides
Sézary syndrome
Primary cutaneous CD30⁺ T-cell lymphoproliferative disorders
• Lymphomatoid papulosis
• Primary cutaneous anaplastic large cell lymphoma
• Primary cutaneous gamma-delta T-cell lymphoma
• Primary cutaneous CD8⁺ aggressive epidermotropic cytotoxic T-cell lymphoma*
• Primary cutaneous CD4⁺ small/medium T-cell lymphoma*
Peripheral T-cell lymphoma, NOS
Angioimmunoblastic T-cell lymphoma
Anaplastic large cell lymphoma, ALK⁺
Anaplastic large cell lymphoma, ALK⁻

Hodgkin Lymphoma
Nodular lymphocyte-predominant Hodgkin lymphoma
Classic Hodgkin lymphoma
• Nodular sclerosis classic Hodgkin lymphoma
• Lymphocyte-rich classic Hodgkin lymphoma
• Mixed cellularity classic Hodgkin lymphoma
• Lymphocyte-depleted classic Hodgkin lymphoma

Posttransplantation Lymphoproliferative Disorders
Early lesions
Plasmacytic hyperplasia
Infectious mononucleosis-like
Polymorphic
Monomorphic (B- and T/NK-cell types)†
Classic Hodgkin lymphoma type†

*Provisional entities for which the WHO Working Group felt there was insufficient evidence to recognize as distinct diseases at this time.
†These lesions are classified according to the leukemia or lymphoma to which they correspond.
Abbreviations: EBV = Epstein-Barr virus; HHV = human herpesvirus; NK = natural killer; NOS = not otherwise specified; WHO = World Health Organization.

---

therapy given once every 3–4 weeks typically for 6–8 cycles) for patients with high tumor burden is associated with median progression-free survival rates of approximately 4 to 5 years.

Treatment options for relapsed indolent lymphoma include repeating rituximab without or without a different chemotherapy regimen, radioimmunotherapy, or stem-cell transplantation. Autologous stem-cell transplantation is an option for patients with relapsed disease, although an improvement in overall survival is debated. Allogeneic stem cell transplantation is a potential curative modality for patients with relapsed or refractory disease, although patient selection is critical owing to potential morbidity and mortality related to this therapeutic option.

Special Considerations
Localized gastric MALT lymphoma cases often may be managed with therapy for *H. pylori* infection; radiation is typically reserved for failure to eradicate *H. pylori*. Patients with lymphoplasmacytic lymphoma (Waldenström's macroglobulinemia) can present clinically with hyperviscosity or cryoglobulinemia, which may be managed acutely with plasmapheresis, but ultimately systemic therapy similar to that for other indolent NHLs is warranted.

Aggressive or High-Grade Non-Hodgkin Lymphomas
High-grade B- and T-cell NHLs are typically aggressive lymphomas that are fatal in weeks to a few months if not treated. However, many of these NHLs are curable with multiagent chemotherapy.

General Principles
DLBCL, the most common aggressive NHL, is curable in all stages in the majority of patients (60%–70%). A key to treatment is anti-CD20 monoclonal antibody combined with anthracycline-based chemotherapy: rituximab-CHOP (R-CHOP) (cyclophosphamide, doxorubicin, vincristine, prednisone). The number of treatment cycles depends on stage of disease and response to treatment. Standard therapy for advanced-stage disease is 6 R-CHOP cycles, whereas patients with early-stage disease may receive 3 or 4 cycles followed by involved field radiation. There are emerging data regarding the prognostic importance of *MYC* in the tumor as a single finding and especially in conjunction with *BCL-2* and/or *BCL6* (i.e., double hit) by molecular studies as well as with immunohistochemical staining. Outcomes with R-CHOP for DLBCL patients with a molecular double hit (e.g., presence of MYC and BCL-2) are modest; more intensive and novel therapeutic options are needed. Therapy for relapsed

TABLE 1	Clinical Prognostic Classification of Adult Immunocompetent Non-Hodgkin Lymphomas*

LYMPHOMA TYPE	PERCENTAGE OF ALL NON-HODGKIN LYMPHOMAS
Indolent or Low-Grade Non-Hodgkin Lymphomas	
Follicular lymphoma	20–25
Small lymphocytic lymphoma	7
MALT-type marginal zone lymphoma	7
Nodal-type marginal zone lymphoma	<2
Lymphoplasmacytic lymphoma	<2
Aggressive or High-Grade Non-Hodgkin Lymphomas	
Diffuse large B-cell lymphoma	30–35
T-cell lymphomas: peripheral or systemic (multiple subtypes)	10–12
Mantle cell lymphoma	6
Lymphoblastic lymphoma	<2
Burkitt's lymphoma	<1

Abbreviation: MALT = mucosa-associated lymphoid tissue.
*Subtypes are listed in order of most to least common.

Box 3	Enhanced International Prognostic Index (NCCN-IPI) Risk Factors and Associated Approximate Cure Rates for Diffuse Large B-Cell Lymphoma

Factors/Scoring
Age, years
    >40 to ≤60: 1
    >60 to ≤75: 2
    >75: 3
LDH, normalized
    >1 to ≤3: 1
    >3: 2
Ann Arbor stage III-IV: 1
*Extranodal disease: 1
Performance status ≥2: 1

Five-Year Progression-Free Survival Rates Based on Score at Diagnosis
Score 0-1: 91%
Score 2-3: 74%
Score 4-5: 51%
Score =/> 6: 30%

---

*Disease in bone marrow, CNS, liver/GI tract, or lung.

DLBCL typically includes abbreviated salvage non–cross resistant chemotherapy followed by autologous stem-cell transplantation (autoSCT), which is curative in approximately 35% to 45% of patients.

Mantle cell lymphoma is a B-cell NHL with initial high remission rates (>90–95%), but it has more modest long-term outcomes, and it is difficult to cure. With standard chemotherapy regimens (e.g., R-CHOP), the median progression-free survival rates are only 18 to 20 months. With more-intensive chemotherapy regimens (e.g., R-hyperCVAD/R-MA [rituximab, cyclophosphamide, vincristine, doxorubicin, dexamethasone/rituximab, methotrexate]), 5-year progression-free survival rates are near 70%. Some groups induction therapy with aggressive high-dose cytarabine[1] (Cytosar-U)-based chemotherapy followed by consolidative autologous stem-cell transplantation in first remission. As noted later, there has been

[1]Not FDA approved for this indication.

the integration of several novel therapeutic agents into the treatment paradigm of mantle-cell lymphoma.

Burkitt's lymphoma and related high-grade NHLs (e.g., lymphoblastic lymphomas) are often rapidly growing malignancies with a doubling time of 24 hours. Prompt initiation of therapy, including aggressive supportive care measures, is often warranted. With aggressive chemotherapy regimens, including prophylactic intrathecal chemotherapy, the majority of Burkitt's patients younger than age 50 years are cured (>70%–80%). In addition, there are data showing high efficacy using lower intensity treatment consisting of infused etoposide (Toposar[1]), doxorubicin, and cyclophosphamide with vincristine, prednisone, and rituximab (EPOCH-R) for patients with untreated Burkitt's lymphoma.

Systemic (i.e., non-cutaneous) T-cell NHLs are treatable; however, cure rates are lower compared with most aggressive B-cell NHLs. Standard therapy consists typically of CHOP-based chemotherapy with or without autologous SCT in first remission as consolidation. Associated five-year disease-free survival rates are approximately 20% to 30%. Novel targeted agents have also been FDA approved over the last several years for the treatment of T-cell NHL.

Special Considerations

There are several clinical subtypes of DLBCL that present as primary extranodal manifestations such as primary testicular DLBCL and primary gastric DLBCL. If these lymphomas are localized, treatment typically consists of abbreviated cycles (3–4) of R-CHOP followed by involved field radiation. In addition, intrathecal chemotherapy prophylaxis is warranted for testicular DLBCL given the predilection of CNS involvement.

Primary central nervous system lymphoma is typically DLBCL; high-dose methotrexate chemotherapy is a key component of therapy.

A long-standing therapeutic maneuver for PTLDs has been reduction of immunosuppression, although using this approach alone, mortality rates have ranged from 50% to 60% in most series. Recent evidence with use of initial rituximab-based therapy suggests significantly improved outcomes in the modern era.

The majority of AIDS-related NHLs are aggressive or high-grade types: DLBCL or Burkitt's lymphoma. Similar therapy as immunocompetent NHL is often recommended. Response to therapy, including cure rate, has improved significantly with better control of opportunistic infections and highly active antiretroviral therapy (HAART).

Mycosis fungoides and Sézary syndrome are cutaneous T-cell lymphomas that initially might show eczematous lesions. It is often difficult to establish diagnosis, but eventually the lesions develop into plaques and tumors. Lymph nodes, spleen, and visceral organs may be involved. Sézary syndrome is a variant of mycosis fungoides and shows peripheral blood involvement; patients usually have diffuse erythroderma. Skin-targeted modalities for treatment of early-stage mycosis fungoides include psoralens with ultraviolet A light (PUVA), narrowband-ultraviolet light, skin electron-beam radiation, and topical steroids, retinoids, carmustine (BiCNU), and nitrogen mustard (Mustargen).[1] Treatment goals in advanced stages are to reduce tumor burden and to relieve symptoms. Treatment options also include mono- or polychemotherapy including CHOP, extracorporeal photopheresis, interferons, retinoids, monoclonal antibodies, and recombinant toxins.

During therapy for aggressive/high-grade NHLs, attention should be paid to preventing tumor lysis syndrome. Measures to prevent this complication include aggressive hydration, allopurinol (Zyloprim), alkalinization of the urine, and frequent monitoring of electrolytes, uric acid, and creatinine. Rasburicase (Elitek), a recombinant urate oxidase enzyme, is an expensive but potent agent for treating hyperuricemia.

Novel Treatment Options and Modalities

Many new agents targeting specific molecular targets such as the ubiquitin-proteasome pathway are available for the treatment of lymphoma. Novel agents in lymphoma include bortezomib (Velcade) and lenalidomide (Revlimid), which are FDA approved

[1]Not FDA approved for this indication.

for relapsed or refractory mantle-cell lymphoma, and histone deacetylase inhibitors, which are approved for cutaneous T-cell lymphoma and peripheral T-cell NHLs as well. In addition, bortezomib was recently FDA approved for untreated mantle-cell lymphoma patients (in combination with immunochemotherapy). Other new agents which are showing promising activity include idelalisib (Zydeliq), an inhibitor of PI3K delta, which is now FDA approved for the treatment of patients with relapsed follicular lymphoma or small lymphocytic lymphoma and a novel inhibitor of Bruton's Tyrosine Kinase (BTK), ibrutinib (Imbruvica), FDA approved for patients with chronic lymphocytic leukemia (CLL) and mantle cell lymphoma (MCL) who have received at least one prior therapy. New anti-CD20 antibodies have been approved for the treatment of CLL (e.g., obinutuzumab (Gazyva)) and antibody drug conjugates have shown promise, including brentuximab vedotin (Adcetris), which is FDA approved for relapsed anaplastic (T-cell) large-cell lymphoma.

Follow-Up of Long-Term Survivors
Relapse
Among patients with aggressive lymphomas, such as DLBCL, most recurrences are seen within the first 2 years after the completion of therapy, although later relapses occur uncommonly. Physical examination and laboratory testing at 2- to 3-month intervals and follow-up CT scans at 6-month intervals for the first 2 years following diagnosis are recommended. Early detection of recurrent disease is important in part because these patients may be candidates for potentially curative therapy (e.g., stem-cell transplantation). Patients with advanced low-grade NHL are at a constant risk for relapse, as discussed before.

Secondary Malignancies
Long-term NHL survivors are at an increased risk for second cancers. Generally, the risk is increased with history of radiation use, but it is also seen with chemotherapy. In a survey of 28,131 Dutch registry patients with NHL who survived 2 years or longer, significant excesses of second cancers were seen for nearly all solid tumors as well as acute myelogenous leukemia (AML) and Hodgkin's lymphoma. The standardized incidence ratio (SIR) for solid tumors after NHL was 1.65. The SIRs for solid tumors are increased for up to 30 years after NHL diagnosis, with the highest relative risk of developing a secondary malignancy occurring more than 21 to 30 years after original diagnosis.

Late Treatment Complications
There has been more selective use of radiation as part of therapy for NHL. Thus, the risk of certain radiation-induced complications has been reduced in patients treated more recently. Nevertheless, the risk still exists. Transplant recipients are at increased risk for secondary myelodysplasia and AML, regardless of whether they received radiation. All chemotherapy agents may cause long-term morbidity; in particular, patients who received an anthracycline (e.g., doxorubicin [Adriamycin]) are at a long-term increased risk of cardiovascular disease. Among Dutch and Belgian NHL patients treated with at least six cycles of doxorubicin-based chemotherapy, cumulative incidence of cardiovascular disease was 12% at 5 years and 22% at 10 years. Risk of coronary artery disease matched that of the general population; however, risk of chronic heart failure was significantly increased (SIR, 5.4) as was stroke (SIR, 1.8). Risk factors associated with excess risk included younger age at start of NHL treatment (<55 years), preexisting hypertension, any salvage treatment, and use of radiotherapy; risk relating to radiotherapy was dose-dependent. Continued studies are needed to develop optimal secondary prevention strategies.

References
Byrd JC, Brown JR, O'Brien S, et al. Ibrutinib versus ofatumumab in previously treated chronic lymphoid leukemia. N Engl J Med 2014;371(3):213–23.

Dave SS, Wright G, Tan B, et al. Prediction of survival in follicular lymphoma based on molecular features of tumor-infiltrating immune cells. N Engl J Med 2004;351:2159–69.

Dunleavy K, Pittaluga S, Shovlin M, et al. Low-intensity therapy in adults with Burkitt's lymphoma. N Engl J Med 2013;369(20):1915–25.

Evens AM, David KA, Helenowski IB, et al. Multicenter analysis of 80 solid organ transplant recipients with posttransplantation lymphoproliferative disease (PTLD): Outcomes and prognostic factors in the modern era. Jan 19 J Clin Oncol 2010;28(6):1038–46.

Gopal AK, Kahl BS, de Vos S, Wagner-Johnston ND, et al. PI3Kδ inhibition by idelalisib in patients with relapsed indolent lymphoma. N Engl J Med 2014;370(11):1008–18.

Hemminki K, Lenner P, Sundquist J, Bermejo JL. Risk of subsequent solid tumors after non-Hodgkin's lymphoma: Effect of diagnostic age and time since diagnosis. J Clin Oncol 2008;26(11):1850–7.

Morton LM, Curtis RE, Linet MS, et al. Second malignancy risks after non-Hodgkin's lymphoma and chronic lymphocytic leukemia: differences by lymphoma subtype. J Clin Oncol 2010;28:4935–44.

Moser EC, Noordijk EM, van Leeuwen FE, et al. Long-term risk of cardiovascular disease after treatment for aggressive non-Hodgkin lymphoma. Blood 2006;107:2912–9.

Moskowitz AJ, Lunning MA, Horwitz SM. How I treat the peripheral T-cell lymphomas. Blood 2014;123(17):2636–44.

Robak T, Huang H, Jin J, et al. Bortezomib-based therapy for newly diagnosed mantle-cell lymphoma. N Engl J Med 2015;372(10):944–53.

Shipp MA. for The International Non-Hodgkin's Lymphoma Prognostic Factors Project: A predictive model for aggressive non-Hodgkin's lymphoma. N Engl J Med 1993;329:987–94.

Swerdlow SH, Campo E, Harris NL, et al. WHO Classification of Tumours of Haematopoietic and Lymphoid Tissues. 4th ed. Lyons, France: International Agency for Research on Cancer; 2008.

Wang ML, Rule S, Martin P, et al. Targeting BTK with ibrutinib in relapsed or refractory mantle-cell lymphoma. N Engl J Med 2013;369(6):507–16.

Younes A, Bartlett NL, Leonard JP, et al. Brentuximab vedotin (SGN-35) for relapsed CD30-positive lymphomas. N Engl J Med 2010;363:1812–21.

Zhou Z, Sehn LH, Rademaker AW, et al. An enhanced International Prognostic Index (NCCN-IPI) for patients with diffuse large B-cell lymphoma treated in the rituximab era. Blood 2014;123(6):837–42.

PERNICIOUS ANEMIA AND OTHER MEGALOBLASTIC ANEMIAS

Method of
Emmanuel Andrès, MD, PhD

CURRENT DIAGNOSIS

- Megaloblastic anemia is a macrocytic anemia characterized by macroovalocytes and hypersegmented neutrophils on the peripheral smear.
- In adults, many underlying conditions lead to megaloblastic anemia, but the most common ones are folate (folic acid, vitamin B_9) deficiency, vitamin B_{12} (cobalamin) deficiency, and pernicious anemia.
- In the adult population, folate deficiency usually develops as a result of inadequate dietary intake or as an adverse effect of several drugs (methotrexate [Trexall], cotrimoxazole [Bactrim], sulfasalazine [Azulfidine], anticonvulsants) or alcohol intake.
- In adults and the elderly, vitamin B_{12} deficiency is mainly due to cobalamin malabsorption from food and to pernicious anemia.

CURRENT THERAPY

- Recognition of the condition causing megaloblastic anemia is a prerequisite of successful therapy.
- Treatment of nutrient-deficiency megaloblastic anemia is easy with nutrient replacement.
- Vitamin B_{12} deficiency can be treated with both oral and parenteral therapy.
- If vitamin B_{12} deficiency is untreated, folate repletion will correct the megaloblastic anemia but not the associated neuropathic changes that occur with B_{12} deficiency.

Anemia is a common condition, especially in adults, and its prevalence increases with age. It affects quality of life, physical function, and even cognitive function in elderly patients. Anemia is a comorbid condition that affects other diseases (e.g., heart disease, cerebrovascular insufficiency) and is associated with a risk of death. Thus, anemia should not be accepted as a benign condition or a consequence of aging. In adults, many underlying conditions lead to megaloblastic anemia, but the most common ones are nutrient deficiencies, especially folate (folic acid, vitamin B_9) deficiency, vitamin B_{12} (cobalamin) deficiency, and pernicious anemia. Recognition of these conditions is a prerequisite of successful therapy.

Although low hemoglobin levels are often seen with advancing age, anemia should not be assumed to be a normal consequence of aging. Age may be associated with compromised hematopoietic reserve, and the elderly can be more susceptible to anemia in the presence of hematopoietic stress induced by an underlying disorder. Consequently, it is important to identify the underlying disorder. In practice, a hemoglobin (Hb) level less than 10 g/dL is considered a trigger for the investigation of the cause of anemia.

Definition

The World Health Organization (WHO) defines anemia as a hemoglobin concentration less than 12 g/dL for nonpregnant women and less than 13 g/dL for men. Megaloblastic anemia is characterized by many large immature and dysfunctional red blood cells (megaloblasts) in the bone marrow and by hypersegmented or multisegmented neutrophils. Megaloblastic anemia includes nutrient deficiencies related to folate and vitamin B_{12} and pernicious anemia. Megaloblastic anemia is included in the group of macrocytic anemias (mean corpuscular volume [MCV] >100 fL). Macrocytic anemia also includes anemia related to chronic alcohol use (with or without liver disease), thyroid failure, and myelodysplastic syndromes.

Epidemiology

In adults, the prevalence of anemia varies by country, ethnic group, and the health status of the patients. Living conditions can also influence this prevalence. Nevertheless, the prevalence of anemia increases with advancing age, especially after age 60 to 65 years, and rises sharply after the age of 80 years. Results from the third National Health and Nutrition Examination Survey (NHANES III) carried out in the United States indicates that the prevalence of anemia was 11% in community-dwelling men and 10.2% among women 65 years or older. Survey findings also indicate that most anemia among the elderly is mild; only 2.8% of women and 1.6% of men have a hemoglobin less than 11 g/dL.

Results from the Framingham cohort indicate a slightly lower prevalence of anemia among older people living in the United States compared to the NHANES IIII survey. In the Framingham group of 1016 subjects 67 to 96 years of age, the prevalence of anemia in men and women is 6.1% and 10.5%, respectively.

In adults, causes of anemia are divided into three broad groups: nutrient-deficiency anemia, including iron deficiency, folate deficiency, and B_{12} deficiency anemia; anemia of chronic disease, perhaps better termed anemia of chronic inflammation; and unexplained anemia. Table 1 presents the cause of anemia in 300 consecutive patients hospitalized in an internal medicine department.

In the NHANES III study, 34% of all anemia in elderly patients is caused by deficiencies of nutrients including folate, vitamin B_{12}, and iron, alone or in combination. About 60% of nutrient-deficiency anemia is associated with iron deficiency, and most of those cases are the result of chronic blood loss from gastrointestinal lesions. The remaining cases of nutrient-deficiency anemia are usually associated with vitamin B_{12} or folate deficiency (or both) and are easily treated. Twelve percent of anemias were associated with renal insufficiency, 20% were due to chronic diseases, and in 34% the cause remained unexplained.

Etiology

Folate Deficiency Anemia in Adults

A balanced diet contains 500 to 700 μg of folate. On average, 50% to 60% of dietary folate is absorbed in the duodenum and jejunum. Folate deficiency usually develops as a result of inadequate dietary intake. The body stores very little folate, only enough to last 4 to 6 months. Patients usually have a history of weight loss,

ETIOLOGY	PREVALENCE (%)
Chronic inflammation (chronic disease)	23.0
Iron deficiency	18
Renal failure	9
Liver disease and endocrine disease (chronic disease)	7
Posthemorrhagic	7
Folate deficiency	6*
Myelodysplasia	5
Vitamin B_{12} deficiency	4†
Unexplained causes	21

TABLE 1 Etiology of Anemia in 300 Consecutive Patients Older than 65 Years Hospitalized in a Department of Internal Medicine in a Tertiary Reference Center

Adapted from Andrès E, Federici L, Serraj K, Kaltenbach G: Update of nutrient-deficiency anemia in elderly patients. Eur J Intern Med 2008;19:488–93.
*10% of these patients have megaloblastic anemia.
†Vitamin B_{12} deficiency is defined as a serum cobalamin level <200 pg/mL (<150 pmol/L) in 2 samples.

poor weight gain, and weakness. In addition, several drugs (methotrexate [Trexall], cotrimoxazole [Bactrim], sulfasalazine [Azulfidine], and anticonvulsants) and alcohol can cause deficiency of folate by inhibiting absorption or by affecting folate metabolism.

Vitamin B_{12} Deficiency Anemia in Adults

Deficiency of vitamin B_{12} and folate are common, especially among the elderly, each occurring in at least 5% of patients. In these patients, the etiologies of cobalamin deficiency are represented primarily by food-cobalamin malabsorption, other causes of malabsorption such as surgical resection of the stomach or ileum, pernicious anemia, and, more rarely, by intake deficiency. In our work, in which we followed more than 200 elderly patients with a proven deficiency, food-cobalamin malabsorption accounted for about 60% to 70% of the etiologies of cobalamin deficiency, and pernicious anemia accounted for 15% to 25%. Figure 1 presents the principal causes of cobalamin deficiency in 172 patients hospitalized in an internal medicine department.

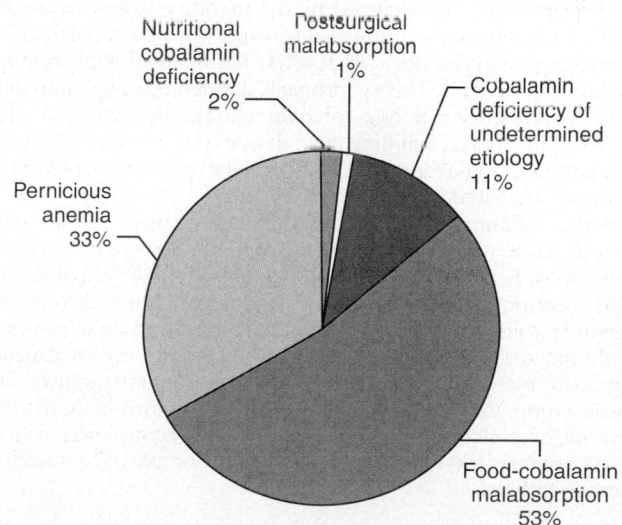

Figure 1. Etiologies of cobalamin deficiency in 172 elderly patients hospitalized in the university hospital of Strasbourg, France. (Adapted from Andrès E, Loukili NH, Noel E, et al: Vitamin B_{12} (cobalamin) deficiency in elderly patients. Can Med Assoc J 2004;171:251-260; and Andrès E, Vidal-Aluball J, Federici L, et al: Clinical aspects of cobalamin deficiency in elderly patients. Epidemiology, causes, clinical manifestations, treatment with special focus on oral cobalamin therapy. Eur J Intern Med 2007;18:456–62.)

Box 1   Food-Cobalamin Malabsorption Syndrome

Criteria for Food-Cobalamin Malabsorption

Low serum cobalamin (vitamin B_{12}) levels

Normal results of Schilling test using free cyanocobalamin labeled with cobalt-58, or abnormal results of derived Schilling test*

No anti-intrinsic factor antibodies

No dietary cobalamin deficiency

Associated Conditions or Agents

Gastric disease
- Atrophic gastritis
- Type A atrophic gastritis
- Gastric disease associated with *Helicobacter pylori* infection
- Partial gastrectomy
- Gastric bypass
- Vagotomy

Pancreatic insufficiency
- Alcohol abuse

Gastric or intestinal bacterial overgrowth
- Achlorhydria
- Tropical sprue
- Ogylvie's syndrome
- HIV

Drugs
- Antacids (H_2-receptor antagonists and proton-pump inhibitors)
- Biguanides (metformin [Glucophage])

Alcohol abuse

Sjögren's syndrome, systemic sclerosis

Haptocorrin deficiency

Aging or idiopathic

---

*Derived Schilling tests use food-bound cobalamin (e.g., egg yolk, chicken, and fish proteins).

Adapted from Andrès E, Affenberger S, Vinzio S, et al: Food-cobalamin malabsorption in elderly patients: Clinical manifestations and treatment. Am J Med 2005;118:1154-1159.

Food-Cobalamin Malabsorption

Initially described by Carmel in the 1990s, food-cobalamin malabsorption is characterized by the inability to release bound cobalamin from food or intestinal transport proteins, particularly in the setting of hypochlorhydria, where the absorption of unbound cobalamin is normal. This syndrome is defined by cobalamin deficiency despite sufficient food-cobalamin intake and a normal Schilling test. The normal Schilling test rules out pernicious anemia and other causes of malabsorption. The principal characteristics of this syndrome are listed in Box 1.

Food-cobalamin malabsorption is caused primarily by atrophic gastritis. More than 40% of patients older than 80 years have gastric atrophy. Factors that commonly contribute to food-cobalamin malabsorption include *Helicobacter pylori* infection, chronic carriage of *H. pylori*, intestinal microbial proliferation (in which case, cobalamin deficiency can be corrected by antibiotic treatment); long-term ingestion of antacids, H_2-receptor antagonists and proton-pump inhibitors, and biguanides (metformin [Glucophage]); chronic alcoholism; surgery or gastric reconstruction (e.g., bypass surgery for obesity); and complete or partial pancreatic exocrine failure.

Pernicious Anemia

Pernicious anemia, also known as Biermer's anemia or Addison's anemia, is caused by impaired absorption of vitamin B_{12} owing to the neutralization of intrinsic factor action in the setting of immune atrophic gastritis. In elderly patients, this form of megaloblastic anemia is one of the leading causes of cobalamin deficiency. Pernicious anemia has a genetic component. In practice, the diagnosis of pernicious anemia is based on the presence of intrinsic factor antibodies in serum (specificity, >98%; sensitivity, around 50%) or biopsy-proven autoimmune atrophic gastritis. The presence of *H. pylori* infection in gastric biopsies is an exclusion factor. Pernicious anemia is associated with other immunologic diseases such as Sjögren's syndrome, Hashimoto's disease, type 1 diabetes mellitus, and celiac disease.

Other Causes of Cobalamin Deficiency

Cobalamin deficiency caused by dietary deficiency or malabsorption is rare. Dietary causes of deficiency are limited to elderly people who are already malnourished. This mainly concerns elderly patients living in institutions or in psychiatric hospitals. Since the 1980s, the malabsorption of cobalamin has become rare, owing mainly to the decreasing frequency of gastrectomy and surgical resection of the terminal small intestine. Other disorders associated with cobalamin malabsorption include deficiency in the exocrine function of the pancreas after chronic pancreatitis (usually alcoholic), lymphomas or tuberculosis of the intestine, Crohn's disease, Whipple's disease, and celiac disease. Uncommon etiology also includes nitrous oxide anesthesia and abuse.

Clinical Features

Box 2 presents features related to vitamin B_{12} deficiency. It should be noted that vitamin B_{12} deficiency may be present in the absence of anemia. The symptoms of folate deficiency are nearly indistinguishable from those of cobalamin deficiency. Box 3 presents the other hematologic manifestations of cobalamin deficiency.

Diagnosis

Patients with nutrient-deficiency anemia often have mild to moderate anemia with hemoglobin levels between 8 and 10 g/dL. In anemia of exclusive folate and/or vitamin B_{12} deficiency, the erythrocytes are usually macrocytic (MCV >100 fL). Megaloblastic processes are characterized on the peripheral smear by macroovalocytes and hypersegmented neutrophils. Bone marrow aspiration, which is rarely required for diagnosis, demonstrates large immature and dysfunctional red blood cells (megaloblasts) and hypersegmented or multisegmented neutrophils. In cobalamin deficiency (<150 pmol/L), serum vitamin B_{12} level is low (<200 pg/mL), serum methylmalonic acid is increased, and homocysteine levels are increased. In folate deficiency, testing the red cell folate concentration is more reliable than the serum level.

Prevention

Providing food sources of nutrients is best for preventing megaloblastic anemia. Food source supplementation may be necessary, especially for the very old. The National Academy of Sciences recommends that folate and vitamin B_{12} be supplemented for the elderly in the form of fortified cereal.

Treatment

Treatment of megaloblastic anemia requires particular attention to discerning the cause. In adult patients, vitamin B_{12} deficiency anemia may be treated by vitamin B_{12} supplementation, parenterally or orally. Our working group has developed an effective oral treatment regimen for food-cobalamin malabsorption and pernicious anemia using crystalline cobalamin (cyanocobalamin)[1] (Figure 2). The effect of oral cobalamin treatment in patients presenting with severe neurologic manifestations has not yet been adequately documented.

For folate deficiency anemia, therapeutic doses of folic acid vary between 1 and 5 mg/day. Usually, these various therapies are continued for at least 3 to 6 months, provided that the underlying causes of the deficiency have been corrected.

---

[1]Not FDA approved for this indication.

Box 2   Nonhematologic Manifestations of Vitamin B_{12} Deficiency

Neuropsychiatric
Common
Polyneuritis (especially sensitive ones)
Ataxia
Babinski's phenomenon

Classic
Combined sclerosis of the spinal cord

Rare
Cerebellar syndromes affecting the cranial nerves including optic neuritis, optic atrophy
Urinary incontinence
Fecal incontinence

Under Study
Changes in higher cognitive functions, including dementia
Stroke and atherosclerosis (hyperhomocysteinemia)
Parkinsonian syndromes
Depression
Multiple sclerosis

Digestive
Classic
Hunter's glossitis
Jaundice
Lactate dehydrogenase and bilirubin elevation (intramedullary destruction)

Debatable
Abdominal pain
Dyspepsia
Nausea, vomiting
Diarrhea
Disturbances in intestinal functioning

Rare
Resistant and recurring mucocutaneous ulcers

Other
Under Study
Atrophy of the vaginal mucosa
Chronic vaginal and urinary infections (especially mycosis)
Venous thromboembolic disease
Angina (hyperhomocysteinemia)

Adapted from Andrès E, Loukili NH, Noel E, et al: Vitamin B_{12} (cobalamin) deficiency in elderly patients. Can Med Assoc J 2004;171:251–60; and Andrès E, Vidal-Alaball J, Federici L, et al: Clinical aspects of cobalamin deficiency in elderly patients. Epidemiology, causes, clinical manifestations, treatment with special focus on oral cobalamin therapy. Eur J Intern Med 2007;18:456–62.

Box 3   Hematologic Manifestations of Vitamin B_{12} Deficiency

Common
Macrocytosis
Hypersegmentation of neutrophils
Aregenerative macrocytic anemia
Megaloblastic anemia

Rare
Isolated thrombocytopenia and neutropenia
Pancytopenia

Uncommon
Hemolytic anemia
Pseudothrombotic microangiopathy

Adapted from Andrès E, Loukili NH, Noel E, et al: Vitamin B_{12} (cobalamin) deficiency in elderly patients. Can Med Assoc J 2004;171:251-260; and Andrès E, Vidal-Alaball J, Federici L, et al: Clinical aspects of cobalamin deficiency in elderly patients. Epidemiology, causes, clinical manifestations, treatment with special focus on oral cobalamin therapy. Eur J Intern Med 2007;18:456–62.

Parenteral administration
(Regardless of the etiology of the vitamin deficiency)

Intensification treatment:
Cyanocobalamin: 1000 µg per day for one week, then 1000 µg per week for 1 month

Maintenance treatment:
Cyanocobalamin: 1000 µg per month until the cause is corrected, or for life in the case of pernicious anemia

Oral administration
(for intake deficiency, food-cobalamin malabsorption, and pernicious anemia)

Intensification treatment:
Cyanocobalamin: 1000 µg per day for 1 month

Maintenance treatment:
Cyanocobalamin 125 to 500 µg per day for intake deficiency and food-cobalamin malabsorption and
Cyanocobalamin: 1000 µg per day for pernicious anemia

Figure 2. Therapeutic schema for vitamin B_{12} deficiency. (Adapted from Andrès E, Affenberger S, Vinzio S, et al: Food-cobalamin malabsorption in elderly patients: Clinical manifestations and treatment. Am J Med 2005;118: 1154–59; Andrès E, Federici L, Serraj K, Kaltenbach G: Update of nutrient-deficiency anemia in elderly patients. Eur J Intern Med 2008;19:488–93; Andrès E, Loukili NH, Noel E, et al: Vitamin B_{12} (cobalamin) deficiency in elderly patients. Can Med Assoc J 2004;171: 251–60; and Andrès E, Vidal-Alaball J, Federici L, et al: Clinical aspects of cobalamin deficiency in elderly patients. Epidemiology, causes, clinical manifestations, treatment with special focus on oral cobalamin therapy. Eur J Intern Med 2007;18:456–62.)

If vitamin B_{12} deficiency is present but undiagnosed, folate repletion will correct the megaloblastic anemia, but not the possible neuropathic changes that occur with B_{12} deficiency.

References

Andrès E, Affenberger S, Vinzio S, et al. Food-cobalamin malabsorption in elderly patients: Clinical manifestations and treatment. Am J Med 2005;118:1154–9.

Andrès E, Federici L, Serraj K, Kaltenbach G. Update of nutrient-deficiency anemia in elderly patients. Eur J Intern Med 2008;19:488–93.

Andrès E, Loukili NH, Noel E, et al. Vitamin B_{12} (cobalamin) deficiency in elderly patients. Can Med Assoc J 2004;171:251–60.

Andrès E, Vidal-Alaball J, Federici L, et al. Clinical aspects of cobalamin deficiency in elderly patients. Epidemiology, causes, clinical manifestations, treatment with special focus on oral cobalamin therapy. Eur J Intern Med 2007;18:456–62.

Carmel R. Malabsorption of food-cobalamin. Baillieres Clin Haematol 1995;8:639–55.

McDowell MA, Fryar CD, Ogden CL. Anthropometric reference data for children and adults: United States, 1988–1994. Vital Health Stat 2009;11(249):1–68.

Vidal-Alaball J, Butler CC, Cannings-John R, et al. Oral vitamin B_{12} versus intramuscular vitamin B_{12} for vitamin B_{12} deficiency. Cochrane Database Syst Rev 2005;(20) CD004655.

Wickramasinghe SN. Diagnosis of megaloblastic anaemias. Blood Rev 2006;20: 299–318.

PLATELET-MEDIATED BLEEDING DISORDERS

Method of
Eric H. Kraut, MD

CURRENT DIAGNOSIS

- Platelet-mediated bleeding disorders commonly present with bleeding from mucosal surfaces and/or skin. Bleeding caused by reduced platelet counts may present with petechiae or purpura, while abnormalities of function are more likely to present with bleeding after injury or menstruation.
- Evaluation of platelet function used to be measured by the bleeding time. However, it is now more commonly evaluated by the PFA-100 and/or platelet aggregation studies.
- Thrombocytopenia is most commonly caused by deficient production of platelets from the bone marrow, decreased platelet survival in the circulation, or sequestration of platelets by an enlarged spleen.
- Patients may bleed after trauma at platelet counts under 50,000/μL and develop petechiae or purpura at platelet counts under 20,000/μL, but usually do not have severe bleeding unless platelet counts drop below 10,000/μL
- The most common causes of new thrombocytopenia in the hospitalized patient are drugs or infection, whereas the usual cause of new platelet function abnormalities are medications.
- Patients in the hospital and placed on heparin should have their platelet counts monitored, and a reduction of 50% should be evaluated for heparin-induced thrombocytopenia.
- Immune thrombocytopenic purpura (ITP) usually presents in outpatients as new-onset mucocutaneous bleeding associated with only a reduced platelet count or unexplained asymptomatic isolated thrombocytopenia.
- Drugs that inhibit platelet activation and aggregation, such as aspirin, clopidogrel (Plavix), and dipyridamole (Persantine) can lead to significant bleeding, especially after surgery or procedures. This effect may last for 7 to 10 days.
- Patients presenting with a lifetime history of easy bruising and or heavy menses should have careful evaluation of their bleeding history and family history of bleeding. If positive, studies to rule out Von Willebrand disease or hereditary disorders of platelet granules such as storage pool disorder should be done.

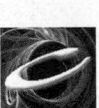

CURRENT THERAPY

- Patients with severe thrombocytopenia (platelet counts <10,000/μL) that is due to impaired production are at risk of severe bleeding and should be considered for platelet transfusions. The benefit of transfusing platelets when the platelet count reaches this level and the patient is not bleeding is currently under investigation.
- Standard practice for platelet transfusions is to maintain platelet counts above 50,000/μL for patients with gastrointestinal bleeding and 75,000-100,000/μL for neurosurgical procedures.
- Patients with immune thrombocytopenia should not receive platelet transfusions unless they are having significant bleeding since response to platelet transfusion occurs in less than 10% of patients and is short lasting.
- Patients with ITP who have no bleeding and platelet counts >30,000/μL can be followed without treatment since the risk of bleeding is low.
- In patients with ITP and thrombocytopenia less than 10,000/μL, initial treatment with high doses of corticosteroids in combination with IVIG (Gamunex) induces a rapid rise in platelets, usually within 24 hours.

- Current treatment for patients with ITP who fail prednisone treatment include splenectomy, rituximab (Rituxan),[1] or thrombopoietin agonists (romiplostim [Nplate] or eltrombopag [Promacta]).
- Patients with chronic renal failure can develop severe bleeding diathesis which appears to be multifactorial including platelet dysfunction. Dialysis can reduce bleeding but not completely correct it. Other treatment which may help include desmopressin (DDAVP),[1] tranexamic acid (Lysteda),[1] and synthetic erythropoietin.[1]
- Patients with drug induced platelet dysfunction who may need to undergo surgery or who are bleeding may require platelet transfusions.
- Patients with inherited platelet disorders and mild bleeding can be treated with desmopressin (DDAVP) but if severe may require platelet transfusions.

[1]Not FDA approved for this indication.

Platelets Role in Hemostasis

Platelets are small non-nucleated blood cells which are derived from bone marrow megakaryocytes. Their production is controlled by the hormone thrombopoietin produced in the liver and they survive in the circulation for 8 to 10 days. Upon blood vessel injury, they form a seal or plug at the site of injury to limit bleeding. This initial event, termed primary hemostasis, occurs after endothelial injury when the subendothelial surface is exposed to circulating blood. Platelets are drawn to the site via von Willebrand factor (vWF), which, in combination with other proteins including fibrillar collagen, fibronectin and laminin, leads to platelet adhesion. After platelets adhere to the vessel wall, they are activated, undergo a shape change and release products from their granules. These platelet granule products, including ADP and thromboxane A_2, further potentiate this process. Fibrinogen then binds to platelets via GPIIb/IIIa on the platelet surface causing firm platelet aggregation. The platelet secretory release reaction and aggregation recruits other platelets forming a firm hemostatic plug. Platelets also support the coagulation phase by interacting with circulating clotting factors and providing a surface for generation of thrombin. Secondary hemostasis occurs and thrombin mediated fibrin mesh stabilizes the platelet plug.

Clinical Manifestations

The hallmark of platelet-mediated bleeding disorders is mucocutaneous bleeding such as nose bleeds, prolonged bleeding after tooth extractions, and heavy menstrual bleeding. When the platelet count drops below 30.000/μL one may also see petechiae or purpuric lesions, especially on lower extremities.

Quantitative Platelet Disorders (Thrombocytopenia)

Primary hemostasis depends on an adequate number of platelets to prevent bleeding. A significant reduction in platelets or thrombocytopenia is usually defined as <100,000/μL. However, bleeding usually does not occur until the platelet count drops much lower. For example, spontaneous bleeding may only occur only when the platelet count is below 20,000/μL and severe life-threatening bleeding occurs only below 10,000/μL. Thrombocytopenia can develop due to inadequate platelet production from the bone marrow, reduced platelet survival in the circulation, or sequestration of platelets in the spleen. Differentiating the cause requires evaluation of the patients associated medical problems, physical findings, drug history, blood chemistry analysis, and possibly bone-marrow sampling.

Decreased platelet production is often the result of chemotherapeutic drugs for cancer, some antibiotics and antivirals (Table 1), or radiation therapy. These drugs may cause bone-marrow injury including damage to the megakaryocytes. Complete recovery may occur after stopping the offending agent. One common agent that can induce thrombocytopenia is alcohol. Thrombocytopenia

TABLE 1	Drugs Commonly Implicated as Causes of Drug-Induced Thrombocytopenia

CATEGORY	IMPLICATED IN SEVERAL REPORTS
Heparin	Unfractionated and LMWH
Cinchona alkaloids	Quinidine, quinine
Platelet inhibitors	Abciximab, eptifibinate, tirofiban
Antirheumatic agents	Gold salts
Antimicrobial agents	Linezolid, rifampin, sulfonamides, vancomycin
Sedative and anticonvulsants	Valproic acid, phenytoin, carbamazepine
Histamine receptor antagonists	Cimetidine
Diuretic agents	Chlorothiazide
Analgesic agents	Acetaminophen, naproxen, diclofenac
Chemotherapy agents	Oxaliplatin, fludarabine, and others

associated with reduction in the white blood cell count and or red blood cell count should alert physicians to the possibility of a bone marrow disorder such as forms of leukemia or aplastic anemia. In cases where the cause is not evident, a bone marrow biopsy may be necessary to demonstrate whether there is a malignancy that may require urgent treatment.

Patients with reduced platelet production can often be observed without intervention depending on the severity of the thrombocytopenia, presence of bleeding, or the need to perform invasive procedures. Guidelines for transfusion of platelets to prevent bleeding (prophylactic transfusion) have changed in the last few years. With evidence that severe bleeding may not occur in most patients until the platelet count is below 10,000/µL, limited platelet resources, and potential for development of alloimmunization to platelets, transfusions are not usually given unless sustained platelet counts are below 10,000/µL. When platelets are transfused it is appropriate to measure the response with a platelet count 1 hour post-transfusion. The platelet count should rise 30,000 to 40,000/µL for the usual four-pack of platelet transfusion. Patients requiring frequent transfusions may require single donor apheresis or HLA-matched platelets to obtain a good response.

Thrombocytopenia Resulting from Increased Platelet Destruction

Normally, platelets live in the circulation for 10 days, and the bone marrow replenishes them at the same rate that they are destroyed. Platelet survival may be altered by both nonimmune and immune processes. Severe infections will often lead to increased platelet destruction, and the platelet count returns to normal when the infection is adequately treated. Consumption of platelets also can occur in association with microangiopathic hemolytic anemia, as seen in disseminated intravascular coagulation (DIC) and thrombotic thrombocytopenic purpura and hemolytic uremic syndrome (TTP/HUS). It is important to review the blood smear to document fragmented red blood cells and evaluate coagulation parameters to help differentiate DIC from TTP/HUS and other causes of consumption. TTP/HUS may require specific and urgent treatment to prevent life-threatening complications. Platelet transfusions are not usually given for TTP as there are reports of patients deteriorating after transfusions.

Immune-mediated platelet destruction is seen in response to several common drugs, including the sulfonamides and vancomycin. The characteristic pattern of immune-mediated platelet destruction is a sharp drop in the platelet count 7 to 10 days after starting the drug. The platelet count may drop to 5000/µL or less. Recognition is important because significant bleeding may occur and the platelet count will only improve after discontinuation of the drug. Glycoprotein IIa/IIIb inhibitors, which are often used after cardiac stent placement, may cause a dramatic drop in the platelet count to as low as 1000/µL within hours of administration. This is important to recognize because this is one case where platelet transfusions may be necessary to prevent severe bleeding and it can be easily confused with other causes of low platelet counts.

Heparin-induced thrombocytopenia (HIT) is a unique drug reaction for several reasons. First, although thrombocytopenia is the initial sign of this entity, the major and feared complication is arterial and venous thromboses. It appears to affect 4% to 5% of patients exposed to unfractionated heparin and about 0.5% of patients exposed to low-molecular-weight heparin. Those at highest risk are female surgical patients who receive a minimum of 4 days of either type of heparin. The classic pattern is exposure to heparin at any dose with development of antibodies to heparin at day 4 and a 50% reduction in platelet count by day 6. The antibodies responsible are to the heparin–platelet factor 4 complex (IgG-PF4). A suspicious clinical pattern and a high antibody titre measured by an ELISA assay are often diagnostic. Patients suspected of having HIT are at a high risk of thromboembolic disease within the first 24 hours of the drop in platelet count, and the heparin should be immediately stopped. However, despite the reduced platelet count, bleeding is unusual. Patients should be placed on an alternative anticoagulant, usually a direct thrombin inhibitor. The platelet count takes about 2 weeks to return to normal, and warfarin (Coumadin) should not be started until the platelet count returns to normal to avoid warfarin-associated necrosis. By reducing protein C and protein S, warfarin creates a temporary hypercoagulable state and places the patient at risk for warfarin-associated necrosis during the time when patients are most susceptible to thrombosis from HIT.

Immune thrombocytopenic purpura (ITP), previously termed *idiopathic thrombocytopenic purpura* affects 1 to 3 people per 100,000, but is probably the most common cause of severe isolated thrombocytopenia seen in the outpatient setting. It affects all ages, although ITP in childhood has a unique natural history. Childhood ITP is often associated with viral illness, is commonly transient, and may not need treatment. In adults, 40% of patients may have protracted or recurrent episodes of ITP, and the majority of patients need treatment. It was demonstrated in the 1950s that ITP is caused by circulating antiplatelet antibodies, and, like many autoimmune diseases, it is more common in women. When ITP presents in association with other diseases such as systemic lupus erythematosus or chronic lymphatic leukemia, or in patients with HIV, management of the underlying disease is important. The clinical presentation of ITP depends on the degree of thrombocytopenia. Mild thrombocytopenia of 20,000 to 80,000/µL is often asymptomatic, whereas platelet counts under 20,000/µL may present with mucocutaneous bleeding and diffuse petechiae and purpura. Thrombocytopenia, an otherwise normal blood count and peripheral blood smear without evidence of splenomegaly in a patient with no other illness helps make a tentative diagnosis. A bone marrow biopsy is no longer considered necessary to confirm the diagnosis.

Treatment of ITP has changed over the last several years, and initial treatment after the diagnosis requires evaluation of the platelet count, whether it is increasing or decreasing, and the presence or absence of bleeding. Patients who have counts above 20,000/µL without bleeding and who are not in need of an invasive procedure can be observed without intervention. Patients with counts between 10,000 and 20,000/µL may be started on oral prednisone at 1 mg/kg. Patients with severe thrombocytopenia less than 10,000/µL and those who are bleeding can receive high-dose dexamethasone (Decadron) at 40 mg daily for 4 days and IVIG (Gamunex). There is usually a response to treatment within 24 hours. Although usually not helpful or required, about 10% of patients will have a response to platelet transfusion, and this can be considered for patients presenting with low platelet counts and bleeding.

Refractory or recurrent ITP is a common problem in these patients, and recommendations for treatment include splenectomy, rituximab (Rituxan),[1] or thrombopoietin agonists. The choice of which to use depends on the patient and his or her clinical condition.

Thromocytopenia Due to Hypersplenism

The platelet mass is distributed 70% in the circulation and 30% in the spleen. Enlargement of the spleen and/or alteration of blood flow in portal hypertension may increase platelet sequestration in the spleen and reduce the platelet count in the peripheral blood circulation. Patients' counts rarely drop below 20,000/µL. Thus, thrombocytopenia caused by hypersplenism does not usually need any intervention. Patients with hepatitis C and cirrhosis may present with low platelet counts, and this may represent both hypersplenism and secondary immune thrombocytopenia. A trial of steroids may be used if these patients' clinical situation requires therapy.

Qualitative Platelet Function Disorders

Acquired Qualitative Platelet Function Disorders

Acquired disorders of platelet function are commonly seen, because platelets are the target of medications used to prevent arterial and cardiac stent thrombosis. Spontaneous bleeding is not common, but bleeding resulting from trauma or surgery can be a significant clinical problem. Because many patients may be on multiple antiplatelet agents or anticoagulants at the same time, the risk of bleeding needs to be recognized. Acquired qualitative disorders of platelet function may be due to drugs, hematologic diseases, or medical illnesses.

Drugs are the most common cause of acquired platelet dysfunction with differing risks of bleeding due to different targets. Aspirin causes irreversible acetylation of cyclooxygenase I (COX-1) and inhibits generation of prostaglandin A2. Although it is considered a weak antiplatelet agent with up to 25% resistance, aspirin increases the risk of bleeding in otherwise normal patients. Major bleeding was seen in up to 3.7% of patients and, when aspirin is used in combination with other antiplatelet agents or in patients with underlying bleeding disorders, the bleeding risk is higher. Clopidogrel (Plavix) is a thienopyridine prodrug, and the active metabolite irreversibly inhibits the surface receptor $P2Y_{12}$ on platelets. In clinical trials the risk of major bleeding in patients taking clopidogrel was similar to what is described with aspirin. Clopidogrel may significantly increase bleeding after surgery. GPIIb/IIIa receptor antagonists used after cardiac stent placement inhibit platelet aggregation and can induce severe thrombocytopenia.

Malignancies of the bone marrow may produce abnormally functioning platelets or alter platelet function by affecting vWF. The myeloproliferative and myelodysplastic disorders may produce platelets with reduced numbers of granules and may have associated increased risk of gastrointestinal bleeding and bleeding after invasive procedures. Acquired von Willebrand disease an infrequent cause of abnormal bleeding, can be seen in patients with lymphoproliferative disease, multiple myeloma, and Waldestrom macroglobulinemia.

Systemic illness can alter platelets and increase the bleeding risk. Acute and chronic renal failure are common causes of platelet-function abnormalities. In uremia, hemorrhagic complications include upper gastrointestinal bleeding, pericardial bleeding, and intracranial bleeding. Bleeding in renal failure is thought to be multifactorial and includes impaired release of platelet granules, decreased prostaglandin formation, vWF dysfunction, and presence of severe anemia. Effective treatment includes improvement of the anemia with erythropoietin[1] and/or desmopressin (DDAVP)[1] or conjugated estrogens (Premarin).[1]

Hereditary Qualitative Platelet Function Disorders

Inherited abnormalities of platelet function are infrequent disorders that give rise to bleeding of varying severity. Inherited

---

[1]Not FDA approved for this indication.

---

abnormalities of platelet function are often classified according to the type of genetic defect. Bernard-Soulier syndrome (BSS) is a severe bleeding disorder with autosomal recessive inheritance characterized by thrombocytopenia, decreased platelet adhesion, reduced platelet survival, and giant platelets on blood smear. Patients with BSS have defects in the GPIb-IX-V complex leading to reduced binding to vWF. Glanzmann thrombasthenia is an autosomal recessive disorder with defects of integrin αIIbβ3, a receptor on activated platelets that normally binds platelets during aggregation. Platelet aggregation to ADP and thrombin is abnormal. Patients with BSS and Glanzmann thrombasthenia who need treatment require platelet transfusions.

Hereditary disorders of platelet secretion are common reasons patients present to clinicians for evaluation of mucocutaneous bleeding. Defects in platelet dense granules (δ storage pool disease) are suspected in patients with bleeding and a negative workup for von Wilebrand disease. Diagnosis is made by platelet electron microscopy and or platelet aggregation studies. Granule deficiency associated with abnormalities of other lysosome-related organelles may lead to specific phenotypes such as Hermansky-Pudlak and Chediak Higashi disease. Gray platelet syndrome (GPS), or alpha granule deficiency, is an autosomal recessive disorder with mild bleeding. GPS patients may also be thrombocytopenic. Treatment for bleeding or in preparation for surgery includes desmopressin (DDAVP)[1] or platelet transfusions.

---

[1]Not FDA approved for this indication.

References

Aster RH, Curtis BR, McFarland JG, Bougie DW. Drug-induced immune thrombocytopenia: pathogenesis, diagnosis, and management. J Thromb Haemost 2009;7:911–8.

Barbour T, Johnson S, Cohney S, Hughes P. Thrombotic microangiopathy and associated renal disorders. Nephrol Dial Transplant 2012;27:2673–85.

Cuker A, Gimotty PA, Crowther MA, Warkentin TE. Predictive value of the 4Ts scoring system for heparin-induced thrombocytopenia: a systematic review and meta-analysis. Blood 2012;120:4160–7.

Estcourt L, Stanworth S, Doree C, et al. Prophylactic platelet transfusion in prevention of bleeding in patients with hematologic disorders and stem cell transplantation. Cochrane Database Syst Rev 2012 May 16;5. http://dx.doi.org/10.1002/14651858.CD004269.pub3, CD004269.

Hedges SJ, Dehoney SB, Hooper JS, et al. Evidence-based treatment recommendations for uremic bleeding. Nat Clin Pract Nephrol 2007;3:138–53.

Jackson S. Arterial thrombosis: insidious, unpredictable, and deadly. Nat Med 2011;17:1423–36.

Lakshmanan S, Cuker A. Contemporary management of immune thrombocytopenic purpura in adults. J Thromb Haemost 2012;10:1988–98.

Nurden A, Nurden P. Advances in our understanding of the molecular basis of disorders of platelet function. J Thromb Haemost Suppl 2011;1:76–91.

Provan D, Stasi R, Newland AC, et al. International consensus report on the investigation and management of primary immune thrombocytopenia. Blood 2010;115:168–86.

Tsantes AE, Nikolopoulos GK, Tsirigotis P, et al. Direct evidence for normalization of platelet function resulting from platelet count reduction in essential thrombocytosis. Blood Coagul Fibrinolysis 2011;22:457–62.

Warkentin AE, Donadni MP, Spencer FA, et al. Bleeding risk in randomized controlled trials comparing warfarin and aspirin: a systemic review and meta-analysis. J Thromb Haemost 2012;10:512–20.

Zucker ML, Hagedorn CH, Murphy CA, et al. Mechanism of thrombocytopenia in chronic hepatitis C as evaluated by the immature platelet fraction. Int J Lab Hematol 2012;34:525–32.

POLYCYTHEMIA VERA

Method of
Peter R. Duggan, MD; and Sonia Cerquozzi, MD

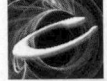

CURRENT DIAGNOSIS

- Polycythemia vera should be considered when there is persistent elevation of hemoglobin (>185 g/L in men and >165 g/L in women).

- *JAK-2* mutation testing and erythropoietin levels should be performed when polycythemia is suspected.
- Bone marrow biopsy and aspiration may be necessary in some cases to confirm the diagnosis of polycythemia and to distinguish polycythemia from other myeloproliferative disorders.
- Polycythemia is highly likely when *JAK2* mutation is present and erythropoietin level is subnormal. When *JAK2* mutation is seen with normal erythropoietin level, polycythemia is possible; bone marrow biopsy is recommended to differentiate polycythemia from other myeloproliferative diseases. When *JAK2* is normal and erythropoietin is low, consider *JAK2* exon 12 mutational analysis or alternative diagnosis of congenital polycythemia. Unmutated *JAK2* and normal or high erythropoietin level make polycythemia very unlikely, and patients should be investigated for secondary causes of erythrocytosis.
- Secondary causes of polycythemia should be ruled out, especially when *JAK2* is not mutated or erythropoietin level is high. Investigations for secondary polycythemia that may be indicated include:
  - Red cell mass and plasma volume measurement
  - Chest x-ray
  - Pulse oximetry
  - Arterial blood gas including carboxyhemoglobin and methemoglobin levels
  - Kidney and liver function tests
  - Abdominal imaging studies (ultrasound or CT scan)
  - Oxyhemoglobin dissociation curve
  - Sleep studies

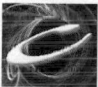

CURRENT THERAPY

- All patients should be treated with phlebotomy and/or cytoreductive therapy with target hematocrit less than 45%.
- Low-dose aspirin[1] should be used in all patients without a contraindication.
- In patients with high-risk polycythemia vera, hydroxyurea (Hydrea)[1] should be used, with dose titrated to maintain a white blood cell count greater than $3.0 \times 10^9/L$ and platelets in the normal range.
- Alkylating agents should be avoided as cytoreductive therapy owing to the risk of acute leukemia.
- Conventional cardiovascular risk factors (diabetes, hypertension, hyperlipidemia) should be aggressively managed, and cigarette smoking should be discouraged.
- Thromboembolic events should be managed according to accepted management guidelines. Thromboprophylaxis should be used after surgery and in other high-risk situations.

[1]Not FDA approved for this indication.

Polycythemia vera (PV) is a clonal stem cell disorder characterized by an increase in red cell production independent of the stimulation by erythropoietin. PV is the most common of the chronic myeloproliferative diseases, occurring in approximately 2 to 3 people per 100,000 annually. The median age at diagnosis is 70 years, and it is rare in patients younger than 40 years.

A mutation of the tyrosine kinase Janus kinase 2 (JAK2) is consistently found in PV. This sheds some light on the pathogenesis of the disease and is useful in the diagnosis of PV and other myeloproliferative disorders. A single acquired mutation (V617F) of the gene for the JH-2 domain of JAK2 can be found in 90% to 95% of PV patients. The JH-2 domain functions to inhibit JAK2 activity. In normal erythropoiesis, binding of erythropoietin to its receptor lifts this inhibition and allows JAK2 stimulation of cell division and differentiation. In mutated JAK2, this inhibitory function is absent, leading to constitutive activity of the tyrosine

kinase. This mutation is also present in about half of patients with essential thrombocytosis and primary myelofibrosis. The small number of patients with PV who are negative for the common JAK2 mutation have another functionally similar mutation.

Presentation

Many patients with PV are asymptomatic, and PV is diagnosed after the incidental finding of an elevated hemoglobin on routine complete blood count. Up to half of patients experience such nonspecific symptoms as weight loss, sweating, headache, fatigue, epigastric discomfort, visual disturbances, and dizziness. Many of these symptoms are likely caused by decreased blood flow due to an increased blood viscosity from polycythemia.

Generalized pruritus is often described, often after a warm bath or shower. Although the cause of this is unknown, it is thought to be due to the degranulation of increased numbers of mast cells in the skin of patients, releasing histamine and other inflammatory mediators. However, the symptom responds poorly to antihistamines, and it does not always resolve with treatment of PV.

Venous and arterial thromboembolic events are a major cause of morbidity and mortality in PV. Thrombosis at presentation occurs in up to 40% of patients. Ischemic stroke, transient ischemic attack, and myocardial infarction are common, especially among elderly patients. These, along with deep venous thrombosis and pulmonary embolus, are the most common thrombotic events and often result in serious morbidity, disability, and even death. Thrombotic events that are considered unusual in the general population, such as Budd-Chiari syndrome and portal, mesenteric, and other abdominal vein thrombosis and cerebral venous thrombosis, occur more among PV patients. The possibility of an underlying myeloproliferative disorder should be considered when a patient presents with such an event.

PV can manifest with symptoms of peripheral vascular disease. Patients with erythromelalgia describe a painful burning sensation of the hands and feet; pallor, erythema, or cyanosis of the extremities; and sometimes cutaneous ulceration. Erythromelalgia results from microvascular thrombosis and ischemia due to platelet activation and aggregation and responds well to platelet reduction and antiplatelet agents such as aspirin (acetylsalicylic acid [ASA]).[1]

Almost all patients with PV are iron deficient at diagnosis, even before the onset of therapeutic phlebotomy. Other manifestations include acute gouty arthritis, peptic ulcer disease, erosive gastritis, and hypertension.

Diagnosis and Differential Diagnosis

The 2008 World Health Organization (WHO) diagnostic criteria for PV are shown in Box 1. The JAK2 V617F mutation is present in about 95% of cases of PV. Erythropoietin level is decreased in more than 90% and is rarely elevated. Most JAK2 assays are negative in the few PV patients with a mutation of exon 12 of the *JAK2* gene instead of the more common JAK2 V617F mutation. A JAK2 mutation can also be found in about half of patients with essential thrombocytosis and primary myelofibrosis.

Leukocytosis and thrombocytosis are present in the majority of cases of PV. Red cell mass is increased. A nuclear medicine study measuring red cell mass and plasma volume is rarely required with the availability of JAK2 testing, but it may be useful when relative polycythemia is suspected. Bone marrow biopsy and aspiration are not often needed for a diagnosis of PV, but they remain minor diagnostic criteria in the WHO classification. Bone marrow examination can be important for diagnosing PV in the rare cases where JAK2 is negative and to differentiate PV from other JAK2-positive myeloproliferative disorders when the distinction cannot be made based on peripheral blood counts.

Erythrocytosis can occur as a result of a number of other conditions in the absence of PV (Box 2). A careful history and physical with selected investigations can usually distinguish PV from secondary polycythemia and relative polycythemia (see Current

[1]Not FDA approved for this indication.

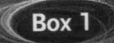

2008 World Health Organization Diagnostic Criteria for Polycythemia Vera

Diagnosis requires two major criteria and one minor criterion, or one major criterion with at least two minor criteria.

Major Criteria

Hemoglobin >18.5 g/d/L in men, 16.5 g/dL in women, or other evidence of increased red cell volume*

Presence of JAK2 V617F or other functionally similar mutation such as JAK2 exon 12 mutation

Minor Criteria

Bone marrow biopsy showing hypercellularity for age with trilineage proliferation

Subnormal serum erythropoietin level

Endogenous erythroid colony formation in vitro

*Unexplained, sustained increase in hemoglobin of at least 2 g/dL, to >17 g/dL in men or >15 g/dL in women, or elevated red cell mass >25% above normal.

Box 2 Differential Diagnosis of Polycythemia

Normal Red Cell Mass
Relative polycythemia
Gaisböck's syndrome

Elevated Red Cell Mass
Primary Polycythemia
Polycythemia vera

Secondary Polycythemia
Congenital
- EPO receptor mutations
- Chuvash polycythemia
- High-affinity hemoglobin
Appropriately elevated EPO (hypoxia driven)
- Chronic hypoxic lung disease
- Cardiac shunts or cyanotic heart disease
- Sleep apnea
- Methemoglobinemia
- High altitude
- Chronic carbon monoxide poisoning
- Cigarette smoking
- Renal artery stenosis
Inappropriately elevated EPO
- Renal cell carcinoma
- Hepatocellular carcinoma
- Hemangioblastoma
- Uterine fibroids
Other causes
- EPO (Epogen) administration
- Androgens (testosterone)
- Kidney transplant

Abbreviation: EPO = erythropoietin.

Diagnosis). In relative (apparent, spurious) polycythemia, there is usually only a modest increase in the hematocrit, because of a decrease in plasma volume rather than a true increase in red cell mass. Thrombocytosis, leukocytosis, and splenomegaly should be absent. Causes include smoking, dehydration, and use of diuretics, and it is also described in middle-aged, obese, hypertensive men (Gaisböck's syndrome).

Red cell mass can be elevated owing to increased stimulation of erythropoiesis by high levels of erythropoietin. Erythropoietin can be increased as an appropriate response to chronic hypoxia (sleep apnea, right-to-left cardiac shunts, chronic lung diseases, high altitude, smoking, methemoglobinemia), and it can be inappropriately elevated owing to erythropoietin-secreting tumors (renal cell carcinoma, hepatocellular carcinoma, cerebellar hemangioma, uterine fibroids) or decreased kidney perfusion (renal artery stenosis). Familial causes of polycythemia include high-affinity hemoglobins, erythropoietin receptor mutations, and Chuvash polycythemia. Polycythemia occurs in 10% to 15% of patients following kidney transplantation, and this may be due to erythropoietin secretion by the native kidneys or increased sensitivity to erythropoietin. Polycythemia can be drug induced, such as with the use of performance-enhancing drugs (erythropoietin [Epogen], androgens) in athletes and testosterone replacement in men.

Prognosis

When PV is left untreated, the outlook for patients is poor, with median survival reported to be as low as 18 months. This improves considerably with treatment, though annual mortality remains almost twice as high as in the general population.

Despite therapy, thrombosis remains an important cause of mortality. Cardiac disease, ischemic stroke, pulmonary embolus, and other thrombotic events account for 40% of deaths among PV patients. Nonfatal thrombosis is common, occurring in almost 4% of patients annually. Age and a history of prior thromboembolic events are independent risk factors for thrombosis and can be used to predict a patient's risk of future events (Box 3). Low-risk patients are younger than 60 years and have no history of thrombosis. They experience new events at a rate of 2% per year. For patients older than 60 years or with a past history of thrombosis this rate is 5% annually, but it can be as high as 11% when both risk factors are present.

The contribution of other cardiovascular risk factors (smoking, diabetes, hypertension, hyperlipidemia) to thrombotic risk in PV has been studied, with inconclusive results. However, because these are major contributors to the development of cardiovascular disease in the general population, they should also be considered when assessing risk in patients with PV.

The risk of major hemorrhage is low, with fatal bleeding causing less than 5% of all deaths. However, there is considerable excess mortality from malignancy, in particular transformation to a myelodysplastic syndrome, myelofibrosis, or acute leukemia. The risk of transformation is highest in those older than 70 years and in patients treated with cytoreductive agents other than hydroxyurea (Hydrea)[1] or interferon alfa-2b (Intron A).[1]

Treatment

The goals of treatment in PV are to lower the risk of thrombosis while minimizing toxicity. This is achieved by a combination of

[1]Not FDA approved for this indication.

Box 3 Thrombotic Risk in Polycythemia Vera

Low Risk
Age younger than 60 years
No history of thromboembolism
No cardiovascular risk factors
Less than 2% risk per year for thrombotic events

Intermediate Risk
Age younger than 60 years
No history of thromboembolism
Presence of cardiovascular risk factors

High Risk
Age older than 60 years
Prior thrombosis
Risk is 5% per year for thrombotic events, 11% if both risk factors are present

phlebotomy, aspirin,[1] and hydroxyurea[1] or other cytoreductive agents. The use of these therapies can be individualized based on a patient's risk of developing future thromboembolic events.

Phlebotomy

As the hematocrit increases in PV, there is a dramatic increase in blood viscosity. Phlebotomy is the fastest, most effective way to normalize a patient's hematocrit, and it should be initiated immediately in those with newly diagnosed or suspected PV. Blood volume should be reduced as rapidly as possible. Usually, 500 mL of blood is removed every 1 or 2 days until the hematocrit is less than 45%. The frequency of phlebotomy or volume of blood removed can be decreased in elderly patients, those with cardiovascular disease, or others who do not tolerate this schedule. The optimal target in PV patients, is to maintain a hemocrit less than 45% in order to lower the risk of major thrombotic events and death from cardiovascular causes. Regular phlebotomy eventually results in iron deficiency, at which point most patients' phlebotomy needs decrease dramatically. Iron replacement should be avoided.

Aspirin

Previous studies did not support the routine use of aspirin to prevent thrombosis in PV. However, high doses of aspirin were used, resulting in excess bleeding in the treatment arm. The results of a recent large randomized trial show that low-dose aspirin reduces major thrombotic events (nonfatal myocardial infarction, nonfatal stroke, pulmonary embolism, major venous thrombosis). This was accomplished without an increase in bleeding risk. Although there was a trend suggesting more minor bleeding events in those receiving aspirin, the rates of major bleeding were identical for those receiving aspirin or placebo. The benefit from aspirin was seen even though this study included many low-risk patients without a prior history of thromboembolism. Low-dose aspirin (75–100 mg daily) should be started in all patients without a contraindication to the drug (history of bleeding or intolerance). Because of the risk of bleeding from acquired von Willebrand's disease that can occur with extreme thrombocytosis, aspirin should be held when platelets are more than 1500×10^9/L until the count can be lowered with hydroxyurea.

Cytoreductive Therapy

Hydroxyurea is the cytoreductive agent most commonly used to treat PV. Hydroxyurea can safely control blood counts and decreases spleen size in PV and other myeloproliferative disorders. Randomized data are limited, but hydroxyurea also appears to reduce thrombotic complications. It is recommended for patients with high-risk PV and should be considered in those with intermediate-risk disease. A starting dosage of 15 to 20 mg/kg daily (1000–1500 mg daily) is used. Occasional phlebotomy is still required to maintain hematocrit less than 45%, but the frequency usually decreases. Myelosuppression is the main toxicity. The lowest dosage that provides therapeutic effect should be used, and excess myelosuppression should be avoided. The dosage can be titrated to ensure that the white cell count remains higher than 3.0×10^9/L, neutrophils are higher than 2.0×10^9/L, and platelets are in the normal range.

Hydroxyurea has been associated with leg ulcers and other skin changes, especially after long-term use. There is growing evidence that hydroxyurea does not contribute to the excess rates of acute leukemia seen in PV; rates are no different than in those treated with phlebotomy alone. However, transformation is clearly associated with the use of other chemotherapeutic agents such as chlorambucil (Leukeran),[1] busulfan (Myleran),[1] and pipobroman (Vercyte),[2] accounting for one third of the deaths among PV patients treated with these agents. The use of these agents should be avoided.

JAK Inhibitors

Ruxolitinib (Jakafi), a JAK-1/2 inhibitor, showed clinical benefit in small Phase II studies resulting in reduction of hemocrit, spleen size and significant symptom control, with 10 mg twice daily established as an effective starting dose. A follow-up Phase III study (RESPONSE) illustrated that Ruxolitinb was effective at controlling Hct (<45%), reducing spleen size (≥35%) and improving symptoms in PV patients, who have been intolerant to or had inadequate response to Hydrea. Ruxolitinib has been approved for use in patients with myelofibrosis, including myelofibrosis evolving from PV. In these patients there was a significant reduction in spleen size and constitutional symptoms in almost half of patients.

Other Treatment Issues

Hyperuricemia is common in myeloproliferative disorders and occasionally results in kidney stones or gout. Allopurinol (Zyloprim) 300 mg daily can be used to reduce uric acid levels in patients with these complications. For those with intractable pruritus, several agents have been used with variable success. Some patients respond to aspirin,[1] hydroxyurea,[1] cimetidine (Tagamet),[1] or cyproheptadine (Periactin).[1] Interferon alfa-2b, 3 million units subcutaneously three times per week, is successful in the majority of cases, and success is also reported with paroxetine (Paxil)[1] 20 mg daily.

Less than 60% of pregnancies occurring in PV patients are successful. First trimester loss is the most common complication, and third trimester fetal loss, preterm birth, and intrauterine growth restriction are also common. Phlebotomy should be used to keep the hematocrit at less than 45%. Interferon alfa-2b[1] is recommended for those requiring cytoreductive therapy; other cytoreductive agents are contraindicated due to possible teratogenic effects. There is some evidence that the use of low-dose aspirin[1] throughout pregnancy improves live birth rate. It is recommended that prophylactic low molecular-weight heparin (LMWH) be used for 6 weeks after delivery.

Surgery in patients with PV has a high risk of both operative bleeding and postoperative thromboembolism. Elective surgeries should be delayed until cytoreductive measures and phlebotomy can be used to achieve good control of blood counts. Aspirin should be held for 1 week before surgery to reduce the risk of hemorrhage. LMWH should be given after surgery to prevent deep venous thrombosis. Mechanical compression stockings are an option for patients with bleeding that prevents the use of anticoagulation.

Because cerebrovascular and cardiovascular disease are among the main causes of morbidity and mortality for these patients, careful attention should be paid to the management of conventional cardiovascular risk factors. Hypertension, diabetes, and hyperlipidemia should be controlled with standard measures, and patients should be encouraged to stop smoking.

When thromboembolic events do occur, treatment should be according to current management guidelines. Venous thromboembolism is treated with LMWH and warfarin (Coumadin). Indefinite anticoagulation should be considered because of the high risk of recurrent events. Low-dose aspirin is indicated in those with a history of arterial events such as stroke and myocardial infarction.

---

[1]Not FDA approved for this indication.

References

Baxter EJ, Scott LM, Campbell PJ, et al. Acquired mutation of the tyrosine kinase JAK2 in human myeloproliferative disorders. Lancet 2005;365:1054–61.

Finazzi G, Barbui T. How I treat patients with polycythemia vera. Blood 2007;109:5104–11.

Finazzi G, Caruso V, Marchioli R, et al. for the ECLAP Investigators: Acute leukemia in polycythemia vera: An analysis of 1638 patients enrolled in a prospective observational study. Blood 2005;105(7):2664–70.

Fruchtman SM, Mack K, Kaplan ME, et al. From efficacy to safety: A polycythemia vera study group report on hydroxyurea in patients with polycythemia vera. Semin Hematol 1997;34:17–23.

---

[1]Not FDA approved for this indication.
[2]Not available in the United States.

Landolfi R, Marchioli R, Kutti J, et al. Efficacy and safety of low-dose aspirin in polycythemia vera. N Engl J Med 2004;350:114–24.

Marchioli R, Finazzi G, Landolfi R, et al. Vascular and neoplastic risk in a large cohort of patients with polycythemia vera. J Clin Oncol 2005;23(10):2224–32.

Marchioli R, Finazzi G, Specchia G, et al. Cardiovascular events and intensity of treatment in polycythemia vera. N Engl J Med 2013;368:22–33.

Najean Y, Mugnier P, Dresch C, Rain JD. Polycythemia vera in young people: An analysis of 58 cases diagnosed before 40 years. Br J Haematol 1987;67:285–91.

Robinson S, Bewley S, Hunt BJ, et al. The management and outcome of 18 pregnancies in women with polycythemia vera. Haematologica 2005;90(11):1477–83.

Ruggeri M, Rodeghiero F, Tosetto A, et al. Postsurgery outcomes in patients with polycythemia vera and essential thrombocythemia: a retrospective survey. Blood 2008;111:666–71.

Silver RT. Long-term effects of the treatment of polycythemia vera with recombinant interferon-alpha. Cancer 2006;107(3):451–8.

Swerdlow S, Campo E, Lee Harris N, et al., WHO Classification of Tumors of Hematopoietic and Lymphoid Tissues. 4th ed. Lyon, France: IARC; 2008.

Verstovsek S, Passamonti F, Rambaldi A, et al. A phase 2 study of ruxolitinib, an oral JAK1 and JAK2 inhibitor, in patients with advanced polycythemia vera who are refractory or intolerant to hydroxyurea. Cancer 2014:513–20.

Verstovsek S, Mesa RA, Gotlib J, et al. A double-blind, placebo-controlled trial of ruxolitinib for myelofibrosis. N Engl J Med 2012;366:799–807.

PORPHYRIAS

Method of
Claus A. Pierach, MD

CURRENT DIAGNOSIS

- There is not just one porphyria; there are at least six types (and a few very rare ones because of homozygosity and dual porphyrias).
- There is not one single test covering all porphyrias. For suspected acute porphyria, screening for excessive porphobilinogen in the urine is the test of choice.
- If cutaneous porphyria is in the differential diagnosis, quantitative measurements of porphyrins in urine and stool are recommended.
- Family studies and genetic counseling are always indicated in these hereditary diseases.

CURRENT THERAPY

- Prophylaxis is mandatory and depends on the type of porphyria.
- Abstinence from alcohol is always indicated.
- The drug list should be respected in the acute porphyrias.
- Glucose therapy for the acute attack has been superseded by the more effective, definitive treatment with hematin (hemin, Panhematin), to be instituted as soon as possible once the diagnosis has been ascertained.

The *porphyrias* present a group of mostly inherited diseases where disturbances along the biosynthetic pathway to heme lead to accumulations of metabolic intermediaries. Porphyria cutanea tarda usually occurs without discernible inheritance; it can also be induced by chemicals. All steps of heme synthesis are enzymatically regulated and all porphyrias are a result of specific impasses along these transitions. Not all enzymatic defects result in clinically relevant or recognizable disease manifestations in every patient. On the one hand, the severity of the enzymatic defect plays a role. On the other, some poorly understood revealing or unveiling cofactors are operational; enzyme cofactors are likely contributing as well. The prevalence of the porphyrias is not known and fluctuates in different parts of the world; for example, variegate porphyria is most common in South Africa, whereas porphyria cutanea tarda is the most common porphyria in the United States.

The porphyrias can be divided between neurovisceral (acute) and cutaneous manifestations. Two types, the very rare delta-aminolevulinic acid-dehydratase deficiency porphyria and acute intermittent porphyria (AIP), have only neurologic symptoms (acute attacks and possibly chronic manifestations). Hereditary coproporphyria and variegate porphyria can have both neurologic and dermatologic signs and symptoms. Congenital erythropoietic porphyria, porphyria cutanea tarda, and erythropoietic protoporphyria exhibit only skin lesions but can be complicated by other problems, such as anemia or hepatic insufficiency.

Heme Synthesis

Succinyl coenzyme-A and glycine are the initial building blocks, subsequently transformed through eight enzymatic steps to the end product, heme, in itself essential not only for hemoglobin but also for other hemoproteins such as cytochromes, myoglobin, and other enzymes including catalase, nitric oxide synthase, and tryptophan pyrrolase. Heme synthesis happens in all cells but mostly in the liver and in the bone marrow. It is controlled by heme through feedback inhibition of the first step, delta-aminolevulinic acid synthase. Figure 1 shows the various steps, intermediaries, and resulting porphyrias. Porphyrins and their precursors, delta-aminolevulinic acid (ALA) and porphobilinogen (PBG), are only generated during heme synthesis and not during heme catabolism toward bilirubin.

Specific enzymatic defects result in specific patterns of heme precursors and are of high diagnostic value when determining the type of porphyria. The ultimate step in ruling in or out if a

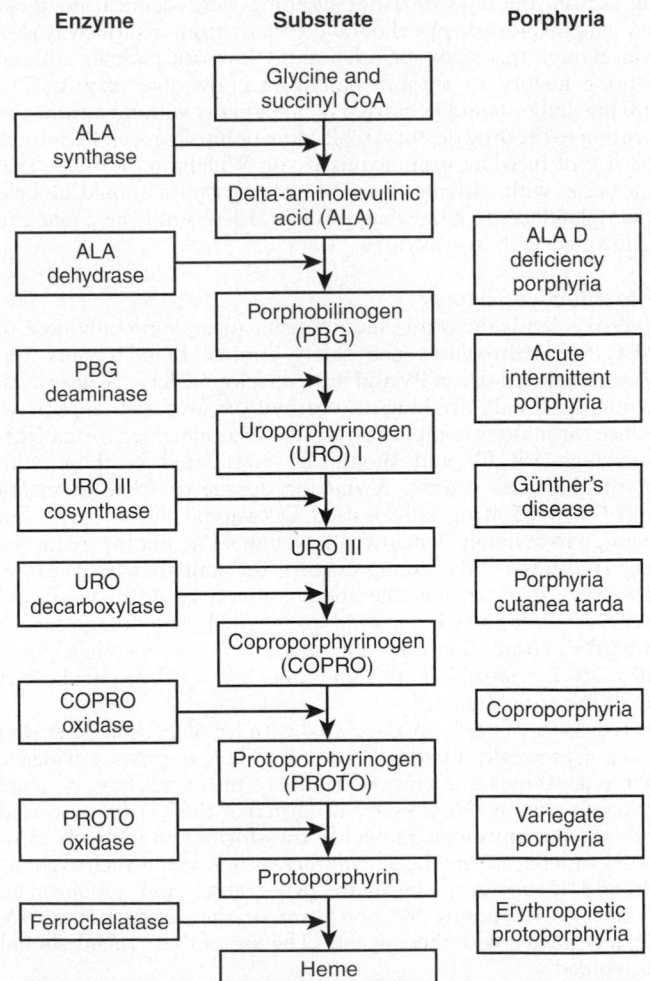

Figure 1. Heme biosynthetic pathway. Enzymes that have defects or deficiencies that cause the various porphyries are listed on the left side, heme and precursors are in the middle, and the resulting porphyrias are on the right side. *Abbreviation:* CoA = coenzyme A.

person has the genetic defect for a specific porphyria is DNA testing, currently offered by the Mount Sinai Genetic Testing Laboratory (porphyria@mssm.edu). However, these specific tests are not necessary in the clinical evaluation of a patient in whom porphyria is suspected. Here, quick and simple tests are sufficient. The excretory pattern of heme precursors is influenced by their water solubility, which decreases toward heme; ALA and PBG are highly water soluble and measured in urine, whereas protoporphyrin is so hydrophobic that it is only excreted in stool and not in urine.

There is no single test that can reveal all types of porphyrias. The porphyric symptomatology can differ from type to type and there is considerable overlap among the various porphyrias. For this reason, highly specific and sensitive laboratory tests are necessary. All porphyrias with acute manifestations manifest with similar attacks and respond to similar treatment, but they exhibit different biochemical patterns according to their specific enzyme defect. A clinically useful grouping splits the porphyrias between acute (neurovisceral) and cutaneous.

The Acute Porphyrias

There are four types of acute porphyria to consider:
- The very rare ALA-dehydratase deficiency porphyria is inherited in an autosomal recessive fashion.
- AIP, an autosomal dominant disorder, is the most common of the acute porphyrias (except in South Africa where variegate porphyria is more common).
- Hereditary coproporphyria, an autosomal dominant disease, is commonly misdiagnosed because coproporphyrin is often moderately and nonspecifically increased in many disorders.
- Variegate porphyria is autosomal dominant and probably the mildest of the acute porphyrias.

All acute porphyrias are sensitive to a multitude of drugs and circumstances (a short list is included in Box 1). Hereditary coproporphyria and variegate porphyria can also have skin lesions resembling porphyria cutanea tarda. Skin lesions and acute attacks can happen at the same time or one after the other, or only one manifestation may ever be present in a given patient.

Diagnosis

Diagnosis of the porphyric attack hinges mainly on a keen sense of suspicion. Any inexplicable symptom complex involving abdominal pain, tachycardia, and psychological findings should be suspect for porphyria. However, no clinical presentation can be called *porphyric* without biochemical support. Small deviations from the narrow normal range for heme precursors are fairly common and nonspecific. PBG or ALA must be markedly elevated, at least fivefold above the normal range, and, if not, porphyria is an unlikely explanation for a patient's acute symptoms.

Older screening mechanisms such as the Watson-Schwartz test and the Hoesch test have been replaced by easier, more specific, semiquantitative tests such as the Trace PBG kit (Thermo Fisher Scientific), but they still rely on the color reaction with Ehrlich's aldehyde. This or a similar test must be available in all emergency departments and in all acute care hospitals. A *random* urine sample is sufficient for the initial diagnostic evaluation, and if it is positive it must be later followed up by more-detailed tests such as quantitative measurements of porphyrins and precursors in a 24-hour urine collection. Fecal porphyrin measurements may also be called for. Enzyme measurements and genetic testing are rarely indicated, but they are used when more routine tests fail. Because the porphyrias are almost always hereditary, family studies are highly appropriate. The proper interpretation of any test result is best done in the context of available clinical information.

Clinical Presentation

Clinical presentations of porphyric attacks vary so much that the term *the little imitator* has been used. Not all signs or symptoms

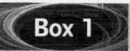
are always present, but severe and poorly localized abdominal pain and unexplained tachycardia are so prevalent that their absence further complicates the diagnosis of an acute porphyric attack. The genesis of the attack is not well understood, but acutely increased demand for heme and production of toxic intermediary products are considered to be the culprit. Increased demand for heme and increased production of intermediary products can be due to a wide variety of circumstances, from drugs through hormones (premenstrual phase) to stress, infection, fasting, and starvation. However, most carriers of the genetic defect for an acute porphyria remain asymptomatic all their lives. Some have only one or two attacks, and only a few suffer from many attacks.

The clinical picture with pain, fast heart rate, and neurovisceral symptoms can be complicated by, at times, severe hyponatremia, heralding seizures with therapeutic dilemmas (see Box 1) and respiratory paralysis necessitating ventilatory support. Death is rare nowadays, especially when the diagnosis is made early. The recovery is usually complete, but at times it is prolonged, up to 1 year after a severe attack.

Superb nursing care, initially preferable in an intensive care unit, is necessary, and meticulous attention has to be paid to *all* problems. Dehydration from vomiting is common and ileus and urinary retention are not infrequent; hyponatremia occurs in approximately half of the porphyric attacks. Muscle strength must be tested frequently. Twice-daily measurement of vital capacity helps to assess the necessity for respiratory assistance. High blood pressure and tachycardia deserve careful attention and, if appropriate, cautious treatment with a β-blocker. A negative caloric balance must be avoided, and if present initially it is best treated with carbohydrates (if necessary, intravenously with glucose, up to 300 g/day), and then later with a balanced diet.

Treatment

Therapy must always start with a careful look at the drugs recently taken by the patient. It is best to discontinue as many drugs as possible, especially those deemed unsafe (see Box 1). Appropriate lists of safe and unsafe drugs in porphyria are readily available from websites (www.porphyriafoundation.com and www.porphyria-europe.com). An infection must be diligently searched for and treated at once. Seizure precautions are especially indicated if hyponatremia is found. Analgesics should be adequately dispensed; opiates are often necessary in fairly large doses.

Specific therapy was introduced a generation ago in the form of hematin (hemin, Panhematin), available from Lundbeck Inc. (847-282-1000 or www.lundbeckinc.com). This has largely replaced glucose (300 g/day), which had the main advantages of availability, relatively low cost, and the possibility of curbing an early or mild attack.

But one must not wait for quick improvement in a patient's condition and should at once take steps to obtain the definitive medication, hematin. This represents the equivalent to the end product, heme, and exerts its beneficial effect through repression of the deranged, and in the porphyric attack, markedly activated pathway to heme. It is still unclear whether the quick suppression of potentially toxic heme precursors (in 1–2 days) or a postulated replenishment of an assumed heme deficiency is the effective mechanism. *Early* administration of hematin is strongly advocated because the course of a porphyric attack is unpredictable, and a point of no return can unfortunately be reached quickly. Thus, the infusion of hematin must start as soon as possible.

A daily dose of 2 to 4 mg/kg body weight is recommended for up to 4 days. Longer treatment periods are of questionable value but may be tried in severe cases for up to 2 weeks. The infusion must be strictly intravenous and with ample flushing because hematin can cause thrombosis and phlebitis. Because it is a procoagulant and anticoagulant, frequent measurements of coagulation parameters are advisable. Anticoagulants such as warfarin (Coumadin) should if possible be avoided. Admixture of 5% human serum albumin (Albuminar-5) has been advocated to stabilize the final hematin solution and to lessen side effects. Hematin is available in many countries as heme arginate (Normosang).[2]

A beneficial clinical effect can be expected in 1 to 2 days, accompanied by a decrease in all heme precursors, most notably ALA and PBG. Many patients have received many treatment courses with hematin without apparent loss of effectiveness. Prophylactic use of hematin can be helpful in the treatment of women with frequent premenstrual exacerbations of their acute porphyria. Hematin should never be given as a diagnostic test to see if unexplained symptoms reminiscent of porphyria lessen. The diagnosis of a porphyric attack must be as quick, precise, and certain as possible, especially in new cases.

Partial liver transplantation has been successfully undertaken and found to be curative in patients with unrelenting porphyric attacks.

Prophylaxis of porphyric attacks is of great importance and can be accomplished to a large extent by avoidance of unsafe drugs, by stable caloric intake, and by prompt attention to intercurrent illnesses. It is a difficult decision if unsafe drugs have to be administered for a vital indication such as seizures. Here, consultation with an expert in porphyria is strongly advised.

The Cutaneous Porphyrias

The symptomatology of cutaneous porphyrias is mainly photosensitivity, often combined with skin fragility and blisters. All these findings occur because of porphyrin toxicity, resulting in cutaneous light absorption at the wavelength of 400 to 410 nm and subsequent formation of damaging reactive oxygen species. Thus, two therapeutic approaches are plausible: decrease of porphyrins and protection of the skin from sunlight. The usual sunscreens are, however, ineffective, and reflective agents containing zinc or titanium, although better, are less popular because of their appearance.

In three porphyrias—porphyria cutanea tarda, hereditary coproporphyria, and variegate porphyria—the skin lesions are rather similar, but erythropoietic protoporphyria and congenital erythropoietic porphyria can lead to very painful nonblistering skin lesions, and, in congenital erythropoietic porphyria, even to mutilations.

Porphyria Cutanea Tarda

Porphyria cutanea tarda is the most common porphyria and occurs because of uroporphyrinogen-decarboxylase deficiency and accumulation of mostly uroporphyrin. It can be inherited autosomal dominantly but more often occurs sporadically. It can also be due to toxins such as halogenated aromatic hydrocarbons.

The most prominent skin manifestations are seen on the dorsa of the hands and on the face, consisting of blisters filled with mostly clear fluid; shallow, slow-healing ulcers; whitish plaques; and tiny inclusion bodies, *milia.* Hypertrichosis and hyperpigmentation are often seen.

Unveiling factors promote the manifestation of the disease and consist mainly of liver disease, often due to alcohol. Hepatitis, often type C, and HIV infections are also common revealers. The drug list (see Box 1) is *not* applicable to the cutaneous porphyrias. The diagnosis is easily suspected at inspection and confirmed by measurement of urinary uroporphyrin excretion, typically manifold increased above the normal range.

There are two treatment options with different principles but rather similar effectiveness. Repeat phlebotomies of 350 to 450 mL at 1- to 2-week intervals are performed and followed by hemoglobin and ferritin measurements. Overt anemia should be avoided. Ferritin usually reaches the lower end of the normal range after approximately 8 to 10 phlebotomies, and clinical remission can be expected after approximately half a year. Remission can be long lasting, especially when unveiling factors are avoided; total abstinence from alcohol is advocated. Patients should not take iron-enriched vitamins because iron plays a critical role in porphyria cutanea tarda.

If phlebotomies are contraindicated (due to anemia or pulmonary or cardiac disease) or are very inconvenient, low-dose chloroquine (Aralen)[1] (125 mg twice weekly) can be given orally. This flushes porphyrins from the liver and can be continued until remission is reached. In such low doses, the drug is virtually free from side effects.

Patients on chronic dialysis can develop porphyria cutanea tarda and also *pseudoporphyria.* Here, plasma porphyrin measurements establish the correct diagnosis. Patients with porphyria cutanea tarda and end-stage renal disease respond well to erythropoietin (Epogen, Procrit),[1] probably via iron depletion through incorporation of iron into hemoglobin. Pseudoporphyria is also seen as a side effect of many drugs, mostly nonsteroidal antiinflammatory drugs and diuretics. Although it is phenotypically identical to porphyria cutanea tarda, pseudoporphyria does not respond to phlebotomies or chloroquine.

Patients with porphyria cutanea tarda have a much higher incidence of hepatocellular carcinoma and should be checked twice annually with hepatic imaging and measurement of alpha fetoprotein.

Congenital Erythropoietic Porphyria (Günther Disease)

Congenital erythropoietic porphyria (Günther disease), a rare autosomal recessive disorder, is usually apparent shortly after

[2]Not available in the United States.

[1]Not FDA approved for this indication.

birth when brick-colored urine in diapers is observed because of excessive amounts of uroporphyrin (even more impressive under UV light). This porphyria and the rare homozygous porphyria cutanea tarda, hepatoerythropoietic porphyria, can be progressive and severely mutilating. Therapy is limited to sun protection and blood transfusion if hemolytic anemia is present.

Erythropoietic Protoporphyria

Erythropoietic protoporphyria is an autosomal dominant disorder due to a deficiency of ferrochelatase, the last enzyme in heme biosynthesis. Urinary porphyrins are normal, but protoporphyrin is markedly elevated in red cells and in stool. These patients suffer from instantly painful sun sensitivity, followed by edema and wrinkles in the thickened, light-exposed skin. In contrast to porphyria cutanea tarda, blisters are not seen here. Approximately one fifth of these patients develop progressive liver disease secondary to hepatic accumulation of protoporphyrin. Liver transplantation can become necessary.

Therapy is often beneficial with oral β-carotene[1] (up to 400 mg/day for adults). This leads to a harmless slight orange-yellow discoloration of the skin and often effective sun protection. Ideally, the β-carotene dose should be adjusted to a plasma level between 11 and 15 mmol/L.

---

[1]Not FDA approved for this indication.

References

American Porphyria Foundation Home page. Available at: http://www.porphyriafoundation.com (accessed August 5, 2015).
Anderson KE, Bonkovsky HL, Bloomer JR, Shedlofsky SI. Reconstitution of hematin for intravenous infusion. Ann Intern Med 2006;144:537–8.
Anderson KE, Bloomer JR, Bonkovsky HL, et al. Recommendations for the diagnosis and treatment of the acute porphyrias. Ann Intern Med 2005;142:439–50.
Anderson KE, Sassa S, Bishop DF, et al. Disorders of heme biosynthesis: X linked sideroblastic anemia and the porphyrias. In: Scriver CR, Beaudet AL, Sly WS, et al., 8th ed. The Molecular and Metabolic Bases of Inherited Disease, vol. 1. New York: McGraw-Hill; 2001. p. 2961–3062.
Badminton MN, Elder GH. Management of acute and cutaneous porphyrias. Int J Clin Pract 2002;56:272–8.
Balwani M, Desnick RJ. The porphyrias: advances in diagnosis and treatment. Blood 2012;120(23):4496–504. http://dx.doi.org/10.1182/blood-2012-05-423186. Epub 2012 Jul 12. Review. Erratum in: Blood, 2013;122(17);3090.
Chemmanur AT, Bonkovsky HL. Hepatic porphyrias: Diagnosis and management. Clin Liver Dis 2004;8;807–38.
European Porphyria Initiative. Home page. Available at: http://www.porphyria-europe.com/ (accessed August 5, 2015).
Kauppinen R. Porphyrias. Lancet 2005;365:241–52.
Puy H, Gouya L, Deybach JC. Porphyrias. Lancet 2010;375:924–37.

SICKLE CELL DISEASE

Method of
Enrico M. Novelli, MD; Mark T. Gladwin, MD; and Lakshmanan Krishnamurti, MD

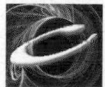

CURRENT DIAGNOSIS

- Sickle cell disease (SCD) is diagnosed by neonatal screening in the United States
- Persons with congenital hemolytic anemia should be tested for SCD by hemoglobin electrophoresis regardless of their ethnic background.
- Infection with parvovirus B19 should be suspected in children presenting with acute anemia and reticulocytopenia.
- Human leukocyte antigen (HLA) class I and II testing should be performed in all patients with SCD and unaffected siblings to identify candidates for hematopoietic stem-cell transplant.
- Transcranial Doppler screening for primary prevention of stroke is indicated in children with SCD.
- Acute chest syndrome is diagnosed in patients presenting with fever, hypoxemia, and a radiographic pulmonary infiltrate.

- Screening for iron overload by ferritin, quantitative liver MRI, cardiac MRI, or liver biopsy is indicated in all patients who have received more than 10 lifetime transfusions.
- Pulmonary hypertension screening by transthoracic echocardiogram is indicated in all patients with homozygous SCD.

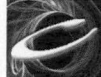

CURRENT THERAPY

- All children with sickle cell disease (SCD) should receive penicillin prophylaxis.
- High fever should be treated empirically with coverage for *Streptococcus pneumoniae* pending results of blood cultures.
- Children with high transcranial Doppler velocity need to be placed on a chronic transfusion regimen to keep the hemoglobin (Hb) S <30%, indefinitely.
- Painful vaso-occlusive episodes warrant prompt treatment with an individualized intravenous opiate regimen, as well as supportive care and incentive spirometry.
- Preoperative transfusion should aim at a target hemoglobin level of 10 g/dL regardless of the HbS percentage and is indicated in all patients with SCD undergoing major surgery.
- Therapy with hydroxyurea is indicated in all patients at all ages with HbSS disease and HbSβ-thalassemia, and in patients with HbSC with a severe phenotype on a case-by-case basis.
- Erythropoietin-stimulating agents can be used in conjunction with hydroxyurea to prevent or ameliorate reticulocytopenia and in patients with underlying renal insufficiency.
- Iron chelation is indicated in all patients with findings of iron overload.
- Treatment of acute chest syndrome includes parenteral antibiotics to cover atypical microorganisms and transfusion, with exchange transfusion reserved for the most severe cases.
- Patients with pulmonary hypertension should receive optimal hematologic care (maximal hydroxyurea and/or chronic transfusion therapy) and specific therapy for pulmonary hypertension in severe cases, with coordination and referral to a pulmonary hypertension specialist.
- Bone marrow transplantation should be offered to all patients who have a matched donor and display a severe phenotype.

Epidemiology

Sickle cell disease (SCD) affects 70,000 to 100,000 persons in the United States and millions worldwide. The hemoglobin (Hb) S mutation arose from four geographic areas in Africa and Asia approximately 10,000 years ago and then propagated to vast tropical and subtropical areas due to the selective pressure of malaria infection. It is predominantly found in persons of African, Mediterranean, Arab, or Indian ancestry. In the United States, approximately 1 in 15 African Americans harbors the HbS (sickle hemoglobin) mutation and 1 in 400 is affected by the disease. Most patients with SCD in the United States are homozygous for HbS (SS), with heterozygous HbSC being the second most common abnormality. Conversely, in Mediterranean countries, HbS/β-thalassemia is the most common SCD syndrome, and in the Arab peninsula HbSS in combination with hereditary persistence of fetal hemoglobin (HPFH) is particularly prevalent.

Pathophysiology

SCD consists of a group of inherited hemoglobinopathies characterized by a qualitatively abnormal hemoglobin molecule that affects the structure and integrity of the red blood cells (RBCs). SCD is an autosomal recessive disease due to homozygosity for HbS, characterized by a single base substitution in the β-globin gene of the hemoglobin tetramer, leading to an amino acid substitution (valine to glutamic acid), or coinheritance of HbS with other abnormal hemoglobins such as hemoglobin C or β-thalassemia.

HbS is less soluble than normal hemoglobin (HbA) in the deoxygenated state and polymerizes when sickle RBCs are exposed to hypoxic conditions in the microcirculation. In the classic pathophysiologic explanation of SCD, sickled RBCs containing HbS polymers are less deformable and remain trapped in the microcirculation, causing end-organ ischemia and necrosis. Compounding this mechanism, more recent literature has emphasized the role of cellular adhesion, abnormal cytokine levels, ischemia-reperfusion injury, oxidative damage and an abnormal endothelial milieu. HbS polymers also lead to deformity and fragility of the RBC membrane, with resulting intra- and extravascular hemolysis.

Patients with SCD suffer from severe chronic hemolytic anemia and acute episodes of RBC trapping and destruction in the microvasculature (vaso-occlusive episodes). Vaso-occlusive episodes are the hallmark of SCD and are characterized by more intense episodic vaso-occlusion, often with increasing hemolysis, and are due to exogenous or endogenous factors that acutely alter the rheologic properties of the RBCs. The main determinants of RBC sickling and vaso-occlusion are hypoxemia, RBC dehydration, RBC concentration, high HbS relative to fetal hemoglobin (HbF), and blood viscosity; these can occur in a multitude of clinical settings. Most common clinical inciting events leading to vaso-occlusive episodes are dehydration due to inadequate replacement of fluid losses, thermal changes, surgical stress, exposure to low oxygen tension, infections, and psychological stressors.

Epidemiologic studies indicate that the risk of vaso-occlusive episodes and acute chest syndrome is related to high steady-state hemoglobin levels, leukocytosis, and low HbF levels. These findings are consistent with pathogenic mechanisms of altered red cell rheology, higher viscosity, HbS polymerization, and inflammatory cellular adhesion. Interestingly, the epidemiologic risk factors associated with chronic vascular complications such as pulmonary hypertension, cutaneous leg ulceration, priapism, systemic systolic hypertension, renal failure with proteinuria, and possibly stroke are different and include a low steady-state hemoglobin level, increased hemolytic intensity, iron overload, and markers of low nitric oxide bioavailability. One hypothesis is that SCD is driven by two overlapping but different mechanisms of disease: on one hand, vaso-occlusion causes vaso-occlusive episodes and acute chest syndrome, and on the other hand, hemolytic anemia leads to endothelial dysfunction and chronic vasculopathy. Both are caused fundamentally by HbS polymerization.

Prevention

"Evidence-Based Management of Sickle Cell Disease: Expert Panel Report, 2014" at http://www.nhlbi.nih.gov/health-pro/guidelines/sickle-cell-disease-guidelines for detailed, consensus guidelines on prevention and treatment.

Bacterial Infections

Before the antibiotic era, most patients with SCD succumbed to bacterial sepsis from encapsulated organisms. A landmark multicenter, randomized, double-blind, placebo-controlled clinical trial of prophylaxis with oral penicillin in children with sickle cell anemia published in 1986 showed that bacterial prophylaxis started at birth reduced by about 80% the incidence of infection in the penicillin group, as compared with the group given placebo. This study became the foundation for universal screening of SCD. Results of the Penicillin Prophylaxis in Sickle Cell Study II (PROPS 2) trial show that prophylaxis can be safely discontinued at age 5 years as long as there is no history of prior serious pneumococcal infection or surgical splenectomy and in the setting of appropriate comprehensive care. All children should also receive both the 7-valent pneumococcal conjugate (Prevnar) and 23-valent pneumococcal polysaccharide (Pneumovax) vaccines, and adults should receive Pneumovax.[3] Vaccinations for *H. influenzae* and *N. meningitidis* are also indicated.

Neurologic Events

Stroke is a devastating complication of SCD and affects predominantly children with HbSS and abnormal transcranial Doppler

(TCD) results. Silent cerebral infarcts are asymptomatic MRI-detectable abnormalities that also carry a high risk of morbidity, including overt stroke and cognitive impairment. There is conclusive evidence that chronic transfusions are effective in the primary and secondary prevention of both overt and silent strokes in SCD. A first landmark trial (STOP) published in 1995 showed that the first stroke can be prevented by placing children with abnormal TCD on prophylactic monthly transfusions with a target HbS of <30%. Transfusions were later found to also have a beneficial effect on reducing the incidence of the recurrence of silent cerebral infarcts, as shown by the SIT trial. The importance of continuing transfusions for more than 30 months was underscored by the STOP2 trial, where TCD abnormalities recurred and the incidence of silent cerebral infarctions on MRI was higher in the transfusion-halted group. Thus, the enthusiasm over the beneficial effects of transfusions was tempered by the concerns about the obvious side effects of long term, possibly indefinite use of this therapeutic strategy. There has been, therefore, an interest in exploring whether hydroxyurea could be an alternative to transfusion in high risk children. Specifically, the SWiTCH trial explored the hypothesis that hydroxyurea and phlebotomy could maintain an acceptable stroke recurrence rate and significantly reduce the hepatic iron burden as compared to a prophylactic chronic transfusion regimen, but was terminated early because of a significantly higher stroke recurrence rate in the hydroxyurea arm compared to the transfusion arm, with equivalent hepatic iron burden in both groups. Thus the issue of when, if ever, it is safe to discontinue transfusions for the secondary prevention of stroke is still unknown. Conversely, as shown by the results of the TWiTCH trial, another study halted prematurely by the NIH, hydroxyurea is not inferior to chronic transfusions in lowering TCD velocities in children at high risk but without a history of stroke, thereby suggesting that this drug may be equally effective in the primary prevention of neurologic complications.

Clinical Manifestations

Multiple genetic and epigenetic factors affect the SCD phenotype. Patients homozygous for HbS (SS) or compound heterozygous for HbS and a nonfunctional β^0-thalassemia allele tend to display the most severe manifestations. On the other end of the spectrum, hereditary persistence of HbF (HPFH), particularly common in Saudi Arabia, or coinheritance of β-thalassemia mitigates the phenotype. Although the net effect of high HbF levels on the phenotype of SCD is beneficial, coinheritance of one or two α-thalassemia alleles has a more complex effect. α-Thalassemia is present in approximately 30% of patients with SCD and is associated with higher hemoglobin, lower mean corpuscular volume (MCV), and decreased rate of hemolysis. These effects are protective toward cerebrovascular accident (CVA) and leg ulcers, but lead to increased rates of vaso-occlusive episodes, osteonecrosis, and acute chest syndrome because of increased blood viscosity related to the higher hemoglobin level. Patients with HbSC and HbS/β^+-thalassemia have an intermediate severity phenotype (Table 1). Haplotypes of polymorphic sites in the β-globin gene cluster in chromosome 11, which correspond and are linked to defined geographic regions of origin of the HbS gene, have been

TABLE 1 Severity of the Main Sickle Cell Syndromes

GENOTYPE	CLINICAL SEVERITY	HEMOGLOBIN (g/dL)
HbSS	Usually marked	6–10
HbS-β^0-thalassemia	Moderate to marked	6–10
HbS-β^+-thalassemia	Mild to moderate	9–12
HbSC	Mild to moderate	10–15
HbSS-HPFH	Mild	

Abbreviations: HbSC = heterozygous phenotype; HbSS = homozygous phenotype; HPFH = hereditary persistence of fetal hemoglobin.

---

[3]Exceeds dosage recommended by the manufacturer.

associated with different disease severity and rates of complications. Other yet unidentified genetic factors predispose certain patients to develop a particularly severe hemolysis with brisk reticulocytosis and a high rate of specific complications that include leg ulcers, priapism, and pulmonary hypertension.

Hematology

This section describes the main clinical manifestations of SCD in each organ system (Figure 1 and Table 2).

Baseline or Steady-State Hematologic Abnormalities

Chronic intravascular and extravascular hemolysis causes a chronic anemia of moderate to severe intensity in HbSS and

HbS/β^0-thalassemia, with a hemoglobin range of 6 to 9 g/dL. In HbSC and HbS/β^+-thalassemia, the anemia may be mild or absent. The anemia of SCD is usually normocytic in HbSS, with anisocytosis and poikilocytosis and a population of small dehydrated dense cells, irreversibly sickled cells, numerous reticulocytes, and schistocytes. Reticulocytosis is common but not compensatory, and nucleated RBCs are seen in acute exacerbations of the anemia such as in splenic or hepatic sequestration. Baseline leukocytosis with neutrophilia is also common and is a poor prognostic sign associated with acute chest syndrome in adults and frequent vaso-occlusive episodes in children. Preclinical studies have shown that leukocytes are not simply a marker of disease activity and acute phase but also have a direct pathogenic role in cellular

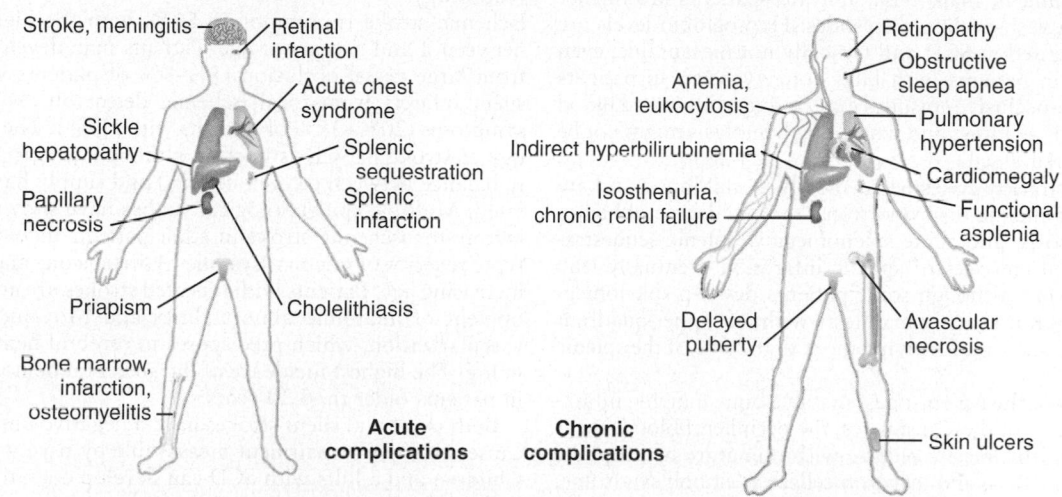

Figure 1. Acute and chronic complications of sickle cell disease.

TABLE 2	Landmark Randomized Clinical Trials in Sickle Cell Disease	
YEAR OF PUBLICATION	**TITLE**	**MAIN FINDINGS**
1986	Prophylaxis with oral penicillin in children with sickle cell anemia: A randomized trial	84% reduction in incidence of infection and no deaths from pneumococcal septicemia in the penicillin group
1995	Multicenter Study of Hydroxyurea in Sickle Cell Anemia (MSH)	Reduced incidence of painful crises, ACS, and transfusion in the hydroxyurea group Survival benefit in follow-up study
1995	Preoperative Transfusion in Sickle Cell Disease Study	A conservative transfusion regimen was as effective as an aggressive regimen in preventing perioperative complications in patients with sickle cell anemia
1996	Multicenter investigation of bone marrow transplantation for sickle cell disease	HCT is safe in SCD with survival and event-free survival at 4 y of 91% and 73% and can lead to cure
1998	Stroke Prevention Trial in Sickle Cell Anemia (STOP)	Transfusion reduces the risk of a first stroke by 92% in children with sickle cell anemia who have abnormal results on transcranial Doppler ultrasonography
2005	Optimizing Primary Stroke Prevention in Sickle Cell Anemia (STOP 2)	Discontinuation of transfusion for the prevention of stroke in children with sickle cell disease results in a high rate of reversion to abnormal blood-flow velocities on Doppler studies and stroke
2009	Improving the Results of Bone Marrow Transplantation for Patients with Severe Congenital Anemias	Nine of 10 adults who received nonmyeloablative allogeneic hematopoietic stem-cell transplantation for severe sickle cell disease achieved stable, mixed donor–recipient chimerism and reversal of the sickle cell phenotype, without acute or chronic GVHD.
2011	Pediatric Hydroxyurea Phase III Clinical Trial (BABY HUG).	Children ages 9–18 mo randomized to receive hydroxyurea irrespective of disease severity for 2 y had decreased pain episodes, dactylitis, ACS, hospitalization, leukocyte count, and transfusion and increased hemoglobin as compared to children receiving placebo.
2014	Silent Infarct Trial (SIT).	Children with silent cerebral infarcts and normal TCD velocity who were randomized to chronic transfusion therapy had a 58% relative risk reduction in the recurrence of silent cerebral infarct or stroke as compared to those in the observation arm.

Abbreviations: ACS = acute chest syndrome; GVHD = graft-versus-host disease; HCT = hematopoietic cell transplantation; SCD = sickle cell disease; VOE = vaso-occlusive crisis.

adhesion and vaso-occlusion. The platelet count is commonly elevated in SCD, particularly in patients who are autosplenectomized as a result of repeated splenic infarction, and platelet activation is increased. In the subset of patients with HbSC and and HbS/β⁺-thalassemia who retain a functional spleen and develop splenomegaly, features of hypersplenism may instead be observed with resulting mild pancytopenia.

Hematologic Indices during Vaso-occlusive Episodes

In acute vaso-occlusive episodes the Hb decreases as a result of hemolysis (by 1.6 g/dL in acute chest syndrome) and sickle cells are observed in the peripheral smear. The lactate dehydrogenase (LDH), reticulocyte count, and other markers of hemolysis such as aspartate transaminase (AST) and indirect bilirubin are elevated in steady state, and in many—but not all—patients are further increased during vaso-occlusive episodes. Haptoglobin levels are chronically depressed in SCD and typically not measurable, even in steady state, in patients with HbS homozygosity. In patients with HbSC, vaso-occlusive episodes may be due to increased blood viscosity and RBC sickling, and worsening hemolysis might not be readily appreciated.

Splenic sequestration crises occur mostly in childhood and are characterized by anemia disproportionate to the degree of hemolysis, reticulocytosis, and acute splenomegaly. Splenic sequestration and repeated episodes of splenic infarction eventually lead to autosplenectomy, although some patients develop splenomegaly. Splenic infarction usually manifests with left upper-quadrant pain and may be massive, involving more than 50% of the splenic tissue.

In severe vaso-occlusive episodes, massive bone marrow infarction can also occur. In these instances, the peripheral blood smear reveals a leukoerythroblastic picture with immature neutrophilic forms, nucleated RBCs, and teardrop cells. Fat emboli syndrome, a life-threatening complication of vaso-occlusive episodes, can then develop as bone marrow fat embolizes to peripheral capillary beds, leading to multiorgan failure.

Red Blood Cell Alloimmunization

RBC alloimmunization is a common complication of transfusional therapy in SCD and occurs in approximately 30% of patients. It is primarily due to the disparate expression of RBC antigens in African Americans as compared to the donor pool, which is mostly composed of Caucasians. Alloimmunization complicates RBC matching and leads to delayed hemolytic transfusion reactions. Alloantigens that become undetectable by indirect Coombs test 2 months after exposure to mismatched blood have the potential to result in future false-negative cross-matching results. A subset of heavily alloimmunized patients with SCD undergoes life-threatening hemolytic reactions upon exposure to mismatched RBC units. In these hyperhemolytic crises, there is intense hemolysis of transfused and nontransfused RBCs and acute anemia. Treatment of hyperhemolytic crises is empirical and includes erythropoietin-stimulating agents (ESA), parenteral steroids, and intravenous immunoglobulins (Gammagard).[1]

Iron Overload

Hemosiderosis is the other major complication of transfusional therapy in SCD and is characterized by iron deposition in the heart, liver, and endocrine glands, leading to organ failure and significant morbidity and mortality. It commonly occurs in patients who have received more than 10 lifetime transfusions or more than 20 packed RBC units. Liver biopsy is the gold standard for diagnosis but it is an invasive and uncomfortable procedure. Noninvasive imaging methods such as quantitative liver and myocardial MRI and superconducting quantum interference device (SQUID) are not always available, and therefore diagnosis often rests on the finding of an elevated ferritin and transferrin saturation in the appropriate clinical setting.

---

[1]Not FDA approved for this indication.

Hemostatic Activation and Thrombosis

Numerous studies have shown that arterial and venous thrombosis are common in SCD and include pulmonary embolism, in situ pulmonary thrombosis, and stroke. In SCD, alterations at all levels of the hemostatic system have been described: patients with sickle cell disease exhibit increased basal and stimulated platelet activation, increased markers of thrombin generation and fibrinolysis, increased tissue factor activity, and increased von Willebrand factor (vWF) antigen and thrombogenic ultralarge vWF multimers. Interestingly, hemostatic activation is amplified during vaso-occlusive episodes, as shown by increases in multiple markers of thrombosis as compared to steady state, suggesting a link between hemolysis and thrombosis.

Neurology

Ischemic stroke is common in SCD, with the highest incidence between 2 and 5 years of age. Patients may develop overt CVAs from large vessel occlusion (5%–8% of patients with HbSS) or silent infarcts from focal ischemia detectable by MRI without symptoms (20%–35% of patients with HbSS). The pathophysiology of stroke in SCD is unclear, although genetic factors and an unbalance between oxygen demand and supply have been postulated. Multiple epidemiological studies have shown that the risk factors for ischemic stroke in adult patients include HbSS genotype, severity of anemia, systolic hypertension, male gender, and increasing age. Patients with repeated strokes are at risk for development of anatomic abnormalities and Moyamoya pattern of vascularization, which predisposes to cerebral hemorrhages later in life. The highest incidence of intracerebral hemorrhages occurs in patients older than 20 years.

Both overt and silent strokes have a negative impact on IQ and cause cognitive impairment measurable by psychometric testing. Children and adults with SCD can develop cognitive impairment and subtle signs of accelerated brain aging and vascular dementia even in the absence of focal ischemia by MRI, with a low hematocrit being a predictor of neuropsychological dysfunction. These abnormalities are probably due to chronic and diffuse, as opposed to focal, cerebral anoxia and may be unmasked by psychometric testing. In patients who do have MRI abnormalities without a history of CVA, the gray matter is predominantly affected.

Ophthalmology

Retinal abnormalities are common in SCD and are often asymptomatic until the occurrence of ophthalmologic emergencies. Retinal disease is due to arteriolar occlusion, with subsequent vascular proliferation, neovascularization, retinal hemorrhage (stage IV) and detachment (stage V). Patients with HbSC are more prone to retinal complications, possibly as a result of increased blood viscosity.

Nephrology

Renal abnormalities are common in SCD and manifest primarily as hematuria, proteinuria, and renal tubular acidosis. Hematuria is usually due to papillary necrosis and is an acute finding that requires supportive care and carries a good prognosis. Rarely, gross hematuria requires urologic consultation. Tubular functional defects include inability to concentrate the urine (hyposthenuria) and renal tubular acidosis. Hyposthenuria often manifests with enuresis in childhood, and it is clinically relevant because it predisposes patients to an increased risk of dehydration. Renal tubular acidosis similar to type IV renal tubular acidosis is a common finding in SCD and may lead to hyperkalemia, an important consideration in patients already predisposed to hyperkalemia with intravascular hemolysis and whenever therapy with angiotensin-converting enzyme inhibitors is entertained.

Hyperphosphatemia and hyperuricemia are also often observed in SCD. Microalbuminuria may be detected in early adulthood and tends to progress to nephrotic range proteinuria. Focal segmental glomerulosclerosis is the most common glomerular abnormality and it is probably due to glomerular sickling and infarction. There are currently no approved therapies to prevent progression to end-stage renal disease, which occurs in up to 20% of patients and at a median age of 37 years. Renal replacement therapy is therefore often needed in older adults with SCD. Serum creatinine and 24-hour creatinine clearance are not adequate for screening and monitoring of progression of kidney disease, because tubular secretion of creatinine is preserved and glomerular hyperfiltration is common in SCD, leading to a relatively low creatinine and a high glomerular filtration rate even in patients with underlying kidney impairment. The albumin or protein-to-creatinine ratio and plasma cystatin C levels may instead be used as a screening tool of glomerulopathy in SCD, as they can predict development of chronic kidney disease.

Leg Ulcers

Leg ulcers occur in 10% to 20% of patients with HbSS and have been associated with a chronically high hemolytic rate. They are usually located over the malleolar areas and are exquisitely painful, debilitating, disfiguring, and nonhealing. Vascular and plastic surgery consultation are recommended and aim at excluding local vascular problems that can complicate management of the ulcers and at providing prompt débridement and skin grafting. Although hydroxyurea is associated with development of leg ulcers in patients with myeloproliferative disorders, a review of the literature has failed to show an association with leg ulcers in SCD. Whereas wound healing may be impaired with hydroxyurea use, patients who develop an increase in fetal hemoglobin and have reduced sickling as a result of hydroxyurea therapy might have a net benefit in terms of tissue oxygenation and perfusion. Transfusional therapy, including exchange transfusional therapy, topical nitrates, and nutritional zinc or L-arginine supplementation, have shown benefit in anecdotal reports, but the evidence is inconclusive.

Gastroenterology

Nausea, vomiting, and dyspepsia in SCD are related to delayed gastric emptying and gastrointestinal motility disorders, autonomic neuropathy, or medical therapy. Opiates are often responsible for acute nausea and vomiting, whereas other medications such as hydroxyurea and deferasirox (Exjade) are occasionally responsible for chronic symptoms. Gastroparesis may be due to damage of the microvasculature of autonomic nerves (vasa vasorum) from repeated episodes of sickling.

The liver may be episodically affected by hepatic sequestration crises, heralded by direct hyperbilirubinemia, right upper quadrant pain from distention of the hepatic capsule, acute anemia, and reticulocytosis. Supportive therapy and exchange transfusion, rather than simple transfusion, are indicated for this vaso-occlusive complication. Elevation of liver injury tests may be drug induced (hydroxyurea, deferasirox), but also related to hepatic sickling, particularly if it occurs during a vaso-occlusive episode. Hepatitis C has a higher prevalence than in the general population and may compound the hepatic manifestations of SCD.

Diarrhea is a common side effect of therapy with deferasirox, particularly in lactose-intolerant patients, and where it is usually self-limited.

Infectious Disease

Patients homozygous for HbSS develop functional asplenia during childhood. This is due to repeated episodes of splenic infarction leading to fibrosis and autosplenectomy. As a result, children are susceptible to overwhelming bacterial sepsis from encapsulated organisms such as *S. pneumoniae, H. influenzae,* and *N. meningitidis.* High pediatric mortality from sepsis was therefore common before a landmark study published in 1986 demonstrated the benefit of penicillin prophylaxis instituted at birth. Vaccination for encapsulated organisms is also standard of care in children and adults. In spite of preventive measures, the incidence of life-threatening bacterial infections is increased in SCD, and high fever should be treated empirically as in splenectomized patients, with coverage for penicillin-resistant *S. pneumoniae* pending blood culture results. Patients with indwelling venous catheters are at risk of catheter-related bacteremia.

Viral infections with bone marrow–tropic viruses such as Epstein–Barr virus, citomegalovirus, and predominantly parvovirus

B19 place patients at risk for bone marrow suppression, which can further worsen chronic anemia. In children, infections with parvovirus B19 are responsible for transient red cell aplasia and severe aplastic crises, characterized by acute anemia and reticulocytopenia due to intra marrow destruction of erythroid precursors. Treatment of these episodes includes transfusion and intravenous immunoglobulins,[1] besides supportive measures.

Pulmonology

A subset of patients with vaso-occlusive episodes develop acute chest syndrome, the major pulmonary complication of SCD. Acute chest syndrome is a lung injury syndrome defined by fever, pleuritic chest pain, oxygen desaturation, and multilobar radiographic infiltrates associated with severe vaso-occlusive episodes, infection, and bone marrow fat embolization (Figure 2). It usually develops a few days after hospitalization for vaso-occlusive episodes and is often misdiagnosed as nosocomial pneumonia or aspiration pneumonia, particularly because it displays a predilection for the lower lobe of the lungs. Although pneumonia often accompanies acute chest syndrome, proper diagnosis is important because acute chest syndrome warrants simple or exchange transfusion in addition to antibiotic therapy and supportive measures. Common infectious pathogens identified in cases of acute chest syndrome include *Chlamydia pneumoniae, Mycoplasma pneumoniae,* and *Legionella pneumophyla,* thus dictating inclusion of a macrolide in the antibiotic cocktail. Pulmonary embolism with resulting infarct is also in the differential diagnosis of acute chest syndrome and may occur concurrently in 17% of patients according to a recent French study. If not recognized and treated promptly, acute chest syndrome leads to pulmonary failure and carries a high mortality.

Reactive airways disease is common in children with SCD and needs to be actively diagnosed and aggressively treated. Children with chronic respiratory symptoms need to be tested for bronchial hyperresponsiveness.

Chronic complications of SCD include pulmonary fibrosis and pulmonary hypertension. Pulmonary hypertension (PH) is an emergent complication of SCD, and is associated with a high morbidity and mortality. Multiple epidemiologic studies have shown that a high baseline hemolysis rate, low hemoglobin, increasing age, a history of leg ulcers, liver dysfunction, iron overload, and kidney failure are risk factors for the development of pulmonary hypertension. Noninvasive transthoracic Doppler echocardiography is recommended as a screening test in this population due to its safety, low cost, and availability to identify patients at high risk for having PH and at high risk for early death. The definitive diagnosis of PH requires a confirmatory right heart catheterization (RHC). Three epidemiologic studies and a randomized clinical trial have shown that an elevated tricuspid regurgitant jet velocity (TRV) measured by Doppler-echocardiography is a common occurrence in SCD, with 30% of the patients having a TRV of 2.5 m/sec (2 SD above the normal mean) or higher, and 10% of the patients having a TRV of 3.0 m/sec (3 SD above the normal mean) or higher. These have proved to be valuable cut-off values, as a TRV of less than 2.5 m/sec, when combined with an N-terminal pro B-type natriuretic peptide (NT-proBNP) value less than 160 has a high negative predictive value for PH. A TRV of 3.0 m/sec or higher confers a positive predictive value for having PH by RHC of 60% to 75% and a relative risk for death of 10.6. Controversy exists on the significance of an intermediate TRV value of 2.5 to 2.9 m/sec, as it is unclear how accurately it predicts RHC-diagnosed PH. In three recently published studies, patients with intermediate or high TRV values had a prevalence of PH by RHC ranging from 25% to 65% depending on what specific cutoff value was used as criteria to perform a RHC (2.5 vs. 2.8) and on whether patients with evidence of end-organ damage were included or excluded. It is, however, worrisome that regardless of the prevalence of PH,

---

[1]Not FDA approved for this indication.

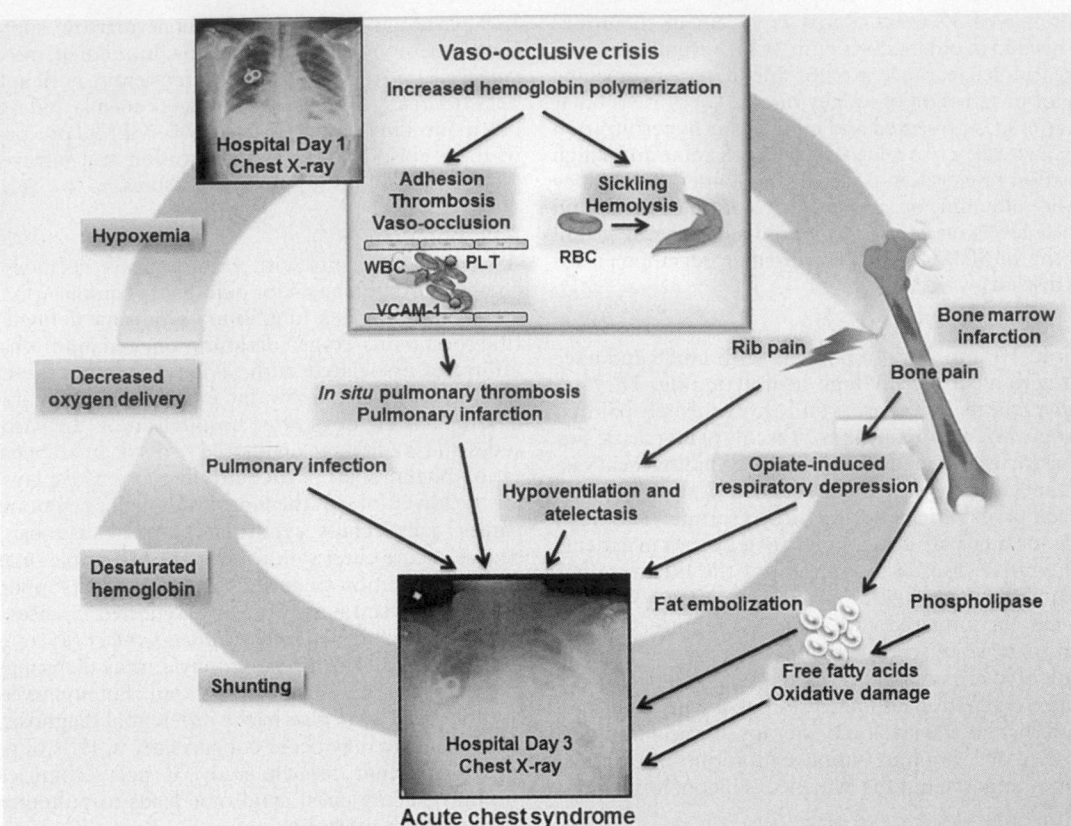

Figure 2. Vicious cycle of acute chest syndrome (ACS). Vaso-occlusive crises are characterized by increased intraerythrocytic polymerization of deoxygenated hemoglobin S, leading to red blood cell sickling, cellular hyperadhesion, hemolysis, and vaso-occlusion in the microvasculature. These processes are responsible for acute pain (pain crisis) and bone marrow necrosis. ACS typically occurs in a subset of patients 2-3 days after hospitalization for a vaso-occlusive episode, and radiographically may present as new multilobar, basilar infiltrates on a chest x-ray. Fat embolization from the necrotic marrow is a recognized cause of ACS and is diagnosed by identifying lipid-laden macrophages in the bronchoalveolar lavage. Pulmonary infection is, however, the most common trigger of ACS and may be superimposed over existing pulmonary infarction. Hypoventilation and molecular pathogens such as reactive oxygen species from ischemia-reperfusion injury and by-products of hemolysis may also play a role in inducing or exacerbating lung injury. Finally, in situ pulmonary thrombosis has been frequently identified as a co-morbid condition in patients with ACS and may be caused by endothelial and hemostatic activation. As a result of lung injury, ventilation-perfusion mismatches and shunting ensues, with subsequent hemoglobin desaturation and hypoxemia. Tissue hypoxia in turn triggers further hemoglobin S polymerization and sickling in a vicious cycle.

patients with an intermediate TRV are as a whole at increased risk of death (RR 4.4). One screening approach is to consider RHC in all patients with TRV of 3.0 or higher and in patients with intermediate TRV values of 2.5 to 2.9 m/sec if the NT-proBNP is greater than 160 pg/mL or the 6 minute walk is less than 333 meters or there is a high clinical pretest probability of having PH (mosaic perfusion pattern on CT scan, low DLCO, significant dyspnea on exertion, etc.). It is likely that intermediate TRV values will need to be combined with other measures of right ventricular function and functional capacity such as NT-proBNP, and 6 minute walk to derive a highly predictive composite biomarker of PH. All studies have been concordant on the high risk of death conferred by PH in SCD whether measured by echocardiography, NT-proBNP, or RHC.

Right heart catheterization studies of patients with SCD and pulmonary hypertension reveal a hyperdynamic state similar to the hemodynamics characteristic of portopulmonary hypertension. It is increasingly clear that pulmonary pressures rise acutely in vaso-occlusive episodes and even more during acute chest syndrome. This suggests that acute pulmonary hypertension and right heart dysfunction represent a major comorbidity during acute chest syndrome, and right heart failure should be considered in patients presenting with acute chest syndrome.

Cardiology

Similarly to other conditions with chronic anemia, SCD is associated with a hyperdynamic state, low peripheral vascular resistance, and normal blood pressure or hypotension. In this setting, even mild elevation of the blood pressure can indicate relative hypertension and represent a risk factor for stroke. Because there are no studies on the treatment of hypertension in SCD, general guidelines on antihypertensive therapy are applied.

Coronary artery disease is rarely observed in SCD, although many patients complain of chest pain during vaso-occlusive episodes. In these instances, the usual work-up for acute coronary syndrome is recommended. It is possible that myocardial microvascular occlusions are the predominant ischemic event in SCD.

Left-sided heart disease in SCD is primarily due to diastolic dysfunction (present in approximately 13% of patients), although systolic dysfunction and mitral or aortic valvular disease (2% of patients) can also occur. The presence of diastolic dysfunction alone in SCD patients is an independent risk factor for mortality. Patients with both pulmonary vascular disease and echocardiographic evidence of diastolic dysfunction are at a particularly high risk for death (OR, 12.0; 95% CI, 3.8-38.1; $P <0.001$).

Cardiac dysfunction is a late complication and the major cause of death in patients with iron overload. Heart failure and conduction defects are the most common abnormalities and warrant emergent iron chelation treatment. Both deferoxamine (Desferal) and deferasirox reduce cardiac iron content and may be used in combination in severe cases.

Methadone (Dolophine) is associated with a risk of QTc prolongation, which carries a risk of arrhythmias and sudden death, particularly in the setting of pulmonary hypertension and iron overload. Frequent electrocardiographic (ECG) monitoring, as well as dosage reduction or discontinuation, are warranted in this group, particularly if the QTc is greater than 500 msec.

Endocrinology

Iron overload is a common cause of endocrinopathy in SCD and thalassemia, with the hypophysis, gonads, and thyroid glands being particularly affected. Patients with iron overload should therefore undergo screening for endocrine dysfunction as it is routinely mandated in thalassemia.

Patients with SCD are, however, at risk for specific endocrine problems regardless of their iron status. Delayed growth and puberty are relatively common, presenting in females with delayed age of menarche by 2 to 3 years and in males with small testicular size and hypospermia. Likely pathogenic factors include increased catabolism, chronic hpoxemia, hospitalizations with prolonged immobility, ischemic insults during vasooclusive episodes, and chronic use of opiates.

Priapism

Priapism is the most common urogenital complication in patients with the HbSS genotype. It is a sustained, painful erection in the absence of sexual stimulation from occlusion of the penile blood return. It is defined as stuttering if it lasts from minutes to less than 3 hours, and as prolonged if it lasts more than 3 hours. The latter is considered a urologic emergency because of the risk of permanent fibrosis and impotence, and requires a urologic consultation. Pseudoephedrine (Sudafed)[1] may lead to detumescence in nonemergency settings, whereas aspiration of the corpus cavernosum is required in the emergency setting and is performed under conscious sedation and local anesthesia. This is usually accompanied by installation of epinephrine.[1] Other supportive measures, such as intravenous fluids and parenteral opiates, are usually indicated.

A rare neurologic syndrome known as ASPEN syndrome (association of sickle cell disease, priapism, exchange transfusion, and neurologic events) has been described in patients with priapism who have undergone exchange transfusion. It is characterized by headache and seizures occasionally progressing to obtundation requiring mechanical ventilation, and may be caused by high postexchange hematocrits.

Penile shunts are employed as a last resort to prevent further episodes of priapism by increasing the cavernous blood flow using native vessels or by creating an arteriovenous shunt. They invariably result in impotence, which can be ameliorated by implantation of an inflatable penile prosthesis. An ongoing clinical trial is assessing whether sildenafil (Viagra)[1] therapy can prevent priapism by altering vascular smooth muscle tone through inhibition of phosphodiesterase 2 activity.

Diagnosis

The diagnosis of SCD rests on the hemoglobin electrophoresis or high-performance liquid chromatography (HPLC), which allow detection of most hemoglobin variants. In patients with microcytosis α-globin gene sequencing may reveal coinheritance of an α-thalassemia trait.

Neonatal Screening

Children with SCD have an increased susceptibility to bacteremia due to S. pneumoniae, which can occur as early as 4 months of age and carries a case fatality rate as high as 30%. Acute splenic sequestration crises also contribute to mortality in infancy. Diagnosis by newborn screening and immediate entry into programs of comprehensive care, including the provision of effective pneumococcal prophylaxis, can reach infants who might otherwise be lost to the health care system and has been demonstrated to decrease morbidity and improve survival. Currently, newborn screening

---

[1]Not FDA approved for this indication.

and follow-up of SCD are carried out in all 50 states in the United States as well as in most developed countries.

Late Diagnoses and Misdiagnoses

Rarely, patients who were born before universal screening was introduced or who were lost at the time of follow-up of positive neonatal screening are only diagnosed late in life. This is particularly the case of patients with HbSC, who might have normal hemoglobin and hematocrit and a mild disease phenotype. Occasionally, the disease is misdiagnosed as iron deficiency in patients with HbS/β[+]-thalassemia on account of their microcytosis, and they undergo futile and potentially harmful prolonged trials of iron supplementation. Patients who have a low HbS level (<40%) due to recent transfusion or who have only mildly decreased hemoglobin (HbSC or HbS/β[+]-thalassemia) may receive an erroneous diagnosis of sickle cell trait (carrier state).

Treatment

From the original description of SCD in 1910 to the 1970s, there was no efficacious therapy for SCD, and most patients died within the first 2 decades of life, with infectious complications being responsible for the majority of pediatric fatalities. Several preventive and pharmacologic milestones since then, and the realization that care has to occur in a multidisciplinary setting, have profoundly affected the natural history of the disease (Table 3). Median age at death in resource-rich countries was 42 years in male patients and 48 years in female patients with HbSS, according to data from the Cooperative Study of Sickle Cell Disease in the 1980s (a pre-hydroxyurea setting), thereby still lagging approximately 2 to 3 decades behind that of the general African American population. The following sections summarize the therapeutic approach to the most important complications of SCD.

Vaso-Occlusive Episodes

Acute pain from vaso-occlusive episodes in SCD is extremely intense, affects both children and adults, and is due to ischemia or necrosis of the vascular beds. Most patients report severe pain in the bones and joints of the extremities, as well as lower back, although acute ischemia and pain can affect unusual sites such as the mandibular area. Occasionally, an affected limb displays the typical signs of inflammation, such as edema, warmth, and erythema, but a paucity of signs is the norm. Imaging studies such as MRI and bone scan can reveal signs of acute bone marrow infarction in a painful bony area, but they are not routinely employed in the work-up of a pain episode.

High-dose IV opiates, as well as nonsteroidal antiinflammatory drugs (NSAIDs), are the mainstay of treatment of a pain episode. Even in opiate-naive patients with SCD, opioid dosages often exceed those required for other indications. For instance, doses of intravenous hydromorphone (Dilaudid) of 1 to 2 mg are typical in adult patients. Most patients, however, are on an oral pain regimen at home and have a history of multiple admissions for vaso-occlusive episodes, thereby dictating individualized care based on what has been effective in the past and the patient's own perception of the intensity of pain. After an attempt at controlling the pain with three or four closely spaced narcotic boluses is made, patients who are in persistent discomfort or have evidence of underlying complications triggering the vaso-occlusive episode should be admitted and placed on patient-controlled analgesia. The American Pain Society has published guidelines for the treatment of acute and chronic pain in SCD, followed by other institutions in the past decade.

Common obstacles to prompt and effective care in SCD are the health professional's fear of overdosing the patient, as well as misconceptions about addiction and pseudoaddiction. In general, health care professionals tend to overestimate the prevalence of opioid abuse and addiction in SCD, and tend to undertreat patients significantly, leading to patients' frustration and anger when their pain demands are not met (pseudoaddiction).

TABLE 3	Manifestations of Sickle Cell Disease with Key Prevention and Treatment Strategies		
MANIFESTATION	**PREVENTION**	**TREATMENT**
Pneumococcal sepsis	Penicillin, Prevnar/Pneumovax vaccination	Antibiotic therapy for penicillin-resistant *Streptococcus pneumoniae*
Splenic or liver sequestration	—	Exchange transfusion
Painful vaso-occlusive episode	Hydroxyurea (Droxia), prevention of exposure to triggers	Intravenous fluids, parenteral opiates, supplemental oxygen
Acute chest syndrome	Incentive spirometry during VOE, hydroxyurea	Transfusion, broad-spectrum antibiotics with atypical coverage
Iron overload	Optimization of transfusion therapy	Iron chelation with deferasirox (Exjade) or deferoxamine (Desferal)
RBC alloimmunization	Transfusion with leukoreduced RBCs	—
CVA	Chronic transfusion in children with high transcranial Doppler velocity	Exchange transfusion and thrombolytics in selected cases
Pulmonary hypertension	Hydroxyurea?, treatment of predisposing conditions such as obstructive sleep apnea, hypoxemia, thromboembolism	Hydroxyurea, chronic transfusion therapy, specific therapy
Kidney disease	Antihypertensive therapy?, hydroxyurea?, ACE inhibitors?	ACE inhibitors?, renal replacement therapy, kidney transplant
Priapism	Hydroxyurea?	Pseudoephedrine (Sudafed),[1] aspiration of corpus cavernosum, sildenafil (Viagra)[1]?
Leg ulcers	Hydroxyurea?, chronic transfusion?	Surgical débridement, surgical grafting

Abbreviations: ACE = angiotensin-converting enzyme; CVA = cerebrovascular accident; RBC = red blood cells; TCD = transcranial Doppler; VOE = vaso-occlusive crisis.
[1]Not FDA approved for this indication.

Nonpharmacologic therapies such as biofeedback, relaxation, localized heat, and acupuncture may be effective and should be incorporated in the management of pain episodes whenever possible. Care for vaso-occlusive episodes should also include management of possible precipitating factors: dehydration and hypovolemia should be corrected with hypotonic crystalloids, and an infection work-up should be initiated in patients with fever, hypoxemia, or leukocytosis above baseline. Antiemetics and antipruritus therapy are also usually needed.

Prior experiences such as that of the Bronx Comprehensive Sickle Cell Center have shown that a dedicated facility for effective and rapid management of uncomplicated vaso-occlusive episodes reduces hospitalizations and length of stay and facilitates integration of care—psychological, socioeconomic, and nutritional—in a multidisciplinary approach. This experience is at the basis of the concept of day hospital in SCD and relies on the need to provide prompt assessment and treatment of pain, safe dose titration to relief, monitoring of adverse effects, and adequate disposition (emergency department, inpatient admission, home) in a clinical environment familiar with SCD and the individual patient.

Chronic Pain
Chronic pain is common, and recent literature based on pain diaries compiled by patients shows that most patients with SCD experience pain on an almost daily basis (PiSCES study). Patients who have successfully transitioned from pediatric to adult care, have a good support system, and are distracted by their work or school schedules tend to cope better and require less pharmacologic support. In most cases, though, short-acting and long-acting opiates are required to empower the patient to manage pain at home and minimize use of the emergency department. Drugs for neuropathic pain, such as gabapentin, may also be used in combination with opiates.

Because analgesic care is life-long, consultation with pain specialists is often valuable, particularly in patients for whom more-sophisticated pain regimens are needed. For instance, the mu-opioid receptor partial agonist buprenorphine (Buprenex), opioid rotation, and methadone used as analgesic can help reduce the total opiate requirements. Urine toxicology screens are indicated and should be scheduled at regular intervals both to document adherence with the therapy and to screen for use of illicit substances.

Transfusional Therapy
In SCD, the benefits of transfusion in terms of improved hemodynamics and oxygenation need to be balanced with the risks of iron overload, alloimmunization, transfusion reactions, and viral transmission of infectious agents. Leukoreduced, sickle-negative RBCs with extended phenotypic matching for Rh Cc, Ee, and Kell, which account for 80% of detected antibodies, are required. By employing extended phenotypic matching, the rate of alloimmunization decreased from 3% to 0.5% per unit, and the rate of delayed hemolytic transfusion reactions decreased by 90% in the STOP study. In previously immunized patients, a full RBC match also inclusive of matching for the Duffy, Kidd, and S antigens is recommended. Indications for transfusion include hemoglobin less than 5 g/dL or less than 6 g/dL with symptoms and any severe complication such as stroke, aplastic anemia, splenic or hepatic sequestration, or acute chest syndrome.

Prophylactic transfusions have been considered standard of care before surgery (with the exclusion of minor procedures such as intravenous port placement). The benefit of preoperative transfusions in preventing SCD-related complications in HbSS patients has been recently confirmed in a small randomized clinical trial (the TAPS study). As to the type of transfusion strategy to be used, a clinical trial published in 1995 showed that a conservative prophylactic transfusion regimen to achieve a target hemoglobin of 10 g/dL and any HbS value was as effective as an aggressive regimen to achieve a hemoglobin of 10 g/dL and a target HbS value of <30% in preventing postsurgical complications such as acute chest syndrome.

Exchange transfusion (erythrocytapheresis with RBC exchange) is usually reserved for the most severe complications, which include acute chest syndrome with impending pulmonary failure, acute stroke and its prevention in children, multiorgan failure and sepsis. Box 1 summarizes the main indications for simple and exchange transfusion in SCD as well as the areas of uncertainty.

Box 1   Indications for Transfusion

No Indication
Chronic steady-state anemia
Uncomplicated painful episode
Infections
Minor surgery without general anesthesia
Aseptic necrosis of hip or shoulder
Uncomplicated pregnancy

Unclear Indication
Intractable or frequent painful episodes
Leg ulcers
Before receiving IV contrast dye
Complicated pregnancy
Cerebrovascular accident in adults
Chronic organ failure

Simple Transfusion
Symptomatic anemia
• High output cardiac failure
• Dyspnea
• Angina
• Central nervous system dysfunction
Sudden decrease in hemoglobin
• Aplastic crisis
• Acute splenic sequestration
Severe anemia (Hb ~5 g/dL) with fatigue or dyspnea
Preparation for surgery with general anesthesia

Exchange Transfusion
Acute cerebrovascular accident
Multiple organ system failure
Acute chest syndrome
Hepatic sequestration
Retinal surgery

Iron Chelation

Patients who have received more than 10 transfusions or 20 units of packed RBCs should be screened for iron overload. Most authorities recommend initiation of iron chelation based on a ferritin level consistently greater than 1000 ng/mL, based on data from the thalassemia literature, although liver iron quantitation by MRI or biopsy should be obtained, when available, prior to therapy and to monitor its effectiveness. In the United States, the oral chelating agents deferasirox and deferiprone and the parenteral deferoxamine are available and should be administered until the ferritin level is less than 500 ng/mL for three consecutive measurements. Patients on iron chelation with deferasirox and defereoxamine need to be monitored for hepatic, renal, auditory, and visual toxicity, and particular caution has to be exercised in the setting of renal disease, because transient, reversible increases in serum creatinine as well as rare instances of irreversible acute kidney injury have been reported in patients with underlying renal insufficiency. In most patients, however, deferasirox is well tolerated, and dyspepsia and diarrhea are the most common side effects. Deferiprone (ferriprox) was recently approved for the treatment of transfusional iron overload in thalassemia and may have a role as a third iron chelator in SCD. Deferiprone has been associated with agranulocytosis and neutropenia, mandating close monitoring of the absolute neutrophil count during therapy.

Erythropoietic Stimulating Agents

Whereas a brisk reticulocytic response is common in SCD, patients who develop renal failure or aplastic crises or who receive therapy with hydroxyurea may experience a relative or absolute reticulocytopenia (<100,000 reticulocytes/mL) and a worsening of their baseline anemia. In these situations, therapy with erythropoietic stimulating agents (ESAs) is indicated. Occasionally, ESAs are used to allow upward titration of hydroxyurea and are used in combination with this medication. A review of the literature and of the experience at the NIH shows that ESAs are safe in patients with SCD, particularly when used in combination with hydroxyurea and when the target hemoglobin is no more than 10 g/dL.

Because of bone marrow expansion in patients with HbSS, higher starting doses of erythropoietin (Epogen, Procrit)[1] than in patients without SCD and on the order of 300 U/kg three times per week (or alternatively as a single dose of 900 U/kg once weekly) may be considered. For darbepoetin (Aranesp),[1] a reasonable starting dose is 100 to 200 μg/weekly or every 2 weeks. ESAs can be titrated by 20% to 25% increases in dose per week in patients who do not respond adequately. Weekly monitoring of hematocrit is essential to avoid overdosage and relative erythrocytosis, which can lead to hyperviscosity and vaso-occlusive episodes.

Nutritional Considerations

Malnutrition, growth retardation, and stunting with findings of low lean and fat body mass have a high prevalence in children and adolescents with SCD due to their increased caloric demands and a hypermetabolic state. Macronutrient and micronutrient deficiencies are common, and nutritional counseling is therefore warranted. Hypovitaminosis D and low bone mineral density are also prevalent in children and adults. Folic acid[1] is indicated at the dose of 1 mg daily as in other hemolytic diseases. Strategies aimed at decreasing iron intake and absorption should be implemented early. There is also growing interest in antioxidant nutrients, although there are no clear guidelines at present. The small subset of patients who are overweight or obese is at risk for exacerbating or precipitating common orthopedic problems in SCD such as avascular necrosis of the femoral heads and their resulting disability. These patients should also receive targeted nutritional counseling.

Hydroxyurea

Since the pediatric hematologist Janet Watson suggested in 1948 that the paucity of sickle cells in the peripheral blood of newborns was due to the presence of increased HbF, there has been interest in developing therapies to modulate the hemoglobin switch from fetal to newborn life. Several antineoplastic agents, including 5-azacytidine and hydroxurea, became the focus of attention after they were found to increase HbF levels in nonhuman primates and individuals with SCD.

The landmark Multicenter Study of Hydoxyurea in Sickle Cell Disease (MSH) showed that the incidence of painful crises was reduced from a median of 4.5 per year to 2.5 per year in hydroxyurea-treated patients with SCD. The rates of acute chest syndrome and blood transfusion were also reduced significantly. A follow-up for up to 9 years of 233 of the original 299 subjects showed a 40% reduction in mortality among those who received hydroxyurea. This study led to the approval of hydroxyurea (Droxia) as the only disease-modifying therapy in adults with SCD. More recent studies showed that hydroxyurea is safe and effective in children with adults with SCD. The recently concluded Baby-HUG study showed that children 9–18 months with HbSS disease randomized to receive 2 years of hydroxyurea therapy, irrespective of the disease severity, had less dactilytis and fewer pain episodes, hospitalizations, and transfusions than children receiving placebo.

On a molecular and cellular level, the benefits of hydroxyurea are mostly related to increased intracellular HbF, which prevents the formation of HbS polymers and sickling. In addition to this mechanism, some patients on hydroxyurea who do not adequately increase their HbF levels also display clinical benefits, suggesting that hydroxyurea might have other beneficial rheologic properties.

Although the MSH study only included patients with HbSS, its findings traditionally have been extrapolated to other sickle cell

---

[1]Not FDA approved for this indication.

syndromes such as HbSC and HbS/β-thalassemia. A report from Greece, where S/β-thalassemia is highly prevalent, has confirmed that hydroxyurea similarly reduces complications and mortality in patients with HbS/β[0]-thalassemia, with a nonsignificant benefit also observed in HbS/β[+]thalassemia. Although the NIH guidelines on SCD do recommend hydroxyurea in patients with HbSC disease, there is still no direct published evidence of benefit in this population, and some authorities contend it should not be used in HbSC disease because the main pathophysiologic alteration in this subset of patients is increased viscosity rather than hemolysis and sickling.

Hydroxyurea has been indicated at a dosage of 15 mg/kg (7.5 mg/kg in patients with renal disease) in patients with frequent pain episodes, history of acute chest syndrome, other severe vaso-occlusive episodes, or severe symptomatic anemia, although a newer approach is to prescribe it to all patients with HbSS regardless of their phenotype. Endpoints are less pain, increase in HbF to 15% to 20%, increased hemoglobin level to 7 to 9 g/dL in severely anemic patients, improved well-being, and acceptable myelotoxicity. The dosage can be increased by 500 mg every other day every 8 weeks to a maximum of 35 mg/kg if no toxicity is encountered. Considering the potential myelotoxicity, hepatotoxicity, and nephrotoxicity of this medication, laboratory monitoring needs to be performed every 2 weeks at the time of initiation or escalation and monthly during maintenance therapy. Laboratory studies should include a complete blood cell count (CBC), differential and reticulocyte count, and serum chemistries. Measurements of HbF can be performed every 3 months. An elevated MCV is a marker of adherence to the therapy.

Criteria for holding hydroyurea are listed in Figure 3. Patients need to be counseled on the teratogenic potential, as demonstrated in animal studies, as well as the risks of infertility and leukemogenesis, although to date no increase in baseline risk of leukemia in patients with SCD on hydroxyurea has been reported.

Other side effects that can affect compliance include, but are not limited to, weight gain, alopecia, skin and nail hyperpigmentation (melanonychia), nausea and vomiting, and mucosal ulcerations. Because of the toxicity concerns as well as factors intrinsic to long-term preventive therapy, hydroxyurea therapy has had low effectiveness in spite of high efficacy, with underprescribing by health care professionals and poor patient compliance being major obstacles to its widespread adoption.

Therapy of Pulmonary Hypertension

Because evidence-based guidelines for managing pulmonary hypertension in patients with SCD are not available, recommendations are based upon the pulmonary arterial hypertension literature, case reports, small open-label studies, and expert opinion. For patients with mild pulmonary hypertension (tricuspid regurgitant velocity [TRV], 2.5-2.9 m/sec), it is important to identify and treat risk factors associated with pulmonary hypertension such as rest, exercise or nocturnal hypoxemia, sleep apnea, pulmonary thromboembolic disease, restrictive lung disease or fibrosis, left ventricular systolic and diastolic dysfunction, severe anemia, and iron overload. These patients may benefit from aggressive SCD management, including optimization of hydroxyurea dosage and initiation of a chronic transfusion program in those who do not tolerate or respond poorly to hydroxyurea. Consultation with a pulmonologist or cardiologist experienced in pulmonary hypertension is also recommended.

For patients with TRV 3 m/sec or more, we recommend following the guidelines for TRV 2.5 to 2.9 m/sec. In addition, right heart catheterization is necessary to confirm diagnosis and to directly assess left ventricular diastolic and systolic function. We would consider specific therapy with selective pulmonary vasodilator and remodeling drugs if the patient has pulmonary arterial hypertension defined by right heart catheterization and exercise limitation defined by a low 6-minute walk distance.

FDA-approved drugs for primary pulmonary arterial hypertension include the endothelin receptor antagonists (bosentan [Tracleer] and ambrisentan [Letairis]), prostaglandin-based therapy (epoprostenol [Flolan], treprostinil [Remodulin, Tyvaso], and iloprost [Ventavis]), the phosphodiesterase-5 inhibitors (sildenafil [Revatio]), and riociguat, the first member of a new class of drugs, the soluble guanylate cyclase (sGC) stimulators. No published randomized studies in the SCD population exist for any of these agents, although a multicenter placebo-controlled trial of sildenafil for pulmonary hypertension of SCD was stopped early because of an unexpected increase in hospitalizations for vaso-occlusive crisis in the treatment group receiving sildenafil.

Anticoagulation is indicated in patients who have evidence of pulmonary thromboembolic complications and is supported by evidence of benefit in other populations with pulmonary hypertension.

Hematopoietic Stem Cell Transplantation

Despite improvement of supportive care in SCD, life expectancy remains lower than for those not affected. In addition, quality of life for patients with SCD is usually significantly impaired. Although hydroxyurea can decrease acute complications of SCD such as vaso-occlusive episodes and acute chest syndrome, no satisfactory measures exist to prevent the development of irreversible organ damage in adults. Further, therapy with hydroxyurea is lifelong, and only 20% to 30% of eligible patients are prescribed or actually take the drug.

Currently, allogeneic hematopoietic stem cell transplantation (HCT) remains the only curative treatment. Indications for HCT have been empirically determined from prognostic factors derived from studies of the natural history of SCD. The most common indications for which patients with SCD have undergone HCT are a history of stroke, recurrent acute chest syndrome, or frequent vaso-occlusive episodes.

Allogeneic HCT after myeloablative therapy has been performed in hundreds of pediatric and numerous adult patients with SCD. The backbone of the preparative regimens have consisted of busulfan (Busulfex)[1] 14 to 16 mg/kg and cyclophosphamide (Cytoxan)[1] 200 mg/kg. Additional immunosuppressive agents used have

---

Start therapy if one or more of the following conditions are present:
- frequent pain episodes
- history of acute chest syndrome
- other severe VOE
- severe symptomatic anemia

Starting dose: 15 mg/kg or 7.5 mg/kg if the patient has kidney disease

Endpoints:
- less pain
- increase in HbF to 15%–20%
- increased hemoglobin level to 7–9 g/dL
- improved well-being
- acceptable myelotoxicity

Dose escalation: increase dose by 500 mg every other day every 8 weeks if no toxicity encountered to a maximum of 35 mg/kg

Lab monitoring:
- At time of initiation or escalation: check CBC/differential/reticulocyte count every 2 weeks; serum chemistries every 2–4 weeks, percent HbF every 6–8 weeks
- During maintenance: check CBC/differential/reticulocyte count chemistries monthly, percent HbF every 3 months

Criteria to hold:
- ANC <2000
- Hb <9.0 g/dL and reticulocyte count <80,000 (alternatively start Epo)
- Platelet count <80,000
- Raising creatinine
- 2-fold elevation of AST or ALT over baseline
- 2 months prior to planned conception/pregnancy

Figure 3. Protocol for hydroxyurea treatment.

---

[1]Not FDA approved for this indication.

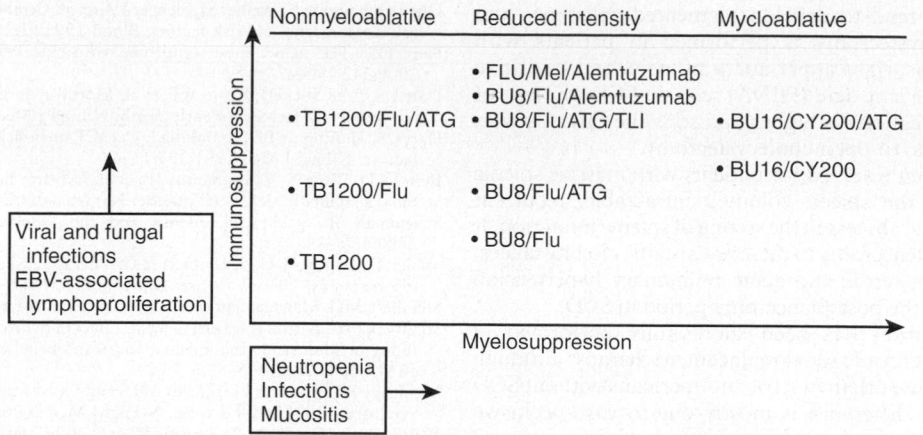

Figure 4. Spectrum of immunosuppression and myelosuppression in preparative regimens in hematopoietic stem cell transplantation (HCT) in sickle cell disease (SCD). Most preparative regimens for HCT in SCD have employed a backbone of busulfan (BU) (Busulfex)[1] and cyclophosphamide (CY) (Cytoxan).[1] Additional immunosuppressive agents include equine antithymocyte globulin (Atgam) or leporine antithymocyte globulin (Thymoglobulin) (ATG), antilymphocyte globulin, total lymphoid or total body irradiation (TLI or TBI), fludarabine (Flu) (Fludara),[1] and alemtuzumab (Campath).[1] Attempts to reduce the intensity of preparative regimens for patients with SCD have been based on one of two approaches. The first is the use of reduced-intensity conditioning regimens to produce less myeloablation. These require donor marrow infusion for hematopoietic recovery. The second is the use of nonmyeloablative regimens, which do not eradicate host hematopoiesis and allow hematopoietic recovery even without donor stem cell infusion. (Adapted with permission from Krishnamurti L: Hematopoietic cell transplantation: A curative option for sickle cell disease. Pediatr Hematol Oncol 2007;24:569–75.)

included antithymocyte globulin (Atgam),[1] rabbit antithymocyte globulin (Thymoglobulin),[1] antilymphocyte globulin, or total lymphoid irradiation (Figure 4). Cyclosporine A (Neoral),[1] alone or with mercaptopurine (Purinethol)[1] or methotrexate,[1] has been used for post-transplant graft-versus-host disease prophylaxis.

The outcome of HCT for patients with SCD from matched siblings is excellent, with an overall survival of 93% to 97% and an event-free survival of 85%. Stabilization or reversal of organ damage from SCD has been documented after HCT. In patients who have stable donor engraftment, complications related to SCD resolve, and there are no further episodes of pain, stroke, or acute chest syndrome. Patients who successfully receive allografts do not experience sickle-related central nervous system complications and have evidence of stabilization of central nervous system disease by cerebral MRI. However, the impact of successful HCT on reversal of cerebral vasculopathy has been variable. Current research is focused on improving the applicability of HCT to a greater proportion of patients with SCD by the development of novel conditioning regimens minimizing myeloablation (see Figure 4) and the use of novel sources of hematopoietic stem cells such as umbilical cord blood. A report published in JAMA in 2014 showed that of 30 SCD patients with and without thalassemia receiving nonmyeloablative HCT, 87% had stable long-term donor engraftment and none had acute or chronic graft-versus-host disease, even after withdrawal of immunosuppression.

Experimental Therapies
Modulation of Cellular Dehydration
Cellular dehydration plays a key role in HbS polymerization and sickling and is caused by water loss through the Ca^{2+}-activated K^+ channel (IK1 or Gardos channel) and the K-Cl cotransport (KCC). The Gardos channel inhibitor senicapoc was tested in phase II and phase III clinical trials, where it led to increased hemoglobin and decreased hemolysis but did not result in a reduction in the rate of pain episodes. There is hope that strategies aiming at reducing cellular dehydration may be used in combination with other therapies to prevent vaso-occlusive episodes.

Modulation of Nitric Oxide and Arginine
Nitric oxide (NO) is an active biogas and a free radical species that mediates arterial relaxation, cellular adhesion to endothelium, hemostasis, and blood viscosity. In SCD, NO bioactivity is reduced

as a result of decreased production due to endothelial perturbation and NO scavenging by cell-free hemoglobin generated during intravascular hemolysis. Dietary supplementation with arginine,[7] a precursor of NO, and delivery of exogenous NO or NO bioactivity to the microvasculature in SCD, should promote dilatation of the terminal arterioles where obstruction to flow and tissue damage occurs, improvement of lung ventilation and perfusion matching, decrease in pulmonary artery pressures, and inhibition of platelet aggregation and cellular adhesion. Although two recent clinical trials on arginine supplementation and inhaled NO (DeNOVO trial) for vaso-occlusive episodes failed to show a clinical benefit, optimization of timing and dosing might lead to valuable NO therapeutics in the future.

Modulation of cellular adhesion
Adhesive interactions between red blood cells, white blood cells and platelets and between cells and endothelium are implicated in the pathogenesis of vaso-occlusive episodes. Recently, several compounds have been developed to target specific adhesion molecules such as E-selectin and P-selectin. A small molecule inhibitor of E-selectin and a monoclonal antibody against P-selectin are being investigated in Phase 1 and 2 clinical trials and single-stranded oligonucleotides (aptamers) against selectins have shown promise in pre-clinical models.

Surgical Issues
Preoperative patient optimization includes prophylactic transfusion, close monitoring of pulse oximetry, adequate analgesia based on the patient's opiate tolerance, and monitoring for sickle cell–related complications.

Avascular necrosis (AVN) of the femoral heads, and more rarely of the humeral heads, is the most common orthopedic problem in SCD. Surgery is usually deferred until the pain and disability from AVN become intolerable and usually involves total hip or shoulder arthroplasty. This is usually a more involved procedure than in the general population on account of the altered bone anatomy in SCD. Patients with bone marrow expansion may experience thinning of the cortical bone and prosthetic instability, whereas some may suffer from the opposite problem of obliteration of the medullary shaft by sclerotic bone in response to multiple necrotic events.

---

[1]Not FDA approved for this indication.

[7]Available as dietary supplement.

Patients with SCD tend to develop pigmented gallstones and cholelithiasis. Cholecystectomy is performed in patients with SCD with cholelithiasis, right upper quadrant pain, and a positive hepatobiliary iminodiacetic acid (HIDA) scan. In SCD, the rate of intraoperative complications is higher and so is the rate of reversion from laparoscopic to open cholecystectomy.

Splenectomy has been reserved for patients with massive splenic infarction (>50% of the spleen volume); intractable, recurrent splenic pain; and splenic abscess in the setting of splenic infarction. It is important to limit splenectomy to these few specific circumstances, because overwhelming sepsis and acute pulmonary hypertension have been reported in the postsplenectomy period in SCD.

Kidney transplantation has been successfully performed in patients with SCD on chronic renal replacement therapy, although survival at 7 years is lower than in African Americans without SCD (67% vs. 83%). This difference is mostly due to vaso-occlusive complications in the transplanted kidney, possibly exacerbated by the higher hematocrit in the postoperative period from resumption of endogenous erythropoietin production and increased blood viscosity. It is therefore critical to closely monitor ESA therapy in the post-transplantation period to prevent overdosing and relative erythrocytosis. A chronic transfusion program to prevent intrarenal sickling and maximization of hydroxyurea therapy should also be entertained, although its benefits need to be balanced against the risk of HLA alloimmunization and rejection. Combined solid organ and HCT protocols are being developed to overcome these complications. Recently, lung transplantation has been successfully performed in a SCD patient with severe pulmonary arterial hypertension and pulmonary veno-occlusive disease.

References

Adams RJ, Brambilla D. Discontinuing prophylactic transfusions used to prevent stroke in sickle cell disease. N Engl J Med 2005;353:2769–78.

Adams RJ, Brambilla DJ, Granger S, et al. Stroke and conversion to high risk in children screened with transcranial Doppler ultrasound during the STOP study. Blood 2004;103:3689–94.

Bunn HF. Pathogenesis and treatment of sickle cell disease. N Engl J Med 1997;337:762–9.

Charache S, Terrin ML, Moore RD, et al. Effect of hydroxyurea on the frequency of painful crises in sickle cell anemia. Investigators of the Multicenter Study of Hydroxyurea in Sickle Cell Anemia. N Engl J Med 1995;332:1317–22.

DeBaun MR, et al. Controlled trial of transfusions for silent cerebral infarcts in sickle cell anemia. N Engl J Med 2014;371(8):699–710.

Falletta JM, Woods GM, Verter JI, et al. Discontinuing penicillin prophylaxis in children with sickle cell anemia. Prophylactic Penicillin Study II. J Pediatr 1995;127:685–90.

Gaston MH, Verter JI, Woods G, et al. Prophylaxis with oral penicillin in children with sickle cell anemia. A randomized trial. N Engl J Med 1986;314:1593–9.

Gladwin MT, Sachdev V. Cardiovascular abnormalities in sickle cell disease. J Am Coll Cardiol 2012;59:1123–33.

Gladwin MT, Sachdev V, Jison ML, et al. Pulmonary hypertension as a risk factor for death in patients with sickle cell disease. N Engl J Med 2004;350:886–95.

Gladwin MT, Vichinsky E. Pulmonary complications of sickle cell disease. N Engl J Med 2008;359:2254–65.

Howard J, Malfroy M, Llewelyn C, et al. The Transfusion Alternatives Preoperatively in Sickle Cell Disease (TAPS) study: a randomised, controlled, multicentre clinical trial. Lancet 2013;381:930–8.

Hsieh MM, Fitzhugh CD, Weitzel RP, et al. Nonmyeloablative HLA-matched sibling allogeneic hematopoietic stem cell transplantation for severe sickle cell phenotype. JAMA 2014;312(1):48–56.

Jeong GK, Ruchelsman DE, Jazrawi LM, Jaffe WL. Total hip arthroplasty in sickle cell hemoglobinopathies. J Am Acad Orthop Surg 2005;13:208–17.

Krishnamurti L, Kharbanda S, Biernacki MA, et al. Stable long-term donor engraftment following reduced-intensity hematopoietic cell transplantation for sickle cell disease. Biol Blood Marrow Transplant 2008;14:1270–8.

Lee MT, Piomelli S, Granger S, et al. Stroke Prevention Trial in Sickle Cell Anemia (STOP): Extended follow-up and final results. Blood 2006;108:847–52.

Little JA, McGowan VR, Kato GJ, et al. Combination erythropoietin-hydroxyurea therapy in sickle cell disease: Experience from the National Institutes of Health and a literature review. Haematologica 2006;91:1076–83.

Mehari A, Alam S, Tian X, et al. Hemodynamic predictors of mortality in adults with sickle cell disease. Am J Respir Crit Care Med 2013;187:840–7.

Merkel KH, Ginsberg PL, Parker JC, Post MJ. Cerebrovascular disease in sickle cell anemia: A clinical, pathological and radiological correlation. Stroke 1978;9:45–52.

Morris CR, Kato GJ, Poljakovic M, et al. Dysregulated arginine metabolism, hemolysis-associated pulmonary hypertension, and mortality in sickle cell disease. JAMA 2005;294:81–90.

Noguchi CT, Rodgers GP, Serjeant G, Schechter AN. Levels of fetal hemoglobin necessary for treatment of sickle cell disease. N Engl J Med 1988;318:96–9.

Novelli EM, Huynh C, Gladwin MT, et al. Pulmonary embolism in sickle cell disease: a case-control study. J Thrombosis and Hemostasis 2012;10:760–6.

Ohene-Frempong K, Weiner SJ, Sleeper LA, et al. Cerebrovascular accidents in sickle cell disease: rates and risk factors. Blood 1998;91:288–94.

Platt OS. The acute chest syndrome of sickle cell disease. N Engl J Med 2000;342:1904–7.

Platt OS, Brambilla DJ, Rosse WF, et al. Mortality in sickle cell disease. Life expectancy and risk factors for early death. N Engl J Med 1994;330:1639–44.

Platt OS, Thorington BD, Brambilla DJ, et al. Pain in sickle cell disease. Rates and risk factors. N Engl J Med 1991;325:11–6.

Reiter CD, Wang X, Tanus-Santos JE, et al. Cell-free hemoglobin limits nitric oxide bioavailability in sickle-cell disease. Nat Med 2002;8:1383–9.

Scheinman JI. Sickle cell disease and the kidney. Nat Clin Pract Nephrol 2009;5:78–88.

Smiley D, Dagogo-Jack S, Umpierrez G. Therapy insight: Metabolic and endocrine disorders in sickle cell disease. Nat Clin Pract Endocrinol Metab 2008;4:102–9.

Steinberg MH. Management of sickle cell disease. N Engl J Med 1999;340:1021–30.

Steinberg MH, Barton F, Castro O, et al. Effect of hydroxyurea on mortality and morbidity in adult sickle cell anemia: Risks and benefits up to 9 years of treatment. JAMA 2003;289:1645–51.

Vichinsky EP, Neumayr LD, Earles AN, et al. Causes and outcomes of the acute chest syndrome in sickle cell disease. N Engl J Med 2000;342:1855–65.

Walters MC, Patience M, Leisenring W, et al. Bone marrow transplantation for sickle cell disease. N Engl J Med 1996;335:369–76.

Walters MC, Storb R, Patience M, et al. Impact of bone marrow transplantation for symptomatic sickle cell disease: An interim report. Multicenter investigation of bone marrow transplantation for sickle cell disease. Blood 2000;95:1918–24.

Yawn BP, et al. Management of sickle cell disease: summary of the 2014 evidence-based report by expert panel members. JAMA 2014;312(10):1033–48.

THALASSEMIA

Method of
Sarah A. Holstein, MD, PhD; and Raymond J. Hohl, MD, PhD

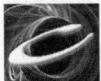

CURRENT DIAGNOSIS

- Complete blood count: anemia (very severe in β-thalassemia major, mild in β-thalassemia minor and α-thalassemia trait), low mean corpuscular volume, variable leukocytosis, thrombocytopenia (secondary to splenomegaly) or thrombocythemia (after splenectomy)
- Peripheral blood smear: hypochromia, microcytosis, anisocytosis, poikilocytosis, target cells, Heinz bodies, nucleated red blood cells
- Evidence of hemolytic anemia: indirect hyperbilirubinemia, elevated lactate dehydrogenase, decreased haptoglobin
- Hemoglobin electrophoresis pattern:
  β-Thalassemia minor: elevated HbA2 ($\alpha_2\delta_2$)
  β-Thalassemia intermedia: elevated HbA2, elevated HbF ($\alpha_2\gamma_2$), and decreased HbA ($\alpha_2\beta_2$)
  β-Thalassemia major: absence of HbA, markedly elevated HbF, and elevated HbA2
  α-Thalassemia trait: normal
  Hemoglobin H disease: decreased HbA, presence of HbH (β_4) and HbBart (γ_4)
  Hemoglobin Barts hydrops fetalis: HbBart, absence of HbA, HbA2, and HbF
- Timing of symptomatic disease:
  β-Thalassemia minor: asymptomatic
  β-Thalassemia intermedia: variable
  β-Thalassemia major: within first year of life
  α-Thalassemia trait: asymptomatic
  Hemoglobin H disease: symptomatic at time of birth
  Hemoglobin Barts hydrops fetalis: death during gestation

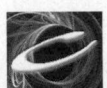

CURRENT THERAPY

- Chronic packed red blood cell transfusions for β-thalassemia major (1–3 units of packed leukoreduced erythrocytes every 3–5 weeks) with a target hemoglobin concentration of 9 to

- 10.5 g/dL; variable transfusion needs for β-thalassemia intermedia and hemoglobin H disease
- Splenectomy with antibiotic prophylaxis and vaccination
- Iron chelation: deferoxamine (Desferal) or deferasirox (Exjade); deferiprone (Ferriprox) does not have FDA approval in the United States
- Osteoporosis management: calcium with vitamin D supplementation; bisphosphonates
- Allogeneic hematopoietic cell transplantation for β-thalassemia major

Globin Gene Arrangements

Thalassemia syndromes encompass a spectrum of hemoglobin disorders that arise from impaired production of globin chains. The genes that encode globins are located in two clusters: the β gene cluster on chromosome 11 and the α gene cluster on chromosome 16 (Figure 1). The β gene cluster includes the adult globin genes (β and δ) as well as the fetal Aγ and Gγ genes and the embryonic ε gene. The arrangement of the 5' to 3' sequence of these genes parallels the order of their developmental expression. Functional hemoglobin is a tetramer that includes two α and two β globin units. The α gene cluster includes two fetal/adult α genes (α1 and α2) and the embryonic ζ genes. In the embryo, three hemoglobins are found ($\zeta_2\varepsilon_2$, $\alpha_2\varepsilon_2$, and $\zeta_2\gamma_2$). Fetal hemoglobin (HbF) is

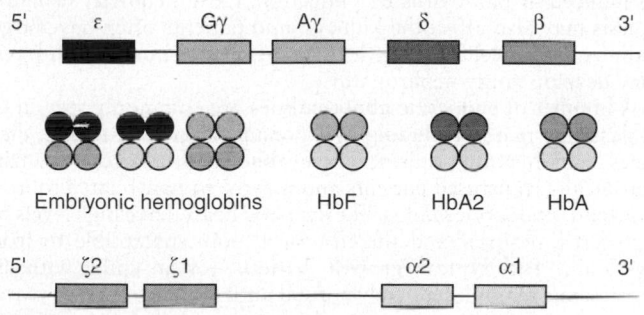

Figure 1. Representation of the β and α globin gene clusters. Also shown are the globin tetramers produced during embryonic development.

Chromosome 11: Beta globin gene cluster

Embryonic hemoglobins   HbF   HbA2   HbA

Chromosome 16: Alpha globin gene cluster

composed of two α chains and two γ chains ($\alpha_2\gamma_2$). In adults, the predominant hemoglobin is hemoglobin A (HbA), consisting of two α chains and two β chains ($\alpha_2\beta_2$) (see Figure 1). Hemoglobin A2, consisting of two α chains and two δ chains ($\alpha_2\delta_2$), is a normal variant in adults and typically represents less than 3% of the total hemoglobin (see Figure 1).

In β-thalassemia, there is diminished production of β globin genes, resulting in an excess of α globin chains. Conversely, in α-thalassemia there is impaired production of α globin genes, resulting in an excess of β globin chains. This imbalance of globin production is variable, and the degree of accumulation of unpaired globin chains is directly related to the severity of the disease phenotype. The genetic basis of thalassemia is heterogeneous, and several hundred mutations have been identified. These mutations may affect any level of globin gene expression, including arrangement of the globin gene complex, gene deletion, splicing, transcription, translation, and protein stability. In general, β-thalassemia occurs as a result of mutations, whereas α-thalassemia occurs as a result of gene deletion.

It has been estimated that there are 270 million carriers of thalassemia in the world, including 80 million β-thalassemia carriers. The frequency of β-thalassemia carriers is highest in the malarial tropical and subtropical regions of Asia, the Mediterranean, and the Middle East. The term thalassemia, derived from Greek, refers to the Mediterranean Sea. This distribution is secondary to the selective advantage of heterozygotes against malaria. β-Thalassemia is subdivided into major, intermedia, and minor types (Table 1). α-Thalassemia is classified into four syndromes: α-thalassemia trait 2 (loss of one α globin gene [αα/α−]); α-thalassemia trait 1, also referred to as α-thalassemia minor (loss of two α globin genes [αα/−− or α−/α−]); hemoglobin H (HbH) disease (loss of three alleles [α−/−−]); and hemoglobin Barts hydrops fetalis (loss of all four α globin loci [−−/−−]).

Pathophysiology

The clinical manifestations of thalassemia and their severity are a consequence of the relative excess of unpaired globin chains. In particular, excess α globin chains are unstable and insoluble and therefore precipitate inside the red blood cell (RBC). These inclusions (precipitated hemoglobin) may be visualized as Heinz bodies. The accumulation of α globin chains leads to a variety of insults to the erythrocyte, including changes in membrane deformability and increased fragility. Free β chains are more soluble than free α chains and are able to form a homotetramer (HbH). The

TABLE 1   Summary of Hematologic and Clinical Features of the Thalassemias

TYPE	HEMATOLOGIC FINDINGS	HEMOGLOBIN ELECTROPHORESIS PATTERN	CLINICAL FEATURES
β-Thalassemia major	Severe anemia, microcytosis, hypochromia, target cells, nucleated RBCs	Absence of HbA, markedly elevated HbF, elevated HbA2	Splenomegaly, jaundice, skeletal abnormalities, abnormal facies; transfusion dependent
β-Thalassemia intermedia	Mild to moderate anemia, microcytosis, hypochromia	Elevated HbA2, elevated HbF, decreased HbA	Splenomegaly; variable transfusion dependence
β-Thalassemia minor	Mild anemia, microcytosis, target cells	Elevated HbA2	None
Hemoglobin Barts hydrops fetalis	Severe anemia, anisopoikilocytosis, hypochromia, nucleated RBCs	HbBart; absence of HbA, HbA2, and HbF	Death during gestation; fetus with massive hepatosplenomegaly, generalized edema
Hemoglobin H disease	Moderately severe anemia, anisopoikilocytosis, microcytosis, Heinz bodies	Decreased HbA; HbH and HbBart present	Splenomegaly, jaundice; generally transfusion-dependent
α-Thalassemia trait 1	Mild anemia, hypochromia, microcytosis, target cells	Normal	None
α-Thalassemia trait 2	Normal	Normal	None

Abbreviations: Hb = hemoglobin; RBCs = red blood cells.

hallmark of thalassemia is an anemia that is a consequence of both increased destruction (i.e., hemolysis) and decreased production (i.e., ineffective erythropoiesis). The bone marrow typically displays erythroid hyperplasia.

Oxidant injury is closely linked with the pathology of thalassemia. Under normal conditions, a small amount of methemoglobin (Fe^{3+}) is formed via oxidation and can then be reduced back to hemoglobin (Fe^{2+}). However, isolated globin chains can be oxidized to hemichromes, some forms of which are irreversibly oxidized. The hemichromes can then generate reactive oxygen species, which can oxidize membrane components, leading to cell injury. There is an increase in membrane rigidity in β-thalassemia, and this appears to be secondary to the binding of partially oxidized α globin chains to components of the membrane skeleton. Increased membrane rigidity in turn leads to decreased membrane deformability and increased destruction. In α-thalassemia, HbH has a left-shifted oxygen disassociation curve and therefore does not readily transport oxygen. HbH erythrocytes have increased rigidity, which is thought to be secondary to interactions between excess β globin chains and the membrane. Unlike with β-thalassemia, HbH erythrocytes have increased membrane stability. Inclusion bodies have been identified in HbH cells, and there appears to be a correlation between RBC age and solubility of HbH. As cells age, the amount of soluble HbH decreases, and the level of inclusions increases.

It has also been recognized that there is increased phagocytosis of thalassemia RBCs compared to normal controls. The etiology is not completely understood, but it may be a consequence of reduction in surface levels of sialic acid, increase in surface immunoglobulin G binding, and changes in phosphatidylserine localization.

Despite the pronounced hemolysis and marrow erythroid hyperplasia, patients with thalassemia generally do not display the compensatory reticulocytosis that is indicative of the other basis for anemia, ineffective erythropoiesis. Accumulation of α chain aggregates is thought to lead to death of erythrocyte precursors. Furthermore, abnormal assembly of membrane proteins in erythroid precursors has been demonstrated.

Iron overload is one of the primary causes of morbidity. Even without transfusion, the long-standing anemia, however mild, leads to increased iron absorption in the gut and eventual chronic iron overload. Excessive iron deposition causes devastating damage to multiple organs, particularly affecting the heart, liver, and endocrine organs.

β-Thalassemia Major

Symptoms of β-thalassemia major are not present at birth, because HbF ($\alpha_2\gamma_2$) is present. However, as HbF levels decline over the first year, the signs and symptoms of severe hemolytic anemia begin to manifest. Affected individuals display hepatosplenomegaly from expansion of the reticuloendothelial system as well as extramedullary hematopoiesis, pallor, growth retardation, and abnormal skeletal development. If left untreated, 80% of children with β-thalassemia major will die before the age of 5 years.

Laboratory Features

Thalassemia major is characterized by a severe microcytic anemia. Hemoglobin levels may be as low as 3 to 4 g/dL. The peripheral blood smear is markedly abnormal and is notable for hypochromia, microcytosis, anisocytosis, poikilocytosis, target cells, and tear drop cells. Routine stains show the presence of precipitated α globin chains as Heinz bodies. The reticulocyte count is often low. The white blood cell count is often high but may be artifactually elevated as a consequence of automated inclusion of high numbers of circulating nucleated RBCs. The platelet count is typically normal, but progressive hypersplenism can result in decreased platelet counts. Patients who have undergone splenectomy often have increased white blood cell and platelet counts. Iron studies reveal elevated serum iron, transferrin saturation, and ferritin. Consistent with hemolysis and ineffective erythropoiesis, indirect bilirubin and lactate dehydrogenase levels are increased and haptoglobin levels are low.

Clinical Features

Unique to β-thalassemia major is the development of extramedullary erythropoiesis. This may be so severe that the masses of bone marrow lead to broken bones and spinal cord compression. Sites of involvement include the sinuses and the thoracic and pelvic cavities. The expansion of the erythroid bone marrow can lead to a number of skeletal changes. In particular, characteristic changes in the facial bones and skull result in frontal bossing, overgrowth of the maxillae, and malocclusion. This has sometimes been referred to as chipmunk facies. Other bones are also affected, and premature fusion of the epiphyses results in shortened limbs. Compression fractures of the spine may occur. Even if the disease is managed appropriately with transfusions and iron chelation, patients will still suffer from osteopenia and osteoporosis. Possible mechanisms include changes secondary to hypogonadism or increased bone resorption secondary to vitamin D deficiency.

Hepatomegaly and splenomegaly, secondary to extramedullary erythropoiesis and RBC destruction, are prominent. Injury to Kupffer cells and hepatocytes from chronic overload leads to fibrosis and end-stage liver disease. Hepatic iron overload is probably caused in part by comparatively high levels of transferrin receptors. Iron overload, and perhaps other factors, increase susceptibility to viral hepatitis. Laboratory studies show indirect hyperbilirubinemia, hypergammaglobulinemia, and elevated liver markers. The chronic hemolysis leads to formation of bilirubin gallstones, although cholecystitis or cholangitis is not common. Splenic dysfunction results in immune dysfunction. The shortened erythrocyte survival time leaves patients susceptible to aplastic crisis induced by parvovirus B19 infection. Extramedullary hematopoiesis may also affect the kidneys, and patients often have large kidneys. Rapid cell turnover leads to hyperuricemia, and children may develop gouty nephropathy.

A number of endocrine abnormalities are commonly seen in β-thalassemia major, including hypogonadism, growth failure, diabetes, and hypothyroidism. These abnormalities occur even in chronically transfused patients and may be in part related to iron overload. Endocrine glands, like liver and heart, have high levels of transferrin-receptor and therefore are more susceptible to iron overload. The typical growth pattern for a child with β-thalassemia major is relatively normal until the age of 9 to 10 years. After that time, the growth velocity slows, and the pubertal growth spurt is either absent or reduced. Although secretion of growth hormone does not appear to be altered in thalassemic patients, a reduction in peak amplitude and nocturnal levels of growth hormone has been observed. Amenorrhea is quite common, with 50% of girls presenting with primary amenorrhea. Secondary amenorrhea also develops, particularly in patients who do not receive regular chelation therapy. In males, impotence and azoospermia is common. Primary hypothyroidism typically appears during the second decade of life. The prevalence of diabetes mellitus and impaired glucose intolerance has been estimated at 4% to 20%. Unlike type 1 diabetes mellitus, diabetes associated with thalassemia is rarely complicated by diabetic ketoacidosis. The risk of diabetic retinopathy is lower, but the risk of diabetic nephropathy is higher. Patients with a high ferritin level (above 1800 μg/L) experience a faster progression to hypothyroidism, hypogonadism, and other endocrinopathies.

Thalassemic patients suffer from extensive cardiac abnormalities. Chronic anemia causes cardiac dilatation. Although chronic transfusion can help prevent cardiac dilatation, the resulting iron overload leads to cardiac hemosiderosis. Pericarditis, ventricular and supraventricular arrhythmias, and end-stage cardiomyopathy can develop. Ventricular arrhythmia is a common cause of death. Patients may also develop pulmonary hypertension. The degree of iron overload in the heart has traditionally been assessed by cardiac biopsy, but cardiac magnetic resonance imaging (MRI) is increasingly being used.

Vitamin and mineral deficiencies may occur. Folic acid deficiency may develop in patients, presumably as a consequence of increased cell turnover. Although the cause is unknown, patients with β-thalassemia major often have very low serum zinc levels. Serum levels of vitamin E and vitamin C may also be low.

Management of β-Thalassemia Major

Transfusion

The key intervention for the management of β-thalassemia major is chronic transfusion therapy. In particular, during the first decade of life, regular transfusion results in improvements in hepatosplenomegaly, skeletal abnormalities, and cardiac dilatation. Patients typically require 1 to 3 units of packed RBCs every 3 to 5 weeks. The optimal target total hemoglobin level has yet to be determined. Alloimmunization does occur, and some blood centers try to leukodeplete their products, match donors by ethnicity, and limit the donor pool for any particular patient. Although the risk of blood-borne infections is now quite small, regular transfusion of blood products still carries a risk for infections such as HIV and hepatitis C.

Splenectomy

The general indication for splenectomy is an increase of more than 50% in the RBC transfusion requirement over the period of 1 year. Splenectomy may initially yield a decrease in the RBC transfusion requirement. It has been noted that thalassemia patients are at higher risk for infection after splenectomy than are those patients splenectomized for other reasons. The bacteria that most frequently cause infections in these patients include *Streptococcus pneumoniae*, *Haemophilus influenzae*, *Neisseria meningitidis*, *Klebsiella*, *Escherichia coli*, and *Staphylococcus aureus*. The increased susceptibility to infection compared with other splenectomized patients is thought to be a result of greater immune dysfunction secondary to iron overload. In particular, it has been reported that iron-overloaded macrophages lose the ability to kill intracellular pathogens. Antibiotic prophylaxis with penicillin, amoxicillin, or erythromycin is recommended for children up to the age of 16 years. In addition, patients should receive immunizations, including the pneumococcal, influenza, and *Haemophilus influenzae* vaccines.

Iron Chelation Therapy

Because of increased iron absorption and chronic transfusion therapy, iron overload develops. As noted earlier, iron overload causes damage to multiple organs. Because iron is poorly excreted, removal must be accomplished by phlebotomy (not an option in thalassemic patients) or by chelation therapy. Historically, deferoxamine (Desferal) has been the most widely used chelator. This agent may be administered subcutaneously, intramuscularly, or intravenously. The dosing for chronic iron overload is 20 to 40 mg/kg/day SQ or 500 to 1000 mg/day IM + 2 g IV per unit transfused blood. The IV-only route is indicated for patients with cardiovascular collapse. Multiple studies have shown that deferoxamine therapy improves long-term survival. In addition, intensive therapy with deferoxamine has been shown to improve cardiac function in patients with severe iron overload. However, compliance with daily injections has been a particular problem, and, unless regular therapy is given, iron will reaccumulate.

Deferiprone (Ferriprox)[2] was the first orally active chelator to be introduced. It is given three times daily (total of 75 mg/kg/day). Studies have indicated that deferiprone may be as effective as deferoxamine in lowering iron levels. A recent Cochrane Review concluded that deferiprone is indicated in the treatment of iron overload in thalassemia major if deferoxamine therapy is contraindicated or inadequate. Agranulocytosis associated with deferiprone has been reported, and, because of this risk, the drug is currently not available in the United States except through the FDA Treatment Use Program. Deferiprone is available in Europe and Asia. There has also been interest in combined therapy with deferiprone and deferoxamine, and one study showed that the combination was more effective in removing cardiac and hepatic iron but did not further improve cardiac function.

Deferasirox (Exjade) is the first orally active agent approved for use in the United States. Its longer half-life in comparison to deferiprone allows this drug to be given once daily (total of 20–40 mg/kg/day). A phase III trial comparing deferasirox to deferoxamine in patients with thalassemia revealed similar decreases in liver iron

concentrations. Side effects include gastrointestinal complaints (abdominal pain, nausea, vomiting, diarrhea) and skin rash. There have been postmarketing reports of acute renal failure, hepatic failure, and cytopenias. It is recommended that serum creatinine, ferritin, and alanine aminotransferase be monitored monthly during therapy. A prospective, randomized study comparing deferipronre and deferoxamine vs deferipronre and deferasirox in 96 patients with β-thalassemia major demonstrated that both regimens reduced iron overload. However, the latter regimen was found to be superior with respect to improving cardiac iron, patient compliance, and patient satisfaction.

The gold standard for measurement of liver iron concentration has been liver biopsy with iron measurement by atomic absorption spectrometry. More recently, there has been increasing use of MRI technology to measure liver iron levels. In general, iron content determined by MRI methodology correlates with liver iron concentration determined by biopsy. However, the precision of liver MRI measurement appears to be dependent on iron levels, liver fibrosis, and calibration. Hepatic iron concentration has also been measured using a superconducting quantum interference device (SQUID), although reported consistency has varied and widespread use of this technique has been limited by expense and complexity.

Management of Osteoporosis

Even with calcium and vitamin D supplementation, iron chelation, transfusion therapy, and hormonal therapy, bone loss continues to be a significant problem for thalassemia patients. Recently, there has been interest in the use of bisphosphonates. This class of drugs, which includes clodronate (Bonefos),[2] alendronate (Fosamax), pamidronate (Aredia), zoledronate (Zometa), and neridronate (Nerixia),[2] inhibit osteoclastic bone resorption and have found extensive use in the management of Paget's disease, osteoporosis, and skeletal metastases. Small studies performed in thalassemia patients have failed to show benefit with clodronate 100 mg IM every 10 days or 300 mg IV every 3 weeks. A very small study using alendronate (Fosamax)[1] 10 mg PO daily revealed an increase in bone mineral density only at the femoral level. Conversely, in a study involving pamidronate (Aredia)[1] 30 or 60 mg IV every month, there was an increase in bone density only at the lumbar level. The most promising results have been achieved with the most potent member of the class, zoledronate. Several trials demonstrated that zoledronate (Zometa)[1] 4 mg IV every 3 or 4 months results in significant improvement in femoral and lumbar bone mineral density and reduces bony pain. The largest randomized trial involved 118 β-thalassemia patients who received calcium plus vitamin D with or without neridronate (given every 90 days). At 6 and 12 months, there was increased bone mineral density as well as decreased back pain and analgesic use in the neridronate arm. Larger, long-term trials are necessary before this agent finds widespread use in the management of thalassemia-induced osteoporosis.

Hematopoietic Cell Transplantation

Hematopoietic cell transplantation is the only curative strategy for patients with hemoglobinopathies. Patients are assigned to a risk class (Pesaro class) based on adherence to regular iron chelation therapy, presence or absence of hepatomegaly, and presence or absence of portal fibrosis. Those children with no or little hepatomegaly, no portal fibrosis, and regular iron chelation therapy (class I) have a better than 90% chance of cure, whereas those with both hepatomegaly and portal fibrosis (class III) have long-term survival rates of about 60% in older studies. More recent reports indicate that class III survival has improved to 80%.

The use of human leukocyte antigen (HLA)-identical sibling donors has been preferred, because the use of HLA-mismatched donors has produced inferior results and is associated with increased graft rejection, graft-versus-host disease, and infection.

---

[2] Not available in the United States.

---

[1] Not FDA approved for this indication.

[2] Not available in the United States.

The use of unrelated donors has been explored, and initial studies showed poorer outcomes. However, more recent data suggest that matched unrelated donors might be a viable option if a suitable sibling donor is lacking, thanks to improved donor selection and transplantation techniques. The use of partially HLA-matched unrelated cord blood has been reported, although 4 out of 9 children did not engraft.

Another emerging technique is the use of reduced-intensity conditioning regimens, although long-term success has yet to be achieved. However, no randomized controlled studies have been performed evaluating the role of transplant in thalassemia patients.

Gene Therapy

Globin gene therapy, achieved through manipulation of autologous stem cells, is an attractive alternative to allogeneic transplantation. There are three major scientific hurdles that must be overcome: design of vectors that yield therapeutic levels of globin gene expression, ability to isolate and transduce autologous stem cells, and development of transplantation conditions that will permit host repopulation. In addition, the safety of viral and nonviral transfection is an issue. At this point, there has been some success in murine models of β-thalassemia. One patient was treated with lentiviral gene therapy and become transfusion independent. This remains an active area of research.

Pharmacologic Induction of Fetal Hemoglobin

Induction of HbF expression has been proposed as a therapeutic strategy. For β-thalassemia, induced γ globin gene expression would be predicted to decrease globin chain imbalance by complexing with free α chains. Hydroxyurea (Hydrea)[1] is an antimetabolite thought to interfere with DNA synthesis. It is well established in the management of sickle cell disease, where it has been shown to increase levels of HbF. The use of hydroxyurea in β-thalassemia is much less well established. In the United States, hydroxyurea has been approved for use in sickle cell disease but not for thalassemia. Studies published elsewhere in the world have generally shown improvements in hemoglobin levels in thalassemia intermedia patients, with some patients becoming transfusion independent. A recent meta-analysis on the use of hydroxyurea in patients with transfusion dependent β-thalassemia concluded that this agent might offer some benefit but that double-blinded placebo-controlled studies are lacking.

5-Azacytidine (azacitidine [Vidaza]),[1] an inhibitor of DNA methyltransferase, has been shown to induce HbF. However, concerns regarding long-term use have prevented further evaluation in thalassemia. Decitabine (Dacogen),[1] an analogue of 5-azacytidine, has been shown to increase HbF levels in patients with sickle cell disease refractory to hydroxyurea. A small pilot study of low-dose decitabine in β-thalassemia intermedia patients demonstrated an increase in total hemoglobin and hemoglobin F levels. Butyrate,[5] an inhibitor of histone deacetylases, is another agent capable of inducing HbF. However, butyrate and its derivatives (arginine butyrate,[5] sodium isobutyramide,[5] and sodium phenylbutyrate [Buphenyl][1]) have failed to show significant clinical benefit in thalassemia patients. Therefore, at this time, no agent has been approved for use in thalassemia patients. A number of hypotheses have been proposed to explain the lack of success of inducers of HbF in thalassemia: there is simply too little γ globin production to significantly affect globin chain balance; these agents decrease expression of partially active β-thalassemia genes; these agents increase expression of α-globin genes; chronic transfusions appear to reduce HbF levels; and these agents suppress erythropoiesis.

Antioxidants

Oxidative damage is believed to be an important cause of tissue damage, and there has been interest in the use of antioxidants in thalassemia patients. A variety of substances have been investigated, including ascorbate,[1] vitamin E,[1] N-acetylcysteine (Mucomyst),[1] flavonoids, and indicaxanthin.[5] A variety of antioxidant effects have been observed in vitro with these agents, but none has been shown to improve anemia in patients with thalassemia.

[1]Not FDA approved for this indication.
[5]Investigational drug in the United States.

β-Thalassemia Intermedia

Given the underlying genetic heterogeneity, it is not surprising that the clinical manifestations of β-thalassemia intermedia are also quite varied. Some patients with more mild forms of β-thalassemia intermedia do not require chronic transfusion therapy. There is not a clear consensus as to when chronic transfusion should be initiated. Factors that are considered for children include growth patterns, spleen size, and bone development. Transfusion may be necessary during infection-induced aplastic crises. In some instances, transfusions are begun in childhood to help with growth and then discontinued after puberty. Some adults gradually become more anemic and eventually require transfusion. Some authors have argued that starting transfusions early in life is advantageous, because the prevalence of alloimmunization appears to increase if transfusion is started after the first few years of life.

Splenomegaly usually develops in all patients, including those who do not require transfusion. With progression of splenomegaly and the accompanying sequestration and hemolysis, there is usually worsening of anemia, to the point at which transfusions may be required. Most patients achieve transfusion independence after splenectomy. Gallstones may develop, and a prophylactic cholecystectomy is sometimes performed at the same time as the splenectomy. As with β-thalassemia major patients, intermedia patients are at increased risk for infection and should be appropriately vaccinated.

For reasons that are not entirely clear, there is an increased risk of thromboembolic complications in intermedia patients compared with thalassemia major patients. An Italian study reported that 10% of thalassemia intermedia and 4% of thalassemia major patients experienced a thromboembolic event. Another study reported that thromboembolism occurred four times more frequently in patients with intermedia versus major disease. This report noted that venous events were more common in the thalassemia intermedia population, whereas arterial events were more common in the thalassemia major population. An even higher rate of venous thrombotic events (29%) was reported in a population of splenectomized patients with thalassemia intermedia. It has been suggested that exposed anionic phospholipids on the surface of damaged RBCs may induce a procoagulant effect. There is no consensus regarding the prophylactic use of antiplatelet agents or anticoagulants in this population.

Patients with thalassemia intermedia may develop iron overload, although it is less severe than in patients with thalassemia major. Even those that are not regularly transfused may develop a degree of iron overload, because there is increased iron absorption. Iron overload may be managed with the iron chelating agents as described earlier. Cardiac toxicity, including congestive heart failure, valvular problems, and pulmonary hypertension (leading to secondary right-sided heart failure), resulting from iron overload is not infrequent in the thalassemia intermedia population.

Bone abnormalities and osteoporosis may develop in thalassemia intermedia patients. In a North American study, the prevalence of fractures in these patients was 12%. Leg ulcers involving the medial malleolus are common and are often difficult to treat. Hypogonadism, hypothyroidism, and diabetes may occur, with frequency related to the severity of anemia and iron overload. Pseudoxanthoma elasticum, a syndrome consisting of skin lesions, angioid streaks in the retina, calcified retinal walls, and aortic valve disease, is more common in thalassemia intermedia than in thalassemia major. Currently, no effective therapy exists, although it has been reported that aluminum hydroxide (Alternagel)[1] reduces skin calcification.

β-Thalassemia Minor

Most patients with β-thalassemia minor are asymptomatic. However, they have an abnormal complete blood count that may sometimes lead to the misdiagnosis of iron deficiency. Although these patients have a microcytic anemia, it is much less severe than in

[1]Not FDA approved for this indication.

patients with β-thalassemia major. In general, the hematocrit is greater than 30%. The mean corpuscular volume is typically less than 75 fL and the RBC distribution width index is normal, in contrast to iron deficiency, in which the degree of microcytosis is less and the distribution width index is usually increased. The peripheral blood smear shows the presence of target cells. Hemoglobin electrophoresis typically reveals an increase in HbA2. The normal anemia experienced during pregnancy may sometimes be exacerbated in patients with β-thalassemia minor, necessitating transfusion. Otherwise, no long-term effects of β-thalassemia minor have been described, and no interventions are required.

α-Thalassemia

Laboratory and Clinical Features

Patients with α-thalassemia trait 2 are asymptomatic and have normal laboratory values, including complete blood count, peripheral smear, and hemoglobin electrophoresis. Individuals with α-thalassemia trait 1 are asymptomatic, and the disease resembles β-thalassemia minor. The peripheral smear shows a hypochromic microcytic anemia with the presence of target cells. Hemoglobin electrophoresis is normal.

HbH disease does produce symptoms. Unlike β-thalassemia major, in which HbF production protects the fetus, individuals with HbH disease develop hemolytic anemia during gestation and are symptomatic at birth. This is because α globin production is required for HbF ($\alpha_2\gamma_2$). As with β-thalassemia major, patients with HbH disease suffer from the consequences of chronic hemolytic anemia, although the severity is somewhat less. The transfusion requirements for HbH patients resemble those for patients with β-thalassemia intermedia, with transfusion support initiated in the second and third decades of life. These patients also develop iron overload, necessitating treatment with chelation therapy.

Hydrops fetalis with hemoglobin Barts is usually fatal in utero. The utter lack of α globin chain production results in absence of HbF. Hemoglobin Barts, a homotetramer consisting of four γ globin genes, is unable to deliver oxygen to tissues. Severe tissue hypoxia develops, leading to widespread tissue ischemia. High cardiac output failure leads to massive edema (hydrops). In most cases, death occurs in the third trimester or late second trimester. There have been reports of live births after intrauterine transfusion, but survival beyond the perinatal period is exceedingly rare. Prenatal diagnosis of hemoglobin Barts hydrops fetalis may be achieved through DNA-based testing using amniocytes from amniocentesis or chorionic villi sampling. Noninvasive testing is under development, including methods that isolate circulating fetal DNA in maternal peripheral blood.

Management

Patients with α-thalassemia 2 and 1 traits do not require treatment. The management of HbH disease is similar to that described for β-thalassemia.

References

Angelucci E, Matthes-Martin S, Baronciani D, et al. Hematopoietic stem cell transplantation in thalassemia major and sickle cell disease: indications and management recommendations from an international expert panel. Haematologica 2014;99:811–20.

Bayanzay K, Khan R. Meta-analysis on effectiveness of hydroxyurea to treat transfusion-dependent beta-thalassemia. Hematology 2014; (epub ahead of print).

Finotti A, Gambari R. Recent trends for novel options in experimental biological therapy of β-thalassemia. Expert Opin Biol Ther 2014;14:1443–54.

Giusti A. Bisphosphonates in the management of thalassemiaassociated osteoporosis: a systematic review of randomized controlled trials. J Bone Miner Metab 2014;32:606–15.

Jagannath VA, Fedorowicz Z, Al Hajeri A, et al. Hematopoietic stem cell transplantation for people with β-thalassaemia major. Cochrane Database Syst Rev 2014;10:CD008708.

Karimi M, Cohan N, De Sanctic V, et al. Guidelines for diagnosis and management of beta-thalassemia intermedia. Pediatr Hematol Oncol 2014;31:583–96.

Marsella M, Borgna-Pignatti C. Transfusional iron overload and iron chelation therapy in thalassemia major and sickle cell disease. Hematol Oncol Clin North Am 2014;28:703–27.

Neufeld EJ. Update on iron chelators in thalassemia. Hematology Am Soc Hematol Educ Program 2010;451–5.

Payen E, Leboulch P. Advances in stem cell transplantation and gene therapy in the β-hemoglobinopathies. Hematology Am Soc Hematol Educ Program 2012;2012:276–83.

Quek L, Thein SL. Molecular therapies in β-thalassemia. Br J Haematol 2006;136:353–65.

Terpos E, Voskaridou E. Treatment options for thalassemia patients with osteoporosis. Ann N Y Acad Sci 2010;1202:237–43.

Toumba M, Sergis A, Kanaris C, et al. Endocrine complications in patients with thalassaemia major. Pediatr Endocrinol Rev 2007;5:642–8.

THROMBOTIC THROMBOCYTOPENIC PURPURA

Method of
Ravi Sarode, MD

CURRENT DIAGNOSIS

- In the past, the diagnosis of thrombotic thrombocytopenic purpura (TTP) was made based on a pentad that included microangiopathic hemolytic anemia (MAHA), thrombocytopenia, neurologic involvement, nonoliguric renal insufficiency, and fever. Clinically, waiting for development of the pentad may delay the diagnosis of TTP, delay treatment, and result in a fatal outcome. Currently, unexplained MAHA and thrombocytopenia in the absence of oliguric renal failure are sufficient to make a working diagnosis of TTP and initiate emergent plasma exchange (PLEX).
- These laboratory tests are recommended for patient evaluation:
  - Complete blood count (shows anemia and moderately to severely decreased "platelet count").
  - Peripheral blood smear (shows "schistocytes/fragmented red cells", a hallmark of thrombotic microangiopathy [TMA]).
  - Reticulocyte count (is elevated).
  - Haptoglobin (is usually undetectable in TTP).
  - "Lactate dehydrogenase" (LDH) (usually more than twice the upper limit of normal in TTP).
  - Blood urea nitrogen, serum creatinine (determines nonoliguric renal insufficiency).
  - Liver function tests, including direct and indirect bilirubin.
  - Plasma "ADAMTS13 activity" (<10% is diagnostic of TTP) and inhibitor level (usually detected in 90% of cases of TTP).
  - Prothrombin time, partial thromboplastin time, fibrinogen, and d-dimers (to rule out DIC).
  - Direct antiglobulin test (to rule out autoimmune hemolytic anemia).
  - Urinalysis.

CURRENT THERAPY

- Daily plasma exchange (PLEX) using plasma as a replacement fluid (1–1.5 total body plasma volume) until platelet count is normal for 2 days, then taper PLEX to three times a week, then twice a week, and then once a week. Discontinue when platelets remain greater than 150,000/mcL.
- Prednisone 1 mg/kg/day taper *pari passu* with PLEX.
- Plasma (10–15 cc/kg) or cryoprecipitate (one dose = 10 units of pooled cryoprecipitate) infusion if PLEX will be delayed >6 hours.
- Exacerbation or relapsing TTP.
  - Rituximab (Rituxan)[1] (375 mg/m² weekly for 2–4 weeks).
  - Cyclosporine (Neoral)[1] (2–3 mg/kg/day up to 6 months).
  - Vincristine (Oncovin)[1] (1.4 mg/m² once a week for 4 weeks).
  - Bortezomib (Velcade)[1] (1.3 mg/m² 1–2 cycles).
- Splenectomy as a last resort.

---

[1]Not FDA approved for this indication.

Thrombotic thrombocytopenic purpura (TTP) is a rare (1–2 cases/ million) but life-threatening thrombotic microangiopathy (TMA) disorder characterized by the presence of microthrombi in microcirculation of various organs, including the brain, kidneys, heart, and abdominal viscera. Microthrombi consist of platelets and von Willebrand factor (VWF), resulting in microangiopathic hemolytic anemia (MAHA) and thrombocytopenia. MAHA refers to the fragmentation of red blood cells (schistocytes) during their passage through partially occluded arterioles and capillaries by microthrombi. TTP diagnosis requires a high degree of suspicion, because a delay in initiating PLEX, the current standard of care, could result in a poor response or fatal outcome. In the past, diagnosis of TTP was made based on a pentad that included MAHA, thrombocytopenia, neurologic involvement, renal affection, and fever. This pentad was found in patients who had died of TTP indicating advanced disease; therefore, one should not wait for development of a pentad, which could delay TTP diagnosis with a potentially fatal outcome. Currently, unexplained MAHA and thrombocytopenia in the absence of oliguric renal failure are sufficient to make a working diagnosis of TTP and initiate emergent PLEX.

Pathophysiology

In congenital TTP (Upshaw Shulman syndrome), ultra large (UL) multimers of VWF were detected during remission and were absent during relapse. Later, a VWF cleaving protease (ADAMTS13, a *disintegrin and metalloproteinase with thrombospondin 1 motif*, 13th member of the family) was identified that was responsible for cleaving UL multimers secreted from endothelium into normal sized VWF multimers seen in normal plasma. This cleavage occurs under high shear rate flow conditions in smaller blood vessels where the UL-VWF undergoes unfolding, exposing the cleavage site for ADAMTS13. ADAMTS13 is severely deficient (<10%) in patients with both congenital and acquired TTP. Persistence of UL-VWF multimers in microcirculation results in the complete unfolding of the molecule, enabling it to bind to platelets at GPIb, producing platelet-VWF microthrombi in capillaries and arterioles causing end organ ischemic damage. Elevated lactate dehydrogenase (LDH) reflects not only MAHA but also tissue damage. Thus, the higher the LDH, the more severe the disease.

Classification

TTP can be divided into (1) a congenital form resulting from a genetic defect in the ADAMTS13 gene and (2) an acquired form secondary to the presence of an autoantibody against ADAMTS13 enzyme, reducing its activity <10% (Figure 1). Congenital TTP can present in the neonatal period; early childhood; or later in life, when it is usually associated with an inciting trigger in the form of pregnancy, severe infection, surgery, or other stress. Acquired TTP is usually idiopathic without underlying disorder, whereas it is secondary when associated with an underlying autoimmune disorder such as SLE, HIV, and use of ticlopidine, etc. Other clinical conditions that present with MAHA and thrombocytopenia with nonsevere ADAMTS13 deficiency are grouped under a broader term called TMA.

Clinical Presentation

Idiopathic TTP is a disease of young adults (20–50 years, F:M ratio 2:1) with the majority being African American. Most patients present in the emergency department with an acute onset of vague, anemia-like symptoms (malaise, fatigue, weakness) and thrombocytopenia (petechiae, gum bleed). Detailed evaluation reveals the onset of these symptoms several days before presentation. Up to 70% to 80% of patients have some neurologic features, including severe headaches, visual disturbances, focal neurologic deficits, transient ischemic attack, memory deficits, unusual behavior, confusion, seizures, paraparesis, stupor, and coma. Mild renal insufficiency is seen in <50% and fever in <15%. As a result of the generalized nature of the disease, any organ system could be affected.

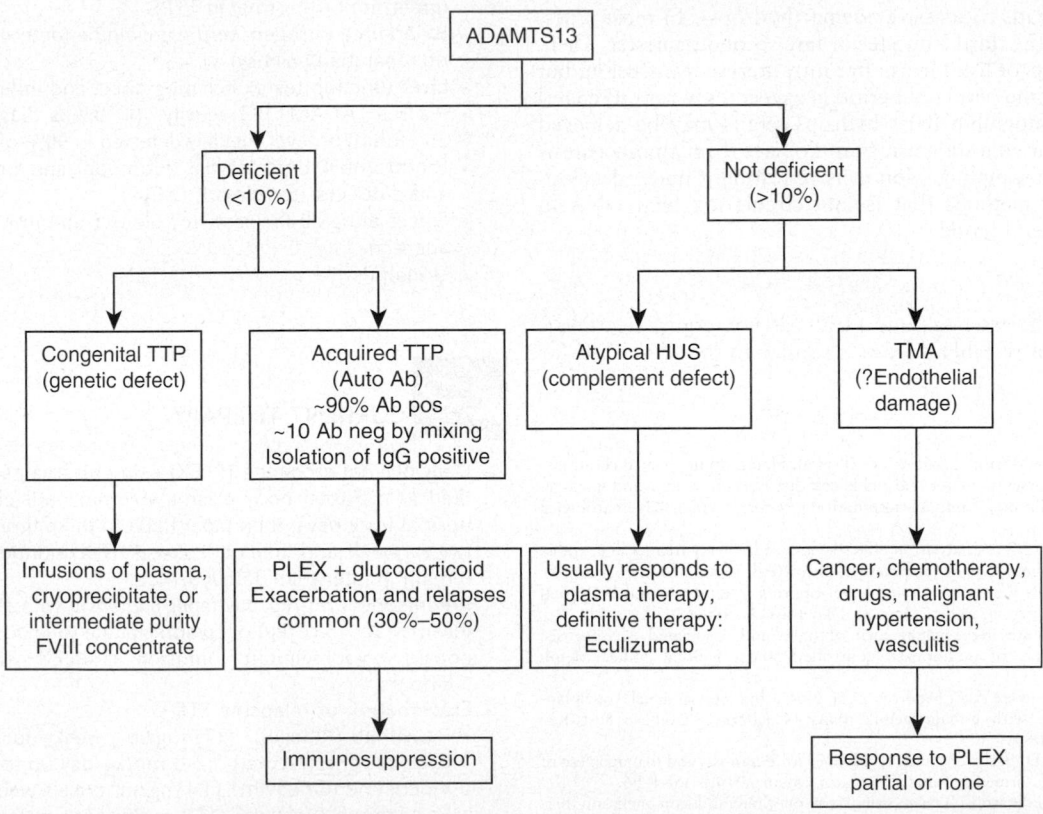

Figure 1. Classification of TTP. *Abbreviations:* MAHA, microangiopathic hemolytic anemia; TTP, thrombotic thrombocytopenic purpura; ADAMTS13, a disintegrin and metalloproteinase with thrombospondin motif 1, 13th member of the family; TMA, thrombotic microangiopathy; HUS, hemolytic uremic syndrome; PLEX, plasma exchange; Ab, antibody.

Diagnosis

Unexplained MAHA and thrombocytopenia constitute the diagnostic features and are associated with elevated LDH, reticulocytosis, undetectable haptoglobin, elevated bilirubin, and nonoliguric renal insufficiency in some patients. A severe deficiency of ADAMTS13 (<10% activity with a detectable inhibitor in up to 90% of patients) confirms the diagnosis. Because this is usually a test that is sent to a reference laboratory, this measurement is unavailable in most places at the time of clinical diagnosis. Based on the initial clinical and laboratory features, PLEX should be initiated emergently, as a delay could increase not only morbidity but also mortality. A sample for ADAMTS13 must be drawn before initiating PLEX or plasma/cryoprecipitate infusion to avoid measuring enzyme from transfused products. ADAMTS13 is a stable enzyme; if a sample for ADAMTS13 could not be drawn before plasma therapy, a routine coagulation test sample may be used. In congenital TTP, there is persistent severe deficiency of ADAMTS13 (without an inhibitor) associated with ADAMTS13 gene defect. However, this diagnosis is at times made difficult because many patients, especially children and young adults, are often misdiagnosed as immune thrombocytopenia or anemia of unknown origin or Hemolysis Elevated Liver enzymes and Low Platelets (HELLP) syndrome in pregnancy.

Differential Diagnosis

The differential diagnosis of TTP includes clinical conditions that present with MAHA and thrombocytopenia but without severe ADAMTS13 deficiency, that is, TMA. These conditions include hematopoietic stem cell transplantation, drug toxicities (mitomycin, clopidogrel [Plavix], cyclosporine A [Neoral], etc.), malignant hypertension, HELLP syndrome with severe preeclampsia, mechanical cardiac devices, for example, (left ventricular assist devices, intraaortic balloon pump and mechanical heart valves), disseminated intravascular coagulation (DIC), vasculitis, and both diarrheaassociated and atypical hemolytic uremic syndrome (HUS).

Treatment

PLEX is the standard of care therapy. Its use has reduced mortality from >90% to <20%. Ideally, it should be initiated within 4 to 6 hours of suspected diagnosis. The patient's plasma (which contains autoantibody) is selectively removed during PLEX (1.0–1.5 plasma volume processed) and replaced with donor plasma containing ADAMTS13. Neurologic symptoms usually disappear within 24 to 48 hours. The platelet count is the most useful laboratory parameter to follow because LDH and hemoglobin lag behind. Complete clinical response, defined as normalization of platelet count for at least 2 days with near normal LDH, generally is achieved with seven to nine daily PLEX in most patients. Thereafter, a gradual taper, that is, PLEX every other day in the first week, twice in the next week, and once in the third week, may be performed. Given the autoimmune nature of the disease, glucocorticoid therapy is often given from the beginning. Approximately 30% to 50% of patients will have exacerbation of the disease (worsening of clinical or laboratory features after initial response) or relapses (recurrence of the disease 30 days after discontinuation of PLEX). Such patients require additional PLEX and other immunomodulatory therapies, e.g., rituximab (Rituxan),[1] cyclosporine (Neoral),[1] vincristine (Oncovin),[1] bortezomib (Velcade),[1] or splenectomy as a last resort. A dialysis-type catheter is required for PLEX and can be placed with ultrasound guidance in patients with platelet counts as low as 10,000/mcL. With the exception of a life-threatening bleed, platelet transfusion is contraindicated in TTP because it is a thrombotic disorder of platelet consumption, and transfused platelets may worsen the condition (appearance of new neurological symptoms, myocardial infarction, etc.). If initiation of PLEX is likely to be delayed, either plasma or cryoprecipitate can be infused temporarily to supplement ADAMTS13. Congenital TPP is treated with plasma infusions (10–15 ml/kg); however, cryoprecipitate and intermediate purity factor FVIII concentrate that contain adequate ADAMTS13 have been used successfully to avoid volume overload in susceptible patients.

Monitoring

Considering the relatively high frequency of cardiac involvement, cardiac monitoring should be performed initially. While PLEX is an otherwise safe procedure, complications related to catheter infection and line thrombosis are not uncommon and should be identified as soon as possible to avoid exacerbation of the disease. If the ADAMTS13 is >10%, then TTP diagnosis is generally ruled out and PLEX may be discontinued depending upon underlying conditions.

Prognosis

Although PLEX has reduced the mortality in last two decades, most deaths occur within 24 to 48 hours of presentation and are due to delay in administration of PLEX for a variety of reasons, including a delay in diagnosis or the line placement or nonavailability of PLEX at the institution. After one PLEX, survival rates can increase to >90%. Importantly, no clinical and laboratory parameter exists to predict outcome. At this stage, ADAMTS13 has a diagnostic but not prognostic value.

---

[1]Not FDA approved for this indication.

References

Fujimura Y, Matsumoto M, Isonishi A, et al. Natural history of Upshaw-Schulman syndrome based on ADAMTS13 gene analysis in Japan. J Thromb Haemost 2011;9(Suppl 1):283–301.

Rock GA, Shumak KH, Buskard NA, et al. Comparison of plasma exchange with plasma infusion in the treatment of thrombotic thrombocytopenic purpura. Canadian Apheresis Study Group. N Engl J Med 1991;325:393–7.

Sarode R, Bandarenko N, Brecher ME, et al. Thrombotic thrombocytopenic purpura: 2012 American Society for Apheresis (ASFA) consensus conference on classification, diagnosis, management, and future research. J Clin Apher 2013; http://dx.doi.org/10.1002/jca.21302.

Shah N, Rutherford C, Matevosyan K, et al. Role of ADAMTS13 in the management of thrombotic microangiopathies including thrombotic thrombocytopenic purpura (TTP). Br J Haematol 2013;163:514–9.

Tsai HM. Thrombotic thrombocytopenic purpura and atypical hemolytic uremic syndrome—An update. Hematol Oncol Clin North Am 2013;27:565–84.

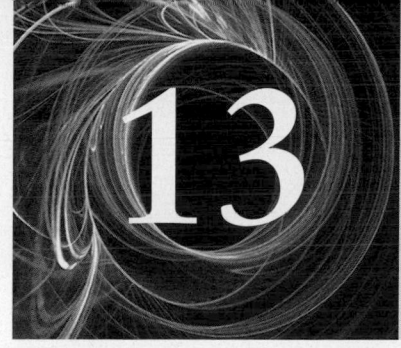

13

The Urogenital Tract

ACUTE RENAL FAILURE

Method of
Kevin Schroeder, MD

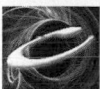

CURRENT DIAGNOSIS

- Prerenal azotemia may be associated with a BUN-to-creatinine ratio >20:1 and a FE_{Na} <1%.
- Intrarenal ARF (ATN) may be associated with a BUN-to-creatinine ratio <20:1 and a FE_{Na} >1%.
- Postrenal ARF can manifest with frank anuria.
- Follow the trends of serum chemistries, BUN, creatinine, and urine output on a daily basis.

Abbreviations: ARF = acute renal failure; ATN = acute tubular necrosis; BUN = blood urea nitrogen; FE_{Na} = fractional excretion of sodium.

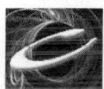

CURRENT THERAPY

- Hemodynamic support and maintenance of euvolemic state
- Correction of electrolyte and acid–base imbalances
- Removal of all offending agents and correction of underlying causes
- Adjustment of all medications for decreased glomerular filtration rate
- Renal replacement when needed on an individual basis

Epidemiology and Definitions

Acute renal failure (ARF), increasingly called acute kidney injury, is a clinical syndrome that can include decreased urine output, retention of nitrogenous metabolic waste products normally excreted by the kidney, retention of sodium and extracellular fluid resulting in peripheral and sometimes central edema, and various electrolyte and acid-base disturbances that may be associated with elevations in the blood urea nitrogen (BUN) and serum creatinine concentrations. Typically these changes occur rapidly over hours to days. Acute renal failure may further be described by the decrement in urine output: polyuric failure, indicating greater than 3 L urine output per 24 hours; nonoliguric failure, indicating 0.4 to 3L urine output per 24 hours; oliguric failure, indicating less than 400 mL urine output per 24 hours; and anuric failure, with less than 50 mL urine output per 24 hours.

Currently accepted definitions of ARF include a rise in the serum creatinine concentration by more than 0.5 mg/dL or a relative increase in the serum creatinine concentration by more than 25% for patients with preexisting chronic kidney disease (CKD) and a reduction in the glomerular filtration rate (GFR) by 50%. Note that these definitions are very operational and based on laboratory data

readily available to practicing physicians, but consensus regarding a single, more sensitive measure of ARF is lacking.

Traditionally, ARF has been subclassified mechanistically into three categories. *Prerenal azotemia* refers to conditions that cause a fall in GFR because of reduced glomerular perfusion pressure. *Intrinsic renal failure* refers to conditions that directly damage any of the four main structural components of the kidney, including the afferent and efferent arterioles, glomeruli, tubules, and interstitium. *Postrenal failure* commonly refers to any condition that causes obstruction of either the upper or lower urinary tract. From a practical standpoint, clinicians must also consider the situation in which ARF occurs (in an ambulatory patient, at hospital admission, during hospitalization, or after discharge) and the rapidity of deterioration, because some diagnoses are more likely depending on the clinical context.

The reported incidence of ARF varies by clinical situation and patient population, occurring in about 2% of all inpatient admissions. Varying definitions of disease and methodologic characteristics of epidemiologic studies also affect the reported incidence. General surgical patients undergoing nonemergent, noncardiac surgery had ARF at a reported incidence of 0.8%, and critically ill surgical patients undergoing noncardiac surgery experienced ARF at a rate nearly 80 times higher. Several scoring systems have been developed to predict the risk of ARF in patients undergoing cardiac surgery, which can vary from 5% to 25%. General medicine patients can experience ARF during a hospitalization at a rate of up to 7%, but the incidence may be in the 30% to 50% range for patients in critical care units. It may be possible that the true incidence of ARF in the United States will increase substantially as the baby boom generation enters its seventh decade.

Despite advances in medical technology, pharmacotherapeutics, and dialysis modalities in the critical care setting, mortality associated with ARF remains largely untouched at 20% to 80%. Recent studies have detected an increased mortality with even a slight rise in serum creatinine (increase <0.5 mg/dL). ARF adds to length of stay by about 4 days and can easily increase the cost of admission by more than $10,000.

Classification

Causes of ARF (Box 1) are elucidated chiefly from the history and physical examination. In particular, the history should focus first on symptoms causing volume depletion, second on symptoms relating to obstruction, and third on systemic symptoms including unexplained malaise, weight loss, fever, sinopulmonary bleeding, joint pain or swelling, rashes, myalgias, and neuropathies. All these factors must be considered in light of the patient's comorbid conditions, especially cardiovascular disease, hypertension, diabetes, liver disease, and peripheral vascular disease. Medications including antihypertensives, diuretics, analgesics, and over-the-counter supplements should be reviewed carefully. The physical examination serves to confirm the patient's volume status (e.g., frank hypotension or orthostatic change in blood pressure with tachycardia), to identify signs of cardiovascular disease and cardiopulmonary decompensation, to assess the status of the urinary bladder, and to detect signs of systemic disease. In addition to routine serum chemistries, BUN, and serum creatinine levels, all

Box 1 Causes of Acute Renal Failure

Prerenal Azotemia
Effective Arterial Blood Volume and Hypotension
Emesis or diarrhea
Hemorrhage
Nephrotic syndrome
Sepsis
Third spacing
- Acute abdomen
- Bowel infarct
- Burns
- Cirrhosis or hepatorenal syndrome
- *Clostridium difficile* colitis
- Pancreatitis
- Peritonitis
- Postoperative abdomen

Pump Failure
- Acute myocardial infarction
- Congestive heart failure
- Tamponade

Overmedication
- Anesthetics
- Diuretics
- Nonsteroidal antiinflammatory drugs (including cyclooxygenase-2 inhibitors)

Intrinsic Acute Renal Failure
Acute Tubular Necrosis
Toxins
- Aminoglycosides
- Cyclosporine (Neoral)
- Ethylene glycol
- Heavy metals
- Hemoglobinuria
- Iodinated dye
- Myoglobinuria
- Nonsteroidal antiinflammatory drugs (including cyclooxygenase-2 inhibitors)
- Pentamidine (Pentam)
- Tumor lysis syndrome
Ischemia
- Cardiovascular surgery
- Dissection
- Embolism

- Severe hypotension
- Trauma
Septic
- Gram-positive or Gram-negative sepsis

Interstitial Nephritis
Allopurinol (Zyloprim)
Antibiotics
- Cephalosporins
- Penicillins
- Rifampin (Rifadin)
- Sulfonamides
Diuretics
Nonsteroidal antiinflammatory drugs
Phenytoin (Dilantin)

Macrovascular Disease
Atheroembolic disease
Malignant hypertension

Microvascular Disease
HELLP syndrome
Hemolytic-uremic syndrome and thrombotic thrombocytopenic purpura
Hepatorenal syndrome
Rapidly progressive glomerulonephritis
Vasculitis

Postrenal Obstruction
Intratubular Obstruction
Crystals
Myeloma casts

Ureteral Obstruction
Ligation
Retroperitoneal fibrosis
Stones/papillae
Tumor compression

Bladder Outlet Obstruction
Anticholinergic medicines
Benign prostatic hyperplasia
Diabetic autonomic dysfunction
Stones and papillae
Urethral valves

Abbreviations: HELLP = hemolysis, elevated liver enzymes, low platelets.

---

patients with nonanuric ARF must have a urinalysis. The clinician must observe the urine sediment for the presence of protein, blood, dysmorphic red cells, and cellular and noncellular casts. Finally, for oliguric patients, calculation of the fractional excretion of sodium (FE_{Na}) might prove useful. Serologic testing regarding acute glomerulonephritis should be obtained when the history and physical examination suggest sufficient pretest probability.

Prerenal Azotemia

Prerenal azotemia is the most common cause of ARF among patients admitted to general medicine services. It is commonly observed in cases of volume depletion or decreased effective arterial blood volume. These include profuse emesis or diarrhea, hemorrhage, and overzealous diuresis, especially in the face of poor oral intake. In these cases, peripheral and central edema is often absent. Decompensated CHF, decompensated cirrhosis leading to the hepatorenal syndrome, and the nephrotic syndrome all lead to effective decreases in circulating arterial volume. Commonly,

patients with these conditions have peripheral edema and sometimes central edema with low albumin states. In the former case, diuretics often improve not only the heart failure but also the renal dysfunction concomitantly. Recalling the principles of vascular autoregulation (Figure 1), the clinician must realize that the kidneys of elderly patients and patients with chronic hypertension are especially susceptible to intravascular volume changes. This is particularly true when patients are medicated with angiotensin converting enzyme inhibitors and angiotensin receptor blockers, nonsteroidal antiinflammatory drugs and cyclooxygenase-2 inhibitors, and calcineurin inhibitors, all of which effectively paralyze the kidney's ability to regulate glomerular perfusion.

Typical laboratory findings in prerenal azotemia include an elevated BUN:creatinine ratio (>20:1) and a FE_{Na} of less than 1%. However, if the patient had been taking diuretics, the FE_{Na} may be falsely elevated. Metabolic alkalosis and hypokalemia might or might not be present. The urinalysis is expected to show a high specific gravity with no blood, no protein, and bland sediment; there

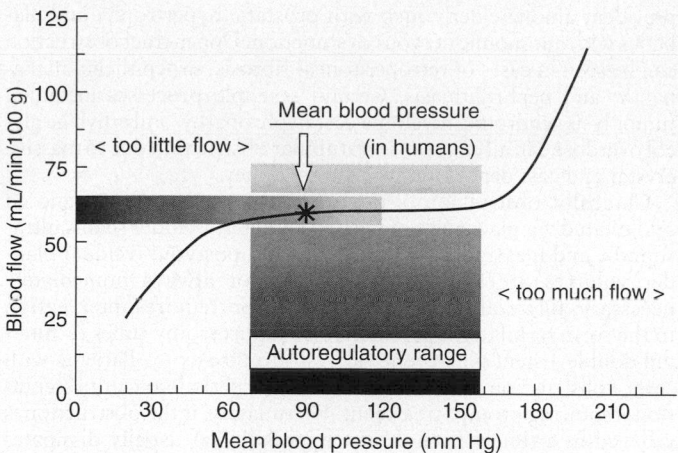

Figure 1. Principle of vascular autoregulation.

may be a few hyaline casts. Clinically, pure prerenal azotemia often responds quickly to restoration of euvolemia with increased urine output and a falling creatinine within 24 hours. Therapy for prerenal azotemia should be aimed at restoring clinical euvolemia and eliminating the cause of the azotemia. Infusion of isotonic saline is the norm, with supplemental oral rehydration where possible, and use of colloids or blood products when needed. In the case of decompensated left heart failure with pulmonary embarrassment, it is often necessary to employ an inotrope (e.g., dobutamine [Dobutrex]) in combination with a diuretic, whereas with hepatorenal syndrome, combinations of midodrine (Proamatine)[1] and octreotide (Sandostatin)[1] have been employed with some success.

Intrinsic renal failure may be subdivided into diseases that affect the renal microvasculature, glomeruli, tubules, and interstitium. Although the pharmacologic effects of certain medications (e.g., angiotensin-converting enzyme inhibitors [ACEIs] and nonsteroidal antiinflammatory drugs [NSAIDs]) directly affect the renal microvasculature, renal dysfunction associated with their use physiologically produces a prerenal picture. However, cholesterol emboli syndrome and small vessel vasculitis represent two diseases whose impact on the renal microvasculature is pathologic. In the former case, cholesterol-laden debris dislodged from the abdominal aorta or aortic arch showers distal vascular beds. The classic scenario involves a patient who, having recently undergone an endovascular procedure, presents with abdominal colic, ARF, livedo reticularis, and evidence of ischemic toes. Depending on the size of the embolus, the patient can have frank intestinal or renal infarction or an acutely ischemic lower extremity, necessitating emergent intervention. Eosinophiluria and hypocomplementemia may be noted. The elevation in creatinine can progress in a stepwise fashion for several days to weeks after the original event. Magnetic resonance imaging (MRI) can show evidence of wedge-shaped infarcts in the renal parenchyma. Optimal therapy with regard to antiplatelet agents versus anticoagulants remains uncertain.

Glomerular Disease

Glomerular disease accounts for roughly 10% of ARF among hospitalized patients. The hallmarks of rapidly progressive acute glomerulonephritis (RPGN) include an active urine sediment (dysmorphic red blood cells (RBCs) and cellular casts), hypertension, some edema, and a rapid decline in renal function over days. World Health Organization (WHO) class IV systemic lupus erythematosus (SLE) nephritis, anti-neutrophil cytoplasmic antibodies (ANCA)-mediated disease, and anti-GBM (glomerular basement membrane) disease are examples. Serologic testing is often useful, but a renal biopsy is almost always indicated for definitive diagnosis. Treatment usually involves some combination of corticosteroids and cytotoxic medications. Because of the severe increase in

morbidity and mortality when these diseases are untreated, RPGN should be considered a medical emergency, with prompt attempts to diagnose and treat. It is important to recognize that whereas diseases that primarily manifest as the nephritic syndrome commonly cause ARF, entities associated more with a nephrotic-syndrome picture—including membranous disease, minimal change disease, or focal sclerosis—can certainly produce ARF as well. This usually occurs in the setting of massive nephrotic-range proteinuria (10–20 g/24 hours) and associated marked hypoalbuminemia.

Acute Tubular Necrosis

Acute tublar necrosis (ATN) accounts for fully 50% of ARF among hospitalized patients; depending on the scenario, this figure can rise to as much as 75%. ATN has three common causes: ischemic, toxic, and septic. ATN has been described by its phases: Injury, during which time the insult causes direct damage to the tubules, is manifested as a progressive increase in the serum creatinine and possibly the development of oliguria. In the plateau phase, the creatinine, urinary output, and volume status are relatively stable. Recovery is marked by a spontaneous decline in serum creatinine and increase in urinary output, perhaps even into a polyuric range. The time course of ATN from injury to recovery is variable. Depending on the severity of the injury and the preexistence of renal disease, ATN can reverse within 1 to 3 weeks, although a small percentage of patients with ATN remain dialysis dependent after months. ATN is typically associated with a loss of urinary concentration, elevated urinary sodium excretion, and an elevated FE_{Na} of greater than 2%. The BUN and creatinine tend to rise proportionally. The urinary sediment can reveal tubular epithelial cell casts that have a coarsely granular or muddy brown appearance.

Ischemic ATN typically occurs during periods of prolonged hypotension and represents an evolution of prerenal azotemia. Ischemic ATN is commonly observed to varying degrees after cardiovascular and major orthopedic or trauma surgery. Careful attention must be paid to urine output and volume status. High-dose diuretics may be employed to avoid pulmonary edema, and if a suboptimal response is seen, the dosage should be doubled after the first dose. Patients who rapidly become oliguric have a high mortality rate, which is unaffected by diuretics and can therefore require early initiation of dialysis. Specific risk factors for developing ischemic ATN in the postoperative setting include advanced age (older than 70 years), preexisting CKD, diabetes, emergent surgery, preexisting vascular disease, and the need for valvular, particularly aortic valve, heart surgery in addition to bypass grafting. The degree and duration of intraoperative hypotension as well as time spent on cardiopulmonary bypass can also play roles.

Toxic ATN is proximal tubular cell death as a consequence of drugs or other endogenous chemicals. Drugs that classically cause toxic ATN include aminoglycosides, amphotericin B (Fungizone), radiocontrast, platinum-based chemotherapy, and NSAIDs. Endogenous chemicals known to cause toxic ATN include uric acid, myoglobin, and heme. Clinically, it is worthwhile noting that although the onset of ATN after a single dose of NSAID or iodinated radiocontrast material may be rapid (24–72 hours) especially in volume-depleted patients, in the case of aminoglycosides the onset of injury may be a bit slower, consistent with cumulative dose exposure. In general, ATN is best avoided by limiting the dose of potentially toxic medications (e.g., once-daily dosing of aminoglycosides), maintenance of adequate volume status, and close attention to the serum creatinine and urinary output.

In the case of radiocontrast agents, low osmolar and isosmolar agents are thought to be less toxic, and dose limitation (or elimination) to less than 100 mL are helpful strategies. Although prospective randomized, controlled trial data are inconclusive, and meta-analyses are equivocal, in cases of elective contrast exposure it remains common practice at many centers to administer N-acetylcysteine (Mucomyst)[1] in a dosage of 600 mg orally every

12 hours on the day before and the day of exposure. This, along with intravenous fluid administration for up to 6 hours before elective procedures (some authors use bicarbonate-containing solutions) seem to be reasonably safe, low-cost measures that can offer some protection against ATN in patients with known renal disease. After contrast-enhanced procedures, serum creatinine should be measured daily in hospitalized patients and at 48 hours after the procedure in outpatients.

Septic ATN often manifests in the critical care setting in patients with multisystem organ failure. Patients are typically hypotensive with either Gram-positive or Gram-negative bacteremia and anuria, often with severe acidemia. Unlike patients with prerenal azotemia whose urine output responds to volume resuscitation, patients with septic ATN do not produce urine in response to substantial volume resuscitation (Table 1). The clinical picture is difficult to distinguish from ischemic ATN because the two disease processes can coexist. Clinically, ischemic and toxic ATN are thought to show signs of resolution within 14 days of removal of the insult, whereas the sequelae of septic ATN can persist for one or several months after the infection requiring prolonged hospitalization and dialysis support. Mortality in this setting can be as high as 80%, and patients who survive their initial illness are particularly susceptible to nosocomial infections, catheter-related bacteremia, and malnutrition.

Interstitial Disease

Interstitial disease represents the third most common cause of ARF among hospitalized patients after prerenal azotemia and ATN. Acute interstitial nephritis is usually the effect of either drugs or pyelonephritis. In the case of medications, key diagnostic points include a delayed onset after medication exposure, as much as 7 days, and the co-incidence of fever and a central rash in about 30% of patients. The diagnosis may be suspected in the presence of sterile pyuria, eosinophiluria, and eosinophilia. Because the disease is of nonglomerular and nontubular origin, the urine sediment should be relatively bland, with minimal hematuria or proteinuria. Renal biopsy confirming the presence of increased numbers of eosinophils in the interstitium remains the gold standard. Antibiotics that are particularly notorious for causing acute interstitial nephritis include penicillins, particularly methicillin (Staphcillin); sulfa-containing drugs; rifampin (Rifadin); and quinolones. Typically, cessation of the suspected agent results in improved renal function within 5 days; however, in severe, prolonged cases, a course of corticosteroids can hasten improvement. Importantly, if the patient is re-exposed to the offending agent, acute interstitial nephritis can develop much more rapidly.

Obstructive Disease

Obstructive renal disease, although relatively uncommon, should be highly suspected in any patient with otherwise unexplained anuria, especially in those with a known pelvic malignancy or recent pelvic surgery. Obstruction of the lower tract and bladder outlet is more prevalent among elderly men with prostatic hypertrophy and diabetics with autonomic nervous dysfunction. Upper-tract obstruction can be seen in cases of retroperitoneal fibrosis, uroepithelial malignancy, and nephrolithiasis. Certain systemic processes including tumor lysis syndrome, myeloma cast nephropathy, and ethylene glycol overdose can all cause an intratubular obstruction due to massive crystal and cast deposition within the kidney.

Clinically, obstruction of the bladder outlet may be diagnosed and treated via placement of a Foley catheter. Bladder scans, ultrasounds, and measurement of the pre- and postvoid residual bladder volumes are also important but not always immediately necessary. Bilateral upper tract obstruction requires intervention in the form of bilateral percutaneous nephrostomy tubes or internal double-J stent placement via cystourethroscopy. Patients with severe obstruction may be significantly hyperkalemic at presentation, requiring prompt treatment. Fortunately, if the obstruction is relieved in a timely fashion, the hyperkalemia usually dissipates without emergent dialysis.

Treatment

Management of hospitalized patients is generally supportive. Specific measures include a thorough daily review of the medication list to ensure that all possible toxic medications have been eliminated and that all drugs excreted via the kidneys have been dose adjusted for the level of renal dysfunction. The patient's volume status should be assessed frequently, with appropriate adjustments in intravenous fluids or diuretics. Similarly, electrolytes, BUN, and creatinine should be checked daily. In general, hospitalized patients should remain hospitalized until the clinical course has at least stabilized and close outpatient follow-up is ensured. Outpatients with acute renal failure can require urgent hospitalization if the cause is not immediately apparent and reversible, or if significant hyperkalemia or volume overload exists, or if the patient has significant comorbidities.

The decision to initiate renal replacement therapy is made by the nephrologist on a patient-by-patient basis. Some absolute clinical indications for dialysis exist, such as severe hyperkalemia; peaked T waves or prolongation of the QRS complex by electrocardiogram; volume overload or acidosis refractory to medical therapy; certain intoxications or electrolyte abnormalities; and symptomatic uremia with pericarditis, neurologic changes, or bleeding diatheses. Depending on the clinical setting, the two most common are hyperkalemia and volume overload; rarely will the nephrologist let ARF with either of these conditions progress to the point of cardiac arrhythmia or intubation undialyzed.

Patients who require urgent or emergent dialysis can typically be dialyzed via standard intermittent hemodialysis. This method is more effective for acute correction of electrolyte, toxin, and acid–base aberrations as well as pulmonary edema. Controversy exists as to the proper dose of dialysis for patients with ARF, particularly those in the critical care setting. Clinical practice varies by center, but studies have shown a survival benefit favoring daily hemodialysis to keep the BUN less than 100 mg/dL.

Continuous renal replacement therapy (CRRT) or continuous veno-venous hemofiltration is usually reserved for critically ill patients, particularly those with hypotension requiring vasopressor support or those with sufficiently poor cardiac performance and volume overload who cannot tolerate acute intravascular volume shifts associated with conventional hemodialysis.

Acute peritoneal dialysis, although certainly a viable modality, is practiced much less commonly in the United States partly due to the widespread availability of hemodialysis.

Emerging Issues

In clinical practice, the diagnosis and treatment of ARF rest on the ability to recognize it in a timely fashion. The two universally available indicators—urinary output and serum creatinine measurement—are limited in their sensitivity and specificity; however, new urinary and plasma biomarkers are emerging that can allow earlier identification of ARF. Urinary neutrophil gelatinase–associated

TABLE 1 Laboratory Differentiation of Prerenal Azotemia from Acute Tubular Necrosis

| TEST | RESULT | |
	PRERENAL AZOTEMIA	ACUTE TUBULAR NECROSIS
U_{Na}	<10–20	>40
FE_{Na}	<1	>1
Urine SG	>1.020	<1.010
BUN:Cr	>20:1	≈10:1
Fe_{Ur}	>60:1	<20:1
$U_{Cr}:P_{Cr}$	>40:1	<10:1

Abbreviations: BUN = blood urea nitrogen; Cr = creatinine; FE_{Ur} = fractional excretion of urea; FE_{Na} = fractional excretion of sodium; SG = specific gravity; $U_{Cr}:P_{Cr}$ = ratio of urine creatinine to serum creatinine; U_{Na} = urine sodium.

lipocalin (NGAL), kidney injury molecule-1 (KIM-1), and interleukin-18 (IL-18), in combination with plasma NGAL and cystatin C measurements, are all currently being evaluated in ARF clinical trials. These assays hold the promise of earlier detection and perhaps more specific anatomic localization of the injury within the kidney. Whether these biomarkers are used alone, serially, or in combination as an acute kidney injury panel remains to be seen as they transition from primarily clinical trial–based application to widespread clinical use. Questions regarding their ability to help predict which patients with ARF will spontaneously recover renal function and which will require dialysis remain to be answered.

Nephrotoxicity associated with gadolinium-containing contrast media has risen to the front of discussion among radiologists and nephrologists. Originally thought to be non-nephrotoxic, gadolinium has been implicated in a number of well-documented cases. Perhaps more striking are the mounting reports of gadolinium-related nephrogenic systemic fibrosis, which is characterized by brawny epidermal fibrotic plaques developing over several weeks after exposure. It is important to recognize that other organs including the subcutaneous tissues, skeletal musculature, lungs, and heart may be involved. Although the pathogenesis of this disease has not been fully elucidated, epidemiologically, 90% of cases have been described among end-stage renal disease patients requiring dialysis, and fully 10% have occurred among patients with CKD stages 3 and 4. Because there is no cure for this disease and its clinical consequences are potentially devastating, clinicians now must consider the risk-to-benefit ratio of exposing a patient to gadolinium-enhanced MRI procedures and weigh that risk against the well-established risk of iodinated contrast used in CT scans.

References

Coca SG, Peixoto AJ, Garg AX, et al. The prognostic importance of a small acute decrement in kidney function in hospitalized patients: A systematic review and meta-analysis. Am J Kidney Dis 2007;50(5):712–20.

Dennen P, Parikh CR. Biomarkers of acute kidney injury: Can we replace serum creatinine? Clin Nephrol 2007;68(5):269–78.

Devarajan P. Proteomics for biomarker discovery in acute kidney injury. Semin Nephrol 2007;27(6):637–51.

Eachempati SR, Wang JC, Hydo LJ, et al. Acute renal failure in critically ill surgical patients: Persistent lethality despite new modes of renal replacement therapy. J Trauma 2007;63(5):987–93.

Greenberg A, Cheung A, Coffman T, et al. Primer on Kidney Diseases. 2nd ed. San Diego: Academic Press; 1998.

Johnson J, Feehally J. Comprehensive Clinical Nephrology. 1st ed. St Louis: Mosby; 2000.

Kheterpal S, Tremper KK, Englesbe MJ, et al. Predictors of postoperative acute renal failure after noncardiac surgery in patients with previously normal renal function. Anesthesiology 2007;107(6):892–902.

Nagle PC, Warner MA. Acute renal failure in a general surgical population: Risk profiles, mortality, and opportunities for improvement. Anesthesiology 2007;107(6):869–70.

Rakel R, Bope E. Conn's Current Therapy 2007. Philadelphia: Elsevier; 2007.

CHRONIC KIDNEY DISEASE

Method of
Jeffrey A. Kraut, MD

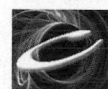

CURRENT DIAGNOSIS

The following lists the optimal care of patients with chronic kidney disease:

- Test for albuminuria and estimate glomerular filtration rate using MDRD formula yearly for early diagnosis and stratification of CKD.
- If possible, determine cause of kidney disease.
- Initiate treatment to delay or prevent progression of disease including use of converting enzyme inhibitors and/or angiotensin receptor blockers to reduce BP to less than 130/80 mm Hg and urine protein excretion to as low as possible but at least less than 1 g/24 hours.
- Control or prevent biochemical or clinical abnormalities including those of serum potassium, serum bicarbonate, serum phosphorus, parathyroid hormone, and hemoglobin.
- Evaluate patients for presence of and treat important co-morbid conditions, particularly heart disease.
- If the GFR is less than 30 mL/min, consider referral to a nephrologist.

Abbreviations: BP = blood pressure; CKD = care of patients with chronic kidney disease; GFR = glomerular filtration rate; MDRD = modification of diet in renal disease.

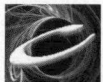

CURRENT THERAPY

The recommendations for the treatment of patients with renal failure is as follows:

RECOMMENDATION	GOAL
Control BP.	130/80 mm Hg
Reduce proteinuria by administering angiotensin converting enzyme inhibitors or angiotensin receptor blockers. In some cases both agents may have to be given concomitantly.	Decrease urine protein excretion as low as possible but at least less than 1 g per day
Control phosphate concentrations with phosphate binders with noncalcium containing binders when possible.	Serum phosphate <4.5 mg/dL
Maintain vitamin D by administration of ergocalciferol.	Maintain 25 OH vitamin D levels at 30 ng/mL by administration of ergocalciferol
Prevent hyperparathyroidism with vitamin D or calcimimetics.	Maintain PTH <150 pg/mL
Correct anemia with erythropoietin and iron replacement as needed.	Maintain Hg between 10 and 11 mg/dL
Administer diuretics to control hypertension and volume overload.	Maintain euvolemia when possible
Control serum potassium with dietary restriction, diuretics, and/or potassium exchange resin as necessary.	Maintain serum potassium <5.0 mEq/L
Keep protein intake at 0.6 to 0.8 g/kg body weight per day.	Slow progression of renal disease while preventing protein depletion
Control metabolic acidosis with administration of sodium citrate (Citra pH).	Maintain serum HCO₃ >20 mEq/L but <24 mEq/L

Abbreviations: BP = blood pressure; HCO₃ = bicarbonate; Hg = mercury; PTH = parathyroid hormone.

Chronic renal failure is defined as a reduction in glomerular filtration rate (GFR) below the normal values of approximately 120 to 130 mL/minute developing over months to years. Its incidence has increased significantly over the last several years, but this probably reflects more accurate estimations of GFR. However, there is an increased prevalence of type II diabetes mellitus, a frequent cause of renal disease, in Western societies that could contribute to a higher incidence of chronic renal failure. When renal failure is severe (GFR <10 mL/minute), renal replacement therapy, either dialysis or renal transplantation, is required to preserve life. However, even before several renal failure ensues, the presence of chronic renal failure has an important impact on organ function and can contribute to the development of significant electrolyte derangements, important hormonal abnormalities, and anemia. Also, its presence can alter the metabolism and therefore the blood concentrations and tissue concentrations of drugs administered for the treatment of various diseases. Moreover, a reduced GFR is associated with an increased risk of death, increased incidence of cardiovascular events, and hospitalizations independent of known risk factors or a history of cardiovascular diseases. Finally, the mortality of several surgical procedures is substantially increased by the presence of chronic renal failure. Therefore, detecting and treating patients with chronic renal failure is extremely important.

Causes of Chronic Renal Failure

Many disorders can cause chronic renal failure. However, epidemiologic studies indicate that diabetes mellitus and hypertension account for the majority of cases (>60%). Chronic glomerulonephritis, polycystic kidney disease, obstructive uropathy, and ischemic nephropathy caused by atherosclerotic renal artery stenosis are less common, but important causes of renal impairment. The latter disorder is postulated to be more frequent than previously believed and is an important undiagnosed cause of chronic renal impairment.

Recent studies have indicated that a reduction in GFR occurs with aging in the absence of factors known to produce renal injury such as hypertension or diabetes. Indeed, the average GFR of subjects in the 8th decade of life in one large study was 40 to 50 mL/minute. Pathologic examination of these individuals, when available, may reveal only benign nephrosclerosis.

Importantly, because a majority of individuals older than 60 years of age have lower muscle mass, the reduced GFR is not accompanied by a rise in serum creatinine concentration. Therefore, renal failure is not detected unless the physician considers other variables such as the patient's age and muscle mass in assessing GFR (see the following section).

Approach to the Diagnosis of Chronic Renal Failure

The first step in the diagnosis of chronic renal failure is, of course, to detect a reduction in GFR. In the past, estimations of GFR were based on the measurement of serum creatinine concentration alone. In adults, the normal serum creatinine ranges between 0.6 and 1.3 mg/dL. Individuals with values greater than this are said to have renal failure. However, there is a wide range of normal values. Also, creatinine production, which is dependent on muscle mass, is a critical variable affecting serum creatinine concentration. Thus, a large group of individuals with reduced muscle mass can have serum creatinine values within the normal range, but a decreased GFR. The most common situation in which this paradox is encountered is in the elderly and in individuals with malignancy or chronic liver disease.

Precise measurement of GFR is accomplished by calculating the clearance of creatinine in a timed urine collection, generally 24 hours in duration:

$$\text{Creatinine clearance (mL/minute)}$$
$$= \text{Ucr (mg/dL)} \times \text{volume (mL)/Scr (mg/dL)}/1440$$

where Ucr = urine creatinine concentration,
Scr = plasma creatinine concentration

However, timed urine collections are often inaccurate because of errors in collection. Moreover, as renal function progresses and serum creatinine rises, or in the presence of nephrotic range proteinuria, GFR tends to be overestimated by creatinine clearance. Most recently, formulas derived from studies of large groups of patients—such as those by Cockroft and Gault and the Modification of Diet in Renal Disease (MDRD) in which GFR was correlated with other factors (e.g., body weight, age, and serum albumin)—are sufficiently accurate to use for clinical purposes:

$$\text{Cockroft} - \text{Gault}: \text{CrCl (mL/minute)}$$
$$= \{(140 - \text{age}) \times \text{wt} \times [1 - (0.15 \times \text{gender})]\}/(0.814 \times \text{Scr})$$

$$\text{MDRD}: \text{GFR} = 170 \times [\text{PCr}]^{-0.999} \times [\text{Age}]^{-0.176}$$
$$\times [0.762 \text{ female}] \times [1.180 \text{ if patient is black}]$$
$$\times [\text{SUN}]^{-0.170} \times [\text{Alb}]^{+0.318}$$

Newer biomarkers such as cystatin C whose blood concentration might not be as affected by body composition as creatinine have been introduced and might better reflect true GFR. The value of these biomarkers in detecting early CKD and following its progress are being investigated, and it is possible that it or other biomarkers might supplant serum creatinine as the means of monitoring renal function in the future.

Once renal function is depressed, the physician determines whether this represents acute or chronic renal failure. When previous measurements of GFR are available, it is relatively easy to determine if the renal failure is chronic in nature. However, if these studies are not available, demonstration that the kidneys are small in size (less than 8 to 9 cm when they are normally approximately 10 to 12 cm) by renal ultrasound will confirm the chronicity of the disease. Evidence of increased echogenicity reflecting augmented fibrous deposits is also suggestive of chronic disease. However, several disorders associated with chronic renal failure have normal kidney size such as diabetes mellitus, polycystic kidney disease, and amyloidosis. Therefore, normal kidney size does not exclude chronic renal failure. If individuals have normal kidney size, the presence of anemia and/or certain abnormalities of divalent ion metabolism can also suggest the disease is chronic in nature.

Once impaired renal function is recognized, measurements of blood urea nitrogen (BUN), sodium, potassium, chloride, bicarbonate, hemoglobin and hematocrit, and calcium and phosphorus are obtained. A urinalysis is obtained looking for increased excretion of protein, presence of blood in the urine, and abnormal cellular elements. In patients with diabetes, studies to find microalbuminuria (albumin urine concentrations less than 300 mg per day) are important to detect the early stages of renal disease. A 24-hour or spot urine protein and creatinine determination to assess the urine's protein-to-creatinine ratio is obtained to quantitate the amount of protein being excreted. Urine protein excretion in excess of 3.5 g daily indicates the presence of glomerular pathology, whereas interstitial disease is characterized by values below 2 g. However, urine protein excretion can vary with glomerular disease so values below 3.5 g are still consistent with this diagnosis. Assessment of urine protein excretion is important for diagnostic purposes, but also because urine protein excretion is often followed to assess effectiveness of therapy.

Obstruction uropathy, an important cause of chronic renal failure and exacerbation of renal failure, can be excluded in the majority of cases by ultrasound of the kidneys. Doppler ultrasound of the renal arteries performed at the same time is helpful in excluding obstruction of the renal arteries. The necessity of obtaining other diagnostic studies such as measurement of serum complement, blood and urine eosinophils, serum and urine and protein electrophoresis, antiglomerular basement membrane antibodies, anti–double-stranded DNA (dsDNA) antibodies, hepatitis B and C antibodies, sedimentation rate, and HIV studies depends on the context of the renal failure.

Finally, a renal biopsy may be required in certain situations to make a definitive diagnosis. Because treatment of specific diseases can vary, making a precise pathologic diagnosis can be extremely important for proper management. Unfortunately, once the renal failure is moderate to severe in nature, renal pathologic examination may not always be helpful in determining the cause.

Clinical and Laboratory Abnormalities in Chronic Renal Failure

Because the kidney plays a critical role in the regulation of the serum concentrations of sodium, potassium, bicarbonate, chloride, calcium, and phosphorus as well as the levels of hemoglobin

TABLE 1 Clinical and Electrolyte Abnormalities Noted with Chronic Renal Failure

CLINICAL OR LABORATORY DISORDER	GFR OR STAGE OF RENAL FAILURE*
Hypertension	GFR <60 mL/min (stage 3)
Hyponatremia or hypernatremia	GFR <30 mL/min (stage 4)
Hyperkalemia*	GFR <30 mL/min (stage 4)
Hyperphosphatemia*	GFR <30 mL/min (stage 4)
Metabolic acidosis	GFR <30 mL/min (stage 4)
Anemia	GFR <60 mL/min (stage 3)
Uremic symptoms	GFR <15 mL/min (stage 5)
Nausea, vomiting, disturbances in sleep	

*Descriptions of the various stages are presented in the text. These electrolyte abnormalities can be seen at higher levels of GFR.
Abbreviation: GFR = glomerular filtration rate.

and hematocrit, blood pressure and extracellular volume, chronic renal injury can lead to derangements in these parameters as summarized in Table 1.

Hyponatremia and Hypernatremia

The kidney plays an essential role in excreting water by producing a dilute urine (less than 1/6 plasma osmolality) or retaining water by producing a concentrated urine (three to four times plasma osmolality). The ability to concentrate or dilute the urine in the majority of cases is usually retained until GFR falls to less than 30% of normal, and therefore hyponatremia or hypernatremia are uncommon until that time. If the disease is primarily interstitial in nature, alterations in urine concentrating ability can appear prior to significant reductions in GFR. However, even with higher levels of GFR the patient can be at risk for either of these electrolyte abnormalities should they ingest large quantities of fluid or be deprived of appropriate fluid intake.

Hyperkalemia

The kidney plays the most critical role in the regulation of potassium balance. Adaptive changes in renal tubular function and possible colonic function enable the kidney to maintain serum potassium within the normal range until GFR falls below 20% to 25% of normal (serum creatinine of 4 mg/dL or greater). Recent studies indicate a tendency for elevations in serum potassium to appear at even modest reductions in GFR (<60 mL/min). When disease of the kidney involves the medullary portion or hormonal derangements such as hyporeninemic hypoaldosterinism are present, hyperkalemia can be observed prior to significant declines in GFR. In addition, patients with even moderate renal failure have a reduced reserve to eliminated potassium and therefore can develop hyperkalemia if potassium load is increased dramatically.

Metabolic Acidosis

A fall in plasma bicarbonate concentration in association with a reduced blood pH (metabolic acidosis) is frequently observed when GFR falls below 20% to 25% of normal. The acidosis results from acid excretion falling below acid production leading to positive proton balance. Recent studies have documented that a tendency to the development of metabolic acidosis can be seen with mild reductions in GFR (<60 mL/min).

The electrolyte pattern seen with the metabolic acidosis of renal failure is often of the high anion gap variety, but frequently a hyperchloremic (normal anion gap) or combined anion gap and hyperchloremic pattern can be observed. The degree of acidosis is usually mild to moderate with plasma bicarbonate concentration ranging from 12 to 22 mEq/L. Of interest, at any given level of GFR, the acidosis is often not progressive, but plasma bicarbonate concentration remains stable unless renal function declines further or there is an increment in acid production.

Abnormal Divalent in Metabolism

Serum phosphorus is regulated by the kidney but in most cases remains within the normal range until GFR falls below 20% to 25% of normal. This stabilization of serum phosphorus is attributed to increased tubular excretion of phosphorus as a result of increased parathyroid hormone secretion. As with potassium and bicarbonate, recent studies demonstrate a tendency for elevation in serum phosphorus can be observed with mild renal failure (<50 to 60 mL/min). Serum calcium is usually in the normal range, but varies reciprocally with serum phosphorus. Because of derangements in divalent ion metabolism bone disease with increased tendency to fractures and disordered soft tissue structures can be observed.

Hyperparathyroidism is a common occurrence in patients with renal failure, the values usually being higher with a greater degree of renal impairment. The elevated PTH values are usually induced by hypocalcemia, although increased serum phosphorus concentrations independent of serum calcium values can also play a role. The increased parathyroid hormone levels can induce damage to bone and soft tissue structures, but also may affect other functions such as cardiac function and the production of red blood cells.

Anemia

The kidney is the source of erythropoietin, the hormone that regulates bone marrow production of red blood cells. Thus, with the development of renal impairment, there is a fall in red blood cell production. A fall in red cell survival also contributes to development of anemia. Anemia generally appears when GFR falls below 60 mL/minute. There is a rough correlation between the severity of renal failure and the degree of anemia: the more severe the renal failure the greater the degree of anemia. However, this relationship is not invariable, and many patients have only mild reductions in hemoglobin and hematocrit.

Anemia initially was believed to contribute only to changes in oxygen delivery. However, recent studies show that anemia can contribute to the genesis of left ventricular hypertrophy and other cardiomyopathies noted with chronic renal failure and can raise mortality in patients with chronic renal failure.

Hypertension

Recent studies emphasize the importance of the kidneys in the regulation of blood pressure, and the bulk of patients with diabetes or other glomerular disease will develop hypertension in the course of their renal failure. In many instances, hypertension does not develop until GFR is below 40% to 50% of normal. The type of renal disease underlying chronic renal failure appears to be important, as hypertension is less common with pyelonephritis. Hypertension might be observed earlier in the course of renal failure, however, in patients with polycystic kidney disease or ischemic nephropathy. Because hypertension is one of the most critical factors in the genesis of cardiovascular disease and can accelerate the progression of renal failure, careful attention of control of hypertension is important.

Volume Overload

Salt retention often accompanies chronic renal failure even when GFR is not severely compromised. The degree of salt retention can be profound if significant albuminuria with resultant hypoalbuminemia is seen and is more severe as GFR falls below 20% to 25% of normal. Salt retention is a critical factor in the development of hypertension and can promote congestive heart failure.

Symptoms and Signs of Renal Failure

Patients with chronic renal failure are often asymptomatic with little evidence of disease other than laboratory abnormalities until late in the course of renal failure. If anemia is present, patients may complain of fatigue; and if significant elevations in parathyroid hormone levels are noted, bone pain, ruptured tendons or other disorders of soft tissue structures can be noted. Once moderate to severe renal failure appears, symptoms of the electrolyte abnormalities can be observed. Hyperkalemia, if severe, can lead to arrhythmias or heart block and muscle weakness. Metabolic acidosis can contribute to fatigue. Anemia can contribute to fatigue and changes in mentation and physical stamina. Weight loss related to metabolic acidosis and or retention of various uremic toxins may occur. Sexual dysfunction characterized by reduced libido and reduced fertility are common with moderate to severe renal failure.

Once severe renal failure develops (stage 4 or 5), the uremic syndrome can be observed characterized by a decreased appetite, nausea, vomiting, and subtle changes in mental status including changes in sleep patterns. However, even with severe renal failure many patients feel surprisingly well.

Management of Chronic Renal Failure

Staging of Chronic Renal Failure

As noted earlier, within the last several years, a great deal of effort has been expended into developing guidelines for the evaluation, monitoring, and treatment of patients with chronic renal failure. To this end, experts working with the National Kidney Foundation have divided chronic renal failure into different states based on measurements or estimations of GFR. The value of staging to the physician is that the studies necessary to monitor patients and the complications of chronic renal failure are often different depending on the stage of renal failure.

Stage 0 (GFR Greater Than 90 mL/Minute with Risk Factors for Renal Disease)

Patients at stage 0 have increased risk for development of chronic renal failure, such as those with diabetes or hypertension but who have GFR greater than 90 mL/minute in the absence of proteinuria or urinary sedimentary abnormalities. These patients should have their blood pressure and diabetes controlled. Estimates of GFR should be obtained approximately every 6 months from measurement of serum creatinine, and qualitative tests for urine protein excretion should be obtained. In diabetics measurement of microalbumin should also be obtained. Because control of disease may forestall progression glycosylated hemoglobin (HbA1C) values should also be obtained.

Stage 1 (GFR Greater Than 90 mL/Minute with Albuminuria)

Once evidence of renal damage is obtained, as reflected by microalbuminuria or proteinuria, but GFR is either normal or increased, patients are said to be in stage 1. These individuals should be monitored more closely and strict attention must be given to maintain blood pressure below 130/80. Furthermore, angiotensin converting enzyme inhibitor (ACEI) or angiotensin receptor blocker (ARB) should be given to prevent evolution of microalbuminuria to full-blown proteinuria (see the following). No clinical or laboratory abnormalities are observed at this stage.

Stage 2: Mild Renal Failure (GFR 60 to 90 mL/Minute)

When GFR is mildly reduced to values from 60 to 90 mL/minute, patients are in stage 2. These patients should also be carefully monitored and blood pressure tightly controlled. If diabetes is present, strict attention to maintaining HbA1C within recommended guidelines should be given. Again, it is rare at this stage for any significant clinical abnormalities other than hypertension to be present.

Stage 3: Moderate Renal Failure (GFR 30 to 59 mL/Minute)

When GFR ranges between 30 to 59 mL/minute, patients are in stage 3. As indicated, this is often broken up into stages 3A (45–59 mL/min) and 3B (30–44 mL/min). At this point hypertension may appear, mild abnormalities in serum phosphorus might be observed, and anemia can be seen. Also in some patients an elevation in serum potassium can be noted, particularly if they are ingesting a relatively high potassium diet. These patients need to be followed more closely, and it is recommended that patients at the lower end of this stage (i.e., close to 30 mL/min) be monitored by a nephrologist.

Stage 4: Moderate to Severe (GFR 15 to 29 mL/Minute)

Once GFR falls to values from 15 to 29 mL/minute, patients have severe renal failure, or stage 4 disease. At this level of GFR, significant electrolyte abnormalities such as metabolic acidosis, hyperkalemia, and hyperphosphatemia are frequent. Anemia is common and the patient may begin to note reductions in appetite and have a fall in muscle mass. However, there is great variability in the appearance of symptoms or laboratory derangements.

Stage 5: Severe (GFR Less Than 15 to 29 mL/Minute)

When GFR falls below 15 mL/minute, severe electrolyte abnormalities are often present and anemia is common. Clinical symptoms can develop. Renal replacement therapy, either dislysis or transplantation, is usually required at this stage.

Recommendations for treatment of patients are summarized below. The frequency of patient visits, of course, largely depends on the complications of renal disease present and co-morbid conditions. Therefore, these are only general recommendations for frequency of examination.

When patients are in stage 0, they should be seen once per year for renal evaluation. When GFR remains normal or elevated, but proteinuria is present, renal evaluation should be performed every 6 months. When stage 3 develops, we usually repeat renal evaluation every 3 months. Patients in stage 4 are seen more frequently, usually at the minimum of once per month. Patients with end-stage disease require renal replacement therapy.

General Approach to Treatment of Chronic Renal Failure

Treatment of chronic renal failure can be divided into the modalities that are specific to the underlying disorder and those that are used to treat all patients with chronic renal failure. Thus, patients with systemic lupus erythematosus or other immune-mediated or inflammatory disease may benefit from treatment with steroids and immunosuppressive agents. Treatments specific for individual disorders are beyond the scope of this article.

The physician treating the patient with renal failure has two goals: preventing or delaying progression of renal failure, and alleviating the electrolyte and hormonal abnormalities that can lead to symptoms or complications of the disease. Understanding the methods to accomplish the former requires knowledge of those factors that are integral to progression of the disease.

Factors Causing Progression of Chronic Renal Failure

It has been recognized for several years that once renal failure has developed, renal function can decline at a predictable rate in the absence of further insults to the kidney. Essential to the optimal approach used to treat chronic renal failure, therefore, is an understanding of those factors that can cause progression of renal failure, including:

- Systemic and intraglomerular hypertension
- Glomerular hypertrophy
- Intrarenal precipitation of calcium and phosphorus
- Hyperlipidemia
- Altered metabolism of prostanoids
- Metabolic acidosis
- Anemia
- Tubulointerstitial disease
- Proteinuria

Intraglomerular Hypertension and Glomerular Hypertrophy

As nephrons are lost, changes are induced in the kidney to preserve GFR such as renal vasodilatation, an increase in glomerular capillary pressure, and an increment in size of individual glomeruli raising wall stress. These adaptive mechanisms probably induce damage by causing endothelial cell damage with detachment of epithelial cells allowing enhanced flux of water and solutes that might cause narrowing of capillary lumens. Also, strain on mesangial cells causes them to produce cytokines and extracellular matrix with resultant expansion of the mesangium and glomerular sclerosis.

Proteinuria

Although proteinuria has traditionally been a marker of glomerular injury, with greater amounts of urinary protein excretion being associated with more severe injury, recent studies indicate that proteinuria can induce mesangial and tubular damage. Therefore, treatments to reduce proteinuria may be beneficial in limiting further renal damage.

Tubulointerstitial Disease

Some component of tubulointerstitial disease is generally found in individuals with chronic renal failure even when the primary process affects the glomerulus. It has been postulated that the tubulointerstitial disease can produce atrophy of tubules or obstruction destroying individual nephrons. Even when tubular inflammation is treated, progressive scarring can continue unabated. Thus, treatments designed to reduce interstitial fibrosis may be important for preventing progression of disease. At present, only experimental drugs not available for human use have been examined for this purpose.

Hyperlipidemia

Hyperlipidemia is frequently observed in disorders associated with nephrotic range proteinuria, but is also noted in a large percentage of the general population without renal disease. Experimental evidence obtained from animal studies shows hyperlipidemia can promote progression of renal failure. Thus, loading with cholesterol augments renal injury and treatment with cholesterol-lowering drugs slows the rate of progression. This effect is synergistic to that achieved by lowering blood pressure.

The mechanisms underlying the effects of lipids are not well understood, but possible explanations include mesangial lipid deposition leading to glomerular injury or tubular injury. A few studies performed in human subjects have demonstrated benefit from lipid lowering on the progression of renal injury, although they are not conclusive. Because patients with chronic renal failure have a high prevalence of cardiovascular disease, it is reasonable to inititate therapy with statin drugs to lower serum cholesterol and lipid levels.

Calcium-Phosphate Deposition

A rise in serum phosphorus, usually seen at the later stages of renal failure, can lead to precipitation of calcium phosphate in the renal interstitium. The deposits can then induce an inflammatory response producing interstitial fibrosis and tubular atrophy. Some have indicated that the deposits may form prior to detectable elevations in serum phosphorus concentrations.

Increased Glomerular Prostaglandin Production

An increment in glomerular prostaglandin production has been found in several studies of chronic renal failure. The increased prostanoids produce renal vasodilatation and a rise in intraglomerular pressure, factors that augment progression of disease.

Metabolic Acidosis

Metabolic acidosis commonly develops in the course of chronic renal failure. Recent studies in humans have demonstrated that correction of the acidosis by administration of base slows the progression of renal failure and delays the development of end-stage renal failure. Recent studies also indicate that a reduction in the interstitial pH of the kidney can be observed even in the absence of a depressed bicarbonate concentration and that administration of base might be indicated with CKD at all stages of renal impairment.

Specific Treatment Measures

Treatment of patients with chronic renal failure should be designed to ameliorate those factors that can cause progression of renal injury, treat or prevent important complications, and normalize important laboratory abnormalities that contribute to symptoms of the disease.

Measures Designed to Reduce the Rate of Progression of Renal Failure

Control of Systemic and Intraglomerular Hypertension

Experimental and human studies demonstrate that control of systemic hypertension can slow the rate of progression of renal disease substantially. Recent evidence indicates that target blood pressure levels should be lower than recommended for the general population (<130/80 mmHg). Control of hypertension with the use of myriad agents can benefit the patient with renal failure. However, as indicated previously, reduction in intraglomerular hypertension may be the most important factor underlying the benefits from blood pressure control. Therefore, when possible, treatment with ACEIs, ARBs, or the combination of these agents should be first-line antihypertensive therapy in these patients. Patients who do not tolerate these drugs might benefit from administration of non-dihydropyridine calcium channel blockers. In patients with proteinuria, even if blood pressure is controlled or they are normotensive, the doses of ACEIs or ARBs should be raised to levels even greater than recommended to reduce urine protein excretion to levels less than 500 mg. This reduction in proteinuria is the most optimal in protecting the kidney.

Potentially serious complications with ACEIs or ARBs include acute reduction in GFR and hyperkalemia. If these complications occur, a reduction in dose or even discontinuation of these agents might be required. It is recommended that these agents be continued even when GFR is less than 20 mL/min. Given the potential severity of these complications, patients should be monitored closely.

Protein Restriction

The benefits of protein restriction in preventing progression are unclear, but it has suggested that reducing protein intake to 0.8 to 1.0 g/kg body weight of high biologic value is beneficial. Others have indicated that 0.6 g/kg body weight should be used. In patients with substantial proteinuria, the quantity of protein recommended will have to be adjusted to prevent hypoalbuminemia. Once patients reached later stage 4, protein restriction may be useful to prevent expression of uremic symptoms. Reducing protein intake will have the added benefit of decreasing acid, potassium, and phosphate production.

Control of Lipids

Control of cholesterol with statins may help prevent progression and should reduce the burden of cardiovascular disease, which remains the most lethal disorder for patients with chronic renal failure. Adherence to the newly proposed aggressive recommendation appears reasonable.

Measures Designed to Treat Significant Laboratory Abnormalities

Anemia

Patients with renal anemia should be treated with erythropoietin (Procrit). Although this requires subcutaneous injection once per week, newer, long-lasting forms (darbepoetin [Aranesp]) enable patients to be treated every 3 weeks. Because iron stores need to be repleted for anemia to be successfully treated, these should be monitored and iron given. Because of the vagaries of ferritin measurements, we use serum iron and iron binding capacity with the goal of maintaining saturation above 20% and near 30%. At present, the target hemoglobin and hematocrit vary between 10 mg/dL and 11 mg/dL and between 30 and 33, respectively. Given the recent concern about vascular complications with

EPO therapy, the clinican must be vigilant in preventing Hg values from exceeding 12 mg/dL.

Metabolic Acidosis

Controversy exists as to the target value of bicarbonate for patients with chronic renal failure. Some experts recommend raising plasma bicarbonate to levels above 20 mEq/L, whereas others recommend complete normalization of plasma bicarbonate. To properly raise plasma bicarbonate concentration, the deficit should be calculated from the formula:

$$\text{Desired} - \text{prevailing level of plasma bicarbonate}$$
$$\times 50\% \text{ body weight} = \text{Total bicarbonate deficit}$$

The deficit should be corrected slowly over several days.

Because patients experience gas when the base is given as bicarbonate, the base is usually administered as Shohl's solution sodium citrate,* the citrate being metabolized to bicarbonate in the liver. Each milliliter of Shohl's solution represents 1 mEq of the base. As noted previously, recent studies suggest that at all stages of CKD, base supplementation could be beneficial in slowing progression of CKD. Therefore, consideration of administration of base in patients with CKD 2 should be given even in the absence of hypobicarbonatemia.

Divalent Ion Metabolism

Serum phosphorus is controlled by administration of phosphate binders usually starting with calcium citrate (Citracal) or acetate (PhosLo). If these are not successful or if patients have elevated serum calcium levels, then sevelamar (Renagel) or lanthanum (Fosrenol) can be used alone or in combination with calcium binders. Physicians should aim to maintain serum phosphorus levels below 5 mg/dL and keep serum calcium phosphorus product below 60.

Parathyroid hormone (PTH) levels should be maintained below 150 pg/mL, or less depending on stage; levels associated with proper bone remodeling but not to values observed in patients without kidney disease. Suppression of parathyroid hormone secretion can be achieved by administration of various vitamin D analogues. The recent recognition of the calcium-sensing receptor and development of calcimimetic drugs that are extremely effective in lowering PTH secretion may make using vitamin D compounds obsolete in the future.

Low 25 OH D levels have been documented in a large number of individuals both with and without renal failure. In patients with renal impairment this can contribute to the abnormal 1,25 OH vitamin D levels. Measurement of 25-hydroxy vitamin D levels should be obtained in all patients with CKD and EGFR <60 mL/min. If levels are below 30 ng/mL, they should be supplemented with ergocalciferol sufficient to maintain levels above this level.

Hyperkalemia

As this is the most serious electrolyte disorder encountered, patients should be monitored closely. Serum potassium concentrations should be maintained below 5 mEq/L. If hyperkalemia develops during treatment with ACEIs or ARBs, the doses of these agents should be reduced or discontinued. Diuretic administration, often given for control of hypertension, can help control hyperkalemia, but if it should develop, particularly when GFR falls below 20% of normal, it can be treated with the potassium exchange resin, sodium polystyrene sulfonate (Kayexalate). Recent studies have shown new exchange resins are effective without adverse effects and these might supplant Kayexalate in the future.

Elevated Blood Urea Nitrogen Concentration

The precise solutes that are retained, which are important for the pathogenesis of the uremic syndrome, are not clear. However, BUN is a marker for other retained solutes and is roughly correlated with development of uremic symptoms. When the BUN is greater than 100 mg/dL and serum creatinine concentration is greater than 8 mg/dL uremic symptoms may develop. These symptoms will often abate merely with protein restriction and reduced production of these compounds. Protein restriction is usually not instituted until GFR is less than 15% to 20% of normal. Prior to that time, it is important to maintain protein intake to keep serum albumin within the normal range.

Volume Overload

Because salt retention is an essential component of the development of hypertension and underlies volume overload, diuretic administration is usually necessary in the treatment of chronic renal failure. Thiazides frequently used in the treatment of hypertension or volume overload in subjects with normal renal function may not be efficacious once GFR is less than or equal to 33% of normal. Therefore, loop diuretics, such as furosemide (Lasix) or a combined loop and proximal tubule diuretic such as metolozone (Zaroxolyn), are generally indicated. Because the effectiveness of both agents requires access to the tubule lumen, the effective dose is often higher than in those with normal renal function. Once patients are in stage 4 renal failure, use of diuretics is hampered by worsening of renal failure and often must be used cautiously.

References

Beco JA, Bansal VK. Medical nutrition therapy in chronic kidney failure: integrating clinical practice guidelines. J Am Diet Assoc 2004;104:404–9.

Clase CM, Garg AX, Kiberd BA. Prevalence of low glomerular filtration rate in non-diabetic Americans: Third National Health and Nutrition Examination Survey (NHANES III). J Am Soc Nephrol 2002;13.

Cleveland DR, Jindal KK, Hirsch DJ, et al. Quality of pre-referral care in patients with chronic renal insufficiency. Am J Kidney Dis 2002;40:30–6.

Curtin RB, Becker B, Kimmel PL, Schatell D. An integrated approach to care for patients with chronic kidney disease. Semin Dial 2003;16:399–402.

Djamali A, Kendziorski C, Brazy PC, Becker BN. Disease progression and outcomes in chronic kidney disease and renal transplantation. Kidney Int 2003;64:1800–7.

Fox CH, Voleti V, Khan LS, et al. A quick guide to evidence-based chronic kidney disease care for the primary care physician. Postgrad Med 2008;120:E01–6.

James MT, Hemmelgarn BR, Tonelli M. Early recognition and prevention of chronic kidney disease. Lancet 2010;10(375):1296–309.

KDOQI. Clinical practice guidelines and clinical practice recommendations for diabetes and chronic kidney disease. Am J Kidney Dis 2007;49:S1–54.

Kopple JD. National Kidney Foundation K/DOQI clinical practice guidelines for nutrition in chronic renal failure. Am J Kidney Dis 2001;37:S66–70.

Kraut JA. Effect of metabolic acidosis on the progression of chronic kidney disease. Am J Physiol 2011;300:F828–29.

Maschio G, Alberti D, Janin G, et al. Effect of the angiotensin-convering-enzyme inhibitor benazepril on the progression of chronic renal insufficiency. N Engl J Med 1996;334:939–45.

Quaseem A, et al. Screening, monitoring, and treatment of stage 1 to 3 chronic kidney disease: A clinical practice guideline from the American College of Physicians. Ann Int Med 2013;159:835–47.

Tonelli M, Gill J, Pandeya S, et al. Slowing the progression of chronic renal insufficiency. Can Med Assoc J 2002;166:906–7.

MALIGNANT TUMORS OF THE UROGENITAL TRACT

Method of
Peter E. Clark, MD

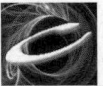

CURRENT DIAGNOSIS

Carcinoma of the Prostate
- Average-risk patients can be offered screening with prostate-specific antigen (PSA) testing and digital rectal examination (DRE) at 55 years of age, high-risk patients with a strong family history, and African American patients at age 40 years.
- Patients with an elevated PSA or abnormal DRE are referred for discussion regarding risks, benefits, and alternatives to biopsy of the prostate.
- Diagnosis is made with transrectal ultrasound-guided biopsy of the prostate.

---

*Investigational drug in the United States.

- Staging with bone scan is done for patients with high-grade tumors (Gleason grade 4 or 5), PSA levels greater than 20 µg/mL, elevated alkaline phosphatase levels, or bone pain.

Renal Cell Carcinoma
- Hematuria is the single most common sign, occurring in up to 60% of cases. Flank pain and a palpable mass can also occur, but the classic triad of hematuria, flank pain, and a palpable abdominal mass is present in only 10% of cases. Other common signs and symptoms are fever, anemia, thrombocytosis, hypercalcemia, and an elevated sedimentation rate.
- Most tumors are asymptomatic and are detected incidentally on radiographic imaging (renal ultrasonography, computed tomography [CT] scanning, or magnetic resonance imaging).

Benign Renal Tumors
- Angiomyolipomas have a characteristic appearance of fat within the lesion on CT scans.
- Angiomyolipomas may occur sporadically or as part of the tuberous sclerosis complex.
- Tuberous sclerosis is characterized by benign tumors within the cerebellum, mental retardation, epilepsy, and adenoma sebaceum. Angiomyolipomas occur in half of these patients and are typically bilateral and multifocal, making management more challenging.
- Oncocytomas are benign renal tumors that account for 5% to 10% of solid renal lesions.
- Oncocytomas can be more round and of uniform density, or they may have a central scar or spoke-wheel appearance on CT scan. However, no feature can reliably distinguish these tumors from a malignant renal tumor.
- Oncocytomas should be diagnosed only histologically; they are characterized by eosinophilic granular, mitochondria-laden cells.
- In general, a non–fat-containing, solid renal mass should be considered malignant until proven otherwise.

Tumors of the Renal Pelvis and Ureter
- Tumors arising in the renal pelvis account for 10% of all renal tumors and approximately 5% of all urothelial carcinomas.
- Ureteral tumors account for 25% of upper tract urothelial carcinomas.
- These tumors are more common in men than in women.
- Cigarette smoking is strongly associated with an increased risk, as are analgesic abuse and cyclophosphamide (Cytoxan).
- The most common presenting symptom is hematuria.
- Diagnostic work-up usually includes CT urography, urinary cytology, and cystoscopy.
- Cytologic examination of the urine has a high specificity but poor sensitivity, particularly for low-grade lesions.
- Between 3% and 5% of patients with bladder cancer have associated upper tract urothelial carcinoma. This risk is increased in patients with carcinoma in situ (CIS) or high-grade disease, in whom the risk can be as high as 20%.
- Patients with upper tract urothelial carcinoma have a 30% to 70% risk of developing bladder cancer.

Urothelial Carcinoma of the Bladder
- Painless, gross hematuria is the most common presenting symptom.
- Twenty percent of patients present with only microscopic hematuria.
- Irritative voiding symptoms such as frequency, urgency, or dysuria may also suggest a malignancy, particularly CIS.
- Patients with suspected bladder cancer should undergo an evaluation of their upper tracts (typically by CT), cystoscopy, and cytologic examination of the urine (or another urine-based tumor marker study).
- Transurethral biopsy or resection confirms the diagnosis.
- Ninety percent of bladder cancers are urothelial carcinoma, and 75% are non–muscle-invasive (superficial) at presentation.

Urethral Carcinoma
- Urethral carcinoma is the only urologic malignancy that is more common in females than in males.
- Fifty percent of cases are associated with urethral stricture.
- Urethral carcinoma may manifest as hematuria, obstructive voiding, or a palpable mass.
- Transurethral biopsy is usually required for diagnosis.

Penile Cancer
- Squamous cell carcinoma of the penis occurs most commonly in the sixth decade of life.
- Symptoms are related to ulceration, necrosis, suppuration, and hemorrhage of the penile lesion.
- The diagnosis is established by biopsy.
- Clinical evaluation of patients with penile cancer includes physical examination with palpation of the inguinal region, chest radiography, CT of the abdomen and pelvis.

Testicular Cancer
- Testicular cancer is relatively rare overall, but it is the most common malignancy in men between the ages of 15 and 35 years, with 8090 new cases occurring annually.
- Testicular cancer often manifests as a painless, enlarging testicular mass.
- Malignant tumors of the testis can be divided into those originating from the germinal cells (seminomatous and nonseminomatous germ cell tumors), rare tumors from the supporting cells (Leydig cells and Sertoli cells), and rare metastases from another primary site.
- Ninety-five percent of tumors originating in the testis are germ cell tumors. Fewer than 10% of all germ cell tumors arise from extragonadal primary sites such as the mediastinum or retroperitoneum.
- Human β-chorionic gonadotropin and α-fetoprotein are accurate and relatively specific tumor markers for testicular cancer.

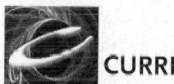

CURRENT THERAPY

Carcinoma of the Prostate
- Potentially curative treatment is generally offered to men with at least a 10-year life expectancy.
- Treatment options for clinically localized T1c and T2 tumors include active surveillance/watchful waiting, radiation therapy (external irradiation and brachytherapy), cryotherapy, and surgery (open and laparoscopic).
- Treatments for locally advanced tumors (T3/T4) or high-risk cancer patients include surgery and external irradiation in combination with androgen-deprivation therapy (ADT).
- Treatment for patients with metastatic disease (N1–2 or M1) includes initial ADT and later potentially chemotherapy, alternate forms of ADT, and/or immunotherapy.
- Follow-up includes history, physical examination, and monitoring of prostate-specific antigen at least every 6 months for 2 years and then annually. Any abnormalities may be more fully evaluated with appropriate imaging.

Renal Cell Carcinoma
- Treatment for localized masses is almost always surgical excision via radical or partial nephrectomy. Both operations may be performed with an open or a laparoscopic approach.
- Partial nephrectomy should be attempted in patients who have a solitary kidney, bilateral disease, or renal insufficiency. Partial nephrectomy is the preferred operation for patients who have lesions 4 cm or smaller and a normal contralateral kidney, with local recurrence rates of less than 5%.

- Minimally invasive approaches including percutaneous radio-frequency ablation and cryotherapy are acceptable alternatives to carefully selected patients.
- Up to 25% of patients have metastatic disease at diagnosis. Sites of metastasis, in decreasing frequency, include lungs, lymph nodes, liver, bone, and adrenal gland.
- Chemotherapy and radiation therapy provide little to no survival benefit, with radiation only palliating painful metastases.
- The mainstay of treatment in the past was immunotherapy, with 5-year survival rates of 10% to 20%.
- Modern therapies for advanced or metastatic RCC include targeted therapies such as the oral tyrosine kinase inhibitors such as suniti-nib (Sutent), votrient (Pazopanib), axitinib (Inlyta), and sorafenib (Nexavar), and the mammalian target of rapamycin (mTOR) inhib-itors, temsirolimus (Torisel) and everolimus (Afinitor).
- Evidence suggests improved survival for those undergoing nephrectomy before systemic immunotherapy for metastatic disease.

Benign Renal Tumors

- For angiomyolipomas, management should be individualized. With asymptomatic lesions smaller than 4 cm, observation with annual imaging is reasonable.
- For patients with a symptomatic angiomyolipoma or one larger than 4 cm, surgical excision should be considered, although angioembolization is another option. Angioembolization can be used to stabilize a patient with acute hemorrhage secondary to an angiomyolipoma.

Tumors of the Renal Pelvis and Ureter

- Distal ureteral tumors can be managed with distal ureterectomy and ureteroneocystostomy.
- High-grade, multifocal, or high-stage tumors are optimally trea-ted by nephroureterectomy with removal of a cuff of bladder at the ureteral orifice.
- Laparoscopic (with or without hand assist) nephroureterectomy is the preferred surgical approach, allowing for complete tumor removal and often quicker convalescence.
- Carefully selected patients, especially those who have bilateral disease or a functionally solitary kidney, can be managed with endoscopic tumor ablation.

Urothelial Carcinoma of the Bladder

- Treatment depends on tumor stage.
- Superficial (Ta) low-grade cancers are managed with transure-thral resection, with or without a single, immediate postresec-tion instillation of a chemotherapeutic agent, typically mitomycin-C (Mutamycin).
- Carcinoma in situ or high-grade stage Ta tumors that involve the lamina propria (stage T1) and recurrent tumors are managed with transurethral resection and intravesical agents such as thio-tepa (Thioplex), doxorubicin (Adriamycin), and mitomycin-C[1] or intravesical bacillus Calmette-Guérin (Tice BCG).
- Bladder surveillance is mandatory, because the recurrence rate in the bladder can be as high as 50% at 5 years.
- Surveillance protocols vary but typically include cystoscopy and urinary tumor studies (usually cytology) every 3 months for the first 2 years, semiannually in years 3 to 5, and annually thereafter.
- Periodic evaluation of the upper tracts should be performed, usually by computed tomographic (CT) urography.
- Superficial disease that progresses or is refractory to conserva-tive management, as well as tumors that invade the bladder muscle (stages T2–4), is best managed by radical cystectomy and urinary diversion.
- Urinary diversion may be either incontinent (conduit) or conti-nent (orthotopic or continent cutaneous).
- Five-year recurrence-free survival rates are 60% to 85% after cystectomy for organ-confined disease (stages T2a–T2b). For extravesical disease (stages T3a to T4), the 5-year survival decreases to 40% to 60%; for node-positive disease it is less than 30%.

- Patients with T2–T4 disease should be strongly considered for combination therapy with surgery plus chemotherapy, either in the neoadjuvant or the adjuvant setting. Recent randomized trials have suggested an approximately 5% survival advantage for neoadjuvant chemotherapy plus surgery, compared with sur-gery alone.
- Patients with M1 disease are usually treated with chemotherapy.
- The standard regimen over the past decade has been MVAC: methotrexate (Trexall),[1] vinblastine (Velban),[1] doxorubicin (Adriamycin), and cisplatin (Platinol); however, durable com-plete response rates are less than 15%.
- Newer agents such as gemcitabine (Gemzar)[1] along with cis-platin appear to offer similar response rates and reduced toxicity.

Urethral Carcinoma

- Treatment of the primary tumor is surgical excision and varies based on the location and stage of the tumor.
- In men, urethrectomy can be performed via a perineal incision.
- Proximal tumors of the bulbar urethra are often managed with cystoprostatectomy and en bloc urethrectomy.
- Among women, for tumors of the proximal urethra and tumors with extension into adjacent structures, cystectomy with en bloc urethrectomy and anterior vaginectomy along with pelvic lym-phadenectomy is usually required.
- Radiation therapy is also reported to provide local control in selective cases.

Penile Cancer

- Small penile cancers limited to the prepuce can be treated by circumcision alone.
- Partial penectomy is used to treat smaller (2–5 cm) distal penile tumors. The remaining penis should be long enough to permit voiding in the standing position. The 5-year cure rate for patients treated with partial penectomy is 70% to 80%.
- Larger distal penile lesions and proximal tumors require total penectomy and perineal urethrostomy. If the scrotum, pubis, or abdominal wall is involved, radical en bloc excision may be necessary.
- Many patients have inguinal lymphadenopathy at presentation. However, inguinal lymph node enlargement before excision of the primary tumor may be the result of infection and not met-astatic disease. Therefore, clinical assessment of the inguinal region should be delayed 4 to 6 weeks, during which time the patient is treated with antibiotics.
- If inguinal lymphadenopathy persists or with high risk features, there is a high likelihood of metastatic disease, and ilioinguinal lymphadenectomy should be performed. The procedure is per-formed on the contralateral side if the initial side contains tumor and could be simultaneously performed or staged.
- Irradiation of the primary tumor and regional lymph nodes is an alternative to surgery in patients with small (≤2 cm), low-stage tumors.
- Mohs' surgery is another alternative for small lesions (≤2 cm).

Testicular Cancer

- All patients with suspected testicular tumors should undergo a radical orchiectomy through an inguinal approach and early, high ligation of the spermatic cord.
- Serum tumor markers should be measured before surgery and are used for disease staging and to monitor for recurrence.
- Radiographic staging should include, at a minimum, a CT scan of the abdomen and pelvis and chest radiography.
- Seminoma is the most common histologic form of germ cell tumor and generally carries a better prognosis than other vari-ants. Standard therapy for low-stage (T1, 2a, or 2b) disease is orchiectomy with active surveillance, short course chemother-apy, or adjuvant radiation therapy to the retroperitoneum. Relapse is relatively rare, occurring in 4% of patients with stage 1 and 10% of patients with stage 2 disease. Relapses after radi-ation therapy can be salvaged in more than 90% of cases

- through systemic chemotherapy. The long-term cure rate for low-stage seminoma is approximately 99%.
- Nonseminomatous germ cell tumors (NSGCTs) include embryonal cell carcinomas, choriocarcinomas, yolk sac carcinomas, teratomas, and mixed germ cell tumors. As with pure seminoma, the cure rate for low-stage NSGCTs is high (>95%) in patients with stage 1 disease.
- Surveillance and retroperitoneal lymph node dissection (RPLND) are both standard treatment options for stage 1 NSGCT. In select cases, adjuvant chemotherapy may be an option. Twenty percent of these patients have lymph node involvement, and those with vascular invasion or predominance of embryonal cell carcinoma are at increased risk (>30%).
- RPLND is a major abdominal operation in which lymph nodes from the retroperitoneum are removed, from the renal hilum down to the level of the common iliac artery, with lateral margins being confined by the ureters.
- Adjuvant chemotherapy after RPLND should be considered if any lymph node is larger than 2 cm in diameter, if at least six nodes are involved, or if there is extranodal invasion.
- Patients with persistently increased concentrations of α-fetoprotein, human β-chorionic gonadotropin, or both but without other clinical evidence of disease after orchiectomy usually have systemic disease and are treated with chemotherapy.
- Approximately one third of patients require up-front chemotherapy. Those with clinical stage 2c disease (or higher), primary retroperitoneal germ cell tumors, or mediastinal seminomas treated with radiation therapy should undergo systemic, cisplatin-based, multiagent chemotherapy.
- Postchemotherapy RPLND for seminoma is typically reserved for patients with residual masses larger than 3 cm. For NSGCT, some groups reserve postchemotherapy RPLND for patients who do not have substantial tumor shrinkage (>90% shrinkage of retroperitoneal nodes and no residual nodes >1.5 cm) and those with teratomatous elements in the primary tumor. Others advocate surgery for all patients with initial bulky retroperitoneal disease. All agree that a clear, residual mass after chemotherapy in the setting of NSGCT warrants postchemotherapy RPLND.
- Multimodal therapy has allowed 90% to 95% of testicular cancer patients to be cured, even in the face of metastatic disease.

[1]Not FDA approved for this indication.

Carcinoma of the Prostate

Prostate cancer is the most common noncutaneous solid malignancy among men in the United States, and it is second only to lung cancer with respect to cancer-related mortality. In 2008, there were an estimated 186,320 new cases of prostate cancer and 28,660 deaths due to this disease. Because prostate cancer is predominantly a disease of the elderly, its incidence may be expected to rise over time as the U.S. population ages.

There is a familial predisposition to prostate cancer, which is more common among those with a first-degree relative who also has the disease, and it appears to be more common among African American men than among Caucasian men. Environmental factors that have been associated with an increased risk of prostate cancer include a high-fat Western-style diet, as compared with a high-soy Asian diet, and low levels of vitamin D.

Hereditary prostate cancer is relatively rare but may account for up to 40% of tumors among young men with the disease. One of several genes found in families with hereditary prostate cancer is hereditary prostate cancer 1 (*HPC1*), which is located on the long arm of chromosome 1. Translocations leading to fusion of two genes (TMPRSS2:ERG gene fusion) has also been implicated in a large number of sporadic prostate cancers.

Diagnosis

The vast majority of prostate cancers are adenocarcinomas. There is a large discrepancy between the risk of finding incidental prostate cancer at autopsy (estimated to be as high as 75% by age 80 or older) and the risk of having the disease clinically diagnosed (lifetime risk, approximately 1 in 6). Most men with early-stage prostate cancer diagnosed in the modern era have no specific disease-related symptoms. Benign prostatic hypertrophy is often found in association with prostate cancer and is also more common in men as they age, but there is no known causal relationship between the two. Prostate cancer can rarely manifest with pelvic pain, bladder outlet obstruction, or ureteral obstruction from locally advanced disease or with bone pain from distant metastatic disease.

The advent and widespread use of the serum prostate-specific antigen (PSA) test as a screening tool for prostate cancer has resulted in a stage migration, with most men now diagnosed with early-stage disease. This has been associated with better recurrence-free survival rates after definitive local therapy. Certain groups, such as the American Urologic Association and the American Cancer Society, have advocated that physicians offer screening with a serum PSA determination and digital rectal examination for men older than 55 years of age and for African American men and those with a family history of prostatic cancer starting at age 40 years. However, these recommendations are not uniformly accepted; the U.S. Preventive Services Task Force recently gave a grade D recommendation for routine screening with PSA for prostate cancer. It is generally accepted that the decision to screen for prostate cancer should be made in individuals with at least 10 years of life expectancy.

Serum PSA is specific for the prostate but is not specific for cancer. It is secreted by both benign and malignant prostatic epithelial cells. The PSA may be elevated in men with a variety of prostate-related conditions, such as prostatitis, benign prostatic hypertrophy, urinary tract infection, or prostatic cancer. Until recently, a PSA level lower than 4.0 ng/mL was considered normal, and in younger men a value of greater than 2.5 ng/mL could perhaps be considered abnormal. More recently, it has become clear that there is no true cutoff value for PSA. Instead, the association between PSA and prostate cancer risk is a continuum. Even at a PSA of essentially zero, there is still a 6% chance of having prostate cancer on biopsy.

The majority of the serum PSA is bound to protease inhibitors such as α_1-antichymotrypsin, whereas a fraction is unconjugated or free. The relative proportion of free serum PSA can be used to improve the specificity of PSA for diagnosis of prostate cancer by biopsy. Benign prostatic hypertrophy is associated with a higher proportion of free PSA, and patients with greater 25% free serum PSA are less likely to harbor prostate cancer. The precise cutoff point associated with prostate cancer is controversial and ranges from 10% to 20% or higher. Development of new tests to improve PSA specificity, such as measurement of complexed PSA or early pro-forms of PSA, is an area of ongoing investigation.

The most common method used to diagnose prostate cancer is a transrectal ultrasonography (TRUS)-guided prostate biopsy. TRUS allows for accurate localization of the zonal anatomy of the prostate and can accurately measure its size. It therefore acts as a guide for the biopsy, because prostatic cancers typically reside in the peripheral zone, and biopsies are concentrated within that zone. Although prostate cancer can manifest as hypoechoic lesions on TRUS, the tumors usually are not visible. TRUS lacks both sensitivity and specificity and should not be used as a screening test.

The most common grading system used to estimate the degree of tumor differentiation is the Gleason grading system. The two most common Gleason grade patterns (on a scale of 1 to 5) are summed to give a score between 2 and 10. Tumors with Gleason scores between 2 and 6 are well differentiated and have a better prognosis, whereas those with Gleason scores between 8 and 10 are poorly differentiated and have a worse prognosis. Gleason score 7 is associated with intermediate differentiation and prognosis. The majority of cancers found in the modern era are well to intermediately differentiated (Gleason score 5 to 7).

Staging of prostatic cancer defines the local, regional, and distant extent of disease. The tumor-node-metastasis (TNM) staging system is the most commonly used method. The most common clinical stage in the modern era is that of nonpalpable tumors detected because of a concerning PSA result (stage T1c). The primary staging modality for local disease is the digital rectal examination. This may be supplemented by pelvic magnetic resonance imaging in selected cases where there is significant concern for locally advanced disease based on the digital rectal examination. Although PSA only roughly correlates with the overall disease burden, bone metastasis is quite uncommon among patients whose PSA value is less than 20 ng/mL. Therefore, a radionucleotide bone scan in the absence of symptoms is not required routinely if the PSA value is less than 10 ng/mL and the Gleason sum is 7 or less. Computed tomography (CT) scanning is not routinely used, because grossly positive nodes are detected rarely with a clinically localized tumor.

Lymph node staging is important in selecting patients for therapy. CT scanning may show enlarged lymph nodes in patients with high-volume or high-grade primary tumor but has poor sensitivity and specificity. Laparoscopic pelvic lymphadenectomy can provide adequate sampling of the pelvic lymph nodes in those patients not selecting surgery. More commonly, lymph node dissection is performed concomitantly at the time of radical prostatectomy.

Treatment

There is no one optimal treatment for clinically localized prostatic cancer, so therapy must be individualized. Among men with a life expectancy of less than 10 years, observation alone may be appropriate. Carefully selected men with low-risk prostate cancer may choose active surveillance rather than curative treatment but must be rigorously monitored for evidence of worsening disease.

Surgery and radiation therapy are the most commonly used curative modalities. For low-risk, organ-confined tumors, the 15-year disease-free survival rates are greater than 90% among patients treated with surgery. Moreover, the survival outcome is similar after radiation therapy and after surgery. However, properly done prospective, randomized comparisons among similarly staged patients have not been done. Radiation therapy can be delivered as external-beam radiotherapy or as brachytherapy using radioactive seeds (iodine 125 or palladium 103) implanted directly into the prostate. Cryotherapy (i.e., freezing of the prostate) is another approved treatment for men with prostatic carcinoma that is becoming more widely accepted as an alternative treatment option.

Radical prostatectomy, or surgical removal of the prostate, may be performed via an open incision or by a laparoscopic technique. Traditionally, an open surgery is performed through an anterior, retropubic approach or, less commonly, through a perineal incision. Laparoscopic and, in particular, robot-assisted radical prostatectomy is being performed with increasing frequency. The benefits of a robot-assisted approach may include reduced blood loss, sooner return to normal function, and possibly better functional outcomes and better surgical margin rates (although the latter two have not been definitively demonstrated to this point). In patients who were sexually active before therapy, preservation of the neurovascular bundles is often undertaken in an attempt to maintain postoperative sexual function. For patients with organ-confined disease, the prognosis is excellent, with a life expectancy similar to that of men without prostatic cancer. For those patients with positive surgical margins or positive lymph nodes on final pathology, consideration can be given to delivering, respectively, adjuvant irradiation or androgen-deprivation therapy (ADT).

Serum PSA should rapidly become undetectable after radical prostatectomy, because, in theory, all PSA-producing tissue has been removed. After radiation therapy or cryotherapy, the PSA is expected to reach low levels over time and then remain stable. An increasing serum PSA is evidence of tumor recurrence. There is controversy about when to initiate ADT in men with a rising PSA level after treatment.

Prostatic cancer, at least initially, is an androgen-sensitive disease. Therefore, the primary first-line treatment for metastatic prostate cancer is ADT. Suppression of serum testosterone can be achieved by orchiectomy (i.e., surgical castration).

Alternatively, medical castration may be considered. Luteinizing hormone–releasing hormone analogues effectively suppress testosterone to the castrate range within 1 month after administration by suppressing central nervous system secretion of luteinizing hormone. There is increasing awareness that ADT can be associated with significant long-term morbidity, including vasomotor reflex changes (hot flushes), loss of libido, erectile dysfunction, osteoporosis, anemia, muscle wasting, gynecomastia, and possibly cognitive changes and increased risk of cardiovascular disease. The choice to use ADT must, therefore, be carefully balanced based on the individual patient's overall risk of prostate cancer–related morbidity and mortality versus ADT-related morbidity.

Most patients with metastatic disease initially respond to ADT, but almost inexorably the disease progresses despite ongoing ADT, to become castrate-resistant prostate cancer (CRPC). At that point, the median survival time is less than 2 years. There is enzalutamide (Xtandi). The standard chemotherapy for CRPC is docetaxel (Taxotere) plus prednisone, and prospective randomized trials have demonstrated a modest survival benefit among patients so treated. An alternative for asymptomatic or minimally symptomatic men with metastatic CRPC include sipuleucel-T (Provenge), a novel cellular immunotherapy-based intervention, and abiraterone acetate (Zytiga). Several options now exist for men with metastatic CRPC who have failed prior docetaxel therapy including cabazitaxel (Jevtana), abiraterone acetate (Zytiga), enzalutamide (Xtandi), and Radium-223 dichloride (Xofigo). Another approved drug is mitoxantrone (Novantrone) for palliative relief of symptomatic bone pain from CRPC. Radiation therapy can be used effectively to palliate focal sites of bone metastases. The mechanisms by which prostatic carcinoma escapes hormonal control and becomes castrate resistant represent an area of ongoing intensive research.

Tumors of the Renal Parenchyma

Malignant tumors of the renal parenchyma are of either primary or metastatic origin. Primary renal tumors may be benign or malignant. The most common tumor of primary renal cell carcinoma (RCC) is conventional (clear cell) RCC; other tumor types, such as papillary, chromophobe, collecting duct, and medullary carcinomas and sarcomas, occur infrequently. The most common benign renal tumors are angiomyolipomas and oncocytomas. The latter, in particular, are generally indistinguishable from malignant lesions on radiographic imaging. Metastatic lesions (e.g., from lung, breast, melanoma, or ovary) may occur, and primary lymphoma may be present in the kidney.

Renal Cell Carcinoma

RCC is the most common primary neoplasm of the kidney, accounting for more than 85% of all primary renal tumors. There were an estimated 54,390 newly diagnosed cases of RCC in the United States in 2008, and an estimated 13,010 people died of this disease. RCC represents approximately 3% of all adult malignancies and usually manifests between 40 and 60 years of age, although it can be found in younger age groups. It has a 2:1 male-to-female preponderance and in both sporadic and familial forms is associated with aberrations of the von Hippel–Lindau (VHL) gene and protein.

RCC is thought to arise from cells of the proximal convoluted tubule. The most consistent genetic aberration found in most cases of sporadic, conventional RCC are aberrations in the VHL gene. No specific agent has been implicated as the cause of RCC, although tobacco products are associated with an approximately twofold increased risk of being diagnosed with the disease. Patients, and particularly younger patients, with end-stage renal disease who develop acquired cystic disease of the kidney also have an increased risk of RCC. Between 1% and 2% of these patients develop RCC, so annual renal ultrasonography is reasonable as a screening tool in this population, with confirmatory studies such as CT for complex or suspicious lesions.

Diagnosis

The most common sign associated with RCC in 29% to 60% of cases is hematuria. The classic triad of flank pain, hematuria, and a palpable abdominal mass is relatively rare, occurring in fewer than 10% of cases. Other common symptoms and signs include fever, anemia, hypercalcemia, thrombocytosis, and elevated erythrocyte sedimentation rate, lactate dehydrogenase, or alkaline phosphatase. Currently, there are no reliable, commercially available tumor markers for RCC. Most often, these tumors are incidentally diagnosed on radiographic imaging performed for unrelated or nonspecific purposes.

The most commonly used staging system for RCC is the TNM staging system. It allows for a distinction between venous involvement and nodal invasion and stratifies the extent of each stage. RCC can involve the renal vein and vena cava and may even extend into the right atrium. Locally, it can directly invade surrounding structures such as the adrenal gland and colon. Five-year survival rates range from 80% to 90% for stages T1 N0 M0 (<7 cm) and T2 N0 M0 (>7 cm), 40% to 60% for stage T3 N0 M0, and 10% to 20% for N1–3 and M1 disease.

Treatment

Surgical excision of the tumor is the primary treatment for RCC. The classic procedure was a radical nephrectomy, in which the kidney was removed en bloc within Gerota's fascia and the ipsilateral adrenal gland and lymph nodes. This was routinely performed as an open procedure (flank, transabdominal, or thoracoabdominal incision). Adrenalectomy is now generally reserved for upper-pole tumors, very large tumors, or lesions that directly extend into the adrenal gland. Although these operations are increasingly performed through a laparoscopic approach, an open approach is usually preferred if there is extensive involvement of the inferior vena cava. In rare cases with supradiaphragmatic tumor extension within the cava, cardiopulmonary bypass may be required for tumor extraction.

A partial nephrectomy has become a standard approach for surgical excision of renal parenchymal tumors, particularly for individuals with solitary kidneys, those with bilateral masses, and those with compromised renal function. It has become the preferred operation for patients who have lesions of 4 cm or smaller and a normal contralateral kidney, because local recurrence rates are less than 5%, and partial (rather than radical) nephrectomy is associated with a lower long-term risk of chronic renal failure. As with radical nephrectomy, there is a growing experience with laparoscopic approaches to partial nephrectomy. There are also several, minimally invasive approaches that are being utilized with increasing frequency including radiographically guided, percutaneous thermal tumor ablation using radiofrequency ablation or cryotherapy. These modalities are typically reserved for older patients or poor surgical candidates.

Up to 25% of patients initially present with metastatic disease. Sites of metastasis of RCC, in decreasing frequency of occurrence, include lung, lymph nodes, liver, bone, and adrenal gland. Chemotherapy and irradiation have little to no survival benefit, with radiation therapy only palliating painful metastases. The mainstay of treatment in the past was immunotherapy, with 5-year survival rates of 10% to 20%. Modern therapies for advanced or metastatic RCC now include the so-called targeted therapies, such as the oral tyrosine kinase inhibitors, sunitinib (Sutent), votrient (Pazopanib), axitinib (Inlyta), and sorafenib (Nexavar), and the mammalian target of rapamycin (mTOR) inhibitors, temsirolimus (Torisel) and everolimus (Afinitor). Evidence suggests improved survival among those patients who undergo nephrectomy before systemic immunotherapy.

Benign Renal Tumors

Although they are not as frequent as malignant tumors, benign solid masses are also seen in the kidney. Angiomyolipomas can often be diagnosed radiographically based on the appearance of fat by CT scan. They can occur sporadically or as part of an inherited familial syndrome, tuberous sclerosis. The latter entity is characterized by mental retardation, benign tumors of the cerebellum, epilepsy, adenoma sebaceum, and angiomyolipomas. Approximately 50% of patients with tuberous sclerosis develop angiomyolipomas, most of which are bilateral and multifocal. The management of angiomyolipoma is controversial and should be individualized. Asymptomatic tumors smaller than 4 cm can generally be observed with annual radiographic imaging. Symptomatic lesions (bleeding, pain, rapid growth) and lesions larger than 4 cm should be considered for surgical excision, although angioembolization is another option. Acute hemorrhage from an angiomyolipoma can often be managed or at least stabilized by angioembolization.

Oncocytomas are the most common solid, benign renal tumors and account for 5% to 10% of solid renal lesions. Although these lesions tend to have a more uniform density than RCC and can have a characteristic central scar or spoke-wheel appearance on CT, there is no radiographic feature that reliably distinguishes an oncocytoma from a malignant renal lesion. Oncocytoma is therefore a diagnosis that should be made only on histologic analysis. The tumors characteristically exhibit eosinophilic, granular cells packed with mitochondria. Oncocytomas are thought to arise from the distal portion of the renal tubule.

Metastatic Renal Lesions

The most common primary malignancy to metastasize to the kidney is lung cancer, although cancers of the ovary, breast, or bowel, melanoma, and lymphoma can do so as well. Lymphoma of the kidney is almost always a manifestation of systemic disease. The management is therefore grounded in systemic chemotherapy, with surgery reserved for palliative symptom relief. However, approximately 15% of renal lymphomas manifest with a solitary renal mass as the sole radiographic manifestation. These lesions can be challenging to manage and difficult to distinguish from RCC preoperatively.

Tumors of the Renal Pelvis and Ureter

Approximately 10% of all renal tumors originate in the renal pelvis rather than the renal parenchyma. These account for 5% of all urothelial carcinomas (the majority of which arise in the bladder). Of the upper tract urothelial carcinomas, approximately one fourth arise in the ureter and the remainder in the renal pelvis. Urothelial carcinoma of the upper urinary tract is more common in men than in women and more common in whites than in blacks. Environmental exposures associated with a higher risk of developing upper tract urothelial carcinoma include analgesic abuse, cyclophosphamide (Cytoxan), and a strong association with tobacco abuse.

Among patients with bladder cancer, approximately 3% to 5% develop upper tract urothelial carcinoma. This can increase to as high as 20% among those with carcinoma in situ (CIS) or high-grade disease. Conversely, approximately 30% to 70% of patients with a history of upper tract urothelial carcinoma go on to develop bladder cancer. As a consequence, these patients require ongoing periodic cystoscopic surveillance. The incidence of bilateral upper tract tumors is 2% to 5%. Other histologic tumor types that can manifest in the upper urinary tract include squamous cell carcinoma (SCC) and adenocarcinoma. Although they are rare, the risk is increased among patients with a history of recurrent, refractory urinary tract infections or staghorn calculi.

Diagnosis

The most common presenting symptom for upper tract urothelial tumors is hematuria. For patients with adequate renal function, the evaluation for hematuria includes CT urography, urinary cytology (or another urinary-based tumor marker), and cystoscopy. Urinary cytology has a high specificity but a generally poor sensitivity, particularly for low-grade disease. Other urinary tumor markers, such as NMP-22, and fluorescent in situ hybridization approaches typically have better sensitivity but are not as specific.

A retrograde ureteropyelogram may be helpful in patients with poor renal function who cannot receive intravenous contrast agents. In general, if a suspicious mass is seen on CT or other imaging, a ureteroscopy is typically performed with biopsy or brushings to establish the diagnosis. The TNM system is the standard for staging.

Treatment

Disease isolated to the distal ureter is most often managed with distal ureterectomy and ureteroneocystostomy. High-grade or high stage disease and multifocal disease isolated to one side are optimally managed in most cases by excision of that upper tract system via a radical nephroureterectomy, including excision of the distal portion of the ureter and complete excision of the ureteral orifice together with a cuff of bladder. Traditionally, these procedures were done via open incisions (one or two separate incisions, depending on the surgeon), but laparoscopy is increasingly being used to decrease patient morbidity and improve surgical recovery. In selected patients who have low-grade, low-stage disease with a small overall disease burden, an endoscopic approach using laser or electrocautery to destroy the tumors may be considered. This is also a strong consideration for those patients with bilateral disease or involvement of a functionally solitary renal unit. Most often, retrograde endoscopic approaches via ureteroscopy are employed, although in highly selected cases antegrade percutaneous approaches can be utilized.

Carcinoma of the Bladder
Urothelial Carcinoma of the Bladder

Bladder carcinoma is the fifth most common malignancy in the United States, with more than 68,810 new cases diagnosed annually. It is almost three times more common in men than in women, in whom it is the fourth most common cancer. Because of its propensity to recur, particularly in patients with superficial disease, it is the second most prevalent cancer. High-grade bladder cancer is a deadly disease and is the fifth most common cause of cancer deaths among men. There is a well-established relationship between the development of bladder cancer and a variety of carcinogens. Perhaps the most widespread factor is tobacco abuse. Cigarette smoking is thought to account for up to half of all bladder cancers in men. Bladder cancer is also associated with other, less frequent occupational exposures, such as in the rubber and oil refinery industries. It is also associated with exposure to the chemotherapeutic agent, cyclophosphamide (Cytoxan); exposed patients have up to a ninefold increased risk of developing bladder cancer, most likely related to a urinary metabolite of cyclophosphamide, acrolein.

Approximately 90% of bladder malignancies are urothelial carcinomas. Of these, the majority (70%) are papillary, 10% are sessile, and 20% demonstrate mixed morphology. Although roughly three quarters of bladder cancer patients present with superficial disease, approximately 20% to 25% progress to muscle invasion over time. Nevertheless, 80% to 90% of patients with muscle-invasive disease had it at initial presentation. A strong correlation exists between tumor grade and stage; most well-differentiated tumors are superficial, and most poorly differentiated tumors are invasive. CIS is a poorly differentiated urothelial carcinoma that grows as a sheet confined to the urothelium. CIS may be found as a solitary or multifocal process and is associated with invasive carcinoma in 25% of cases, where it portends a poor prognosis. Between 10% and 20% of patients treated with cystectomy for diffuse or refractory CIS are found to have microscopic muscle-invasive disease.

Diagnosis

Gross painless hematuria is the most common presenting sign of bladder cancer. However, approximately 1 in 5 patients have only microscopic hematuria. Other symptoms that can be indicative of urothelial carcinoma (in particular, CIS) include irritative voiding symptoms such as frequency, urgency, and dysuria. Patients who present with symptoms and signs concerning for urothelial carcinoma should undergo an evaluation that includes cystoscopy, urinary tumor marker study (typically, urinary cytology), and evaluation of the upper tracts (typically by CT urography). The diagnosis is usually confirmed at the time of transurethral resection or biopsy.

Treatment

The management options for urothelial carcinoma are heavily dependent on the stage and grade of disease. The TNM system is recommended for staging. For most superficial, low-grade tumors, transurethral resection, with or without a single, immediate instillation of a chemotherapeutic agent such as mitomycin-C (Mutamycin),[1] is all that is required. This must then be followed by careful, ongoing surveillance by cystoscopy, urinary tumor studies (typically cytology), and periodic upper tract imaging. For patients with high-grade disease (including CIS) and tumors that superficially invade the lamina propria (stage T1) or are rapidly recurrent tumors, adjuvant treatment with intravesical agents such as thiotepa (Thioplex), doxorubicin (Adriamycin), and mitomycin-C (Mutamycin)[1] or intravesical bacillus Calmette-Guérin (Tice BCG) may be indicated. In the United States, the most frequently used agent for this purpose, particularly for CIS, is intravesical BCG.

Patients with superficial disease must undergo regular surveillance, because the recurrence rate is as high as 50% at 5 years. Surveillance protocols vary but typically include cystoscopy and urinary tumor studies (usually urinary cytology) every 3 months for 2 years, then every 6 months for 3 years, and annually thereafter. Periodic evaluation of the upper tracts, typically by CT urography, is warranted, because there is a 3% to 5% incidence of development of upper tract urothelial carcinoma among patients with bladder urothelial carcinoma.

The risk of disease progression in patients with low-grade, low-stage (Ta) urothelial carcinoma is less than 5% to 10%. This risk increases as the stage and grade of the tumor increase. Patients who have muscle-invasive disease (stage T2 or higher), either at presentation or with progression after therapy for superficial disease, are best treated by radical cystectomy and urinary diversion. A thorough pelvic lymphadenectomy should be performed at the time of surgery. The precise limits of dissection for the lymphadenectomy remain somewhat controversial, although the latest data suggest that patients who have more lymph nodes removed fare better.

High-grade bladder cancer is a potentially lethal disease. There are an estimated 14,100 deaths due to bladder cancer annually. Among patients with organ-confined (pT2a-pT2b), muscle-invasive disease who undergo cystectomy, the 5-year recurrence-free survival rates are between 60% and 85%. For patients undergoing radical cystectomy who have extravesical extension of their disease (pT3-pT4 disease), the 5-year recurrence-free survival rates are lower, 40% to 60%. Patients with lymph node–positive disease fare the worst, with 5-year recurrence-free survival rates of 20% to 30%.

Patients with muscle-invasive bladder cancer should be considered for multimodal therapy (i.e., chemotherapy in addition to surgery). The standard regimen over the past decade has been MVAC: methotrexate (Trexall),[1] vinblastine (Velban),[1] doxorubicin (Adriamycin), and cisplatin (Platinol). This can be delivered either before surgery (neoadjuvant) or in the postsurgery setting (adjuvant). There is level 1 evidence to support MVAC chemotherapy combined with cystectomy for muscle-invasive bladder cancer, although the survival benefit across studies is only on the order of 5% to 10%. Newer agents, such as gemcitabine (Gemzar)[1] along with cisplatin, appear to offer similar response rates and reduced toxicity and are often used currently in lieu of MVAC. Cytotoxic chemotherapy produces response rates of 50% to

---

[1]Not FDA approved for this indication.

70% in patients with advanced or metastatic disease; however, the durable, long-term, complete response rates at 5 years are no more than 15% across series.

Urinary diversion may be accomplished after cystectomy in several ways, but the fundamental categories are incontinent and continent forms. Incontinent forms of diversion include ileal and colon conduits, both of which require that the patient wear an external collection appliance. Continent forms of diversion include the continent cutaneous diversion, which requires creation of a low-pressure reservoir (often of colon) and a catheterizable efferent limb with an associated valve mechanism to prevent urine leakage. More recently, emphasis has shifted to continent diversions in which the low-pressure reservoir is anastomosed to the native urethra. These orthotopic neobladders may be crafted from colon or ileum and offer the opportunity to avoid any external collection devices and, usually, any need for catheterization. Such devices may improve patients' quality of life after surgery, although this has not been formally demonstrated in a randomized trial.

Adenocarcinoma of the Bladder
Adenocarcinomas account for fewer than 2% of bladder cancers. They can be found in three settings: as primary lesions in the bladder, as metastases or local extensions from another site, or as primary urachal carcinomas. They are typically invasive and poorly differentiated and carry a poor prognosis. Adenocarcinomas may be found in association with bladder augmentation cystoplasties and are the most common form of bladder cancer in patients born with bladder exstrophy. The treatment of choice is typically radical cystectomy, pelvic lymphadenectomy, and urinary diversion.

Squamous Cell Carcinoma of the Bladder
SCC accounts for approximately 6% of bladder cancers in the United States but more than 75% of bladder cancers in Egypt. SCC is associated with chronic bladder inflammation from a variety of sources. These include chronic indwelling Foley catheters, recurrent or refractory bladder infections, and bladder diverticula or stones. In Egypt, approximately 80% of SCCs are associated with *Schistosoma haematobium* infestation. These bilharzia-associated SCCs of the bladder tend to occur in patients 10 to 20 years earlier than in the United States.

SCC of the bladder often carries a poor prognosis and is usually best treated by radical cystectomy. After surgery, this form of bladder cancer has a higher propensity for local recurrence, compared with urothelial carcinomas. SCC of the bladder is typically resistant to cytotoxic chemotherapy, particularly the regimens frequently used for urothelial carcinoma. The benefit of neoadjuvant radiation therapy before cystectomy remains to be proven, at least for the non-bilharzial SCC typically found in the United States.

Urethral Carcinoma
Diagnosis
Urethral carcinoma is unusual in that it is more common in women than in men. It is a disease of the elderly, typically occurring after 60 years of age. The etiology remains to be determined, but approximately half of the cases are associated with urethral stricture disease. In women, there is an association with urethral malakoplakia and urethral caruncles. The usual presenting symptom in this circumstance is a papillary or fungating urethral mass and hematuria. A number of scenarios warrant a more thorough evaluation for possible urethral carcinoma, including a palpable urethral mass, an obstruction that does not respond to conventional management, development of a urethral abscess or fistula, presence of microscopic or gross hematuria, and the development of inguinal adenopathy.

Treatment
The primary treatment of urethral carcinoma is most often surgical excision, with the approach and the extent of surgery driven by both gender and the location of the mass relative to the sphincteric complex (likelihood of postoperative continence). For example, cystectomy with en bloc urethrectomy and anterior vaginectomy along with pelvic lymphadenectomy is usually required for tumors located in the proximal urethra or tumors with extension into adjacent structures. In selected cases, radiation therapy can provide local control. In locally advanced disease, multimodality treatment with chemotherapy and either surgical excision or radiation therapy provides the optimal chance for long-term cure, although there is no standard regimen to date.

Penile Cancer
Diagnosis
Penile cancer is relatively rare in the United States. Penile carcinoma has been associated with retained phimotic foreskin and poor personal hygiene. It is rare among men who are circumcised before puberty and occurs most commonly in the sixth decade of life. The symptoms relate directly to the mass itself and can include ulceration, pain, necrosis, foul odor, hemorrhage, and suppuration of the lesion. The clinical evaluation of patients with penile cancer involves a thorough physical examination including of the phallus and careful attention to palpation of the inguinal lymph nodes. Additional studies may include radiographic testing with chest radiography, CT scan of the abdomen and pelvis, and bone scan.

Treatment
Treatment is usually dictated by the tumor stage (TNM system), size, and location. Small tumors that are confined to the prepuce can often be managed by circumcision alone. Smaller tumors on the distal shaft can be treated by partial penectomy, provided that a normal tissue margin can be achieved and there is enough penile length remaining to permit voiding in the standing position. Among patients treated by partial penectomy, the 5-year recurrence-free survival rate is 70% to 80%. Large lesions and tumors on the proximal shaft may require total penectomy and perineal urethrostomy to achieve adequate local tumor control. If there is involvement of local structures such as the scrotum or pubis, radical en bloc resection may be required. Achieving negative margins is critical, because local recurrence of the disease can rarely be salvaged by radiation or chemotherapy.

Although many patients have inguinal lymphadenopathy at presentation, inguinal lymph node enlargement before excision of the primary tumor may be the result of infection and not metastatic disease. Clinical assessment of the inguinal region is therefore typically delayed for 4 to 6 weeks, during which time the patient receives antibiotic treatment. Lymphadenopathy that persists or develops de novo raises the strong possibility of lymph node metastases, and an ilioinguinal lymphadenectomy should be performed. If inguinal lymphadenopathy resolves on antibiotics, prophylactic lymph node dissection may not be necessary. It is often necessary to perform bilateral inguinal lymphadenectomy, particularly in patients with high-risk disease, for whom this should be considered regardless of the presence or absence of palpable nodes. Radiation of the primary tumor and regional lymph nodes is an alternative to surgery in carefully selected patients with small (≤2 cm), low-stage tumors. Similarly, Mohs' surgery is an option for small tumors, particularly ones at the base that otherwise might require a total penectomy.

Testicular Cancer
Malignant tumors of the male gonads can be divided into neoplasms originating from the germinal cells, rare tumors from the supporting cells (Leydig cells and Sertoli cells), and rare metastases from another primary site. The germinal neoplasms include seminomatous and nonseminomatous germ cell tumors (NSGCTs). Ninety-five percent of tumors originating in the testis are germ cell tumors. Fewer than 10% of all germ cell tumors arise from extragonadal primary sites such as the mediastinum and retroperitoneum. Testicular cancer is relatively rare overall, but it is the most common malignancy in men between the ages of 15 and 35 years, with 8090 new cases occurring annually.

Testicular cancer represents one of the great success stories in modern medicine. The mortality rates for testis cancer have decreased from more than 50% before the 1970s to less than 10% in the modern age. This is the result of a variety of advances, including more effective multiagent chemotherapy, improved surgical techniques, and better methods to diagnose and monitor the disease (e.g., CT scans, tumor markers). Testicular cancer currently serves as a paradigm for the multimodal treatment of malignancies.

Germ cell tumors are substantially more prevalent in Caucasians than in African Americans, by a margin of at least 5:1. Indeed, a report from the U.S. military indicated a relative incidence of 40:1. The exact etiology of germ cell tumors is not fully understood. Familial clustering has been demonstrated, particularly among siblings. Two conditions associated with a higher risk for germ cell tumors are cryptorchidism and Klinefelter's syndrome, the latter associated with disease arising from the mediastinum. Orchidopexy for cryptorchidism does not appear to reduce the risk of neoplasia, but it does improve the ability to monitor the testis.

Diagnosis

A painless testicular mass in a patient of the appropriate age group should be considered a primary testicular tumor until proven otherwise. A substantial number of testicular tumors manifest with less specific symptoms, including diffuse testicular pain, swelling, hardness, or some combination of these findings. A tumor can be difficult to distinguish from an infectious epididymo-orchitis. However, because the latter is more common than a testicular tumor, a short trial of antibiotics is often undertaken. If symptoms do not abate or the findings do not revert to normal within 2 to 4 weeks, testicular sonography is indicated to identify any underlying testicular mass. A radical inguinal orchiectomy with early, high ligation of the spermatic cord at the internal ring is required for all patients with a suspected testicular tumor.

Testicular cancers typically first spread to regional, retroperitoneal lymph nodes below the level of the renal vessels. The primary nodal landing zone for right-sided tumors lies between the aorta and the inferior vena cava (interaortocaval nodes), whereas for left-sided tumors it is lateral to the aorta (para-aortic). Other frequent sites of metastases include the left supraclavicular lymph nodes and the lungs. Standard initial metastatic evaluation should include a CT scan of the abdomen and pelvis and chest radiography. Enlarged lymph nodes (>1–2 cm) in the primary lymphatic drainage areas (landing zones) of the affected side are involved by metastatic disease in approximately 70% of cases. CT imaging of the chest is required if mediastinal, hilar, or lung parenchymal disease is suspected. Serum tumor markers should be measured before orchiectomy and should include human β-chorionic gonadotropin (β-hCG), α-fetoprotein (AFP), and the less specific marker, lactate dehydrogenase.

Treatment

All suspected testicular tumors should be treated with a radical orchiectomy through an inguinal approach and early, high ligation of the spermatic cord. β-hCG and AFP are relatively specific tumor markers for testicular cancer. They have substantially improved the ability to monitor the disease and to intervene early in the event of recurrence. They, along with lactate dehydrogenase, should be measured before orchiectomy. AFP production is restricted to NSGCTs, specifically tumors that contain at least a component of embryonal carcinoma or yolk sac tumor. Patients with an increased AFP and pure seminoma on pathologic examination of the orchiectomy specimen are still considered to have an NSGCT. Increased serum β-hCG can occur with seminomatous and nonseminomatous tumors. Increased concentrations of β-hCG are seen in 40% to 60% of patients with metastatic NSGCT and in 15% to 20% of patients with metastatic seminomas. Lactate dehydrogenase is less specific but has independent prognostic value in patients with advanced germ cell tumors. Serum lactate dehydrogenase is increased in approximately 60% of patients with NSGCT and in 80% of those with seminomatous germ cell tumors.

Persistently elevated concentrations of AFP and β-hCG, even in the absence of radiographic or clinical findings, implies active disease and is sufficient cause to initiate systemic therapy, provided that false-positive elevations have been ruled out. The serum half-life of β-hCG is 5 to 7 days, and that for AFP is 30 hours. A slow decrease in serum levels after orchiectomy also implies metastatic disease.

Seminoma is the most common histologic form of germ cell tumor and generally carries a better prognosis than other variants. Standard therapy for low-stage (T1, 2a, or 2b) disease is orchiectomy followed by active surveillance, chemotherapy, or radiation therapy to the retroperitoneal and possibly the ipsilateral pelvic lymph nodes, depending on clinical stage and patient preference. Relapse is relatively rare, occurring in 4% of patients with stage 1 and 10% of patients with stage 2 disease. Relapses can be salvaged in more than 90% of cases by systemic chemotherapy. The long-term cure rate for low-stage seminoma is approximately 99%.

NSGCTs include embryonal cell carcinomas, choriocarcinomas, yolk sac carcinomas, teratomas, and mixed germ cell tumors. As with pure seminoma, the cure rate is high (>95%) in patients with stage 1 disease. Retroperitoneal lymphatic metastases may be found in 20% of patients who have no lymphatic or vascular invasion or invasion into the tunica albuginea, spermatic cord, or scrotum at the time of orchiectomy, even if CT scans are negative for lymphadenopathy. There are two options for low-stage NSGCT after orchiectomy in the absence of radiographic evidence of lymphadenopathy and with normalized serum tumor markers: surveillance and nerve-sparing retroperitoneal lymph node dissection (RPLND). Patients with clinical stage 1 disease but embryonal histology or the presence of lymphovascular invasion or extension beyond the tunica albuginea have a higher risk of relapse (>30%) with surveillance and should be considered for primary RPLND.

Although RPLND is a major abdominal operation, it offers the best way to control disease within the retroperitoneum. Lymph nodes are removed from the level of the renal hilum caudad to the level of the aortic bifurcation. The lateral margins are the ureters. Historically, this operation was associated with loss of ejaculatory function due to ligation of the sympathetic nerve fibers in the region. With modern, nerve-sparing techniques, ejaculatory function can be preserved in more than 95% of patients. Patients with persistently elevated AFP or β-hCG after orchiectomy most likely have metastatic disease, even in the absence of radiographically detectable lesions. These patients usually should go on to systemic chemotherapy first, rather than RPLND.

Clinical stage 2 NSGCTs can be managed by either RPLND or primary chemotherapy, depending on several factors. Those patients who are without marker elevation, are asymptomatic, and have small-volume retroperitoneal-only disease can be offered primary RPLND. Those with persistently elevated tumor markers, symptomatic disease, or more bulky retroperitoneal disease usually undergo systemic chemotherapy. Local recurrence in the retroperitoneum after a properly performed RPLND is rare (<10%).

Adjuvant chemotherapy after RPLND should be considered if any lymph node is more than 2 cm in diameter, if six or more nodes are involved, or if there is extranodal invasion. Cure rates are not different in those who do or do not receive adjuvant chemotherapy, but the former group require fewer cycles of chemotherapy and fewer additional surgeries.

Approximately one third of patients require up-front chemotherapy. Those patients with clinical stage 2c disease (or higher), primary retroperitoneal germ cell tumor, or mediastinal seminomas treated with radiation therapy should all undergo systemic, cisplatin-based, multiagent chemotherapy.

Postchemotherapy RPLND for seminoma is typically reserved for patients with residual masses more than 3 cm in size and/or a positive PET scan. For NSGCT, this issue is more controversial. Some groups reserve this treatment for patients who do not have substantial tumor shrinkage (>90% shrinkage of retroperitoneal nodes and no residual nodes >1.5 cm) and for those with teratomatous elements in the primary tumor. Others advocate surgery for all patients with initial bulky retroperitoneal disease, regardless of the response to chemotherapy. All agree that a clear residual mass after chemotherapy in the setting of NSGCT warrants a postchemotherapy RPLND.

The first successful combination chemotherapy regimens for testicular cancer included cisplatin, vinblastine, and bleomycin (Blenoxane) and resulted in complete remission in 70% to 80% of patients with metastatic disease. Studies have shown that prolonged maintenance chemotherapy is unnecessary, and etoposide (VePesid) has largely replaced vinblastine (because it is less toxic and probably more efficacious). Serious adverse effects of chemotherapy include neuromuscular toxic affects, myelosuppression, bleomycin-induced pulmonary fibrosis, Raynaud's phenomenon, and secondary malignancy.

Leydig cell tumors are generally benign tumors that make up between 1% and 3% of all testicular tumors. The majority of cases occurs in men aged 20 to 60 years old, although roughly one fourth are diagnosed before puberty. After radical orchiectomy, the prognosis is usually good, with recurrences rarely reported.

Gonadoblastoma is a rare tumor that occurs almost exclusively in patients with a history of gonadal dysgenesis. They account for fewer than 1% of all testicular neoplasms and can occur at any age from infancy to beyond 70 years, although most patients are diagnosed before age 30. Initial management is with radical orchiectomy. Because of a 50% incidence of bilateral disease, a contralateral gonadectomy is generally warranted. The prognosis after orchiectomy is usually excellent.

Lymphoma is the most common secondary neoplasm of the testicle and the most common testicular neoplasm in men older than 50 years of age, with a median age at presentation of 60 years. Although survival is often poor for patients with bilateral disease and those presenting with lymphoma at other sites who later experience a testicular relapse, the prognosis is substantially better for patients presenting with primary testicular lymphoma confined to the testicle.

Disclaimer

The views expressed in this article are those of the author and do not reflect the official policy or position of the United States Army, the Department of Defense, or the U.S. government.

References

Barocas DA, Clark PE. Bladder cancer. Curr Opin Oncol 2008;20:307–14.
Damber JE, Aus G. Prostate cancer. Lancet 2008;371:1710–21.
Flechon A, Rivoire M, Droz JP. Management of advanced germ-cell tumors of the testis. Nat Clin Pract Urol 2008;5:262–76.
Jemal A, Siegel R, Ward E, et al. Cancer statistics, 2008. CA Cancer J Clin 2008;58:71–96.
Rini BI, Rathmell WK, Godley P. Renal cell carcinoma. Curr Opin Oncol 2008;20:300–6.

PRIMARY GLOMERULAR DISEASES

Method of
Manuel Praga, MD; and Enrique Morales, MD

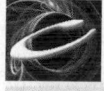

CURRENT DIAGNOSIS

- Clinical presentations of glomerular diseases range from asymptomatic urinary abnormalities (proteinuria, microhematuria) to severe forms of rapidly progressive glomerulonephritis (gross hematuria, edema, acute renal function worsening, hypertension).
- Secondary causes of glomerular disease should be excluded by means of history, physical examination, and appropriate laboratory tests.
- Renal biopsy establishes the diagnosis and classification of primary glomerular diseases.

CURRENT THERAPY

- Appropriate treatment should be instituted as early as possible.
- Blood pressure should be lower than 130/80 mm Hg (<125/75 mm Hg in patients with proteinuria >1 g/24 h).
- Angiotensin-converting enzyme inhibitors and angiotensin receptor blockers are indicated in most cases of chronic proteinuric glomerular diseases due to their antiproteinuric, antihypertensive, and renoprotective effects.
- Specific therapy of primary glomerular diseases includes steroids, anticalcineurinic agents, and cytotoxics. Due to the potential risks of these therapies, the likelihood of progression and the presence of chronic irreversible parenchymal damage must be carefully assessed.
- Primary or idiopathic glomerular diseases comprise a wide variety of glomerular histologic lesions, with different clinical presentations and variable prognosis. Although some entities portend a favorable long-term prognosis, a considerable fraction of untreated patients who have other glomerular entities reach end-stage renal failure.

Clinical Presentation and Diagnosis

The clinical manifestations of primary glomerular diseases are very variable, ranging from asymptomatic urinary abnormalities to severe forms of rapidly progressive glomerulonephritis. The different clinical presentations are summarized and defined in Box 1.

Most milder forms of glomerular diseases are diagnosed by a positive dipstick test for microhematuria or proteinuria. All these patients should have quantitative estimations of proteinuria (24-hour proteinuria or protein-to-creatinine ratio in a random sample of urine), urinary microscopic examination, and serum creatinine. Glomerular disorders can be the renal manifestation of systemic diseases of different causes (e.g., malignancies, infections, autoimmune disorders), as discussed later. Therefore, medical history and physical examination should carefully investigate data suggesting such diseases. In addition to general laboratory analysis and assessment of renal morphology (renal echography), more specific determinations should be performed in all patients with suspected glomerular diseases: protein electrophoresis, serum levels of immunoglobulins, serum complement fractions C3 and C4, antinuclear antibody (ANA), anti-DNA antibodies, antineutrophilic cytoplasmic antibodies (ANCA), and tests for hepatitis B virus (HBV), hepatitis C virus (HCV), and HIV infections.

Renal biopsy is the conclusive method for establishing the diagnosis and classification of primary glomerular disorders. Indications for renal biopsy include the nephrotic syndrome in adults (except cases attributed to diabetic nephropathy) and steroid-resistant nephrotic syndrome in children, rapidly progressive nephritis, persistent nephritic syndrome with deteriorating renal function, and, usually, recurrent macroscopic hematuria. The need for renal biopsy in patients with asymptomatic urinary abnormalities should be individualized. The most characteristic pathologic findings of the main primary glomerulonephritis are summarized in Box 2, and their commonest clinical presentations are summarized in Box 3.

Treatment

Conservative Therapy

Hypertension is a common finding in patients with primary glomerulonephritis. Current guidelines recommend blood pressure targets lower than 130/80 mm Hg in these patients and lower than 125/75 mm Hg in patients with proteinuria greater

Box 1   Clinical Presentations of Glomerular Diseases

Nephrotic Syndrome
- Proteinuria >3.5 g/d in adults and >40 mg/h/m^2 in children
- Hypoalbuminemia
- Hyperlipidemia
- Edema

Nephritic Syndrome
- Hypertension
- Oliguria
- Edema
- Hematuria (usually macroscopic)
- Red cell casts
- Non-nephrotic proteinuria
- Mild and nonprogressive GFR decrease

Rapidly Progressive Glomerulonephritis
- Acute or subacute progressive worsening of renal function
- Hematuria (usually macroscopic)
- Red cell casts
- Proteinuria (usually <3.5 g/d)
- Blood pressure often normal

Persistent Asymptomatic Urinary Abnormalities
- Non-nephrotic proteinuria (<3.5 g/d in adults and <40 mg/h/m^2 in children)
- Persistent microscopic hematuria

Recurrent Macroscopic Hematuria
- Bouts of gross hematuria, usually triggered by infections
- Persistent microhematuria between the episodes of gross hematuria

Chronic Renal Insufficiency
- Persistent proteinuria and/or microhematuria
- Hypertension
- Small kidneys

Hypocomplementemia
The C3 and C4 fractions of serum complement are characteristically reduced in some types of glomerular diseases. This is an important clue for diagnosis.

Abbreviation: GFR = glomerular filtration rate.

Box 2   Main Histologic Findings of Primary Glomerular Diseases

Minimal Change Disease
- Normal glomeruli on light microscopy
- Negative immunofluorescence and diffuse effacement of epithelial foot processes on electron microscopy

Focal and Segmental Glomerulosclerosis
- Focal (some glomeruli) and segmental (parts of affected glomeruli) scarring of the glomerular tuft

Membranous Nephropathy
- Thickening of glomerular capillary walls with projections of glomerular basement membrane ("spikes")
- Subepithelial immune deposits detected by immunofluorescence and electron microscopy

Membranoproliferative Glomerulonephritis
- Increase of mesangial cells and mesangial matrix
- Widening (double contoured appearance) of capillary loops
- IgG, C3, and IgM on immunofluorescence and subendothelial (type I) or intra-GBM (type II) deposits on electron microscopy

IgA Nephropathy
- Predominant deposition of mesangial IgA on immunofluorescence
- Proliferation of mesangial cellularity and mesangial matrix on light microscopy
- Mesangial electron-dense deposits on electron microscopy

Acute Postinfectious (Diffuse Proliferative) Glomerulonephritis
- Marked hypercellularity due to mesangial and endothelial cell proliferation and glomerular influx of neutrophils
- Hump-like subepithelial dense deposits on electron microscopy

Crescentic Glomerulonephritis
- Cellular or fibrocellular crescents in a variable percentage of glomeruli
- Immunofluorescence pattern distinguishes the main three types:
  - Type I: Linear IgG staining of the GBM (anti-GBM disease)
  - Type II: Granular deposits along GBM (immune complex deposition)
  - Type III: Negative immunofluorescence (pauci-immune glomerulonephritis)

Abbreviations: GBM = glomerular basement membrane; Ig = immunoglobulin.

---

than 1 g/24 hours. Any antihypertensive drug or drug combinations are useful, and they should be selected on the basis of the patient's characteristics. However, blockade of the renin-angiotensin system either with an angiotensin-converting enzyme inhibitor (ACEI) or an angiotensin receptor blocker (ARB) should be the main basis of antihypertensive treatment because of their demonstrated renoprotective effect (slowing or preventing loss of renal function) in patients with chronic renal diseases. The beneficial effects of ACEIs and ARBs appear to be similar and are also observed in proteinuric patients with normal blood pressure. Renal protection induced by ACEIs and ARBs is closely related to the significant reduction in proteinuria that these agents induce. The level of proteinuria is the best way to monitor the efficacy of ACEIs and ARBs. Aldosterone antagonists (spironolactone, eplerenone) have also shown a remarkable antiproteinuric efficacy. Nevertheless, serum creatinine and potassium should be monitored after ACEI, ARB, or antialdosteronic agents are initiated, particularly in patients with reduced renal function.

Hyperlipidemia is a common finding in patients with glomerular diseases, particularly in those with the nephrotic syndrome. Prospective clinical studies have demonstrated that treatment of hyperlipidemia decreases proteinuria and prevents renal function loss. Statins such as atorvastatin (Lipitor) (10–40 mg after the evening meal) are the most commonly used lipid-lowering drugs. A level of LDL cholesterol lower than 100 mg/dL is recommended.

Weight loss in obese patients induces a significant reduction in proteinuria, and smoking should be strictly forbidden, because smoking is associated with a more rapid progression toward renal failure in any type of renal disease.

All these measures (blood pressure lowering, treatment with ACEIs or ARBs, treatment of hyperlipidemia, weight loss, cessation of smoking) are also beneficial for the global cardiovascular risk that is significantly higher in proteinuric patients (mainly in those with renal insufficiency) than in the normal population.

The complications of the nephrotic syndrome require specific treatment. Edema is usually managed with a low-sodium diet plus furosemide (Lasix) in doses carefully adjusted to the severity of edema. Daily weight measurement is very important, because excessive diuretic doses can lead to volume depletion and functional worsening of renal function. In resistant cases, combinations of different types of diuretics (furosemide plus a thiazide diuretic, or furosemide plus a potassium-sparing diuretic such as spironolactone [Aldactone] in patients with hypokalemia) are needed. More severe cases require albumin infusions followed by high-dose intravenous furosemide (although intravenous

Box 3 — Commonest Presentations of the Main Primary Glomerular Diseases

Minimal Change Disease
- Nephrotic syndrome

Focal and Segmental Glomerulosclerosis
- Nephrotic syndrome in more than two thirds of patients
- Non-nephrotic proteinuria in the remaining patients
- Renal insufficiency (20%–40%), hypertension (50%), and microhematuria (40%)

Membranous Nephropathy
- Nephrotic syndrome in >80% of patients
- Non-nephrotic proteinuria in the remaining patients

Membranoproliferative Glomerulonephritis
- Nephrotic syndrome in 50%
- Nephritic syndrome in 20%–30%
- Asymptomatic urinary abnormalities in 20%–30%
- Hypocomplementemia is common.

IgA Nephropathy
- Asymptomatic urinary abnormalities (microhematuria ± proteinuria) in >75%
- Intercalated recurrent or isolated episodes of macroscopic hematuria in >40%
- Nephritic or nephrotic syndrome in <10%

Acute Postinfectious Glomerulonephritis
- Nephritic syndrome
- Hypocomplementemia

Crescentic Glomerulonephritis
- Rapidly progressive glomerulonephritis

Abbreviation: Ig = immunoglobulin.

---

albumin [Albuminar][1] increases proteinuria) or even removal of fluids by hemodialysis. Nephrotic patients are at increasing risk for thrombotic events. Prophylactic treatment (subcutaneous low-molecular-weight heparin) is indicated in conditions of high risk, such as immobilization.

Specific Therapy
Box 4 summarizes the immunosuppressive treatment of primary glomerular diseases.

Minimal Change Disease
Minimal change disease (MCD) is most common in children but also causes 10% to 15% of nephrotic syndrome in adults. Corticosteroid therapy is a very effective treatment for MCD. For children, the dose of prednisone is 60 mg/m^2/day and for adults 1 mg/kg/day (up to 80 mg/day). About 75% of patients respond (complete proteinuria disappearance) within 2 weeks, and more than 90% respond within 8 weeks, but adults show in general a slower response than children. Initial steroid dose is continued for 4 weeks and then changed to alternate-day prednisone (40 mg/m^2 on alternate days) or to daily prednisone, slowly tapering off over 6 to 10 weeks. Keeping patients on steroids for more than 3 months is associated with a lower 1-year relapse rate.

Up to 75% of children and many adults have nephrotic syndrome relapses. Isolated relapses are re-treated with steroids as in the first episode. Frequent relapsers (two or more relapses within a 6-month period) are treated with a low-dose steroid course plus cyclophosphamide (Cytoxan) (1.5–2 mg/kg/day) or chlorambucil (Leukeran)[1] (0.1–0.2 mg/kg/day) in an 8-week course. After these short-term cytotoxic courses, a considerable fraction of patients remain free of proteinuria for prolonged periods, with a low rate

[1]Not FDA approved for this indication.

Box 4 — Immunosuppressive Treatment of Primary Glomerular Disease

Minimal Change Disease
First Line
- Steroids

Second Line
- Cytotoxics (frequent relapsers)
- Anticalcineurinics or mycophenolate mofetil (CellCept)[1] (steroid-dependent)

Focal Segmental Glomerulosclerosis
First Line
- Steroids
- ACEIs
- ARBs

Second Line
- Anticalcineurinics
- Mycophenolate mofetil[1]
- Rituximab (steroid dependent)

Membranous Nephropathy
First Line
- Anticalcineurinics
- Steroids plus cytotoxics
- ACEIs
- ARBs

Second Line
- Mycophenolate mofetil
- Intramuscular ACTH (Synacthen)[1,2]
- Rituximab (Rituxan)[1]

Membranoproliferative Glomerulonephritis
- Steroids
- ACEIs
- ARBs

IgA Nephropathy
First Line
- ACEIs
- ARBs

Second Line
- Steroids
- Fish oil

Acute Postinfectious Glomerulonephritis
- Conservative therapy

Crescentic Glomerulonephritis
Type I (anti-GBM)
- Steroids
- Cyclophosphamide (Cytoxan)[1]
- Plasmapheresis

Type II and III Induction
- Steroids
- Cyclophosphamide[1]
- Plasmapheresis in severe acute renal failure
- Rituximab in ANCA-positive type III crescentic GN

Maintenance
- Low-dose steroids
- Azathioprine (Imuran)[1]

[1]Not FDA approved for this indication.
[2]Not available in the United States.

Abbreviations: ACEI = angiotensin-converting enzyme inhibitor; ACTH = adrenocorticotropic hormone; ARB = angiotensin receptor blocker; GBM = glomerular basement membrane; Ig = immunoglobulin.

of serious complications. Longer or repeated courses can induce severe side effects and are not recommended.

The response of steroid-dependent patients (reappearance of the nephrotic syndrome during or immediately after steroid withdrawal) to cytotoxics is poorer than that of frequent relapsers. Steroid-dependent patients and frequent relapsers unresponsive to cytotoxics are commonly treated with cyclosporine (Neoral)[1] given in an initial dose of 3 to 4 mg/kg in two divided doses, then adjusting for serum levels of 100–175 ng/mL. Most steroid-dependent patients transform into cyclosporine-dependent, and the risk of cyclosporine-induced nephrotoxicity should be considered. Mycophenolate mofetil (MMF, CellCept)[1] (600 mg/m^2/12 h in children, 500–1000 mg/12 h in adults) is a very useful alternative. Rates of response and relapse are similar to those of cyclosporine, but tolerance is better and there is no risk of nephrotoxicity. Therapy with cyclosporine or MMF if the patient responds is continued for up to 12 months before slow and careful tapering. Rituximab[1] (four weekly intravenous doses of 375 mg/m^2) has been used in some patients with steroid-dependent nephrotic syndrome and frequent relapsers, inducing a significant decrease in the number of relapses in many of them. However, randomized controlled trials or observational studies with longer follow-up are needed.

Less than 10% of MCD patients are steroid resistant. Because most of them subsequently have focal segmental glomerulosclerosis (FSGS) on biopsy, their therapeutic approach is the same as for FSGS.

Focal and Segmental Glomerulosclerosis

Causes of secondary FSGS (obesity, reflux nephropathy, reduction in renal mass) should be carefully excluded. Treatment with an ACEI or ARB is the first option in patients with non-nephrotic proteinuria or in patients with nonaggressive nephrotic syndrome (proteinuria <5 g/day, serum albumin >3 g/dL, normal renal function), mainly if hypertension coexists. Patients with severe nephrotic syndrome or nephrotic proteinuria after ACEI or ARB introduction should be treated with prednisone 1 mg/kg/day. Several retrospective studies have shown that steroid treatment maintained for at least 6 months is followed by more than 50% partial or complete remissions. However, in responsive patients, proteinuria starts to decrease after 2 to 3 months of treatment.

If proteinuria did not show significant changes within this period, introduction of an anticalcineurinic agent together with steroid tapering is recommended. Cyclosporine (doses and blood levels as in MCD) has been the most commonly used drug, and prospective studies have shown more than 70% partial or complete remission after 6 months of treatment. Tacrolimus (Prograf)[1] (0.05–0.10 mg/kg/day in two divided doses, then adjusted for serum levels of 4–7 ng/mL) is proved to be effective in some cyclosporine-resistant FSGS cases.

In patients with complete or partial response to cyclosporine or tacrolimus, these drugs should be maintained at the lowest effective doses for at least 1 year before slowly tapering off. In some patients resistant to steroids and cyclosporine, or in those with mild degrees of renal insufficiency, MMF[1] (same doses as in MCD) has decreased proteinuria and stabilized renal function for prolonged periods in some patients, but there are no prospective controlled studies. Sirolimus (Rapamune)[1] has induced complete (19%) or partial (38%) remission in a series of patients, although other studies have failed to confirm these beneficial effects and have shown a remarkable number of serious side effects.

About 20% to 25% of children with aggressive forms of FSGS have mutations in the genes coding for several podocyte proteins, mainly podocin. Most of these patients are unresponsive to any kind of treatment.

Membranous Nephropathy

More than one third of MGN patients have a spontaneous remission, and most remissions take place during the first 2 years of the disease. Conservative therapy should be maintained during the first 9 to 12 months, unless renal function starts to deteriorate.

ACEIs or ARBs, or both, can induce partial remission (non-nephrotic proteinuria) in a considerable percentage of cases.

In patients with an aggressive presentation (massive nephrotic syndrome and deteriorating renal function) a 6-month course of alternating monthly prednisone 0.5 mg/kg/day with a month of chlorambucil[1] 0.2 mg/kg/day or cyclophosphamide[1] 2 mg/kg/day is recommended. Other clinicians simultaneously use prednisone starting with 1 mg/kg/day and tapering off over 6 months plus chlorambucil or cyclophosphamide for 14 weeks.

In patients maintaining normal renal function and persistent nephrotic proteinuria beyond 9 to 12 months, immunosuppressive therapy should be initiated, mainly in the presence of markers of poor outcome, which include male gender, older age, and proteinuria persistently higher than 8 g/day after ACEI or ARB treatment. Alternating prednisone and chlorambucil (as indicated earlier), prednisone and cyclophosphamide, and cyclosporine[1] 3–4 mg/kg/day, targeting blood levels of 100–175 ng/mL are beneficial, inducing complete or partial remission in most patients.

Side effects (diabetes, bone necrosis, infections) are more serious with steroids plus cytotoxic treatments; trimethoprim-sulfamethoxazole (TMP-SMX, Bactrim) (80 mg/400 mg/day) should be concurrently administered for *Pneumocystis jirovecii* prophylaxis. Cyclosporine, administered for 6 months, is followed by approximately 50% of recurrences after drug withdrawal.

No studies comparing anticalcineurinic and cytotoxics have been published for MGN. Tacrolimus,[1] another anticalcineurinic agent, can also induce partial response in more than 80% of treated patients, although recurrence after withdrawal is the same (50%) as with cyclosporine. A recent randomized pilot trial reported that tetracosactide (Synacthen),[1,2] an analogue of ACTH (1 mg IM twice a week for 1 year) induced remissions in the same percentage as a regimen of steroids plus cyclophosphamide.

Uncontrolled studies reported that MMF[1] (1000–2000 mg/day) reduced proteinuria and stabilized renal function in some MGN patients unresponsive to other therapies. Rituximab (Rituxan),[1] a monoclonal antibody against CD20-lymphocytes, has induced complete (15%–20%) or partial (35%–40%) remission in several series of patients, although no prospective controlled studies have been published. On the other hand, rituximab has been effective to avoid nephrotic syndrome relapse after tacrolimus withdrawal in patients successfully treated with this drug but showing anticalcineurin dependence.

Membranoproliferative Glomerulonephritis

The incidence of idiopathic membranoproliferative glomerulonephritis (MPGN) has progressively decreased over the last decades, being currently an uncommon disease in developed countries. Most cases of MPGN are now secondary to HCV infection and concurrent cryoglobulinemia. No prospective studies about the treatment of idiopathic MPGN have been carried out in the last several years. Uncontrolled series of patients suggested that prolonged (>2 years) prednisone treatment is beneficial in terms of proteinuria reduction and renal survival. Prospective randomized trials with aspirin[1] and dipyridamole (Persantine)[1] showed a significant reduction in proteinuria some decades ago, but later analysis did not demonstrate long-term benefits on renal survival.

Conservative therapy, including ACEIs and ARBs, should be prescribed in all cases. In patients with the nephrotic syndrome after an observation period or in those with more aggressive presentations (deteriorating renal function, crescents), a 6- to 12-month course of prednisone could be indicated. Some small series of patients suggested that cyclophosphamide[1] is effective in aggressive cases of MPGN, but conclusive evidence is lacking.

MMF has been suggested as a possible therapeutic alternative, based on some observational studies. In MPGN with isolated deposits of C2 on immunofluorescence (so-called C3 glomerulopathy), a dysregulation in the complement system has been demonstrated, and eculizumab, a specific inhibitor of the complement system, has been effective in some cases.

---

[1]Not FDA approved for this indication.

---

[1]Not FDA approved for this indication.
[2]Not available in the United States.

Immunoglobulin A Nephropathy

As in all types of primary glomerular diseases, the aggressiveness of therapeutic approaches in patients with immunoglobulin A (IgA) nephropathy should be graded according to the severity of the presentation. In patients with microhematuria and normal renal function, only regular follow-up is required. If slowly increasing proteinuria appears, an ACEI or ARB, or a combination of both drugs, should be started, even in the absence of hypertension, targeting for proteinuria less than 1 g/day and blood pressure lower than 125/75 mm Hg.

In patients with increasing proteinuria greater than 1–1.5 g/day in spite of these measures, other therapies should be contemplated. Steroids were proven to be beneficial in patients with normal renal function and proteinuria greater than 1 g/day in a prospective randomized trial: methylprednisolone (Solu-Medrol) pulses, 1 g/day for 3 days in the beginning of months 1, 3, and 5, and oral prednisone 0.5 mg/kg every other day for 6 months reduced proteinuria and increased renal survival in comparison with untreated patients.

Treatment with fish oil supplements[1] in this type of patient remains controversial. Although eicosapentaenoic acid (1.8 g/day) or docosahexaenoic acid (1.2 g/day) demonstrated beneficial effects in some trials, these effects were not reproduced in others.

In patients with more aggressive presentations (proteinuria and deteriorating renal function), a prospective trial demonstrated that prednisone 40 mg/day tapering to 10 mg/day within 2 years plus cyclophosphamide[1] 1.5 mg/kg/day for 3 months followed by azathioprine (Imuran)[1] 1.5 mg/kg/day for at least 2 years significantly improved renal survival in comparison with untreated patients.

MMF (1000–2000 mg/day) has been tested by means of several randomized controlled trials in IgA nephropathy, obtaining disparate results. Although some studies suggested a positive influence, others have failed to confirm these results.

Acute Postinfectious (Diffuse Proliferative) Glomerulonephritis

As in MPGN, the incidence of diffuse proliferative glomerulonephritis has drastically decreased in recent years in developed countries. The prognosis is generally good, and signs and symptoms of the disease (nephritic syndrome) resolve sporadically within 2 to 6 weeks in a great majority of cases. Treatment should be focused on adequate control of blood pressure, salt restriction, and diuretics to prevent fluid excess and the risks of cardiac failure. The triggering infection should be investigated and treated if it has not disappeared spontaneously.

Some patients present with more aggressive courses, developing progressive renal insufficiency. In these cases, crescents involving a large proportion of glomeruli can be observed in a second biopsy. No controlled studies have been carried out in these aggressive cases, but some series of patients recommend high-dose intravenous pulse steroid, followed by oral prednisone 1 mg/kg/day, tapering off over 2 to 3 months. There is no evidence that more aggressive immunosuppressive therapy is beneficial.

Crescentic Glomerulonephritis

Treatment of crescentic glomerulonephritis (CGN) should be promptly instituted because of the rapid transformation of cellular crescents into irreversible fibrotic crescents that collapse the glomerular tufts. Prognosis of type I (anti-GBM disease) CGN is poorer than that of types II and III, particularly in the presence of oligoanuria, dialysis requirement, or a large fraction of glomeruli with crescents.

Treatment of type I CGN includes steroids, cyclophosphamide,[1] and plasmapheresis. Pulse intravenous methylprednisolone (500–1000 mg daily for 3–4 days) is followed by oral prednisone (1 mg/kg/day for 3–4 weeks, then slowly tapering off over 6 months). Oral cyclophosphamide (2 mg/kg/day) is usually maintained for 2 to 3 months. Plasmapheresis (daily or alternate-day 4-liter exchanges) using albumin as replacement fluid or fresh frozen plasma if bleeding risk is high, is usually performed for 2 to 3 weeks.

---

[1]Not FDA approved for this indication.

The duration of plasmapheresis, as well as the intensity and the duration of immunosuppressive therapy, should be guided by the clinical status and the titers of anti-GBM antibodies. In patients without pulmonary hemorrhage and with very advanced renal involvement (massive presence of glomerular fibrotic crescents), aggressive immunosuppression is not indicated.

The precise etiology of type II CGN (e.g., systemic lupus erythematosus, cryoglobulinemia) should be identified and the therapy guided by the diagnosis. If no apparent diagnosis is available, treatment is similar to that for type III (pauci-immune) CGN.

Induction treatment of type III CGN consists of steroids (oral prednisone, 1 mg/kg/day for 3–4 weeks, slowly tapered to a maintenance dose of 10–20 mg), and intravenous monthly pulses of cyclophosphamide (initial dose 0.5 to 1 g/m^2, adjusted for renal function and age), which has proved to be as effective and less toxic than oral administration. Once remission is achieved (recovery of renal function, absence of extrarenal symptoms), usually within 3 to 6 months, cyclophosphamide is replaced by azathioprine[1] 1 to 2 mg/kg/day for 12 to 18 months plus prednisone 5 to 10 mg daily or every other day. Positive titers of ANCA, particularly p-ANCA, can indicate more prolonged, low-dose, maintenance treatment, because the risk of recurrence is high. Plasmapheresis (similar to that in type I CGN) is proven to add benefits in type III CGN manifesting with severe renal failure. In two recent trials, rituximab (375 mg/m^2 per week for 4 weeks) was as effective as cyclophosphamide as induction therapy in ANCA-positive vasculitis. Interestingly, rituximab was more effective than cyclophosphamide in relapsing cases. Although not tested in prospective trials, MMF[1] (1500–3000 mg/day) has been shown effective and well tolerated, even as induction therapy in some series of patients.

---

[1]Not FDA approved for this indication.

References

Cattran DC, Alexopoulos E, Heering P, et al. Cyclosporin in idiopathic glomerular disease associated with the nephrotic syndrome: workshop recommendations. Kidney Int 2007;72:1429–47.

Cattran DC, Appel GB, Hebert LA, et al. A randomized trial of cyclosporine in patients with steroid-resistant focal segmental glomerulosclerosis. Kidney Int 1999;56:2220–6.

Jayne D, Rasmussen N, Andrassy K, et al. A randomized trial of maintenance therapy for vasculitis associated with antineutrophil cytoplasmic autoantibodies. N Engl J Med 2003;349:36–44.

Polanco N, Gutierrez E, Covarsi A, et al. Spontaneous remission of nephrotic syndrome in idiopathic membranous nephropathy. J Am Soc Nephrol 2010;21:697–704.

Ponticelli C, Altieri P, Scolari F, et al. A randomized study comparing methylprednisolone plus chlorambucil versus methylprednisolone plus cyclophosphamide in idiopathic membranous nephropathy. J Am Soc Nephrol 1998;9:444–50.

Pozzi C, Bolasco PG, Fogazzi GB, et al. Corticosteroids in IgA nephropathy: A randomized controlled trial. Lancet 1999;13:883–7.

Praga M, Barrio V, Juarez FG, et al. Tacrolimus monotherapy in idiopathic membranous nephropathy: A randomized controlled trial. Kidney Int 2007;71:924–30.

Praga M, Gutiérrez E, González E, et al. Treatment of IgA nephropathy with ACE inhibitors: A randomized and controlled trial. J Am Soc Nephrol 2003;14:1578–83.

Sethi S, Fervenza FC. Membranoproliferative glomerulonephritis: A new look at an old entity. N Engl J Med 2012;366:1119–31.

PYELONEPHRITIS

Method of
Patricia D. Brown, MD

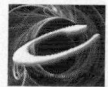

CURRENT DIAGNOSIS

- Abrupt onset of fever, flank pain, and costovertebral angle tenderness with or without symptoms of cystitis are classic presenting features.
- Patients with lower UTI symptoms or laboratory evidence of UTI accompanied by flank pain, fever, or signs of systemic toxicity such as GI complaints should be managed as having APN.

- Urinalysis with microscopic examination should be performed in all patients with suspected APN. Absence of pyuria is strong evidence against the diagnosis.
- A urine culture should be obtained in all patients with APN. Blood cultures should be obtained in those who are hospitalized.
- Patients should be categorized into those with uncomplicated and those with complicated infections.

Abbreviations: APN = acute pyelonephritis; GI = gastrointestinal; UTI = urinary tract infection.

CURRENT THERAPY

- Hospitalization is recommended for patients unable to tolerate oral intake, those with severe pain, and those with signs of severe sepsis. Hospitalization is generally recommended for patients with complicated infections and for all pregnant women.
- Parenteral regimens for hospitalized patients include an aminoglycoside, third-generation cephalosporin, or fluoroquinolone, with oral switch therapy selected on the basis of culture and susceptibility data.
- Initial empiric therapy for outpatients is a fluoroquinolone.
- Imaging is not recommended for patients with uncomplicated infections. Pre- and postcontrast computed tomographic scans should be obtained in those who fail to respond within 72 hours to appropriate antibiotic therapy.

Acute pyelonephritis (APN) is a urinary tract infection (UTI) that involves the renal parenchyma, also referred to as *upper tract UTI*. Most episodes of APN occur as a result of ascending infection from the bladder; patients with APN might or might not have symptoms of concomitant cystitis. Rarely, pyelonephritis occurs secondary to hematogenous seeding of the kidney as a result of infection elsewhere, most commonly endocarditis due to *Staphylococcus aureus* or disseminated fungal infection.

Epidemiology

Surprisingly little is known about the epidemiology of APN. Similar to cystitis, APN (and hospitalization for APN) is more common in women than men; men have been reported to have higher in-hospital mortality. In contrast to cystitis, risk factors for pyelonephritis are not well defined. One recent study of nonpregnant women 18 to 49 years of age found risk factors for APN included factors known to be risk factors for acute cystitis, including frequency of sexual intercourse, recent UTI, diabetes, and maternal UTI history. The incidence of bacteremia in patients with APN is reported to be 11% to 53% in various studies; risk factors for bacteremia are not well established. In a recent study, age greater than 65 years, vomiting, pulse greater than 110 beats per minute, segmented neutrophils greater than 90%, and pyuria with greater than 50 leukocytes per high-powered field were independent risk factors for bacteremia in women with uncomplicated APN.

Similar to lower UTI, APN can be further classified into complicated or uncomplicated infection. The factors that make an episode of APN a complicated UTI are outlined in Box 1.

Clinical Presentation

The classic presenting features of APN include abrupt onset of fever, flank pain, and costovertebral angle tenderness with or without symptoms of lower UTI including dysuria, urgency, and frequency. Unfortunately, there is no single constellation of signs or symptoms that is pathognomonic for APN. When localization studies have been performed on patients with symptoms of acute cystitis, 30% to 50% have been shown to have APN. Women who present with symptoms that have been present more than 7 days and those with a recent history of UTI are more likely to have APN. Flank pain is reported in approximately one half of patients

---

Box 1   Factors Associated with Complicated Pyelonephritis

- Diabetes
- Foreign body (catheter, stent)
- Health care–associated infections
- Immunocompromise
- Incomplete voiding (detrusor muscle dysfunction due to neurologic disease or medications)
- Infections due to multidrug-resistant pathogens
- Obstruction (including stones)
- Pregnancy
- Recent history of instrumentation
- Renal transplant recipient
- UTI in a male patient
- Vesicoureteral reflux

Abbreviation: UTI = urinary tract infection.

---

with APN but also occurs in almost 20% of patients with cystitis. Fever is present in one half of patients with APN, but less than 5% of patients with cystitis. Nausea, vomiting, and diarrhea occur commonly in patients with APN, and gastrointestinal (GI) symptoms can dominate the presenting complaints.

In general, patients who present with lower urinary tract symptoms or laboratory evidence of urinary tract infection accompanied by fever, flank pain or tenderness, or signs of systemic toxicity, such as GI symptoms, should be treated for APN.

The diagnosis can be particularly challenging in the frail elderly patient, because symptoms such as frequency, urgency, and incontinence are often chronic in this patient population and unrelated to active UTI. Change in mental status may be the only presenting complaint. Because the prevalence of bacteriuria in this patient population is high, particularly among those with chronic indwelling catheters, UTI must be a diagnosis of exclusion.

Acute pelvic inflammatory disease can have a presentation similar to APN. Pelvic examination should be performed on all sexually active women to exclude this diagnosis.

The differential diagnosis of APN is outlined in Box 2.

Diagnosis

Urinalysis, ideally with microscopic examination, using a clean-catch, midstream specimen, should be performed in all patients with suspected APN. Pyuria is a key finding in the diagnosis of UTI, and the absence of pyuria is strong evidence against a diagnosis of APN. Direct microscopic examination under high power of the urinary sediment from a centrifuged specimen should reveal more than 10 leukocytes per high-powered field. The presence of white blood cell (WBC) casts is highly specific for localization of the infection to the kidney, but it is inadequately sensitive to exclude the diagnosis of APN. The dipstick test for leukocyte esterase is used as a rapid screening test to detect significant pyuria; the sensitivity is reported to be 75% to 96%, with a specificity of 94% to 98%. Because of the

---

Box 2   Differential Diagnosis of Acute Pyelonephritis

- Appendicitis
- Cholecystitis
- Diverticulitis
- Gastroenteritis
- Herpes zoster
- Musculoskeletal pain, including vertebral disorders
- Ovarian cysts, tumors
- Pancreatitis
- Perforated viscus
- Pelvic inflammatory disease
- Pneumonia
- Renal stones, renal vein thrombosis, renal infarction

lower range of the reported sensitivity of the dipstick test, microscopic examination to exclude significant pyuria should be obtained in patients with suspected APN.

The presence of nitrite in the urine, detected by a dipstick test, has a reported sensitivity of 35% to 85% and a specificity of 92% to 100% for UTI. Microscopic examination of a Gram-stained, centrifuged urine specimen revealing at least one bacterium per oil-immersion field correlates with more than 10^5 colony-forming units (cfu)/mL of bacteria, with a sensitivity of 95%. Although this is the standard definition of significant bacteriuria, it has been shown that women with UTI can have levels of bacteriuria as low as 10^2 cfu/mL.

Although the microbiology of APN has remained predictable, significant changes in antimicrobial susceptibility patterns have occurred. Therefore, in contrast to recommendations for acute uncomplicated cystitis, a urine culture should be obtained in all patients with suspected APN. The need to obtain blood cultures has been debated, because blood cultures rarely yield a pathogen different from what was isolated from the urine. Bacteremia has been reported in 11% to 53% of patients hospitalized with APN. Bacteremic patients have a longer length of stay, and one recent report suggests that this is due to a longer time to resolution of fever. Many experts continue to recommend that blood cultures be obtained as part of the diagnostic evaluation of patients who are ill enough to require hospitalization; blood cultures are not necessary for those who will be managed as outpatients.

The role of diagnostic imaging in the management of APN is discussed later. In some cases with an atypical presentation, imaging may be helpful to confirm the diagnosis of APN. In this setting, pre- and postcontrast computed tomography (CT) is the imaging procedure of choice in adults.

Microbial Etiology

Most cases of APN are caused by *Escherichia coli*. Other enterobacteriaceae, including *Klebsiella* species and *Proteus* species, are also occasionally implicated. Other gram-negative pathogens such as *Pseudomonas*, *Serratia*, *Enterobacter*, and *Acinetobacter* should be considered in health care–associated infections. *Enterococcus* is an uncommon pathogen in community-acquired infections, but it must be considered in health care associated infections, including vancomycin resistant enterococci. Other gram-positive pathogens include *Streptoccocus agalactiae* and *Staphylococcus* species. Although a common cause of acute cystitis in young women, *Staphylococcus saprophyticus* is a rare cause of pyelonephritis; the finding of *Staphylococcus aureus* in a urine culture should always prompt a search for an extrarenal source of infection that might have served as a source of hematogenous seeding. A Gram stain of the urine is a simple and rapid test to exclude a gram-positive pathogen as the etiology of APN and guide the initial selection of empiric therapy.

The emergence of resistance to trimethoprim-sulfamethoxazole (TMP-SMX [Bactrim]) among *E. coli* has had a major impact on the approach to initial empiric antimicrobial therapy for APN. It is clear that the prevalence of resistance varies depending on geographic region, and clinicians often do not have access to meaningful local resistance data. Recent reports of increasing fluoroquinolone resistance among uropathogens are of great concern, although overall resistance rates in North America remain low. Also concerning is the increasing prevalence of extended-spectrum β-lactamase (ESBL) E.coli and Klebsiella species, although these are mainly a concern in health care-associated infections in the U.S. Risk factors for infection with ESBL producing organisms are poorly defined however recent infection or colonization with an ESBL producing organism should be considered a risk factor for this pathogen.

Treatment

The first decision in the management of patients with APN is whether or not the patient requires hospitalization. Although prospective randomized trials are lacking, several retrospective studies as well as several prospective nonrandomized trials suggest that outpatient management is safe for many patients. Hospitalization should be considered for patients who cannot tolerate oral intake or who have severe pain or signs of severe sepsis. A strategy of initial management in the emergency department or an observation unit with an initial dose of parenteral antibiotic therapy, intravenous fluids, and symptomatic treatment of nausea and pain may be used in select patients to avoid hospital admission. Patients who will be treated as outpatients should have a stable social situation and the ability to contact the physician and return promptly if their symptoms worsen. Hospitalization is generally recommended for patients with complicated infections. Most experts believe that pregnant women with APN should always be hospitalized.

There are surprisingly few prospective randomized trials of the treatment of pyelonephritis. For patients who require hospitalization, parenteral therapy with an aminoglycoside, a third-generation cephalosporin, or a fluoroquinolone is recommended. At my institution, we discourage fluoroquinolones for this indication because there are other effective alternatives and we wish to minimize the use of these very broad-spectrum agents in the hospital setting. Although resistance to TMP-SMX among uropathogenic *E. coli* appears to have leveled off and might actually be decreasing, this agent should not be used for empiric therapy of APN. If a ESBL-producing organism is suspected, empiric therapy should include a carbapenem.

If a gram-positive pathogen is suspected or suggested by the results of urine Gram stain, ampicillin or ampicillin-sulbactam (Unasyn) with or without an aminoglycoside can be used. Patients should receive intravenous therapy until they are clinically improving and able to reliably tolerate oral intake; oral therapy can be chosen based on the results of urine culture and susceptibility data. TMP-SMX, a fluoroquinolone, and ampicillin are all potential candidates for oral switch therapy. The narrowest spectrum, least expensive agent to which the isolated pathogen is susceptible should be chosen. Despite in vitro susceptibility data, first- and second-generation cephalosporins have a poor track record in the treatment of APN and are generally not recommended, with the exception of pyelonephritis in pregnancy.

Bacteremic patients might take longer to respond but do not require more prolonged parenteral therapy. The total duration of therapy for pyelonephritis is generally 14 days. Seven days of therapy with ciprofloxacin for uncomplicated APN has been shown to be effective as has 5 days of therapy with high-dose (750 mg daily) levofloxacin, and these regimens are endorsed by the current guidelines. Longer courses of therapy may be required for select patients with complicated pyelonephritis. For outpatients, initial empiric therapy with a fluoroquinolone is recommended, with adjustment of therapy, if needed, based on the results of urine culture. All of the currently available fluoroquinolones can be used, with the exception of moxifloxacin (Avelox), which does not achieve adequate levels in the urine. Although it is useful in the treatment of cystitis, norfloxacin (Noroxin) is not recommended for the treatment of APN because it does not achieve sustained tissue or serum levels. Suggested antimicrobial dosing regimens for APN are outlined in Box 3.

| **Box 3** | Antimicrobial Therapy for the Management of Acute Pyelonephritis |

Parenteral Regimens
- Ampicillin 2 g q4h–q6h
- Ampicillin-sulbactam (Unasyn) 3 g q6h
- Ceftriaxone (Rocephin) 2 g q24h
- Ciprofloxacin (Cipro) 400 mg q12h
- Gentamicin (Garamycin) 3–5 mg/kg q24h
- Levofloxacin (Levaquin) 500 mg q24h

Oral Regimens
- Amoxicillin 500 mg q8h
- Ciprofloxacin 500 mg q12h
- Ciprofloxacin XR 1000 mg q24h
- Levofloxacin 250 mg q24h
- Trimethoprim-sulfamethoxazole DS (Bactrim DS) 160/800 mg q12h

Imaging

Imaging is generally not needed in patients with uncomplicated APN. For patients with complicated infections (e.g., history of stones, prior renal surgery), renal ultrasound with abdominal plain films is considered an acceptable alternative to excretory urography. For patients with diabetes or other immunocompromise and for patients who fail to respond after 72 hours of appropriate antibiotic therapy, pre- and postcontrast CT is the imaging procedure of choice.

Follow-up

Most patients will respond to appropriate antibiotic therapy. Follow-up urine cultures to document microbiological response are not recommended in patients who have responded clinically.

References

Foxman B, Klemstine KL, Brown PD. Acute pyelonephritis in US hospitals in 1997: Hospitalization and in-hospital mortality. Ann Epidemiol 2003;13:144–50.

Gupta K, Hooton TN, Naber K, et al. International clinical practice guidelines for the treatment of acute uncomplicated cystitis and pyelonephritis in women: a 2010 update by The Infectious Diseases Society of America and the European Society for Microbiology and Infectious Diseases. Clin Infect Dis 2010;52:e103–20.

Kim KS, Kim K, Jo YH, et al. A simple model to predict bacteremia in women with acute pyelonephritis. J Infect 2011;63:124–30.

Pappas PG. Laboratory in the diagnosis and management of urinary tract infections. Med Clin North Am 1991;75:313–25.

Sandberg T, Skoog G, Hermansson AB, et al. Ciprofloxacin for 7 days versus 14 days in women with acute pyelonephritis: a randomised, open-label and double-blind, placebo-controlled, non-inferiority trial. Lancet 2012;380:484–90.

Sandler CM, Amis Jr ES, Bigongiari LR, et al. Imaging in acute pyelonephritis. American College of Radiology. ACR appropriateness criteria. Radiology 2000;215(Suppl):677–81.

Scholes D, Hooton TM, Roberts PL, et al. Risk factors associated with acute pyelonephritis in healthy women. Ann Intern Med 2005;142:20–7.

RENAL CALCULI

Method of
Michael E. Karellas, MD

According to the Urologic Diseases in America Project, a renal calculus will be diagnosed in approximately 13% of U.S. men and 7% of women during their lifetime. Moreover, up to 50% of these patients will experience a recurrent stone within 5 years of their original episode. Most stone patients have their first stone between the ages of 20 and 60 years of age, with peak incidence in the fourth to sixth decade of life. These ages coincide with the years of peak employment and productivity, which can be affected significantly by kidney stones. An employee with kidney stones files roughly $3500 more in medical claims than a coworker who does not have kidney stones. Overall, adjusted for 2012 levels, it is estimated that the U.S. health care system will spend approximately $3 billion dollars this year on direct medical costs associated with urinary stone disease.

Risk Factors

The risk of developing a stone depends on many factors including sex, fluid intake, diet, geographic location, obesity, and the presence of inflammatory bowel disease or other systemic medical conditions. Ethnic European men are more likely than Hispanic, Asian, or African American men to develop a stone. Patients who live in the southeastern United States have the highest rates of kidney stones when compared to residents of other regions, with the highest incidence of stones peaking 1 to 2 months after the hottest months of the year. Persons with occupations exposing them to continual high temperatures have been found to have an approximately eightfold increased rate of forming a kidney stone compared to other workers. Simply being adequately hydrated by increasing water intake has been shown to decrease stone recurrence rates by almost a third. Being obese also increases a person's chance to form kidney stones as, reflected by increased amounts urinary excretion of stone-forming elements (oxalate, uric acid). Patients with inflammatory bowel disease or with history of gastric bypass procedures also have an increased risk for stone formation.

Pathophysiology

Renal calculi are broadly classified into two major categories of calcareous (calcium containing) or noncalcareous stones based on the presence or absence of calcium. Calcareous stones account for approximately 80% of urinary calculi, with the most common stone composition being calcium oxalate (70%), followed by calcium phosphate (5% to 10%). Commonly occurring noncalcareous stones include struvite or infection stones (15% to 20%) uric acid (10%) and less-common cystine stones (1%). Calcareous stones are radiopaque on plain-film radiographic imaging, and noncalcareous calculi are radiolucent on these types of examinations but can be visualized by computed tomography (CT).

The process of stone formation starts when urine within the nephron becomes supersaturated with stone-forming salts that ultimately precipitate out of solution as crystals. This is a complex process, with interplay between the urinary solutes and stone inhibitors. Natural stone inhibitors such as citrate, Tamm–Horsfall glycoprotein, and nephrocalcin attempt to block this process, but once the concentration of stone-forming crystals reaches a certain threshold (concentration product), stone crystals can form. Small crystals are often unstable and can dissolve; however, if the supersaturated state exists along with low levels of citrate, then the stone crystals form by homogenous aggregation. Once formed, the crystal structure continues to grow through a process of heterogeneous aggregation by adsorption of other types of crystals or cellular debris.

Hypercalciuria (more than 200 mg per 24 hours) is the most common urinary abnormality associated with the formation of calcium stones. Increased urinary levels of calcium could be the result of increased intestinal absorption of calcium (absorptive), which is further subdivided into types I and II. Type I absorptive hypercalciuria occurs in approximately 55% of stone formers and is diagnosed with high urinary calcium (more than 200 mg per 24 hours) in the presence of a low-calcium diet (400 mg/day). This is in contrast to type II absorptive hypercalciuria, where the urinary calcium normalizes with a low-calcium diet. Other, less-common forms of hypercalciuria include increased calcium leakage from the kidney (renal hypercalciuria) or as a result of increased bone resorption from excess parathyroid hormone (primary hyperparathyroidism). Primary hyperparathyroidism is present in less than 5% of patients with stone disease, but it should be considered in any stone patient with serum calcium greater than 10mg/dL.

Hyperoxaluria (more than 45 mg per 24 hours) can also contribute to stone formation. Enteric hyperoxaluria is the most common reason for increased urinary oxalate and is found in patients with chronic diarrhea. Malabsorption of enteric fat leads to saponification of divalent cations (calcium and magnesium), leading to increased oxalate absorption. This is commonly seen in patients with short-bowel syndrome, following bariatric surgery, or resulting from inflammatory bowel disease. Increased dietary consumption of oxalate (nuts, chocolate, tea, rhubarb, broccoli, spinach) can also lead to hyperoxaluria. Primary hyperoxaluria is the result of an autosomal recessive inborn error of metabolism that can lead to early end-stage renal failure (by age 15 years) and death without a combined liver and kidney transplant. Lastly, a low level of the oxalate-degrading bacteria *Oxalobacter formigenes* has been shown to increase the risk of forming oxalate stones.

Hyperuricosuria (more than 600 mg per 24 hours) along with a urinary pH less than 5.5 is the cause of radiolucent uric acid stones. However, at a pH greater than 5.5, sodium urate promotes heterogeneous nucleation and the formation of calcium oxalate stones. High uric acid is often the result of a high-protein diet but it can also occur in patients with end-ileostomies, gout, or myeloproliferative diseases.

Struvite (infection) stones are composed of magnesium, ammonium, and calcium phosphate and are the leading cause of large stones that occupy the entire renal pelvis (staghorn calculi). These stones are caused by urea-splitting bacteria, which result in alkalization of the urine. The most common organisms associated with struvite stones are *Klebsiella pneumoniae, Proteus mirabilis,* and

Ureaplasma urealyticum. Failure to treat these stones carries an increased risk of renal damage, sepsis, and possibly death.

Cystinuria (more than 250 mg per 24 hours) leads to stone formation as a result of an autosomal recessive disorder of dibasic amino acid transport. Homozygous patients usually present with their first stone during childhood, which may be pure cystine or may be mixed with calcium oxalate. Pure cystine stones are radiolucent on plain radiographic imaging and are yellow in appearance.

Clinical Manifestations

Patients with renal calculi generally present for evaluation when the stone begins to move down the urinary tract. Acute renal or ureteral colic from an obstructive calculus is described as intermittent crampy pain that is severe and often debilitating. The pain starts in the flank and generally radiates down the patient's side and into the groin area as the calculus travels down the ureter. Some patients also experience nausea and vomiting during these episodes and can have varying amounts of blood in the urine. Patients with staghorn calculi can present with signs and symptoms of a systemic infection and are at risk for progression to sepsis.

Diagnosis

A thorough history should be taken during the initial evaluation, with questions focusing on the nature and location of the pain, radiation of the pain, duration of pain, and presence of nausea, vomiting, dysuria, and hematuria. Questions directly related to stone disease should be asked, such as personal or family history of stone disease, age of first stone, and history of recurrent urinary tract infections. If the patient has had prior stones, it is important to ask how the stone was managed, did it pass spontaneously or was an intervention required?

The physical examination usually demonstrates significant costovertebral angle or flank tenderness to palpation. Peritoneal signs are not common with renal calculi, and an alternative diagnosis should be pursued if these are found. Patients with fevers, tachycardia, or labile blood pressure and flank pain should be considered to have an obstructing stone and should be treated emergently.

Laboratory and Radiographic Work-Up

The typical work-up for a stone patient consists of laboratory studies, which include a comprehensive metabolic panel, complete blood count, urinalysis with microscopic analysis, urine culture, and pregnancy test for premenopausal women. Attention should be paid to the urinalysis for presence of crystals, hematuria, signs of infection, and pH. An elevated white blood cell count could indicate systemic infection. An elevated creatinine could indicate obstruction of the kidney or dehydration from nausea and vomiting.

Initial imaging studies usually consist of a plain abdominal radiograph to examine for the presence and location radiopaque stones. Noncontrast CT scans of the abdomen and pelvis (stone protocol) are now becoming the imaging modality of choice. This type of scan can visualize any stone regardless of its composition. CT can also determine if there is evidence of renal obstruction and can evaluate the surrounding structures for unexpected pathology.

Treatment

Once a stone has been discovered, treatment depends on multiple factors including size, location, presence of obstruction, evidence of systemic illness or fevers, and presence of nausea and vomiting. For patients who are clinically stable, outpatient expectant management is generally possible with a combination of oral hydration, pain control, and antiemetics. Medical expulsive therapy with the addition of an α-blocker such as tamsulosin[1] (Flomax

0.4 mg daily) increases the rate of stone passage by 29% compared to patients not taking the medication. Ultimately, approximately 98% of stones 5 mm or less pass spontaneously, taking an average time of 12 days to dislodge.

Invasive Treatment

If the patient has signs of sepsis, intractable pain, or nausea and vomiting, then immediate procedural intervention should be considered. Options include cystoscopy with placement of a ureteral stent to temporarily decompress the obstruction, or placement of a percutaneous nephrostomy tube. Septic patients should be emergently decompressed with a ureteral stent or a nephrostomy tube.

The decision to recommend a procedural intervention is often multifactorial, involving factors such as chance for spontaneous passage, absolute indications for intervention, and patient preference and work and family requirements. Treatment options depend on the size and location of the ureteral stone. Ureteral stones larger than 1 cm have a minimal chance of passing and require surgical treatment in most cases.

Appropriate initial treatment options include extracorporeal shock wave lithotripsy (ESWL) or ureteroscopic extraction with or without holmium laser lithotripsy. Both procedures are generally performed as a same-day surgical procedure. ESWL is less invasive, but stone-free rates are variable (45% to 92%) and repeat procedures can be needed. Contraindications to ESWL include pregnancy, bleeding diathesis, anticoagulation treatment, sepsis, and ureteral obstruction distal to the stone. Ureteroscopic management is more invasive than ESWL, but it has been shown to be more effective in rendering the patient stone-free in one setting compared to ESWL, with stone-free rates ranging from 88% to 100%. After ureteroscopy a ureteral stent may be left in place, which is generally removed in the office in 1 to 2 weeks. Stents are usually well tolerated, but some patients do experience bothersome urinary symptoms including urgency, frequency, and bladder pain at the end of urination.

Renal calculi larger than 1.5 cm and staghorn calculi are best treated by percutaneous nephrolithotomy (PNL). Percutaneous access is obtained by either interventional radiology or by the urologist, and a 30-F working tract is created. The calculus is then fragmented by ultrasonic or pneumatic lithotripsy devices, and fragments are removed. PNL is the most invasive approach, requires hospitalization, and can have complications such as bleeding, pneumothorax, or injury to the colon.

Medical Treatment

Patients with recurrent renal calculi should undergo a metabolic work-up, which consists of two separate 24-hour urine collections obtained after the acute stone episode has resolved. These samples should be analyzed for urine volume, pH, calcium, creatinine, sodium, phosphate, oxalate, uric acid, citrate, and cystine levels. General recommendations to prevent recurrent stones include increasing water intake to make at least 2 L of urine per day and adhering to a low-salt, low-meat, moderate-calcium diet.

Hypercalciuria is treated by thiazide diuretics (hydrochlorothiazide)[1] 25 mg daily and/or potassium citrate (Urocit-K) 10 to 20 mEq twice daily. Hyperoxaluria is treated by decreasing dietary intake of oxalate with oral calcium supplementation. Hyperuricosuria is treated by the addition of potassium citrate to increase the urinary pH plus allopurinol (Zyloprim) to decrease serum uric acid.

Patients with cystine stones are best managed by a low-methionine diet and alkalization of the urine with potassium citrate. If these measures are not sufficient, cystine binders such as tiopronin (Thiola) or D-penicillamine (Cuprimine) can help prevent recurrent cystine stones.

---

[1]Not FDA approved for this indication.

[1]Not FDA approved for this indication.

References

Atan L, Andreoni C, Ortiz V, et al. High kidney stone risk in men working in steel industry at hot temperatures. Urology 2005;65:858–61.

Borghi L, Meschi T, Amato F, et al. Urinary volume, water and recurrences in idiopathic calcium nephrolithiasis: A 5-year randomized prospective study. J Urol 1996;155:839–43.

Broadus AE, Horst RL, Littledike ET, et al. Primary hyperparathyroidism with intermittent hypercalcaemia: serial observations and simple diagnosis by means of an oral calcium tolerance test. Clin Endocrinol 1980;12:225–35.

Kaufman DW, Kelly JP, Curhan GC, et al. Oxalobacter formigenes may reduce the risk of calcium oxalate kidney stones. J Am Soc Nephrol 2008;19:1197–203.

Kok DJ. Intratubular crystallization events. World J Urol 1997;15:219–28.

Pak CY. Should patients with single renal stone occurrence undergo diagnostic evaluation? J Urol 1982;127:855–8.

Park H, Park M, Park T. Two-year experience with ureteral stones: Extracorporeal shockwave lithotripsy v ureteroscopic manipulation. J Endourol 1998;12:501–4.

Pearle MS, Calhoun EA, Curhan GC. Urologic diseases in America project: Urolithiasis. J Urol 2005;173:848–57.

Pietrow PK, Karellas ME. Medical management of common urinary calculi. Am Fam Physician 2006;74:86–894.

Prince CL, Scardino PL. A statistical analysis of ureteral calculi. J Urol 1960;83:561–5.

Saigal CS, Joyce G, Timilsina AR. Direct and indirect costs of nephrolithiasis in an employed population: Opportunity for disease management? Kidney Int 2005;68:1808–14.

Soucie JM, Thun MJ, Coates RJ, et al. Demographic and geographic variability of kidney stones in the United States. Kidney Int 1994;46:893–9.

Sur RL, Scales Jr CD, Preminger GM, Dahm P. Evidence-based medicine: A survey of American Urological Association members. J Urol 2006;176:1127–34.

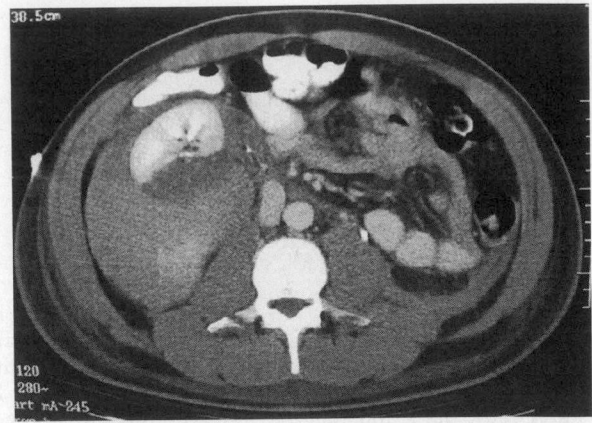

Figure 1. Computed tomography scan demonstrating large right perirenal hematoma and thrombosed posterior segmental artery. This was classified as a grade IV renal injury.

TRAUMA TO THE GENITOURINARY TRACT

Method of
Sean P. Elliott, MD, MS; and Bahaa S. Malaeb, MD

The genitourinary tract is involved in 3% to 10% of trauma cases. The kidney, followed by the bladder and urethra, are the most commonly involved genitourinary organs. In most cases, injury to the genitourinary tract is not isolated, and the initial evaluation of the urologic injuries should emphasize the context of the patient's associated injuries that might be more pressing or life-threatening. Still, early involvement of the urologist is prudent to help plan further interventions. The spectrum of genitourinary injuries is widespread, and management can range from immediate repair to temporization with delayed reconstruction. The goal of a urologist in the trauma setting is to establish urinary drainage in order to optimize kidney function, minimize hemorrhage, and control urinary extravasation to reduce associated complications such as infection or ileus.

Renal Trauma

Renal injury occurs in 1% to 5% of all trauma cases. Blunt impact accounts for the majority of renal injuries (90%–95%) and causes damage secondary to direct organ injury or disruption of the kidney from its attachments (e.g., renal hilum and ureteropelvic junction). Penetrating trauma most commonly is caused by stabbing or gunshot wounds. The damage from penetrating injury can be limited to the tract of the stab wound, or it can be more extensive secondary to necrosis from energy transfer and the blast effect of high-velocity bullets. The history is crucial in the diagnosis of renal injury and should include the mechanism of trauma as well as any preexisting kidney disease or condition that might contribute to worsening renal function. Hematuria has a very poor correlation with degree of injury, because disruption of the ureteropelvic junction, arterial disruption or thrombosis, and other severe injuries can exist in a setting with no hematuria.

The American Association for the Surgery of Trauma (AAST) classifies renal injuries into five grades (Figures 1 and 2):

- Grade 1: Nonexpanding subcapsular hematoma/contusion with absence of parenchymal injury
- Grade 2: Less than 1 cm laceration into the renal cortex, not extending into the collecting system, with a nonexpanding hematoma confined to the perirenal fascia

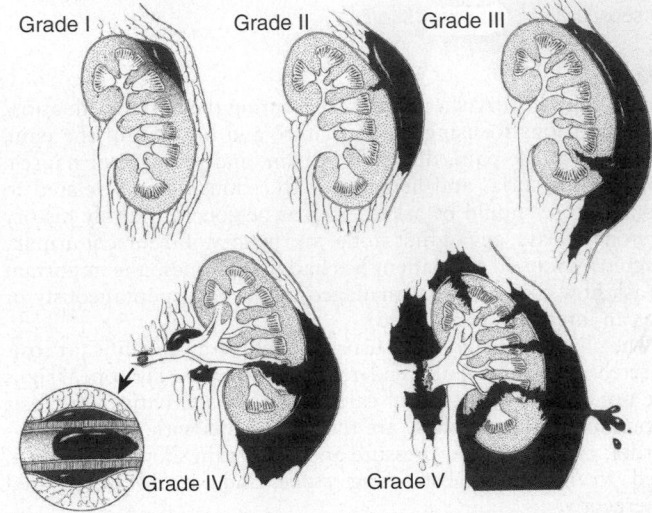

Figure 2. American Association for the Surgery of Trauma grading system for traumatic renal injuries: grade I, renal contusion and subcapsular hematoma; grade II, cortical laceration and perirenal hematoma; grade III, laceration into medulla or segmental renal artery thrombosis without a parenchymal injury; grade IV, laceration involving the collecting system, with or without a devascularized segment and contained vascular injury; grade V, renal artery thrombosis, avulsion of the renal pedicle, and shattered kidney. (From McAninch JW [ed]: Traumatic and Reconstructive Urology. Philadelphia, WB Saunders, 1996.)

- Grade 3: Greater than 1 cm laceration, extending through the renal cortex and medulla but not the collecting system
- Grade 4: Laceration extending to the collecting system with urinary extravasation or a segmental vascular injury with contained hematoma; renal artery thrombosis
- Grade 5: Shattered kidney or renal pedicle avulsion

Renal injury should be suspected in any trauma patient who has a penetrating injury with gross or microscopic hematuria (>2 red blood cells per high-power field), a blunt injury with gross hematuria, or a blunt injury with microscopic hematuria and shock (systolic blood pressure <90 mm Hg). In addition, imaging of the urinary tract should be obtained in children who have more than 50 red blood cells per high-power field even in the absence of hypotension.

In a stable patient, radiographic evaluation should consist of computed tomographic (CT) scanning with intravenous contrast and delayed images showing opacification of the collecting system and ureters. In the absence of a CT scan in a patient who is transported directly to the operating room for exploration, an intraoperative single-film intravenous pyelogram can be performed to confirm that two functioning kidneys are present; however, the poor quality of the images makes them unreliable for staging purposes.

Kidney exploration is indicated for the unstable patient in whom renal injury is thought to be the reason for a life-threatening and persistent hemorrhage. Another absolute indication for renal exploration and revascularization is renal artery hilar avulsion or renal artery thrombosis, if bilateral or in a solitary kidney. In patients undergoing exploratory laparotomy for associated injuries, renal exploration should be performed only in the presence of an expanding or pulsatile hematoma. Exploration of a nonexpanding, nonpulsatile hematoma is associated with a higher rate of nephrectomy and should be avoided. Almost all other injuries can be managed conservatively or with minimally invasive methods.

Nonoperative management consists of supportive care with intravenous hydration, antibiotics, bedrest, and serial measurements of hemoglobin and hematocrit. Patients can ambulate after they are clinically stable, gross hematuria has resolved, and the hemoglobin and hematocrit have been relatively constant over 24 hours.

Routine early follow-up imaging for grades 1 to 3 blunt renal injury is unnecessary. Any imaging should be motivated by a change in the patient's clinical situation or laboratory values. Grade 4 renovascular injuries can be followed up clinically. Follow-up imaging is indicated for patients with grade 4 or 5 injuries with urinary extravasation to assess for worsening urinoma or hematoma that might require further intervention.

Ureteral Trauma

Trauma to the ureter is rare, most likely because of its retroperitoneal and bony pelvis location, its relatively small caliber, and its mobility. The etiology of ureteric trauma is mostly iatrogenic (75% of all ureteric injuries); 73% of iatrogenic injuries occur secondary to gynecologic procedures, and the remainder are divided between general surgery and urologic procedures. Ureteral injury should be suspected in all cases of penetrating trauma to the abdomen, especially with high-velocity projectiles, because of the blast effect.

The AAST has classified ureteric injuries into five grades of severity:
- Grade 1: Hematoma only
- Grade 2: Injury involving less than 50% of the circumference of the ureter
- Grade 3: Injury involving more than 50% of the circumference of the ureter
- Grade 4: Complete transsection with less than 2 cm of devascularization
- Grade 5: Complete transsection with more than 2 cm of devascularization

The diagnosis usually is made intraoperatively if a high suspicion of ureteric injury is present or postoperatively by imaging obtained for investigation of fistula formation or clinical signs of upper tract obstruction. For noniatrogenic injuries, imaging should be obtained in patients who had rapid deceleration or penetrating injuries to the flank. Imaging modalities used are usually intravenous pyelography, CT scanning with intravenous contrast and delayed images, and retrograde pyelography. Findings indicative of ureteral injury include contrast extravasation, ureteral narrowing, and delayed peristalsis (Figure 3). Alternatively, the ureters may be interrogated intraoperatively by using direct inspection, by injecting intravenous methylene blue[1] and watching for leakage of dye, or by passing a ureteral catheter (if it passes easily, an injury is unlikely).

Grade 1 and 2 injuries can be managed initially by placement of a ureteral stent. If grade 2 or 3 injuries are identified immediately during exploration for a suspected ureteric injury, they can be managed by primary closure of the ureteric injury over an internal stent and placement of a nonsuction abdominal drain, as long as there is no associated thermal injury or necrosis. Grade 3 to

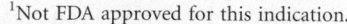
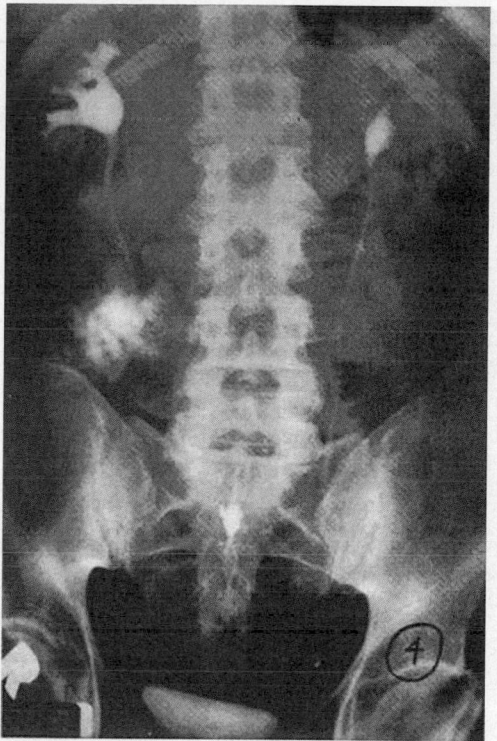

Figure 3. Intravenous pyelogram demonstrating extravasation of urine from right mid-ureter.

5 injuries usually require débridement of nonviable ends with reanastomosis over an internal ureteral stent or more complicated surgical procedures involving mobilization of the bladder and reimplantation of the ureter into the bladder. The type of ureteral repair depends on the amount of devitalized tissues and the location of the injury (proximal, middle, or distal ureter). Ureteroureterostomy, transureteroureterostomy, ureterocalicostomy, renal autotransplantation, ureteroneocystostomy with or without Boari flap or psoas hitch, and bowel interposition are all treatment options for various degrees of ureteral injuries.

Bladder Trauma

Blunt trauma accounts for 67% to 86% of bladder injuries resulting from external trauma, and up to 97% of those patients have associated pelvic fractures. The most common cause of blunt trauma is motor vehicle crashes. Penetrating trauma accounts for 14% to 33% of traumatic bladder injuries. The incidence of iatrogenic injury varies by procedure but is highest for hysterectomy and other obstetric and gynecologic procedures (up to 61 per 1000 cases). In cases of blunt trauma, injury should be suspected in patients who have pelvic fractures, suprapubic pain and inability to void, ileus, absent bowel sounds, or abdominal distention. For iatrogenic injuries, any urine in the field, visible laceration in bladder, or gas distention of the urinary drainage bag in laparoscopic surgery warrants further investigation. It is important to delineate whether a bladder injury involves intraperitoneal or extraperitoneal rupture. Intraperitoneal rupture occurs at the level of the bladder dome, where the muscular support is weakest (Figures 4 and 5).

The diagnostic test of choice is a CT cystogram, in which the bladder is filled with contrast to capacity (350–400 mL instilled by gravity). In children, the volume instilled is 60 mL plus 30 mL per year of age up to a maximum of 300 mL. Passive filling of the bladder by clamping of the catheter is associated with unacceptably high rates of false-negative tests. Plain film cystography is an alternative, but a single anteroposterior film is insufficient; postdrainage films and, preferably, oblique views should be obtained as well. In both settings, retrograde urethrography should be performed, if there is a suspicion of urethral injury, before placement of a Foley catheter.

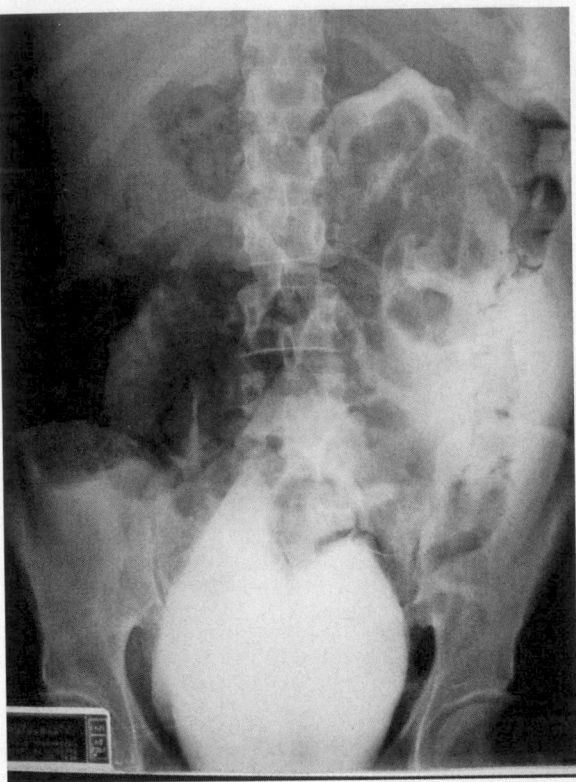

Figure 4. Intraperitoneal bladder rupture. Note contrast extravasating from the dome of the bladder and outlining the small intestine as well as the left colon.

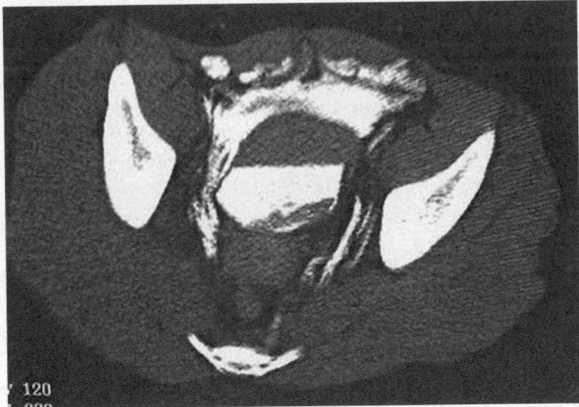

Figure 5. Extraperitoneal bladder rupture seen on computed tomographic cystogram.

Most extraperitoneal bladder ruptures can be managed with Foley catheter drainage for 7 to 10 days. Bladder neck involvement, concomitant vaginal or rectal injuries, presence of bone fragments in the bladder, or bladder wall entrapment necessitates surgical intervention. Intraperitoneal ruptures should be managed with surgical exploration because of the associated ileus and peritonitis caused by urine leak. In contrast, all penetrating bladder injuries should be explored and repaired because of the risk of necrosis and nonhealing. Bladder repair is performed with a multiple-layer closure and catheter drainage for 7 to 10 days.

Urethral Trauma

Traumatic injury to the urethra occurs in 10% of patients who sustain a pelvic fracture. Female urethral injuries are very rare. The male urethra is anatomically divided into a posterior part (prostatic and membranous urethra) and an anterior part (bulbous urethra, penile/pendulous urethra, and fossa navicularis). Injury to the anterior urethra occurs mostly from blunt trauma, penetrating

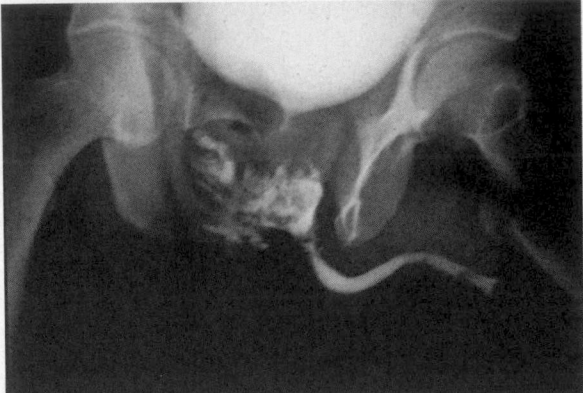

Figure 6. Retrograde urethrogram diagnostic of partial bulbar urethral transaction resulting from straddle injury.

injuries, or instrumentation. Posterior urethral injuries are usually associated with pelvic fractures but can occur secondary to blunt, penetrating, or iatrogenic injury.

Classic signs of urethral injury include blood at the meatus, a high-riding prostate on rectal examination, and perineal or scrotal ecchymosis. Imaging is indicated with any of these signs. The imaging study of choice is a retrograde urethrogram, and it should be performed before placement of a urethral catheter is attempted. In the absence of any signs, the diagnosis is most frequently made when retrograde urethrography is performed to investigate difficulty with urethral catheter placement (Figure 6).

The AAST grading system does not distinguish between anterior or posterior injury but classifies urethral injuries as follows:
- Grade 1: Contusion and blood at the meatus with normal urethrogram
- Grade 2: Stretch injury with no extravasation of contrast
- Grade 3: Partial disruption with contrast extravasating at the injury site but still reaching the bladder
- Grade 4: Complete disruption with contrast not reaching the bladder; urethral defect of less than 2 cm
- Grade 5: Complete disruption with urethral defect greater than 2 cm or complex injury involving the bladder neck, prostate, rectum, or vagina

Grade 1 and 2 injuries can be managed conservatively by placement of a urethral catheter. Management of grade 3 urethral injury should initially emphasize stabilization of the patient, because extensive bleeding could be present in cases of severe injury to the pelvis. Placement of a catheter may be attempted even if there is a suspicion of partial urethral injury. If this is met with difficulty, a suprapubic tube may be placed.

In cases of complete disruption, evidence supports early endoscopic realignment performed within the initial hospitalization if the patient is stable. This involves endoscopic passage of a guidewire across the defect and placement of a catheter over the guidewire, with the purpose of reestablishing urethral continuity. An alternative method is placement of a suprapubic tube and delayed reconstruction; the latter approach is associated with a 100% rate of stricture formation. Early endoscopic alignment has been shown to decrease the rate of stricture formation and the severity of strictures when they do occur, compared with suprapubic tube placement and delayed urethral reconstruction. Immediate open repair is rarely indicated unless complex injury extends into the bladder, rectum, or vagina and the patient is undergoing surgery for associated injuries. Immediate exploration is recommended for anterior urethral injuries associated with penetrating trauma or penile fractures.

Trauma to the External Genitalia

Injury to the scrotum is most frequently secondary to blunt trauma and can cause subcutaneous hematoma, hematocele, or testicular injury. Scrotal swelling and patient discomfort can make

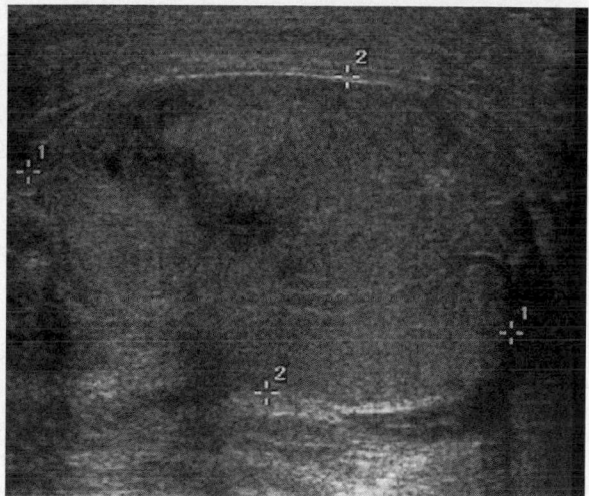

Figure 7. Testis ultrasound image demonstrating heterogeneous architecture characteristic of testicular rupture.

separation of testicular injury from extratesticular scrotal trauma difficult on physical examination. Therefore, one should have a low threshold for further investigation with ultrasound. A heterogeneous echo pattern in the testicular parenchyma on ultrasonography suggests testicular injury (Figure 7). Visualization of a tear in the tunica albuginea is less accurate. Ultrasound studies additionally provide information about any compromise in testicular blood flow.

Scrotal exploration should be performed whenever testicular injury is suspected. If the tunica is ruptured and there is extrusion of seminiferous tubules, the extruded tubules should be débrided, hemorrhage controlled, and the tunica closed. Testicular salvage rates are high (90%) when the scrotum is explored acutely but drop by half if exploration is delayed. Another indication for scrotal exploration is a large hematocele; evacuation of the hematoma can decrease the morbidity associated with protracted recovery and resolution of the hematoma and can occasionally identify a manageable source of bleeding. Scrotal exploration should also be performed in cases of inconclusive ultrasound findings or whenever the clinical suspicion for testicular injury is high.

Trauma to the penis can range in severity from a contusion to complete amputation. In cases of penile amputation, stabilization of the patient is important, and the need for transfusion should be addressed. Immediate microreimplantation is the management technique of choice if available. Penile fracture occurs after blunt injury to the erect penis, usually incurred during sexual intercourse. Patients often report a "crack" or a "pop" followed by severe pain and detumescence. Penile fractures involve rupture of the tunica albuginea. The hematoma is usually limited to the penis, unless the injury also involves Buck's fascia, causing ecchymosis and bruising that involves the scrotum as well. It is important to rule out associated urethral injury, which occurs in 10% of the cases. Surgical exploration, closure of the fascial defect, and repair of any associated urethral injury should be done acutely.

In females, blunt trauma to the vulva is rare. Injuries to genitalia can be associated with sexual assault and must be evaluated in that context. Consequently, vaginal smears should be taken, and the vagina should be thoroughly inspected with a speculum and with the patient under anesthesia.

Trauma resulting in skin loss, such as burns, large abrasions, and avulsions, the lesions should be explored and débrided in an effort to stage the injury and decrease the risk of complications such as Fournier's gangrene and urinoma. Delayed reconstruction can be performed after stabilization and proper delineation of viable versus nonviable tissues. The reconstructive options include mobilization of local flaps or skin grafts.

An understanding of the mechanism of injury is important to establish clinical suspicion of urologic trauma. Radiologic imaging is essential in making the correct diagnosis and managing it appropriately. Early diagnosis minimizes patient morbidity.

Studies of prospective design are clearly lacking for urologic trauma. Consolidation of the experience of major trauma institutions nationwide in a consortium for multi-institutional protocols could be the answer to this lack of prospective data.

References

Brandes S, Coburn M, Armenakas N, McAninch J. Diagnosis and management of ureteric injury: An evidence-based analysis. BJU Int 2004;94(3):277–89.

Chapple C, Barbagli G, Jordan G, et al. Consensus statement on urethral trauma. BJU Int 2004;93(9):1195–202.

Gomez RG, Ceballos L, Coburn M, et al. Consensus statement on bladder injuries. BJU Int 2004;94(1):27–32.

Lynch TH, Martínez-Piñeiro L, Plas E, et al. European Association of Urology: EAU guidelines on urological trauma. Eur Urol 2005;47(1):1–15.

Malcolm JB, Derweesh IH, Mehrazin R, et al. Nonoperative management of blunt renal trauma: Is routine early follow-up imaging necessary? BMC Urol 2008;8:11.

Morey AF, Metro MJ, Carney KJ, et al. Consensus on genitourinary trauma: External genitalia. BJU Int 2004;94(4):507–15.

Phonsombat S, Master VA, McAninch JW. Penetrating external genital trauma: A 30-year single institution experience. J Urol 2008;180(1):192–5 discussion 195–196.

Santucci RA, Fisher MB. The literature increasingly supports expectant (conservative) management of renal trauma: A systematic review. J Trauma 2005;59(2):493–503.

Santucci RA, Wessells H, Bartsch G, et al. Evaluation and management of renal injuries: Consensus statement of the renal trauma subcommittee. BJU Int 2004;93(7):937–54.

URETHRAL STRICTURES

Method of
Brian J. Flynn, MD; and Paul Knoll, MD

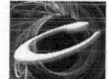

CURRENT DIAGNOSIS

- Retrograde urethrography is essential in the diagnosis and management of urethral stricture disease.
- Obstructive voiding complaints are the most common presentation in patients with urethral stricture disease.
- Patients with recurrent urinary tract infections, prostatitis, or epididymitis should be evaluated for urethral stricture.

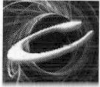

CURRENT THERAPY

- The patient and doctor should have a good understanding of the goals, limitations, and definitions of success before treatment of urethral stricture disease is undertaken.
- Office-based dilation is the most common and accepted initial treatment for urethral strictures.
- Dilation and urethrotomy are equivalent in terms of long-term success and are more likely to succeed in short, bulbar strictures with minimal fibrosis.
- Open surgical therapy is based on the length, location, and cause of the urethral stricture.

Urethral stricture occurs when scar tissue in the epithelium contracts and subsequently narrows the urethral lumen. The scarring process is induced by trauma, inflammation, or ischemia, with more severe strictures involving progressive fibrosis into the corpus spongiosum (spongiofibrosis). By definition, urethral strictures may involve the anterior urethra (fossa navicularis, pendulous urethra, and bulbous urethra), the posterior urethra (membranous or prostatic urethra), or both. Anterior urethral injuries commonly result from direct penile or perineal trauma, instrumentation, catheterization, infections, or lichen sclerosis.

Posterior urethral strictures may represent an actual defect in the membranous urethra after a distraction injury or a complication from prostate cancer treatment (surgery, irradiation, cryosurgery, or brachytherapy).

The prevalence of urethral strictures has been reported to be as high as 0.6% in the male population, and they have been a recognized problem throughout history, usually in relation to trauma and infection. Antibiotics for gonococcal urethritis have significantly reduced the incidence of strictures after infection, but iatrogenic injuries from urologic instrumentation and urethral catheterization have significantly increased as a cause of urethral stricture disease.

Evaluation and Diagnosis

Men with a urethral stricture may present acutely in the emergency department with urinary retention or may be referred to the clinic with chronic obstructive voiding symptoms. Patients complain of decreased force of the urinary stream, hesitancy, inability to empty, nocturia, postvoid dribbling, and difficulty emptying the bladder. Irritative symptoms can also occur, including frequency, urgency, and dysuria. Patients are typically 16 to 40 years of age and tend to live an active lifestyle (e.g., mountain biking, riding motorcycles or all-terrain vehicles, horseback riding), which may cause chronic perineal trauma. Often a hallmark event such as urethral trauma or urethral instrumentation resulting in blood per urethra occurs immediately before the onset of symptoms.

Physical examination should include a standard genital examination for any abnormalities, specifically evaluating the meatus for stenosis and the penile shaft for any fibrosis or stigmata of lichen sclerosis. Laboratory evaluation should include urinalysis, urine culture for infection, and a basic metabolic panel for renal function. Basic urodynamic studies, including simple uroflowmetry and measurement of the postvoid residual with ultrasound, can assess for obstruction and ability to empty. Inability to pass a catheter should further raise suspicion for a urethral stricture and prompt an evaluation of the urethra with endoscopy and retrograde urethrography.

Retrograde urethrography remains the gold standard for diagnosis and evaluation of urethral strictures, defining the length, location, caliber, and number of strictures. A voiding cystourethrogram (VCUG) obtained by means of a suprapubic cystotomy tube should outline the proximal urethra in cases of complete urethral occlusion. Alternative imaging modalities include magnetic resonance imaging and ultrasonography. These studies are better able to image a urethral cancer or diverticulum.

Cystourethroscopy complements the radiologic findings, confirming the anatomic location of the stricture and its caliber, and can rule out other urethral pathology such as stones, necrosis, fistula, or cancer. Urethral dilation, if planned, can also be performed by initially placing a wire under direct vision across the stricture and into the bladder.

Management

Once the diagnosis has been made, the first step is to treat the acute issues such as urinary retention and concomitant genitourinary infections. Urinary retention is treated with urethral catheterization or with a suprapubic cystotomy tube if urethral catheterization is unsuccessful. Once the acute issues are resolved, future management is based on the length, location, degree, and cause of the stricture and patient preference. Absolute indications for intervention include urinary retention, azotemia, recurrent infections, stone formation, and pain.

Urethrotomy and Dilation

Urethral dilation or urethrotomy is often the initial treatment, because it is less invasive than open surgical management. Dilation may be performed with filiforms and followers, serial dilators, or a balloon in the clinic or the emergency room. Urethrotomy is performed in the operating room with the patient under general regional anesthesia, with the use of an endoscopic knife or a laser to incise the scar under direct vision.

Strictures amenable to dilation are short (<1.0 cm) and are associated with minimal spongiofibrosis. Typically, dilation is performed initially, and urethrotomy is reserved for denser strictures in the bulbar or posterior urethra. In general, there is no statistical difference in success rate between dilation and urethrotomy. Recurrent strictures, long strictures, and those associated with significant fibrosis reoccur in more than 80% of cases and therefore require self-dilation or open urethral reconstruction (urethroplasty).

Stents

Urethral stents such as the UroLume (American Medical Systems, Minnetonka, MN) are made with titanium and are considered permanent. Introduced with much enthusiasm, stents have fallen out of favor secondary to problems of migration, encrustation, postvoid dribbling, and perineal and penile pain. Overall, long-term success is less than 30%, and these devices are best reserved for patients who are not candidates for open reconstruction.

Open Reconstruction

Surgical excision of the diseased segment with primary anastomosis (EPA) remains the gold standard for short strictures in the bulbous or posterior urethra, with long-term success rates greater than 95% in most studies. Keys to a successful repair include complete excision of the spongiofibrosis and a widely spatulated, tension-free anastomosis. Typically, strictures smaller than 2 cm are amenable to EPA, although longer stricture repair has been reported, especially in the posterior urethra (Figure 1). Whereas significant bulbar urethral mobilization can create length in men with longer strictures, this may compromise penile length and cosmesis.

If the stricture is located in the pendulous urethra or its length exceeds the limits of EPA (>2 cm), substitution urethroplasty with a graft or a flap may be performed (Figures 2 and 3). The graft or flap is onlayed ventrally or dorsally after a longitudinal incision is made in the diseased segment, thereby increasing the urethral caliber. A hybrid technique involves stricture excision of the worst disease with onlay to the less severe adjacent segments. If there are long obliterative segments, a two-stage repair is necessary.

Multiple sources of graft material have been successfully used in urethroplasty, including preputial skin, split-thickness skin from the thigh, bladder epithelium, rectal mucosa, and buccal mucosa. Buccal mucosa has emerged as the graft of choice, with excellent short-term results. Buccal mucosa has the ideal histologic characteristics, is non–hair bearing, leaves no visible scar, and is water

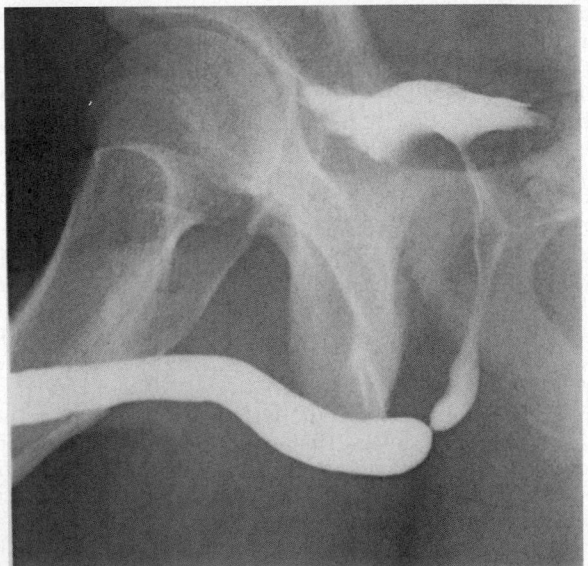

Figure 1. Retrograde urethrogram demonstrating a short bulbar urethral stricture amenable to excision with primary anastomosis.

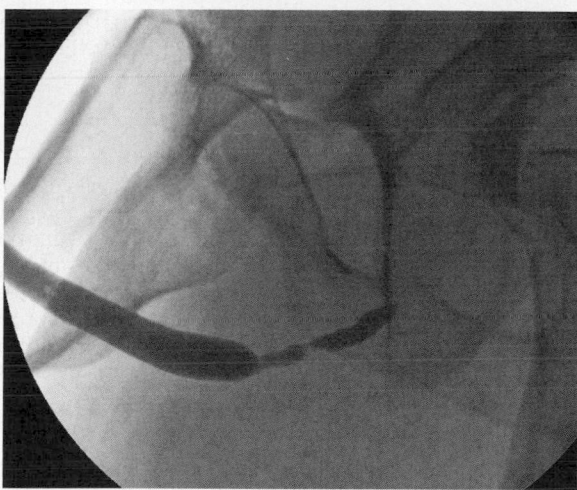

Figure 2. Retrograde urethrogram demonstrating a longer bulbar urethral stricture requiring excision of the most significant area of stricture and onlay of the remaining stricture: the excisional, augmented anastomotic urethroplasty.

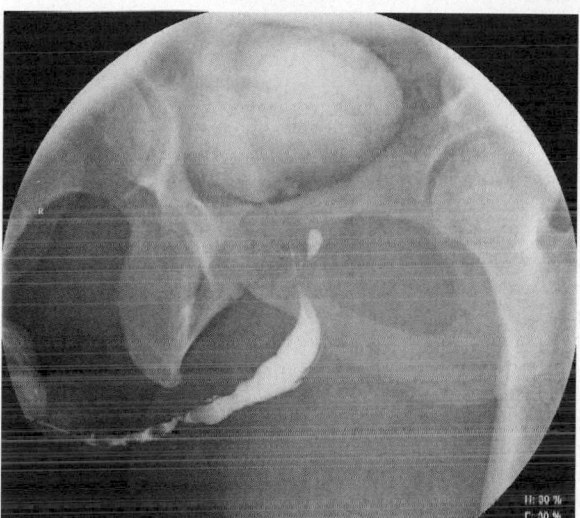

Figure 3. Retrograde urethrogram showing a panurethral stricture from lichen sclerosis. These may be repaired with complex staged reconstruction or perineal urethrostomy.

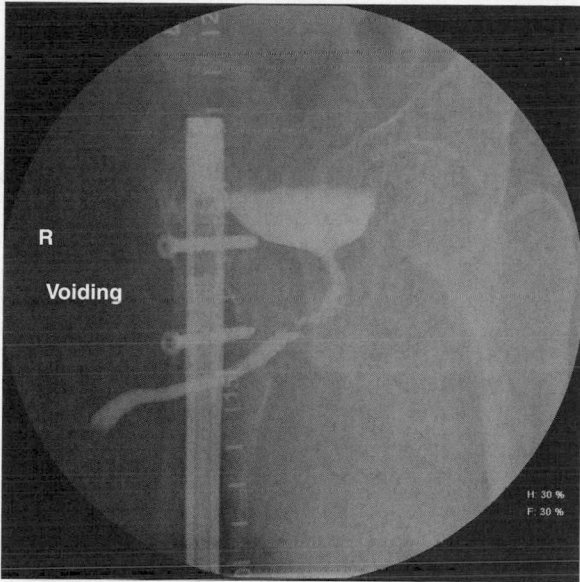

Figure 4. Retrograde urethrogram may be combined with a voiding cystourethrogram (the bladder is filled via a suprapubic catheter) to demonstrate a posterior urethral disruption due to pelvic fracture. These defects are usually amenable to excision with primary anastomosis.

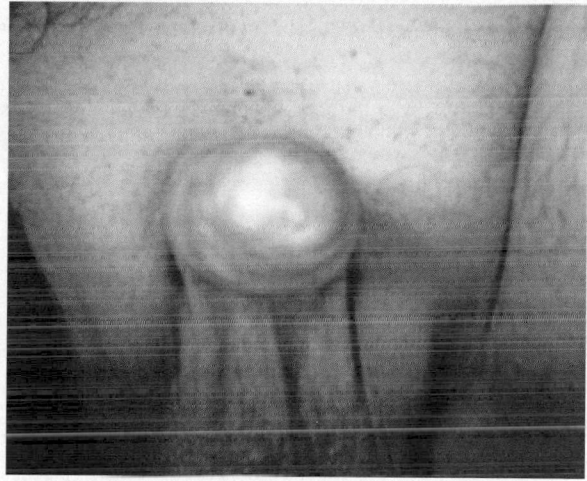

Figure 5. Picture of the glans penis afflicted with lichen sclerosis.

resistant and hence does not appear to have has much contracture as other graft materials.

Posterior urethral distraction injuries are a result of pelvic fracture and occur in up to 10% of cases. At the time of pelvic fracture, if there is blood at the meatus, a high index for suspicion, or inability to void, a RUG should be performed (Figure 4). In some cases, a partial disruption may have occurred, with a small portion of epithelium left intact. An endoscopically placed urethral catheter can facilitate stricture-free healing. If complete transection has occurred or a urethral catheter cannot be placed, the patient can be taken to the operating room, where a suprapubic cystotomy tube is placed. An antegrade-retrograde two-team approach using cystoscopy and fluoroscopy is then performed in an effort to place a catheter across the defect. Recent literature has suggested that early realignment decreases the need for subsequent urethroplasty without compromising erectile or sphincter function. However, if a primary realignment is not feasible, a suprapubic catheter is used for drainage, and delayed repair (3 months after the injury) is indicated. A progressive perineal anastomotic repair in these cases has a success rate of more than 95%. Complex posterior urethral injuries (e.g., with a concomitant bladder neck injury, rectal injury, or fistula) usually require an abdominal-perineal approach.

A variant of lichen sclerosis, balanitis xerotica obliterans, is an idiopathic, lymphocyte-mediated inflammatory skin disease that affects the anogenital region. A sclerotic white ring around the prepuce or glans penis is diagnostic in the early stage (Figure 5) and can lead to phimosis or meatal stenosis and urethral stricture in as many as 20% of patients. The use of genital tissue for reconstruction is contraindicated because it has a failure rate of more than 90%. Surgical options include a two-stage repair with buccal mucosa or extended meatotomy and perineal urethrostomy for more severe disease. In some cases, penile biopsy for diagnosis and to rule out squamous cell carcinoma is necessary preoperatively.

References

Abouassaly R, Angermeier KW. Augmented anastomotic urethroplasty. J Urol 2007;177(6):2211–5 discussion 2215–16.

Armitage JN, Cathcart PJ, Rashidian A, et al. Epithelializing stent for benign prostatic hyperplasia: A systematic review of the literature. J Urol 2007;177 (5):1619–24.

Dubey D, Vijjan V, Kapoor R, et al. Dorsal onlay buccal mucosa versus penile skin flap urethroplasty for anterior urethral strictures: Results from a randomized prospective trial. J Urol 2007;178(6):2466–9.

Eltahawy EA, Virasoro R, Schlossberg SM, et al. Long-term followup for excision and primary anastomosis for anterior urethral strictures. J Urol 2007;177 (5):1803–6.

Flynn BJ, Webster GD. Urethral stricture and disruption. In: Graham SD, Keane TE, Glenn J, editors. Glenn's Urologic Surgery. 6th ed. Philadelphia: Lippincott Williams & Wilkins; 2003. p. 394–407.

Heyns CF, Steenkamp JW, Kock MLSD, et al. Treatment of male urethral strictures: Is repeated dilation of internal urethrotomy useful? J Urol 1998;160(2):356–8.

Jordan GH. Imaging of the penis and male urethra. AUA Update Series 2008;27: [Lesson 23].

Jordan GH, Schlossberg SM. Surgery of the penis and urethra. In: Wein AJ, Kavoussi LR, et al., editors, Campbell-Walsh Urology. 9th ed Philadelphia: Saunders/Elsevier; 2007. p. 1054–87.

Levine LA, Strom KH, Lux MM. Buccal mucosa graft urethroplasty for anterior urethral stricture repair: Evaluation of the impact of stricture location and lichen sclerosis on surgical outcome. J Urol 2007;178(5):2011–5.

Mouraviev VB, Coburn M, Santucci RA. The treatment of posterior urethral disruption associated with pelvic fractures: Comparative experience of early realignment versus delayed urethroplasty. J Urol 2005;173(3):873–6.

Pugliese JM, Morey AF, Peterson AC. Lichen sclerosis: Review of the literature and current recommendations for management. J Urol 2007;178(6):2268–76.

Santucci RA, Joyce GF, Wise M. Male urethral stricture disease. J Urol 2007;177 (5):1667–74.

URINARY INCONTINENCE

Method of
Toby C. Chai, MD; and Leslie Rickey, MD, MPH

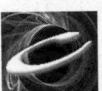

CURRENT DIAGNOSIS

- Determine whether stress or urge is the predominant urinary incontinence.
- Assess for reversible causes of incontinence.
- Rule out infection, hematuria, and glycosuria with a urinalysis.
- Consider measurement of postvoid residual to rule out urinary retention.

CURRENT THERAPY

Behavioral Modifications for Stress Incontinence and Urgency Incontinence
- Pelvic floor muscle exercises
- Fluid titration, timed voids
- Weight loss

Office Therapies
- Anticholinergic medication for urgency incontinence
- Pessary or incontinence ring for stress incontinence
- Posterior tibial nerve stimulation for refractory urgency incontinence

Surgical Treatments
- Suburethral sling for stress incontinence
- Sacral neuromodulation for refractory urgency incontinence
- OnabotulinumtoxinA injection (Botox) into bladder for refractory urgency incontinence

Epidemiology

Urinary incontinence, as a symptom, is defined by two international societies, the International Continence Society (ICS) and the International Urogynecological Association (IUGA) as "complaint of any involuntary leakage of urine." Urinary incontinence can be further categorized into stress incontinence (loss of urine with cough, Valsalva, straining, increased abdominal pressures), urgency incontinence (loss of urine preceded by urgency, which is the sudden compelling desire to pass urine that is difficult to defer), or mixed (loss of urine characterized by elements of both stress and urgency incontinence). From several epidemiologic studies, the prevalence of urinary incontinence is significantly higher in women than in men in community-dwelling adults: approximately 30% versus 17%.

Risk Factors

Various risk factors for urinary incontinence have been described, including age, increasing body mass index (BMI), pregnancy, childbirth, smoking, diabetes, hysterectomy, functional and cognitive impairment, pelvic radiation and surgery, and possible heritable factors. In male patients, other risk factors include prostate surgery and bladder outlet obstruction from an enlarged prostate. Although urgency incontinence is often idiopathic, lower urinary tract symptoms in general are common among people with neurologic disease such as multiple sclerosis, spinal cord injury, or spinal dysraphism.

Pathophysiology and Clinical Presentation

The lower urinary tract (bladder and urethra) has two functions: storing and evacuating urine. During the storage phase, the sympathetic and somatic nerves work in concert to keep the urethra contracted and the detrusor muscle relaxed, allowing urine to fill the bladder at low bladder pressures (the bladder has high compliance during storage). Once the voiding reflex is activated, sympathetic and somatic neural activity is diminished, resulting in relaxation at the urethral sphincter and pelvic floor, and parasympathetic activity increases via cholinergic neurotransmission, resulting in detrusor contraction and bladder emptying.

Failure to store urine normally can manifest as urinary incontinence, urinary frequency, and/or nocturia secondary to bladder and/or urethral dysfunction. Alternatively, urine leakage can result from a nonurologic cause (functional incontinence) and can sometimes be reversible when the underlying cause is identified (Box 1).

Stress incontinence occurs when increases in intraabdominal pressure overcome the ability of the urethral sphincter to stay closed. The patient complains of leakage with activity, cough, lifting, and other stressors. Stress incontinence can result from urethral neuromuscular injury, urethral vascular changes, or lack of proper pelvic floor support in some women with associated pelvic organ prolapse. Stress incontinence in a male patient is most commonly due to a radical prostatectomy performed for treatment of prostate cancer.

Urgency incontinence is less well understood, but it can be due to uninhibited bladder contractions (detrusor overactivity) and can result in large-volume urine loss. It is unclear whether the etiology for urgency incontinence or "overactive bladder" originates in the central nervous system, the peripheral nervous system, or the bladder. In the neurogenic population, a poorly compliant bladder can develop, which results in a steady increase in storage bladder pressures that eventually results in leakage in addition to neurologically induced uninhibited bladder contractions (neurogenic detrusor overactivity). Urgency incontinence can be unpredictable,

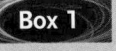
Box 1 Transient/Reversible Causes of Incontinence (DIAPPERS)

Delirium
Infection (urinary tract infection)
Atrophic urethritis and/or vaginitis
Pharmaceuticals
Psychological problem, depression
Excess urine output (congestive heart failure, hyperglycemia, increased intake)
Restricted mobility
Stool impaction

From Resnick NM. Urinary incontinence in the elderly. Med Grand Rounds 1984;3:281–90.

leading to a more negative impact on quality of life compared to pure stress incontinence.

Bladder outlet obstruction or decreased bladder contractility can result in overflow incontinence due to incomplete bladder emptying. Patients report constant dribbling of urine and sometimes extreme frequency. Bladder outlet obstruction can result from prostatic obstruction or bladder neck or urethral stricture in male patients and, less commonly, from advanced prolapse or as a side effect from surgical correction of stress incontinence in women.

Prevention

Because of the association of urinary incontinence with diabetes and obesity, it is likely that efforts to prevent these disease states would lower the incidence of urinary incontinence. Indeed, weight loss is an effective treatment option for urinary incontinence, and this has been demonstrated scientifically. Additionally, a behavioral modification program that included pelvic floor muscle training resulted in improved continence status in postmenopausal women in a randomized, controlled trial. There are conflicting data on the effect of preoperative and/or postoperative pelvic floor muscle training on the continence status of men undergoing radical prostatectomy. Pelvic floor muscle exercises during the antepartum and postpartum period can prevent development of urinary incontinence in women after childbirth, at least in the short term. Further long-term studies are necessary to investigate the true potential of lifestyle and behavioral modifications to prevent urinary incontinence.

Diagnosis

There are barriers that prevent men and women from seeking care for their urinary incontinence. These include embarrassment, fear of invasive testing, and a belief that urinary incontinence is a normal part of aging. A simple screening questionnaire such as the 3IQ (3 Incontinence Questions) can help primary care providers identify patients who might benefit from further inquiry.

Urinary incontinence is categorized into stress incontinence, urgency incontinence and mixed incontinence, and the history and physical examination are therefore used to help with stratifying the type of incontinence. After determining instigating factors for leakage (activity, urge, lack of mobility), associated symptoms such as urgency, frequency, nocturia, dysuria, straining to void, and incomplete emptying should be queried as well. The onset, severity, and pattern of leakage are important to ascertain, as is

the degree of bother to the patient and how he or she is managing the symptoms. Common comorbidities that may be pertinent to a patient's incontinence include diabetes, stroke, cognitive impairment, weight gain, neurologic disease, parity, prior pelvic surgery (e.g., hysterectomy in women, prostatectomy in men), and pelvic radiation. Many medications can affect bladder and urethral function, resulting in exacerbation of urinary retention or urinary incontinence (Table 1).

During the physical examination, some basic components can help assess the patient's incontinence. Measurement of a postvoid residual by bladder scan or catheter can help rule out urinary retention, and a urine specimen should be obtained to assess for infection, hematuria, and glycosuria. Transurethral loss of urine observed with a standing cough stress test is likely to indicate stress incontinence. In female patients, degree of pelvic organ prolapse and pelvic floor muscle strength can be assessed when the pelvic examination is being performed.

Certain situations can lead a clinician to pursue additional evaluation with urodynamics and/or cystoscopy. These situations include inability to make a definitive diagnosis based on symptoms and the initial evaluation; prior lower urinary tract surgery, including failed anti-incontinence procedures; known or suspected neurogenic bladder (e.g., patient with comorbid neurologic diagnoses); abnormal urinalysis, such as unexplained hematuria or pyuria; recurrent urinary tract infections; excessive residual urine volume; and pelvic organ prolapse beyond the introitus.

Differential Diagnosis

Lower urinary tract symptoms of urgency, frequency, and urgency incontinence can result from or be aggravated by other conditions that should be evaluated before treatment. A urinary tract infection (UTI), polyuria from uncontrolled diabetes, and sometimes even bladder cancer can also cause these symptoms. A urinalysis will help diagnose a UTI, glycosuria, or isolated hematuria that would prompt further work-up or referral. A patient who reports continuous incontinence should have formal measurement of postvoid residual to rule out urinary retention, and in a female patient, investigation for a genitourinary fistula should be considered, especially if she has had recent pelvic surgery such as a hysterectomy.

Treatment

Once the history and physical have been obtained, treatment can be directed at the predominant or most bothersome leakage symptoms. In addition, 80% of women with incontinence and other

TABLE 1	Drugs that May Affect Lower Urinary Tract		
CLASS OF DRUGS	**SIDE EFFECT**	**IMPACT ON LUT**
Psychotropic Agents		
Antidepressants	Anticholinergic	Urinary retention
Antipsychotics	Anticholinergic, sedation	Urinary retention
Sedatives/hypnotics	Sedation, muscle relaxation	Urinary retention
Alcohol, caffeine	Diuresis	Polyuria, urgency, frequency
Other Types of Medication		
Diuretics		Polyuria, urgency, frequency
Narcotics	Sedation, confusion Decrease detrusor contraction central effects?	Urinary retention
Angiotensin-converting enzyme inhibitors	Cough	Aggravate preexisting stress incontinence
Antihistamines	Anticholinergic	Urinary retention
α-Adrenergic agonists	Increase urethral tone	Urinary retention

lower urinary tract symptoms report an additional pelvic floor disorder, so defecation function should be assessed as well.

Stress Incontinence
Nonsurgical Therapies
Behavioral modifications can include weight loss, bladder training, and pelvic floor muscle therapy. Obesity is a known risk factor for urinary incontinence, and weight loss of 5% to 10% results in 60% decrease in incontinence episodes (compared to 15% decrease in controls). Often bladder training and pelvic floor rehabilitation are incorporated into a treatment regimen. These therapies can be carried out under the supervision of a physical therapist, and there are good data that a home pelvic floor exercise regimen augmented by intermittent monitoring can provide significant improvements in episode frequency. A Cochrane review supported pelvic floor muscle training as first-line therapy for symptoms of urinary incontinence. Another nonsurgical option for treating female stress incontinence is an incontinence ring, a type of pessary. A pessary is a removable device that is placed in the vagina to provide support to the bladder neck and therefore prevent leakage.

Urethral Bulking Agents
The goal of urethral bulking is augmentation of the urinary sphincter, which is achieved by bulking the bladder neck and/or proximal urethra and thus increasing coaptation and resistance. The procedure is usually performed in a periurethral or transurethral fashion though a cystoscope, and the material is injected in the suburothelial space to achieve coaptation of the tissue. In general, the injectable material should not cause an immune response or significant inflammatory reaction and should be durable. Because women are more commonly affected by stress incontinence, most trials involve female stress incontinence. Approximately 20% to 40% of patients are "dry" at 1 year, and overall 50% of patients are improved, with many patients undergoing two or three injections to achieve improvement.

Surgical Treatment
The mainstay of surgical treatment for female stress incontinence is the suburethral sling. Either a biological or synthetic sling is placed underneath the urethra to provide resistance to increases in abdominal pressure that can lead to loss of urine in symptomatic patients.

The current pubovaginal sling procedure involves harvesting a piece of rectus fascia or fascia lata (or alternatively, using a cadaveric or other biological graft) and passing the sling up bilaterally through the retropubic space to the abdominal incision. The suture arms are then tied over the rectus fascia so that the sling lies under the proximal urethra. A more minimally invasive procedure was introduced in 1996, the midurethral sling, which uses a synthetic mesh placed under the midurethra and avoids the incision necessary to harvest the autologous fascia. The procedure can be performed via a retropubic or transobturator route.

For a male patient with stress incontinence, surgical options include placing an occlusive polypropylene sling under the bulbar urethra or implanting an artificial urinary sphincter, which is a multicomponent prosthesis that uses a hydraulically activated cuff around the bulbar urethra to prevent stress incontinence.

Future Therapies
Studies are under way to evaluate the optimal methods to harvest and inject autologous adult stem cells into the urethral sphincter. Muscle-derived and adipose-derived stem cells have been described. The stem cells have the advantage of being able to differentiate into functional muscle cells within the urethra, but there is also evidence of release of growth factors that promote nerve ingrowth and possible improvement of neural function as well. Further work in this area will better characterize the efficacy as well as the role of stem cell injection for treating stress incontinence.

Urgency Incontinence
Treatment for urge incontinence usually involves anticholinergic medication; however, it is recommended that education regarding fluid intake, voiding interval, and urge suppression techniques be included in the treatment plan. Other effective therapies include neuromodulation and intradetrusor injection of onabotulinumtoxinA into the bladder wall.

Pharmacotherapy
Anticholinergic (or antimuscarinic) agents work by blocking cholinergic muscarinic receptors at the postsynaptic neuromuscular junction of the detrusor smooth muscle cell, and therefore decrease the ability of the bladder to respond to acetylcholine released by the parasympathetic nerves. Inhibition of the muscarinic receptors can result in decreased bladder contraction and decreased detrusor pressure and therefore can help relieve the symptoms of urge incontinence. Incontinence episodes can be reduced by 60% to 70%, and improvements in urinary urgency and frequency are seen as well, though at lower rates (20% to 40%).

Muscarinic receptors are also involved in the function of other muscles such as gastrointestinal smooth muscle and well as saliva production, which can lead to unwanted symptoms while taking antimuscarinic medication. Common side effects include dry mouth (10% to 30%) and constipation (10% to 20%), and there is a relatively high discontinuation rate in part because of bothersome side effects. Contraindications to taking an antimuscarinic medication are untreated narrow-angle glaucoma, gastric retention, and urinary retention.

Neuromodulation
For patients who are refractory to or unable to tolerate medication, another option to treat urgency incontinence is neuromodulation. The exact mechanism is not well understood, but it is thought that by stimulating the afferent input to the sacral cord, efferent outflow to the bladder can be modulated.

Sacral nerve stimulation with the InterStim device has been successfully used on refractory urgency incontinence patients for more than a decade and is FDA approved for urgency incontinence as well as urinary urgency and frequency. A lead is placed through the third sacral foramen and is connected to an external stimulator. If the patient experiences greater than 50% improvement in symptoms, the lead is attached to an implantable pulse generator.

Posterior tibial nerve stimulation is another form of neuromodulation. Posterior tibial nerve stimulation involves placement of a 34-gauge needle over the posterior tibial nerve as it crosses the medial malleolus of the ankle. The needle is then attached to an electrical stimulator, and a treatment of 30 minutes is given usually once a week for 10 to 12 weeks.

OnabotulinumtoxinA Intradetrusor Injection
OnabotulinumtoxinA, produced by *Clostridium botulinum*, is a potent neurotoxin that inhibits release of acetylcholine from presynaptic nerve terminals at the neuromuscular junction, causing flaccid muscle paralysis. Intradetrusor injection was originally described in patients with neurogenic urgency incontinence, and it has been approved by the FDA for use in this population. In patients with refractory idiopathic urgency incontinence, continence rates range from 50% to 80% and generally last from 6 to 9 months. Areas of current study include clarification of treatment dosage and dose-related complications as well as comparative efficacy trials to evaluate the role of onabotulinumtoxinA in the treatment of urgency incontinence.

Overflow Incontinence
In a patient with urinary retention that leads to urinary incontinence, self-catheterization can be recommended. In a male patient with lower urinary tract symptoms and urinary retention due to prostatic enlargement, pharmacotherapy using α-agonists or 5α-reductase inhibitors can be used. If medications fail to improve

symptoms, transurethral resection of the prostate or other minimally invasive approaches such as microwave or radiofrequency ablation of the prostate may be required.

Complications

Urinary incontinence incurs a high individual and societal cost. Annual costs are estimated at $23 billion, and consequences can include rashes, pressure ulcers, increased risk of falls, low self-esteem, social isolation, anxiety, and depression. The prevalence of urinary incontinence will continue to grow as the percentage of older Americans increases; therefore, it is important that primary care physicians are able to recognize urinary incontinence and provide adequate diagnosis and treatment for their patients.

References

Brown J, Bradley CS, Subak LL, et al. The sensitivity and specificity of a simple test to distinguish between urge and stress urinary incontinence. Ann Intern Med 2006;141:715–23.

Diokno AC, Sampselle CM, Herzog AR, et al. Prevention of urinary incontinence by behavioral modification program: A randomized, controlled trial among older women in the community. J Urol 2004;171:1165–71.

Dumoulin C, Hay-Smith J. Pelvic floor muscle training versus no treatment, or inactive control treatments, for urinary incontinence in women. Cochrane Database Syst Rev 2010;(1) CD005654.

Schmid DM, Sauermann P, Werner M, et al. Experience with 100 cases treated with botulinum-A toxin injections in the detrusor muscle for idiopathic overactive bladder syndrome refractory to anticholinergics. J Urol 2006;176: 177–1785.

Subak LL, Wing R, West DS, et al. Weight loss to treat urinary incontinence in overweight and obese women. N Engl J Med 2009;360:481–90.

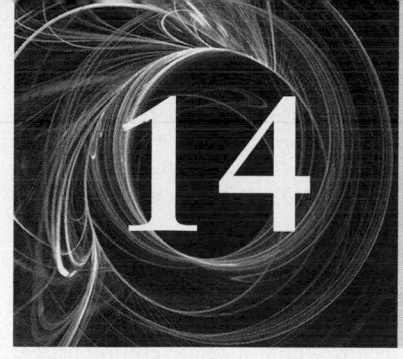

14 The Sexually Transmitted Diseases

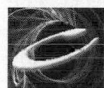

CHLAMYDIA TRACHOMATIS

Method of
Tracy L. Williams, MD

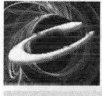

CURRENT DIAGNOSIS

- Screen all sexually active woman 25 years of age or younger for *C. trachomatis* annually regardless of symptoms per the CDC recommendations.
- Symptomatic patients should be tested regardless of gender.
- Reinfection with *C. trachomatis* is common.
  - Retest all patients who have a history of *C. trachomatis* or *N. gonorrhea* at 3 to 6 months following treatment, regardless of whether their partner(s) were treated.
  - If the patient does not follow up at 3 to 6 months, then retest upon presentation for medical care within the first 12 months posttreatment.
- Patients who screen positive for *C. trachomatis* need to be screened for gonorrhea, syphilis, and HIV.
- Perform test of cure on pregnant patients at 3 to 4 weeks posttreatment and repeat in 3 to 6 months, preferably in the third trimester if the pregnant woman was diagnosed during the first trimester.
- Rescreen pregnant patients for other sexually transmitted infections (STIs) 3 months posttreatment including gonorrhea, syphilis, and HIV.

CURRENT THERAPY

- Azithromycin (Zithromycin) 1 g orally in a single dose or doxycycline (Vibramycin) 100 mg orally twice a day for 7 days are the recommended regimens for nonpregnant patients and for presumptive treatment for *C. trachomatis*.
- All of the patient's recent sexual partners need referral and treatment.
  - The patient's last sexual contact should be referred and treated if it has been more than 60 days since the patient had a sexual partner.
  - The partner needs to be treated for *C. trachomatis* even if his or her personal STI results are negative.
- Counsel patients and their partners to abstain from sexual contact until 7 days after one-dose therapy or after the final dose of the 7-day regimen.
- The CDC recommends that patients who test positive for gonorrhea should also receive presumptive treatment for *C. trachomatis* because coinfection is common.

Epidemiology

Chlamydia trachomatis is the most common notifiable sexually transmitted infection (STI) in the United States, with an incidence of over 1.2 million cases per year according to the Centers for Disease Control and Prevention (CDC) in 2009. Women age 15 to 19 years are the most commonly affected, followed by women age 20 to 24. The incidence of *C. trachomatis* has steadily climbed yearly since it became a federally mandated notifiable disease; part of this is an artifact of improved screening practices that are discovering disease in asymptomatic patients.

C. trachomatis costs an estimated $2.4 billon annually. Cost-benefit analyses have consistently shown prioritizing screening efforts in asymptomatic women to be cost-effective.

Risk Factors

The risk of contracting *C. trachomatis* increases with: multiple sexual partners; unprotected sex including vaginal, oral, and anal intercourse; anal-receptive intercourse; and men having sex with men. The risk increases in the presence of other coinfections including human immunodeficiency virus (HIV) or Herpes simplex virus (HSV). African Americans have a fourfold higher incidence compared to their white counterparts (13% versus 2.4%, respectively).

Pathophysiology

Chlamydia trachomatis is an obligate intracellular parasite. It is found only in human cells, but can live on fomites for up to 30 hours. Previous infections do not yield protection against future infections with *C. trachomatis*. *C. trachomatis* does not infect the squamous epithelium of the vaginal vault, but can infect the urethra, the squamocolumnar junction of the cervix, the rectal mucosa, and the oropharynx.

Prevention

Prevention depends on screening of asymptomatic patients, who make up a large portion of the infected population. The CDC updated its recommendations for screening in 2010, with emphasis continuing to be on annual screening of all sexually active women age 25 years and younger. The United States Preventive Services Task Force (USPTF) has similar recommendations but uses age 24 years and younger.

The CDC and the USPTF found insufficient evidence to recommend routine screening of men based on cost-effectiveness, efficacy, and practicality, but screening of symptomatic men or men in areas with high prevalence of *Chlamydia*, including men having sex with men, men in correctional facilities, and men visiting STI clinics, is recommended. Overall, screening of men is recommended so long as it does not detract resources from the screening of women. Symptomatic patients should be tested regardless of gender.

Men who have sex with other men are at high risk for bacterial and viral STI. The CDC STI screening recommendation in this group is an annual test for urethral infection with *C. trachomatis* and *N. gonorrhea*. The preferred methodology is testing the urine using nucleic acid amplification technique (NAAT). Men who have receptive anal intercourse are recommended to have annual anal screening for both *C. trachomatis* and *N. gonorrhea*. Men who have oral receptive sex are also advised to have pharyngeal screening for *N. gonorrhea* but not *C. trachomatis*. The NAAT is only Food and Drug Administration (FDA)–approved on urine in the above scenarios but is used off-label in laboratories that have met all regulatory requirements.

Patients who screen positive for *Chlamydia* need to be screened for other STIs, including gonorrhea, syphilis, and HIV.

Abstinence and monogamous relationships are ideal to help prevent the transmission of *C. trachomatis*. Safer sex practices to limit the spread of *C. trachomatis* include the consistent use of condoms. Epidemiologic studies show that people often base their decision to use condoms on their perception of their partner's risk. Given the high prevalence of asymptomatic *C. trachomatis* infections in certain American populations, selective condom use is not an effective strategy.

Clinical Manifestations

Most infections are asymptomatic. However, some women will report vaginal discharge, postcoital or intermenstrual bleeding, or lower abdominal pain. Men are more commonly symptomatic than women and may report dysuria or urethral discharge.

Untreated *C. trachomatis* in women has significant health sequelae. Approximately 40% of women with untreated *Chlamydia* go on to develop pelvic inflammatory disease (PID). Women with PID may become infertile (20%), develop debilitating chronic pelvic pain (18%), or suffer ectopic pregnancy (9%).

Men do not tend to suffer as severe sequelae from *C. trachomatis*. The most common illness is urethritis, but men may also suffer epididymitis, proctitis, and conjunctivitis. Reactive arthritis is also more common in men.

Diagnosis

Tests used for detection of *C. trachomatis* can be divided into molecular (NAAT, DNA probing, and hybrid capture), antigen detection (direct immunofluorescence and enzyme immunoassay), and cell culture.

The most reliable method of testing for *C. trachomatis* is NAAT. It is FDA-approved for use on vaginal/endocervical secretions, male intraurethral swabs, and urine. It is not FDA-approved for rectal or orophyngeal use but is used off label in laboratories as described above. The primary benefit of NAAT is the lack of a need for viable organisms to induce a positive test result; this increases its sensitivity to more than 95% because of the ability to detect *C. trachomatis* even if only one copy of the targeted RNA or DNA is present. Its specificity is also desirable at 99%.

C. trachomatis cell culture is used as the reference standard for all testing but has many limitations, including expense, long turnaround time (72 hours), and transport and specimen storage requirements. Its sensitivity is 80% to 85%. It is not readily available.

Limiting barriers to screening is important. If testing in the clinic is difficult to arrange, self-collected vaginal swab specimens perform at least as well as other approved specimens using NAAT. Urine NAAT testing is also more acceptable to many patients, particularly asymptomatic men and women who do not otherwise need a pelvic examination.

Differential Diagnosis

Infection with *Chlamydia* is often asymptomatic but is included in the differential diagnosis of various organ system complaints. It should be ruled out in any sexually active patient presenting with urethritis, mucopurulent cervicitis, epididymitis, and proctitis. There is significant overlap in the symptoms caused by *C. trachomatis* with *N. gonorrhea*, so testing for both bacteria with NAAT is preferred. Other agents that are included in the differential diagnosis after *C. trachomatis* and *N. gonorrhea* have been ruled out include: *Trichomonas vaginalis*, HSV, adenovirus, *Mycoplasma* species, and *Ureaplasma*. More specifically, persistent urethritis after treatment with doxycycline (Vibramycin) can be caused by infection with *T. vaginalis* or doxycycline-resistant *Urea urealyticum* or *Mycoplasma genitalium*.

C. trachomatis should be ruled out in newborn infants with conjunctivitis in the first 30 days of life or pneumonia at 1 to 3 months of life, especially if they were born to mothers with untreated chlamydial infections.

Treatment

Recommendations for treatment regimens are summarized in Box 1. The benefit of using single-dose azithromycin (Zithromycin) is the ability to directly observe the patient taking the therapy. The 7-day course of doxycycline (Vibramycin) has comparable cure rates to azithromycin, but decreased compliance.

Presumptive treatment for *C. trachomatis* should be considered for high-risk patients with cervicitis. High-risk patients include women up to 25 years old, those with new or multiple sexual partners, those who engage in unprotected sex, especially if follow-up cannot be ensured, and those for whom a relatively insensitive diagnostic test is used in place of NAAT.

The CDC also recommends presumptive treatment for patients being treated for *N. gonorrhea*. Coinfection is common, as illustrated in a study that found 20% of men with *N. gonorrhea* and 42% of women with *N. gonorrhea* were also infected with *C. trachomatis*. Cotreatment is also recommended in the hope that it will impede the development of antimicrobial-resistant *N. gonorrhea*.

Chlamydia trachomatis is a reportable infectious disease. The patient is instructed to refer all of his or her sexual partners for testing and treatment if they have had sexual contact during the previous 60 days. If the patient has not been sexually active for the last 60 days, then the patient is to refer his or her most recent sexual contact. The patient's recent sexual partners should be treated empirically even if their personal STI evaluation returns negative results. The patient and his or her sexual partners should be counseled to abstain from sexual activity for 7 days post treatment. Reinfection, rather than recurrence, is the more common etiology of repeat *C. trachomatis* infection.

Expedited partner therapy is an option in certain cases. This entails the patient delivering the antibiotic to his or her partner(s) without a physician first seeing the patient. Patients are to give their partners written materials on the importance of following up with a physician if any signs of complications occur (e.g., pelvic pain in women or testicular pain in men). It can be used effectively in certain situations but is not routinely recommended in men who have sex with men because of the high risk for coexisting infections, especially undiagnosed HIV infection, in their partners. Please refer to the CDC website (www.cdc.gov/std/ept) to check on legality in individual states. In general, utilizing the traditional patient-physician model is preferred.

Infants born to women with untreated *C. trachomatis* infection are at increased risk for vertical transmission. Prophylactic treatment with oral erythromycin (E-Mycin) for *C. trachomatis* is not recommended. The state-mandated standard erythromycin eye ointment (Ilotycin) that all newborns receive is still indicated. Overall, infants born to infected mothers need to be closely monitored for any signs and symptoms of infection and treated appropriately.

Intrauterine devices (IUDs) have regained popularity in the United States after they were implicated in causing PID in the 1970s. The IUD has evolved and now the risk of PID appears increased only in the first three weeks postinsertion. If *C. trachomatis* or PID is contracted with an IUD in place, practitioners must decide if the IUD should be removed. Research has found insufficient evidence to mandate removal, but close follow-up is mandatory.

Monitoring

Repeat testing is recommended for all patients treated for *C. trachomatis* at 3 to 6 months regardless of the treatment status of the patient's partner(s) because reinfection is so common. If the patient does not follow up at 3 to 6 months, he or she should be retested upon presentation for medical care within the first 12 months posttreatment.

Test of cure, which is testing at 3 to 4 weeks posttreatment, is recommended only for pregnant patients. Testing for cure earlier than 3 to 4 weeks increases the rate of false positive results. If the initial diagnosis was in the first trimester of pregnancy, testing should be

Box 1   *Chlamydia trachomatis:* Recommended Treatment Regimens by Clinical Syndrome

Cervicitis or urethritis or for presumptive treatment in nonpregnant patient*
- Azithromycin (Zithromycin) 1 g orally in a single dose

or
- Doxycycline (Vibramycin) 100 mg orally twice a day for 7 days

Alternative regimens (one of the following)
- Erythromycin base (E-Mycin) 500 mg orally four times a day for 7 days

or
- Erythromycin ethylsuccinate (EES) 800 mg orally four times a day for 7 days

or
- Levofloxacin (Levaquin)[1] 500 mg orally once daily for 7 days

or
- Ofloxacin (Floxin) 300 mg orally twice a day for 7 days

Pregnant patient with cervicitis or urethritis*
- Azithromycin 1 g orally in a single dose

or
- Amoxicillin 500 mg orally three times a day for 7 days

Alternative regimens
- Erythromycin base 500 mg orally four times a day for 7 days

or
- Erythromycin base[†] 250 mg orally four times a day for 14 days

or

- Erythromycin ethylsuccinate 800 mg orally four times a day for 7 days

or
- Erythromycin ethylsuccinate[†] 400 mg orally four times a day for 14 days
- Epididymitis
  - Ceftriaxone (Rocephin) 250 mg IM in a single dose

plus
- Doxycycline 100 mg orally twice a day for 10 days
- Ophthalmia neonatorum or *C. trachomatis* pneumonia
- Erythromycin base or ethylsuccinate 50 mg/kg/day orally divided into 4 doses daily for 14 days[‡]

Recommended regimen for children who weigh <45 kg
- Erythromycin base or ethylsuccinate 50 mg/kg/day orally divided into 4 doses daily for 14 days

Recommended regimen for children who weigh ≥45 kg but who are <8 years old
- Azithromycin 1 g orally in a single dose

Recommended regimens for children aged ≥8 years
- Azithromycin 1 gram orally in a single dose

or
- Doxycycline 100 mg orally twice a day for 7 days

Inpatient and outpatient PID
- Please refer to PID chapter for treatment regimens

Providers should consult the Centers for Disease Control and Prevention's website at http://cdc.gov/std/treatment for up-to-date treatment recommendations.
[1]Not FDA approved for this indication.
*Consider concurrent treatment for gonococcal infection if prevalence of gonorrhea is high in the patient population under assessment.
[†]The lower-dose and longer-treatment option with erythromycin can be considered if gastrointestinal tolerance is an issue.
[‡]Infants <6 weeks of age who are treated with erythromycin should be followed for signs and symptoms of infantile hypertrophic pyloric stenosis.

---

repeated in 3 to 6 months, preferably in the third trimester. Rescreening for other STIs should be performed upon retesting for *Chlamydia*.

Complications

C. trachomatis is a major public health concern because it results in serious health complications and sequelae. In women it can cause PID, endometritis, ectopic pregnancy, infertility, salpingitis, and perihepatitis (Fitz-Hugh-Curtis Syndrome). In men it is associated with postgonococcal or nongonococcal urethritis and epididymitis. Reactive arthritis can occur in both men and women.

C. trachomatis is especially problematic in pregnancy because it is associated with an increased risk of preterm labor and preterm premature rupture of membranes. Infants born to women infected with *Chlamydia* risk suffering pneumonia and conjunctivitis.

C. trachomatis pneumonia can present as an afebrile pneumonia often with a staccato cough without wheezing between 1 and 3 months of life. *C. trachomatis* conjunctivitis, also known as ophthalmia neonatorum, is uncommon in the United States, but worldwide it is the number one cause of blindness. It usually presents within the 5th and 12th day of life but can present at up to 1 month of age. State-mandated prophylactic eye ointment given to babies at birth mainly helps prevent gonococcal ophthalmia; it does not prevent perinatal transmission of *Chlamydia* from mother to infant. Therefore the screening of pregnant women and ultimate treatment of their *Chlamydia* during pregnancy is the best method of preventing complications in newborn infants.

References

Bebear C, de Barbeyrac B. Genital *Chlamydia trachomatis* infections. Clin Microbiol Infect 2009;15:4–10.
Blas MM, Canchihuaman FA, Alva IE, et al. Pregnancy outcomes in women infected with *Chlamydia trachomatis*: a population-based cohort study in Washington State. Sex Transm Infect 2007;83:314–8.
Centers for Disease Control and Prevention (CDC). Sexually Transmitted Disease Surveillance 2009. Available at: http://www.cdc.gov/std/stats09/ [accessed August 6, 2015].
Centers for Disease Control and Prevention (CDC). Sexually transmitted diseases treatment guidelines 2010. MMWR 2010;59(No. RR 12):43–9 63 67.
Honey E, Augood C, Templeton A, et al. Cost effectiveness of screening for *Chlamydia trachomatis*: a review of published studies. Sex Transm Infect 2002;78:406–12.
Johnson RE, Newhall WJ, Papp JR, et al. Screening tests to detect *Chlamydia trachomatis* and *Neisseria gonorrhoeae* infections—2002. MMWR Recomm Rep 2002;51(RR-15):1–38.
Kramer A, Schwebke I, Kampf G. How long do nosocomial pathogens persist on inanimate surfaces? A systematic review. BMC Infect Dis 2006;6:130.
Lyss SB, Kamb ML, Peterman TA, et al. *Chlamydia trachomatis* among patients infected with and treated for *Neisseria gonorrhoeae* in sexually transmitted clinics in the United States. Ann Intern Med 2003;139:178–85.

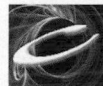

CONDYLOMA ACUMINATA

Method of
M. Chantel Long, MD

CURRENT DIAGNOSIS

- Condyloma acuminata are usually flesh-colored, brown, or gray and can be flat, plaquelike, or exophytic papules, giving them the classic "cauliflower" appearance.
- The lesions may be single or multiple and can range in size from minute to several centimeters in diameter.
- When the appearance of the lesion is typical, confirmatory tests are usually unnecessary.
- Suspicious lesions or uncertain diagnoses warrant biopsy to rule out malignancy.

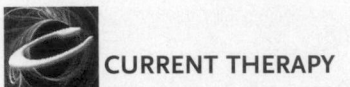

CURRENT THERAPY

- In the absence of dysplasia, treatment of subclinical human papilloma virus infection is not recommended.
- The goal of therapy is to eliminate symptoms, namely clinically apparent warts, rather than address the underlying HPV infection.
- Common treatment options include podofilox (Condylox), imiquimod (Aldara, Zyclara), sinecatechins (Veregen), podophyllin resin (Podocon-25), trichloroacetic acid (Tri-Chlor), cryotherapy, and surgery.

Epidemiology

Condyloma acuminata, commonly known as genital warts, is a sexually transmitted disease caused by the human papilloma virus (HPV). It is estimated that 20 million people are infected with HPV in the United States, with the highest prevalence in adolescents and young adults. Lifetime incidence of HPV infection is greater than 50% and appears to be increasing, making it the most common sexually transmitted disease.

Risk Factors

Risk factors associated with HPV infection include sex with an infected partner, early age at first sexual intercourse, multiple sexual partners, history of sexually transmitted infections, cigarette smoking, and lack of condom use. The majority of patients whose sexual partner has condyloma will themselves develop condyloma within 3 months. An even larger percentage of people are believed to develop subclinical infection.

Pathophysiology

About 90% of warts are caused by HPV types 6 and 11; condyloma can be coinfected with types 16, 18, 31, 33, 35, and 45, which have oncogenic potential. Genital skin appears to be less susceptible to the oncogenic potential of HPV compared to the transformation zones of the cervix and anal canal.

The virus is easily transmitted via sexual contact. Vertical transmission and autoinoculation are possible. The average incubation period between infection and appearance of condyloma ranges from 3 months to several years. Condyloma can persist or recur after therapy, undergo malignant transformation, or spontaneously regress.

Prevention

Prevention options include HPV vaccination, abstinence, routine condom use, and limiting sexual partners. Once patients have condyloma, they should be encouraged to use condoms consistently. Educate patients that condoms can decrease transmission but might not completely prevent infection.

Two HPV vaccine series are currently available in the United States. Gardasil is a quadrivalent HPV vaccine indicated for male and female patients aged 9 to 25 years for prevention of cervical cancer and genital warts. Cervarix is the bivalent vaccine indicated for female patients aged 9 to 25 years for prevention of cervical cancer.

Clinical Manifestations

Most genital warts are asymptomatic on presentation, although patients can present with complaints of a "bump." Localized irritation, pruritus, pain, or bleeding can occur, and symptoms may vary based on the location and size of the lesions. Usually, the warts appear flesh-colored, brown, or gray and can be flat, plaque-like, or exophytic papules, giving them the classic "cauliflower" appearance. The lesions may be single or multiple and range in size from minute to several centimeters in diameter. Flat HPV lesions might not be grossly visible.

The majority of HPV infections are either subclinical or unrecognized. Clinically apparent disease might represent only a small portion of the actual infected area.

Diagnosis

When the clinical appearance of the lesion is typical, confirmatory tests are usually unnecessary. The entire anogenital tract should be examined because of the widespread nature of HPV. A magnifying glass and anoscopy may be helpful for thorough detection and examination. Application of dilute 3% to 5% acetic acid solution to the skin surface can help detect subtle HPV lesions by producing an acetowhitening of the condyloma; however, this is not a specific test and is not routinely recommended. Pap smears or tissue biopsy can provide histopathologic confirmation of the diagnosis. Biopsy is recommended to rule out malignancy in any suspicious lesions, such as large or rapidly growing condyloma; pigmented, atypical, friable, bleeding, or ulcerated lesions; sites of previous treatment failure; areas of recurrence; acetowhite lesions; or lesions in immunocompromised patients. Although costly and not recommended, HPV identification via DNA testing can be performed.

Differential Diagnosis

Table 1 outlines the differential diagnosis for condyloma acuminata.

Treatment

In the absence of dysplasia, the Centers for Disease Control and Prevention recommends no treatment of subclinical HPV infection. The goal of treatment is to eliminate symptoms, namely clinically apparent warts, rather than address the underlying HPV infection. Current treatments do not eradicate the virus.

Ideally, treatment of condyloma should continue until all warts are gone. A repeated course of therapy is often required to achieve a wart-free state. Recurrence may be due to latent HPV in the surrounding normal tissue, HPV reinfection, or improper selection or use of a therapy modality. Nearly all treatment regimens have similar efficacy and rates of intolerance and toxicity. All are known to cause local pain and irritation. Any given treatment has a 40% to 80% rate of wart clearance and up to a 50% recurrence rate. It is unknown whether eliminating warts will decrease infectivity of current or future sexual partners.

The factors to consider when deciding on treatment include location and size of the warts, the patient's tolerance and preference, cost, convenience, and the clinician's preference. Patient-applied options allow the patient greater control; however, this requires good compliance, and the warts must be accessible by the patient or caregiver. Provider-applied treatments are good choices for large treatment areas. Data regarding the efficacy of using more than one modality at a time are lacking. It is common

TABLE 1	Differential Diagnosis
LESION	**APPEARANCE**
Verruca vulgaris	Occurs anywhere Tends to be thicker, drier, and hyperkeratotic
Molluscum contagiosum	Occurs anywhere Smooth, round papules with central umbilication
Seborrheic keratoses	Occurs anywhere Multiple waxy, rough, hyperpigmented papules
Condyloma latum	Moist, rounded, white papules of syphilis
Pearly penile papules	Smooth, uniform, small, 1–2 mm at corona, benign
Vestibular papillae	Both sides of vulva, female equivalent of pearly penile papules
Lichen planus	Purplish, pruritic rash or flat-topped polygonal papules
Nonpigmented nevi	Occurs anywhere Flat or raised, reddish or flesh colored

TABLE 2 Treatment Regimens

DRUG	USE ON	ADVANTAGES	DISADVANTAGES	INSTRUCTIONS
Patient Applied				
Podofilox 0.5% gel or solution (Condylox)	Moist warts	Relatively inexpensive	Avoid in pregnancy Avoid on mucous membranes Do not exceed 10 cm² area Do not exceed 0.5 mL daily; can have systemic side effects	Apply bid × 3 d, then 4 d off Repeat weekly May use for 4–6 cycles
Imiquimod 5% cream (Aldara)	Dry or moist warts		Avoid with large warts >10 cm² Requires compliance Hypo- or hyperpigmentation of treated skin can occur	Apply nightly on dry warts Apply every other night on moist warts Use up to 16 wk Wash off after 6–10 h
Sinecatechins 15% ointment (Veregen)	Dry warts		Avoid in pregnancy Avoid in immunocompromised patients	Apply tid Use up to 16 wk Do not wash off
Provider Applied				
Podophyllin resin (Podocon-25, Podofilm)	Moist warts	Use on large warts May use on urethral meatus	Avoid in pregnancy Do not exceed 10 cm² area Do not exceed 0.5 mL daily; can have systemic side effects	Apply thin layer with cotton tip Allow to air dry Repeat weekly Leave on for 4 h Do not cover May leave on overnight if tolerated
Trichloroacetic acid (TCA) (Tri-Chlor 80%)	Small, few Moist warts	May use on vagina, cervix May use on anal warts May use in pregnancy	Avoid with dry and large warts	Apply sparingly with cotton tip Air dry Repeat weekly to every other week Do not allow to "run" on normal skin Neutralize with soap or sodium bicarbonate
Cryotherapy	Small, few, flat Dry or moist	May use in pregnancy May use liquid nitrogen in vagina, meatus, anus	Avoid with large warts Avoid cryoprobe use in vagina or anus	Freeze q1–2wk Freeze 1–2 mm border May offer/need local anesthesia
Surgery	Small or large Dry or moist	May use on anal warts Use on large warts and large treatment areas	Avoid in patients with bleeding disorder	Scissors, shave biopsy, punch excision, curettage, cautery, laser
Interferon-α-2b injections (Intron A)	Refractory warts		Expensive Flulike side effects	Multiple intralesional injections Several times a week Often requires specialty referral
Laser vaporization	Refractory warts	May use on intraurethral and large warts as well as large treatment areas	Expensive	Requires specialty referral

practice for health care providers to combine treatment modalities. Table 2 outlines current therapy regimens. Topical fluorouracil (Efudex)[1] is no longer recommended. Failure to respond after four treatments or failure to clear within 3 months warrants a change in therapy modality and possible reevaluation of the diagnosis.

Advise patients to abstain from sexual activity while undergoing treatment for genital warts.

Monitoring
Counseling of patients regarding prevention and recognition of condyloma as well as screening and treatment of sexual partners should be part of the comprehensive management plan. One should consider testing for other sexually transmitted diseases because they often coexist with HPV. Encourage patients to discuss their HPV diagnosis with sexual partners. Asymptomatic partners likely harbor a subclinical infection, and examination for genital warts is appropriate if lesions are suspected. Discuss the need for smoking cessation and regular physician examinations, including Pap smears, as ways to prevent early HPV-related neoplasm.

Complications
Anogenital HPV infection with high-risk genotypes is associated with squamous cell carcinoma of the cervix, vagina, vulva, penis, and anus. Persistent HPV infection is the most important risk factor for development of cervical intraepithelial neoplasia and cancer.

[1]Not FDA approved for this indication.

References

American Academy of Pediatrics. Human papillomavirus. In: Pickering LK, Baker CJ, Kimberlin DW, Long SS, editors. Red Book: 2009 Report of the Committee on Infectious Diseases. 28th ed. Elk Grove Village, IL: American Academy of Pediatrics; 2009. p. 477–83.

Centers for Disease Control and Prevention. Epidemiology and Prevention of Vaccine-Preventable Diseases. The Pink Book. 12th ed Washington, DC: Public Health Foundation; 2011.

Centers for Disease Control and Prevention. 2010 Sexually Transmitted Diseases Treatment Guidelines. MMWR 2010;59:1–5 69–78.

Centers for Disease Control and Prevention. Human papillomavirus: HPV information for clinicians. Available at www.cdc.gov/std/hpv/Provider6-2005/ApF1-DesignA.pdf [accessed August 6, 2015].

Gilbert SM, Lambert SM, Weiner D. Extensive condylomata acuminata of the penis: Medical and surgical management. Infect Urol 2003;16:65–76.

Kodner CM, Nasrat S. Management of genital warts. Am Fam Physician 2004;70:2335–42.

GENITAL ULCER DISEASE: CHANCROID, GRANULOMA INGUINALE, AND LYMPHOGRANULOMA

Method of
Todd Stephens, MD

Chancroid, granuloma inguinale, and lymphogranuloma venereum (LGV) are important genital ulcer diseases that should be included in the differential diagnosis of patients presenting with anal or genital ulcers with or without inguinal adenopathy. Syphilis and herpes simplex virus testing should be considered on all such patients because of similarities in clinical presentation. Testing or treatment for other potential sexually transmitted infections (STIs), including HIV, should be considered given the high risk for concomitant infection.

Chancroid

History

Chancroid, also called soft sore, was first distinguished from the hard chancre of syphilis by Ricord in 1838. Ducrey, in Naples, demonstrated that inoculation of material from the chancroid ulcer into the skin of the forearm could reproduce the ulcer, and he went on to identify the causative organism, which bears his name.

Epidemiology

Chancroid is an important cause of genital ulceration in most countries of the developing world, accounting for about 10 million cases annually. Chancroid was diagnosed in 60% of patients who had genital ulcers and who presented to STI clinics in Africa before the HIV epidemic. Now, herpes simplex lesions represent a higher percentage. The prevalence of this disease is highest among commercial sex workers, and the presence of chancroid lesions significantly increases the risk of transmission of HIV. Although generally rare in industrialized countries, there have been several well-documented outbreaks in urban centers of North America, particularly among men who have sex with men.

Etiology

Chancroid is caused by *Haemophilus ducreyi*, a small anaerobic Gram-negative bacillus that forms streptobacillary chains on Gram stain and grows only on enriched media.

Clinical Features

After an incubation of 3 to 7 days, a papule appears that soon ulcerates, leaving a soft ulcer with an undermined edge and a purulent base. Vesicles are not seen. About half of patients develop unilateral inguinal adenopathy (Figure 1). Both the adenopathy and the lesions are very painful. Lesions can be single or multiple, and atypical presentations occur. Kissing lesions often occur on adjacent cutaneous surfaces. Not infrequently, a giant ulcer develops

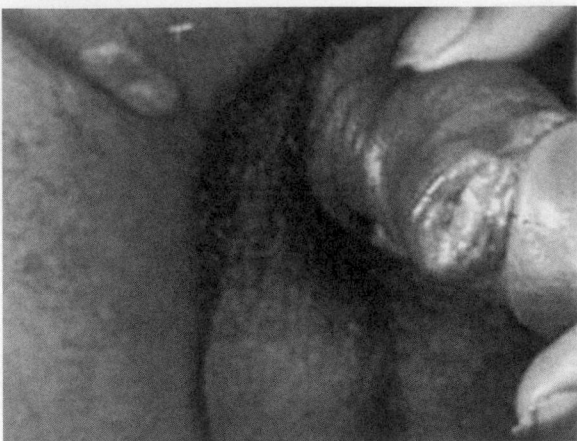

Figure 1. Chancroid. This photo shows an early chancroid ulcer on the penis along with accompanying regional inguinal adenopathy. (Courtesy of Dr. Pirozzi, Centers for Disease Control and Prevention.)

with several smaller satellite ulcers around the periphery, which can mimic the ulcerative phase of herpes simplex. More than half of the lesions occur on the prepuce, particularly in uncircumcised men. In women, the majority of lesions are on the fourchette, labia, and perianal area. Adenopathy can progress to bubo formation with tender, overlying erythema. These buboes can rupture and produce inguinal abscesses.

Diagnosis

Gram stain of smears obtained from the ulcer base has been advocated in the past for diagnosis, but this lacks both sensitivity and specificity. The preferred diagnostic modality is swabs for culture from the ulcer base or undermined edge. These are plated directly on enriched media (GC agar and Mueller-Hinton agar base) and incubated for 72 hours in an atmosphere of 5% carbon dioxide at 33°C. Polymerase chain reaction (PCR) and immunochromatography tests are also available.

Treatment

The Centers for Disease Control and Prevention (CDC) recommend a syndromal management approach in which a positive diagnosis is suggested if the patient has one or more painful ulcers and no evidence of syphilis or herpes simplex virus. Ulcers with painful adenopathy are pathognomonic (Table 1 lists antimicrobial treatment). The safety and efficacy of azithromycin (Zithromax) for pregnant and lactating women have not been established. Ciprofloxacin (Cipro)[1] is contraindicated during pregnancy and lactation. No adverse effects of chancroid on pregnancy outcome have been reported. Serologic testing for syphilis, HIV, and other appropriate STIs should be performed. Chancroidal ulcers should be kept clean with regular washing in soapy water and kept dry. Fluctuant buboes might require incision and drainage, which is preferable over needle aspiration. Treatment of all sexual partners within 60 days should be pursued, and treatment is similar to that for the source patient. Patients should not engage in sexual activity until the ulcers are healed.

Granuloma Inguinale (Donovanosis)

History

Granuloma inguinale was first recognized in India, where Donovan observed, in an oral lesion of the disease, the bodies that bear his name. There is considerable confusion about terminology between this disease and LGV, because various similar synonyms have been used inconsistently. Adding to the confusion, Donovan's name is associated with two tropical diseases that he discovered: leishmaniasis, with the discovery of intracellular protozoan

---

[1]Not FDA approved for this indication.

TABLE 1 Clinical Features and Treatment Summary of Chancroid, Granuloma Inguinale, and Lymphogranuloma Venereum

FEATURES AND TREATMENT	CHANCROID	GRANULOMA INGUINALE	LYMPHOGRANULOMA VENEREUM
Clinical Features			
Incubation period	3–7 days	3–40 days	1–28 days
Primary lesion	Papule	Papule	Papule or vesicle
Ulcerative lesion painful	Yes	No	No
Lymphadenopathy	Yes (unilateral)	No	Yes (unilateral or bilateral)
Base	Purulent	Raised, easily bleeds	Nonvascular
Border	Round, raised, undermined edges	Irregular, expansion along skin folds	Irregular, ragged
Treatment			
Treatment of choice (any of the options listed)	Azithromycin (Zithromycin) 1 g Ciprofloxacin (Cipro)[1] 500 mg bid × 3 d Ceftriaxone (Rocephin)[1] 250 mg IM once	Azithromycin 1 g PO on day 1 followed by 500 mg PO daily for 3 weeks Doxycycline (Vibramycin) 100 mg bid × 3 wks	Azithromycin[1] 1 g weekly × 3 wk Doxycycline 100 mg bid × 3 wk
Alternative treatment (any of the options listed)	Erythromycin (Ery-Tab)[1] 500 mg qid × 7 d	Azithromycin 1 g PO qwk × 3 wk Erythromycin[1] 500 mg qid × 3 wk Ciprofloxacin[1] 750 mg bid × 3 wk Trimethoprim/Sulfamethoxazole: One double-strength (160 mg/ 800 mg) tablet PO bid × 3 wk	Erythromycin[1] 500 mg qid × 3 wk

[1]Not FDA approved for this indication.

inclusions that bear his name (Leishman-Donovan bodies), and granuloma inguinale (whose intracellular inclusions were believed to be caused by protozoa but are now known to be caused by bacteria).

Epidemiology
Endemic areas are localized to a few specific areas of the tropics, particularly India, Papua New Guinea, Brazil, and the eastern part of South Africa, particularly Durban. Commercial sex workers and men are primarily involved.

Etiology
The disease is caused by an encapsulated Gram-negative coccobacillus *Klebsiella granulomatis* (previously known as *Calymmatobacterium* or *Donovania granulomatis*).

Clinical Features
A firm, painless papule or nodule is the presenting sign of granuloma inguinale. The incubation period is variable from 3 to 40 days from inoculation. This nodule quickly ulcerates, and the base is highly vascular, is beefy red, and bleeds easily. Lymphadenopathy is not part of the clinical presentation of this disease, distinguishing granuloma inguinale from chancroid and LGV. However, the ulcer can be easily confused with chancroid, condyloma lata, ulcerated verrucous warts, and squamous carcinoma. Untreated, the ulcers slowly expand, particularly along skin folds toward the inguinal region or anus (Figure 2). The ulcers are flat and raised and have slightly hypertrophic margins, but the bases are typically free of pus and necrotic debris. Less-common presentations include extragenital lesions involving the neck and mouth; cervical lesions that resemble carcinoma; and involvement of the uterus, tubes, and ovaries, producing hard masses, abscesses, or frozen pelvis.

Diagnosis
Diagnosis requires the demonstration of intracellular Donovan bodies from Giemsa or Wright staining of smears taken from a swab of the ulcer base or from biopsy material.

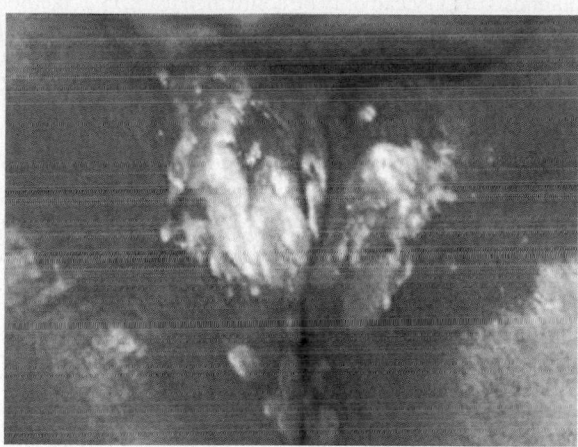

Figure 2. Granuloma inguinale. (Source: NEHC http://www.nhec.med.navy.mil/hp/sharp/std_pictures.htm)

Treatment
See Table 1 for antimicrobial treatment. Treatment should be continued until lesions are resolved and, if possible, a little longer to reduce the risk of relapse.

Lymphogranuloma Venereum
History
LGV was first differentiated from syphilis in 1906 by Wasserman, though the first full description of the disease was given by Durand, Nicolas, and Favre in 1913. In 1925, Frei developed an intradermal skin test that gave positive responses in most LGV patients. The term "tropical bubo" was associated with the disease later.

Epidemiology
LGV is largely confined to the tropics and is not a common STI. The global overall incidence is in a decline. It is seen more commonly in men, but since 2004, there has been a resurgence manifesting as proctitis in North America and Europe among HIV-positive men who have sex with men.

Etiology

LGV is a chlamydial infection caused by the invasive L1, L2, and L3 serovars of *Chlamydia trachomatis*, an intracellular gram-negative bacterium.

Clinical Features

LGV is essentially a systemic disease whose natural course is divided into three distinct phases. The initial phase of LGV is normally an inconspicuous genital lesion beginning as a typically small, painless papule or vesicle occurring 1 to 28 days after inoculation. This papule or vesicle quickly ulcerates and heals without a scar, and it often goes unrecognized by the patient (Figure 3). However, the second phase of LGV is the development of increasingly painful lymphadenopathy, often with fever and malaise. The lymphadenopathy progresses to bubo formation over 1 to 2 weeks. When a sexually active adult patient presents with an inguinal bubo not associated with genital ulcers, LGV is an important diagnosis to consider. The infected nodes are usually unilateral (bilateral in a third of cases) and often coalesce into a matted mass that can project outwards above or below the inguinal ligament, producing the pathognomonic groove sign present in 20% of patients with LGV. The buboes are likely to rupture, forming multiple sinuses. Untreated, LGV can cause extensive lymphatic damage, resulting in elephantiasis of the genitalia. Anal involvement, likewise, can lead to perirectal abscesses, fistulas, and rectal strictures. These complications represent the late phase of LGV.

Diagnosis

The diagnosis of LGV can only be confirmed using PCR methods of smears, scrapings, or aspirated material. Alternatively, the ability to perform micro-immunofluorescence serology testing using a fluorescein-conjugated monoclonal antibody and viewing the slide with a fluorescence microscope can demonstrate the inclusion bodies within the cytoplasm of macrophages. Gram staining by itself lacks appropriate sensitivity or specificity. Additional laboratory findings include leukocytosis, elevated erythrocyte sedimentation rate, and increases in immunoglobulin G and cryoglobulins.

Treatment

Antimicrobial treatment is summarized in Table 1. Needle aspiration or incision and drainage of fluctuant buboes may be required for symptomatic relief but are not routinely recommended for treatment because drainage can delay healing. Fistula openings should receive sterile dressings. One of the primary goals of treatment of LGV is to prevent long-term complications such as anogenital strictures or fistulas. Plastic surgical operations may be of benefit in cases with extensive rectal strictures or elephantiasis of the genitalia. However, these surgical interventions should only be performed after a prolonged course of antibiotics. Scars should be monitored to detect malignant change.

References

Centers for Disease Control and Prevention, Workowski KA, Berman SM. Sexually transmitted diseases treatment guidelines, 2006, MMWR Recomm Rep Aug 4;2006;55(RR-11):1–94. Available at http://www.cdc.gov/std/treatment/default.htm [accessed August 6, 2015].

Habif T. Clinical Dermatology. 4th ed. Philadelphia: Mosby; 2004. p. 325–9.

Leppard B. An Atlas of African Dermatology. Oxon, UK: Radcliffe Medical Press; 2002. pp. 69, 151, 237.

Ndinya-Achola JO, Kihara AN, Fisher LD, et al. Presumptive specific clinical diagnosis of genital ulcer disease (GUD) in a primary health care setting in Nairobi. Int J STD AIDS 1996;7(3):201–5.

Richens J, Mabey DC. Sexually transmitted infections (excluding HIV). In: Cook GC, Zumla AI, editors. Manson's Tropical Diseases. 22nd ed. London: Saunders; 2009. p. 403–34.

Ronald A. Chancroid. In: Hunter GW, Strickland GT, Magill AJ, editors. Hunter's Tropical Medicine and Emerging Infectious Diseases. 8th ed. Philadelphia: WB Saunders; 2000. p. 367–9.

GONORRHEA

Method of
Khalil G. Ghanem, MD, PhD

CURRENT DIAGNOSIS

- Gonorrhea is caused by the gram-negative diplococcus *Neisseria gonorrhoeae*.
- Asymptomatic genital gonococcal infections are common in men and women.
- Most cases of rectal and pharyngeal infections are asymptomatic.
- Culture and molecular tests are available for diagnosis, depending on the specimen type and anatomic site tested.
- All patients diagnosed with gonorrhea should be tested for other sexually transmitted infections, including HIV.

CURRENT THERAPY

- Ceftriaxone (Rocephin) 250 mg IM × 1 plus azithromycin (Zithromax) 1 g PO × 1 *or* doxycycline (Vibramycin) 100 mg PO bid × 7 days is the first-line treatment for gonorrhea.
- In the United States, single done ceftriaxone should no longer be used to treat gonorrhea.

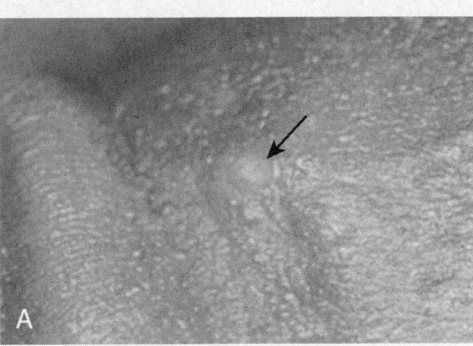
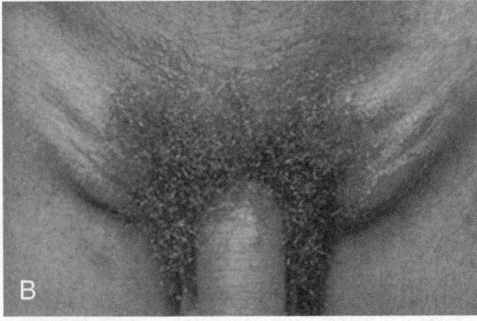

Figure 3. Lymphogranuloma venereum. **A,** Small ulcerative lesion near corona of penis *(arrow)*. **B,** Bilateral inguinal adenopathy, with developing groove sign as adenopathy expands above and below the inguinal ligament. (**A** courtesy Ronald Ballard, Reproduced with permission from The Diagnosis and Management of Sexually Transmitted Infections in South Africa, 3rd ed., Johannesburg, South African Institute for Medical Research, 2000. **B** courtesy Connexions (http://cnx.org/content/m14883/latest/Case_10-pres1-1.jpg).

Gonorrhea is caused by the gram-negative diplococcus *Neisseria gonorrhoeae*, an obligate parasite of humans that has no other natural host and to which no animal is naturally susceptible. In 2013, 333,004 cases were reported to the Centers for Disease Control and Prevention (CDC). This number is likely an underestimate because many cases are asymptomatic and others go unreported. Rates of gonorrhea in the United States declined sharply starting in the 1970s after the institution of gonorrhea control programs. It remains, however, the second most commonly reported communicable disease. Worldwide, more than 60 million new cases are estimated to occur every year.

In 2013, in the United States, the gonorrhea rate among women was 102.4 and the rate among men was 109.5 cases per 100,000 people in the general population; the rate among African Americans was 12.4 times greater than the rate for whites, although this is a decrease from 2001, when there was a 26-fold difference. Risk factors for infection include young age, unprotected intercourse, multiple sexual partners, new sexual partners, and sexual activity associated with illicit drug use. Gonococcal infection increases the rate of HIV transmission fivefold.

N. gonorrhoeae infects noncornified epithelia, including urethral, endocervical, rectal, oropharyngeal, and conjunctival cells. It is transmitted through contact with infected secretions, most often sexually, although vertical transmission from mother to infant is well described. Sexual transmission is efficient; a man who has intercourse 2.5 times with an infected female partner has a 22% chance of becoming symptomatically infected. The transmission from men to women is thought to be even more efficient.

Clinical Manifestations

Asymptomatic urethral infections occur in at least 30% of men and asymptomatic cervical infections occur in at least 50% of women. More than 50% of rectal and up to 90% of pharyngeal gonorrhea in men and women may be asymptomatic. These numbers highlight the importance of a thorough sexual history in all at-risk patients that focuses on a history of exposure rather than symptoms.

In men, urethritis is the most common manifestation of gonococcal infection. Urethral discharge and dysuria are the most frequent signs occurring 2 to 5 days after exposure. Acute epididymitis manifesting as unilateral scrotal pain is the most common local complication. In young men, 30% of cases of acute epididymitis are caused by *N. gonorrhoeae*. Rarely, cellulitis, lymphangitis, or periurethral abscesses may complicate local infections. Differential diagnosis of urethritis in men includes *Chlamydia trachomatis, Mycoplasma genitalium,* and *Trichomonas vaginalis* infections.

Among women, the most common manifestation of local gonococcal infection is cervicitis, which tends to occur 5 to 10 days after exposure. When patients are symptomatic, common complaints include a vaginal discharge, dysuria, and genital itching. Concomitant infection of the urethra may occur in up to 90% of women and accounts for some of these symptoms. *N. gonorrhoeae* may also infect Skene's and Bartholin's glands. The differential diagnosis of cervicitis includes infection with *C. trachomatis, T. vaginalis, M. genitalium,* or herpes simplex virus and bacterial vaginosis. An important complication of gonococcal infections in women is pelvic inflammatory disease (PID). PID is the result of ascending infection involving the uterus, fallopian tubes, ovaries, or peritoneum. Sequelae of PID include infertility, ectopic pregnancy, and chronic pelvic pain. All women presenting with cervicitis should undergo a bimanual examination. The diagnosis of PID is made when one or more of the following signs are present: uterine tenderness, cervical motion tenderness, or adnexal tenderness.

Among men and women with rectal gonorrhea, those who are symptomatic may complain of rectal discharge, pain, and tenesmus. Most cases of rectal gonorrhea in men result from receptive anal intercourse; some cases in women may result from perineal contamination. The differential diagnosis includes *C. trachomatis* (including lymphogranuloma venereum strains), *Treponema pallidum,* and herpes simplex virus infections. Most cases of pharyngeal gonorrhea are asymptomatic; when present, signs and symptoms may include acute pharyngitis, tonsillitis, and cervical lymphadenopathy.

The pharynx may be the only infected site in up to 30% of patients. A careful history, including past oral-genital contact, is mandatory. Conjunctivitis is rare in adults and usually is a result of self-inoculation from anogenital infections.

Disseminated gonococcal infections may occur in up to 2% of untreated patients. Certain gonococcal strains are more likely to cause disseminated gonococcal infections. Although patients are bacteremic, many appear nontoxic. Symptoms and signs may include fevers, myalgias, arthralgias, asymmetrical polyarthritis, and a characteristic dermatitis consisting of a small number (<30) of skin lesions on the distal extremities that begin as papules and progress to pustules and ulcerations. Rarely, meningitis and endocarditis may occur.

Vertical transmission to neonates may result in ophthalmia neonatorum, sepsis, arthritis, meningitis, rhinitis, vaginitis, urethritis, and inflammation at the sites of fetal monitoring. Gonococcal infections diagnosed in preadolescent children usually indicate sexual abuse.

Diagnosis

Gram's stain of urethral discharge among symptomatic men is 90% sensitive and 95% specific. It is only 70% sensitive in asymptomatic men. Endocervical Gram's stain is only 50% to 70% sensitive, and anal swabs are only 60% sensitive. Culture (usually on Thayer-Martin medium) is 95% sensitive in symptomatic men but is less so for asymptomatic men and women (80%–90%). The sensitivity of culture in detecting gonococcal infections from urine is low. Culture may be used to diagnose pharyngeal and rectal infections (but has low sensitivity) and is the only FDA-approved test to diagnose gonococcal infections in children. Antibiotic susceptibility testing can be performed only on cultured specimens.

Definitive diagnosis of gonorrhea by culture from any genital or extragenital site requires confirmation of isolates by biochemical, enzymatic, serologic, or nucleic acid testing (e.g., carbohydrate use, rapid enzyme substrate tests, serologic methods such as coagglutination or fluorescent antibody tests) supplemented with additional tests that can ensure accurate identification of isolates or a DNA probe technique for confirmation. After the culture is submitted, this type of identification is usually performed by the laboratory without requesting it, and when these methods are used, there should be no pitfalls in interpreting the extragenital culture data.

Nucleic acid amplification tests (e.g., polymerase chain reaction, transcription-mediated amplification, etc.) are the most sensitive (>95%) and specific (>95%), and most can be performed on urethral or cervical specimens in addition to first-catch urine and clinician or self-collected vaginal swabs. Among women, vaginal swabs are the preferred collection specimen. Urine is the preferred collection specimen among men. Nucleic acid amplification tests are not FDA cleared for pharyngeal and rectal specimens, although data demonstrate that some are far more sensitive than culture in detecting gonococcal infections at these sites. The CDC currently recommends nucleic acid amplification tests as the method of choice for detecting extragenital gonococcal infections. Most commercial laboratories now offer testing of extragenital specimens using nucleic acid amplification. Serologic tests have been used for epidemiologic studies, but they should not be used for diagnosis. All patients tested for gonorrhea should also be tested for Chlamydia trachomatis, syphilis, and HIV.

Antimicrobial Resistance and Therapy

For 40 years, penicillin was the drug of choice for treating gonorrhea. Tetracyclines were also highly effective. By the 1980s, widespread resistance to both of these drug classes rendered them all but useless. Subsequently, drug resistance to aminoglycosides, spectinomycin,[2] macrolides, trimethoprim-sulfamethoxazole (Bactrim),[1] and fluoroquinolones has made the treatment of gonorrhea more challenging.

Fluoroquinolone resistant *N. gonorrhoeae* (FQRNG) strains emerged in the 1990s. In April 2007, the CDC recommended that fluoroquinolones not be used to treat gonococcal infections in the United States.

---

[1]Not FDA approved for this indication.
[2]Not available in the United States.

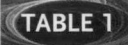

TABLE 1 Centers for Disease Control and Prevention 2006 Treatment Recommendations for Complicated and Uncomplicated Gonorrhea

DISEASE	TREATMENT
Uncomplicated infections of the cervix, urethra, and rectum*	Ceftriaxone (Rocephin) 250 mg IM × 1 *plus* Azithromycin (Zithromax) 1 g PO × 1 *or* Doxycycline (Vibramycin) 100 mg PO bid × 7 d
Infections of the pharynx	*As above*
Epididymitis	Ceftriaxone (Rocephin) 250 mg IM × 1 *plus* Doxycycline (Vibramycin) 100 mg PO bid × 10 d
Gonococcal conjunctivitis	Ceftriaxone (Rocephin) 1 g IM × 1
Disseminated gonococcal infections[†]	Ceftriaxone (Rocephin) 1 g IM or IV q24h

*Alternative regimens are: (1) azithromycin (Zithromax) 2 g PO × 1 or (2) Cefixime 400 mg PO plus azithromycin (Zithromax) 1 g PO or doxycycline (Vibramycin) 100 mg PO bid × 7d.

[†]Should be treated with a parenteral regimen until 24 hours after clinical improvement; can complete a 7-day course of therapy with oral cefixime if antimicrobial susceptibility testing results confirm susceptibility to cefixime.

Table 1 summarizes the current CDC recommendations for treating gonococcal infections. There have been no reports of ceftriaxone-resistant strains in the United States, although strains resistant to oral cephalosporins have been reported. Increasing MICs to cephalosporins prompted the CDC to recommend dual therapy for gonorrhea using cephalosporins and either azithromycin (Zithromax) or doxycycline (Vibramycin)—even if concomitant infection with *Chlamydia trachomatis* is excluded. Ceftriaxone (Rocephin), the preferred cephalosporin, is given intramuscularly and is effective for infections at all sites. Cefixime (Suprax) is effective for anogenital infections, but it may have lower efficacy than ceftriaxone for pharyngeal infections. Cephalosporins and macrolides are safe to use in pregnancy. All sexual contacts in the preceding 60 days of index patients should also be treated.

For penicillin-allergic patients, treatment of gonorrhea has become more challenging. Initially, spectinomycin was recommended as a second-line agent. Spectinomycin has only 80% efficacy in treating pharyngeal gonococcal infections, but spectinomycin is no longer available in the United States.

Alternative regimens include a single dose of azithromycin (Zithromax) 2 g PO. This regimen has excellent activity against anogenital and pharyngeal infections. Azithromycin has been used in pregnant women without evidence of teratogenicity. Cases of high-level resistance to azithromycin have been described recently in the United States. Another approved alternative regimen is cefixime 400 mg PO plus either 1 g of azithromycin or 1 week of oral doxycycline.

If any alternative regimen is used, a test of cure within 2 weeks following therapy is currently recommended by the CDC. Suspected treatment failures should prompt clinicians to obtain cultures and antimicrobial susceptibility testing. Treatment failures following therapy with an alternative regimen must be treated with ceftriaxone 250 mg IM plus azithromycin 2 g PO. Confirmed treatment failures using the preferred ceftriaxone-based regimen should be treated based on antimicrobial susceptibility testing results in consultation with an infectious diseases specialist.

To prevent gonococcal ophthalmia neonatorum, 1% silver nitrate aqueous solution, 0.5% erythromycin ophthalmic ointment (Ilotycin), or 1% tetracycline ophthalmic ointment[1] should be instilled into the eyes of all newborns. Treatment of gonococcal ophthalmia requires hospitalization, evaluation for evidence of disseminated infection, and ceftriaxone (Rocephin) 25 to 50 mg/kg IM or IV × 1 dose.

---

[1]Not FDA approved for this indication.

Prevention and Screening

Abstinence from sexual intercourse is the single most reliable method of preventing infection. Male condoms, when used correctly and consistently, are highly effective in preventing infection. Diaphragms may help prevent gonococcal infections in women. There have not been any successful vaccine candidates.

The CDC does not recommend universal screening for *N. gonorrhoeae*. All sexually active men who have sex with men should be screened annually at all sites of exposure. High-risk women (e.g., multiple sexual partners, illicit drug use, history of gonorrhea or other sexually transmitted infection, commercial sex worker, inconsistent condom use) should be screened. Up to 20% persons diagnosed with gonorrhea become reinfected in the next few months. Rescreening 3 months after infection is treated is recommended in both men and women. High-risk pregnant women should be screened during the first prenatal visit. Repeat testing during the third trimester for those at continued risk is recommended.

References

Centers for Disease Control and Prevention. Update to CDC's sexually transmitted diseases treatment guidelines, 2010: oral cephalosporins no longer a recommended treatment for gonococcal infections. MMWR 2012;61:590–4.

Deguchi T, et al. Management of pharyngeal gonorrhea is crucial to prevent the emergence and spread of antibiotic-resistant *Neisseria gonorrhoeae*. Antimicrob Agents Chemother 2012;56:4039–40.

Katz KA, Pierce EF, Aiem H, et al. *Neisseria gonorrhoeae* with reduced susceptibility to azithromycin—San Diego County, CA, 2009. MMWR 2011;60:579–81.

Kircaldy RD, et al. Cephalosporin-resistant gonorrhea in North America. JAMA 2013;309:185–7.

Workowski KA. Chlamydia and gonorrhea. Ann Int Med 2013;158:ITC2–1.

Workowski KA, Berman SM. For the Centers for Disease Control and Prevention. Sexually transmitted diseases treatment guidelines, 2010. MMWR Morb Mortal Wkly Rep 2010;59(RR-2):1–114.

NONGONOCOCCAL URETHRITIS

Method of
Robert S. Freelove, MD

CURRENT DIAGNOSIS

- Urethritis is diagnosed by the presence of mucopurulent/purulent urethral discharge, >5 WBC/hpf on Gram stain of urethral secretions, a positive leukocyte esterase test or ≥10 WBC/hpf on microscopic examination of first-void urine.
- Testing first-void urine/urethral discharge using NAAT has replaced culture as the "gold standard" in diagnosis of chlamydial NGU.
- Test for cure is indicated in pregnant women and should wait at least 3 to 4 weeks after treatment.
- Patients with confirmed *Chlamydia* infection should be rescreened 3 to 6 months after treatment.

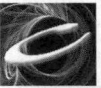

CURRENT THERAPY

- Treatment of choice is azithromycin (Zithromax) 1 g orally in a single dose.
- Other first-line treatment is doxycycline (Vibramycin) 100 mg orally twice a day for 7 days.
- If test results are not immediately available, patients should receive concurrent treatment for gonorrhea with ceftriaxone (Rocephin) 250 mg IM.
- Expedited partner therapy should be offered where allowed.

- Persistent symptoms in compliant patients who have not been reexposed can be treated with metronidazole (Flagyl) 2 g orally in a single dose.

Epidemiology

Chlamydia trachomatis is the most common pathogen identified in nongonococcal urethritis (NGU) in men. Other potential causes include *Mycoplasma genitalium*, *Trichomonas vaginalis*, herpes simplex virus, adenovirus, and urethral trauma. Chlamydia is the most commonly reported sexually transmitted infection (STI) in the United States. Determining the exact prevalence of *C. trachomatis* infection is difficult, because most infected individuals are asymptomatic. Additionally, although screening commonly occurs in women, empiric treatment without confirmatory testing is routinely extended to sexual partners of those who test positive. While 1,307,893 cases were reported to the CDC in 2010, the estimated prevalence is 2.8 million.

Risk Factors

C. trachomatis infection is associated with young age (less than 25 years), multiple sex partners, history of prior STI, low condom use, cervical ectopy, lower socioeconomic status, and low/intermediate education. Insertive oral sex among men who have sex with men is associated with urethritis caused by HSV or adenovirus. Posttraumatic urethritis is 10 times more likely in patients using latex catheters than silicone catheters for intermittent catheterization.

Pathophysiology

Urethritis is inflammation of the urethra caused by infection or traumatic injury. The term *nongonococcal urethritis* is typically reserved to describe an STI of the male urethra with a negative Gram stain of urethral discharge, most commonly due to *Chlamydia*. In women, urethral infection often accompanies chlamydial cervicitis.

C. trachomatis is an obligate intracellular parasite with a two-phase life cycle: an extracellular, nonreplicating, infectious elementary body; and an intracellular, replicating, noninfectious reticulate body. A cycle can take 3 to 5 days, requiring prolonged courses of treatment. Immunity to infection is relatively short-lived, contributing to reinfection or persistent infection.

Prevention

Primary prevention of NGU relies on education regarding chlamydial infection targeted at adolescents and young adults. Education should include promotion of behavioral changes aimed at reducing the risk of acquiring and transmitting STIs such as abstinence from sexual activity, delaying coitarche, reducing the number of sexual partners, and consistent and correct condom use.

Because most infections in males and females are asymptomatic, screening at-risk individuals is a cornerstone of secondary prevention. As most reproductive complications of *Chlamydia* infection occur in women, the CDC recommends annual screening of all sexually active, nonpregnant women 25 years old or younger and sexually active older women with a new partner or multiple partners. Because of the potential for maternal complications and transmission to the neonate, the CDC also recommends screening all pregnant women regardless of age. The CDC reserves screening of males for those at highest risk, including men attending STI clinics, under age 30 in the military, in correctional facilities, whose partners test positive, and who have sex with men. The United States Preventive Services Task Force recommends screening all sexually active and pregnant women age 24 or younger; recommends screening women age 25 or older only if they are at increased risk, whether or not they are pregnant; and concludes that there is insufficient evidence to assess benefits and harms of screening in men.

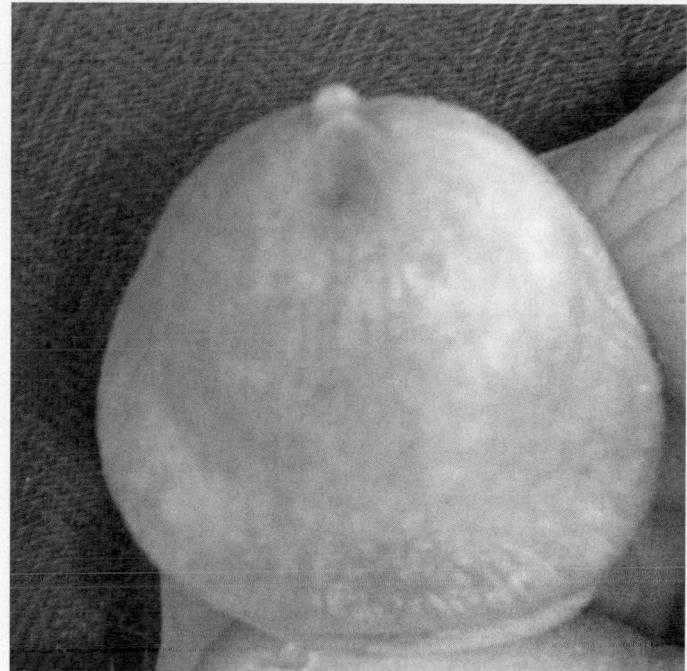

Figure 1. Mucopurulent urethral discharge in patient with NGU.

Clinical Manifestations

Many patients with NGU are asymptomatic, including up to 42% of men and 75% of women. The most common complaints are urethral discharge and/or dysuria, usually appearing 1 to 3 weeks after exposure. The discharge can be watery, mucoid, or mucopurulent (Figure 1). The dysuria is commonly described as a burning sensation. Men may also have some itching and/or redness at the urethral meatus. Symptoms appear 1 to 3 weeks after exposure. Physical examination should include inspection for inguinal lymphadenopathy, ulcers, and/or urethral discharge.

Diagnosis

Urethritis is diagnosed clinically based on the presence of mucopurulent or purulent urethral discharge, greater than 5 WBC/hpf on Gram stain of urethral secretions, a positive leukocyte esterase test on first-void urine or 10 WBC/hpf or greater on microscopic examination of first-void urine sediment. All patients who have confirmed or suspected urethritis should be tested for both gonorrhea and chlamydia, and consideration should be given to check for other STIs. *C. trachomatis* cannot be cultured on artificial media and instead requires a tissue culture. However, nucleic acid amplification techniques (NAAT) are both sensitive and specific and have replaced culture as the "gold standard" in diagnosis of chlamydial NGU. Testing can be performed on urethral specimens or on urine. Performing the testing on urine avoids invasive sampling of the urethra and may improve patient acceptance. Testing first-morning void improves detection rate.

Differential Diagnosis

The differential diagnoses include gonococcal urethritis, urinary tract infection (UTI), and urethritis caused by *M. genitalium*, HSV, and *T. vaginalis*. The incubation period for gonococcal urethritis is typically shorter and the discharge is more copious and purulent. UTIs usually cause more dysuria as well as other urinary symptoms, and bacteria can often be identified on Gram stain during urinalysis.

Therapy (or Treatment)

Treatment for chlamydial urethritis should be initiated immediately after diagnosis, ideally observed and in the health-care provider's office to ensure compliance. Recommended first-line agents are azithromycin (Zithromax) 1 g orally in a single dose or doxycycline (Vibramycin) 100 mg orally twice a day for 7 days.

Alternative regimens include erythromycin base (Ery-Tab) 500 mg orally four times a day for 7 days; or erythromycin ethylsuccinate (E.E.S.) 800 mg orally four times a day for 7 days; or ofloxacin (Floxin) 300 mg orally twice a day for 7 days; or levofloxacin (Levaquin) 500 mg orally once daily for 7 days. Patients with confirmed urethritis in whom test results are not already known or immediately available should also be treated empirically for gonorrhea with ceftriaxone (Rocephin) 250 mg intramuscularly in a single dose. All sexual partners should be referred for evaluation and treatment. Alternatively, expedited partner therapy (EPT), providing prescriptions or medications to the patient to take to his/her partner, should be offered where allowed; EPT has been shown to increase partner treatment and reduce reinfection. Patients with symptoms of persistent or recurrent infection can be re-treated with the initial regimen if they were not compliant with treatment or have been reexposed to an untreated partner. If the patient was compliant and was not reexposed, he or she should be treated with metronidazole (Flagyl) 2 g orally in a single dose; or tinidazole (Tindamax) 2 g orally in a single dose plus azithromycin (Zithromax) 1 g orally in a single dose.

Monitoring

Testing for cure is not recommended except in pregnant women or those in whom therapeutic compliance is in question, and must wait for at least 3 to 4 weeks after treatment, because NAAT may be positive in the presence of dead organisms. All patients with *Chlamydia* infection should be screened again 3 to 6 months after treatment.

Complications

In men, untreated chlamydial NGU can lead to epididymitis and/or prostatitis. Reactive arthritis is an uncommon complication in men, as is Reiter syndrome (arthritis, conjunctivitis/uveitis, urethritis, mucocutaneous lesions). In women, concurrent cervicitis can lead to PID. Transmission to newborns can result in conjunctivitis or pneumonia.

References

Workowski KA, Berman S. Centers for Disease Control and Prevention. Sexually transmitted diseases treatment guidelines, 2010. MMWR 2010;59(RR-12):1–110.

Centers for Disease Control and Prevention. STD trends in the United States: 2010 national data for gonorrhea, chlamydia, and syphilis. Table. http://www.cdc.gov/std/stats10/tables/trends-table.htm; [accessed 05.08.13].

Centers for Disease Control and Prevention. Expedited partner therapy in the management of sexually transmitted diseases. Atlanta, GA: US Department of Health and Human Services; 2006.

U.S. Preventive Services Task Force. Screening for chlamydial infection: U.S. Preventive Services Task Force Recommendation Statement. Ann Intern Med 2007;147:128–33.

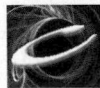 **SYPHILIS**

Method of
Jennifer Frank, MD

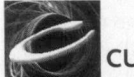 **CURRENT DIAGNOSIS**

- Serologic testing includes both nontreponemal-specific testing (VDRL and RPR) and treponemal-specific testing (FTA-Abs [fluorescent treponemal antibody absorption] and TP-PA [*Treponema pallidum* particle agglutination]).
- Cerebrospinal fluid testing (VDRL [Venereal Disease Research Laboratory], protein, cell count) is performed to diagnose neurosyphilis.

CURRENT THERAPY

- Penicillin is first-line therapy for all types and stages of syphilis.
- Penicillin is the only recommended treatment for pregnant women and for congenital syphilis. Penicillin-allergic patients should undergo desensitization.

Epidemiology

Primary and secondary syphilis rates have increased since 2000 when they reached the lowest-ever rate of 2.1 cases per 100,000. Rates peaked in 2009 but have increased from 2005 through 2013. While rates in men have increased from 2005–2013, rates in women initially rose from 2005–2008 but have declined since 2009. Men who have sex with men (MSM) account for the majority of those with primary and secondary syphilis with a 50–75% rate of HIV coinfection. Historically, the majority of cases occurred in the South but in 2013 the Western region had the highest case rate.

Risk Factors

MSM and HIV-positive persons are at highest risk for primary and secondary syphilis. Other risk factors include living in the southern part of the United States or an urban area, young age (20 to 29 years), and being born to a mother infected with syphilis.

Pathophysiology

Syphilis is caused by infection with the spirochete *Treponema pallidum* subspecies *pallidum* (Figure 1). Primary infection manifests with signs and symptoms at the site of infection; secondary and tertiary syphilis manifest with systemic signs and symptoms. Syphilis is primarily sexually transmitted but may be transmitted perinatally or through nonsexual cutaneous transmission.

Prevention

Prevention includes both avoiding initial infection and preventing disease progression through early detection and treatment. Transmission of syphilis can be reduced (although not eliminated) by using condoms. Screening for syphilis in pregnancy combined with treatment of infected women reduces perinatal transmission.

Clinical Manifestations

Primary syphilis manifests as a chancre at the site of inoculation. The chancre, a painless ulcer with sharp borders, is usually solitary and associated with regional lymphadenopathy. Atypical presentations include extragenital location (most commonly oral or anal) and the presence of pain or multiple lesions. Secondary syphilis characteristically manifests with a generalized rash with variable

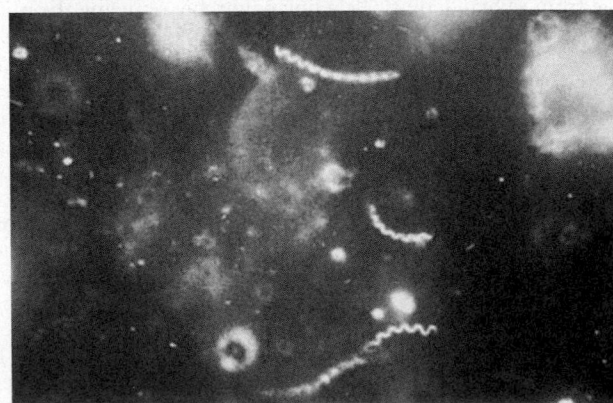

Figure 1. *Treponema pallidum* on darkfield microscopy.

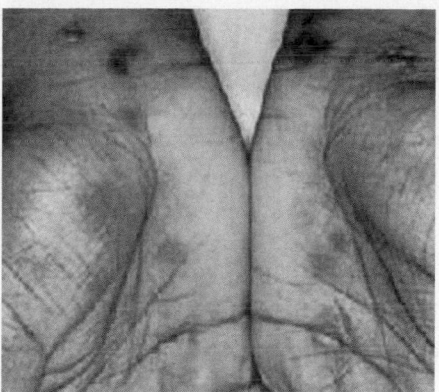

Figure 2. Syphilis skin lesion.

features (Figure 2). The palms and soles are affected in the majority of patients. Typically, the rash is maculopapular or papulosquamous and nonpruritic. Other clinical manifestations include highly infectious flat lesions (condyloma lata), fever, malaise, sore throat, headache, myalgias, alopecia, and, rarely, renal, bone, eye, or liver involvement. Latent syphilis, by definition, has no clinical manifestations.

Tertiary syphilis is a late manifestation in untreated people and includes neurosyphilis, cardiovascular, and gummatous disease. Gummas are nodular lesions that vary in size and location. They can ulcerate and cause local tissue destruction. Other skin lesions include granulomas and plaque formation. Cardiovascular syphilis most commonly manifests as aortitis of the ascending aorta. The clinical manifestations of neurosyphilis are numerous and include meningitis with or without vascular involvement, dementia, tabes dorsalis (posterior column involvement with ataxia and bowel and bladder dysfunction), and ocular or otologic involvement.

Congenital syphilis has early (birth to 2 years) and late (2 to 20 years) clinical manifestations. Early signs include hepatosplenomegaly, rash, fever, neurosyphilis, pneumonitis, rhinitis, generalized lymphadenopathy, hepatitis, ascites, hematologic disease, renal disease, periostitis, and osteochondritis. Late manifestations (present in 40% of untreated patients) include skeletal deformities, neurologic disease (deafness), dental abnormalities, and ocular abnormalities.

Diagnosis

Diagnostic evaluation of syphilis depends on the stage and location of suspected infection. Darkfield microscopy or direct fluorescent antibody testing is done on tissue or exudates obtained from an ulcer or chancre (primary infection). Serologic testing is done using nontreponemal (VDRL or RPR) and treponemal testing (FTA-ABS or TP-PA) because both tests have limitations. Nontreponemal testing may be falsely positive with other medical conditions, but antibody titers correlate with disease activity and therefore can indicate response to treatment. Nontreponemal tests usually become nonreactive after successful treatment. A serofast reaction can occur in which the nontreponemal test stays reactive. Treponemal tests are specific for syphilitic infection but usually stay reactive regardless of treatment or disease status. Treponemal test antibody titers do not match the level of disease activity and therefore cannot be used to monitor treatment response.

Neurosyphilis is diagnosed based on clinical signs and symptoms using laboratory testing to support a clinical diagnosis. No single test can be used to diagnose all patients with neurosyphilis, which means that neurosyphilis is usually diagnosed by a combination of serologic testing, testing of cerebrospinal fluid (CSF), and clinical evaluation. Laboratory testing includes reactive serologic testing; cerebrospinal fluid (CSF) VDRL (Venereal Disease Research Laboratory) testing, which is specific but not sensitive; and CSF positive for white blood cells or protein, or both. The CSF FTA-Abs (fluorescent treponemal antibody absorption) test is sensitive but less specific than CSF VDRL testing.

Differential Diagnosis

Syphilis, which can affect every organ system, has historically been called the great mimicker. Syphilis is on the differential diagnosis of, most commonly, conditions causing genital ulcers or lesions, conditions causing systemic rashes affecting the palms and soles, conditions causing ocular and otologic manifestations (uveitis, sudden visual changes, hearing loss), and conditions causing dementia, meningitis, or ataxia.

Treatment

Penicillin G is the preferred treatment for all stages of syphilis. The stage and extent of clinical disease determine which preparation is used, the dosage, and the length of treatment (Table 1). In penicillin-allergic patients, antibiotic alternatives exist for all types and stages of syphilis except for syphilis in pregnancy and congenital syphilis.

Neurosyphilis is ideally treated with penicillin. Alternative treatment of primary and secondary syphilis and early latent syphilis includes doxycycline (Vibramycin) 100 mg orally twice a day or tetracycline 500 mg orally four times daily for 14 days. Ceftriaxone (Rocephin)[1] 1 g daily IM or IV for 10 to 14 days is also used, although data is limited regarding optimal dose and treatment duration. Azithromycin (Zithromax)[1] 2 g orally as a single dose may be used when treatment with both penicillin and doxycycline is contraindicated, although treatment failures have been reported and azithromycin is not appropriate treatment for MSM or in pregnancy. Penicillin-allergic patients with late latent syphilis can be treated with doxycycline 100 mg orally twice daily or tetracycline 500 mg orally four times daily for 28 days, recognizing that there is limited data to support this treatment. Treatment of penicillin-allergic patients with tertiary syphilis should be done is consultation with a specialist. Ceftriaxone[1] 2 g given IV or IM daily for 10 to 14 days has been described for the treatment of neurosyphilis in penicillin-allergic patients.

The Jarisch-Herxheimer reaction is an acute febrile reaction (with accompanying headache, myalgias, and other symptoms) occurring within 24 hours of treatment of syphilis. It is more common in early stages of syphilis and rare in newborns.

Monitoring

No definite criteria exist for either cure of syphilis or treatment failure. It is recommended that nontreponemal antibody titers be followed every 6 months, and patients should be periodically reexamined for clinical signs or symptoms of syphilitic infection. Treatment failure is probable in patients with either persistent or recurrent clinical signs or symptoms or a sustained fourfold increase in nontreponemal antibody titer (compared to maximum titer at time of treatment). Treatment failure is possible if nontreponemal antibody titers fail to decline fourfold within 6 months after treatment. Suspected treatment failure warrants retesting for neurosyphilis and HIV infection. Patients with HIV infection, with congenital syphilis, who are pregnant, or who have neurosyphilis warrant closer and more-specific laboratory and clinical follow-up. Full recommendations can be found in the Centers for Disease Control and Prevention (CDC) treatment guidelines (http://www.cdc.gov/std/treatment/2010/default.htm).

---

[1]Not FDA approved for this indication.

TABLE 1 CDC Recommendations for Treatment of Syphilis

STAGE	RECOMMENDED PENICILLIN TREATMENT	
	PENICILLIN	*DOSAGE*
Primary and secondary syphilis	Benzathine penicillin G (Bicillin LA)	2.4 million U IM once
Early latent syphilis (acquired within previous 12 mo)	Benzathine penicillin G	2.4 million U IM once
Late latent syphilis	Benzathine penicillin G	2.4 million U IM weekly × 3 doses
Tertiary syphilis	Benzathine penicillin G	2.4 million units IM weekly × 3 doses
Neurosyphilis	Aqueous crystalline penicillin G *or*	3–4 million U q4h
	Continuous infusion *or*	18–24 U daily IV × 10–14 d (preferred)
	Procaine penicillin (Wycillin) *plus*	2.4 million U IM
	Probenecid	500 mg PO qid
Congenital Syphilis		
Proven or highly probable disease	Aqueous crystalline penicillin G *or*	100,000–150,000 U/kg/d (divided 50,000 U/kg/dose) IV q12h × first 7 d of life, then q8h for total of 10 d of treatment
	Procaine penicillin G	50,000 U/kg/dose IM daily × 10 d
Normal examination but mother inadequately treated	Aqueous crystalline penicillin G *or*	100,000–150,000 U/kg/d (divided 50,000 U/kg/dose) IV q12h × first 7 d of life, then q8h for total of 10 days of treatment
	Procaine penicillin G *or*	50,000 U/kg/dose IM daily × 10 d
	Benzathine penicillin G	50,000 U/kg/dose IM once
Normal examination, serologic titers ≤4× the maternal titer, and mother adequately treated during pregnancy	Benzathine penicillin G	50,000 U/kg/dose IM once

Abbreviation: CDC = Centers for Disease Control and Prevention.

Complications

Complications of syphilis are primarily related to neurologic involvement, tertiary syphilis, or late manifestations of congenital syphilis.

References

Centers for Disease Control and Prevention. Secually transmitted diseases treatment guidelines 2010. MMWR 2010; 59(N. RR-12):26–39.

Centers for Disease Control and Prevention, WorkowskiKA. Berman SM. Sexually transmitted diseases treatment guidelines, 2006, MMWR Recomm Rep Aug 4;2006;55(RR-11):1–94. Available at: http://www.cdc.gov/std/treatment/default.htm; (accessed August 6, 2015).

Kent ME, Romanelli F. Reexamining syphilis: An update on epidemiology, clinical manifestations, and management. Ann Pharmacother 2008;42:226–36.

Koss CA, Dunne EF, Warner L. A systematic review of epidemiologic studies assessing condom use and risk of syphilis. Sex Trans Dis 2009;36:401–5.

Lautenschlager S. Cutaneous manifestations of syphilis. Am J Clin Dermatol 2006;7:291–304.

Morbidity and Mortality Weekly Report. Primary and secondary syphilis – United States, 2005–2013. Available at: http://www.cdc.gov/mmwr/preview/mmwrhtml/mm6318a4.htm; (accessed August 6, 2015).

Marra CM. Update on neurosyphilis. Curr Infect Dis Rep 2009;11:127–34.

Woods CR. Congenital syphilis—persisting pestilence. Pediatr Infect Dis 2009;28:536–7.

15 Psychiatric Disorders

ALCOHOLISM

Method of
Richard N. Rosenthal, MD

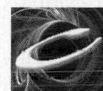

CURRENT DIAGNOSIS

Risky or Hazardous Drinking (Need Further Evaluation)
- Men who drink more than four standard drinks per day or 14 standard drinks per week
- Women and those older than 65 years who drink more than three standard drinks per day or more than seven standard drinks per week
- Drinking concurrent with any medical condition where alcohol is contraindicated

Alcohol Use Disorder
- Repeated failure to fulfill obligations at home, school, or work
- Increased risk of physical harm
- Drinking despite causing social or interpersonal problems
- Episodes of alcohol craving or strong urges
- Cannot cut down or stop
- Decreased time spent in other usual activities
- Drinking despite physical or psychological consequences
- Drinking more than intended
- Physical tolerance
- Preoccupied with drinking
- Withdrawal episodes

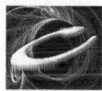

CURRENT THERAPY

All At-Risk Patients
- Assess: Screen patients with standard instruments and compute average standard drinks per week.
- Advise: Give feedback, express concern, present findings and conclusions, and recommend specific behavioral changes.
- Agree: Determine the patient's readiness to change, encourage reflection, listen empathically, elicit patient concerns, avoid arguing, express optimism, set a specific reduction or abstinence goal.
- Assist: Formulate concrete implementation plan, including avoiding high-risk situations, recording alcohol intake, and eliciting family and community support for patient goals.
- Arrange: Set up follow-up visits and refer patients meeting dependence criteria for specialty treatment.

Additionally for Alcohol-Dependent Patients
- Offer or arrange for detoxification if indicated.
- Offer or arrange for specialty alcoholism treatment and/or mutual help groups.
- Offer pharmacotherapy to support maintenance of abstinence: naltrexone, acamprosate, or disulfiram.
- Offer medication management support during follow-up visits.

Epidemiology
Alcohol use disorders are among the most prevalent mental disorders in the population, occurring at frequencies that rival those of mood and anxiety disorders. In any year, almost 8.5% of the U.S. population older than 18 years meets criteria for a formal alcohol use disorder (alcohol abuse or dependence), and almost 4% meets criteria for alcohol dependence.

Economic and Medical Sequelae
Alcohol use disorders are important to identify and treat for several reasons. The first is the direct negative impact of chronic heavy alcohol exposure on cognitive, physical, social, and vocational functioning. The second is the well-described long-term medical sequelae of alcohol dependence such as hepatic cirrhosis, pancreatitis, and dementia. Chronic heavy drinking, even in the absence of a formal diagnosis of alcohol dependence, is associated with an increased risk of diabetes mellitus, hypertension, gastrointestinal bleeding, hemorrhagic stroke, and several forms of carcinoma. The third reason for identification and treatment is the public impact of alcohol use disorders, which covers associated traumatic injuries from motor vehicle and job-related accidents, alcohol related crime, and their associated economic costs. More than $180 billion is lost to the U.S. economy each year as a result of alcohol-related crime, injury, health care costs, and lost productivity in the workplace.

Screening
Screening Rationale
Screening for alcohol problems arrays patients on a continuum from abstinence to dependence and is a highly efficient way to identify patients who are at acute risk for the effects of alcohol abuse and dependence as well as those who do not currently meet formal alcohol-related diagnoses but who are at risk for long-term medical and social consequences of heavy alcohol exposure (Box 1). The U.S. Preventative Services Task Force (USPSTF) found that screening could accurately identify patients whose levels or patterns of alcohol consumption do not meet criteria for alcohol dependence but that place them at risk for increased morbidity and mortality. The USPSTF also found good evidence that brief interventions that consist of behavioral counseling and follow-up can reduce alcohol consumption for 6 to 12 months or longer and that the benefits outweigh any potential harms. Thus, it is recommended that alcohol screening and brief interventions be performed in primary care settings to reduce alcohol problems for adults, including pregnant women.

Brief Screening
Every patient should be asked about alcohol use. Because drinking is normative in the United States, if drinking is denied, it is useful to determine if the patient used to drink but has stopped because of a past problem. After determining if a patient currently uses any

Abstinence
- No alcohol use

Moderate Drinking
- Men: No more than 2 standard drinks per drinking d
- Women: No more than 1 standard drink per drinking d
- Elderly persons (>65 y): No more than 1 standard drink per drinking d

Risky or Hazardous Drinking
- Men
  - More than 4 standard drinks per drinking d
  - More than 14 standard drinks per wk
- Women
  - More than 3 standard drinks per drinking d
  - More than 7 standard drinks per wk
- Elderly persons (>65 y):
  - More than 3 standard drinks per drinking d
  - More than 7 standard drinks per wk

Box 2 Standard Drinks

Each equivalent drink contains about 14 g of pure alcohol:
- 12 oz of beer or wine cooler
- 8–9 oz of malt liquor
- 5 oz of wine
- 3–4 oz of fortified wine (e.g., port)
- 1½ oz of 80-proof distilled spirits (or 1 jigger of liquor before mixing)

The Alcohol Use Disorders Identification Test (AUDIT) (Table 1) is a 10-item screen developed by the World Health Organization. Given its length, the AUDIT can be used as a self-report screener that patients can fill out in the waiting area before seeing the clinician. The minimum score is 0 and the maximum score is 40. A score of 8 or more for men or 4 or more for women, adolescents, and persons older than 65 years, like a positive endorsement of any heavy drinking days, indicates the need for further evaluation of alcohol use and an increased risk of an alcohol use disorder. For brevity, the AUDIT-C, a truncated version of the AUDIT consisting of the first three AUDIT questions focused on alcohol consumption, can be used as a part of a waiting-room health history form. A score of 6 or more for men or 4 or more for women on the AUDIT-C indicates a need for further evaluation.

Asking about alcohol consumption during a routine clinical interview is best bundled with other questions about lifestyle and health, such as diet, smoking, and exercise. In addition to giving the patient a pre-examination questionnaire to fill out such as the AUDIT, another screening strategy is to ask the CAGE

alcohol, the simplest strategy is to ask about the number of heavy drinking days in the past year, where heavy drinking is defined as more than four drinks for men and more than three drinks for women in one day. If that threshold is reached, which corresponds to at-risk or hazardous drinking, then further evaluation of alcohol-related problems is indicated through the use of screening instruments. A standard drink is the same amount of alcohol contained in different volumes of alcoholic beverages (Box 2).

TABLE 1 Alcohol Use Disorders Identification Test (AUDIT)

QUESTIONS	SCORING				
	0	1	2	3	4
Consumption (AUDIT-C)					
How often do you have a drink containing alcohol?	Never	Monthly or less	2 to 4 times a month	2 to 3 times a week	4 or more times a week
How many drinks containing alcohol do you have on a typical day when you are drinking?	1 or 2	3 or 4	5 or 6	7 to 9	10 or more
How often do you have five or more drinks on one occasion?	Never	Less than monthly	Monthly	Weekly	Daily or almost daily
Personal Consequences					
How often during the last year have you found that you were not able to stop drinking once you had started?	Never	Less than monthly	Monthly	Weekly	Daily or almost daily
How often during the last year have you failed to do what was normally expected of you because of drinking?	Never	Less than monthly	Monthly	Weekly	Daily or almost daily
How often during the last year have you needed a first drink in the morning to get yourself going after a heavy drinking session?	Never	Less than monthly	Monthly	Weekly	Daily or almost daily
How often during the last year have you had a feeling of guilt or remorse after drinking?	Never	Less than monthly	Monthly	Weekly	Daily or almost daily
How often during the last year have you been unable to remember what happened the night before because of your drinking?	Never	Less than monthly	Monthly	Weekly	Daily or almost daily
Social Consequences					
Have you or someone else been injured because of your drinking?	No		Yes, but not in the last year		Yes, during the last year
Has a relative, friend, doctor, or other health care worker been concerned about your drinking or suggested you cut down?	No		Yes, but not in the last year		Yes, during the last year
Scoring and Interpretation					

Add all scores to obtain a total: >8 points for men or >4 points for women indicates a high risk of alcohol use disorder.

AUDIT-C (first three AUDIT questions): >6 points for men or >4 points for women indicates a need for further evaluation.

Box 3 — CAGE Questionnaire

- Have you ever felt that you should *Cut down* on your drinking?
- Have people *Annoyed* you by criticizing your drinking?
- Have you ever felt bad or *Guilty* about your drinking?
- Have you ever taken a drink *(Eye opener)* first thing in the morning to steady your nerves or to get rid of a hangover?
  One yes response indicates need for further assessment. Two yes responses indicate risk of an alcohol use disorder.

Box 4 — CRAFFT Questionnaire

- Have you ever ridden in a **C**ar driven by someone (including yourself) who was high or had been using alcohol or drugs?
- Do you ever use alcohol or drugs to **R**elax, feel better about yourself, or fit in?
- Do you ever use alcohol or drugs while you are **A**lone?
- Do you ever **F**orget things you did while using alcohol or drugs?
- Do your **F**amily or **F**riends ever tell you that you should cut down on your drinking or drug use?
- Have you ever gotten into **T**rouble while you were using alcohol or drugs?
  One yes response indicates need for further assessment. Two yes responses indicate risk of alcohol use disorder.

Box 5 — S-MAST-G Questionnaire

- When talking with others, do you ever underestimate how much you actually drink?
- After a few drinks, have you sometimes not eaten or been able to skip meals because you didn't feel hungry?
- Does having a few drinks help decrease your shakiness or tremors?
- Does alcohol sometimes make it hard for you to remember parts of the day or night?
- Do you usually take a drink to relax or calm your nerves?
- Do you drink to take your mind off your problems?
- Have you ever increased your drinking after experiencing a loss in your life?
- Has a doctor or nurse ever said that he or she was worried or concerned about your drinking?
- Have you ever made rules to manage your drinking?
- When you feel lonely, does having a drink help?
  Two or more yes responses indicate a probable alcohol problem.

Abbreviation: S-MAST-G = Short Michigan Alcoholism Screening Test—Geriatric.

questions (Box 3) during the clinical examination. A positive answer to any of these questions also indicates the need for further evaluation of alcohol use. Two or more CAGE questions answered affirmatively identifies a patient at high risk for alcohol dependence. Because the CAGE screens for consequences, it is not as sensitive for risky drinking.

There are other question sets that are more sensitive than the CAGE in specific demographic subsets, and these can also be easily asked during a routine history. The five-item TWEAK questionnaire (Table 2) may be a more optimal screening questionnaire for identifying women (including pregnant women) with risky drinking or alcohol use disorders in racially mixed populations. The CRAFFT (Box 4) is a 6-item question set that has high sensitivity in screening adolescents for alcohol and other substance-abuse problems. For patients older than 65 years, the Short Michigan Alcoholism Screening Test—Geriatric (S-MAST-G) (Box 5) is useful in identifying those at risk for alcohol problems, because these patients might not need the same volumes of alcohol intake as others to develop alcohol-related problems. To complete the initial screening, one should compute the average number of drinks per week by multiplying the days per week on average that the patient drinks by the number of drinks consumed on a typical drinking day.

Laboratory testing for elevations of alanine aminotransferase (ALT), aspartate aminotransferase (AST), γ-glutamyltransferase (GGT), or carbohydrate-deficient transferrin (CDT) have no incremental sensitivity over those of validated screening instruments, and they may be better suited to monitoring patients already in treatment for alcohol use disorders. The patient must still be asked about quantity and frequency of alcohol use. However, laboratory testing can provide indicators of covert heavy drinking (e.g., elevated GGT and CDT) when the patient does not reveal the extent of alcohol intake. CDT, which is perturbed less than other indices by nonalcoholic liver disease, may be a more specific and sensitive indicator of heavy drinking.

Diagnosis

Screening can identify those who are at risk for the sequelae of risky or hazardous drinking and who might benefit from a brief intervention conducted in the primary care office, but only a diagnostic evaluation can confirm the clinician's suspicion that the patient's use of alcohol meets syndromal criteria and warrants specific medical and psychosocial treatment beyond the brief intervention. According to Diagnostic and Statistical Manual of Mental Disorders, fifth edition (DSM-5) criteria (Table 3), the patient has a diagnosis of an alcohol use disorder if he or she has two or more of the following criteria over a 12-month period related to alcohol use: physical tolerance, symptoms of withdrawal, repeatedly drinking more than intended, unsuccessful reduction or quit attempts, repeated episodes of failure to fulfill obligations at home, school or work, episodes of increased risk of physical harm, recurrent problems with significant others, increased time drinking or recovering from drinking, reduced time in other pleasurable or important activities, and continued drinking despite physical or psychological problems. With DSM-5, the term alcohol dependence describes the symptoms of physical tolerance and withdrawal, not the use disorder syndrome. Severity is defined as: Mild 2-3 symptoms; Moderate 4-5 symptoms; and, Severe 6 or more symptoms.

TABLE 2 — TWEAK Questionnaire

FEATURE	QUESTION	ANSWER	SCORE
Tolerance	How many drinks does it take before you begin to feel the first effects of alcohol?	≥3	2
Worry	Have your friends or relatives worried or complained about your drinking in the past year?	Yes	2
Eye-opener	Do you sometimes take a drink in the morning when you first get up?	Yes	1
Amnesia	Are there times when you drink and afterward you can't remember what you said or did?	Yes	1
Kut	Do you sometimes feel the need to cut down on your drinking?	Yes	1

Scoring and interpretation: Two or more points indicate a possible alcohol problem.

TABLE 3 Diagnosis of Alcohol Use Problems

CRITERIA	TYPICAL SYMPTOMS AND HISTORY
Alcohol Use Disorder (≥2 in the last 12 mo)	
Alcohol has caused or contributed to repeated:	
Failure to fulfill obligations at home, school, or work	Hangovers at work, truancy at school, missing appointments
Episodes of increased risk of physical harm	Driving, swimming, or operating machinery under the influence of alcohol
Craving, or a strong desire or urge to use alcohol	Inability to refrain from drinking due to strong impulses
Problems with significant others	Spousal strife, physical fights
Development of physical tolerance	Drinks more for the same effect
Episodes of withdrawal syndrome (see below)	Morning shakes, nausea, anxiety
Drinking more than intended repeatedly	Binging episodes
Unsuccessful efforts to cut down or stop drinking	Failed New Year's resolution
Increased time planning for drinking, drinking, or recovering from drinking	Instead of being with kids, spends weekend mornings sleeping in
Reduced time in other pleasurable or important activities	Stopped socializing with friends, withdrew from hobby group
Drinking persists despite physical or psychological problems	Developed depressed mood, but kept on drinking
Alcohol Withdrawal (≥2 within hours to days after lowered blood alcohol levels)	
Autonomic hyperactivity	Heart rate ≥100 bpm, diaphoresis
Hand tremor	Hands shake when extended
Insomnia	Difficulty falling asleep
Nausea or vomiting	Feels queasy
Anxiety	Spontaneous report of fear
Psychomotor agitation	Inability to keep still, pacing
Hallucinations or illusions	Reports visual disturbances
Seizures	Tonic-clonic movements

Rates of co-occurring mood and anxiety disorders are especially high among those with alcohol use disorders. Untreated mood and anxiety disorders tend to have a negative impact on alcoholism recovery. Among treatment-seeking patients in the National Epidemiologic Survey on Alcohol and Related Conditions (NESARC) sample with a current alcohol use disorder, 40% had at least one current independent mood disorder, and more than one third had at least one current independent anxiety disorder. Heavy alcohol intake can also induce symptoms of mood and other mental disorders. To differentiate alcohol-induced symptoms from independent disorders, it is optimal to reassess symptoms of a mental disorder several weeks after cessation or significant reduction of alcohol intake.

Brief Intervention
Intention
Although risky or hazardous drinking is not a formal diagnosis, it describes a group with a higher likelihood to develop alcohol problems with risk for accidents, injuries, and social and health problems compared with the general population (see Box 1). Thus, even without a formal diagnosis, it is beneficial to help the patient with risky drinking to change his or her drinking behavior. Several well-described short interchanges between the clinician and the patient, organized under the rubric of *brief interventions*, have been validated in randomized trials as decreasing alcohol intake in those who drink too much but do not have a diagnosis of alcohol dependence. Brief intervention has been demonstrated to reduce weekly alcohol use, frequency of binging, liver enzymes associated with heavy drinking, blood pressure, emergency department visits, hospital days, and psychosocial problems, typically for

6 to 12 months, and to reduce drinking and hospital days at up to 4 years in one study. Because most at-risk patients seen in primary care settings are subsyndromal for alcohol use disorders, the typical clinical interaction related to alcohol will be that of screening and then a brief intervention for positive cases. The two are typically referred to together under the acronym SBI (screening and brief intervention).

The basic intention of a brief intervention is to educate the patient about the risks of heavy alcohol use in such a way as to motivate him or her to reduce weekly alcohol consumption. The standard initial brief intervention takes about 15 minutes and consists of feedback, advice, and goal setting. It can be performed wholly in the primary care setting by the physician or other members of the health delivery team. Including alcohol screening, the USPSTF suggests five A's to conducting SBI: *assess* the patient's alcohol consumption with a screening tool and clinical evaluation as indicated; *advise* reduction of alcohol consumption to appropriate levels, including abstinence if indicated; *agree* on individual goals for reducing alcohol use, including abstinence if indicated; *assist* patients in obtaining the motivation, skills, or supports needed to institute changes in drinking; and *arrange* for follow-up support, including specialty treatment referral for dependent patients. The most effective interventions are multicontact ones that provide ongoing assistance and follow-up.

Procedure
Assess
Screen patients with the AUDIT or with the CAGE, TWEAK, CRAFFT, or S-MAST-G questionnaires as appropriate, and compute average drinks per week.

Advise

Give feedback in the form of expression of concern, direct conclusions, and recommendations. Present medical findings, such as elevated liver enzymes, to back up conclusive statements such as "I'm concerned that your alcohol intake exceeds safe limits." Show the patient information comparing use with population norms and the associated health risks. Educate the patient about how alcohol can lead to medical, psychosocial, and legal consequences. Where possible, link the patient's current symptoms to alcohol use. Recommend appropriate and specific changes in behavior, such as "I strongly recommend you cut down your drinking," or in the case in which any drinking places the patient at high risk, "I strongly suggest you quit drinking."

Agree

Determine the patient's readiness to change drinking behavior, such as asking, "Do you think that cutting down on your drinking is something you are willing to talk about?" If the patient is ambivalent, avoid labeling the patient's behavior with a diagnosis at this stage, which can increase resistance to change, but encourage the patient to reflect on the positive reasons for drinking and the negative consequences of drinking. Offer concerns that continued drinking at the same level will impede the patient's achievement of goals such as decreased gastric distress or improved sleep patterns.

Empathic listening is generally more effective than a confrontational approach, and it is useful to express optimism about the patient's capacity to change. Elicit what the patient's concerns are about cutting down or quitting. Avoid arguing or challenging when the patient is unready to change, but schedule a follow-up visit to continue the dialogue and reassess drinking behavior. Restate your commitment to help when the patient is ready and that you remain open to questions.

When the patient concurs that a change in drinking would be beneficial, agree on a specific goal to cut down to particular daily and weekly limits for low-risk drinking or to stop drinking, if indicated, for a specific period of time. The agreement should be recorded and a copy given to the patient both as a reminder and motivator for behavioral change.

Assist

Work with the patient to formulate concrete steps to implement the drinking reduction plan. These steps include how to avoid high-risk drinking situations, how to keep a record of alcohol intake, and who can support the patient in meeting his or her goals. Provide resources in the form of patient educational materials, examples of which can be downloaded from the National Institute of Alcohol Abuse and Alcoholism (NIAAA) website (www.niaaa.nih.gov).

Arrange

Set up follow-up support and counseling visits or refer patients meeting dependence criteria for specialty treatment. Advise the patient to seek immediate medical treatment if withdrawal symptoms occur.

Treatment

Detoxification

Put simply, detoxification is medical stabilization that offers an opportunity to engage patients in alcoholism treatment, but it is not in itself treatment for alcohol dependence. Patients who drink more than 250 grams of alcohol daily are likely to experience physiologic withdrawal symptoms on cessation of drinking, but volume is not the only predictor of withdrawal severity. Although often mild, untreated alcohol withdrawal can result in seizures or delirium tremens (DTs), with increased risk of mortality.

Assessment

The Clinical Institute Withdrawal Assessment for Alcohol scale, Revised (CIWA-Ar) is a public domain scale that scores 10 signs and symptoms of withdrawal by severity ranging from not present to severe (Box 6). A score of less than 8 indicates mild withdrawal, characterized by increased autonomic activity with low-grade anxiety, diaphoresis, agitation, nausea, and elevated blood pressure, temperature, and heart rate. Scores of 8 to 15 indicate moderate withdrawal, and scores of 15 or more indicate more severe withdrawal states. In severe withdrawal, in the context of autonomic hyperarousal, the patient can become disoriented and have a clouded sensorium, the hallmarks of delirium.

Prior history of severe withdrawal, such as DTs, is a reasonable predictor of similar future responses to alcohol withdrawal. Risk for withdrawal delirium is increased if the patient has a heart rate of greater than 120 bpm before treatment, a current infectious disease, withdrawal symptoms in the context of a blood alcohol concentration greater than 100 mg/dL, a prior history of either delirium or seizures, or a high CIWA-Ar score, indicating severe autonomic hyperactivity. Patients who have severe withdrawal symptoms, who are at high risk for seizures, or who have a medical condition likely to be exacerbated by withdrawal, such as type 1 diabetes or coronary artery disease, should have medically supervised inpatient detoxification.

Pharmacologic Therapy

Alcohol withdrawal is best treated with sedative hypnotic medications that are cross-tolerant with alcohol, such as benzodiazepines. Longer-acting benzodiazepines such as diazepam (Valium) and chlordiazepoxide (Librium) are easier to titrate against withdrawal symptoms and give a gradual offset in plasma concentration, but shorter-acting benzodiazepines such as lorazepam (Ativan)[1] are less likely to oversedate the patient. Rapid-onset benzodiazepines have a higher abuse liability and are generally best avoided. However, patients with severe hepatic impairment (elevated total bilirubin) are best treated with benzodiazepines that are not oxidized by the liver, such as oxazepam (Serax) or lorazepam.

Typical dosing is chlordiazepoxide 50 to 100 mg, diazepam 10 to 20 mg, oxazepam 20 to 40[3] mg, or lorazepam[1] 2 to 4 mg. The typical front-loading style of dosing is to administer medication at the higher end of the dose range every 1 to 2 hours so that the CIWA-Ar score is less than 8 for 24 hours.

With long-acting medications, once symptoms subside, there is often no need to taper doses. The short-acting benzodiazepines and long-acting benzodiazepines given to patients at high-risk for seizures or DTs are best given on a fixed-dose regimen of four times daily for the first 24 hours, with the patient reassessed 1 to 2 hours after each dose, and additional medication given as needed. On days 2 and 3, 50% of the dose can be given four times daily.

Long acting barbiturates, such as phenobarbital,[1] can be also used on a fixed-dose regimen of 60 mg every 4 to 6 hours, with a loading dose of 120 mg orally or intramuscularly every hour for acute withdrawal symptoms (e.g., pulse >110 bpm) or a CIWA-Ar score of 10 or more.

Anticonvulsants such as carbamazepine (Tegretol),[1] valproate (Depakote),[1] or gabapentin (Neurontin)[1] have also been used effectively in uncomplicated withdrawal, but they are unproved in preventing withdrawal-related seizures and in treating DTs.

Although phenothiazines and haloperidol are somewhat effective compared with benzodiazepines in reducing withdrawal symptoms such as agitation, they are not as protective against seizures or delirium and thus are not recommended.

Thiamine (vitamin B_1) supplementation of 100 mg/day for 3 days can counteract the thiamine deficiencies that are common in alcoholic patients.

Psychosocial Interventions for Alcohol Use Disorder

In addition to brief interventions for risky alcohol use, the most opportune and practical psychosocial intervention that the primary care office can provide is clinical behavioral support for pharmacotherapy for alcohol dependence. Simply put, medication

---

[1]Not FDA approved for this indication.
[3]Exceeds dosage recommended by the manufacturer.

Patient:_____ Date:_____ Time:_____ (24-hour clock, midnight = 00:00)

Pulse or heart rate, taken for one minute:_____ Blood pressure:_____ mm Hg

Nausea and Vomiting – Ask, "Do you feel sick to your stomach? Have you vomited?" Observation:
0 no nausea and no vomiting
1 mild nausea with no vomiting
2
3
4 intermittent nausea with dry heaves
5
6
7 constant nausea, frequent dry heaves, and vomiting

Tactile Disturbances – Ask, "Have you any itching, pins and needles sensations, any burning, any numbness, or do you feel bugs crawling on or under your skin?" Observation:
0 none
1 very mild itching, pins and needles, burning, or numbness
2 mild itching, pins and needles, burning, or numbness
3 moderate itching, pins and needles, burning, or numbness
4 moderately severe hallucinations
5 severe hallucinations
6 extremely severe hallucinations
7 continuous hallucinations

Tremor – Arms extended and fingers spread apart. Observation:
0 no tremor
1 not visible, but can be felt fingertip to fingertip
2
3
4 moderate, with patient's arms extended
5
6
7 severe, even with arms not extended

Auditory Disturbances – Ask, "Are you more aware of sounds around you? Are they harsh? Do they frighten you? Are you hearing anything that is disturbing to you? Are you hearing things you know are not there?" Observation:
0 not present
1 very mild harshness or ability to frighten
2 mild harshness or ability to frighten
3 moderate harshness or ability to frighten
4 moderately severe hallucinations
5 severe hallucinations
6 extremely severe hallucinations
7 continuous hallucinations

Paroxysmal Sweats – Observation:
0 no sweat visible
1 barely perceptible sweating, palms moist
2
3
4 beads of sweat obvious on forehead
5
6
7 drenching sweats

Visual Disturbances – Ask, "Does the light appear to be too bright? Is its color different? Does it hurt your eyes? Are you seeing anything that is disturbing to you? Are you seeing things you know are not there?" Observation:
0 not present
1 very mild sensitivity
2 mild sensitivity
3 moderate sensitivity
4 moderately severe hallucinations
5 severe hallucinations
6 extremely severe hallucinations
7 continuous hallucinations

Anxiety – Ask, "Do you feel nervous?" Observation:
0 no anxiety, at ease
1 mild anxious
2
3
4 moderately anxious, or guarded, so anxiety is inferred
5
6
7 equivalent to acute panic states as seen in severe delirium or acute schizophrenic reactions

Headache, Fullness in Head – Ask, "Does your head feel different? Does it feel like there is a band around your head?" Do not rate for dizziness or lightheadedness. Otherwise, rate severity:
0 not present
1 very mild
2 mild
3 moderate
4 moderately severe
5 severe
6 very severe
7 extremely severe

Agitation – Observation:
0 normal activity
1 somewhat more than normal activity
2
3
4 moderately fidgety and restless
5
6
7 paces back and forth during most of the interview or constantly thrashes about

Orientation and Clouding of Sensorium – Ask, "What day is this? Where are you? Who am I?"
0 oriented and can do serial additions
1 cannot do serial additions or is uncertain about date
2 disoriented for date by no more than 2 calendar days
3 disoriented for date by more than 2 calendar days
4 disoriented for place or person

Total CIWA-Ar Score_____
Rater's Initials_____
Maximum Possible Score: 67

The CIWA-Ar *is not* copyright and may be reproduced freely. This assessment for monitoring withdrawal symptoms requires approximately 5 minutes to administer.

From Sullivan JT, et al: Assessment of alcohol withdrawal: The revised Clinical Institute Withdrawal Assessment for Alcohol scale (CIWA-Ar). Br J Addiction 1989;84:1353–57.

management support consists initially of feedback to the patient of screening and medical evaluation results and the negative health effects of continued heavy drinking, as in a brief intervention. The patient is then given the basis for the diagnosis of alcohol dependence, the rationale for abstinence, and recommendation for pharmacotherapy. The patient is given information about medication and the appropriate prescriptions and is encouraged to seek community support for sobriety in mutual help groups such as Alcoholics Anonymous or to follow a plan such as Rational Recovery. Follow-up visits consist of assessment of medication side effects, patient adherence to the medication regimen, assessment of abstinence or quantity and pattern of alcohol intake, and assessment of overall functioning. Problems with medication adherence are identified and addressed.

There are evidence-based psychosocial interventions that are typically performed in the context of specialty programs for alcohol dependence, but they can be offered by clinical personnel in the context of the physician's office. Cognitive behavior therapy, network therapy, behavioral family therapy, and motivational interviewing are effective approaches for the treatment of alcohol dependence. Motivational interviewing is especially adaptable for use in primary care settings in that it is an approach to interacting with the alcohol-dependent patient that can be learned quickly and executed by any staff with clinical contact. A motivational enhancement manual can be accessed at the NIAAA website (http://www.niaaa.nih.gov/).

Medication Management of Alcohol Dependence

There are currently four FDA-approved medications for the treatment of alcohol dependence. Any of these medications can and should be given concurrently with other interventions such as psychosocial treatment or mutual help groups.

Disulfiram (Antabuse) works by inhibiting the metabolism of ethyl alcohol, causing a buildup of acetaldehyde, a noxious substance, which causes a strong stereotypic aversive response (flushing, diaphoresis, nausea, tachycardia) in the patient. Standard dosing is 250 mg/day (range, 125–500 mg). The major clinical concern with disulfiram is patient noncompliance with the medication regimen. Thus, it is most likely to be effective when there is a concrete method for supporting compliance in place, such as directly observed therapy by a spouse or in a clinic.

More recently, the opioid antagonist naltrexone (ReVia, Depade) was approved for the treatment of alcohol dependence. It is dosed at 50 mg once daily. Naltrexone reduces days of heavy drinking and can reduce alcohol craving. Naltrexone in a long-acting intramuscular formulation (Vivitrol) allows once-monthly dosing (380 mg) and reduces the risk of noncompliance. It reduces heavy drinking overall and helps maintain abstinence in those who are abstinent at initial drug administration. Both oral and IM naltrexone formulations carry FDA black-box warnings related to findings of reversible elevations of liver enzymes at three to six times the standard dosage; however, naltrexone is safe at the recommended dose.

Acamprosate (Campral) is a taurine analogue that has been demonstrated to reduce relapse to any drinking as well as reducing heavy drinking in nonabstinent patients. It is dosed as two 333-mg tablets three times a day to patients who have ceased alcohol intake. It is excreted unchanged through the kidneys and has no interactions with other medications. Side effects are benign, and the most frequent is loose stools, which are mild to moderate and self-limited.

Topiramate[1] (Topamax) titrated over 5 weeks between 50 mg and 300 mg daily appears to reduce heavy drinking and days of any drinking over the short term (12 weeks) in alcohol-dependent patients who have not established abstinence prior to treatment. Common side effects include paresthesias, taste perversion, decreased appetite, and difficulty concentrating.

---

[1]Not FDA approved for this indication.

References

American Psychiatric Association. American Psychiatric Association: Diagnostic and statistical manual of mental disorders, 5th ed. (DSM-5). Washington, DC, American Psychiatric Publishing, 2013.

Bertholet N, Daeppen J-B, Wietlisbach V, et al. Reduction of alcohol consumption by brief alcohol intervention in primary care systematic review and meta-analysis. Arch Intern Med 2005;165:986–95.

Bradley KA, Boyd-Wickizer J, Powell SH, Burman ML. Alcohol screening questionnaires in women: A critical review. JAMA 1998;280:166–71.

Fleming MF, Mundt MP, French MT, et al. Brief physician advice for problem drinkers: Long-term efficacy and cost-benefit analysis. Alcohol Clin Exp Res 2002;26:36–43.

Grant BF, Stinson FS, Dawson DA, et al. Prevalence and co-occurrence of substance use disorders and independent mood and anxiety disorders: Results from the National Epidemiologic Survey on Alcohol and Related Conditions. Arch Gen Psychiatry 2004;61:807–16.

Johnson BA, Rosenthal N, Capece JA, et al. Topiramate for treating alcohol dependence: A randomized controlled trial. JAMA 2007;298:1641–51.

Knight JR, Sherritt L, Shrier LA, et al. Validity of the CRAFFT substance abuse screening test among adolescent clinic patients. Arch Pediatr Adolesc Med 2002;156(6):607–14.

Kranzler HR, Knapp CM, Ciraulo DA. Alcohol. In: Kranzler HR, Ciraulo DA. Zindel LR, editors. Clinical Manual of Addiction Psychopharmacology. Washington, DC: American Psychiatric Publishing; 2014. p. 1–69.

Maisto SA, Saitz R. Alcohol use disorders: Screening and diagnosis. Am J Addict 2003;12(Suppl. 1):S12–S25.

McCaul ME, Petry NM. The role of psychosocial treatments in pharmacotherapy for alcoholism. Am J Addict 2003;12(Suppl. 1):S41–52.

National Institute on Alcohol Abuse and Alcoholism. Helping patients who drink too much: a clinician's guide, Rockville, MD: National Institute on Alcohol Abuse and Alcoholism; 2005. Available at http://pubs.niaaa.nih.gov/publications/Practitioner/CliniciansGuide2005/guide.pdf (accessed July 20, 2014).

Saitz R. Unhealthy alcohol use. N Engl J Med 2005;352:596–607.

Saunders JB, Aasland OG, Babor TF, et al. Development of the Alcohol Use Disorders Screening Test (AUDIT) WHO collaborative project on early detection of persons with harmful alcohol consumption. Addiction 1993;88:791–804.

Sullivan JT, Sykora K, Schneiderman J, et al. Assessment of alcohol withdrawal: The revised Clinical Institute Withdrawal Assessment for Alcohol scale (CIWA-Ar). Br J Addict 1989;84:1353–7.

U.S. Preventive Services Task Force. Screening and behavioral counseling interventions in primary care to reduce alcohol misuse: Recommendation statement. Ann Intern Med 2004;140:554–6.

ANXIETY DISORDERS

Method of
Natalie C. Dattilo, PhD; and Andrew W. Goddard, MD

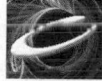

CURRENT DIAGNOSIS

- A thorough history is required to ensure the patient meets DSM-5-TR criteria for an anxiety disorder. Symptoms that persist and are associated with significant distress and impairment of functioning are likely caused by an anxiety disorder that warrants treatment.
- Anxiety is characterized by subjective feelings of worry, dread, or anticipation and can include hypervigilance and avoidance of anxiety-producing situations. Physical symptoms often include jitteriness, restlessness, muscle aches and tension, sweating, dizziness, fatigue, racing heart, hyperventilation, dry mouth, nausea, decreased sexual desire, and sleep and appetite disturbances.
- Relevant medical examination and laboratory work may be indicated to rule out organic causes, substance abuse, or withdrawal.

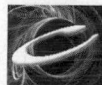

CURRENT THERAPY

- Educate the patient and family members about treatment options as well as realistic treatment expectations and reassure them of the absence of medical causes.

- First-line treatment is a selective serotonin reuptake inhibitor (SSRI), starting at low doses with careful titration so as not to exacerbate anxiety symptoms.
- Initiate cognitive-behavioral therapy (CBT) along with medication to significantly increase response rates.
- Consider short-term, high-potency benzodiazepine use in more severe cases. Use medications with longer half-lives to minimize withdrawal effects.
- Refer to a psychiatrist in difficult cases or for patients with a less-than-expected response to treatment.

Epidemiology

Anxiety disorders are among the most prevalent psychiatric disorders in the world. In the United States, it is estimated that an anxiety disorder is diagnosed in approximately 16 million adults each year and approximately 30 million meet criteria for an anxiety disorder over the course of their lifetimes. Second to depression, anxiety disorders are the most common mental health problems seen by physicians in the general medical setting. In fact, patients with anxiety are more likely to present initially to a general practitioner's office than to a mental health care provider.

Anxiety disorders tend to be chronic and disabling, and they impose a high individual and social burden. It has been estimated that the United States spends approximately $40 billion to $60 billion per year for costs associated with anxiety disorders. These include not only direct costs associated with treatment but also indirect costs associated with lost productivity. Thus, the importance of early detection and treatment is critically important.

Risk Factors

Risk factors found to be associated with anxiety disorders include past personal or family history of anxiety; recent increase in stressful life events; lack or perceived lack of social support; ineffective emotional coping strategies; being female; experiencing childhood adversity, including trauma or witnessing a traumatic event; having a chronic health condition or serious illness; having an acute or chronic pain condition; and substance abuse. Although a genetic predisposition to developing an anxiety disorder is likely, environmental stressors clearly play a role. Research has also shown that patients suffering from anxiety are generally more sensitive to physiologic changes than nonanxious patients. This heightened sensitivity leads to diminished autonomic flexibility, which may be the result of faulty central information processing in anxiety-prone persons.

Pathophysiology

Anxiety symptoms and the resulting disorders are believed to be due to dysregulation of neuronal activity with the CNS fear circuit. Physical and emotional manifestations of this dysregulation are the result of a state of hyperarousal. Several neurotransmitter systems have been implicated in the genesis of this state.

The most commonly considered are the serotoninergic and noradrenergic neurotransmitter systems. Very simply, it is believed that an underactivation of the serotoninergic system and an overactivation of the noradrenergic system are involved. These systems regulate and are regulated by other pathways and neuronal circuits in various regions of the brain, including the locus caeruleus and limbic structures, resulting in dysregulation of physiologic arousal and the emotional experience of this arousal. Disruption of the γ-aminobutyric acid (GABA) system has also been implicated because of the response of many of the anxiety-spectrum disorders to treatment with benzodiazepines.

There has also been some interest in the role of corticosteroid regulation and its relation to symptoms of fear and anxiety. Corticosteroids might increase or decrease the activity of certain neural pathways, affecting not only behavior under stress but also the brain's processing of fear-inducing stimuli. The stress response is hardwired into the brain and is most often triggered when survival of the organism is threatened. The stress response, however, can be triggered not only by a physical challenge or threat but also by the mere anticipation (or fear) of threat. As a result, when humans chronically and erroneously believe that a threatening event is about to occur, they begin to experience the physical and psychological symptoms of anxiety and panic.

Finally, a subcortical neural structure, the amygdala, serves an important role in coordinating the cognitive, affective, neuroendocrine, cardiovascular, respiratory, and musculoskeletal components of fear and anxiety responses (fear expression). It is central to registering the emotional significance of stressful stimuli and creating emotional memories. The amygdala receives input from neurons in the sensory cortex. When activated, the amygdala stimulates regions of the midbrain and brain stem, causing autonomic hyperactivity, which can be correlated with the physical symptoms of anxiety.

Prevention

No biological markers are specific enough yet to detect anxiety early, and there is no available evidence to suggest that current medications prove efficacious in preventing these disorders. Therefore, it is important to screen for specific risk factors, such as family history and substance abuse. If a person is anxiety-prone, he or she should first be encouraged to adopt healthy lifestyle habits. Physical activity has been shown to relieve tension and anxiety. These patients should also be encouraged to avoid stimulants such as caffeine and nicotine, which can exacerbate symptoms. It is also recommended that anxiety-prone persons reduce subjective levels of stress by learning effective methods of relaxation and other stress-management skills.

Clinical Manifestations

Anxiety is characterized by subjective feelings of worry, dread, or anticipation and can include hypervigilance and avoidance of anxiety-producing situations. The physical symptoms can include jitteriness or shakiness, trembling, muscle aches and tension, sweating, cold or clammy hands, dizziness, or vertigo; fatigue; racing or pounding heart, hyperventilation; sensation of a lump in the throat, choking sensation, dry mouth; numbness and tingling in hands, feet, or other body part; upset stomach, nausea, vomiting, or diarrhea; decreased sexual desire; and sleep and appetite disturbances.

Psychological symptoms include unrealistic or excessive worry, apprehension, exaggerated startle response, hypervigilance, and distractibility. Patients often express feelings of impatience, irritability, and fear. Some patients exhibit phobias such as fear of being far from home or fear of social contact. Others express fear of falling asleep owing to recurrent nightmares. These symptoms cause significant distress and impairment of function.

Diagnosis

An anxiety disorder diagnosis is arrived at when a patient meets the specific diagnostic criteria outlined in the *Diagnostic and Statistical Manual of Mental Disorders*, Fifth Edition (DSM-5). The four most common anxiety disorders seen in primary care are generalized anxiety disorder, panic disorder, social anxiety disorder, and posttraumatic stress disorder.

Generalized Anxiety Disorder

Persons with generalized anxiety disorder (GAD) experience uncontrollable, excessive anxiety and worry involving several areas of functioning on most days for at least 6 months. The anxiety must be associated with at least three of the following symptoms: restlessness, fatigue, impaired concentration, irritability, muscle tension, or sleep problems. Patients tend to express chronic excessive nervousness, exaggerated worry, tension, and irritability that appear to have no cause or are more intense than the situation warrants. Physical signs such as headaches, trembling, twitching, or sweating often develop, which lead to further worries. GAD symptoms tend to wax and wane over time, with short-term exacerbations of acute anxiety in response to stress. Symptoms show substantial overlap with those of other medical and psychological disorders, particularly major depressive disorder, substance abuse disorders, and other anxiety disorders, which tends to complicate diagnosis.

Panic Disorder

Panic disorder is marked by recurrent, unexpected panic attacks with persistent concern about future attacks or worries about their implications or consequences. A panic attack is a period of intense fear, developing abruptly and peaking within 10 minutes. Diagnosis requires at least four of the following: chest pain or discomfort; chills or hot flushes; derealization (feeling of unreality) or depersonalization (being detached from oneself); fear of losing control; feeling dizzy, unsteady, lightheaded, or faint; feeling of choking; nausea; palpitations; paresthesias; sensations of shortness of breath or smothering; sense of impending doom; sweating; or trembling or shaking.

Patients with panic disorder often seek medical treatment because they fear that their physical symptoms are caused by a heart attack. The anticipatory anxiety and intense fear of future attacks can lead to phobic avoidance. The combination of panic symptoms and the phobic avoidance can impair the patient's occupational, social, and family functioning. Sometimes, panic disorder leads to agoraphobia, which can be disabling. Patients with agoraphobia often refuse to leave their home for fear of being in a situation in which they might experience anxiety or panic and from which escape might be difficult or embarrassing.

Social Anxiety Disorder

Social phobia or social anxiety disorder is manifested by excessive, persistent fear of social and performance situations that is so severe that it disrupts daily life and relationships. Persons with social anxiety have a persistent, intense, and ongoing fear of being extremely embarrassed or being watched, judged by others, or humiliated by their own actions. Exposure to the feared social situation provokes anxiety, which can take the form of a panic attack. The person recognizes that the fear is excessive or unreasonable.

Posttraumatic Stress Disorder

Posttraumatic stress disorder (PTSD) develops after a person experiences, witnesses, or confronts a physically or psychologically traumatic event. The event might involve actual or threatened death, serious injury, or sexual violence. PTSD is diagnosed in a person who displays symptoms associated with re-experiencing the traumatic event, including recurrent and intrusive distressing recollections, nightmares, or a sense of reliving the experience through flashbacks. The person must also display a consistent pattern of avoidance of themes associated with the traumatic event (thoughts, feelings, conversations, activities, places, or people), negative alterations in cognitions and mood (e.g., inability to remember important aspects of the trauma, persistent negative emotional state, feelings of detachment from others, markedly diminished interest or participation in activities), hyperarousal and autonomic hyperactivity that can manifest in difficulties with sleep or concentration, irritability, hypervigilance, and an exaggerated startle response, as well as angry outbursts with little or no provocation and reckless or self-destructive behavior. The diagnosis is made if the symptoms have been present for at least 1 month and cause clinically significant distress or impairment in functioning.

Differential Diagnosis

It is important to perform a thorough medical workup when initially assessing the patient with anxiety symptoms. The differential diagnosis can include several organic causes, such as endocrine dysfunction, intoxication or withdrawal, hypoxia, metabolic abnormalities, and neurologic disorders. It is also important to rule out other comorbid psychiatric disorders. Severe depression, bipolar disorder, prodromal schizophrenia, delusional disorder, and adjustment disorder can often be accompanied by severe anxiety. Many organic causes can be ruled out by a thorough history and basic laboratory work, including thyroid-stimulating hormone, urine toxicology, electrocardiogram, complete blood count, and metabolic panel. The most common medical conditions associated with anxiety are presented in Box 1.

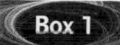 **Box 1** Medical Conditions Often Associated with Anxiety Symptoms

Cardiopulmonary
Angina
Mitral valve prolapse
Pulmonary embolism
Chronic obstructive pulmonary disease (COPD)
Asthma

Endocrine
Hyperthyroidism
Pheochromocytoma
Cushing's syndrome
Menopause

Gastrointestinal
Gastroesophageal reflux
Irritable bowel syndrome (IBS)
Gastritis

Neurologic
Dementia
Substance intoxication or withdrawal
Seizure disorder
Migraine

The list of drugs suspected of causing anxiety is extensive. Drugs commonly associated with anxiety include stimulants such as amphetamine, cocaine, methamphetamine, and caffeine. Drugs such as lysergic acid diethylamide (LSD) and 3,4-methylenedioxymethamphetamine (MDMA, or "ecstasy") can also cause acute and chronic anxiety. Prescription medications to consider include sympathomimetics, antihypertensives, and nonsteroidal antiinflammatory drugs (NSAIDs).

Treatment and Monitoring

Treatment for a patient with an anxiety disorder begins with education. The practice guidelines for panic disorder recommend education of the family as well. Many people are confused by the symptoms and behavior and are reassured to know they are not alone and that there are effective interventions. The patient should receive an appropriate medical work up, such as a physical examination, and studies (e.g., electrocardiogram, thyroid-stimulating hormone) when indicated. After ruling out a medical condition, developing a working alliance with the patient provides a basis for ongoing management and prevents further inappropriate use of the medical system.

A combination of psychotherapy and medication management is recommended in all of the anxiety disorders. Cognitive-behavioral therapy (CBT) has the strongest empiric support of all the psychotherapies, but it requires commitment to treatment on the part of the patient. Its efficacy is also contingent on the ability of the therapist and the length of therapy, with a 78% response rate in panic-disorder patients who have committed to 12 to 15 weeks of therapy. Studies show that when compared with patients undergoing monotherapy, patients treated with a combination of CBT and medication experience nearly twice the remission rate.

The selective serotonin reuptake inhibitors (SSRIs) have been shown to be the best-tolerated medications, and response rates are significantly higher than placebo for panic disorder, PTSD, social anxiety disorder, and GAD. This class of medication includes fluoxetine (Prozac), fluvoxamine (Luvox), citalopram (Celexa), escitalopram (Lexapro), paroxetine (Paxil), and sertraline (Zoloft). Some improvement should be noted within 3 or 4 weeks, and the dose should be increased if no improvement is seen. In all of the anxiety disorders, SSRIs should be started at low doses and gradually titrated up to therapeutic levels to avoid an initial exacerbation of anxiety. Pharmacotherapy options for the treatment of GAD are presented in Table 1.

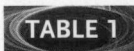

TABLE 1 Pharmacotherapy for the Treatment of Generalized Anxiety Disorder

DRUG	STARTING DOSE	TARGET DOSE
Selective Serotonin Reuptake Inhibitors		
Paroxetine (Paxil)*	10 mg qd	10–60 mg qd
Escitalopram (Lexapro)*	5–10 mg qd	10–20 mg qd
Sertraline (Zoloft)	12.5–25 mg qd	50–200 mg qd
Fluoxetine (Prozac)	10 mg qd	20–40 mg qd
Serotonin-Norepinephrine Reuptake Inhibitors		
Venlafaxine (Effexor XR)*	37.5 mg qAM	150–300 mg qAM[3]
Duloxetine (Cymbalta)*	30 mg qd	60–90 mg qd
Other		
Buspirone (BuSpar)	5 mg bid-tid	10 mg tid

[3]Exceeds dosage recommended by the manufacturer.
*FDA indication for GAD.

Benzodiazepines, which have been used commonly in the past to treat anxiety disorders, continue to be useful in the short-term management of symptoms until acceptable reduction of symptoms is achieved with an SSRI or CBT. The tolerability and lack of addiction potential make the SSRIs more desirable for long-term management, but the delay in response makes short-term symptom relief with a benzodiazepine desirable for those with the greatest impairment. Because of the risk for rebound anxiety when withdrawing from benzodiazepines with short half-lives, such as alprazolam (Xanax), many prefer the longer-acting benzodiazepines, such as clonazepam (Klonopin).

If the patient does not respond to the combination of CBT and medication, a reevaluation of symptoms might reveal a comorbid disorder missed on the first examination. Comorbid psychiatric disorders significantly lower the likelihood of recovery from anxiety and increase recurrence rates. Many clinicians try switching between SSRIs before considering the next step in treatment. A referral to a psychiatrist for further evaluation and management may be necessary if none of these strategies works. Treatment-refractory anxiety can be extremely frustrating for both the patient and clinician. This can lead to increased dependence on benzodiazepines and an escalation of doses required for the same effect.

When approaching the start of therapy, the clinician should reassure the patient that effective treatment is available, but that patience may be necessary until the right combination of modalities is found. Although all of the anxiety disorders display a significant amount of chronicity, most patients have an improved outcome with appropriate treatment. Response rates improve when comorbidity is low. Patients with an earlier onset of symptoms (childhood or adolescence) can generally expect a more chronic course and may be more difficult to treat. In some of the disorders (e.g., PTSD, panic disorder), patients can have a spontaneous remission of symptoms or can continue to function despite the symptoms. However, time to resolution of symptoms is shortened and overall functioning can improve with treatment.

Pharmacotherapy often helps to prevent relapse, and rates are improved when effective treatment is continued for 12 months. When considering termination of pharmacologic treatment, the risk for relapse in all of the disorders should be discussed with the patient. When discontinuing the SSRIs, a slow taper is recommended, with close monitoring for withdrawal symptoms (e.g., headache, gastrointestinal upset, restlessness, and other flulike symptoms). Also monitor for rebound anxiety symptoms. If relapse occurs, reinstituting treatment is indicated, and many patients opt for indefinite treatment to maintain remission of symptoms. Lifelong management with pharmacotherapy or psychotherapy, or both, is not unusual for many patients. For many,

TABLE 2 Helpful Resources for Patients with Anxiety Disorders

ORGANIZATION	WEBSITE
Anxiety Disorders Association of America	www.adaa.org
Association for Behavioral and Cognitive Therapies	www.abct.org
National Institute of Mental Health	www.nimh.nih.gov/index.shtml

a maximum reduction of symptoms, rather than a full remission, is an acceptable outcome.

Complications

Untreated anxiety disorders can lead to, or worsen, other mental and physical health conditions, including bruxism (teeth grinding), cognitive impairment, depression, gastrointestinal disorders, headache, insomnia, heart disease, substance abuse, and significantly impaired quality of life.

Conclusion

Anxiety disorders are highly prevalent. These conditions can be disabling and costly to the patient and to the health care system. Despite the prevalence of anxiety disorders, patients often remain undiagnosed and untreated, and patients with unrecognized anxiety disorders tend to be high users of general medical care. Patients with anxiety disorders can present with multiple somatic complaints and comorbid disorders, causing great effort and expense in identifying the cause of unexplained symptoms. Once anxiety disorders are identified, patients may be treated using well-tested and efficacious pharmacologic and psychotherapeutic treatments. Helpful resources for patients and families are listed in Table 2.

References

American Psychiatric Association. Diagnostic and statistical manual of mental disorders. 5th ed. Washington, DC: American Psychiatric Association; 2013.

American Psychiatric Association. Practice guideline for the treatment of patients with panic disorder. 2nd ed. Washington, DC: American Psychiatric Association; 2009.

Campbell-Sills L, Stein MB. Guideline watch: Practice guidelines for the treatment of patients with panic disorder. Arlington, VA: American Psychiatric Association; 2006.

Gabbard GO. 3rd ed. Treatment of psychiatric disorders, vols. 1–2. Washington, DC: American Psychiatric Publishing; 2001.

Goddard AW, Coplan JD, Shekhar A, et al. Principles of the pharmacotherapy of anxiety disorders. In: Charney DS, Nestler EJ, editors. The Neurobiology of Mental Illness. 2nd ed. New York: Oxford University Press; 2004. p. 661–82.

Kessler RC, Berglund P, Demler O, et al. Lifetime prevalence and age-of-onset distributions of DSM-IV disorders in the National Comorbidity Survey Replication. Arch Gen Psychiatry 2005;62:593–602.

Kroenke K, Spitzer RL, Williams JBW, et al. Anxiety disorders in primary care: Prevalence, impairment, comorbidity, and detection. Ann Intern Med 2007;146: 317–25.

Lépine JP. The epidemiology of anxiety disorders: Prevalence and societal costs. J Clin Psychiatry 2002;63(Suppl. 14):4–8.

Sadock BJ, Sadock VA. Kaplan and Sadock's synopsis of psychiatry: Behavioral sciences/clinical psychiatry. 10th ed. Philadelphia: Lippincott Williams & Wilkins; 2007.

Stein MB. Attending to anxiety disorders in primary care. J Clin Psychiatry 2003;64 (Suppl. 15):35–9.

DELIRIUM

Method of
Inna D'Empaire, MD; and E. Wesley Ely, MD, MPH

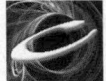

CURRENT DIAGNOSIS

- Delirium is an "acute" and "fluctuating" disruption of "attention" and "cognition."
- Delirium is characterized by a reduced ability to direct, focus, and shift attention, and a reduced orientation to the environment.
- Important signs and symptoms of delirium include inattention, disorientation, impaired memory, visuospatial impairment,

perceptual disturbances, language impairment, sleep cycle disturbance, and agitation/lethargy.
• Symptoms develop over a short period of time.

CURRENT THERAPY

The mnemonic TREAT summarizes the evaluation and management of delirium.
• T—take time to notice change from baseline and diagnose delirium.
• R—review all medications, including recent changes, errors in administration/delivery, side effect profile, and possible drug-drug interactions.
• E—ensure effective communication between all healthcare providers, staff, and patient's family.
• A—address possible underlying causes.
• T—therapeutics (reevaluate all medications and consider which ones could be removed before adding new ones).

Epidemiology

Delirium is one of the most common conditions in the hospital, with prevalence rates ranging from 15% to 20% on medical floors to 60% in surgical patients and 80% in the intensive care units.

Risk Factors

Several predisposing, precipitating, and perpetuating factors for delirium have been well described. Medication exposure and polypharmacy have been associated with strong predication of delirium. Table 1 provides examples of possible contributing risk factors.

Pathophysiology

Delirium is a complex neurobehavioral syndrome with multifactorial etiology. Many theories have been postulated regarding the development of delirium without a single compelling explanation of this complex neurobehavioral syndrome. Knowledge of contributing factors and pathophysiologic mechanisms can assist clinicians in addressing, correcting, and possibly preventing delirium. The following hypotheses summarize current knowledge of the neuropathogenesis of delirium: (1) acute inflammatory processes, that is, infection, surgery, trauma leading to increased neuroinflammatory response in the central nervous system, and increased activity of proinflammatory cytokines and inflammatory mediators; (2) neuronal aging processes and dementia are independent risk factors for the development of delirium resulting from changes in vascularization, neuronal loss, and decrease in physiological reserve; (3) association of changes in oxygen requirements and availability and decreased brain oxygenation, decreased metabolism, and increase in oxidative stress; (4) decreased central cholinergic neurotransmission and subsequent increased dopaminergic transmission, that is, medications with anticholinergic effects; (5) activation of the hypothalamic-pituitary axis leading to increased catabolic activity of glucocorticoid hormones and subsequent neuronal injury; (6) sleep fragmentation, sleep-cycle disruption, and sleep deprivation leading to memory deficits; (7) neurotransmitter and brain connectivity dysfunction related to the combined effect of baseline resiliency, underlying level of cognitive functioning, and environmental modifiable risk factors (i.e., inflammation, infection, trauma, medications).

Diagnosis

According to the DSM-5, delirium is characterized by a reduced ability to direct, focus, and shift attention, and a reduced orientation to the environment. Important diagnostic features of delirium include development of the disturbance over a short period of time; its fluctuating nature; and the noticeable change from baseline attention, awareness, and cognition. Dysregulation of neuronal activity is accompanied by sleep-cycle disturbance, conceptual disorganization, lability of affect, thought process abnormalities, and evidence of systemic disturbance in physical condition. Table 2 provides a summary of diagnostic criteria for delirium.

Monitoring

Early identification, appropriate management, and system-wide efforts at prevention can improve treatment outcome and quality of patient care. Systematic implementation and routine use of validated delirium screening tools have a significant impact on healthcare delivery, quality measures, and patient satisfaction. A wide variety of screening instruments have been described in the literature: Confusion Assessment Method (CAM), Confusion Assessment Method modified for ICU (CAM-ICU), Delirium Rating Scale-Revised-98 (DRS-R-98), Memorial Delirium Assessment Scale, Intensive Care Delirium Screening Checklist (ICDSC), and the Nursing Delirium Screening Scale. The ICDSC and the CAM ICU are the two scales that are well studied, validated, reliable, widely implemented, and recommended by clinical practice guidelines. CAM-ICU offers ease of administration with detailed instructions and training at http://www.icudelirium.org/delirium. Improved care of patients with delirium could be achieved through the implementation of effective screening tools, incorporation of delirium assessments into nursing and physician documentation, and improved communication between team members. See http://www.iculiberation.org/Pain-Agitation-Delirium.

TABLE 1 Risk Factors for Developing and Prolonging Delirium

PREDISPOSING FACTORS	PRECIPITATING FACTORS	PERPETUATING FACTORS
Impairments in: Cognition Vision Hearing function	Sleep deprivation Dehydration Oxidative stress Recent acute illness/ surgery Substance intoxication/ withdrawal Polypharmacy Medication adverse effect	Severe disease (morbidity) CNS pathology Immobility Excessive sedation Poorly controlled pain

---

TABLE 2 American Psychiatric Association (APA) Diagnostic and Statistical Manual DSM-5 Criteria for Delirium

A. Disturbance in attention (i.e., reduced ability to direct, focus, sustain, and shift attention) and awareness (reduced orientation to the environment)

B. The disturbance develops over a short period of time (usually hours to a few days), represents a change from baseline attention and awareness, and tends to fluctuate in severity during the course of the day

C. An additional disturbance in cognition (e.g., memory deficit, disorientation, language, visuospatial ability, or perception)

D. The disturbance in criteria A and C are not better explained by another preexisting, established, or evolving neurocognitive disorder and do not occur in the context of a severely reduced level of arousal, such as coma

E. There is evidence from the history, physical examination, or laboratory findings that the disturbance is a direct physiological consequence of another medical condition, substance intoxication or withdrawal (i.e., resulting from a drug of abuse or to a medication), or is from exposure to a toxin, or is due to multiple etiologies

Clinical Manifestations

Several subtypes of delirium have been described without clear, distinguishing etiology. Subjective assessment is most commonly based on the clinical manifestations of the patient's motor activity. The patient may be hyperactive (agitated) or hypoactive (lethargic) or may demonstrate a mixed pattern. Symptoms develop acutely over a short period of time. The patient demonstrates a reduced ability to direct, focus, and shift his or her attention, and a reduced orientation to their environment. Important signs and symptoms of delirium include inattention, disorientation, impaired memory, visuospatial impairment, perceptual disturbances, language impairment, and sleep-cycle disturbance. Symptoms may fluctuate.

Differential Diagnosis

Delirium can be mistaken for many clinical conditions and is frequently missed or misdiagnosed. Early recognition, identification, and adequate treatment of underlying medical conditions will help demystify this common syndrome. The "I WATCH DEATH" and "Dr. DRE" mnemonics are helpful in developing a comprehensive differential diagnosis in patients with delirium (see http://www.icudelirium.org/terminology).

I WATCH DEATH

Infection	UTI, HIV, sepsis, pneumonia
Withdrawal	Alcohol, barbiturate, sedative-hypnotic, possibly nicotine
Acute metabolic	Acidosis, alkalosis, electrolyte disturbance, hepatic, renal failure, dehydration
Trauma	Closed-head injury, heat stroke, postoperative state, burns
CNS pathology	Abscess, hemorrhage, subdural hematoma, infection, seizures, stroke, tumors, metastases, vasculitis, encephalitis, meningitis
Hypoxia	Hypotension, respiratory/cardiac failure, anemia, severe illness
Deficiencies	Vitamin B12, folate, niacin, thiamine
Endocrinopathies	Adrenal, thyroid, parathyroid, hypo/hyperglycemia
Acute vascular	Hypertensive encephalopathy, arrhythmia, stroke
Toxins/drugs	Anticholinergic medications, illicit drugs, bath salts
Heavy metals	Lead, manganese, mercury

Dr. DRE

Diseases	Sepsis, CHF
Drug Removal	Stop deliriogenic medications (benzodiazepines, antihistamines, opioids)
Environment	Remove restraints, provide orientation, reduce isolation, mobilize the patient, restore day/night light pattern, reduce noise, promote sleep

Complications

The most significant complications of delirium include increased morbidity; mortality; lengths of ICU and hospital stay; cognitive and/or functional impairment; risk of institutional placement; patient, family, and caregiver distress; and the overall burden of the illness.

Treatment

The treatment of delirium consists of early awareness, identification, and treatment of underlying medical conditions. The consideration of risk factors is an essential component of a comprehensive interdisciplinary approach to the treatment of acute delirium. Careful assessment of the patient's current medical condition and early recognition of modifiable risk factors is essential. Even though antipsychotic medications may be widely available for the treatment of acute agitation, it is imperative to use a detail-oriented approach to the workup of the etiology of delirium. The following table outlines a nonpharmacologic approach to the management of patients with delirium.

Nonpharmacologic Treatment

1. Etiologic—identification of all possible risk factors and disease etiology;
2. Behavioral interventions—early mobilization, sleep enhancement, noise reduction, frequent reorientation, assistance with visual/hearing aids;
3. Environmental controls—private room, night lights, personal objects within view/reach, clock, calendar, daily schedule, familiar objects;
4. Family support—provide reassurance, education and support for family members.

Pharmacological treatment of delirium is not a substitute for instituting nonpharmacologic treatment modalities. The following table outlines pharmacologic treatments that have been used as an adjunct to nonpharmacologic treatment.

Pharmacologic Treatment

1. Antipsychotics: **None of the antipsychotic medications are FDA approved for treatment or prevention of delirium.** Haloperidol (Haldol), PO, IM, or IV administration, is the most commonly chosen antipsychotic based on extensive empirical evidence over the last several decades with evidence base from placebo controlled trials still being gathered. MIND-USA (Modifying the Impact of ICU-Induced Neurological Dysfunction-USA) trial is currently underway with the long-term objective to define the role of the antipsychotics in the management of delirium: www.clinicaltrials.gov. Atypical antipsychotis have been used for symptomatic management of delirium with variable comparable efficacy: risperidone (Risperdal), olanzapine (Zyprexa), quetiapine (Seroquel), ziprasidone (Geodon), and aripiprazole (Abilify). Choice of the medication should always be based on the patient-medication related factors and side-effect profile with caution advised due to the risk of QTc prolongation.
2. α-2 receptor agonists: clonidine (Catapres)[1] should be considered for patients with suspected opioid/alcohol withdrawal. Dexmedetomidine (Precedex),[1] a selective alpha-2 adrenergic agonist, offers the advantage of controlled sedation in management of patients with severe agitation and treatment refractory delirium.
3. Benzodiazepines: benzodiazepines have been used widely in ICUs for treatment of agitation and are FDA approved for alcohol withdrawal delirium. Recent publications emphasize an increased risk of delirium and unfavorable side effects profile of benzodiazepines as well as an increased risk of falls and cognitive impairment.
4. Cholinesterase inhibitors: cholinesterase inhibitors (i.e., rivastigmine [Exelon]), are not indicated for treatment or prevention of delirium in critically ill patients.

Prevention

Prevention of delirium is based on identification of at-risk individuals and minimization of risk factors. Although still experimental, with evidence yet to be solidified, there is an increasing role of using low doses of familiar (i.e., haloperidol,[1] risperidone,[1] olanzapine[1]) medications utilized for the treatment of delirium in patients at high risk of delirium who are undergoing elective surgeries. Additionally, medications such as melatonin[2] could be considered as sleep-promoting agents for patients at risk for delirium. The safety and clinical efficacy of other agents such as gabapentin (Neurontin),[1] ketamine,[1] and cholinesterase inhibitors (rivastigmine[1]) are yet to be determined.

---

[1]Not FDA approved for this indication.
[2]Not available in the United States.

References

http://www.icudelirium.org. Accessed December 15, 2013.
http://www.iculiberation.org/Pain-Agitation-Delirium/Pages/Delirium (accessed December 19, 2013).
http://www.apm.org/library/monographs/delirium (accessed December 12, 2013).
http://publications.nice.org.uk/delirium-cg103 (accessed December 10, 2013).

American Psychiatric Association. Desk Reference to the Diagnostic Criteria from DSM-5. Arlington, VA: American Psychiatric Association; 2013.

Maldonado JR. Neuropathogenesis of delirium: Review of current etiologic theories and common pathways. Am J Geriatr Psychiatry 2013;21:12.

Bledowski J, Trutia A. A review of pharmacological management and prevention strategies for delirium in the intensive care unit. Psychosomatics 2012;53:203–11.

Devlin JW, Al-Qadhee NS, Skrobik Y. Pharmacologic prevention and treatment of delirium in critically ill and non-critically ill hospitalized patients: A review of data from prospective, randomized studies. Best Pract Res Clin Anaesthesiol 2012;26:289–309.

Teslyar P, Stock VM, Wilk CM, et al. Prophylaxis with antipsychotic medication reduces the risk of post-operative delirium in elderly patients: A meta-analysis. Psychosomatics 2013;54:124–31.

Barr J, Fraser GL, Puntillo K, et al. Clinical practice guidelines for the management of pain, agitation, and delirium in adult patients in the intensive care unit. Crit Care Med 2013;41:263–306.

Brummel NE, Vasilevskis EE, Han JH, et al. Implementing delirium screening in the ICU: Secrets to success. Crit Care Med 2013;41(9):1–13.

DRUG ABUSE

Method of
William M. Greene, MD; and Mark S. Gold, MD

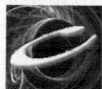

CURRENT DIAGNOSIS

- Screen for substance use in all primary care and emergency settings.
- The clinical interview remains the mainstay of diagnosis.
- Clinicians should have a low threshold for ordering a urine drug test.
- Collateral information should be obtained from family or other sources.
- DSM-V offers current diagnostic criteria for substance use disorders (see Box 1).

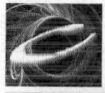

CURRENT THERAPY

- Effective pharmacologic and psychosocial treatments exist.
- Formal detoxification is indicated for dangerous withdrawal states or in patients with serious medical comorbidity.
- Pharmacologic relapse prevention treatment options are substance-specific, and particularly useful options exist for nicotine and opioids.
- Psychosocial treatments remain the mainstay of substance treatment, and these range along a continuum of intensity from outpatient counseling to long-term residential treatment.
- Patients should be referred to self-help groups (e.g., Narcotics Anonymous) to complement other therapies.
- Indefinite remission is an attainable goal for many—a relapse does not constitute total failure but gives opportunity to reevaluate the treatment approach.

Epidemiology

Widespread pathologic use of intoxicating substances, both legal and illegal, remains one of the greatest public health concerns facing our nation. According to the 2010 National Survey on Drug Use and Health, 22.6 million Americans (8.9% of the population) aged 12 years and older used an illicit drug within the past month. By order of frequency, these include marijuana, nonmedical use of prescription drugs, cocaine, hallucinogens, inhalants, and heroin. In addition, 69.6 million Americans (27.4%) aged 12 years and older used tobacco within the past month, mostly in the form of cigarettes. Each year in the United States, approximately 443,000 people die of an illness attributable to cigarette smoking, making this the foremost cause of preventable death.

The estimated annual economic cost of drug abuse is over $600 billion in the United States alone: $185 billion for illicit drugs, $235 billion for alcohol, and $193 billion for tobacco. These costs include only direct health-related, crime-related, and lost-productivity costs, thus underestimating the full impact of drug abuse on society.

From 2002 to 2010, the rate of past-month cigarette use among 12- to 17-year-olds has steadily dropped from 13.0% to 8.3%. The 2010 Monitoring the Future survey data confirm that cigarette smoking has continued to fall to the lowest rate in the survey's history (i.e., past month use among 12th graders is now at 19%). Since 2000, overall rates of illicit drug use have slowly dropped, but use of marijuana has recently slowed its rate of decline and initiation of illicit prescription drugs is now on the rise. In 2006, new users of illicit prescription drugs caught up with new users of marijuana for the first time; however, since then, first-time use of marijuana has regained its ascendancy, with 2.4 million first-time users estimated in 2010. As of 2010, 48.2% of 12th graders still report having used an illicit drug at some point in their life. Despite advances in our understanding and treatment of substance use disorders, drug abuse remains an epidemic, especially in the areas of drugged driving and drug use (including tobacco) in pregnancy.

Diagnosis

With the publication of the DSM-V in 2013, the diagnostic categories of substance abuse and substance dependence have been entirely eliminated. In the interest of consistency and clarity, and based on large population data, these have been replaced with a new diagnostic entity: "substance use disorder" (Box 1). It is no longer necessary for the clinician to decide between two different diagnoses. Those familiar with DSM-IV terminology will find the new criteria quite familiar, as they essentially represent a combination of the old abuse and dependence criteria, with two notable

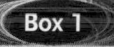

Box 1 DSM-V Diagnostic Criteria for "Substance Use Disorder"

A problematic pattern of use leading to clinically significant impairment or distress as manifested by two or more of the following in a 12-month period:
1. Often taken in larger amounts or longer period than intended.
2. Persistent desire or unsuccessful efforts to cut down or control use.
3. Great deal of time spent in activities necessary to obtain, use, or recover from effects.
4. Craving, or strong desire or urge to use.
5. Recurrent use resulting in failure to fulfill major role obligations at work, school, or home.
6. Continued use despite having persistent/recurrent social or interpersonal problems caused or exacerbated by the substance.
7. Important social, occupational, or recreational activities are given up or reduced because of use.
8. Recurrent use in situations in which it is physically hazardous.
9. Continued use despite knowledge of having a persistent/recurrent physical or psychological problem likely to have been caused or exacerbated by the substance.
10. Tolerance (needing increased amounts for desired effect, or diminished effect with same amount).
11. Withdrawal (manifested by characteristic syndrome or taking more to relieve/avoid withdrawal).

Specify current severity:

Mild: Two to three criteria are met

Moderate: Four to five criteria are met

Severe: Six or more criteria are met

exceptions: one, legal problems has been eliminated; and two, a craving criterion has been added. When diagnosing a substance use disorder, the specific substance for which criteria are met must be listed. In addition, it is also important to document the severity of the disorder based on the number of symptoms present. Examples of specific diagnoses using the new nomenclature would be "alcohol use disorder, moderate" or "alprazolam use disorder, severe." This simpler, evidence-based, diagnostic schema should eliminate some of the confusion previously surrounding the term "dependence," which was often mistaken to be synonymous with "physiological dependence." It has long been understood, in the context of certain prescribed drugs, that the presence of tolerance and withdrawal is not pathological in nature; rather, these represent an expected state of neuroadaptation. This fact is reflected in the new criteria for opioid use disorder; stimulant use disorder; and sedative, hypnotic, or anxiolytic use disorder. For these three categories, the tolerance and withdrawal criteria are not considered to be met if present when the substance is taken solely under appropriate medical supervision. It should be noted this exception does not apply to cannabis, even if it is "prescribed."

Despite the importance and usefulness of the DSM-V, many patients (and clinicians) may still be left wondering if the problem at hand would appropriately be characterized as "addiction." In a 2011 public policy statement, the American Society of Addiction Medicine offered the following short definition of addiction, which has been well received: *"Addiction is a primary, chronic disease of brain reward, motivation, memory and related circuitry. Dysfunction in these circuits leads to characteristic biological, psychological, social and spiritual manifestations. This is reflected in an individual pathologically pursuing reward and/or relief by substance use and other behaviors. Addiction is characterized by inability to consistently abstain, impairment in behavioral control, craving, diminished recognition of significant problems with one's behaviors and interpersonal relationships, and a dysfunctional emotional response. Like other chronic diseases, addiction often involves cycles of relapse and remission. Without treatment or engagement in recovery activities, addiction is progressive and can result in disability or premature death."*

Tobacco and Nicotine

Nicotine is the main addictive component in tobacco, which is administered via smoking (e.g., cigarettes, cigars, pipes, bidis, hookah) or in smokeless formulations (e.g., dip, snuff, snus, chew). However, smoking tobacco is clearly not equivalent to taking nicotine. Cigarette smoking causes nicotine, brain monoamine oxidase (MAO), and other effects in the smoker, some resulting from the smoke and others resulting from the nicotine.

Following administration, nicotine rapidly binds to nicotinic acetylcholine receptors in the central nervous system (CNS), where it acts as a mild psychostimulant and mood modulator in a non-impairing, yet profoundly addictive manner. When the user is tired, smoking has a stimulating effect. When the user is anxious or stressed, smoking exerts a calming effect. Smoking is like an injection without the needle, and given its short half-life, repeated self-administration serves to effectively relieve unpleasant withdrawal symptoms from the nicotine itself. Repeated use quickly leads to both physiologic and psychological dependence.

As with other drugs of abuse, cue-induced cravings play an important role in maintaining the addiction. For example, the smell of the smoke, the sound of a lighter, and the feel of a cigarette on the lips all contribute to an overall process addiction beyond just addiction to the nicotine itself. Tobacco use is also strongly associated with alcohol use, with which it has synergistic toxic effects.

Toxicities from tobacco use are well described and include severe pulmonary disease, cardiovascular disease, and carcinomas of the upper aerodigestive tract and bladder. Even secondhand smoke, previously considered harmless, is now correctly regarded as a serious health risk to the nonsmoker and a "drug" itself. Cigarette smoke contains more than nicotine (up to 4700 components, all of which affect the smoker). Additionally, secondhand tobacco exposure in utero can cause addiction and lead to serious health-related consequences.

Although quitting remains difficult for even the most motivated tobacco users, effective treatments for nicotine dependence now exist. Clinical trials indicate a combination of counseling and medications offers the best chance for success and should be offered to patients who are willing to make a quit attempt. A wide range of FDA-approved nicotine replacement therapies are readily available and have similar rates of efficacy (Table 1). Patches

TABLE 1 Pharmacotherapy for Nicotine Dependence

DRUG	MECHANISM OF ACTION	DOSAGE	INSTRUCTIONS	COMMENTS
Nicotine patch (Nicoderm CQ)	NRT	7 mg, 14 mg, 21 mg	1 patch daily	Tapering doses recommended to discontinue
Nicotine gum (Nicorette)	NRT	2 mg, 4 mg	Chew slightly then "park" on oral mucosa	Tapering doses recommended to discontinue
Nicotine lozenge (Commit)	NRT	2 mg, 4 mg	Absorbed through oral mucosa; minimize swallowing	Tapering doses recommended to discontinue
Nicotine inhaler (Nicotrol Inhaler)	NRT	4 mg/cartridge	6–16 cartridges/day	By prescription only; tedious administration
Nicotine nasal spray (Nicotrol NS)	NRT	0.5 mg/spray	1–2 sprays each nostril q1h; max 80 sprays/day	By prescription only
Bupropion HCl (Wellbutrin,[1] Zyban)	Inhibits reuptake of NE and DA	150 mg SR tab, 300 mg XL tab	300 mg PO (divided qd [XL tab]-bid [SR tab]) daily × 7–12 wk	Helps with comorbid depression; can help prevent weight gain
Varenicline (Chantix)	Partial agonist at $\alpha_4\beta_2$ nicotinic acetylcholine receptor	0.5 mg, 1 mg	0.5 mg PO qd × 3 d, then 0.5 mg PO bid × 4 d, then 1 mg PO bid × 11 wk	May smoke during 1st wk; may continue additional 12 wk
Nicotine vaccine (NicVAX)	Antibody sequestration of nicotine	n/a	n/a	In clinical trials

[1]Not FDA approved for this indication.

Abbreviations: DA = dopamine; max = maximum; n/a = not applicable; NE = norepinephrine; NRT = nicotine replacement therapy; SR = sustained release; XL = extended release.

(Nicoderm CQ), gums (Nicorette), and lozenges (Commit) are available over the counter, but the nasal spray (Nicotrol NS) and inhaler (Nicotrol Inhaler) are available by prescription only. Recently, "electronic cigarettes" have gained in popularity, but unlike other nicotine products are not regulated as a drug by the FDA.

Non-nicotine prescription medications with proven efficacy are available. Bupropion HCl (Wellbutrin) is an antidepressant that was serendipitously noted to dramatically reduce nicotine cravings in some patients, and it is now widely used for this purpose (as Zyban). Varenicline (Chantix) was specifically developed to treat nicotine dependence and represents a considerable advancement, with improved smoking cessation rates. It acts as a partial agonist at the nicotine receptor and effectively serves to satisfy cravings while simultaneously blocking the effects of exogenously administered nicotine. Although probably the most effective agent, varenicline carries significant risk of psychiatric side effects. The "nicotine vaccine" (NicVAX),[1] a novel approach, is currently in phase III clinical trials, and appears promising.

Nicotine replacement, bupropion, and varenicline are all considered first-line pharmacotherapy. Bupropion, but not varenicline, may also be used in combination with nicotine-replacement therapies. All pharmacotherapy options are enhanced with coadministration of counseling or behavioral therapies. Helpful resources for patients interested in quitting include www.smokefree.gov (a government website dedicated to helping people quit smoking), 1-800-QUIT-NOW (a free phone-based services with coaches and educational materials), and a variety of resources available through the American Cancer Society and American Heart Association.

Cannabis

Cannabis (marijuana, pot, weed, grass, ganja, hash) remains the most-used illicit drug in the world. In Americans older than 12 years, 45% have used cannabis at least once, and 7.4% have used it in the past month. Cannabis is readily harvested from *Cannabis sativa*, and typically it is smoked, although it may also be ingested or vaporized. Despite a recent trend advocating legitimate medicinal use, it is still listed in Schedule I by the Drug Enforcement Agency (DEA), with high potential for abuse and no currently accepted medical use. Delta-9-tetrahydrocannabinol (THC) is the active ingredient, which exerts its desired psychoactive effects at CB_1 receptors diffusely throughout the CNS. Marijuana's THC concentration has been steadily increasing as a result of selective plant breeding. Annual analysis of DEA seizures indicates average THC concentrations increased from approximately 1% in 1975 to approximately 10% in 2008. To what extent this makes the drug more dangerous or more addictive remains unclear.

Acute psychoactive effects of cannabis include euphoria, relaxation, heightened sensations, increased appetite, distorted sense of time, slowed reaction time, illusions and hallucinations, paranoia, and anxiety. Acute somatic effects include conjunctival injection, xerostomia, increased heart rate and blood pressure, muscle relaxation, and reduced intraocular pressure. There is no known risk of dangerous overdose, and withdrawal symptoms are generally mild but include irritability, cravings, diminished appetite, and insomnia. Cannabis is now recognized as unequivocally addictive. Abusers of this drug rapidly develop tolerance, and commonly demonstrate loss of control and continued use despite negative consequences—the hallmarks of addiction. It is estimated that 1 million Americans sought treatment for cannabis as their primary drug of choice in 2010.

Not surprisingly, with more than 400 chemicals identified in its smoke, cannabis is dangerous with respect to long-term health. Chronic cannabis use is associated with lung cancer, chronic obstructive pulmonary disease, cardiovascular disease, impaired immunity, persistent disruption of memory and attention, and various psychiatric disorders, most commonly anxiety disorders and depressive

disorders. There is a growing body of evidence that cannabis abuse can lead to lasting psychosis (i.e., schizophrenia) in predisposed persons.

Currently, treatment of cannabis dependence remains entirely psychosocial. Various existing drugs (including fluoxetine [Prozac],[2] lithium,[2] buspirone [Buspar][2]) have been investigated. However, well-controlled clinical trials to support their use are lacking. Preliminary data suggest that dronabinol (Marinol)[2] may be of some utility in relieving cravings and withdrawal symptoms without causing intoxication. Rimonabant (Acomplia),[3] a CB_1 antagonist previously prescribed for weight loss in Europe, showed promise but has failed to achieve FDA approval because of psychiatric side effects.

Cocaine Methamphetamine, and Other Stimulants

As a class, cocaine and other stimulants work primarily by enhancing dopamine transmission in a dose-dependent fashion, either directly (amphetamines) or by blocking reuptake (cocaine). Cocaine and a variety of amphetamines (e.g., amphetamine/dextroamphetamine [Adderall], dextroamphetamine [Dexedrine], methamphetamine [Desoxyn], methylphenidate [Methylin, Ritalin]) are available for legitimate medical use as Schedule II drugs. Cocaine (in solution) is still used as a topical anesthetic, and amphetamine derivatives are used to treat attention-deficit/hyperactivity disorder (ADHD), narcolepsy (amphetamine and methylphenidate), and obesity (methamphetamine only). Any of these agents may be abused and carry significant potential for addiction. Even newer "safer" agents such as modafinil (Provigil) and armodafinil (Nuvigil) are associated with abuse and dependency, albeit less commonly than with traditional stimulants.

Prescription stimulant abuse can involve using excessive doses to achieve a euphoric high, or via nonmedical use or diversion of prescriptions (e.g., students sharing medication to facilitate studying). When taken at prescribed doses for an appropriate condition, even methamphetamine is generally safe and effective. In contrast, when it is synthesized in clandestine laboratories and smoked or injected in extreme quantities, methamphetamine (crystal meth, ice, crank, speed) is alarmingly dangerous. No other commonly abused drug is so strongly associated with permanent brain damage, resembling that seen in traumatic brain injury victims. As ADHD becomes more recognized and treated, physicians must be aware of the potential for abuse of their well-intentioned prescriptions. To this end, several recent pharmacologic developments have introduced improved options for treatment. Time-released formulations of methylphenidate (e.g., Concerta) and amphetamine/dextroamphetamine (Adderall XR) are considered to have less abuse potential than the short-acting formulations. Better still, the formulation of lisdexamfetamine (Vyvanse) includes the amino acid lysine coupled with the amphetamine molecule, consequently acting as a prodrug with the least abuse potential of all ADHD stimulants.

Cocaine and other stimulants induce sympathomimetic effects including tachycardia, hypertension, mydriasis, and diaphoresis. These drugs are commonly associated with seizures, myocardial infarction, hemorrhagic strokes, dyskinesias and dystonias, and psychosis when taken at the doses typically used to achieve euphoria. Withdrawal is generally experienced as a crash and includes fatigue, depressed mood, increased appetite, and cravings. Considered nonaddictive until about 1980, cocaine is now widely recognized as one of the most addictive drugs, particularly in the base form (crack or freebase). MDMA (methylenedixoymethylamphetamine), or ecstasy, shares the pharmacodynamic properties of the stimulants, combined with serotoninergic effects of the hallucinogens.

Currently, no medication has demonstrated efficacy in treating cocaine or stimulant dependence. Pharmacologic treatment remains symptomatic during the acute withdrawal phase. Stimulant-induced

---

[1]Not FDA approved for this indication.

[2]Not available in the United States.
[3]Exceeds dosage recommended by the manufacturer.

psychosis and mania respond well to traditional psychotropics when warranted; however, to date, no medications have reliably demonstrated efficacy in preventing relapse. A "cocaine vaccine,"[2] which enlists the immune system to develop antibodies rendering cocaine useless, is currently in phase II clinical trials and holds promise for the future. In the meantime, traditional psychosocial treatments remain the mainstay of clinical care.

Opioids

Opioids are categorized as endogenous (endorphins, enkephalins, dynorphins), opium alkaloids (morphine, codeine), semisynthetic (heroin, oxycodone [Roxicodone, OxyContin]), or synthetic (methadone [Dolophine], fentanyl [Sublimaze, Duragesic]). The last three categories have a wide range of clinical uses including analgesia, anesthesia, antidiarrhea, cough suppression, and detoxification and maintenance therapy.

Opioids exert their clinical effect at mu, delta, and kappa opioid receptors. The effect on mu receptors is considered the most important, with its activation directly linked to both analgesic and euphoric effects. Most humans subjectively experience opioids with a neutral to aversive response. However, when used in sufficient quantities by genetically vulnerable persons, some users experience energy, relief of emotional pain, and a euphoria many describe as a "total body orgasm." Intoxication manifests with miosis, impaired consciousness, slurred speech, bradycardia, and depressed respiration. Overdose is potentially fatal via respiratory depression, but it is quite amenable to treatment with repeated doses of intravenous naloxone (Narcan). The withdrawal syndrome is characterized by a constellation of miserable, but not life-threatening, symptoms including mydriasis, piloerection, muscle cramps, diaphoresis, vomiting, lacrimation, rhinorrhea, chills, insomnia, cravings, and autonomic hyperactivity.

Since pain was recognized as "the fifth vital sign" in the 1990s, concurrent with heavy marketing campaigns from pharmaceutical companies, the United States has experienced a veritable explosion of widespread opioid prescribing for nonmalignant pain. An entire industry of pain management has developed, with the unfortunate side effect of having a sizable proportion of its output being used nonmedically. It is important for prescribers to recognize that the abuse potential of prescription opioids matches, or in some cases even exceeds, that of heroin. Today, oxycodone has a street value of approximately $1.00 per milligram.

The most common method of abuse involves simply taking more than prescribed, usually by the appropriate route of administration. Alternatively, opioid abusers commonly take their medications via nasal insufflation or inject them intravenously. The time-release property of certain medications, such as oxycodone (OxyContin), is easily circumvented by crushing the pills, which greatly enhances the euphoric effect. Even transdermal fentanyl patches (Duragesic) are abused via any number of methods, such as applying heat to a worn patch, employing complex extraction techniques described on the Internet, or simply sucking on the patch itself (a common finding by the coroner). Once the prescription is finished early, the user must either supplement the supply or face the unpleasant effects of withdrawal.

There is no shortage of easy methods to obtain opiates illegally. These include seeing multiple prescribers (doctor shopping), purchasing online at foreign "pharmacies," and general trade or purchase on the black market. Also alarming is the growing problem of diversion from hospitals and pharmacies by health care professionals, who are not immune to the disease of addiction. Many states are implementing controlled substance databases aimed to curb the problem of abuse of opioids and other prescription drugs.

Acute detoxification from opioids is achieved via one of two basic strategies: symptomatic treatment with unrelated medications, or substitution with a cross tolerant (opioid) drug with less abuse potential (Table 2). The first strategy may employ the use of clonidine (Catapres),[2] an α_2-adrenergic agonist, to help with the autonomic component of withdrawal. This is commonly done in combination with other symptomatic treatments on an as-needed basis, such as diazepam (Valium) for anxiety, loperamide (Imodium) for diarrhea, and promethazine (Phenergan)[2] or ondansetron (Zofran)[2] for nausea.

The second strategy typically involves either methadone or buprenorphine (Subutex). Methadone, a pure mu agonist with a half-life of about 36 hours, is usually started in the 20- to 30-mg range and titrated cautiously by 10 mg every 4 to 7 days. Maintenance therapy with methadone occurs only in highly regulated methadone clinic settings. Buprenorphine, a partial agonist at the mu receptor (and kappa antagonist) is administered sublingually and has a half-life similar to that of methadone. It was approved in 2002 for office-based treatment of opioid addiction, making pharmacotherapy much more widely available. Caution should be used to not administer buprenorphine too soon (before onset of withdrawal syndrome), or acute withdrawal can actually be precipitated. Buprenorphine is available either alone or in combination with naloxone (Suboxone). Here, the role of naloxone is solely to deter intravenous abuse, because naloxone is inactive when taken as sublingually as prescribed.

[2]Not available in the United States.

[2]Not available in the United States.

TABLE 2	Useful Medications in Treating Opioid Use Disorders				
DRUG	**UTILITY**	**FORMS**	**ADMINISTRATION**	**NOTES**	
Naloxone (Narcan)	Overdose; additive to prevent abuse[1]	SC, IM, IV	0.4–2 mg q2–3 min prn	$T_{1/2} = 1$ h, wears off quickly	
Naltrexone (ReVia, Vivitrol)	Prevention of relapse	PO, IM	ReVia: 50–100 mg PO daily; Vivitrol: 380 mg IM q4wk	Potential for hepatotoxicity; precipitates withdrawal; useful for ETOH as well	
Clonidine (Catapres, Catapres-TTS patch)[1]	Withdrawal	PO, transdermal	0.1–0.2 mg PO tid prn; 0.1–0.3 mg/24 h transdermal via weekly patch	Monitor for hypotension	
Methadone (Dolophine)	Withdrawal; maintenance	PO	Start 20–30 mg PO qd Target 80–120 mg PO qd	Restricted to methadone clinics	
Buprenorphine (Subutex, Suboxone [with naloxone], Buprenex injection[1])	Withdrawal; maintenance	SL IM, IV	Start 2–4 mg SL qd-bid Target 4–32 mg SL daily divided qd-tid	Requires special DEA certification	

[1]Not FDA approved for this indication.
Abbreviations: DEA = Drug Enforcement Administration; ETOH = ethanol.

Buprenorphine and methadone are useful in managing acute withdrawal as well as long-term (months to years) maintenance therapy for preventing relapse to heroin or the opioid of choice. As maintenance therapy, these agents serve to block euphoria, satisfy cravings, and reduce illicit use, with consequent verifiable harm reduction. Buprenorphine, with a built-in ceiling effect because of its unique pharmacology, is much safer than methadone, which is often fatal in overdose. Increasingly, buprenorphine is being used as an analgesic as well (Butrans), and it may be an ideal choice in patients with comorbid pain and addiction who have demonstrated an inability to safely use other opioids.

Also approved for prevention of opioid relapse is naltrexone, an opioid antagonist, which is available in oral (ReVia) and intramuscular depot formulations (Vivitrol).

Sedative-Hypnotics

This class of drugs includes a wide array of compounds (benzodiazepines, barbiturates, and various related compounds) (Table 3), most of which have at least some potential for abuse. Overall, these medications do much more good than harm, and are useful in treating anxiety disorders, insomnia, seizures, and muscle spasms. They are also important in managing withdrawal states and as a component of surgical anesthesia. These drugs act as CNS depressants, and their primary mechanism of action is to enhance inhibitory GABA neurotransmission.

TABLE 3	Common Sedative-Hypnotics, Equivalent Dose Conversions		
GENERIC NAME	**TRADE NAME**	**DOSE (mg)**
Benzodiazepines		
Diazepam	Valium	10
Alprazolam	Xanax, Niravam	0.5–1
Lorazepam	Ativan	2
Clonazepam	Klonopin	1–2
Chlordiazepoxide	Librium	25
Clorazepate	Tranxene	7.5
Oxazepam	Serax	10–15
Temazepam	Restoril	15
Triazolam	Halcion	0.25
Flurazepam	Dalmane	15
Barbiturates		
Phenobarbital	n/a	30
Pentobarbital	Nembutal	100
Secobarbital	Seconal	100
Butalbital (with caffeine and aspirin or acetaminophen)	Fiorinal, Fioricet	100
Amobarbital	Amytal	100
Related Compounds		
Carisoprodol	Soma	700
Meprobamate	Miltown, Equanil	1200
Chloral hydrate	Noctec	500
Methaqualone[1]	Quaalude	300
Ethchlorvynol[1]	Placidyl	500
Zolpidem	Ambien	20
Zaleplon	Sonata	20
Eszopiclone	Lunesta	3

[1]Not FDA approved for this indication.
n/a, not applicable.

The risk of toxicity is by respiratory depression, which is magnified by concomitant use of opioids or other CNS depressants, such as alcohol.

Sedative-hypnotic intoxication and withdrawal states closely resemble those of alcohol, except for a more protracted time course of withdrawal. Anxiety, restlessness, insomnia, tremor, nystagmus, tachycardia, and hypertension usually appear 2 to 12 hours after the last dose, and symptoms gradually resolve over 1 to 2 weeks. Withdrawal seizures, psychosis, and delirium are fairly common. Detoxification is best accomplished on an inpatient basis and typically involves tapering doses of a long-acting benzodiazepine (e.g., clonazepam [Klonopin], diazepam, clorazepate [Tranxene]) at a rate of about 10% of initial daily requirement per day. Acute sedative overdose is managed primarily with supportive care and airway management. Flumazenil (Romazicon) 0.2 to 0.5 mg/min IV may be used with caution for acute overdose of benzodiazepines, because it can precipitate severe acute withdrawal symptoms.

Since their introduction in the 1960s, benzodiazepines have largely replaced barbiturates, given their enhanced safety profile. However, barbiturates still in common use include phenobarbital and butalbital. Phenobarbital, used mainly for treating seizures, is considered to have low potential for abuse. Butalbital, compounded with caffeine plus acetaminophen or aspirin (Fioricet, Fiorinal), has moderate abuse potential, typically in combination with other drugs. Carisoprodol (Soma), although not a barbiturate, is metabolized into meprobamate, a barbiturate-like drug. Commonly taken in combination with opioids and other sedatives, carisoprodol is highly abused.

Alprazolam (Xanax) stands out among its peers as the single most abused, most addictive, and yet currently most prescribed sedative-hypnotic. Its rapid onset (T_{max} 1–2 h) and relatively short half-life (6–14 h) contribute to its abuse liability and propensity for withdrawal seizures. Diazepam, historically the most prescribed sedative, also has relatively rapid onset and significant abuse potential, but its long half-life makes it an ideal agent for use in treating withdrawal from other sedatives. Flunitrazepam (Rohypnol, "roofies") is a benzodiazepine that causes anterograde amnesia and is now illegal in the United States because of its use in drug-facilitated sexual assaults.

γ-Hydroxybutyric acid (GHB) and baclofen (Lioresal) also act as GABAergic CNS depressants, with intoxication and withdrawal states consistent with the class. Oddly, GHB is considered a Schedule I drug with high abuse potential and no accepted medical use, but marketed as sodium oxybate (Xyrem), GHB is available as a Schedule III drug (with special restrictions) when used to treat narcolepsy. Baclofen, on the other hand, appears to have rather low abuse potential and may actually play a role in the treatment of alcoholism.[1]

Relatively new drugs such as zolpidem (Ambien), zaleplon (Sonata), and eszopiclone (Lunesta) are benzodiazepine-like drugs with CNS depressant activity, approved for short-term treatment of insomnia, and have at least some potential for abuse and dependence. Clonazepam is generally considered to have the lowest potential for euphoria and abuse and is the agent of choice if a benzodiazepine must be given to patients with a relative contraindication, such as a history of any drug abuse or dependence.

Conclusion

Despite intensive supply-reduction strategies, improved primary prevention efforts, and the many recent pharmacotherapy advances, drug abuse remains largely unchanged in its overall scale, with the exceptions of increasing use, abuse, and dependence of both marijuana and prescription opioids. Another notable exception is the significant reduction in tobacco use since the turn of the century. It is estimated that 25% of patients seen in office settings and 50% of those seen in emergency department settings have active problems related to substance abuse. All patients

[1]Not FDA approved for this indication.

in primary care settings must be screened for tobacco, alcohol, and illicit drug abuse. Patients should be asked directly about substance use at the initial point of contact (e.g., emergency departments, primary care offices), and clinicians should maintain a healthy degree of skepticism toward patients' responses, remembering that most patients minimize substance use. When any suspicion exists, urine drug screens should be readily utilized without hesitation or fear of communicating mistrust. A variety of affordable quick screen kits are available, which can be sent out for laboratory confirmation of positive results if necessary.

Physicians and other health care professionals are in a unique position to intervene with drug abuse at the individual level, because it is encountered commonly in clinical practice. The problem must first be identified, and depending on the skill set of the primary provider, patients should be treated or referred to an appropriate treatment provider. There is an initiative to incorporate formal SBIRT (screening, brief intervention, and referral to treatment) into routine clinical practice. Current procedural terminology (CPT) codes and a reimbursement schedule for screening and brief intervention may be located online at http://www.samhsa.gov/prevention/sbirt/coding.aspx. Screening may involve the written or verbal assessment of substance use to determine whether the patient exhibits problematic levels of use. The brief intervention aspect of SBIRT targets those with milder substance use problems and provides effective strategies for intervention before the need for more extensive or specialized treatment arises. Referral to specialized treatment is recommended for patients with moderate-to-severe substance use disorders. Data suggest this approach is successful in modifying problematic substance-use behavior. In addition to formal treatment, physician referral to local 12-step recovery meetings (Alcoholics Anonymous, Narcotics Anonymous) has proved beneficial. Local chapters provide physicians with names and telephone numbers of members willing to welcome newcomers (www.aa.org).

Physicians are usually well equipped to treat the sequelae of drug abuse, but they often forget that addiction is a treatable disease entity itself. Treatment ranges in intensity along a continuum including medically managed inpatient detoxification, partial hospitalization, intensive outpatient treatment, and outpatient care. The American Society of Addiction Medicine provides patient placement criteria that dictate the appropriate level of treatment based on a multidimensional assessment. Health care professionals should be familiar with the treatment centers in their area, which can place the patient in the appropriate level of care.

It is important to remember that relapse is a characteristic of addiction and does not equate to treatment failure, but rather indicates a need for an adjustment in the treatment level or monitoring. Other chronic diseases, such as diabetes or hypertension, necessitate the ongoing monitoring and adjustment of treatment interventions as needed, and so is the case with addiction. Recently published data on the treatment and monitoring of recovering physicians (a subgroup of addicts that boasts a 5-year success rate greater than 78%) teaches us the lesson that adequate initial treatment coupled with ongoing monitoring is critical. Sustained recovery from substance use disorders is attainable and is characterized by voluntary sobriety, improved personal health, and improved citizenship.

References

American Psychiatric Association. Diagnostic and Statistical Manual of Mental Disorders. 5th ed. Washington, DC: American Psychiatric Publishing; 2013.

Bailey JA, Hurley RW, Gold MS. Crossroads of pain and addiction. Pain Med 2010;11:1803–18.

Centers for Disease Control, Prevention. Annual smoking-attributable mortality, years of potential life lost, and productivity losses—United States, 1997–2001. MMWR Morb Mortal Wkly Rep 2005;54:625–8.

DuPont RL, McLellan AT, White WL, et al. Setting the standard for recovery: Physicians health programs. J Subst Abuse Treat 2009;36:159–71.

Fowler JS, Volkow ND, Wang GJ, et al. Neuropharmacological actions of cigarette smoke: Brain monoamine oxidase B (MAO B) inhibition. J Addict Dis 1998;17:23–4.

Gold MS, Kobeissy FH, Wang KK, et al. Methamphetamine- and trauma-induced brain injuries: Comparative cellular and molecular neurobiological substrates. Biol Psychiatry 2009;66:118–27.

Haney M, Hart CL, Foltin RW. Effects of baclofen on cocaine self-administration: Opioid- and nonopioid-dependent volunteers. Neuropharmacology 2006;31:1814–21.

Johnston LD, O'Malley PM, Bachman JG, et al. Monitoring the Future: National Results on Adolescent Drug Use: Overview of Key Findings, 2010. Ann Arbor: Institute for Social Research, The University of Michigan; 2011.

Office of National Drug Control Policy. The Economic Costs of Drug Abuse in the United States: 1992–2002. Washington, DC: Executive Office of the President; 2004 [Publication No. 207303].

Small E, Shah HP, Davenport JJ, et al. Tobacco smoke exposure induces nicotine dependence in rats. Psychopharmacology (Berl) 2010;208:143–58.

American Society of Addiction Medicine. Public policy statement: Definition of addiction, August 15, Available at http://www.asam.org/docs/publicy-policy-statements/1definition_of_addiction_long_4-11.pdf; 2011.

EATING DISORDERS

Method of
Sarah Forsberg, PsyD; and James Lock, MD, PhD

Bulimia Nervosa

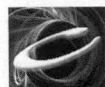

CURRENT DIAGNOSIS

- Binge eating episodes occur at least once per week for 3 months (eating objectively large quantities of food accompanied by a loss of control while eating).
- Compensatory purging episodes occur at least once per month for a period of 3 months (e.g., self-induced vomiting, laxatives, diuretics, excessive and driven exercise, enemas).
- Shape and weight are overvalued in self-worth and self-esteem.
- Weight is at or above expected range given age, height, and historical growth curves.

CURRENT TREATMENT

- Cognitive behavioral therapy (CBT) is the best evidence-based treatment for bulimia nervosa (BN).
- Interpersonal psychotherapy (IPT) is an appropriate alternative.
- Family-based treatment (FBT) is useful for adolescents with BN.
- Antidepressant treatment (selective serotonin reuptake inhibitors [SSRIs]) may be useful in augmenting psychotherapy, or as an alternative in the event that psychotherapy is not effective, is refused, or is unavailable. It is not as effective as CBT and thus not a front-line approach.

Diagnosis

To diagnose BN, an individual must engage in recurrent binge episodes with compensatory behaviors (e.g., self-induced vomiting, diuretic or laxative use, excessive exercise). A binge is a discrete episode of eating a quantity of food that is more than the average person would eat in the same setting. While binging, there is a loss of control or sense of being unable to stop eating. A disproportionate emphasis on weight and shape in one's self-evaluation is also required in diagnosing BN. DSM-V criteria require that these episodes occur at a minimum of once weekly for 3 months. Unlike individuals with anorexia nervosa (AN), who may binge and purge, individuals with BN are within or above a normal weight range.

Significant health consequences may accompany BN. Laboratory studies often reveal electrolyte abnormalities, which can lead to cardiac arrhythmias and cardiac arrest in severe cases. Physical examination may detect enamel decay and parotid gland enlargement because of recurrent vomiting. When ipecac[1] is used to

---

[1]Not FDA approved for this indication.

induce vomiting, severe cardiac and skeletal myopathies may develop. Laxative abuse is associated with metabolic acidosis and elevated serum amylase levels. BN has an elevated risk for mortality (crude mortality rate is estimated at 2% per decade) and suicide. Most common comorbid psychiatric diagnoses are mood, anxiety, personality disorders (specifically borderline personality), and substance use disorders.

Epidemiology

BN behaviors typically first occur in middle adolescence (ages 14–16), with onset of full syndrome BN in later adolescence and early adulthood (ages 17–24). The 12-month prevalence estimate of DSM-V BN for young females is 2.6%, and while less is known about males, at minimum, they are estimated to account for approximately 10% of all cases. Symptoms may persist for a number of years, with intermittent periods of remission. A recent review of existing treatment studies suggests that approximately 45% of patients fully recover, with 27% improving considerably and the remaining 23% exhibiting a chronic course.

Etiology

BN can be explained by a confluence of biological, sociocultural, psychological, and familial factors. From a biological standpoint, BN clusters in families; in twin studies, about half of the variance in heritability can be explained by genetic factors. Serotonin levels may be reduced, and imaging studies show abnormal serotonergic circuitry in the orbital-frontal cortex. Internalization of cultural ideals of beauty may present as a focus on thinness for women, where for males there is often pressure to be muscular with low body fat. Participation in sports where weight and appearance are tied to performance (e.g., gymnastics, wrestling) may increase risk in males. Early puberty and childhood obesity are common precipitants, as are experiences with peer weight-related teasing. Personality characteristics of individuals with BN may include perfectionism, impulsivity, and instability in interpersonal relationships. Childhood sexual and physical abuse increases the risk for BN.

Treatment

Given the significant physical, social, and emotional consequences associated with BN, effective treatment requires addressing wide-ranging difficulties. Over 70 randomized controlled treatment trials (RCTs) exist for adults with BN, yet only two focus on adolescents. Most studies have examined behavioral therapies, medications, or a combination thereof. CBT is established as the treatment of choice for adults with BN and has been subjected to a large number of RCTs. The underlying assumption of CBT is that bulimic behaviors are maintained by dysfunctional attitudes about shape, weight, and physical appearance, which thereby lead to an overemphasis of these aspects in self-evaluation. Excessive dieting typically ensues, resulting in physiologic and psychologic deprivation that increases vulnerability to binge eating. Feelings of guilt and fear about weight gain are mitigated through engaging in purging behaviors. CBT targets this cycle through the use of self-monitoring to increase an awareness of patterns in behaviors, thoughts, and emotions that maintain BN.

CBT is found to be more effective than no treatment, pill placebo, nondirective supportive psychotherapy, nutritional counseling, stress management, and antidepressant medication therapy. Response to CBT is good, with approximately 50% recovered and 20% with significant reductions in symptoms at the end of treatment. CBT is acceptable and feasible with adolescents with 56% in a case series and 36% in a guided self-help (GSH) version recovered at the end of treatment. When compared to an alternative intervention, IPT, CBT demonstrates a greater probability of remission and reduction in symptoms at the end of treatment. However, these initial differences appear to diminish at a 1-year follow-up, suggesting that while less efficient, IPT is a viable alternative. IPT was adapted for BN to target interpersonal factors thought to contribute to the development and maintenance of the disorder. IPT has yet to be studied with adolescents.

More recently, CBT has been expanded to address other maintaining features of eating disorders more broadly (e.g., interpersonal difficulties, clinical perfectionism, low self-esteem, and mood intolerance). Enhanced CBT (CBT-E) addresses these features and is delivered in a focused or broad (addressing aforementioned maintaining features) format. For individuals with more complex psychopathology, the broad version may be more effective.

Other interventions show promise in the treatment of BN and require further examination. For adolescents, FBT may be helpful, demonstrating higher rates of abstinence (40%) than supportive psychotherapy (18%). Derived from FBT for AN, parents are supported to directly change dysfunctional eating behaviors. For adults, dialectical behavior therapy (DBT) has been shown to significantly decrease binge/purge episodes when delivered in an individual format. Similar effects were found when an appetite-awareness component was added to standard DBT.

Antidepressants (SSRIs) are the most studied medication treatment for BN. Fluoxetine (Prozac) demonstrates greater reductions in binge eating, purging, and eating-related cognitions than placebo when prescribed at higher doses (60 mg/day). A small pilot study of fluoxetine with adolescents suggests it is acceptable and may decrease BN symptoms. Antidepressants alone are not as effective as when combined with CBT, or as CBT alone.

Binge Eating Disorder

CURRENT DIAGNOSIS

- Recurrent episodes of binge eating, defined as eating an objectively large amount of food in a discrete period of time with an experience of loss of control.
- Binge eating is associated with at least three of the following: eating rapidly; eating until uncomfortably full; eating outside of physical hunger; eating alone because of embarrassment; and subsequent feelings of disgust, depression, or guilt.
- There is marked distress associated with binge eating.
- These episodes occur at least once per week over 3 months.
- There is no associated compensatory behavior (e.g., purging), and binging does not occur in the context of another eating disorder diagnosis (anorexia or bulimia nervosa [BN]).

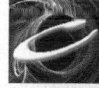

CURRENT TREATMENT

- CBT and IPT have good evidence of efficacy among adults.
- GSH CBT may be effective for those with less psychopathology.
- DBT requires further study to determine if good outcomes are sustained over time.
- There is no evidence-based treatment for young patients with binge eating disorder (BED).

Diagnosis

Binge episodes are characterized by eating quantities that are larger than others would eat in a similar setting and are accompanied by a feeling of being out of control. Individuals with BED do not engage in compensatory behaviors (e.g., self-induced vomiting, excessive exercise) as in BN. DSM-V criteria require that the episodes occur at a minimum frequency of once per week over a 3-month period. Binge eating (BE) is commonly associated with feelings of guilt and embarrassment and may result in attempts to hide eating. Further, during binge episodes, eating is often rapid, and results in feeling uncomfortably full.

Epidemiology

Lifetime prevalence of BE among adults is 3.5% and 2% in females and males respectively. It occurs at equal rates across ethnic and racial groups. BE most typically onsets in later adolescence or early adulthood, although it does occur in children and is often associated with overweight and obesity as well as psychological symptoms. Among obese adolescents, an estimated 1% meet the criteria for BED and 9% experience BE. In BED, dieting typically occurs after the onset of BE, where in BN this pattern is reversed. Remission rates in BED are higher than in other eating disorders, although duration and severity is similar to BN.

Etiology

The etiology of BED is unknown. Restrictive dieting, body image dissatisfaction, pressure to be thin, low self-esteem, depressive symptoms, and limited social support increase the risk for the onset of adolescent BE. Increased rates of BE in families suggests there may be a genetic link. Potential medical causes for BE include CNS tumors, Kleine-Levin syndrome, Kluver-Bucy syndrome, Prader-Willi syndrome, and gastrointestinal pathology, and these causes should be ruled out during assessment. Comorbid psychiatric disorders are common among adults with BED, including mood disorders, anxiety disorders, and, at lesser frequency, substance use disorders and personality disorders. There are high rates of obesity among individuals with BED; however, psychiatric symptoms are linked to the severity of BE rather than obese status.

Treatment

Treatment for adults with BED has received considerable attention in RCTs compared to other eating disorder diagnoses. Most treatments target reduction in BE, psychological symptoms, and weight loss for those who are overweight. CBT has been applied in multiple formats (group, GSH, CD-ROM delivered, and in combination with medication) and appears to have the highest rates of abstinence. Individual CBT outperformed group CBT in one trial, and a GSH version was more effective in reducing BE than behavioral weight-loss (BWL). CBT targets underlying dysfunctional attitudes and behaviors that maintain BE. An alternative treatment, IPT, is a time-limited psychodynamic therapy targeting interpersonal difficulties that underlie the disorder. IPT is helpful in reducing the frequency of BE. IPT, CBT, and motivational intervention (MI) all lead to improvements in cognitive restraint, disinhibition, shape and weight concerns thought to maintain BE.

Dialectical behavior therapy (DBT) is another treatment adapted for BED with the aim of targeting affect regulation difficulties formulated to be a maintaining mechanism of BE. Women in a small trial comparing group DBT to a waitlisted group had significantly greater decreases in BE and related eating disorder thoughts and behaviors, with over half abstinent from BE at follow-up. However, when compared to supportive psychotherapy, the rate of abstinence, while achieved more quickly in the DBT group, did not differ between the groups at follow-up. Pilot data suggest comprehensive DBT (individual, group, and skills coaching) may be effective.

Pharmacologic treatments targeting binge eating and weight loss have been tested alone and in combination with psychotherapy. There may be improvement in weight loss with addition of pharmacotherapy. The combination of CBT with topiramate (Topamax)[1] resulted in greater weight loss and better psychosocial outcomes than CBT with fluoxetine.[1] A high dose of the SSRI escitalopram (Lexapro),[1] anticonvulsants topiramate[1] and zonisamide (Zonegran),[1] Lisdexamfetamine (Vyvanse) at a dose of 50 mg or 70 mg, and the selective norepinephrine reuptake inhibitor atomoxetine (Strattera),[1] were each associated with significantly decreased binge eating and weight in separate placebo-controlled trials.

---

[1]Not FDA approved for this indication.

Anorexia Nervosa

CURRENT DIAGNOSIS

- Persistent restriction of energy (caloric) intake relative to requirements, leading to significantly low weight (e.g., accounting for age, sex, developmental trajectory, and physical health).
- Fear of becoming fat, or ongoing behavior interferes with weight gain.
- Disturbance in the perception of shape, weight, overvaluation of weight, and shape in self-evaluation, or lack of acknowledgment of seriousness of low weight.
- Either meets criteria for restricting type—with absence of binge or purge behaviors, or binge-eating/purging type.

CURRENT TREATMENT

- FBT for adolescents with AN is the best evidentially based approach.
- Adolescent-focused therapy (AFT) may be a helpful alternative.
- There are no first-line treatments for adults with AN.
- CBT may prevent relapse in weight-restored individuals.

Diagnosis

AN is characterized by dietary restriction that is severe enough to lead to seriously low weight, fear of weight gain, and difficulty or inability to accurately perceive shape or weight. Secondary amenorrhea is no longer required for a diagnosis of AN in DSM-V. Individuals may be classified as AN-restricting type or AN-binge/purge subtype. The definition of low weight is less than "minimally normal" among adults, or "minimally expected" among children and adolescents. Growth charts normed by age and gender are necessary to calculate expected BMI for individuals under 18 and growth curves may help detect deviations from an individual's growth trajectory. A BMI at or below the 10th percentile is a benchmark reflecting malnourishment associated with AN, and BMI below 18.5 kg/m^2 may be used as guidelines.

A wide variety of medical and psychiatric symptoms accompany AN. Potentially life-threatening medical conditions may develop as a result of semistarvation. Vital sign abnormalities (bradycardia, orthostasis, hypothermia), and amenorrhea are common consequences of malnutrition. Bone loss resulting in osteopenia and in more severe cases, osteoporosis, may occur. Abnormal laboratory findings may occur in some patients with AN who use laxatives, diuretics, and diet pills and who engage in self-induced vomiting.

The lifetime rate of comorbid psychiatric diagnoses among adolescents with AN is approximately 55%. Most commonly, these comorbidities include anxiety disorders (social anxiety, separation anxiety, generalized anxiety and obsessive compulsive disorder [OCD]), depression, and substance abuse. There is significant overlap in OCD symptoms and AN, thus careful consideration must be given to the content of obsessions and compulsions in diagnosis. In AN, obsessional preoccupations are related to eating, food, weight, and shape, and compulsions may appear as calorie counting, excessive exercise routines, and mealtime rituals. Depressive symptoms such as dysphoric thought, low energy, difficulty concentrating, and low self-esteem also manifest in AN and may not indicate a separate depressive disorder.

Epidemiology

Peak age of onset for AN is between 14 and 18 years. Lifetime prevalence of females with DSM-IV diagnosis of AN in the United States is between 1% and 2%, and DSM-V AN was estimated at .8% among adolescent females before age 20. The incidence of AN among males is less studied, and the previously estimated ratio of 1 male to every 10 female cases is now known to be a gross underestimate. Little is known about the prevalence of AN across racial and ethnic groups. A recent study did not reflect significantly higher rates of AN among non-Hispanic white adolescents as compared to Hispanic and non-Hispanic black peers; however, other evidence suggests that it is less common among persons of African origin.

AN has the highest mortality rate of any psychiatric illness, with reports as high as 5% per decade. Rates of chronicity obtained from long-term adult follow-up studies (AN diagnosis persisting greater than 5 years) are estimated between 7% and 15%. Death occurs most commonly secondary to medical complications of starvation or suicide. Prognosis for adolescents with short-duration (less than 3 years) is better than adults.

Etiology

The causal mechanisms of AN are multiply determined through the interface of biological/genetic, psychological, and sociocultural factors. Heritability estimates from twin studies range from 30% to 75%, and family aggregation studies report that AN occurs at about five times the expected rate in affected families. The interactional effect between genes and developmental processes is reflected in studies demonstrating greater heritability among 17-year-old twins as compared to 11-year-old twins. Hormonal changes during adolescence could mediate gene expression during puberty, explaining this difference.

Perfectionistic and avoidant personality features are associated with AN, and are likely heritable. Neurocognitive features including cognitive rigidity and an overly detailed style of information processing are common and may represent an endophenotype as those who are recovered as well as unaffected siblings who demonstrate similar cognitive styles. Common developmental challenges associated with adolescence may also precipitate or emerge as a consequence of AN—these include navigating issues of autonomy, self-efficacy, and intimacy. Sociocultural factors including exposure to a Westernized "thin ideal" of beauty for females and an overly muscular ideal for males may be internalized, thereby triggering extreme dieting or exercise. Further, activities where weight or appearance is intertwined with performance may also elevate risk (e.g., gymnastics, ballet, wrestling, figure skating).

Treatment

Given the severity of psychological, social, and health consequences of AN, both close medical monitoring and psychotherapy are the standard of care. In severe cases, inpatient medical monitoring may be required, and standard criteria for hospitalization are available for physicians. Findings from RCTs among adults are inconclusive because of dropout rates as high as 50%. Medication trials of antidepressants (serotonin reuptake inhibitors and tricyclics) have high dropout rates and little to no improvement in weight or eating disorder behaviors. Therefore, these should not be used independent of psychotherapy. CBT may help prevent relapse for individuals who are already weight-restored. For underweight individuals, findings are mixed, and nonspecific therapies such as nonspecific supportive clinical management (NSCM) showed better outcomes compared to IPT and CBT at end of treatment. However, improvements in NSCM appear to decline over time, and IPT may catch up to CBT.

Recent treatment studies have focused on improving retention. For example, an enhanced version of outpatient CBT (CBT-E), which employs motivational enhancement strategies, retained 64% of the original sample, improving on previous trends in attrition. Individuals completing treatment had clinically significant improvements in weight and eating disorder psychopathology. When CBT-E was compared to focal psychodynamic therapy and treatment as usual (TAU) in the community, weight gain and improvements in eating disorder symptoms were more rapid. However, focal psychodynamic treatment had the highest rates of recovery at follow-up (35%), though these were only significantly higher than the TAU group.

FBT, otherwise known as Maudsley family therapy, has been studied in six RCTs with superior outcome to other individual therapies. This outpatient treatment empowers parents to disrupt self-starvation and other behaviors that maintain AN. In the initial phase of treatment, parents take full control over managing eating-related behaviors. FBT demonstrates rates of remission ranging from 49% (full remission in weight and eating disorder thoughts and behaviors) to 89% for partial remission. Rates of relapse are about 10% and there is minimal dropout, suggesting it is acceptable to families.

AFT may be an alternative approach for individuals whose family members are unable to participate. The focus in AFT is on helping an adolescent move towards healthy individuation and increased self-efficacy. AN is conceptualized as an ineffective strategy that the adolescent has adopted in managing common developmental challenges. In AFT, adolescents learn new skills to support eating and weight gain and parents are involved in separated collateral sessions. CBT has also been studied in adolescents; when compared to TAU and hospitalization, it appeared to be the most cost-effective approach.

Avoidant-Restrictive Food Intake Disorder

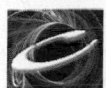

CURRENT DIAGNOSIS

- Disturbance in eating/feeding resulting in persistent failure to meet nutritional and/or energy needs.
- The disorder must result in one of the following consequences: significant weight loss or faltering growth; significant nutritional deficiency; dependence on nutritional supplements or enteral feeding; and interference with psychosocial functioning.
- The eating/feeding disturbance is not better explained by another medical or psychiatric condition or by cultural or religious practices.

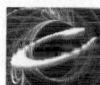

CURRENT TREATMENT

- There are no established treatments for this new diagnosis.
- CBT or family interventions that employ behavioral strategies are being explored as potential treatment options.

Diagnosis

Avoidant-restrictive food intake disorder (ARFID) is a new diagnosis included in the DSM-V, which reflects the recognition of "food neophobia" or extreme picky eating as challenges. Individuals with ARFID can be of any age and exhibit clinically significant feeding/eating difficulties, which result in failure to meet energy (caloric) or nutritional needs. In response, individuals have low weight or failure to meet expectations for growth, significant nutritional deficiency, a need for enteral feeding or oral nutritional supplementation, or impairment in psychosocial functioning. Although there may be failure to thrive or to make expected weight gain/weight loss, it is distinguished from AN by the absence of body image disturbance. Low weight can be determined through clinical judgment and examination of developmental trajectory using growth charts. Nutritional deficiency may be assessed through dietary history as well as physical examination. Related medical consequences may follow those seen in malnourished individuals with AN (e.g., bradycardia, anemia, hypothermia), and can be life threatening. If limited food intake is better explained by cultural or religious practice, an eating disorder in which there is disturbance in experience of shape/weight, or current physiologic or psychiatric condition, ARFID is not diagnosed. Further, in the event of a coexisting medical diagnosis, food refusal is serious enough to warrant separate clinical attention. Thorough assessment should include examination of feeding and eating history, psychiatric symptoms, development, and underlying medical causes must be ruled out before making a diagnosis.

Individuals with ARFID often exhibit selective eating, food neophobia, and hypersensitivity to sensory features of food (texture, taste, temperature, appearance). Similar clinical presentations may have varying etiology, requiring individualized treatment plans. In some, development of food avoidance can be traced to a specific aversive event, trauma, or related gastrointestinal problem, or may arise out of a choking, swallowing, or vomiting phobia. Individuals may also have a lack of drive or interest in eating or heightened textural sensitivity, which is common in autism spectrum disorders.

Epidemiology

No data exist on prevalence, course, and outcome of this disorder. Surveillance studies are underway in the UK and Canada for related "food avoidance emotional disorder," with overlap in clinical features. ARFID appears to arise most commonly in infancy and early childhood, but can occur at any age and last into adulthood. Preliminary data suggest ARFID occurs at equal rates in males and females. There is no evidence to guide for whom clinical intervention is warranted versus those whose symptoms resolve over time.

Treatment

There are no systematically studied treatments to date for ARFID; however, behavioral interventions with contingency management have been successfully utilized among children who have food neophobia in the context of a developmental disability. Given limited data, individualized treatment plans are best derived through assessment of medical history, temperament, psychiatric symptoms, and development. Food avoidance may be treated through use of behavioral strategies (e.g., shaping, chaining, contingency management, extinction) that systematically desensitize individuals to a wider range of foods. Related anxiety management techniques (relaxation training, visualization for mastery), and cognitive strategies derived from CBT may address maintaining psychiatric features. CBT was successfully applied in a case study of young adults with food neophobia. In most severe cases of malnutrition, hospitalization may be needed before outpatient therapy.

References

Bulik CM, Berkman ND, Brownley KA, et al. Anorexia nervosa treatment: A systematic review of randomized controlled trials. Int J Eat Disord 2007;40:310–20.
Call C, Walsh B, Attia E. From DSM-IV to DSM-5: Changes to eating disorder diagnoses. Curr Opin Psychiatry 2013;26:532–6.
Hay P. A systematic review of evidence for psychological treatments in eating disorders: 2005-2012. Int J Eat Disord 2013;46:462–9.
Kreipe R, Palomski A. Beyond picky eating: Avoidant/restrictive food intake disorder. Curr Psychiatry Rep 2012;14:421–31.
Le Grange D, Lock J, editors. Eating Disorders in Children and Adolescents: A Clinical Handbook. New York: The Guilford Press; 2011.
Peat C, Brownley K, Berkman N, et al. Binge eating disorder: Evidence-based treatments. Curr Psychiatry 2013;11:32–9.
Shapiro J, Berkman N, Brownley K, et al. Bulimia nervosa treatment: A systematic review of randomized controlled trials. Int J Eat Disord 2007;40:321–36.
Smink F, van Hoeken D, Hoek H. Epidemiology of eating disorders: Incidence, prevalence and mortality rates. Curr Psychiatry Rep 2012;14:406–14.
Steinhausen H, Weber S. The outcome of bulimia nervosa: Findings from one-quarter century of research. Am J Psychiatry 2009;166:1331–41.

MOOD DISORDERS: DEPRESSION, BIPOLAR DISEASE, AND MOOD DYSREGULATION

Method of
Andrei Novac, MD

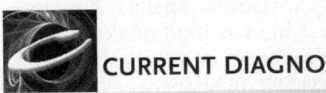

CURRENT DIAGNOSIS

- Clinical evaluation of mood disorders starts with a thorough psychosocial and medical history.
- Identify symptoms and patterns of the appearance of mood changes.
- Differentiate between unipolar and bipolar symptom patterns.
- Use collateral history, if possible.
- For recent-onset disorder, rule out new medical disorders. Always check thyroid function.

CURRENT THERAPY

- Any underlying medical conditions must be treated simultaneously.
- The mainstay of treatment for all mood disorders remains the combination of pharmacology and psychotherapy.
- Monitor frequently for suicidality.
- Allow for at least 2 to 4 weeks for response before a medication switch.
- Switch medication early in cases of intense side effects.
- Monitor for hypomanic switch on medications in undiagnosed bipolarity.

Mood disorders and mood dysregulation encompass a broad range of human experiences. They can be divided into three types of manifestations: (1) psychiatric disorders, which make up a major chapter in medical texts; (2) a variety of mood syndromes, often comorbid, less well classified, that coexist with medical and psychiatric disorders alike; (3) an aggregate of reactive transient behavioral manifestations outside the pathologic realm, inherent to human nature. Only the first two areas will be the focus of this chapter. Mood disorders and mood dysregulation are among the most common manifestations of human suffering. They are not mutually exclusive; dysregulation of mood may be present both as an independent symptom and as part of a mood disorder. They all deserve particular attention because they can gravely impact the level of functioning, compliance, treatment outcome, and quality of life.

Mood Disorders*

Both the *Diagnostic and Statistical Manual*, Fifth Edition (DSM-5) (2013), and the ICD-10 classify mood disorders into similar types. These include: major depressive disorders (unipolar, single episodes, and recurrent), persistent depressive disorder (dysthymia), bipolar I disorder, bipolar II disorder, cyclothymic disorder, mood disorder due to medical conditions, substance-induced mood disorders, and the "unspecified" unipolar and bipolar disorders. In addition, the DSM-5 has included new clinical entries, such as disruptive mood dysregulation disorder, persistent depressive disorder (dysthymia) with intermittent major depressive disorders and premenstrual dysphoric disorder. The previously entitled "not otherwise specified" syndromes are now called "unspecified mood disorders." New to the DSM-5 are the following *specifiers* that apply to *both* bipolar and unipolar disorders: (a) with anxious distress (a mixture of mood disorder and anxiety disorder); (b) with mixed features; (c) with melancholic features; (d) with atypical features; (e) with psychotic features; (f) with catatonia; (g) with peripartum onset; and (h) with seasonal pattern.

Epidemiology

Most recent data regarding prevalence comes from the National Comorbidity Survey, which has exposed in detail the rates of subtypes of mood disorders: unipolar, bipolar, and the subthreshold disorders. The lifetime prevalence of any mood disorder was found to be 21.4% (female 24.9%, male 17.5%), with major depression occurring at a lifetime prevalence of 16.9% (female 20.2%, male

---

*In this chapter, no DSM-5 or ICD-10 diagnostic codes are included. The clinician is advised to consult the DSM-5 for specific diagnostic codes.

13.2%) and 12-month prevalence of 6.8%. Persistent depressive disorder (dysthymia) occurs at a lifetime prevalence of 2.5% (female 3.1%, male 1.8%) and 12-month prevalence of 1.5%. The DSM-5 specifies the prevalence for dysthymia as being approximately 0.5% and for the chronic form of major depressive disorder, 1.5%. Bipolar disorders present with a lifetime prevalence of 4.4% (female 4.5%, male 4.3%). If broken down, bipolar I disorder occurs at a lifetime prevalence of 1.0%, and 0.6% of new cases over 12 months. Bipolar II disorder occurs at the prevalence of 1.1% and 0.8%, respectively. Subthreshold bipolar disorder is twice as common at 2.4% lifetime and 1.4% new cases over 12 months.

Risk Factors

For unipolar major depressive disorders, risk factors include: gender (women at greater risk), age (18–44 years of age at greater risk), marital status (separated and divorced at greater risk), family history (relatives with depression), early parental death, life events (negative stressful events, chronic exposure to stress), low confidence, and urban environments. For bipolar disorder, risk factors are similar. In addition, for bipolar disorder, higher rather than lower socioeconomic status and suburban environments have been cited as risk factors.

Individuals with anxiety disorder, chronic exposure to stress and trauma, substance abuse, psychotic disorders, and chronic medical conditions are all known to be at risk for mood disorders.

Depressive Disorder (Unipolar Mood Disorder)

Major Depression

The mainstay of major depressive disorder is a major depressive episode. The DSM-5 provides criteria according to a threshold of symptoms, yet all mood disorders have to be understood as lying on a continuum. Therefore, even individuals who do not meet all criteria have to be carefully followed, and in many cases preventive treatment is warranted.

At least five or more of the following symptoms during the same 2-week period are required: (1) depressed mood most of the day, nearly every day (sadness, feelings of emptiness, tearfulness); (2) marked diminished interest or pleasure in almost all activities; (3) significant weight loss or weight gain or fluctuations in appetite; (4) insomnia or hypersomnia; (5) psychomotor retardation or agitation nearly every day; (6) fatigue or loss of energy; (7) feelings of worthlessness and/or inappropriate guilt; (8) inability to concentrate, think, and make decisions; and (9) recurrent thoughts of death and/or suicidal ideations. These symptoms: (1) cause significant distress or impairment in social, occupational, and/or personal functions; and (2) are not due to a general medical condition. In the DSM-5, contrary to previous classifications, the bereavement and depression are not mutually exclusive. In fact, bereaved individuals can also develop major depression, which would warrant additional medical treatment (see Table 3.)

Following are some forms of manifestations:

- Major depressive disorder, single episode: Episodes may occur only one time in life or may occur again years later, usually triggered by major stressful events.
- Major depressive disorder, recurrent type: Episodes reoccur at shorter intervals. Often the distance between episodes shortens with advancement in age. The first few episodes are more likely to be triggered by stressful life events, while in time the condition becomes self-maintained and self-triggered.
- Depressive disorder with catatonic features (motoric immobility, catalepsy, stupor, extreme opposition, posturing, echolalia).
- Major depression occurring after giving birth may predict further depressive episodes years later. Postpartum depression has also been associated with bipolar disorder.

Depressive disorder can also take a chronic course. Some patients present with *melancholic features* (profound loss of pleasure, depression worse in the morning, early morning awakening, severe psychomotor retardation, severe anorexia and weight loss). Melancholia may be a predictor of relatively good response to medications. *Atypical depression* features are characterized by inverted functional shift (weight gain and increased appetite, craving for sweets, hypersomnia, leaden paralysis, long-standing interpersonal rejection sensitivity). Table 1 presents the subtypes (specifiers) of mood disorders according to the DSM-5. These subtypes are encountered both in unipolar and bipolar mood disorders. Under these new DSM-V classifications, conditions such as catatonia, seasonal affective disorders, and atypical depression may occur both in individuals with unipolar and bipolar disorders.

Persistent Depressive Disorder (Dysthymia)

Persistent depressive disorder, the new designation for dysthymic disorder, is a chronic form of depression in which the depressed mood has persisted for at least 2 years (in children for at least

TABLE 1 Subtypes of Mood Disorders (Specifiers) Common to Both Unipolar and Bipolar Mood Disorders

SUBTYPE WITH	PRESENTATION	FEATURES
Anxious distress (with elements of mood disorder and anxiety disorder)	During the majority of days of depressive, manic or hypomanic episode	Feeling keyed-up or tense, feeling restless, unable to concentrate, fear that something awful may happen, etc.
Mixed features	Meets criteria for either mania, hypomania, or depression	With mixed symptoms (if manic, there is associated dysphoria and depression), observable by others
Melancholic features	During the most severe period	Severe anhedonia, worse in the morning, early morning awakening, psychomotor retardation or agitation, weight loss or gain
Typical features	During majority of days of a major depressive episode	Inverted functional shift (hypersomnia, hyperphasia, weight gain), leaden paralysis, long-standing pattern of interpersonal rejection sensitivity
Psychotic features	The presence of delusions and/or hallucinations	- Mood-congruent psychosis (delusion/hallucinations include themes consistent with the type of mood [manic or depressed]) - (b) Mood-incongruent psychosis
Catatonia	The presence of catatonia	Catatonic features are present during most of depressive or manic episodes
Peripartum onset	Mania, hypomania, major depression in bipolar I or II disorders	During pregnancy or in the 4 weeks following delivery
Seasonal pattern	At least one type of episode (mania, hypomania or depression) within a seasonal pattern	Temporal relationship between an episode and a particular time of the year (fall or winter, in bipolar I or II)

1 year), as manifested by at least two of the following symptoms: (1) poor appetite or overeating; (2) insomnia or hypersomnia; (3) low energy or fatigue; (4) low self-esteem; (5) poor concentration or difficulty making decisions; (6) feelings of hopelessness. These manifestations are distinct from any major depressive episode, there have been no manic symptoms, and there is significant distress or impairment in social, occupational, or personal functioning. Dysthymia can occur in any age and can co-occur with major depressive disorder.

The following clinical forms have been identified: (1) with pure dysthymic syndrome: no full criteria of major depression have been met in the past 2 years; (2) with persistent major depressive episode: full criteria of a major depressive episode have been present in the past 2 years; (3) with intermittent major depressive episodes, with current episode: full criteria for major depressive episodes are currently met but there have been periods of at least 8 weeks in the last 2 years when major depression criteria have not been met; (4) with intermittent major depressive episodes, without current episode: no current major depression is identified (only symptoms of dysthymia) but there has been one or more major depressive episode in the past 2 years. Persistent depressive disorder may also qualify for any of the specifiers described in Table 1. (Note: Table 1 specifiers can apply to any of the unipolar and bipolar form of mood disorders.)

Disruptive Mood Dysregulation Disorder

This condition occurs in childhood or adolescence between the ages of 6 and 18. It is characterized by (1) severe recurrent temper outbursts manifested verbally (verbal rages) and/or behaviorally (physical aggression toward people or property) that are grossly out of proportion in intensity or duration to the situation or provocation; (2) temper outbursts that are inconsistent with developmental level; (3) temper outbursts that occur on average three or more times per week; (4) a mood between temper outbursts that is persistently irritable or angry most of the day, nearly every day, and is observable by others; (5) the above criteria, which have been present for 12 or more months (with no lapse in symptoms for a duration of 3 or more months); (6) an age of onset that is before 10. Diagnosis should not be made before age 6 or after 18.

Pre-menstrual Dysphoric Disorder

- The condition is characterized by the majority of menstrual cycles that include five symptoms. The following symptoms occur in the final week before the onset of menses and begin to improve within a few days after the onset of menses.
- One or more of the following symptoms must be present: (1) marked affective lability (mood swings; feeling suddenly sad or tearful; increased sensitivity to rejection); (2) marked irritability or anger or increased interpersonal conflict; (3) marked depressed mood, feelings of hopelessness or self-deprecating thoughts; (4) marked anxiety, tension, and/or feelings of being keyed-up or on edge.
- One or more of the following symptoms must be present to reach a total of five symptoms: decreased interest in usual activities; subjective difficulty in concentration; lethargy; easily fatigued; marked changes in appetite, overeating, specific food cravings; hypersomnia or insomnia; a sense of being overwhelmed or out of control; physical symptoms such as breast tenderness or swelling, joint or muscle pain, bloating or weight gain.

Substance/Medication Induced Depressive Disorder

This diagnosis is used when persistent disturbance in mood predominates the clinical picture and is characterized by depression and diminished interest or pleasure in activities. These symptoms occur during or soon after substance intoxication or withdrawal or after exposure to a medication. The substance in question has to be known to cause symptoms of depression.

Depressive Disorder Due to Another Medical Condition

This diagnosis is used when a depressive disorder is triggered by a medical condition (diagnosed by physical examination and laboratory findings) known to cause symptoms of depression. These may include disorder of the CNS, systemic disorders (Lupus, cancer), etc.

Other Specified Depressive Disorders

These are depressions that do not fully meet criteria of the above-described conditions. However, they may appear in one of the following forms:

- recurrent brief depression (symptoms of depression lasting from 2–13 days at least once per month) not associated with menstrual cycles;
- short duration depressive episode (lasting from 4–13 days), with at least four symptoms of major depressive episode associated with clinical distress and impaired functioning that persist but never meets criteria of major depression;
- depressive episode with insufficient symptoms (at least one of the symptoms of major depression associated with distress and impairment persisting for at least 2 weeks with no prior history of major depression).

These "other specified depressive disorders" are helpful to clinicians in refining the description of a clinical pattern exhibited by a particular patient.

Unspecified Depressive Disorder

Finally, the previously used designation of "not otherwise specified" now reads "unspecified depressive disorder" (when none of the criteria are fully met, yet the patient is suffering from a mood disorder).

Bipolar Mood Disorders
Manic Episode

A manic episode is characterized by a period of at least 1 week with abnormal and persistently elevated, expansive, or irritable mood. At least three of the following should be also present: (1) inflated self-esteem or grandiosity; (2) decreased need for sleep (yet still feeling rested); (3) more talkative than usual or inability to stop talking; (4) flight of ideas or racing thoughts; (5) distractibility; (6) increase in goal-oriented activities (socially, sexually) or psychomotor agitation; (7) excessive involvement in pleasurable activities with little regard for consequences (e.g., sexual indiscretions, unwise investments). These symptoms (1) result in marked impairment in most areas of life, and (2) are not due to substance abuse or general medical conditions.

Hypomania

A hypomanic episode is similar to, but less intense, than a manic episode. At least three symptoms from the same symptom cluster (inflated self-esteem, decreased need for sleep, excessive talking, racing thoughts, hyperactivity, increased involvement in pleasurable activities) are required, but the condition is not severe enough to cause marked impairment in social, occupational, and personal functioning, and it does not necessitate hospitalization. However, functional impairment is noticeable over time.

"Bipolar I" disorder requires only one full manic episode for the diagnosis. Usually, individuals with bipolar I disorder also have both manic and depressive episodes, but the depressions can range from severe and disabling to very brief and unnoticed. Therefore, a history of a depressive episode is not required for the diagnosis.

"Bipolar II" disorder is characterized by long periods of hypomania, with occasional major depressive episodes. Such individuals are usually not hospitalized for their hypomania and tend to function relatively well between depressive episodes. Hypomanic states are episodic and exhibit an unequivocal change in functioning that is uncharacteristic for the individual when not symptomatic. These changes are observable by others. Depressions tend to be severe and disabling. Bipolar II disorders do not include full manic episodes.

Mixed States and Rapid Cycling

The particular specifiers for bipolar disorder are mixed states and rapid cycling. "Mixed states" refers to manic or hypomanic episodes with at least three of the following depressive symptoms: prominent dysphoria or depressed mood, diminished interest in activities, psychomotor retardation, fatigue or loss of energy, feelings of worthlessness, recurrent thoughts of death. Often there is a rapid alternation between mania and depression (rapid cycling). Contingent upon severity, mixed states are usually accompanied by severe impairment. "Rapid cycling" refers to bipolar disorder that includes at least four episodes of illness per year. In addition, bipolar disorders may include any of the specifiers described in Table 1, under the section titled unipolar depression.

Cyclothymic Disorder

Cyclothymic disorder is a cycling mood disorder lasting for 2 years or more and is characterized by numerous periods with hypomanic symptoms and depressive symptoms that do not meet criteria for bipolar disorder or major depression. During a 2-year period (1 year in children and adolescents), hypomanic and depressive periods have been present for at least half the time, and the individual has not been without symptoms for more than 2 months at a time. Criteria for major depression, mania, or hypomanic episodes have never been met. However, in the long run, some patients may develop symptoms of bipolar affective disorder. These symptoms should not be attributable to the effect of a substance (drug abuse, medication) or another medical condition (hyperthyroidism, Cushing's disease, etc.). The condition is significantly impairing and includes psychological distress. Cyclothymia has the specifier (subtype) "cyclothymia with anxious distress." This condition comprises cyclothymia and features of anxious distress as outlined in Table 1. A variety of subclinical forms of subthreshold cyclothymia may be encountered in clinical practice. Such patients tend to develop overt symptoms of cyclothymia, or even bipolar disorder, when exposed to a variety of psychosocial stressors, substance abuse, and/or a variety of medications. Finally, Table 2 presents subtypes of bipolar disorder currently listed in the DSM-5 as: "Other specified bipolar and related disorders" and "unspecified bipolar and related disorder."

Specifiers for Bipolar and Related Disorders

Please refer to Table 1 for specifiers of depressive disorders that apply to bipolar disorders as well.

Diagnosis

When faced with symptoms of mood disorder, a clinician has to decide whether these are transient manifestations related to life circumstances or symptoms of treatable psychopathology. The clinical evaluation of patients with mood disorders starts with a thorough history of the present illness. A thorough medical history is paramount given the numerous medical disorders that present with depression or mania. Mood disorders are, in general, recurrent conditions. Past history will provide not only a suspicion toward a diagnosis, but also clues toward clinical manifestations, which, in the cases of depression and mania, are often similar to previous episodes. An early history of childhood behavioral problems can constitute a precursor of mood disorders. The Mental Status Examination provides further clues to the diagnosis. For depressive states, patients often exhibit psychomotor retardation; slow speech; constricted affect; and slow, observable mental activity. For mania and hypomania, the opposite can be observed. Patients show increased psychomotor activity, pressured speech, full or labile affect, and elevated mood. Often, they will appear unrealistically optimistic. In general, the diagnosis of mood disorder is aided significantly by obtaining a collateral history from friends or family members. The value of the Mental Status Examination is enhanced if the clinician knows the patient from before the mood disorder episode. A variety of psychological tests and depression rating scales exist, including the Beck Depression Inventory, the Hamilton Depression Rating Scale, and the Profile of Mood States (POMS) Depression Scale. While extremely useful in quantifying symptoms of depression, psychological testing is time-consuming and not necessary for the initial diagnosis of a mood disorder.

A thorough account of all symptoms present in a patient can point to treatment choice and outcome. Depression symptoms can be classified into at least three major groups:

- Emotional symptoms: sadness, dysphoria, emotional numbness
- Physical symptoms: low energy, sluggishness with difficulties in initiating activities, difficulties concentrating, sleep and appetite problems
- Cognitive (mental) symptoms: pessimism, loss of enthusiasm, hopelessness, thoughts of death

Not all three groups of symptoms are present from the beginning. In many individuals, the presence of cognitive symptoms may be a sign of chronicity. At other times, it may have been a premorbid feature or a constant presence between episodes. Cognitive symptoms tend to respond both to medication and psychotherapy (cognitive-behavioral techniques), and their monitoring is paramount to suicide prevention. If a mood disorder is secondary to a medical condition, the diagnosis will be made both by monitoring for mood symptoms and pathognomonic medical findings.

993

TABLE 2 Other Specified and Unspecified Bipolar Disorders

SUBTYPE	PRESENTATION	FEATURES
Substance/medication-induced bipolar and related disorder	Persistent disturbance of mood characterized by manic, hypomanic, with or without depressed mood, which occurs soon after substance intoxication or withdrawal or after administration of a medication	• Substance involved is capable of producing described mood symptoms • Does not occur in the course of delirium • There is significant stress or impairment
Bipolar and related disorder due to another medical condition	• Persistent period of abnormally elevated expansive or irritable mood • Evidence from history, physical examination, laboratory findings that disturbance is a direct pathophysiologic consequence of another medical condition	• With manic features • With manic or hypomanic-like episode • With mixed features (depression is also present)
Other specified bipolar and related disorder	Symptoms of bipolar disorder, but do not meet full criteria	• Short duration hypomanic episodes (2–3 days) and major depressive episodes • Hypomanic episodes with insufficient symptoms and major depressive episodes • Hypomanic episode without prior major depressive episode • Short duration cyclothymia (less than 24 mo)
Unspecified bipolar and related disorders	Patients with bipolar symptoms and clinical distress and impairment; however, the clinician chooses not to specify the reason that the criteria are not met	

Differential Diagnosis

Given the multitude of clinical manifestations, both a differential diagnosis between subtypes of mood disorders and mood and other psychiatric disorders is necessary. Table 3 presents comparisons and differences between subtypes of mood disorders and guidelines to the differential diagnoses.

Given the frequent overlap of anxiety and mood disorders, it is useful to inquire about the presence of anxiety disorder in a systematic manner. Anxiety disorder symptoms can also be classified into at least three major groups:

- Emotional symptoms: anxiety and/or fear, either fluctuating or in form of attacks
- Physical symptoms: palpitations, tachycardia, diaphoresis, sweaty palms, sensation of a knot in the throat, muscle tension, shortness of breath, GI symptoms, insomnia, etc.
- Cognitive symptoms: (a) intrusive thoughts (such as, "What if…," "I should have…," other specific exaggerated worries); (b) racing thoughts; (c) ruminative thoughts, etc.

Because of the long-term, chronic, egosyntonic nature of these symptoms, they are often not readily volunteered by the patient unless specifically asked about. Between mood disorders and anxiety disorders, there is a comorbidity of over 50% with generalized anxiety, panic disorders, and posttraumatic stress disorders constituting both a risk factor for and a possible complication of mood disorders. Please note that the DSM-5 allows for a specifier "with anxious distress" that can be applied to both unipolar and bipolar mood disorders. Depending on the primary diagnosis, the clinician may choose between adding this specifier or the comorbid separate diagnosis of "anxiety disorder" in addition to mood disorder.

Treatment

As a general rule, the treatment approach to mood disorders relies on the combination of psychopharmacology and psychotherapy. An accurate initial diagnosis directs the first choice of treatment. Close monitoring of treatment with frequent visits usually predicts better outcome. In general, response is considered to be a 50% reduction of symptoms, while remission refers usually to the absence or only minimal symptoms for 6 months or more. By Tohen and colleagues' opinion, relapse is considered a return of symptoms within 6 months, while recurrence is after 6 months of remission.

Treatment of Unipolar Depression (Major Depression and Dysthymia)

Given the fact that many depressive disorders occur along a spectrum, the treatment of major depression and dysthymia will be covered together.**

Psychopharmacology

First, a thorough medical work-up should be performed in any new case of mood disorder. The NIH-sponsored STAR*D study (Sequenced Treatment Alternatives to Relieve Depression) recommends the initial choice of an SSRI (citalopram [Celexa]). In the study, nonresponders were then switched to sertraline (Zoloft) and/or venlafaxine XR (Effexor XR). In clinical practice, other factors have to be weighed when choosing the first antidepressant. Prior response history to a specific antidepressant or to an overall treatment modality should take precedence in the first choice of treatment. If such a history is unavailable, any family history of response to a specific treatment should be considered. Response to treatment seems to be similar among blood relatives. Table 4 includes a list of the more common medications used in clinical

---

**The newly introduced DSM-5 diagnosis, Disruptive Mood Dysregulation Disorder, is a condition of childhood and adolescence. Prior to the publication of the DSM-5, many of these patients were diagnosed as bipolar. Many clinicians prefer to initiate treatment with psychotherapy, which includes addressing a variety of family issues, before initiating psychopharmacological intervention. Premenstrual Dysphoric Disorder, also newly introduced in the DSM-5, is treated, depending upon the intensity of symptoms, by using protocols similar to those utilized in the treatment of dysthymic and/or cyclothymic disorders.

---

practice for the treatment of unipolar and bipolar disorder. Given the possibility of manic switch with antidepressants, it is recommended that in bipolar depression, mood stabilizers be started concomitantly with antidepressants.

Although a myriad of side effects are known to exist for each medication, all selective serotonin reuptake inhibitors (SSRIs) and serotonin norepinephrine reuptake inhibitors (SNRIs) are generally well tolerated. Any trial of medications should be continued for 4 to 6 weeks before failure is declared. However, clinical judgment in assessing each circumstance, especially regarding suicide risk, is crucial. Often in the initial phase of response, the physical symptom of low energy remits first while cognitive symptoms of depression (persistent thoughts of death) persist. The coexistence of higher energy and thoughts of death may constitute a temporary suicide risk in the initial phase of antidepressant treatment. Currently, biological markers for the prediction of treatment response and side effects are being considered. Reference EEG (rEEG), renamed Psychiatric EEG Evaluation Registry (PEER), compares variations of normal awake EEG readings with a large database of medication responders. Results are available for antidepressants, mood stabilizers, stimulants, second-generation antipsychotics, etc. The AmpliChip CYP450 Test is a method that predicts side effects by measuring the activity of genes that control the P450 hepatic enzyme system and implicitly the ability to metabolize a specific drug. Both methods are promising, but high cost has so far prevented general use.

Given the risk of suicide, close monitoring during treatment of major depression is required. The choice of medication and adjustment has to be tailored according to the most dominant initial presentation. For patients with severe insomnia, an SSRI is indicated. If the initial choice (e.g., citalopram [Celexa], escitalopram [Lexapro], or sertraline [Zoloft]) shows little impact in improving sleep, the temporary addition of a sleep aid is a reasonable choice. Alternatively, some clinicians prefer to avoid hypnotics, which may allow close monitoring of the natural improvement in sleep during the first 2 weeks of SSRI treatment. This in turn may predict a good response. For many years, in patients with hypersomnia and hyperphagia—a variant known as "atypical depression"—the first choice was a monoamine oxidase inhibitor (MAOI). Currently, for atypical depression, clinicians prefer as a first choice a norepinephrine/serotonin reuptake inhibitor (venlafaxine [Effexor], desvenlafaxine [Pristiq]), or a norepinephrine/dopamine active medication (bupropion [Wellbutrin]). Response to medications is often difficult to predict. Again, early in treatment, a thorough medical work-up, which should always include a thyroid panel, should be the norm. Sometimes switches to other classes of antidepressants (dopamine enhancers, tricyclics) are necessary before a result is obtained. Pharmacologic augmentation with mood stabilizers, neuroleptics, and thyroid hormone has been used in cases of treatment-resistant depression. In cases where severe anxiety, insomnia, and poor appetite dominate the picture, the early addition of a second-generation neuroleptic (olanzapine [Zyprexa], quetiapine [Seroquel], risperidone [Risperdal],[1] and aripiprazole [Abilify]) is recommended. Medication resistance (after several failed trials) dictates the reassessment of diagnosis to further rule out psychiatric and medical comorbidity. For medication-resistant mood disorders, Table 5 presents a list of further biological treatments. Some of these treatments are promising, but have yet to be included as routine choices in some of the most difficult-to-treat patients.

Psychotherapy

For mood disorders, cognitive-behavioral and interpersonal psychotherapy have been considered therapies of choice. The former directly addresses the negative, pessimistic bias of the depressive thinking, which is a maintenance factor of depressed mood. The latter addresses social and interpersonal functioning by enhancing coping abilities. Their popularity has been increasing; however, they require special training and supervision. In clinical practice, though, the most readily available therapies remain supportive and insight-

---

[1]Not FDA approved for this indication.

TABLE 3 Guidelines to the Differential Diagnoses

DIAGNOSIS	SIMILARITIES	DIFFERENTIATING DETAILS	CLINICAL CLUES	TREATMENT RESPONSE
Major depression (MDD) versus persistent depressive disorder (dysthymia) (PDD)	Depressed mood; depressive cognition (pessimism); vegetative symptoms (physical)	MDD: Acute or subacute onset; possible recent life stressors; often more numerous symptoms PDD: May overlap with MDD; chronic, fluctuating course	MDD: Usually a marked drop in functionality PDD: Significant chronic impairment; often symptoms are ego-syntonic; "personality disorder" flavor	MDD: Antidepressants and/or initial antianxiety medications; consider psychotherapy PDD: Cognitive-behavioral psychotherapy; antidepressants (often long term); sometimes enhancement pharmacology
Mixed mania versus agitated depression	Psychomotor agitation; dysphoria; mood swings	Mixed mania: Labile affect; often rapid switch with brief euphoric states Agitated depression: No euphoric states; severe anxiety, including sympathetic symptoms	Mixed mania: Personal and family history Agitated depression: Anxiety symptoms, often subtle, precede depressive symptoms	Mixed mania: Mood stabilizers; caution regarding antidepressants: can cause worsening Agitated depression: Antidepressants and sedating mood stabilizers; avoid long-term tranquilizers
Mania versus cyclothymia	Intermittent states of high energy and euphoria with or without recurrent depression	Mania: Distinct states of high energy; depression is sometimes unnoticed Cyclothymia: Distinct cycling from depression to hypomania	Mania: More often severe insomnia without fatigue; severity of mania and insomnia directly related Cyclothymia: May take unpredictable forms; fluctuation of mood and sleep	Mania: Mood stabilizers; caution about antidepressants; atypical antipsychotics if needed Cyclothymia: Same as above, according to clinical judgment
Substance abuse disorder versus cyclothymia	Intermittent use of stimulant abuse may mimic cycling mood disorder; may coexist	Substance abuse: Substance abuse tends to escalate Cyclothymia: Cyclothymia may remain constant for years (even lifelong)	Substance abuse: Look for specific syndromes; drug screen Cyclothymia: Negative drug screens; no withdrawals; no drug culture history	Substance abuse: Rehabilitation; treat underlying psychiatric symptoms Cyclothymia: Mood stabilizers and/or antidepressants and/or atypical antipsychotics
Personality disorder versus mood disorder	More often overlap; requires concomitant treatment	Personality disorder: Long-term pervasive history since adolescence Mood disorder: More often episodic	Personality disorder: Borderline personality disorder includes mood lability/depressive episodes; often narcissistic personality, includes grandiose/hypomanic states Mood disorder: More often symptoms are egodystonic	Personality disorder: Acute decompensation; long-term psychotherapy; mood stabilizers; atypical antipsychotics Mood disorder: See treatment of mood disorders
Bereavement versus MDD	May overlap; attention to recent major loss; sometimes similar picture; bereavement and MDD may co-occur	Bereavement: Tends to improve over time MDD: Tends to worsen over time	Bereavement: Preoccupation with loss persists MDD: Duration of average major depressive episode is 9 mo	Bereavement: Social support; grief counseling; psychotherapy; if MDD present, treat as MDD MDD: See treatment of MDD
Primary mood disorder versus mood disorder arising from medical condition	Clinical picture may be identical	Primary mood disorder: May be triggered by external stressful events Medical condition: Often onset is insidious; sometimes precedes medical condition	Neurological, endocrine, infectious, systemic, and blood disorders*	Treat both primary medical condition and mood disorder; treatment same as for primary mood disorder

*Medical conditions complicated by mood disorders: Addison's disease, AIDS, anemia, brain tumors, chronic pain, complex partial seizures, Cushing's disease, CVA, dementia, diabetes mellitus, encephalitis, head trauma, hepatitis, hyperparathyroidism, hyperthyroidism, hypopituitarism, hypothyroidism, infectious mononucleosis, influenza, lupus erythematosus disseminatus, meningitis, multiple sclerosis, pneumonia, porphyria, rheumatoid arthritis, scleroderma, sleep apnea, toxoplasmosis, and others.

TABLE 4 Medications Used for the Treatment of Unipolar and Bipolar Depression

MEDICATION GROUP	MEDICATION	USUAL DAILY DOSE	CAUTIONS
SSRI	Fluoxetine (Prozac) Sertraline (Zoloft) Paroxetine (Paxil) Citalopram (Celexa) Escitalopram (Lexapro) Fluvoxamine (Luvox)[1]	10–80 mg 25–200 mg 5–60 mg 10–40 mg 5–20 mg 100–300 mg	All can cause sedation, agitation, insomnia, GI side effects, sexual dysfunction
SSRIs with combined action	Vilazodone (Viibryd) Functions of SSRI and a 5-HT_{1A} Receptor Agonist Vortioxetine (Brintellix) Functions of SSRI and multiple Serotonin Receptor Agonists and Antagonist	10–40 mg 5–20 mg	Same as above
NSRI	Venlafaxine XR (Effexor XR) Desvenlafaxine (Pristiq) Levomilnacipran ER (Fetzima)	37.5–225 mg 50–100 mg 40–120 mg	Insomnia, sedation, possible HTN Mydrasis, urinary hesitation
Dopamine/norepinephrine agonist	Bupropion SR, XL (Wellbutrin SR, XL)	100–450 mg	Agitation, GI side effects, possible HTN
Stimulants (usually used to enhance effects of other antidepressants)	Methylphenidate (Ritalin)[1] Dextroamphetamine (Dexedrine)[1] Amphetamine/dextroamphetamine mixed (Adderall)[1]	10–60 mg 5–60 mg 5–60 mg	Agitation, insomnia, psychosis, HTN, seizures
Second-generation neuroleptics	Olanzapine (Zyprexa) Quetiapine (Seroquel) Aripiprazole (Abilify) Risperidone (Risperdal)[1]	2.5–20 mg (in unipolar depression, olanzapine 5 mg, plus fluoxetine 20 mg [Symbyax]) 50–300 mg (up to 800 mg in bipolar disorder) 2–30 mg 0.5–6 mg	Metabolic syndrome, sedation Over-sedation, metabolic syndrome, cardiovascular complications in elderly Oversedation, metabolic syndrome, hyperprolactinemia
Tricyclic antidepressants	Amitriptyline (Elavil) Imipramine (Tofranil) Doxepin (Sinequan) Desipramine (Norpramin) Nortriptyline (Pamelor) Maprotiline (Ludiomil) Protriptyline (Vivactil)	50–300 mg 50–300 mg 50–300 mg 50–300 mg 20–200 mg[3] 100–225 mg 20–60 mg	All can cause anticholinergic effects, sedation; occasional agitation, weight gain
Mixed action (presynaptic and postsynaptic, multiple neurotransmitter action)	Mirtazapine (Remeron) Trazodone (Desyrel) Clomipramine (Anafranil)[1]	15–30 mg 150–600 mg 50–300 mg[3]	Sedation, weight gain
MAOI (Dietary restrictions are obligatory)	Phenelzine (Nardil) Tranylcypromine (Parnate)	15–90 mg 30–60 mg	Hypertensive crisis, occasional sedation/activation
Mood stabilizers	Lithium Carbonate/Citrate/ER[1] Valproate (Valproic Acid, Depakote ER)[1] Lamotrigine (Lamictal)/ER[1] Carbamazepine (Tegretol)[1]	600–1800 mg (attaining blood level from 0.6–1.2 mEq/L) 250–1500 mg (attaining blood level from 50–100 mcg/ml) 50–300 mg 200–1000 mg (attaining blood level from 5–12 mdg/mL)	Signs of toxicity: tremor, nausea, vomiting, staggering gait; monitor kidney and thyroid function Oversedation, GI side effects, may affect blood levels of other medications, weight gain A variety of severe skin rashes, Stevens-Johnson syndrome Monitor blood count for aplastic anemia/agranulocytosis, possible Stevens-Johnson syndrome, sedation

[1]Not FDA approved for this indication.
[3]Exceeds dosage recommended by the manufacturer.
Abbreviations: ER = extended release; GI = gastrointestinal; HTN = hypertension; MAOI = monoamine oxidase inhibitor; SSRI = selective serotonin reuptake inhibitor.

TABLE 5 Biological Treatments for Medication-Resistant Mood Disorders

TYPE OF INTERVENTION	REPORTED RESPONSE	CURRENT AVAILABILITY
Electroconvulsive therapy (ECT)	50.9%–53.2% remission rate	Common
Transcranial magnetic stimulation (TMS)	41.5%–56.4% response rate, 26.5%–28.7% remission rate	Rare
Vagal nerve stimulation (VNS)	53% response rate, 33% remission after 1 year	Rare (neurosurgical)
Deep brain stimulation (DBS)	29% response rate at 1 year	Rare (neurosurgical)
Ketamine (Ketalar) infusion[1]	79% response rate	Very rare (only in selective institutions)
Anterior cingulotomy	33.3% response rate, after 30 mo	Very rare (only in selective institutions, neurosurgical)

[1]Not FDA approved for this indication.

oriented psychotherapy. They too complement the effect of pharmacology. Brain imaging studies have revealed that the activity of the subgenual anterior cingulate cortex (Brodmann area 25) predicts the outcome of response to cognitive-behavioral psychotherapy in depression. As a general rule, therapies should have specific goals that need to be discussed with patients at onset of treatment. This needs to be part of an overall "informed consent" approach to treatment. Given the availability of a variety of clinicians with different levels of expertise that provide psychotherapy, it is important to monitor results and coordinate care. If "split" treatment (pharmacology and psychotherapy provided by different clinicians) is chosen, communication between parties of the treatment team remains a crucial requirement for rapid response and recovery. Other therapeutic measures, such as an increase in physical activity, normalization of sleep, and improvement of social support, are particularly important in promoting recovery.

Treatment of Bipolar Disorders (Bipolar Type-I, Type-II, Mixed Type, and Cyclothymia)

The treatment of bipolar disorder has been well refined over the years by a large body of literature. For acute mania, the treatment with mood stabilizers and/or antipsychotics has remained the main approach for the past several decades. Severe forms of mania and psychosis usually require hospitalization. Table 6 indicates intervention options for different phases of bipolar disorder.

As indicated in the table, some of the medication choices overlap between different clinical presentations. For chronic forms of bipolarity, such as mixed bipolar and cyclothymic disorder, a variety of new approaches has been developed, including social rhythm therapy. The latter includes monitoring and optimization of social interactions, sleep, and circadian rhythms that seem to

benefit bipolar patients. Chronic bipolarity, with its significant impairment and suicide risk, remains a major problem, often requiring multidisciplinary consultations and referral to a tertiary institution. In treatment-resistant cases, employment of electroconvulsive therapy and other novel biological approaches can be lifesaving. Even with partial treatment response, maintenance is paramount. Lifelong maintenance treatment is likely to prevent suicide and further functional deterioration. More recently, suicide prevention both in chronic mood disorders and/or personality disorders has been reported with maintenance treatment of lithium carbonate and clozapine (Clozaril).[1]

Mood Dysregulation

Mood dysregulation is a broad phenomenon encountered both in clinical and nonclinical settings. For clinicians, a variety of difficult-to-classify syndromes remain relevant (referred to here as "mood syndrome variants"). These mood syndrome variants present anecdotal but clinically pertinent manifestations collected from the medical literature of the past century. Psychiatric and medical disorders often coexist with different degrees of mood dysregulation. A more detailed description of each clinical entity in Table 7 is beyond the scope of this chapter. As seen from the table, different forms of mood dysregulation can occur both within and outside DSM diagnoses. For instance, atypical depression has been included in the DSM whereas other syndromes, such as neurasthenia, remain unclassified. When encountered, any of the listed syndromes should raise suspicion of an underlying mood disorder. A diagnosis of "unspecified depressive disorder" (311) can be made, and the entire mood disorder treatment armamentarium should be considered.

Clinical Course and Prognosis of Mood Disorders

Given the heterogeneity of mood disorders, there is great variation in clinical outcome. Clinical course and outcome depend on whether treatment was available, whether an individual is sensitive or resistant to the treatment, and the degree of compliance. Many individuals with mild and subsyndromal disorders remain undiagnosed, whereas others with severe forms of mood disorders refuse treatment. As a general rule, most untreated mood disorders tend to become chronic. Episodic disorders, such as bipolar I and II and depression, recurrent type, may show more frequent recurrences with advancement in age. Other patients with hyposymptomatic presentations and infrequent episodes may show long-term remissions. Such remissions are favored by stable, low-stress lifestyles. Table 8 demonstrates the severe impact on life expectancy of bipolar disorder. Mortality comes from suicide, cardiovascular disease, and respiratory disorders. However, treatment can at least partially reverse these trends.

---

[1]Not FDA approved for this indication.

TABLE 6	Intervention Options for Phases of Bipolar Disorder
PHASE OF DISORDER	**INTERVENTIONS**
Acute	Hospitalization if necessary Antipsychotics, tranquilization, start mood stabilizers
Subacute	Antipsychotics/neuroleptics, mood stabilizers If already medicated, adjust dose
Rapid cycling/mixed	As in acute phase; check thyroid; medical work-up Rule out substance abuse May require treatment indefinitely
Cyclothymia	Mood stabilizers, long-term, with or without antidepressants based on history Close initial monitoring May need treatment indefinitely

---

TABLE 7	Examples of Mood Syndrome Variants (MSV) with Different Degrees of Mood Dysregulation as Encountered in the Literature over the Past Century

I MSV WITH MANIFESTATIONS OF OTHER PSYCHIATRIC DISORDERS	**II MSV WITH UNUSUAL SYMPTOMS (MASKED DEPRESSION)**	**III MSV AS PART OF OTHER CONDITIONS**
Atypical depression	Mood dysregulation and thrill-seeking behavior (gambling, racing, substance abuse, hypersexuality)	Postpartum depression
Subaffective dysthymia		Depression secondary to chronic pain
Hysteroid dysphoria	Reactive overeating	Substance- and medication-induced mood dysregulation*
Pseudodementia	Isolated sleep disturbance and mood dysregulation	"Organic" mood disorders (due to CNS disorders)
Pseudoborderline	Atypical facial pain	Vicarious traumatization†
Somatic depression	Dysphagia	
Underground depression	Monosymptomatic hypochondriasis	
Neurasthenia	Monosymptomatic delusions	
Mood syndrome as part of personality disorders		
Mood syndromes and depression in schizophrenia		

Source: Novac and Djenderedjian, unpublished data.

*Medications more often associated with depression are, among others are: Reserpine, alpha-methyldopa (Aldomet), some alpha- and beta-blockers, sedative hypnotics, cimetidine (Tagamet), indomethacin (Indocin), anticancer medications, oral contraceptives, and corticosteroids.
†It has been described as a form of secondary trauma in mental health professionals who treat victims of trauma.

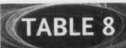

TABLE 8 Causes of Mortality in Patients with Bipolar Disease: Index Group Compared to the General Population

CAUSE OF DEATH	OBSERVED DEATHS (% STUDY GROUP)	EXPECTED DEATHS (% REGISTRAR GENERAL'S* FIGURES)	MORTALITY RATIO (ACTUAL STUDY)
Suicide	15.7	0.67	23.4
Cardiovascular system	42.1	14	3.0
Respiratory system	33.3	1.08	30.8

Data from Sharma and Markar (1994).
*Edinburgh Registrar General's Office.

Prevention

Primary prevention of mood disorders requires a concerted effort to educate the public and policymakers for funding of prevention. "Depression Awareness Week" and other community efforts enhance awareness and decrease stigma. Primary prevention may also include the promotion of general health and healthy work environments and addressing of major social problems, including the avoidance of early trauma and family problems as well as prevention of excessive stress and trauma in adults. These are all known to be associated with mental illness. Populations at risk need to be identified in primary care settings. Secondary prevention requires availability of mental health services, including early detection, education about the need for adequate treatment, and continuity of care to prevent impairment. Tertiary prevention would include continuation of treatment to prevent comorbidity of other psychiatric disorders and catastrophic complications, including suicide. Finally, in the case of mood disorders, quaternary prevention would include long-term follow-up, monitoring of recurrences, and medical comorbidity (accidents, cardiovascular, respiratory, and other medical conditions), to avoid the overburdening of the health system.

The high medical comorbidity rate recently found among patients with mood disorders varies by medical diagnosis and socioeconomic background. Chronic pain, neurological conditions, gastrointestinal, cardiovascular disorders and the metabolic syndrome are the most common medical conditions associated with mood disorders. Except for thyroid disorders, the seriousness of the comorbid condition seems to be even higher among lower socioeconomic patients. This poses a significant medical and socioeconomic burden of untreated mood disorders.

References

American Psychiatric Association. Diagnostic and Statistical Manual of Mental Disorders (DSM-5). 5th ed. Washington, DC: American Psychiatric Publishing; 2013.

Connolly KR, Thase ME. If at first you don't succeed: A review of the evidence for antidepressant augmentation, combination and switching strategies. Drugs 2011;71:43–64. http://dx.doi.org/10.2165/11587620-000000000-00000.

Dobson KS, Dozois DJA, editors. Risk Factors in Depression. San Diego, California: Academic Press (Elsevier); 2008.

Frank E, Kupfer DJ, Thase ME, et al. Two-year outcomes for interpersonal and social rhythm therapy in individuals with bipolar I disorder. Arch Gen Psychiatry 2005;62:996.

Lamers F, van Oppen P, Comijs HC, et al. Comorbidity patterns of anxiety and depressive disorders in a large cohort study: The Netherlands Study of Depression and Anxiety (NESDA). J Clin Psychiatry 2011;72:341–8. http://dx.doi.org/10.4088/JCP.10m06176blu.

Merikangas KR, Akiskal HS, Angst J, et al. Lifetime and 12-month prevalence of bipolar spectrum disorder in the national comorbidity survey replication. Arch Gen Psychiatry 2007;64:543–52. http://dx.doi.org/10.1001/archpsyc.64.5.543.

National Comorbidity Survey-Replication, Appendix Tables: Table 1 and 2. http://www.hcp.med.harvard.edu/ncs/publications.php; 2011 (accessed 13.08.13).

Sachs GS, Dupuy JM, Wittmann CW. The pharmacologic treatment of bipolar disorder. J Clin Psychiatry 2011;72:704–15.

Sharma R, Markar HR. Mortality in affective disorder. J Affect Disord 1994;31:91–6.

Siegle GJ, Thompson WK, Collier A, et al. Toward clinically useful neuroimaging in depression treatment: Prognostic utility of subgenual cingulate activity for determining depression outcome in cognitive therapy across studies, scanners, and patient characteristics. Arch Gen Psychiatry 2012;69:913–24. http://dx.doi.org/10.1001/archgenpsychiatry.2012.65.

Smith D, Court H, McLean G, Martin D, Langan Martin J, Guthrie B, et al. Depression and multimorbidity in psychiatry and primary care. J Clin Psychiatry 2014;75 (11):1202–8.

Tohen M, Frank E, Bowden CL, et al. The International Society for Bipolar Disorders (ISBD) Task Force report on the nomenclature of course and outcome in bipolar disorders. Bipolar Disord 2009;11:453–73.

Weissman M. The psychological treatment of depression. Arch Gen Psychiatry 1979;36:1261–9.

PANIC DISORDER

Method of
Cheryl Wehler, MD

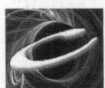

CURRENT DIAGNOSIS

- Panic disorder (PD) is characterized by the presence of multiple untriggered panic attacks.
- These unexpected panic attacks are associated with significant anticipatory anxiety and/or changes in behavior to minimize the consequences or avoid another panic attack.
  - Patients worry about being negatively judged due to visible panic symptoms.
  - Patients worry about dying or "going crazy."
- The panic attacks are not attributable to another medical condition or to the effects of a substance (medication or drug of abuse).
- The panic attacks are not better explained by another mental disorder.
- Patients frequently present with concern about somatic symptoms (e.g., fear of heart attack because of shortness of breath and chest discomfort).
- Assess patients for suicidality, as suicide risk increases with panic attacks or recent diagnosis of panic disorder.

CURRENT THERAPY

- Pharmacology and psychotherapy are effective treatments for PD.
- Selective serotonin reuptake inhibitors (SSRIs), serotonin norepinephrine reuptake inhibitors (SNRIs), tricyclic antidepressants (TCAs), and benzodiazepines have demonstrated efficacy for the treatment of PD.
- The favorable safety profile of SSRIs and SNRIs make them first-line monotherapy agents.
- While TCAs are effective, their side effects and greater toxicity in overdose limit their clinical utility.
- Monoamine oxidase inhibitors (MAOIs) also appear effective but are reserved for patients who are nonresponders to multiple first-line treatments because of their safety profile limitations.
- Benzodiazepines are not first-line monotherapy but are useful adjuncts to antidepressants if residual anxiety requires additional treatment.
- While the more rapid response of benzodiazepines (compared with SSRIs/SNRIs) make them attractive, the inevitable physiological dependence make them less so.
- Patients with PD can be sensitive to medication side effects; therefore, the adage "start low and go slow" is applicable to dosing.
- Cognitive behavioral therapy (CBT) or CBT with medications are first-line treatments for children and adults with PD.

Epidemiology

The 12-month prevalence estimate for panic disorder (PD) in the general population of the United States and Europe is approximately 2% to 3% in adults and adolescents. Non-Latino Caucasians and Native Americans have significantly higher rates than Latinos, African Americans, and Asian Americans. Adolescent and adult females are approximately twice as likely as males to be affected (although the clinical features of PD do not differ between males and females).

The prevalence is highest in adult females. Prevalence rates decline in older individuals. The overall prevalence of PD is low in children (<14 years). PD is associated with the highest number of medical visits among all anxiety disorders.

Risk Factors

Risks factors for PD include a disposition to negativity, experience of childhood physical and sexual abuse, and family history, indicating genetic vulnerability. Respiratory disorders such as asthma are associated with panic disorder. Smoking is a risk factor for panic attacks and PD. PD is associated with social and occupational/physical disability and high economic cost. PD may be comorbid with a variety of other psychiatric diagnoses, such as depression, bipolar affective disorder, and other anxiety disorders.

Diagnosis

PD is defined by the *Diagnostic and Statistical Manual of Mental Disorders*, fifth edition (DSM-V) as recurrent unexpected panic attacks followed by at least 1 month of anticipatory anxiety about having another attack, and/or a significant change in behavior to avoid another panic attack. A panic attack, the core feature of panic disorder, is an abrupt surge of intense fear/anxiety with concurrent physical and cognitive symptoms (Box 1). To be diagnosed as having PD, a patient must have more than one panic attack that is not the result of an obvious trigger or cue. The best example might be a nocturnal panic attack in which the individual is waking from sleep, with no external cues, in a state of intense fear (panic) and experiencing physical and cognitive symptoms. Expected panic attacks, that is, those for which there is an obvious cue or trigger, also occur in patients with PD. In the United States and Europe, approximately half of individuals with PD experience expected panic attacks as well as unexpected panic attacks. The presence of expected panic attacks does not rule out the diagnosis but is insufficient to make the diagnosis of this disorder.

A thorough diagnostic evaluation, including a complete history and thorough physical examination, is necessary to rule out medical or substance-induced panic attacks and establish the diagnosis of PD. Atypical symptoms or features of a panic attack may be suggestive of a medical illness or pharmacologic substance as the precipitant. A work-up that includes laboratory tests such as complete blood cell count, complete chemistry panel (including calcium level), thyroid-stimulating hormone (TSH) level, and urine drug screen may be helpful in determining a medical or substance-related cause. These tests may be followed by a chest radiograph, an electrocardiogram, and cardiac enzymes, as warranted. If the clinical examination or history is suggestive, a Holter monitor, EEG, CT scan, or urine catecholamine assay may be performed.

Box 1 | DSM-V Criteria for Panic Disorder

- Recurrent unexpected panic attacks. A panic attack is an abrupt surge of intense fear or intense discomfort that reaches a peak within minutes, and during which time four (or more) of the following symptoms occur:
  Note: The abrupt surge can occur from a calm state or an anxious state.
  - Palpitations, pounding heart, or accelerated heart rate
  - Sweating
  - Trembling or shaking
  - Sensations of shortness of breath or smothering
  - Feelings of choking
  - Chest pain or discomfort
  - Nausea or abdominal distress
  - Feeling dizzy, light-headed, faint, or unsteady
  - Chills or heat sensations
  - Parenthesis (numbness or tingling sensations)
  - Depersonalization (being detached from oneself) or derealization (feelings of unreality)
  - Fear of "going crazy" or losing control
  - Fear of dying
  Note: Culture-specific symptoms (e.g., tinnitus, neck soreness, headache, uncontrollable screaming or crying) may be seen. Such symptoms should not count as one of the four required symptoms [to diagnose PD].
- At least one of the attacks has been followed by 1 month (or more) of one or both of the following:
  - Persistent concern or worry about additional panic attacks or their consequences (e.g., losing control, having a heart attack, "going crazy")
  - A significant maladaptive change in behavior related to the attacks (e.g., behaviors designed to avoid having panic attacks, such as avoidance of exercise or unfamiliar situations)
- The disturbance is not attributable to the physiological effects of a substance (e.g., a drug of abuse, a medication) or another medical condition (e.g., hyperthyroidism, cardiopulmonary disorders)
- The disturbance is not better explained by another mental disorder (e.g., the panic attacks do not occur only in response to feared social situations, as in social anxiety disorder; in response to circumscribed phobic objects or situations, as in specific phobia; in response to obsessions, as in obsessive-compulsive disorder; in response to reminders of traumatic events, as in posttraumatic stress disorder; or in response to separation from attachment figures, as in separation anxiety disorder)

Clinical Manifestations

In the United States, the median age of onset for PD is 20 to 24 years. PD is rare in childhood but occurs in adolescents; their symptoms are similar to those in adults. Onset after age 45 is unusual. If untreated, the usual course is chronic, and attacks may wax and wane. Some individuals have a chronic course complicated by frequent attacks while others have rare episodic symptoms. A minority of individuals have full remission. Caffeine and several other substances can provoke a panic attack.

The severity and frequency of panic attacks vary widely. Individuals who have infrequent panic attacks resemble individuals with more frequent panic attacks with regard to symptoms, demographics, and family history. To be diagnosed with PD, an individual must have more than one full-symptom attack with more than four of the symptoms listed in Box 1. Individuals may, however, have limited-symptom attacks with fewer than four symptoms.

There are three symptomatic facets of PD: acute panic, anticipatory anxiety, and phobic avoidance. Phobic avoidance often includes restricting daily activities to minimize or avoid panic attacks. Panic disorder is associated with other psychopathology, such as other anxiety disorders, particularly agoraphobia.

While medical illness can precipitate a panic attack, individuals with anxiety, particularly PD, may be hypervigilant and misinterpret mild physical symptoms as harbingers of a catastrophic or fatal illness. Individuals with PD often report feelings of anxiety that are associated with health or mental health concerns.

Panic attacks often contribute to the presentation of other psychiatric illnesses, such as other anxiety disorders and major depression. A thorough history that documents the onset of symptoms, possible triggers, and context of symptoms is critical to establishing the diagnosis of PD. In addition to the history of the present illness and current symptoms, a psychiatric review of symptoms, past psychiatric history, general medical history and current medications, substance use history, family history, and mental status exam are valuable in constructing a psychiatric differential diagnosis and then a final working diagnosis. For instance, an individual with a history of a past trauma presenting with flashbacks, nightmares, and triggered panic attacks may have posttraumatic stress disorder (versus panic disorder).

Suicidal behavior in individuals with anxiety disorders has long been attributed to co-occurring risk factors, such as depression. New research suggests that an anxiety disorder is associated with suicidal ideation and suicide attempts beyond the effects of co-occurring mental disorders. Panic attacks and a recent diagnosis of PD are associated with a higher rate of suicide attempts and suicidal ideation.

TABLE 1	Differential Diagnosis of Panic Attacks
SYSTEM	**POSSIBLE DIAGNOSES**
Psychiatric	Mood disorder (panic attacks associated with depression or bipolar disorder)
	Anxiety disorders (panic attacks associated with social anxiety, specific phobia, posttraumatic stress disorder, generalized anxiety disorder, obsessive compulsive disorder)
	Agoraphobia
	Psychotic disorder (panic attacks associated with psychosis)
	Somatoform disorder
	Factitious disorder
Cardiac	Myocardial infarction
	Angina
	SVT or other arrhythmia
	Mitral valve prolapse
	Labile hypertension
Respiratory	Asthma
	COPD
	Pulmonary embolus
Neurologic	Seizure disorder
	Vestibular dysfunction
Endocrine	Thyroid disorder
	Hypoglycemia
	Adrenal dysfunction
	Hyperparathyroidism
	Pheochromocytoma
Substance	Excess caffeine
Use	Psychostimulants
Substance	Caffeine
Withdrawal	Nicotine
	Alcohol or sedative
	Opioid

TABLE 2	Pharmacologic Treatments of Panic Disorder		
MEDICATION (TRADE NAME)		**INITIAL DOSE (mg/DAY)**	**DOSE RANGE (mg/DAY)**
SSRIs			
Citalopram (Celexa)[1]		10–20	20–40
Escitalopram (Lexapro)[1]		5–10	10–20
Fluoxetine (Prozac)		10–20	20–80
Fluvoxamine (Luvox)[1]		50	100–300[†]
Fluvoxamine CR (Luvox CR)[1]		100	100–300
Paroxetine (Paxil)		10–20	20–60
Paroxetine CR (Paxil CR)		12.5–25	25–75
Sertraline (Zoloft)		25	50–200
SNRIs			
Duloxetine (Cymbalta)[1]		30	60–120
Venlafaxine (Effexor)[1]		25–50	150–225
Venlafaxine ER (Effexor ER)		37.5	75–225
TCAs			
Desipramine (Norpramin)		25–50	100–200
Clomipramine (Anafranil)[1]		25	50–150
Imipramine (Tofranil)[1]		25	50–150
Nortriptyline (Pamelor)[1]		10–25	75–150
MAOIs			
Phenelzine* (Nardil)[1]		45[†]	45-75[§]
Benzodiazepines			
Alprazolam (Xanax)		0.25–0.5 tid	5–6
Alprazolam XR (Xanax XR)		0.5–1	3–6
Lorazepam (Ativan)[1]		0.25 tid	2–8[‡]
Clonazepam (Klonopin)		0.25 bid	0.5–2[†]

[1]Not FDA approved for this indication.
*Dietary restrictions required (low-tyramine diet); 2-week washout required before initiation and after termination of monoamine oxidase inhibitor (MAOI) trial.
[†]Divided doses may be given.
[‡]Total daily dosage divided across 2–4 doses/day.
[§]Usually administered tid.

Differential Diagnosis

The differential diagnosis of PD is wide ranging (Table 1). PD is not diagnosed if panic attacks are the direct physiologic consequence of another medical condition or substance. Medical conditions that can cause panic attacks include cardiopulmonary conditions such as arrhythmias and asthma or chronic obstructive pulmonary disease (COPD). Endocrine and neurologic disorders such as hyperthyroidism, pheochromocytoma, vestibular dysfunction, and seizures may also cause panic attacks. In addition, central nervous system (CNS) stimulants and withdrawal from CNS depressants may precipitate a panic attack. On the other hand, a panic attack may mimic a wide variety of medical disorders.

Treatment

PD is a common mental disorder. It is associated with social and occupational/physical disability and high economic cost. When symptoms cause significant distress or interfere with functioning, treatment is warranted. Regardless of the modality chosen, the goal of treatment is a reduction in the frequency and severity of panic attacks as well as the resultant anticipatory anxiety and avoidance behaviors.

Research has confirmed the efficacy of multiple psychosocial and pharmacologic interventions in treating PD. Choice of treatment depends on multiple factors, including patient preference; risks and benefits for an individual patient; cost; past treatment history; and co-occurring medical, psychiatric, or substance abuse issues.

Selective serotonin reuptake inhibitors (SSRIs), serotonin norepinephrine reuptake inhibitors (SNRIs), tricyclic antidepressants (TCAs), and benzodiazepines have demonstrated efficacy for the treatment of PD. The favorable safety profile of SSRIs and SNRIs makes them first-line monotherapy agents. While TCAs are effective, their side effects and toxicity in overdose limit their clinical utility. Monoamine oxidase inhibitors (MAOIs) also appear effective but are reserved for patients who are nonresponders to multiple first-line treatments because of their safety profile. Benzodiazepines are not first-line monotherapy but are useful adjuncts to antidepressants if residual anxiety requires additional treatment (Table 2).

An important consideration when using psychopharmacologic treatments in PD is the side-effect profile of a particular agent. Because patients with PD can be acutely sensitive to medication side effects, it is prudent to start medications at low doses and gradually increase them to therapeutic doses as tolerated. An effective dose is patient dependent—the goal is to prevent (versus respond to) panic attacks. If a decision is made to discontinue a SSRI, SNRI, or TCA, the medication should be gradually tapered when feasible.

Cognitive behavioral therapy (CBT) and CBT with medications are first-line treatments for children and adults with PD. CBT presents the most evidence of efficacy from random control trials. CBT for panic disorder generally includes psychoeducation, episode monitoring and response, self-awareness of anxious automatic thoughts and beliefs, controlled exposure to fear cues, modification of anxiety-reducing behaviors, and prevention of relapse. Psychosocial interventions, such as CBT, may enhance long-term outcomes by reducing the likelihood of relapse.

References

American Psychiatric Association. Diagnostic and Statistical Manual of Mental Disorders. 5th ed. Arlington, VA: American Psychiatric Association; 2013.

American Psychiatric Association. Practice Guideline for the Treatment of Patients with Panic Disorder. 2nd ed. Arlington, VA: American Psychiatric Association; 2010.

Craske MG, Kircanski K, Epstein A, et al. Panic disorder: A review of DSM-IV panic disorder and proposals for DSM-V. Depress Anxiety 2010;27:93–112.

Thibodeau MA, Welch PG, Sareen J, Asmundson GJG. Anxiety disorders are independently associated with suicide ideation and attempts: Propensity score matching in two epidemiological samples. Depress Anxiety 2013;30:947–54.

Locke AB, Kirst N, Shultz CG. Diagnosis and management of generalized anxiety disorder and panic disorder in adults. Am Fam Physician 2015;91(9):617–24.

Marchesi C. Pharmacological management of panic disorder. Neuropsychiatr Dis Treat 2008;4:93–106.

Milrod B, Chambless DL, Gallop R, et al. Psychotherapies for panic disorder: a tale of two sites. J Clin Psychiatry 2015 Jun 9; [Epub ahead of print].

Stahl SM. Stahl's Essential Psychopharmocology: The Prescriber's Guide. 4th ed. New York: Cambridge University Press; 2011.

Andrisano C, Chiesa A, Serretti A. Newer antidepressants and panic disorder: A meta-analysis. Int Clin Psychopharmacol 2013;28:33–45.

SCHIZOPHRENIA

Method of
Brian Miller, MD, PhD, MPH; and Peter Buckley, MD

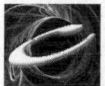

CURRENT DIAGNOSIS

- There are three primary symptom domains in schizophrenia:
  - Positive symptoms (i.e., hallucinations, delusions, disorganized thought, and abnormal psychomotor behavior)
  - Negative symptoms (i.e., restricted affect or avolition/asociality)
  - Cognitive symptoms (i.e., attention, language, memory, and processing speed)
- Symptoms last ≥ 1 month and there are continuous signs of illness for > 6 months.
- There is significant impairment one or more major areas of functioning (work, interpersonal relations, or self-care).
- Rule out that psychosis is not due to a primary mood disorder, schizoaffective disorder, substance intoxication or withdrawal, or a general medical condition.

CURRENT THERAPY

- Antipsychotic medication, with monitoring for medication adherence and side effects.
- Adjunctive medications as needed, including antidepressants, mood stabilizers, benzodiazepines, beta-blockers, and anticholinergics.
- Aggressive monitoring for and management of medical comorbidities, substance use disorders, and suicidality, including collaboration with primary care physician.
- Psychosocial interventions.
- Involvement of family/support system in care.
- Long-term treatment, including outpatient medication management and therapy, with inpatient care for acute crisis intervention/illness exacerbation.

Schizophrenia is a complex, chronic, and often severe psychiatric disorder that is a leading cause of disability worldwide. Although the literal translation of the word schizophrenia is "split mind," patients with this disorder do not have a "split personality" or "multiple personality disorder" (known as dissociative identity disorder). Rather, schizophrenia is a psychotic disorder that interferes with a person's thinking, mood, behavior, and/or interpersonal relations. Schizophrenia often has devastating, lifelong consequences for affected individuals and their families and is associated with an increased risk of premature mortality, including deaths from suicide and cardiovascular disease. In this chapter, the epidemiology and diagnosis of schizophrenia are reviewed. We then discuss pharmacologic and psychosocial treatments for schizophrenia in the context of a chronic disease model. The risks of medical and substance-use comorbidity and suicidality are also highlighted.

Epidemiology and Risk Factors

The etiology of schizophrenia is not known, but is thought to involve interactions between genetic (or epigenetic) and environmental factors, including developmental problems that occur during gestation. The lifetime prevalence of schizophrenia is approximately 1% and is equal in men and women. The usual age of onset is in the late teens or early 1920s to late 1930s, although schizophrenia can have onset before age 10 (early onset) or after age 45 (late onset). The age of onset is usually younger for men than women.

Several lines of evidence support a genetic contribution to the risk of schizophrenia. There is a 40% lifetime risk of schizophrenia in a child of two parents with schizophrenia. Twin-twin concordance is 50% in monozygotic twins, and 12% in dizygotic twins. A recent genome-wide association study and meta-analysis found that schizophrenia is significantly associated with single nucleotide polymorphisms in the major histocompatibility complex region on chromosome 6p22.1 (which includes several immunity-related genes), although numerous other genes have been implicated. There are likely multiple candidate genes that increase the risk of schizophrenia, each with small effect size.

Replicated environmental risk factors for schizophrenia include season of birth (winter), advanced paternal age, prenatal stress throughout gestation (famine and acute maternal stress in the first trimester, prenatal infections with a myriad of different agents, loss of the father in the second or third trimester), obstetric complications (including gestational diabetes, low birth weight, asphyxia), severe childhood abuse, and cannabis use. It remains unclear whether some of these risk factors are causal to schizophrenia or represent early manifestations of disease.

Diagnosis

There are three primary symptom domains in schizophrenia: positive, negative, and cognitive symptoms. Positive symptoms are abnormalities of thought content, including hallucinations (abnormal sensory perceptions in the absence of external stimuli) and delusions (fixed, false beliefs), formal thought disorder (also called disorganized thinking), and abnormal psychomotor behavior (such as catatonia). Hallucinations are most commonly auditory, but can occur in any sensory modality. Negative symptoms include impairments in emotional expression (blunted affect), motivation (avolition), social behavior (asociality), speech (alogia), and the ability to experience pleasure (anhedonia). Cognitive symptoms include impairments in attention, language, memory, processing speed, and executive function.

The most commonly used diagnostic criteria for schizophrenia are derived from the *Diagnostic and Statistical Manual of Mental Disorders*, Fifth Edition (DSM-V). These criteria include the presence of two or more characteristic symptoms—delusions, hallucinations, disorganized speech, grossly abnormal psychomotor behavior (such as catatonia), or negative symptoms (i.e., restricted affect or avolition/asociality)—for a significant portion of time during a 1-month period (or less if successfully treated), with continuous signs of the disturbance persisting for at least 6 months. At least one of these two characteristic symptoms should include delusions, hallucinations, or disorganized speech. During this period, there is significant impairment in one or more major areas of functioning, including work, interpersonal relations, or self-care. It must also be established that the disorder is not better accounted for by a primary mood disorder, schizoaffective disorder, substance intoxication or withdrawal, or other general medical condition. From these criteria, it is important to note that delusions and hallucinations, although common, are not required for the diagnosis. Furthermore, although cognitive symptoms are also not required for the diagnosis, they are a tremendous cause of illness-related disability. A diagnosis of schizophrenia is most definitively made by interviewing the patient, obtaining collateral history from family and/or friends, and completing a medical work-up (physical examination, routine blood and urine tests). According to DSM-V (released May 2013), the diagnostic criteria no longer identify subtypes of schizophrenia, primarily because of a lack of utility for clinicians. Also of note, the Psychoses Workgroup for DSM-V considered the addition of "attenuated psychosis syndrome" (i.e., prodromal or high-risk psychosis) as a diagnostic category, echoing increased attention and efforts at identifying individuals with an increased risk for developing schizophrenia for early intervention. Ultimately, attenuated psychosis syndrome is listed in DSM-V among conditions that require further research before consideration as formal disorders, as more study is needed for reliable diagnosis.

Treatment

At present there is no cure for schizophrenia. Although there is significant clinical heterogeneity within the disorder, schizophrenia is usually a chronic condition that requires long-term treatment. Comprehensive treatment involves outpatient medication management and psychotherapy, psychosocial interventions, involvement of the family/support system, inpatient care for acute crisis intervention/illness exacerbation, and collaboration with primary care physicians.

Antipsychotic medications play an important role in the pharmacologic management of schizophrenia. So-called first-generation antipsychotics (FGAs) have been in clinical use since the introduction of chlorpromazine (Thorazine) in the 1950s. These agents block the dopamine D2 receptor, and common side effects include extrapyramidal side effects (EPS) (e.g., Parkinsonism, dystonia). The newer or "second-generation antipsychotics" (SGAs), in addition to D2 receptor blockade, are also serotonin 5-HT2 receptor antagonists. While the risk of EPS is lower for SGAs than FGAs, SGAs are associated with a heightened risk of weight gain and the metabolic syndrome. Table 1 provides a more detailed description of antipsychotic medications. The Texas Medication Algorithm Project (TMAP) currently recommends a trial of a single (non-clozapine) SGA for newly diagnosed patients with schizophrenia, or patients never before treated with an SGA. However, neither the TMAP nor the American Psychiatric Association (APA) guidelines for the treatment of schizophrenia preferentially endorse a particular antipsychotic. Clozapine (Clozaril) is primarily used for "treatment-refractory" schizophrenia, usually defined as a lack of/partial response to an adequate trial of monotherapy with two or three different antipsychotics.

Adjunctive medications may also play an important role in the pharmacologic treatment of some patients with schizophrenia. These include antidepressants for depression and anxiety, mood stabilizers for depression or mood elevation, benzodiazepines for anxiety or agitation, beta-blockers for akathisia, and anticholinergics for EPS.

Medication nonadherence is a major treatment issue in patients with schizophrenia at all phases of the illness. Reasons for nonadherence are complex and multifaceted, but may include medication side effects, impaired insight into illness, psychopathology in all three symptom domains, lack of efficacy, and comorbid substance use. Over 70% of patients in the Clinical Antipsychotic Trials of Intervention Effectiveness (CATIE) Schizophrenia Trial discontinued medication within the first 18 months of treatment. Medication nonadherence leads to dramatically increased risk of illness relapse, hospitalization, and suicidal behavior and should be routinely assessed in clinical visits. The use of rapid-dissolving oral or long-acting injectable medications may improve adherence in some patients.

Psychosocial interventions are also a cornerstone of the comprehensive treatment of patients with schizophrenia, and when utilized in combination with medication, are more effective than antipsychotics alone. Psychotherapy, including cognitive-behavioral therapy, supportive therapy, and group therapy, promotes improved illness management and medication adherence. Involvement of the patient's family/support system in care, including family-based therapies and psychoeducation, has been shown to increase medication adherence and decrease illness relapse rates. Psychosocial rehabilitation, which may include assertive community treatment, social skills training, vocational rehabilitation, and cognitive remediation, can help maximize patients' psychosocial functioning. There is growing evidence that cognitive remediation therapy in combination with other psychosocial interventions, particularly vocational rehabilitation, can improve "real-world" functioning for patients with schizophrenia in a relatively short time period.

Although there is no "typical" patient with schizophrenia, the clinical course is often characterized by acute relapses of the illness with the interepisode absence or attenuation of symptoms. Multiple factors increase a patient's risk of illness relapse, including medication nonadherence, psychosocial stressors, substance use, medical illnesses such as infections, and the natural history of the disorder itself. Hospitalization may be required for acute exacerbations of psychotic symptoms, including hallucinations, delusions, and impaired self-care. Hospitalization may also be required if a patient represents an acute danger to self or others.

The concept of the recovery model and recovery-oriented care is a movement that is currently transforming the delivery of mental health services. Integral to the recovery model are certified peer specialists (CPS). A CPS is a licensed professional who has progressed in their own recovery from mental illness and works to assist patients with schizophrenia and other mental illness in regaining control over their own lives and over their own recovery process. CPSs provide peer support services, serve as consumer advocates, are resources for psychoeducation, and offer the unique perspectives based on their individual experiences.

Comorbidity

Schizophrenia is associated with an increased risk of premature mortality, and cardiovascular disease is a leading cause of death in this patient population. Multiple factors contribute to this risk, including a high prevalence of smoking, poor health habits, poor health care, medication side effects, and (perhaps) the pathophysiology of the disorder itself. SGAs as a class are associated with weight gain and an increased risk of metabolic syndrome. Over 40% of the 1460 patients in the CATIE Schizophrenia Trial met the criteria for metabolic syndrome at baseline. Recommendations for monitoring of patients on SGAs, based on a consensus statement from the American Diabetes Association and the APA, are described in Table 2. Primary care physicians play an important collaborative role with psychiatrists in the detection and management of metabolic disturbances in patients with schizophrenia, in order to minimize the cardiovascular risks associated with these comorbidities.

Patients with schizophrenia are also at an increased risk of suicide, which is also a leading cause of premature mortality. The prevalence of completed suicide in patients with schizophrenia is about 10%, and suicide attempts occur with even greater frequency. Clinicians should routine assess patients for suicidal ideation, and if present, explore risk factors for completed suicide, which include a suicidal plan and intent, previous suicide attempts, a family history of suicide, age, sex, access to lethal means, social isolation, and comorbid substance use. Medications, psychotherapy, and/or hospitalization may be required.

Comorbid substance use disorders predominate in patients with schizophrenia, with an estimated prevalence of 40% to 50%. Common substances of abuse include alcohol, marijuana, and cocaine. Patients with schizophrenia and comorbid substance use are at increased risk of medication nonadherence, illness

| TABLE 1 | Antipsychotic Medications |

AGENT	MECHANISM OF ACTION*	TYPICAL DOSING	SIDE EFFECTS†	SIDE EFFECTS†	NOTES
First Generation					
Haloperidol (Haldol)	D_2-antagonist	1.5–15 mg/day	EPS/TD Akathisia	NMS Hyperprolactinemia	PO, IM, IV, and long-acting injection formulations
Loxapine (Adasuve)	D_2-antagonist	10 mg/day	Dysgeusia Sedation	Throat irritation	INH formulation; for treatment of acute agitation
Second Generation					
Aripiprazole (Abilify)	Partial D_2-agonist and antagonist	10–30 mg/day	Weight gain (+) Dyslipidemia (+) Glucose dysregulation (+)	Headache EPS/TD Akathisia	PO, rapid-dissolving PO, IM, and long-acting injection formulations
Asenapine (Saphris)	D_2-antagonist/5-HT_2 antagonist	10–20 mg/day	Weight gain (+) Dyslipidemia (+) Glucose dysregulation (+)	Sedation EPS/TD Akathisia	Rapid-dissolving PO formulation
Clozapine (Clozaril)	D_2-antagonist/5-HT_2 antagonist	300–900 mg/day	Weight gain (+++) Dyslipidemia (+++) Glucose dysregulation (++) Agranulocytosis Sedation	Orthostatic hypotension Seizures Myocarditis EPS/TD	PO and rapid-dissolving PO formulations
Iloperidone (Fanapt)	D_2-antagonist/5-HT_2 antagonist	12–24 mg/day	Weight gain (++) Dyslipidemia (+) Glucose dysregulation (+)	Dizziness Tachycardia Sedation EPS/TD	PO formulation
Lurasidone (Latuda)	D_2-antagonist/5-HT_2 antagonist	40–80 mg/day	Weight gain (+) Dyslipidemia (+) Glucose dysregulation (+)	Sedation Akathisia Nausea EPS/TD	PO formulation
Olanzapine (Zyprexa)	D_2-antagonist/5-HT_2 antagonist	5–30 mg/day	Weight gain (+++) Dyslipidemia (+++) Glucose dysregulation (++)	Sedation Dizziness Hyperprolactinemia EPS/TD	PO, rapid-dissolving PO, IM, and long-acting injection formulations
Paliperidone (Invega)	D_2-antagonist/5-HT_2 antagonist	6–12 mg/day	Weight gain (+) Dyslipidemia (+) Glucose dysregulation (+)	Tachycardia Headache EPS/TD	PO and long-acting injection formulations Active metabolite of Risperidone (Risperdal)
Quetiapine (Seroquel)	D_2-antagonist/5-HT_2 antagonist	200–800 mg/day	Weight gain (++) Dyslipidemia (+) Glucose dysregulation (+)	Sedation Headache Orthostatic hypotension EPS/TD	PO and extended-release PO formulations
Risperidone (Risperdal)	D_2-antagonist/5-HT_2 antagonist	2–6 mg/day	Weight gain (++) Dyslipidemia (+) Glucose dysregulation (+)	Sedation Hyperprolactinemia EPS/TD	PO, PO liquid, rapid-dissolving PO, and long-acting injection formulations
Ziprasidone (Geodon)	D_2-antagonist/5-HT_2 antagonist	80–160 mg/day	Weight gain (+) Dyslipidemia (+) Glucose dysregulation (+)	Sedation QTc prolongation EPS/TD	PO and IM formulations

*All first-generation and second-generation antipsychotics have an FDA black box warning for an "association with an increased risk of mortality in elderly patients treated for dementia-related psychosis." All second-generation agents are D_2 and 5-HT_2 antagonists; however, many act on multiple receptors, including alpha-adrenergic, beta-adrenergic, histaminergic, muscarinic cholinergic, and D_1, and 5-HT_1 receptors.

†EPS and TD are possible side effects with all antipsychotics, but they occur less frequently with second-generation than first-generation drugs.

Abbreviations: D_2 = dopamine D_2 receptor; +++, severe risk; EPS = extrapyramidal side effects; 5-HT_2 = serotonin 5-HT_2 receptor; ++ = moderate risk; TD = tardive dyskinesia; + = mild or low risk; NMS = neuroleptic malignant syndrome.

TABLE 2 Monitoring Second-Generation Antipsychotic (Excluding Clozapine)

	BASELINE	4 WEEKS	8 WEEKS	12 WEEKS	QUARTERLY	ANNUALLY	IF SYMPTOMS ARISE	EVERY 5 YEARS	OTHER
Personal/family history*	X					X			
Pregnancy test†	X						X		
Weight/BMI	X	X	X	X	X				
Waist circumference	X					X			
Blood pressure	X			X		X			
Fasting glucose/HgbA1C	X			X		X			
Fasting lipid panel	X			X				X	
EKG‡	X						X		
Prolactin	X						X		
CBC with differential§									X

*Including obesity, diabetes, hypertension, and dyslipidemia.
†In all women of childbearing age.
‡For patients taking Ziprasidone (Geodon), which may prolong the QTc interval, and Clozapine (Clozaril).
§For patients taking Clozapine (Clozaril). CBC with differential required at baseline, then weekly for 6 months, then every other week for 6 months, then monthly thereafter. WBC count must be $\geq 3500/mm^3$, and absolute neutrophil count (ANC) must be $\geq 2000/mm^3$ due to risk of agranulocytosis.
More frequent assessments may be warranted based on clinical status.

relapse, hospitalization, suicidal and violent behavior, and an overall poor response to treatment. Furthermore, up to 70% to 90% of patients with schizophrenia are tobacco users, which contribute to the increased risk of medical comorbidity. Clinicians are encouraged to routinely screen for and address substance use in their treatment plans.

Conclusions

Schizophrenia is a complex, heterogeneous, and chronic psychiatric disorder. Comprehensive treatment usually involves long-term medication management and therapy, education for patients and their families, and psychosocial interventions. Primary care physicians play an important collaborative role in the detection and management of medical comorbidities, substance use disorders, and suicidality. Physicians, patients, and families are encouraged to become involved in the National Alliance on Mental Illness (NAMI; www.nami.org), which is a tremendous resource for help, support, education, and advocacy for patients with schizophrenia and other mental illness.

References

American Diabetes Association, American Psychiatric Association, American Association of Clinical Endocrinologists, et al. Consensus development conference on antipsychotic drugs and obesity and diabetes. J Clin Psychiatry 2004;65:267.

American Psychiatric Association. Practice guideline for the treatment of patients with schizophrenia, 2nd edition. Am J Psychiatry 2004;161(Suppl):1717.

Buchanan RW, Carpenter WT. Schizophrenia and other psychotic disorders. In: Sadock BJ, Sadock VA, editors. Kaplan and Sadock's Comprehensive Textbook of Psychiatry. 8th ed. Philadelphia: Lippincott Williams and Wilkins; 2005. p. 1329–45.

Buckley PF, Miller BJ, Lehrer DS, et al. Psychiatric comorbidities and schizophrenia. Schizophr Bull 2009;35:383.

Laursen TM, Munk-Olsen T, Vestergaard M. Life expectancy and cardiovascular mortality in persons with schizophrenia. Curr Opin Psychiatry 2012;25:83.

Leucht S, Corves C, Arbter D, et al. Second-generation versus first-generation antipsychotic drugs for schizophrenia: A meta-analysis. Lancet 2009;373:31.

Lieberman JA, Stroup TS, McEvoy JP, et al. Effectiveness of antipsychotic drugs in patients with chronic schizophrenia. N Engl J Med 2005;353:1209.

McEvoy JP, Meyer JP, Goff DC, et al. Prevalence of the metabolic syndrome in patients with schizophrenia: Baseline results from the clinical antipsychotic trials of intervention effectiveness (CATIE). Schizophr Res 2005;80:19.

Messias EL, Chen CY, Eaton WW. Epidemiology of schizophrenia: Review of findings and myths. Psychiatr Clin North Am 2007;30:323.

Shi J, Levinson DF, Duan J, et al. Common variants on chromosome 6p22.1 are associated with schizophrenia. Nature 2009;460:753.

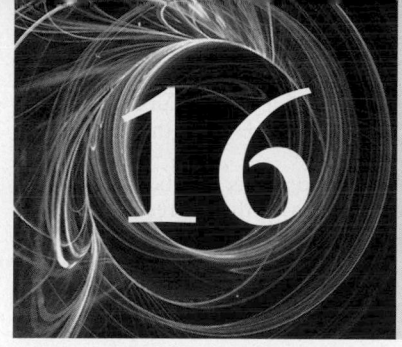

16 Men's Health

BACTERIAL INFECTIONS OF THE MALE URINARY TRACT

Method of
John N. Krieger, MD

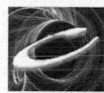

CURRENT DIAGNOSIS

- UTIs include a wide clinical spectrum.
- Infection at any site in the urinary tract places the entire system at risk.
- The critical clinical issue is to distinguish uncomplicated (medical) from complicated (surgical) infections.
- Anatomic evaluation and imaging studies are seldom indicated for patients with uncomplicated UTIs.
- Well-documented UTIs in boys require urologic investigation because of the high prevalence of structural urinary tract abnormalities.
- We recommend culture and sensitivity testing of urine specimens for any male patient with symptoms or signs suggesting a UTI.
- We discourage routine screening of urine cultures in long-term care patients who have no localizing signs or symptoms suggesting a UTI.

CURRENT THERAPY

- The optimal goal of therapy is to eliminate the infecting organism from the urinary tract.
- Antimicrobial therapy alone is less effective for patients with complicated UTIs than for patients with uncomplicated UTIs.
- Managing patients with complicated UTIs often requires anatomic evaluation and imaging studies.
- For patients with complicated UTIs it is often necessary to eliminate or control predisposing factors.
- Rapid eradication of the infection can limit the potential for infection of adjacent structures.
- Ensure elimination of the infection by repeating urine cultures.
- A prolonged course of antimicrobial therapy might prove necessary for patients with persistent infections.

Urinary tract infections (UTIs) include a wide clinical spectrum whose common denominator is bacterial invasion of the genitourinary organs and tissues. UTI can involve any part of the urinary tract from the renal cortex to the urethral meatus. UTI can predominate at a single site, such as the bladder (cystitis), prostate (prostatitis), epididymis (epididymitis), kidneys (pyelonephritis), or perinephric space (perinephric abscess). When any of its parts has become infected, the entire urinary tract is placed at risk for bacterial invasion.

The great majority of UTIs occur by the ascending route. Bacteria from the fecal flora colonize the perineum and then ascend via the urethra to involve the bladder, the ureter, and the kidneys. On occasion, hematogenous dissemination results in bacterial seeding of the urinary tract. Classic examples of such hematogenous infection are genitourinary tuberculosis or staphylococcal infection of a renal cyst (historically known as a renal carbuncle). On rare occasions, the urinary tract is involved by infection from contiguous structures. For example, patients with diverticulitis or appendicitis occasionally develop abscesses or fistulas that involve the urinary tract.

Distinguishing Complicated from Uncomplicated Infections

The first step in evaluating a patient is to distinguish uncomplicated (medical) infections from complicated (surgical) infections. Uncomplicated UTIs occur in the absence of underlying structural, functional, or neurologic disorders of the urinary tract. Uncomplicated UTIs usually respond promptly to appropriate antimicrobial therapy. Anatomic evaluation and imaging studies are seldom indicated in patients with uncomplicated UTIs.

Complicated UTIs occur when the urinary tract has been repeatedly invaded by bacteria, leaving residual inflammation, in some cases accompanied by obstruction, stones, foreign bodies, or neurologic conditions that interfere with urinary drainage. Antimicrobial therapy alone is markedly less effective in complicated UTIs than in uncomplicated UTIs. Managing patients with complicated infections often requires anatomic evaluation and imaging studies. An important differential point is that patients with complicated UTIs tend to have persistence of bacteria within the urinary tract in the face of antimicrobial agents to which the bacteria appear to be sensitive in laboratory tests. Often, it is necessary to correct an underlying obstructive lesion, improve voiding, drain an abscess, or remove a stone or foreign body to clear the infection.

Total elimination of the infecting organism from the urinary tract represents the ideal goal of UTI therapy. This is a realistic goal for patients with uncomplicated UTIs. However, achieving this goal can prove difficult in patients with complicated UTIs whose underlying abnormalities cannot be corrected. For example, it is often impossible to achieve long-standing resolution of bacteriuria in patients who require indwelling catheters or who have functional obstruction of their voiding mechanisms. In such cases, resolution of symptoms directly related to UTI is the only practical therapeutic goal.

Natural History

During infancy, the incidence of symptomatic UTIs is higher in boys than in girls. In part, this has been related to male circumcision status. It appears that bacteria can adhere to the prepuce of uncircumcised boys, providing access to the urinary tract. Neonatal circumcision appears to reduce the UTI rate in boys by about 90%. After the neonatal period, symptomatic UTIs in boys and men are distinctly uncommon until middle age. This contrasts dramatically with UTI rates in girls and women, who experience increasing rates of both symptomatic and asymptomatic infections, with a marked increase following initiation of sexual activity, then a continued gradual rise with increasing age. Asymptomatic bacteriuria is also distinctly unusual in male patients compared with female patients.

Well-documented UTIs in boys mandate thorough urologic investigation. This is because of the high prevalence of structural urinary tract abnormalities in boys with UTIs. Often, UTI represents the key diagnostic presentation for major abnormalities of the urinary tract. For example, vesicoureteral reflux of urine, posterior urethral valves, and other major structural abnormalities often manifest initially with bacterial UTIs. Early diagnosis and appropriate therapy offer the best chance for preservation of maximal kidney function. Unfortunately, the developing kidneys are especially susceptible to continued scarring that can progress despite appropriate treatment.

Structural urinary tract abnormalities remain a major cause of renal failure in children. Morbidity may be minimized by appropriate evaluation and therapy. The optimal radiologic approach for children with UTI is controversial. The traditional choice for evaluation of a boy with a UTI is the combination of renal ultrasound to evaluate the upper urinary tract plus a voiding cystourethrogram to evaluate the lower urinary tract. Voiding cystourethrography should be obtained after resolution of the initial infection, because dilation of the upper urinary tract may be exaggerated after a recent UTI. More recent approaches focus on confirming the diagnosis of acute pyelonephritis before invasive imaging is considered, often starting with a nuclear medicine scan. In my opinion this is an attractive approach to minimize unnecessary interventions and to improve compliance with recommended testing.

Because UTIs are unusual in young men, there are few well-done natural history studies in this population. In young men with UTIs who have no obvious neurologic or structural abnormalities, sexual intercourse, particularly among homosexual men or heterosexual men who practice insertive anal intercourse, may be a risk factor. The overall contribution of these practices to bacterial UTIs in men is uncertain.

Traditional urologic teaching is to recommend thorough evaluation for structural abnormalities in such patients, including radiographic studies and cystourethroscopy. However, our published experience suggests that previously healthy college-age men with well-documented UTIs have a low rate of structural genitourinary tract abnormalities. A uroflow study and postvoid residual urine determination by ultrasound are adequate to screen for structural abnormalities in young men whose UTIs resolve. We reserve imaging studies and cystoscopy for patients at risk for significant abnormalities on the basis of these screening studies and a thorough physical examination. Recent studies indicate that bacterial pathogens require an exceptional repertoire of virulence factors to cause UTIs in previously healthy young men. The other major risk factors for UTIs in men are instrumentation of the urinary tract and bacterial prostatitis.

Diagnosis and Localization

Accurate diagnosis is prerequisite for appropriate UTI therapy. Therefore, we recommend culture and sensitivity testing of urine specimens from any male patient with symptoms or signs suggesting a UTI. In patients who do not have obstructive lesions, stasis, stones, or foreign bodies, recurrent and persistent bacterial UTIs are often related to bacterial prostatitis. Segmented localization cultures can be used to differentiate cystitis and urethritis from bacterial prostatitis. The procedure should be carried out at a time when the patient does not have bacteriuria.

My procedure for lower urinary tract localization is outlined briefly. After cleaning the glans with sterile water, the first-void urine (initial 5–10 mL of voided urine) is collected in a sterile container. Next, a midstream specimen is obtained. The patient is asked to stop voiding. Prostatic fluid is expressed by digital rectal prostate massage. The post–prostate massage urine (next 5–10 mL voided after the massage) is then collected. Culture and sensitivity testing are then carried out on each of these four specimens. It is

critical to ensure that the clinical microbiology laboratory is aware of the purpose of these studies so that they will evaluate low concentrations of uropathogens that may be present in the localization cultures.

Diagnosis of chronic bacterial prostatitis can be made if the post–prostate-massage urine specimen or the expressed prostatic secretion contains a 10-fold or greater increase in the concentration of the uropathogen compared with that in the first-void urine specimen. In patients with well-documented bacterial prostatitis, the causative organism is identical to the uropathogen causing recurrent UTI episodes.

It is important to recognize that only a small minority of men presenting with symptoms of prostatitis fit into the acute or chronic bacterial prostatitis categories. The great majority of patients with symptoms of prostatitis are classified in the chronic prostatitis/chronic pelvic pain category. In contrast to the recognized benefit of therapy for patients with acute and chronic bacterial prostatitis, the role of antimicrobial therapy and other treatments has not been defined for men with symptoms of chronic prostatitis/chronic pelvic pain syndrome.

Treatment

There are three keys to successful UTI therapy. First, eliminate or control predisposing factors, if possible. For example, we are often asked to manage resistant UTIs in long-term care patients with indwelling catheters. One approach is to change their bladder management from a chronic indwelling catheter to an intermittent self- or assisted-catheterization program. Other examples include removing or correcting obstructing lesions, stones, or strictures to improve drainage of the urinary tract. These measures may be successful in eliminating the focus of infection, even with no antimicrobial therapy. Second, eradicate the infection as soon as possible to prevent colonization of the prostate and other structures. Third, ensure resolution of the UTI by obtaining cultures during or immediately after therapy and at follow-up 1 to 2 months after therapy.

Uncomplicated Infections

Uncomplicated infections generally manifest with symptoms of bacterial cystitis, such as the combination of urinary frequency, urgency, dysuria, nocturia, suprapubic discomfort, low-back pain, or hematuria. Systemic symptoms of fever, chills, and rigor are absent. Urine culture confirms the diagnosis, with *Escherichia coli* representing the most common pathogen. Uncomplicated infections, including those introduced by a single or short course of indwelling urethral catheterization, generally respond promptly to a short course of antimicrobial therapy. The infection can persist and become difficult to eradicate if the prostate becomes colonized or if the patient has a stone or structural abnormality of the urinary tract. Thus, an effort should be made to eliminate predisposing factors while routine therapy is guided by in vitro susceptibility tests.

I prefer oral therapy with one of the agents listed in Table 1. In the Pacific Northwest, bacteria causing UTIs have developed substantial resistance to trimethoprim–sulfamethoxazole (Bactrim). Therefore, I usually initiate empiric therapy with a quinolone. Nitrofurantoin (Macrodantin) remains highly effective and is an attractive alternative drug. In general, I recommend that the duration of therapy be at least 2 weeks, although only limited data address this point in male patients.

Complicated Infections

Patients with systemic signs or those with a history of structural or neurologic abnormalities merit anatomic and functional investigation of the urinary tract. Antimicrobial therapy alone might fail to cure infection, and urosepsis can develop unless there is specific management of the underlying problem. My initial choice for evaluating these patients is usually computed tomography (CT) with IV contrast. If a renal or retroperitoneal abscess is suspected, CT scanning has proved superior to the other modalities for

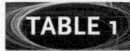

TABLE 1	Oral Antimicrobial Agents Prescribed for Urinary Tract Infections In Men
AGENT	**DOSAGE**
Fluoroquinolones	
Ciprofloxacin (Cipro)	250–500 mg bid
Ciprofloxacin extended release (CiproXR)	500–1000 mg qd
Levofloxacin (Levaquin, Levaquin LEVA-pak)	250–750 mg qd
Ofloxacin (Floxin)	200–400 mg bid[3]
Norfloxacin (Noroxin)	400 mg bid
Combination Agents	
Trimethoprim–sulfamethoxazole (Bactrim, Septra, Bactrim DS, Septra DS)	160 mg trimethoprim, 800 mg sulfamethoxazole bid
Amoxicillin–clavulanate (Augmentin)	500–875 mg amoxicillin, 125 mg clavulanate bid
Other Antimicrobials	
Trimethoprim (Proloprim)	100–200 mg bid
Nitrofurantoin monohydrate (Macrobid)	100 mg bid
Nitrofurantoin (Macrodantin)	50–100 mg qid

[3]Exceeds dosage recommended by the manufacturer.

diagnosis. The exception is that I prefer transrectal ultrasound for evaluation of possible prostatic abscesses.

Prolonged courses of therapy are indicated for patients with persistent infections. Often, I use 3 to 4 months of therapy in this situation. In patients with chronic bacterial prostatitis, elderly patients, or those in nursing homes, continuous therapy may be necessary to suppress bacteriuria, even though eradication can prove impossible. Thus, for patients with recurrent or complicated infections, I recommend an attempt to eradicate the focus of infection, following thorough evaluation of the urinary tract. The therapy is usually with the drugs listed in Table 1. My first choice for curative therapy is usually a quinolone. For patients with persistent or frequently relapsing infections, I consider long-term therapy (months or years) using low dosages of antimicrobial drugs for prophylaxis or suppression. In this situation, my choice is usually either trimethoprim–sulfamethoxazole or nitrofurantoin.

Prostatitis

Acute and chronic bacterial prostatitis can manifest with local urinary tract symptoms characteristic of bacterial cystitis or with systemic signs and symptoms. Acute bacterial prostatitis can manifest with the sudden onset of chills, fever, malaise, and low back and perineal pain, as well as difficulty with urination. On rectal examination, the prostate is tense and exquisitely tender. Excessive palpation can induce septicemia.

For patients who require hospitalization, my initial choice is the combination of a β-lactam drug with an aminoglycoside until the results of antimicrobial sensitivity testing are available. Following parenteral therapy, the patient is managed with continued antimicrobial therapy for at least 4 weeks, usually employing a quinolone. Patients with acute bacterial prostatitis usually respond well to a variety of antimicrobial agents that penetrate an acutely inflamed prostate. Many of these agents are not effective in chronic bacterial prostatitis.

In contrast to acute bacterial prostatitis, chronic bacterial prostatitis is often insidious in onset. Patients usually have recurrent symptomatic UTIs and, sometimes, recurrent episodes of acute prostatitis. Between symptomatic episodes, patients may be totally asymptomatic. Diagnosis depends on the localization cultures described earlier. Treatment must be prolonged, because diffusion of many antimicrobial agents into the uninflamed prostate is poor.

My initial choice is usually a quinolone, with trimethoprim–sulfamethoxazole as a second-choice agent. Other agents may be indicated based on culture and susceptibility test results.

It is important to avoid confusing bacterial prostatitis with chronic prostatitis/chronic pelvic pain syndrome. This is the most common category of symptomatic prostatitis. A critical distinguishing point is that patients with chronic prostatitis/chronic pelvic pain syndrome do not have bacteriuria and they have negative bacterial localization cultures.

Long-Term Care Patients

My approach to managing UTI differs in long-term care patients, including those with incontinence and indwelling urinary catheters or other devices. In such patients, chronic asymptomatic bacterial colonization should not be treated. It is impossible to sterilize the urine permanently in such men. Furthermore, resistant organisms will likely emerge, making subsequent therapy difficult. I treat such patients only if they develop acute symptoms referable to the urinary tract or before genitourinary tract procedures. I strongly recommend against obtaining screening cultures in long-term care patients because these cultures often lead to unnecessary therapy that selects resistant bacterial flora. Further, there is evidence that bacterial colonization with relatively benign strains can inhibit establishment of symptomatic infections caused by more-virulent bacteria. If UTI treatment is necessary for a patient who requires an indwelling catheter, then it is best to change the catheter before starting treatment.

References

Abarbanel J, Engelstein D, Lask D, et al. Urinary tract infection in men younger than 45 years of age: Is there a need for urologic investigation? Urology 2003;62: 27–9.

Andrews SJ, Brooks PT, Hanbury DC, et al. Ultrasonography and abdominal radiography versus intravenous urography in investigation of urinary tract infection in men: Prospective incident cohort study. BMJ 2002;324:454–6.

Griebling TL. Urologic diseases in America project: Trends in resource use for urinary tract infections in men. J Urol 2005;173:1288–94.

Hooton TM, Bradley SF, Cardenas DD, et al. Diagnosis, prevention, and treatment of catheter-associated urinary tract infection in adults: 2009 International Clinical Practice Guidelines from the Infectious Diseases Society of America. Clin Infect Dis 2010;50:625–63.

Johansen TE. The role of imaging in urinary tract infections. World J Urol 2004;22:392–8.

Koyle MA, Elder JS, Skoog SJ, et al. Febrile urinary tract infection, vesicoureteral reflux, and renal scarring: Current controversies in approach to evaluation. Ped Surg Int 2011;27:337–46.

Krieger JN, Dobrindt U, Riley DE, Oswald E. Acute Escherichia coli prostatitis in previously healthy young men: Bacterial virulence factors, antimicrobial resistance, and clinical outcomes. Urology 2011;77:1420–5.

Krieger JN, Nyberg L, Nickel JC. NIH consensus definition and classification of prostatitis. JAMA 1999;282:236–7.

Krieger JN, Ross SO, Simonsen JM. Urinary tract infections in healthy university men. J Urol 1993;149:1046–48.

Merguerian PA, Sverrisson EF, Herz DB, McQuiston LT. Urinary tract infections in children: Recommendations for antibiotic prophylaxis and evaluation. An evidence-based approach. Curr Urol Rep 2010;11:98–108.

Naber KG. Levofloxacin in the treatment of urinary tract infections and prostatitis. J Chemother 2004;16(Suppl. 2):18–21.

Nicolle LE. Symptomatic urinary tract infection in nursing home residents. J Am Geriatr Soc 2009;57:1113–4.

Singh-Grewal D, Macdessi J, Craig J. Circumcision for the prevention of urinary tract infection in boys: A systematic review of randomised trials and observational studies. Arch Dis Child 2005;90:853–8.

Sundén F, Hakansson L, Ljunggren E, et al. Bacterial interference—is deliberate colonization with Escherichia coli 83972 an alternative treatment for patients with recurrent urinary tract infection? Int J Antimicrob Agents 2006;1(28 Suppl): S26–9.

Ulleryd P, Zackrisson B, Aus G, et al. Selective urological evaluation in men with febrile urinary tract infection. BJU Int 2001;88:15–20.

van Nieuwkoop C, Hoppe BP, Bonten TN, et al. Predicting the need for radiologic imaging in adults with febrile urinary tract infection. Clin Infect Dis 2010;51:266–72.

Wagenlehner FM, Wullt B, Perletti G. Antimicrobials in urogenital infections. Int J Antimicrob Agents 2011;(38 Suppl):3–10.

Method of
Judd W. Moul, MD

Epidemiology

Benign prostatic hyperplasia (BPH) was generally a topic only of interest to urologists up to about 20 years ago, when several classes of medical therapy became available. Once widespread direct-to-consumer medical advertising hit the airwaves, the public's lexicon included "BPH" and men and their families were being educated about it. When combined with the aging population, the obesity epidemic, and subsequent health consequences, we have a very important disease process. As other countries improve their standards of living, BPH has become one of the most common health conditions of the aging man worldwide.

From a practical standpoint, BPH and its symptoms are very uncommon before the age of 40 years. By ages 60 years and 85 years, the histologic prevalence of BPH at autopsy is 50% and 90%, respectively. The symptoms of BPH are now referred to as lower urinary tract symptoms (LUTS). At age 70 years, about 40% of men report LUTS and by age 75 years, the incidence of LUTS increases to 50%.

The diagnosis and treatment of BPH has always been in the realm of the specialty of urology, and this remains the case. However, as more medical therapies have been introduced and prostate-specific antigen (PSA) testing for prostate cancer has become commonplace, urologists are working more closely with internists, family physicians, generalists, and physician extenders to jointly manage these patients.

Pathophysiology

Even though BPH is common, we know very little about the true pathophysiology. However, we do know that men who were castrated before puberty do not develop BPH, and we also know that it is a progressive disease of aging. Before the 1980s, BPH was generally thought of as a static condition of a gradually growing prostate gland that caused progressive bladder outlet obstruction. In fact, it was common to use the "donut hole" analogy with patients, explaining to them that the prostate is like a donut surrounding the bladder neck and outlet. With aging and prostate growth, the donut hole gets smaller, causing progressive obstruction. In the era when transurethral resection of the prostate (TURP) was the only effective treatment, this simple static explanation was sufficient.

However, from the 1980s onward, our understanding has advanced to recognize that BPH has both a static obstructive and a dynamic component under neural control. The donut hole now has to have electrical wires attached to it with the ability to adjust the current. In addition, the contribution of the bladder to LUTS has been well recognized as a key contributor to the dynamic component of BPH and LUTS.

The static growth and proliferation of the periurethral tissue into BPH is under androgenic stimulation. Specifically, the main male hormone testosterone is converted to the more active metabolite dihydrotestosterone by the enzyme 5α-reductase in the prostatic stromal and epithelial cells of the prostate. 5α-Reductase occurs in two forms, type 1 and type 2. Only type 2 is present in the prostate and genitalia. This is critical for the understanding of one of the two main classes of medical therapy for BPH, the 5α-reductase inhibitors (5-ARIs).

The dynamic component of BPH and LUTS is based on autonomic input to the smooth muscles in the lower urinary tract, including the bladder, prostate, and urethra. These areas have a large concentration of α_1-adrenergic receptors that, when stimulated by various stressors, cause increasing smooth muscle tone. This increased smooth muscle tone leads to increased urethral resistance and contributes to the bladder outlet obstructive symptoms of BPH. This physiology leads to the basis for the other main class of drugs to treat BPH, the α_1-adrenergic blockers.

Symptoms

LUTS include urinary frequency, decreased force and caliber of the urinary stream, hesitancy, straining, urgency, and nocturia. The severity can range from the stoic man who refuses to acknowledge any symptoms to the man in frank urinary retention. Most urologists now use a standardized patient-self-administered questionnaire, such as the International Prostate Symptom Score (IPSS) (Figure 1). This is very useful to elicit symptoms and bother in a typical male population with suboptimal health-seeking behavior.

It is now very common for men to be referred to urology for a collection of age-related issues including elevated PSA, LUTS, BPH, or erectile dysfunction. Commonly, the PSA or the erectile dysfunction brings the patient to the attention of the health care system for the first time in years and may be the first opportunity to influence men on healthy living and health maintenance as they enter middle or older vulnerable ages. Recognizing this, all health care providers should keep this in mind and try to perform a broader men's health assessment while the patient is captive.

Diagnosis

The diagnosis of BPH is generally made based on symptoms or the IPSS standardized patient-self-administered questionnaire combined with a digital rectal examination, PSA blood test, urinalysis, and, in some cases, a cystoscopy. The differential diagnosis can include urinary tract infection (UTI), prostatitis, urinary stones in the lower urinary tract, urethral stricture disease, neurogenic or overactive bladder, prostate or bladder cancer, and even congestive heart failure. Some common medications, such as over-the-counter cold medicines containing α-adrenergic agents, can exacerbate LUTS and can even put a man into acute urinary retention if he has underlying BPH.

A properly performed digital rectal examination is critical to master in the diagnosis of BPH. Because the posterior prostate gland is located adjacent to the rectum and about 3 to 5 cm internal to the anus, the experienced clinician can gain valuable information. I prefer the patient to bend over the examining table with toes pointed slightly inward, the knees bent slightly forward and the forehead and arms resting on the table. The examiner uses a liberally lubricated gloved index finger to palpate the posterior side of the prostate for size estimate and for any induration or nodularity that might indicate the presence of prostate cancer. In this case, referral to an urologist is mandatory.

The size of the prostate is measured either by estimating the weight in grams or the volume in cubic centimeters. Models have been developed to teach clinicians how to gauge size and consistency. In general, a normal size prostate is 20 to 25 g (or cm^3) in middle-aged men. A size of 25 to 30, 30 to 50, and greater than 50 g (or cm^3) is a general guide to mild, moderate, and severe BPH. However, size does not necessarily correlate to symptoms, and both symptom score and size estimate should be reported. The size gauges the histologic condition and the symptoms indicate the LUTS and the bother index, which are both important for individualized treatment.

The laboratory assessment should include a urinalysis to rule out hematuria. Like an abnormal digital rectal examination, a urinalysis that shows persistent red blood cells should prompt referral to a urologist for cystoscopic and upper urinary tract assessment. A urinalysis suggesting UTI should be followed up with a urine culture. If the patient presents in acute or chronic urinary retention and especially if there is a high postvoid or post-catheter residual bladder volume, a serum creatinine and blood urea nitrogen should be obtained. Severe BPH sometimes causes hydronephrosis and renal insufficiency, and rarely it causes renal failure. In-office bladder ultrasound scanners are very useful to quickly assess residual urine.

Contemporary diagnosis of BPH involves obtaining a PSA result. The latest guidelines from the American Urological Association (http://www.auanet.org) regarding the use of PSA testing are very helpful. Although the traditional upper limit of normal for

International Prostate Symptom Score (I-PSS)

Patient Name: _____ Date of birth: _____ Date completed _____

In the past month:	Not at all	Less than 1 in 5 times	Less than half the time	About half the time	More than half the time	Almost always	Your score
1. Incomplete emptying How often have you had the sensation of not emptying your bladder?	0	1	2	3	4	5	
2. Frequency How often have you had to urinate less than every two hours?	0	1	2	3	4	5	
3. Intermittency How often have you found you stopped and started again several times when you urinated?	0	1	2	3	4	5	
4. Urgency How often have you found it difficult to postpone urination?	0	1	2	3	4	5	
5. Weak stream How often have you had a weak urinary stream?	0	1	2	3	4	5	
6. Straining How often have you had to strain to start urination?	0	1	2	3	4	5	
	None	**1 Time**	**2 Times**	**3 Times**	**4 Times**	**5 Times**	
7. Nocturia How many times did you typically get up at night to urinate?	0	1	2	3	4	5	
Total I-PSS score							

Score   1–7: *Mild*   8–19: *Moderate*   20–35: *Severe*

Quality of life due to urinary symptoms	Delighted	Pleased	Mostly satisfied	Mixed	Mostly dissatisfied	Unhappy	Terrible
If you were to spend the rest of your life with your urinary condition just the way it is now, how would you feel about that?	0	1	2	3	4	5	6

Figure 1. International Prostate Symptom Score (IPSS) questionnaire. (Available from the Urological Sciences Research Foundation at http://www.usrf.org/questionnaires/AUA_SymptomScore.html [accessed August 29, 2014].)

PSA testing has been 4.0 ng/mL, recent guidelines base more on changes in PSA levels over time, considering that most men with BPH will have prior PSA results. In the specific setting of using PSA to help manage BPH, the best data come from the PLESS trial (Proscar Long-Term Efficacy and Safety Study), where a PSA of 0 to 1.3 ng/mL, 1.4 to 3.2 ng/mL, and greater than 3.2 ng/mL was associated with small, medium, and large prostate glands (assuming prostate cancer has been ruled out) and predicted therapeutic response to finasteride (Proscar) (see later section).

Treatment

Treatment of BPH is always individualized to the patient and involves evaluation of symptoms and bother along with objective findings from examination and laboratory results. Current treatments range from periodic monitoring without treatment to treatment of extreme cases with open enucleative surgery.

Active Surveillance and Watchful Waiting

For many men, especially those with lower symptom scores and little bother, annual monitoring with digital rectal examination, PSA, urinalysis and symptom assessment are all that is required. Many men are happy to be reassured that they do not have clinically significant prostate cancer and are glad to hear that no immediate treatment is necessary.

Complementary and Alternative Medicine

The use of complementary and alternative medicine supplements is very common and physicians should ask patients about their use just as they ask about prescription medications. There are now many "prostate" and "men's health" supplements containing a variety of chemicals that include zinc, saw palmetto, vitamin E,[1] vitamin

_____

[1]Not FDA approved for this indication.

D,[1] and selenium, among others. Aside from a few European clinical trials of saw palmetto, the use of supplements to help BPH is speculative. One challenge is quality assurance of dose and ingredients of these agents that are not FDA-regulated. Although not for BPH, the NIH-funded SELECT trial (Selenium and Vitamin E Cancer Prevention Trial) to determine whether vitamin E or selenium, or both, would prevent prostate cancer is illustrative. Neither supplement had any effect on prostate cancer (or BPH to my knowledge). With the lack of robust trial data for the plethora of supplements, the evidence-based medicine answer to patients is clear.

Medical Therapy
α-Blocker Medications
The use of α-adrenergic blocking oral agents to treat BPH has been commonplace since the 1980s. These agents are directed at the dynamic component of BPH and LUTS by relaxing the smooth muscle tissue in the bladder neck and prostate. In simple terms, they relax the bladder outlet, resulting in better urinary flow.

Initial agents, such as prazosin (Minipress),[1] were not selective blockers and were also used to treat hypertension. Furthermore, these early agents were not long-acting and had to be taken multiple times per day, which severely limited their practical clinical utility. The next generation in the class were doxazosin (Cardura) and terazosin (Hytrin), which were longer-acting agents only dosed once a day. However, they were not selective and also lowered blood pressure, so titration was necessary. The third and current generation agents are selective blockers that treat BPH but do not lower blood pressure when used at recommended doses. The three in this class are tamsulosin (Flomax), alfuzosin (Uroxatral), and silodosin (Rapaflo).

In general, clinicians use α-blockers in men with smaller prostate glands (≤30–35 g or cm^3), in younger men, and in patients where rapid effect is needed. Side effects of this class include headache, dizziness, asthenia, drowsiness, and retrograde ejaculation. Alfuzosin is reported to have the lowest rate of retrograde ejaculation. α-Blockers lower urinary tract muscular relaxation properties and are also now employed for ureteral urinary calculi (kidney stones) to facilitate spontaneous passage. α-Blockers are often used to treat prostatitis as well. In this setting, the agents can relieve dysfunctional voiding that contributes to some cases of prostatitis.

5α-Reductase Inhibitors
The 5α-reductase inhibitors have been available since the early 1990s. Finasteride (Proscar) was the first agent in this class (5 mg/daily) and is a type 1 inhibitor. Dutasteride (Avodart; 0.5 mg/daily) is a type 1 and type 2 inhibitor and was approved in 2002. Both drugs prevent the conversion of testosterone to the more active metabolite dihydrotestosterone in the prostate. This inhibition results in involution of BPH tissue and prostate shrinkage. On average, most men achieve 20% to 40% reduction in prostate size after at least 6 months of use. In general, these agents are most effective in men with prostate glands more than 30 g (or cm^3). Both drugs lower PSA levels by about 50% after 6 months of use. This is critical to take into account when screening for prostate cancer. If the PSA level does not fall by one half and the patient has been compliant with medication, the patient should be referred to a urologist for a work-up. In follow-up of men, PSA is generally doubled in assessing risk for prostate cancer. However, the use of PSA velocity or doubling-time and other prostate cancer screening tools are still valid as long as the effect on PSA is appreciated. There are two key clinical trials that are important. The MTOPS trial (Medical Therapy of Prostate Symptoms) showed that the combination of an α-blocker (doxazosin) and a 5α-reductase inhibitor (finasteride) was more effective than either alone or placebo in treatment of BPH and LUTS. The PCPT (Prostate Cancer Prevention Trial) showed that finasteride[1] lowered the rate of prostate cancer by 25% over placebo in a large 7-year study. Recently, the REDUCE trial (Reduction by Dutasteride of Prostate Cancer

Events) confirmed the prostate chemoprevention benefit of this class of drugs, showing that dutasteride[1] also lowered the rate of prostate cancer by 23% over placebo. In 2010 the FDA ruled that dutasteride would not be approved for prostate cancer prevention, citing safety concerns in this prevention setting. In 2013, the long term follow up of the PCPT showed that there was no excess mortality associated with long-term finasteride use compared to placebo, proving the long term safety of this therapy.

Urologists also use 5α-reductase inhibitors to treat chronic hematuria due to an enlarged prostate and sometimes prescribe these agents before transurethral resection of the prostate (TURP) to lessen surgical bleeding.

Minimally Invasive Procedures
Since the 1980s, a series of transurethral procedures have been evaluated to shrink or non-obstruct the prostate using heat, pressure, or direct pharmacotherapy. Balloon dilation of the prostate was the first to come and go as it was proved not to be durable. Then came microwave energy delivered either transurethrally (transurethral microwave thermotherapy [TUMT]) or via the rectum using transrectal ultrasound guidance. The microwaves create heat in the prostate gland, which can shrink the prostate and improve BPH and LUTS symptoms and flow rates. A number of these therapies are FDA approved; however, their popularity has waned a bit because long-term follow-up is lacking and results are thought not to be as durable as the gold standard TURP.

Heat energy to the prostate can also be delivered via radiofrequency energy in the form of the transurethral needle ablation (TUNA) procedure. A transurethral cystoscope-like device deploys several radiofrequency needles into the prostate to deliver the heat and shrinkage or cavitation effect. Clinical trials were also conducted with transurethral ethanol injection into the prostate to cause shrinkage; however, this therapy has yet to be FDA approved. High-intensity focused ultrasound (HIFU) is also used in some countries to treat prostate cancer, but it is not approved in the United States to treat cancer or BPH as of 2014.

Surgical Therapy
Surgical therapy for BPH was the mainstay of treatment until about 1990, when medical and minimally invasive treatments came on the scene. Currently, surgical therapy, mostly consisting of TURP, is generally reserved for men who fail medical or minimally invasive therapy or men who present with advanced or complicated BPH. The classic indications to proceed directly to TURP include bladder calculi, severe BPH causing renal insufficiency, or urinary retention in cases of severe BPH. It is also reasonable to proceed to TURP in the man who does not desire medical therapy.

A TURP has become safer in the era of improved fiberoptic and endoscopic equipment now employed by urologists. This new generation of equipment allows improved visualization during the operation, especially when combined with microchip endoscopic cameras and large flat-screen technology available in modern endoscopic suites. The removal of prostate tissue has traditionally been accomplished using resectoscopes equipped with electrocautery. Today, this tissue removal can be accomplished using new button electrodes and saline irrigation solution making TURP safer and more precise and efficient. In addition, lasers, such as the Green Light system, can be used to vaporize or enucleate the BPH tissue. The key as far as TURP technology is having a urologic surgeon that is experienced in his/her preferred technique. In other words, experience trumps one TURP technique over another and patients should not assume "laser" is necessarily better just because it is newer.

A variation of TURP is the transurethral incision of the prostate (TUIP). In this operation, the laser or resectoscope is used to make longitudinal cuts or incisions along the course of the prostate urethra from the bladder neck out to the apex of the prostate. This effective treatment can be used in men with smaller prostate glands who have significant LUTS.

---

[1]Not FDA approved for this indication.

---

[1]Not FDA approved for this indication.

Finally, for men with severe BPH and gland sizes 80 to 100 g/mL or more, open prostatectomy is still a valuable and highly effective surgical treatment. A small suprapubic incision is used to remove the prostate adenoma. As with radical prostatectomy used for prostate cancer, open prostatectomy for BPH should be performed by urologic surgeons who are experienced in this area.

References

Barkin J. Benign prostatic hyperplasia and lower urinary tract symptoms: evidence and approaches for best case management. Can J Urol 2011;(18 Suppl):14–9.

Biester K, Skipka G, Jahn R, et al. Systematic review of surgical treatments for benign prostatic hyperplasia and presentation of an approach to investigate therapeutic equivalence (non-inferiority). BJU Int 2012;109:722–30.

Chughtai B, Te A. Photoselective vaporization of the prostate for treating benign prostatic hyperplasia. Expert Rev Med Devices 2011;8:591–5.

Djavan B, Kazzazi A, Bostanci Y. Revival of thermotherapy for benign prostatic hyperplasia. Curr Opin Urol 2012;22:16–21.

Gravas S, Bachmann A, Reich O, et al. Critical review of lasers in benign prostatic hyperplasia (BPH). BJU Int 2011;107:1030–43.

Lepor H, Kazzazi A, Djavan B. α-Blockers for benign prostatic hyperplasia: the new era. Curr Opin Urol 2012;22:7–15.

Nicholson TM, Ricke WA. Androgens and estrogens in benign prostatic hyperplasia: past, present and future. Differentiation 2011;82:184–99.

Slater S, Dumas C, Bubley G. Dutasteride for the treatment of prostate-related conditions. Expert Opin Drug Saf 2012;11:325–30.

EPIDIDYMITIS

Method of
Robin A. Walker, MD

CURRENT DIAGNOSIS

- Subacute or gradual onset of scrotal pain and swelling that occasionally radiates to lower abdomen. Typically unilateral; however, inflammation can spread to opposite testicle.
- Fever and urinary tract symptoms (e.g., dysuria, frequency, urgency, hematuria) may be present
- Testicle should be in normal position with cremasteric reflex intact (rule out torsion).
- Pain is relieved by elevation of testicle (Prehn sign).
- Ultrasound with Doppler is readily available and has high sensitivity and specificity for ruling out testicular torsion; however, referral to urology should not be delayed if torsion is suspected.
- Urinalysis should be obtained, preferably on first-void urine.
- Send urine for culture, especially when sexually transmitted disease (STD) is not suspected.
- Nucleic acid amplification assays for Gonorrhea and Chlamydia can be run on urine or urethral specimens.

CURRENT THERAPY

- Sexually active men 14 to 35 years old: ceftriaxone (Rocephin) 250 mg IM once and doxycycline (Vibromycin) 100 mg twice daily for 10 days. Azithromycin (Zithromax) 1 g PO for one dose may be substituted for doxycycline if compliance is questionable.
- Oral cephalosporins and fluoroquinolones are no longer recommended for gonococcal infections.
- For older men or when enteric organisms are thought to be the most likely cause: levofloxacin (Levaquin) 500 mg orally twice daily for 10 days, or ofloxacin (Floxin) 300 mg orally twice daily for 10 days.
- Cultures, if obtained, should be followed and treatment adjusted accordingly.

- Patients should follow up in 2 to 3 days. Pain should improve in 1 to 3 days with treatment. Failure to improve should elicit reevaluation of the diagnosis and therapy, and consideration should be given to other causes such as a testicular tumor/cancer, abscess, infarction, and tuberculosis (TB) or fungal pathogens.
- Sexual partners should be referred for evaluation and treatment if there was intercourse in the preceding 60 days from onset of symptoms.
- Education should occur regarding prevention of STDs.

Epidemiology

Epididymitis is most common in males 18 to 35 years of age, but can occur in all ages. There are approximately 600,000 cases per year in the United States and these accounted for 1 in 144 outpatient visits in men (2002 data).

In men 35 years of age or younger who are sexually active, the most common pathogens are *Chlamydia trachomatis* and *Neisseria gonorrhoeae*. In those older than 35, the cause is most likely urinary tract pathogens such as *Escherichia coli*. In men who perform insertive anal intercourse, coliform bacteria are common causative agents. Other less common pathogens include TB, fungal infections, and viruses. Cytomegalovirus has been identified as a cause in HIV patients.

In boys ages 2 to 13 the incidence is approximately 1.2 per 1000 and is most commonly a postinfectious inflammatory reaction to pathogens such as enteroviruses, adenoviruses, and mycoplasma pneumonia. If a bacterial pathogen is isolated, a urologic workup for any anatomic abnormalities is warranted.

Other uncommon noninfectious causes include vasculitides and medications such as amiodarone (Pacerone).

Risk Factors

The predominant risk factor for epididymitis is unprotected sexual intercourse. Additionally, trauma from strenuous physical activity, bicycle or motorcycle riding, and prolonged sitting can predispose to epididymitis. Risk factors in prepubertal boys and men over age 35 are related to anatomic abnormalities (e.g., prostatic obstruction, posterior urethral valves, meatal stenosis), recent instrumentation, or urogenital tract surgery (e.g., vasectomy). In prepubertal boys, recent infections can predispose to a postinfectious inflammatory reaction in the epididymis.

Pathophysiology

Infective epididymitis is usually caused by retrograde ascent of pathogens, most commonly bacterial. Noninfectious epididymitis can be autoimmune or can be associated with known syndromes (e.g., Behçet's disease) or a side effect of medications, most notably amiodarone (Pacerone). If symptoms last longer than 3 months, the patient meets the diagnostic criteria for chronic epididymitis.

Clinical Manifestations

The typical presentation is subacute onset of unilateral scrotal pain. Any acute onset of pain requires careful consideration of possible testicular torsion. The pain in epididymitis can radiate to the lower abdomen. Fever and urinary tract symptoms such as increased frequency, dysuria, and hematuria are frequently present. The cremasteric reflex is preserved and the testicle should be in its normal anatomic position. The epididymis is tender, swollen, and often indurated. Pain is relieved on testicular elevation (Prehn sign). Over time, scrotal wall erythema and a reactive hydrocele may appear and infection can spread from the epididymis to the testicle (orchitis), as well as to the opposite testicle.

Epididymitis secondary to noninfectious causes tends to have a more gradual onset of symptoms.

Diagnosis

Diagnosis can be made by a careful history and physical examination; however, laboratory testing can help confirm epididymitis. Urine should be obtained for analysis and culture, preferably from a first-void sample. The presence of leukocyte esterase and 10 or more white blood cells (WBCs) per high-power field is suggestive for urethritis, helping to differentiate from testicular torsion.

Nucleic acid amplification tests for *N. gonorrhoeae* and *C. trachomatis* should be run on all sexually active men 35 years of age or younger, and those over 35 who are at increased risk. These can be run on urine or urethral samples. A Gram stain of urethral discharge should demonstrate 5 or more WBCs per high-power field. Gonococcal infection is established by the presence of WBCs containing intracellular gram-negative diplococci. Depending on risks, consideration should be given to testing for the presence of other STDs.

Color Doppler ultrasound is a readily available study with a sensitivity and specificity for testicular torsion ranging between 89% and 100%. However, imaging should not delay immediate referral to a specialist if torsion is clinically suspected.

Differential Diagnosis

- Testicular torsion: duration less than 6 hours, absence of cremasteric reflex, diffuse testicular tenderness. Elevation of the testis usually exacerbates discomfort.
- Orchitis: testicular tenderness and swelling, normal cremasteric reflex.

Therapy/Treatment

In sexually active men ages 14 to 35, empiric treatment should be started for suspected epididymitis before laboratory results are available. The current recommended regimen is ceftriaxone (Rocephin) 250 mg IM once plus doxycycline (Vibromycin) 100 mg orally twice daily for 10 days. If compliance is questionable or the patient is allergic to doxycycline, azithromycin (Zithromax) 1 g orally once can be substituted. The Centers for Disease Control and Prevention (CDC) no longer recommends fluoroquinolones or oral cephalosporins for the treatment of gonococcal infections.

For men 35 years of age or older, and when coliform pathogen is suspected, treatment consists of levofloxacin (Levaquin) 500 mg orally for 10 days or ofloxacin (Floxin) 300 mg orally twice daily for 10 days.

Most patients can be treated in the outpatient setting. Inpatient treatment is recommended for suspicion of abscess, intractable pain, signs of sepsis, or failure of outpatient care. Symptomatic care consists of pain control with supportive garments, analgesics, rest, and cold packs.

Complications

Complications include sepsis, abscess formation, extension of infection, and infertility.

References

Centers for Disease Control and Prevention. Sexually transmitted diseases treatment guidelines; 2010. Available at http://www.cdc.gov/std/treatment/2010/epididymitis.htm[accessed 09.08.14].

Centers for Disease Control and Prevention. Update to CDC's sexually transmitted diseases treatment guidelines, 2010: oral cephalosporins no longer recommended treatment for gonococcal infections. MMWR Morb Mortal Wkly Rep 2012;61:590–4.

Centers for Disease Control and Prevention. Update to CDC's sexually transmitted diseases treatment guidelines, 2006: fluoroquinolones no longer recommended for treatment of gonococcal infections. MMWR Morb Mortal Wkly Rep 2007;56:332–6.

Remer EM, Casalino DD, Arellano RS, et al. ACR appropriateness criteria: acute onset of scrotal pain—without trauma, without antecedent mass. Ultrasound Q. 2012;28:47–51.

Trojian TH, Lishnak TS, Meiman D. Epididymitis and orchitis: an overview. Am Fam Physician 2009;79:583–7.

ERECTILE DYSFUNCTION

Method of
Maurice Duggins, MD

The 1992 National Institutes of Health (NIH) Consensus Development Conference on Impotence defined *erectile dysfunction* (ED) as "any male patient with an inability to achieve an erect penis as part of the overall multifaceted process of male sexual function." Compared to the previous term of *impotence*, the NIH definition is more descriptive, more inclusive, and less pejorative. Impotence suggests that a man is unable to perform sexually, whereas ED allows for better understanding of the varying degrees of sexual dysfunction that can result in ED. The NIH conference also highlighted that many men with ED were not diagnosed, probably because of embarrassment in discussing the issue. In the decades since the consensus conference, widespread advertising of ED therapies has encouraged more men to discuss ED with their physicians.

Epidemiology

According to the most recent survey, about 18 million men in the United States over age 20 are affected by ED. The prevalence ranges from 20% to above 50% with increasing age. The prevalence is also increased threefold in men with diabetes. Because not all patients report ED or seek therapy, the true prevalence may be significantly higher. A large study in which family physicians screened for and investigated ED symptoms found that nearly half of male patients over 40 had problems, with the prevalence strongly linked to age, diabetes, and cardiovascular disease. According to current estimates, over 152 million men worldwide experience ED. This estimate is projected to reach over 300 million by 2035 and may be even higher due to increasing levels of diabetes and obesity.

In about 80% of patients, an organic cause can be identified for ED. The remaining 20% are attributed to psychogenic causes. Although traditionally organic and psychogenic have been regarded as distinct types of ED, cases with organic causes are often confounded by psychogenic factors.

Besides the personal and emotional burden, ED is one of the most costly urologic conditions. Treatment costs in the United States are estimated at $328 million annually. Even with insurance, a patient may spend from $119 to $30,000 for ED therapy in 1 year.

Risk Factors

Risk factors for ED include age, cardiovascular disease, diabetes, psychiatric disorders, unhealthy lifestyle choices, low education level, and pelvic trauma or surgery. Many men have multiple risk factors. As men age, libido decreases, probably due to decline in testosterone levels. Cardiovascular diseases encompass vascular damage associated with diabetes, hypertension, coronary heart disease, and dyslipidemia. Any history of psychological or psychiatric problems including depression, anxiety, sexual abuse, or stress predisposes to developing ED. Endocrine conditions also indicate potential risk for ED. Thyroid or gonadal diseases put men at especially high risk. Lifestyle choices associated with ED include being sedentary, obese, smoking, and abuse of either illicit substances (e.g., cocaine) or alcohol. Lower education levels are also associated with higher prevalence of ED. The correlation between ED and surgery or trauma to the pelvis is not surprising. Patients undergoing pelvic or prostatic radiation, transurethral resection of the prostate (TURP), or radical prostatectomy are at increased risk for ED.

Pathophysiology

Sexual performance in men has four stages: libido (desire), erection (arousal or engorgement), ejaculation, and detumescence. Problems in any stage can result in male sexual dysfunction. The basic mechanical or primary focus of erectile dysfunction is in stage 2. Erection is a complex neuroendocrine psychophysiological event. Erection can occur during sleep, indicating that sexual stimulation is not required.

Nitric oxide (NO) is essential for erection. The release of NO in the cells of the corpus cavernosa following parasympathetic stimulation leads to the conversion of guanylate cyclase to cyclic guanosine monophosphate (cGMP). This causes smooth muscle relaxation that permits the influx of blood causing engorgement of the penis. This mechanism also slows the outflow of venous blood from the penis thus enhancing penile engorgement. Other contributors to vasodilation during erection include vasoactive intestinal peptide (VIP) and prostaglandins E1 and E2 (PGE1 and PGE2).

Prevention

The prevention of ED is mainly directed at modifying risk factors. Patients should be encouraged to quit smoking to reduce vascular damage. Regular exercise, weight management, reducing or stopping alcohol, and abstaining from illicit drugs are important in preventing ED. Family physicians can review medications to identify those with potential to induce ED. Similarly, family physicians can work with patients to identify and manage psychological, hormonal, or neurologic conditions associated with ED.

Clinical Manifestation

Not all men readily admit to ED. Some patients assume that sexual dysfunction is part of the aging process. Others may be embarrassed by the topic. It is important for physicians to anticipate and proactively ask about ED, especially in men with risk factors. In addition to medical conditions such as hypertension, diabetes, or depression, men dealing with difficult personal relationships or major life stresses such as divorce, illness of spouse or partner, bereavement, or work-related stress should be asked about sexual function and ED.

Diagnosis

Establishing the diagnosis of ED begins with a comprehensive history and physical examination. The patient should be asked about risk factors as well as any sexual concerns. The interview must be open, welcoming, and nonjudgmental. Sexual problems can be identified and documented using validated questionnaires such as the International Index of Erectile Function Questionnaire (IIEF), the Sexual Encounter Profile (SEP), or the Global Assessment Questions (GAQ). Though these tools are helpful, they are not necessary to make the diagnosis. Their usefulness may be noted when assessing the patient's response to therapy. A history of sudden, situational, or complete immediate loss of erection during sexual activity (but otherwise experiencing normal erections while awake) may indicate a psychogenic source. Conversely, gradual onset of poor or absent erections suggests an organic cause of ED. The history should address symptoms of conditions associated with ED, especially diabetes, hypertension, cardiovascular disease, and depression or other psychological problems. Medications should be reviewed.

The physical examination should include the genitalia and the cardiac, vascular, endocrine, and neurologic systems. Any anatomic anomaly may be significant. The testicles, penis, and prostate should be palpated and any atrophy or abnormality noted. The cardiovascular examination should document any findings of heart failure or problems in perfusion.

Differential Diagnosis

Erectile dysfunction may be primary or a manifestation of another medical problem. Endocrinopathies such as hypogonadism, thyroid disorders, and hyperprolactinemia must be ruled out. Drug abuse, alcoholism, renal disease, spinal cord injury, multiple sclerosis, and prostate diseases may all masquerade as ED. Stress-related conditions and sleeping disorders such as sleep apnea should be considered. The condition may also be an adverse effect of medication.

Therapy

In addition to modifying risk factors and any exacerbating conditions, several strategies are available to treat ED. The principal current options are behavioral therapy, medication, hormone replacement or supplement, assistive devices, and surgery.

Phosphodiesterase type 5 (PDE5) inhibitor medications have become the most reliable and acceptable oral therapy for treating ED. This class of medication includes sildenafil (Viagra), vardenafil (Levitra), and tadalafil (Cialis). The mechanism of action is identical but the drugs differ in pharmacokinetic properties. Both sildenafil and vardenafil have an action window of 4 to 6 hours whereas tadalafil is effective for up to 36 hours. The common adverse effects with this group of medications are limited to brief headache, flushing, dyspepsia, rhinitis, and vision changes. They are contraindicated with the use of nitrates. Because the onset of action varies with PDE5 inhibitors, they should be taken on an empty stomach at least 1 hour before sexual activity. Trazodone (Desyrel)[1] may be helpful in men whose ED has significant depression/anxiety basis. Yohimbine[7] has fallen out of favor because of its low level of predictable erection response coupled with its adverse side effects.

Testosterone replacement is most appropriately used in hypogonadal patients, but may enhance other therapy in men with ED. The oral formulation is not highly recommended or used in the United States. Gels, patches, and injections are preferred methods of administering testosterone. Testosterone may be used with PDE5 inhibitors. Potential adverse effects include exacerbation of sleep apnea, prostatic hyperplasia, and the unmasking of occult prostate cancer. Care must also be given to avoiding gel-skin contact with women and children. Testosterone should never be used in men with breast or prostate cancer.

Other medications are administered as injectable or intraurethral suppositories. Alprostadil (Caverject), papaverine,[1] vasoactive intestinal polypeptide (VIP),[5] and phentolamine[1] began as individual penile injections and evolved into combination injections over time. These are usually given initially by a urologist to quantify the optimal safe dose that is required for a full erection. The lowest effective dose is the goal of titration.

Vacuum-assisted devices are effective and have the benefit of being considered the most cost-effective therapy for ED. They are not, however, convenient or acceptable for some patients and/or their sexual partners. These devices draw blood into the penis and then maintain the erection with the use of a special constrictive band placed at the base of the penis to prevent the blood from leaving the penis. These devices should never be used in patients with blood dyscrasias or sickle cell anemia.

Surgical therapies are mainly limited to correction of a traumatic penile injury, repair of Peyronie's deformity or other abnormality, or prosthesis insertion. Some surgical interventions attempt arterial revascularization. Procedures for venous revascularization are considered experimental therapy for ED. Prostheses can be rigid, malleable, or inflatable. They are mostly inserted as a final and permanent treatment for ED.

No therapy for ED is complete without counseling. This may be limited to a physician-patient discussion on appropriate and responsible use of therapy plus self-education or physician-directed readings on ED; however, referral to a psychiatrist and/or psychologist may be appropriate. Psychosexual counseling in addition to medication has being shown to benefit patients suffering from ED and should be seen as an integrative part of overall therapy.

Complementary and alternative therapies do not have enough data to support recommendation at this stage. Many treatments are promoted as nutritional cures and have not been scientifically evaluated or have insufficient evidence to support use. Ginkgo biloba,[7] ginseng,[7] human chorionic gonadotropin (HCG),[7] and L-arginine[7] are some of the popular supplements advertised for ED. Patient should be asked about use of these therapies, and those patients who choose to continue use should be monitored for adverse effects and potential drug-drug interactions.

Monitoring

Monitoring is based on patient needs and the therapy selected. The PDE5 inhibitors may only need routine follow-up to assess efficacy and to make dosage adjustments. Warning and education on appropriate response to priapism should be discussed with the patient. Signs of hemodynamic changes should also be reviewed such as dizziness, arrhythmias, tachycardia, or syncope. These occur less often with PDE5 inhibitors and most commonly with

---

[1]Not FDA approved for this indication.
[5]Investigational drug in the United States.
[7]Available as dietary supplement.

injectable therapies. Patients taking testosterone replacement need annual prostate examinations and blood testing to monitor hormone, liver enzymes, hemoglobin, and prostate-specific antigen (PSA) levels. The frequency of testing should be increased for those patients at higher risk for prostate cancer such as African Americans and those with a family history of prostate cancer.

Complications

Complications from ED and its treatment must always be considered and appropriately addressed. They include depression, anxiety, schizoid behavior, and deviant or violent behavior. Sildenafil can cause a blue or green halo visual effect. Musculoskeletal pain is a common side effect of vardenifil and tadalafil. The PDE5 inhibitors should never be taken with nitrates or other vasodilators because severe or fatal hypotensive response may occur. Priapism may result from any of the medicated forms of therapy. Hormonal replacement therapy can lead to elevated liver enzymes, exacerbation of sleep apnea, and either prostatic hypertrophy or enhanced growth of prostate cancer. Pain, hematomas, or plaques may occur as a result of penile injections. Topical agents can cause skin irritation, urethral bleeding, or dysuria. ED has a significant effect on patients' families, self-esteem, and quality of life; therefore patients, their partners, and family members should be treated with respect and compassion.

References

American Urological Association. The management of erectile dysfunction: an update; June 2007. Available at http://www.auanet.org/common/pdf/education/clinical-guidance/Erectile-Dysfunction.pdf.

Burnett AL. Evaluation and management of erectile dysfunction. In: Wein AJ, Kavoussi LR, Novick AC, Partin AW, editors. Campbell-Walsh Urology. 10th ed. Philadelphia: Saunders Elsevier; 2010. p. 721–48.

Carroll P, Albertsen PC, Greene K, et al. Prostate-specific antigen best practice statement: 2009 update. American Urological Association Education and Research; 2009. Available at www.auanet.org.

Chew K, Bremmer A, Jamrozik K. Male erectile dysfunction and cardiovascular disease: is there an intimate nexus? J Sex Med 2008;5:928–34.

Feldman H, Goldstein I, Hatzichristou D, et al. Impotence and its medical and psychosocial correlates: results of the Massachusetts male ageing study. J Urol 1994;151:54–61.

Goldstein I. Screening for erectile dysfunction: rationale. Int J Impot Res 2000;12 (Suppl 4):S147–S151.

Grover S, Lowensteyn I, Mohammed K, et al. The prevalence of erectile dysfunction in the primary care setting. Arch Intern Med 2006;166:213–9.

Heidelbaugh JJ. Management of erectile dysfunction. Am Fam Physician 2010;81:305–12.

Jackson G, Rosen RC, Kloner RA, et al. The second Princeton consensus on sexual dysfunction and cardiac risk: New guidelines for sexual medicine. J Sex Med 2006;3:28.

Johannes CB, Araujo AB, Feldman HA, et al. Incidence of erectile dysfunction in men 40 to 69 years old: longitudinal results from the Massachusetts male aging study. J Urol 2000;163:460.

Miller T. Diagnostic evaluation of erectile dysfunction. Am Fam Physician 2000;61:95–104.

NIH Consensus Development Panel on Impotence. NIH consensus conference: importance. J Am Med Assoc 1993;270:83–90.

Rosen R, Leiblum S, Spector I. Psychologically based treatment for male erectile disorder: a cognitive-interpersonal model. J Sex Marital Ther. 1994;20:67–85.

Saigal C, Wessells H, Pace J, et al. Predictors and prevalence of erectile dysfunction in a racially diverse population. Arch. Intern. Med. 2006;166:207.

Selvin E, Burnett AL, Platz EA. Prevalence and risk factors for erectile dysfunction in the US. Am J Med 2007;120:151–7.

PROSTATITIS

Method of
Charles R. Powell, MD

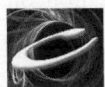

CURRENT DIAGNOSIS

- The workup for prostatitis begins with a thorough history and physical as well as a urinalysis and urine culture. Diagnosis is based on symptoms (Figure 1) and tenderness on digital rectal examination.
- Urinalysis and midstream urine culture are important to distinguish bacterial from nonbacterial causes, but are not necessary for the diagnosis of prostatitis.
- Prostatitis is categorized as acute or chronic. It has been further characterized by the National Institutes of Health (NIH) into four categories: acute bacterial, chronic bacterial, chronic pelvic pain syndrome (also called chronic nonbacterial prostatitis), and asymptomatic (Table 1).
- Chronic prostatitis is defined as duration longer than 3 months and typically manifests with pelvic pain and lower urinary tract symptoms.

Urinary retention (feelings of incomplete voiding)
Straining to void
Urinary hesitancy
Urinary intermittency (interrupted stream)

Sepsis (hypotension, tachycardia)
Fevers
Malaise
Nausea, vomiting

Pain on sitting for long periods
Pain shooting to the tip of the penis
Pain with defecation
Pain with ejaculation
Dysuria

Prostatitis

Figure 1. Symptoms associated with prostatitis.

TABLE 1 National Institutes of Health Consensus Classification of Prostatitis

CATEGORY	DESCRIPTION
I. Acute bacterial prostatitis	Acute infection of the prostate gland with positive urine or semen cultures. Symptoms present for less than 3 months.
II. Chronic bacterial prostatitis	Chronic infection of the prostate gland with positive urine or semen cultures. Symptoms present for greater than 3 months.
III. Chronic pelvic pain syndrome	Chronic pelvic pain in the absence of bacterial infection localized to the prostate. Symptoms present for greater than 3 months.
A. Inflammatory	Significant white blood cell (WBC) count in the prostatic secretions, urine, or semen.
B. Noninflammatory	Insignificant WBC count in the prostatic secretions, urine, or semen.
IV. Asymptomatic prostatitis	WBC count elevated and/or bacteria in the prostatic secretions, urine, semen, or histologic specimens of prostate tissue.

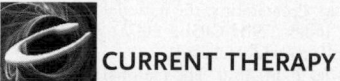

CURRENT THERAPY

- Fluoroquinolone antibiotics are first-line therapy for acute and chronic bacterial prostatitis.
- Trimethoprim/sulfamethoxazole (Bactrim)[1] can be considered first-line therapy, but local antibiotic resistance patterns should be considered before empiric treatment.
- First-generation cephalosporins, doxycycline (Vibramycin), tetracycline, azithromycin (Zithromax),[1] and clarithromycin (Biaxin)[1] are all second-line agents.
- Acute prostatitis may require inpatient admission and intravenous (IV) antibiotics depending on severity and presence of sepsis. Urinary retention may require suprapubic tube urinary drainage because a Foley catheter may worsen prostate inflammation.
- The role of antibiotics in the treatment of chronic pelvic pain syndrome is less clear. Treatment directed at specific phenotypes has improved outcomes recently.

[1]Not FDA approved for this indication.

Epidemiology

The prevalence of prostatitis is approximately 8.2% (range 2.2%–9.7%). It accounts for 8% of visits to urologists and up to 1% of visits to primary care physicians. In 2000, the estimated cost to diagnose and treat prostatitis was $84 million, not including pharmaceutical spending.

Risk Factors

The risk factors for prostatitis include urinary tract infection, elevated postvoid residual (urinary retention), recent history of prostate biopsy, urinary catheterization, unprotected anal intercourse, recent urethral instrumentation such as cystoscopy, and condom catheter use.

Pathophysiology

The causes for acute and chronic bacterial prostatitis include prior genitourinary infections such as epididymitis/orchitis, infection resulting from prostate needle biopsy, and recent urinary tract infection. Other predisposing factors include obstruction of urine from urethral stricture, benign prostatic hypertrophy (BPH), or neurogenic causes. The causative organisms include *Escherichia coli* (most common at 65%–80% of infections), *Pseudomonas aeruginosa*, *Serratia* species, *Klebsiella* species, and *Enterobacter aerogenes*. Gram-positive organisms include enterococci. Organisms isolated from patients with recent history of lower urinary tract instrumentation or manipulation exhibit more resistance to ciprofloxacin (Cipro) and cephalosporins. For these patients ciprofloxacin is often inadequate. A combination of cephalosporins and aminoglycosides is appropriate. Patients with a history of HIV infection should prompt investigation for atypical pathogens. The cause of chronic pelvic pain syndrome/chronic nonbacterial prostatitis (NIH category 3) is less well understood, as is asymptomatic prostatitis (NIH category 4).

Prevention

Prophylactic antibiotic dose before urologic procedures, particularly prostate needle biopsy, according to the American Urological Association Best Practice Statement for Urologic Surgery (http://www.auanet.org).

Clinical Manifestations

Figure 1 details some symptoms of prostatitis, separated by domain.

Diagnosis

Diagnosis of acute and chronic bacterial prostatitis is primarily based on history, physical examination, urine culture, and urine specimen testing before and after prostatic massage. If acute bacterial prostatitis is suspected prostatic massage should not be performed because this might be harmful. Sexually active men younger than 35 years and older men who engage in high-risk sexual behaviors should be tested for *Neisseria* gonococcus and *Chlamydia trachomatis* as well. The presence of leukocytes in the semen, first voided urine, midstream urine, expressed prostatic secretions, or post–prostatic massage urine did not correlate with symptoms when studied in a prospective manner. Bacterial localization studies, such as the Meares-Stamey four-glass test, are useful in subcategorizing type 3 chronic pelvic pain syndrome but have unclear significance in the acute clinical setting.

Differential Diagnosis

The differential diagnosis of prostatitis includes acute cystitis, benign prostatic hyperplasia, prostate cancer, urinary tract stones, bladder cancer, prostatic abscess, enterovesical fistula, foreign body within the urinary tract, voiding dysfunction, and inflammatory conditions of the bladder such as interstitial cystitis/painful bladder syndrome.

Therapy (or Treatment)

Treatment depends on the NIH Prostatitis Classification Category. For those with acute prostatitis, oral ciprofloxacin (Cipro)[1] 500 mg orally twice daily for 4 to 6 weeks or levofloxacin (Levaquin)[1] 500 mg orally once daily for 4 to 6 weeks is appropriate for nonseptic-appearing patients. Trimethoprim/sulfamethoxazole (Bactrim, Septra)[1] 160 mg/800 mg orally twice daily for 4 to 6 weeks is also appropriate, depending on local antibiotic resistance patterns. Patients appearing septic (hypotension, tachycardia, high fevers) should be admitted to the hospital and started on broad-spectrum antibiotics such as ampicillin (Principen) 2 g IV every 6 hours and an aminoglycoside such as gentamicin 1 mg/kg IV every 8 hours. Aminoglycosides should be monitored and adjusted for azotemia. Prostatic abscess should be considered if patients do not improve within 24 to 48 hours. Prostatic abscesses are urologic emergencies and can be drained with transurethral resection of the prostate, transrectal ultrasound drainage, or computed tomography (CT)–guided needle drainage. Urinary retention should be treated with suprapubic catheter drainage in cases of acute prostatitis and alpha blockers. Chronic bacterial prostatitis is treated with the same oral agents as acute bacterial prostatitis. For the treatment of chronic pelvic pain syndrome antibiotics play a less clear role, but fluoroquinolone antibiotics used empirically for 4 to 6 weeks have been effective in previously untreated patients. There is little value to repeated courses of antibiotics if the first course is not effective. There is conflicting evidence for alpha blockers such as tamsulosin (Flomax 0.4 mg orally once per night).[1] The interested reader is referred to a review article by Nickel and Shoskes (2010), wherein a multidisciplinary approach is advocated taking into account a more detailed six-domain phenotype with therapy directed at the relevant phenotype(s).

Monitoring

Monitoring is based on symptoms. In cases of acute prostatitis treated with appropriate antibiotics, persistent fevers should prompt a workup for prostatic abscess. The NIH Chronic Prostatitis Symptom Index (CPSI) patient-reported questionnaire can be used to quantify symptoms over time. It is available online at http://www.prostatitis.org/symptomindex.html.

[1]Not FDA approved for this indication.

Complications

Acute prostatitis can progress to urosepsis and hypotension. Chronic bacterial prostatitis might have the ability to progress to chronic pelvic pain syndrome and become a source of pain for years.

References

Collins MM, Stafford RS, O'Leary MP, et al. How common is prostatitis? A national survey of physician visits. J Urol 1998;159:1224–8.

Ha US, Kim ME, Kim CS, et al. Acute bacterial prostatis in korea: clinical outcome, including symptoms, management, microbiology and course of disease. Int J Antimicrob Agents 2008;31(Suppl 1):S96–S101.

Krieger JN, Lee SW, Jeon J, et al. Epidemiology of prostatitis. Int J Antimicrob Agents 2008;31(Suppl 1):S85–S90.

Litwin MMC, Fowler Jr F, Nickel JC, et al. Prostatatitis: the national institutes of health chronic prostatitis symptoms index (NIH-CPSI); 2002. Available at http://www.prostatitis.org/nih-cpsi.html[accessed 26.12.12].

Litwin MS, McNaughton-Collins M, Fowler Jr FJ, et al. The national institutes of health chronic prostatitis symptom index: development and validation of a new outcome measure. Chronic Prostatitis Collaborative Research Network. J Urol 1999;162:369–75.

Nickel JC, Shoskes DA. Phenotypic approach to the management of the chronic prostatitis/chronic pelvic pain syndrome. BJU Int 2010;106:1252–63.

Pontari MA, Joyce GF, Wise M, et al. Prostatitis. J Urol 2007;177:2050–7.

Schaeffer AJ, Knauss JS, Landis JR, et al. Leukocyte and bacterial counts do not correlate with severity of symptoms in men with chronic prostatitis: the national institutes of health chronic prostatitis cohort study. J Urol 2002;168:1048–53.

Sharp VJ, Takacs EB, Powell CR. Prostatitis: diagnosis and treatment. Am Fam Physician 2010;82:397–406.

Wolf JSB, Carol J, Dmochowski RR, et al. Urologic surgery antimicrobial prophylaxis. Transrectal prostate biopsy; 2008. Available at http://www.auanet.org/content/media/antimicroprop08.pdf [accessed 29.08.14].

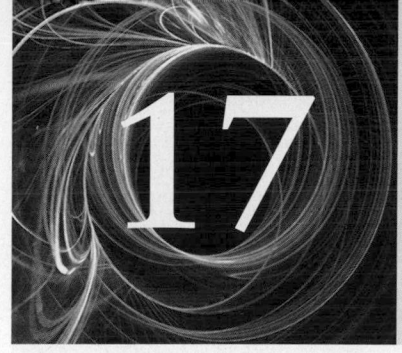

17 Women's Health

ABNORMAL UTERINE BLEEDING

Method of
Sarina Schrager, MD, MS

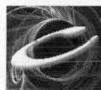

CURRENT DIAGNOSIS

- Anovulation and pelvic structural abnormalities are the most common causes of abnormal vaginal bleeding in reproductive-age women.
- All women with abnormal bleeding should have a pregnancy test.
- A pelvic ultrasound will detect many structural causes of abnormal bleeding.
- Either a pelvic ultrasound or endometrial biopsy is appropriate for evaluation of postmenopausal bleeding.

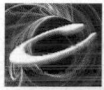

CURRENT THERAPY

- Unstable women with acute heavy vaginal bleeding should be admitted to hospital for intravenous (IV) estrogen therapy (Premarin) or surgical intervention.
- Treatment of anovulatory bleeding includes ovulation induction if a woman desires pregnancy and hormonal cycle control if she does not.
- Anovulatory women are at risk for endometrial hyperplasia or carcinoma due to unopposed estrogen and should have regular progesterone-induced withdrawal bleeds.
- Treatment of menorrhagia can include nonsteroidal anti-inflammatory drugs (NSAIDs), tranexamic acid (Lysteda), or insertion of a levonorgestrel intrauterine device (IUD) (Mirena).

Epidemiology

Abnormal vaginal bleeding is a common complaint in primary care. The prevalence of some type of abnormal bleeding is between 10% and 30% among women of reproductive age. Anovulatory bleeding is more common in women who are perimenopausal and who are overweight. The estimated direct and indirect costs of abnormal bleeding are $1 billion and $12 billion annually, respectively. Abnormal bleeding is also a common reason for women to be referred to gynecologists and is an indication for up to 25% of all gynecologic surgery.

Pathophysiology

Normal menstrual bleeding is defined as regular vaginal bleeding that occurs at intervals from every 21 to 35 days. A normal menstrual cycle is ovulatory, with two distinct phases: the follicular phase and the luteal phase. The follicular phase is the first half of the cycle. The luteal phase occurs after ovulation, when the corpus luteum develops in anticipation of a possible pregnancy. Table 1 defines vocabulary to describe different patterns of abnormal bleeding.

The pathologic abnormality in anovulatory cycles is a lack of ovulation, which produces an unopposed estrogen state. The luteal phase of the menstrual cycle is dominated by progesterone, which is only produced after ovulation. This lack of progesterone contributes to irregular endometrial growth and nonuniform bleeding. In a normal cycle, the entire endometrium sloughs off during menstruation. In an anovulatory cycle, different sections of endometrium outgrow their blood supply at different times and bleed erratically. Anovulatory bleeding (also referred to as dysfunctional uterine bleeding) is unpredictable in timing and amount of bleeding.

The most common structural abnormalities that cause abnormal bleeding are endometrial polyps, leiomyomas, adenomyosis, and hyperplasia or malignancy.

Abnormal bleeding is also common in women who use hormonal contraception, usually due to endometrial abnormalities from exogenous hormones. Women who take combination estrogen/progestin contraception often have intermenstrual bleeding for the first 3 months of treatment. Missed pills are a very frequent cause of abnormal bleeding. In women using progestin-only methods, the abnormal bleeding usually is caused by progestin-induced endometrial atrophy.

Diagnosis

All women with abnormal bleeding should have a thorough history and physical examination and a pregnancy test. If the pregnancy test is negative, the next step is to determine whether her cycles are ovulatory or anovulatory. Table 2 describes characteristics of ovulatory cycles. Laboratory evaluation includes looking for causes of anovulation (Table 3), assessing for anemia with a hemoglobin and hematocrit level, and consideration of getting a pelvic ultrasound to look for structural abnormalities.

In menorrhagia, evaluation for a coagulation disorder (most commonly von Willebrand disease), liver failure, or chronic renal failure is also indicated. Evaluation in an acute bleeding episode (usually due to anovulatory bleeding) should include a hemoglobin and hematocrit if the bleeding is heavy, assessment of volume status, and an endometrial biopsy. Postmenopausal bleeding is related to an increased risk of endometrial hyperplasia and cancer and should be evaluated with a transvaginal ultrasound to look at the endometrial thickness (under 4 mm is reassuring) or an office endometrial biopsy. Table 4 describes the steps in evaluation of a woman with abnormal bleeding.

Treatment

If a woman presents with heavy bleeding and exhibits any signs or symptoms of hypovolemia, she should be admitted to the hospital and either treated with IV estrogen (Premarin) to stop the bleeding or have a surgical procedure (such as dilation and curettage). If the bleeding is heavy, but the woman is stable and her hemoglobin and

1017

| TABLE 1 | Causes of Abnormal Uterine Bleeding (ACOG) |

Palm (structural causes)	**COEIN (non-structural causes)**
Polyp	Coagulopathy
Adenomyosis	Ovulatory dysfunction
Leiomyoma	Endometrial
Malignancy and hyperplasia	Iatrogenic
	Not yet classified

| TABLE 2 | Signs and Symptoms of Ovulatory Cycles |

Regular cycle length	Presence of premenstrual stress (PMS) symptoms
Dysmenorrhea	Mittelschmerz (pain at ovulation)
Changes in cervical mucus	Biphasic temperature curve
Premenstrual breast tenderness	Positive test result from luteinizing hormone (LH) predictor kit

| TABLE 3 | Causes of Anovulatory Cycles |

Hypothalamic
- Weight loss
- Eating disorders
- Female athlete triad
- Chronic illness
- Stress
- Excessive exercise

Polycystic ovary syndrome

Thyroid disorders

Hyperprolactinemia

Idiopathic chronic anovulation

Medication-induced (i.e., after discontinuation of hormonal contraceptives)

| TABLE 4 | Clinical Evaluation of a Woman with Abnormal Bleeding |

OVULATORY BLEEDING	ANOVULATORY BLEEDING
History, physical examination, pregnancy test	History, physical examination, pregnancy test
In menorrhagia: • Consideration of liver function tests, BUN/Cr, CBC, coagulation profile • Pelvic ultrasound to exclude uterine fibroids • Sonohysterogram to exclude polyps or adenomyosis • Endometrial biopsy (especially if age >40) to exclude endometrial hyperplasia	Laboratory studies: • TSH • Prolactin • CBC (if acute bleeding episode or frequent heavy bleeding) • Consideration of endometrial biopsy (especially if age >40) to exclude hyperplasia or malignancy • Evaluation for other symptoms of PCOS
In intermenstrual bleeding: • Pap smear, cervical cultures	Screen for eating disorder, stress, female athlete triad

Abbreviations: BUN/Cr = blood urea nitrogen/creatinine; CBC = complete blood count; Pap = Papanicolaou smear; PCOS = polycystic ovary syndrome; TSH = thyroid-stimulating hormone.

| TABLE 5 | Treatment Options for Abnormal Vaginal Bleeding |

Anovulation: cycle control with estrogen/progestin contraception, DMPA, levonorgestrel IUD (Mirena), or scheduled progestin-induced withdrawal bleeds, ovulation induction with clomiphene citrate (Clomid), and referral to gynecologist if pregnancy desired

Acute bleeding episode—outpatient: administration of high-dose OCPs (up to 4 per day) for 5–7 days with subsequent continuous cycling with OCPs for at least 1 month, administration of oral estrogen to acutely stop bleeding, or administration of oral progesterone to acutely stop bleeding

Acute bleeding episode—inpatient: IVF, supportive care, IV estrogen therapy, consultation for surgical intervention

Menorrhagia—treatment with NSAIDs, tranexamic acid (Lysteda), insertion of levonorgestrel IUD, referral for endometrial ablation or surgical treatment of structural abnormality

On combination estrogen/progestin contraception: supportive care for first 3 months, assessment of adherence to pill regimen, add supplemental estrogen, change to a method with a higher dose of estrogen or a different class of progestin

On progestin-only contraception: add supplemental estrogen or combination oral contraceptive pill and NSAID to decrease bleeding

Abbreviations: DMPA = depot medroxyprogesterone acetate (Depo-Provera); IUD = intrauterine device; IV = intravenous; IVF = in vitro fertilization; NSAID = nonsteroidal antiinflammatory drug; OCP = oral contraceptive pill.

hematocrit are close to normal, outpatient treatment with high-dose oral contraceptive pills (OCPs), estrogen, cyclic progesterone, NSAIDs, or tranexamic acid (Lysteda) is indicated. Women with structural abnormalities causing menorrhagia should be referred for possible surgical treatment.

Treatment of women with ovulatory bleeding is indicated if the woman is anemic or is bothered by her bleeding pattern. However, treatment of anovulation with some type of progesterone is necessary to reduce the risk of endometrial hyperplasia or carcinoma. All women with chronic anovulation should have regular progesterone-induced withdrawal bleed. OCPs, monthly cycling of progesterone, and continuous administration of progestin contraception (e.g., depot medroxyprogesterone acetate [Depo-Provera] or levonorgestrel IUD [Mirena]) are all effective treatments (Table 5).

Treatment of women with abnormal bleeding on OCPs involves education and support to try to get them through the first 3 months on the pills. After that, consideration of supplemental estrogen, changing to a higher dose of an estrogen pill, changing to a pill with a different class of progestin, use of a supplemental NSAID to decrease the amount of bleeding, decreasing the hormone free interval, or changing to a nonhormonal type of contraception are all potential treatments.

References

Abdel-Aleem H, d'Arcangues C, Vogelsong KM, et al. Treatment of vaginal bleeding irregularities induced by progestin only contraceptives. Cochrane Database Syst Rev 2007;(4), CD003449.

ACOG. Practice bulletin no 128: Diagnosis of abnormal uterine bleeding in reproductive-aged women. Obstet Gynecol 2012;120:197–206.

ACOG Practice Bulletin No. 136. Management of abnormal uterine bleeding associated with ovulatory dysfunction. Obstet Gynecol 2013;122(1):176–85.

Ely JW, Kennedy CM, Clark EC, et al. Abnormal uterine bleeding: A management algorithm. J Am Board Fam Med 2006;19:590–602.

Liu Z, Doan QV, Blumenthal P, et al. A systematic review evaluating health-related quality of life, work impairment, and health-care costs and utilization in abnormal uterine bleeding. Value Health 2007;10:183–94.

Naoulou B, Tsai MC. Efficacy of tranexamic acid in the treatment of idiopathic and non-functional heavy menstrual bleeding: A systematic review. Acta Obstet Gynecol 2012;91:529–37.

Schrager S. Abnormal bleeding associated with hormonal contraception. Am Fam Physician 2002;65:2073–802083.

Sweet MG, Schmidt-Dalton TA, Weiss PM, et al. Evaluation and management of abnormal uterine bleeding in premenopausal women. Am Fam Physician 2012;85:35–43.

AMENORRHEA

Method of
Vickie Martin, MD; and Robert L. Reid, MD

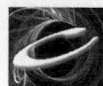

CURRENT DIAGNOSIS

- Always consider the possibility of pregnancy in any woman presenting with secondary amenorrhea.
- Secondary amenorrhea is most commonly the result of some significant lifestyle change (weight gain or loss, stress, excessive exercise) or illness (with marked weight loss) in the preceding 6 months.
- Obesity and features of androgen excess are most often related to polycystic ovary syndrome (PCOS).
- Because constitutional delay of puberty is found in only one third of girls presenting with delayed menarche, an investigation should be initiated at the time of presentation rather than waiting until the girl is 16 years old (meeting the definitional criteria).
- Primary amenorrhea, particularly with the absence of other features of pubertal development (breasts and pubic and axillary hair), suggests ovarian failure.
- When amenorrhea due to ovarian failure (high FSH) occurs before age 35 years, a karyotype is indicated. If Y chromosome material is identified on karyotype, gonadectomy is required to reduce the risk of malignancy in the gonadal tissues.

Amenorrhea, simply put, is the absence of menses. It can be classified as either primary (when a woman of reproductive age has never had menstruation) or secondary (when amenorrhea occurs after menstruation has been established). There are normal situations in which amenorrhea is expected (physiologic amenorrhea): during pregnancy, during lactation, and at the onset of menopause. Approximately 5% of reproductive-age women experience amenorrhea at times other than these, which warrants investigation. Women with amenorrhea often present with significant apprehension and anxiety. Thus, an appropriate but timely workup and diagnosis are required. The clinician must have a systematic approach for evaluating such women to ensure that important causes of amenorrhea are identified. As always, a detailed history, a targeted physical examination, and selective use of simple diagnostic tests are required.

Definition

Amenorrhea may be defined as the absence of menstruation for 3 or more months in women with past menses (secondary amenorrhea) or the absence of menarche by the age of 16 years in girls who have never menstruated (primary amenorrhea). Infrequent menstruation, termed *oligomenorrhea*, may have similar causes and also warrants investigation.

Menstrual Cycle

A clear working knowledge of the menstrual cycle and its physiology is mandatory for the clinician in these circumstances. Menstruation normally results when a cascade of hormonal signals from the hypothalamus (gonadotropin-releasing hormone [GnRH]) cause pituitary release of luteinizing hormone (LH) and follicle-stimulating hormone (FSH). These in turn stimulate the development of an egg-containing ovarian follicle. Estrogen from this follicle results in steady growth of the endometrial lining over a 2-week period (follicular phase). When ovulation occurs, the follicle (now called the corpus luteum) develops the ability to produce a second hormone, progesterone.

The secretion of estrogen and progesterone for the next 2-week period causes the endometrial lining to become lush (decidualized) in preparation for implantation of a pregnancy. If pregnancy fails to occur, the corpus luteum undergoes a spontaneous demise, the endometrium no longer has adequate hormonal support to survive, and the tissue is sloughed synchronously over the next 5 to 7 days as menstrual flow. The final steps of this process require a means of egress for blood, implying a normal uterus with a patent cervix and vagina (the outflow tract).

Etiology

Different classification systems have been employed. One system defines the type of amenorrhea based on the level of FSH in circulation. For example, high FSH levels indicate that the hypothalamus and pituitary are fully functioning but that the ovary is not responding (similar to menopause). The gonadotropin (FSH) levels are high and the ovary (gonad) is not functioning, which is termed *hypergonadotropic hypogonadism. Hypogonadotropic hypogonadism* refers to the situation where FSH levels are very low due to some central disturbance of hypothalamic or pituitary function. The problem with this classification is that normal FSH levels are often low and the distinction between hypogonadotropic and eugonadotropic causes of amenorrhea can be difficult.

A simple way to consider causes of amenorrhea is to divide the processes that regulate menstruation (the hypothalamic-pituitary-ovarian axis [HPO axis]) into compartments (Figure 1) and then consider possible contributory factors for disruption of normal processes at each of these levels. Always consider the possibility that amenorrhea may be due to unexpected pregnancy before moving on to a full investigation.

Hypothalamic Compartment

The hypothalamus integrates a wide variety of signals from the brain and is ultimately responsible for turning on or off the hormonal cascade necessary for triggering ovulatory and menstrual function. In adolescents, the development of breasts (thelarche) between ages 8 and 10 years is usually the first sign that the HPO axis has turned on and first menstruation (menarche) typically follows within 3 to 5 years. All girls with primary amenorrhea by age 14 years, particularly if 5 or more years have passed since the first evidence of pubertal development, warrant careful investigation, because girls with primary amenorrhea on the basis of constitutional delay cannot readily be differentiated on clinical history from the two thirds of patients with primary amenorrhea who have irreversible causes of reproductive failure.

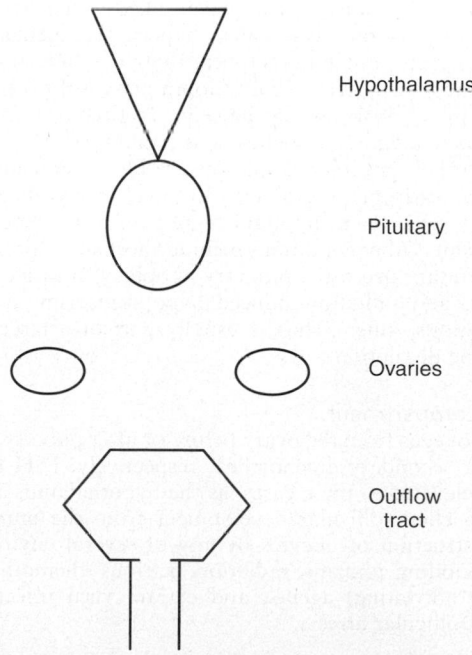

Figure 1. The four compartments to consider when evaluating amenorrhea.

Constitutional Delay

One third of young women presenting with primary amenorrhea have constitutional delay of puberty, meaning that they are undergoing a normal sequence of pubertal development at a rate that falls 2.5 standard deviations behind the mean. Girls with constitutional delay often present between ages 13 and 16 with primary amenorrhea and only early signs of breast development. Investigation reveals low to low-normal levels of gonadotropins and an otherwise negative workup.

Congenital Causes

A variety of unusual congenital conditions result in hypogonadotropic hypogonadism and primary amenorrhea. These conditions may be caused by deficiency of GnRH production or by abnormalities of the GnRH receptor. A Kallman's-like syndrome has been identified in some affected women who present with anosmia and a complete lack of pubertal development.

Acquired Causes

Acquired diseases can lead the hypothalamus to shut down the reproductive hormonal cascade, resulting in amenorrhea, which may be primary or secondary, depending on when they develop. Nutritional deprivation (including eating disorders), excessive caloric demand due to participation in demanding sports, and extreme psychological stress are common reasons for delayed activation of reproductive processes by the hypothalamus. Less commonly, systemic illnesses, including malabsorption states, active autoimmune diseases, and rare hypoxemic states related to congenital heart malformations or severe anemias (sickle cell disease), can lead to amenorrhea.

Pituitary Compartment

Lesions of the pituitary stalk that interrupt normal delivery of GnRH to the pituitary include those resulting from head trauma, rare stalk tumors such as craniopharyngiomas, or from the surgery to remove these.

Pituitary causes of amenorrhea are almost always due to over secretion of prolactin. Hyperprolactinemia resulting in amenorrhea, if associated with central retro-orbital headache and bitemporal hemianopia, can result from a prolactin-producing tumor.

Other causes of hyperprolactinemia originate outside the pituitary. For example, primary hypothyroidism, breast or chest wall lesions (or piercings) in the T4-6 dermatome, renal failure, and a variety of medications have all been linked to hyperprolactinemia. Medications that can cause hyperprolactinemia include dopamine receptor antagonists (phenothiazines, butyrophenones, thioxanthenes, risperidone, metoclopramide, sulpiride,[2] pimozide), dopamine-depleting agents (e.g., methyldopa, reserpine), H_2-blockers (cimetidine), opiates, and cocaine.

Rarely, other pituitary conditions result in amenorrhea. In empty sella syndrome, radiologic examination reveals an apparently empty sella due to pituitary regression from some vascular or other insult. Other conditions include Sheehan syndrome (postpartum pituitary necrosis), pituitary apoplexy (massive pituitary infarction), and radiation-induced hypopituitarism. In each of these situations, amenorrhea is usually part of a larger picture of endocrine disruption.

Ovarian Compartment

Depletion of eggs from the ovary before or after puberty results in primary or secondary amenorrhea, respectively. FSH levels are markedly elevated in these cases, as the hypothalamus and pituitary try to elicit follicular development from the unresponsive ovary. Destruction of oocytes by any of several environmental insults, including ionizing radiation, various chemotherapeutic (especially alkylating) agents, and certain viral infections can accelerate follicular atresia.

---

[2]Not available in the United States.

Primary amenorrhea in a woman with evidence of gonadal failure should elicit a search for a chromosomal abnormality. It is known that two intact X chromosomes are needed for maintenance of ovarian function. A variety of X chromosome structural abnormalities have been identified in women with premature ovarian failure, including complete absence of one X chromosome (Turner's syndrome).

Elevated FSH occurs in association with a normal karyotype. These women have normal 46,XY or 46,XX karyotypes without the phenotypic abnormalities of Turner's syndrome. Those with a Y chromosome should have their gonads removed because of the potential for malignant transformation.

Several rare inherited enzymatic defects also may be associated with premature ovarian failure. These include partial deficiencies in four enzymes in the steroidogenic pathway—17α-hydroxylase, 17,20-desmolase, 20,22-desmolase, and aromatase—and galactosemia.

Premature ovarian failure may be associated with a number of autoimmune disorders. Most commonly associated with thyroiditis, ovarian failure also occurs in women with polyglandular failure, including hypoparathyroidism, hypoadrenalism, and mucocutaneous candidiasis.

Though it is not exclusively an ovarian disorder, it is useful to consider polycystic ovary syndrome (PCOS) in the ovarian compartment for the purpose of completeness in considering possible diagnoses. PCOS is one of the most common causes of secondary amenorrhea. Typically, women suffering from this condition are overweight (although one third have normal body weight) and have clinical features of hyperandrogenism (acne and hirsutism), hyperinsulinism (acanthosis nigricans), and hyperestrogenism (watery cervical mucus). Months of amenorrhea may be punctuated by episodes of heavy and prolonged menstrual bleeding as an estrogen-thickened endometrium sheds irregularly over several weeks.

Outflow Tract Compartment

Congenital abnormalities of development of the reproductive outflow tract can cause amenorrhea. Complete absence of a uterus can be due to isolated müllerian agenesis or it can manifest in phenotypic females with a 46,XY karyotype who have complete androgen insensitivity. Developmental abnormalities can include cervical atresia, tranverse vaginal septum, and imperforate hymen. These latter abnormalities may be associated with cyclic menstrual pain in the absence of bleeding (cryptomenorrhea). Similarly, monthly cramps can occur with cervical stenosis following trachelectomy or conization. Uterine synechiae due to a vigorous curettage in the face of a postpartum or postabortion endometritis can result in obliteration of the uterine cavity and secondary amenorrhea with or without monthly menstrual-like cramps.

Other Causes

Pregnancy must always be considered in a sexually active female patient presenting with secondary amenorrhea. Hormonal suppression of the endometrium can be accomplished with a variety of medications. The progestin component of the cyclic oral contraceptive gradually results in a thinner and thinner endometrium, which can ultimately result in pill-withdrawal amenorrhea. Other medications, including danazol, medroxyprogesterone, and long-acting GnRH agonists can result in amenorrhea.

Diagnosis

History

A search for clues as to the etiology should start with a personal developmental history in the amenorrheic teen and with a menstrual and reproductive history in the older amenorrheic woman. Events in the 3 to 6 months preceding the onset of amenorrhea are often critical. Rapid weight gain or loss or a marked change in energy expenditure through exercise may be important. Systems review should examine possible disruption to any of the compartments (Box 1). Inquiry about general health, risk of pregnancy, and use of medication (including illicit drugs) is important.

Box 1 | A Compartmental Approach to Systems Review

Hypothalamic Compartment
- Changes in temperature regulation, sleep, appetite, thirst
- Headache or visual field defects

Pituitary Compartment
- Central retro-orbital headache, bitemporal hemianopia
- Galactorrhea
- Features of hypothyroidism
- Medications affecting prolactin

Ovary Compartment
- Hot flushes
- Insomnia
- Night sweats
- Vaginal dryness

Outflow Compartment
- Cyclic cramps
- Possibility of pregnancy
- Recent gynecologic procedures (dilation and curettage, cervical laser or conization)

Physical Examination

Height, weight, and body mass index (BMI) should be determined. Body habitus often provides an important clue to which patients are amenorrheic due to excessive physical or nutritional stress (eating disorder or malnutrition). In primary amenorrhea, examination for the stage of breast and pubic hair development (Tanner staging) can indicate whether there has been delay or disruption to the entire process of pubertal development. Restriction of later visual fields to examination by confrontation, the presence of galactorrhea, or evidence of recent scars or lesions in the region of the breast (such as zoster) can implicate hyperprolactinemia. The thyroid gland should be palpated and features of hypothyroidism sought. A lower abdominal mass may be due to pregnancy, hematocolpos, or hematometra.

The gynecologic examination should be tailored to the patient. The external genitalia should be evaluated for pubic hair, acanthosis nigricans, and clitoral size. The hymen should be visualized; an imperforate hymen usually shows a bluish central bulge. Estrogenization of the tissues (presence of leukorrhea, thickened mucosa, or watery cervical mucus) can be assessed with speculum examination (choosing a speculum size appropriate to the sexual maturity of the patient). Visualization of the cervix in most circumstances is sufficient to rule out an outflow compartment problem.

Investigations

Initial Investigations

Initial investigation for any patient with amenorrhea or oligomenorrhea includes follicle-stimulating hormone (FSH), prolactin (PRL), thyroid stimulating hormone (TSH), and a sensitive pregnancy test if pregnancy is a possibility.

Ultrasonography can be helpful when an internal examination cannot be performed. When a congenital anomaly is considered, magnetic resonance imaging (MRI) can provide more definitive information.

Follow-up Investigations

A low normal FSH in the presence of a normal outflow tract should elicit a more detailed search for hypothalamic disruptors (such as nutritional, physical, or psychological stress). In a patient who has low FSH in conjunction with an elevated PRL and who is not taking medications known to increase PRL and whose TSH is normal, lesions of the hypothalamus or pituitary should be excluded with CT or MRI.

An elevated FSH indicates ovarian failure and should elicit a search for possible explanations such as past surgery, exposure to radiation or chemotherapy, or genetic causes. With an elevated

FSH, a karyotype is usually indicated unless there is some obvious cause for loss of ovarian function. If the karyotype reveals any Y chromosome material, then, at the appropriate age, referral to a gynecologist is necessary for counseling and gonadectomy to reduce the risk of gonadoblastoma and dysgerminoma.

Evidence of outflow tract obstruction on pelvic examination or the possibility of cervical stenosis (cyclic dysmenorrhea without bleeding after a cervical surgical procedure such as a loop excision, cone biopsy, or trachelectomy) or Asherman's syndrome (obliteration of the endometrial cavity following a postpregnancy or postabortion dilation and curettage) merits referral to a gynecologist for further assessment and management.

Secondary amenorrhea related to weight gain or obesity, particularly when associated with features of acne and hirsutism, suggests the polycystic ovary syndrome. Management depends on whether the patient is seeking menstrual cycle regulation and relief from hirsutism (cyclic progestational therapy or an oral contraceptive plus an anti-androgen) or pregnancy (weight loss and fertility medication such as clomiphene citrate [Clomid]).

References

Rebar RW. Evaluation of amenorrhea, anovulation and abnormal bleeding. March 26, 2006. Available at http://endotext.org/female/female4/female-frame4.htm [accessed October 10, 2013].

Reid RL. Amenorrhea. In: Copeland L, Jarrell J, McGregor J, editors. Textbook of Gynecology. 2nd ed. Philadelphia: WB Saunders; 1997. p. 365–90.

Reindollar R, Lalwani S. Abnormalities of female pubertal development. November 21, 2002. Available at http://endotext.org/female/female2/femaleframe2.htm [accessed August 12, 2013].

BACTERIAL INFECTIONS OF THE URINARY TRACT IN WOMEN

Method of
Kinder Fayssoux, MD

CURRENT DIAGNOSIS

- Acute cystitis is the most common urologic disorder in women.
- *Escherichia coli* and *Staphylococcus saprophyticus* are the causative agents for 80% of community acquired urinary tract infections (UTIs).
- *E. coli* is also the most common uropathogen in the nosocomial setting.
- Anatomic risk factors include short urethra, the proximity of the urethra to the anus, and the colonization of the periurethral mucosa with bowel flora.
- Other risk factors include previous UTI, sexual intercourse, and, separately, the use of spermicide, pregnancy, diabetes, incontinence, cystocoele, and incomplete emptying of the bladder and dysfunctional voiding (defined as abnormal bladder emptying in the absence of neurologic disease).
- Postmenopausal women are also at increased risk if they are estrogen deficient.
- Acute cystitis typically presents with abrupt onset of dysuria, increased frequency, and/or urgency. Less frequently a patient will present with hematuria, suprapubic discomfort, or back/costovertebral angle pain. If a fever is present, it is usually less than 38.9°C (102°F).
- Acute pyelonephritis can evolve from either asymptomatic bacteriuria or from an ascending bladder infection.
- Symptoms usually include fever usually greater than 38.9°C (102°F) with chills, nausea/vomiting, dysuria, increased frequency, urgency, and costovertebral angle (CVA) tenderness (usually unilateral).
- *E. coli* is the major pathogen in acute pyelonephritis and treatment depends on severity and pregnancy status.

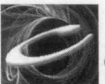

CURRENT TREATMENT

- Empiric therapy for uncomplicated UTIs should be dependent on the most recent antibiotic guidelines and the uropathogen resistance patterns in a community.
- In a community with >20% incidence of resistant *E. coli*, nitrofurantoin (Macrobid) 100 mg bid for 7 days is the treatment of choice with quinolones as second-line therapy.
- In a community with <20% *E. coli* resistance, trimethoprim/sulfamethoxazole 160/800 (Bactrim DS) PO twice daily for 3 days is also acceptable as first-line therapy with quinolones still considered as second-line therapy.
- Phenazopyridine (Pyridium), a smooth muscle relaxant, can be prescribed for spasm relief.
- Fungal UTIs or candiduria should be treated with fluconazole (Diflucan) 200 mg daily for 2 weeks.
- Outpatient treatment guidelines for acute pyelonephritis are the same as for uncomplicated UTI except the duration of antimicrobial therapy is longer (10–14 days).
- Inpatient treatment for acute pyelonephritis is typically IV levofloxacin (Levaquin) (750 mg daily) or ampicillin (1 g every 6 h).
- Acute pyelonephritis should resolve in 48 to 72 hours, if patients are not getting better, imaging should be undertaken with ultrasound or CT scan to assess for renal abscess or urethral obstruction.

Acute Cystitis (Urinary Tract Infection)

Acute cystitis is the most common urologic disorder among women. It represents 4% of all outpatient visits. Of these visits, 52% present to a primary care clinic and 23% to the emergency department. The annual health care costs associated with urinary tract infections (UTIs) are roughly 1.6 billion and climbing. Antimicrobial prescriptions for UTIs account for 15% of all outpatient prescriptions. One-third of all women will have at least one symptomatic UTI by age 24, with more than half of all women having at least one during their lifetime.

Acute cystitis can be defined as uncomplicated or complicated. Uncomplicated cystitis is defined as a UTI in patients with normal urinary tract anatomy without a contributing medical condition such as diabetes mellitus, neurogenic bladder, pregnancy, renal insufficiency, immune deficiency, recent antibiotic use, recent genitourinary instrumentation, spinal cord injury, ureteral obstruction, or nephrolithiasis. Complicated cystitis is defined as a UTI in patients with abnormal urinary tract anatomy or with one of the aforementioned medical conditions. These patients generally require urine culture as part of the initial work-up to guide antimicrobial therapy and often additional condition specific evaluation and treatment.

Acute cystitis is caused by ascending bacteria of perineal/urethral/fecal origin through the urethra into the bladder and renal systems. *Escherichia coli* and *Staphylococcus saprophyticus* are the causative agents for 80% of community acquired UTIs (complicated and uncomplicated). *E. coli* is also the most common uropathogen in the nosocomial setting. Other known uropathogens include *Pseudomonas spp*, *Klebsiella spp*, *Proteus*, *Corynebacterium urealyticum*, and *Providencia*. Fungal UTIs caused by *Candida spp*, *Aspergillus spp*, and *Cryptococcus neoformans* are also increasingly encountered. These are usually caused by indwelling urinary devices and seen more frequently in diabetics. Other populations prone to fungal UTIs include patients who are immunocompromised, hospitalized, or elderly.

There are numerous risk factors for acute cystitis, several specific to women. Risk factors unique to women include several related to their anatomy. These anatomic differences are the primary reason for the increased incidence of UTI in women when compared to men and include the female's relatively short urethra (when compared to the male counterpart), the proximity of the urethra to the anus, and the colonization of the periurethral mucosa with bowel flora.

Other risk factors include previous UTI, sexual intercourse, and, separately, the use of spermicide, pregnancy, diabetes, incontinence, cystocoele, and incomplete emptying of the bladder and dysfunctional voiding (defined as abnormal bladder emptying in the absence of neurologic disease). Postmenopausal women are also at increased risk if they are estrogen deficient.

Dysfunctional voiding has an unknown etiology and results in increased external sphincter activity during voluntary voiding which results in reflux, increasing chances of UTI.

Commonly advised behavioral modifications thought to decrease the risk of UTI (e.g., postcoital voiding, increased fluid intake, avoidance of urinary holding, douching, front-to-back wiping, proper tampon/sanitary napkin use, and loose/cotton underwear) have been supported by the literature.

Acute cystitis typically appears as an abrupt onset of dysuria, increased frequency, and/or urgency. Less frequently a patient will present with hematuria, suprapubic discomfort, or back/costovertebral angle pain. If a fever is present, it is usually less than 38.9°C (102°F).

Obtaining a good history that assesses for risk factors and symptoms is important in diagnosing acute cystitis. In a woman who presents with one or more symptoms of UTI (dysuria, frequency, urgency, hematuria), the probability of infection is already 50%. A urine dipstick is a useful diagnostic test, with a positive (+) nitrite or leukocyte esterase result increasing the chances of infection. The combination of positive nitrite *and* leukocyte esterase results has the highest diagnostic correlation with UTI. Physical examination findings may include suprapubic tenderness or costovertebral angle tenderness, although these are unlikely in an uncomplicated UTI scenario.

The gold standard for diagnosis of acute cystitis is a culture that has 10^2 to 10^3 colony-forming units of a single uropathogen from a clean catch or catheterized urine specimen. However, research has shown that, for uncomplicated cystitis, ordering cultures and sensitivities makes little difference in treatment while increasing cost of care. Thus, it is reasonable to start empiric treatment without a culture and sensitivities in a patient presenting with uncomplicated UTI.

The differential diagnosis for an uncomplicated UTI includes:
- Vaginitis/vaginal infections: can cause dysuria
  - *Gardnerella*, *Candida albicans*, and *Trichomonas*
- Urethritis: can cause dysuria/frequency
  - STDs (*Chlamydia trachomatis*, gonorrhea, herpes simplex)
  - Pelvic floor spasm (leads to urethral spasm/irritability)
- Interstitial cystitis
- Malignancy
- Renal tuberculosis

Differentiating between sexually transmitted infections (STI), vaginal infections, and UTIs can be difficult because symptoms and signs commonly overlap. History elements that should prompt a pelvic examination and laboratory evaluation for pathogens are complaints of a vaginal discharge or vaginal irritation/pruritus. Persistent hematuria should raise the concern for underlying malignancy or renal tuberculosis, and further evaluation should be done.

Empiric therapy for uncomplicated UTIs should be dependent on the most recent antibiotic guidelines and the uropathogen resistance patterns in a community. In a community with >20% incidence of resistant *E. coli*, nitrofurantoin (Macrobid) 100 mg bid for 7 days is the treatment of choice with quinolones as second-line therapy. In a community with <20% *E. coli* resistance, trimethoprim/sulfamethoxazole 160/800 (Bactrim DS) PO twice daily for 3 days is also acceptable as first-line therapy with quinolones still considered as second-line therapy. Phenazopyridine (Pyridium), a smooth muscle relaxant, can be prescribed for spasm relief and is usually only necessary for the first 24 hours after treatment is initiated. Fungal UTIs or *candiduria* should be treated with fluconazole (Diflucan) 200 mg daily for 2 weeks.

For a complicated UTI, a culture must always be obtained and the patient should be evaluated in the context of his or her specific comorbid condition before treatment.

Acute Pyelonephritis

Acute pyelonephritis can evolve from either asymptomatic bacteruria or from an ascending bladder infection. Although it can progress from an uncomplicated cystitis, it more commonly presents from a complicated cystitis in the setting of other medical conditions such cholelithiasis, urinary obstruction, malformations, or pregnancy.

Symptoms usually include fever usually greater than 38.9°C (102°F) with chills, nausea/vomiting, dysuria, increased frequency, urgency, and CVA tenderness (usually unilateral). These symptoms can present on a spectrum from mild to severe. *E. coli* is the major pathogen, and treatment depends on severity and pregnancy status. Pregnant patients or patients with moderate to severe nausea/vomiting that would interfere with oral antibiotic treatment should be hospitalized and have blood cultures done in addition to urine culture. Patients with mild symptoms and the ability to tolerate oral antibiotics can be treated as on an outpatient basis with a urine culture obtained before initializing treatment. Outpatient treatment guidelines are the same as for uncomplicated UTI, except the duration of antimicrobial therapy is longer (10–14 days). Inpatient treatment is typically IV levofloxacin (Levaquin 750 mg daily) or ampicillin (1 g every 6 h). Once the inpatient is able to tolerate oral antibiotics and the infection is felt to be controlled, he or she can be switched to oral antibiotics and discharged to complete a 14-day course of treatment as an outpatient.

Symptoms should resolve in 48 to 72 hours; if patients are not getting better, imaging should be undertaken with ultrasound or CT scan to assess for renal abscess or urethral obstruction.

Urethritis

Urethritis usually has a gradual onset and is accompanied with milder symptoms of dysuria, frequency, urgency, or hematuria. It can also occur with a vaginal discharge and complaints of dyspareunia and vaginal pruritus depending on cause. Chalmydial, gonorrheal, candidal and trichomonal urethritis is usually accompanied by a vaginal discharge. Candidal urethritis can also be associated with pruritus and dyspareunia. If urethritis is suspected, a pelvic examination and further laboratory work-up is necessary.

Asymptomatic Bacteruria

Asymptomatic bacteruria is defined as the presence of 100,000 microorganisms/milliliter of urine without any symptoms of cystitis.

No screening should be performed in healthy nonpregnant women, elderly living in the community, diabetic women, institutionalized elderly, or persons with spinal cord injury. Pregnant women are the exception. They should be screened; positive cultures need to be treated, as there is an increased likelihood of asymptomatic bacteruria turning into UTI or pyelonephritis because of vesicoureteral reflux and urinary stasis resulting from increased progesterone levels.

Recurrent Cystitis

Recurrent cystitis is defined as at least three episodes of uncomplicated UTI with one or more documented positive (+) cultures in 12 months. It can be due to relapse or reinfection. Relapse is defined as infection occurring with the same organism as a previous UTI. Reinfection is when symptoms return after treatment and a completely symptom-free interval along with a negative urine culture or when the second infection is caused by a different organism. Most recurrent cystitis tends to be caused by reinfection.

In patients presenting with recurrent cystitis, an age-based evaluation is a good place to start. Adolescents who are not sexually active should be evaluated for congenital abnormalities. Premenopausal females should be questioned about the temporal relationship of the onset of UTI to increased frequency/recent sexual intercourse, spermicide use (with or without condom or diaphragm), or renal stones. Postmenopausal females should be

evaluated for decreased estrogen/vaginal atrophy, incontinence, incomplete bladder emptying, cystocoeles, and prolapse.

If a complete and thorough evaluation is done, complicating factors are ruled out, modifiable factors are treated, and recurrent cystitis still remains a problem, then treatment should be considered. Treatment options include continuous antibiotics, postcoital therapy, or self- initiated treatment at the first sign or symptom of an infection.

Gross hematuria or persistent microscopic hematuria should increase suspicion for an underlying malignancy. Also, recurrent cystitis symptoms in a setting of negative cultures may suggest mycobacterial infection or interstitial cystitis.

Catheter Associated Urinary Tract Infection

Catheter-associated UTI is defined as a UTI in a patient who had an indwelling urethral catheter within 48 hours of onset of infection. Indwelling urinary catheters and clean intermittent catheterization are associated with the highest rates of bacteriuria; after 1 month of either there is almost 100% risk of bacteriuria. Formation of a bacterial biofilm on the catheter is thought to be the mechanism of infection in this setting.

No treatment is recommended for asymptomatic patients, and neither prophylactic antibiotics nor routine UA and culture are recommended for this population. For symptomatic patients, the first step is to determine whether the catheter can be removed. If it cannot, then it should be replaced. In addition, a blood and urine culture (taken from a new catheter) should be obtained. Initial treatment is the same as for an uncomplicated UTI as discussed earlier. Confirmation of susceptibility should be confirmed with culture results.

References

Litza JA, Brill JR. Urinary tract infection. Primary Care Clinical Office Practice 2010;37:491–507.

Minardi D, d'Anzeo G, Cantoro D, et al. Urinary tract infections in women: Etiology and treatment options. Int J Gen Med 2011;4:333–43.

Finer G, Landau D. Pathogenesis of urinary tract infections with normal female anatomy. Lancet 2004;4:631–4.

Foster RT: Office gynecology uncomplicated urinary tract infections in women. Obstet Gynecol Clin 35:235–48.

Berek JS. Berek and Novak's Gynecology. Philadelphia: Lippincott; 2012 p. 570–71.

Essentials evidence plus: Urinary tract infection (adults), Available at http://essentialevidenceplus.com, accessed December 28, 2013.

Essentials evidence plus: Urethritis (female), http://essentialevidenceplus.com, Accessed December 28, 2013.

Bent SN, Nallamothu BK, Simel DL, et al. Does this woman have an acute uncomplicated urinary tract infection? JAMA 2002;287:2701–10.

Wagenlehner F, Weidner W, Naber K. An updated on uncomplicated urinary tract infections in women. Curr Opin Urol 2009;19:368–74.

Dielubaza EJ, Schaeffer AJ: Urologic issues for the internist- urinary tract infections in women. Med Clin North Am 95:27–41.

Giesen LG, Cousins G, Dimitrov DD, et al. Predicting acute uncomplicated urinary tract infections in women: A systematic review of the diagnostic accuracy of symptoms and signs, BMC Fam Pract 2010;11:78. Available at http://www.biomedcentral.com/1471-2296/11/78, Accessed December 28, 2013.

BREAST DISEASE

Method of
Jana Lewis, MD; and Patrick Borgen, MD

Benign diseases of the breast historically are subdivided into proliferative and nonproliferative lesions (Table 1). In a study by Dupont and Page, patients with breast biopsies yielding nonproliferative lesions had no increased risk for subsequent breast cancer. In contrast, proliferative lesions were associated with a minimal to a fivefold increased risk for breast cancer. In clinical practice, of the proliferative lesions, only atypical epithelial lesions increase breast cancer risk significantly. Appropriate treatment and counseling of patients depend on the risk for breast cancer associated with these benign diseases.

TABLE 1	Benign Diseases of the Breast

LESION	INCREASE IN BREAST CANCER RISK
Nonproliferative Lesions	
Mild hyperplasia without atypia	None
Squamous or apocrine metaplasia	None
Duct ectasia	None
Mastitis	None
Cysts	None
Proliferative Lesions	
Fibroadenoma	None
Moderate or florid hyperplasia	Minimal
Microglandular adenosis	Minimal
Sclerosing adenosis	Minimal
Papilloma	Minimal
Atypical ductal hyperplasia	4-fold to 5-fold
Atypical lobular hyperplasia	5.8-fold

Nonproliferative Lesions

Nonproliferative lesions include mild hyperplasia without atypia, squamous or apocrine metaplasia, duct ectasia, mastitis, and fibrocystitc disease. In the study of 3303 patients by Dupont and Page, only 2.2% of patients with nonproliferative lesions had breast cancer following a benign breast biopsy with a mean follow-up time of 17 years.

Breast Cysts and Fibrocystic Breast Disease

Fibrocystic breast disease is a benign process in which generalized microcystic formation with stromal proliferation leads to increased breast nodularity. Cysts within the breast are most common in perimenopausal women 50 to 59 years of age but may present in premenopausal women as well. Postmenopausal women on hormone replacement therapy may develop cysts in their breasts. Benign cysts are often tender and fluctuate in size with the menstrual cycle. Cysts may be detected either on physical examination as a palpable, smooth, mobile nodule or by breast ultrasound. They may appear as a solitary nodule or in a cluster. Ultrasonographic appearance of simple benign cysts is that of an anechoic, round or oval, well-circumscribed mass with posterior enhancement. If the mass meets all four criteria, the accuracy of ultrasound is close to 100% for the diagnosis of a simple benign cyst. Cysts that appear complex, with internal echoes, thick septations, and irregular walls are suspicious for breast carcinoma and should be examined surgically or with an ultrasound-guided biopsy. Confirmation of the diagnosis can be made by fine-needle aspiration (FNA) of the cystic fluid. Bloody fluid may be an indication for a biopsy. In a study of 6782 cyst aspirates, Ciatto and colleagues found that cytologic examination identified atypical cells in 1677 specimens. Of these specimens, only 0.3% of these cases had clinically and radiologically negative intracystic papillomas. Cytologic examination was positive in only 0.1% of these cases. Thus fluid from cyst aspirations is not routinely sent for cytologic examination. Figure 1 describes the management of suspected cysts.

Mastitis and Duct Ectasia

Mastitis is divided into lactational and nonlactational. Lactational mastitis can occur from the reflux of bacteria into the breast during breast-feeding. The causative bacteria are usually gram-positive cocci. Patients should be treated with antibiotics with the appropriate coverage and can continue to nurse or pump the breast to

Figure 1. Algorithm for the management of suspected cysts.

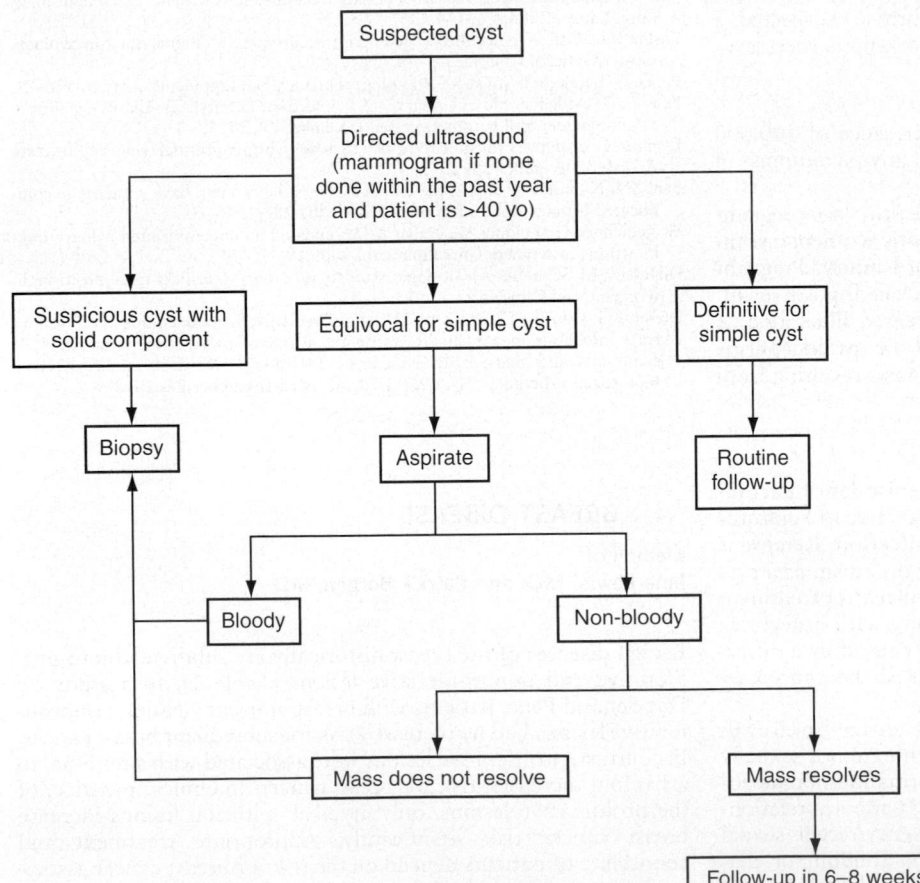

prevent engorgement. Nursing mothers can continue to breast-feed because the infant is not at risk for infection. Nonlactational (periductal) mastitis can be caused by duct ectasia, which occurs when the milk ducts become congested with secretions and debris, resulting in a periductal inflammation. These patients may present with greenish nipple discharge, nipple retraction, and subareolar noncyclical pain. The treatment of nonlactational mastitis includes broad-spectrum antibiotics to cover for Gram-positive cocci and skin anaerobes. Total duct excision and eversion of the nipple may be necessary to treat recurrent periductal mastitis.

Proliferative Benign Breast Diseases

Proliferative breast diseases include moderate or florid hyperplasia, microglandular and sclerosing adenosis, papilloma, fibroadenoma, atypical ductal hyperplasia (ADH), and atypical lobular hyperplasia (ALH). All proliferative lesions have an increased risk for subsequent breast cancer after biopsy except for fibroadenoma. This risk is 1.9 times higher in the presense of proliferative disease without atypia and increases to 5.3 times higher with atypia. Patients with moderate or florid hyperplasia, sclerosing adenosis, and solitary papilloma without atypia carry a minimal increase in risk for developing breast cancer over the general population. These patients are not classified as high risk. However, the risk for subsequent breast cancer is increased by fourfold to fivefold in the presence of atypia. ALH carries a higher risk than ADH, with a relative risk as high as 5.8. This increased risk applies to the contralateral breast as well because subsequent breast carcinomas are evenly divided between both breasts.

Proliferative Lesions with No Increased Risk for Subsequent Cancer: Fibroadenoma

Fibroadenomas are the most common breast tumor in women, as well as the most common benign tumor found in young women (less than 30 years of age with a peak incidence at 21 to 25 years of age). They are characteristically detected on physical examination as well-circumscribed, rubbery, highly mobile, palpable masses. On mammograms, these lesions may appear as a well-circumscribed mass. Involution of fibroadenomas in the elderly can lead to hyalinization and dense popcorn-like calcification on mammograms. Fibroadenomas pose no increased risk for breast cancer and do not mandate surgical removal unless desired by the patient. Pregnancy can increase the size of these lesions; thus it may be reasonable to remove them prior to a planned pregnancy. Removal may facilitate follow-up, given the inability to follow breast masses adequately during pregnancy. Other types of fibroadenomas include juvenile and giant fibroadenomas. Juvenile fibroadenomas occur in adolescent women and can grow larger than 5 cm in diameter. These lesions are not malignant; given their large size, however, surgical excision may be needed to prevent asymmetry of the breasts. Giant fibroadenomas are large fibroadenomas found in the lactating breast or in the breasts of pregnant patients. These lesions may regress in size once hormonal stimulation subsides. Lesions that remain large can be excised surgically. Fibroadenomas and phyllodes tumors may be linked. Any rapidly enlarging fibroadenoma should be considered for surgical excision to rule out phyllodes tumor because it is difficult clinically to differentiate the two.

Proliferative Lesions with Minimal Increased Risk for Subsequent Breast Cancer
Multiple Peripheral Papillomas

Multiple peripheral papillomas are lesions that occur in the peripheral ducts. They most commonly present as a mass but may also present with nipple discharge. Complete excisional removal may be considered to rule out a papillary carcinoma of the breast. In the era of larger-gauge biopsy devices it is easier to classify a lesion as a benign intraductal papilloma, which may be observed.

Sclerosing and Microglandular Adenosis

Sclerosing adenosis occurs as result of the proliferation of stromal tissue along with small terminal ductules. Often these lesions are picked up incidentally, but they may also present as microcalcifications on mammogram or as a mass (termed *adenosis tumor*). Sclerosing adenosis may be confused with a tubular carcinoma.

Proliferative Lesions with a Fourfold to Fivefold Risk for Subsequent Breast Cancer: Atypical Ductal Hyperplasia and Atypical Lobular Hyperplasia

ADH and ALH are very similar to their in situ counterparts. These lesions are termed *atypical hyperplasia* because they lack some of the microscopic features of in situ disease. The distinction between atypical hyperplasia and carcinoma in situ may be difficult to discern. In a study by Rosai, five expert breast cancer pathologists reviewed 17 cases of ductal or lobular lesions. In no case did all five agree on a diagnosis. Four of the five were able to agree on a diagnosis in three cases (18%). In one third of the patients, the diagnosis ran the gamut from hyperplasia without atypia to carcinoma in situ. Despite such difficulty, the diagnosis of atypical hyperplasia is on the rise as mammographic screening becomes more routine. Atypical hyperplasia, which is detected secondary to microcalcifications or by serendipity, carries the highest risk for subsequent breast carcinoma among all proliferative lesions of the breast, with a fourfold to fivefold increased risk over the general population. ALH carries a higher risk than ADH, with a relative risk as high as 5.8. This risk applies to the contralateral breast as well as the ipsilateral breast. Surgical excision of atypical hyperplasia on a core biopsy is recommended because 20% of patients are found to have breast cancer at time of surgical excision for atypical hyperplasia. It is not necessary to achieve negative margins for these lesions.

Other Benign Breast Lesions: Fat Necrosis, Hamartoma, Mondor's Disease, Radial Scars, and Pseudoangiomatous Stromal Hyperplasia

Other benign lesions of the breast include fat necrosis, hamartoma, Mondor's disease, radial scars, and pseudoangiomatous stromal hyperplasia (PASH). Trauma to the breast may lead to fat necrosis and can be mistaken for carcinomas on clinical examination. Fat necrosis lesions present clinically as painless, irregular masses with or without associated skin changes such as skin thickening. These lesions can be normal or may have rim calcifications on mammograms. No further treatment is needed when a core biopsy definitively makes the diagnosis of fat necrosis.

Hamartomas are benign lesions that are often picked up on a mammogram. The fatty composition of the mass makes these lesions clinically occult. They can be mistaken for fibroadenomas on mammograms. Hamartomas can be left alone without histologic confirmation if diagnosed definitively on a mammogram.

Mondor's disease is a thrombophlebitis of the superficial breast veins that presents as a palpable tender cord leading to the axilla. In a study of 63 cases, 8 patients (25%) had an underlying malignancy; thus a mammogram should be done to rule out the presence of breast carcinoma.

Radial scars are benign lesions whose etiology is unknown. They are often mistaken for breast carcinoma on mammograms because of their stellate appearance. Radial scars may also mimic breast carcinoma histologically. Staining for myoepithelial cells can help distinguish between invasive carcinoma and a radial scar. Radial scars carry a 1.5-fold increase in risk for subsequent breast carcinoma, so these lesions should be considered markers of future disease.

First described in 1986, PASH is a benign proliferative lesion that may present as an incidental finding or a mobile breast mass. It can occur in all ages and also in men. On a mammogram, PASH appears as a round noncalcified mass. Histologically, PASH may be mistaken for low-grade angiosarcoma. Unlike angiosarcoma, however, there should be no evidence of mitosis or cytologic atypia in PASH specimens. The role of hormones in the pathogenesis of PASH is controversial. Although these lesions tend to occur in young patients or in elderly patients on hormone therapy, most cases tend to be negative for estrogen receptors. The treatment for symptomatic PASH is complete surgical excision. Approximately 7% of cases recur despite adequate treatment.

Risk Factors for Breast Cancer

An estimated 80% of women in whom breast cancer develops have no documented risk factors or determinants. Risk factors cannot be changed, whereas risk determinants can be altered to decrease a person's risk for subsequent breast cancer. Common risk factors include a familial history of breast cancer, personal breast biopsy history, menarche before 12 years of age, menopause after 55 years of age, increasing age, geographic location, and mutations of the *BRCA1* or *BRCA2* genes. The risk determinants for breast cancer include reproductive factors such as nulliparity and first pregnancy after the age of 30 years and previous radiation exposure. Previous radiation therapy for lymphoma, especially during adolescence, elevates a woman's risk for subsequent breast cancer.

BRCA Gene Mutations

BRCA1 and *BRCA2* (breast cancer susceptibility gene) are tumor suppressor genes that normally ensure DNA stability and prevent uncontrolled cell growth. Mutations in these genes may lead to the development of hereditary breast and/or ovarian cancer in affected individuals, and less commonly to other cancers such as pancreatic, uterine, and colon. It is estimated that these inherited mutations account for 3% to 5% of all breast cancers and 10% to 15% of all ovarian cancers among white women in the United States. Men with a mutated *BRCA2* gene also have an increased risk for breast cancer. The likelihood that a breast and/or ovarian cancer is associated with a *BRCA* mutation is increased in families with history of multiple cases of breast cancer, cases of both breast and ovarian cancer, one or more family members with two primary cancers, or an Ashkenazi Jewish background. Roughly 10% of women in the general population will develop breast cancer sometime in their life, compared to 60% to 80% of women with a harmful *BRCA* mutation. For ovarian cancer, 1.4% of unaffected women will develop the disease, while 15% to 40% of affected women will.

To test for *BRCA1* and *BRCA2* mutations, a DNA sample (blood is currently required for full-length gene sequencing) is needed. There are currently no universally agreed-upon criteria for screening patients with a suspected *BRCA* mutation, and each case should be assessed individually. Genetic counseling is recommended before and after the workup. Options for further management after a positive *BRCA* test include close surveillance, prophylactic (risk reducing) surgery, and chemoprevention. A discussion between physician and patient should include all options and be adjusted to the patient's needs.

Screening Techniques

Screening for breast cancer includes mammography, ultrasound, breast self-examination (BSE), and physical examination by a physician. Multiple studies, such as the Gothenburg and Malmö trials, show a reduction in breast cancer mortality from 30% to 40% in patients 40 to 49 years of age who undergo screening mammograms. A meta-analysis of six randomized trials revealed a 30% reduction in breast cancer mortality in patients 50 to 69 years of age. The sensitivity of mammograms depends on the patient's age and ranges from 53% to 81% in women 40 to 49 years of age to 73% to 81% in patients 50 years of age or older. An estimated 10% to 15% of breast cancer cases are not detectable on screening mammography, thus emphasizing the importance of physical breast examination by a physician and BSE that include both visual inspection and manual examination of the breast. On inspection, signs of breast malignancy include skin or nipple retraction or discoloration, nipple discharge/crusting, or peau d'orange edema of the breast. On palpation, any asymmetric mass

of the breast or axilla may be regarded as a potential malignancy that deserves further evaluation.

Screening for a woman with an average risk for developing breast cancer should start with routine BSEs at 18 years of age, yearly physical examinations, and initiation of annual mammography at 40 years of age in accordance with the American Cancer Society's recommendations. In November 2009, the U.S. Preventative Services Task Force (USPSTF) updated their own breast-cancer screening recommendations by recommending that screening mammograms begin at age 50 instead of the previous recommended age 40, and that biannual screening is sufficient. They also advised against teaching BSEs, stating that BSEs do not reduce the risk of death from breast cancer. Further evaluation of the analysis and opinion statement of the USPSTF led all concerned parties (including the United States Senate, the American Cancer Society, the American College of Surgeons and the American Society of Clinical Oncology) to reject the USPTF guideline changes.

In patients who have a very high risk for breast cancer development, such as *BRCA* carriers, screening should start 10 years earlier than the age of onset of an affected relative or at the age of 35. Krieger screened 1909 patients (including 358 *BRCA* mutation carriers) who had more than a 15% lifetime risk for developing breast cancer. These patients had a biannual breast examination as well as annual mammogram and breast magnetic resonance imaging (MRI). In this population, mammograms had a sensitivity of 33% with a specificity of 95%. Breast MRI had significantly higher rates of sensitivity and specificity at 80% and 90%, respectively. Given these findings, breast MRI should be a part of the screening examination for these high-risk patients. Moreover, MRI is recommended as a standard screening test in BRCA heterozygotes.

Patients with a history of mantle radiation for lymphoma should start annual screening at 25 years of age and biannual screening 10 years after receiving radiation therapy.

Workup of a Breast Mass
Dominant Palpable Mass

The workup of a dominant palpable breast mass depends on the patient's menopausal status and age, and on the degree of suspicion. It is reasonable to follow a premenopausal patient with a nonsuspicious mass over one menstrual cycle and then reexamine her. Suspicious lesions present as a hard, nontender, irregular mass or as a mass in a high-risk patient. Palpable masses in postmenopausal patients may also warrant a workup. In general, certain benign lesions on core biopsy should be excised, including lobular carcinoma in situ (LCIS), ADH, radial scars, sclerosing papillary lesions, columnar cell hyperplasia with atypia, and symptomatic PASH (Figure 2). Patients with a high-risk proliferative lesion should have close follow-up after surgery including physical examinations. Negative findings on a mammogram do not preclude the diagnosis of cancer because 10% of cancers are occult mammographically. This number drops to 3% when a lesion is occult both mammographically and ultrasonographically. An alternative to core biopsies in younger women is the use of the triple test: a physical examination in conjunction with breast imaging (mammogram or ultrasound) and FNA. When all three components indicate the mass is benign, the negative predictive value approaches 100%.

Masses Revealed on Screening Mammograms

The American College of Radiology's classification lexicon, the Breast Imaging Reporting and Data System (BI-RADS), is used in breast imaging to universally characterize lesions found on mammography (Table 2). BI-RADS 0 means the assessment is incomplete and repeat workup is needed. BI-RADS 1 indicates a normal mammogram. Mammograms with BI-RADS 2 signify benign findings. Patients with BI-RADS 3 have a 1% to 2% risk for malignancy and should have short-term follow-up with another mammogram in 6 months. BI-RADS 4 indicates the presence of suspicious lesions with a 20% to 40% probability of

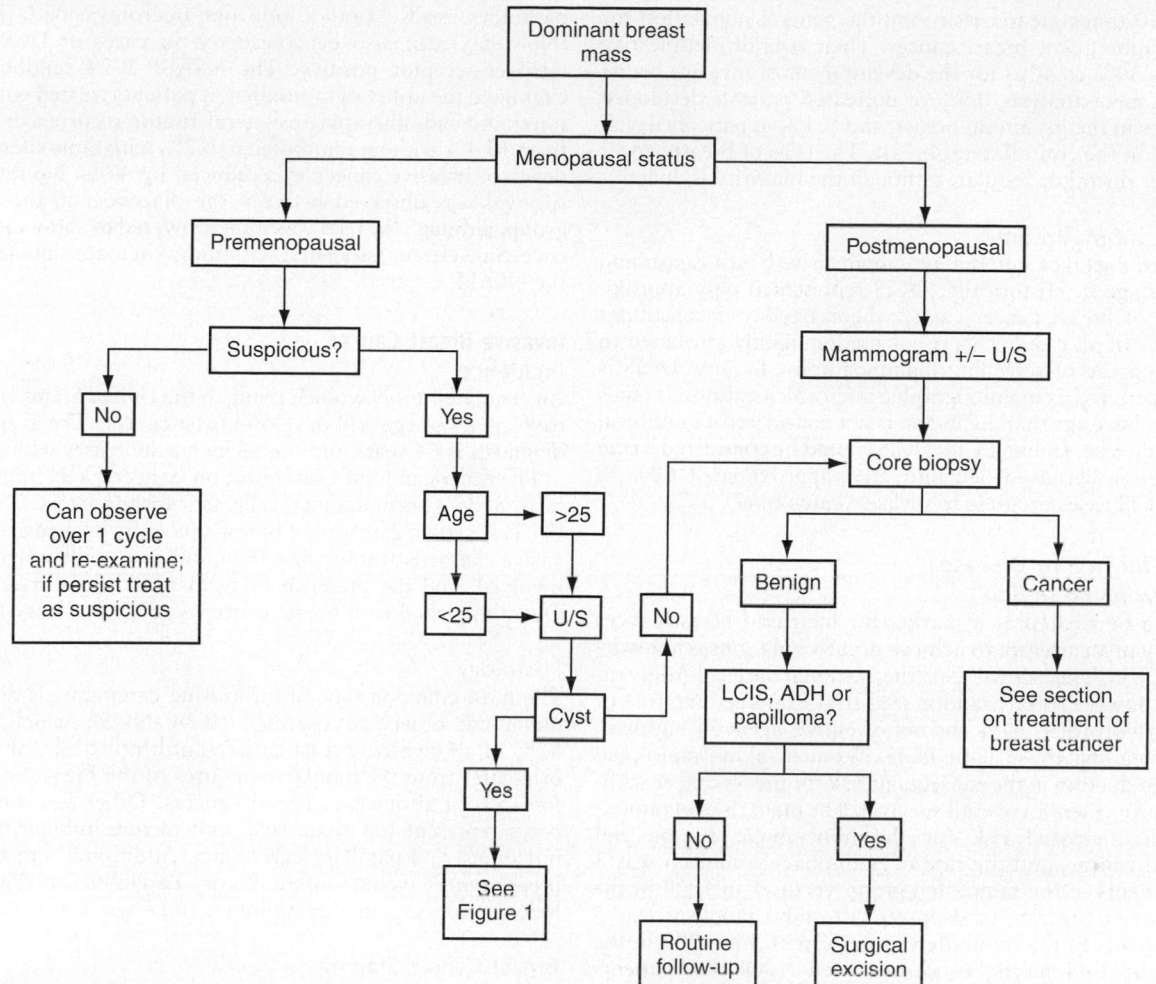

Figure 2. Algorithm for workup of a breast mass. *Abbreviations:* ADH = atypical ductal hyperplasia; LCIS = lobular cancer in situ; U/S = ultrasound.

TABLE 2	BI-RADS Mammography Classification		
BI-RADS CATEGORY	**DEFINITION**	**RISK FOR MALIGNANCY**	**RECOMMENDED FOLLOW-UP**
0	Incomplete assessment	N/A	Further workup
1	Negative study	N/A	Repeat mammogram in 1 y
2	Benign	N/A	Repeat mammogram in 1 y
3	Probably benign	<2%	Repeat mammogram in 6 mo
4	Suspicious	20%	Biopsy should be considered
5	Highly suggestive of malignancy	90%	Appropriate action should be taken
6	Known biopsy-proven malignancy	N/A	Appropriate action should be taken

Abbreviation: BI-RADS = Breast Imaging Reporting and Data System.

a malignant lesion. BI-RADS 5 is highly suggestive of cancer with a greater than 95% chance of harboring an underlying malignant lesion. BI-RADS 6, recently added as a category, indicates known malignant disease. BI-RADS 4 and 5 both indicate the need for a biopsy.

A core biopsy via ultrasound guidance may be attempted first. A stereotactic core biopsy should be considered if the lesion is occult on ultrasound (such as calcifications). Stereotactic biopsies may be impossible in patients with lesions that are very superficial or close to the chest wall or in patients with very small breasts that compress to less than 3 cm or who are unable to lie still for the procedure. In such situations, surgical excision with needle localization is warranted. In studies comparing surgical excision to core biopsies, the concordance rate is close to 100%. The surgeon

can obviate the need for multiple surgeries in the same patient by performing a core biopsy for diagnosis.

In Situ Diseases
Lobular Carcinoma In Situ
LCIS is considered a marker for future breast cancer risk and not an early, noninvasive lobular cancer. This disease is most commonly seen in premenopausal women, with a peak incidence in women 40 to 50 years of age. Only 10% of LCIS occurs in postmenopausal women. Unlike ductal carcinoma in situ (DCIS), LCIS is often found incidentally because typically no clinical or radiologic abnormalities are seen at time of diagnosis. In 50% of patients, LCIS is a multifocal finding. In 30% of patients, it can also be found in the contralateral breast. Patients with LCIS are

at an 8 to 10 times greater risk than the general population for developing subsequent breast cancer. Their overall lifetime risk is as high as 30% to 40% for the development of invasive breast cancer. In a meta-analysis, 15% of untreated patients developed breast cancer in the ipsilateral breast, and 9.3% of patients developed cancer in the contralateral breast. The type of breast cancer can be either ductal or lobular, although the majority is ductal.

Ductal Carcinoma In Situ

DCIS, or intraductal carcinoma, is a noninvasive breast cancer and designated stage 0. Historically, DCIS represented only approximately 5% of breast cancer cases, whereas today it constitutes 20% to 30% of all cases. This rise is predominantly attributed to the increasing use of screening mammography, because DCIS is most often detected as mammographic microcalcifications. It tends to occur at a later age than LCIS and is not considered a multifocal or bilateral disease. Unlike LCIS, DCIS should be considered a true precursor lesion because if left untreated, approximately 60% to 100% of DCIS cases progress to invasive carcinoma.

Treatment for In Situ Disease
Lobular Carcinoma In Situ

LCIS should be treated as a marker for increased breast cancer risk. Surgery in an attempt to achieve negative margins is not warranted for LCIS. The NSABP P-1 (the National Surgical Adjuvant Breast and Bowel Project) randomized trial examined the role of tamoxifen (Nolvadex) as a chemopreventive agent in high-risk patients, including those with LCIS. Women taking tamoxifen had a 50% reduction in the subsequent risk for breast cancer without any improvement in overall survival. The main risks of tamoxifen include increased risk for thromboembolic disease and endometrial cancer, and the rate of pulmonary embolism was 3 in 1000 patients in the tamoxifen group versus 1 in 1000 in the placebo group. The rate of deep-vein thromboembolism was 5 in 1000 patients in the tamoxifen group versus 3 in 1000 in the placebo group. Endometrial cancer was seen in 9 in 1000 patients in the tamoxifen group versus 3.5 in 1000 in the placebo group. The decision to use tamoxifen as a chemopreventive agent should be made on an individual basis given these side effects. The highest reduction in breast cancer occurred in the LCIS group with a 70% reduction in risk. Despite this, no difference in survival was seen between the tamoxifen and placebo group. A patient with LCIS may opt for a prophylactic bilateral mastectomy or to continue with close observation.

Ductal Carcinoma In Situ

Treatment of DCIS has evolved from simple mastectomy to lumpectomy with radiation therapy. A simple mastectomy is associated with a 1% local recurrence rate. Thus it is still considered a viable option in patients who do not desire or are ineligible for breast conservation therapy (BCT). No difference in survival is seen in patients treated with mastectomy versus BCT. The NSABP B-17 randomized trial examined the role of lumpectomy with and without radiotherapy for the treatment of DCIS. The addition of radiotherapy decreased the recurrence rate from 16.4% to 7% with 8 years of follow-up. More importantly, it decreased the rate of invasive carcinoma from 8% to 2%. The 5-year event-free survival with lumpectomy and radiation is 84%. Silverstein showed in retrospective studies that the recurrence rate in such patients is approximately 4%. Routine axillary lymph node dissection (ALND) is not recommended for DCIS because only 1% of patients have positive axillary nodes. Recent studies, however, show that sentinel lymph node biopsy may have a role in the management of selected patients with DCIS. This is especially true in patients receiving mastectomy as definitive treatment or if there is a question of microinvasion on the core biopsy. Patients with DCIS and microinvasion can have anywhere from a 3% to 20% incidence of nodal involvement. Indications for a sentinel node biopsy include extensive calcifications, a palpable lesion, patients undergoing mastectomy as treatment for DCIS, and lesions for which the

pathology reads "cannot rule out microinvasion." Tamoxifen (Nolvadex) can also be considered in cases of DCIS that are estrogen-receptor positive. The NSABP B-24 randomized trial examined the utility of tamoxifen in patients treated with lumpectomy and radiotherapy. Ipsilateral tumor recurrences decreased from 13.4% without tamoxifen to 8.2% with tamoxifen. The incidence of invasive cancer was reduced by 47%. No difference in survival was observed between the placebo and the tamoxifen group, although the trial was underpowered to show such a difference. Side effects associated with tamoxifen are similar to that of the NSABP P-1 trial.

Invasive Breast Cancer
Incidence

An estimated 1 in 9 women living in the United States who survive to 90 years of age will develop breast cancer. The average age at diagnosis is 64 years and the incidence increases with age.

The American Joint Committee on Cancer TMN (tumor, metastasis, node) system designates breast cancer as stage 0, I, II, III, or IV. This system categorizes breast cancer by its invasive or noninvasive character, tumor size, the number of axillary lymph nodes involved, and the presence of metastatic disease (see Table 2). Overall survival with breast cancer is related to stage (Table 3).

Histology

The most common type of infiltrating carcinoma is ductal carcinoma–not otherwise specified (IFDC-NOS), which represents 85% of all invasive breast cancer. Infiltrating lobular carcinoma originates from the lobular structures of the breast and accounts for 15% of all invasive breast cancers. Other less-common subtypes represent less than 10% and include tubular, medullary, mucinous, and papillary carcinoma. Additional rare subtypes of breast cancer include inflammatory carcinoma, malignant phyllodes tumor, sarcoma, lymphoma, and Paget's disease.

Breast Cancer Staging

In 2010 the American Joint Committee on Cancer (AJCC) revised their staging system on breast cancer. This latest revision made important additions and changes to the TNM staging system. Major changes to the staging system include the following:
- All invasive cancers should be assigned a histologic tumor grade using the Elston-Ellis modification of the Scarff-Bloom- Richardson grading system (Nottingham combined histologic grade). The grade is based on morphologic features and is defined as GX if grade cannot be assessed, G1 as low grade (favorable), G2 as intermediate (moderately favorable), and G3 as high grade (unfavorable).

TABLE 3	Overall Survival in Breast Cancer Patients	
STAGE	**10-YEAR OVERALL SURVIVAL**	**15-YEAR OVERALL SURVIVAL**
I	74%–95%	64%
II	76%	62%
IIA	81%	72%
IIB	70%	52%
III	50%	40%
IIIA	59%	49%
IIIB	36%	18%
IIIC	36%	18%
IV	18%	18%

Adapted from Rosen PP, et al. A long-term follow-up study of survival in stage I (T1N0M0) and stage II (T1N1M0) breast carcinoma. J Clin Oncol 1989;355–66; Woodward WA, Strom EA, Tucker SL, et al. Changes in the 2003 American Joint Committee on Cancer staging for breast cancer dramatically affect stage-specific survival. J Clin Oncol 2003;21:3244–8.

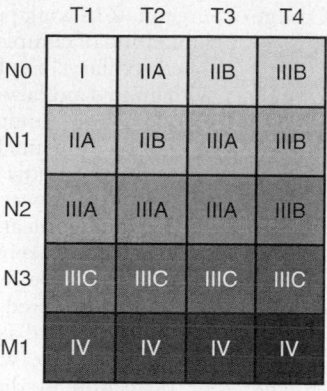

	T1	T2	T3	T4
N0	I	IIA	IIB	IIIB
N1	IIA	IIB	IIIA	IIIB
N2	IIIA	IIIA	IIIA	IIIB
N3	IIIC	IIIC	IIIC	IIIC
M1	IV	IV	IV	IV

Figure 3. Pathologic staging of breast cancer.

- Provides clarification of the classification of isolated tumor cells (ITCs) in axillary lymph node staging. ITCs are defined as single-tumor cells or small cell clusters not greater than 0.2 mm, usually detected only by immunohistochemical or molecular methods.
- Subdivides stage I into IA and IB based on the presence or absence of nodal micrometastatis (N0 vs. N0mi$^+$).
- Defines the category M0(i$^+$), referring to tumor cells detectable in bone marrow or circulating tumor cells or found incidentally in other tissues if not greater than 0.2 mm.
- Recommends the collection of prognostic factors including tumor grade, estrogen receptor status, progesterone receptor status, and HER2 status. These characteristics do not specifically influence the assigned stage of the disease.

Staging of breast cancer can be divided into clinical staging versus pathologic staging. Factors used for clinical staging include the size of the tumor within the breast, presence or absence of pathologically confirmed lymph nodes, and presence or absence of distant metastasis. There are five stages for breast cancer (Figure 3). Stage 0 is defined as the presence of in situ disease only, without evidence of nodal or distant metastasis. Stage I is considered breast cancer confined to the breast, which is 2 cm or less in size. Exceptions to this general characterization include tumors with extension to the chest wall or skin and inflammatory breast cancers. These tumors are at least stage IIIB. Stage IIA is a breast cancer that is 2 cm or less in size with pathologically positive ipsilateral mobile axillary nodes or less than 5 cm with negative lymph node status. A stage IIB cancer is defined as a tumor less than 5 cm with pathologically positive ipsilateral mobile axillary nodes or a tumor greater than 5 cm without lymph node involvement. Stage IIIA is considered a breast cancer of any size with pathologically positive ipsilateral fixed axillary nodes or clinically apparent internal mammary nodes in the absence of positive axillary nodes. Stage IIIB tumors are breast tumors with extension to the skin or chest wall or inflammatory breast cancer. Involvement of the pectoralis major or minor muscle does not constitute chest wall involvement. Stage IIIC tumors are breast cancers of any size with either positive infraclavicular or supraclavicular nodes or positive internal mammary nodes in the presence of positive axillary nodes. Stage IV connotes any breast cancers with distant metastasis.

Pathologic staging of breast cancer is more complicated and differs from clinical staging in that the number of nodes involved as well as how nodal metastasis is detected are used in stage designation of nodal status (see Figure 3).

Surgical Treatment of the Breast

A significant paradigm shift in the treatment of breast cancer has occurred over the past several decades. The Halsted paradigm, popularized at the beginning of the 20th century, hypothesized that breast cancer spreads in a contiguous fashion from the breast to the axillary lymph nodes and then to distant sites elsewhere in the body. The Fisher paradigm, which views breast cancer as systemic from very early in the course of the disease, modified this theory; according to this hypothesis the axillary lymph nodes act not as a barrier but as indicators of disease aggressiveness. Both paradigms are correct and incorrect. At a certain point in the evolution of a breast cancer, the disease changes from a local disease to a systemic disease. The Halsted paradigm promotes more intensive local treatment to eradicate the cancer, whereas the Fisher paradigm promotes less aggressive local treatment with the addition of systemic treatment in most women, even with relatively early disease. Because of this philosophy change and the detection of earlier disease through diligent screening techniques, surgical treatment of breast cancer is progressing toward less radical surgery and more adjuvant therapy, with equal or better outcomes.

Breast Conservation Therapy

Most small noninvasive and invasive breast cancers are treated by BCT, which consists of wide local excision with negative surgical margins and irradiation of the breast. The NSABP B-06, Milan I and Milan II, as well as other clinical trials, show no statistically significant difference in patient survival with mastectomy or BCT.

The addition of radiation treatment to wide local excision in patients with noninvasive and invasive carcinoma is currently the standard of treatment. The NSABP B-06 randomized trial evaluated local recurrence of small invasive tumors with and without irradiation after lumpectomy. Patients who did not undergo radiation therapy had significantly higher rates of local recurrence. With BCT, incidence of recurrence in the treated breast is widely variable. Local recurrence rate is lower in patients treated with mastectomy. The majority of recurrences occur in the first 3 years after surgery. Absolute contraindications to BCT include first- or second-trimester pregnant patients, multicentric disease, history of previous radiation therapy to the chest wall, and persistent positive margins after reasonable surgical attempts. Relative contraindications include a tumor of any size that cannot be adequately excised without significant deformity to the breast, a noncompliant patient, and history of significant collagen vascular disease. If both BCT and mastectomy are viable options, the patient's preference should also play a role in the decision to proceed with BCT versus a mastectomy.

Mastectomy

A patient with contraindications to breast conservation should have a mastectomy with or without immediate reconstruction. Total mastectomy surgically removes the breast parenchyma, pectoral fascia, nipple, and the areola complex. A modified radical mastectomy includes axillary dissection. A radical mastectomy, rarely done today, includes removal of the pectoralis major and minor muscles and axillary dissection.

Breast Reconstruction

Any patient recommended to have a mastectomy should be offered the option of immediate or delayed reconstruction and referred to a plastic and reconstructive surgeon to discuss which techniques are appropriate. One commonly used method of breast reconstruction is a tissue expander breast implant. A tissue expander is placed beneath the pectoralis muscles, and expansions are performed over a period of several weeks to months to stretch the subpectoral pocket to accommodate the permanent implant. The permanent saline or silicone implant is then inserted as a secondary procedure.

Another method of breast reconstruction is the transverse rectus abdominis myocutaneous (TRAM) flap, which involves the transfer of skin, fat, and muscle from the lower part of the abdomen to create a reconstructed breast. This procedure can be performed as a free flap with the arterial and venous supply anastomosed to vessels in the axilla or as a pedicle flap with the arterial and venous supply from the superior epigastric vessels. Other types of flap reconstructions include latissimus dorsi or gluteal flaps. Reconstruction of the nipple and areola is often performed as a later procedure.

Surgical Treatment of the Axilla

The status of the axilla should be assessed for metastases in any patient with invasive breast cancer for several reasons. The status of the axillary lymph nodes is important in determining the patient's stage of disease. The presence or absence of axillary lymph node metastases is predictive of the prognosis and facilitates decisions by the medical oncology team regarding adjuvant therapy. Relapse-free survival is closely related to the number of lymph nodes that are positive. In a study of 2873 patients, Hilsenbeck found that the relapse-free survival at 5 years was 80% in patients with node-negative disease. This number decreased to 70%, 60%, and 40% with 1 to 3 positive nodes, 4 to 9 positive nodes, and more than 10 positive nodes, respectively. Nodal tumor burden (number of involved axillary lymph nodes) is now incorporated into the sixth revision of the AJCC staging system. Surgical removal of metastatic nodes in the axilla significantly decreases the possibility of axillary recurrence. ALND may improve overall survival, but this issue is debated in the medical literature.

Sentinel Lymph Node Biopsy

Axillary dissection traditionally was performed on all patients with invasive breast cancer. Today, sentinel lymphadenectomy, or sentinel lymph node (SLN) biopsy, identifies the first, or sentinel, lymph node or nodes in the axillary chain to receive drainage from the breast cancer and thus the most likely to contain metastases. The SLN biopsy is performed by injecting isosulfan blue dye and/or radioactive isotope to localize the SLN.

The SLN can be identified in 95% of all cases. Multiple studies show that SLN biopsy can predict accurately the presence of axillary metastases in T1-2 breast cancer with a false-negative rate of 5% and an accuracy rate of 95%. The false-negative rate of SLN biopsy can be decreased to 1% to 3% if any palpable node is removed along with any hot or blue nodes. The SLN biopsy, a less invasive way to assess the status of the axilla, is associated with fewer complications than an axillary node dissection. Areas of controversy in SLN biopsy include T3, palpable suspicious axillary lymph nodes, and previous neoadjuvant therapy. In a study by Specht, 25% of palpable suspicious axillary lymph nodes proved benign on final pathology. Previous axillary dissection is not a strict contraindication per se because 75% of these patients can still have an identifiable sentinel node. The success rate depends on the number of nodes previously removed, with a success rate of 87% when fewer than 10 nodes are removed versus a success rate of 47% when more than 10 nodes are removed. Contraindications to SLN biopsy include T4 breast cancer and pregnancy. SLN biopsy is contraindicated in pregnancy because of the lack of data regarding fetal safety, although computer models suggest the amount of radiation exposure to the fetus is negligible.

Axillary Dissection

Patients who have metastatic cells on SLN biopsy typically undergo complete ALND. Alternatively, if a patient is not a candidate for SLN biopsy or if the attempt at the procedure fails, ALND should be considered. Axillary dissection involves the removal of 10 to 30 lymph nodes from the axilla. The potential risk of axillary dissection includes the accumulation of a seroma, ipsilateral arm lymphedema, and numbness around the area of the intercostal brachial innervation if the nerve is sacrificed at the time of surgery. Because of the lifetime increased chance of arm lymphedema and possible infection, patients should avoid any trauma or procedures such as venipuncture or blood pressure measurements on the ipsilateral arm.

Currently, the decision to undergo a completion axillary lymph node dissection following a positive SLN biopsy is determined by the level of physician and patient preference for or against it. Wasif reported that only 23% of 537 American Society of Clinical Oncology surgeons and medical oncologists "always" perform an axillary dissection for findings of micrometastatese in the sentinel node.

The American College of Surgeons Z11 trial, published in 2011, attempted to prove that the elimination of completion axillary dissection in patients with involved axillary lymph nodes was not harmful to patients. Women with limited axillary nodal metastases and generally favorable index lesions were randomized to a complete dissection or no further axillary treatment. The study opened in 1999 and closed in 2004 after accruing only 891 of the 1900 patients needed to obtain statistical significance. (In point of fact, based upon the trialists projected number of death events required to answer the question and the observed survival of the overall group, the trial needed to accrue some 5000 patients.) After failing to reach accrual goals the trial was reconsidered using an alternative "salvage" hypothesis that labeled the trial as a "non-inferiority" study. The authors reported that there was no benefit to performing the axillary node dissection in the control group, although the median number of nodes that contained breast cancer was the same in both arms. Also, the intent to treat group was included in the treated group, which meant that over 100 patients who were simply lost to follow-up were included in the analysis. These factors allied themselves to render this trial underpowered to adequately address the question that it was ostensibly asking. As a non-inferiority trial (in which we reverse the null hypothesis and the alternative hypothesis) this represents a type 1 statistical error. Despite these important caveats, the authors concluded that a completion axillary dissection can be avoided in these patients. For women with positive SLN biopsies, axillary dissection provides locoregional control, offers prognostic information, and may increase survival. Until further studies show otherwise, completion axillary dissection should remain our standard practice.

Adjuvant Therapy

Historically, adjuvant cytotoxic chemotherapy was used to treat patients with a significant likelihood for the development of metastatic disease. Randomized clinical trials in patients with negative axillary lymph nodes suggested that the risk was sufficient in virtually all patients whose index tumor was greater than 1 cm in diameter. Today, in patients with estrogen receptor positive breast cancer and negative axillary nodes it is highly preferable to obtain a genomic profile of the primary cancer to determine the risk for recurrence. (OncoType DX, Genomic Health Inc.; see below.)

The most commonly used cytotoxic regimens include CMF (cyclophosphamide [Cytoxan], methotrexate, and 5-FU [fluorouracil]) for 6 cycles or AC-T for 8 cycles (4 cycles of doxorubicin [Adriamycin] and cyclophosphamide followed by 4 cycles of paclitaxel [Taxol]). Patients whose tumors show overexpression or amplification of the HER-2/neu oncogene benefit from the addition of trastuzumab (Herceptin). Trastuzumab, an immunotherapeutic agent, is a monoclonal antibody that is used in early-stage breast cancer patients who are Human Epidermal growth factor Receptor 2 positive. Herceptin can be given in conjunction with the chemotherapy agents Adriamycin, Cytoxan, and either Taxol or docetaxel (Taxotere). This treatment course is known as "AC→TH". It can also be given with the chemotherapy drugs Taxotere and carboplatin (Paraplatin)[1] or alone after treatment with multiple other therapies, including an anthracycline (Adriamycin)-based therapy. In women with HER2-positive breast cancers being treated with neoadjuvant chemotherapy, the addition of neoadjuvant Herceptin to paclitaxel followed by combination chemotherapy was associated with an increase in pathologic complete response rate from 26% to 65.2%. As an adjuvant treatment, NSABP B-31 and NCCTG N9831 trials were combined to show a 52% reduction in the risk for recurrence and a 35% reduction in the risk for death with the addition of trastuzumab. The results were reproduced when each trial was analyzed separately. Several other studies looking at risk for recurrence and death have shown supporting evidence of the benefits of Herceptin use.

In the elderly population, the CMF regimen may be easier to tolerate than the AC-T regimens. A dose-dense regimen of AC-T

---

[1]Not FDA approved for this indication.

results in a slight improvement of disease-free and overall survival. A dose-dense regimen involves giving the chemotherapy in cycles every 2 weeks, with bone marrow support such as G-CSF (Neupogen), as opposed to the traditional cycles every 3 weeks. In the Early Breast Cancer Trialists' Collaborative Group (EBCTCG) meta-analysis from Oxford, England, adjuvant chemotherapy appears the most beneficial for women younger than 50 years of age. Combination chemotherapy resulted in the improvement of 10-year-overall survival from 71% in node-negative patients not receiving chemotherapy to 78% in those who did receive chemotherapy. This increase was even more dramatic in node-positive patients, with an improvement of overall survival from 42% to 53%. A much smaller effect was seen in patients older than 50 years of age. In this group of patients, survival was increased from 67% to 69% when node-negative patients not receiving chemotherapy were compared to those receiving chemotherapy. In node-positive elderly patients, improvement in overall survival was also minimal, with an increase of survival from 47% to 49% with chemotherapy.

Breast cancers are somewhat unique in their propensity to be dependent upon steroid binding hormones (such as estrogen). Estrogen blockade therapy is a mainstay in the treatment of these breast cancers. Estrogen ablative therapy can be achieved via a wide range of strategies, including the use of selective estrogen receptor modulators (tamoxifen citrate, raloxifene [Evista][1], aromatase inhibitors (anastrozole [Arimidex], letrozole [Femara], exemestane [Aromasin]) or estrogen receptor downregulators (fulvestrant [Faslodex]). Ablation in premenopausal women can also be achieved surgically via bilateral salpingo-oophorectomy.

The EBCTCG meta-analysis looking at the role of tamoxifen in the premenopausal patients found that tamoxifen results in an absolute improvement of 10-year overall survival of 5.6% in node-negative patients and 10.9% in node-positive patients. This effect is even greater in the postmenopausal population, with a 26% proportional reduction in 10-year mortality rates. The recommended length of treatment for node-negative patients is 5 years. Additionally, tamoxifen can be used as a chemopreventive agent to decrease the chance of an additional ipsilateral tumor developing in patients undergoing breast conservation or to decrease the possibility of contralateral breast cancer.

Three large randomized trials of aromatase inhibitors, such as anastrozole (Arimidex), exemestane (Aromasin), and letrozole (Femara), were published. In the ATAC (Arimidex, Tamoxifen, Alone or in Combination) trial, patients on anastrozole had a statistically significant longer disease-free interval when compared with patients on tamoxifen alone (hazard ratio of 0.83). No difference in survival was seen between the two groups. In another large study, patients on tamoxifen for 2 to 3 years were randomized to continuing tamoxifen versus switching to exemestane for a total of 5 years of therapy. There appeared to be an improvement in disease-free survival in the aromatase inhibitor arm (hazard ratio of 0.68). No difference in survival was seen, and given the early stoppage and crossover of patients, no survival data will be obtainable from this study. Yet another large, double-blind, randomized trial involved patients who had finished a 5-year course of tamoxifen and were then randomized to receiving letrozole versus placebo. The trial was stopped at a mean follow-up of 2.4 years secondary to a significant improvement in disease-free survival in the letrozole arm (hazard ratio of 0.57). Again, no difference in survival was seen. Aromatase inhibitors are useful only in postmenopausal patients. Premenopausal patients may benefit from an aromatase inhibitor only after ovarian ablation.

Disease Subsetting and Personalized Breast Cancer Treatment

One of the fundamental conceptual advances in the field of breast cancer in the past 100 years centers on the fact that breast cancer is not a single disease entity but rather is a large, complex family of diseases. Monolithic treatment approaches have been the hallmark of breast cancer care until very recently, when disease subsetting through genomic profiling has become a reality. The first approved and validated assay in estrogen receptor positive, node negative breast cancer is known as the Oncotype DX recurrence score.

Oncotype DX is the most commonly used genomic profiling tool for breast cancer in the United States. This test evaluates and scores the status of expression of 21 genes within a tumor sample. The results are reported as a quantitative Recurrence Score, which correlates with the likelihood that a particular tumor will recur within the next 10 years following appropriate hormonal ablative therapy. Indirectly, the data suggest which patients may benefit the most from cytotoxic chemotherapy (and may be refractory to hormonal therapy). This assay has been incorporated into evidence-based patient management algorithms supported by both ASCO and the NCCN.

Surveillance after a Diagnosis of Breast Cancer

Surveillance should continue after diagnosis and treatment of breast cancer to detect local recurrence or a new primary breast cancer in either the ipsilateral or contralateral breast. The National Comprehensive Cancer Network guidelines recommend that patients continue diligent monthly self-examinations and that a physician perform a physical examination at 6-month intervals to assess for evidence of local recurrence and symptoms of metastatic disease. The ipsilateral arm should be evaluated to detect early signs of lymphedema and initiate appropriate management. Bilateral mammograms should be obtained every year. Bone and computed tomographic scans and other tumor markers should be performed only on patients with symptomatic systemic disease because of the lack of evidence of improved survival with early detection of distant metastases.

Special Topics in Breast Disease
Phyllodes Tumor

Phyllodes tumor (cystosarcoma phyllodes) is a fibroepithelial lesion that can be either benign or malignant. It is a rare tumor of the breast accounting for 1% of all cases. The mean age of patients is 54 years of age. These tumors often present as a breast mass on clinical and mammographic examination, and they are considered benign or malignant depending on stromal cellularity, mitotic activity, presence of necrosis, and type of borders. Treatment is complete excision without axillary node dissection. Metastases secondary to malignant phyllodes are hematogenous and primarily travel to the lungs. It is important to obtain negative margins. A mastectomy occasionally may be warranted for large lesions. Patients with malignant phyllodes have an 80% chance of 5-year survival as opposed to more than 95% for benign phyllodes.

Nipple Discharge

Nipple discharge can occur at any age and presents as a bloody, serous, or milky discharge. Only 6% to 12% of patients with a nipple discharge are found to have an underlying malignancy. This risk is slightly elevated if the discharge is bloody. The most common cause of serous or serosanguinous nipple discharge is a benign intraductal papilloma. Numerous drugs can also cause nipple discharge, such as phenothiazine, tricyclic antidepressants, reserpine, butyrophenones, cimetidine (Tagamet), verapamil (Calan), metoclopramide (Reglan), thiazides, and hormone replacement therapy. The most common underlying malignancy is DCIS. Ductograms may be useful in locating the papilloma. When the nipple discharge is unilaterally persistent, spontaneous, or postmenopausal, further workup may be considered. Other suspicious nipple discharges are those confined to one duct and those that are bloody or serous. In general, the evaluation of nipple discharge should begin with a clinical examination and a mammogram. Cytologic examination of the discharge has a low sensitivity for detection of underlying malignancy and should not be used in the workup. Treatment consists of a major duct excision.

[1]Not FDA approved for this indication.

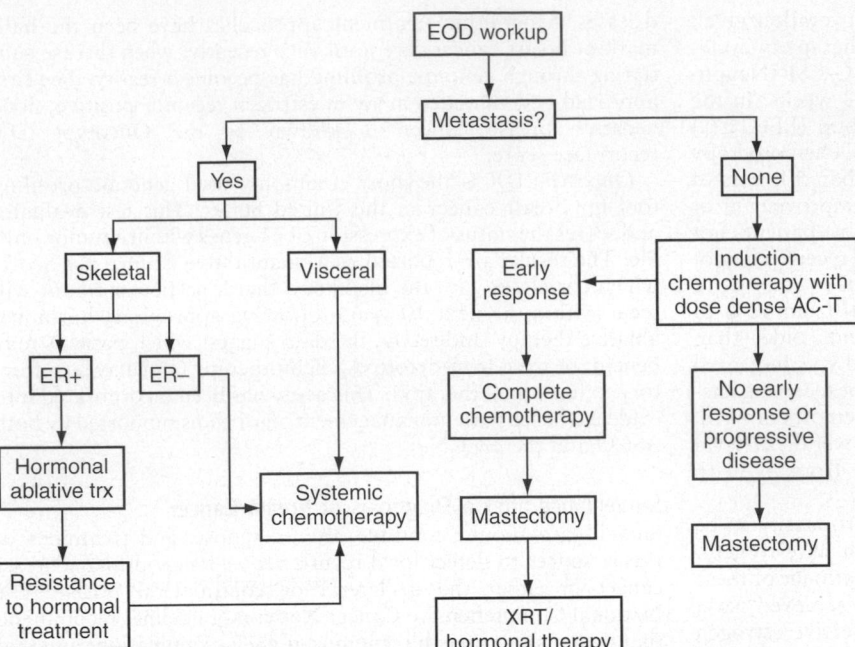

Figure 4. Algorithm for treatment of locally advanced breast cancer (LABC). *Abbreviations:* AC-T = Adriamycin and cyclophosphamide plus Taxol; EOD = extent-of-disease; trx = treatment; XRT = x-radiation therapy.

Gynecomastia

Gynecomastia is the unilateral or bilateral benign enlargement of male breast tissue. The etiology is often related to various substances, including exogenous hormones, cimetidine (Tagamet), thiazides, digoxin, theophylline, phenothiazines, alcohol, and marijuana use; it may also be idiopathic. The main concern is to rule out the diagnosis of male breast cancer. Once breast cancer is excluded, no treatment is indicated. If medication and lifestyle etiologies are eliminated without remission of the gynecomastia, the excess breast tissue may be surgically removed for cosmetic considerations or for breast pain.

Male Breast Cancer

Carcinoma of the male breast represents 1% of all breast cancers. Because men are not routinely screened for breast cancer, the diagnosis is often delayed. The most common manifestation of male breast cancer is a painless, firm, subareolar breast mass. The differential diagnosis includes gynecomastia. Breast imaging with mammography and/or ultrasound may be helpful in rendering a diagnosis inasmuch as the appearance of male breast cancer is a stellate, irregular solid mass. Any suspicious breast mass in a male patient should undergo diagnostic biopsy. If a malignancy is diagnosed, standard treatment is mastectomy with assessment of the axillary nodes by SLN biopsy or ALND. Most cases of male breast cancer are estrogen-receptor positive, and recommendations for adjuvant chemotherapy or hormonal therapy should be based on criteria similar to those for breast cancer in female patients. Any male with the diagnosis of breast cancer should undergo *BRCA* testing.

Breast Cancer in Pregnancy

Pregnancy-associated breast cancer represents less than 2% of all breast cancer diagnoses. The breast cancer frequently is diagnosed at a late stage because of the difficulty of examining the breast in pregnant women and the avoidance of mammography during pregnancy. Any suspicious lesion noted during pregnancy should be subjected to biopsy in the same fashion as in a nongravid woman. Radiation therapy should not be administered during pregnancy, so breast conservation is generally contraindicated unless the diagnosis is made within a few weeks of delivery. Surgical treatment with mastectomy and ALND is the standard treatment of breast cancer during pregnancy. Adjuvant chemotherapy can be delivered with selective agents during the second and third trimesters. The prognosis is similar to that of nongravid women in whom breast cancer is diagnosed at a comparable stage.

Inflammatory Breast Cancer

The classic manifestation of inflammatory breast cancer is erythema, edema, peau d'orange, and color of the breast resembling an infectious process. Malignant cells within the dermal lymphatic vessels of the breast confirm the diagnosis. The usual pathology of the associated carcinoma is IFDC-NOS. Inflammatory carcinoma is a very aggressive type of breast cancer, with over 90% of patients having positive axillary lymph nodes at diagnosis. The recommended treatment is multimodality therapy, with chemotherapy preceding surgery. Surgical treatment is mastectomy followed by radiation therapy and often additional chemotherapy.

Locally Advanced Breast Cancer

Patients with N2 or N3 nodal status or those with four or more positive axillary nodes, T3 or T4 tumors, or involvement of the pectoralis fascia have locally advanced breast cancer (LABC). The recommended treatment for patients is neoadjuvant chemotherapy, which is administered before surgical treatment, although it has no impact on overall survival. An extent-of-disease workup should be done in patients with LABC and includes computed tomography of the chest, abdomen, and pelvis along with a bone scan. Figure 4 provides an algorithm for the treatment of LABC.

CANCER OF THE ENDOMETRIUM

Method of
Dan-Arin Silasi, MD; and Masoud Azodi, MD

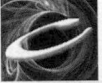

CURRENT DIAGNOSIS

- Most patients with uterine cancer are postmenopausal, and bleeding occurs early in the course of the disease.
- Postmenopausal vaginal bleeding is evaluated by endometrial biopsy.

- In premenopausal patients, especially obese women, irregular bleeding, including absence of menses, requires diagnostic evaluation.
- The presence of endometrial cells on a Papanicolaou (Pap) smear in premenopausal women is an indication for biopsy only when they are abnormal.
- The biopsy can be performed in the office and requires no sedation or analgesia.
- When it is not possible to obtain an adequate sample because of severe genital atrophy, obesity, or pain, operative dilation and curettage should be performed.

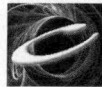

CURRENT THERAPY

- Most patients with endometrial cancer present with stage I disease and surgery is the mainstay of therapy.
- Conventional or robotic laparoscopic approaches have faster postoperative recovery.
- The current standard is pelvic and periaortic lymphadenectomy in addition to hysterectomy and adnexectomy.
- Controversy exists regarding the need and extent of lymph node dissection, especially for patients with low-grade endometrioid cancers.
- Adjuvant radiation therapy is recommended for type I cancers when the tumors are high-grade, penetrate deep into the myometrium, involve the cervix, or show evidence of lymphovascular space invasion.
- Platinum-based chemotherapy is indicated for uterine papillary serous and clear cell cancers, even for stage IA.

Epidemiology

In the United States, endometrial cancer is the most common malignancy of the female reproductive tract. In 2008, the American Cancer Society estimated that endometrial cancer was diagnosed in 40,100 women, and 7470 deaths were caused by this disease. Endometrial cancer ranks eighth in cause of cancer deaths for women.

Although it has been described to occur as early as age 16 years, it is primarily a disease of the postmenopausal woman. Only 25% of the cases occur in premenopausal patients.

Classification

Two types of endometrial cancer have been described.

Type I Cancer

Type I has endometrioid histology and is the more common form. These tumors often arise in the background of chronically estrogen-stimulated endometrium; progesterone has a protective effect. Most commonly, an excess estrogenic environment occurs when steroid hormone precursors are converted by aromatase in adipose cells into estrone, a weak estrogen. This explains why type I uterine cancer is strongly linked to obesity. Other conditions related to a hyperestrogenic status are chronic anovulation, nulliparity, late menopause, iatrogenic estrogen administration, and estrogen-secreting tumors such as granulosa-cell tumors. Tamoxifen (Nolvadex) is a selective-estrogen receptor (ER) modulator that exhibits antiestrogenic properties on the breast tissue and estrogenic effects on the endometrium. Its use in the treatment of ER–positive breast cancers is an established risk factor for uterine cancer.

Type I cancers have a more indolent course when compared to type II, are better differentiated, and have a better prognosis. Seventy-five percent of patients with type I cancers present with stage I disease.

Type I endometrioid carcinomas are diploid in 80% of cases, and they often exhibit a mutation of the PTEN tumor suppressor gene, microsatellite instability, and ER and progesterone-receptor (PR) positivity.

A genetic predisposition for uterine cancer accounts for less than 5% of all cases. The most common is the hereditary nonpolyposis colorectal syndrome, which is caused by a germline mutation of the DNA repair genes. Members of families with these mutations are affected mostly by colorectal adenocarcinomas, but endometrial cancer is second in incidence.

Type II Cancer

Type II cancers encompass clear cell carcinoma and papillary serous carcinoma. Endometrioid carcinomas with architectural grade 3 are also classified as type II. Obesity and exposure to excess estrogen are not established risk factors. These cancers occur at ages older than type I, are characterized by aggressive behavior, and occur commonly in a background of atrophic endometrium.

Less than 10% of all endometrial cancers are of the papillary serous variety, but they cause 40% of deaths from endometrial cancer. Metastatic disease can occur even when the primary tumor is confined to an endometrial polyp. Only 55% of patients present with stage I disease, and 40% present with metastatic disease.

Uterine papillary serous carcinoma has a histologic appearance similar to ovarian serous papillary cancer and has the same pattern of spread. However, ovarian cancer has a much better response to chemotherapy.

At the molecular level, $p53$ overexpression is encountered in 90% of tumors, $PTEN$ mutations are rare, and half exhibit $HER-2/neu$ overexpression. They are ER and PR negative. Type II tumors are often aneuploid.

Clear cell carcinomas are characterized by aggressive behavior and account for 4% of all uterine cancers and 8% of deaths. $PTEN$ or $p53$ mutations are present in less than 20%.

Clinical Presentation

The majority of patients with endometrioid cancer present with abnormal vaginal bleeding. This is often the only symptom, but fortunately it appears early in the course of the disease, especially for the type I carcinomas. For most women, postmenopausal bleeding prompts them to seek medical attention, and this accounts for the diagnosis at stage I in 75% of the patients.

For menstruating women, a change in the bleeding pattern, spotting, or frank intermenstrual bleeding requires investigation. In anovulatory patients, of whom a significant proportion are obese or morbidly obese, the absence of menses for long periods of time, interspersed with spotting or episodes of heavy vaginal bleeding, can be an indicator of endometrial pathology, including malignancy.

Advanced disease, with spread to and beyond the pelvic organs, can manifest with pelvic pressure, pain, or urinary and bowel symptoms.

Diagnosis

No screening methods for endometrial cancer exist.

Abnormal vaginal bleeding, whether it is postmenopausal, irregular, or the absence of menses in a nonpregnant premenopausal woman, is routinely assessed by endometrial biopsy. This can be performed in the office using a small-bore rigid or flexible catheter and is 95% as accurate as dilation and curettage (D&C). Fractional D&C with or without hysteroscopic guidance is another approach used to obtain an endometrial and endocervical specimen.

The finding of endometrial cells on cytologic examination of the cervix (Papanicolaou [Pap] smear) in a postmenopausal woman can be an indicator of uterine carcinoma and requires endometrial sampling. For premenopausal women, an endometrial biopsy is indicated only when the endometrial cells on the Pap smear are abnormal.

When the endometrial biopsy detects changes of endometrial hyperplasia with nuclear atypia, up to 25% of patients harbor an undetected uterine carcinoma. This is invariably well differentiated and early stage.

Rarely, carcinoma is discovered in the surgical specimen after hysterectomy was performed for other indications.

Imaging techniques are of limited value for the diagnosing endometrial cancer. Carcinoma is unlikely to be present when the endometrial thickness in a postmenopausal woman measures less than 5 mm by transvaginal ultrasound.

Staging

Uterine cancer is staged surgically. In 2009, the Committee on Gynecologic Oncology of the International Federation of Gynecology and Obstetrics revised the 1988 staging system for endometrial cancer (Table 1).

Treatment

Surgical Treatment

Comprehensive surgical staging for carcinoma of the corpus uteri includes exploration of the peritoneal cavity, hysterectomy, resection of the ovaries and fallopian tubes, and pelvic and periaortic lymph node dissection. At the beginning of each operation, a cytologic evaluation of the abdominal cavity is performed. In addition to these procedures, omentectomy and peritoneal biopsies are often performed for type II uterine cancers. When intraabdominal metastatic disease is encountered, resection of all masses is indicated.

Controversy exists regarding the necessity and extent of lymph node dissection, especially for early type I cancers. There is consensus, however, that the most accurate evaluation of lymph node involvement is by lymphadenectomy and pathologic review. Two large prospective trials conducted in Europe randomized patients to hysterectomy and lymphadenectomy or hysterectomy only and found no difference in survival and recurrence rate. However, all patients were treated with radiation postoperatively. In the

United States, a retrospective study of 12,000 patients found a survival benefit for patients who underwent lymph node dissection.

The surgical staging can be performed by laparotomy or laparoscopy. A body of literature exists that recognizes minimally invasive surgery as a better treatment option where applicable. A Gynecologic Oncology Group (GOG) study has shown that the number of lymph nodes and the incidence of lymph node metastases were similar for both operative approaches. Laparoscopy has the advantage of a shorter hospital stay, less postoperative pain, lesser incidence of incisional hernias, faster recovery, and faster return to regular activities.

Main deterrents to a laparoscopic approach are obesity, prior abdominal surgeries, and long learning curve for the operator. In our experience, since the introduction of the robotic surgical system in clinical practice, these factors have had no impact on the patients' care. At Yale New Haven Hospital, the hospital course and postoperative outcomes of obese and morbidly obese patients who underwent robotic surgery was no different than that of patients with a body mass index in the normal range. The median postoperative hospital stay for patients with malignant obesity was 1.2 days.

Adjuvant Therapy
Early-Stage Disease

Adjuvant radiation therapy is recommended for type I cancers when the tumors are high-grade, penetrate deep into the myometrium, involve the cervix, or show evidence of lymphovascular space invasion. The treatment can be in the form of external beam pelvic radiation or brachytherapy to the vaginal apex and superior vagina.

Platinum-based chemotherapy is indicated for uterine papillary serous and clear cell cancers, even for stage IA.

Metastatic Disease

Cytotoxic chemotherapy is the mainstay of therapy for metastatic carcinoma of the endometrium. Systemic therapy was found to be superior to whole abdominal radiation. Regardless of the regimen chosen, response rates are modest. Median values of progression-free intervals do not exceed 6 months, and overall survival does not exceed 12 months.

Single-Agent Therapies. Single-agent therapies with doxorubicin (Adriamycin),[1] cisplatin (Platinol),[1] carboplatin (Paraplatin),[1] and paclitaxel (Taxol)[1] have response rates of 20% and higher. Pegylated liposomal doxorubicin (Doxil)[1] has poor activity against metastatic endometrial cancer.

Combination Chemotherapy. Both the GOG and EORTC (European Organisation for Research and Treatment of Cancer) have completed phase III trials that investigated differences in responses to doxorubicin versus doxorubicin and cisplatin. The response rates were 25% versus 42% for GOG and 17% versus 43% for EORTC. Although these differences were statistically significant, no benefit in overall survival was noted.

In another GOG trial, the response rate of patients treated with a three-drug regimen, doxorubicin, cisplatin, and paclitaxel, was 57%, whereas the doxorubicin and cisplatin arm showed a response rate of 34%. Toxicity was higher in the three-drug arm, and the GOG final statistical report in January 2007 showed that the addition of paclitaxel to doxorubicin and cisplatin following surgery and volume-directed radiation did not increase survival.

The combination of carboplatin and paclitaxel is often prescribed for metastatic and recurrent endometrial cancer. Response rates range from 46% to 78%. In the current phase III GOG protocol for recurrent endometrial cancers, the combination of doxorubicin, cisplatin, and paclitaxel (control arm) is being compared to carboplatin and paclitaxel.

Progestin Treatment. Endometrial cancers with low histologic grade, the presence of PR, and a longer interval to develop metastases after treatment of the primary tumor are more likely to

TABLE 1	Staging System for Endometrial Cancer
STAGE	**DESCRIPTION**
Stage I	
I*	Tumor confined to the corpus uteri
IA*	No or less than half myometrial invasion
IB*	Invasion equal to or more than half of the myometrium
Stage II	
II*	Tumor invades cervical stroma but does not extend beyond the uterus†
Stage III	
III*	Local and/or regional spread of the tumor
IIIA*	Tumor invades the serosa of the corpus uteri and/or adnexae‡
IIIA*	Tumor invades the serosa of the corpus uteri and/or adnexae‡
IIIB*	Vaginal and/or parametrial involvement‡
IIIC*	Metastases to pelvic and/or para-aortic lymph nodes‡
IIIC1*	Positive pelvic nodes
IIIC2*	Positive para-aortic lymph nodes with or without positive pelvic lymph nodes
Stage IV	
IV*	Tumor invades bladder and/or bowel mucosa, and/or distant metastases
IVA*	Tumor invasion of bladder and/or bowel mucosa
IVB*	Distant metastases, including intra-abdominal metastases and/or inguinal lymph nodes

*G1, G2, or G3.
†Endocervical glandular involvement only should be considered as stage I and no longer as stage II.
‡Positive cytology must be reported separately without changing the stage.

[1]Not FDA approved for this indication.

respond to progesterone treatment, usually administered as oral megestrol acetate (Megace).

Other Treatments

From the selective estrogen-receptor modulators, tamoxifen[1] alone has modest efficacy in the treatment of metastatic endometrial cancer. Tamoxifen was also added to progestins to prevent downregulation of PR that occurs with progesterone treatment. Response rates were higher than for progesterone alone, but progression-free intervals and overall survival were similar.

Two aromatase inhibitors, anastrozole (Arimidex)[1] and letrozole (Femara),[1] were investigated in phase II trials and demonstrated minimal activity.

A gonadotropin-releasing hormone agonist, goserelin acetate (Zoladex),[1] has shown insufficient activity.

Molecular Therapy

Trastuzumab (Herceptin)[1] has not shown activity in a GOG study investigating its efficacy in the treatment of *HER-2/neu*-positive endometrial cancer.

Erlotinib (Tarceva),[1] an epidermal growth factor receptor (EGFR) inhibitor, demonstrated some activity, and cetuximab (Erbitux)[1] is currently being investigated.

A GOG phase II trial of the antiangiogenic agent bevacizumab (Avastin)[1] has been completed; results are pending. Sorafenib (Nexavar)[1] has shown modest activity.

Other agents investigated that have shown clinical responses were the fusion protein VEGF-Trap, and mTOR (mammalian target of rapamycin) inhibitors such as everolimus (RAD-001 [Afinitor])[1] and AP23573.

Recurrent Disease

The most common site for recurrence, especially for type I cancers, is at the vaginal apex. When the recurrent cancer occurs in the form of surgically resectable masses, surgery is followed by systemic chemotherapy. Unresectable metastatic disease is treated with systemic therapy.

---

[1]Not FDA approved for this indication.

References

FIGO Committee on Gynecologic Oncology. Revised FIGO staging for carcinoma of the vulva, cervix, and endometrium. Int J Gynecol Obstet 2009;105:103–4.

Fowler W, Mutch D. Management of endometrial cancer. Women's Health 2008;4 (5):479–89.

Lowe MP, Johnson PR, Kamelle SA, et al. A multiinstitutional experience with robotic-assisted hysterectomy with staging for endometrial cancer. Obstet Gynecol 2009;114.236–43.

Mendivil A, Schuler KM, Gehrig PA. Non-endometrioid adenocarcinoma of the uterine corpus: A review of selected histological subtypes. Cancer Control 2009;16 (1):46–52.

Writing Committee on behalf of the ASTEC Study Group. Efficacy of systematic pelvic lymphadenectomy in endometrial cancer (MRC ASTEC trial): A randomised study. Lancet 2009;373:125–36.

CANCER OF THE UTERINE CERVIX

Method of
Lucybeth Nieves-Arriba, MD; and Peter G. Rose, MD

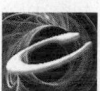

CURRENT DIAGNOSIS

- New recommendations for cytology screening recommend starting screening at 21 years of age.
- Initial workup must include a biopsy.
- Imaging techniques including magnetic resonance imaging and positron emission tomography–computed tomography can assist in treatment planning.

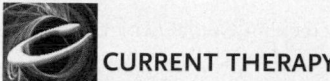

CURRENT THERAPY

- Despite recent availability of human papilloma virus (HPV) vaccination (Gardasil, Cervarix) and advances in screening, cervical cancer remains a significant global health problem, especially in underserved populations.
- Improved understanding of the disease has allowed more conservative treatment of selected patients with early-stage disease.
- For advanced and high-risk cervical cancer, chemoradiation has had a significant impact on survival.

Epidemiology

Worldwide, cervical cancer is the second most common cancer in women. It is the greatest cancer killer of young women and the most common cause of death from cancer in women in the developing world. Worldwide in 2008, among the 530,000 new cases of cervical cancer, the highest incidence rates were in Africa, Central and South America, and Asia. In the United States, it is estimated that approximately 12,200 new cases were diagnosed and 4,210 patients died from cervical cancer in 2010. Significant disparities in incidence and stage at time of diagnosis have been identified among different ethnic groups—African Americans, Asian Americans, European Americans, and Latin Americans—in the United States. Factors that increase the risk of cervical cancer include early age at first coitus, multiple sexual partners, history of sexually transmitted diseases, low socioeconomic status, cigarette smoking, immunosuppression, and Fanconi's syndrome.

Pathophysiology

Cervical cancer occurs secondary to viral transformation of the surface (epithelial) cells by high-risk types of the human papillomavirus (HPV), and it is the only gynecologic cancer that can be prevented by regular screening. Persistent infection with high-risk HPV has been identified as the essential factor in the pathogenesis of the majority of cervical cancers. The virus's ability to transform human epithelium has been associated with the expression of two viral gene products, E6 and E7, which interact with p53 (a tumor-suppressor protein) and retinoblastoma protein (pRB), respectively, and affect control mechanisms of the cell cycle.

The prevalence of genital HPV infection in the world is estimated to be 400 million. Data from the National Health and Nutrition Examination Survey (NHANES) estimate the prevalence of HPV infection among girls and women in the United States aged 14 to 59 years is 26.8%. In about 90% of cases, the high-risk HPV infection is cleared by the immune system within 16 months. HPV infections in girls and younger women are more likely transient and therefore less likely to be associated with significant cervical lesions.

Prevention and Screening

Recent advances in molecular biology have allowed the development of viral-like particles using the L1 protein (major immunogenic capsid protein) of the HPV virus. Current vaccines, Gardasil (approved 2006) and Cervarix (approved 2009) contain two high-risk genotypes, HPV-16 and HPV-18, and could theoretically prevent 70% of cervical cancer cases. The Gardasil vaccine also contains two low-risk genotypes, HPV-6 and HPV-11, to prevent viral genital warts. The vaccines were FDA approved to use in girls and women between the ages of 9 and 26 years. If all children younger than 12 years were vaccinated, the most optimistic predictions expect a major effect on the cancer incidence will not be seen for 30 years. In 2009 HPV vaccination of males in the same age group was approved.

The current standard screening algorithm in the United States for preventing cervical cancer is presented in Table 1. Women with abnormal cytology are referred for a colposcopic examination.

TABLE 1	Cervical Cytologic Screening Guidelines from the American College of Obstetricians and Gynecologists	
AGE (Y)	RECOMMENDATION FOR CYTOLOGIC SCREENING	COMMENTS
Younger than 21	Avoid screening	
21 to 29	Screen every 3 y	
30 to 65 or 70	May screen every 3 y*	This recommendation applies only to women with 3 consecutive cytologic tests; exceptions include women with HIV infection, compromised immunity, a history of cervical intraepithelial neoplasia grade 2 or 3, or exposure to DES in utero.
	Screen every 5 y	If HPV co-testing use
Between 65 and 70	May discontinue screening	This recommendation applies only to women with ≥3 consecutive negative cytologic tests and no abnormal tests in the preceding 10 y; exceptions include women with multiple sexual partners.

Abbreviation: DES = diethylstilbestrol.
Adapted from American College of Obstetricians and Gynecologists (ACOG). Cervical cytology screening. Washington (DC): American College of Obstetricians and Gynecologists (ACOG); 2012 Nov. (ACOG practice bulletin; no.131); 2009 Dec. 12 (ACOG practice bulletin; no. 109).

TABLE 2	Revised FIGO Staging for Carcinoma of the Cervix
STAGE	CRITERIA
Stage I	
I	The carcinoma is strictly confined to the cervix
IA	Invasive carcinoma, which can be diagnosed only by microscopy, with deepest invasion ≤5 mm and largest extension ≥7 mm
IA1	Measured stromal invasion of ≤3 mm in depth and extension of ≤7 mm
IA2	Measured stromal invasion of >3 mm in depth and extension of >7 mm
IB	Clinically visible lesions limited to the cervix or preclinical cancers greater than stage IA
IB1	Clinically visible lesion ≤4 cm in greatest dimension
IB2	Clinically visible lesion >4 cm in greatest dimension
Stage II	
II	Cervical carcinoma invades beyond the uterus, but not to the pelvic wall or to the lower third of the vagina
IIA	Without parametrial invasion
IIA1	Clinically visible lesion ≤4 cm in greatest dimension
IIA2	Clinically visible lesion >4 cm in greatest dimension
IIB	With obvious parametrial invasion
Stage III	
III	The tumor extends to the pelvic wall and/ or involves lower third of the vagina and/ or causes hydronephrosis or nonfunctioning kidney
IIIA	Tumor involves lower third of the vagina, with no extension to the pelvic wall
IIIB	Extension to the pelvic wall and/ or hydronephrosis or nonfunctioning kidney
Stage IV	
IV	The carcinoma has extended beyond the true pelvis or has involved (biopsy proven) the mucosa of the bladder or rectum; a bullous edema, as such, does not permit a case to be allotted as stage IV
IVA	Spread of the growth to adjacent organs
IVB	Spread to distant organs

Adapted from Pecorelli S: Revised FIGO staging for carcinoma of the vulva, cervix, and endometrium. Int J Gynaecol Obstet 2009;105(2):103-4. Erratum in Int J Gynaecol Obstet 2010;108(2):176.

The colposcopic examination is used to guide biopsies of the exocervix, and in most cases an endocervical biopsy is also performed. The biopsy results then determine the type of follow-up and or therapy required.

Staging

The International Federation of Gynecology and Obstetrics (FIGO) defined the most commonly accepted staging of cervical cancer. This staging is based on a careful clinical examination and the results of specific radiologic studies and procedures. FIGO's latest update (2009) is summarized in Table 2.

In cervical cancer, primary lesions initially progress to lymphatics in the parametrium and pelvic nodes and then extend laterally to the pelvic side wall, bladder, and rectum. The two major spread patterns identified in cervical cancer include direct extension and lymphatic spread.

Diagnosis

The initial workup for cervical cancer depends on whether a cervical lesion is visible. Patients without a visible cervical lesion require a cone biopsy to diagnose stage IA1 or IA2 tumor. Patients with a cervical lesion are assessed by history and physical examination and possibly by examination under anesthesia for biopsy, cystoscopy, sigmoidoscopy, and conventional imaging (chest x-ray, intravenous pyelogram). Other imaging modalities including computed tomography (CT), magnetic resonance imaging (MRI), and fluorodeoxyglucose positron emission tomography (FDG-PET) are useful in evaluating nodal or other metastatic sites but are not incorporated in the FIGO staging system owing to their limited availability worldwide. MRI performed significantly better than CT in detecting parametrial invasion, presence of bladder or rectal invasion, and identification of women suitable for fertility-preserving surgery. PET-CT is the most sensitive modality in identifying nodal metastasis or metastatic disease assisting with radiotherapy planning and evaluation of metabolic response to therapy. A 3-month post-therapy PET scan is highly predictive of long-term survival outcome.

Treatment

Multiple factors including tumor stage, size, histologic features (lymphovascular space invasion [LVSI], nonsquamous components, and depth of cervical stromal invasion), and evidence of lymph node metastasis influence the choice of treatment for cervical cancer. Patients with stage IA1 cervical cancer have undergone a cone biopsy and pathology demonstrates 3 mm of invasion or less, less than 7 mm width, no LVSI, and negative margins. Patients with this extent of disease can safely be treated with a less-radical hysterectomy, an extrafascial hysterectomy. Pelvic lymphadenectomy is not recommended owing to the low risk of pelvic node metastasis (<1%). In patients who desire to retain fertility, a cone biopsy may be considered. Wright and colleagues reported on 1409 women from the SEER database who were younger than 40 years and had stage IA1 cancer. The 5-year survival was 98% among 568 who underwent cone biopsy alone versus 99% among 841 who underwent hysterectomy.

Patients with stage IA2 to IB1 are generally treated with radical hysterectomy; in patients who are not candidates for surgery owing to comorbidities, radiation therapy is used. In patients with high-risk criteria after surgery—positive surgical margin, parametrial involvement, and positive pelvic nodes—cisplatin-based[1] chemoradiation, based on a positive randomized trial, is recommended. Those with intermediate risk factors including tumor size, cervical stromal invasion, and lymphovascular invasion had an improved progression-free survival with adjuvant radiation.

Radical trachelectomy—laparoscopic, vaginal or open—in conjunction with lymphadenectomy is a reasonable alternative treatment for select young patients with stage IA2 and IB1 who desire to maintain their childbearing capacity. The criteria used for patient selection include early-stage cervical cancer with a lesion less than 2 cm, no lymphovascular invasion, and no lymph node metastasis. Reports comparing radical trachelectomies with matched controls identified increased complications (25% vs. 3%) and overall less-radical dissection.

Treatment of stage IB2 cancer of the cervix varies depending on the bulkiness and shape of the lesion. Surgery and chemoradiation therapy have advantages and disadvantages. Finan and colleagues reported that up to 72% of patients with stage IB2 disease who were treated with surgery received adjuvant radiation owing to high-risk factors identified in pathologic evaluation of specimens. In a randomized Gynecologic Oncology Group trial, 94% of patients with IB2 cervical cancer who underwent radical hysterectomy had high or intermediate risk factors warranting adjuvant radiation.

[1]Not FDA approved for this indication.

In 1999 the National Cancer Institute (NCI) initiated a clinical alert recommending that concurrent cisplatin-based[1] chemotherapy be given with radiotherapy to women with cervical cancer based on five randomized studies, and this established a new standard of care (Table 3).

It is estimated that approximately 35% of patients with invasive cervical cancer will have recurrent or persistent disease, with most recurrences occurring in the first 2 years following primary therapy. Recurrence can be expected in 10% to 20% of patients treated with radical hysterectomy in contrast to 30% to 50% treated for more-advanced disease primarily with radiation plus concurrent chemotherapy. The site of the recurrence can direct further treatment. Patients with central pelvic recurrences after surgery are candidates for curative radiation; after primary treatment with radiation therapy patients may be candidates for curative radical surgery (exenteration). Prognosis is more favorable for patients undergoing exenteration when there is a small (<3 cm) central recurrence, no sidewall involvement, and longer than 2 years of disease-free interval. Those with small recurrences limited to the cervix or upper vagina can occasionally be treated with radical hysterectomy and upper vaginectomy.

However, most recurrences are distant, involving the lung, bone, abdominal cavity, and supraclavicular lymph nodes. Recurrences within irradiated areas have a poor response to therapy (0% to 5%). Recurrences in the nonirradiated areas respond better to chemotherapy, with response rates of 25% to 70%. The use of chemotherapy in the treatment of recurrent cervical cancer is challenging because agents are only moderately active and patients can present with renal impairment secondary to obstructive uropathy, resulting in altered excretion with increased toxicity from chemotherapeutic agents. Table 4 compares results of randomized chemotherapy trials for the treatment of recurrent cervical cancer.

TABLE 3 Randomized Trials of Cisplatin-based Chemoradiation

| TREATMENT | STAGE | SURVIVAL | | SIGNIFICANCE |
		TYPE	PERCENTAGE	
Gynecology Oncology Group 85				
RT/5-FU[1] infusion/bolus cisplatin[1]	IIB-IVA	3 y PFS	67%	$P = 0.033$
RT/oral HU[1]			57%	
Gynecology Oncology Group 109				
Rad hyst/RT	IA2-IIA	Est. 4-y	63%	$P = 0.003$
Rad hyst/RT/cisplatin[1]/5-FU[1]			80%	
Radiation Therapy Oncology Group 9001				
RT	IIB-IVA	DFS	40%	$P < 0.001$
RT/5-FU[1]/cisplatin[1]			67%	
Gynecology Oncology Group 120				
RT + cisplatin[1]	IIB-IVA	3-y PFS	67%	$P < 0.001$
RT + cisplatin[1]/5-FU[1]/HU[1]			64%	
RT + HU[1]			47%	
Gynecology Oncology Group 123				
RT + TAH	IB2	3 y PFS	74%	$P < 0.001$
RT + cisplatin[1] + TAH			83%	
Di Silvestro et al				
RT + cisplatin	IB2- IVA	3 y PFS	64%	$P = 0.7869$
RT + cisplatin+TPZ			63%	
Pearcey et al				
RT + cisplatin[1]	IB-IVA >5 cm	5-y DFS	62%	$P = 0.42$
RT			58%	

[1]Not FDA approved for this indication.
Abbreviations: DFS = disease-free survival; 5-FU = fluorouracil (Adrucil); HU = hydroxyurea; PFS = progression free survival; rad hyst = radical hysterectomy; RT = radiotherapy; TAH = total abdominal hysterectomy.

TABLE 4 — Phase III Trials Comparing Cisplatin Doublets and Cisplatin Alone to Treat Metastatic or Recurrent Cervical Carcinoma

STUDY	STAGE	RESPONSE RATE (%)	PROGRESSION-FREE SURVIVAL (MO)	OVERALL SURVIVAL (MO)
Gynecology Oncology Group 110				
Cisplatin[1]	IVB or recurrent	18	3.2	8
Cisplatin/mitolactol[8]		21	3.3	7.3
Cisplatin/ifosfamide (Ifex)[1]		31	8.3	4.6
Significance		$P = 0.004$	$P = 0.003$	$P = 0.835$
Gynecology Oncology Group 149				
Cisplatin/bleomycin[1]/ifosfamide	IVB or recurrent	31	5.1	8.4
Cisplatin/ifosfamide		32	4.6	8.5
Significance		$P = 0.42$	$P = 0.495$	$P = 0.79$
Gynecology Oncology Group 169				
Cisplatin	IVB or recurrent	19	2.8	8.8
Cisplatin/paclitaxel (Taxol)[1]		36	4.8	9.7
Significance		$P = NS$	$P = NS$	$P = NS$
Gynecology Oncology Group 179				
Cisplatin	IVB or recurrent	13	2.9	6.5
Cisplatin/topotecan (Hycamtin)[1]		27	4.6	9.4
Cisplatin/methotrexate[1]/vinblastine (Velban)[1]/doxorubicin (Adriamycin)[1]				
Significance		$P = 0.004$	$P = 0.014$	$P = 0.017$
Gynecology Oncology Group 204				
Cisplatin/paclitaxel versus cisplatin/vinorelbine (Navelbine)[1]			$HR^† = 1.35$	NR
Cisplatin/gemcitabine (Gemzar)[1]			$HR^† = 1.43$	NR
Cisplatin/topotecan	IVB or recurrent		$HR^† = 1.28$	NR
Gynecology Oncology Group 240				
Cisplatin/paclitaxel	IVB or recurrent	45%	5.9	13.3
Paclitaxel/topotecan		27%		
Cisplatin/paclitaxel/Bevacizumab		50%	8.2	17.0
Paclitaxel/topotecan/Bevacizumab		47%		
			HR = 0.67	HR = 0.71

[1]Not FDA approved for this indication.
[8]Orphan drug in the United States.
[†]Hazard ratio for PFS for experimental arms to cisplatin/paclitaxel.
Abbreviations: NR = not reported; NS = not significant.

Conclusion

Adherence to current screening guidelines should allow early cervical cancer or precancerous detection. However, most patients with cervical cancer have not participated in regular screening and present with a variety of disease extents.

References

American Cancer Society. Cancer facts and figures, Available at http://www.cancer.org/Research/CancerFactsFigures/CancerFactsFigures/index [accessed July 28, 2014].

American College of Obstetricians and Gynecologists (ACOG). Dec.Cervical cytology screening. Washington (DC): American College of Obstetricians and Gynecologists (ACOG); 2012 Nov. (ACOG practice bulletin:no.131).

Bloss JD, Blessing JA, Behrens BC, et al. Randomized trial of cisplatin and ifosfamide with or without bleomycin in squamous carcinoma of the cervix: A Gynecologic Oncology Group study. J Clin Oncol 2002;20:1832–7.

Covens A, Shaw P, Murphy J, et al. Is radical trachelectomy a safe alternative to radical hysterectomy for patients with stage IA-B carcinoma of the cervix? Cancer 1999;86:2273–9.

DiSilvestro PA, Ali S, Craighed PS, et al. Phase III randomized trial of weekly cisplatin and irradiation versus cisplatin and tirapazamine and irradiation in stages IB2, IIA, IIB, IIIB and IVA cervical carcinoma limited to the pelvis: a Gynecologic Oncology Group study. J Clin Oncol 2014;32(5):458–64.

Dunne EF, Unger ER, Sternberg M, et al. Prevalence of HPV infection among females in the United States. JAMA 2007;297(8):813–9.

Finan MA, Decesare S, Fiorica JV, et al. Radical hysterectomy for stage IB1 vs IB2 carcinoma of the cervix: does the new staging system predict morbidity and survival? Gynecol Oncol 1996;62(2):139–47.

Keys HM, Bundy BN, Stehman FB, et al. Cisplatin, radiation, and adjuvant hysterectomy compared with radiation and adjuvant hysterectomy for bulky stage IB cervical carcinoma. N Engl J Med 1999;340(15):1154–61 Erratum in N Engl J Med 1999;341(9):708.

Long 3rd HJ, Bundy BN, Grendys EC, et al. Randomized phase III trial of cisplatin with or without topotecan in carcinoma of the uterine cervix: A Gynecologic Oncology Group study. J Clin Oncol 2005;23(21):4626–33.

Monk BJ, Sill MW, McMeekin DS, et al. Phase III trial of four cisplatin-containing doublet combinations in stage IVB, recurrent, or persistent cervical carcinoma: A Gynecologic Oncology Group study. J Clin Oncol 2009;27(28):4649–55.

Moore DH, Blessing JA, McQuellon RP, et al. Phase III study of cisplatin with or without paclitaxel in stage IVB, recurrent, or persistent squamous cell carcinoma of the cervix: A Gynecologic Oncology Group study. J Clin Oncol 2004;22(15):3113–9.

Morris M, Eifel PJ, Lu J, et al. Pelvic radiation with concurrent chemotherapy compared with pelvic and para-aortic radiation for high-risk cervical cancer. N Engl J Med 1999;340(15):1137–43.

National Cancer Institute. Cervical cancer, Available at: http://www.cancer.gov/cancertopics/types/cervical [accessed August 10, 2015].

Omura GA, Blessing JA, Vaccarello L, et al. Randomized trial of cisplatin versus cisplatin plus mitolactol versus cisplatin plus ifosfamide in advanced squamous carcinoma of the cervix: A Gynecologic Oncology Group study. J Clin Oncol 1997;15(1):165–71.

Pearcey R, Brundage M, Drouin P, et al. Phase III trial comparing radical radiotherapy with and without cisplatin chemotherapy in patients with advanced squamous cell cancer of the cervix. J Clin Oncol 2002;20(4):966–72.

Pecorelli S. Revised FIGO staging for carcinoma of the vulva, cervix, and endometrium. Int J Gynaecol Obstet 2009;105(2):103–4, Erratum in Int J Gynaecol Obstet 2010;108(2):176.

Peters 3rd WA, Liu PY, Barrett 3rd. RJ, et al. Concurrent chemotherapy and pelvic radiation therapy compared with pelvic radiation therapy alone as adjuvant therapy after radical surgery in high-risk early-stage cancer of the cervix. J Clin Oncol 2000;18(8):1606–13.

Rose PG, Bundy BN, Watkins EB, et al. Concurrent cisplatin-based radiotherapy and chemotherapy for locally advanced cervical cancer. N Engl J Med 1999;340(15):1144–53.

Tewari KS, Sill MW, Long HR, et al. Improved survival with bevacizumab in advance cervical cancer. N Engl J Med 2014;370(8):734–43.

Whitney CW, Sause W, Bundy BN, et al. Randomized comparison of fluorouracil plus cisplatin versus hydroxyurea as an adjunct to radiation therapy in stage IIB-IVA carcinoma of the cervix with negative para-aortic lymph nodes: A Gynecologic Oncology Group and Southwest Oncology Group study. J Clin Oncol 1999;17(5):1339–48.

Wright JD, Nathavithrana R, Lewin SN, et al. Fertility-conserving surgery for young women with stage IA1 cervical cancer: Safety and access. Obstet Gynecol 2010;115(3):585–90.

CONTRACEPTION

Method of
Rachel A. Bonnema, MD, MS; and Abby L. Spencer, MD, MS

CURRENT THERAPY

- Combined estrogen and progesterone methods (e.g., pills, patch, ring) are effective and commonly used. They provide excellent cycle control and decreased rates of ectopic pregnancy, pelvic inflammatory disease, and endometrial and ovarian cancer, and they can be used in extended-cycle methods for patients who desire fewer than 12 periods per year.
- The use of estrogen has been associated, albeit rarely, with the development of deep vein thrombosis, myocardial infarction, and stroke; estrogen should not be used in smokers older than 35 years, in patients with diabetes with end-organ damage, coronary artery disease, migraines with aura, or a known hypercoagulable condition.
- For women with a contraindication to estrogen, progestin-only methods are safe to use.
- Long-acting reversible contraception (LARC) such as an implant or intrauterine device (IUD) is safe and extremely effective and should be considered in all women, including nulliparous women.

Nearly half of all pregnancies in the United States are unplanned, a rate higher than the rate in other developed countries. Primary care physicians need up-to-date knowledge on contraceptive counseling for women in order to provide the best match between patient and contraceptive method, in part because providers frequently need to supply contraceptives to women who have particular medical comorbidities. Newer contraceptive preparations are now available, including long-acting implants and altered oral formulations, which differ from traditional oral contraceptives in their hormonal dosages, cycle length, and hormone-free intervals.

Nonhormonal Methods

Nonhormonal methods of contraception include barrier methods and the copper IUD. These methods are safe, easily available, inexpensive, and reversible. Common barrier methods include male and female condoms, spermicides, vaginal sponges, diaphragms, and cervical caps (Table 1). Only condom use has been consistently found to protect against sexually transmitted diseases including HIV, and condom use may reduce risks of cervical cancer as well. Barrier methods have the lowest efficacy rates of all contraceptive methods, and users should also be counseled about emergency contraception. The copper IUD is an extremely effective form of LARC and is a particularly attractive option for a woman with contraindications to hormone use desiring effective contraception.

Combined Hormonal Contraception

Combined hormonal contraception (CHC) contains estrogen (ethinyl estradiol) and a progestin and works primarily by preventing the surge of luteinizing hormone and thereby preventing ovulation. CHC can be delivered as an oral contraceptive pill (OCP), as a vaginal ring (NuvaRing), or as a transdermal patch (Ortho Evra). Risks, benefits, side effects, and contraindications of CHC are thought to be largely similar across delivery methods.

There are many noncontraceptive benefits to CHC, including first-line treatment for dysfunctional uterine bleeding, dysmenorrhea, and menorrhagia. Benefits in addition to menstrual control include reduction in the risks for, and symptoms of, endometriosis, ovulatory pain, ovarian cysts, benign breast disease, premenstrual syndrome, and premenstrual dysphoric disorder. CHC also reduces risk of ovarian and endometrial cancers; these risk reductions extend for years after stopping CHC. The most common side effects of CHC are outlined in Table 2. The risk of venous thromboembolism (VTE) may be higher in obese women, smokers, and those who use certain progestins such as desogestrel or

---

TABLE 1 Nonhormonal Contraception

	BARRIER METHODS			INTRAUTERINE DEVICE
	CONDOM (MALE/FEMALE)	*DIAPHRAGM OR CERVICAL CAP*	*SPONGE*	*COPPER IUD*
Duration	Female condom can be inserted up to 8 hours before intercourse; male condoms must be changed with each act of intercourse	Can be placed up to 6 hours before intercourse and should be removed within 6 hours after	Can be left in for 30 hours and through multiple acts of intercourse	Approved for up to 10 years
Typical-use failure rate*	15%	15%	15%	Less than 0.1%
Side effects and considerations	High failure rates: condom can break, slip. Acceptability by partner may be limited	Requires expert fitting. Needs to be refitted after childbirth. Requires dexterity and self-placement by patient. Use with spermicide increases efficacy but can lead to risk of UTIs, increased risk of toxic shock syndrome, and potential increased risk of HIV transmission	May increase risk of UTIs. Use with spermicide increases efficacy but can lead to risk of UTIs, increased risk of toxic shock syndrome, and potential increased risk of HIV transmission	Bleeding and cramping with menses initially. Low risk of ectopic pregnancy, premature delivery, perforation, or expulsion. Avoid with active infection, undiagnosed genital bleeding, cervical cancer, or Wilson's disease
Consider in:	Patients at risk for STIs. Patients without access to medical care and who are looking for nonhormonal, reversible, and convenient methods of contraception	Women who are looking for nonhormonal, reversible, and convenient methods of contraception	Women who are looking for nonhormonal, reversible, and convenient methods of contraception. Patients without access to medical care	Women with contraindication to hormones or who desire hormone-free, long-acting, reversible contraception. Women in need of EC followed by long-term effective contraception

*Trussel 2011.
Abbreviations: EC = emergency contraception; HIV = human immunodeficiency virus; IUD = intrauterine device; UTI = urinary tract infection.

TABLE 2 Hormonal Contraception

| | COMBINATION ESTROGEN-PROGESTIN | | PROGESTIN-ONLY | | |
	TRADITIONAL OCPs	*EXTENDED-CYCLE OCPs*	*PILL*	*INJECTION*	*IMPLANT/IUD*
Duration Reversibility	Daily pill Immediate	Daily pill Immediate	Daily pill with no hormone-free interval Immediate	3 months Variable	3–5 years Immediate
Cost*	≥$20/month	≥$60/month	$36/month	Average $10–$30/month	Average $10–$20/month
Typical-use failure rate†	9%	9%	9%	6%	0.05%–0.8%
Side effects‡	Spotting, nausea, headache, breast tenderness, breakthrough bleeding, VTE, stroke, MI	Spotting, increased unscheduled bleeding, nausea, VTE, stroke, MI	Spotting, unscheduled bleeding, or absence of bleeding; headaches, nausea, mood changes, breast tenderness, depression, enlarged ovarian follicles	Spotting, unscheduled bleeding, or absence of bleeding; weight gain, depression, reversible decrease in BMD	Spotting, unscheduled bleeding, or absence of bleeding
Consider in:	Women with dysmenorrhea, menorrhagia, irregular menstrual periods, acne, hirsutism, or polycystic ovary syndrome.	Women who do not desire monthly periods. Fewer withdrawal bleeds per year and shorter placebo may offer particular benefit for women with estrogen withdrawal symptoms, dysmenorrhea, or endometriosis.	Women with contraindication to estrogen, hypercoagulable states, dysmenorrhea, migraine with aura, or breast-feeding.	Women with contraindication to estrogen, seizure disorder, hypercoagulable states, dysmenorrhea, migraine with aura, or breast-feeding.	Women with contraindication to estrogen, seizure disorder, hypercoagulable states, dysmenorrhea, migraine with aura, or breast-feeding.

*http://birth-control-pills-compared.lifescript.com/, http://www.plannedparenthood.org/ (accessed March 28, 2013).
†Trussell J: Contraceptive failure in the United States. Contraception 2011;83:397–404.
‡Note: For all combination methods, must have no contraindication to estrogen.
Abbreviations: BMD = bone mineral density; IUD = intrauterine device; MI = myocardial infarction; OCP = oral contraceptive pill; VTE = venous thromboembolism.

drospirenone. This risk is lower, however, than the risk of VTE associated with pregnancy, and the absolute risk of VTE among CHC users remains small.

CHCs can be used safely by women who have a range of medical conditions, including well-controlled hypertension, uncomplicated diabetes, migraines *without* aura in women less than age 35, and a family history of breast cancer, to name a few. CHC use is contraindicated in women who have a history of migraine headache with aura at any age, or in women over age 35 with any migraine, due to elevated risk for stroke. Due to the increased risk of a cardiovascular event, CHC is also contraindicated in women with moderate hypertension, diabetes with end-organ damage, or known cardiovascular disease and in women who smoke after age 35 years. Other contraindications include a personal history of breast cancer, an estrogen-dependent tumor, unexplained vaginal bleeding, stroke, known thromboembolic disorder, or known VTE. Elevated risk of VTE and negative effect on lactation restrict use of CHC in the first 6 weeks after delivery.

Combined Oral Contraceptive Pills
There are dozens of formulations of OCPs, which differ by their estrogen dosage, progestin type and dosage, and hormone delivery schedule. OCPs can be monophasic, where each pill contains the same amount of hormones, or multiphasic, where pills contain different amounts of hormones throughout the monthly cycle. The different formulations offer patients options in cycle length, hormone levels, duration of withdrawal bleeding, and side-effect profile. Women should be educated to take their pill at the same time each day; this becomes even more critical in OCPs containing lower dosages of estrogen (20 mcg). If a pill is missed, it should be taken as soon as the woman remembers. If 2 days of pills are missed, she should take two pills daily for 2 days in a row and use a backup method. If 3 days of pills are missed, she should discard the pill pack and use a backup method. At that point, it should be discussed whether to start a new pack or to change contraceptive methods.

Traditional OCP regimens include 21 days of hormones, followed by 7 days of placebo pills during which women get their menses. Other women desire fewer days of menses or fewer than 12 menses per year. For these women, extended-cycle OCP regimens can be offered that shorten the placebo period to 4 days, offer a placebo week every 4 months, or eliminate the placebo week altogether. Extended-cycle regimens have other benefits, including decreased hormone withdrawal symptoms such as headaches, tiredness, bloating, excessive bleeding, or menstrual pain.

In addition to estrogen dose and scheduling, it is also important to consider the progestin component, which theoretically may affect libido, weight gain, acne, and hirsutism. But these choices must be balanced with potential increased risk for VTE; levonorgestrel-containing OCPs have a long track record and are associated with a lower risk of VTE than other progestins such as desogestrel, gestodene, and drospirenone.

Contraceptive Patch
Norelgestromin/ethinyl estradiol (Ortho Evra) is a thin transdermal patch containing 75 mcg of ethinyl estradiol and 6 mg of norelgestromin; it delivers a daily dose of about 20 mcg of estrogen and 150 mcg of progesterone daily. Patches should be changed weekly for 3 weeks on "patch change day" followed by a patch-free week during which menses occur. Only one patch should be worn at a time, and no more than 7 days should pass during the patch-free week. The patch has decreased efficacy in women who weigh more than 90 kg. Most of the noncontraceptive benefits, side effects, cardiovascular risks, and contraindications are similar to those of other forms of CHC, but there may be an increased risk of VTE in patch users as compared to users of OCPs. Studies are controversial as to the actual increase in risk associated with patch use, but did prompt the updating of the drug label to indicate a higher risk of VTE. Of note, the VTE risk associated with patch use is lower than that associated with pregnancy.

Vaginal Ring

Etonogestrel/ethinyl estradiol (NuvaRing) is a soft plastic ring that is inserted vaginally by the patient, usually for 3 weeks, and then removed for 1 week at which time menses occur. A new ring is inserted 7 days after the last was removed even if bleeding is not complete. The ring releases 15 mcg of ethinyl estradiol and 0.12 mg of etonogestrel daily for 3 to 5 weeks, so it can be kept in longer than 3 weeks for women who desire the benefits of extended-cycling use discussed above. Each ring releases about half the level of hormones as the average OCP without affecting efficacy. If the ring falls out (as occurs in 2.5% of women per year), it can be rinsed and reinserted without a change in efficacy. Unlike the patch, the ring is not affected by excess weight. Most women find the ring easy to insert and remove and comfortable to retain during intercourse. The vaginal ring has been associated with an increase in leukorrhea. Otherwise, its noncontraceptive benefits, side effects, cardiovascular risks, and contraindications are similar to those of other forms of CHC.

Progestin-Only Contraceptives

Progestin-only contraceptives are of particular benefit for women who have a contraindication to estrogen, because progestin-only methods have decreased medical risks associated with their use including no increased risk of stroke, myocardial infarction, or VTE. All progestin-only methods have a similar method of action: ovulation is variably inhibited, cervical mucus is thickened, and the endometrial lining undergoes histologic alterations making implantation less likely. Because many of the progestin-only methods are long acting, they tend to have lower failure rates as opposed to CHCs (see Table 2). All progestin-only methods are appropriate for breast-feeding women.

Pill

Progestin-only pills (POPs) are taken without a hormone-free interval and fertility returns immediately on discontinuation. In fact, most experts believe fertility can return in as little as 3 hours after a missed dose; thus a woman should be counseled to use a backup method if she is 3 or more hours late in taking her dose. Given this small window for error, this method should be prescribed only to patients who can adhere closely to a daily pill schedule. Additionally, women should be counseled that while taking the POP, normal menstrual patterns may include anything from amenorrhea to menometrorrhagia. This unpatterned bleeding is likely one of the greatest obstacles to wider use of progestin-only oral contraception. Because POPs have demonstrated no significant negative effects on breastfeeding, POPs are most commonly used in the postpartum period and can be prescribed immediately postpartum. POPs may have similar effects as other progestin-only methods in decreasing the frequency of sickle cell crises; however, unlike depot medroxyprogesterone acetate (DMPA, Depo-Provera) injections, certain anticonvulsants may lower effectiveness of the POP so other methods may be more beneficial in women with seizure disorders.

Injectable

The intramuscular DMPA injection (Depo-Provera) is given every 12 weeks and has a typical-use failure rate of 6%. A lower dose of DMPA (104 mg in Depo-SubQ Provera) has been approved for subcutaneous injection. Women with seizure disorders are particularly good candidates for DMPA injections because, unlike other forms of contraception, DMPA's efficacy is not affected by enzyme-inducing antiepileptic drugs. Depo-Provera may also decrease seizure frequency, providing additional benefit for patients who have a seizure disorder. DMPA reduces serum estradiol levels, which can adversely affect bone health. In 2004, the FDA issued a black box warning that women who use Depo-Provera may lose significant bone mineral density (BMD) and recommended that use be limited to less than 2 years unless other methods are inadequate. Since that time, data have shown that although there is a clear association between DMPA use and decreased BMD, the BMD loss was reversible with discontinuation of use and there is no increased risk of fracture with use of DMPA. The World Health Organization has recommended that

there be no restriction on the use of Depo-Provera in women ages 18 to 45. According to recent consensus guidelines, clinicians should advise patients about the risk for BMD loss but can reassure them about reversibility with discontinuation.

Intrauterine System

The levonorgestrel intrauterine system (LNG-IUS) is a highly effective contraceptive method long considered to be reversible sterilization due to its excellent efficacy in preventing pregnancy and quick return to fertility after its removal. Mirena is an IUD that releases approximately 20 mcg/day of LNG and is effective for 5 years. Skyla is a new "lower dose" LNG-IUS that releases approximately 14 mcg/day of LNG and is effective for 3 years. The LNG-IUS is ideal for women who require highly effective contraception and is particularly beneficial for women requiring a progestin-only contraception. Its relatively low cost over time is another factor for patients to consider. Numerous studies have confirmed the effectiveness of the LNG-IUS for reduction of menstrual blood loss in menorrhagia, leiomyomas, and pain due to endometriosis. In fact, the LNG-IUS (Mirena) recently received FDA approval for the indication of menorrhagia and has also been shown to decrease menorrhagia even in women on anticoagulation. Insertion of the LNG-IUS requires a trained provider. At the time of placement, women may have cramping and pain; a rare complication of placement is uterine wall rupture. Though women will likely develop amenorrhea, they should be counseled about initial irregular bleeding and spotting.

Implant

There is one single-rod subdermal implant available in the United States (formerly Implanon, now called Nexplanon) that is a highly effective long-term contraceptive containing the progestin etonogestrel (ENG). The rod is implanted in the upper arm and remains active for 3 years. ENG does not cause a hypoestrogenic state, thus this method is not considered to have any significant effect on BMD. ENG implantation can be done as a simple office procedure by a trained provider under local anesthetic with a preloaded, disposable applicator. Women experience a quick return to normal cycles after implant removal, and there have been no reports of infertility after removal. Similar to other progestin-only forms of contraception, irregular bleeding is the major side effect of the ENG implant. The most common bleeding pattern associated with the implant is infrequent, irregular bleeding. Unfortunately, there is no method to predict bleeding response for an individual patient after ENG implantation, so this is an important counseling point, particularly since the highest rate of discontinuation is during the first 8 to 9 months of use, primarily due to frequent bleeding.

Permanent

Permanent birth control methods include vasectomy and female sterilization by various procedures. These methods are highly effective (typical failure rate 0.15% to 0.5%); however, they are permanent, and can be associated with regret. Each sterilization procedure has advantages and disadvantages that should be considered by the patient before choosing which one to use.

Emergency Contraception

Familiarity with emergency contraception (EC) is critical both for women who are having unprotected sex and for those who are using methods with higher failure rates. EC use has not been shown to reduce compliance with other first-line methods. EC primarily acts by inhibiting or delaying ovulation, and works before implantation; if a fertilized egg has already implanted, EC will not work. EC includes pills (comprised of estrogen-+ progestin, progestin only, and anti-progestins) and copper IUD placement (inserted up to 5 days after unprotected intercourse); EC pills are most effective when taken in the first 12 hours, but have gradually decreasing effectiveness for up to 120 hours after intercourse. The most commonly used and most accessible form of EC in the United States contains levonorgestrel only (Plan B, Plan B One Step) and is dispensed as two 75 mcg pills either together or 12 hours apart. EC is available at most pharmacies over the counter to women 17 years and older and by prescription to younger women.

Counseling

When counseling patients about their contraceptive choices, it is important that providers are aware of their role in giving information and allowing patients to make informed decisions. The only effective contraceptive is one that a patient is willing to use consistently and correctly, and the choice of contraception is ultimately the patient's decision. Providers must educate patients regarding the advantages and disadvantages of each method that is medically appropriate for them. Discussing a patient's preferences for menstrual frequency and tolerance for scheduled and unscheduled bleeding will be important in deciding which contraceptive will best fit her needs. Providers should counsel patients on expected side effects as well as expectant management strategies. Every effort should be made to remove barriers to initiation, including having no requirement for a pelvic examination or Pap smear before initiation. Using the conversation about contraceptives to also discuss safe sex is ideal.

References

ACOG Committee on Practice Bulletins—Gynecology. ACOG practice bulletin. No. 73: use of hormonal contraception in women with coexisting medical conditions. Obstet Gynecol 2006;107:1453–72.

Association of Reproductive Health Professionals. Available at http://www.arhp.org/Publications-and-Resources/Quick-Reference-Guide-for-Clinicians/choosing/Progestin-Only-OCs; [accessed 19.03.13].

Department of Reproductive Health, World Health Organization. Medical eligibility criteria for contraceptive use. 4th ed. Geneva, Switzerland: WHO Press; 2009.

Finer LB, Zolna MR. Unintended pregnancy in the United States: incidence and disparities, 2006. Contraception 2011;84:478–85.

Lanza LL, McQuay LJ, Rothman KJ, et al. Use of depot medroxyprogesterone acetate contraception and incidence of bone fracture. Obstet Gynecol 2013;121:593–600.

Parkin L, Sharples K, Hernandez RK, et al. Risk of venous thromboembolism in users of oral contraceptives containing drospirenone or levonorgestrel: nested case control study based on UK General Practice Research Database. BMJ 2011;340:d2139.

Petitti DB. Combination estrogen-progestin oral contraceptives. N Engl J Med 2003;349:1443–50.

Spencer AL, Bonnema RA, McNamara MC. Helping women choose appropriate hormonal contraception: update on risks, benefits, and indications. Am J Med 2009;122:497–506.

Trussel J. Contraceptive failure in the United States. Conception 2011;83:397–404.

World Health Organization. Cardiovascular disease and use of oral and injectable progestogen-only contraceptives and combined injectable contraceptives. Results of an international, multicenter, case-control study. World Health Organization Collaborative Study of Cardiovascular Disease and Steroid Hormone Contraception. Contraception 1998;57:315–24.

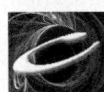

DYSMENORRHEA

Method of
Linda Speer, MD

CURRENT DIAGNOSIS

- Primary dysmenorrhea (painful menses without underlying pathology) is common among adolescents and young women. It usually begins shortly after menarche.
- Diagnosis of primary dysmenorrhea can be made based on typical history of crampy pelvic pain during the first 1 to 3 days of the menstrual cycle. Pelvic examination is not required.
- Secondary dysmenorrhea (with underlying pathology) should be considered in cases that do not match the typical history, begin later in life, and/or are refractory to treatment.
- The most common cause of secondary dysmenorrhea is endometriosis. The clinical standard for diagnosis of endometriosis is laparoscopic confirmation. Ultrasound imaging is useful in some cases.

CURRENT THERAPY

- Nonsteroidal antiinflammatory drugs (NSAIDs) are well-established first-line therapy for treatment of primary dysmenorrhea. None has been confirmed as superior to others.
- Cyclooxygenase-2 (COX-2) inhibitors are effective and have fewer gastrointestinal side effects but may be less effective than NSAIDs.
- Oral contraceptives and the levonorgestrel intrauterine system (Mirena)[1] reduce dysmenorrhea.
- Other effective therapies include topical heat, high-frequency transcutaneous electrical nerve stimulation (TENS), and several herbal preparations.
- Treatments for endometriosis as a secondary cause of pelvic pain and dysmenorrhea include hormonal suppression of the endometrial tissue, conservative laparoscopic surgical debulking, and hysterectomy in selected cases.

[1]Not FDA approved for this indication.

Dysmenorrhea is defined as painful menses. Primary dysmenorrhea occurs without underlying pathology, typically beginning soon after menarche. It is common in adolescent girls, with prevalence ranging from 20% to 90% depending on measurement methods; about 15% of adolescents describe their dysmenorrhea as severe. The median duration of each episode is 2 days beginning with the onset of menses. During adolescence, dysmenorrhea leads to high rates of school absence and activity nonparticipation. According to representative national survey data in the United States, 14% of adolescent girls aged 12 to 17 years frequently miss school because of menstrual cramps.

A prospective cohort study showed that the prevalence and severity of dysmenorrhea was lower at 24 years of age than at 19 years of age. At 24 years of age, 67% of the women still experienced dysmenorrhea, and 10% reported pain severity that limited daily activity. The prevalence and severity of dysmenorrhea were reduced in women who were parous at 24 years and nulliparous at 19 years, but they were unchanged in women who were still nulliparous or women who had had a miscarriage or abortion.

There is a significant correlation between the severity of dysmenorrhea and the amount of menstrual flow. Survey data demonstrate that depression and anxiety are associated with menstrual pain and suggest that loss of social support is a significant contributor to menstrual symptoms. The severity of dysmenorrhea is not associated with height, weight, or regularity of the menstrual cycle. A relationship to smoking has been found inconsistently. Physical activity has been studied and found not to be associated with any pain parameter.

Secondary dysmenorrhea typically starts later in life after the onset of an underlying causative condition, most often endometriosis. The association between dysmenorrhea and endometriosis is uncertain for women with minimal disease. However, based on a study of more than 1000 women with laparoscopically confirmed endometriosis, chronic pelvic pain, dyspareunia, and dysmenorrhea are in fact related to the extent of endometriosis.

Diagnosis

For adolescents who present with complaints typical for primary dysmenorrhea, treatment may be started empirically without a pelvic examination or diagnostic studies. Sexually active adolescents and young women should be screened for chlamydia and gonorrhea, which can be done with either urine or a genital sampling.

For adolescents and women who do not have a history consistent with primary dysmenorrhea or who are refractory to treatment, endometriosis may be suspected. The gold standard for diagnosis is laparoscopy and biopsy. Ultrasound may also be useful, especially to identify endometriomas.

Treatment

Nonsteroidal Antiinflammatory Drugs

A Cochrane review of randomized, controlled trials (RCTs) concluded that among women with primary dysmenorrhea, NSAIDs were significantly more effective for pain relief than placebo or acetaminophen (Tylenol). No specific NSAID was shown to be superior to others for either pain relief or safety. However, the available evidence had little power to detect such differences, because most individual comparisons were based on few small trials. In one study in which diclofenac (Voltaren) 100 mg was compared with placebo for treatment of primary dysmenorrhea, the authors found that leg strength and aerobic capacity were maintained at the level found during luteal phase when women took diclofenac for dysmenorrhea, but they were reduced during menses in the placebo group.

COX-2 Inhibitors

Several COX-2 inhibitors have been evaluated for treatment of dysmenorrhea in RCTs. Celecoxib (Celebrex) 200 mg was compared with naproxen sodium (Naprosyn) 550 mg and placebo for treatment of dysmenorrhea and found to be superior to placebo but not as effective as naproxen. Etoricoxib (Arcoxia)[5] 120 mg daily was found to be better than placebo and equivalent to mefenamic acid (Ponstel) for treatment of primary dysmenorrhea with less nausea and epigastric pain than mefenamic acid. Lumiracoxib (Prexige)[5] 200 mg daily was compared with naproxen 500 mg twice daily and placebo for treatment of primary dysmenorrhea and found to reduce pain more than placebo and similar to naproxen.

Oral Contraceptives

In a systematic review of NSAIDs and oral contraceptives (OCs) for treatment of dysmenorrhea that included 10 placebo-controlled RCTs of NSAIDs, two RCTs of OCs and six prospective observational studies of OCs, the authors concluded that both are effective. In a study of women with laparoscopically proven endometriosis, low-dose ethinyl estradiol and norethisterone (norethindrone) decreased dysmenorrhea associated with endometriosis as compared with placebo (with pain assessment on a verbal rating scale from 0 to 3). There was also a significant reduction in volume of endometriomas with OCs but not placebo.

Levonorgestrel Intrauterine System

The levonorgestrel intrauterine system[1] (LNG-IUS; Mirena) reduces menstrual bleeding and dysmenorrhea, which can be a desirable side effect for women desiring long-term contraception. In an uncontrolled case series of women treated with LNG-IUS for adenomyosis, dysmenorrhea diminished continuously during the 3-year study from a mean 78 mm to a mean 12 mm on a 100-mm visual analog scale. Overall satisfaction with treatment was 73%. Depot medroxyprogesterone acetate[1] (Depo-Provera) is similarly effective, but it is less likely to be well tolerated owing to unpredictable bleeding, weight gain, and mood changes.

Nifedipine

In one uncontrolled study, nifedipine[1] (Procardia) 20 to 40 mg given orally reduced myometrial activity and relieved dysmenorrhea. This drug could be considered as an adjunct in severe cases of primary dysmenorrhea after ruling out endometriosis.

Transcutaneous Electrical Nerve Stimulation

In a study comparing transcutaneous electrical nerve stimulation (TENS) with interferential current for treatment of dysmenorrhea, each group received application of the modality for 20 minutes while experiencing dysmenorrhea. Both groups improved significantly from baseline without significant difference between them.

High-frequency TENS has been found to be effective for the treatment of dysmenorrhea in a number of small trials. Low-frequency TENS does not appear to be effective.

Topical Heat and Infrared Light

Continuous low-level topical heat therapy has been shown to be as effective as ibuprofen (Advil) for the treatment of dysmenorrhea in one RCT. In a trial comparing far-infrared emitting belt versus placebo belt for treatment of primary dysmenorrhea, both with concurrent application of topical heat, both groups improved, and the duration of the analgesic effect was significantly longer in the group treated with the infrared belt.

Complementary and Alternative Medicine Approaches

Herbal

Several herbal remedies have been studied in RCTs for treatment of dysmenorrhea and found to be effective as compared with placebo or NSAIDs. They include *Psidii guajava* extract[7] 6 mg/day, French maritime pine bark extract (pycnogenol),[7] and ginger root powder[7] 250 mg 4 times daily.

Acupressure and Acupuncture

The evidence for the effectiveness of acupuncture is not conclusive. In unblinded studies women experience clinically relevant reduction in pain scores, a mean of more than 10 points on a 100-point scale, which could be due to placebo effect. In fact, in a well-designed RCT of electro-acupuncture at the Sanyinjiao point (the point expected to be related to uterine pain) compared to an unrelated nonacupoint or no acupuncture, the only significant differences were with the no-acupuncture group as measured with a visual analogue rating scale.

Adequate blinding is also an issue among studies of acupressure. For example, in an RCT comparing auricular seed acupressure versus adhesive tape only for treatment of primary dysmenorrhea the acupressure group (but not the tape only group) had instructions to massage the seed 15 times, three times daily for 20 days. Menstrual pain decreased significantly in the acupressure group. Several other studies suggest that acupressure at the Sanyinjiao point or Taichong point is more effective than no intervention or inadequately blinded control groups. Because acupressure is a low-cost and harmless intervention, it may be worth considering even if the pain reduction is a placebo response.

Yoga

Yoga is another alternative approach with low cost and little risk that may be worth considering despite weak evidence for effectiveness. In one unblinded RCT, three yoga poses (cat, cobra, and fish) were studied for treatment of primary dysmenorrhea. Participants randomized to the intervention group were told to do the yoga poses during luteal phase and complete a questionnaire regarding menstrual characteristics. The control group was asked to complete the questionnaire only. There was significant reduction in intensity and duration of pain in the yoga group compared with baseline and with the control group.

Spinal Manipulation

Overall there is no evidence to suggest that spinal manipulation is effective in the treatment of primary and secondary dysmenorrhea.

Surgical Treatment

Surgical treatment may be considered in severe and refractory cases of pelvic pain including dysmenorrhea. Laparoscopic utero-sacral nerve ablation (LUNA, n = 35) alone has been compared with LUNA plus presacral neurectomy (n = 32). There were no differences between groups for relief of dysmenorrhea at 3-, 6-, and 12-month follow-up, but more surgical complications were experienced with neurectomy.

Treatment of Endometriosis

Treatment of endometriosis may start with use of NSAIDs, hormonal contraceptives, and/or LNG-IUS.[1] However, often endometriosis is diagnosed after those first-line therapies have failed. Debulking of the ectopic endometrial tissue during laparoscopy can relieve pain.

Other treatments involve hormonal suppression of endometrial tissue. Danazol is a 19-nortestosterone derivative with a long history of use for treatment of endometriosis pain at a dosage of 400 to 800 mg daily for 6 months, but it is often poorly tolerated owing to androgenic side effects. Oral progestin regimens (medroxyprogesterone acetate[1] [Depoprovera] up to 100 mg daily[3] or norethindrone [Aygestin] up to 15 mg daily) may be used to suppress menses for a 6-month course. Other accepted therapies include gonadotropin-releasing hormone (GnRH) agonist analogues such as leuprolide (Lupron). Aromatase inhibitors have been shown to be effective in a systematic review of several small RCTs. Etonogestrel subdermal implant[1] (Implanon, Nexplanon) has been evaluated in an uncontrolled case series and found to be associated with pain relief.

In severe refractory cases, hysterectomy may be considered.

---

[1]Not FDA approved for this indication.
[3]Exceeds dosage recommended by the manufacturer.

References

Akin MD, Weingand KW, Hengehold DA, et al. Continuous low-level topical heat in the treatment of dysmenorrhea. Obstet Gynecol 2001;97:343–9.

Alonso C, Coe CL. Disruptions of social relationships accentuate the association between emotional distress and menstrual pain in young women. Health Psychol 2001;20:411–6.

Andersch B, Milsom I. An epidemiologic study of young women with dysmenorrhea. Am J Obstet Gynecol 1982;144:655–60.

Andersson KE, Ulmsten U. Effects of nifedipine on myometrial activity and lower abdominal pain in women with primary dysmenorrhoea. Br J Obstet Gynaecol 1978;85:142–8.

Bazarganipour F, Lamyian M, Heshmat R, et al. A randomized clinical trial of the efficacy of applying a simple acupressure protocol to the Taichong point in relieving dysmenorrhea. Int J Gynaecol Obstet 2010;111:105–9.

Brown J, Pan A, Hart RJ. Gonadotrophin-releasing hormone analogues for pain associated with endometriosis. Cochrane Database Syst Rev 2010;(12), CD008475.

Chantler I, Mitchell D, Fuller A. Diclofenac potassium attenuates dysmenorrhea and restores exercise performance in women with primary dysmenorrhea. J Pain 2009;10:191–200.

Daniels S, Robbins J, West CR, Nemeth MA. Celecoxib in the treatment of primary dysmenorrhea: Results from two randomized, double-blind, active- and placebo-controlled, crossover studies. Clin Ther 2009;31:1192–208.

Daniels S, Gitton X, Zhou W, et al. Efficacy and tolerability of lumiracoxib 200 mg once daily for treatment of primary dysmenorrhea: Results from two randomized controlled trials. J Womens Health (Larchmt) 2008;17:423–37.

Davis AR, Westhoff CL. Primary dysmenorrhea in adolescent girls and treatment with oral contraceptives. J Pediatr Adolesc Gynecol 2001;14:3–8.

Doubova SV, Morales HR, Hernández SF, et al. Effect of a *Psidii guajavae folium* extract in the treatment of primary dysmenorrhea: A randomized clinical trial. J Ethnopharmacol 2007;110:305–10.

Harada T, Momoeda M, Taketani Y, et al. Low-dose oral contraceptive pill for dysmenorrhea associated with endometriosis: A placebo-controlled, double-blind, randomized trial. Fertil Steril 2008;90:1583–8.

Harlow SD, Park M. A longitudinal study of risk factors for the occurrence, duration and severity of menstrual cramps in a cohort of college women. Br J Obstet Gynaecol 1996;103:1134–42.

Jensen JT. Noncontraceptive applications of the levonorgestrel intrauterine system. Curr Womens Health Rep 2002;2:417–22.

Juang CM, Chou P, Yen MS, et al. Laparoscopic uterosacral nerve ablation with and without presacral neurectomy in the treatment of primary dysmenorrhea: A prospective efficacy analysis. J Reprod Med 2007;52:591–6.

Kashefi F, Ziyadlou S, Khajehei M, et al. Effect of acupressure at the Sanyinjiao point on primary dysmenorrhea: A randomized controlled trial. Complement Ther Clin Pract 2010;16:198–202.

Klein JR, Litt IF. Epidemiology of adolescent dysmenorrhea. Pediatrics 1981;68:661–4.

Lee CH, Roh JW, Lim CY, et al. A multicenter, randomized, double-blind, placebo-controlled trial evaluating the efficacy and safety of a far infrared-emitting sericite belt in patients with primary dysmenorrhea. Complement Ther Med 2011;19:187–93.

Liu CZ, Xie JP, Wang LP, et al. Immediate analgesia effect of single point acupuncture in primary dysmenorrhea: A randomized controlled trial. Pain Med 2011;12:300–7.

Marjoribanks J, Proctor M, Farquhar C, Derks RS. Nonsteroidal anti-inflammatory drugs for dysmenorrhoea. Cochrane Database Syst Rev 2010;(1), CD001751.

Mirbagher-Ajorpaz N, Adib-Hajbaghery M, Mosaebi F. The effects of acupressure on primary dysmenorrhea: A randomized controlled trial. Complement Ther Clin Pract 2011;17:33–26.

Moen MH, Stokstad T. A long-term follow-up study of women with asymptomatic endometriosis diagnosed incidentally at sterilization. Fertil Steril 2002; 78:773–6.

Momoeda M, Taketani Y, Terakawa N, et al. Is endometriosis really associated with pain? Gynecol Obstet Invest 2002;54(Suppl. 1):18–21.

Nawathe A, Patwardhan S, Yates D, et al. Systematic review of the effects of aromatase inhibitors on pain associated with endometriosis. BJOG 2008;115: 818–22.

Ozgoli G, Goli M, Moattar F. Comparison of effects of ginger, mefenamic acid, and ibuprofen on pain in women with primary dysmenorrhea. J Altern Complement Med 2009;15:129–32.

Proctor ML, Smith CA, Farquhar CM, Stones RW. Transcutaneous electrical nerve stimulation and acupuncture for primary dysmenorrhoea. Cochrane Database Syst Rev 2 2002;(1), CD002123.

Proctor ML, Hing W, Johnson TC, Murphy PA. Spinal manipulation for primary and secondary dysmenorrhoea. Cochrane Database Syst Rev 2006;(3), CD002119.

Rakhshaee Z. Effect of three yoga poses (cobra, cat and fish poses) in women with primary dysmenorrhea: A randomized clinical trial. J Pediatr Adolesc Gynecol 2011;24:192–6.

Ranong CN, Sukcharoen N. Analgesic effect of etoricoxib in secondary dysmenorrhea: A randomized, double-blind, crossover, controlled trial. J Reprod Med 2007;52:1023–9.

Selak V, Farquhar C, Prentice A, Singla A. Danazol for pelvic pain associated with endometriosis. Cochrane Database Syst Rev 2007;(4), CD000068.

Sheng J, Zhang WY, Zhang JP, Lu D. The LNG-IUS study on adenomyosis: A 3-year follow-up study on the efficacy and side effects of the use of levonorgestrel intrauterine system for the treatment of dysmenorrhea associated with adenomyosis. Contraception 2009;79:189–93.

Strinić T, Buković D, Pavelić L, et al. Anthropological and clinical characteristics in adolescent women with dysmenorrhea. Coll Antropol 2003;27:707–11.

Sundell G, Milsom I, Andersch B. Factors influencing the prevalence and severity of dysmenorrhoea in young women. Br J Obstet Gynaecol 1990;97:588–94.

Suzuki N, Uebaba K, Kohama T, et al. French maritime pine bark extract significantly lowers the requirement for analgesic medication in dysmenorrhea: A multicenter, randomized, double-blind, placebo-controlled study. J Reprod Med 2008;53: 338–46.

Telimaa S, Puolakka J, Rönnberg L, Kauppila A. Placebo-controlled comparison of danazol and high-dose medroxyprogesterone acetate in the treatment of endometriosis. Gynecol Endocrinol 1987;1:13–23.

Tugay N, Akbayrak T, Demirtürk F, et al. Effectiveness of transcutaneous electrical nerve stimulation and interferential current in primary dysmenorrhea. Pain Med 2007;8:295–300.

Wang MC, Hsu MC, Chien LW, et al. Effects of auricular acupressure on menstrual symptoms and nitric oxide for women with primary dysmenorrhea. J Altern Complement Med 2009;15:235–42.

Witt CM, Reinhold T, Brinkhaus B, et al. Acupuncture in patients with dysmenorrhea: A randomized study on clinical effectiveness and cost-effectiveness in usual care. Am J Obstet Gynecol 2008;198:166, e1–8.

Wong CL, Lai KY, Tse HM. Effects of SP6 acupressure on pain and menstrual distress in young women with dysmenorrhea. Complement Ther Clin Pract 2009;16:64–9.

Yisa SB, Okenwa AA, Husemeyer RP. Treatment of pelvic endometriosis with etonogestrel subdermal implant (Implanon). J Fam Plann Reprod Health Care 2005;31:67–70.

Zahradnik HP, Hanjalic-Beck A, Groth K. Nonsteroidal anti-inflammatory drugs and hormonal contraceptives for pain relief from dysmenorrhea: A review. Contraception 2010;81:185–96.

ENDOMETRIOSIS

Method of
David L. Olive, MD

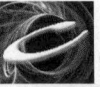

CURRENT DIAGNOSIS

- Symptoms associated with endometriosis are primarily those of pain and infertility, although site-specific symptoms and signs may exist when the disease is in unusual locations.
- The standard for diagnosis is laparoscopic visualization; however, this method has a high false-positive and false-negative rate. The only method to confirm the disease absolutely is excisional biopsy.

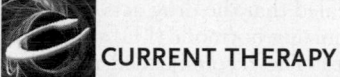

CURRENT THERAPY

- Both medical and surgical therapies are efficacious in the treatment of endometriosis-associated pain. It is unclear which offers the better approach.
- Combined medical/surgical therapy may offer an advantage over surgery alone, if the medication is used at least 6 months postoperatively.
- Medical therapy has no role in the treatment of endometriosis-associated infertility.
- Surgical therapy for endometriosis-associated infertility appears to be of value for all stages of disease, but its relative value compared to assisted reproduction is not yet determined.

Endometriosis is one of the most common diseases encountered by the practicing gynecologist, yet it is also one of the most vexing. Researchers have been searching for answers to even the most fundamental questions regarding this disease for well over a century; even today huge gaps remain in the understanding of this disorder.

Definition

Endometriosis is defined as the presence of endometrial glands and stroma outside the endometrial cavity and uterine musculature. The requirement for both glands and stroma is an arbitrary standard, and it is unclear whether either component of endometrium alone, if placed ectopically, can result in the symptoms and signs of endometriosis.

Two related diseases are also frequently observed. Adenomyosis is the presence of endometrial glands and stroma within the myometrium. This disorder is epidemiologically and pathogenically distinct from endometriosis, but the resulting symptoms (and medical treatments) are similar. Endosalpingiosis is identical to endometriosis in location and appearance but histologically resembles tubal glands and stroma. This latter abnormality has been poorly studied, and to date, little is known regarding the distinction between endometriosis and endosalpingiosis.

Genetics

Evidence continues to accumulate that endometriosis has a genetic basis. Evidence for this includes familial clustering, concordance in monozygotic twins, and increased prevalence among first-degree relatives. A search was recently undertaken to identify the gene or genes responsible for susceptibility to endometriosis. Although suggestive linkages were discovered, no genes have been firmly identified as instrumental in this disorder. It is hoped, however, that genetic research will eventually uncover information critical to understanding the molecular and cellular basis of this disease.

Pathogenesis

The pathogenesis of endometriosis is a controversial subject inspiring many researchers to investigate it. Over the last 25 years considerable advancement has been made, providing solid clues to the understanding of the disease process. Today, a clear picture is beginning to emerge regarding how women develop endometriosis.

Histogenesis

Leading researchers in the field have proposed numerous theories of histogenesis. The primary theory of histogenesis is transplantation of shed uterine endometrium to ectopic locations. A number of routes of dissemination of the tissue are proposed, including lymphatic dissemination, vascular spread, iatrogenic transplantation, and retrograde menstruation.

A critical aspect of this theory is that cast-off endometrium cells remain viable and capable of implanting. Furthermore, it proposes that the tissue distribution has the capacity to sustain implantation. Considerable research has established that shed endometrial cells are viable in vitro. In vitro studies of endometrial attachment to peritoneum also support the concept of transplantation, attachment, and invasion.

Additional theories of histogenesis include coelomic metaplasia and induction of endometriosis. However, little scientific evidence indicates that either route is a viable etiology of the disease, much less a common method for development.

Etiology and Maintenance

Retrograde menstruation is a well-established phenomenon. Data available from women undergoing peritoneal dialysis and laparoscopy at the time of menses suggest that 76% to 90% of women have retrograde flow. This mechanism is considered a critical first step in the initiation of much if not most endometriosis by a wide variety of epidemiologic and anatomic data. However, the majority of women do not have endometriosis. The question that arises is "Why not?"

Because the placement of menstrual debris into the peritoneal cavity happens with each menses, a mechanism must exist to eliminate this tissue. The prime candidate for removal of endometrial cells is cell-mediated cytotoxicity. Deficient cytotoxic response to ectopic endometrium is suggested as a mechanism for allowing implantation and growth. It is also postulated that factors positively affecting growth and maintenance may be altered to enhance the risk of endometriosis. Current evidence suggests that a variety of cytokines, including monocyte chemotactic protein-1, interleukin-8, and regulated on activation, T-cell expressed and secreted (RANTES) are overexpressed in women with endometriosis, resulting in the attraction and activation of macrophages. The source of this cytokine increase could be one or more of several tissues: Endometrium, peritoneal mesothelium, and macrophages themselves could be the primary aberrancy by which this cascade is begun.

Other abnormalities are speculated to promote endometriosis. These include abnormal expression of matrix metalloproteinases and the enzyme aromatase, which could locally produce a hyperestrogenic proimplantation environment. The mechanisms by which these abnormalities may cause disease as well as the source of such alterations are under investigation.

Prevalence and Epidemiology

Endometriosis is a disease found almost exclusively in reproductive-age women. The mean age at diagnosis is reported to be from 25 to 29 years, although this figure depends on the diagnostic method. Because traditional diagnosis requires laparoscopy, it is likely that the disease is frequently present in even younger patients for whom many gynecologists do not readily schedule surgery.

Although rare in the premenarcheal female, adolescent endometriosis is a relatively common entity. Endometriosis is found in 47% to 65% of women younger than 20 years with chronic pelvic pain or dyspareunia.

Endometriosis is associated with increased exposure to menstruation typified by earlier menarche, more frequent menses, longer menses, fewer pregnancies, later initial pregnancy, and less breast-feeding. In addition, factors known to decrease the amount of menses or lower estrogen levels also reduce the risk: oral contraceptive use, irregular menses/oligomenorrhea, stress, exercise, and cigarette smoking (Box 1).

Postmenopausal endometriosis seldom occurs; this age group represents only 2% to 4% of all women requiring laparoscopy for endometriosis. The majority of such cases are a sequela to reactivation of disease by hormone replacement therapy; this is not true in all cases.

Clinical Presentation

Endometriosis is associated with a wide array of presenting signs and symptoms, although many women with physical manifestations of the disease remain completely asymptomatic. Commonly, the severity of symptoms does not correlate with the stage of

Box 1   Epidemiology of Endometriosis

Increased risk with:
- Menses >6 d
- More menses

Decreased risk with:
- Increased parity
- Irregular menses
- Oral contraceptives
- Late menarche
- Exercise
- Smoking

endometriosis; extensive disease sometimes causes only minimal symptoms, and in others, minimal disease can be associated with severe symptoms. Some symptoms may strongly suggest the presence of endometriosis, but none are pathognomonic of this disorder. Because endometriosis most commonly involves the pelvis, infertility, dysmenorrhea, pelvic pain, dyspareunia, and menstrual dysfunction are common clinical presentations. When the ovary is severely involved, an ovarian cyst or pelvic mass may be the initial sign of endometriosis.

Pelvic pain is the most frequent complaint for endometriosis patients. This generally presents as secondary dysmenorrhea, worsening primary dysmenorrhea, dyspareunia, or even noncyclic lower abdominal pain, chronic pelvic pain, and backaches. In addition, pain may be site specific when endometriosis is found in unusual locations outside of the pelvis.

Only rarely are physical findings specific for endometriosis. Localized cul-de-sac and uterosacral ligament tenderness may frequently be detected. Thickened, nodular uterosacral ligaments or rectovaginal masses may be palpable. Adnexal enlargement or tenderness may reflect ovarian involvement. Retroverted fixation of the uterus may be noted with posterior cul-de-sac obliteration by the disease.

Cutaneous manifestations may be present, with apparent lesions on the perineum or vagina, or, less commonly, in the inguinal region, the umbilical area, or at the site of surgical scars. They should be suspected whenever a scar or lesion is associated with cyclical pain, tenderness, swelling, or bleeding.

Diagnosis

The current gold standard for the definitive diagnosis of endometriosis is laparoscopy. However, because of the heterogeneity in appearance of endometriosis lesions, the accuracy of laparoscopic diagnosis is variable and depends on the ability of the surgeon to recognize the disease. Although histologic confirmation would be ideal to ensure the presence of disease, this is infrequently accomplished because of the reticence of surgeons to excise endometriosis lesions.

Ultrasound is most useful for the detection of ovarian endometriomas, although the appearance of a cystic structure with heightened echogenicity is certainly not limited to this form of endometriosis. Structures often confused with endometriomas include corpora lutea, hemorrhagic cysts, unilocular dermoid cysts, and other benign cystic neoplasias. Ultrasound is not currently useful for identifying focal implants.

Magnetic resonance imaging (MRI) demonstrates significant potential in the diagnosis of endometriosis. MRI is clearly of value in diagnosing the ovarian endometrioma, and as technology improves, the potential for detecting peritoneal lesions will increase.

Treatment

Medical Therapy

The first drug to be approved for the treatment of endometriosis in the United States was danazol (Danocrine), a derivative of testosterone. It was originally thought to produce a pseudomenopause,

but subsequent studies have revealed that the drug acts primarily by diminishing the midcycle luteinizing hormone (LH) surge, creating a chronic anovulatory state. The recommended dosage of danazol for the treatment of endometriosis is 600 to 800 mg/day; however, these doses have substantial androgenic side effects such as increased hair growth, mood changes, adverse serum lipid profiles, deepening of the voice (possibly irreversible), and, rarely, liver damage (possibly irreversible and life threatening) and arterial thrombosis. Studies of lower doses as primary treatment for endometriosis-associated pain have been uncontrolled or with small numbers and thus contain information of limited value.

Progestogens are a class of compounds that produce progesterone-like effects on endometrial tissue. A large number of progestogens exist, ranging from those chemically derived from progesterone (progestins), such as medroxyprogesterone acetate (MPA), to 19-nortestosterone derivatives such as norethindrone and norgestrel. The proposed mechanism of action of these compounds causes initial shedding of endometrial tissue followed by eventual atrophy. The most extensively studied progestational agent for the treatment of endometriosis is medroxyprogesterone (dep-subQ Provera 104), which is currently approved by the Food and Drug Administration (FDA) for use in treating endometriosis in a depot subcutaneous form. A common side effect is transient breakthrough bleeding, which occurs in 38% to 47% of patients. This is generally well tolerated and, when necessary, can be adequately treated with supplemental estrogen or an increase in the progestogen dose. Other side effects include nausea (0% to 80%), breast tenderness (5%), fluid retention (50%), and depression (6%). A recent approach to treating endometriosis with progestogen is the use of a progestogen-containing intrauterine contraceptive device[1] (Mirena).

The combination of estrogen and progestogen for therapy of endometriosis, the so-called pseudopregnancy regimen, has been used for 40 years. The most commonly used pseudopregnancy regimen today is the oral contraceptive pill[1] (OCP); in fact, it is the most commonly prescribed treatment for endometriosis symptoms. Like progestational therapy, pseudopregnancy is believed to produce initial decidualization and growth of endometrial tissue, followed in several months by atrophy.

Gonadotropin-releasing hormone (GnRH) agonists are analogues of the hormone GnRH. This hypothalamic hormone is responsible for stimulating the pituitary gland to secrete follicle-stimulating hormone (FSH) and LH, two hormones necessary for normal ovarian function. GnRH is secreted in a pulsatile manner; the correct pulse results in stimulation of FSH and LH release, whereas too high or too low a pulse rate results in a decrease in pituitary hormone secretion. GnRH agonists are modified forms of GnRH that bind to the pituitary receptors and remain for a lengthy period. Thus, they are identified by the pituitary as rapidly pulsatile GnRH, and after initial stimulation of FSH and LH secretion, result in a shutdown (down-regulation) of the pituitary and no stimulation of the ovary. The result is a hypoestrogenic state similar to that of menopause, producing endometrial atrophy and amenorrhea. The agonist can be given intranasally (naferelin [Synarel]), subcutaneously (goserelin [Zoladex]), or intramuscularly (IM) (leuprolide acetate [Lupro Depot]), depending on the specific product, with frequency of administration ranging from twice daily to every 3 months. The side effects are those of hypoestrogenism such as transient vaginal bleeding, hot flashes, vaginal dryness, decreased libido, breast tenderness, insomnia, depression, irritability and fatigue, headache, osteoporosis, and decreased skin elasticity; these are dose dependent.

A recent modification of GnRH agonist treatment is to add back small amounts of steroid hormone in a manner similar to that used in the treatment of postmenopausal women. The theory is that the requirement for estrogen is greater for endometriosis than is needed by the brain (to prevent hot flashes), the bone (to prevent osteoporosis), and other tissues deprived of this hormone. With

---

[1]Not FDA approved for this indication.

this approach there is an equivalent rate of pain relief with far fewer side effects than GnRH agonist alone. Estrogen as a solitary add-back, however, is less effective and thus not indicated.

Surgical Therapy

Most surgeons performing surgery for endometriosis must choose one of two possibilities: conservative surgery, where the patient's future fertility remains an option, or definitive surgery. The latter procedure generally involves removal of the female gonads, a hysterectomy, or a combination of the two. The general perception is that definitive surgery is more effective over time than conservative treatment, but it must be reserved for patients in whom fertility or continued endocrine function is deemed less important than relief of pain symptoms.

When conservative surgery is desired, the first technical issue confronted is method of access. Traditionally, laparotomy was used for endometriosis surgery. However, recently, most surgeons performing extensive surgery for endometriosis have favored a laparoscopic approach because of improved magnification of disease with a resulting increase in surgical precision.

Surgical destruction of endometriosis lesions can be accomplished in a variety of ways: Excision, vaporization, and fulguration/desiccation have all been used. Excision is generally thought to be the most complete of these techniques, but no comparative trials have assessed the relative efficacy of each approach.

Endometriomas, or ovarian cysts formed from endometriosis, are commonly present in the patient with endometriosis. The ovaries should first be freed of all adhesions when operating on endometriomas. The endometrioma may open spontaneously during this process; if not, incision and drainage is indicated. At this point, the cyst wall may be stripped, excised, or drained.

Treatment Results

Medical therapy is effective against endometriosis-associated pain. Placebo-controlled randomized clinical trials (RCTs) have proven that danazol and medroxyprogesterone reduce pain significantly better than no treatment for up to 6 months following discontinuation of the drug. No good data exist for longer follow-up periods. Numerous randomized trials have compared medical therapies to one another. In 15 RCTs comparing danazol to GnRH agonists, no difference was demonstrated between the two as first-line drugs. Similarly, little difference was seen when GnRH agonists were compared to oral contraceptives, progestogens, or gestrinone.

Several trials have addressed the efficacy of combined add-back therapy and GnRH agonist treatment during 6-month treatment periods. In general, pain was relieved as effectively with the combination as with GnRH agonist alone, and it significantly reduced the side effects of the GnRH agonist. The results were similar in three longer trials of approximately 1-year duration (Figure 1). The amelioration of side effects with maintenance of efficacy seems to be even when the add-back therapy is begun during the first month of treatment, suggesting that an add-back-free interval at the beginning of a treatment cycle is unnecessary.

Although the studies just described randomize patients for initial therapy of endometriosis-associated pain, one study examined the value of GnRH agonist in patients failing primary therapy. Ling and colleagues treated women having failed to obtain relief with OCPs with either GnRH agonist or placebo. Those treated with active drug responded significantly better than those given placebo, with more than 80% experiencing pain relief in 3 months (Figure 2). Of interest is the fact that the therapy seemed to be beneficial whether or not endometriosis was seen at laparoscopy.

Most of the established medical therapies used to treat endometriosis have been applied to the problem of subfertility in women with this disease. These medications inhibit ovulation, and thus they are used to treat the disease for a period of time prior to allowing an attempt at conception. Five randomized trials with six treatment arms have compared one of these medical treatments for endometriosis to placebo or no treatment with fertility as the outcome measure. Another eight RCTs compared danazol to a second

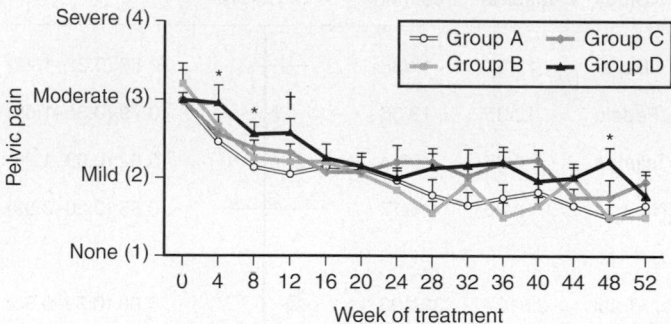

MEAN PELVIC PAIN SCORE AT EACH VISIT

* $P \le 0.05$ ⎱ Change from baseline
† $P \le 0.01$ ⎰ compared with Group A

Figure 1. Pain relief from gonadotropin-releasing hormone (GnRH) agonist (Group A) and three different add-back therapies. (High-dose progestin, low-dose estrogen/progestin, higher-dose estrogen/progestin). No difference is seen among the groups in the amount of pain relief. (From Hornstein MD, Surrey ES, Weisberg GW, Casino LA: et al: Leuprolide acetate depot and hormonal add-back in endometriosis: A 12-month study. Lupron Add-Back Study Group. Obstet Gynecol 1998;91[1]:16–24.)

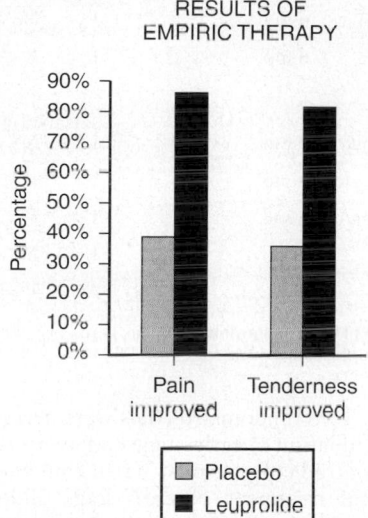

RESULTS OF EMPIRIC THERAPY

Figure 2. Patients with pain relief from empirical gonadotropin-releasing hormone (GnRH) agonist or placebo.

medication. These latter trials were summarized by a meta-analysis by Hughes et al. and modified by Olive and Pritts to include loss of fertility while on the medications (Figure 3). The data clearly show that medical therapy for endometriosis has not proven to be of value, and in fact may be counterproductive, to the subfertile patient.

Only two studies have investigated surgery for endometriosis-associated pain versus sham surgery. Sutton and colleagues assessed the efficacy of laser laparoscopic surgery in the treatment of pain associated with minimal, mild, or moderate endometriosis. They found that there was no difference in pain at 3 months follow-up, but by 6 months a clear-cut advantage was seen for surgery. Abbott and colleagues evaluated excision of endometriosis versus diagnostic laparoscopy and had nearly identical results at 6 months. Thus, both techniques were proven better than no therapy.

Conservative surgery was used extensively in an attempt to enhance fertility. Most studies, however, are uncontrolled and

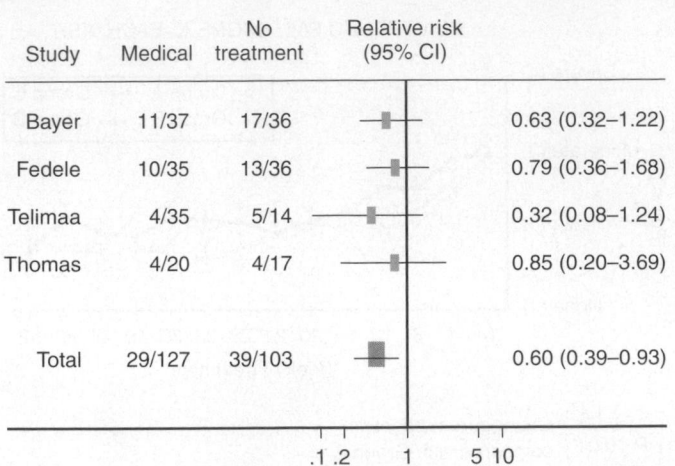

Study	Medical	No treatment	Relative risk (95% CI)
Bayer	11/37	17/36	0.63 (0.32–1.22)
Fedele	10/35	13/36	0.79 (0.36–1.68)
Telimaa	4/35	5/14	0.32 (0.08–1.24)
Thomas	4/20	4/17	0.85 (0.20–3.69)
Total	29/127	39/103	0.60 (0.39–0.93)

Figure 3. Meta-analysis of all randomized trials comparing medical therapy versus no treatment or placebo for endometriosis-associated infertility. Note that the untreated group has a significantly better pregnancy rate.

 TABLE 1 Postoperative Medical Therapy

DRUG	DURATION OF TREATMENT	STUDIES	FINDINGS
OCPs	6 mo	1	NS at 24, 36 mo
Medroxy-progesterone, 100 mg/d	6 mo	1	$P < 0.05$ at 6 mo
Danazol, 600 mg/d	3 mo	1	NS at 6 mo
Danazol, 600 mg/d	6 mo	1	$P < 0.05$ at 6 mo
Danazol, 100 mg/d	6 mo	1	$P < 0.05$ at 24 mo
GnRH-a	3 mo	1	NS at 6 mo
GnRH-a	6 mo	2	$P = 0.008$ at 12 mo

Abbreviations: GnRH = gonadotropin-releasing hormone; NS = not significant; OCPs = oral contraceptive pills.

of poor quality. Two randomized trials were performed to examine the value of ablation of early-stage endometriosis versus sham surgery, with contradictory results. When combined into a meta-analysis, surgical treatment of early-stage endometriosis still appears to provide a significant improvement in pregnancy rates. No such trials exist for more extensive disease; expert opinion would suggest that surgery will enhance fertility but may be inferior to advanced reproductive technologies.

The use of medical therapies for endometriosis is not restricted to their use as stand-alone agents. Clinicians frequently have used drugs in combination with surgical treatment of the disease. Numerous trials have examined the issue of postoperative medical therapy as an effective adjunct for pain. Those that have treated patients for at least 6 months after surgery showed efficacy, but in those studies where only 3 months of postoperative treatment was performed, no benefit was seen. Results are similar for all medications (Table 1).

In summary, endometriosis is an enigmatic disease that has long frustrated clinicians and patients. However, great strides in the understanding of this disorder are being made. The coming years are likely to produce a plethora of new treatment approaches targeting the biologic basis of this disease. In this regard, better understanding will undoubtedly result in renewed hope for the patient suffering from the ravages of endometriosis.

References

Abbott JA, Hawe J, Hunter D, et al. Laparoscopic excision of endometriosis: A randomized, placebo controlled trial. Fertil Steril 2004;82:878–84.

Hornstein MD, Surrey ES, Weisberg GW, Casino LA. Lupron Add-Back Study Group. Leuprolide acetate depot and hormonal add-back in endometriosis: a 12-month study. Obstet Gynecol 1998;91:16–24.

Hughes E, Ferorkow D, Collins J, Vandekerckhone P. Ovulation suppression for endometriosis (Cochrane review). In: The Cochrane Library (issue 1). Oxford, England: Update Software; 2000.

Jacobson TZ, Barlow DH, Koninclex PR, et al. Laparoscopic surgery for sub-fertility associated with endometriosis. Cochrane Database Syst Rev 2002;(4), CD001398.

Jansen RPS, Russel P. Nonpigmented endometriosis: Clinical, laparoscopic and pathologic definition. Am J Obstet Gynecol 1986;155:1154.

Ling FW. Randomized controlled trial of depot leuprolide in patients with chronic pelvic pain and clinically suspected endometriosis. Obstet Gynecol 1999;93:51–8.

Moghissi KS, Schlaff WD, Olive DL, et al. Goserelin acetate (Zoladex) with or without hormone replacement therapy for the treatment of endometriosis. Fertil Steril 1998;69:1056–62.

Olive DL, Pritts EA. The treatment of endometriosis: a review of the evidence. Ann NY Acad Sci 2002;955:360–72.

Olive DL, Pritts EA. Treatment of endometriosis. N Engl J Med 2001;345:266–75.

Sampson JA. Perforating hemorrhagic (chocolate) cysts of the ovary. Arch Surg 1921;3:245.

Sutton CJG, Ewen SP, Whitelaw N, Haines P. Prospective, randomized, double-blind, controlled trial of laser laparoscopy in the treatment of pelvic pain associated with minimal, mild, or moderate endometriosis. Fertil Steril 1994;62:696.

INFERTILITY

Method of
Keith A. Frey, MD

 ## CURRENT DIAGNOSIS

- Infertility occurs in approximately 15% to 20% of couples, many of whom present to their primary care physician for initial evaluation.
- A thorough evaluation of both partners is necessary, because 25% of couples have more than one etiologic factor.
- The causes of infertility include abnormalities of any portion of the male or female reproductive system.

CURRENT THERAPY

- Treatment should not be initiated until the diagnostic evaluation is completed.
- The male and female partners should be treated as a couple whenever possible.
- Emotional support for the couple is an important aspect of their care.

Epidemiology

Infertility is defined as 1 year of unprotected intercourse in which a pregnancy has not been achieved. From 15% to 20% of all couples in the United States are infertile, with high rates seen in older couples. This rate has remained relatively stable since the early 1980s.

Risk Factors

The causes of infertility include abnormalities of any portion of the male or female reproductive system. Although infertility results from a single cause in the majority of couples, more than one factor contributes to infertility in as many as 25% of couples. "Unexplained" infertility, in which no specific cause is identified, occurs in approximately 25% of infertile couples. Specific causes for infertility generally distribute as follows: male factors (approximately 25%), ovulatory dysfunction (approximately 20%), tubal pathology (approximately 15%), and other categories (including endometriosis, uterine, or cervical factors; approximately 15%).

Prevention

The Centers for Disease Control and Prevention (CDC) recommends that all men, women, and couples have a reproductive life plan. This is defined as a set of goals about having children, or not having children based on personal values and resources, and a plan to achieve these goals. Couples should be questioned regarding any previous children, desire to have any more children, whether there has ever been trouble conceiving, and what timeframe the couple has for conception.

Clinical Manifestations

Infertility is a common condition seen in a primary care practice and is defined as 1 year of unprotected intercourse in which a pregnancy has not been achieved. Fecundability is the probability of achieving a pregnancy within one menstrual cycle, and the fecundability of a "normal" couple (under age 35) is approximately 25%. Infertility is considered primary if neither partner has achieved a successful pregnancy. Secondary infertility relates to those couples where there has previously been a pregnancy but there is current difficulty with conception. It is estimated that approximately 25% of women will have an episode of infertility during their childbearing years.

Diagnosis

The physician should arrange a meeting with the couple early in the diagnostic workup. This provides an important opportunity to review reproductive biology and the rationale for subsequent laboratory test results. Because infertility may arise from one or more areas of the reproductive system, it requires a comprehensive diagnostic evaluation. The initial assessment of both the male and the female partner consists of a thorough history and physical examination. In addition to a comprehensive history and physical examination, each couple must be evaluated by a series of routine laboratory tests (complete blood count, urinalysis, semen analysis, or Pap smear) and appropriately timed studies to evaluate each major reproductive factor that may be the cause of infertility. This comprehensive diagnostic survey should be completed for most couples in 6 to 12 months. Each couple's evaluation must be individualized based on the findings of the history and the physical examination. However, an initial survey of each major reproductive factor is necessary in all couples and can be coordinated by the primary care physician.

Male Factors

The male is evaluated with a complete blood count, urinalysis, and at least two semen analyses. Each semen analysis is performed on a fresh (within 2 hours), warm specimen obtained by masturbation after at least 2 days of abstinence.

Ovulatory Dysfunction

Anovulation or inconsistent ovulation may be suggested by history (irregular menses), and confirmed by an abnormally low serum progesterone levels in the luteal phase, or persistently negative home luteinizing hormone testing. If the patient is not ovulating, further laboratory evaluation is needed (serum prolactin and thyroid-stimulating hormone). Those patients with a diminished ovarian reserve (day 3 follicle-stimulating hormone >10) should be referred to an infertility specialist.

Tubal Factors

The female partner must undergo an evaluation for tubal patency. A hysterosalpingogram is obtained if the history and physical examination show no evidence of tubal damage. Otherwise, the patient is referred for laparoscopy.

Differential Diagnosis

Male Factors

The most commonly encountered cause of male infertility is oligospermia or azoospermia secondary to varicocele. Other causes of male infertility include primary hypogonadism (e.g., congenital or acquired testicular disorders, orchitis), altered sperm transport (e.g., absent vas deferens), and secondary hypogonadism (e.g., androgen excess or pharmacologic effects). These disorders manifest as oligospermia or azoospermia, disorders of sperm function or motility (asthenospermia), and abnormalities of sperm morphology (teratospermia).

Ovulatory Dysfunction

Ovulation disorders account for 40% of female factor infertility. The possible causes of anovulation may be grouped into several major categories: aging, diminished ovarian reserve, endocrine disorders (e.g., hypothalamic amenorrhea, hyperprolactinemia, thyroid disease, adrenal disease), polycystic ovary syndrome (PCOS), premature ovarian failure, and tobacco use.

Tubal and Pelvic Pathology

Infertility may be associated with tubal damage or adnexal adhesions. Tubal obstruction may result from scarring secondary to acute salpingitis, although many cases of tubal occlusion are encountered in which no episodes of salpingitis are recalled. The chronic inflammation associated with endometriosis may disrupt normal conception by causing tubal damage or by secretion of toxic substances.

Unusual Problems

Cervical mucus abnormalities occur if at the time of ovulation the mucus is either insufficient in quantity or poor in quality. Factors contributing to the formation of such unreceptive cervical mucus include cervical infections, previous cervical surgery or cautery, and clomiphene therapy.

Treatment

Generally, treatment should not be initiated until the diagnostic evaluation is completed. The male and female partners should be treated as a couple whenever possible. Therapy should proceed at a rate that the couple finds comfortable.

Male Factors

Specific antibiotics are used to treat infections such as prostatitis and epididymitis. Men with findings on physical examination that suggest hormonal or testicular abnormalities should be referred to an infertility expert. Male patients should also be counseled regarding the growing evidence of increased risks associated with advanced paternal age. The risk of a child with schizophrenia is twice as likely if the father is 45 or older compared to those in their twenties and three times more likely after paternal age 50. Autism is 5.75 times more likely if the paternal age is 40 or older, compared to those men who father a child when they are younger than 40.

Ovulatory Dysfunction

Underlying causes of ovulatory dysfunction such as thyroid abnormalities or hyperprolactinemia should be corrected. If anovulation is diagnosed, consider treatment with clomiphene (Clomid). Metformin (Glucophage)[1] has been found to increase the rate of ovulation in patients who have anovulation secondary to PCOS. However, there was no increase in the rate of pregnancy in women who received metformin alone. Clomiphene plus metformin may increase the rate of pregnancy in women with resistant PCOS compared to clomiphene alone.

Tubal and Pelvic Pathology

Tubal blockage or deformity may necessitate surgical correction. The management of endometriosis in a woman desiring to achieve pregnancy depends on the degree and location of endometrial deposits. Conservative surgical treatment may enhance fertility potential by destroying endometrial implants and endometriomas. Laparoscopic conservative surgical treatment should be

---

[1]Not FDA approved for this indication.

Box 1 — Management Strategies

- Help the couple understand their motives for parenting, which may include desires (1) to parent, (2) to experience a pregnancy, (3) to meet the expectations of others, and (4) to promote genetic continuity.
- Assist the couple in the development of mutual support and an adaptive "couple-coping" style. Discuss sexual issues, and encourage the couple to nurture their intimacy; they will need its strength to deal with the problems associated with infertility. Periodic meetings with the couple to review diagnostic progress provide further opportunity to reinforce coping skills.
- Help the couple broaden their support systems, including self-help groups, such as Resolve, Inc.

considered as a treatment option for mild endometriosis-associated infertility. Patients with endometriosis may also benefit from ovulation induction with or without other assisted-reproduction techniques. For patients with more severe tubal and pelvic pathology, referral for assisted reproductive technologies is warranted.

Unusual Problems

For cervical mucus abnormalities, antibiotics should be used to treat the specific bacterial cause of the problem. Low-dose estrogens can be used for poor cervical mucus that does not result from infectious causes. However, intrauterine insemination (IUI) is the best treatment option for a cervical factor.

Management Strategies

The workup, diagnosis, and treatment of infertility can precipitate intense emotional reactions. The sensitive physician should discuss such emotions as anger, guilt, self-doubt, depression, and grief with the couple. The actions described in Box 1 may also prove beneficial.

References

Files JA, Frey KA, David PS, et al. Developing a reproductive life plan. J Midwife Women's Health 2011;56:468–74.
Frey KA. Male reproductive health and infertility. Prim Care 2010;37:643–52.
Jose-Miller AB, Boyden JW, Frey KA. Infertility. Am Fam Physician 2007;75:849–56.
Kolettis PN. Evaluation of the subfertile man. Am Fam Physician 2003;67:2165–72.
Malaspina D, Harlap S, Fennig S, et al. Advancing paternal age and the risk of schizophrenia. Arch Gen Psychiatry 2001;58:361–7.
Reichenberg A, Gross R, Weiser M, et al. Advancing paternal age and autism. Arch Gen Psychiatry 2006;63:1026–32.
Warner JN, Frey KA. The well man visit: addressing a man's health to optimize pregnancy outcomes. J Am Board Fam Med 2013;26:196–202.

MENOPAUSE

Method of
Irina Burd, MD, PhD; Stacey A. Scheib, MD; and Krystene I. Boyle, MD

CURRENT DIAGNOSIS

- For women older than 45 years who have menopausal symptoms, no further workup is necessary unless there are symptoms of hyperthyroidism.
- For women younger than 45 years, proceed with an oligomenorrhea or amenorrhea workup: Check serum hCG, prolactin, TSH, and FSH.
- Women younger than 40 years should have a complete evaluation for premature ovarian failure.

- Common symptoms of menopause include abnormal bleeding, hot flushes, genitourinary complaints, sleep disturbances, mood disturbances, joint pain, and difficulty concentrating.
- FSH and estradiol levels can be misleading and so should not be used to make the diagnosis.

Abbreviations: FSH = follicle-stimulating hormone; hCG = human chorionic gonadotropin; TSH = thyroid-stimulating hormone.

CURRENT THERAPY

- CEE or 17-β estradiol plus MPA, as either continuous or cyclic short-term therapy lasting no more than 5 years is a first-line treatment for vasomotor symptoms in a patient with no contraindications.
- Locally active estrogen-containing compounds are available for treating urogenital symptoms.
- SERMs provide an alternative for treating menopausal symptoms, specifically osteoporosis. Raloxifene has less antiresorptive action than the bisphosphonates (e.g., alendronate) and should be given to patients who do not tolerate bisphosphonates.
- Alendronate increases BMD in the vertebral spine and femoral neck more than raloxifene, but patients taking both alendronate and raloxifene increased their BMD the most.
- More research is needed in the use of androgen replacement in menopause, although some evidence suggests that it might improve libido.

Abbreviations: BMD = bone mineral density; CEE = conjugated equine estrogen; MPA = medroxyprogesterone acetate; SERM = selective estrogen-receptor modulator.

Menopause is the physiologic process characterized by a marked decrease in the number of oocytes, subsequent follicular depletion, decreased ovarian estrogen secretion, and finally cessation of menses. For 95% of women, menopause occurs between the ages of 45 and 55, with a mean age of 51. Time of menopause is influenced by genetic as well as environmental factors (Box 1). Menopause before age 40 years is considered premature ovarian failure.

Diagnosis

Menopause is defined clinically as 12 months of amenorrhea following the last menstrual period in the absence of other causes. The Staging of Reproductive Aging Workshop (STRAW) has

Box 1 — Factors That Influence the Timing of Menopause

- Alcohol abuse
- Chemotherapy
- Cigarette smoking
- Contraception
- Family history of early menopause
- Galactose consumption
- Obesity
- Parity
- History of pelvic irradiation
- Physiologic and psychological stresses (e.g., living at high altitudes, depression)
- Race
- Shorter cycle length during adolescence
- Type 1 diabetes mellitus

---

provided a beneficial staging system to help categorize patients (Box 2).

The differential diagnosis for menopause includes thyroid disease, pregnancy, hyperprolactinemia, medications, carcinoid, pheochromocytoma, or underlying malignancy, which are important in considering the diagnosis algorithm (Box 3). Follicle-stimulating hormone (FSH) and estradiol are commonly measured to diagnose menopause and are often misleading because they can fluctuate vastly in the perimenopausal period.

Systemic Manifestations of Menopause

Vasomotor Symptoms
Hot flushes are the most common symptom associated with menopause. They are self-limited sensations of generalized heat that last 2 to 4 minutes and vary widely among people and across cultures. Without treatment, they resolve within 1 to 5 years.

Sleep Disturbances
Sleep disturbances often occur in menopause as a result of hot flushes arousing the woman from sleep. When the hot flushes are treated, sleep usually improves. Persistent sleep disturbances can lead to more serious symptoms such as difficulty concentrating, fatigue, mood disturbances, depression, and other psychological symptoms.

Genitourinary Symptoms
Estrogen deficiency leads to atrophy of the urethral and vaginal epithelium. Vaginal atrophy can result in vaginal dryness, itching, irritation, and dyspareunia. The pH in the vagina also increases and, with vaginal atrophy, can lead to recurrent vaginal infections. Decreasing elasticity of the vaginal wall elasticity can result in a shorter and narrower vagina, especially without continued sexual activity. The lack of estrogen affects blood flow to the vagina and vulva, which in turn causes decreased lubrication and neuropathy. These are both reversible with estrogen replacement therapy, especially vaginal therapy.

Incontinence incidence increases with age but has not been clearly associated with menopause. The theory is that atrophy of the urethral epithelium results in diminished urethral mucosal seal, loss of compliance, and irritation. These are believed to contribute to stress and urge incontinence. These patients also report recurrent urinary tract infections; this is probably related to the increase in vaginal pH.

Abnormal Bleeding
Even though most postmenopausal bleeding is due to atrophy, during the perimenopausal period the endometrium may be exposed to unopposed estrogen that can result in anovulatory bleeding or endometrial hyperplasia. If this occurs, endometrial biopsy is needed to rule out endometrial hyperplasia or cancer. A transvaginal ultrasound can also be used as a screening tool first and then be followed by an endometrial biopsy if the endometrial thickness is greater than 4 mm.

Mood Disturbances
In the Study of Women's Health Across the Nation (SWAN), higher risks of mood symptoms were found in perimenopausal women. The strongest risks of depression associated with menopause are a prior history of depression and premenstrual syndrome. Depression might not be entirely related to the physiology of menopause but may be a result of stressors concomitantly occurring around the time of menopause, such as children leaving home, dealing with aged parents, and midlife adjustment.

Menstrual Migraines
Menstrual migraines are believed to be related to decreased estrogen levels around the time of menses. Because menopause is related to a decrease in estrogen, menstrual migraines can increase in intensity and frequency.

Balance and Osteoporosis
Estrogen deficiency can have an effect on the central nervous system by impairing balance. Along with osteoporosis, loss of balance remains one of the big causes of fractures in menopausal women. There are multiple risk factors for osteoporosis, modifiable and nonmodifiable (Box 4).

Other Effects
Other long-term issues that are believed to be related to menopause include cardiovascular disease and dementia.

Treatment

Hormone Replacement Therapy
Until relatively recently, long-term estrogen and combined estrogen and progestin therapy was routinely given to postmenopausal

women. Hormone replacement therapy (HRT) was believed to prevent cardiovascular disease and osteoporosis. The Women's Health Initiative (WHI) was a set of clinical trials, whose results were first published in 2002, that resulted in a dramatic change in clinical practice. The study was designed to see if there was a decrease in cardiovascular risk with conjugated equine estrogen (CEE [Premarin]) in patients without a uterus or in combination with medroxyprogesterone acetate (MPA [Provera]). The CEE-MPA (Prempro) arm of the trial was stopped early after 5 years because of the increased risks for breast cancer, coronary heart disease (CHD) (29%), stroke (41%) and venous thromboembolism (VTE) (33%), even though there was a reduction in risk of hip and vertebral fractures and colon cancer. There was also an increased risk of stroke (39%) and VTE (33%) in the CEE-alone arm after 7-year follow-up, but there was no difference in heart disease.

The Heart and Estrogen/progestin Replacement Studies (HERS I and II trials) looked at secondary prevention in postmenopausal women with known CHD, which showed that there was not a reduction of CHD events with CEE-MPA. Both the WHI and HERS studies revealed an increase in the number of VTEs.

In the WHI Memory Study (WHIMS), with CEE and CEE-MPA there was an increased risk of dementia compared with placebo, but this was in an older postmenopausal population. Epidemiologic studies indicate that estrogen may be neuroprotective if initiated earlier. Therefore, therapy should not initiated after age 65 years.

As a result of these studies and the recommendations of the North American Menopause Society, the only use for estrogen therapy, either alone or combined with progestin, is for control of menopausal symptoms, particularly hot flushes, vaginal dryness, urinary symptoms, joint pain, skin changes, and emotional lability. Studies are inconclusive whether CEE alone or CEE-MPA is beneficial for incontinence. Contraindications to estrogen therapy are a history of endometrial cancer, liver disease, breast cancer, CHD, history of VTE or stroke, or high risk of any of the above. In the Nurses' Health Study, an increased incidence of new onset of asthma that

may be dose related and development of systemic lupus erythematosus might result from estrogen therapy.

The absolute risk of an adverse event is extremely low. For a 50-year-old woman on combined estrogen-progestin, estimated risk is 1:1000 at 1 year and 1:200 at 5 years. This absolute risk doubles for a 60 year-old woman. The goal of treatment is a short-term therapy, lasting no more than 5 years. Therapy should be tapered, decreasing by one pill every 1 or 2 weeks, so that there is no rebound in menopausal symptoms.

Progestin should be added to HRT for any woman with a uterus in order to prevent endometrial hyperplasia and cancer. The Postmenopausal Estrogen/Progestin Interventions (PEPI) trial showed a statistically significant reduction in the incidence of simple, complex, and atypical endometrial hyperplasia with CEE-MPA therapy compared with CEE alone. The only recommended progestin at this time is MPA 2.5 mg/day. Alternative progestin doses, less frequent administration, and alternative routes of administration have not been studied and thus might not be able to prevent endometrial hyperplasia or cancer; if these are used, closer endometrial surveillance is necessary.

Women with premature ovarian failure should be given hormonal therapy, and risks and benefits should be reassessed at age 50 years.

More research is needed in the use of androgen replacement in menopause, although some evidence suggests that it might improve libido.

Alternative therapy has been proposed for menopausal symptoms (Table 1 and Box 5).

Bisphosphonates

Bisphosphonates impair osteoclastic bone resorption and are used to treat osteoporosis (Box 6). The most common side effects are bone pain and upper gastrointestinal disorders such as dysphagia, esophagitis, and esophageal or gastric ulcer. They are contraindicated in patients with renal impairment, uncorrected hypocalcemia,

TABLE 1 Treatment of Vasomotor Symptoms

TREATMENT	SUGGESTED DOSE	POSSIBLE SIDE EFFECTS
Hormones		
CEE (Premarin) or 17-β estradiol, plus MPA (Provera), either continuous or cyclic	CEE 0.3 mg/d *or* Estradiol 0.5 mg PO qd *or* Estradiol 0.05 mg patch qd *plus* MPA 2.5 mg/d or for 12–14 d/mo	See text
MPA	20 mg/d[3] oral or 150 mg IM (Depo-Provera)[1] q3 mo	Mood disturbances, breast tenderness, alopecia
Megestrol acetate (Megace)[1]	20 mg bid	Vomiting, diarrhea, flatulence
Selective Serotonin Reuptake Inhibitors		
Paroxetine (Paxil, Paxil CR)[1] Fluoxetine (Prozac)[1] Venlafaxine (Effexor, Effexor XR)[1]	10–20 mg/d or 12.5–25 mg CR/d 20 mg/d 37.5–75 mg XR/d	Fatigue, dry mouth, nausea, decreased libido
Other Medications		
Gabapentin (Neurontin)[1] Clonidine (Catapres TTS)[1]	300–900 mg/d 0.1 mg/24 h wk patch	Dizziness, somnolence, peripheral edema Orthostatic hypotension, drowsiness
Dietary Supplements		
Vitamin E[1] Black cohosh[7] Evening primrose oil[7]	800 IU/d	Fatigue, weakness, diarrhea Gastrointestinal complaints, dizziness
Other Interventions		
Acupuncture or acupressure Exercise Lifestyle interventions (e.g., layered clothing, fans, air conditioners)		

[1]Not FDA approved for this indication.
[3]Exceeds dosage recommended by the manufacturer.
[7]Available as a dietary supplement.
Abbreviations: CEE = conjugated equine estrogen; MPA = medroxyprogesterone acetate.

or sensitivity to the drug components. There have been no randomized, controlled studies comparing one type of bisphosphonate with another.

Selective Estrogen Receptor Modulators

Selective estrogen receptor modulators (SERMs) provide an alternative for treating menopausal symptoms, specifically osteoporosis (Box 6). SERMs bind to the estrogen receptor, but they have tissue-specific properties. The two SERMs that have been studied the most are raloxifene (Evista) and tamoxifen (Nolvadex). Raloxifene's mechanism for tissue-specific activity is not fully clear. Tamoxifen probably works by variable gene expression in different cell types.

Raloxifene

Two major double-blinded, placebo-controlled trials, one in the United States and one in Europe, have looked at raloxifene versus placebo, measuring bone mineral density (BMD), markers of bone turnover, and serum lipid levels. In all treatment arms in both studies, BMD was significantly increased and serum concentrations of both total and low-density lipoprotein (LDL) cholesterol were significantly decreased compared with placebo. In both trials there was no difference in complaints of breast pain or vaginal bleeding and no difference in endometrial thickness.

In the longer-term Multiple Outcomes of Raloxifene Evaluation (MORE) study, there was a relative risk reduction in vertebral fractures but not for nonvertebral fractures. The risk of invasive, but not noninvasive, breast cancer appeared to decrease, most likely due to the antagonistic effect of raloxifene. There was no increase in endometrial cancer. The relative risk of thromboembolic disease was 3.1 compared with placebo, but it appears that the risk is less than that with tamoxifen. There was no difference in cardiovascular events, except there was a decrease in the subset of women at greatest risk.

In a study looking at osteoporosis in postmenopausal women, patients on alendronate (Fosamax) increased their BMD in the vertebral spine and femoral neck more than patients on raloxifene, but patients taking both medications increased their BMD the most. CEE had a better effect on BMD compared with raloxifene in hysterectomized postmenopausal women. Raloxifene has less antiresorptive action than the bisphosphonates (e.g., alendronate) and should be given to patients who do not tolerate bisphosphonates.

Raloxifene significantly increased the occurrence of hot flushes compared with placebo in all the studies. Other side effects of raloxifene noted were influenza-like symptoms, peripheral edema, and leg cramps. It does not appear to affect vaginal symptoms, urinary symptoms, gallbladder disease, cognitive decline, or cataracts. The recommended starting dose is 60 mg/day.

Tamoxifen

Tamoxifen[1] has demonstrated some benefit for osteoporosis, but estrogen and bisphosphonates have shown a greater increase in lumbar spine BMD. In the National Surgical Adjuvant Breast and Bowel Project (NSABP) P-1 Trial, women on tamoxifen had fewer hip, wrist, and vertebral fractures at 7-year follow-up. In this study there was not a significant difference in the occurrence of cardiovascular events. Total and LDL cholesterol were significantly decreased on tamoxifen.

In combination with adjuvant therapy for estrogen receptor–positive breast cancer, tamoxifen can decrease the risk of recurrence and death and aid those with metastatic disease.

As with raloxifene, patients taking tamoxifen have a greater risk for VTE. This association is found particularly in patients who are concomitantly receiving chemotherapy.

The main difference between raloxifene and tamoxifen is that tamoxifen use is associated with a greater risk of endometrial cancers, especially uterine sarcoma. This risk depended on length of treatment. As a result, the American College of Obstetrics and Gynecologists (ACOG) has recommendations regarding monitoring women taking tamoxifen (Box 7), but these are not evidence based. For prevention, an intrauterine levonorgestrel could be placed. Even though there is evidence to suggest that tamoxifen is effective in preventing and treating osteoporosis, it is not approved by the FDA except for the prevention and treatment of breast cancer.

---

[1] Not FDA approved for this indication.

References

American College of Obstetricians and Gynecologists. Tamoxifen and endometrial cancer. ACOG Committee Opinion 232. Washington, DC: American College of Obstetricians and Gynecologists; 2000.

American College of Obstetricians and Gynecologists Task Force. Hormone Therapy. Obstet Gynecol 2004;104(Suppl. 4):S1–S129.

Barnabei VM, Cochrane BB, Aragaki AK, et al. Menopausal symptoms and treatment-related effects of estrogen and progestin in the Women's Health Initiative. Obstet Gynecol 2005;105:1063–73.

Barrett-Connor E, Cauley JA, Kulkarni PM, et al. Risk-benefit profile for raloxifene: 4-Year data from the Multiple Outcomes of Raloxifene Evaluation (MORE) randomized trial. J Bone Miner Res 2004;19:1270–5.

Grady D, Herrington D, Bittner V, et al. Cardiovascular disease outcomes during 6.8 years of hormone therapy: Heart and Estrogen/Progestin Replacement Study follow-up (HERS-II). JAMA 2002;288:49–57.

Hulley S, Grady D, Bush T, et al. for the Heart and Estrogen/Progestin Replacement Study (HERS) Research Group. Randomized trial of estrogen plus progestin for secondary prevention of coronary heart disease in postmenopausal women. JAMA 1998;280:605–13.

North American Menopause Society. Treatment of menopause-associated vasomotor symptoms: Position statement of The North American Menopause Society. Menopause 2004;11:11–33.

Soules MR, Sherman S, Parrott E, Rebar R. Executive summary: Stages of Reproductive Aging Workshop (STRAW). Fertil Steril 2001;76:874–8.

Women's Health Initiative Steering Committee. Effects of conjugated equine estrogen in postmenopausal women with hysterectomy. JAMA 2004;291:1707–12.

Writing Group for the PEPI Trial. Effects of estrogen or estrogen/progestin regimens on heart disease risk factors in postmenopausal women. The Postmenopausal Estrogen/Progestin Interventions (PEPI) Trial. JAMA 1995;273:199–208.

Writing Group for the Women's Health Initiative Investigators. Risks and benefits of estrogen plus progestin in healthy postmenopausal women: Principal results from the Women's Health Initiative randomized controlled trial. JAMA 2002;288:321–33.

OVARIAN CANCER

Method of
Michelle A. Roett, MD, MPH

CURRENT DIAGNOSIS

- The U.S. Preventive Services Task Force (USPSTF) recommends against routine screening for ovarian cancer in asymptomatic women. Screening for ovarian cancer may lead to significant harms, including invasive surgical interventions for women without cancer.
- The USPSTF recommends that women with family history associated with increased risk for deleterious mutations in *BRCA1* and *BRCA2* should be referred for genetic counseling and evaluation for *BRCA* testing.

CURRENT THERAPY

- Cancer antigen 125 (CA-125) and transvaginal ultrasound are indicated for known adnexal mass.
- Ovarian cancer is treated with surgical debulking and adjuvant chemotherapy.
- Prophylactic bilateral salpingo-oophorectomy should be considered in women with a mutation in the *BRCA1* or *BRCA2* gene, or hereditary nonpolyposis colorectal cancer syndrome.

Epidemiology

Ovarian cancer accounts for only 3% of cancers in women in the United States but results in more deaths than any other gynecologic cancer. Ovarian cancer has an age-adjusted incidence of 12.1 per 100,000 women, slightly decreased in recent years. In women over 50, incidence rates have declined by as much as 2.4%. In 2012, 192,446 women were living with ovarian cancer. According to the American Cancer Society 21,290 new cases of ovarian cancer and 14,180 were expected in the United States in 2015.

Caucasian women have the highest incidence rate of ovarian cancer followed by Hispanic, Asian/Pacific Islander, African American, and American Indian/Alaska Native women. Caucasian women are more likely to die of ovarian cancer than any other group. African American and AI/AN women have the second highest rates of death from ovarian cancer, followed by Hispanic and Asian/Pacific Islander women. African American women with advanced epithelial ovarian cancer are more likely to die than their Caucasian counterparts (Hazard Ratio 1.27). Hispanic women have intermediate incidence and death rates compared to non-Hispanic women. Similar to other cancers affecting women, incidence of ovarian cancer and associated mortality increase with age, with women over 50 years of age experiencing the highest incidence. However, varying types of ovarian cancer may be diagnosed at any age, from infancy onward.

Risk Factors

Women at highest risk of ovarian cancer have a family history, associated genetic syndrome, or specific genetic mutation. For women of Ashkenazi Jewish descent increased-risk family history refers to having one first-degree relative with breast or ovarian cancer or two second-degree relatives on the same side of the family. For other women increased-risk family history refers to having two or more first- or second-degree relatives with a history of ovarian cancer, a combination of breast and ovarian cancer among first- or second-degrees relatives, breast cancer in a male relative, one first-degree relative with bilateral breast cancer, or three or more first- or second-degree relatives with breast cancer.

Women with hereditary breast and ovarian cancer syndrome have an autosomal dominant mutation in the *BRCA1* or *BRCA2* gene. This occurs in one in every 500 women. Hereditary breast and ovarian cancer syndrome increases the risk of breast, ovarian, pancreatic, and prostate cancers, and is associated with up to 54% lifetime risk of ovarian cancer. Hereditary nonpolyposis colorectal cancer syndrome (Lynch II) is also autosomal dominant, increases risk of breast, colorectal, endometrial and ovarian cancers, and is associated with up to 12% lifetime risk of ovarian cancer.

Early age of menarche and later age at menopause are both associated with increased risk of ovarian cancer. Current smoking status increases risk of mucinous epithelian ovarian cancer (RR 2.22), along with former smoking (RR 2.02). Other risk factors including 7-fold increased risk from taking 12 or more monthly cycles of clomiphene, or taking fertility drugs used in in-vitro fertilization (RR 1.59).

Pathophysiology

Ovarian cancer arises from epithelial, stromal, and germ cells, with up to 95% of cases arising from epithelial cells, 5% to 8% stromal cells, and 3% to 5% germ cells. The age distribution of patients with ovarian cancer corresponds with the type of ovarian tumor. Germ cell tumors commonly occur in adolescents or patients under 1 year of age. Stromal cell tumors may occur at any age but include types more common in adolescence, such as androblastomas. Epithelial cell tumors commonly affect patients 50 years of age and older.

Ovarian cancer primarily spreads based on proximity to the uterus and opposite ovary, followed by intraperitoneal metastasis. Death usually arises from complications associated with local spread. Rare distant metastases may spread to the lungs, liver, adrenal glands, or spleen. In 2014 the International Federation of Gynecology and Obstetrics redefined stages of ovarian cancer to include ovarian, peritoneal and fallopian tube cancers because of similarities in their origins and treatment. FIGO staging guides treatment and prognosis to complement tumor-node-metastasis (TNM) staging defined by the American Joint Committee on Cancer. Stage II inlcudes pelvic extension of an ovarian tumor, with a 60% to 80% 5-year survival rate. The 5-year survival rate is greatly diminished for stages III and IV. Some 85% of ovarian cancer cases are diagnosed in Stage III, which is associated with 20% survival. Stage III includes metastasis to the peritoneum outside the pelvis, primary peritoneal cancer, and/or metastasis to retroperitoneal lymph nodes. Stage IV is associated with less than 10% survival and includes distant metastases.

Prevention

The U.S. Preventive Services Task Force recommends again routine screening for ovarian cancer in asymptomatic women. The USPSTF also recommends that primary care clinicians screen women who have any family members with breast, ovarian, tubal or peritoneal with a validated screening tool to identiry a significant family history with increased risk for PRCA-1 or BRCA-2 mutations. If the screening is positive the patient should be referred for genetic counseling, and if indicated by counseling, BRCA testing. Screening with serum cancer antigen 125 (CA-125) level or transvaginal ultrasound does not reduce deaths from ovarian cancer and may lead to significant harms, including possibly unnecessary major surgical interventions in women without cancer. The most protective factors decreasing risk of ovarian cancer include older age at menarche, hormonal contraceptive use, multiparity, and younger age at menopause, primarily by decreasing the frequency of ovulation. Oral contraceptives (OR 0.75) and tubal ligation (OR 0.63) both decrease risk with longer duration. IUD use for up to 4 years is also protective (OR 0.53), but risk increases with IUD in place for more than 10 years (OR 1.4). Statin use for more than 5 years also reduces risk (RR 0.48). Multiple dietary interventions may be associated with lower risk of ovarian cancer. Drinking two or more cups of tea per day is associated with lower risk of ovarian cancer compared to one cup or less per day. A low-fat, high-fiber diet and a diet with increased vegetable consumption are both associated with decreased risk of ovarian cancer. Ovarian cancer is effectively reduced in women with *BRCA* mutations (NNT = 36) and hereditary nonpolyposis colorectal cancer syndrome (NNT=28) by prophylactic bilateral salpingo-oophorectomy (BSO). Given the risk of ovarian cancer and 60% lifetime risk of endometrial cancer, total abdominal hysterectomy with BSO may be considered for patients with hereditary nonpolyposis colorectal cancer syndrome.

Clinical Manifestations

Although presenting symptoms for ovarian cancer may be nonspecific, the most common symptom is abdominal pain. Children and teenagers may also present with irregular menses, precocious puberty, or hirsutism. Any one of six symptoms for more than 12 days per month for less than 1 year has a 56.7% sensitivity for early ovarian cancer and 79.5% sensitivity for advanced stage ovarian cancer. These symptoms include abdominal pain, pelvic pain, increased abdomen size, bloating, difficulty eating, and early satiety. For patients with a pelvic mass, an irregular or enlarged ovary more than 10 cm, a nodular or fixed pelvic mass, or bilateral lesions more significantly increase suspicion of ovarian cancer. For women more than 3 years postmenopausal, ovaries are normally significantly diminished in size and often nonpalpable.

Diagnosis

Ovarian cancer patients with primarily gastrointestinal symptoms such as nausea, vomiting, diarrhea, and constipation tend to be diagnosed at a later stage than patients presenting with primarily gynecologic symptoms such as abnormal vaginal bleeding or pain. Diagnostic evaluation involves consideration of nonspecific signs and symptoms (Table 1). Women over 40 with persistent or unexplained symptoms should undergo laboratory evaluation including complete blood count, comprehensive metabolic panel, and CA-125. Pelvic inflammatory disease, endometriosis, functional ovarian cysts, menstruation, pregnancy, ascites, and other malignancies may cause elevated CA-125 levels.

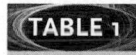

| **TABLE 1** | Diagnostic Findings Associated with Ovarian Cancer |

History
- Abdominal fullness
- Back pain
- Constipation
- Diarrhea
- Early satiety
- Fatigue
- Nausea
- Pelvic pain
- Urinary symptoms

Family History
- Bilateral breast cancer
- Early-onset breast cancer (younger than 50 years)
- Male breast cancer
- Personal or family history of colon or endometrial cancer
- Two or more first- or second-degree relatives with ovarian cancer

Physical Examination
- Abdominal mass
- Inguinal lymphadenopathy
- Pelvic or adnexal mass
- Sister Mary Joseph nodule
- Laboratory tests for patient with known adnexal mass:
  - CA-125 levels >200 U/mL (200 arb U/L) in premenopausal women
  - CA 125 >35 U/mL (35 arb U/L) in postmenopausal women
  - Increased β–human chorionic gonadotropin*
  - Increased serum alpha-fetoprotein*
  - Increased neuron-specific enolase*
  - Increased lactate dehydrogenase*

*Primarily used to evaluate adnexal masses during adolescence.

Unfortunately, early detection is limited because CA-125 is elevated in only 50% of stage I tumors, but 90% of advanced stage ovarian cancer. Highest estimates of sensitivities, specificities, and positive predictive values are most applicable to postmenopausal women with known adnexal mass. An elevated CA-125 level (more than 200 U/mL in a premenopausal women, more than 35 U/mL in postmenopausal women) with an adnexal mass warrants evaluation by a gynecologic oncologist. OVA-1 is an FDA-approved panel measuring five biomarkers: CA-125, transferrin, prealbumin, apolipoprotein A1, and beta-2 microglobulin. Scored results identify ovarian cancer with 93% sensitivity and 43% specificity. Doppler transvaginal ultrasound for patients with adnexal masses has up 86% sensitivity and up to 91% specificity for ovarian cancer. Suspicious findings include a complex mass with both solid and cystic areas, extramural fluid, echogenicity, wall thickening, septa, or papillary projections, or an increased number and tortuosity of vessels on Doppler evaluation. Gadolinium-enhanced magnetic resonance imaging is useful for further delineation of indeterminate masses seen on ultrasonography.

Differential Diagnosis

The differential diagnosis for the signs and symptoms is broad, based on the nonspecific nature of presenting complaints. The differential for an adnexal mass may include a benign ovarian tumor, metastatic lesion, ovarian cyst or torsion, tubo-ovarian abscess, endometrioma or endometriosis, and rarely a pelvic kidney or pedunculated uterine fibroid.

Therapy or Treatment

Treatment for ovarian cancer is surgical debulking followed by chemotherapy. Chemotherapy before debulking surgery is associated with similar outcomes. Radiation may be used for palliative therapy or postchemotherapy localized disease. Surgical staging involves total abdominal hysterectomy, BSO, and the removal of pelvic and para-aortic lymph nodes and omentum.

Monitoring

Ovarian cancer of low malignant potential presents at stage I in 82% of cases typically between 30 and 50 years old, allowing for consideration of fertility-sparing measures, such as unilateral salpingo-oophorectomy. Adjuvant chemotherapy is reserved for patients with postoperative residual disease. Surgical treatment completion with total abdominal hysterectomy and unilateral salpingo-oophorectomy should be considered after the reproductive years. Positron emission tomography scans are useful for evaluation of increased CA-125 in known ovarian cancer in combination with computed tomography.

References

American Cancer Society. Cancer facts and figures 2015. Atlanta: American Cancer Society; 2015.

American College of Obstetricians and Gynecologists. ACOG committee opinion: number 280, December 2002. The role of the generalist obstetrician-gynecologist in the early detection of ovarian cancer. Obstet Gynecol 2002; 100:1413–6.

American College of Obstetricians and Gynecologists. ACOG practice bulletin. Management of adnexal masses. Obstet Gynecol 2007;110:201–14.

Barney SP, Muller CY, Bradshaw KD. Pelvic masses. Med Clin North Am 2008;92:1143–61.

Ellenson LH, Pirog EC. The female genital tract. In: Kumar V, Abbas AK, Aster AC, et al., editors. Robbins and Cotran pathologic basis of disease. 9th ed. Philadelphia: Elsevier; 2005.

Finch A, Beiner M, Lubinski J, et al. for the Hereditary Ovarian Cancer Clinical Study Group. Salpingo-oophorectomy and the risk of ovarian, fallopian tube, and peritoneal cancers in women with a BRCA1 or BRCA2 mutation. JAMA 2006;296:185–92.

Funt SA, Hann LE. Detection and characterization of adnexal masses. Radiol Clin North Am 2002;40:591–608.

Goff BA, Mandel LS, Drescher CW, et al. Development of an ovarian cancer symptom index: possibilities for earlier detection. Cancer 2007;109:221–7.

Han LY, Coleman RL. Ovarian cancer staging. Oper Tech Gen Surg 2007;9:53–60.

Howell EA, Egorova N, Hayes MP, Wisnivesky J, Franco R, Bickell N. Racial disparities in the treatment of advanced epithelial ovarian cancer. Obstet Gynecol 2013;122(5):1025–32.

Larsson SC, Holmberg L, Wolk A. Fruit and vegetable consumption in relation to ovarian cancer incidence: the Swedish mammography cohort. Br J Cancer 2004;90:2167.

Larsson SC, Wolk A. Tea consumption and ovarian cancer risk in a population-based cohort. Arch Intern Med 2005;165:2683.

Li LL, Zhou J, Qian XJ, Chen YD. Meta-analysis on the possible association between in vitro fertilization and cancer risk. Int J Gynecol Cancer 2013;23(1):16–24.

Liu Y, Qin A, Li T, Qin X, Li S. Effect of statin on risk of gynecologic cancers: a meta-analysis of observational studies and randomized controlled trials. Gynecol Oncol 2014;133(3):647–55.

Morrison J, Swanton A, Collins S, et al. Chemotherapy versus surgery for initial treatment in advanced ovarian epithelial cancer. Cochrane Database Syst Rev 2007;4, CD005343.

Moyer VA. Risk assessment, genetic counseling, and genetic testing for BRCA-related cancer in women: U.S. preventive services task force recommendation statement. Ann Intern Med 2014;160(4):271–82.

Moyer VA. Screening for ovarian cancer: U.S. Preventive Services Task Force reaffirmation recommendation statement. Ann Intern Med 2012;157:900–4.

Ness RB, Dodge RC, Edwards RP, et al. Contraception methods, beyond oral contraceptives and tubal ligation, and risk of ovarian cancer. Ann Epidemiol 2011;21(3):188–96.

Prentice RL, Thomson CA, Caan B, et al. Low-fat dietary pattern and cancer incidence in the Women's health initiative dietary modification randomized controlled trial. J Natl Cancer Inst 2007;99:1534.

Roett MA, Evans P. Ovarian cancer: an overview. Am Fam Physician 2009;80:609–16.

Ryerson AB, Eheman C, Burton J, et al. Symptoms, diagnoses, and time to key diagnostic procedures among older U.S. women with ovarian cancer. Obstet Gynecol 2007;109:1053–61.

Sanner K, et al. Ovarian epithelial neoplasia after hormonal infertility treatment: long-term follow-up of a historical cohort in Sweden. Fertil Steril 2009 Apr;91 (4):1152–8.

SEER Cancer Statistics Factsheets: Vulvar Cancer. Bethesda MD: National Cancer Institute. Available at http://seer.cancer.gov/statfacts/html/vulva.html. [Accessed June 12, 2015].

Smith LH, Morris CR, Yasmeen S, et al. Ovarian cancer: can we make the clinical diagnosis earlier? Cancer 2005;104:1398–407.

Tworoger SS, Gertig DM, Gates MA, et al. Caffeine, alcohol, smoking, and the risk of incident epithelial ovarian cancer. Cancer 2008;112:1169.

U.S. Cancer Statistics Working Group. United States Cancer Statistics: 1999–2009. Incidence and mortality web-based report, Atlanta: Department of Health and Human Services, Centers for Disease Control and Prevention, and National Cancer Institute; 2013. Available at http://www.cdc.gov/uscs, [accessed 29.01.12].

Ueland FR, Desimone CP, Seamon LG, Miller RA, Goodrich S, Podzielinski I, et al. Effectiveness of a multivariate index assay in the preoperative assessment of ovarian tumors. Obstet Gynecol 2011;117(6):1289–97.

Yang HP, Anderson WF, Rosenberg PS, et al. Ovarian cancer incidence trends in relation to changing patterns of menopausal hormone therapy use in the United States. J Clin Oncol 2013;31:2146–51.

Young RH, Clement PB, Scully RE. The ovary. In: Sternberg SS, Antonioli DA, Mills SE, et al., editors. Diagnostic surgical pathology. 2nd ed. New York: Raven Press; 1994.

PELVIC INFLAMMATORY DISEASE

Method of
Amy E. Curry, MD

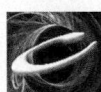

CURRENT DIAGNOSIS

- Pelvic inflammatory disease is a clinical diagnosis based on suspicious clinical findings in a woman who is at risk.
- Patients may be asymptomatic. Symptoms may range from nonspecific complaints including lower abdominal pain, vaginal discharge, dyspareunia, and irregular uterine bleeding to high fever, vomiting, and lower abdominal tenderness with rebound.
- Physical examination findings may include vaginal and endocervical discharge, as well as cervical motion, uterine and adnexal tenderness, and adnexal fullness.
- Cultures should be performed for *Chlamydia trachomatis* and *Neisseria gonorrhoeae*, the two most commonly implicated organisms, though a variety of infectious agents may be causative.

CURRENT THERAPY

Empiric treatment for pelvic inflammatory disease (PID) should be initiated in any woman at risk for sexually transmitted infections if:
- Pelvic or lower abdominal pain is present;
- Cervical motion tenderness *OR* uterine tenderness *OR* adnexal tenderness is found on pelvic examination;
- No other cause for the pain can be identified.

Inpatient therapy for PID:
- Regimen A: either cefotetan (Cefotan) 2 g IV every 12 hours *OR* cefoxitin (Mefoxin) 2 g IV every 6 hours *PLUS* doxycycline (Vibramycin) 100 mg PO/IV every 12 hours.
- Regimen B: clindamycin (Cleocin) 900 mg IV every 8 hours *PLUS* gentamicin (Garamycin) 2 mg/kg of body weight loading dose followed by 1.5 mg/kg of body weight IV/IM every 8 hours. A single daily dose of 3 to 5 mg/kg of body weight IV/IM can also be used.
- Alternate regimen: ampicillin/sulbactam (Unasyn) 3 g IV every 6 hours *PLUS* doxycycline (Vibramycin) 100 mg PO/ IV every 12 hours.

Outpatient therapy for PID:
- Ceftriaxone (Rocephin) 250 mg IM single dose *PLUS* doxycycline (Vibramycin) 100 mg PO every 12 hours for 14 days *WITH/WITHOUT* metronidazole (Flagyl) 500 mg PO every 12 hours for 14 days.
- *OR*
- Cefoxitin (Mefoxin) 2 g IM and probenecid (Benemid) 1 g PO both given concurrently as a single dose *PLUS* doxycycline (Vibramycin) 100 mg PO every 12 hours for 14 days *WITH/ WITHOUT* metronidazole (Flagyl) 500 mg PO every 12 hours for 14 days.
- *OR*
- Other parenteral third-generation cephalosporins: either ceftizoxime (Cefizox) 1 g IM single dose *OR* cefotaxime (Claforan) 1 g IM single dose *PLUS* doxycycline (Vibramycin) 100 mg PO every 12 hours for 14 days *WITH/WITHOUT* metronidazole (Flagyl) 500 mg PO every 12 hours for 14 days.
- Alternative treatment options are available for those who have penicillin or cephalosporin allergy.

Pelvic inflammatory disease (PID) is a polymicrobial infection of any or all of the upper genital tract organs in women. It is initiated by a community-acquired sexually transmitted agent and can involve the uterus, fallopian tubes, and ovaries, as well as adjacent pelvic structures.

Epidemiology
In the United States, the diagnosis of PID accounted for 110,000 initial visits to physician offices and over 35,000 admissions to the hospital in 2009 among women 15 to 44 years of age.

Risk Factors
The single greatest risk factor for PID is a history of multiple sex partners. Other risk factors include 15 to 25 years of age, a male partner with symptoms of a sexually transmitted infection (STI) such as dysuria or urethral discharge, history of previous PID, inconsistent use of condoms, African American ethnicity, and use of vaginal douching. Any phenomenon that disrupts the mucus barrier of the endocervical canal can also potentially facilitate PID, such as menses, bacterial vaginosis, or intrauterine instrumentation. Accordingly, the risk of an intrauterine device causing PID usually occurs during the first 3 weeks following insertion and rarely thereafter.

Pathophysiology
PID occurs when bacteria from the vagina ascend into the normally sterile environment of the upper genital tract. This typically

occurs in the setting of a *Neisseria gonorrhoeae* or *Chlamydia trachomatis* infection. Ascending bacteria can include anaerobes, especially those implicated in bacterial vaginosis, group A and B *Streptococcus*, *Escherichia coli*, *Klebsiella*, *Proteus mirabilis*, *Haemophilus influenzae*, *Peptococcus*, genital *Mycoplasma*, *Actinomycosis*, and cytomegalovirus. Methicillin-resistant *Staphylococcus aureus* has been reported to cause PID, but rarely. Once present, this polymicrobial infection can remain asymptomatic or cause endometritis, salpingitis, oophoritis, peritonitis, perihepatitis, or tubo-ovarian abscesses.

Clinical Presentation

PID may be asymptomatic. It may have an indolent presentation of low-grade fever, weight loss, and nonspecific abdominal pain. A more symptomatic presentation of PID includes bilateral lower quadrant abdominal pain, recent onset of dyspareunia, abnormal vaginal bleeding, and vaginal discharge. On physical examination, the patient may have fever, decreased bowel sounds, diffuse lower abdominal tenderness with rebound tenderness, and/or right upper quadrant tenderness. During the pelvic examination, purulent vaginal or endocervical discharge, vaginal mucosa redness, and cervical irritation or friability may be noted. Cervical motion pain or tenderness of the adnexa or uterus during the bimanual examination is strongly suggestive of PID.

There are several diagnostic findings that support the diagnosis of PID: the presence of abundant white blood cells or clue cells in vaginal or cervical mucus; the presence of an STI, especially gonorrhea or chlamydia; an elevated erythrocyte sedimentation rate or C-reactive protein; an elevated serum white blood cell count; evidence of endometritis on endometrial biopsy; findings of thickened, fluid-filled fallopian tubes, free fluid in the pelvis, or a tubo-ovarian abscess on transvaginal sonography or magnetic resonance imaging; or evidence of pelvic organ inflammation on laparoscopic exploration.

Diagnosis

Unfortunately, no single element of the history, finding on physical examination, laboratory test result, or diagnostic procedure has both the sensitivity and the specificity to help the clinician accurately diagnose PID. Consequently, PID remains a diagnosis based primarily on clinical suspicion in at-risk women.

Differential Diagnosis

The differential diagnosis of PID includes ectopic pregnancy, inflammatory bowel disorders, ovarian cysts and cyst rupture, ovarian torsion, appendicitis, endometriosis, proctitis, urinary tract infections, diverticulitis, constipation, or functional pain related to current or past abuse.

Treatment

The 2010 Centers for Disease Control and Prevention (CDC) treatment guidelines for STIs are outlined in the Current Diagnosis and Current Treatment boxes. These guidelines recommend empiric treatment for PID in all at-risk women who meet the criteria listed and encourage health care providers to "maintain a low threshold for the diagnosis" and treatment of PID due to "the potential for significant damage to the reproductive health of women."

Treatment guidelines are based on the patient's need for inpatient versus outpatient care. The Pelvic Inflammatory Disease Evaluation and Clinical Health (PEACH) trial demonstrated no difference in the reproductive outcomes of women with mild-to-moderate PID who were randomized to inpatient treatment versus those randomized to outpatient treatment.

Indications for inpatient treatment of PID include the following: pregnancy; failed trial or intolerance to oral medications; signs of severe PID such as high fever, nausea, vomiting, or intractable abdominal pain; complicated PID (e.g., peritonitis, perihepatitis); and pelvic abscesses. The need for surgical intervention or diagnostic exploration to rule out other abdominal pathology would also mandate inpatient treatment. In those patients requiring inpatient treatment, any one of the parenteral antibiotic regimens as outlined above may be administered, depending on the patient's history of allergies and the cost and availability of treatment options. When possible, the use of oral doxycycline (Vibramycin) is preferred over intravenous (IV) infusion due to the complications of IV infusion and the similar bioavailability of the oral form as compared to IV administration. Treatment should also include appropriate analgesia, antiemetics, antipyretics, IV fluids, and rest. Patients may be transitioned from parenteral to oral therapy after 24 hours of sustained clinical improvement including lack of fever. Further completion of a total of 14 days of treatment with oral medications is recommended. Those patients treated with either regimen A or the alternative regimen should be transitioned to oral doxycycline (Vibramycin) 100 mg every 12 hours. Those treated with regimen B should be transitioned to oral doxycycline (Vibramycin) 100 mg every 12 hours or oral clindamycin (Cleocin) 450 mg every 6 hours. If a tubo-ovarian abscess is present, the patient should be transitioned preferably to oral clindamycin (Cleocin) 450 mg every 6 hours for a total of 14 days of treatment. Alternatively, oral doxycycline (Vibramycin) 100 mg every 12 hours with oral metronidazole (Flagyl) 500 mg every 8 hours for a total of 14 days of treatment may also be used.

In patients not meeting criteria for inpatient treatment, any of the outpatient treatment regimens as outlined above may be used, the choice being again dependent on the cost and availability of treatment options. The addition of metronidazole (Flagyl) is recommended due to cephalosporin limitations in anaerobic coverage and in the case of *Trichomonas* or bacterial vaginosis infections. The addition of metronidazole (Flagyl) is also recommended if there is a history of recent uterine instrumentation.

In patients who are at a high risk for gonorrheal infection and who have a history of anaphylaxis to penicillin (urticaria, angioedema, stridor, hypotension, or desquamation), recommended treatment options include the following: hospitalization for regimen B parenteral antibiotic treatment; azithromycin (Zithromax) 2 g PO administered as a single dose along with either levofloxacin (Levaquin) 500 mg PO every 24 hours for 14 days or moxifloxacin (Avelox) 400 mg PO every 24 hours for 14 days. If these patients are at a low risk of gonorrhea, either levofloxacin (Levaquin) 500 mg PO every 24 hours or ofloxacin (Floxin) 400 mg PO every 24 hours with or without metronidazole (Flagyl) 500 mg PO every 12 hours for 14 days may be used.

In patients with a history of mild, nonanaphylactic reaction to penicillin, a 25 mg test dose IM of ceftriaxone (Rocephin) can be administered, followed by the remaining 225 mg dose if the patient has no signs of reaction after 2 hours of observation. The patient should be observed for another 1 hour after the second dose.

Regardless of the treatment regimen used, patients should be advised to abstain from intercourse until treatment is completed and they are free of symptoms. In patients with an intrauterine device (IUD), there are inconclusive data to recommend its removal, unless clinical improvement does not occur, but close clinical follow-up is warranted. There is no difference in the treatment regimens for PID in women with a history of HIV.

Patient Monitoring and Counseling

Patients treated with an outpatient regimen should be evaluated for clinical improvement within 48 to 72 hours. If no improvement is noted, the patient should be hospitalized for parenteral antibiotics and further diagnostic evaluation. All patients should be counseled on the need to complete the full course of antibiotic treatment to decrease the potential complications of PID. Patients should be informed of the cause of their infection, if known, and the need for any sexual partners to be tested and treated. Testing for HIV, syphilis, and hepatitis B and C should also be offered. If the patient is an appropriate candidate, immunization against hepatitis B (Engerix-B, Recombivax HB) and human papillomavirus (Cervarix, Gardasil) should also be offered. In order to decrease future PID episodes, patients should be advised on the need for safe sex practices and the recommendation for future routine screening for chlamydia and gonorrhea.

Complications

Complications of PID include recurrence of the infection, infertility secondary to fallopian tube scarring, chronic pelvic pain, and ectopic pregnancy. Extension of the infection can also occur, potentially causing pelvic abscesses, peritonitis, and perihepatitis (Fitz-Hugh-Curtis syndrome).

References

Buitrago MI, Crompton JA, Bertolami S, et al. Extremely low excretion of daptomycin into breast milk of a nursing mother with methicillin-resistant *Staphylococcus aureus* pelvic inflammatory disease. Pharmacotherapy 2009;29:347–51.

Centers for Disease Control and Prevention. STD surveillance 2010—STDs in women and infants—public health impact, pelvic inflammatory disease. Available at http://www.cdc.gov/std/PID/stats.htm; [accessed 06.08.12].

Centers for Disease Control and Prevention. STDs treatment guidelines, 2010. MMWR Morb Mortal Wkly Rep 2010;59/RR-12:63–7.

Crossman SH. The challenge of pelvic inflammatory disease. Am Fam Physician 2006;73:859–64.

Grimes DA. Intrauterine device and upper-genital-tract infection. Lancet 2000;356:1013.

Ness RB, Soper DE, Holley RL, et al. Effectiveness of inpatient and outpatient treatment strategies for women with pelvic inflammatory disease: results from the pelvic inflammatory disease evaluation and clinical health (PEACH) randomized trial. Am J Obstet Gynecol 2002;186:929–37.

Ross J, Judlin P, Nilas L. European guideline for the management of pelvic inflammatory disease. Int J STD AIDS 2007;18:662–6.

PREMENSTRUAL SYNDROME

Method of
Ellen W. Freeman, PhD

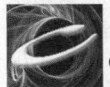

CURRENT DIAGNOSIS

- Confirm that symptoms occur premenstrually and abate following menses.
- Confirm that symptoms are clinically significant and impair daily activities and/or cause problems for the woman.
- Obtain a medical history and conduct a physical examination to determine that other disorders are not causing the symptoms.
- Assess depression, stress, substance abuse, and other diagnoses that could cause the symptoms.
- Ask the woman to maintain a daily symptom report for two or more menstrual cycles to confirm the reported symptoms and their relation to the menstrual cycle.
- Perform laboratory tests only as needed to confirm general good health or rule out other suspected conditions.

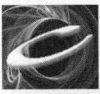

CURRENT THERAPY

SSRI	Range Studied (mg)	Mean Dose (mg/d)
Citalopram (Celexa[1])	10–30	20
Escitalopram (Lexapro[1])	10–20	15
Fluoxetine (Prozac,[1] Sarafem*)	10–60	20
Paroxetine (Paxil[1])	10–30	20
Paroxetine-CR* (Paxil-CR)	12.5, 25	NA[†]
Sertraline (Zoloft*)	50–150	75
SNRI		
Venlafaxine (Effexor[1])	37.5–200	112.5

[1]Not FDA approved for this indication.
*FDA approved for the indication of premenstrual dysphoric disorder (PMDD).
[†]Not applicable because of fixed-dose study.

The premenstrual syndromes (PMS) are characterized by mood, behavioral, and physical symptoms that occur from several days to 2 weeks before menses and remit with the menstrual flow. The term *PMS* as used by clinicians and the general public is generic, imprecise, and commonly applied to numerous symptoms. Included symptoms range from the mild and normal physiologic changes of the menstrual cycle to clinically significant symptoms that limit or impair normal functioning. In recent years, randomized controlled trials and other well-designed studies have defined diagnostic criteria for PMS and identified effective treatments for this disorder.

Based on scientific evidence at this time, serotonergic antidepressants are considered the primary treatment for clinically significant PMS, and particularly its severe form termed *premenstrual dysphoric disorder* (PMDD). This review focuses on PMS and its treatment with serotonergic antidepressants. It is not a comprehensive review of all treatments or associated literature. Other recent reviews may guide the reader to further information and other treatments for PMS and PMDD.

Symptoms

Numerous symptoms were traditionally attributed to PMS. This plethora is related in part to the absence of a clear diagnosis that distinguishes PMS from other co-morbid conditions. Many disorders, both physical and psychiatric, are exacerbated premenstrually or occur as a co-morbid disorder with PMS. When a careful diagnosis is made to distinguish PMS from other conditions, a much smaller group of symptoms appear to be typical of the disorder (Box 1).

Mood symptoms are usually the main complaint (irritability, anxiety, tension, mood swings, feeling out of control, depression), but behavioral symptoms (e.g., decreased interest, fatigue, poor concentration, poor sleep) and physical symptoms, most commonly breast tenderness and abdominal swelling, are also present. Several recent studies suggest that irritability is the cardinal symptom of PMS. Although depressive symptoms such as low mood, fatigue, sleep difficulties, and poor concentration are frequent complaints of women with PMS, the growing evidence indicates that PMS is not a simple variant of depression but has distinct mechanisms that differ from those of depressive disorders.

Prevalence

Surveys indicate that PMS is among the most common health problems reported by reproductive-age women. Current estimates from epidemiologic data indicate that approximately 25% of women experience severe and clinically significant premenstrual symptoms, although only 6% to 8% of menstruating women meet the stringent and predominantly dysphoric criteria for PMDD.

Box 1	Symptoms of Premenstrual Syndrome

Affective
- Irritability
- Anxiety
- Angry outbursts
- Confusion
- Social withdrawal
- Depression

Somatic
- Bloating
- Swelling
- Breast tenderness
- Headache

From American College of Obstetricians and Gynecologists (ACOG) Practice Bulletin 15, 2001.

Morbidity

The morbidity of PMS is related to its severity, chronicity, and resulting distress that affect work, personal relationships, or daily activities. The level of impairment is significantly above community norms and similar to that of other health problems such as major depressive disorder. Studies consistently demonstrate that the greatest impairment or distress resulting from PMS is in relationships with the partner or children and in the effectiveness of work.

Etiology

The etiology of PMS remains undefined, although the monthly cycling of the reproductive hormones appears to have an essential role in the disorder. While circulating levels of the hormones are in normal range, the dominant theory is that some women have an underlying vulnerability to the normal fluctuations of one or more of these hormones. It is further believed that PMS involves central nervous system–mediated interactions of the reproductive steroids with neurotransmitters. The principal research evidence at this time supports the involvement of reproductive hormones, serotonergic dysregulation, and possibly dysregulation of GABAergic receptor functioning.

Diagnosis

A diagnosis of PMS is determined primarily by the *timing* and the *severity* of the symptoms. These factors, together with an assessment of whether other physical or psychiatric disorders may account for the symptoms, are more important for the diagnosis than the particular symptoms, which are typically nonspecific and must be assessed for their relationship to the menstrual cycle.

Box 2 lists the diagnostic criteria for PMS presented by the American College of Obstetricians and Gynecologists in 2000. These criteria indicate that PMS symptoms must be experienced during the 5 days before menses and abate during the menstrual flow. The symptoms should cause identifiable impairment or distress, be confirmed by prospective reports recorded daily by the woman for at least two menstrual cycles, and not be accounted for by other disorders.

The diagnostic criteria for PMDD are listed in the *Diagnostic and Statistical Manual of Mental Disorders, Fifth Edition (DSM-IV)*. Importantly, the Food and Drug Administration (FDA) has approved medications only for the indication of PMDD and not for the indication of PMS at the present time. The PMDD criteria are intended to diagnose a severe, dysphoric form of PMS and require 5 of 11 listed symptoms including at least one of the mood symptoms. Physical symptoms, regardless of the number, are considered a single symptom in meeting the diagnostic criteria. The 11 PMDD symptoms are depressed mood, anxiety or tension, mood swings, anger or irritability, decreased interest, concentration difficulties, fatigue, appetite change or food cravings, sleep disturbance, feeling overwhelmed, and physical symptoms. At least five of these symptoms must each be severe premenstrually and abate with the menstrual flow. The symptoms must markedly interfere with functioning, be confirmed by daily symptom reports for at least two menstrual

cycles, and not be an exacerbation of another physical or mental disorder.

To diagnose PMS, a medical history should be obtained and a complete physical with gynecologic examination performed. PMS is understood to occur in ovulatory menstrual cycles; cycles that are irregular or outside the normal range are an indication for further gynecologic investigation. Co-morbid conditions such as dysmenorrhea, endometriosis, uterine fibroids, pelvic inflammatory disease, thyroid disorders, migraine, diabetes, mood disorders, substance abuse, and numerous other possibilities should be identified. It may be difficult to determine whether the symptoms under investigation are an exacerbation of a co-morbid condition or superimposed on another condition. In either case, the usual recommendation is to treat the ongoing condition first, then reassess and possibly add treatment for the symptoms that arise premenstrually.

No laboratory test identifies PMS and none should be routinely performed for diagnosis. Laboratory tests that indicate or confirm other possible disorders are useful if suggested by the individual woman's symptom presentation or medical findings.

The key diagnostic tool for evaluating premenstrual symptoms is the daily symptom report. The diagnostic criteria for both PMS and PMDD include a daily symptom report that is kept by the woman for at least two menstrual cycles to confirm that the woman's reported symptoms are linked to the menstrual cycle in the requisite pattern. Numerous symptom reports appropriate for this diagnosis are identified in the medical literature on PMS and PMDD. It is important that the ratings indicate the severity of each symptom (and not simply check the presence or absence of symptoms).

It is informative to use two visits for the diagnostic evaluation. Although counterintuitive, seeing the patient following menses when PMS symptoms have abated is instructive. If symptoms are absent, it provides strong evidence for the diagnosis. If symptoms are present in the follicular phase, the type and severity of the symptoms are important diagnostic information for identifying other physical or mental disorders that may be the primary focus of treatment.

Treatment

Selective Serotonin Reuptake Inhibitors

Serotonergic antidepressants are the primary treatment for severe PMS and PMDD at this time. Modulating serotonergic function is consistent with a leading theoretical view that the normal gonadal steroid fluctuations of the menstrual cycle are associated with an abnormal serotonergic response in vulnerable women. A meta-analysis of randomized controlled trials of selective serotonin reuptake inhibitors (SSRIs) in treatment of PMS and PMDD determined that these drugs were an effective first-line therapy, with both a statistically significant and clinically meaningful difference from placebo. The FDA has approved fluoxetine (Sarafem), sertraline (Zoloft), and paroxetine (Paxil) for the indication of PMDD. Other randomized, placebo-controlled, double-blind trials showed efficacy for citalopram (Celexa[1]), escitalopram (Lexapro[1]), venlafaxine (Effexor[1]) (a selective serotonin-norepinephrine reuptake inhibitor [SNRI]), and clomipramine (Anafranil[1]) (a tricyclic antidepressant) for treatment of PMS and PMDD.

Effective doses of SSRIs are consistently at the low end of the dose range for depressive disorders in all reports of PMS and PMDD treatments. Significant response is often seen in the first menstrual cycle of treatment, with smaller increments with or without dose adjustments in the second and third treatment cycles. If there is not sufficient response in the first treated menstrual cycle, the dose should be increased in the next cycle unless precluded by side effects.

Side effects are common with the initiation of an SSRI but are usually transient and abate within 1 to 2 weeks of continued

---

| **Box 2** | Diagnosis of Premenstrual Syndrome |

Presenting symptoms:
- Consistent with premenstrual syndrome
- Restricted to the luteal phase
- Cause impairment or distress
- Not an exacerbation of another disorder
- Confirmed by 2 cycles of daily symptom rating

From American College of Obstetricians and Gynecologists (ACOG) Practice Bulletin 15, 2001.

---

[1]Not FDA approved for this indication.

treatment. The most common side effects include headache, nausea, insomnia, fatigue or lethargy, diarrhea, decreased concentration, dizziness, and decreased libido or delayed orgasm. The sexual side effects of SSRIs have received considerable attention, although it is often difficult to determine the extent to which sexual effects are related to the medication or to preexisting conditions. The incidence of decreased sexual interest or delayed orgasm in the few published reports of PMS patients is approximately 9% to 16%, which is notably lower than the rates reported with the use of SSRIs by depressed patients. Another important issue is the lack of any well-controlled clinical trials of SSRI treatment for PMS and PMDD in adolescents. Whether SSRIs are safe and effective for this indication in women younger than 18 years is not demonstrated.

Luteal Phase Dosing

The use of medication only in the symptomatic luteal phase of the menstrual cycle is particularly important in PMS because of the cyclic pattern of the symptoms, which occur only in the premenstrual phase and abate following menses. Efficacy of luteal phase administration of the SSRIs is demonstrated in multiple trials: three large multicenter, randomized, placebo-controlled trials that examined fluoxetine (Sarafem), paroxetine (Paxil), and sertraline (Zoloft); a trial that directly compared continuous and luteal phase administration of sertraline; and multiple preliminary studies.

Luteal phase administration of an SSRI is typically initiated 14 days prior to the expected onset of menstrual bleeding and concluded within several days of bleeding, using a taper for increased doses. As with continuous dosing, the SSRI doses are usually at the low end of the dose range.

One preliminary study compared symptom-onset dosing (mean of 6 days before menses) to luteal phase dosing and found no difference between the two dosing regimens in improvement overall, although there was suggestion that women with more severe symptoms may respond better to full luteal phase dosing.

Side effects may be less frequent with an intermittent dosing regimen because they may not occur when not taking the medication. However, some women experience recurring side effects when dosing is resumed, and discontinuation symptoms might also occur with the stop-start dosing pattern. At this time, no systematic data confirm discontinuation symptoms with the intermittent dosing regimen.

Insufficient Response to Selective Serotonin Reuptake Inhibitors

Approximately 60% of PMS and PMDD patients in controlled studies respond well to an SSRI. There are no clear predictors of response. An adequate trial of an SSRI for PMS and PMDD is at least two menstrual cycles at a dose level of demonstrated efficacy, with a third cycle when there is partial response. If a woman has an insufficient response or unacceptable side effects, it is reasonable to try another SSRI. Although the SSRIs are similar in their structure and have similar response rates and side-effect profiles, an individual patient may respond better to one SSRI versus another.

Other approaches to a poor treatment response include augmenting the SSRI with another medication to address the nonresponding symptoms, but there is no systematic information on this in PMS or PMDD treatment. Switching to another class of medication, such as anxiolytics, is suggested, but no data indicate whether nonresponders to SSRIs will respond to another class of medication. Nonresponse may also be related to other co-morbid disorders. A thorough review of the diagnosis and adjustments of the premenstrual doses of medication for both the primary disorder and PMS should be considered before pursuing other treatments.

Other Treatments

Hormonal

In spite of the evidence for hormonal involvement in PMS and PMDD, traditional oral contraceptives (OCs) do not show efficacy for the disorder. However, recent data indicate that shortening or omitting the placebo week in the traditional OC pill pack may effectively treat PMS and PMDD. The FDA has approved the oral contraceptive YAZ, a 24/4-day combination pill, to treat PMDD. The continuous daily use of an OC (without a hormone-free interval) suppresses ovulation-related hormone cyclicity. Continuous daily levonorgestrel 90 mcg/ethinyl estradiol 20 mcg (Amethyst)[1] has been evaluated for continuous use up to one year and may be useful for managing the symptoms of PMDD.

Gonadotropin-releasing hormone (GnRH) agonists such as depot leuprolide[1] (Lupron) and buserelin[2] (Suprefact) are effective for PMS and PMDD but are of limited usefulness because of the risks associated with low estrogen levels that result from these treatments. Although add-back therapy using low-lose estrogen and progesterone together with the GnRH agonist did not appear to reduce efficacy in a meta-analysis, there are no definitive data on the safety and efficacy of this approach in long-term treatment. The historic use of progesterone has failed to show efficacy for the mood and behavioral symptoms of PMS in numerous controlled trials.

Anxiolytics

Alprazolam[1] (Xanax) and buspirone[1] (Buspar) showed modest efficacy for PMS in some studies but not others. Although these medications offer an alternative to antidepressants, the response rates appear much lower, and it is not known whether a PMS patient who does not respond to antidepressants will respond to an anxiolytic. The risk of dependency with alprazolam should be considered. Dosing should be strictly limited to the luteal phase, and the patient should have no history of substance abuse.

Nonpharmacologic

Calcium supplementation[1] (600 mg twice daily) reduced PMS symptoms significantly more than placebo. Calcium offers a dietary supplement approach that may be beneficial for some women with PMS, although there are no predictors of which women will respond well to this therapy. Other complementary and alternative therapies may be helpful for some women, but there is no convincing evidence of their efficacy for PMS.

Behavioral treatments that facilitate coping or reduce stress may reduce PMS symptoms. Cognitive-behavioral therapy is effective for PMS, and in one study it was as effective as the SSRI fluoxetine after 6 months of treatment.

Treatment Duration

All published studies of treatment efficacy for PMS and PMDD are based on acute treatment of 2 to 3 months' duration. Several small pilot investigations suggest that PMS symptoms are likely to return within several months after medication is stopped. It also appears that PMS symptoms do not resolve spontaneously but continue for many years. These observations of PMS as a chronic condition and the swift return of symptoms following the cessation of medication suggest that treatment can be expected to be long term. In a controlled study that compared 4 months to 1 year of SSRI treatment, approximately half of the patients who improved with SSRI treatment relapsed within 6 to 8 months after discontinuing medication. Longer treatment was marginally better at preventing relapse. Patients with more severe symptoms before treatment were the most likely to relapse, while patients who experienced symptom remission with treatment were least likely to relapse.

The SSRIs are currently the first-line treatment for severe PMS and PMDD. Continuous dosing and luteal phase dosing regimens are similarly effective for these disorders when the symptoms are clearly limited to the luteal phase of the menstrual cycle. Hormonal treatments have lacked consistent scientific evidence of their efficacy or safety or both for PMS treatment. Several new oral contraceptives that decrease or omit the placebo interval may provide an effective alternative to antidepressant medications. Evidence indicates that long-term maintenance of the medication may be required for PMS and PMDD.

---

[1]Not FDA approved for this indication.
[2]Not available in the United States.

References

ACOG Practice Bulletin. Premenstrual syndrome. Int J Gynecol Obstet 2001;73 (2):183–90.

Brown J, O'Brien PM, Marjoribanks J, Wyatt K. Selective serotonin reuptake inhibitors for premenstrual syndrome. Cochrane Database Syst Rev 2009;2: CD001396.

Dell DL. Premenstrual syndrome, premenstrual dysphoric disorder, and premenstrual exacerbation of another disorder. Clin Obstet Gynecol 2004;47(3):568–75.

Freeman EW. Luteal phase administration of agents for the treatment of premenstrual dysphoric disorder. CNS Drugs 2004;18(7):453–68.

Freeman EW, Rickels K, Sammel MD, et al. Time to relapse after short-term or long-term treatment of severe premenstrual syndrome with sertraline. Arch Gen Psychiatry 2009;66(5):537–44.

Girman A, Lee R, Kligler B. An integrative medicine approach to premenstrual syndrome. Am J Obstet Gynecol 2003;188(5 Suppl.):S56–S65.

Grady-Weliky TA. Premenstrual dysphoric disorder. N Engl J Med 2003;348 (5):433–8.

Halbreich U. The etiology, biology, and evolving pathology of premenstrual syndromes. Psychoneuroendocrinology 2003;28(Suppl. 3):55–99.

Johnson SR. Premenstrual syndrome, premenstrual dysphoric disorder, and beyond: A clinical primer for practitioners. Obstet Gynecol 2004;104(4):845–59.

Whelan AM, Jurgens TM, Naylor H. Herbs, vitamins and minerals in the treatment of premenstrual syndrome: A systematic review. Can J Clin Pharmacol 2009;16: c407–c429.

UTERINE LEIOMYOMAS

Method of
Patricia Evans, MD; and Susan C. Brunsell, MD*

CURRENT DIAGNOSIS

- Most leiomyomas are asymptomatic.
- Most common clinical manifestations include menorrhagia, pelvic pain, obstructive symptoms, and infertility.
- Physical examination findings are enlarged and/or irregular shaped uterus.
- Transvaginal sonography is the initial imaging modality.
- Magnetic resonance imaging (MRI) is used for precise mapping of the leiomyoma.
- Sonohysterography and hysteroscopy can diagnose submucosal leiomyomas.

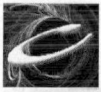

CURRENT THERAPY

- Expectant management is the treatment of choice for asymptomatic leiomyomas.
- Myomectomy is used to treat symptoms and preserve fertility.
- Hysterectomy provides a definitive treatment for symptoms.
- Uterine artery embolization and myolysis are nonsurgical treatment options.
- Hormone treatments are treatment options in a limited number of clinical scenarios.

Epidemiology

Uterine leiomyomas (also referred to as leiomyomas or myomas) are benign smooth-muscle tumors. They are classified according to their position in the uterus: subserous (just beneath the serosa), interstitial (within the myometrium), and submucous (just below the endometrium). Subserosal leiomyomas can grow in a pedunculated fashion from the uterus as they enlarge. Leiomyomas arise during the reproductive years, can enlarge during pregnancy, and regress following menopause. The incidence of leiomyomas identified via ultrasound is about 5% in young adults, 15% in middle-aged women, and 30%

*The views expressed in this publication are those of the author and do not reflect the official policy of the Department of Defense or of the U.S. government.

in women older than 40 years. In postmortem examinations the incidence has been found to be even higher.

Risk Factors

Factors associated with increased risk of leiomyomas include early age of menarche, alcohol intake, nulliparity, obesity, family history, age, hypertension, and African descent. Factors associated with decreased risk for leiomyomas include depot medroxyprogesterone (Depo Provera) use, increased parity, and menopause.

Pathophysiology

Leiomyomas arise from a unicellular origin in the smooth muscle of the myometrium. Leiomyomas have a relatively poor vascular supply of one or two arteries at the base of the leiomyoma, which can result in a tumor outgrowing its blood supply. Their growth rate is influenced by estrogen, growth hormone, and progesterone. Estrogen exposure is associated with an increased incidence of leiomyomas. Growth hormones act synergistically with estradiol in affecting the growth of leiomyomas. Conversely, progesterone appears to inhibit their growth. Leiomyomas produce a dysregulation of growth factors and their receptors, causing vascular abnormalities that can contribute to the symptom of menorrhagia.

Clinical Manifestations

Leiomyomas are most commonly asymptomatic. They can also be found in association with menorrhagia, dysmenorrhea, pelvic pain and pressure, obstructive symptoms, infertility, and pregnancy loss. Many women with symptomatic myomas present with more than one symptom.

Menstrual abnormalities are the most common symptoms associated with the presence of myomas. Menorrhagia is the most common bleeding pattern and can result in an iron deficiency anemia. Pelvic pain and pressure can be the result of a large leiomyoma alone or from vascular compromise. Chronically, women can experience the sensation of pressure from an enlarged uterus. Acute pain from vascular compromise can occur when pedunculated myomas torse, when hemorrhage occurs within a myoma (usually in association with pregnancy), or when a myoma outgrows its blood supply.

Obstructive symptoms affect the urinary system (urinary frequency or urgency) more commonly, but they can also cause rectal symptoms like constipation. These manifestations are more common during pregnancy in the setting of large leiomyomas and uterine enlargement.

The role of leiomyomas in infertility is controversial. Current evidence suggests that submucosal and intramural leiomyomas that distort the uterine cavity can impair in vitro fertilization (IVF) outcomes. Submucosal leiomyomas, intramural leiomyomas distorting the uterine cavity, leiomyomas larger than 5 cm, and multiple leiomyomas are commonly treated in a patient with otherwise unexplained infertility.

There is uncertainty regarding the possible role leiomyomas play in early miscarriage.

Diagnosis

The bimanual examination finding of an enlarged and irregularly shaped uterus is often the first indication that a patient has leiomyomas. A number of studies can be helpful in evaluating a patient for the presence of leiomyomas, including transvaginal sonography, sonohysterography, hysteroscopy, and magnetic resonance imaging (MRI). Transvaginal sonography has the lowest sensitivity and specificity, but it is the best initial test based on its noninvasiveness and cost-efficiency. MRI is preferred when precise leiomyoma mapping is required (usually for surgical purposes), but it is the most expensive modality for evaluating leiomyomas. Sonohysterography and hysteroscopy can be used to evaluate the extent of submucosal leiomyomas, but these methods are invasive.

Differential Diagnosis

Patients consult physicians because of symptoms related to leiomyomas or when the lesions are diagnosed incidentally during physical or radiologic examinations. Attributing symptoms to uterine leiomyoma with certainty is complicated owing to their high prevalence and because the differential diagnosis for symptoms related to leiomyomas is wide. For example, possible causes of menorrhagia include pregnancy, infection, carcinoma, and endocrine, hematologic, physiologic, systemic, structural, and iatrogenic causes. Pelvic pain causes include endometriosis, adenomyosis, pelvic adhesions, pelvic inflammatory disease (PID), cystitis, ovarian diseases, and bowel disease.

One of the biggest challenges is identifying malignant leiomyosarcomas, because rapid growth alone is not an adequate marker. There is evidence that combining dynamic MRI (MRI enhanced by gadopentetate dimeglumine [Magnevist]) and serum lactate dehydrogenase levels is useful in distinguishing leiomyosarcoma from leiomyoma. This approach may be useful in evaluating selected patients such as the postmenopausal patient with an enlarging leiomyoma.

Treatment

Expectant Management

Expectant management is the treatment of choice for women with asymptomatic leiomyomas regardless of size. Early intervention may be an option for asymptomatic young women desiring future fertility because leiomyoma tumors can become larger with the passage of time, thereby complicating treatment in the future.

Medical Treatments

Hormone therapy with cyclic or noncyclic estrogen–progestin combinations is ineffective in alleviating the symptoms of leiomyoma tumors or limiting tumor growth. There is no evidence that low-dose contraceptives cause the growth of uterine leiomyoma tumors; thus, leiomyomas are not a contraindication to their use. The use of the levonorgestrel-releasing IUD[1] (Mirena) can reduce heavy menstrual bleeding in symptomatic women with uterine leiomyomas. However, the presence of leiomyomas increases the risk of expulsion of the IUD.

Treatment with mifepristone (Mifeprex),[1] a synthetic steroid with potent antiprogesterone activity, has been shown to reduce the volume of leiomyomas by about 50% and improve bleeding symptoms. Currently mifepristone is only available via restricted access to registered prescribers in the United States.

[1]Not FDA approved for this indication.

The aromatase inhibitor letrozole (Femara) has been shown to decrease leiomyoma size and reduce bleeding without causing vasomotor symptoms or changing bone density. Larger clinical trials are needed to fully evaluate safety and efficacy of letrozole for this indication.

Gonadotropin-releasing hormone (GnRH) agonists (leuprolide [Lupron]) are the most well-established therapy for medical management, causing amenorrhea and a rapid reduction in the size of the tumor. This therapy is best suited for women in the perimenopausal or preoperative periods owing to significant side effects resulting from hypoestrogenism (e.g., hot flushes, vaginal dryness, bone demineralization).

Surgical Treatments

Selected patients can benefit from surgery: those with persistent abnormal uterine bleeding or symptoms resulting from uterine bulk that do not respond to conservative measures or when the diagnosis of leiomyosarcoma is being considered (e.g., a menopausal woman with an enlarging tumor) (Table 1). Abdominal or vaginal hysterectomy is the definitive treatment for *symptomatic uterine leiomyomas*. There is no chance for recurrence and there is less blood than with other procedures such as myomectomy.

Myomectomy (i.e., surgical removal of leiomyoma tumors while preserving the uterus) is performed via laparotomy, endoscopy, or hysteroscopy. The choice of surgical approach largely depends on the expertise of the physician. When myomectomies are performed to preserve fertility, care must be taken to avoid adhesions, which can compromise the goal of the operation. Currently, many clinicians recommend cesarean section for all pregnancies following myomectomy despite limited data to support this recommendation.

Uterine artery embolization uses interventional radiology to occlude the uterine arteries with polyvinyl alcohol microspheres positioned by a catheter passed through the femoral artery. Postprocedure pain is significant, generally requiring admission at least overnight for narcotic analgesia. Postprocedure complications include postembolization syndrome (pain accompanied by fever, nausea, and vomiting); injury to the ovary, ureter, or other structures (misembolization); and infection. Short-term outcomes demonstrate that uterine artery embolization has lower morbidity than hysterectomy, but readmission rates are high: 5% to 10%. Long-term outcomes have been encouraging: 73% of women had continued symptom control at 5 years in one study. The issue

TABLE 1 Treatment Options

TREATMENT	DESCRIPTION	ADVANTAGES AND USES	DISADVANTAGES AND RISKS	FERTILITY PRESERVED?
Hysterectomy	Surgical removal of the uterus (transabdominal, transvaginal, or laparoscopic)	Definitive treatment for women who do not wish to preserve fertility	Surgery and anesthesia risks	No
Myomectomy	Excision of leiomyomas via laparotomy or endoscopy	Resolution of symptoms with preservation of fertility; perioperative morbidity similar to hysterectomy	Recurrence of leiomyomas (up to 50% at 5 y) Success of procedure determined by number and extent of leiomyomas	Yes
Uterine artery embolization	Interventional radiology procedure to occlude uterine arteries	Minimally invasive Avoids surgery Short hospital stay (24–36 h)	Symptom recurrence (20% at 5 y) Risk of rehospitalization for postprocedure pain Bleeding	No (limited experience)
Myolysis	In situ destruction of leiomyomas by ultrasound, laser, or cryotherapy	Ease and rapidity of procedure Low blood loss Rapid recovery time	Delay in reduction of uterine size Unknown risk for recurrence Prolonged vaginal bleeding	No (unknown)
Gonadotropin-releasing hormone agonists (Leuprolide [Lupron])	Preoperative treatment to decrease size of leiomyomas before hysterectomy, myomectomy, or myolysis, or at perimenopause	Decreases blood loss, operative time, recovery time	Long-term treatment associated with high cost, menopausal symptoms, and bone loss Possible increased recurrence risk with myomectomy	Depends on subsequent procedure

of fertility following uterine artery embolization is still under investigation.

Myolysis involves techniques designed to destroy rather than remove leiomyoma tumors. Techniques under development include hypothermic ablation (liquid nitrogen) and hyperthermic ablation (laser, radiofrequency electricity, or focused ultrasound). Available data are promising, with a decrease in myoma volume of about 50%. Ablation using focused ultrasound energy, guided either by MRI or ultrasound, is the only technique that delivers energy to the tissue without direct contact with the treated tissue. This approach offers the potential for incisionless surgery. The FDA has approved the ExAblate 2000 device, which uses MRI to focus the ultrasound beam, for treatment of symptomatic uterine leiomyomas.

References

Bajekal N, Li TC. Leiomyomas, infertility and pregnancy wastage. Hum Reprod Update 2000;6:614–20.

Gorny KR, Woodrum DA, Brown DL, et al. Magentic resonance–guided focused ultrasound of uterine leiomyomas: A review of a 12-month outcome of 130 clinical patients. J Vasc Interv Radiol 2011;22:857–64.

Griffin KW, Ellis MR, Wilder L. What is the appropriate diagnostic evaluation of leiomyomas? J Fam Pract 2005;54:458–62.

Gupta S, Jose J, Manyonda I. Clinical presentation of leiomyomas. Best Pract Res Clin Obstet Gynaecol 2008;22:615–26.

Laughlin SK, Schroeder JC, Baird DD. New directions in the epidemiology of uterine leiomyomas. Semin Reprod Med 2010;28:204–17.

Lurie S, Piper I, Woliovitch I, Glezerman M. Age-related prevalence of sonographically confirmed uterine myomas. J Obstet Gynecol 2005;25:42–3.

Munro MG. Uterine leiomyomas, current concepts: Pathogenesis, impact on reproductive health, and medical, procedural, and surgical management. Obstet Gynecol Clin North Am 2011;38:703–31.

Schwartz PE, Kelly MG. Malignant transformation of myomas: Myth or reality? Obstet Gynecol Clin North Am 2006;33:183–98.

Van der Kooji SM. Uterine artery embolization versus surgery in the treatment of symptomatic leiomyomas: A systematic review and metaanalysis. Am J Obstet Gynecol 2011;205:317, e1–18.

Viswanathan M, Hartmann K, McKoy N, et al. Management of Uterine Leiomyomas: An Update of the Evidence. Evidence Report/Technology Assessment No. 154 (Prepared by RTI International–University of North Carolina Evidence-based Practice Center under Contract No. 290-02-0016). AHRQ Publication No. 07-E011, Rockville, MD: Agency for Healthcare Research and Quality; 2007.

VULVAR NEOPLASIA

Method of
Susan A. Davidson, MD

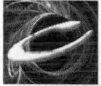

CURRENT DIAGNOSIS

- Most cystic lesions are benign. Excision is reserved for symptomatic cysts and suspicious Bartholin's gland cysts, especially in women older than 40 years of age.
- All solid lesions should be biopsied for diagnostic purposes.
- Multifocal disease requires multiple biopsies to rule out invasive disease.
- Most premalignant and malignant lesions cause pruritus, discomfort, or a noticeable lesion.
- The vagina and cervix in women with dysplastic or malignant vulvar lesions should be evaluated.

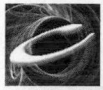

CURRENT THERAPY

- Benign solid lesions should be excised.
- After ablative treatment of vulvar intraepithelial neoplasia (VIN), excise any residual lesions to rule out occult invasive disease.
- Avoid podophyllin and 5-fluorouracil in women of reproductive potential.
- Rule out synchronous neoplasms in women with Paget's disease.
- Invasion more than 1 mm requires radical excision and lymph node evaluation.

The female external genitalia includes the mons pubis, labia majora, labia minora, clitoris, perineal body, and the structures of the vaginal introitus or vestibule. Whether benign or malignant, vulvar neoplasms are uncommon, occur at all ages, and have varying characteristics. Therefore liberal use of biopsies is usually required for diagnosis and to guide treatment.

Benign Cystic Neoplasms

Benign cystic lesions of the vulva include Bartholin's duct cyst, sebaceous and epidermal inclusion cysts, mucinous cysts, Skene duct cysts, and cysts of the canal of Nuck. Bartholin's duct cyst, located in the posterior labia near the vaginal introitus, is most common. Treatment is usually not required in asymptomatic young women (<40 years). If the cyst is symptomatic or infected, however, drainage by marsupialization or use of a Word catheter, is indicated. Bartholin's gland carcinomas are rare, especially in women younger than 40 years of age. But if the mass feels firm or nodular, it should be biopsied.

Sebaceous and epidermal inclusion cysts are also common. They are prone to infection but rarely malignant. If an infection develops, they should be incised and drained. Mucinous cysts are rare and possibly arise from the minor vestibular glands. They are located anteriorly on the vulva, typically on the inner labia minora. Skene duct cysts are located next to the urethra. Excision of these cysts is necessary only if symptomatic.

Cysts of the canal of Nuck are located in the anterior portion of the labia majora at the termination of the insertion of the round ligament. These cysts represent herniation of the peritoneum through the inguinal canal and contain peritoneal fluid. If symptomatic, excision must be accompanied by closure of the fascial defect to prevent recurrence.

Benign Solid Neoplasms

The benign solid tumors of the vulva include fibromas, myomas, lipomas, hidradenomas, syringomas, myoblastomas, vestibular adenomas, and angiomas, among others. Benign pigmented lesions, such as nevi and seborrheic keratoses, may occasionally be found. Malignancy is rare, but most should be excised for diagnostic and therapeutic purposes.

Condyloma Acuminatum

Vulvar condyloma acuminatum is a sexually transmitted verrucous lesion of the vulva caused by human papilloma virus (HPV), most frequently types 6 and 11. These lesions are warty growths that frequently cover large areas of the vulva. Smoking and immunosuppression are risk factors. Representative biopsies should be obtained to document disease and rule out malignancy. Wide local excision can be used for small lesions, although these growths are usually best treated by ablation.

Chemical ablative techniques include topical application of trichloroacetic acid (Tri-Chlor), podofilox (0.5%, Condylox), 5-fluorouracil[1] (1%, Fluoroplex or 5%, Efudex),[1] or imiquimod (5%, Aldara). Podophyllin can be applied twice daily for 3 days, repeated weekly for 4 weeks. Imiquimod can be applied three times per week for up to 16 weeks. Podophyllin and 5-fluorouracil should not be used in women who could become pregnant. Surgical ablative therapies include CO_2 laser vaporization and use of the Cavitron ultrasonic aspirator (CUSA), especially for extensive disease.

Intraepithelial Neoplasms of the Vulva
Vulvar Intraepithelial Neoplasia

Vulvar intraepithelial neoplasia (VIN) is a dysplastic condition of the squamous epithelium whose incidence is increasing, especially in younger women. There are two pathologically distinct types of VIN, usual and differentiated types. The usual type has a strong association with HPV infections and thus shares similar risk factors with cervical intraepithelial neoplasias (CIN). These risk factors include early first intercourse, multiple sexual partners, smoking, and immunosuppression. Up to 22% of women have concurrent CIN lesions and up to 71% have had a previous,

---

[1]Not FDA approved for this indication.

TABLE 1	Recurrence of Vulvar Intraepithelial Neoplasia III
TREATMENT METHOD	**% RECURRENCE**
Chemical ablation	20–40
Mechanical ablation	20–40

Wide local excision
    Negative margin
    Positive margin
	
	15–25
	30–45

concominant or subsequent history of vaginal intraepithelial neoplasia. Differentiated VIN is not associated with HPV and is found in relation to vulvar dermatoses such as lichen sclerosus. Differentiated VIN typically occurs in older women with a mean age of 67 years compared to 47.8 years in usual type VIN. Symptoms of both types include pruritus (most common), pain, a noticeable lesion, and discoloration. Most patients with HPV-related disease have multifocal lesions. Typical findings are raised white, gray, red, or mottled lesions; application of 4% acetic acid for several minutes can help identify faint lesions and outline abnormal vascular patterns. Diagnosis of VIN is made by punch biopsies through full thickness of the epithelium to rule out invasion. Usual and differentiated VIN have very different cancer progression risks, 5.7% for HPV-mediated VIN and 32.8% for differentiated VIN. Differentiated VIN, also, has a shorter time to progression, 22.8 months compared to 41.4 months.

Treatment of VIN can be categorized into excisional and ablative therapies. Management should be individualized to each patient taking into account risk of progression, distribution of disease and histologic features on biopsy. Often a combination of medical and surgical management is appropriate. Patients at risk for microinvasion (unifocal disease, raised lesions, older age, and prior radiation) should have the lesion excised completely if possible. Skinning vulvectomy is rarely used because of psychological and sexual consequences related to scarring and disfigurement.

The ablative therapies can be divided into mechanical and chemical. The mechanical method most commonly used is the CO_2 laser, although use of the CUSA is also described. Both can ablate large or multifocal lesions successfully with an excellent cosmetic and functional outcome. The chemical method most commonly used is topical 5-fluorouracil (5%, Efudex).[1] Because of its teratogenic potential, it should not be used in women who could become pregnant. It can be applied on two consecutive nights weekly for 10 weeks. An alternative ablative therapy is use of imiquimod[1] (Aldara), as described earlier. Because of the irritation caused by these topical therapies, many patients have problems with treatment compliance. Residual disease should be excised to rule out invasion.

Patients with VIN frequently have recurrent disease, regardless of the treatment method used (Table 1). Continued smoking increases this risk, so patients should be counseled in smoking cessation. In those patients whose cancers recur and are retreated, subsequent 5-fluorouracil prophylaxis, with a single application biweekly, is used successfully to minimize further recurrences.

Paget's Disease
Paget's disease of the vulva is an uncommon condition characterized by a patchy, eczematoid lesion that frequently covers much of the vulva. Most patients are postmenopausal and present with complaints of pruritus. Although Paget's disease is an in situ disease process, 15% to 25% of patients have an underlying malignancy, usually an adenocarcinoma of the apocrine glands but occasionally an invasive Paget's. In addition, up to 30% of patients have a synchronous adenocarcinoma of the breast, colon, rectum, or upper genital tract. Screening for these cancers is therefore recommended. To assess for invasion, the lesion should be excised via wide local excision or simple vulvectomy with at least 5 mm of the adjacent subcutaneous tissue. Achieving negative margin

[1]Not FDA approved for this indication.

status is frequently difficult. However, the risk of recurrence is approximately 30% whether margins are negative or positive. Thus expectant management, reserving treatment for symptomatic recurrences, is usually recommended.

Invasive Vulvar Lesions
Less than 5% of gynecologic cancers arise on the vulva. Over 90% are squamous cell carcinomas. The etiology of this type appears mixed. The differentiated type is more common, occurs in older women (age 60–69) and is associated with vulvar dystrophies. The classic or usual type is predominantly associated with HPV-16. These women are slightly younger (age 45–52 years). Most arise in older women (age 60–69 years), and suggested risk factors include immunosuppression, hypertension, diabetes mellitus, obesity, and chronic vulvar inflammation. Other histologic types are melanomas (5%–10%), basal cell carcinomas (2%–3%), adenocarcinomas (1%), and sarcomas (1%–2%). Most patients present with a combination of symptoms, including pruritus, discomfort, and complaints of a mass. Examination frequently reveals a suspicious lesion, which should be biopsied for diagnosis. Vulvar cancers typically spread by local extension and lymphatic dissemination. Factors that influence dissemination include tumor size (Table 2), depth of invasion (Table 3), lymphovascular space invasion, and tumor grade. Staging is surgical and classified using the tumor, nodes, and metastasis (TNM) system (Box 1) as well as the International Federation of Gynecology and Obstetrics (FIGO) system (Box 2).

TABLE 2	Incidence of Regional Node Metastases by Tumor Diameter
TUMOR DIAMETER (cm)	**% POSITIVE INGUINAL NODES**
<1 5–20 25–35 35–50 ≥50	1–15 ≥50

TABLE 3	Incidence of Regional Node Metastases by Depth of Tumor Invasion
DEPTH OF INVASION (mm)	**% POSITIVE INGUINAL NODES**
<1	1–5
1–3	10–15
3–5	15–30
5–10	30–45

Box 1	TNM Classification of Vulvar Carcinoma
T	Primary tumor
Tis	Carcinoma in situ
T1	Confined to vulva, diameter ≤2 cm
T2	Confined to vulva, diameter >2 cm
T3	Adjacent spread to urethra, vagina, perineum, or anus (any size)
T4	Infiltration of upper urethral mucosa, bladder, rectum, or bone
N	Regional lymph nodes
N0	No lymph node metastases
N1	Unilateral regional lymph node metastasis
N2	Bilateral regional lymph node metastasis
M	Distant metastases
M0	No clinical metastases
M1	Distant metastasis (including pelvic lymph node metastasis)

Abbreviation: TNM = tumor, node, metastasis.

Box 2 — FIGO Classification (With Corresponding TNM Classification) for Vulvar Carcinoma

Stage I (T1N0M0)	Tumor confined to vulva and/or perineum, 2 cm in greatest dimension; nodes are negative
Stage IA	Stromal invasion no greater than 1 mm
Stage IB	Stromal invasion >1 mm
Stage II (T2N0M0)	Tumor confined to the vulva and/or perineum, >2 cm in greatest dimension; nodes are negative
Stage III	
T3N0M0	Tumor of any size with adjacent spread to the lower urethra and/or the vagina or the anus
T3N1M0	Unilateral regional lymph node metastasis
T2N1M0	
Stage IVA	
T1N2M0	Tumor invades any of the following: upper urethra, bladder mucosa, rectal mucosa, pelvic bone, and/or bilateral regional node metastasis
T2N2M0	
T3N2M0	
T4 any N M0	
Stage IVB	
Any T any N M1	Any distant metastasis including pelvic lymph nodes

Abbreviations: FIGO = International Federation of Gynecology and Obstetrics; TNM = tumor, node, metastasis.

Squamous Cell Carcinomas and Adenocarcinomas

Surgical management of squamous cell carcinomas and adenocarcinomas depends on the size, depth of invasion, and location of the lesion. The vulvar lesion is managed with a radical excision. Management of the groins is based on depth of invasion. Lesions with invasion of less than 1 mm (Stage IA) have minimal risk of lymphatic spread (<1%) and do not require lymphadenectomy. All others require surgical assessment of the lymph nodes. Lesions less than 2 cm in size of the primary tumor, greater than 2 cm from the vulvar midline and are of squamous histology require only unilateral lymphadenectomy. Those without these characteristics or have palpable lymph nodes of the contralateral side require bilateral assessment. This surgical approach is associated with significant morbidity including disfigurement, wound breakdown, and problems with lymphocysts and chronic lymphedema. For patients with very large lesions or lesions in sensitive areas such as the clitoris, preoperative radiation, followed by less radical excision of residual disease, may minimize problems with the vulvar wound. Current investigations are ongoing in the use of sentinel lymph node dissections as a method of minimizing the groin morbidity without sacrificing survival. Positive vulvar margins or metastases to lymph nodes are managed with postoperative radiation. Survival depends on stage at diagnosis (Table 4).

Malignant Melanoma

Malignant melanoma is the second most common vulvar malignancy. Most patients have disease on the mucosal surfaces of the vulvar introitus, clitoris, and labia minora. The vulvar lesion is treated by radical excision, but management of the groins is controversial. The risk of spread is significant with a tumor thickness greater than 0.75 mm, but survival at 5 years is only approximately 10% with groin node metastases. Some argue against node dissection for this reason. However, given some long-term survivors with modern melanoma therapy, either lymphadenectomy or sentinel lymph node dissection, as is done for other cutaneous melanomas, appears indicated.

Verrucous Carcinoma

Verrucous carcinoma is a large exophytic tumor that resembles giant condyloma acuminatum. It is a variant of squamous carcinomas but has an excellent prognosis because of the lack of metastases. Verrucous carcinomas have a high tendency to recur and should be managed with radical local excision.

Basal Cell Carcinoma

Basal cell carcinomas typically occur in elderly white women, are commonly located on the labia majora, and have characteristics similar to basal cell carcinomas at other sites. Treatment is wide local excision only because metastases are rare. Basal cell carcinomas are prone to local recurrence, however. A malignant squamous component must be ruled out because it should be managed as a squamous cell carcinoma.

Sarcomas

Leiomyosarcoma is the most common vulvar sarcoma and usually arises in the labia majora. Malignant fibrous histiocytoma is the second most common. Management of these lesions is radical vulvar excision.

References

Beller U, Quinn MA, Benedet JL, et al. Carcinoma of the vulva. Int J Gynaecol Obstet 2006;95:S7.

Garland SM. Imiquimod. Curr Opin Infect Dis 2003;16.85–9.

Homesley HD, Bundy BN, Sedlis A, et al. Prognostic factors for groin node metastasis in squamous cell carcinoma of the vulva (a Gynecologic Oncology Group study). Gynecol Oncol 1993;49:279–83.

Hørding U, Junge J, Lundvall F. Vulvar intraepithelial neoplasia III: a viral disease of undetermined progressive potential. Gynecol Oncol 1995;56(2):276.

Krebs HB. The use of topical 5-fluorouracil in the treatment of genital condylomas. Obstet Gynecol Clin North Am 1987;14(2):559–68.

Modesitt SC, Waters AB, Walton L, et al. Vulvar intraepithelial neoplasia III: Occult cancer and the impact of margin status on recurrence. Obstet Gynecol 1998;92(6):962–6.

Phillips GL, Bundy BN, Okagaki T, et al. Malignant melanoma of the vulva treated by radical hemivulvectomy, a prospective study of the Gynecologic Oncology Group. Cancer 1994;73:2626–32.

Tebes S, Cardosi R, Hoffman M. Paget's disease of the vulva. Am J Obstet Gynecol 2002;187:281–4.

Trimble CL, Trimble EL, Woodruff JD. Diseases of the vulva. In: Hernandez E, Atkinson BE, editors. Clinical Gynecologic Pathology. Philadelphia: WB Saunders; 1995. p. 1–90.

Van de Nieuwehnof, et al. Vulvar squamous cell carcinoma development after diagnosis of VIN increases with age. Eur J Canc 2009;45:851.

Wright VC, Chapman WB. Colposcopy of intraepithelial neoplasia of the vulva and adjacent sites. Obstet Gynecol Clin North Am 1993;20(1):231–55.

Table 4 — Survival Rate by FIGO Stage for Patients With Invasive Squamous Cell Vulvar Cancer

FIGO STAGE	OVERALL SURVIVAL (PERCENT)		
	One year	Two years	Five years
I	96.4	90.4	78.5
II	87.6	73.2	58.8
III	74.7	53.8	43.2
IV	35.3	16.9	13.0

Abbreviation: FIGO = International Federation of Gynecology and Obstetrics.

VULVOVAGINITIS

Method of
Michael A. Malone, MD

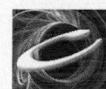

CURRENT DIAGNOSIS

- Bacterial vaginosis: pH >4.5; 20% clue cells, malodorous "fishy" discharge.
- Vulvovaginal candidiasis: pH 4–4.5; pseudohyphae, blastospores, Thick curd-like discharge, vulvar inflammation.
- Trichomonas vaginitis: pH 5–6; motile, flagellated trichomonads, many white blood cells (WBCs), purulent discharge, vulvovaginal inflammation.

Vulvovaginitis is the general term for disorders of the vulva and vagina caused by infection, inflammation, or changes in the normal vaginal flora. Common symptoms include vulvovaginal erythema, discomfort, odor, and vaginal discharge. From a medical perspective, vaginitis is considered a relatively benign problem. However, it can be cause physical discomfort, potential pregnancy risks, and with chronic vaginitis, body image problems and sexual dysfunction can occur. Despite a large percentage of patients who self-treat with over-the-counter treatments, vaginal symptoms are one of the most common reasons for gynecological consultation. A health care provider is consulted in the majority of women with vaginitis symptoms accounting for 10 million office visits a year in the United States.

This article addresses the most common causes of vaginitis which account for over 90% of cases. The common causes include bacterial vaginosis (40%–50% of cases), candidiasis (20%–25%), and trichomoniasis (15%–20%). Less common causes of these symptoms include vaginal atrophy, cervicitis, foreign body, irritants and allergens, and desquamative inflammatory vaginitis. History can help differentiate the cause of the vaginitis. For example, a patient's lack of itching makes candidiasis less likely while lack of perceived odor makes bacterial vaginosis unlikely and candidiasis more likely. However, none of the findings from the history alone allows a definitive diagnosis as there is considerable overlap in symptoms among the different etiologies. Inspecting the vulva on examination can also be helpful in determining the diagnosis. The vulva is often inflamed by candidiasis and trichomoniasis, but not by bacterial vaginosis. The characteristics of the vaginal discharge may help distinguish the type of infection, if present. (Table 1) However, the appearance of the discharge is unreliable and should not be the sole basis for diagnosis.

Identifying the etiology of vaginitis is primarily based on patient history, pelvic examination, vaginal pH measurement (Table 2), whiff test, speculum examination, and microscopic evaluation of the discharge. Microscopic examination is used to look for hyphae, motile trichomonads, epithelial cells studded with adherent coccobacilli (clue cells), and increased numbers of polymorphonuclear leukocytes (PMNs). Initial office evaluation correctly diagnoses 60% of *Candida* vulvovaginitis, 70% of trichomoniasis, and 90% of bacterial vaginosis. If microscopy is negative, culture for *Candida* species or polymerase chain reaction (PCR) testing for *Trichomonas vaginalis* (the choice is dictated by the clinical findings) is important because **microscopy is not sufficiently sensitive to exclude these diagnoses in symptomatic patients.** Bacterial cultures are not indicated in women with vaginal discharge. In fact, they are frequently misleading since a large variety of bacterial species colonize the vagina.

Trichomoniasis

Trichomoniasis is caused by the protozoan *T. vaginalis* and most men and women who are infected do not have any symptoms. Symptomatic disease is characterized by purulent, malodorous, greenish-yellow discharge, which may be accompanied by burning, pruritus, dysuria, and/or dyspareunia, and postcoital bleeding. Although all of the common causes of vulvovaginitis have been associated with other sexually transmitted infections, trichomoniasis is the only one that is actually sexually transmitted. *T. vaginalis* can be identified in 70% of the male sexual partners of infected women, although carriage in men is often self-limited.

Trichomonas infection increases the risk of complications in pregnancy. In a 2014 systematic review and meta-analysis of the association between *T. vaginalis* and perinatal outcomes, the risk of preterm birth was increased by 42% among infected women. The risks of premature rupture of membranes and delivery of a small for gestational age infant also increased. Although it should be treated when identified, whether the successful treatment of trichomonas in pregnancy affects or decreases these risks is unclear.

The diagnosis of trichomonas is based on laboratory testing including motile trichomonads on wet mount, positive culture, positive nucleic acid amplification test, and positive rapid antigen test (Box 1). As with other types of vaginitis, none of the clinical features of trichomoniasis is sufficiently sensitive or specific to allow a diagnosis based upon signs and symptoms alone. The presence of motile trichomonads on wet mount is diagnostic of infection, but they are identified in only 50% to 70% of culture-confirmed cases. There should not be significant delay in viewing the wet prep slide for trichomonas as they only remain motile for 10 to 20 minutes after collection. Other findings suggestive, but not diagnostic, of trichomonas include an elevated vaginal pH (>4.5) and an increase in PMNs on saline microscopy. Fixation and staining is not useful as trichomonads may lose morphologic characteristics during this process.

Culture (sensitivity over 80%) can be useful with a high clinical suspicion, but an absence of motile trichomonads on wet mount. However, **PCR detection has become the new gold standard for diagnosis of trichomoniasis** and can be used with a urine or vaginal specimen. Papanicolaou (Pap) smear should not be used as a diagnostic test or screen for trichomoniasis. However, asymptomatic women with trichomonads identified on a Pap smear can be treated empirically or further evaluated by wet mount, PCR detection, or culture.

The nitroimidazoles, metronidazole (Flagyl) and tinidazole (Tindamax), are the only medications approved by the FDA for the treatment of trichomoniasis. In randomized clinical trials, the recommended metronidazole regimens have resulted in cure rates of approximately 90% to 95%, and the recommended tinidazole regimen has resulted in cure rates of approximately 86% to 100%. Topically applied antimicrobials such as metronidazole gel (MetroGel Vaginal)[1] are unlikely to achieve therapeutic levels in

---

[1]Not FDA approved for this indication.

TABLE 1	Characteristics for Different Causes of Vaginitis	
	TYPICAL PH	**DISCHARGE CHARACTERISTICS**
Bacterial vaginosis	>4.5	Thin, homogeneous, "fishy smelling" gray discharge.
Trichomonas	5–6	Greenish-yellow purulent malodorous discharge
Vulvovaginal candidiasis	4–4.5	Thick, white, adherent, "cottage cheese-like" discharge

TABLE 2	Common Findings With Each Cause of Vaginitis		
FINDING	**DISCHARGE WITH AN ODOR**	**INFLAMMATION**	**VULVAR INVOLVEMENT**
Bacterial vaginosis	Yes	No	No
Candidiasis	No	Yes	Yes
Trichomonas	Yes	Yes	Yes

Box 1	Treatment of Trichomoniasis

Recommended Regimens
Metronidazole (Flagyl) 2 g orally in a single dose
OR
Tinidazole (Tindamax) 2 g orally in a single dose

Alternative Regimen
Metronidazole 500 mg orally twice a day[3] for 7 days

[3]Exceeds dosage recommended by the manufacturer.

the urethra or perivaginal glands and are not recommended. **Sex partners of patients with _T. vaginalis_ should be treated.** Treatment of patients and sex partners results in relief of symptoms, microbiologic cure, and reduction of transmission.

Bacterial Vaginosis (BV)

Bacterial vaginosis is caused by a shift in the normal bacterial vaginal flora with a decrease of lactobacilli and overgrowth of _Gardnerella vaginalis_, _Mycoplasma hominus_, and anaerobes. The normal acidic (pH 4–4.5) vaginal environment helps maintain the normal vaginal flora and inhibits growth of pathogenic organisms. Disruption of the normal ecosystem can lead to conditions favorable for development of bacterial vaginosis. Factors that are associated with bacterial vaginosis include multiple sex partners, a new sex partner, sexual activity, phase of the menstrual cycle, contraceptive choice, pregnancy, foreign bodies, estrogen level, sexually transmitted diseases, antibiotics, and douching.

In contrast to trichomonas and candidiasis, bacterial vaginosis is associated with only minimal inflammation and minimal irritative symptoms. Clinical indicators of bacterial vaginosis include Amsel's criteria (Box 2). If two or three of the criteria are present, the clinical diagnosis of bacterial vaginosis can be made with a 90% sensitivity and 77% specificity. The presence of >20% clue cells on microscopy is the most reliable single finding predictor of BV. **The use of culture for the diagnosis of bacterial vaginosis is not useful or recommended because the organisms that tend to overgrow are normal vaginal flora.**

Use of a Gram-stained smear of vaginal discharge is the diagnostic gold standard for diagnosis of BV, but is typically performed only in research studies. In clinical practice, the diagnosis of BV is usually based on Amsel criteria, which is easy to use at the point-of-care. Using Gram's stain as the standard for diagnosing BV, the sensitivity of Amsel criteria is over 90% and has a specificity of 77%. **It may have false positives with trichomonas, as the first three Amsel criteria findings are sometimes present in patients with trichomoniasis, as well.** Commercial tests for diagnosis of BV are not commonly used, given the reliability and ease of Amsel criteria, but can be useful when microscopy is not available.

Changes suggesting bacterial vaginosis reported on a Pap smear do have good specificity, but do not require treatment unless the patient is symptomatic (sensitivity 49%, specificity 93%). BV has been diagnosed using a swab of vaginal discharge obtained by the patient or clinician without speculum examination. However, omission of the speculum examination results in under-diagnosis and, therefore, is not ideal.

In pregnant patients, bacterial vaginosis has been associated with premature rupture of membranes (PROM), prematurity, chorioamnionitis, and low birth weight. In symptomatic patients, the treatment of bacterial vaginosis decreases those risks. In asymptomatic pregnant women, however, the effectiveness of treatments in reducing pregnancy-related risk is uncertain. There conflicting data on treatment of bacterial vaginosis in high-risk women and no evidence of risk reduction in low-risk women. Therefore, the current data does not support universal screening and treatment of asymptomatic patients during pregnancy.

| Box 2 | Amsel Criteria for Diagnosis of BV |

At least 3 of the 4 criteria must be present:
1. Homogeneous, thin, grayish-white discharge that smoothly coats the vaginal walls
2. Vaginal pH >4.5
3. Positive whiff-amine test, defined as the presence of a fishy odor when a drop of 10% potassium hydroxide (KOH) is added to a sample of vaginal discharge.
4. Clue cells: At least 20% of the epithelial cells clue cells (vaginal epithelial cells with adherent coccobacilli at the edge of the cell)

| Box 3 | Treatment of Bacterial Vaginosis |

Recommended Treatment Regimens
Metronidazole 500 mg orally twice a day for 7 days[1]
Metronidazole gel (MetroGel-Vaginal) 0.75%, one full applicator (5 g) intravaginally, once a day for 5 days
Clindamycin (Cleocin) cream 2%, one full applicator (5 g) intravaginally at bedtime for 7 days

Alternative Regimens
Tinidazole (Tindamax) 2 g orally once daily for 2 days
Tinidazole 1 g orally once daily for 5 days
Clindamycin 300 mg orally twice daily for 7 days[1]
Clindamycin ovules 100 mg intravaginally once at bedtime for 3 days

Recommended Regimens for Pregnant Women
Metronidazole 500 mg orally twice a day for 7 days
Metronidazole 250 mg orally three times a day for 7 days
Clindamycin 300 mg orally twice a day for 7 days

[1]Not FDA approved for this indication.

Bacterial Vaginosis Treatment

Treatment is recommended for women with symptoms (Box 3). Besides relief of symptoms, potential benefits to treatment include reduction in the risk of acquiring sexually transmitted diseases (STDs). Because of positive results for much of the Amsel criteria with both BV and trichomonas (and lack of microscopy sensitivity for trichomonas), using a metronidazole regimen that covers both of these diagnoses (500 mg twice a day × 7 days)[1] may be reasonable when a patient meets the Amsel criteria. Treatment of male sex partners has not been beneficial in preventing the recurrence of BV. No data support the use of douching for treatment or symptomatic relief and it may increase the risk for relapse. Metronidazole appears to be safe in pregnancy, as multiple studies and meta-analyses have shown no association between its use during pregnancy and teratogenic or mutagenic effects in newborns. Several studies have evaluated the clinical and microbiologic efficacy of using intravaginal lactobacillus formulations to treat BV and restore normal flora, but further research is needed to determine possible utility.

Vulvovaginitis Candidiasis (VVC)

Candida is considered part of the normal vaginal flora, but overgrowth of the organism and penetration of superficial epithelial cells can result in vulvovaginitis. Vulvovaginal candidiasis often presents with marked inflammation, scant discharge, itching, dysuria, and dyspareunia (Box 4). Vulvar pruritus is typically the

---

[1]Not FDA approved for this indication.

| Box 4 | Classification of Vulvovaginal Candidiasis (VVC) |

Uncomplicated VVC
Sporadic or infrequent vulvovaginal candidiasis
Mild-to-moderate vulvovaginal candidiasis
Likely to be _C. albicans_
Non-immunocompromised women

Complicated VVC (if any of below apply)
Recurrent vulvovaginal candidiasis (>4 episode in 1yr)
Severe vulvovaginal candidiasis (extensive vulvar erythema, edema, excoriation, and fissure formation)
Non-albicans candidiasis
Women with uncontrolled diabetes, debilitation, or immunosuppression

Box 5	Recommended Regimens for Uncomplicated VVC

Over-the-Counter Intravaginal Agents:

Butoconazole (Femstat, Mycelex), clotrimazole (Gyne-Lotrimin), miconazole (Monistat), tioconazole (Vagistat)

Prescription Intravaginal Agents:

Butoconazole (Gynazole-1) 2% cream 5 g intravaginally for 1 day

Nystatin 100,000-unit vaginal tablet, one tablet for 14 days

Terconazole (Terazol-7, Zazole): 0.4% cream 5 g intravaginally for 7 days

Terconazole (Terazol-3, Zazole): 0.8% cream 5 g intravaginally for 3 days

Terconazole (Terazol-3, Zazole) 80 mg vaginal suppository, one suppository for 3 days

Oral Agent:

Fluconazole (Diflucan) 150 mg oral tablet, one tablet in single dose

Box 6	Treatment Regimens of Complicated VVC:

Recurrent VVC Initial Regimen:

Any topical agent 7 to 14 days

OR

Fluconazole: 100, 150, or 200 mg orally once daily every third day for three doses[3]

Maintenance Regimens

Fluconazole 100- or 200-mg tab: 1 tab PO every week for 6 months[3]

Alternative Maintenance Regimens:

Clotrimazole 200-mg suppository (Gyne-Lotrimin 3): 1 suppository intravaginally qhs 2 × /week[3]

Butoconazole 2% cream (Femstat-3, Mycelex-3): 1 applicator (5 g) intravaginally qhs for 3 days

Severe VVC:

Any topical azole intravaginally once daily for 7 to 14 days

OR

Fluconazole 150 mg in two sequential doses (second dose 72 hours after initial dose)[3]

[3]Exceeds dosage recommended by the manufacturer.

dominant symptom and erythema, excoriations, and fissures of the vulva and vagina may be present. There is often little or no discharge; when present, it is classically white, thick, adherent, and clumpy (cottage cheese-like) with no or minimal odor. The diagnosis of vulvovaginal candidiasis is based on history, examination findings, and the presence of *Candida* on wet mount or culture.

Candida albicans accounts for 80% to 92% of episodes of vulvovaginal candidiasis; *Candida glabrata* is the next most common species. For the diagnosis of a specific *Candida* species, a culture must be obtained, but culture is not necessary for diagnosis if microscopy shows yeast. A culture should be obtained in women with clinical features of vulvovaginal candidiasis, normal vaginal pH, and negative microscopy and in women with persistent or recurrent symptoms. Many of the women with recurrent symptoms have non-albicans infection resistant to azoles. If the wet mount is negative and *Candida* cultures cannot be done, empiric treatment can be considered for symptomatic women with any sign of VVC on examination.

Treatment of Vaginal Candidiasis

Asymptomatic women and sexual partners do not require treatment. The treatment regimen is based on whether the woman has an uncomplicated infection (90% of patients) or complicated infection (Box 5). Treatment with oral or topical azoles results in symptom relief in 80% to 90% of patients who complete therapy, and are more effective than nystatin. Intravaginal antifungals are available over the counter, although unnecessary or inappropriate use of these preparations is common and can lead to a delay in appropriate treatment. In pregnant women, topical azole therapies, applied for 7 days, are recommended. Oral azole therapy should be avoided in pregnancy, as case reports have described a pattern of birth defects after first trimester exposure to high dose oral azole therapy.

Candida glabrata should be considered in those who do not respond to recommended therapy or have multiple recurrences. *Candida glabrata* does not form pseudohyphae or hyphae and is not easily recognized on microscopy, making diagnosis difficult without culture. The optimal treatment of non-albicans vulvovaginal candidiasis, such as *C. glabrata*, remains unknown but recommended regimens include an azole drug for a longer duration of therapy (7–14 days) (Box 6). If recurrence occurs, 600 mg of boric acid in a gelatin capsule[2] administered vaginally once daily for 2 weeks is recommended.

---

[2]Not available in the United States.

Severe vulvovaginitis is characterized by extensive vulvar erythema, edema, excoriation, and fissure formation. It is associated with lower clinical response rates in patients treated with short courses of topical or oral therapy. Recurrent vulvovaginal candidiasis (RVVC) is usually defined as four or more symptomatic episodes in 1 year. Routine treatment of sex partners in women with RVVC is controversial and does not appear effective. Vaginal cultures should be obtained from patients with RVVC to confirm the clinical diagnosis and to identify unusual species (including non-albicans species), particularly *Candida glabrata*. Each episode of RVVC caused by *Candida albicans* tends to respond well to short-duration oral or topical azole therapy. However, for recurrent infections, some specialists recommend a longer duration of therapy before initiating a maintenance antifungal regimen. Suppressive maintenance antifungal therapies are effective in preventing episodes, but 30% to 50% of women will have recurrent disease when maintenance therapy is stopped.

References

Anderson MR, Klink K, Cohrssen A. Evaluation of vaginal complaints. JAMA 2004;291:1368–79.

Centers for Disease Control and Prevention. Sexually transmitted diseases treatment I guidelines, 2010. MMWR 2010;59(RR12):1–110. Available at: http://www.cdc.gov/std/treatment/2010 (accessed August 10, 2015).

Edwards T, Burke P, Smalley H, Hobbs G. *Trichomonas vaginalis*: clinical relevance, pathogenicity and diagnosis. Crit Rev Microbiol 2014;10:1–12.

Hainer BL, Gibson MV. Vaginitis. Am Fam Physician 2011;83:807–15.

Huppert JS, Hesse EA, Bernard MC. Accuracy and trust of self-testing for bacterial vaginosis. J Adolesc Health 2012;51:400–5.

Landers DV, Wiesenfeld HC, Heine RP. Predictive value of the clinical diagnosis of lower genital tract infection in women. Am J Obstet Gynecol 2004;190:1004–10.

Nyirjesy P. Management of persistent vaginitis. Obstet Gynecol 2014;124 (6):1135–46.

Seña AC, Miller WC, Hobbs MM, et al. *Trichomonas vaginalis* infection in male sexual partners: implications for diagnosis, treatment, and prevention. Clin Infect Dis 2007;44:13–22.

Senok AC, Verstraelen H, Temmerman M, Botta GA. Probiotics for the treatment of bacterial vaginosis. Cochrane Database Syst Rev 2009:CD006289.

Silver BJ, Guy RJ, Kaldor JM, et al. *Trichomonas vaginalis* as a cause of perinatal morbidity: a systematic review and meta-analysis. Sex Transm Dis 2014;41:369–76.

Singh RH, Zenilman JM, Brown KM, et al. The role of physical examination in diagnosing common causes of vaginitis: a prospective study. Sex Transm Infect 2013;89:185–90.

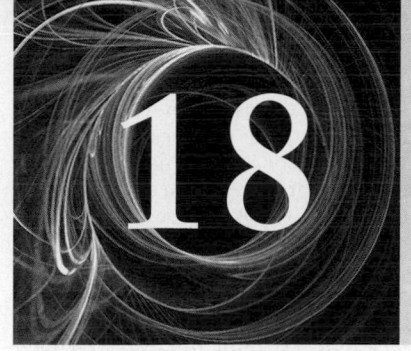

18 Pregnancy and Antepartum Care

ANTEPARTUM CARE

Method of
Stoney Abercrombie, MD; and Matthew Cline, MD

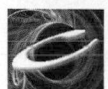

CURRENT DIAGNOSIS

- Pregnancy evaluation should begin 3 to 6 months before conception with optimization of underlying medical conditions, update of immunizations, and commencement of prenatal vitamins with 400 μg of folic acid.[1]
- Preconception counseling with a specialist in high-risk pregnancies should be considered in all patients with underlying medical conditions, such as diabetes and hypertension.
- The first prenatal visit should include a review of the medical and obstetric histories, current medications, allergies, herbal remedies, supplements, and tobacco, alcohol, and drug use.
- Prenatal laboratory studies should be done at the first visit after a pregnancy is confirmed with a urine pregnancy test. These studies include hemoglobin, platelet count, type and screen, rubella status, hepatitis B screening, rapid plasma reagin, and a urine culture. All women should be offered screening for HIV. High-risk patients should be screened for hepatitis C, gonorrhea, and chlamydia.
- Genetic screening should be offered based on ethnic background and family history.
- Either first-trimester screening (nuchal translucency combined with maternal serum pregnancy-associated plasma protein A [PAPP-A]/free β–human chorionic gonadotropin [β-hCG]) or second-trimester quadruple screen should be offered to all patients. These tests aid in diagnosis of chromosome abnormalities. If a patient opts for a first-trimester screen, it is important to perform an alpha-fetoprotein (AFP) screen in the second trimester to screen for neural tube defects. Women 35 years and older should be offered amniocentesis for genetic screening.
- Appropriate weight gain in pregnancy depends on maternal body mass index (BMI) before pregnancy. In patients with a normal BMI, a 25- to 30-pound weight gain is recommended. Underweight patients are encouraged to gain 30 to 35 pounds, and overweight patients are encouraged to gain no more than 20 pounds.
- Prenatal visits should begin at 8 to 12 weeks' gestation and continue monthly until 28 weeks. Visits should then be every 2 weeks until 36 weeks and then weekly. Each visit should include assessment of maternal weight, blood pressure (BP), urinalysis for protein and glucose, fundal height measurement, documentation of fetal heart tones, and review of symptoms of preterm labor and preeclampsia.
- All patients should undergo a glucose challenge test at 24 to 28 weeks. This is done nonfasting by administering a 50-g load of glucose and obtaining a serum sample 1 hour after administration. A level greater than 140 mg/dL is considered abnormal, and a 3-hour glucose tolerance test is indicated (which is done after a 12-hour fast with a 100-g oral glucose load). If a woman demonstrates abnormalities in two of the four values, gestational diabetes is diagnosed.

[1]Not FDA approved for this indication.

CURRENT THERAPY

- Administration of the inactivated influenza vaccine (Fluzone, Fluvirin, Fluvarix) is recommended in all pregnant patients, regardless of trimester, who will be pregnant (or up to 3 months postpartum) during the flu season.
- Additionally, recent recommendations support Tdap vaccine (Adacel, Boostrix) in each pregnancy given between 27 and 36 weeks or immediately postpartum in order to decrease rates of pertussis in this age group.
- An updated listing of vaccination recommendations throughout pregnancy (including international travel) can be found at http://www.cdc.gov/vaccines/pubs/preg-guide.htm#12.
- Folic acid supplementation should begin before conception. The recommended dose is 400 μg daily and is usually given as a prenatal vitamin. In patients with a previous pregnancy complicated by a neural tube defect, 4 mg daily is recommended to decrease the chance of recurrence of a neural tube defect.
- Pyelonephritis requires hospitalization and intravenous (IV) antibiotics in all pregnant patients. IV antibiotics should be continued until the patient is afebrile for longer than 24 hours. Oral antibiotics should then be commenced to complete a 14-day course. All patients should continue on suppressive antibiotic therapy until delivery after a diagnosed single episode of pyelonephritis or two episodes of cystitis.
- All patients with HIV should be treated with antiretroviral therapy regardless of gestation.
- Intrapartum zidovudine (Retrovir) is recommended for all patients with HIV and consideration of cesarean delivery is appropriate based on viral load evaluation.

Antepartum Care

Ideally, antepartum care commences 3 months before conception with the recommendation that women who are sexually active and not using contraception should begin taking daily multivitamin or folic acid supplements.[1] The most convincing trials of this were performed in Europe and China when it was concluded that women of reproductive age should take multivitamin supplements containing 0.4 mg of folate daily to reduce the incidence of neural tube defects. Women with histories of children with neural tube

[1]Not FDA approved for this indication.

| Box 1 | Potential Indications for High-Risk Referral |

- Current disease involving renal, cardiac, or endocrine systems
- Fetal anomalies (in previous pregnancies or first-degree family relatives)
- History of preterm delivery
- Incompetent cervix
- Isoimmunization
- Known carrier of genetic disorder
- Multiple gestation
- Placenta previa after 28 weeks
- Prior intrauterine fetal demise or stillbirth
- Systemic diseases such as hypertension, diabetes, or asthma
- Third-trimester bleeding

defects or other anomalies should increase this dose to 4 mg^3 of folate in the periconceptional period to reduce risks of recurrence.

Preconception counseling should also include an accurate assessment of preexisting maternal medical conditions. This is the ideal time to stress changes in factors that respond to early intervention: quitting smoking, refraining from alcohol or drug abuse, treating gum disease, and avoiding teratogens. Alcohol is a known teratogen. Immunization status should be reviewed and vaccines should be administered as appropriate. Special consideration is given to patients with thyroid disease. Concern focuses on associations with low intelligence quotients (IQs) in children conceived by hypothyroid mothers. Patients with diabetes should be counseled that the increased risk of birth defects is directly related to the level of glucose control at conception.

High-risk obstetric referrals may be offered to women with potential for obstetric complications suggested by conditions listed in Box 1. Identification of the high-risk patient is critical to avoiding adverse outcomes.

In most cases, a woman's pregnancy is a normal event that is complicated by potentially dangerous disease in a minority of cases. The physician who manages pregnant patients must follow the normal changes that occur during antepartum care, so that abnormalities can be recognized and treated appropriately. Additionally, routine prenatal care offers multiple opportunities for patient education, primary intervention, and appropriate monitoring of the low-risk pregnancy in the setting of the family and community. For some women, antepartum care is part of their own continuum in a long-term primary care relationship with caregivers.

Timeline of Routine Antepartum Care
First Visit and Early Care
History
After pregnancy is confirmed, it is extraordinarily important to determine the duration of pregnancy and the estimated date of confinement (EDC). Further care is heavily predicated on this estimate. The history begins with ascertaining the first day of the last normal menstrual period and calculating the EDC by assuming duration of pregnancy averages 280 days (40 weeks). Because a first-trimester dating ultrasound (US) is accurate to within 5 days at confirmation or determination of an accurate EDC, its value cannot be overestimated.

The documentation of prior obstetric history includes prior complications, route of delivery, and estimated birth weights. Maternal medical disorders are often exacerbated by pregnancy; cardiovascular, renal, and endocrine disorders require evaluation and counseling concerning possible treatments required. A history of previous gynecologic surgery, including cesarean delivery, is

---

^{3}Exceeds dosage recommended by the manufacturer.

---

important to consider. A family history of twinning, diabetes mellitus, familial disorders, or hereditary disease is relevant.

Current medications (prescription and nonprescription) are reviewed, along with any herbals or supplements. Certain prescription medications are known teratogens and should be discontinued. Examples include isotretinoin (Accutane), tetracycline (Sumycin), quinolone antibiotics (ciprofloxacin [Cipro], levofloxacin [Levaquin]), and warfarin (Coumadin). Angiotensin-converting enzyme (ACE) inhibitors should not be used in pregnancy because they can be associated with renal agenesis.

Open discussion of substance abuse (alcohol, tobacco, and illicit drugs) is an integral part of the patient interview. Counseling patients about smoking cessation is vital in early pregnancy. Smoking increases the risk of fetal death or damage in utero. It is also associated with increased risk of placental abruption and placenta previa, each of which put both mother and child at risk, along with premature birth. The interest that pregnant women have in delivering a healthy infant can be a potent motivator for change at this point.

Domestic Violence Screening and Counseling
Pregnancy is also a time of increased incidence of domestic or intimate partner violence, and because of this, it is appropriate to screen patients about the safety of their homes and relationships starting at the first prenatal visit. Although the U.S. Preventive Services Task Force (USPSTF) gives screening for domestic violence an "I" rating (inconclusive), a large evidence review supports benefit to patients being screened with one of many possible screening tools. The Personal Violence Screen consists of three "Yes" or "No" questions that can be quickly administered to a patient in private, and a positive result is one or more "Yes" responses:
1. Have you been hit, kicked, punched, or otherwise hurt by someone in the past year?
2. Do you feel unsafe in your current relationship?
3. Is there a partner from a previous relationship who is making you feel unsafe now?

A positive screen should be followed by specific referral to local resources for the patient to reach a safe environment and continued support. Each office should evaluate local resources and have a prepared contact list for these patients to use as their next step to safety.

Examination
Physical examination begins with a thorough general examination to assess maternal well-being, including BMI and BP. The BMI is calculated by dividing weight in kilograms by height in meters squared. The BMI of a patient is categorized as underweight (under 19.8), normal weight (19.8 to 25), overweight (25 to 30), or obese (over 30).

Breast examination may be significant for changes in pregnancy that result from hormonal responses by the mammary ducts. These changes include engorgement and vascular prominence, occasionally resulting in mastodynia. Enlargement of areolar sebaceous glands (Montgomery's tubercles) occurs between 6 and 8 weeks' gestation.

A pelvic examination is performed with attention to the adequacy of pelvis and evaluation for adnexal masses. Numerous changes in the pelvic organs occur in pregnancy. For example, congestion of the pelvic vasculature (Chadwick's sign) causes bluish discoloration of the vagina and cervix. Softening of the cervix due to increased vascularity of the cervical tissue (Goodell's sign) can occur as early as 4 weeks.

Portable devices using Doppler will reliably detect fetal heart tones at a normal rate of 120 to 160 beats per minute as early as 10 to 11 weeks.

Laboratory Studies
Routine laboratory studies and screenings in pregnancy are listed in Table 1, along with their USPSTF level of recommendation.

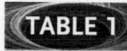

TABLE 1 U.S. Preventive Services Task Force Recommendations for Pregnancy

Grade A = The USPSTF recommends the service. There is high certainty that the net benefit is substantial. Screening/actions in pregnancy in this category include the following:

- Screen for asymptomatic bacteriuria at 12–16 weeks or at first prenatal visit.
- Screen for hepatitis B infection in all pregnant women.
- Screen for HIV infection in all pregnant women.
- Screen for Rh (D) blood typing and antibody testing at first prenatal visit.
- Screen for syphilis in all pregnant women.
- Screen for cervical cancer all women between 21 and 65 who have a uterus.
- Ask about smoking and provide augmented, pregnancy-tailored counseling for those who smoke and are pregnant.
- All women planning or capable of pregnancy should take 400–800 µg of folic acid daily.

Grade B = The USPSTF recommends the service. There is high certainty that the net benefit is moderate or there is moderate certainty that the net benefit is moderate to substantial. Screening/actions in pregnancy in this category include the following:

- Screen for chlamydia in pregnant women 24 and younger or at high risk.
- Screen for gonorrhea if at high risk of infection.
- Screen for iron deficiency anemia in asymptomatic pregnant women.
- Provide intervention during pregnancy and after birth to support breast-feeding.
- Repeat Rh (D) antibody testing for all unsensitized Rh (D) negative women at 24–28 weeks unless it is certain that father is Rh (D) negative.
- Screen for alcohol misuse and provide behavioral counseling interventions to reduce its misuse.
- For women at high risk of preeclampsia, start low dose aspirin[1] at 81 mg/day after 12 weeks of gestation.

Grade C = Clinicians may provide this service to selected patients depending on individual circumstances. However, for most individuals without signs or symptoms there is likely to be only a small benefit from this service.

- Screen for chlamydia in all patients 25 and over.

Grade D = The USPSTF recommends against the service. There is moderate or high certainty that the service has no net benefit or that the harms outweigh the benefits.

- Screen for bacterial vaginosis in asymptomatic pregnant women at low risk for preterm birth.
- Screen for herpes simplex with serology in asymptomatic pregnant women.

Grade I = The USPSTF concludes that the current evidence is insufficient to assess the balance of benefits and harms of the service.

- Screen for gestational diabetes mellitus before or after 24 weeks' gestation.
- Screen for gonorrhea in all patients.

Listing of all topics is available at http://www.uspreventiveservicestaskforce.org/uspstopics.htm.
Abbreviation: USPSTF = U.S. Preventive Services Task Force.

Other Studies

Special-purpose studies are also considered in early gestation. First-trimester screening with nuchal translucency should be offered to all women between 11 and 14 weeks' gestation. The first-trimester screen uses the nuchal translucency and maternal serum-free β-hCG and PAPP-A and detects up to 85% of Down syndrome and trisomy 18 cases with a false-positive rate of 5%.

Chorionic villus sampling (CVS) (done at 10–12 weeks' gestation) or amniocentesis (performed at 14–16 weeks' gestation) should be offered to women older than 35 years, to those with abnormal first-trimester screens or second trimester "quad" screens, and to those with significant family history of genetic disease. From either test, fetal cells grown in culture may be subjected to chromosomal, metabolic, or DNA study for trisomy 13, 18, or 21 or abnormal numbers of sex chromosomes. CVS cannot be used for diagnosis of neural tube defects, but amniocentesis can accurately diagnose open neural tube defects or open abdominal defects by measuring amniotic fluid AFP.

Patients with tuberculosis exposure may be assessed for active tuberculosis with skin testing (if not vaccinated with bacille Calmette-Guérin [BCG]) and chest x-ray with abdominal shielding. Serologic assessment for toxoplasmosis, cytomegalovirus, and varicella immunity are not routinely indicated.

Screening for genetic disorders should be undertaken if concern exists based on racial or ethnic background (hemoglobinopathies, β-thalassemia, α-thalassemia, Tay-Sachs disease) or familial background (cystic fibrosis, fragile X, Duchenne's muscular dystrophy).

Education

Several areas are appropriate for routine education during the first prenatal visit, and may be provided by handouts, nursing instruction, or directly by the physician. These will vary based on the patient's individual knowledge and prior experience, but at a minimum should include discussions of the following:

- Common discomforts of pregnancy and safe methods to relieve them
- Foods to avoid during pregnancy and safe food preparation
- Avoidance of tobacco, ethanol, and nonprescribed drugs throughout pregnancy
- Limitations on travel and importance of proper seatbelt use
- Danger signs of pregnancy and reasons to call or be seen after hours
- Availability of birth education classes, tours, and other educational resources

Follow-up

Follow-up visits are scheduled once monthly until 28 weeks' gestation, and then patients are followed twice monthly until 36 weeks. Visits are then scheduled at weekly intervals until delivery. At each visit, weight gain, edema, BP, fundal height, Leopold's maneuvers, and fetal heart tones are recorded.

Interval history includes questions about diet, sleeping patterns, and fetal movement. Warning signs such as bleeding, contractions, leaking of fluid, headache, or visual disturbances are reviewed.

15 to 20 Weeks' Gestation

Interval History

At each visit, it is appropriate to ask about specific symptoms: headache, dysuria, swelling, vaginal discharge, any bleeding, pelvic pain, and nausea or vomiting. The nausea and vomiting of the first trimester usually begins to decrease after 12 to 14 weeks. By this point in the pregnancy, the patient is usually feeling well. The other items above, if present, may indicate reasons for a targeted examination to evaluate for the cause, such as a speculum examination with wet prep for an increased symptomatic discharge (though the physiologic discharge of pregnancy has often become evident by this point, it should be asymptomatic).

Alpha-Fetoprotein and Aneuploidy Testing

For patients who received first-trimester aneuploidy screening, maternal serum AFP testing should be offered for all pregnancies at 16 to 20 weeks as a means of screening for open neural tube defects. High levels of AFP are associated with various fetal anomalies, including neural tube defects, multiple gestations, and ventral wall defects. Unexplained elevation of AFP has been associated with poor fetal growth, fetal loss, and preeclampsia. In cases with unexplained elevation of AFP, maternal and fetal surveillance should be increased. Low levels of AFP are associated with increased risk of Down syndrome.

For those who did not have the first trimester screen, a "quad screen" with multiple analytes can be done at this time to screen for aneuploidy such as trisomy 21, 18, and 13 as well. The interpretation of this test depends on the gestational age; even if timed correctly, it is known to have a moderate level of false-positive results. Therefore, the first step after an abnormal AFP or quad screen is to refer for a detailed ultrasound to confirm gestational age. If the results of the screening remain abnormal, definitive testing via amniocentesis is recommended.

The above screening tests are recommended for screening for aneuploidy in low-risk women. For those women at increased risk, such as maternal age over 35, history of a previous baby with a trisomy, or a positive first trimester or quad screen for trisomy, the use of cell-free fetal DNA testing has a role as a screening test. It detects fetal DNA in the maternal circulation and then assesses relative amounts of chromosomes 21, 18, and 13 compared to other fetal chromosomes to evaluate the risk of trisomy of these 3 chromosomes. Its detection rate for these three trisomies is over 98% with a false positive rate of less than 0.5%. This test can be drawn as early as the 10th week of gestation and the results are usually available within a week. Its limitations are that it currently can only test for these specific trisomies, and requires invasive diagnosis (such as amniocentesis) to confirm the results. Appropriate pre-test counseling is important due to the limitations of this test and its evolving role in screening during pregnancy.

Physical Findings

Interval changes in the physical examination now include the start of colostrum secretion, which can begin as early as 16 weeks' gestation. The mother might detect fetal movements (quickening) at around 18 to 20 weeks. The uterus is palpable at 20 weeks at the umbilicus.

Chloasma is darkening of the skin over the forehead, bridge of the nose, or cheekbones and is more obvious in those with dark complexions. It can begin to manifest at this time, and is intensified by exposure to sunlight. Darkening of the skin in the areolae and nipples becomes more accentuated. A darkened line appears in the lower midline of the abdomen from the umbilicus to the pubis (linea nigra). The basis of these changes is stimulation of melanophores by increased melanocyte-stimulating hormone.

At 15 to 20 weeks, abdominal enlargement can appear more rapid as the uterus rises out of the pelvis and into the abdomen.

Ultrasonography

Sonography has long established itself as the single most useful technology in monitoring pregnancy and diagnosing complications. It is for this reason that an anatomic US is offered at 18 to 20 weeks to evaluate growth, placentation, amniotic fluid volume, and fetal anatomy. If earlier dating of the pregnancy is uncertain, this is an opportunity to confirm or refute prior estimates. If anomalous conditions are discovered or the patient has a history of diabetes, advanced maternal age, or has prior children with anomalies, more comprehensive US becomes necessary.

20 to 35 Weeks' Gestation
Interval History
This period in the middle trimester of the pregnancy is often the time when patients feel their best: the challenges of nausea and vomiting from the first trimester are usually past. Patients should be asked about diet and activity, fetal activity (which should continue to increase throughout this period), and any symptoms that might suggest preeclampsia, such as hand or face swelling, visual changes, or severe headaches. Vaginal secretions do increase during this period but any bleeding or leakage of a large amount of fluid, along with any uterine rhythmic contractions, should also prompt a call or evaluation of the patient.

Physical Findings
The uterus should be palpable at the umbilicus at 20 weeks, and from this period until 34 weeks the measurement in centimeters from the fundus to the symphysis pubis should correspond to the gestational age in weeks. Measurements that are more than 2 cm below the expected size should raise suspicion for oligohydramnios, intrauterine growth restriction, fetal anomalies, or an abnormal fetal position. Conversely, measurements more than 2 cm larger than expected may indicate multiple gestation, polyhydramnios, or fetal macrosomia. These rules apply for the gestational ages of 20 to 32 weeks. Either situation can be better

evaluated with maternal US examination and consultation with a maternal-fetal-medicine specialist.

New physical examination findings at this time include the onset of stretch marks (striae) of the breasts and abdomen. These are caused by separation of underlying collagen tissue, a response to increased adrenocorticosteroid. The ligamentous structures of the pelvis also undergo slight but definite relaxation of the joints, a progesterone effect. As the uterus enlarges, it often rotates to the right. Braxton-Hicks contractions, characterized as painless uterine tightening, increase in regularity. The fetal outline can be easily palpated through the maternal abdominal wall.

Laboratory Studies
Increased surveillance for preeclampsia includes testing for urine protein in patients with BP 140/90 mm Hg or higher or in those with weight gains greater than 3 pounds/week. Evaluation is also necessary for clinical signs of upper extremity or facial edema, right upper quadrant tenderness, headaches, or vision changes. Proteinuria of more than 300 mg in 24 hours can indicate renal dysfunction or the onset of preeclampsia.

A complete blood count (to screen for anemia) and a nonfasting 1-hour glucose tolerance test (after ingestion of 50 g of glucose) are scheduled to detect patients at risk for developing gestational diabetes at 24 to 28 weeks. If the screening test is abnormal, a 3-hour test is performed with 100 g of glucose to confirm the diagnosis. Two or more abnormal values on this test are considered diagnostic of gestational diabetes mellitus.

A repeat Rh antibody is checked at 28 weeks' gestation in Rh-negative mothers. Those who remain unsensitized at 28 weeks' gestation receive a first dose of Rho(D) immune globulin (RhoGAM) of 300 µg to prevent maternal isoimmunization to fetal red blood cells. (This should also be given at any point after the first 12 weeks of pregnancy in the setting of significant maternal trauma in an Rh-negative mother. If there is suspicion of a significant fetal-maternal hemorrhage, a Kleihauer-Betke test can be used to quantitate the amount of fetal blood in the maternal circulation in order to increase the dose of RhoGAM appropriately.)

Follow-up
Return visits at 2-week intervals are initiated beginning at 28 weeks, and the patient is oriented to the labor and delivery ward. Precautions are given regarding the onset of conditions listed in Box 2. The onset of any of these should prompt immediate medical attention.

36 to 41 Weeks' Gestation
Physical Findings
Patients often note increased vaginal discharge at this time in their pregnancy, a physiologic consequence of hormone stimulation. The discharge consists mainly of epithelial cells and cervical mucus and is treated with reassurance. Discharge accompanied by itching, burning, or malodor should be evaluated with a wet prep and any abnormalities treated.

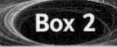 **Box 2** — Warning Signs and Symptoms Prompting Medical Attention

- Burning with urination
- Chills or fever
- Prolonged vomiting or inability to keep liquids down
- Pronounced decrease in fetal movements
- Rhythmic cramping pains (>4/hr)
- Rupture of membranes
- Severe abdominal, pelvic, or back pain
- Signs of preeclampsia (headache, edema, right upper quadrant pain, visual changes)
- Vaginal bleeding (though spotting may occur after any pelvic examination)

Laboratory Studies

Vaginal and rectal cultures are collected to evaluate for the presence of group B streptococci (GBS) at 35 to 37 weeks. GBS organisms are implicated in preterm labor, amnionitis, endometritis, and wound infection. If cultures are positive, the patient will be given antibiotic prophylaxis during active labor to protect the newborn against vertical transmission and the resulting infection that could occur. If a patient has a positive urine culture during the pregnancy of over 100,000 colony-forming units of GBS, she is treated at the time of that culture but also assumed to be heavily colonized and given intrapartum antibiotics without performing the vaginal/rectal cultures at 35 to 37 weeks.

Follow-up

Follow-up visits are planned on a weekly basis with emphasis on weight gain, BP, and signs of preeclampsia. Review of precautions regarding infection, pregnancy loss, and symptoms of preeclampsia completes the visit.

Postterm Gestation

About 3% to 12% of pregnancies continue beyond 42 weeks' gestation and are considered postterm. Although some of these may be due to inaccurate dating, some patients clearly progress to excessively long gestations that are a significant risk to the fetus. Increased antepartum surveillance by cervical examination, fetal heart rate testing (such as nonstress testing [NST]), and biophysical profile should be initiated between 41 and 42 weeks. Even if fetal testing is reassuring, patients with reliable dating greater than 41 weeks are candidates for induction of labor.

Common Concerns of the Antenatal Period
Bleeding

About one half of pregnant women experience some form of bleeding during the pregnancy; often this is benign. Patients also have a heightened awareness of symptoms that previously may have gone unnoticed in the nonpregnant state. Efficient and competent evaluation, followed by compassion and reassurance when prudent, allays many fears and provides clear direction. Spotting due to bleeding at the implantation site occurs from the time of implantation (about 6 days after fertilization) until 29 to 35 days after the last menstrual period in many women. Usually, cardiac activity on US and appropriate β-hCG levels confirm a viable early pregnancy. First-trimester bleeding may be a sign of spontaneous miscarriage or ectopic pregnancy and deserves further evaluation, often with a pelvic examination and US. Vaginal bleeding in late pregnancy is covered in other articles.

Nausea

Nausea is a common symptom that occurs in most pregnancies. It is heightened before 14 weeks' gestation and is largely benign. The etiology is not well understood but likely is related to elevating levels of β-hCG. Nausea of pregnancy can occur at any time during the day. Aggravating factors vary with the individual patient; success varies with interventions designed to reduce symptoms.

Uncomplicated nausea may be responsive to small nonfatty portions at mealtime. Pyridoxine (vitamin B₆)[1] tablets 12.5 mg three times daily with 12.5 mg of doxylamine (Unisom)[1] twice a day are safe in pregnancy and may be helpful. A combination product of doxylamine 10 mg and pyridoxine 10 mg (Diclegis) has recently been approved by the FDA for the treatment of nausea and vomiting of pregnancy in women who do not respond to conservative management. Antiemetic drugs in the outpatient setting are the next step; ondansetron[1] (Zofran, FDA category B) 4 to 8 mg up to three times a day and meclizine[1] (Antivert, FDA category B) 12.5 to 25 mg three times a day are agents with the best safety profile. A small study comparing pyridoxine + doxylamine to ondansetron for treatment of nausea in pregnancy showed that ondansetron was more effective that than pyridoxine + doxylamine in decreasing nausea and vomiting over 5 days, with similar side effects.

[1]Not FDA approved for this indication.

Inability to control protracted vomiting in conjunction with clinical dehydration can require hospitalization for IV fluids and treatment of hyperemesis gravidarium. Extreme nausea and vomiting that persists beyond 18 to 20 weeks' gestation may be a sign of multiple gestation, thyroid disease, molar pregnancy, or liver or pancreatic disease.

Nutrition and Weight Gain

The mother's nutrition is a vital factor in the development of the fetus from preconception through the postpartum period. Therefore, the pregnant woman should be advised to eat a balanced diet and should be informed of the additional 300 kcal/day needed during pregnancy. The American College of Obstetricians and Gynecologists (ACOG) recommends a target weight gain of 22 to 27 pounds (10–12 kg) during pregnancy. It also advises that underweight women might need to gain more and obese women should gain less. Nutritional requirements for protein are 80 g/day, for calcium are 1500 mg/day, for iron are 30 mg/day, and for folate are 0.4 mg/day (4 mg/day in some cases, such as those patients with previous baby with neural tube defects). Patients with seizure disorders managed with valproic acid (Depakene) or carbamazepine (Tegretol) are also at risk for birth defects and might benefit from the higher dose of folate.

Heartburn

Heartburn in the form of reflux esophagitis is caused by the enlarging uterus displacing the stomach and by progesterone's relaxation of the lower esophageal sphincter. Treatment consists of taking antacids, decreasing exacerbating factors such as spicy foods, eating more frequently but in smaller quantities, limiting eating before bedtime, and taking H₂-receptor inhibitors.

Urinary Symptoms

Urinary frequency, nocturia, and bladder irritability are common complaints due to progesterone-mediated relaxation of smooth muscle and subsequent altered bladder function. Later in pregnancy, urinary frequency becomes even more prominent from pressure on the bladder by the enlarging uterus and the fetal presenting parts, such as when the fetal head descends into the pelvis.

Dysuria, however, is often a sign of infection that requires antibiotic treatment. Bacteriuria combined with urinary stasis from altered bladder function predisposes the patient to pyelonephritis. Although simple urinary tract infections are treated on an outpatient basis, pyelonephritis remains the most common nonobstetric cause for hospitalization during antenatal care.

Patients with a diagnosis of pyelonephritis require hospitalization, aggressive fluid replacement, and IV antibiotics until they remain afebrile for longer than 24 hours. Close monitoring of maternal respiratory status is important because these women are at risk for acute respiratory distress syndrome (ARDS) and renal failure. All patients should complete a 14-day course of antibiotic treatment. After treatment has been completed, suppressive therapy should be continued until delivery.

Infection

Two infections of special note are HIV and bacterial vaginosis (BV). HIV transmission to the newborn can be reduced significantly with appropriate infectious disease and maternal-fetal medicine specialty management. Appropriate treatment of BV in women at high risk for preterm delivery or recurrent loss can significantly reduce either of these untoward outcomes. Debate exists as to whether or not low-risk women should be screened for BV; should the patient be symptomatic, appropriate treatment is metronidazole (Flagyl) 500 mg twice daily for 7 days orally.

Chlamydia trachomatis is an obligate intracellular bacterium and is the most common sexually transmitted bacterial infection in women of reproductive age. It may be associated with urethritis, mucopurulent cervicitis, and acute salpingitis, or it may be clinically silent. Perinatal transmission is clearly associated with neonatal conjunctivitis (leading to blindness) and pneumonia and is likely associated with preterm delivery, premature rupture of membranes, and perinatal mortality. Diagnosis is confirmed by polymerase chain reaction (PCR) during routine screening. Doxycycline should be avoided in pregnancy, and erythromycin is associated with gastrointestinal upset, so treatment with azithromycin (Zithromax 1000 mg as single dose) is often the best choice in pregnancy.

Gonococcal infection is associated with concomitant chlamydia infection in about 40% of infected pregnant women. It is usually limited to the lower genital tract, including the cervix, urethra, and periurethral or vestibular glands. Because of an association between gonococcal cervicitis and septic spontaneous abortion, and because preterm delivery, premature rupture of membranes, and postpartum infection are more common with gonococcal infection, routine cultures are appropriate at the first antenatal visit. Because some strains have rendered some β-lactam drugs ineffective for therapy, the recommendation for uncomplicated gonococcal infection is intramuscular ceftriaxone (Rocephin) 250 mg.

Vaginosis due to *Candida albicans* can become symptomatic with caseous white discharge and vaginal itching or burning, and it may be associated with red satellite lesions on the vulva. Marked inflammation of the vagina and introitus may be noted. Topical application of over-the-counter antifungal creams such as miconazole nitrate (Monistat) or nystatin (Mycostatin) is generally helpful in controlling the imbalance of vaginal flora, but this requires a 7-day regimen to achieve adequate cure rates. A single dose of fluconazole (Diflucan), 150 mg by mouth, is another appropriate choice after the first trimester.

Trichomonas vaginalis can be found in 20% to 30% of pregnant patients, but only a small number complain of discharge or irritation. This flagellated, oval, motile organism can be seen on normal saline wet prep and is evident clinically by presence of a foamy or greenish discharge accompanied by multiple cervical petechiae. Treatment is oral metronidazole (Flagyl) as a single 2-g dose for the patient and her partner (though most states support expedited partner treatment, each practitioner will need to individualize this approach).

Rubella, also known as German measles, is directly responsible for spontaneous miscarriage and severe congenital malformations. Although large epidemics of rubella are nonexistent in the United States because of immunization, the disease can still affect up to 25% of susceptible women. Absence of rubella antibody indicates susceptibility. Vaccination involves an attenuated live virus (MMR) and therefore is avoided in pregnancy. Vaccination of nonpregnant susceptible women (including those during the postpartum period) and hospital personnel continues to be the mainstay of therapy. Detection by immunoglobulin M (IgM)–specific antibody confirms recent infection.

Varicella-zoster virus, the etiologic agent of childhood chickenpox, is a DNA herpes virus that remains latent in the dorsal root ganglia and may be reactivated years later to cause herpes zoster or shingles. Infection early in pregnancy can lead to severe congenital malformations, including chorioretinitis, cerebral cortical atrophy, hydronephrosis, and cutaneous and bony leg defects. Varicella-zoster immunoglobulin (VZIg) 125 U/10 kg can attenuate varicella infection if given to an exposed, nonimmune pregnant woman within 96 hours of her exposure to a patient with active varicella.

Genital herpes simplex virus (HSV) may be confirmed by tissue culture if active lesions are present in pregnant patients at term or in labor. In this event, cesarean delivery is indicated because the fetus is at risk for acquiring the virus during passage through the birth canal. For HSV outbreaks remote from term, acyclovir (Zovirax) and its derivatives can shorten the course of an outbreak. For those with a history of active herpes during or preceding pregnancy, prophylaxis with acyclovir from 36 weeks onward can decrease the chance of an outbreak at term and the need for a cesarean delivery.

Influenza can occur during pregnancy, and because the risk of secondary complication such as pneumonia is increased during the antepartum period, influenza vaccination is recommended for all patients in any trimester who are pregnant or up to 3 months postpartum during the local influenza season. Rapid testing of nasal or throat swabs can ascertain the diagnosis of influenza. Though oseltamivir (Tamiflu) and zanamivir (Relenza) are both FDA category C in pregnancy, no toxic effects have been observed in animal trials, so these are the preferred agents. These agents need to be started within 72 hours of the onset of symptoms to provide benefit, and they provide the greatest improvement in symptom duration and severity if started in the first 24 hours.

Varicose Veins

Pressure by the enlarged uterus on venous return from the legs and progesterone-mediated vasodilation can lead to prominent varicosities and edema of the legs or vulva. Any concern for deep vein thrombosis should be ruled out with duplex ultrasound imaging. Benign varicosities almost invariably return to normal after delivery, thus limiting the need for intervention in the antepartum period, though their symptoms may be decreased through the wearing of support hose. Edema of the lower extremities is common, responds to elevation, and must be differentiated from facial or hand edema accompanying preeclampsia. Hemorrhoids are manifestations of the varicosities of the rectal veins. Treatment focuses on stool softeners, sitz baths, and over-the-counter topical preparations. If a hemorrhoid becomes firm and tender, evaluation for possible treatment by opening and removing the thrombus can provide immediate relief.

Constipation

Bowel transit time and relaxation of intestinal smooth muscle are both increased due to progesterone effects, resulting in overall slowing of bowel function. If pronounced, this can lead to constipation. Dietary management of this condition is centered on recommendations for increased fluids and high-fiber foods; stool softeners, such as docusate (Colace), can also be used in pregnancy. Enemas and laxatives are not recommended.

Upper Extremity Discomfort

Periodic numbness and tingling of the fingers is due to exacerbations of carpal tunnel compression exacerbated by tissue edema. Splinting of the affected hand at night may help, along with stretching exercises of the wrist and neck that can be done throughout the day. Most of these symptoms resolve after delivery.

Backache and Pelvic Discomfort

Endocrine relaxation of ligamentous structures coupled with an offset center of gravity create exaggerated lordotic spinal curve, joint instability, and back pain. Most women experience some form of this discomfort as pregnancy progresses. Advice given for improvements in posture, local heat, acetaminophen (Tylenol), and massage may be helpful. Minimizing the time spent standing can have a positive effect. Round ligament pain usually occurs during the second trimester and is described as sharp bilateral or unilateral groin pain. It may be exacerbated by change in position or rapid movement and might respond to similar measures. These routine aches and pains of pregnancy must be differentiated from rhythmic cramping pains originating in the back or uterus. The latter may be a sign of preterm labor requiring appropriate evaluation.

Leg Cramps

Leg cramps in the form of recurrent muscle spasms in pregnancy are believed to be due to lower levels of serum calcium or higher levels of serum phosphorus. The calves are most commonly involved and attacks are more frequent at night and in the third trimester. There are no data from controlled trials to show benefit over placebo for treatment targeted toward reduced phosphate and increased calcium or magnesium intake. Local heat, putting the affected muscle on stretch, acetaminophen, and massage can be helpful in acute events.

Intercourse

In general, intercourse is considered safe in pregnancy. The exception to this rule is found in patients who have a known placenta previa, are experiencing uterine bleeding, or have postcoital cramps and spotting. It may be wise to avoid intercourse in couples who are at risk for special circumstances. Firmer recommendations can be made in instances of placenta previa or known rupture of membranes; in these instances intercourse should not occur.

Dental Care

Ideally, women should have dental care completed before conception. However, dental procedures under local anesthesia may be carried out at any time during the pregnancy. Use of nitrous oxide inhalants is to be avoided, however. Long procedures should be postponed until the second trimester. Antibiotics are appropriate as needed for dental infections and in cases of rheumatic heart disease or mitral valve prolapse with regurgitation.

X-rays, Ionizing Radiation, and Imaging

The adverse effects of ionizing radiation are dose dependent, but there is no single diagnostic procedure that results in a dose of radiation high enough to threaten the fetus or embryo. Diagnostic radiation of less than 5000 mrad is considered by ACOG to have minimal teratogenic risk, and if medically indicated, x-ray imaging may be performed safely (with appropriate abdominal shielding). Patients receiving dental x-rays are additionally protected by a lead apron. Still, the need for x-ray films should be evaluated for risks and potential benefits in the individual pregnant patient to conservatively protect the mother and fetus from theoretical genetic or oncogenic risk. Magnetic resonance imaging (MRI) is considered safe due to its mechanism of action, which is a nonionizing form of radiation. Radioactive iodine (^{131}I) is contraindicated in pregnancy.

Immunization

Live virus vaccines must be avoided during pregnancy because of possible effects on the fetus. These include measles, mumps, rubella (MMR), yellow fever (YF-Vax), and varicella (Varivax) vaccinations. The risks to the fetus from the administration of rabies vaccine (RabAvert, IMOVAX) are unknown.

Diphtheria and tetanus toxoid with pertussis (Tdap) may be administered in pregnancy safely. The hepatitis B vaccine (Engerix B, Recombivax HB) series is safe and may be given in pregnancy to women at risk. The inactivated influenza vaccine (Fluzone, Fluvirin, Fluvarix) is also recommended in all women during any trimester they will be pregnant during the flu season (or up to 3 months postpartum during flu season).

Tests of Fetal Well-Being

A primary goal in antepartum care is the competent management of patient care extended to both mother and baby in order to reduce the risk of fetal demise after 24 weeks, ensure optimal conditions for term delivery after 37 weeks, and intervene for evolving conditions threatening the well-being of either patient. Any pregnancy that may be at increased risk for antepartum fetal compromise is a candidate for tests of fetal well-being performed weekly, beginning at 28 to 32 weeks. Some conditions requiring antepartum testing are listed in Box 3.

Box 3	Conditions that Prompt Enhanced Fetal Surveillance

- Decreased fetal movements
- Fetal growth restriction
- Hypertensive disorders
- Insulin-dependent diabetes mellitus
- Multiple gestation with discordant fetal growth
- Oligohydramnios or polyhydramnios
- Postterm pregnancy
- Prior loss or stillbirth

Nonstress Test

The nonstress test (NST) consists of fetal heart rate monitoring in the absence of uterine contractions. A reactive tracing is one in which heart rate accelerations of 15 beats/min above the baseline of 120 to 160 beats/min are of at least 15 seconds' duration. Two of these accelerations must be observed in a 20-minute period. False-positive nonreactive tracings are more common before 28 weeks' gestation.

Biophysical Profile

The biophysical profile (BPP) consists of an NST with ultrasound observations. A total of 10 points is given for the following elements (2 points each):

- Reactive NST
- Presence of fetal breathing movements of 30 seconds or more in 30 minutes
- Fetal movement defined as three or more discrete body or limb movements within 30 minutes
- Fetal tone defined as one or more episodes of fetal extremity extension and return to flexion
- Quantification of amniotic fluid volume, defined as a pocket of fluid that measures at least 2 cm by 2 cm

The results of a BPP are usually reported out of 8 points if done without the NST, and out of 10 points if done with an NST. Scores of 8 or 10 points (out of 10) are considered reassuring, with retesting indicated in 4 to 7 days depending on the original indication for the testing. A score of 6 points is borderline; testing should be repeated in 24 hours. Scores of 4 or 2 points are nonreassuring and should prompt additional testing, treatment, or planning for delivery depending on the setting.

References

American College of Obstetricians and Gynecologists. Compendium of selected publications. Atlanta: American College of Obstetricians and Gynecologists; 2012.

Centers for Disease Control and Prevention. Influenza: information for health professionals. Available at http://www.cdc.gov/flu/; [accessed November 23, 2012].

Centers for Disease Control and Prevention. Updated recommendations for use of tetanus toxoid, reduced diphtheria toxoid and acellular pertussis vaccine (Tdap) in pregnant women and persons who have or anticipate having close contact with an infant aged <12 months—Advisory Committee on Immunization Practices (ACIP), 2011. MMWR Morb Mortal Wkly Rep 2011;60:1426.

Gabbe SG, Niebyl JR, Simpson JL, et al. Obstetrics: Normal and Problem Pregnancies. 6th ed. Philadelphia: Saunders Elsevier; 2012.

Kirkham C, Harris S, Grzybowski S. Evidence-based prenatal care: part I. General prenatal care and counseling issues. Am Fam Physician 2005a;71:1307–16.

Kirkham C, Harris S, Grzybowski S. Evidence-based prenatal care: part II. Third-trimester care and prevention of infectious diseases. Am Fam Physician 2005b;71:1555–60.

Nelson HD, Bougatsos C, Blazina I. Screening women for intimate partner violence: a systematic review to update the U.S. Preventive Services Task Force Recommendation. Ann Intern Med 2012;156:796–808, W279–82.

Noninvasive prenatal testing for fetal aneuploidy. Committee Opinion No. 545, American College of Obstetricians and Gynecologists. Obstet Gynecol 2012; 120:1532–4.

Oliveira LG, Cap SM, You WB, et al. Ondansetron compared with doxylamine and pyridoxine for treatment of nausea in pregnancy: a randomized controlled trial. Obstet Gynecol 2014;124:735–42.

ECTOPIC PREGNANCY

Method of
Samantha F. Butts, MD; and Kurt T. Barnhart, MD

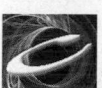

CURRENT DIAGNOSIS

- Vaginal bleeding and abdominal pain in pregnancy suggest the possibility of ectopic pregnancy but may also be present in normal intrauterine pregnancies and early miscarriage.
- Transvaginal ultrasound and measurement of serum β–human chorionic gonadotropin (β-hCG) are the best initial steps in determining if a pregnancy is ectopic; if the β-hCG is above the discriminatory zone (3000 mIU/mL), a normal pregnancy should be visualized in the uterus.
- If the initial β-hCG is below the discriminatory zone and there is no ultrasound evidence of ectopic pregnancy, patients should

be followed with serial β-hCG every 48 hours; updated guidelines about the appropriate β-hCG patterns help guide decision making and determine whether additional diagnostic interventions (i.e., dilation and curettage) are needed.

CURRENT THERAPY

- Both surgical and medical approaches to treating ectopic pregnancy are effective; the best option depends on clinical features of the ectopic pregnancy, stability of the patient, future fertility plans, and additional patient characteristic that would preclude one approach or the other.
- Conservative, tube-sparing therapies require patient follow-up until β-hCG levels are undetectable.
- Medical management with methotrexate[1] is most effective when ectopic pregnancies are small (less than 3.5 cm) and not producing abundant β-hCG (less than 5000 mIU/mL); empiric treatment of pregnancies of unknown location with methotrexate is not advised.

[1]Not FDA approved for this indication.

The development of an ectopic pregnancy is a potentially serious threat to the general and reproductive health of a woman. Despite vast improvements in the clinical care of women with ectopic pregnancy over recent years, diagnostic challenges and therapeutic controversies regarding this condition still exist. The objective of this chapter is to provide an overview of the epidemiology, diagnosis, and contemporary management of ectopic pregnancy. The focus is on ectopics that implant in the fallopian tube, which represent greater than 95% of all ectopic pregnancies.

Epidemiology
Ectopic pregnancies comprise 1% to 2% of all conceptions in the United States. Between 1970 and 1992, the rate of ectopic pregnancy increased from 4.5 to 19.7 per 1000 pregnancies, and has remained stable recently. This rise in ectopic pregnancy incidence is likely due to enhanced capability to detect early ectopic pregnancies, the rising incidence of gonorrhea and chlamydial infections, and the growing use of infertility treatments.

Ectopic pregnancy is a source of serious maternal morbidity and mortality in the United States. Complications of ectopic pregnancy are responsible for 6% of all pregnancy-related deaths, making this condition the leading cause of maternal mortality in the first trimester of pregnancy. Fortunately, the risk of ectopic-related mortality appears to be declining despite the increase in incidence of this condition.

Pathophysiology
Damage to the fallopian tube and fallopian tube dysfunction are the primary factors associated with development of ectopic pregnancy. Normal embryo transport can be disrupted by damage to the structural integrity of the mucosal portion of the fallopian tube. Intratubal scarring secondary to infection or trauma could lead to trapping of a conceptus within intratubal adhesions or diverticula.

Alteration of the hormonally mediated events leading to implantation—as sometimes occurs in treatments for infertility—offers another mechanism for consideration. A change in the estrogen-to-progesterone ratio could theoretically affect smooth muscle activity in the fallopian tube, immobilizing ciliary activity.

Risk Factors
The most important risk factors for the development of ectopic pregnancy include history of prior ectopic pregnancy, history of pelvic inflammatory disease (PID), prior fallopian tube surgery, and a history of infertility. Eliciting a history of such risk factors affects clinical suspicion of ectopic pregnancy diagnosis; however, half of all women with ectopic pregnancy will not report any known risk factors.

Prior Ectopic Pregnancy
A history of ectopic pregnancy confers a 7- to 13-fold increased risk of subsequent ectopic pregnancy compared to those with no such prior history. On average, after one ectopic pregnancy the odds of recurrence range from 9% to 27%. After two ectopic pregnancies, a repeat ectopic pregnancy occurs in 36% to 40% of subsequent pregnancies.

Pelvic Infection
PID can lead to tubal deciliation, intratubal and extratubal adhesions, and fimbrial injury. The offending organisms are most likely chlamydia, gonorrhea, or mixed anaerobic and aerobic organisms. In a study of 415 women with PID, the incidence of tubal occlusion after one, two, and three episodes was 13%, 35%, and 75%, respectively.

Contraception and Surgical Sterilization
In general, the risk of ectopic pregnancy in women using any form of contraception is diminished compared to women who do not use contraception. Nevertheless, different forms of birth control have very distinct degrees of risk of ectopic pregnancy if they fail. When contraceptive failure occurs with an intrauterine device (IUD) in place, 6% to 50% of pregnancies are ectopic. Data from the U.S. Collaborative Review of Sterilization demonstrated that tubal ligation failure results in an ectopic pregnancy in one-third of cases. The risk of ectopic pregnancy after tubal sterilization is inversely proportional to the age of the patient at the time of surgery and is increased with tubal fulguration techniques. Most ectopic pregnancies associated with failed tubal ligations occur several years after the procedure.

Prior Surgery
Prior tubal surgery results in an increased risk of ectopic implantation. Examples of reported rates of ectopic pregnancies following distal salpingostomy range between 12% and 18%, and approach 5% following a tubal anastomosis. Except for appendectomy of a ruptured appendix, a history of nontubal abdominal surgery does not appear to increase ectopic pregnancy risk.

Infertility and Infertility Treatment
Infertility alone or in combination with fertility treatments is a risk factor for ectopic pregnancy even in women with normal tubal integrity. One possible explanation for this association could reside in the influence of higher-than-normal preovulatory levels of estradiol in these patients, which might adversely affect tubal function. Several descriptive studies have described the incidence of ectopic pregnancy to range from 5% to 7% after in vitro fertilization (IVF). It has been postulated that reverse embryo migration toward an abnormal fallopian tube following embryo transfer is associated with the development of ectopic pregnancies after IVF. In addition, heterotopic pregnancies, considered extremely rare in the general population, occur with greater frequency (0.3%–1% of pregnancies) in women who conceive with infertility treatments, especially IVF.

Smoking
Smoking has emerged in recent years as an important risk factor for ectopic pregnancy, with a relative risk of 2.5. Chemicals in cigarettes are believed to cause abnormal tubal motility and increase the odds of tubal implantation. A dose response has been observed such that women who smoke heavily have the greatest risk of ectopic pregnancy.

Diagnosis and Clinical Manifestations
Although some patients present acutely with a ruptured ectopic pregnancy and hemoperitoneum, the vast majority (up to 80%) of ectopic pregnancies are diagnosed in stable outpatients. Many

of these patients will present with symptoms of light vaginal bleeding and/or abdominal discomfort and thus need to be differentiated from women with at-risk, nonectopic gestations. The use of high-resolution transvaginal sonography and sensitive quantitative human chorionic gonadotropin (β-hCG) assays represents the current standard for accurate and timely diagnosis of ectopic pregnancy.

Transvaginal Ultrasonography

To conduct the ultrasound evaluation of a patient with suspected ectopic pregnancy properly requires an understanding of the findings typical of normal and abnormal pregnancies. The earliest ultrasonographic finding of a normal intrauterine pregnancy is the gestational sac surrounded by a thick echogenic ring, located eccentrically within the endometrial cavity. On average, the gestational sac is seen on transvaginal ultrasound scan 5 weeks after the last menstrual period (LMP). As the gestational sac grows, a yolk sac is then seen within it (5.5 weeks following the LMP) followed by an embryonic pole (6 weeks following the LMP) with cardiac activity (6.5 weeks following the LMP). The appearance of a normal gestational sac can be simulated by a pseudogestational sac and intrauterine fluid collection, which occurs in 8% to 29% of patients with ectopic pregnancy. The pseudogestational sac likely represents bleeding into the endometrial cavity by the decidual cast.

The demonstration of an adnexal gestational sac with a fetal pole and cardiac activity is the most specific but least sensitive sign of ectopic pregnancy, occurring in only 10% to 17% of cases. Adnexal rings (fluid sacs with thick echogenic rings) that have a yolk sac or nonliving embryo are accepted as specific signs of ectopic pregnancy and are visualized in ectopic pregnancies 33% to 50% of the time.

A critical concept in the evaluation of early pregnancy by transvaginal ultrasound is that of the β-hCG discriminatory value (zone), or the level at or above which an examiner should see a normal intrauterine gestation, if present. In the setting of a β-hCG level above the discriminatory zone and no intrauterine pregnancy on ultrasound, an ectopic pregnancy or an abnormal intrauterine pregnancy is highly likely. The exact β-hCG discriminatory value varies somewhat from institution to institution, depending on the experience of the ultrasonographer and the β-hCG assay used. The value should be approximately 3000 mIU/mL.

Hormonal Assays

Many patients with suspected ectopic pregnancy will present with a β-hCG below the discriminatory zone and have an ultrasound that does not provide a definitive diagnosis (7%–20%). These patients require repeat β-hCG measures at least every 48 hours to evaluate the appropriateness of hormonal trends. Comparing serial measures of β-hCG from an individual patient to accepted patterns of β-hCG trends in early pregnancy helps distinguish an ectopic pregnancy from a viable intrauterine pregnancy or a spontaneous miscarriage. Current data show that approximately 99% of viable intrauterine pregnancies are associated with a 53% or greater increase in β-hCG values every 2 days. This rate is slower than the previously accepted rule of a 66% increase in β-hCG at 2 days; the updated rules support a more conservative approach to incorporating invasive diagnostic procedures when following β-hCG values to prevent the interruption of normal pregnancies.

Patients with symptomatic first-trimester pregnancies, nondiagnostic ultrasound, and a β-hCG level that is declining (when the initial value is below the discriminatory zone) should also be followed with serial β-hCG levels until resolution to distinguish a resolving miscarriage from an ectopic pregnancy. Fifty percent of women with ectopic pregnancies will present with declining β-hCG levels. Rules describing the expected elimination of β-hCG in spontaneous miscarriage indicate that the minimum rate of decline ranges from 12% to 35% at 2 days to 34% to 84% at 7 days. Faster rates of decline occur with higher initial β-hCG levels. When the serial decline in β-hCG is in the range associated with spontaneous miscarriage, continued follow-up surveillance is indicated. If the β-hCG decline is slower than expected for a miscarriage, an ectopic pregnancy must be highly suspected.

Surgical Diagnosis

The patient presenting with either (1) initial β-hCG below the discriminatory zone followed by an abnormal rise or decline or (2) initial β-hCG value at or above the discriminatory zone with no detectable intrauterine pregnancy has an abnormal pregnancy. The only exception to the rule for scenario 2 would be if a multiple gestation had been conceived. The challenge for the clinician is to then determine whether the pregnancy is an abnormal intrauterine pregnancy or an ectopic pregnancy. At this point, additional interventions are typically employed to differentiate the two possibilities. The most common approaches are listed below and each is discussed in turn.

- Dilation and curettage followed by β-hCG measurement the day after surgery. If the β-hCG level plateaus or increases, medical management of ectopic pregnancy with methotrexate[1] is implemented.
- Dilation and curettage followed by full pathologic evaluation of endometrial curettings. If no products of conception are detected, either medical management with methotrexate[1] is implemented or a diagnostic laparoscopy is performed.
- Diagnostic laparoscopy outright to evaluate the fallopian tubes and pelvis for the presence of an ectopic pregnancy; if no ectopic pregnancy is found, a dilation and curettage may be performed to evacuate the uterus.
- Empiric medical management of ectopic pregnancy with methotrexate[1] without dilation and curettage.

The option of medical treatment without dilation and curettage is the least desirable owing to the risk of overtreating women without verified ectopic pregnancy. Empiric treatment of suspected ectopic pregnancy without the performance of a dilation and curettage could result in inappropriate treatment of up to 40% of women. In addition to lacking clinical utility, this treatment option is not cost-effective.

Treatment and Therapeutic Monitoring

Surgery has long been the mainstay of treatment for ectopic pregnancy, but medical management is a widely used alternative. The choice of any treatment option depends on factors such as clinical presentation, the risks of either surgery or medical management to the patient, and future fertility plans.

Surgical Management

Patients with hemodynamic instability caused by a ruptured ectopic pregnancy require laparotomy and salpingectomy of the involved fallopian tube owing to extensive tubal damage. The majority of women with ectopic pregnancy who are stable can be safely treated with laparoscopy. For a woman with an unruptured ectopic pregnancy, surgical options include tube-sparing salpingostomy or removal of the fallopian tube (salpingectomy). Ideal candidates for linear salpingostomy include patients who have an ectopic pregnancy in the ampulla or infundibulum of the fallopian tube. Persistent ectopic pregnancy after linear salpingostomy ranges in frequency from 3% to nearly 30% of procedures so patients must be followed with serial β-hCG to resolution. Prophylactic methotrexate[1] has been proposed as a means of reducing the odds of a persistent ectopic pregnancy following conservative surgery. A suggested approach to reducing the risk of persistent ectopic after salpingostomy would be to incorporate a postoperative day 1 β-hCG into the monitoring strategy using a drop of less than 50% to help predict a persistent ectopic pregnancy and need for prophylactic methotrexate.

Salpingectomy is reserved for patients with isthmic ectopic pregnancies, tubal rupture, or an ipsilateral recurrent ectopic pregnancy. Salpingectomy is more appropriate for isthmic ectopic pregnancies because the narrowness of the isthmic lumen of the fallopian tube can predispose to tubal obstruction and scarring after salpingostomy. Women who have completed childbearing might be better candidates for salpingectomy than salpingostomy.

With respect to future fertility, much of the published data supports higher odds of intrauterine conception following

---

[1]Not FDA approved for this indication.

salpingostomy compared to salpingectomy; some studies, however, suggest no difference in the odds of intrauterine pregnancy based on method of ectopic surgery. The most important determinant of normal conception following surgical treatment is the presence of a healthy contralateral fallopian tube. The odds of recurrent ectopic pregnancy appear to be higher in women after conservative rather than radical surgical treatment.

Medical Management

Methotrexate (MTX)[1] therapy for ectopic pregnancy is a widely used medical alternative to surgery. Methotrexate is a folic acid antagonist that impairs DNA synthesis and cellular replication targeting rapidly proliferating cells such as trophoblasts. Although medical treatment of ectopic pregnancy is an appealing option for many patients, certain absolute contraindications exist to the use of the drug and are listed in Table 1. Among the most important of the contraindications to MTX therapy is the inability of the

---

[1]Not FDA approved for this indication.

patient to comply with follow-up after initiation of therapy. Without the ability to monitor response to medication and provide additional doses if deemed appropriate, opportunities to prevent ectopic rupture could be missed. To ascertain whether a patient is eligible for MTX therapy, a comprehensive laboratory and medical evaluation should first be performed, including tests of renal and liver function, as well as a complete blood count. Treatment failure occurs when decline in β-hCG levels is deemed inadequate and surgery is required. In some cases, medication failure presents as tubal rupture requiring emergent surgery.

Relative contraindications to MTX treatment pertain to patient characteristics that reduce the odds of successful treatment. These include β-hCG levels of 5000 mIU/mL or greater and ultrasonographic evidence of an ectopic pregnancy with fetal heart activity and an ectopic gestational mass measuring 3.5 cm or more in diameter. The strongest predictor for the efficacy of MTX treatment is the β-hCG concentration.

Three methotrexate treatment regimens exist: single-dose, two-dose, and multidose regimens (Table 2). These designations refer more to the number of intended doses in the protocol rather than

---

TABLE 1   Contraindications to Medical Management of Ectopic Pregnancy with Methotrexate

	ACOG*	ASRM†
Absolute contraindications	Breast-feeding; laboratory evidence of immunodeficiency; preexisting blood dyscrasias (bone marrow hypoplasia, leukopenia, thrombocytopenia, or clinically significant anemia); known sensitivity to methotrexate; active pulmonary disease; peptic ulcer disease; hepatic, renal, or hematologic dysfunction; alcoholism; alcoholic or other chronic liver disease	Breast-feeding; evidence of immunodeficiency; moderate-to-severe anemia, leukopenia, or thrombocytopenia; sensitivity to methotrexate; active pulmonary or peptic ulcer disease; clinically important hepatic or renal dysfunction; intrauterine pregnancy
Relative contraindications	Ectopic mass >3.5 cm; embryonic cardiac motion	Ectopic mass >4 cm detected by transvaginal ultrasonography; embryonic cardiac activity detected by transvaginal ultrasonography; patient declines blood transfusion; patient is not able to participate in follow-up; high initial hCG level (>5000 mIU/mL)

*Data are from the American College of Obstetricians and Gynecologists (ACOG).
†Data are from the American Society for Reproductive Medicine (ASRM).

TABLE 2   Methotrexate[1] Protocols for Treatment of Ectopic Pregnancy

	SINGLE DOSE	TWO DOSE	MULTIDOSE
Day 1	Check β-hCG value. Administer first dose of MTX 50 mg/m² IM.	Check β-hCG value. Administer first dose of MTX 50 mg/m² IM.	Check β-hCG value. Administer first dose of MTX 1 mg/kg IM followed by leucovorin[1] 0.1 mg/kg IM on day 2. Check β-hCG on day 2.
Day 4	Check β-hCG value.	Check β-hCG value. Administer second dose of MTX 50 mg/m² IM.	Administer second dose of MTX (day 3) and leucovorin (day 4) Check β-hCG on day 4.
Day 7	Check β-hCG value looking for 15% decrease between days 4 and 7. If >15% fall, check β-hCG weekly until not detectable in serum. If <15% fall, administer second dose of MTX 50 mg/m² IM.	Check β-hCG value for 15% decrease between days 4 and 7. If >15% fall, check β-hCG weekly until not detectable in serum. If <15% fall, administer third dose of MTX 50 mg/m² IM	Continue administering doses of MTX and leucovorin (i.e., course 3 days 5 and 6 and course 4 days 7 and 8) until β-hCG values have declined by 15%. Do not exceed 4 courses. If >15% decline, check β-hCG weekly until not detectable in serum.
Day 11		Check β-hCG value for 15% decrease between days 7 and 11. If >15% decline, check β-hCG weekly until not detectable in serum. If <15%, administer fourth dose of MTX 50 mg/m² IM.	
Weekly surveillance	If follow-up β-hCG value plateau or rise, consider surgical intervention or repeat dose of MTX as additional therapy.	If follow-up β-hCG value plateau or rise, consider surgical intervention or repeat dose of MTX as additional therapy.	If follow-up β-hCG value plateau or rise, consider surgical intervention or repeat dose of MTX as additional therapy.

[1]Not FDA approved for this indication.
Abbreviations: β-hCG = β–human chorionic gonadotropin; IM = intramuscular; MTX = methotrexate.

the actual number or doses received by all patients. For any of the protocols, once β-hCG levels have declined by at least 15% between interval assessments, no additional doses of medication are required, but β-hCG must still be followed until complete resolution to ensure treatment efficacy. Although each regimen has demonstrated efficacy, only one small, randomized trial of comparative efficacy exists in which no significant difference between protocols was observed. A recent meta-analysis demonstrated that the risk of treatment failure was nearly five times higher in women receiving single-dose MTX than in those receiving multidose MTX (adjusted for confounders). Of note, the meta-analysis demonstrated that patients designated to receive single-dose therapy often received more than one dose and that patients getting multidose therapy often required fewer than four doses to be cured. The two-dose protocol aims to address these considerations, improving on the efficacy of single-dose MTX while not requiring more visits than are typically required for the single-dose protocol.

Side effects of MTX therapy occur in up to 30% of women; however, most of these resolve rapidly and are generally of minor consequence. Abdominal pain is common early in treatment and is of concern as a possible indicator of tubal rupture. A potential cause of this pain in nonacute patients can be tubal miscarriage. Additional potential side effects include nausea, vomiting, diarrhea, gastritis, stomatitis, and liver transaminitis. Serious side effects such as alopecia and neutropenia can occur but are extremely rare.

Reproductive success following successful MTX therapy appears similar to that following conservative surgery. The most critical predictors of fertility after ectopic pregnancy treated by any conservative means are the condition of the contralateral fallopian tube and the presence of additional ectopic risk factors.

Expectant Management

Based on the fact that numerous ectopic pregnancies resolve spontaneously, there has been great interest in considering expectant management in selected patients. Expectant management includes close monitoring of symptoms, determination of β-hCG levels, and transvaginal ultrasound scanning. The likelihood of successful ectopic resolution is highest in the presence of a nondiagnostic ultrasound and β-hCG values less than 1000 mIU/mL.

References

ACOG Practice Bulletin No. 94. Medical management of ectopic pregnancy. Obstet Gynecol 2008;111:1479.

Ailawadi M, Lorch SA, Barnhart KT. Cost-effectiveness of presumptively medically treating women at risk for ectopic pregnancy compared with first performing a dilatation and curettage. Fertil Steril 2005;83:376.

Alleyassin A, Khademi A, Aghahosseini M, et al. Comparison of success rates in the medical management of ectopic pregnancy with single-dose and multiple-dose administration of methotrexate: A prospective, randomized clinical trial. Fertil Steril 2006;85:1661.

Barnhart K, Hummel AC, Sammel MD, et al. Use of "2-dose" regimen of methotrexate to treat ectopic pregnancy. Fertil Steril 2007;87:250.

Barnhart K, Sammel MD, Chung K, et al. Decline of serum human chorionic gonadotropin and spontaneous complete abortion: Defining the normal curve. Obstet Gynecol 2004;104:975.

Barnhart KT. Clinical practice. Ectopic pregnancy. N Engl J Med 2009;361:379.

Barnhart KT, Gosman G, Ashby R, et al. The medical management of ectopic pregnancy: a meta-analysis comparing "single dose" and "multidose" regimens. Obstet Gynecol 2003;101:778.

Barnhart KT, Katz I, Hummel A, et al. Presumed diagnosis of ectopic pregnancy. Obstet Gynecol 2002;100:505.

Berek J. Berek and Novak's Gynecology. 15th ed. Philadelphia: Lippincott Williams & Wilkins; 2011.

Butts S, Sammel M, Hummel A, et al. Risk factors and clinical features of recurrent ectopic pregnancy: a case control study. Fertil Steril 2003;80:1340.

Chow WH, Daling JR, Weiss NS, et al. Maternal cigarette smoking and tubal pregnancy. Obstet Gynecol 1988;71:167.

Ectopic pregnancy—United States, 1990–1992. MMWR Morb Mortal Wkly Rep 1995;44:46.

Furlong L. Ectopic pregnancy risk when contraception fails: a review. J Reprod Med 2001;47:881.

Gervaise A, Masson L, de Tayrac R, et al. Reproductive outcome after methotrexate treatment of tubal pregnancies. Fertil Steril 2004;82:304.

Graczykowski JW, Mishell Jr DR. Methotrexate prophylaxis for persistent ectopic pregnancy after conservative treatment by salpingostomy. Obstet Gynecol 1997;89:118.

Henderson SR. The reversibility of female sterilization with the use of microsurgery: a report on 102 patients with more than one year of follow-up. Am J Obstet Gynecol 1984;149:57.

Herman A, Ron-El R, Golan A, et al. The role of tubal pathology and other parameters in ectopic pregnancies occurring in in vitro fertilization and embryo transfer. Fertil Steril 1990;54:864.

In vitro fertilization–embryo transfer (IVF-ET) in the United States: 1990 results from the IVF-ET Registry. Medical Research International. Society for Assisted Reproductive Technology (SART), the American Fertility Society. Fertil Steril 1992;57:15.

Kirk E, Papageorghiou AT, Condous G, et al. The diagnostic effectiveness of an initial transvaginal scan in detecting ectopic pregnancy. Hum Reprod 2007;22:2824.

Medical treatment of ectopic pregnancy. Fertil Steril 2006;86:S96.

Ni HY, Daling JR, Chu J, et al. Previous abdominal surgery and tubal pregnancy. Obstet Gynecol 1990;75:919.

Ory SJ, Nnadi E, Herrmann R, et al. Fertility after ectopic pregnancy. Fertil Steril 1993;60:231.

Pauerstein CJ, Croxatto HB, Eddy CA, et al. Anatomy and pathology of tubal pregnancy. Obstet Gynecol 1986;67:301.

Peterson HB, Xia Z, Hughes JM, et al. The risk of pregnancy after tubal sterilization: findings from the U.S. Collaborative Review of Sterilization. Am J Obstet Gynecol 1996;174:1161.

Robertson JN, Hogston P, Ward ME. Gonococcal and chlamydial antibodies in ectopic and intrauterine pregnancy. Br J Obstet Gynaecol 1988;95:711.

Russell JB, DeCherney AH, Laufer N, et al. Neosalpingostomy: comparison of 24- and 72-month follow-up time shows increased pregnancy rate. Fertil Steril 1986;45:296.

Seifer DB, Gutmann JN, Doyle MB, et al. Persistent ectopic pregnancy following laparoscopic linear salpingostomy. Obstet Gynecol 1990;76:1121.

Spandorfer SD, Sawin SW, Benjamin I, et al. Postoperative day 1 serum human chorionic gonadotropin level as a predictor of persistent ectopic pregnancy after conservative surgical management. Fertil Steril 1997;68:430.

Speroff L, Fritz M. Clinical gynecologic endocrinology and infertility. 8th ed. Philadelphia: Lippincott Williams & Wilkins; 2010.

Svensson L, Mardh PA, Ahlgren M, et al. Ectopic pregnancy and antibodies to Chlamydia trachomatis. Fertil Steril 1985;44:313.

Tulandi T, Saleh A. Surgical management of ectopic pregnancy. Clin Obstet Gynecol 1999;42:31, quiz 55.

Uotila J, Heinonen PK, Punnonen R. Reproductive outcome after multiple ectopic pregnancies. Int J Fertil 1989;34:102.

Westrom L. Effect of acute pelvic inflammatory disease on fertility. Am J Obstet Gynecol 1975;121:707.

HYPERTENSIVE DISORDERS OF PREGNANCY

Method of
Brenda Stokes, MD

CURRENT DIAGNOSIS

- Hypertensive disorders of pregnancy are the most common medical disorder in pregnancy.
- Hypertensive disorders of pregnancy are a major cause of maternal and fetal morbidity and mortality.
- Clinicians providing care for pregnant patients should be aware of the signs and symptoms of preeclampsia and screen for them at every visit.

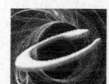

CURRENT THERAPY

- Mild to moderate hypertension in pregnancy does not require treatment.
- Antihypertensive drug selection should be based on the clinician's familiarity with the medication.
- Angiotensin-converting enzyme (ACE) inhibitors, angiotensin receptor blockers, and direct renin inhibitors are contraindicated in pregnancy.
- Low-dose aspirin[1] is beneficial in the prevention of preeclampsia in selected high-risk women.

Hypertensive disorders of pregnancy are the most common medical disorder in pregnancy. Hypertension is estimated to occur in 5% to 12% percent of all pregnancies. It is a major cause of maternal and fetal morbidity and mortality. The hypertensive disorders of pregnancy are classified as shown in Box 1.

Gestational hypertension is the most common cause of hypertension in pregnancy. It is defined as a systolic blood pressure of more than 140 mm Hg and diastolic blood pressure of more than 90 mm Hg on two different measurements at least 4 hours apart. The measurements should be done no more than 1 week apart. This is further classified as mild or severe disease. Mild disease usually develops after 20 weeks gestation with no proteinuria. The pregnancy outcomes with mild disease usually are good. Severe disease is associated with a higher morbidity in pregnancy than is mild preeclampsia. Women with severe disease have rates of preterm delivery, small-for-gestational-age infants, and abruption similar to those for women with severe preeclampsia.

Clinical Characteristics and Diagnosis

Preeclampsia is classically defined as hypertension developing after 20 weeks' gestation and with proteinuria. Hypertension is defined the same for preeclampsia as for gestational hypertension. Proteinuria is defined as excretion of 300 mg or more of protein in a 24-hour urine collection or protein:creatinine ratio equal to or exceeds 0.3. Women who present with hypertension with signs of end-organ dysfunction should be considered to have preeclampsia. Preeclampsia is further divided into mild or severe disease. Multiple risk factors have been associated with the development of preeclampsia. Box 2 lists some of the common risk factors.

There are many theories about the cause of preeclampsia. For example, ongoing investigations suggest that preeclampsia may be an autoimmune disorder caused by pregnancy-induced autoantibodies that activate the angiotensin II receptor type 1a (AT1 receptor). Women with preeclampsia have been found to have autoantibodies that bind and stimulate AT1 receptors. In one study, injection of these AT1 autoantibodies into pregnant mice caused all of the main features of preeclampsia, including hypertension, glomerular endotheliosis, proteinuria, placental abnormalities, and reduced fetal size. There is definitely a relationship between abnormal placentation and preeclampsia, but it is unclear if this is a cause or an effect. For example, a genetic deficiency of an estradiol metabolite, 2-methoxyestradiol (2-ME), may underlie the placental effects in preeclampsia, suggesting that therapeutic supplementation may prevent or treat the disorder. Serum levels

of 2-ME were greatly reduced in a model of preeclampsia, resulting from a lack of placental catechol-O-methyltransferase (COMT) expression. In normal pregnant women, levels of 2-ME are elevated during the third trimester, but in women with preeclampsia, 2-ME levels are lower, and placental expression of COMT protein expression is reduced. This suggests that the actions of COMT and 2-ME are central to proper vascular function in the placenta.

Preeclampsia affects multiple maternal organ systems. It causes proteinuria and can rarely lead to renal failure. Hyperreflexia, grand mal seizures, hemorrhagic stroke (rare), and visual disturbances, including transient blindness, can occur. The vascular system becomes contracted, which increases the hematocrit. Thrombocytopenia, coagulation abnormalities, and hemolysis can occur. Heart failure and pulmonary edema are late complications. Abnormal liver transaminase levels with hepatic congestion and hepatic rupture can also occur.

Preeclampsia also affects the developing fetus. Decreased placental perfusion leads to an increased incidence of intrauterine growth restriction and placental abruption. Oligohydramnios can develop as a result of the poor placental perfusion.

The initial signs and symptoms of preeclampsia vary. Patients typically present with increased blood pressure and proteinuria. Peripheral nondependent edema is common, as is weight gain. Symptoms may include epigastric or right upper quadrant abdominal pain, headaches, and visual disturbances. Most patients present with mild preeclampsia. However, some present with severe disease, which requires prompt diagnosis and treatment. Preeclampsia can manifest antepartum, intrapartum, or postpartum.

An increased rate of maternal and fetal morbidity and mortality is associated with preeclampsia. The rate depends on the severity of maternal disease and the gestational age of the fetus at diagnosis. Mild preeclampsia has been associated with fetal outcomes similar to those for normotensive patients. Patients with mild preeclampsia have a higher rate of cesarean delivery. Severe disease is associated with an increased risk of maternal morbidity and mortality and a higher rate of premature delivery, abruption, and small-for-gestational-age infants. Because of the potential morbidity and mortality associated with preeclampsia, there is interest in early diagnosis and primary prevention in patients at high risk for the disease.

Prevention and Treatment

Many different therapies have been studied for primary prevention of preeclampsia in patients who are at high risk for the disease. Calcium[1] supplementation of 2 g/day or less has been studied, and the incidence of preeclampsia and gestational hypertension has been reduced. The benefit is seen more in patients at high risk for gestational hypertension and in women with a low dietary intake of calcium. Antioxidant supplementation, mostly with vitamins C[1] and E,[1] has been evaluated for preventing preeclampsia. A Cochrane systematic review of many studies failed to show

[1]Not FDA approved for this indication.

any benefits for using antioxidants in pregnancy to prevent preeclampsia or its complications. A prospective cohort study showed a reduction in preeclampsia with supplementation of a multivitamin with folic acid[1] in the second trimester. Antiplatelet therapy, mainly low-dose aspirin,[1] has been moderately effective in reducing the incidence of preeclampsia and its complications in women at high risk for the disease. Physical activity has been studied for the prevention of preeclampsia, but the results have been inconclusive.

Preeclampsia can occur as mild or severe disease. Table 1 shows the clinical manifestations for each type. Disease is considered mild unless any of the criteria for severe disease is met.

The management of preeclampsia, especially severe disease, is controversial. Suggested management plans for mild and severe disease are presented in Figure 1. The recommendations are based on the best available data of maternal and fetal outcomes. The management of preeclampsia depends on the gestational age of the fetus at diagnosis and the severity of illness in the mother. Although some cases can occur in the postpartum period, delivery of the fetus is the definitive treatment for preeclampsia in other situations. Conservative management is recommended in pregnancies at less than 37 weeks' gestation and mothers with mild disease. Bedrest is not recommended for mild disease. Care

includes daily fetal kick counts and blood pressure measurement at least twice a week. Patients with mild disease can be managed on an inpatient or outpatient basis. Laboratory evaluation, which includes urine evaluation for protein, platelet count and liver function testing, should be obtained for all patients at least weekly. Daily fetal kick counts are advised with antenatal fetal testing twice weekly. Serial obstetric ultrasound evaluations are recommended to monitor fetal growth at baseline and then every 3 weeks.

Severe preeclampsia is managed aggressively because of the increased risk of maternal and fetal morbidity. The primary goal in management is the health and well-being of the mother and then the delivery of a mature fetus. All patients with severe preeclampsia require immediate hospitalization. Intravenous magnesium sulfate infusion is recommended for seizure prophylaxis. Antihypertensive medications are recommended to treat systolic blood pressure higher than 160 mm Hg and diastolic blood pressure higher than 110 mm Hg. Corticosteroids are recommended for patients at gestational ages between 22 and 34 weeks. Daily maternal and fetal evaluations with laboratory testing and antepartum fetal testing are recommended. Obstetric ultrasound scans are used to evaluate intrauterine fetal growth restriction (IUGR), oligohydramnios, and abruption.

Choice of the mode of delivery of the fetus is based on the gestational age and the maternal and fetal status. Vaginal delivery is the preferred route of delivery in a patient with preeclampsia.

---

[1]Not FDA approved for this indication.

TABLE 1 Classification of Preeclampsia

FEATURE	MILD DISEASE	SEVERE DISEASE
CNS symptoms	Headache, hyperreflexia	Seizures, blurred vision, scotomas, headache, clonus, irritability
Proteinuria	≥300 mg/24 hours or protein: creatinine ratio > or equal to 0.3	>5 g/24 hours
Liver function	Normal transaminase levels	Elevated transaminase levels, epigastric pain, liver rupture
Platelet level	>100,000/hpf	<100,000/hpf
Hemoglobin level	Normal	Elevated level, hemolysis, DIC
Blood pressure	<160/110 mm Hg	>160/110 mm Hg
Fetal status	Normal AFI, fetal testing, and growth	IUGR, oligohydramnios, signs of fetal distress, abruption, fetal demise

Abbreviations: AFI = amniotic fluid index; CNS = central nervous system; DIC = disseminated intravascular coagulation; hpf = high-power field; IUGR = intrauterine growth restriction.

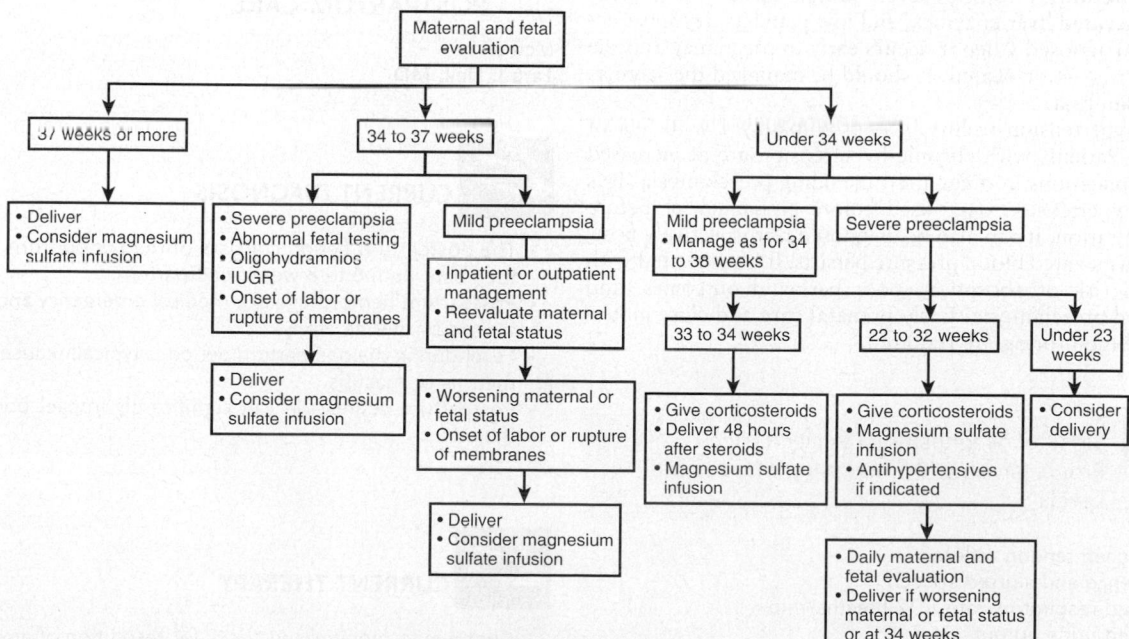

Figure 1. Management of preeclampsia. *Abbreviation:* IUGR = intrauterine growth restriction.

Cesarean delivery should be considered for premature infants, for severe IUGR, and for severe disease with an unfavorable cervix. Continuous fetal monitoring should be instituted intrapartum. Epidural or spinal anesthesia is preferred for cesarean delivery. If necessary, maternal transfer should be considered to an institution that has the ability to care for the newborn infant, who may be premature, and the mother, who may need intensive care monitoring after delivery.

Intravenous magnesium sulfate infusion is typically initiated for seizure prophylaxis intrapartum and continued postpartum. Its use in mild preeclampsia is controversial because the data are not clear about whether the benefits outweigh the risks. The total intravenous fluid rate needs to be monitored closely and usually does not exceed 150 mL/hour. Magnesium sulfate is started as a bolus infusion of 4 to 6 g over 15 to 20 minutes and then continued at a rate of 1 to 2 g/hour. Magnesium toxicity needs to be monitored. Box 3 lists clinical signs of magnesium toxicity. Therapeutic levels are 4 to 8 mg/dL. Urine output should be monitored closely. Calcium gluconate should be available to reverse toxicity if needed. It is administered intravenously as 1 g over 2 minutes. The magnesium sulfate infusion is usually continued for 24 hours postpartum but should be continued longer if clinically indicated.

Blood pressure is monitored closely in the patient with preeclampsia. Treatment is indicated for systolic blood pressure higher than 160 mm Hg and diastolic blood pressure higher than 110 mm Hg. Traditionally, intravenous hydralazine (Apresoline) or labetalol (Trandate) have been used. Oral nifedipine (Procardia) also has been effective.

Eclampsia occurs in the setting of preeclampsia when seizures or coma develop without other identified causes. It can be associated with mild or severe disease, and it can occur antepartum, intrapartum, or postpartum. The pathophysiology is unknown but is thought to include cerebral edema, ischemia, hemorrhage, or transient cerebral arterial vasospasm.

Eclampsia is managed by controlling blood pressure and preventing recurrent seizures. Intravenous magnesium sulfate infusion is the agent of choice for treatment of eclampsia and prevention of recurrent seizures. The maternal airway should be protected and supplemental oxygen given. Fetal heart rate abnormalities, usually fetal bradycardia, may occur but heart rate typically returns to baseline after the seizure. Immediate delivery is not always necessary if the infant and mother are stabilized. Polypharmacy to treat the seizures should be avoided because it only increases maternal side effects.

HELLP syndrome, a form of severe preeclampsia, is defined as hemolysis, elevated liver enzymes, and low platelets. It can sometimes be misdiagnosed when it occurs early in pregnancy and the blood pressure is not elevated. It should be managed the same as severe preeclampsia.

Chronic hypertension occurs in approximately 1% to 5% of pregnancies. Patients with chronic hypertension are at increased risk for complications in pregnancy, including preeclampsia. It is defined as hypertension diagnosed before pregnancy or before 20 weeks' gestation. It can also be diagnosed retrospectively postpartum when elevated blood pressure persists. It is associated with an increased risk of abruption, poor perinatal outcomes, and superimposed preeclampsia. Early prenatal care and close maternal and fetal monitoring are required.

It is unclear whether treatment of chronic hypertension affects pregnancy outcomes, especially for women with mild hypertension. Maternal and fetal outcomes are generally good despite mild hypertension. Antihypertensive medications can reduce the risk of severe hypertension but do not reduce other complications. Medications usually can be discontinued in early pregnancy. Antihypertensive medication is chosen based on the clinician's preference and experience if indicated. Angiotensin-converting enzyme (ACE) inhibitors, direct renin inhibitors and angiotensin receptor blockers are contraindicated in pregnancy.

Hypertensive disorders of pregnancy are the most common medical problems encountered during pregnancy. Hypertension is associated with increased maternal and fetal morbidity and mortality. Close monitoring and appropriate timing of delivery are required to ensure the best possible maternal and fetal outcomes.

References

Abalos E, Duley L, Steyn DW, Henderson-Smart DJ. Antihypertensive drug therapy for mild to moderate hypertension during pregnancy. Cochrane Database Syst Rev 2014;(1): CD002252.

ACOG Task Force on Hypertension in Pregnancy. Hypertension in Pregnancy. ACOG, Washington D.C., 2013.

Askie LM, Duley L, Henderson-Smart DJ, Stewart L. For the PARIS Collaborative Group. Antiplatelet agents for prevention of preeclampsia: A meta-analysis of individual patient data. Lancet 2007;369:1791–8.

Duley L, Henderson-Smart DJ, Meher S. Drugs for treatment of very high blood pressure during pregnancy. Cochrane Database Syst Rev 2013;(3):CD001449.

Duley L, Meher S, Abalos E. Management of preeclampsia. BMJ 2006;332:463–538.

Hofmeyr GJ, Atallah AN, Duley L. Calcium supplementation during pregnancy for preventing hypertensive disorders and related problems. Cochrane Database Syst Rev 2014;(3):CD001059.

Kanasaki K, Palmsten K, Sugimoto H. Deficiency in catechol-O-methyltransferase and 2-methoxyoestradiol is associated with pre-eclampsia. Nature 2008;453: 1117–21.

Leeman L, Fontaine P. Hypertensive disorders of pregnancy. Am Fam Physician 2008;78:93–100.

Meher S, Duley L. Exercise or other physical activity for preventing preeclampsia and its complications. Cochrane Database Syst Rev 2006;(2):CD005942.

Roberts JM, Pearson G, Cutler J, Lindheimer M. Summary of the NHLBI working group on research on hypertension during pregnancy. Hypertension 2003;41: 437–45.

Rumbold A, Duley L, Crowther CA, Haslam RR. Antioxidants for preventing pre-eclampsia. Cochrane Database Syst Rev 2008;(1):CD004227.

Sabai B, Dekker G, Kupferminc M. Pre-eclampsia. Lancet 2005;365:785–99.

Wen SW, Chen XK, Rodger M, et al. Folic acid supplementation in early second trimester and the risk of preeclampsia. Am J Obstet Gynecol 2008;198:45.

Zhou CC, Zhang Y, Irani RA, et al. Angiotensin receptor agonistic autoantibodies induce pre-eclampsia in pregnant mice. Nat Med 2008;14:810–2.

POSTPARTUM CARE

Method of
Tara J. Neil, MD

CURRENT DIAGNOSIS

- The postpartum period consists of the period from delivery of the infant until 6 to 8 weeks postpartum.
- Postpartum hemorrhage is a medical emergency and is usually caused by uterine atony.
- Fever during the postpartum period is typically caused by endometritis or mastitis.
- Postpartum depression can significantly impact bonding with the infant.

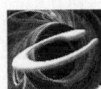

CURRENT THERAPY

- Continue to monitor and check for resolution of any complications or medical conditions that arise during pregnancy.

Box 3 Signs of Magnesium Toxicity, Listed Progressively with Increasing Magnesium Levels

- Loss of deep tendon reflexes
- Somnolence and slurred speech
- Decreased respiratory rate <12 breaths/min
- Decreased urine output
- Pulmonary edema

- Postpartum depression can be treated with psychotherapy and medications.
- Uterine atony responds to massage and medications. Providers should be familiar with the medications and their dosages.
- Postpartum contraception counseling should be started immediately and all forms can be used by 6 weeks postpartum.
- Breast-feeding is the preferred nutrition for newborns and success is dependent on provider counseling and encouragement.

Postpartum care encompasses the period after delivery of infant and placenta until 6 to 8 weeks after delivery. The hormonal and physiologic systems that underwent changes during pregnancy return to normal during this time. During the initial 24 to 48 hours, most patients are monitored in the hospital for possible complications after delivery. Patients should have an appointment 6 weeks after discharge focusing on this period. This chapter addresses postpartum care and complications that can arise.

Postpartum Hemorrhage

Postpartum hemorrhage is defined as blood loss greater than 500 mL after vaginal delivery or greater than 1000 mL after cesarean section. It is the major cause of maternal morbidity and mortality worldwide. Practitioners should be prepared to diagnose and treat the cause.

Some common causes of hemorrhage are identified in Box 1, including the most common cause: uterine atony. Once abnormal bleeding is identified, resuscitation measures should be started, including IV access, nursing assistance, starting fluid resuscitation with crystalloids or blood products, and anesthesia if needed. The uterus should be examined using a bimanual examination and vigorous massage. If the uterus is boggy, the medications listed in Table 1 can be used to improve uterine tone and decrease bleeding. If the bladder is full, a catheter should be placed. Careful inspection of the cervix, vaginal walls, and perineum should be performed to identify other sources of hemorrhage. If bleeding is not slowed or the cause of hemorrhage not identified, manual exploration of the uterus can be performed with proper anesthesia to check for retained products. Surgical treatment with dilation and curettage and hysterectomy can also be used if manual

exploration and medical management do not control bleeding. If the patient is hemodynamically stable and the resources are available, embolization of the uterine arteries can also control bleeding.

Fever and Infection

Fever above 38°C (100.4°F) should be evaluated and a source identified. Box 2 lists the most common causes of postpartum fever. Evaluation should include a physical examination to include the uterus and breasts, with attention to any lacerations or incisions. Laboratory testing should include urinalysis, CBC, and blood cultures if appropriate.

Endometritis, a polymicrobial infection of the endometrium of the uterus, typically causes fever in the first 1 to 2 weeks postpartum. Diagnostic criteria include fever and uterine pain with palpation. Endometritis is treated with intravenous broad-spectrum antibiotics until fever and uterine pain resolves. No oral antibiotics are needed. If there is no clinical improvement after several days of treatment, imaging with computed tomography (CT) or ultrasound of the pelvis can be used to look for complications, including pelvic abscess and septic pelvic thrombophlebitis.

Mastitis causes fever in breast-feeding mothers. It is caused by the introduction of skin flora through cracks in the nipple and skin and infects milk ducts and surrounding soft tissues in areas of stasis. Treatment includes frequent feeding or pumping to alleviate the stasis. There is inadequate evidence to support antibiotic use, but if symptoms persist after effectively emptying breasts, most practitioners treat with a 10- to 14-day course of oral narrow-spectrum antibiotics. Complications can include breast abscesses, which are usually diagnosed by ultrasound.

Immunization

Immunizations should be updated during the postpartum period. Rubella status is routinely checked during the prenatal period and immunization should be given if indicated. Tdap (tetanus toxoid, reduced diphtheria toxoid, and acellular pertussis vaccine [Adacel, Boostrix]) should be given to the patient and offered to other members of the family if they have not received a pertussis booster to help protect the infant from contracting pertussis. Influenza vaccine (Fluzone) should be given if it was not given during pregnancy.

| Box 1 | Causes of Postpartum Hemorrhage |

- Uterine atony
- Vaginal or cervical laceration
- Coagulation disorder
- Uterine inversion
- Retained placenta/products

| Box 2 | Causes of Postpartum Fever |

- Mastitis
- Urinary tract infection
- Wound infection (perineal or abdominal)
- Septic thrombophlebitis
- Deep vein thrombosis

| TABLE 1 | Medications Used to Treat Uterine Atony |

MEDICATION	ADMINISTRATION	FREQUENCY	SPECIAL CONSIDERATIONS
Oxytocin (Pitocin)	10 units IM 10–40 units in 1000 mL of IV solution	Once Continuous to maintain uterine tone	Should not be given directly in IV
Methylergonovine maleate (Methergine)	0.2 mg IM/IV 0.2 mg PO	Repeat every 2–4 hours as needed 3–4 times daily for maximum of 7 days	Contraindicated in hypertension
Carboprost tromethamine (Hemabate)	0.25 mg IM	Repeat every 15–90 minutes. Maximum dose 2 mg	Contraindicated in active cardiac, renal, pulmonary, and liver disease. Use cautiously in asthmatics.
Misoprostol (Cytotec)[1]	800–1000 μg rectally[3]	One time dose	

[1]Not FDA approved for this indication.
[3]Exceeds dosage recommended by the manufacturer.

Rh(D) negative mothers should receive anti-D immune globulin if their infants are Rh(D) positive.

Breast-feeding

Breast milk is universally recognized as the best nutrition for newborns. Infants who are breast-fed have fewer ear, lower respiratory, and gastrointestinal infections. They are also less likely to develop asthma, diabetes, and obesity. Contraindications to breast-feeding include HIV, active herpetic lesions on breasts, maternal drug abuse, and certain medications. Any medications prescribed during breast-feeding should be checked for safety. It is currently recommended, when possible, for infants to be exclusively breast-fed until 6 months and supplemented with foods between the ages of 6 months and one year. Clinicians play a crucial role in educating mothers about the importance of breast-feeding and supporting them during breast-feeding.

Postpartum Depression

Postpartum depression has an incidence as high as 15 percent in the 3 months postpartum. Risk factors include history of depression or postpartum depression, poor social support, family history of postpartum depression, depressed symptoms during pregnancy, and major life events during pregnancy. Baby blues symptoms are less severe and start 2 to 3 days after delivery and resolve within 10 days of delivery. Postpartum depression is seen during the 3 months after delivery, and diagnostic criteria are the same as for depression. Treatment includes psychotherapy and antidepressants. The best choices for breast-feeding mothers include paroxetine (Paxil), fluoxetine (Prozac), and citalopram (Celexa). If not lactating, the choice of medications is similar to those for treating depression. The best screening tool is the Edinburgh postnatal depression scale. Postpartum psychosis is rare but requires inpatient treatment.

Contraception

Discussing contraception after delivery is important for spacing healthy pregnancies. Many women resume intercourse before their scheduled 6 week postpartum appointment so this discussion should begin at the time of discharge. Breast-feeding mothers can use lactational amenorrhea during this period if they are exclusively breast-feeding. They can also use progesterone-only contraception (Micronor) starting 6 weeks postpartum. Combined estrogen-progesterone formulations can be started as early as 3 weeks postpartum in non–breast-feeding mothers. Starting estrogen-containing formulations before this can increase the risk for thromboembolism. Tubal ligation can be done immediately postpartum. Intrauterine devices and diaphragms are typically placed at 6 weeks after the uterus has returned to its normal size. Medroxyprogesterone (Depo-Provera) and etonogestrel (Implanon) may be given in the first 5 days postpartum if a patient is not breast-feeding, and at 6 weeks if breast-feeding.

Other Considerations

Close evaluation and continued management of medical conditions that develop during pregnancy, including thyroid disease, gestational diabetes, and preeclampsia, should be continued.

The postpartum period is an important time for new mothers. Open communication with their providers during this time helps support them and helps them to recognize conditions that are important for their health and the health of their newborn.

References

American College of Obstetricians and Gynecologists. Compendium of Selected Publications. Atlanta: American College of Obstetricians and Gynecologists; 2007.

Breastfeeding, Family Physicians Supporting. Available at: http://www.aafp.org/online/en/home/policy/policies/b/breastfeedingpositionpaper.html; [accessed August 14, 2015].

Centers for Disease Control. Pertussis (Whooping Cough) Vaccination. Available at: http://www.cdc.gov/vaccines/vpd-vac/pertussis/default.htm; [accessed August 14, 2015].

French LM, Smaill FM. Antibiotic regimens for endometritis after delivery. Cochrane Database Syst Rev 2004;(4):CD001067.

Hirst KP, Moutier CY. Postpartum Major Depression. Am Fam Physician 2010;82: 926–33.

Jahanfar S, Ng C-J, Teng CL. Antibiotics for mastitis in breastfeeding women. Cochrane Database Syst Rev 2009;(1):CD005458.

Truitt ST, Fraser AB, Gallo MF, et al. Combined hormonal versus nonhormonal versus progestin-only contraception in lacation. Cochrane Database Syst Rev 2003; (2):CD003988.

VAGINAL BLEEDING LATE IN PREGNANCY

Method of
Jennifer Frank, MD

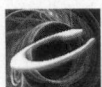

CURRENT DIAGNOSIS

- A patient with late-pregnancy bleeding should only be evaluated with a vaginal examination once placenta previa is excluded by ultrasound.
- A patient can have more than one serious cause of late-pregnancy bleeding.
- Vaginal bleeding with rupture of membranes should prompt consideration of vasa previa.

CURRENT THERAPY

- Complete placenta previa requires cesarean section; however, with a placental edge more than 2 cm from the cervical os, vaginal delivery may be attempted in a stable patient.
- Antenatal diagnosis of vasa previa allowing delivery between 34 and 37 weeks of gestation is associated with significantly reduced perinatal mortality.
- Management of placental abruption ranges from outpatient management of a stable patient to immediate cesarean section in an unstable patient or with nonreassuring fetal heart tones.

Bleeding in the second half of pregnancy complicates 2% to 5% of pregnancies. Placenta previa, placental insertion into the lower uterine segment covering all or part of the internal cervical os, is the most common serious diagnosis, causing 30% of late-pregnancy bleeds and occurring in 0.5% of all pregnancies. Other serious causes include placental abruption (20% of antepartum hemorrhages and 1% of all pregnancies), uterine rupture (occurring in approximately 0.7% of women with a history previous low-transverse cesarean section), and vasa previa (0.5% of late-pregnancy bleeding and approximately 0.0002–0.0008% of all pregnancies). About 2% to 3% of such cases go undiagnosed.

Risk Factors

Higher parity and maternal age, smoking or cocaine use, history of the same condition, and multifetal gestation are risk factors for both placenta previa and abruption. Risk factors for placenta previa also include uterine abnormalities, assisted reproductive technology (ART), and history of uterine surgery, including cesarean section. Additional risk factors for abruption include blunt abdominal trauma, polyhydramnios, and external cephalic version. The greatest risk factor for uterine rupture is a trial of labor following previous cesarean section. A uterine scar increases risk; spontaneous uterine rupture rarely occurs in an unscarred uterus. Other risk factors include uterine abnormalities, maternal connective tissue disease, abnormal placental implantation, and uterine hyperstimulation during labor. Shortened interpregnancy interval (less than 18 to 24 months between pregnancies) can also increase risk. Risk factors for vasa previa include artificial reproductive techniques, bilobed or succenturiate lobed placenta (odds ratio [OR] = 22.11), placenta previa (OR = 22.86), certain fetal anomalies, and velamentous cord insertion.

Pathophysiology
The cause of placenta previa is unknown but may be related to impaired placental attachment in a uterus with a previous scar. Placental abruption, defined as premature separation of the placenta from the uterus, is caused by hemorrhage where the placenta and decidua meet. Abruption is often preceded by vasospasm (such as that induced by cocaine), thrombosis, or shearing forces. Some cases are acute, but many cases could represent a chronic process in which abruption is the end result. Uterine rupture most often occurs in a uterus with a previous scar and is a dehiscence of the scar. Vasa previa occurs when fetal blood vessels are present in the membranes, traversing the cervix beneath the fetal presenting part. The pathophysiology of vasa previa is unknown, although it is theorized to be caused by abnormal development or growth of the umbilical cord secondary to velamentous insertion or reduced intrauterine space.

Prevention
Because previous cesarean section is a risk factor for both placenta previa and uterine rupture, reducing unnecessary cesarean section might prevent these conditions. Patients who have had a cesarean section might decrease the risk of uterine rupture by spacing out the next pregnancy by at least 24 months. Uterine rupture may also be prevented by limiting or avoiding certain agents to induce or augment labor in women undergoing a trial of labor after cesarean section. Although vasa previa cannot be prevented, fetal morbidity and mortality are reduced by early diagnosis and delivery. Placental abruption is associated with smoking and cocaine use; counseling directed to cessation theoretically reduces risk. Seat belts are recommended for all pregnant women; trauma sustained during a motor vehicle accident is a potential cause of abruption. Control of hypertension and treatment of thrombophilia have not been proved to prevent abruption, although both interventions are recommended.

Clinical Manifestations
Placenta previa classically manifests with painless vaginal bleeding, whereas placental abruption and uterine rupture are typically associated with pain and bleeding. Because these conditions are not mutually exclusive, it is important to consider the possibility of more than one serious cause of antepartum hemorrhage. Bleeding secondary to placenta previa may be heavy or light, can recur, and is not associated with the degree of previa or prognosis. Thirty percent of women with placental abruption may have a retroplacental clot concealing an abruption. Approximately one half of women with placental abruption present in labor, and 30% of cases are complicated by fetal death. Monitoring can reveal uterine irritability or hypertonicity. Uterine rupture can manifest with loss of fetal station or palpable uterine defect. Pain and bleeding might not occur until after uterine rupture, when both maternal and fetal status are compromised. Vasa previa is detectable on ultrasound and color Doppler imaging, but it still most commonly occurs as vaginal bleeding with rupture of membranes. Placental abruption, uterine rupture, and vasa previa can manifest with nonreassuring fetal heart tracings.

Diagnosis
Ultrasound can detect placenta previa and vasa previa. In contrast, ultrasound is not reliable in establishing the diagnosis of placental abruption or uterine rupture. Transvaginal ultrasonography (TVU) is recommended to establish placental location because transabdominal ultrasonography has a false-positive rate for placenta previa up to 25%. TVU has a sensitivity of 87.5% and a specificity of 98.8% for placenta previa and is safe in the presence of vaginal bleeding.

Placental abruption has variable appearance on ultrasound, including absence of any abnormality. Diagnosis is made clinically in a patient with bleeding and a hard or tender uterus, uterine irritability, and often a nonreassuring fetal heart tracing, although bleeding may be absent. Vasa previa can be diagnosed using TVU and color Doppler.

High-risk women may be screened in order to plan for cesarean delivery at 34 to 37 weeks of gestation. Vasa previa may also be detected on magnetic resonance imaging (MRI; rarely used), amnioscopy, palpation of vessels during vaginal examination, or identifying fetal blood cells in vaginal blood, although tests to detect fetal hemoglobin cannot be performed quickly enough to be clinically useful.

Differential Diagnosis
In addition to placenta previa, placental abruption, uterine rupture, and vasa previa, diagnostic considerations include bloody show, cervical trauma, cervical polyp, cervical cancer, or infection.

Therapy
Women with placenta previa and active bleeding are managed expectantly in the hospital, although outpatient management may be a reasonable approach in women who are not bleeding, have adequate support at home, and are able to get to the hospital quickly. Cervical cerclage in women with placenta previa and bleeding before term is not currently recommended.

Treatment of women with placental abruption depends on multiple factors including severity of clinical presentation, gestational age, fetal status, and maternal status. In the most severe case in which there has been fetal death, vaginal delivery is acceptable if the maternal status is reassuring. Because of risk for disseminated intravascular coagulopathy (DIC) and blood loss, women should be carefully monitored, proceeding to cesarean section for worsening maternal status or failed vaginal delivery. In mild cases of placental abruption before term, steroids should be administered between 24 and 34 weeks of gestation; preterm birth is the leading reason for perinatal death. With a stable abruption in a preterm patient with reassuring fetal and maternal status, outpatient management may be reasonable after a period of inpatient observation. When placental abruption is known or suspected in a term patient, delivery should proceed. Labor may progress towards a goal of vaginal delivery if both maternal and fetal status are reassuring, although cesarean section should be performed expeditiously for any fetal or maternal compromise. Longer decision-to-incision intervals are associated with worse perinatal outcomes.

Uterine rupture is associated with high perinatal morbidity and mortality as well as potential maternal morbidity and mortality. When rupture is recognized or suspected, delivery should proceed rapidly.

Vasa previa is managed with immediate cesarean section if diagnosed during labor and with planned cesarean section if diagnosed antenatally. Administration of steroids is recommended at 28 to 32 weeks of gestation, and hospitalization should be considered at around 30 to 32 weeks of gestation because approximately 10% of women have premature rupture of membranes and could need urgent cesarean section. Certain patients are appropriate candidates for outpatient management. Optimal time for planned cesarean section is not definitively established and has been recommended between 34 and 37 weeks, with the largest study supporting delivery at 35 to 36 weeks of gestation. Neonatal resuscitation, including transfusion, may be required and should be anticipated.

Monitoring
In placenta previa, the distance between the placental edge and cervical os is monitored during pregnancy because the placental location can change with advancing pregnancy. After 35 weeks' gestation, women with a placental edge more than 20 mm from the internal cervical os may be offered a trial of labor because they are likely to achieve vaginal delivery. Women with any degree of

placental overlap should be delivered by cesarean section. When the placental edge is greater than 0 mm but less than 20 mm from the internal cervical os, vaginal delivery might still be possible, although the likelihood of cesarean section is much higher. Women at increased risk of vasa previa should be screened with TVU and color Doppler. When vasa previa is identified, serial ultrasound is indicated because abnormal vessels regress in up to 15% of women.

Complications

Maternal risks associated with placenta previa include need for cesarean section, postpartum hemorrhage, and blood transfusion. Women who have a history of cesarean section and who have placenta previa are at increased risk for placenta accreta. Fetal risks are primarily associated with prematurity. Placental abruption can cause hypovolemic shock, postpartum hemorrhage, and DIC. Perinatal complications include prematurity, intrauterine growth restriction, anemia, coagulopathy, and death. Uterine rupture can be catastrophic for both mother and baby. Maternal risks include surgical risk associated with cesarean section, hypovolemic shock and hemorrhage, and hysterectomy. Perinatal

morbidity can include hypoxic–ischemic encephalopathy. Stillbirth and neonatal death are possible as well. When undiagnosed prior to labor, vasa previa carries a fetal mortality rate of 55% to 95%. Antenatal diagnosis with planned cesarean section decreases fetal mortality to 3% and reduces the need for transfusion from 60% to 3%. Because the hemorrhage is fetal blood, maternal risk from vasa previa is complications related to cesarean section.

References

Gagnon R, Morin L, Bly S, et al. Guidelines for the management of vasa previa. J Obstet Gynaecol Can 2009;31:748–60.

Magann EF, Cummings JE, Niderhauser A. Antepartum bleeding of unknown origin in the second half of pregnancy: A review. Obstet Gynecol Surv 2005;60:741–5.

Oppenheimer L, Armson A, Farine D, et al. Diagnosis and management of placenta previa. J Obstet Gynaecol Can 2007;29:261–66.

Oyelese Y, Ananth C. Placental abruption. Obstet Gynecol 2006;108:1005–16.

Sinha P, Kuruba N. Ante-partum hemorrhage: An update. J Obstet Gynaecol 2008;28:377–81.

Smith JG, Mertz HL, Merrill DC. Identifying risk factors for uterine rupture. Clin Perinatol 2008;35:85–99.

Zlatnik MG, Cheng YW, Norton ME, et al. Placenta previa and the risk of preterm delivery. J Matern Fetal Neonatal Med 2007;20:719–23.

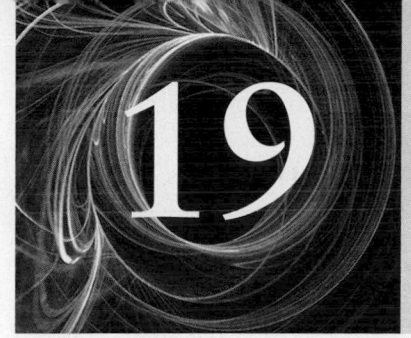

Children's Health

ACUTE LEUKEMIA IN CHILDREN

Method of
Patrick Brown, MD; and Stephen P. Hunger, MD

The word "leukemia" is derived from the Greek roots *leukos* (white) and *haima* (blood). Leukemia, cancer of the blood-forming cells, is characterized by a marked proliferation of abnormal leukocytes in the bone marrow and blood that may be associated with widespread infiltration in extramedullary sites including the central nervous system (CNS), testes, thymus, liver, spleen, and lymph nodes.

Classification

The first level of classification of leukemia is *acute* versus *chronic*. Acute leukemia is characterized by the predominance of very immature white blood cell precursors, or blasts, and is an aggressive, rapidly fatal disease if left untreated. Chronic leukemia is characterized by proliferation of relatively mature white blood cells and is typically an indolent disease.

The second level of classification is *lymphoid* versus *myeloid*, depending on whether the leukemic cells display characteristics of lymphocyte precursors or myelocyte (granulocyte, erythrocyte, monocyte, or megakaryocyte) precursors. Acute lymphoblastic leukemia (ALL) and acute myeloid leukemia (AML) account for the overwhelming majority of pediatric leukemias. Chronic leukemias are uncommon in pediatrics.

ALL and AML are further subclassified by morphology and expression of cell surface antigens using flow cytometry. For ALL, classification is largely based on cell surface and cytoplasmic marker expression (Table 1). AML cases are classified by characteristic chromosomal abnormalities (if present) or by light microscopic morphology in cases where these specific chromosomal changes are absent (Box 1).

Epidemiology

The incidence of childhood cancer is 14 cases per 100,000 children younger than 16 years of age per year, which translates into approximately 11,000 new cases per year in the United States. Leukemia accounts for approximately 30% of childhood cancers, making it the most common form of childhood cancer. The distribution of the major forms of leukemia is vastly different in children than in adults (Figure 1). In general, children are far more likely to have acute leukemia, and ALL is much more common than AML. In adults, most cases of leukemia are chronic, and AML is much more common than ALL.

The incidence of the various forms of leukemia varies by age in both children and adults (Figure 2). This is especially true for childhood ALL, for which there is a marked incidence peak in the 2- to 4-year-old age group. This ALL age peak is primarily found in children living in industrialized nations, leading to speculation that a common environmental exposure, coupled with age-related immunologic susceptibility, is at least partially responsible for many cases of ALL. Except for a small peak in infants, the incidence of AML is fairly constant in childhood but rises quickly in later adulthood.

Prognosis

One of the most dramatic success stories in modern medicine is the improvement in survival of children with ALL over the past four decades. Leukemia was once a uniformly fatal diagnosis, with less than a 5% to 10% cure rate until the mid to late 1960s. Today, approximately 85% of children with ALL are cured. The improved prognosis has been built on pioneering observations on the efficacy of multiagent systemic therapy and the importance of presymptomatic CNS treatment in the late 1960s and early 1970s. Further successive, incremental improvements in outcome have been achieved due to clinical trials conducted by large single centers and national and international cooperative groups that have successfully enrolled a high percentage of eligible children.

Similar approaches have unfortunately not been quite so successful in improving the prognosis of children with AML. Although approximately one half of children with AML are cured today, this has been accomplished by intensifying therapy to the point that the toxic death rate in the early phases of therapy is about 10%. Current research in AML is therefore focusing on developing novel molecularly targeted agents that hold the promise of improving efficacy and limiting toxicity.

Etiology

The question "What is the cause of leukemia?" can be considered on a few different levels. First, what is wrong with *this child* that caused the child to develop leukemia? Second, what is wrong with *the leukemia cell* that causes it to behave so badly? Third, what is wrong with *the leukemia cell's genes* that cause the cell to behave that way?

Predispositions

The answer to the first question is unknown in the vast majority of cases. Attempts to correlate various genetic features or environmental or infectious exposures with risk of childhood leukemia have been largely uninformative. It is presumed that children are particularly susceptible to ALL because of the marked expansion and genetic rearrangement of lymphocytes that occurs during early childhood as the result of exposure to a multitude of immunogenic antigens for the first time. The proliferation required to meet the constant demand for granulocytes, erythrocytes, and platelets is likely a setup for the development of AML in children.

Although a number of constitutional and single-gene disorders are known to confer an increased risk of childhood leukemia (Table 2), in total, these are involved in only a very small minority of cases. The most common of these is Down syndrome. Children with Down syndrome have a 10- to 20-fold increased risk of leukemia, with an approximately equal incidence of ALL and AML. The peak age at onset of leukemia for children with Down syndrome is earlier than for other children. Approximately 30% of Down syndrome children with AML have the megakaryoblastic form (M7AML), a subtype that is extremely rare in children without Down syndrome. In the newborn period, Down syndrome patients can present with transient myeloproliferative disease, a disorder distinguishable from congenital AML primarily by its spontaneous resolution within 3 months. Children with Down syndrome tend to present with biologically favorable subtypes of leukemia, but they also suffer increased toxicity from therapy.

TABLE 1		Classification of Childhood Acute Lymphoblastic Leukemia					
	PHENOTYPIC MARKER					
ALL SUBTYPE	**CD19**	**CD10**	**clg**	**slg**	**%**	**COMMENT**
Pre-pre B	+	−	−	−	5	Mostly infants, poor prognosis, frequent *MLL* 11q23 rearrangements
Early pre-B	+	+	−	−	63	Common ALL, young children, good prognosis
Pre-B	+	+	+	−	16	Older children, good prognosis with intense therapy
B-cell	+	+	+	+	4	Burkitt leukemia, *MYC/Ig* fusion genes, good prognosis with lymphoma-type therapy
T-cell	−	−	−	−	12	Adolescents, anterior mediastinal mass, CNS involvement, good prognosis with intense therapy

Abbreviations: ALL = acute myeloid leukemia; clg = cytoplasmic immunoglobulin; slg = surface immunoglobulin; CNS = central nervous system.

Box 1 — Classification of Childhood Acute Myeloid Leukemia (World Health Organization Criteria)

Acute Myeloid Leukemia with Recurrent Genetic Abnormalities

Acute myeloid leukemia with t(8;21)(q22;q22), *(AML1/ETO)*

Acute myeloid leukemia with abnormal bone marrow eosinophils and inv(16)(p13q22) or t(16;16)(p13;q22), *(CBFβ/MYH11)*

Acute promyelocytic leukemia with t(15;17)(q22;q12), *(PML/RARα)*, and variants

Acute myeloid leukemia with 11q23 *(MLL)* abnormalities

Acute Myeloid Leukemia, Not Otherwise Categorized

Acute myeloid leukemia, minimally differentiated (FAB M0)

Acute myeloid leukemia without maturation (FAB M1)

Acute myeloid leukemia with maturation (FAB M2)

Acute myelomonocytic leukemia (FAB M4)

Acute monoblastic/acute monocytic leukemia (FAB M5)

Acute erythroid leukemia (FAB M6)

Acute megakaryoblastic leukemia (FAB M7)

Abbreviation: FAB = French–American–British classification.

On balance, the prognosis of leukemia in Down syndrome patients is similar to that in other children.

The only environmental exposures that are known to predispose to leukemia are ionizing radiation (such as was seen with atomic bomb survivors) and prior exposure to certain chemotherapy drugs (cyclophosphamide [Cytoxan], etoposide [Vepesid]). There is good evidence that in utero exposure to maternal diagnostic radiation also increases the risk of childhood cancer (including leukemia), particularly if the exposure is in the first trimester. Other environmental or infectious exposures remain unproved as risk factors for childhood leukemia, including electromagnetic fields from power lines.

Cellular Pathogenesis

Three major characteristics of leukemia cells distinguish them from normal hematopoietic cells. They proliferate rapidly, they do not differentiate, and they have defects in apoptosis. This results in a growth advantage for leukemia cells, leading to progressive replacement of the normal bone marrow with a massive clonal population of poorly differentiated leukemic blasts. Another characteristic of leukemia cells is their tendency to spread throughout the body and infiltrate organs other than the bone marrow. This is discussed in more detail in the section on clinical presentation.

Molecular Pathogenesis

As is true of most human cancers, development of leukemia is a multihit process. The initiating or permissive mutation (first hit) in childhood ALL often occurs in utero or early infancy, which is the peak of lymphocyte expansion and recombinase activity.

The initiating events are typically chromosomal rearrangements that activate expression of cellular proto-oncogenes by fusing them to transcriptionally active immunoglobulin or T-cell receptor genes or by joining two genes from different chromosomes to create a new fusion gene that encodes a chimeric protein with unique functional properties. The most common of these sentinel chromosomal rearrangements are translocations (exchanges of genetic material between chromosomes), which can serve as a unique marker of the malignant clone. Retrospective studies of blood obtained at birth and preserved on filter paper used for diagnosis of genetic disorders (Guthrie cards) of children who developed leukemia in early childhood have shown that leukemia-associated fusion genes were present at birth in a large percentage of children, including some who did not develop leukemia for one or more years.

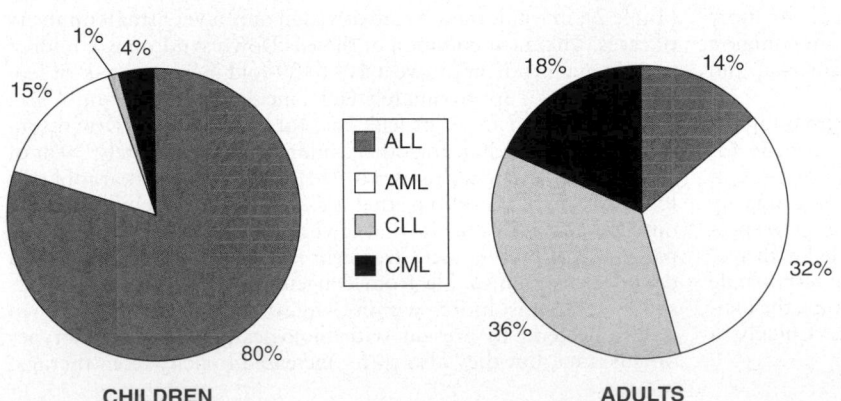

Figure 1. Relative incidence of four major leukemia subtypes in children and adults. *Abbreviations:* ALL = acute lymphoblastic leukemia; AML = acute myeloid leukemia; CLL = chronic lymphoblastic leukemia; CML = chronic myeloid leukemia.

Figure 2. Age-specific incidence of acute lymphoblastic leukemia *(ALL)* and acute myeloid leukemia *(AML)* in children and in adults *(inset)*.

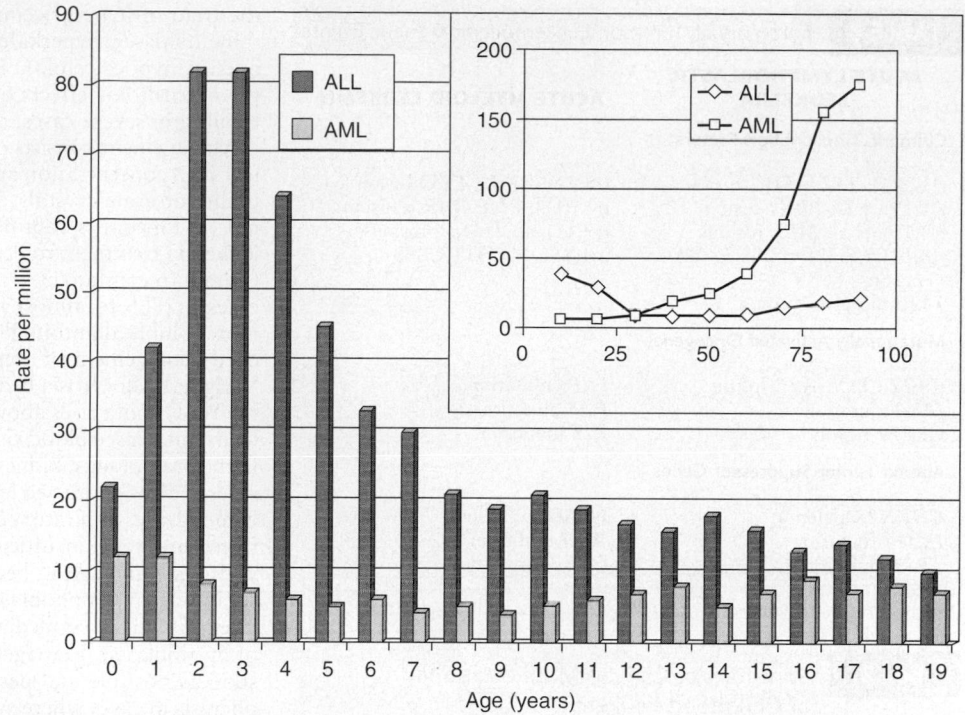

TABLE 2 Summary of Known Constitutional and Heritable Childhood Leukemia Predispositions

DISORDER	INHERITANCE	MALIGNANCY TYPE	COMMENTS
Ataxia-telangiectasia	AR	ALL, NHL	*ATM* gene mutations lead to defective DNA repair
Bloom's syndrome	AR	AML, ALL	Chromosomal instability, sister chromatid exchanges
Down syndrome	Sporadic	AML, ALL	See text
Li-Fraumeni syndrome	AD	AML, ALL, many others	*p53* mutations; leukemias less common than solid tumors
Fanconi's anemia	AR	AML	Chromosomal instability, increased sensitivity to DNA damage
Kostmann's syndrome	AR	AML	G-CSF receptor mutations lead to agranulocytosis
Neurofibromatosis type 1	AD	AML, JMML, MPNST	*NF1* gene mutations lead to enhanced *RAS* signaling

Abbreviations: AD = autosomal dominant; ALL = acute lymphoblastic leukemia; AML = acute myeloid leukemia, AR = autosomal recessive; G-CSF = granulocyte colony-stimulating factor; JMML = juvenile myelomonocytic leukemia; MPNST = malignant peripheral nerve sheath tumor; NHL = non-Hodgkin's lymphoma.

In ALL, the promotional mutation (second hit) likely occurs during the proliferative stress generated by immune responses to exogenous antigens. Because these are maximal in the 2- to 4-year-old age group, this is thought to explain the age peak of childhood ALL during these years. The lack of such a peak in AML suggests that the promotional mutations can occur at any time or are not triggered by immune stimulation. Examples of specific genetic hits known to be associated with the development of childhood leukemia are summarized in Table 3.

Clinical Presentation

Most symptoms and signs of childhood leukemia are the result of the propensity of leukemia cells to replace the bone marrow and infiltrate multiple other organs throughout the body. It is estimated that approximately 10^9 (1 trillion) leukemia cells are present in the child's body at diagnosis.

The replacement of normal bone marrow is responsible for the characteristic abnormal blood counts, which in most cases include the triad of neutropenia, anemia, and thrombocytopenia. Depending on the number of circulating leukemic blasts in the peripheral blood, the total white blood cell count may be low, normal, or high. The neutropenia is often profound (absolute neutrophil count < 500/µL), and is associated with an increased risk of serious infection. Blood cultures and broad-spectrum intravenous antibiotic coverage are indicated in any patient with newly diagnosed leukemia and fever. Anemia is often manifested by fatigue, lethargy, headache, pallor, and, in extreme cases, congestive heart failure that may be precipitated by vigorous transfusion or intravenous hydration. Thrombocytopenia often leads to bruising and petechiae; however, clinically significant hemorrhage is uncommon in industrialized countries. Platelet transfusion is indicated for bleeding or for very low platelet counts (<10,000–20,000/µL).

Infiltration of organs other than the bone marrow with leukemia cells is responsible for additional presenting clinical features. Box 2 summarizes the organ systems most often involved in leukemia and the typical clinical manifestations.

Medical Emergencies in Childhood Leukemia

Newly diagnosed leukemia in a child is a medical emergency. There are several potentially life-threatening complications that may be present at diagnosis or can develop within a short time after diagnosis. The need to diagnose and treat potential infection in patients who are febrile and neutropenic was discussed earlier.

TABLE 3 Summary of Common Leukemogenic Genetic Events

ACUTE LYMPHOBLASTIC LEUKEMIA	ACUTE MYELOID LEUKEMIA
Chimeric Transcription Factors	
t(12;21): *TEL-AML1* fusion	t(8;21): *AML1-ETO* fusion
t(1;19): *E2A-PBX1* fusion	t(15;17): *PML-RAR α* fusion
t(4;11), et al: *MLL* fusions	t(9;11), et al: *MLL* fusions
t(8;14), t(8;22), t(2;8): *Ig-MYC* fusions	inv(16): MYH11-CBFB
T-cell receptor fusions	
Mutationally Activated Oncogenes	
t(9;22): *BCR-ABL* fusion	*FLT3* mutation
JAK2 mutation	*RAS* mutation
CRLF2 fusion	*KIT* mutation
Altered Tumor-Suppressor Genes	
CDKN2A deletion	*NPM1* mutation
IKZF1 mutation	*WT1* mutation
TP53 mutation	*CEBPA* mutation

Box 2 Summary of Clinical Manifestations of Childhood Leukemia*

Bone Marrow
Pancytopenia, bone pain

Reticuloendothelial System
Lymphadenopathy
Hepatosplenomegaly

Thymus
Anterior mediastinal mass (T-cell leukemia)

Bones
Bone pain is common
Fractures and chloromas are rare

Gums
Gingival hypertrophy (M4 and M5 AML)

Skin
Leukemia cutis and chloromas (M2, M4, and M5 AML, infant ALL)

Central Nervous System
Meningitis
Cranial nerve palsies
Rarely intracranial epidural or orbital chloromas (M4 and M5 AML, T-cell ALL)

Kidneys
Often infiltrated or enlarged
Rarely acute renal failure (except in tumor lysis syndrome)

Genitourinary
Testicular enlargement (T-cell ALL)

*See Box 1 for descriptions of classifications.
Abbreviations: ALL = acute lymphoblastic leukemia; AML = acute myeloid leukemia; TBSA = total body surface area.

Tumor lysis syndrome (TLS) is a complication resulting from the rapid lysis of large numbers of tumor cells, releasing intracellular contents. Although TLS is seen most often after initial treatment with chemotherapy, it can also be present before therapy is initiated due to spontaneous lysis. Risk factors include high white blood cell (WBC) count, lymphadenopathy, hepatosplenomegaly, high mitotic index, and a diagnosis of ALL (especially Burkitt's leukemia or lymphoma and T-cell ALL). TLS is characterized by the triad of hyperuricemia (from breakdown of purines by xanthine oxidase), hyperkalemia, and hyperphosphatemia (with secondary hypocalcemia). Renal insufficiency can develop due to the nephrotoxic effects of precipitated urate crystals in the renal tubules; in severe cases, dialysis may be necessary.

Management consists of aggressive hydration to reduce tubular uric acid concentration and alkalinization of urine to promote solubility of urate crystals. The xanthine oxidase inhibitor allopurinol (Zyloprim) is routinely used during the first 3 to 7 days of leukemia treatment to decrease uric acid production. Rasburicase (Elitek) (recombinant urate oxidase) is a new agent used in severe cases of TLS to almost instantaneously convert uric acid to the more soluble allantoin. Frequent electrolyte monitoring with standard management of abnormal levels is essential.

Hyperleukocytosis becomes a potential clinical problem when the WBC count rises above $100,000/\mu L$. Markedly elevated WBCs lead to increased blood viscosity that can produce sludging of blood in the brain, lungs, kidneys, and other organs, causing clinical features such as depressed level of consciousness, stroke, intracranial hemorrhage, respiratory distress, hypoxia, diffuse pulmonary infiltrates, and renal insufficiency. The risk of hyperviscosity is higher with AML than ALL, because myeloblasts are generally larger and stickier than lymphoblasts (likely due to increased expression of integrins and other mediators of cell–cell adherence on the surface of myeloblasts). Management consists of treating the leukemia as soon as possible and performing exchange transfusion or leukopheresis in cases where symptoms are prominent.

Life-threatening bleeding is another potential complication of leukemia. Although all patients with thrombocytopenia are at risk, patients with concomitant coagulopathy due to disseminated intravascular coagulation (DIC) are at particularly high risk. The leukemia subtype most commonly complicated by DIC and serious bleeding is acute promyelocytic leukemia (APL). This association results from the release of thromboplastin from the cytoplasmic granules in promyelocytic blasts. Aggressive blood product support and early treatment with the differentiation-inducing agent all-*trans* retinoic acid (ATRA) has been shown to decrease the risk of bleeding in APL. Despite these measures, up to 10% of patients die of bleeding complications during the initial weeks of therapy, and additional patients suffer lasting morbidity from retinal hemorrhages and nonfatal central nervous system hemorrhages.

Tracheal compression and superior vena cava syndrome can result from large anterior mediastinal masses, which are commonly present in T-cell ALL but are rare in other forms of leukemia. Patients can present with respiratory distress, cough, orthopnea, headaches, syncope, dizziness, facial swelling, or plethora. A chest x-ray should be performed to assess the mediastinum in any patient suspected to have ALL. If the mediastinum is enlarged, a CT is indicated to assess airway patency. This evaluation must precede any attempts at sedation for diagnostic procedures, because even light sedation can precipitate acute airway collapse. Diagnostic material should be obtained by the least invasive method possible before treatment. If necessary, emergent airway compromise can be treated with radiation or steroids, or both.

Differential Diagnosis

Although leukemia should be considered in cases of isolated neutropenia, anemia, or thrombocytopenia, the vast majority of leukemia patients present with depressions in more than one cell line. In suspected cases of immune thrombocytopenic purpura (ITP), for example, a careful review of the peripheral blood smear should be performed to rule out the presence of circulating leukemic blasts. Routine bone marrow aspiration is not necessary for children with ITP, but it should be performed in patients with atypical features, such as concomitant anemia or neutropenia, hepatosplenomegaly, bone pain, or significant weight loss. Treatment of ITP with corticosteroids should only be instituted after evaluation by an experienced hematologist.

Pancytopenia can be caused by diseases other than leukemia. Some viral infections have a propensity to suppress bone marrow function and cause low peripheral blood cell counts, including Epstein-Barr virus (EBV), herpes simplex virus (HSV), influenza, hepatitis viruses, and HIV. Infectious mononucleosis from EBV infection can be particularly difficult to differentiate from leukemia, because patients often have hepatosplenomegaly and circulating atypical lymphocytes (which can appear very similar to leukemic blasts). Pancytopenia on the basis of bone marrow failure (from acquired aplastic anemia or rare inherited bone marrow failure syndromes) can be distinguished from leukemia by bone marrow biopsy for assessment of overall marrow cellularity. Certain solid tumors have a tendency to metastasize to the bone marrow and cause cytopenias, including neuroblastoma, rhabdomyosarcoma, and retinoblastoma, but it is rare for pancytopenia to be the primary presenting feature in these cases.

Joint pain, fever, hepatosplenomegaly, and pallor are common presenting features in both systemic-onset juvenile rheumatoid arthritis (JRA) and leukemia. A bone marrow aspirate should be performed to rule out leukemia before treatment with steroids in suspected cases of systemic-onset JRA.

Risk Stratification

In the last several years, treatment decisions for children with newly diagnosed acute leukemia have been based on the concept of risk stratification. Using factors identified during clinical trials to predict a high or low risk of relapse, patients are separated into risk groups before the start of treatment or at the end of the first month of induction therapy. The treatment plan is then tailored to the degree of risk. The desired result is that patients with relatively low-risk disease can be treated with less toxic therapy without compromising cure rates, and patients with high-risk disease receive more-intensive, potentially toxic therapy. The risk groups are currently defined based on several criteria and differ for ALL and AML. Different centers and cooperative groups typically employ different risk-stratification strategies.

In ALL, the initial risk assessment is based on two simple clinical parameters that are available immediately at the time of diagnosis (the National Cancer Institute [NCI] or Rome criteria): WBC count (>50,000/μL is high risk), and age (<1 year or >9 years is high risk). Further refinement of risk assignment is often based on a combination of leukemia phenotype (B- vs T-lineage), the presence of certain sentinel cytogenetic lesions, and how quickly the patient's leukemia responds to the first few weeks of therapy (rapid clearance of leukemia cells from the blood or marrow is associated with a lower risk of relapse).

Low-risk cytogenetic features include hyperdiploidy (≥50 chromosomes in the leukemia cells) or trisomies of specific chromosomes and the presence of a t(12;21) that results in TEL/AML1 fusion. High-risk cytogenetic features include hypodiploidy (<44 chromosomes in the leukemia cells) and the presence of either an 11q23 (MLL gene) rearrangement or a t(9;22), or Philadelphia chromosome, that creates a BCR/ABL fusion gene.

Early response has historically been measured by the response to a prednisone prophase that includes a single dose of intrathecal methotrexate and 7 days of prednisone, or by the percentage of blast cells remaining in the bone marrow after 7 to 14 days of multiagent therapy. Over the past 10 to 15 years, measures of tumor burden remaining in the marrow at the end of induction therapy (minimal residual disease) have been shown to be highly predictive of outcome and have been integrated into risk-stratification schemata of all of the major leukemia cooperative groups.

In AML, risk stratification is based largely on cytogenetics. Low-risk features include a t(8;21), which results in the AML1/ETO fusion, and either inv(16) or a t(16;16), both of which create the CBFβ/MYH11 fusion. High-risk features include monosomy 7 and abnormalities in the long arm of chromosome 5. In addition to these cytogenetic abnormalities, failure to achieve remission with induction chemotherapy is another high-risk feature in AML. All other cytogenetic abnormalities, as well as normal cytogenetics (which are seen in approximately 60% of cases), are considered intermediate risk. More recently, a specific type of genetic mutation in the tyrosine kinase gene FLT3 has been identified as another high-risk feature. This type of FLT3 mutation (called an internal tandem duplication [ITD]) occurs in 10% to 15% of childhood AML.

Treatment

There are significant differences in the specific treatments for ALL and AML, so they will be discussed separately. Table 4 summarizes the most salient features of the treatment for each.

TABLE 4	Summary of Treatment for Childhood Leukemia	
CHARACTERISTICS	**ACUTE LYMPHOBLASTIC LEUKEMIA**	**ACUTE MYELOID LEUKEMIA**
Remission Induction		
Chemotherapy	4 wk with prednisone or dexamethasone, vincristine, L-asparaginase, doxorubicin (not all cases)	Two courses (6–8 wk) with cytarabine (Ara-C), doxorubicin, others (e.g., etoposide, thioguanine)
Toxic death rate	Low (<3%)	High (>10%)
Remission rate	>98%	75%–85%
CNS Preventive Therapy		
Intrathecal chemotherapy	Methotrexate	Cytarabine
Cranial irradiation	For high risk (blasts in CSF at diagnosis and/or high WBC count)	None
Consolidation		
Chemotherapy	Combinations of various drugs (not cross-resistant) Intensity/duration based on risk stratification	Based on cytogenic/molecular risk group and minimal residual disease (MRD) Low risk: 2–3 additional courses Intermediate risk: If MRD-negative, treat as low risk; if MRD positive, treat as high risk High risk: BMT for patients with best available donor
Maintenance		
Chemotherapy	Low-dose oral (6-mercaptopurine and methotrexate) Total duration of therapy 2–3 y	No maintenance therapy (does not improve survival)

Abbreviations: BMT = bone marrow transplant; CNS = central nervous system; CSF = cerebrospinal fluid; HLA = human leukocyte antigen; WBC = white blood cell.

Acute Lymphoblastic Leukemia

Treatment for ALL generally occurs in four phases: remission induction, CNS preventive therapy, consolidation, and maintenance. Remission induction in ALL typically lasts 4 to 6 weeks and includes three to five systemic agents. Common to almost all regimens are a corticosteroid (either prednisone [Deltasone] or dexamethasone [Decadron]), vincristine (Vincasar), and L-asparaginase (Elspar), which compose the three-drug induction. An anthracycline, typically doxorubicin (Adriamycin), is also included in many regimens (four-drug induction), with other agents such as cyclophosphamide (Cytoxan) or etoposide (VePesid) used in a small minority of centers. More than 98% of children enter remission by the end of 4 weeks of induction therapy, and the mortality rate from toxicity during induction therapy is generally less than 2% to 3% in industrialized countries.

The concept that the CNS could be a sanctuary site for leukemia emerged in the mid 1960s when the introduction of multiagent systemic chemotherapy led to high remission rates, but a majority of patients relapsed within 6 to 12 months, with many of these recurrences being limited to the CNS. Routine introduction of presymptomatic CNS radiation in the late 1960s and early 1970s led to substantial increases in cure rates to approximately 50%. Modern CNS preventive therapy includes periodic administration of intrathecal chemotherapy (usually methotrexate) starting at the time of the first diagnostic lumbar puncture. Systemic agents with improved CNS penetration (dexamethasone rather than prednisone, higher doses of intravenous methotrexate) might also play an important role in CNS control. Cranial irradiation is currently reserved for patients at the highest risk for CNS relapse (e.g., those with high diagnostic WBC count or leukemic blasts in CSF at diagnosis). Over time, CNS radiation has been given to fewer and fewer ALL patients; some groups believe that it can be eliminated for all patients. With these modern strategies, the risk of isolated CNS relapse is less than 5%.

Following the induction of remission, patients receive additional chemotherapy designed to consolidate the remission. The intensity and duration of the consolidation phase are risk based, and alternating cycles of non–cross-resistant chemotherapy drugs are typically used. These consolidation or intensification phases typically last about 6 months and often include a reinduction phase similar to the first month of treatment.

It has been clearly demonstrated that the risk of relapse in ALL can be reduced with an extended phase of continuous low-dose chemotherapy (maintenance) that lasts until 2 to 3 years from the time of diagnosis. Oral 6-mercaptopurine (Purinethol) and methotrexate are used universally, with variable administration of intrathecal chemotherapy. Some centers or groups also employ periodic doses of vincristine and 5- to 7-day pulses of prednisone or dexamethasone. The optimal frequency of intrathecal chemotherapy treatments and vincristine and steroid pulses is uncertain and might depend on the intensity of therapy delivered during the induction and consolidation phases.

Acute Myeloid Leukemia

Remission induction in AML typically consists of two courses of very intensive chemotherapy with cytarabine (Tarabine) and doxorubicin, often combined with thioguanine (Tabloid) or etoposide. Remission rates are 75% to 85%, with about one half of the failures due to resistant leukemia and the others to mortality from toxicity (usually infection).

Similar to ALL, CNS preventive therapy in AML begins at diagnosis with intrathecal chemotherapy (usually cytarabine) and continues with additional periodic intrathecal treatments during consolidation. High-dose cytarabine, which is a key component of most AML treatment regimens, also contributes to CNS treatment. Cranial radiation is not typically administered by most groups to children with AML, except for treatment of chloromas (solid masses of leukemia cells) that do not resolve with chemotherapy.

Consolidation in AML is risk dependent. High-risk patients can be identified who have less than a 20% to 25% chance of cure with intensive chemotherapy. Most groups consider these patients to be candidates for BMT. If a matched sibling is unavailable, then alternative donor sources (e.g., matched unrelated bone marrow or umbilical cord blood) are usually offered. For low-risk patients, for whom the cure rate with chemotherapy alone approaches 70%, BMT is usually not offered in first remission, even for patients with a matched sibling donor. In addition, relapses in low-risk patients, unlike relapses in intermediate-risk or high-risk patients, can often be successfully treated with BMT in second remission, justifying reservation of BMT for use as a salvage therapy for low-risk patients. Consolidation in these cases consists of two to three additional chemotherapy courses that are slightly less intense and usually consist of cytarabine combined with drugs not used in induction, such as mitoxantrone (Novantrone) and L-asparaginase. For intermediate-risk patients, minimal residual disease (MRD) testing at the end of induction is increasingly being used to determine whether to consolidate with chemotherapy or BMT. Unlike ALL, most groups have found no benefit to extended maintenance therapy in children with AML.

Relapse

The most common site of relapsed leukemia is the bone marrow (with or without concomitant CNS involvement). Less common are isolated extramedullary relapses (CNS or testicular relapse

---

TABLE 5 Summary of Late Effects of Leukemia Treatment

LATE EFFECT	TREATMENT-RELATED RISK FACTORS	DIAGNOSTIC APPROACH
Bone	Avascular necrosis, osteonecrosis	X-ray and/or MRI of major joints for persistent pain
Cardiac dysfunction	Anthracyclines: cardiomyopathy (risk related to cumulative dose, higher risk in AML)	ECG or echocardiogram every 3 y (cardiomyopathy can occur decades after treatment)
Cataracts	CNS RT	Yearly eye examination
CNS and psychosocial	CNS RT, IT chemotherapy: learning problems, neurocognitive dysfunction	Yearly educational assessment, neurocognitive testing
Dental abnormalities	CNS RT	Dental examination at age 5
Endocrine and reproductive	CNS RT: pituitary dysfunction Alkylators: primary gonadal failure	Yearly growth curves, TSH, LH, FSH LH, FSH, estradiol or testosterone, semen analysis
Hepatic dysfunction	Methotrexate, 6-mercaptopurine, 6-thioguanine: late hepatic fibrosis	Yearly LFTs
Secondary neoplasms	CNS RT: brain tumors Alkylators or epipodophyllotoxins: secondary AML	MRI for symptoms Yearly CBC

Abbreviations: ALL = acute lymphoblastic leukemia; AML = acute myeloid leukemia; CNS = central nervous system; ECG = electrocardiogram; FSH = follicle stimulating hormone; IT = Intrathecal; LFT = liver function test; LH = luteinizing hormone; MRI = magnetic resonance imaging; RT = radiation therapy; TSH = thyroid-stimulating hormone.

in ALL, chloromas in AML). For both ALL and AML, a critical determinant of outcome following relapse is the time from diagnosis to relapse.

ALL patients who relapse within 18 months of initial diagnosis have a dismal outcome, with only about one half able to attain a second remission and less than 10% overall cure rate; the outcome is marginally better for those who relapse between 18 and 36 months after diagnosis. ALL patients with such early relapses are typically treated with 3 to 4 months of intensive therapy in an attempt to achieve a second remission and attain further cytoreduction, followed by BMT using a matched sibling or unrelated donor. In contrast, children with ALL who relapse more than 3 years after initial diagnosis have an approximately 95% chance of entering a second remission, and 40% to 45% can be cured with intensive chemotherapy; these patients are generally considered to be candidates for matched sibling, but not unrelated donor, BMT in second remission.

Overall, relapsed AML has a dismal outcome (long-term survival approximately 20%), and the approach is to attempt to reinduce remission and then proceed to BMT or investigational treatments. Even in this setting, there is clearly an improved outcome for patients who relapse after a prolonged initial remission (>12 months from the end of remission-induction therapy) compared with patients who have refractory disease or who relapse after a shorter period of remission.

New treatment strategies are urgently needed for patients with relapsed ALL and AML, because the current regimens produce poor results and are associated with a great deal of toxicity. The major clinical trial groups are testing novel and targeted therapies in these patient populations.

Late Effects

Approximately 70% of children with leukemia are cured of their disease. As the numbers of long-term survivors of childhood leukemia has grown, there has been increasing interest in assessing the late effects of leukemic therapy. In childhood ALL, with cure rates of 85%, a major effort is being made in ongoing clinical trials to reduce the intensity of therapy for lower-risk patients, with the hope of reducing late effects of therapy without compromising high cure rates. The most common late effects of leukemia therapy, with the known treatment-related risk factors and recommended diagnostic approach for each, are summarized in Table 5. Many pediatric oncology centers have developed late-effects programs to conduct surveillance for the development of these problems and provide follow-up care to patients who develop late complications of therapy.

References

Brown P, Small D. FLT3 inhibitors: A paradigm for the development of targeted therapeutics for paediatric cancer. Eur J Cance 2004;40:707–21.

Gaynon PS, Qu RP, Chappell RJ, et al. Survival after relapse in childhood acute lymphoblastic leukemia: Impact of site and time to first relapse—the Children's Cancer Group Experience. Cancer 1998;82:1387–95.

Gibson BE, Wheatley K, Hann IM, et al. Treatment strategy and long-term results in paediatric patients treated in consecutive UK AML trials. Leukemia 2005;19:2130–8.

Greaves MF, Wiemels J. Origins of chromosome translocations in childhood leukaemia. Nat Rev Cancer 2003;3:639–49.

Hitzler JK, Zipursky A. Origins of leukaemia in children with Down syndrome. Nat Rev Cancer 2005;5:11–20.

Meshinchi S, Alonzo TA, Stirewalt DL, et al. Clinical implications of FLT3 mutations in pediatric AML. Blood 2006;108:3654–61.

Moghrabi A, Levy DE, Asselin B, et al. Results of the Dana—Farber Cancer Institute ALL Consortium Protocol 95–01 for children with acute lymphoblastic leukemia. Blood 2007;109:896–904.

Mrozek K, Heinonen K, Bloomfield CD. Clinical importance of cytogenetics in acute myeloid leukaemia. Best Pract Res Clin Haematol 2001;14:19–47.

Pinkel D, Simone J, Hustu HO, Aur RJ. Nine years' experience with "total therapy" of childhood acute lymphocytic leukemia. Pediatrics 1972;50:246–51.

Pui CH, Cheng C, Leung W, et al. Extended follow-up of long-term survivors of childhood acute lymphoblastic leukemia. N Engl J Med 2003;349:640–9.

Pui CH, Evans WE. Treatment of acute lymphoblastic leukemia. N Engl J Med 2006;354:166–78.

Pui CH, Mahmoud HH, Rivera GK, et al. Early intensification of intrathecal chemotherapy virtually eliminates central nervous system relapse in children with acute lymphoblastic leukemia. Blood 1998;92:411–5.

Pui CH, Sandlund JT, Pei D, et al. Improved outcome for children with acute lymphoblastic leukemia: Results of Total Therapy Study XIIIB at St Jude Children's Research Hospital. Blood 2004;104:2690–6.

Ries LAG, Melbert D, Krapcho M, et al. SEER Cancer Statistics Review, 1975–2004. Bethesda, Md: National Cancer Institute; 2007.

Schrappe M, Reiter A, Zimmermann M, et al. Long-term results of four consecutive trials in childhood ALL performed by the ALL-BFM study group from 1981 to 1995. Berlin–Frankfurt–Munster. Leukemia 2000;14:2205–22.

Stahnke K, Boos J, Bender-Gotze C, et al. Duration of first remission predicts remission rates and long-term survival in children with relapsed acute myelogenous leukemia. Leukemia 1998;12:1534–8.

Wakeford R, Little MP. Risk coefficients for childhood cancer after intrauterine irradiation: A review. Int J Radiat Biol 2003;79:293–309.

Woods WG, Kobrinsky N, Buckley JD, et al. Timed-sequential induction therapy improves postremission outcome in acute myeloid leukemia: A report from the Children's Cancer Group. Blood 1996;87:4979–89.

Woods WG, Neudorf S, Gold S, et al. A comparison of allogeneic bone marrow transplantation, autologous bone marrow transplantation, and aggressive chemotherapy in children with acute myeloid leukemia in remission. Blood 2001;97:56–62.

ADOLESCENT HEALTH

Method of
Kari R. Harris, MD

CURRENT DIAGNOSIS

- In addition to general medical care, it is important to identify psychosocial health concerns at all adolescent visits.
- The key components of a psychosocial history are addressed in the HEADS private and confidential interview.
- Conducting a Home/Education/Employment/Activities/Accident Prevention/Diet/Disordered Eating/Drugs/Depression/Suicide/Self-harm/Sex/Sleep/Social Media (HEADS) interview is standard practice for adolescent care: it should be part of all adolescent well-checks and used, as time permits, in acute visits for teens who have high-risk behaviors or have no regular health care.
- High acuity areas identified from the HEADS interview include substance use, disordered eating, sexual activity, and mental health.
- Depression screening should be part of well visits for all patients between 11 and 21 years of age.
- Substance use screening should be included in all adolescent well visits.
- HIV screening should be completed initially between 16 and 18 years of age and the need for re-screening reassessed annually.

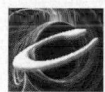

CURRENT THERAPY

- Long acting reversible contraception (LARC) provides safe and effective contraception for teenagers.
- Emergency contraception should be offered within 5 days of unprotected sexual activity.
- Treatment for teens is often multidisciplinary involving subspecialists, mental health providers, medical or psychiatric inpatient units, and county welfare or health departments.

Setting the Stage for the Adolescent Visit

Comprehensive care for adolescents includes screening for high-risk behaviors in addition to routine medical care. To facilitate open communication, providers should be clear about consent and confidentiality policies in their practices. This can be achieved by discussing policies with patients and parents/caretakers during young adolescent visits (11–14 years) and by providing materials documenting the policies and practices such as a standard letter to parents. Policies can also be displayed in the office, provided in practice newsletters and materials, and available through patient access portals.

Adolescent visits differ from early childhood visits in several important respects. At the beginning of the visit, time should be spent with both the teen and his/her parent or caregiver clarifying medical history and current concerns. The adolescent should then be offered time without the parent or caregiver present in order to discuss sensitive issues, including reproductive and mental health. At the end of the visit, the parent/caregiver should be provided with a summary of the visit, limited to the nonconfidential portion, and including recommendations and arrangements for follow-up appointments.

Consent and Confidentiality Laws—Consent does not Equal Confidential

Consent and confidentiality laws vary by state. Most states allow minors to consent for reproductive health care, including testing and treatment for sexually transmitted infections. Most states also allow providers to prescribe contraceptives to minors. Many states have a "mature minor" statute that allows physicians to provide care if they deem the adolescent patient mature and capable of understanding the medical care. These laws give teens autonomy to consent to their own health care and they also enable care to be provided when a parent is unable to attend the appointment.

While consent and confidentiality laws are related, they are separate entities. Many states allow minors to consent for specific health services but do not prohibit a provider from informing the teen's parent/caretaker about that service. Even if allowed by law, expert consensus holds that such disclosures should only be made when in the best interest of the minor patient. The disclosure should not compromise future health care. Many teens will not seek reproductive health care if they have to involve a parent, making confidentiality necessary for comprehensive adolescent health care.

Confidentiality is limited when a minor patient is in direct harm such as intimate partner violence, sexual coercion or rape, certain pregnancy, suicidality, or self-harm. In such instances, a parent/caretaker should become involved, unless he/she is the perpetrator or some other extraordinary circumstances exist. Local authorities or social welfare agencies may also need to be contacted. These necessary breeches in confidentiality to protect safety must be explained beforehand to the patient and be included in written policies. Any breach of confidentiality must be carried out in a professional manner, explained sensitively to the patient and others, and well documented. Every attempt must be made not to compromise future care.

Information on consent and confidentiality laws for each state is available at the Guttmacher Institute website (guttmacher.org) and from Physicians for Reproductive Health (http://prh.org/resources/minors-access-cards/).

The HEADS Interview

The HEADS acronym provides a structured psychosocial history-taking tool that also screens for high-risk behaviors (Table 1). Although several variations of HEADS have been described, they all cover the most common risk categories for adolescents. Progressing from the least invasive topics to the most sensitive issues, HEADS covers all essential categories (see Table 1).

When using the HEADS interview tool, it is important to build rapport with the patient. The teen deserves explanation of why they are being asked personal questions and every attempt should be made to increase patient comfort and trust. The interview begins with questions regarding hobbies, school, and home life. Once rapport is established, questions proceed to more sensitive issues. Questioning should be open-ended, nonassuming and nonjudgmental. This allows for honest answers and does not discriminate among patients.

TABLE 1		HEADS Acronym
H	Home	Who lives with you at home? Tell me about your relationships at home. Are you safe at home? Do you have a trusted adult to confide in at home? Do you have your own space at home? Have there been any changes at home?
E	Education	What grade are you in and what school? Is your school safe? Tell me about your friends. Does anyone bother you at school? How are your grades? Do you have any problems with school? Have you ever gotten in trouble for missing school? Do you plan to graduate? What do you want to do after graduation?
	Employment	Are you working? Do you like your job? Do you help your family with finances? Do you feel stressed because of work; is your family stressed by your work? How many hours a week do you work?
A	Activities	What do you do for fun? Who do you hang out with? Tell me what you do after school. Are you in any organized after-school or summer activities? Tell me about your hobbies.
	Accident prevention	Tell me about your activities. Do you wear a seatbelt? Do you wear a helmet while biking or using an all-terrain vehicle? Have you ever ridden with someone while they were under the influence of drugs or alcohol, or have you ever driven under the influence?
D	Diet/Disordered eating	Tell me about your diet. Do you eat breakfast daily? How many fruits and vegetables do you eat? How do you feel about your weight? Do you like the way you look? Have you ever not eaten to try to lose weight? Do you ever feel guilty about what you have eaten? Have you ever skipped meals or thrown up on purpose after you have eaten?
	Drugs	Have you seen drugs at your school? Do any of your friends smoke, drink alcohol, or use other drugs? Have you ever tried drugs? Have you ever been in trouble because of drug use?
	Depression	Do you ever feel sad, down, or depressed? Have you ever felt like you had nothing to look forward to? Do you still like to do the things you used to do?
S	Suicide/self-harm	Have you ever been so upset you have wanted to hurt yourself? Have you ever cut yourself? Have you ever thought about killing yourself or someone else?
	Sex	Are you in a relationship? When is the last time you had sex? Did you use a condom? Are you using anything to prevent pregnancy? Have you ever been tested for STIs? How many partners have you had? Tell me about your partner (age, gender, etc). Do you feel safe with your partner? Have you ever been forced to have sex or do something you were not comfortable with?
	Sleep	What time do you go to bed? Where is your cell-phone when you go to sleep? When do you wake up in the morning?
	Social Media	What social media sites do you have profiles on? Are you friends with people you do not know in real life? How much time do you spend on social media? Does this affect your grades? Tell me about your privacy settings. Do you have any trusted adults that can access your social media sites?

Adapted from: Klein, DA, Goldenring, JM. HEEADSSS 3.0: The psychosocial interview for adolescents updated for a new century fueled by media. Contemporary Pediatrics. 2014. Available at http://contemporarypediatrics.modernmedicine.com/contemporary-pediatrics/news/probing-scars-how-ask-essential-questions?page=full [accessed Oct 13, 2014].

Home/Education/Employment/Activities/Accident Prevention

These topics begin the confidential interview with the least risky activities for adolescents. Although grouped together in this text, each category deserves its own time and questions (see Table 1). All adolescents should have a trusted adult with whom they can discuss concerns. Safety at home and school safety, including any bullying or coercion regardless of site or circumstances, should be discussed and addressed. Current school performance, concerns, grades and post-graduation goals should be discussed. After school employment has benefits, but can also negatively impact academic performance, mood, or family dynamics. These should be screened for and addressed if present. Healthy after-school activities should be encouraged. Predictably, adolescent illegal activity, drug use, and sexual activity, peak during after-school hours. Participation in organized, supervised, extracurricular activities has been shown to decrease these risky behaviors and confer positive health and emotional benefits. Accidents remain the leading cause of death for this age group and prevention should be emphasized. Safety should be assessed at this time as well as throughout the course of the interview as it applies to each topic.

Diet/Disordered Eating

Nutritional health problems are of concern with adolescents. Many lifestyle habits, especially regarding nutrition, are formed during this period. Asking the teen to describe his/her typical diet provides insight on potential areas for improvement. Limiting portion sizes, avoiding excessive or late night snacking, and replacing sugary drinks with water is common advice for teens. This portion of the interview provides opportunity to screen for body image distortion or disordered eating. The growth chart should be reviewed and any significant weight changes discussed.

Drugs (Substance Use)

When asking about riskier behaviors, it is important to have rapport and trust. The subject of substance use can be broached by asking if peers use substances. Because alcohol, marijuana, and tobacco use is so prevalent among high school students (reported by 65%, 40%, and 40%, respectively), this initial question can make a teen more comfortable moving on to talk about personal use. The CRAFFT acronym is a brief and effective screening tool designed specifically for use with adolescents and helps the provider determine if further conversation or evaluation regarding substance use is warranted. The questions are broken into part A and B. If a patient answers "yes" to any questions in A, then part B questions are asked. If the patient answers "yes" to two or more questions of part B, the screen is positive and further evaluation is recommended (Table 2). If necessary, referral should be made to a qualified mental health provider for treatment. Substance use is a leading cause of morbidity and mortality for teens in the United States and teens who use substances at an early age are more likely to become addicted. Substance use should not be ignored or minimized by providers. Counseling on prevention should contain a clear message of nonuse.

Depression/Suicide/Self-Harm

Depression screening is recommended at all well-visits. Several screening tools are available. Questions covering loss of interest in normal activities and feeling depressed, down, or hopeless, open the door to more specific questions regarding signs and symptoms of depression. In addition to depressive feelings, teens should be explicitly screened for suicidal intention, past attempts, plans, self-harm, and safety. If a teen discloses an unsafe environment, law enforcement should be included in immediate plan of care. If a teen is actively suicidal then immediate inpatient treatment is warranted. Outpatient treatment for mental health disorders in teens includes cognitive therapy with or without medication. For most teens, parental involvement is necessary when treating mental health disorders. If the provider feels the teen is unsafe due to their own actions or those of others, then the confidential

 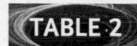
interview is no longer appropriate and the caretaker must be included in the next stage of management.

Sex

Nearly half of high school students have had sex. Of those, only about a quarter used reliable contraception at their last intercourse. Adolescents and young adults account for the majority of gonorrhea and chlamydia cases each year. Risk factors for morbidity related to sexual activity include early sexual initiation, increasing number of partners, substance use prior to sex, and unprotected sexual acts. Teenagers and men who have sex with men are the highest population groups at risk for sexually transmitted infections (STIs). STI screening should be discussed. Recommendations are outlined in Table 3.

When discussing the sensitive issue of sex with teens it is important to use neutral terms and remain nonjudgmental. Sexual history should include age of first sexual encounter, age of partner (s), gender of partner, number of partners, type of sexual activities, date of last sexual activity, contraceptive and barrier use. Quality of relationships should also be assessed as 10% of high school students report that they have experienced sexual dating violence including sexual coercion and rape. As with substance use, providers should relay a clear message of abstinence as the safest method to prevent morbidity. Even for patients who are already sexually active, delaying future sex should be recommended.

Teens should be counseled on contraceptive options, emphasizing that LARC (intrauterine contraception and implants) is safe and the most reliable contraception available for teens. Quick start contraception (prescribing or providing contraception at the current appointment) should be strongly considered to improve adherence in sexually active teens. The possibility of pregnancy should be reasonably ruled out prior to providing contraception by lab work and a careful sexual history including last menstrual period, date of last sex, and method of contraception. If a patient has been recently sexually active, most contraception has not been shown to harm an existing pregnancy. Nevertheless, counseling regarding this risk is important prior to initiating contraception. For patients who have had unprotected sex in the past 5 days, emergency contraception should be discussed and offered at the time of quick start contraception. Concurrent barrier contraception should be stressed. Aside from abstinence, male condoms are the most effective way of preventing STIs.

TABLE 3 Screening recommendations

SCREENING	AGE	TEST	COMMENTS
Dyslipidemia	9–11 17–21	Nonfasting lipid profile	Once between 9 and 11 years and again between 17 and 21 years with annual risk assessment (NHLBI, AAP) Insufficient evidence for screening (USPSTF)
Hemoglobin/hematocrit	11–21	Verbally screen for risk	No routine testing recommended
Human immunodeficiency virus (HIV)	16–18	HIV 1–2 immunoassay	At least once if >15 years with more frequent screening if high-risk. (CDC, USPSTF) Screen MSM at least annually (CDC)
Chlamydia	Females ≤25	NAAT at site of potential infection	Screen all sexually active women ≤25 years at risk (USPSTF) or annually and MSM at least annually. (CDC)
Gonorrhea	Females ≤25	NAAT at site of potential infection	Screen all sexually active women ≤25 years at risk (USPSTF) and MSM at least annually (CDC)
Syphilis	MSM	Serology with confirmatory testing if positive	Screen persons at increased risk (USPSTF). Screen MSM at least annually (CDC)
Cervical dysplasia screening	21 years	Pap smear	Other indications for pelvic exam still apply but routine Pap testing <21 years is not recommended (USPSTF, AAP)

Abbreviations: AAP = American Academy of Pediatrics; CDC = Center for Disease Control and Prevention; MSM = Men who have sex with men; NAAT = nucleic acid amplification testing; NIHLB = National Heart, Lung, and Blood Institute; Pap smear = Papanicolaou smear; USPSTF = US Preventive Services Task Force.

Sleep/Social Media

The conclusion of this format of the HEADS interview concerns less sensitive topics and allows for a comfortable close to the interview. Sleep is problematic for many teens and can usually be improved with better sleep hygiene. Encourage all teens to have a consistent sleep and wake time and 8 to10 hours of sleep daily. Caffeinated beverages should be limited. Daily exercise should be recommended. The teen's bedroom should be free from distractions including radios, TVs, computers, and phones.

Social media and cell phones are now integral to popular culture. While these offer benefits to teens, use should be limited. Both social media and cell phones contribute to unintentional injuries, especially with distracted driving. In addition, personal information being shared on the internet and electronic media opens the teen up to vulnerability. Lastly, both can act as significant distractions from academic work, family time, and sleep. Discuss safe and appropriate use of social media and cell phones with patients and summarize to parents.

Summary

In addition to providing routine health care to teens, providers should focus on the psychosocial history. The HEADS acronym provides a tool for providers to approach these sensitive topics systematically. This interview should take place privately, respecting the teen's ability to consent for certain care, and when able, keeping care confidential. Providers should be familiar with the laws regarding consent and confidentiality of minors in their state. Although teens should be allowed access to confidential health care, providers must be aware that often the best care includes a trusted adult. Parents should be involved in their teen's care when appropriate. Once teens have been assessed for high-risk behaviors, problematic behaviors should be addressed and low-risk behaviors should be commended and encouraged.

References

American Academy of Pediatrics Committee on Practice and Ambulatory Medicine, Bright Futures. 2014 Recommendations of pediatric preventive health care, Pediatrics 2014;133:568–70. Available at http://pediatrics.aappublications.org/content/133/3/568.full?sid=f34dab63-1372-4765-bdbb-0b41a3b24a15 [accessed 03.10.14].

Center for Disease Control and Prevention. Fact sheet, Reported STDs in the United States: 2012 National Data for Chlamydia, Gonorrhea, and Syphilis; January 2014. Available athttp://www.cdc.gov/nchhstp/newsroom/docs/std-trends-508.pdf [accessed 03.11.14].

Cohen DA, Farley TA, Taylor SN, et al. When and where do youths have sex? The potential role of adult supervision, Pediatrics 2001;110:e66. Available at http://pediatrics.aappublications.org/content/110/6/e66.long [accessed 28.10.14].

Daniels SR, Benuck I, Christakis DA, et al. Expert panel on integrated guidelines for cardiovascular health and risk reduction in children and adolescents: summary report. National Heart, Lung, and Blood Institute. Available at http://www.nhlbi.nih.gov/health-pro/guidelines/current/cardiovascular-health-pediatric-guidelines/summary.htm [accessed 03.10.14].

Guttmacher Institute. State policies in brief: an overview of minors' consent law; Oct 1, 2014. Available at https://www.guttmacher.org/statecenter/spibs/spib_OMCL.pdf [accessed 13.10.14].

Klein DA, Goldenring JM. HEEADSSS 3.0: the psychosocial interview for adolescents updated for a new century fueled by media. Contemp Pediatr 2014. Available at http://contemporarypediatrics.modernmedicine.com/contemporary-pediatrics/news/probing-scars-how-ask-essential-questions?page=full [accessed 13.10.14].

Levy SJL, Kokotailo PK. Substance use screening, brief intervention, and referral to treatment for pediatricians, Pediatrics 2011;128:e1330–40. Available at http://pediatrics.aappublications.org/content/128/5/e1330.full.pdf+html [accessed 28.10.14].

Performing preventive services: a bright futures handbook. American Academy of Pediatrics; 2010. Available at http://brightfutures.aap.org/pdfs/preventive%20services%20pdfs/physical%20examination.pdf [accessed 13.10.14].

The CRAFFT Screening Tool, The Center for Adolescent Substance Abuse Research (CeASAR), Children's Hospital Boston, 2009. Available at http://www.ceasar.org/CRAFFT/index.php [accessed 28.10.14].

U.S. Preventive Services Task Force. The guide to clinical preventive services 2014; 2014. Available at http://www.uspreventiveservicestaskforce.org/Page/Name/tools-and-resources-for-better-preventive-care [accessed 03.11.14].

Workowski K, Berman S. Sexually transmitted diseases treatment guidelines 2010. Morb Mortal Wkly Rep 2010;59(RR12). Available at http://www.cdc.gov/mmwr/preview/mmwrhtml/rr5912a1.htm [accessed 03.11.14].

Youth risk behavior surveillance – 2013. Morb Mortal Wly Rep Surveillance Summaries 2014;63:4.

ASTHMA IN CHILDREN

Method of
Susan M. Pollart, MD, MS; and Amanda Kolb, MD

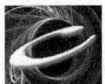

CURRENT DIAGNOSIS

- Recurrent wheeze, cough, and shortness of breath are typical asthma symptoms.
- A personal or family history of atopy is associated with an increased risk of developing asthma.
- Atopy, allergic rhinitis, eczema, or nasal polyps are common comorbidities in patients with asthma.
- Specifically elicit symptom triggers such as allergens, irritants, exercise, stress, cold, or infection.
- At initial diagnosis, outline symptom frequency, intensity, and timing to classify severity.
- Physical examination of asthmatic children is often normal, but mucosal edema of nasal turbinates, eczematous skin rashes, tachypnea, tachycardia, expiratory wheezes, and lung hyperexpansion may be observed.

- In children older than 5 years spirometry revealing an obstructive pattern at least partially reversible with bronchodilators confirms the diagnosis. In children younger than 5 years, diagnosis is based on history, physical examination, and a trial of anti-asthma medications.
- Chest x-ray, complete blood count (CBC), and IgE levels are not routinely recommended but may be useful in certain situations.

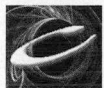 **CURRENT THERAPY**

- The goal of asthma management is to reduce impairment of activities and decrease risk of exacerbations.
- Initial assessment of asthmatics should focus on symptom frequency, timing, and effect on activities to classify the degree of severity as intermittent, mild persistent, moderate persistent, or severe persistent.
- The four central components of management are continual assessment and monitoring, patient education, controlling environmental triggers, and appropriate use of medication.
- Short-acting inhaled β_2-adrenergic receptor agonists such as albuterol (Proventil HFA) are the mainstay of acute therapy in an episode of bronchoconstriction. Anticholinergics such as ipatropium bromide (Atrovent HFA)[1] and systemic steroids are important components of managing an acute exacerbation. Magnesium sulfate,[1] epinephrine (Adrenalin), and terbutaline (Brethine)[1] are reserved for refractory cases, and terbutaline is only approved for children 12 years and older.
- Inhaled corticosteroids are the most effective daily controller medications for children. Long-acting β_2-agonists, leukotriene-receptor antagonists, and mast cell stabilizers are commonly used adjunctive therapies.
- Visits should be scheduled frequently in the outpatient setting to reassess symptom severity, adjust medications accordingly, and emphasize patient education.
- Consider increasing medication therapy only after assessing the patient's adherence and technique with medications. Consider a step down in therapy only after 3 months of adequate control of symptoms.
- Involve both children and their caregivers in designing a written asthma action plan to empower patients in recognizing and managing escalating symptoms.
- Refer to a pulmonologist or allergist if there is any question regarding diagnosis or if symptoms are not adequately controlled with standard treatment.

[1]Not FDA approved for this indication.

Epidemiology

Asthma prevalence in the United States has been on the rise since the 1990s. It is currently estimated that 9.6% of children younger than 18 years (7.1 million children) carry the diagnosis of asthma. Male sex, African American or Puerto Rican ethnicity, and lower socioeconomic status are associated with an increased risk of developing asthma. Prevalence estimates for these groups are as high as 11% to 16%.

Asthma has a significant impact on both school attendance and health care expenditures. According to the National Health Statistic Report in 2007, children made 640,000 emergency department visits and were hospitalized 157,000 times as a result of asthma. In 2008 it was estimated that there were 10.5 million missed school days, and about 5% of children reported long-term limitations on their usual activities due to asthma symptoms.

Although no significant difference in asthma prevalence between urban areas and suburban or rural areas has been found, there do seem to be broader geographic trends with higher prevalence in the Northeast and Midwest. Mortality rates remain low, but preventable deaths attributable to asthma exacerbations persist.

Risk Factors

No clear precipitating factors have been associated with the onset of asthma in children, but multiple risk factors for the development of this disease have been identified. Perhaps the strongest link is that between a family history of atopy, atopic dermatitis in infancy, or elevated serum immunoglobulin (Ig)E levels and subsequent sensitization to aeroallergens at 5 years of age. Other associations including sensitization to dust mites, preterm birth, exposure to tobacco smoke, and certain respiratory infections such as respiratory syncytial virus (RSV) have been identified.

Pathophysiology

Asthma is a chronic disease with recurrent episodes of reversible airway obstruction. It is thought to consist of three major pathophysiologic components: bronchoconstriction, airway inflammation, and bronchial hyperresponsiveness. Bronchoconstriction results from bronchial smooth muscle contraction in response to exposure to allergens, irritants, stress, infection, exercise, or certain medications such as aspirin and nonsteroidal antiinflammatory drugs (NSAIDs). Inflammation occurs via the T helper 2- (T_H2) and IgE-mediated pathways. Examination of the airways of asthmatics reveals inflammatory infiltrates consisting of neutrophils, eosinophils, lymphocytes, and activated mast cells. These mast cells release histamine along with other inflammatory mediators, causing airway edema, mucous hypersecretion, and airway hyperresponsiveness to environmental stimuli. Over time remodeling can occur, with airway thickening and smooth muscle hyperplasia, with a resulting decline in lung function and reduced response to therapeutic interventions.

Long-term observational studies have suggested that declining lung function is most commonly seen in children with symptom onset before 3 years of age. It still remains unclear whether older children or adults experience the same reductions in lung function.

Prevention

Primary prevention of asthma is a well-studied topic, yet few studies have successfully identified effective strategies for preventing asthma. The effect of breast-feeding on asthma prevalence has been a focus of extensive research. Much of the literature regarding breast-feeding as primary prevention for asthma suggests a protective effect of breast-feeding, but this has not been borne out consistently. One study of 952 patients showed no evidence that avoidance of antigens (milk, eggs, nuts) by breast-feeding mothers during pregnancy or lactation decreased asthma or eczema in children.

Although reducing exposure to inhalant allergens such as mites and pet dander can improve symptoms in patients with diagnosed asthma, there is conflicting evidence regarding allergen avoidance to prevent the onset of asthma. In the randomized, controlled Childhood Asthma Prevention Study, dust mite avoidance and dietary fatty acid modifications from 0 to 5 years of age did not decrease the prevalence of asthma or atopy at 8 years.

Other studies combining a reduction in exposure to multiple allergens have been more hopeful. One study demonstrated that in infants with at least one first-degree relative with atopy, decreasing dust mite exposure and following a diet that includes hydrolyzed milk formula (not cow's milk), and avoiding cow's milk (both mother and child) for 4 months decreased the risk of wheezing in the first 12 months of life. A systematic review of multifaceted interventions to reduce or avoid allergen exposure in high-risk children found a decreased rate of asthma diagnosis later in childhood; however, the reliability of the data was limited by subjective reporting of symptoms and by potentially confounding variables. The topic of primary prevention of asthma warrants further study to clearly establish feasible preventive measures.

Clinical Manifestations

Asthma is characterized by recurrent episodes of wheezing, chest tightness, and shortness of breath. Asthma can also manifest as a chronic dry cough, especially if occurring at night. Young children commonly present with chronic cough alone, a form of asthma called cough-variant asthma. Wheezing that recurs in the setting of specific, predictable triggers is also a manifestation of asthma.

Diagnosis

A focused history revealing recurrent episodes of wheezing, shortness of breath, or cough suggests asthma and merits further investigation. In infants, the symptoms of asthma can involve difficulty feeding. Parents might also report intermittent grunting or loud breathing.

When taking the history it is important to ask about symptom triggers, time course, and frequency of symptoms to assess severity. It is also important to discuss any family history of atopy, asthma, eczema, or nasal polyps. Triggers such as exposure to inhalant allergens (mold, dust, pollen, pet dander), irritants (chemicals, cigarette smoke), weather changes, intense emotion, physical activity, and viral illnesses should be elicited specifically (Box 1).

Begin the physical examination with measurements of height and weight and inspection of the growth chart. Most children do not have a significant growth or height reduction as a result of asthma. If a child's growth chart demonstrates a marked decrease in growth velocity it is prudent to seriously consider alternative diagnoses.

Owing to the intermittent nature of asthma symptoms, children with asthma often have an entirely normal examination. Upper airway findings can include nasal polyps or mucosal edema of nasal turbinates. The skin examination might reveal signs of atopic dermatoses such as eczema or urticaria. Lung examination may be remarkable for wheezing, hyperexpanded barrel chest, increased respiratory rate, or tachycardia, depending on severity of symptoms.

In children older than 5 years, spirometry is a useful means of obtaining objective data on lung function and presence of obstructive disease. Assessment with spirometry before and after short-acting β-agonist inhalation should show reversibility of obstruction. A rise in forced expiratory volume in 1 second (FEV_1) of 200 mL and 12% above baseline after bronchodilator is consistent with reversible obstruction. In children younger than 5 years such studies might not be feasible. In these cases diagnosis is based on history and physical. A trial of bronchodilator is helpful in establishing the diagnosis as well as ruling out other possible etiologies of symptoms.

A common presenting symptom of asthma in children is chronic cough. In cough-variant asthma, spirometry may be entirely normal. A trial of antiasthma medication that results in resolution of cough confirms the diagnosis.

Peak flow meters are useful in monitoring symptom severity but should not be used to make a diagnosis owing to wide variations in individual results and normal values.

Chest x-ray should be considered when ruling out alternative diagnoses but is not recommended in routine diagnostic testing for asthma. Allergy skin testing can identify potentially avoidable inhalant indoor allergens and, when appropriate, guide immunotherapy. Finally, checking a complete blood count with differential and serum IgE levels is not clearly indicated in making a diagnosis but may be useful in guiding treatment. Eosinophilia (greater than 4%) can indicate the need for controller medications, and patients with high levels of IgE have been shown to have a particularly good response to inhaled corticosteroids.

Differential Diagnosis

The differential diagnosis of recurrent respiratory symptoms is broad and must be considered when initiating diagnostic work-up. When creating a list of other diagnoses it can be useful to consider the airway from the top down, as is shown in Box 2. Also keep in mind that the age of the patient and the chronicity of symptoms can point to certain diagnoses in your differential.

Treatment

To treat asthma in children appropriately, the severity of symptoms must first be assessed. This initial evaluation should be followed by an ongoing assessment that monitors response to therapy. The general tenets of asthma treatment are to reduce the functional limitations caused by asthma symptoms and decrease the risk of exacerbations, decline in lung function, and side effects of medications. The Expert Panel Report 3 on the National Asthma Education and Prevention Program released in 2007 describes a patient-oriented and clinically relevant approach to asthma management. Emphasis is placed on organized primary care visits and patient education. It is important to plan routine visits with a child's pediatrician or family doctor until symptoms are adequately controlled.

Once the diagnosis of asthma is made in a child, symptom severity should be assessed. Symptoms are classified as intermittent, mild persistent, moderate persistent, or severe persistent. To determine severity, the frequency of daytime symptoms, nighttime

---

Box 1 Asthma Triggers

Allergens
- Animal dander
- Pollen
- Dust mites
- Mold

Chemical irritants
- Tobacco smoke
- Wood stove smoke
- Air pollution
- Cleaning chemicals
- Gases

Medications
- Aspirin
- Nonsteroidal antiinflammatory drugs
- β-Blockers

Other
- Gastroesophageal reflux
- Exercise
- Respiratory infection
- Extremes of emotion
- Stress
- Changes in weather
- Cold air

Box 2 Differential Diagnosis

Upper Airway
Allergic rhinitis
Sinusitis

Large Airway Obstruction
Vocal cord dysfunction
Laryngotracheomalacia (infants)
Tracheal stenosis (infants)
Vascular rings
Tracheal webs
Inhaled foreign body
Tumor or enlarged lymph nodes compressing airway

Small Airway Obstruction
Viral bronchiolitis
Pneumonia
Obliterative bronchiolitis
Cystic fibrosis
Bronchopulmonary dysplasia
Heart failure

Other
Gastroesophageal reflux disease
Swallowing mechanism dysfunction leading to aspiration

Adapted from National Heart, Lung, and Blood Institute, National Asthma Education and Prevention Program. Expert Panel Report 3: Guidelines for the diagnosis and management of asthma. Summary report 2007. http://www.nhlbi.nih.gov/guidelines/asthma/asthgdln.htm (accessed July 22, 2012).

TABLE 1 Classification of Asthma Severity

| COMPONENTS OF SEVERITY | AGE (Y) | INTERMITTENT | PERSISTENT | | |
			MILD	MODERATE	SEVERE
Impairment					
Symptoms	All	≤2 d/wk	>2 d/wk but not daily	Daily	Throughout the day
Nighttime awakenings	0–4	0	1–2 ×/mo	3–4 ×/mo	>1 ×/wk
	≥5	≤2 ×/mo	3–4 ×/mo	>1 ×/wk but not nightly	Often 7 ×/wk
SABA for symptom control	All	≤2 d/wk	>2 d/wk but not daily	Daily	Several ×/day
Interference with normal activity	All	None	Minor limitation	Some limitation	Extremely limited
Lung Function		Normal FEV$_1$ between exacerbations			
FEV$_1$ (predicted) or PEF (personal best)	≥5	>80%	>80%	60%–80%	<60%
FEV$_1$/FVC	5–11	>85%	>80%	75%–80%	<60%
	≥12	Normal	Normal	Reduced 5%	Reduced >5%
Risk					
Exacerbations requiring oral corticosteroids	0–4	≤1/y	≥2× in 6 mo or ≥4 wheezing episodes/y lasting >1 d *and* risk factors for persistent asthma		
	5–11	≤1/y	≥ 2 ×/y*		
	≥12	≤1/y			
Starting Treatment					
Recommended step	0–4	Step 1	Step 2	Step 3	Step 3
	5–11	Step 1	Step 2	Step 3	Step 3 or 4
	≥12	Step 1	Step 2	Step 3	Step 4 or 5
	All			Consider short course of oral corticosteroids	
	All	In 2–6 wk, evaluate level of asthma control and adjust therapy accordingly. For children 0–4 yr, if no clear benefit is observed in 4–6 wk, stop treatment and consider alternative diagnosis or adjusting therapy			

Abbreviations: FEV$_1$ = forced expiratory volume in 1 second; FVC = forced vital capacity; PEF = peak expiratory flow; SABA = short-acting β$_2$-adrenergic receptor agonist.
Adapted from National Heart, Lung, and Blood Institute. National Asthma Education and Prevention Program Expert Panel Report 3: Guidelines for the Diagnosis and Management of Asthma. NIH Publication Number 08-5846. Washington, D.C., National Heart, Lung, and Blood Institute, 2007.
*Consider severity and interval since last exacerbation. Frequency and severity can fluctuate over time for patients in any severity category. Relative annual risk of exacerbations may be related to FEV1.

symptoms, frequency of using short acting β$_2$-agonists, impairment of activities, frequency of exacerbations requiring oral steroids, and lung function must be considered (Table 1). Once severity has been classified, treatment can be started based on the stepwise approach outlined in Table 2. This stepwise approach is intended to be a guideline only. Clinical judgment is necessary when applying these guidelines to the individual patient. Children 12 years and older may be assessed and treated according to the guidelines described for adults.

Assessing adequacy of symptom control is essential to the management of asthma. At each follow-up visit, discussion should focus on how often the patient is having asthma symptoms and how much those symptoms are interfering with normal activities. Tools such as the Asthma Control Test (ACT) or the Childhood Asthma Control Test are helpful in measuring symptom control in a standardized fashion. Symptom assessment determines adequacy of control and guides changes in treatment, as shown in Table 2 and 3. Frequency of primary care visits depends on severity of symptoms and can initially occur every 2 to 6 weeks. As control improves, visits may be decreased to every 1 to 6 months. At each visit, medications can be reviewed, doses adjusted, and education reiterated on recognizing symptoms and using medication and spacers.

Only after at least 3 months of adequate control should a decrease in therapy be considered. When stepping down, do so gradually, with frequent reassessment for reemerging symptoms. In the same way, therapy should be increased only after ensuring that the patient has been adherent with medications and is using the inhaler properly and that comorbid conditions have been addressed.

Referral to a pulmonologist or allergist is recommended if there is any question about the accuracy of diagnosis or if symptoms are difficult to control. The National Heart, Lung, and Blood Institute (NHLBI) recommends consultation if a child older than 5 years requires step 4 or higher level of therapy (step 3 or higher therapy in children younger than 5 years).

Allergen avoidance is currently recommended in the management of all asthmatics, but there is limited evidence that these interventions are effective. Various studies have analyzed the effects of controlling dust mite exposure with specially designed mattress and pillow covers and the use of air filtration units to reduce the burden of airborne pet dander. None of these studies have demonstrated clear benefits in decreasing symptoms.

Influenza vaccination is of questionable benefit. Although it is clear that giving the vaccine does not increase the risk of an exacerbation immediately after vaccination (except in infants receiving live intranasal vaccine [FluMist]), a Chochrane review showed that following vaccination there was no significant reduction in the number of cases of influenza related asthma exacerbation or their severity or duration. The same study did show that children who had received the vaccine had better symptoms ratings during illness than unvaccinated children.

Finally, management of comorbid conditions has been implicated in improving asthma control. Sinusitis, allergic rhinitis, gastroesophageal reflux disease (GERD), and obesity are thought to contribute to asthma symptoms. Research has shown, however, that treatment of GERD with lansoprazole (Prevacid) in children with poorly controlled asthma not only had no effect on asthma symptoms but also led to a significant increase in respiratory infections.

| TABLE 2 | Levels of Asthma Control |

COMPONENTS OF CONTROL	AGE (Y)	WELL CONTROLLED	NOT WELL CONTROLLED	VERY POORLY CONTROLLED
Impairment				
Symptoms	0–4	≤2 d/wk but ≤1 ×/day	>2 d/wk or multiple times on ≤2 d/wk	Throughout the day
	5–11			
	≥12	≤2 d/wk	>2 d/wk	
Nighttime awakenings	0–4	≤1 ×/mo	>1 ×/mo	>1 ×/wk
	5–11	≤1 ×/mo	≥2 ×/mo	≥2 ×/wk
	≥12	≤2 ×/mo	1–3 ×/wk	≥4 ×/wk
Interference with normal activity	All	None	Some limitation	Extremely limited
SABA for symptoms	All	≤2 d/wk	>2 d/wk	Several ×/d
Lung Function				
FEV$_1$ (predicted) or PEF (personal best)	≥5	>80%	60%–80%	<60%
FEV$_1$/FVC	5–11	<80%	75%–80%	<75%
Validated Questionnaires				
ATAQ	≥12	0	1–2	3–4
ACQ	≥12	≤0.75	≥1.5	N/A
ACT	≥12	≥20	16–19	≤15
Risk				
Exacerbations requiring oral corticosteroids	0–4	≤1 ×/year	2–3 ×/yr	>3 ×/yr
	5–11	≤1 ×/year	≤2 ×/yr	
	≥12	≤1 ×/year	Consider severity and interval since last exacerbation	
Reduction in lung growth	5–11	Evaluation requires long-term follow-up care		
Loss of lung function	≥12	Evaluation requires long-term follow-up care		
Treatment-related adverse effects	All	Medication side effects can vary in intensity from none to very troublesome and worrisome		
Recommended Treatment				
Recommended treatment actions	All	Maintain current step Regular follow-up q1–6 mo Consider stepping down if well controlled for ≥3 mo	Step up 1 step Before stepping up, review adherence to medication, inhaler technique, environmental control, comorbid conditions If an alternative treatment option was used in a step, discontinue and use the preferred treatment for that step Reevaluate the level of asthma control in 2–6 wk and adjust therapy accordingly For side effects, consider alternative treatment options	Step up 1–2 steps and consider short course of oral corticosteroids

Abbreviations: ACQ = Asthma Control Questionnaire; ACT = Asthma Control Test; ATAQ = Asthma Therapy Assessment Questionnaire; FEV$_1$ = forced expiratory volume in 1 second; FVC = forced vital capacity; ICS = inhaled corticosteroid; PEF = peak expiratory flow; SABA = short-acting β$_2$-adrenergic receptor agonist.
Adapted from National Heart, Lung, and Blood Institute: National Asthma Education and Prevention Program Expert Panel Report 3: Guidelines for the Diagnosis and Management of Asthma. NIH Publication Number 08-5846. Washington, D.C., National Heart, Lung, and Blood Institute, 2007.

Medications

Asthma management requires both fast-acting rescue medications and long-term controller medications. The goal of therapy is to find a daily controller medicine that reduces symptoms to such a degree that rescue medications are needed only rarely. Patients and their caretakers must be educated regarding the different roles of these two classes of medication to ensure the best possible outcome and the patient's safety.

Rescue Medications

Fast-acting bronchodilators are important in both the mildest and the most-severe forms of asthma. Short-acting β$_2$-adrenergic receptor agonists lead to smooth muscle relaxation and airway dilation. Racemic albuterol (Proventil) is a commonly used member of this group, but levalbuterol (Xopenex) is an alternative. Initially levalbuterol was thought to have fewer side effects, but studies have shown similar tolerability between racemic albuterol and levalbuterol. There is no significant difference in efficacy between these medications. Short-acting β$_2$-adrenergic receptor agonists should be reserved for relief of acute symptoms. Frequent use is discouraged and can indicate inadequate control of symptoms. See Table 4 for usual dosing of rescue medications.

Controller Medications

Inhaled corticosteroids are the most effective long-term controller medications. Some commonly used inhaled corticosteroids are fluticasone (Flovent), budesonide (Pulmicort), beclomethasone (Qvar), mometasone (Asmanex), and funisolide (Aerobid).[2] No single formulation of inhaled corticosteroid is superior to another. These medications reduce frequency of exacerbations and hospitalizations and are superior to leukotriene receptor antagonists and mast cell stabilizers. They are available as both metered-dose inhalers and dry-powder inhalers. A significant concern related to their use in children, however, is their effect on bone density and growth. High-dose inhaled corticosteroids have been linked to reduced growth velocity, but several studies have shown that at low doses they do not consistently or significantly affect growth. High and medium dose inhaled corticosteroids have been linked to reduced growth velocity, but several studies have shown that at low doses they do no consistently

---

[2]Not available in the United States.

TABLE 3 Stepwise Treatment of Asthma in Children Younger than 12 Years

STEP	0–4 YEARS OLD	5–11 YEARS OLD
Step 1: Intermittent	SABA as needed	SABA as needed
Step 2: Mild persistent	Add low-dose daily ICS or cromolyn or montelukast (Singulair)	Add low-dose daily ICS or cromolyn, LTRA, nedocromil (Tilade)[2] or theophyllline
Step 3: Moderate persistent	Increase ICS to medium dose	Increase ICS to medium dose or continue low dose ICS plus either LTRA, LABA or theophylline
Step 4: Severe persistent	Medium-dose ICS plus either LABA or montelukast	Medium-dose ICS plus LABA, or medium-dose ICS plus either LTRA or theophylline
Step 5: Severe persistent	High dose ICS plus either LABA or montelukast	High-dose ICS plus LABA, or high-dose ICS plus LTRA or theophylline
Step 6: Severe persistent	Step 5 plus oral glucocorticoids	Step 5 plus oral glucocorticoids

Step-Down Therapy	Step-Up Therapy
If control is adequate for 3 mo, may consider gradual decrease in treatment Reassess every 1–3 mo	SABA use >2 ×/wk can indicate inadequate control Check for triggers, medication adherence, medication technique, comorbid disease before increasing therapy

Children ≥12 years: May be treated according to adult guidelines.
Children 5–11 years: Consider subcutaneous allergen immunotherapy if the child has allergic asthma in steps 2 to 6.
All children: Treat comorbid conditions to improve asthma control.
For exacerbations that occur at all levels:
SABA 2–4 puffs every 4–6 h for 24 h with physician consultation.
Consider 3- to 10-day course of oral glucocorticoids for moderate to severe exacerbation.

Abbreviations: ICS = inhaled corticosteroid; LABA = long-acting β-agonist; LTRA = leukotriene receptor antagonist; SABA = short-acting β$_2$-adrenergic receptor agonist.
Adapted from National Heart, Lung, and Blood Institute: National Asthma Education and Prevention Program Expert Panel. Report 3: Guidelines for the Diagnosis and Management of Asthma. NIH Publication Number 08-5846. Washington, D.C., National Heart, Lung, and Blood Institute, 2007.
[2]Not available in the United States.

TABLE 4 Usual Dosing of Rescue Medications

DRUG	BRONCHOSPASM*	ACUTE EXACERBATION†
Albuterol (Proventil HFA, AccuNeb)	>4 yr old: 2 inhalations q4–6 h prn >2 yr old (min 15 kg): 0.083% nebulized soln (AccuNeb) inhaled over 5–15 min 3–4 × daily prn	4–8 inhalations q20 min × 3 doses, then q1–4 h prn; add mask in children <4 yr 0.15 mg/kg (min 2.5 mg) q20min × 3 doses, then 0.15–0.3 mg/kg up to 10 mg q1–4 h prn
Levalbuterol (Xopenex)	Age 0–4 yr: 0.31–1.25 mg nebulized soln q4–6 h prn Age 5–11 yr: 0.31–0.63 mg q8h prn	0.075 mg/kg (min 1.25 mg) q20min × 3 doses, then 0.075–0.15 mg/kg up to 5 mg q1–4 h prn

*Symptoms of obstruction, cough, wheeze, breathlessness.
†Symptoms of obstruction not responsive to initial SABA use.
Abbreviations: SABA = short-acting β$_2$-adrenergic receptor agonist; soln = solution.
Information from Micromedex Healthcare Series. http://www.micromedex.com.

or significantly affect growth. The effect of the inhaled corticosteroid on growth velocity has also been linked to the specific ICS molecule but more study is required to clarify this relationship. To minimize potential side effects, continuous monitoring, reevaluation, and consideration of step-down treatment is imperative.

Long-acting β-agonists include salmeterol (Serevent) and formoterol (Foradil). They are an adjunctive therapy to inhaled corticosteroids and should be considered in step 3 of management of symptoms in children aged 5 to 11 years and in step 4 in children 0 to 4 years old. Long-acting β-agonists carry a risk of increased asthma-related deaths, intubations, and hospitalizations when used alone. This risk was most prominent in children 4 to 11 years of age. Long-acting β-agonists should never be used as monotherapy and are not recommended for use during exacerbations. In combination with inhaled corticosteroids, however, long-acting β-agonists reduce exacerbations, increase asthma control days, and improve lung function. For children younger than 5 years, data are lacking.

Leukotriene receptor antagonists, including montelukast (Singulair) and zafirlukast (Accolate), are another adjunctive therapy to inhaled corticosteroids. They reduce symptoms by blocking the inflammatory cascade initiated by mast cells. In the mildest forms of asthma they may be used as an alternative to inhaled corticosteroids if the steroids are not well tolerated or there is difficulty with administration. They are also effective in decreasing symptoms of exercise-induced asthma.

Mast cell stabilizers such as cromolyn sodium (Intal) or nedocromil (Tilade)[2] have a role similar to that of the leukotriene-receptor antagonists. They reduce inflammation by preventing mast cells from initiating the inflammatory cascade. They are safe and well tolerated in children but the efficacy of inhaled sodium cromoglycate (Intal) has been brought into question after a systematic review found insufficient evidence to demonstrate sodium cromoglycate's superiority over placebo. The nedocromil inhaler has been discontinued owing to difficulties with manufacturing inhaler propellant.

Immunotherapy consists of subcutaneous injections of extracts from allergens intended to desensitize a patient to specific allergic triggers. This should occur in consultation with an allergist and may be considered at steps 2 through 6 of asthma treatment in children ages 5 to 11 years if asthma symptoms are predominantly allergic.

Immunomodulators are reserved for the most refractory cases of asthma. Omalizumab (Xolair, an anti-IgE agent) functions by blocking the binding of IgE to mast cells and basophils. It is effective in children with allergic triggers for their asthma but carries a risk of anaphylaxis and the FDA as of 2014 has associated its use with an increase in cardiovascular and cerebrovascular events. In 2013 the National Institute for Health and Care Excellence (NICE) issues a recommendation that omalizumab be reserved for children age 6 and older who have frequent need for oral steroids (more

[2]Not available in the United States.

TABLE 5 Usual Dosing of Controller Medications

DRUG	FORMAT	DOSING
Fluticasone (Flovent)	MDI: 44, 110, 220 μg/puff Dry powder: 50, 100, 250 μg/inhalation	Low: 88–176 μg Medium: 176–440 μg High: >440 μg
Budesonide (Pulmicort)	200 μg/puff	Low: 100–200 μg Medium: 200–400 μg High: >400 μg
Beclomethasone (Qvar)	40 or 80 μg/puff	Low: 80–160 μg Medium: 160–320 μg High: >320 μg
Mometasone fumarate (Asmanex)	110, 220 μg/puff	110 μg daily is max per guidelines for 4–11 y
Flunisolide (Aerospan)[2]	80 μg/puff	6–11 y: 80–160 μg bid >12 y: 160–320 μg bid
Triamcinolone acetonide (Azmacort)[2]	100 μg/puff	Low: 400–800 μg Medium: 800–1200 μg High: >1200 μg
Salmeterol (Serevent)	Dry powder inhaler 50 μg/blister	>5 y: 1 blister q12
Formoterol (Foradil)	Dry powder inhaler 12 μg/cap	>5 y: 1 cap q12h
Montelukast (Singulair)		<5 y: 4 mg hs 6–14 y: 5 mg hs
Zafirlukast (Accolate)		Ages 5–11 y: 10 mg bid
Cromolyn sodium (Intal)	nebulized soln (20 mg/2 mL), MDI 800 μg	>2 y: nebulized soln: inhale 20 mg qid Age >2: MDI: 2 puffs qid
Theophylline		Starting dose: 10 mg/kg/d <1 y: max dose $0.2 \times$ (age in weeks) $+5 =$ mg/kg/d ≥1 y: max dose 16 mg/kg/day

[2]Not available in the United States.
Abbreviations: cap = capsule; MDI = metered-dose inhaler; soln = solution.
Information from Micromedex Healthcare Series. http://www.micromedex.com.

than three courses in prior 12 months) and who have failed optimized therapy. Optimized therapy is defined as a full trial of inhaled high dose corticosteroid, long acting B2 agonist, leukotriene receptor antagonist, theophyllines and oral steroids.

Theophylline (Theochron) was previously a mainstay of asthma management but is no longer a first-line medication. With the development of alternative treatments and because of theophylline's risk for toxicity, theophylline now has a smaller role in asthma management. Currently it is used as an alternative treatment in the chronic management of patients with symptoms refractory to or intolerant of standard therapies. Use of this medication requires frequent monitoring of drug serum levels. It can cause nausea, vomiting, or tachyarrhythmias if dosing is too high. See Table 5 for usual dosing of controller medications.

Acute Asthma Exacerbations

Exacerbations consist of worsening wheezing, cough, or shortness of breath. They can vary in severity from mild to life threatening. When deciding how to treat a patient in an exacerbation, use the history and physical examination to determine severity. As in all emergency situations first assess airway, breathing, and circulation. In a life-threatening exacerbation the patient can appear confused or obtunded, may be bradycardic, and can have minimal respiratory effort, indicating imminent respiratory arrest. A child in a severe exacerbation can appear short of breath even at rest, may be agitated, and might only be speaking one word at a time. The child is likely tachycardic and tachypneic, with obvious use of accessory muscles. In certain cases, lung examination might not reveal wheezing owing to severe impairment of aeration; only after treatment does the wheezing become audible as air movement improves. In mild to moderate exacerbations the patient might only be short of breath with walking, might speak in short phrases or full sentences, and can appear anxious but not necessarily agitated. Lung examination can reveal wheezing.

The cornerstone of treatment of asthma exacerbations is rapid recognition of symptoms, correction of hypoxemia, and early initiation of short-acting β2-adrenergic receptor agonists and corticosteroids. Oxygen administration should be employed to maintain oxygen saturation at greater than 94%. Short-acting β-agonists are essential to relieve bronchoconstriction and may be combined with ipratropium (Atrovent),[1] especially if the patient is not responsive to initial therapy with a short-acting β2-adrenergic receptor agonist alone. Ipatropium should not be used as single agent as it is less efficacious than B2 agonists alone as well as combined b2 agonist - ipatropium. In 2006 a systematic review showed that metered-dose inhalers with a spacer are as effective in administering β-agonists as nebulizers are in children older than 2 years. It was noted in the same study that length of stay in the emergency department was reduced in those using the spacers.

Corticosteroids given systemically are also considered rescue medications, although onset of action is 1 to 2 hours and duration of action is 18 to 36 hours. They work primarily as antiinflammatories and are an important treatment in exacerbations. Early use of systemic steroids, either oral or intravenous, reduced rates of relapse and decreased admissions to the hospital. The greatest benefit of systemic steroids was seen in patients having a severe attack and those who were not already on a course of steroids. Studies have shown that oral steroids are as effective as intravenous or intramuscular preparations. Even a short course of oral steroids can reduce relapse and decreases the need for rescue inhalers. Systemic corticosteroids should be continued for 3 to 10 days after an exacerbation. A taper is not necessary if the course is less than 1 week or less than 10 days in a patient who is also using an inhaled corticosteroid. Prolonged use of systemic corticosteroids carries significant risk for side effects such as adrenal suppression, osteoporosis, reduced growth, and cataracts, and thus their use should be minimized. Despite some evidence that use of inhaled corticosteroids in acute exacerbations can reduce admission rates, it is unclear how much benefit they have when used in conjunction with systemic steroids.

---

[1]Not FDA approved for this indication.

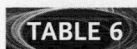

TABLE 6 Usual Dosing of Medications Used in Exacerbations

DRUG	DOSING
Chronic Management	
Corticosteroids (methylprednisolone, prednisolone, prednisone)	0.25–2 mg/kg daily or every other day
Acute Exacerbation	
Ipratropium bromide (Duoneb)[1]	Age 0–5 y: 250 µg nebulized × 2, then q4h prn Age 5–11: 500 µg nebulized × 2, then q4h prn
Corticosteroids (methylprednisolone, prednisolone, prednisone)	1–2 mg/kg/day (max 60 mg/day) in 2 divided doses × 3–10 d
Severe Acute Exacerbation	
Not Responding to SABAs	
Magnesium sulfate[1]	25–50 mg/kg IV up to 2 g over 10–20 min
Terbutaline[1]	0.01 mg/kg SC q20min for 3 doses, then every 2–6 hr prn
Epinephrine	0.01 mg/kg up to 0.3–0.5 mg SC q20min for 3 doses
Related to Allergic Reaction	
Epinephrine	1:1000: 0.01 mL/kg SC (max 0.3 mL)

[1]Not FDA approved for this indication.

Abbreviation: SABA = short-acting β₂-adrenergic receptor agonist.

Use of intravenous magnesium sulfate[1] (a smooth muscle relaxer) should be reserved for severe exacerbations only. Its use has not been shown to reduce admission rates in milder exacerbations but can improve lung function in those with only a partial response to short-acting β-agonists. Similarly, subcutaneous epinephrine, and subcutaneous terbutaline[1] should be reserved for emergency department settings when patients are not responding to short-acting β₂-adrenergic receptor agonists, anticholinergics, or corticosteroids or when air entry is so diminished that inhaled medications are not effective.

Finally, not enough evidence exists to make a recommendation regarding routine use of antibiotics during an acute asthma exacerbation. In some circumstances when there are findings consistent with bacterial infections (such as consolidation on chest x-ray) their use may be warranted. See Table 6 for usual dosing of medications used in acute exacerbations.

Monitoring

Asthma is a dynamic disease whose symptoms fluctuate based on a number of variables. Routine scheduled appointments with a pediatrician or family physician are essential to monitor symptoms and adjust therapy. Initial management can require visits every 2 to 6 weeks; as control of symptoms improves the interval may be increased to every 3 to 6 months.

Patient education is essential to successfully controlling this disease. Education should be focused on the theory behind controller and rescue medications as well as how to administer these medications properly. The National Asthma Education and Prevention Program Expert Panel 3 emphasizes the importance of asthma action plans to empower patients in recognizing and treating escalating symptoms of asthma. Action plans also provide recommendations on reducing exposure to irritants, allergens, and triggers. Some plans are based on peak flow levels, but studies show that symptom-based written action plans are better at decreasing acute care visits. Examples of asthma actions plans can be found on the National Heart Lung and Blood Institute website.

---

[1]Not FDA approved for this indication.

Complications

The most worrisome complications of asthma include reduced lung function, pneumonia, pneumothorax, and death. More-common complications include chronic cough, fatigue due to poor sleep, missed school days and worse academic performance, and limited ability to participate in sports.

References

Bacharier LB, Boner A, Carlsen KH, et al. Diagnosis and treatment of asthma in childhood: A PRACTALL consensus report. Allergy 2008;63:5–34.

Brightling CE, Bradding P, Symon FA, et al. Mast-cell infiltration of airway smooth muscle in asthma. N Engl J Med 2002;346:1699–705.

Cates CJ, Jefferson T, Rowe BH. Vaccines for preventing influenza in people with asthma. Cochrane Database Syst Rev 2008;(2):CD000364.

Courtney U, McCarter D, Pollart S. Childhood asthma: Treatment update. Am Fam Physician 2005;71:1959–68.

Dicpinigaitis PV. Chronic cough due to asthma: ACCP evidence-based clinical practice guidelines. Chest 2006;129:75S–79S.

Elward K, Pollart S. Medical therapy for asthma: Updates from the NAEPP guidelines. Am Fam Physician 2010;82(10):1242–51.

Holbrook JT, Wise RA, Gold BD. Lansoprazole for children with poorly controlled asthma: A randomized controlled trial. JAMA 2012;307(4):373–81.

Kramer MS, Kakuma R. Maternal dietary antigen avoidance during pregnancy or lactation, or both, for preventing or treating atopic disease in the child. Cochrane Database Syst Rev 2006;(3):CD000133.

Lemanske RF, Mauger DT, Sorkness CA, Jackson DJ. Step up therapy for children with uncontrolled asthma receiving inhaled corticosteroids. N Engl J Med 2010;362(11):975–85.

Maas T, Kaper J, Sheikh A, et al. Mono and multifaceted inhalant and/or food allergen reduction interventions for preventing asthma in children at high risk of developing asthma. Cochrane Database Syst Rev 2009;(3):CD006480.

McCowan C, Neville R, Thomas G, et al. Effect of asthma and its treatment on growth: Four year follow up of cohort of children from general practices in Tayside, Scotland. BMJ 1998;316(7132):668–72.

McIvor RA, Kaplan A, Koch C. Montelukast as an alternative to low dose inhaled corticosteroids in the management of mild asthma(the SIMPLE trial): An open label effectiveness trial. Can Respir J 2009;16:11A–21A.

National Heart, Lung, and Blood Institute. Asthma action plan. Available at http://www.nhlbi.nih.gov/health/public/lung/asthma/asthma_actplan.pdf; [accessed August 14, 2015].

National Heart, Lung, and Blood Institute, National Asthma Education and Prevention Program. Expert Panel Report 3: Guidelines for the diagnosis and management of asthma. Summary report 2007. http://www.nhlbi.nih.gov/guidelines/asthma/asthgdln.htm; [accessed August 14, 2015].

Pollart S, Compton R, Elward K. Management of acute asthma exacerbations. Am Fam Physician 2011;84:40–7.

Pollart S, Elward K. Overview of changes to asthma guidelines: Diagnosis and screening. Am Fam Physician 2009;79:761–7.

Prevention strategies for asthma—primary prevention. CMAJ 2005;173(Suppl. 6): S20–24.

Ram FS, Ducharme FM, Scarlett J. Cow's milk protein avoidance and development of childhood wheeze in children with a family history of atopy. Cochrane Database Syst Rev 2002;3:CD003795Review. Update in Cochrane Database Syst Rev 2007; (2).CD003795.

Toelle B, Ng K. Eight year outcomes of the Childhood Asthma Prevention Study. J Allergy Clin Immunol 2010;126:388–9.

ATTENTION-DEFICIT/HYPERACTIVITY DISORDER

Method of
Harris Strokoff, MD; and Craig L. Donnelly, MD

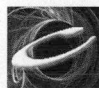

CURRENT DIAGNOSIS

- Patients with ADHD have several impairing inattentive symptoms or hyperactive/impulsive symptoms, or both.
- The DSM-IV inattentive core symptoms of ADHD include difficulty sustaining attention, making careless mistakes, increased distractibility, forgetfulness, not seeming to listen when spoken to, not following through on instructions, difficulties with organization, reluctance to engage in schoolwork, and a tendency to lose things.
- The DSM-IV hyperactive/impulsive core symptoms of ADHD include being fidgety; running or climbing excessively; having difficulty awaiting a turn, staying seated, or being quiet; acting as if "driven by a motor"; talking excessively, blurting out answers, and interrupting others.

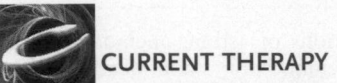

- Stimulant medications (e.g., methylphenidate [Ritalin, Methylin, Concerta] and amphetamine preparations) are the primary treatments for ADHD in children and adults when not contraindicated.
- Nonstimulants such as atomoxetine (Strattera), guanfacine (Intuniv), clonidine (Kapvay), and bupropion (Wellbutrin)1 are useful medication treatments for ADHD as well.
- Medication should be implemented collaboratively, with the child's parents and teachers providing feedback about treatment efficacy and tolerability.
- Psychosocial therapies can add benefit to pharmacotherapy and may be necessary for patients who cannot use pharmacotherapy due to intolerability or preference.
- There is growing evidence that Psychotherapies can also be useful in trying to reduce ADHD symptoms in children and adults.

Attention-deficit/hyperactivity disorder (ADHD) is among the most commonly diagnosed illnesses in pediatric medicine. Approximately 4% to 8% of children are diagnosed with ADHD. ADHD is most commonly diagnosed in children between the ages of 6 and 12 years, but it is also diagnosed and treated in children as young as age 3. Although previously thought to largely abate in adolescence and adulthood, ADHD is now considered to be a chronic condition. More than 60% of children with ADHD have impairing symptoms well into adolescence and adulthood. ADHD can cause social problems, academic and learning problems, emotional problems, delinquency, and increased risk-taking behavior, including substance abuse.

ADHD is highly heritable. Approximately 10% to 35% of immediate family members of children with ADHD have ADHD themselves, and approximately 30% of siblings of children with ADHD also have the disorder. Parents of children with ADHD are at high risk for ADHD themselves, and appropriate assessment and potential treatment of ADHD in the parents can improve the child's environment. ADHD is thought to reflect decreased dopamine and norepinephrine transmission in the brain. Maternal smoking and alcohol use, low birth weight, and lead exposure are associated with increased rates of ADHD. Social factors are not thought to play a major role in the development of ADHD.

Diagnosis

Children with ADHD tend to have profound difficulties in maintaining or sustaining attention, and/or they are hyperactive or impulsive. The core inattentive and hyperactive/impulsive symptoms of ADHD are defined by the *Diagnostic and Statistical Manual of Mental Disorders*, Fifth Edition (DSM-V). ADHD is classified according to three subtypes: predominantly inattentive type, predominantly hyperactive/impulsive type, and combined type, which is the most common subtype.

The predominantly inattentive type of ADHD is characterized by at least six of the inattention core symptoms but fewer than six of the hyperactive/impulsive symptoms (see Current Diagnosis box). The predominantly hyperactive/impulsive type of ADHD involves six of nine hyperactive/impulsive symptoms but fewer than six of the inattention symptoms. If a patient has at least six of the inattention and six of the hyperactive/impulsive symptoms, the diagnosis is combined-type ADHD. These symptoms must also cause significant impairment in the child's life in more than one domain (e.g., in school and home settings) to meet the criteria for ADHD. Symptoms of ADHD must have been present before the age of 12 years to meet the full criteria.

ADHD is diagnosed by clinical interviews of the child and parents and from information from outside sources, especially from the child's school or daycare. Standardized assessment tools and rating scales, such as the Vanderbilt, Medium SNAP IV (developed by Swanson, Nolan, and Pelham), the Behavior Assessment System for Children (BASC), the Achenbach Child Behavior Checklist (CBCL), the Achenbach Teacher Report Form (TRF), the Achenbach Youth Self-Report (YSR), and the Connor's rating scale are useful for the diagnosis of ADHD, for monitoring of symptoms over time, and as broader indicators of psychopathology in children and adolescents with ADHD. It is important to rule out underlying conditions (e.g., absence seizures, sleep apnea, learning disorder, anxiety) when making a diagnosis of ADHD. PTSD and substance use disorders are also known to cause many symptoms consistent with those of ADHD.

Comorbidity is the rule in childhood ADHD. It is estimated that only 30% of children with ADHD have the disorder alone. Up to 60% of children with ADHD may have learning disorders, 30% to 40% of children with ADHD also have oppositional defiant disorder or conduct disorder, approximately 30% of children with ADHD have a comorbid anxiety disorder, and approximately 25% of these children have a comorbid major depressive disorder. ADHD is typically diagnosed three or four times more often in boys than in girls, and girls tend to have more predominant inattentive symptoms that may not be noticed as easily in classroom or home settings.

In adults with ADHD, hyperactivity commonly found in children tends to change into a sense of internal restlessness, and impaired attention and distractibility tend to evolve into difficulties with organization and planning. An estimated 4.4% of adults in the United States meet the diagnostic criteria for ADHD. Adults with ADHD tend to be underdiagnosed and have a higher incidence of criminal behavior, injuries, accidents, and employment and marital difficulties compared with adults without ADHD. Untreated symptoms of inattention or hyperactivity often cause or exacerbate anxious and depressive disorders, which may manifest in adulthood in complex comorbid patterns along with ADHD.

Treatment

The gold standard for treatment of ADHD is pharmacotherapy. Treatment with a stimulant medication or atomoxetine (Strattera) is most effective for ADHD, regardless of ADHD subtype. Psychosocial interventions can be a useful adjunct in many children with ADHD, especially those for whom poor tolerability or comorbid diagnoses could be better addressed with psychotherapy.

Stimulants

For approximately 75% of children with ADHD, treatment with stimulants decreases their symptoms. As a class, stimulants are fast acting (i.e., improvements are usually evident in the first few days of treatment) and usually well tolerated. Several types of stimulant medications are available. No stimulant has consistently proved to be more effective than another. Choice of a first stimulant medication for the treatment of ADHD is typically based on the desired duration of effect, frequency of dosing, percentage of short-acting medication versus long-acting medication, and the desired delivery system.

The two major classes of stimulant medications are methylphenidate (e.g., Ritalin, Methylin, Concerta) and amphetamine-type preparations. Figure 1 summarizes the medications FDA approved for the treatment of ADHD. Because the data equally support short-acting (immediate-release) and longer-acting stimulant preparations, most clinicians begin with longer-acting preparations, which are thought to offer a smoother level of medication effect and need to be dosed only once daily, which tends to improve compliance. Reasons to consider a shorter-acting medication include wanting to give a test dose before beginning a longer-acting stimulant, wanting to use a very low dose (e.g., in very young children or children with a pervasive developmental disorder), or attempting to minimize potential side effects, such as insomnia and anorexia. Stimulants given twice daily are typically given once in the morning and once at lunchtime. Stimulant medications are available in tablet, capsule, liquid, chewable, and transdermal patch forms.

Like all medications, stimulants have side effects. Stimulants commonly cause appetite suppression, which can lead to weight loss. Stimulants also can decrease linear growth rates, and children with ADHD who are managed with stimulant medication over time may have decreases in projected maximum height of approximately 0.4 to 1 inch. However, after stimulant pharmacotherapy is discontinued, children's linear growth velocity usually accelerates. In the past, drug holidays (e.g., having a child with ADHD off medication for the summer) were common, but it is currently thought that these holidays interrupt optimal treatment and that untreated symptoms during drug holidays can be difficult for the child psychologically

Drug	Dosing	Typical starting dose	Comments
Methylphenidate preparations			
Methylphenidate (generic name)			
(Brand name formulations)			
Ritalin	bid to tid	5 mg bid	
Methylin	bid to tid	5 mg bid	available in both liquid and chewable tablet forms
Methylin ER	once daily	10 mg qam	capsule can be opened and contents can be sprinkled into food, longer-acting formulation
Metadate ER	once daily	10 mg qam	capsule can be opened and contents can be sprinkled into food, longer-acting formulation
Metadate CD	once daily	20 mg qam	
Ritalin SR	once daily	10 mg qam	
Ritalin LA	once daily	20 mg qam	capsule can be opened and contents can be sprinkled into food, longer-acting formulation
Concerta	once daily	18 mg qam	uses osmotic pump mechanism, longer-acting formulation
Daytrana patch	apply once daily, then remove at end of the day	10 mg patch	
D-Methylphenidate (generic name)			
(Brand name formulations)			
Focalin	bid to tid	2.5 mg bid	
Focalin XR	once daily	5 mg qam	capsule can be opened and contents can be sprinkled into food, longer-acting formulation
Amphetamine preparations			
Mixed amphetamine salts [D-amphetamine and amphetamine] (generic name)			
(Brand name formulations)			
Adderall	qd to bid	3–5 y: 2.5 mg qam ≥6 y: 5 mg qd to bid	
Adderall XR	once daily	≥6 y: 10 mg qam	capsule can be opened and contents can be sprinkled into food, longer-acting formulation
D-Amphetamine (generic name)			
(Brand name formulations)			
Dexedrine	qd to bid	3–5 y: 2.5 mg qam ≥6 y: 5 mg qd to bid	capsule can be opened and contents can be sprinkled into food
Dextrostat	qd to bid	3–5 y: 2.5 mg qam ≥6 y: 5 mg qd to bid	capsule can be opened and contents can be sprinkled into food
Dexedrine Spansule	qd to bid	≥6 y: 5–10 mg qd to bid	capsule can be opened and contents can be sprinkled into food, longer-acting formulation
Lisdexamphetamine (generic name)			
(Brand name formulations)			
Vyvanse	once daily	30 mg qam	is a pro-drug, thus must be enzymatically cleaved in the gastrointestinal tract in order to yield active D-amphetamine. Not thought to be abusable intranasally
Non-stimulant medication			
Atomoxetine (generic name)			
(Brand name formulations)			
Strattera	once daily (also can be given divided bid)	patients <70 kg: 0.5 mg/kg/day for 4 days; then 1 mg/kg/day for 4 days; then 1.2 mg/kg/day	less likely to exacerbate anxiety in some children, not thought to be abusable
Guanfacine (generic name)			
(Brand name formulations)			
Intuniv	once daily	1 mg/day increasing by 1 mg each week to a max of 4 mg/day	little abuse potential, may cause somnolence
Clonidine (generic name)			
(Brand name formulations)			
Kapvay	once daily	1 mg/day	little abuse potential, may cause somnolence

Figure 1. Medications commonly used to treat ADHD. *Abbreviations:* bid = twice daily; ER = extended release; LA = long acting; qam = every morning; qd = once daily; SR = sustained release; tid = three times daily; XR = extended release.

and socially. If weight loss and decreased linear growth velocity remain concerns despite attempts at optimizing the psychopharmacologic regimen, drug holidays could be considered.

Stimulants can cause or exacerbate vocal and motor tics. Stimulants may also cause insomnia. α-Blocking agents such as clonidine (Catapres)[1] or guanfacine (Tenex)[1] are sometimes used in addition to stimulant medication to treat the side effects of insomnia or tics. Insomnia can sometimes be managed by decreasing the dose of the stimulant, changing the timing of the dose, or changing to a different stimulant preparation. Melatonin[1,7] is commonly used as an adjunct therapy for the treatment of stimulant-induced insomnia.

Headaches and stomachaches are side effects of stimulants, although they are usually transient in nature. In some patients, stimulants can cause or worsen anxiety in patients with comorbid anxiety disorders, and in these cases, switching to a more anxiety-neutral ADHD treatment (e.g., atomoxetine) or the addition of a selective serotonin reuptake inhibitor (SSRI) should be considered. Rarely, stimulants can cause mood changes and psychotic reactions.

Stimulant treatment in preschool-age children (3–5.5 years old) with ADHD is effective, but it is not as effective as using stimulants to treat school-age children with ADHD. Side effects commonly include emotional lability and aggression in this population, and stimulants should be dosed lower and monitored carefully.

Stimulants have the potential to exacerbate preexisting cardiac conditions, and children should be screened for cardiac disease and a history of premature cardiac death in the family. Patients on stimulant medication should have their heart rate and blood pressure monitored, although the average predictable increases in heart rate (1–2 beats/min) and blood pressure (3–4 mm Hg) are thought to be clinically insignificant. In April 2008, the American Heart Association (AHA) released a statement recommending that children receiving stimulant treatment for ADHD receive screening electrocardiograms (ECGs), and in May 2008, the AHA released a clarification stating that screening ECGs for patients with ADHD are reasonable to consider but not mandatory. In summary, children on stimulants should have their height, weight, blood pressure, and heart rate monitored while receiving therapy.

Stimulants are potential drugs of abuse and are class II schedule medications. Stimulant abuse can cause euphoria, enhance academic and athletic performance, cause weight loss, and induce desired insomnia. ADHD alone is associated with increased rates and severity of substance abuse, and most studies show no change in substance abuse rates in adolescents with ADHD treated with stimulants compared with those left untreated. Longer-acting and alternative formulations (e.g., patch, prodrug, osmotic pump mechanism) of stimulants are more difficult to abuse (e.g., intranasally, intravenously) than are immediate-release agents.

Nonstimulants

Atomoxetine (Strattera) is an FDA-approved medication used to treat children, adolescents, and adults with ADHD. Although the degree of effect tends to be somewhat lower than those found with stimulant treatments of ADHD, it is typically effective and well tolerated. Atomoxetine works less quickly than stimulants (peak effectiveness usually apparent around weeks 4 to 6), but it may provide longer duration (i.e., 24-hour) coverage. Atomoxetine is less likely to exacerbate anxiety or cause tics compared with stimulant medications. Atomoxetine has no abuse liability and is not a controlled substance.

Side effects include increased heart rate and blood pressure, and it should be used with caution in children with structural or conductive cardiac abnormalities. Atomoxetine carries an FDA black box warning recommending monitoring for the potential emergence of suicidality in patients taking this medication. Atomoxetine can markedly elevate hepatic enzymes and bilirubin, although hepatic failure is thought to be a rare event. Patients who exhibit symptoms such as jaundice or other indices of liver disease should stop taking this medication and receive medical work-up. Other potential side effects of atomoxetine include agitation, gastrointestinal upset, and headaches, although overall, this medication is thought to be well tolerated.

α-Adrenergic agonists such as clonidine[1] and guanfacine[1] are antihypertensive agents that have been used off-label for many years for the treatment of ADHD, and in recent years have become FDA-approved for the treatment of ADHD. Although these medications can improve functioning in patients with ADHD, clinical response is usually less robust than with stimulants. Clonidine and guanfacine are often times useful in the treatment of inattentive and hyperactive/impulsive symptoms and are most commonly used adjunctively with stimulants in children with ADHD to treat stimulant-induced tics and insomnia. Clonidine requires three to four doses throughout the day, and guanfacine is typically dosed twice daily, although extended release versions of these medications are now available that allow for less frequent dosing, and are Kapvay and Intuniv, respectively. These medications should be used with caution because they carry risks of sedation, orthostasis, potential cardiac side effects, and rare reports of sudden cardiac death with overdose. They should be started at low doses and then titrated slowly. These medications should not be discontinued without a gradual taper over the course of 1 to 2 weeks because of the potential of rebound hypertension and irritability.

Certain antidepressant medications are used to treat children and adults with ADHD, although they do not carry FDA approval for this purpose. Some studies have shown that the antidepressant bupropion (Wellbutrin)[1] improves symptoms of ADHD in children and adults, and it is efficacious in treating depression and ADHD in children and adults who suffer from these comorbid conditions. Potential side effects of bupropion include increases in pulse and blood pressure and potential lowering of a person's seizure threshold. Bupropion, like all antidepressants, carries an FDA black box warning about the potential of these medications to increase suicidality in youths and young adults.

Although rarely used for this purpose and not FDA approved, the tricyclic antidepressants desipramine (Norpramin),[1] imipramine (Tofranil),[1] and nortriptyline (Pamelor)[1] are thought to have some efficacy in the treatment of ADHD. These medications are used less commonly because of significant side effects such as ECG changes (prolonged QTc), sedation, and risk of sudden cardiac death with overdose.

Modafinil (Provigil)[1] is FDA approved for the treatment of narcolepsy, shift-work sleep disorder, and obstructive sleep apnea/hypopnea syndrome, and it is thought to improve vigilance and decrease distractibility. It is sometimes used to treat ADHD. Modafinil is not thought to be as easily abused as the stimulant medications.

Stimulant pharmacotherapy should be the initial treatment for most cases of ADHD. Formal dosing guidelines of stimulants should be followed. Titration of the dose until sufficient improvement is gained or limiting side effects emerge is the best way to optimize stimulant treatment outcome. There is sufficient evidence to suggest switching to another stimulant if treatment with the initial agent is suboptimal (e.g., switching from an amphetamine preparation to a methylphenidate preparation), and if the second stimulant trial fails, consideration should be given to a third stimulant trial. If there is a partial response to a stimulant trial, consider augmentation with atomoxetine or the addition of an α-blocking agent if insomnia or tics are mitigating side effects.

Although ADHD tends to be a chronic condition, not all children with ADHD progress to become adults with ADHD. Children who are being treated for ADHD should be reassessed yearly to determine if treatment for ADHD is still indicated. In the treatment of adults with ADHD, the same treatment strategies apply, although adults may require higher doses of medication. Stimulants and atomoxetine are the primary treatments for adults with ADHD. Because of higher rates of substance abuse comorbidities in adults, the risks of potential stimulant abuse and diversion may be higher in this population.

Psychosocial Treatments

Psychosocial therapies can be a useful and sometimes necessary adjunct to pharmacotherapy for the treatment of ADHD. Behavior therapy can be effective in helping to manage symptoms of ADHD, and parents and teachers are essential for implementing behavioral strategies and for continually assessing ADHD symptoms and treatment side effects. Parent training groups are effective at maximizing children's compliant behaviors, and several books (e.g., Barkley's *Your Defiant Child*, Forehand and Long's *Parenting the Strong-Willed Child*) are available for training parents and clinicians to teach and reinforce behavioral therapy.

Classroom management techniques are an important part of any psychosocial approach to the treatment of ADHD in children and adolescents. Teachers of students with ADHD have found it helpful to increase the structure in classrooms, use consistent rewards and punishments, and use daily report cards to communicate school performance to parents at home.

Although medication treatment remains the hallmark treatment for most cases of ADHD, it is also very important to improve modifying factors in therapy. There is also growing opinion that optimizing exercise, sleep, healthy eating, and engaging in pro-social activities may also help ADHD symptoms improve over time.

References

Adler LA. From childhood into adulthood: The changing face of ADHD. CNS Spectr 2007;12(Suppl. 23):12.
American Academy of Pediatrics/American Heart Association. Clarification of statement on cardiovascular evaluation and monitoring of children and adolescents with heart disease receiving medications for ADHD, Available at http://newsroom.heart.org/news/american-academy-of-pediatrics-218228 [accessed September 3, 2014].
American Psychiatric Association Task Force on DSM-IV. Diagnostic and Statistical Manual of Mental Disorders: DSM-IV-TR. Washington, DC: American Psychiatric Association; 2000.
Barkley R. Attention-Deficit Hyperactivity Disorder: A Handbook for Diagnosis and Treatment. 3rd ed New York: Guilford Press; 2006.
Clinical Pharmacology Online. Drug and toxicology information, Available at http://www.clinicalpharmacology.com [accessed September 3, 2014].
Gilchrist RH, Arnold EL. Long-term efficacy of ADHD pharmacotherapy in children. Pediatr Ann 2008;37:46.
Greenhill L, Kollins S, Abikoff H, et al. Efficacy and safety of immediate-release methylphenidate treatment for preschoolers with ADHD. J Am Acad Child Adolesc Psychiatry 2006;45:11.
Jensen PS, Arnold LE, Swanson JM, et al. 3-Year follow-up of the NIMH MTA study. J Am Acad Child Adolesc Psychiatry 2007;46:8.
Kessler RC, Adler L, Barkley R, et al. The prevalence and correlates of adult ADHD in the United States: Results from the National Comorbidity Survey Replication. Evid Based Ment Health 2006;9:116.
Newcorn JH. Nonstimulants and emerging treatments in adults with ADHD. CNS Spectr 2008;13(Suppl. 13):9.
Palumbo DR, Sallee FR, Pelham WE. Clonidine for attention-deficit/hyperactivity disorder. I. Efficacy and tolerability outcomes. J Am Acad Child Adolesc Psychiatry 2008;47:2.
Pliszka S. AACAP Work Group on Quality Issues: Practice parameter for the assessment and treatment of children and adolescents with attention-deficit/hyperactivity disorder. J Am Acad Child Adolesc Psychiatry 2007;46:7.
Towbin K. Paying attention to stimulants: Height, weight, and cardiovascular monitoring in clinical practice. J Am Acad Child Adolesc Psychiatry 2008;47:9.

CARE OF THE HIGH-RISK NEONATE

Method of
Paul S. Kingma, MD, PhD

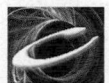

CURRENT DIAGNOSIS

- Evaluation of the high-risk infant begins with the prenatal and perinatal history.
- Initial assessment in the delivery room should focus on the status of airway, breathing, and circulation.
- Neonatal signs are often systemic, nonspecific, and overlapping.
- Common neonatal problems involve prematurity, abnormal transition, infection, intestinal malformations, or pulmonary hypoplasia.

CURRENT THERAPY

- Most neonatal respiratory problems are treated with gentle supportive therapy.
- Ampicillin and gentamicin remain the most effective first-line therapy against most organisms responsible for sepsis in neonates.
- Selective pulmonary vasodilators have significantly improved the outcome in infants with pulmonary hypertension.
- Cooling therapy should be considered in infants with hypoxic brain injury.
- Initial therapy of intestinal obstruction requires decompression of proximal bowel and stabilization with intravenous fluids.

The maturation of the fetus and transition to neonatal life requires the precise coordination of an immensely complex cascade of biochemical and physiologic events. As a result, the late fetal and early neonatal period is also the time of life exhibiting the highest mortality rate of any pediatric age interval. The infant mortality rate includes both the neonatal (days 1–28) and the postneonatal (days 28–365) periods and is expressed as the number of deaths per 1000 live births. Despite considerable advances in neonatal and obstetrics care over the past few decades, the infant mortality rate in the United States in 2011 was 6.05 per 1000 live births, with congenital malformations and prematurity or low birth weight as the top two causes of infant death. Early identification and initiation of appropriate care of these high-risk neonates is essential to improving their outcome.

Care of the high-risk neonate begins with appropriate delivery, management, and resuscitation of the infant. The goals of resuscitation are to maintain or establish effective ventilation and oxygenation, maintain or restore adequate cardiac output and tissue perfusion, and maintain or restore normal body temperature. The steps needed to achieve these goals are based on the common ABC (airway, breathing, circulation) principles that are relevant to all infants. However, after adequate resuscitation, the care of the high-risk neonate is dictated by the diagnosis of the infant's problem. Most of these diagnoses and the treatment approach for each can be categorized into prematurity, abnormal transition, infection, intestinal malformations, and pulmonary hypoplasia.

Prematurity

Epidemiology
The mean duration of a spontaneous singleton pregnancy is 40 postmenstrual weeks. An infant delivered before the completion of the 37th week is considered preterm. Preterm infants can be further classified according to birth weight: low birth weight (LBW) if less than 2500 g, very low birth weight (VLBW) if less than 1500 g, and extremely low birth weight (ELBW) if less than 1000 g. The rate of preterm births increased to 12.3 in 2008, up 20% since 1990. This is a result mostly of increases in late preterm births, which, in turn, can be attributed to a significant rise in both indicated preterm births and multifetal gestations associated with assisted reproductive technology.

Clinical Manifestations and Treatment
Besides the risk for death, prematurity is also associated with an increased risk of morbidity in nearly every organ system, and this risk increases dramatically as both the gestational age and birth weight decrease. The approach to the common problems associated with the premature neonate is presented in Box 1.

Complications
One of the most difficult decisions faced by families and health care professionals regards the treatment of infants at the threshold of viability. Although this threshold has decreased since the 1970s, most neonatologists recognize 22 to 24 weeks' gestation as the limit of viability. Survival rates for infants born at 23 weeks'

Box 1 Common Problems and Treatment in Premature Infants

Delivery Room

Anticipation and preparation are key. The delivery team should include a neonatologist, neonatal nurse, and respiratory therapists. Dry and warm the infant immediately. Ventilate with a bag mask if the heart rate is low or there is no respiratory effort. Use mask continuous positive airway pressure (CPAP) if the heart rate is good and the infant has good respiratory effort. Intubate if there is no response from bag mask ventilation. Avoid high pressures.

Pulmonary

Respiratory distress syndrome owing to surfactant deficiency is common in preterm infants. Care is supportive with supplemental oxygen, CPAP, or gentle ventilation as needed. To reduce risk of chronic lung disease, use the lowest support needed to achieve oxygen saturations of 91% to 95% and $Paco_2$ of 50 to 65 mm Hg. Use exogenous surfactant when indicated. Apnea is common and is treated with caffeine citrate (Cafcit) 20 mg/kg bolus, 5 mg/kg every 24 hours maintenance.

Cardiovascular

Hypotension can require inotropic (epinephrine or dopamine) support. Avoid large fluid boluses in extremely-low-birth-weight (ELBW) infants. Some hypotensive preterm infants are adrenal deficient and might respond to hydrocortisone (Solu-Cortef). Patent ductus arteriosus (PDA) occurs in 50% of ELBW infants. Medical treatment consists of fluid restriction and indomethacin (Indocin IV, 0.2 mg/kg/dose for four doses[3]). Surgical ligation of the PDA may be needed.

Nutrition

Parenteral nutrition is required in most infants younger than 32 weeks' gestation while enteral feedings are increased and will require placement of a percutaneous central venous catheter. Premature infants require higher-calorie (24 to 30 calories/ounce) preterm formula or human milk supplemented with preterm fortifiers.

Fluids and Electrolytes

Total fluid requirements for premature infants start at 80 mL/kg/day on day 1 of life and increase by 20 mL/kg/day each day to a maximum of 140 to 160 mL/kg/day. Fluid intake needs can vary depending on the clinical status of the infant. Sodium and potassium supplements are added on day 2. Hypernatremia is caused by increased free water loss.

Gastrointestinal

Necrotizing enterocolitis is a devastating complication of prematurity and is characterized by abdominal distention, feeding intolerance, bloody stools, and evidence of pneumatosis intestinalis, portal venous gas, and/or free air on abdominal radiographs. Early medical management includes decompressing the bowel, stopping enteral feedings, and giving intravenous antibiotics. Surgery is indicated in patients with intestinal perforation or failed medical treatment.

Anemia

Because of frequent blood draws and delayed activation of erythropoiesis, most ELBW infants require a transfusion of packed red blood cells (10 to 20 mL/kg) during their hospital stay.

Hyperbilirubinemia

Bilirubin central nervous system toxicity occurs at a lower level in preterm infants, and as a result phototherapy needs to be initiated sooner in this population.

Central Nervous System

Intraventricular hemorrhage remains a significant problem in premature infants. The risk increases with decreasing gestational age, stress, sepsis, birth asphyxia, rapid shifts in volume status, and hypotension. A head ultrasound should be obtained at 7 to 10 days of age to evaluate for intraventricular hemorrhage and afterward as needed depending on the severity of the findings.

---

[3]Exceeds dosage recommended by the manufacturer.

---

gestation (23 0/7 to 23 6/7 days) range from 15% to 30%, whereas survival increases to between 30% and 55% for infants born at 24 weeks' gestation. Within this group of survivors, 30% to 50% will have moderate to severe disability, including blindness, deafness, developmental delays, and cerebral palsy. Up-to-date preterm birth outcome estimates are available at the National Institute of Child Health and Human Development (www. nichd.nih.gov/about/org/cdbpm/pp/prog_epbo/index.cfm). The American Academy of Pediatrics recommends that decisions regarding life-sustaining treatment of these infants should be based on the best interests of the newborn, and the Academy also recognizes that parents should have the primary role in choosing aggressive versus palliative care of their infant. Making decisions within this gestational range requires accurate information regarding the mortality and morbidity risks for this population and thorough communication with the family.

Abnormal Transition

The transition from fetal to neonatal life involves a dramatic process of pulmonary adaptation that includes evacuation of fluid from the lungs, expansion of the lungs with air, decreasing pulmonary vascular resistance, and initiating respiratory effort. Often,

this transition is delayed or disrupted and the respiratory status of the newborn is compromised. A few conditions associated with an abnormal transition are reviewed.

Transient Tachypnea of the Newborn
Epidemiology

Transient tachypnea of the newborn (TTN) is a mild condition affecting term and late preterm infants and is the most common respiratory cause of admission to the special care nursery. By definition, TTN is self-limiting, rarely causes hypoxic respiratory failure (hypoxia requiring ventilator support), and has no increased risk of pulmonary dysfunction later in life.

Risk Factors

TTN is classically seen in term or late preterm infants, especially after cesarean birth before the onset of spontaneous labor.

Pathophysiology

Traditional explanations for the pathophysiology of TTN involve impaired fluid clearance from the lungs because of decreased Starling forces and pulmonary squeeze normally encountered during movement through the birth canal. However, the bulk of pulmonary fluid clearance during labor is mediated by activation of sodium channels in the respiratory epithelial cells. In addition, some studies suggest TTN might also involve a mild surfactant deficiency.

Clinical Manifestation
TTN usually manifests with significant grunting along with tachypnea, nasal flaring, mild retractions, and mild hypoxia.

Diagnosis
TTN is primarily a clinical diagnosis. Chest x-rays often demonstrate mild pulmonary congestion, with small accumulations of extrapleural fluid, especially in the minor fissure on the right side. Symptoms usually improve rapidly and resolve within the first 24 to 36 hours.

Differential Diagnosis
TTN is a diagnosis of exclusion and it is important that other potential causes of respiratory distress in the newborn such as infection, pneumothorax, meconium aspiration, polycythemia, and congenital heart disease are excluded.

Treatment
Management is mainly supportive. Supplemental oxygen is provided to keep the O_2 saturations greater than 91%. Continuous positive airway pressure is rarely needed and may increase the risk of pneumothorax in this population. If symptoms last longer than 2 to 3 hours, infants are usually given intravenous fluids and not fed orally until their tachypnea resolves.

Meconium Aspiration
Epidemiology
Meconium stained amniotic fluid occurs in 12% to 15% of all deliveries, and this rate increases in postterm gestation and in African American infants. In contrast to meconium-stained amniotic fluid, meconium aspiration syndrome is rare, occurring in 2% of deliveries with meconium stained amniotic fluid, although the reported incidence varies and trends suggest this incidence is decreasing.

Risk Factors
Risk factors for meconium aspiration include meconium stained fluid, in utero stress, and postterm gestation.

Pathophysiology
Traditional explanations for the pathophysiology of meconium aspiration syndrome suggest that fetal stress leads to passage of meconium in utero. Once this meconium is aspirated, it can cause airway obstruction, pneumothorax, chemical pneumonitis, and pulmonary hypertension. However, recent reports that describe infants born through clear amniotic fluid with respiratory distress and other clinical findings similar to meconium aspiration syndrome suggest this traditional explanation may be incorrect.

Clinical Manifestation
Meconium aspiration syndrome manifests as severe respiratory failure and pulmonary hypertension.

Diagnosis
By definition, the diagnosis of meconium aspiration syndrome includes delivery through meconium-stained amniotic fluid along with respiratory distress and a characteristic chest x-ray appearance of patchy infiltrates with areas of hyperlucency throughout the lung fields.

Differential Diagnosis
Other potential causes of respiratory distress in the newborn such as infection, surfactant deficiency, pneumothorax, and congenital heart disease must be considered.

Treatment
Until recently, aggressive suctioning of the airway in infants delivered through meconium stained fluid was considered the key to preventing meconium aspiration syndrome. Now the Neonatal Resuscitation Program protocol for delivery room management no longer recommends tracheal suctioning for vigorous infants (depressed infants should have their airways cleared as needed), implying that establishment of ventilation should take precedence over attempting to suction an unobstructed airway.

The treatment of meconium aspiration syndrome has dramatically improved in recent years, leading to decreases in morbidity, mortality, and the use of extracorporeal membrane oxygenation (ECMO). Most of these advances have come from treatment of pulmonary hypertension with selective pulmonary vasodilators such as inhaled nitric oxide (iNO). These agents improve oxygenation, which in turn decreases the need for ventilator support and the risk of air leak and chronic lung disease. Administration of exogenous surfactant (Survanta) may be another useful treatment modality.

Persistent Pulmonary Hypertension of the Newborn
Epidemiology
Persistent pulmonary hypertension of the newborn (PPHN) occurs when the normal cardiopulmonary transition of the delivered infant fails. Estimates indicate that severe PPHN occurs in 2 per 1000 liveborn term infants, but PPHN complicates the clinical course of up to 10% of all neonates with respiratory failure.

Risk Factors
Risk factors for developing PPHN include sepsis, pneumonia, congenital malformations, and all conditions associated with pulmonary hypoplasia.

Pathophysiology
At delivery, the normal decrease in pulmonary vascular resistance requires relaxation of pulmonary arteriolar smooth muscle, distention of alveoli, and a change in endothelial cell shape. When pulmonary development is hypoplastic or the fetus experiences significant intrauterine stress or hypoxemia, there is an increase in both pulmonary arteriole reactivity and proliferation of medial smooth muscle of the pulmonary vessels. When these vessels are subjected to hypoxemia or acidosis, they are more prone to constriction, which subsequently induces right-to-left shunting of deoxygenated blood.

Clinical Manifestation
PPHN typically manifests with severe hypoxemia in the setting of respiratory failure with a more than 5% differential in preductal and postductal oxygen saturations. Often, hypotension secondary to right heart failure and decreased left ventricular filling is also present. PPHN symptoms may be isolated or occur in combination with the primary cause of stress or respiratory failure.

Diagnosis
PPHN is diagnosed with an echocardiogram, which reveals elevated right ventricular pressures and right-to-left shunting across the foramen ovale and ductus arteriosus. In severe PPHN, right ventricular pressures are equal to or greater than systemic pressures.

Differential Diagnosis
The primary cause of stress or respiratory failure in PPHN such as sepsis, pneumonia, and pulmonary hypoplasia must always be considered. In addition, congenital heart disease must be excluded.

Treatment
The first goal of PPHN therapy is optimal oxygenation and ventilation. However, care must be taken not to induce significant overdistention of alveoli and pulmonary injury. Often the short-term benefit of improving carbon dioxide levels or oxygen saturations

by a few points is not worth the risk of lung injury and broncho-pulmonary dysplasia. As a result, targeting an oxygen saturation of 91% to 95%, arterial pH levels of 7.25 to 7.35, and carbon dioxide levels of 50 to 65 mm Hg usually achieves a good balance between short-term and long-term goals.

The treatment of PPHN has significantly improved since the turn of the 21st century owing to pharmacologic interventions that specifically reduce pulmonary vascular resistance. Of these, iNO (dose 5-20 ppm) is the best studied and has demonstrated a clear benefit in the setting of PPHN caused by meconium aspiration syndrome or sepsis. Other pulmonary vasodilators, including sildenafil (Revatio),[1] bosentan (Tracleer),[1] and prostacyclin (epoprostenol, Flolan)[1] are increasing in use. When adequate ventilation and pulmonary vasodilators fail in patients with PPHN, ECMO may be considered.

Hypoxic-Ischemic Encephalopathy
Epidemiology
Despite significant advances in obstetric and neonatal care, the incidence of hypoxic-ischemic encephalopathy (HIE) remains at 1 to 2 infants per 1000 term births. Although HIE was once thought to result from brain injury sustained only during the perinatal period, recent data show that most brain injury occurs well before labor and only 10% of neonatal brain injury is related to perinatal or intrapartum events.

Risk Factors
Several clinical measures such as fetal heart rate abnormalities, meconium-stained amniotic fluid, low Apgar scores, large size for gestational age, and the need for resuscitation in the delivery room suggest an increased risk for developing HIE. However, all of these indicators have a very high false-positive rate and therefore do not reliably identify infants who will develop HIE.

Pathophysiology
The brain injury referred to as HIE occurs when oxygen delivery to the brain is insufficient to meet the metabolic demands, resulting in hypoxia, hypercarbia, and metabolic acidosis. This asphyxia is due most often to an interruption of placental blood flow or gas exchange. Although HIE is initiated by a hypoxic event, a growing body of evidence now suggests that there is also a reperfusion phase of brain injury, and several emerging neuroprotective therapies are targeting this phase of injury.

Clinical Manifestation
HIE is clinically characterized by a depressed level of consciousness, seizures and abnormalities in muscle tone (hypotonia initially followed by hypertonia), reflexes (usually decreased initially), and respiratory effort. If other organ systems are involved, infants can also present with signs of heart, kidney, and liver failure.

Diagnosis
HIE is a clinical diagnosis. The Sarnat staging system is often used to classify the severity of the brain injury. Sarnat stage 1 infants have a good prognosis. Sarnat stage 2 infants have long-term neurologic impairment in 20% to 25% of cases, and more than 80% of Sarnat stage 3 infants develop long-term neurologic sequelae. Although brain imaging studies such as magnetic resonance imaging (MRI) are often used to assess the location and severity of brain injury, correlating MRI findings with long-term neurologic outcome is difficult.

Differential Diagnosis
The findings of HIE usually result from hypoxic injury, but they can also result from exposure to toxins or from metabolic, neuromuscular, and chromosomal abnormalities.

Treatment
First-line therapy in infants with HIE is supportive. Adequate ventilation and systemic perfusion should be established using ventilator and inotropic support as needed. If seizures occur, phenobarbital is a good first-line antiepileptic agent in these infants.

Cooling therapy is recommended in infants with HIE. In infants with moderate to severe HIE, whole-body cooling decreased the risk of death or moderate to severe disability by 18%. Current recommendations suggest the following clinical parameters in order to qualify for cooling: gestational age 36 weeks or older, umbilical artery pH less than 7.00 or a base deficit at least 16 mEq/L, and evidence of an abnormal neurologic examination, seizures, or abnormal electroencephalogram (EEG).

Infection
Epidemiology
Neonatal sepsis is a significant cause of morbidity and mortality in term and preterm infants, and the risk of infection increases as the gestational age decreases. Neonatal sepsis is generally divided into two categories: early and late onset. Early-onset sepsis occurs in the first 3 days of life at a rate of approximately 1.9% of VLBW infants. Early-onset sepsis is caused by bacteria residing in the mother's genitourinary tract such as *Escherichia coli*, group B *Streptococcus* (GBS), and *Listeria monocytogenes*. The incidence of GBS disease has significantly decreased since the institution of screening and treatment for GBS colonization in mothers during the third trimester. Late-onset sepsis occurs between days 3 and 28 and is more common, with an incidence of 21% of VLBW infants. Late-onset sepsis is caused by a variety of bacteria including *Staphylococcus epidermidis*, *Staphylococcus aureus*, *Escherichia coli*, *Klebsiella*, *Enterococcus*, *Pseudomonas*, and *Streptococcus pneumoniae*. Ultimately 18% to 36% of infected VLBW infants die; those who survive have a significantly prolonged hospital stay and increased morbidity when compared to uninfected infants.

Risk Factors
The risk for neonatal infection is inversely proportional to gestational age. African American race and male sex are additional risk factors for neonatal infection. Specific risk factors for early-onset sepsis include prolonged rupture of membranes (>24 hours), chorioamnionitis, maternal infection, and prematurity. The risk for late-onset sepsis is increased by the presence of central venous catheters, peripheral intravenous catheters, endotracheal tubes, umbilical vessel catheters, and electronic monitoring devices.

Pathophysiology
Although infants are protected by maternal antibodies transferred across the placenta during the third trimester, compared with older children or adults, the neonatal immune system is still deficient. Innate immunity is defective at several levels. Skin and mucosal barriers are poorly developed, and bacterial translocation across these barriers is common. Antibacterial proteins such as lysozyme, lactoferrin, and lectins are decreased. Neutrophil chemotaxis, phagocytosis, and intracellular killing are limited. In addition to these defects in innate immunity, humoral and cell-mediated immune functions are also poorly developed.

Clinical Manifestation
Neonatal sepsis can manifest with a variety of nonspecific signs including lethargy, poor feeding, temperature instability, decreased tone, increased work of breathing, apnea, cyanosis, bradycardia, tachycardia, abdominal distention, and altered perfusion. Petechiae and purpura may be present during disseminated intravascular coagulation. Although fever and localizing symptoms are common in older children and adults with infection, neonatal sepsis rarely manifests with these symptoms.

Diagnosis
The gold standard for diagnosing sepsis is a positive blood culture. However, the sensitivity of a blood culture in an infected neonate is between 30% and 60% depending on the volume of blood used for

---

[1]Not FDA approved for this indication.

the culture. Therefore, the diagnosis of sepsis in the neonate is more often based on clinical suspicion than laboratory evaluation.

All infants in whom sepsis is suspected should have a thorough clinical examination to evaluate the infant for signs of infection and assess his or her clinical stability. A complete blood count (CBC), cerebrospinal fluid (CSF) culture, and urine culture can also be sent as part of the work-up for neonatal infection, but the value of each of these tests is uncertain. A white blood cell count less than 5000 or greater than 40,000, a total neutrophil count less than 1000, and a band-neutrophil-to-total-neutrophil ratio of greater than 0.2 all correlate with an increased risk of infection, but these tests have a sensitivity for detecting infection that is less than 50%. In addition, because CBC values are often abnormal in healthy neonates, the positive predictive value of an abnormal CBC is less than 18%. Therefore, a normal CBC only weakly supports that the infant is uninfected, and likewise an abnormal CBC only weakly supports the diagnosis of infection.

Many institutions send a CSF for culture, Gram stain, cell count, and protein and glucose levels as part of the evaluation of every infant with suspected sepsis. In contrast, some institutions only send CSF for analysis if the blood culture is positive. The latter method is based on the assumption that because of the inability to isolate infections and the poorly developed blood–brain barrier in the neonate, all neonates with meningitis also have positive blood cultures. This approach is refuted by studies that demonstrate negative blood cultures in up to 50% of infants with meningitis. However, there is still uncertainty regarding the benefit to subjecting every neonate with suspected sepsis to a lumbar puncture.

Differential Diagnosis

The differential diagnosis of neonatal sepsis includes respiratory distress syndrome, TTN, PPHN, metabolic disorders, and congenital heart disease.

Treatment

Ampicillin and gentamicin for 10 to 14 days remains the most effective first-line therapy against most organisms responsible for early-onset sepsis. The antibiotic choice can be tailored once the identity of the organism and antibiotic sensitivities are determined. If meningitis is present, improved penetration of the blood–brain barrier with a third-generation cephalosporin is recommended. Late-onset sepsis is treated with a similar approach but the antibiotic choice may be modified depending on the exposure history of the infant and the indigenous microbiologic flora of the hospital. If methicillin-resistant *Staphylococcus* species are common, vancomycin (Vancocin) may be warranted as a first-line agent in late-onset sepsis. If signs of infection persist despite aggressive antibacterial treatment, a fungal infection may be present, which is treated with amphotericin B (Fungizone).

After initiating appropriate antibiotic coverage, the remaining therapy for neonatal sepsis is supportive. Adequate oxygenation and ventilation can require ventilator support. Blood pressure and urine output are monitored to determine the need to treat septic shock with fluids or inotropic agents. Pulmonary vasodilators may be needed to treat exacerbations of pulmonary hypertension associated with sepsis.

Intestinal Malformations

Intestinal Obstruction

Epidemiology

Obstruction of the gastrointestinal tract can be complete (atresia) or partial (stenosis) and occur at any point from the esophagus to the anus. Obstruction of the intestinal tract occurs in 1 out of 1500 live births.

Esophageal atresia occurs in 1 out of 4000 live births. Of infants with esophageal atresia, 85% have a tracheoesophageal fistula and approximately 40% of infants with tracheoesophageal fistula have other associated anomalies as part of the VACTERL syndrome, which includes vertebral, anal, cardiac, tracheal, esophageal, renal, and limb anomalies.

Duodenal atresia occurs in 1 out of 5000 live births and is often associated with trisomy 21. Seventy percent of duodenal atresia cases are associated with other malformations such as cardiac anomalies, intestinal malrotation, annular pancreas and imperforate anus. In the jejunum and ileum, atresia is more common than stenosis, and ileal lesions are more common than jejunal lesions. Malrotation is associated with other gastrointestinal lesions including duodenal atresia, gastroschisis, omphalocele, and congenital diaphragmatic hernia.

Hirschsprung's disease occurs in 1 out of 5000 live births and is the most common cause of large bowel obstruction in neonates. It is more common in boys, siblings of infants with Hirschsprung's disease, and infants with trisomy 21.

Imperforate anus occurs in 1 out of 5000 live births.

Pathophysiology

All intestinal atresia or stenosis occurs as a result of either an incomplete formation during development or a vascular accident in utero. Regardless of the location or cause, the obstruction will lead to dilation of the bowel proximal to the narrowing and atrophy of the bowel distally. If the proximal bowel is not decompressed, distention can lead to injury and necrosis.

Malrotation is caused by the incomplete rotation and fixation of the bowel as it returns to the abdominal cavity during development, with abnormally fixed bands crossing the duodenum. Malrotated intestine is at increased risk for volvulus, which causes strangulation of the superior mesenteric artery and occlusion of blood flow to the intestine.

Hirschsprung's disease is caused by defective migration of neural crest cells to the distal colon, resulting in a distal segment of colon that is aganglionic and dysfunctional.

Clinical Manifestation

Infants with atresia or stenosis of the intestinal tract present with signs of obstruction. Infants with esophageal atresia present with excessive oral secretions, inability to feed, gagging, and respiratory distress when feeding is attempted. Infants with duodenal atresia present with abdominal distention and vomiting shortly after the first feeding. Patients with jejunal and ileal atresia also present with abdominal distention and vomiting, but the emesis may be delayed until the second or third feeding.

Malrotation and volvulus manifest as abdominal distention and bilious emesis. As this condition rapidly progresses, hematochezia, hypotension, and disseminated intravascular coagulation can develop.

Hirschsprung's disease can manifest with failure to pass meconium in the first 24 hours of life, constipation, abdominal distention, explosive stool output with rectal examination, vomiting, and poor feeding.

Imperforate anus manifests with abdominal distention, lack of stool output, and the finding of imperforate anus on clinical examination.

Diagnosis

The diagnosis of esophageal fistula is often suggested by clinical symptoms and the inability to pass a feeding catheter into an infant with poor feeding skills. The diagnosis is then confirmed by chest radiographs with a feeding catheter looped in the obstructed proximal esophagus.

Duodenal atresia is diagnosed by the characteristic duodenal gaseous distention on radiograph (the double bubble sign) and contrast radiographic study of the upper gastrointestinal tract. Malrotation, jejunal atresia, and ileal atresia are all suggested by plain radiographs showing distention of the proximal small bowel and confirmed by contrast radiographic study of the upper gastrointestinal tract. If true bilious emesis occurs and malrotation is suspected, these patients are considered a medical emergency because the integrity of the bowel will be quickly compromised by vascular occlusion and these patients will rapidly progress to a fulminant and even fatal condition without surgical intervention.

Hirschsprung's disease is suggested by clinical history and examination, plain radiograph revealing intestinal distention, and contrast radiograph of the distal bowel revealing proximal dilation and distal narrowing of the aganglionic segment. The diagnosis is confirmed by rectal biopsy revealing the absence of ganglia.

Imperforate anus is diagnosed by clinical examination.

Treatment

The first stage of therapy in all intestinal obstructions is to decompress the tract proximal to the obstruction with a repogle and stabilize the infant with intravenous fluids. The infant should be evaluated for associated anomalies, when indicated, by echocardiogram and renal ultrasound. Once the infant is stable, the obstruction is repaired by surgical removal of the lesion or dysfunctional bowel and reanastomosis. Often the defect can be repaired primarily, but in certain severe cases a diverting ostomy is required until the final repair can be completed.

Complications

In severe cases, intestinal obstruction is complicated by compromise of significant segments of bowel, requiring removal of large portions of the intestinal tract. When large sections are removed, absorption of nutrients is deficient and long-term parental nutrition may be needed.

Gastroschisis and Omphalocele

Epidemiology

The combined incidence of omphalocele and gastroschisis is 1 in 4000 live births. Of these two defects, gastroschisis is more common. In infants with omphalocele, 35% have other gastrointestinal defects and 20% have congenital heart defects. Other anomalies including trisomies 13 and 18, urinary tract anomalies, and Beckwith-Wiedemann syndrome are associated with omphalocele. In contrast, associated congenital or chromosomal anomalies are rare in gastroschisis patients, but these patients do have higher rates of malrotation, intestinal atresia, and necrotizing enterocolitis.

Risk Factors

Pregnancies complicated by infection, young maternal age, smoking, or drug abuse can increase the rate of gastroschisis. Interestingly, owing to unknown causes, the incidence of gastroschisis has increased in recent years.

Pathophysiology

Gastroschisis is caused by a cleft in the abdominal wall to the right of the umbilical cord that allows abdominal contents to herniate into the amniotic fluid. By definition, gastroschisis is not covered by a sac. In addition to being at risk for torsion and necrosis during this herniated state, the prolonged exposure of the bowel to the amniotic fluid causes a severe inflammatory response that results in intestinal injury and ileus.

Omphalocele results when the abdominal contents herniate through the base of the umbilical cord into a sac covered by peritoneum and amniotic membrane. The sac covering the defect is thin and can rupture in utero or during delivery. The size of the defect can range from small (containing only a small amount of intestine), to large (containing most of the abdominal organs), to giant (containing the majority of the liver). Giant omphaloceles are rare (1 in 10,000 births) and are often associated with pulmonary hypoplasia.

Clinical Manifestation and Diagnosis

Polyhydramnios is noted in utero in both conditions. Ten percent of infants with omphalocele and 60% of those with gastroschisis are born prematurely. Diagnosis of gastroschisis and omphalocele is initially made by prenatal ultrasound and confirmed by physical examination after delivery. Early prenatal diagnosis allows proper counseling of the family and referral to a tertiary care center for further management. Infants with omphalocele are also at risk for congenital heart defects and should be evaluated by echocardiogram. Infants with gastroschisis should be evaluated for areas of intestinal torsion, necrosis, or atresia at the time of their initial physical examination.

Treatment

Cesarean section is recommended in giant omphalocele to decrease the risk of rupture of the omphalocele sac, but cesarean section does not improve the outcome in smaller omphaloceles or gastroschisis. If the infant is stable, small omphalocele defects can be closed primarily, but larger defects require a staged repair and can be postponed as long as the sac is intact. Treatment of the intact omphalocele before closure includes intestinal decompression with a repogle to minimize gastrointestinal distention. Although protocols for topical care of the omphalocele sac vary, many cover the sac with petroleum-impregnated gauze and then wrap the sac with gauze to support the viscera on the abdominal wall. Prognosis worsens if the sac is ruptured; therefore there should be no attempt to reduce the omphalocele.

Initial treatment of gastroschisis involves placement of a nasogastric tube to suction, covering the exposed intestine with saline-soaked gauze, and wrapping the exposed intestine and lower half of the infant with a sterile bag to minimize fluid loss and injury to the bowel. Aggressive fluid management is required to compensate for extra fluid loss from the exposed bowel. Many institutions place the infant on antibiotics to cover for infection caused by bowel flora.

In 10% of infants with gastroschisis, single-stage primary closure is possible. In most infants with gastroschisis, a silicone elastic silo is placed over the exposed bowel, allowing gradual reduction of the intestine into the abdomen over a period of several days. Once the bowel is completely reduced, the defect is surgically closed. Postsurgical care of infants with gastroschisis involves a prolonged recovery phase of the bowel during which the infants will require parenteral nutrition and a gradual advancing of enteral feeds.

Pulmonary Hypoplasia

Epidemiology

Lung development begins during the first trimester, progresses through several rounds of branching morphogenesis during the remaining months of gestation, and is not completed until the second or third year of life. Perturbation of lung development during any phase of gestation can result in pulmonary hypoplasia. Because of the variety of conditions associated with pulmonary hypoplasia, the true incidence is unknown.

Risk Factors

The most common risk factors for pulmonary hypoplasia include prolonged rupture of membranes, fetal renal dysplasias and obstructive uropathies, congenital diaphragmatic hernia, and congenital cystic lung lesions.

Pathophysiology

For lung development to proceed normally, the volume of the thorax must be adequate for lung expansion, and amniotic fluid must enter the lung through fetal breathing. Conditions that externally compress the lung (congenital diaphragmatic hernia, cystic lung lesions, pleural effusions with fetal hydrops, malformations of the thorax, abdominal mass lesions) or conditions that decrease amniotic fluid levels (prolonged rupture of membranes, renal agenesis, cystic kidney disease, and urinary tract obstruction) inhibit the branching morphogenesis of the lung and development of the gas exchange interface. As a result, hypoplastic lungs have reduced lung weight and alveolar number, fewer branchings of airways, fewer pulmonary arteries, and an increase in both pulmonary arteriole reactivity and proliferation of medial smooth muscle in pulmonary vessels.

Clinical Manifestation

In addition to the manifestations associated with the primary disease, infants with pulmonary hypoplasia also present with significant respiratory and cardiac signs. The presentation is highly dependent on the severity of the pulmonary hypoplasia. Most infants with pulmonary hypoplasia present with increased work of breathing and significant hypoxia and acidosis. Shunting across the ductus arteriosus is evident on pre- and postductal oxygen saturations. Hypotension secondary to right heart failure and decreased left ventricular filling is often present.

Diagnosis

The diagnosis is based on a clinical history of an anomaly associated with pulmonary hypoplasia. Chest radiographs reveal small bell-shaped lungs or space-occupying chest mass depending on the cause of the hypoplasia. Pulmonary hypertension is often evident on echocardiogram.

Differential Diagnosis

The differential diagnosis of pulmonary hypoplasia includes pneumonia, cyanotic congenital heart disease, primary PPHN, and sepsis.

Treatment

In the fetus with pulmonary hypoplasia, a few interventions can improve prognosis. These include serial amnioinfusions in the setting of prolonged rupture of membranes and nephrostomy tubes in obstructive uropathy.

A portion of these infants have relatively mild disease and require only minimal support; however, many have profound hypoxia as a result of severe pulmonary hypertension. In these infants, the first goal is to establish adequate oxygenation and ventilation. However, care must be taken not to induce significant overdistention of alveoli and pulmonary injury. Targeting an oxygen saturation of 91% to 95%, arterial pH levels of 7.25 to 7.35, and carbon dioxide levels of 50 to 65 mm Hg usually achieves a good balance between short-term benefit and long-term pulmonary injury. Pulmonary vasodilators have significantly improved the care of infants, with pulmonary hypertension associated with pulmonary hypoplasia. Of these, inhaled nitric oxide, 5 to 20 ppm, is the best studied. Other pulmonary vasodilators, including sildenafil,[1] bosentan,[1] and prostacyclin,[1] are increasing in use. Often long-term pulmonary vasodilators are needed to promote lung remodeling and growth.

In patients with congenital diaphragmatic hernia, distention of the bowel that is herniated into the thorax can significantly compromise the respiratory status of the infant. Therefore, at delivery, the infant should be intubated immediately and have a repogle placed to facilitate decompression of the bowel. In addition, bag-mask ventilation in infants with unrepaired congenital diaphragmatic hernia should be avoided.

References

Greenberg JM, Donovan EF, Warner BB, et al. Neonatal morbidities of prenatal and perinatal origin. In: Creasy R, Resnik R, Iams J, editors. Creasy and Resnik's Maternal-Fetal Medicine: Principles and Practice. 6th ed. Philadelphia: Saunders; 2009. p. 1197–2228.

Klaus MH, Fanaroff AA. Care of the High-Risk Neonate. 5th ed Philadelphia: WB Saunders; 2001.

Ledbetter DJ. Gastroschisis and omphalocele. Surg Clin North Am 2006;86 (2):249–60, vii.

Orford J, Cass DT, Glasson MJ. Advances in the treatment of esophageal atresia over three decades: the 1970s and the 1990s. Pediatr Surg Int 2004;20(6):402–7.

Shankaran S, Johnson Y, Langer JC, et al. Outcome of extremely-low-birth-weight infants at highest risk: Gestational age ≤24 weeks, birth weight ≤750 g, and 1-minute Apgar ≤3. Am J Obstet Gynecol 2004;191(4):1084–91.

Steinhorn RH. Neonatal pulmonary hypertension. Pediatr Crit Care Med 2010;11 (Suppl. 2):S79–S84.

Stoll BJ, Hansen N, Fanaroff AA, et al. Late-onset sepsis in very low birth weight neonates: the experience of the NICHD neonatal research network. Pediatrics 2002;110(2 Pt 1):285–91.

[1]Not FDA approved for this indication.

DIABETES MELLITUS IN CHILDREN

Method of
Lori M.B. Laffel, MD, MPH; and Jamie R.S. Wood, MD

CURRENT DIAGNOSIS

ADA Recommendations for the Diagnosis of Diabetes

- Symptoms (polyuria, polydipsia, unexplained weight loss) and a casual plasma glucose (any time of day without regard to time since last meal) ≥200 mg/dL (11.1 mmol/L) or
- Fasting (no caloric intake for at least 8 h) plasma glucose ≥126 mg/dL (7.0 mmol/L) or
- 2-hour plasma glucose ≥200 mg/dL (11.1 mmol/L) during an oral glucose tolerance test (glucose load of 75 g anhydrous glucose dissolved in water or 1.75 g/kg body weight if weight <43 kg).
- A1C ≥6.5%

Note: Criteria 2 and 3 should be confirmed on a second day if child/adolescent is asymptomatic. The OGTT is not recommended for routine clinical use and should be reserved for the asymptomatic child with incidental glucosuria/hyperglycemia or in the child with suspected diabetes but normal fasting plasma glucose. Criteria 4 should be confirmed with a repeat A1C laboratory test (not point-of-care device).
Adapted from American Diabetes Association: Care of children and adolescents with type 1 diabetes. Diabetes Care 2005;28(1):186–212; Diabetes Care 2009;32: 1327–34.

CURRENT THERAPY

Examples of Insulin Regimens

Injections bid:
- Premixed insulin (70/30, 75/25) given at breakfast and dinner
- NPH and rapid- or short-acting insulin given at breakfast and dinner

Injections tid:
- NPH and rapid- or short-acting insulin given at breakfast, rapid- or short-acting insulin given at dinner, and NPH given at bedtime
- NPH and rapid- or short-acting insulin given at breakfast, rapid- or short-acting insulin given at dinner, and NPH or glargine (Lantus) or detemir (Levemir) given at bedtime

Injections qid:
- NPH and rapid-acting insulin given at breakfast, rapid-acting insulin given at lunch and dinner, and rapid-acting insulin and NPH given at bedtime
- NPH and rapid-acting insulin given at breakfast and lunch, rapid-acting insulin given at dinner, and NPH given at bedtime
- Rapid-acting insulin given at breakfast, lunch, dinner, and snacks, and glargine (Lantus) or detemir (Levemir) given at breakfast, dinner, or bedtime

Continuous subcutaneous insulin infusion (CSII)
- Rapid-acting insulin given for basal requirements and as bolus at every meal/snack and periodically to correct hyperglycemia (no more frequent than q2–3h)

Diabetes mellitus is a group of metabolic disorders that have hyperglycemia as a common feature caused by inadequate insulin secretion, insulin action, or both. Chronic hyperglycemia and its numerous downstream effects lead to micro- and macrovascular complications involving the eyes, kidneys, nerves, and blood vessels. Childhood and adolescent years are periods of rapid physical growth and psychosocial change, and these two factors make the care of children and adolescents with diabetes both challenging and rewarding. The health care professional must balance the important goals of optimal glycemic control and normal growth and development along with the risks of hypoglycemia and the challenges of expected glycemic excursions during childhood.

Multidisciplinary care is the hallmark of successful diabetes management for the child and adolescent with diabetes and for family members.

The American Diabetes Association (ADA) classifies diabetes mellitus into four main types: type 1 diabetes (T1D), type 2 diabetes (T2D), other specific types, and gestational diabetes mellitus (Table 1). T1D is caused by insulin deficiency, which results from the autoimmune destruction of the pancreatic β cells. There are multiple genetic loci in the major histocompatibility region of chromosome 6 that predispose (DR 3/4, DQ 0201/0302, DR 4/4, and DQ 0300/0302) or protect against (DQB1*0602, DQA1*0102) the development of T1D. T2D is caused by the combination of insulin resistance and relative insulin deficiency. Type 1 diabetes is most common in pediatrics.

Genetic forms of diabetes include maturity-onset diabetes in the young (MODY), neonatal diabetes, mitochondrial diabetes, and certain syndromes of insulin resistance. MODY is characterized by young age of onset, autosomal dominant inheritance, the lack of association with obesity, and a variable phenotype. The most common disease of the exocrine pancreas that causes diabetes in children and adolescents is cystic fibrosis. Glucocorticoids used in the treatment of systemic illnesses are also commonly associated with hyperglycemia and diabetes. Certain genetic syndromes, such as Down syndrome, Klinefelter's syndrome, and Turner's syndrome, increase the risk for diabetes.

Diagnosis

The diagnosis of T1D in children and adolescents is typically straightforward. The classic symptoms of polyuria, polydipsia, polyphagia, and weight loss over a several-week period are common. A thorough history and physical exam may reveal perineal candidiasis or thrush. Such symptoms may be followed by nausea, abdominal pain, vomiting, lethargy, and Kussmaul respirations if diabetic ketoacidosis (DKA) and lactic acidosis develop. The presentation of T2D in children and adolescents can be more subtle and sometimes even clinically silent. However, approximately a third of adolescents with T2D have ketosis and a quarter have ketoacidosis at presentation.

The Current Diagnosis box outlines the diagnosis of diabetes mellitus. In the asymptomatic child or adolescent, diabetes is diagnosed when a fasting plasma glucose is 126 mg/dL or more, a 2-hour plasma glucose during an oral glucose tolerance test (OGTT) is 200 mg/dL or more, or a random plasma glucose is 200 mg/dL or more with confirmation on a second day. The symptomatic child or adolescent with a random plasma glucose of 200 mg/dL or more does not need repeat testing to confirm the diagnosis. Measurement of islet cell autoantibodies consistent with T1D (GAD, insulin, IA2, zinc transporter) at diagnosis may help distinguish between T1D and T2D. Care must be taken to avoid delay in the diagnosis and initiation of treatment because of the risk of rapid metabolic deterioration with insulin deficiency.

Initial Management

The goals of initial management of the child or adolescent newly diagnosed with diabetes mellitus are to correct fluid and electrolyte imbalances, reverse hepatic gluconeogenesis and ketogenesis by halting lipolysis with insulin replacement, and begin the process of diabetes education. The location of this initial management depends on the severity of the clinical presentation, the age of the patient, the psychosocial assessment of the child or adolescent and caregiver, and the diabetes-related resources available in the family's geographic location (availability of an outpatient education program).

Diabetic Ketoacidosis

Approximately 25%–30% of children with newly diagnosed T1D present with diabetic ketoacidosis (DKA). Children who are younger (less than 4 years), without a first-degree relative with T1D, and from a family of lower socioeconomic status are at higher risk of DKA at onset of T1D. The majority of DKA episodes occur in patients with established diabetes, not in those newly diagnosed. Children or adolescents with established T1D are at higher risk for DKA if they are in poor metabolic control, have had a previous episode of DKA, are peripubertal/adolescent girls, have a psychiatric disorder, or are from a disadvantaged background.

Management of DKA in children and adolescents is based on the same principles used in adults and therefore is covered in a separate chapter in this book. The development of cerebral edema, however, warrants discussion because this complication is seen primarily in children and is associated with both high morbidity and mortality. Risk factors for the development of cerebral edema include lower initial partial pressure of carbon dioxide, higher initial serum urea nitrogen concentrations, treatment with bicarbonate, and an attenuated rise in measured serum sodium concentrations during therapy. Current recommendations endorse fluid rehydration (generally 10 mL/kg NS bolus) followed by initiation of an insulin drip (0.05–0.1 U/kg/h) without an insulin bolus and continued cautious rehydration. In addition, children who are younger (less than 5 years), have new-onset T1D, and longer duration of symptoms may also be at an increased risk. A high index of suspicion is needed with mannitol (Osmitrol) or 3% NS nearby to allow for timely intervention.

Initiation of Insulin Replacement Therapy

Subcutaneous insulin is initiated in the patient who does not present in DKA or following intravenous insulin therapy in the child with resolved DKA who is tolerating oral intake (pH >7.3, tCO$_2$ >18, anion gap 12 ± 2 mEq/L). The starting dose of insulin replacement therapy depends on the age, weight, and pubertal status of the patient, as well as the presence or absence of DKA. For the prepubertal child without DKA, the starting dose is usually 0.25 to 0.5 U/kg/day. For the prepubertal child with resolved

TABLE 1	Classification of Diabetes Mellitus*

Type 1 diabetes
Type 2 diabetes
Other specific types:
- Genetic defects of β-cell function
  - MODY 1: chromosome 20, HNF-4α
  - MODY 2: chromosome 7, glucokinase
  - MODY 3: chromosome 12, HNF-1α
  - MODY 4: chromosome 13, IPF-1
  - MODY 5: chromosome 17, HNF-1β
  - MODY 6: chromosome 2, NeuroD1
  - Mitochondrial diabetes
  - Neonatal diabetes
- Genetic defects in insulin action
  - Leprechaunism
  - Rabson-Mendenhall syndrome
- Diseases of the exocrine pancreas
  - Pancreatitis
  - Cystic fibrosis
  - Pancreatectomy
- Endocrinopathies
  - Acromegaly
  - Cushing's syndrome
  - Glucagonoma
  - Pheochromocytoma
- Drug or chemical induced
  - Glucocorticoids
- Infections
  - Congenital rubella
  - Cytomegalovirus
- Other genetic syndromes associated with diabetes
  - Down's syndrome
  - Klinefelter's syndrome
  - Turner's syndrome
Gestational diabetes mellitus (GDM)

*Table is not all-inconclusive and gives examples of each subtype of diabetes mellitus. For complete list, see American Diabetes Association: Diagnosis and classification of diabetes mellitus. Diabetes Care 2010;33:S62–69.
Abbreviation: MODY = maturity-onset diabetes in the young.

DKA, the usual starting dose is 0.5 to 0.75 U/kg/day. For the pubertal child without DKA, the starting dose is 0.5 to 0.75 U/kg/day and for the pubertal child with resolved DKA, 0.75 to 1 U/kg/day. This total daily dose (TDD) of insulin is typically divided into a multiple daily injection program with basal bolus insulin therapy or occasionally two injections per day, with the former the preference for implementation of intensive therapy (Figure 1). The twice-daily regimen may be selected if the psychosocial assessment determines that fewer injections per day would be beneficial. The use of an insulin pump at diagnosis remains within the research realm currently.

When the patient is metabolically stable, the focus turns to the psychosocial assessment of the child or adolescent and caregiver(s) and the initiation of diabetes education. A licensed social worker or other mental health professional evaluates each family and screens for circumstances that might complicate diabetes management: family composition, alternative caregiver(s), financial concerns, lack of health insurance, psychiatric or medical illness in a family member, or severe emotional distress of caregiver secondary to the diabetes diagnosis.

Diabetes education can be provided in the inpatient or outpatient setting by a certified diabetes nurse educator (CDE) and focuses on the set of essential skills needed to keep a child or adolescent with diabetes safe at home and school. These survival skills include techniques of blood glucose monitoring, urine or blood ketone measurement, drawing up and administration of subcutaneous insulin and glucagon, recognition and treatment of hypoglycemia and hyperglycemia, basics of sick day management, and indications for and methods of contacting the child's diabetes team. In addition to the survival skills, the child or adolescent and family should meet with a registered dietician who will assist them in developing an individualized meal plan and introduce the family to the concept of carbohydrate counting or exchanges. Once the child or adolescent (if developmentally appropriate) and caregiver(s) demonstrate the knowledge and skills needed, they are discharged with the expectation of daily phone contact with a member of their diabetes team to further titrate insulin doses and answer questions. When available and clinically indicated, a visiting nurse may assist with ongoing home-based education and support in the short term.

Outpatient Diabetes Care

The management of children and adolescents with diabetes requires a multidisciplinary team approach. Members of this team include either a pediatric endocrinologist or pediatrician with training in diabetes, a pediatric CDE, a dietician, and a mental health professional (social worker and psychologist). Members of this team need to be easily accessible to the family in times of illness or metabolic crisis. Another member of the child/adolescent's team is a pediatrician or family doctor who will continue to provide routine well child care including anticipatory guidance, immunizations, and general medical care.

In the first few months of outpatient diabetes care, patients are seen frequently by members of the diabetes team to assess the family's adaptation to the new diagnosis, reinforce skills and knowledge learned during the first few days, and expand on the skills and knowledge needed for intensive diabetes management. Patients are subsequently seen at a minimum frequency of every 3 months, alternating between their CDE and their pediatric endocrinologist. Visits with the dietician are recommended yearly or more frequently if circumstances warrant (e.g., young child or toddler, desired weight loss, initiating pump therapy, etc.).

Diabetes Education

Diabetes education is an ongoing process with continuous need for review of previously learned material and introduction of new concepts as the family develops a more sophisticated understanding of intensive diabetes management. The educator should evaluate the patient and his or her caregiver's knowledge and skills regularly. In addition, age-appropriate issues need to be discussed as the patient matures (e.g., driving guidelines, issues related to alcohol and smoking, etc.). Diabetes education needs to be tailored to each family taking into account their educational level and cultural practices. The educator must be sensitive to the age and developmental stage of the child or adolescent, and shift his or her educational efforts from the caregiver(s) to the adolescent when it is developmentally appropriate. Continued parental involvement and supervision of the adolescent with diabetes is crucial to good metabolic control.

The health care provider should complete a focused interval history at each visit that includes recent illnesses, visits to the emergency department, hospitalizations, medications prescribed other than insulin, types of insulin and current doses, daily routine including meal plan, dietary pattern, and activity level, self-care behaviors and identifying who performs them, episodes of hypoglycemia and their precipitants, school performance, emotional health, and a review of systems focusing on symptoms of hyperglycemia (polyuria, polydipsia, polyphagia, weight loss, candidal infections) and the possible development of other autoimmune disorders. If appropriate, a history of tobacco, alcohol, recreational drugs, and sexual activity should be elicited. A focused physical examination that includes measurement of blood pressure and heart rate, weight, height, body mass index (BMI), and examination of the thyroid gland, sites of blood glucose monitoring, and insulin injections should be completed at each visit. A more

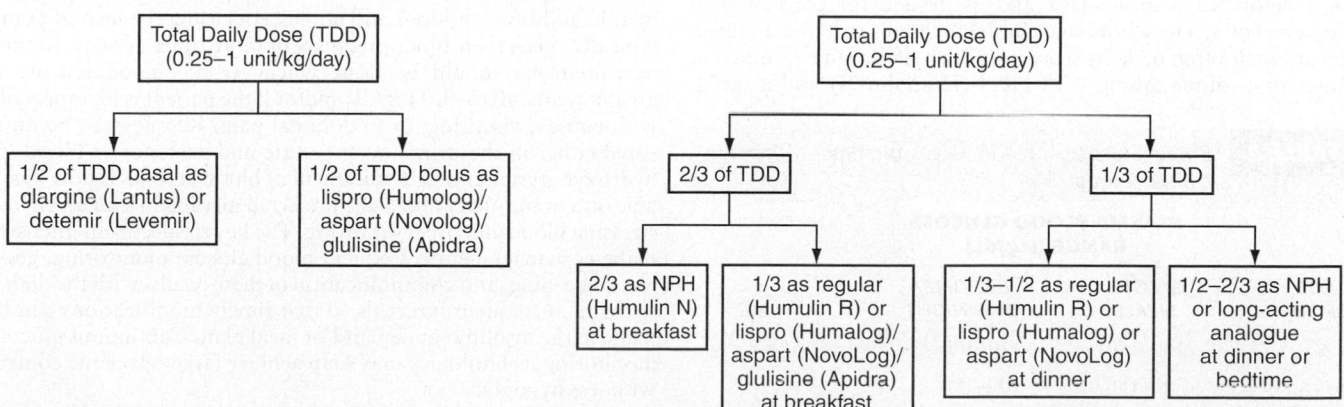

Figure 1. Initiation of insulin replacement therapy. Half of the daily dose (TDD) is given as basal insulin (usually long-acting insulin analogue) and half is given as bolus insulin (usually rapid-acting analogue) before meals and snacks. Two thirds of the total daily dose (TDD) is given at breakfast and further divided into NPH (two thirds) and short/rapid-acting insulin (one third). The remaining one third is either given in one injection at dinner (in a twice-daily regimen) or divided between dinner and bedtime (in a thrice-daily regimen), and should also be divided into NPH or long-acting analogue (two thirds) and short/rapid-acting insulin (one third). Short/rapid-acting insulin can be regular (Humulin R), lispro (Humalog), aspart (NovoLog), or glulisine (Apidra).

thorough physical examination including Tanner staging should be performed once per year or more frequently if indicated.

The hemoglobin A1C, the fraction of hemoglobin that has glucose attached to it, is a measure of the average level of blood glucose over the preceding 2 to 3 months. It should be measured every 3 months and serves as an objective measure of blood glucose control. A discrepancy between the hemoglobin A1C and the average blood glucose levels from self-monitoring records suggests that the patient needs to monitor at different times of day (including use of a 3-day blinded continuous glucose-monitoring device) and may benefit from a review of blood glucose monitoring technique and equipment, or that there may be fabrication of results. Obtaining computer downloaded data helps eliminate the latter possibility. The International Society of Pediatric and Adolescent Diabetes (ISPAD) recommends a single pediatric goal of less than 7.5%.

Goals of Therapy

The Diabetes Control and Complications Trial (DCCT) demonstrated that the incidence of microvascular complications was reduced with improved blood glucose control (hemoglobin A1C approximately 7%). The reduction in complications, however, was accompanied by an increased risk of severe hypoglycemia. Because young children are more vulnerable to hypoglycemia (reduced catecholamine response to hypoglycemia, decreased ability to communicate symptoms of hypoglycemia, and risk for neuropsychologic impairment from hypoglycemia), the ADA has developed age-specific glycemic targets (Table 2).

Insulin Therapy

The ideal insulin replacement therapy would be one that mirrors the basal and prandial insulin secretion in individuals without diabetes. Numerous insulin preparations are available that vary in time to onset, peak, and duration of action (Table 3). No single regimen is superior to another; thus individualization of the insulin regimen to the child or adolescent and family remains a major determinant. Important factors for consideration include blood glucose monitoring frequency, number of daily injections the family can perform, the need for flexibility in meal planning, and the unique family schedule. Regimens range in intensity from twice-a-day injections with a set dose of premixed insulin to intensive diabetes management with multiple injections per day of two or more types of insulin or use of an insulin pump (continuous subcutaneous insulin infusion [CSII]).

Typical regimens that children or adolescents begin at diagnosis were described previously (Figure 1). Some centers initiate a basal-bolus regimen in which insulin is replaced in a manner that attempts to mimic physiologic insulin release. Basal-bolus regimens include the insulin pump and glargine (Lantus) given once a day with rapid-acting insulin (lispro [Humalog] or aspart [NovoLog]) before each meal/snack and as needed for correction of hyperglycemia. The school-age child who hopes to avoid an injection at lunch often benefits from a regimen of glargine (Lantus) at dinner or bedtime, along with NPH (Humulin N) and a rapid-

acting insulin at breakfast, plus a rapid-acting insulin at dinner. The peak of the NPH covers carbohydrate intake at lunch. The use of basal insulin analogues glargine (Lantus) or detemir (Levemir) in the evening is associated with less nocturnal hypoglycemia.

Patients on a basal-bolus regimen determine their insulin doses based on an insulin-to-carbohydrate ratio and a correction factor or sensitivity index (CF or SI). The insulin-to-carbohydrate ratio is the number of grams of carbohydrate covered by 1 U of insulin (roughly 450 divided by TDD) for each meal and snack. The CF/SI is the expected decrement in glucose following 1 U of rapid-acting insulin (roughly 1650 divided by TDD). The CF/SI is applied no more than every 2 to 3 hours to lower an elevated blood glucose toward the target range to avoid so-called stacking of insulin action and subsequent hypoglycemia. For patients on a combination of intermediate-acting insulin (NPH) and rapid- or short-acting insulin, meals typically contain a certain amount of carbohydrates (e.g., 60 g or 4 carbohydrate exchanges) and require consistency in timing to avoid hypoglycemia.

The CSII, otherwise known as insulin pump therapy, comes the closest to mimicking the basal and prandial insulin secretion of an individual without diabetes. The insulin pump is steadily becoming a commonly used method to replace insulin, especially in the pediatric population. There are many advantages to the insulin pump including the elimination of multiple daily injections, increased flexibility in meal planning, ease of decreasing insulin for physical activity, fewer hypoglycemic events, and the ability to deliver very small amounts of insulin. The disadvantages are more frequent blood glucose monitoring, always being tethered to the pump, and increased risk for the development of DKA. Because only rapid-acting insulin (lispro [Humalog], aspart [NovoLog], or glulisine [Apidra]) is used in the insulin pump, discontinuation of insulin delivery can result in ketone production within hours. Increased vigilance, therefore, is necessary to ensure proper functioning of the insulin pump with frequent blood glucose monitoring and checking for ketones if hyperglycemia develops.

Self-Monitoring

One of the main goals of diabetes education is to teach and empower the patient and family in the self-management of diabetes. Self-management of diabetes includes measuring blood glucose and blood/urine ketone levels, recording the results along with amount of carbohydrate intake and amount of insulin administered, and the ability to make insulin dosing decisions based on the interpretation of these records. Monitoring blood glucose four or more times daily is recommended in children with T1D. Additional monitoring may be necessary postprandially, overnight, or during periods of increased physical activity to help optimize control and prevent severe hypoglycemia. Preschool or early school-age children may require more frequent monitoring because of their inability to recognize symptoms or to communicate during episodes of hypoglycemia. In addition, children and adolescents using the insulin pump typically check their blood sugar six or more times per day. Ketone measurements should be done whenever the blood glucose is greater than 250 to 300 mg/dL and/or if the patient is ill, especially with nausea, vomiting, or abdominal pain. Ketones can be measured either in the urine (acetoacetate and acetone) or blood (β-hydroxybutyric acid). Measurement of blood ketones is now available on a home meter and is the preferred method in the current era stressing blood glucose monitoring. The key to successful intensive diabetes management is frequent blood glucose monitoring, good record keeping, and communication of these results with the diabetes team at frequent intervals so that timely modifications can be made to the insulin regimen and/or meal plan. Continuous glucose monitoring technologies may help achieve target glycemic control with less hypoglycemia.

Medical Nutrition Therapy

The meal plan remains an important component of management aimed at good glycemic control, although it is often the most difficult aspect of intensive diabetes management for families. A dietician trained in pediatric nutrition and diabetes should meet with the family at the time of T1D diagnosis and periodically

TABLE 2 Blood Glucose and A1C Goals for Type 1 Diabetes by Age Group

AGE GROUP	PLASMA BLOOD GLUCOSE RANGE (mg/dL)		A1C
	BEFORE MEALS	*BEDTIME/ OVERNIGHT*	
<6 y	100–180	110–200	7.5%–8.5%
6–12 y	90–180	100–180	<8%
13–19 y	90–130	90–150	<7.5%

Adapted from American Diabetes Association: Care of children and adolescents with type 1 diabetes. Diabetes Care 2005;28(1):186–212.

Goals should be individualized; lower goals may be reasonable and achievable without hypoglycemia.

Goals should be higher in patients with frequent hypoglycemia or hypoglycemia unawareness.

TABLE 3 Insulin Analogues

INSULIN PREPARATION	ONSET OF ACTION	PEAK ACTION	EFFECTIVE DURATION
Rapid Acting			
Insulin lispro	5–15 min	30–90 min	2–4 h
Insulin aspart	5–10 min	60–180 min	3–5 h
Insulin glulisine	5–15 min	30–90 min	3–5 h
Short Acting			
Regular	30–60 min	2–3 h	3–6 h
Intermediate Acting			
NPH (isophane insulin)	2–4 h	4–10 h	10–16 h
Long Acting			
Insulin glargine	1.1 h	None	24 h
Insulin detemir	2–3 h	6–14 h	16–24 h
Insulin Mixtures			
70/30 human mix* (70% NPH, 30% regular)	30–60 min	Dual	10–16 h
70/30 aspart analog mix (70% intermediate, 30% aspart)*	5–15 min	Dual	10–16 h
75/25 lispro analogue mix* (75% intermediate, 25% lispro)	5–15 min	Dual	10–16 h
50/50 lispro analogue mix (50% intermediate, 50% lispro)	30–60 min	Dual	10–16 h
50/50 lispro analogue mix (50* intermediate, 50% lispro)	5–15 min	Dual	10–16 h

In many countries, including the United States, insulin preparations contain 100 U/mL and are referred to as U-100 insulin. Highly concentrated U-500 short-acting insulin is available and used primarily in adults with severe insulin resistance.

Profiles for each insulin preparation are reasonable estimates only, based on data from adult study participants. There is variation between individuals, and time of onset, peak, and duration are also affected by size of dose, site and depth of injection, dilution, exercise, and temperature. Some studies include children.

*Typically used in fixed doses in twice-a-day insulin regimens.

thereafter. The dietician should help develop a meal plan that is individualized to the patient's daily schedule, food preferences, cultural influences, and physical activity. The meal plan is more likely to be successful if it is designed to fit into the family's already established schedule and preferences. The patient and family should also be instructed on carbohydrate counting so that either carbohydrate exchanges or insulin-to-carbohydrate ratios can be used. Like the child without diabetes, the total number of recommended calories follows the child's growth requirements along with consideration of the need for weight gain or loss. Growth velocity, weight gain, and BMI should be monitored at every visit to ensure that the meal plan is sufficient to meet the energy requirements of the patient. Unexpected weight loss or poor weight gain should prompt consideration of suboptimal metabolic control, as well as eating disorders, thyroid dysfunction, or gastrointestinal disease.

The ADA does not have pediatric specific guidelines for medical nutrition therapy, but the recommendations for adults can be extrapolated to children. The ADA recommends that carbohydrates provide 45% to 65% of total calories, with protein and fat contributing 15% and 30%, respectively. The patient and family should be educated to avoid foods high in cholesterol, saturated fat, and concentrated sweets and select foods high in complex carbohydrate and dietary fiber.

All children and adolescents are recommended to have three meals per day. If they receive intermediate-acting insulin preparations, they should also receive three snacks per day (morning, afternoon, and bedtime) to match anticipated peaks of insulin action. If the child or adolescent is on a basal-bolus regimen, snacks are optional and require insulin coverage based on insulin-to-carbohydrate ratios.

Exercise

Exercise, or periods of sustained physical activity, can be beneficial to the patient by contributing to a sense of well-being, helping achieve the recommended BMI, improving glycemic control (exercise enhances insulin sensitivity), improving the lipid panel (increasing HDL), and lowering blood pressure and improving cardiovascular fitness. All children and adolescents, especially those with diabetes, should be encouraged to participate in routine physical activity.

The child or adolescent with diabetes needs to take precautions to avoid hypoglycemia during periods of increased physical activity.

The patient and family need to check blood glucose before the initiation of activity, every hour during sustained activity, and at the completion of physical activity. For the first several days of increased activity, the child should also check his or her blood glucose frequently during the 12-hour postexercise period because there is often a delayed drop in the blood glucose following exercise (i.e., the lag effect). Some children require additional carbohydrate before, during, and after activity; lower insulin doses on the days of increased physical activity; or both. It is suggested that the child take 5 to 15 g of carbohydrates, depending on age and exercise intensity, before exercise if the blood sugar is below target, and repeat the 5 to 15 g of carbohydrate for every 30 minutes of sustained activity. Rapid-acting carbohydrate should be readily available, and coaches and trainers should be aware of the diagnosis of diabetes and trained in the treatment of hypoglycemia.

Psychosocial Support

The mental health professional is an important member of the diabetes team. A thorough family assessment generally accompanies the diabetes diagnosis with appropriate referrals for additional services as needed. Thereafter, children or adolescents should be referred back to a mental health professional if social, emotional, or economic barriers to the achievement of good glycemic control are identified. Family conflict, especially conflict over diabetes care, can be associated with deterioration in glycemic control. Encouragement of ongoing family teamwork in the management of childhood diabetes promotes successful outcomes with respect to glycemic control, reducing diabetes-specific conflict, and preventing acute complications and emergency assessments.

Sick Day Management

The goals for the management of children and adolescents during sick days are never omit insulin, prevent dehydration and hypoglycemia, monitor blood glucose frequently (every 2 to 4 hours), monitor for ketosis, provide supplemental rapid- or short-acting insulin doses (5% to 20% of TDD) depending on degree of hyperglycemia and ketosis, treat underlying illness, and have frequent contact with the diabetes team. The majority of DKA among children or adolescents with established diabetes is caused by insulin omission or errors in administration of insulin. Inadequate insulin therapy in the context of an intercurrent illness accounts for the remaining small percentage. Although it is more common for children to require more insulin during illnesses, some children require a reduction of the basal and/or rapid-acting insulin dose if he or she is unable to eat and the blood glucose is less than 150 to 180 mg/dL.

Families need to be educated about symptoms that warrant immediate medical attention, including signs of dehydration (dry mouth, sunken eyes, cracked lips, weight loss, dry skin), persistent vomiting for more than 2 to 4 hours, persistence of blood glucose levels greater than 300 mg/dL or ketones for more than 12 hours, or symptoms of DKA (nausea, abdominal pain, chest pain, vomiting, ketotic breath, hyperventilation, or altered consciousness). It is helpful for the diabetes team to review sick day management annually with the family (can accompany flu immunization) to avoid metabolic decompensation during intercurrent illness.

Hypoglycemia

Fear of hypoglycemia can be a common occurrence in the management of childhood diabetes, especially among caregivers, and can be a barrier to optimal glycemic control. Recognition and treatment of hypoglycemia are important topics for diabetes education. Families are trained to treat hypoglycemia with 10 to 15 g of rapid-acting carbohydrate, recheck blood glucose in 15 minutes, repeat treatment with 10 to 15 g if blood glucose remains below target, and follow with a protein-containing snack if a meal will not follow within 1 to 2 hours. This technique avoids the natural tendency to overtreat low blood glucose levels. Caregivers should also receive glucagon training (20 to 30 µg/kg; maximum 1 mg) for severe hypoglycemia and low-dose glucagon (1 U on an insulin syringe for every year of life up to 15 years) for impending hypoglycemia, for example, in the context of a gastrointestinal illness or inadvertent insulin administration (lispro given instead of NPH). A member of the diabetes team should assess frequency, treatment, awareness, and circumstances of hypoglycemia at each visit.

Screening for Diabetes-Related Complications

Patients, families, and caregivers worry about the risk of diabetes-related complications, and therefore the diabetes team must educate families and screen for complications with sensitivity and optimism, emphasizing prevention of complications and the maintenance of health. Screening for nephropathy, hypertension, dyslipidemia, and retinopathy are indicated.

Microalbuminuria (MA) is the first sign of diabetic nephropathy, and patients who develop persistent MA are at increased risk of progression to macroalbuminuria. Poor glycemic control, smoking, and a family history of essential hypertension are risk factors for the development of MA and nephropathy. Identification of persistent MA provides an opportunity for intervention and prevention of progressive renal disease through improvements in glycemic control and/or therapy with angiotensin-converting enzyme (ACE) inhibitors. There are currently no pediatric data on the use of angiotensin receptor blockers (ARBs). Table 4 outlines definitions, screening recommendations, and treatment.

Hypertension is an important predictor of the progression of diabetic nephropathy to end-stage renal disease. Hypertension in children and adolescents may go unrecognized because providers are not familiar with the gender-, age-, and height-specific definitions. Blood pressure should be measured every 3 months with standardized technique, using the proper size cuff. If elevated blood pressures are detected and confirmed, the first step is to exclude causes not related to diabetes. Table 4 outlines the definitions, screening recommendations, and treatment.

Dyslipidemia and diabetes are established risk factors for cardiovascular disease, and recent research suggests that a significant proportion of adolescents with diabetes already have evidence of atherosclerosis. Low-density lipoprotein (LDL) cholesterol is most closely associated with cardiovascular disease, and therefore, the ADA has developed guidelines for LDL cholesterol. Screening may be delayed until puberty if family history is negative for cardiovascular disease. A lipid profile should be performed on prepubertal children with diabetes who are older than 2 years if there is a positive family history of cardiovascular disease hyperlipidemia, or if the family history is unknown. If the LDL cholesterol is less than 100 mg/dL, screening can be repeated every 5 years. The mainstay of therapy for dyslipidemia is dietary management (saturated fat less than 7% of calories and less than 200 mg/day of cholesterol). Children with levels between 130 and 159 mg/dL should be started on medication if diet and lifestyle modification are unsuccessful after 6 months or if the child has additional risk factors for cardiovascular disease, such as obesity or hypertension. Pharmacotherapy is recommended if the LDL cholesterol is more than 160 mg/dL. The LDL goal for children with diabetes is less than 100 mg/dL.

Diabetic retinopathy is a feared complication because it is the leading cause of vision loss. According to the ADA, the first ophthalmologic examination should be performed when the child is 10 years or older within 5 years after the onset of diabetes. Examinations with an eye care professional with expertise in diabetic retinopathy should occur early.

TABLE 4 Screening for Diabetes-Related Complications

COMPLICATION	HOW TO SCREEN	DEFINITION	WHEN TO SCREEN	THERAPY
Microalbuminuria	Spot urine sample, timed overnight, or 24-h collection	Spot urine albumin/creatinine ratio 30–299 µg/g or AER 20–199 µg/min from timed collection	Annual screening begins at 10 y or after >5 y duration of diabetes	Optimize glucose control, smoking cessation, normalize BP
Persistent microalbuminuria		2/3 of urine samples meet above criteria		Above, plus addition of ACE inhibitor
High-normal BP	Manual BP measurement with standard technique	Systolic or diastolic BP within the 90th–95th percentile for age, gender, and height	At every clinic visit	Dietary intervention, weight control, and exercise; if target BP not reached within 3–6 mo, then initiate pharmacologic therapy
Hypertension		Systolic or diastolic BP above the 95th percentile for age, gender, and height, or >130/80 on >3 occasions (whichever is lower)		Above, plus pharmacologic therapy titrated to achieve target BP

Note: Urine collection should not be performed following vigorous exercise, during an acute infection, during a female patient's menstrual cycle, or following an episode of severe hypoglycemia. Once angiotensin-converting enzyme (ACE) inhibitor is started, microalbumin excretion should be monitored q3–6 mo.
Target BP is <130/80 or <90th percentile for age, gender, and height. Initial drug treatment is ACE inhibition. Angiotensin II receptor blockers (ARBs) are FDA approved to treat hypertension in pediatric patients >6 years old.
Abbreviations: AER = albumin excretion rate; BP = blood pressure.

Screening for Other Autoimmune Diseases

Children and adolescents with T1D are at an increased risk for other autoimmune diseases and should be screened accordingly. Approximately 15% of patients with T1D also have autoimmune thyroid disease. All children and adolescents should be screened for autoimmune thyroid disease at the time of diabetes diagnosis once metabolic control is established. TSH measurement is a useful initial screen, along with measuring the presence of thyroid autoantibodies. Screening should be repeated yearly or if there is any clinical suspicion of thyroid disease (abnormal growth rate, symptoms of hypo- or hyperthyroidism, goiter on examination, erratic blood glucose control).

Another commonly associated disorder is celiac disease. Nearly 6% of patients with T1D have elevated levels of circulating autoantibodies to tissue transglutaminase. Celiac disease can cause diarrhea, weight loss or failure to gain weight, abdominal pain, fatigue, and unexplained hypoglycemia or erratic blood glucose secondary to malabsorption. Patients with T1D should be screened with circulating IgA autoantibody to tissue transglutaminase. A quantitative serum IgA level should be drawn at the same time to rule out IgA deficiency as a cause for falsely low IgA tissue transglutaminase levels. Positive antibodies should be confirmed with a second measurement, and if positive, a referral should be made to a gastroenterologist for small bowel biopsy. If the diagnosis is confirmed, celiac disease is treated with a gluten-free diet with recommendations and support from a registered dietician with pediatric expertise in diabetes and celiac management.

Type 2 Diabetes Mellitus in Youth

With the increasing prevalence of childhood obesity during the last two decades, there is an increased occurrence of T2D in youth. Based on National Health and Nutrition Examination survey data, the prevalence of obese children (defined as a body mass index greater than the 95th percentile for children and youth) increased from 5% in the 1970s to more than 15% by 1999. The epidemic of obesity follows the increased consumption of fast foods, increased consumption of soft drinks, increased sedentary behavior with more television watching, video games, and decreased physical activity. Mirroring this epidemic of childhood obesity is the occurrence of T2D in children and adolescents. Before 1990, T2D in youth was a rare occurrence. By 2000, between 8% and 45% of all newly diagnosed cases of childhood diabetes were caused by T2D. T2D occurs most commonly in those with a family history of T2D; individuals from certain racial and ethnic minority groups including Native Americans, Hispanics, African Americans, and Asian and Pacific Islanders; those with overweight/obesity falling above the 85th percentile for BMI based on age and gender; and in association with markers of insulin resistance (Table 5). Markers of insulin resistance include

---

TABLE 5 Risk Factors and Screening for Type 2 Diabetes in Children

CRITERIA	AGE OF INITIATION	FREQUENCY	METHOD
Overweight (BMI ≥85th percentile for age and gender), weight for height ≥85th percentile, or weight ≥120% of ideal for height	10 y or at pubertal onset if puberty occurs at a younger age	q2y	Fasting plasma glucose and/or A1C
Plus 2 of the following risk factors:			
Family history of T2D in 1st- or 2nd-degree relative			
Race/ethnicity (Native American, African American, Hispanic, Asian/Pacific Islander)			
Signs of or conditions associated with insulin resistance (acanthosis nigricans, PCOS, HTN, dyslipidemia)			

Abbreviations: BMI = body mass index; T2D = type 2 diabetes; HTN = hypertension; PCOS = polycystic ovarian syndrome.
Adapted from American Diabetes Association: Type 2 diabetes in children. Diabetes Care 2000;23(3):381–89.
Note: Clinical judgment should be used to test for diabetes in high-risk patients who do not meet these criteria.

TABLE 6 Medications to Treat Type 2 Diabetes

CLASS	MECHANISM OF ACTION	ADVERSE EFFECTS
Biguanides (metformin)*	Decrease hepatic glucose production Increase peripheral glucose disposal	Gastrointestinal upset Lactic acidosis
Sulfonylureas (glimepiride, glyburide, glipizide)	Insulin secretagogues	Hypoglycemia Weight gain
Meglitinides (repaglinide, nateglinide)	Insulin secretagogues	Hypoglycemia Weight gain
α-Glucosidase inhibitors (acarbose)	Decrease gut carbohydrate absorption	Gastrointestinal upset
Thiazolidinediones (rosiglitazone and pioglitazone)[†]	Decrease hepatic glucose production Increase peripheral glucose disposal	Weight gain Edema Increased liver enzymes Anemia
GLP-1 analogues	Increase insulin response Decrease glucagon response to eating Slow down gastric emptying	Gastrointestinal upset Acute pancreatitis Possible increased thyroid cancer risk
DPP-4 inhibitors	Increase insulin response Decrease glucagon response to eating Slow down gastric emptying	Possible interference with immune function

*Metformin (Glucophage) is the only medication with FDA approval for use in children.
[†]Thiazolidinediones have restricted use and/or safety concerns; thus their use in pediatric patients should be avoided at this time, pending additional studies or FDA recommendations.

the occurrence of acanthosis nigricans and polycystic ovarian syndrome (PCOS). In addition, other well-known risk factors include hypertension and hyperlipidemia.

As noted earlier, the diagnosis of T2D is based on elevated fasting plasma glucose (FPG), 2-hour glucose value during an OGTT, and a casual glucose level or A1C determined in a laboratory on two occasions. Because T2D often goes without symptoms, individuals who are overweight, have a positive family history of T2D, come from one of the high-risk racial and ethnic minority groups, and/or have markers of insulin resistance warrant screening for T2D. Screening can be performed with a FPG or OGTT when clinical concerns are high and the FPG is normal.

Currently one oral medication is approved for the treatment of T2D in youth. This medication is metformin (Glucophage), which is also available in a liquid formulation. The maximum recommended daily dose of metformin (Glucophage) in youth is 2000 mg/day divided as 1000 mg twice daily. Often patients with T2D present in ketoacidosis and require initial insulin therapy. The goal of management of the child with T2D is initial stabilization often with insulin therapy, metformin (Glucophage) directed at managing the insulin resistance, and education. Once glucose levels are stabilized, insulin dosage may be lowered along with continued treatment with metformin (Glucophage) and approaches to lifestyle management. Lifestyle management involves a healthy diet, increasing exercise, and decreasing sedentary behaviors.

Other medications used to treat T2D include second-generation sulfonylureas, meglitinides, thiazolidinediones, α-glucosidase inhibitors, GLP-analogues, and DPP-4 inhibitors, none of which is currently approved for use in pediatric patients. There are ongoing studies to assess the efficacy and safety of these medications (Table 6).

References

American Diabetes Association. Diagnosis and classification of diabetes mellitus. Diabetes Care 2005;28(Suppl 1):S37–42.

American Diabetes Association. Type 2 diabetes in children. Diabetes Care 2000;23 (3):381–9.

Barroso I. Genetics of type 2 diabetes. Diabet Med 2005;22:517–35.

Borus JS, Laffel L. Adherence challenges in the management of type 1 diabetes in adolescents: prevention and intervention. Curr Opin Pediatr 2010;22:405–11.

Dunger DB, Sperling MA, Acerini CL, et al. ESPE/LWPES consensus statement on diabetic ketoacidosis in children and adolescents. Arch Dis Child 2004;89: 188–94.

Fox LA, Buckloh LM, Smith SD, et al. A randomized controlled trial of insulin pump therapy in young children with type 1 diabetes. Diabetes Care 2005;28:1277–81.

Glaser N, Barnett P, McCaslin 1, et al. The Pediatric Emergency Medicine Collaborative Research Committee of the American Academy of Pediatrics. N Engl J Med 2001;344(4):264–9.

Goodwin G, Volkening LK, Laffel LM. Younger age at onset of type 1 diabetes in concordant sibling pairs is associated with increased risk for autoimmune thyroid disease. Diabetes Care 2006;29(6):1397–8.

Hannon TS, Rao G, Arslanian SA. Childhood obesity and type 2 diabetes mellitus. Pediatrics 2005;116(2):473–80.

Hirsch IB. Insulin analogues. N Engl J Med 2005;352:174–83.

Laffel LM, Vangsness L, Connell A, et al. Impact of ambulatory, family-focused teamwork intervention on glycemic control in youth with type 1 diabetes. J Pediatr 2003;142(4):409–16.

Mehta SN, Wolfsdorf JI. Contemporary management of patients with type 1 diabetes. Endocrinol Metab Clin North Am 2010;39:573–93.

Nathan DM, Buse JB, Davidson MB, et al. Medical management of hyperglycemia in type 2 diabetes: a consensus algorithm for the initiation and adjustment of therapy: a consensus statement of the American Diabetes Association and the European Association for the Study of Diabetes. Diabetes Care 2009;32:193–203.

Rewers M, Pihoker C, Donaghue K, et al. Assessment and monitoring of glycemic control in children and adolescents with diabetes. Pediatr Diabetes 2009;10(Suppl 12):71–81.

Rosenbloom AL. Cerebral edema in diabetic ketoacidosis and other acute devastating complications: Recent observations. Pediatr Diabetes 2005;6:41–9.

Silverstein J, Klingensmith G, Copeland K, et al. American Diabetes Association: Care of children and adolescents with type 1 diabetes. Diabetes Care 2005;28 (1):186–212.

Wysocki T, Harris MA, Mauras N, et al. Absence of adverse effects of severe hypoglycemia on cognitive function in school-aged children with diabetes over 18 months. Diabetes Care 2003;26(4):1100–5.

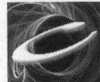

ENCOPRESIS

Method of
Sarah Houssayni, MD

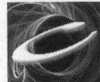

CURRENT DIAGNOSIS

- Voluntary or involuntary passage of stools into inappropriate places at least once a month for 3 consecutive months once a chronologic or developmental age of 4 years has been reached.
- Encopresis can be primary when it persists from infancy onward or secondary when it appears after toilet training.
- The behavior is not due to the direct effects of a substance such as a laxative or a general medical condition except those associated with constipation.
- Distinguishing subtypes is essential because treatment differs:
  - Retentive encopresis: occurs as a result of involuntary leakage of liquid stools due to severe constipation and impaction.
  - Nonretentive encopresis: children pass bowel movements into their underwear due to their refusal to use the toilet.
- Children occasionally fail to wipe after bowel movements and the secondary soiling should be distinguished from encopresis.

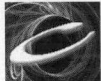

CURRENT THERAPY

Retentive Encopresis
Initial Disimpaction
- Hyperphosphate enemas (Pedia-Lax Enema) (one daily for 2 or 3 days):
  - Less than 1 year old: 60 mL.[3]
  - Greater than 1 year old: 6 mL/kg, up to 135 mL twice.[3]
- Glycerin suppositories (Glycerin Pediatric Suppositories) for infants and toddlers.

Older Children—Slow Disimpaction
- Polyethylene glycol with electrolytes (Golytely, Colyte)[1] ingested over 2–3 days: 25 mL/kg/hr up to 1 L/hr until stooling clear bowel movements. (This is not approved for bowel cleansing for children.)
- Over 5–7 days:
  - Mineral oil[1] 3 mL/kg twice a day for 1 week. (Mineral oil is not approved for use in children younger than 6 years of age.)
  - Lactulose[1] 2 mL/kg twice a day for 1 week.
  - Magnesium hydroxide (Milk of Magnesia) 2 mL/kg twice a day for 1 week.
  - Polyethylene glycol without electrolyte (MiraLax)[1] 1.5 g/kg/day for 3 days.

Maintenance Therapy
- Polyethylene glycol 3350 (MiraLax)[1] age greater than 1 month: 0.7 g/kg divided into 1–2 doses daily.
- Lactulose or sorbitol 70% solution age greater than 1 month: 1–3 mL/kg/day divided into 1–2 doses daily for 1–3 months.
- Sennosides (Senna, Senna-GRX, Senexon) are habit forming, doses vary greatly in the different available formulations, and they can only be used for short-term treatment. Give at bedtime for a morning bowel movement. Dose is 5 mL (1 tablet) for 1-[1] to 5-year-olds and 2 tablets for 5- to 15-year-olds for a maximum of three tablets daily. (Sennosides are not approved for use in children younger than 2 years of age.)
- Glycerin enemas and bisacodyl suppositories (Dulcolax) can be used for short-term constipation treatment.
- Glycerin/saline enema in patients greater than 10 years of age: 20–30 mL/day (solution of 1/2 glycerin and 1/2 normal saline).
- Bisacodyl suppositories in patients greater than 10 years of age: 10 mg daily.

Nonretentive Encopresis
- **NO** medical treatment.
- Clean up soiling immediately, involve the child.
- Ensure adequate water and dietary fiber intake.
- Avoid use of stool softeners and laxatives.
- **STOP** all reminders, make child responsible for own toilet habits.
- Use rewards when child defecates in toilet.
- Refer to health care professional when refractory (refuses to sit on toilet and older than 5 years of age, refuses to take medication, is older than 8 years of age with nonretentive encopresis).

Encopresis is the voluntary or involuntary passage of stools at least once a month for 3 consecutive months once a chronologic or developmental age of 4 years has been reached. Encopresis is classified as primary when it persists from infancy onward or secondary when it appears after toilet training. Retentive encopresis occurs as a result of involuntary leakage of liquid stools due to severe constipation and fecal impaction. Nonretentive encopresis occurs in children who pass stool into their underwear due to their refusal to use the toilet. It is important to distinguish between the types of encopresis, because treatment differs.

Epidemiology

The prevalence of encopresis is reported to be 4% in 5- to 6-year-olds and 1.5% in 11- to 12-year olds. Affected boys outnumber girls by a factor of anywhere from 3:1 to 5:1 depending on the source. Encopresis tends to decrease with age. A large number of children with encopresis go unreported due to the shame associated with the condition and underdiagnosis of the condition.

Diagnosis

The diagnosis of encopresis includes the following four criteria: (1) Repeated passage of feces into inappropriate places such as in clothing or on the floor, whether intentional or involuntary. (2) At least one event a month for at least 3 months. (3) A chronologic age of at least 4 years or an equivalent developmental level. (4) The behavior is not due exclusively to the direct physiologic effects of a substance such as a laxative or a general medical condition other than constipation.

Differential Diagnosis

Retentive encopresis is organic in less than 5% of the affected patients. Organic causes include hypothyroidism, hypercalcemia, cerebral palsy, abnormal anatomy of the anus, Hirschsprung's disease, cystic fibrosis, and neuropathy with secondary impaired voiding sensation. Spinal cord conditions such as tethered cord, spina bifida occulta, and spinal cord dysplasia affect stooling through diminished bowel sensation and secondary fecal retention.

Pathophysiology

Patients who are severely constipated hold stools back because of the pain associated with defecation. This becomes a vicious cycle of constipation, rectal dilation, and secondary encopresis. Frequently, emotional problems emerge due to the fear and shame associated with the problem. Control issues with parents trying to take the stooling issues at hand may worsen the constipation problem.

From 10% to 20% of encopretic patients are not constipated. They are frequently preschoolers or school-age children who are postponing their bowel movements too long because they are distracted or because they associate the bathroom with an unpleasant experience (i.e., fear or disgust).

Clinical Manifestations

History

The history should assess for size and consistency of stools, as well as stooling intervals. Families often confuse soiling with stooling, leading to inaccurate reporting of the frequency of bowel

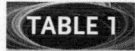

TABLE 1 Characteristic Symptoms of Retentive and Nonretentive Encopresis

Retentive Encopresis

- Constipation
- Stained underwear
- Fewer than three bowel movements per week
- Large-caliber or hard stools
- Abdominal pain, reports of bloated sensation
- Odor of feces from leakage onto underwear
- Difficult or painful defecation
- Enuresis
- Overflow incontinence
- Anorexia

Nonretentive Encopresis

- Passage of stools in inappropriate places without presence of constipation
- Refusal to sit on toilet even though old enough to (older than 5 years, even older than 8 years at times)
- Refusal to take medications
- Child may be depressed

movements. Characteristic symptoms of retentive and nonretentive encopresis differ (Table 1).

In retentive encopresis the physician may elicit a history of difficult or painful defecation, crying with bowel movements, and posturing that suggests the child is deliberately holding back stools due to the pain associated with passage.

Children may suddenly become still or hide during play, cross their legs, grimace, or shift their position in an attempt to retain stools. The physician should assess for a history of enuresis and urinary tract infections, anorexia, sensations of bloating, fullness, and abdominal pain leading to the patient's avoidance of food and weight loss. Obtain a dietary history including fiber, fluid, and dairy intake. The historian needs to inquire about streaks of blood on toilet paper and underwear. With retentive encopresis, when the child does pass stool, it may be of large caliber and hard, indicative of constipation.

With nonretentive encopresis, the history often reveals bowel movements of normal size and consistency passed into the underwear once or twice a day. Symptoms of constipation are usually absent. A history of behavioral problems, child-parent struggles, and history of abuse may be elicited. Toilet avoidance is common.

Patients with encopresis eventually develop secondary emotional problems, which can be elicited from the history taking.

Physical Examination

Retentive Encopresis

In retentive soiling the physical examination should assess for abdominal distention and tenderness on palpation. A mass can be occasionally felt in the midline in the suprapubic area. This mass of hardened fecal matter most commonly involves the rectosigmoid area and can sometimes extend throughout the entire colon. If the patient is anxious or in pain and tightens the rectus abdominis, this mass can be missed. Rectal examination is a must; it can be done with minimal discomfort. Rectal examination assesses the dilation of the rectum, which may be 6 to 10 cm wide. It is usually packed with stools with clay-like consistency. Visually inspect the anal opening for tone, fissure, and hemorrhoids.

Nonretentive Encopresis

The child with nonretentive encopresis typically has a normal abdominal examination, is likely to have a rectal vault that is not dilated, and the stool will be of normal caliber and consistency. The rectal vault may be empty if the child has just passed a bowel movement. The anal opening may reveal protruding fecal material in children who are deliberate stool holders.

Treatment

Encopresis is treated through a multistep approach. First, clearing the colon of fecal material will allow the dilated rectal vault and rectosigmoid colon to return to normal. The rectal cleanout can be achieved in different ways (see Current Therapy). Enemas and stool softeners are often used in combination.

Maintenance is achieved by keeping stools soft and ensuring daily bowel movements with mineral oil and hyperosmolar agents (e.g., Miralax[1]) that are very safe and can be used from a very young age and are not habit forming. The goal is painless stools once or twice a day with no associated withholding behavior.

Education is key for families so that they understand the physiology and process of stool elimination. Frustration is associated with failure, guilt, and depression and should be replaced with a positive attitude if success is to be achieved.

- Patients should sit daily on the toilet for 5 minutes after meals twice a day.
- Families need to keep a record of the events, as well as a record for success.
- Soiled underwear should be changed as soon as noticed and the child should be cleaned and changed in a timely, emotionally neutral fashion.
- As soon as compliance wanes, the problem is expected to return and is sometimes worse than the previous episode.
- The care provider's continued involvement in titrating medication with the patient's symptoms is necessary.
- Pain-related impaction can be cured in the majority of cases with medical management of the initial presentation. The success rate is reported to be about 70% with psychogenic impaction.
- With nonretentive encopresis, behavioral modification is essential. Stress reduction, effective coping techniques, relaxation training, and a combination of individual and family therapy is sometimes indicated.

---

[1]Not FDA approved for this indication.

References

Baker SS, et al. Clinical practice guideline. Evaluation and treatment of constipation in infants and children: recommendations of the North American Society for Pediatric Gastroenterology, Hepatology and Nutrition. J Pediatr Gastroenterol Nutr 2006;43:e1–e13.

Becker A, Ruby M, El Khatib D, et al. Central nervous system processing of emotions with faecal incontinence. Acta Paediatr 2011;100:e267–747.

Boris NM, Dalton R, et al. Encopresis. Nelson textbook of pediatrics. 19th ed. Philadelphia: Saunders; 2011.

Brazzelli M, Griffiths P. Behavioral and cognitive interventions with or without other treatments for the management of faecal incontinence in children. Art. No. CD002240Cochrane Database Syst Rev 2006;(2) http://dx.doi.org/10.1002/14651858.CD002240.pub3.

Coelho DP. Encopresis. A medical and family approach. Pediatr Nurs 2011;37:107–12.

Har AF, Groffie JM. Encopresis. Pediatr Rev 2010;31:368–74.

Raghumath N, Glassman MS, Halata MS, et al. Anorectal motility abnormalities in children with encopresis and chronic constipation. J Pediatr 2011;158:293–6.

EPILEPSY IN INFANTS AND CHILDREN

Method of
Adam L. Hartman, MD

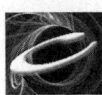

CURRENT DIAGNOSIS

- At initial diagnosis, determine whether the event was a seizure or not.
- The most critical diagnostic finding is to determine whether the seizure had a focal or generalized onset.
- If appropriate, diagnose an epilepsy *syndrome*.
- Age of onset aids in the development of a differential diagnosis.

CURRENT THERAPY

- Selection of an anticonvulsant should be made based on the type of seizure.
- General principles include the use of a single agent at the lowest effective dosage with the goal of no side effects.
- Epilepsy can be associated with comorbidities such as depression and anxiety. Successful management includes referrals and/or management of these and associated psychosocial issues.

A seizure can be defined as clinical signs or symptoms resulting from abnormal neuronal firing. Epilepsy is defined as either: (1) at least two unprovoked seizures occurring >24 hours apart; (2) one unprovoked seizure and a probability of further seizures similar to the general recurrence risk (at least 60%) after two unprovoked seizures, occurring over the next 10 years; or (3) diagnosis of an epilepsy syndrome. There may be associated psychological, social, and cognitive consequences. Approximately 3% to 5% of the U.S. population has had a seizure (mostly febrile seizures). Nearly 1% of the U.S. population is being treated actively for seizures at any given time. Infants and children represent one of the two major peaks in seizure incidence, making this a very common diagnosis in pediatric practice.

Risk Factors

The primary risk factors for epilepsy in any age group include a history of meningitis, encephalitis, brain trauma, complicated perinatal course, and febrile seizures. Other risk factors for seizures include cortical or developmental malformations, certain inborn errors of metabolism, congenital infections, stroke, intracranial hemorrhage, acute metabolic abnormalities, and drug withdrawal.

Pathophysiology

Because the primary abnormality is abnormal neuron firing, many different types of pathology can lead to seizures. Abnormalities in neuronal networks (e.g., cortical malformations), structure (e.g., abnormal dendrite structure in trisomy 21), or ion channels (e.g., *KCNQ2*) can lead to seizures. In many cases, an underlying cause of seizures cannot be identified. Some forms of epilepsy have been linked to various genetic mutations, although the exact relationship between specific genotypes and phenotypes is unclear for most.

Clinical Manifestations

Broadly speaking, the clinical manifestations of seizures vary depending on which brain structures are involved. Although most people think of seizures only as generalized tonic–clonic seizures (GTCS), a wide variety of signs and symptoms can be caused by seizures. Furthermore, a GTCS may be the initial manifestation of a seizure (i.e., as seen in primary generalized epilepsy) or it may be the end result of a seizure that started in one brain location and then spread to the rest of the brain (e.g., a focal-onset seizure with generalization). These two broad categories (generalized versus focal) are approached somewhat differently from a diagnostic and therapeutic perspective.

Signs of a generalized seizure (i.e., those involving abnormal synchronized firing in both sides of the brain) include loss of interaction or staring (absence seizures), myoclonus, tonic posturing, and/or tonic–clonic seizures. Signs of focal-onset seizures can involve specific regions controlling motor, sensory, or autonomic function, a loss of interaction, or automatisms (chewing, lip smacking, repetitive hand motions), to name a few. Patients with focal seizures might have an aura (a warning sign just prior to the seizure). The aura is an altered sensory function that can include salty or metallic taste, tingling sensations, rising sensation in the abdomen, déjà vu, jamais vu, sense of fear, or a nonspecific feeling that something is about to happen. After a seizure, patients also can have a period of postictal lethargy or confusion.

The initial symptoms or signs of a seizure are the most important in determining whether a seizure is generalized or focal in origin because they often localize the anatomic site of pathology. Thus, it is the beginning of a seizure, rather than its end, that is most useful in making a specific diagnosis.

Diagnosis and Management

History and Physical Examination

A detailed history is usually more valuable than any expensive test in diagnosing a seizure or epilepsy. In addition to a description of the actual event, it is useful to inquire about subtle signs that might not be recognized by observers as a seizure, including staring spells, myoclonic jerks, loss of time, and unexplained nocturnal tongue biting, enuresis, or emesis. The presence of postictal weakness can help localize the region of onset after a focal seizure, even if secondarily generalized. Making the diagnosis of a specific epilepsy syndrome allows the clinician to develop a plan for further diagnosis and treatment and to counsel about prognosis. On physical examination, any signs of focal neurologic deficits can indicate an underlying lesion. A skin examination might identify a neurophakomatosis, such as tuberous sclerosis complex or neurofibromatosis.

Diagnostic Studies

In selected cases, typical clinical findings in the right clinical context strongly support the diagnosis of epilepsy, but an electroencephalogram (EEG) may be required to confirm the diagnosis. Even if the patient does not have a seizure during the EEG recording, interictal findings (when the patient is not having a seizure) can provide enough evidence to make the diagnosis of epilepsy. Under ideal circumstances, a single EEG can detect epileptiform activity in a patient with untreated generalized epilepsy about 75% of the time, making it a very sensitive test. In contrast, an EEG can detect epileptiform activity in a patient with focal-onset seizures only 70% of the time (although this number increases to about 90% after three EEGs have been done). Conversely, a normal interictal EEG (particularly one that includes sleep and provocative maneuvers such as intermittent photic stimulation and hyperventilation) in an untreated patient suggests, but is not necessarily diagnostic of, a focal rather than generalized onset.

Other ancillary studies can show underlying structural lesions that lead to epilepsy or provide physiologic information. Magnetic resonance imaging (MRI) can be useful in detecting lesions such as tumors, cortical dysgenesis, and strokes (both ischemic and hemorrhagic). Magnetic resonance spectroscopy also can provide information about metabolites in a specific region, which can aid in determining the nature of a lesion before resection (e.g., tumor versus inflammation). Positron-emission tomography (PET) scans may show regions of abnormal metabolism that might not be evident on MRI. Another nuclear medicine study, single photon emission tomography (SPECT), can be used to identify the region of onset of a seizure. Functional MRI (fMRI) studies show regions involved in a specific task.

Magnetoencephalography, when combined with MRI, can be useful in detecting areas of abnormal electrical activity that might not be evident on a scalp EEG recording. Neuropsychology evaluations can aid in localization of regions of dysfunction and also aid in determining risk for loss of function if surgery is performed. The intracarotid amobarbital (Amytal)[1] test (Wada test) or intracarotid methohexital (Brevital)[1] test is used to lateralize language function and memory; fMRI is being investigated as a replacement for aspects of this invasive test. Some institutions use intracranial electrodes to localize the onset of a seizure prior to a surgical resection and to identify regions of eloquent neurologic function (regions where critical function would be lost if they were resected).

Specific Epilepsy Syndromes

Some of the more common syndromes are described here, listed by typical age at presentation.

Neonatal Seizures

Seizures in neonates can be caused by any type of neurologic pathology, including infections (prenatal or postnatal), strokes, hemorrhages, electrolyte abnormalities, cortical dysgenesis, inborn errors of metabolism (including vitamin B_6 dependency), withdrawal, and medications. Some neonatal seizure syndromes (benign idiopathic neonatal seizures and benign familial neonatal seizures) are benign; early infantile epileptic encephalopathy (Ohtahara syndrome) and early myoclonic encephalopathy frequently are refractory to medical treatment and have a poor prognosis for development. Neonatal seizures should be managed in conjunction with specialists.

Febrile Seizures

Febrile seizures are the most common type of seizure, occurring in 3% to 5% of people in the United States. Febrile seizures, even though they can recur, are not diagnostic of epilepsy because they are provoked (i.e., by fever). With an onset between 1 month and 5 years of age (and almost always outgrown by 6 to 7 years of age), these seizures can be generalized or focal in onset. Meningitis and encephalitis also can manifest with seizures and fever and thus are exclusion criteria for febrile seizures because the prognosis and treatment are completely different. Febrile seizures that last longer than 15 minutes have a focal onset, or occur more than once in a febrile illness are complex febrile seizures; only one of the three criteria are needed to make the diagnosis. Patients with complex febrile seizures are at a higher risk for developing epilepsy, although the overall risk still is low (4%). In patients who lack all three of these factors (i.e., simple febrile seizures), routine imaging, blood work, lumbar puncture, and EEG are not necessary for diagnosing the cause of the seizure. Rather, the work-up should be guided by other concerns, such as dehydration, concern for occult bacteremia, or in the appropriate clinical context, meningitis.

Approximately one third of patients have a recurrence of a febrile seizure. Factors that increase the recurrence risk include very young age at onset, family history of febrile seizures, low-grade fever at onset of the seizure, frequent febrile illnesses, or the occurrence of the seizure in the first hour of the fever. Febrile seizures always are outgrown, so typically, long-term seizure prophylaxis is not used. Oral diazepam (Valium) prophylaxis, started at the onset of fever, prevents febrile seizures but can produce excessive sedation. Patients who have prolonged febrile seizures can benefit from rectal diazepam gel (Diastat) or other benzodiazepines given soon after the onset of a febrile seizure to prevent additional prolonged seizures or febrile status epilepticus. A similarly good prognosis is seen in infants and children who have febrile seizures in the setting of acute gastroenteritis (whether febrile or not). The risk of epilepsy is increased after a febrile seizure in the setting of a complex febrile seizure, abnormal development, frequent febrile seizures, or a family history of epilepsy.

Infantile Spasms

With an onset typically around 4 to 8 months of age, infantile spasms consist of a triad of typical seizures (head drops and brief flexor and/or extensor spasms occurring in clusters around sleep transitions), a highly disorganized multifocal EEG pattern called hypsarrhythmia, and developmental delays. Between 70% and 90% of patients have identifiable underlying neurologic pathology associated with this syndrome. This is one of the most medically intractable epilepsy syndromes, and the prognosis for seizure control and development are very poor, except in a small subset of patients with no identifiable underlying pathology. Treatment typically is hormonal with prednisolone (Orapred)[1] or ACTH (Acthar HP), dietary with a ketogenic diet, or medical with vigabatrin

[1]Not FDA approved for this indication.

[1]Not FDA approved for this indication.

(Sabril), which is commonly the first-line treatment in infants with tuberous sclerosis complex (Box 1).

Dravet Syndrome

The typical presentation for Dravet syndrome is a prolonged febrile seizure involving one side of the body (hemiclonic) or recurrent GTCS in a previously normal infant. After a relatively quiescent period, seizures (including myoclonic, focal, and absence) appear in the second year of life. Additional features include developmental abnormalities, ataxia, and extrapyramidal signs. Seizures induced by heat (either with fevers or exogenous) may be noted.

Genetic testing for mutations in the *SCN1A* gene is recommended, because this eliminates the need for other extensive testing for an underlying diagnosis and allows the clinician to prognosticate. The EEG may be normal initially but later shows generalized spike-and-wave complexes. Treatment typically is with anticonvulsant medications; some recommend avoiding drugs that block sodium channels, although direct evidence for this is limited. The ketogenic diet may be useful.

Lennox–Gastaut Syndrome

Typically occurring between the ages of 1 and 8 years, Lennox–Gastaut syndrome is characterized by mixed seizure types, a markedly abnormal EEG, and abnormal development. Virtually any type of brain pathology can be seen as an antecedent of Lennox–Gastaut syndrome. Patients with Lennox–Gastaut syndrome typically have combinations of tonic, atonic, and absence seizures, although focal-onset seizures and GTCS also occur. The EEG shows slow (less than 2.5 Hz) spike-and-wave complexes and occasionally a paroxysmal fast pattern, although background slowing also is very common. The vast majority of patients have developmental delays. Diagnosis is made in the setting of typical findings. Seizures are very difficult to control but treatment commonly includes medicines and/or nonpharmacologic options (see Box 1). The prognosis for seizure control and development are poor. The differential diagnosis of Lennox–Gastaut syndrome also includes Doose syndrome, characterized by myoclonic and astatic seizures (although other seizure types can occur), which often includes patients with normal development and a good prognosis once seizures are controlled.

Childhood and Juvenile Absence Epilepsy

Most clinicians are familiar with childhood and juvenile absence epilepsy. The typical age of onset is 4 to 14 years of age, and there is a slight female predominance. The most common type of seizure is an absence seizure, characterized by staring and loss of interaction lasting 5 to 20 seconds, occurring tens to hundreds of times per day. Patients also can have GTCS (particularly if they present later in childhood) and/or myoclonic seizures. There is no aura and there are no postictal behavior changes. Absence seizures can be induced with 3 to 4 minutes of hyperventilation at the bedside. The interictal EEG shows a 3 Hz generalized spike-and-wave pattern. Treatment includes ethosuximide (Zarontin) if the patient has not had a GTCS (see Box 1). Valproate (Depakene) is the first choice if the patient has had a GTCS. Nearly two thirds of patients grow out of their seizures by young adulthood.

Benign Epilepsy with Centrotemporal Spikes and Benign Occipital Epilepsy

One of the more-common epilepsies in childhood, benign epilepsy with centrotemporal spikes (benign Rolandic epilepsy) first occurs between the ages of 3 and 13 years. The typical seizure involves the face and/or hand, but GTCS also are common. The most common time for a seizure is within the first few hours of sleep, but a minority of patients only have daytime seizures. The diagnosis is made based on a typical seizure history and EEG (which shows spikes over bilateral central and temporal regions). Learning disabilities are fairly common in patients with this syndrome, so extra vigilance is warranted.

Benign occipital epilepsy (also known as Panayiotopoulos syndrome) can occur between the ages of 1 and 14 years (with a peak at 4 to 5 years) with autonomic symptoms such as emesis, pallor, flushing, or tachycardia, as well as focal-onset or generalized seizures. Patients also can have visual symptoms. The EEG can show sharp waves in the occipital regions, but abnormal activity has been reported in other brain regions as well.

> ### Box 1   Recommendations for Treatment
>
> **Infantile Spasms, West Syndrome**
> Oral steroids[1]
> Ketogenic diet
> Adrenocorticotropic hormone
> Topiramate[1]
> Valproate[1]
> Zonisamide[1]
> Pyridoxine[1]
> Benzodiazepines[1]
> Surgery (if there is a lesion)
> Vigabatrin (may use first if patient has tuberous sclerosis)
>
> **Dravet Syndrome**
> Valproate[1]
> Topiramate[1]
> Ketogenic diet
> Benzodiazepines[1]
>
> **Lennox–Gastaut Syndrome**
> Valproate
> Clobazam
> Lamotrigine
> Topiramate
> Benzodiazepines
> Rufinamide
> Felbamate
> Ketogenic diet
> Vagus nerve stimulator
> Surgery
>
> **Doose Syndrome**
> Valproate
> Ketogenic diet
> Lamotrigine[1]
> Ethosuximide[1]
> Vagus nerve stimulator
>
> **Childhood Absence Epilepsy**
> Ethosuximide
> Valproate
> Lamotrigine[1]
>
> **Juvenile Absence Epilepsy**
> Valproate
> Ethosuximide
> Lamotrigine[1]
>
> **Benign Epilepsy with Centrotemporal Spikes**
> Levetiracetam
> Carbamazepine
> Valproate
> Oxcarbazepine
>
> **Juvenile Myoclonic Epilepsy**
> Valproate
> Levetiracetam
> Topiramate
> Zonisamide[1]
> Lamotrigine
>
> ---
> [1]Not FDA approved for this indication.
> Adapted Muthugovindan D, Hartman AL: Pediatric epilepsy syndromes. Neurologist 2010;16:223–37.

Because most patients have fewer than six seizures in both syndromes, medicine usually is not prescribed. Seizures typically are outgrown by adolescence. Patients with frequent seizures are treated with medicine. Gastaut occipital epilepsy (not to be confused with Lennox–Gastaut syndrome) occurs in older children and can require anticonvulsant treatment because of seizure recurrence.

Juvenile Myoclonic Epilepsy

The most common form of generalized seizures in adolescents, juvenile myoclonic epilepsy first occurs between the ages of 12 and 20 years. Most patients have brief myoclonic seizures that tend to cluster in the early morning hours (but may occur at any time of day). Patients often are unaware that these are seizures but on careful questioning report loss of control of a toothbrush or spoon. Many patients also have absence seizures. The interictal EEG typically shows a 4 to 5 Hz generalized spike-and-wave pattern. The prognosis for lifelong remission of seizures is poor, although most patients' seizures are controlled easily with medicines (see Box 1). There is a subgroup of patients (many of whom previously had childhood absence epilepsy) whose seizures are very challenging to control.

Other Epilepsy Syndromes with a Poor Prognosis

Landau–Kleffner syndrome and epileptic encephalopathy with continuous spike-and-wave during sleep are syndromes characterized by mild seizures, nearly continuous epileptiform activity during sleep, and neuropsychological deterioration. Progressive myoclonus epilepsy represents a family of disorders characterized by medically intractable epilepsy (commonly including myoclonic seizures) and significant neurologic deterioration. Underlying diagnoses include myoclonus epilepsy with ragged red fibers (MERRF), Unverricht–Lundborg disease and Lafora's disease, among others. Gelastic (laughing) seizures can be caused either by hypothalamic hamartomas or temporal lobe seizures. The prognosis depends on response to medication and/or surgery but is not always bad. Rasmussen syndrome is characterized by medically intractable epilepsy, progressive unilateral neurologic deficits, and cortical atrophy on MRI. Because they are so rare, any suspicion of these diagnoses should prompt referral to a pediatric epilepsy center with expertise in diagnosing and managing these conditions.

Tumors

Brain tumors can manifest with seizures and are covered in a separate chapter. Certain developmental tumors are seen with an increased frequency in pediatric epilepsy clinics, including dysembryoplastic neuroepithelial tumors (DNET) and gangliogliomas. These tumors typically manifest with seizures and can be associated with malformations of cortical development. EEG can show abnormalities over the involved region but can be falsely localizing, as well. MRI shows the location of the tumor but can underestimate the extent of surrounding abnormal tissue. If seizures are not controlled with medicine, or if there is progression in tumor size, resection surgery is recommended.

Cortical Dysgenesis

Abnormal brain development can lead to inappropriately wired brain circuitry, which can be the underlying substrate for seizures. Two forms of abnormal cortical development include lissencephaly (abnormally smooth, or simplified, gyral pattern) and polymicrogyria. Another form of cortical dysgenesis, the malformations of cortical development, is graded based on both dyslamination of the normal six-layer cortex and the occurrence of abnormal cell types (including balloon cells). EEG shows epileptiform abnormalities over the involved region. MRI shows the anatomic location of the involved tissue in more-severe cases but may be normal if the abnormality is mild. In patients with focal abnormalities, if seizures are not controlled with medicine, resection surgery is an option. Patients with more-extensive abnormalities can try nonpharmacologic options if medicines do not work.

Mesial Temporal Lobe Epilepsy with Hippocampal Sclerosis

The mesial temporal structures (particularly the hippocampus) can become scarred and remaining neurons develop abnormal connections (i.e., mossy fiber sprouting). This can lead to medically intractable seizures. EEG shows interictal epileptiform activity over the temporal regions. Imaging studies show atrophic mesial temporal structures with increased signal on T2-weighted FLAIR (fluid-attenuated inversion recovery) images. A temporal lobectomy should be considered as an option for patients who do not respond to two medications for seizure control.

Comorbidities

The definition of epilepsy includes comorbidities, which in turn can have a significant impact on quality of life. Clinicians must actively probe for these underlying conditions in order to optimize outcomes. People with epilepsy have increased rates of depression and anxiety compared to the general population. Developmental disorders and learning disabilities are more common in children with epilepsy, as are attention-deficit/hyperactivity disorder and migraines. Once identified, these conditions should be managed by clinicians experienced with their treatment.

Differential Diagnosis

The differential diagnosis of seizures depends largely on age. In infants, opisthotonic posturing can be seen in gastroesophageal reflux disease (Sandifer's syndrome). Some infants have benign myoclonus or shuddering attacks. The EEG in all these disorders is normal, but the diagnosis can be made based on the history. Apparent life-threatening events can appear to be seizures, although apnea rarely is the only manifestation of a seizure. Hyperekplexia is an exaggerated startle response that can be due to abnormal glycine receptor subunits in the spinal cord. Because of potential involvement of the diaphragm, this disorder can be lethal. In children, stereotypies can be paroxysmal and persistent, but the behaviors during these episodes are typical enough that the diagnosis usually is made based on the history.

Breath-holding spells may be associated with an older infant or toddler who is upset, followed by unresponsiveness and either facial pallor or mild cyanosis, lasting less than 1 to 3 minutes. These episodes are typical enough that the history is all that is usually needed to make the diagnosis. Children with pallid breath-holding spells are at higher risk for vasovagal syncope in the adolescent and young adult ages.

Night terrors, one of the parasomnias, occur in toddlers and young children. Persistent screaming (lasting minutes to 1 hour) and lack of memory for the event are seen commonly; the latter raises a question of whether the child had a seizure. Most commonly, these are outgrown by the late preschool years.

Patients with syncope may have a few mild clonic twitches, but this typically does not represent epilepsy. Screening orthostatic blood pressures should be done to rule out one of the orthostatic syndromes. Consideration also should be given to an electrocardiogram or a cardiology consultation in the appropriate clinical context.

Older children and adolescents can have psychogenic nonepileptic events, also known as psychogenic nonepileptic seizures. Considered to be a form of a conversion disorder, the diagnosis is made by noting a normal EEG during a typical clinical episode (and thus should be referred to a neurologist for diagnosis). Cognitive behavioral therapy is helpful in some patients.

In all age groups, focal lesions such as infarctions, hemorrhages, and infections should be considered in the differential diagnosis, although the diagnostic work-up should be guided by the history and physical examination.

Treatment

The goals for treatment are to maximize efficacy and minimize side effects. Medication is the first line of therapy for most patients. Nearly 70% to 80% of patients are treated successfully by one of the first two medications tried. Practically speaking, neurologists try to use a single agent at the lowest tolerated dosage.

Suggested medicines for the epilepsy syndromes discussed previously are listed in Box 1. Details about specific medicines are listed in Table 1. If one of the first two medicines tried do not work, there are three major options.

Trials of Additional Medication

Although the first two medicines might not work, new medicines often are introduced into the market. Clinical trials often show that a modest number of patients respond well to newer medicines, although the positive response to newer medicines is no greater overall than response to older medicines, despite lower rates of adverse effects and drug–drug interactions.

Surgery

Any patient who fails to respond to two medications should be assessed for surgery. In patients with a potentially resectable lesion, surgery offers the greatest chance of seizure freedom. Ideal surgical candidates have identifiable lesions on imaging studies and an epileptogenic zone that is distinct from eloquent cortex. Patients without identifiable lesions or those with multifocal or generalized seizures are poor candidates for resection surgery. Options for these patients include the vagus nerve stimulator, which has outstanding compliance and adherence because it is surgically implanted. Although this device significantly decreases seizure frequency in some patients, it rarely leads to seizure freedom. In the future, neurostimulation devices, some of which also include seizure detectors, will become more widely available.

Diet Therapy

The concept of fasting to improve seizure control dates back to Hippocrates, but in modern times, dietary management of epilepsy is implemented using a high-fat, low-carbohydrate (adequate protein) ketogenic diet. More recently, a modified Atkins diet and a low glycemic index treatment have been used successfully, as well. These diets require varying degrees of supervision at a center experienced in their implementation.

TABLE 1 Summary of New Commonly Used Antiseizure Drugs

DRUG	MAINTENANCE DOSAGE* (mg/kg/d)	STARTING DOSAGE*	HALF-LIFE (h)	COMMON SIDE EFFECTS	SERIOUS IDIOSYNCRATIC SIDE EFFECTS
Clobazam (Onfi)	>2 y, <30 kg: 10 mg bid >2 y, >30 kg: 20 mg bid	>2 y, <30 kg: 5 mg/d >2 y, >30 kg: 5 mg bid	Parent drug: 36–42 Active metabolite: 71–82	Sedation irritability Needs to be tapered off slowly	Respiratory depression, benzodiazepine withdrawal, Stevens–Johnson syndrome
Lacosamide (Vimpat)	>17 y, 100–200 mg bid	>17 y 50 mg bid	13	Somnolence, fatigue, headache	Cardiac conduction abnormalities, Stevens-Johnson syndrome, cytopenias
Lamotrigine (Lamictal)	5–15 Dosage depends on other drugs used w/enzyme inducers: 10–15 W/valproate: 1–3 Non-valproate noninducer: 4.5–7.5	W/valproate: 2–12 y: 0.15 mg/kg/d >12 y: 25 mg qod W/enzyme inducer: 2–12 y: 0.6 mg/kg div bid >12 y: 50 mg qd Non-valproate noninducer: 2–12 y: 0.3 mg/kg div bid >12 y: 25 mg qd	14–59 (depending on concomitant seizure medications)	Rash, lethargy, irritability, tremor	Stevens–Johnson syndrome, cytopenias
Levetiracetam (Keppra)	20–60	10 mg/kg/d, incr in 10-mg/kg increments	6–8	Agitation, behavioral disinhibition, rashes	Suicidal ideation
Oxcarbazepine (Trileptal)	30–60	8–10 mg/kg/d, incr by 10–15 mg/kg increments	Parent drug: 2 Metabolite: 9	Hyponatremia, somnolence, lethargy, dizziness, blurred vision	Rash
Perampanel (Fycompa)	> 12 y, 8–12 mg qhs	> 12 y, 2–4 mg qhs	105 h	Somnolence, headaches	Serious psychiatric and behavior reactions
Rufinamide (Banzel)	45 mg/kg/d	10 mg/kg/d	6–10	Nausea, vomiting, somnolence	Seizures, QT shortening
Topiramate (Topamax)	5–9	1–2 mg/kg/d (not to exceed 25 mg)	21	Irritability, hyperactivity, cognitive slowing, weight loss, kidney stones, metabolic acidosis, oligohydrosis	Rash
Vigabatrin (Sabril)	50–150	50	7.5 (5.7 in infants)	Headache, dizziness, fatigue, tremor, swallowing problems, T2-weighted or DWI hyperintensities	Vision loss
Zonisamide (Zonegran)	>16 y: 100–600	>16 y: 100 mg qd	63	Somnolence, irritability, cognitive slowing, weight loss, renal stones, oligohidrosis	Rash

*Dosages should not exceed maximum adult dosages.
Abbreviations: DWI = diffusion-weighted imaging; incr = increase.

Monitoring

Seizure calendars (which can take the form of notebooks or Internet-based tools) are very useful for tracking frequency of events, especially if they are completed on a daily basis. Monitoring for medication-related adverse effects and comorbidities should continue during treatment. In addition, some comorbidities can occur even if seizures have stopped; there is good evidence for this in patients with childhood absence epilepsy, which typically is considered a benign syndrome. Patients taking certain medicines are screened periodically for evidence of renal and/or hepatic abnormalities and abnormal blood cell counts. Scenarios for testing drug levels include the following:

- Assessing adherence to a prescribed drug regimen
- Testing whether symptoms result from drug toxicity
- Determining whether a patient could tolerate higher amounts of medicine when the administered doses are already high

Reminders about seizure-related safety (i.e., what to do in the event of a GTCS) should be reinforced periodically. This counseling typically includes instructions about safety for the patient, including protecting the head and airway (putting the patient on his or her side to prevent aspiration), and not putting anything in the patient's mouth. Periodic assessments of bone health should be considered for patients taking enzyme-inducing or enzyme-inhibiting medicines. Patients of an appropriate age should seek counseling regarding local driving laws. Adolescent girls should be counseled about the effect of anticonvulsants on hormonal forms of contraception (and vice versa). Consideration should be given to prescribing folate in this group, as well.

Complications

Single GTCS can lead to trauma (e.g., from a fall), tongue biting, pneumothorax, fractures of the vertebrae or limbs, and joint dislocations. A brief physical examination can rule out the more-serious complications of a single GTCS. Adverse effects of medications are listed in Table 1. Surgical resections can lead to a variety of neurologic deficits, depending on which tissue is involved. Vagus nerve stimulator surgery can lead to hoarseness and coughing. Unsupervised diet therapy also can have adverse effects and should be undertaken only by centers with experience. Rarely, patients with epilepsy can die unexpectedly from no apparent cause; this is called sudden unexplained death in epilepsy (SUDEP). The cause is unknown, but most (not all) patients have epilepsy that is resistant to medications. Counseling about this condition should be provided by an epilepsy expert.

References

Baldin E, Hauser WA, Buchhalter JR, et al. Yield of epileptiform electroencephalogram abnormalities in incident unprovoked seizures: a population-based study. Epilepsia 2014;55:1389–98.

Berg AT, Berkovic SF, Brodie MJ, et al. Revised terminology and concepts for organization of seizures and epilepsies: Report of the ILAE Commission on Classification and Terminology, 2005–2009. Epilepsia 2010;51:676–85.

Chu-Shore CJ, Thiele EA. New drugs for pediatric epilepsy. Semin Pediatr Neurol 2010;17:214–23.

Ferrie CD, Patel A. Treatment of Lennox–Gastaut syndrome (LGS). Eur J Paediatr Neurol 2009;13:493–504.

Fisher RS, Acevedo C, Arzimanoglou A, et al. ILAE official report: a practical clinical definition of epilepsy. Epilepsia 2014;55:475–82.

Glauser TA, Cnaan A, Shinnar S, et al. Ethosuximide, valproic acid, and lamotrigine in childhood absence epilepsy. N Engl J Med 2010;362:790–9.

Go CY, Mackay MT, Weiss SK, et al. Child Neurology Society; American Academy of Neurology. Evidence-based guideline update: medical treatment of infantile spasms. Report of the Guideline Development Subcommittee of the American Academy of Neurology and the Practice Committee of the Child Neurology Society. Neurology 2012;78:1974–80.

Muthugovindan D, Hartman AL. Pediatric epilepsy syndromes. Neurologist 2010;16:223–37.

Ottman R, Hirose S, Jain S, et al. Genetic testing in the epilepsies—report of the ILAE Genetics Commission. Epilepsia 2010;51:655–70.

Panayiotopoulos CP, Michael M, Sanders S, et al. Benign childhood focal epilepsies: Assessment of established and newly recognized syndromes. Brain 2008;131:2264–86.

Subcommittee on Febrile Seizures, American Academy of Pediatrics. Neurodiagnostic evaluation of the child with a simple febrile seizure. Pediatrics 2011;127:389–94.

HEMOLYTIC DISEASE OF THE FETUS AND NEWBORN

Method of
Michael A. Posencheg, MD; and Phyllis A. Dennery, MD

CURRENT DIAGNOSIS

- The direct antiglobulin, or Coombs, test (DAT) on neonatal blood is the cornerstone for differentiating isoimmune from non–immune-mediated hemolysis.
- The presence of a positive antibody screen in maternal blood should raise suspicion for hemolytic disease resulting from minor antibody-antigen reactions.
- In utero monitoring for severe fetal anemia includes maternal antibody screen titers, △OD450 measurement, middle cerebral artery peak systolic velocity, and cordocentesis.
- Serial and frequent measurements of bilirubin levels and complete blood counts postnatally can aid the practitioner in determining whether therapy should be escalating.

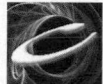

CURRENT THERAPY

- Intrauterine transfusion may be indicated in the setting of severe fetal anemia with or without edema or hydrops fetalis.
- Phototherapy, the mainstay of postnatal management of hyperbilirubinemia, converts unconjugated bilirubin in a nonenzymatic fashion to a polar, water-soluble form that is more readily excretable.
- Intravenous immunoglobulin (Gammagard)[1] is indicated in infants who have isoimmune hemolytic disease and bilirubin levels approaching the threshold for double-volume exchange transfusion.
- Double-volume exchange transfusion is reserved for infants who fail phototherapy and intravenous immunoglobulin (if indicated). It replaces and removes approximately 86% of the infant's own blood. In the setting of isoimmune hemolytic disease, double-volume exchange transfusion has the added benefit of removing offending maternal antibodies, which contribute to the hemolysis from the infant's circulation.

[1]Not FDA approved for this indication.

Epidemiology

Early-onset hyperbilirubinemia, anemia with or without edema in the fetus or newborn, was previously synonymous with hemolytic disease resulting from Rh-isoimmunization. With the onset of the use of Rh-immunoglobulin (RhIg [RhoGAM]) in pregnant Rh-negative women in 1968, the landscape of this disorder has changed dramatically. The differential diagnosis of hemolytic disease of the fetus and newborn is broad and can be subdivided into isoimmune and nonimmune categories (Box 1). In this article, we discuss various diseases that result in fetal and neonatal hemolysis, along with recent improvements in diagnosis and management.

Isoimmune hemolytic disease in the fetus and newborn manifests when maternal antibodies cross the placenta and bind to antigens present on the baby's red blood cells. These antigens include Rh factor (D antigen), leading to Rh isoimmunization, the major blood group antigens (e.g., A, B) leading to ABO incompatibility, or minor blood group antigens (e.g., Kell, Kidd, Duffy). The incidence of Rh isoimmunization has now fallen from nearly 14% of pregnancies in the pre-RhIg era to between 1 and 6 per 1000 live births. Incomplete eradication is due to inadvertent failures of RhIg administration, poor prenatal care, or earlier sensitization. Rh-isoimmunization can lead to severe complications, with up

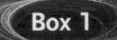

Box 1 Causes of Hemolytic Disease of the Fetus and Newborn

Isoimmune Hemolysis
Rh Isoimmunization
ABO Incompatibility
Antibody-mediated hemolysis due to minor antigens

Non–Immune Mediated
RBC membrane disorders (e.g., hereditary spherocytosis)
RBC enzyme defects (e.g., G6PD deficiency)
Hemoglobinopathies (e.g., α-thalassemia)

Abbreviations: G6PD = glucose-6-phosphate dehydrogenase; RBC = red blood cell.

to 20% of fetuses having significant anemia and evidence of hydrops in utero.

ABO incompatibility occurs nearly exclusively in fetuses and newborns with type A or B blood born to mothers with type O blood. Although nearly one quarter of pregnancies result in ABO incompatibility, only approximately 1% to 5% of ABO-incompatible infants demonstrate significant hemolytic disease. The incidence of hemolytic disease from minor antigens is more difficult to estimate due to the large number of antigen-antibody reactions that can result in disease. Of the minor antigens, Kell and Duffy antigens are associated with the most severe disease, and Lewis and Lutheran are more likely associated with mild or insignificant hemolysis.

The group of disorders that is nonimmune in nature results in red blood cell destruction in the absence of an antibody-antigen reaction. These include red blood cell membrane defects such as hereditary elliptocytosis or spherocytosis, red blood cell enzyme defects such as glucose-6-phosphate dehydrogenase (G6PD) deficiency and pyruvate kinase deficiency, and hemoglobinopathies such as α-thalassemia. With rates up to 1 in 5000 live births, hereditary spherocytosis is the most common of the RBC membrane defects, occurring most commonly in infants of Northern European descent.

Of the enzyme defects, G6PD is the most common, especially in infants of African or Mediterranean descent. It is an X-linked disorder that is most commonly seen in male infants, but females can also manifest the disease. Interestingly, this disease accounts for a disproportionately large percentage of infants who develop kernicterus. α-Thalassemia is a rare hemoglobinopathy in which all α-globin chain genes are deleted. It is most common in Asian infants and is nearly uniformly fatal, with severe fetal anemia and hydrops fetalis, especially when intrauterine transfusions have not been performed.

Risk Factors

Several elements of the maternal, fetal, and neonatal histories can assist in determining a fetus's or infant's risk of developing one of these hemolytic processes. The results of the maternal blood type and antibody screen are useful to evaluate this risk. Infants born to mothers with type O blood are at risk for ABO incompatibility, whereas infants born to mothers with Rh-negative blood are at risk for Rh isoimmunization. The antibody screen that is performed on maternal blood is specifically searching for antibodies associated with the minor antigen groups that can also be found on red blood cells. Selected minor antigens are listed in Table 1. The presence of a positive direct Coombs' test should raise suspicion of an isoimmune hemolytic process. This test is not always available or warranted.

Assessing the risk of nonimmune disease is based almost entirely on a complete family history. Many of these disorders are associated with certain ethnic or geographic backgrounds. As examples, G6PD deficiency is found more commonly in persons of African or Mediterranean descent, and a family history of persistent anemia requiring splenectomy is often seen in hereditary spherocytosis.

Pathophysiology

The isoimmune forms of fetal and neonatal hemolysis have a similar pathophysiology in that all of them involve the passage of specific maternal IgG antibodies across the placenta, which then interact with their corresponding antigens on the fetal red blood cells. Red cell destruction results when the antibody-coated cells are scavenged by the mononuclear phagocytic system. The production of maternal antibodies is usually the result of previous exposure of the maternal system to fetal red blood cells, which is common during labor or abortion. The initial response of the maternal immune system is to produce IgM antibodies, but repeat exposure elicits an IgG response. This is especially true for Rh isoimmunization, and therefore explains why first-born Rh-positive infants born to Rh-negative mothers are not affected.

In ABO incompatibility, antibodies to A or B antigens already exist, but they are normally IgM antibodies. They do not cross the placenta and therefore do not result in disease. It is only when the antigenicity results in the production of IgG antibodies that passage across the placenta can occur and disease can result. This is exceedingly uncommon in blood type A with B incompatibility (mother is type A, baby is type B), but is more common in mothers with blood type O who have a fetus with either blood type A or B. This can occur in first-born infants. As to hemolysis from antibodies to minor antigens, IgG antibody production may be the result of prior exposure to fetal cells such as during a previous pregnancy or via prior blood transfusion.

The pathophysiology of the nonimmune group of hemolytic disease is unique to the specific disease process. Red blood cell membrane defects, such as hereditary spherocytosis, have specific abnormalities of red blood cell membrane proteins that result in abnormal red blood cell shapes. These cells are more prone to destruction from mechanical forces. The enzyme defects such as G6PD and pyruvate kinase deficiency result in an inability of the red blood cell to protect itself from oxidant stress (G6PD) or to produce energy (pyruvate kinase). This makes the cell more prone to hemolysis. Hemoglobinopathies result in anemia from decreased production of stable hemoglobin chains. Specifically, α-thalassemia major involves the lack of production of the α chain of hemoglobin and leads to early fetal anemia, severe hydrops, and death unless intrauterine transfusions are instituted.

TABLE 1 Selected Minor Antigens Associated with Fetal or Neonatal Hemolytic Disease

BLOOD GROUP	SEVERE DISEASE	RARELY SEVERE DISEASE	MILD DISEASE	USUALLY NO DISEASE
Rh	D, c	C, E, f, Evans, G, Rh29, Rh32, Rh42, Rh46, and others	E,e,f	
Lutheran			Lu^a, Lu^b	
Kell	K	k, Kp^a, Kp^b, Ku, Js^a, Js^b, K11, K22	Ku, Js^a, K11	K23, K24
Lewis				Le^a, Le^b
Duffy		Fy^a	Fy^b, Fy3	
Kidd		Jk^a	Jk^b, Jk3	

Adapted from Eder AF: Update on HDFN: New information on long-standing controversies. Immunohematology 2006;22(4):188-195; and Moise KJ: Fetal anemia due to non–Rhesus-D red-cell alloimmunization. Semin Fetal Neonatal Med 2008;13:207-214.

Prevention

The administration of Rh-immunoglobulin (RhIg) to mothers who are Rh-negative has dramatically decreased the incidence of hemolytic disease resulting from Rh-isoimmunization. The current recommendation of the American College of Obstetrics and Gynecology (ACOG) is to administer 300 µg of RhIg intramuscularly at 28 weeks' gestation and within 72 hours of delivery of an Rh-positive infant to an Rh-negative mother. RhIg should also be administered to Rh-negative mothers if the mother undergoes amniocentesis, chorionic villus sampling, or cordocentesis, or in the event of maternal bleeding due to placental abruption, placental previa, partial molar pregnancy, spontaneous abortion, or elective termination.

Controversy exists regarding the use of RhIg in the first trimester. As early as 7 weeks of gestation, fetal blood cells can express the D antigen, and women with threatened abortion in the first trimester have been shown to become Rh-sensitized, although this is a rare event. Some advocate for administration of RhIg 50 µg (MICRhoGAM) intramuscularly in the first trimester in the setting of spontaneous abortion, elective termination, ectopic pregnancy, or threatened abortion.

The proposed mechanism of action for RhIg involves binding to Rh-positive fetal cells with resultant scavenging by the maternal mononuclear phagocytic system before sensitization and production of maternal antibody against the Rh-D antigen. Sadly, the other forms of hemolytic disease do not have specific preventive strategies.

Clinical Manifestations

The clinical presentation of hemolytic disease in the fetus and newborn varies according to the timing and severity of the disease. Significant and early hemolysis in utero results in fetal anemia, and, as oncotic pressure decreases in the fetal blood vessels, edema forms in the soft tissues and potential spaces. Hydrops fetalis results when there is edema or fluid accumulation in at least two of these spaces: skin, pleura, pericardium, or peritoneum. If this continues unabated, fetal death can result. Of all of the diseases discussed here, Rh-isoimmunization and α-thalassemia are those most commonly associated with fetal anemia and the most severe disease.

Most commonly, hemolytic disease results in early neonatal onset anemia and significant hyperbilirubinemia. Often, infants present with clinical jaundice in the first 24 hours of life and have a significant rate of rise of their serum bilirubin levels or a prolonged course of hyperbilirubinemia. Neonatal anemia with significant hyperbilirubinemia is a common manifestation of ABO incompatibility, hemolysis due to minor antigens, and red blood cell enzyme and membrane defects. The degree of anemia in each, however, is quite variable even within a given diagnosis.

Diagnosis

The assessment of maternal blood type and antibody screen can provide valuable insight into the risk of isoimmune hemolytic anemia. Ultrasound techniques and amniocentesis for the antenatal monitoring of fetal anemia are reviewed later.

In the neonate, concern for hemolytic anemia results from a rapidly rising bilirubin level, especially in the first 24 hours of life, a positive direct Coombs' test, hemolysis detected on a blood smear with anemia detected on a complete blood count (CBC), or prolonged hyperbilirubinemia, individually or in combination. In addition to following serial bilirubin levels, in this setting the practitioner should include a neonatal blood type, Coombs' (DAT) test, and complete blood count with reticulocyte count to determine whether hemolysis is occurring. A positive DAT in the appropriate clinical setting suggests isoimmune hemolysis, and a negative DAT nearly rules it out. However, in the setting of ABO incompatibility a significant number of infants can have a positive Coombs' test and not have significant hemolysis. If umbilical cord blood is used to perform a Coomb's test, contamination with Wharton's jelly can produce a false positive result.

A G6PD level can be helpful in establishing a diagnosis in infants with the appropriate ethnic background or geographic location. Many states have adopted universal newborn screening for G6PD deficiency. Serum albumin, the primary protein transporter for bilirubin in the blood, can also be measured. Low serum levels of albumin increase the risk of developing neurologic sequelae from the subsequent increased amount of free, unbound bilirubin crossing the blood-brain barrier.

Differential Diagnosis

The differential diagnosis of hemolytic disease starts with determining whether or not the hemolysis is antibody-mediated (see Box 1).

Isoimmune hemolytic disease involves the production of maternal IgG antibodies against antigens on fetal red blood cells, resulting in hemolysis. The major diseases in this group include Rh isoimmunization, ABO incompatibility, and hemolysis resulting from the production of antibodies to minor red blood cell antigens. Examples of these include the broad groups Kell, Duffy, Lutheran, Lewis, and Kidd.

The non–immune mediated hemolytic diseases result from inherent defects in the neonatal red blood cells or hemoglobin productions. Examples of these include the red blood cell membrane defects such as hereditary spherocytosis and hereditary elliptocytosis; red blood cell enzyme defects, including G6PD deficiency and pyruvate kinase deficiency; and hemoglobinopathies, most notably α-thalassemia. Descriptions of these have been included elsewhere in this article.

Treatment

The goals of therapy are different depending on the timing of disease. When significant hemolysis occurs in utero, the fetus becomes progressively anemic. In the fetus, bilirubin is normally processed and excreted through the placenta. Therefore, the primary concern is to treat the anemia and, in doing so, prevent or reverse any signs of edema or hydrops fetalis. In this circumstance, percutaneous umbilical blood sampling (PUBS) and intrauterine blood transfusion can diagnose and treat fetal anemia, respectively. In a recent cohort study, 291 children who received intrauterine transfusions (IUT) for alloimmune hemolytic disease were assessed at ages 2 to 17 years for neurodevelopmental impairment (NDI: cerebral palsy, severe developmental delay, or bilateral deafness). The overall incidence of NDI was 4.8%. Evaluating only prenatally known risk factors, severe hydrops (OR 11.2; 95% CI 1.7-92.7, $p = 0.011$) was significantly associated with NDI.

In the neonate, the problem is somewhat different. In the absence of placental transfer and maternal clearance of bilirubin, the neonate must now take on this task. However, in the first days of life infants are ill equipped to do so owing to inadequate activity of the glucuronyl-transferase enzyme that conjugates bilirubin produced from the high heme load resulting from significant hemolysis. This leads to accumulation of bilirubin because it must be conjugated to be excreted (Figure 1). Therefore, the more pressing problem faced by the pediatrician is the hyperbilirubinemia.

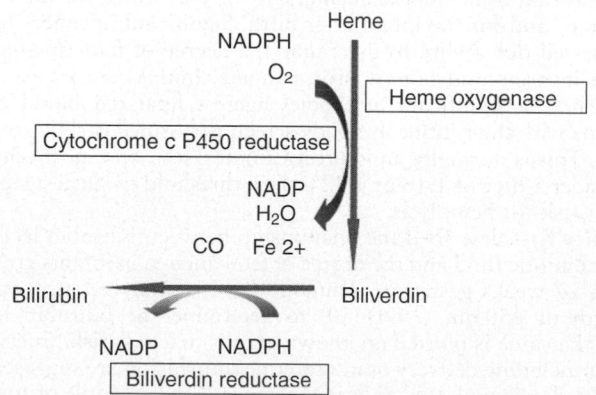

Figure 1. Enzymatic pathway leading to the production of bilirubin. Heme is degraded in a rate-limiting, oxygen (O_2) and energy-requiring (NADPH) step by heme oxygenase. This process results in the generation of carbon monoxide (CO) and iron (Fe) and biliverdin. Biliverdin is then converted to bilirubin by biliverdin reductase in another energy-requiring step.

The mainstay of treatment for hyperbilirubinemia is phototherapy. Unconjugated bilirubin absorbs light maximally in the blue portion of the visible spectrum (approximately 450 nm). Phototherapy with a light source that approximates this spectrum results in the photoisomerization of unconjugated bilirubin into a polar, water-soluble, and more readily excretable form. As a result, both configurational and structural isomers are formed; the most common structural isomer is called lumirubin. The efficacy of phototherapy is related to the spectrum of light used, irradiance of light, exposed surface area of the skin, and the distance of the light source from the infant.

In the setting of isoimmune (or antibody-associated) hemolysis, the use of intravenous immune globulin (IVIg [Gammagard])[1] has been shown to decrease the need for exchange transfusion and is a helpful adjunctive therapy. The current recommendation from the American Academy of Pediatrics (AAP) is to administer IVIg 0.5 to 1 g/kg over 2 hours if the total serum bilirubin is rising despite phototherapy or if the total serum bilirubin is within 2 to 3 mg/dL of the exchange transfusion level. This dose may be repeated in 12 hours.

For some infants, the use of phototherapy and IVIg, if indicated, is not sufficient to control the rising bilirubin level. Alternatively, some infants have neurologic manifestations of bilirubin toxicity despite bilirubin levels lower than suggested therapeutic levels. In these instances, a double-volume exchange transfusion is indicated. This procedure involves removing double the infant's blood volume with simultaneous isovolemic replacement of reconstituted whole blood. This process achieves two separate but related goals. First, it removes bilirubin and, second, in the setting of isoimmune hemolytic disease, it removes offending maternal antibodies. Criteria for performing a double-volume exchange transfusion are clearly outlined in the guidelines from the AAP published in 2004, but some experts suggest performing a double-volume exchange transfusion at even lower levels when significant antibody-mediated hemolysis is occurring owing to the added benefit provided by removing maternal antibodies.

Two pharmacologic therapies have been proposed in the treatment of neonatal hyperbilirubinemia. Phenobarbital,[1] when given to mothers just before birth, has been shown to decrease the need for exchange transfusion in their newborn infants. Synthetic metalloporphyrins (e.g., tin-mesoporphyrin, stannsoporfin [Stanate][5]) decrease the production of bilirubin by inhibiting heme oxygenase, the rate-limiting enzyme in the degradation of heme to biliverdin (which is then converted to bilirubin by biliverdin reductase, see Figure 1). Both of these therapies are still considered experimental because the safety profile of both remains in question.

Monitoring

Monitoring of hemolytic anemia may be performed for the fetus in utero and for the infant after birth. Significant advances have improved our ability to determine the degree of fetal anemia in both invasive and noninvasive manners. Initial concern for the presence of significant antibodies against fetal red blood cells begins with the routine antibody screen performed early in gestation. This is normally an indirect Coombs' test, and most centers consider a titer of 1:16 or 1:32 to be a threshold to suggest significant risk for hemolysis.

Liley first described the relationship between bilirubin level in the amniotic fluid and the degree of fetal anemia in infants greater than 27 weeks gestation. Amniotic fluid is analyzed at a wavelength of 450 nm (ΔOD450) to determine the bilirubin level and the value is plotted on known graphs to assess risk. Interventions including delivery or intrauterine transfusion are suggested if the level, when plotted, falls in the upper 20th percentile of zone II or in zone III. An expanded form of the Liley curve as well as the development of the Queenan curve has provided practitioners

with tools to determine the risk of Rh isoimmune fetal anemia as early as 14 weeks' gestation. However, these methods may be less useful when antibodies to the Kell antigens are involved.

The measurement of middle cerebral artery peak systolic velocity (MCA-PSV) by Doppler ultrasonography gives practitioners a noninvasive alternative to amniocentesis for monitoring fetal anemia. Theoretically, as a fetus becomes more anemic, the blood flow velocity increases due to increased cardiac output and vasodilatation, resulting in increased MCA-PSV. The measurement is specific for gestational age and can be charted to determine if it is more than 1.5 multiples of the median (MoM), suggesting moderate to severe anemia. The effect of intrauterine transfusions on this measurement is unclear owing to the presence of adult red blood cells, and they can alter the interpretation of MCA-PSV. Large randomized, controlled trials are needed to determine if measurement of MCA-PSV or ΔOD450 are equivalent in assessing the risk of anemia. This would give practitioners a noninvasive way to monitor fetuses at risk for severe anemia.

Cordocentesis is the gold standard for measuring fetal anemia, but it comes with severe risks including fetal and perinatal death, cord bleeding, hematomas, further maternal sensitization from fetal-maternal hemorrhage, infection, and placental abruption.

After birth, the neonate at risk for hemolytic anemia must be monitored for degree of anemia and for the development of significant hyperbilirubinemia. In utero, bilirubin is transferred to the maternal circulation via the placenta and processed in the maternal liver, which explains why hyperbilirubinemia is a postnatal event. Early and frequent bilirubin levels and complete blood counts allow the practitioner to evaluate the need for intervention. The availability of hour-specific nomograms that plot the risk of severe hyperbilirubinemia based on the level of bilirubin can be used in term infants to guide therapy and timing of outpatient follow-up. These are published in the AAP position statement from 2004.

Complications

Complications of phototherapy, IVIg,[1] and double-volume exchange transfusions are all possible. Side effects of phototherapy include disruption of mother-baby bonding, increased insensible water loss (less common with modern bilirubin lights), retinal injury from UV light, and, in the setting of an elevated conjugated fraction, a brown discoloration of the skin called "bronze-baby syndrome." The presence of an elevated conjugated fraction or bronzing of the skin is not a contraindication for phototherapy. This is of cosmetic concern only and is usually reversible after removal of the phototherapy.

Complications involving the use of IVIg are rare but include renal dysfunction, necrotizing enterocolitis (NEC), increased incidence of thrombotic events, transfusion reactions, and transmission of infections that can occur with transfusion of any blood product, because blood products are derived from pooled plasma.

Many potential complications are associated with double-volume exchange transfusion. These include electrolyte disturbances, arrhythmias, cardiac arrest, thrombotic or embolic sequelae, metabolic acidosis, thrombocytopenia, disseminated intravascular coagulation, infection, necrotizing enterocolitis, temperature instability, and blood transfusion–related complications such as hepatitis, HIV infection, or transfusion reaction.

---

[1]Not FDA approved for this indication.

References

American Academy of Pediatrics. Subcommittee on Hyperbilirubinemia: Management of hyperbilirubinemia in the newborn infant 35 or more weeks of gestation. Pediatrics 2004;114(1):297–316.

Dennery PA, Seidman DS, Stevenson DK. Neonatal hyperbilirubinemia. N Engl J Med 2001;344(8):581–90.

Eder AF. Update on HDFN: New information on long-standing controversies. Immunohematology 2006;22(4):188–95.

Harkness UF, Spinnato JA. Prevention and management of RhD isoimmunization. Clin Perinatol 2004;31:721–42.

---

[1]Not FDA approved for this indication.
[5]Investigational drug in the United States.

Lindenburg IT, Smits-Wintjens VE, van Klink JM, et al. on behalf of the LOTUS study group. Long-term neurodevelopmental outcome after intrauterine transfusion for hemolytic disease of the fetus/newborn: the LOTUS study. Am J Obstet Gynecol 2012;206:141. e1–141.e8.

Moise KJ. Fetal anemia due to non–Rhesus-D red-cell alloimmunization. Semin Fetal Neonatal Med 2008;13:207–14

Murray NA, Roberts IAG. Haemolytic disease of the newborn. Arch Dis Child Fetal Neonatal Ed 2007;92:F83–88.

Watchko JF. Identification of neonates at risk for hazardous hyperbilirubinemia: Emerging clinical insights. Pediatr Clin North Am 2009;56:671–87.

NOCTURNAL ENURESIS

Method of
Alexander K.C. Leung, MBBS

Note: This chapter has been published in part in *Common Problems in Ambulatory Pediatrics: Specific Clinical Problems,* volume 1, with permission from Nova Science Publishers, Inc.

CURRENT DIAGNOSIS

- Nocturnal enuresis is defined as involuntary nighttime bedwetting in a child at least 5 years of age.
- Primary nocturnal enuresis is present when the child has never achieved a period of nighttime dryness greater than 6 consecutive months. Secondary nocturnal enuresis is present when the child has experienced a period of nighttime dryness of at least 6 consecutive months.
- The most common causes of primary nocturnal enuresis are a deep sleep pattern, nocturnal polyuria, and a small-capacity bladder or nocturnal detrusor overactivity.
- A urinalysis is warranted to rule out urinary tract infection, glycosuria, and a defect in the ability to concentrate urine.
- Ultrasound examination of the bladder (prevoid and postvoid) can be used to evaluate bladder dysfunction and functional bladder capacity.

CURRENT THERAPY

- Desmopressin (DDAVP, 1-desamino-8-arginine vasopressin) is indicated as a first-line therapy for children with monosymptomatic nocturnal enuresis associated with nocturnal polyuria and normal bladder function.
- Enuretic alarm is indicated as a first-line therapy for children with monosymptomatic nocturnal enuresis associated with a small bladder capacity or in children with severe enuretic symptoms refractory to desmopressin therapy.
- Behavioral therapy such as encouraging the child to urinate frequently during the daytime, emptying the bladder before bedtime, and restricting fluid in the evening may increase the success rate of pharmacologic therapy or enuretic alarm therapy.

Nocturnal enuresis is defined as involuntary nighttime bedwetting in a child at least 5 years of age. Primary nocturnal enuresis is present when the child has never achieved a period of nighttime dryness greater than 6 consecutive months. Secondary nocturnal enuresis is present when the child has experienced a period of nighttime dryness of at least 6 consecutive months. For the majority of children with secondary nocturnal enuresis, the pathogenesis is no different from that of primary nocturnal enuresis.

Nocturnal enuresis is a common problem that is frustrating for children, parents, and physicians alike. The condition may affect the child's self-esteem and may lead to reduced social interaction and behavioral problems.

Epidemiology

It has been estimated that 15% to 25% of 5-year-old children and 5% to 10% of 7-year-old children have nocturnal enuresis. Without specific treatment, approximately 15% of affected children become dry each year. The male-to-female ratio is approximately 3:1.

Risk Factors

Encopresis, daytime wetting (diurnal enuresis), and male gender are significant risk factors. Constipation, emotional stress, developmental delay, bladder dysfunction, sleep deprivation, adenotonsillar hypertrophy, and attention-deficit/hyperactivity disorder also play a role.

Pathogenesis

The most common causes of primary nocturnal enuresis are a high arousal threshold, nocturnal polyuria, and a small-capacity bladder or nocturnal detrusor overactivity. Although these causes may overlap, it is important to conceptualize them separately, because this differentiation will help the physician to understand the problem, to educate both the parents and child, and to plan an appropriate treatment program.

It has been shown that enuretic children have a high arousal threshold and a reduced prepulse inhibition of startle. In most children, arousability from sleep improves with maturation of the central nervous system.

In most circumstances, the rate of secretion of antidiuretic hormone from the posterior pituitary gland is increased at night. This circadian variation is usually established when the child is 3 to 4 years old. Some children with primary nocturnal enuresis have a lack of this circadian variation with an abnormally low nocturnal secretion of antidiuretic hormone with resultant nocturnal polyuria. Other causes of nocturnal polyuria include fluid and solute overload in the evening.

Children with a small-capacity bladder or nocturnal detrusor overactivity often have primary nocturnal enuresis. Conditions that may reduce the functional bladder capacity include cystitis and constipation.

There is a strong genetic component to nocturnal enuresis. The child of parents who were both enuretic has a 77% chance of developing enuresis. If one parent was enuretic, there is up to a 44% occurrence rate. If neither parent was enuretic, the occurrence rate is only 15%. Twin studies also support a genetic basis for nocturnal enuresis: the concordance rate is much higher in monozygotic twins (68%) when compared with dizygotic twins (36%). Linkage studies have suggested possible genetic markers for primary nocturnal enuresis located on chromosomes 12, 13, and 22.

A neurogenic bladder is one of the few anatomic abnormalities that can cause primary nocturnal enuresis. Congenital urethral obstruction is another infrequent anatomic cause of primary nocturnal enuresis. The enuresis in these children is due to an overflow phenomenon from a poorly compliant bladder. The most common cause of urethral obstruction in the male is posterior urethral valves. Girls and boys with significant congenital urethral stenosis may also present with this problem. An ectopic ureter or vesicovaginal fistula is an infrequent anatomic cause of primary nocturnal enuresis in girls.

A defect in the ability of the kidney to concentrate urine can cause primary nocturnal enuresis. The causes of concentrating defects include any cause of chronic renal failure and diabetes insipidus.

Diagnosis

History

Onset and Frequency

The timing of the onset and the frequency of nocturnal enuresis are important historical clues to the etiology. Secondary nocturnal enuresis and intermittent nocturnal enuresis are not usually associated with structural abnormalities in the urinary tract. Nocturnal enuresis due to a structural abnormality of the urinary tract is usually present from birth and is not associated with periods of remission.

Timing, Frequency, and Volume per Episode

A history of soaking absorbent underpants in the morning suggests nocturnal polyuria. Parents of children with nocturnal polyuria often remark that the volume of urine associated with the enuretic episode or the first morning void is very large. Frequent episodes of nocturnal enuresis with a small volume of urine suggest bladder dysfunction such as may occur with a urethral obstruction or a neurogenic bladder. Several episodes of nocturnal enuresis with a large volume suggest diabetes mellitus or diabetes insipidus. Constant wetting suggests an ectopic ureter or vesicovaginal fistula.

Associated Symptoms

Nocturnal enuresis associated with daytime urinary frequency, urgency, incontinence, and difficulties in initiating the urinary stream suggests urethral obstruction. Daytime urinary frequency, urgency, incontinence, squatting behavior, constipation, encopresis, gait disturbance, and a history of spina bifida or spinal trauma suggest a neurogenic bladder. Constant dampness in the underwear by day and night in a female suggests an ectopic ureter or vesicovaginal fistula. Secondary nocturnal enuresis associated with dysuria, urinary frequency, urgency, fever, suprapubic/loin pain, or cloudy, foul-smelling urine suggests a urinary tract infection. Polyuria, polydipsia, polyphagia, and weight loss suggest diabetes mellitus. Polyuria, polydipsia, and episodes of dehydration in a child with a history of central nervous system disease suggest diabetes insipidus. A history of constipation is important because the condition is associated with a reduced functional bladder capacity.

Volume of First Morning Void

Most children with nocturnal enuresis void only a small or average amount of urine in the morning after an enuretic episode. A large volume of urine voided following a significant episode of nocturnal enuresis may be a clue to the presence of low nocturnal secretion of antidiuretic hormone.

Soundness of Sleep

Children with nocturnal enuresis often sleep more deeply than other family members. Some children only wet when they are overtired. Conversely, children who are usually enuretic may be continent during periods of wakeful sleep such as during intercurrent illnesses.

Past Health

A child with a history of a structural abnormality of the urinary tract or neurogenic bladder may have nocturnal enuresis due to these causes. A history of spinal trauma may indicate a neurogenic bladder as a cause of enuresis. A history of central nervous system disorder may indicate neurogenic diabetes insipidus. Certain medications such as methylxanthines and caffeine may be associated with nocturnal enuresis.

Family History

A family history of nocturnal enuresis should be sought because nocturnal enuresis tends to run in the family. A family history of diabetes mellitus, diabetes insipidus, or kidney disease suggests the corresponding disorder. Any stressful events in the family such as birth of a sibling and parental disharmony should be explored, especially in children with secondary nocturnal enuresis.

Physical Examination

Height and weight should be measured and plotted onto standard growth charts. All children should have their blood pressure checked, which, if elevated, might indicate renal disease. A thorough physical examination should include examination of the abdomen and genitalia and a complete neurologic examination. In chronic constipation, fecal masses are often palpable in the left lower quadrant of the abdomen and in the suprapubic area.

In the majority of children with primary nocturnal enuresis, the physical examination is unremarkable. An abnormal physical examination is only present when primary nocturnal enuresis is due to a structural cause. A myelomeningocele is usually obvious at birth; however, subtle spinal defects may also be associated with primary nocturnal enuresis. A midline tuft of hair, an exaggerated dimple, or a birthmark in the area of the lumbosacral spine; a gait abnormality; absence of anal wink; or abnormal motor power, tone, reflexes, or sensation in the lower extremities suggests a neurogenic bladder. A palpably enlarged bladder or kidney and a weak or dribbling urinary stream suggests urinary obstruction, such as may result from posterior urethral valves.

Laboratory and Imaging Studies

A urinalysis is warranted to rule out urinary tract infection, diabetes mellitus, and a defect in the ability to concentrate urine. Ultrasound examination of the bladder (prevoid and postvoid) can be used to evaluate bladder dysfunction and functional bladder capacity.

Treatment

One essential part of the treatment plan of every child with primary nocturnal enuresis should be compassion and support from both the family and physician. It is important to clarify to parents that the child is not at fault and to specify that punishment for bedwetting is inappropriate. The child and family can be reassured that in the absence of structural defect, primary nocturnal enuresis tends to resolve with time.

Simple behavioral strategies such as encouraging the child to urinate frequently during the daytime, emptying the bladder before bedtime, and limiting fluid and solute intake in the evening are often recommended. Caffeinated beverages should be avoided, particularly in the evening. Some authors recommend waking the child 1.5 to 2 hours after bedtime to go to the bathroom. Star charts and reward systems need to reinforce positive behavior. Behavioral therapy may increase the success rate of pharmacologic therapy or enuretic alarm therapy.

Desmopressin (DDAVP, 1-desamino-8-arginine vasopressin) is an analogue of vasopressin that has a profound antidiuretic activity without pressor activity. The medication acts on the V2 receptors of the renal tubules and increases the reabsorption of fluid from the renal tubules, thereby decreasing the amount of urine produced. The medication is indicated as a first-line therapy for children with monosymptomatic nocturnal enuresis associated with nocturnal polyuria and normal bladder function. Desmopressin is available in a sublingual lyophilisate (melt) preparation,[2] as well as a tablet. The bioavailability of the lyophilisate (melt) preparation is approximately 60% greater than that of the tablet formulation. The recommended dose of desmopressin is 120 to 240 µg melt and 200 to 400 µg tablet. The former is usually given 30 minutes to 1 hour before bedtime, and the latter is usually given 1 hour before bedtime. Side effects are rare and include symptomatic hyponatremia with water intoxication. When desmopressin is prescribed, patients should be instructed to avoid high fluid intake in the evening.

Imipramine (Tofranil), a tricyclic agent with antimuscarinic property, may be helpful in children who have not responded to desmopressin alone. Presumably, the medication decreases the amount of time spent in rapid eye movement sleep, stimulates antidiuretic hormone secretion, and relaxes the detrusor muscle. The recommended starting dose is 25 mg for children 6 to 12 years of age and 50 mg for those older than 12 years, given 1 to 2 hours before bedtime. If necessary, the dose may be increased gradually to a maximum of 50 mg in children 6 to 12 years of age and 75 mg for those older than 12 years. However, potential side effects (anxiety, depression, dizziness, headache, drowsiness, lethargy, sleep disturbance, dry mouth, anorexia, vomiting, skin rashes) and serious adverse effects (hepatotoxicity, cardiotoxicity) with overdose limit their use.

---

[2]Not available in the United States.

Monotherapy with oxybutynin (Ditropan),[1] an anticholinergic and antispasmodic agent that decreases uninhibited bladder contraction, is not effective in treating monosymptomatic nocturnal enuresis. The medication can be added, however, as a second-line drug in the treatment of children with both diurnal and nocturnal enuresis. The dose is 5 mg administered 1 hour before bedtime.

Enuretic alarm is indicated as a first-line therapy for children with monosymptomatic nocturnal enuresis associated with a small bladder capacity or nocturnal detrusor overactivity. Randomized controlled trials have demonstrated that the enuretic alarm has greater efficacy than other forms of treatment. The enuretic alarm is triggered when a sensor in the sheets or night clothes gets wet; a bell or buzzer is thereby activated. Presumably, alarm therapy startles the child and improves arousal from sleep either by classical conditioning or avoidance conditioning. A disadvantage of alarm therapy is that it takes a couple of weeks to take effect. As such, alarms should be used for at least 6 weeks in children who do not respond before discontinuing their use. Because success depends on a cooperative, motivated child, conditioning therapy with an alarm device is generally used in children over 6 years of age.

It has been shown that combination of alarm and desmopressin works better than either treatment alone. Such treatment may be considered for children with refractory nocturnal enuresis.

When an anatomic abnormality or defect in urinary concentration ability is present, the underlying problem may require specific dietary, pharmacologic, or surgical treatment. Any underlying constipation should also be treated.

---

[1]Not FDA approved for this indication.

References

Brown ML, Pope AW, Brown EJ. Treatment of primary nocturnal enuresis in children: a review. Child Care Health Dev 2011;37:153–60.

Glazener CM, Evans JH. Desmopressin for nocturnal enuresis in children. Cochrane Database Syst Rev 2002;3, CD002112.

Glazener CM, Evans JH, Pero RE. Alarm interventions for nocturnal enuresis in children. Cochrane Database Syst Rev 2005;2, CD002911.

Kamperis K, Hagstroem S, Rittig S, et al. Combination of the enuresis alarm and desmopressin: Second line treatment for nocturnal enuresis. J Urol 2008;179:1128–31.

Leung AK. Nocturnal enuresis. In: Leung AK, editor. Common Problems in Ambulatory Pediatrics: Specific Clinical Problems, vol 1. New York: Nova Science Publishers; 2011. p. 161–71.

Lottmann H, Froeling F, Alloussi S, et al. A randomized comparison of oral desmopressin lyophilisate (MELT) and tablet formulations in children and adolescents with primary nocturnal enuresis. Int J Clin Pract 2007;61:1454–60.

Nevéus T. Nocturnal enuresis—theoretic background and practical guidelines. Pediatr Nephrol 2011;26:1207–14.

Robson WL. Evaluation and management of enuresis. N Engl J Med 2009;360:1429–36.

Robson WL, Leung AK, van Howe R. Primary and secondary nocturnal enuresis: similarities in presentation. Pediatrics 2005;115:956–9.

Robson WL, Leung AK, Norgaard JP. The comparative safety of oral versus intranasal desmopressin in the treatment of children with nocturnal enuresis. J Urol 2007;178:24–30.

Van de Walle J, Rittig S, Bauer S, et al. Practical consensus guidelines for the management of enuresis. Eur J Pediatr 2012;171:971–83.

NORMAL INFANT FEEDING

Method of
Amy Seery, MD

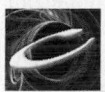

CURRENT THERAPY

- Breast milk is considered the best nutritional source for all infants including preterm infants.
- Breast-feeding is strongly encouraged but many mothers require support from a multidisciplinary medical team to achieve success.
- There are few absolute contraindications to breast-feeding but these include maternal HIV, infant galactosemia, herpetic lesions on the breast, maternal use of illicit drugs, and mothers undergoing some types of chemotherapy.
- Maternal medications should be individually reviewed for safety during breast-feeding.
- Newborns should be fed at least every 3 hours during the day and every 4 hours during the night.
- Breast-fed infants can go up to 10 days between stools. This is a normal stooling pattern so long as the infant shows no signs of distress or illness.

The newborn period is defined as birth through the 28th day of life. During this time, newborns primarily feed, grow, and sleep. Therefore, adequate nutrition carries special significance during this phase of life. This chapter focuses on available options for newborn nutrition (e.g., breast milk and commercial formulas), information medical caregivers can use when counseling families, definitions of adequate quality and quantity of nutritional sources, and assessing for appropriate intake in terms of growth.

Breast-feeding and Breast Milk

Breast-feeding is the nutritional source of choice as recommended by the American Academy of Pediatrics (AAP), the Canadian Pediatric Society, and the American Academy of Family Physicians. Caregivers should always respect the choice of the mother and support her during her bonding period with her newborn infant. However, because many misconceptions exist regarding breast-feeding, it is practical for caregivers to inquire about a mother's reasons if she chooses to use formula to feed her infant. She may have several concerns about breast-feeding including returning to work, the logistics of pumping, or her modesty, or she may consider breast-feeding to be "antiquated." Breast-feeding may be contrary to cultural and ethnic beliefs of the mother. For example, some Hispanic women are concerned that when breast-feeding they might inadvertently pass on negative emotions to their newborn. Because Somalian mothers attribute special powers to Western medicine and infant formulas, they often breast-feed but supplement with formula to ensure their infant gets everything that modern medicine can offer. With proper education and support, many mothers find breast-feeding to be a more reasonable option than they first thought.

Thanks to the efforts of several organizations promoting the health benefits of breast-feeding, even mothers who choose to formula feed recognize breast milk as the best nutritional option for their infant. But even after making the decision to breast-feed, some mothers continue to struggle with the actual undertaking of breast-feeding. There remains in our culture the inaccurate belief that something so "natural" must be easy to do. Many first-time mothers are easily frustrated and discouraged during the first few attempts at breast-feeding because they have unreasonable expectations based on the media and popular culture. With more and more women willing to try breast-feeding after delivery, adequate support and teaching should be provided by the entire medical team.

Healthy People 2010 established a national breast-feeding initiation goal of 75% and in 2003 and 2004 reported rates for all U.S. women were at 70.9% and 70.3%, respectively. These rates are the highest reported since before World War II and are largely the result of improved public knowledge. Unfortunately, other *Healthy People 2010* breast-feeding goals fell short. Despite a goal of 50% breast-feeding at 6 months, only 36% of infants were still receiving any human milk at this age and only 14% were exclusively being breast-fed. Only 17% of babies are breast-fed at 1 year, despite a goal of 25%. The biggest disparities in breast-feeding rates are among racial and ethnic minorities. Special attention should be made by medical teams to provide sufficient support and education to these women.

Breast milk is considered the ideal source of nutrition for all newborns, including premature infants, in a large part owing to its contents. There is a greater ratio of whey to casein in breast milk than in formula. Whey is associated with better absorption and digestion as well as faster gastrointestinal transit times. There are also several specific proteins found only in breast milk, such as lactoferrin, lysosyme, and secretory immunoglobulin A, that aid in immune defense in the gut. Breast milk also contains long-chain polyunsaturated fatty acids (PUFAs) that aid in neural and visual development. Infants given formulas that contain long-chain PUFAs have serum concentrations that never match those of breast milk-fed infants, but there is also no known minimum amount needed to achieve benefit.

There is also a difference in the intestinal microflora seen in infants fed breast milk versus those fed formula. Larger percentages of *Lactobacillus* and *Bifidobacterium* species are found in infants fed breast milk, whereas *Bacteroides* spp and enterobacteria are in more abundance in formula-fed counterparts. Newer evidence suggests this difference in the diversity of gut microflora accounts for the stronger immune systems seen in breast-fed infants.

Breast milk has the benefit of containing several nonnutritive substances that are advantageous for young infants including maternal antibodies, growth regulators, digestive enzymes, and hormones. Breast milk has been associated with a reduced risk for many chronic illnesses including asthma, food and environmental allergies, diabetes mellitus, eczema, cardiovascular disease, and obesity. There is a reduction in the number of short-term illnesses of childhood including acute respiratory and gastrointestinal illnesses as well as otitis media.

Newer research shows an association between being fed breast milk and having higher IQ scores later in childhood.

The act of breast-feeding offers several benefits to the infant. There is a sense of security and closeness that comes from skin-to-skin contact and the resultant interaction between infant and mother. Nursing can also reduce the opportunities and risk for bottle-propping and overfeeding. Breast-feeding allows nutrition to be more immediately available with minimal preparation work compared to the mixing and warming of formula. Breast milk is a much cheaper alternative to supplemental formulas. Breast-feeding can also lead to health benefits for the mother such as decreased risk of ovarian and breast cancers as well as diabetes mellitus type II.

There are very few contraindications to breast-feeding. Contraindications include maternal HIV, active herpetic lesions on the breast (herpetic lesions elsewhere are not a contraindication), maternal use of illicit drugs, women undergoing chemotherapy with antimetabolite agents, and mothers with active tuberculosis. Nearly all over-the-counter medications are safe to take during breast-feeding. Some prescription medications are contraindicated, though safe substitutes are usually available. Providers can use the online National Library of Medicine's Drugs and Lactation Database (LactMed) to check safety and provide up-to-date counseling. Infants with galactosemia should not be breast-fed or bottle fed with milk products.

Infant Formulas

Commercially available infant formulas became widely used during World War II when there was a large influx of women into the national workforce. Since that time, infant formulas have been continuously improved upon and contain all the necessary energy and nutrient requirements for full-term infants up to the age of 6 months. According to the AAP there are three indications for the use of formulas:

- An alternative primary nutritional source for infants whose mothers choose not to or are unable to breast-feed
- A supplementary nutritional source for mothers with an inadequate supply of breast milk
- A nutritional source in infants with a medical condition in which breast-feeding is contraindicated (e.g., galactosemia)

Commercial formulas usually come in three distinct preparations including ready-to-feed, concentrated liquid, and powder. All three preparations yield 20 kcal per fluid ounce when prepared correctly, the same amount of energy per volume found in breast milk. Powder preparations are generally the least expensive. An advantage to formulas over breast-feeding is the ability to increase caloric density for an infant with increased metabolic needs (e.g., infants with congenital heart defects). Breast-feeding mothers have the option to breast pump and add a fortifier if needed to achieve similar increases in caloric density.

Formulas carry the risk of improper preparation, whether intentional or accidental. Caregivers might choose to dilute the formula secondary to financial pressures or to concentrate formula preparations in a desire to have a larger infant, because some cultures equate larger infant size and weight with better health. Either change can be dangerous to the infant. Diluting leads to an excess of free water with an insufficient solute load (e.g., hyponatremia) and concentrating can conversely lead to hypernatremia. Nevertheless, formulas remain an appropriate alternative when desired by the infant's mother or when medically indicated (Table 1).

Micronutrients

Both breast milk and formula contain most of the micronutrients needed by infants. Calcium and phosphorus are found in lower concentrations in breast milk but are more bioavailable than the minerals present in formulas. Therefore there is no difference in bone mineral concentrations in both sets of infants. Iron, zinc, and copper serum levels are sufficient during the first 6 months of life in breast-fed infants, though tissue stores are gradually depleted. After 6 months breast-feeding should be supplemented with complementary foods to prevent outcomes such as iron deficiency anemia.

Vitamin K, necessary to prevent hemorrhagic disease, is produced by the digestive actions of intestinal flora. For this reason, most infants at the time of birth are given a single intramuscular dose to provide adequate amounts until intestinal flora concentrations are more mature and dietary supplementation with solid food begins at 6 months.

Vitamin D needs historically have been achieved with adequate sunlight exposure. However, with appropriate use of sunscreens and sunlight avoidance, most infants are at risk for vitamin D deficiency. Vitamin D is not passed in sufficient quantities in breast milk, and the content in formulas is so low that the daily recommended amount of 400 IU is only achieved when infants are consuming a volume typical of a 6-month old. Therefore, supplementation should be recommended for all infants regardless of skin color and nutritional source to help prevent rickets. The recommendation is 400 IU of vitamin D for all pediatric age groups beginning after the first 2 weeks of life.

Neither formula-fed nor breast-fed infants usually require supplementation with water. In fact, providing infants with excess free water can lead to hyponatremia, seizures, and death. If there is concern that the infant is constipated or overheated, caregivers can provide up to a tablespoon of water daily to infants younger than 4 months old.

Defining Adequate Intake

To determine if a newborn is receiving adequate nutrition physicians should ask the caregiver how often feedings are occurring, for how long (for breast-fed infants), and how much is eaten (for formula-fed infants) and should assess the number of wet diapers and stools daily. Initially infants should consume 10 to 15 mL per feeding for the first 24 to 36 hours, gradually increasing to 30 to 45 mL by the fourth day of life. Breast-fed infants should feed 15 to 20 minutes each side. At the time of discharge to home, all newborns should be feeding 8 to 12 times a day, or every 2 to 3 hours. This interval can be increased to every 4 hours at night, and parents should be encouraged to wake any infants who sleep for longer than this duration. If an infant has lost more than 10% of his or her birth weight, the care team should consider delaying discharge to review the infant's nutritional status and feeding habits. Caregivers should be attentive to infant cues of hunger and satiety to provide an ideal feeding pattern for each infant.

TABLE 1   Infant Formulas and their Indications

CLASS	BRAND NAMES	CALORIES (KCAL PER OZ)	CARBOHYDRATE SOURCE	PROTEIN SOURCE	INDICATIONS
Breast milk	—	20	Lactose	Human milk	Preferred for all infants
Term formula	Gerber Good Start Gentle	20	Lactose	Cow's milk	Appropriate for most infants
Term formula with DHA and ARA	Enfamil Premium Infant; Good Start Protect; Similac Advanced	20	Lactose	Cow's milk	Marketed to promote eye and brain development
Preterm formula	Enfamil Premature; Similac Special Care 24 with Iron	24	Lactose	Cow's milk	<34 wk gestational age Weight <1800 g
Enriched formula	Enfacare; Similac Neosure	22	Lactose	Cow's milk	34–36 wk gestational age Weight ≥1800 g
Soy formula	Enfamil Prosobee; Good Start Soy; Similac Isomil	20	Corn-based	Soy	Congenital lactase deficiency, galactosemia
Lactose-free formula	Similac Sensitive	20	Corn-based	Cow's milk	Congenital lactase deficiency, primary lactase deficiency, galactosemia
Hypoallergenic formula	Similac Alimentum; Enfamil Nutramigen; Enfamil Pregestimil	20	Corn or Sucrose	Hydrolyzed proteins	Milk protein allergy
Nonallergenic formula	Elecare; Neocate Infant; Nutramigen AA	20	Corn or Sucrose	Amino acids	Milk protein allergy
Antireflex formula	Enfamil AR; Similac Senstive for Spit-Up	20	Lactose (thickened with rice starch)	Cow's milk	Gastroesophageal reflux

Abbreviations: ARA = arachidonic acid; DHA = docosahexaenoic acid.
Adapted from O'Connor NR. Infant formula. Am Fam Physician 2009;79:565–70.

Voiding and stooling patterns change with age and can also be influenced by the infant's diet. All newborns should have at least one wet diaper and one stool within the first 24 hours of life. If this does not occur, close observation and further work-up is indicated to rule out structural or metabolic abnormalities. During the first week of life, infants usually void and stool with every feeding or even more often. Beyond the first week, infants should have at least 4 to 6 voids daily regardless of diet. Formula-fed infants might have one stool every other day up to 2 to 3 stools daily. Because of the higher percentage of protein that is absorbed in breast milk, breast-fed infants can go up to 10 days between stools. Physicians should review with families the signs and symptoms (emesis, refusal to feed, lethargy, inconsolability, and abdominal distention) that indicate an infant with infrequent stooling should be medically evaluated. Breast-fed infants also have stools that are described as loose, yellow, and seedy. Caregivers should be educated that this is a normal stool color and consistency and is not considered diarrhea.

Medical providers can also calculate an infant's nutritional needs and compare to the actual intake. Nutritional needs are represented as kcal/kg per day (KKD). The following formula can be used:

$$KKD = \frac{Volume\ in\ mL\ consumed\ in\ 24\,h}{Weight\ in\ kg} \times \frac{20\,kcal/oz}{30}$$

During the first 3 months of life, infants should consume an intake that equals 90 to 135 kcal/kg per day. This intake goal should lead to a weight gain of approximately 25 to 30 g daily. From 3 to 6 months of age, infants gain at a slightly slower rate of approximately 15 to 20 g per day (Table 2). For example, a 2-month-old who weighs 6 kg should consume between 810 mL to 1215 mL daily.

At subsequent visits an infant can be assessed for adequate growth using standardized, gender-specific growth curves. Attention should be paid to growth parameters including weight, length, head circumference, and weight-for-length. Weight-for-length charts are used during the first 2 years of life as a gross equivalent

TABLE 2   Expected Growth Velocities during Infancy

AGE	WEIGHT GAIN (g/d)	LENGTH (cm/mo)	HEAD CIRCUMFERENCE (cm/wk)
0–3 mo	25–30	2.5	0.5
3–6 mo	15–20	2.5	0.5
6–12 mo	10	1.25	0.25

to body-mass-index charts used for children older than 2 years. For years, practices defined adequate weight gain using growth charts as designed by the National Center for Health Statistics (NCHS), a branch of the Centers for Disease Control and Prevention (CDC). These charts were last updated in 2000 and unfortunately still reflect means for a population with a predominance of formula-fed infants. The World Health Organization (WHO) has since completed the Multi-Centre Growth Reference Study to better establish growth norms for infants and children who are breast-fed throughout the first year of life. A provider who is uncertain if an exclusively breast-fed infant is meeting minimum growth requirements should refer to these charts before automatically encouraging caregivers to begin formula supplementation. Growth failure is usually considered a weight less than the third percentile or a drop of two or more percentiles in a short time (Figures 1 to 8, available on Expert Consult).

Overfeeding of newborns is unfortunately common, though bottle-fed infants are at a greater risk compared to breast-fed infants. Several factors can contribute to overfeeding including lack of caregiver experience and support, as well as cultural biases such as the desire to have a chubbier infant. Many caregivers are unable to recognize infant cues for hunger and satiety and misinterpret cries or other vocalizations as a request for food. Medical providers should teach families about the rooting and sucking reflex and explain that some forms of sucking provide the infant

Head circumference-for-age BOYS

Birth to 2 years (percentiles)

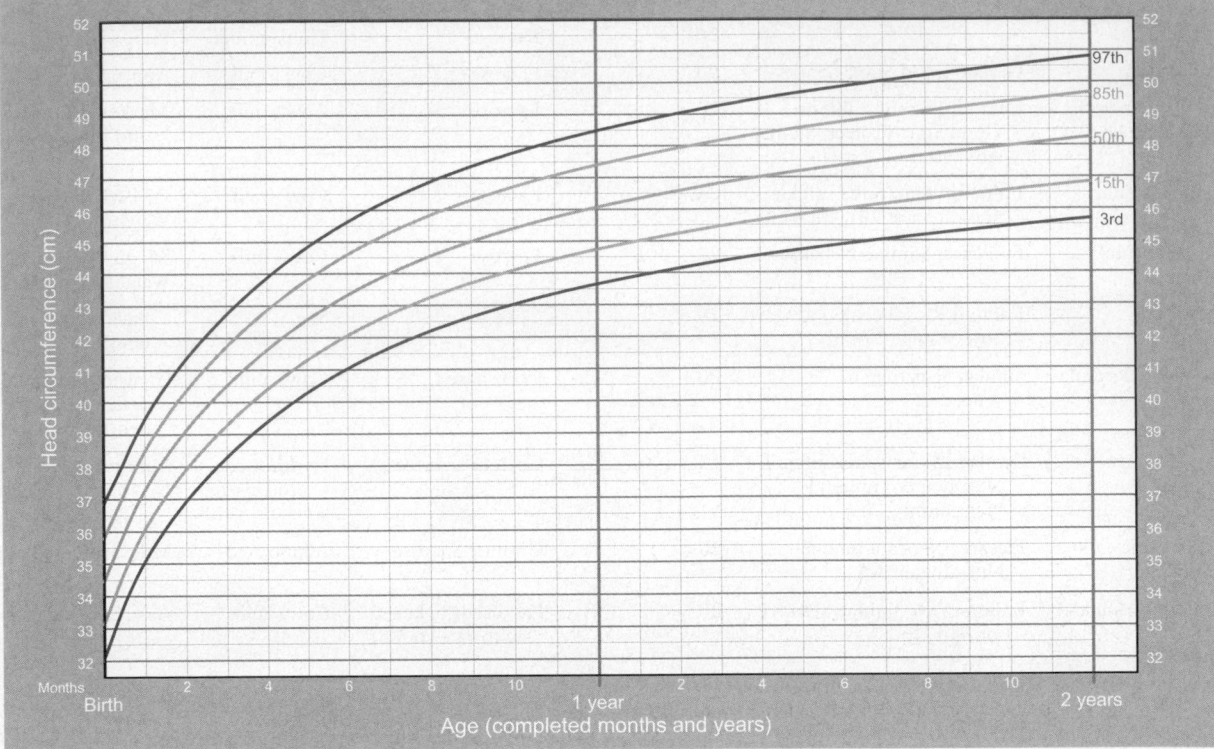

Figure 1. Head circumference for age: boys.

Length-for-age BOYS

Birth to 2 years (percentiles)

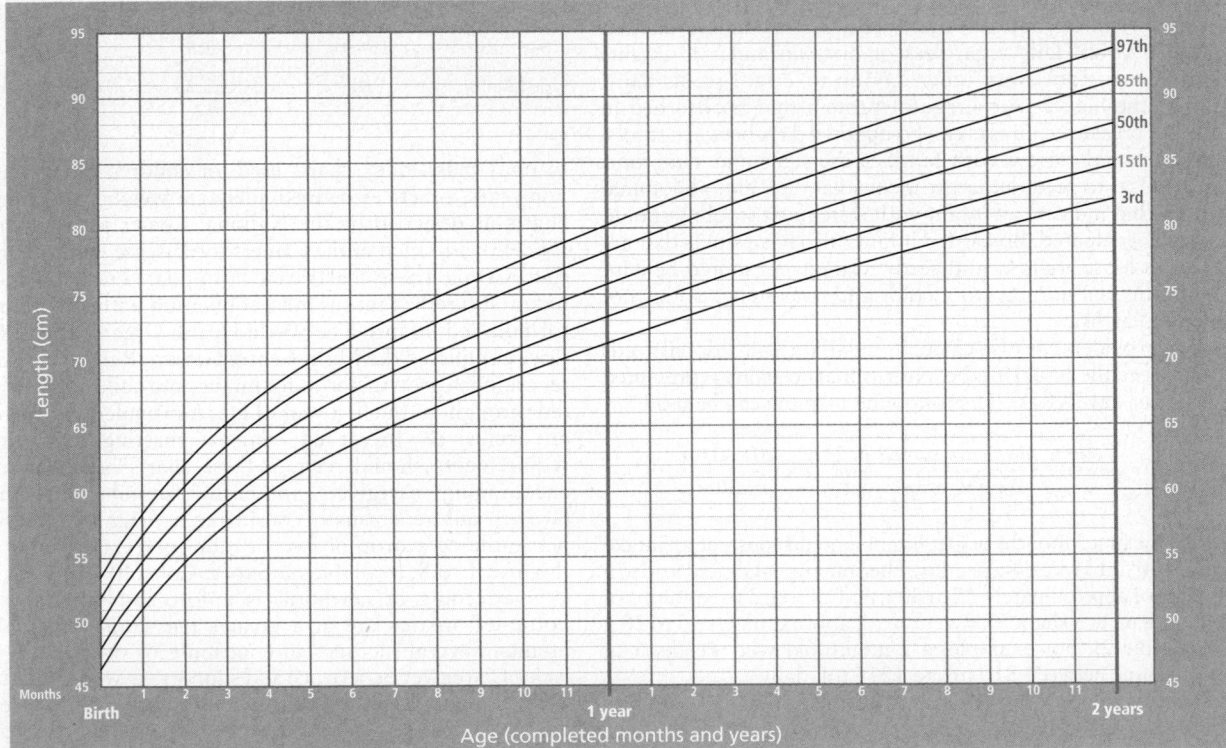

Figure 2. Length for age: boys.

Weight-for-age GIRLS
Birth to 2 years (percentiles)

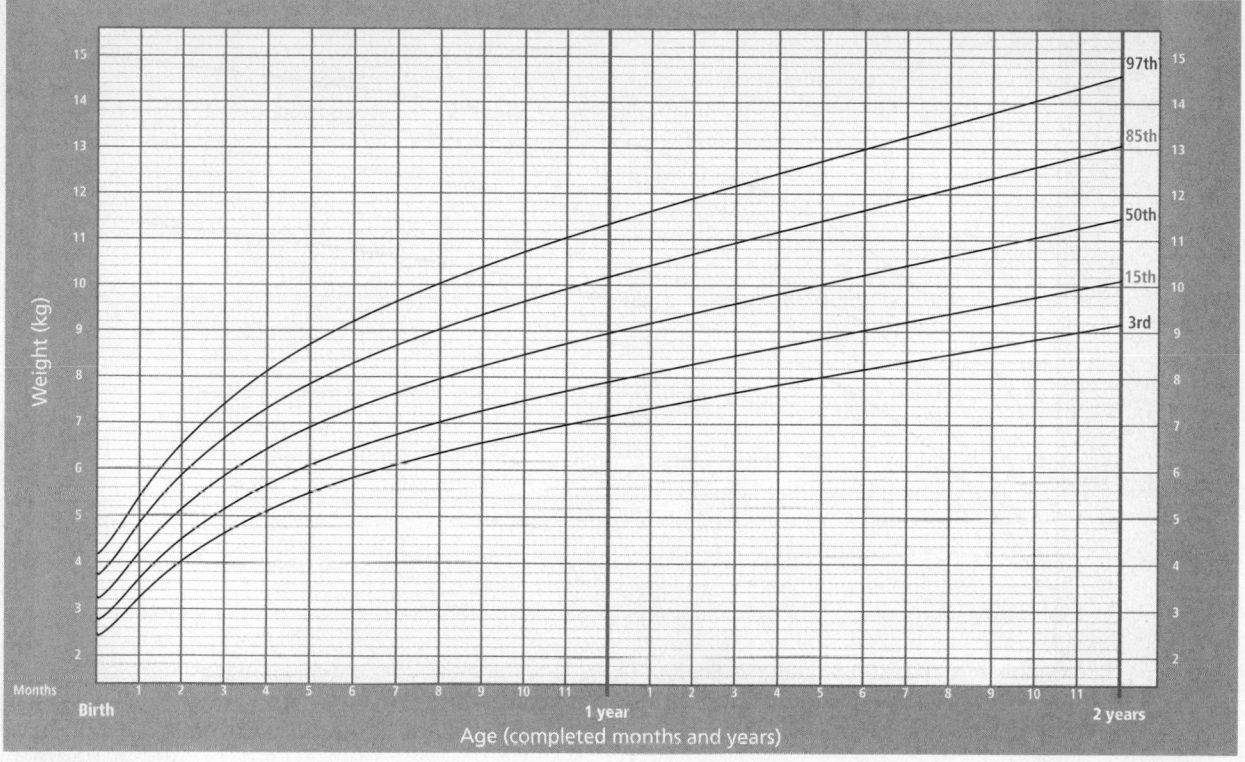

WHO Child Growth Standards

Figure 3. Weight for age: girls.

Weight-for-length GIRLS
Birth to 2 years (percentiles)

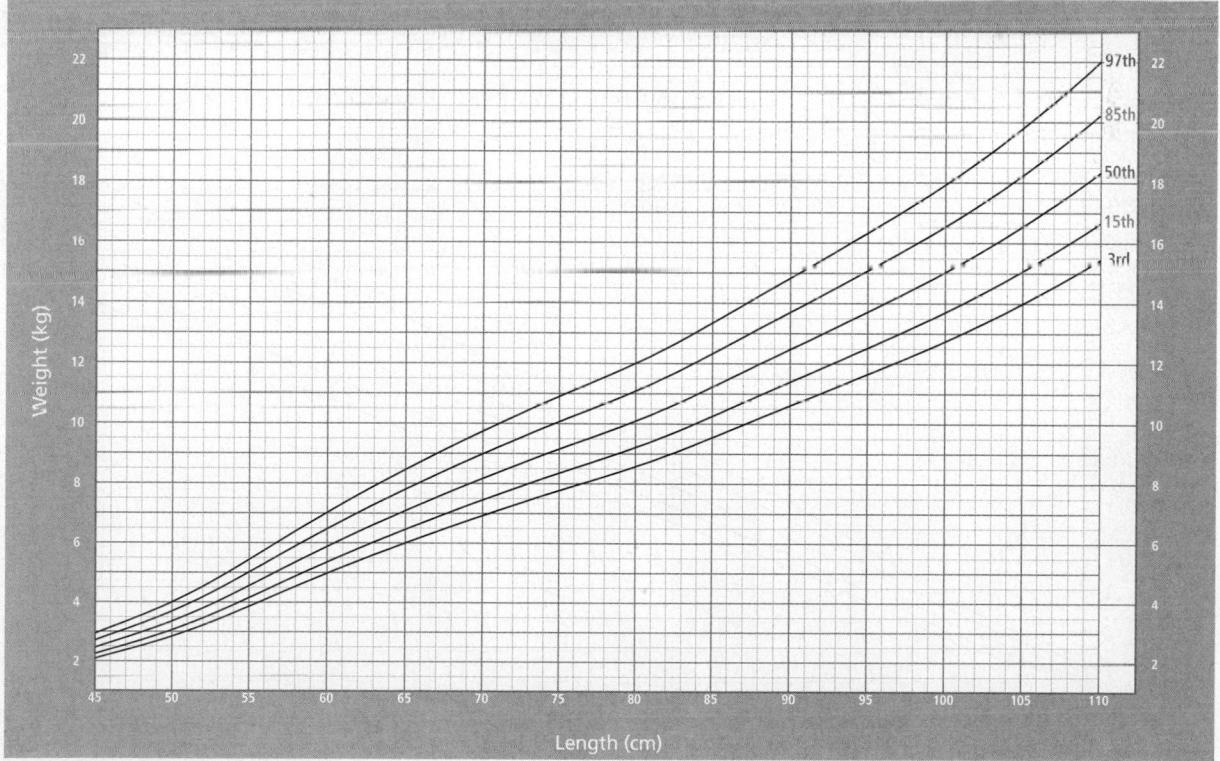

WHO Child Growth Standards

Figure 4. Weight for length: girls.

Head circumference-for-age GIRLS

Birth to 2 years (percentiles)

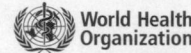

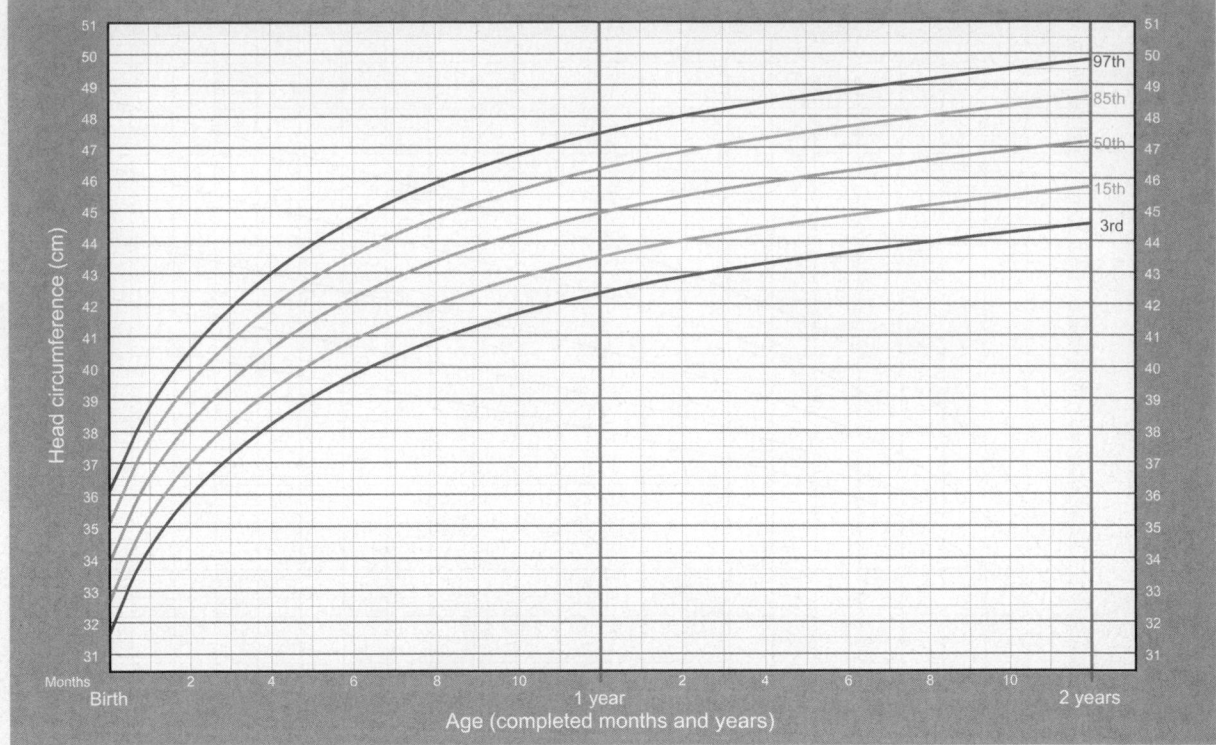

WHO Child Growth Standards

Figure 5. Head circumference for age: girls.

Weight-for-length BOYS

Birth to 2 years (percentiles)

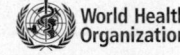

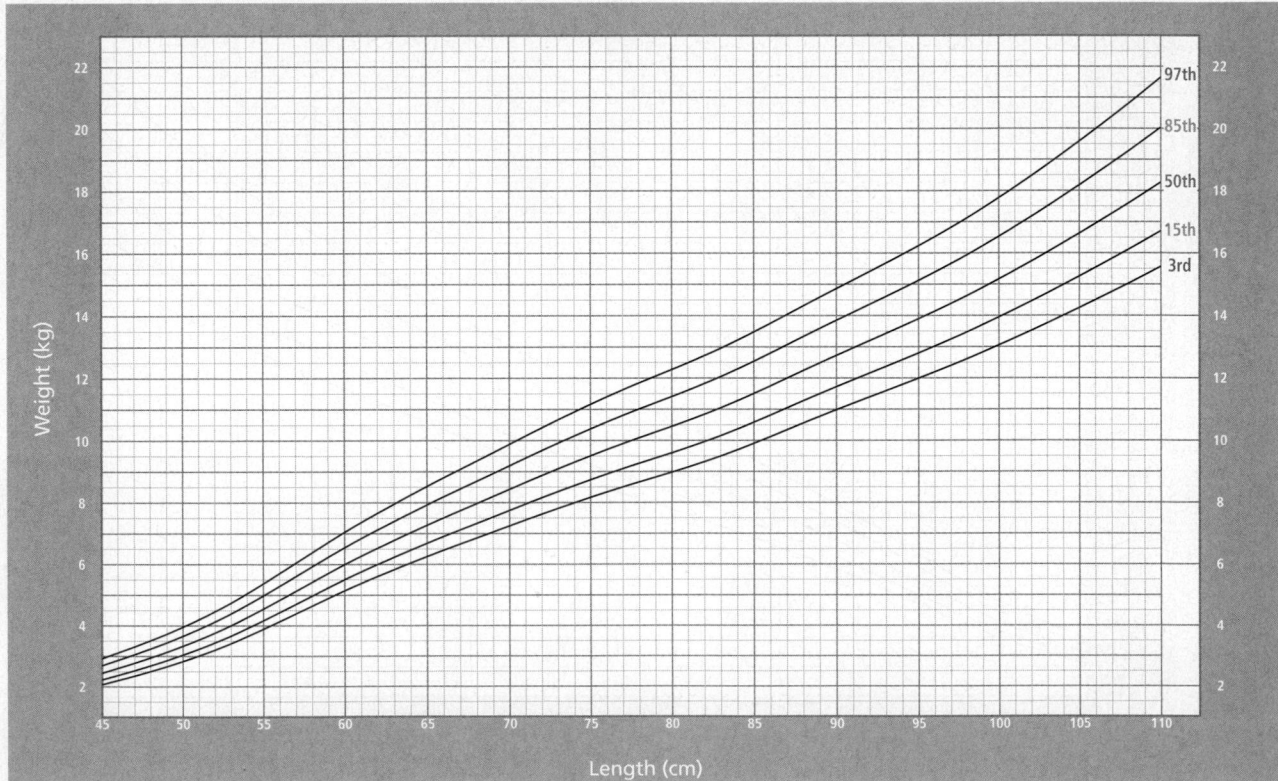

WHO Child Growth Standards

Figure 6. Weight for length: boys.

Weight-for-age BOYS
Birth to 2 years (percentiles)

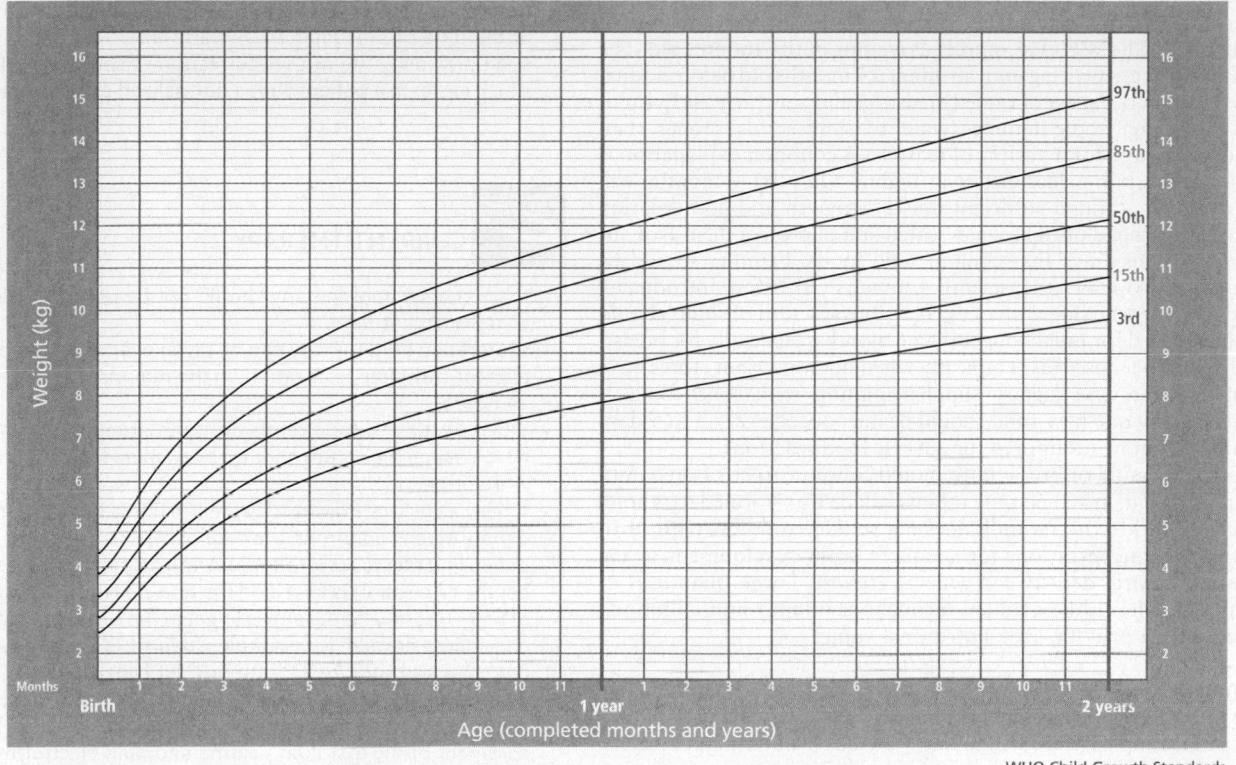

WHO Child Growth Standards

Figure 7. Weight for age: boys.

Length-for-age GIRLS
Birth to 2 years (percentiles)

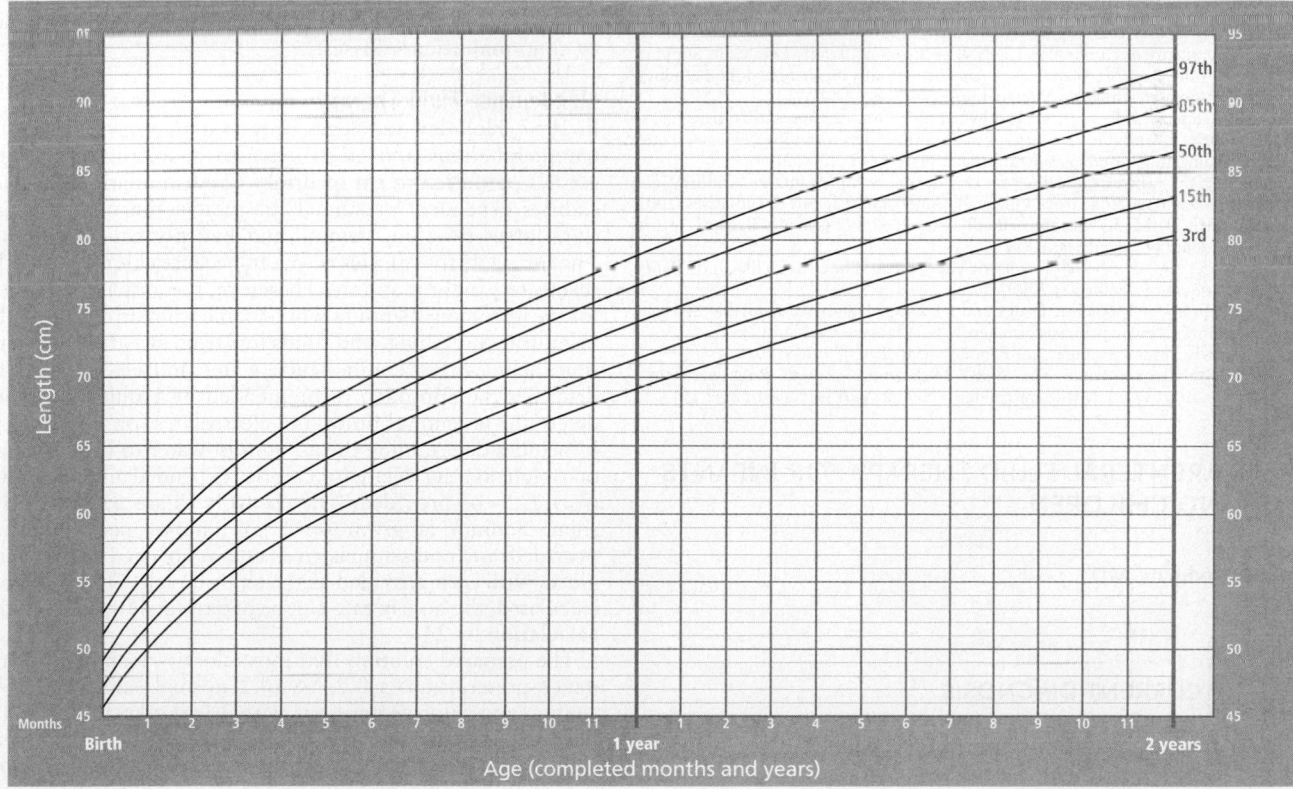

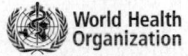

WHO Child Growth Standards

Figure 8. Length for age: girls.

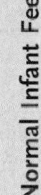

Normal Infant Feeding

1139

with a means for self-soothing and are not signals that the infant is hungry (nonnutritive versus nutritive sucking).

Introduction of Complementary Foods

It remains controversial when solid foods should be added to the diet of an infant. The WHO recommends waiting until 6 months old. The AAP encourages waiting until an infant is 4 months old before adding solids and encourages continued breast-feeding until at least 1 year of age. However, some families want to start solids sooner than 4 months of age for a variety of reasons. A common explanation is "helping the baby sleep better at night." Only by 4 months will infants have attained sufficient muscle strength and coordination to keep their head upright when seated and to protect their own airway during feedings that contain solid foods. Families should be encouraged to wait at least until 4 months old before introducing solids, usually starting with rice cereal. Introduction of solids should not be delayed for much longer than 6 months, especially for breast-fed infants, because this is typically when micronutrient stores have been depleted and dietary supplementation with solid foods is needed. Only one new solid should be introduced every 3 to 5 days so infants can be monitored for adverse food reactions.

Either formula or breast milk should continue to be offered until 12 months old, at which time infants can be transitioned to whole-fat cow's milk. Low-fat milk does not provide toddlers with sufficient lipid concentrations for adequate brain development or the required caloric density for general growth. Large quantities of fruit juices should be avoided throughout infancy and childhood because they provide little nutritional value.

Summary

The majority of term infants are born ready and able to begin feeding, but it is up to providers to know available nutritional options, normal feeding patterns, and means for measuring adequate intake and growth. Providers and other members of the care team also need to be able to counsel caregivers about best practices when feeding infants. When infants are suspected to be overfed or underfed, it may take a multidisciplinary approach by physicians, nurses, dieticians, speech therapists, lactation counselors, and social workers to help patients and their families.

References

American Academy of Family Physicians. Breastfeeding, Family Physicians Supporting (Position Paper). Available at http://www.aafp.org/online/en/home/policy/policies/b/breastfeedingpositionpaper.htm; [accessed 22.07.12].

American Academy of Pediatrics, HealthyChildren.Org. Feeding and Nutrition, 0 to 12 Months. Available at http://www.healthychildren.org/English/ages-stages/baby/feeding-nutrition/Pages/default.aspx; [accessed 22.07.12].

Duncan P. Bright Futures: Guidelines for Health Supervision of Infants, Children, and Adolescents. 3rd ed. Elk Grove Village, IL: American Academy of Pediatrics; 2007.

Kleinmann RE. Pediatric Nutrition Handbook. 6th ed. Elk Grove Village, IL: American Academy of Pediatrics; 2008.

McInerny TK. AAP Textbook of Pediatric Care. 1st ed. Elk Grove Village, IL: American Academy of Pediatrics; 2009.

National Library of Medicine. Drugs and Lactation Database. Available at http://toxnet.nlm.nih.gov/cgi-bin/sis/htmlgen?LACT; [accessed 22.07.12].

O'Connor NR. Infant formula. Am Fam Physician 2009;79:565–70.

World Health Organization. The WHO Multicentre Growth Reference Study. Available at http://www.who.int/childgrowth/mgrs/en/; [accessed 22.07.12].

PARENTERAL FLUID THERAPY FOR INFANTS AND CHILDREN

Method of
Aaron Friedman, MD

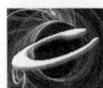

CURRENT DIAGNOSIS

- Maintenance fluid therapy is designed to replace the next 24 hours' anticipated losses from sensible and insensible losses in an otherwise healthy, euvolemic patient with normal kidney function.

- In a patient with extracellular volume loss, the percentage of body weight lost should be used as a guide to the volume needed for restoration.
- Serum sodium in patients with dehydration should be measured at the time of presentation and also after restoration fluid has been provided. The further correction of serum sodium will be much easier in a patient with a normalized extracellular volume.

CURRENT THERAPY

- Maintenance fluid therapy should not be used as a restoration or replacement fluid.
- Restoration fluid therapy can be given over short periods with a plan for complete restoration, in the majority of patients, within 24 hours.
- When treating hyponatremia or hypernatremia, the goal should be to change the serum sodium by *no more than* 10 mmol/L in a 24-hour period.
- When calculating how much water (in the case of hypernatremia) or how much sodium (in the case of hyponatremia) to provide a patient in order to restore sodium into the normal range, remember the calculation is based on the *total body water*, which is 60% of body weight, and the aim is to get to the closest serum sodium considered normal; for example, sodium 135 mmol/L for hyponatremia and sodium 145 mmol/L for hypernatremia.
- Replacement fluid therapy for patients with abnormal losses—gastrointestinal or urinary losses—should be based on measurement of the lost fluid volume and fluid electrolyte content.

Children receive three types of parenteral fluid therapy: maintenance therapy, restoration therapy, and replacement therapy. Maintenance fluid therapy provides the typical anticipated fluid and electrolyte losses seen in otherwise normal, euvolemic children. Restoration fluid therapy restores fluid volume previously lost. Replacement fluid therapy keeps up with ongoing abnormal fluid losses, such as ongoing losses from the gastrointestinal tract or abnormal urinary losses.

Maintenance Fluid Therapy

In 1957, Holliday and Segar proposed an approach to providing parenteral fluids and electrolytes to hospitalized children who are not permitted to eat or drink. The formulation was based on calories expended, presumed the patient did not have previous fluid losses (was euvolemic), and had normal kidney function. The surrogate for calories is weight because calories expended correlates to weight in grams. Therefore, the anticipated fluid losses for the upcoming 24 hours would come from urine excreted, water lost during breathing, and fluids lost from sweating. The prescription includes two components: water and electrolytes. Table 1 describes the approach recommended by Holliday and Segar to determine parenteral fluids and electrolytes for a 24-hour period. It includes determining the amount of water to be provided based on weight as a surrogate for calories expended and it includes electrolytes to be provided. The electrolytes are sodium and potassium. Sodium is given at 2 to 3 mmol per 100 mL water provided, and potassium is given at 2 mmol per 100 mL water provided, with each provided as the chloride salt. Once the amount is calculated, the hourly rate can be determined by dividing the final calculation by 24.

The prepared solution that most closely resembles this maintenance prescription is 0.2 NS (0.2 normal saline, or 154 mmol sodium and chloride per liter) with 20 mEq KCl/L of fluid. Often glucose is added at 50 g/L (D_5W) or 5 g/100 mL. This provides some readily available calories to reduce catabolism. Note also that D_5W has an osmolality of nearly 300 mOsm/kg H_2O, essentially the same as plasma. This allows safe administration of the

TABLE 1 Approach to Determine Parenteral Fluids and Electrolytes for a 24-Hour Period

WEIGHT (KG)	WATER (mL)	NA (mEq/L)	K (mEq/L)
0–10	100/kg	3/100 mL	2/100 mL
11–20	1000 + 50/kg 11–20 kg	3/100 mL	2/100 mL
>20	1500 + 20/kg >20 kg	3/100 mL	2/100 mL
Examples			
15-kg child	1250	37 mEq/1250 mL	25 mEq/1250 mL
30-kg child	1700	51	34

Note: For sodium, potassium, and chloride, milliequivalents (mEq) and milliosmoles (mOsm) are the same.

solution, because a markedly hypotonic solution administered into a vein could result in lysis of cells (especially red cells) in the vicinity of the infused hypotonic solution.

Another approach for calculating the water with the appropriate electrolytes to be provided is 1500 mL/m²/24 hours. This approach requires measuring the child's height and weight to determine square meters and is less convenient. The volume provided by the approach in Table 1 and the 1500 mL/m² calculation are equivalent.

Another approach is to determine the hourly need of water bearing the electrolytes to be provided, the same as Holliday and Segar. The hourly approach to determining volume is shown in Table 2. Using this approach, maintenance fluid therapy for a 15-kg child would be infused at a rate of 50 mL/hour:

$$(4\,mL/kg/h \times 10\,kg) + (2\,mL/kg/h \times 5\,kg)$$

Maintenance fluid therapy was designed to provide water and electrolytes to cover *future* (anticipated) loss, particularly from urine, expired air, and sweat. Unfortunately, since the publication of maintenance fluid therapy guidelines by Holliday and Segar, the formulation has often been misused. Maintenance fluid therapy should *not* be used as a fluid prescription for *restoring* extracellular fluid volume previously lost, for example, as a result of vomiting, diarrhea, or burns. It is almost always *not* an appropriate solution for *replacing* abnormal losses from the gastrointestinal tract, urinary tract, and so on. The volume calculation and the electrolyte concentrations are *not* appropriate to calculate a restoration solution or replacement solution.

The primary reason that a hypotonic solution such as maintenance fluids, as described by Holliday and Segar, is problematic for use as a restoration solution is the nonosmotic release of antidiuretic hormone (ADH, also called AVP [arginine vasopressin]). Since the mid 1950s it has been known that ADH is released from the hypothalamus under two different physiologic stimuli. One is an increase in serum and extracellular osmolality, usually greater than 290 mOsm/kg H₂O, termed *osmotic stimulus*. The other is a nonosmotic stimulus, usually the result of a fall in extracellular fluid volume or the perception of such a fall by volume receptors mainly in the thorax.

Since the 1950s we have come to learn that a large number of other stimuli can act as a nonosmotic stimulus to ADH release. These include, but are not limited to, a wide range of medications

(antihypertensives, some antineoplastics, barbiturates), stress, central nervous system (CNS) injury or surgery, positive pressure ventilation, malignancy, and intrathoracic infection or malignancy. Under these conditions, ADH levels will be high and the administration of a hypotonic solution even at calculated maintenance doses could result in a fall in serum sodium and serum osmolality, on occasion to levels that might cause serious CNS injury, seizures, and even CNS herniation and death. Even in the early 1960s, when the precise reasons for the nonosmotic release of ADH were not well known, the risk of developing hyponatremia when providing the full volume prescribed in maintenance fluid therapy in the face of a concentrated urine and low urine volumes (signaling ADH release) was well known. The recommendation was to reduce the volume of fluid provided to approximately 50% of the standard calculated amount.

More recently, some have recommended, to prevent the development of hyponatremia, that all maintenance fluid therapy should be delivered as isotonic (normal) saline. The volume portion of the Holliday–Segar formulation is not altered, but the solution recommended in this approach is isotonic saline. The full impact of this approach on all types of hospitalized children is still unknown. It seems clear that patients in the perioperative period should receive normal saline in anticipation of the potential need for extracellular volume restoration. This approach does not guarantee that hyponatremia or hypernatremia will be totally prevented.

Restoration Fluid Therapy

Many children require parenteral fluids because of an inability to take fluids by mouth or due to abnormal fluid losses, such as from vomiting and diarrhea, excessive urinary losses, burns (excessive fluid losses from skin), or third spacing (the extravasation of fluid from the extracellular spaces such as the abdominal or thoracic cavity). In these situations, patients are at risk for serious extracellular volume depletion and even plasma volume depletion, which, left untreated, can result in hypotension or shock.

The parenteral fluid therapy for volume depletion should aim to first replace extracellular volume depletion. How much fluid to provide can be estimated by a long-standing approach using clinical signs to estimate the percentage of reduction in body weight associated with fluid losses (Table 3). In general, these losses can be replaced with a solution that restores extracellular fluid (isotonic saline or lactated Ringer's solution). In situations of prolonged fluid losses (more than 7 days), partial replacement with isotonic saline followed by a slower replacement with a more hypotonic solution with added potassium may be warranted. Table 3 outlines the clinical approach to assessing a patient's degree of volume depletion as a percentage of body weight.

Once the percentage of volume depletion is determined and the decision is made to use parenteral fluids based on moderate to severe volume depletion and ongoing vomiting, thus decreasing the effectiveness of oral rehydration, then rapid parenteral volume repletion is usually safe and effective. Replacing 50% of the determined volume depletion in 1 to 4 hours is appropriate, with the remaining replacement in the subsequent 4 to 16 hours. This should result in restored volume and improvement in the signs

TABLE 2 Hourly Administration of Fluids

CHILD'S WEIGHT (kg)	VOLUME OF WATER PER HOUR
≤10	4 ml/kg
11–20	40 mL + 2 mL/kg for every kilogram 11–20
>20	60 mL + 1 mL/kg for every kilogram >20

TABLE 3 Signs of Volume Depletion

SIGN	DEGREE OF DEPLETION		
	MILD (1%–4%)	MODERATE (5%–7%)	SEVERE (>7%)
Skin	Normal	Cool	Cool, mottled
Capillary refill	Normal	Decreased	Markedly decreased
Skin turgor	Normal	Loose	Tenting
Buccal mucosa	Slightly dry	Dry	Parched
Eyes	Normal	Sunken	Markedly sunken
Fontanel*	Normal	Sunken	Markedly sunken
Pulse	Normal (full)	Rapid	Rapid, thready
Urine output	Normal	Decreased	Oliguria (<1 mL/kg/h)
Systolic blood pressure	Normal	Normal, low	Low, shock

*Infants <9 mo of age.

and symptoms demonstrated or reported by the patient. Often, partial restoration of extracellular volume depletion improves gastrointestinal symptoms and allows a switch to the oral route for completing volume restoration.

Example: A 15-kg patient presents with a 3-day history of vomiting and diarrhea. Physical examination suggests 5% volume depletion. The patient has ongoing vomiting, and parenteral fluids will be started. Volume depletion of 5% is 750 mL of fluid:

$$0.5 \times 15\,kg\,(body\,weight)$$

A commonly used volume expansion technique is to provide isotonic saline, 20 mL/kg, in a bolus (over 30 minutes to 1 hour). This amount of 300 mL (15 kg × 20 mL/kg) is approximately 2% of body weight and in this example is less than 50% of the determined volume depletion. The plan, therefore, is 375 mL (50%) over 1 to 2 hours of isotonic saline (or lactated Ringer's solution) parenterally, then 375 mL of the same solution over the next 4 to 6 hours.

Replacement Fluids

As a general rule of thumb, unusual losses—gastrointestinal or renal, for example—should be replaced with a solution of comparable electrolyte concentration and of comparable volume. The most precise way to determine the needed solution is to measure the concentration of solutes such as sodium, potassium, chloride, or bicarbonate lost in emesis, diarrhea, or urine. Emesis contains sodium at 10 to 40 mmol/L and even less potassium (5–20 mmol/L) but large amounts of chloride (90–150 mmol/L). Diarrheal fluid typically contains sodium at 40 to 90 mmol/L, potassium at 10 to 50 mmol/L, and up to 40 or 50 mmol/L of bicarbonate. Cholera patients can excrete sodium up to 140 mmol/L. When possible, the volume of loss should be measured so a replacement fluid solution volume can be planned.

The safe approach to the patient with ongoing losses is first to restore extracellular volume to normal using normal saline or lactated Ringer's solution as noted earlier. During extracellular volume restoration, measure the output and electrolyte content of abnormal losses, preferably over a 12- to 24-hour period. Once this is known, then replacement of ongoing losses should be provided as a separate solution, the volume and electrolyte concentration determined by the measurements of each. Provide the replacement solution over the next 12 to 24 hours. For example, a patient with diarrhea is found to be producing 300 mL of diarrheal fluid over 12 hours. The measured sodium concentration is 80 mmol/L, potassium is 20 mmol/L, and bicarbonate is 40 mmol/L. The solution that will nearly approximate the losses is 0.2 NS (34 mmol/L of sodium and of chloride) with 20 mmol/L of potassium and 40 mmol/L of sodium bicarbonate. The solution will contain 74 mmol/L of Na, 20 mmol/L of K and 40 mmol/L of bicarbonate. The solution would be infused at a rate of 25 mL/hour. The advantage of providing this separately from maintenance or restoration fluids is that the rate of infusion or even the electrolyte content can be changed to address just the replacement needs without having to change all the intravenous solutions.

Hyponatremia and Hypernatremia

Hyponatremia (serum sodium <135 mmol/L) and hypernatremia (serum sodium >145 mmol/L) are often associated with volume depletion. Hypernatremia is nearly exclusively associated with volume depletion, and hyponatremia can be seen in situations of volume expansion such as vasopressin excess (syndrome of inappropriate antidiuretic hormone [SIADH]) or congestive heart failure, kidney failure, or liver failure. At times, the need to normalize the serum sodium concentration requires parenteral intervention.

Approach to Hyponatremia

Symptomatic hyponatremia can occur if the serum sodium falls rapidly, but usually not until the serum sodium falls below 125 mmol/L. The symptoms associated with hyponatremia include anorexia, anxiety, agitation, ataxia, weakness, lethargy, disorientation, depressed deep tendon reflexes, seizures, coma, and death (usually the result of CNS herniation).

In situations where hyponatremia is associated with volume depletion, restoration of volume with isotonic saline often raises the serum sodium. When extracellular fluid volume is normal or expanded (such as situations when SIADH is at play), a four-fold approach to hyponatremia should be considered:
1. Treat the underlying condition.
2. Reduce water intake. In particular, if parenteral fluids are being provided, reduce or eliminate the use of hypotonic fluids.
3. Increase water excretion. This is usually done with loop diuretics such as furosemide (Lasix 0.5–1 mg/kg IV) to achieve a more rapid response.
4. Hypertonic saline IV is a step reserved for symptomatic patients. The most readily available hypertonic saline solution is 3% normal saline (sodium concentration of 513 mmol/L or approximately 0.5 mmol/mL). The desired outcome is to raise the serum sodium sufficiently to improve symptoms, but never more than 10 mmol/L in a 24-hour period. There is no need to raise the serum sodium beyond the lower limit of normal or 135 mmol/L. The desired increase in the serum sodium concentration should not exceed a maximum of 10 mmol/L.

The addition of sodium into the extracellular space will result in a shift of water from the intracellular to the extracellular space. Thus, the entire water space will be affected. The following example demonstrates how to calculate the amount of hypertonic saline to infuse in the face of severe hyponatremia:

A patient weighing 15 kg has a serum sodium of 125 mmol/L and experiences a seizure. The patient is felt to be euvolemic. Thus, hypertonic saline infusion is being considered. How should this be prescribed? Raise the serum sodium to 135 mmol/L from 125 mmol/L:

$$\text{Change in serum sodium (mmol/L)} \times \text{body weight (kg)}$$
$$\times 0.6 \text{(total body water space)}$$
$$= 10 \times 15 \times 0.6 = 90\,mmol$$

Because hypertonic saline is approximately 0.5 mmol/mL, if 90 mmol is the amount of sodium calculated to raise the serum sodium and osmolality, then 180 ml of 3% saline is needed.

An alternative way to calculate the maximum 3% saline to use is: The maximum change in serum sodium is 10, the body weight is 15 kg, the water space is 1.2 (0.6 × 2 = 1.2; i.e., 2 ml/mmol sodium in 3% saline), so:

$$10 \times 15 \times 1.2 = 180\,mL\,of\,3\%\,saline$$

Once the amount is calculated, the rate of administration should be no more than 2 to 4 mL/kg/hour, with measurements of the serum sodium at 2-hour intervals. Usually symptoms improve before there is a full 10-mmol rise in serum sodium. This rate should not result in a change of greater than 1 to 2 mmol/hour. If a change faster than this is seen, slow or stop the infusion immediately.

Approach to Hypernatremia

Hypernatremia (serum sodium >145 mmol/L) is seen with volume depletion. The extremely rare situation of pure salt overload is seen in babies receiving improperly mixed formula or intensive care patients receiving concentrated blood products and IV solutions. In these situations the patients do not show evidence of volume depletion, and urinary sodium excretion (and fractional excretion of sodium) is very high. In the overwhelming majority of patients who are volume depleted, hypernatremia signals volume losses of *at least* 10% of body weight. The classic teaching is that hypernatremic patients appear less-severely volume depleted than they actually are. This is attributed to the increased osmolality protecting the extracellular space at the cost of intracellular space. Intracellular volume contains two thirds of total body water, and the decreased volume in the intracellular space means nearly all cells in the body (importantly, including in the brain) are smaller than normal.

The approach to hypernatremia is first to restore volume using isotonic saline. Providing 40 to 50 mL/kg of isotonic saline over 4 hours will improve extracellular volume and is unlikely to markedly reduce the serum sodium. Restoring extracellular volume will improve organ perfusion, especially perfusion of the gut and the kidney. This will improve the likelihood of being able to use the gut for fluid replacement and improve glomerular filtration rate and overall kidney function so as to be able to restore volume and safely return serum sodium and osmolality to normal. The major consequence of a too-rapid fall in serum sodium or osmolality is cerebral edema, the result of smaller-than-normal cell volume too rapidly expanded by IV (especially hypotonic) fluids.

Following the first infusion, as noted earlier, consider providing 30 to 40 mL/kg of isotonic fluid over the next 20 hours (to complete a 24-hour treatment plan) to continue replenishing extracellular volume. Check the serum sodium and serum osmolality frequently, at 2- to 4-hour intervals in the first 24 to 48 hours if the serum sodium is greater than 155 mmol/L at presentation. As with hyponatremia, it is important not to change (in this case, drop) the serum sodium by more than 10 mmol/L in 24 hours or to change the serum osmolality by more than 20 mOsm/kg H_2O in 24 hours. To determine how much water is necessary to lower the serum sodium, the following formula is often used:

Actual serum sodium − desired serum sodium (not to exceed 10)
× body weight in kg × 4 mL

For a 15-kg child with a serum sodium of 155:

$$10 \times 15 \times 4 = 600 \text{ mL of water}$$

The safe approach to reducing the water deficit is to provide no more than half of the water deficit in the first 24 hours as a solution of 5% dextrose (D_5W) with potassium of 20 to 30 mmol/L. The intracellular fluid compartment is rich in potassium, and patients with hypernatremic dehydration have had considerable intracellular volume loss and have lost potassium, usually through urinary losses. The same approach may be considered in day 2 and following. Certain caveats are important here. First, as noted earlier, frequent measurements of serum sodium and serum osmolality are necessary to prevent too rapid a decline. Because the maintenance prescription is very hypotonic in the first 24 hours, at least, replacing volume loss should be the first priority. Once the patient approaches a normal volume status and serum sodium, providing maintenance *may* be appropriate. Patients with hypertonicity (hypernatremic dehydration) are very thirsty. Any fluid they consume by mouth must be measured and monitored lest their oral consumption along with parenteral fluids exceed the safe amount recommended.

Intravenous Electrolyte Replacements

At times, IV replacement of other electrolytes may be necessary. The IV replacement of potassium, in situations where the serum potassium concentration falls below 2.5 mmol/L or where oral replacement cannot be used, can be given as potassium chloride or potassium phosphate at a dose of no more than 0.5 mmol/kg/hour. The concentration of potassium in the solution infused should not exceed 40 mmol/L in a peripheral vein because potassium infusions are painful and sclerosing. Higher concentrations under the appropriate circumstances could be given through a central vein.

On occasion, IV administration of calcium or phosphate (or both) is clinically indicated. IV calcium is considered in patients with tetany, usually a serum calcium <6.5 mg/dL with a normal serum albumin. For IV calcium administration to correct symptomatic hypocalcemia, in older children the recommendation is 10 to 20 mL of a 10% calcium gluconate solution over 15 minutes to reduce or stop symptoms such as tetany or seizures. In neonates and young children, 10 to 20 mg/kg or 1 to 2 mL/kg of a 10% calcium gluconate solution administered at a rate of 1 mL/min with cardiac monitoring is recommended. For more chronic administration, 50 to 75 mg/kg/24 hours of calcium gluconate is recommended. Rapid calcium administration temporarily lowers the serum phosphate and can lead to arrhythmia, hence the cardiac monitoring.

Hypophosphatemia might require parenteral administration of phosphate. This approach is usually reserved for patients with a serum phosphate less than 1 mg/dL. The recommended dosage of elemental phosphorus is 2.5 to 5 mg/kg (0.08 to 0.16 mmol/kg) over 6 to 8 hours. This administration can lower serum calcium, so frequent testing of both the serum phosphorus and calcium is appropriate.

Finally, bicarbonate may be given intravenously. Usually the IV solution of bicarbonate should not exceed a concentration of 45 mmol/L. For example, in certain clinical conditions alkalinization of the urine is desired to prevent crystal or stone formation. The usual prescription is 1 to 2 mmol/kg body weight in 24 hours. Higher infused concentrations of bicarbonate (seen in patients with proximal tubule disease or injury as noted with certain chemotherapeutic agents) should be given into a central vein under careful monitoring. Calcium and bicarbonate should not be given in the same solution.

References

Feld LG, Friedman AL, Massengil SF. Disorders of water metabolism in fluid and electrolytes. In: Feld LG, Kaskel FJ, editors. Pediatrics. Totowa, NJ: Humana Press; 2010. p. 3–47.

Friedman AL, Ray PE. Maintenance fluid therapy. What it is and what it is not. Pediatr Nephrol 2008;23:677–80.

Gauer OH, Henry JP. Circulatory basis of fluid volume control. Physiol Rev 1963;43:423–81.

Holliday MA, Segar WE. The maintenance need for water in parenteral fluid therapy. Pediatrics 1957;19:823–32.

Moritz ML, Ayus JC. Prevention of hospital acquired hyponatremia, a case for using isotonic saline. Pediatrics 2003;111:227–30.

Nelville KA, Sondeman DJ, Rubenstein A, et al. Prevention of hyponatremia during maintenance intravenous fluid administration: A prospective, randomized study of fluid type versus fluid rate. J Pediatr 2010;156:313–9.

Robertson GL. Antidiuretic hormone. Normal and disordered function. Endocrinol Metab Clin North Am 2001;30:671–84.

PEDIATRIC SLEEP DISORDERS

Method of
Julie M. Baughn, MD

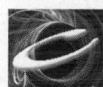 **CURRENT DIAGNOSIS**

- Sleep disorders are common in children.
- Evaluation of pediatric sleep disorders in children begins with a thorough sleep history.

- Overnight polysomnography is most commonly used to evaluate for sleep-disordered breathing
- Other diagnostic tools include the multiple sleep latency test (MSLT), oximetry, sleep logs, and actigraphy.
- Common sleep disorders in children include obstructive sleep apnea, insomnia, restless legs syndrome, and delayed sleep phase syndrome.

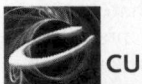 CURRENT THERAPY

- For most children tonsillectomy and adenoidectomy are an effective treatment for obstructive sleep apnea.
- Behavioral therapy is essential to treating insomnia.
- Only in select circumstances are medications used to treat children with sleep disorders.

Introduction

Pediatric sleep medicine has grown as the importance of sleep in the developing child has been recognized along with the impact that insufficient or disrupted sleep can have on cognitive development and behavior. The American Academy of Sleep Medicine (AASM) and the American Academy of Pediatrics (AAP) have recently published guidelines and practice parameters addressing several aspects of pediatric sleep medicine. Pediatric sleep disorders have unique societal impact; both the child's and the family's sleep can be affected when a disorder is present. The aim of this chapter is to offer a practical approach to the diagnosis and treatment of the most common pediatric sleep disorders, discuss diagnostic tools available, and discuss recommended treatment. A comprehensive list of sleep disorders from the *International Classification of Sleep Disorders, Second Edition* (ICSD-2) can be found in Box 1.

Developmental Aspects of Sleep

Pediatric sleep disorders also have the unique challenge of dealing with sleep issues that are subject to change based on the child's developmental age. The amount of sleep and its characteristics vary from birth to adolescence (Table 1). The sleep architecture of the child characteristically changes as he or she develops. The portion of rapid eye movement (REM) sleep declines from 50% at birth to 25% to 30% in adolescence. The proportion of slow-wave sleep is highest in early childhood and continues to decline throughout life. The pattern of sleep and sleep requirement also change. Neonates may not develop a regular sleep-wake pattern until about 3 months of age. Most infants are capable of sleeping through the night by about 6 months of age, but many may continue to waken. Naps are typically given up somewhere between 3 and 5 years of age. Most adolescents, due to many societal and social constraints, do not get a requisite 9 hours of sleep at night.

Clinical Approach

Taking a Sleep History

There are several key elements to obtaining a sleep history in children. The mnemonic BEARS (*B*edtime problems, *E*xcessive daytime sleepiness, *A*wakenings during the night, *R*egularity and duration of sleep, and *S*leep-disordered breathing) has been offered as a practical starting point for obtaining a history, tailoring questions to both parent and child where appropriate (Table 2).

The primary sleep complaint should be obtained in the child's or parent's own words. Once the primary complaint is detailed, the presence/absence of snoring, the presence of restlessness at sleep initiation and during sleep, and the child's sleep-wake patterns during school should be gathered. The presence or absence of a bedtime routine and the details of that routine should be noted. A child's sleep environment should be carefully queried. A child

who shares his or her bedroom, sleeps in his or her parents' bed, or ends up sleeping on a couch in front of the television may lead to specific sleep complaints. A history of whether there is more than one household involved (i.e., shared custody) is particularly important.

Sleepiness in children can be a particularly challenging symptom to evaluate. It is normal physiologically for children to nap until age 5. Other clues to daytime sleepiness that can be obtained in children include behavior issues, hyperactivity, excessive napping, or napping after age 5 years (intentionally or unintentionally). School-age children often display symptoms of behavioral problems or inattentiveness rather than sleepiness. Sleep-wake patterns on school days, weekends, and vacations need to be detailed. Often the child's most natural sleep pattern will emerge over the summer months.

Determining the child's sleep hygiene or good sleep practices is important in diagnosing and treating sleep disorders. Principles of good sleep hygiene are listed in Table 3.

Past Medical History/Family History

A history of prematurity, trisomy 21, velopharyngeal cleft palate repair, or hypotonia is each associated with an increased risk of sleep-disordered breathing. A past history of adenotonsillectomy for snoring is important information to obtain. Chronic nasal obstruction can cause maxillary hypoplasia. Arnold-Chiari malformation, myelomeningocele, or a brainstem lesion can predispose to central sleep apnea due to impaired central respiratory drive. Chronic health issues can also be associated with sleep disruption and consequently with behavioral problems associated with sleep.

A family history of obstructive sleep apnea (OSA), insomnia, or restless legs syndrome (RLS) is important; a family history of RLS can be used to support a diagnosis of RLS in the child. In particular, questioning the mother if she had symptoms of RLS during any of her pregnancies can be helpful because this is a common time for RLS to present or worsen. Morning or evening preferences (i.e., "night-owl" or "lark" tendencies) can also have a familial element. In addition, sleepwalking can be found to occur in families.

Focused Physical Examination

The physical examination in a child presenting with a sleep complaint should include a general assessment. Presence/absence of sleepiness, fatigue, and irritability/hyperactivity are all important. Height, weight, and body mass index (BMI) should be recorded. Children with OSA can have poor growth and even failure to thrive. Obesity is a risk factor for OSA. Special attention to a child's craniofacial features is important because these may make a child more at risk for sleep-disordered breathing. Assessment of tonsil size, oropharyngeal crowding (using the Mallampati or Friedman classification systems can be useful), and presence of maxillary/mandibular hypoplasia can all offer clues to an airway that may predispose to OSA. The practitioner should evaluate for evidence of nasal obstruction by noting mouth breathing and signs of allergy (i.e., allergic shiners, nasal crease).

Diagnostic Tools

Polysomnography

The AASM has published practice parameters on both the respiratory and nonrespiratory indications for polysomnography (PSG) in pediatric patients. In this chapter, a sleep study or PSG will refer only to an in-laboratory attended study, because home monitoring currently has not been sufficiently evaluated in the pediatric population. PSG in children entails spending the night at a sleep center. A parent or caregiver must also spend the night. During the night, the child's sleep characteristics, respiratory function, and movement are analyzed. This is done by the following measures: electroencephalography (EEG), electromyography (EMG) of chin and limbs, airflow by thermistor and nasal pressure, end-tidal or transcutaneous carbon dioxide measurements, and induction plethysmography to measure respiratory effort. Scoring of a PSG

Insomnia and Inadequate Sleep Hygiene

Primary Insomnias

Idiopathic insomnia

Psychophysiological insomnia

Paradoxical insomnia

Secondary Insomnias

Insomnia due to mental disorder

Inadequate sleep hygiene

Behavioral insomnia of childhood

Adjustment insomnia

Insomnia due to drug or substance (alcohol)

Insomnia due to medical condition

Insomnia not due to substance or known physiologic condition, not organic

Physiologic (organic) insomnia, unspecified

Sleep-Related Breathing Disorders

Continuum of obstructive sleep-disordered breathing: snoring, upper airway resistance syndrome, and obstructive sleep apnea

Central sleep apnea

- Primary central sleep apnea
- Due to Cheyne-Stokes breathing pattern
- Due to high-altitude periodic breathing
- Due to medical condition not Cheyne-Stokes
- Due to drug or substance

Primary sleep apnea of infancy

Complex sleep apnea syndrome

Sleep-related hypoventilation

- Sleep-related nonobstructive alveolar hypoventilation, idiopathic
- Congenital central alveolar hypoventilation syndrome
- Due to lower airways obstruction, neuromuscular and chest wall disorders, or pulmonary parenchymal or vascular pathology
- Unspecified

Narcolepsy and Primary CNS Hypersomnias

Narcolepsy

- With cataplexy
- Without cataplexy
- Due to medical condition
- Unspecified

Recurrent hypersomnia

- Kleine-Levin syndrome
- Menstrual-related hypersomnia

Idiopathic hypersomnia

- With long sleep time
- Without long sleep time

Behaviorally induced insufficient sleep syndrome

Hypersomnia due to medical condition, drug, or substance (alcohol)

Hypersomnia not due to substance or known physiologic condition

Physiologic hypersomnia (unspecified)

Circadian Sleep Disorders

Delayed sleep phase syndrome

Advanced sleep phase syndrome

Irregular sleep-wake type

Nonentrained type (free running)

Jet lag type

Shift work type

Circadian sleep disorder due to medical condition

Circadian sleep disorder due to drug or substance (alcohol)

Parasomnias

Disorders of Arousal from NREM Sleep

Confusional arousals

Sleepwalking

Sleep terrors

Parasomnias Usually Associated with REM Sleep

REM sleep behavior disorder

Recurrent isolated sleep paralysis

Nightmare disorder

Other Parasomnias

Sleep-related dissociative disorders

Sleep enuresis

Sleep-related groaning (catathrenia)

Exploding head syndrome

Sleep-related hallucinations

Sleep-related eating disorder

Parasomnias due to drug or substance (alcohol)

Parasomnias due to medical condition

Sleep-Related Movement Disorders

Restless legs syndrome

Periodic limb movement disorder

Sleep-related leg cramps

Sleep-related bruxism

Sleep-related rhythmic movement disorder

Sleep-related movement disorder, unspecified, due to drug or substance, due to medical condition

Isolated Symptoms, Apparently Normal Variants, and Unresolved Issues

Long sleeper

Short sleeper

Snoring

Sleep talking

Sleep starts (hypnic jerks)

Benign sleep myoclonus of infancy

Hypnagogic foot tremor and alternating leg muscle activation during sleep

Propriospinal myoclonus at sleep onset

Excessive fragmentary myoclonus

Other Sleep Disorders

Physiologic sleep disorder, unspecified

Environmental sleep disorder

Fatal familial insomnia

Abbreviations: CNS = central nervous system; NREM = non–rapid eye movement (sleep); REM = rapid eye movement (sleep).

From St Louis EK, Morgenthaler TI: Sleep disorders. In Bope E, Kellerman R (eds): Conn's Current Therapy 2013. Philadelphia: Saunders Elsevier, 2013.

performed on a child is done using pediatric scoring rules set forth by the AASM.

The most common indication for a sleep study in children is OSA. PSG can be used to both diagnose OSA and treat sleep apnea with continuous positive airway pressure (CPAP). PSG can also be used to evaluate for elevated periodic limb movements of sleep, and in rare cases to characterize abnormal nocturnal behavior such as evaluation of parasomnias or nocturnal seizures.

Overnight Oximetry

The gold standard for diagnosis of pediatric OSA is PSG. Overnight oximetry has been suggested as an alternative screening tool for pediatric sleep-disordered OSA. Although an abnormal oximetry will suggest OSA, a normal oximetry does not rule out OSA. Children can have sleep apnea that is severe and still maintain normal oxygenation. In a study by Brouillette and colleagues (2000), when a positive oximetry graph was present (defined by three or

TABLE 1 — Sleep Characteristics across Development

AGE	AVERAGE SLEEP DURATION IN 24 HOURS	NORMAL DEVELOPMENTAL CHANGES IN CHILDREN'S SLEEP ARCHITECTURE
Newborn	13–14.5 hours Sleep periods separated by 1–2 hours awake	Three sleep states (active or "REM-like," quiet or "non-REM-like," and indeterminant) Enter sleep through active state (50% of sleep)
Infant (0–1 year)	9–10 hours overnight and 3–4 hours during naps	Development of the four sleep stages Sleep cycles every 50 minutes Enter sleep through non-REM
Toddler (1–3 years)	11–13 hours between nighttime and naps	REM-sleep amounts continue to decline
Preschool (2–5 years)	9–10 hours Most give up naps between 3 and 5 years	REM sleep continues to decline Sleep cycles every 90 minutes High levels of slow-wave sleep
School-age (6–12 years)	9–10 hours	High sleep efficiency (time in bed spent sleeping)
Adolescent (>12 years)	9 hours	40% decline in slow-wave sleep Amount of REM sleep has declined to adult levels (25%–30%)

Abbreviations: NREM = non–rapid eye movement (sleep); REM = rapid eye movement (sleep).
From Mindell JA, Owens J: A Clinical Guide to Pediatric Sleep: Diagnosis and Management of Sleep Problems. Philadelphia: Lippincott Williams & Wilkins, 2003; Mindell JA, Owens J: A Clinical Guide to Pediatric Sleep: Diagnosis and Management of Sleep Problems, 2nd ed. Philadelphia: Lippincott Williams & Wilkins, 2010. Table from first edition, revised based on second edition.

TABLE 2 — BEARS Mnemonic: A Screening Tool for Sleep Disorders in Children

	PRESCHOOL (2–5 YEARS)	SCHOOL-AGE (6–12 YEARS)	ADOLESCENT (13–18 YEARS)
Bedtime problems	Does your child have any problems going to bed? Falling asleep?	Does your child have any problems at bedtime? (P) Do you have any problems going to bed? (C)	Do you have any problems falling asleep at bedtime? (C)
Excessive daytime sleepiness	Does your child seem overly tired or sleepy during the day? Does your child still take naps?	Does your child have difficulty waking in the morning, seem sleepy during the day, or take naps? (P) Do you feel tired a lot? (C)	Do you feel sleepy a lot during the day? In school? While driving? (C)
Awakenings during the night	Does your child wake up a lot at night?	Does your child seem to wake up a lot at night? Any sleepwalking or nightmares? (P) Do you wake up a lot at night? Have trouble getting back to sleep? (C)	Do you wake up a lot at night? Have trouble getting back to sleep? (C)
Regularity and duration of sleep	Does your child have a regular bedtime and wake time? What are they?	What time does your child go to bed and get up on school days? Weekends? Do you think your child is getting enough sleep? (P)	What time do you usually go to bed on school nights? Weekends? How much sleep do you usually get? (C)
Sleep-disordered breathing	Does your child snore a lot or have difficulty breathing at night?	Does your child have loud or nightly snoring or any breathing difficulties at night? (P)	Does your teenager snore loudly or nightly? (P)

Abbreviations: C = child; P = parent.
From Owens JA, Dalzell V: Use of the "BEARS" sleep screening tool in a pediatric residents' continuity clinic: A pilot study. Sleep Med 2005;6:63–9.

more desaturation clusters and at least three desaturations <90%) in a referred population, the positive predictive value for OSA on PSG was 97%. A negative or inconclusive oximetry by this definition did not rule out OSA and there was still a 47% chance OSA was present on PSG.

Sleep Logs/Actigraphy
Sleep logs can be effective in demonstrating a child's sleep-wake patterns. Actigraphy is often done in conjunction with a sleep log. Actigraphy is a portable wristband that measures movement. The absence of movement over a certain time period is used as a surrogate marker of sleep, and the presence of movement over a certain time period is used as a surrogate for wakefulness. Some devices also measure ambient light exposure. Used in conjunction with actigraphy sleep logs can be extremely helpful in demonstrating discrepancies between perceived and actual sleep, and are helpful in demonstrating insufficient sleep and circadian rhythm disorders. Those that measure light as well can aid in uncovering sleep hygiene issues.

Multiple Sleep Latency Test
The multiple sleep latency test (MSLT) is a daytime study used to objectively measure sleepiness. It is often used to aid in the diagnosis of narcolepsy or hypersomnia. It is a set of four to five scheduled naps that typically occur the day after an overnight sleep study. Often 2 weeks of actigraphy are done before the MSLT to determine sleep-wake patterns.

Common Pediatric Sleep Diagnoses and Treatment
Obstructive Sleep Apnea
Epidemiology
Up to one-fifth of children can have intermittent snoring. Prevalence rates of OSA range from 1.2% to 5.7%. OSA is most common in children 2 to 8 years of age corresponding to the peak

TABLE 3 — Principles of Sleep Hygiene in Children

The child's bedroom should be dark and quiet.

Bedtime routines should be strictly enforced. Routines should be relaxing and only 20 to 30 minutes in length.

The time of morning awakening should be firmly and consistently structured.

Bedroom temperatures should be kept comfortably cool (<75 °F).

Environmental noise should be minimized as much as possible.

Background music and/or white noise may inhibit extraneous noise.

Children should not go to bed hungry and may have a snack before bedtime.

Excessive fluids before bedtime may result in bladder distention and arousal and disrupt sleep.

Children should learn to fall asleep alone (i.e., without their parents' presence in the room).

Vigorous activity should be avoided before bedtime.

A bath is often a stimulating activity for children. If bedtime struggles are present after a child's bath, it may be moved to the morning or separated from the child's bedtime by at least 2 hours.

Methylxanthine-containing beverages and food (e.g., caffeinated beverages/colas, tea, chocolate) should be avoided several hours before bedtime.

Parents should read labels on all over-the-counter and prescription medications. Some may contain alcohol or caffeine and may disrupt sleep.

Naps should be developmentally appropriate. Brief naps may be refreshing, but prolonged naps or napping too frequently may result in significant accumulation of sleep during the day and make it more difficult to fall asleep at night.

Modified from Sheldon SH, Ferber R, Kryger M (eds): Principles and Practice of Pediatric Sleep Medicine. Philadelphia: Elsevier Saunders, 2005.

age of adenotonsillar hypertrophy. Due to the rise in childhood obesity there is now a corresponding rise in older children diagnosed with OSA.

Pathophysiology

The pharynx has many roles, including swallowing, speaking, and maintaining airway patency. Pharyngeal size is determined by the bones and soft tissue. The soft tissue is affected by the size of the tonsils and adenoids, as well as adipose tissue. Airway patency is maintained during wakefulness; a small airway can become vulnerable during sleep resulting in partial or total closure of the airway, hypoxemia, hypercapnia, and an arousal that results in opening of the airway and termination of the obstructive event. This leads to sleep disruption and daytime consequences. OSA in children likely results from a combination of narrowing of the upper airway, abnormal upper airway tone, and genetic factors.

Clinical Manifestation

OSA in adults is typically associated with daytime sleepiness. Associations have been made with hypertension, stroke, and metabolic syndrome. In children, OSA may not present with daytime sleepiness. Children may present with daytime inattention and/or neurocognitive and behavioral issues. Symptoms include snoring with or without apneic pauses or gasps. Restless sleep or secondary enuresis may also be noted. Parents may comment on increased work of breathing while sleeping. Other associations include poor growth, obesity, hypertension, and systemic inflammation.

Diagnosis

The gold standard for diagnosis of pediatric OSA is an in-laboratory attended PSG by an accredited sleep laboratory. History and physical examination lack sensitivity and specificity in predicting which children with snoring have OSA. However, a history of loud snoring, tonsillar hypertrophy, and abnormal oximetry is strongly suggestive of the diagnosis of OSA (see above). History alone cannot distinguish children with OSA from those with primary snoring. Criteria for the diagnosis of OSA in children are met when there is one or more apnea or hypopnea events per hour identified using scoring criteria by the AASM.

Differential Diagnosis

Other forms of sleep-disordered breathing are not as common as OSA. Sleep-related hypoventilation can occur in patients with neuromuscular weakness. Central hypoventilation syndromes are rare, but should be considered in children with persistent gas exchange abnormalities without additional explanation. Sleep-related hypoxemia can be present in pediatric patients with chronic lung disease. Central sleep apnea should be thought of in patients with brainstem abnormalities or Arnold-Chiari malformation. Sleep-related seizures may be difficult to differentiate from OSA in infants and an extended EEG montage may be necessary during their sleep study. Normal breathing patterns of infants and children should also be identified; brief (less than 10 seconds), central respiratory pauses that are self-resolving (and without significant desaturation) are common in normal children in either REM sleep or post-arousal/post-sigh.

Treatment

Treatment of OSA in most children is adenotonsillectomy. Recent guidelines from the AAP recommend an overnight sleep study in children where the practitioner had a clinical suspicion of OSA before adenotonsillectomy. Children with mild OSA preoperative can be monitored clinically postoperatively. Children with moderate to severe OSA, as well as children with craniofacial abnormalities, neurologic disorders, and obesity, should have a follow-up PSG to demonstrate resolution of OSA after surgery. Children who are not candidates for adenotonsillectomy may be treated with CPAP and use may have an impact on neurobehavioral outcomes. Treatment with CPAP therapy in children requires close follow-up because pressure needs may change with growth.

Difficulty with Sleep Initiation and Night Wakings

Epidemiology

Bedtime problems and night wakings occur in up to 30% of children.

Clinical Manifestations

The diagnosis of insomnia includes difficulty going to sleep and/or staying asleep, the complaint that sleep is not of good quality, and the report of poor daytime functioning. The sleep complaints of infants and young children are often in the words of their parent or caregiver.

In preschool age children both bedtime problems and night wakings are common and characterized by two types of behavioral insomnia of childhood: sleep-onset association type and limit-setting type. The definition of the *sleep-onset association type*, as defined in the ICSD-2, includes the following: sleep initiation is an extended process, associations are demanding, if the associations are not present sleep onset is delayed, and awakenings require caregiver intervention. The *limit-setting type* involves difficulty initiating or maintaining sleep, there is bedtime stalling or refusal, and the caregiver does not set sufficient and appropriate limits around this behavior. Children with frequent and prolonged night wakings have the sleep-onset association type. They often require an intervention by the caretaker to reinitiate sleep. Both problems can be present at once. Children who have difficulty going to sleep and provide resistance to bedtime have the limit-setting type. Parents of these children may complain of daytime behavioral issues due to the parent's inability to set limits during the day as well.

Diagnosis

Diagnosis is made from the history in the majority of cases. An overnight sleep study may be indicated in cases where another sleep disorder is suspected.

Differential Diagnosis

The differential diagnosis of insomnia or behavioral insomnia of childhood includes sleep disorders such as OSA, RLS, or nocturnal seizures. These disorders can prompt nocturnal awakenings or make sleep initiation difficult. If there is clinical suspicion of one of these disorders, an overnight sleep study may be indicated.

Treatment
Behavioral interventions have been shown to be effective in treating all forms of insomnia. In older children, primary and secondary insomnia can be effectively treated with cognitive-behavioral therapy. This often includes stimulus control and sleep restriction. Stimulus control includes maintaining a regular sleep-wake pattern and using the bed and bedroom only for sleeping. It involves getting out of bed if sleep is not initiated within about 20 minutes. Sleep restriction includes minimizing the time in bed to be only sleeping. It often includes delaying bedtime to the child's actual sleep onset, and then over time gradually advancing the bedtime. Sleep hygiene should be effectively addressed, including development of a relaxing bedtime routine, maintaining a regular sleep-wake pattern, and eliminating electronic use before bedtime.

There are several treatments of behavioral insomnia of childhood sleep-onset association type. No one treatment has been found to be superior. The goal of all of these methods is for the child to fall asleep in his or her crib or bed on the child's own. These include extinction (i.e., "cry it out"), which is often not palatable to caregivers. There is the graduated extinction method, which has parents ignoring crying or protests for specified periods of increasingly longer intervals. Some prefer an even more gradual approach of sitting next to the child's bed in a chair and over several days to weeks moving that chair across the room and out of the room. A consistent bedtime routine should also be implemented. Use of a transitional object can be helpful. Treatment of the limit-setting type includes firm limit setting. Positive reinforcement and limiting negative reinforcement should be used. The use of a reward system can be helpful. Effectively addressing behavioral treatment of sleep issues can be challenging for the primary care provider because of time constraints.

Restless Legs Syndrome
Epidemiology
Prevalence rates for pediatric RLS have ranged from 1% to 6%.

Risk Factors
Risk factors include a family history and a history of anemia or iron deficiency. Attention-deficit/hyperactivity disorder (ADHD) is associated with RLS.

Pathophysiology
Decreased dopamine has been suggested in the pathophysiology of RLS. Iron is a cofactor in the synthesis of dopamine and treatment of iron deficiency or low ferritin, if present, may improve symptoms.

Diagnosis
Diagnosis of pediatric RLS is a clinical diagnosis. It is made using the adult criteria set forth in the ICSD-2 but with some modification for children due to developmental issues. It consists of the child reporting an urge to move the legs, usually accompanied by an uncomfortable sensation; this urge or sensation worsens during rest or inactivity; the sensations are improved or resolved by movement; the sensations are present or worsen in the evening or night. If a child cannot express a description in his or her own words, diagnosis can be made using two out of the following three criteria: a sleep disturbance for age, a family history of RLS, and a periodic limb movement index on PSG of >5 per hour. Because of this last criterion, a sleep study can be helpful in children to make this diagnosis. There can be an association with sleep initiation and maintenance difficulties.

Differential Diagnosis
Differential diagnosis of RLS should include insomnia, sleep-disordered breathing, or neurologic or musculoskeletal etiologies for the discomfort.

Treatment
Nonpharmacologic treatment of RLS includes good sleep hygiene, moderate exercise a few hours before bedtime, and avoidance of substances that are associated with worsening of RLS symptoms, including caffeine, alcohol, antihistamines, and antiemetics. A serum ferritin should be drawn in all children with RLS and if <50 ng/mL, treatment with 6 mg/kg/day of oral elemental iron should be considered. Oral iron absorption is enhanced by vitamin C and impaired by calcium. Gastrointestinal upset and constipation can be common side effects. Compliance can be difficult. A serum ferritin should be rechecked at 3 months to evaluate therapy. Referral to a sleep medicine specialist should be made if lifestyle and oral iron therapy have been unsuccessful. There are no FDA-approved medications for the treatment of RLS in children. Dopamine agonists, gabapentin (Neurontin),[1] clonazepam (Klonopin),[1] and clonidine (Catapres)[1] have been used to treat pediatric RLS.

Delayed Sleep Phase Syndrome
Epidemiology
Delayed sleep phase syndrome (DSPS) occurs most commonly in adolescents and young adults.

Clinical Manifestations
Symptoms usually present in adolescents but can occur in younger children. Adolescents with DSPS consistently have sleep onset at a later time, typically after midnight. They have difficulty initiating sleep earlier. They do not have difficulty maintaining sleep. They have difficulty waking in the morning unless able to sleep until their preferred time, which is typically after 10 AM. They may have sleepiness during the daytime if forced to rise early (i.e., for school); however, during long vacations or summer breaks when allowed to sleep to preferred wake time they feel refreshed. Children who already have a preferred evening preference may find this exacerbated in adolescence. Poor school performance can be present.

Diagnosis
Diagnosis is made from history; actigraphy and sleep logs are also useful. An overnight sleep study may be indicated if another sleep disorder is suspected (e.g., OSA).

Differential Diagnosis
The differential diagnosis includes insomnia, poor sleep hygiene, insufficient sleep, mood disorder, OSA, and RLS.

Treatment
Treatment is typically behavioral and includes good sleep hygiene. Typically either the patient's sleep-wake schedule is advanced (if there is less than 3 hours between actual and desired bedtime) by 15 minutes every 2 to 3 days until the goal bedtime is achieved. Rise time is advanced as well and if set at the desired wake time initially it should facilitate the advancement of the bedtime by increasing sleep drive. If the desired bedtime of the adolescent is greater than 3 hours from the current bedtime, phase delay can be considered. Bedtime is delayed by 2 to 3 hours each day until the target bedtime is reached. Timing of this therapy should be considered, because it will interfere with school or other daytime activities. Parental or caregiver support is necessary, as well as commitment by the adolescent.

Once the new pattern is established weekends must not differ from weekdays by more than 1 to 2 hours. This is particularly important for the rise time. Relapse is common if strict sleep-wake patterns are not adhered to, a problem common on vacations.

Both bright light exposure and melatonin[7] have been used to help reset the circadian rhythm. Exposure to bright light in the morning is encouraged and can be as simple as increasing sun

---

[1]Not FDA approved for this indication.
[7]Available as a dietary supplement.

exposure in the morning. Light boxes using 2500 to 10,000 lux can be used in the morning for 20 to 30 minutes. Exposure to light in the evening should be limited. A small dose of melatonin (0.5 mg) can be used in the early evening (about 5 hours before desired bedtime) to attempt to physiologically advance sleep onset. If the timing is not optimal for both light and melatonin, the phase delay can be worsened; consultation with a sleep physician should be considered.

Parasomnias

Parasomnias can occur out of both non-REM (NREM) and REM sleep. Those occurring out of NREM sleep include sleepwalking, sleep terrors, and confusional arousals. They typically occur in the first one-third of the night, when NREM-3 sleep is most prevalent, and are not recalled the next day. They can be part of normal development, but depending on their nature, they can be distressing to caregiver and child. Parasomnias occurring out of REM sleep include nightmares and REM-sleep behavior disorder (RBD). Nightmares are commonly recalled and have been associated with anxiety in children. Nightmares typically peak in the school-age child. RBD is rare in children but has been reported; it involves the loss of atonia that occurs in REM sleep and consequently dreams are "acted out."

Risk Factors

Poor sleep hygiene, insufficient sleep, irregular sleep-wake patterns, and a positive family history are all risk factors. Sleep disruption from sleep-disordered breathing or periodic limb movements of sleep can exacerbate parasomnias.

Differential Diagnosis

The differential diagnosis should include nocturnal seizures. In addition, if another sleep disorder is present, parasomnias can be exacerbated.

Treatment

Safety is most important in children with parasomnias, and it is important that the child's sleep environment is kept clear of things that could cause injury. Door alarms can be effective. The child should not be awakened during the episode. The event should not be referred to the next morning because this can cause distress for the child. Maintaining good sleep hygiene and regular sleep-wake patterns is important. If the events occur at a predictable time each night, the caregiver can do planned awakenings 30 minutes before the event typically occurs for several weeks. This may abolish the episodes. It can also have the effect of pushing the episode to later in the night. Pharmacologic treatment with a small dose of a benzodiazepine (e.g., 0.5 mg of clonazepam [Klonopin][1] at bedtime) may be indicated in severe cases with the drug tapered slowly after episodes are suppressed.

Hypersomnias

A full discussion of primary hypersomnias (including narcolepsy) in children is beyond the scope of this chapter. Consideration for a primary hypersomnia should be made in a child who is sleepy after common causes of sleepiness such as insufficient sleep and obstructive sleep apnea have been ruled out. Symptoms of narcolepsy include disrupted nocturnal sleep, hallucinations on going to sleep or waking up, and sleep paralysis. Daytime sleepiness is present with "sleep attacks" both during quiet activities and while active. Cataplexy may also be present and is defined by loss of muscle tone without loss of consciousness. It should be noted that onset of narcolepsy is often in adolescence or as a young adult. Diagnosis is often delayed because the symptoms are attributed to other conditions. Treatment of pediatric hypersomnia is done under the supervision of a sleep specialist and often involves use of stimulants.

---

[1]Not FDA approved for this indication.

References

Aurora RN, Lamm CI, Zak RS, et al. Practice parameters for the non-respiratory indications for polysomnography and multiple sleep latency testing for children. Sleep 2012;35:1467–73.

Aurora RN, Zak RS, Karippot A, et al. Practice parameters for the respiratory indications for polysomnography in children. Sleep 2011;34:379–88.

Berry RB, Brooks R, Gamaldo C, et al. The AASM manual for the scoring of sleep and associated events. Westchester, Illinois: American Academy of Sleep Medicine; 2012.

Brouillette RT, Morielli A, Leimanis A, et al. Nocturnal pulse oximetry as an abbreviated testing modality for pediatric obstructive sleep apnea. Pediatrics 2000;105:405–12.

Kaditis A, Kheirandish-Gozal L, Gozal D. Algorithm for the diagnosis and treatment of pediatric OSA: a proposal of two pediatric sleep centers. Sleep Med 2012;13:217–27.

Kotagal S, Nichols CD, Grigg-Damberger MM, et al. Non-respiratory indications for polysomnography and related procedures in children: an evidence-based review. Sleep 2012;35:1451–66.

Lloyd R, Tippmann-Peikert M, Slocumb N, et al. Characteristics of REM sleep behavior disorder in childhood. J Clin Sleep Med 2012;8:127–31.

Marcus CL, Brooks LJ, Draper KA, et al. Diagnosis and management of childhood obstructive sleep apnea syndrome. Pediatrics 2012a;130:576–84.

Marcus CL, Brooks LJ, Draper KA, et al. Diagnosis and management of childhood obstructive sleep apnea syndrome. Pediatrics 2012b;130:e714–55.

Marcus CL, Radcliffe J, Konstantinopoulou S, et al. Effects of positive airway pressure therapy on neurobehavioral outcomes in children with obstructive sleep apnea. Am J Respir Crit Care Med 2012c;185:998–1003.

Mindell JA, Barrett KM. Nightmares and anxiety in elementary-aged children: is there a relationship? Child Care Health Dev 2002;28:317–22.

Mindell JA, Owens J. A clinical guide to pediatric sleep: diagnosis and management of sleep problems. Philadelphia: Lippincott Williams & Wilkins; 2003.

Mindell JA, Owens J. A clinical guide to pediatric sleep: diagnosis and management of sleep problems. 2nd ed. Philadelphia: Lippincott Williams & Wilkins; 2010.

Morgenthaler T, Alessi C, Friedman L, et al. Practice parameters for the use of actigraphy in the assessment of sleep and sleep disorders: an update for 2007. Sleep 2007;30:519–29.

Morgenthaler T, Kramer M, Alessi C, et al. Practice parameters for the psychological and behavioral treatment of insomnia: an update. An American Academy of Sleep Medicine report. Sleep 2006;29:1415–9.

Owens JA, Dalzell V. Use of the "BEARS" sleep screening tool in a pediatric residents' continuity clinic: a pilot study. Sleep Med 2005;6:63–9.

Picchietti D, Allen RP, Walters AS, et al. Restless legs syndrome: prevalence and impact in children and adolescents—the Peds REST study. Pediatrics 2007;120:253–66.

Sateia MJ, editor. The International Classification of Sleep Disorders. Westchester, Illinois: American Academy of Sleep Medicine; 2005.

Sheldon SH, Ferber R, Kryger M, editors. Principles and Practice of Pediatric Sleep Medicine. Philadelphia: Elsevier Saunders; 2005.

St Louis EK, Morgenthaler TI. Sleep disorders. In: Bope E, Kellerman R, editors. Conn's Current Therapy 2013. Philadelphia: Saunders Elsevier; 2013.

RESUSCITATION OF THE NEWBORN

Method of
Stacey A. Hinderliter, MD; and David Gregory, MD

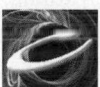

CURRENT DIAGNOSIS

- The transition from intrauterine to extrauterine life at birth requires effective breathing by the infant to expand the lungs and oxygenate the blood. All newborn infants are at risk for delays in this process, prompting a need for resuscitation.
- The fetal and newborn response to hypoxia is to develop apnea. If primary apnea is diagnosed, it can be corrected by gentle stimulation and oxygen delivery. If hypoxia persists, secondary apnea will occur. It is not readily apparent whether a newborn has primary or secondary apnea, and the approach to resuscitation therefore requires that any apneic event be treated using the same sequence of interventions.
- The initial steps of newborn resuscitation include drying the infant, providing warmth, suctioning the airway, and providing gentle stimulation. Infants who do not respond to these interventions need more assistance. Establishment of effective ventilation spontaneously by the newborn or with assistance by positive-pressure ventilation is the most important step in newborn resuscitation.

- Reassessment of the infant's heart rate, respiratory effort or pulse oximeter reading, color, and tone every 30 seconds during resuscitation is crucial to determine the next appropriate intervention. Apgar scoring should *not* be used to guide newborn resuscitation. Pulse oximetry in the delivery room should be used to guide oxygen therapy.
- If application of positive-pressure ventilation does not improve the infant's heart rate, chest compressions or drug therapy, or both, may be required. A team approach is needed to coordinate these interventions, and ongoing reassessment is necessary to determine cardiorespiratory and hemodynamic status. Subsequent assessment and treatment should be performed in an intensive care setting.

CURRENT THERAPY

- Term gestation infants who are breathing and crying with good muscle tone do not need newborn resuscitation.
- Initial resuscitation includes drying the infant, providing warmth, suctioning the nose and mouth, and giving gentle stimulation.
- If the infant is breathing vigorously but has central cyanosis, oxygen should be administered. Pulse oximetry should be used to guide oxygen therapy.
- If the infant is apneic, breathing slowly, or gasping, positive-pressure ventilation (PPV) with a mask and bag should be administered. Infants with meconium-stained amniotic fluid who are apneic should receive suctioning of the trachea by endotracheal intubation before PPV.
- If the infant's heart rate drops below 60 beats/min, chest compressions should be initiated using the thumb or two-finger technique.
- If the heart rate remains less than 60 beats/min despite PPV and chest compressions, IV epinephrine (Adrenalin) should be given using an umbilical venous catheter.
- Reassessment of the newborn every 30 seconds during resuscitation is required to adjust therapy as indicated.

The changes that occur in the transition from fetus to newborn are unmatched in any other time of life. Most newborns manage to make this transition on their own, but about 10% require some assistance. Approximately 1% of newborns require extensive resuscitative measures to survive. The approach to resuscitation in infants is similar to that in adults, consisting of evaluation and intervention when needed for the infant's airway, breathing, and circulation. Every birth should be attended by personnel trained in neonatal resuscitation. Specific training and certification are offered by the American Heart Association's Neonatal Resuscitation Provider (NRP) course.

Transition from Fetal to Extrauterine Life

The environment of the fetus differs greatly from that of the infant after birth. The fetus depends on receiving oxygen and nutrients from the mother through the placental circulation. The fetus experiences relative hypoxia and almost constant body temperature in the amniotic fluid. The fetal lungs are filled with fluid and do not participate in the exchange of oxygen and carbon dioxide. Several adaptations in the fetus permit survival in this environment.

Oxygenated blood from the mother enters the fetus by means of the placenta through the umbilical vein. Most of this oxygenated blood bypasses the liver through the ductus venosus and enters the inferior vena cava. On entering the right atrium, this oxygenated blood is directed toward the patent foramen ovale into the left atrium, bypassing the fetal lungs. Fetal blood also passes through the right atrium into the right ventricle and then into the pulmonary artery. The vascular resistance and blood pressure of the pulmonary vessels in the fetal lung are higher than in the aorta and systemic circulation; most of the blood is therefore shunted away from the lungs through the ductus arteriosus into the ascending aorta. Only a small amount of fetal blood passes through the lungs to the left atrium and then to the left ventricle. The umbilical arteries branch off from the internal iliac arteries and return fetal blood to the placenta. The functional organ for gas exchange of oxygen and carbon dioxide in the fetus is the placenta.

At birth, the newborn is no longer connected to the placenta, and the lungs become the only source of oxygen. The first breaths of the infant cause the fluid in the lung alveoli to be replaced with air. The umbilical arteries and veins constrict at birth and are eventually clamped. This increases the vascular resistance and blood pressure of the systemic circulation. As the oxygen level in the alveoli increases, the blood vessels in the lung start to relax, decreasing pulmonary vascular resistance. Blood in the pulmonary artery travels toward the lung and away from the ductus arteriosus because the blood pressure in the systemic circulation is higher than that in the pulmonary circulation. Increased blood flow to the lungs allows the oxygen from the alveoli to enter the infant's blood, increasing the P_{O_2}. Oxygenated blood enters the left heart through the pulmonary vein and is delivered to the rest of the infant's tissues through the aorta.

Although the initial steps in this transition occur within a few minutes of birth, the entire process may not be completed for several hours to days. The ductus venosus, foramen ovale, and ductus arteriosus remain potentially patent and do not completely involute for days or weeks. Changes in the infant's systemic and pulmonary pressures can result in blood flow through these channels in the infant.

Transition can be prevented or delayed in several circumstances. The infant may not breathe adequately, in which case the lung fluid is not forced out of the alveoli. Material such as meconium may block air from entering the alveoli. If the lungs do not fill with air, hypoxia will quickly develop. Systemic hypotension due to excessive blood loss, poor cardiac function, or bradycardia prevents the change in the direction of blood flow that is necessary to promote blood flow into the lungs. Failure of the lungs to expand or hypoxia can prevent relaxation of the pulmonary blood vessels, resulting in a high pulmonary vascular resistance. This leads to decreased blood flow to the lungs and worsening of hypoxia.

Risk Factors for Newborn Resuscitation

A number of prenatal and intrapartum factors are associated with a higher chance that the infant will have a delay in transition and require resuscitation (Table 1). However, some infants *with no risk factors* need resuscitation; therefore, preparations for neonatal resuscitation should be made during all deliveries.

Reaction to Hypoxia and Asphyxia

Normally at birth, the newborn makes vigorous efforts to breathe. The process of leaving the warm, dark, and liquid environment in utero is replaced by cold air, dryness, and bright lights. Drying the infant with towels and wiping the mouth and nose are all the assistance that most newborns require. The end result of any mechanism that delays transition is a period of hypoxia for the fetus or newborn infant. Laboratory studies have shown that the first sign of oxygen deprivation in the newborn is a change in the breathing pattern. After an initial period of rapid breathing attempts, cessation of breathing occurs. This is called *primary apnea*. Stimulation by drying the infant or slapping the feet can cause breathing to resume. If hypoxia continues after primary apnea has occurred, the infant will make attempts at gasping and then stop breathing. This is called *secondary apnea*. Stimulation does not affect secondary apnea. Assisted ventilation is necessary to provide breaths to the newborn to reverse the hypoxia. The infant's heart rate starts to decrease when primary apnea occurs. The heart rate increases with stimulation if the infant has primary apnea, and blood pressure is maintained. With continued hypoxia, the heart rate continues to drop, and hypotension develops. If assisted ventilation is not adequate to increase the infant's heart rate, chest compressions will be required.

When a newborn becomes apneic, it is not readily apparent whether the infant has primary or secondary apnea. The approach

TABLE 1 — Risk Factors for Newborn Resuscitation

PRENATAL FACTORS	INTRAPARTUM FACTORS
Maternal	Placental
Diabetes, preexisting	Placenta previa
Chronic hypertension	Abruption of the placenta
Infection	Premature or prolonged
Cardiac, renal, pulmonary,	rupture of membranes
thyroid, or neurologic	Chorioamnionitis
disease	Fetal
Drug therapy	Macrosomia
Substance use	Low birth weight
Lack of prenatal care	Breech or other abnormal
Age <16 or >35 years	presentation
Previous fetal or neonatal	Persistent fetal bradycardia
death	Non-reassuring fetal heart
Pregnancy	rate patterns
Bleeding in second or	Labor
third trimester	Premature labor
Pregnancy-induced	Precipitous labor
hypertension	Prolonged labor (>24 h)
Toxemia	Prolonged second stage of
Gestational diabetes	labor (>2 h)
Fetal anemia or	Prolapsed cord
isoimmunization	Emergency cesarean section
Polyhydramnios	Forceps or vacuum-assisted
Oligohydramnios	delivery
Fetal hydrops	Other
Postterm gestation	Meconium-stained amniotic
Multiple gestation	fluid
Size-date discrepancy	General anesthesia
Diminished fetal activity	Narcotics given within 4 h of
Fetal malformation or	delivery
abnormality	Uterine hyperstimulation
	Severe intrapartum bleeding

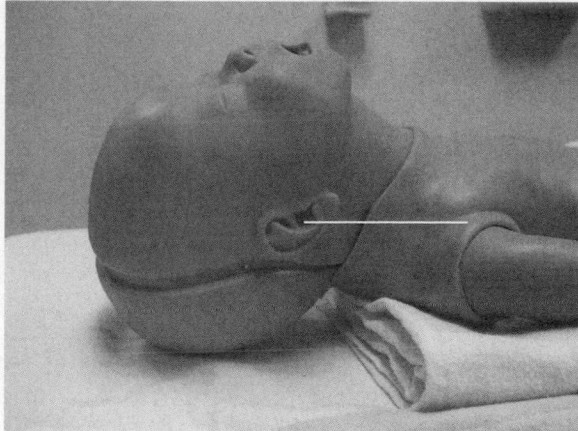

Figure 1. The sniffing position. Positioning the infant on the back with the neck slightly extended brings the posterior pharynx, larynx, and trachea in line (*white line*) to facilitate air entry into the lungs.

to resuscitation therefore requires that any apneic event in a newborn be treated using the same sequence of interventions. If the apneic infant responds to simple stimulation, the diagnosis is primary apnea, and no further intervention is required. If the infant does not improve with stimulation, secondary apnea has occurred, and more intensive intervention is needed.

Sequence of Newborn Resuscitation

Initial Steps and Basic Resuscitation

Resuscitation of the newborn starts the rapid assessment of three characteristics: Is the infant at term gestation, is the infant crying and breathing, and does the infant have good muscle tone? The answers to these questions will affect the approach to care. Resuscitation when fluid is meconium stained is discussed later in this chapter. The information presented here refers to term infants with clear amniotic fluid. More information regarding the care of premature infants is discussed in a later section.

The infant at term who is crying and breathing with good muscle tone does not need resuscitation and should not be separated from the mother. The baby should be dried, placed skin-to-skin with the mother, and covered with dry linen to maintain temperature. Ongoing observation for breathing, activity, and color should continue while the infant is with the mother. If the infant is not term, is not crying and breathing, or does not have good muscle tone, newborn resuscitation should begin with the initial steps: providing warmth, positioning and clearing (if needed) the airway, drying and stimulating the infant.

The newborn should be placed under a radiant warmer to prevent heat loss and to allow easy observation. Although warm blankets or towels can be used to dry the infant, they should not be left in place to cover the infant. The newborn should be placed on the back with the neck slightly extended in the "sniffing" position (Figure 1). This facilitates air entry into the lungs by lining up the posterior pharynx, larynx, and trachea. Hyperextension or hyperflexion of the neck can obstruct air entry into the lungs.

If the newborn is crying vigorously, secretions can be removed by wiping the nose and the mouth with a towel. Gentle suctioning of the mouth and nose with a bulb syringe or suction catheter is only indicated when there is obvious obstruction to spontaneous breathing or when there is a need for positive-pressure ventilation. Deep or vigorous suctioning can be detrimental to the infant because of stimulation of the vagus nerve, causing bradycardia or apnea. The mouth should be suctioned before the nose to prevent aspiration if the infant gasps during suctioning.

Drying the infant, slapping the feet, and rubbing the back are appropriate forms of stimulation. More forceful methods of stimulation can harm the infant. Primary apnea, if present, will respond to stimulation in less than 30 seconds. Prolonged apnea will require positive-pressure ventilation (PPV).

Evaluating the infant's response to resuscitation is essential. The Apgar score is a traditional method for evaluating newborn status at 1 and 5 minutes after delivery. However, effective resuscitation demands that evaluation of the newborn's status not be delayed until 1 minute of age, and Apgar scores therefore should *not* be used to guide resuscitative efforts. Within 30 seconds of delivery, the infant's need for PPV must be assessed. Establishment of effective ventilation spontaneously by the newborn or with assistance by PPV is the most important step in newborn resuscitation. The respiratory status, heart rate, and color or oximetry reading should be determined. The chest wall should move with each breath, and the newborn should be breathing spontaneously. Heart rate can be assessed by feeling for a pulse at the base of the umbilical cord. If this pulse cannot be felt, a stethoscope can be used to listen for the heartbeat. The heart rate should be greater than 100 beats/min. Peripheral cyanosis (i.e., blueness of the hands and feet) is acceptable in the initial period after delivery. Central cyanosis in which the lips and trunk are blue indicates hypoxemia and the need for more resuscitation efforts. A pulse oximeter can provide continuous assessment of the pulse and oxygen saturation and is the optimal method for monitoring the infant's state of oxygenation. The initial steps of stabilization, reassessment, and establishing ventilation should be completed within the first minute of life (the "Golden Minute"). The oximeter probe should be placed on the newborn's right wrist or hand to detect preductal saturation. A pulse oximeter should be used to confirm the perception of central cyanosis.

Respiratory Support and Positive-Pressure Ventilation

If the infant is breathing with a heart rate higher than 100 beats/min but has central cyanosis, free-flowing oxygen delivery is indicated. This can be administered with a facemask or by holding oxygen tubing or a flow-inflating bag and mask close to the infant's face. *A self-inflating bag and mask cannot be used to give free-flowing oxygen.* If the newborn is apneic, not breathing effectively, or has a heart rate less than 100 beats/min, PPV using a self-inflating bag, flow-inflating (or anesthesia) bag, or a T-piece resuscitator is required. Use of a flow-inflating bag requires a

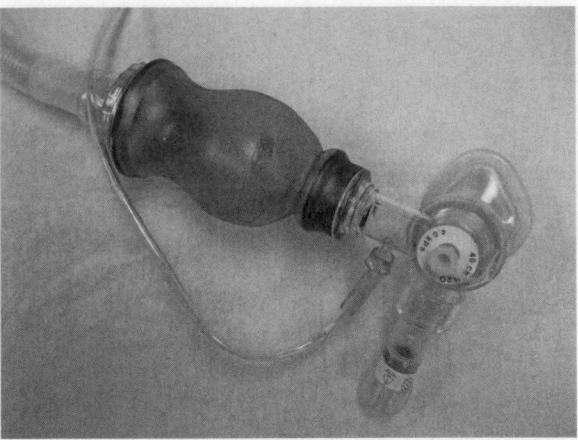

Figure 2. Self-inflating bag with infant mask and reservoir. This type of device is available in most delivery rooms.

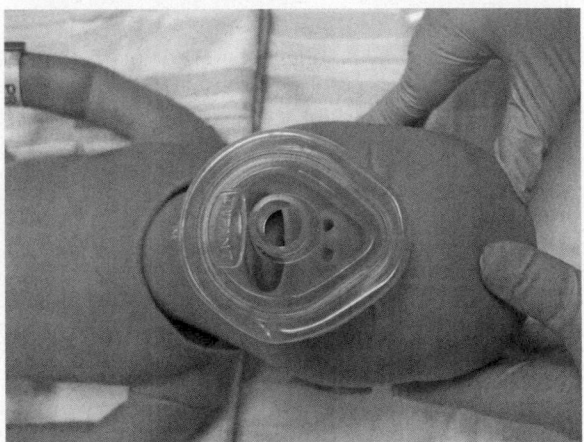

Figure 3. Facemask. Choose a size that covers the infant's mouth and nose.

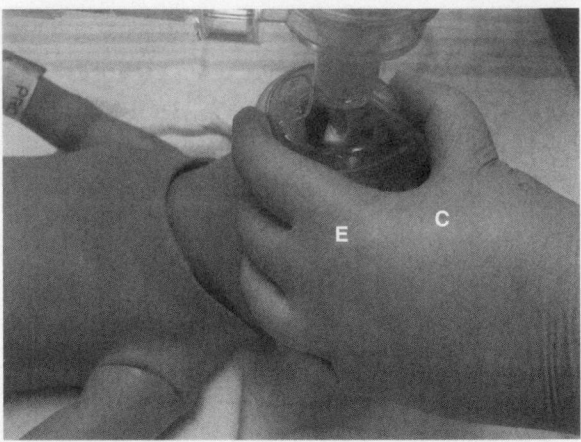

Figure 4. Facemask placement. The thumb and index finger are held in a C-shaped position on top of the mask, and the remaining fingers are held in an E-type position under the chin.

TABLE 2	Titrated Oxygen Saturations After Birth
1 minute	60-65%
2 minutes	65-70%
3 minutes	70-75%
4 minutes	75-80%
5 minutes	80-85%
10 minutes	85-90%

compressed gas source and considerable practice to be used effectively. A T-piece resuscitator needs special equipment and a compressed gas source. Most delivery rooms are equipped with self-inflating bags (Figure 2) because they are easy to use and can be fitted with a pressure-release valve to decrease overinflation. A reservoir must be used with a self-inflating bag to provide 100% oxygen.

The facemask should cover the infant's nose, mouth, and tip of chin, but not the eyes (Figure 3). Multiple sizes should be available. A tight seal between the infant's skin and the facemask is needed, but excessive pressure can bruise the face. The mask can be held in place using the thumb and index finger in a C-shaped position on top of the mask, with the remaining fingers in an E-shaped position below the infant's chin (Figure 4). Inspiratory pressures of 20 to 30 cm H_2O are usually needed when squeezing the bag to make the infant's chest rise. A pressure gauge can be connected to the self-inflating bag for monitoring inspiratory pressure. The heart rate and color of the infant should rapidly improve if enough pressure is being given. An assistant can also use a stethoscope to listen to breath sounds for air movement. Breaths should be given at a rate of 40 to 60 breaths/min.

Traditionally, 100% oxygen has been used in newborn resuscitation. However, several randomized, controlled studies enrolling term and near-term infants have shown that room air can be used initially with oxygen as a backup if room air fails. A meta-analysis of these trials showed a benefit for the use of room air. Providing oxygen at concentrations between room air and 100% requires the use of compressed air, oxygen, and blenders by experienced personnel. A pulse oximeter with a probe designed for use in newborns can be used to guide oxygen administration during newborn resuscitation. It will take 1 to 2 minutes to apply the pulse oximeter probe to the infant's right palm or wrist (preductal site) and get

a consistent reading. The pulse oximeter may not function during states of very poor cardiac output or perfusion. In these situations, observation for central cyanosis will be necessary. The infant's oxygen saturation may remain in the 70% to 80% range for several minutes after birth. Oxygen may be titrated to the interquartile range of preductal saturations measured in healthy babies following vaginal birth at sea level (see Table 2). If blended oxygen is not available, room air should be used for resuscitation. If the infant's heart rate does not respond to positive pressure ventilation with room air after 90 seconds, 100% oxygen should then be used.

After 30 seconds of PPV, the infant should be reevaluated. Ventilation with a bag and mask can be stopped when the newborn has a heart rate higher than 100 beats/min, spontaneous breathing, improved color, and good muscle tone. Supplemental oxygen should still be given to the infant. If the newborn is not improving, use the acronym "MR SOPA" to correct the technique of PPV: M=mask adjustment to check seal, R=reposition head in sniffing position, S=suction mouth and nose, O=open mouth with infant's jaw lifted forward, P=increase pressure up to 30-40 cm H_2O, A=consider using an alternative airway such as endotracheal (ET) intubation.

ET intubation is a technical skill that must be learned and practiced to maintain competency. Effective ventilation can be given with a bag and mask approach to most newborns. This skill is easily mastered and maintained. If an infant is responding well to bag and mask ventilation, it can be continued for longer periods; however, some air may escape into the esophagus and into the stomach. This may cause gastric distention, which can prevent full expansion of the lungs and cause vomiting and aspiration. An orogastric tube can be placed in the stomach and left open to air to vent any air introduced into the infant's stomach during bag and mask ventilation.

Chest Compressions

After 30 seconds of effective PPV, the heart rate should be assessed. If the heart rate dips below 60 beats/min, chest compressions are needed to support the circulation. The thumb technique (Figure 5) is preferred, but the two-finger technique (Figure 6) can be used, especially when placement of an umbilical venous catheter is required. Two people are required to give PPV and chest compressions effectively. To coordinate the breaths and chest

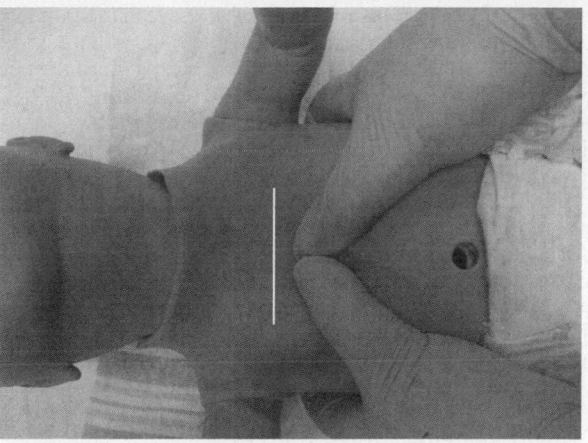

Figure 5. Thumb technique. The hands encircle the torso, and the thumbs are placed on top of the lower sternum above the xyphoid process and below a line drawn between the nipples *(white line)*.

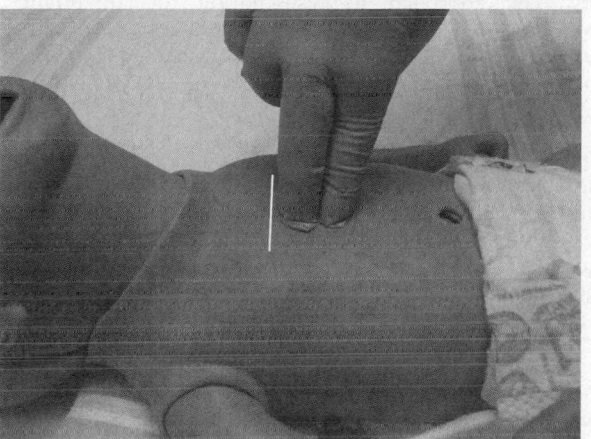

Figure 6. Two-finger technique. The index and middle finger are used to apply pressure on the lower third of the sternum above the xyphoid process and below a line drawn between the nipples *(white line)*

compressions, three compressions are given followed by one breath, and this sequence is repeated to give the infant 90 compressions and 30 breaths/min. The thumb or fingers are placed on the lower third of the infant's sternum but above the xyphoid process. The sternum is depressed to a depth of one third of the infant's anteroposterior chest diameter. The purpose of chest compressions is to squeeze the heart between the sternum and the spine, forcing blood in and out of the heart and to the body. The direction of the compressions should be perpendicular to the chest surface, and the fingers should not be lifted off of the chest after the correct placement is obtained. Incorrect methods during chest compressions can cause rib fracture and liver laceration.

After 45-60 seconds of chest compressions, the infant's heart rate, color, breathing or pulse oximeter reading, and tone are reassessed. If the heart rate is higher than 60 beats/min, chest compressions can be stopped, although PPV may still be needed. If the heart rate is not improving, the following problems must considered: ventilation is not adequate, 100% oxygen concentration is not being given, or the compressions may not be deep enough or well coordinated with the breaths. If the arrest is suspected to be of primary cardiac etiology, a compression ratio of 15 compressions to 2 breaths or 30 compressions to 2 breaths may be more effective.

Medications for Newborn Resuscitation

If the newborn heart rate remains below 60 beats/min despite PPV and chest compressions, epinephrine (Adrenalin) can be used to stimulate the newborn heart. Fewer than 2 of 1000 infants will require this step in resuscitation. *IV administration of epinephrine is preferred.*

A catheter can be quickly inserted into the umbilical vein for intravenous access. A 3.5 or 5 F catheter prefilled with saline and connected to a 3-way stopcock is inserted about 2 to 4 cm into the umbilical vein using sterile technique. After blood is aspirated, insertion of the catheter is stopped, and the epinephrine is given rapidly, followed by a saline flush. The concentration of epinephrine used in neonatal resuscitation is 1:10,000. The intravenous dose is 0.01 to 0.03 mg/kg (0.1 to 0.3 mL/kg) (Table 3). A dose of epinephrine may be considered through the ET tube during the umbilical vein catheterization. The ET dose of epinephrine is 0.05 to 0.1 mg/kg (0.5 to 1 mL/kg).[1] *These higher doses are for ET use only.* Because lung absorption of epinephrine varies, the intravenous route using the umbilical vein is preferred.

During umbilical vein cannulation, PPV and chest compressions are continued. More personnel will be needed to place the catheter and draw up the medications and saline flushes. After an intravenous dose of epinephrine, the infant's heart rate, respirations, color or oximeter reading, and tone are reevaluated. The heart rate should increase to more than 60 beats/min. If the heart rate does not respond, the dose of epinephrine can be repeated every 3 to 5 minutes. The effectiveness of ventilation and compressions should be reassessed. If the infant appears pale, has delayed capillary refill, or decreased pulses, shock may be present. Infant blood loss might have occurred during delivery from placental problems or other sources. Administration of an isotonic crystalloid solution such as normal saline or Ringer's lactate at 10 mL/kg over 5 to 10 minutes can improve circulation. Volume expansion should be used cautiously because there is evidence from animal studies for poorer outcomes when it is used in the absence of hypovolemia. Rapid infusion of large volumes has been associated with intraventricular hemorrhage in premature infants.

Newborns, especially premature infants, are at risk for hypoglycemia. Blood from the infant's heel or the umbilical vein can be tested at the bedside and intravenous 10% dextrose (2 to 5 mL/kg) given for low blood glucose. No specific glucose level has been associated with a poorer outcome. There is no evidence that use of sodium

---

[1]Not FDA approved for this indication.

TABLE 3	Drugs for Newborn Resuscitation			
DRUG	**CONCENTRATION**	**DOSE**	**INDICATIONS**	**COMMENTS**
Epinephrine	1:10,000	0.01–0.03 mg/kg IV = 0.1–0.3 mL/kg IV route preferred 0.05–0.1 mg/kg ETT[1]	Asystole Bradycardia that does not improve with PPV and chest compressions Shock	May repeat every 3–5 min
Volume expanders	Normal saline Ringer's lactate O negative blood	10 mL/kg IV	Hypovolemia	Crossmatch blood to mother if possible Repeat if needed
Glucose	10% Dextrose	2–5 mL/kg IV	Hypoglycemia	Monitor glucometer or venous glucose levels

[1]Not FDA approved for this indication.
Abbreviations: ETT = endotracheal tube; IV = intravenous.

bicarbonate benefits the neonate, and its use during resuscitation in the delivery room is not recommended.

After resuscitation, newborns should be monitored in an intensive care setting. These infants are at risk for several complications, such as infection, metabolic abnormalities, and seizures. Infants of 36 weeks' gestation or older with moderate to severe hypoxic-ischemic encephalopathy may benefit from induced hypothermia.

Special Considerations

Some newborns do not respond to resuscitation because of specific problems. Infants with upper airway obstruction from micrognathia can be helped by a nasopharyngeal airway and placement of the infant in the prone position. Choanal atresia can be treated by placing an oral airway. Absence of breath sounds on one side of the chest can indicate a pneumothorax, requiring needle aspiration of the chest. An infant with a scaphoid abdomen and decreased breath sounds may have a diaphragmatic hernia. These infants should be intubated, and PPV by mask and bag should not be used. If the mother has received narcotics shortly before the delivery, the narcotic may be the cause of respiratory depression in the infant. These infants need *PPV and respiratory support*. Naloxone is no longer recommended as part of initial resuscitative efforts in the delivery room. Heart rate and oxygenation should be supported by PPV.

Endotracheal Intubation

During neonatal resuscitation, endotracheal intubation may be indicated in the following circumstances: initial endotracheal suctioning of a nonvigorous meconium-stained infant, cases in which bag and mask ventilation is ineffective or prolonged, if chest compressions are performed, and in special situations such as congenital diaphragmatic hernia or extremely low birth weight infants. Intubation of the newborn requires preparation that can be performed while the infant is being ventilated by bag and mask. The ET tube should not be placed unless the glottis is visualized by direct laryngoscopy. To ensure that the tube is in the trachea, a carbon dioxide (CO_2) detector should be used. Listening for equal breath sounds and looking for vapor condensation in the ET tube during exhalation can help, but an increase in the infant's heart rate or a positive detection of CO_2 is most reliable. It should be noted that poor or absent pulmonary blood flow may result in the absence of CO_2 detection despite tube placement in the trachea.

Intubation should be performed as quickly as possible, with a goal of 30 seconds from insertion of the laryngoscope to the connection of the ET tube to the resuscitation bag. Complications of intubation include worsening of hypoxia and bradycardia, pneumothorax, contusions, perforation of the trachea or esophagus, and infection. After the infant has been intubated, deterioration in the infant's status should prompt an organized sequence to assess the adequacy of ventilation using the mnemonic DOPE: *Dislodged* (D): Is the tube in the right bronchus or out of the trachea? *Obstructed* (O): Is the tube obstructed by secretions or blood? *Pneumothorax* (P) and *esophagus* (E): Is the tube in the esophagus?

An alternative to intubation is placement of a laryngeal mask airway. This type of airway does not require laryngoscopy. A soft inflatable mask that is attached to a flexible airway tube is placed in the hypopharynx such that the air in the tube is directed into the larynx and away from the esophagus. However, this type of airway cannot be used to suction meconium from the trachea nor to give endotracheal drugs. Its use has not been evaluated during chest compressions.

Premature Infants

Infants born before 37 weeks' gestation are at increased risk for complications and the need for resuscitation. Premature lungs may lack surfactant, making ventilation difficult. Very low birth weight (less than 1500 g) infants will need additional warming techniques such as prewarming the delivery room, covering the baby in plastic wrapping, and placing the baby under a radiant warmer and/or an exothermic mattress; however, iatrogenic hyperthermia should be avoided. Immature brain development may decrease the drive to breathe. Weak muscles make respiratory

efforts less effective. Thin skin and decreased subcutaneous fat make temperature regulation a challenge. Premature infants often have infections such as pneumonia or sepsis. The blood vessels in their brains are fragile and can easily bleed during periods of blood pressure variation. The lower birth weights of premature newborns also require smaller sizes of equipment for resuscitation such as facemasks, suction catheters, endotracheal tubes, and umbilical catheters. Oxygen concentrations less than 100% are often used to protect the premature infant from oxygen toxicity. The use of continuous positive airway pressure (CPAP) in premature infants who are breathing spontaneously but with difficulty following birth may reduce the need for intubation, mechanical ventilation, and surfactant use. Many personnel trained in newborn resuscitation should be present at the delivery of a high-risk premature infant.

Meconium Staining of the Amniotic Fluid

Meconium is formed in the newborn gastrointestinal system during gestation. Intrauterine stress can cause release of meconium into the amniotic fluid. Aspiration of meconium-stained amniotic fluid into the lungs can result in severe pneumonitis and lung injury. The approach to resuscitation for an infant with meconium-stained fluid depends on the *condition of the infant immediately after birth*. There is no evidence that the consistency of meconium-stained fluid (i.e., thick or thin) should change these approaches.

Crying and Vigorous Infant

If the newborn with meconium-stained amniotic fluid has normal respiratory effort and muscle tone with a heart rate higher than 100 beats/min, *gentle* mouth and nose suctioning can be performed using a bulb syringe or suction catheter. Deep and prolonged suctioning should be avoided. ET intubation is not required for vigorous infants with meconium-stained amniotic fluid.

Nonvigorous Infant

Newborns who are gasping or apneic, have poor muscle tone, and have a heart rate less than 100 beats/min may benefit from direct suctioning of the trachea. A laryngoscope is inserted, and a 12- or 14-F catheter is used to suction the mouth and posterior pharynx. After visualizing the glottis, an ET tube is inserted and attached to a suction source. Suction is applied as the ET tube is withdrawn (Figure 7). This maneuver may be repeated until the suctioned fluid is clear unless the infant requires resuscitation (e.g., apneic, heart rate <100 beats/min, decreased muscle tone, cyanotic). After ET suctioning, a bag and mask can be used to provide PPV for the infant if needed. The usual sequence of newborn resuscitation is then followed. If attempted intubation is difficult and prolonged,

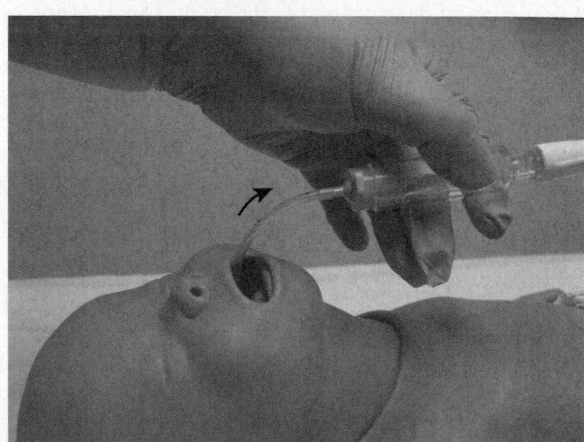

Figure 7. The meconium aspirator is attached to a suction source and connected to the endotracheal (ET) tube inserted into the infant's trachea. The thumb is used to occlude the suction-control port to apply suction to the ET tube while gradually withdrawing the ET tube from the trachea *(arrow)*.

TABLE 4 Equipment for Newborn Resuscitation

TYPE OF USE	EQUIPMENT
General	Sterile towels Radiant warmer or heat lamps Pulse oximeter Cardiorespiratory monitor Sterile gowns, gloves
Airway	Bulb syringe Suction catheters (5, 8, 10, 12, 14 F) Suction source with manometer Oral and nasopharyngeal airways (newborn sizes) Laryngoscope and straight blades sizes 0 and 1 Endotracheal tubes (sizes 2.5, 3.0, 3.5, 4.0) Meconium suction device
Ventilation	Face masks (premature, newborn, and infant sizes) Self-inflating bag (450–750 mL) with oxygen reservoir and manometer Oxygen source Orogastric tubes (8, 10 F) Carbon dioxide (CO_2) indicator Chest tubes (8 and 10 F)
Circulation	Umbilical catheters (3.5 and 5 F) Umbilical catheter tray (sterile scissors, scalpel, forceps, umbilical tape) Three-way stopcock Syringes (1, 3, 5, 10 mL) Normal saline Epinephrine 1:10,000 10% Dextrose Ringer's lactate

bag and mask ventilation should be started without tracheal suctioning, especially if there is persistent bradycardia.

Newborn Resuscitation Outside of the Delivery Room

Resuscitation of infants born at home, in an emergency room, in an ambulance, or otherwise outside of a delivery room setting should proceed according to the same principles as in the delivery room. Providing warmth, wiping the airway, and providing stimulation are usually adequate measures. Establishing effective ventilation using a bag and mask is the most important step if the infant fails to breathe on its own. Emergency providers should be familiar with resuscitation of the newborn, and basic equipment (Table 4) should be available.

Withholding and Withdrawing Newborn Resuscitation

Newborns should be offered resuscitation at delivery except in extreme circumstances. Newborn resuscitation should not be used if the infant has a condition that is incompatible with survival, such as a confirmed gestational age of less than 23 completed weeks, birth weight less than 400 g, or congenital anomalies associated with certain death or extreme morbidity.

In most situations, initial resuscitation can provide time to observe the infant's response to interventions and to discuss the infant's condition with the parents. Techniques for obstetric dating of pregnancies are accurate only to ±1 to 2 weeks, and estimates of fetal weight are accurate only to ±100 to 200 g. Care must be taken before deciding to withhold resuscitation from a newborn. Ongoing conversation between parents and medical caregivers allows mutual decision making. Withdrawal of care is indicated if continued support is futile. After 10 minutes of asystole (heart rate of 0), newborns are very unlikely to survive.

References

American Academy of Pediatrics Committee on Fetus and Newborn. EF Bel. Noninitiation or withdrawal of intensive care for high-risk newborns. Pediatrics 2007;119:401.
American Heart Association. American Heart Association guidelines for cardiopulmonary resuscitation and emergency cardiovascular care. Part 15: Neonatal Resuscitation. Circulation 2010;122(Suppl 3):S909–S919 2010.

Aschner JL, Poland RL. Sodium bicarbonate: Basically useless therapy. Pediatrics 2008;122:831.
Bassam H, Mercer BM, Livingston JC, et al. Outcome after successful resuscitation of babies born with Apgar scores of 0 at both 1 and 5 minutes. Am J Obstet Gynecol 2000;182:1210.
Escobedo M. Moving from experience to evidence: Changes in US Neonatal Resuscitation Program based on International Liaison Committee on Resuscitation Review. J Perinatol 2008;28:835.
Field DJ, Dorling JS, Manktelow BN, et al. Survival of extremely premature babies in a geographically defined population: Prospective cohort study of 1994–99 compared with 2000–05. BMJ 2008;336:1221.
Halliday HL. Endotracheal intubation at birth for preventing morbidity and mortality in vigorous, meconium-stained infants born at term. Cochrane Database Syst Rev 2001;(1) CD000500.
Jain L, Ferre C, Vidyasagar D, et al. Cardiopulmonary resuscitation of apparently stillborn infants: Survival and long-term outcome. J Pediatr 1991;118:778.
Kattwinkel J, Perlman J. The neonatal resuscitation program: the evidence evaluation process and anticipating edition 6. Neoreviews 2010;11:e673.
Textbook of neonatal resuscitation. 6th ed. American Academy of Pediatrics; 2011.
Wiswell TE, Gannon CM, Jacob J, et al. Delivery room management of the apparently vigorous meconium-stained neonate: Results of the multicenter, international collaborative trial. Pediatrics 2000;105:1.

TRAUMATIC BRAIN INJURY IN CHILDREN

Method of
Peter D. Patrick, PhD

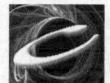

CURRENT DIAGNOSIS

Acute:
- Comorbid medical complications.

Rehabilitation:
- Functional activities of daily living.
- Neuropsychological status.

Community:
- School-based/learning issues.
- Social learning problems.
- Neuropsychiatric disorders.
- Monitor for mood disorders/anxiety.
- Monitor for personality changes.

CURRENT THERAPY

Acute:
- Need for Level I trauma services.

Rehabilitation:
- Multidisciplinary team, organized rehabilitation program.
- Functional therapies for communication, self-care, and self-protection.
- Organized comprehensive rehabilitation program.
- Neuropsychological baseline assessment.
- Cognitive remediation.
- Neurobehavioral monitoring.

Community:
- Psychoeducational assessment.
- Group participation/socialization opportunities.
- Longitudinal neuropsychological or neuropsychiatric monitoring.

Epidemiology and Risk Factors

Pediatric traumatic brain injury (TBI) has been called the "silent epidemic." Each year TBI accounts for more mortality and morbidity in children from birth to young adulthood than any other childhood illness or disease. TBI accounts for more deaths, emergency department visits, and hospitalizations than any other disorder confronting children and teenagers. According to the Centers for Disease Control and Prevention, children from birth to 4 years of age and adolescents from 15 to 19 years of age represent the highest-incidence groups. Children from birth to 14 will account for 473,947 emergency department visits. Of these visits, approximately 35,000 will be hospitalized and over 2,000 will die. With age comes the higher likelihood (percentage) of a death resulting from TBI, with the senior citizen population most at risk. Between 2002 and 2006 children 0 to 4 years had the highest rate of TBI with approximately 1300/100,000, with teenagers second with approximately 800/100,000. The rate of TBI then declines until ages 60 to 65 where there is once again an increase in emergency department visits. Males tend to outnumber females at all three peak episodes. By comparison, TBI causes 6 times the death rate of HIV/AIDS, 20 times the death rate of asthma, and 38 times the death rate of cystic fibrosis.

Causes of TBI vary over the life span. During infancy and early childhood falls are the number one cause, followed by "be struck by/against," and then automobile accidents. During the adolescent years motor vehicle accidents are first, followed by assaults. Likelihood of death from a TBI also rises with age, with the senior citizen most likely to die from a TBI. Although automobile accidents are the leading cause of death due to TBI, falls overall contribute to the highest number of emergency department visits. From 2002 to 2006 there was an increase in emergency department visits due to TBI overall and more specifically there was an increase in fall-related TBIs in children 14 years of age and younger. The literature would also suggest that the earlier the injury, the more significant the mortality and morbidity. Based on Levin's 1992 study, children from birth to 4 years have the lowest survival rate and highest morbidity, followed by 11- to 15-year-olds. Interestingly, the children injured from 5 to 10 years of age tended to have better survivor rates over the first year, and also may have less morbidity.

Pathophysiology

Pediatric brain injury is made up of a heterogeneous array of injuries that can be classified according by severity, location, and nature of insults, with each injury existing within the context of a person's array of premorbid characteristics and talents. Some insults to the brain are localized/focal and others are diffuse/generalized. The scope of injuries can range from alteration in anatomic structures to the alteration in physiologic functioning at the microscopic level.

Structural changes at the time of injury are due to the biomechanics of blunt trauma to the head and/or acceleration/deceleration shear forces. The child's, especially the very young child's, biomechanics are magnified due to head–to–body size ratios, as well as lack of neck and shoulder girdle strength. In addition, the child may be more vulnerable to "rotational forces" that have been associated with greater likelihood of unconsciousness. Resulting changes include immediate and delayed/prolonged edema. Intracranial pressure is a significant result of edema, as well as inflammatory response, which sets up the conditions for brainstem herniation. In addition, supporting blood vessels and glial cells are compromised. Blood vessel compromise can lead to hemorrhagic events or subdural and subarachnoid hematomas (which can be fast or slow developing). Hydrocephalus or isolated compromise to cerebrospinal flow can also be more immediate or slow to develop.

Microscopic and secondary injury is associated with the alteration in cellular environment. Cytotoxic cascade includes excessive neurotransmitter release (e.g., glutamate cascade) or "neurotransmitter storm," as well as alteration in electrolyte balances, magnesium, sodium/potassium balance, and calcium influx. Furthermore, there is an "energy crisis" in the brain based on reduction/compromise in oxygenation/perfusion rates, as well as metabolic changes, resulting in both hypoglycemic and hyperglycemic episodes. The microscopic crisis taking place can extend the primary injury over hours and days and set up the conditions for further cell injury and/or cell death.

Clinical Manifestations and Diagnosis

The clinical picture of injury is dictated by severity, location, and nature of the brain injury, as well as presence or absence of multiple trauma. The clinical picture in moderate to severe injuries is an unfolding presentation that starts prehospital and continues through return to home and community.

Acute Trauma Care

During the acute phase the primary goals are to preserve life and prevent/minimize secondary injury. Moderate to severe TBI can directly and indirectly affect every organ system of the body negatively. Trauma services with emphasis on managing intracranial pressure, monitoring for herniation, and maintaining oxygenation/perfusion rates to vital organs/brain are all seen as contributing to improved outcomes. In some children surgical intervention for evacuation of hematoma, decompression, and/or managing hydrocephalus are important in effecting long-term outcomes. In addition, addressing seizures, hypoglycemic and hyperglycemic episodes ("energy crisis"), and hyponatremia and anemia are equally important. Anti-inflammatory management, including steroid treatments, and hypothermia have been used effectively, and the literature continues to grow regarding their utility and impact. Management of hyperglycemic episodes is important and is associated with improved outcomes. During acute care, seizure management and other comorbid conditions are addressed as the team works toward establishing medical stability. This is especially true for children with multiple trauma. In addition to addressing structural lesions and injury, the trauma team prevents secondary injury by addressing physiologic changes at the microscopic level. Managing sodium/potassium balance and calcium levels has become a part of managing secondary injury, which is also addressed by reducing free radical and excitotoxicity ("glutamate cascade"). The role of adenosine metabolite has become more understood as a possible "retaliatory metabolite" against cytotoxic reaction. Adenosine levels appear to be higher in children and especially in severely injured children. The pediatric intensive care unit then takes over, further addressing primary injuries, preventing secondary injuries, and further supporting a road back to medical stability.

During the acute phase, measures that are associated with later outcomes are (1) length of unconsciousness (Box 1), (2) Glasgow Coma Scale scores, and (3) measures of posttraumatic amnesia. Disorders of consciousness (DOC) applies to those children with prolonged low-response states that include coma, vegetative state, and minimally conscious state. Although no one instrument is available for the infant with DOC, the Coma–Near-Coma Scale, Coma Recovery Scale, and Western NeuroSensory Profile have all been used with children to serially assess the slow to recover.

The Glasgow Coma Scale for Infants and Children is composed of a score for each of three domains (Table 1): eye opening, best verbal response, and best motor response. In younger children their ability to communicate and respond to instructions requires a modified reading that includes response to consoling and use of facial grimace in place of the older child's ability to talk and respond to instruction. Based on the total score of 15, 3 to 8 is severe, 9 to 13 is moderate, and 14 to 15 is mild.

As a neuropsychological marker associated with severity of cognitive injury, the serial assessment of posttraumatic amnesia (PTA) has been used. Following the lead from adult literature, the Children's Orientation and Amnesia Test (COAT) was published and is composed of 16 items that assess orientation, temporal

Box 1	Length of Unconsciousness
Mild	15–30 minutes
Moderate	15 min–24 hours
Severe	1–90 days
Profound	90 days or longer

TABLE 1   Glasgow Coma Scale

EYE OPENING		VERBAL RESPONSE			MOTOR RESPONSE	
		Infant and young child	Older child/adolescent			
Spontaneous	4	Oriented to sound, visual stimuli; interacts	Oriented to person, place, and time	5	Normal spontaneous movement/ follows commands	6
To verbal or touch	3	Cries but consolable	Converses but may be confused	4	Withdraws to touch	5
To painful stimuli	2	Inconsistent consolable, moaning	Replies with inappropriate words	3	Withdraws to pain	4
None	1	Inconsolable, agitated	Makes incomprehensible sounds	2	Flexion to pain	3
		None	None	1	Extension to pain	2
					None	1

orientation, and memory for children 3 to 15 years old. At the younger age temporal orientation items may not be age appropriate so a prorated score can be used. An early study by Ewing-Cobbs concluded that the COAT was a better predictor of verbal and nonverbal memory skills at 6 and 12 months after injury than the Glasgow Coma Scale. In a related study the number of days until a score of 75% accuracy was reached further strengthened the prognostic powers of the COAT when assessing neurocognitive return. Even the use of the COAT in later stages of recovery has been positive. A 1994 article by Iverson and colleagues found that the COAT score was associated with special services in school and rating the student as "impaired."

Medical Aspects during Inpatient Rehabilitation

Once medically stable and the child's survival is established, most children with moderate to severe TBI will move on to inpatient rehabilitation. The new focus will be around skill reacquisition, remedial care that strongly emphasizes mobility (physical therapy), activities of daily living (occupational therapy), and communication (speech/language therapy). In addition, neuropsychological monitoring will continue and cognitive return will be monitored. However, there continues to be a significant need for medical intervention that addresses primary problems (e.g., spasticity, seizures) and secondary/comorbid (e.g., fractures) medical conditions. Delayed seizure onset is of particular importance given that seizure onset can occur over the next 2 to 5 years of life. The younger child is reportedly more vulnerable to seizure onset. During inpatient rehabilitation the therapists begin to address relearning skills while the medical team addresses medical and health care needs (Table 2).

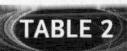 **TABLE 2**   Common Medical Aspects to Moderate/Severe TBI during Rehabilitation

REVIEW BY SYSTEMS	CONDITIONS
Neurologic	Seizures, pain, hydrocephalus, movement disorders
Respiratory	Tracheotomy care
Cardiovascular	Autonomic instability/"storming"
Fluid, electrolytes, and nutrition/gastrointestinal	Nutrition
Head/eyes/ears/nose/throat	Neuro-optomomoly examination, vision, hearing acuity disorders
Hematology	Deep vein thrombosis prophylaxis
Muscular/skeletal	Heterotopic ossification, spasticity, rigidity
Endocrine	Hypopituitary, growth hormone deficiency, diabetes insipidus
Genitourinary	Incontinence
Skin	Decubitus ulcers
Psychiatric	Delirium, agitation, depression, anxiety, neurobehavioral disorders

Differential Diagnosis and Interventions

During inpatient and outpatient rehabilitation, sensory/motor deficits continue to be addressed. However, over time with moderate to severe TBI neurocognitive and neurobehavioral issues require diagnostic attention and services.

Neurocognitive Consequences of TBI

We now know that changes in mental skills for problem solving, learning, and adaptive skills can be transient or enduring consequences of TBI in children. Mental support skills such as attention/concentration, processing speed, mental fluency, and working memory can all be affected and in some cases in spite of preserved intellectual skills. Some children will demonstrate an acquired form of attention-deficit/hyperactivity disorder (ADHD) called secondary attention-deficit/hyperactivity disorder (SADHD). In addition to being inattentive, the child will present as impulsive and hyperactive, thereby meeting the diagnostic criteria for ADHD. Preinjury characteristics can contribute to risk factors for SADHD. Also, unlike primary ADHD, SADHD typically occurs within the context of other cognitive and neuropsychological difficulties. Treatments include environmental management, cognitive remediation, and use of psychostimulant medications (however, there is a lack of clinical trials in children with TBI).

We also know that memory deficits are common. Early assessment and monitoring of retrograde and posttraumatic amnesia has become standard even in the young child. Resolution of PTA is a milestone in recovery, setting the stage for cognitive return. Short-term memory deficits in some children and historical memory deficits can persist beyond the inpatient hospitalization. The disturbances in memory make new learning difficult if not impossible. Consequently, over time not only does the child struggle with memory limitations, but also suffers the consequences of poor achievement of basic educational skills and knowledge due to poor learning. The natural course of memory disorder starts with early assessment of retrograde amnesia and serial assessment of PTA. As the amnesia resolves and/or shrinks the child is left with a permanent loss of recall for specific events surrounding the injury. Many times the child will have a disturbance to short-term memory recall, with retrieval error and lesser decline in historical memory (although in severe injuries there can be a loss of historical memory, and more specifically memory of personal history). Global memory disturbance is less likely; instead, more specific changes in domains of memory may occur, such as auditory/verbal short-term memory or visual/perceptual short-term memory. Typically the memory disorder is characterized by poor storage and retrieval of main ideas and details. Those factors appear to benefit from cueing and prompting techniques in order to assist recall.

Children on examination can have an array of information processing deficits that, on examination, profile much like verbal and nonverbal learning disability. In most children the learning disability occurs in parallel to difficulties with mental support skills, memory, and behavior problems.

Complex reasoning is frequently affected due to poor mental organization skills, lack of ability to sequence information, and poor mental abstraction skills. Also, in addition to specific compromise within learning domains, the child's "mental support skills" can be limited and have a more global impact on problem solving. For example, poor processing speed, poor working memory, and limitations in mental fluency can all undermine preserved and at times average intellectual skills following injury.

Executive, self-guiding skills are among the most complex of injuries. Poor goal maintenance and limits in initiation, persistence, and follow-through can be severe. Also, the child's loss of age-appropriate self-control and inability to set problem-solving strategies or maintain mental set contribute to both academic and social learning problems (Figure 1).

Neurobehavioral/Neuropsychiatric Limitations following Moderate and Severe TBI

"Socialization behavior is the supreme achievement of the cortex."

—FLOYD ALLPORT

In 1978 Muriel Lezak brought to light the "characterological alterations following traumatic brain injury." She made clear that alterations in complex behaviors, temperament, and personality could be direct sequelae of TBI and not a reaction to or premorbid characteristics of the person injured. With this came a greater appreciation that TBI alters who people are. Children also suffer these changes in "nature" (personality/temperament). Changes in behavior and "nature" limit successful social reentry and result in the child's being marginalized and excluded from group

RANCHO LOS AMIGOS MEDICAL CENTER
PEDIATRIC LEVELS OF CONSCIOUSNESS
INFANT TO 2 YEARS

V.   NO RESPONSE TO STIMULI
- A. Complete absence of observable change in behavior to visual, auditory, or painful stimuli.

IV.   GIVES GENERALIZED RESPONSE TO SENSORY STIMULI
- A. Gives generalized startle to loud sound.
- B. Responds to repeated auditory stimulation with increased or decreased activity.
- C. Gives generalized reflex response to painful stimuli.

III.   GIVES LOCALIZED RESPONSE TO SENSORY STIMULI
- A. Blinks when strong light crosses visual field.
- B. Follows moving object passed within visual field.
- C. Turns toward or away from loud sound.
- D. Gives specific, localized response to painful stimuli.
- E. Spontaneous, nonpurposeful movement of extremities.

II.   RESPONSIVE TO ENVIRONMENT
- A. Responds to name.
- B. Recognizes mother or other family members.
- C. Enjoys imitative vocal play.
- D. Giggles or smiles when talked to or played with.
- E. Fussing is quieted by soft voice or touch.

I.   INTERACTS WITH ENVIRONMENT
- A. Shows active interest in toys; manipulates or examines before mouthing or discarding.
- B. Watches other children at play; may move toward them purposefully.
- C. Initiates social contact with adults; enjoys socializing.
- D. Shows active interest in bottle.
- E. Reaches or moves toward person or object.

Copyright 1980. Brink, J.D.; Imbus, C.; Woo-Sam, J.
Physical Recovery After Severe Closed Head Trauma in Children and Adolescents.
Journal of Pediatrics, 97(5) pp 721-727, Nov. 1980

Figure 1. Rancho Los Amigos Cognitive Levels.

Continued

RANCHO LOS AMIGOS MEDICAL CENTER
PEDIATRIC LEVELS OF CONSCIOUSNESS
PRE-SCHOOL AGE 2-5 YEARS

V.	NO RESPONSE TO STIMULI	A. Complete absence of observable change in behavior to visual, auditory, or painful stimuli.
IV.	GIVES GENERALIZED RESPONSE TO SENSORY STIMULI	A. Gives generalized startle to loud sound. B. Responds to repeated auditory stimulation with increased or decreased activity. C. Gives generalized reflex response to painful stimuli.
III.	GIVES LOCALIZED RESPONSE TO SENSORY STIMULI	A. Blinks when strong light crosses visual field. B. Follows moving object passed within visual field. C. Turns toward or away from loud sound. D. Gives specific, localized response to painful stimuli. E. Spontaneous, nonpurposeful movement of extremities.
II.	RESPONSIVE TO ENVIRONMENT	A. Follows simple commands. B. Initiates purposeful activity. C. Refuses to follow commands by shaking head or saying "no". D. Imitates examiner's gestures or facial expressions. E. Responds to name. F. Recognizes mother or other family members.
I.	ORIENTED TO SELF AND SURROUNDINGS	A. Provides accurate information about self. B. Knows he is away from home. C. Knows where toys, clothes, etc. are kept. D. Actively participates in treatment program. E. Recognizes own room, knows way to bathroom, nuring station, etc. F. Is potty-trained. G. Initiates social contact with adult. Enjoys socializing.

Copyright 1980. Brink, J.D.; Imbus, C.; Woo-Sam, J.
Physical Recovery After Severe Closed Head Trauma in Children and Adolescents.
Journal of Pediatrics, 97(5) pp 721-727, Nov. 1980

Figure 1—cont'd.

membership. Ultimately the changes in conduct disqualify full participation as a citizen. These changes included impaired social perceptiveness, impaired capacity for self-regulation (limited reflective thought, limited self-critical capacity, stimulus-bound behavior), emotional alterations (apathy, silliness, lability, irritability, altered libido), and the inability to profit from learning (poor use of feedback). Prigatano in later years published a report regarding changes in conduct due to "frustration and limitations" versus changes due to neurologic injury.

In 2001 Max and colleagues studied a sample of 94 children 5 to 14 years of age. These children were diagnosed with mild/moderate (57) and severe (37) TBI. Personality changes were reported in 59% of those with severe TBI (22/37), but in only 5% of those with mild/moderate TBI (3/57). Children with severe TBI were most likely to have the "labile subtype" (49% of severe), with aggressive (38%) and disinhibited (38%) most likely next and apathy subtype at 14%.

A follow-up study looked at predictors of personality change in children and adolescents. The report concluded that severity of injury predicted the initial changes in personality and that preinjury adaptive skills predicted changes in the second year after injury. There were also findings to magnetic resonance imaging (MRI) localization of injury. The study revealed that lesions of the superior dorsal lateral frontal gyrus were associated with personality changes taking place from 6 months to 1 year after injury. Changes in the second year were more closely associated with lesions of the frontal white matter.

Interventions

Treatment intervention for the array of cognitive changes includes cognitive remediation and special education services. Cognitive remediation is an instructional intervention that attempts to isolate specific skills and then practice, strengthen, and/or restore them. These efforts depend on the brain's ability to compensate, learn, and utilize underlying inherent plasticity. Review of the literature on cognitive remediation has evolved, but it is still in need of investigation for the young and very young child with TBI.

Currently the literature supports cognitive remediation for mild memory disturbance and recommends compensatory training for more severe forms of memory disturbance. Severe forms of memory disorder have been studied regarding psychopharmacologic intervention (e.g., donepezil/Aricept[1]) in children and adults. There is class II support for attention retraining, and auditory processing training is frequently mentioned. Disorders of executive function have been addressed programmatically with multimodal techniques, including social discourse training, coupled with cognitive remediation and neurobehavioral care. Specific programmatic elements include self-managing skills, goal setting, and strategic problem-solving skills for social transactions. Feeney and Ylvisaker's work has greatly contributed to the positive behavioral intervention strategies used across multiple environments. The works of Lucia Braga (Brazil) and Jennie Ponsford (Australia) included family training and education, which appeared to greatly improve outcomes.

Mental Health Services

Psychotherapy

Traditional modes of counseling and psychotherapy may need adaptation, due to cognitive and communication limitations. Emphasis on complex skills that require self-reflection, self-assessment, and the ability to identify deficits may not be available for therapy either due to developmental appropriateness of these skills and/or due to consequences of brain injury. Also, social discourse skills may not be strong enough to support maximum participation in counseling or psychotherapeutic exchange. In addition, impulsivity and adynamic/areactivity (poor initiation, persistence, and follow-through) can undermine full participation in psychotherapy. It is not uncommon for there to be a need for "precounseling" training that addresses needed cognitive and emotional skills in order to participate in counseling/psychotherapy.

Medications

Much of the literature about medications following TBI is in the adult population. There is no level I class evidence for children or the very young. However, increasing interest and research over the last 5 to 10 years has explored the relationship between recovery in children and medication use. In general, case studies, retrospective studies, and small observational trials have begun to explore effectiveness/safety and what the rules of application would look like with children following TBI. Currently medications are typically used off label to address arousal, agitation, cognitive impairment, and depression/anxiety. Impaired arousal has focused on the use of dopamine agonist agents (e.g., amantadine [Symmetrel],[1] methylphenidate [Ritalin],[1] bromocriptine [Parlodel][1]), and for a small group of individuals with impaired arousal omega-1 specific indirect GABA agonists (e.g., Zolpidem [Ambien][1], intrathecal baclofen [Lioresal][1]) have been reported to have clinical benefit.

The medications for agitation have included benzodiazepines, β-blockers (e.g., propranolol [Inderal][1]), some antidepressants (selective serotonin reuptake inhibitors [SSRIs]) and second-generation antipsychotic agents (e.g., risperidone [Risperidal][1]), and even anticonvulsant agents (e.g., valproic acid [Depakene][1]). Anxiety and depression have been treated with SSRIs in children (with some indication of increased side effects and tendency toward activation). In general with children, older tricyclic medications are not as effective and have a more negative side-effect profile. In the area of cognitive enhancement the dopamine agonists have been again included but acetylcholine agonists (e.g., nAch-r) have been explored, including donepezil (Aricept).[1] Much still needs to be learned regarding use of psychotropic agents with this population of children. However, increasing effort and

resources are being committed to the safe exploration of agents and possible uses with children.

Educational Service

The child with TBI presents a unique combination of learning problems, behavior problems, and emotional reactivity. Poor reading, writing, and arithmetic skills, as well as poor communication skills, all undermine speed of learning and the rate, pace, and load of academic challenge the child can tolerate. Unique disturbances to memory skills are most noteworthy, wherein short-term memory problems, difficulty encoding, and retrieval of new learning add to the poor achievement. Although special education services provide remedial services, there is also a significant need to manage educational exchange between child and instructor. In particular, there is a need for guiding and supporting positive instruction, utilizing strengths, and compensating for limitations in order to make best use of existing skills while remedial services progress. Behavior management programs that focus on improving social discourse, pragmatic language, and communications would be most beneficial to establishing positive and productive exchange between student and instructor.

At an organizational level, improved communication and synergy of action between medical/rehabilitative community and educational institutions is important. Savage and DePompei recommended the following: (1) Involve special education and school-based team in the hospital or rehabilitation center. (2) Train all school-based staff who will have contact with the child with TBI. (3) Plan for the short- and long-term support and services needed. (4) Continue follow-up and coordination with the rehabilitation team.

Family Reentry

Successful return to home and community depends on multiple factors. Both clinical and nonclinical factors play a part in success. There are child-specific factors, family-specific factors, and community-specific factors.

Child-Specific Factors

Reentry to home and community is a major milestone in recovery. Successful reentry is due to an interaction of child-specific factors, family-specific factors, and community-specific factors. Child-specific factors include the severity of cognitive changes. More important, family and educators report changes in behaviors, personality, and emotional regulation that mostly disqualify children for participation opportunities. Prigatono reported that changes in personality/behaviors in part are due to the child's reaction to limitation and loss of function. He suggested that irritability, increased distress, and increased sensitivity to distress that affects the child's psychological resilience may contribute to the "catastrophic reaction" (Goldstein, 1952). The child's neuropsychological profile of poor awareness of deficits, poor episodic dyscontrol/aggression/anger, and emotional lability are neurobiologic factors that negatively affect participation. In some children the inability to initiate, lack of persistence, and lack of follow-through create an adynamic/areactive profile that also undermines participation.

Family-Specific Factors

Family-specific factors include health of remaining members of the family, family style of coping, patterns of communication, and available resources (financial, social resources) and innovativeness. Characteristics that appear to predict positive family outcomes include the family's resilience and preinjury traits. Higher levels of communication, expressiveness, and role flexibility and a greater orientation to activities are all associated with successful return home. Low levels of family control also appear to be related to positive outcomes. Other factors predicting a successful living environment include age of injury (younger children more successful), similarity to preinjury living environment, time after injury, and family educational level, as well as current monthly income.

---

[1]Not FDA approved for this indication.

Community-Specific Factors

Community-specific factors are also important to supporting and encouraging social participation. For example, how good is the community at recognizing the needs of children with TBI? Can the community provide a pattern of support beyond the family's ability? Can the community provide "meaningful activities"? Do community members sponsor group membership and help "bring children into the group"? And ultimately, how does the community support full citizenship as much as it is possible for the individual with TBI?

Monitoring

Moderate to severe TBI is a chronic condition that extends over years. Prolonged health concerns, cognitive factors, and emotional factors change over the years as the child meets increasing demands. Routine health monitoring might include a developmental pediatrics consultation, as well as the conventional medical point of view (e.g., delayed onset of seizures). School-based monitoring for delayed onset of cognition and neurobehavior may be helpful. Extended surveillance is necessary given delayed onset of difficulties and the emergence of late-onset problems. Late onset of difficulties is particularly important when monitoring frontal cortex injuries. Injuries to the body and white matter frontal lobe are particularly important, bilateral injury being higher risk than unilateral. This is especially true in the lack of detection of late-onset behavior and cognitive problems in children injured very early in life. When there is relative lack of sensory motor or communication difficulties, the original brain injury event is not apparent and goes underappreciated over time. Instead, late-onset cognitive and neurobehavioral problems are mislabeled and given a new diagnosis such as bipolar disorder, ADHD, or personality disorder, when in fact this is a late expression of the early brain injury. Conceptually and in terms of what resources are mobilized, it is important to understand the child in terms of the contribution that childhood and infant brain injury brings.

Complications

Medical complications can burden the recovery process from the first. Given the incidence of comorbid medical conditions (e.g., diabetes insipidus, seizures, pituitary disorders), ongoing medical monitoring and treatment is common. Later complications typically emerge as the child reenters home, school, and community. The increased challenge the community brings can unmask latent or late-stage limitations that the pediatricians or family practice physicians need to be aware of. In addition, the interaction of negative life events, family stress, and the challenge of meeting developmental demands can all negatively interact with a child who has cognitive and neurobehavioral limitations. Late-onset mental health needs, neuropsychiatric and neuropsychological services, and special education and medical specialties may be needed over time as the child and family confront long-term recovery challenges.

References

Cantore L, Norwood K, Patrick P. Medical aspects of pediatric rehabilitation after moderate to severe traumatic brain injury. NeuroRehabilitation 2012;30:325–34.

Ewing-Cobbs L, Levin HS, Fletcher JM, et al. The children's orientation and amnesia test: relationship to severity of acute head injury and the recovery of memory. Neurosurgery 1990;27:683–91.

Faul M, Xu L, Wald MM, Coronado VG. Traumatic brain injury in the united states: emergency departments visits, hospitalizations and deaths. Atlanta: Centers for Disease Control and Prevention, National Center for Injury Prevention and Control; 2010.

Guilliams K, Madikians A, Pineda J, Giza C. Pediatric neurocritical care: special considerations. In: Zasler N, Katz D, Zafonte R, et al., editors, Brain injury medicine. New York: Demos Medical Publications; 2012. p. 1591–2.

Iverson GL, Iverson AM, Barton EA. The children's orientation and amnesia test: educational status is a moderator variable in tracking recovery from TBI. Brain Inj 1994;8:685–8.

Kurowski BG, Michaud L, Babcock L, Rhine T. Pediatric traumatic brain injury: special considerations. In: Zasler N, Katz D, Zafonte R, et al., editors, Brain injury medicine. New York: Demos Medical Publishing; 2012. p. 448–62.

Levin HS, Aldrich EF, Saydjari C, et al. Severe head injury in children: experience of the traumatic coma data bank. Neurosurgery 1992;32:435–44.

Max JE, Levin HS, Schachar RJ, et al. Predictors of personality change due to traumatic brain injury in children and adolescents six to twenty four months after injury. J Neuropsychiatry Clin Neurosci 2006;18:21–32.

McDonald CM, Jaffe KM, Fay GC, et al. Comparison of indices of traumatic brain injury severity as predictors of neurobehavioral outcome in children. Arch Phys Med Rehabil 1999;75:328–37.

Prigatono GP, Schachter DL, editors. Awareness of deficits after brain injury: clinical and theoretical issues. New York: Oxford Press; 1991.

Ross B, Patrick P. Pediatric neuropsychological issues and cognitive rehabilitatation. In: Zasler N, Katz D, Zafonte R, et al., editors, Brain injury medicine. New York: Demos Medical Publications; 2012. p. 586–601.

Savage, DePompei, Tyler J, Lash M. Integrating rehabilitation and education services for school-aged children with brain injury. J Head Trauma Rehabil 1997;12:11–20.

Stanford LD, Dorflinger JM. Pediatric brain injury: mechanism and amelioration. In: Reynolds CR, Fletcher-Janzen E, editors. Handbook of clinical child neuropsychology. 3rd ed. New York: Springer; 2009. p. 169–86.

URINARY TRACT INFECTIONS IN INFANTS AND CHILDREN

Method of
Ellen R. Wald, MD

The urinary tract is the most common site for serious bacterial infections in infants and young children. Urinary tract infections (UTIs) are more common than bacterial meningitis, bacterial pneumonia, and bacteremia.

Infection of the urinary tract may involve only the bladder, or only the kidney, or both. In general, infections of the bladder (cystitis), while causing substantial morbidity, are not regarded as serious bacterial infections. In contrast, infections that involve the kidney (pyelonephritis) can cause acute morbidity and lead to scarring with the consequences of hypertension, preeclampsia, and chronic renal disease.

Diagnosis

The diagnosis of UTI may be suggested by certain signs and symptoms, but culture of the urine is the gold standard. Because culture results are not available for at least 24 hours, there has been considerable interest in evaluating tests that may predict the results of urine culture, so that appropriate therapy can be initiated at the first encounter with the symptomatic patient. The tests that have received the most attention are urine microscopy for white cells and bacteria and biochemical analysis of leukocyte esterase and nitrite, which can be assessed rapidly by dipstick.

Several studies have concluded that both the presence of any bacteria on Gram staining of an uncentrifuged urine sample and dipstick analysis for leukocyte esterase perform similarly in children from birth through 12 years of age and are helpful in identifying individuals with UTI. Other recent studies done involving young infants (<2 months of age) and older infants (<12 months and 1–24 months) concluded that a hemocytometer white blood cell count of 10 or more cells per microliter provides the most valuable cutoff point for identifying infants for whom urine culture is warranted.

The definition of a positive urine culture depends on the method used to collect the specimen. This variable definition reflects the fact that urine which has passed through the urethra may be contaminated by bacteria present in the distal urethra. If the urine is obtained by the clean-catch method, a positive culture is defined as equal to or greater than 10^5 colony-forming units (CFU)/mL. If the specimen is obtained by catheterization of the urethra, a positive culture is defined as equal to or greater than 5×10^4 CFU/mL. Finally, if a urine culture is obtained by suprapubic aspiration, a method that bypasses the potential source of contamination, a positive culture is defined as recovery of any bacteria from the urine.

Imaging

Imaging studies have been the standard of care for young children with a first UTI for the past decade. Commonly, a renal ultrasound study is performed to evaluate the gross anatomy of the urinary tract (size and shape of the kidneys, duplication or dilatation of the ureters). A voiding cystourethrogram (VCUG) is done to determine whether vesicoureteral reflux is present. This practice has rested on the assumption that continuous prophylactic antimicrobial therapy is effective in reducing the incidence of reinfection of the kidney and renal scarring that may occur in children with vesicoureteral reflux. The 2011 guidelines on diagnosis and management of urinary tract infection in infants and children 2–24 months of age issued by the American Academy of Pediatrics recommend postponing performance of the VCUG until the second infection (unless there is a major abnormality of the renal ultrasound).

Treatment

In general, there are many choices for the antibiotic treatment of UTIs in children. If a child is toxic in appearance or vomiting (thereby precluding oral antimicrobials), admission to the hospital for parenteral therapy is appropriate. Many would recommend a third-generation cephalosporin, such as ceftriaxone (Rocephin) 50 mg/kg/day given once daily or cefotaxime (Claforan) 25 mg/kg/dose every 6 hours, until the emesis has resolved and the patient can be treated orally. Otherwise, children, even those with presumed pyelonephritis, do well on oral therapy.

For the child who is to receive oral therapy, the choices are amoxicillin potassium clavulanate (Augmentin) 30 mg/kg/dose given every 12 hours[3]; a second- or third-generation cephalosporin such as cefuroxime (Ceftin) 50 mg/kg/dose twice daily,[3] cefpodoxime (Vantin)[1] 5 mg/kg/dose given twice daily, cefdinir (Omnicef)[1] 7 mg/kg/dose given twice daily, or cefixime (Suprax)[1] 10 mg/kg/dose once daily[3]; or sulfamethoxazole-trimethoprim (Bactrim) 6 mg/kg/day[3] or trimethoprim given once daily. There has been a tendency during the past several years for the prevalence of antimicrobial resistance to increase. The overall resistance to antibiotics varies geographically, and it is essential for the practitioner to be familiar with local antibiotic resistance patterns. In patients with suspected acute pyelonephritis, amoxicillin (Amoxil), cephalexin (Keflex), and sulfamethoxazole-trimethoprim should be avoided because of the potentially high rate of antibiotic resistance.

The optimal duration of therapy for children with UTI has been somewhat controversial. If the diagnosis of pyelonephritis is known or suspected, 10 days of treatment is conventional. Shorter courses of therapy have been successful in adult women with infection of the lower urinary tract. A recent meta-analysis conducted by the Cochrane Database of Systematic Reviews evaluated 10 trials (652 children) with lower-tract UTI. There was no significant difference in frequency of positive urine cultures between short-term (2–4 days) and standard (7–14 days) duration of oral antibiotic therapy for cystitis in children, either early after treatment or at 1 to 15 months after treatment. Furthermore, there was no difference between groups in the development of resistant organisms at the end of treatment or in the incidence of recurrent UTIs. Accordingly, in cases in which the diagnosis of cystitis is assured, 4 days of antimicrobial therapy is sufficient.

Voiding Dysfunction

Voiding dysfunction is a broad term indicating a voiding pattern that is abnormal for the child's age. This is a condition that should be considered in all children who are diagnosed as having a UTI after toilet training has been accomplished. Constipation plays a significant role in some children with voiding dysfunction, and attention to this comorbidity sometimes results in resolution of recurrent UTIs.

Prophylaxis

For children who are thought to be at very high risk for recurrent UTIs and potential scarring, prophylactic treatment with sulfamethoxazole-trimethoprim or nitrofurantoin (Macrodantin) should be considered. These groups include children with high degrees of vesicoureteral reflux (grades 4 and 5), those with frequent and closely spaced UTIs without reflux, and, occasionally, those who have urologic abnormalities.

The RIVUR study, Randomized Intervention for Children with Vesicoureteral Reflux (VUR), was undertaken in 2007 to determine whether antimicrobial prophylaxis with SMX-TMP is effective in preventing recurrent UTI in infants and children with reflux of any grade. The study showed a modest benefit of prophylaxis with regard to febrile episodes of UTI but no difference in scarring. There is no question of the biologic plausibility of prophylactic antimicrobial therapy in preventing recurrent UTI; however, adverse effects, emergence of antimicrobial resistance, and difficulties with long-term adherence to prophylactic strategies present barriers to effectiveness.

References

Gorelick MH, Shaw KN. Screening tests for urinary tract infection: A meta-analysis. Pediatrics 1999;104:e54.

Hellerstein S, Linebarger JS. Voiding dysfunction in pediatric patients. Clin Pediatr 2003;42:43–49.

Hellerstein S, Nickell E. Prophylactic antibiotics in children at risk for urinary tract infection. Pediatr Nephrol 2002;17:506–10.

Hoberman A, Charron M, Hickey RW, et al. Imaging studies after a first febrile urinary tract infection in young children. N Engl J Med 2003;348:195–202.

Hoberman A, Keren R. Antimicrobial prophylaxis for urinary tract infection in children. N Engl J Med 2009;361:1804–6.

Hoberman A, Wald ER, Hickey RW, et al. Oral versus initial intravenous therapy for urinary tract infections in young febrile children. Pediatrics 1999;104:79–86.

Hoberman A, Wald ER, Reynolds EA, et al. Pyuria and bacteriuria in urine specimens obtained by catheter from young children with fever. J Pediatr 1994;124:513–19.

Huicho L, Campos-Sanchez M, Alamo C. Metaanalysis of urine screening tests for determining the risk of urinary tract infection in children. Pediatr Infect Dis J 2002;21:1–11 88.

Lin D-S, Huang F-Y, Chui N-C, et al. Comparison of hemocytometer leukocyte counts and standard urinalyses for predicting urinary tract infection in febrile infants. Pediatr Infect Dis J 2000;19:223–27.

Michael M, Hodson EM, Craig JC, et al. Short versus standard duration oral antibiotic therapy for acute urinary tract infection in children. Cochrane Database Syst Rev 2009;(1) CD003966 [First published in 2003].

RIVUR Trial Investigators, Hoberman A, Greenfield SP, Mattoo TK, et al. Antimicrobial prophylaxis for children with vesicoureteral reflux. N Engl J Med 2014;370:2367–76.

Subcommittee on Urinary Tract Infection. Steering Committee on Quality Improvement and Management, Roberts KB. Urinary tract infection: clinical practice guideline for the diagnosis and management of the initial UTI in febrile infants and children 2 to 24 months. Pediatrics 2011;128:595–610.

---

[1]Not FDA approved for this indication.
[3]Exceeds dosage recommended by the manufacturer.

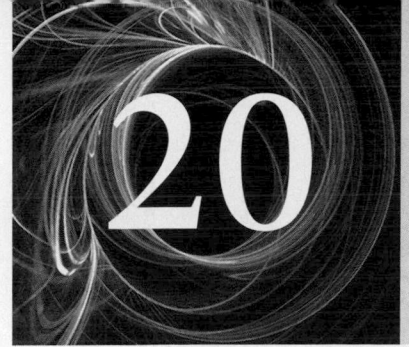

20 Preventive Health

IMMUNIZATION PRACTICES

Method of
Beth A. Damitz, MD

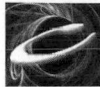

CURRENT DIAGNOSIS

- Single-agent and poly-agent variety vaccines are available in the United States.
- Vaccine-preventable diseases are occurring in the United States despite efforts.
- Vaccine registries and office-based strategies can increase vaccination rates.

CURRENT THERAPY

- Vaccination schedules are available through various sources such as the CDC, including catch-up dosing.
- Vaccines can prevent diseases that are still occurring in the United States.
- Vaccination registry participation can increase vaccination rates.
- Each office visit should be used as an opportunity to review and offer vaccines.
- Providers need to be aware of special populations such as breast-feeding and pregnant women, immunosuppressed persons, and health care workers who could need different vaccines.

Definitions and Background

Vaccination is one of the most successful and cost-effective ways to prevent infectious diseases. Immunization is the process of inducing immunity artificially by either active immunization or passive immunization. It also occurs naturally through transplacental transmission of antibodies to a fetus, which provides protection against many infectious diseases for the first few months of life.

Physiology of Vaccines

Vaccines prevent disease in the people who receive them and protect those who come into contact with unvaccinated individuals such as children too young to receive vaccines, those who cannot be immunized for medical reasons, and those who cannot make an adequate response to vaccination. Vaccines are preparations of proteins, polysaccharides, or nucleic acids of pathogens that are delivered to the immune system as single entities, as part of complex particles, or by live, attenuated agents to induce specific responses that inactivate, destroy, or suppress the pathogen.

Immunization Recommendations

The Advisory Committee on Immunization Practices (ACIP) sponsored by the Centers for Disease Control (CDC), the American Academy of Pediatrics (AAP), and the American Academy of Family Practice (AAFP) work together to issue a national schedule for routinely recommended vaccinations. They recommend routine vaccination to prevent 17 vaccine-preventable diseases that occur in infants, children, adolescents, or adults. These recommendations are reviewed and revised periodically. These immunization schedules give ranges of target ages for vaccines to be given. They include single and combination vaccine products. Catch-up dosing and special-population schedules are also available (Figures 1 to 6).

Disease Prevention

Since the development of vaccines, we have seen a dramatic decrease in both cases and deaths from vaccine-preventable diseases. For example, in 1950, there were 319,124 cases and 468 deaths from measles. This dramatically decreased to 43 cases and zero deaths in 2007. Obviously, decrease in disease and death is paramount, but in addition is the decrease in cost burden to our health care system. For every $1 spent on measles, mumps, and rubella (MMR) vaccine, $21 is saved in direct medical costs of treating a case of measles.

Immunization Responsibility

Appropriate vaccination is the responsibility of the health care team and patient (and parents). Education is critical. This can be done through various dissemination techniques such as one-on-one counseling, posters in the office, health fairs, and handouts at school and work. An office-based strategy consists of nursing and physician education of updates and changes in vaccines, the ability to track patient immunization records through registries, sending reminder letters to patients that there are vaccines they are recommended to have, and adopting standing orders to take advantage of appropriate office visits to maximize vaccination opportunities.

There are many sources for keeping current on immunizations and vaccines including the CDC's *Morbidity and Mortality Weekly Report* (MMWR). For parents and patients, the vaccine information statement (VIS), which is made available by the CDC to inform patients about the risks and benefits of immunizations, is very helpful and by law must be distributed before administering any vaccine. After the patient reads the VIS, the physician can then give any further information or answer questions before administering the vaccine. This discussion should be documented in the patient's medical record, including the refusal to receive certain vaccines (i.e., informed refusal).

General Principles for Vaccine Scheduling

Optimal response to a vaccine depends on several factors, including the type of vaccine, age of the recipient, and immune status of the recipient. Simultaneous administration of vaccines increases the probability that a patient will be vaccinated fully by the appropriate age. Simultaneous administration of all age-appropriate doses of vaccines is recommended by the MMWR for children for whom no specific contraindications exist at the time of the visit. The use of combination vaccine preparations greatly reduces

1163

(FOR THOSE WHO FALL BEHIND OR START LATE, SEE THE CATCH-UP SCHEDULE [FIGURE 2]).

These recommendations must be read with the footnotes that follow. For those who fall behind or start late, provide catch-up vaccination at the earliest opportunity as indicated by the green bars in Figure 1. To determine minimum intervals between doses, see the catch-up schedule (Figure 2). School entry and adolescent vaccine age groups are shaded.

Vaccine	Birth	1 mo	2 mos	4 mos	6 mos	9 mos	12 mos	15 mos	18 mos	19–23 mos	2-3 yrs	4-6 yrs	7-10 yrs	11-12 yrs	13–15 yrs	16-18 yrs
Hepatitis B¹ (HepB)	1ˢᵗ dose	←—— 2ⁿᵈ dose ——→			←———————— 3ʳᵈ dose ————————→											
Rotavirus² (RV) RV1 (2-dose series); RV5 (3-dose series)			1ˢᵗ dose	2ⁿᵈ dose	See footnote 2											
Diphtheria, tetanus, & acellular pertussis³ (DTaP: <7 yrs)			1ˢᵗ dose	2ⁿᵈ dose	3ʳᵈ dose		←——————— 4ᵗʰ dose ———————→					5ᵗʰ dose				
Tetanus, diphtheria, & acellular pertussis⁴ (Tdap: ≥7 yrs)														(Tdap)		
Haemophilus influenzae type b⁵ (Hib)			1ˢᵗ dose	2ⁿᵈ dose	See footnote 5		←— 3ʳᵈ or 4ᵗʰ dose, See footnote 5 —→									
Pneumococcal conjugate⁶ (PCV13)			1ˢᵗ dose	2ⁿᵈ dose	3ʳᵈ dose		←—— 4ᵗʰ dose ——→									
Pneumococcal polysaccharide⁶ (PPSV23)																
Inactivated poliovirus⁷ (IPV: <18 yrs)			1ˢᵗ dose	2ⁿᵈ dose	←———————— 3ʳᵈ dose ————————→							4ᵗʰ dose				
Influenza⁸ (IIV; LAIV) 2 doses for some: See footnote 8					See footnote 9		Annual vaccination (IIV only) 1 or 2 doses				Annual vaccination (LAIV or IIV) 1 or 2 doses		Annual vaccination (LAIV or IIV) 1 dose only			
Measles, mumps, rubella⁹ (MMR)							←——— 1ˢᵗ dose ———→					2ⁿᵈ dose				
Varicella¹⁰ (VAR)							←——— 1ˢᵗ dose ———→					2ⁿᵈ dose				
Hepatitis A¹¹ (HepA)							←—— 2-dose series, See footnote 11 ——→									
Human papillomavirus¹² (HPV2: females only; HPV4: males and females)											See footnote 13			(3-dose series)		
Meningococcal¹³ (Hib-MenCY ≥ 6 weeks; MenACWY-D ≥9 mos; MenACWY-CRM ≥ 2 mos)														1ˢᵗ dose		Booster

Legend:
- Range of recommended ages for all children
- Range of recommended ages for catch-up immunization
- Range of recommended ages during which catch-up is encouraged and for certain high-risk groups
- Range of recommended ages for certain high-risk groups
- Not routinely recommended

This schedule includes recommendations in effect as of January 1, 2015. Any dose not administered at the recommended age should be administered at a subsequent visit, when indicated and feasible. The use of a combination vaccine generally is preferred over separate injections of its equivalent component vaccines. Vaccination providers should consult the relevant Advisory Committee on Immunization Practices (ACIP) statement for detailed recommendations, available online at http://www.cdc.gov/vaccines/hcp/acip-recs/index.html. Clinically significant adverse events that follow vaccination should be reported to the Vaccine Adverse Event Reporting System (VAERS) online (http://www.vaers.hhs.gov) or by telephone (800-822-7967). Suspected cases of vaccine-preventable diseases should be reported to the state or local health department. Additional information, including precautions and contraindications for vaccination, is available from CDC online (http://www.cdc.gov/vaccines/recs/vac-admin/contraindications.htm) or by telephone (800-CDC-INFO [800-232-4636]).

This schedule is approved by the Advisory Committee on Immunization Practices (http://www.cdc.gov/vaccines/acip), the American Academy of Pediatrics (http://www.aap.org), the American Academy of Family Physicians (http://www.aafp.org), and the American College of Obstetricians and Gynecologists (http://www.acog.org).

NOTE: The above recommendations must be read along with the footnotes of this schedule.

Figure 1. Recommended immunization schedule for persons aged 0 through 18 years. Be sure to also read the footnotes (Figure 3).

The figure below provides catch-up schedules and minimum intervals between doses for children whose vaccinations have been delayed. A vaccine series does not need to be restarted, regardless of the time that has elapsed between doses. Use the section appropriate for the child's age. Always use this table in conjunction with Figure 1 and the footnotes that follow.

Vaccine	Minimum Age for Dose 1	Minimum Interval Between Doses			
		Dose 1 to Dose 2	Dose 2 to Dose 3	Dose 3 to Dose 4	Dose 4 to Dose 5
Children age 4 months through 6 years					
Hepatitis B[1]	Birth	4 weeks	8 weeks *and* at least 16 weeks after first dose. Minimum age for the final dose is 24 weeks.		
Rotavirus[2]	6 weeks	4 weeks	4 weeks[2]		
Diphtheria, tetanus, and acellular pertussis[3]	6 weeks	4 weeks	4 weeks	6 months	6 months[3]
Haemophilus influenzae type b[5]	6 weeks	4 weeks if first dose was administered before the 1st birthday. 8 weeks (as final dose) if first dose was administered at age 12 through 14 months. No further doses needed if first dose was administered at age 15 months or older.	4 weeks[5] if current age is younger than 12 months **and** first dose was administered at younger than age 7 months, **and** at least 1 previous dose was PRP-T (ActHib, Pentacel) or unknown. 8 weeks (as final dose) *and* age 12 through 59 months (as final dose) if current age is younger than 12 months **and** first dose was administered at age 7 through 11 months; OR if current age is 12 through 59 months **and** first dose was administered before the 1st birthday, **and** second dose administered at younger than 15 months; OR if both doses were PRP-OMP (PedvaxHIB, Comvax) **and** were administered before the 1st birthday. No further doses needed if previous dose was administered at age 15 months or older.	8 weeks (as final dose) This dose only necessary for children age 12 through 59 months who received 3 doses before the 1st birthday.	
Pneumococcal[6]	6 weeks	4 weeks if first dose administered before the 1st birthday. 8 weeks (as final dose for healthy children) if first dose was administered at the 1st birthday or after. No further doses needed for healthy children if first dose administered at age ≥24 months or older.	4 weeks if current age is younger than 12 months and previous dose given at <7months old 8 weeks (as final dose for healthy children) if previous dose given between 7–11 months (wait until at least 12 months old); OR if current age is 12 months or older and at least 1 dose was given before age 12 months. No further doses needed for healthy children if previous dose administered at age ≥24 months or older.	8 weeks (as final dose) This dose only necessary for children aged 12 through 59 months who received 3 doses before age 12 months or for children at high risk who received 3 doses at any age.	
Inactivated poliovirus[7]	6 weeks	4 weeks[7]	4 weeks[7]	6 months[7] (minimum age 4 years for final dose).	
Meningococcal[13]	6 weeks	8 weeks[13]	See footnote 13	See footnote 13	
Measles, mumps, rubella[8]	12 months	4 weeks			
Varicella[10]	12 months	3 months			
Hepatitis A[11]	12 months	6 months			
Children and adolescents age 7 through 18 years					
Tetanus, diphtheria; tetanus, diphtheria, and acellular pertussis[4]	7 years[4]	4 weeks	4 weeks if first dose of DTaP/DT was administered before the 1st birthday. 6 months (as final dose) if first dose of DTaP/DT was administered at or after the 1st birthday.	6 months if first dose of DTaP/DT was administered before the 1st birthday.	
Human papillomavirus[12]	9 years	Routine dosing intervals are recommended.[12]			
Hepatitis A[11]	Not applicable (N/A)	6 months			
Hepatitis B[1]	N/A	4 weeks	8 weeks **and** at least 16 weeks after first dose.		
Inactivated poliovirus[7]	N/A	4 weeks	4 weeks[7]	6 months[7]	
Meningococcal[13]	N/A	8 weeks[13]			
Measles, mumps, rubella[8]	N/A	4 weeks			
Varicella[10]	N/A	3 months if younger than age 13 years. 4 weeks if age 13 years or older.			

NOTE: The above recommendations must be read along with the footnotes of this schedule.

Figure 2. Recommended immunization schedule for persons aged 7 through 18 years.

Footnotes — Recommended immunization schedule for persons aged 0 through 18 years—United States, 2015

For further guidance on the use of the vaccines mentioned below, see: http://www.cdc.gov/vaccines/hcp/acip-recs/index.html.

For vaccine recommendations for persons 19 years of age and older, see the Adult Immunization Schedule.

Additional information

- For contraindications and precautions to use of a vaccine and for additional information regarding that vaccine, vaccination providers should consult the relevant ACIP statement available online at http://www.cdc.gov/vaccines/hcp/acip-recs/index.html.
- For purposes of calculating intervals between doses, 4 weeks = 28 days. Intervals of 4 months or greater are determined by calendar months.
- Vaccine doses administered 4 days or less before the minimum interval are considered valid. Doses of any vaccine administered ≥5 days earlier than the minimum interval or minimum age should not be counted as valid doses and should be repeated as age-appropriate. The repeat dose should be spaced after the invalid dose by the recommended minimum interval. For further details, see *MMWR, General Recommendations on Immunization and Reports / Vol. 60 / No. 2; Table 1. Recommended and minimum ages and intervals between vaccine doses* available online at http://www.cdc.gov/mmwr/pdf/rr/rr6002.pdf.
- Information on travel vaccine requirements and recommendations is available at http://wwwnc.cdc.gov/travel/destinations/list.
- For vaccination of persons with primary and secondary immunodeficiencies, see Table 13, *"Vaccination of persons with primary and secondary immunodeficiencies,"* in *General Recommendations on Immunization* (ACIP), available at http://www.cdc.gov/mmwr/pdf/rr/rr6002.pdf; and American Academy of Pediatrics. "Immunization in Special Clinical Circumstances," in Pickering LK, Baker CJ, Kimberlin DW, Long SS eds. *Red Book: 2012 report of the Committee on Infectious Diseases. 29th ed.* Elk Grove Village, IL: American Academy of Pediatrics.

1. Hepatitis B (HepB) vaccine. (Minimum age: birth)

Routine vaccination:

At birth:

- Administer monovalent HepB vaccine to all newborns before hospital discharge.
- For infants born to hepatitis B surface antigen (HBsAg)-positive mothers, administer HepB vaccine and 0.5 mL of hepatitis B immune globulin (HBIG) within 12 hours of birth. These infants should be tested for HBsAg and antibody to HBsAg (anti-HBs) 1 to 2 months after completion of the HepB series at age 9 through 18 months (preferably at the next well-child visit).
- If mother's HBsAg status is unknown, within 12 hours of birth administer HepB vaccine regardless of birth-weight. For infants weighing less than 2,000 grams, administer HBIG in addition to HepB vaccine within 12 hours of birth. Determine mother's HBsAg status as soon as possible and, if mother is HBsAg-positive, also administer HBIG for infants weighing 2,000 grams or more as soon as possible, but no later than age 7 days.

Doses following the birth dose:

- The second dose should be administered at age 1 or 2 months. Monovalent HepB vaccine should be used for doses administered before age 6 weeks.
- Infants who did not receive a birth dose should receive 3 doses of a HepB-containing vaccine on a schedule of 0, 1 to 2 months, and 6 months starting as soon as feasible. See Figure 2.
- Administer the second dose 1 to 2 months after the first dose (minimum interval of 4 weeks), administer the third dose at least 8 weeks after the second dose AND at least 16 weeks after the **first** dose. The final (third or fourth) dose in the HepB vaccine series should be administered **no earlier than age 24 weeks.**
- Administration of a total of 4 doses of HepB vaccine is permitted when a combination vaccine containing HepB is administered after the birth dose.

Catch-up vaccination:

- Unvaccinated persons should complete a 3-dose series.
- A 2-dose series (doses separated by at least 4 months) of adult formulation Recombivax HB is licensed for use in children aged 11 through 15 years.
- For other catch-up guidance, see Figure 2.

2. Rotavirus (RV) vaccines. (Minimum age: 6 weeks for both RV1 [Rotarix] and RV5 [RotaTeq])

Routine vaccination:

Administer a series of RV vaccine to all infants as follows:

1. If Rotarix is used, administer a 2-dose series at 2 and 4 months of age.
2. If RotaTeq is used, administer a 3-dose series at ages 2, 4, and 6 months.
3. If any dose in the series was RotaTeq or vaccine product is unknown for any dose in the series, a total of 3 doses of RV vaccine should be administered.

Catch-up vaccination:

- The maximum age for the first dose in the series is 14 weeks, 6 days; vaccination should not be initiated for infants aged 15 weeks, 0 days or older.
- The maximum age for the final dose in the series is 8 months, 0 days.
- For other catch-up guidance, see Figure 2.

3. Diphtheria and tetanus toxoids and acellular pertussis (DTaP) vaccine. (Minimum age: 6 weeks. Exception: DTaP-IPV [Kinrix]: 4 years)

Routine vaccination:

- Administer a 5-dose series of DTaP vaccine at ages 2, 4, 6, 15 through 18 months, and 4 through 6 years. The fourth dose may be administered as early as age 12 months, provided at least 6 months have elapsed since the third dose. However, the fourth dose of DTaP need not be repeated if it was administered at least 4 months after the third dose of DTaP.

3. Diphtheria and tetanus toxoids and acellular pertussis (DTaP) vaccine (cont'd)

Catch-up vaccination:

- The fifth dose of DTaP vaccine is not necessary if the fourth dose was administered at age 4 years or older.
- For other catch-up guidance, see Figure 2.

4. Tetanus and diphtheria toxoids and acellular pertussis (Tdap) vaccine. (Minimum age: 10 years for both Boostrix and Adacel)

Routine vaccination:

- Administer 1 dose of Tdap vaccine to all adolescents aged 11 through 12 years.
- Tdap may be administered regardless of the interval since the last tetanus and diphtheria toxoid-containing vaccine.
- Administer 1 dose of Tdap vaccine to pregnant adolescents during each pregnancy (preferred during 27 through 36 weeks' gestation) regardless of time since prior Td or Tdap vaccination.

Catch-up vaccination:

- Persons aged 7 years and older who are not fully immunized with DTaP vaccine should receive Tdap vaccine as 1 dose (preferably the first) in the catch-up series; if additional doses are needed, use Td vaccine. For children 7 through 10 years who receive a dose of Tdap as part of the catch-up series, an adolescent Tdap vaccine dose at age 11 through 12 years should NOT be administered. Td should be administered instead 10 years after the Tdap dose.
- Persons aged 11 through 18 years who have not received Tdap vaccine should receive a dose followed by tetanus and diphtheria toxoid (Td) booster doses every 10 years thereafter.
- Inadvertent doses of DTaP vaccine:
  - If administered inadvertently to a child aged 7 through 10 years may count as part of the catch-up series. This dose may count as the adolescent Tdap dose, or the child can later receive a Tdap booster dose at age 11 through 12 years.
  - If administered inadvertently to an adolescent aged 11 through 18 years, the dose should be counted as the adolescent Tdap booster.
- For other catch-up guidance, see Figure 2.

5. *Haemophilus influenzae* type b (Hib) conjugate vaccine. (Minimum age: 6 weeks for PRP-T [ACTHIB, DTaP-IPV/Hib (Pentacel) and Hib-MenCY (MenHibrix)], PRP-OMP [PedvaxHIB or COMVAX], 12 months for PRP-T [Hiberix])

Routine vaccination:

- Administer a 2- or 3-dose Hib vaccine primary series and a booster dose (dose 3 or 4 depending on vaccine used in primary series) at age 12 through 15 months to complete a full Hib vaccine series.
- The primary series with ActHIB, MenHibrix, or Pentacel consists of 3 doses and should be administered at 2, 4, and 6 months of age. The primary series with PedvaxHib or COMVAX consists of 2 doses and should be administered at 2 and 4 months of age; a dose at age 6 months is not indicated.
- One booster dose (dose 3 or 4 depending on vaccine used in primary series) of any Hib vaccine should be administered at age 12 through 15 months. An exception is Hiberix vaccine. Hiberix should only be used for the booster (final) dose in children aged 12 months through 4 years who have received at least 1 prior dose of Hib-containing vaccine.
- For recommendations on the use of MenHibrix in patients at increased risk for meningococcal disease, please refer to the meningococcal vaccine footnotes and also to *MMWR* February 28, 2014 / 63(RR01):1-13, available at http://www.cdc.gov/mmwr/PDF/rr/rr6301.pdf.

Figure 3. Catch-up immunization schedule for persons aged 4 months through 18 years who start late or who are more than 1 month behind.

5. *Haemophilus influenzae* type b (Hib) conjugate vaccine (cont'd)

Catch-up vaccination:

- If dose 1 was administered at ages 12 through 14 months, administer a second (final) dose at least 8 weeks after dose 1, regardless of Hib vaccine used in the primary series.
- If both doses were PRP-OMP (PedvaxHIB or COMVAX), and were administered before the first birthday, the third (and final) dose should be administered at age 12 through 59 months and at least 8 weeks after the second dose.
- If the first dose was administered at age 7 through 11 months, administer the second dose at least 4 weeks later and a third (and final) dose at age 12 through 15 months or 8 weeks after second dose, whichever is later.
- If first dose is administered before the first birthday and second dose administered at younger than 15 months, a third (and final) dose should be given 8 weeks later.
- For unvaccinated children aged 15 months or older, administer only 1 dose.
- For other catch-up guidance, see Figure 2. For catch-up guidance related to MenHibrix, please see the meningococcal vaccine footnotes and also *MMWR* February 28, 2014 / 63(RR01);1–3, available at http://www.cdc.gov/mmwr/PDF/rr/rr6301.pdf.

Vaccination of persons with high-risk conditions:

- Children aged 12 through 59 months who are at increased risk for Hib disease, including chemotherapy recipients and those with anatomic or functional asplenia (including sickle cell disease), human immunodeficiency virus (HIV) infection, immunoglobulin deficiency, or early component complement deficiency, who have received either no doses or only 1 dose of Hib vaccine before 12 months of age, should receive 2 additional doses of Hib vaccine 8 weeks apart; children who received 2 or more doses of Hib vaccine before 12 months of age should receive 1 additional dose.
- For patients younger than 5 years of age undergoing chemotherapy or radiation treatment who received a Hib vaccine dose(s) within 14 days of starting therapy or during therapy, repeat the dose(s) at least 3 months following therapy completion.
- Recipients of hematopoietic stem cell transplant (HSCT) should be revaccinated with a 3-dose regimen of Hib vaccine starting 6 to 12 months after successful transplant, regardless of vaccination history; doses should be administered at least 4 weeks apart.
- A single dose of any Hib-containing vaccine should be administered to unimmunized* children and adolescents 15 months of age and older undergoing an elective splenectomy; if possible, vaccine should be administered at least 14 days before procedure.
- Hib vaccine is not routinely recommended for patients 5 years or older. However, 1 dose of Hib vaccine should be administered to unimmunized* persons aged 5 years or older who have anatomic or functional asplenia (including sickle cell disease) and unvaccinated persons 5 through 18 years of age with human immunodeficiency virus (HIV) infection.

Patients who have not received a primary series and booster dose or at least 1 dose of Hib vaccine after 14 months of age are considered unimmunized.

6. Pneumococcal vaccines. (Minimum age: 6 weeks for PCV13, 2 years for PPSV23)

Routine vaccination with PCV13:

- Administer a 4-dose series of PCV13 vaccine at ages 2, 4, 6 months and at age 12 through 15 months.
- For children aged 14 through 59 months who have received an age-appropriate series of 13-valent PCV (PCV7), administer a single supplemental dose of 13-valent PCV (PCV13).

Catch-up vaccination with PCV13:

- Administer 1 dose of PCV13 to all healthy children aged 24 through 59 months who are not completely vaccinated for their age.
- For other catch-up guidance, see Figure 2.

Vaccination of persons with high-risk conditions with PCV13 and PPSV23:

- All recommended PCV13 doses should be administered prior to PPSV23 vaccination if possible.
- For children 2 through 5 years of age with any of the following conditions: chronic heart disease (particularly cyanotic congenital heart disease and cardiac failure); chronic lung disease (including asthma if treated with high-dose oral corticosteroid therapy); diabetes mellitus; cerebrospinal fluid leak; cochlear implant; sickle cell disease and other hemoglobinopathies; anatomic or functional asplenia; HIV infection; chronic renal failure; nephrotic syndrome; diseases associated with immunosuppressive drugs or radiation therapy, including malignant neoplasms, leukemias, lymphomas, and Hodgkin's disease; solid organ transplantation; or congenital immunodeficiency:

  1. Administer 1 dose of PCV13 if any incomplete schedule of 3 doses of PCV (PCV7 and/or PCV13) were received previously.
  2. Administer 2 doses of PCV13 at least 8 weeks apart if unvaccinated or any incomplete schedule of fewer than 3 doses of PCV (PCV7 and/or PCV13) were received previously.
  3. Administer 1 supplemental dose of PCV13 if 4 doses of PCV7 or other age-appropriate complete PCV7 series was received previously.
  4. The minimum interval between doses of PCV (PCV7 or PCV13) is 8 weeks.
  5. For children with no history of PPSV23 vaccination, administer PPSV23 at least 8 weeks after the most recent dose of PCV13.

6. Pneumococcal vaccines (cont'd)

- For children aged 6 through 18 years who have cerebrospinal fluid leak; cochlear implant; sickle cell disease and other hemoglobinopathies; anatomic or functional asplenia; congenital or acquired immunodeficiencies; HIV infection; chronic renal failure; nephrotic syndrome; diseases associated with treatment with immunosuppressive drugs or radiation therapy, including malignant neoplasms, leukemias, lymphomas, and Hodgkin's disease; generalized malignancy; solid organ transplantation; or multiple myeloma:

  1. If neither PCV13 nor PPSV23 has been received previously, administer 1 dose of PCV13 now and 1 dose of PPSV23 at least 8 weeks later.
  2. If PCV13 has been received previously but PPSV23 has not, administer 1 dose of PPSV23 at least 8 weeks after the most recent dose of PCV13.
  3. If PPSV23 has been received but PCV13 has not, administer 1 dose of PCV13 at least 8 weeks after the most recent dose of PPSV23.

- For children aged 6 through 18 years with chronic heart disease (particularly cyanotic congenital heart disease and cardiac failure), chronic lung disease (including asthma if treated with high-dose oral corticosteroid therapy), diabetes mellitus, alcoholism, or chronic liver disease, who have not received PPSV23, administer 1 dose of PPSV23. If PCV13 has been received previously, then PPSV23 should be administered at least 8 weeks after any prior PCV13 dose.
- A single revaccination with PPSV23 should be administered 5 years after the first dose to children with sickle cell disease or other hemoglobinopathies; anatomic or functional asplenia; congenital or acquired immunodeficiencies; HIV infection; chronic renal failure; nephrotic syndrome; diseases associated with treatment with immunosuppressive drugs or radiation therapy, including malignant neoplasms, leukemias, lymphomas, and Hodgkin's disease; generalized malignancy; solid organ transplantation; or multiple myeloma.

7. Inactivated poliovirus vaccine (IPV). (Minimum age: 6 weeks)

Routine vaccination:

- Administer a 4-dose series of IPV at ages 2, 4, 6 through 18 months, and 4 through 6 years. The final dose in the series should be administered on or after the fourth birthday and at least 6 months after the previous dose.

Catch-up vaccination:

- In the first 6 months of life, minimum age and minimum intervals are only recommended if the person is at risk of imminent exposure to circulating poliovirus (i.e., travel to a polio-endemic region or during an outbreak).
- If 4 or more doses are administered before age 4 years, an additional dose should be administered at age 4 through 6 years and at least 6 months after the previous dose.
- A fourth dose is not necessary if the third dose was administered at age 4 years or older and at least 6 months after the previous dose.
- If both OPV and IPV were administered as part of a series, a total of 4 doses should be administered, regardless of the child's current age. IPV is not routinely recommended for U.S. residents aged 18 years or older.
- For other catch-up guidance, see Figure 2.

8. Influenza vaccines. (Minimum age: 6 months for inactivated influenza vaccine [IIV], 2 years for live, attenuated influenza vaccine [LAIV])

Routine vaccination:

- Administer influenza vaccine annually to all children beginning at age 6 months. For most healthy, nonpregnant persons aged 2 through 49 years, either LAIV or IIV may be used. However, LAIV should NOT be administered to some persons, including 1) persons who have experienced severe allergic reactions to LAIV, any of its components, or to a previous dose of any other influenza vaccine; 2) children 2 through 17 years receiving aspirin or aspirin-containing products; 3) persons who are allergic to eggs; 4) pregnant women; 5) immunosuppressed persons; 6) children 2 through 4 years of age with asthma or who had wheezing in the past 12 months; or 7) persons who have taken influenza antiviral medications in the previous 48 hours. For all other contraindications and precautions to use of LAIV, see *MMWR* August 15, 2014 / 63(32);691-697 [40 pages] available at http://www.cdc.gov/mmwr/pdf/wk/mm6332.pdf.

For children aged 6 months through 8 years:

- For the 2014-15 season, administer 2 doses (separated by at least 4 weeks) to children who are receiving influenza vaccine for the first time. Some children in this age group who have been vaccinated previously will a so need 2 doses. For additional guidance, follow dosing guidelines in the 2014-15 ACIP influenza vaccine recommendations, *MMWR* August 15, 2014 / 63(32);691-697 [40 pages] available at http://www.cdc.gov/mmwr/pdf/wk/mm6332.pdf.
- For the 2015-16 season, follow dosing guidelines in the 2015 ACIP influenza vaccine recommendations.

For persons aged 9 years and older:

- Administer 1 dose.

Figure 3—cont'd

Continued

For further guidance on the use of the vaccines mentioned below, see: http://www.cdc.gov/vaccines/hcp/acip-recs/index.html.

9. **Measles, mumps, and rubella (MMR) vaccine. (Minimum age: 12 months for routine vaccination)**

Routine vaccination:
- Administer a 2-dose series of MMR vaccine at ages 12 through 15 months and 4 through 6 years. The second dose may be administered before age 4 years, provided at least 4 weeks have elapsed since the first dose.
- Administer 1 dose of MMR vaccine to infants aged 6 through 11 months before departure from the United States for international travel. These children should be revaccinated with 2 doses of MMR vaccine, the first at age 12 through 15 months (12 months if the child remains in an area where disease risk is high), and the second dose at least 4 weeks later.
- Administer 2 doses of MMR vaccine to children aged 12 months and older before departure from the United States for international travel. The first dose should be administered on or after age 12 months and the second dose at least 4 weeks later.

Catch-up vaccination:
- Ensure that all school-aged children and adolescents have had 2 doses of MMR vaccine; the minimum interval between the 2 doses is 4 weeks.

10. **Varicella (VAR) vaccine. (Minimum age: 12 months)**

Routine vaccination:
- Administer a 2-dose series of VAR vaccine at ages 12 through 15 months and 4 through 6 years. The second dose may be administered before age 4 years, provided at least 3 months have elapsed since the first dose. If the second dose was administered at least 4 weeks after the first dose, it can be accepted as valid.

Catch-up vaccination:
- Ensure that all persons aged 7 through 18 years without evidence of immunity (see MMWR 2007 / 56 [No. RR-4], available at http://www.cdc.gov/mmwr/pdf/rr/rr5604.pdf) have 2 doses of varicella vaccine. For children aged 7 through 12 years, the recommended minimum interval between doses is 3 months (if the second dose was administered at least 4 weeks after the first dose, it can be accepted as valid); for persons aged 13 years and older, the minimum interval between doses is 4 weeks.

11. **Hepatitis A (HepA) vaccine. (Minimum age: 12 months)**

Routine vaccination:
- Initiate the 2-dose HepA vaccine series at 12 through 23 months; separate the 2 doses by 6 to 18 months.
- Children who have received 1 dose of HepA vaccine before age 24 months should receive a second dose 6 to 18 months after the first dose.
- For any person aged 2 years and older who has not already received the HepA vaccine series, 2 doses of HepA vaccine separated by 6 to 18 months may be administered if immunity against hepatitis A virus infection is desired.

Catch-up vaccination:
- The minimum interval between the two doses is 6 months.

Special populations:
- Administer 2 doses of HepA vaccine at least 6 months apart to previously unvaccinated persons who live in areas where vaccination programs target older children, or who are at increased risk for infection. This includes persons travelling to or working in countries that have high or intermediate endemicity of infection; men having sex with men; users of injection and non-injection illicit drugs; persons who work with HAV-infected primates or with HAV in a research laboratory; persons with clotting-factor disorders; persons with chronic liver disease; and persons who anticipate close personal contact (e.g., household or regular babysitting) with an international adoptee during the first 60 days after arrival in the United States from a country with high or intermediate endemicity. The first dose should be administered as soon as the adoption is planned, ideally 2 or more weeks before the arrival of the adoptee.

12. **Human papillomavirus (HPV) vaccines. (Minimum age: 9 years for HPV2 [Cervarix] and HPV4 [Gardasil])**

Routine vaccination:
- Administer a 3-dose series of HPV vaccine on a schedule of 0, 1-2, and 6 months to all adolescents aged 11 through 12 years. Either HPV4 or HPV2 may be used for females, and only HPV4 may be used for males.
- The vaccine series may be started at age 9 years.
- Administer the second dose 1 to 2 months after the first dose (minimum interval of 4 weeks); administer the third dose 24 weeks after the first dose and 16 weeks after the second dose (minimum interval of 12 weeks).

Catch-up vaccination:
- Administer the vaccine series to females (either HPV2 or HPV4) and males (HPV4) at age 13 through 18 years if not previously vaccinated.
- Use recommended routine dosing intervals (see Routine vaccination above) for vaccine series catch-up.

13. **Meningococcal conjugate vaccines. (Minimum age: 6 weeks for Hib-MenCY [MenHibrix], 9 months for MenACWY-D [Menactra], 2 months for MenACWY-CRM [Menveo])**

Routine vaccination:
- Administer a single dose of Menactra or Menveo vaccine at age 11 through 12 years, with a booster dose at age 16 years.
- Adolescents aged 11 through 18 years with human immunodeficiency virus (HIV) infection should receive a 2-dose primary series of Menactra or Menveo with at least 8 weeks between doses, see below.
- For children aged 2 months through 18 years with high-risk conditions, see below.

Catch-up vaccination:
- Administer Menactra or Menveo vaccine at age 13 through 18 years if not previously vaccinated.
- If the first dose is administered at age 13 through 15 years, a booster dose should be administered at age 16 through 18 years with a minimum interval of at least 8 weeks between doses.
- If the first dose is administered at age 16 years or older, a booster dose is not needed.
- For other catch-up guidance, see Figure 2.

Vaccination of persons with high-risk conditions and other persons at increased risk of disease:
- Children with anatomic or functional asplenia (including sickle cell disease):
  1. Menveo
     o *Children who initiate vaccination at 8 weeks through 6 months:* Administer doses at 2, 4, 6, and 12 months of age.
     o *Unvaccinated children 7 through 23 months:* Administer 2 doses, with the second dose at least 12 weeks after the first dose AND after the first birthday.
     o *Children 24 months and older who have not received a complete series:* Administer 2 primary doses at least 8 weeks apart.
  2. MenHibrix
     o *Children 6 weeks through 18 months:* Administer doses at 2, 4, 6, and 12 through 15 months of age.
     o If the first dose of MenHibrix is given at or after 12 months of age, a total of 2 doses should be given at least 8 weeks apart to ensure protection against serogroups C and Y meningococcal disease.
  3. Menactra
     o *Children 24 months and older who have not received a complete series:* Administer 2 primary doses at least 8 weeks apart. If Menactra is administered to a child with asplenia (including sickle cell disease), do not administer Menactra until 2 years of age and at least 4 weeks after the completion of all PCV13 doses.

- Children with persistent complement component deficiency:
  1. Menveo
     o *Children who initiate vaccination at 8 weeks through 6 months:* Administer doses at 2, 4, 6, and 12 months of age.
     o *Unvaccinated children 7 through 23 months:* Administer 2 doses, with the second dose at least 12 weeks after the first dose AND after the first birthday.
     o *Children 24 months and older who have not received a complete series:* Administer 2 primary doses at least 8 weeks apart.
  2. MenHibrix
     o *Children 6 weeks through 18 months:* Administer doses at 2, 4, 6, and 12 through 15 months of age.
     o If the first dose of MenHibrix is given at or after 12 months of age, a total of 2 doses should be given at least 8 weeks apart to ensure protection against serogroups C and Y meningococcal disease.
  3. Menactra
     o *Children 9 through 23 months:* Administer 2 primary doses at least 12 weeks apart.
     o *Children 24 months and older who have not received a complete series:* Administer 2 primary doses at least 8 weeks apart.

- For children who travel to or reside in countries in which meningococcal disease is hyperendemic or epidemic, including countries in the African meningitis belt or the Hajj, administer an age-appropriate formulation and series of Menactra or Menveo for protection against serogroups A and W meningococcal disease. Prior receipt of MenHibrix is not sufficient for children traveling to the meningitis belt or the Hajj because it does not contain serogroups A or W.
- For children at risk during a community outbreak attributable to a vaccine serogroup, administer or complete an age- and formulation-appropriate series of MenHibrix, Menactra, or Menveo.
- For booster doses among persons with high-risk conditions, refer to MMWR 2013 / 62(RR02);1-22, available at http://www.cdc.gov/mmwr/preview/mmwrhtml/rr6202a1.htm.

For other catch-up recommendations for these persons, and complete information on use of meningococcal vaccines, including guidance related to vaccination of persons at increased risk of infection, see MMWR March 22, 2013 / 62[RR02];1-22, available at http://www.cdc.gov/mmwr/pdf/rr/rr6202.pdf.

Figure 3—cont'd

Recommended Adult Immunization Schedule—United States - 2015

Note: These recommendations must be read with the footnotes that follow containing number of doses, intervals between doses, and other important information.

Figure 1. Recommended adult immunization schedule, by vaccine and age group[1]

VACCINE ▼ / AGE GROUP ►	19-21 years	22-26 years	27-49 years	50-59 years	60-64 years	≥ 65 years
Influenza[*,2]	1 dose annually					
Tetanus, diphtheria, pertussis (Td/Tdap)[*,3]	Substitute 1-time dose of Tdap for Td booster; then boost with Td every 10 yrs					
Varicella[*,4]	2 doses					
Human papillomavirus (HPV) Female[*,5]	3 doses					
Human papillomavirus (HPV) Male[*,5]	3 doses					
Zoster[6]					1 dose	
Measles, mumps, rubella (MMR)[*,7]	1 or 2 doses					
Pneumococcal 13-valent conjugate (PCV13)[*,8]					1-time dose	
Pneumococcal polysaccharide (PPSV23)[8]	1 or 2 doses					1 dose
Meningococcal[*,9]	1 or more doses					
Hepatitis A[*,10]	2 doses					
Hepatitis B[*,11]	3 doses					
Haemophilus influenzae type b (Hib)[*,12]	1 or 3 doses					

*Covered by the Vaccine Injury Compensation Program

For all persons in this category who meet the age requirements and who lack documentation of vaccination or have no evidence of previous infection; zoster vaccine recommended regardless of prior episode of zoster

Recommended if some other risk factor is present (e.g., on the basis of medical, occupational, lifestyle, or other indication)

No recommendation

Report all clinically significant postvaccination reactions to the Vaccine Adverse Event Reporting System (VAERS). Reporting forms and instructions on filing a VAERS report are available at www.vaers.hhs.gov or by telephone, 800-822-7967.

Information on how to file a Vaccine Injury Compensation Program claim is available at www.hrsa.gov/vaccinecompensation or by telephone, 800-338-2382. To file a claim for vaccine injury, contact the U.S. Court of Federal Claims, 717 Madison Place, N.W., Washington, D.C. 20005; telephone, 202-357-6400.

Additional information about the vaccines in this schedule, extent of available data, and contraindications for vaccination is also available at www.cdc.gov/vaccines or from the CDC-INFO Contact Center at 800-CDC-INFO (800-232-4636) in English and Spanish, 8:00 a.m. - 8:00 p.m. Eastern Time, Monday - Friday, excluding holidays.

Use of trade names and commercial sources is for identification only and does not imply endorsement by the U.S. Department of Health and Human Services.

The recommendations in this schedule were approved by the Centers for Disease Control and Prevention's (CDC) Advisory Committee on Immunization Practices (ACIP), the American Academy of Family Physicians (AAFP), the America College of Physicians (ACP), American College of Obstetricians and Gynecologists (ACOG) and American College of Nurse-Midwives (ACNM).

Figure 2. Vaccines that might be indicated for adults based on medical and other indications[1]

VACCINE ▼ / INDICATION ►	Pregnancy	Immuno-compromising conditions (excluding human immunodeficiency virus [HIV])[4,6,7,8,13]	HIV infection CD4+ T lymphocyte count[4,6,7,8,13] < 200 cells/µL	HIV infection CD4+ T lymphocyte count[4,6,7,8,13] ≥ 200 cells/µL	Men who have sex with men (MSM)	Kidney failure, end-stage renal disease, receipt of hemodialysis	Heart disease, chronic lung disease, chronic alcoholism	Asplenia (including elective splenectomy and persistent complement component deficiencies)[8,12]	Chronic liver disease	Diabetes	Healthcare personnel
Influenza[*,2]	1 dose IIV annually				1 dose IIV or LAIV annually	1 dose IIV annually					1 dose IIV or LAIV annually
Tetanus, diphtheria, pertussis (Td/Tdap)[*,3]	1 dose Tdap each pregnancy	Substitute 1-time dose of Tdap for Td booster; then boost with Td every 10 yrs									
Varicella[*,4]	Contraindicated			2 doses							
Human papillomavirus (HPV) Female[*,5]	3 doses through age 26 yrs				3 doses through age 26 yrs						
Human papillomavirus (HPV) Male[*,5]	3 doses through age 26 yrs				3 doses through age 21 yrs						
Zoster[6]	Contraindicated			1 dose							
Measles, mumps, rubella (MMR)[*,7]	Contraindicated			1 or 2 doses							
Pneumococcal 13-valent conjugate (PCV13)[*,8]	1 dose										
Pneumococcal polysaccharide (PPSV23)[8]	1 or 2 doses										
Meningococcal[*,9]	1 or more doses										
Hepatitis A[*,10]	2 doses										
Hepatitis B[*,11]	3 doses										
Haemophilus influenzae type b (Hib)[*,12]	post-HSCT recipients only	1 or 3 doses									

*Covered by the Vaccine Injury Compensation Program

For all persons in this category who meet the age requirements and who lack documentation of vaccination or have no evidence of previous infection; zoster vaccine recommended regardless of prior episode of zoster

Recommended if some other risk factor is present (e.g., on the basis of medical, occupational, lifestyle, or other indications)

No recommendation

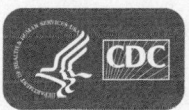

U.S. Department of Health and Human Services
Centers for Disease Control and Prevention

These schedules indicate the recommended age groups and medical indications for which administration of currently licensed vaccines is commonly recommended for adults ages 19 years and older, as of February 1, 2015. For all vaccines being recommended on the Adult Immunization Schedule: a vaccine series does not need to be restarted, regardless of the time that has elapsed between doses. Licensed combination vaccines may be used whenever any components of the combination are indicated and when the vaccine's other components are not contraindicated. For detailed recommendations on all vaccines, including those used primarily for travelers or that are issued during the year, consult the manufacturers' package inserts and the complete statements from the Advisory Committee on Immunization Practices (www.cdc.gov/vaccines/hcp/acip-recs/index.html). Use of trade names and commercial sources is for identification only and does not imply endorsement by the U.S. Department of Health and Human Services.

Figure 4. The 2015 Adult Immunization Schedule approved by the Centers for Disease Control and Prevention's (CDC) Advisory Committee on Immunization Practices (ACIP), American Academy of Family Physicians (AAFP), the American College of Physicians (ACP), the American College of Obstetricians and Gynecologists (ACOG), and the American College of Nurse-Midwives (ACNM).

1. Additional information
- Additional guidance for the use of the vaccines described in this supplement is available at www.cdc.gov/vaccines/hcp/acip-recs/index.html.
- Information on vaccination recommendations when vaccination status is unknown and other general immunization information can be found in the General Recommendations on Immunization at www.cdc.gov/mmwr/preview/mmwrhtml/rr6002a1.htm.
- Information on travel vaccine requirements and recommendations (e.g., for hepatitis A and B, meningococcal, and other vaccines) is available at wwwnc.cdc.gov/travel/destinations/list.
- Additional information and resources regarding vaccination of pregnant women can be found at www.cdc.gov/vaccines/adults/rec-vac/pregnant.html.

2. Influenza vaccination
- Annual vaccination against influenza is recommended for all persons aged 6 months or older.
- Persons aged 6 months or older, including pregnant women and persons with hives-only allergy to eggs can receive the inactivated influenza vaccine (IIV). An age-appropriate IIV formulation should be used.
- Adults aged 18 years or older can receive the recombinant influenza vaccine (RIV) (FluBlok). RIV does not contain any egg protein and can be given to age-appropriate persons with egg allergy of any severity.
- Healthy, nonpregnant persons aged 2 to 49 years without high-risk medical conditions can receive either intranasally administered live, attenuated influenza vaccine (LAIV) (FluMist) or IIV.
- Health care personnel who care for severely immunocompromised persons who require care in a protected environment should receive IIV or RIV; health care personnel who receive LAIV should avoid providing care for severely immunosuppressed persons for 7 days after vaccination.
- The intramuscularly or intradermally administered IIV are options for adults aged 18 through 64 years.
- Adults aged 65 years or older can receive the standard-dose IIV or the high-dose IIV (Fluzone High-Dose).
- A list of currently available influenza vaccines can be found at www.cdc.gov/flu/protect/vaccine/vaccines.htm.

3. Tetanus, diphtheria, and acellular pertussis (Td/Tdap) vaccination
- Administer 1 dose of Tdap vaccine to pregnant women during each pregnancy (preferably during 27 to 36 weeks' gestation) regardless of interval since prior Td or Tdap vaccination.
- Persons aged 11 years or older who have not received Tdap vaccine or for whom vaccine status is unknown should receive a dose of Tdap followed by tetanus and diphtheria toxoids (Td) booster doses every 10 years thereafter. Tdap can be administered regardless of interval since the most recent tetanus or diphtheria-toxoid containing vaccine.
- Adults with an unknown or incomplete history of completing a 3-dose primary vaccination series with Td-containing vaccines should begin or complete a primary vaccination series including a Tdap dose.
- For unvaccinated adults, administer the first 2 doses at least 4 weeks apart and the third dose 6 to 12 months after the second.
- For incompletely vaccinated (i.e., less than 3 doses) adults, administer remaining doses.
- Refer to the ACIP statement for recommendations for administering Td/Tdap as prophylaxis in wound management (see footnote 1).

4. Varicella vaccination
- All adults without evidence of immunity to varicella (as defined below) should receive 2 doses of single-antigen varicella vaccine or a second dose if they have received only 1 dose.
- Vaccination should be emphasized for those who have close contact with persons at high risk for severe disease (e.g., health care personnel and family contacts of persons with immunocompromising conditions) or are at high risk for exposure or transmission (e.g., teachers; child care employees; residents and staff members of institutional settings, including correctional institutions; college students; military personnel; adolescents and adults living in households with children; nonpregnant women of childbearing age; and international travelers).
- Pregnant women should be assessed for evidence of varicella immunity. Women who do not have evidence of immunity should receive the first dose of varicella vaccine upon completion or termination of pregnancy and before discharge from the health care facility. The second dose should be administered 4 to 8 weeks after the first dose.
- Evidence of immunity to varicella in adults includes any of the following:
  — documentation of 2 doses of varicella vaccine at least 4 weeks apart;
  — U.S.-born before 1980, except health care personnel and pregnant women;
  — history of varicella based on diagnosis or verification of varicella disease by a health care provider;
  — history of herpes zoster based on diagnosis or verification of herpes zoster disease by a health care provider; or
  — laboratory evidence of immunity or laboratory confirmation of disease.

5. Human papillomavirus (HPV) vaccination
- Two vaccines are licensed for use in females, bivalent HPV vaccine (HPV2) and quadrivalent HPV vaccine (HPV4), and one HPV vaccine for use in males (HPV4).
- For females, either HPV4 or HPV2 is recommended in a 3-dose series for routine vaccination at age 11 or 12 years and for those aged 13 through 26 years, if not previously vaccinated.

- For males, HPV4 is recommended in a 3-dose series for routine vaccination at age 11 or 12 years and for those aged 13 through 21 years, if not previously vaccinated. Males aged 22 through 26 years may be vaccinated.
- HPV4 is recommended for men who have sex with men through age 26 years for those who did not get any or all doses when they were younger.
- Vaccination is recommended for immunocompromised persons (including those with HIV infection) through age 26 years for those who did not get any or all doses when they were younger.
- A complete series for either HPV4 or HPV2 consists of 3 doses. The second dose should be administered 4 to 8 weeks (minimum interval of 4 weeks) after the first dose; the third dose should be administered 24 weeks after the first dose and 16 weeks after the second dose (minimum interval of at least 12 weeks).
- HPV vaccines are not recommended for use in pregnant women. However, pregnancy testing is not needed before vaccination. If a woman is found to be pregnant after initiating the vaccination series, no intervention is needed; the remainder of the 3-dose series should be delayed until completion or termination of pregnancy.

6. Zoster vaccination
- A single dose of zoster vaccine is recommended for adults aged 60 years or older regardless of whether they report a prior episode of herpes zoster. Although the vaccine is licensed by the U.S. Food and Drug Administration for use among and can be administered to persons aged 50 years or older, ACIP recommends that vaccination begin at age 60 years.
- Persons aged 60 years or older with chronic medical conditions may be vaccinated unless their condition constitutes a contraindication, such as pregnancy or severe immunodeficiency.

7. Measles, mumps, rubella (MMR) vaccination
- Adults born before 1957 are generally considered immune to measles and mumps. All adults born in 1957 or later should have documentation of 1 or more doses of MMR vaccine unless they have a medical contraindication to the vaccine or laboratory evidence of immunity to each of the three diseases. Documentation of provider-diagnosed disease is not considered acceptable evidence of immunity for measles, mumps, or rubella.

Measles component:
- A routine second dose of MMR vaccine, administered a minimum of 28 days after the first dose, is recommended for adults who:
  — are students in postsecondary educational institutions,
  — work in a health care facility, or
  — plan to travel internationally.
- Persons who received inactivated (killed) measles vaccine or measles vaccine of unknown type during 1963–1967 should be revaccinated with 2 doses of MMR vaccine.

Mumps component:
- A routine second dose of MMR vaccine, administered a minimum of 28 days after the first dose, is recommended for adults who:
  — are students in a postsecondary educational institution,
  — work in a health care facility, or
  — plan to travel internationally.
- Persons vaccinated before 1979 with either killed mumps vaccine or mumps vaccine of unknown type who are at high risk for mumps infection (e.g., persons who are working in a health care facility) should be considered for revaccination with 2 doses of MMR vaccine.

Rubella component:
- For women of childbearing age, regardless of birth year, rubella immunity should be determined. If there is no evidence of immunity, women who are not pregnant should be vaccinated. Pregnant women who do not have evidence of immunity should receive MMR vaccine upon completion or termination of pregnancy and before discharge from the health care facility.

Health care personnel born before 1957:
- For unvaccinated health care personnel born before 1957 who lack laboratory evidence of measles, mumps, and/or rubella immunity or laboratory confirmation of disease, health care facilities should consider vaccinating personnel with 2 doses of MMR vaccine at the appropriate interval for measles and mumps or 1 dose of MMR vaccine for rubella.

8. Pneumococcal (13-valent pneumococcal conjugate vaccine [PCV13] and 23-valent pneumococcal polysaccharide vaccine [PPSV23]) vaccination
- General information
  — When indicated, only a single dose of PCV13 is recommended for adults.
  — No additional dose of PPSV23 is indicated for adults vaccinated with PPSV23 at or after age 65 years.
  — When both PCV13 and PPSV23 are indicated, PCV13 should be administered first; PCV13 and PPSV23 should not be administered during the same visit.
  — When indicated, PCV13 and PPSV23 should be administered to adults whose pneumococcal vaccination history is incomplete or unknown.
- Adults aged 65 years or older who
  — Have not received PCV13 or PPSV23: Administer PCV13 followed by PPSV23 in 6 to 12 months.
  — Have not received PCV13 but have received a dose of PPSV23 at age 65 years or older: Administer PCV13 at least 1 year after the dose of PPSV23 received at age 65 years or older.

(Continued on next page)

Figure 5. The footnotes for the immunization schedule for adults.

8. Pneumococcal vaccination (continued)

— Have not received PCV13 but have received 1 or more doses of PPSV23 before age 65: Administer PCV13 at least 1 year after the most recent dose of PPSV23; administer a dose of PPSV23 6 to 12 months after PCV13, or as soon as possible if this time window has passed, and at least 5 years after the most recent dose of PPSV23.

— Have received PCV13 but not PPSV23 before age 65 years: Administer PPSV23 6 to 12 months after PCV13 or as soon as possible if this time window has passed.

— Have received PCV13 and 1 or more doses of PPSV23 before age 65 years: Administer PPSV23 6 to 12 months after PCV13, or as soon as possible if this time window has passed, and at least 5 years after the most recent dose of PPSV23.

• Adults aged 19 through 64 years with immunocompromising conditions or anatomical or functional asplenia (defined below) who

— Have not received PCV13 or PPSV23: Administer PCV13 followed by PPSV23 at least 8 weeks after PCV13; administer a second dose of PPSV23 at least 5 years after the first dose of PPSV23.

— Have not received PCV13 but have received 1 dose of PPSV23: Administer PCV13 at least 1 year after the PPSV23; administer a second dose of PPSV23 at least 8 weeks after PCV13 and at least 5 years after the first dose of PPSV23.

— Have not received PCV13 but have received 2 doses of PPSV23: Administer PCV13 at least 1 year after the most recent dose of PPSV23.

— Have received PCV13 but not PPSV23: Administer PPSV23 at least 8 weeks after PCV13; administer a second dose of PPSV23 at least 5 years after the first dose of PPSV23.

— Have received PCV13 and 1 dose of PPSV23: Administer a second dose of PPSV23 at least 5 years after the first dose of PPSV23.

• Adults aged 19 through 64 years with cerebrospinal fluid leaks or cochlear implants: Administer PCV13 followed by PPSV23 at least 8 weeks after PCV13.

• Adults aged 19 through 64 years with chronic heart disease (including congestive heart failure and cardiomyopathies, excluding hypertension), chronic lung disease (including chronic obstructive lung disease, emphysema, and asthma), chronic liver disease (including cirrhosis), alcoholism, or diabetes mellitus: Administer PPSV23.

• Adults aged 19 through 64 years who smoke cigarettes or reside in nursing home or long-term care facilities: Administer PPSV23.

• Routine pneumococcal vaccination is not recommended for American Indian/Alaska Native or other adults unless they have the indications as above; however, public health authorities may consider recommending the use of pneumococcal vaccines for American Indians/Alaska Natives or other adults who live in areas with increased risk for invasive pneumococcal disease.

• Immunocompromising conditions that are indications for pneumococcal vaccination are: Congenital or acquired immunodeficiency (including B- or T-lymphocyte deficiency, complement deficiencies, and phagocytic disorders excluding chronic granulomatous disease), HIV infection, chronic renal failure, nephrotic syndrome, leukemia, lymphoma, Hodgkin disease, generalized malignancy, multiple myeloma, solid organ transplant, and iatrogenic immunosuppression (including long-term systemic corticosteroids and radiation therapy).

• Anatomical or functional asplenia that are indications for pneumococcal vaccination are: Sickle cell disease and other hemoglobinopathies, congenital or acquired asplenia, splenic dysfunction, and splenectomy. Administer pneumococcal vaccines at least 2 weeks before immunosuppressive therapy or an elective splenectomy, and as soon as possible to adults who are newly diagnosed with asymptomatic or symptomatic HIV infection.

9. Meningococcal vaccination

• Administer 2 doses of quadrivalent meningococcal conjugate vaccine (MenACWY [Menactra, Menveo]) at least 2 months apart to adults of all ages with anatomical or functional asplenia or persistent complement component deficiencies. HIV infection is not an indication for routine vaccination with MenACWY. If an HIV-infected person of any age is vaccinated, 2 doses of MenACWY should be administered at least 2 months apart.

• Administer a single dose of meningococcal vaccine to microbiologists routinely exposed to isolates of *Neisseria meningitidis*, military recruits, persons at risk during an outbreak attributable to a vaccine serogroup, and persons who travel to or live in countries in which meningococcal disease is hyperendemic or epidemic.

• First-year college students up through age 21 years who are living in residence halls should be vaccinated if they have not received a dose on or after their 16th birthday.

• MenACWY is preferred for adults with any of the preceding indications who are aged 55 years or younger as well as for adults aged 56 years or older who a) were vaccinated previously with MenACWY and are recommended for revaccination, or b) for whom multiple doses are anticipated. Meningococcal polysaccharide vaccine (MPSV4 [Menomune]) is preferred for adults aged 56 years or older who have not received MenACWY previously and who require a single dose only (e.g., travelers).

• Revaccination with MenACWY every 5 years is recommended for adults previously vaccinated with MenACWY or MPSV4 who remain at increased risk for infection (e.g., adults with anatomical or functional asplenia, persistent complement component deficiencies, or microbiologists).

10. Hepatitis A vaccination

• Vaccinate any person seeking protection from hepatitis A virus (HAV) infection and persons with any of the following indications:

— men who have sex with men and persons who use injection or noninjection illicit drugs;

— persons working with HAV-infected primates or with HAV in a research laboratory setting;

— persons with chronic liver disease and persons who receive clotting factor concentrates;

— persons traveling to or working in countries that have high or intermediate endemicity of hepatitis A; and

— unvaccinated persons who anticipate close personal contact (e.g., household or regular babysitting) with an international adoptee during the first 60 days after arrival in the United States from a country with high or intermediate endemicity. (See footnote 1 for more information on travel recommendations.) The first dose of the 2-dose hepatitis A vaccine series should be administered as soon as adoption is planned, ideally 2 or more weeks before the arrival of the adoptee.

• Single-antigen vaccine formulations should be administered in a 2-dose schedule at either 0 and 6 to 12 months (Havrix), or 0 and 6 to 18 months (Vaqta). If the combined hepatitis A and hepatitis B vaccine (Twinrix) is used, administer 3 doses at 0, 1, and 6 months; alternatively, a 4-dose schedule may be used, administered on days 0, 7, and 21 to 30 followed by a booster dose at month 12.

11. Hepatitis B vaccination

• Vaccinate persons with any of the following indications and any person seeking protection from hepatitis B virus (HBV) infection:

— sexually active persons who are not in a long-term, mutually monogamous relationship (e.g., persons with more than 1 sex partner during the previous 6 months); persons seeking evaluation or treatment for a sexually transmitted disease (STD); current or recent injection drug users; and men who have sex with men;

— health care personnel and public safety workers who are potentially exposed to blood or other infectious body fluids;

— persons with diabetes who are younger than age 60 years as soon as feasible after diagnosis; persons with diabetes who are age 60 years or older at the discretion of the treating clinician based on the likelihood of acquiring HBV infection, including the risk posed by an increased need for assisted blood glucose monitoring in long-term care facilities, the likelihood of experiencing chronic sequelae if infected with HBV, and the likelihood of immune response to vaccination;

— persons with end-stage renal disease, including patients receiving hemodialysis, persons with HIV infection, and persons with chronic liver disease;

— household contacts and sex partners of hepatitis B surface antigen–positive persons, clients and staff members of institutions for persons with developmental disabilities, and international travelers to countries with high or intermediate prevalence of chronic HBV infection; and

— all adults in the following settings: STD treatment facilities, HIV testing and treatment facilities, facilities providing drug abuse treatment and prevention services, health care settings targeting services to injection drug users or men who have sex with men, correctional facilities, end-stage renal disease programs and facilities for chronic hemodialysis patients, and institutions and nonresidential day care facilities for persons with developmental disabilities.

• Administer missing doses to complete a 3-dose series of hepatitis B vaccine to those persons not vaccinated or not completely vaccinated. The second dose should be administered 1 month after the first dose; the third dose should be given at least 2 months after the second dose (and at least 4 months after the first dose). If the combined hepatitis A and hepatitis B vaccine (Twinrix) is used, give 3 doses at 0, 1, and 6 months; alternatively, a 4-dose Twinrix schedule, administered on days 0, 7, and 21 to 30 followed by a booster dose at month 12 may be used.

• Adult patients receiving hemodialysis or with other immunocompromising conditions should receive 1 dose of 40 mcg/mL (Recombivax HB) administered on a 3-dose schedule at 0, 1, and 6 months or 2 doses of 20 mcg/mL (Engerix-B) administered simultaneously on a 4-dose schedule at 0, 1, 2, and 6 months.

12. *Haemophilus influenzae* type b (Hib) vaccination

• One dose of Hib vaccine should be administered to persons who have anatomical or functional asplenia or sickle cell disease or are undergoing elective splenectomy if they have not previously received Hib vaccine. Hib vaccination 14 or more days before splenectomy is suggested.

• Recipients of a hematopoietic stem cell transplant (HSCT) should be vaccinated with a 3-dose regimen 6 to 12 months after a successful transplant, regardless of vaccination history; at least 4 weeks should separate doses.

• Hib vaccine is not recommended for adults with HIV infection since their risk for Hib infection is low.

13. Immunocompromising conditions

• Inactivated vaccines generally are acceptable (e.g., pneumococcal, meningococcal, and inactivated influenza vaccine) and live vaccines generally are avoided in persons with immune deficiencies or immunocompromising conditions. Information on specific conditions is available at www.cdc.gov/vaccines/hcp/acip-recs/index.html.

Immunization Practices

1171

Figure 5—cont'd

Vaccine	Contraindications	Precautions
Influenza, inactivated (IIV)[2]	• Severe allergic reaction (e.g., anaphylaxis) after previous dose of any influenza vaccine; or to a vaccine component, including egg protein	• Moderate or severe acute illness with or without fever • History of Guillain-Barré Syndrome within 6 weeks of previous influenza vaccination • Adults who experience only hives with exposure to eggs may receive RIV or, with additional safety precautions, IIV[2]
Influenza, recombinant (RIV)	• Severe allergic reaction (e.g., anaphylaxis) after previous dose of RIV or to a vaccine component. RIV does not contain any egg protein[2]	• Moderate or severe acute illness with or without fever • History of Guillain-Barré Syndrome within 6 weeks of previous influenza vaccination

Influenza, live attenuated (LAIV)[2,3]	• Severe allergic reaction (e.g., anaphylaxis) to any component of the vaccine, or to a previous dose of any influenza vaccine
	• In addition, ACIP recommends that LAIV not be used in the following populations:
	  — pregnant women
	  — immunosuppressed adults
	  — adults with egg allergy of any severity
	  — adults who have taken influenza antiviral medications (amantadine, rimantadine, zanamivir, or oseltamivir) within the previous 48 hours; avoid use of these antiviral drugs for 14 days after vaccination
		• Moderate or severe acute illness with or without fever.
		• History of Guillain-Barré Syndrome within 6 weeks of previous influenza vaccination
		• Asthma in persons aged 5 years and older
		• Other chronic medical conditions, e.g., other chronic lung diseases, chronic cardiovascular disease (excluding isolated hypertension), diabetes, chronic renal or hepatic disease, hematologic disease, neurologic disease, and metabolic disorders

Tetanus, diphtheria, pertussis (Tdap); tetanus, diphtheria (Td)	• Severe allergic reaction (e.g., anaphylaxis) after a previous dose or to a vaccine component • For pertussis-containing vaccines: encephalopathy (e.g., coma, decreased level of consciousness, or prolonged seizures) not attributable to another identifiable cause within 7 days of administration of a previous dose of Tdap, diphtheria and tetanus toxoids and pertussis (DTP), or diphtheria and tetanus toxoids and acellular pertussis (DTaP) vaccine	• Moderate or severe acute illness with or without fever • Guillain-Barré Syndrome within 6 weeks after a previous dose of tetanus toxoid-containing vaccine • History of Arthus-type hypersensitivity reactions after a previous dose of tetanus or diphtheria toxoid-containing vaccine; defer vaccination until at least 10 years have elapsed since the last tetanus toxoid-containing vaccine • For pertussis-containing vaccines: progressive or unstable neurologic disorder, uncontrolled seizures, or progressive encephalopathy until a treatment regimen has been established and the condition has stabilized
Varicella[3]	• Severe allergic reaction (e.g., anaphylaxis) after a previous dose or to a vaccine component • Known severe immunodeficiency (e.g., from hematologic and solid tumors, receipt of chemotherapy, congenital immunodeficiency, or long-term immunosuppressive therapy,[4] or patients with human immunodeficiency virus [HIV] infection who are severely immunocompromised) • Pregnancy	• Recent (within 11 months) receipt of antibody-containing blood product (specific interval depends on product)[5] • Moderate or severe acute illness with or without fever • Receipt of specific antivirals (i.e., acyclovir, famciclovir, or valacyclovir) 24 hours before vaccination; avoid use of these antiviral drugs for 14 days after vaccination
Human papillomavirus (HPV)	• Severe allergic reaction (e.g., anaphylaxis) after a previous dose or to a vaccine component	• Moderate or severe acute illness with or without fever • Pregnancy
Zoster[3]	• Severe allergic reaction (e.g., anaphylaxis) to a vaccine component • Known severe immunodeficiency (e.g., from hematologic and solid tumors, receipt of chemotherapy, or long-term immunosuppressive therapy,[4] or patients with HIV infection who are severely immunocompromised) • Pregnancy	• Moderate or severe acute illness with or without fever • Receipt of specific antivirals (i.e., acyclovir, famciclovir, or valacyclovir) 24 hours before vaccination; avoid use of these antiviral drugs for 14 days after vaccination
Measles, mumps, rubella (MMR)[3]	• Severe allergic reaction (e.g., anaphylaxis) after a previous dose or to a vaccine component • Known severe immunodeficiency (e.g., from hematologic and solid tumors, receipt of chemotherapy, congenital immunodeficiency, or long-term immunosuppressive therapy,[4] or patients with HIV infection who are severely immunocompromised) • Pregnancy	• Moderate or severe acute illness with or without fever • Recent (within 11 months) receipt of antibody-containing blood product (specific interval depends on product)[5] • History of thrombocytopenia or thrombocytopenic purpura • Need for tuberculin skin testing[6]
Pneumococcal conjugate (PCV13)	• Severe allergic reaction (e.g., anaphylaxis) after a previous dose or to a vaccine component, including to any vaccine containing diphtheria toxoid	• Moderate or severe acute illness with or without fever
Pneumococcal polysaccharide (PPSV23)	• Severe allergic reaction (e.g., anaphylaxis) after a previous dose or to a vaccine component	• Moderate or severe acute illness with or without fever
Meningococcal, conjugate (MenACWY); meningococcal, polysaccharide (MPSV4)	• Severe allergic reaction (e.g., anaphylaxis) after a previous dose or to a vaccine component	• Moderate or severe acute illness with or without fever
Hepatitis A	• Severe allergic reaction (e.g., anaphylaxis) after a previous dose or to a vaccine component	• Moderate or severe acute illness with or without fever
Hepatitis B	• Severe allergic reaction (e.g., anaphylaxis) after a previous dose or to a vaccine component	• Moderate or severe acute illness with or without fever
Haemophilus influenzae Type b (Hib)	• Severe allergic reaction (e.g., anaphylaxis) after a previous dose or to a vaccine component	• Moderate or severe acute illness with or without fever

1. Vaccine package inserts and the full ACIP recommendations for these vaccines should be consulted for additional information on vaccine-related contraindications and precautions and for more information on vaccine excipients. Events or conditions listed as precautions should be reviewed carefully. Benefits of and risks for administering a specific vaccine to a person under these circumstances should be considered. If the risk from the vaccine is believed to outweigh the benefit, the vaccine should not be administered. If the benefit of vaccination is believed to outweigh the risk, the vaccine should be administered. A contraindication is a condition in a recipient that increases the chance of a serious adverse reaction. Therefore, a vaccine should not be administered when a contraindication is present.

2. For more information on use of influenza vaccines among persons with egg allergies and a complete list of conditions that CDC considers to be reasons to avoid receiving LAIV, see CDC. Prevention and control of seasonal influenza with vaccines: recommendations of the Advisory Committee on Immunization Practices (ACIP) — United States, 2014–15 Influenza Season. *MMWR* 2014;63(32):691–97.

3. LAIV, MMR, varicella, or zoster vaccines can be administered on the same day. If not administered on the same day, live vaccines should be separated by at least 28 days.

4. Immunosuppressive steroid dose is considered to be ≥2 weeks of daily receipt of 20 mg of prednisone or the equivalent. Vaccination should be deferred for at least 1 month after discontinuation of such therapy. Providers should consult ACIP recommendations for complete information on the use of specific live vaccines among persons on immune-suppressing medications or with immune suppression because of other reasons.

5. Vaccine should be deferred for the appropriate interval if replacement immune globulin products are being administered. See CDC. General recommendations on immunization: recommendations of the Advisory Committee on Immunization Practices (ACIP). *MMWR* 2011;60(No. RR-2). Available at www.cdc.gov/vaccines/pubs/pinkbook/index.html.

6. Measles vaccination might suppress tuberculin reactivity temporarily. Measles-containing vaccine may be administered on the same day as tuberculin skin testing. If testing cannot be performed until after the day of MMR vaccination, the test should be postponed for at least 4 weeks after MMR vaccination. If an urgent need exists to skin test, do so with the understanding that reactivity might be reduced by the vaccine.

* Adapted from CDC. Table 6. Contraindications and precautions to commonly used vaccines. General recommendations on immunization: recommendations of the Advisory Committee on Immunization Practices. MMWR 2011;60(No. RR-2):40–41 and from Atkinson W, Wolfe S, Hamborsky J, eds. Appendix A. Epidemiology and prevention of vaccine preventable diseases. 12th ed. Washington, DC: Public Health Foundation, 2011. Available at www.cdc.gov/vaccines/pubs/pinkbook/index.html.

† Regarding latex allergy, consult the package insert for any vaccine administered.

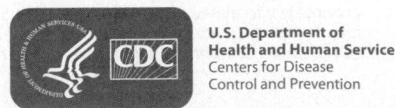

U.S. Department of Health and Human Services
Centers for Disease Control and Prevention

CS244083-F

Figure 6. Contraindications and precautions to commonly used vaccines in adults.

the overall number of injections a child or patient will receive. However, care must be taken to ensure that the individual vaccine entities are not administered too early and are not administered too many at once. This can be a challenge when patients switch clinics or in times of vaccine shortages.

More often, dosing intervals longer than recommended are encountered in the office. With the exception of oral live typhoid vaccine (Vivotif Berna), an interruption in the vaccination schedule does not require restarting the entire series of a vaccine or toxoid or addition of extra doses. When an unknown or uncertain vaccination status is encountered, every effort should be made to access records. If this cannot be done in a reasonable amount of time, these persons should be considered susceptible and started on the age-appropriate vaccination schedule. Serologic testing for immunity is an alternative to vaccination; however, commercial serologic testing might not always be sufficiently sensitive or standardized for detection of vaccine-induced immunity, and research laboratory testing might not be readily available.

Route of Administration

There are two orally administered vaccines in the United States: rotavirus (Rotarix, RotaTeq) and typhoid vaccines. Rotavirus is licensed for infants and does not need to be repeated if the vaccine is spit up or vomited. Typhoid vaccine capsules should be taken as directed by the manufacturer. Live, attenuated influenza vaccine (LAIV, FluMist) is the only intranasal vaccine available. It does not need to be repeated if the person coughs or sneezes immediately after administration. With the exception of bacille Calmette-Guerin (BCG) vaccine and smallpox vaccine,[10] injectable vaccines are administered by the intramuscular or subcutaneous route.

Storage

In general, vaccines need to be stored in a refrigerator or freezer. When vaccines are inappropriately stored, they can lose potency. Refrigerator and freezer storage units must be properly monitored and maintained to assure vaccine integrity. Temperature logs should be maintained for 3 years unless state or local authorities require a longer time. Vaccines that have been stored at inappropriate temperatures should not be administered. An office protocol should be established for handling inappropriately stored vaccines, procedures for follow-up when these vaccines are inadvertently given, emergency vaccine retrieval and storage, handling vaccine shipments, maintaining a vaccine inventory log, and rotating vaccine stock to avoid expiration. Care should be taken to store similar vaccine products (sound-alike or lookalike) away from each other (on different shelves) or by color-coding labels. Diphtheria toxoid-, tetanus toxoid-, and acellular pertussis-containing vaccines are easily confused.

Vaccine Safety

Vaccines in the United States undergo extensive safety and efficacy evaluations through the FDA licensing process. Despite this rigorous process, adverse reactions can and do occur. Adverse reactions are reportable to the Vaccine Adverse Event Reporting System (VAERS). VAERS is a national reporting system created in 1990 to unify the collection of all reports of adverse events after vaccination. Its primary purpose is detecting new or rare vaccine adverse events, increases in rates of known side effects, and risk factors for particular types of adverse events.

In 1986, the National Childhood Vaccine Injury Act established the Vaccine Injury Compensation Program (VICP). It is a no-fault program that covers all routinely recommended childhood vaccines. Those claims may be based on a vaccine injury table, which lists the adverse events associated with vaccines and provides a rebuttable presumption of causation, or by proving by preponderant evidence that the vaccine caused an injury not on the table. The table was created to provide swift compensation to those possibly injured by vaccines.

The provider's role to help ensure safety of vaccination includes proper vaccine storage and administration, timing and spacing of vaccine doses, observation of contraindications and precautions, and reporting adverse events to the VAERS.

Contraindications and Adverse Events

A contraindication is a condition in a recipient that increases the chance of a *serious* adverse reaction. A precaution is a condition in a recipient that *might* increase the chance or severity of an adverse reaction or compromise the ability of the vaccine to produce immunity. Situations do arise when the benefits outweigh the risks of a side effect. The only contraindication applicable to all vaccines is a history of a severe allergic reaction (anaphylaxis) after a previous dose of vaccine or to a vaccine component unless the recipient has been desensitized. Children who experienced encephalopathy within 7 days after administration of a previous dose of DTP,[2] DTaP (Daptacel, Infanrix), or Tdap (Adacel, Boostrix) not attributable to another identifiable cause should not receive additional doses of a vaccine that contains pertussis. The following are *not* contraindications to vaccination:
- Minor illness
- Diarrhea
- Mild or moderate local reaction or fever following a prior dose
- Antimicrobial therapy
- Disease exposure or convalescence
- Pregnant or immunosuppressed person in the household
- Premature birth
- Breast-feeding

Vaccination should be deferred for persons with a moderate or severe acute illness. This precaution avoids causing diagnostic confusion between manifestations of the underlying illness and possible adverse effects of vaccination or superimposing adverse effects of the vaccine on the underlying illness.

Vaccine adverse reactions are classified as local, systemic, or allergic. Allergic reactions might be caused by the vaccine antigen, residual animal protein, antimicrobial agents, preservatives, stabilizers, or other vaccine components. Anaphylaxis is rare and usually begins within minutes of vaccine administration. Children who have had an apparent severe allergic reaction to a vaccine should be evaluated by an allergist to determine the responsible allergen and to make recommendations regarding future vaccination.

Barriers

Barriers to appropriate and timely vaccination include patients' misconceptions, false contraindications, complexity of the immunization schedules, religious or philosophical beliefs, and cost. The Vaccines for Children Program (VCP) is a federally funded program that provides free ACIP-recommended vaccines to adolescents and children younger than 19 years old. This program has reduced the barrier of cost.

Recording Vaccinations

Health care providers who administer vaccines covered by the National Childhood Vaccine Injury Act are required to ensure that the permanent medical record of the recipient indicates the date the vaccine was administered, the vaccine manufacturer, the vaccine lot number, and the name, address, and title of the person administering the vaccine. In addition, the provider is required to record the edition date of the VIS distributed and the date those materials were provided. Patients should also keep a record of the immunizations they receive, when they were received, and at what facility they received them. A permanent vaccination record card should be established for each newborn infant and maintained by the parent or guardian.

[10]Available in the United States from the Centers for Disease Control and Prevention.

[2]Not available in the United States.

Immunization information systems (IIS), formerly referred to as immunization registries, are confidential population-based computerized information systems that collect and consolidate vaccination data from multiple health care providers within a geographic area. The CDC oversees a network of 64 IIS programs distributed throughout all 50 states, the District of Columbia, and eight U.S. territories. A fully operational IIS can prevent duplicate vaccinations, provide a complete record of immunizations if the patient has received vaccines from multiple sites, and offer catch-up and needed vaccine information. Although participation of a provider is voluntary, it is highly encouraged.

Special Populations
Children
Although infants are born with some level of immunoglobulin (Ig) G that is contributed from the mother via passive immunity, these levels generally decrease by 9 months of age, leaving them vulnerable to many infectious diseases. Infants begin developing IgG shortly after birth and continue to increase these levels throughout the first year of life, but they remain generally susceptible to infection until they achieve adult levels of IgG at 10 years of age. Therefore, this age group is especially important to vaccinate.

Breast-feeding
Neither inactivated nor live virus vaccines administered to a lactating woman affect the safety of breast-feeding for women or their infants. Breast-feeding is a contraindication for smallpox vaccination of the mother because of the theoretical risk for contact transmission from mother to infant. Yellow fever vaccine (YF-VAX) should be avoided. Breast-fed infants should be vaccinated according to the recommended schedule.

Pregnancy
No evidence exists of risk to the fetus from vaccinating pregnant women with inactivated virus or bacterial vaccines or toxoids. Live vaccines, such as smallpox, MMR, and varicella (Varivax), pose a theoretical risk to the fetus and therefore are generally contraindicated during pregnancy. New recommendations from ACIP advise to give all pregnant women a Tdap in every pregnancy. New data indicate that maternal antipertussis antibodies are short-lived; therefore, Tdap vaccination in one pregnancy will not provide high levels of antibodies to protect newborns during subsequent pregnancies. Alternatively, if Tdap is not administered during pregnancy, the woman should receive a dose of Tdap as soon as possible after delivery to ensure pertussis immunity and reduce the risk for transmission to the newborn regardless of when she last received a tetanus booster. Routine influenza vaccination is recommended for all women who are or will be pregnant (in any trimester) during influenza season, which usually occurs early October through late March.

Altered Immunocompetence
Persons with altered immunocompetence include those with primary and secondary causes of immunodeficiency as well as those with asplenia, chronic kidney disease, treatments with therapeutic monoclonal antibodies, and prolonged administration of high-dose corticosteroids. In general they should receive trivalent inactivated influenza virus (TIV, Fluzone) and age-appropriate polysaccharide-based vaccines (pneumococcal conjugate vaccine [PCV, Prevnar], pneumococcal polyvalent [PPSV, Pneumovax 23], meningococcal conjugate [MCV4, Menactra], meningococcal polysaccharide [MPSV4, Menomune] and haemophilus B conjugate [Hib, ActHib, PedvaxHib]). Persons with most forms of altered immunocompetence should not receive live vaccines (MMR, varicella, MMRV [ProQuad], LAIV, zoster [Zostavax], yellow fever, oral typhoid, BCG, and rotavirus).

Health Care Personnel
Health care personnel are considered to be at substantial risk for acquiring or transmitting hepatitis B, influenza, measles, mumps, rubella, pertussis, and varicella and should be counseled on appropriate vaccinations.

TRAVEL MEDICINE

Method of
Edward Dick, MD, MPH

Travelers increasingly seek out new destinations entailing health risks unfamiliar to most western physicians. Travel-acquired illness is no respecter of country of origin, age, sex, and social class. Although travel medicine typically involves prevention of infectious diseases, it is much more. Injuries and cardiovascular disease combined constitute the most common causes of mortality in foreign travelers. Travel medicine encompasses tropical, wilderness, adventure, occupational, and preventive medicine.

The goal of a travel medicine consultation is to maximize health while avoiding unneeded side effects and costs of drugs and immunizations. The goal should be to perform a risk assessment of individual patients based on their health status, risk aversion, all planned destinations, and purpose of visit. For example, a visitor to La Paz, Bolivia, might need very basic immunizations, advice on acclimatization, and prevention of traveler's diarrhea. However, if the person had a serious cardiac condition, a high-altitude stay might be contraindicated. If the same person took a side trip to the Amazon basin, malaria prophylaxis would be needed. If the patient were working on a medical team, a completed hepatitis B series would be needed.

A consultation includes six elements: general medical advice for all travelers, routine immunizations, routine travel vaccinations, geographically specific vaccines, vaccines for special circumstances, and drug prophylaxis, if indicated, for malaria, traveler's diarrhea (TD), and altitude illness.

Because local health conditions and appropriate prophylaxis change frequently, the travel medicine provider must use current resources to offer appropriate therapy. Standard sources include U.S. State Department Travel Advisories, Centers for Disease Control and Prevention (CDC) Traveler's Health Section, and commercial packages with broadly sourced recommendations such as Travax or TravelCare (Box 1).

The travel medicine consultation, like all medical visits, is a conversation regarding the patient's risks, benefits, alternatives in light of their own goals, health status, and resources. The inter-

---

Box 1 Pretrip Travel Itinerary Risk Assessment

Association for Safe International Road Travel
Road hazard travel reports: www.asirt.org

Centers for Disease Control and Prevention
Comprehensive travel reports and travel vaccination and preparation information including the online Yellow Book with information on country-specific risks and travel advice: www.cdc.gov/travel/

Travax
Commercial software-generated reports combining itinerary-specific recommendations on recommended travel vaccines and risks. Offers other services and resources for travel medicine providers. Shoreland, Inc., telephone: 800–433–5256, www.shoreland.com

Travel Care
Commercial software-generated reports with vaccine, prophylaxis, risk assessment, and other itinerary-specific advice. Travel Care International, telephone: 800–385–8560, https://www.travelcare.com/en/index.cfm

U.S. Department of State
Travel warnings: http://travel.state.gov/travel warnings

World Health Organization
General travel health information and access to their international travel guide and alerts: www.who.int/ith/en/

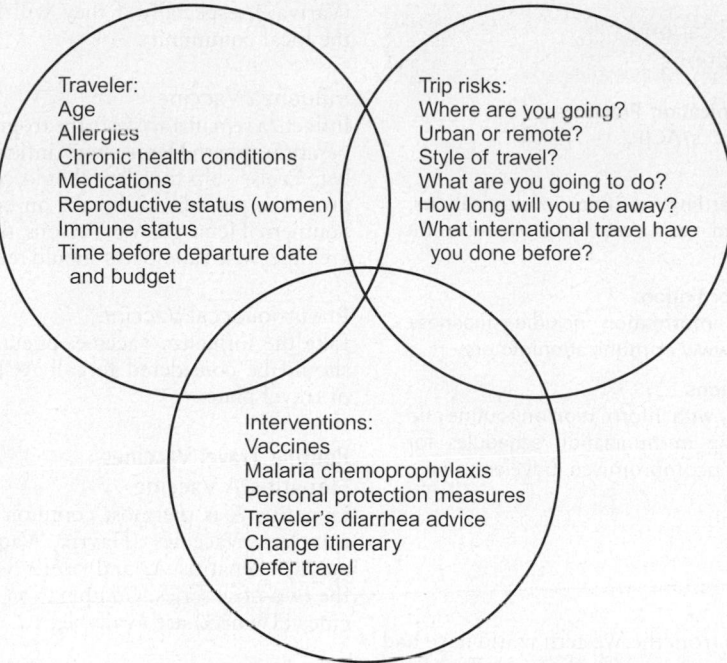

Figure 1. Pretravel decision matrix.

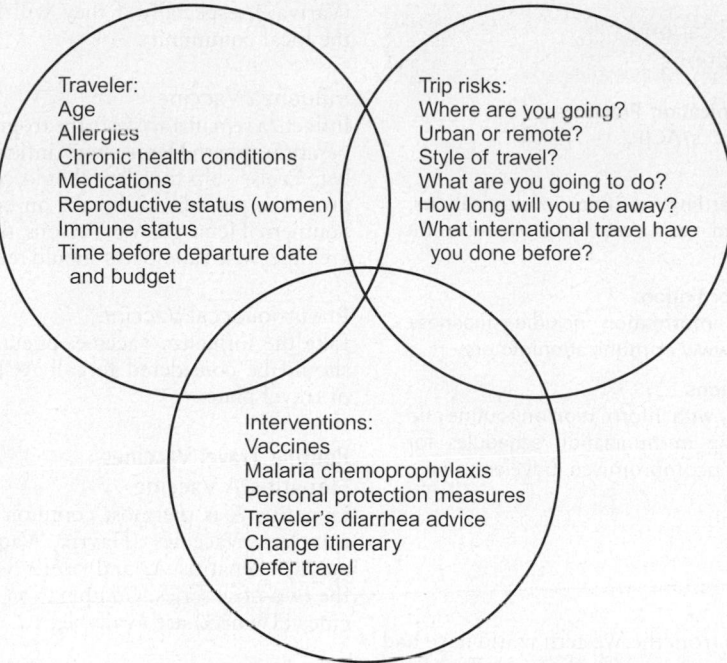

Traveler:
Age
Allergies
Chronic health conditions
Medications
Reproductive status (women)
Immune status
Time before departure date
    and budget

Trip risks:
Where are you going?
Urban or remote?
Style of travel?
What are you going to do?
How long will you be away?
What international travel have
    you done before?

Interventions:
Vaccines
Malaria chemoprophylaxis
Personal protection measures
Traveler's diarrhea advice
Change itinerary
Defer travel

Box 2   Traveler's Health History

International travelers should assemble the following information in a concise and clearly written form to carry with them.
- An up-to-date immunization record (preferably the International Certificates of Vaccination).
- A list of current medications giving both trade name and generic name and the actual dose.
- A list of all medical problems, such as hypertension, diabetes, asthma, and heart disease (cardiac patients should carry a copy of the most recent electrocardiogram).
- A list of known drug allergies.
- ABO blood type and Rh factor type.
- Name and telephone number (and fax number, if available) of his or her regular doctor (attach a business card to the health history document).
- Name and telephone number of the closest relative or friend in the United States who might assist if the traveler incurs serious illness while out of the country.

Adapted with permission from Jong E, Sanford C (eds): The Travel and Tropical Medicine Manual, 4th ed. Philadelphia, Saunders, 2008.

Box 3   Pretravel Preparation Recommendations

- Consult personal physician, local public health department, or travel clinic about recommendations for immunizations and malaria chemoprophylaxis after selecting the travel itinerary, but preferably 4 to 6 weeks before departure.
- Prepare a traveler's health history (see Box 2) and a traveler's medical kit (see Box 5).
- Carry a telephone credit card that can be used for international telephone calls, or make sure that the friends or relatives listed in the health history would accept an international collect call in case of an emergency.
- Make sure to have the telephone number of your personal physician, including office and after-hours numbers, and a fax number if available. A business card attached to the traveler's health history is a handy way to carry this information.
- Check the medical insurance policy or health plan for coverage for illness or accidents occurring outside the country of origin (home country).
- Specifically inquire if the regular insurance policy or health plan will cover emergency medical evacuation by an air ambulance.
- Arrange for additional medical insurance coverage or for a line of credit as necessary for a medical emergency situation.

Adapted with permission from Jong E, Sanford C (eds): The Travel and Tropical Medicine Manual, 4th ed. Philadelphia, Saunders, 2008.

---

section of these elements is illustrated by the Venn diagram in Figure 1. A useful tool for collecting the pretravel history is the International Travel Medical Questionnaire found in Shoreland's *Travel and Routine Immunization* text (see Box 1). Box 2 lists items that travelers should have at the consultation and carry with them while traveling.

General Medical Advice

As many as one third of travelers on a 14-day stay experience some form of illness. Most are self-limited, such as upper respiratory illnesses or diarrhea. Patients should have acute and chronic illnesses controlled, dental examinations current, medical and evacuation insurance that will cover them while abroad, a basic first aid kit, and enough of their prescription medicines for the entire trip.

Persons with chronic heart disease should bring a current electrocardiogram (ECG). Cruise ship travelers should follow the same advice because cruise ship infirmaries remain limited in their onboard resources. Box 3 outlines general pretravel steps the traveler should complete. Travelers returning to their country of origin should be aware that they retain similar risks as other nonnative travelers and should be prepared accordingly. Consult the sources in Box 4 for the details of the vaccines indications, contraindications, administration, storage, and accelerated schedules if approved or tested.

Advisory Committee on Immunization Practices
http://www.cdc.gov/vaccines/recs/ACIP/

Immunization Action Coalition
Comprehensive website regarding routine immunizations, patient education, and related resources: http://www.immunize.org/

Network for Immunization Information
Patient handouts and vaccine information including Japanese encephalitis and yellow fever: www.immunizationinfo.org

Travel and Routine Immunizations
Print resource updated annually with information on routine and travel immunizations including immunization schedules for special situations and immunocompromised travelers: www.shoreland.com, 800–433–5256

Routine Immunizations

It is assumed that most travelers from the Western world have had their routine childhood vaccinations or the illness itself and are immune. However, some destinations require a booster immunization. Also, one should be aware that some travelers born in the nonwestern world might not have had the same immunization schedules. Box 4 provides information about routine vaccinations. Travelers should have their vaccinations updated according to the current Advisory Committee on Immunization Practices (ACIP) recommendations, with attention to travel advisories and special circumstances. Shoreland's *Travel and Routine Immunizations* provides helpful summaries on routine and travel vaccines including accelerated schedules, if applicable. Checks of the CDC website or commercial travel software will alert the clinician to periodic outbreaks in the country of interest. Routine vaccinations are also covered elsewhere in this volume.

Measles–Mumps–Rubella Vaccine (MMR)

Measles remains a serious cause of morbidity and mortality in the non-Western world. Persons born in the United States in or before 1957 usually have measles immunity. All other persons should have had two doses of the MMR vaccine after age 12 months. Children traveling to endemic areas might need a first dose of MMR vaccine at age 9 months (some authors recommend age 6 months), but these children still need the standard two-dose schedule after age 12 months to ensure immunity.

Poliovirus Vaccine

The Western Hemisphere is polio-free, but polio remains active in the rest of the developing world, especially Africa. Outbreaks occur sporadically, including in mainland China. A single booster of poliovirus vaccine is recommended for travelers to endemic areas. The inactivated, injectable poliovirus vaccine (IPV, IPOL) is available for adults and children.

Tetanus–Diphtheria–Pertussis Vaccine

Outbreaks of diphtheria emerge periodically worldwide. Follow ACIP recommendations regarding use of the tetanus vaccine booster and the diphtheria toxoid, tetanus toxoid, and acellular pertussis (Tdap [Adacel, Boostrix]) vaccine boosters.

Varicella Vaccine

Varicella remains prevalent worldwide. The morbidity and mortality associated with varicella increases with age. Pregnant women and their unborn or newborn children may be especially prone to severe sequelae. Travelers without a history of the disease or documented immunity should consider receiving the series (Varivax), especially if they will be living in close proximity to the local community.

Influenza Vaccine

Influenza remains active in the tropical world year round. In the temperate Southern Hemisphere, influenza peaks from May to September. Cruise ship travelers should consider influenza immunization given the periodic outbreaks on board ships in the Northern and Southern Hemispheres. Persons traveling during flu season who are otherwise candidates should receive the vaccine if it is available.

Pneumococcal Vaccine

Like the influenza vaccine, pneumococcal vaccine (Pneumovax) should be considered for all ACIP-indicated persons regardless of travel plans.

Routine Travel Vaccines

Hepatitis A Vaccine

Hepatitis A is the most common vaccine-preventable disease of travelers. Vaccines (Havrix, Vaqta) provide 100% protection against hepatitis A, and protection lasts at least 10 years with the two-dose series. Combination hepatitis A and hepatitis B vaccines (Twinrix) are available.

Typhoid Vaccine

Although hepatitis A and typhoid are both spread by contaminated food and water, hepatitis A is 100 times more common than typhoid in travelers, with the developing world a particular foci. The efficacy of typhoid vaccines range from 40% to 90% in various published studies. Travelers staying in endemic areas longer than 3 weeks can benefit from the vaccine. The Indian subcontinent seems to be a focus of typhoid in travelers and might merit special consideration for the vaccine. The oral live, attenuated typhoid vaccine (Ty21A, Vivotif Berna) and injectable typhoid V1 polysaccharide vaccine (Typhim Vi) are preferred in terms of side-effect profiles.

Geographically Required Vaccines

Yellow Fever Vaccine (YF-VAX)

Under World Health Organization (WHO) rules, yellow fever vaccination is the only one that a country may routinely require for entry. Valid yellow fever vaccinations must be given at an authorized site, recorded on the WHO standardized yellow card, and completed 10 days before entry. Areas at risk for yellow fever transmission are in South America and Africa. WHO has updated its maps and recommendations. Periodically, unvaccinated Western travelers have contracted yellow fever after visiting at-risk areas. Infected mosquitoes spread yellow fever, so protection against insect bites should be stressed as well (see personal protection below). The WHO Strategic Advisory Group of Experts (SAGE) on Immunization now states that a booster dose of yellow fever vaccine may not be needed.

Cholera Vaccine

Vaccination against cholera can no longer be routinely required by any country under WHO rules. No cholera vaccine is currently licensed in the United States.

Japanese Encephalitis Vaccine

Japanese encephalitis (JE) is a mosquito-borne arbovirus disease. It is transmitted by mosquitoes and found primarily in China, Korea, the Indian subcontinent, and Southeast Asia. Areas of pig and rice farming hold the highest prevalence of JE. Although JE encephalitis has a mortality rate of up to 30%, only 55 cases of travel-associated JE were reported between 1973 and 2008, with most cases reported from Thailand and Bali. A killed-cell vaccine, IXIARO, is licensed in the United States for use for persons 17 years and older. ACIP and CDC have maps of at-risk areas and indications for use, especially options for pediatric travelers. Advise personal protection against mosquitoes.

Meningococcal Vaccine

Meningococcal meningitis has a May to July surge in the meningitis belt of Africa from May to July each year. Meningitis vaccine (Menactra, Menveo, Menomune) is required for haj pilgrims to Saudi Arabia. In the United States, outbreaks occur sporadically in close living quarters such as dormitories, and meningitis vaccines are included in ACIP recommendations for some U.S. populations. The vaccine protects only against the A, C, Y, and W-135 serogroups of meningitis. Serogroup B accounts for 40% of meningococcal cases.

Special Circumstances Vaccines

Hepatitis B Vaccine

Traditional risk factors for hepatitis B infection include receipt of contaminated blood products, intravenous drug use, tattooing, mother-to-child vertical transmission, and sexual intercourse. Studies of missionary families living for long periods in highly endemic areas demonstrate an as-yet poorly explained increased risk of hepatitis B in expatriates apart from traditional risk factors. Persons whose occupation or personal behavior places them at risk for contracting hepatitis B need the three-dose series (Engerix B, Recombivax HB). Long-term or frequent travelers to endemic areas should also consider the vaccine, because the local blood supply might not be screened. Combinations with hepatitis A vaccines are available.

Rabies Vaccine

Rabies exists worldwide, with only small pockets of the world being rabies-free. Dogs remain the primary vector, but bats are increasingly important sources. Persons such as veterinarians or mammologists whose work puts them into regular contact with animals should receive the three-dose series (Imovax rabies) and test of titers or booster immunizations. The decision to vaccinate travelers remains controversial. Persons with the three-dose preexposure series still require a two-dose postexposure series as soon as possible. Persons vaccinated before exposure do not need human rabies immune globulin (HRIG [HyperRab, Imogam Rabies]), which may be expensive, unavailable, or unreliable in the traveler's locale.

Children may be at higher risk for rabies exposure because of more-frequent contact with dogs and their failure to inform parents of incidental bites or scratches. If one is living, jogging, hiking, or biking through endemic areas, one can either confirm the availability of appropriate vaccines and rabies immune globulin and the funds to purchase them, or receive the three-dose preexposure series. The first strategy does not address unreported bites or scratches of children by rabid animals. The second strategy still requires a two-dose postexposure series. Rabies is also addressed elsewhere in this text.

Other Vaccines

A vaccine against tick-borne encephalitis (TBE) is available in Europe for travelers to endemic areas of Europe and Asia. The most active season is April through November in forested areas up to 4600 feet (1400 m) in altitude. Protection against tick exposure and avoiding unpasteurized milk is recommended. Current endemic maps and information on the vaccine can be found at http://www.tbe-info.com/tbe.aspx.

Malaria Prophylaxis

Malaria continues to kill millions of people worldwide. There are some 1500 cases of imported malaria in the United States every year. Malaria is transmitted by mosquitoes and involves four species of the parasite *Plasmodium*, with *Plasmodium falciparum* and *Plasmodium vivax* being the most common. First- and second-generation immigrants to the United States from their home countries are a major source of imported malaria because they do not use prophylaxis when returning to the endemic country. The CDC maintains a web page devoted to travelers and malaria (http://www.cdc.gov/malaria/) that includes a list of countries and regions with recommendations about prophylaxis. Further details and information on consultations with malaria experts is also listed on the website.

Because malaria is such an important and complex topic, the reader is referred to the malaria article in this text and encouraged to seek expert advice if there is any doubt about the approach to take with a patient. The Travax and TravelCare software also help map zones with likelihood of malaria transmission and choice of prophylaxis. In addition to the options recommended for each country, the CDC malaria site provides helpful tables for choosing among the particular chemoprophylaxis regimens and details on each drug. The decision tools are regularly updated and should be consulted before deciding on the best chemoprophylaxis options.

The traveler should be briefed on common and serious side effects of the drugs as well as when to start the medication before travel and how long to continue it once outside the endemic malarial zone. Travelers should be instructed if the drug is to be taken once daily (e.g., doxycycline [Doryx], atovaquone–proguanil [Malarone]) or once a week (e.g., mefloquine [Lariam] or chloroquine) because serious toxicities or drug failures have occurred when these drugs are taken improperly.

Personal protection against mosquito bites remains essential in addition to drug prophylaxis. Travelers to endemic areas who have symptoms of malaria should seek medical attention and note the areas of travel and prophylaxis used. Other drugs may be available in other countries or on the Internet, but they should be discouraged owing to lack of reliability or drug resistance. Special considerations for pediatric and pregnant travelers are on the CDC site as well.

Personal Protection

Drug prophylaxis against malaria is important, but reducing exposure to mosquitoes remains an integral part of disease prevention. Studies of permethrin-coated bed nets demonstrated significant reductions in malaria cases in African communities using no other prophylaxis. Travelers can protect themselves by sleeping under well-made, treated bed nets and employing a knock-down aerosol to treat the room.

A strategy of using diethyltoluanide (DEET) containing insecticides on exposed areas of skin and wearing clothing impregnated with permethrin significantly reduces mosquito bites. Picaridin (KBR 3023) is an acceptable DEET alternative. Concentrations of DEET up to 30% are safe for children and infants older than 2 months when eyes, hands, and mouth and mucous membranes are avoided. The concentration of DEET determines the length of protection; 35% DEET is effective from 6 to 8 hours. The mosquitoes that spread malaria are most active from dusk to dawn, but the mosquitoes that transmit dengue and yellow fever feed in the daytime. Use of permethrin-impregnated clothing can provide some protection when it is impractical to use a mosquito repellant applied to the skin.

Traveler's Diarrhea

The standard advice to "boil it, cook it, peel it, or forget it" may be inadequate to prevent traveler's diarrhea in all persons. The risk of acquiring diarrhea varies by location, person, and length of stay but ranges from 20% to 83% in travelers to the developing world. Most cases of traveler's diarrhea are self-limited, lasting no longer than 5 days. Nonetheless, traveler's diarrhea can force otherwise healthy persons to change or limit their travel activities. Depending on the region, season, and sensitivity of the testing used, *E. coli, Campylobacter, Salmonella, Shigella,* and Noroviruses tend to be the most common causes of traveler's diarrhea.

Prevention

Traveler's diarrhea is linked to contaminated food, beverages, and hands. Foods more often linked to diarrhea include reheated foods (such as quiche or casseroles), raw vegetables, raw meats (especially shellfish), unpasteurized milk products (also a source of brucellosis), buffet services, and raw berries. The key to food safety is keeping hot foods hot and cold foods cold. Water may be a less-important source of traveler's diarrhea than foods, but consuming pure water remains important. Carbonated beverages, alcoholic beverages without ice, and properly bottled water are safest. Ice from contaminated water can contaminate any drink, carbonated or alcoholic.

Water may be made safer at any altitude by bringing it to a boil and allowing it to cool covered. Various filtration devices are available commercially and must now meet Environmental Protection Agency (EPA) standards for their claims. Halogenation with iodine or chlorine is also an acceptable means to treat water. Frequent hand washing should be stressed regardless. Taking two 262-mg tablets of bismuth subsalicylate[1] (BSS [Pepto Bismol]) four times a day, preferably with a meal, can reduce the risk of traveler's diarrhea by 50%. Side effects of BSS include black tongue and stool and tinnitus. BSS should not be used with other salicylates or for longer than 3 weeks. Prophylactic antibiotic use offers few cost–benefit advantages, especially because treatment with antibiotics offers relief to most patients within 24 hours.

Treatment

At the onset of a loose bowel movement, a quinolone antibiotic plus loperamide (Imodium) provides relief to most persons within 24 hours. Because of increasing drug resistance to antibiotics worldwide, alternatives should be considered as well (Table 1) Adult travelers with traveler's diarrhea rarely lose significant electrolytes; therefore, specific replacement is rarely indicated. Children may have more-severe fluid and electrolyte losses, so oral rehydration remains paramount to any pediatric drug therapy. Packets of oral rehydration salts (ORS) are available in most pharmacies in the developing world, or a rice-based ORS called Ceralyte may be purchased before travel (available from Travel Medicine Inc., Box 5).

Adults with traveler's diarrhea should drink nonalcoholic beverages as often as desired and may benefit from a diet of rice, bananas, potatoes, and other complex carbohydrates. Probiotics have proved promising for reducing the risk or duration and severity of diarrhea but the they are likely more adjuvant than primary prevention or treatment. Persons with high fever, mucoid or bloody stools, or significant abdominal pain should seek medical attention as soon as possible.

Sexually Transmitted Diseases

Few travelers volunteer their intent of having sex while abroad, but sexual encounters with local inhabitants and other foreign nationals while traveling is not uncommon. Travelers need to be reminded of the higher incidence of sexually transmitted diseases

TABLE 1 Drugs for Treatment of Traveler's Diarrhea		
DRUG	**ADULT DOSAGE**	**COMMENTS**
Symptomatic Medications		
Bismuth subsalicylate (Pepto-Bismol)	30 mL (or 2 tabs) q30min × 8 doses	The maximum recommended dose is 240 mL/d (16 tabs)
Diphenoxylate + atropine (Lomotil)	2 tabs first dose; then 1 after each loose stool Do not exceed 8 tabs in 24 h	Antiperistaltic drug Do not use in dysentery Available by prescription
Loperamide (Imodium)	Take 2 caplets (2 mg each) for first dose, then 1 after each loose stool Do not exceed 8 caplets (16 mg) in 24 h	Antiperistaltic drug Do not use in dysentery Sold over the counter
Antibiotics		
Trimethoprim–Sulfamethoxazole (Bactrim, Septra)	160 mg/800 mg tab (1 DS tab) q12h × 3 d	Do not use in sulfa-allergic patients Less effective against TD in many areas of the world because of drug-resistance Drug of choice for *Cyclospora* (treat for 7 days)
Norfloxacin[1] (Noroxin)	400 mg tab q12h × 3 d	Do not use in pregnant women Do not use in children <18 y
Ciprofloxacin (Cipro)	500 mg tab q12h × 3 d *or* 750 mg tab once at start of diarrhea symptoms	Do not use in pregnant women Do not use in children <18 y
Levofloxacin[1] (Levaquin)	500 mg tab once Need for a 2nd or 3rd dose once daily determined by clinical response	Do not use in pregnant women Do not use in children <18 y
Azithromycin[1] (Zithromax)	1 g as a single oral dose *or* 500 mg once daily × 3 d	Drug of choice for quinolone-resistant *Campylobacter* strains Use for TD in persons unable to use fluoroquinolones
Rifaximin (Xifaxin)	200 mg tab tid × 3 d	Effective drug treatment for pathogen-negative TD in patients ≥ 12 y Poorly absorbed following an oral dose
Tetracycline[1]	2.5 g as a single oral dose *or* 500 mg qid × 3–5 d	Do not use in pregnant women Do not use in children <8 y Multiday regimen is less effective against TD in many areas of the world because of drug resistance
Doxycycline[1] (Vibramycin, Doryx)	100 mg tab bid–tid × 3–5 d	Less effective against TD in many areas of the world because of drug resistance Do not use in pregnant women or in children <8 y
Furazolidone[2]	100 mg tab q6h × 7–10 d	Alternative treatment for cholera

Abbreviations: DS = double strength; tab = tablet; TD = traveler's diarrhea.
Adapted with permission from Jong E, Sanford C (eds). The Travel and Tropical Medicine Manual, 4th ed. Philadelphia, Saunders, 2008.
[1]Not FDA approved for this indication.
[2]Not available in the United States.

> **Box 5** Prevention of Venous Thromboembolism in Long-Distance Travelers

- For long-distance travelers at increased risk of VTE (including previous VTE, recent surgery or trauma, active malignancy, pregnancy, estrogen use, advanced age, limited mobility, severe obesity, or known thrombophilic disorder), we suggest:
  - Frequent ambulation, calf muscle exercise, or sitting in an aisle seat if feasible (Grade 2C)
  - Use of properly fitted below-knee GCS providing 15 to 30 mm Hg of pressure at the ankle during travel (Grade 2C)
- For all other long-distance travelers, we suggest against the use of GCS (Grade 2C).
- For all long-distance travelers, we suggest against the use of aspirin or anticoagulants to prevent VTE (Grade 2C).

From Guyatt GH, Akl EA, Crowther M, et al. Executive summary: Antithrombotic Therapy and Prevention of Thrombosis, 9th ed: American College of Chest Physicians Evidence-Based Clinical Practice Guidelines. Chest. 2012;141:7S–47S. *Abbreviations:* GCS = graduated compression stockings; VTE = venous thromboembolism.

abroad, especially human immunodeficiency virus (HIV) infection and acquired immunodeficiency syndrome (AIDS). Condoms and oral contraceptives might not be readily available in some locations. Travelers free of familiar surroundings and restraints may be more likely to engage in risky sexual behavior. Encouragement of abstinence and "safer sex" may be indicated for travelers.

Other Travel Medicine Issues

Infectious diseases constitute the bulk of travel medicine visits. However, a number of other potential threats to a traveler's health merit attention for some travelers.

Altitude Sickness

Air travel makes rapid ascents in altitude possible with little time for acclimatization. Rapid ascent (less than 24 hours) to altitudes to over 2400 meters is associated with altitude sickness. Ideally, ascent rates less than 300 meters per day to altitudes over 2400 meters may reduce the risk of altitude sickness. A 2- to 4-day stay at an "intermediate" altitude of 6000–8000 feet may reduce but not eliminate the risk of altitude illness.

Acute mountain sickness is characterized by headache, dyspnea, nausea, vomiting, and mental status changes. It may be reduced or prevented in adults by taking acetazolamide (Diamox), 125 mg orally twice a day, for 1 day before ascent and continuing for 2 to 3 days on arrival at altitude. The safety of taking infants and children to altitude remains controversial because acute mountain sickness can be harder to diagnose, with only nonspecific symptoms such as irritability, poor feeding, and sleeplessness. Increasing hydration and rest and limiting exertion in the first few days of arrival help acclimatization. The definitive treatment of all forms of altitude sickness is descent to a lower altitude. All travelers experiencing difficulty at altitude should be ready to abandon the trip if symptoms persist or worsen.

Motion Sickness

Watercraft and motor vehicle travel can precipitate the nausea and light-headedness of motion sickness. Traveling on larger, modern cruise ships reduces motion sickness for some. Medications such as meclizine (Antivert), dimenhydrinate (Dramamine), or transdermal scopolamine (Transderm Scop) reduce symptoms of motion sickness but can induce sedation or dry mouth.

Air Travel

Various over-the-counter supplements, prescription drugs, special diets, and various sleep–wake recipes have been prescribed to combat jet lag, but none works sufficiently and consistently enough to recommend it. Avoidance of alcohol, frequent stretching or standing, and generous hydration make air travel more comfortable. Assuming the local time for activities may help the time-change adjustment. Venous thromboembolism (VTE) is increasingly recognized as an increased risk for long-distance travelers. The American College of Chest Physicians has released new guidelines for reducing the risk of VTE (2012) for long distance travelers (see Box 5).

Motor Vehicle Safety

Motor vehicles probably injure or kill more foreign travelers than most infectious diseases. When possible, use of available safety devices and avoidance of overcrowded vehicles and night driving reduce injury from motor vehicles. Driving a car or motorcycle abroad requires more vigilance than at home and should not be viewed as the opportunity to go native in manner or fail to use safety rules and equipment.

Sun, Heat, Water

Broad-spectrum sunscreens with protection against ultraviolet A and B should be used liberally as indicated. A sun protection factor (SPF) of 15 is probably sufficient. Sunscreens should be applied first and mosquito repellents applied second to preserve efficacy of both. A combination insect repellent and sunscreen product is available from Sawyer Products. Moderation in activities, frequent rehydration, and rest minimize risk of heat exhaustion and heat stroke.

Beaches may be contaminated with larvae. Wearing shoes and sunbathing with a towel can reduce cutaneous larval migrans. Marine environments pose their own threat of envenomations and decompression illnesses. Travelers should be properly trained, outfitted, and cautious in all water activities. Fresh water may be infested with schistosomes, especially in Africa.

Conclusion

The scope of travel medicine continues to expand and requires effort by the physician to maintain currency. In addition to providing pretravel advice, the travel medicine practitioner must be prepared to follow traveler's post-travel concerns. Space does not permit detailed discussion, but a few items merit discussion. First, one should consider the diagnosis of malaria in returned travelers who develop a fever 7 or more days after the start of travel, regardless of prophylactic measures taken. Second, most acute cases of diarrhea do not need extensive work-up unless the patient is severely ill or has failed appropriate self-treatment or if diarrhea persists beyond 7 days. Additional assistance with travel medicine questions may be obtained from travel medicine providers and organizations (Box 6).

> **Box 6** General Travel Medicine Resources

American Society of Tropical Medicine and Hygiene
Training and certification of travel medicine providers. The website has a listing of travel medicine clinics and clinicians: www.astmh.org

International Association for Medical Assistance to Travelers
Worldwide listing of medical doctors and travel clinics that may be of assistance to travelers while abroad: http://www.iamat.org

International Society of Travel Medicine
Training in travel medicine and travel medicine clinicians: www.istm.org

Wilderness Medical Society
Adventure and remote medicine training and clinicians: http://www.wms.org

Travel Medicine, Inc.
Travel supplies including permethrin-treated clothing, water purification, and mosquito repellents: http://www.travmed.com

References

Bazemore A, Huntington M. The pretravel consultation. Am Fam Physician 2009;80:583–90.

Chen LH, Hill DR, Wilder-Smith A. Vaccination of travelers: How far have we come and where are we going? Expert Rev Vaccines 2011;10:1609–20.

Guyatt GH, Akl EA, Crowther M, et al. Executive summary: Antithrombotic Therapy and Prevention of Thrombosis, 9th ed: American College of Chest Physicians Evidence-Based Clinical Practice Guidelines. Chest 2012;141:7S–47S.

Jong E, Sanford C, editors. The Travel and Tropical Medicine Manual. 4th ed. Philadelphia: Saunders; 2008.

LaRocque RC, Jentes ES. Health recommendations for international travel: a review of the evidence base of travel medicine. Curr Opin Infect Dis 2011;24:403–9.

Shoreland. Travel and Routine Immunizations. Milwaukee: Shoreland; 2012.

Tonellato DJ, Guse CE, Hargarten SW. Injury deaths of US citizens abroad: New data source, old travel problem. J Travel Med 2009;16:304–10.

World Health Organization. Revised recommendations for yellow fever vaccination for international travellers, 2011. Wkly Epidemiol Rec 2011;86:401–11.

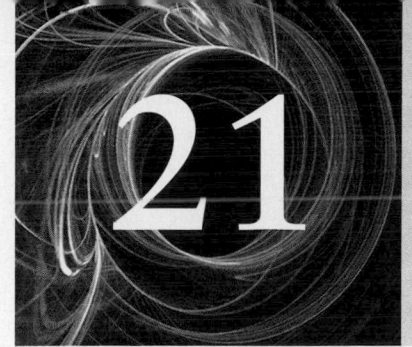# 21 Physical and Chemical Injuries

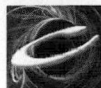# BURN TREATMENT GUIDELINES

Method of
Barbara A. Latenser, MD

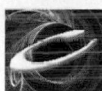# CURRENT DIAGNOSIS

- Have a high index of suspicion.
- Remember the ABCs.
- Rule out concomitant trauma.
- Establish size and depth of the burn.
- Chemical and electrical burns may be misleading.
- Establish resuscitation requirements.

CURRENT THERAPY

- Communicate with your burn center early and often.
- Remember the ABCs.
- Cover the wound with plastic wrap.
- Prevent hypothermia.
- Transport to the burn center.

The initial management of the severely burned patient follows guidelines established by the American College of Surgeons. It is crucial that the patient be managed properly in the early hours after injury because the initial management of a seriously burned patient can significantly affect the long-term outcome. Optimal burn-care criteria have been established and refined by the American Burn Association over the past 20 years.

Because of regionalization, it is common for the initial care of the seriously burned patient to occur outside the burn center. Burns are a specialized form of trauma. Therefore, the ABCDE is the same as for the trauma patient: airway with cervical spine immobilization if appropriate, breathing, circulation, disability, and exposure. Also remember that the burn patient could be a victim of associated trauma. It is easy to be sidetracked by the obvious thermal injury. Only after the primary and secondary surveys have been performed should you evaluate the severity of the burn injury. Obtain as much information as possible regarding the incident and about the patient. An easy way to remember the information is the mnemonic AMPLE: *a*llergies, *m*edications, *p*ast medical history, *l*ast meal, *e*vents. Universal precautions appropriate for each burn patient must be implemented by every member of the health care team.

The most commonly used guide for making an initial estimate of the second- and third-degree burns is the rule of nines (Figure 1). Various anatomic regions are roughly 9% of the total body surface area (TBSA) or multiples thereof. To calculate scattered burn areas, the patient's palm, including fingers, represents approximately 1%

of the TBSA. A much more precise estimate of burn area is provided by the Lund–Browder diagram (Figure 2).

By drawing in the areas that are burned, the burn area necessary for calculating resuscitation requirements can be determined. The Parkland formula for the first 24 hours following a burn is

$$4 \text{ mL Ringer's lactate} \times \text{body weight in kg} \times \% \text{ BSA burned}$$

Half the calculated amount is given in the first 8 hours and the rest over the remaining 16 hours. Patients with burns more than 10% TBSA likely require resuscitation. Patients with burns more than 20% TBSA are prone to gastric dilatation and should have a nasogastric tube. If you are considering the hourly urine output, then a urinary catheter is necessary.

Intravenous fentanyl or morphine sulfate is indicated for control of pain associated with burns. Drugs should not be administered by IM or SC routes because absorption is erratic. To calculate fluid needs, weigh the patient or estimate the preinjury weight. Reliable peripheral veins should be used to establish an IV line. Use vessels underlying burned skin if necessary. If it is impossible to establish peripheral IV access, an intraosseous line may be necessary and may be used in patients of any age. If you are unable to insert an intraosseous line, central venous access may be necessary using a short fluid infusion line made specifically for large-volume resuscitations.

The burn wound should be covered with a clean, dry sheet to prevent air currents from causing pain in the burned areas and to decrease fluid losses and hypothermia. Although there are many common topical antimicrobials in use, the optimal dressing before transferring the patient to the burn center is plastic wrap such as Saran Wrap. Topical antimicrobials are washed off upon arrival to the burn center, causing patient discomfort and mechanical trauma to the wound. Cold applications are appropriate only in small burns because they rapidly lead to hypothermia. Ice should never be applied because it will deepen the zone of ischemia in a thermal injury.

Escharotomies and/or fasciotomies are rarely required before transfer to the burn center, unless transfer is delayed beyond 24 hours. Patients most at risk are those with very large TBSA burns, circumferential full-thickness burns, and those with electrical injury. Circumferential chest and abdominal burns can restrict ventilatory excursion. A child has a more pliable rib cage and might need an escharotomy earlier than an adult burn patient. If you are considering performing an escharotomy, discuss it with the accepting burn physician before proceeding.

How do you know which patients should be referred to a burn center? To guide your decision making, there are currently 10 burn unit referral criteria. You should have a written transfer agreement in place with a referral burn unit. The agreement should specify which patients will be referred, what stabilization is expected, who arranges transportation, and what the patient will need during transport.

Partial-Thickness Burns More than 10% Total Body Surface Area

Second-degree, or partial-thickness, burns involve a variable portion of dermis. The skin may be red, blistered, and edematous. Because sensory nerves are damaged and/or exposed, these wounds are typically very painful. Healing time is proportional to the depth of dermal injury. Scarring is minimal if healing occurs

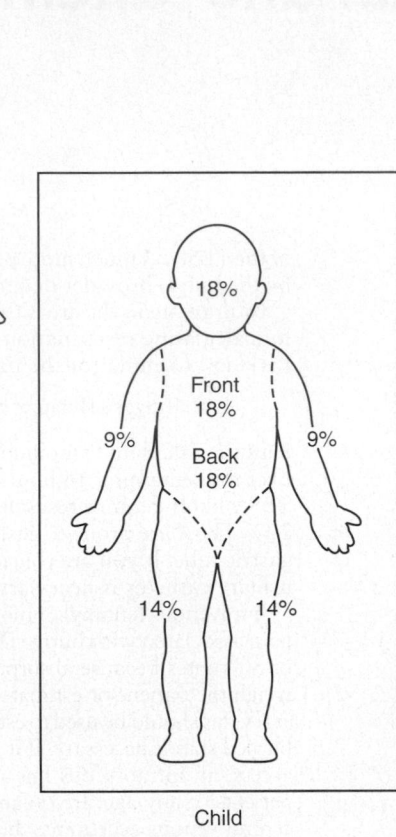

Figure 1. Rule of nines.

9%

1%

Front
18%

Back
18%

9%   9%

18%   18%

Adult

18%

Front
18%

Back
18%

9%   9%

14%   14%

Child

in 14 days or less. With closure time beyond 3 weeks, scarring will occur, the degree being greater in darker-skinned patients.

Proper fluid management is critical to the survival of patients with extensive burns. Fluid resuscitation is aimed at maintaining tissue perfusion and organ function while avoiding the complications of inadequate or excessive fluid therapy. Shock and organ failure, most commonly acute renal failure, can occur as a consequence of hypovolemia in a patient who has an extensive burn and who is inadequately resuscitated. The increase in capillary permeability caused by the burn is greatest in the immediate post-burn period, and diminution in effective blood volume is most rapid at that time. A marked increase in peripheral vascular resistance accompanied by a decrease in cardiac output occurs in the first 18 to 24 hours after injury.

In the presence of increased capillary permeability, colloid content of the resuscitation fluid exerts little influence on intravascular retention during the initial hours after the burn. Crystalloid fluid is the initial resuscitation of burn patients. Always remember, estimates are inexact. Each patient reacts differently to burn injury and resuscitation. The actual volume of fluid infused should be varied from the calculated volume as indicated by physiologic monitoring. The patient's general condition reflects the adequacy of fluid resuscitation and should be assessed and reassessed. Mental status, anxiety, and restlessness may be signs of hypoxemia, hypovolemia, or pain.

Although urine output does not guarantee tissue perfusion, it remains the most readily available and generally reliable guide to resuscitation. Adults should produce 0.5 mL/kg of urine per hour. Children should produce urine at the rate of 1.0 mL/kg per hour, and infants 12 months or younger should produce 2.0 mL/kg per hour. Oliguria is most commonly the result of inadequate fluid administration. Diuretics are contraindicated; the rate of resuscitation should be increased by 10% of the initial rate for 1 hour and reassessed. During the first 24 hours, neither the

hemoglobin nor hematocrit is a reliable guide to resuscitation, and using either leads to overresuscitation. For resuscitation failures or patients with burns greater than 25% TBSA, colloid should be added at the start of resuscitation. One method is hetastarch (Hespan) at 20 mL/kg per day for adults and 15 mL/kg per day for children. Hetastarch should be given only for 24 hours owing to the increased bleeding risks.

Measuring blood pressure (BP) by a sphygmomanometer may be misleading in a burned limb with progressive edema formation. As the swelling increases, the signal becomes diminished. If fluid infusion is increased based on this finding, edema formation may be exaggerated. Even intraarterial monitoring may be unreliable in patients with massive burns because of peripheral vasoconstriction secondary to marked elevation of catecholamines. Heart rate is also of limited usefulness in monitoring fluid therapy. The level of tachycardia depends upon the normal heart rate in each child.

Burns that Involve the Face, Hands, Feet, Genitalia, Perineum, or Major Joints

Facial burns are considered a serious injury. The possibility of respiratory tract damage must be considered. Because of the rich blood supply and loose areolar tissue of the face, facial burns are associated with extensive edema formation. To minimize this edema, keep the head of the bed elevated at 30 degrees. Cool saline compresses on the face can also help. Careful examination of the eyes should be completed as soon as possible because the rapid onset of eyelid swelling will make this difficult. Fluorescein (Fluorets) should be used to identify corneal injury. Chemical burns to the eyes should be rinsed with copious amounts of saline. Burns of the ears require examination of the external auditory canal and eardrum before swelling occurs.

Minor burns of the hands might result in only temporary disability and inconvenience. More-extensive thermal injury can

Figure 2. Lund–Browder classification of burn size.

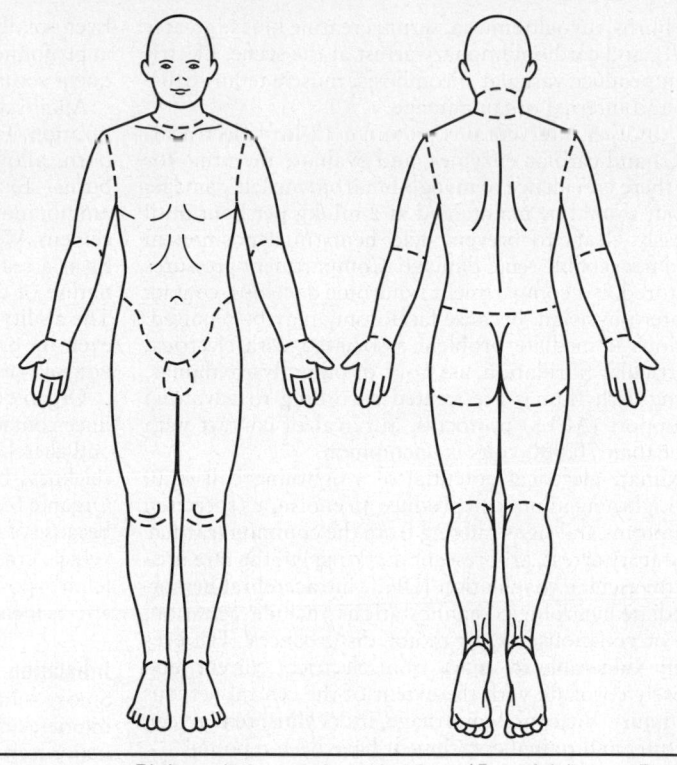

	Birth 1 yr.	1–4 yrs.	5–9 yrs.	10–14 yrs.	15 yrs.	Adult	Burn size estimate
Head	19	17	13	11	9	7	
Neck	2	2	2	2	2	2	
Anterior trunk	13	13	13	13	13	13	
Posterior trunk	13	13	13	13	13	13	
Right buttock	2.5	2.5	2.5	2.5	2.5	2.5	
Left buttock	2.5	2.5	2.5	2.5	2.5	2.5	
Genitalia	1	1	1	1	1	1	
Right upper arm	4	4	4	4	4	4	
Left upper arm	4	4	4	4	4	4	
Right lower arm	3	3	3	3	3	3	
Left lower arm	3	3	3	3	3	3	
Right hand	2.5	2.5	2.5	2.5	2.5	2.5	
Left hand	2.5	2.5	2.5	2.5	2.5	2.5	
Right thigh	5.5	6.5	8	8.5	9	9.5	
Left thigh	5.5	6.5	8	8.5	9	9.5	
Right leg	5	5	5.5	6	6.5	7	
Left leg	5	5	5.5	6	6.5	7	
Right foot	3.5	3.5	3.5	3.5	3.5	3.5	
Left foot	3.5	3.5	3.5	3.5	3.5	3.5	

Total BSAB _____

cause permanent loss of function. Monitoring the digital and palmar pulses with an ultrasonic flowmeter is the most accurate means of assessing perfusion of the tissues in the hand. The burned extremity should be elevated above the heart to minimize edema formation. Digital escharotomies are not indicated before transfer to a burn center. Contact the accepting burn center physician if you are concerned about the extent of the digital injury. As with burns of the upper extremity, it is important to assess the circulation and neurologic function of the feet on an hourly basis.

Third-Degree Burns in Any Age Group
A full-thickness, or third-degree, burn occurs with destruction of the entire epidermis and dermis, leaving no dermal elements to repopulate. A characteristic initial appearance is a waxy white color. Full-thickness injuries require emergent management. In most cases, treatment of the wound requires surgical skin grafting.

Deep partial-thickness and full-thickness burns heal with severe scarring if not treated by surgical excision and skin grafting for optimal recovery. There is also a high risk of infection, because an unexcised deep partial- or full-thickness burn behaves like an undrained abcess. Even with skin grafting, disfigurement is common, and long-term functional problems can persist for years.

Electric Burns, Including Lightning Injury
Electrical burns can be divided into flash (typical thermal injury) and high-tension injury. The latter, caused by more than 1000 volts, produces clinically characteristic entry and exit wounds. They are usually ischemic, painless, and dry; wounds of entry might appear charred and the exit wound explosive. Deep muscle injury may be present even when skin appears normal. Findings that suggest electrical injury include loss of consciousness, paralysis or mummification of an extremity, loss of peripheral pulses,

flexor surface burns, myoglobinuria, serum creatine kinase greater than 1000 IU/L, and cardiopulmonary arrest at the scene. Electrical injuries can produce vascular thrombosis, muscle tetany causing fractures, and internal organ damage.

In addition to other interventions, obtain a 12-lead electrocardiogram (ECG) and cardiac enzymes, and evaluate the urine for myoglobin. If there is evidence of myoglobin from muscle damage, the urine output should be maintained at 2 mL/kg per hour until the urine grossly clears to prevent acid hematin deposition in the kidney and irreversible renal damage. Compartment pressures must be monitored. If a compartment syndrome develops, contact your burn center physician, because fasciotomy may be required. The most serious immediate problem associated with electrical injuries is ventricular fibrillation, asystole, or other dysrhythmias. Life-threatening arrhythmias are treated according to advanced cardiac life support (ACLS) protocols. Survival of contact with voltage greater than 70,000 volts is uncommon.

The approximate electrical potential of a lightning bolt is 20 million volts. Lightning injury can produce an enormous spectrum of clinical symptoms and signs ranging from the common (cardiac asystole, respiratory arrest, arborescent markings) to the rare (disseminated intravascular coagulation [DIC], intracerebral hemorrhage). Immediate neurologic manifestations include agitation, amnesia, loss of consciousness, or motor disturbances. The eyes are particularly vulnerable to injury from electrical current, and symptoms closely correlate with the extent of the central nervous system (CNS) injury. Vitreous hemorrhage, iridocyclitis, retinal tear, macular puncture, and retinal detachment have been reported.

Lightning injuries are not usually associated with deep burns but most often with superficial injury to the skin and underlying soft tissue called ferning. The feathering type of burn appears as an arborescent, branching skin marking that disappears within a few days. Pathognomonic of lightning injury, ferning may be of great diagnostic value in a comatose patient. Often the respiratory arrest lasts longer than the cardiac arrest. Severely injured victims often present in asystole or ventricular fibrillation. Cardiac resuscitation is, on occasion, successful, but direct brain trauma as well as blunt trauma, skull fracture, and intracranial injuries are common in these patients. The prognosis for neurologic recovery in these patients is usually poor.

Chemical Burns

Health care providers must wear protective clothing when caring for patients with potential chemical injury. The initial appearance of a chemical burn is usually deceptively benign. The severity of a chemical injury is related to the agent, concentration, volume, duration of contact, and mechanisms of action of the agent. Immediate irrigation decreases the concentration and duration of contact, reducing the severity of injury. If the agent is a powder, brush it off and then irrigate with water. Irrigation should continue through emergency evaluation in the hospital and, in general, until evaluation in a burn center, especially for an alkali or an unknown agent. Neutralizing agents are contraindicated owing to the potential for heat generation, thereby giving the patient both a chemical and a thermal injury.

Acid burns are usually less severe than alkali burns. Acids are found in many household products including bathroom cleansers, drain cleaners, and swimming pool acidifiers. Tissue is damaged by coagulation necrosis and protein precipitation. Once a layer of eschar is formed, the burning process is self-limiting.

The exception to this rule is hydrofluoric acid, used to etch glass, make Teflon, and remove rust. The pathogenesis of tissue damage in hydrofluoric acid burns is distinct from other acids. Hydrofluoric acid readily crosses lipid membranes and has a potent diffusing capacity into the tissues. The molecule releases the freely dissociable fluoride ion, which produces extensive liquefactive necrosis of the soft tissues. Fluoride rapidly binds free calcium in the blood, and death from hypocalcemia can occur. Treatment for small surface area burns from dilute hydrofluoric acid is 10 mg calcium gluconate diluted in 30 mL K-Y jelly. For nondilute hydrofluoric acid, treatment is intravenous calcium gluconate administered until the characteristic pain out of proportion to the burn has resolved.

Even small areas of nondilute hydrofluoric acid contact can result in profound hypocalcemia and death. Cardiac monitoring and frequent serum calcium determinations are indicated.

Alkalis damage tissue by liquefaction necrosis and protein denaturation. Tissue pH abnormalities can persist for 12 hours after the burn, allowing deeper spread of the chemical and more-severe burns. Examples include the hydroxides, caustic sodas, and ammonium compounds found in oven cleaners, fertilizer, and cement. Wet cement damages skin in three ways: allergic dermatitis as a reaction to chromate ions, abrasions caused by the gritty nature of the cement, and burns as an alkali with a pH of 12.5. The ability of cement to cause such injury is not well recognized, even by professional users. With the increased interest in do-it-yourself projects, it is likely that this problem will increase.

Organic compounds such as creosote and petroleum products produce contact chemical burns as well as systemic toxicity. Gasoline and diesel fuel are petroleum products that can produce a full-thickness burn that initially appears to be only partial thickness. Organic compounds cause cutaneous damage by delipidation because of their fat solvent action on cell membranes. After a motor vehicle crash involving petroleum products, always look for petroleum exposure in the lower extremities, back, and buttocks. Systemic effects include elevated liver enzymes and decreased urinary output.

Inhalation Injury

Smoke-inhalation injuries are the leading cause of fatalities from burn injuries, accounting for some 80% of all fire-related deaths. The major forms of inhalation injuries are carbon monoxide (CO) toxicity, injury to the upper airway, and pulmonary parenchymal damage. Each has different symptoms and signs, treatment, and prognosis.

The compromised airway is protected by tracheal intubation, and respiratory failure is treated with assisted ventilation. Inhalation injury is manifested by the pathology and dysfunction that rapidly become evident in the airways, lungs, and respiratory system after inhaling the products of incomplete combustion. Patients receiving massive fluid resuscitation can develop upper airway edema with subsequent asphyxiation.

Immediate medical attention and diagnosis depend on a high index of suspicion, an appropriate history, careful examination of the upper airway, the presence of clinical symptoms, and suggestive arterial blood gases. An inhalation injury is suspected in any patient with full-thickness facial burns or with any burns combined with a history of being confined within an enclosed space. Other classic signs are soot or carbonaceous sputum, stridor or hoarseness, or blistering of the pharynx or vocal cords. Late signs include grunting, nasal flaring, retractions, wheezes, and rales. Use of prophylactic antibiotics and steroids is discouraged.

The effect of CO poisoning may be exhibited by respiratory symptoms and CNS findings such as altered level of consciousness, seizures, or coma. Cardiovascular effects include diminished cardiac output evidenced by decreased perfusion and hypotension. There is much controversy regarding hyperbaric oxygen therapy, but there are no objective data proving the efficacy of hyperbaric oxygen in CO poisoning. At this time, hyperbaric oxygen treatment for acute CO toxicity should be restricted to randomized prospective studies. The correct treatment is administering 100% oxygen, thereby decreasing the CO half-life from 4 hours to 45 minutes.

Burn Injury in Patients with Preexisting Medical Disorders that could Complicate Management, Prolong Recovery, or Affect Mortality

Peripheral vascular disease can lead to a decrease in wound blood flow. Diabetes, through high blood glucose, impedes capillary flow. Optimum control of the blood glucose is needed to optimize blood flow. A local decrease in wound tissue oxygen tension is recognized to be a major impediment to wound healing because all phases of healing are oxygen dependent, including local infection control. The most common causes are a decrease in systemic blood volume and oxygen delivery, decrease in hemoglobin saturation, eschar on the wound surface, or infection. Treatment modalities need to focus first on correction of systemic abnormalities:

correcting cardiovascular and lung function, correcting large-vessel obstructive disease impeding wound flow, aggressive wound débridement, and eliminating tissue exudates. Patients with preexisting cardiac disease are particularly sensitive to fluids and might tolerate the necessary fluid resuscitation poorly.

Patients with Burns and Concomitant Trauma

In patients with burns and concomitant trauma (such as fractures) in which the burn injury poses the greatest risk of morbidity and mortality, if the trauma poses the greater immediate risk, the patient may be initially stabilized in a trauma center before being transferred to a burn unit. Physician judgment is necessary in such situations and should be in concert with the regional medical control plan and triage protocols.

Most burn–trauma publications cite a 5% incidence of burn and trauma. Because burn–trauma is rare outside of a major conflict or disaster, most centers see only a few patients annually. By definition, child abuse falls into the burn–trauma category. It may be the burn injury that prompts relatives or neighbors to bring the child to the hospital or report the family to authority. The visibility of the injury can instigate corrective action. In a 44-month review, we saw 120 cases of burns and trauma. Although motor vehicle crashes can result in fracture, soft tissue, and thermal injury, unique to this burn–trauma population was that the crash injury was often a result of assault. With the graying of America, elder abuse could also become a larger societal problem.

Burned Children in Hospitals without Qualified Personnel or Equipment for the Care of Children

Each year more than 2500 children die and 10,000 more sustain permanent disability from thermal injury. Children are not just little adults! They respond differently than adults do to severe trauma, maintaining normal vital signs longer but then decompensating rapidly. Owing to the smaller cross-sectional diameter of the pediatric airway, it takes much less edema to compromise a child's airway. If intubation is required, the most experienced pediatric airway manager should intubate the child because repeated attempts may create sufficient airway edema to cause obstruction. Anatomic airway differences make intubation by the inexperienced even more difficult.

The greater surface area per unit body mass of children necessitates the administration of relatively greater amounts of resuscitation fluid. The surface area–to–body mass relationship of the child also defines a lesser intravascular volume per unit surface area burned. This makes the burned child more susceptible to fluid overload and hemodilution. Hypoglycemia can occur if the limited glycogen stores of the child are rapidly exhausted by the early postburn elevation of circulating levels of steroids and catecholamines. Children under 10 kg or 12 months of age should receive maintenance fluids with 5% dextrose in addition to the resuscitation fluids outlined in the consensus formula. Children younger than 2 years have disproportionately thin skin so that exposures that would produce only partial-thickness burns in older patients produce full-thickness injuries. Children have a relatively small muscle mass, hampering intrinsic heat generation. Children younger than 6 months are unable to shiver and thus are even more prone to develop hypothermia.

Stress for the burned child not only includes the TBSA burn and the pain that is involved but also the separation from parents and loved ones. This escalates, especially if the parents were also burned in the fire. Emergency management of each pediatric burn patient requires an individualized care plan. Early consultation with the burn center physician is advised.

Burn Injury in Patients Who Require Special Intervention

Some patients with burn injuries require special social, emotional, and/or long-term rehabilitative intervention. Failure to recognize the thermal manifestations of child abuse not only negates protection of the child but also predicates potential lethal injury. Awareness of the patterns of abuse, the behavior patterns of the parents, and the physical manifestations will protect the child by early recognition and reporting. Children who are victims of physical abuse often present with thermal injuries of varying degrees. The history of injury should correlate with the physical findings. The history

also becomes important in identifying repetitious hospital visits for accidental injury. Not infrequently, the hospital visits are made to different hospitals to avoid disclosure and identification.

The events leading to an injury are extremely important in the initial evaluation of an infant or child. Always consider the potential for child abuse. The incidence of child abuse is approximately 10% of all children presenting to an emergency department, with a mortality rate less than 1%. Abused children present with a higher median Injury Severity Score, more-severe injuries of the head and integument, longer hospital lengths of stay, and a higher mortality rate than if the burns were accidentally incurred.

Summary

A burn of any magnitude can be a serious injury. Health care providers must be able to assess the injuries rapidly and develop a priority-based plan of care. The plan of care is determined by the type, extent, and degree of burn as well as by available resources.

Burn care is complex. It involves a multisystem assessment and appropriate intervention. The first 24 hours of management are perhaps the most critical for the patient's survival. Burn centers provide optimal care in a cost-effective, multidisciplinary manner. Every health care provider must know how and when to contact the closest burn center. If the attending physician determines that the patient should be treated at the burn center, the extent of treatment provided at the referring hospital—and the method of transport to the burn center—should be decided in consultation with the burn center physician. A complete list of verified burn centers is available at http://ameriburn.org.

References

American Burn Association. Advanced Burn Life Support Course. Chicago: American Burn Association; 2001.

American College of Surgeons, Committee on Trauma. Resources for Optimal Care of the Injured Patient. Chicago: American College of Surgeons; 2006.

Andrews CJ, Cooper MA, Darveniza M, Mackerras D, editors. Lightning Injuries: Electrical, Medical, and Legal Aspects. Boca Raton: CRC Press; 1992.

Burd A. Hydrofluoric acid—revisited. Burns 2004;30:720–2.

Chang DC, Knight V, Ziegfeld S, et al. The tip of the iceberg for child abuse: The critical roles of the pediatric trauma service and its registry. J Trauma 2004;57:1189–98.

Chung JY, Kowal-Vern A, Latenser BA, et al. Cement-related injuries: Review of a series, the National Burn Repository, and the prevailing literature. J Burn Care Res 2007;28:827–34.

Hayek SN, Wibbenmeyer LA, Kealey LD, et al. The efficacy of hair and urine toxicology screening on the detection of child abuse by burning. J Burn Care Res 2009;30:587–92.

Heimbach DM. Regionalization of burn care—a concept whose time has come. J Burn Care Rehabil 2003;24(3):173–4.

Latenser BA. Critical care of the burn patient: The first 48 hours. Crit Care Med 2009;37:2819–26.

Latenser BA, Iteld L. Smoke inhalation injury. Semin Respir Crit Care Med 2001;22:13–22.

Luce EA. guest editor. Special issue: Burn care and management. Clin Plast Surg 2000;27(1).

Varghese TK, Kim AW, Kowal-Vern A, et al. Frequency of burn-trauma patients in an urban setting. Arch Surg 2003;138.1292–6.

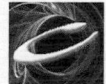

DISTURBANCES DUE TO COLD*

Method of
Jerrold B. Leikin, MD; Scott M. Leikin, BA; Frederick K. Korley, MD; and Ernest Wang, MD

CURRENT DIAGNOSIS

- Accidental hypothermia may be classified as mild, moderate, or severe.
- The measured temperature should be the core body temperature.
- The method of rewarming depends on the severity of the temperature drop.

---

*Portions of this chapter have been previously printed in *Conn's Current Therapy* 2009–2012. The content of this chapter has also appeared in *Disease-a-Month* 2012;58(1)6–32.

- The complications of rewarming include arrhythmias, rewarming-related hypotension, core temperature after drop, and rhabdomyolysis.
- Patients can be declared dead only after they are warm.

CURRENT THERAPY

Mild Hypothermia: 32.2 °C (90 °F) to 35 °C (95 °F)
- Start passive external rewarming; remove wet clothing.
- Ambient temperature should exceed 21.0 °C (70.0 °F).
- Cover patient with insulating material.

Moderate Hypothermia: 28 °C (82.4 °F) to 32.2 °C (90 °F)
- Start active external rewarming; use radiant heat.
- Use thermal mattresses and electric heating blankets.
- Use forced-air heating blankets.
- Perform active core rewarming; use warmed humidified oxygen.
- Give warmed intravenous saline.
- Give bladder, colonic, and gastric irrigation.
- Start pleural cavity lavage.
- Avoid alcohol, caffeine, and nicotine (tobacco).

Severe Hypothermia: Less than 28 °C (82.4 °F)
- Begin aggressive active core rewarming; use warmed, humidified oxygen.
- Give warmed intravenous saline.
- Give bladder, colonic, and gastric irrigation.
- Start pleural cavity lavage.
- Perform peritoneal lavage or dialysis.
- Perform extracorporeal warming or heated cardiopulmonary bypass.

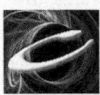

CURRENT THERAPY

Frostnip
- Gentle rewarming, generally in a water bath of 104 °F to 108 °F (40 °C to 42 °C).
- It is usually self-resolving.

Frostbite
- Immerse in warm (not hot) water.
- Débride broken vesicles.
- Do not débride hemorrhagic or intact blisters
- Apply topical aloe vera[7] or antibiotic ointment.
- Use NSAIDs for pain.
- Update tetanus status.
- Do not rub or massage the affected area.
- Do not use a heating pad or heat lamp; affected areas can be easily burned.
- Avoid alcohol and tobacco products.

Chilblain
- Rewarm gently.
- Nifedipine (Procardia)[1] may be useful.

Trench foot
- Dry the foot.
- Rewarm gently.
- Use NSAIDs for pain.

---

[1]Not FDA approved for this indication.
[7]Available as dietary supplement.

Accidental Hypothermia

Hypothermia is classically defined as a reduction in the body's core temperature below 95.0 °F (35.0 °C). Most reported cases of hypothermia are due to environmental exposure to low ambient temperatures (accidental hypothermia). Other causes of hypothermia include sepsis, severe hypothyroidism (myxedema coma), acute spinal cord injury, diabetic ketoacidosis, multisystem trauma, and prolonged cardiac arrest.

Epidemiology

Risk factors for developing hypothermia include extremes of age (elderly people might not be able to remove themselves from cold environments, and young children lose heat more rapidly because of their increased total body surface area), major trauma, homelessness, psychiatric illness, and drug and alcohol abuse (Box 1). Cold-related deaths also are reported in military combatants

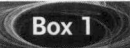

Box 1 Factors Predisposing to Hypothermia or Frostbite

Physiologic
Decreased Heat Production
Age extremes (infants, elderly)
Dehydration or malnutrition
Diaphoresis or hyperhidrosis
Endocrinologic insufficiency
Hypoxia
Insufficient fuel
Overexertion
Physical conditioning
Prior cold injury
Trauma (multisystem or extremity)

Increased Heat Loss
Burns
Dermatologic malfunction
Cold infusions
Emergency resuscitation
Poor acclimatization or conditioning
Shock
Vascular diseases

Impaired Thermoregulation
Central nervous system trauma or disease
Metabolic disorders
Pharmacologic or toxicologic agents
Sepsis
Spinal cord injury

Psychological
Fatigue
Fear or panic
Hunger
Intense concentration on tasks
Intoxicants
Mental status or attitude
Peer pressure

Environmental
Altitude with or without associated conditions
Ambient temperature or humidity
Duration of exposure
Heat loss (conductive, evaporative, radiative, convective)
Quantity of exposed surface area
Wind chill factor

Mechanical
Constricting or wet clothing or boots
Inadequate insulation
Immobility or cramped positioning

and outdoor winter sports participants. Several drugs and chemicals can predispose to hypothermia (Box 2). Alcohol is the most common intoxicant associated with hypothermia because of its ability to cause cutaneous vasodilation, impairment of shivering, and impairment of adaptive behavior.

Between 1979 and 2002, 16,555 deaths in the United States, an average of 689 per year, were attributed to exposure to low environmental temperatures. In 2002, of the 646 hypothermia-related deaths reported, 66% occurred in male patients, 52% of all decedents were aged 65 years or younger, 45% of the deaths occurred among white male patients, and 14% occurred among black male patients. The states of Alaska, New Mexico, North Dakota, and Montana had the largest overall death rates from hypothermia in 2002. The lowest recorded core temperature in a pediatric survivor of accidental hypothermia is 57.9 °F (14.4 °C) and the lowest in an adult survivor is 56.7 °F (13.7 °C).

Pathophysiology

The normal range of human core temperature is 97.5 °F (36.4 °C) to 99.5 °F (37.5 °C). Humans are thus warm-blooded and are normally able to maintain their body temperature by heat-generating mechanisms and heat-conserving behavior. These compensatory responses, however, can be overwhelmed under extreme environmental conditions, leading to hypothermia.

The anterior hypothalamus coordinates the nonshivering heat conservation and dissipation mechanisms, and the posterior hypothalamus coordinates shivering thermogenesis. Heat loss usually occurs by four mechanisms: About 55% to 65% of heat is lost by radiation, 25% to 30% by evaporation from the skin and respiratory tract, and 10% to 15% by conduction and convection. The amount of heat lost via conduction is markedly increased in cold-water immersion (by about 32-fold). Each organ system is affected uniquely by hypothermia.

Skin

Cutaneous blood flow is regulated by the individual's thermoregulatory needs, modulated by neural control through the arteriovenous anastomoses located in the extremities. Sympathetic tone is increased, which leads to arteriovenous constriction, which is maximum at 59 °F (15 °C). Cold-induced vasodilatation can occur at 50 °F (10 °C).

Cardiovascular System

One of the initial heat-conserving mechanisms is peripheral vasoconstriction to decrease blood flow to the skin. There are also initial increases in heart rate and blood pressure owing to a catecholamine surge. At core temperatures below 82.4 °F (28.0 °C), bradycardia can result from a decrease in spontaneous depolarization of the pacemaker cell firing. The myocardium also becomes irritable, predisposing it to bradyarrhythmias and hypotension.

Atrial arrhythmias can occur with a slow ventricular response and they can precede ventricular arrhythmias and asystole at core temperatures below 77.0 °F (25.0 °C). The characteristic Osborn or J waves (a hump seen at the QRS-ST junction) may be seen on the electrocardiogram (ECG) at core temperatures below 89.6 °F (32.0 °C). Orthostasis also commonly occurs.

Renal System

Renal blood flow is increased by peripheral vasoconstriction, leading to cold-induced diuresis. Antidiuretic hormone activity is usually inhibited. This results in intravascular volume depletion, subsequent vasodilation, to increase renal blood flow and, ultimately, acute renal failure. Urinary output can increase threefold and this may be accentuated with concomitant ethanol use.

Respiratory System

At core temperatures below 82.4 °F (28 °C), minute ventilation is reduced; bronchorrhea can occur, with a loss of cough and gag reflexes leading to an increased risk for aspiration. Carbon dioxide production drops by one-half for every 14 °F (8 °C) drop in temperature, and oxygen consumption is reduced by 75% at 72 °F (22 °C). Apnea can then result.

Central Nervous System

Cerebral metabolism is depressed 6% to 7% per 1 °C decrease in core temperature. Cerebrovascular autoregulation remains intact until below 77.0 °F (25.0 °C), which helps maintain cortical blood flow. Electroencephalographic activity is clearly not prognostic, but it is abnormal below 92 °F (33 °C) and it silences around 66.2 °F to 68.0 °F (19.0 °C to 20.0 °C).

Coagulation

Because of depression of enzymatic activity of the activated clotting factors, clotting time (particularly partial thromboplastin time [PTT]) is prolonged. At 84 °F (29 °C), a 50% increase of PTT can be expected. Thrombocytopenia also commonly occurs due to bone marrow suppression along with splenic and hepatic platelet sequestration, which can be exacerbated by cryoglobinemia.

Clinical Presentation

Accidental hypothermia is classified as mild at body temperatures of 90 °F (32.2 °C) to 95 °F (35 °C), moderate at body temperatures of 82.4 °F (28.0 °C) to 90 °F (32.2 °C), or severe at body temperatures less than 82.4 °F (28 °C).

In general, a patient's symptoms depend on the severity of the temperature drop. Patients with mild hypothermia can develop vigorous shivering and cold diuresis. Those with moderate hypothermia can have a paradoxical decrease in shivering, slurred speech, hyporeflexia, and confusion. They might have Osborn J waves on the ECG. They are also at risk for intravascular thrombosis. Splanchnic vasoconstriction, gastric erosions, hepatic necrosis, and pancreatitis can occur. Prominent laboratory abnormalities include leukopenia (from splenic sequestration), thrombocytopenia (during rewarming), hypoglycemia, respiratory or metabolic acidosis, and hyperkalemia. Fetal bradycardia can occur in response to maternal hypothermia, but long-term sequelae are unknown.

During severe hypothermia, shivering gives way to rigor, minute ventilation decreases, and heart rate and cardiac output decrease. Cardiac instability can be seen at this stage and can manifest in the form of arrhythmias, heart blocks, and eventually asystole. Neurologically, the patient's mental status declines. The patient might attempt to undress (paradoxical undressing) and might respond only to painful stimuli, have decreased gag reflexes, and eventually become apenic. Generally, at about 68.0 °F (20.0 °C), patients become totally neurologically unresponsive, lose corneal and ocular reflexes, and can have a flat electroencephalogram (EEG).

Emergency Department Evaluation

Typically, the source of hypothermia is revealed from the patient's history; however, it is very important to rule out secondary causes of hypothermia, such as sepsis, hypothyroidism, central nervous system lesions, and hypoglycemia, among others. All patients arriving in the emergency department with hypothermia need a complete evaluation to rule out traumatic injuries and drug or toxin ingestion or overdose.

As in all resuscitation, attention should be paid to the ABCs (airway, breathing, and circulation). Successful neurologic recovery has been documented following five hours of cardiopulmonary resuscitation in the setting of profound accidental hypothermia (62.4 °F or 16.9 °C). Respiratory failure should be treated with endotracheal intubation and mechanical ventilation. Hypotension can be treated initially with warmed fluids. Placing the patient in a warm environment, removing all cold and wet clothes, and remembering to cover up the patient after he or she has been exposed should help prevent further heat loss.

The temperature should be confirmed by checking a core temperature (e.g., rectal, bladder, or esophageal), using a thermometer

Box 2   Drugs and Chemicals that can cause Hypothermia

Medicinals
Acetaminophen (Tylenol)
N-Acetylcysteine (Mucomyst)
β-Adrenergic blocking agents
Alprostadil (Caverject, Muse)
Amphotericin B (Fungizone)
Atropine
Azithromycin (Zithromax)
Baclofen (Lioresal)
Barbiturates
Benzodiazepines
Bethanechol (Urecholine)
Biperiden (Akineton)
Bromocriptine (Parlodel)
Carbamazepine (Tegretol)
Chloral hydrate (Noctec)
Chlorpromazine (Thorazine)
Clonidine (Catapres)
Colchicine (Colcrys)
Delorazepam (Dadumir)[2]
Diazepam (Valium)
Diltiazem (Cardizem)
Enfluran[2]
Erythromycin
Ethchlorvynol (Placidyl)[2]
Ethyl alcohol
Fenoprofen (Nalfon)
Fluphenazine (Prolixin)
Fosphenytoin (Cerebyx)
Gallium nitrate (Ganite)
Glutethimide (Doriden)[2]
Guanabenz (Wytension)
Guanfacine (Tenex)
Haloperidol (Haldol)
Halothane (Fluothane)
Heroin
γ-Hydroxybutyrate (as sodium salt [Xyrem])
Ibuprofen (Advil, Motrin)
Immune globulin
Insulin preparations
Interferon β-1b (Betaseron)
Iobitridol (Xenetix)[2]
Iopanic acid (Telepaque)
Ipsapirone[2]
Isoflurane (Forane)
Lincomycin (Lincocin)
Lithium (Eskalith, Lithobid)
Lormetazepam[2]
Loxapine (Loxitane)
Magnesium sulfate
Maprotiline (Ludiomil)
Mefenamic acid (Ponstel)
Melatonin
Methyldopa (Aldomet)
Methyprylon (Noludar)[2]

Moricizine (Ethmozine)
Morphine sulfate
Naphazoline (Naphcon)
Nitrofurantoin (Macrodantin)
Nitrous oxide
Olanzapine (Zyprexa)
Omeprazole (Prilosec)
Oseltamivir (Tamiflu)
Oxcarbazepine (Trileptal)
Oxymetazoline (Afrin)
Penicillin V
Phencyclidine (PCP)
Phenol
Phenytoin (Dilantin)
Pilocarpine (Salagen)
Prazosin (Minipress)
Propoxyphene (Darvon)[2]
Procarbazine (Matulane)
Propylthiouracil (PTU)
Quinine (Quinamm)
Rauwolfia serpentine
Reserpine
Risperidone (Risperdal)
Salicylate
Spectinomycin (Trobicin)[2]
Terazosin (Hytrin)
Tetracycline (Sumycin)
Tetrahydrozoline (Visine, Opti-Clear)
Thioridazine (Mellaril)
Topiramate (Topamax)
Tretinoin (topical) (Retin-A)
Triazolam (Halcion)
Tricyclic antidepressants
Valproic acid and derivatives (Depakene)
Zinc sulfate

Nonmedicinals
Acrylamide
Aldicarb
Amitraz
Ashwagandha
Barium
Bis(chloromethyl) ether
Boron hydrides
Bromophos
Cadmium oxide
Carbon disulfide
Carbon monoxide
Castor pornace
Chloralose
Chlorfenvinphos
Chloryrifos
Copper fumes
Coumaphos
Cyanide
Diazinon Dichlorvos

Dicrotophos
Dioxathion
Disulfoton
Ether
Ethion
Fensulfothion
Fenthion
Hexachlorobenzene
Hyaluronidase (Hylenex)
Hydrochloric acid
Hydrogen sulfide
Isopropyl alcohol
Lewisite
Lobelia
Mace
Malathion
Metal fume fever
Methidathion
Methiocarb
Methomyl
Methyl bromide
Methylene chloride
Methylparathion
Nickel carbonyl
Parathion
Profenofos
Pyrimidifen
Sarin
Sodium azide
Terbufos
Tetraethyl pyrophosphate
Tetrafluoroethylene
Thiocyanates
Vacor
Zinc fumes (zinc oxide)

Biologicals
Ackee fruit poisoning
Brown recluse spider
Ciguatera food poisoning
Clostridium perfringens
Clupeotox
Copperhead envenomation
Cotton mouth envenomation
Delphinium
Lobelia
Marijuana (Cannabis)
Monkshood
Nutmeg
Salmonella food poisoning
Selenious acid fume
Star of Bethlehem (Hippobroman longiflora)
Streptococcus food poisoning
Tetrodotoxin food poisoning
White chameleon

[2]Not available in the United States.

capable of recording very low temperatures. Patients should be placed on a cardiac monitor and an ECG should be obtained. Laboratory testing is especially useful in the postresuscitative period, when complications begin. Laboratory tests should include a complete blood count (CBC), a chemistry panel, creatine phosphokinase (CPK) to evaluate for rhabdomyolysis, a coagulation profile, blood type and screen, an arterial blood gas, and a drug screen. A Foley catheter should be placed to assess urinary output.

Rewarming Strategies

There are several methods of rewarming. The method of choice usually depends on the severity of hypothermia. During rewarming, the patient should be placed on a cardiac monitor with frequent measurements of blood pressure and temperature (via a rectal probe) for easy detection of complications of rewarming, such as rewarming-related hypotension, arrhythmias, and core temperature after-drop. It should be noted that the human body is capable of raising the body temperature through heat generation by approximately one degree centigrade per hour.

Passive External Warming
Passive external warming is ideal for patients with mild hypothermia (greater than 93 °F or 34 °C) who are otherwise healthy. It uses the patient's endogenous heat production for rewarming and it involves simple, logical passive maneuvers that minimize heat dissipation. When using this method, all wet clothing should be removed and the patient should be covered with insulating materials. Patients warmed easily using this method can be safely discharged.

Active External Rewarming
Active external rewarming should be considered for patients with core temperatures between 86 °F and 92 °F (30 °C to 34 °C). It involves exposing the patient's skin to exogenous heat sources. Radiant heat, thermal mattresses, electric heating blankets, and forced-air heating blankets are some of the available techniques.

This method has several disadvantages. First, burn injuries can occur to the vasoconstricted skin. Second, any sort of immersion can hinder monitoring and other resuscitative activities. Finally and most important, active external rewarming produces a phenomenon called *core-temperature after drop*. This refers to a drop in core temperature resulting from sudden peripheral vasodilation. This causes cold, acidic blood to return to the core. Hypotension and potentially fatal dysrhythmias can result. Focusing on rewarming the trunk only (rather than the trunk and extremities) can prevent these temperature gradients. In general, active external rewarming is used in conjunction with active core rewarming.

Active Core Rewarming
Active core rewarming involves techniques to deliver direct heat internally. It should be used in patients with moderate to severe hypothermia (under 86 °F or 30 °C). The simplest method entails the administration of heated, humidified oxygen at 107.6 °F to 114.8 °F (42.0 °C to 46.0 °C) and intravenous saline solution warmed to 109.4 °F (43.0 °C). Saline should be administered via a central line at 150 to 200 mL/h. Gastric, bladder, and colonic irrigations have been used, but their relatively small surface areas usually limit their effect.

Another method of active core rewarming is pleural irrigation using two large-bore (36 °F or greater) thoracostomy tubes. One tube is placed at the midclavicular line and is connected to saline at 107.6 °F (42.0 °C). The other tube is placed at the posterior axillary line and connected to a chest tube drainage kit.

A more-aggressive method of active core rewarming is via peritoneal lavage and dialysis. This can be accomplished using a standard diagnostic peritoneal lavage kit and introducing an 8-F catheter into the peritoneum using Seldinger's technique. The crystalloid dialysate should be warmed at 104.0 °F to 113.0 °F (40.0 °C to 45.0 °C). This method affords the added advantage of allowing the serum potassium level to be adjusted.

The most efficient and physiologic active core rewarming method is via extracorporeal warming or heated cardiopulmonary bypass. This is the method of choice for the most-severe cases, patients with severe rhabdomyolysis, and patients who require cardiopulmonary resuscitation.

Most arrhythmias are corrected by rewarming. Atropine is typically ineffective for cold-associated bradydysrhythmias. Ventricular tachycardia and fibrillation require electrocardioversion and the use of bretylium (not available in the United States) if it is available. Dopamine, epinephrine,[1] and vasopressin (Pitressin)[1] may be effective vasopressors. Empiric antibiotics may be given. However, the empiric use of levothyroxine (Synthroid)[1] and corticosteroids may be hazardous. Phenytoin (Dilantin) might have cardiacdepressant qualities in the moderately hypothermic patient. Box 3 demonstrates drugs with possible decreased metabolism or clearance with resultant increase in toxicity in hypothermia.

---

[1]Not FDA approved for this indication.

Indicators of grave prognosis include development of profound hyperkalemia (serum potassium greater than 10 mEq/L), underlying medical conditions, intravascular thrombosis (fibrinogen less than 59 mg/dL), pH less than 6.5, and a core temperature less than 50.0 °F to 53.6 °F (10.0 °C to 12.0 °C).

Peripheral Cold Injuries
Peripheral cold injuries span a spectrum ranging from minimal to severe tissue damage. Freezing and nonfreezing syndromes can cause these injuries. Frostnip and frostbite are caused by exposure to freezing temperatures. *Frostnip* refers to the numbness and blue-white discoloration of the face and extremities that occur during exposure to freezing temperatures. It is a precursor to frostbite. It is characterized by reversible skin changes, including blanching and numbness with no permanent tissue damage, unlike frostbite. Nonfreezing injuries depend on whether the ambient environment during exposure was wet (trench or immersion foot) or dry (pernio or chilblain).

Pathophysiology
During exposure to cold temperatures, the core body temperature is preserved to the detriment of the extremities. Frostbite occurs in four stages: prefreeze, freeze–thaw, vascular stasis, and late ischemic stages. The prefreeze phase occurs when the temperature of the extremities falls below 50.0 °F (10.0 °C) and cutaneous sensation is lost. Vasoconstriction also occurs along with leakage of intracellular fluid into the interstitium.

The freeze–thaw phase begins at the freezing point of water (32.0 °F or 0 °C) with the formation of ice crystals extracellularly. This further enhances the exit of water from the intracellular space under osmotic forces, resulting in cell shrinkage and, ultimately, damage. During the vascular stasis phase, plasma leakage and formation of ice crystals continue. Arachidonic acid breakdown products are then released from underlying damaged tissue. Both prostaglandin $F_{2\alpha}$ and thromboxane A_2 produce platelet aggregation, leukocyte immobilization, and vasoconstriction.

Endothelial cells are sensitive to cold injury, and the microvasculature becomes distorted and clogged, leading to tissue ischemia. The late ischemic phase is characterized by ischemia, thrombosis, continued shunting, gangrene, autonomic dysfunction, and denaturation of tissue proteins. The tissue can eventually mummify and demarcate more than 60 to 90 days later.

Clinical Presentation of Local Extremity Issues
Frostnip and Frostbite
The face and ears are the most common sites prone to cold injury, followed by the hands and feet. Patients with frostnip usually have blanching and numbness of their fingertips. The skin has a firm or waxy texture. Often the patient is unaware of these changes. Frostnip is usually reversible. Frostbite has been classified as superficial, affecting the skin and subcutaneous tissue, or deep, affecting the bones, joints, and tendons. When a superficial frostbite is rewarmed, the skin can form a clear blister; however, when a deep frostbite is rewarmed, it can form a hemorrhagic blister. This

classification, however, has no therapeutic or prognostic value given that frostbites can initially appear benign. Many weeks can pass before the demarcation between viable and nonviable tissues becomes apparent. Facial frostbite, with skin blistering, can also occur following halogenated (especially fluorinated) hydrocarbon inhalation abuse. This can appear initially as angioneurotic edema if it involves the oral mucosa membranes.

Although no prognostic factors can be entirely predictive, favorable factors include retained sensation, normal skin color, and clear rather than cloudy fluid in the blisters, if present. Poor prognostic features include nonblanching cyanosis, firm skin, and dark, fluid-filled blisters. Patients can present with pain, numbness, and a clumsy "chunk of wood" sensation in the affected extremity. The pain is initially described as a dull ache and evolves to become a throbbing sensation in about 48 to 72 hours.

Chilblain

Chilblain, also referred to as perniosis, results from repetitive exposure to cold, dry air. It manifests as painful erythematous nodules or cyanotic lesions often referred to as cold sores. These lesions usually develop on exposed surfaces after a delay of 12 to 14 hours and are characterized by pruritus and burning paresthesias. Young women, especially those with Raynaud's phenomenon and/or a low body mass index, are at risk.

Chilblains are located on acral skin associated with cold exposure. They are usually located on the dorsum of the fingers, toes, and thighs, where blisters or ulcerations can develop in very severe cases. Perivascular lymphocytic infiltration with vacuolation of the basal layer is often seen on histologic analysis, especially when it is associated with an autoimmune disease (particularly lupus erythematosus).

Susceptibility to chilblains increases when the ambient temperature is less than 10 °C and relative humidity is 60%.

Trench Foot and Immersion Foot

Trench foot occurs as a result of prolonged exposure to a damp, cold, nonfreezing environment (with temperature as high as 60 °F). It has been classically described among soldiers in World War I, many of whom were confined to cold and damp trenches for prolonged periods. Symptoms include numbness and painful paresthesias that can progress to a throbbing and burning sensation. Initial evaluation reveals a cold, pale extremity, with or without vesicles or bullae.

Immersion foot may be considered the sailor's counterpart to trench foot. It occurs after prolonged immersion in cold water at temperatures above freezing.

Treatment

Treatment of frostbite should begin with removing all wet or frozen clothing. For patients with moderate or severe hypothermia, initial resuscitative efforts should be geared toward raising their core temperature. The patient should be moved to a warm environment and all wet clothing should be removed. The frozen extremity should be rewarmed by immersion in circulation water at 104.0 °F to 108.0 °F (40.0 °C to −42.0 °C) for about 15 to 30 minutes. Given the risks of thermal injury, the frozen parts should not be exposed to direct or dry heat (such as hair dryers, heating pads, or heat lamps). Do not rub or massage the affected area. The process should be continued until the extremity appears warm and well perfused. Because of the pain associated with reperfusion, there may be the temptation to abruptly abort the rewarming process. This can, however, promote further tissue damage.

Because the pain is usually prominent at night, amitriptyline (Elavil)[1] at an initial dosage of 10 to 25 mg and a maximum of 100 mg may be helpful. Gabapentin (Neurontin)[1] also may be an alternative therapy. Parenteral analgesic medications—nonsteroidal antiinflammatory drugs (NSAIDs) and opioids—may be administered as needed to make this process more tolerable.

Almost all authors agree that hemorrhagic blisters should not be débrided because of the risk of secondary desiccation of deep dermal layers, extending the injury. Débriding broken vesicles or bullae is also widely accepted; however, clear, intact vesicles may be broken and débrided or left intact. Topical aloe vera ointment (Dermaide Aloe)[7] or topical antibiotic ointments may be applied.

The injured tissue should be loosely covered with sterile, dry, nonadherent dressing. Hands and feet may be splinted and elevated to reduce edema. Because the damaged tissue is tetanus prone, patients whose tetanus status has not been updated may require a tetanus booster (Td).

Adjunctive agents that have been used for their antithrombotic and vasodilative properties with varying success include heparin,[1] steroids,[1] NSAIDs,[1] dimethylsulfoxide (DMSO, Rimso-50),[1] nonionic detergents,[1] dipyridamole (Persantine),[1] calcium channel blockers,[1] pentoxifylline (Trental),[1] and phenoxybenzamine (Dibenzyline).[1] Surgical consultation is appropriate for guiding long-term management, because some patients might need débridement of infections or skin grafts for nonhealing wounds. A sympathetic nerve block can relieve painful and refractory vasospasms.

For hypothermia due to myxedema coma, levothyroxine (Synthroid) should be administered intravenously (at a dose of 250 to 500 µg over 30 to 60 seconds). Daily intravenous injections of 100 µg may be required for up to 7 days. A familial association of chilblain (associated with contractual arachnodactyly) has been described in Italy.

Chilblain (pernio) may be treated with nifedipine at an oral dose of 20 to 60 mg daily. Oral prednisolone (Millipred),[1] 0.5 mg/kg in two divided doses over 2 weeks, and topical glucocorticoids have been used to treat perniosis; pentoxyfylline[1] (1200 mg/day in three divided doses for 2 weeks) has also been demonstrated to be effective.

Sequelae

Late sequelae of frostbite include cold hypersensitivity, numbness, pain, and decreased sensation. This is a result of early neuronal damage and abnormal sympathetic tone. Patients with chronic symptoms should be advised to avoid nicotine and cold exposure while using NSAIDs. Tissue demarcation can occur 60 to 90 days after initial injury. Amputation decisions should be deferred unless there is supervening sepsis or gangrene. The ultimate tissue salvage after a spontaneous slough usually far exceeds the most optimistic initial estimates. A simulation flow diagram is presented in Figure 1.

Therapeutic Hypothermia Considerations

Inducing hypothermia to reduce anoxic brain injuries has now become common practice. Permanent neurologic issues as a result of anoxia from cardiac arrest are a prominent concern. Studies have shown that hypothermia can reduce oxygen use rate in the brain by 6% for every 1°C reduction in brain temperature. Neuroprotection induced by hypothermia involves inhibition of molecular pathways that can result in cerebral edema and inflammatory responses. This modality is also being studied for use in encephalopathies, cardiogenic shock, and traumatic brain injury.

A patient must meet a few criteria to be eligible for induced hypothermia. The first is the patient should be comatose, meaning the patient should not be able to follow commands and have no speech or eye opening and no purposeful movements to noxious stimuli. This is equivalent to a Richmond Agitation Sedation Score of −4 or −5. Next, the patient must be resuscitated to a cardiac perfusing rhythm (with or without pressors) following a cardiac arrest that resulted from nonperfusing ventricular tachycardia or fibrillation. Any evidence of a head trauma of any kind needs to be ruled out before induced hypothermia can be used. The best time frame for inducing hypothermia is still not clear; however, it is strongly suggested that it be initiated within in the first 6 hours (but one can still start it at 12 hours). The desired temperature for induced hypothermia is 32 °C to 34 °C, with the optimal duration being 12 hours to 24 hours in adults. It has even been suggested that

---

[1]Not FDA approved for this indication.

---

[1]Not FDA approved for this indication.
[7]Available as a dietary supplement.

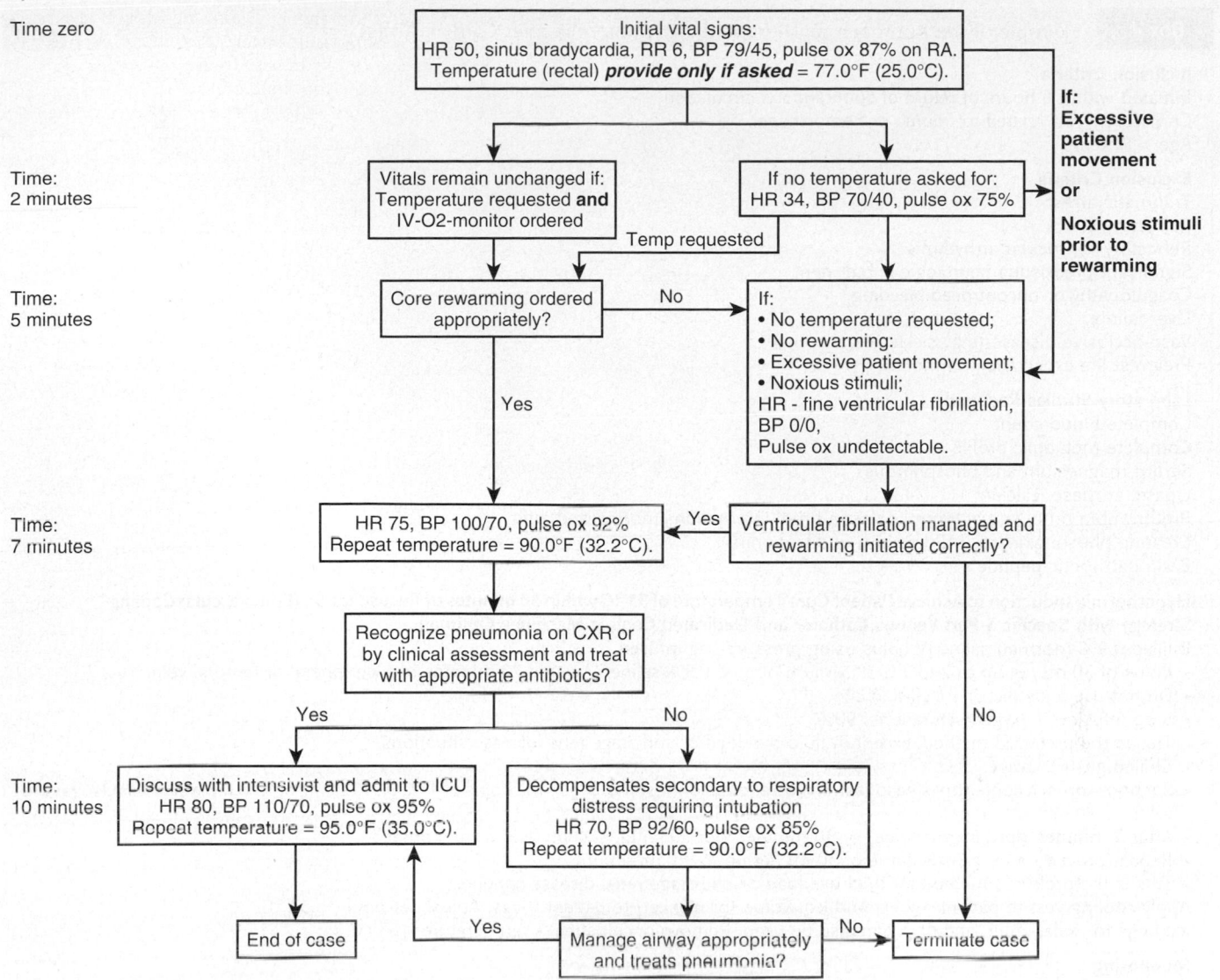

Figure 1. Hypothermia simulation flow diagram.

the infusion of 4 °C normal saline can improve the rate of return of spontaneous circulation.

In some cases, the cooling is done with ice bags and intravenous cold saline. If ice bags are used, the proper placement is groin, chest, axilla, and side of the neck. The type of cooling usually depends on where the patient is and what is available. For example, in the critical care unit, an endovascular catheter into the inferior vena cava via the femoral vein might be best. However, in the emergency department, it might be best to use cold intravenous saline with ice bags. The patient should usually be transferred to a temperature-management system to help keep the temperature constant. Two methods to measure temperature should be used for every patient whether it is esophageal, bladder, rectal, central, tympanic, or nasal. Axillary and oral temperature measurements are not reliable. Potential complications of cooling include hyperglycemia, coagulopathy, and arrhythmias. Sepsis and pneumonia can also occur because of depression of immune function.

The rewarming should be done at a temperature rate of 0.25 °C to 0.5 °C every hour for 6 to 8 hours. The patient could develop hypotension, hyperkalemia, or hyperthermia during the rewarming period. It is also important to check the blood pressure every 30 minutes during the rewarming period. It is important while the patient is under induced hypothermia to avoid shivering because shivering can also create heat, thereby increasing the oxygen demands. For the shivering, administering a neuromuscular blockade can help. First-line treatment for this is cisatracurium

(Nimbex),[1] 0.15 mg/kg IV bolus followed by 0.5 g/kg per minute. The lowest possible dose that eliminates shivering is recommended.

Sedation is recommended for patients; propofol (Diprivan) 1 mg/kg per hour, with maximum of 5 mg/kg per hour is the first-line agent. Midazolam (Versed) 0.125 mg/kg per hour is the second-line agent. All patients should receive a low-dose opioid for analgesic purposes. Fentanyl (Sublimaze) 25 mcg/h IV as needed is the first-line drug in this category. Hydromorphone (Dilaudid) may be considered as a second-line treatment. A sample approach is documented in Box 4.

The implementation of hypothermia in a patient following cardiac arrest could reduce neurologic deficits and thereby increase survival. The presence of at least two independent outcome predictors indicates a poor neurologic recovery at 3 to 6 months. Predictors of poor outcome include incomplete brain stem reflexes, presence of myoclonus, unreactive electroencephalography, and absent cortical somatosensory-evoked potentials. EEG background reactivity is probably the most important determinant in prognosis. It does not appear that patients who required active rewarming intervention exhibited a higher risk for poor outcome. Furthermore, neither rewarming speed nor fever development has a potential effect on outcome. There should be a 24-hour moratorium on any "withdrawal of care" decisions.

---

[1]Not FDA approved for this indication.

Inclusion Criteria
Initiated within 6 hours of return of spontaneous circulation
Comatose—not related to trauma or hemorrhage
Age >12 years

Exclusion Criteria
Traumatic arrest
Refractory shock
Refractory ventricular arrhythmia
Significant preexisting neurologic impairment
Coagulopathy or uncontrolled bleeding
Liver failure
Vaso-occlusive disease (e.g., sickle cell anemia)
Prearrest life expectancy <6 months

Laboratory Studies Required
Complete blood count
Complete metabolic profile
Serum magnesium and phosphorous
Lipase, amylase, calcium
Prothrombin time, partial thromboplastin time, international normalized ratio
Creatine phosphokinase (MB fraction) and troponin
Brain natriuretic peptide

Hypothermia Induction to Achieve Patient Core Temperature of 33 °C within 90 minutes of Resuscitation (Endovascular Cooling Strategy with Specific 5-Port Venous Catheter and Dedicated Cooling Machines Optimal)
Chilled 0.9% (normal) saline IV bolus using pressure-bag infuser:
- Bolus of 30 mL/kg up to 2 to 3 L, maximum of 4 °C 0.9% saline IV within 20 minutes in a peripheral or femoral vein.
- Do not use a jugular or subclavian site.
- Stop infusion if oxygen saturation <90%.
- This is the preferred method, except in fluid overload or end-stage renal disease situations.
- Chilled gastric lavage:
- Suction stomach contents via nasogastric tube and rapidly instill 250–500 mL bolus of 4 °C 0.9% saline or iced tap water via nasogastric tube.
- After 5 minutes (for 250 mL bolus) or 10 minutes (for 500 mL), suction fluid from stomach.
- Repeat procedure to target volume of 30 mL/kg up to 3 L maximum.
- This is the preferred method for fluid overload or end-stage renal disease patients.
Apply cooling vest to patient's chest and leg wraps (or blanket) to patient's legs. Adjust set point to 34 °C.
Ice bags to axilla, groin, and neck can also be used. Remove once patient's temperature ≤33 °C.

Monitoring
Monitor and document temperature (esophageal or bladder) every 15 minutes until temperature ≤34 °C, and then hourly.
Place arterial line to monitor blood pressure. Mean arterial pressure >90 mm Hg is the target. Dopamine (10–20 μg/kg/min) can be used to support blood pressure.
Sedation to deep sedation (no response to voice, but movement or eye opening to physical stimulation) to prevent shivering.
Maintain patient temperature at 32 °C–34 °C for 24 h using a cooling blanket.
Monitor CPK-MB, troponin, basic metabolic profile, serum magnesium, CBC with platelets, PT/PTT/INR at 6, 12, 18, and 24 hours. Obtain blood sugar and whole blood potassium level when target temperature is reached. Obtain blood cultures at 12 h.
Neurologic checks every 2 h to monitor for decerebrate or decorticate posturing, pupil size and asymmetry, or seizure.
Monitor skin for burns every 6 hours if a cooling vest is used.
2:1 nursing care for at least the first 12 hours.

Rewarming
Avoid active rewarming techniques.
Maintain sedation until temperature of 36 °C is attained.
Monitor for hypotension due to vasodilation.
Monitor potassium results and discontinue potassium replacement therapy at least 1 hour before rewarming.
Monitor blood sugar (by finger stick) every 2 hours during rewarming if receiving insulin therapy.
Increase patient's temperature by 0.5 °C/h until temperature is 36.5 °C (usually over 6–7 h).
Monitor esophageal and bladder temperature every 30 minutes during rewarming.
If temperature exceeds 38 °C within 12 hours after rewarming, use antipyretics and cooling blanket to maintain temperature <38 °C.

Abbreviations: CPK = creatine phosphokinase; INR = international normalized ratio; PT = prothrombin time; PTT = partial thromboplastin time.

References

Albright JT, Lebovitz BL, Lipson R, et al. Upper aerodigestive tract frostbite complicating volatile substance abuse. Int J Pediatr Otorhinolaryngol 1999; 1:63–7.

Boada A, Bielsa I, Frenandez-Figueras MT, et al. Perniosis: Clinical and histopathological analysis. Am J Dermatopathol 2010;32(1):19–23.

Bottie Y, Lavolaine J, Bouzat P, et al. Neurologic recovery from profound accidental hypothermia after 5 hours of cardiopulmonary resuscitation. Crit Care Med 2014;42:e167–e170.

Bouwes A, Robillard LB, Binnekade JM, et al. The influence of rewarming after therapeutic hypothermia on outcome after cardiac arrest. Resuscitation 2012;83:996–1000.

Bright F, Gilbert JD, Winskog C, Byard RW. Additional risk factors for lethal hypothermia. Journal of Forensic and Legal Medicine 2013;20:(6):595–97.

Centers for Disease Control and Prevention (CDC). Hypothermia-related deaths—United States, 2003–2004. MMWR Morb Mortal Wkly Rep 2005;54:173–5.

Danzl D. Hypothermia Semin Respir Crit Care Med 2002;23:57–68.

Danzl DF. Accidental hypothermia. In: Auerbach PS, editor. Wilderness Medicine. 5th ed. St. Louis: Mosby; 2007. p. 125–60.

Garrett JS, Studnek JR, Blackwell T, et al. The association between intra-arrest therapeutic hypothermia and return of spontaneous circulation among individuals experiencing out of hospital cardiac arrest. Resuscitation 2011;82:21–5.

Gilbert M, Busund R, Skagseth A, et al. Resuscitation from accidental hypothermia of 13.7°C with circulatory arrest. Lancet 2000;355:375–6.

Gomez CR. Disorders of body temperature. Handbook of Clinical Neurology 2014;120:947–57.

Heise L, Campo TM. Implementing the hypothermia protocol: A case study. Adv Emerg Nurs J 2011;33(2):137–44.

Herzog E, Shapiro J, Aziz EF, et al. Pathway for the management of survivors of out-of-hospital cardiac arrest. Crit Pathw Cardiol 2010;9:49–54.

Imray CH, Richards P, Greeves J, et al. Nonfreezing cold-induced injuries. J R Army Med Corps 2011;157:79–84.

Kurbat RS, Pollack Jr CV. Facial injury and airway threat from inhalant abuse: A case report. J Emerg Med 1998;16(2):167–9.

Lloyd EL. Accidental hypothermia. Resuscitation 1996;32:111–24.

McCauley RD, Killyon GW, Smith Jr DJ, et al. Frostbite and other cold-induced injuries. In: Auerbach PS, editor. Wilderness Medicine. 5th ed. St. Louis: Mosby; 2007. p. 195–210.

McDonagh DL, Allen IN, Keifer JC, et al. Induction of hypothermia after intraoperative hypoxic brain insult. Anesth Analg 2006;103:180–1.

Mikkelsen ME, Christie JD, Abella BS, et al. Use of therapeutic hypothermia after in-hospital cardiac arrest. Crit Care Med 2013;41:1385–95.

Mommse P, Andruszkow H, Fromke C, et al. Effects of accidental hypothermia on posttraumatic complications and outcome in multiple trauma patients. Injury 2013;44:86–90.

Noaimi AA, Fadheel BM. Treatment of perniosis with oral pentoxyfylline in comparison with oral prednisolone plus topical clobetasol ointment in Iraqi patients. Saudi Med J 2008;29:1762–4.

Parna SL, Wisco OJ. What is your diagnosis? Perniosis (chilblain). Cutis 2009;84:27–9.

Peberdy MA, Callaway CW, Neumar RW, et al. Part 9: Post–cardiac arrest care: 2010 American Heart Association Guidelines for Cardiopulmonary Resuscitation and Emergency Cardiovascular Care. Circulation 2010;122:S768–86.

Piga M, Vacca A, Cauli A, et al. Familial chilbain and late contractual arachnodactyly: A novel association? Joint Bone Spine 2009;7:205–8.

Plumb J, Thomas RG, Corneli HM. Facial frostbite associated with intentional inhalation of a commercial dusting product. Clin Toxicol 2011;49:529.

Raza N. Sajid MD, Suhail M. Haroun-ur-Rashid Onset of chilblains in relation to weather conditions J Ayub Med Coll Abbottabad 2008;20:17–20.

Rossetti AO, Oddo M, Logroscino G, et al. Prognostication after cardiac arrest and hypothermia: A prospective study. Ann Neurol 2010;67:301–7.

Szumita PM, Baroletti S, Avery KR, et al. Implementation of a hospital-wide protocol for induced hypothermia following successfully resuscitated cardiac arrest. Crit Pathw Cardiol 2010;9:216–20.

Tsai MS, Chen JY, Chen WJ, et al. Do we need to wait longer for cardiac arrest survivor to wake up in hypothermia era? Am J Emerg Med 2013;31:888.e5–6.

Ulrich AS, Rathlev NK. Hypothermia and localized cold injuries. Emerg Med Clin North Am 2004;22:281–98.

University of Chicago. Therapeutic hypothermia protocol. Available at http://erc.uchicago.edu/html/overviewmission/hypothermiaprotocols.html; [accessed 22.07.12].

Urbanic RC, Mazzaferri EL. Thyrotoxic crisis and myxedema coma. Heart Lung 1978;7:435–47.

Vanden Hoek TT, Morrison LJ, Shuster M, et al. Part 12: Cardiac arrest in special situations: 2010 American Heart Association Guidelines for Cardiopulmonary Resuscitation and Emergency Cardiovascular Care, part 12. Circulation 2010;122:S829–S861

Varon J, Marik PE, Einav S. Therapeutic hypothermia: A state-of-the-art emergency medicine perspective. Am J Emerg Med 2012;30:800–10.

Wang CJ, Yang SH, Lee CH, et al. Therapeutic hypothermia application vs standard support care in post resuscitated out-of-hospital cardiac arrest patients. Am J Emerg Med 2013;31:319–25.

Xiao G, Guo Q, Shu M, et al. Safety profile and outcome of mild therapeutic hypothermia in patients following cardiac arrest: Systemic review and meta-analysis. Emerg Med J 2013;30:91–100

Zhao H, Li CS, Gong P, et al. Molecular mechanisms of therapeutic hypothermia on neurological function in a swine model of cardiopulmonary resuscitation. Resuscitation 2012;83:913–20.

Zobel C, Adler C, Kranz A, et al. Mild therapeutic hypothermia in cardiogenic shock syndrome. Crit Care Med 2012;40:1715–23.

HEAT-RELATED ILLNESS

Method of
Ryan Lasota, MD; and Nathan Krug, MD

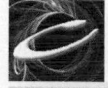

CURRENT DIAGNOSIS

- Heat illness is a spectrum of disorders that can occur when an individual is exposed to warm environments during exercise and at rest.
- Risk factors for heat illness include lack of acclimatization, extremes of age, dehydration, prolonged exposure to heat, high intensity exercise, and obesity.

- Core body temperature must be determined by rectal temperature.
- Heat stroke is a life-threatening illness and is defined as a core body temperature greater than 104°F (40°C) accompanied by central nervous system dysfunction.
- Heat exhaustion is the fatigue-induced inability to continue an activity because of extremes of exertion or environmental heat stress. Temperature is commonly elevated; however, no central nervous system dysfunction is observed.
- Exercise-associated muscle cramping involves intense, painful muscle spasms occurring after or during prolonged intense exercise.

CURRENT THERAPY

- The most effective management for heat-related illness is prevention.
- Immediate recognition of heat illness signs and symptoms is critical for preventing morbidity and mortality.
- Effective heat illness prevention principles include appropriate acclimatization, maintenance of adequate hydration status, proper electrolyte replacement, and modification of activity during times of increased heat stress.
- Heat stroke requires immediate initiation of body cooling methods after addressing airway, breathing, and circulation. Cold-water immersion most effectively lowers core body temperature, but other methods such as fans and ice packs on the neck, axilla, and groin are acceptable alternatives.
- Patients should be monitored and treated for complications of heat stroke including seizures, rhabdomyolysis, hepatic injury, and acute renal injury.
- Treatment of heat exhaustion follows similar treatment principles of heat stroke and includes the following: transfer from warm environment, remove excess clothing, place in supine or Trendelenburg position, begin oral hydration with cold electrolyte beverages, and monitor for signs of progression to heat stroke.
- Exercise-associated muscle cramping is best managed by discontinuation of activity, stretching of the involved muscle group at full length, and oral sodium replacement. Refractory cases may require IV normal saline or benzodiazepines.

Heat-related illness is a spectrum of pathologic states that occurs when an individual is exposed to elevated temperatures. These maladies affect a diverse patient population. Mortality is common, but can be prevented with early recognition and treatment.

Under normal circumstances, a body at rest produces heat through metabolic functions. Physical activity increases heat generation. While heat production depends on body mass, heat dissipation depends on body surface area. Core body temperature is regulated by the hypothalamus through input from peripheral and central heat receptors. A rise in body temperature of less than 1°C (1.8°F) triggers thermoregulatory cooling mechanisms. Cutaneous vasodilation shunts blood to the body surface. Sweating occurs, leading to cooling through evaporation. Hyperthermia also results in tachycardia, increased cardiac output, and increased minute ventilation, all with the goal of decreasing body temperature.

Understanding the pathophysiology and treatment of heat-related illness requires understanding the thermoregulatory concepts of conduction, convection, radiation, and evaporation. While conduction, convection, and radiation direct treatment of heat illness, evaporation is the primary mechanism of cooling under normal circumstances. Sweat produced by the body releases heat as it is converted from liquid to vapor form. Heat loss is inversely related to environmental humidity and directly related to salt content of sweat produced.

Heat-related illness occurs when heat is produced faster than heat is dissipated through physiologic mechanisms. Cellular damage occurs when core temperatures rise above 104°F (40°C). This damage triggers a systemic inflammatory response, which leads to increased cellular permeability, release of endotoxins, tissue hypoxia, metabolic acidosis, cellular death, and organ dysfunction in severe cases. Heat damage usually affects the nervous system first, but may also cause hepatic, renal, or muscle damage.

The damage induced by heat illness can be diminished through proper acclimatization. Incremental increases in heat stress lead to physiologic changes that allow a person to work safely at heat levels that were previously intolerable. Acclimatization requires 10 to 14 days of exposure to occur. With gradual heat exposure, the body improves sodium retention, increases glomerular filtration rate, and enhances cardiac performance. Heat stress leads to production of heat shock proteins that allow cells to be more tolerant of heat. Heat illness prevention hinges on these physiologic changes of acclimatization.

Heat-related illness is the third most common cause of death among high school athletes; however, morbidity and mortality associated with these illnesses can be prevented. Proper hydration slows the rate of body temperature rise and should be emphasized during extremes of heat and humidity, especially for athletes participating in these conditions. Electrolyte-containing solutions should be used, as sodium depletion can lead to muscle cramping and salt loss hyponatremia. Acclimatization and activity modification are key elements to heat illness prevention during high-risk environmental conditions. High-risk environmental conditions can be assessed using online heat index charts.

Heat Stroke

Heat stroke is defined as core body temperature greater than 104°F (40°C) accompanied by central nervous system dysfunction. Multiple organ system failure may also be present. Clinically, heat stroke is subdivided into *classic heat stroke* (also known as nonexertional heat stroke), which results from prolonged exposure to elevated environmental temperatures, and *exertional heat stroke*, which occurs with prolonged strenuous physical activity. Classic heat stroke generally occurs during the hot, humid months of summer. Onset is insidious in nature. Exertional heat stroke generally affects a younger, healthier, more active cohort. While exertional heat stroke is generally associated with elevations in ambient temperature, it can also occur at cooler temperatures with prolonged physical activity and in times of high relative humidity. The incidence of heat stroke varies based on season, geographic location, and form of physical activity, but has been shown to increase with rising ambient temperature and relative humidity.

Risk factors for heat stroke vary based on the form of heat stroke encountered. Classic heat stroke generally occurs because of a lack of access to adequate air conditioning. Affected individuals tend to be at the extremes of age, of lower socioeconomic status, and/or with other medical and psychiatric comorbidities. Primary risk factors for exertional heat stroke include exercise in a hot, humid environment, lack of acclimatization, and poor physical fitness. Other risk factors include obesity, dehydration, a previous history of exertional heat stroke, sleep deprivation, sweat gland dysfunction, sunburn, viral illness, and diarrhea. Medications that affect the body's ability to dissipate heat also increase risk of both forms of heat stroke (Table 1). Children are at increased risk for heat-related illness. A higher surface area to body mass ratio allows for the transfer of more heat from the environment than in adults. Children also have slower sweat rates, higher temperature thresholds for the initiation of sweating, and produce more dilute sweat, all of which diminish the body's ability to dissipate heat.

The clinical presentation of heat stroke is often nonspecific. Signs and symptoms can include confusion, dizziness, altered mental status, headache, collapse, fatigue, vomiting, seizures, and coma. Therefore, any clinical status change should prompt evaluation for heat stroke, especially in hot, humid conditions. Sweating may or may not be present. Hypotension, tachycardia, hyperventilation, and shock-like appearance are common at the time of initial evaluation.

The diagnosis of heat stroke requires measurement of core body temperature. A rectal temperature greater than 104°F (40°C) in

TABLE 1	Medications that May Increase the Risk of Heat-Related Illness

- Amphetamines
- Anticholinergic agents
- Antiepileptic agents
- Antihistamines
- Benzodiazepines
- Beta blockers
- Calcium channel blockers
- Cocaine
- Decongestants
- Diuretics
- Ergogenic stimulants
- Ethanol
- Laxatives
- Lithium
- Phenothiazines
- Tricyclic antidepressants

Data from Becker and Stewart (2011) and Wexler (2002).

the presence of altered mental status or multiorgan dysfunction confirms the diagnosis. Rectal temperature is preferred over other methods, as the reported temperature can be falsely lowered because of air temperature, liquids on the skin and in the mouth, hyperventilation, fanning, and other factors.

The differential diagnosis for heat stroke includes any process that causes altered mental status and/or elevation in core body temperature. Metabolic causes such as hypoglycemia, hypoxia, sodium disturbances, or thyroid abnormalities should be considered. Use of prescription and recreational drugs should be assessed (see Table 1). Infectious causes should be ruled out by history or laboratory/radiographic testing. Vascular abnormalities such as stroke, intracranial hemorrhage, and acute myocardial infarction should be considered and further evaluated if history is suggestive as the cause of clinical deterioration. Seizure should also be considered in the differential diagnosis.

Heat stroke is a medical emergency and requires immediate initiation of body cooling. Prolonged elevation of core body temperature results in more severe injuries. In the absence of life-threatening conditions, cooling treatment should be completed on-site before EMS transfer. Treatment begins with assessing airway, breathing, and circulation. Methods to lower core body temperature occur immediately after these elements are secure. Moving patients to shaded environments reduces the effect of radiant heat. Cold-water and ice-water immersion therapy produces the most rapid whole-body cooling rate through conduction of body heat to the surrounding cooler water. This method has been found to have the lowest morbidity and mortality rates for exertional heat stroke. When whole-body immersion is not available, placement of ice packs on the neck, axilla, and groin combined with rapid rotation of ice-water-soaked towels to the head, trunk, and extremities provides an effective, albeit slower, method of whole-body cooling. Warm air mist and fanning utilize evaporation to cool the body. While effective, these methods are slower at reducing body temperature and depend heavily on relative humidity.

Core temperature-lowering efforts continue until rectal temperature is ≤101°F (38.3°C) and mental status normalizes. Patients with rapid return to normal state have the best prognosis. Even with rapid improvement of clinical condition, injury to hepatic, musculoskeletal, and renal tissue can occur, as evidenced by laboratory abnormalities. Patients recovering from heat stroke should refrain from physical activity for at least 7 days. Physician follow-up should occur during this time and should include reevaluation of laboratory abnormalities and discussion regarding return to activity. Once cleared for activity, exercise should be initiated in a cool environment. Acclimatization and heat tolerance occur over a 2-week period with gradual increases in exercise duration, intensity, and heat exposure. Patients may return to full competition if heat tolerance exists after 2 to 4 weeks of training. Those who have difficulty with a return to activity at 1 month should be evaluated with a laboratory exercise-heat tolerance test.

Heat Exhaustion

Heat exhaustion is the fatigue-induced inability to continue an activity because of extremes of exertion or environmental heat stress. Core temperature is commonly elevated. However, central nervous system dysfunction is not observed, differentiating this condition from heat stroke. Heat exhaustion is the most common type of heat illness observed in active populations and is often a precursor to heat stroke and end organ damage. Risk factors for heat exhaustion are similar to those for heat stroke and clinical manifestations are similar to other forms of heat illness. Heat exhaustion prevention is best accomplished by adequate hydration, avoiding exercise in the hottest part of the day, exercising in light/loose clothing, and proper acclimatization.

Treatment of heat exhaustion should be initiated as soon as signs are apparent, as delay can lead to increased morbidity. Most patients will improve with conservative therapy. Move the patient to a shaded or air conditioned area, remove excess clothing, and place in the supine position with legs elevated. Correct dehydration with cold electrolyte beverages orally if the patient is conscious and able to swallow. If the patient is unable to take oral fluids or shows signs of hemodynamic instability, IV normal saline will rapidly restore intravascular volume. D5NS should be used in patients with documented or suspected low blood glucose. Vital signs, rectal temperature, and neurologic status should be monitored with rapid transport to an emergency facility if symptoms do not improve within 20 to 30 minutes of conservative therapy.

Exercise-Associated Muscle Cramps

Exercise-associated muscle cramps, also known as heat cramps, are defined by intense, painful muscle spasms occurring after or during prolonged intense exercise. The incidence of exercise-associated muscle cramps is not well defined, but has been reported as 1.2 cases per 1,000 marathon runners. Exercise-associated muscle cramps are more prevalent in hot or humid climates, but can be seen in cooler environments as well. Risk factors mirror those observed in other heat-related illnesses. Although the pathophysiology is not fully elucidated or agreed upon, it is generally accepted that large-volume sweating and subsequent sodium loss predisposes patients to exercise-associated muscle cramps. It is important to evaluate the patient's medical history and other symptoms to avoid missing an underlying pathologic process. Other diagnoses to consider when evaluating a patient with exercise-associated muscle cramps include sickle cell disease or trait, rhabdomyolysis, medication side effects, or musculotendinous injury. Physical examination reveals tight, contracted muscles, helping to differentiate exercise-associated muscle cramps from these other processes.

The treatment for exercise-associated muscle cramps is similar to other forms of heat illness as outlined above. Management includes rest from the current activity, stretching of the involved muscle group at full length, and oral sodium ingestion via electrolyte beverages or salty snack foods. For refractory cases, IV normal saline may be used as well as an IV benzodiazepine to effectively and rapidly relieve cramping. If possible, obtaining a serum sodium level before the initiation of IV normal saline is recommended, as both hypernatremia and hyponatremia can cause cramping. As with all heat illnesses, prevention is the key principal and is achieved by maintaining adequate hydration status, avoiding exercise in extreme heat conditions, ensuring adequate acclimation, and monitoring for early signs of heat illness throughout the activity.

References

American College of Sports Medicine, Armstrong LE, Casa DJ, et al. American College of Sports Medicine position stand. Exertional heat illness during training and competition. Med Sci Sports Exerc 2007;39:556–72.

Becker JA, Stewart LK. Heat-related illness. Am Fam Physician 2011;83:1325–30.

Bouchama A, Knochel JP. Heat stroke. N Engl J Med 2002;346:1978–88.

DeFranco MJ, Baker 3rd CL, DaSilva JJ, et al. Environmental issues for team physicians. Am J Sports Med 2008;36:2226–37.

Noonan B, Bancroft RW, Dines JS, et al. Heat- and cold-induced injuries in athletes: Evaluation and management. J Am Acad Orthop Surg 2012;20:744–54.

Wexler RK. Evaluation and treatment of heat-related illnesses. Am Fam Physician 2002;65:2307–14.

HIGH-ALTITUDE SICKNESS

Method of
Adrienne N. Kovalsky, DO, MPH

CURRENT DIAGNOSIS

Acclimatization
- Symptoms include exertional dyspnea, increased respiratory rate, polyuria, peripheral edema, and insomnia.

High-Altitude Headache (HAH)
- New onset headache that fulfils at least two of the following:
  - Develops in temporal relation to altitude gain above 2500 m
  - Worsens in conjunction with continued ascent and/or resolves within 24 hours of descent below 2500 m
  - Includes at least two of the following characteristics: bilateral; mild or moderate intensity; aggravated by exertion, movement, straining, coughing, and/or bending

Acute Mountain Sickness (AMS)
- New-onset headache occurs within 12 hours of altitude gain above 2500 m.
- Anorexia, nausea, vomiting, fatigue, weakness, dizziness, lightheadedness, or difficulty sleeping (see Box 3).

High-Altitude Cerebral Edema
- Mental status changes or ataxia with preexisting AMS.
- Mental status changes and ataxia without a prodrome of AMS.

High-Altitude Pulmonary Edema
- Relative hypoxemia in the setting of at least two signs or symptoms from each of the following lists:
  - Resting dyspnea, cough, weakness, decreased exercise performance, and chest tightness or congestion
  - Wheezing, rales, tachypnea, tachycardia, or central cyanosis

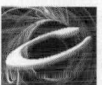

CURRENT THERAPY

Insomnia or Sleep Disturbance
- Acetazolamide (Diamox)[1] 125 mg PO at bedtime is recommended.
- Consider diphenhydramine (Benadryl) 50 mg at bedtime, zolpidem (Ambien) 5–10 mg at bedtime, or temazepam (Restoril) 15 mg at bedtime for patients with no history of altitude illness.

High-Altitude Headache
- Medications for headache include ibuprofen (Advil) 600–800 mg PO every 8 hours, acetaminophen (Tylenol) 650–1000 mg PO every 6 hours, enteric-coated aspirin (Ecotrin) 325–650 mg PO every 4 hours, oxygen by nasal cannula at 1–2 L/min, or acetazolamide[1] 125 mg PO twice daily.

Acute Mountain Sickness, Mild (Lake Louise Score <5)
- Avoid respiratory depressants, strenuous activity, or further ascent until the patient is asymptomatic.
- Acetazolamide 125–250 mg PO twice daily may be tried.
- Symptomatic treatment as for headache and nausea.

Acute Mountain Sickness, Moderate to Severe (Lake Louise Score 5–15)
- Stop ascent and rest until asymptomatic AND:
  - Administer acetazolamide 125–250 mg PO twice daily.
  - Oxygen (1–2 L) or hyperbaric chamber 2–4 psi may be used if available.
  - Consider dexamethasone (Decadron)[1] 4 mg PO or IM every 6 hours as an adjunct or if acetazolamide is contraindicated.
  - Monitor for mental status changes, confusion, or ataxia and descend immediately at onset.
- If symptoms are severe, or if there is no response to 24 hours of therapy, immediate descent of at least 500 m or to last asymptomatic altitude is the definitive treatment;

High-Altitude Cerebral Edema
- Prepare for evacuation or emergent descent of at least 1000 m.
- Administer dexamethasone[1] 8 mg PO, IM, or IV once followed by 4 mg every 6 hours.
- Consider adding acetazolamide[1] 250 mg PO twice daily as an adjunct.
- Early recognition and treatment are essential.

High-Altitude Pulmonary Edema
- Bed rest with oxygen 4–6 L by nasal cannula.
- If the patient is not improving or if HAPE is severe, descend at least 500 m, avoiding exertion.
- Use a hyperbaric chamber at 2–4 psi if oxygen is unavailable or the patient is unable to descend.
- If oxygen is unavailable or the patient is unable to descend, or if the patient is not responding to either:
  - Give nifedipine (Procardia)[1] 10 mg PO once and 30 mg extended-release PO every 12[3] to 24 hours (contraindicated in HACE).
  - Consider adding salmeterol[1] 125 μg[3] inhaled twice daily, tadalafil (Adcirca, Cialis)[1] 10 mg PO twice daily,[3] or sildenafil (Revatio, Viagra)[1] 50 mg PO thrice daily[3] (these are not yet well studied for treatment).
  - It is not advisable to use both nifedipine and a phosphodiesterase inhibitor; if this becomes necessary, carefully monitor blood pressure and stagger doses to prevent potential cerebral hypoperfusion.

Concurrent High-Altitude Pulmonary and Cerebral Edema
- As always, immediate descent and supplemental oxygen therapy are critical
- Treatment as for HAPE with the addition of dexamethasone.

---

[1]Not FDA approved for this indication.
[3]Exceeds dosage recommended by the manufacturer.

The appeal of travel to high altitude is vast. For many it is tourism, skiing, or mountaineering, but for others it is far more fundamental, as increasing numbers travel to high altitudes for work. Any elevation greater than 1500 m is considered high altitude (Denver, for example, is 1609 m), but most high-altitude illness occurs at higher than 2500 m. It is at these altitudes that the effects of hypoxia and decreasing barometric pressure start to be seen. Many persons become symptomatic during the adaptive process known as acclimatization, and some develop acute high-altitude syndromes, including acute mountain sickness (AMS), high-altitude cerebral edema (HACE), and high-altitude pulmonary edema (HAPE). These syndromes are often preventable, but they have the potential to cause significant morbidity and mortality for the patient and for those involved in risky rescue efforts by land or air.

Epidemiology and Risk Factors
The incidence of altitude illnesses is highly variable and commonly idiosyncratic. At 3000 m the incidence of AMS ranges from 4% to 58%, whereas the incidence of HAPE and HACE generally is less than 1%. The occurrence of altitude illness depends on the rate of ascent, altitude of residence, exertion, prior history of altitude illness, and individual susceptibility. Physical fitness does not alter susceptibility, whereas obesity is a risk factor. Tobacco smoking, asthma, and diabetes do not confer any additional risk. Certain medical conditions including chronic obstructive pulmonary disease, pulmonary hypertension, congestive heart failure, coronary artery disease, sickle cell disease, and sleep apnea increase risk of developing altitude illness. A more-detailed discussion of some of these diseases is included later in the text.

Physiologic Adaptation and Pathophysiology
Hypoxia and its effects are much more pronounced with increasing elevation owing to concomitant decreases in barometric pressure. In the first few hours at high altitude, the body responds to hypoxia with an increased respiratory rate. The subsequent respiratory alkalosis also improves oxygen-binding in the lung but ultimately slows respiration. After 24 to 48 hours the kidneys excrete excess bicarbonate, normalizing the elevated pH that would otherwise prevent an adequate increase in respiration. This is the basis for acclimatization.

Periodic breathing is also more likely to occur at higher elevations owing to hypoxia and resulting respiratory alkalosis. Altitude-dependent diuresis causes transient hemoconcentration in the first 1 to 2 days, with true erythropoiesis starting at 4 to 5 days. Chronic residence at altitude can cause polycythemia, increasing risk for tissue infarction. The most complex effects of hypobaric hypoxia are seen in the lung and the brain and are not completely understood.

The physiologic response to altitude rests along one end of a spectrum of compensatory mechanisms that can evolve into to high-altitude syndromes. In the brain, hypoxia causes vasodilation and fluid retention, which is suspected to be the basis for AMS and HACE. In the lung the fluid retention results from vasoconstriction rather than vasodilation and is the basis for HAPE. With exposure to ambient hypoxia, the normally protective mechanism of focal shunting from a poorly oxygenated segment occurs throughout the lung. This diffuse pulmonary vasoconstriction causes a reversible pulmonary hypertension and a noncardiogenic pulmonary edema.

Prevention
The most reliable way to prevent altitude illness is through graded ascent, thereby allowing sufficient time for acclimatization. A conservative guideline for activities above 2500 m is increasing sleep altitude by no more than 300 m in a 24-hour period. If symptoms of AMS are noted, no further ascent should be attempted until they resolve in order to prevent more-severe illness or evolution of HACE or HAPE. Additional preventive measures should be taken and are of particular importance for persons planning rapid ascent, whether on foot or flying directly into altitudes of 2500 m or greater. Light activity can accelerate acclimatization, but strenuous exertion should be avoided in the first 2 days. Preexposure of 5 days of comparable altitude within 2 months of ascent is protective. CNS depressants such as alcohol are thought to worsen effects of altitude, particularly overnight when respiration is already more depressed, and they should be avoided. Refer to Box 1 for a summary.

Medical prophylaxis should be considered when graded ascent is not possible, whether on foot or flying directly into altitudes of 2500 m or greater, and for persons with a history of prior altitude

---

Box 1 — Prevention of High-Altitude Sickness

Ascent above 2500 m should be at a gradual rate of 300 m per 24 hours, with an additional rest day for every 1000 m gain.

With rapid ascent above 2500 m, light activity may be helpful with acclimatization, but strenuous activity should be avoided for at least 48 hours.

Avoid respiratory depressants such as alcohol until acclimatized.

Five days of comparable altitude exposure should be undertaken within 2 months of ascent.

For AMS or HACE, begin prophylaxis 1 or 2 days before starting ascent:
- Acetazolamide 125 mg PO bid
- Dexamethasone[1] 4 mg PO q6h for patients with sulfa allergy.
- Prophylaxis is strongly recommended for patients with a history of AMS or HACE or for rapid ascent.

For persons with a history of HAPE, begin prophylaxis 1 day before starting ascent:
- Salmeterol[1] 125 μg[3] inhaled bid
- Dexamethasone 8 mg PO bid
- Tadalafil (Adcirca, Cialis)[1] 10 mg PO bid[3]
- Sildenafil (Revatio, Viagra)[1] 50 mg PO tid[3]
- Nifedipine[1] 20 mg extended release PO tid[3]

Stop ascent with onset of even mild AMS to prevent evolution to HACE.

---

[1]Not FDA approved for this indication.
[3]Exceeds dosage recommended by the manufacturer.
Abbreviations: AMS=acute mountain sickness; HACE=high-altitude cerebral edema; HAPE=high-altitude pulmonary edema.

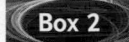

Box 2 Medications for Acute Mountain Sickness and High-Altitude Cerebral Edema

Acetazolamide

Acetazolamide is a central-acting respiratory stimulant that causes a metabolic acidosis and ultimately facilitates acclimatization. It is effective in preventing and treating AMS and HACE.[1] Patients should be warned about side effects, including paresthesias, flat taste of carbonated beverages, and polyuria, particularly at night. Persons with a history of asthma, sulfonamide allergy, anaphylaxis, or penicillin allergy should try this medication under the supervision of a medical professional prior to departure.

Dexamethasone

Dexamethasone[1] is also effective in the prevention and treatment of AMS and HACE, though its mechanism is not completely understood. Unlike with acetazolamide, symptoms can recur after stopping treatment, and it does not facilitate acclimatization. It is not recommended for prophylaxis of AMS unless acetazolamide is contraindicated, though it is the drug of choice for treatment of HACE.

---

[1]Not FDA approved for this indication.
Abbreviations: AMS = acute mountain sickness; HACE = high-altitude cerebral edema.

---

illness. This should begin the day prior to starting ascent and continue until at a stable altitude for at least 2 to 4 days. If further ascent is undertaken, or if symptoms recur, prophylaxis can be restarted at any point.

The most effective medication for prophylaxis of AMS and HACE is acetazolamide (Diamox) 125 mg PO twice daily. This is a central-acting respiratory stimulant that causes a metabolic acidosis and ultimately facilitates acclimatization. Patients should be warned about side effects and possible allergy (Box 2). Dexamethasone (Decadron)[1] 4 mg every 6 hours also is effective, though its mechanism is not completely understood. Unlike with acetazolamide, symptoms can recur after stopping dexamethasone, and it does not facilitate acclimatization. It is not recommended for prophylaxis unless acetazolamide is contraindicated, and it is best saved for treatment of severe AMS or HACE. Ginkgo biloba[7] and oral ibuprofen (Advil)[1] as prophylaxis are ongoing and inconclusive at this time. Inhaled budesonide (Pulmicort)[1] has recently been evaluated and shows promise.

Prophylaxis of HAPE has been studied in preventing recurrence in persons with a history of HAPE, though it also would be prudent to consider prophylaxis for anyone undertaking very rapid ascent. Numerous agents have been evaluated in patients with history of HAPE and are listed in Box 1. Nifedipine (Procardia)[1] is the preferred medication for prevention, with salmeterol (Serevent)[1] as a potential adjunct if there is significant history of HAPE and anticipated rapid ascent profile.

Symptomatic Acclimatization and Disrupted Sleep

Many people experience symptoms of normal adaptation that do not always herald illness, but they should nonetheless always be completely evaluated. Expected symptoms include exertional dyspnea, polyuria, peripheral and facial edema, and nocturnal awakenings and insomnia. The most common side effects of normal acclimatization are disrupted sleep and mild peripheral edema. Acetazolamide[1] 125 mg at bedtime has been shown to decrease nocturnal oxygen saturation and lessen awakenings (see Box 2). Diphenhydramine (Benadryl)[1] 25 to 50 mg may also be used, but it does not have the same benefits. Studies have showed that zolpidem (Ambien)[1] 10 mg and temazepam (Restoril)[1] 15 mg are probably safe, but because studies have been small and targeted, these medications probably should be avoided whenever possible, particularly in persons with a history of altitude illness.

---

[1]Not FDA approved for this indication.
[7]Available as a dietary supplement.

High-Altitude Headache

Headache is a common occurrence and does not always evolve into AMS. The headache is generally bilateral and throbbing is exacerbated with coughing, bending, straining and exertion, and is often worst early in the morning. There should be no other associated symptoms. Onset can occur within 1 hour but usually begins within 6 to 10 hours. Numerous medications are effective for treatment, including analgesics and medications used in prophylaxis of AMS. See the Current Therapy box for a complete listing.

High-Altitude Syndromes

Acute Mountain Sickness

In the setting of a recent gain in altitude, AMS is defined as headache with at least one of the following: anorexia, nausea, or vomiting; fatigue or weakness; dizziness or lightheadedness; or difficulty sleeping. As with high-altitude headache, onset can occur within 1 hour but usually begins within 6 to 10 hours. Other symptoms can include decreased urine output, lassitude, and ataxia. All symptoms typically resolve within 2 to 3 days, though on occasion at higher altitudes symptoms can persist for days or weeks without progression or resolution. Examination is normal and no diagnostic studies are indicated. The differential includes dehydration, exhaustion, hangover, viral illness, carbon monoxide poisoning, caffeine withdrawal, migraine, and meningitis. Recognition of AMS is essential in order to begin appropriate measures that might help prevent evolution to the potentially fatal HACE, which exists along the same spectrum.

If mild, AMS can be monitored at a stable altitude with no further ascent undertaken. Analgesics and antiemetics are effective for managing symptoms. Acetazolamide may be considered for mild AMS and is recommended for moderate to severe symptoms. Dexamethasone[1] may be added, or used in substitution if intolerant of or allergic to acetazolamide, for a short course (less than five days) while acclimatizing. Low-flow supplemental oxygen and hyperbaric chambers can be used as an adjunct for moderate to severe symptoms. Descent is advised for symptoms that progress after 24 hours of rest or treatment or for symptoms that are severe or stable but prolonged in order to prevent evolution to HACE. Immediate descent should be undertaken for ataxia, altered mental status, or any signs or symptoms of pulmonary edema. Refer to the Current Therapy box for dosing and summary.

High-Altitude Cerebral Edema

In the setting of a recent gain in altitude, HACE is defined as a change in mental status and/or ataxia in a person with AMS, or both mental status changes and ataxia in a person without AMS. There may be changes in mood or hallucinations. It generally progresses over 1 to 3 days, but it can also cause loss of consciousness within 12 hours. Examination has nonfocal neurologic findings with confusion. Papilledema may be seen, and rales are often present from concurrent HAPE. If computed tomography (CT) or magnetic resonance imaging (MRI) is available acutely, findings would be consistent with vasogenic edema.

Differential diagnosis is similar to that for AMS but should be expanded to include diabetic ketoacidosis, hypoglycemia, electrolyte imbalances, brain tumor, stroke, and seizure. After long term at altitude or any length of time at very high altitudes blood can become hyperviscous and increasingly thrombogenic, so in these circumstances stroke should rise on the differential.

Early recognition is crucial in management of HACE to prevent evolution to irreversible disease. The most important element of treatment is descent of at least 1000 m. Supplemental oxygen and hyperbaric bags may be used during descent and are imperative if descent is not possible. Dexamethasone[1] should be initiated, and should be continued after descent if symptoms persist. Acetazolamide[1] may be added. Dosages are listed in the Current Therapy box.

High-Altitude Pulmonary Edema

In the setting of a recent gain in altitude, HAPE is diagnosed with at least two of resting dyspnea, cough, weakness or decreased exercise performance, and chest tightness or congestion and two of

---

[1]Not FDA approved for this indication.

wheezing or rales, tachypnea, tachycardia, or central cyanosis. There may also be an associated low-grade temperature elevation. Cough is initially dry but in late stages is productive of pink or bloody sputum. Onset often occurs during sleep, usually the second night at altitude, and often after the use of sleep aids that cause respiratory depression. It rarely occurs after 4 or 5 days at a stable altitude and should resolve within 48 hours of descent.

Examination is significant for rales that can begin in the right axilla and progress diffusely and for low-grade temperature elevation. Hypoxia, often very pronounced, is noted on pulse oximetry; oxygen levels will be disproportionately low for given elevation. If available, chest radiography typically demonstrates bilaterally diffuse patchy opacities without pulmonary vascular changes, though initially they may be seen in the right middle lobe. Ultrasound may be more readily available than radiography in remote locations and through the use of the comet-tail technique may be helpful in identifying HAPE and differentiating from pneumonia or other conditions.

HAPE can occur in conjunction with severe AMS or HACE. Differential includes heart failure, acute myocardial ischemia, pulmonary embolus, asthma, bronchitis, and pneumonia. Among the altitude illnesses, HAPE is associated with the highest rate of mortality but, unlike HACE, it is unlikely to cause long-term sequelae if treated appropriately. As with all altitude illness, removing the hypoxic stimulus is the central principle in management, and with HAPE it is also the most effective. This can be done with descent, supplemental oxygen, or a hyperbaric chamber. If available, supplemental oxygen and bed rest may be sufficient. If the pulmonary edema is severe, descent is the definitive treatment and should be undertaken without delay. Exertion and cold stress should be avoided. Nifedipine (Adalat, Procardia)[1] and salmeterol (Serevent)[1] may be of benefit in treatment of HAPE, but they are not as effective as oxygen or descent and should be used as an adjunct or if no other alternatives exist. Dual vasodilating agent use (nifedipine and a phosphodiesterase inhibitor) is not recommended, but if attempted when no alternatives exist, doses should be staggered and blood pressure carefully monitored to prevent potentially disastrous hypotension and cerebral hypoperfusion. Refer to the Current Therapy box for dosing. Reascent may be considered 2 to 3 days after resolution, but risk of recurrence becomes significantly higher.

Special Populations

Children and Pregnant Women

Susceptibility of the pediatric population to altitude illness is no different from that of the adult population. Diagnostic criteria, management, and prevention all apply as noted earlier, with the following dosage adjustments: acetazolamide* 2.5 mg/kg every 12 hours can be used for prevention and treatment of both AMS and HACE,[1] and dexamethasone[1] 0.15 mg/kg every 6 hours should be used only for treatment of AMS and HACE. Medications to prevent and treat HAPE have not been adequately studied in the pediatric population. Data are limited on acute effects of altitude on pregnancy, but it is generally accepted that women with low-risk pregnancies can safely travel to high altitude.

Patients with Cardiopulmonary Disease

Patients with allergic asthma are likely to see improvement in their symptoms, though asthma induced by exercise or cold may be made worse at high altitudes. An optimized pretravel medical regimen should be continued, and these patients should travel with additional rescue medications, including bronchodilators and corticosteroids.

Patients with mild to moderate chronic obstructive pulmonary disease (COPD) might not be more predisposed to high-altitude illness. However, data are limited in these populations, and these patients should avoid remote settings without supplemental oxygen or medical care. Patients should continue an optimized home medical regimen, and those already on home oxygen should anticipate using more oxygen and should travel with a pulse oximeter (typically pocket-sized and inexpensive) to titrate accordingly.

---

[1]Not FDA approved for this indication.
*Acetazolamide is approved for use in children aged 12 years and older only.

Patients with pulmonary hypertension are at increased risk for developing HAPE and should avoid travel to high altitudes if mean pulmonary arterial pressure is 35 mm Hg or above, or if systolic pulmonary arterial pressure is 50 mm Hg or above. Any patient with pulmonary hypertension should use medical prophylaxis for HAPE.

Patients with obstructive sleep apnea tend to do better at high altitudes than those with central sleep apnea, but both of these populations should continue CPAP while at altitude. In patients not using CPAP, acetazolamide prophylaxis is recommended.

Patients with obesity hypoventilation or bilateral carotid body resection should avoid travel to high altitudes. If such travel is unavoidable, supplemental oxygen should be used and any home use of CPAP should be continued while at altitude.

Travel to high altitude for any patient with coronary artery disease is a complex issue that should take into account severity of disease and exercise tolerance. These patients should be assessed by their cardiologists before undertaking travel to high altitudes.

References

Bartsch P, Maggiorini M, Ritter M, et al. Prevention of high-altitude pulmonary edema by nifedipine. N Engl J Med 1991;325:1284–9.

Gertsch JH, Basnyat B, Johnson EW, et al. Randomised, double blind, placebo controlled comparison of ginkgo biloba and acetazolamide for prevention of acute mountain sickness among Himalayan trekkers: The Prevention of High Altitude Illness Trial (PHAIT). BMJ 2004;328:797.

Ghofrani HA, Reichenberger F, Kohstall M, et al. Sildenafil increased exercise capacity during hypoxia at low altitudes and at Mount Everest base camp: A randomized, double-blind, placebo-controlled crossover trial. Ann Intern Med 2004;141:169–77.

Hackett PH, Roach RC. High-altitude medicine and physiology. In: Auerbach PS, editor. Wilderness Medicine. 6th ed. Philadelphia: Mosby; 2012 p. 2–33.

Maggiorini M. Brunner-La Rocca HP, Peth S, et al. Both tadalafil and dexamethasone may reduce the incidence of high-altitude pulmonary edema Ann Intern Med 2006;145:497–6.

Nickol AH, Leverment J, Richards P, et al. Temazepam at high altitude reduces periodic breathing without impairing next-day performance: A randomized cross-over double-blind study. J Sleep Res 2006;15:445–54.

Oelz O, Maggiorini M, Ritter M, et al. Nifedipine for high altitude pulmonary oedema. Lancet 1989;2:1241–4.

Sartori C, Allemann Y, Duplain H, et al. Salmeterol for the prevention of high-altitude pulmonary edema. N Engl J Med 2002;346:1631–6.

Schneider M, Bernasch D, Weymann J, et al. Acute mountain sickness: Influence of susceptibility, pre-exposure and ascent rate. Med Sci Sports Exerc 2002;34:1886–91.

Zafren K, Reeves JT, Schoene R. Treatment of high-altitude pulmonary edema by bed rest and supplemental oxygen. Wilderness Environ Med 1996;7(2):127–32.

MARINE POISONINGS, ENVENOMATIONS, AND TRAUMA

Method of
Allen Perkins, MD, MPH

CURRENT DIAGNOSIS

- History of exposure is necessary for diagnosis.
- Ingested toxins can cause unusual symptoms, predominately gastrointestinal.
- Jellyfish envenomation is very painful but almost always self-limited.
- Trauma management follows principles of dirty wounds.
- Specific marine pathogens should be covered if contamination is suspected.

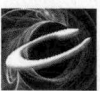

CURRENT THERAPY

Ingestions

- Avoidance is the best strategy.
- Early decontamination with activated charcoal (Actidose-Aqua) can reduce duration of symptoms.
- Symptomatic care is generally sufficient.

Jellyfish
- Remove visible stingers.
- Control pain with topical analgesia.

Trauma
- Avoiding water at feeding time can help to avoid injury.
- If envenomation is suspected, consider hot water immersion.
- Tetanus status should be checked.
- Antibiotic coverage should take marine pathogens into account.

The United States has more than 80,000 miles of coastline, and more people are enjoying water-dependent recreation activities such as scuba diving, snorkeling, and surfing. As a consequence, people are more likely to suffer trauma, envenomation, or poisoning related to an encounter with a marine creature, which will come to the attention of a physician. The science of marine medicine is limited; hence, treatment of these conditions is largely based on case reports and expert opinion; very few randomized, controlled studies are available. Misdiagnosis is common, especially when the patient has returned from vacationing or when the patient has been poisoned by improperly handled seafood. This article describes common ailments and injuries occurring as a consequence of direct contact with sea creatures and discusses management and prevention.

Ingestions
Ciguatera
Epidemiology
Ciguatera poisoning is the most commonly reported marine toxin disease in the world. It is caused by human ingestion of reef fish that have bioaccumulated sufficient amounts of the dinoflagellate *Gambierdiscus toxicus*, either through direct ingestion or through ingestion of smaller reef fish. Although limited to tropical regions, it is heat and cold tolerant, is lipid soluble, and can survive transport to other areas. The toxin becomes more concentrated as it passes up the food chain; fish such as amberjack, grouper, and snapper pose less of a risk than predatory fish such as barracuda and moray eel. Ciguatera poisoning affects at least 50,000 people worldwide annually, and there are several thousand cases of poisoning in Puerto Rico, the U.S. Virgin Islands, Hawaii, and Florida each year.

Clinical Features
Patients can exhibit a primarily gastrointestinal (diarrhea, abdominal cramps, and vomiting), neurologic (parasthesias, diffuse pain, blurred vision), cardiac (bradycardia), or mixed pattern of symptoms. Additionally, a cold sensation reversal, in which a patient perceives the cold temperatures as a hot sensation and vice versa, occurs in 80% of patients and is considered pathognomonic for ciguatera poison (Box 1).

The attack rate is high. As many as 80% to 100% of people who ingest affected fish develop symptoms depending on the size of the fish and the toxin load. Ingestion of internal organs where the toxin accumulates (e.g., liver, roe) is associated with more severe symptoms, but avoiding these organs is not protective. The symptoms are also related to the number of exposures over time, and patients typically have more severe symptoms with subsequent exposures. There is no age-related susceptibility, and no immunity is acquired through exposure.

Symptoms typically begin 1 to 6 hours after ingestion, although a delay of 12 to 24 hours can occur. Duration is 7 to 14 days, and neurologic symptoms occasionally persist for months to years. Chronic ciguatera syndrome can also occur as a constellation of symptoms such as general malaise, depression, headaches, muscle aches, and dysesthesias in the extremities. Patients with chronic disease report recurrences with ingestion of fish, ethanol, caffeine, and nuts up to 6 months after the acute illness resolves.

Diagnosis
The diagnosis should be entertained in any patient who has neurologic, gastrointestinal, or cardiac symptoms and a history of ingesting predatory fish within the past 24 hours. The symptom constellation can be similar to other ingestions, such as certain shellfish toxins, and differentiation requires knowledge of the

---

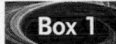

Box 1   Symptom Patterns Associated With Ciguatera Poisoning

Gastrointestinal Pattern
Onset 15 minutes to 24 hours, typically worsens, lasts 1–2 days and resolves
- Nausea and/or vomiting
- Profuse, watery diarrhea
- Abdominal pain

Neurologic Pattern
Onset up to 24 hours after ingestion, commonly nonphysiologic pattern, can last several months
- Numbness and paresthesias
- Vertigo
- Ataxia
- Severe weakness or lethargy
- Severe myalgia
- Decreased vibration and pain sensations
- Diffuse pain pattern
- Cold sensation reversal
- Coma

Cardiovascular Pattern
Onset up to 24 hours after ingestion is uncommon but occurs rapidly
- Bradycardia
- Hypotension
- Cardiovascular collapse

---

patient's diet for the previous day. Additionally, scombroid and type E botulinum poisoning should be considered, but these are unlikely if the patient did not ingest ill-appearing game. Other poisonings, such as organophosphates, can produce a similar symptom complex. There are no currently available clinical assays to assist in making the diagnosis, which is based on clinical suspicion and knowledge of the patient's diet history.

Treatment
If ciguatera poisoning is suspected soon after ingestion, I would consider gut decontamination with activated charcoal (Actidose Aqua) because it can reduce the toxin load and subsequent symptoms. Initial symptomatic treatment typically consists of fluid replacement to replace gastrointestinal losses.

Atropine (AtroPen) is used in patients who have bradycardia. Temporary electrical pacing may be used for refractory symptoms, and pressors may be needed in cases of severe hypotension. Neurologic symptoms are problematic because of their extended course as well as their severity. Mannitol (Osmitrol)[1] is often cited as effective in reducing the duration of neurologic symptoms, but I would use it with caution because the only double-blind trial failed to show any benefit. Nifedipine (Procardia)[1] (adult dose 10–20 mg three times daily) shows some theoretical promise in this regard, but there have been no studies in humans at this time. There are many local remedies used throughout the world that are said to be successful, which likely attests to the self-limited course of the ingestion in most cases. Table 1 offers more details regarding treatments currently used for ciguatera poisoning.

Prevention
Prevention is difficult except by avoiding ingestion of affected reef fish. The toxin is not deactivated by cooking, freezing, smoking, or salting. There are no outward signs of ciguatera: The fish look, taste, and smell normal. Although several commercial assays are available, they are neither sensitive nor specific enough to be relied on to prevent ciguatera poisoning.

To decrease the risk of ciguatera poisoning, I recommend the following steps: Avoid warm-water reef fish, especially those caught where ciguatera poisoning is known to occur; avoid moray eel injection; avoid ingesting large game fish; avoid consuming the

---

[1]Not FDA approved for this indication.

TABLE 1 Treatment for Ciguatera Poisoning

DRUG	DOSE	INDICATION
Activated charcoal (Actidose-Aqua)	Children <1 y: 1 g/kg Children 1–12 y: 25–50 g Adults: 25–100 g	Gut emptying and decontamination More effective in first hour
Antiemetics (no preference)	Administer per dosing recommendations	Intractable nausea and/or vomiting
Intravenous fluid bolus and infusion (normal saline or lactated Ringer's as initial)	Per volume replacement protocols	Hypovolemia
Atropine (AtroPen)	0.5–1.0 mg IV every 3–5 min to a maximum dose of 0.04 mg/kg per episode Maximum total dose: 3 mg for adults, 2 mg for adolescents, 1 mg for young children	Bradycardia
Pressors: Dopamine (Intropin), dobutamine (Dobutrex), epinephrine	Varies with clinical response	Hypotension, shock
Antihistamines (no preference)	Administer per dosing recommendations	Pruritus
Mannitol (Osmitrol)[1]	1 g/kg of a 20% solution given IV over several h Adult dose: 25–100 g, titrate to urinary output of 100 mL/h	Neurologic symptoms, double-blind study did not show benefit
Amitriptyline (Elavil)[1]	25–75 mg PO bid for patients >25 kg	Pruritus, dysesthesias

[1]Not FDA approved for this indication.

internal organs; and limit the amount of initial ingestion if you are in an area where ciguatera is known to occur. Additionally, patients travelling to distant locales should be made aware that, although the vast majority of cases result from direct ingestion, there have been cases of ciguatera passed through sexual contact and through breast milk, so they should be wary of body fluid contact if ciguatoxin is endemic to the area, if for no other reasons.

Scombroid
Epidemiology
Scombroid poisoning (also known as histamine fish poisoning) results from improper handling of certain fish between the time the fish is caught and the time it is cooked. In the United States it is most common in Hawaii and California. Improper preservation and refrigeration lead to histamine and histamine-like substances being produced in the dark meat of certain fish through a conversion of histadine to histamine by bacterial decarboxylases. Members of the family Scombridae, such as tuna and mackerel, contain the highest amounts of this substance, but both scombroid and nonscombroid fish have been associated with the disease. The production of toxins requires the introduction of bacteria during the handling process, primarily during storage at high temperatures. It is the total amount of histamine, the presence of other biogenic amines, and individual susceptibility that determine the severity of the symptoms.

Clinical Features
The patient develops a histamine reaction 20 to 30 minutes after ingestion. Symptoms can be cutaneous, gastrointestinal, neurologic, or hemodynamic or any combination of these. Cutaneous symptoms include flushing, urticaria and conjunctival injection, and localized edema; gastrointestinal symptoms include dry mouth, nausea, vomiting, diarrhea, and abdominal cramping; neurologic symptoms include severe headache and dizziness; and hemodynamic symptoms include palpitations and hypotension. In severe cases there can be bronchospasm and respiratory distress. These symptoms typically come on rapidly (within several minutes) and last less than 6 to 8 hours. Flushing is the most consistent clinical sign, occurring on exposed areas so it typically resembles sunburn. Diarrhea is also very common, occurring in 75% of symptomatic patients.

Diagnosis
As with ciguatera, the diagnosis is one of history. If the time between ingestion and illness is short and the patient has ingested a type of fish previously implicated in scombroid, then a tentative diagnosis can be made. The diagnosis is often confused with an allergic reaction. It can be distinguished from allergy by the lack of a previous allergic reaction as well as by testing the remaining fish for histamine, although testing is rarely warranted.

Treatment
Treatment is the same as for any histamine reaction, the cornerstone of which is antihistamine. Diphenhydramine (Benadryl) 50 mg for adults and 0.5–1 mg/kg/dose for children, repeated every 4 hours until symptoms abate, is delivered either intravenously or intramuscularly in severe cases and orally for milder cases. For severe cases, cimetidine (Tagamet)[1] 300 mg for adults, 20 mg/kg for children, either orally or intravenously, might be added for more complete histamine-receptor blockade. In cases where ingestion was recent, consider induced emesis using syrup of ipecac: 15 mL for children younger than 12 years or 30 mL otherwise. Most patients require only reassurance, and pharmacologic treatment will be unnecessary. It should be stressed to the patient that this is not an *allergic* reaction to fish, because the histamine is exogenous. Prevention is possible in regions where food storage and preparation are monitored through identification and removal of suspect fish.

Other Ingested Toxins
In addition to the toxins just discussed, ingestion of certain other marine creatures can lead to problems.

Ingestion of bivalves harvested from contaminated waters has been associated with hepatitis A, Norwalk virus, *Vibrio parahaemolyticus* and *Vibrio vulnificans* infections, the latter two particularly problematic and occasionally fatal in immunocompromised patients. I counsel patients likely to be immunocompromised, including diabetics and those with known liver disease, to avoid uncooked bivalves.

Shellfish are occasionally known to contain one or more of several toxins acquired through bioaccumulation of certain algae. These dinoflagellates tend to bloom in summer months. The symptoms occur immediately after ingestion and last several hours and are typically neurologic or gastrointestinal, or both. The shellfish poisoning syndromes are known as paralytic, neurologic, diarrheal, or amnestic depending on the predominant symptom. The care is typically supportive. Public health officials typically monitor local mollusk populations fairly carefully and alert the public to possible hazards.

Ingestion of the flesh of certain puffer fish has been associated with tetrodotoxin poisoning. The flesh of the fish (fugu) is considered a delicacy. The toxin builds up in internal organs such as the liver and the roe. If the toxin is ingested, it is likely to be fatal but there are certified chefs who are trained in avoiding the toxin when preparing the dish. Despite this precaution, as many as 50 deaths occur in

[1]Not FDA approved for this indication.

Japan annually from exposure to this toxin. Avoiding this puffer fish and avoiding the ingestion of certain other exotic animals (such as the blue-ringed octopus) eliminate the risk of acquiring this toxin.

Envenomations

Many marine creatures are venomous, and beachgoers experience clinically significant envenomations with some regularity. Jellyfish and related creatures (Cnidarians), sea urchins (Echinodermata), and stingrays (Chondrichthyes) are some of the more commonly identified marine animals involved with envenomations.

Jellyfish

These invertebrates have stinging cells called *nematocytes*, which carry nematocysts that continue to function when separated from the larger organism. For example, jellyfish nematocysts can sting if the tentacle is separated and after the jellyfish is dead. The venom is antigenic and causes a reaction of a dermatonecrotic, hemolytic, cardiopathic, or neurotoxic nature. The severity of the reaction depends on several variables, including the number of nematocysts that discharge, the toxicity of the coelenterate involved, and each patient's unique antigenic response.

Clinical Features

Although occasionally fatal as a consequence of an anaphylactic response in the United States and Caribbean, the primary concern in these areas with contact is pain, which is almost always self-limiting. Other less common symptoms include parasthesias, nausea, headaches, and chills. The symptoms may last up to 2 to 3 days. Certain Pacific jellyfish primarily found in the waters around Australia have a more potent toxin and are much more likely to cause death (which is still very uncommon). Additionally, the Irukandji syndrome, which occurs in the Pacific, is a suite of symptoms including muscle spasms, vomiting, hypertension, incessant coughing, and occasionally heart failure and brain hemorrhage. Almost all exposed people, regardless of the geographic location, do not have a severe reaction, and the principles of first aid are primarily the same throughout the world.

Treatment

In my experience, treatment is mostly concerned with limiting pain and neurologic symptoms, because anaphylaxis and other severe reactions are rare, and the following general guidelines can be applied. In the field, either the victim or a companion should remove any visible tentacles. To do so requires using care, with gloves or forceps being optimal to prevent further stings. If a towel is used, any nematocysts remaining on the towel can still discharge. Salt water can be used to wash off the nematocysts. Urine, household vinegar, fresh water, and rubbing with sand should be avoided.

Should the victim present to the physician's office or emergency department, topical lidocaine (4%)[1] should be liberally applied for 30 minutes or until the pain subsides followed by removal of the nematocysts, usually through use of the gloved hand or with forceps. Another method for removing the nematocysts is to apply shaving cream or baking soda slurry to the area and scrape off the nematocysts with a razor. Applications of cold, in the form of an ice pack, and immesion in hot water have variously been shown to improve pain, but because of the self-limited nature of the discomfort it is hard to gauge an optimum therapy. Either is probably acceptable until the patient is comfortable. Meat tenderizer has been found to be ineffective. Local anesthetics, antihistamines, and steroids are all used to control prolonged symptoms based on anecdotal experience. Antibiotics are not generally necessary. In the rare cases of cardiovascular collapse, supportive care and principles of treatment of anaphylaxis should be followed. A delayed hypersensitivity reaction can occur 1 to 3 days out, which will almost certainly be self-limited and can be treated with oral antihistamines and topical steroids if symptoms are severe.

Sea bather's itch is a form of jellyfish sting caused by the larvae of the thimble jellyfish. It is characterized by a painful, itchy rash under the edges of the bathing suit or wet suit. It can occasionally progress to a papular rash. Topical steroids can be used to relieve symptoms.

[1]Not FDA approved for this indication.

Prevention

Prevention is mostly a matter of common sense. Staying away from the organism (the tentacles can extend several meters from the body of the organism) and staying out of the water when jellyfish are known to be present are the most effective. There is a commercially available product, Safe Sea, which has been shown to reduce the number of nematocyst discharges and thus the severity of the sting should a swimmer need to be in the water when jellyfish are present. Wetsuits and other protective gear are ineffective.

Echinoderms

The Echinoderm family includes sea urchins. Urchins have toxin-coated spines that break off, leaving calcareous material in the wound, which can potentially cause infection. Symptoms include local pain, burning, and local discoloration. The discoloration is thought to be a temporary tattooing of the skin resulting from dye in the spines; absence of a spine is indicated if the discoloration spontaneously resolves within 48 hours. Theoretically, hot water disables the toxin, although there is no evidence in humans that it is effective. If a spine is present and easily accessible, it should be removed with fingers or forceps. If it is close to a joint or neurovascular structure it should be surgically removed. If the spines do not cause symptoms, retained pieces will likely reabsorb into the skin.

Stingrays

Although many fish are venomous, stingrays are the most clinically important, accounting for an estimated 1500 mostly minor injuries in the United States annually. These creatures partially bury themselves in the shallow, sandy bottom of the ocean, leading water enthusiasts to accidentally step on them or grab at what they think is a seashell.

Clinical Features

Stingrays have a spine at the base of their tail, which contains a venom gland. The spine, including the venom gland, is broken off and may be left in the resulting wound. The venom has vasoconstrictive properties that can lead to cyanosis and necrosis with poor wound healing and infection. Symptoms can include immediate and intense pain, salivation, nausea, vomiting, diarrhea, muscle cramps, dyspnea, seizures, headaches, and cardiac arrhythmias. Fatalities are rare and mostly a consequence of exsanguination at the scene or penetration of a vital organ.

Treatment

Home care should include rinsing the area thoroughly with fresh water if available (salt water if not) and removing any foreign body. If the damage is minimal the victim may soak the wound in warm water at home. The victim should watch for signs of infection and seek care for excessive bleeding, retained foreign body, or infection.

For severe wounds that lead the victim to seek medical attention, treatment should include achieving hemostasis followed by submersion of the affected region in hot but not scalding water (42–45°C, 108–113°F) for 30 to 90 minutes or until the pain resolves. Spines and stingers are typically radiopaque, so radiographs or an ultrasound should be obtained if a retained spine is suspected. The wound should be thoroughly cleansed, and delayed closure should be allowed. Tetanus immunization status should be reviewed and updated as appropriate. Surgical exploration may be necessary to remove residual foreign bodies. Prophylactic antibiotics are typically not necessary unless there is a residual foreign body or if the patient is immunosuppressed. If the wound becomes infected, *Staphylococcus* and *Streptococcus* species are the most common pathologic organisms. Unique to the marine environment are *Vibrio vulnificus* and *Mycobacterium marinum*, and antibiotic coverage should include coverage for all of these (Table 2).

Other Venomous Sea Creatures

Seasnakes are venomous creatures found most commonly in the Indo-Pacific area. Bites are uncommon (and envenomation is even less common), but should they occur, the toxin is very potent. The care is supportive. There is antivenom, which may be available in areas where the snakes are endemic.

Certain other fish and octopi have been associated with envenomation and occasional death. Most are tropical such as the stonefish,

TABLE 2 Antibiotic Choices in Marine Injuries

DRUG	DOSAGE	
	PEDIATRIC	ADULT
Outpatient Management		
Ciprofloxacin (Cipro)	20–30 mg/kg/day PO × 14 d[1]	500 mg PO bid × 14 d
Levofloxin (Levaquin)		750 mg PO qd × 14 d
Doxycycline (Vibramycin, Doryx)	>8 y: 2.2 mg/kg PO qd × 14 d	100 mg bid × 14 d
Inpatient Management		
Preferred		
Ceftazidime (Fortaz, Tazicef) *plus*	150 mg/kg/d q8h	1 g IV q8h
PO or IV quinolone or doxycycline	150 mg/kg/d q8h	1 g IV q8h
Alternative		
Gentamicin *plus*	Typically based on institutional protocol and adjusted based on serum levels	Typically based on institutional protocol and adjusted based on serum levels
TMP-SMX (Bactrim, Cotrim, Septra)	8–10 mg/kg/d TMP	8–10 mg/kg (lean body mass)/d TMP

[1]Not FDA approved for this indication.
Abbreviation: TMP-SMX = trimethoprim-sulfamethoxazole.

scorpionfish, and rabbitfish and the blue-ringed octopus. Certain varieties of catfish have venom as well. Envenomations, are rare and if they occur, treatment is based on good first-aid principles and antivenom where available (mostly in tropical areas).

Certain cone shells contain a toxin that can be fatal. This toxin is injected by the mollusk into the victim from a proboscis, which it extends from the small end of the cone. Treatment is primarily supportive.

Trauma

Abrasions, bites, and lacerations are usually the result of a marine animal's instinct to protect itself against a perceived danger. The most commonly involved marine animals are octopi, sharks, moray eels, and barracuda. The trauma alone creates problems for patients but the trauma can be further complicated by envenomation. It is often difficult to identify the marine animal involved in the attack. Treatment is for the most part symptomatic, with local cleansing and topical dressing usually sufficing. If the wound becomes infected, antibiotics should cover common organisms (see Table 2).

Environmental Hazards

Abrasions from the ambient environment are also common. These wounds should be thoroughly cleansed with soap and water and a topical antibiotic applied, because the wounds can contain toxins and are commonly contaminated with bacteria. Coral contains nematocysts and also has very sharp edges. Scuba divers in particular suffer from coral cuts in the course of their recreational diving. If these wounds become infected, coverage for *Vibrio* species should be included as well.

Sharks

Although shark attacks receive a lot of publicity, there are only around 50 such attacks worldwide annually and they result in fewer than 10 deaths. The majority of the deaths are in South Africa. Typically these attacks involve the tiger, great white, gray reef, and bull sharks. Attacks occur in shallow water within 100 feet of shore during the evening hours when sharks tend to feed. Common sense dictates avoiding areas where aggressive shark feeding has been noted.

Sequelae of a shark attack range from abrasions to death from hemorrhage. Abrasions and lacerations can occur when sharks brush or aggressively investigate humans. Soft tissue damage, fractures, and neurovascular damage result from such attacks. The majority of attacks result in minor injuries that require simple suturing. Morbidity increases in wounds that are greater than 20 cm or where more than one myofascial compartment is lost. General principles of first aid in marine animal injuries are found in Box 2. Although it would seem self-evident, practices such as urinating on the injury, applying oil or gasoline to injuries, and application of any strong oxidizing

Box 2 Management of Marine Trauma

Remove the victim from the water.
Ensure airway control.
Control bleeding.
Do not remove the wet suit if the victim is wearing one.
Attempt to identify the animal involved in the injury.
If the injury is severe, transport the victim to a hospital.
If envenomation is suspected, consider hot water immersion.
Irrigate the wound with normal saline.
Perform surgical débridement of the wound as appropriate.
If sutures must be placed, place them loosely and allow drainage. Primary suturing should be avoided in puncture wounds, crush injuries, and wounds in the distal extremities.
Start appropriate antibiotics if indicated.

agents, such as strong bases or acids should be counseled against when doing patient education regarding self-care.

References

Birsa L, Verity P, Lee R. Evaluation of the effects of various chemicals on discharge of and pain caused by jellyfish nematocysts. Comp Biochem and Physiol Part C: Toxicology & Pharmacology 2010;151:426–30.

Centers for Disease Control and Prevention. *Vibrio vulnificans* after a disaster. Available at http://emergency.cdc.gov/disasters/vibriovulnificus.asp (accessed August 19, 2015).

Edmonds C. Marine animal injuries. In: Bove AA, editor. Bove and Davis' Diving Medicine. 4th ed Philadelphia: Saunders; 2004. p. 287–318.

Fleming LE. Ciguatera fish poisoning. In: National Institute of Environmental Health Sciences, Marine and Freshwater Biomedical Sciences Center; 2006.

Isbister GK. Venomous fish stings in tropical northern Australia. Am J Emerg Med 2001;19:561–5.

Lahey T. Invasive *Mycobacterium marinum* infections, Emerg Infect Dis [serial online] 2003. November; Available at http://wwwnc.cdc.gov/eid/article/9/11/03-0192_article.htm (accessed August 19, 2015).

Lehane L, Olley J. Histamine (scombroid) fish poisoning: A review in a risk-assessment framework. Canberra, Australia: National Office of Animal and Plant Health; 1999.

Lynch PR, Bove AA. Marine poisonings and intoxications. In: Bove AA, editor. Bove and Davis' Diving Medicine. 4th ed. Philadelphia: Saunders; 2004. p. 287–318.

Perkins A, Morgan S. Poisonings, envenomations, and trauma from marine creatures. Am Fam Physician 2004;69:885–90.

Thomas C, Scott SA. All Stings Considered: First Aid and Medical Treatment of Hawaii's Marine Injuries. Honolulu: University of Hawaii Press; 1997.

Thomas CS, Scott SA, Galanis DJ, Goto RS. Box jellyfish *Carybdea alata* in Waikiki. The analgesic effect of Sting-Aid, Adolph's meat tenderizer and fresh water on their stings: A double-blinded, randomized, placebo-controlled clinical trial. Hawaii Med J 2001;60:205–10.

Thomas CS, Scott SA, Galanis DJ, Goto RS. Box jellyfish *Carybdea alata* in Waikiki. Their influx cycle plus the analgesic effect of hot and cold packs on their stings to swimmers at the beach: A randomized, placebo-controlled, clinical trial. Hawaii Med J 2001;60:100–7.

MEDICAL TOXICOLOGY

Method of
Howard C. Mofenson, MD; Thomas R. Caraccio, Pharm D;
Michael McGuigan, MD; and Joseph Greensher, MD

Introduction and Epidemiology

According to the national Toxic Exposure Surveillance System (TESS), over 2.4 million potentially toxic exposures were reported last year to Poison Control Centers throughout the United States. Poisonings were responsible for 1183 deaths and more than 500,000 hospitalizations. Poisoning accounts for 2% to 5% of pediatric hospital admissions, 10% of adult admissions, 5% of hospital admissions in the elderly (>65 years of age), and 5% of ambulance calls. In one urban hospital, drug-related emergencies accounted for 38% of the emergency department visits. An evaluation of a medical intensive care unit and step-down unit over a 3-month period indicated that poisonings accounted for 19.7% of admissions.

The largest number of fatalities resulting from poisoning reported to the TESS are caused by analgesics. The other principal toxicologic causes of fatalities are antidepressants, sedative hypnotics/antipsychotics, stimulants/street drugs, cardiovascular agents, and alcohols. Less than 1% of overdose cases reaching the hospitals result in fatality. However, patients presenting in deep coma to medical care facilities have a fatality rate of 13% to 35%. The largest single cause of coma of inapparent etiology is drug poisoning.

Pharmaceutical preparations are involved in 50% of poisonings. The number one pharmaceutical agent involved in exposures is acetaminophen. The severity of the manifestations of acute poisoning exposures varies greatly depending on whether the poisoning was intentional or unintentional. Unintentional exposures make up 85% to 90% of all poisoning exposures. The majority of cases are acute, occurring in children younger than 5 years of age, in the home, and resulting in no or minor toxicity. Many are actually ingestions of relatively nontoxic substances that require minimal medical care. Intentional poisonings, such as suicides, constitute 10% to 15% of exposures and may require the highest standards of medical and nursing care and the use of sophisticated equipment for recovery. Intentional ingestions are often of multiple substances and frequently include ethanol, acetaminophen, and aspirin. Suicides make up 54% of the reported fatalities. About 25% of suicides are attempted with drugs. Sixty percent of patients who take a drug overdose use their own medication and 15% use drugs prescribed for close relatives. The majority of the drug-related suicide attempts involve a central nervous system (CNS) depressant, and coma management is vital to the treatment.

Assessment and Maintenance of the Vital Functions

The initial assessment of all patients in medical emergencies follows the principles of basic and advanced cardiac life support. The adequacy of the patient's airway, degree of ventilation, and circulatory status should be determined. The vital functions should be established and maintained. Vital signs should be measured frequently and should include body core temperature. The assessment of vital functions should include the rate numbers (e.g., respiratory rate) and indications of effectiveness (e.g., depth of respirations and degree of gas exchange). Table 1 gives important measurements and vital signs.

Level of consciousness should be assessed by immediate AVPU (Alert, responds to Verbal stimuli, responds to Painful stimuli, and Unconscious). If the patient is unconscious, one must assess the severity of the unconsciousness by the Glasgow Coma Scale (Table 2).

If the patient is comatose, management requires administering 100% oxygen, establishing vascular access, and obtaining blood for pertinent laboratory studies. The administration of glucose, thiamine, and naloxone, as well as intubation to protect the airway, should be considered. Pertinent laboratory studies include arterial blood gases (ABG), electrocardiography (ECG), determination of blood glucose level, electrolytes, renal and liver tests, and acetaminophen plasma concentration in all cases of intentional ingestions. Radiography of the chest and abdomen may be useful. The severity of a stimulant's effects can also be assessed and should be documented to follow the trend.

The examiner should completely expose the patient by removing clothes and other items that interfere with a full evaluation. One should look for clues to etiology in the clothes and include the hat and shoes.

Prevention of Absorption and Reduction of Local Damage

Exposure

Poisoning exposure routes include ingestion (76.8%), dermal (8%), ophthalmologic (5%), inhalation (6%), insect bites and stings (4%), and parenteral injections (0.5%). The effect of the toxin may be local, systemic, or both.

TABLE 1 Important Measurements and Vital Signs

AGE	BODY SURFACE AREA (m²)	WEIGHT (kg)	HEIGHT (cm)	PULSE (BPM) RESTING	BLOOD PRESSURE HYPOTENSION	HYPERTENSION SIGNIFICANT	HYPERTENSION SEVERE	RESPIRATORY RATE (rpm)
Newborn	0.19	3.5	50	70–190	<60/40	>96	>106	30–60
1 mo–6 mo	0.30	4–7	50–65	80–160	<70/45	>104	>110	30–50
6 mo–1 y	0.38	7–10	65–75	80–160	<70/45	>104	>110	20–40
1–2 y	0.50–0.55	10–12	75–85	80–140	<74/47	>112/74	>118/82	20–40
3–5 y	0.54–0.68	15–20	90–108	80–120	<80/52	>116/76	>124/84	20–40
6–9 y	0.68–0.85	20–28	122–133	75–115	<90/60	>122/82	>130/86	16–25
10–12 y	1.00–1.07	30–40	138–147	70–110	<90/60	>126/82	>134/90	16–25
13–15 y	1.07–1.22	42–50	152–160	60–100	<90/60	>136/86	>144/92	16–20
16–18 y	1.30–1.60	53–60	160–170	60–100	<90/60	>142/92	>150/98	12–16
Adult	1.40–1.70	60–70	160–170	60–100	<90/60	>140/90	>210/120	10–16

Data from Nadas A: Pediatric Cardiology, 3rd ed. Philadelphia, WB Saunders, 1976; Blumer JL (ed): A Practice Guide to Pediatric Intensive Care. St Louis, Mosby, 1990; AAP and ACEP: Respiratory Distress in APLS Pediatric Emergency Medicine Course, 1993; Second Task Force: Blood pressure control in children–1987, Pediatr 79:1, 1987; Linakis JG: Hypertension. In Fliesher GR, Ludwig S (eds); Textbook of Pediatric Emergency Medicine, 3rd ed. Baltimore, Williams & Wilkins, 1993.

TABLE 2	Glasgow Coma Scale			
SCALE	**ADULT RESPONSE**	**SCORE**		**PEDIATRIC, 0–1 YEARS**
Eye opening	Spontaneous	4		Spontaneous
	To verbal command	3		To shout
	To pain	2		To pain
	None	1		No response
Motor response				
To verbal command	Obeys	6		
To painful stimuli	Localized pain	5		Localized pain
	Flexion withdrawal	4		Flexion withdrawal
	Decorticate flexion	3		Decorticate flexion
	Decerebrate extension	2		Decerebrate flexion
	None	1		None
Verbal response: adult	Oriented and converses	5		Cries, smiles, coos
	Disoriented but converses	4		Cries or screams
	Inappropriate words	3		Inappropriate sounds
	Incomprehensible sounds	2		Grunts
	None	1		Gives no response
Verbal response: child	Oriented	5		
	Words or babbles	4		
	Vocal sounds	3		
	Cries or moans to stimuli	2		
	None	1		

Data from Teasdale G, Jennett B: Assessment of coma impaired consciousness. Lancet 2:83, 1974; Simpson D, Reilly P: Pediatric coma scale. Lancet 2:450, 1982; Seidel J: Preparing for pediatric emergencies. Pediatr Rev 16:470, 1995.

Local effects (skin, eyes, mucosa of respiratory or gastrointestinal tract) occur where contact is made with the poisonous substance. Local effects are nonspecific chemical reactions that depend on the chemical properties (e.g., pH), concentration, contact time, and type of exposed surface.

Systemic effects occur when the poison is absorbed into the body and depend on the dose, the distribution, and the functional reserve of the organ systems. Shock and hypoxia are part of systemic toxicity.

Delayed Toxic Action
Therapeutic doses of most pharmaceuticals are absorbed within 90 minutes. However, the patient with exposure to a potential toxin may be asymptomatic at this time because a sufficient amount has not yet been absorbed or metabolized to produce toxicity at the time the patient presents for care.

Absorption can be significantly delayed under the following circumstances:

1. Drugs with anticholinergic properties (e.g., antihistamines, belladonna alkaloids, diphenoxylate with atropine [Lomotil], phenothiazines, and tricyclic antidepressants).
2. Modified release preparations such as sustained-release, enteric-coated, and controlled-release formulations have delayed and prolonged absorption.
3. Concretions may form (e.g., salicylates, iron, glutethimide, and meprobamate [Equanil]) that can delay absorption and prolong the toxic effects. Large quantities of drugs tend to be absorbed more slowly than small quantities.

Some substances must be metabolized into a toxic metabolite (acetaminophen, acetonitrile, ethylene glycol, methanol, methylene chloride, parathion, and paraquat). In some cases, time is required to produce a toxic effect on organ systems (*Amanita phalloides* mushrooms, carbon tetrachloride, colchicine, digoxin [Lanoxin], heavy metals, monoamine oxidase inhibitors, and oral hypoglycemic agents).

Initial Management
1. Stabilization of airway, breathing, and circulation and protection of same.
2. Identification of specific toxin or toxic syndrome.
3. Initial treatment: D50W; consider thiamine, naloxone (Narcan), oxygen, and antidotes if needed.
4. Physical assessment.
5. Decontamination: Gastrointestinal tract, skin, eyes.

Decontamination
In the asymptomatic patient who has been exposed to a toxic substance, decontamination procedures should be considered if the patient has been exposed to potentially toxic substances in toxic amounts.

Ocular exposure should be immediately treated with water irrigation for 15 to 20 minutes with the eyelids fully retracted. One should not use neutralizing chemicals. All caustic and corrosive injuries should be evaluated with fluorescein dye and by an ophthalmologist.

Dermal exposure is treated immediately with copious water irrigation for 30 minutes, not a forceful flushing. Shampooing the hair, cleansing the fingernails, navel, and perineum, and irrigating the eyes are necessary in the case of an extensive exposure. The clothes should be specially bagged and may have to be discarded. Leather goods can become irreversibly contaminated and must be abandoned. Caustic (alkali) exposures can require hours of irrigation. Dermal absorption can occur with pesticides, hydrocarbons, and cyanide.

Injection exposures (e.g., snake envenomation) can be treated with venom extractors. Venom extractors can be used within minutes of envenomation, and proximal lymphatic constricting bands or elastic wraps can be used to delay lymphatic flow and immobilize the extremity. Cold packs and tourniquets should not be used and incision is generally not recommended. Substances of abuse may be injected intravenously or subcutaneously. In these cases, little decontamination can be done.

Inhalation exposure to toxic substances is managed by immediate removal of the victim from the contaminated environment by protected rescuers.

Gastrointestinal exposure is the most common route of poisoning. Gastrointestinal decontamination historically has been done by gastric emptying: induction of emesis, gastric lavage, administration of activated charcoal, and the use of cathartics or whole bowel irrigation. No procedure is routine; it should be individualized for each case. If no attempt is made to decontaminate the patient, the reason should be clearly documented on the medical record (e.g., time elapsed, past peak of action, ineffectiveness, or risk of procedure).

Gastric Emptying Procedures

The gastric emptying procedure used is influenced by the age of the patient, the effectiveness of the procedure, the time of ingestion (gastric emptying is usually ineffective after 1 hour postingestion), the patient's clinical status (time of peak effect has passed or the patient's condition is too unstable), formulation of the substance ingested (regular release versus modified release), the amount ingested, and the rapidity of onset of CNS depression or stimulation (convulsions). Most studies show that only 30% (range, 19% to 62%) of the ingested toxin is removed by gastric emptying under optimal conditions. It has not been demonstrated that the choice of procedure improved the outcome.

A mnemonic for gathering information is STATS:

S—substance
T—type of formulation
A—amount and age
T—time of ingestion
S—signs and symptoms

The examiner should attempt to obtain AMPLE information about the patient:

A—age and allergies
M—available medications
P—past medical history including pregnancy, psychiatric illnesses, substance abuse, or intentional ingestions
L—time of last meal, which may influence absorption and the onset and peak action
E—events leading to present condition

The intent of the patient should also be determined.

The Regional Poison Center should be consulted for the exact ingredients of the ingested substance and the latest management. The treatment information on the labels of products are notoriously inaccurate.

Ipecac Syrup

Syrup of ipecac–induced emesis has virtually no use in the emergency department. Although at one time it was considered most useful in young children with a recent witnessed ingestion, it is no longer advised in most cases. Current guidelines from the American Association of Poison Control Centers have significantly limited the indications for inducing emesis because the risk most often exceeds the benefit derived from this procedure. The Poison Control Center should be called if inducing emesis is being considered.

Contraindications or situations in which induction of emesis is inappropriate include the following:

- Ingestion of caustic substance
- Loss of airway protective reflexes because of ingestion of substances that can produce rapid onset of CNS depression (e.g., short-acting benzodiazepines, barbiturates, nonbarbiturate sedative-hypnotics, opioids, tricyclic antidepressants) or convulsions (e.g., camphor [Ponstel], chloroquine [Aralen], codeine, isoniazid [Nydrazid], mefenamic acid, nicotine, propoxyphene [Darvon], organophosphate insecticides, strychnine, and tricyclic antidepressants)
- Ingestion of low-viscosity petroleum distillates (e.g., gasoline, lighter fluid, kerosene)
- Significant vomiting prior to presentation or hematemesis
- Age under 6 months (no established dose, safety, or efficacy data)
- Ingestion of foreign bodies (emesis is ineffective and may lead to aspiration)
- Clinical conditions including neurologic impairment, hemodynamic instability, increased intracranial pressure, and hypertension
- Delay in presentation (more than 1 hour postingestion)

The dose of syrup of ipecac in the 6- to 9-month-old infant is 5 mL; in the 9- to 12-month-old, 10 mL; and in the 1- to 12-year-old, 15 mL. In children older than 12 years and in adults, the dose is 30 mL. The dose can be repeated once if the child does not vomit in 15 to 20 minutes. The vomitus should be inspected for remnants of pills or toxic substances, and the appearance and odor should be documented. When ipecac is not available, 30 mL of mild dishwashing soap (not dishwasher detergent) can be used, although it is less effective.

Complications are very rare but include aspiration, protracted vomiting, rarely cardiac toxicity with long-term abuse, pneumothorax, gastric rupture, diaphragmatic hernia, intracranial hemorrhage, and Mallory-Weiss tears.

Gastric Lavage

Gastric lavage should be considered only when life-threatening amounts of substances were involved, when the benefits outweigh the risks, when it can be performed within 1 hour of the ingestion, and when no contraindications exist.

The contraindications are similar to those for ipecac-induced emesis. However, gastric lavage can be accomplished after the insertion of an endotracheal tube in cases of CNS depression or controlled convulsions. The patient should be placed with the head lower than the hips in a left-lateral decubitus position. The location of the tube should be confirmed by radiography, if necessary, and suctioning equipment should be available.

Contraindications to gastric lavage include the following:

- Ingestion of caustic substances (risk of esophageal perforation)
- Uncontrolled convulsions, because of the danger of aspiration and injury during the procedure
- Ingestion of low-viscosity petroleum distillate products
- CNS depression or absent protective airway reflexes, without endotracheal protection
- Significant cardiac dysrhythmias
- Significant emesis or hematemesis prior to presentation
- Delay in presentation (more than 1 hour postingestion)

Size of Tube. The best results with gastric lavage are obtained with the largest possible orogastric tube that can be reasonably passed (nasogastric tubes are not large enough to remove solid material). In adults, a large-bore orogastric Lavacuator hose or a No. 42 French Ewald tube should be used; in young children, orogastric tubes are generally too small to remove solid material and gastric lavage is not recommended.

The amount of fluid used varies with the patient's age and size. In general, aliquots of 50 to 100 mL per lavage are used in adults. Larger amounts of fluid may force the toxin past the pylorus. Lavage fluid is 0.9% saline.

Complications are rare and may include respiratory depression, aspiration pneumonitis, cardiac dysrhythmias as a result of increased vagal tone, esophageal-gastric tears and perforation, laryngospasm, and mediastinitis.

Activated Charcoal

Oral activated charcoal adsorbs the toxin onto its surface before absorption. According to recent guidelines set forth by the American Academy of Clinical Toxicology, activated charcoal should not be used routinely. Its use is indicated only if a toxic amount of substance has been ingested and is optimally effective within 1 hour of the ingestion. Because of the slow absorption of large quantities of toxin, activated charcoal may be beneficial after 1 hour postingestion.

Activated charcoal does not effectively adsorb small molecules or molecules lacking carbon (Table 3). Activated charcoal adsorption may be diminished by milk, cocoa powder, and ice cream.

There are a few relative contraindications to the use of activated charcoal:

1. Ingestion of caustics and corrosives, which may produce vomiting or cling to the mucosa and falsely appear as a burn on endoscopy.
2. Comatose patient, in whom the airway must be secured prior to activated charcoal administration.
3. Patient without presence of bowel sounds.

Note: Activated charcoal was shown not to interfere with effectiveness of *N*-acetylcysteine in cases of acetaminophen overdose, so it is no longer contraindicated as was thought in the past.

The usual initial adult dose is 60 to 100 g and the dose for children is 15 to 30 g. It is administered orally as a slurry mixed

TABLE 3	Substances Poorly Adsorbed by Activated Charcoal
C	Caustics and corrosives
H	Heavy metals (arsenic, iron, lead, mercury)
A	Alcohols (ethanol, methanol, isopropanol) and glycols (ethylene glycols)
R	Rapid onset of absorption (cyanide and strychnine)
C	Chlorine and iodine
O	Others insoluble in water (substances in tablet form)
A	Aliphatic hydrocarbons (petroleum distillates)
L	Laxatives (sodium, magnesium, potassium, and lithium)

with water or by nasogastric or orogastric tube. *Caution:* Be sure the tube is in the stomach. Cathartics are not necessary.

Although repeated dosing with activated charcoal may decrease the half-life and increases the clearance of phenobarbital, dapsone, quinidine, theophylline, and carbamazepine (Tegretol), recent guidelines indicate there is insufficient evidence to support the use of multiple-dose activated charcoal unless a life-threatening amount of one of the substances mentioned is involved. At present there are no controlled studies that demonstrate that multiple-dose activated charcoal or cathartics alter the clinical course of an intoxication. The dose varies from 0.25 to 0.50 g/kg every 1 to 4 hours, and continuous nasogastric tube infusion of 0.25 to 0.5 g/kg/h has been used to decrease vomiting.

Gastrointestinal dialysis is the diffusion of the toxin from the higher concentration in the serum of the mesenteric vessels to the lower levels in the gastrointestinal tract mucosal cell and subsequently into the gastrointestinal lumen, where the concentration has been lowered by intraluminal adsorption of activated charcoal.

Complications of treatment with activated charcoal include vomiting in 50% of cases, desorption (especially with weak acids in intestine), and aspiration (at least a dozen cases of aspiration have been reported). There are many cases of unreported pulmonary aspirations and "charcoal lungs," intestinal obstruction or pseudoobstruction (three case reports with multiple dosing, none with a single dose), empyema following esophageal perforation, and hypermagnesemia and hypernatremia, which have been associated with repeated concurrent doses of activated charcoal and saline cathartics. Catharsis was used to hasten the elimination of any remaining toxin in the gastrointestinal tract. There are no studies to demonstrate the effectiveness of cathartics, and they are no longer recommended as a form of gastrointestinal decontamination.

Whole-Bowel Irrigation

With whole-bowel irrigation, solutions of polyethylene glycol (PEG) with balanced electrolytes are used to cleanse the bowel without causing shifts in fluids and electrolytes. The procedure is not approved by the U.S. Food and Drug Administration for this purpose.

Indications. The procedure has been studied and used successfully in cases of iron overdose when abdominal radiographs reveal incomplete emptying of excess iron. There are additional indications for other types of ingestions, such as with body-packing of illicit drugs (e.g., cocaine, heroin).

The procedure is to administer the solution (GoLYTELY or Colyte), orally or by nasogastric tube, in a dose of 0.5 L per hour in children younger than 5 years of age and 2 L per hour in adolescents and adults for 5 hours. The end point is reached when the rectal effluent is clear or radiopaque materials can no longer be seen in the gastrointestinal tract on abdominal radiographs.

Contraindications. These measures should not be used if there is extensive hematemesis, ileus, or signs of bowel obstruction, perforation, or peritonitis. Animal experiments in which PEG was added to activated charcoal indicated that activated charcoal-salicylates and activated charcoal-theophylline combinations resulted in decreased adsorption and desorption of salicylate and theophylline and no therapeutic benefit over activated charcoal alone. Polyethylene solutions are bound by activated charcoal in vitro, decreasing the efficacy of activated charcoal.

Dilutional treatment is indicated for the immediate management of caustic and corrosive poisonings but is otherwise not useful. The administration of diluting fluid above 30 mL in children and 250 mL in adults may produce vomiting, reexposing the vital tissues to the effects of local damage and possible aspiration.

Neutralization is not proven to be either safe or effective.

Endoscopy and surgery have been required in the case of body-packer obstruction, intestinal ischemia produced by cocaine ingestion, and iron local caustic action.

Differential Diagnosis of Poisons on the Basis of Central Nervous System Manifestations

Neurologic parameters help to classify and assess the need for supportive treatment as well as provide diagnostic clues to the etiology. Table 4 lists the effects of CNS depressants, CNS stimulants, hallucinogens, and autonomic nervous system anticholinergics and cholinergics.

CNS depressants are cholinergics, opioids, sedative-hypnotics, and sympatholytic agents. The hallmarks are lethargy, sedation, stupor, and coma. In exception to the manifestations listed in Table 4, (a) barbiturates may produce an initial tachycardia; (b) convulsions are produced by codeine, propoxyphene (Darvon), meperidine (Demerol), glutethimide, phenothiazines, methaqualone, and tricyclic and cyclic antidepressants; (c) benzodiazepines rarely produce coma that will interfere with cardiorespiratory functions; and (d) pulmonary edema is common with opioids and sedative-hypnotics.

The CNS stimulants are anticholinergic, hallucinogenic, sympathomimetic, and withdrawal agents. The hallmarks of CNS stimulants are convulsions and hyperactivity.

There is considerable overlapping of effects among the various hallucinogens, but the major hallmark manifestation is hallucinations.

Guidelines for In-Hospital Disposition

Classification of patients as high risk depends on clinical judgment. Any patient who needs cardiorespiratory support or has a persistently altered mental status for 3 hours or more should be considered for intensive care.

Guidelines for admitting patients older than 14 years of age to an intensive care unit, after 2 to 3 hours in the emergency department, include the following:

1. Need for intubation
2. Seizures
3. Unresponsiveness to verbal stimuli
4. Arterial carbon dioxide pressure greater than 45 mm Hg
5. Cardiac conduction or rhythm disturbances (any rhythm except sinus arrhythmia)
6. Close monitoring of vital signs during antidotal therapy or elimination procedures
7. The need for continuous monitoring
8. QRS interval greater than 0.10 second, in cases of tricyclic antidepressant poisoning
9. Systolic blood pressure less than 80 mm Hg
10. Hypoxia, hypercarbia, acid-base imbalance, or metabolic abnormalities
11. Extremes of temperature
12. Progressive deterioration or significant underlying medical disorders

Use of Antidotes

Antidotes are available for only a relatively small number of poisons. An antidote is not a substitute for good supportive care. Table 5 summarizes the commonly used antidotes, their indications, and their methods of administration. The Regional Poison Control Center can give further information on these antidotes.

TABLE 4 Agents with Central Nervous System (CNS) Effects

AGENTS	GENERAL MANIFESTATIONS	AGENTS	GENERAL MANIFESTATIONS
CNS Depressants Alcohols and glycols (S-H) Anticonvulsants (S-H) Antidysrhythmics (S-H) Antihypertensives (S-H) Barbiturates (S-H) Benzodiazepines (S-H) Butyrophenones (Syly) β-Adrenergic blockers (Syly) Calcium channel blockers (Syly) Digitalis (Syly) Opioids Lithium (mixed) Muscle relaxants Phenothiazines (Syly) Nonbarbiturate/benzodiazepine glutethimide, methaqualone, methyprylon, sedative-hypnotics (chloral hydrate, ethchlorvynol, bromide) Tricyclic antidepressants (late Syly)	Bradycardia Bradypnea Shallow respirations Hypotension Hypothermia Flaccid coma Miosis Hypoactive bowel sounds	**Hallucinogens** Amphetamines‡ Anticholinergics Cardiac glycosides Cocaine Ethanol withdrawal Hydrocarbon inhalation (abuse) Mescaline (peyote) Mushrooms (psilocybin) Phencyclidine	Tachycardia and dysrhythmias Tachypnea Hypertension Hallucinations, usually visual Disorientation Panic reaction Toxic psychosis Moist skin Mydriasis (reactive) Hyperthermia Flashbacks
CNS Stimulants Amphetamines (Sy) Anticholinergics* Cocaine (Sy) Camphor (mixed) Ergot alkaloids (Sy) Isoniazid (mixed) Lithium (mixed) Lysergic acid diethylamide (H) Hallucinogens (H) Mescaline and synthetic analogs Metals (arsenic, lead, mercury) Methylphenidate (Ritalin) (Sy) Monoamine oxidase inhibitors (Sy) Pemoline (Cylert) (Sy) Phencyclidine (H)† Salicylates (mixed) Strychnine (mixed) Sympathomimetics (Sy) (phenylpropanolamine, theophylline, caffeine, thyroid) Withdrawal from ethanol, β-adrenergic blockers, clonidine, opioids, sedative–hypnotics (W)	Tachycardia Tachypnea and dysrhythmias Hypertension Convulsions Toxic psychosis Mydriasis (reactive) Agitation and restlessness Moist skin Tremors	**Anticholinergics** Antihistamines Antispasmodic gastrointestinal preparations Antiparkinsonian preparations Atropine Cyclobenzaprine (Flexeril) Mydriatic ophthalmologic agents Over-the-counter sleep agents Plants (*Datura* spp)/mushrooms Phenothiazines (early) Scopolamine Tricyclic/cyclic antidepressants (early)	Tachycardia, dysrhythmias (rare) Tachypnea Hypertension (mild) Hyperthermia Hallucinations ("mad as a hatter") Mydriasis (unreactive) ("blind as a bat") Flushed skin ("red as a beet") Dry skin and mouth ("dry as a bone") Hypoactive bowel sounds Urinary retention Lilliputian hallucinations ("little people")
		Cholinergics Bethanechol (Urecholine) Carbamate insecticides (Carbaryl) Edrophonium Organophosphate insecticides (Malathion, parathion) Parasympathetic agents (physostigmine, pyridostigmine) Toxic mushrooms (*Clitocybe* spp.)	Bradycardia (muscarinic) Tachycardia (nicotinic effect) Miosis (muscarinic) Diarrhea (muscarinic) Hypertension (variable) Hyperactive bowel sounds Excess urination (muscarinic) Excess salivation (muscarinic) Lacrimation (muscarinic) Bronchospasm (muscarinic) Muscle fasciculations (nicotinic) Paralysis (nicotinic)

*Anticholinergics produce dry skin and mucosa and decreased bowel sounds.

†Phencyclidine may produce miosis.

‡The amphetamine hybrids are methylene dioxymethamphetamine (MDMA, ecstasy, "Adam") and methylene dioxyamphetamine (MDA, "Eve"), which are associated with deaths.

Abbreviations: H = hallucinogen; S-H = sedative–hypnotic; Sy = sympathomimetic; Syly = sympatholytic; W = withdrawal.

TABLE 5 Initial Doses of Antidotes for Common Poisonings

ANTIDOTE	USE	DOSE	ROUTE	ADVERSE REACTIONS/COMMENTS
N-Acetyl Cysteine (NAC, Mucomyst): Stock level to treat 70 kg adult for 24 h: 25 vials, 20%, 30 mL	Acetaminophen, carbon tetrachloride (experimental)	140 mg/kg loading, followed by 70 mg/kg q4h for 17 doses 150 mg/kg in 200 mL of D_5W over 1 h, then 50 mg/kg in 1 liter D_5W over 16 h	PO IV	Nausea, vomiting. Dilute to 5% with sweet juice or flat cola. Useful for those who cannot tolerate oral route.
Atropine: Stock level to treat 70 kg adult for 24 h: 1 g (1 mg/mL in 1, 10 mL)	Organophosphate and carbamate pesticides: bradydysrhythmics, β-adrenergics, calcium channel blockers/nerve agents	*Child:* 0.02–0.05 mg/kg repeated q5–10 min to max of 2 mg as necessary until cessation of secretions *Adult:* 1–2 mg q5–10 min as necessary. Dilute in 1–2 mL of 0.9% saline for ET instillation. *IV infusion dose:* Place 8 mg of atropine in 100 mL D_5W or saline. Conc. = 0.08 mg/mL; dose range = 0.02–0.08 mg/kg/h or 0.25–1 mL/kg/h. Severe poisoning may require supplemental doses of IV atropine intermittently in doses of 1–5 mg until drying of secretions occurs.	IV/ET	Tachycardia, dry mouth, blurred vision, and urinary retention. Ensure adequate ventilation before administration.
Calcium Chloride (10%): Stock level to treat 70 kg adult for 24 h: 10 vials 1 g (1.35 mEq/mL)	Hypocalcemia, fluoride, calcium channel blockers, β-blockers, oxalates, ethylene glycol, hypermagnesemia	0.1–0.2 mL/kg (10–20 mg/kg) slow push q10 min up to max 10 mL (1 g). Since calcium response lasts 15 min, some may require continuous infusion 0.2 mL/kg/h up to maximum of 10 mL/h while monitoring for dysrhythmias and hypotension.	IV	Administer slowly with BP and ECG monitoring and have magnesium available to reverse calcium effects. Tissue irritation, hypotension, dysrhythmias from rapid injection. Contraindications: digitalis glycoside intoxication.
Calcium Gluconate (10%): Stock level to treat 70 kg adult for 24 h: 20 vials 1 g (0.45 mEq/mL)	Hypocalcemia, fluoride, calcium channel blockers, hydrofluoric acid; black widow envenomation	0.3–0.4 mL/kg (30–40 mg/kg) slow push; repeat as needed to max dose 10–20 mL (1–2 g).	IV	Same comments as calcium chloride.
Infiltration of Calcium Gluconate	Hydrofluoric acid skin exposure	Dose: Infiltrate each square cm of affected dermis/subcutaneous tissue with about 0.5 mL of 10% calcium gluconate using a 30-gauge needle. Repeat as needed to control pain.	Infiltrate	
Intra-arterial Calcium Gluconate	Hydrofluoric acid skin exposure	Infuse 20 mL of 10% calcium gluconate (not chloride) diluted in 250 mL D_5W via the radial or brachial artery proximal to the injury over 3–4 h.		Alternatively, dilute 10 mL of 10% calcium gluconate with 40–50 mL of D_5W.
Calcium Gluconate Gel: Stock level: 3.5 g	Hydrofluoric acid skin exposure	2.5 g USP powder added to 100 mL water-soluble lubricating jelly, e.g., K-Y Jelly or Lubifax (or 3.5 mg into 150 mL). Some use 6 g of calcium carbonate in 100 g of lubricant. Place injured hand in surgical glove filled with gel. Apply q4h. If pain persists, calcium gluconate injection may be needed (above).	Dermal	Powder is available from Spectrum Pharmaceutical Co. in California: 800-772-8786. Commercial preparation of Ca gluconate gel is available from Pharmascience in Montreal, Quebec: 514-340-1114.
Cyanide Antidote Kit: Stock level to treat 70 kg adult for 24 h: 2 Lilly Cyanide Antidote kits	Cyanide Hydrogen sulfide (nitrites are given only) Do not use sodium thiosulfate for hydrogen sulfide Individual portions of the kit can be used in certain circumstances (consult PCC)	Amyl nitrite: 1 crushable ampule for 30 sec of every min. Use new amp q3 min. May omit step if venous access is established.	Inhalation	If methemoglobinemia occurs, do not use methylene blue to correct this because it releases cyanide.

Antidote	Indication	Route	Dose	Adverse Effects/Comments
	Cyanide Hydrogen sulfide (nitrites are given only) Do not use sodium thiosulfate for hydrogen sulfide Individual portions of the kit can be used in certain circumstances (consult PCC) Do not use sodium thiosulfate for hydrogen sulfide Individual portions of the kit can be used in certain circumstances (consult PCC)	IV IV	Sodium nitrite: *Child:* 0.33 mL/kg of 3% solution if hemoglobin level is not known, otherwise based on tables with product. *Adult:* up to 300 mg (10 mL). Dilute nitrite in 100 mL 0.9% saline, administer slowly at 5 mL/min. Slow infusion if fall in BP. Sodium thiosulfate: *Child:* 1.6 mL/kg of 2.5% solution, may be repeated q30–60 min to a maximum of 12.5 g or 50 mL in adult. Administer over 20 min.	If methemoglobinemia occurs, do not use methylene blue to correct this because it releases cyanide. Nausea, dizziness, headache. Tachycardia, muscle rigidity, and bronchospasm (rapid administration).
Dantrolene Sodium (Dantrium): Stock level to treat 70 kg adult for 24 h: 700 mg, 35 vials (20 mg/vial)	Malignant hyperthermia	IV/PO	2–3 mg/kg IV rapidly. Repeat loading dose every 10 min. If necessary up to a maximum total dose of 10 mg/kg. When temperature and heart rate decrease, slow the infusion 1–2 mg/kg q6h for 24–28 h until all evidence of malignant hyperthermia syndrome has subsided. Follow with oral doses 1–2 mg/kg four times a day for 24 h as necessary.	Hepatotoxicity occurs with cumulative dose of 10 mg/kg. Thrombophlebitis (best given in central line). Available as 20 mg lyophilized dantrolene powder for reconstruction, which contains 3 g mannitol and sodium hydroxide in 70-mL vial. Mix with 60 mL sterile distilled water without a bacteriostatic agent and protect from light. Use within 6 hours after reconstituting.
Deferoxamine (Desferal): Stock level to treat 70 kg adult for 24 h: 17 vials (500 mg/amp)	Iron	Preferred IV: avoid therapy >24 h	IV infusion of 15 mg/kg/h (3 mL/kg/h: 500 mg in 100 mL D_5W) max 6 g/d Rates of >45 µg/kg/h if conc >1000 µg/dL.	Hypotension (minimized by avoiding rapid infusion rates) DFO challenge test 50 mg/kg is unreliable if negative.
Diazepam (Valium): Stock level to treat 70 kg adult for 24 h: 200 mg, 5 mg/mL; 2, 10 mL	Any intoxication that provokes seizures when specific therapy is not available (e.g., amphetamines, PCP, barbiturate and alcohol withdrawal) Chloroquine poisoning	IV	Adult, 5–10 mg IV (max 20 mg) at a rate of 5 mg/min until seizure is controlled. May be repeated 2 or 3 times. Child, 0.1–0.3 mg/kg up to 10 mg IV slowly over 2 min.	Confusion, somnolence, coma, hypotension. Intramuscular absorption is erratic. Establish airway and administer 100% oxygen and glucose.
Digoxin-Specific Fab Antibodies (Digibind): Stock level to treat 70 kg adult for 24 h: 20 vials	Digoxin, digitoxin, oleander tea with the following: (1) Imminent cardiac arrest or shock (2) Hyperkalemia >5.0 mEq/L (3) Serum digoxin >5 ng/mL (child) at 8–12 h post ingestion in adults (4) Digitalis delirium (5) Ingestion over 10 mg in adults or 4 mg in child (6) Bradycardia or second- or third-degree heart block unresponsive to atropine (7) Life-threatening digitoxin or oleander poisoning	IV	(1) If amount ingested is known total dose × bioavailability (0.8) = body burden. The body burden ÷ 0.6 (0.5 mg of digoxin is bound by 1 vial of 38 mg of Fab) = # vials needed. (2) If amount is unknown but the steady state serum concentration is known in ng/mL: Digoxin: ng/mL: (5.6 L/kg Vd) × (wt kg) = µg body burden. Body burden ÷ 100 = mg body burden/0.5 = # vials needed. Digitoxin body burden = ng/mL × (0.56 L/kg Vd) × (wt kg) Body burden ÷ 1000 = mg body burden/0.5 = # vials needed. (3) If the amount is not known, it is administered in life-threatening situations as 10 vials (400 mg) IV in saline over 30 min in adults. If cardiac arrest is imminent, administer 20 vials (adult) as a bolus.	Allergic reactions (rare), return of condition being treated with digitalis glycoside. Administer by infusion over 30 min through a 0.22-µ filter. If cardiac arrest is imminent, may administer by bolus. Consult PCC for more details.

Continued

TABLE 5 Initial Doses of Antidotes for Common Poisonings—cont'd

ANTIDOTE	USE	DOSE	ROUTE	ADVERSE REACTIONS/COMMENTS
Dimercaprol (BAL in Peanut Oil):Stock level to treat 70 kg adult for 24 h: 1200 mg (4 amps—100 mg/mL 10% in oil in 3 mL amp)	Chelating agent for arsenic, mercury, and lead	3–5 mg/kg q4h usually for 5–10 d	Deep IM	Local infection site pain and sterile abscess, nausea, vomiting, fever, salivation, hypertension, and nephrotoxicity (alkalinize urine).
2,3 Dimercaptosuccinic Acid (DMSA Succimer): 100 mg/capsule:20 capsules	Used as a chelating agent for lead, especially blood lead levels >45 µg/dL. May also be used for symptomatic mercury exposure	10 mg/kg 3 × daily for 5 days followed by 10 mg/kg 2 × daily for 14 days	PO	Precautions: monitor AST/ALT; use with caution in G6PD-deficient patients. Avoid concurrent iron therapy. Relatively safe antidote, rarely severe, uncommon minor skin rashes may occur.
Diphenhydramine (Benadryl): Antiparkinsonian action. Stock level to treat a 70 kg adult for 24 h: 5 vials (10 mg/mL, 10 mL each)	Used to treat extrapyramidal symptoms and dystonia induced by phenothiazines, phencyclidine, and related drugs	*Children:* 1–2 mg/kg IV slowly over 5 min up to maximum 50 mg followed by 5 mg/kg/24 h orally divided every 6 h up to 300 mg/24 h *Adults:* 50 mg IV followed by 50 mg orally four times daily for 5–7 d. *Note:* Symptoms abate within 2–5 min after IV.	IV	Fatal dose: 20–40 mg/kg. Dry mouth, drowsiness.
Ethanol (Ethyl Alcohol): Stock level to treat 70 kg adult for 24 h: 3 bottles 10% (1 L each)	Methanol, ethylene glycol	10 mL/kg loading dose concurrently with 1.4 mL/kg (average) infusion of 10% ethanol (consult PCC for more details)	IV	Nausea, vomiting, sedation. Use 0.22-µ filter if preparing from bulk 100% ethanol.
Flumazenil (Romazicon): Stock level to treat 70 kg adult for 24 h: 4 vials (0.1 mg/mL, 10 mL)	Benzodiazepines (may also be beneficial in the treatment of hepatic encephalopathy)	Administer 0.2 mg (2 mL) IV over 30 sec (pediatric dose not established, 0.01 mg/kg), then wait 3 min for a response, then if desired consciousness is not achieved, administer 0.3 mg (3 mL) over 30 sec, then wait 3 min for response, then if desired consciousness is not achieved, administer 0.5 mg (5 mL) over 30 sec at 60-sec intervals up to a maximum cumulative dose of 3 mg (30 mL) (1 mg in children). Because effects last only 1–5 h, if patient responds, monitor carefully over next 6 h for resedation. If multiple repeated doses, consider a continuous infusion of 0.2–1 mg/h.	IV	Nausea, vomiting, facial flushing, agitation, headache, dizziness, seizures, and death. It is not recommended to improve ventilation. Its role in CNS depression needs to be clarified. It should not be used routinely in comatose patients. It is **contraindicated** in cyclic antidepressant intoxications, stimulant overdose, long-term benzodiazepine use (may precipitate life-threatening withdrawal), if benzodiazepines are used to control seizures, in head trauma.
Folic Acid (Folvite): Stock level to treat 70 kg adult for 24 h: 4 100-mg vials	Methanol/ethylene glycol (investigational)	1 mg/kg up to 50 mg q4h for 6 doses	IV	Uncommon
Fomepizole (4-MP, Antizol): Stock level to treat 70 kg adult for 24 h: 4 1.5-mL vials (1 g/mL)	Ethylene glycol Methanol	Loading dose: 15 mg/kg (0.015 mL/kg) IV followed by maintenance dose of 10 mg/kg (0.01 mL/kg) q12h for 4 doses, then 15 mg/kg q12h until ethylene glycol levels are <20 mg/dL. Fomepizole can be given to patients undergoing hemodialysis (dose q4h).	IV	Suggested: co-administer folate 50 mg IV (child 1 mg/kg), thiamine 100 mg/d (child 50 mg), and pyridoxine 50 mg IV/IM q6h until intoxication is resolved. Monitor for urinary oxalate crystals. Adverse reactions include headache, nausea, and dizziness. Antizole should be diluted in 100 mL 0.9% saline or D5W and mixed well. Antizole should not be given undiluted.
Glucagon: Stock level to treat 70 kg adult for 24 h: 10 vials, 10 units	β-Blocker, calcium channel blocker	3–10 mg in adult, then infuse 2–5 mg/h (0.05–0.1 mg/kg in child, then infuse 0.07 mg/kg/h) Large doses up to 100 mg/24 h used	IV	Use D5W, not 0.9% saline, to reconstitute the glucagon (rather than diluent of Eli Lilly, which contains phenol). Vomiting precautions.

Drug (Stock level)	Indication	Route	Dose	Comments
Magnesium Sulfate: Stock level to treat 70 kg adult for 24 h: approx 25 g (50 mL of 50% or 200 mL of 12.5%)	Torsades de pointes	IV	*Adult:* 2 g (20 mL or 20%) over 20 min. If no response in 10 min, repeat and follow by continuous infusion 1 g/h. *Children:* 25–50 mg/kg initially and maintenance is 30–60 mg/kg/24 h (0.25–0.5 mEq/kg/24 h) up to 1000 mg/24 h. (Dose not studied in controlled fashion.)	Use with caution if renal impairment is present.
Methylene Blue: Stock level to treat 70 kg adult for 24 h: 5 amps (10 mg/10 mL)	Methemoglobinaemia	IV	0.1–0.2 mL/kg of 1% solution, slow infusion, may be repeated q30–60 min	Nausea, vomiting, headache, dizziness.
Naloxone (Narcan): Stock level to treat 70 kg adult for 24 h: 3 vials (1 mg/mL, 10 mL)	Comatose patient; decreased respirations <12; opioids	IV, ET	In postoperative opioid depression reversal, IV 0.1–0.5 µg/kg q2 min as needed and may repeat up to a total dose of 1 µg/kg In suspected overdose, administer IV 0.1 mg/kg in a child younger than 5 years of age up to 2 mg; in older children and adults administer 2 mg every 2 min up to a total of 10–20 mg. Can also be administered into the endotracheal tube. If no response by 10 mg, a pure opioid intoxication is unlikely. If opioid abuse is suspected, **restraints** should be in place before administration; **initial dose** 0.1 mg to avoid withdrawal and violent behavior. The initial dose is then doubled every minute progressively to a total of 10 mg. A **continuous infusion** has been advocated because many opioids outlast the short half-life of naloxone (30–60 min). The **naloxone infusion hourly rate** to produce a response is equal to the effective dose required (improvement in ventilation and arousal). An additional dose may be required in 15–30 min as a bolus.	**Larger doses** of naloxone may be required for more poorly antagonized synthetic opioid drugs: buprenorphine (Buprenex), codeine, dextromethorphan, fentanyl, pentazocine (Talwin), propoxyphene (Darvon), diphenoxylate, nalbuphine (Nubain), new potent "designer" drugs, or long-acting opioids such as methadone (Dolophine). **Complications.** Although naloxone is safe and effective, there are rare reports of complications (<1%) of pulmonary edema, seizures, hypertension, cardiac arrest, and sudden death. The infusions are titrated to avoid respiratory depression and opioid withdrawal manifestations. Tapering of infusions can be attempted after 12 h and when the patient is stable.
Physostigmine (Antilirium): Stock level to treat 70 kg adult for 24 h: 2–4 mg (2 mL each)	Anticholinergic agents (not routinely used, only indicated if life-threatening complications)	IV	*Child:* 0.02 mg/kg slow push to max 2 mg q30–60 min *Adult:* 1–2 mg q5 min to max 6 mg.	Bradycardia, asystole, seizures, bronchospasm, vomiting, headaches. Do not use for cyclic antidepressants.
Pralidoxime (2PAM, Protopam): Stock level to treat 70 kg adult for 24 h: 12 vials (1 g per 20 mL)	Organophosphates/nerve agents	IV	Child ≤12 y, 25–50 mg/kg max (4 mg/min); >12 y, 1–2 g/dose in 250 mL of 0.9% saline over 5–10 min. Max 200 mg/min. Repeat q6–12h for 24–48h. Max adult 6 g/d. Alternative: Maintenance infusion 1 g in 100 mL, of 0.9% saline at 5–20 mg/kg/h (0.5–12 mL/kg/h) up to max 500 mg/h or 50 mL/h. Titrate to desired response. End point is absence of fasciculations and return of muscle strength.	Nausea, dizziness, headache; tachycardia, muscle rigidity, bronchospasm (rapid administration).

Continued

TABLE 5 Initial Doses of Antidotes for Common Poisonings—cont'd

ANTIDOTE	USE	DOSE	ROUTE	ADVERSE REACTIONS/COMMENTS
Pyridoxine (Vitamin B6): Stock level to treat 70 kg adult for 24 h: 100 mg/mL 10% solution. For a 70 kg patient, 10 g = 10 vials	Seizures from isoniazid or *Gyromitra* mushrooms, ethylene glycol	*Isoniazid: Unknown amount ingested:* 5 g (70 mg/kg) in 50 mL D5W over 5 min + diazepam 0.3 mg/kg IV at rate of 1 mg/min in child or 10 mg dose at rate up to 5 mg/min in adults. Use different site (synergism). May repeat q5–20 min until seizure controlled. Up to 375 mg/kg have been given (52 g). *Known amount:* 1 g for each gram isoniazid ingested over 5 min with diazepam (dose above) *Gyromitra mushroom:* Child 25 mg/kg or 2–5 g, adults IV over 15–30 min to max 20 g	IV	After seizure is controlled, administer remainder of pyridoxine 1 g/1 g isoniazid total 5 g as infusion over 60 min. Adverse reactions uncommon; do not administer in same bottle as sodium bicarbonate. For *Gyromitra* mushrooms, some use PO 25 mg/kg/d early when mushroom ingestion is suspected.
Sodium Bicarbonate (NaHCO3): Stock level to treat 70 kg adult for 24 h: 10 ampules or syringes (500 mEq)	Tricyclic antidepressant cardiotoxicity (QRS >0.12 sec; ventricular tachycardia, severe conduction disturbances); metabolic acidosis: phenothiazine toxicity *Salicylate:* to keep blood pH 7.5–7.55 (not >7.55) and urine pH 7.5–8.0. Alkalinization recommended if salicylate conc. >40 mg/dL in acute poisoning and at lower levels if symptomatic in chronic intoxication, 2 mEq/kg will raise blood pH 0.1 unit	*Ethylene glycol:* 100 mg IV daily. 1–2 mEq/kg undiluted as a bolus. If no effect on cardiotoxicity, repeat twice a few minutes apart *Adult* with clear physical signs and laboratory findings of acute moderate or severe salicylism: Bolus 1–2 mEq/kg followed by infusion of 100–150 mEq NaHCO3 added to 1 L of 5% dextrose at rate of 200–300 mL/h *Child:* Bolus same as adult followed by 1–2 mEq/kg in infusion of 20 mL/kg/h 5% dextrose in 0.45% saline Add potassium when patient voids Rate and amount of the initial infusion, if patient is volume depleted: 1 h to achieve urine output of 2 mL/kg/h and urine pH 7–8 In mild cases without acidosis and urine pH >6, administer 5% dextrose in 0.9% saline with 50 mEq/L or 1 mEq/kg NaHCO3 as maintenance to replace ongoing renal losses. If acidemia is present and pH <7.2, add 2 mEq/kg as loading dose followed by 2 mEq/kg q3–4h to keep pH at 7.5–7.55. If acidemia is present, recommend isotonic NaHCO3, 3 ampules to 1 L of D5W at 10–15 mL/kg/h or sufficient to produce normal urine flow and a urine pH of 7.5 or higher NaHCO3: 2 mEq/kg during the first hour or 100 mEq in 1 L of D5W with 40 mEq/L potassium at a rate of 100 mL/h in adults Adequate potassium is necessary to accomplish alkalinization	IV	Monitor sodium, potassium, and blood pH because fatal alkalemia and hyponatremia have been reported. Monitor both urine and blood pH. Do not use the urine pH alone to assess the need for alkalinization because of the paradoxical aciduria that may occur. Adjust the urine pH to 7.5–8 by NaHCO3 infusion. After urine output established, add potassium 40 mEq/L.
	Long-acting barbiturates: Phenobarbital and primidone (Mysoline). *Note:* Alkalinization is ineffective for the short- or intermediate-acting barbiturates		IV	Additional sodium bicarbonate and potassium chloride may be needed. Adjust the urine pH to 7.5–8 by NaHCO3 infusion.
Thiamine: 100 mg/mL, 2 vials	Thiamine deficiency, ethylene glycol poisoning, alcoholism	100 mg IV followed with 100 mg V/IM for 5–7 days in an alcoholic and followed by 100 mg/d orally	IV/IM	
Vitamin K1 (Aqua Mephyton): 10 mg/ 1–5 mL; 5-mg tablets	Warfarin anticoagulant or rodenticide toxicity	Oral 0.4 mg/kg/dose child, 10–25 mg adults. If evidence of bleeding, administer vitamin K1 SC, IV 0.6 mg/kg/dose child and up to 2.5–50 mg adults for 6 hours depending on severity	PO/SC, IV	Give vitamin K daily until PT/INR are normal. Examine stools and urine for evidence of bleeding.

Abbreviations: ALT = alanine aminotransferase; amp = ampule; AST = aspartate aminotransferase; BAL = British anti-Lewisite; BP = blood pressure; conc. = concentration; ECG = electrocardiogram; ET = endotracheal; G6PD = glucose-6-phosphate dehydrogenase; IM = intramuscular; IV = intravenous; PCC = poison control center; PO = oral; PT = prothrombin time; SC = subcutaneous.

Enhancement of Elimination

The acceptable methods for elimination of absorbed toxic substances are dialysis, hemoperfusion, exchange transfusion, plasmapheresis, enzyme induction, and inhibition. Methods of increasing urinary excretion of toxic chemicals and drugs have been studied extensively, but the other modalities have not been well evaluated.

In general, these methods are needed in only a minority of cases and should be reserved for life-threatening circumstances when a definite benefit is anticipated.

Dialysis

Dialysis is the extrarenal means of removing certain substances from the body, and it can substitute for the kidney when renal failure occurs. Dialysis is not the first measure instituted; however, it may be lifesaving later in the course of a severe intoxication. It is needed in only a minority of intoxicated patients.

Peritoneal dialysis uses the peritoneum as the membrane for dialysis. It is only 1/20 as effective as hemodialysis. It is easier to use and less hazardous to the patient but also less effective in removing the toxin; thus it is rarely used except in small infants.

Hemodialysis is the most effective dialysis method but requires experience with sophisticated equipment. Blood is circulated past a semipermeable extracorporeal membrane. Substances are removed by diffusion down a concentration gradient. Anticoagulation with heparin is necessary. Flow rates of 300 to 500 mL/min can be achieved, and clearance rates may reach 200 or 300 mL/min.

Dialyzable substances easily diffuse across the dialysis membrane and have the following characteristics: (a) a molecular weight less than 500 daltons and preferably less than 350; (b) a volume of distribution less than 1 L/kg; (c) protein binding less than 50%; (d) high water solubility (low lipid solubility); and (e) high plasma concentration and a toxicity that correlates reasonably with the plasma concentration. Considerations for hemodialysis and hemoperfusion are cases of serious ingestions

(the nephrologist should be notified immediately), and cases involving a compound that is ingested in a potentially lethal dose and the rapid removal of which may improve the prognosis. Examples of the latter are ethylene glycol 1.4 mL/kg 100% solution or equivalent and methanol 6 mL/kg 100% solution or equivalent. Common dialyzable substances include alcohol, bromides, lithium, and salicylates.

The patient-related criteria for dialysis are (a) anticipated prolonged coma and the likelihood of complications; (b) renal compromise (toxin excreted or metabolized by kidneys and dialyzable chelating agents in heavy metal poisoning); (c) laboratory confirmation of lethal blood concentration; (d) lethal dose poisoning with an agent with delayed toxicity or known to be metabolized into a more toxic metabolite (e.g., ethylene glycol, methanol); and (e) hepatic impairment when the agent is metabolized by the liver, and clinical deterioration despite optimal supportive medical management. Table 6 gives plasma concentrations above which removal by extracorporeal measures should be considered.

The contraindications to hemodialysis include the following: (a) substances are not dialyzable; (b) effective antidotes are available; (c) patient is hemodynamically unstable (e.g., shock); and (d) presence of coagulopathy because heparinization is required.

Hemodialysis also has a role in correcting disturbances that are not amenable to appropriate medical management. These are easily remembered by the "vowel" mnemonic:

A—refractory acid-base disturbances
E—refractory electrolyte disturbances
I—intoxication with dialyzable substances (e.g., ethanol, ethylene glycol, isopropyl alcohol, methanol, lithium, and salicylates)
O—overhydration
U—uremia

Complications of dialysis include hemorrhage, thrombosis, air embolism, hypotension, infections, electrolyte imbalance, thrombocytopenia, and removal of therapeutic medications.

| **TABLE 6** | Plasma Concentrations Above Which Removal by Extracorporeal Measures Should Be Considered |

DRUG	PLASMA CONCENTRATION	PROTEIN BINDING (%)	VOLUME DISTRIBUTION (L/kg)	METHOD OF CHOICE
Amanitin	NA	25	1.0	HP
Ethanol	500–700 mg/dL	0	0.3	HD
Ethchlorvynol	150 µg/mL	35–50	3–4	HP
Ethylene glycol	25–50 µg/mL	0	0.6	HD
Glutethimide	100 µg/mL	50	2.7	HP
Isopropyl alcohol	400 mg/dL	0	0.7	HD
Lithium	4 mEq/L	0	0.7	HD
Meprobamate (Equanil)	100 µg/mL	0	NA	HP
Methanol	50 mg/dL	0	0.7	HD
Methaqualone	40 µg/dL	20–60	6.0	HP
Other barbiturates	50 µg/dL	50	0–1	HP
Paraquat	0.1 mg/dL	poor	2.8	HP > HD
Phenobarbital	100 µg/dL	50	0.9	HP > HD
Salicylates	80–100 mg/dL	90	0.2	HD > HP
Theophylline		0	0.5	
Chronic	40–60 µg/mL			HP
Acute	80–100 µg/mL			HP
Trichlorethanol	250 µg/mL	70	0.6	HP

Abbreviations: HD = hemodialysis; HP = hemoperfusion; HP > HD = hemoperfusion preferred over hemodialysis.
Data from Winchester JF: Active methods for detoxification. In Haddad LM, Winchester JF (eds). Clinical Management of Poisoning and Drug Overdose, 2nd ed. Philadelphia, WB Saunders, 1990; Balsam L, Cortitsidis GN, Fienfeld DA: Role of hemodialysis and hemoperfusion in the treatment of intoxications. Contemp Manage Crit Care 1:61, 1991.
Note: Cartridges for charcoal hemoperfusion are not readily available anymore in most locations. So hemodialysis may be substituted in these situations. In mixed or chronic drug overdoses, extracorporeal measures may be considered at lower drug concentrations.

Hemoperfusion

Hemoperfusion is the parenteral form of oral activated charcoal. Heparinization is necessary. The patient's blood is routed extracorporeally through an outflow arterial catheter through a filter-adsorbing cartridge (charcoal or resin) and returned through a venous catheter. Cartridges must be changed every 4 hours. The blood glucose, electrolytes, calcium, and albumin levels; complete blood cell count; platelets; and serum and urine osmolarity must be carefully monitored. This procedure has extended extracorporeal removal to a large range of substances that were formerly either poorly dialyzable or nondialyzable. It is not limited by molecular weight, water solubility, or protein binding, but it is limited by a volume distribution greater than 400 L, plasma concentration, and rate of flow through the filter. Activated charcoal cartridges are the primary type of hemoperfusion that is currently available in the United States.

The patient-related criteria for hemoperfusion are (a) anticipated prolonged coma and the likelihood of complications; (b) laboratory confirmation of lethal blood concentrations; (c) hepatic impairment when an agent is metabolized by the liver; and (d) clinical deterioration despite optimally supportive medical management.

The contraindications are similar to those for hemodialysis.

Limited data are available as to which toxins are best treated with hemoperfusion. Hemoperfusion has proved useful in treating glutethimide intoxication, phenobarbital overdose, and carbamazepine, phenytoin, and theophylline intoxication.

Complications include hemorrhage, thrombocytopenia, hypotension, infection, leukopenia, depressed phagocytic activity of granulocytes, decreased immunoglobulin levels, hypoglycemia, hypothermia, hypocalcemia, pulmonary edema, and air and charcoal embolism.

Hemofiltration

Continuous arteriovenous or venovenous hemodiafiltration (CAVHD or CVVHD, respectively) has been suggested as an alternative to conventional hemodialysis when the need for rapid removal of the drug is less urgent. These procedures, like peritoneal dialysis, are minimally invasive, have no significant impact on hemodynamics, and can be carried out continuously for many hours. Their role in the management of acute poisoning remains uncertain, however.

Plasmapheresis

Plasmapheresis consists of removal of a volume of blood. All the extracted components are returned to the blood except the plasma, which is replaced with a colloid protein solution. There are limited clinical data on guidelines and efficacy in toxicology. Centrifugal and membrane separators of cellular elements are used. It can be as effective as hemodialysis or hemoperfusion for removing toxins that have high protein binding, and it may be useful for toxins not filtered by hemodialysis and hemoperfusion.

Plasmapheresis has been anecdotally used in treating intoxications with the following agents: paraquat (removed 10%), propranolol (removed 30%), quinine (removed 10%), L-thyroxine (removed 30%), and salicylate (removed 10%). It has been shown to remove less than 10% of digoxin, phenobarbital, prednisolone, and tobramycin. Complications include infection; allergic reactions including anaphylaxis; hemorrhagic disorders; thrombocytopenia; embolus and thrombus; hypervolemia and hypovolemia; dysrhythmias; syncope; tetany; paresthesia; pneumothorax; acute respiratory distress syndrome; and seizures.

Supportive Care, Observation, and Therapy for Complications

Altered Mental Status

If airway protective reflexes are absent, endotracheal intubation is indicated for a comatose patient or a patient with altered mental status. If respirations are ineffective, ventilation should be instituted, and if hypoxemia persists, supplemental oxygen is indicated. If a cyanotic patient fails to respond to oxygen, the practitioner should consider methemoglobinemia.

Hypoglycemia

Hypoglycemia accompanies many poisonings, including with ethanol (especially in children), clonidine (Catapres), insulin, organophosphates, salicylates, sulfonylureas, and the unripe fruit or seed of a Jamaican plant called ackee. If hypoglycemia is present or suspected, glucose should be administered immediately as an intravenous bolus. Doses are as follows: in a neonate, 10% glucose (5 mL/kg); in a child, 25% glucose 0.25 g/kg (2 mL/kg); and in an adult, 50% glucose 0.5 g/kg (1 mL/kg).

A bedside capillary test for blood glucose is performed to detect hypoglycemia, and the sample is sent to the laboratory for confirmation. If the glucose reagent strip visually reads less than 150 mg/dL, one administers glucose. Venous blood should be used rather than capillary blood for the bedside test if the patient is in shock or is hypotensive. Large amounts of glucose given rapidly to nondiabetic patients may cause a transient reactive hypoglycemia and hyperkalemia and may accentuate damage in ischemic cerebrovascular and cardiac tissue. If focal neurologic signs are present, it may be prudent to withhold glucose, because hypoglycemia causes focal signs in less than 10% of cases.

Thiamine Deficiency Encephalopathy

Thiamine is administered to avoid precipitating thiamine deficiency encephalopathy (Wernicke-Korsakoff syndrome) in alcohol abusers and in malnourished patients. The overall incidence of thiamine deficiency in ethanol abusers is 12%. Thiamine 100 mg intravenously should be administered around the time of the glucose administration but not necessarily before the glucose. The clinician should be prepared to manage the anaphylaxis that sometimes is caused by thiamine, although it is extremely rare.

Opioid Reactions

Naloxone (Narcan) reverses CNS and respiratory depression, miosis, bradycardia, and decreased gastrointestinal peristalsis caused by opioids acting through μ, κ, and δ receptors. It also affects endogenous opioid peptides (endorphins and enkephalins), which accounts for the variable responses reported in patients with intoxications from ethanol, benzodiazepines, clonidine (Catapres), captopril (Capoten), and valproic acid (Depakote) and in patients with spinal cord injuries. There is a high sensitivity for predicting a response if pinpoint pupils and circumstantial evidence of opioid abuse (e.g., track marks) are present.

In cases of suspected overdose, naloxone 0.1 mg/kg is administered intravenously initially in a child younger than 5 years of age. The dose can be repeated in 2 minutes, if necessary up to a total dose of 2 mg. In older children and adults, the dose is 2 mg every 2 minutes for five doses up to a total of 10 mg. Naloxone can also be administered into an endotracheal tube if intravenous access is unavailable. If there is no response after 10 mg, a pure opioid intoxication is unlikely. If opioid abuse is suspected, restraints should be in place before the administration of naloxone, and it is recommended that the initial dose be 0.1 to 0.2 mg to avoid withdrawal and violent behavior. The initial dose is then doubled every minute progressively to a total of 10 mg. Naloxone may unmask concomitant sympatho-mimetic intoxication as well as withdrawal.

Larger doses of naloxone may be required for more poorly antagonized synthetic opioid drugs: buprenorphine (Buprenex), codeine, dextromethorphan, fentanyl and its derivatives, pentazocine (Talwin), propoxyphene (Darvon), diphenoxylate, nalbuphine (Nubain), and long-acting opioids such as methadone (Dolophine).

Indications for a continuous infusion include a second dose for recurrent respiratory depression, exposure to poorly antagonized opioids, a large overdose, and decreased opioid metabolism, as with impaired liver function. A continuous infusion has been advocated because many opioids outlast the short half-life of naloxone (30 to 60 minutes). The hourly rate of naloxone infusion is equal to the effective dose required to produce a response (improvement in ventilation and arousal). An additional dose may be required in 15 to 30 minutes as a bolus. The infusions are titrated to avoid respiratory depression and opioid withdrawal manifestations. Tapering of infusions can be attempted after 12 hours and when the patient's condition has been stabilized.

Although naloxone is safe and effective, there are rare reports of complications (less than 1%) of pulmonary edema, seizures, hypertension, cardiac arrest, and sudden death.

Agents Whose Roles Are Not Clarified

Nalmefene (Revex), a long-acting parenteral opioid antagonist that the Food and Drug Administration has approved, is undergoing investigation, but its role in the treatment of comatose patients and patients with opioid overdose is not clear. It is 16 times more potent than naloxone, and its duration of action is up to 8 hours (half-life 10.8 hours, versus naloxone 1 hour).

Flumazenil (Romazicon) is a pure competitive benzodiazepine antagonist. It has been demonstrated to be safe and effective for reversing benzodiazepine-induced sedation. It is not recommended to improve ventilation. Its role in cases of CNS depression needs to be clarified. It should not be used routinely in comatose patients and is not an essential ingredient of the coma therapeutic regimen. It is contraindicated in cases of co-ingestion of cyclic antidepressant intoxication, stimulant overdose, and long-term benzodiazepine use (may precipitate life-threatening withdrawal) if benzodiazepines are used to control seizures. There is a concern about the potential for seizures and cardiac dysrhythmias that may occur in these settings.

Laboratory and Radiographic Studies

An electrocardiogram (ECG) should be obtained to identify dysrhythmias or conduction delays from cardiotoxic medications. If aspiration pneumonia (history of loss of consciousness, unarousable state, vomiting) or noncardiac pulmonary edema is suspected, a chest radiograph is needed. Electrolyte and glucose concentrations in the blood, the anion gap, acid-base balance, the arterial blood gas (ABG) profile (if patient has respiratory distress or altered mental status), and serum osmolality should be measured if a toxic alcohol ingestion is suspected. Table 7 lists appropriate testing on the basis of clinical toxicologic presentation. All laboratory specimens should be carefully labeled, including time and date. For potential legal cases, a "chain of custody" must be established. Assessment of the laboratory studies may provide a clue to the etiologic agent.

Electrolyte, Acid-Base, and Osmolality Disturbances

Electrolyte and acid-base disturbances should be evaluated and corrected. Metabolic acidosis (usually low or normal pH with a low or normal/high $PaCO_2$ and low HCO_3) with an increased anion gap (AG) is seen with many agents in cases of overdose.

The AG is an estimate of those anions other than chloride and HCO_3 necessary to counterbalance the positive charge of sodium. It serves as a clue to causes, compensations, and complications. The AG is calculated from the standard serum electrolytes by subtracting the total CO_2 (which reflects the actual measured bicarbonate) and chloride from the sodium: $(Na - [Cl + HCO_3]) = AG$. The potassium is usually not used in the calculation because it may be hemolyzed and is an intracellular cation. The lack of anion gap does not exclude a toxic etiology.

The normal gap is usually 7 to 11 mEq/L by flame photometer. However, there has been a "lowering" of the normal AG to 7 ± 4 mEq/L by the newer techniques (e.g., ion selective electrodes or colorimetric titration). Some studies have found AGs to be relatively insensitive for determining the presence of toxins.

It is important to recognize anion gap toxins, such as salicylates, methanol, and ethylene glycol, because they have specific antidotes, and hemodialysis is effective in management of cases of overdose with these agents.

Table 8 lists the reasons for increased AG, decreased anion gap, or no gap. The most common cause of a decreased AG is laboratory error. Lactic acidosis produces the largest AG and can result from any poisoning that results in hypoxia, hypoglycemia, or convulsions.

Table 9 lists other blood chemistry derangements that suggest certain intoxications.

Serum osmolality is a measure of the number of molecules of solute per kilogram of solvent, or mOsm/kg water. The osmolarity is molecules of solute per liter of solution, or mOsm/L water at a specified temperature. Osmolarity is usually the calculated value and osmolality is usually a measured value. They are considered interchangeable where 1 L equals 1 kg. The normal serum osmolality is 280 to 290 mOsm/kg. The freezing point serum osmolality measurement specimen and the serum electrolyte specimens for calculation should be drawn simultaneously.

The serum osmolal gap is defined as the difference between the measured osmolality determined by the freezing point method and the calculated osmolarity. It is determined by the following formula (BUN is blood urea nitrogen):

$$(Sodium \times 2) + (BUN/3) + (Glucose/20)$$

This gap estimate is normally within 10 mOsm of the simultaneously measured serum osmolality. Ethanol, if present, may be included in the equation to eliminate its influence on the osmolal gap (the ethanol concentration divided by 4.6; Table 10).

The osmolal gap is not valid in cases of shock and postmortem state. Metabolic disorders such as hyperglycemia, uremia, and dehydration increase the osmolarity but usually do not cause gaps greater than 10 mOsm/kg. A gap greater than 10 mOsm/mL suggests that unidentified osmolal-acting substances are present: acetone, ethanol, ethylene glycol, glycerin, isopropyl alcohol, isoniazid, ethanol, mannitol, methanol, and trichloroethane. Alcohols and glycols should be sought when the degree of obtundation exceeds that expected from the blood ethanol concentration or when other clinical conditions exist: visual loss (methanol), metabolic acidosis (methanol and ethylene glycol), or renal failure (ethylene glycol).

A falsely elevated osmolar gap can be produced by other low molecular weight un-ionized substances (dextran, diuretics, sorbitol, ketones), hyperlipidemia, and unmeasured electrolytes (e.g., magnesium).

TABLE 7	Patient Condition/Systemic Toxin and Appropriate Tests
CONDITION	**TESTS**
Comatose	Toxicologic tests (acetaminophen, sedative-hypnotic, ethanol, opioids, benzodiazepine), glucose.
Respiratory toxicity	Spirometry, FEV_1, arterial blood gases, chest radiograph, monitor O_2 saturation
Cardiac toxicity	ECG 12-lead and monitoring, echocardiogram, serial cardiac enzymes (if evidence or suspicion of a myocardial infarction), hemodynamic monitoring
Hepatic toxicity	Enzymes (AST, ALT, GGT), ammonia, albumin, bilirubin, glucose, PT, PTT, amylase
Nephrotoxicity	BUN, creatinine, electrolytes (Na, F, Mg, Ca, PO_4), serum and urine osmolarity, 24-hour urine for heavy metals if suspected, creatine kinase, serum and urine myoglobin, urinalysis and urinary sodium
Bleeding	Platelets, PT, PTT, bleeding time, fibrin split products, fibrinogen, type and match

Abbreviations: ALT = alanine transaminase; AST = aspartate transaminase; BUN = blood urea nitrogen; ECG = electrocardiogram; FEV_1 = forced expiratory volume in 1 second; GGT = γ-glutamyltransferase; PT = prothrombin time; PTT = partial thromboplastin time.

| TABLE 8 | Etiologies of Metabolic Acidosis |

NORMAL ANION GAP HYPERCHLOREMIC	INCREASED ANION GAP NORMOCHLOREMIC	DECREASED ANION GAP
Acidifying agents	Methanol	Laboratory error[†]
Adrenal insufficiency	Uremia*	Intoxication—bromine, lithium
Anhydrase inhibitors	Diabetic ketoacidosis*	Protein abnormal
Fistula	Paraldehyde,* phenformin	Sodium low
Osteotomies	Isoniazid	
Obstructive uropathies	Iron	
Renal tubular acidosis	Lactic acidosis[†]	
Diarrhea, uncomplicated*	Ethanol,* ethylene glycol*	
Dilutional	Salicylates, starvation solvents	
Sulfamylon		

*Indicates hyperosmolar situation. Studies have found that the anion gap may be relatively insensitive for determining the presence of toxins.
[†]Lactic acidosis can be produced by intoxications of the following: carbon monoxide, cyanide, hydrogen sulfide, hypoxia, ibuprofen, iron, isoniazid, phenformin, salicylates, seizures, theophylline.

| TABLE 9 | Blood Chemistry Derangements in Toxicology |

DERANGEMENT	TOXIN
Acetonemia without acidosis	Acetone or isopropyl alcohol
Hypomagnesemia	Ethanol, digitalis
Hypocalcemia	Ethylene glycol, oxalate, fluoride
Hyperkalemia	β-Blockers, acute digitalis, renal failure
Hypokalemia	Diuretics, salicylism, sympathomimetics, theophylline, corticosteroids, chronic digitalis
Hyperglycemia	Diazoxide, glucagon, iron, isoniazid, organophosphate insecticides, phenylurea insecticides, phenytoin (Dilantin), salicylates, sympathomimetic agents, thyroid vasopressors
Hypoglycemia	β-Blockers, ethanol, insulin, isoniazid, oral hypoglycemic agents, salicylates
Rhabdomyolysis	Amphetamines, ethanol, cocaine, or phencyclidine, elevated creatine phosphokinase

| TABLE 10 | Conversion Factors for Alcohols and Glycols |

ALCOHOLS/ GLYCOLS	1 mg/dL IN BLOOD RAISES OSMOLALITY mOsm/L	MOLECULAR WEIGHT	CONVERSION FACTOR
Ethanol	0.228	40	4.6
Methanol	0.327	32	3.2
Ethylene glycol	0.190	62	6.2
Isopropanol	0.176	60	6.0
Acetone	0.182	58	5.8
Propylene glycol	not available	72	7.2

Example: Methanol osmolality. Subtract the calculated osmolality from the measured serum osmolarity (freezing point method) = osmolar gap × 3.2 (one-tenth molecular weight) = estimated serum methanol concentration.
Note: This equation is often not considered very reliable in predicting the actual measured blood concentration of these alcohols or glycols.

Note: A normal osmolal gap may be reported in the presence of toxic alcohol or glycol poisoning, if the parent compound is already metabolized. This situation can occur when the osmolar gap is measured after a significant time has elapsed since the ingestion. In cases of alcohol and glycol intoxication, an early osmolar gap is a result of the relatively nontoxic parent drug and delayed metabolic acidosis, and an anion gap is a result of the more toxic metabolites. The serum concentration is calculated as

$$mg/dL = mOsm \text{ gap} \times MW \text{ of substance divided by } 10.$$

Radiographic Studies

Chest and neck radiographs are useful for suspected pathologic conditions such as aspiration pneumonia, pulmonary edema, and foreign bodies and to determine the location of the endotracheal tube. Abdominal radiographs can be used to detect radiopaque substances.

The mnemonic for radiopaque substances seen on abdominal radiographs is CHIPES:

C—chlorides and chloral hydrate
H—heavy metals (arsenic, barium, iron, lead, mercury, zinc)
I—iodides
P—PlayDoh, Pepto-Bismol, phenothiazine (inconsistent)
E—enteric-coated tablets
S—sodium, potassium, and other elements in tablet form (bismuth, calcium, potassium) and solvents containing chlorides (e.g., carbon tetrachloride)

Toxicologic Studies

Routine blood and urine screening is of little practical value in the initial care of the poisoned patient. Specific toxicologic analyses and quantitative levels of certain drugs may be extremely helpful. One should always ask oneself the following questions: (a) How will the result of the test alter the management? and (b) Can the result of the test be returned in time to have a positive effect on therapy?

Owing to long turnaround time, lack of availability, factors contributing to unreliability, and the risk of serious morbidity without supportive clinical management, toxicology screening is estimated to affect management in less than 15% of cases of drug overdoses or poisonings. Toxicology screening may look specifically for only 40 to 50 drugs out of more than 10,000 possible drugs or toxins and more than several million chemicals. To detect many different drugs, toxic screens usually include methods with broad specificity, and sensitivity may be poor for some drugs, resulting in false-negative or false-positive findings. On the other hand, some drugs present in therapeutic amounts may be detected on the screen, even though they are causing no clinical symptoms. Because many agents are not sought or detected during a toxicologic screening, a negative result does not always rule out poisonings. The specificity of toxicologic tests is dependent on the method and the laboratory. The presence of other drugs, drug metabolites, disease states, or incorrect sampling may cause erroneous results.

For the average toxicologic laboratory, false-negative results occur at a rate of 10% to 30% and false-positives at a rate of 0% to 10%. The positive screen predictive value is approximately 90%. A negative toxicology screen does not exclude a poisoning. The negative predictive value of toxicologic screening is approximately 70%. For example, the following benzodiazepines may not be detected by some routine immunoassay benzodiazepine screening tests: alprazolam (Xanax), clonazepam (Klonopin), temazepam (Restoril), and triazolam (Halcion).

The "toxic urine screen" is generally a qualitative urine test for several common drugs, usually substances of abuse (cocaine and metabolites, opioids, amphetamines, benzodiazepines, barbiturates, and phencyclidine). Results of these tests are usually available within 2 to 6 hours. Because these tests may vary with each hospital and community, the physician should determine exactly which substances are included in the toxic urine screen of his or her laboratory. Tests for ethylene glycol, red blood cell cholinesterase, and serum cyanide are not readily available.

For cases of ingestion of certain substances, quantitative blood levels should be obtained at specific times after the ingestion to avoid spurious low values in the distribution phase, which result from incomplete absorption. The detection time for drugs is influenced by many variables, such as type of substance, formulation, amount, time since ingestion, duration of exposure, and half-life. For many drugs, the detection time is measured in days after the exposure.

Common Poisons

Acetaminophen (Paracetamol, N-Acetyl-Paraaminophenol)

Toxic Mechanism

At therapeutic doses of acetaminophen, less than 5% is metabolized by P450-2E1 to a toxic reactive oxidizing metabolite, N-acetyl-p-benzoquinoneimine (NAPQI). In a case of overdose, there is insufficient glutathione available to reduce the excess NAPQI into nontoxic conjugate, so it forms covalent bonds with hepatic intracellular proteins to produce centrilobular necrosis. Renal damage is caused by a similar mechanism.

Toxic Dose

The therapeutic dose of acetaminophen is 10 to 15 mg/kg, with a maximum of five doses in 24 hours for a maximum total daily dose of 4 g. An acute single toxic dose is greater than 140 mg/kg, possibly greater than 200 mg/kg in a child younger than age 5 years. Factors affecting the P450 enzymes include enzyme inducers such as barbiturates and phenytoin (Dilantin), ingestion of isoniazid, and alcoholism. Factors that decrease glutathione stores (alcoholism, malnutrition, and HIV infection) contribute to the toxicity of acetaminophen. Alcoholics ingesting 3 to 4 g/d of acetaminophen for a few days can have depleted glutathione stores and require N-acetylcysteine therapy at 50% below hepatotoxic blood acetaminophen levels on the nomogram.

Kinetics

Peak plasma concentration is usually reached 2 to 4 hours after an overdose. Volume distribution is 0.9 L/kg, and protein binding is less than 50% (albumin).

Route of elimination is by hepatic metabolism to an inactive nontoxic glucuronide conjugate and inactive nontoxic sulfate metabolite by two saturable pathways; less than 5% is metabolized into reactive metabolite NAPQI. In patients younger than 6 years of age, metabolic elimination occurs to a greater degree by conjugation via the sulfate pathway.

The half-life of acetaminophen is 1 to 3 hours.

Manifestations

The four phases of the intoxication's clinical course may overlap, and the absence of a phase does not exclude toxicity.

- Phase I occurs within 0.5 to 24 hours after ingestion and may consist of a few hours of malaise, diaphoresis, nausea, and vomiting or produce no symptoms. CNS depression or coma is not a feature.
- Phase II occurs 24 to 48 hours after ingestion and is a period of diminished symptoms. The liver enzymes, serum aspartate aminotransferase (AST) (earliest), and serum alanine aminotransferase (ALT) may increase as early as 4 hours or as late as 36 hours after ingestion.

- Phase III occurs at 48 to 96 hours, with peak liver function abnormalities at 72 to 96 hours. The degree of elevation of the hepatic enzymes generally correlates with outcome, but not always. Recovery starts at about 4 days unless hepatic failure develops. Less than 1% of patients with a history of overdose develop fulminant hepatotoxicity.
- Phase IV occurs at 4 to 14 days, with hepatic enzyme abnormalities resolving. If extensive liver damage has occurred, sepsis and disseminated intravascular coagulation may ensue.

Transient renal failure may develop at 5 to 7 days with or without evidence of hepatic damage. Rare cases of myocarditis and pancreatitis have been reported. Death can occur at 7 to 14 days.

Laboratory Investigations

The therapeutic reference range is 10 to 20 µg/mL. For toxic levels, see the nomogram presented in Figure 1.

Appropriate and reliable methods for analysis are radioimmunoassay, high-pressure liquid chromatography, and gas chromatography. Spectroscopic assays often give falsely elevated values: bilirubin, salicylate, salicylamide, diflunisal (Dolobid), phenols, and methyldopa (Aldomet) increase the acetaminophen level. Each 1 mg/dL increase in creatinine increases the acetaminophen plasma level 30 µg/mL.

If a toxic acetaminophen level is reached, liver profile (including AST, ALT, bilirubin, and prothrombin time), serum amylase, and blood glucose must be monitored. A complete blood cell count (CBC); platelet count; phosphate, electrolytes, and bicarbonate level measurements; ECG; and urinalysis are indicated.

Management

Gastrointestinal Decontamination. Although ipecac-induced emesis may be useful within 30 minutes of ingestion of the toxic substance, we do not advise it because it could result in vomiting of the activated charcoal. Gastric lavage is not necessary. Studies have indicated that activated charcoal is useful within 1 hour after ingestion. Activated charcoal does adsorb N-acetylcysteine (NAC) if given together, but this is not clinically important. However, if activated charcoal needs to be given along with NAC, separate the administration of activated charcoal from the administration of NAC by 1 to 2 hours to avoid vomiting.

N-Acetylcysteine (Mucomyst). NAC (Table 11), a derivative of the amino acid cysteine, acts as a sulfhydryl donor for glutathione synthesis, as surrogate glutathione, and may increase the nontoxic sulfation pathway resulting in conjugation of NAPQI. Oral NAC should be administered within the first 8 hours after a toxic amount of acetaminophen has been ingested. NAC can be started while one awaits the results of the blood test for acetaminophen plasma concentration, but there is no advantage to giving it before 8 hours. If the acetaminophen concentration result after 4 hours following ingestion is above the upper line on the modified Rumack-Matthew nomogram (see Figure 1), one should continue with a maintenance course. Repeat blood specimens should be obtained 4 hours after the initial level is measured if it is greater than 20 mg/mL, which is below the therapy line, because of unexpected delays in the peak by food and co-ingestants. Intravenous NAC (see Table 11) is approved in the United States.

There have been a few cases of anaphylactoid reaction and death by the intravenous route.

Variations in Therapy

In patients with chronic alcoholism, it is recommended that NAC treatment be administered at 50% below the upper toxic line on the nomogram.

If emesis occurs within 1 hour after NAC administration, the dose should be repeated. To avoid emesis, the proper dilution from 20% to 5% NAC must be used, and it should be served in a palatable vehicle, in a covered container through a straw. If this administration is unsuccessful, a slow drip over 30 to 60 minutes through a nasogastric tube or a fluoroscopically placed nasoduodenal tube can be used. Antiemetics can be used if necessary:

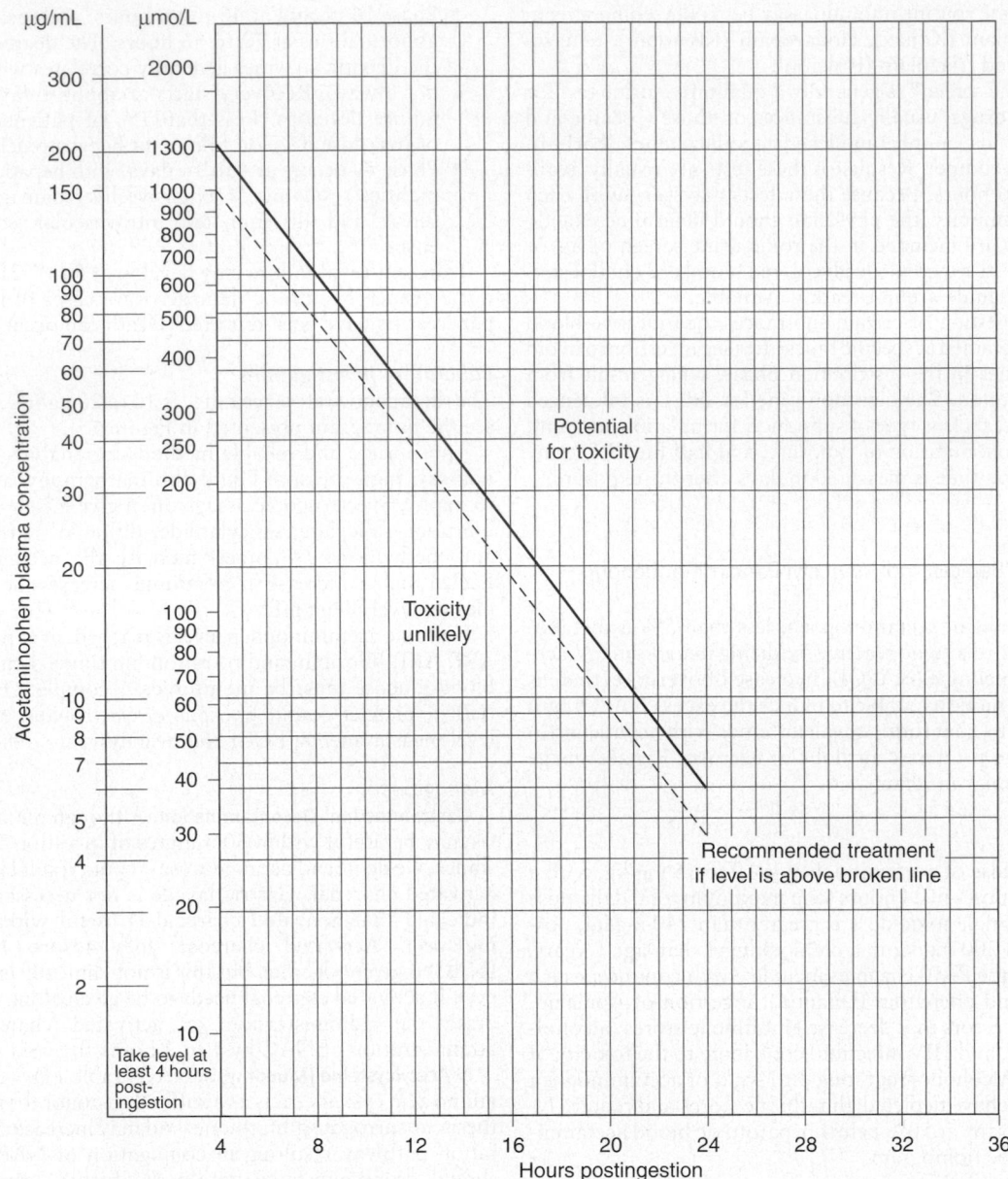

Figure 1. Nomogram for acetaminophen intoxication. *N*-acetylcysteine therapy is started if levels and time coordinates are above the lower line on the nomogram. Continue and complete therapy even if subsequent values fall below the toxic zone. The nomogram is useful only in cases of acute single ingestion. Levels in serum drawn before 4 hours may not represent peak levels. (From Rumack BH, Matthew H: Acetaminophen poisoning and toxicity. Pediatrics 55:871, 1975.)

TABLE 11	Protocol for *N*-Acetylcysteine Administration				
ROUTE	**LOADING DOSE**	**MAINTENANCE DOSE**	**COURSE**	**FDA APPROVAL**
Oral	140 mg/kg	70 mg/kg every 4 h	72 h	Yes
Intravenous	150 mg/kg over 15 min	50 mg/kg over 4 h followed by 100 mg/kg over 16 h	20 h	Yes

metoclopramide (Reglan) 10 mg per dose intravenously 30 minutes before administration of NAC (in children, 0.1 mg/kg; maximum, 0.5 mg/kg/d) or ondansetron (Zofran) 32 mg (0.15 mg/kg) by infusion over 15 minutes and repeated for three doses if necessary. The side effects of these antiemetics include anaphylaxis and increases in liver enzymes.

Some investigators recommend variable durations of NAC therapy, stopping the therapy if serial acetaminophen blood concentrations become nondetectable and the liver enzyme levels (ALT and AST) remain normal after 24 to 36 hours.

There is a loss of efficacy if NAC is initiated 8 or 10 hours post-ingestion, but the loss is not complete, and NAC may be initiated 36 hours or more after ingestion. Late treatment (after 24 hours) decreases the rates of morbidity and mortality in patients with fulminant liver failure caused by acetaminophen and other agents.

Extended relief formulations (*ER* embossed on caplet) contain 325 mg of acetaminophen for immediate release and 325 mg for delayed release. A single 4-hour postingestion serum acetaminophen concentration can underestimate the level because ER formulations can have secondary delayed peaks. In cases of overdose of the ER formulation, it is recommended that additional acetaminophen levels be obtained at 4-hour intervals after the initial level is measured. If any level is in the toxic zone, therapy should be initiated.

It is recommended that pregnant patients with toxic plasma concentrations of acetaminophen be treated with NAC to prevent hepatotoxicity in both fetus and mother. The available data suggest no teratogenicity to NAC or acetaminophen.

Indications for NAC therapy in cases of chronic intoxication are a history of ingestion of 3 to 4 g for several days with elevated liver enzyme levels (AST and ALT). The acetaminophen blood concentration is often low in these cases because of the extended time lapse since ingestion and should not be plotted on the Rumack-Matthew nomogram. Patients with a history of chronic alcoholism or those on chronic enzyme inducers may also present with elevated liver enzyme levels and should be considered for NAC therapy if they have a history of taking acetaminophen on a chronic basis, because they are considered to be at a greater risk for hepatotoxicity despite a low acetaminophen blood concentration.

Specific support care may be needed to treat liver failure, pancreatitis, transient renal failure, and myocarditis.

Liver transplantation has a definite but limited role in patients with acute acetaminophen overdose. A retrospective analysis determined that a continuing rise in the prothrombin time (4-day peak, 180 seconds), a pH of less than 7.3 2 days after the overdose, a serum creatinine level of greater than 3.3 mg/dL, severe hepatic encephalopathy, and disturbed coagulation factor VII/V ratio greater than 30 suggest a poor prognosis and may be indicators for hepatology consultation for consideration of liver transplantation.

Extracorporeal measures are not expected to be of benefit.

Disposition

Adults who have ingested more than 140 mg/kg and children younger than 6 years of age who have ingested more than 200 mg/kg should receive therapy within 8 hours postingestion or until the results of the 4-hour postingestion acetaminophen plasma concentration are known.

Amphetamines

The amphetamines include illicit methamphetamine ("Ice"), diet pills, and formulations under various trade names. Analogues include MDMA (3,4 methylenedioxymethamphetamine, known as "ecstasy," "XTC," or "Adam") and MDA (3,4-methylenedioxyamphetamine, known as "Eve"). MDA is a common hallucinogen and euphoriant "club drug" used at "raves," which are all-night dances. Use of methamphetamine and designer analogues is on the rise, especially among young people between the ages of 12 and 25 years. Other similar stimulants are phenylpropanolamine and cocaine.

Toxic Mechanism

Amphetamines have a direct CNS stimulant effect and a sympathetic nervous system effect by releasing catecholamines from α- and β-adrenergic nerve terminals but inhibiting their reuptake.

Hallucinogenic MDMA has an additional hazard of serotonin effect (refer to serotonin syndrome in the SSRI section). MDMA also affect the dopamine system in the brain. Because of its effects on 5-hydroxytryptamine, dopamine, and norepinephrine, MDMA can lead to serotonin syndrome associated with malignant hyperthermia and rhabdomyolysis, which contributes to the potentially life-threatening hyperthermia observed in several patients who have used MDMA.

Phenylpropanolamine stimulates only the β-adrenergic receptors.

Toxic Dose

In children, the toxic dose of dextroamphetamine is 1 mg/kg; in adults, the toxic dose is 5 mg/kg. The potentially fatal dose of dextroamphetamine is 12 mg/kg.

Kinetics

Amphetamine is a weak base with pKa of 8 to 10. Onset of action is 30 to 60 minutes, and peak effects are 2 to 4 hours. The volume distribution is 2 to 3 L/kg.

Through hepatic metabolism, 60% of the substance is metabolized into a hydroxylated metabolite that may be responsible for psychotic effects.

The half-life of amphetamines is pH dependent—8 to 10 hours in acid urine (pH <6.0) and 16 to 31 hours in alkaline urine (pH >7.5). Excretion is by the kidney—30% to 40% at alkaline urine pH and 50% to 70% at acid urine pH.

Manifestations

Effects are seen within 30 to 60 minutes following ingestion.

Neurologic manifestations include restlessness, irritation and agitation, tremors and hyperreflexia, and auditory and visual hallucinations. Hyperpyrexia may precede seizures, convulsions, paranoia, violence, intracranial hemorrhage, psychosis, and self-destructive behavior. Paranoid psychosis and cerebral vasculitis occur with chronic abuse.

MDMA is often adulterated with cocaine, heroin, or ketamine, or a combination of these, to create a variety of mood alterations. This possibility must be taken into consideration when one manages patients with MDMA ingestions, as the symptom complex may reflect both CNS stimulation and CNS depression.

Other manifestations include dilated but reactive pupils, cardiac dysrhythmias (supraventricular and ventricular), tachycardia, hypertension, rhabdomyolysis, and myoglobinuria.

Laboratory Investigations

The clinician should monitor ECG and cardiac readings, ABG and oxygen saturation, electrolytes, blood glucose, BUN, creatinine, creatine kinase, cardiac fraction if there is chest pain, and liver profile. Also, one should evaluate for rhabdomyolysis and check urine for myoglobin, cocaine and metabolites, and other substances of abuse. The peak plasma concentration of amphetamines is 10 to 50 ng/mL 1 to 2 hours after ingestion of 10 to 25 mg. The toxic plasma concentration is 200 ng/mL. When the rapid immunoassays are used, cross-reactions can occur with amphetamine derivatives (e.g., MDA, "ecstasy"), brompheniramine (Dimetane), chlorpromazine (Thorazine), ephedrine, phenylpropanolamine, phentermine (Adipex-P), phenmetrazine, ranitidine (Zantac), and Vicks Inhaler (L-desoxyephedrine). False-positive results may occur.

Management

Management is similar to management for cocaine intoxication. Supportive care includes blood pressure and temperature control, cardiac monitoring, and seizure precautions. Diazepam (Valium) can be administered. Gastrointestinal decontamination can be undertaken with activated charcoal administered up to 1 hour after ingestion.

Anxiety, agitation, and convulsions are treated with diazepam. If diazepam fails to control seizures, neuromuscular blockers can be used and the electroencephalogram (EEG) monitored for nonmotor seizures. One should avoid neuroleptic phenothiazines and butyrophenone, which can lower the seizure threshold.

Hypertension and tachycardia are usually transient and can be managed by titration of diazepam. Nitroprusside can be used for hypertensive crisis at a maximum infusion rate of 10 µg/kg/minute for 10 minutes followed with a lower infusion rate of 0.3 to 2 mg/kg/minute. Myocardial ischemia is managed by oxygen, vascular access, benzodiazepines, and nitroglycerin. Aspirin and thrombolytics are not routinely recommended because of the danger of intracranial hemorrhage. It is important to distinguish between angina and true ischemia. Delayed hypotension can be treated with fluids and vasopressors if needed. Life-threatening tachydysrhythmias may respond to an α-blocker such as phentolamine (Regitine) 5 mg IV for adults or 0.1 mg/kg IV for children and a short-acting β-blocker such as esmolol (Brevibloc) 500 µg/kg IV over 1 minute for adults, or 300 to 500 µg/kg over 1 minute for children. Ventricular dysrhythmias may respond to lidocaine or, in a severely hemodynamically compromised patient, immediate synchronized electrical cardioversion.

Rhabdomyolysis and myoglobinuria are treated with fluids, alkaline diuresis, and diuretics. Hyperthermia is treated with external cooling and cool 100% humidified oxygen. More extensive therapy may be needed in severe cases. If focal neurologic symptoms are present, the possibility of a cerebrovascular accident should be considered and a CT scan of the head should be obtained.

Paranoid ideation and threatening behavior should be treated with rapid tranquilization using a benzodiazepine. One should observe for suicidal depression that may follow intoxication and may require suicide precautions.

Extracorporeal measures are of no benefit.

Disposition

Symptomatic patients should be observed on a monitored unit until the symptoms resolve and then observed for a short time after resolution for relapse.

Anticholinergic Agents

Drugs with anticholinergic properties include antihistamines (H_1 blockers), neuroleptics (phenothiazines), tricyclic antidepressants, antiparkinsonism drugs (trihexyphenidyl [Artane], benztropine [Cogentin]), ophthalmic products (atropine), and a number of common plants.

The antihistamines are divided into the sedating anticholinergic types, and the nonsedating single daily dose types. The sedating types include ethanolamines (e.g., diphenhydramine [Benadryl], dimenhydrinate [Dramamine], and clemastine [Tavist]), ethylenediamines (e.g., tripelennamine [Pyribenzamine]), alkyl amines (e.g., chlorpheniramine [Chlor-Trimeton], brompheniramine [Dimetane]), piperazines (e.g., cyclizine [Marezine], hydroxyzine [Atarax], and meclizine [Antivert]), and phenothiazine (e.g., Phenergan). The nonsedating types include astemizole (Hismanal), terfenadine (Seldane), loratadine (Claritin), fexofenadine (Allegra), and cetirizine (Zyrtec).

The anticholinergic plants include jimsonweed (*Datura stramonium*), deadly nightshade (*Atropa belladonna*), henbane (*Hyoscyamus niger*), and antispasmodic agents for the bowel (atropine derivatives).

Toxic Mechanism

By competitive inhibition, anticholinergics block the action of acetylcholine on postsynaptic cholinergic receptor sites. The toxic mechanism primarily involves the peripheral and CNS muscarinic receptors. H_1 sedating-type agents also depress or stimulate the CNS, and in large overdoses some have cardiac membrane–depressant effects (e.g., diphenhydramine [Benadryl]) and α-adrenergic receptor blockade effects (e.g., promethazine [Phenergan]). Nonsedating agents produce peripheral H_1 blockade but do not possess anticholinergic or sedating actions. The original agents terfenadine (Seldane) and astemizole (Hismanal) were recently removed from the market because of the severe cardiac dysrhythmias associated with their use, especially when used in combination with macrolide antibiotics and certain antifungal agents such as ketoconazole (Nizoral), which inhibit hepatic metabolism or excretion. The newer nonsedating agents, including loratadine (Claritin), fexofenadine (Allegra), and cetirizine (Zyrtec), have not been reported to cause the severe drug interactions associated with terfenadine and astemizole.

Toxic Dose

The estimated toxic oral dose of atropine is 0.05 mg/kg in children and more than 2 mg in adults. The minimal estimated lethal dose of atropine is more than 10 mg in adults and more than 2 mg in children. Other synthetic anticholinergic agents are less toxic, and the fatal dose varies from 10 to 100 mg.

The estimated toxic oral dose of diphenhydramine (Benadryl) in a child is 15 mg/kg, and the potential lethal amount is 25 mg/kg. In an adult, the potential lethal amount is 2.8 g. Ingestion of five times the single dose of an antihistamine is toxic.

For the nonsedating agents, an overdose of 3360 mg of terfenadine was reported in an adult who developed ventricular tachycardia and fibrillation that responded to lidocaine and defibrillation.

A 1500-mg overdose produced hypotension. Cases of delayed serious dysrhythmias (torsades de pointes) have been reported with doses of more than 200 mg of astemizole. The toxic doses of fexofenadine (Allegra), cetirizine, and loratadine (Claritin) need to be established.

Kinetics

The onset of absorption of intravenous atropine is in 2 to 4 minutes. Peak effects on salivation after intravenous or intramuscular administration are at 30 to 60 minutes.

Onset of absorption after oral ingestion is 30 to 60 minutes, peak action is 1 to 3 hours, and duration of action is 4 to 6 hours, but symptoms are prolonged in cases of overdose or with sustained-release preparations.

The onset of absorption of diphenhydramine is in 15 minutes to 1 hour, with a peak of action in 1 to 4 hours. Volume distribution is 3.3 to 6.8 L/kg, and protein binding is 75% to 80%. Ninety-eight percent of diphenhydramine is metabolized via the liver by N-demethylation. Interactions with erythromycin, ketoconazole (Nizoral), and derivatives produce excessive blood levels of the antihistamine and ventricular dysrhythmias.

The half-life of diphenhydramine is 3 to 10 hours.

The chemical structure of nonsedating agents prevents their entry into the CNS. Absorption begins in 1 hour, with peak effects in 4 to 6 hours. The duration of action is greater than 24 hours.

These agents are metabolized in the gastrointestinal tract and liver. Protein binding is greater than 90%. The plasma half-life is 3.5 hours. Only 1% is excreted unchanged; 60% of that is excreted in the feces and 40% in the urine.

Manifestations

Anticholinergic signs are hyperpyrexia ("hot as a hare"), mydriasis ("blind as a bat"), flushing of skin ("red as a beet"), dry mucosa and skin ("dry as a bone"), "Lilliputian type" hallucinations and delirium ("mad as a hatter"), coma, dysphagia, tachycardia, moderate hypertension, and rarely convulsions and urinary retention. Other effects include jaundice (cyproheptadine [Periactin]), dystonia (diphenhydramine [Benadryl]), rhabdomyolysis (doxylamine), and, in large doses, cardiotoxic effects (diphenhydramine).

Overdose with nonsedating agents produces headache and confusion, nausea, and dysrhythmias (e.g., torsades de pointes).

Laboratory Investigations

Monitoring of ABG (in cases of respiratory depression), electrolytes, glucose, and the ECG should be undertaken. Anticholinergic drugs and plants are not routinely included on screens for substances of abuse.

Management

For patients in respiratory failure, intubation and assisted ventilation should be instituted. Gastrointestinal decontamination can be instituted. Caution must be taken with emesis in cases of diphenhydramine (Benadryl) overdose because of the drug's rapid onset of action and risk of seizures. If bowel sounds are present for up to 1 hour after ingestion, activated charcoal can be given. Seizures can be controlled with benzodiazepines (diazepam [Valium] or lorazepam [Ativan]).

The administration of physostigmine (Antilirium) is not routine and is reserved for life-threatening anticholinergic effects that are refractory to conventional treatments. It should be administered with adequate monitoring and resuscitative equipment available. The use of physostigmine should be avoided if a tricyclic antidepressant is present because of increased toxicity. Urinary retention should be relieved by catheterization to avoid reabsorption of the drug and additional toxicity.

Supraventricular tachycardia should be treated only if the patient is hemodynamically unstable. Ventricular dysrhythmias can be controlled with lidocaine or cardioversion. Sodium bicarbonate 1 to 2 mEq/kg IV may be useful for myocardial depression and QRS prolongation. Torsades de pointes, especially when associated with terfenadine and astemizole ingestion, has been treated with magnesium sulfate 4 g or 40 mL 10% solution intravenously over 10 to 20 minutes and countershock if the patient fails to respond.

Hyperpyrexia is controlled by external cooling. Hemodialysis and hemoperfusion are not effective.

Disposition

Antihistamine H₁ Antagonists. Symptomatic patients should be observed on a monitored unit until the symptoms resolve, then observed for a short time (3 to 4 hours) after resolution for relapse.

Nonsedating Agents. All asymptomatic children who acutely ingest more than the maximum adult dose and all symptomatic children should be referred to a health care facility for a minimum of 6 hours' observation as well as cardiac monitoring. Asymptomatic adults who acutely ingest more than twice the maximum adult daily dose should be monitored for a minimum of 6 hours. All symptomatic patients should be monitored for as long as there are symptoms present.

Barbiturates

Barbiturates have been used as sedatives, anesthetic agents, and anticonvulsants, but their use is declining as safer, more effective drugs become available.

Toxic Mechanism

Barbiturates are γ-aminobutyric acid (GABA) agonists (increasing the chloride flow and inhibiting depolarization). They enhance the CNS depressant effect of GABA and depress the cardiovascular system.

Toxic Dose

The shorter-acting barbiturates (including the intermediate-acting agents) and their hypnotic doses are as follows: amobarbital (Amytal), 100 to 200 mg; aprobarbital (Alurate), 50 to 100 mg; butabarbital (Butisol), 50 to 100 mg; butalbital, 100 to 200 mg; pentobarbital (Nembutal), 100 to 200 mg; secobarbital (Seconal), 100 to 200 mg. They cause toxicity at lower doses than long-acting barbiturates and have a minimum toxic dose of 6 mg/kg; the fatal adult dose is 3 to 6 g.

The long-acting barbiturates and their doses include mephobarbital (Mebaral), 50 to 100 mg, and phenobarbital, 100 to 200 mg. Their minimum toxic dose is greater than 10 mg/kg, and the fatal adult dose is 6 to 10 g. A general rule is that an amount five times the hypnotic dose is toxic and an amount 10 times the hypnotic dose is potentially fatal. Methohexital and thiopental are ultrashort-acting parenteral preparations and are not discussed.

Kinetics

The barbiturates are enzyme inducers. Short-acting barbiturates are highly lipid-soluble, penetrate the brain readily, and have shorter elimination times. Onset of action is in 10 to 30 minutes, with a peak at 1 to 2 hours. Duration of action is 3 to 8 hours. The volume distribution of short-acting barbiturate is 0.8 to 1.5 L/kg; pKa is about 8. Mean half-life varies from 8 to 48 hours.

Long-acting agents have longer elimination times and can be used as anticonvulsants. Onset of action is in 20 to 60 minutes, with a peak at 1 to 6 hours. In cases of overdose, the peak can be at 10 hours. Usual duration of action is 8 to 12 hours. Volume distribution is 0.8 L/kg, and half-life is 11 to 120 hours. The pKa of phenobarbital is 7.2. Alkalinization of urine promotes its excretion.

Manifestations

Mild intoxication resembles alcohol intoxication and includes ataxia, slurred speech, and depressed cognition. Severe intoxication causes slow respirations, coma, and loss of reflexes (except pupillary light reflex).

Other manifestations include hypotension (vasodilation), hypothermia, hypoglycemia, and death by respiratory arrest.

Laboratory Investigations

Most barbiturates are detected on routine drug screens and can be measured in most hospital laboratories. Investigation should include barbiturate level; ABG; toxicology screen, including acetaminophen; glucose, electrolyte, BUN, creatinine, and creatine kinase levels; and urine pH. The minimum toxic plasma levels are greater than 10 µg/mL for short-acting barbiturates and greater than 40 µg/dL for long-acting agents. Fatal levels are 30 µg/mL for short-acting barbiturates and 80 to 150 µg/mL for long-acting agents. Both short-acting and long-acting agents can be detected in urine 24 to 72 hours after ingestion, and long-acting agents can be detected up to 7 days.

Management

Vital functions must be established and maintained. Intensive supportive care including intubation and assisted ventilation should dominate the management. All stuporous and comatose patients should have glucose (for hypoglycemia), thiamine (if chronically alcoholic), and naloxone (Narcan) (in case of an opioid ingestion) intravenously and should be admitted to the intensive care unit. Emesis should be avoided especially in cases of ingestion of the shorter-acting barbiturates. Activated charcoal followed by MDAC (0.5 g/kg) every 2 to 4 hours has been shown to reduce the serum half-life of phenobarbital by 50%, but its effect on clinical course is undetermined.

Fluids should be administered to correct dehydration and hypotension. Vasopressors may be necessary to correct severe hypotension, and hemodynamic monitoring may be needed. The patient must be observed carefully for fluid overload. Alkalinization (ion trapping) is used only for phenobarbital (pKa 7.2) but not for short-acting barbiturates. Sodium bicarbonate, 1 to 2 mEq/kg IV in 500 mL of 5% dextrose in adults or 10 to 15 mL/kg in children during the first hour, followed by sufficient bicarbonate to keep the urinary pH at 7.5 to 8.0, enhances excretion of phenobarbital and shortens the half-life by 50%. Diuresis is not advocated because of the danger of cerebral or pulmonary edema.

Hemodialysis shortens the half-life to 8 to 14 hours, and charcoal hemoperfusion shortens the half-life to 6 to 8 hours for long-acting barbiturates such as phenobarbital. Both procedures may be effective in patients with both long-acting and short-acting barbiturate ingestion. If the patient does not respond to supportive measures or if the phenobarbital plasma concentration is greater than 150 µg/mL, both procedures may be tried to shorten the half-life.

Bullae are treated as a local second degree skin burn. Hypothermia should be treated.

Disposition

All comatose patients should be admitted to the intensive care unit. Awake and oriented patients with an overdose of short-acting agents should be observed for at least 6 asymptomatic hours; overdose of long-acting agents warrants observation for at least 12 asymptomatic hours because of the potential for delayed absorption. In the case of an intentional overdose, psychiatric clearance is needed before the patient can be discharged. Chronic use can lead to tolerance, physical dependency, and withdrawal and necessitates follow-up.

Benzodiazepines

Benzodiazepines are used as anxiolytics, sedatives, and relaxants.

Toxic Mechanism

The GABA agonists produce CNS depression and increase chloride flow, inhibiting depolarization.

Flunitrazepam (Rohypnol; street name "roofies") is a long-acting benzodiazepine agonist sold by prescription in more than 60 countries worldwide, but it is not legally available in the United States.

Toxic Dose

The long-acting benzodiazepines (half-life >24 hours) and their maximum therapeutic doses are as follows: chlordiazepoxide (Librium), 50 mg; clorazepate (Tranxene), 30 mg; clonazepam (Klonopin), 20 mg; diazepam (Valium), 10 mg in adults or 0.2 mg/kg in children; flurazepam (Dalmane), 30 mg; and prazepam, 20 mg.

The short-acting benzodiazepines (half-life 10 to 24 hours) and their doses include the following: alprazolam (Xanax), 0.5 mg, and lorazepam (Ativan), 4 mg in adults or 0.05 mg/kg in children, which act similar to the long-acting benzodiazepines.

The ultrashort-acting benzodiazepines (half-life <10 hours) are more toxic and include temazepam (Restoril), 30 mg; triazolam (Halcion), 0.5 mg; midazolam (Versed), 0.2 mg/kg; and oxazepam (Serax), 30 mg.

In cases of overdose of short- and long-acting agents, 10 to 20 times the therapeutic dose (>1500 mg diazepam or 2000 mg chlordiazepoxide) have been ingested with resulting mild coma but without respiratory depression. Fatalities are rare, and most patients recover within 24 to 36 hours after overdose. Asymptomatic unintentional overdoses of less than five times the therapeutic dose can be seen. Ultrashort-acting agents have produced respiratory arrest and coma within 1 hour after ingestion of 5 mg of triazolam (Halcion) and death with ingestion of as little as 10 mg. Midazolam (Versed) and diazepam (Valium) by rapid intravenous injection have produced respiratory arrest.

Kinetics
Onset of CNS depression is usually in 30 to 120 minutes; peak action usually occurs within 1 to 3 hours when ingestion is by the oral route. The volume distribution varies from 0.26 to 6 L/kg (LA, 1.1 L/kg); protein binding is 70% to 99%. For flunitrazepam, the onset of action is in 0.5 to 2 hours, oral peak is in 2 hours, and duration 8 hours or more. The half-life of flunitrazepam is 20 to 30 hours, volume distribution is 3.3 to 5.5 L/kg, and 80% is protein bound. Flunitrazepam can be identified in urine 4 to 30 days after ingestion.

Manifestations
Neurologic manifestations include ataxia, slurred speech, and CNS depression. Deep coma leading to respiratory depression suggests the presence of short-acting benzodiazepines or other CNS depressants. In elderly persons, the therapeutic doses can produce toxicity and can have an additive effect with other CNS depressants. Chronic use can lead to tolerance, physical dependency, and withdrawal.

Laboratory Investigations
Most benzodiazepines can be detected in urine drug screens. Quantitative blood levels are not useful. Some of the immunoassay urinary screens cannot detect all of the new benzodiazepines currently available. A consultation with the laboratory analyst is warranted if a specific case occurs in which the test result is negative but benzodiazepine use is suspected by the patient's history. Situations in which benzodiazepines may not be detected include ingestion of a low dose (e.g., <10 mg), rapid elimination, and a different or no metabolite. Some immunoassay methods can produce a false-positive finding for the benzodiazepines when nonsteroidal antiinflammatory drugs (tolmetin [Tolectin], naproxen [Aleve], etodolac [Lodine], and fenoprofen [Nalfon]) are used. If this is a concern, the laboratory analyst should be consulted.

In cases in which "date rape" drugs such as flunitrazepam are suspected, a police crime or reference laboratory should be consulted for testing.

Management
Emesis and gastric lavage should be avoided. Activated charcoal can be useful only if given early before the peak time of absorption occurs. Supportive treatment should be instituted but rarely requires intubation or assisted ventilation.

Flumazenil (Romazicon) is a specific benzodiazepine receptor antagonist that blocks the chloride flow and inhibitor of GABA neurotransmitters. It reverses the sedative effects of benzodiazepines, zolpidem (Ambien), and endogenous benzodiazepines associated with hepatic encephalopathy. It is not recommended to reverse benzodiazepine-induced hypoventilation. The manufacturer advises that flumazenil be used with caution in cases of overdose with possible benzodiazepine dependency (because it can precipitate life-threatening withdrawal), if cyclic antidepressant use is suspected, or if a patient has a known seizure disorder.

Disposition
If the patient is comatose, he or she must be admitted to the intensive care unit. If the overdose was intentional, psychiatric clearance is needed before the patient can be discharged.

β-Adrenergic Blockers (β-Blockers)
β-Blockers are used in the treatment of hypertension and of a number of systemic and ophthalmologic disorders. Properties of β-blockers include the factors listed in Table 12.

Lipid-soluble drugs have CNS effects, active metabolites, longer duration of action, and interactions (e.g., propranolol). Cardioselectivity is lost in overdose. Intrinsic partial agonist agents (e.g., pindolol) may initially produce tachycardia and hypertension. Cardiac membrane depressive effect (quinidine-like) occurs in cases of overdose but not at therapeutic doses (e.g., with metoprolol or sotalol). α-Blocking effect is weak (e.g., with labetalol or acebutolol).

Toxic Mechanism
β-Blockers compete with the catecholamines for receptor sites and block receptor action in the bronchi, the vascular smooth muscle, and the myocardium.

Toxic Dose
Ingestions of greater than twice the maximum recommended daily therapeutic dose are considered toxic (see Table 12). Ingestion of 1 mg/kg propranolol in a child may produce hypoglycemia. Fatalities have been reported in adults with 7.5 g of metoprolol. The most toxic agent is sotalol, and the least toxic is atenolol.

Kinetics
Regular-release formulations usually cause symptoms within 2 hours. Propranolol's onset of action is 20 to 30 minutes and peak is at 1 to 4 hours, but it may be delayed by co-ingestants. The onset of action with sustained-release preparations may be delayed to 6 hours and the peak to 12 to 16 hours. Volume distribution is 1 to 5.6 L/kg. Protein binding is variable, from 5% to 93%.

Metabolism
Atenolol (Tenormin), nadolol (Corgard), and santalol (Betapace) have enterohepatic recirculation. The duration of action for regular-acting agents is 4 to 6 hours, but in cases of overdose it may be 24 to 48 hours. The duration of action for sustained-release agents is 24 to 48 hours.

The regular preparation with the longest half-life is nadolol, at 12 to 24 hours, and the one with the shortest half-life is esmolol, at 5 to 10 minutes.

Manifestations
See "Toxic Properties" and Table 12.

Highly lipid soluble agents produce coma and seizures. Bradycardia and hypotension are the major cardiac symptoms and may lead to cardiogenic shock. Intrinsic partial agonists initially may cause tachycardia and hypertension. ECG changes include atrioventricular conduction delay or asystole. Membrane-depressant effects produce prolonged QRS and QT interval, which may result in torsades de pointes. Sotalol produces a very prolonged QT interval. Bronchospasm may occur in patients with reactive airway disease with any β-blocker because the selectivity is lost in overdose. Other manifestations include hypoglycemia (because β-blockers block catecholamine counter-regulatory mechanisms) and hyperkalemia.

Laboratory Investigations
Measurements of blood levels are not readily available or useful. ECG and cardiac monitoring should be maintained, and blood glucose and electrolytes, BUN, and creatinine levels should be monitored, as well as ABG if there are respiratory symptoms.

Management
Vital functions must be established and maintained. Vascular access, baseline ECG, and continuous cardiac and blood pressure monitoring should be established. A pacemaker must be available.

TABLE 12 Pharmacologic and Toxic Properties of β-Blockers

β-BLOCKER	MAXIMUM SOLUBILITY	THERAPEUTIC PLASMA LEVEL	LIPID SOLUBILITY	INTRINSIC SYMPATHOMIMETIC ACTIVITY (PARTIAL AGONIST)	MEMBRANE STABILIZING EFFECT / β-SELECTIVE β1	β2	CARDIAC SELECTIVITY / α-SELECTIVE
Acebutolol (Sectral)	800 mg	200–2000 ng/mL	Moderate	+	+	+	+
Alprenolol[2]	800 mg	50–200 ng/mL	Moderate	2+	+	−	−
Atenolol (Tenormin)	100 mg	200–500 ng/mL	Low	−	−	2+	−
Betaxolol (Kerlone)	20 mg	NA	Low	+	−	+	−
Carteolol (Cartrol)	10 mg	NA	No	+	−	−	−
Esmolol (Brevibloc) (Class II antidysrhythmic, IV only)			Low	−	−	+	−
Labetalol (Trandate)	800 mg	50–500 ng/mL	Low	+	+/−	−	+
Levobunolol (AKBeta eyedrop) (Eye drops 0.25% and 0.5%)	20 mg	NA	No				
Metoprolol (Lopressor)			Moderate	−	−	2+	
Nadolol (Corgard)	320 mg	20–40 ng/mL	Low	−	−	−	−
Oxyprenolol[2]	480 mg	80–100 ng/mL	Moderate	2+	+	−	−
Pindolol (Visken)	60 mg	50–150 ng/mL	Moderate	3+	+/−	−	−
Propranolol (Inderal) (Class II antidysrhythmic)	360 mg	50–100 ng/mL	High	−	2+	−	−
Sotalol (Betapace) (Class II antidysrhythmic)	480 mg	500–4000 ng/mL	Low	−	−	−	−
Timolol (Blocadren)	60 mg	5–10 ng/mL	Low	−	+/−	−	−

[2]Not available in the United States.

Gastrointestinal decontamination can be undertaken initially with activated charcoal up to 1 hour after ingestion. MDAC is no longer recommended, based on the latest guidelines. Whole-bowel irrigation can be considered in cases of large overdoses with sustained-release preparations, but there are no studies evaluating the efficacy of intervention.

If there are cardiovascular disturbances, a cardiac consultation should be obtained. Class IA antidysrhythmic agents (procainamide, quinidine) and III (bretylium) are not recommended. Hypotension is treated with fluids initially, although it usually does not respond. Frequently, glucagon and cardiac pacing are needed. Bradycardia in asymptomatic, hemodynamically stable patients requires no therapy. It is not predictive of the future course of the disease. If the patient is unstable (has hypotension or a high-degree atrioventricular block), atropine 0.02 mg/kg (up to 2 mg) in adults, glucagon, and a pacemaker can be used. In case of ventricular tachycardia, overdrive pacing can be used. A wide QRS interval may respond to sodium bicarbonate. Torsades de pointes (associated with sotalol) may respond to magnesium sulfate and overdrive pacing. Prophylactic magnesium for prolonged QT interval has been suggested, but there are no data. Epinephrine must not be used because an unopposed α effect may occur.

Hypotension and myocardial depression are managed by correction of dysrhythmias, Trendelenburg position, fluids, glucagon, or amrinone (Inocor), or a combination of these. Hemodynamic monitoring with a Swan-Ganz catheter or arterial line may be necessary to manage fluid therapy.

Glucagon is the initial drug of choice. It works through adenyl cyclase and bypasses catecholamine receptors; therefore, it is not affected by β-blockers. Glucagon increases cardiac contractility and heart rate. It is given as an intravenous bolus of 5 to 10 mg[3] over 1 minute and followed by a continuous infusion of 1 to 5 mg/h (in children, 0.15 mg/kg followed by 0.05 to 0.1 mg/kg/h). In large doses and in infusion therapy D_5W, sterile water, or saline should be used as a diluant to reconstitute glucagon in place of the 0.2% phenol diluent provided with some drugs. Effects are seen within minutes. It can be used with other agents such as amrinone.

Amrinone (Inocor) inhibits phosphodiesterase enzyme, which metabolizes cyclic AMP. It is administered as a bolus of 0.15 to 2 mg/kg (0.15 to 0.4 mL/kg) intravenously, followed by infusion of 5 to 10 µg/kg/min.

Hypoglycemia should be treated with intravenous glucose. Life-threatening hyperkalemia is treated with calcium (avoid if digoxin is present), bicarbonate, and glucose or insulin. Convulsions can be controlled with diazepam or phenobarbital. If bronchospasm is present, β2 nebulized bronchodilators are given.

Extraordinary measures such as intra-aortic balloon pump support can be instituted. Extracorporeal measures can be undertaken. Hemodialysis for cases of atenolol, acebutolol, nadolol, and sotalol (low volume distribution, low protein binding) ingestion may be helpful, particularly when there is evidence of renal failure. Hemodialysis is not effective for propranolol, metoprolol, and timolol.

Prenalterol[2] has successfully reversed both bradycardia and hypotension but is not currently available in the United States.

[2]Not available in the United States.
[3]Exceeds dosage recommended by the manufacturer.

Disposition

Asymptomatic patients with history of overdose require baseline ECG and continuous cardiac monitoring for at least 6 hours with regular-release preparations and for 24 hours with sustained-release preparations. Symptomatic patients should be observed with cardiac monitoring for 24 hours. If seizures or abnormal rhythm or vital signs are present, the patient should be admitted to the intensive care unit.

Calcium Channel Blockers

Calcium channel blockers are used in the treatment of effort angina, supraventricular tachycardia, and hypertension.

Toxic Mechanism

Calcium channel blockers reduce influx of calcium through the slow channels in membranes of the myocardium, the atrioventricular nodes, and the vascular smooth muscles and result in peripheral, systemic, and coronary vasodilation, impaired cardiac conduction, and depression of cardiac contractility. All calcium channel blockers have vasodilatory action, but only bepridil, diltiazem, and verapamil depress myocardial contractility and cause atrioventricular block.

Toxic Dose

Any ingested amount greater than the maximum daily dose has the potential of severe toxicity. The maximum oral daily doses in adults and toxic doses in children of each are as follows: amlodipine (Norvasc), 10 mg for adults and more than 0.25 mg/kg for children; bepridil (Vascor), 400 mg for adults and more than 5.7 mg/kg for children; diltiazem (Cardizem), 360 mg for adults (toxic dose >2 g) and more than 6 mg/kg for children; felodipine (Plendil), 40 mg for adults and more than 0.56 mg/kg for children; isradipine (DynaCirc), 40 mg for adults and more than 0.4 mg/kg for children; nicardipine (Cardene), 120 mg for adults and more than 0.85 mg/kg for children; nifedipine (Procardia), 120 mg for adults and more than 2 mg/kg for children; nimodipine (Nimotop), 360 mg for adults and more than 0.85 mg/kg for children; nitrendipine (Baypress),[1] 80 mg for adults and more than 1.14 mg/kg for children; and verapamil (Calan), 480 mg for adults and 15 mg/kg for children.

Kinetics

Onset of action of regular-release preparations varies: for verapamil it is 60 to 120 minutes, for nifedipine 20 minutes, and for diltiazem 15 minutes after ingestion. Peak effect for verapamil is 2 to 4 hours, for nifedipine 60 to 90 minutes, and for diltiazem 30 to 60 minutes, but the peak action may be delayed for 6 to 8 hours. Duration of action is up to 36 hours. The onset of action for sustained-release preparations is usually 4 hours but may be delayed, and peak effect is at 12 to 24 hours. In cases of massive overdose, concretions and prolonged toxicity can develop.

Volume distribution varies from 3 to 7 L/kg. Hepatic elimination half-life varies from 3 to 7 hours. Patients receiving digitalis and calcium channel blockers run the risk of digitalis toxicity, because calcium channel blockers increase digitalis levels.

Manifestations

Cardiac manifestations include hypotension, bradycardia, and conduction disturbances occurring 30 minutes to 5 hours after ingestion. A prolonged PR interval is an early finding and may occur at therapeutic doses. Torsades de pointes has been reported. All degrees of blocks may occur and may be delayed up to 16 hours. Lactic acidosis may be present. Calcium channel blockers do not affect intraventricular conduction, so the QRS interval is usually not affected.

Hypocalcemia is rarely present. Hyperglycemia may be present because of interference in calcium-dependent insulin release. Mental status changes, headaches, seizures, hemiparesis, and CNS depression may occur.

[1] Not FDA approved for this indication.

Laboratory Investigations

Specific drug levels are not readily available and are not useful. Monitor blood sugar, electrolytes, calcium, ABG, pulse oximetry, creatinine, and BUN, and also use hemodynamic monitoring, ECG, and cardiac monitoring.

Management

Vital functions must be established and maintained. Baseline ECG readings should be obtained and continuous cardiac and blood pressure monitoring maintained. A pacemaker should be available. Cardiology consultation should be sought.

Gastrointestinal decontamination with activated charcoal is recommended. If a large dose of a sustained-release preparation was ingested, whole-bowel irrigation can be considered, but its effectiveness has not been investigated.

If the patient is symptomatic, immediate cardiology consult must be obtained, because a pacemaker and hemodynamic monitoring may be needed. In the case of heart block, atropine is rarely effective and isoproterenol (Isuprel) may produce vasodilation. The use of a pacemaker should be considered early.

Hypotension and bradycardia can be treated with positioning, fluids, and calcium gluconate or chloride, glucagon, amrinone (Inocor), and ventricular pacing. Calcium salts must be avoided if digoxin is present. Calcium usually reverses depressed myocardial contractility but may not reverse nodal depression or peripheral vasodilation. Calcium chloride can be given in a 10% solution, 0.1 to 0.2 mL/kg up to 10 mL in an adult, or calcium gluconate in a 10% solution 0.3 to 0.4 mL/kg up to 20 mL in an adult. Administration is intravenous, over 5 to 10 minutes. One should monitor for dysrhythmias, hypotension, and the serum ionized calcium. The aim is to increase calcium 4 mg/dL to a maximum of 13 mg/dL. The calcium response lasts 15 minutes and may require repeated doses or a continuous calcium gluconate infusion 0.2 mL/kg/h up to maximum of 10 mL/h.

If calcium fails, glucagon can be tried for its positive inotropic and chronotropic effect, or both. Amrinone (Inocor), an inotropic agent, may reverse the effects of calcium channel blockers. An effective dose is 0.15 mg to 2 mg/kg (0.15–0.4 mL/kg) by intravenous bolus followed by infusion of 5 to 10 μg/kg/min.

In case of hypotension, fluids, norepinephrine (Levophed), and epinephrine may be required. Amrinone and glucagon have been tried alone and in combination. Dobutamine and dopamine are often ineffective.

Extracorporeal measures (e.g., hemodialysis and charcoal hemoperfusion) are not useful, but extraordinary measures such as intra-aortic balloon pump and cardiopulmonary bypass have been used successfully.

For cases of calcium channel blocker toxicity that fail to respond to aggressive management, recent studies demonstrate that insulin and glucose have therapeutic value. The suggested dose range for insulin is to infuse regular insulin at 0.5 IU/kg/h with a simultaneous infusion of glucose 1 g/kg/h, with glucose monitoring every 30 minutes for at least the first 4 hours of administration and subsequent glucose adjustment to maintain euglycemia (70 to 100 mg/dL). Potassium levels should be monitored regularly, as they may shift in response to the insulin.

Disposition

Patients who have ingested regular-release preparations should be monitored for at least 6 hours and those who have ingested sustained-release preparations should be monitored for 24 hours after the ingestion. Intentional overdose necessitates psychiatric clearance. Symptomatic patients should be admitted to the intensive care unit.

Carbon Monoxide

Carbon monoxide is an odorless, colorless gas produced from incomplete combustion; it is also an in vivo metabolic breakdown product of methylene chloride used in paint removers.

Toxic Mechanism

Carbon monoxide's affinity for hemoglobin is 240 times greater than that of oxygen. It shifts the oxygen dissociation curve to the left, which impairs hemoglobin release of oxygen to tissues and inhibits the cytochrome oxidase enzymes.

Toxic Dose and Manifestations

Table 13 describes the manifestations of carbon monoxide toxicity. Exposure to 0.5% for a few minutes is lethal. Sequelae correlate with the patient's level of consciousness at presentation. ECG abnormalities may be noted. Creatine kinase is often elevated, and rhabdomyolysis and myoglobinuria may occur.

The carboxyhemoglobin (CoHB) expresses in percentage the extent to which carbon monoxide has bound with the total hemoglobin. This may be misleadingly low in the anemic patient with less hemoglobin than normal. The patient's presentation is a more reliable indicator of severity than the CoHB level. The manifestations listed in Table 13 for each level are in addition to those listed at the level above. The CoHB may not correlate reliably with the severity of the intoxication, and linking symptoms to specific levels of CoHB frequently leads to inaccurate conclusions. A level of carbon monoxide greater than 40% is usually associated with obvious intoxication.

Kinetics

The natural metabolism of the body produces small amounts of CoHB, less than 2% for nonsmokers and 5% to 9% for smokers.

Carbon monoxide is rapidly absorbed through the lungs. The rate of absorption is directly related to alveolar ventilation. Elimination also occurs through the lungs. The half-life of CoHB in room air (21% oxygen) is 5 to 6 hours; in 100% oxygen, it is 90 minutes; in hyperbaric pressure at 3 atmospheres oxygen, it is 20 to 30 minutes.

Laboratory Investigations

An ABG reading may show metabolic acidosis and normal oxygen tension. In cases of significant poisoning, the ABG, electrolytes, blood glucose, serum creatine kinase and cardiac enzymes, renal function tests, and liver function tests should be monitored. A urinalysis and test for myoglobinuria should be obtained. Chest radiograph can be useful in cases of smoke inhalation or if the patient is being considered for hyperbaric chamber. ECG monitoring should be maintained, especially if the patient is older than

40 years, has a history of cardiac disease, or has moderate to severe symptoms. Which toxicology studies are used is based on symptoms and circumstances. CoHB should be monitored during and at the end of therapy. The pulse oximeter has two wavelengths and overestimates oxyhemoglobin saturation in carbon monoxide poisoning. The true oxygen saturation is determined by blood gas analysis, which measures the oxygen bound to hemoglobin. The co-oximeter measures four wavelengths and separates out CoHB and the other hemoglobin binding agents from oxyhemoglobin. Fetal hemoglobin has a greater affinity for carbon monoxide than adult hemoglobin and may falsely elevate the CoHB as much as 4% in young infants.

Management

The first step is to adequately protect the rescuer. The patient must be removed from the contaminated area, and his or her vital functions must be established.

The mainstay of treatment is 100% oxygen via a non-rebreathing mask with an oxygen reservoir or endotracheal tube. All patients receive 100% oxygen until the CoHB level is 5% or less. Assisted ventilation may be necessary. ABG and CoHB should be monitored and the present CoHB level determined. *Note:* A near-normal CoHB level does not exclude significant carbon monoxide poisoning, especially if the measurement is taken several hours after termination of exposure or if oxygen has been administered prior to obtaining the sample.

The exposed pregnant woman should be kept on 100% oxygen for several hours after the CoHB level is almost 0, because carbon monoxide concentrates in the fetus and oxygen is needed longer to ensure elimination of the carbon monoxide from fetal circulation. The fetus must be monitored, because carbon monoxide and hypoxia are potentially teratogenic.

Metabolic acidosis should be treated with sodium bicarbonate only if the pH is below 7.2 after correction of hypoxia and adequate ventilation. Acidosis shifts the oxygen dissociation curve to the right and facilitates oxygen delivery to the tissues.

The decision to use the hyperbaric oxygen chamber must be made on the basis of the ability to handle other acute emergencies that may coexist in the patient and of the severity of the poisoning. The standard of care for persons exposed to carbon monoxide has yet to be determined, but most authorities recommend using the hyperbaric oxygen chamber under any of the following conditions:

- If the patient is in a coma or has a history of loss of consciousness or seizures
- If there is cardiovascular dysfunction (clinical ischemic chest pain or ECG evidence of ischemia)
- If the patient has metabolic acidosis
- If symptoms persist despite 100% oxygen therapy
- In a child, if the initial CoHB is greater than 15%
- In symptomatic patients with preexisting ischemia
- If there are signs of maternal or fetal distress regardless of CoHB level (infants and fetus are a special problem because fetal hemoglobin has greater affinity for carbon monoxide)

Although controversial, a neurologic-cognitive examination has been used to help determine which patients with low carbon monoxide levels should receive more aggressive therapy. Testing should include the following: general orientation memory testing involving address, phone number, date of birth, and present date; and cognitive testing, involving counting by 7s, digit span, and forward and backward spelling of three-letter and four-letter words. Patients with delayed neurologic sequelae or recurrent symptoms up to 3 weeks may benefit from hyperbaric oxygen chamber treatment.

Seizures and cerebral edema must be treated.

Disposition

Patients with no or mild symptoms who become asymptomatic after a few hours of oxygen therapy and have a carbon monoxide level less than 10%, and normal physical and neurologic-cognitive examination findings can be discharged, but they should be

TABLE 13	Carbon Monoxide Exposure and Possible Manifestations

CoHB SATURATION (%)	MANIFESTATIONS
3.5	None
5	Slight headache, decreased exercise tolerance
10	Slight headache, dyspnea on vigorous exertion, may impair driving skills
10–20	Moderate dyspnea on exertion, throbbing, temporal headache
20–30	Severe headache, syncope, dizziness, visual changes, weakness, nausea, vomiting, altered judgment
30–40	Vertigo, ataxia, blurred vision, confusion, loss of consciousness
40–50	Confusion, tachycardia, tachypnea, coma, convulsions
50–60	Cheyne-Stokes, coma, convulsions, shock, apnea
60–70	Coma, convulsions, respiratory and heart failure, death

instructed to return if any signs of neurologic dysfunction appear. Patients with carbon monoxide poisoning requiring treatment need follow-up neuropsychiatric examinations.

Caustics and Corrosives

The terms *caustic* and *corrosive* are used interchangeably and can be divided into acids and alkalis. The U.S. Consumer Product Safety Commission Labeling Recommendations on containers for acids and alkalis indicate the potential for producing serious damage, as follows:

- Caution—weak irritant
- Warning—strong irritant
- Danger—corrosive

Some common acids with corrosive potential include acetic acid, formic acid, glycolic acid, hydrochloric acid, mercuric chloride, nitric acid, oxalic acid, phosphoric acid, sulfuric acid (battery acid), zinc chloride, and zinc sulfate. Some common alkalis with corrosive potential include ammonia, calcium carbide, calcium hydroxide (dry), calcium oxide, potassium hydroxide (lye), and sodium hydroxide (lye).

Toxic Mechanism

Acids produce mucosal coagulation necrosis and may be absorbed systemically; they do not penetrate deeply. Injury to the gastric mucosa is more likely, although specific sites of injury for acids and alkalis are not clearly defined.

Alkalis produce liquefaction necrosis and saponification and penetrate deeply. The esophageal mucosa is likely to be damaged. Oropharyngeal and esophageal damage is more frequently caused by solids than by liquids. Liquids produce superficial circumferential burns and gastric damage.

Toxic Dose

The toxicity is determined by concentration, contact time, and pH. Significant injury is more likely with a substance that has a pH of less than 2 or greater than 12, with a prolonged contact time, and with large volumes.

Manifestations

The absence of oral burns does not exclude the possibility of esophageal or gastric damage. General clinical findings are stridor; dysphagia; drooling; oropharyngeal, retrosternal, and epigastric pain; and ocular and oral burns. Alkali burns are yellow, soapy, frothy lesions. Acid burns are gray-white and later form an eschar. Abdominal tenderness and guarding may be present if perforation has happened.

Laboratory Investigations

If acid ingestion has taken place, the patient's acid-base balance and electrolyte status should be determined. If pulmonary symptoms are present, a chest radiograph, ABG measurement, and pulse oximetry are called for.

Management

It is recommended that the container be brought to the examination, as the substance must be identified and the pH of the substance, vomitus, tears, or saliva tested.

If the acid or alkali has been ingested, all gastrointestinal decontamination procedures are contraindicated except for immediate rinse, removal of substance from the mouth, and dilution with small amounts (sips) of milk or water. The examiner should check for ocular and dermal involvement. Contraindications to oral dilution are dysphagias, respiratory distress, obtundation, or shock. If there is ocular involvement one should immediately irrigate the eye with tepid water for at least 30 minutes, perform fluorescein stain of eye, and consult an ophthalmologist. If there is dermal involvement, one should immediately remove contaminated clothes and irrigate the skin with tepid water for at least 15 minutes. Consultation with a burn specialist is called for.

In cases of acid ingestion, some authorities advocate a small flexible nasogastric tube and aspiration within 30 minutes after ingestion.

Patients should receive only intravenous fluids following dilution until endoscopic consultation is obtained. Endoscopy is valuable to predict damage and risk of stricture. The indications are controversial, with some authorities recommending it in all cases of caustic ingestions regardless of symptoms, and others selectively using clinical features such as vomiting, stridor, drooling, and oral or facial lesions as criteria. We recommend endoscopy for all symptomatic patients or patients with intentional ingestions. Endoscopy may be performed immediately if the patient is symptomatic, but it is usually done 12 to 48 hours postingestion.

The use of corticosteroids is considered controversial. Some feel they may be useful for patients with second-degree circumferential burns. They recommend starting with hydrocortisone sodium succinate (Solu-Cortef) intravenously 10 to 20 mg/kg/d within 48 hours and changing to oral prednisolone 2 mg/kg/d for 3 weeks before tapering the dose. We do not usually recommend using corticosteroids because they have not been shown to be effective.

Tetanus prophylaxis should be provided if the patient requires it for wound care. Antibiotics are not useful prophylactically. Contrast studies are not useful in the first few days and may interfere with endoscopic evaluation; later, they can be used to assess the severity of damage.

Emergency medical therapy includes agents to inhibit collagen formation and intraluminal stents. Esophageal and gastric outlet dilation may be needed if there is evidence of stricture. Bougienage of the esophagus, however, has been associated with brain abscess. Interposition of the colon may be necessary if dilation fails to provide an adequate-sized passage.

Management of inhalation cases requires immediate removal from the environment, administration of humid supplemental oxygen, and observation for airway obstruction and noncardiac pulmonary edema. Radiographic and ABG evaluation should be obtained when appropriate. Intubation and respiratory support may be required.

Certain caustics produce systemic disturbances. Formaldehyde causes metabolic acidosis, hydrofluoric acid causes hypocalcemia and renal damage, oxalic acid causes hypocalcemia, phenol causes hepatic and renal damage, and picric acid causes renal injury.

Disposition

Infants and small children should be medically evaluated and observed. All symptomatic patients should be admitted. If they have severe symptoms or danger of airway compromise, they should be admitted to the intensive care unit. After endoscopy, if no damage is detected, the patient may be discharged when he or she can tolerate oral feedings. Intentional exposures require psychiatric evaluation before the patient can be discharged.

Cocaine (Benzoylmethylecgonine)

Cocaine is derived from the leaves of *Erythroxylum coca* and *Truxillo coca*. "Body packing" refers to the placement of many small packages of contraband cocaine for concealment in the gastrointestinal tract or other areas for illicit transport. "Body stuffing" refers to spontaneous ingestion of substances for the purpose of hiding evidence.

Toxic Mechanism

Cocaine directly stimulates the CNS presynaptic sympathetic neurons to release catecholamines and acetylcholine, while it blocks the presynaptic reuptake of the catecholamines; it blocks the sodium channels along neuronal membranes; and it increases platelet aggregation. Long-term use depletes the CNS of dopamine.

Toxic Dose

The maximum mucosal local anesthetic therapeutic dose of cocaine is 200 mg or 2 mL of a 10% solution. Although CNS effects can occur at relatively low local anesthetic doses (50 to 95 mg), they are more common with doses greater than 1 mg/kg; cardiac effects can occur with doses greater than 1 mg/kg. The potential fatal dose is 1200 mg intranasally, but death has occurred with 20 mg parenterally.

Kinetics

Cocaine is well absorbed by all routes, including nasal insufflation, and oral, dermal, and inhalation routes (Table 14). Protein binding is 8.7%, and volume distribution is 1.5 L/kg.

Cocaine is metabolized by plasma and liver cholinesterase to the inactive metabolites ecgonine methyl ester and benzoylecgonine. Plasma pseudocholinesterase is congenitally deficient in 3% of the population and decreased in fetuses, young infants, the elderly, pregnant people, and people with liver disease. These enzyme-deficient individuals are at increased risk for life-threatening cocaine toxicity.

Ten percent of cocaine is excreted unchanged. Cocaine and ethanol undergo liver synthesis to form cocaethylene, a metabolite with a half-life three times longer than that of cocaine. It may account for some of cocaine's cardiotoxicity and appears to be more lethal than cocaine or ethanol alone.

Manifestations

The CNS manifestations of cocaine ingestion are euphoria, hyperactivity, agitation, convulsions, and intracranial hemorrhage. Mydriasis and septal perforation can occur, as well as cardiac dysrhythmias, hypertension, and hypotension (with severe overdose). Chest pain is frequent, but only 5.8% of patients have true myocardial ischemia and infarction. Other manifestations include vasoconstriction, hyperthermia (because of increased metabolic rate), ischemic bowel perforation if the substance is ingested, rhabdomyolysis, myoglobinuria, and renal failure. In pregnant users, premature labor and abruptio placentae can occur.

Body cavity packing should be suspected in cases of prolonged toxicity.

Mortality can result from cerebrovascular accidents, coronary artery spasm, myocardial injury, or lethal dysrhythmias.

Laboratory Investigations

Monitoring of the ECG and cardiac rhythms, ABG, oxygen saturation, electrolytes, blood glucose, BUN, creatinine, and creatine kinase levels should be maintained. One should monitor cardiac fraction if the patient has chest pain, as well as the liver profile, and the urine for myoglobin. Intravenous drug users should have HIV and hepatitis virus testing.

Urine should be tested for cocaine and metabolites and other substances of abuse, and abdominal radiographs or ultrasonogram should be ordered for body packers. If the urine sample was collected more than 12 hours after cocaine intake, it will contain little or no cocaine. If cocaine is present, cocaine has been used within the past 12 hours. Cocaine's metabolite benzoylecgonine may be detected within 4 hours after a single nasal insufflation and for up to 114 hours. Cross-reactions with some herbal teas, lidocaine, and droperidol (Inapsine) may give false-positive results by some immunoassay methods.

Management

Supportive care includes blood pressure, cardiac, and thermal monitoring and seizure precautions. Diazepam (Valium) is the drug of choice for treatment of cocaine toxicity agitation, seizures, and dysrhythmias; doses are 10 to 30 mg intravenously at 2.5 mg per minute for adults and 0.2 to 0.5 mg/kg at 1 mg per minute up to 10 mg for a child.

Gastrointestinal decontamination should be instituted, if the cocaine was ingested, by administration of activated charcoal. MDAC may adsorb cocaine leakage in body stuffers or body packers. Whole-bowel irrigation with polyethylene glycol solution (PEG) has been used in body packers and stuffers if the contraband is in a firm container. If the packages are not visible on plain radiographs of the abdomen, a contrast study or CT scan can help to confirm successful passage. Cocaine in the nasal passage can be removed with an applicator dipped in a non–water-soluble product (lubricating jelly) if this is done within a few minutes after application.

In body packers and stuffers, venous access must be secured, and drugs must be readily available for treating life-threatening manifestations until the contraband is passed in the stool. Surgical removal may be indicated if the packet does not pass the pylorus, in an asymptomatic body packer, or in the case of intestinal obstruction.

Hypertension and tachycardia are usually transient and can be managed by careful titration of diazepam. Nitroprusside may be used for severe hypertension. Myocardial ischemia is managed by oxygen, vascular access, benzodiazepines, and nitroglycerin. Aspirin and thrombolysis are not routinely recommended because of the danger of intracranial hemorrhage.

Dysrhythmias are usually supraventricular (SVT) and do not require specific management. Adenosine is ineffective. Life-threatening tachydysrhythmias may respond to phentolamine (Regitine) 5 mg IV bolus in adults or 0.1 mg/kg in children at 5- to 10-minute intervals. Phentolamine also relieves coronary artery spasm and myocardial ischemia. Electrical synchronized cardioversion should be considered for patients with hemodynamically unstable dysrhythmias. Lidocaine is not recommended initially but may be used after 3 hours for ventricular tachycardia. Wide complex QRS ventricular tachycardia may be treated with sodium bicarbonate 2 mEq/kg as a bolus. β-Adrenergic blockers are not recommended.

Anxiety, agitation, and convulsions can be treated with diazepam. If diazepam fails to control seizures, neuromuscular blockers can be used. The EEG should be monitored for nonmotor seizure activity. For hyperthermia, external cooling and cool humidified 100% oxygen should be administered. Neuromuscular paralysis to control seizures will reduce temperature. Dantrolene and antipyretics are not recommended. Rhabdomyolysis and myoglobinuria are treated with fluids, alkaline diuresis, and diuretics.

If the patient is pregnant, the fetus must be monitored and the patient observed for spontaneous abortion.

Paranoid ideation and threatening behavior should be treated with rapid tranquilization. The patient should be observed for suicidal depression that may follow intoxication and may require suicide precautions. If focal neurologic manifestations are present, one should consider the possibility of a cerebrovascular accident and obtain a CT scan.

Extracorporeal clearance techniques are of no benefit.

Disposition

Patients with mild intoxication or a brief seizure that does not require treatment who become asymptomatic may be discharged after 6 hours with appropriate psychosocial follow-up. If cardiac

TABLE 14	The Different Routes and Kinetics of Cocaine					
TYPE	**ROUTE**	**ONSET**	**PEAK (min)**	**HALF-LIFE (min)**	**DURATION (min)**
Cocaine leaf	Oral, chewing	20–30 min	45–90	—	240–360
Hydrochloride	Insufflation	1–3 min	5–10	78	60–90
	Ingestion	20–30 min	50–90	54	Sustained
	Intravenous	30–120 sec	5–11	36	60–90
Freebase/crack	Smoking	5–10 sec	5–11	—	Up to 20
Coca paste	Smoking	Unknown	—	—	—

or cerebral ischemic manifestations are present, the patient should be monitored in the intensive care unit. Body packers and stuffers require care in the intensive care unit until passage of the contraband.

Cyanide

Hydrogen cyanide is a byproduct of burning plastic and wools in residential fires. Hydrocyanic acid is the liquefied form of hydrogen cyanide. Cyanide salts can be found in ore extraction. Nitriles, such as acetonitrile (artificial nail removers), are metabolized in the body to produce cyanide. Cyanogenic glycosides are present in some fruit seeds (such as amygdalin in apricots, peaches, and apples). Sodium nitroprusside, the antihypertensive vasodilator, contains five cyanide groups.

Toxic Mechanism

Cyanide blocks the cellular electron transport mechanism and cellular respiration by inhibiting the mitochondrial ferricytochrome oxidase system and other enzymes. This results in cellular hypoxia and lactic acidosis. *Note:* Citrus fruit seeds form cyanide in the presence of intestinal β-glucosidase (the seeds are harmful only if the capsule is broken).

Toxic Dose

The ingestion of 1 mg/kg or 50 mg of hydrogen cyanide can produce death within 15 minutes. The lethal dose of potassium cyanide is 200 mg. Five to 10 mL of 84% acetonitrile is lethal. Infusions of sodium nitroprusside in rates above 2 µg/kg per minute may cause cyanide to accumulate to toxic concentrations in critically ill patients.

Kinetics

Cyanide is rapidly absorbed by all routes. In the stomach, it forms hydrocyanic acid. Volume distribution is 1.5 L/kg. Protein binding is 60%. Cyanide is detoxified by metabolism in the liver via the mitochondrial thiosulfate-rhodanase pathway, which catalyzes the transfer of sulfur donor to cyanide, forming the less toxic irreversible thiocyanate that is excreted in the urine. Cyanide is also detoxified by reacting with hydroxocobalamin (vitamin B_{12a}) to form cyanocobalamin (vitamin B_{12}).

The cyanide elimination half-life from the blood is 1.2 hours. The elimination route is through the lungs.

Manifestations

Hydrogen cyanide has the distinctive odor of bitter almonds or silver polish. Manifestations of cyanide intoxication include hypertension, cardiac dysrhythmias, various ECG abnormalities, headache, hyperpnea, seizures, stupor, pulmonary edema, and flushing. Cyanosis is absent or appears late.

Laboratory Investigations

The examiner should obtain and monitor ABGs, oxygen saturation, blood lactate, hemoglobin, blood glucose, and electrolytes. Lactic acidemia, a decrease in the arterial-venous oxygen difference, and bright red venous blood occurs. If smoke inhalation is the possible source of cyanide exposure, CoHB and methemoglobin (MetHb) concentrations should be measured.

Cyanide levels in whole blood, red blood cells, or serum are not useful in the acute management because the determinations are not readily available. Specific cyanide blood levels are as follows: smokers have less than 0.5 µg/mL; a patient with flushing and tachycardia has 0.5 to 1.0 µg/mL, one with obtundation has 1.0 to 2.5 µg/mL, and one in coma or who has died has more than 2.5 µg/mL.

Management

If the cyanide was inhaled, the patient must be removed from the contaminated atmosphere. Attendants should not administer mouth-to-mouth resuscitation. Rescuers and attendants must be protected. Immediate administration of 100% oxygen is called for and oxygen should be continued during and after the administration of the antidote. The clinician must decide whether to use any or all components of the cyanide antidote kit.

The mechanism of action of the antidote kit is twofold: to produce methemoglobinemia and to provide a sulfur substrate for the detoxification of cyanide. The nitrites make methemoglobin, which has a greater affinity for cyanide than does the cytochrome oxidase enzymes. The combination of methemoglobin and cyanide forms cyanomethemoglobin. Sodium thiosulfate provides a sulfur substrate for the rhodanese enzyme, which converts cyanide into the relatively nontoxic sodium thiocyanate, which is excreted by the kidney.

The procedure for using the antidote kit is as follows:

Step 1: Amyl nitrite inhalant perles is only a temporizing measure (forms only 2% to 5% methemoglobin) and it can be omitted if venous access is established. Alternate 100% oxygen and the inhalant for 30 seconds each minute. Use a new perle every 3 minutes.

Step 2: Sodium nitrite ampule is indicated for cyanide exposures, except for cases of residential fires, smoke inhalation, and nitroprusside or acetonitrile poisonings. It is administered intravenously to produce methemoglobin of 20% to 30% at 35 to 70 minutes after administration. A dose of 10 mL of 3% solution of sodium nitrite for adults and 0.33 mL/kg of 3% solution for children is diluted to 100 mL 0.9% saline and administered slowly intravenously at 5 mL/min. If hypotension develops, the infusion should be slowed.

Step 3: Sodium thiosulfate is useful alone in cases of smoke inhalation, nitroprusside toxicity, and acetonitrile toxicity and should not be used at all in cases of hydrogen sulfide poisoning. The administration dose is 12.5 g of sodium thiosulfate or 50 mL of 25% solution for adults and 1.65 mL/kg of 25% solution for children intravenously over 10 to 20 minutes.

If cyanide symptoms recur, further treatment with nitrites or the perles is controversial. Some authorities suggest repeating the antidotes in 30 minutes at half of the initial dose, but others do not advise this for lack of efficacy. The child dosage regimen on the package insert must be carefully followed.

One hour after antidotes are administered, the methemoglobin level should be obtained and should not exceed 20%. Methylene blue should not be used to reverse excessive methemoglobin.

Gastrointestinal decontamination of oral ingestion by activated charcoal is recommended but is not very effective because of the rapidity of absorption. Seizures are treated with intravenous diazepam. Acidosis should be treated with sodium bicarbonate if it does not rapidly resolve with therapy. There is no role for hyperbaric oxygen or hemodialysis or hemoperfusion.

Other antidotes include hydroxocobalamin (vitamin B_{12a}) (Cyanokit), which has proven effective when given immediately after exposure in large doses of 4 g (50 mg/kg) or 50 times the amount of cyanide exposure with 8 g of sodium thiosulfate. Hydroxocobalamin has FDA orphan drug approval.

Disposition

Asymptomatic patients should be observed for a minimum of 3 hours. Patients who ingest nitrile compounds must be observed for 24 hours. Patients requiring antidote administration should be admitted to the intensive care unit.

Digitalis

Cardiac glycosides are found in cardiac medications, common plants, and the skin of the Bufo toad.

Toxic Mechanism

Cardiac glycosides inhibit the enzyme sodium/potassium-adenosine triphosphatase ($Na^+,K^+,ATPase$), leading to intracellular potassium loss and increased intracellular sodium, and producing phase 4 depolarization, increased automaticity, and ectopy. There is increased intracellular calcium and potentiation of contractility. Pacemaker cells are inhibited, and the refractory period is prolonged, leading to atrioventricular blocks. There is increased vagal tone.

Toxic Dose

Digoxin total digitalizing dose, the dose required to achieve therapeutic blood levels of 0.6 to 2.0 ng/mL, is 0.75 to 1.25 mg or 10 to 15 µg/kg for patients older than 10 years of age; 40 to 50 µg/kg for patients younger than 2 years of age; and 30 to 40 µg/kg for patients 2 to 10 years of age.

The acute single toxic dose is greater than 0.07 mg/kg or greater than 2 or 3 mg in an adult, but 2 mg in a child or 4 mg in an adult usually produces only mild toxicity. One to 3 mg or more may be found in a few leaves of oleander or foxglove. Serious and fatal overdoses are more than 4 mg in a child and more than 10 mg in an adult.

Acute digitoxin ingestion of 10 to 35 mg has produced severe toxicity and death. Digitoxin therapeutic steady state is 15 to 25 ng/mL. In cases of chronic or acute-on-chronic ingestions in patients with cardiac disease, more than 2 mg may produce toxicity; however, toxicity can develop within therapeutic range on chronic therapy.

Patients at greatest risk of overdose include those with cardiac disease, those with electrolyte abnormalities (low potassium, low magnesium, low T_4, high calcium), those with renal impairment, and those on amiodarone (Cordarone), quinidine, erythromycin, tetracycline, calcium channel blockers, and β-blockers.

Kinetics

Digoxin is a metabolite of digitoxin. In cases of oral overdose, the typical onset is 30 minutes, with peak effects in 3 to 12 hours. Duration is 3 to 4 days. Intravenous onset is in 5 to 30 minutes; peak level is immediate, and peak effect is at 1.5 to 3 hours.

Volume distribution is 5 to 6 L/kg. The cardiac-to-plasma ratio is 30:1. After an acute ingestion overdose, the serum concentration is not reflective of tissue concentration for at least 6 hours or more, and steady state is 12 to 16 hours after last dose.

Sixty percent to 80% of the parent compound is excreted unchanged in the urine. The elimination half-life is 30 to 50 hours.

Manifestations

Onset of manifestations is usually within 2 hours but may be delayed up to 12 hours.

Gastrointestinal effects of nausea and vomiting are frequently present in cases of acute ingestion but may also occur in cases of chronic ingestion. The "digitalis effect" on ECG is scooped ST segments and PR prolongation; in cases of overdose, any dysrhythmia or block is possible but none are characteristic. Bradycardia occurs in patients with acute overdose with healthy hearts; supraventricular tachycardia occurs in patients with existing heart disease or chronic overdose. Ventricular tachycardia is seen only in cases of severe poisoning.

The CNS effects include headaches, visual disturbances, and colored halo vision. Hyperkalemia occurs following acute overdose and correlates with digoxin level and outcome. Among patients with serum potassium levels of less than 5.0 mEq/L, all survive. If the level is 5 to 5.5, 50% survive, and if the level is greater than 5.5, all die. Hypokalemia is commonly seen with chronic intoxication. Patients with normal digitalis levels may have toxicity in the presence of hypokalemia.

Chronic intoxications are more likely to produce scotoma, color perception disturbances, yellow vision, halos, delirium, hallucinations or psychosis, tachycardia, and hypokalemia.

Laboratory Investigations

Continuous monitoring of ECG, pulse, and blood pressure is called for. Blood glucose, electrolytes, calcium, magnesium, BUN, and creatinine levels should also be monitored. An initial digoxin level should be measured on patient presentation and repeated thereafter. Levels should be measured more than 6 hours postingestion because earlier values do not reflect tissue distribution. Digoxin clinical toxicity is usually associated with serum digoxin levels of greater than 3.5 ng/mL in adults.

An endogenous digoxin-like substance cross-reacts in most common immunoassays (not with high-pressure liquid chromatography) and values as high as 4.1 ng/mL have been reported in newborns, patients with chronic renal failure, patients with abnormal immunoglobulins, and women in the third trimester of pregnancy.

Management

A cardiology consult should be obtained and a pacemaker should be readily available.

In undertaking gastrointestinal decontamination, excessive vagal stimulation should be avoided (e.g., emesis and gastric lavage). Activated charcoal should be administered, and if a nasogastric tube is required for the activated charcoal, pretreatment with atropine (0.02 mg/kg in children and 0.5 mg in adults) should be considered.

Digoxin-specific antibody fragments (Fab, Digibind) 38 mg binds 0.5 mg digoxin and then is excreted through the kidneys. The onset of action is within 30 minutes. Problems associated with Fab therapy are mainly from withdrawal of digoxin and worsening heart failure, hypokalemia, decrease in glucose (if the patient has low glycogen stores), and allergic reactions (very rare). Digitalis administered after Fab therapy is bound and may be inactivated for 5 to 7 days.

Absolute indications for Fab therapy include the following:
- Life-threatening malignant (hemodynamically unstable) dysrhythmias
- Ventricular dysrhythmias, unstable severe bradycardia, or second- or third-degree blocks unresponsive to atropine or rapid deterioration in clinical status
- Life-threatening digitoxin and oleander poisonings
- Relative indications for Fab therapy include the following:
- Ingestions greater than 4 mg in a child and 10 mg in an adult
- Serum potassium level greater than 5.0 mEq/L
- Serum digoxin level greater than 10 ng/mL in adults or greater than 5 ng/mL in children 6 hours after an acute ingestion
- Digitalis delirium and thrombocytopenia response

Digoxin-specific Fab fragments therapy can be administered as a bolus through a 22-µm filter if the case is a critical emergency. If the case is less urgent, then it can be administered over 30 minutes. An empiric dose is 10 vials in adults and 5 vials in a child for an unknown amount ingested in a symptomatic patient with history of a digoxin overdose.

To calculate the dose in the case of a known ingestion, the following equation is used:

$$\text{Amount (total mg)} \times (0.8) \text{ body burden}$$

If liquid capsules were taken or the substance was given intravenously the 80% bioavailability figure is not used. Instead, the body burden divided by 0.5 (0.5 mg digoxin is bound by 1 vial of 38 mg of Fab) equals the number of vials needed.

If the amount is unknown but the steady state serum concentration is known, the following equations are used:

For digoxin:

$$\text{Digitoxin ng/mL} \times (5.6 \text{ L/kg Vd}) \times (\text{wt kg}) = \text{mg body burden}$$
$$\text{Body burden} \div 1000 = \text{mg body burden}$$
$$\text{Body burden}/0.5 = \text{number of vials needed}$$

For digitoxin:

$$\text{Digitoxin ng/mL} \times (0.56 \text{ L/kg Vd}) \times (\text{wt kg}) = \text{mg body burden}$$
$$\text{Body burden} \div 1000 = \text{mg body burden}$$
$$\text{Body burden}/0.5 = \text{number of vials needed}$$

Antidysrhythmic agents or a pacemaker should be used only if Fab therapy fails. For ventricular tachydysrhythmias, electrolyte disturbances should be corrected by the administration of lidocaine or phenytoin. For torsades de pointes, magnesium sulfate 20 mL 20% IV can be given slowly over 20 minutes (or 25 to 50 mg/kg in a child), titrated to control the dysrhythmia. Magnesium should be discontinued if hypotension, heart block, or decreased deep tendon reflexes are present. Magnesium is used with caution if the patient has renal impairment.

Unstable bradycardia and second-degree and third-degree atrioventricular block should be treated by Fab first. A pacemaker should be available if necessary. Isoproterenol should be avoided because it causes dysrhythmias. Cardioversion is used with caution, starting at a setting of 5 to 10 joules. The patient should be pretreated with lidocaine, if possible, because cardioversion may precipitate ventricular fibrillation or asystole.

Potassium disturbances are caused by a shift, not a change, in total body potassium. Hyperkalemia (>5.0 mEq/L) is treated with Fab only. Calcium must never be used, and insulin/glucose and sodium bicarbonate should not be used concomitantly with Fab because they may produce severe life-threatening hypokalemia. Sodium polystyrene sulfonate (Kayexalate) should not be used. Hypokalemia must be treated with caution because it may be cardioprotective. Treatment can be administered if the patient has ventricular dysrhythmias or a serum potassium level less than 3.0 mEq/L and atrioventricular block.

Extracorporeal procedures are ineffective. Hemodialysis is used for severe or refractory hyperkalemia.

One must never use antidysrhythmic types Ia (procainamide, quinidine, disopyramide [Norpace], amiodarone [Cordarone]), Ic (propafenone [Rythmol], flecainide [Tambocor]), II (β-blockers), or IV (calcium channel blockers). Class Ib drugs (lidocaine, phenytoin [Dilantin], mexiletine [Mexitil], and tocainide [Tonocard]) can be used.

Disposition
Consultation with a poison control center and a cardiologist experienced with digoxin-specific Fab fragments is warranted. All patients with significant dysrhythmias, symptoms, elevated serum digoxin concentration, or elevated serum potassium level should be admitted to the intensive care unit.

Ethanol
Table 15 lists the features of alcohols and glycols.

Toxic Mechanism
Ethanol has CNS depressant and anesthetic effects. Ethanol stimulates the γ-aminobutyric acid (GABA) system. It promotes cutaneous vasodilation (contributes to hypothermia), stimulates secretion of gastric juice (gastritis), inhibits the secretion of the antidiuretic hormone, inhibits gluconeogenesis (hypoglycemia), and influences fat metabolism (lipidemia).

Toxic Dose
A dose of 1 mL/kg of absolute ethanol (100% ethanol, or 200 proof) gives a blood ethanol concentration of 100 mg/dL. A potentially fatal dose is 3 g/kg for children or 6 g/kg for adults. Children are more prone to developing hypoglycemia than adults.

Kinetics
Onset of action is 30 to 60 minutes after ingestion; peak action is 90 minutes on empty stomach. Volume distribution is 0.6 L/kg. The major route of elimination (>90%) is by hepatic oxidative metabolism. The first step is by the enzyme alcohol dehydrogenase, which converts ethanol to acetaldehyde. Alcohol dehydrogenase metabolizes ethanol at a constant rate of 12 to 20 mg/dL/h (12 to 15 mg/dL/h in nondrinkers, 15 to 30 mg/dL/h in social drinkers, 30 to 50 mg/dL/h in heavy drinkers, and 25 to 30 mg/dL/h in children). At very low blood ethanol concentration (>30 mg/dL), the metabolism is by first-order kinetics. In the second step, acetaldehyde is metabolized by acetaldehyde dehydrogenase to acetic acid, which is metabolized by the Krebs cycle to carbon dioxide and water. The enzyme steps are nicotinamide adenine dinucleotide-dependent, which interferes with gluconeogenesis. Less than 10% of ethanol is excreted unchanged by the kidneys. The relationship between blood ethanol concentration (BEC) and dose (amount ingested) can be calculated as follows:

$$BEC\,(mg/dL) = amount\ ingested\,(mL) \times$$
$$\%\ ethanol\ product \times SG\,(0.79)/Vd\,(0.6\ L/kg) \times body\ wt\,(kg)$$
$$Dose\,(amount\ ingested) = BEC\,(mg/dL) \times$$
$$Vd\,(0.6) \times body\ wt\,(kg)/\%\ ethanol \times$$
$$specific\ gravity\,(0.79)$$

Manifestations
Table 16 lists the clinical signs of acute ethanol intoxication.

Chronic alcoholic patients tolerate higher blood ethanol concentration, and correlation with manifestations is not valid. Rapid interview for alcoholism is the CAGE questions:
- C—Have you felt the need to Cut down?
- A—Have others Annoyed you by criticism of your drinking?
- G—Have you felt Guilty about your drinking?
- E—Have you ever had a morning Eye-opening drink to steady your nerves or get rid of a hangover?

Two affirmative answers indicate probable alcoholism.

Laboratory Investigations
The blood ethanol concentration should be specifically requested and followed. Gas chromatography or a breathalyzer test gives rapid reliable results if no belching or vomiting is present. Enzymatic methods do not differentiate between the alcohols. ABG, electrolytes, and glucose should be measured, the anion and osmolar gaps determined (measure by freezing point depression, not vapor pressure), and a check for ketosis made.

TABLE 15	Summary of Alcohol and Glycol Features			
	METHANOL	**ISOPROPANOL**	**ETHANOL**	**ETHYLENE GLYCOL**
Principal uses	Gas line antifreeze, Sterno, windshield de-icer	Solvent jewelry cleaner, rubbing alcohol	Beverage, solvent	Radiator antifreeze, windshield de-icer
Specific gravity	0.719	0.785	0.789	1.12
Fatal dose	1 mL/kg 100%	3 mL/kg 100%	5 mL/kg 100%	1.4 mL/kg
Inebriation	±	2+	2+	1+
Metabolic change		Hyperglycemia	Hypoglycemia	Hypocalcemia
Metabolic acidosis	4+	0	1+	2+
Anion gap	4+	±	2+	4+
Ketosis	Ketobutyric	Acetone	Hydroxybutyric	None
Gastrointestinal tract	Pancreatitis	Hemorrhagic gastritis	Gastritis	
Osmolality*	0.337	0.176	0.228	0.190

*1 mL/dL of substances raises freezing point osmolality of serum. The validity of the correlation of osmolality with blood concentrations has been questioned.

TABLE 16	Clinical Signs in the Nontolerant Ethanol Drinker
ETHANOL BLOOD CONCENTRATION (mg/dL)*	**MANIFESTATIONS**
>25	Euphoria
>47	**Mild incoordination,** sensory and motor impairment
>50	Increased risk of motor vehicle accidents
>100	Ataxia (legal toxic level in many localities)
>150	**Moderate incoordination,** slow reaction time
>200	Drowsiness and confusion
>300	Severe incoordination, stupor, blurred vision
>500	**Flaccid coma,** respiratory failure, hypotension; may be fatal

*Ethanol concentrations sometimes reported in %.
Note: mg% is not equivalent to mg/dL because ethanol weighs less than water (specific gravity 0.79). A 1% ethanol concentration is 790 mg/dL and 0.1% is 79 mg/dL. There is great variation in individual behavior at different blood ethanol levels. Behavior is dependent on tolerance and other factors.

Management

The examiner should inquire about trauma and disulfiram use. The patient must be protected from aspiration and hypoxia. Vital functions must be established and maintained. The patient may require intubation and assisted ventilation.

Gastrointestinal decontamination plays no role in the management of ethanol intoxication.

If the patient is comatose, glucose should be administered intravenously, 1 mL/kg 50% glucose in adults and 2 mL/kg 25% glucose in children. Thiamine, 100 mg intravenously, is administered if the patient has a history of chronic alcoholism, malnutrition, or suspected eating disorders to prevent Wernicke-Korsakoff syndrome. Naloxone (Narcan) has produced a partial inconsistent response but is not recommended for known alcoholics.

General supportive care includes administration of fluids to correct hydration and hypotension and correction of electrolyte abnormalities and acid-base imbalance. Vasopressors and plasma expanders may be necessary to correct severe hypotension. Hypomagnesemia is frequent in chronic alcoholics. In case of hypomagnesemia, a loading dose of 2 g magnesium sulfate 10% is administered by intravenous solution over 5 minutes in the intensive care unit with blood pressure and cardiac monitoring and calcium chloride 10% on hand in case of overdose. This is followed with constant infusion of 6 g of 10% solution over 3 to 4 hours. Caution must be taken with the use of magnesium if renal failure is present.

Hypothermic patients should be warmed. See the section on disturbances caused by cold.

Hemodialysis can be used in severe cases when conventional therapy is ineffective (rarely needed).

Repeated or prolonged seizures should be treated with diazepam (Valium). The brief "rum fits" do not need long-term anticonvulsant therapy. Repeated seizures or focal neurologic findings may warrant skull radiographs, lumbar puncture, and CT scan of the head, depending on the clinical findings. Withdrawal is treated with hydration and large doses of chlordiazepoxide (Librium) 50 to 100 mg or diazepam (Valium) 2 to 10 mg intravenously; these doses may be repeated in 2 to 4 hours. Very large doses of benzodiazepines may be required for delirium tremens. Withdrawal can occur in presence of elevated blood ethanol concentration and can be fatal if left untreated.

Chest radiograph is warranted to determine whether aspiration pneumonia is present. Renal and liver function tests and bilirubin level measurement should be made.

Disposition

Clinical severity (e.g., intubation, assisted ventilation, aspiration pneumonia) should determine the level of hospital care needed. Young children with significant unintentional exposure to ethanol (calculated to reach a blood ethanol concentration of 50 mg/dL) should have blood ethanol concentration obtained and blood glucose levels monitored for hypoglycemia frequently for 4 hours after ingestion. Patients with acute ethanol intoxication seldom require admission unless a complication is present. However, intoxicated patients should not be discharged until they are fully functional (can walk, talk, and think independently), have suicide potential evaluated, have proper disposition environment, and have a sober escort.

Ethylene Glycol

Ethylene glycol is found in solvents, de-icers, radiator antifreeze (95%), and air-conditioning units. Ethylene glycol is a sweet-tasting, colorless, water-soluble liquid with a sweet aromatic fragrance.

Toxic Mechanism

Ethylene glycol is oxidized by alcohol dehydrogenase to glycolaldehyde, which is metabolized to glycolic acid and glyoxylic acid. Glyoxylic acid is metabolized to oxalic acid via a pyridoxine-dependent pathway to glycine and by thiamine and magnesium-dependent pathways to α-hydroxy-ketoadipic acid. The metabolites of ethylene glycol produce a profound metabolic acidosis, increased anion gap, hypocalcemia, and oxalate crystals, which deposit in tissues (particularly the kidney).

Toxic Dose

The ingestion of 0.1 mL/kg 100% ethylene glycol can result in a toxic serum ethylene glycol concentration of 20 mg/dL. Ingestion of 3.0 mL (less than 1 teaspoonful or swallow) of a 100% solution in a 10-kg child or 30 mL of 100% ethylene glycol in an adult produces a serum ethylene glycol concentration of 50 mg/dL, a concentration that requires hemodialysis. The fatal amount is 1.4 mL/kg of 100% solution.

Kinetics

Absorption is via dermal, inhalation, and ingestion routes. Ethylene glycol is rapidly absorbed from the gastrointestinal tract. Onset is usually in 30 minutes but may be delayed by co-ingestion of food and ethanol. The usual peak level is at 2 hours. Volume distribution is 0.65 to 0.8 L/kg.

For metabolism, see *Toxic Mechanism.*

The half-life of ethylene glycol without ethanol is 3 to 8 hours; with ethanol, it is 17 hours, and with hemodialysis it is 2.5 hours. Renal clearance is 3.2 mL/kg/minute. About 20% to 50% is excreted unchanged in the urine. The relationship between serum ethylene glycol concentration (SEGC) and dose (amount ingested) can be calculated as follows:

$$0.12 \, mL/kg \, of \, 100\% = SEGC \, 10 \, mg/dL$$

Manifestations

Phase I. The onset of manifestations is 30 minutes to several hours longer after ingestion with concomitant ethanol ingestion. The patient may be inebriated. Hypocalcemia, tetany, and calcium oxalate and hippuric acid crystals in urine can be seen within 4 to 8 hours but are not always present. Early, before metabolism of ethylene glycol, an osmolal gap may be present (see *Laboratory Investigations*). Later, the metabolites of ethylene glycol produce changes starting 4 to 12 hours following ingestion, including an anion gap, metabolic acidosis, coma, convulsions, cardiac disturbances, and pulmonary and cerebral edema. Because fluorescein is added to some antifreeze, the presence of fluorescence may be a clue to ethylene glycol exposure. However, it has been shown that fluorescent urine is not a reliable indicator of ethylene glycol ingestion and should not be used as a screen.

Phase II. After 12 to 36 hours, cardiopulmonary deterioration occurs, with pulmonary edema and congestive heart failure.

Phase III. Phase III occurs 36 to 72 hours after ingestion, with pulmonary edema and oliguric renal failure from oxalate crystal deposition and tubular necrosis predominating.

Phase IV. Neurologic sequelae may occur rarely, especially in patients who fail to receive early antidotal therapy. The onset ranges from 6 to 10 days after ingestion. Findings include facial diplegia, hearing loss, bilateral visual disturbances, elevated cerebrospinal fluid pressure with or without elevated protein levels and pleocytosis, vomiting, hyperreflexia, dysphagia, and ataxia.

Laboratory Investigations

Blood glucose and electrolytes should be monitored. Urinalysis should look for oxalate ("envelope") and monohydrate ("hemp seed") crystals. Urine fluorescence is not reliable as a screen. ABG, ethylene glycol, and ethanol levels, plasma osmolarity (using freezing point depression method), calcium, BUN, and creatinine should be measured. A serum ethylene glycol concentration of 20 mg/dL is toxic (ethylene glycol levels are very difficult to obtain). If possible, a glycolate level should be obtained. Cross-reactions with propylene glycol, a vehicle in many liquids and intravenous medications (phenytoin [Dilantin], diazepam [Valium]), other glycols, and triglycerides may produce spurious ethylene glycol levels. False-positive ethylene glycol values may occur with colorimetric or gas chromatography using an OV-17 column in the presence of propylene glycol.

The following equations can be used to calculate the osmolality, osmolal gap, and ethylene glycol level:

$$2(Na + mEq/L) + (Blood\ glucose\ mg/dL)/20 + (BUN\ mg/dL)/3 =$$
$$Total\ calculated\ osmolality (mOsm/L)$$
$$Osmolar\ Gap = measured\ osmolality\ (by\ freezing\ point\ depression$$
$$method) - calculate\ osmolality$$

A gap greater than 10 is abnormal. *Note:* if ethanol is involved, add ethanol level/4.6 to the calculated equation.

An increased osmolal gap is produced by the following common substances: acetone, dextran, dimethyl sulfoxide, diuretics, ethanol, ethyl ether, ethylene glycol, isopropanol, paraldehyde, mannitol, methanol, sorbitol, and trichloroethane. Table 10 gives the conversion factors for these substances.

Although a specific blood level of ethylene glycol in milligrams per deciliter can be estimated using the equation below, this is not considered to be a reliable method and should not take the place of obtaining a measured ethylene glycol blood concentration.

$$osmolar\ gap \times conversion\ factor = serum\ concentration$$

Caution: The accuracy of the ethylene glycol estimated decreases as the ethylene glycol levels decrease. The toxic metabolites are not osmotically active, and patients presenting late may show signs of severe toxicity without an elevated osmolar gap.

The anion gap can be calculated using the following equation:

$$Na - (Cl + HCO_3) = anion\ gap$$

The normal gap is 8 to 12. Potassium is not used because it is a small amount and may be hemolyzed. Table 8 lists factors that may account for an increased or a decreased anion gap.

Management

Vital functions should be established and maintained. The airway must be protected, and assisted ventilation can be used, if necessary. Gastrointestinal decontamination has a limited role. Only gastric aspiration can be used within 60 minutes after ingestion. Activated charcoal is not effective.

Baseline measurements of serum electrolytes and calcium, glucose, ABGs, ethanol, serum ethylene glycol concentration (may be difficult to obtain readily in some institutions), and methanol concentrations should be obtained. In the first few hours, the measured serum osmolality should be determined and compared to calculated osmolality (see osmolality equation, earlier). If seizures occur, one should measure serum calcium (preferably ionized calcium) and treat with intravenous diazepam. If the patient has hypocalcemic seizures, he or she should also be treated with 10 to 20 mL 10% calcium gluconate (0.2 to 0.3 mL/kg in children) slowly intravenously, with the dose repeated as needed. Metabolic acidosis should be corrected with intravenous sodium bicarbonate.

Ethanol therapy should be initiated immediately if fomepizole (Antizol) is unavailable (see next paragraph). Alcohol dehydrogenase has a greater affinity for ethanol than ethylene glycol. Therefore, ethanol blocks the metabolism of ethylene glycol. Ethanol therapy is called for if there is a history of ingestion of 0.1 mL/kg of 100% ethylene glycol, serum ethylene glycol concentration is greater than 20 mg/dL, there is an osmolar gap not accounted for by other alcohols or factors (e.g., hyperlipidemia), metabolic acidosis is present with an increased anion gap, or there are oxalate crystals in the urine. Ethanol should be administered intravenously (the oral route is less reliable) to produce a blood ethanol concentration of 100 to 150 mg/dL. The loading dose is 10 mL/kg of 10% ethanol intravenously, administered concomitantly with a maintenance dose of 10% ethanol of 1.0 mL/kg/h. This dose may need to be increased to 2 mL/kg/h in patients who are heavy drinkers. The blood ethanol concentration should be measured hourly and the infusion rate should be adjusted to maintain a blood ethanol concentration of 100 to 150 mg/dL.

Fomepizole (Antizol, 4-methylpyrazole) inhibits alcohol dehydrogenase more reliably than ethanol and it does not require constant monitoring of ethanol levels and adjustment of infusion rates. Fomepizole is available in 1 g/mL vials of 1.5 mL. The loading dose is 15 mg/kg (0.015 mL/kg) IV; maintenance dose is 10 mg/kg (0.01 mL/kg) every 12 hours for four doses, then 15 mg/kg every 12 hours until the ethylene glycol levels are less than 20 mg/dL. The solution is prepared by being mixed with 100 mL of 0.9% saline or D5W (5% dextrose in water). Fomepizole can be given to patients requiring hemodialysis but should be dosed as follows:

Dose at the beginning of hemodialysis:
* If <6 hours since last Antizol dose, do not administer dose
* If >6 hours since last dose, administer next scheduled dose

Dosing during hemodialysis:
* Dose every 4 hours

Dosing at the time hemodialysis is completed:
* If <1 hour between last dose and end of dialysis, do not administer dose at end of dialysis
* If 1 to 3 hours between last dose and end of dialysis, administer one half of next scheduled dose
* If >3 hours between last dose and end of dialysis, administer next scheduled dose

Maintenance dosing off hemodialysis:
* Give the next scheduled dose 12 hours from the last dose administered

Hemodialysis is indicated if the ingestion was potentially fatal; if the serum ethylene glycol concentration is greater than 50 mg/dL (some recommend at levels of >25 mg/dL); if severe acidosis or electrolyte abnormalities occur despite conventional therapy; or if congestive heart failure or renal failure is present. Hemodialysis reduces the ethylene glycol half-life from 17 hours on ethanol therapy to 3 hours. Therapy (fomepizole and hemodialysis) should be continued until the serum ethylene glycol concentration is less than 10 mg/dL, the glycolate level is nondetectable (not readily available), the acidosis has cleared, there are no mental disturbances, the creatinine level is normal, and the urinary output is adequate. This may require 2 to 5 days.

Adjunct therapy involving thiamine, 100 mg/d (in children, 50 mg), slowly over 5 minutes intravenously or intramuscularly and repeated every 6 hours and pyridoxine, 50 mg IV or IM every 6 hours, has been recommended until intoxication is resolved, but these agents have not been extensively studied. Folate, 50 mg IV (child 1 mg/kg), can be given every 4 hours for 6 doses.

Disposition

All patients who have ingested significant amounts of ethylene glycol (calculated level above 20 mg/dL), have a history of a toxic dose, or are symptomatic should be referred to the emergency department and admitted. If the serum ethylene glycol concentration cannot be obtained, the patient should be followed for 12 hours, with monitoring of the osmolal gap, acid-base parameters, and electrolytes to exclude development of metabolic acidosis with an anion gap. Transfer should be considered for fomepizole therapy or hemodialysis.

Hydrocarbons

The lower the viscosity and surface tension of hydrocarbons or the greater the volatility, the greater the risk of aspiration. Volatile substance abuse has produced the "Sudden Sniffing's Death Syndrome," most likely caused by dysrhythmias.

Toxicologic Classification and Toxic Mechanism

All systemically absorbed hydrocarbons can lower the threshold of the myocardium to dysrhythmias produced by endogenous and exogenous catecholamines.

Aliphatic hydrocarbons are branched straight chain hydrocarbons. A few aspirated drops are poorly absorbed from the gastrointestinal tract and produce no systemic toxicity by this route. However, aspiration of very small amounts can produce chemical pneumonitis. Examples of aliphatic hydrocarbons are gasoline, kerosene, charcoal lighter fluid, mineral spirits (Stoddard's solvent), and petroleum naphtha. Mineral seal oil (signal oil), found in furniture polishes, is a low-viscosity and low-volatility oil with minimum absorption that never warrants gastric decontamination. It can produce severe pneumonia if aspirated.

Aromatic hydrocarbons are six carbon ring structures that are absorbed through the gastrointestinal tract. Systemic toxicity includes CNS depression and, in cases of chronic abuse, multiple organ effects such as leukemia (benzene) and renal toxicity (toluene). Examples are benzene, toluene, styrene, and xylene. The seriously toxic ingested dose is 20 to 50 mL in adults.

Halogenated hydrocarbons are aliphatic or aromatic hydrocarbons with one or more halogen substitutions (Cl, Br, Fl, or I). They are highly volatile and are abused as inhalants. They are well absorbed from the gastrointestinal tract, produce CNS depression, and have metabolites that can damage the liver and kidneys. Examples include methylene chloride (may be converted into carbon monoxide in the body), dichloroethylene (also causes a disulfiram [Antabuse] reaction known as "degreaser's flush" when associated with consumption of ethanol), and 1,1,1-trichloroethane (Glamorene Spot Remover, Scotchgard, typewriter correction fluid). An acute lethal oral dose is 0.5 to 5 mL/kg.

Dangerous additives to the hydrocarbons can be summed up with the mnemonic CHAMP: C, camphor (demothing agent); H, halogenated hydrocarbons; A, aromatic hydrocarbons; M, metals (heavy); and P, pesticides. Ingestion of these substances may warrant gastric emptying with a small-bore nasogastric tube.

Heavy hydrocarbons have high viscosity, low volatility, and minimal gastrointestinal absorption, so gastric decontamination is not necessary. Examples are asphalt (tar), machine oil, motor oil (lubricating oil, engine oil), home heating oil, and petroleum jelly (mineral oil).

Laboratory Investigations

The ECG, ABG, pulmonary function, serum electrolytes, and serial chest radiographs should be continuously monitored. Liver and renal function should be monitored in cases of inhalation of aromatic hydrocarbons.

Management

Asymptomatic patients who ingested small amounts of aliphatic petroleum distillates can be followed at home by telephone for development of signs of aspiration (cough, wheezing, tachypnea, and dyspnea) for 4 to 6 hours. Inhalation of any hydrocarbon vapors in a closed space can produce intoxication. The victim must be removed from the environment, have oxygen administered, and receive respiratory support.

Gastrointestinal decontamination is not advised in cases of hydrocarbon ingestion that usually do not cause systemic toxicity (aliphatic petroleum distillates, heavy hydrocarbons). In cases of ingestion of hydrocarbons that cause systemic toxicity in small amounts (aromatic hydrocarbons, halogenated hydrocarbons), the clinician should pass a small-bore nasogastric tube and aspirate if the ingestion was within 2 hours and if spontaneous vomiting has not occurred. Some toxicologists advocate ipecac-induced emesis under medical supervision instead of small-bore nasogastric gastric lavage; we do not.

Patients with altered mental status should have their airway protected because of concern about aspiration. The use of activated charcoal has been suggested, but there are no scientific data as to effectiveness and it may produce vomiting. Activated charcoal may, however, be useful in adsorbing toxic additives such as pesticides or co-ingestants.

The symptomatic patient who is coughing, gagging, choking, or wheezing on arrival has probably aspirated. The clinician should provide supportive respiratory care and supplemental oxygen, while monitoring pulse oximetry, ABG, chest radiograph, and ECG. The patient should be admitted to the intensive care unit. A chest radiograph for aspiration may be positive as early as 30 minutes after ingestion, and almost all are positive within 6 hours. Negative chest radiographs within 4 hours do not rule out aspiration.

Bronchospasm is treated with a nebulized β-adrenergic agonist and intravenous aminophylline if necessary. Epinephrine should be avoided because of susceptibility to dysrhythmias. Cyanosis in the presence of a normal arterial PaO_2 may be a result of methemoglobinemia that requires therapy with methylene blue. Corticosteroids and prophylactic antimicrobial agents have not been shown to be beneficial. (Fever or leukocytosis may be produced by the chemical pneumonitis itself.)

Most infiltrations resolve spontaneously in 1 week; lipoid pneumonia may last up to 6 weeks. It is not necessary to surgically treat pneumatoceles that develop because they usually resolve. Dysrhythmias may require α- and β-adrenergic antagonists or cardioversion.

There is no role for enhanced elimination procedures.

Methylene chloride is metabolized over several hours to carbon monoxide. See treatment of carbon monoxide poisoning. Halogenated hydrocarbons are hepatorenal toxins; therefore, hepatorenal function should be monitored. N-acetylcysteine therapy may be useful if there is evidence of hepatic damage.

Extracorporeal membrane oxygenation (ECMO) has been used successfully for a few patients with life-threatening respiratory failure. Surfactant used for hydrocarbon aspiration was found to be detrimental.

Disposition

Asymptomatic patients with small ingestions of petroleum distillates can be managed at home. Symptomatic patients with abnormal chest radiographic, oxygen saturation, or ABG findings should be admitted. Patients who become asymptomatic and have normal oxygenation and a normal repeat radiograph can be discharged.

Iron

There are more than 100 iron over-the-counter preparations for supplementation and treatment of iron deficiency anemia.

Toxic Mechanism

Toxicity depends on the amount of elemental iron available in various salts (gluconate 12%, sulfate 20%, fumarate 33%, lactate 19%, chloride 21% of elemental iron), not the amount of the salt. Locally, iron is corrosive and may cause fluid loss, hypovolemic shock, and perforation. Excessive free unbound iron in the blood is directly toxic to the vasculature and leads to the release of vasoactive substances, which produces vasodilation. In cases of overdose, iron deposits injure mitochondria in the liver, the kidneys, and the myocardium. The exact mechanism of cellular damage is not clear but is thought to be related to free radical formation.

Toxic Dose
The therapeutic dose is 6 mg/kg/d of elemental iron. An elemental iron dose of 20 to 40 mg/kg may produce mild self-limited gastrointestinal symptoms, 40 to 60 mg/kg produces moderate toxicity, more than 60 mg/kg produces severe toxicity and is potentially lethal, and more than 180 mg/kg is usually fatal without treatment. Children's chewable vitamins with iron have between 12 and 18 mg of elemental iron per tablet or 0.6 mL of liquid drops. These preparations rarely produce toxicity unless very large quantities are ingested and have never caused death.

Kinetics
Absorption occurs chiefly in the upper small intestine. Ferrous ($+2$) iron is absorbed into the mucosal cells, where it is oxidized to the ferric ($+3$) state and bound to ferritin. Iron is slowly released from ferritin into the plasma, where it binds to transferrin and is transported to specific tissues for production of hemoglobin (70%), myoglobin (5%), and cytochrome. About 25% of iron is stored in the liver and spleen. In cases of overdose, larger amounts of iron are absorbed because of direct mucosal corrosion. There is no mechanism for the elimination of iron (elimination is 1 to 2 mg/d) except through bile, sweat, and blood loss.

Manifestations
Serious toxicity is unlikely if the patient remains asymptomatic for 6 hours and has a negative abdominal radiograph. Iron intoxication can produce five phases of toxicity. The phases may not be distinct from one another.

Phase I. Gastrointestinal mucosal injury occurs 30 minutes to 12 hours postingestion. Vomiting starts within 30 minutes to 1 hour of ingestion and is persistent; hematemesis and bloody diarrhea may occur; abdominal cramps, fever, hyperglycemia, and leukocytosis may occur. Enteric-coated tablets may pass through the stomach without causing symptoms. Acidosis and shock can occur within 6 to 12 hours.

Phase II. A latent period of apparent improvement occurs over 8 to 12 hours postingestion.

Phase III. Systemic toxicity phase occurs 12 to 48 hours postingestion with cardiovascular collapse and severe metabolic acidosis.

Phase IV. Two to 4 days postingestion, hepatic injury associated with jaundice, elevated liver enzymes, and prolonged prothrombin time occur. Kidney injury with proteinuria and hematuria occur. Pulmonary edema, disseminated intravascular coagulation, and *Yersinia enterocolitica* sepsis can occur.

Phase V. Four to 8 weeks postingestion, pyloric outlet or intestinal stricture may cause obstruction or anemia secondary to blood loss.

Laboratory Investigations
Iron poisoning produces anion gap metabolic acidosis. Monitoring should include complete blood cell counts, blood glucose level, serum iron, stools and vomitus for occult blood, electrolytes, acid-base balance, urinalysis and urinary output, liver function tests, and BUN and creatinine levels. Blood type and match should be obtained.

Serum iron measurements taken at the proper time correlate with the clinical findings. The lavender top Vacutainer tube contains EDTA, which falsely lowers serum iron. One must obtain the serum iron measurement before administering deferoxamine. Serum iron levels of less than 350 µg/dL at 2 to 6 hours predict an asymptomatic course; levels of 350 to 500 µg/dL are usually associated with mild gastrointestinal symptoms; those greater than 500 µg/dL have a 20% risk of shock and serious iron toxicity. A follow-up serum iron measurement after 6 hours may not be elevated even in cases of severe poisoning, but a serum iron measurement taken at 8 to 12 hours is useful to exclude delayed absorption from a bezoar or sustained-release preparation. The total iron-binding capacity is not necessary.

Adult iron tablet preparations are radiopaque before they dissolve by 4 hours postingestion. A "negative" abdominal radiograph more than 4 hours postingestion does not exclude iron poisoning.

Patients who develop high fevers and signs of sepsis following iron overdose should have blood and stool cultures checked for *Yersinia enterocolitica*.

Management
Gastrointestinal decontamination should involve immediate induction of emesis in cases of ingestions of elemental iron of greater than 40 mg/kg if vomiting has not already occurred. Activated charcoal is ineffective. An abdominal radiograph should be obtained after emesis to determine the success of gastric emptying. Children's chewable vitamins and liquid iron preparations are not radiopaque. If radiopaque iron is still present, whole-bowel irrigation with polyethylene glycol solution should be considered. In extreme cases, removal by endoscopy or surgery may be necessary because coalesced iron tablets produce hemorrhagic infarction in the bowel and perforation peritonitis.

Deferoxamine (Desferal) in a dose of about 100 mg binds 8.5 to 9.35 mg of free iron in the serum. The deferoxamine infusion should not exceed 15 mg/kg/h or 6 g daily, but faster rates (up to 45 mg/kg) and larger daily amounts have been administered and tolerated in extreme cases of iron poisoning (>1000 mg/dL). The deferoxamine-iron complex is hemodialyzable if renal failure develops.

Indications for chelation therapy are any of the following:
- Very large, symptomatic ingestions
- Serious clinical intoxication (severe vomiting and diarrhea [often bloody], severe abdominal pain, metabolic acidosis, hypotension, or shock)
- Symptoms that persist or progress to more serious toxicity
- Serum iron level greater than 500 mg/dL

Chelation should be performed as early as possible within 12 to 18 hours to be effective. One should start the infusion slowly and gradually increase to avoid hypotension.

Adult respiratory distress syndrome has developed in patients with high doses of deferoxamine for several days; infusions longer than 24 hours should be avoided.

The endpoint of treatment is when the patient is asymptomatic and the urine clears if it was originally a positive "vin rosö" color.

For supportive therapy, intravenous bicarbonate may be needed to correct the metabolic acidosis. Hypotension and shock treatment may require volume expansion, vasopressors, and blood transfusions. The physician should attempt to keep the urinary output at greater than 2 mL/kg/h. Coagulation abnormalities and overt bleeding require blood products or vitamin K. Pregnant patients are treated in a fashion similar to any other patient with iron poisoning.

Hemodialysis and hemoperfusion are ineffective. Exchange transfusion has been used in single cases of massive poisonings in children.

Disposition
The asymptomatic or minimally symptomatic patient should be observed for persistence and progression of symptoms or development of toxicity signs (gastrointestinal bleeding, acidosis, shock, altered mental state). Patients with mild self-limited gastrointestinal symptoms who become asymptomatic or have no signs of toxicity for 6 hours are unlikely to have a serious intoxication and can be discharged after psychiatric clearance, if needed. Patients with moderate or severe toxicity should be admitted to the intensive care unit.

Isoniazid
Isoniazid is a hydrazide derivative of vitamin B_3 (nicotinamide) and is used as an antituberculosis drug.

Toxic Mechanism
Isoniazid produces pyridoxine deficiency by increasing the excretion of pyridoxine (vitamin B_6) and by inhibiting pyridoxal 5-phosphate (the active form of pyridoxine) from acting with

L-glutamic acid decarboxylase to form γ-aminobutyric acid (GABA), the major CNS neurotransmitter inhibitor, resulting in seizures. Isoniazid also blocks the conversion of lactate to pyruvate, resulting in profound and prolonged lactic acidosis.

Toxic Dose

The therapeutic dose is 5 to 10 mg/kg (maximum 300 mg) daily. A single acute dose of 15 mg/kg lowers the seizure threshold; 35 to 40 mg/kg produces spontaneous convulsions; more than 80 mg/kg produces severe toxicity. A fatal dose in adults is 4.5 to 15 g. The malnourished patients, those with a previous seizure disorder, alcoholic patients, and slow acetylators are more susceptible to isoniazid toxicity. In cases of chronic intoxication, 10 mg/kg/d produces hepatitis in 10% to 20% of patients but less than 2% at doses of 3 to 5 mg/kg/d.

Kinetics

Absorption from intestine occurs in 30 to 60 minutes, and onset is in 30 to 120 minutes, with peak levels of 5 to 8 µg/mL within 1 to 2 hours. Volume distribution is 0.6 L/kg, with minimal protein binding.

Elimination is by liver acetylation to a hepatotoxic metabolite, acetyl-isoniazid, which is then hydrolyzed to isonicotinic acid. In slow acetylators, isoniazid has a half-life of 140 to 460 minutes (mean 5 hours), and 10% to 15% is eliminated unchanged in the urine. Most (45% to 75%) whites and 50% of African blacks are slow acetylators, and, with chronic use (without pyridoxine supplements), they may develop peripheral neuropathy. In fast acetylators, isoniazid has a half-life of 35 to 110 minutes (mean 80 minutes), and 25% to 30% is excreted unchanged in the urine. About 90% of Asians and patients with diabetes mellitus are fast acetylators and may develop hepatitis on chronic use.

In patients with overdose and hepatic disease, the serum half-life may increase. Isoniazid inhibits the metabolism of phenytoin (Dilantin), diazepam, phenobarbital, carbamazepine (Tegretol), and prednisone. These drugs also interfere with the metabolism of isoniazid. Ethanol may decrease the half-life of isoniazid but increase its toxicity.

Manifestations

Within 30 to 60 minutes, nausea, vomiting, slurred speech, dizziness, visual disturbances, and ataxia are present. Within 30 to 120 minutes, the major clinical triad of severe overdose includes refractory convulsions (90% of overdose patients have one or more seizures), coma, and resistant severe lactic acidosis (secondary to convulsions), often with a plasma pH of 6.8.

Laboratory Investigations

Isoniazid produces anion gap metabolic acidosis. Therapeutic levels are 5 to 8 µg/mL and acute toxic levels are greater than 20 µg/mL. These levels are not readily available to assist in making decisions in acute overdose situations. One should monitor the blood glucose (often hyperglycemia), electrolytes (often hyperkalemia), bicarbonate, ABGs, liver function tests (elevations occur with chronic exposure), BUN, and creatinine.

Management

Seizures must be controlled. Pyridoxine and diazepam should be administered concomitantly through different IV sites. Pyridoxine (vitamin B_6) is given in a dose of 1 g for each gram of isoniazid ingested. If the dose ingested is unknown, at least 5 g of pyridoxine should be given intravenously. Pyridoxine is administered in 50 mL D_5W or 0.9% saline over 5 minutes intravenously. It must not be administered in the same bottle as sodium bicarbonate. Intravenous pyridoxine is repeated every 5 to 20 minutes until the seizures are controlled. Total doses of pyridoxine up to 52 g have been safely administered; however, patients given 132 and 183 g of pyridoxine have developed a persistent crippling sensory neuropathy.

Diazepam is administered concomitantly with pyridoxine but at a different site. They work synergistically. Diazepam should be administered intravenously slowly, 0.3 mg/kg at a rate of 1 mg/min in children or 10 mg at a rate of 5 mg/min in adults. After the seizures are controlled, the remainder of the pyridoxine is administered (1 g/1 g isoniazid) or a total dose of 5 g.

Phenobarbital or phenytoin is ineffective and should not be used.

In asymptomatic patients or patients without seizures, pyridoxine has been advised by some toxicologists prophylactically in gram-for-gram doses in cases of large overdoses (<80 mg/kg per dose) of isoniazid, although there are no studies to support this recommendation. In comatose patients, pyridoxine administration may result in the patient's rapid regaining of consciousness. Correction of acidosis may occur spontaneously with pyridoxine administration and correction of the seizures. Sodium bicarbonate should be administered if acidosis persists.

Hemodialysis is rarely needed because of antidotal therapy and the short half-life of isoniazid, but it may be used as an adjunct for cases of uncontrollable acidosis and seizures. Hemoperfusion has not been adequately evaluated. Diuresis is ineffective.

Disposition

Asymptomatic or mildly symptomatic patients who become asymptomatic can be observed in the emergency department for 4 to 6 hours. Larger amounts of isoniazid may warrant pyridoxine administration and longer periods of observation. Intentional ingestions necessitate psychiatric evaluation before the patient is discharged. Patients with convulsions or coma should be admitted to the intensive care unit.

Isopropanol (Isopropyl Alcohol)

Isopropanol can be found in rubbing alcohol, solvents, and lacquer thinner. Coma has occurred in children sponged for fever with isopropanol. See Table 10 for ethanol features of alcohols and glycols.

Toxic Mechanism

Isopropanol is a gastric irritant. It is metabolized to acetone, a CNS and myocardial depressant. It inhibits gluconeogenesis. Normal propyl alcohol is related to isopropyl alcohol but is more toxic.

Toxic Dose

A toxic dose of 0.5 to 1 mg/kg of 70% isopropanol (1 mL/kg of 70%) produces a blood isopropanol plasma concentration of 70 mg/dL. The CNS depressant potency is twice that of ethanol.

Kinetics

Onset of action is within 30 to 60 minutes, and peak is 1 hour postingestion. Volume distribution is 0.6 kg/L. Isopropyl alcohol metabolizes to acetone. Its excretion is renal.

Note. The serum isopropyl concentration and amount ingested can be estimated using the same equation as is used in ethanol kinetics and substituting the specific gravity of 0.785 for isopropyl alcohol.

Manifestations

Ethanol-like inebriation occurs, with an acetone odor to the breath, gastritis, occasionally with hematemesis, acetonuria, and acetonemia without systemic acidosis.

Depression of the CNS occurs: lethargy at blood isopropyl alcohol levels of 50 to 100 mg/dL, coma at levels of 150 to 200 mg/dL, potentially death in adults at levels greater than 240 mg/dL.

Hypoglycemia and seizures may occur.

Laboratory Investigation

Monitoring of blood isopropyl alcohol levels (not readily available in all institutions), acetone, glucose, and ABG should be maintained. The osmolal gap increases 1 mOsm per 5.9 mg/dL of isopropyl alcohol and 1 mOsm per 5.5 mg/dL of acetone. The absence of excess acetone in the blood (normal is 0.3 to

2 mg/dL) within 30 to 60 minutes or excess acetone in the urine within 3 hours excludes the possibility of significant isopropanol exposure.

Management

The airway must be protected with intubation, and assisted ventilation administered if necessary. If the patient is hypoglycemic, glucose should be administered. Supportive treatment is similar to that for ethanol ingestions.

Gastrointestinal decontamination has no role in the treatment of isopropanol ingestion. Hemodialysis is warranted in cases of life-threatening overdose but is rarely needed. A nephrologist should be consulted if the blood isopropanol plasma concentration is greater than 250 mg/dL.

Disposition

Symptomatic patients with concentrations greater than 100 mg/dL require at least 24 hours of close observation for resolution and should be admitted. If the patient is hypoglycemic, hypotensive, or comatose, he or she should be admitted to the intensive care unit.

Lead

Acute lead intoxication is rare and usually occurs by inhalation of lead, resulting in severe intoxication and often death. Lead fumes can be produced by burning of lead batteries or use of a heat gun to remove lead paint. Acute lead intoxication also occurs from exposure to high concentrations of organic lead (e.g., tetraethyl lead).

Chronic lead poisoning occurs most often in children 6 months to 6 years of age who are exposed in their environment and in adults in certain occupations (Table 17). In the United States, the prevalence in children aged 1 to 5 years with a venous blood lead greater than 10 µg/dL decreased from 88.2% in a 1976–1980 survey to 8.9% in a 1988–1991 survey as a consequence of measures to reduce lead in the environment, particularly leaded gasoline. However, an estimated 1.7 million children between 1 and 5 years of age and more than 1 million workers in over 100 different occupations still have blood lead levels greater than 10 µg/dL.

Toxic Dose

In cases of chronic lead poisoning, a daily intake of more than 5 µg/kg/d in children or more than 150 µg/d in adults can give a positive lead balance. In 1991, the Centers for Disease Control and Prevention (CDC) recommended routine screening for all children younger than 6 years of age. In children a venous blood level greater than 10 µg/dL was determined to be a threshold of concern. The average venous blood level in the United States is 4 µg/dL. In cases of occupational exposure (see Table 17), a venous blood level greater than 40 µg/dL is indicative of increased lead absorption in adults.

Toxic Mechanism

Lead affects the sulfhydryl enzyme systems, the immature CNS, the enzymes of heme synthesis, vitamin D conversion, the kidneys, the bones, and growth. Lead alters the tertiary structure of cell proteins by denaturing them and causing cell death. Risk factors are mouthing behavior of infants and children and excessive oral behavior (pica), living in the inner city, a poorly maintained home, and poor nutrition (e.g., low calcium and iron). The CDC questionnaire given in Table 18 is recommended at every pediatric visit. If any answers to the CDC questionnaire are "positive," a blood screening test for lead should be administered. To be more accurate, however, identifying lead exposure studies have suggested that the questionnaire will have to be modified for each individual community because it has had poor sensitivity (40%) and specificity (60%) as it stands.

Table 19 lists sources of lead. The number one source is deteriorating lead-based paint, which forms leaded dust. Lead concentrations in indoor paint were not reduced to safer (0.06%) levels until 1978. Lead can also be produced by improper interior or exterior home renovation (scraping or demolition). It is found in pre-1960 built homes. The use of leaded gasoline (limited in 1973) resulted in residue from leaded motor vehicle emissions. Lead persists in the soil near major highways and in deteriorating homes and buildings. Vegetables grown in contaminated soil may contain lead.

Oil refineries and lead-processing smelters produce lead residue. Food cans produced in Mexico contain lead solder (95% do not in United States). Lead water pipes (until 1950) and lead solder (until 1986) deliver lead-containing drinking water (calcium deposits, however, may offer some protection). Water at a consumer's tap should contain less than 15 parts per billion (ppb) of lead (Table 20).

TABLE 18 CDC Questionnaire: Priority Groups for Lead Screening

1. Children age 6–72 months (was 12–36 months) who live in or are frequent visitors to older, deteriorated housing built before 1960.

2. Children age 6–72 months who live in housing built prior to 1960 with recent, ongoing, or planned renovation or remodeling.

3. Children age 6–72 months who are siblings, housemates, or playmates of children with known lead poisoning.

4. Children age 6–72 months whose parents or other household members participate in a lead-related industry or hobby.

5. Children age 6–72 months who live near active lead smelters, battery recycling plants, or other industries likely to result in atmospheric lead release.

TABLE 19 Sources of Lead

PRODUCT	LEAD CONTENT (%) BY DRY WEIGHT
Paint	0.06
Solder	0.6
Plastic additives	2.0
Priming inks	2.0
Plumbing fixtures	2.0
Pesticides	0.1
Stained glass panes	0.1
Wine bottle foils	0.1
Construction material	0.1
Fertilizers	0.1
Glazes, enamels	0.06
Toys/recreational games	0.1
Curtain weights	0.1
Fishing weights	0.1

TABLE 17 Occupations Associated With Lead Exposure

Lead production or smelting	Demolition of ships and bridges
Production of illicit whiskey	Battery manufacturing
Brass, copper, and lead foundries	Machining/grinding lead alloys
Radiator repair	Welding of old painted metals
Scrap handling	Thermal paint stripping of old
Sanding of old paint	buildings
Lead soldering	Ceramic glaze/pottery mixing
Cable stripping	
Worker or janitor at a firing range	

Modified from Rempel D: The lead-exposed worker. JAMA 262:533, 1989.

TABLE 20	Agency Regulations and Recommendations Concerning Lead Content		
AGENCY	**SPECIMEN**	**LEVEL**	**COMMENTS**
CDC	Blood (child)	10 µg/dL	Investigate community
OSHA	Blood (adult)	60 µg/dL	Medical removal from work
OSHA	Air	50 µg/m³	PEL*
	Air	0.75 µg/m³	Tetraethyl or tetramethyl
ACGIH	Air	150 µg/m³	TWA†
EPA	Air	1.5 µg/m³	Three-month average
EPA	Water	15 µg/L (ppb)	5 ppb circulating
EPA	Food	100 µg/d	Advisory
FDA	Wine	300 ppm	Plan to reduce to 200 ppm
EPA	Soil/dust	50 ppm	
CPSC	Paint	600 ppm (0.06%) by dry weight	

*PEL = permissible exposure limit (highest level over an 8-hour workday).
†TWA = time-weighted average (air concentration for 8-hour workday and 40-hour workweek).
Abbreviations: ACGIH = American Conference of Governmental Industrial Hygienists; CDC = Centers for Disease Control and Prevention; CPSC = Consumer Product Safety Commission; EPA = Environmental Protection Agency; FDA = Food and Drug Administration; OSHA = Occupational Safety and Health Administration.

For occupational exposure, see Table 17. The Occupational Safety and Health Administration (OSHA) standards require employers to provide showering and clothes changing facilities for personnel working with lead; however, businesses with fewer than 25 employees are exempt from the regulation. The OSHA lead standard of 1978 set a limit of 60 µg/dL for occupational exposure to lead. At a blood lead level of 60 µg/dL, a worker should be removed from lead exposure and not allowed back until his or her lead level is below 40 µg/dL. Many authorities believe that this level should be lower. The lead residue on the clothes of the workers may represent a hazard to the family. Other occupations that are potential sources of lead exposure include plumbers, pipe fitters, lead miners, auto repairers, ship-builders, printers, steel welders and cutters, construction workers, and rubber product manufacturers.

Leaded pots to make molds for "kusmusha" tea represent lead exposure. Imported pottery lined with ceramic glaze can leach large amounts of lead into acids (e.g., citrus fruit juices).

Hobbies associated with lead exposure are listed in Box 1. Some "traditional" folk remedies or cosmetics that contain lead include the following:

Box 1	Hobbies Associated With Lead Exposure

Casting of ammunition
Collecting antique pewter
Collecting/painting lead toys (e.g., soldiers and figures)
Ceramics or glazed pottery
Refinishing furniture
Making fishing weights
Home renovation
Jewelry making, lead solder
Glass blowing, lead glass
Bronze casting
Print making and other fine arts (when lead white, flake white, chrome yellow pigments are involved)
Liquor distillation
Hunting and target shooting
Painting
Car and boat repair
Burning/engraving lead-painted wood
Making stained leaded glass
Copper enameling

- "Azarcon por empacho" ("Maria Louisa" 90% to 95% lead trioxide): a bright orange powder used in Hispanic culture, especially Mexican, for digestive problems and diarrhea.
- "Greta" (4% to 90% lead): a yellow powder "por empacho" ("empacho" refers to a variety of gastrointestinal symptoms), used in Hispanic cultures, especially Mexican.
- "Pay-loo-ah": an orange-red powder used for rash and fever in Southeast Asian cultures, especially among Northern Laos Hmong immigrants.
- "Alkohl" (Al-kohl, kohl, suma 5% to 92% lead): a black powder used in Middle Eastern, African, and Asian cultures as a cosmetic and an umbilical stump astringent.
- "Farouk": an orange granular powder with lead used in Saudi Arabian culture.
- "Bint Al Zahab": used to treat colic in Saudi Arabian culture.
- "Surma" (23% to 26% lead): a black powder used in India as a cosmetic and to improve eyesight.
- "Bali goli": a round black bean that is dissolved in "grippe water," used by Asian and Indian cultures to aid digestion.

Cases of substance abuse involving lead poisoning have been reported, in which the patient sniffs leaded gasoline or uses improperly synthesized amphetamines.

Kinetics
Absorption of lead is 10% to 15% of the ingested dose in adults; in children, up to 40% is absorbed, especially in cases of iron deficiency anemia. With inhalation of fumes, absorption is rapid and complete. Volume distribution in blood (0.9% of total body burden) is 95% in red blood cells. Lead passes through the placenta to the fetus and is present in breast milk.

Organic lead is metabolized in the liver to inorganic lead. Its half-life is 35 to 40 days in blood; in soft tissue, the half-life is 45 days and in bone (99% of the lead), the half-life is 28 years. The major elimination route is the stool, 80% to 90%, and then renal 10% (80 g/d) and hair, nails, sweat, and saliva. Nine percent of organic lead is excreted in the urine per day.

Manifestations
Adverse health effects are given in Table 21 and include the following.

Hematologic. Lead inhibits γ-aminolevulinic acid dehydratase (early in the synthesis of heme) and ferrochelatase (transfers iron to ferritin for incorporation of iron into protoporphyrin to produce heme). Anemia is a late finding. Decreased heme synthesis starts at >40 µg/dL. Basophilic stippling occurs in 20% of severe lead poisoning.

TABLE 21	Summary of Lead-Induced Health Effects in Adults and Children	
BLOOD LEAD LEVEL (μG/DL)	**AGE GROUP**	**HEALTH EFFECT**
>100	Adult	Encephalopathic signs and symptoms
>80	Adult	Anemia
	Child	Encephalopathy
		Chronic nephropathy (e.g., aminoaciduria)
>70	Adult	Clinically evident peripheral neuropathy
	Child	Colic and other gastrointestinal symptoms
>60	Adult	Female reproductive effects
		CNS disturbance symptoms (i.e., sleep disturbances, mood changes, memory and concentration problems, headaches)
>50	Adult	Decreased hemoglobin production
		Decreased performance on neurobehavioral tests
	Adult	Altered testicular function
		Gastrointestinal symptoms (i.e., abdominal pain, constipation, diarrhea, nausea, anorexia)
	Child	Peripheral neuropathy*
>40	Adult	Decreased peripheral nerve conduction
		Hypertension, age 40–59 years
		Chronic neuropathy*
>25	Adult	Elevated erythrocyte protoporphyrin in males
15–25	Adult	Elevated erythrocyte protoporphyrin in females
>10	Child	Decreased intelligence and growth
		Impaired learning
		Reduced birth weight*
		Impaired mental ability
	Fetus	Preterm delivery

From Anonymous: Implementation of the Lead Contamination Control Act of 1988. MMWR Morb Mortal Wkly Rep 41:288, 1992.
*Controversial.

Neurologic. Segmental demyelination and peripheral neuropathy, usually of the motor type (wrist and ankle drop), occurs in workers. A venous blood level of lead greater than 70 μg/dL (usually >100 μg/dL), produces encephalopathy in children (symptom mnemonic "PAINT": P, persistent forceful vomiting and papilledema; A, ataxia; I, intermittent stupor and lucidity; N, neurologic coma and refractory convulsions; T, tired and lethargic). Decreased cognitive abilities have been reported with a venous blood level of lead greater than 10 μg/dL, including behavioral problems, decreased attention span, and learning disabilities. IQ scores may begin to decrease at 15 μg/dL. Encephalopathy is rare in adults.

Renal. Nephropathy as a result of damaged capillaries and glomerulus can occur at a venous blood level of lead greater than 80 μg/dL, but recent studies show renal damage and hypertension with low venous blood levels. A direct correlation between hypertension and venous blood level over 30 μg/dL has been reported. Lead reduces excretion of uric acid, and high-level exposure may be associated with hyperuricemia and "saturnine gout," Fanconi's syndrome (aminoaciduria and renal tubular acidosis), and tubular fibrosis.

Reproductive. Spontaneous abortion, transient delay in the child's development (catch up at age 5 to 6 years), decreased sperm count, and abnormal sperm morphology can occur with lead exposure. Lead crosses the placenta and fetal blood levels reach 75% to 100% of maternal blood levels. Lead is teratogenic.

Metabolic. Decreased cytochrome P450 activity alters the metabolism of medication and endogenously produced substances. Decreased activation of cortisol and decreased growth is caused by interference in vitamin conversion (25-hydroxyvitamin D to 1,25-hydroxyvitamin D) at venous blood levels of 20 to 30 μg/dL.

Other Manifestations. Abnormalities of thyroid, cardiac, and hepatic function occur in adults. Abdominal colic is seen in children at doses greater than 50 μg/dL. "Lead gum lines" at the dental border of the gingiva can occur in cases of chronic lead poisoning.

Laboratory Investigations

Serial venous blood lead measurements are taken on days 3 and 5 during treatment and 7 days after chelation therapy, then every 1 to 2 weeks for 8 weeks, and then every month for 6 months. Intravenous infusion should be stopped at least 1 hour before blood lead levels are measured. Table 22 gives a classification of blood lead concentrations in children.

One should evaluate CBC, serum ferritin, erythrocyte protoporphyrin (>35 μg/dL indicates lead poisoning as well as iron deficiency and other causes), electrolytes, serum calcium and phosphorus, urinalysis, BUN, and creatinine. Abdominal and long bone radiographs may be useful in certain circumstances to identify radiopaque material in bowel and "lead lines" in proximal tibia (which occur after prolonged exposure in association with venous blood lead levels greater than 50 μg/dL).

Neuropsychological tests are difficult to perform in young children but should be considered at the end of treatment, especially to determine auditory dysfunction.

Management

The basis of treatment is removal of the source of lead. Cases of poisoning in children should be reported to local health department and cases of occupational poisoning should be reported to OSHA. The source must be identified and abated, and dust controlled by wet mopping. Cold water should be let to run for

TABLE 22	Classification of Blood Lead Concentrations in Children
BLOOD LEAD (μG/DL)	**RECOMMENDED INTERVENTIONS**
<9	None
10–14	Community intervention
	Repeat blood lead in 3 months
15–19	Individual case management
	Environmental counseling
	Nutritional counseling
	Repeat blood lead in 3 months
20–44	Medical referral
	Environmental inspection/abatement
	Nutritional counseling
	Repeat blood lead in 3 months
45–69	Environmental inspection/abatement
	Nutritional counseling
	Pharmacologic therapy
	DMSA succimer oral or CaNa₂EDTA parenteral
	Repeat every 2 weeks for 6–8 weeks, then monthly for 4–6 months
>70	Hospitalization in intensive care unit
	Environmental inspection/abatement
	Pharmacologic therapy
	Dimercaprol (BAL in oil) IM initial alone
	Dimercaprol IM and CaNa₂EDTA together
	Repeat every week

Abbreviations: BAL = British anti-Lewisite; CaNa$_2$EDTA = edetate calcium disodium; DMSA = dimercaptosuccinic acid; IM = intramuscular.

2 minutes before being used for drinking. Planting shrubbery (not vegetables) in contaminated soil will keep children away.

Supportive care should be instituted, including measures to deal with refractory seizures (continued antidotal therapy, diazepam, and possibly neuromuscular blockers), with the hepatic and renal failure, and intravascular hemolysis in severe cases. Seizures are treated with diazepam followed by neuromuscular blockers if needed.

Lead does not bind to activated charcoal. One must not delay chelation therapy for complete gastrointestinal decontamination in severe cases. Whole-bowel irrigation has been used prior to treatment. Some authorities recommend abdominal radiographs followed by gastrointestinal decontamination if necessary before switching to oral therapy. Chelation therapy can be used for patients in whom venous blood level of lead is greater than 45 µg/dL in children and greater than 80 µg/dL in adults or in adults with lower levels who are symptomatic or who have a "positive" lead mobilization test result (not routinely performed at most centers) (Table 23).

Succimer (dimercaptosuccinic acid, DMSA, Chemet), a derivative of British anti-Lewisite (BAL), is an oral agent for chelation in children with a venous blood level of greater than 45 µg/dL. The recommended dose is 10 mg/kg every 8 hours for 5 days, then every 12 hours for 14 days. DMSA is under investigation to determine its role in children with a venous blood level less than 45 µg/dL. Although not approved for adults, it has been used in the same dosage. Monitoring should be maintained by CBC, liver transaminases, and urinalysis for adverse effects.

D-Penicillamine (Cuprimine) is another oral chelator that is given in doses of 20 to 40 mg/kg/d not to exceed 1 g/d. However, it is not FDA approved and has a 10% adverse reaction rate. Nevertheless, D-penicillamine has been used infrequently in adults and children with elevated venous blood lead levels.

Edetate calcium disodium (ethylene diaminetetra-acetic acid or CaNa₂EDTA Versenate) is a water soluble chelator given intramuscularly (with 0.5% procaine) or intravenously. The calcium in the compound is displaced by divalent and trivalent heavy metals, forming a soluble complex, which is stable at physiologic pH (but not at acid pH) and enhances lead clearance in the urine. EDTA usually is administered intravenously, especially in severe cases. It must not be administered until adequate urine flow is established. It may redistribute lead to the brain; therefore, BAL may be given first at a venous blood lead level of greater than 55 µg/dL in children and greater than 100 µg/dL in adults. Phlebitis occurs at a concentration greater than 0.5 mg/mL. Alkalinization of the urine may be helpful. CaNa₂EDTA should not be confused with sodium EDTA (disodium edetate), which is used to treat hypercalcemia; inadvertent use may produce severe hypocalcemia.

Dimercaprol (BAL) is a peanut oil–based dithiol (two sulfhydryl molecules) that combines with one atom of lead to form a heterocyclic stable ring complex. It is usually reserved for patients in whom venous blood lead is greater than 70 µg/dL, and it chelates red blood cell lead, enhancing its elimination through the urine and bile. It crosses the blood-brain barrier. Approximately 50% of patients have adverse reactions, including bad metallic taste in the mouth, pain at the injection site, sterile abscesses, and fever.

A venous blood lead level greater than 70 µg/dL or the presence of clinical symptoms suggesting encephalopathy in children is a potentially life-threatening emergency. Management should be accomplished in a medical center with a pediatric intensive care unit by a multidisciplinary team including a critical care specialist, a toxicologist, a neurologist, and a neurosurgeon. Careful monitoring of neurologic status, fluid status, and intracranial pressure should be undertaken if necessary. These patients need close monitoring for hemodynamic instability. Hydration should be maintained to ensure renal excretion of lead. Fluids, renal and hepatic function, and electrolyte levels should be monitored.

While waiting for adequate urine flow, therapy should be initiated with intramuscular dimercaprol (BAL) only (25 mg/kg/d divided into 6 doses). Four hours later, the second dose of BAL should be given intramuscularly, concurrently with CaNa₂EDTA 50 mg/kg/d as a single dose infused over several hours or as a continuous infusion. The double therapy is continued until the venous blood level is less than 40 µg/dL.

As long as the venous blood level is greater than 40 µg/dL, therapy is continued for 72 hours and followed by two alternatives: either parenteral therapy with two drugs (CaNa₂EDTA and BAL) for 5 days or continuation of therapy with CaNa₂EDTA alone if a good response is achieved and the venous blood level of lead is less than 40 µg/dL. If one cannot get the venous blood lead report back, one should continue therapy with both BAL and EDTA for 5 days. In patients with lead encephalopathy, parenteral chelation should be continued with both drugs until the patient is clinically stable before changing therapy. Mannitol and dexamethasone can reduce the cerebral edema, but their role in lead encephalopathy is not clear. Surgical decompression is not recommended to reduce cerebral edema in these cases.

If BAL and CaNa₂EDTA are used together, a minimum of 2 days with no treatment should elapse before another 5-day course of therapy is considered. The 5-day course is repeated with CaNa₂EDTA alone if the blood lead level rebounds to greater than 40 µg/dL or in combination with BAL if the venous blood level is greater than 70 µg/dL. If a third course is required, unless there are compelling reasons, one should wait at least 5 to 7 days before administering the course.

Following chelation therapy, a period of equilibration of 10 to 14 days should be allowed and a repeat venous blood lead

TABLE 23	Pharmacologic Chelation Therapy of Lead Poisoning				
DRUG	**ROUTE**	**DOSE**	**DURATION**	**PRECAUTIONS**	**MONITOR**
Dimercaprol (BAL in oil)	IM	3–5 mg/kg q4–6h	3–5 days	G6PD deficiency Concurrent iron therapy	AST/ALT enzymes
CaNa₂EDTA (calcium disodium versenate)	IM/IV	50 mg/kg per day	5 days	Inadequate fluid intake Renal impairment Penicillin allergy	Urinalysis, BUN Creatinine Urinalysis, BUN
D-Penicillamine (Cuprimine)	PO	10 mg/kg per day increase 30 mg/kg over 2 weeks	6–20 weeks	Concurrent iron therapy; lead exposure Renal impairment	Creatinine, CBC
2,3-Dimercaptosuccinic acid (DMSA; succimer)	PO	10 mg/kg per dose 3 times daily 10 mg/kg per dose twice daily for 14 days	19 days	AST/ALT Concurrent iron therapy G6PD deficiency lead exposure	AST/ALT

Abbreviations: ALT = alanine aminotransferase; AST = aspartate transaminase; BAL = British anti-Lewisite; bid = twice daily; BUN = blood urea nitrogen; CBC = complete blood count; G6PD = glucose-6-phosphate dehydrogenase; IM = intramuscular; IV = intravenous; PO = oral; tid = three times daily.

concentration should be obtained. If the patient is stable enough for oral intake, oral succimer 30 mg/kg/d in three divided doses for 5 days followed by 20 mg/kg/d in two divided doses for 14 days has been suggested, but there are limited data to support this recommendation. Therapy should be continued until venous blood lead level is less than 20 µg/dL in children or less than 40 µg/dL in adults.

Chelators combined with lead are hemodialyzable in the event of renal failure.

Disposition
All patients with a venous blood lead level of greater than 70 µg/dL or who are symptomatic should be admitted. If a child is hospitalized, all lead hazards must be removed from the home environment before allowing the child to return. The source must be eliminated by environmental and occupational investigations. The local health department should be involved in dealing with children who are lead poisoned, and OSHA should be involved with cases of occupational lead poisoning. Consultation with a poison control center or experienced toxicologist is necessary when chelating patients. Follow-up venous blood lead concentrations should be obtained within 1 to 2 weeks and followed every 2 weeks for 6 to 8 weeks, then monthly for 4 to 6 months if the patient required chelation therapy. All patients with venous blood level greater than 10 µg/dL should be followed at least every 3 months until two venous blood lead concentrations are 10 µg/dL or three are less than 15 µg/dL.

Lithium (Eskalith, Lithane)
Lithium is an alkali metal used primarily in the treatment of bipolar psychiatric disorders. Most intoxications are cases of chronic overdose. One gram of lithium carbonate contains 189 mg (5.1 mEq) of lithium; a regular tablet contains 300 mg (8.12 mEq) and a sustained-release preparation contains 450 mg or 12.18 mEq.

Toxic Mechanism
The brain is the primary target organ of toxicity, but the mechanism is unclear. Lithium may interfere with physiologic functions by acting as a substitute for cellular cations (sodium and potassium), depressing neural excitation and synaptic transmission.

Toxic Dose
A dose of 1 mEq/kg (40 mg/kg) of lithium will give a peak serum lithium concentration about 1.2 mEq/L. The therapeutic serum lithium concentration in cases of acute mania is 0.6 to 1.2 mEq/L, and for maintenance it is 0.5 to 0.8 mEq/L. Serum lithium concentration levels are usually obtained 12 hours after the last dose. The toxic dose is determined by clinical manifestations and serum levels after the distribution phase.

Acute ingestion of twenty 300-mg tablets (300 mg increases the serum lithium concentration by 0.2 to 0.4 mEq/L) in adults may produce serious intoxication. Chronic intoxication can be produced by conditions listed below that can decrease the elimination of lithium or increase lithium reabsorption in the kidney.

The risk factors that predispose to chronic lithium toxicity are febrile illness, impaired renal function, hyponatremia, advanced age, lithium-induced diabetes insipidus, dehydration, vomiting and diarrhea, and concomitant use of other drugs, such as thiazide and spironolactone diuretics, nonsteroidal antiinflammatory drugs, salicylates, angiotensin-converting enzyme inhibitors (e.g., captopril), serotonin reuptake inhibitors (e.g., fluoxetine [Prozac]), and phenothiazines.

Kinetics
Gastrointestinal absorption of regular-release preparations is rapid; serum lithium concentration peaks in 2 to 4 hours and is complete by 6 to 8 hours. The onset of toxicity may occur at 1 to 4 hours after acute overdose but usually is delayed because lithium enters the brain slowly. Absorption of sustained-release preparations and the development of toxicity may be delayed 6 to 12 hours.

Volume distribution is 0.5 to 0.9 L/kg. Lithium is not protein bound. The half-life after a single dose is 9 to 13 hours; at steady state, it may be 30 to 58 hours. The renal handling of lithium is similar to that of sodium: glomerular filtration and reabsorption (80%) by the proximal renal tubule. Adequate sodium must be present to prevent lithium reabsorption. More than 90% of lithium is excreted by the kidney, 30% to 60% within 6 to 12 hours.

Manifestations
The examiner must distinguish between side effects, acute intoxication, acute or chronic toxicity, and chronic intoxications. Chronic is the most common and dangerous type of intoxication.

Side effects include fine tremor, gastrointestinal upset, hypothyroidism, polyuria and frank diabetes insipidus, dermatologic manifestations, and cardiac conduction deficits. Lithium is teratogenic.

Patients with acute poisoning may be asymptomatic, with an early high serum lithium concentration of 9 mEq/L, and deteriorate as the serum lithium concentration falls by 50% and the lithium distributes to the brain and the other tissues. Nausea and vomiting may occur within 1 to 4 hours, but the systemic manifestations are usually delayed several more hours. It may take as long as 3 to 5 days for serious symptoms to develop. Acute toxicity and acute on chronic toxicity are manifested by neurologic findings, including weakness, fasciculations, altered mental state, myoclonus, hyperreflexia, rigidity, coma, and convulsions with limbs in hypertension. Cardiovascular effects are nonspecific and occur at therapeutic doses, flat T or inverted T waves, atrioventricular block, and prolonged QT interval. Lithium is not a primary cardiotoxin. Cardiogenic shock occurs secondary to CNS toxicity. Chronic intoxication is associated with manifestations at lower serum lithium concentrations. There is some correlation with manifestations, especially at higher serum lithium concentrations. Although the levels do not always correlate with the manifestations, they are more predictive in cases of severe intoxication. A serum lithium concentration greater than 3.0 mEq/L with chronic intoxication and altered mental state indicates severe toxicity. Permanent neurologic sequelae can result from lithium intoxication.

Laboratory Investigations
Monitoring should include CBC (lithium causes significant leukocytosis), renal function, thyroid function (chronic intoxication), ECG, and electrolytes. Serum lithium concentrations should be determined every 2 to 4 hours until levels are close to therapeutic range. Cross-reactions with green-top Vacutainer specimen tubes containing heparin will spuriously elevate serum lithium concentration 6 to 8 mEq/L.

Management
Vital function must be established and maintained. Seizure precautions should be instituted and seizures, hypotension, and dysrhythmias treated. Evaluation should include examination for rigidity and hyperreflexia signs, hydration, renal function (BUN, creatinine), and electrolytes, especially sodium. The examiner should inquire about diuretic and other drug use that increase serum lithium concentration, and the patient must discontinue the drugs. If the patient is on chronic therapy, the lithium should be discontinued. Serial serum lithium concentrations should be obtained every 4 hours until serum lithium concentration peaks and there is a downward trend toward almost therapeutic range, especially in sustained-release preparations. Vital signs should be monitored, including temperature, and ECG and serial neurologic examinations should be undertaken, including mental status and urinary output. Nephrology consultation is warranted in case of a chronic and elevated serum lithium concentration (>2.5 mEq/L), a large ingestion, or altered mental state.

An intravenous line should be established and hydration and electrolyte balance restored. Serum sodium level should be determined before 0.9% saline fluid is administered in patients with chronic overdose because hypernatremia may be present from diabetes insipidus. Although current evidence supports an initial 0.9% saline infusion (200 mL/h) to enhance excretion of lithium, once hydration, urine output, and normonatremia are established, one should administer 0.45% saline and slow the infusion (100 mL/h) for all patients.

Gastric lavage is often not recommended in cases of acute ingestion because of the large size of the tablets, and it is not necessary after chronic intoxication. Activated charcoal is ineffective. For sustained-release preparations, whole-bowel irrigation may be useful but is not proven. Sodium polystyrene sulfonate (Kayexalate), an ion exchange resin, is difficult to administer and has been used only in uncontrolled studies. Its use is not recommended.

Hemodialysis is the most efficient method for removing lithium from the vascular compartment. It is the treatment of choice for patients with severe intoxication with an altered mental state, those with seizures, and anuric patients. Long runs are used until the serum lithium concentration is less than 1 mEq/L because of extensive re-equilibration. Serum lithium concentration should be monitored every 4 hours after dialysis for rebound. Repeated and prolonged hemodialysis may be necessary. A lag in neurologic recovery can be expected.

Disposition

An acute asymptomatic lithium overdose cannot be medically cleared on the basis of single lithium level. Patients should be admitted if they have any neurologic manifestations (altered mental status, hyperreflexia, stiffness, or tremor). Patients should be admitted to the intensive care unit if they are dehydrated, have renal impairment, or have a high or rising lithium level.

Methanol (Wood Alcohol, Methyl Alcohol)

The concentration of methanol in Sterno fuel is 4% and it contains ethanol, in windshield washer fluid it is 30% to 60%, and in gasoline antifreeze it is 100%.

Toxic Mechanism

Methanol is metabolized by alcohol dehydrogenase to formaldehyde, which is metabolized to formate. Formate inhibits cytochrome oxidase, producing tissue hypoxia, lactic acidosis, and optic nerve edema. Formate is converted by folate-dependent enzymes to carbon dioxide.

Toxic Dose

The minimal toxic amount is approximately 100 mg/kg. Serious toxicity in a young child can be produced by the ingestion of 2.5 to 5.0 mL of 100% methanol. Ingestion of 5-mL 100% methanol by a 10 kg child produces estimated peak blood methanol of 80 mg/dL. Ingestion of 15 mL 40% methanol was lethal for a 2-year-old child in one report. A fatal adult oral dose is 30 to 240 mL 100% (20 to 150 g). Ingestion of 6 to 10 mL 100% causes blindness in adults. The toxic blood concentration is greater than 20 mg/dL; very serious toxicity and potential fatality occur at levels greater than 50 mg/dL.

Kinetics

Onset of action can start within 1 hour but may be delayed up to 12 to 18 hours by metabolism to toxic metabolites. It may be delayed longer if ethanol is ingested concomitantly or in infants. Peak blood methanol concentration is 1 hour. Volume distribution is 0.6 L/kg (total body water).

For metabolism, see *Toxic Mechanism*.

Elimination is through metabolism. The half-life of methanol is 8 hours; with ethanol blocking it is 30 to 35 hours; and with hemodialysis 2.5 hours.

Manifestations

Metabolism creates a delay in onset for 12 to 18 hours or longer if ethanol is ingested concomitantly. Initial findings are as follows:

- 0 to 6 hours: Confusion, ataxia, inebriation, formaldehyde odor on breath, and abdominal pain can be present, but the patient may be asymptomatic. Note: Methanol produces an osmolal gap (early), and its metabolite formate produces the anion gap metabolic acidosis (see later). Absence of osmolar or anion gap does not always exclude methanol intoxication.
- 6 to 12 hours: Malaise, headache, abdominal pain, vomiting, visual symptoms, including hyperemia of optic disc, "snow vision," and blindness can be seen.

- More than 12 hours: Worsening acidosis, hyperglycemia, shock, and multiorgan failure develop, with death from complications of intractable acidosis and cerebral edema.

Laboratory Investigation

Methanol can be detected on some chromatography drug screens if specified. Methanol and ethanol levels, electrolytes, glucose, BUN, creatinine, amylase, and ABG should be monitored every 4 hours. Formate levels correlate more closely than blood methanol concentration with severity of intoxication and should be obtained if possible.

Management

One should protect the airway by intubation to prevent aspiration and administer assisted ventilation as needed. If needed, 100% oxygen can be administered. A nephrologist should be consulted early regarding the need for hemodialysis.

Gastrointestinal decontamination procedures have no role.

Metabolic acidosis should be treated vigorously with sodium bicarbonate 2 to 3 mEq/kg intravenously. Large amounts may be needed.

Antidote therapy is initiated to inhibit metabolism if the patient has a history of ingesting more than 0.4 mL/kg of 100% with the following conditions:

- Blood methanol level is greater than 20 mg/dL
- The patient has osmolar gap not accounted for by other factors
- The patient is symptomatic or acidotic with increased anion gap and/or hyperemia of the optic disc.

The ethanol or fomepizole therapy outlined below can be used.

Ethanol Therapy. Ethanol should be initiated immediately if fomepizole is unavailable (see *Fomepizole Therapy*). Alcohol dehydrogenase has a greater affinity for ethanol than ethylene glycol. Therefore, ethanol blocks the metabolism of ethylene glycol.

Ethanol should be administered intravenously (oral administration is less reliable) to produce a blood ethanol concentration of 100 to 150 mg/dL. The loading dose is 10 mL/kg of 10% ethanol administered intravenously concomitantly with a maintenance dose of 10% ethanol at 1.0 mL/kg/h. This dose may need to be increased to 2 mL/kg/h in patients who are heavy drinkers. The blood ethanol concentration should be measured hourly and the infusion rate should be adjusted to maintain a concentration of 100 to 150 mg/dL.

Fomepizole Therapy. Fomepizole (Antizol, 4-methylpyrazole) inhibits alcohol dehydrogenase more reliably than ethanol and it does not require constant monitoring of ethanol levels and adjustment of infusion rates. Fomepizole is available in 1 g/mL vials of 1.5 mL. The loading dose is 15 mg/kg (0.015 mL/kg) IV, maintenance dose is 10 mg/kg (0.01 mL/kg) every 12 hours for 4 doses, then 15 mg/kg every 12 hours until the ethylene glycol levels are less than 20 mg/dL. The solution is prepared by being mixed with 100 mL of 0.9% saline or D_5W. Fomepizole can be given to patients requiring hemodialysis but should be dosed as follows:

Dose at the beginning of hemodialysis:
- If less than 6 hours since last Antizol dose, do not administer dose
- If more than 6 hours since last dose, administer next scheduled dose

Dosing during hemodialysis:
- Dose every 4 hours

Dosing at the time hemodialysis is completed:
- If less than 1 hour between last dose and end dialysis, do not administer dose at end of dialysis
- If 1 to 3 hours between last dose and end dialysis, administer one half of next scheduled dose
- If more than 3 hours between last dose and end dialysis, administer next scheduled dose

Maintenance dosing off hemodialysis:
- Give the next scheduled dose 12 hours from the last dose administered

Hemodialysis increases the clearance of both methanol and formate 10-fold over renal clearance. A blood methanol concentration greater than 50 mg/dL has been used as an indication for hemodialysis, but recently some toxicologists from the New York City Poison Center recommended early hemodialysis in patients with blood methanol concentration greater than 25 mg/dL because it may be able to shorten the course of intoxication if started early. One should continue to monitor methanol levels and/or formate levels every 4 hours after the procedure for rebound. Other indications for early hemodialysis are significant metabolic acidosis and electrolyte abnormalities despite conventional therapy and if visual or neurologic signs or symptoms are present.

A serum formate level greater than 20 mg/dL has also been used as a criterion for hemodialysis, although this is often not readily available through many laboratories. If hemodialysis is used, the infusion rate of 10% ethanol should be increased 2.0 to 3.5 mL/kg/h. The blood ethanol concentration and glucose level should be obtained every 2 hours.

Therapy is continued with both ethanol and hemodialysis until the blood methanol level is undetectable, there is no acidosis, and the patient has no neurologic or visual disturbances. This may require several days.

Hypoglycemia is treated with intravenous glucose. Doses of folinic acid (Leucovorin) and folic acid have been used successfully in animal investigations to enhance formate metabolism to carbon dioxide and water. Leucovorin 1 mg/kg up to 50 mg IV is administered every 4 hours for several days.

An initial ophthalmologic consultation and follow-up are warranted.

Disposition
All patients who have ingested significant amounts of methanol should be referred to the emergency department for evaluation and blood methanol concentration measurement. Ophthalmologic follow-up of all patients with methanol intoxications should be arranged.

Monoamine Oxidase Inhibitors
Nonselective monoamine oxidase inhibitors (MAOIs) include the hydrazines phenelzine (Nardil) and isocarboxazid (Marplan), and the nonhydrazine tranylcypromine (Parnate). Furazolidone (Furoxone) and pargyline (Eutonyl)[2] are also considered nonselective MAOIs. Moclobemide,[2] which is available in many countries but not the United States, is a selective MAO-A inhibitor. MAO-B inhibitors include selegiline (Eldepryl), an antiparksonism agent, which does not have similar toxicity to MAO-A and is not discussed. Selectivity is lost in an overdose. MAOIs are used to treat severe depression.

Toxic Mechanism
Monoamine oxidase enzymes are responsible for the oxidative deamination of both endogenous and exogenous catecholamines such as norepinephrine. MAO-A in the intestinal wall also metabolizes tyramine in food. MAOIs permanently inhibit MAO enzymes until a new enzyme is synthesized after 14 days or longer. The toxicity results from the accumulation, potentiation, and prolongation of the cate-cholamine action followed by profound hypotension and cardiovascular collapse.

Toxic Dose
Toxicity begins at 2 to 3 mg/kg and fatalities occur at 4 to 6 mg/kg. Death has occurred after a single dose of 170 mg of tranylcypromine in an adult.

Kinetics
Structurally, MAOIs are related to amphetamines and catecholamines. The hydrazine peak levels are at 1 to 2 hours; metabolism is hepatic acetylation; and inactive metabolites are excreted in the

urine. For the nonhydrazines, peak levels occur at 1 to 4 hours, and metabolism is via the liver to active amphetamine-like metabolites.

The onset of symptoms in a case of overdose is delayed 6 to 24 hours after ingestion, peak activity is 8 to 12 hours, and duration is 72 hours or longer. The peak of MAO inhibition is in 5 to 10 days and lasts as long as 5 weeks.

Manifestations
Manifestations of an acute ingestion overdose of MAO-A inhibitors are as follows:

Phase I. An adrenergic crisis occurs, with delayed onset for 6 to 24 hours, and may not reach peak until 24 hours. The crisis starts as hyperthermia, tachycardia, tachypnea, dysarthria, transient hypertension, hyperreflexia, and CNS stimulation.

Phase II. Neuromuscular excitation and sympathetic hyperactivity occur with increased temperature greater than 40°C (104°F), agitation, hyperactivity, confusion, fasciculations, twitching, tremor, masseter spasm, muscle rigidity, acidosis, and electrolyte abnormalities. Seizures and dystonic reactions may occur. The pupils are mydriatic, sometimes nonreactive with "ping-pong gaze."

Phase III. CNS depression and cardiovascular collapse occur in cases of severe overdose as the catecholamines are depleted. Symptoms usually resolve within 5 days but may last 2 weeks.

Phase IV. Secondary complications occur, including rhabdomyolysis, cardiac dysrhythmias, multiorgan failure, and coagulopathies.

Biogenic interactions usually occur while the patient is on therapeutic doses of MAOI or shortly after they are discontinued (30 to 60 minutes), before the new MAO enzyme is synthesized. The following substances have been implicated: indirect acting sympathomimetics such as amphetamines, serotonergic drugs, opioids (e.g., meperidine, dextromethorphan), tricyclic antidepressants, specific serotonin reuptake inhibitors (SSRIs; e.g., fluoxetine [Prozac], sertraline [Zoloft], paroxetine [Paxil]), tyramine-containing foods (e.g., wine, beer, avocados, cheese, caviar, chocolate, chicken liver), and L-tryptophan. SSRIs should not be started for at least 5 weeks after MAOIs have been discontinued.

In mild cases, usually caused by foods, headache and hypertension develop and last for several hours. In severe cases, malignant hypertension and severe hyperthermia syndromes consisting of hypertension or hyperthermia, altered mental state, skeletal muscle rigidity, shivering (often beginning in the masseter muscle), and seizures may occur.

The serotonin syndrome, which may be a result of inhibition of serotonin metabolism, has similar clinical findings to those of malignant hyperthermia and may occur with or without hyperthermia or hypertension.

Chronic toxicity clinical findings include tremors, hyperhidrosis, agitation, hallucinations, confusion, and seizures and may be confused with withdrawal syndromes.

Laboratory Investigations
Monitoring of the ECG, cardiac monitoring, CPK, ABG, pulse oximeter, electrolytes, blood glucose, and acid-base balance should be maintained.

Management
In the case of MAOI overdose, ipecac-induced emesis should not be used. Only activated charcoal alone should be used.

If the patient is admitted to the hospital and is well enough to eat, a nontyramine diet should be ordered.

Extreme agitation and seizures can be controlled with benzodiazepines and barbiturates. Phenytoin is ineffective. Nondepolarizing neuromuscular blockers (not depolarizing succinylcholine) may be needed in severe cases of hyperthermia and rigidity. If the patient has severe hypertension (catecholamine mediated), phentolamine (Regitine), a parenteral β-blocking agent, 3 to 5 mg intravenously, or labetalol (Normodyne), a combination of an α-blocking agent and a β-blocker, 20-mg intravenous bolus, should be given. If malignant hypertension with rigidity is present, a short-acting nitroprusside and benzodiazepine can be used. Hypertension is often followed by severe hypotension, which

---

[2]Not available in the United States.

should be managed by fluid and vasopressors. *Caution:* Vasopressor therapy should be administered at lower doses than usual because of exaggerated pharmacologic response. Norepinephrine is preferred to dopamine, which requires release of intracellular amines.

Cardiac dysrhythmias are treated with standard therapy but are often refractory, and cardioversion and pacemakers may be needed.

For malignant hyperthermia, dantrolene (Dantrium), a nonspecific peripheral skeletal relaxing agent, is administered, which inhibits the release of calcium from the sarcoplasm. Dantrolene is reconstituted with 60 mL sterile water without bacteriostatic agents. Glass equipment must not be used, and the drug must be protected from light and used within 6 hours. Loading dose is 2 to 3 mg/kg intravenously as a bolus, and the loading dose is repeated until the signs of malignant hyperthermia (tachycardia, rigidity, increased end-tidal CO_2, and temperature) are controlled. Maximum total dose is 10 mg/kg to avoid hepatotoxicity.

When malignant hyperthermia has subsided, 1 mg/kg IV is given every 6 hours for 24 to 48 hours, then orally 1 mg/kg every 6 hours for 24 hours to prevent recurrence. There is a danger of thrombophlebitis following peripheral dantrolene, and it should be administered through a central line if possible. In addition one should administer external cooling and correct metabolic acidosis and electrolyte disturbances. Benzodiazepine can be used for sedation. Dantrolene does not reverse central dopamine blockade; therefore, bromocriptine mesylate (Parlodel) 2.5 to 10 mg should be given orally or through a nasogastric tube three times a day.

Rhabdomyolysis and myoglobinuria are treated with fluids. Urine alkalinization should also be treated.

Hemodialysis and hemoperfusion are of no proven value.

Biogenic amine interactions are managed symptomatically, similar to cases of overdose. For the serotonin syndrome cyproheptadine (Periactin), a serotonin blocker, 4 mg orally every hour for three doses, or methysergide (Sansert), 2 mg orally every 6 hours for three doses, should be considered. The effectiveness of these drugs has not been proven.

Disposition

All patients who have ingested more than 2 mg/kg of an MAOI should be admitted to the hospital for 24 hours of observation and monitoring in the intensive care unit because the life-threatening manifestations may be delayed. Patients with drug or dietary interactions that are mild may not require admission if symptoms subside within 4 to 6 hours and the patients remain asymptomatic. Patients with symptoms that persist or require active intervention should be admitted to the intensive care unit.

Opioids (Narcotic Opiates)

Opioids are used for analgesia, as antitussives, and as antidiarrheal agents and are illicit agents (heroin, opium) used in substance abuse. Tolerance, physical dependency, and withdrawal may develop.

Toxic Mechanism

At least four main opioid receptors have been identified. The μ receptor is considered the most important for central analgesia and CNS depression. The κ and δ receptors predominate in spinal analgesia. The σ receptors may mediate dysphoria. Death is a consequence of dose-dependent CNS respiratory depression or secondary to pulmonary aspiration or noncardiac pulmonary edema. The mechanism of noncardiac pulmonary edema is unknown.

Dextromethorphan can interact with MAOIs, causing severe hyperthermia, and may cause the serotonin syndrome (see *Selective Serotonin Reuptake Inhibitors*). Dextromethorphan inhibits the metabolism of norepinephrine and serotonin and blocks the reuptake of serotonin. It is found as a component of a large number of non-prescription cough and cold remedies.

Toxic Dose

The toxic dose depends on the specific drug, route of administration, and degree of tolerance. For therapeutic and toxic doses, see Table 24. In children, respiratory depression has been produced by 10 mg of morphine or methadone, 75 mg of meperidine, and 12.5 mg of diphenoxylate. Infants younger than 3 months of age

TABLE 24   Doses and Onset and Duration of Action of Common Opioids

DRUG	ADULT ORAL DOSE	CHILD ORAL DOSE	ONSET OF ACTION	DURATION OF ACTION	ADULT FATAL DOSE
Camphored tincture of opium	25 mL	0.25–0.50 mL/kg (0.4 mg/mL)	15–30 min	4–5 h	NA
Codeine	30–180 mg	0.5–1 mg/kg	15–30 min	4–6 h	800 mg
	>1 mg/kg is toxic in a child, above 200 mg in adult >5 mg/kg fatal in a child				
Dextromethorphan	15 mg 10 mg/kg is toxic	0.25 mg/kg	15–30 min	3–6 h	NA
Diacetylmorphine; street heroin is less than 10% pure	60 mg	NA	15–30 min	3–4 h	100 mg
Diphenoxylate atropine (Lomotil)	5–10 mg	NA	120–240 min	14 h	300 mg
	7.5 mg is toxic in a child, 300 mg is toxic in adult				
Fentanyl (Duragesic)	0.1–0.2 mg	0.001–0.002 mg/kg	7–8 min	Intramuscular: ½–2 h	1.0 mg
Hydrocodone with APAP (Lortab)	5–30 mg	0.15 mg/kg	30 min	3–4 h	100 mg
Hydromorphone (Dilaudid)	4 mg	0.1 mg/kg	15–30 min	3–4 h	100 mg
Meperidine (Demerol)	100 mg	1–1.5 mg/kg	10–45 min	3–4 h	350 mg
Methadone (Dolophine)	10 mg	0.1 mg/kg	30–60 min	4–12 h	120 mg
Morphine	10–60 mg	0.1–0.2 mg/kg	<20 min	4–6 h	200 mg
	Oral dose is 6 times parenteral dose, MS Contin sustained-release prep				
Oxycodone APAP (Percocet)	5 mg	NA	15–30 min	4–5 h	NA
Pentazocine (Talwin)	50–100 mg	NA	15–30 min	3–4 h	NA
Propoxyphene (Darvon)	65–100 mg	NA	30–60 min	2–4 h	700 mg

are more susceptible to respiratory depression. The dose should be reduced by 50%.

Kinetics

Oral onset of analgesic effect of morphine is 10 to 15 minutes; the action peaks in 1 hour and lasts 4 to 6 hours. With sustained-release preparations, the duration is 8 to 12 hours. Opioids are 90% metabolized in the liver by hepatic conjugation and 90% excreted in the urine as inactive compounds. Volume distribution is 1 to 4 L/kg. Protein binding is 35% to 75%. The typical plasma half-life of opiates is 2 to 5 hours, but that of methadone is 24 to 36 hours. Morphine metabolites include morphine-3-glucuronide (inactive) and morphine-6-glucuronide (active) and normorphine (active). Meperidine (Demerol) is rapidly hydrolyzed by tissue esterases into the active metabolite normeperidine, which has twice the convulsant activity of meperidine. Heroin (diacetylmorphine) is deacetylated within minutes to 6-monacetylmorphine and morphine. Propoxyphene (Darvon) has a rapid onset of action, and death has occurred within 15 to 30 minutes after a massive overdose. Propoxyphene is metabolized to norpropoxyphene, an active metabolite with convulsive, cardiac dysrhythmic, and heart block properties. Symptoms of diphenoxylate overdose appear within 1 to 4 hours. It is metabolized into the active metabolite difenoxin, which is five times more active as a regular respiratory depressant agent. Death has been reported in children after ingestion of a single tablet.

Manifestations

Initially, mild intoxication produces miosis, dull face, drowsiness, partial ptosis, and "nodding" (head drops to chest then bobs up). Larger amounts produce the classic triad of miotic pupils (exceptions below), respiratory depression, and depressed level of consciousness (flaccid coma). The blood pressure, pulse, and bowel activity are decreased.

Dilated pupils do not exclude opioid intoxication. Some exceptions to the miosis effect include dextromethorphan (paralyzes iris), fentanyl, meperidine, and diphenoxylate (rarely). Physiologic disturbances including acidosis, hypoglycemia, hypoxia, and post-ictal state, or a co-ingestant may also produce mydriasis.

Usually, the muscles are flaccid, but increased muscle tone can be produced by meperidine and fentanyl (chest rigidity). Seizures are rare but can occur with ingestion of codeine, meperidine, propoxyphene, and dextromethorphan. Hallucinations and agitation have been reported.

Pruritus and urticaria are caused by histamine release by some opioids or by sulfite additives.

Noncardiac pulmonary edema may occur after an overdose, especially with intravenous heroin abuse. Cardiac effects include vasodilation and hypotension. A heart murmur in an intravenous addict suggests endocarditis. Propoxyphene can produce delayed cardiac dysrhythmias.

Fentanyl is 100 times more potent than morphine and can cause chest wall muscle rigidity. Some of its derivatives are 2000 times more potent than morphine.

Laboratory Investigations

For patients with overdose, one should obtain and monitor ABG, blood glucose, and electrolyte levels; chest radiographs; and ECG. For drug abusers, one should consider testing for hepatitis B, syphilis, and HIV antibody (HIV testing usually requires consent). Blood opioid concentrations are not useful. They confirm diagnosis (morphine therapeutic dose, 65 to 80 ng/mL; toxic, <200 ng/mL), but are not useful for making a therapeutic decision. Cross-reactions can occur with Vick's Formula 44, poppy seeds, and other opioids (codeine and heroin are metabolized to morphine). Naloxone 4 mg IV was not associated with a positive enzyme multiplied immunoassay technique urine screen at 60 minutes, 6 hours, or 48 hours.

Management

Supportive care should be instituted, particularly an endotracheal tube and assisted ventilation. Temporary ventilation can be provided by a bag-valve mask with 100% oxygen. The patient should be placed on a cardiac monitor, have intravenous access established, and have specimens for ABG, glucose, electrolytes, BUN, and creatinine levels, CBC, coagulation profile, liver function, toxicology screen, and urinalysis taken.

For gastrointestinal decontamination, emesis should not be induced, but activated charcoal can be administered if bowel sounds are present.

If it is suspected that the patient is an addict, he or she should be restrained first and then 0.1 mg of naloxone (Narcan) should be administered. The dose should be doubled every 2 minutes until the patient responds or 10 to 20 mg has been given. If the patient is not suspected to be an addict, then 2 mg every 2 to 3 minutes to total of 10 to 20 mg is administered.

It is essential to determine whether there is a complete response to naloxone (mydriasis, improvement in ventilation), because it is a diagnostic therapeutic test. A continuous naloxone infusion may be appropriate, using the "response dose" every hour. Repeat doses of naloxone may be necessary because the effects of many opioids can last much longer than naloxone does (30 to 60 minutes). Methadone ingestions may require a naloxone infusion for 24 to 48 hours. Half of the response dose may need to be repeated in 15 to 20 minutes, after the infusion has been started.

Acute iatrogenic withdrawal precipitated by the administration of naloxone to a dependent patient should not be treated with morphine or other opioids. Naloxone's effects are limited to 30 to 60 minutes (shorter than most opioids) and withdrawal will subside in a short time.

Nalmefene (Revex), an FDA-approved long-acting (4 to 8 hours) pure opioid antagonist, is being investigated, but its role in cases of acute intoxication is unclear and it could produce prolonged withdrawal. It may have a role in place of naloxone infusion.

Noncardiac pulmonary edema does not respond to naloxone, and the patient needs intubation, assisted ventilation, positive end-expiratory pressure, and hemodynamic monitoring. Fluids should be given cautiously in patients with opioid overdose because opioids stimulate the antidiuretic hormone.

If the patient is comatose, 50% glucose (3% to 4% of comatose opioid overdose patients have hypoglycemia) and thiamine should be given prior to naloxone. If the patient has seizures that are unresponsive to naloxone, one administers diazepam and examines for metabolic (hypoglycemia, electrolyte disturbances) causes and structural disturbances.

Hypotension is rare and should direct a search for another etiology. If the patient is agitated, hypoxia and hypoglycemia must be excluded before opioid withdrawal is considered as a cause. Complications to consider include urinary retention, constipation, rhabdomyolysis, myoglobinuria, hypoglycemia, and withdrawal.

Disposition

If a patient responds to intravenous naloxone, careful observation for relapse and the development of pulmonary edema is required, with cardiac and respiratory monitoring for 6 to 12 hours. Patients requiring repeated doses of naloxone or an infusion, or those who develop pulmonary edema, require intensive care unit admission and cannot be discharged from the intensive care unit until they are symptom free for 12 hours. Intravenous overdose complications are expected to be present within 20 minutes after injection, and discharge after 4 symptom-free hours has been recommended. Adults with oral overdose have delayed onset of toxicity and require 6 hours of observation. Children with oral opioid overdose should be admitted to the hospital for observation because of delayed toxicity. Some toxicologists advise restraining a patient who attempts to sign out against medical advice after treatment with naloxone, at least until the patient receives psychiatric evaluation.

Organophosphates and Carbamates

Cholinergic intoxication sources are insecticides (organophosphates or carbamates), some medications, and some mushrooms. Examples of organophosphate insecticides are malathion (low toxicity, median lethal dose [LD_{50}] 2800 mg/kg), chlorpyrifos, which has been removed from market (moderate toxicity), and parathion (high toxicity, LD$_{50}$ 2 mg/kg). Carbamate insecticides include carbaryl (low toxicity, LD$_{50}$ 500 mg/kg), propoxur (moderate toxicity, LD$_{50}$ 95 mg/kg), and aldicarb (high toxicity, LD$_{50}$ 0.9 mg/kg). Pharmaceuticals with carbamate properties include neostigmine (Prostigmin) and physostigmine (Antilirium). Cholinergic compounds also include the "G" nerve war weapons tabun (GA), sarin (GB), soman (GB), and venom X (VX).

Toxic Mechanism

Organophosphates phosphorylate the active site on red cell acetylcholinesterase and pseudocholinesterase in the serum, neuromuscular and parasympathetic neuroeffector junctions, and in the major synapses of the autonomic ganglia, causing irreversible inhibition. There are two types of organophosphate intoxication: (a) direct action by the parent compound (e.g., tetraethylpyrophosphate), or (b) indirect action by the toxic metabolite (e.g., parathoxon or malathoxon).

Carbamates (esters of carbonic acid) cause reversible carbamylation of the active site of the enzymes. When a critical amount, greater than 50%, of cholinesterase is inhibited, acetylcholine accumulates and causes transient stimulation at cholinergic synapses and sympathetic terminals (muscarinic effect), the somatic nerves, the autonomic ganglia (nicotinic effect), and CNS synapses. Stimulation of conduction is followed by inhibition of conduction.

The major differences between the carbamates and the organophosphates are as follows: (a) carbamate toxicity is less and the duration is shorter; (b) carbamates rarely produce overt CNS effects (poor CNS penetration); (c) carbamate inhibition of the acetylcholinesterase enzyme is reversible and activity returns to normal rapidly; (d) pralidoxime, the enzyme regenerator, may not be necessary in the management of mild carbamate intoxication (e.g., carbaryl).

Toxic Dose

Parathion's minimum lethal dose is 2 mg in children and 10 to 20 mg in adults. The lethal dose of malathion is greater than 1375 mg/kg and that of chlorpyrifos is 25 g; the latter compound is unlikely to cause death.

Kinetics

Absorption is by all routes. The onset of acute ingestion toxicity occurs as early as 3 hours, usually before 12 hours and always before 24 hours. Lipid-soluble agents absorbed by the dermal route (e.g., fenthion) may have a delayed onset of more than 24 hours. Inhalation toxicity occurs immediately after exposure. Massive ingestion can produce intoxication within minutes.

Metabolism is via the liver. With some pesticides (e.g., parathion, malathion), the effects are delayed because they undergo hepatic microsomal oxidative metabolism to their toxic metabolites, the oxons (e.g., paroxon, malaoxon).

The half-life of malathion is 2.89 hours and that of parathion is 2.1 days. The metabolites are eliminated in the urine and the presence of p-nitrophenol in the urine is a clue up to 48 hours after exposure.

Manifestations

Many organophosphates produce a garlic odor on the breath, in the gastric contents, or in the container. Diaphoresis, excessive salivation, miosis, and muscle twitching are helpful clues to diagnosis.

Early, a cholinergic (muscarinic) crisis develops that consists of parasympathetic nervous system activity. DUMBELS is the mnemonic for defecation, cramps, and increased bowel motility; urinary incontinence; miosis (mydriasis may occur in 20%); bronchospasm and bronchorrhea; excess secretion; lacrimation; and seizures. Bradycardia, pulmonary edema, and hypotension may be present.

Later, sympathetic and nicotinic effects occur, consisting of MATCH: muscle weakness and fasciculation (eyelid twitching is often present), adrenal stimulation and hyperglycemia, tachycardia, cramps in muscles, and hypertension. Finally, paralysis of the skeletal muscles ensues.

The CNS effects are headache, blurred vision, anxiety, ataxia, delirium and toxic psychosis, convulsions, coma, and respiratory depression. Cranial nerve palsies have been noted. Delayed hallucinations may occur.

Delayed respiratory paralysis and neurologic and neurobehavioral disorders have been described following certain organophosphate ingestions or dermal exposure. The "intermediate syndrome" is paralysis of proximal and respiratory muscles developing 24 to 96 hours after the successful treatment of organophosphate poisoning. A delayed distal polyneuropathy has been described with ingestion of certain organophosphates, such as triorthocresyl phosphate, bromoleptophos, and methomidophos.

Complications include aspiration, pulmonary edema, and acute respiratory distress syndrome.

Laboratory Investigations

Monitoring should include chest radiograph, blood glucose (nonketotic hyperglycemia is frequent), ABG, pulse oximetry, ECG, blood coagulation status, liver function, hyperamylasemia (pancreatitis reported), and urinalysis for the metabolite alkyl phosphate paranitrophenol. Blood should be drawn for red blood cell cholinesterase determination before pralidoxime is given. The red blood cell cholinesterase activity roughly correlates with clinical severity. Mild poisoning is 20% to 50% of normal, moderate poisoning is 10% to 20% of normal, and severe poisoning is 10% of normal (>90% depressed). A postexposure rise of 10% to 15% in the cholinesterase level determined at least 10 to 14 days after the exposure confirms the diagnosis.

Management

Protection of health care personnel with clothing (masks, gloves, gowns, goggles) and respiratory equipment or hazardous material suits, as necessary, is called for. General decontamination consists of isolation, bagging, and disposal of contaminated clothing and other articles. Vital functions should be established and maintained. Cardiac and oxygen saturation monitoring are needed. Intubation and assisted ventilation may be needed. Secretions should be suctioned until atropinization drying is achieved.

Dermal decontamination involves prompt removal of clothing and cleansing of all affected areas of skin, hair, and eyes. Ocular decontamination involves irrigation with copious amounts of tepid water or 0.9% saline for at least 15 minutes. Gastrointestinal decontamination, if the ingestion was recent, involves the administration of activated charcoal.

Atropine sulfate can be given as an antidote. It is both a diagnostic and a therapeutic agent. Atropine counteracts the muscarinic effects but is only partially effective for the CNS effects (seizures and coma). Preservative-free atropine (no benzyl alcohol) should be used. If the patient is symptomatic (bradycardia or bronchorrhea), a test dose should be administered, 0.02 mg/kg in children or 1 mg in adults, intravenously. If no signs of atropinization are present (tachycardia, drying of secretions, and mydriasis), atropine should be administered immediately, 0.05 mg/kg in children or 2 mg in adults, every 5 to 10 minutes as needed to dry the secretions and clear the lungs. Beneficial effects are seen within 1 to 4 minutes and maximum effect in 8 minutes. The average dose in the first 24 hours is 40 mg, but 1000 mg or more has been required in severe cases. Glycopyrrolate (Robinul) can be used if atropine is not available. The maximum dose should be maintained for 12 to 24 hours, then tapered and the patient observed for relapse. Poisoning, especially with lipophilic agents (e.g., fenthion, chlorfenthion), may require weeks of atropine therapy. An alternative is a continuous infusion of atropine 8 mg in 100 mL 0.9% saline at rate of 0.02 to 0.08 mg/kg/h (0.25 to 1.0 mL/kg/h) with additional 1 to 5 mg boluses as needed to dry the secretions.

Pralidoxime chloride (Protopam) has both antinicotinic and antimuscarinic effects and possibly also CNS effects. Successful treatment with pralidoxime chloride may allow a reduction in the dose of atropine. Pralidoxime acts to reactivate the phosphorylated cholinesterases by binding the phosphate moiety on the esteritic site and displacing it. It should be given early before "aging" of phosphate bond produces tighter binding. However, recent reports indicate that pralidoxime chloride is beneficial even several days after the poisoning. Improvement is seen within 10 to 40 minutes. The initial dose of pralidoxime chloride is 1 to 2 g in 250 mL 0.89% saline over 5 to 10 minutes, maximum 200 mg/minute, in adults or 25 to 50 mg/kg, maximum 4 mg/kg/minute, in children younger than 12 years of age. The dose can be repeated every 6 to 12 hours for several days. An alternative is a continuous infusion of 1 g in 100 mL 0.89% saline at 5 to 20 mg/kg/h (0.5 to 12 mL/g/h) up to 500 mg/h and titrated to desired response. Maximum adult daily dose is 12 g. Cardiac and blood pressure monitoring are advised during and for several hours after the infusion. The end point is absence of fasciculations and return of muscle strength.

Contraindicated drugs include morphine, aminophylline, barbiturates, opioids, phenothiazine, reserpine-like drugs, parasympathomimetics, and succinylcholine.

Noncardiac pulmonary edema may require respiratory support. Seizures may respond to atropine and pralidoxime chloride but often require anticonvulsants. Cardiac dysrhythmias may require electrical cardioversion or antidysrhythmic therapy if the patient is hemodynamically unstable. Extracorporeal procedures are of no proven value.

Disposition
Asymptomatic patients with normal examination findings after 6 to 8 hours of observation may be discharged. In cases of intentional poisoning, the patients require psychiatric clearance for discharge. Symptomatic patients should be admitted to the intensive care unit. Observation of milder cases of carbamate poisoning, even those requiring atropine, for 6 to 8 hours symptom-free may be sufficient to exclude significant toxicity. In cases of workplace exposure, OSHA should be notified.

Phencyclidine (Angel Dust)
Phencyclidine is an arylcyclohexylamine related to ketamine and chemically related to the phenothiazines. Originally a "dissociative" anesthetic banned in United States since 1979, it is now an illicit substance, with at least 38 analogs. It is inexpensively manufactured by "kitchen chemists" and is mislabeled as other hallucinogens. Improper phencyclidine synthesis may release cyanide when heated or smoked and can cause explosions.

Toxic Mechanism
The mechanism of phencyclidine is complex and not completely understood. It inhibits some neurotransmitters and causes a loss of pain sensation without depressing the CNS respiratory status. It stimulates α-adrenergic receptors and may act as a "false neurotransmitter." The effects are sympathomimetic, cholinergic, and cerebellar.

Toxic Dose
The usual dose of phencyclidine mixed with marijuana joints is 100 to 400 mg of phencyclidine. Joints or leaf mixtures contain 0.24% to 7.9% of PCP, 1 mg of PCP/150 leaves. Tablets contain 5 mg (the usual street dose). CNS effects at doses of 1 to 6 mg include hallucinations and euphoria, 6 to 10 mg produces toxic psychosis and sympathetic stimulation, 10 to 25 mg produces severe toxicity, and more than 100 mg has resulted in fatalities.

Kinetics
Phencyclidine is a lipophilic weak base, with a pKa of 8.5 to 9.5. It is rapidly absorbed when smoked and snorted, poorly absorbed from the acid stomach, and rapidly absorbed from the alkaline middle small intestine. It has an enterogastric secretion and is reabsorbed in the small intestine. The onset of action when smoked is 2 to 5 minutes, with a peak in 15 to 30 minutes. With oral ingestion, the onset is in 30 to 60 minutes and when taken intravenously it is immediate. Most adverse reactions in cases of overdose begin within 1 to 2 hours. Its duration of action at low doses is 4 to

6 hours and normality returns in 24 hours; in large overdoses, fluctuating coma may last 6 to 10 days.

Volume distribution is 6.2 L/kg. Phencyclidine concentrates in brain and adipose tissue. Protein binding is 70%. The route of elimination is by gastric secretion, liver metabolism, and 10% urinary excretion of conjugates and free phencyclidine. Renal excretion may be increased 50% with urinary acidification. The half-life is 1 hour (in cases of overdose, it is 11 to 89 hours).

Manifestations
The classic picture is bursts of horizontal, vertical, and rotary nystagmus, which is a clue to diagnosis (occurs in 50% of cases), miosis, hypertension, and fluctuating altered mental state. There is a wide spectrum of clinical presentations.

Mild intoxication with 1 to 6 mg produces drunken and bizarre behavior, agitation, rotary nystagmus, and blank stare. Violent behavior and sensory anesthesia make these patients insensitive to pain, self-destructive, and dangerous. Most are communicative within 1 to 2 hours, are alert and oriented in 6 to 8 hours, and recover completely in 24 to 48 hours.

Moderate intoxication with 6 to 10 mg produces excess salivation, hypertension, hyperthermia, muscle rigidity, myoclonus, and catatonia. Recovery of consciousness occurs in 24 to 48 hours and complete recovery in 1 week.

Severe intoxication with 10 to 25 mg results in opisthotonus, decerebrate rigidity, convulsions, prolonged fluctuating coma, and respiratory failure. Patients in this category have a high rate of medical complications. Recovery of consciousness occurs in 24 to 48 hours, with complete normality in a month. Medical complications include apnea, aspiration pneumonia, cardiac arrest, hypertensive encephalopathy, hyperthermia, intracerebral hemorrhage, psychosis, rhabdomyolysis and myoglobinuria, and seizures. Loss of memory and "flashbacks" last for months. Phencyclidine-induced depression and suicide have been reported.

Fatalities occur with ingestions of greater than 100 mg and with serum levels greater than 100 to 250 ng/mL.

Laboratory Investigations
Marked elevation of creatine kinase level may occur. Values greater than 20,000 units have been reported. Urinalysis should be monitored and urine tested for myoglobin. One should monitor the blood for creatine kinase, uric acid (an early clue to rhabdomyolysis), BUN, creatinine, electrolytes (hyperkalemia), blood glucose (20% of patients have hypoglycemia), urinary output, liver function tests, ECG, and ABG if the patient has any respiratory manifestations. Measurement of phencyclidine in the gastric juice is called for because concentrations are 10 to 50 times higher than in blood or urine. Phencyclidine blood concentrations are not helpful. Phencyclidine may be detected in the urine of the average user for 10 days to 3 weeks after the last dose. In chronic users, it can be detected for over 1 month. The analogs of phencyclidine may not produce positive test results for phencyclidine in the urine. Cross-reactions with bleach and dextromethorphan may cause false-positive urine test results on immunoassay, and cross-reaction with doxylamine may produce a false-positive finding on gas chromatography.

Management
The patient should be observed for violent, self-destructive, bizarre behavior and paranoid schizophrenia. Patients should be placed in a low sensory environment and dangerous objects should be removed from the area.

Gastrointestinal decontamination is not effective because phencyclidine is rapidly absorbed from intestines. Overtreating the mild intoxication should be avoided. There is insufficient evidence to support the use of MDAC. In cases of severe toxicity (stupor or coma), continuous gastric suction can be tried (with protection of the airway) because the drug is secreted into the gastric juice. The value of this procedure is controversial because of limited data.

The patient must be protected from harming himself or herself or others. Physical restraints may be necessary, but they should be used sparingly and for the shortest time possible because they increase risk of rhabdomyolysis. Metal restraints such as handcuffs should be avoided. For behavioral disorders and toxic psychosis, diazepam is the agent of choice. Pharmacologic intervention includes diazepam (Valium) 10 to 30 mg orally or 2 to 5 mg intravenously initially and titrated upward to 10 mg; however, up to 30 mg may be required. "Talk down" technique is usually ineffective and dangerous. Phenothiazines and butyrophenones should be avoided in the acute phase because they lower the convulsive threshold; however, they may be needed later for psychosis. Haloperidol (Haldol) administration has been reported to produce catatonia.

Seizures and muscle spasm are managed with diazepam, from 2.5 mg up to 10 mg. Hyperthermia (>38.5°C [101.3°F]) is treated with external cooling measures. Hypertension is usually transient and does not require treatment. In the case of emergent hypertensive crisis (blood pressure >200/115 mm Hg) nitroprusside can be used in a dose of 0.3 to 2 μg/kg/min. Maximum infusion rate is 10 μg/kg/min for only 10 minutes.

Acid ion trapping diuresis is not recommended because of the danger of myoglobin precipitation in the renal tubules. Rhabdomyolysis and myoglobinuria are treated by correcting volume depletion and insuring a urinary output of greater than 2 mL/kg/h. Alkalinization is controversial because of reabsorption of phencyclidine.

Hemodialysis is beneficial if renal failure occurs; otherwise, the extracorporeal procedures are not beneficial.

Disposition
All patients with coma, delirium, catatonia, violent behavior, aspiration pneumonia, sustained hypertension greater than 200/115, and significant rhabdomyolysis should be admitted to the intensive care unit until asymptomatic for at least 24 hours. If patients with mild intoxication are mentally and neurologically stable and become asymptomatic (except for nystagmus) for 4 hours, they may be discharged in the company of a responsible adult. All patients must be assessed for suicide risk before discharge. Drug counseling and psychiatric follow-up should be arranged. Patients should be warned that episodes of disorientation and depression may continue intermittently for 4 weeks or more.

Phenothiazines and Nonphenothiazines (Neuroleptics)
Toxic Mechanism
Neuroleptics have complex mechanisms of toxicity, including (a) block of the postsynaptic dopamine receptors; (b) block of peripheral and central α-adrenergic receptors; (c) block of cholinergic muscarinic receptors; (d) quinidine-like antidysrhythmic and myocardial depressant effect in cases of large overdose; (e) lowering of the convulsive threshold; (f) effect on hypothalamic temperature regulation (Table 25).

Toxic Dose
Extrapyramidal reactions, anticholinergic effects, and orthostatic hypotension may occur at therapeutic doses. The toxic amount is not established, but the maximum daily therapeutic dose may result in significant side effects, and twice this amount may be potentially fatal. Chlorpromazine (Thorazine), the prototype, may produce serious hypotension and CNS depression at doses greater than 200 mg (17 mg/kg) in children and 3 to 5 g in an adult. Fatalities have been reported after 2.5 g of loxapine (Loxitane) and mesoridazine (Serentil) and 1.5 g of thioridazine (Mellaril).

Kinetics
These agents are lipophilic and have unpredictable gastrointestinal absorption. Peak levels occur 2 to 6 hours postingestion and have enterohepatic recirculation.

The mean serum half-life in phase 1 is 1 to 2 hours and the biphasic half-life is 20 to 40 hours. Volume distribution is 10 to 40 L/kg; protein binding is 92% to 98%. Chlorpromazine taken orally has an onset of action in 30 to 60 minutes, peak in 2 to 4 hours, and duration of 4 to 6 hours. With sustained-release preparations, the onset is in 30 to 60 minutes and duration is 6 to 12 hours.

Elimination is by hepatic metabolism, which results in multiple metabolites (some are active). Metabolites can be detected in urine months after chronic therapy. Only 1% to 3% is excreted unchanged in the urine.

TABLE 25 Neuroleptics and Properties

COMPOUND	ANTIPSYCHOTIC	ANTICHOLINERGIC	EXTRAPYRAMIDAL	HYPOTENSIVE AND CARDIOTOXIC	SEDATIVE
Phenothiazine					
Aliphatic Chlorpromazine (Thorazine) Promethazine (Phenergan)	1+	3+	2+	2+	3+
Piperazine Fluphenazine (Prolixin) Perphenazine (Trilafon) Prochlorperazine (Compazine) Trifluoperazine (Stelazine)	3+	1+	3+	1+	1+
Piperidine Mesoridazine (Serentil) Thioridazine (Mellaril)	1+	2+	1+	3+	3+
Nonphenothiazine					
Butyrophenone Haloperidol (Haldol)	3+	1+	3+	1+	1+
Dibenzoxazepine Loxapine (Loxitane)	3+	1+	3+	1+	2+
Dihydroindolone Molindone (Moban)	3+	1+	3+	1+	1+
Thioxanthenes Thiothixene (Navane) Chlorprothixene (Taractan)	3+	1+	3+	3+	1+

1+ = very low activity; 2+ = moderate activity; 3+ = very high activity.

Manifestations

In cases of phenothiazine overdose, anticholinergic symptoms may be present early but are not life-threatening. Miosis is usually present (80%) if the phenothiazine has strong α-adrenergic blocking effect (e.g., chlorpromazine), but anticholinergic activity mydriasis may occur. Agitation and delirium rapidly progress into coma. Major problems are cardiac toxicity and hypotension. The cardiotoxic effects are seen more commonly with thioridazine and its metabolite mesoridazine. These agents have produced the largest number of fatalities in patients with phenothiazine overdose. Cardiac conduction disturbances include prolonged PR, QRS, and QTc intervals, U- and T-wave abnormalities, and ventricular dysrhythmias, including torsades de pointes. Seizures occur mainly in patients with convulsive disorders or with administration of loxapine. Sudden death in children and adults has been reported.

Idiosyncratic dystonic reactions are most common with the piperidine group. Reactions are not dose-dependent and consist of opisthotonos, torticollis, orolingual dyskinesia, or oculogyric crisis (painful upward gaze). These reactions are more frequent in children and women. Neuroleptic malignant syndrome occurs in patients on chronic therapy and is characterized by hyperthermia, muscle rigidity, autonomic dysfunction, and altered mental state. There is one case reported with acute overdose. The loxapine syndrome consists of seizures, rhabdomyolysis, and renal failure.

Laboratory Investigations

Monitoring should include arterial blood gases, renal and hepatic function, electrolytes, blood glucose, and creatine kinase and myoglobinemia in neuroleptic malignant syndrome. Most of these agents are detected on routine screening. Quantitative serum levels are not useful in management. Cross-reactions with enzyme multiplied immunoassay technique tests occur with cyclic antidepressants. Phenothiazines give false-negative results on pregnancy urine tests using human chorionic gonadotropin as an indicator, and give false-positive results for urine porphyrins, indirect Coombs test, urobilinogen, and amylase.

Management

Vital functions must be established and maintained. All overdose patients require venous access, 12-lead ECG (to measure intervals), cardiac and respiratory monitoring, and seizure precautions. One should monitor core temperature to detect poikilothermic effect. If the patient is comatose, intubation and assisted ventilation may be required, as well as 100% oxygen, intravenous glucose, naloxone (Narcan), and thiamine.

Emesis is not recommended. Activated charcoal can be administered if ingestion was within 1 hour. MDAC has not been proven beneficial. A radiograph of the abdomen may be useful, if the phenothiazine is radiopaque. Haloperidol (Haldol) and trifluoperazine (Stelazine) are most likely to be radiopaque. Whole-bowel irrigation may be useful when a large number of pills are visualized on radiograph or if sustained-release preparations were taken, but whole-bowel irrigation has not been evaluated in patients with phenothiazine overdose.

Convulsions are treated with diazepam or lorazepam (Ativan). Loxapine (Loxitane) overdose may result in status epilepticus. If nondepolarizing neuromuscular blockade is required, pancuronium (Pavulon) or vecuronium (Norcuron) should be used (not succinyl-choline [Anectine], which may cause malignant hyperthermia), and EEG should be monitored during paralysis.

Patients with dysrhythmias should be monitored with serial ECGs. Unstable rhythms can be treated with electrical cardioversion. Class 1a antidysrhythmics (procainamide, quinidine, and disopyramide [Norpace]) must be avoided.

Hypokalemia predisposes to dysrhythmias and should be corrected aggressively. Supraventricular tachycardia with hemodynamic instability is treated with electrical cardioversion. The role of adenosine has not been defined. Calcium channel and β-blockers should be avoided.

Prolongation of the QRS interval is treated with sodium bicarbonate 1 to 2 mEq/kg by intravenous bolus over a few minutes.

Torsades de pointes is treated with magnesium sulfate IV 20% solution 2 g over 2 to 3 minutes. If there is no response in 10 minutes, the dose is repeated and followed by a continuous infusion of 5 to 10 mg/minute or given as an infusion of 50 mg/minute for 2 hours followed by 30 mg/minute for 90 minutes twice a day for several days, as needed. The dose in children is 25 to 50 mg/kg initially and maintenance dose is 30 to 60 mg/kg per 24 hours (0.25 to 0.50 mEq/kg per 24 hours) up to 1000 mg per 24 hours. Serum magnesium levels should be monitored.

To treat ventricular tachydysrhythmias in a stable patient, lidocaine is used. If the patient is unstable, electrical cardioversion is used. Patients with heart block with hemodynamic instability should be managed with temporary cardiac pacing.

Hypotension is treated with the Trendelenburg position and 0.9% saline. If the condition is refractory to treatment or there is a danger of fluid overload, vasopressors are administered. The vasopressor of choice is α-adrenergic agonist norepinephrine (Levophed), titrated to response. Epinephrine and dopamine should not be used because β-receptor stimulation in the presence of α-receptor blockade may provoke dysrhythmias and phenothiazines are antidopaminergic.

Hypothermia and hyperthermia are treated with external warming and cooling measures, respectively. Antipyretic drugs must not be used.

Management of the neuroleptic malignant syndrome includes the following actions:

- Immediately discontinuing the offending agent
- Hyperventilating the patient, using 100% humidified, cooled oxygen at high gas flows (at least 10 L/min) because of rapid breathing
- Administering a benzodiazepine to control convulsions and facilitate cooling measures
- Initiating appropriate mechanical cooling measures, which may include intravenous cold saline (not lactated Ringer's), ice baths, cold lavage of the stomach, bladder, and rectum, and a hypothermic blanket
- Correcting acid-base and electrolyte disturbances and treating significant hyperkalemia with hyperventilation, calcium, sodium bicarbonate, intravenous glucose, and insulin; hemodialysis may be necessary

In addition, dysrhythmias usually respond to correction of the underlying acid-base disturbances and hyperkalemia. If antidysrhythmic agents are required, calcium channel blockers must be avoided because they may precipitate hyperkalemia and cardiovascular collapse. Dantrolene sodium (Dantrium), which is a phenytoin derivative, inhibits calcium release from the sarcoplasmic reticulum and results in decreased muscle contraction. Dantrolene acts peripherally and does not reverse the rigidity or psychomotor disturbances resulting from the central dopamine blockade; it therefore is often used in combination with bromocriptine. Bromocriptine mesylate (Parlodel) acts centrally as a dopamine agonist, as does amantadine hydrochloride (Symmetrel). Bromocriptine and dantrolene have been reported to be successful in combination with cooling and good supportive measures in malignant hyperthermia.

Dosing for these agents is as follows: dantrolene sodium at 2 to 3 mg/kg IV as a bolus, then 1 mg/kg/minute to a maximum of 10 mg/kg or until the tachycardia, rigidity, increased end-tidal CO_2, and temperature elevation are controlled. *Note:* Hepatotoxicity occurs with doses greater than 10 mg/kg. To prevent symptom recurrence, 1 mg/kg should be administered every 6 hours for 24 to 48 hours after the episode. After that time, oral dantrolene can be used at a dose of 1 mg/kg every 6 hours for 24 hours as necessary. The patient should be observed for thrombophlebitis following intravenous dantrolene. It is best administered via a central line. Bromocriptine mesylate at 2.5 to 10 mg orally or via a nasogastric tube, three times a day, should be used in combination with dantrolene.

Idiosyncratic dystonic reaction can be treated with diphenhydramine (Benadryl) 1 to 2 mg/kg/dose intravenously over 5 minutes up to maximum of 50 mg intravenously; a response is noted within 2 to 5 minutes. This can be followed with oral doses for 4 to 6 days to prevent recurrence.

Extracorporeal measures (hemodialysis, hemoperfusion) are not effective in removing these agents.

Disposition

Asymptomatic patients should be observed for at least 6 hours after gastric decontamination. Symptomatic patients with cardiotoxicity, hypotension, and convulsions should be admitted to the intensive care unit and monitored for 48 hours.

Salicylates (Acetylsalicylic Acid, Salicylic Acid)

Toxic Mechanism

The primary toxic mechanisms include (a) direct stimulation of the medullary chemoreceptor trigger zone and respiratory center; (b) uncoupling oxidative phosphorylation; (c) inhibition of the Krebs cycle enzymes; (d) inhibition of vitamin K dependent and independent clotting factors; (e) alteration of platelet function; and (f) inhibition of prostaglandin synthesis.

Toxic Dose

Acute mild intoxication occurs at a dose of 150 to 200 mg/kg, moderate intoxication at 200 to 300 mg/kg, and severe intoxication at 300 to 500 mg/kg. Acute salicylate plasma concentration greater than 30 mg/dL (usually >40 mg/dL) may be associated with clinical toxicity. Chronic intoxication occurs at ingestions greater than 100 mg/kg/d for more than 2 days because of accumulation kinetics. Methyl salicylate (oil of wintergreen) is the most toxic form of salicylate. A dose of 1 mL of 98% contains 1.4 g of salicylate. Fatalities have occurred with ingestion of 1 teaspoonful in children and 1 ounce in adults. It is found in topical ointments and liniments (18% to 30%).

Kinetics

Acetylsalicylic acid and salicylic acid are weak acids with a pKa of 3.5 and 3.0, respectively. Acetylsalicylic acid is absorbed from the stomach, from the small bowel, and dermally. Onset of action is within 30 minutes. Methyl salicylate and effervescent tablets are absorbed more rapidly. Salicylate plasma concentration is detectable within 15 minutes after ingestion and peaks in 30 to 120 minutes. The peak may be delayed 6 to 12 hours in cases of large overdose, overdose with enteric-coated or sustained release preparations, and development of concretions. The therapeutic duration of action is 3 to 4 hours but is markedly prolonged in cases of overdose.

Volume distribution is 0.13 L/kg for salicylic acid but increases as the salicylate plasma concentration increases. Protein binding is greater than 90% for salicylic acid at pH 7.4 and a salicylate plasma concentration of 20 to 30 mg/dL, 75% at a salicylate plasma concentration greater than 40 mg/dL, 50% at a salicylate plasma concentration of 70 mg/dL, and 30% at a salicylate plasma concentration of 120 mg/dL.

The half-life for salicylic acid is 3 hours after a 300 mg dose, 6 hours after a 1 g overdose, and greater than 10 hours after a 10-g overdose. Elimination includes Michaelis-Menten hepatic metabolism by three saturable pathways: (a) glycine conjugation to salicyluric acid (75%); (b) glucuronyl transferase to salicyl phenol glucuronide (10%); and (c) salicyl aryl glucuronide (4%). Nonsaturable pathways are hydrolysis to gentisic acid (<1%). Ten percent is excreted unchanged.

Acidosis increases the severity of the intoxication by increasing the non-ionized salicylate that can cross membranes and enter the brain cells. In kidneys, the unionized salicylic acid undergoes glomerular filtration, and the ionized portion undergoes tubular secretion in proximal tubules and passive reabsorption in the distal tubules. Renal excretion of salicylate is enhanced by alkaline urine.

Manifestations

The ingestion of concentrated topical salicylic acid preparations (e.g., wart remover) can cause mucosal caustic injury to the gastrointestinal tract. Occult salicylate overdose should be considered in any patient with unexplained acid-base disturbance.

The manifestations of acute overdose of salicylates are as follows:

Minimal Symptoms. Tinnitus, dizziness, and deafness may occur at high therapeutic salicylate plasma concentrations of 20 to 30 mg/dL. Nausea and vomiting may occur immediately because of local gastric irritation.

Phase I. Mild manifestations occur at 1 to 12 hours after ingestion with a 6-hour salicylate plasma concentration of 45 to 70 mg/dL. Nausea and vomiting followed by hyperventilation are usually present within 3 to 8 hours after acute overdose. Hyperventilation, an increase in both rate (tachypnea) and depth (hyperpnea), is present but it may be subtle. It results in a mild respiratory alkalosis with a serum pH greater than 7.4 and urine pH greater than 6.0. Some patients may have lethargy, vertigo, headache, and confusion. Diaphoresis may be noted.

Phase II. Moderate manifestations occur at 12 to 24 hours after ingestion with a 6-hour salicylate plasma concentration of 70 to 90 mg/dL. Serious metabolic disturbances, including a marked respiratory alkalosis with anion gap metabolic acidosis, dehydration, and urine pH less than 6.0, may occur. Other metabolic disturbances include hypoglycemia or hyperglycemia, hypokalemia, decreased ionized calcium, and increased BUN, creatinine, and lactate. Mental disturbances (confusion, disorientation, hallucinations) may occur. Hypotension and convulsions have been reported.

Phase III. Severe intoxication occurs more than 24 hours after ingestion with a 6-hour salicylate plasma concentration of 90 to 130 mg/dL. In addition to the above clinical findings, coma and seizures develop and indicate severe intoxication. Pulmonary edema may occur. Metabolic disturbances include metabolic acidemia (pH <7.4) and aciduria (pH <6.0). In adults, alkalosis may persist until terminal respiratory failure.

In children younger than 4 years of age, a mixed metabolic acidosis and respiratory alkalosis develop earlier (within 4 to 6 hours) than in adults because children have less respiratory reserve and accumulate lactate and other organic acids. Hypoglycemia is more common in children.

Fatalities occur at 6-hour salicylate plasma concentrations greater than 130 to 150 mg/dL and result from CNS depression, cardiovascular collapse, electrolyte imbalance, and cerebral edema.

Chronic salicylism is more serious than acute intoxication and the 6-hour salicylate plasma concentration does not correlate well with the manifestations in both acute and chronic cases of intoxication. Chronic intoxication usually occurs with therapeutic errors in young children or the elderly with underlying illness, and the diagnosis is delayed because it is not recognized. Noncardiac pulmonary edema is a frequent complication in the elderly. The mortality rate is about 25%. Chronic salicylate poisoning in children may mimic Reye syndrome. It is associated with exaggerated CNS findings (hallucinations, delirium, dementia, memory loss, papilledema, bizarre behavior, agitation, encephalopathy, seizures, and coma). Hemorrhagic manifestations, renal failure, and pulmonary and cerebral edema may occur. The metabolic picture is hypoglycemia and mixed acid-base derangements. A chronic salicylate plasma concentration greater than 60 mg/dL with metabolic acidosis and an altered mental state is very serious.

Laboratory Investigations

All patients with intentional salicylate overdoses should have acetaminophen plasma level measured after 4 hours.

One should continuously monitor ECG, urine output, urine pH, and specific gravity. Every 2 to 4 hours in cases of severe intoxication, salicylate plasma concentration, glucose (in a case of salicylism, CNS hypoglycemia may be present despite normal serum glucose), electrolytes, ionized calcium, magnesium and phosphorus, anion gap, ABGs, and pulse oximeter should be monitored. Daily monitoring of BUN, creatinine, liver function tests, and prothrombin time should take place.

The therapeutic salicylate plasma concentration is less than 10 mg/dL for analgesia and 15 to 30 mg/dL for antiinflammatory effect. Cross-reaction with diflunisal (Dolobid) will give a falsely high salicylate plasma concentration. The Done nomogram is not considered accurate in evaluating acute or chronic salicylate intoxications.

Management

Treatment is based on clinical and metabolic findings, not on salicylate levels. Continuous monitoring of the urine pH is essential for successful alkalinization treatment. One should always obtain an acetaminophen plasma level.

Vital functions must be established and maintained. If the patient is in an altered mental state, glucose, naloxone, and thiamine are administered in standard doses. Depending on the severity, the initial studies include an immediate and a 6-hour postingestion salicylate plasma concentration, ECG and cardiac monitoring, pulse oximeter, urine (analysis, pH, and specific gravity), chest radiograph, ABGs, blood glucose, electrolytes and anion gap calculation, calcium (ionized), magnesium, renal and liver profiles, and prothrombin time. Gastric contents and stool should be tested for occult blood. Bismuth and magnesium salicylate preparations may be radiopaque on radiographs. Consultation with a nephrologist is warranted in cases of moderate, severe, or chronic intoxication.

For gastrointestinal decontamination, activated charcoal is useful (each gram of activated charcoal binds 550 mg of salicylic acid) if a toxic dose was ingested up to 4 hours postingestion. MDAC is not recommended for salicylate intoxication.

Concretions may occur with massive (usually >300 mg/kg) ingestions. If blood levels fail to decline, prompt contrast radiography of the stomach may reveal concretions that have to be removed by repeated lavage, whole-bowel irrigation, endoscopy, or gastrostomy.

Fluids and electrolyte treatment of salicylate poisonings is given in Table 26. For shock, perfusion and vascular volume should be established with 5% dextrose in 0.9% saline, then the treatment can proceed with correction of dehydration and alkalinization.

For cases of acute moderate or severe salicylism (see Table 26), adults should receive a bolus of 1 to 2 mEq/kg of sodium bicarbonate ($NaHCO_3$) followed by an infusion of 100 to 150 mEq $NaHCO_3$ added to 500 to 1000 mL of 5% dextrose and administered over 60 minutes. Children should receive a bolus of 1 to 2 mEq/kg of $NaHCO_3$ followed by an infusion of 1 to 2 mEq/kg added to 20 mL/kg of 5% dextrose administered over 60 minutes. Potassium is added after the patient voids. The goal is to achieve a urine output of greater than 2 mL/kg/hr and a urine pH of greater than 8. The initial infusion is followed by subsequent infusions (two to three times normal maintenance) of 200 to 300 mL/h in adults or 10 mL/kg/h in children. If the patient is acidotic and has a serum pH of less than 7.15, an additional 1 to 2 mEq/kg of $NaHCO_3$ is given over 1 to 2 hours; persistent acidosis may

require 1 to 2 mEq/kg of bicarbonate every 2 hours. The infusion rate, the amount of bicarbonate, and the electrolytes should be adjusted to correct serum abnormalities and to maintain the targeted urine output and urinary pH. Diuresis is not as important as the alkalinization. Careful monitoring for fluid overload should take place for patients at risk of pulmonary and cerebral edema (e.g., the elderly) and because of inappropriate secretion of the antidiuretic hormone.

In patients with mild intoxication who are not acidotic and have a urine pH greater than 6, 5% dextrose in 0.45% saline should be administered as maintenance to replace ongoing fluid loss. Some toxicologists may consider adding sodium bicarbonate 50 mEq/L or 1 mEq/kg in some cases.

To achieve alkalinization, sodium bicarbonate is administered to produce a serum pH 7.4 to 7.5 and a urine pH greater than 8. Carbonic anhydrase inhibitors (acetazolamide [Diamox]) should not be used. If the patient is acidotic, additional bicarbonate may be required. About 2 mEq/kg raises the blood pH 0.1. In children, alkalinization may be a difficult problem because of the organic acid production and hypokalemia. Hypokalemic and fluid-depleted patients cannot be adequately alkalinized. Alkalinization is usually discontinued in asymptomatic patients with a salicylate plasma concentration less than 30 to 40 mg/dL but is continued in symptomatic patients regardless of the salicylate plasma concentration. A decreased serum bicarbonate but normal or high blood pH indicates respiratory alkalosis predominating over metabolic acidosis, and the bicarbonate should be administered cautiously. An alkalemic pH of 7.40 to 7.50 is not a contraindication to bicarbonate therapy because these patients have a significant base deficit in spite of elevated blood pH.

Potassium is added, 20 to 40 mEq/L, to the infusion after the patient voids. In cases of severe, late, and chronic salicylism, 60 mEq/L of potassium may be needed. When the serum potassium is below 4.0 mEq/L, 10 mEq/L should be added over the first hour. If the patient has hypokalemia less than 3 mEq/L and flat T waves and U waves, 0.25 to 0.5 mEq/kg up to 10 mEq/h is administered. Potassium should be administered under ECG monitoring. Serum potassium is rechecked after each rapidly administered dose. A paradoxical urine acidosis (alkaline serum pH and acid urine pH) indicates that potassium is probably needed.

Convulsions are treated with diazepam or lorazepam, but hypoglycemia, low ionized calcium, cerebral edema, and hemorrhage should first be excluded with a CT scan. If tetany develops, the $NaHCO_3$ therapy is discontinued and calcium gluconate 0.1 to 0.2 mL/kg 10% administered.

Pulmonary edema management consists of fluid restriction, high FiO_2, mechanical ventilation, and positive end-expiratory pressure.

Cerebral edema management consists of fluid restriction, elevation of the head, hyperventilation, osmotic diuresis, and

---

TABLE 26 Fluid and Electrolyte Treatment of Salicylate Poisoning

TYPE OF SALICYLISM	METABOLIC DISTURBANCE	BLOOD pH	URINE pH	HYDRATING SOLUTION	AMOUNT OF NAHCO₃ (mEq/L)	AMOUNT OF POTASSIUM (mEq/L)
Mild	Respiratory alkalosis	>7.4	>6.0	5% Dextrose, 0.45% saline	50 (adult) 1 mEq/kg (child)	20
Moderate Chronic Child <4 years	Respiratory alkalosis Metabolic acidosis	>7.4 or <7.4	<6.0	5% Dextrose in water	100 (adult) 1–2 mEq/kg (child)	40
Severe Chronic Child <4 years	Metabolic acidosis Respiratory alkalosis	<7.4	<6.0	5% Dextrose in water	150 (adult) 2 mEq/kg (child)	60
CNS Depressant Co-ingestant	Respiratory acidosis	<7.4	<6.0	5% Dextrose in water	100–150*	60

Modified from Linden CH, Rumack BH: The legitimate analgesics, aspirin and acetaminophen. In Hansen Jr W (ed): Toxic Emergencies. New York, Churchill Livingstone, 1984.
*Correct hypoventilation.

administration of dexamethasone. Vitamin K_1 is administered parenterally to correct an increased prothrombin time (>20 seconds) and coagulation abnormalities. If the patient has active bleeding, fresh plasma and platelets are administered as needed. Hyperpyrexia is managed by external cooling measures, not antipyretics.

Hemodialysis is the choice for removal of salicylates because it corrects the acid-base, electrolyte, and fluid disturbances as well. The indications for hemodialysis include the following:

- Acute poisoning with salicylate plasma concentration greater than 100 mg/dL without improvement after 6 hours of appropriate therapy
- Chronic poisoning with cardiopulmonary disease and a salicylate plasma concentration as low as 40 mg/dL with refractory acidosis, severe CNS manifestations (coma and seizures), and progressive deterioration, especially in elderly patients
- Impairment of vital organs of elimination
- Clinical deterioration in spite of good supportive care and alkalinization
- Severe refractory acid-base or electrolyte disturbances despite appropriate corrective measures

Disposition

There are limitations of salicylate plasma levels and patients are treated on the basis of clinical and laboratory findings. Patients who are asymptomatic should be monitored for a minimum of 6 hours, and longer if enteric-coated tablets or massive overdose was taken or if there is suspicion of concretions. Those who remain asymptomatic with a salicylate plasma concentration less than 35 mg/dL may be discharged following psychiatric evaluation, if indicated. Chronic salicylate-intoxicated patients with acidosis and an altered mental state should be admitted to the intensive care unit. Patients with acute ingestion and a salicylate plasma concentration less than 60 mg/dL and mild symptoms may be able to be treated in the emergency department. Patients with moderate and severe intoxications should be admitted to the intensive care unit.

Selective Serotonin Reuptake Inhibitors

Selective serotonin reuptake inhibitors (SSRIs) are primarily prescribed as antidepressants. SSRIs include fluoxetine (Prozac), paroxetine (Paxil), and sertraline (Zoloft).

Toxic Mechanism

The SSRIs interfere with the neuron reuptake of serotonin (5-hydroxytryptamine) at the presynaptic ganglia sites in the brain, increasing the activity of serotonin. SSRIs should not be used within 5 weeks of when a MAOI is given, nor should MAOI therapy be initiated or discontinued within 5 weeks of SSRI therapy.

Toxic Dose

The therapeutic oral dose of fluoxetine is 20 to 80 mg/d. No toxicity is seen in children with up to 3.5 mg/kg/dose orally. A fatal dose for adults is 6 g. The therapeutic dose for paroxetine is 20 to 50 mg/d. In 35 adult patients, none developed serious side effects after the ingestion of 10 to 1000 mg, and a study involving 35 children failed to demonstrate serious adverse effects at doses less than 180 mg. The therapeutic dose for sertraline is 50 mg to 200 mg/d. Patients have ingested up to 2.6 g without serious side effects. Overdose involving children who ingested less than 100 mg failed to cause adverse events.

Kinetics

Fluoxetine is well absorbed from the gastrointestinal tract, and has a peak plasma concentration at 6 to 8 hours. Volume distribution is 20 to 42 L/kg; 95% is protein bound. The half-life is 4 days (for the demethylated active metabolite norfluoxetine, the half-life is 7 to 15 days). Elimination is 80% renal. Fluoxetine and other serotonin inhibitors are inhibitors of the cytochrome P450, CYP 2D6 enzyme. Therefore interactions may occur with many other medications, such as antidysrhythmic class IC drugs (quinidine),

phenytoin (Dilantin), haloperidol, lithium, tricyclic antidepressants (TCAs), β-blockers, codeine, and carbamazepine (Tegretol).

Paroxetine is almost completely absorbed from the gastrointestinal tract, with a peak in 2 to 8 hours. Protein binding is greater than 90%; volume distribution is 13 L/kg. Paroxetine undergoes extensive first-pass liver metabolism by oxidation and methylation to inactive metabolites. It inhibits the P450 system (see fluoxetine metabolism). The average half-life is 21 hours.

Sertraline peaks in 8 to 12 hours. Its volume distribution is 20 L/kg and protein binding is 98%. The average half-life of sertraline is 26 hours. It is metabolized to form a less-active metabolite, N-desmethylsertraline (half-life of 62 to 104 hours).

Manifestations

All SSRIs may cause serotonin syndrome, a potentially life-threatening reaction, if they are administered concurrently with an MAOI. Serotonin syndrome is caused by cerebral serotonergic stimulation and can cause severe hyperthermia, myoclonus, rhabdomyolysis, confusion, tremors, and a variety of psychological disturbances. In addition, cardiovascular complications and extrapyramidal side effects, including akathisia, dyskinesia, and Parkinson-like syndromes may occur. Also, increased suicidal ideation, seizures, sexual disorders, and hematologic disorders (platelet serotonin activity blockade leading to prolonged bleeding times) may develop. Inappropriate secretion of antidiuretic hormone resulting in hyponatremia may occur when SSRIs are administered to the elderly. This effect is usually seen within the first week of therapy.

Overdose effects are similar to the serotonin syndrome.

Laboratory Investigations

One should obtain a complete blood count (CBC), electrolytes, glucose levels, a coagulation profile, liver function tests, creatine kinase level, and an ECG.

Management

There is no specific antidote to SSRI intoxication.

Initial management consists of stabilizing vital functions, including thermoregulation. Supportive therapy and anticipation of potential life-threatening manifestations (hypotension, hyperthermia, seizures, coma, disseminated intravascular coagulation, ventricular tachycardia, and metabolic acidosis), are essential. Vital signs, EEG, creatine kinase, and blood chemistry should be monitored.

Benzodiazepines are administered to prevent and control muscle hyperactivity (diazepam [Valium] for seizures, clonazepam [Klonopin] for myoclonus). If benzodiazepine therapy fails to control muscle activity or seizures, anesthesia or nondepolarizing neuromuscular blockade may be necessary.

Electrolyte abnormalities and acid-base balance should be corrected. Fluids are used to maintain a urine output of greater than 2 mL/kg/h if there is a risk of myoglobinuria.

There are no data to support the use of gastrointestinal decontamination, although activated charcoal may be used if an ingestion has occurred within 1 hour. Hemodialysis and charcoal hemoperfusion are unlikely to be beneficial. Haloperidol (Haldol), phenothiazines, and other highly protein-bound drugs are to be avoided.

Benzodiazepine and cooling therapy can be used for hyperthermia. Serotonin antagonists, such as cyproheptadine (Periactin), may be useful in treating serotonin syndrome, although there are no controlled data. Dantrolene (Dantrium) and bromocriptine (Parlodel) are not recommended and may actually precipitate serotonin syndrome.

Disposition

Cases of ingestions in children up to 5 years of age of less than 180 mg of paroxetine (Paxil), less than 3.5 mg/kg of fluoxetine (Prozac), or less than 100 mg of sertraline (Zoloft) can be observed at home. Symptomatic patients should be admitted to the intensive care unit until asymptomatic for 24 hours. Asymptomatic patients should be observed for 6 hours. All patients should be assessed for risk of suicide before discharge. When taken chronically, SSRIs may increase cholesterol and triglycerides and decrease uric acid, so these test results should be followed.

Theophylline

Theophylline (Slo-Phyllin) is a methylxanthine alkaloid similar to caffeine and theobromine. Aminophylline is 80% theophylline. Theophylline is used in the acute treatment of asthma, pulmonary edema, chronic obstructive pulmonary disease, and neonatal apnea.

Toxic Mechanism

The proposed mechanisms of action include phosphodiesterase inhibition, adenosine receptor antagonism, inhibition of prostaglandins, and increase in serum catecholamines. Theophylline stimulates the central nervous, respiratory, and emetic centers and reduces the seizure threshold. It has positive cardiac inotropic and chronotropic effects, acts as a diuretic, relaxes smooth muscle, and causes peripheral vasodilation but cerebral vasoconstriction. Gastric secretions, gastrointestinal motility, lipolysis, glycogenolysis, and gluconeogenesis are all increased.

Toxic Dose

A single dose of 1 mg/kg produces a theophylline plasma concentration of approximately 2 µg/mL. The therapeutic range usually is 10 to 20 µg/mL. An acute, single dose greater than 10 mg/kg causes mild toxicity, a dose greater than 20 mg/kg causes moderate toxicity, and a dose greater than 50 mg/kg causes serious, possibly fatal toxicity. Fatalities occur at lower doses in patients with chronic toxicity, especially those with risk factors (see *Kinetics*).

Kinetics

The pKa is 9.5. Absorption from the stomach and upper small intestine is complete and rapid, with onset in 30 to 60 minutes. Peak theophylline plasma concentration occurs within 1 to 2 hours after ingestion of liquid preparations, 2 to 4 hours after ingestion of regular tablets, and 7 to 24 hours after ingestion of slow-release formulations. Volume distribution is 0.3 to 0.7 L/kg. Protein binding is 40% to 60% in adults, mainly to albumin (low albumin increases free active theophylline).

Elimination is 90% by hepatic metabolism to an active metabolite, 2-methyl xanthine. The half-life is 3.5 hours in a child and 4 to 6 hours in an adult. The half-life is shorter in smokers and patients taking enzyme-inducing drugs. Only 8% to 10% of the drug is excreted unchanged in the urine.

Risk factors that produce a longer half-life include age younger than 6 months or older than 60 years, use of enzyme-inhibitor drugs (calcium channel blockers, oral contraceptives, cimetidine [Tagamet], ciprofloxacin [Cipro], erythromycin, macrolide antibiotics, isoniazid), illness (persistent fever >38.9°C [>102°F]), viral illness, liver impairment, heart failure, chronic obstructive pulmonary disease, and influenza vaccination.

Manifestations

Acute toxicity generally correlates with blood levels; chronic toxicity does not (Table 27).

In the case of an acute, single, regular-release overdose, vomiting and occasionally hematemesis occur at low theophylline plasma concentrations. CNS stimulation includes restlessness, muscle tremors, and protracted tonic–clonic seizures, but coma is rare. Convulsions are a sign of severe toxicity and usually are preceded by gastrointestinal symptoms (except with sustained-release and chronic intoxications). Cardiovascular disturbances include cardiac dysrhythmias (supraventricular tachycardia) and transient hypertension with mild overdoses, but hypotension and ventricular dysrhythmias with severe intoxications. Rhabdomyolysis and renal failure are occasionally seen. Children tolerate higher serum levels, and cardiac dysrhythmias and seizures occur at theophylline plasma concentrations greater than 100 µg/mL. Possible metabolic disturbances include hyperglycemia, pronounced hypokalemia, hypocalcemia, hypomagnesemia, hypophosphatemia, increased serum amylase, and elevation of uric acid.

TABLE 27 Theophylline Blood Concentrations and Acute Toxicity

PLASMA CONCENTRATION (µg/mL)	TOXICITY DEGREE	MANIFESTATIONS
8–10	None	Bronchodilation
10–20	Mild	Therapeutic range: nausea, vomiting, nervousness, respiratory alkalosis, tachycardia
15–25		35% have mild manifestations of toxicity
20–40	Moderate	Gastrointestinal complaints and central nervous system stimulation Transient hypertension, tachypnea, tachycardia; 80% will have some manifestations of toxicity
60–100	Severe	Convulsions, dysrhythmias Hypokalemia, hyperglycemia Ventricular dysrhythmias, protracted convulsions, hypotension, acid-base abnormalities

Reprinted and modified from Linden CH, Rumack BH: In Hansen Jr W (ed): Toxic Emergencies. New York, Churchill Livingstone, 1984. With permission from Elsevier.

Chronic intoxication, defined as multiple doses of theophylline over 24 hours, or cases in which interacting drugs or illness interfere with theophylline metabolism are more serious and difficult to treat. Cardiac dysrhythmias and convulsions may occur at theophylline plasma concentrations of 40 to 60 µg/mL and there is no correlation with TPC. The seizures occur without warning and are protracted and repetitive and may produce status epilepticus. Vomiting and typical metabolic disturbances do not occur.

Differences with slow-release preparations are that few or no gastrointestinal symptoms occur, peak concentrations and convulsions may be delayed 12 to 24 hours postingestion, and convulsions occur without warning.

Laboratory Investigations

Monitoring includes vital signs, pulse oximeter, ABG, hemoglobin, hematocrit (for gastrointestinal hemorrhage), ECG and cardiac monitor, renal and hepatic function, electrolytes, blood glucose, acid-base balance, and serum albumin. Gastric contents and stools should be tested for occult blood. Samples for theophylline plasma concentration measurement should be drawn within 1 to 2 hours after ingestion of liquid preparations, 2 to 4 hours after ingestion of regular-release formulations, and 4 hours after ingestion of slow-release formulations. One should check the serum albumin level because a decrease in albumin levels may cause manifestations of toxicity despite normal theophylline plasma concentration. A single theophylline plasma concentration reading may be misleading; therefore, theophylline plasma concentration measurement should be repeated every 2 to 4 hours to determine the trend until a declining trend is reached and then monitored every 4 to 6 hours until it is below 20 µg/mL.

Management

Vital functions must be established and maintained. If the patient is in a coma or has convulsions or vomiting, he or she should be intubated immediately. The theophylline plasma concentration is obtained and repeated every 2 to 4 hours to determine peak absorption, and a theophylline bezoar should be considered if the theophylline plasma concentration fails to decline. Consultation with a nephrologist about charcoal hemoperfusion is recommended.

Gastrointestinal decontamination is warranted in the case of an acute overdose, but emesis must not be induced. Activated charcoal is the choice decontamination procedure in a dose of 1 g/kg to all patients, followed with MDAC 0.5 g/kg every 2 to 4 hours until the theophylline plasma concentration is less than 20 µg/mL. MDAC is effective in treating acute, chronic, and intravenous overdoses. Activated charcoal shortens the half-life of theophylline by about 50% and may be indicated up to 24 hours following ingestion.

Whole-bowel irrigation with polyethylene-electrolyte solution has been recommended for cases of massive overdose, possible concretions, and ingestion of sustained-release preparations. If intractable vomiting occurs, the antiemetic metoclopramide (Reglan) (0.1 mg/kg adult dose), droperidol (Inapsine) (2.5 to 10 mg IV), or ondansetron (Zofran) (8 to 32 mg IV) is administered. Ondansetron, however, inhibits metabolism of theophylline after a few doses.

Convulsions are controlled with lorazepam (Ativan) or diazepam (Valium) and phenobarbital. Phenytoin (Dilantin) is ineffective. The convulsions in patients with chronic intoxication are often refractory and may require, in addition to anticonvulsants, neuromuscular paralyzing agents, sedation, assisted ventilation, and EEG monitoring.

Hypotension is treated with fluids and vasopressors, if necessary. Norepinephrine (Levophed) 0.05 µg/kg/minute is preferred as the vasopressor over dopamine.

Supraventricular tachycardia with hemodynamic instability requires cardioversion. Low-dose β-blockers may be used but should not be used in patients with reactive airway disease or hypotension. Adenosine (Adenocard) is ineffective. For ventricular dysrhythmias, electrolyte disturbances should be corrected. Lidocaine is the treatment of choice but has the potential to cause seizures at toxic concentrations. Cardioversion may be needed.

Hematemesis is managed with sucralfate (Carafate) 1 g four times daily and/or Maalox TC 30 mL every 2 hours and blood replacement, if necessary. H_2 antihistamine blockers that are enzyme inhibitors are not used.

Fluid and metabolic disturbances should be corrected. Hyperglycemia does not require insulin therapy. Hypokalemia should be corrected cautiously, as it may be largely an intracellular shift and not total body loss. Usually adding 40 mEq potassium to a liter of fluid will suffice. The serum potassium level must be monitored closely.

Charcoal hemoperfusion is the management of choice for patients with serious intoxications. Hemoperfusion can increase the clearance twofold to threefold over hemodialysis, but hemodialysis can be used if hemoperfusion is not available. Criteria for charcoal hemoperfusion are as follows:

- Life-threatening events such as convulsions or dysrhythmias
- Intractable vomiting refractory to antiemetics
- Acute intoxications with a theophylline plasma concentration greater than 80 µg/mL or greater than 70 µg/mL 4 hours after overdose with a sustained-release formulation and greater than 40 µg/mL in the case of chronic intoxication
- Acute or chronic overdoses with a theophylline plasma concentration greater than 40 µg/mL, especially if the patient has risk factors that lengthen the half-life of the drug (see Kinetics).

Disposition

Patients with mild symptoms and a theophylline plasma concentration less than 20 µg/mL can be treated in emergency department and discharged when asymptomatic for a few hours. Any patient with acute ingestion and a theophylline plasma concentration greater than 35 µg/mL should be admitted to a monitored bed with seizure precautions and suicide precautions, if needed. If neurologic or cardiotoxic effects or a theophylline plasma concentration greater than 50 µg/mL is present, the patient should be admitted to the intensive care unit. A patient with an overdose of a sustained-release preparation, regardless of symptoms or initial theophylline plasma concentration, requires admission, monitoring, activated charcoal, and MDAC. In patients on chronic therapy, toxicity

may occur at a lower theophylline plasma concentration, and these patients should not be discharged until they are asymptomatic for several hours.

Tricyclic and Cyclic Antidepressants

Historically, tricyclic antidepressants are an important cause of pharmaceutical overdose fatalities. The mortality rate was reduced from 15% in the 1970s to less than 1% in the 1990s because of a better understanding of the pathophysiology of these agents and improvements in management (Table 28).

Toxic Mechanism

The major mechanisms of toxicity of the tricyclic antidepressants are (a) central and peripheral anticholinergic effects; (b) peripheral α-adrenergic blockade; (c) quinidine-like cardiac membrane stabilizing action blockade of the fast inward sodium channels; and (d) inhibition of synaptic neurotransmitter reuptake in the CNS presynaptic neurons. The tetracyclics, monocyclic aminoketones, and dibenzoxazepines possess convulsive activity and less cardiac toxicity in overdose than the older tricyclic antidepressants. Triazolopyridine has less serious cardiac and CNS toxicity.

Toxic Dose

The therapeutic dose of imipramine (Tofranil) is 1.5 to 5 mg/kg; a dose greater than 5 mg/kg may be mildly toxic; 10 to 20 mg/kg may be life threatening, although less than 20 mg/kg has produced few fatalities; greater than 30 mg/kg carries a 30% mortality rate; and at a dose greater than 70 mg/kg, patients rarely survive. In children 375 mg and in adults as little as 500 mg have been fatal. In adults, five times the maximum daily dose is toxic and 10 times is potentially fatal. Although major overdose symptoms are associated with plasma concentrations greater than 1 µg/mL (>1000 ng/mL), plasma tricyclic levels do not correlate well with toxicity; clinical signs and symptoms should guide therapy.

The relative dosage or potency equivalents are as follows: amitriptyline (Elavil) 100 mg = amoxapine (Asendin) 125 mg = desipramine (Norpramin) 75 mg = doxepin (Sinequan) 100 mg = imipramine (Tofranil) 75 mg = maprotiline (Ludiomil) 75 mg = nortriptyline (Pamelor) 50 mg = trazodone (Desyrel) 200 mg. This allows one to determine an equivalent dosage of an agent compared with another (see Table 28).

Kinetics

The tricyclic and cyclic antidepressants are lipophilic. They are rapidly absorbed from the alkaline small intestine, but absorption may be prolonged and delayed in cases of massive overdose owing to anticholinergic action. Onset varies from less than 1 hour (30 to 40 minutes) to, rarely, 12 hours. The peak serum levels are reached in 2 to 8 hours and the peak effect is in 6 hours but may be delayed 12 hours because of erratic absorption. The clinical effects correlate poorly with plasma levels.

Cyclic antidepressants are highly protein-bound to plasma glycoproteins, 98% at a pH 7.5 and 90% at 7.0. Volume distribution is 10 to 50 L/kg. The elimination route is by hepatic metabolism. The tertiary amines are metabolized into active demethylated secondary amine metabolites. The active secondary amine metabolites undergo a 15% enterohepatic recirculation and are metabolized over a period of days into nonactive metabolites. The intestinal bacterial flora may reconstitute the metabolites, which are active.

The half-life varies from 10 hours for imipramine to 81 hours for amitriptyline and 100 hours for nortriptyline. The active metabolites have longer half-lives.

Only 3% of the ingested dose is excreted in the urine unchanged.

Manifestations

There are reports of asymptomatic patients who, upon arrival to an emergency department, suddenly have a seizure, develop hemodynamically unstable dysrhythmias, and die shortly thereafter

TABLE 28 — Cyclic Antidepressants: Daily Dose and Their Major Properties

GENERIC NAME (TRADE NAME)	ADULT DAILY DOSE (mg)	THERAPEUTIC RANGE (ng/mL)	HALF-LIFE (HOURS)	TOXICITY ANTICHOL	CNS	CARDIAC
Tertiary Amines						
Amitriptyline (Elavil)	75–300	120–250	31–46	3+	3+	3+
Imipramine (Tofranil)	75–300	125–250	9–24	3+	3+	2+
Doxepin (Sinequan)	75–300	30–150	8–24	3+	3+	2+
Trimipramine (Surmantil)	75–200	10–240	16–18	3+	3+	2+
Secondary Amines						
Nortriptyline (Pamelor)	75–150	50–150	18–93	2+	3+	3+
Desipramine (Norpramin)	75–200	75–160	14–62	1+	3+	3+
Protriptyline (Vivactil)	20–60	70–250	54–198	2+	3+	3+
Newer Cyclic Antidepressants						
Teracyclic			30–60	1+	2+	3+
Maprotiline (Ludiomil)	75–300	—	30–60	1+	2+	3+
Trizolopyridine, a noncyclic, produces less serious cardiac and CNS toxicity						
Trazodone (Desyrel)	50–600	700	4–7	1+	1+	1+
Monocyclic Aminoketones						
Bupropion (Wellbutrin)	200–400	—	8–24	1+	3+	1+
Dibenzazepine						
Clomipramine (Anafranil)	100–250	200–500	21–32	2+	2+	2+
Dibenoxazepine						
Amoxapine (Ascendin)	150–300	200–500	6–10	1+	3+	2+

Abbreviations: Antichol = anticholinergic effect; CNS = central nervous system effect primarily seizures; Cardiac = cardiac effect.
Other drugs with similar structures are cyclobenzaprine, a muscle relaxant (similar to amitriptyline), and carbamazepine, an anticonvulsant (similar to imipramine); however, they cause less cardiac toxicity.

from ingestion of a tricyclic antidepressant. Most patients with severe toxicity develop symptoms within 1 to 2 hours, but symptoms may be delayed 6 hours after overdose.

Small overdoses produce early anticholinergic effects, agitation, and transient hypertension, which are not life-threatening. Large overdoses produce depression of the CNS and myocardium, convulsions, and hypotension. Death can occur within the first 2 to 6 hours following ingestion.

Some ECG screening tools for predicting cardiac or neurologic toxicity from ingestion of a tricyclic antidepressant have been developed: (a) A QRS greater than 0.10 second may produce seizures, and if greater than 0.16 second, 50% of patients may develop ventricular dysrhythmias (20% of these may be life-threatening) and seizures; (b) a terminal 40 msec of the QRS axis greater than 120 degrees in the right frontal plane may be associated with toxicity; or (c) a large R wave greater than 3 mm in ECG lead aVR may predispose the patient to toxicity. The quinidine cardiac membrane stabilizing effect produces depression of myocardium, conduction, and ECG changes. The peripheral α-adrenergic blockade produces hypotension.

The secondary amines are metabolized to inactive metabolites. The tetracyclics produce a high incidence of cardiovascular disturbances and seizures. Monocyclic aminoketones produce seizures in doses greater than 600 mg. Dibenzoxazepines produce a syndrome of convulsions, rhabdomyolysis, and renal failure.

Laboratory Investigations
If the patient has altered mental status or ECG abnormalities, ABG, ECG, chest radiograph, blood glucose, serum electrolytes, calcium, magnesium, blood urea nitrogen, and creatinine levels, liver profile, creatine kinase level, urine output, and, in severe cases, hemodynamic monitoring are indicated. Levels of the tricyclic and cyclic antidepressants less than 300 ng/mL are therapeutic; levels greater than 500 ng/mL indicate toxicity, and levels greater than 1000 ng/mL indicate serious poisoning and are associated with QRS widening.

Management
Vital functions must be established and maintained. Even if the patient is asymptomatic, intravenous access should be established, vital signs and neurologic status monitored, and baseline 12-lead ECG and continuous cardiac monitoring obtained for at least 6 hours from admission or 8 to 12 hours postingestion. QRS interval should be measured on a limb lead ECG every 15 minutes for 6 hours postingestion.

For gastrointestinal decontamination, emesis should not be induced and gastric lavage should not be used. Activated charcoal is preferable. If the patient is in an altered mental state, the airway must be protected. Activated charcoal 1 g/kg is recommended up to 1 hour postingestion. Benefit from MDAC has not been demonstrated.

Alkalinization does not control seizures; diazepam or lorazepam should be used. Status epilepticus may require high-dose barbiturates or neuromuscular blockers with intravenous diazepam. If not successful, the patient can be paralyzed with short-term nondepolarizing neuromuscular blockers such as vecuronium (Norcuron), intubation, and assisted ventilation. A bolus of sodium bicarbonate is recommended as an adjunct to correct the acidosis produced by the seizures.

Sodium bicarbonate is administered in a dose of 1 to 2 mEq/kg undiluted as a bolus and repeated twice a few minutes apart, if needed, for "sodium loading" and alkalinization, which may increase protein binding from 90% to 98%. The sodium loading overcomes the sodium channel blockage and is more important than the alkalinization. Indications include (a) a QRS complex greater than 0.12 second, (b) ventricular tachycardia, (c) severe conduction disturbances, (d) metabolic acidosis, (e) coma, and (f) seizures. A continuous infusion of sodium bicarbonate is of

21 Physical and Chemical Injuries

1254

limited usefulness for controlling dysrhythmias. Bolus therapy should be used as needed.

Hyperventilation alone has been recommended, but the pH elevation is not as instantaneous and there is compensatory renal excretion of bicarbonate; therefore, we do not recommend it. The combination of hyperventilation and sodium bicarbonate has produced fatal alkalemia and is not recommended. One should monitor serum potassium level (the sudden increase in blood pH can aggravate or precipitate hypokalemia), serum sodium, and ionized calcium levels (hypocalcemia may occur with alkalinization) and blood pH.

Specific cardiovascular complications should be treated as follows: Hypotension is treated with norepinephrine, a predominantly α-adrenergic drug, which is preferred over dopamine. Hypertension that occurs early rarely requires treatment. Sinus tachycardia usually does not require treatment. Supraventricular tachycardia in a patient who is hemodynamically unstable requires synchronized electrical cardioversion, starting at 0.25 to 1.0 watt-second per kg, after sedation. Ventricular tachycardia that persists after alkalinization requires intravenous lidocaine or countershock if the patient is hemodynamically unstable. Ventricular fibrillation should be treated with defibrillation. Torsades de pointes is treated with magnesium sulfate IV 20% solution, 2 g over 2 to 3 minutes, followed by a continuous infusion of 1.5 mL 10% solution or 5 to 10 mg per minute. For the treatment of bradydysrhythmias, atropine is contraindicated because of the anticholinergic activity. Isoproterenol 0.1 μg/kg/minute, used with caution, may produce hypotension. If the patient is hemodynamically unstable, a pacemaker is used.

Extraordinary measures, such as aortic balloon pump and cardiopulmonary bypass, have been successful.

Investigational treatments include FAB fragments specific for tricyclic antidepressant, which have been successful in animals. Prophylactic $NaHCO_3$ to prevent dysrhythmias is also being investigated.

Physostigmine has produced asystole, and flumazenil has produced seizures. Both are contraindicated.

Disposition

A patient with an antidepressant overdose who meets any of the following criteria should be admitted to the intensive care unit for 12 to 24 hours: (a) ECG abnormalities except sinus tachycardia, (b) altered mental state, (c) seizures, (d) respiratory depression, and (e) hypotension. Low-risk patients include those in whom the above symptoms are absent at 6 hours postingestion, those who present with minor transient manifestations such as sinus tachycardia who subsequently become and remain asymptomatic for a 6-hour period, and asymptomatic patients who remain asymptomatic for 6 hours. These patients may be discharged if the ECG remains normal, they have normal bowel sounds, and they undergo psychiatric disposition.

Even if the patient is asymptomatic upon presentation to the health care facility, intravenous access should be established, vital signs and neurologic status monitored, a baseline 12-lead ECG obtained, and cardiac monitoring continued for at least 6 hours. *Caution:* in 25% of fatal cases, the patients were initially alert and awake at presentation. However, in most cases of fatality initially deemed as sudden cardiac death, the patient, upon reexamination, actually had symptoms that were missed.

Children younger than 6 years of age with non-intentional (accidental) exposures to amitriptyline (Elavil), desipramine (Norpramin), doxepin (Sinequan), imipramine (Tofranil), or nortriptyline (Aventyl) in a dose less than 5 mg/kg, who are asymptomatic and have what are deemed reliable caregivers, can be observed at home, with close poison control follow-up for 6 hours. Parents or caregivers should be given instructions regarding signs and symptoms to be alert for. Children who are symptomatic, or who ingested greater than 5 mg/kg, should be referred to the emergency department for monitoring, observation, and activated charcoal treatment.

SPIDER BITES AND SCORPION STINGS

Method of
Anne-Michelle Ruha, MD

CURRENT DIAGNOSIS

Black Widow Bite
- Target lesion, not always present
- Generalized pain and muscle cramps
- Hypertension, regional diaphoresis

Brown Recluse Bite
- Unlikely to occur outside of endemic areas
- Cyanotic or blistering wound within area of pallor surrounded by erythema
- Systemic loxoscelism associated with rash, fever, hemolysis, renal failure

Bark Scorpion Sting
- Absence of lesion or local inflammatory reaction
- Painful paresthesias
- Disconjugate, roving eye movements are characteristic
- Restlessness, agitation, and involuntary jerking of muscles

CURRENT THERAPY

Black Widow Bite
- Opioid analgesics to control pain
- Benzodiazepines to control muscle cramping and anxiety
- Anti-*Latrodectus* antivenom (Antivenin) for persistent severe symptoms

Brown Recluse Bite
- General wound care
- If surgical excision is required, perform after 6 to 8 weeks
- Antibiotics only if infected

Bark Scorpion Sting
- Close attention to airway
- Opioid analgesics to control pain
- Benzodiazepines to control agitation
- *Centruroides* (scorpion) Immune F(ab')$_2$

Spider Bites

The majority of spiders native to the United States are incapable of envenomating humans. Important exceptions are *Latrodectus* and *Loxosceles* spiders, which produce clinical envenomations that, on rare occasion, are life-threatening.

Brown Recluse Spider

The most famous and abundant *Loxosceles* spider in the United States is *Loxosceles reclusa*, known as the brown recluse or fiddleback spider, due to the violin-shaped marking on its cephalothorax. The brown recluse inhabits the midwestern United States, with a range extending from east Texas to west Georgia and reaching north to southern Iowa. Bites from this nonaggressive spider are defensive, and they generally occur when spiders become trapped in clothes or bedsheets. The risk of a bite, even in heavily infested homes, appears to be very small. Most diagnoses of brown recluse bites, including many published in the medical literature, are likely erroneous, occurring in nonendemic areas without identification of the spider. Other *Loxosceles* species found in the United States are even less likely to bite because they avoid human dwellings. Evidence supporting an association between other native spider species and necrotic wounds is weak.

Although the majority of brown recluse bites do not produce significant injury, some result in loxoscelism, which ranges from minor dermonecrosis to, very rarely, life-threatening illness. The venom component thought responsible for loxoscelism is sphingo-myelinase D, which affects platelets and cell membranes and activates inflammatory mediators. The first signs of dermonecrosis are often erythema, pruritus, and pain at the bite site. Over hours the site becomes pale and edematous. Erythema can progress and spread gravitationally. A vesicle can develop, form an eschar, and slough over days to weeks. In the first days after the bite, a sunken bluish wound surrounded by a ring of pallor and then erythema is characteristic. Some patients develop a generalized maculopapular rash. Although most necrotic lesions are not serious, some can enlarge to 40 cm and leave a significant scar. Obese persons are at risk for more-severe lesions.

Very rarely, systemic loxoscelism develops within 48 hours of the bite, characterized by fever, myalgias, and hemolysis. Vomiting and diarrhea can occur, and some patients develop a diffuse erythroderma. Renal failure, disseminated intravascular coagulation, and death can result. Death from massive hemolysis is rare and is more likely to occur in children.

Diagnosis of loxoscelism depends on recognition of signs and symptoms in combination with positive identification of the spider when possible. Alternative etiologies for necrotic wounds are much more common than necrotic arachnidism, especially in nonendemic areas. The differential diagnosis of brown recluse bite is large and includes infectious causes, neoplastic disease, and vascular disease.

Treatment is supportive. Most wounds heal without intervention, although a scar might remain. Early surgical excision, dapsone,[1] hyperbaric oxygen, or prophylactic antibiotics cannot be recommended owing to lack of convincing evidence. Patients should receive tetanus prophylaxis (Td) and general wound care. In severe cases, healing can take months and require surgical intervention, which should occur 6 to 8 weeks following the bite after the wound is fully demarcated.

Black Widow Spiders

Latrodectus, or widow, spiders are, medically, the most important group of spiders in the world. Native black widow spiders are shiny black with a red hourglass pattern on their ventral surface. They can reside in or near human structures, leading to contact with humans and subsequent bites.

α-Latrotoxin in venom causes neurotransmitters to be released from synaptic vesicles. This results in a combination of neuromuscular and autonomic effects unique to *Latrodectus* bites, termed *latrodectism*. Bites are inconsistently felt, and they might or might not leave visible puncture marks and a target-like lesion. Pain can progress locally or become generalized within several hours. Severe muscle pain, particularly involving the abdomen and back, is common. Other findings include hypertension, tachycardia, tremor, localized or diffuse diaphoresis, periorbital edema, and urinary retention. Less commonly, vomiting, fever, priapism, paresthesias, and fasciculations occur. Rhabdomyolysis can result from increased muscle activity. Rarely, acute cardiomyopathy, cardiac ischemia, and pulmonary edema occur. Deaths are uncommon but reported.

Diagnosis of latrodectism is based on history of a spider bite and consistent clinical findings. In the absence of a witnessed bite, diagnosis can be difficult. Sudden onset and rapid progression of symptoms should raise suspicion. Infectious and surgical etiologies must be considered in a febrile or vomiting patient. Similar neuromuscular and autonomic findings might also be seen with intoxication by stimulant drugs and scorpion envenomations, and these should be considered in the differential.

Latrodectism typically resolves within 2 to 7 days. Opioid analgesics are often required to treat pain. Severe symptoms require intravenous opioids for adequate pain control and benzodiazepines for muscle spasms and anxiety. If symptoms are life-threatening or not controlled with these therapies, antivenom (Antivenin [*Latrodectus mactans*, equine origin], Merck, Boston, Mass.) should be considered. One vial reverses symptoms of envenomation. This whole-immunoglobulin product can produce acute hypersensitivity and should be administered in a monitored setting. Risks and benefits must be weighed before using this product. If antivenom is not an option or the patient is critically ill, care is supportive, including oxygen and airway support as needed, antihypertensives, antiemetics, and other symptomatic treatment.

Tarantulas

Tarantulas are common pets and are generally harmless. Bites may be painful, but envenomation by native species has not been reported. Most injury to humans resulting from interaction with tarantulas is secondary to trauma and inflammation caused by barbed abdominal hairs that the spiders eject defensively when threatened. If the hairs embed in the skin, a rash and pruritus can result. They can also embed in the cornea or be transferred there by rubbing the eyes after handling a tarantula. Ophthalmia nodosa, iritis, and keratouveitis have all been reported following exposure to tarantula hairs.

Treatment of embedded corneal hairs entails referral to an ophthalmologist and removal of the hairs if possible. Topical steroids are generally recommended, and some authors also recommend topical antibiotics.

Scorpion Stings

The bark scorpion, *Centruroides sculpturatus*, is the only native scorpion capable of producing a life-threatening envenomation. This small (<3 inches), yellowish-brown scorpion is found throughout Arizona and in bordering areas of surrounding states.

The scorpion seeks cool, dark environments and commonly enters homes. It injects venom by thrusting its stinger, located at the tip of its tail, toward the victim. The neurotoxic venom increases release of neurotransmitters that act at the neuromuscular junction and autonomic nerve endings.

Most stings are minor, producing local pain and paresthesias. Less than 5% of stings result in neurotoxicity, and the majority of these occur in children. Stings typically do not produce a visible skin lesion, although on rare occasion a small red mark is noted. Pain is immediate, and in a grade 1 envenomation remains local and resolves quickly. Grade 2 envenomations involve pain and paresthesias distal from the sting site, which can persist for days to weeks.

Most severe envenomations affect children younger than 5 years. Symptoms develop within 5 to 45 minutes and can progress for 4 hours. Infants and toddlers can exhibit sudden agitation and crying and transient vomiting, and they might rub their face and ears in response to paresthesias. If the child is verbal, complaints of burning pain and sensation of tongue swelling are common. Sinus tachycardia, hypertension, low-grade fever, and hypersalivation are common, and some children develop stridor. Restlessness, agitation, and twisting of the trunk with thrashing of the extremities is typical, as are tongue fasciculations and dysconjugate eye movements, or opsoclonus. Patients are conscious but often keep their eyes closed owing to diplopia. Presence of cranial nerve findings or neuromuscular agitation constitute a grade 3 envenomation; both are present in grade 4 envenomation. Severe envenomation may be associated with pulmonary edema, rhabdomyolysis, and aspiration pneumonia. Respiratory failure can occur due to several factors, including loss of tongue and respiratory muscle control, hypersalivation, and use of respiratory depressant medications.

---

[1]Not FDA approved for this indication.

Diagnosis often relies on recognition of symptoms, because children might not report a sting. Characteristic findings in regions inhabited by this scorpion usually make diagnosis straightforward. Differential diagnosis includes seizures or amphetamine toxicity. If a suspected envenomation does not follow the expected clinical course, a urine drug screen should be obtained.

Patients with grade 4 envenomation must be monitored for respiratory compromise in an emergency department or intensive care unit. If available, treatment with the antivenom Centruroides (Scorpion) Immune F(ab')2 (Equine) Injection (Anascorp) should be considered. Anascorp reverses neurotoxicity within hours and often allows discharge home from the emergency department. In clinical trials Anascorp had an excellent safety profile; however, acute hypersensitivity reactions are possible, so antihistamines and epinephrine (Adrenalin) must be accessible. Serum sickness can also develop up to 3 weeks after receiving antivenom.

If antivenom is not an option, longer-acting medications (morphine and lorazepam [Ativan][1]) may be used to control pain and agitation. Intubation and mechanical ventilation is sometimes necessary owing to venom effects and respiratory depression from the medications used to control symptoms. While the patient is intubated, continuous infusion of sedative, analgesic, and muscle relaxing agents may be necessary until signs and symptoms of envenomation resolve. This typically occurs within 24 hours, although residual medication effects can require prolonged observation.

---

[1]Not FDA approved for this indication.

References

Anascorp package insert: http://www.fda.gov/downloads/BiologicsBloodVaccines/BloodBloodProducts/ApprovedProducs/LicensedProductsBLAs/FractionatedPlasmaProducts/UCM266725.pdf.

Bernardino CR, Rapuano C. Ophthalmia nodosa caused by casual handling of a tarantula. CLAO 2000;26(2):111–12.

Boyer LV, Theodorou AA, Berg RA, et al. Antivenom for critically ill children with neurotoxicity from scorpion stings. N Engl J Med 2009;360(20):2090–98.

Clark RF, Wethern-Kestner S, Vance MV, Gerkin R. Clinical presentation and treatment of black widow spider envenomation: A review of 163 cases. Ann Emerg Med 1992;21(7):782–87.

Curry SC, Vance MV, Ryan PJ, et al. Envenomation by the scorpion Centruroides sculpturatus. J Toxicol Clin Toxicol 1983-1984;21(4–5):417–49.

Furbee RB, Kao LW, Ibrahim D. Brown recluse spider envenomation. Clin Lab Med 2006;26:211–26.

Vetter RS. Spiders of the genus Loxosceles (Araneae, Sicariidae): A review of biological, medical and psychological aspects regarding envenomations. J Arachnol 2008;36:150–63.

Vetter RS, Isbister GK. Medical aspects of spider bites. Annu Rev Entomol 2008;53:409–29.

Vetter RS, Isbister GK. Do hobo spider bites cause dermonecrotic injuries? Ann Emerg Med 2004;44(6):605–7.

Watts P, Mcpherson R, Hawksworth NR. Tarantula keratouveitis. Cornea 2000;19(3):393–94.

VENOMOUS SNAKEBITE

Method of
Steven A. Seifert, MD

Two families of venomous snakes are native to the United States. The Viperidae family (viperids) is composed of three genera and more than 30 species of rattlesnakes, copperheads, and cottonmouths. The Elapidae family (elapids) is composed of two genera and several species of coral snakes.

Each year, there are approximately 4750 venomous bites by native species reported to U.S. poison centers, with fewer than 10 deaths. Ninety-eight percent of these bites are from viperids, and a single Crotalidae polyvalent immune FAB (ovine) antivenom (CroFab, Protherics, Brentwood, Tenn.) is effective against all native species in this family. There is also a single antivenom (Antivenin [Micrurus fulvius], equine origin, Wyeth Laboratories, Marietta, Pa.) against coral snakes, which are usually easily recognized by their distinctive markings. After a bite, it is not necessary to capture or further identify the snake, because this will only increase the likelihood of additional envenomations and victims.

There are approximately 50 additional bites per year by a wide variety of nonnative venomous species of snakes housed in zoos, academic institutions, and private collections. Identification of the biting species in these cases is usually not an issue.

Diagnostic and Management Overview
Taking Action
Only a few actions can be undertaken in the field to reduce morbidity or mortality from a venomous snakebite. Most "treatments" that have been advocated—cutting, sucking, or applying tourniquets, heat, cold, or electricity—have no proven efficacy and are much more likely to result in additional tissue injury and delay of definitive therapy. Appropriate local injury management—primarily removal of jewelry, splinting of the extremity, and measures to retard venom entry into central circulation until definitive therapy can be undertaken in carefully selected cases—and expeditious transport to a health care facility can produce optimal outcomes.

Definitive management for native venomous snakes in the United States is achieved with appropriate local wound care and antivenom, which is composed of antibodies raised in a host animal (i.e., horses or sheep) against snake venom components. Because native viperids inhabit every state except Maine, every hospital should stock or have ready access to this antivenom.

No FDA-approved elapid antivenom is currently being manufactured in the United States. Older stocks of a previously produced antivenom (Antivenin) are still available at many hospitals in endemic areas (e.g., Florida, Georgia, Alabama, Louisiana, Texas), but they are rapidly being depleted, and existing stocks eventually will be consumed or pass their expiration dates. Foreign-produced antivenoms against related coral snake species may have efficacy against U.S. snakes.

An even more difficult situation results from exotic envenomations, for which the appropriate antivenom (if one exists) is certain to be a non–FDA-approved product and may be located at a zoo or other non–health care source quite distant from the location of the envenomation.

Antivenom, local wound care, and symptomatic and supportive care are the mainstays of envenomation management. A regional poison center should be contacted for information and assistance in managing any venomous snake exposure, including locating an appropriate antivenom. Poison centers have personnel who are experienced at assessing and managing envenomations and have access to a database, the Antivenom Index, which lists sources of non–FDA-approved antivenoms. Poison centers can be contacted from anywhere in the United States by calling 800-222-1222.

Snake Identification
Beyond determining whether the victim has been bitten by a coral snake or a viperid, it is relatively immaterial to know the species of the offending snake. A photo taken with a cell phone may be of some value to the treating physician, but it should be obtained only if it can be done safely and without causing a delay in transporting the patient. Viperid snakes are easily differentiated from coral snakes by virtue of the latter's distinctive color pattern of red, yellow, and black bands. It can be difficult to differentiate a coral snake from nonvenomous snakes that have similar markings. The ditty "red on yellow, kill a fellow; red on black, venom lack," which describes the red band being surrounded on either side by yellow or black, is accurate only for North American coral snakes. South American coral snakes may have the opposite pattern.

Because all viperid envenomations are currently treated with a single product and the physical findings or laboratory evaluation is all that is required to determine that the snake is venomous, attempting to kill or capture the snake is unlikely to add additional information to treatment decisions but is likely to result in the individual being bitten a second time or other individuals becoming bite victims. Differences in the appearance of the bite wound (e.g., fang punctures, swelling, ecchymosis) and the observation of signs and symptoms are usually sufficient to determine whether the biting snake was venomous and to guide therapy.

For future reference, remember this advice: "Red on yellow, leave it alone. Red on black, leave it alone. Slithers on the ground, LEAVE IT ALONE."

Factors Affecting Toxicity and the Severity of Envenomation

Many factors govern whether an envenomation occurs after a bite, the signs and symptoms that develop, and the overall severity of effects. Up to 25% of viperid bites and up to 50% of elapid bites do not result in an envenomation. Barriers to fang penetration and other factors may result in no venom being injected. Patients must be watched for a sufficient length of time (i.e., 8 hours in a viperid bite and 24 hours in a coral snakebite) to ensure that this has been the case.

If an envenomation has occurred, the family and species of snake generally determines the spectrum of symptoms and signs. The amount of venom, specific venom components, and the underlying health status of the victim determine severity.

Viperid Envenomations
Epidemiology and Recognition

Viperid snakes are distributed throughout North America, with the apparent exception of Maine. Bites are more common in southern states and during summer months, but they occur year-round and may occur at any time and in any location with captive collections. The various genera and species of viperids in the United States have relatively stable geographic ranges, with much overlap. Many different species of venomous snakes may inhabit any given area. Nonvenomous or mildly venomous colubrid snakes are also native to the United States. Viperids, also called pit vipers (i.e., rattlesnakes, copperheads, and cottonmouths), may be recognized by a generally triangular-shaped head, the so-called pit (an infrared heat-detection organ) located approximately midway between the nostril and the eye, and pupils shaped like those of a cat (not round).

Pit vipers have large, movable fangs through which venom is injected into the victim. Because fangs are curved, venom is usually injected subcutaneously, rather than into deeper muscle compartments. Because of anatomic and other physical factors, bite wounds may appear as scratches or as one or more punctures. Envenomation may occur with a break in the skin.

Viperid venom is complex, consisting of dozens of proteolytic enzymes, small peptides, phospholipases, and other elements responsible for the spectrum of clinical effects seen. There is a great variability in this complex poison between species, within species, and even within a single specimen over the course of a season and lifespan.

Clinical Effects

The spectrum of clinical effects is based on the specific genus or species of viperid and is unpredictable, ranging in any given event from a nonenvenomation (up to 25% of bites) to life-threatening reactions. Viperid snake envenomation invariably results in tissue injury, manifested by pain and progressive swelling, and it may include ecchymosis, elevated tissue and compartment pressures, tissue necrosis, and tissue loss. The complete absence of local effects can be used as a reliable marker of nonenvenomation in a viperid bite as long as a sufficient period (8–10 hours) of observation has occurred.

Systemic effects may occur, including hematologic, neurologic, cardiovascular, and nonspecific findings. Rattlesnake envenomations are more likely to result in hematologic effects, such as thrombocytopenia, hypofibrinogenemia, or prolongation of the prothrombin time (PT) or activated partial thromboplastin time (aPTT), and are more likely to produce neurologic effects, such

as muscle fasciculation or weakness, compared with copperhead or cottonmouth envenomations, but these effects can be seen with any viperid snake. Hypotension from direct myocardial depression or from type 1 hypersensitivity (i.e., anaphylactic or anaphylactoid) reactions may occur with any viperid exposure. Nausea, vomiting, diaphoresis, anxiety, and other nonspecific effects may be seen.

Duration of Clinical Effects

Local effects may develop rapidly or may not be apparent for many hours. Progression may occur for 24 to 36 hours, with resolution of tissue injury occurring over 3 to 6 weeks. Complications of tissue necrosis or infection have their own time frame of resolution. Hematologic effects usually begin within 1 to 2 hours of envenomation. If antivenom is given within this time frame, the detection of those effects may be masked and become apparent only after unbound antivenom has been eliminated from the body, usually 2 to 4 days after treatment. Hematologic effects may persist for 1 to 3 weeks after an envenomation. Neurologic and other systemic effects tend to occur within a few hours of envenomation and resolve over 24 to 36 hours.

Severity of Envenomation

Untreated, local injury worsens over time, with proximal progression of tissue injury. Hematologic effects can be profound, resulting in spontaneous hemorrhage. Hypotension may be profound and can result in death. Neurologic and other systemic effects are rarely life-threatening events. Because of changes in basic medical care and health care systems, it is not directly applicable to compare case-fatality rates before the introduction of antivenom (1950) with what can be expected today. However, at that time, there were several hundred deaths per year in the United States from viperid envenomations.

Management
Determining Whether Envenomation Has Occurred and Its Severity

Because of the unpredictability of envenomation and the variability of possible clinical effects, each viperid bite must be assessed and responded to individually (Box 1). It is important to determine whether an envenomation has occurred. If there are no signs or symptoms of envenomation, there is no indication for antivenom or other specific treatment. The severity of the envenomation helps to determine the amount of antivenom required to counter and neutralize venom effects, but this may not be immediately apparent, because envenomations tend to progress over time, and what may at first appear to be mild venom effects may progress to a severe envenomation.

Initial Hospital Management

On arrival at the hospital, jewelry should be removed and the bitten extremity loosely splinted. The wound should be cleaned, and a radiograph should be obtained to rule out a foreign body (Box 2). Tetanus status should be updated if needed. In the absence of other factors, the extremity should be maintained slightly below heart level until antivenom is started and then should be elevated. If

---

Box 1 Prehospital Management of Viperid Envenomation

- Remove jewelry.
- Splint the extremity and maintain just below heart level.
- Expeditiously transport to a health care facility.
- Consider use of lymphatic constriction band (blood pressure cuff at 15–25 mm Hg) *for life-threatening effects only.*
- Obtain intravenous access if possible.
- Do not use cutting, sucking, heat, cold, or other local "therapies."

- Remove jewelry.
- If an arterial or venous tourniquet has been placed, convert to a lymphatic constriction band.
- Obtain intravenous access, and use crystalloid as indicated.
- Obtain CBC with platelet count, PT or INR, aPTT, and fibrinogen level q6–12h for 1 day and then daily if values are abnormal. An initial D-dimer value (or fibrin degradation products) should be obtained to detect fibrinogenolytic activity that may not yet have produced hypofibrinogenemia.
- Determine whether an envenomation has occurred.
- Determine severity based on the family or species of snake, age and health status of the victim, and development and rate of progression of signs and symptoms (e.g., local injury, hematologic abnormalities, hypotension and other systemic effects).
- Determine the tetanus vaccination status and update if necessary.
- Seek consultation from a poison center: 800-222-1222.
- If a pressure immobilization or lymphatic constriction band was placed before arriving at the hospital, determine whether antivenom is indicated, and remove the band after the antivenom infusion is started.
- If there are minimal or no signs of envenomation or if the bands are placed inappropriately, remove them under close observation.
- Determine whether antivenom is indicated, and administer per protocol.
- Provide basic wound care (i.e., cleaning and radiograph), and determine whether local injury requires specific management.
- Determine whether hematologic or other systemic effects require specific management.

Abbreviations: aPTT = activated partial thromboplastin time; CBC = complete blood cell count; INR = international normalized ratio; PT = prothrombin time.

---

there are immediate life-threatening effects (e.g., anaphylaxis, hypotension), the extremity should be placed in an interior position and consideration given to impeding venom entry into central circulation by means of a lymphatic constriction band or pressure immobilization bandage, weighing the potential benefit against the possible risk of increased local tissue injury from increasing venom concentration and duration in the tissues. Patients often require opioid-level pain relief.

At least one large intravenous line should be initiated and crystalloid infused as needed. Initial hospital therapy, including a first dose of antivenom, should be provided in an area capable of close monitoring of vital signs and capable of managing life-threatening reactions; this usually is an emergency department. Whether an intensive care unit (ICU) or similar patient care area is used for subsequent management depends on the clinical situation.

Indications for Antivenom

Because of the safety of the current FDA-approved antivenom and its ability to stop proximal progression of local tissue injury, all patients with signs of progressive local envenomation effects and those with significant systemic effects are candidates for treatment with antivenom.

Depending on the original indication for treatment, initial control of envenomation effects is the goal of the loading dose of antivenom. The only FDA-approved viperid antivenom for North American pit viper envenomation is Crotalidae Polyvalent Immune Fab (Ovine) Antivenin (CroFab), which is an ovine-based Fab antivenom. The incidence of type 1 hypersensitivity reactions is approximately 6%. There are rare reports of IgE-mediated type 1 hypersensitivity reactions on repeat exposure in individuals who

were previously treated with CroFab, but most people who have been previously treated do not develop an adverse reaction to subsequent administrations. The incidence of type 3 hypersensitivity reactions ("serum sickness") is also approximately 6%. Pretreatment sensitivity testing is not required or recommended. The half-life of this antivenom is approximately 18 to 24 hours, which is considerably shorter than IgG or F(ab′)2 antivenoms, and it is responsible for the recurrence of hematologic effects in approximately 70% of patients with an initial coagulopathy.

For moderate to severe envenomations, antivenom is administered as an intravenous solution, with 4 to 6 vials diluted into 250 to 500 mL of D_5W or normal saline. Treatment of life-threatening envenomations may be started with 10 to 12 vials. The infusion should be run slowly for the first 5 to 10 minutes, and the patient should be observed closely for a type 1 hypersensitivity reaction. If such a reaction occurs, the infusion should be slowed or stopped, depending on the severity, and appropriate symptomatic treatment should be started with H_1- and H_2-blockers, epinephrine, corticosteroids, and other supportive measures, as needed. It should be determined whether antivenom is still required, and if so, it should be restarted at a slower rate or higher dilution, or both. If a reaction does not occur, the infusion is concluded over 1 hour.

Treatment of Local Tissue Injury

If the antivenom is given exclusively for local findings, the syndromic response to envenomation is deemed to be controlled if there is cessation of proximal progression of edema at the end of the infusion. There is often some redistribution of existing tissue edema, and continued proximal progression is usually distinguishable by a raised, tender, and perhaps erythematous leading edge of edema. If antivenom is being given for hematologic effects, cessation of worsening or reversal should be seen. Often, thrombocytopenia rebounds dramatically. Hypofibrinogenemia may not rebound as quickly or merely stabilize, because the liver must manufacture new fibrinogen. Although an elevated D-dimer value indicates fibrinogenolytic activity, it is not an independent indicator for antivenom treatment.

Other systemic effects may serve as indicators for antivenom use, and they should show control by the end of the initial infusion. If initial control is not deemed to have occurred, additional doses of antivenom should be administered until initial control is determined to have occurred. Most patients achieve initial control with 4 to 12 vials of antivenom, although more may be required.

Maintenance Doses

Because of the rapid decline of antivenom levels resulting from the larger volume of distribution of Fab antivenoms, after initial control is achieved, maintenance dosing of 2 vials every 6 hours for three doses is commenced. This usually maintains adequate antivenom serum levels to prevent recurrence of local tissue injury progression. If progression does recur, an additional 2 vials of antivenom usually are sufficient to control local worsening. Tissue pressures may be increased, and elevated muscle compartment pressures may be identified when measured directly. My colleagues and I do not routinely measure tissue or compartment pressures. When pressures are measured and demonstrated to be elevated, it should be remembered that the mechanisms of these phenomena are different from other muscle compartment syndromes. For example, extensive edema in the subcutaneous space circumferentially in an extremity may elevate compartment pressures by extrinsic compression. Case reports and series suggest that additional antivenom and extremity elevation result in reduced tissue and compartment pressures. Intracompartmental injection of venom can result in a true compartment syndrome. However, there is no evidence that fasciotomy is beneficial in this setting, and there are animal data to suggest that it may result in worse clinical outcomes.

Bleb formation at the site of a bite is not an important sign in and of itself, although it may suggest significantly elevated tissue pressures resulting in dermal-epidermal separation or the presence of tissue necrosis. Bleb fluid may contain unneutralized venom. It is reasonable to unroof blebs at or near the bite site and to débride obviously necrotic tissue that usually becomes apparent several days after the bite.

Antibiotics

The incidence of culture-proven infection in U.S. viperid bites is low, probably less than 5%. There are no data to support the use of prophylactic antibiotics, and it is best to limit the opportunities for adverse drug effects. It is often difficult to distinguish inflammatory venom effects from infection starting on the second day after an envenomation. If antibiotics are prescribed, a first-generation, broad-spectrum agent should be used.

Long-Term Local Tissue Effects

The edema and tissue injury produced by most North American viperid envenomations usually resolves within 1 to 2 months, and a return to normal function can be anticipated. However, tissue necrosis or deep tissue injury may result in longer-term or even permanent structural and functional disability. Loss of tissue may occur, including digits and other parts of extremities, although this is rare and may be associated with prehospital application of tourniquets or other imprudent surgical interventions, delayed care, or complications such as infections. Some victims engage in behaviors that result in multiple envenomations, and this may increase the risks of long-term tissue injury.

Hematologic Abnormalities and Bleeding

One or more hematologic abnormalities may occur with native viperid envenomation (Box 3). Significant decreases in platelet count or fibrinogen concentrations are independent indications for antivenom treatment. Isolated, mild prolongations of PT or aPTT may not require antivenom treatment. However, these effects may be progressive or indicate an impending hypofibrinogenemia, and early antivenom treatment may prevent severe abnormalities. Even if platelets, fibrinogen, and intrinsic and extrinsic clotting systems are involved, the end result is not a true disseminated intravascular coagulopathy, because there is no true intravascular coagulation. Sufficient platelets, fibrinogen, and thrombin are usually available for hemostasis, and clinically significant bleeding is rarely seen. However, severe depletion of individual clotting elements or a combination of hematologic abnormalities can result in bleeding.

The management of initial or persistent laboratory abnormalities is achieved with additional antivenom. Administration of blood products (e.g., fresh-frozen plasma [FFP], platelet concentrates, other blood products) should be reserved for clinically significant bleeding and be given in conjunction with additional antivenom, because transfused elements are similarly likely to be consumed by venom activity. Ecchymoses in damaged tissues, expansion of the vascular volume from crystalloid administration, and red blood cell hemolysis from hemolytic venom factors may produce an anemia that may rarely require a red blood cell transfusion.

Recurrence of Hematologic Effects

Approximately 70% of patients who develop an initial hematologic effect will have a recurrence of those effects 2 to 4 days after initial treatment. The severity of the recurrence is usually similar to the initial effects. A person who presented with a severe thrombocytopenia is likely to return with recurrent severe thrombocytopenia. The mechanism is recurrent unneutralized venomemia after elimination of unbound Fab antivenom. The recurrent effects may be milder, because there is less venom in the body and severity is a function of venom effect and the body's ability to produce factors such as platelets or fibrinogen in excess of their rate of consumption. Recurrent effects may be more severe, however, or even appear to be occurring de novo if the patient was treated soon after envenomation, blunting the acute effects of the venom and masking the true severity of the envenomation.

Patients who present with severe early hematologic effects, an elevated D-dimer, an increase in the platelet count of more than 20% within 4 hours of the initial antivenom dose, or who are treated with antivenom within 1 to 2 hours of envenomation are at risk for severe recurrent effects and should be followed closely after discharge. Although the incidence of significant bleeding is low, even with profound laboratory abnormalities, it seems prudent to administer additional antivenom if the platelet count is less than 25,000, the fibrinogen level is less than 50 mg/dL, the PT or PTT values indicate nonclotting, there is a combination of significant defects in coagulation, or there are underlying medical conditions that make hemorrhage more likely, such as advanced age, hypertension, or a bleeding diathesis. Additional antivenom may be given for severe hematologic effects or abnormalities associated with significant bleeding. In patients who have been discharged and who are not actively bleeding, 2 to 4 vials IV may be given and the patient followed daily. Additional such doses may be needed for more than 2 weeks. For patients who remain hospitalized or are readmitted, antivenom has been given by continuous IV infusion in a small case series. An infusion initiated at 3 vials over 24 hours and titrated to clinical effect (up to 4 vials per 24 hours) was successful in reversing recurrent hematologic effects in all five cases reported. Sterility and stability data for this product during prolonged administration is not currently available, however. If used in this way, infusing 1 vial continuously over no more than 8 hours (3 vials per 24 hours) would be prudent.

Disposition

Patients whose local effects are regressing and do not have complications, such as infection or necrosis, and whose hematologic and other systemic effects are controlled may be discharged. Typically, this occurs between 36 and 48 hours after envenomation. Patients with any venom-related hematologic abnormality during

---

Box 3 | Management of Hematologic Effects and Recurrence in Viperid Envenomation

- Administer 4 to 6 vials of antivenom (Crotalidae Polyvalent Immune Fab [Ovine]) for significant abnormalities of platelet count, PT or INR, aPTT, or fibrinogen. An elevated D-dimer value indicates accelerated fibrinogen breakdown and should prompt close monitoring of the fibrinogen concentrations, but it is not an independent indication to treat with antivenom.
- Administer additional antivenom in 4- to 6-vial increments until there is reversal of hematologic abnormalities. Replacement of platelets, clotting factors, or fibrinogen may be gradual, and a positive trend indicates neutralization of venom or replacement in excess of venom effect.
- Patients with initial hematologic effects or who were treated within 1 to 2 hours of envenomation are at risk for recurrent effects 2 to 4 days after treatment and should be followed closely: every other day until no recurrence at 4 days or daily for declining parameters.
- Consider treating recurrent hematologic abnormalities with additional antivenom. Indications include platelets <25,000/mm^3; fibrinogen <50 mg/dL; INR >5; aPTT >150 seconds; and lesser abnormalities involving more than one parameter.
- Consider readmission for severe abnormalities, other risk factors (e.g., uncontrolled hypertension, advanced age, other bleeding diatheses), or clinically significant bleeding.
- Administer blood products *plus* additional antivenom for significant bleeding.

Abbreviations: aPTT = activated partial thromboplastin time; INR = international normalized ratio; PT = prothrombin time.

hospitalization (thrombocytopenia, hypofibrinogenemia, elevated D-dimer, or prolonged PT/INR or PTT) should have at least one repeat set of labs within 5 days of treatment, as there is a risk of recurrent effects or late, new onset of hematologic abnormalities. Patients without any of these abnormalities and who also did not have an increase of more than 20% in platelet count within 4 hours of antivenom administration may constitute a group at very low risk of late effects, although confirmatory studies are needed. Ongoing pain relief may be required, with an effort to transition to nonopioid agents during the first week, and the patient should be warned to watch for signs of serum sickness. Occupational or physical therapy should be arranged to maximize return of function, and follow-up for local and systemic effects should be arranged.

Elapid Envenomations
Epidemiology and Recognition
U.S. coral snakes can be recognized by their distinctive band pattern, with a red band seeming to be placed on top of a larger yellow band. This color pattern applies only to North American coral snakes. Each year, there are approximately 75 to 100 bites by coral snakes in the United States. Two genera and several species inhabit the United States, with the *Micrurus* genus responsible for most bites in Florida, Texas, Georgia, Louisiana, Alabama, and some neighboring states. A smaller genus, *Micruroides*, is found in Arizona and New Mexico, but it is responsible for very few bites, and there have been no reports of serious envenomations in recent years. Bites are more common during the warmer months.

Elapids have relatively short, fixed fangs, which may decrease the rate of envenomation. More than one puncture, deep punctures, and a history of the snake hanging on increases the risk of envenomation.

Clinical Effects
Envenomation by the coral snake produces primarily neurologic toxicity from presynaptic toxins initially producing bulbar muscle weakness, ptosis, diplopia, and dysphagia. These effects can begin within 15 to 30 minutes or may be delayed up to 24 hours after an envenomation. Muscle weakness and paralysis progress to include respiratory muscles, and they can result in respiratory arrest and death. Typical of presynaptic toxins, effect progression can be arrested with the use of antivenom, but the effects are not rapidly reversed. Typically, there is no or little local tissue injury, and the absence of local injury cannot be used to exclude envenomation. Likewise, there is usually no effect on hematologic function, and other systemic effects are rare. Patients cannot be assumed to have eluded envenomation by a coral snake because they lack these symptoms, and patients should be observed for at least 24 hours before concluding that an envenomation has not occurred.

Because of changes in basic medical care and health care systems, it is not directly applicable to compare case fatality rates before the introduction of antivenom (1967) with what can be expected today. However, at that time, the case-fatality rate was approximately 10%.

Management
Because of the potential for rapid progression of motor paralysis and respiratory compromise, the difficulty of reversing paralysis after it is established, and the lack of local effects, it is reasonable to attempt to retard venom progression into the circulation until a decision regarding antivenom can be made. A pressure immobilization band (i.e., elastic bandage wrapped from an extremity's tip to trunk with the degree of tension used for sprains) is used for this purpose for elapid envenomations elsewhere in the world (Boxes 4 and 5). In Australian studies, a pressure immobilization bandage has been shown to slow venom absorption and in those studies, bandage pressures have been between 40–70 mmHg in the upper extremity and 55–70 mm Hg in the lower extremity. However, the proper technique requires training, and the infrequency of these bites makes teaching and retention of such skills

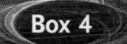

Box 4 Prehospital Management of Elapid Envenomation

- Remove jewelry.
- Splint the extremity and maintain just below heart level.
- Expeditiously transport to a health care facility.
- Apply a pressure immobilization bandage (i.e., 3- to 4-inch crepe bandage at lymphatic pressure from the tip of the extremity to the trunk) or a lymphatic constriction band (i.e., wide rubber band or blood pressure cuff at 15–25 mm Hg) proximal to the bite site.
- Obtain intravenous access if possible.
- Do not use cutting, sucking, heat, cold, or other local "therapies."

Box 5 Hospital Diagnosis and Initial Management of Elapid Envenomation

- Remove jewelry.
- If an arterial or venous tourniquet has been placed, convert to a lymphatic constriction band.
- Obtain intravenous access, and use crystalloid as indicated.
- Determine whether an envenomation has occurred.
- Determine severity based on the family or species of snake, the age and health status of the victim, and the rate of progression of signs or symptoms (i.e., paralysis and other neurologic effects).
- Determine the tetanus vaccination status and update if necessary.
- Seek consultation from a poison center: 800-222-1222.
- If a pressure immobilization band or lymphatic constriction band has been placed before arrival at the hospital, determine whether antivenom is needed, and begin antivenom infusion before removing the band.
- Determine whether antivenom is indicated, and administer per protocol.
- Provide basic wound care (i.e., cleaning and radiograph), and determine whether local injury requires specific management.
- Determine whether other systemic effects require specific management.

problematic. A blood pressure cuff inflated to similar pressures may also retard venom entry into circulation, and it can be a more reliable and easily taught technique, although it has not been validated in clinical studies.

Standard wound care should be performed, including cleansing the wound, obtaining a radiograph, and updating the tetanus status, if needed. Wound infection is uncommon, and prophylactic antibiotics are not recommended.

Because the first signs of envenomation can be rapidly progressive neurotoxicity and because of the difficulty of reversing paralysis, some authorities have proposed administering antivenom in cases in which an envenomation is possible, before the appearance of any clinical symptoms. Others have pointed to the infrequency of respiratory muscle paralysis resulting in the need for intubation and respiratory support and to possible geographic differences in snake toxicity, and they have counseled observation and antivenom treatment only after envenomation has been confirmed by progressive symptoms. Recent analysis of the national database has not demonstrated a significant difference in clinical severity between Florida and Texas coral snake envenomations, which supports early treatment. However, the impending loss of an FDA-approved coral snake antivenom (Antivenin)[2] is likely to result in delays of many hours before antivenom can be administered, if it is available at all. The expiration date for Coral snake (Micrurus fulvius) antivenom Lots #4030024 and #4030026 has

---

[2]Not available in the United States.

been extended to April 30, 2015. Updated information can be obtained from the FDA website on Vaccines, Blood and Biologics (http://www.fda.gov/BiologicsBloodVaccines/). The designated poison center (1-800-222-1222) will have information on antivenom availability in the region. Aggressive and meticulous respiratory support, including intubation and ventilation that may be needed for days to weeks, should ultimately result in survival of even severe neurotoxic envenomations. If an FDA-approved coral snake antivenom is not available, there may be a clinical trial of an investigational coral snake antivenom in progress. Clinical trials can be located at: www.clinicaltrials.gov.

Exotic Snakebite

Epidemiology and Clinical Effects

In the United States, most exotic snake envenomations occur in private collections. These are not usually known to authorities or health care providers until an envenomation occurs, and they may involve the collection owner or family members, including children. They may occur in any locale, and victims may present to any health care facility.

Viperid and elapid snakes, which account for the bulk of venomous bites worldwide, have patterns of venom activity similar to those of their North American counterparts, with some variation and with generally greater toxicity for some non-U.S. species. Some nonnative elapids, such as cobras, mambas, black snakes, or taipans, produce much higher rates of respiratory paralysis and may produce much greater local tissue injury than U.S. coral snakes. Similarly, envenomation from some nonnative viperids, such as *Bothrops, Echis*, or *Bitis* species, or from an African colubrid, such as the boomslang, results in a greater risk of bleeding. Some of these species may directly activate prothrombin (e.g., *Echis* species, *Bothrops* species) and factor X (e.g., *Vipera* species, *Dispholidus* species), leading to a true disseminated intravascular coagulopathy with intravascular thrombosis, marked organ dysfunction, and potentially, death.

Management

The specific management of exotic envenomations is beyond the scope of this chapter. Not all venomous exotic snakes have antivenoms, and even for snakes with antivenoms, none may be available in the United States, but zoos stock antivenoms for snakes in their collections. An updateable online database, the Antivenom Index, lists these antivenoms and is accessible by regional poison centers. For information on exotic antivenoms and assistance in managing an exotic snake envenomation, the regional poison center should be contacted (1-800-222-1222).

References

Boyer LV, Seifert SA, Cain JS. Recurrence phenomena after immunoglobulin therapy for snake envenomations. Part 2. Guidelines for clinical management with Crotaline Fab antivenom. Ann Emerg Med 2001;37:196–1.

Boyer LV, Seifert SA, Clark RF, et al. Recurrent and persistent coagulopathy following pit viper envenomation. Arch Intern Med 1999;159(7):706–10.

Bush SP, Seifert SA, Oakes J, et al. Continuous IV crotalidae polyvalent immune fab (ovine) (FabAV) for selected North American rattlesnake bite patients. Toxicon 2013;69:29–37. http://dx.doi.org/10.1016/j.toxicon.2013.02.008. Epub 2013 Mar 6.

Gold BS, Barish RA, Dart RC. North American snake envenomation: Diagnosis, treatment, and management. Emerg Med Clin North Am 2004;22 (2):423–43 ix.

Kitchens CS, Van Mierop LH. Envenomation by the Eastern coral snake (*Micrurus fulvius fulvius*). A study of 39 victims. JAMA 1987;258(12):1615–8.

Seifert SA, Boyer LV. Recurrence phenomena after immunoglobulin therapy for snake envenomations. Part 1. Pharmacokinetics and pharmacodynamics of immunoglobulin antivenoms and related antibodies. Ann Emerg Med 2001;37 (2):189–95.

Seifert SA, Boyer LV, Dart RC, et al. Relationship of venom effects to venom antigen and antivenom serum concentrations in a patient with *Crotalus atrox* envenomation treated with a Fab antivenom. Ann Emerg Med 1997;30(1):49–53.

Seifert SA, Kirschner RI, Martin N. Recurrent, persistent, or late, new-onset hematologic abnormalities in crotaline snakebite. Clin Toxicol (Phila) 2011;49:324–9. http://dx.doi.org/10.3109/15563650.2011.566883.

Seifert SA, Oakes JA, Boyer LV. Toxic Exposure Surveillance System (TESS)-based characterization of U.S. non-native venomous snake exposures, 1995–2004. Clin Toxicol (Phila) 2007;45(5):571–8.

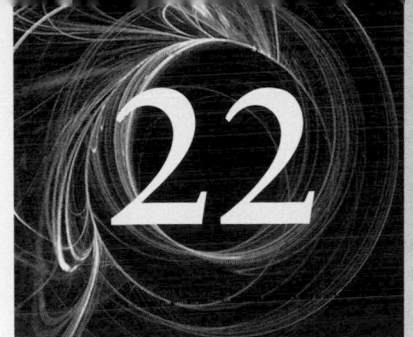

22 Appendices

BIOLOGIC AGENTS REFERENCE CHART

Method of
James J. James, MD; and James M. Lyznicki, MS, MPH

Biological weapons are devices used intentionally to cause disease or death through dissemination of microorganisms or toxins in food and water, by insect vectors, or by aerosols. Potential targets include human beings, food crops, livestock, and other resources essential for national security, economy, and defense. Unlike nuclear, chemical, and conventional weapons, the onset of a biological attack will probably be insidious. For some infectious agents, secondary and tertiary transmission could continue for weeks or months after the initial attack.

Initial detection of an unannounced biological attack will likely occur when an astute health professional notices an unusual case or disease cluster and reports his or her concerns to local public health authorities. Physicians and other health professionals should be alert to the following:
- Unusual temporal or geographic clustering of illnesses
- Sudden increase of illness in previously healthy persons
- Sudden increase in nonspecific illnesses such as pneumonia; flu-like illness; bleeding disorders; unexplained rashes, particularly in adults; neuromuscular illnesses; and diarrhea

To enhance detection and treatment capabilities, physicians and other health professionals in acute care settings should be familiar with the clinical manifestations, diagnostic techniques, isolation precautions, treatment, and prophylaxis for likely causative agents (e.g., smallpox, pneumonic plague, anthrax, viral hemorrhagic fevers). Table 1 provides a quick summary of diagnostic and treatment considerations for various infectious and toxic biological agents. For some of these agents, delay in medical response could result in a potentially devastating number of casualties. To mitigate such consequences, early identification and intervention are imperative. Frontline physicians must have an increased level of suspicion regarding the possible intentional use of biological agents as well as an increased sensitivity to reporting those suspicious to public health authorities, who, in turn, must be willing to evaluate a predictable increase in false-positive reports.

Medical response efforts require coordination and planning with emergency management agencies, law enforcement, health care facilities, and social services agencies. Health care agencies should ensure that physicians know whom to call with reports of suspicious cases and clusters of infectious diseases, and they should work to build a good relationship with the local medical community. Resource integration is absolutely necessary to
- Establish adequate capacity to initiate rapid investigation of an outbreak
- Educate the public
- Begin mass distribution of antibiotics and vaccines
- Ensure mass medical care
- Control public anger and fear

In an epidemic, overwhelming numbers of critically ill patients will require acute and follow-up medical care. Both infected persons and the worried well will seek medical attention, with a corresponding need for medical supplies, diagnostic tests, and hospital beds. The impact—or even the threat—of an attack can elicit widespread panic and civil disorder, overwhelm hospital resources, and disrupt social services.

Any suspicious or confirmed exposure to a biological weapons agent should be reported immediately to the local health department, local Federal Bureau of Investigation office, and the Centers of Disease Control and Prevention (770–488–7100).

1263

TABLE 1 Quick Reference Chart on Biological Weapon Agents

DISEASE AND AGENT	DIAGNOSTIC CONSIDERATIONS — SIGNS AND SYMPTOMS	INCUBATION PERIOD	DIAGNOSIS	LETHALITY	TREATMENT CONSIDERATIONS* — TREATMENT	PROPHYLAXIS	COMMENTS
Bacteria							
Anthrax *Bacillus anthracis* (all forms)		1–5 d (perhaps ≤60 d)[†]	Gram stain and culture of blood, pleural fluid, cerebrospinal fluid, ascitic fluid, vesicular fluid, or lesion exudate. Confirmatory serologic and PCR tests are available through public health laboratory network		Steroids may be considered for severe edema and for meningitis. Penicillin[1] should be considered if strain is susceptible and does not possess inducible β-lactamases	Ciprofloxacin or doxycycline with or without vaccination. If strain is susceptible, penicillin[1] or amoxicillin[1] (Amoxil) should be considered. Inactivated vaccine (licensed but not readily available): six injections and annual booster	If meningitis is suspected, doxycycline may be less optimal because of poor CNS penetration
Cutaneous	Evolving skin lesion (face, neck, arms), progresses to vesicle, depressed ulcer, and black necrotic lesions			20% if untreated, otherwise rarely fatal			
Gastrointestinal	Nausea, vomiting, abdominal pain, bloody diarrhea, sepsis. Widened mediastinum on chest radiograph is occasionally seen[‡]			Approaches 100% if untreated, but data are limited. Rapid, aggressive treatment can reduce mortality			
Inhalational	Abrupt onset of flulike symptoms, fever with or without chills, sweats, fatigue or malaise, non- or minimally productive cough, nausea, vomiting, dyspnea, headache, chest pain, followed in 2–5 d by severe respiratory distress, mediastinitis, hemorrhagic meningitis, sepsis, shock[§]. Widened mediastinum on chest radiograph is characteristic[‡]		Sputum is rarely positive	Once respiratory distress develops, mortality rates approach 90%. Begin treatment when inhalational anthrax is suspected; do not wait for confirmatory testing[‖]	Combination therapy of ciprofloxacin or doxycycline plus one or two other antimicrobials should be considered[¶]		

Agent	Incubation	Clinical features	Diagnosis	Mortality	Treatment	Prophylaxis/vaccine	Comments
Brucellosis *Brucella abortus, B. canis, B. mellitensis, B. suis*	5–60 d, usually 1–2 mo	Nonspecific flulike symptoms: fever, headache, profound weakness and fatigue; GI symptoms such as anorexia, nausea, vomiting, diarrhea, or constipation	Blood and bone marrow culture (can require 6 wk to grow *Brucella*); Confirmatory culture and serologic testing available through public health laboratory network	Less than 5% even if untreated; Tends to incapacitate rather than kill	Doxycycline plus streptomycin or rifampin; *Alternative therapies:* Ofloxacin[1] plus rifampin[1]; Doxycycline plus gentamicin (Garamycin); TMP-SMX[1] plus gentamicin	Doxycycline plus streptomycin or rifampin; No approved human vaccine	Osteoarticular complications are common
Inhalational (pneumonic) tularemia *Francisella tularensis*	3–5 d; Range, 1–21 d	Sudden onset of acute febrile illness, weakness, chills, headache, generalized body aches, elevated WBCs; Pulmonary symptoms such as dry cough, chest pain or tightness with or without objective signs of pneumonia; Progressive weakness, malaise, anorexia, and weight loss, potentially leading to sepsis and organ failure	Largely clinical; Culture of blood, sputum, biopsies, pleural fluid, bronchial washings (culture is difficult and potentially dangerous); confirmatory testing available through public health laboratory network	~30%–60%; Fatal if untreated	Streptomycin or gentamicin (Garamycin); *Alternative therapies:* Ciprofloxacin[1]; Doxycycline; Chloramphenicol[1] (Chloromycetin)	Tetracycline; Doxycycline; Ciprofloxacin[1]; Live, attenuated vaccine (USAMRIID, IND) given by scarification; currently under FDA review, limited availability	
Pneumonic plague *Yersinia pestis*	1–10 d, typically 2–3 d	Acute onset of flulike prodrome: fever, myalgia, weakness, headache; within 24 h of prodrome, chest discomfort, cough with bloody sputum, and dyspnea; By day 2 to 4 of illness, symptoms progressing to cyanosis, respiratory distress, and hemodynamic instability	Gram stain and culture of blood, CSF, sputum, lymph node aspirates, bronchial washings; Confirmatory serologic and bacteriologic tests available through public health laboratory network	Almost 100% if untreated; 20%–60% if appropriately treated within 18–24 h of symptoms	Streptomycin, gentamicin (Garamycin); *Alternative therapies:* Doxycycline; Tetracycline; Ciprofloxacin[1]; Chloramphenicol[1] (Chloromycetin) is first choice for meningitis except for pregnant women	Tetracycline; Doxycycline; Ciprofloxacin[1]; Inactivated whole-cell vaccine licensed but not readily available; injection with boosters; Vaccine not effective against aerosol exposure	Begin treatment when diagnosis of plague is suspected; do not wait for confirmatory testing

Continued

Biologic Agents Reference Chart

TABLE 1 Quick Reference Chart on Biological Weapon Agents—cont'd

DISEASE AND AGENT	DIAGNOSTIC CONSIDERATIONS				TREATMENT CONSIDERATIONS*		
	SIGNS AND SYMPTOMS	INCUBATION PERIOD	DIAGNOSIS	LETHALITY	TREATMENT	PROPHYLAXIS	COMMENTS
Rickettsia Q-fever *Coxiella burnetii*	Nonspecific febrile disease, chills, cough, weakness and fatigue, pleuritic chest pain Pneumonia is possible	2–14 d May be ≤40 d	Isolation of organism may be difficult; confirmatory testing via serology or PCR available through public health laboratory network	1%–3% Fatalities are uncommon even if untreated Relapsing symptoms can occur	Tetracycline Doxycycline	Tetracycline Doxycycline Inactivated whole-cell[2] vaccine (IND)	Skin test to determine prior exposure to *C. burnetii* is recommended before vaccination

DISEASE AND AGENT	SIGNS AND SYMPTOMS	INCUBATION PERIOD	DIAGNOSIS	LETHALITY	TREATMENT	PROPHYLAXIS	COMMENTS
Viruses							
Smallpox Variola major virus	Prodrome of high fever, malaise, prostration, headache, vomiting, delirium followed in 2–3 d by maculopapular rash uniformly progressing to pustules and scabs, mostly on extremities and face	7–17 d	Pharyngeal swab, vesicular fluid, biopsies, scab material for electron microscopy and PCR testing through public health laboratory network	30% in unvaccinated persons	Supportive care Cidofovir (Vistide) shown to be effective in vitro and in experimental animals infected with surrogate orthopox virus	Live, attenuated vaccinia vaccine derived from calf lymph; given by scarification (licensed, restricted supply) New vaccine being developed from tissue culture Vaccination given within 3–4 d following exposure can prevent or decrease the severity of disease	Requires astute clinical evaluation; may be confused with chickenpox, erythema multiforme with bullae, or allergic contact dermatitis Notify CDC Poxvirus Section at 404-639-2184
Viral Encephalitis							
All forms	Systemic febrile illness, with encephalitis developing in some populations Generalized malaise, spiking fevers, headache, myalgia		Clinical and epidemiologic diagnosis WBC count can show striking leukopenia and lymphopenia Confirmatory test and viral isolation available through public health laboratory network		Supportive care Analgesics, anticonvulsants as needed	Several IND vaccines, poorly immunogenic, highly reactogenic	Incidence of seizures and/or focal neurologic deficits may be higher after biological attack
Eastern equine encephalitis		7–14 d		50%–75%			
Western equine encephalitis		7–14 d		10%			
Venezuelan equine encephalitis		2–6 d		<10%			

Viral Hemorrhagic Fevers

DISEASE AND AGENT	SIGNS AND SYMPTOMS	SYMPTOM ONSET	DIAGNOSIS	LETHALITY	TREATMENT	PROPHYLAXIS	COMMENTS
Arenaviruses (Lassa, Junin, and related viruses) Bunyaviruses (Hanta, Congo–Crimean, Rift Valley) Filoviruses (Ebola, Marburg) Flaviviruses (yellow fever, dengue, various tick-borne disease viruses)	Fever with mucous membrane bleeding, petechiae, thrombocytopenia, and hypotension in patients without underlying malignancies Malaise, myalgias, headache, vomiting, diarrhea possible	4–21 d	Confirmatory testing and viral isolation available through public health laboratory network	Variable depending on viral strain; 15%–25% with Lassa fever to ≤90% with Ebola	Supportive therapy Ribavirin (Virazole) may be effective for Lassa fever, Rift Valley fever, Argentine hemorrhagic fever, and Congo–Crimean hemorrhagic fever	Ribavarin (Virazole)[1] is suggested for Congo–Crimean hemorrhagic fever and Lassa fever Yellow fever vaccine is the only licensed vaccine available Vaccines for some of the other VHFs exist but are for investigational use only	Call CDC Special Pathogens Office at 404-639-1115

Biological Toxins

DISEASE AND AGENT	SIGNS AND SYMPTOMS	SYMPTOM ONSET	DIAGNOSIS	LETHALITY	TREATMENT	PROPHYLAXIS	COMMENTS
Botulism *Clostridium botulinum* toxin	Blurred vision, diplopia, dry mouth, ptosis, fatigue As disease progresses, acute bilateral descending flaccid paralysis, respiratory paralysis resulting in death	1–5 d, typically 12–36 h	Clinical Serum and stool should be assayed for toxin by mouse neutralization bioassay, which can take several days	60% without ventilatory support	Intensive and prolonged supportive care; ventilation may be necessary Trivalent equine antitoxin (serotypes A, B, E, – licensed, available from the CDC) should be administered immediately after clinical diagnosis	Pentavalent toxoid (A–E), yearly booster (IND, CDC) Not available to the public Antitoxin may be sufficient to prevent illness following exposure but is not recommended until patient is showing symptoms	Anaphylaxis and serum sickness are potential complications of antitoxin Aminoglycosides and clindamycin (Cleocin) A must not be used
Enterotoxin B *Staphylococcus aureus*	Acute onset of fever, chills headache, nonproductive cough	3–12 h	Clinical Normal chest radiograph Serology on acute and convalescent serum can confirm diagnosis	Probably low (few data available for respiratory exposure)	Supportive care	No vaccine available	
Ricin toxin *Ricinus communis*	Weakness, nausea, chest tightness, fever, cough, pulmonary edema, respiratory failure, circulatory collapse, hypoxemia resulting in death (usually within 36–72 h)	≤6–24 h	Clinical and epidemiologic Confirmatory serological testing available through public health laboratory network	Mortality data are not available, but likely to be high with extensive exposure	Supportive care Treatment for pulmonary edema Gastric decontamination if toxin is ingested	No vaccine available	

Continued

TABLE 1 Quick Reference Chart on Biological Weapon Agents—cont'd

DISEASE AND AGENT	DIAGNOSTIC CONSIDERATIONS				TREATMENT CONSIDERATIONS*		COMMENTS
	SIGNS AND SYMPTOMS	SYMPTOM ONSET	DIAGNOSIS	LETHALITY	TREATMENT	PROPHYLAXIS	
T-2 Mycotoxins *Fusarium Myrothecium Trichoderma Stachybotrys*	Abrupt onset of mucocutaneous and airway irritation and pain Can include skin, eyes, and GI tract; systemic toxicity can follow	Minutes to hours			Clinical support	No vaccine available	Soap and water washing within 4–6 h reduces dermal toxicity; washing within 1 h can eliminate toxicity entirely
Other filamentous fungi			Confirmation requires testing blood, tissue, and environmental samples	Severe exposure can cause death in hours to days			Consult with local health department regarding specimen collection and diagnostic testing procedures

Adapted from Lyznicki JL: AMA quick reference guide: Biological emergencies. In American Medical Association: Management of Public Health Emergencies. A Resource Guide for Physicians and Other Community Responders. Chicago, American Medical Association, 2005.

[1] Not FDA approved for this indication.

[2] Not available in the United States.

*Different situations can require different dosage and treatment regimens. Please consult other references and an infectious disease specialist for definitive dosage information, especially dosages for pregnant women and children.

†Data from 22 patients infected with anthrax in October and November 2001 indicate a median incubation period of 4 days (range, 4–7 days) for inhalational anthrax and a mean incubation of 5 days (range, 1–10 days) for cutaneous anthrax.

‡Chest radiograph abnormalities include paratracheal and hilar fullness and may be subtle. Consider chest computed tomography if diagnosis is uncertain.

§Limited data from the October and November 2001 anthrax infections indicate hemorrhagic pleural effusions to be strongly associated with inhalational anthrax; rhinorrhea was present in only 1/10 patients.

‖Limited data from the 2001 terrorist-related anthrax infections indicate that early treatment significantly decreased the mortality rate.

•Other agents with in vitro activity suggested for use in conjunction with ciprofloxacin or doxycycline for treatment of inhalational anthrax include rifampin, vancomycin (Vancocin), imipenem (Primaxin), chloramphenicol (Chloromycetin), penicillin and ampicillin, clindamycin (Cleocin), and clarithromycin (Biaxin).

Abbreviations: CDC = Centers for Disease Control and Prevention; CNS = central nervous system; CSF = cerebrospinal fluid; GI = gastrointestinal; IND = investigational new drug; PCR = polymerase chain reaction; TMP-SMX = trimethoprim-sulfamethoxazole; USAMRIID = U.S. Army Medical Research Institute of Infectious Diseases; VHF = viral hemorrhagic fever; WBC = white blood cell.

Method of
Miriam Chan, BSc Pharm, PharmD

Popular Herbs and Nutritional Supplements

HERB OR NUTRITIONAL SUPPLEMENT	COMMON USES	REASONABLE ADULT ORAL DOSAGE*	PRECAUTIONS AND DRUG INTERACTIONS
Aloe vera	Commonly found in skin products as a moisturizer Used topically to treat burns, wounds, skin infections, and inflammation Approved in Germany to use orally as a laxative Used orally for a variety of conditions, including diabetes, asthma, epilepsy, and osteoarthritis	For external use, apply aloe gel on the skin tid to qid For constipation, 40–170 mg of dried aloe juice or latex (corresponds to 10–30 mg hydroxyanthracene derivatives) taken in the evening For other conditions, no established dosage documented	Aloe gel is generally well tolerated and safe when used topically Aloe gel taken orally can cause hypoglycemia in patients who are concomitantly taking antidiabetic drugs Aloe juice or latex contains anthraquinone, a cathartic laxative and should not be taken by people with intestinal obstruction, acute intestinal inflammation, and ulcers Pregnant women should not take aloe latex because it may cause uterine contractions Oral use of aloe latex can cause abdominal cramps and diarrhea. Long-term use or abuse can cause electrolyte imbalances, albuminuria, hematuria, and pseudomelanosis coli. Prolonged use of high doses (≥ 1 g/d) can cause nephritis, acute renal failure, and death In 2002, the FDA banned the sale of aloe-containing laxative products in the United States because of the lack of safety data Aloe can decrease platelet aggregation and should be avoided at least 2 wk before surgery
Astragalus	Used in combination with other herbs to support and enhance the immune system Used to prevent and treat common colds and upper respiratory infections Used for heart disease Widely used in China for chronic hepatitis and as an adjunctive therapy in cancer	Extract: 250–500 mg tid to qid standardized to 0.4% 4-hydroxy-3-methoxyisoflavone 7-sug Powdered root: 500–1000 mg tid Tincture (1:5) in 30% ethanol: 3–5 mL tid Decoction: 3–6 g of dried root per 12 oz water tid	Avoid using astragalus in organ transplant patients and those with autoimmune disorders Side effects include mild stomach upset and allergic reactions Astragalus can decrease the effects of cyclophosphamide and other immunosuppressants
Bilberry fruit	Often used orally to improve visual acuity and to treat degenerative retinal conditions Used orally to treat chronic venous insufficiency, varicose veins, and hemorrhoids Approved in Germany to use orally for acute diarrhea and topically for mild inflammation of the mucous membranes of mouth and throat	For eye conditions and circulation, 80–160 mg tid of the extract standardized to at least 25% anthocyanosides For diarrhea, 20–60 g/d of the dried, ripe berries or as a tea preparation (5–10 g of crushed dried berries in 150 mL water, brought to a boil for 10 min, then strained) For external use, 10% decoction	No known side effects reported with bilberry fruit and extract However, bilberry leaf taken in large quantities or used long term has been shown to cause wasting, anemia, jaundice, acute excitation, disturbances of tonus, and death in animals The anthocyanidin extracts from bilberry can increase the risk of bleeding in those taking warfarin or other blood thinners
Black cohosh root	Commonly used to relieve hot flashes and other menopausal symptoms Used to treat premenstrual discomfort and dysmenorrhea	20 mg bid of the rhizome extract standardized to triterpene glycosides Remifemin is the proprietary brand used in a number of clinical trials The German guidelines do not recommend its use for >6 mo	Black cohosh may have an estrogen-like effect and should be avoided in women with breast cancer Large doses may induce miscarriage and it is contraindicated during pregnancy It may cause GI disturbances, headache, and hypotension International case reports of liver dysfunction suspected to be associated with its use
Black haw	To relieve uterine cramps and painful periods To prevent miscarriage and ease pain that followed childbirth	For menstrual pain, 5 mL of tincture in water, taken 3–5 times daily	Black haw should not be used in pregnancy because of its uterine relaxant effects The salicylate constituent in black haw could trigger allergic reactions in individuals with aspirin allergies or asthma Black haw may aggravate tinnitus

Continued

HERB OR NUTRITIONAL SUPPLEMENT	COMMON USES	REASONABLE ADULT ORAL DOSAGE	PRECAUTIONS AND DRUG INTERACTIONS
Black haw, cont'd		For prevention of miscarriage, 1–2 cups of tea per day (1 tsp of dried herb in 1 cup of boiling water, steeped for 10 min)	Large doses of black haw can prolong bleeding time The oxalic acid component of black haw can increase kidney stone formation in susceptible individuals Black haw can interact with warfarin and increase risk of bleeding
Cat's claw	Used primarily to reduce pain in osteoarthritis and rheumatoid arthritis Used for a variety of health conditions, including viral infections (e.g., herpes, HIV), Alzheimer's disease, and cancer Used to support the immune system and promote kidney health Used to prevent and abort pregnancy	For osteoarthritis, 100 mg/d of the dry encapsulated extract For rheumatoid arthritis, 20 mg tid of the dry extract standardized to 1.3% pentacyclic oxindole alkaloids free of tetracyclic oxindole alkaloids For general uses, 1–3 cups of tea per day (1 g root bark boiled for 15 min in 250 mL of water) or 1 mL of tincture 2–3 ×/d	Avoid using cat's claw during pregnancy or breastfeeding People with autoimmune diseases and transplant recipients should avoid cat's claw because of its immune stimulating effects Side effects include headaches, dizziness, and vomiting Cat's claw can lower blood pressure and cause hypotension when use with antihypertensive drugs Cat's claw can inhibit CYP3A4 enzyme and increase levels of drugs metabolized by this enzyme
Chamomile flower	Used orally to calm nerves and treat GI spasms and inflammatory diseases of the GI tract Used topically to treat wounds, skin infections, and skin or mucous membrane inflammation	1 cup of freshly made tea 3–4 times daily (1 tbsp or 3 g of dried flower in 150 mL boiling water for 5–10 min)	Chamomile can cause an allergic reaction, especially in people with severe allergies to ragweed or other members of the daisy family (e.g., echinacea, feverfew, and milk thistle) It should not be taken concurrently with other sedatives, such as alcohol or benzodiazepines
Chaste tree berry (Chasteberry, Vitex)	For normalizing irregular menstrual periods and relieving premenstrual complaints For relieving menopausal symptoms For restoring fertility in women For treating acne associated with menstrual cycles For increasing breast milk production in lactating women	For menstrual irregularities and premenstrual complaints, 30–40 mg/d of the dried berries or an equivalent amount of aqueous-alcoholic extracts (50%–70% v/v) Dried fruit extract, standardized to 0.6% agnusides, is used in doses of 175–225 mg/d For other conditions, no established dosage documented	Chaste tree berry can have uterine stimulant properties and should be avoided in pregnancy Women with hormone-dependent conditions (e.g., breast, uterine, and ovarian cancers, and endometriosis and uterine fibroids) and men with prostate cancer should avoid chaste tree berry because it contains progestins Side effects include intramenstrual bleeding, dry mouth, headache, nausea, rash, alopecia, and tachycardia High doses ($\geq$ 480 mg/d extract) can paradoxically decrease lactation Chaste tree berry is thought to have dopaminergic effects and can interact with dopamine antagonists, such as antipsychotics and metoclopramide Chaste tree berry can decrease the effects of oral contraceptives and hormone therapy
Chondroitin	Orally, used frequently in combination with glucosamine for osteoarthritis Topically, in combination with sodium hyaluronate, as a viscoelastic agent in cataract surgery	Oral: 200–400 mg tid	Occasional mild side effects include nausea, indigestion, and allergic reactions Chondroitin derived from bovine cartilage carries a potential risk of contamination with diseased animals
Chromium	For diabetes For hypercholesterolemia Commonly found in weight-loss products Also promoted for body building	For diabetes, 100 mcg bid for $\leq$4 mo or 500 mcg bid for 2 mo For hypercholesterolemia, 200 mcg tid or 500 mcg bid for 2–4 mo For body building, 200–400 mcg/d Chromium picolinate has been used in most studies, even though the chloride form is also available	Adverse effects are rare, but they include headaches, insomnia, sleep disturbances, irritability and mood changes; some patients may also experience cognitive, perceptual, and motor dysfunction Long-term use of high doses (600–2400 mcg/d) can cause anemia, thrombocytopenia, hemolysis, hepatic dysfunction, and renal failure Interstitial nephritis has been reported A few studies suggest that chromium can cause DNA damage Chromium competes with iron for binding to transferrin and can cause iron deficiency Antacids, H_2 blockers, and proton pump inhibitors can decrease the absorption of chromium

HERB OR NUTRITIONAL SUPPLEMENT	COMMON USES	REASONABLE ADULT ORAL DOSAGE	PRECAUTIONS AND DRUG INTERACTIONS
Coenzyme Q10	As adjunctive treatment for congestive heart failure, angina, hypertension, and diabetes Used for reducing cardiotoxicity associated with doxorubicin Used to treat statin-induced myopathy	For heart failure, 100 mg/d in 2 or 3 divided doses For angina, 50 mg tid For hypertension, 60 mg bid For diabetes, 100–200 mg/d	Mild adverse events include gastric distress, nausea, vomiting, and hypotension Doses >300 mg/d can cause elevated liver enzyme levels Coenzyme Q10 can reduce the anticoagulation effects of warfarin Oral hypoglycemic agents and HMG-CoA reductase inhibitors can reduce serum coenzyme Q10 levels
Cranberry	To prevent and treat UTIs or *Helicobacter pylori* infections that can lead to stomach ulcers To prevent dental plaque As an antioxidant to prevent cardiovascular disease and cancer	For UTIs, 150–600 mL of cranberry juice daily or 300–400 mg of standardized extract bid For other conditions, no dosage determined	Drinking excessive amounts of juice could cause GI upset or diarrhea Prolonged use of cranberry juice in large doses increases the risk of kidney stones formation because of its high oxalate content Cranberry can interact with warfarin and cause an increase in INR The effectiveness of proton pump inhibitors can be reduced by cranberry because of its acidity
Creatine	To enhance muscle performance, especially during short-duration, high-intensity exercise	Loading dose of 20 g/d for 5–7 d followed by a maintenance dose of ≥2 g/d An alternative dosing of 3 g/d for 28 d has been suggested	Creatine can cause gastroenteritis, diarrhea, heat intolerance, muscle cramps, and elevated serum creatinine levels Creatine is contraindicated in patients taking diuretics Concurrent use with cimetidine, probenecid, or nonsteroidal anti-inflammatory drugs increases the risk of adverse renal effects Caffeine can decrease creatine's ergogenic effects
Dehydroepi-androsterone (DHEA)	Replace low serum DHEA levels in adrenal insufficiency Treat SLE Reverse aging Used in many other conditions, including Alzheimer's disease, depression, diabetes, menopause, osteoporosis, impotence, and AIDS Used to promote weight loss Used by bodybuilders to increase muscle mass	For replacement therapy, 25–50 mg/d For SLE, 200 mg/d For antiaging and osteoporosis, 50 mg/d For other conditions, no established dosage documented	Most common side effects are androgenic in nature and include acne, hair loss, hirsutism, and deepening of the voice Cases of hepatitis have been reported When used in high doses, DHEA can cause insomnia, manic symptoms, and palpitations DHEA at physiologic doses increases circulating androgens in women, but not in men; it also increases circulating estrogens in both men and women Avoid use of DHEA in individuals with a history of sex hormone–dependent malignancy Safety of DHEA in individuals <30 y unknown DHEA inhibits CYP3A4 enzyme and could increase serum concentrations of drugs metabolized by this enzyme (e.g., lovastatin, ketoconazole, itraconzaole, and triazolam)
Dong quai root	Commonly used for the relief of premenstrual and menopausal symptoms Used as a "blood tonic" and a strengthening treatment for the heart, spleen, liver, and kidneys	For premenstrual and menopausal symptoms, 3–4 g/d in 3 divided doses For other conditions, no established dosage documented	Dong quai should not be used in pregnant women because of its uterine stimulant and relaxant effects Women with hormone sensitive conditions (e.g., breast, uterine, and ovarian cancers, and endometriosis and uterine fibroids) should avoid dong quai because of its estrogenic effects Drinking the essential oil of dong quai is not recommended because it contains a small amount of carcinogenic constituents Dong quai contains psoralens that can cause photosensitivity and photodermatitis Dong quai contains natural coumarin derivatives that can increase the risk of bleeding in those who are taking anticoagulant or antiplatelet drugs
Echinacea	As an immune stimulant, particularly for the prevention and treatment of the common cold and influenza Supportive therapy for lower urinary tract infections Used topically to treat skin disorders and promote wound healing	300 mg tid of *Echinacea pallida* root or 2–3 mL tid of expressed juice of *Echinacea purpurea* herb Do not use for >8 wk because echinacea may suppress immunity if used long term	Echinacea should not be used in transplant patients and those with autoimmune disease or liver dysfunction Allergic reactions have been reported Adverse events are rare and include mild GI effects It should be discontinued as far in advance of surgery as possible Echinacea can decrease effectiveness of the immunosuppressants

Continued

HERB OR NUTRITIONAL SUPPLEMENT	COMMON USES	REASONABLE ADULT ORAL DOSAGE	PRECAUTIONS AND DRUG INTERACTIONS
Ephedra (ma huang)	For diseases of the respiratory tract with mild bronchospasm Promoted for weight loss and performance enhancement	1 tsp or 2 g of dried herb (15–30 mg of ephedrine) in 240 mL boiling water for 10 min In Canada, the maximum allowable dosage of ephedrine is 8 mg per dose or 32 mg/d	Ephedra contains ephedrine, which has sympathomimetic activities; consequently, it should not be used in patients who have cardiovascular disease, diabetes, glaucoma, hypertension, hyperthyroidism, prostate enlargement, psychiatric disorders, or seizures Serious adverse effects, including seizures, arrhythmias, heart attack, stroke, and death, have been associated with the use of ephedra; as a result, the FDA has banned the sale of ephedra products in the United States Because of the cardiovascular effects of ephedrine, patients taking ephedra should discontinue use at least 24 h before surgery Concurrent use of ephedra and digitalis, guanethidine, monoamine oxidase inhibitors, or other stimulants, including caffeine, is not recommended
Evening primrose oil	For PMS, especially if mastalgia is present For treatment of atopic eczema Used for other medical conditions, including rheumatoid arthritis, menopausal symptoms, Raynaud's phenomenon, Sjögren's syndrome, and diabetic neuropathy	For PMS, 2–4 g/d For atopic eczema, 6–8 g/d For rheumatoid arthritis, 2.8 g/d These doses are based on products standardized to 9% γ-linolenic acid Daily dose can be given in divided doses	Evening primrose oil can increase the risk of pregnancy complications Side effects include indigestion, nausea, soft stools, and headache Seizures have been reported in patients with schizophrenia who were taking phenothiazines and evening primrose oil concomitantly Evening primrose oil can interact with anesthesia and cause seizures Concomitant use of evening primrose oil with anticoagulant and antiplatelet drugs can increase the risk of bleeding
Fenugreek seed	For diabetes and hypercholesterolemia For constipation, dyspepsia, gastritis, and kidney ailments Approved in Germany for use orally for loss of appetite and topically as a poultice for local inflammation	For loss of appetite, 1–2 g of the seed tid or 1 cup of tea (500 mg seed in 150 mL cold water for 3 h) several times a day Maximum 6 g/d For other conditions, no established dosage documented For topical use, 50 g powdered seed in 0.25 L of hot water to form a paste	Fenugreek can cause uterine contractions and should be avoided in pregnancy Individuals who have allergies to peanuts or soybeans might also be allergic to fenugreek Fenugreek can cause diarrhea and flatulence; it can also make urine smell like maple syrup Hypoglycemia can occur if fenugreek is taken in large amounts Repeated external applications can result in undesirable skin reactions Fenugreek contains small amounts of coumarins and can interact with anticoagulants and antiplatelet drugs High mucilage content of fenugreek can affect the absorption of oral drugs; therefore, fenugreek should not be taken within 2 h of other drugs
Feverfew	For migraine headache prophylaxis For treatment of fever, menstrual problems, and arthritis	25–75 mg bid of the encapsulated dried leaf extract standardized to 0.2% parthenolide	Feverfew can induce menstrual bleeding and is contraindicated in pregnancy Fresh leaves can cause oral ulcers and GI irritation Sudden discontinuation of feverfew can precipitate rebound headache Feverfew can interact with anticoagulants and potentiate the antiplatelet effect of aspirin
Fish oils (omega-3 fatty acids)	Commonly used in the treatment of hypertriglyceridemia Used to prevent CHD and stroke Used in many noncardiac conditions, including depression, diabetes, dysmenorrhea, rheumatoid arthritis, and IgA nephropathy	For hypertriglyceridemia, 3–5 g/d For cardioprotection, 1 g/d for patients with CHD; oily fish at least twice a week, or about 0.5 g/d for people with no known heart disease For other conditions, no established dosage documented	Common side effects include fishy aftertaste, GI disturbances, belching, halitosis, and heartburn High doses can cause nausea and loose stools Doses >3 g/d can inhibit platelet aggregation, suppress immune function, worsen glycemic control, and raise LDL cholesterol levels Long-term use may be associated with weight gain Less well-controlled preparations can contain appreciable amount of organochloride contaminants

HERB OR NUTRITIONAL SUPPLEMENT	COMMON USES	REASONABLE ADULT ORAL DOSAGE	PRECAUTIONS AND DRUG INTERACTIONS
Fish oils (omega-3 fatty acids), cont'd	Used to reduce the risk of developing age-related maculopathy, Alzheimer's disease, and cancer Promotes visual and mental development in children	Fish oils are composed of EPA and DHA; fish oil capsules vary widely in amounts and ratios of EPA and DHA; the most common fish oil capsules in the United States provide 180 mg of EPA and 120 mg DHA per capsule, and three capsules will provide about 1 g/d of omega-3 fatty acids	Fish oil can increase the risk of bleeding in patients taking warfarin, an antiplatelet agent, or herbs that have antiplatelet constituents (e.g., garlic, ginkgo, and red clover) Fish oils can lower blood pressure and can have additive effects with antihypertensive agents Oral contraceptives can interfere with the triglyceride lowering effects of fish oils
Flaxseed	Orally, approved in Germany for chronic constipation, irritable bowel and other colon disorders Often used orally for hypercholesterolemia and atherosclerosis Topically, approved in Germany for painful skin inflammation	For constipation, 1 tbsp (5 g) of whole or "bruised" seeds (not ground) in 150 mL of liquid 2–3 times daily For bowel inflammation, soak 2–3 tbsp of milled flaxseed soaked in 200–300 mL water and strain after 30 min For hypercholesterolemia, 1–2 tbsp flaxseed oil daily Topical: 30–50 g flaxseed flour as poultice or compress for a moist-heat direct application directly to the skin	Flaxseed should be taken with plenty of water to prevent possible intestinal blockage Patients with ileus should not take flaxseed High mucilage content of flaxseed can delay absorption of other drugs taken at the same time
Garlic	To lower blood pressure and serum cholesterol To prevent atherosclerosis	Fresh clove: one 4 g clove per day Tablet: 300 mg bid to tid standardized to 0.6%–1.3% allicin	Intake of large quantities can lead to stomach complaints Garlic has antiplatelet effects, so patients should discontinue use of garlic at least 7 d before surgery Concomitant use of garlic and anticoagulants can increase the risk of bleeding
Ginger root	As an antiemetic For prevention of motion sickness	Fresh rhizome: 2–4 g/d Powdered ginger: 250 mg 3–4 times daily Tea: 1 cup of tea tid (0.5–1 g dried root in 150 mL boiling water for 5–10 min)	Ginger should not be used by patients with gallstones because of its cholagogic effect It can inhibit platelet aggregation; cases of postoperative bleeding have been reported Large doses of ginger can increase bleeding time in patients taking antiplatelet agents
Ginkgo biloba leaf	To slow cognitive deterioration in dementia To increase peripheral blood flow in claudication To treat sexual dysfunction associated with the use of SSRIs	60–120 mg bid of extract Egb/61 standardized to 24% flavonoids and 6% terpenoids	Adverse effects are rare and can include mild stomach or intestinal upset, headache, or allergic skin reaction Ginkgo can inhibit platelet aggregation; reports of spontaneous bleeding have been published Patients should discontinue ginkgo at least 36 h before surgery Concurrent use of ginkgo and anticoagulants, antiplatelet agents, vitamin E, or garlic can increase the risk of bleeding
Ginseng root	As a tonic during times of stress, fatigue, disability, and convalescence To improve physical performance and stamina	Root: 1–2 g/d Tablet: 100 mg bid of extract standardized to 4%–7% ginsenosides A 2- to 3-wk period of using ginseng followed by a 1- to 2-wk "rest" period is generally recommended Ginseng is commonly adulterated, especially Siberian ginseng (eleuthero) products	Ginseng has a mild stimulant effect and should be avoided in patients with cardiovascular disease Tachycardia and hypertension can occur Overdosages can lead to ginseng abuse syndrome, characterized by insomnia, hypotonia, and edema Ginseng has estrogenic effects and can cause vaginal bleeding and breast tenderness Ginseng has been shown to inhibit platelets, so patients should discontinue ginseng use at least 7 d before surgery Ginseng should not be used with other stimulants Patients taking antidiabetic agents and ginseng should be monitored to avoid the hypoglycemic effects of ginseng

Continued

HERB OR NUTRITIONAL SUPPLEMENT	COMMON USES	REASONABLE ADULT ORAL DOSAGE	PRECAUTIONS AND DRUG INTERACTIONS
Ginseng root, cont'd			Ginseng can interact with warfarin and cause a decreased INR Siberian ginseng can increase digoxin levels Ginseng can interact with phenelzine (a MAOI) resulting in insomnia, headache, tremulousness, and manic-like symptoms
Glucosamine	For osteoarthritis	500 mg tid with meals Glucosamine is available in the form of sulfate, hydrochloride, or N-acetyl salt; glucosamine sulfate is the form that has been used in most clinical studies	Side effects are generally limited to mild GI symptoms, including stomach upset, heartburn, diarrhea, nausea, and indigestion Glucosamine derived from marine exoskeletons may cause reactions in people allergic to shellfish Glucosamine may raise blood glucose level in patients with diabetes
Goldenseal	Often combined with echinacea to treat colds and other upper respiratory infections Used for diarrhea, dyspepsia, and gastritis Used topically as an eyewash, mouthwash, feminine cleansing product, and skin remedy	Oral: 0.5–1 g of the dried rhizome/root or 2–4 mL tincture (1:10, 60% ethanol) or 0.3–1 mL fluid extract (1:1, 60% ethanol) tid Eyewash: For trachoma infections, 2 drops of a 0.2% aqueous berberine solution tid × 3 wk	Avoid using goldenseal during pregnancy and breast feeding; berberine, the principle constituent in goldenseal, can cause uterine contractions and neonatal jaundice Avoid using goldenseal in kidney failure because of inadequate urinary excretion of its alkaloids High dosages or long-term usage can lead to nausea, vomiting, headache, hypotension, bradycardia, leucopenia, and mucosal irritation Berberine can increase the risk of bleeding in patients taking warfarin or an antiplatelet agent Be aware that other herbs containing berberine, including Chinese goldthread and Oregon grape, are sometimes substituted for goldenseal
Grape seed	For conditions related to the heart and blood vessels, such as atherosclerosis, high blood pressure, high cholesterol, and poor circulation For vision problems, diabetic neuropathy or retinopathy, and swelling after an injury or surgery For cancer prevention and wound healing	For general health purposes, 100–300 mg daily of a standardized extract (95% oligomeric proanthocyanidin complexes)	Side effects include headache, dizziness, nausea, and dry, itchy scalp Concomitant use with warfarin or antiplatelet agents can increase risk of bleeding because of the tocopherol content of grape seed oil
Hawthorn leaf with flower	Commonly used in Germany to increase cardiac output in patients with New York Heart Association stage I and II heart failure	160–900 mg water-ethanol extract (30–169 mg procyanidins or 3.5–19.8 mg flavonoids) divided into 2–3 doses	Side effects include GI upset, palpitations, hypotension, headache, dizziness, and insomnia Concomitant use with CNS depressants can have additive CNS effects Hawthorn can potentiate effects of digoxin and vasodilators
Hops	For mood disturbances such as restlessness and anxiety For sleep disturbances Commonly found in combination products with other herbal sedatives	0.5 g of cut or powdered strobile in a single dose; can be taken as tea (0.5 g in 150 mL water), fluid extract 1:1 (0.5 mL), tincture 1:5 (2.5 mL), or dry extract 6–8:1 (60–80 mg) The preparation contains at least 0.35% (v/w) essential oil	Side effects are rare but include drowsiness and allergic reactions Hops is not recommended for use during pregnancy and lactation It can potentiate the sedative effect of CNS depressants (e.g., benzodiazepines, alcohol) and other herbal tranquilizers
Horse chestnut seed	To relieve symptoms of chronic venous insufficiency	250 mg bid of extract standardized to 50 mg aescin in delayed-release form Unsafe to ingest the raw seed, which contains significant amounts of the most toxic constituent, esculin	Mild GI symptoms, headache, dizziness, and pruritis have been reported Ingestion of high doses can cause renal, hepatic, and hematologic toxicity Concomitant use with anticoagulants can increase the risk of bleeding Horse chestnut can potentiate the effects of hypoglycemic drugs

HERB OR NUTRITIONAL SUPPLEMENT	COMMON USES	REASONABLE ADULT ORAL DOSAGE	PRECAUTIONS AND DRUG INTERACTIONS
Kava kava	As an anxiolytic for nervous anxiety, stress, and restlessness As a sedative to induce sleep	Herb and preparations equivalent to 60–120 mg/d of kava pyrones Most clinical trials have used 100 mg tid of extract standardized to 70% kava pyrones for anxiety disorders	Kava should not be used by patients with depression Kava should be avoided in pregnant or nursing women Kava can affect motor reflexes and judgment, so it should not be taken while driving and/or operating heavy machinery Accommodative disturbances have been reported; kava can exacerbate Parkinson's disease Extended use can cause a temporary yellow discoloration of skin, hair, and nails Reports have linked kava use to at least 25 cases of severe liver toxicity; sale of products containing kava has been banned in Canada and several European countries Kava has been shown to have additive CNS depressant effects with benzodiazepines, alcohol, and herbal tranquilizers Kava can potentiate the sedative effects of anesthetics, so kava should be discontinued at least 24 h before surgery
Lutein	Commonly used to prevent AMD and cataracts Used to prevent skin cancer, breast cancer, and colon cancer Used to protect against cardiovascular disease	For AMD and cataracts, 6–20 mg/d of lutein from diet For other uses, no established dosage documented Foods containing high concentrations of lutein include kale, spinach, broccoli, and romaine lettuce Not known if supplemental lutein is as effective as natural lutein Supplemental lutein in the form of esters might require a higher fat intake for effective absorption than purified lutein	No major adverse effects and drug interactions have been reported
Lycopene	Commonly used to prevent and treat prostate cancer Used for cancer prevention, arthrosclerosis prevention, and reduction of asthma symptoms	For decreasing the growth of prostate cancer, 15 mg supplement bid For prostate cancer prevention, at least 6 mg/d from tomato products (or ≥ 10 servings/wk) For other uses, no established dosage documented Heat processing converts lycopene in fresh tomatoes from the *trans* to the *cis*-configuration. The *cis* isomer has better bioavailability Lycopene supplements usually do not specify the type and amount of isomers in their product labeling	Lycopene, when consumed in amounts found in foods, is generally considered to be safe Concomitant ingestion of beta-carotene can increase lycopene absorption Lycopene may reduce cholesterol levels and potentiate the effects of statins
Melatonin	For jet lag, insomnia, shift-work disorder, and circadian rhythm disorders For other medical conditions, including depression, multiple sclerosis, tinnitus, headache, and cancer	For jet lag, 5 mg at bedtime for 2–5 d beginning the day of return For sleep disorders, 0.3–5 mg taken 2 h before bedtime Avoid melatonin from animal pineal gland because of the possibility of contamination.	Avoid use in pregnancy because melatonin decreases serum luteinizing hormone concentrations and increases serum prolactin levels The common adverse reactions include headache, transient depressive symptoms, daytime fatigue and drowsiness, dizziness, abdominal cramps, irritability, and reduced alertness Concomitant use of melatonin with alcohol, benzodiazepines, or other CNS depressants can cause additive sedation Melatonin can affect immune function and may interfere with immunosuppressive therapy Concomitant use with other herbs that have sedative properties (e.g., chamomile, goldenseal, hop, kava, valerian) can produce additive CNS-impairing effects

Continued

Popular Herbs and Nutritional Supplements

1275

HERB OR NUTRITIONAL SUPPLEMENT	COMMON USES	REASONABLE ADULT ORAL DOSAGE	PRECAUTIONS AND DRUG INTERACTIONS
Milk thistle fruit	As a hepatoprotectant and antioxidant, particularly for treatment of hepatitis, cirrhosis, and toxic liver damage Used in Europe for the treatment of hepatotoxic mushroom poisoning from *Amanita phalloides*	Average daily dose is 12–15 g of crude drug or formulations equivalent to 200–400 mg of silymarin	Adverse effects are rare but include diarrhea and allergic reactions Milk thistle can potentiate the hypoglycemic effect of antidiabetic agents
Peppermint	Commonly used for indigestion and irritable bowel syndrome (IBS) Used externally for myalgia and neuralgia	Indigestion: 1 tsp dried leaves in 1 cup of boiling water, steeped for 10 min; drink 4–5 ×/d between meals IBS: 1–2 enteric coated cap (0.2 mL of peppermint oil/cap) 2–3 ×/d. Take peppermint ≥2 h before or after an acid-reducing drug to ensure adequate absorption	Peppermint, in amounts normally found in food, is likely to be safe Larger supplemental amounts can cause side effects including heartburn, flushing, headache, and mouth sores Hypersensitivity reactions, contact dermatitis, and exacerbations of asthma may occur Peppermint can exacerbate symptoms in patients with GERD because it can relax the lower esophageal sphincter Peppermint tea has been shown to reduce free testosterone levels in men Peppermint can decrease the blood levels of cyclosporine and drugs that metabolized by the CYP3A4 isoenzyme
Probiotics	Prevent and treat antibiotic-associated diarrhea and acute infectious diarrhea Relieve symptoms of irritable bowel syndrome Treat atopic dermatitis for at-risk infants	Dosage varies based on preparations *Lactobacillus* sp., *Bifidobacterium* sp., *Saccharomyces boulardii* are the most widely used organisms For *Lactobacillus* sp., 10 billion CFUs/d For *Lactobacillus* sp./ *Bifidobacterium* sp., 100 million to 35 billion CFUs/d For *Saccharomyces boulardii*, 250–500 mg/d Quality of products varies among brands Refrigeration is required to maintain potency	Avoid use in short-gut syndrome and severe immunocompromised condition Common adverse effects include flatulence, mild abdominal discomfort, and, rarely, septicemia
Red clover flower	Commonly used for conditions associated with menopause, such as hot flashes, cardiovascular health, and osteoporosis Used for PMS, benign prostate hyperplasia, and cancer prevention Used topically to treat psoriasis, eczema, and other rashes	For hot flashes, 40 mg/d of the isoflavones extract (Promensil™) For other conditions, no established dosage documented	Red clover has estrogenic activity and should be avoided during pregnancy and lactation Women with hormone-dependent conditions (e.g., breast, uterine, and ovarian cancer, and endometriosis and uterine fibroids) and men with prostate cancer should also avoid taking red clover Side effects include headache, myalgia, nausea, and rash Red clover contains coumarin derivatives and can increase the risk of bleeding in those who are taking anticoagulants or antiplatelet drugs Preliminary report suggests that red clover might antagonize the effects of tamoxifen Some evidence suggests that red clover can increase the levels of drugs that metabolized by the cytochrome P450 3A4 isoenzyme (e.g., lovastatin, ketoconazole, itraconzaole, fexofenadine, and triazolam)
SAMe (S-adenosyl-L-methionine)	For treatment of osteoarthritis, depression, fibromyalgia, and liver disease	For osteoarthritis, 200 mg tid For depression and fibromyalgia, 800 mg bid For liver disease, 600–800 mg bid	Common side effects include flatulence, nausea, vomiting, and diarrhea SAMe can cause anxiety in people with depression and hypomania in people with bipolar disorder Concurrent use of SAMe and other antidepressants can cause serotonin syndrome

HERB OR NUTRITIONAL SUPPLEMENT	COMMON USES	REASONABLE ADULT ORAL DOSAGE	PRECAUTIONS AND DRUG INTERACTIONS
Saw palmetto berry	To treat symptomatic benign prostatic hyperplasia and irritable bladder	160 mg bid of extract standardized to 85%–95% fatty acids and sterols	Adverse effects are rare but include headache, nausea, and upset stomach High doses can cause diarrhea
Soy	Commonly used for cholesterol reduction in combination with a low fat diet Used for menopausal symptoms and for prevention of osteoporosis and cardiovascular disease in postmenopausal women	For lowering cholesterol, 25–50 g/d of soy protein For hot flashes, 20–60 g/d of soy protein For osteoporosis, 40 g/d of soy protein containing 90 mg isoflavones	Soy, when consumed as whole foods (e.g., tofu or soy milk), has minimal adverse effects Consumption of large amounts of soy can cause gastric complaints such as constipation, bloating, and nausea Long-term use of soy tablets containing isoflavones (150 mg/d for 5 y) has been shown to cause endometrial hyperplasia
St. John's wort	Used for treatment of mild to moderate depression May have anti-inflammatory and antiinfective activities	300 mg tid of hypericum extract standardized to 0.3% hypericin	St. John's wort should not be used in pregnancy Side effects include dry mouth, GI upset, dizziness, fatigue, and constipation St. John's wort can induce photosensitivity, especially in fair-skinned individuals It can cause serotonin syndrome if used with other antidepressants, including SSRIs, or other serotonergic drugs It has been shown to induce CYP3A4 and decrease blood levels of many drugs such as indinavir, nevirapine, cyclosporine, digoxin, theophylline, simvastatin, oral contraceptive pills, and warfarin St. John's wort should be discontinued at least 5 d before surgery to avoid any potential drug interactions
Stinging nettle root	Approved in Germany for difficulty in urination in BPH stage 1 and 2	4–6 g per day of cut root; can be taken as tea (1.5 g in 150 mL boiling water for 10–20 min, tid), fluidextract 1:1 (1.5 mL tid), tincture 1:5 (5–7.5 mL tid), or dry extract 5.4–6.6:1 (0.22–0.33 g tid)	Occasionally, mild GI upsets may occur No known interactions with drugs
Valerian root	Used as a mild sedative for insomnia and anxiety	2–3 g of dried root or 1–3 mL of tincture, up to several times per day Two clinical trials found 400–450 mg of the root extract effective for insomnia	Valerian has a bad odor and can cause morning drowsiness Long-term administration can lead to paradoxical stimulation, including restlessness and palpitations Because of the risk of benzodiazepine-like withdrawal, valerian should be tapered over a period of several weeks before surgery It can potentiate the sedative effect of CNS depressants (e.g., benzodiazepines, alcohol) and other herbal tranquilizers

*Doses presented in the table are adapted from the German Commission E Monographs and/or data from clinical trials. Products from different manufacturers vary considerably. A reliable product should have a label clearly stating the botanical name of the herb and milligram amount contained in the product. Standardized extracts should be used whenever possible and are often disclosed on the label of quality products.

Abbreviations: AMD = age-related macular degeneration; BPH = benign prostatic hyperplasia; CFU = colony-forming unit; CHD = coronary heart disease; CNS = central nervous system; CYP3A4 = cytochrome P450 3A4; DHE = docosahexaenoic acid; EPA = eicosapentaenoic acid; FDA = Food and Drug Administration; GI = gastrointestinal; HMG-CoA = 3-hydroxy-3-methylglutaryl coenzyme A; INR = international normalized ratio; LDL = low-density lipoprotein; MAOI = monoamine oxidase inhibitor; PMS = premenstrual syndrome; SLE = systemic lupus erythematosus; SSRIs = selective serotonin reuptake inhibitors; UTIs = urinary tract infections.

References

Ang-Lee MK, Moss J, Yuan C. Herbal medicines and perioperative care. JAMA 2001;286:208–16.

Barnes J, Anderson LA, Phillipson JD. PDR for Herbal Medicines. 3rd ed. Montvale: Medical Economics Co.; 2004

Bent S. Herbal medicine in the United States: Review and efficacy, safety, and regulation. J Gen Intern Med 2008;23:854–9.

Blumenthal M, editor. Herbal Medicines: Expanded Commission E monographs. Austin, TX: American Botanical Council; 2000.

Blumenthal M, editor. The ABC Clinical Guide to Herbs. Austin, TX: American Botanical Council; 2003.

Cupp MJ. Herbal remedies: Adverse effects and drug interactions. Am Fam Physician 1999;59:1239–44.

Ernst E. The risk-benefit profile of commonly used herbal therapies: Ginkgo, St John's wort, ginseng, Echinacea, saw palmetto, and kava. Ann Intern Med 2002;136:42–53.

Jellin JM, Gregory P, Batz F, et al., editors. Available from Pharmacist's Letter/Prescriber's Letter Natural Medicines Comprehensive Database (Internet). Stockton, CA: Therapeutic Research Faculty; 1995-2011. Available from, www.naturaldatabase.com.

Klepser TB, Klepser ME. Unsafe and potentially safe herbal therapies. Am J Health Syst Pharm 1999;56:125–38.

Kligler B, Cohrssen A. Probiotics. Am Fam Physician 2008;78:1073–8.

Kronenberg F, Fugh-Berman A. Complementary and alternative medicine for menopausal symptoms: A review of randomized controlled trials. Ann Intern Med 2002;137:805–13.

Mar C. An evidence-based review of the 10 most commonly used herbs. West J Med 1999;171:169.

O'Hara MA, Kiefer D, Farrell K, et al. A review of 12 commonly used medicinal herbs. Arch Fam Med 1998;7:523–36.

Rotblatt MD. Cranberry, feverfew, horse chestnut, and kava. West J Med 1999;171:195–8.

Smet P. Herbal remedies. N Engl J Med 2002;347:2046–56.

REFERENCE INTERVALS FOR THE INTERPRETATION OF LABORATORY TESTS

Method of
Lindsay R. Simon, MD; Douglas F. Stickle, PhD; and Laura J. McCloskey, PhD

Most of the tests performed in a clinical laboratory are quantitative; that is, the amount of a substance present in blood or serum is measured and reported in terms of concentration, activity (e.g., enzyme activity), or counts (e.g., blood cell counts). The laboratory must provide reference intervals to assist the clinician in the interpretation of laboratory results. These reference intervals represent the physiologic quantities of a substance (concentrations, activities, or counts) to be expected in healthy persons. Deviation above or below the reference range may be associated with a disease process, and the severity of the disease process may be associated with the magnitude of the deviation. Unfortunately, a sharp demarcation rarely exists to distinguish between physiologic and pathologic values, and the time of transition between the two is often gradual as the disease process progresses.

Defining Normal Values

The terms "normal" and "abnormal" have been used to describe laboratory values that fall inside and outside the reference range, respectively. Use of these terms is inappropriate because no good definition of normality exists in the clinical sense, and the term "normal" may be confused with the statistical term "gaussian." Reference ranges are established from statistical studies in groups of healthy volunteers. These study subjects must be free of disease, but they may have lifestyles or habits that result in variations in certain laboratory values. Examples of these variables include diet, body mass, exercise, and geographic location. Age and gender can also affect reference values.

When the data from a large cohort of healthy subjects fit a gaussian distribution, the usual statistical approach is to define the reference limits as 2 standard deviations (SD) above and below the mean. By definition, the reference range excludes the 2.5% of the population with the lowest values and the 2.5% with the highest values. Nongaussian distributions are handled by different statistical methods, but the result is similar, in that the reference range is defined by the central 95% of the population. In other words, the probability that a healthy person has a laboratory result falling outside the reference range is 1 in 20. If 12 laboratory tests are performed, the probability that at least one of the results is outside the reference range increases to about 50%, which means that all healthy persons are likely to have a few laboratory results that are unexpected. The clinician must then integrate these data with other clinical information, such as the history and physical examination, to arrive at an appropriate clinical decision.

The reference intervals for many tests (especially enzyme and immunochemical measurements) vary with the method used. Accordingly, each laboratory must establish its own reference intervals that are appropriate for the methods used.

International System of Units

During the 1980s, a concerted effort was made to introduce the International System of Units (Système International d'Unités; SI units). The rationale for conversion to SI units is sound. Laboratory data are scientifically more informative when the units are

Conventional Units	SI Units
1.0 g of hemoglobin:	1.0 mmol of hemoglobin:
Combines with 1.37 mL of oxygen	Combines with 4.0 mmol of oxygen
Contains 3.4 mg of iron	Contains 4.0 mmol of iron
Forms 34.9 mg of bilirubin	Forms 4.0 mmol of bilirubin

based on molar concentration rather than on mass concentration. For example, the conversion of glucose to lactate and pyruvate or the binding of a drug to albumin is more easily understood in units of molar concentration. Another example is illustrated as follows:

The use of SI units would also enhance the standardization of nomenclature to facilitate global communication of medical and scientific information. The units, symbols, and prefixes used in the international system are shown in Tables 1, 2, and 3.

TABLE 1 Base SI Units

PROPERTY	UNIT	SYMBOL
Length	Meter	m
Mass	Kilogram	kg
Amount of substance	Mole	mol
Time	Second	s
Thermodynamic temperature	Kelvin	K
Electrical current	Ampere	A
Luminous intensity	Candela	cd
Catalytic amount	Katal	kat

Abbreviation: SI = International System of Units.

TABLE 2 Derived SI Units and Non-SI Units Retained for Use with SI Units

PROPERTY	UNIT	SYMBOL
Area	Square meter	m^2
Volume	Cubic meter / Liter	m^3 / L
Mass	Kilograms per cubic meter / Grams per liter	kg/m^3 concentration / g/L
Substance concentration	Moles per cubic meter	mol/m^3 / mol/L
Temperature	Degree Celsius	C = K − 273.15
Dynamic viscosity	Pascal-second	$Pa\text{-}s = 1 \, kg \cdot m^{-1} \cdot s^{-1}$

Abbreviation: SI = International System of Units.

TABLE 3	Standard Prefixes		
PREFIX	MULTIPLICATION FACTOR	SYMBOL	
yocto	10^{-24}	y	
zepto	10^{-21}	z	
atto	10^{-18}	a	
femto	10^{-15}	f	
pico	10^{-12}	p	
nano	10^{-9}	n	
micro	10^{-6}	μ	
milli	10^{-3}	m	
centi	10^{-2}	c	
deci	10^{-1}	d	
deca	10^{1}	da	
hecto	10^{2}	h	
kilo	10^{3}	k	
mega	10^{6}	M	
giga	10^{9}	G	
tera	10^{12}	T	

Unfortunately, problems have arisen with the implementation of SI units in the United States. The introduction of this system in 1987 prompted many medical journals to report laboratory values in both SI and conventional units in anticipation of complete conversion to SI units in the early 1990s. The lack of a coordinated effort toward this goal forced a retrenchment on the issue. Physicians continue to think and practice with laboratory results expressed in conventional units, and few, if any, hospitals or clinical laboratories in the United States use SI units exclusively. Complete conversion to SI units is not likely to occur in the foreseeable future, but most medical journals will probably continue to publish both sets of units. For this reason, the values in the tables of reference ranges in this appendix are given in both conventional units and SI units.

Tables of Reference Intervals

Some of the values included in the tables that follow have been established by the Clinical Laboratories at the Thomas Jefferson University Hospital in Philadelphia and have not been published elsewhere. Other values have been compiled from the sources cited in the suggested readings. These tables are provided for information and educational purposes only. Laboratory values must always be interpreted in the context of clinical data derived from other sources, including the medical history and physical examination. One must exercise individual judgment when using the information provided in this appendix.

Reference Intervals* for Hematology

TEST	CONVENTIONAL UNITS	SI UNITS
Acid hemolysis (Ham test)	No hemolysis	No hemolysis
Alkaline phosphatase, leukocyte	Total score, 14–100	Total score, 14–100
Cell counts		
Erythrocytes		
Males	4.5–6.0 T/L	$4.5–6.0 \times 10^{12}$/L
Females	3.7–5.2 T/L	$3.7–5.2 \times 10^{12}$/L
Children (varies with age)	3.9–5.2 T/L	$3.9–5.2 \times 10^{12}$/L
Leukocytes, total	$4–11 \times 10^{3}/\mu$L	$4.0–11.0 \times 10^{6}$/L
Leukocytes, differential counts[1]		
Myelocytes	0%	0/L
Band neutrophils	0.0%–0.7%	$0.0–70 \times 10^{6}$/L
Segmented neutrophils	40%–73%	$1800–8000 \times 10^{6}$/L
Lymphocytes	20%–44%	$900–4800 \times 10^{6}$/L
Monocytes	3%–13%	$300–1400 \times 10^{6}$/L
Eosinophils	0%–6%	$0–660 \times 10^{6}$/L
Basophils	0%–3%	$15–50 \times 10^{6}$/L
Platelets	140–400 B/L	$140–400 \times 10^{9}$/L
Reticulocytes	24–84 10^{9}/L	$24–84 \times 10^{9}$/L
Coagulation tests		
Bleeding time (template)	2–9 min	2–9 min
Coagulation time (glass tube)	5–15 min	5–15 min
D dimer	<0.49 μg/mL	<0.49 mg/L
Factor VIII and other coagulation factors	50–150% of normal	0.5–1.5 of normal
Fibrin split products (Thrombo-Welco test)	<5 μg/mL	<5 mg/L
Fibrinogen	140–476 mg/dL	1.4–4.8 g/L
Partial thromboplastin time, activated (aPTT)	20–38 s	20–38 s
Prothrombin time (PT)	11.2–14.8 s	11.2–14.8 s
Coombs' test		
Direct	Negative	Negative
Indirect	Negative	Negative
Corpuscular values of erythrocytes		
Mean corpuscular hemoglobin (MCH)	26–34 pg/cell	26–34 pg/cell
Mean corpuscular volume (MCV)	80–99 mm³	80–99 fL/cell
Mean corpuscular hemoglobin concentration (MCHC)	32–37.5 g/dL	320–375 g/L
Haptoglobin	16–200 mg/dL	0.16–2.00 g/L

Continued

TEST	CONVENTIONAL UNITS	SI UNITS
Hematocrit		
Males	42%–52%	0.42–0.52
Females	36%–46%	0.36–0.46
Newborns	42%–65%	0.42–0.65
Children (varies with age)	28%–44%	0.28–0.44
Hemoglobin		
Males	14–17 g/dL	8.7–10.6 mmol/L
Females	12.5–15.0 g/dL	7.6–9.3 mmol/L
Newborns	9.4–20.5 g/dL	5.8–2.7 mmol/L
Children (varies with age)	10.3–16.0 g/dL	6.4–9.9 mmol/L
Hemoglobin, fetal	<2.0% of total	<0.02 of total
Hemoglobin A1c	<5.7% of total	<0.057 of total
Hemoglobin A2	1.7–3.4% of total	0.017–0.034 of total
Hemoglobin, plasma	≤6.9 mg/dL	<4.28 mmol/L
Methemoglobin	0.06–0.24 g/dL	9.3–37.2 mmol/L
Erythrocyte sedimentation rate (ESR)		
Westergren		
Males	0–20 mm/h	0–20 mm/h
Females	0–30 mm/h	0–30 mm/h
Wintrobe		
Males	(0–5 mm/h) 0–9 mm/h	0–9 mm/h
Females	(0–15 mm/h) 0–20 mm/h	0–20 mm/h

*Reference values can vary depending on the method and sample source used.
†Conventional units are percentages; SI units are absolute cell counts.
Abbreviations: B/L = billions per liter; fL = femtoliter; T/L = trillions per liter.

Reference Intervals* for Clinical Chemistry (Blood, Serum, and Plasma)

ANALYTE	CONVENTIONAL UNITS	SI UNITS
Acetoacetate plus acetone		
Qualitative	Negative	<0.1 mmol/L
Quantitative	<2.0 mg/dL	20–200 mol/L
Acid phosphatase, serum (thymolphthalein monophosphate substrate)	0.1–0.6 U/L	0.1–0.6 U/L
ACTH (see Corticotropin)		
Alanine aminotransferase (ALT), serum (SGPT)	1–45 U/L	1–45 U/L
Albumin, serum	3.2–4.9 g/dL	32–49 g/L
Aldolase, serum	1.0–8.0 U/L	1.0–8.0 U/L
Aldosterone, plasma		
Standing (8:00–10:00 AM)	≤28 ng/dL	<776 pmol/L
Standing (4:00–6:00 PM)	83–280 U/L 21 ng/dL	<582 pmol/L
Recumbent (8:00–10:00 AM)	3–16 ng/dL	80–443 pmol/L
Alkaline, phosphatase (ALP), serum		
Adult	25–160 IU/L	25–160 IU/L
Adolescent	91–400 IU/L	91–400 IU/L
Child	83–280 U/L	83–280 U/L
Ammonia nitrogen, plasma	11–35 umol/L	10–35 mmol/L
Amylase, serum	28–100 U/L	28–100 U/L
Anion gap, serum calculated	4–16 mmol/L	4–16 mmol/L
Ascorbic acid, blood	0.20–1.90 mg/dL	11–108 mmol/L
Aspartate aminotransferase (AST), serum (SGOT)	7–42 IU/L	7–42 U/L
Base excess, arterial blood, calculated		
Male	0.0–2.3 mmol/L	0.0–2.3 mmol/L
Female	0.0–1.2 mmol/L	0.0–1.2 mmol/L
Bicarbonate		
Venous plasma	22–27 mmol/L	22–27 mmol/L
Arterial blood	21–27 mEq/L	21–27 mmol/L
Bile acids, serum	0.3–3.0 mg/dL	0.8–7.6 mmol/L
Bilirubin, serum		
Conjugated	0.0–0.3 mg/dL	0.0–5.1 mmol/L
Total	0.1–0.9 mg/dL	1.7–15.4 mmol/L
Calcium, serum	8.5–10.5 mg/dL	2.10–2.65 mmol/L

ANALYTE	CONVENTIONAL UNITS	SI UNITS
Calcium, ionized, serum	4.5–5.3 mg/dL	1.1–1.30 mmol/L
Carbon dioxide, total, serum or plasma	23–31 mEq/L	23–31 mmol/L
Carbon dioxide tension (PCO2), blood	31–45 mm Hg	31–45 mm Hg
β-Carotene, serum	10–85 µg/dL	0.19–1.58 mmol/L
Ceruloplasmin, serum	18–45 mg/dL	180–450 mg/L
Chloride, serum or plasma	96–106 mEq/L	96–106 mmol/L
Cholesterol, serum or EDTA plasma		
Desirable range	<200 mg/dL	<5.20 mmol/L
Low-density lipoprotein (LDL) cholesterol, optimal	<100 mg/dL	<2.85 mmol/L
High-density lipoprotein (HDL) cholesterol desirable	40–60 mg/dL	1.04–1.55 mmol/L
Copper	70–175 µg/dL	11–27 mmol/L
Corticotropin (ACTH), plasma, 8:00 AM	9–46 pg/mL	2–10 pmol/L
Cortisol, plasma		
8:00 AM	5–23 µg/dL	138–635 mmol/L
4:00 PM	3–16 µg/dL	83–441 mmol/L
8:00 PM	<50% of 8:00 AM value	<50 of 8:00 AM value
Creatine, serum		
Males	0.2–0.5 mg/dL	15–40 mmol/L
Females	0.3–0.9 mg/dL	25–70 mmol/L
Creatine kinase (CK), serum		
Males	20–200 U/L	20–200 U/L
Females	20–180 U/L	20–180 U/L
Creatine kinase MB isoenzyme, serum	<5% of total CK activity <5% of ng/mL by immunoassay	<5% of total CK activity <5% of ng/mL by immunoassay
Creatinine, serum		
Males	0.7–1.4 mg/dL	61.9–123.8 µmol/L
Females	0.7–1.4 mg/dL	61.9–123.8 µmol/L
Erythrocytes	145–540 ng/mL	330–120 nmol/L
Estradiol-17β, adult		
Males	7.6–42.0 pg/mL	28–150 pmol/L
Females		
Follicular	12.5–166 pg/mL	46–609 pmol/L
Ovulatory	85.8–498 pg/mL	315–1830 pmol/L
Luteal	43.8–211 pg/mL	160–775 pmol/L
Ferritin, serum	30–400 ng/mL	30–400 µg/L
Fibrinogen, plasma	140–476 mg/dL	1.4–4.8 g/L
Folate, serum	4.6–35.0 ng/mL	10.41–79.28 mmol/L
Follicle-stimulating hormone (FSH), plasma		
Males	1.5–12.4 mIU/mL	1.5–12.4 U/L
Females, premenopausal	1.7–21 mIU/mL	1.7–21 U/L
Females, postmenopausal	26–135 mIU/mL	26–135 U/L
Gastrin, fasting, serum	0–100 pg/mL	0–100 mg/L
Glucose, fasting, plasma or serum	70–100 mg/dL	3.9–5.6 nmol/L
γ-Glutamyltransferase (GGT), serum	6–71 IU/L	6–71 U/L
Growth hormone (hGH), plasma, adult, fasting	≤10 ng/mL	<10 mg/L
Haptoglobin, serum	16–200 mg/dL	0.16–2.00 g/L
Immunoglobulins, serum (see table, Reference Intervals for Tests of Immunologic Function)		
Iron, serum	40–160 µg/dL	7–29 mmol/L
Iron-binding capacity, serum		
Total	250–400 µg/dL	45–73 mmol/L
Saturation	20%–55%	0.20–0.55
Lactate (enzymatic)		
Venous whole blood	4.5–19.8 mg/dL	0.5–2.2 mmol/L
Arterial whole blood	4.5–14.4 mg/dL	0.5–1.6 mmol/L
Lactate dehydrogenase (LD), serum	125–240 IU/L	125–240 U/L
Lipase, serum	13–60 U/L	13–60 U/L

Continued

ANALYTE	CONVENTIONAL UNITS	SI UNITS
Lutropin (LH), serum		
Males	No normal range	No normal range
Females		
Follicular phase	2.4–12.6 mU/mL	2.4–12.6 U/L
Midcycle peak	14.0–96 mU/mL	14–96 U/L
Luteal phase	1.0–11.4 mU/mL	1–11.4 U/L
Postmenopausal	7.7–58.5 mU/mL	7.7–58.5 U/L
Magnesium, serum	1.3–2.1 mEq/L	0.65–1.05 mmol/L
Osmolality	275–295 mOsm/kg H_2O	275–295 mOsm/kg H_2O
Oxygen, blood, arterial, room air		
Partial pressure (PaO_2)	83–108 mm	Hg 83–108 mm Hg
Saturation (SaO_2)	95%–99%	95%–99%
pH, arterial blood	7.35–7.45	7.35–7.45
Phosphate, inorganic, serum		
Adult	2.4–4.5 mg/dL	0.78–1.5 mmol/L
Child	3.1–7.5 mg/dL	1.0–2.4 mmol/L
Potassium		
Serum	3.5–5.0 mmol/L	3.5–5.0 mmol/L
Plasma	3.5–4.5 mEq/L	3.5–4.5 mmol/L
Progesterone, serum, adult		
Males	0.2–1.4 ng/mL	0.6–4.5 mmol/L
Females		
Follicular phase	0.2–1.5 ng/mL	0.6–4.8 mmol/L
Luteal phase	1.7–27.0 ng/mL	5.4–86.0 mmol/L
Prolactin, serum		
Males	0–19 ng/mL	1.0–19.0 mg/L
Females	0–29 ng/mL	1.0–29.0 mg/L
Protein, serum, electrophoresis		
Total 6.0–8.5 g/dL	60–85 mg/L	
Albumin	3.3–5.2 g/dL	33–52 mg/L
Globulins		
α_1	0.1–0.3 g/dL	1.0–3.0 g/L
α_2	0.5–0.9 g/dL	5.0–9.0 g/L
β	0.5–1.2 g/dL	5.0–12.0 g/L
γ	0.5–1.6 g/dL	5.0–16.0 g/L
Pyruvate, blood	0.30–1.50 mg/dL	0.03–0.17 mmol/L
Rheumatoid factor (nephelometry)	<30.0 IU/mL	<30.0 kIU/L
Sodium, serum or plasma	135–146 mmol/L	135–146 mmol/L
Testosterone, plasma		
Men	190–840 ng/dL	6.6–29 nmol/L
Women	2.9–48 ng/dL	0.1–1.7 nmol/L
Pregnant	3–4× adult level	
Thyroglobulin	3–40 ng/mL	3–40 mg/L
Thyrotropin (hTSH), serum	0.3–5.0 μU/mL	0.3–5.0 μU/L
Thyroxine, free (FT_4), serum	0.7–1.7 ng/dL	9–22 pmol/L
Thyroxine (T_4), serum	4.5–11.0 mg/mL	59–142 nmol/L
Thyroxine-binding globulin (TBG)	1.2–3.0 mg/mL	12–30 mg/L
Transferrin	212–360 mg/dL	2.1–3.6 g/L
Triglycerides, serum (after 12-h fast)	<150 mg/dL	<1.7 mmol/L
Triiodothyronine (T_3), serum	90–180 mg/dL	1.4–2.8 nmol/L
Triiodothyronine uptake, resin (T_3RU)	22%–32%	22–32 AU
(Troponin I) troponin T	<0.01 ng/mL	<0.01 ng/mL
Urate		
(FT_4) Males	3.5–9.0 mg/dL	210–540 mmol/L
(FT_4) Females	2.5–6.0 mg/dL	150–360 mmol/L
Urea, serum or plasma	24–49 mg/dL	4.0–8.2 nmol/L
Urea nitrogen, serum or plasma	7–27 mg/dL	2.5–9.6 mmol/L
Viscosity, serum	1.00–1.24 cP	1.00–1.24 mPas-s
Vitamin A, serum	30–80 μg/mL	1.05–2.80 μmol/L
Vitamin B_{12}, serum	210–950 pg/mL	155–701 pmol/L

*Reference values can vary depending on the method and sample source used.
Abbreviations: AU=average uptake; cP=centipoise; EDTA=ethylenediaminetetraacetic acid; SI=International System of Units.

ANALYTE	THERAPEUTIC RANGE	TOXIC CONCENTRATIONS	PROPRIETARY ANALYTE NAME
Analgesics			
Acetaminophen	10–25 µg/mL	>150 µg/mL	Tylenol, Datril
Salicylate	100–300 mg/mL	>300 mg/mL	Aspirin, Bufferin
Antibiotics			
Amikacin	25–35 mg/mL	Peak >35–40 µg/mL Trough >10–15 µg/mL	Amkin
Gentamicin	5–10 mg/mL	5–10 mg/mL <4 mg/L	Garamycin
Tobramycin	5–10 mg/mL	Peak >10–12 µg/mL Trough <2–4 µg/mL	Nebcin
Vancomycin	5–40 µg/mL Peak 20–40 µg/L Trough 5–10 µg/L	>80–100 µg/mL	Vancocin
Anticonvulsants			
Carbamazepine	4–12 mg/L	>15 mg/mL	Tegretol
Ethosuximide	40–100 mg/mL	>150 mg/mL	Zarontin
Phenobarbital	15–40 mg/mL	35–100 mg/mL (varies widely)	Luminal
Phenytoin	10–20 mg/mL	>20 mg/mL	Dilantin
Primidone	5–12 mg/mL	>15 mg/mL	Mysoline
Valproic acid	50–100 mg/mL	>100 mg/mL	Depakene
Antineoplastics and Immunosuppressives			
Cyclosporine A	100–400 ng/mL	>400 ng/mL	Sandimmune
Methotrexate, high-dose, 48 h	Variable	>0.5 mmol/L, 48 h after dose	
Sirolimus (within 1 h of 2-mg dose)	5–15 ng/mL	Variable	Rapamune
Sirolimus (within 1 h of 5-mg dose)	10–28 ng/mL	Variable	Rapamune
Tacrolimus (FK-506), whole blood	5–20 mg/L	>20 mg/L	Prograf
Bronchodilators and Respiratory Stimulants			
Caffeine	5–25 µg/mL	>50 µg/mL	
Theophylline (aminophylline)	10–20 mg/mL	>20 mg/mL	Quibron
Cardiovascular Drugs			
Amiodarone (obtain specimen more than 8 h after last dose)	1.0–2.0 mg/mL	>2.0 mg/mL	Cordarone
Digoxin (obtain specimen more than 6 h after last dose)	0.8–2.0 ng/mL	>2.4 ng/mL	Lanoxin
Disopyramide	2.8–7.5 mg/mL	>7 mg/mL	Norpace
Flecainide	0.2–1.0 mg/mL	>1 mg/mL	Tambocor
Lidocaine	2.0–6.0 mg/mL	>6 mg/mL	Xylocaine
Mexiletine	0.5–2.0 mg/mL	>2 mg/mL	Mexitil
Procainamide	4–8 mg/mL	>10 mg/mL	Pronestyl
Procainamide plus NAPA (N-acetyl procainamide)	5–30 mg/mL	>30 mg/mL	
Propranolol	50–100 ng/mL	Not defined	Inderal
Quinidine	2–5 µg/mL	>6 mg/mL	Cardioquin, Quinaglute
Tocainide	4–10 µg/mL	Not defined	Tonocard
Psychopharmacologic Drugs			
Amitriptyline	100–250 ng/mL	>500 ng/mL	Elavil, Triavil
Bupropion	25–100 ng/mL	>1200 ng/mL	Wellbutrin

Continued

ANALYTE	THERAPEUTIC RANGE	TOXIC CONCENTRATIONS	PROPRIETARY ANALYTE NAME
Desipramine	50–300 ng/mL	>400 ng/mL	Norpramin
Imipramine	150–250 ng/mL	>500 ng/mL	Tofranil
Lithium (obtain specimen 12 h after last dose)	0.5–1.5 mmol/L	>1.5 mEq/L	Lithobid
Nortriptyline	50–150 ng/mL	>500 ng/mL	Aventyl, Pamelor

*Values can vary depending on the method and sample collection device used. Always consult the reference values provided by the laboratory performing the analysis.

Reference Intervals* for Clinical Chemistry (Urine)

ANALYTE	CONVENTIONAL UNITS	SI UNITS
Acetone and acetoacetate, qualitative	Negative	Negative
Albumin		
Qualitative	Negative	10–140 mg/L (24 h)
Quantitative	Negative	10–140 mg/L (24 h)
Aldosterone	1–80 mg/24 h	3–222 nmol/d
δ-Aminolevulinic acid (δ-ALA)	1.5–7.5 mg/24 h	11.4–57.2 mmol/d
Amylase	1–17 U/h	<17 U/h
Amylase-to-creatinine clearance ratio	<0.3 IU/mg	<0.3 IU/mg
Bilirubin, qualitative	Negative	Negative
Calcium (regular diet)	<300 mg/24 h	<7.5 nmol/d
Catecholamines		
Epinephrine	<24 µg/24 h	<131 nmol/d
Norepinephrine	<100 µg/24 h	<546 nmol/d
Total free catecholamines	26–121 µg/24 h	142–660 nmol/d
Total metanephrines	49–741 µg/24 h	0.27–4.04 mmol/d
Copper	2–80 µg/L	0.03–1.26 µmol/L
Cortisol, free	20–90 mg/24 h	0.6–2.5 mmol/d
Creatine		
Males	0–40 mg/24 h	0.0–0.30 mmol/d
Females	0–80 mg/24 h	0.0–0.60 mmol/d
Creatinine	800–2000 mg/24 h	7.1–17.7 mmol/kg/d
Creatinine clearance (endogenous)		
Males	70–130 mL/min	70–130 mL/min/1.73 m^2
Females	60–120 mL/min	60–120 mL/min/1.73 m^2
Cystine or cysteine	Negative	Negative
Dehydroepiandrosterone		
Males	<3.1 mg/24 h	<10.7 mmol/d
Females	<1.5 mg/24 h	<4.1 mmol/d
Estrogens, total		
Males	4–25 mg/24 h	14–90 nmol/d
Females	5–100 mg/24 h	18–360 nmol/d
Glucose (as reducing substance)	0–500 mg/24 h	0–500 mg/d
Hemoglobin and myoglobin, qualitative	Negative	Negative
Homogentisic acid, qualitative	Negative	Negative
17-Hydroxycorticosteroids		
Males	3–9 mg/24 h	8.3–25 mmol/d
Females	2–8 mg/24 h	5.5–22 mmol/d
5-Hydroxindoleacetic acid		
Qualitative	Negative	Negative
Quantitative	(2–6 mg/24 h) <8.0 mg/24 h	<19 mmol/d
17-Ketogenic steroids		
Males	5–23 mg/24 h	17–80 mmol/d
Females	3–15 mg/24 h	10–52 mmol/d
17-Ketosteroids		
Males	8–22 mg/24 h	28–76 mmol/d
Females	6–15 mg/24 h	21–52 mmol/d

Reference Intervals* for Clinical Chemistry (Urine)—cont'd

ANALYTE	CONVENTIONAL UNITS	SI UNITS
Magnesium	1–24 mEq/24 h	0.4–10 mmol/d
Metanephrines	0.05–1.2 ng/mg creatinine	0.03–0.70 mmol/mmol creatinine
Osmolality	38–1400 mOsm/kg water	38–1400 mOsm/kg water
pH	5.0–8.0	5.0–8.0
Phenylpyruvic acid, qualitative	Negative	Negative
Phosphate	0.4–1.3 g/24 h	13–42 mmol/d
Porphobilinogen		
Qualitative	Negative	Negative
Quantitative	<2.4 mg/24 h	<11 mmol/d
Porphyrins		
Coproporphyrin	52–163 µg/ 24 h	80–250 nmol/d
Uroporphyrin	17–52 µg/ 24 h	20–62 nmol/d
Potassium	25–120 mmol/24 h	25–120 mmol/d
Pregnanediol		
Males	0.0–1.9 mg/24 h	0.0–6.0 mmol/d
Females		
Follicular phase	0.0–2.6 mg/24 h	0.0–8.0 mmol/d
Luteal phase	2.6–10.6 mg/24 h	8–33 mmol/d
Postmenopausal	0.2–1.0 mg/24 h	0.6–3.1 mmol/d
Pregnanetriol	0.1–2.5 mg/24 h	0.3–7.5 mmol/d
Protein, total		
Qualitative	Negative	Negative
Quantitative	<150 mg/24 h	<150 mg/d
Protein-to-creatinine ratio	<0.2	<0.2
Sodium (regular diet)	40–220 mmol/24 h	40–220 mmol/d
Specific gravity		
Random specimen	(1.003–1.030) 1.010–1.025	1.010–1.025
24-h collection	1.015–1.025	1.015–1.025
Urate (regular diet)	250–750 mg/24 h	1.5–4.4 mmol/d
Urobilinogen	(0.5–4.0 mg/24 h) Normal	0.6–6.8 mmol/d
Vanillylmandelic acid (VMA)	<6.0 mg/24 h	<30 mmol/d

*Values can vary depending on the method used.
Abbreviation: SI = International System of Units

Reference Intervals for Toxic Substances

ANALYTE	CONVENTIONAL UNITS	SI UNITS
Arsenic, urine	5–50 mg/24 h	0.07–0.7 mmol/d
Bromides, serum, inorganic	<100 mg/dL	<10 mmol/L
Toxic symptoms	140–1000 mg/dL	14–100 mmol/L
Carboxyhemoglobin, blood	0.1–2.0%	
Urban environment	<5%	<0.05
Smokers	8%–9%	0.08–0.09
Symptoms		
Headache	>15%	>0.15
Nausea and vomiting	>25%	>0.25
Potentially lethal	>50%	>0.50
Ethanol, blood	<0.05 mg/dL, <0.005%	<1.0 mmol/L
Intoxication >100 mg/dL, >0.1%	>22 mmol/L	
Marked intoxication	300–400 mg/dL, 0.3%–0.4%	65–87 mmol/L
Alcoholic stupor	400–500 mg/dL, 0.4%–0.5%	87–109 mmol/L
Coma	>500 mg/dL, >0.5%	>109 mmol/L
Lead, blood		
Adults	<25 mg/dL	<1.3 mmol/L
Children	<10 mg/dL	<0.5 mmol/L
Lead, urine	<80 µg/L/24 h	<0.4 µmol/L/24 h
Mercury, urine	<20 mg/24 h	<0.1 mmol/L/24 h

Reference Intervals for Tests Performed on Cerebrospinal Fluid

TEST	CONVENTIONAL UNITS	SI UNITS
Cells	<5 mm^3; all mononuclear	<5 × 10^6 L, all mononuclear
Protein electrophoresis	Albumin predominant	Albumin predominant
Glucose	40–70 mg/dL	2.8–4.2 mmol/L (1.1 mmol/L less than in serum)

IgG
  Children <14 y
  Adults
	
	<8% of total protein
	5%–15% of total protein
		
		<0.08 of total protein
		0.05–0.15 of total protein

IgG index	0.34–0.66	0.34–0.66
Oligoclonal banding on electrophoresis	Absent	Absent
Pressure, opening	70–180 mm H$_2$O	70–180 mm H$_2$O
Protein, total	15–45 mg/dL	150–450 mg/L

Abbreviations: Ig=immunoglobulin; SI=International System of Units.

Reference Intervals for Tests of Gastrointestinal Function

TEST	CONVENTIONAL UNITS
Bentiromide	6-h urinary arylamine excretion >57% excludes pancreatic insufficiency
β-Carotene, serum	10–85 μg/dL

Fecal fat estimation
  Qualitative
  Quantitative
	
	No fat globules seen by high-power microscope
	<7 g/24 h

Gastric acid output
  Basal
    Males
    Females
  Maximum (after histamine or pentagastrin)
    Males
    Females
  Ratio: basal/maximum
    Males
    Females
	
	0.0–10.5 mmol/h
	0.0–5.6 mmol/h
	
	9.0–48.0 mmol/h
	6.0–31.0 mmol/h
	
	0.0–0.31
	0.0–0.29

Secretin test, pancreatic fluid
  Volume
  Bicarbonate
	
	>1.8 mL/kg/h
	>80 mEq/L

D-Xylose	>25 mg/dL (25-g dose)

Reference Intervals for Lymphocyte Subsets, Whole Blood, Heparinized

ANTIGEN(S)	CELL TYPES	LIGANDS	PERCENTAGE	ABSOLUTE CELL COUNT
CD2	T cells, B cells, NK cells	CD58, CD48, CD58 CD15, LFA-3	73%–87%	1040–2160
CD3	Total T cells	T cell receptor (TCR)	56%–77%	860–1880
CD3 and CD4	Helper-inducer cells	TCR/MHC Class II, gp 120, IL-16, Lck	32%–54%	550–1190
CD3 and CD8	Suppressor-cytotoxic cells	TCR/MHC Class I, Lck	24%–37%	430–1060
CD3 and DR	Activated T cells	TCR/MHC Class II	5%–14%	70–310
CD56	T cells, NK cells	Leu-19, NKH-1, Neural Cell Adhesion Molecule (NCAM)	8%–22%	130–500
CD19 and CD20	B cells	CD19: co-receptor with CD21 and CD81 CD20: antigenic target of therapeutic monoclonal antibody drugs rituximab, ibritumomab, tiuxetan, tositumomab, and ofatumumab	7%–17%	140–370

Reference Intervals for Tests of Immunologic Function

TEST	CONVENTIONAL UNITS	SI UNITS
Autoantibodies, Serum, Adult		
Anti-CCP antibody	0–19 U	
Anti-dsDNA antibody	0–41 IU	0–41 IU
Antinuclear antibody	<1:40, Negative	
Rheumatoid factor (total IgG, IgA, IgM)	<14 IU/mL	
Complement, Serum		
C3	88–201 mg/dL	0.88–2.01 g/L
C4	10–44 mg/dL	100–440 mg/L
Total hemolytic (CH$_{50}$)	31–60 U/mL	150–250 U/mL
Immunoglobulins, Serum, Adult		
IgA	70–380 mg/dL	0.70–3.8 g/L
IgD	<179 mg/dL	<0.179 mg/L
IgE	1–180 IU/mL	0.0–430 mg/L
IgG	723–1685 mg/dL	7.2–16.9 g/L
IgM	40–230 mg/dL	0.40–2.3 g/L

Helper-to-suppressor ratio: 0.8–1.8.
Abbreviations: anti-CCP = anticyclic citrullinated peptide; dsDNA = double-stranded DNA; Ig = immunoglobulin; SI = International System of Units.

Reference Values for Semen Analysis

TEST	CONVENTIONAL UNITS	SI UNITS
Volume	2–6 mL	2–6 mL
Liquefaction	Complete in 30 min	Complete in 30 min
pH	7.2–7.8	7.2–7.8
Leukocytes	<2000	$<2 \times 10^9$/L
Spermatozoa		
Count	60–150 $\times 10^6$ mL	>80 $\times 10^6$ mL
Fructose	>150 mg/dL	8.3–33.3 mmol/L
Morphology	80%–90% normal forms	>0.80–0.90 normal
Motility	>80% motile	>0.80 motile

Abbreviation: SI = International System of Units.

References

American Medical Association. Drug evaluations annual. Chicago: American Medical Association; 1994.

Bick RL, editor. Hematology: Clinical and laboratory practice. St Louis: Mosby—Year Book; 1993.

Borer WZ. Selection and use of laboratory tests. In: Tietz NW, Conn RB, Pruden E, editors. Applied laboratory medicine. Philadelphia: WB Saunders; 1992. p. 1–5.

Burtis CA, Ashwood EA, Bruns DE, editors. Tietz textbook of clinical chemistry and molecular diagnostics. 5th ed. St. Louis: Elsevier Saunders; 2012.

Campion EW. A retreat from SI units. N Engl J Med 1992;327:49.

Colantonio DA, et al. Closing the gaps in pediatric laboratory reference intervals: a CALIPER database of 40 biochemical markers in a healthy and multiethnic population of children. Clin Chem 2012;58:854–68.

Friedman RB, Young DS. Effects of disease on clinical laboratory tests. 3rd ed. Washington, DC: American Association for Clinical Chemistry Press; 1997.

Henry JB. Clinical diagnosis and management by laboratory methods. 19th ed. Philadelphia: WB Saunders; 1996.

Hicks JM, Young DS. DORA 97-99: Directory of rare analyses. Washington, DC: American Association for Clinical Chemistry Press; 1997.

Horowitz GL, et al. Defining, Establishing and verifying reference intervals in the clinical laboratory; approved guideline. 3rd ed. Wayne PA: Clinical Laboratory Standards Institute; 2008.

Jacob DS, Demott WR, Grady HJ, et al., Laboratory test handbook. 4th ed. Baltimore: Williams & Wilkins; 1996.

Kaplan LA, Pesce AJ. Clinical chemistry: Theory, analysis, and correlation. 3rd ed. St. Louis: Mosby—Year Book; 1996.

Kjeldsberg CR, Knight JA. Body fluids: laboratory examination of amniotic, cerebrospinal, seminal, serous and synovial fluids. 3rd ed. Chicago: ASCP Press; 1993.

Laposata M. SI Unit Conversion Guide. Boston: NEJM Books; 1992.

Scully RE, McNeely WF, Mark EJ, McNeely BU. Normal reference laboratory values. N Engl J Med 1992;327:718–24.

Speicher CE. The right test: A physician's guide to laboratory medicine. 3rd ed. Philadelphia: WB Saunders; 1998.

Wallach J. Interpretation of diagnostic tests: A synopsis of laboratory medicine. 6th ed. Boston: Little, Brown; 1996.

Wu AHB, editor. Tietz clinical guide to laboratory tests. 4th ed. Philadelphia: WB Saunders; 2006.

Young DS. Effects of preanalytical variables on clinical laboratory tests. 2nd ed. Washington, DC: American Association for Clinical Chemistry Press; 1997.

Young DS. Effects of drugs on clinical laboratory tests. 4th ed. Washington, DC: American Association for Clinical Chemistry Press; 1995.

Young DS. Determination and validation of reference intervals. Arch Pathol Lab Med 1992;116:704–9.

Young DS. Implementation of SI units for clinical laboratory data. Ann Intern Med 1987;106:114–29.

TOXIC CHEMICAL AGENTS REFERENCE CHART: SYMPTOMS AND TREATMENT

Method of
James J. James, MD; and James M. Lyznicki, MS, MPH

Toxic chemical agents are poisonous vapors, aerosols, gases, liquids, or solids that have toxic effects on people, animals, or plants. Most of these agents are liquid at room temperature and are disseminated as vapors and aerosols. They may be released as bombs, sprayed from aircraft and boats, or disseminated by other means to intentionally create a hazard to people and the environment. Some of these agents are highly toxic and persistent, features that can render a site uninhabitable and require costly and potentially hazardous decontamination and remediation. Health effects range from irritation and burning of skin and mucous membranes to rapid cardiopulmonary collapse and death.

Efficient deployment of hazardous materials (HazMat) teams is critical to control a chemical agent attack. Although all major cities and emergency medical systems have plans and equipment in place to address this situation, physicians and other health professionals must be aware of principles involved in managing a patient or multiple patients exposed to these agents. Chemical-weapon agents have a high potential for secondary contamination from victims to responders. This requires that medical treatment facilities have clearly defined procedures for handling contaminated casualties, many of whom will transport themselves to the facility. Precautions must be used until thorough decontamination has been performed or the specific chemical agent is identified. Health care professionals must first protect themselves (e.g., by using protective suits, respiratory protection, and chemical-resistant gloves) because secondary contamination with even small amounts of these substances (particularly nerve agents such as VX) may be lethal.

Primary detection of exposure to chemical agents is based on the signs and symptoms of the potential victim (Table 1). Confirmation of a chemical agent, using detection equipment or laboratory analyses, takes considerable time and will not likely contribute to the early management of mass casualty victims. Several patients presenting with the same symptoms should alert physicians and hospital staff to the possibility of a chemical attack. If a chemical attack occurs, most victims will likely arrive within a short time. This situation differentiates a chemical attack from a biological attack involving infectious microorganisms. Additional diagnostic clues include the following:

- Unusual temporal or geographic clustering of illness
- Any sudden increase in illness in previously healthy persons
- Sudden increase in nonspecific syndromes (e.g., sudden unexplained weakness in previously healthy persons; dimmed or blurred vision; hypersecretion, inhalation, or burnlike syndrome)

A coordinated communication network is critical for transmitting reliable information from the incident scene to treatment facilities. Any suspicious or confirmed exposure to a chemical weapons agent should be reported to the local health department, local Federal Bureau of Investigation office, and the Centers for Disease Control and Prevention (770–488–7100).

TABLE 1 Quick Reference Chart on Chemical Weapon Agents

CHEMICAL AGENT	DIAGNOSTIC CONSIDERATIONS				TREATMENT CONSIDERATIONS*			COMMENTS
	SIGNS AND SYMPTOMS	SYMPTOM ONSET	ODOR	ACTION	TESTING	TREATMENT	ANTIDOTE	

Cyanides

| Cyanogen chloride (CK) Hydrogen cyanide (AC) | Nonspecific hypoxic and hypoxemic symptoms Resp: SOB, chest tightness, hyperventilation, resp arrest GI: nausea, vomiting CV: ventricular arrhythmias, hypotension, cardiac arrest, shock CNS: anxiety, headache, drowsiness, weakness, apnea, convulsions, seizure, coma Metabolic acidosis and increased concentration of venous oxygen (possibly also cyanosis) | Rapid, seconds to minutes | Bitter almond, musty, or chlorine-like | Binds cellular cytochrome oxidase, causing chemical asphyxia | Cyanide, thiocyanate, serum lactate levels Venous and arterial partial oxygen pressure | Immediate treatment of symptomatic patients is critical Hydroxycobalamin (vitamin B$_{12a}$) administered with thiosulfate[5,†] Activated charcoal[1] for oral exposure Mechanical ventilation as needed Circulatory support with crystalloids and vasopressors Metabolic acidosis corrected with IV sodium bicarbonate Seizures controlled with benzodiazepines | Sodium nitrite and sodium thiosulfate; repeat one-half initial doses of both agents in 30 min if inadequate clinical response; amyl nitrate capsules are available for first aid until intravenous access is achieved Hydroxycobalamin (vitamin B$_{12a}$, Cyanokit) | Cyanide antidote kits are commercially available CNS effects may be confused with carbon monoxide and hydrogen sulfide poisoning |

Incapacitating Agents

| Agent 15 3-quinuclidinyl benzilate (3Z) | Mydriasis, blurred vision, dry mouth, dry skin, possible atropine-like flush, initial rise in heart rate, decreased level of consciousness, confusion, disorientation, visual hallucinations, impaired memory | Hours 0–4 h: parasympathetic blockade and mild CNS effects 4–20 h: stupor with ataxia and hyperthermia 20–96 h: full-blown delirium Resolution phase: paranoia, deep sleep, reawakening, crawling, climbing automatism, eventual reorientation | Odorless | Competitive inhibitor of acetylcholine muscarinic receptor | | Support, intravenous fluids | Physostigmine salicylate (Antilirium)[1] | |

Nerve Agents

| Cyclohexyl sarin (GF) Sarin (GB) Soman (GD) Tabun (GA) VX | Most toxic of known chemical agents May be confused with organophosphate and carbamate pesticide poisoning Eyes: excessive lacrimation, miosis may be present | Vapor: seconds Liquid: minutes or hours Symptom onset may be delayed up to 18 h, particularly for localized exposures | GB, VX: none GA: fruity GD: camphor-like | Irreversible acetylcholinesterase inhibitors | Erythrocyte or serum cholinesterase activity to confirm exposure | Rapid establishment of patent airway Early administration of 2-PAM is critical to minimize permanent agent inactivation of acetylcholinesterase (i.e., "aging") | Atropine,[1] and 2-PAM[1] Additional doses until bronchial secretions are cleared and ventilation improved | Atropine,[1] 2-PAM,[1] and diazepam[1] are available in autoinjector kits through the U.S. military |

Continued

TABLE 1 Quick Reference Chart on Chemical Weapon Agents—cont'd

CHEMICAL AGENT	DIAGNOSTIC CONSIDERATIONS				TREATMENT CONSIDERATIONS*			COMMENTS
	SIGNS AND SYMPTOMS	SYMPTOM ONSET	ODOR	ACTION	TESTING	TREATMENT	ANTIDOTE	
	Resp: rhinorrhea, bronchospasm, resp failure GI: hypersalivation, nausea, vomiting, diarrhea Skin: localized sweating Cardiac: sinus bradycardia Skeletal muscles: fasciculations followed by weakness, flaccid paralysis CNS: loss of consciousness, convulsions, apnea, seizures					Benzodiazepines to control nerve agent–induced seizures Airway and ventilatory support as needed		
Pulmonary or Choking Agents								
Acrolein Ammonia (NH_3) Chlorine (Cl) Chloropicrin (PS) Diphosgene (DP) Nitrogen oxides (NO_x) Perfluoroisobutylene (PFIB) Phosgene (CG) Sulfur dioxide (SO_2)	Degree of water solubility of the agent influences onset and severity of respiratory injury Eye and airway irritation, dyspnea, chest tightness, rhinorrhea, hypersalivation, cough, wheezing High-dose inhalation can cause laryngospasm, pneumonitis, and acute lung injury with delayed onset (≤48 h) of acute resp distress syndrome Chest radiograph: hyperinflation, noncardiogenic pulmonary edema	Rapid or delayed 1–24 h; rarely up to 72 h	CG: freshly mown hay or grass			Supportive measures Specific treatment depends on the agent IV fluids for hypotension; no diuretics Ventilation with or without positive airway pressure Bronchodilators for bronchospasm Methylprednisolone[1] may be effective in preventing noncardiogenic pulmonary edema	No specific antidote	Easily absorbed via mucous membranes of eyes, nose, oropharynx May be confused with inhalation exposure to industrial chemicals (e.g., HCl, Cl_2, NH_3)
Riot Control Agents								
Mace (CN) Tear gas (CS)	Metallic taste Burning and pain on mucosal membranes and skin Eyes: irritation, pain, tearing, blepharospasm Airways: burning in nose and mouth, respiratory discomfort, bronchospasm (may be delayed 36 h) Skin: tingling, erythema Nausea and vomiting are common CN can cause corneal opacification	Immediate	CN: apple blossom CS: pepper	SN2 alkylating agents	No specific laboratory tests	Supportive care Irrigation as necessary Persons with asthma, emphysema might need oxygen, inhaled bronchodilators, steroids, assisted ventilation Lotions, such as calamine[1] for persistent erythema		

Vesicant or Blister Agents

General	Clinical effects depend on extent and route of exposure	Effects may be delayed, appearing hours after exposure		Intracellular enzyme and DNA alkylating agents	Immediate decontamination; Supportive care; Thermal burn–type treatment; Symptomatic management of lesions		Primary liquid hazard; May be confused with skin exposure to caustic irritants (e.g., NaOH, NH₃)
Sulfur mustard (H) Distilled mustard (HD)	Skin: erythema and blisters (may be delayed ≤8 h), pruritus; Eye: irritation, conjunctivitis, corneal damage, lacrimation, pain, blepharospasm; Resp: mild to marked acute airway damage, pneumonitis within 1–3 d, respiratory failure; GI effects (nausea, vomiting, diarrhea) may be present; Bone marrow stem cell suppression leading to pancytopenia and increased susceptibility to infection; Fever, sputum production	Delayed 2–48 h	Garlic, horseradish, or mustard		Skin: silver sulfadiazine[1]; Eye: homatropine[1] ophthalmic ointment; Pulmonary: antibiotics, bronchodilators, steroids; Colony-stimulating factor may be helpful for leukopenia; Systemic analgesic and antipruritics; Early use of PEEP or CPAP; Maintain fluid and electrolyte balance (do not excessively fluid resuscitate as in thermal burns)	No specific antidote	Combination with lewisite (called mustard-Lewisite or HL) results in rapid effects of lewisite and delayed effects of mustard agents
Lewisite (L)	Skin: gray area of dead skin within 5 min, erythema within 30 min, blistering 2–3 h, immediate irritation or burning pain on contact, severe tissue necrosis; Eye: pain, blepharospasm, conjunctival and lid edema; Airway: pseudomembrane formation, nasal irritation; Intravascular fluid loss, hypovolemia, shock, organ congestion, leukocytosis	Immediate	Fruity or geranium			British anti-lewisite (BAL or dimercaprol)	More volatile than mustard; Damages eyes, skin, and airways by direct contact

Continued

TABLE 1 Quick Reference Chart on Chemical Weapon Agents—cont'd

CHEMICAL AGENT	DIAGNOSTIC CONSIDERATIONS				TREATMENT CONSIDERATIONS*			
	SIGNS AND SYMPTOMS	SYMPTOM ONSET	ODOR	ACTION	TESTING	TREATMENT	ANTIDOTE	COMMENTS
Phosgene oxime (CX)	Burning, irritation, wheal-like skin lesions, eye and airway damage, conjunctivitis, lacrimation, lid edema, blepharospasm	Immediate	Freshly mown hay	Urticant, nonvesicant agent	No distinctive laboratory findings	Parenteral methylprednisolone[1] may be effective in preventing noncardiogenic pulmonary edema Experimental: aerosolized dexamethasone[1] and theophylline[1] for pulmonary involvement	No antidote	Vapor extremely irritating; vapor and liquid cause tissue damage upon contact
Vomiting (Arsine-Based) Agents								
Adamsite (DM) Diphenylchlorarsine (DA) Diphenylcyanoarsine (DC)	Eyes: conjunctival irritation, tearing, and blepharospasm Airways: sneezing, mucosal lung irritation, edema, progressive cough, wheezing Cardiac: tachypnea, tachycardia GI: intestinal cramps, emesis, diarrhea Skin: erythema, edema at the site of dermal contact CNS: depression, syncope	All rapidly acting within minutes	DA: none DC: garlic DM: burning fireworks	Arsine gas depletes erythrocyte glutathione and causes hemolysis	Chest radiograph to rule out chemical pneumonitis	Supportive care Monitor for hemolysis Wheezing or dyspnea: may need albuterol inhalation Eye irrigation (water, normal saline, lactated Ringer's) in patients with ocular exposure Treat repetitive emesis with IV hydration and antiemetics Blood transfusion may be required Exchange transfusion may be required Hemodialysis may be useful in decreasing arsenic level and treating renal failure		Primary route of absorption is through respiratory system

Adapted from Lyznicki JL: AMA quick reference guide: Exposure to toxic chemical agents. In American Medical Association: Management of Public Health Emergencies. A Resource Guide for Physicians and Other Community Responders. Chicago, American Medical Association, 2005.

[1]Not FDA approved for this indication.

[5]Investigational drug in the United States.

*Different situations can require different treatment and dosage regimens. Please consult other references as well as a regional poison control center (800–222–1222), medical toxicologist, clinical pharmacologist, or other drug information specialist for definitive dosage information, especially dosages for pregnant women and children.

†Available in Europe.

Abbreviations: CNS = central nervous system; CPAP = continuous positive airway pressure; CV = cardiovascular; GI = gastrointestinal; 2-PAM = pralidoxime (2-pyridine aldoxime methyl chloride); PEEP = positive end-expiratory pressure; resp = respiratory; SOB = shortness of breath.

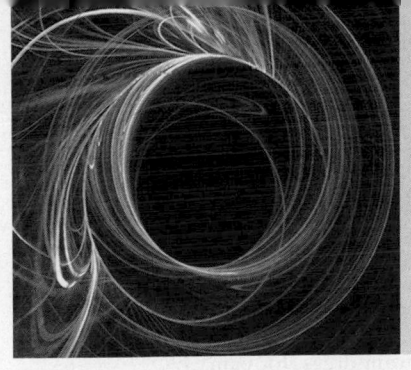

Index

Note: Page numbers followed by *b* indicate boxes, *f* indicate figures and *t* indicate tables.

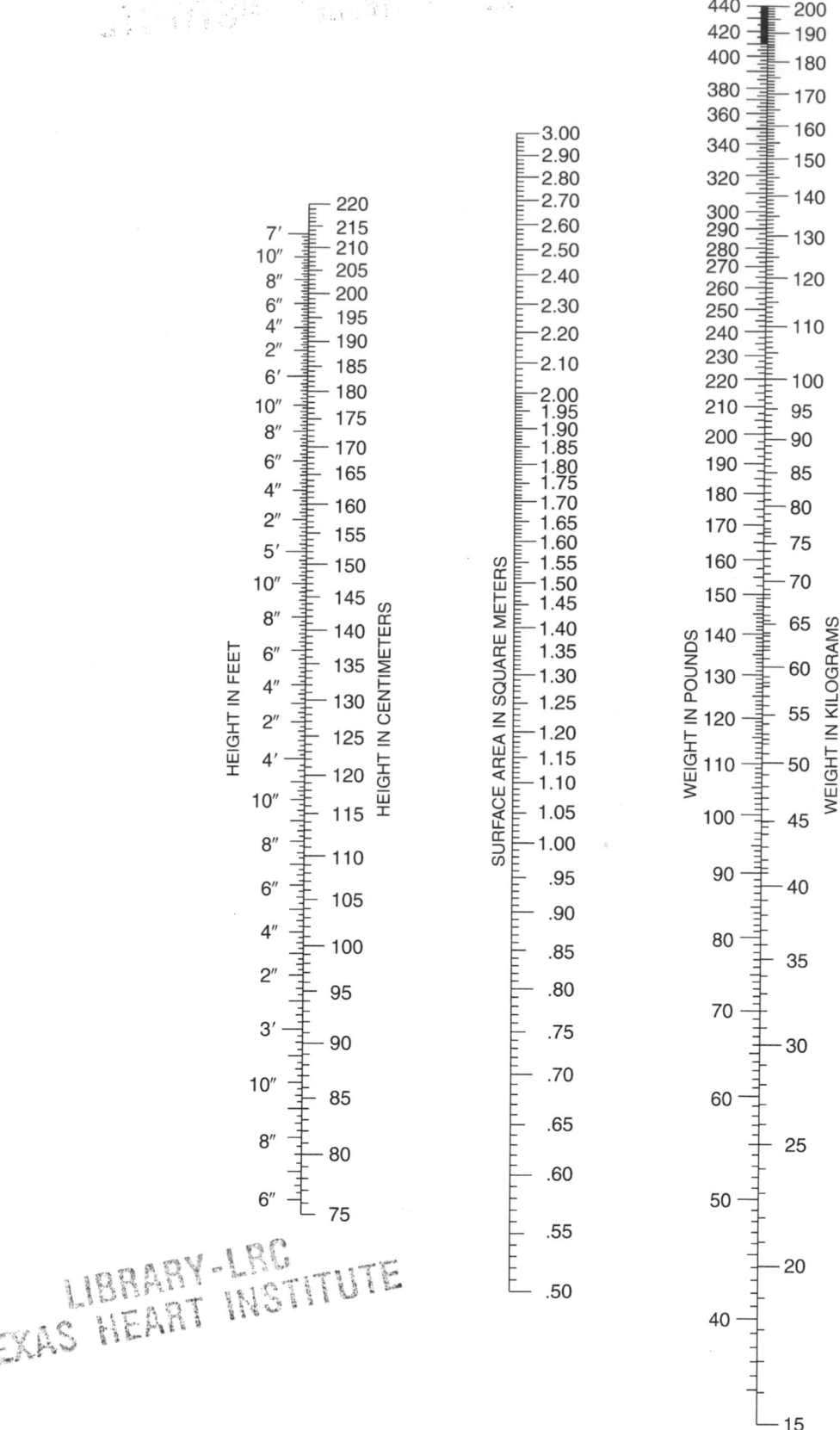

HEIGHT IN FEET

HEIGHT IN CENTIMETERS

SURFACE AREA IN SQUARE METERS

WEIGHT IN POUNDS

WEIGHT IN KILOGRAMS